A REFERENCE GUIDE TO FETAL AND NEONATAL RISK

Drugs in **Pregnancy** and **Lactation,** Tenth Edition

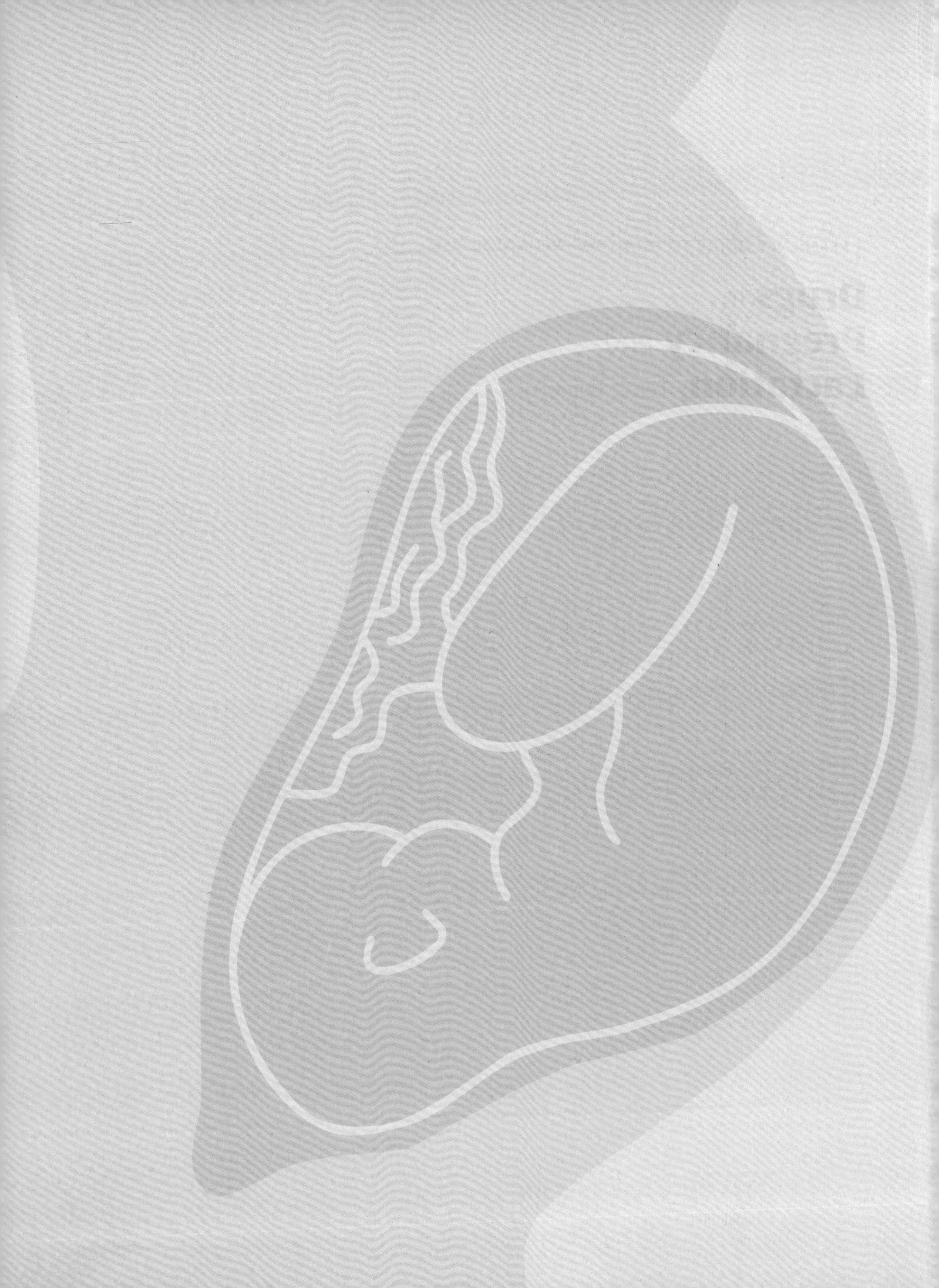

A REFERENCE GUIDE TO FETAL AND NEONATAL RISK

Drugs in Pregnancy and Lactation, Tenth Edition

Gerald G. Briggs, BPharm, FCCP
Pharmacist Clinical Specialist (Obstetrics) (Retired)
MemorialCare Center for Women
Miller Children's Hospital
Long Beach Memorial Medical Center
Long Beach, California
Clinical Professor of Pharmacy
University of California, San Francisco
Adjunct Professor of Pharmacy Practice
University of Southern California, Los Angeles
Adjunct Professor, Department of Pharmacotherapy
Washington State University, Spokane, Washington

Roger K. Freeman, MD
MemorialCare Center for Women
Miller Children's Hospital
Long Beach Memorial Medical Center
Long Beach, California
Director Mednax Medical Group
Clinical Professor of Obstetrics and Gynecology
University of California, Irvine

Wolters Kluwer

Philadelphia • Baltimore • New York • London
Buenos Aires • Hong Kong • Sydney • Tokyo

Acquisitions Editor: Jamie M. Elfrank
Marketing Manager: Stephanie Manzo
Product Development Editor: Ashley Fischer
Production Project Manager: Marian Bellus
Senior Manufacturing Coordinator: Beth Welsh
Design Coordinator: Doug Smock
Production Service: Integra Software Services Pvt. Ltd.

Two Commerce Square
2001 Market Street
Philadelphia, PA 19103

Printed in China

Library of Congress Cataloging-in-Publication Data

Briggs, Gerald G., author.
Drugs in pregnancy and lactation: a reference guide to fetal and neonatal risk / Gerald G. Briggs, Roger K. Freeman, Sumner J. Yaffe. — Tenth edition.
p. ; cm.
Includes bibliographical references.
ISBN 978-1-4511-9082-3 — ISBN 1-60831-708-0
I. Freeman, Roger K., 1935- author. II. Yaffe, Sumner J., 1923-2011, author. III. Title.
[DNLM: 1. Infant, Newborn, Diseases—chemically induced—Handbooks. 2. Drug-Related Side Effects and Adverse Reactions—Handbooks. 3. Lactation—drug effects—Handbooks. 4. Maternal-Fetal Exchange—drug effects—Handbooks. 5. Milk, Human—drug effects—Handbooks. 6. Pregnancy—drug effects—Handbooks. WS 39]
RG627.6.D79
618.3'2—dc23

2014012988

Care has been taken to confirm the accuracy of the information presented and to describe generally accepted practices. However, the authors, editors, and publisher are not responsible for errors or omissions or for any consequences from application of the information in this book and make no warranty, expressed or implied, with respect to the currency, completeness, or accuracy of the contents of the publication. Application of the information in a particular situation remains the professional responsibility of the practitioner.

The authors, editors, and publisher have exerted every effort to ensure that drug selection and dosage set forth in this text are in accordance with current recommendations and practice at the time of publication. However, in view of ongoing research, changes in government regulations, and the constant flow of information relating to drug therapy and drug reactions, the reader is urged to check the package insert for each drug for any change in indications and dosage and for added warnings and precautions. This is particularly important when the recommended agent is a new or infrequently employed drug.

Some drugs and medical devices presented in the publication have Food and Drug Administration (FDA) clearance for limited use in restricted research settings. It is the responsibility of the health care provider to ascertain the FDA status of each drug or device planned for use in their clinical practice.

To purchase additional copies of this book, call our customer service department at (800) 638-3030 or fax orders to (301) 223-2320. International customers should call (301) 223-2300. Visit Lippincott Williams & Wilkins on the Internet: at LWW.com. Lippincott Williams & Wilkins customer service representatives are available from 8:30 am to 6 pm, EST.

10 9 8 7 6 5 4 3 2 1

In Memory

Sumner J. Yaffe, M.D.

May 9, 1923–August 10, 2011

On August 10, 2011, Dr. Sumner J. Yaffe, often regarded as the father of pediatric clinical pharmacology, passed away. He had a long and distinguished career as a renowned researcher and expert in pediatric pharmacology.

Dr. Yaffe was our friend, colleague, and co-author for 31 years. In 1980, he enthusiastically accepted our offer to co-author this book. At that time, he was the Director of the Center for Research for Mothers and Children at the National Institute of Child Health and Human Development. Over the years, he authored and/or contributed to nearly 300 scientific articles and books, including ours. His comments on our reviews were always on target. Our readers and ourselves have reaped the benefits of his vast experience. We were indeed fortunate to have received his wise advice and counsel over three decades.

Foreword

This book is now in its 10th edition and continues to enjoy great success with physicians and other professionals involved in the care of pregnant and lactating patients. Many of the reviews are exhaustive but pertinent to the management of pregnant and lactating patients who have already ingested a drug or who are in need of drug therapy where a cost–benefit analysis may be necessary for appropriate counseling. There are seldom absolute answers to questions a woman may have when she ingests a drug when pregnant or nursing because human experience is usually, of necessity, somewhat anecdotal. Even with all the information in this publication, there are risks that are yet unknown that may apply to a small number of people making the dictum of not using drugs in pregnancy without good cause still important. The effect of drugs in animals, the importance of timing and dose, and the effect of environmental factors are all involved in the risks and benefits of drugs in pregnant and/or lactating women and their fetuses/neonates. These factors are considered when data are available, but we must admit that in no individual case is the understanding of risks and benefits absolute.

Because many pregnant and lactating women take substances, both legal and illegal, without the knowledge of their caregivers, the challenge to understand the risks/benefits of any drug and its interactions with these substances is daunting. Today, we are just beginning to understand the specific genetic influences on the action, toxicity, and teratogenicity of drugs in an individual. I expect in the future there will be many identified genetic factors that will influence therapeutic decisions.

The contributions of Dr. Sumner J. Yaffe, who died after the last edition, will be greatly missed. His vast experience and expertise regarding the use of drugs in pregnancy and lactation were significant contributions to all editions of this book.

It is our hope that the 10th edition will continue to provide the practitioner appropriate assistance with questions regarding drugs in pregnancy and lactation.

Roger K. Freeman, MD
MemorialCare Center for Women
Miller Children's Hospital
Long Beach Memorial Medical Center
Long Beach, California
Director Mednax Medical Group
Clinical Professor of Obstetrics and Gynecology
University of California, Irvine

Preface

In 2011, our co-author, Dr. Sumner J. Yaffe, MD, passed away. Our tribute to this great man is shown on the In Memory page.

We have been writing this book for 34 years. The first edition was released in 1983, 31 years ago. With each new edition, we have tried to make improvements that would benefit our readers. The same is true for this edition.

Not only is the 10th edition in a print version, it is now completely online for those who prefer that method to acquire information. We have attempted to reduce the size of the book by removing 161 reviews of drugs no longer marketed. If information is needed for these agents, it can be obtained by referring to the 9th edition. There are 124 new drugs in this edition. Unfortunately, the majority have no reported human pregnancy experience. Consequently, to estimate the embryo–fetal risk, we had to rely on information from other drugs that had the same mechanism of action (if they had human data) and/or on animal data. Finally, 201 drug reviews have been revised with new information, but no new relevant data were found for an additional 300 drugs. However, the search for new data on all drugs in this edition is an ongoing process. Although new or revised drug reviews published in future quarterly Updates will not be in the print version of this edition, they will be available online. We believe this will be a significant benefit for our readers.

The revision focus has been on drugs with no human pregnancy data and those where new information would change our pregnancy or breastfeeding recommendation. Nevertheless, there are still a large number of drugs that have little or no published human pregnancy experience, thus making the counseling function difficult.

As in previous editions, some drug reviews have toll-free telephone numbers for the use of health care professionals or patients to enroll in observational studies. These studies are an important method for gathering prospective data on pregnancy exposures for high-risk drugs. In fact, such studies are often the only human pregnancy experience available for new drugs and pharmacologic drug classes. The data generated by these studies and registries can be valuable for the raising of hypotheses of major teratogenicity or providing some assurance that the agent is not a significant teratogen. Because their importance is so high, health care professionals and patients are encouraged to call for information about patient enrollment.

We take great pleasure for the opportunity to thank the many individuals who have helped us. To those who have sent us references, know that your efforts are sincerely appreciated. We also appreciate those who have commented on our work because it identifies areas that may need modification or topics that we need to cover. In addition, the questions we received served to keep us informed of your information needs and often lead to the preparation of new reviews. On the following page, we have listed the names of those who have been particularly helpful in the preparation of this edition.

It also is a pleasure to announce that we have two new co-authors who will assist us in the next edition. Dr. Craig Towers, M.D., is a Maternal-Fetal Specialist and a professor at the University of Tennessee Medical Center, Knoxville. We have had the pleasure of working with Dr. Towers in the past and look forward to renewing that relationship. Dr. Alicia Forinash, Pharm.D, FCCP, BCPS, BCACP, is an Associate Professor, Saint Louis College of Pharmacy, and a Clinical Pharmacy Specialist in the Maternal-Fetal Care Clinic at Saint Mary's Health Center in Saint Louis. We believe both will have a significant and beneficial impact on future editions of this book.

Gerald G. Briggs, BPharm, FCCP
Pharmacist Clinical Specialist (Obstetrics) (Retired)
MemorialCare Center for Women
Miller Children's Hospital
Long Beach Memorial Medical Center
Long Beach, California
Clinical Professor of Pharmacy
University of California, San Francisco
Adjunct Professor of Pharmacy Practice
University of Southern California, Los Angeles
Adjunct Professor, Department of Pharmacotherapy
Washington State University, Spokane, Washington

Preface

Acknowledgment

It is a pleasure to acknowledge the assistance of Dr. Christine Chambers, PhD, MPH, for her help in the preparation of several drug reviews. In addition, we want to thank Elizabeth Mason-Renteria, Parks Medical Library, Long Beach Memorial Medical Center, who retrieved numerous references for us during the preparation of this edition. Without her assistance, this edition would have been much harder to prepare.

We also are pleased to acknowledge the assistance of our former students in the preparation of some of the reviews contained in this edition. The students came from five schools of pharmacy. During their clerkship training in obstetrics/gynecology, each researched and wrote two drug reviews. It was their first experience in how to assess the reproductive toxicity of drugs, and they did very well.

University of California, San Diego
Samantha Luk, PharmD
Natalie Nguyen, PharmD
Esther Park, PharmD
Teri Phan, PhD, PharmD
Linda Tang, PharmD
Caroline Wesemuller, PharmD

University of California, San Francisco
Sam Chung, PharmD
Martha Prieto, MPH, PharmD
Julia Zhu, PharmD

University of Southern California, Los Angeles
Rebecca Myung, PharmD
Sherehan Salib, PharmD
Chandra Smallwood, PharmD

Midwestern University, Glendale, Arizona
Tu Tran, PharmD

University of Washington, Seattle
Maridith Yoshida, PharmD

Contents

Introduction, 9th Edition

Sumner J. Yaffe, MD

It is now generally accepted that the developing fetus may be adversely affected by exposure to drugs and environmental chemicals. The stage of development of the intrauterine host is a major determinant of the resultant effect as well as the nature and the concentration of the drug or chemical agent. On a more positive side, fetal therapy (i.e., treatment of fetal disease in utero by administering the drug to the mother or directly to the fetus) has been recognized recently as a rational approach to treat fetal disease.

Forty years ago, the thalidomide catastrophe (limb defects) occurred when this drug was administered to pregnant women as an antianxiety and hypnotic agent during the 1st trimester. Thalidomide had been evaluated for safety in several animal species, had been given a clean bill of health, and had come to be regarded as a good pharmacologic agent (hypnotic/sedative). It is of interest that this drug is being reevaluated today for use in leprosy and approval for this use has been given by the FDA.

It is important to note that, even though thalidomide produces a distinct cluster of anatomic defects that are virtually pathognomonic for this agent, it required several years of thalidomide use and the birth of many thousands of grossly malformed infants before the cause-and-effect relationship between thalidomide administration in early pregnancy and its harmful effects was recognized. This serves to emphasize the difficulties that exist in incriminating drugs and chemicals that are harmful when administered during pregnancy. Hopefully, we will never have another drug prescribed for use during pregnancy whose teratogenicity is as potent as thalidomide (about one-third of women taking this agent during the 1st trimester gave birth to infants with birth defects).

Concern about the safety of foreign compounds administered to pregnant women has been increasingly evident since thalidomide. The direct response to this misadventure led to the promulgation of the drug regulations of 1962 in the United States. According to these regulations, a drug must be demonstrated to be safe and effective for the conditions of use prescribed in its labeling. The regulations concerning this requirement state that a drug should be investigated for the conditions of use specified in the labeling, including dosage levels and patient populations for whom the drug is intended. In addition, appropriate information must be provided in the labeling and be available when the drug is prescribed. The intent of the regulations is not only to ensure adequate labeling information for the safe and effective administration of the drug by the physician but also to ensure that marketed drugs have an acceptable benefit:risk ratio for their intended uses.

It is clear that any drug or chemical substance administered to the mother is able to cross the placenta to some extent unless it is destroyed or altered during passage, or its molecular size and low lipid solubility limit transplacental transfer. Placental transport of maternal substrates to the fetus and of substances from the fetus to the mother is established at about the 5th week of embryo life. Substances of low molecular weight diffuse freely across the placenta, driven primarily by the concentration gradient. It is important to note, therefore, that almost every substance used for therapeutic purposes can and does pass from the mother to the fetus. Of greater importance is whether the rate and extent of transfer are sufficient to result in significant concentrations within the fetus. Today, the concept of a placental barrier must be discarded.

Experiments with animals have provided considerable information concerning the teratogenic effects of drugs. Unfortunately, these experimental findings cannot be extrapolated with certainty from species to species, or even from strain to strain within the same species, much less from animals to humans. Research in this area and the prediction of toxicity in the human are further hampered by a lack of specificity between cause and effect.

Traditionally, teratogenic effects of drugs have been noted as anatomic malformations. It is clear that these are dose and time related and that the fetus is at greater risk during the first 3 months of gestation. However, it is possible for drugs and chemicals to exert their effects upon the fetus at other times during pregnancy. Functional and behavioral changes are much more difficult to identify as to cause and effect. Consequently, they are rarely recognized. A heightened awareness on the part of health care providers and recipients will make this task easier.

The use of dietary supplements as well as complementary or alternative medicine products has been increasing markedly in the Western industrialized world. This use continues unabated during pregnancy and lactation. The efficacy of these compounds is generally unknown, with rare exception, and their safety poorly studied. In particular, little is known about the interaction between the use of a broad range of dietary supplements, alternative medicine products, and health outcomes in women, developing fetuses and nursing neonates. Such knowledge is essential to the evaluation of both the justification and safety of the use of these products during these critical periods of development. Until this occurs, women should be advised about current lack of knowledge and cautioned as to their use. A notable exception is folic acid supplementation during pregnancy to prevent neural tube defects.

It is crucial that concern also be given to events beyond the narrow limits of congenital anatomic malformations; evidence exist that intellectual, social, and functional development can also be adversely affected by drug administration during pregnancy. There are examples that toxic manifestations of intrauterine exposure to environmental agents may be subtle, unexpected, and delayed. Concern for the delayed effects of drugs, following intrauterine exposure, was first raised following the tragic discovery that female fetuses exposed to diethylstilbestrol (DES) are at an increased risk for adenocarcinoma of the vagina. This type of malignancy is not discovered until after puberty. Many of the drugs prescribed to pregnant women have been evaluated in the following pages as to their propensity to produce congenital anatomic malformations. During the past several decades, awareness that many of these compounds may act after the period of organogenesis, through birth and into lactation, has increased. We now realize that drugs considered safe (i.e., not producing anatomic malformations) can still produce more subtle yet permanent alterations in the physiology and biochemistry of the developing perinate. Furthermore, many of these subtle hitherto unrecognized defects are not present at birth and may be dormant and latent until years later after the time of administration. The teratogen appears to produce a programming or imprinting defect in the developing tissue or organ. This defect need not be expressed until adulthood, because the program may not be required until that time. Consequently, in the absence of anatomical defects readily recognized, there is the danger that these late-onset dysfunctions will either be unrecognized or will be attributed to some other cause.

The purpose of the above paragraph is to raise the concept of a little known but potentially serious health hazard in children and adults. This refers to the ability of perinatally consumed drugs and food additives and nonprescription alternative agents to produce the subtle biochemical defects undetectable or unrecognized in the neonate but expressed years or even decades after birth. How serious a problem is the in utero exposure to drugs and chemicals to the delayed latent defect? The answer may in lie in the use of animals for these fetal origins of adult disease.

The physician is confronted with two imperatives in treating the pregnant woman: alleviate maternal suffering and do no harm to the fetus. Until now, the emphasis has been on the amelioration of suffering, but the time has come to concentrate on not harming the fetus. The simple equation to be applied here is to weigh the therapeutic benefits of the drug to the mother against its risk potential to the developing fetus. Since fetal ova may also be exposed to drugs given to the mother, effects may be evident in future generations.

When one considers that more than a billion drug prescriptions are written each year, that there is unlimited self-administration of over-the-counter drugs, and that approximately 500 new pharmaceutical products are introduced annually, the need for prudence and caution in the administration of pharmaceuticals has reached a critical point. Pregnancy is a symptom-producing event. Pregnancy has the potential of causing women to increase their intake of drugs and chemicals, with the potential being that the fetus will be nurtured in a sea of drugs.

In today's society, the physician cannot stand alone in the therapeutic decision-making process. It has now become the responsibility of each woman of childbearing age to consider her use of drugs carefully. In a pregnant woman, the decision to administer a drug should be made only after a collaborative appraisal between the woman and her physician of the risk:benefit ratio.

BREASTFEEDING AND DRUGS

Between 1930 and the late 1960s, there was a dramatic decline in the percentage of American mothers who breastfed their babies. This was also accompanied by a reduction in the length of breastfeeding for those who did nurse. The incidence of breastfeeding declined from approximately 80% of the children born between 1926 and 1930 to 49% of children born some 25 years later. For children born between 1966 and 1970, 28% were breastfed. Indeed, in 1972 only 20% of newborns were breastfed. As data have become available for the following years, it is clear the decline has been reversed. By 1975, the percentage of first-born babies who were breastfed rose to 37%. At the present time in the United States, a number of surveys indicate that more than 50% of babies discharged from the hospital are breastfed, and the number is increasing. Breastfeeding is difficult to contemplate, as more than 50% of mothers work and return to work soon after delivery. New solutions must be found by employers to encourage breastfeeding and develop the logistics to enable employees to breastfeed on the job.

Breast milk is known to possess nutritional and immunologic properties superior to those found in infant formulas. An American Academy of Pediatrics position paper emphasizes breastfeeding as the best nutritional mode for infants for the first 6 months of life. In addition to those qualities, studies also suggest significant psychologic benefits of breastfeeding for both the mother and the infant.

The upswing in breastfeeding, together with a markedly increased concern about health needs on the part of parents, has led to increased questioning of the physician, pharmacist, and other health professionals about the safety and potential toxicity of drugs and chemicals that may be excreted in breast milk. Answers to these questions are not very apparent. Our knowledge concerning the long- and short-term effects and safety of maternally ingested drugs on the suckling infant is meager. We know more now than Soranus did in 150 AD, when he admonished wet nurses to refrain from the use of drugs and alcohol, lest it have an adverse effect on the nursing infant. We must know more! The knowledge to be acquired should be specific with respect to dose administered to the mother, amount excreted in breast milk, and amount absorbed by the suckling infant. In addition, effects on the infant should be determined (both acute and chronic).

It would be easy to recommend that the medicated mother not nurse, but it is likely that this recommendation would be ignored by the mother and may offend many health providers, as well as their patients, on both psychosocial and physiologic grounds.

It must be emphasized that many of the investigations concerned with milk secretion and synthesis have been carried out in animals. The difficulty in studying human lactation using histologic techniques and the administration of radioactive isotopes is obvious. There are considerable differences in the composition of milk in different species. Some of these differences in composition would obviously bring about changes in drug elimination. Of great importance in this regard are the differences in the pH of human milk (pH usually >7.0) compared with the pH of cow's milk (pH usually <6.8) where drug excretion has been extensively studied.

A number of reviews give tables of the concentration of drugs in breast milk. Often, these tables also give the milk:plasma ratio. Most of the values from which the tables are derived consist of a single measurement of the drug concentration. Important information, such as the maternal dose, the frequency of dose, the time from drug administration to sampling, the frequency of nursing, and the length of lactation, is not given.

The significance of these concentration tables only means that the drug is present in the milk, and they offer no advice to the physician. Because the drug in the nursing infant's blood or urine is not measured, we have little information about the amount that is actually absorbed by the infant from the milk and, therefore, have no way of determining the possible pharmacologic effects on the infant. In fact, a critical examination of the tables that have been published reveals that much of the information was gathered decades ago when analytic methodology was not as sensitive as it is today. Because the discipline of pharmacokinetics was not developed until recently, many of the studies quoted in the tables of the review articles do not precisely look at the time relationship between drug administration and disposition.

Certain things are evident with regard to drugs administered during lactation. It is necessary that physicians become aware of the results of animal studies in this area and of the potential risk of maternal drug ingestion to the suckling infant. Many drugs prescribed to the lactating woman need to be studied more so that their safety during lactation can be assessed. It is clear that if the mother needs a drug that has a moderate-to-high potential to cause infant harm, then she should consider not nursing. The ultimate decision must be individualized according to the specific illness and the therapeutic modality. Nursing should be avoided following the administration of radioactive pharmaceuticals that are usually given to the mother for diagnostic purposes.

CONCLUSIONS

Two basic situations are dealt with throughout this book: (a) risk potential to the fetus of maternal drugs ingested during the course of pregnancy, and (b) risk potential to the infant of drugs taken by the mother while nursing.

The obvious solution to fetal and nursing infant risk avoidance is maternal abstinence. However, from a pragmatic standpoint, that would be impossible to implement. Another solution is to disseminate knowledge, in an authoritative manner, to all those involved in the pregnancy and breastfeeding processes: physician, mother, midwife, nurse, father, and pharmacist.

This book helps to fill a communication and information gap. We have carefully evaluated the research literature, animal and human, applied and clinical. Each of the more than 1180 drugs has a risk factor assigned by the manufacturer or ourselves in keeping with the FDA guidelines. We have also assigned our own recommendations for use of these drugs in pregnancy and lactation. We believe that this book will be helpful to all concerned parties in developing the risk:benefit decision.

This is but a beginning. It is our fervent hope that the information gained from the use of this book will cause the concerned parties to be more trenchant in their future decision-making, either before prescribing or before ingesting drugs during pregnancy and lactation.

Instructions for Use of the Reference Guide

The Reference Guide is arranged so that the user can quickly locate a monograph. If the American generic name is known, go directly to the monographs, which are listed in alphabetical order. If only the trade or foreign name is known, refer to the Index for the appropriate American generic name. Foreign trade names have been included in the Index. To the best of our knowledge, all trade and foreign generic names are correct as shown, but because these may change, the reader should check other reference sources if there is any question as to the identity of an individual drug. Some prescription combination products are listed in the Index. If not listed, the user should refer to the manufacturer's product information for the specific ingredients, and then use the Reference Guide as for single entities.

Each monograph contains eight parts:

Generic Name (United States)
Pharmacologic Class
Pregnancy Recommendation
Breastfeeding Recommendation
Pregnancy Summary
Fetal Risk Summary
Breastfeeding Summary
References

PREGNANCY SUMMARY

The Pregnancy Summary is intended as a brief overview of the reported data in pregnancy, both animal and human, whereas the Fetal Risk Summary provides the specific details of the data. Both the Pregnancy Summary and the Fetal Risk Summary support the Pregnancy Recommendation.

FETAL RISK SUMMARY

The Fetal Risk Summary is an analysis of the literature concerning use of the drug in pregnancy. The intent is to provide clinicians and others with sufficient data to counsel patients and to arrive at conclusions as to the risk:benefit ratio a particular drug poses for the embryo, fetus, and newborn. The molecular weight of most drugs has been included in the reviews because they help determine if a drug can reach the embryo or fetus, but this value, by itself, may not predict the amount crossing the placenta. The major determinant of the drug concentration in the embryo or fetus is the blood concentration of the drug in the mother. Other important factors include the elimination half-life, metabolism, placental blood flow, the placental surface area available for crossing (i.e., correlated to the gestational age), and the lipid solubility, protein binding, and the amount of ionization of the drug at physiologic pH.

Because few absolutes are possible in the area of human teratology, the reader must carefully weigh the evidence, or lack thereof, before utilizing any drug in a pregnant woman. Readers who require more details than are presented should refer to the specific references listed at the end of the monograph. See Definitions for recommendations.

BREASTFEEDING SUMMARY

The Breastfeeding Summary is a brief review of the literature concerning excretion of the drug into human breast milk and the effects, if any, on a nursing infant. Unfortunately, in many cases, there is no published information about use of the drug during lactation. Moreover, when studies do exist, infants often were not allowed to breastfeed. Readers should pay close attention to this distinction (i.e., excretion into milk vs. effects on the nursing infant) when using a Summary. Those who require more details than are presented should refer to the specific references listed at the end of the monograph. See Definitions for recommendations.

PREGNANCY AND BREASTFEEDING RECOMMENDATIONS

The pregnancy recommendations are intended to assist the reader in determining the level of risk of a specific drug. They only apply to the usual therapeutic dose of the drug in a typical patient. Because the genetic makeup of a specific patient may significantly alter the risk, the recommendations may not apply to the entire population. In addition to the animal reproduction data and known human pregnancy outcomes, the assessment of risk includes, when relevant, other major factors such as route of administration, metabolism to active metabolites, species differences, type of defects, pharmacokinetics, effects of other agents in the drug class, and the embryo–fetal effects of untreated or undertreated maternal disease. Moreover, drug exposures represent different levels of risk depending on the stage of pregnancy and, thus, timing of the exposure is critical in determining risk. Because short statements of risk may not always adequately assess the risk throughout the pregnancy, readers are encouraged to review the entire monograph before estimating the risk for a specific patient.

The risks also change during breastfeeding because nearly all reported adverse effects in nursing infants have occurred in infants <6 months of age. The neonate and very young infant are most at risk for toxic effects from drugs present in breast milk. The recommendations for breastfeeding are based on the known toxicity of the drug or similar drugs in adults or children (when known) and the amount of drug excreted into breast milk (if known). Although most drugs taken by the mother are probably present in milk, the milk concentrations are usually unknown. Fortunately, the amounts are usually too low to cause toxicity. However, the therapeutic dose for infants of most drugs is rarely known. Therefore, we used a proposal from the literature (Ito S. N Engl J Med 2000;343:118–28) to classify exposures as clinically insignificant if, in the absence of data suggesting otherwise, the estimated dose ingested by a nursing infant was no more than 10% of the mother's weight-adjusted dose. In some cases, this classification may not be relevant. For example, the potential for neurotoxicity in a nursing infant from long-term maternal use of psychotropic medications continues to be a concern.

DEFINITIONS OF PREGNANCY RECOMMENDATIONS

COMPATIBLE

The human pregnancy experience, either for the drug itself or drugs in the same class or with similar mechanisms of action, is adequate to demonstrate that the embryo–fetal risk is very low or nonexistent. Animal reproduction data are not relevant.

NO (LIMITED) HUMAN DATA—PROBABLY COMPATIBLE

There may or may not be human pregnancy experience, but the characteristics of the drug suggest that it does not represent a significant risk to the embryo–fetus. For example, other drugs in the same class or with similar mechanisms are compatible or the drug does not obtain significant systemic concentrations. Any animal reproduction data are not relevant.

COMPATIBLE—MATERNAL BENEFIT >> EMBRYO–FETAL RISK

There may or may not be human pregnancy experience, but the potential maternal benefit far outweighs the known or unknown embryo–fetal risk. Animal reproduction data are not relevant.

HUMAN DATA SUGGEST LOW RISK

There is limited human pregnancy experience, either for the drug itself or drugs in the same class or with similar mechanisms of action, including the 1st trimester, suggesting that the drug does not represent a significant risk of developmental toxicity (growth restriction, structural anomalies, functional/behavioral deficits, or death) at any time in pregnancy. The limited human pregnancy data outweigh any animal reproduction data.

NO (LIMITED) HUMAN DATA—ANIMAL DATA SUGGEST LOW RISK

Either there is no human pregnancy experience or the few pregnancy exposures have not been associated with developmental toxicity (growth restriction, structural anomalies, functional/behavioral deficits, or death). The drug does not cause developmental toxicity (at doses that did not cause maternal toxicity) in all animal species studied at doses $\leq$10 times the human dose based on body surface area (BSA) or AUC*.

NO (LIMITED) HUMAN DATA—ANIMAL DATA SUGGEST MODERATE RISK

Either there is no human pregnancy experience or the few pregnancy exposures have not been associated with developmental toxicity (growth restriction, structural anomalies, functional/behavioral deficits, or death). The drug causes developmental toxicity (at doses that did not cause maternal toxicity) in one animal species at doses $\leq$10 times the human dose based on body surface area (BSA) or AUC*.

NO (LIMITED) HUMAN DATA—ANIMAL DATA SUGGEST RISK

Either there is no human pregnancy experience or the few pregnancy exposures have not been associated with developmental toxicity (growth restriction, structural anomalies, functional/behavioral deficits, or death). The drug causes developmental toxicity (at doses that did not cause maternal toxicity) in two animal species at doses $\leq$10 times the human dose based on body surface area (BSA) or AUC*.

NO (LIMITED) HUMAN DATA—ANIMAL DATA SUGGEST HIGH RISK

Either there is no human pregnancy experience or the few pregnancy exposures have not been associated with developmental toxicity (growth restriction, structural anomalies, functional/behavioral deficits, or death). The drug causes developmental toxicity (at doses that did not cause maternal toxicity) in three or more animal species at doses $\leq$10 times the human dose based on body surface area (BSA) or AUC*.

CONTRAINDICATED—1ST TRIMESTER

Human exposures in the 1st trimester, either to the drug itself or to drugs in the same class or with similar mechanisms of action, have been associated with developmental toxicity (growth restriction, structural anomalies, functional/behavioral deficits, or death). The drug should not be used in the 1st trimester.

CONTRAINDICATED—2ND AND 3RD TRIMESTERS

Human exposures in the 2nd and 3rd trimesters, either to the drug itself or to drugs in the same class or with similar mechanisms of action, have been associated with developmental toxicity (growth restriction, structural anomalies, functional/behavior deficits, or death). The drug should not be used in the 2nd and 3rd trimesters.

CONTRAINDICATED

Human exposures at any time in pregnancy, either to the drug itself or to drugs in the same class or with similar mechanisms of action, have been associated with developmental toxicity (growth restriction, structural anomalies, functional/behavioral deficits, or death). Animal reproduction data, if available, confirm the risk. The drug should not be used in pregnancy.

NO (LIMITED) HUMAN DATA—NO RELEVANT ANIMAL DATA

There is no human pregnancy data or relevant data in animals, or the human pregnancy experience, that may or may not include the 1st trimester, is limited. The risk in pregnancy cannot be assessed.

HUMAN DATA SUGGEST RISK IN 1ST TRIMESTER

Evidence (for the drug or similar drugs) suggests that there may be an embryo–fetal risk for developmental toxicity (growth restriction, structural anomalies, functional/behavioral deficits, or death) in the 1st trimester but not in the 2nd and 3rd trimesters. The human pregnancy data outweigh any animal reproduction data.

**AUC = area under the plasma concentration vs. time curve; a measure of the systemic exposure of a drug*

HUMAN DATA SUGGEST RISK IN 1ST AND 3RD TRIMESTERS

Evidence (for the drug or similar drugs) suggests that there may be an embryo–fetal risk for developmental toxicity (growth restriction, structural anomalies, functional/behavioral deficits, or death) in the 1st and 3rd trimesters but not in the 2nd trimester. The human pregnancy data outweigh any animal reproduction data.

HUMAN DATA SUGGEST RISK IN 2ND AND 3RD TRIMESTERS

Evidence (for the drug or similar drugs) suggests that there may be a fetal risk for developmental toxicity (growth restriction, structural anomalies, functional/behavioral deficits, or death) in the 2nd and 3rd trimesters but not in the 1st trimester. The human pregnancy data outweigh any animal reproduction data.

HUMAN DATA SUGGEST RISK IN 3RD TRIMESTER

Evidence (for the drug or similar drugs) suggests that there may be a fetal risk for developmental toxicity (growth restriction, structural anomalies, functional/behavioral deficits, or death) in the 3rd trimester, or close to delivery but not in the 1st or 2nd trimesters. The human pregnancy data outweigh any animal reproduction data.

HUMAN (AND ANIMAL) DATA SUGGEST RISK

The human data for the drug or drugs in the same class or with the same mechanism of action, and animal reproduction data if available, suggest there may be a risk for developmental toxicity (growth restriction, structural anomalies, functional/behavioral deficits, or death) throughout pregnancy. Usually, pregnancy exposure should be avoided, but the risk may be acceptable if the maternal condition requires the drug.

DEFINITIONS OF BREASTFEEDING RECOMMENDATIONS

COMPATIBLE

Either the drug is not excreted in clinically significant amounts into human breast milk or its use during lactation does not, or is not expected to, cause toxicity in a nursing infant.

HOLD BREASTFEEDING

The drug may or may not be excreted into human breast milk, but the maternal benefit of therapy far outweighs the benefits of breast milk to an infant. Breastfeeding should be held until maternal therapy is completed and the drug has been eliminated (or reaches a low concentration) from her system.

NO (LIMITED) HUMAN DATA—PROBABLY COMPATIBLE

Either there is no human data or the human data are limited. The available data suggest that the drug does not represent a significant risk to a nursing infant.

NO (LIMITED) HUMAN DATA—POTENTIAL TOXICITY

Either there is no human data or the human data are limited. The characteristics of the drug suggest that it could represent a clinically significant risk to a nursing infant. Breastfeeding is not recommended.

HUMAN DATA SUGGEST POTENTIAL TOXICITY

Human data suggest a risk to a nursing infant. The drug is best avoided during breastfeeding. Depending on the drug, short-term use by the mother may be possible, but the infant should be closely monitored for potential adverse effects.

NO (LIMITED) HUMAN DATA—POTENTIAL TOXICITY (MOTHER)

Either there is no human data or the human data are limited. The characteristics of the drug suggest that breastfeeding could represent a clinically significant risk to the mother such as further loss of essential vitamins or nutrients. Breastfeeding is not recommended.

CONTRAINDICATED

There may or may not be human experience, but the combined data suggest that the drug may cause severe toxicity in a nursing infant, or breastfeeding is contraindicated because of the maternal condition for which the drug is indicated. Women should not breastfeed if they are taking the drug or have the condition.

COMPARISON OF AGENTS WITHIN THE SAME PHARMACOLOGIC CLASS

The Appendix arranges the drugs by their pharmacologic category. This allows the reader to identify all of the drugs that have been reviewed within a specific category, thus allowing, if desired, a comparison of the drugs. For example, the subsection *Antihypertensives* lists together those agents used for this purpose under the general heading *Cardiovascular Drugs*. To assist the reader in locating an agent in the Appendix, page numbers (in parentheses) referring to the location in the Appendix have been added to the generic names (shown in **bold**) in the Index.

FDA RISK CATEGORIES DEFINITIONS

Although the FDA risk categories have been excluded from this edition, readers wanting this information can obtain it from the manufacturer's product information.

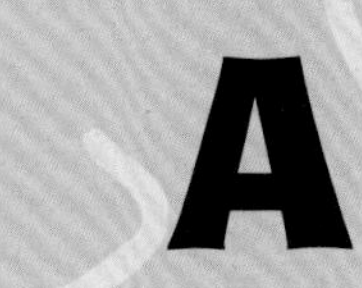

ABACAVIR

Antiviral

PREGNANCY RECOMMENDATION: Compatible—Maternal Benefit >> Embryo–Fetal Risk
BREASTFEEDING RECOMMENDATION: Contraindicated

PREGNANCY SUMMARY

The animal data suggest moderate risk. Although the human pregnancy experience does not suggest a risk of structural anomalies, other potential developmental toxicities require study. Antiretroviral nucleosides have been shown to have a direct dose-related cytotoxic effect on preimplantation mouse embryos (see Didanosine, Stavudine, Zalcitabine, and Zidovudine). This toxicity has not been studied in humans. Mitochondrial dysfunction in offspring exposed in utero or postnatally to nucleoside reverse transcriptase inhibitors (NRTIs) has been reported (see Lamivudine and Zidovudine), but these findings are controversial and require confirmation. However, if indicated, the drug should not be withheld because of pregnancy.

FETAL RISK SUMMARY

Abacavir is a synthetic carbocyclic nucleoside analog that is converted by cellular enzymes to the active metabolite, carbovir triphosphate. It is an NRTI used for the treatment of HIV type 1 (HIV-1). Other drugs in this class are didanosine, lamivudine, stavudine, zalcitabine, and zidovudine (1).

In reproduction studies, doses of abacavir up to 8 times the human therapeutic dose (HTD) based on BSA had no effect on the fertility or mating performance of male and female rats. However, embryo toxicity (increased resorptions, decreased body weight) was observed. During organogenesis, doses up to 35 times the human exposure based on AUC (about 16 times the HTD) resulted in fetal growth restriction (reduced body weight and crown–rump length), as well as increased incidences of fetal anasarca and skeletal malformations. Offspring exposed from implantation through weaning had an increased incidence of stillbirth and survivors had decreased body weights throughout life. In contrast, no developmental toxicity or malformations were observed in rabbits at doses up to 8.5 times the human exposure based on AUC (1).

Abacavir crosses the human placenta. In four women being treated for multiple agents for HIV infection, the mean abacavir cord:maternal blood ratio was 1.03 at a mean of 3.5 hours (range 0.4–9.0 hours) after a dose (dose not specified) and the amniotic fluid concentration in one woman was 1.6 mg/L (2). These results are consistent with the relatively low molecular weight (about 671) and high lipophilic properties of abacavir. In an ex vivo human placental model, the antiviral agent readily crossed to the fetal side with a high clearance index of about 50% that of antipyrine (3). No accumulation of the drug was found on the fetal side.

The Antiretroviral Pregnancy Registry reported, for the period January 1989 through July 2009, prospective data (reported before the outcomes were known) involving 4702 live births that had been exposed during the 1st trimester to one or more antiretroviral agents (4). Congenital defects were noted in 134, a prevalence of 2.8% (95% confidence interval [CI] 2.4–3.4). In the 6100 live births with earliest exposure in the 2nd/3rd trimesters, there were 153 infants with defects (2.5%, 95% CI 2.1–2.9). The prevalence rates for the two periods did not differ significantly. There were 288 infants with birth defects among 10,803 live births with exposure anytime during pregnancy (2.7%, 95% CI 2.4–3.0). The prevalence rate did not differ significantly from the rate expected in a nonexposed population. There were 1547 outcomes exposed to abacavir (628 in the 1st trimester and 919 in the 2nd/3rd trimesters) in combination with other antiretroviral agents. There were 45 birth defects (19 in the 1st trimester and 26 in the 2nd/3rd trimesters). In reviewing the birth defects of prospective and retrospective (pregnancies reported after the outcomes were known) registered cases, the Registry concluded that except for isolated cases of neural tube defects with efavirenz exposure in retrospective reports, there was no other pattern of anomalies (isolated or syndromic) (4). (See Lamivudine for required statement.)

Two reviews, one in 1996 and the other in 1997, concluded that all women receiving antiretroviral therapy should continue to receive therapy during pregnancy and that treatment of the mother with monotherapy should be considered inadequate therapy (5,6). The same conclusion was reached in a 2003 review with the added admonishment that therapy must be continuous to prevent emergence of resistant viral strains (7). In 2009, the updated U.S. Department of Health and Human Services guidelines for the use of antiretroviral agents in HIV-1-infected patients continued the recommendation that therapy, with the exception of efavirenz, should be continued during pregnancy (8). If indicated, abacavir should not be withheld in pregnancy because the expected benefit to the HIV-positive mother outweighs the unknown risk to the fetus. Updated guidelines for the use of antiretroviral drugs to reduce perinatal HIV-1 transmission were also released in 2010 (9). Women receiving antiretroviral therapy during pregnancy should continue the therapy but, regardless of the regimen, zidovudine administration is recommended during the intrapartum period to prevent vertical transmission of HIV to the newborn (9).

BREASTFEEDING SUMMARY

No reports have been located that describe the use of abacavir during human lactation. The molecular weight (about 671) suggests that the drug will be excreted into breast milk. The effect on a nursing infant is unknown.

Reports on the use of abacavir during human lactation are unlikely because the drug is used in the treatment of HIV-1 infections. HIV-1 is transmitted in milk, and in developed countries, breastfeeding is not recommended (5,6,8,10–12). In developing countries, breastfeeding is undertaken despite the risk because there are no affordable milk substitutes available. Until 1999, no studies had been published that examined the effect of any antiretroviral therapy on HIV-1 transmission in milk. In that year, a study involving zidovudine was published that measured a 38% reduction in vertical transmission of HIV-1 infection despite breastfeeding when compared with controls (see Zidovudine).

References

1. Product information. Ziagen. Glaxo Wellcome, 2000.
2. Chappuy H, Treluyer JM, Jullien V, Dimet J, Rey E, Fouche M, Firtion G, Pons G, Mandelbrot L. Maternal–fetal transfer and amniotic fluid accumulation of nucleoside analogue reverse transcriptase inhibitors in human immunodeficiency virus-infected pregnant women. Antimicrob Agents Chemother 2004;48:4332–6.
3. Bawdon RE. The *ex vivo* human placental transfer of the anti-HIV nucleoside inhibitor abacavir and the protease inhibitor amprenavir. Infect Dis Obstet Gynecol 1998;6:244–6.
4. Antiretroviral Pregnancy Registry Steering Committee. *Antiretroviral Pregnancy Registry International Interim Report for 1 January 1989 through 31 July 2009*. Wilmington, NC: Registry Coordinating Center; 2009. Available at http://www.apregistry.com. Accessed May 29, 2010.
5. Carpenter CCJ, Fischi MA, Hammer SM, Hirsch MS, Jacobsen DM, Katzenstein DA, Montaner JSG, Richman DD, Saag MS, Schooley RT, Thompson MA, Vella S, Yeni PG, Volberding PA. Antiretroviral therapy for HIV infection in 1996. JAMA 1996;276:146–54.
6. Minkoff H, Augenbraun M. Antiretroviral therapy for pregnant women. Am J Obstet Gynecol 1997;176:478–89.
7. Minkoff H. Human immunodeficiency virus infection in pregnancy. Obstet Gynecol 2003;101:797–810.
8. Panel on Antiretroviral Guidelines for Adults and Adolescents. *Guidelines for the Use of Antiretroviral Agents in HIV-1-Infected Adults and Adolescents*. Department of Health and Human Services. December 1, 2009:1–161. Available at http://www.aidsinfo.nih.gov/ContentFiles/AdultandAdolescentGL.pdf. Accessed September 17, 2010:60, 96–8.
9. Panel on Treatment of HIV-Infected Pregnant Women and Prevention of Perinatal Transmission. *Recommendations for Use of Antiretroviral Drugs in Pregnant HIV-1-Infected Women for Maternal Health and Interventions to Reduce Perinatal HIV Transmission in the United States*. May 24, 2010:1–117. Available at http://aidsinfo.nih.gov/ContentFiles/PerinatalGL.pdf. Accessed September 17, 2010:30, 39–44 (Table 5).
10. Brown ZA, Watts DH. Antiviral therapy in pregnancy. Clin Obstet Gynecol 1990;33:276–89.
11. De Martino M, Tovo P-A, Pezzotti P, Galli L, Massironi E, Ruga E, Floreea F, Plebani A, Gabiano C, Zuccotti GV. HIV-1 transmission through breast-milk: appraisal of risk according to duration of feeding. AIDS 1992; 6:991–7.
12. Van de Perre P. Postnatal transmission of human immunodeficiency virus type 1: the breast feeding dilemma. Am J Obstet Gynecol 1995; 173:483–7.

ABATACEPT

Immunologic Agent (Immunomodulator)/Antirheumatic Agent

PREGNANCY RECOMMENDATION: Limited Human Data—Animal Data Suggest Low Risk
BREASTFEEDING RECOMMENDATION: No Human Data—Potential Toxicity

PREGNANCY SUMMARY

Although the animal data suggest low risk, the human pregnancy experience is too limited to assess the embryo–fetal risk. Several reviews have discussed the potential risk of abatacept in human pregnancy (1–5). Some recommend discontinuing the drug 10–18 weeks before pregnancy because the drug has a long elimination half-life (2,4,5). It is not known if in utero exposure could result in autoimmune diseases in later life (6). Moreover, use in pregnancy is contraindicated if abatacept is combined with methotrexate or leflunomide. Until more data are available, the safest course is to avoid abatacept during gestation. If abatacept is used in pregnancy for the treatment of rheumatoid arthritis, health care professionals are encouraged to call the toll-free number (877-311-8972) for information about patient enrollment in the Organization of Teratology Information Specialists (OTIS) Rheumatoid Arthritis study.

FETAL RISK SUMMARY

Abatacept, a soluble fusion protein, is a selective costimulation modulator that inhibits T-lymphocyte activation, thereby decreasing T-cell proliferation and inhibiting the production of the cytokines tumor necrosis factor-α, interferon-γ, and interleukin-2. It is administered as an IV infusion. Abatacept is indicated, either as monotherapy or in combination with other agents, for the treatment of rheumatoid arthritis in patients with moderately to severely active rheumatoid arthritis that has not responded to other drug therapy. The elimination half-life after a single 10 mg/kg IV dose in a healthy subject was 16.7 days (range 12–23 days), whereas in rheumatoid arthritis patients after multiple 10 mg/kg IV infusions, it was 13.1 days (range 8–25 days) (6).

Reproduction studies have been conducted in mice, rats, and rabbits. In these species, daily doses (*route not specified but assumed to be SC*) were not teratogenic. The dose comparisons were about 29 times the maximum recommended human dose of 10 mg/kg dose based on AUC (MRHD). There were no adverse effects in the offspring when rats were treated every 3 days from early gestation and throughout lactation with doses up to 3 times the MRHD. However, at a dose 11 times the MRHD, alterations of immune function were observed in female pups and one female pup (of 10 male and 10 female pups evaluated) had inflammation of the thyroid (6).

In carcinogenicity studies, weekly SC doses of abatacept for about 2 years in mice were associated with increased incidences of malignant lymphomas and mammary gland tumors at doses ≤3 times the HD. However, the mice were infected with viruses known to cause these cancers in immunosuppressed mice. In cynomolgus monkeys, an IV dose given once weekly that was 9 times the HD was not associated with any significant adverse effects. No evidence of lymphomas or preneoplastic morphologic changes was observed despite the presence of a virus known to cause these lesions in immunosuppressed monkeys. Abatacept was not mutagenic and did not cause chromosomal aberrations, nor did it impair the fertility of male and female monkeys given doses every 3 days up to 11 times the HD (6).

Abatacept crosses the human placenta, despite its high molecular weight (about 92,000) (6). However, the amount reaching the embryo and/or fetus was not quantified.

Several reviews have discussed the potential risks of abatacept in pregnancy (1–5). As discussed in a 2012 review, eight patients became pregnant while receiving abatacept during clinical trials in rheumatoid arthritis, seven of whom were also receiving methotrexate and one was also receiving leflunomide (4). A spontaneous abortion (SAB) occurred during the 1st trimester in three (two had a prior history of SAB) and two had an elective abortion (EAB). The remaining three women were still pregnant. In another case, the wife of a man treated with abatacept became pregnant and gave birth to a healthy baby. In a phase II trial of abatacept in multiple sclerosis, two women became pregnant and a third women became pregnant by a abatacept-treated man. The outcomes of these pregnancies were a healthy baby, an EAB, and a SAB (4).

A 2013 case report described the outcome of a pregnancy exposed to abatacept in the 1st trimester (7). A 33-year-old woman with rheumatoid arthritis conceived while receiving abatacept (10 mg/kg every 4 weeks) and methotrexate (15 mg/week). The dose given in pregnancy occurred at 2.5 weeks'. Both drugs were stopped, but a daily 5 mg dose of an unspecified corticosteroid was allowed. At 40 weeks', the woman gave birth vaginally to a healthy 3180-g infant (sex not specified) with Apgar scores of 10 and 10 at 5 and 10 minutes, respectively. The child was doing well at 3.5-year follow-up (7).

BREASTFEEDING SUMMARY

No reports describing the use of abatacept during human lactation have been located. Although the molecular weight is high (about 92,000), excretion into breast milk is a possibility, especially because of the long elimination half-life (13 days; range 8–25 days). However, the amount in milk and the systemic bioavailability are unknown as are the effects on a nursing infant, but the potential for adverse effects on an infant's developing immune system should be considered.

References

1. Ostensen M, Lockshin M, Doria A, Valesini G, Meroni P, Gordon C, Brucato A, Tincani A. Update on safety during pregnancy of biological agents and some immunosuppressive anti-rheumatic drugs. Rheumatology 2008;47(Suppl 3):iii28–31.
2. Ostensen M, Förger F. Management of RA medications in pregnant patients. Nat Rev Rheumatol 2009;5:382–90.
3. Makol A, Wright K, Amin S. Rheumatoid arthritis and pregnancy—safety considerations in pharmacological management. Drugs 2011;71:1973–87.
4. Pham T, Bachelez H, Barthelot JM, Blacher J, Claudepierre P, Constantin A, Fautrel B, Gaujoux-Viala C, Goeb V, Gossec L, Goupille P, Guillaume-Czitrom S, Hachulla E, Lequerre T, Marolleau JP, Martinez V, Masson C, Mouthon L, Puechal X, Richette P, Saraux A, Schaeverbeke T, Soubrier M, Viguier M, Vittecoq O, Wendling D, Mariette X, Sibilia J. Abatacept therapy and safety management. Joint Bone Spine 2012;72(Suppl 1):3–84.
5. Furst DE, Keystone EC, So AK, Braun J, Breedveld FC, Burmester GR, De Benedetti F, Dorner T, Emery P, Fleischmann R, Gibofsky A, Kalden JR, Kavanaugh A, Kirkham B, Mease P, Rubbert-Roth A, Sieper J, Singer NG, Smolen JS, VanRiel PLCM, Weisman MH, Winthrop KI. Updated consensus statement on biological agents in the treatment of rheumatic disease, 2012. Ann Rheum Dis 2013;72(Suppl 2):ii2–34.
6. Product information. Orencia. Bristol-Myers Squibb, 2011.
7. Ojeda-Uribe M, Afif N, Dahan E, Sparsa L, Haby C, Sibilia J, Ternant D, Ardizzone M. Exposure to abatacept or rituximab in the first trimester of pregnancy of three women with autoimmune diseases. Clin Rheumatol 2013;32:695–700.

ABCIXIMAB

Hematologic Agent (Antiplatelet)

PREGNANCY RECOMMENDATION: Compatible—Maternal Benefit >> Embryo–Fetal Risk
BREASTFEEDING RECOMMENDATION: Compatible

PREGNANCY SUMMARY

Two case reports have described the use of abciximab during human pregnancy. In addition, the reproduction effects of the drug, if any, have not been studied in animals. However, a placental perfusion study suggests that abciximab does not reach the fetus in clinically significant amounts. The primary risk, therefore, appears to be from maternal hemorrhage during drug administration. If this is adequately controlled, the benefits of the drug to the mother appear to far outweigh the unknown risks to the embryo–fetus.

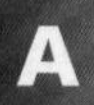

FETAL RISK SUMMARY

Abciximab, the Fab fragment of the chimeric human-murine monoclonal antibody 7E3, binds to the GP IIb/IIIa receptor on human platelets and inhibits platelet aggregation. It also binds to vessel wall endothelial and smooth muscle cells. It is in the same subclass of antiplatelet agents as eptifibatide and tirofiban. Abciximab is indicated as an adjunct to percutaneous coronary intervention for the prevention of cardiac ischemic complications. It increases the risk of bleeding, especially when used with heparin and other anticoagulants or thrombolytics (1).

Animal reproduction studies have not been conducted with abciximab. No mutagenicity was observed with in vitro and in vivo tests, but long-term animal studies to detect carcinogenicity or adverse effects on fertility have not been conducted (1).

Using an in vitro perfused human placenta, researchers found that only pharmaceutically insignificant amounts of abciximab could be detected in the fetal circuit. Minute amounts of abciximab were found on fetal platelets, but not on the endothelium or smooth muscle of fetal blood vessels, indicating that some transfer had taken place (2).

A 1998 case described the treatment of an acute myocardial infarction (AMI) in a 30-year-old woman at 38 weeks' gestation (3). Because her condition did not improve with aspirin, heparin, nitrates, or balloon angioplasty after an abciximab infusion was started, a stent was placed in the partially occluded left anterior descending coronary artery. The drug infusion was continued for 12 hours. Adequate blood flow was reestablished in the artery. Postoperatively, the woman was treated with ticlopidine, aspirin, and an unspecified β-blocker. Two weeks later, she delivered a healthy baby boy vaginally, with no evidence of bleeding and a normal ductus arteriosus. No excessive maternal bleeding was observed (3).

A brief 2009 case report described a 39-year-old woman at 6 weeks' who developed an AMI and was started on clopidogrel, aspirin, and heparin (4). Following placement of a stent, the woman again experienced chest pain and thrombus were discovered in three coronary arteries that were removed under coverage of abciximab (dose not specified) and intracoronary adenosine. She was maintained on clopidogrel and aspirin throughout the pregnancy. At 41 weeks', she was given platelet concentrates and a cesarean section delivered a female infant with appropriate weight (weight not specified). Defects in the infant included a patent foramen ovale, a muscular ventricular septal defect, and moderate mitral regurgitation. The authors considered the anomalies relatively common with a benign prognosis (4).

BREASTFEEDING SUMMARY

No reports describing the use of abciximab during lactation have been located. Because of the indications for abciximab, it is doubtful that such reports will be forthcoming. The very high molecular weight of the drug (about 48,000) suggests that it will not be excreted into milk in clinically significant amounts. Therefore, the risk to a nursing infant appears to be nil.

References

1. Product information. ReoPro. Eli Lilly, 2004.
2. Miller RK, Mace K, Polliotti B, DeRita R, Hall W, Treacy G. Marginal transfer of ReoPro™ (abciximab) compared with immunoglobulin G (F105), inulin and water in the perfused human placenta in vitro. Placenta 2003;24:727–38.
3. Sebastian C, Scherlag M, Kugelmass A, Schechter E. Primary stent implantation for acute myocardial infarction during pregnancy: use of abciximab, ticlopidine, and aspirin. Cathet Cardiovasc Diagn 1998;45:275–9.
4. Santiago-Diaz P, Arrebola-Moreno AL, Ramirez-Hernandez JA, Melgares-Moreno R. Use of antiplatelet drugs during pregnancy. Rev Exp Cardiol 2009;62:1197–8.

ABIRATERONE ACETATE

Antineoplastic

PREGNANCY RECOMMENDATION: Contraindicated
BREASTFEEDING RECOMMENDATION: Contraindicated

PREGNANCY SUMMARY

Abiraterone acetate, given in combination with prednisone, is indicated for the treatment of prostate cancer. No reports describing its use in human pregnancy have been located, but such reports are unlikely because of the indication. Reproduction studies in pregnant animals have not been conducted. Because of the risk of embryo and fetal harm, the drug is classified as contraindicated in pregnancy.

FETAL RISK SUMMARY

Abiraterone acetate is converted in vivo to abiraterone, an inhibitor of the enzyme (CYP17) that is expressed in testicular, adrenal, and prostatic tumor tissues and is required for androgen biosynthesis. It is indicated for use in combination with prednisone for the treatment of patients with metastatic castration-resistant prostate cancer who have received prior chemotherapy containing docetaxel. The active metabolite abiraterone is further metabolized to inactive metabolites. Abiraterone is highly bound (>99%) to human plasma proteins, albumin, and α_1-acid glycoprotein and the mean terminal half-life is 12 hours (1).

Reproduction and carcinogenesis studies with abiraterone acetate in animals have not been conducted. However, neither abiraterone acetate nor abiraterone was mutagenic or clastogenic in multiple assays. In rats and monkeys, abiraterone caused atrophy, aspermia/hypospermia, and hyperplasia in the reproductive system at doses that were 1.14 and 0.6 times, respectively, the human clinical exposure based on AUC. These effects were consistent with the antiandrogenic pharmacologic action of the agent (1).

It is not known if abiraterone acetate or its active metabolite abiraterone crosses the human placenta. The molecular weight of abiraterone acetate (about 392) and abiraterone (about 333) and the long terminal half-life of abiraterone suggest that both agents will cross to the embryo–fetus, but the high plasma protein binding of abiraterone might limit the exposure.

BREASTFEEDING SUMMARY

No reports describing the use of abiraterone acetate during human lactation have been located. Because of the indication, it is unlikely that such reports will occur. The molecular weight of abiraterone acetate (about 392) and the active metabolite abiraterone (about 333), and the long terminal half-life of abiraterone (12 hours) suggest that the both agents will be excreted into breast milk. However, the high plasma protein binding (>99%) of abiraterone might limit the exposure. The effects of exposure to the drug on a nursing infant are unknown but, because of the potential for severe toxicity, breastfeeding is classified as contraindicated.

Reference

1. Product information. Zytiga. Janssen Biotech, 2012.

ACAMPROSATE

Antialcoholic Agent

PREGNANCY RECOMMENDATION: Limited Human Data—Animal Data Suggest High Risk
BREASTFEEDING RECOMMENDATION: No Human Data—Probably Compatible

PREGNANCY SUMMARY

Although no published reports describing the use of acamprosate in human pregnancy have been located, there are human data from a Teratology Information Service (TIS) in France. The animal data suggest high risk, but the very limited human pregnancy experience prevents an assessment of the embryo–fetal risk. However, the use of ethanol (alcohol) in pregnancy is well known to cause dose-related developmental toxicity (see Ethanol). Even in the absence of obvious structural defects, alcohol use during gestation is associated with marked neurotoxicity in the offspring. Therefore, in pregnant women with alcohol dependency, the risk:benefit ratio may favor the use of acamprosate.

FETAL RISK SUMMARY

The synthetic compound acamprosate has a chemical structure similar to that of the endogenous amino acid homotaurine, a structural analog of the amino acid neurotransmitter γ-aminobutyric acid and the amino acid neuromodulator taurine. Acamprosate is indicated to maintain abstinence from alcohol in patients with alcohol dependence who are abstinent at treatment initiation. The mechanism of action is not completely understood, but acamprosate is thought to act differently than disulfiram, another agent in the class. Moreover, acamprosate and disulfiram have completely different chemical structures. Acamprosate is not metabolized and protein binding is negligible. It has a long elimination half-life ranging from about 20 to 33 hours (1).

Reproduction studies have been conducted in rats, rabbits, and mice. In rats, acamprosate was teratogenic at doses about equal to the maximum recommended human daily dose based on BSA (MRHDD). The dose-related defects were hydronephrosis, malformed iris, retinal dysplasia, and retroesophageal subclavian artery. The no-effect dose in rats was about 0.2 times the MRHDD. In Burgundy Tawny rabbits, hydronephrosis was observed at about 3 times the MRHDD. However, no defects were observed in New Zealand white rabbits at doses about 8 times the MRHDD. In mice, a dose about 2 times the MRHDD administered from day 15 of gestation through the end of lactation on postnatal day 28 was associated with an increased incidence of stillbirths. The no-effect dose in mice was about 0.5 times the MRHDD (1).

No carcinogenicity was observed in studies with rats, and no evidence of mutagenicity or clastogenicity was noted in several tests and assays. Acamprosate had no effect on the fertility of male and female rats at doses up to about 4 times the MRHDD, or in female mice at doses up to about 5 times the MRHDD (1).

It is not known ifacamprosate crosses the human placenta. The molecular weight (about 400), lack of metabolism and protein binding, and long elimination half-life suggest that it will cross to the embryo and/or fetus.

A TIS in France has gathered information on 18 pregnancies exposed to acamprosate during the 1st trimester (T. Vial, personal communication, Teratology Information Service, Lyon, France, 2010). The outcomes of these pregnancies included 2 spontaneous abortions, 3 elective abortions, 10 normal newborns (1 premature and 1 died at 1 month of age probably from sudden infant death syndrome), 1 newborn with minor facial anomalies, and a fetus and a newborn with major malformations. The fetus was electively aborted because of an omphalocele and found also to have micro-retrognathism, cleft palate, and a ventricular septal defect.

The major defect in the infant was a cleft lip. Concomitant exposure to alcohol and other drugs occurred in several of the pregnancies.

BREASTFEEDING SUMMARY

No reports describing the use of acamprosate during human lactation have been located. The molecular weight (about 400), lack of metabolism and protein binding, and prolonged elimination half-life (20–33 hours) suggest that the drug will be excreted in breast milk. The effect on a nursing infant from exposure in milk is unknown. However, alcohol is excreted into milk and is known to be a neurotoxin (see Ethanol). Thus, if a lactating woman requires acamprosate to refrain from drinking, the benefit to the nursing infant appears to outweigh the unknown risk from the drug.

Reference

1. Product information. Campral. Forest Pharmaceuticals, 2012.

ACARBOSE

Antidiabetic Agent

PREGNANCY RECOMMENDATION: Limited Human Data—Animal Data Suggest Low Risk
BREASTFEEDING RECOMMENDATION: No Human Data—Probably Compatible

PREGNANCY SUMMARY

Less than 2% of acarbose is absorbed systemically, but several metabolites are absorbed in much greater proportions, and the embryo or fetal risk from any of these is unknown. Acarbose is normally used in combination with oral hypoglycemic agents, and these hypoglycemic drugs might not be indicated for the pregnant diabetic. Carefully prescribed insulin therapy will provide better control of the mother's blood glucose, thereby preventing the fetal and neonatal complications that occur with this disease. High maternal glucose levels, as may occur in diabetes mellitus, are closely associated with a number of maternal and fetal effects, including fetal structural anomalies if the hyperglycemia occurs early in gestation. To prevent this toxicity, the American College of Obstetricians and Gynecologists recommends that insulin be used for type 1 and type 2 diabetes occurring during pregnancy and, if diet therapy alone is not successful, for gestational diabetes (1,2).

FETAL RISK SUMMARY

Acarbose is an oral α-glucosidase inhibitor that delays the digestion of ingested carbohydrates within the gastrointestinal tract, thereby reducing the rise in blood glucose after meals. It is used in the management of non–insulin-dependent diabetes mellitus (type 2). Less than 2% of a dose is absorbed as active drug in adults, but the systemic absorption of metabolites is much higher (approximately 34% of the dose) (3).

Reproductive studies in rats found no evidence of impaired fertility or reproductive performance. Doses of acarbose up to 9 and 32 times the human dose (HD) in pregnant rats and rabbits, respectively, were not teratogenic in either species or, at 10 times the HD, embryotoxic in rabbits (3).

A 1998 noninterventional observational cohort study described the outcomes of pregnancies in women who had been prescribed 1 or more of 34 newly marketed drugs by general practitioners in England (4). Data were obtained by questionnaires sent to the prescribing physicians 1 month after the expected or possible date of delivery. In 831 (78%) of the pregnancies, a newly marketed drug was thought to have been taken during the 1st trimester with birth defects noted in 14 (2.5%) singleton births of the 557 newborns (10 sets of twins). In addition, two birth defects were observed in aborted fetuses. However, few of the aborted fetuses were examined. Acarbose was taken during the 1st trimester in five pregnancies. The outcomes of these pregnancies included two spontaneous abortions and three normal newborns (one premature) (4).

A 2002 abstract reported the pregnancy outcomes (birth weight and gestational age at delivery) of 91 women at ≥20 weeks' gestation who were treated with either acarbose ($N = 45$) or insulin ($N = 46$) for gestational diabetes mellitus (5). The women had failed to achieve glucose goals with diet alone. In the oral group, 6% were changed to insulin because they were unable to tolerate acarbose (gastrointestinal complaints). There was no difference in the pregnancy outcomes between the groups.

A 2002 report described the use of acarbose (200 mg/day) in early pregnancy (6). A 35-year-old woman with several diseases (hypertension, diabetes mellitus, hypercholesterolemia, anxiety disorder, epilepsia, and morbid obesity) conceived while being treated with multiple drugs: rosiglitazone, gliclazide (a sulfonylurea), atorvastatin, spironolactone, hydrochlorothiazide, carbamazepine, thioridazine, amitriptyline, chlordiazepoxide, and pipenzolate bromide (an antispasmodic). Her pregnancy was diagnosed in the 8th week of gestation and all medications were stopped. She was treated with methyldopa and insulin for the remainder of her pregnancy. At 36 weeks' gestation, a repeat cesarean section delivered a healthy, 3.5-kg female infant with Apgar scores of 7 and 8 at 1 and 5 minutes, respectively. The infant was developing normally after 4 months (6).

BREASTFEEDING SUMMARY

No studies describing the use of acarbose during human lactation have been located. Because the drug acts within the gastrointestinal tract to slow the absorption of ingested

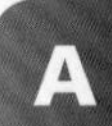

carbohydrates, and <2% of a dose is absorbed systemically, the amount of unmetabolized drug in the mother's circulation available for transfer to the milk is probably clinically insignificant. As with all drugs, however, the safest course while taking acarbose is not to breastfeed until data on its safety during lactation are available.

References

1. American College of Obstetricians and Gynecologists. Pregestational diabetes mellitus. *ACOG Practice Bulletin*. No. 60. March 2005. Obstet Gynecol 2005;105:675–85.
2. American College of Obstetricians and Gynecologists. Gestational diabetes. *ACOG Practice Bulletin*. No. 30. September 2001. Obstet Gynecol 2001;98:525–38.
3. Product information. Precose. Bayer Corporation, 1997.
4. Wilton LV, Pearce GL, Martin RM, Mackay FJ, Mann RD. The outcomes of pregnancy in women exposed to newly marketed drugs in general practice in England. Br J Obstet Gynaecol 1998;105:882–9.
5. De Veciana M, Trail PA, Evans AT, Dulaney K. A comparison of oral acarbose and insulin in women with gestational diabetes mellitus (abstract). Obstet Gynecol 2002;99(Suppl):5S.
6. Yaris F, Yaris E, Kadioglu M, Ulku C, Kesim M, Kalyoncu NI. Normal pregnancy outcome following inadvertent exposure to rosiglitazone, gliclazide, and atorvastatin in a diabetic and hypertensive woman. Reprod Toxicol 2004;18:619–21.

ACEBUTOLOL

Sympatholytic (Antihypertensive)

PREGNANCY RECOMMENDATION: Limited Human Data—Animal Data Suggest Low Risk
BREASTFEEDING RECOMMENDATION: Limited Human Data—Potential Toxicity

PREGNANCY SUMMARY

Some β-blockers may cause growth restriction, including intrauterine growth restriction (IUGR), and reduced placental weight, especially those lacking intrinsic sympathomimetic activity (ISA) (i.e., partial agonist). Treatment beginning early in the 2nd trimester results in the greatest weight reductions, whereas treatment restricted to the 3rd trimester primarily affects only placental weight. Acebutolol does possess ISA. However, IUGR and reduced placental weight may potentially occur with all agents within this class. Although growth restriction is a serious concern, the benefits of maternal therapy with β-blockers, in some cases, might outweigh the risks to the fetus and must be judged on a case-by-case basis.

FETAL RISK SUMMARY

Acebutolol, a cardioselective β-adrenergic blocking agent, has been used for the treatment of hypertension occurring during pregnancy (1–5). The drug undergoes extensive first-pass hepatic metabolism after oral administration (absolute bioavailability about 40%). The major metabolite, diacetolol, is equipotent to acebutolol (6).

In animal reproduction studies, no teratogenic effects were observed in pregnant rats and rabbits with doses up to about 32 times the maximum recommended human dose (MRHD) and up to about 7 times the MRHD, respectively. The maximum dose in rabbits produced slight intrauterine growth restriction that was thought to be secondary to maternal toxicity (6).

Acebutolol crosses the placenta, producing a maternal:cord ratio of 0.8 (3). The corresponding ratio for the active metabolite, diacetolol, was 0.6. Newborn serum levels of acebutolol and the metabolite were <5–244 and 17–663 ng/mL, respectively (3). A cord:maternal ratio of 0.7 for acebutolol has also been reported (4).

No human malformations attributable to acebutolol have been observed, but experience with the drug during the 1st trimester is lacking. In a study comparing three β-blockers, the mean birth weight of 56 newborns was slightly lower than 38 pindolol-exposed infants but higher than 31 offspring of atenolol-treated mothers (3160 vs. 3375 vs. 2745 g) (2). Growth restriction has been associated with β-blockers and the weight reduction may have been drug induced.

In a comparison of 20 pregnant women treated with either acebutolol or methyldopa for mild-to-moderate hypertension, no differences between the drugs were found for pregnancy duration, birth weight, Apgar scores, or placental weight (5). In addition, no evidence of bradycardia, hypoglycemia, or respiratory problems was found in the acebutolol-exposed newborns. In an earlier study, however, 10 newborns exposed to acebutolol near term had blood pressures and heart rates significantly lower than similar infants exposed to methyldopa (7). The hemodynamic differences were still evident 3 days after birth. Mean blood glucose levels were not significantly lower than those of similar infants exposed to methyldopa, but transient hypoglycemia was present 3 hours after birth in four term newborns (5). The mean half-life of acebutolol in the serum of newborns has been calculated to be 10.1 hours, but the half-life based on urinary excretion was 15.6 hours (7). The manufacturer cites the elimination half-life of acebutolol in newborns as 6–14 hours, compared with a half-life for diacetolol of 24–30 hours during the first 24 hours, then 12–16 hours thereafter (6). Therefore, newborn infants of women consuming the drug near delivery should be closely observed for signs and symptoms of β-blockade for at least 3–4 days to allow for elimination of the parent and active metabolite from the infant. Long-term effects of in utero exposure to β-blockers have not been studied but warrant evaluation.

BREASTFEEDING SUMMARY

Acebutolol and its active metabolite, diacetolol, are excreted into breast milk (3,8). Milk:plasma ratios for the two compounds were 7.1 and 12.2, respectively (3). Absorption of

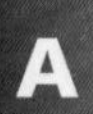

both compounds was demonstrated in breastfeeding infants, but no adverse effects were mentioned (3).

In a study of seven nursing, hypertensive mothers treated with 200–1200 mg/day within 13 days of delivery, milk:plasma acebutolol ratios in three of the mothers varied from 2.3 to 9.2, whereas similar ratios of the metabolite ranged from 1.5 to 13.5 (8). The highest milk concentration of acebutolol, 4123 ng/mL, occurred in a mother taking 1200 mg/day. Two to three days after treatment was stopped, milk:plasma ratios of acebutolol and the metabolite in the seven women were 1.9–9.8 and 2.3–24.7, respectively. Symptoms of β-blockade (hypotension, bradycardia, and transient tachypnea) were observed in one nursing infant, although the time of onset of the adverse effects was not given. Neonatal plasma concentrations of the drug and metabolite (specific data not given), which were already high from in utero exposure, rose sharply after nursing commenced. The mother was taking 400 mg/day, and her milk:plasma ratios of acebutolol and metabolite during treatment were 9.2 and 13.5, respectively, the highest observed in this study (8).

Breastfed infants of mothers taking acebutolol should be closely observed for hypotension, bradycardia, and other signs or symptoms of β-blockade. Long-term effects of exposure to β-blockers from milk have not been studied but warrant evaluation. The American Academy of Pediatrics classifies acebutolol as a drug that has been associated with adverse effects in nursing infants (9).

References

1. Dubois D, Petitcolas J, Temperville B, Klepper A. Beta blockers and high-risk pregnancies. Int J Biol Res Pregnancy 1980;1:141–5.
2. Dubois D, Petitcolas J, Temperville B, Klepper A, Catherine P. Treatment of hypertension in pregnancy with beta-adrenoceptor antagonists. Br J Clin Pharmacol 1982;13(Suppl):375S–8S.
3. Bianchetti G, Dubruc C, Vert P, Boutroy MJ, Morselli PL. Placental transfer and pharmacokinetics of acebutolol in newborn infants (abstract). Clin Pharmacol Ther 1981;29:233–4.
4. Boutroy MJ. Fetal and neonatal effects of the beta-adrenoceptor blocking agents. Dev Pharmacol Ther 1987;10:224–31.
5. Williams ER, Morrissey JR. A comparison of acebutolol with methyldopa in hypertensive pregnancy. Pharmatherapeutica 1983;3:487–91.
6. Product information. Sectral. Wyeth-Ayerst Pharmaceuticals, 2000.
7. Dumez Y, Tchobroutsky C, Hornych H, Amiel-Tison C. Neonatal effects of maternal administration of acebutolol. Br Med J 1981;283:1077–9.
8. Boutroy MJ, Bianchetti G, Dubruc C, Vert P, Morselli PL. To nurse when receiving acebutolol: is it dangerous for the neonate? Eur J Clin Pharmacol 1986;30:737–9.
9. Committee on Drugs, American Academy of Pediatrics. The transfer of drugs and other chemicals into human milk. Pediatrics 2001;108:776–89.

ACETAMINOPHEN

Analgesic/Antipyretic

PREGNANCY RECOMMENDATION: Human Data Suggest Low Risk
BREASTFEEDING RECOMMENDATION: Compatible

PREGNANCY SUMMARY

Acetaminophen is commonly used in all stages of pregnancy. Although originally thought not to cause risk in offspring, some recent reports have questioned this assessment, especially with frequent maternal use or in cases where genetic variability exists. Additional data are needed to confirm these risks but, as with all drug use in pregnancy, routine use of acetaminophen should be avoided.

FETAL RISK SUMMARY

Acetaminophen is routinely used during all stages of pregnancy for pain relief and to lower elevated body temperature. The drug crosses the placenta (1). In therapeutic doses, it is apparently safe for short-term use. However, continuous, high daily dosage in one mother probably caused severe anemia (possibly hemolytic) in her and fatal kidney disease in her newborn (2).

The pharmacokinetics of acetaminophen in pregnancy have been reported (3,4). In six healthy women who ingested a 1000-mg dose at 36 weeks' gestation and again 6 weeks after delivery, the mean serum half-lives were similar, 3.7 and 3.1 hours, respectively (3). The absorption, metabolism, and renal clearance of the drug were similar in the pregnant and nonpregnant states. A 1994 study compared the pharmacokinetics of a single 650-mg acetaminophen oral dose in 10 nonpregnant women (controls) with 8 women at a mean gestational age of 11.1 weeks (4). Among the pharmacokinetic parameters evaluated, significant differences between the pregnant and controls were found for elimination constant (0.431 vs. 0.348/hour), serum half-life (1.62 vs. 2.02 hours), and clearance (7.14 vs. 5.22 L/hour-kg).

The potential for acetaminophen-induced fetal liver toxicity after a toxic maternal dose was first suggested in 1979 (5). Two recent reports have described such toxicity (6,7). A woman, in her 27th–28th week of pregnancy, ingested 29.5 g of acetaminophen over <24 hours for severe dental pain (6). Fetal movements were last felt about 23 hours after the first dose, and on presentation to the hospital 16 hours later, no fetal heart beat was heard. The mother eventually recovered, although her serum levels of acetaminophen by extrapolation were thought to exceed 300 mcg/mL, a toxic level. Autopsy of the 2190-g female fetus revealed a liver acetaminophen concentration of 250 mcg/g of tissue. The extensive lysis of the fetal liver and kidneys, which may have been caused by autolysis before delivery (approximately 3 days after the mother last felt fetal movement), prevented documentation of the characteristic lesions observed in acetaminophen overdose (6).

A 1997 report described the fatal outcomes of a 38-year-old woman and her fetus at 31 weeks' gestation after she consumed an acute 35-g acetaminophen dose (7). The woman presented to the hospital 26 hours after the overdose with signs and symptoms of hepatorenal failure. On admission, she had a toxic acetaminophen serum level (40.43 mcg/mL) that was predictive of a very high risk of hepatocellular damage and subsequent fulminant liver failure (7). IV administration of *N*-acetylcysteine was started 30 minutes after admission. Severe fetal distress was diagnosed 30 minutes later and a cesarean section under spinal anesthesia was performed to deliver a 1620-g female infant who had Apgar scores of 0, 0, and 1 at 1, 5, and 10 minutes, respectively. The infant's acetaminophen serum level was 41.42 mcg/mL. Despite intensive therapy, the infant died 34 hours after birth and the mother died 66 hours after the overdose. Although the infant's laboratory data indicated hepatorenal toxicity, the actual cause of death could not be determined because permission for autopsy was refused (7).

In four other cases of acute overdosage, acetaminophen-induced fetal liver toxicity was apparently not observed, although such damage may have resolved before delivery in some cases (8–11). One woman, at 36 weeks' gestation, consumed a single dose of 22.5 g of acetaminophen, producing toxic blood levels of 200 mcg/mL (8). She delivered a normal infant approximately 6 weeks later. In another case, a woman at 20 weeks' gestation consumed a total of 25 g in two doses during a 10-hour period (9). She gave birth at 41 weeks to a normal infant with an occipital cephalohematoma as a result of birth position. At 24 hours of age, the infant had jaundice that responded to phototherapy. No evidence of permanent liver damage was observed. The jaundice was thought to have been caused by the cephalohematoma. A third case of acute maternal overdose occurred at 15.5 weeks' gestation when a mother ingested 64 g of the drug (10). Her acetaminophen level 10 hours after the ingestion was 198.5 mcg/mL. Marked hepatic necrosis and adult respiratory distress syndrome (because of aspiration pneumonia) ensued and then gradually resolved. The patient was discharged home approximately 3 weeks after ingestion and subsequently delivered a healthy 2000-g male infant at 32 weeks' gestation. The infant had physiologic hyperbilirubinemia with a peak level on the fourth day of life of 10.3 mg/dL, but phototherapy was not required. Follow-up evaluation at 4 months indicated normal development. One case involved a 22-year-old woman in her 31st week of pregnancy who consumed a 15-g dose, followed by a 50-g dose 1 week later (11). Fetal distress was observed 16 hours after the second overdose, as evidenced by a complete lack of fetal movements and breathing, a marked decrease in fetal heart rate beat-to-beat variability with no accelerations, and a falling baseline rate. Because of the fetal condition, labor was induced (cesarean section was excluded because of the mother's incipient hepatic failure). Eighty-four hours after the overdose, a healthy 2198-g female infant was delivered with Apgar scores of 9 and 10 at 1 and 5 minutes, respectively. Except for hypoglycemia, mild respiratory disease, and mild jaundice, the newborn did well. Liver enzymes were always within the normal range, and the jaundice was compatible with immaturity. Acetaminophen was not detected in the cord blood. Follow-up examinations of the infant at 6 weeks and again at 6 months were normal. In each of these instances, protection against serious or permanent liver damage was probably afforded by the prompt administration of IV *N*-acetylcysteine.

A 1993 report described a 25-year-old woman at 27 weeks' gestation who consumed 12.5–15 g of acetaminophen as a single dose 36 hours before admission for premature labor (12). She had also consumed an unknown amount of the drug over a few days before the acute overdose. Because of severe fetal distress, a cesarean section was performed under general anesthesia before her preoperative laboratory tests indicating liver failure were available. A 1300-g male infant was delivered who had Apgar scores of 1, 4, and 4 at 1, 5, and 10 minutes, respectively. No mention was made of hepatic or other toxicity in the infant and his course was thought to be satisfactory for his gestational age. The mother was treated for progressive liver failure and eventually recovered.

The Rocky Mountain Poison and Drug Center reported the results of a nationwide study on acetaminophen overdose during pregnancy involving 113 women (13). Of the 60 cases that had appropriate laboratory and pregnancy outcome data, 19 occurred during the 1st trimester, 22 during the 2nd trimester, and 19 during the 3rd trimester. In those cases with a potentially toxic serum level of acetaminophen, early treatment with *N*-acetylcysteine was statistically associated with an improved pregnancy outcome by lessening the incidence of spontaneous abortion and fetal death. Only one congenital anomaly was observed in the series and that involved a 3rd trimester overdose with nontoxic maternal acetaminophen serum levels (13). Based on these observations, neither acetaminophen nor *N*-acetylcysteine was likely a teratogen, although follow-up data on the infants were not available (13).

A Teratology Information Service in England conducted a prospective study of the pregnancy outcomes of 300 women who had consumed an overdose of acetaminophen, either alone or as a combination product (14). The overdoses occurred in all trimesters: 118 (39.3%), 103 (34.3%), and 79 (26.3%) in the 1st, 2nd, and 3rd trimesters, respectively. Systemic antidote treatment consisted of *N*-acetylcysteine (*N* = 33), ipecac (*N* = 52), and methionine (*N* = 16). In the remaining 199 cases, treatment was not recorded or not given, or a variety of nonsystemic treatments (charcoal, gastric lavage, or miscellaneous) were used. The fetal outcomes included 219 (72%) normal infants (two sets of twins), 16 (5%) spontaneous abortions (10 within 3 weeks of the overdose), 2 (1%) late fetal deaths, 54 (18%) elective abortions (1 with a diaphragmatic hernia), and 11 (4%) newborns with malformations (exposed between 16 and 32 weeks' gestation). All of the spontaneous abortions and one late fetal death occurred after 1st trimester overdoses. The other late fetal death followed a 2nd trimester overdose. The majority of the elective abortions were conducted for "social," rather than medical reasons. Malformations included one each of systolic murmur, small port wine stain on occiput, cleft lip and palate, bilateral inguinal hernia, soft palate defect, spina bifida occulta/bilateral squint, hypospadias, and ptosis of left eye. There were three cases of talipes. The malformation rate was within the expected rate in England and none of the cases, including the one with diaphragmatic hernia, could be related to acetaminophen (14). Seven full-term newborns had neonatal complications (all exposed during the 2nd or

3rd trimester). The complications did not appear to be related to acetaminophen overdose (14). Moreover, evaluations up to at least 6 weeks of age did not demonstrate any clinical signs of renal or hepatotoxicity.

The Collaborative Perinatal Project monitored 50,282 mother–child pairs, 226 of whom had 1st trimester exposure to acetaminophen (15, pp. 286–295). Although no evidence was found to suggest a relationship to large categories of major or minor malformations, a possible association with congenital dislocation of the hip based on three cases was found, but independent confirmation is required (15, p. 471). For use anytime during pregnancy, 781 exposures were recorded (15, p. 434). As with the qualifications expressed for 1st trimester exposure, possible associations with congenital dislocation of the hip (eight cases) and clubfoot (six cases) were found (15, p. 484).

A 1982 report described craniofacial and digital anomalies in an infant exposed in utero to large daily doses of acetaminophen and propoxyphene throughout pregnancy (16). The infant also exhibited withdrawal symptoms as a result of propoxyphene (see also Propoxyphene). The authors speculated with caution that the combination of propoxyphene with other drugs, such as acetaminophen, might have been teratogenic. In a study examining 6509 women with live births, acetaminophen with or without codeine was used by 697 (11%) during the 1st trimester (17). No evidence of a relationship to malformations was observed.

In a surveillance study of Michigan Medicaid recipients conducted between 1985 and 1992 involving 229,101 completed pregnancies, 9146 newborns had been exposed to acetaminophen during the 1st trimester (F. Rosa, personal communication, FDA, 1993). A total of 423 (4.6%) major birth defects were observed (416 expected). Specific data were available for six defect categories, including (observed/expected) 87/91 cardiovascular defects, 16/16 oral clefts, 4/7 spina bifida, 30/27 polydactyly, 14/16 limb reduction defects, and 16/22 hypospadias. These data do not support an association between the drug and the defects.

Using data from the North Jutland Pharmaco-Epidemiological Prescription Database in Denmark, investigators identified 123 women who had received a prescription for acetaminophen during pregnancy and/or 30 days before conception (18). The pregnancy outcomes of these women were compared with 13,329 controls who had received no prescriptions. Among the offspring of the 55 women who had received an acetaminophen prescription up to 30 days before conception and/or during the 1st trimester, there were six (10.9%) infants with congenital malformations compared with 697 (5.2%) from controls. The odds ratio (OR) for malformations was 2.3 (95% confidence interval [CI] 1.0–5.4). The six malformations were ventricular septal defect, two congenital dislocations of the hip, stenosis of tear canal, diaphragmatic hernia, and megalocornea (keratoglobus). The nature of the defects does not indicate a causal relationship to acetaminophen (18). No increased risk of malformation was found when the analysis was restricted to primigravidas (OR 0.7, 95% CI 0.1–5.5) (18). In addition, no effect was observed on fetal growth.

Unlike aspirin, acetaminophen does not affect platelet function, and there is no increased risk of hemorrhage if the drug is given to the mother at term (19,20). In a study examining intracranial hemorrhage in premature infants, the incidence of bleeding after exposure of the fetus to acetaminophen close to birth was no different from that in nonexposed control infants (21) (see also Aspirin).

A 1993 study examined the effect of therapeutic levels of acetaminophen on prostacyclin (PGI_2) production by endothelial cells isolated from human umbilical veins in culture and during the 3rd trimester in women with either hypertension or various complications of pregnancy (22). The drug reduced the production of PGI_2 in culture and during pregnancy, but thromboxane (TxA_2) production was not affected in the women. A balance between PGI_2 and TxA_2 is thought to be critical during pregnancy. PGI_2, derived from endothelial cells, is vasodilatory and antiaggregatory, whereas the platelet-derived TxA_2 is vasoconstrictive and proaggregatory (22). PGI_2 production increases normally during pregnancy, but this increase is markedly inhibited in pregnancy-induced hypertension (PIH) (22). Thus, a significant acetaminophen-induced reduction in PGI_2 production could adversely affect pregnancies complicated by PIH, including those treated with low-dose aspirin (see Aspirin). Because the effects of acetaminophen on PGI_2 are known to be tissue-specific, the authors of this study cautioned that additional studies, such as those measuring the effect of acetaminophen on placental PGI_2 and in patients being treated with low-dose aspirin for PIH, are required before the clinical significance of their findings can be determined (22).

In a prospective study of 1529 pregnant women in the mid-1970s, acetaminophen was used in the first half of pregnancy by 41% (23). A computerized system for stratifying on maternal alcohol and smoking histories was used to select 421 newborns for follow-up. Of this group, 43.5% had been exposed in utero to acetaminophen in the first half of pregnancy. After statistical control of numerous potentially confounding covariates, the data indicated that acetaminophen was not significantly related to child IQ at 4 years of age or to attention variables (see Aspirin for opposite results). Three physical growth parameters (height, weight, and head circumference) were also not significantly related to in utero acetaminophen exposure.

Acetaminophen has been used as an antipyretic just before delivery in women with fever secondary to chorioamnionitis (24). A significant improvement in fetal and newborn status, as measured by fetal heart rate tracings and arterial blood gases, was observed after normalization of the mother's temperature.

In a 2004 case–control study, 168 infants who had a nonsyndromic muscular ventricular septal defect were compared with 692 infants without birth defects (25). No significant associations were found between the occurrence of the ventricular septal defect and maternal use of acetaminophen or nonsteroidal anti-inflammatory agents after adjusting for maternal fever nor were they detected between maternal fever and the defect.

Use of acetaminophen during pregnancy was not associated with an increased risk of congenital anomalies in a 7-year prospective cohort study of 101,041 Danish women (26). Similar results were found in a 2010 report from the National Birth Defects Prevention Study (27). Moreover, use of acetaminophen appeared to decrease the risk of selected malformations when used for febrile illness.

In contrast to the above two studies, male offspring of Danish mothers who had used mild analgesics (acetaminophen, aspirin, ibuprofen) for >2 weeks, especially in the 2nd trimester, had a significant risk of cryptorchidism diagnosed at birth. The greatest risk observed was when more than one mild analgesic was used. The findings of this study were supported by antiandrogenic effects in rat models (28).

An in vitro study was conducted to determine the primary hepatic enzymes responsible for acetaminophen sulfation (29). The study found that the sulfotransferse isoform, SULT1A3/4, was the primary determinant of this activity. Genetic variation in this enzyme could lead to reduced fetal biotransformation of acetaminophen and persistence of the drug in the fetus. The investigators hypothesized that this could be a risk factor for the development of fetal gastroschisis (29).

A 2013 study evaluated the effect of prolonged use of acetaminophen during pregnancy on the neurodevelopment of 3-year-old offspring (30). The cases came from the prospective Norwegian Mother and Child Cohort Study. Data on acetaminophen use were obtained from a follow-up questionnaire sent to the mothers who were asked about their use of acetaminophen at gestational weeks 17 and 30. Among the 48,631 children whose mothers returned the questionnaire, 2919 same-sex sibling pairs were identified. In the sibling-controlled analysis, children exposed to prenatal acetaminophen for >28 days had significantly poorer gross motor development, communication, externalizing behavior, internalizing behavior, and higher activity levels than their nonexposed siblings. In those exposed prenatally to short-term use (1–27 days), poorer gross motor outcomes were found but the effects were smaller than with long-term use. Ibuprofen prenatal exposure was not associated with adverse neurodevelopment outcomes (30).

In a 2009 study, 1505 pregnant women and their children were prospectively followed up until 6 months of life (31). The use of acetaminophen during gestation did not increase the risk of asthma in the children. Use of the drug in the 1st and 3rd trimesters significantly reduced the risk of asthma. There was no evidence of a dose response, even with very high doses, such as >32 tablets (10,400 mg) per month (31).

BREASTFEEDING SUMMARY

Acetaminophen is excreted into breast milk in low concentrations (32–36). A single case of maculopapular rash on a breastfeeding infant's upper trunk and face was described in 1985 (32). The mother had taken 1 g of the drug at bedtime for 2 days before the onset of the symptoms. The rash resolved 24 hours after discontinuing acetaminophen. Two weeks later, the mother took another 1-g dose, and the rash recurred in the infant after breastfeeding at 3, 8, and 12 hours after the dose. Milk levels at 2.25 and 3.25 hours after the dose were 5.78/7.10 (right/left breasts) and 3.80/5.95 mcg/mL (right/left breasts), respectively. These represented milk:plasma ratios of 0.76 and 0.50, respectively (32).

Unpublished data obtained from one manufacturer showed that after an oral dose of 650 mg, an average milk level of 11 mcg/mL occurred (McNeil Laboratories, personal communication, 1979). Timing of the samples was not provided.

In 12 nursing mothers (nursing 2–22 months) given a single oral dose of 650 mg, peak levels of acetaminophen occurred at 1–2 hours in the range of 10–15 mcg/mL (33). Assuming 90 mL of milk were ingested at 3-, 6-, and 9-hour intervals after ingestion, the amount of drug available to the infant was estimated to range from 0.04% to 0.23% of the maternal dose.

After ingestion of a single analgesic combination tablet containing 324 mg of phenacetin, average milk levels of acetaminophen, the active metabolite, were 0.89 mcg/mL (34). Milk:plasma ratios at 1 and 12 hours were 0.91 and 1.42, with a milk half-life of 4.7 hours, as compared with 3.0 hours in the serum. Repeated doses at 4-hour intervals were expected to result in a steady-state concentration of 2.69 mcg/mL (34).

In three lactating women, a mean milk:plasma ratio of 0.76 was reported after a single oral dose of 500 mg of acetaminophen (35). In this case, the mean serum and milk half-lives were 2.7 and 2.6 hours, respectively. Peak milk concentrations of 4.2 mcg/mL occurred at 2 hours. In a more recent study, the calculated milk:plasma ratio was approximately 1.0 (36). Based on a dose of 1000 mg, the estimated maximum dose the infant could ingest was 1.85% of the maternal dose.

Except for the single case of rash, no other adverse effects of acetaminophen ingestion via breast milk have been reported. The American Academy of Pediatrics classifies acetaminophen as compatible with breastfeeding (37).

References

1. Levy G, Garretson LK, Soda DM. Evidence of placental transfer of acetaminophen. Pediatrics 1975;55:895.
2. Char VC, Chandra R, Fletcher AB, Avery GB. Polyhydramnios and neonatal renal failure—a possible association with maternal acetaminophen ingestion. J Pediatr 1975;86:638–9.
3. Rayburn W, Shukla U, Stetson P, Piehl E. Acetaminophen pharmacokinetics: comparison between pregnant and nonpregnant women. Am J Obstet Gynecol 1986;155:1353–6.
4. Beaulac-Baillargeon L, Rocheleau S. Paracetamol pharmacokinetics during the first trimester of human pregnancy. Eur J Clin Pharmacol 1994;46:451–4.
5. Rollins DE, Von Bahr C, Glaumann H, Moldens P, Rane H. Acetaminophen: potentially toxic metabolite formed by human fetal and adult liver microsomes and isolated fetal liver cells. Science 1979;205:1414–6.
6. Haibach H, Akhter JE, Muscato MS, Cary PL, Hoffmann MF. Acetaminophen overdose with fetal demise. Am J Clin Pathol 1984;82:240–2.
7. Wang P-H, Yang M-J, Lee W-L, Chao H-T, Yang M-L, Hung J-H. Acetaminophen poisoning in late pregnancy. A case report. J Reprod Med 1997;42:367–71.
8. Byer AJ, Taylor TR, Semmer JR. Acetaminophen overdose in the third trimester of pregnancy. JAMA 1982;247:3114–5.
9. Stokes IM. Paracetamol overdose in the second trimester of pregnancy. Case report. Br J Obstet Gynaecol 1984;91:286–8.
10. Ludmir J, Main DM, Landon MB, Gabbe SG. Maternal acetaminophen overdose at 15 weeks of gestation. Obstet Gynecol 1986;67:750–1.
11. Rosevear SK, Hope PL. Favourable neonatal outcome following maternal paracetamol overdose and severe fetal distress: case report. Br J Obstet Gynaecol 1989;96:491–3.
12. Friedman S, Gatti M, Baker T. Cesarean section after maternal acetaminophen overdose. Anesth Analg 1993;77:632–4.
13. Riggs BS, Bronstein AC, Kulig K, Archer PG, Rumack BH. Acute acetaminophen overdose during pregnancy. Obstet Gynecol 1989;74:247–53.
14. McElhatton PR, Sullivan FM, Volans GN. Paracetamol overdose in pregnancy analysis of the outcomes of 300 cases referred to the teratology information service. Reprod Toxicol 1997;11:85–94.
15. Heinonen OP, Slone D, Shapiro S. *Birth Defects and Drugs in Pregnancy*. Littleton, MA: Publishing Sciences Group, 1977.
16. Golden NL, King KC, Sokol RJ. Propoxyphene and acetaminophen: possible effects on the fetus. Clin Pediatr 1982;21:752–4.
17. Aselton P, Jick H, Milunsky A, Hunter JR, Stergachis A. First-trimester drug use and congenital disorders. Obstet Gynecol 1985;65:451–5.
18. Thulstrup AM, Sorensen HT, Nielsen GL, Andersen L, Barrett D, Vilstrup H, Olsen J, and the EuroMap Study Group. Fetal growth and adverse birth outcomes in women receiving prescriptions for acetaminophen during pregnancy. Am J Perinatol 1999;16:321–6.

19. Pearson H. Comparative effects of aspirin and acetaminophen on hemostasis. Pediatrics 1978;62(Suppl):926–9.
20. Rudolph AM. Effects of aspirin and acetaminophen in pregnancy and in the newborn. Arch Intern Med 1981;141:358–63.
21. Rumack CM, Guggenheim MA, Rumack BH, Peterson RG, Johnson ML, Braithwaite WR. Neonatal intracranial hemorrhage and maternal use of aspirin. Obstet Gynecol 1981;58(Suppl):52S–6S.
22. O'Brien WF, Krammer J, O'Leary TD, Mastrogiannis DS. The effect of acetaminophen on prostacyclin production in pregnant women. Am J Obstet Gynecol 1993;168:1164–9.
23. Streissguth AP, Treder RP, Barr HM, Shepard TH, Bleyer WA, Sampson PD, Martin DC. Aspirin and acetaminophen use by pregnant women and subsequent child IQ and attention decrements. Teratology 1987;35:211–9.
24. Kirshon B, Moise KJ Jr, Wasserstrum N. Effect of acetaminophen on fetal acid-base balance in chorioamnionitis. J Reprod Med 1989;34:955–9.
25. Cleves MA, Savell VH Jr, Raj S, Zhao W, Correa A, Werler MM, Hobbs CA, and the National Birth Defects Prevention Study. Maternal use of acetaminophen and nonsteroidal anti-inflammatory drugs (NSAIDs), and muscular ventricular septal defects. Birth Defects Res A Clin Mol Teratol 2004;70:107–13.
26. Rebordosa C, Kogevinas M, Horvath-Puho E, Norgard B, Morales M, Czeizel AE, Vilstrup H, Sorensen HT, Olsen J. Acetaminophen use during pregnancy: effects on risk for congenital abnormalities. Am J Obstet Gynecol 2008;198:178e1–7.
27. Feldkamp ML, Meyer RE, Krikov S, Botto LD. Acetaminophen use in pregnancy and risk of birth defects. Findings from the National Birth Defects Prevention Study. Obstet Gynecol 2010;115:109–15.
28. Kristensen DM, Hass U, Lesne L, Lottrup G, Jacobsen PR, Desdoits-Lethimonier C, Boberg J, Petersen JH, Toppari J, Jensen TK, Brunak S, Skakkebaek NE, Nellemann C, Main KM, Jegou B, Leffers H. Intrauterine exposure to mild analgesics is a risk factor for development of male reproductive disorders in human and rat. Human Reprod 2011;26:235–44.
29. Adjei AA, Gaedigk A, Simon SD, Weinshilboum RM, Leeder JS. Interindividual variability in acetaminophen sulfation by human fetal liver: implications for pharmacogenetic investigations of drug-induced birth defects. Birth Defects Res A Clin Mol Teratol 2008;82:155–65.
30. Brandlistuen RE, Ystrom E, Nulman I, Koren G, Nordeng H. Prenatal paracetamol exposure and child neurodevelopment: a sibling-controlled cohort study. Int J Epidemiol 2013;1–12. doi:10.1093/ije/dyt183.
31. Kang EM, Lundsberg LS, Illuzzi JL, Bracken MB. Prenatal exposure to acetaminophen and asthma in children. Obstet Gynecol 2009;114:1295–306.
32. Matheson I, Lunde PKM, Notarianni L. Infant rash caused by paracetamol in breast milk? Pediatrics 1985;76:651–2.
33. Berlin CM Jr, Yaffe SJ, Ragni M. Disposition of acetaminophen in milk, saliva, and plasma of lactating women. Pediatr Pharmacol 1980;1:135–41.
34. Findlay JWA, DeAngelis RL, Kearney MF, Welch RM, Findlay JM. Analgesic drugs in breast milk and plasma. Clin Pharmacol Ther 1981;29:625–33.
35. Bitzen PO, Gustafsson B, Jostell KG, Melander A, Wahlin-Boll E. Excretion of paracetamol in human breast milk. Eur J Clin Pharmacol 1981;20:123–5.
36. Notarianni LJ, Oldham HG, Bennett PN. Passage of paracetamol into breast milk and its subsequent metabolism by the neonate. Br J Clin Pharmacol 1987;24:63–7.
37. Committee on Drugs, American Academy of Pediatrics. The transfer of drugs and other chemicals into human milk. Pediatrics 2001;108:776–89.

ACETAZOLAMIDE

Diuretic (Carbonic Anhydrase Inhibitor)

PREGNANCY RECOMMENDATION: Compatible
BREASTFEEDING RECOMMENDATION: Compatible

PREGNANCY SUMMARY

Although some animal data have shown toxicity in offspring, a comparison to the human dose has not been provided and most studies found no adverse effects. Moreover, despite widespread use, the human data do not suggest a risk of developmental toxicity. The drug can be considered compatible in pregnancy.

FETAL RISK SUMMARY

Acetazolamide is an inhibitor of the enzyme carbonic anhydrase. It is indicated as adjunctive treatment of chronic simple (open-angle) glaucoma, secondary glaucoma, and preoperatively in acute angle-closure glaucoma where delay of surgery is desired in order to lower intraocular pressure. It also is indicated for the prevention or amelioration of symptoms associated with acute mountain sickness despite gradual ascent (1). The drug also is used off-label for idiopathic intracranial hypertension (IIH) (2–5).

Shepard (6) reviewed six reproduction studies using acetazolamide in mice, rats, hamsters, and monkeys. Forelimb defects were observed in the fetuses of rodents, but not in those of monkeys. One of the studies found that potassium replacement reduced the risk of congenital defects in rats (6). A study with pregnant rabbits found that, with doses producing maternal acidosis and electrolyte changes, acetazolamide produced a dose-related increase in axial skeletal malformations (7). The combination of acetazolamide and amiloride was found to produce abnormal development of the ureter and kidney in fetal mice when given at the critical moment of ureter development (8).

It is not known if acetazolamide crosses the human placenta. However, the molecular weight (about 222) suggests that the drug will cross to the embryo–fetus.

Despite widespread usage, no reports linking the use of acetazolamide with congenital defects have been located. A single case of a neonatal sacrococcygeal teratoma has been described (9). The mother received 750 mg daily for glaucoma during the 1st and 2nd trimesters. A relationship between the drug and carcinogenic effects in the fetus has not been supported by other reports. Retrospective surveys on the use of acetazolamide during gestation have not demonstrated an increased fetal risk (10,11).

The Collaborative Perinatal Project monitored 50,282 mother–child pairs, 12 of whom had 1st trimester exposure to acetazolamide (12, p. 372). No anomalies were observed in the exposed offspring. For use anytime during pregnancy, 1024 exposures were recorded (12, p. 441), and 18 infants were found to have malformations (18.06 expected). Thus, no evidence was found to suggest a relationship to large categories of major or minor malformations or to individual defects.

A woman with glaucoma was treated throughout pregnancy with acetazolamide, 250 mg twice daily, and topical pilocarpine and timolol (13). Within 48 hours of birth at 36 weeks' gestation, the infant's condition was complicated by hyperbilirubinemia and asymptomatic hypocalcemia, hypomagnesemia, and metabolic acidosis. The deficiencies of calcium and magnesium resolved quickly after treatment, as did the acidosis, even though the mother continued her medications while breastfeeding the infant. Mild hypertonicity of the lower limbs requiring physiotherapy was observed at 1-, 3-, and 8-month examinations. Two healthy infants of an epileptic mother, treated throughout two pregnancies with acetazolamide 250 mg/day and carbamazepine, were delivered at term and showed no effects of exposure to the drugs (13).

Four reports described the use of acetazolamide for treatment of IIH in a large number of pregnant women (2–5). No embryo or fetal adverse effects attributable to the drug were noted in any of the cases.

BREASTFEEDING SUMMARY

Acetazolamide is excreted into breast milk (14). A mother, 6 days postpartum, was given 500 mg (sustained-release formulation) twice daily for glaucoma, and she breastfed her infant for the following week. Nursing was stopped after that time because of the mother's concerns about exposing the infant to the drug. However, no changes attributable to drug exposure were noted in the infant. Breast milk levels of acetazolamide on the fourth and fifth days of therapy, 1–9 hours after a maternal dose, varied between 1.3 and 2.1 mcg/mL. A consistent relationship between concentration and time from last dose was not apparent. A milk:plasma ratio 1 hour after a dose was 0.25. Three plasma levels of acetazolamide in the infant were 0.2, 0.2, and 0.6 mcg/mL. The authors estimated that the infant ingested about 0.6 mg/day (i.e., 0.06% of the maternal dose) (15).

The American Academy of Pediatrics classifies acetazolamide as compatible with breastfeeding (15).

References

1. Product information. Acetazolamide. Teva Pharmaceuticals, 2009.
2. Lee AG, Pless M, Falardeau J, Capozzoli T, Wall M, Kardon RH. The use of acetazolamide in idiopathic intracranial hypertension during pregnancy. Am J Ophthalmol 2005;139:855–9.
3. Falardeau J, Lobb BM, Golden S, Maxfield SD, Tanne E. The use of acetazolamide during pregnancy in intracranial hypertension patients. J Neuroophthalmol 2013;33:9–12.
4. Kesler A, Kupferminc M. Idiopathic intracranial hypertension and pregnancy. Clin Obstet Gynecol 2013;56:389–96.
5. Golan S, Maslovitz S, Kupferminc MJ, Kesler A. Management and outcome of consecutive pregnancies complicated by idiopathic intracranial hypertension. Isr Med Assoc J 2013;15:160–3.
6. Shepard TH. *Catalog of Teratogenic Agents*. 6th ed. Baltimore, MD: Johns Hopkins University Press, 1989:5–6.
7. Nakatsuka T, Komatsu T, Fujii T. Axial skeletal malformations induced by acetazolamide in rabbits. Teratology 1992;45:629–36.
8. Miller TA, Scott WJ Jr. Abnormalities in ureter and kidney development in mice give acetazolamide–amiloride or dimethadione (DMO) during embryogenesis. Teratology 1992;46:541–50.
9. Worsham GF, Beckman EN, Mitchell EH. Sacrococcygeal teratoma in a neonate. Association with maternal use of acetazolamide. JAMA 1978;240:251–2.
10. Favre-Tissot M, Broussole P, Robert JM, Dumont L. An original clinical study of the pharmacologic–teratogenic relationship. Ann Med Psychol 1964;1:389. As cited in Nishimura H, Tanimura T, eds. *Clinical Aspects of the Teratogenicity of Drugs*. New York, NY: Excerpta Medica, 1976:210.
11. McBride WG. The teratogenic action of drugs. Med J Aust 1963;2:689–93.
12. Heinonen OP, Slone D, Shapiro S. *Birth Defects and Drugs in Pregnancy*. Littleton, MA: Publishing Sciences Group, 1977.
13. Merlob P, Litwin A, Mor N. Possible association between acetazolamide administration during pregnancy and metabolic disorders in the newborn. Eur J Obstet Gynecol Reprod Biol 1990;35:85–8.
14. Soderman P, Hartvig P, Fagerlund C. Acetazolamide excretion into human breast milk. Br J Clin Pharmacol 1984;17:599–600.
15. Committee on Drugs, American Academy of Pediatrics. The transfer of drugs and other chemicals into human milk. Pediatrics 2001;108:776–89.

ACETOHEXAMIDE

[Withdrawn from the market. See 9th edition.]

ACETOPHENAZINE

[Withdrawn from the market. See 8th edition.]

ACETYLCHOLINE

[See 9th edition.]

ACETYLCYSTEINE

Respiratory Agent (Mucolytic), Antidote

PREGNANCY RECOMMENDATION: Compatible—Maternal Benefits >> Embryo–Fetal Risk
BREASTFEEDING RECOMMENDATION: No Human Data—Probably Compatible

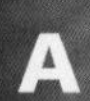

PREGNANCY SUMMARY

Acetylcysteine is not teratogenic or embryotoxic in animals and, although the data are limited, do not appear to represent a risk to the human fetus when IV doses are used as an antidote for acute acetaminophen overdose. After IV administration, the drug crosses the placenta to achieve protective serum levels in the fetus. A 1999 report concluded that acetaminophen overdose in pregnant women should be managed the same way as in nonpregnant patients and that acetylcysteine therapy was protective to both the mother and the fetus (1). There is no reported human pregnancy experience after use of acetylcysteine as a mucolytic agent.

FETAL RISK SUMMARY

Acetylcysteine (*N*-acetyl-L-cysteine) is a mucolytic agent indicated as adjuvant therapy in the treatment of abnormal, viscid, or inspissated mucous secretions in a variety of pulmonary conditions. It is also indicated as an antidote to prevent or lessen hepatic injury following the ingestion of potentially hepatic toxic doses of acetaminophen (2). Acetylcysteine has been used as an ophthalmic solution to treat keratoconjunctivitis sicca (dry eye) and as an enema for bowel obstruction due to meconium ileus (3), although these indications are not approved by the FDA. In mice, the agent has also demonstrated efficacy as a chelating agent to reduce organic mercury-induced developmental toxicity (4).

Reproductive studies with acetylcysteine have been conducted in rats and rabbits. Pregnant rabbits were given oral doses about 3 times the human mucolytic dose on days 6–16 of gestation. Additional pregnant rabbits were exposed to an aerosol of 10% acetylcysteine and 0.05% isoproterenol for 30–35 minutes twice daily from the 16th to the18th day of gestation. No teratogenic effects were observed in either the oral or the aerosol studies. In pregnant rats, an aerosol combination of acetylcysteine and isoproterenol was given in a manner similar to that used in rabbits from the 6th to the 15th day of gestation. Other pregnant rats were exposed to the aerosol from the 15th to the 21st day of gestation. No teratogenic effects or maternal or fetal toxicity was observed in these studies (2).

Consistent with its low molecular weight (about 163), acetylcysteine crosses the human placenta. In a study of three pregnant women who delivered viable infants while undergoing treatment for acetaminophen toxicity, the mean acetylcysteine cord blood concentrations was 9.4 mcg/mL (range 8.6–10.9 mcg/mL) (5). The corresponding maternal serum concentrations (trough levels, 4 hours after a dose) ranged from 7.2–11.8 mcg/mL. In a fourth nonviable infant delivered at 22 weeks' gestation, the acetylcysteine level in a postmortem cardiac blood sample obtained 48 hours after death was 55.8 mcg/mL. The mean cord blood level was within the range associated with therapeutic acetylcysteine doses in adults. No adverse effects attributable to acetylcysteine or acetaminophen were observed in the three viable infants, nor was there evidence of acetaminophen toxicity in the fourth infant (5).

The only published reports describing the use of acetylcysteine during human pregnancy involve the agent's use as an antidote following acute acetaminophen overdose (1,6–10). A case report published in 1982 described a woman at 36 weeks' gestation who took an overdose of acetaminophen (6). A few hours after the ingestion, acetylcysteine was administered (140 mg/kg IV, then 70 mg/kg IV every 4 hours for 17 doses). The mother made an uneventful recovery and 6 weeks later delivered a healthy 3.29-kg female infant with Apgar scores of 9 and 9 (6).

Two other case reports of maternal acetaminophen overdose, at 15 and 32 weeks' gestation, respectively, appeared in 1986 and 1989 (7,8). Both women were successfully treated with IV acetylcysteine. In the first case, a 2.00-kg male infant was eventually delivered at 32 weeks' gestation. He was developing normally at 4 months of age (7). Because of severe toxicity in the second woman and fetal distress, delivery was induced 84 hours after the overdose resulting in the birth of a healthy 2.198-kg female infant (8). Acetaminophen was not detected in the cord blood (no test for acetylcysteine was done). Except for hyperbilirubinemia of prematurity, the infant did well with no evidence of toxicity at follow-up examinations at 6 weeks and 6 months of age (8).

In a 1989 study from the Rocky Mountain Poison and Drug Center, covering 1976–1985, pregnancy outcomes were available for 60 of the 110 women who had an acute acetaminophen overdose during gestation (9). Of the 60 women, 24 were treated with IV acetylcysteine (4 in the 1st trimester) for toxic acetaminophen serum levels. The outcomes of the 24 cases were 14 viable infants (2 premature), 3 spontaneous abortions (SABs), 5 elective abortions, 1 stillbirth, and 1 maternal death. In the stillbirth case, the mother overdosed at 33 weeks' gestation with fetal death occurring 2 days later. An autopsy of the fetus revealed massive centrilobular hepatic necrosis that was consistent with acetaminophen-induced hepatotoxicity. Of the five potential independent variables evaluated, only two were significantly predictive of pregnancy outcome: time to start of acetylcysteine and gestational age. The probability of fetal death increased the longer it took to receive the antidote and the lower the gestational age. One infant was reported to have a mild positional deformity of the feet. No other congenital defects were reported (9).

A 1997 study from a teratology information service in England reported the pregnancy outcomes of 300 cases of acute acetaminophen overdose (10). A total of 33 mothers were treated with IV acetylcysteine. The outcomes of these cases were 24 normal infants, 3 SABs or fetal deaths, 5 elective terminations, and 1 infant with hypospadias. There was no relationship between the defect and either acetaminophen or acetylcysteine due to the timing of exposure. None of the other adverse outcomes were related to acetylcysteine (10).

BREASTFEEDING SUMMARY

No reports have described the use of acetylcysteine during lactation. Although the molecular weight of the drug (about 163) is low enough for excretion into breast milk, the various conditions in which acetylcysteine is used suggest that the drug will rarely be prescribed during breastfeeding. Moreover, IV acetylcysteine has been administered directly to preterm neonates for therapeutic indications, at doses far above those that would be obtained from milk, without causing toxicity (11,12).

References

1. Zed PJ, Krenzelok EP. Treatment of acetaminophen overdose. Am J Health-Syst Pharm 1999;56:1081–91.
2. Product information. Acetylcysteine Solution, USP. Bedford Laboratories, 1999.
3. Acetylcysteine (*N*-Acetylcysteine). *Drug Facts and Comparisons*. St. Louis: Facts and Comparisons, 2000.
4. Domingo JL. Developmental toxicity of metal chelating agents. Reprod Toxicol 1998;12:499–510.
5. Horowitz RS, Dart RC, Jarvie DR, Bearer CF, Gupta U. Placental transfer of *N*-acetylcysteine following human maternal acetaminophen toxicity. Clin Toxicol 1997;35:447–51.
6. Byer AJ, Traylor TR, Semmer JR. Acetaminophen overdose in the third trimester of pregnancy. JAMA 1982;247:3114–5.
7. Ludmir J, Main DM, Landon MB, Gabbe SG. Maternal acetaminophen overdose at 15 weeks of gestation. Obstet Gynecol 1986;67:750–1.
8. Rosevear SK, Hope PL. Favourable neonatal outcome following maternal paracetamol overdose and severe fetal distress. Case report. Br J Obstet Gynaecol 1989;96:491–3.
9. Riggs BS, Bronstein AC, Kulig K, Archer PG, Rumack BH. Acute acetaminophen overdose during pregnancy. Obstet Gynecol 1989;74:247–53.
10. McElhatton PR, Sullivan FM, Volans GN. Paracetamol overdose in pregnancy: analysis of the outcomes of 300 cases referred to the teratology information service. Reprod Toxicol 1997;11:85–94.
11. Ahola TM, Fellman V, Laaksonen R, Laitila J, Lapatto R, Neuvonen PJ, Raivio KO. Pharmacokinetics of intravenous *N*-acetylcysteine in preterm neonates (abstract). Pediatr Res 1998;43(Suppl 2):163.
12. Isbister GK, Bucens IK, Whyte IM. Paracetamol overdose in a preterm neonate. Arch Dis Child Fetal Neonat Ed 2001;85:F70–2.

ACETYLDIGITOXIN

Cardiac Glycoside

[See Digitalis.]

ACITRETIN

Vitamin

PREGNANCY RECOMMENDATION: Contraindicated
BREASTFEEDING RECOMMENDATION: Compatible

PREGNANCY SUMMARY

Like all retinoids, acitretin, the active metabolite of etretinate, is a potent teratogen. It represents not only a significant fetal risk during pregnancy, but also a risk for an unknown time after therapy has ceased. This added fetal risk results because acitretin can be converted back to the parent drug, etretinate, which can persist, along with acitretin and 13-*cis*-acitretin, in SC fat for prolonged periods, perhaps for >3 years. Measuring plasma levels of the retinoids does not appear to be beneficial in determining the risk of fetal harm. Effective contraception must be used for at least 1 month before beginning acitretin, during therapy, and for at least 3 years after acitretin therapy (1). Women of childbearing age who are considering treatment with acitretin must be informed of this very slow elimination and the possibility of adverse pregnancy outcome if they conceive within 3 years of therapy. There apparently is no risk of acitretin-induced developmental toxicity when only the father is being treated (2).

FETAL RISK SUMMARY

Acitretin, an oral active synthetic retinoid and vitamin A derivative, is the active metabolite of etretinate (see also Etretinate). It is used for the treatment of severe psoriasis resistant to other forms of therapy and for severe congenital ichthyosis and keratosis follicularis (Darier disease).

Similar to vitamin A and it derivatives, acitretin may cause congenital defects at human dosage levels in various animal species, including the mouse, rat, and rabbit. Fertility of rats was not impaired at the highest dose tested (about 3 times the maximum recommended human dose [MRHD]). Chronic administration to male dogs (30 mg/kg/day) produced testicular changes: reversible mild-to-moderate spermatogenic arrest and the appearance of multinucleated giant cells (1).

After oral absorption, acitretin undergoes extensive metabolism and interconversion by simple isomerization to 13-*cis*-acitretin. When consumed with alcohol, acitretin may be converted back to etretinate, a retinoid with a very long elimination half-life (mean 120 days, but may be as long as 168 days). Because the prolonged elimination would increase the teratogenic potential for women of childbearing age (see also Etretinate), the manufacturer states that alcohol must not be ingested during therapy with acitretin and for 2 months after cessation of therapy because of the long elimination period of acitretin (1).

In a 1994 reference, the concentrations of etretinate, acitretin, and 13-*cis*-acitretin were measured in plasma and SC fat samples from 37 women of childbearing age (3). Twenty of the women were receiving acitretin and 17 had stopped. Sixteen of the 20 women current acitretin users had taken etretinate but had stopped that drug a mean 45 months before sampling, whereas 4 women had never received etretinate. Among current acitretin users, detectable etretinate levels in the plasma and SC fat were found in 45% and 83%, respectively. The 17 women who had stopped taking acitretin had been off the drug a mean 12 months. Eleven of these women had also used etretinate but had stopped a mean 43 months before sampling. The 6 women who had never taken etretinate stopped acitretin 17 months before testing. Among these 17 women, etretinate was detected in 18% and 86%, respectively, of the plasma and SC fat samples. In some cases, acitretin and/or etretinate were detectable in plasma or SC fat up to 29 months after acitretin therapy had ceased. Thus, plasma concentrations correlated poorly with concentrations in fat. The findings led the authors to conclude that the recommended contraception period of 2 years after acitretin treatment (in 1994) was too short to avoid the risk of teratogenicity (3). Currently, the manufacturer recommends a contraception period of 3 years, but the human threshold concentration of acitretin below which the drug is not teratogenic has not been established (1).

A case report of a pregnancy exposed to acitretin starting 10 days after conception and throughout the 1st trimester was published in 1995 (4). The 34-year-old woman was treated with acitretin (50 mg/day) for severe palmoplantar epidermolytic keratoderma. Pregnancy was diagnosed 6 weeks after stopping acitretin therapy. The pregnancy was terminated at 20 weeks' gestation with delivery of a stillborn, 210-g, 24-cm-long male fetus with severe symmetric defects of the upper and lower limbs and craniofacial malformations. The extremity defects included bilateral short arms with pterygium formation in the elbows, shortened thumbs and little fingers without nails, contractures of both lower limbs in the groins and knees, irregularly thickened femora and tibiae, and point-shaped feet with only two small toes without nails. X-ray of the limbs revealed bilateral humeroradial synostosis and bone defects in the hands and feet. Craniofacial malformations included underdeveloped maxilla and mandibula, a small mouth with a high, arched and narrow palate, low-set ears, bilateral microtia, agenesis of the external ear canals, and bilateral preauricular tags. Except for an atrioventricular septal defect type II, no other anomalies were discovered on autopsy. Concentrations of acitretin, 13-*cis*-acitretin, and etretinate, in the maternal plasma, fetal brain and liver, and amniotic fluid 48 days after stopping therapy, were either undetectable (<0.3 ng/mL) or unquantifiable. An attempted chromosomal analysis of the fetus failed. Because the authors could find no other explanation for the malformations, including potential genetic defects, and the craniofacial malformations were similar to previous cases of retinoic acid embryopathy (e.g., see Isotretinoin), they concluded that the defects were caused by acitretin. In addition, the authors were aware of the poor correlation between plasma and fat concentrations of the vitamin A derivatives (3); thus the failure to detect the retinoids in the plasma did not affect their conclusion (4).

A 1994 study attempted to determine if there was a threshold dose or plasma concentration of acitretin below which there was no teratogenic risk in females (5). In various species, the highest nonteratogenic oral doses (mg/kg/day) were 1 (mouse), 7.5 (rat), and 0.2 (rabbit). No data were available for cynomolgus monkeys or humans. The authors also summarized the outcomes of pregnancies that had occurred during or after acitretin therapy and been reported to the manufacturer since human therapy with the drug began in 1983. A total of 75 women were exposed to acitretin either during pregnancy (*N* = 8) or before pregnancy (*N* = 67) (median time before pregnancy 5 months, range 6 weeks to 23 months). Among those exposed during pregnancy, there were four spontaneous abortions, one induced abortion (no information on the fetus), one induced abortion with typical malformations, one newborn with a nontypical anomaly, and one normal newborn. The mother of the fetus with typical malformations took 50 mg/day of acitretin during the first 19 weeks of gestation. Malformations in the fetus were microtia and defects of the face and extremities. The mother of the infant with a nontypical anomaly took acitretin (20 mg/day) during the first 8 months of pregnancy. The infant had a hearing impairment for high frequencies. The outcomes of the 67 pregnancies exposed before conception were 9 spontaneous abortions, 18 induced abortions (15 fetuses with no information, 3 normal fetuses), 4 newborns with nontypical abnormalities, and 36 normal newborns. One of the mothers who delivered an infant with nontypical malformations had received 1 week of acitretin, 25 mg/day, 18 months before conception. The abnormalities, considered incompatible with life, included macrocephaly, low-set ears, microphthalmia, low-inserted thumb, ventricular and atrial septal defects, total duodenal obstruction, and cystic kidneys. The malformations were thought to be due to a chromosomal abnormality (partial trisomy 1) and a history of maternal drug abuse. The nontypical abnormalities in the other three newborns were transitory neonatal icterus and hypocalcemia, left testis ectopia, and slight transitory hypotonia (5).

In 1999, a report from the manufacturer summarized the worldwide data relating to acitretin and human pregnancy exposures that had been reported to the manufacturer since acitretin became available (6). Some of these data may have also been reported in the study discussed above. There were 123 reports of acitretin exposure either before or during pregnancy, 88 of which were prospective reports. Details on malformations were provided in only one case. Outcomes that did not involve congenital malformations were classified as "other abnormalities," defined as pregnancy-related, placental, perinatal, or neonatal disorders, such as hyperbilirubinemia, abnormal growth, and delayed motor skills. There were 11 exposures during pregnancy, five reported prospectively and six retrospectively. Among the prospective cases, there was one spontaneous abortion (SAB) (no information on the fetus), three elective abortions (EABs) (no information on the fetuses), and one newborn with malformations (no details provided, but reference 3 above was included whereas reference 4 was not). Among those reported retrospectively, there was one SAB (no information), three EABs (two with malformations and one with other adverse conditions), and two newborns with other adverse conditions. For exposures that occurred 0–2 years before pregnancy, there were 97 cases, 77 of them prospective. Outcomes in these cases were 8 SABs (1 normal embryo–fetus, and 7 with no information), 25 EABs (3 normal, 2 with malformations, and 20 with no information), and 44 newborns (41 normal, 1 with an undescended testicle, 1 hypotonic, and 1 with hypocalcemia and jaundice). The outcomes in the 20 retrospective cases were 5 SABs (no information), 4 EABs (1 normal, 1 with malformations, and 2 with no information), and 11 newborns (9 normal, 2 with malformations). Two of the five cases in which exposure occurred more than 2 years before pregnancy were prospective. Their outcomes were one SAB (no information) and one normal newborn. The three retrospective cases all involved newborns with malformations. Finally, 10 cases involved exposure at an unknown time before conception, 4 of which were prospective. The outcomes were one SAB (no information), one EA (no information), and two normal neonates. For the six retrospective cases, there was one SAB (no information), two EABs (one normal and one with no information), and three normal newborns (6).

A 2004 case described the pregnancy outcome of a woman who had taken acitretin 10 mg/day until the 10 completed weeks of pregnancy (7). The 1450-g (25th percentile) female infant was born at 32 weeks' with Apgar scores of 8 and 10 at 1 and 5 minutes, respectively. Evaluation up to 11 months of age revealed growth restriction (length and head circumference <3rd percentile, weight 50th percentile), epicanthal folds, low nasal bridge, high palate, cup-shaped ears, anteverted nostrils, prominent heels, atrial septal defect (closed spontaneously), and bilateral sensorineural deafness. At 18 months of age, the infant was microcephalic, hypotonic, and had neurodevelopmental delay. The pattern of defects resembled those observed with isotretinoin and etretinate (7).

An interaction between acitretin and a very low-dose progestin contraceptive (levonorgestrel 0.03 mg) was observed in one woman undergoing treatment with acitretin 0.4 mg/kg/day (8). Her plasma progesterone level increased from 2.15 ng/mL before acitretin or contraceptive to 3.87–13.46 ng/mL while receiving both drugs. The increase in plasma concentration was thought to indicate failure of contraception and development of a corpus luteum after ovulation. No interaction, as evidenced by a rise in plasma progesterone concentration, was observed in nine other women who received combined oral contraceptives (normal or mini-dose) (8).

Acitretin has been measured in the seminal fluid of men consuming either acitretin or etretinate (1). In men administered 30–50 mg/day for at least 12 weeks, the sperm count, concentration, motility, and morphology were unchanged. In addition, no adverse effects were observed with regard to testosterone production, luteinizing hormone, follicle-stimulating hormone, or on the hypothalamic–pituitary axis. The maximum concentration of acitretin found in seminal fluid was 12.5 ng/mL. The amount of acitretin transferred in semen, assuming an ejaculate volume of 10 mL, would be 125 ng or 1/200,000th of a single 25-mg capsule. Of five pregnancies in which the father was receiving acitretin therapy, two ended in SABs, one fetus had bilateral cystic hygromas and multiple cardiopulmonary anomalies, one normal newborn was delivered, and one was lost to follow-up. The relationship between acitretin and the fetal malformations is unknown. However, no teratogenicity was observed in the offspring of male rats treated with 5 mg/kg/day (about 5 times the MRHD) for 10 weeks (approximate duration of one spermatogenic cycle) before and during mating with untreated females (1).

BREASTFEEDING SUMMARY

Acitretin is excreted into the milk of humans. A woman 8 months postpartum was treated with a single daily 40 mg dose of acitretin (0.65 mg/kg/day) for extensive plaque psoriasis and acral pustulosis (9). Nursing was stopped before the therapy was started. Milk was collected each day by an electric pump before the dose and again 12 hours later. At steady state, milk concentrations of the drug and its main metabolite were 30–40 ng/mL, corresponding to a milk:serum ratio of 0.18. The estimated infant dose was 1.5% of the maternal dose (9).

The plasma elimination half-lives of acitretin and 13-*cis*-acitretin may be as long as 96 and 157 hours, respectively (1). Because of storage in subcutaneous fat, the actual elimination of these compounds may take much longer. The manufacturer recommends a contraception period of 3 year after acitretin therapy is stopped, but a similar recommendation for breastfeeding has not been made. Although there is a potential for toxicity, the American Academy of Pediatrics classifies the drug as compatible with breastfeeding (10).

References

1. Product information. Soriatane. Roche Laboratories, 2000.
2. Geiger JM, Walker M. Is there a reproductive safety risk in male patients treated with acitretin (Neotigason®/Soriatane®)? Dermatology 2002;205:105–7.
3. Sturkenboom MCJM, DeJong-Van Den Berg LTW, Van Voorst-Vader PC, Cornel MC, Stricker BHCH, Wesseling H. Inability to detect plasma etretinate and acitretin is a poor predictor of the absence of these teratogens in tissue after stopping acitretin treatment. Br J Clin Pharmacol 1994;38:229–35.
4. De Die-Smulders CEM, Sturkenboom MCJM, Veraart J, Van Katwijk C, Sastrowijoto P, Van Der Linden E. Severe limb defects and craniofacial anomalies in a fetus conceived during acitretin therapy. Teratology 1995;52:215–9.
5. Geiger JM, Baudin M, Saurat JH. Teratogenic risk with etretinate and acitretin treatment. Dermatology 1994;189:109–16.
6. Maradit H, Geiger JM. Potential risk of birth defects after acitretin discontinuation. Dermatology 1999;198:3–4.
7. Barbero P, Lotersztein V, Bronberg R, Perez M, Alba L. Acitretin embryopathy: a case report. Birth Defects Res A Clin Mol Teratol 2004;70:831–3.
8. Berbis PH, Bun H, Geiger JM, Rognin C, Durand A, Serradimigni A, Hartmann D, Privat Y. Acitretin (RO10-1670) and oral contraceptives: interaction study. Arch Dermatol Res 1988;280:388–9.
9. Rollman O, Pihl-Lundin I. Acitretin excretion into human breast milk. Acta Derm Venereol (Stockh) 1990;70:487–90.
10. Committee on Drugs, American Academy of Pediatrics. The transfer of drugs and other chemicals into human milk. Pediatrics 2001;108:776–89.

ACLIDINIUM BROMIDE

Respiratory (Bronchodilator)

PREGNANCY RECOMMENDATION: No Human Data—Probably Compatible
BREASTFEEDING RECOMMENDATION: No Human Data—Probably Compatible

PREGNANCY SUMMARY

No reports describing the use of aclidinium in human pregnancy have been located. The animal data suggest low risk, but the absence of human pregnancy experience prevents a more complete assessment of embryo–fetal risk. However, the low (unspecified) plasma concentrations suggest that the drug, if indicated, represents a low, if any, risk in pregnancy.

FETAL RISK SUMMARY

Aclidinium bromide, a dry powder for inhalation, is indicated for the long-term, maintenance treatment of bronchospasm associated with chronic obstructive pulmonary disease, including chronic bronchitis and emphysema. It is an antimuscarinic agent that is often referred to as an anticholinergic. Aclidinium is rapidly and extensively hydrolyzed to inactive metabolites so that plasma concentrations (not specified) are low. The estimated effective half-life is 5–8 hours (1).

Reproduction studies have been conducted in rats and rabbits. No evidence of structural anomalies was observed in rats exposed during organogenesis to about 15 times the recommended human daily dose based on summed AUC of aclidinium and its metabolites (RHDD) (based on inhaled doses ≤5 mg/kg/day). However, during lactation, exposures that were about 5 times the RHDD (based on inhaled doses ≥0.2 mg/kg/day) resulted in decreased pup weights. These doses also caused maternal toxicity. In rabbits during organogenesis, no evidence of structural anomalies was observed at exposures that were about 20 times the RHDD (based on inhaled doses ≤3.6 mg/kg/day). Compared with controls, an increased incidence of liver lobes was noted at exposures that were about 1400 times the RHDD (based on oral doses ≥150 mg/kg/day) and decreased fetal body weights occurred at exposures that were about 2300 times the RHDD (based on oral doses ≥300 mg/kg/day). Both exposures caused maternal toxicity (1).

Long-term studies for carcinogenicity in mice and rats were negative. In various tests for mutagenicity, both positive and negative assays were noted. In male and female rats given inhaled doses that were about 15 times the RHDD, impaired fertility and reproductive performance were observed, as well as paternal toxicity. However, in other rat studies (treated males mated with untreated females; treated females mated with untreated males), no effects on fertility were observed at inhaled doses resulting in exposures that were about 30 and 15 times the RHDD, respectively (1).

It is not known if aclidinium or its metabolites cross the human placenta. The molecular weight of the parent drug (about 565) and the long half-life suggest that the drug will cross to the embryo–fetus. However, the low (unspecified) plasma concentrations indicate that the amount crossing will also be low.

BREASTFEEDING SUMMARY

No reports describing the use of aclidinium during human lactation have been located. The molecular weight of the parent drug (about 565) and the long effective half-life (5–8 hours) suggest that the drug will be excreted into breast milk. However, the low (unspecified) plasma concentrations indicate that the amount excreted into milk will also be low. The most common adverse reactions (≥3% incidence) among adults were headache, nasopharyngitis, and cough (1). Although the drug appears to be compatible during breastfeeding, nursing infants of mothers receiving the drug should be monitored for these effects.

Reference

1. Product information. Tudorza Pressair. Forest Pharmaceuticals, 2012.

ACYCLOVIR

Antiviral

PREGNANCY RECOMMENDATION: Compatible
BREASTFEEDING RECOMMENDATION: Compatible

PREGNANCY SUMMARY

No adverse effects in the fetus or newborn attributable to the use of acyclovir during pregnancy have been reported. Congenital malformations have been reported in infants exposed during pregnancy, but they do not appear to be related to the drug. Systemic IV treatment is indicated for life-threatening disseminated herpes simplex virus (HSV) infections to reduce the maternal, fetal, and infant mortality of these infections. Oral acyclovir treatment of primary genital HSV infections also appears to be indicated to prevent adverse fetal outcomes, such as prematurity, intrauterine growth restriction (IUGR), and neonatal HSV infection.

FETAL RISK SUMMARY

Acyclovir is a synthetic acyclic purine nucleoside analog used as an antiviral agent against the herpes viruses. Three studies observed no teratogenic effects in animals at nontoxic doses (1–3). One study, however, observed abnormal thymus development and functional deficits of the immune system in rats exposed in utero to acyclovir (4). Chromosome breaks were observed in some tests with cultured human lymphocytes, but only with prolonged exposure and at doses much higher than those obtainable in clinical use (5). A 1997 publication, however, cited studies that gave SC doses of 100 mg/kg once, twice, or 3 times to pregnant rats on day 10 of gestation (6). Altered development was observed in fetuses examined on day 11.5 (reduced crown–rump length, number of somites, and protein content) or on day 21 (skull, eye, and tail defects). The SC doses caused slight and reversible maternal nephropathia, but this was not thought to have induced the fetal anomalies (6).

Reproduction studies in mice, rats, and rabbits, as reported by the manufacturer, did not observe teratogenic effects (7). The doses used in the three species produced plasma levels that were the same as human levels, 1–2 times human levels, and 4 and 9 times human levels, respectively.

Although there are no approved indications for acyclovir in pregnancy, the principal clinical use of acyclovir during this period is for the treatment of primary genital HSV type 2 infection and for the prophylaxis against recurrent genital HSV infection. The Acyclovir in Pregnancy Registry found that, of the American women reported to the Registry as exposed during pregnancy, 62% and 70% of their prospective and retrospective samples, respectively, had been treated for genital herpes (8). They estimated that as many as 7500 live births per year in the United States may be exposed to acyclovir (8).

The treatment of genital herpes is intended to prevent the adverse outcomes on the fetus and newborn that the primary infection may cause, such as prematurity, IUGR, and neonatal HSV infection, and to reduce the incidence of cesarean section with recurrent disease. Reviews evaluating the various indications for acyclovir in pregnancy concluded that life-threatening maternal HSV infection and varicella pneumonia were the most justifiable indications (9,10). Some evidence was cited that the benefits of treatment of primary genital herpes, under certain conditions, might outweigh the risks, but the lack of controlled studies prevented any conclusion (9,10). Similarly, the treatment of uncomplicated varicella infections and the prophylaxis against recurrent genital HSV were unproven indications because of the absence of supporting data (9,10). Some authors have proposed the use of acyclovir for the prophylaxis of genital HSV during pregnancy, although all qualify their proposals with statements that controlled studies are needed to assess efficacy and safety (11–13).

A 1998 randomized, placebo-controlled study was conducted to determine if oral acyclovir (800 mg/day) could reduce the rate of cesarean section in women with recurrent genital herpes infection at <36 weeks' gestation (14). A total of 63 women were enrolled (acyclovir N = 31, placebo N = 32) in the study. Except for a significant reduction in clinical recurrences (odds ratio [OR] 0.10, 95% confidence interval [CI] 0.00–0.86), the other outcome measures showed no significant difference from placebo: cesarean section (OR 0.44, 95% CI 0.09–1.59), and clinical recurrence or asymptomatic shedding (OR 0.32, 95% CI 0.05–1.56). None of the newborns were infected with HSV and no abnormal findings were detected in the 19 exposed infants examined 1 year later. The investigators concluded that acyclovir should not be used for recurrent genital herpes infection during pregnancy outside of randomized controlled trials (14).

The CDC 1998 Sexually Transmitted Diseases Treatment Guidelines states, in part:

> *The first clinical episode of genital herpes during pregnancy may be treated with oral acyclovir. In the presence of life-threatening maternal HSV infection (e.g., disseminated infection, encephalitis, pneumonitis, or hepatitis), acyclovir administered IV is indicated. Investigations of acyclovir use among pregnant women suggest that acyclovir treatment near term might reduce the rate of abdominal deliveries among women who have frequently recurring or newly acquired genital herpes by decreasing the incidence of active lesions. However, routine administration of acyclovir to pregnant women who have a history of recurrent genital herpes is not recommended at this time.* (15)

The drug readily crosses the placenta to the fetus (16–23). After IV dosing, acyclovir levels in cord blood were higher than those in maternal serum with ratios of 1.4 and 1.25 reported (16,17). A 1992 study concluded that the placental transfer of acyclovir was most consistent with a carrier-dependent, nucleobase-type uptake of the drug, but that the overall net transfer was passive and dependent on solubility characteristics (16).

The pharmacokinetics of oral acyclovir in term pregnant women were reported in 1991 (21). Fifteen women with a history of active recurrent genital HSV type 2 infection antedating and during pregnancy, but without currently active disease, were given either 200 mg (N = 7) or 400 mg (N = 8) orally every 8 hours from 38 weeks' gestation until delivery. The mean steady-state plasma peak and trough levels in the 200-mg group were 1.9 and 0.7 μmol/L, respectively; those in the 400-mg group were 3.3 and 0.8 μmol/L, respectively. Acyclovir was concentrated in the amniotic fluid with concentrations ranging from 1.87 to 6.06 μmol/L in the low-dose group compared with 4.20–15.5 μmol/L in the high-dose group. The maternal:cord plasma ratio was similar in both groups with a mean of 1.3, a value comparable to that observed after IV dosing (21).

Acyclovir has been administered orally and intravenously during all stages of pregnancy (8,9,14,17–61). Topical acyclovir, which may produce low levels of the drug in maternal serum, urine, and vaginal excretions, has been used in pregnancy, and the manufacturer is aware of two women treated topically during the 3rd trimester who delivered normal infants (A. Clark, personal communication, Burroughs-Wellcome, 1985). However, no published reports of these cases have been located.

Favorable maternal and fetal outcomes were observed in two cases of isolated HSV encephalitis treated with IV and oral acyclovir (36,37). Treatment in the two mothers began at 29 and 26 weeks' gestation, respectively, and continued until term. In the only other reported cases occurring during pregnancy, none of whom were treated with acyclovir, four mothers and three fetuses died (37). The onset of the encephalitis in the mother of the surviving fetus was at term. A 1996 case report described the successful treatment with IV acyclovir of a woman with herpes simplex hepatitis at 24 weeks' gestation (38). A viable 1013-g male infant was delivered at 28 weeks because of severe preeclampsia. Both the mother and her infant were doing well at the time of the report.

A 1991 case report and review cited data indicating that varicella pneumonia occurring during pregnancy resulted in a maternal mortality up to 44% (47). In 15 cases treated with IV acyclovir, however, only two (13%) mothers died, one fetus was stillborn, and one infant expired. Another 1991 reference added 5 new cases and a review of 16 cases from the literature to total 21 women treated during pregnancy with acyclovir for varicella pneumonia (48). Twelve women were treated during the 2nd trimester and nine during the 3rd trimester. The mean duration of acyclovir treatment was 7 days. Maternal mortality occurred in four cases, but two of the deaths occurred after delivery. One mother died of multiorgan failure 11 days after delivery, and one mother died after surgery for intestinal obstruction 1 month after delivery. The three maternal deaths directly attributable to varicella pneumonia were in the 3rd trimester at the onset of disease. Two fetal or infant deaths occurred, one from prematurity after birth at 26 weeks' gestation, and one stillborn at 34 weeks' (both cases also described in reference 47). No adverse effects were observed in the surviving infants. None of the infants had features of congenital varicella infection, nor did any develop active perinatal varicella infection. A 1993 abstract briefly described data collected retrospectively (1988–1992) on 14 pregnant women with varicella pneumonia, 11 of whom were treated with acyclovir (58). No specific information was given on the outcome of the 11 treated pregnancies. A 1998 case report described a woman at 32 weeks' gestation that was treated with IV acyclovir for varicella pneumonia (59). A healthy female infant was delivered approximately 3 days later because of fetal distress secondary to cord compression and prolapse into the right uterine segment. The infant was given varicella immunoglobulin and a 5-day course of IV acyclovir and was discharged home at 20 days of age without ever showing signs of varicella.

Data gathered for the period 1984–1999, by the Acyclovir in Pregnancy Registry, a group sponsored by the manufacturer and the CDC, were published in 2004 (8). Excluding 461 patients with exposure to topical acyclovir only, 1234 pregnancies (12 sets of twins; 1246 outcomes) with known outcomes were followed up prospectively. The trimester of initial exposure was as follows: 1st—756 (7 sets of twins), 2nd—197 (2 sets of twins), 3rd—291 (3 sets of twins), and unknown—2. Among the 1st trimester exposures, there were 76 spontaneous abortions (SABs), 1 stillbirth, 83 elective abortions (EABs), 19 infants with birth defects, and 577 live births without birth defects. In the remaining exposures, there were no SABs, 2 EABs, 2 stillbirths, 9 infants with birth defects, and 477 live births without birth defects. For exposures during the 1st trimester with known outcomes (excluding SABs, EABs, and stillbirths), the rate of birth defects was 3.2% (19 of 596). For all trimesters, the rate was 2.6% (28 of 1082). These rates are no different from the rates expected in a nonexposed population (8). As for pregnancies reported retrospectively (i.e., in which the outcome was known before reporting), there were 47 birth defects that, in general, were similar to those reported prospectively. There was no uniqueness or pattern among the malformations, reported prospectively or retrospectively, that suggested a common cause (8).

In a surveillance study of Michigan Medicaid recipients conducted between 1985 and 1992 involving 229,101 completed pregnancies, 478 newborns had been exposed to acyclovir during the 1st trimester (F. Rosa, personal communication, FDA, 1993). A total of 18 (3.8%) major birth defects were observed (20 expected). Specific data were available for six defect categories, including (observed/expected) 5/5 cardiovascular defects, 0/1 oral clefts, 0/0 spina bifida, 1/1 polydactyly, 1/1 limb reduction defects, and 2/1 hypospadia. These data do not support an association between the drug and the defects.

A 1998 noninterventional observational cohort study described the outcomes of pregnancies in women who had been prescribed ≥34 newly marketed drugs by general practitioners in England (60). Data were obtained by questionnaires sent to the prescribing physicians 1 month after the expected or possible date of delivery. In 831 (78%) of the pregnancies, a newly marketed drug was thought to had been taken during the 1st trimester with birth defects noted in 14 (2.5%) singleton births of the 557 newborns (10 sets of twins). In addition, two birth defects were observed in aborted fetuses. However, few of the aborted fetuses were examined. Acyclovir was taken during the 1st trimester in 24 pregnancies. The outcomes of these pregnancies included 1 SAB, 5 EABs, and 18 normal term babies (60).

Because there is more human pregnancy experience with acyclovir than with similar antiviral agents (e.g., valacyclovir or famciclovir) and this experience does not demonstrate a major risk, some authors consider acyclovir to be the drug of choice when indicated (62,63). However, for the management of herpes in pregnancy, either valacyclovir or acyclovir is recommended for primary or first-episode infection (for 7–10 days), symptomatic recurrent episode (for 5 days), and daily suppression (from 36 weeks' gestation until delivery), but only acyclovir is recommended for severe or disseminated disease (64). Long-term follow-up of children exposed in utero to these agents is warranted.

BREASTFEEDING SUMMARY

Acyclovir is concentrated in human milk with levels usually exceeding those found in maternal serum (65–69). In an in vitro experiment, the transfer of acyclovir from the plasma to breast milk was determined to be due to passive diffusion (65).

A woman, breastfeeding a 4-month-old infant, was treated with acyclovir 200 mg orally every 3 hours (5 times daily) for presumed oral herpes (66). She had taken 15 doses of the drug before the study dose. Approximately 9 hours after her 15th dose, she was given another 200-mg dose and paired maternal plasma and breast milk samples were drawn at 0, 0.5, 1.5, 2.0, and 3.0 hours. Breastfeeding was discontinued during the study interval. Milk:plasma ratios ranged from 0.6–4.1. Milk concentrations were greater than those in maternal serum at all times except at 1.5 hours, the time of peak plasma concentration (4.23 μmol/L). (*Note*: 1 μmol/L = 0.225 mcg/mL [9].) The initial level in the milk was 3.3 μmol/L, reflecting the doses taken prior to the study period. The highest level measured in milk was 5.8 μmol/L at 3.2 hours, but this was not the peak concentration because it was still rising at the time of sampling. Acyclovir was demonstrated in the infant's urine. Based on the poor lipid solubility of the drug, the pK_a's, and other known pharmacokinetic parameters, the calculated theoretical milk:plasma ratio was 0.15. Because the actual measured ratio was much greater than this value, it was concluded that acyclovir entered the milk by an active or facilitated process that would make it unique from any other medicinal agent. The maximum ingested dose, based on 750 mL of milk/day, was calculated to be 1500 mcg/day, approximately 0.2 mg/kg/day in the infant, or about 1.6% of the adult dose. This was thought not to represent an immediate risk to the infant, and, in fact, no adverse effects of the exposure were observed in the infant (66).

In a second case, a woman 1 year postpartum was treated with oral acyclovir, 200 mg 5 times a day, for presumed herpes zoster (67). The mean concentrations in the milk and serum were 1.06 and 0.33 mcg/mL, respectively, a milk:plasma ratio of 3.24. Detectable amounts were present in both serum and milk 48 hours after the last dose with an estimated half-life in the milk of 2.8 hours. The estimated amount of acyclovir ingested by the infant consuming 1000 mL/day of milk was about 1 mg (67).

Two recent studies measured the excretion of acyclovir in milk (68,69). In one, a woman 6 weeks postpartum suffering from eczema herpeticum received acyclovir IV 300 mg 3 times daily for 5 days (68). Breastfeeding was interrupted during the treatment. Serum and milk samples were collected after the last dose at 6-hour intervals for 4 days. Acyclovir levels in the milk exceeded those in the serum at every analysis and within the first 72 hours the milk concentration was 2.25 times higher than that in the serum. During the 88 hours that acyclovir was detectable in breast milk, a total of 4.448 mg was excreted (79% was recovered during the first 24 hours) (68).

In the other study, a woman was taking 800 mg 5 times daily for herpes zoster (69). She continued to breastfeed her 7-month-old infant. Three random milk samples were obtained (0.25–9.42 hours after a dose) with acyclovir levels ranging from 18.5 (4.16 mcg/mL) to 25.8 μmol/L (5.81 mcg/mL). The highest level occurred 9.42 hours after a dose. No adverse effects were observed in the infant who had ingested from the milk, what was thought to be, a clinically insignificant amount of acyclovir (0.73 mg/kg/day or about 1% of the maternal dose in mg/kg/day) (69).

Because acyclovir has been used to treat herpes virus infections in the neonate, and because of the lack of adverse effects in reported cases, mothers undergoing treatment with acyclovir can breastfeed safely. The American Academy of Pediatrics classifies acyclovir as compatible with breastfeeding (70).

References

1. Moore HL, Szczech GM, Rodwell DE, Kapp RW Jr, deMiranda P, Tucker WE Jr. Preclinical toxicology studies with acyclovir: teratologic, reproductive, and neonatal tests. Fund Appl Toxicol 1983;3:560–8.
2. Stahlmann R, Klug S, Lewandowski C, Bochert G, Chahoud I, Rahm U, Merker HJ, Neubert D. Prenatal toxicity of acyclovir in rats. Arch Toxicol 1988;61:468–79.
3. Chahoud I, Stahlmann R, Bochert G, Dillmann I, Neubert D. Gross-structural defects in rats after acyclovir application on day 10 of gestation. Arch Toxicol 1988;62:8–14.
4. Stahlmann R, Korte M, Van Loveren H, Vos JG, Thiel R, Neubert D. Abnormal thymus development and impaired function of the immune system in rats after prenatal exposure to aciclovir. Arch Toxicol 1992;66:551–9.
5. Clive D, Turner NT, Hozier J, Batson AGE, Tucker WE Jr. Preclinical toxicology studies with acyclovir: genetic toxicity tests. Fund Appl Toxicol 1983;3:587–602.
6. Stahlmann R, Chahoud I, Thiel R, Klug S, Forster C. The developmental toxicity of three antimicrobial agents observed only in nonroutine animal studies. Reprod Toxicol 1997;11:1–7.
7. Product information. Zovirax. Glaxo Wellcome, 2000.
8. Stone KM, Reiff-Eldridge R, White AD, Cordero JF, Brown Z, Alexander ER, Andrews EB. Pregnancy outcomes following systemic prenatal acyclovir exposure: conclusions from the International Acyclovir Pregnancy Registry, 1984–1999. Birth Defects Res A Clin Mol Teratol 2004;70:201–7.
9. Brown ZA, Baker DA. Acyclovir therapy during pregnancy. Obstet Gynecol 1989;73:526–31.
10. Brown ZA, Watts DH. Antiviral therapy in pregnancy. Clin Obstet Gynecol 1990;33:276–89.
11. Arvin AM, Hensleigh PA, Prober CG, Au DS, Yasukawa LL, Wittek AE, Palumbo PE, Paryani SG, Yeager AS. Failure of antepartum maternal cultures to predict the infant's risk of exposure to herpes simplex virus at delivery. N Engl J Med 1986;315:796–800.
12. Carney O, Mindel A. Screening pregnant women for genital herpes. BMJ 1988;296:1643.
13. Canadian Task Force on the Periodic Health Examination. Periodic health examination, 1989 update: 4. Intrapartum electronic fetal monitoring and prevention of neonatal herpes simplex. Can Med Assoc J 1989;141:1233–40.
14. Brocklehurst P, Kinghorn G, Carney O, Helsen K, Ross E, Ellis E, Shen R, Cowan F, Mindel A. A randomised placebo controlled trial of suppressive acyclovir in late pregnancy in women with recurrent genital herpes infection. Br J Obstet Gynaecol 1998;105:275–80.
15. CDC. 1998 Guideline for treatment of sexually transmitted diseases. MMWR 1998;47:25.
16. Henderson GI, Hu Z-Q, Johnson RF, Perez AB, Yang Y, Schenker S. Acyclovir transport by the human placenta. J Lab Clin Med 1992;120:885–92.
17. Landsberger EJ, Hager WD, Grossman JH III. Successful management of varicella pneumonia complicating pregnancy: a report of three cases. J Reprod Med 1986;31:311–4.
18. Utley K, Bromberger P, Wagner L, Schneider H. Management of primary herpes in pregnancy complicated by ruptured membranes and extreme prematurity: case report. Obstet Gynecol 1987;69:471–3.
19. Greffe BS, Dooley SL, Deddish RB, Krasny HC. Transplacental passage of acyclovir. J Pediatr 1986;108:1020–1.
20. Haddad J, Simeoni U, Messer J, Willard D. Transplacental passage of acyclovir. J Pediatr 1987;110:164.
21. Kingsley S. *Fetal and Neonatal Exposure to Acyclovir (Abstract)*. Second World Congress on Sexually Transmitted Diseases, Paris, June 1986. As cited in Haddad J, Simeoni U, Messer J, Willard D. Transplacental passage of acyclovir. J Pediatr 1987;110:164.
22. Frenkel LM, Brown ZA, Bryson YJ, Corey L, Unadkat JD, Hensleigh PA, Arvin AM, Prober CG, Connor JD. Pharmacokinetics of acyclovir in the term human pregnancy and neonate. Am J Obstet Gynecol 1991;164:569–76.
23. Fletcher CV. The placental transport and use of acyclovir in pregnancy. J Lab Clin Med 1992;120:821–2.
24. Lagrew DC Jr, Furlow TG, Hager WD, Yarrish RL. Disseminated herpes simplex virus infection in pregnancy. JAMA 1984;252:2058–9.
25. Grover L, Kane J, Kravitz J, Cruz A. Systemic acyclovir in pregnancy: a case report. Obstet Gynecol 1985;65:284–7.
26. Berger SA, Weinberg M, Treves T, Sorkin P, Geller E, Yedwab G, Tomer A, Rabey M, Michaeli D. Herpes encephalitis during pregnancy: failure of acyclovir and adenine arabinoside to prevent neonatal herpes. Isr J Med Sci 1986;22:41–4.
27. Anderson H, Sutton RNP, Scarffe JH. Cytotoxic chemotherapy and viral infections: the role of acyclovir. J R Coll Physicians Lond 1984;18:51–5.
28. Hockberger RS, Rothstein RJ. Varicella pneumonia in adults: a spectrum of disease. Ann Emerg Med 1986;15:931–4.
29. Glaser JB, Loftus J, Ferragamo V, Mootabar H, Castellano M. Varicella-zoster infection in pregnancy. N Engl J Med 1986;315:1416.
30. Tschen EH, Baack B. Treatment of herpetic whitlow in pregnancy with acyclovir. J Am Acad Dermatol 1987;17:1059–60.
31. Kundsin RB, Falk L, Hertig AT, Horne HW Jr. Acyclovir treatment of twelve unexplained infertile couples. Int J Fertil 1987;32:200–4.
32. Chazotte C, Andersen HF, Cohen WR. Disseminated herpes simplex infection in an immunocompromised pregnancy: treatment with intravenous acyclovir. Am J Perinatol 1987;4:363–4.
33. Cox SM, Phillips LE, DePaolo HD, Faro S. Treatment of disseminated herpes simplex virus in pregnancy with parenteral acyclovir: a case report. J Reprod Med 1986;31:1005–7.
34. Bernuau J, Caujolle B, Rouzioux C, Degott C, Rueff B, Benhamou JP. Severe acute hepatitis due to herpes-simplex in the third trimester of pregnancy: combatting with acyclovir (abstract). Gastroenterol Clin Biol 1987;11:79.
35. Hankins GDV, Gilstrap LC III, Patterson AR. Acyclovir treatment of varicella pneumonia in pregnancy. Crit Care Med 1987;15:336–7.
36. Hankey GR, Bucens MR, Chambers JSW. Herpes simplex encephalitis in third trimester of pregnancy: successful outcome for mother and child. Neurology 1987;37:1534–7.

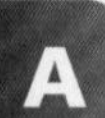

37. Frieden FJ, Ordorica SA, Goodgold AL, Hoskins IA, Silverman F, Young BK. Successful pregnancy with isolated herpes simplex virus encephalitis: case report and review of the literature. Obstet Gynecol 1990;75:511–3.
38. Glorioso DV, Molloy PJ, Van Thiel DH, Kania RJ. Successful empiric treatment of HSV hepatitis in pregnancy. Case report and review of the literature. Dig Dis Sci 1996;41:1273–5.
39. Leen CLS, Mandal BK, Ellis ME. Acyclovir and pregnancy. Br Med J 1987;294:308.
40. Eder SE, Apuzzio JJ, Weiss G. Varicella pneumonia during pregnancy: treatment of two cases with acyclovir. Am J Perinatol 1988;5:16–8.
41. Boyd K, Walker E. Use of acyclovir to treat chickenpox in pregnancy. BMJ 1988;296:393–4.
42. Key TC, Resnik R, Dittrich HC, Reisner LS. Successful pregnancy after cardiac transplantation. Am J Obstet Gynecol 1989;160:367–71.
43. Stray-Pedersen B. Acyclovir in late pregnancy to prevent neonatal herpes simplex. Lancet 1990;336:756.
44. Brocklehurst P, Carney O, Helson K, Kinghorn G, Mercey D, Mindel A. Acyclovir, herpes, and pregnancy. Lancet 1990;336:1594–5.
45. Stray-Pedersen B. Acyclovir, herpes, and pregnancy. Lancet 1990;336:1595.
46. Greenspoon JS, Wilcox JG, McHutchison LB. Does acyclovir improve the outcome of disseminated herpes simplex virus during pregnancy (abstract)? Am J Obstet Gynecol 1991;164:400.
47. Broussard RG, Payne DK, George RB. Treatment with acyclovir of varicella pneumonia in pregnancy. Chest 1991;99:1045–7.
48. Smego RA Jr, Asperilla MO. Use of acyclovir for varicella pneumonia during pregnancy. Obstet Gynecol 1991;78:1112–6.
49. Ciraru-Vigneron N, Nguyen Tan Lung R, Blondeau MA, Brunner C, Barrier J. Interest in the prescription acyclovir in the end of pregnancy in the case of genital herpes: a new protocol of the prevention of risks of herpes neonatal. Presse Med 1987;16:128.
50. Haddad J, Langer B, Astruc D, Messer J, Lokiec F. Oral acyclovir and recurrent genital herpes during late pregnancy. Obstet Gynecol 1993;82:102–4.
51. Esmonde TF, Herdman G, Anderson G. Chickenpox pneumonia: an association with pregnancy. Thorax 1989;44:812–5.
52. Horowitz GM, Hankins GDV. Early-second-trimester use of acyclovir in treating herpes zoster in a bone marrow transplant patient. A case report. J Reprod Med 1992;37:280–2.
53. Gilbert GL. Chickenpox during pregnancy. BMJ 1993;306:1079–80.
54. Moling O, Mayr O, Gottardi H, Mian P, Zanon P, Oberkofler F, Gramegna M, Colucci G. Severe pneumonia in pregnancy three months after resolution of cutaneous zoster. Infection 1994;22:216–8.
55. Greenspoon JS, Wilcox JG, McHutchison LB, Rosen DJD. Acyclovir for disseminated herpes simplex virus in pregnancy. A case report. J Reprod Med 1994;39:311–7.
56. Randolph AG, Hartshorn RM, Washington AE. Acyclovir prophylaxis in late pregnancy to prevent neonatal herpes: a cost-effectiveness analysis. Obstet Gynecol 1996;88:603–10.
57. Scott LL, Sanchez PJ, Jackson GL, Zeray F, Wendel GD Jr. Acyclovir suppression to prevent cesarean delivery after first-episode genital herpes. Obstet Gynecol 1996;87:69–73.
58. Whitty JE, Renfroe YR, Bottoms SF, Isada NB, Iverson R, Cotton DB. Varicella pneumonia in pregnancy: clinical experience (abstract). Am J Obstet Gynecol 1993;168:427.
59. Chandra PC, Patel H, Schiavello HJ, Briggs SL. Successful pregnancy outcome after complicated varicella pneumonia. Obstet Gynecol 1998;92:680–2.
60. Wilton LV, Pearce GL, Martin RM, Mackay FJ, Mann RD. The outcomes of pregnancy in women exposed to newly marketed drugs in general practice in England. Br J Obstet Gynaecol 1998;105:882–9.
61. Anderson R, Lundqvist A, Bergstrom T. Successful treatment of generalized primary herpes simplex type 2 infection during pregnancy. Scand J Infect Dis 1999;31:210–2.
62. Balfour HH Jr. Antiviral drugs. N Engl J Med 1999;340:1255–68.
63. Smith JR, Cowan FM, Munday P. The management of herpes simplex virus infection in pregnancy. Br J Obstet Gynaecol 1998;105:255–60.
64. American College of Obstetricians and Gynecologists. Management of herpes in pregnancy. *ACOG Practice Bulletin*. No. 82, June 2007.
65. Bork K, Kaiser T, Benes P. Transfer of aciclovir from plasma to human breast milk. Drug Res 2000;50:656–8.
66. Lau RJ, Emery MG, Galinsky RE. Unexpected accumulation of acyclovir in breast milk with estimation of infant exposure. Obstet Gynecol 1987;69:468–71.
67. Meyer LJ, de Miranda P, Sheth N, Spruance S. Acyclovir in human breast milk. Am J Obstet Gynecol 1988;158:586–8.
68. Bork K, Benes P. Concentration and kinetic studies of intravenous acyclovir in serum and breast milk of a patient with eczema herpeticum. J Am Acad Dermatol 1995;32:1053–5.
69. Taddio A, Klein J, Koren G. Acyclovir excretion in human breast milk. Ann Pharmacother 1994;28:585–7.
70. Committee on Drugs, American Academy of Pediatrics. The transfer of drugs and other chemicals into human milk. Pediatrics 2001;108:776–89.

ADALIMUMAB

Immunologic Agent (Immunomodulator)

PREGNANCY RECOMMENDATION: Compatible
BREASTFEEDING RECOMMENDATION: Limited Human Data—Probably Compatible

PREGNANCY SUMMARY

The maternal benefits from treatment with adalimumab appear to far outweigh the unknown embryo–fetal risks (1,2). No developmental toxicity attributable to adalimumab has been observed in a limited number of cases and the animal data suggest low risk. In 2011, the World Congress of Gastroenterology stated "Adalimumab in pregnancy is considered low risk and compatible with use during conception and pregnancy in at least the first two trimesters" (3). Theoretically, tumor necrosis factor-alpha (TNF-α) antagonists could interfere with implantation and ovulation, but this has not been shown clinically (4). Because of the long elimination half-life, use before conception may result in inadvertent exposure of an unplanned pregnancy. If adalimumab is used in pregnancy for the treatment of rheumatoid arthritis, health care professionals are encouraged to call the toll-free number (877-311-8972) for information about patient enrollment in the Organization of Teratology Information Specialists (OTIS) Rheumatoid Arthritis study and pregnancy registry.

FETAL RISK SUMMARY

Adalimumab is a recombinant IgG1 monoclonal antibody that binds specifically to human TNF-α to block its action on cell surface TNF receptors. TNF-α is a pro-inflammatory cytokine with a central role in inflammatory processes. Adalimumab is in the same subclass of immunomodulators (blockers of TNF activity) as etanercept, certolizumab pegol, golimumab, and infliximab. It is indicated for reducing the signs and symptoms and inhibiting the progression of structural damage in adult patients with moderate to severe active rheumatoid arthritis who have had an inadequate response to one or more disease-modifying antirheumatic drugs. It has also been used in Crohn's disease. The mean terminal elimination half-life is about 14 days (range 10–20 days) (5).

An animal reproduction study for perinatal development toxicity was conducted in pregnant cynomolgus monkeys. Doses up to 266 times the human AUC (SC 40 mg with methotrexate every week) or 373 times the human AUC (SC 40 mg without methotrexate) revealed no fetal harm (the timing of the exposure was not specified). No clastogenic or mutagenic effects were observed in various tests, but adalimumab has not been tested for carcinogenic or fertility effects (5).

Although the molecular weight is very high (about 148,000), adalimumab crosses the human placenta to the fetus in late gestation (6). As an IgG1 antibody, the drug would be transported actively across the placenta, especially in the 3rd trimester, but with minimal transfer in the 1st trimester. In 10 cases at a mean gestational age of 39 weeks (range 38–41 weeks), the median of infliximab concentrations in cord blood as a percentage of maternal concentration was 179% (range 98%–293%). The last dose was given a median of 5.5 weeks (range 0.14–8 weeks) before birth. Infant or cord blood concentrations were higher than maternal levels in every case. Moreover, infliximab was detected in the infants for at least 11 weeks. No birth defects, infections, or neonatal intensive care unit stays occurred in any infant (6).

A 2005 case report described a 34-year-old woman with long-standing Crohn's disease who was treated throughout gestation with adalimumab and prednisone (7). The woman received 38 weekly SC doses of adalimumab (40 mg/dose). Normal fetal growth was documented during the uncomplicated pregnancy. An elective cesarean section at 38.5 weeks' delivered a normal infant with Apgar scores of 8 and 9, presumably at 1 and 5 minutes, respectively. The infant was growing and developing normally at 6 months of age (7).

The preliminary results of an on-going prospective cohort study and pregnancy registry involving adalimumab that is being conducted by OTIS were reported at an October 2006 meeting (D. Johnson, personal communication, University of California, San Diego, 2006). Of the 95 women enrolled in the study or registry, 26 involved exposure in the 1st trimester. Thirteen outcomes were known, 12 of which resulted in healthy, full-term infants without birth defects. In the 13th case, a woman with twins, one fetus was aborted and the other was delivered prematurely without defects.

A 35-year-old woman with Crohn's disease was treated with adalimumab (SC 40 mg every other week) throughout gestation (8). She delivered a normal infant (details not provided) that had normal growth and development at 6 months of age.

A 34-year-old woman with Crohn's disease was treated with budesonide, then prednisone only from 6 to 20 weeks' gestation (9). At that point, she was started on azathioprine 100 mg/day and adalimumab 80 mg (one dose), then 40 mg every other week. Prednisone was tapered and stopped by the 32nd week. Labor was induced at 38 weeks' and she delivered a healthy, 2.89-kg, male infant who was well and developing normally at 1 year of age (9).

A 2006 communication from England described the pregnancy outcomes of 23 women directly exposed to TNF-α agents at the time of conception (17 etanercept, 3 adalimumab, and 3 infliximab) (10). Additional therapy included methotrexate in nine women and leflunomide in two. There also were nine patients (four etanercept, five infliximab) that discontinued therapy before conception. The outcomes for the 32 pregnancies were 7 spontaneous abortions (SABs), 3 elective abortions (EABs), and 22 live births. No major anomalies were observed in the live births, including one infant exposed to adalimumab and methotrexate early in gestation (10).

A 2007 case report and literature review described the use of adalimumab in a 41-year-old woman with rheumatoid arthritis (11). The woman had received a single dose of 40 mg after conception when an unplanned pregnancy at 5 weeks' was discovered. A healthy 2.6-kg infant was delivered at 32 weeks' gestation. At 25 months of age, the child was growing and developing normally (11).

A 2008 report described a 22-year-old woman with Takayasu arteritis who conceived while taking adalimumab 40 mg SC every 4 weeks, leflunomide 10 mg/day, prednisolone 5 mg/day, and dalteparin 500 IU/day (12). Leflunomide was discontinued by the patient at 8 weeks' gestation but the other agents were continued throughout. At 37 weeks', a cesarean section was performed to deliver a healthy 2550-g male infant with Apgar scores of 9, 9, and 10 at 1, 5, and 10 minutes, respectively (12).

A woman with lupus nephritis took mycophenolate mofetil (1000 mg/day) and adalimumab (40 mg every other week) during the first 8 weeks of pregnancy (13). She underwent a cesarean section for transverse position at 32 weeks' gestation to give birth to a 4422-g female infant with normal karyotype (46,XX). The infant had multiple birth defects including arched eyebrows, hypertelorism, epicanthic folds, micrognathia, thick everted lower lip, cleft palate, bilateral microtia with aural atresia, congenital tracheomalacia, and brachydactyly. Shortly after birth, a tracheostomy was done for respiratory distress and a G-tube was placed because of feeding difficulties. The cleft palate was repaired surgically. At 20 months of age, the infant had normal growth and slightly delayed motor development. The tracheostomy was still required as were G-tube feedings. She seemed to have some hearing, but had significant expressive speech delay. The defects were attributed to mycophenolate (13).

A 2009 study from France reported the outcomes of 15 women who took anti-TNF drugs during pregnancy (10 etanercept, 3 infliximab, and 2 adalimumab) (14). The drugs were given in the 1st, 2nd, and 3rd trimesters in 12, 3, and 2 cases, respectively. The outcomes were 2 SABs, 1 EAB, and 12 healthy babies without malformation or neonatal illness. They also reviewed the literature regarding the use of anti-TNF agents in pregnancy and found more than 300 cases. It was concluded that, although only 29 were treated throughout gestation, the malformation rate was similar to the general population (14).

A 32-year-old woman with Crohn's disease was treated with adalimumab 40 mg every other week for a total of 18 doses (15). Therapy at that time was stopped when her pregnancy was diagnosed. She had received 40 mg doses at 2, 4, and 6 weeks' gestation. She eventually delivered at term a healthy 3360-g female infant with Apgar scores of 10, 10, and 10. The child was doing well at 2 years of age (15).

In 2008, investigators reviewed >120,000 adverse events involving TNF-α agents that had been reported to the FDA in 1999–2005 (16). There were 61 congenital anomalies in

41 children born to mothers taking etanercept or infliximab. There were no cases of birth defects involving adalimumab (16).

In a 2010 case report, a 34-year-old woman was treated for psoriasis with adalimumab from 3 months before conception through 5 weeks of pregnancy (17). An elective cesarean section at 38.5 weeks gave birth to a low-birth-weight infant (weight and sex not specified). The child was developing normally at 12 months of age (17).

A 26-year-old woman with Crohn's ileitis was treated with adalimumab before and during gestation up to week 30 of gestation (18). At that time the drug was discontinued, and she gave birth at 38 weeks' to a healthy infant (weight and sex not specified).

In subfertile women with T helper 1/T helper 2 cytokine elevations undergoing in vitro fertilization, adalimumab and IV immunoglobulin significantly improved the rates of implantation, clinical pregnancies, and live births (19).

BREASTFEEDING SUMMARY

Adalimumab is excreted into breast milk. In a case described above, adalimumab therapy was discontinued at 30 weeks' gestation and the woman gave birth to a healthy infant at term (18). The mother did not require therapy while breastfeeding her infant during the first 4 weeks after birth but, at that time, she experienced a flare-up of Crohn's disease. Nursing was discontinued when a 40-mg SC dose was given. Immediately before the dose, maternal serum and breast milk concentrations of adalimumab were undectable. Postdose, the serum level peaked at 4300 ng/mL at 3 days, whereas the peak milk concentration of 31 ng/mL was reached on day 6 (18).

In another study described above, 9 of 10 mothers continued to take adalimumab after birth and 6 of 10 infants were breastfed (6). No other details were provided.

The very low adalimumab concentration in breast milk is consistent with its high molecular weight (about 148,000). The systemic bioavailability of the drug from milk and any effect of this exposure on a nursing infant are unknown. However, two mothers, described above, did continue adalimumab during breastfeeding and no adverse effects in their infants were mentioned (7,8).

References

1. Gisbert JP. Safety of immunomodulators and biologics for the treatment of inflammatory bowel disease during pregnancy and breast-feeding. Inflamm Bowel Dis 2010;16:881–95.
2. El Mourabet M, El-Hachem S, Harrison JR, Binion DG. Anti-TNF antibody therapy for inflammatory bowel disease during pregnancy: a clinical review. Curr Drug Targets 2010;234–41.
3. Mahadevan U, Cucchiara S, Hyams JS, Steinwurz F, Nuti F, Travis SPL, Sandborn WJ, Colombel IH. The London position statement of the World Congress of Gastroenterology on biological therapy for IBD with the European Crohn's and Colitis Organization: pregnancy and pediatrics. Am J Gastroenterol 2011;106:214–23.
4. Khanna D, McMahon M, Furst DE. Safety of tumour necrosis factor-α antagonists. Drug Saf 2004;27:307–24.
5. Product information. Humira. Abbott Laboratories, 2004.
6. Mahadevan U, Wolf DC, Dubinsky M, Cortot A, Lee SD, Siegel CA, Ullman T, Glover S, Valentine JF, Rubin DT, Miller J, Abreu MT. Placental transfer of anti-tumor necrosis factor agents in pregnant patients with inflammatory bowel disease. Clin Gastroenterol Hepatol 2013;11:286–92.
7. Vesga L, Terdiman JP, Mahadevan U. Adalimumab use in pregnancy. Gut 2005;54:890.
8. Mishkin D, Van Deinse W, Becker J, Farraye FA. Successful use of adalimumab (Humira) for Crohn's disease in pregnancy. Inflamm Bowel Dis 2006;12:827–8.
9. Coburn LA, Wise PE, Schwartz DA. The successful use of adalimumab to treat active Crohn's disease of an ileoanal pouch during pregnancy. Dig Dis Sci 2006;51:2045–7.
10. Hyrich KL, Symmons DPM, Watson KD, Silman AJ. Pregnancy outcome in women who were exposed to anti-tumor necrosis factor agents: results from a national population register. Arthritis Rheum 2006;54:2701–2.
11. Roux CH, Brocq O, Breuil V, Albert C, Euller-Ziegler L. Pregnancy in rheumatology patients exposed to anti-tumour necrosis factor (TNF)-α therapy. Rheumatology 2007;46:695–8.
12. Kraemer B, Abele H, Hahn M, Rajab T, Kraemer E, Wallweiner D, Becker S. A successful pregnancy in a patient with Takayasu's arteritis. Hypertens Pregnancy 2008;27:247–52.
13. Velinov M, Zellers N. The fetal mycophenolate mofetil syndrome. Clin Dysmorphol 2008;17:77–8.
14. Berthelot JM, De Bandt M, Goupille P, Solau-Gervais E, Liote F, Goeb V, Azais I, Martin A, Pallot-Prades B, Maugars Y, Mariette X, on behalf of CRI (Club Rhumatismes et Inflammation). Exposition to anti-TNF drugs during pregnancy: outcome of 15 cases and review of the literature. Joint Bone Spine 2009;76:28–34.
15. Jurgens M, Brand S, Filik L, Hubener C, Hasbargen U, Beigel F, Tillack C. Safety of adalimumab in Crohn's disease during pregnancy: case report and review of the literature. Inflamm Bowel Dis 2010;16:1634–6.
16. Carter JD, Ladhani A, Ricca LR, Valeriano J, Vasey FB. A safety assessment of tumor necrosis factor antagonists during pregnancy: a review of the Food and Drug Administration database. J Rheumatol 2009;36:635–41.
17. Dessinioti C, Stefanaki I, Stratigos AJ, Kostaki M, Katsambas A, Antoniou C. Pregnancy during adalimumab use for psoriasis. J Eur Acad Dermatol Venereol 2011;25:738–9.
18. Ben-Horin S, Yavzori M, Katz L, Picard O, Fudim E, Chowers Y, Lang A. Adalimumab level in breast milk of a nursing mother. Clin Gastroenterol Hepatol 2010;8:475–6.
19. Winger EE, Reed JL, Ashoush S, Ahuja S, El-Toukhy T, Taranissi M. Treatment with adalimumab (Humira) and intravenous immunoglobulin improves pregnancy rates in women undergoing IVF. Am J Reprod Immunol 2009;61:113–20.

ADAPALENE

Dermatologic Agent

PREGNANCY RECOMMENDATION: Limited Human Data—Animal Data Suggest Low Risk
BREASTFEEDING RECOMMENDATION: No Human Data—Probably Compatible

PREGNANCY SUMMARY

Adapalene is not teratogenic in two experimental animal species. After chronic use in humans, trace amounts of adapalene have been detected in the systemic circulation. The adverse pregnancy outcome described below is the only report of adapalene exposure in human pregnancy. The combination of animal data and very low systemic bioavailability suggests that any risk to a fetus from inadvertent exposure would be very low, but the nearly complete absence of human data prevents further assessment. Until more experience in pregnancy has been reported, the safest course is to avoid use of this agent in the 1st trimester.

FETAL RISK SUMMARY

Adapalene is used topically (cream, gel, or solution) for the treatment of acne vulgaris. The agent is a retinoid-like compound that is a modulator of cellular differentiation, keratinization, and inflammatory processes. It binds to specific retinoic acid nuclear receptors. Plasma concentrations are very low after chronic topical application (<0.25 ng/mL) (1).

No teratogenic effects were noted in pregnant rats given oral doses up to 120 times the maximum daily human dose (MDHD). Topical application of adapalene to pregnant rats and rabbits up to 150 times the MDHD demonstrated no fetotoxicity and only minimal increases in supernumerary ribs in rats (1).

It is not known if adapalene crosses the human placenta. The molecular weight (about 413) and low plasma concentrations suggest that minimal amounts of drug would be available to cross the placenta.

Only one report describing the use of adapalene during human pregnancy has been located (2). At 22 weeks' gestation, a small-for-date fetus with anophthalmia was detected by ultrasound examination and the pregnancy was terminated. Anophthalmia and agenesis of the optic chiasma were observed in the aborted fetus. The mother had been treated with adapalene gel (0.3 mg/day) from 1 month before conception until 13 weeks' gestation. The defects were not thought to be typical of retinoid-induced malformations (heart, central nervous system, thymus, limbs, and craniofacial) (2).

BREASTFEEDING SUMMARY

No reports describing the use of adapalene during lactation have been located. The systemic availability of this drug from topical administration is very low (<25 ng/mL) (1). The amount in breast milk, therefore, should also be very low. It is doubtful that this level, if it is excreted in milk, represents any risk to a nursing infant.

References

1. Product information. Differin. Galderma Laboratories, 2002.
2. Autret E, Berjot M, Jonville-Bera AP, Aubry MC, Moraine C. Anophthalmia and agenesis of optic chiasma associated with adapalene gel in early pregnancy. Lancet 1997;350:339.

ADEFOVIR

Antiviral

PREGNANCY RECOMMENDATION: Compatible—Maternal Benefit >> Embryo–Fetal Risk
BREASTFEEDING RECOMMENDATION: No Human Data—Potential Toxicity (Hepatitis B) Contraindicated (HIV)

PREGNANCY SUMMARY

The animal data suggest low risk, but the human data are limited and prevent an assessment of the embryo–fetal risk. If indicated, the drug should not be withheld because of pregnancy.

FETAL RISK SUMMARY

Adefovir, an acyclic nucleotide analog of adenosine monophosphate, is used for the treatment of chronic hepatitis B, especially in patients with clinical evidence of lamivudine-resistant hepatitis B virus. The mechanism involves the inhibition of hepatitis B virus DNA polymerase (reverse transcriptase) (1). It has also been used in patients infected with HIV (1,2). The antiviral agent is available as a prodrug, adefovir dipivoxil, which is rapidly converted to adefovir after oral administration (1). Adefovir is then phosphorylated to the active metabolite, adefovir diphosphate, by cellular kinases. Serum protein binding is very low (≤4%) and the terminal elimination half-life is about 7.5 hours (1).

Reproduction studies have been conducted in rats and rabbits. No evidence of embryotoxicity or teratogenicity was observed in rats after oral dosing that produced systemic exposures up to 23 times the human exposure achieved with the therapeutic dose of 10 mg/day (HE) or in rabbits at 40 times the HE. In rats given maternal toxic IV doses (systemic exposures 38 times the HE), embryotoxicity and an increase in the incidence of fetal malformations (anasarca, depressed eye bulge, umbilical hernia, and kinked tail) were observed. The no-effect exposure from IV doses in pregnant rats was 12 times the HE (1). Intraperitoneal doses of adefovir in mice resulted in dose-related resorptions, low birth weight, neonatal death, and severe lymphoid depletion of the thymus (3).

It is not known if adefovir crosses the human placenta. The molecular weight (about 501) of the prodrug, adefovir dipivoxil, the relative lack of protein binding, and the moderately long terminal elimination half-life suggest that adefovir will cross to the fetal compartment.

The Antiretroviral Pregnancy Registry reported, for the period January 1989 through July 2009, prospective data (reported before the outcomes were known) involving 4702 live births that had been exposed during the 1st trimester

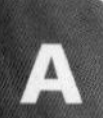

to one or more antiretroviral agents (4). Congenital defects were noted in 134, a prevalence of 2.8% (95% confidence interval [CI] 2.4–3.4). In the 6100 live births with earliest exposure in the 2nd/3rd trimesters, there were 153 infants with defects (2.5%, 95% CI 2.1–2.9). The prevalence rates for the two periods did not differ significantly. There were 288 infants with birth defects among 10,803 live births with exposure anytime during pregnancy (2.7%, 95% CI 2.4–3.0). The prevalence rate did not differ significantly from the rate expected in a nonexposed population. There were 37 outcomes exposed to adefovir all in the 1st trimester in combination with other antiretroviral agents. There were no birth defects. In reviewing the birth defects of prospective and retrospective (pregnancies reported after the outcomes were known) registered cases, the Registry concluded that, except for isolated cases of neural tube defects with efavirenz exposure in retrospective reports, there was no other pattern of anomalies (isolated or syndromic) (4). (See Lamivudine for required statement.)

For HIV infection, two reviews, one in 1996 and the other in 1997, concluded that all women currently receiving antiretroviral therapy should continue to receive therapy during pregnancy and that treatment of the mother with monotherapy should be considered inadequate therapy (5,6). The same conclusion was reached in a 2003 review with the added admonishment that therapy must be continuous to prevent emergence of resistant viral strains (7). In 2009, the updated U.S. Department of Health and Human Services guidelines for the use of antiretroviral agents in HIV type 1 (HIV-1)-infected patients continued the recommendation that therapy, with the exception of efavirenz, should be continued during pregnancy (8). If indicated, adefovir should not be withheld in pregnancy because the expected benefit to the HIV-positive mother outweighs the unknown risk to the fetus. Updated guidelines for the use of antiretroviral drugs to reduce perinatal HIV-1 transmission also were released in 2010 (9). Women receiving antiretroviral therapy during pregnancy should continue the therapy; however, regardless of the regimen, zidovudine administration is recommended during the intrapartum period to prevent vertical transmission of HIV to the newborn (9).

BREASTFEEDING SUMMARY

No reports describing the use of adefovir during lactation have been located. The molecular weight (about 501) of the prodrug, adefovir dipivoxil, the relative lack of protein binding, and the moderately long terminal elimination half-life suggest that the adefovir will be excreted into breast milk. Women infected with hepatitis B can breastfeed without additional risk for the transmission of hepatitis B. However, if adefovir is used during nursing for the treatment of the maternal infection, there is a potential risk of serious toxicity for the nursing infant, such as the nephrotoxicity seen in adults.

Reports on the use of adefovir during human lactation in women infected with HIV are unlikely because HIV-1 is transmitted in milk, and in developed countries, breastfeeding is not recommended (5,6,8,10–12). In developing countries, breastfeeding is undertaken, despite the risk, because there are no affordable milk substitutes available. Until 1999, no studies had been published that examined the effect of any antiretroviral therapy on HIV-1 transmission in milk. In that year, a study involving zidovudine was published that measured a 38% reduction in vertical transmission of HIV-1 infection in spite of breastfeeding when compared with controls (see Zidovudine).

References

1. Product information. Hepsera. Gilead Sciences, 2004.
2. Horowitz HW, Telzak EE, Sepkowitz KA, Wormser GP. Human immunodeficiency virus infection, part II. Dis Mon 1998;44:677–716.
3. Lee JS, Mullaney S, Bronson R, Sharpe AH, Jaenisch R, Balzarini J, De Clercq E, Ruprecht RM. Transplacental antiretroviral therapy with 9-(2-phosphonylmethoxyethyl)adenine is embryotoxic in transgenic mice. J Acquir Immune Defic Syndr 1991;4:833–8.
4. Antiretroviral Pregnancy Registry Steering Committee. *Antiretroviral Pregnancy Registry International Interim Report for 1 January 1989 through 31 July 2009*. Wilmington, NC: Registry Coordinating Center; 2009. Available at www.apregistry.com. Accessed May 29, 2010.
5. Carpenter CCJ, Fischi MA, Hammer SM, Hirsch MS, Jacobsen DM, Katzenstein DA, Montaner JSG, Richman DD, Saag MS, Schooley RT, Thompson MA, Vella S, Yeni PG, Volberding PA. Antiretroviral therapy for HIV infection in 1996. JAMA 1996;276;146–54.
6. Minkoff H, Augenbraun M. Antiretroviral therapy for pregnant women. Am J Obstet Gynecol 1997;176:478–89.
7. Minkoff H. Human immunodeficiency virus infection in pregnancy. Obstet Gynecol 2003;101:797–810.
8. Panel on Antiretroviral Guidelines for Adults and Adolescents. *Guidelines for the Use of Antiretroviral Agents in HIV-1-Infected Adults and Adolescents*. Department of Health and Human Services. December 1, 2009;1–161. Available at http://www.aidsinfo.nih.gov/ContentFiles/AdultandAdolescentGL.pdf. Accessed September 17, 2010:60, 96–8.
9. Panel on Treatment of HIV-Infected Pregnant Women and Prevention of Perinatal Transmission. *Recommendations for Use of Antiretroviral Drugs in Pregnant HIV-1-Infected Women for Maternal Health and Interventions to Reduce Perinatal HIV Transmission in the United States*. May 24, 2010:1–117. Available at http://aidsinfo.nih.gov/ContentFiles/PerinatalGL.pdf. Accessed September 17, 2010:30, 39–44 (Table 5).
10. Brown ZA, Watts DH. Antiviral therapy in pregnancy. Clin Obstet Gynecol 1990;33:276–89.
11. De Martino M, Tovo P-A, Pezzotti P, Galli L, Massironi E, Ruga E, Floreea F, Plebani A, Gabiano C, Zuccotti GV. HIV-1 transmission through breast-milk: appraisal of risk according to duration of feeding. AIDS 1992;6:991–7.
12. Van de Perre P. Postnatal transmission of human immunodeficiency virus type 1: the breast feeding dilemma. Am J Obstet Gynecol 1995;173:483–7.

ADENOSINE

Antiarrhythmic

PREGNANCY RECOMMENDATION: Compatible—Maternal Benefit >> Embryo–Fetal Risk
BREASTFEEDING RECOMMENDATION: No Human Data—Probably Compatible

PREGNANCY SUMMARY

Adenosine has been used in all stages of pregnancy for maternal and embryo–fetal indications without harming the embryo or fetus. If indicated, the drug should not be withheld because of pregnancy.

FETAL RISK SUMMARY

Adenosine, an endogenous purine-based nucleoside found in all cells of the body, is used for the treatment of paroxysmal supraventricular tachycardia. Adenosine phosphate and adenosine triphosphate have been used as vasodilators. Ordinarily, adverse fetal effects secondary to adenosine would not be expected because of the widespread, natural distribution of this substance in the body and its very short (<10 seconds) half-life after IV administration. However, the maternal administration of large IV doses of adenosine may potentially produce fetal toxicity, as has been observed with other endogenous agents (e.g., see Epinephrine).

A reproduction study in chick embryos did not observe teratogenicity (1). Injection into the fourth cerebral ventricle of fetal sheep resulted in depressed fetal respiratory drive (2). In pregnant sheep, constant infusions and single injections of adenosine produced alterations in maternal heart rate and a decrease in diastolic pressure, but no changes in maternal systolic pressure or arterial blood gases, and had no effect on fetal heart rate, arterial pressure, or arterial blood gases (3,4). Another experiment using near-term sheep demonstrated that angiotensin II-induced maternal–placental vasoconstriction could not be reversed by a high-dose infusion of adenosine (5).

Endogenous adenosine cord blood levels, measured in 14 fetuses of 19–34 weeks' gestation, were not related to gestational age, but were significantly increased in anemic fetuses and were positively associated with blood oxygen tension (6). The investigators concluded that the results were compatible with a fetal response to tissue hypoxia.

The first case describing the use of adenosine in human pregnancy appeared in 1991 (7). Recurrent narrow complex tachycardia occurred suddenly in a 40-year-old woman in her 39th week of gestation. She had been hospitalized 6 months before the current episode for a similar condition secondary to mitral valve prolapse and had been taking atenolol for tachyarrhythmia prophylaxis since that occurrence. Maternal blood pressure was 80 mm Hg systolic with a pulse of 240 beats/minute. Fetal heart rate was 140 beats/minute. Two IV bolus doses of adenosine (6 and 12 mg) were administered resulting in conversion to sinus rhythm with a rate of 80 beats/minute. A nonstress test, conducted after stabilization of the mother, was normal. Two weeks later, a healthy 3.6-kg infant was delivered. Both mother and baby were doing well 1 month postpartum.

Since the above case, a number of reports have described the safe use of adenosine to treat maternal or fetal supraventricular tachycardia (8–20) during all phases of gestation, including one woman in active labor (15), eight during the 1st trimester (16), and four cases of direct fetal administration (18–20). The first three of the maternal reports and the first fetal case are described below.

A 19-year-old woman was treated at 38 weeks' gestation for the arrhythmia during labor (8). Conversion to a normal sinus rhythm required two IV bolus doses (6 and 12 mg). No effect was observed on uterine contractions, fetal heart rate, or variability. A cesarean section was required for failure of the labor to progress. The second case occurred in a 34-year-old woman with onset of supraventricular tachycardia at 30 weeks' gestation (9). She responded within 30 seconds to a single 6-mg IV adenosine dose with no changes observed in the fetal heart rate tracing. A normal infant was delivered at term. The third woman was a 26-year-old patient with a history of Wolff-Parkinson-White syndrome who was initially treated successfully with 6 mg IV adenosine at 7 months' gestation (10). She was subsequently treated with atenolol and eventually admitted at term for labor induction. During labor the supraventricular tachycardia recurred and two doses (6 and 12 mg) of adenosine were required to convert to a normal sinus rhythm. During the mother's arrhythmia, fetal distress demonstrated by recurrent, deep variable decelerations with loss of short-term variability was observed, but fetal bradycardia resolved with a return to a fetal heart rate of 130 beats/minute on conversion of the mother. A third recurrence of the mother's tachycardia occurred shortly before a cesarean section and this was successfully converted with a 12-mg dose of adenosine. A male infant was delivered with Apgar scores of 1 and 5 at 1 and 5 minutes, respectively. No adverse effects in the fetus or newborn attributable to adenosine were observed in any of the above cases or in the other cited cases.

A 1995 reference described the direct fetal administration of adenosine for the treatment of persistent supraventricular tachycardia with massive hydrops at 28 weeks' gestation (18). Treatment with digoxin and flecainide for 5 weeks had not been successful in reversing the condition. Based on estimated fetal weight, 0.2 mg/kg of adenosine was given by bolus injection into the umbilical vein and a normal rhythm occurred within seconds. The umbilical serum levels of digoxin and flecainide were determined at the same time and further loading of the fetus with digoxin (0.05 mg/kg) and flecainide (1.0 mg/kg) were administered via the umbilical vein (18). After about 20 minutes of intermittent atrial arrhythmia and tachycardia, the fetal heart converted to a stable, normal rhythm. One week later, the fetus died in utero from what was thought to be a recurrence of the tachycardia or the onset of a drug-induced arrhythmia (18). Massive hydrops fetalis with a structurally normal heart was found at autopsy.

BREASTFEEDING SUMMARY

Because adenosine is used only by IV injection in acute care situations, it is doubtful that any report will be located describing the use of adenosine during human lactation. Moreover, the serum half-life is so short that it is unlikely that any of the drug will pass into milk.

References

1. Shepard TH. *Catalog of Teratogenic Agents*. 6th ed. Baltimore, MD: Johns Hopkins University Press, 1989:194.
2. Bissonnette JM, Hohimer AR, Knopp SJ. The effect of centrally administered adenosine on fetal breath movements. Respir Physiol 1991;84:273–85.

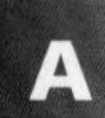

3. Mason B, Ogunyemi D, Punla O, Koos B. Maternal and fetal cardiovascular effects of intravenous adenosine (abstract). Am J Obstet Gynecol 1993;168:439.
4. Mason BA, Ogunyemi D, Punla O, Koos BJ. Maternal and fetal cardiorespiratory responses to adenosine in sheep. Am J Obstet Gynecol 1993;168:1558–61.
5. Landauer M, Phernetton TM, Rankin JHG. Maternal ovine placental vascular responses to adenosine. Am J Obstet Gynecol 1986;154: 1152–5.
6. Ross Russell RI, Greenough A, Lagercrantz H, Dahlin I, Nicolaides K. Fetal anaemia and its relation with increased concentrations of adenosine. Arch Dis Child Fetal Neonatal 1993;68:35–6.
7. Podolsky SM, Varon J. Adenosine use during pregnancy. Ann Emerg Med 1991;20:1027–8.
8. Harrison JK, Greenfield RA, Wharton JM. Acute termination of supraventricular tachycardia by adenosine during pregnancy. Am Heart J 1992;123:1386–8.
9. Mason BA, Ricci-Goodman J, Koos BJ. Adenosine in the treatment of maternal paroxysmal supraventricular tachycardia. Obstet Gynecol 1992;80:478–80.
10. Afridi I, Moise KJ Jr, Rokey R. Termination of supraventricular tachycardia with intravenous adenosine in a pregnant woman with Wolff-Parkinson-White syndrome. Obstet Gynecol 1992;80:481–3.
11. Leffler S, Johnson DR. Adenosine use in pregnancy. Lack of effect on fetal heart rate. Am J Emerg Med 1992;10:548–9.
12. Propp DA, Broderick K, Pesch D. Adenosine during pregnancy. Ann Emerg Med 1992;21:453–4.
13. Adair RF. Fetal monitoring with adenosine administration. Ann Emerg Med 1993;22:1925.
14. Matfin G, Baylis P, Adams P. Maternal paroxysmal supraventricular tachycardia treated with adenosine. Postgrad Med J 1993;69:661–2.
15. Hagley MT, Cole PL. Adenosine use in pregnant women with supraventricular tachycardia. Ann Pharmacother 1994;28:1241–2.
16. Elkayam U, Goodwin TM Jr. Adenosine therapy for supraventricular tachycardia during pregnancy. Am J Cardiol 1995;75:521–3.
17. Hagley MT, Haraden B, Cole PL. Adenosine use in a pregnant patient with supraventricular tachycardia. Ann Pharmacother 1995;29:938.
18. Kohl T, Tercanli S, Kececioglu D, Holzgreve W. Direct fetal administration of adenosine for the termination of incessant supraventricular tachycardia. Obstet Gynecol 1995;85:873–4.
19. Hubinont C, Debauche C, Bernard P, Sluysmans T. Resolution of fetal tachycardia and hydrops by a single adenosine administration. Obstet Gynecol 1998;92(Part 2):718.
20. Dangel JH, Roszkowski T, Bieganowska K, Kubicka K, Ganowicz J. Adenosine triphosphate for cardioversion of supraventricular tachycardia in two hydropic fetuses. Fetal Diagn Ther 2000;15:326–30.

AGALSIDASE ALFA

Endocrine/Metabolic Agent (Enzyme)

See Agalsidase Beta.

AGALSIDASE BETA

Endocrine/Metabolic Agent (Enzyme)

PREGNANCY RECOMMENDATION: Compatible—Maternal Benefit >> Embryo–Fetal Risk
BREASTFEEDING RECOMMENDATION: No Human Data—Probably Compatible

PREGNANCY SUMMARY

The successful use of agalsidase-β or agalsidase-α in human pregnancy has been described in a few reports. The animal data, involving only one species, suggest low risk, but the limited human pregnancy experience prevents a more complete assessment of the embryo–fetal risk. However, Fabry disease is a debilitating condition that can be markedly improved by the use of enzyme replacement therapy. If a woman requires enzyme replacement therapy and gives informed consent, the enzyme should not be withheld because of pregnancy.

FETAL RISK SUMMARY

Agalsidase-β, a glycoprotein, is a recombinant α-galactosidase A enzyme that has the same amino acid sequence as the endogenous enzyme. It is indicated for patients with Fabry disease, an X-linked genetic disorder of glycosphingolipid metabolism. Agalsidase-β reduces globotriaosylceramide deposition in capillary endothelium of the kidney and certain other cells. It is given as an IV infusion every 2 weeks. The terminal plasma half-life of agalsidase-β is dose-dependent with a range of 45–102 minutes (1).

Agalsidase-α is available in Europe and the United States (as an orphan drug). The α- and β-products are produced by different protein expression systems (2). Another commercial product, α-galactosidase A, also is an orphan drug in the United States that is available elsewhere. All three formulations contain the same enzyme, α-galactosidase A.

Reproduction studies have been conducted with agalsidase-β in rats. Doses up to 30 times the human dose were not associated with impaired fertility or embryo–fetal harm. Studies for carcinogenicity and mutagenicity have not been conducted (1).

It is not known if agalsidase-β crosses the human placenta. The molecular weight (about 100,000) and short elimination half-life suggest that the enzyme will not cross to the embryo or fetus.

A 2005 case report described the use of agalsidase-α throughout gestation in a 34-year-old woman (3). Fabry disease had been diagnosed at 15 years of age and treatment with the enzyme, 0.2 mg/kg every 2 weeks infused over 40 minutes, was started 18 months before pregnancy. When pregnancy was diagnosed, the patient requested continuation of the therapy. Analysis of the amniotic fluid showed normal α-galactosidase A activity so the male fetus was not expected to have Fabry disease. After an uneventful pregnancy, the woman gave birth at 37 weeks' to a healthy, 3010-g male infant with Apgar scores of 9, 10, and 10, presumably at 1, 5, and 10 minutes, respectively. The infant's length and head circumference were 52 and 32 cm, respectively (3). A brief 2009 report described two pregnant women with Fabry disease who were treated with agalsidase-α (4). The outcomes of both pregnancies were healthy infants.

Three reports have described successful pregnancy outcomes that were treated with agalsidase-β for Fabry disease (5–7).

BREASTFEEDING SUMMARY

No reports describing the use of agalsidase-β, agalsidase-α, or α-galactosidase A during human lactation have been located. The molecular weight of the enzyme (about 100,000) and short plasma elimination half-life (45–102 minutes) suggest that it will not be excreted into breast milk. Even if excretion does occur, the enzyme probably would be digested in the nursing infant's gut. α-Galactosidase A is a native enzyme and should be present in the infant. Moreover, the indication for enzyme replacement therapy implies that the mother would have received it during pregnancy. Thus, the risk to a nursing infant from maternal use of any of the three formulations appears to be nil.

References

1. Product Information. Fabrazyme. Genzyme, 2007.
2. Lee K, Jin X, Zhang K, Copertino L, Andrews L, Baker-Malcolm J, Geagan L, Qiu H, Seiger K, Barngrover D, McPherson JM, Edmunds T. A biochemical and pharmacological comparison of enzyme replacement therapies for the glycolipid storage disorder Fabry disease. Glycobiology 2003;13:305–13.
3. Wendt S, Whybra C, Kampmann C, Teichmann E, Beck M. Successful pregnancy outcome in a patient with Fabry disease receiving enzyme replacement therapy with agalsidase alfa. J Inherit Metab Dis 2005;28:787–8.
4. Kalkum G, Macchiella D, Reinke J, Kolbl H, Beck M. Enzyme replacement therapy with agalsidase alfa in pregnant women with Fabry disease. Eur J Obstet Gynecol Reprod Biol 2009;144:92–3.
5. Germain DP, Bruneval P, Tran TC, Balouet P, Richalet B, Benistan K. Uneventful pregnancy outcome after enzyme replacement therapy agalsidase beta in a heterozygous female with Fabry disease: a case report. Eur J Med Genet 2010;53:111–2.
6. Politei JM. Treatment with agalsidase beta during pregnancy in Fabry disease. J Obstet Gynaecol Res 2010;36:428–9.
7. Thurberg BL, Politei JM. Histologic abnormalities of placental tissues in Fabry disease: a case report and review of the literature. Hum Pathol 2012;43:610–4.

ALBENDAZOLE

Anthelmintic

PREGNANCY RECOMMENDATION: Compatible
BREASTFEEDING RECOMMENDATION: Limited Human Data—Probably Compatible

PREGNANCY SUMMARY

Albendazole is a broad-spectrum anthelmintic that is used both in humans and in mass treatments of farm animals (1,2). The human use of albendazole is apparently widespread (1). The animal data suggest risk, but the poor oral bioavailability in humans suggests low risk. One source stated that the developmental toxicity of albendazole observed in animals was attributable to the active metabolite, albendazole sulfoxide (1). Moreover, in rats, the bioavailability is much higher than in humans (20%–30% vs. 1%). There is a potential, though, for much higher plasma concentrations of the metabolite if the drug is consumed with a fatty meal. If albendazole is required during pregnancy, avoiding the 1st trimester should be considered (2).

FETAL RISK SUMMARY

Albendazole is an orally administered, benzimidazole class, broad-spectrum anthelmintic used in the treatment of parenchymal neurocysticercosis caused by larval forms of the pork tapeworm, *Taenia solium*. It is also active against the larval forms of *Echinococcus granulosus*. Plasma concentrations of albendazole are negligible or undetectable because of poor systemic absorption attributable to low water solubility and its rapid hepatic metabolism to the active metabolite, albendazole sulfoxide. However, administration of albendazole with a fatty meal will markedly increase the levels of the metabolite in human plasma (up to fivefold on average) (3).

Reproduction studies have been conducted in mice, rats, and rabbits. In rats, albendazole did not adversely affect male or female fertility at oral doses 0.32 times the recommended human dose based on BSA (RHD). The drug was embryotoxic and teratogenic (skeletal malformations) in pregnant rats given oral doses during organogenesis that were 0.10 and 0.32 times the RHD, respectively. Similar toxicity was observed in pregnant rabbits at 0.60 times the RHD, but the dose was maternally toxic (33% mortality). No teratogenicity was observed in mice given oral doses up to 0.16 times the RHD during organogenesis (3).

A reproductive study in rats examined the effect of oral albendazole (0, 10, or 20 mg/kg/day) administered on gestational days 9–11. Compared with controls, the 10 mg/kg dose resulted in a decrease in crown–rump length, a small increase in resorptions, but no teratogenicity. The high dose, however, caused marked fetal growth restriction, an increase in the number of resorptions, and craniofacial and skeletal malformations. Because the severity of the toxic effects differed significantly among the litters, the results suggested that differences in maternal metabolism of albendazole might be involved (4).

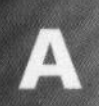

In another report by the above researchers, pregnant rats were administered albendazole 0, 10, 20, or 30 mg/kg/day on gestational days 10–12 (1). Dose-related resorptions and growth restriction were observed in the three groups receiving albendazole. At 10 mg/kg/day, increased development delay of limb buds was observed, but <5% of the embryos had abnormal heads or shapes. At the two higher doses, however, >20% of the embryos had morphologic alterations in head shapes and in the development of forelimb buds, branchial bars, eyes, and telencephalon. As in their initial communication, the researchers concluded that differences in maternal metabolism might have accounted for the observed interlitter differences in adverse fetal outcomes (1).

It is not known if albendazole or its active metabolite, albendazole sulfoxide, cross the placenta. The molecular weight of the parent compound (about 265) is low enough for transfer, but the poor oral bioavailability suggests that little, if any, of this agent reaches the plasma. No information is available on the metabolite other than that portions of it undergo further oxidative metabolism before elimination (3).

A brief 1993 publication reported the "accidental" exposure to "high doses" (specific doses not given) of albendazole for systemic infections during the 1st trimester in 10 women (5). The women were followed up to term, and all delivered normal infants. Moreover, some of the offspring have been followed up for up to 1 year without noting any adverse effects from the exposure (5).

In a randomized, placebo-controlled field trial in western Sierra Leone, anthelmintic treatment was studied as part of a strategy to control maternal anemia caused by parasitic infections (6). A single oral dose of albendazole (400 mg) was given to 61 pregnant women in the 2nd trimester. No adverse pregnancy outcomes attributable to the drug were observed (6).

Several reports have described the use of albendazole during human pregnancy as either single dose or multiple doses. No adverse effects of the drug were observed in the offspring (7–13).

BREASTFEEDING SUMMARY

Consistent with its molecular weight (about 265) and negligible bioavailability, very low amounts of albendazole and its active metabolite are excreted into breast milk. In a 2009 report, 33 women who were breastfeeding healthy full-term infants between 2 weeks and 6 months after birth received a single 400-mg dose of albendazole (14). Milk samples were collected at 6, 12, 24, and 36 hours after the dose and maternal blood samples were obtained at 6 hours. The mean peak milk concentrations of the parent drug and active metabolite, occurred at 6 hours, 31.9 and 312.8 ng/mL, respectively. At 36 hours, the parent drug was not detected in milk. The milk:maternal serum ratios (range) for the parent drug and active metabolite were 0.9 (0.2–6.5) and 0.6 (0.1–1.5), respectively. The authors concluded that the low concentrations in milk were unlikely to cause harm in a nursing infant (14).

A 2002 reference concluded that a single oral dose could be given to pregnant and lactating women (15).

References

1. Mantovani A, Ricciardi C, Stazi AV, Macri C. Effects observed on gestational day 13 in rat embryos exposed to albendazole. Reprod Toxicol 1995;9:265–73.
2. de Silva N, Guyatt H, Bundy D. Anthelmintics. A comparative review of their clinical pharmacology. Drugs 1997;53:769–88.
3. Product information. Albenza. SmithKline Beecham Pharmaceuticals, 2001.
4. Mantovani A, Macri C, Stazi AV, Ricciardi C. Effects of albendazole on the early phases of rat organogenesis in vivo: preliminary results (abstract). Teratology 1992;46:25A.
5. Horton J. The use of antiprotozoan and anthelmintic drugs during pregnancy and contraindications. J Infect 1993;26:104–5.
6. Torlesse H, Hodges M. Anthelmintic treatment and haemoglobin concentrations during pregnancy. Lancet 2000;356:1083.
7. Auer H, Kollaritsch H, Juptner J, Aspock H. Albendazole and pregnancy. Appl Parasitol 1994;35:146–7.
8. Cowden J, Hotez P. Mebendazole and albendazole treatment of geohelminth infections in children and pregnant women. Pediatr Infect Dis J 2000;19:659–60.
9. Torlesse H, Hodges. Albendazole therapy and reduced decline in haemoglobin concentration during pregnancy (Sierra Leone). Trans R Soc Trop Med Hyg 2001;95:195–201.
10. Montes H, Soetkino R, Carr-Locke DL. Hydatid disease in pregnancy. Am J Gastroenterol 2002;97:1553–5.
11. Can D, Oztekin O, Oztekin O, Tinar S, Sanci M. Hepatic and splenic hydatid cyst during pregnancy: a case report. Acta Gynecol Obstet 2003;268:239–40.
12. Elliott AM, Quigley MA, Nampijja M, Muwanga M, Ndibazza J, Whitworth JAG. Helminth infection during pregnancy and development of infantile eczema. JAMA 2005;294:2032–4.
13. Yilmaz N, Kiymaz N, Etlik O, Yazici T. Primary hydatid cyst of the brain during pregnancy—case report. Neurol Med Chir (Tokyo) 2006;46:415–7.
14. Abdel-Tawab AM, Bradley M, Ghazaly EA, Horton J, El-Setouhy M. Albendazole and its metabolites in the breast milk of lactating women following a single oral dose of albendazole. Br Clin Pharmacol 2009;68:737–42.
15. Allen HE, Crompton DWT, de Silva N, LoVerde PT, Olds GR. New policies for using anthelmintics in high risk groups. Trends Parasitol 2002;18:381–2.

ALBUTEROL

Sympathomimetic/Bronchodilator

PREGNANCY RECOMMENDATION: Compatible
BREASTFEEDING RECOMMENDATION: No Human Data—Probably Compatible

PREGNANCY SUMMARY

Albuterol (salbutamol) has not caused structural anomalies, but there is evidence of an association with functional and neurobehavioral toxicity with prolonged use. Similar to other β-mimetics, the drug can cause maternal and fetal tachycardia and hyperglycemia. Nevertheless, the drug should not be withheld because of pregnancy, but excessive use should be avoided. If albuterol is used in pregnancy for the treatment of asthma, health care professionals are encouraged to call the toll-free number (877-311-8972) for information about patient enrollment in an Organization of Teratology Information Specialists (OTIS) study.

FETAL RISK SUMMARY

Albuterol is a β_2-sympathomimetic used to prevent premature labor (see also Terbutaline and Ritodrine) and for the treatment of asthma (1–12). The inhaled formulation is indicated for the relief of bronchospasm in patients with reversible obstructive airway disease and acute attacks of bronchospasm (13). It is in the same subclass of β_2-adrenergic bronchodilators as arformoterol, formoterol, metaproterenol, pirbuterol, salmeterol, and terbutaline.

In twins, however, a double-blind, controlled study involving 144 women (74 treated with albuterol and 70 treated with placebo) observed no difference between the groups in the length of gestation, birth weight, or fetal outcome, except fewer infants in the albuterol group had respiratory distress syndrome (14).

In an in vitro experiment using perfused human placentas, 2.8% of infused drug crossed to the fetal side, but the method only used about 5% of the exchange area of the total placenta (15). Maternal serum concentrations during IV and oral albuterol therapy have been reported (16).

Reproduction studies in mice observed an increase in the incidence of cleft palate at a SC dose 0.4 times the maximum recommended human oral dose (MRHD) and higher (17). Cranioschisis was observed in 37% of the fetuses from pregnant rabbits treated with a dose 78 times the MRHD) (16).

No published reports linking the use of albuterol to human congenital anomalies have been located, but the majority of reports do not involve 1st trimester exposures. However, in a surveillance study of Michigan Medicaid recipients conducted between 1985 and 1992 involving 229,101 completed pregnancies, 1090 newborns had been exposed to albuterol during the 1st trimester (F. Rosa, personal communication, FDA, 1993). A total of 48 (4.4%) major birth defects were observed (43 expected). Specific data were available for six defect categories, including (observed/expected) 9/11 cardiovascular defects, 2/2 oral clefts, 2/0.6 spina bifida, 1/2 limb reduction defects, 0/3 hypospadias, and 6/3 polydactyly. Only with the latter defect is there a suggestion of a possible association, but other factors, including the mother's disease, concurrent drug use, and chance, may be involved.

A brief 1980 report described a patient who was treated with a continuous IV infusion of albuterol for 17 weeks via a catheter placed in the right subclavian vein (10,18,19). A normal male infant was delivered within a few hours of stopping the drug. A 1982 report described the use of albuterol in two women with incompetent cervix from the 14th week of gestation to near term (20). Both patients delivered normal infants.

Adverse reactions observed in the fetus and mother after albuterol treatment are secondary to the cardiovascular and metabolic effects of the drug. Albuterol may cause maternal and fetal tachycardia with fetal rates >160 beats/minute (1–3,12,21). Major decreases in maternal blood pressure have been reported with both systolic and diastolic pressures dropping >30 mmHg (2,4,6). Fetal distress after maternal hypotension was not mentioned. One study observed a maximum decrease in diastolic pressure of 24 mm Hg (34% decrease) but a rise in systolic pressure (21). Other maternal adverse effects associated with albuterol have been acute congestive heart failure, pulmonary edema, and death (22–30).

Like all β-mimetics, albuterol may cause transient fetal and maternal hyperglycemia followed by an increase in serum insulin (4,31–34). Cord blood levels of insulin are about twice those of untreated control infants and are not dependent on the duration of exposure, gestational age, or birth weight (33,34). These effects are more pronounced in diabetic patients, especially in juvenile diabetics, with the occurrence of significant increases in glycogenolysis and lipolysis (21,35,36). Maternal blood glucose should be closely monitored and neonatal hypoglycemia prevented with adequate doses of glucose.

A group of 20 women in premature labor, treated with oral albuterol (4 mg every 4 hours for several weeks), was matched with a control group of women who were not in premature labor (37). The mean gestational ages at delivery for the treated and nontreated patients were 36.4 and 37.0 weeks, respectively. No significant differences were found between the groups for cord blood concentrations of insulin, triiodothyronine (T3), thyroxine (T4), and thyroid-stimulating hormone (TSH). However, growth hormone levels were significantly higher in the treated group than in control patients (36.5 vs. 17.4 ng/mL, respectively, $p < 0.001$). The investigators did not determine the reason for the elevated growth hormone level but speculated that it could be caused by either the use of β-methasone for fetal lung maturation in some women of the albuterol group (and resulting fluctuations in fetal blood glucose and insulin levels) or direct adrenergic stimulation of the fetal pituitary (37). Of interest, of the 12 women who received β-methasone, cord blood growth hormone levels in 11 were compared with those of 8 untreated control women. Although the levels in the treated patients were higher (39.5 vs. 31.4 ng/mL), the difference was not significant.

Albuterol decreases the incidence of neonatal respiratory distress syndrome similar to the way that other β-mimetics do (14,38,39). Long-term evaluation of infants exposed to in utero β-mimetics has been reported but not specifically for albuterol (40,41). No harmful effects were observed in these infants. However, a brief 1994 reference described the use of β-sympathomimetics (albuterol, $N = 1$; ritodrine $N = 7$) in eight infants from a group of 16 with retinopathy of prematurity (42). In a matched control group with retinopathy, only 1 of 16 infants was exposed to ritodrine ($p < 0.008$). The authors speculated that the β-sympathomimetics had compromised retinal perfusion in utero leading to ischemia and eventually to the ophthalmic complication (42).

The effects of inhaled albuterol on maternal and fetal hemodynamics were first published as an abstract (43) and then as a full report (44). Twelve pregnant asthmatic women between 33 and 39 weeks' gestation received two deep inhalations of a 0.05% solution as recommended by the manufacturer. No effects on the mean maternal, uterine, or fetal hemodynamics were observed.

In contrast, a 1997 case report described fetal tachycardia from the inadvertent administration of a double dose of inhaled albuterol over 24 hours (45). The 34-year-old woman at 33 weeks' gestation received a metered-dose inhaler (two 90-mcg actuations every 4–6 hours; five doses over 24 hours) and albuterol nebulizer treatment (2.5 mg) every 4 hours (five doses over 24 hours). Three hours after the last dose, fetal tachycardia (>200 beats/minute) was detected (maternal heart rate was 90–100 beats/minute). Atrial flutter of 420 beats/minute was detected by fetal echocardiography with a predominate 2:1 conduction. Eight hours later, spontaneous

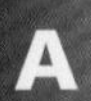

conversion to a normal rate occurred. A normal infant was delivered at term and did well during the 4 days of hospitalization.

A 2009 report examined the evidence for the use and toxicity of β_2-agonists in pregnancy, particularly for terbutaline and ritodrine as tocolytic agents and albuterol for asthma (46). Based on animal and human reports, the authors concluded that there was a biologic plausible basis for associating prolonged in utero exposure to β_2-agonists with functional and behavioral teratogenesis, specifically increased risks for autism spectrum disorders, psychiatric disorders, poor cognitive and motor function, and poor school performance. There also were increased risks in offspring for elevated heart rate and hypertension. The mechanisms for these effects appeared to be a decrease in parasympathetic activity resulting in an increase in sympathetic activity. A genetic predisposition for the toxicity was supported by data. The available data suggested that albuterol use in the 1st and 2nd trimesters was associated with a modest increase in the risk of autism spectrum disorders. The authors concluded that excessive treatment with albuterol should be avoided (46).

BREASTFEEDING SUMMARY

No reports describing the use of albuterol during human lactation have been located. However, the inhaled formulation is probably compatible with breastfeeding because of the low maternal systemic concentrations. Other drugs in the class (see Terbutaline) are considered compatible with breastfeeding and albuterol, most likely, is compatible.

References

1. Liggins GC, Vaughan GS. Intravenous infusion of salbutamol in the management of premature labor. J Obstet Gynaecol Br Commonw 1973;80:29–33.
2. Korda AR, Lynerum RC, Jones WR. The treatment of premature labor with intravenous administered salbutamol. Med J Aust 1974;1:744–6.
3. Hastwell G. Salbutamol aerosol in premature labour. Lancet 1975;2:1212–3.
4. Hastwell GB, Halloway CP, Taylor TLO. A study of 208 patients in premature labor treated with orally administered salbutamol. Med J Aust 1978;1:465–9.
5. Hastwell G, Lambert BE. A comparison of salbutamol and ritodrine when used to inhibit premature labour complicated by ante-partum haemorrhage. Curr Med Res Opin 1979;5:785–9.
6. Ng KH, Sen DK. Hypotension with intravenous salbutamol in premature labour. Br Med J 1974;3:257.
7. Pincus R. Salbutamol infusion for premature labour—the Australian trials experience. Aust NZ Obstet Gynaecol 1981;21:1–4.
8. Gummerus M. The management of premature labor with salbutamol. Acta Obstet Gynecol Scand 1981;60:375–7.
9. Crowhurst JA. Salbutamol, obstetrics and anaesthesia: a review and case discussion. Anaesth Intensive Care 1980;8:39–43.
10. Lind T, Godfrey KA, Gerrard J, Bryson MR. Continuous salbutamol infusion over 17 weeks to pre-empt premature labour. Lancet 1980;2:1165–6.
11. Kuhn RJP, Speirs AL, Pepperell RJ, Eggers TR, Doyle LW, Hutchison A. Betamethasone, albuterol, and threatened premature delivery: benefits and risks. Study of 469 pregnancies. Obstet Gynecol 1982;60:403–8.
12. Eggers TR, Doyle LW, Pepperell RJ. Premature labour. Med J Aust 1979;1:213–6.
13. Product information. Albuterol sulfate inhalant. Actavis Mid Atlantic, 2003.
14. Felicity Ashworth M, Spooner SF, Verkuyl DAA, Waterman R, Ashurst HM. Failure to prevent preterm labour and delivery in twin pregnancy using prophylactic oral salbutamol. Br J Obstet Gynaecol 1990;97:878–82.
15. Sodha RJ, Schneider H. Transplacental transfer of β-adrenergic drugs studied by an in vitro perfusion method of an isolated human placental lobule. Am J Obstet Gynecol 1983;147:303–10.
16. Haukkamaa M, Gummerus M, Kleimola T. Serum salbutamol concentrations during oral and intravenous treatment in pregnant women. Br J Obstet Gynaecol 1985;92:1230–3.
17. Product information. Proventil. Schering Corporation, 2000.
18. Boylan P, O'Discoll K. Long-term salbutamol or successful Shirodkar suture? Lancet 1980;2:1374.
19. Addis GJ. Long-term salbutamol infusion to prevent premature labor. Lancet 1981;1:42–3.
20. Edmonds DK, Letchworth AT. Prophylactic oral salbutamol to prevent premature labour. Lancet 1982;1:1310–1.
21. Wager J, Fredholm B, Lunell NO, Persson B. Metabolic and circulatory effects of intravenous and oral salbutamol in late pregnancy in diabetic and non-diabetic women. Acta Obstet Gynecol Scand Suppl 1982;108:41–6.
22. Whitehead MI, Mander AM, Hertogs K, Williams RM, Pettingale KW. Acute congestive cardiac failure in a hypertensive woman receiving salbutamol for premature labour. Br Med J 1980;280:1221–2.
23. Poole-Wilson PA. Cardiac failure in a hypertensive woman receiving salbutamol for premature labour. Br Med J 1980;281:226.
24. Fogarty AJ. Cardiac failure in a hypertensive woman receiving salbutamol for premature labour. Br Med J 1980;281:226.
25. Davies PDO. Cardiac failure in a hypertensive woman receiving salbutamol for premature labour. Br Med J 1980;281:226–7.
26. Robertson M, Davies AE. Cardiac failure in a hypertensive woman receiving salbutamol for premature labour. Br Med J 1980;281:227.
27. Crowley P. Cardiac failure in a hypertensive woman receiving salbutamol for premature labour. Br Med J 1980;281:227.
28. Whitehead MI, Mander AM, Pettingale KW. Cardiac failure in a hypertensive woman receiving salbutamol for premature labour (reply). Br Med J 1980;281:227.
29. Davies AE, Robertson MJS. Pulmonary oedema after the administration of intravenous salbutamol and ergometrine—case report. Br J Obstet Gynaecol 1980;87:539–41.
30. Milliez, Blot PH, Sureau C. A case report of maternal death associated with betamimetics and betamethasone administration in premature labor. Eur J Obstet Gynaecol Reprod Biol 1980;11:95–100.
31. Thomas DJ, Dove AF, Alberti KG. Metabolic effects of salbutamol infusion during premature labour. Br J Obstet Gynaecol 1977;84:497–9.
32. Wager J, Lunell NO, Nadal M, Ostman J. Glucose tolerance following oral salbutamol treatment in late pregnancy. Acta Obstet Gynecol Scand 1981;60:291–4.
33. Lunell NO, Joelsson I, Larsson A, Persson B. The immediate effect of a B-adrenergic agonist (salbutamol) on carbohydrate and lipid metabolism during the third trimester of pregnancy. Acta Obstet Gynecol Scand 1977;56:475–8.
34. Procianoy RS, Pinheiro CE. Neonatal hyperinsulinism after short-term maternal beta sympathomimetic therapy. J Pediatr 1982;101:612–4.
35. Barnett AH, Stubbs SM, Mander AM. Management of premature labour in diabetic pregnancy. Diabetologia 1980;188:365–8.
36. Wager J, Fredholm BB, Lunell NO, Persson B. Metabolic and circulatory effects of oral salbutamol in the third trimester of pregnancy in diabetic and non-diabetic women. Br J Obstet Gynaecol 1981;88:352–61.
37. Desgranges M-F, Moutquin J-M, Peloquin A. Effects of maternal oral salbutamol therapy on neonatal endocrine status at birth. Obstet Gynecol 1987;69:582–4.
38. Hastwell GB. Apgar scores, respiratory distress syndrome and salbutamol. Med J Aust 1980;1:174–5.
39. Hastwell G. Salbutamol and respiratory distress syndrome. Lancet 1977;2:354.
40. Wallace RL, Caldwell DL, Ansbacher R, Otterson WN. Inhibition of premature labor by terbutaline. Obstet Gynecol 1978;51:387–92.
41. Freysz H, Willard D, Lehr A, Messer J, Boog G. A long term evaluation of infants who received a beta-mimetic drug while in utero. J Perinat Med 1977;5:94–9.
42. Michie CA, Braithwaite S, Schulenberg E, Harvey D. Do maternal β-sympathomimetics influence the development of retinopathy in the premature infant? Arch Dis Child 1994;71:F149.
43. Rayburn WF, Atkinson BD, Gilbert KA, Turnbull GL. Acute effects of inhaled albuterol (Proventil) on fetal hemodynamics (abstract). Teratology 1994;49:370.
44. Rayburn WF, Atkinson BD, Gilbert K, Turnbull GL. Short-term effects of inhaled albuterol on maternal and fetal circulations. Am J Obstet Gynecol 1994;171:770–3.
45. Baker ER, Flanagan MF. Fetal atrial flutter associated with maternal beta-sympathomimetic drug exposure. Obstet Gynecol 1997;89:861.
46. Witter FR, Zimmerman AW, Reichmann JP, Connors SL. In utero beta 2 adrenergic agonist exposure and adverse neurophysiologic and behavioral outcomes. Am J Obstet Gynecol 2009;210:553–9.

ALCAFTADINE

Ophthalmic Antihistamine

PREGNANCY RECOMMENDATION: No Human Data—Probably Compatible
BREASTFEEDING RECOMMENDATION: No Human Data—Probably Compatible

PREGNANCY SUMMARY

No reports describing the use of alcaftadine in human pregnancy have been located. The animal data suggest low risk. Moreover, antihistamines, in general, are considered compatible with pregnancy.

FETAL RISK SUMMARY

Alcaftadine is an antihistamine indicated for the prevention of itching associated with allergic conjunctivitis. It is available as a 0.25% ophthalmic solution. Minimal amounts are measured in the plasma and concentrations of alcaftadine were below the level of detection (10 pg/mL) at 3 hours. The drug is metabolized to an active carboxylic acid metabolite that was undetectable in the plasma 12 hours after a dose. Plasma protein binding for the parent drug and active metabolite were about 39% and 63%, respectively. The elimination half-life of the active metabolite was about 2 hours (1).

Reproduction studies have been conducted in rats and rabbits. No evidence of impaired female reproduction or fetal harm was observed in these species at oral doses that produced plasma exposures that were about 200 and 9000 times, respectively, the human plasma exposure at the recommended human ocular dose (RHOD) (1).

No evidence of mutagenic or genotoxic effects was observed in multiple assays. There also was no evidence of fertility impairment in male and female rats at oral doses producing plasma exposures that were about 200 times the human plasma exposure at the RHOD (1).

It is not known if alcaftadine or its active metabolite crosses the human placenta. The molecular weight of the parent drug (about 307) and moderate protein binding imply that exposure of the embryo and/or fetus is possible, but the minimal amounts in the plasma suggest that any exposure would be clinically insignificant.

BREASTFEEDING SUMMARY

No reports describing the use of alcaftadine during human lactation have been located. The molecular weight of the parent drug (about 307) and moderate protein binding imply that the drug and possibly the active carboxylic acid metabolite will be excreted into breast milk. However, the minimal plasma concentrations that occur after ocular use suggest that the risk to a nursing infant will be nil. Moreover, antihistamines, in general, are considered compatible with breastfeeding.

Reference

1. Product information. Lastacaft. Allergan, 2010.

ALDESLEUKIN

Antineoplastic

PREGNANCY RECOMMENDATION: No Human Data—Animal Data Suggest Low Risk
BREASTFEEDING RECOMMENDATION: No Human Data—Probably Compatible

PREGNANCY SUMMARY

No reports describing the use of aldesleukin in human pregnancy have been located. The limited animal reproduction data, although based on body weight and at doses causing maternal toxicity, suggest low risk. In addition, the biologic effects of aldesleukin are the same as endogenous interleukin-2. Nevertheless, until human pregnancy experience is available, the best course is to avoid use of this agent in pregnancy. However, metastatic renal carcinoma and melanoma are potentially fatal, so if a woman requires aldesleukin and informed consent is obtained, it should not be withheld because of pregnancy. If an inadvertent pregnancy occurs, the woman should be advised of the unknown risk to her embryo–fetus.

FETAL RISK SUMMARY

Aldesleukin, a biologic response modifier, is a human recombinant interleukin product produced by recombinant technology. The protein possesses the biologic activities of human native interleukin-2. Aldesleukin is in the same antineoplastic subclass as denileukin. Aldesleukin is indicated for the treatment of metastatic renal carcinoma and metastatic melanoma. After IV infusion, aldesleukin undergoes rapid distribution into the extravascular space and elimination by metabolism. The distribution and elimination half-lives are 13 and 85 minutes, respectively (1).

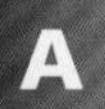

In a reproduction study in rats, embryolethal effects were observed at IV doses that were 27–36 times the human dose based on body weight (HD). However, IV doses 2.1–36 times higher than the HD caused significant maternal toxicity. No evidence of teratogenicity other than that caused by maternal toxicity was observed. Studies for carcinogenicity, mutagenicity, or effects on fertility have not been conducted (1).

It is not known if aldesleukin crosses the human placenta. The molecular weight of the protein, about 15,300, suggests that it does not. However, other proteins, such as the immunoglobulins cross the placenta. Moreover, the protein rapidly distributes into tissues (e.g., into the lung, liver, kidney, and spleen in rats). The very short distribution and elimination half-lives may limit the amount reaching the embryo and fetus.

BREASTFEEDING SUMMARY

No reports describing the use of aldesleukin during human lactation have been located.

The molecular weight, about 15,300, suggests that it will not be excreted into breast milk. However, other proteins, such as the immunoglobulins, are excreted into milk and so may aldesleukin. The very short distribution (13 minutes) and elimination (85 minutes) half-lives may limit the amount reaching the embryo and fetus. Waiting about 4 hours after a dose to breastfeed should limit the potential exposure of the infant even more. The effects, if any, on a nursing infant are unknown.

Reference

1. Product information. Proleukin. Novartis Pharmaceuticals, 2007.

ALEFACEPT

Immunologic Agent (Immunosuppressant)

PREGNANCY RECOMMENDATION: No Human Data—Animal Data Suggest Low Risk
BREASTFEEDING RECOMMENDATION: No Human Data—Potential Toxicity

PREGNANCY SUMMARY

No reports describing the use of alefacept in human pregnancy have been located. The animal data suggest that the human embryo and fetal risk are low, but the absence of human pregnancy experience prevents a full assessment of the risk. Psoriasis is common in women of childbearing potential (1). Combined with the very long elimination half-life, this suggests that exposure of inadvertent pregnancies is highly probable. Although the effects on pregnancy are unknown, there is a potential that alefacept could adversely affect the development of the fetal immune system and the immune function of the infant. Health care professionals are encouraged to enroll women who became pregnant while being treated with alefacept in the Biogen Pregnancy Registry by calling 1-866-263-8483 (1).

FETAL RISK SUMMARY

Alefacept is an immunosuppressive dimeric fusion protein consisting of a portion of the human leukocyte function antigen-3 linked to the Fc portion of immunoglobulin G (IgG1) produced by recombinant DNA technology. Alefacept is indicated for the treatment of moderate to severe chronic plaque psoriasis in patients who are candidates for systemic therapy or phototherapy. The drug is administered either IM or IV. After an IV dose, the mean elimination half-life was about 270 hours (about 11 days) (1).

Reproduction studies with alefacept have been conducted in cynomolgus monkeys. At doses about 62 times the human dose based on body weight (HD), no evidence of impaired fertility or fetal harm was observed. Weekly IV bolus doses administered during organogenesis were not abortifacient or teratogenic. Alefacept crossed the placenta in monkeys producing fetal concentrations that were 23% of the maternal concentrations. No evidence of fetal toxicity or adverse effects on immune system development was observed in the exposed fetuses (1).

In long-term studies in cynomolgus monkeys with weekly IV doses that were 12 or 248 times the HD, one animal in the high-dose group developed a β-cell lymphoma. Other animals in both groups developed β-cell hyperplasia of the spleen and lymph nodes. All animals were positive for an endemic primate gammaherpesvirus. It is known that the immune suppression of animals infected with this virus may lead to β-cell lymphomas (1). Hyperplasia of β-cell-dependent regions in baboon spleens was observed in another low-dose study. Carcinogenicity and fertility studies were not conducted with alefacept, but mutagenicity assays, both in vitro and in vivo, were negative (1).

It is not known if alefacept crosses the human placenta. The monkey and human placentas are classified as hemomonochorial and, since the drug crosses the monkey placenta, it probably crosses the human placenta as well. The human fetal exposure to the drug should be similar to that observed in monkeys.

BREASTFEEDING SUMMARY

No reports describing the use of alefacept during human lactation have been located. As an immune globulin, the drug is probably excreted into breast milk. Moreover, because of the very long elimination half-life (about 11 days), holding breastfeeding after a dose to allow clearance from the mother's system is not practical. The effect of this exposure on a nursing infant is unknown, but the dimeric fusion protein would most likely undergo some degree of digestion in the infant's gut. However, suppression of a nursing infant's immune function is a potential complication. Until data are available, avoiding nursing during the use of alefacept is the safest course.

Reference

1. Product information. Amevive. Biogen Idec, 2005.

ALEMTUZUMAB

Antineoplastic

PREGNANCY RECOMMENDATION: No Human Data—No Relevant Animal Data
BREASTFEEDING RECOMMENDATION: No Human Data—Potential Toxicity

PREGNANCY SUMMARY

No reports describing the use of alemtuzumab in human or animal pregnancies have been located. It is not known if the antibody crosses the placenta but, if it did, a potential fetal consequence of this exposure could be the depletion of B and T lymphocytes (1). Because of the potential for embryo and fetal harm, the antibody should be avoided, if possible, during pregnancy. In addition, based on the very long half-life, a woman should not conceive for several months after the last dose. The manufacturer recommends that men of reproductive potential and women of childbearing potential should use effective contraceptive methods during treatment and for a minimum of 6 months after therapy is stopped (1). However, leukemia can be fatal, so if a woman requires alemtuzumab and informed consent is obtained, it should not be withheld because of pregnancy. If an inadvertent pregnancy occurs, the woman should be advised of the potential risk for severe adverse effects in the embryo and fetus.

FETAL RISK SUMMARY

Alemtuzumab is a recombinant DNA-derived humanized monoclonal antibody (Campath-1H) that is given by IV infusion. It is indicated for the treatment of B-cell chronic lymphocytic leukemia. The mean plasma half-life changes with time, increasing from 11 hours (range 2–32 hours) after the first 30 mg dose to 6 days (range 1–14 days) after the last 30 mg dose (1).

Alemtuzumab may cause severe, infusion-related toxicity, including hypotension and other adverse effects. Premedication with acetaminophen and antihistamines is recommended (1). Hypotension in a pregnant woman could have deleterious effects on placental perfusion resulting in embryo and fetal harm.

Animal reproduction studies have not been conducted with alemtuzumab. Neither have studies been conducted for carcinogenicity, mutagenicity, or fertility (1).

It is not known if alemtuzumab crosses the human placenta. The very high molecular weight (about 150,000 for the Campath-1H antibody) suggests that it will not cross. However, human immunoglobulin G (IgG) does cross and, therefore, alemtuzumab may also cross (1).

BREASTFEEDING SUMMARY

No reports describing the use of alemtuzumab during lactation have been located. The very high molecular weight (about 150,000 for the Campath-1H antibody) suggests that it will not be excreted into breast milk. However, human IgG is excreted into milk and, therefore, alemtuzumab may also be excreted (1). The effects of this potential exposure on a nursing infant are unknown, but immunosuppression and other severe adverse effects are potential complications.

Reference

1. Product information. Campath. Genzyme, 2012.

ALENDRONATE

Bisphosphonate

PREGNANCY RECOMMENDATION: Limited Human Data—Animal Data Suggest Risk
BREASTFEEDING RECOMMENDATION: No Human Data—Probably Compatible

PREGNANCY SUMMARY

Alendronate does not cause structural anomalies in animals but does produce dose-related maternal and fetal toxicity. Several reports have described its use in or near pregnancy. Although one report did find significantly shorter gestations, reduced birth weight, and an increased rate of spontaneous abortions, these outcomes may have been due to the underlying maternal disease and/or the use of corticosteroids (1). Because the oral bioavailability is very low and the plasma clearance is rapid, clinically significant amounts may not cross the placenta. The drug is slowly released from bone; thus, the use before pregnancy may result in low-level, continuous exposure throughout gestation. The use of alendronate in women who may become pregnant or during pregnancy is not recommended. However, inadvertent exposure during early pregnancy does not appear to present a major risk to the embryo or fetus.

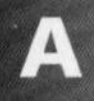

FETAL RISK SUMMARY

Bisphosphonates are synthetic analogs of pyrophosphate that bind to the hydroxyapatite found in bone. Alendronate, a specific inhibitor of osteoclast-mediated bone resorption, is indicated for the treatment and prevention of osteoporosis in postmenopausal women and men. Alendronate is also indicated for the treatment of Paget's disease of bone and for glucocorticoid-induced osteoporosis. The oral bioavailability, relative to an IV reference dose, is very low with only about 0.6% absorbed under fasting conditions. Alendronate is not metabolized in animals or humans. Approximately 78% of the drug is bound to protein in human plasma. After an IV dose, the plasma half-life is about 1 hour (plasma concentrations fell by >95% within 6 hours). However, the terminal elimination half-life is >10 years because of its slow release from bone (2).

In pregnant rats, a dose 0.26 times the maximum recommended daily dose for Paget's disease of 40 mg based on BSA (MRHD) caused decreased body weight in otherwise-normal pups. Decreased postimplantation survival occurred at 0.52 times the MRHD. With higher doses (2.6 times the MRHD), there was an increase in the incidence of incomplete fetal ossification in vertebrae, skull, and sternebrae. (*Note: The daily doses for prevention and treatment of osteoporosis are 5 and 10 mg, respectively.*) None of these adverse effects was observed in pregnant rabbits treated with doses up to 10.3 times the MRHD (2).

Delays and failure of delivery secondary to maternal hypocalcemia (both total and ionized calcium) were observed in pregnant rats at 3.9 times the MRHD. Normal calcium levels were measured in the fetuses. Late maternal pregnancy deaths also were observed at this dose. When the rats were treated from before mating through gestation, doses as small as 0.13 times the MRHD resulted in protracted parturition. Oral calcium supplementation did not prevent the hypocalcemia or prevent maternal and fetal deaths secondary to delays in delivery. However, IV calcium did prevent maternal, though not fetal, deaths (2,3).

In a study published in 1999, pregnant rats were treated with a daily SC dose of alendronate (0.1 mg/kg) during days 11–20 of pregnancy (4). Based on body weight, the dose was comparable to a human oral dose of 10 mg/day, but the systemic bioavailability was much higher than that obtained in humans. The gestational period was chosen because it covered the time of active bone development in rat fetuses. Alendronate passed through the placenta and accumulated in the fetuses. A significant increase in fetal bone calcium content (i.e., bone mass) with an accompanying significant decrease in bone marrow volume was found (4).

It is not known if alendronate crosses the placenta to the human fetus, but the molecular weight (about 325) is low enough that fetal exposure should be expected. Although the low maternal plasma concentration and short plasma half-life should reduce the amount of drug available for passage to the fetus, any drug that crosses the placenta probably will accumulate in fetal bones, as it does in rat fetuses.

A 2003 case report has described the use of alendronate in human pregnancy (5). A 49-year-old woman, who was amenorrheic and thought to be postmenopausal, was treated with oral alendronate 10 mg/day for osteoporosis. Treatment was begun before and continued throughout her gestation. An apparently normal female infant with a birth weight of 2390 g (50th percentile) was born at 36 weeks' gestation. Laboratory tests were within normal limits. X-ray studies of the skull and wrists revealed normal bone structure and density without abnormal calcifications. At 1 year of age, the girl's weight was 8 kg (10th percentile), her height was 73 cm (50th percentile), and her physical examination and psychomotor development were normal (5).

In a 2006 case series, 24 pregnancies were exposed to alendronate, 8 of the women took the drug 1–6 months before pregnancy, 15 before and during the first 3–8 weeks', and 1 through week 21 (1). Because of the long elimination half-life, the three groups were combined and compared with 790 nonexposed controls. In the subjects, there were 19 liveborn infants with a median gestational age of 38 weeks (p = 0.001 vs. controls [40 weeks]). The median birth weight also was significantly lower in subjects, 2910 vs. 3290 g (p = 0.002), and there were more spontaneous abortions 20.8 vs. 7% (p = 0.026). However, 13 of the women were also taking corticosteroids. No major anomalies were observed in the subjects (1).

A 2008 review described 51 cases of exposure to bisphosphonates before or during pregnancy: alendronate (N = 32) pamidronate (N = 11), etidronate (N = 5), risedronate (N = 2), and zoledronic acid (N = 1) (6). The authors concluded that although these drugs may affect bone modeling and development in the fetus, no such toxicity has yet been reported.

BREASTFEEDING SUMMARY

No reports describing the use of alendronate during nursing have been located. The molecular weight (about 325) is low enough for excretion into breast milk, but the low plasma concentrations and rapid plasma clearance suggest that minimal amounts will be excreted into milk. Moreover, since the oral bioavailability of this drug in the nonfasting state is negligible, systemic levels in a nursing infant should also be negligible (2).

References

1. Ornoy A, Wajnberg R, Diav-Citrin O. The outcome of pregnancy following pre-pregnancy or early pregnancy alendronate treatment. Reprod Toxicol 2006;22:578–9.
2. Product information. Fosamax. Merck & Co, 2003.
3. Minsker DH, Manson JM, Peter CP. Effects of the bisphosphonate, alendronate, on parturition in the rat. Toxicol Appl Pharmacol 1993;121:217–23.
4. Patlas N, Golomb G, Yaffe P, Pinto T, Breuer E, Ornoy A. Transplacental effects of bisphosphonates on fetal skeletal ossification and mineralization in rats. Teratology 1999;60:68–73.
5. Rutgers-Verhage AR, deVries TW, Torringa MJL. No effects of bisphosphonates on the human fetus. Birth Defects Res A Clin Mol Teratol 2003;67:203–4.
6. Djokanovic N, Klieger-Grossmann C, Koren G. Does treatment with bisphosphonates endanger the human pregnancy? J Obstet Gynaecol Can 2008;30:1146–8.

ALFENTANIL

Narcotic Agonist Analgesic

PREGNANCY RECOMMENDATION: Human Data Suggest Risk in 3rd Trimester
BREASTFEEDING RECOMMENDATION: Limited Human Data—Probably Compatible

PREGNANCY SUMMARY

Alfentanil is not teratogenic in animals and, based on the experience with similar agents, teratogenicity in humans is unlikely. However, there are no reports describing the use of this drug during organogenesis. As with all opioid agonist analgesics, alfentanil may cause neonatal respiratory depression if used close to delivery.

FETAL RISK SUMMARY

No reports linking the use of alfentanil during pregnancy with congenital abnormalities have been located, but experience in the 1st trimester has not been reported. The narcotic is not teratogenic in rats and rabbits (1,2). An embryocidal effect was observed with doses 2.5 times the upper human dose administered for 10–30 days, but this may have been related to maternal toxicity (1).

Alfentanil rapidly crosses the placenta to the fetus (3–5). A 1986 report described the pharmacokinetics and placental transfer of alfentanil after a single 30-mcg/kg IV dose administered to 5 women scheduled for cesarean section (group A) and during a continuous epidural infusion (30-mcg/kg loading dose followed by 30-mcg/kg/hour infusion) given to five women for vaginal delivery (group B) (3). The ratio of total alfentanil in umbilical vein to maternal blood in the combined 10 women was 0.29 (0.31 and 0.28 for groups A and B, respectively). The fetal:maternal ratio of free (unbound) alfentanil, however, was 0.97, reflecting the decreased α_1-acid glycoprotein (the most important binding protein for the drug) levels in the fetuses compared with the mothers (3).

Alfentanil was administered as a continuous infusion (30 mcg/kg/hour with as-needed bolus doses of 30 mcg/kg) via an extradural catheter to 16 women undergoing vaginal delivery (4). The umbilical vein:maternal ratios in six women varied between 0.221 and 0.576 (mean 0.33). For all 16 newborns, the mean (range) Apgar scores at 1, 3, and 5 minutes were 8.56 (range 7–10), 9.60 (range 8–10), and 9.80 (range 9–10), respectively, and were comparable to a control group. However, neurobehavioral assessment of the newborns using the Amiel-Tison score at 15–30 minutes of life indicated a significant decrease, compared with that of control newborns, in passive and active tone and total score. Primary reflexes and general assessment were not statistically different from those of control newborns. No abnormal feeding habits or behavior changes were noted on later evaluation, presumably after the effects of the narcotic had dissipated.

In 21 women scheduled for elective cesarean section, alfentanil (10 mcg/kg IV) administered before the induction of anesthesia significantly decreased the pressor response to laryngoscopy and endotracheal intubation in comparison to 16 control patients ($p < 0.01$) (5). At delivery, the mean total alfentanil fetal:maternal ratio was 0.32, but based on the lower α_1-acid glycoprotein levels in the newborns (33% of maternal levels), the calculated unbound alfentanil concentrations in the newborns and mothers were approximately equal (5).

Other reports have described the use of IV alfentanil immediately before the induction of anesthesia for cesarean section to lessen the hypertensive effects of tracheal intubation in women with preeclampsia (6–8) or as a single epidural injection (1 mg) in combination with a continuous epidural infusion of bupivacaine before vaginal delivery (9). As with other opioid agonist analgesics, neonatal respiratory depression is a potential complication, but it can be quickly reversed with naloxone.

BREASTFEEDING SUMMARY

Alfentanil is excreted into breast milk. Nine nonbreastfeeding women undergoing postpartum tubal ligation were administered alfentanil, 50 mcg/kg IV (10). An additional 10 mcg/kg was given if needed. Colostrum was collected from the right breast 4 hours after the last injection of alfentanil and from the left breast at 28 hours. The mean level of alfentanil in the colostrum at 4 hours was 0.88 ng/mL (range 0.21–1.56 ng/mL), and the mean level at 28 hours was 0.05 ng/mL (range 0.11–0.26 ng/mL). The clinical significance of the drug level in milk to the nursing infant at either time is unknown but is probably nil.

References

1. Product information. Alfenta. Janssen Pharmaceutica, Inc., 1992.
2. Fujinaga M, Mazze RI, Jackson EC, Baden JM. Reproductive and teratogenic effects of sufentanil and alfentanil in Sprague-Dawley rats. Anesth Analg 1988;67:166–9.
3. Gepts E, Heytens L, Camu F. Pharmacokinetics and placental transfer of intravenous and epidural alfentanil in parturient women. Anesth Analg 1986;65:1155–60.
4. Heytens L, Cammu H, Camu F. Extradural analgesia during labour using alfentanil. Br J Anaesth 1987;59:331–7.
5. Cartwright DP, Dann WL, Hutchinson A. Placental transfer of alfentanil at caesarean section. Eur J Anaesthesiol 1989;6:103–9.
6. Ashton WB, James MFM, Janicki P, Uys PC. Attenuation of the pressor response to tracheal intubation by magnesium sulphate with and without alfentanil in hypertensive proteinuric patients undergoing caesarean section. Br J Anaesth 1991;67:741–7.
7. Rout CC, Rocke DA. Effects of alfentanil and fentanyl on induction of anaesthesia in patients with severe pregnancy-induced hypertension. Br J Anaesth 1990;65:468–74.
8. Batson MA, Longmire S, Csontos E. Alfentanil for urgent caesarean section in a patient with severe mitral stenosis and pulmonary hypertension. Can J Anaesth 1990;37:685–8.
9. Perreault C, Albert JF, Couture P, Meloche R. Epidural alfentanil during labor, in association with a continuous infusion of bupivacaine. Can J Anaesth 1990;37:S5.
10. Giesecke AH Jr, Rice LJ, Lipton JM. Alfentanil in colostrum. Anesthesiology 1985;63:A284.

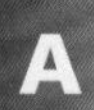

ALGLUCERASE

Endocrine/Metabolic Agent (Gaucher Disease)

PREGNANCY RECOMMENDATION: Limited Human Data—Probably Compatible
BREASTFEEDING RECOMMENDATION: Limited Human Data—Probably Compatible

PREGNANCY SUMMARY

No alglucerase-related adverse effects in embryos and fetuses have been reported in the limited data on pregnancies complicated by type I Gaucher disease. Pregnancy may exacerbate existing disease or result in new disease manifestations, but the data suggest that treatment may reduce the risk of spontaneous abortion and bleeding complications. However, systematic human or animal studies have not been conducted. The manufacturer has replaced alglucerase with imiglucerase and the last commercially available alglucerase expired in March 2011.

FETAL RISK SUMMARY

Alglucerase, an enzyme given by IV infusion, is used in the treatment of patients with type I Gaucher disease. It is in the same pharmacologic subclass as imiglucerase, taliglucerase-α, and velaglucerase-α. Alglucerase replaced the endogenous enzyme β-glucocerebrosidase. Alglucerase is prepared from pooled human placental tissue. After infusion, the terminal elimination half-life ranges from 3.6 to 10.4 minutes (1).

Reproduction studies with alglucerase have apparently not been conducted. Moreover, the carcinogenic and mutagenic potential of alglucerase has not been studied. Histopathology studies to detect effects on spermatogenesis in rats revealed no testicular changes (1).

It is not known if alglucerase crosses the human placenta. The relatively high molecular weight (about 55,600) and the short terminal half-life suggest that exposure of the embryo–fetus will be limited, if it occurs at all.

A 1996 case report and review involved a 24-year-old woman with Gaucher disease who was treated with alglucerase 40 U/kg every 2 weeks (2). She received two doses of the enzyme during the 1st trimester and then additional doses were held until 12 weeks' gestation when therapy was reinstituted. She gave birth at term to 3.65-kg, female infant with Apgar scores of 9 and 9 at 1 and 5 minutes, respectively. No additional information on the condition of the infant was provided (2).

A 1997 report described six pregnancies exposed to alglucerase (3). In one pregnancy, a low-dose, high-frequency regimen (30 U/kg/month, administered 3 times weekly) was discontinued before conception and then restarted at 12 weeks' gestation. At term, a normal, 2.84-kg female infant was delivered. A second pregnancy was similarly treated but with a dose of 60 U/kg/month. This patient gave birth at term to a healthy, 3.65-kg male infant. Two women were treated throughout pregnancy on the low-dose, high-frequency regimen and gave birth at term to healthy, but small-for-gestational-age, female infants (2.56 and 2.50 kg, respectively). In a fifth pregnancy, a low-dose regimen was started at 5 months' gestation but, about 1 month later, the woman delivered a female infant who died within 24 hours. The sixth case involved a woman with symptomatic pulmonary hypertension who had been treated with alglucerase for 3 years. At 10 weeks' gestation, the pregnancy was terminated because of the lung condition. The conceptus was normal and appropriate for gestational age (3).

Another case report described a 25-year-old woman with avascular necrosis of the femur complicating Gaucher disease (4). She conceived 4 months later while receiving alglucerase 3200 U every 2 weeks (body weight not specified). She gave birth at term to a 4.19-kg, male infant who was doing well at 6 months of age (4).

Outcomes of exposed pregnancies treated with either alglucerase or imiglucerase have been summarized from surveys gathered from international treatment centers, from reports in the literature, as well as the manufacturer's pharmacovigilance database. The total number of exposed patients is unclear as there could be overlap between the various sources of reports. However, as reviewed in a 2010 publication, among 43–78 treated pregnancies compared with 71–388 untreated pregnancies with the same disease, the risk of spontaneous abortion, disease-related bleeding complications at delivery, and disease-related complications postpartum was reduced. No evidence of teratogenic risk was noted (5,6).

BREASTFEEDING SUMMARY

Alglucerase has been detected in breast milk even though the relatively high molecular weight (about 55,600) and the short terminal half-life (3.6–10.4 minutes) suggest that excretion will be limited.

In a woman receiving an IV infusion of 60 U/kg, milk concentrations of the enzyme ranged from 69 to 187 ng/mL above baseline for 2–48 hours postinfusion (7). A 1998 case report described successful breastfeeding in a mother being treated with alglucerase (8).

The glycoprotein is largely destroyed in the digestive tract suggesting that even if small amounts are transferred into breast milk, the enzyme is unlikely to reach the systemic circulation of a breastfed infant (1).

References

1. Product information and personal communication. Ceredase. Genzyme, 2011.
2. Rosnes JS, Sharkey MF, Jean-Claude V, Eberhard MH. Gaucher's disease in pregnancy. Obstet Gynecol Surv 1996;51:549–58.
3. Ebstein D, Granovsky-Grisaru S, Rabinowitz R, Kanai R, Abrahamov A, Zimran A. Use of enzyme replacement therapy for Gaucher disease. Am J Obstet Gynecol 1997;177:1509–12.
4. Cleary JE, Burke WM, Baxi LV. Pregnancy after avascular necrosis of the femur complicating Gaucher's disease. Am J Obstet Gynecol 2001;184:233–4.

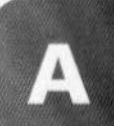

5. Zimran A, Morris E, Mengel E, Kaplan P, Belmatoug N, Hughes DA, Malinova V, Heitner R, Sobreira E, Mrsic M, Granovsky-Frisaru S, Amato D, vom Dahl S. The female gaucher patient: the impact of enzyme replacement therapy around key reproductive events (menstruation, pregnancy and menopause). Blood Cells Mol Dis 2009;43:264–88.
6. Granovsky-Grisaru S, Belmatoug N, vom Dahl S, Mengel E, Morris E, Zimran A. The management of pregnancy in Gaucher disease. Eur J Obstet Gynecol Reprod Biol 2011;156:3–8.
7. Esplin J, Greenspoon JS, Cheng E, Perkins C, Westman JA, Grabowski GA. Alglucerase infusions in pregnant type 1 Gaucher patients (abstract). Blood 1993;82:509a.
8. Aporta Rodriguez R, Escobar Vedia JL, Navarro Castro AM, Aguilar Garcia G, Cabrera Torres A. Alglucerase enzyme replacement therapy used safely and effectively throughout the whole pregnancy of a Gaucher disease patient. Haematologica 1998;83:852–3.

ALGLUCOSIDASE ALFA

Endocrine/Metabolic Agent (Enzyme)

PREGNANCY RECOMMENDATION: Compatible—Maternal Benefit >> Embryo–Fetal Risk
BREASTFEEDING RECOMMENDATION: Limited Human Data—Probably Compatible

PREGNANCY SUMMARY

One report describing the use of alglucosidase alfa in human pregnancy has been located. The animal data suggest low risk, but the dose used was very low. Untreated Pompe disease is a fatal condition with death usually related to respiratory failure (1). If a woman requires alglucosidase alfa, it should not be withheld because of pregnancy.

FETAL RISK SUMMARY

Alglucosidase alfa, a glycoprotein produced by recombinant DNA technology, consists of the enzyme α-glucosidase (GAA) encoded by the most predominant of nine haplotypes of this gene. It is given by IV infusion every 2 weeks. Alglucosidase is indicated for patients with Pompe disease (GAA deficiency). The plasma half-life is dose-dependent ranging from 2.3 to 2.9 hours (1).

Reproduction studies have been conducted in mice. IV doses, given every other day, up to about 0.2 times the recommended bi-weekly human dose based on BSA revealed no evidence of fetal harm. A similar dose had no effect on fertility or reproductive performance in mice. Studies for carcinogenicity and mutagenicity have not been conducted (1).

It is not known if alglucosidase alfa crosses the human placenta. The molecular weight (about 99,377–109,000) and the short plasma half-life suggest that little, if any, of the glycoprotein will cross to the embryo or fetus.

A 2011 case report described the use of alglucosidase alfa (20 mg/kg every other week) throughout pregnancy in 40-year-old woman with adult-onset Pompe disease (2). Because of worsening disease, an elective cesarean section was performed at about 38 weeks' to deliver a healthy male infant with Apgar scores of 8, 9, and 10. The infant's weight, length, and head circumference were normal and there were no congenital anomalies. The infant was developing normally at 1 year of age (2).

BREASTFEEDING SUMMARY

One report describing the use of alglucosidase alfa during lactation has been located. In the above case report, a mother treated throughout pregnancy with the enzyme continued therapy while breastfeeding her infant (2). Before a dose, enzyme activity in her milk was 3 nmol/mL/hr, about 10% of what is measured in the milk of an unaffected mother. After infusion, the highest activity (245 nmol/mL/hr) was reached at 2.5 hours postinfusion (2). As expected, because alglucosidase alfa is a native enzyme and would be present in the infant, no adverse effects were reported in the nursing infant.

If a woman requires alglucosidase alfa for the treatment of Pompe disease, it should not be withheld because of breastfeeding.

References

1. Product information. Myozyme. Genzyme, 2007.
2. de Vries JM, Brugma JDC, Ozkan L, Steegers EAP, Reuser AJJ, van Doorn PA, van der Ploeg AT. First experience with enzyme replacement therapy during pregnancy and lactation in Pompe disease. Mol Genet Metab 2011;104:552–5.

ALISKIREN

Antihypertensive

PREGNANCY RECOMMENDATION: Human Data Suggest Risk in 2nd and 3rd Trimesters
BREASTFEEDING RECOMMENDATION: No Human Data—Probably Compatible

PREGNANCY SUMMARY

Although there is no human pregnancy experience, the animal reproduction data suggest low risk in the 1st trimester. Because aliskiren acts directly on the renin–angiotensin system, exposure in the 2nd and 3rd trimesters should be avoided except in those rare incidences in which the mother requires therapy with this agent. Two other classes of agents that act on this system, angiotensin-converting-enzyme (ACE) inhibitors and angiotensin II receptor antagonists (ARA), are known to cause marked fetal toxicity in the 2nd and 3rd trimesters. (See Captopril and Losartan for representative agents.) Therefore, use of aliskiren during the 2nd and 3rd trimesters may cause teratogenicity and severe fetal and neonatal toxicity identical to that seen with ACE inhibitors and ARA drugs. Fetal toxic effects may include anuria, oligohydramnios, fetal hypocalvaria, intrauterine growth restriction, prematurity, and patent ductus arteriosus. Anuria-associated anhydramnios/oligohydramnios may be associated with fetal limb contractures, craniofacial deformation, and pulmonary hypoplasia. Severe anuria and hypotension, resistant to both pressor agents and volume expansion, may occur in the newborn following in utero exposure to aliskiren. Newborn renal function and blood pressure should be closely monitored.

FETAL RISK SUMMARY

Aliskiren is a nonpeptide renin inhibitor. It is indicated for the treatment of hypertension either alone or in combination with other antihypertensive agents. Aliskiren is partially metabolized to inactive metabolites apparently by the CYP450 isoenzyme CYP3A4. Oral bioavailability is poor with only about 2.5% absorbed systemically (1). The mean elimination half-life is 30 hours (range 23–36 hours) and plasma protein binding is about 50% (2).

Reproduction studies have been conducted in rats and rabbits. In pregnant rats and rabbits, there was no evidence of teratogenicity with oral doses ≤20 and ≤7 times, respectively, the maximum recommended human dose of 300 mg/day (MRHD) on a BSA basis (MRHD-BSA). However, in rabbit offspring fetal birth weights were reduced at 3.2 times the MRHD-BSA. In rabbits, the drug was present in the placenta, amniotic fluid, and fetuses (1).

Carcinogenic studies in mice and rats with doses producing exposures that were about 1.5 and 4 times, respectively, the MRHD based on AUC (MRHD-AUC) observed no significant increases in tumor incidence. However, tumors that are considered rare in the strain of rat studied were observed in two animals; a colonic adenoma in one and a cecal adenocarcinoma in the other. Mucosal epithelial hyperplasia of the lower gastrointestinal tract, with or without erosion/ulceration, was noted in both species at exposures that were about 0.75 and 2 times, respectively, the MRHD-AUC. No genotoxic potential was observed in multiple assays. In addition, no effect on the fertility of male and female rats was observed with doses ≤8 times the MRHD-BSA (1).

Although aliskiren crosses the placenta in rabbits (1), this has not been studied in humans. The molecular weight (about 552 for the free base), long elimination half-life, and moderate plasma protein binding suggest that the drug will cross to the embryo and fetus. However, the low lipid solubility should limit the amount transferred.

No reports have described the use of aliskiren in human pregnancy. However, use of the drug in the 2nd and 3rd trimesters is not recommended because of the potential for severe toxicity in the fetus and newborn.

BREASTFEEDING SUMMARY

No reports describing the use of aliskiren during human lactation have been located. The molecular weight (about 552 for the free base), long elimination half-life (mean 30 hours), and moderate plasma protein binding (about 50%) suggest that the drug will be excreted into breast milk. However, the low lipid solubility should limit the amount excreted. The effect on a nursing infant is unknown. The American Academy of Pediatrics, however, classifies ACE inhibitors, a closely related group of antihypertensive agents, as compatible with breastfeeding. (See Captopril or Enalapril.)

References

1. Product information. Tekturna. Novartis Pharmaceuticals, 2008.
2. Azizi M, Webb R, Nussberger J, Hollenberg NK. Renin inhibition with aliskiren: where are we now, and where are we going? J Hypertens 2006;24:243–56.

ALLOPURINOL

Antineoplastic/Antigout

PREGNANCY RECOMMENDATION: Limited Human Data—No Relevant Animal Data
BREASTFEEDING RECOMMENDATION: Limited Human Data—Potential Toxicity

PREGNANCY SUMMARY

The human pregnancy experience with allopurinol is limited because the conditions for which it is indicated are relatively rare in women of childbearing age. No adverse effects were observed in rats and rabbits but, in one study, severe toxicity was noted in mice. However, the only dose comparisons to the human dose were based on body weight and are not interpretable. In one study, the use of allopurinol throughout gestation was associated with multiple major defects in the newborn. Additional data are needed before the association can be classified as causal.

FETAL RISK SUMMARY

Allopurinol, a xanthine oxidase inhibitor, is used for the treatment of symptomatic primary or secondary hyperuricemias. It is in the same antineoplastic subclass of antimetabolites that reduce uric acid levels as rasburicase. Allopurinol is indicated for the management of patients with (a) signs and symptoms of primary or secondary gout; (b) leukemia, lymphoma, and malignancies who are receiving cancer therapy which causes elevations of serum and urinary uric acid levels; and (c) recurrent calcium oxalate calculi whose daily uric acid excretion exceeds 800 mg/day in male patients and 750 mg/day in female patients. Allopurinol is rapidly metabolized to oxipurinol, an active metabolite. Allopurinol has a plasma half-life of about 1–2 hours, whereas oxipurinol has a half-life of about 15 hours (1).

Reproduction studies by the manufacturer have been conducted in rats and rabbits. At doses up to 20 times the usual human dose based on body weight, no evidence of impaired fertility or fetal harm was observed (1). In a 1972 study, doses of 50 mg/kg and 100 mg/kg of allopurinol were given intraperitoneally to mice (2). The high dose, but not the low dose, resulted in a significant increase in the number of dead offspring. Both doses were associated with cleft palate and skeletal defects (2). However, it was not determined if the toxicity was a fetal effect or an effect secondary to maternal toxicity (1). In studies involving other animal species, no fetal harm was observed (3).

Consistent with the low molecular weight (about 136 for allopurinol), as well as the plasma half-lives for allopurinol and oxipurinol, both cross the placenta. A group of mothers were given allopurinol 500 mg IV 18–190 minutes before birth (4). The median maternal concentration of allopurinol and oxipurinol were 3.8 mcg/mL (1.2–7.9 mcg/mL) and 3.2 mcg/mL (1.5–6.4 mcg/mL), respectively, whereas arterial cord blood levels were 2.0 mcg/mL (0.2–7.3 mcg/mL) and 1.5 mcg/mL (0.6–7.6 mcg/mL), respectively (4).

The manufacturer is aware of two unpublished reports of women receiving the drug during pregnancy who gave birth to normal infants (1).

Allopurinol, in daily doses of 300–400 mg (unspecified dose in one patient), was combined with cancer chemotherapeutic agents in six patients for the treatment of leukemia occurring during pregnancy (5–9). Treatment in each of these cases was begun in the 2nd or 3rd trimester. The outcomes of these pregnancies were as follows: four normal healthy infants (5–7); one intrauterine fetal death probably a result of severe preeclampsia (8); and one growth-restricted infant with absence of the right kidney, hydronephrosis of the left kidney, and hepatic subcapsular calcifications (9). The cause of the defects in the latter infant was unknown but, because drug therapy was not started until the 20th week of gestation, any relationship to allopurinol can be excluded. The intrauterine growth restriction was thought to be caused by the chemotherapeutic agent, busulfan, that the mother received (9).

A 1976 case report described the use of allopurinol in a woman with type I glycogen storage disease (von Gierke's disease) (10). One of the characteristics of this inherited disease is hyperuricemia as a result of decreased renal excretion and increased production of uric acid. The woman was receiving allopurinol, 300 mg/day, at the time of conception and during the early portion of the 1st trimester (exact dates were not specified). The drug was stopped at that time. A term female infant was delivered by cesarean section for failed labor. Phenylketonuria, an autosomal recessive disorder, was subsequently diagnosed in the infant (10).

A woman with primary gout and gouty nephropathy was treated with 300 mg/day of allopurinol throughout gestation (11). She delivered an appropriate-for-gestational-age 2510-g healthy female infant at 35 weeks' gestation. The infant's weight gain was normal at 10 weeks of age, but other developmental milestones were not provided (11).

A 1997 randomized, double-blind, placebo controlled trial, allopurinol (200 mg/day) was combined with vitamin E (800 IU/day) and vitamin C (1000 mg/day) for women with severe preeclampsia diagnosed between 24 and 32 weeks of gestation (12). The outcomes evaluated were prolongation of pregnancy, infant outcomes, and other factors. The results did not suggest a benefit of the therapy (12).

A 2009 feasibility study evaluated whether allopurinol given to mothers with signs of fetal distress immediately before birth would reduce free radical formation in the fetus, a potential first step to reduce or prevent fetal hypoxia-induced brain injury (4). The study found that therapeutic doses of allopurinol reduced cord blood levels of the protein S-100B, a marker of brain injury. Two other reports described the rationale for this intervention and a new study that was just beginning (13,14).

A 2011 case report described multiple major birth defects in an infant born at 41 weeks' (15). Birth weight, length, and head circumference were appropriate for gestational age. The mother had taken allopurinol 300 mg/day for recurrent kidney stones and methyldopa for hypertension throughout gestation. External anomalies were as follows: hypertelorism, left-sided microphthalmia and coloboma of upper eyelid, left-sided microtia and absent left external auditory canal, simplified right ear with a preauricular tag, left-sided cleft lip and palate, and bilateral undescended testes. The infant died at 8 days of age. The following internal defects were found at autopsy: hypoplasia of corpus callosum, left optic nerve atrophy, left microphthalmia, small frontal fossa, agenesis of the left diaphragm with intrusion of liver, stomach, and spleen into the diaphragmatic space, mildly enlarged right-sided kidney, absent left kidney, small accessory spleen, and profound left pulmonary hypoplasia. The cerebellum and gyral pattern of the brain surface appeared to be normal, as was the cardiovascular system and skeleton. The infant's karyotype was a normal 46,XY, but a chromosome microdeletion/duplication syndrome could not be ruled out. Because the anomalies shared some features with those caused by mycophenolate mofetil (see Mycophenolate), and because both allopurinol

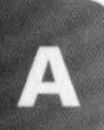

and mycophenolate interrupt purine synthesis, the authors concluded that allopurinol should be considered a potential teratogen (15).

In contrast to the above report, a 2012 case described a 27-year-old woman with ulcerative colitis who was treated throughout pregnancy with allopurinol 100 mg/day, mercaptopurine 25 mg/day, and mesalazine 4 g/day (16). Pregnancy was complicated by diarrhea and blood loss in the 2nd trimester. An elective cesarean section was performed at 39 weeks' to give birth to a healthy 3550-g infant (sex not specified) with Apgar score of 9, 10, and 10 at 1, 5, and 10 minutes, respectively. No anomalies were observed in the infant (16).

BREASTFEEDING SUMMARY

Allopurinol and its active metabolite, oxipurinol, are excreted into human milk. A woman with hyperuricemia was taking allopurinol 300 mg/day for 4 weeks while breastfeeding her 5-week-old infant (17,18). Maternal plasma and milk samples were drawn 2 and 4 hours after a 300-mg dose. Her plasma levels of allopurinol and oxipurinol at these times were 1.0 and 13.8 mcg/mL, and 1.0 and 19.9 mcg/mL, respectively. Milk levels of the drug and metabolite at 2 and 4 hours were 0.9 and 53.7 mcg/mL, and 1.4 and 48.0 mcg/mL, respectively. At these times, the milk:plasma ratios for allopurinol were 0.9 and 1.4, respectively, and for oxipurinol were 3.9 and 2.4, respectively. The mother breastfed her infant 2 hours after her dose and a single infant plasma sample was taken 2 hours later. Allopurinol was not detected (detection limit 0.5 mcg/mL) in the infant's plasma but the concentration of oxipurinol was 6.6 mcg/mL. The average daily dose of allopurinol and oxipurinol ingested by the infant from the milk (based on 150 mL/kg/day) was 0.14–0.20 and 7.2–8.0 mg/kg, respectively. No adverse effects in the nursing infant were observed (18). However, 4 hours after a dose and 2 hours after feeding, the infant's oxipurinol plasma level was 48% and 33% of the mother's levels at 2 and 4 hours. As such, the infant should be monitored for allergic reactions, such as rash, periodic blood counts, and other common toxicities observed in adults.

The American Academy of Pediatrics classifies allopurinol as compatible with breastfeeding (19).

References

1. Product information. Zyloprim. Prometheus Laboratories, 2003.
2. Fujii T, Nishimura H. Comparison of teratogenic action of substances related to purine metabolism in mouse embryos. Jpn J Pharmacol 1972;22:201–6.
3. Chaube S, Murphy ML. The teratogenic effects of the recent drugs active in cancer chemotherapy. In: Woollam DHM, ed. *Advances in Teratology*. New York, NY: Academic Press, 1968;3:181–237. As cited in Shepard TH. *Catalog of Teratogenic Agents*. 6th ed. Baltimore, MD: Johns Hopkins University Press, 1989:58.
4. Torrance HL, Benders MJ, Derks JB, Rademaker CMA, Bos AF, Van Den Berg P, Longini M, Buonocore G, Venegas M, Baquero H, Visser GHA, Van Bel F. Maternal allopurinol during fetal hypoxia lowers cord blood levels of the brain injury marker S-100B. Pediatrics 2009;124:350–7.
5. Awidi AS, Tarawneh MS, Shubair KS, Issa AA, Dajani YF. Acute leukemia in pregnancy: report of five cases treated with a combination which included a low dose of Adriamycin. Eur J Cancer Clin Oncol 1983;19:881–4.
6. Ali R, Kimya Y, Koksal N, Ozkocaman V, Yorulmaz H, Eroglu A, Ozcelik T, Tunali A. Pregnancy in chronic lymphocytic leukemia: experience with fetal exposure to chlorambucil. Leuk Res 2009;33:567–9.
7. AlKindi S, Dennison D, Pathare A. Imatinib in pregnancy. Eur J Haematol 2005;74:535–7.
8. O'Donnell R, Costigan C, O'Connell LG. Two cases of acute leukaemia in pregnancy. Acta Haematol 1979;61:298–300.
9. Boros SJ, Reynolds JW. Intrauterine growth retardation following third-trimester exposure to busulfan. Am J Obstet Gynecol 1977;129:111–2.
10. Farber M, Knuppel RA, Binkiewicz A, Kennison RD. Pregnancy and von Gierke's disease. Obstet Gynecol 1976;47:226–8.
11. Coddington CC, Albrecht RC, Cefalo RC. Gouty nephropathy and pregnancy. Am J Obstet Gynecol 1979;133:107–8.
12. Gülmezoğlu AM, Hofmeyr GJ, Oosthuisen MMJ. Antioxidants in the treatment of severe pre-eclampsia: an explanatory randomized controlled trial. Br J Obstet Gynaecol 1997;104:689–96.
13. Kaandorp JJ, Benders MJNL, Rademaker CMA, Torrance HL, Oudijk MA. Antenatal allopurinol for reduction birth asphyxia induced brain damage (ALLO-Trial); a randomized double blind placebo controlled multicenter study. BMC Pregnancy Childbirth 2010;10:8. [Epub 2010 Feb 18].
14. Boda D. Results of and further prevention of hypoxic fetal brain damage by inhibition of xanthine oxidase enzyme with allopurinol. J Perinat Med 2011;39:441–4.
15. Kozenko M, Grynspan D, Oluyomi-Obi, Sitar D, Elliott AM, Chodirker BN. Potential teratogenic effects of allopurinol: a case report. Am J Med Genet 2011;155:2247–52.
16. Seinen ML, de Boer NKH, van Hoorn ME, van Bodegraven AA, Bouma G. Safe use of allopurinol and low-dose mercaptopurine therapy during pregnancy in an ulcerative colitis patient. Inflamm Bowel Dis 2013;Mar 19(3):E37. doi:10,1002/ibd. 22945.
17. Kamilli I, Gresser U, Schaefer C, Zollner N. Allopurinol in breast milk. Adv Exp Med Biol 1991;309A:143–5.
18. Kamilli I, Gresser U. Allopurinol and oxypurinol in human breast milk. Clin Invest 1993;71:161–4.
19. Committee on Drugs, American Academy of Pediatrics. The transfer of drugs and other chemicals into human milk. Pediatrics 2001;108:776–89.

ALMOTRIPTAN

Antimigraine

PREGNANCY RECOMMENDATION: No Human Data—Animal Data Suggest Low Risk
BREASTFEEDING RECOMMENDATION: No Human Data—Probably Compatible

PREGNANCY SUMMARY

No reports describing the use of almotriptan in human pregnancy have been located. The animal data are suggestive of low risk, but an assessment of the actual risk cannot be determined until human pregnancy experience is available. Although a 2008 review of triptans in pregnancy found no evidence for teratogenicity, the data did suggest a possible increase in the rate of preterm birth (1).

FETAL RISK SUMMARY

Almotriptan is an oral selective serotonin (5-hydroxytryptamine; 5-$HT_{1B/1D}$) receptor agonist that has high affinity for 5-HT_{1B}, 5-HT_{1D}, and 5-HT_{1F} receptors. The drug is closely related to eletriptan, frovatriptan, naratriptan, rizatriptan, sumatriptan, and zolmitriptan (see also Eletriptan, Frovatriptan, Naratriptan, Rizatriptan, Sumatriptan, and Zolmitriptan). It is indicated for the acute treatment of migraine with or without aura in adults. Protein binding is minimal (about 35%). Almotriptan is metabolized to inactive metabolites, but about 40% is excreted unchanged in the urine. The mean elimination half-life is approximately 3–4 hours (2).

Reproduction studies have been conducted in rats and rabbits. Rats were given doses throughout organogenesis that produced maternal exposures up to about 958 times the human exposure from the maximum recommended daily dose (MRDD) of 25 mg based on AUC (MRDD-AUC). At the highest dose (958 times the MRDD-AUC), increased embryo deaths were observed. Doses >80 times the MRDD-AUC resulted in an increased incidence of fetal skeletal variations (decreased ossification). When almotriptan was administered to pregnant rats throughout gestation and lactation, a dose 160 times the MRDD based on BSA (MRDD-BSA) caused an increase in gestational length and a decrease in litter size and pup birth weight. The decreased pup weight persisted throughout lactation. The no-observed-effect-level (NOEL) was 40 times the MRDD-BSA. In pregnant rabbits, a dose 50 times the MRDD-BSA resulted in an increase in embryo deaths (2).

It is not known if almotriptan crosses the human placenta to the fetus. The molecular weight (about 336 for the free base) is low enough that passage to the fetus should be expected. In addition, the minimal plasma protein binding, incomplete metabolism, and moderate elimination half-life suggest that substantial amounts of the drug will be available for transfer at the maternal:fetal interface.

BREASTFEEDING SUMMARY

No reports describing the use of almotriptan during human lactation have been located. The molecular weight (about 336 for the free base) suggests that the drug will be excreted into breast milk. The effect of this exposure on a nursing infant is unknown.

References

1. Soldin OP, Dahlin J, O'Mara DM. Triptans in pregnancy. Ther Drug Monit 2008;30:5–9.
2. Product information. Axert. Ortho-McNeil Pharmaceutical, 2004.

ALOSETRON

Antidiarrheal/Antiemetic

PREGNANCY RECOMMENDATION: No Human Data—Animal Data Suggest Low Risk
BREASTFEEDING RECOMMENDATION: No Human Data—Potential Toxicity

PREGNANCY SUMMARY

No reports describing the use of alosetron in human pregnancy have been located. Because the drug is restricted by the manufacturer to severe diarrhea-predominant irritable bowel syndrome, pregnancy exposures are probably infrequent. The animal data suggest low risk, but the absence of human pregnancy experience prevents an assessment of the embryo–fetal risk. Limited information for other agents in this class (e.g., see Ondansetron) does not suggest a risk of teratogenicity. Therefore, if indicated, alosetron should not be withheld because of pregnancy.

FETAL RISK SUMMARY

Alosetron is a selective antagonist of the serotonin 5-HT_3 receptor type. It is the same pharmacologic class as dolasetron, granisetron, ondansetron, and palonosetron. Although classified as an antiemetic, alosetron is indicated for the treatment of irritable bowel syndrome in women whose primary symptom is severe chronic diarrhea. Alosetron is extensively metabolized to metabolites with unknown biologic activity. About 82% is bound to plasma proteins and the terminal elimination half-life is very short (about 1.5 hours) (1).

Reproduction studies have been conducted in rats and rabbits. In rats, doses up to about 160 times the recommended human dose based on BSA (RHD) revealed no evidence of impaired fertility or fetal harm. Similar findings were observed in rabbits given doses up to about 240 times the RHD. In addition, dose up to about 160 times the RHD had no effect on reproductive performance in male or female rats (1).

It is not known if alosetron crosses the human placenta. The molecular weight of the free base (about 295) and moderate plasma protein binding suggest that the drug will cross to the embryo–fetus, but the very short terminal elimination half-life will limit the amount of drug at the maternal:fetal interface.

BREASTFEEDING SUMMARY

No reports describing the use of alosetron during human lactation have been located. The molecular weight of the free base (about 295) and moderate plasma protein binding suggest that the drug will be excreted into breast milk. However, the very short terminal elimination half-life (about 1.5 hours) suggests that the amount of drug in milk will be minimal. The effects of this exposure on a nursing infant are unknown. However, because of the potential for severe toxicity (e.g., gastrointestinal symptoms that have caused deaths in adults), alosetron should probably not be used in women who are breastfeeding.

Reference

1. Product information. Lotronex. GlaxoSmithKline, 2004.

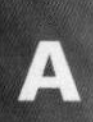

ALPHA-GALACTOSIDASE A

Endocrine/Metabolic Agent (Enzyme)

See Agalsidase Beta.

ALPHAPRODINE

[Withdrawn from the market. See 8th edition.]

ALPRAZOLAM

Sedative

PREGNANCY RECOMMENDATION: Human and Animal Data Suggest Risk
BREASTFEEDING RECOMMENDATION: Limited Human Data—Potential Toxicity

PREGNANCY SUMMARY

No structural anomalies have been attributed to the use of alprazolam during human pregnancy but in some reports, large numbers of patients were lost to follow-up. When used close to delivery, neonatal withdrawal has been reported. The long-term effects of in utero exposure on neurobehavior, especially when the exposure occurs in the latter half of pregnancy, have not been studied but are of concern.

FETAL RISK SUMMARY

Alprazolam, a member of the benzodiazepine class of agents, is used for the treatment of anxiety. Although no congenital anomalies have been attributed to the use of alprazolam during human pregnancies, other benzodiazepines (e.g., see Diazepam) have been suspected of producing fetal malformations after 1st trimester exposure. In pregnant rats, the drug produced thoracic vertebral anomalies and increased fetal death only at the highest dose (50 mg/kg) tested (1).

Researchers described the effects of alprazolam exposure on gestational day 18 (i.e., near term) on the neurodevelopment of mice in a series of reports (2–4). In one strain of mice, exposure induced persistent imbalance in the newborn and hind limb impairment in the adult offspring suggesting a defect in cerebellar development (2). In the second part of this study, in utero exposure to the drug (0.32 mg/kg orally) did not increase anxiety in adult offspring but did reduce motivation (3). A decrease in the tendency to engage in group activity and an increase in male aggression was observed in the third part of the study (4).

No data have been located on the placental passage of alprazolam. However, other benzodiazepines, such as diazepam, freely cross the placenta and accumulate in the fetus (see Diazepam). A similar distribution pattern should be expected for alprazolam.

One manufacturer has received 441 reports of in utero exposure to alprazolam or triazolam, two short-acting benzodiazepines, almost all of which occurred in the 1st trimester (5,6). Although most of the women discontinued the drugs when pregnancy was diagnosed, 24 continued to use alprazolam throughout their gestations (5). At the time of publication, about one-fifth of the 441 cases were still pregnant; one-sixth had been lost to follow-up, and one-sixth had been terminated by elective abortion for various reasons (5). Spontaneous abortion or miscarriage (no congenital anomalies were observed in the abortuses) occurred in 16 women; 2 pregnancies ended in stillbirths; and 1 newborn infant died within 24 hours of birth. Most of the remainder of the reported exposures ended with the delivery of a normal infant. The manufacturer also received two retrospective reports of congenital defects after alprazolam exposure (5). One of the cases involved an infant with Down's syndrome after maternal consumption of a single 5.5-mg dose of alprazolam and an unknown amount of doxepin during pregnancy (5). The second report involved a mother who had ingested 0.5 mg/day of alprazolam during the first 2 months of gestation. She delivered an infant with cat's eye with Pierre Robin syndrome. Neither of these outcomes can be attributed to alprazolam.

A 1992 reference reported the prospective evaluation of 542 pregnancies involving 1st trimester exposure to alprazolam gathered by a manufacturer from worldwide surveillance (7). These data were an extension of the data provided immediately above. Of the total, 131 (24.2%) were lost to follow-up. The outcome of the remaining 411 pregnancies was 42 (10.2%) spontaneous abortions, 5 (1.2%) stillbirths, 88 (21.4%) induced abortions, and 263 (64.0%) infants without and 13 (3.2%) infants with congenital anomalies. A total of 276 live births occurred, but two of these infants, both born prematurely, died shortly after birth. One, included in the group with congenital anomalies, had bilateral hydroceles and ascites, whereas the other died after intraventricular hemorrhage. The type and incidence of defects were comparable to those observed in the Collaborative Perinatal Project with no pattern of defects or excess of defects or spontaneous abortions apparent (7).

A second 1992 study reported on heavy benzodiazepine exposure during pregnancy from Michigan Medicaid data collected during 1980–1983 (8). Of the 2048 women, from a total sample of 104,339, who had received benzodiazepines, 80 had received ≥10 prescriptions for these agents. The records of these 80 women indicated frequent alcohol and substance abuse. Their pregnancy outcomes were 3 intrauterine deaths, 2 neonatal deaths in infants with congenital malformations, and 64 survivors. The outcome for 11 infants was unknown. Six of the surviving infants had diagnoses consistent with congenital defects. The investigators concluded that the high rate of congenital anomalies was suggestive of multiple alcohol and substance abuse. The outcome may not have been related to benzodiazepine exposure (8).

Single case reports of pyloric stenosis, moderate tongue-tie, umbilical hernia and ankle inversion, and clubfoot have been received by the manufacturer after in utero exposure to either alprazolam or triazolam (5). In addition, the manufacturer has received five reports of paternal use of alprazolam with pregnancy outcomes of two normal births, one elective abortion, one unknown outcome, and one stillbirth with multiple malformations (5). There is no evidence that the drug affected any of these outcomes.

Neonatal withdrawal after in utero exposure to alprazolam throughout gestation has been reported in three infants (5,9). In two cases involving maternal ingestion of 3 mg/day and 7–8 mg/day, mild withdrawal symptoms occurred at 2 days of age in the infant exposed to 3 mg/day (5). No details were provided on the onset or severity of the symptoms in the infant exposed to the higher dose. The third neonate was exposed to 1.0–1.5 mg/day (9). The mother continued this dosage in the postpartum interval while breastfeeding. Restlessness and irritability were noted in the infant during the 1st week. The symptoms worsened 2–3 days after breastfeeding was stopped on the seventh day because of concerns over drug excretion into the milk. Short, episodic screams and bursts of crying were observed frequently. Treatment with phenobarbital was partially successful, allowing the infant to sleep for longer periods. However, on awakening, jerking movements of the extremities and crying continued to occur. The infant was lost to follow-up at approximately 3 weeks of age.

BREASTFEEDING SUMMARY

Alprazolam is excreted into breast milk. Eight lactating women, who stopped breastfeeding their infants during the study, received a single 0.5 mg oral dose and multiple milk and serum samples were collected up to 36 hours after the dose (9). Transfer into milk was consistent with passive diffusion. The mean milk:serum concentrations ratio (using area under the drug concentration-time curve) was 0.36, indicating that a nursing infant would have received 0.3–5 mcg/kg/day, or about 3% (body weight adjusted) of the maternal dose (9).

A brief 1989 report citing information obtained from the manufacturer described a breastfed infant whose mother took alprazolam (dose not specified) for 9 months after delivery but not during pregnancy (10). The mother tapered herself off the drug over a 3-week period. Withdrawal symptoms consisting of irritability, crying, and sleep disturbances were noted in the nursing infant. The symptoms resolved without treatment after 2 weeks.

Because of the potent effects, the drug may have on a nursing infant's neurodevelopment, the case of probable alprazolam withdrawal, and the lethargy and loss of body weight observed with the chronic use of other benzodiazepines (see Diazepam), alprazolam should be avoided during lactation. The American Academy of Pediatrics classifies alprazolam as an agent for which the effect on a nursing infant is unknown but may be of concern (11).

References

1. Esaki K, Oshio K, Yanagita J. Effects of oral administration of alprazolam (TUS-1) on the rat fetus: experiment on drug administration during the organogenesis period. Preclin Rep Cent Inst Exp Anim 1981;7:65–77. As cited in Shepard TH. *Catalog of Teratogenic Agents*. 6th ed. Baltimore, MD: Johns Hopkins University Press, 1989:32.
2. Gonzalez C, Smith R, Christensen HD, Rayburn WF. Prenatal alprazolam induces subtle impairment in hind limb balance and dexterity in C57BL/6 mice (abstract). Teratology 1994;49:390.
3. Christensen HD, Pearce K, Gonzalez C, Rayburn WF. Does prenatal alprazolam exposure increase anxiety in adult mice offspring (abstract)? Teratology 1994;49:390.
4. Rayburn W, Gonzalez C, Christensen D. Social interactions of C57BL/6 mice offspring exposed prenatally to alprazolam (Xanax) (abstract). Am J Obstet Gynecol 1995;172:389.
5. Barry WS, St Clair SM. Exposure to benzodiazepines in utero. Lancet 1987;1:1436–7.
6. Ayd FJ Jr, ed. Exposure to benzodiazepines in utero. Int Drug Ther Newslett 1987;22:37–8.
7. St. Clair SM, Schirmer RG. First-trimester exposure to alprazolam. Obstet Gynecol 1992;80:843–6.
8. Bergman U, Rosa FW, Baum C, Wiholm B-E, Faich GA. Effects of exposure to benzodiazepine during fetal life. Lancet 1992;340:694–6.
9. Oo CY, Kuhn RJ, Desai N, Wright CE, McNamara PJ. Pharmacokinetics in lactating women: prediction of alprazolam transfer into milk. Br J Clin Pharmacol 1995;40:231–6.
10. Anderson PO, McGuire GG. Neonatal alprazolam withdrawal—possible effects of breast feeding. DICP Ann Pharmacother 1989;23:614.
11. Committee on Drugs, American Academy of Pediatrics. The transfer of drugs and other chemicals into human milk. Pediatrics 2001;108:776–89.

ALTEPLASE

Thrombolytic

PREGNANCY RECOMMENDATION: Compatible
BREASTFEEDING RECOMMENDATION: Compatible

PREGNANCY SUMMARY

The limited use of alteplase during pregnancy does not suggest a significant fetal risk. Although only one of the reported human exposures occurred during organogenesis, the high molecular weight probably precludes the transfer of alteplase to the embryo. Moreover, teratogenicity was not observed in animals. Hemorrhage is a risk of therapy at any time during gestation, but careful monitoring of the mother can prevent this from becoming a significant risk to the fetus. Therefore, it appears that alteplase may be used during gestation if the mother's condition requires this therapy.

FETAL RISK SUMMARY

Alteplase (tissue plasminogen activator; t-PA; rt-PA), an enzyme formed by recombinant DNA technology, is a thrombolytic agent used for the treatment of acute conditions such as myocardial infarction, pulmonary embolism, and ischemic stroke. The agent is a glycoprotein composed of 527 amino acids (1).

No maternal or fetal toxicity was observed in rats and rabbits dosed with 1 mg/kg (approximately 0.65 times the human dose for acute myocardial infarction [HD]) during organogenesis (1). An embryocidal effect was noted in rabbits administered an IV dose of 3 mg/kg (about 2 times the HD) (1). Shepard (2) cited two studies in which no teratogenicity or other toxicity was observed in the offspring of pregnant rats and rabbits administered t-PA during organogenesis.

Ten case reports have described the use of alteplase in human pregnancy (3–12). A 27-year-old woman in premature labor at 31 weeks' gestation was treated with urokinase and heparin, supplemented with continuous dobutamine to maintain a stable hemodynamic state, for massive pulmonary embolism (3). Because she failed to improve, low-dose alteplase therapy was initiated at 10 mg/hour for 4 hours, followed by 2 mg/hour for 1.5 hours (total dose 43 mg). The patient's clinical condition markedly improved with complete reperfusion of the right upper and middle lobe and partial reperfusion of the left lower lobe. Coagulation tests (prothrombin time, partial thromboplastin time, and thrombin time) during alteplase therapy remained within or close to the normal range. A healthy, premature, 2100-g male infant was delivered 48 hours after thrombolysis. A 38-year-old woman at 32 weeks' gestation developed a superior vena caval thrombosis during total parenteral hyperalimentation (4). Treatment with alteplase, 2 mg/hour for 48 hours resulted in clinical resolution of her symptoms (swelling of face and arms) within 24 hours. No evidence of placental bleeding was observed. Labor was induced 2 days later, and a healthy premature infant was delivered. A 29-year-old woman with severe pulmonary embolism and congenital antithrombin III deficiency was treated at 35 weeks' gestation with 100 mg alteplase for 3 hours followed by IV heparin (5). Nearly complete reperfusion of the right lung and the lower two-thirds of the left lung was observed at the end of the alteplase infusion. No placental bleeding was noted. The male infant, delivered by cesarean section 20 hours later, died at 14 days of age secondary to intracranial hemorrhage, a complication thought to be caused by prematurity and unrelated to the thrombolytic therapy.

Brief details of a case (6) of t-PA therapy during pregnancy were described in a 1995 review (8). A 30-year-old woman in her 11th week of gestation was treated with alteplase for pulmonary embolism. No complications were observed, and she had a normal, term delivery (6). A 30-year-old woman at 21 weeks' gestation had an acute myocardial infarction that was treated with a total dose of 100 mg alteplase given IV for 90 minutes (7). Immediate relief of her chest pain occurred and the other effects of cardiac reperfusion (arrhythmias and hypotension) were successfully treated. A cesarean section was performed at 33 weeks' gestation for premature labor unresponsive to magnesium sulfate, and a 1640-g male infant who has done well was delivered. A 20% abruptio placentae was noted during surgery. The cause of the abruption was thought to be either alteplase or the aspirin (81 mg/day) the mother had received after her initial treatment (7).

A 32-year-old pregnant woman had two episodes of a thrombosed St. Jude mitral valve prosthesis (8). The first event, at 20 weeks' gestation, was successfully treated by clot removal under cardiopulmonary bypass. About 8 weeks later, another clot formed on the valve and it was treated with 50 mg alteplase. An anterior placental hematoma was noted on ultrasound during treatment, but it resolved spontaneously within 2 weeks. At 38 weeks' gestation, the patient delivered vaginally a healthy girl with Apgar scores of 10 at 1 and 5 minutes (8). A 31-year-old patient developed a pulmonary embolism at 12 weeks' gestation (9). The woman was initially treated with IV heparin. However, because of continued hemodynamic deterioration, IV alteplase 100 mg over 2 hours was administered with rapid clinical improvement. SC heparin was given for the remainder of the pregnancy. At 33 weeks' gestation, placental abruption was diagnosed and a cesarean section delivered a normal 2325-g female infant with Apgar scores of 7 and 8 at 1 and 5 minutes, respectively (9). The last case report involved a 28-year-old woman who underwent in vitro fertilization because of long-standing infertility (10). Approximately 7 days after embryo transfer, she experienced a middle cerebral artery thrombosis secondary to ovarian hyperstimulation syndrome induced by the fertility medications. Treatment with 15.5 mg of intra-arterial alteplase over 68 minutes dissolved the clot but a hematoma developed in the right basal ganglia resulting in worsening the stroke. She improved over the next 3 months with only mild residual effects of the stroke and eventually delivered a healthy male infant by spontaneous vaginal delivery at term (10).

A 2005 report described the use of alteplase in an 18-year-old woman with nephritic syndrome who was treated with cyclosporine and prophylactic enoxaparin from 9 weeks' gestation (11). At 26 weeks', a subtotal thrombus of the right main renal vein was found. Enoxaparin was stopped and a continuous infusion of alteplase and low-dose heparin was begun. After 24 hours, the thrombus had decreased by 25%. On hospital day 7 (27 weeks'), a cesarean section performed for a prolonged fetal heart rate deceleration delivered a 720-g female infant with Apgar scores of 5 and 6 at 1 and 5 minutes, respectively. Alteplase and heparin were discontinued intraoperatively. The infant, with repeated normal head ultrasound scans, went home on the 83rd day of life with no evidence of focal neural deficits (11).

A 2006 report described the use of alteplase in a 34-year-old woman at 10 weeks' gestation who developed a fulminate pulmonary thromboembolism (12). Treatment with alteplase removed most of the thrombotic material in the pulmonary arteries. The patient was treated with heparin and then danaparoid and gave birth to a healthy female infant at term (12).

A 1995 review found no increased risk for preterm rupture of membranes, placental hemorrhage, or premature labor from thrombolytic agents (streptokinase, urokinase, or alteplase) (13). In seven women administered thrombolytic therapy before 14 weeks' gestation, pregnancy loss occurred in one case. Because of the small number of exposures, the concern that thrombolytics may interfere with placental implantation cannot be completely excluded and, indeed, one such case has been reported, although the exact cause was not determined (13).

BREASTFEEDING SUMMARY

It is not known whether alteplase (t-PA) crosses into human milk. Because of the nature of the indications for this agent and its very short initial half-life (<5 minutes), the opportunities for its use during lactation or the possibility of exposure of a nursing infant is minimal.

References

1. Product information. Activase. Genentech, 2001.
2. Shepard TH. *Catalog of Teratogenic Agents*. 8th ed. Baltimore, MD: Johns Hopkins University Press, 1995:416.
3. Flossdorf T, Breulmann M, Hopf H-B. Successful treatment of massive pulmonary embolism with recombinant tissue type plasminogen activator (rt-PA) in a pregnant woman with intact gravidity and preterm labour. Intensive Care Med 1990;16:454–6.
4. Barclay GR, Allen K, Pennington CR. Tissue plasminogen activator in the treatment of superior vena caval thrombosis associated with parenteral nutrition. Postgrad Med J 1990;66:398–400.
5. Baudo F, Caimi TM, Redaelli R, Nosari AM, Mauri M, Leonardi G, deCataldo F. Emergency treatment with recombinant tissue plasminogen activator of pulmonary embolism in a pregnant woman with antithrombin III deficiency. Am J Obstet Gynecol 1990;163:1274–5.
6. Seifried E, Gabelmann A, Ellbrück D. Thrombolytische Therapie einer Lungenarterienembolie in der Frühschwangerschaft mit rekombinantem Gewebe-Plasminogen-Aktivator. Geburtshilfe Frauenheilkd 1991;51:655. As cited in Turrentine MA, Braems G, Ramirez MM. Use of thrombolytics for the treatment of thromboembolic disease during pregnancy. Obstet Gynecol Surv 1995;50:534–41.
7. Schumacher B, Belfort MA, Card RJ. Successful treatment of acute myocardial infarction during pregnancy with tissue plasminogen activator. Am J Obstet Gynecol 1997;176:716–9.
8. Fleyfel M, Bourzoufi K, Huin G, Subtil D, Puech F. Recombinant tissue type plasminogen activator treatment of thrombosed mitral valve prosthesis during pregnancy. Can J Anaesth 1997;44:735–8.
9. Huang WH, Kirz DS, Gallee RC, Gordey K. First trimester use of recombinant tissue plasminogen activator in pulmonary embolism. Obstet Gynecol 2000;96:838.
10. Elford K, Leader A, Wee R, Stya PK. Stroke in ovarian hyperstimulation syndrome in early pregnancy treated with intra-arterial rt-PA. Neurology 2002;59:1270–2.
11. Song JY, Valentino L. A pregnant patient with renal vein thrombosis successfully treated with low-dose thrombolytic therapy: a case report. Am J Obstet Gynecol 2005;192:2073–5.
12. Weilbach C, Rahe-Meyer N, Raymondos K, Piepenbrock S. Delivery of a healthy child 30 weeks after resuscitation for thromboembolism and treatment with danaparoid: 5-year follow up. J Perinat Med 2006;34:505–6.
13. Turrentine MA, Braems G, Ramirez MM. Use of thrombolytics for the treatment of thromboembolic disease during pregnancy. Obstet Gynecol Surv 1995;50:534–41.

ALVIMOPAN

Gastrointestinal Agent (Peripheral Opioid Antagonist)

PREGNANCY RECOMMENDATION: No Human Data—Animal Data Suggest Low Risk
BREASTFEEDING RECOMMENDATION: No Human Data—Probably Compatible

PREGNANCY SUMMARY

No reports describing the use of alvimopan in human pregnancy have been located. The animal reproduction data suggest low risk, but the absence of human pregnancy experience prevents further assessment of the risk to the embryo–fetus. Alvimopan is available only for short-term use (15 doses or 7 days) in patients who are in hospitals registered to use the drug. Moreover, the indication suggests that use in pregnancy will be uncommon.

FETAL RISK SUMMARY

Alvimopan, a peripheral-acting selective antagonist with high affinity for the μ-opioid receptor, has no measurable opioid-agonist effects. It is in the same class as methylnaltrexone, a drug used for opioid-induced constipation. It achieves its action without reversing the central analgesic effects of μ-opioid agonists. Alvimopan is indicated to accelerate the time to upper and lower gastrointestinal recovery after partial large- or small-bowel resection surgery with primary anastomosis. The agent is metabolized to an active metabolite. Plasma protein binding to albumin of alvimopan and its metabolite is 80% and 94%, respectively. The mean terminal phase half-lives of the parent drug and metabolite are 10–17 and 10–18 hours, respectively (1).

Reproduction studies have been conducted in rats and rabbits. In pregnant rats, oral and IV doses that were about 68–136 and 3.4–6.8 times, respectively, the recommended human oral dose based on BSA (RHOD) revealed no evidence of fetal harm. Similar findings were observed in pregnant rabbits given IV doses that were about 5–10 times the RHOD (1).

In 2-year carcinogenicity studies, significant increases in the incidences of fibromas, fibrosarcoma and sarcoma in the skin/subcutis, and osteoma/osteosarcoma in bones were observed in female mice. No tumors were observed in rats. Neither alvimopan nor its active metabolite was genotoxic in multiple assays. No adverse effects on fertility in male and female rats were observed with alvimopan IV doses that were about 3.4–6.8 times the RHOD (1).

It is not known if alvimopan or its metabolite crosses the human placenta. The molecular weight of the parent drug (about 425 for nonhydrated molecule), and moderate plasma protein binding and long half-lives for the parent drug and metabolite suggest that both will cross to the embryo and/or fetus.

BREASTFEEDING SUMMARY

No reports describing the use of alvimopan during human lactation have been located. The molecular weight of the parent drug (about 425 for the nonhydrated molecule), moderate plasma protein binding (80% parent drug; 94% active metabolite), and long half-lives (10–17 and 10–18 hours, respectively) suggest that both alvimopan and its active metabolite will be excreted into breast milk. The effect of this exposure on a nursing infant is unknown.

Reference

1. Product information. Entereg. GlaxoSmithKline, 2008.

AMANTADINE

Antiviral/Antiparkinson

PREGNANCY RECOMMENDATION: Limited Human Data—Animal Data Suggest Risk
BREASTFEEDING RECOMMENDATION: Limited Human Data—Potential Toxicity

PREGNANCY SUMMARY

Amantadine is teratogenic and embryotoxic in one animal species, but the human pregnancy data are too limited for a complete risk assessment. However, complex cardiac defects were reported in three cases, and five other outcomes involved various malformations. The drug is best avoided in the 1st trimester.

FETAL RISK SUMMARY

Amantadine is indicated for the treatment of Parkinson disease and for the treatment and prophylaxis of influenza A. The plasma half-life is approximately 16–17 hours (range 10–31 hours) and the drug is moderately (about 67%) bound to plasma proteins (1). In a 1975 correspondence, one author thought the drug was a potential human teratogen and the absence of published reports at the time had more to do with its infrequent use in pregnancy than to its teratogenic potency (2).

Amantadine was teratogenic in pregnant rats at a dose that was equivalent to the estimated human dose based on BSA conversion (EHD) of 7.1 mg/kg/day and embryotoxic at a dose that was equivalent to the EHD of 14.2 mg/kg/day. No embryo or fetal harm was observed at a dose that was equivalent to the EHD of 5.3 mg/kg/day. No teratogenic or embryotoxic effects were seen in pregnant rabbits given a dose that was equivalent to the EHD of 9.6 mg/kg/day (1).

No reports describing the placental passage of amantadine in humans have been located. The low molecular weight (about 152 for the free base), moderate plasma protein binding, and long plasma half-life suggest that the drug will cross to the embryo–fetus.

A cardiovascular defect (single ventricle with pulmonary atresia) has been reported in an infant exposed to amantadine during the 1st trimester (3). The mother was taking 100 mgday for a Parkinson-like movement disorder.

A 1987 retrospective report described the use of amantadine, starting before conception in four women, one of whom had a probable molar pregnancy (4). In the remaining three cases, 1st trimester spotting was observed in one (apparently normal outcome), one newborn had an inguinal hernia (also exposed to levodopa/carbidopa), and one pregnancy aborted a fetus without apparent anomalies at 4 months (also exposed to levodopa) (4).

A 1991 report described the outcomes of consecutive pregnancies in a woman with multiple sclerosis who was treated with amantadine throughout each pregnancy (5). The infants were born at 34 and 36 weeks', respectively, with birth weights of 2640 and 2954 g, respectively. At the time of the report, the ages of the infants were 2.8 years and 3 months, respectively, and both were physically and developmentally normal (5).

Tibial hemimelia and tetralogy of Fallot was reported in an infant born from a mother exposed during early organogenesis to amantadine (6). The 37-year-old mother had taken the drug 100 mg daily for 7 days during the fourth and sixth postconception weeks for a para-influenza virus infection. Chromosome analysis of the infant revealed a normal female karyotype. In addition to this case, the investigators reported two other pregnancies exposed to amantadine throughout, both with normal outcomes. Both children, aged 4.4 and 3.2 years, had normal growth and development (6).

In a surveillance study of Michigan Medicaid recipients involving 229,101 completed pregnancies conducted between 1985 and 1992, 51 newborns had been exposed to amantadine during the 1st trimester (F. Rosa, personal communication, FDA, 1993). Five (9.8%) major birth defects were observed (2 expected). Among six categories of defects for which specific data were available, one cardiovascular defect (0.5 expected) and one limb reduction defect (0 expected) were observed. No cases of oral clefts, spina bifida, polydactyly, or hypospadias were recorded. Although the incidence of defects is high, the number of exposures is too small to draw any conclusions.

Rosa expanded the above communication with additional data in 1994 (7). In addition to the six types of defects surveyed, brain and eye defects were added for a new total of eight defects. Among 333,000 pregnancies, 64 had 1st trimester prescriptions for amantadine. Five defects (same as in his 1993 communication) were now linked to the drug (3.1 expected), including one cardiovascular defect, but no limb reduction defects were found in the new analysis. Because heart defects were common among nonexposed cases in Medicaid data (1 in 98 births), and considering the above reports, he cautioned that if amantadine did cause the cardiac defects, the available data suggested that the risk was not high (7).

A retrospective cohort study, covering the period 2003–2008, described 239 pregnancies that were treated with antiviral agents during pregnancy (8). Of these, 104 women received M2 ion channel inhibitors (rimantadine, amantadine, or both) and 135 received oseltamivir. The pregnancy outcomes of these patients were compared with 82,097 controls from the site's overall obstetric patient population. The exposure timing for the combined treated groups was 13% 1st trimester, 32% 2nd trimester, and 55% 3rd trimester. There were no significant differences between the treated groups and controls in terms of maternal and delivery characteristics except that M2 inhibitors had more multiple gestations. For M2 inhibitors, oseltamivir vs. controls, there were also no differences in stillbirths (0%, 0% vs. 1%), major defects (1% [trisomy 21], 0% vs. 2%), and minor defects (19%, 15% vs. 22%). The only significant finding in the characteristics of liveborn, singleton neonates, after exclusion of twins and major anomalies, was a higher risk of necrotizing enterocolitis in both treatment groups compared to controls—1.0%, 0.8% vs. 0.02%. (8).

BREASTFEEDING SUMMARY

Amantadine is excreted into breast milk in low concentrations (1). This is consistent with its low molecular weight (about 152 for the free base), moderate plasma protein binding, and long plasma half-life. Although no reports of adverse effects in nursing infants have been located, one manufacturer recommended that the drug be used with caution in lactating mothers because of the potential for urinary retention, vomiting, and skin rash in a nursing infant (9). The current manufacturer recommends that amantadine should not be used during breastfeeding (1).

References

1. Product information. Symmetrel. Endo Pharmaceuticals, 2000.
2. Coulson AS. Amantadine and teratogenesis. Lancet 1975;2:1044.
3. Nora JJ, Nora AH, Way GL. Cardiovascular maldevelopment associated with maternal exposure to amantadine. Lancet 1975;2:607.
4. Golbe LI. Parkinson's disease and pregnancy. Neurology 1987;37:1245–9.
5. Levy M, Pastuszak A, Koren G. Fetal outcome following intrauterine amantadine exposure. Reprod Toxicol 1991;5:79–81.
6. Pandit PB, Chitayat D, Jefferies AL, Landes A, Qamar IU, Koren G. Tibial hemimelia and tetralogy of Fallot associated with first trimester exposure to amantadine. Reprod Toxicol 1994;8:89–92.
7. Rosa F. Amantadine pregnancy experience. Reprod Toxicol 1994;8:531.
8. Greer LG, Sheffield JS, Rogers VL, Roberts SW, McIntire DD, Wendel GD Jr. Maternal and neonatal outcomes after antepartum treatment of influenza with antiviral medications. Obstet Gynecol 2010;115:711–6.
9. Product information. Symmetrel. Du Pont Pharmaceuticals, 1985.

AMBENONIUM

[Withdrawn from the market. See 9th edition.]

AMBRISENTAN

Vasodilator

PREGNANCY RECOMMENDATION: Contraindicated
BREASTFEEDING RECOMMENDATION: No Human Data—Potential Toxicity

PREGNANCY SUMMARY

No reports describing the use of ambrisentan in human pregnancy have been located. The animal data suggest risk if the drug is used in human pregnancy. In a black-box warning, the manufacturer classifies ambrisentan as contraindicated in women who are or may become pregnant (1). Pregnancy must be excluded before the initiation of therapy and women of reproductive potential must use two reliable methods of contraception. Monthly pregnancy tests are required. In addition, ambrisentan is available only through a special restricted distribution program because of the dual risk of teratogenicity and the potential for liver injury. Only physicians and pharmacies registered in this program can prescribe and distribute the drug.

FETAL RISK SUMMARY

Ambrisentan is an oral endothelin receptor antagonist in the same class as bosentan. It is indicated for the treatment of pulmonary arterial hypertension (WHO group 1) in patients with WHO class II or III symptoms to improve exercise capacity and delay clinical worsening. The molecule is a carboxylic acid with a pK_a of 4.0 and is water soluble at higher pH. Plasma protein binding is 99%. The terminal elimination half-life is 15 hours but the effective half-life is 9 hours (1).

Animal reproduction studies have been conducted in rats and rabbits, but the doses used were not compared with the human dose. The drug was teratogenic in both species causing abnormalities of the lower jaw and hard and soft palate, malformation of the heart and great vessels, and failure of formation of the thymus and thyroid. The malformations were similar to those observed with other endothelin receptor antagonists and were thought to be a class effect. In rats given doses that were 17, 51, and 170 times, respectively, the maximum oral human dose of 10 mg based on BSA during late gestation and through weaning, decreased newborn pup survival was observed with the middle and high doses. The high dose was also associated with adverse effects on testicle size and fertility of pups (1).

It is not known if ambrisentan crosses the human placenta. Although the molecular weight (about 378) and the elimination half-life suggest that the drug will cross the placenta, the low lipid solubility and the high plasma binding might mitigate the amount reaching the embryo–fetus.

BREASTFEEDING SUMMARY

No reports describing the use of ambrisentan during human lactation have been located. Although the molecular weight (about 378) and the elimination half-life (15 hours) suggest that the drug will be excreted into breast milk, the low lipid solubility and the high plasma binding (99%) might mitigate the amount in milk. The effect of exposure on a nursing infant is unknown, but the potential for toxicity is a concern. Therefore, until human data are available, the safest course is to not breastfeed during treatment with ambrisentan.

Reference

1. Product information. Letairis. Gilead Sciences, 2008.

AMIFOSTINE

Antineoplastic Cytoprotectant

PREGNANCY RECOMMENDATION: Compatible—Maternal Benefit >> Embryo–Fetal Risk
BREASTFEEDING RECOMMENDATION: No Human Data—Probably Compatible

PREGNANCY SUMMARY

No reports describing the use of amifostine in human pregnancy have been located. The animal reproduction data suggest risk, but the absence of human pregnancy experience prevents a more complete assessment. However, one of the indications for amifostine is the prevention of cisplatin-induced renal toxicity in women being treated for ovarian cancer. Thus, if a pregnant woman requires amifostine and gives informed consent, the maternal benefit from amifostine appears to outweigh the potential embryo–fetal risk. If inadvertent exposure occurs during pregnancy, the woman should be advised of the potential risk for adverse effects in the embryo and fetus.

FETAL RISK SUMMARY

Amifostine is an organic thiophosphate cytoprotective agent that is administered as an IV infusion. It is a prodrug that is dephosphorylated by a tissue enzyme to the active free thiol metabolite. Amifostine is indicated to reduce the cumulative renal toxicity associated with repeated doses of cisplatin in patients with ovarian cancer. It also is indicated to reduce the incidence of moderate to severe xerostomia in patients undergoing postoperative radiation treatment for head and neck cancer, where the radiation port includes a substantial portion of the parotid gland. Amifostine is rapidly metabolized to the active metabolite and subsequently to a less active metabolite. The plasma elimination half-life is very short, about 8 minutes.

Reproduction studies have been conducted in rabbits. Amifostine was embryotoxic in pregnant rabbits at a dose that was about 60% of the recommended human dose based on BSA (1).

Long-term studies have not been done to determine the carcinogenic or fertility impairment potential of amifostine, but the agent was not mutagenic in two tests. The active metabolite was mutagenic in some, but not other, tests and was not clastogenic (1).

It is not known if amifostine crosses the human placenta. The molecular weight of the prodrug (about 214) suggests that it will distribute to the embryo and/or fetus, but the very short plasma elimination half-life should limit the amount available for transfer.

BREASTFEEDING SUMMARY

No reports describing the use of amifostine during human lactation have been located. The molecular weight of the prodrug (about 214) suggests that it will be excreted into breast milk, but the very short plasma elimination half-life (about 8 minutes) should limit the amount. The effects of this potential exposure on a nursing infant are unknown. However, because the drug is given as a short IV infusion immediately before chemotherapy or radiation, and breastfeeding would be unlikely at this time, the risk of exposing an infant to amifostine when nursing is later resumed appears to be nil.

Reference

1. Product information. Ethyol. MedImmune Oncology, 2007.

AMIKACIN

Antibiotic (Aminoglycoside)

PREGNANCY RECOMMENDATION: Human Data Suggest Low Risk
BREASTFEEDING RECOMMENDATION: Compatible

PREGNANCY SUMMARY

No reports linking the use of amikacin to congenital defects have been located. Ototoxicity, which is known to occur after amikacin therapy in humans, has not been reported as an effect of in utero exposure. However, eighth cranial nerve toxicity in the human fetus is well known after exposure to other aminoglycosides (see Kanamycin and Streptomycin) and amikacin could potentially cause this.

FETAL RISK SUMMARY

Amikacin is an aminoglycoside antibiotic. The drug causes dose-related nephrotoxicity in pregnant rats and their fetuses (1). Reproduction studies were conducted in mice and rats and no evidence of impaired fertility or teratogenicity was observed (2).

The drug rapidly crosses the placenta into the fetal circulation and amniotic fluid (3–6). Studies in patients undergoing elective abortions in the 1st and 2nd trimesters indicate that amikacin distributes to most fetal tissues except the brain and cerebrospinal fluid (3,5). The highest fetal concentrations were found in the kidneys and urine. At term, cord serum levels were one-half to one-third of maternal serum levels whereas measurable amniotic fluid levels did not appear until almost 5 hours after injection (4).

BREASTFEEDING SUMMARY

Amikacin is excreted into breast milk in low concentrations. After 100- and 200-mg IM doses, only traces of amikacin could be found for 6 hours in two of four patients (4,7). Because oral absorption of this antibiotic is poor, ototoxicity in the infant would not be expected. However, three potential problems exist for the nursing infant: modification of bowel flora, direct effects on the infant, and interference with the interpretation of culture results if a fever workup is required.

References

1. Mallie JP, Coulon G, Billerey C, Faucourt A, Morin JP. In utero aminoglycosides-induced nephrotoxicity in rat neonates. Kidney Inter 1988;33:36–44.
2. Product information. Amikacin. Elkins-Sinn, 2000.
3. Bernard B, Abate M, Ballard C, Wehrle P. *Maternal–Fetal Pharmacology of BB-K8*. Antimicrobial Agents and Chemotherapy 14th Annual Conference, 1974, Abstract 71.
4. Matsuda C, Mori C, Maruno M, Shiwakura T. A study of amikacin in the obstetrics field. Jpn J Antibiot 1974;27:633–6.
5. Bernard B, Abate M, Thielen P, Attar H, Ballard C, Wehrle P. Maternal–fetal pharmacological activity of amikacin. J Infect Dis 1977;135:925–31.
6. Flores-Mercado F, Garcia-Mercado J, Estopier-Jauregin C, Galindo-Hernandez E, Diaz-Gonzalez C. Clinical pharmacology of amikacin sulphate: blood, urinary and tissue concentrations in the terminal stage of pregnancy. J Int Med Res 1977;5;292–4.
7. Yuasa M. A study of amikacin in obstetrics and gynecology. Jpn J Antibiot 1974;27;377–81.

AMILORIDE

Diuretic

PREGNANCY RECOMMENDATION: Limited Human Data—Animal Data Suggest Low Risk
BREASTFEEDING RECOMMENDATION: No Human Data—Probably Compatible

PREGNANCY SUMMARY

Similar to other diuretics, amiloride does not appear to pose a risk to the embryo–fetus when used for indications other than gestational hypertension or preeclampsia.

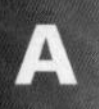

FETAL RISK SUMMARY

Amiloride is a potassium-conserving diuretic. In general, diuretics are not recommended in the treatment of gestational hypertension because of the maternal hypovolemia characteristic of this disease.

Reproduction studies using amiloride alone in mice at 25 times the maximum recommended human dose (MRHD) and in rabbits at 20 times the MRHD found no evidence of fetal harm (1). The combination of acetazolamide and amiloride was found to produce abnormal development of the ureter and kidney in fetal mice when given at the critical moment of ureter development (2).

Amiloride crosses the placenta in modest amounts in mice and rabbits (1). No reports describing the human placenta passage of amiloride have been located. The molecular weight (about 230 for the free base) suggests that drug will cross the placenta.

Seven reports of fetal exposure to amiloride have been located (3–9). In one case, a malformed fetus was discovered after voluntary abortion in a patient with renovascular hypertension (3). The patient had been treated during the 1st trimester with amiloride, propranolol, and captopril. The left leg of the fetus ended at midthigh without distal development and no obvious skull formation was noted above the brain tissue. The authors attributed the defects to captopril (3), but this agent is not thought to cause birth defects in the 1st trimester.

A second case involved a 21-year-old woman with Bartter's syndrome who was maintained on amiloride (20–30 mg/day) and potassium chloride (160–300 mEq/day) throughout pregnancy (4). Progressive therapy with the two agents was required to maintain normal potassium levels. Mild intrauterine growth restriction was detected at 30 weeks' gestation with eventual vaginal delivery of a 2800-g female infant at 41 weeks' gestation. No abnormalities were noted in the infant. A normal 3500-g female infant was delivered by cesarean section at 37 weeks' gestation from a mother who had been treated throughout pregnancy with amiloride, hydrochlorothiazide, and amiodarone for severe chronic atrial fibrillation (5). A second case with Bartter's syndrome was reported in 2004 (6). Amiloride was used throughout the pregnancy and a healthy 3.300-kg female infant was born at term.

Two cases of Gitelman syndrome, an inherited hypokalemic salt-losing renal tubular disorder that is closely related to Bartter's syndrome, that were treated with amiloride have been located (7,8). Both pregnancy outcomes were normal babies born at 37 weeks' gestation.

A woman with primary aldosteronism had two pregnancies that were treated with amiloride (9). Both pregnancies ended with the birth of a healthy infant.

In a surveillance study of Michigan Medicaid recipients involving 229,101 completed pregnancies conducted between 1985 and 1992, 28 newborns had been exposed to amiloride during the 1st trimester (F. Rosa, personal communication, FDA, 1993). Two (7.1%) major birth defects were observed (one expected), one of which was a hypospadias. No anomalies were observed in five other categories of defects (cardiovascular, oral clefts, spina bifida, polydactyly, and limb reduction defects) for which specific data were available.

BREASTFEEDING SUMMARY

No reports describing the use of amiloride during human lactation have been located. The molecular weight (about 230 for the free base) suggests that excretion into breast milk will occur.

References

1. Product information. Midamor. Merck, 2000.
2. Miller TA, Scott WJ Jr. Abnormalities in ureter and kidney development in mice given acetazolamide–amiloride or dimethadione (DMO) during embryogenesis. Teratology 1992;46:541–50.
3. Duminy PC, Burger PT. Fetal abnormality associated with the use of captopril during pregnancy. S Afr Med J 1981;60:805.
4. Almeida OD Jr, Spinnato JA. Maternal Bartter's syndrome and pregnancy. Am J Obstet Gynecol 1989;160:1225–6.
5. Robson DJ, Jeeva Raj MV, Storey GCA, Holt DW. Use of amiodarone during pregnancy. Postgrad Med J 1985;61:75–7.
6. Deruelle P, Dufour P, Magnenant E, Courouble N, Puech F. Maternal Bartter's syndrome in pregnancy treated with amiloride. Eur J Obstet Gynecol Reprod Biol 2004;115;106–7.
7. Mascetti L, Bettinelli A, Simonetti GD, Tagliabue A, Syren ML, Nordio F, Bianchetti MG. Pregnancy in inherited hypokalemic salt-losing renal tubular disorder. Obstet Gynecol 2011;117:512–6.
8. Mathen S, Venning M, Gillham J. Outpatient management of Gitelman's syndrome in pregnancy. BMJ Case Rep. Jan 25;2013. pii:bcr2012007927. doi:10.1136/bcr-2012-007927.
9. Krysiak R, Samborek M, Stojko R. Primary aldosteronism in pregnancy. Acta Clin Belg 2012;67:130–4.

AMINOCAPROIC ACID

Hemostatic

PREGNANCY RECOMMENDATION: Limited Human Data—No Relevant Animal Data
BREASTFEEDING RECOMMENDATION: Hold Breastfeeding

PREGNANCY SUMMARY

The human pregnancy experience with this agent is too limited to assess the embryo–fetal risk. There are no animal reproduction data to assist in an assessment.

FETAL RISK SUMMARY

Aminocaproic acid is used to enhance hemostasis when fibrinolysis contributes to bleeding. Animal reproduction studies have not been conducted with the drug (1).

No reports describing the placental passage of aminocaproic acid have been located. The molecular weight (about 131) is low enough that passage to the fetus should be expected.

Aminocaproic acid was used during the 2nd trimester in a patient with subarachnoid hemorrhage as a result of multiple intracranial aneurysms (2). The drug was given for 3 days preceding surgery (dosage not given). No fetal toxicity was observed.

BREASTFEEDING SUMMARY

No reports describing the use of aminocaproic acid during lactation have been located. Although the molecular weight (about 131) is low enough that excretion into breast milk should be expected, the indication for the drug probably implies that the chance of its use during nursing is very small.

References

1. Product information. Amicar. Immunex, 2000.
2. Willoughby JS. Sodium nitroprusside, pregnancy and multiple intracranial aneurysms. Anaesth Intensive Care 1984;12:358–60.

AMINOGLUTETHIMIDE

[Withdrawn from the market. See 9th edition.]

AMINOPHYLLINE

Respiratory Drug (Bronchodilator)

See Theophylline.

AMINOPTERIN

[Withdrawn from the market. See 9th edition.]

para-AMINOSALICYLIC ACID

Antitubercular

PREGNANCY RECOMMENDATION: Human and Animal Data Suggest Risk
BREASTFEEDING RECOMMENDATION: Limited Human Data—Probably Compatible

PREGNANCY SUMMARY

Reports have associated *para*-aminosalicylic acid with structural anomalies, but confirming studies are required. The best course is to avoid this agent, if possible, in the 1st trimester.

FETAL RISK SUMMARY

para-Aminosalicylic acid is a bacteriostatic agent used for the treatment of *Mycobacterium tuberculosis*. It is most frequently used in combination with other agents for the treatment of multidrug-resistant tuberculosis.

In reproduction studies with rats at doses within the human dose range, occipital malformations were observed (1). No adverse effects on the fetus were observed in rabbits treated with 5 mg/kg/day throughout gestation (1).

No reports describing the placental transfer of *para*-aminosalicylic acid have been located. The molecular weight (approximately 153) is low enough that passage to the fetus should be expected.

The Collaborative Perinatal Project monitored 50,282 mother–child pairs, 43 of whom had 1st trimester exposure to *para*-aminosalicylic acid (4-aminosalicylic acid) (2). Congenital defects were found in five infants. This incidence (11.6%) was nearly twice the expected frequency. No major category of malformations or individual defects were identified.

An increased malformation rate for ear, limb, and hypospadias has been reported for 123 patients taking 7–14 g/day of *para*-aminosalicylic acid with other antitubercular drugs (3). An increased risk of congenital defects has not been found in other studies (4–6).

BREASTFEEDING SUMMARY

para-Aminosalicylic acid is excreted into breast milk. In one non-breastfeeding patient given an oral 4-g dose of the drug, a peak milk concentration of 1.1 mcg/mL was measured at 3 hours with an elimination half-life of 2.5 hours (7). The peak maternal plasma concentration, 70.1 mcg/mL, occurred at 2 hours.

References

1. Product information. Paser. Jacobus Pharmaceutical, 2000.
2. Heinonen OP, Slone D, Shapiro S. *Birth Defects and Drugs in Pregnancy*. Littleton, MA: Publishing Sciences Group, 1977:299.
3. Varpela E. On the effect exerted by first line tuberculosis medicines on the foetus. Acta Tuberc Scand 1964;35:53–69.
4. Lowe CR. Congenital defects among children born to women under supervision or treatment for pulmonary tuberculosis. Br J Prev Soc Med 1964;18:14–6.
5. Wilson EA, Thelin TJ, Ditts PV. Tuberculosis complicated by pregnancy. Am J Obstet Gynecol 1973;115;526–9.
6. Scheinhorn DJ, Angelillo VA. Antituberculosis therapy in pregnancy. Risk to the fetus. West J Med 1977;127;195–8.
7. Holdiness MR. Antituberculosis drugs and breast-feeding. Arch Intern Med 1984;144:1888.

AMIODARONE

Antiarrhythmic

PREGNANCY RECOMMENDATION: Human and Animal Data Suggest Risk
BREASTFEEDING RECOMMENDATION: Contraindicated

PREGNANCY SUMMARY

Fetal adverse effects directly attributable to amiodarone have been observed. Congenital goiter/hypothyroidism and hyperthyroidism may occur after in utero exposure. Newborns exposed to amiodarone in utero should have thyroid function studies performed because of the large proportion of iodine contained in each dose.

FETAL RISK SUMMARY

Amiodarone is an antiarrhythmic agent used for difficult or resistant cases of arrhythmias. The drug contains about 75 mg of iodine per 200 mg dose (1–3).

Amiodarone was maternal and embryo toxic (increased fetal resorptions, decreased live litter size, growth restriction, and restricted sternum and metacarpal ossification) in rats administered an IV infusion about 1.4 times the maximum recommended human dose based on BSA (MRHD) (4). Lower doses, about 0.4 and 0.7 times the MRHD, produced no embryo toxicity (4). In pregnant rabbits administered IV doses about 0.1, 0.3, and 0.7 times the MRHD, embryo toxicity was observed at 0.3 times the MRHD and above. At about 2.7 times the MRHD, >90% of the animals aborted. No teratogenic effects were observed in any of the rabbit groups (4).

Amiodarone and its metabolite, desethylamiodarone, cross the placenta to the fetus (1–3,5–9). In the 10 infants described in these reports, cord blood concentrations of the parent compound were 0.05–0.35 mcg/mL, representing cord:maternal ratios of 0.10–0.28 in nine cases (1–3,5–9) and 0.6 in one case (9). Cord blood concentrations of the metabolite varied between 0.05 and 0.55 mcg/mL, about one-fourth of the maternal levels in 9 of the 10 cases. In one study, the amount of amiodarone crossing the placenta to the fetus was dependent on the degree of hydrops fetalis (10). The expected fetal concentrations of the drug were not achieved until substantial compensation of the fetus had occurred.

In 22 cases of amiodarone therapy during pregnancy, the antiarrhythmic was administered for maternal indications (1–3,5,7–9,11–16). One patient in the last 3 months of pregnancy was treated with 200 mg daily for resistant atrial tachycardia (1). She delivered a 2780-g female infant at 40 weeks' gestation. Both the mother and the infant had a prolonged QT interval on electrocardiogram (ECG). A second woman was also treated by these investigators under similar conditions. Both infants were normal (infant sex, weight, and gestational age were not specified for the second case), including having normal thyroid function. In another report, a woman was treated at 34 weeks' gestation when quinidine failed to control her atrial fibrillation (2). After an initial dose of 800 mg/day for 1 week, the dose was decreased to 400 mg/day and was continued at this level until delivery at 41 weeks' gestation. The healthy 3220-g infant experienced bradycardia during labor induction (104–120 beats/minute [bpm]) and during the first 48 hours after birth. No other adverse effects were observed in the infant, who had normal thyroid and liver function tests. A woman was treated during the 37th–39th weeks of pregnancy with daily doses of 600, 400, and 200 mg, each for 1 week, for atrial tachycardia that was resistant to propranolol, digoxin, and verapamil (3). No bradycardia or other abnormalities were noted in the newborn. The infant's thyroid-stimulating hormone (TSH) level on the 4th day was 9 mU/L, a normal value. Goiter was not observed and the infant was clinically euthyroid.

A 1985 report described the treatment of two women with amiodarone for maternal heart conditions (5). One of these patients, a 31-year-old woman with atrial fibrillation, was treated with amiodarone, 200 mg/day, and diuretics throughout gestation. She delivered a healthy 3500-g female without goiter or corneal changes at 37 weeks' gestation. A cord blood thyroxine (T4) level was elevated (209 nmol/L) and was still elevated 1 week later (207 nmol/L), but TSH concentrations at these times were 3.2 mU/L and <1 mU/L (both normal), respectively. The second woman, a 27-year-old primigravida, was treated with amiodarone, 400–800 mg/day, starting at 22 weeks' gestation. Fetal bradycardia, 100–120 bpm, was observed at approximately 33 weeks' gestation. Spontaneous labor ensued at 39 weeks with delivery of a healthy 2900-g male. Thyroid function studies were not reported, but the neonatal examinations were normal (5).

A woman in her 16th week of pregnancy presented with severe atrial fibrillation (7). She was treated with amiodarone, 800 mg/day for 1 week followed by 200 mg/day for the remainder of her pregnancy (7). She delivered a growth-restricted 2660-g male in the 39th week of gestation who had no goiter and whose free T4 index, serum-free triiodothyronine (T3), and serum TSH concentrations were all within normal limits. An ECG at 1 day of age showed a prolonged QT interval. Follow-up of the infant at 6 months was normal.

A healthy 3650-g male infant was delivered at term from a mother who had taken 200–400 mg/day of amiodarone throughout gestation (8). The infant's thyroid function was normal at birth; no goiter or corneal deposits were noted; and subsequent growth and thyroid function remained within normal limits. In another case, a woman was treated with propranolol and amiodarone, 400 mg/day for 4 days each week, throughout gestation (11). A healthy 2670-g female infant was delivered, but the gestational age was not specified. No goiter or corneal microdeposits were present in the infant and clinically she was euthyroid. The T4 and TSH levels in cord blood were both normal although a total serum iodine level (290 mcg/dL) was markedly elevated (normal 5.5–17.4 mcg/dL).

A 1991 report described the use of amiodarone in one woman with a history of symptomatic ventricular arrhythmia, and mitral and tricuspid valve prolapse through two complete pregnancies (12). She also had a history of right upper lobectomy for drug-resistant pulmonary tuberculosis. She was treated with 400 mg/day of amiodarone during the first 12 weeks of gestation of one pregnancy before the dose was reduced to 200 mg/day. She continued this dose during the remainder of this pregnancy and through a successive pregnancy. One of the newborns, a 2500-g female delivered at 38 weeks' gestation, was growth-restricted. The second infant, a 2960-g male, was delivered prematurely at 35.5 weeks' gestation. Except for the growth restriction in the one infant, the newborns were physically normal and had no clinical or biochemical signs of hypothyroidism (12). The concentrations of amiodarone and its metabolite desethylamiodarone were <0.3 mcg/mL in the first-born infant (not determined in the second newborn).

In two other reports, treatment was begun at 25 and 32 weeks' gestation (13,14). Delivery occurred at 31 weeks in one case (sex and birth weight not given), and the infant died 2 days after delivery (13). In the second report, the infant (sex and birth weight not given) was born at 37 weeks' gestation (14). Amiodarone and desethylamiodarone concentrations in the cord blood were 0.1 and 0.2 mcg/mL, respectively. The drug and its metabolite were not detected in the infant's serum at 3 and 6 days after birth. A prolonged QT interval was observed on the infant's ECG.

Five pregnancies in four women treated with amiodarone for various cardiac arrhythmias were described in a 1992 reference (9). The drug was used throughout gestation in four pregnancies and during the last 6 weeks in a fifth. One infant delivered at 34 weeks' gestation was growth-restricted (birth weight, length, and head circumference were all at the 10th percentile or less), but the other four newborns were of normal size. No adverse effects—such as goiter, corneal microdeposits, pulmonary fibrosis, and dermatologic or neurologic signs—were observed (9). The infants were clinically euthyroid, but one of the five newborns had transient biochemical signs of hypothyroidism (low T4 concentration) that responded to treatment. This latter infant, whose mother had taken the β-blocker, metoprolol, throughout gestation and amiodarone only during the last 6 weeks, had delayed motor development and impaired speech performance at 5 years of age. He had been delivered at 40 weeks' gestation with a birth weight of 2880 g (10th percentile) and a length of 50 cm (50th percentile). The other four infants had normal follow-up examinations at periods ranging from 8 months to 5 years.

Congenital hypothyroidism with goiter was described in a growth-restricted 2450-g male newborn whose mother had taken 200 mg/day of amiodarone from the 13th week of gestation until delivery at 38 weeks for treatment of Wolff-Parkinson-White syndrome (15). The mother had no signs or symptoms of hypothyroidism. Thyroid tests of cord blood revealed a TSH level of >100 mU/L (normal 10–20 mU/L), a T4 level of 35.9 mcg/L (normal 60–170 mcg/L), and no thyroid antibodies. In addition to a homogeneous goiter, the newborn had persistent hypotonia and bradycardia, large anterior and posterior fontanels, and macroglossia, but no corneal microdeposits. The bradycardia resolved after several days. Greater than normal amounts of urinary iodine were measured from birth (144 mcg/dL; normal <15 mcg/dL) until the sixth week of life. The infant's plasma concentrations of amiodarone and desethylamiodarone on day 5 were 140 and 260 ng/mL, respectively, and were still detectable after 1 month. His bone age at birth and at 20 months of age was estimated to be 28 weeks and 12 months, respectively. Treatment with levothyroxine during the first 20 months resulted in the complete disappearance of the goiter at about 3 months of age, but his psychomotor development was held back.

A 1994 report described three pregnancies in two women who were being treated with amiodarone (16). Recurrent ventricular fibrillation was treated in one woman with an implanted defibrillator and amiodarone, 400 mg/day. She became pregnant 4 years after beginning this therapy and eventually delivered a premature, 2540-g male infant at 35 weeks' gestation with a holosystolic murmur and an umbilical hernia. At 2 weeks of age, the infant experienced mild congestive heart failure with labored breathing. A large midmuscular ventricular septal defect, with marked left ventricular and left atrial dilatation and left ventricular hypertrophy, was observed by echocardiogram (16). The defect was still present at 21 months of age. A second pregnancy in this woman, at the same amiodarone dose, was electively terminated at approximately 11 weeks' gestation. The thorax and limbs of the fetus were normal and contained 1.55 and 5.8 mcg/g of amiodarone and desethylamiodarone, respectively. The second woman had been treated with amiodarone, 600 mg/day, for 2 years for recurrent sustained ventricular tachycardia (Chagas disease) before conception. She eventually delivered a term 3300-g male infant with mild bradycardia (110 bpm) at birth. Both liveborn infants were clinically euthyroid without goiter or corneal changes.

Six cases of amiodarone therapy for refractory fetal tachycardia have been described in the literature (6,10,17–20). In the first of these, a fetus at 27 weeks' gestation experienced tachycardia (260 bpm) that was unresponsive to digoxin and propranolol (17). Lidocaine and procainamide lowered the heart rate somewhat but were associated with unacceptable maternal toxicity. Amiodarone combined with verapamil was successful in halting the tachycardia and reversing the signs of congestive heart failure. An amiodarone maintenance dose of 400 mg/day was required for control. Spontaneous labor occurred after 39 days of therapy, with delivery of a 2700-g male infant at 33 weeks' gestation. Atrial flutter with a 2:1 block and a ventricular rate of 200 bpm were converted on the third day by electrical cardioversion. No adverse effects from the drug therapy were mentioned.

A fetus with supraventricular tachycardia (220 bpm) showed evidence of congestive heart failure at 32 weeks' gestation (6). Maternal therapy with digoxin alone or in combination with sotalol (a β-blocker) or verapamil failed to stop the abnormal rhythm. Digoxin was then combined with amiodarone, 1600 mg/day for 4 days, then 1200 mg/day for 3 days, then 800 mg/day for 6 weeks. The fetal heart rate fell to 140 bpm after 14 days of therapy, and the signs of congestive heart failure gradually resolved. Neonatal thyroid indices at birth (about 38 weeks' gestation) and at 1 month were as follows (normal values are shown in parentheses): free T3 index, 3.4 and 5.6 pmol/L (4.3–8.6 pmol/L); free T4 index, 5.4 and 25 pmol/L (9–26 pmol/L); T3, 1.7 and 2.7 nmol/L (1.2–3.1 nmol/L); T4, 196 and 300 nmol/L (70–175 nmol/L); and TSH, 30 and 4.12 mU/L (<5 mU/L). The elevated T4 level returned to normal at a later unspecified time. It was not mentioned whether a goiter was present at birth. At 10 months of age, all thyroid function tests were within normal limits.

A third case involved a fetus at 30 weeks' gestation with tachycardia (220 bpm) and congestive heart failure that had not responded to digoxin and propranolol (18). At 32 weeks' gestation, digoxin and amiodarone lowered the rate to 110–180 bpm with improvement in the congestive failure. Amiodarone was given at 1200 mg/day for 3 days, then 600 mg/day until delivery 3 weeks later. The newborn had tachycardia of up to 200 bpm that was treated with digoxin, furosemide, and propranolol. Hypothyroidism was diagnosed based on the presence of a goiter and abnormal thyroid tests (normal values are in parentheses): T4, 48 mcg/mL (70–180 mcg/mL); free T4, 0.5 mcg/mL (>1.5 mcg/mL); and TSH, >240 mU/L (<30 mU/L). The infant was treated with 10 mcg/day of T4 until 3 months of age, at which time his cardiac and thyroid functions were normal. Follow-up at 15 months was normal.

A 27-week fetus with refractory supraventricular tachycardia and hydrops fetalis was treated with repeated injections of amiodarone into the umbilical vein after maternal therapy with amiodarone, and multiple other antiarrhythmic drugs failed to resolve the fetal condition (10). Subtherapeutic transplacental passage of amiodarone and digoxin was documented that did not improve until substantial resolution of the hydrops had occurred with direct administration of amiodarone to the fetus. A male infant was delivered at 37 weeks' gestation because of growth restriction, but thyroid function and other tests were within normal limits, and no corneal deposits were observed.

In a similar case, a 27-week fetus with severe hydrops secondary to congenital sinoatrial disease-induced sinus bradycardia and atrial flutter was treated with amiodarone via the IV, intraperitoneal, and transplacental routes (19). Prior maternal therapy with oral sotalol and flecainide had failed to reverse the worsening right heart failure. A 15-mg IV dose was administered to the fetus concurrently with initiation to the mother of 200 mg orally every 8 hours. Approximately 24 hours later, an additional 15-mg dose of amiodarone was given intraperitoneally to the fetus. The fetal ascites resolved over the next 3 weeks. A 2686-g female infant in good condition was eventually delivered at 37 weeks' gestation. Cardiac function was normal in the neonatal period and at 3-month follow-up, as were thyroid tests at 6 days of age.

A 1994 report described the use of amiodarone, 1600 mg/day (25 mg/kg/day), for the treatment of fetal supraventricular tachycardia that had failed to respond to flecainide at 33 weeks' gestation (20). The tachycardia recurred 2 weeks later and a cesarean section was performed under epidural anesthesia with lidocaine to deliver a 3380-g male infant (follow-up of the infant not specified).

A historic cohort study, first published as an abstract (21) and then as a full report (22), described the fetal effects of maternal treatment with amiodarone. Twelve women, with various heart conditions requiring amiodarone therapy, were treated with individualized therapeutic doses (mean dose 321 mg/day) during gestation. Seven patients were treated throughout their pregnancies with one suffering a spontaneous abortion at 10 weeks. β-Blockers were used concurrently in the six pregnancies that delivered live newborns, but in one the β-blocker was stopped after 14 weeks. In the other five women, treatment with amiodarone was begun in the 2nd or 3rd trimester, and concurrent β-blockers were used in three for various intervals. The 11 infants were delivered at term (>37 weeks' gestation). Amiodarone was detected in two of three cord blood samples. The level in one was 0.2 mcg/mL (maternal serum not detectable), and the cord blood level in the other was 21.3% of the maternal concentration. One of the newborns was hyperthyroid (asymptomatic, transient) and one was hypothyroid. Fetal bradycardia occurred in three of the infants, two of whom had been exposed to β-blockers (acebutolol and propranolol). Four infants were small for gestational age (<3rd percentile corrected for gestational age) and three of these had been exposed to β-blockers throughout pregnancy. Two infants had birth defects, only one of whom had been exposed during the 1st trimester. This infant had congenital jerk nystagmus with synchronous head titubation (exposed to amiodarone and propranolol throughout, and quinidine during the 1st 3 weeks). The other newborn had hypotonia, hypertelorism, and micrognathia (exposed to amiodarone from the 20th week, atenolol from 18 to 20 weeks, and phenoxybenzamine during week 39), as well as delayed motor development assessed at 18 months (normal speech but milestone delay of about 3 months as indicated by lifting head, sitting unaided, crawling, standing, and walking). The child's birth weight and Apgar scores had been normal for gestational age and his neonatal course, other than a meconium plug, had been unremarkable. Other than this case, the other exposed infants had normal development (mean age at follow-up 30 months, range 0 months to 11.5 years) (22).

Congenital defects have been observed in two newborns, but any association between amiodarone and the defects may be fortuitous. Ventricular septal defects reportedly occur at an incidence of 1–3/1000 live births (16). The transient bradycardia and prolonged QT interval observed in some amiodarone-newborns are direct effects of the drug but apparently lack clinical significance. Intrauterine growth restriction occurs frequently in infants exposed in utero to amiodarone, but it is uncertain whether this is a consequence of amiodarone, the mother's disease, other drug therapy (such as β-blockers), or a combination of these and other factors. Growth restriction has also been observed in animal studies. Because of the above outcomes and the limited data available, the drug should be used cautiously during pregnancy. As a result of the potential for fetal and newborn toxicity, it is not recommended as a first-line drug in uncomplicated cases of fetal supraventricular tachycardia (23).

Following chronic administration, amiodarone has a very long elimination half-life of 14–58 days (24). Therefore, the drug must be stopped several months before conception to avoid exposure in early gestation. A 1987 review of the management of cardiac arrhythmias during pregnancy recommends that amiodarone be restricted to refractory cases (25). Similarly, a 1992 review of maternal drug therapy for fetal disorders suggests caution, if it is used at all, before amiodarone is prescribed during pregnancy (26).

BREASTFEEDING SUMMARY

Amiodarone is excreted into breast milk (2,3,8,9). The drug contains about 75 mg of iodine/200 mg dose (2,3,5). One woman consuming 400 mg/day had milk levels of amiodarone and its metabolite, desethylamiodarone (activity unknown), determined at varying times between 9 and 63 days after delivery (2). Levels of the two substances in milk were highly variable during any 24-hour period. Peak levels of amiodarone and the metabolite ranged from 3.6 to 16.4 and from 1.3 to 6.5 mcg/mL, respectively. The milk:plasma ratio of the active drug at 9 weeks postpartum ranged from 2.3 to 9.1 and that of desethylamiodarone from 0.8 to 3.8. The authors calculated that the nursing infant received about 1.4–1.5 mg/kg/day of active drug. Plasma levels of amiodarone in the infant remained constant at 0.4 mcg/mL (about 25% of maternal plasma) from birth to 63 days. In a second case, a mother taking 200 mg/day did not breastfeed, but milk levels of the drug and the metabolite on the second and third days after delivery were 0.5–1.8 and 0.4–0.8 mcg/mL, respectively (3). A mother taking 400 mg/day had milk concentrations of amiodarone and the metabolite during the first postpartum month ranging from 1.06 to 3.65 and from 0.50 to 1.24 mcg/mL, respectively (8). No adverse effects were observed in her nursing infant.

Mothers of three breastfeeding infants had taken amiodarone, 200 mg/day, during pregnancy and continued the same dose in the postpartum period (9). Milk concentrations of the drug at various times after delivery in the three mothers were 1.70 (2 days postpartum) and 3.04 mcg/mL (3 weeks postpartum), 0.55 (4 weeks postpartum) and 0.03 mcg/mL (6 weeks postpartum), and 2.20 mcg/mL (at birth), respectively. The milk:plasma ratios at these times varied widely from 0.4 to 13.0, as did the milk concentrations of the metabolite (0.002–1.81 mcg/mL). Two of the infants had concentrations of amiodarone in their plasma of 0.01–0.03 mcg/mL.

Although no adverse effects were observed in the one breastfed infant, relatively large amounts of the drug and its metabolite are available through the milk. Amiodarone, after chronic administration, has a very long elimination half-life of 14–58 days in adults (24). Data in pediatric patients suggest a more rapid elimination, but the half-life in newborns has not been determined. The effects of chronic neonatal exposure to this drug are unknown. Because of this uncertainty and because of the high proportion of iodine contained in each dose (see also Potassium Iodide), breastfeeding is not recommended if the mother is currently taking amiodarone or has taken it chronically within the past several months.

The American Academy of Pediatrics, noting that hypothyroidism is a potential complication, classifies amiodarone as a drug for which the effect on nursing infants is unknown but may be of concern (27).

References

1. Candelpergher G, Buchberger R, Suzzi GL, Padrini R. Trans-placental passage of amiodarone: electrocardiographic and pharmacologic evidence in a newborn. G Ital Cardiol 1982;12:79–82.
2. McKenna WJ, Harris L, Rowland E, Whitelaw A, Storey G, Holt D. Amiodarone therapy during pregnancy. Am J Cardiol 1983;51:1231–3.
3. Pitcher D, Leather HM, Storey GAC, Holt DW. Amiodarone in pregnancy. Lancet 1983;1:597–8.
4. Product information. Cordarone. Wyeth-Ayerst Laboratories, 2000.
5. Robson DJ, Jeeva Raj MV, Storey GAC, Holt DW. Use of amiodarone during pregnancy. Postgrad Med J 1985;61:75–7.
6. Arnoux P, Seyral P, Llurens M, Djiane P, Potier A, Unal D, Cano JP, Serradimigni A, Rouault F. Amiodarone and digoxin for refractory fetal tachycardia. Am J Cardiol 1987;59:166–7.
7. Penn IM, Barrett PA, Pannikote V, Barnaby PF, Campbell JB, Lyons NR. Amiodarone in pregnancy. Am J Cardiol 1985;56:196–7.
8. Strunge P, Frandsen J, Andreasen F. Amiodarone during pregnancy. Eur Heart J 1988;9:106–9.
9. Plomp TA, Vulsma T, de Vijlder JJM. Use of amiodarone during pregnancy. Eur J Obstet Gynecol Reprod Biol 1992;43:201–7.
10. Gembruch U, Manz M, Bald R, Rüddel H, Redel DA, Schlebusch H, Nitsch J, Hansmann M. Repeated intravascular treatment with amiodarone in a fetus with refractory supraventricular tachycardia and hydrops fetalis. Am Heart J 1989;118:1335–8.
11. Rey E, Bachrach LK, Burrow GN. Effects of amiodarone during pregnancy. Can Med Assoc J 1987;136:959–60.
12. Widerhorn J, Bhandari AK, Bughi S, Rahimtoola SH, Elkayam U. Fetal and neonatal adverse effects profile of amiodarone treatment during pregnancy. Am Heart J 1991;122:1162–6.
13. Wladimiroff JW, Steward PA. Treatment of fetal cardiac arrhythmias. Br J Hosp Med 1985;34:134–40. As cited by Widerhorn J, Bhandari AK, Bughi S, Rahimtoola SH, Elkayam U. Fetal and neonatal adverse effects profile of amiodarone treatment during pregnancy. Am Heart J 1991;122:1162–6.
14. Foster CJ, Love HG. Amiodarone in pregnancy: case report and review of literature. Int J Cardiol 1988;20:307–16.
15. De Wolf D, De Schepper J, Verhaaren H, Deneyer M, Smitz J, Sacre-Smits L. Congenital hypothyroid goiter and amiodarone. Acta Paediatr Scand 1988;77:616–8.
16. Ovadia M, Brito M, Hoyer GL, Marcus FI. Human experience with amiodarone in the embryonic period. Am J Cardiol 1994;73:316–7.
17. Rey E, Duperron L, Gauthier R, Lemay M, Grignon A, LeLorier J. Transplacental treatment of tachycardia-induced fetal heart failure with verapamil and amiodarone: a case report. Am J Obstet Gynecol 1985;153:311–2.
18. Laurent M, Betremieux P, Biron Y, LeHelloco A. Neonatal hypothyroidism after treatment by amiodarone during pregnancy. Am J Cardiol 1987;60:942.
19. Flack NJ, Zosmer N, Bennett PR, Vaughan J, Fisk NM. Amiodarone given by three routes to terminate fetal atrial flutter associated with severe hydrops. Obstet Gynecol 1993;82:714–6.

20. Fulgencio JP, Hamza J. Anaesthesia for caesarean section in a patient receiving high dose amiodarone for fetal supraventricular tachycardia. Anaesthesia 1994;49:406–8.
21. Magee LA, Taddio A, Downar E, Sermer M, Boulton BC, Cameron D, Rosengarten M, Waxman M, Allen LC, Koren G. Pregnancy outcome following gestational exposure to amiodarone (abstract). Teratology 1994;49:398.
22. Magee LA, Downar E, Sermer M, Boulton BC, Allen LC, Koren G. Pregnancy outcome after gestational exposure to amiodarone in Canada. Am J Obstet Gynecol 1995;172:1307–11.
23. Ito S, Magee L, Smallhorn J. Drug therapy for fetal arrhythmias. Clin Perinatol 1994;21:543–72.
24. Sloskey GE. Amiodarone: a unique antiarrhythmic agent. Clin Pharm 1983;2:330–40.
25. Rotmensch HH, Rotmensch S, Elkayam U. Management of cardiac arrhythmias during pregnancy: current concepts. Drugs 1987;33:623–33.
26. Ward RM. Maternal drug therapy for fetal disorders. Semin Perinatol 1992;16:12–20.
27. Committee on Drugs, American Academy of Pediatrics. The transfer of drugs and other chemicals into human milk. Pediatrics 2001;108:776–89.

AMITRIPTYLINE

Antidepressant

PREGNANCY RECOMMENDATION: Human Data Suggest Low Risk
BREASTFEEDING RECOMMENDATION: Limited Human Data—Potential Toxicity

PREGNANCY SUMMARY

Although occasional reports have associated the therapeutic use of amitriptyline with congenital malformations, the bulk of the evidence indicates that these widely used drugs are relatively safe during pregnancy. The single case of gross overdose is suggestive of an association between amitriptyline, perphenazine, or both, and malformations, but without confirming evidence no conclusions can be determined. Because of the experience with tricyclic antidepressants, one review recommended that they were preferred during gestation over other antidepressants (1).

FETAL RISK SUMMARY

Two reviews found reports of amitriptyline-induced teratogenicity in animals: encephaloceles and bent tails in hamsters (2) and skeletal malformations in rats (1). However, reproduction studies conducted by the manufacturer in mice, rats, or rabbits with oral doses up to 13 times the maximum recommended human dose revealed no evidence of teratogenicity (3). The manufacturer does cite the teratogenicity of amitriptyline in mice, hamsters, rats, and rabbits when higher doses were used (3).

The manufacturer states that amitriptyline crosses the placenta (3). The relatively low molecular weight (approximately 314) is consistent with this finding.

In humans, limb reduction anomalies have been reported with amitriptyline (4,5). However, analysis of 522,630 births, 86 with 1st trimester exposure to amitriptyline, did not confirm an association with this defect (6–13). Reported malformations other than limb reduction defects after therapeutic dosing included: micrognathia, anomalous right mandible, left pes equinovarus (1 case); swelling of hands and feet (1 case); hypospadias (1 case); and bilateral anophthalmia (1 case) (8,12–14).

A case of maternal suicide attempt with a combination of amitriptyline (725 mg) and perphenazine (58 mg) at 8 days' gestation was described in a 1980 abstract (15). An infant was eventually delivered with multiple congenital defects. The abnormalities included microcephaly, "cotton-like" hair with pronounced shedding, cleft palate, micrognathia, ambiguous genitalia, foot deformities, and undetectable dermal ridges (15).

Thanatophoric dwarfism was found in a stillborn infant exposed throughout gestation to amitriptyline (>150 mg/day), phenytoin (200 mg/day), and phenobarbital (300 mg/day) (16). The cause of the malformation could not be determined, but both drug and genetic etiologies were considered.

In a surveillance study of Michigan Medicaid recipients involving 229,101 completed pregnancies conducted between 1985 and 1992, 467 newborns had been exposed to amitriptyline during the 1st trimester (F. Rosa, personal communication, FDA, 1993). A total of 25 (5.4%) major birth defects were observed (20 expected). Specific data were available for six defect categories, including (observed/expected) 6/5 cardiovascular defects, 0/1 oral clefts, 0/0 spina bifida, 2/1 polydactyly, 2/1 limb reduction defects, and 1/1 hypospadias. These data do not support an association between the drug and the defects.

In a 1996 descriptive case series, the European Network of the Teratology Information Services (ENTIS) prospectively examined the outcomes of 689 pregnancies exposed to antidepressants (17). Multiple drug therapy occurred in about two-thirds of the mothers. Amitriptyline (118 exposures; one set of twins) was the second most commonly used tricyclic antidepressant. The outcomes of these pregnancies were 18 elective abortions, 10 spontaneous abortions, 2 stillbirths, 79 normal newborns (including 7 premature infants), 5 normal infants with neonatal disorders, 4 infants with congenital defects, and 1 premature infant with other complications. The defects (all exposed in the 1st trimester or longer) were small ventricular septal defect; single palmar crease and small palpebral fissure; facial microangioma and right hydrocele (exposed also to clobazam, as well as diphtheria, tetanus, and typhoid vaccines); and facial muscle asymmetry and glucose-6-phosphate dehydrogenase (G6PD) deficiency (exposed also to clonazepam and oxazepam) (17).

Neonatal withdrawal after in utero exposure to other antidepressants (see Imipramine), but not with amitriptyline, has been reported. However, the potential for this complication exists because of the close similarity among these compounds. Urinary retention in the neonate has been associated with maternal use of nortriptyline, an amitriptyline metabolite (see Nortriptyline) (18).

A 2002 prospective study compared two groups of mother–child pairs exposed to antidepressants throughout gestation (46 exposed to tricyclics—18 to amitriptyline; 40 to fluoxetine) to 36 nonexposed, not depressed controls (19). Offspring were studied between the ages 15 and 71 months for effects of antidepressant exposure in terms of IQ, language, behavior, and temperament. Exposure to antidepressants did not adversely affect the measured parameters, but IQ was significantly and negatively associated with the duration of depression, and language was negatively associated with the number of depression episodes after delivery (19).

BREASTFEEDING SUMMARY

Amitriptyline and its active metabolites are excreted into breast milk (20–24). A recent study has measured the amount of a second active metabolite, E-10-hydroxynortriptyline, in milk (23).

Serum and milk concentrations of amitriptyline in one patient were 0.14 and 0.15 mcg/mL, respectively, a milk:plasma ratio of 1.0 (20). No drug was detected in the infant's serum. In another patient, it was estimated that the baby received about 1% of the mother's dose (22). No clinical signs of drug activity were observed in the infant.

In another study, the mother was treated with 175 mg/day of amitriptyline (23). Milk and maternal serum samples were analyzed for active drug and active metabolites on postpartum days 1–26. Amitriptyline serum levels ranged from 24 (day 1) to 71 ng/mL (days 3–26), whereas those in the milk ranged from 24 ng/mL (day 1) to only 54% of the serum levels on days 2–26. Nortriptyline serum levels ranged from 17 (day 1) to 87 ng/mL (day 26) with milk levels 74% of those in the serum. Mean concentration of the second metabolite, E-10-hydroxynortriptyline, was 127 ng/mL (days 1–26) in the serum and 70% of that in the milk. The total dose (parent drug plus metabolites) consumed by the male infant on day 26 was estimated to be 35 mcg/kg (80 times lower than the mother's dose). The compounds were not detected in the nursing infant's serum on day 26 and no adverse effects, including sedation, were observed in him (23).

Ten nursing infants of mothers taking antidepressants (two with amitriptyline 100–175 mg/day) were compared with 15 bottle-fed infants of mothers with depression who did not breastfeed (24). Concentrations of clomipramine in fore- and hind-milk were 30 ng/mL (one patient) and 113 and 197 ng/mL (two patients), respectively. The milk:maternal plasma ratios were 0.2 and 0.9, respectively. One infant had a plasma level of 7.5 ng/mL when the mother was taking 100 mg/day. No toxic effects or delays in development were observed in the infants. The estimated daily dose consumed by the infants was about 1% of the mother's weight-adjusted dose (24).

A 1996 review of antidepressant treatment during breastfeeding found no information that amitriptyline exposure of the infant during nursing caused adverse effects (25).

Although amitriptyline and its metabolite have not been detected in infant serum, the effects of exposure to small amounts in the milk are unknown (26). The American Academy of Pediatrics classifies amitriptyline as a drug whose effect on the nursing infant is unknown but may be of concern (27).

References

1. Elia J, Katz IR, Simpson GM. Teratogenicity of psychotherapeutic medications. Psychopharmacol Bull 1987;23:531–86.
2. Shepard TH. *Catalog of Teratogenic Agents*. 6th ed. Baltimore, MD: Johns Hopkins University Press, 1989:44–5.
3. Product information. Elavil. AstraZeneca, 2000.
4. McBride WG. Limb deformities associated with iminodibenzyl hydrochloride. Med J Aust 1972;1:492.
5. Freeman R. Limb deformities: possible association with drugs. Med J Aust 1972;1:606.
6. Australian Drug Evaluation Committee. Tricyclic antidepressants and limb reduction deformities. Med J Aust 1973;1:768–9.
7. Heinonen OP, Slone D, Shapiro S. *Birth Defects and Drugs in Pregnancy*. Littleton, MA: Publishing Sciences Group, 1977:336–7.
8. Idanpaan-Heikkila J, Saxen L. Possible teratogenicity of imipramine/chloropyramine. Lancet 1973;2:282–3.
9. Rachelefsky GS, Glynt JW, Ebbin AJ, Wilson MG. Possible teratogenicity of tricyclic antidepressants. Lancet 1972;1:838.
10. Banister P, Dafoe C, Smith ESO, Miller J. Possible teratogenicity of tricyclic antidepressants. Lancet 1972;1:838–9.
11. Scanlon FJ. Use of antidepressant drugs during the first trimester. Med J Aust 1969;2:1077.
12. Crombie DL, Pinsent R, Fleming D. Imipramine in pregnancy. Br Med J 1972;1:745.
13. Kuenssberg EV, Knox JDE. Imipramine in pregnancy. Br Med J 1972;2:292.
14. Golden SM, Perman KI. Bilateral clinical anophthalmia: drugs as potential factors. South Med J 1980;73:1404–7.
15. Wertelecki W, Purvis-Smith SG, Blackburn WR. Amitriptyline/perphenazine maternal overdose and birth defects (abstract). Teratology 1980;21:74A.
16. Rafla NM, Meehan FP. Thanatophoric dwarfism: drugs and antenatal diagnosis. A case report. Eur J Obstet Gynecol Reprod Biol 1990;38:161–5.
17. McElhatton PR, Garbis HM, Elefant E, Vial T, Bellemin B, Mastroiacovo P, Arnon J, Rodriguez-Pinilla E, Schaefer C, Pexieder T, Merlob P, Dal Verme S. The outcome of pregnancy in 689 women exposed to therapeutic doses of antidepressants. A collaborative study of the European Network of Teratology Information Services (ENTIS). Reprod Toxicol 1996;10:285–94.
18. Shearer WT, Schreiner RL, Marshall RE. Urinary retention in a neonate secondary to maternal ingestion of nortriptyline. J Pediatr 1972;81:570–2.
19. Nulman I, Rovet J, Stewart DE, Wolpin J, Pace-Asciak P, Shuhaiber S, Koren G. Child development following exposure to tricyclic antidepressants or fluoxetine throughout fetal life: a prospective, controlled study. Am J Psychiatry 2002;159:1889–95.
20. Bader TF, Newman K. Amitriptyline in human breast milk and the nursing infants serum. Am J Psychiatry 1980;137;855–6.
21. Wilson JT, Brown D, Cherek DR, Dailey JW, Hilman B, Jobe PC, Manno BR, Manno JE, Redetzki HM, Stewart JJ. Drug excretion in human breast milk. Principles, pharmacokinetics and projected consequences. Clin Pharmacokinet 1980;5:1–66.
22. Brixen-Rasmussen L, Halgrener J, Jorgensen A. Amitriptyline and nortriptyline excretion in human breast milk. Psychopharmacology (Berlin) 1982;76:94–5.
23. Breyer-Pfaff U, Nill K, Entenmann A, Gaertner HJ. Secretion of amitriptyline and metabolites into breast milk. Am J Psychiatry 1995;152:812–3.
24. Yoshida K, Smith B, Craggs M, Kumar RC. Investigation of pharmacokinetics and of possible adverse effects in infants exposed to tricyclic antidepressants in breast-milk. J Affect Disord 1997;43:225–37.
25. Wisner KL, Perel JM, Findling RL. Antidepressant treatment during breastfeeding. Am J Psychiatry 1996;153:1132–7.
26. Erickson SH, Smith GH, Heidrich F. Tricyclics and breast feeding. Am J Psychiatry 1979;136:1483.
27. Committee on Drugs, American Academy of Pediatrics. The transfer of drugs and other chemicals into human milk. Pediatrics 2001;108:776–89.

AMLODIPINE

Calcium Channel Blocker

PREGNANCY RECOMMENDATION: Limited Human Data—Animal Data Suggest Moderate Risk
BREASTFEEDING RECOMMENDATION: Limited Human Data—Probably Compatible

PREGNANCY SUMMARY

Three reports, totaling five pregnancies, have described the use of amlodipine in human pregnancy. The outcomes of these pregnancies were two normal term-infants, one growth-restricted newborn (no relationship to drug because of timing of exposure), one fetal death (cause unknown, but possibly related to other exposures), and one neonate with a rare skin disease (doubtful relationship to drug).

FETAL RISK SUMMARY

Amlodipine is a calcium channel blocking agent used in the treatment of hypertension and angina. It is the same calcium channel blocker subclass as nine other agents (see Appendix). Amlodipine is extensively converted to inactive metabolites. Plasma protein binding is about 93% and the terminal elimination half-life is about 30–50 hours (1).

The drug is not teratogenic or embryotoxic in rats and rabbits given doses up to 8 and 23 times, respectively, the maximum recommended human dose based on BSA (MRHD) during organogenesis. However, rats administered 8 times the MRHD for 14 days before mating and throughout gestation had a significant decrease in litter size (by about 50%), a significant increase in intrauterine deaths (about fivefold), and prolonged labor and gestation. This dose, however, had no effect on fertility in the rat (1).

It is not known if amlodipine crosses the human placenta. The molecular weight (about 567 for the besylate salt) and the long terminal elimination half-life suggest that it will cross to the embryo–fetus.

A 1998 case report described an unusual condition in a neonate whose mother had been treated for hypertension with amlodipine throughout gestation (2). The 3.97-kg male infant had been born at 39 weeks' with meconium staining of the amniotic fluid at Apgar scores of 3 and 8 at 1 and 5 minutes, respectively, and required oxygen therapy. At 24 hours of age, the infant developed firm, red, pea-sized nodular lesions over most of his body. The skin lesions were extremely tender requiring morphine analgesia. A skin biopsy revealed needle-like crystals within adipocytes of the SC fat. On the second day of life, he had two generalized tonic–clonic seizures. Although his general clinical condition improved over the 1st week of life with no further seizures, the skin changes, diagnosed as SC fat necrosis of the newborn, persisted until 9 months of age. The cause of the infant's condition was unknown (2).

A 2007 report described three hypertensive women exposed to amlodipine in the 1st trimester (3). In the first case, the mother took amlodipine 5 mg/day until 7 weeks' gestation and then declined further treatment. Her blood pressure remained in good control throughout gestation. At about 38 weeks, she delivered a healthy, 3750-g female infant with Apgar scores of 9 and 10 at 1 and 5 minutes, respectively. The infant was healthy at 3 months of age with normal development (see also Breastfeeding Summary). The second case involved treatment with amlodipine until about 2 weeks' gestation at which time the therapy was changed to atenolol 50 mg/day. Just before the seventh week the woman declined further treatment. Her blood pressure remained in good control throughout pregnancy. The growth-restricted (2600 g; $<$10th percentile), but otherwise-normal female infant was born at about 39 weeks' with Apgar scores of 8 and 9 at 1 and 5 minutes, respectively. At 20 months of age, the 10-kg child was still growth-restricted, and intellectual delay and weakness in the left arm and hand grasp were noted. The cause of the condition was unknown but not thought to be related to the drug therapy. The third case involved a woman with polycystic kidney disease and hypertension that was being treated with imidapril 5 mg/day (an ACE inhibitor) and barnidipine 10 mg/day (a calcium channel blocker) in an unknown pregnancy. Because of uncontrolled blood pressure, her therapy was changed at about 8 weeks' to amlodipine 5 mg/day. The mother also was taking sucralfate for acute gastritis and lorazepam for anxiety, and reported occasional use of 1 ounce of alcohol. At 12 weeks', an ultrasound revealed no cardiac activity and she underwent dilatation and evacuation of a dead fetus (3).

A 26-year-old woman with pulmonary arterial hypertension conceived while taking amlodipine (dose not specified) and warfarin (4). Warfarin was discontinued (exact gestational timing not specified) and replaced with enoxaparin. The patient remained on amlodipine and enoxaparin throughout pregnancy. At about 38 weeks', a cesarean section was performed to deliver a 3123-g male infant with Apgar scores of 9 and 9. The infant went home with his mother, and no other information was provided on the infant (4).

BREASTFEEDING SUMMARY

The molecular weight (about 567 for the besylate salt) and the long terminal elimination half-life (30–50 hours) suggest that it will be excreted into breast milk. The effect of this exposure on a nursing infant is unknown. However, no adverse effects were reported in the case below.

A mother 2 weeks postpartum, who was exclusively breastfeeding her infant, was restarted on amlodipine 5 mg/day to control her hypertension (3). At 3 months of age, the healthy female infant weighed 6.3 kg (25th–50th percentile) and had normal physical and neurodevelopment.

Although not mentioning amlodipine, the American Academy of Pediatrics classifies nifedipine, another calcium channel blocker, as compatible with breastfeeding (5).

References

1. Product information. Norvasc. Pfizer, 2000.
2. Rosbotham JL, Johnson A, Haque KN, Holden CA. Painful subcutaneous fat necrosis of the newborn associated with intra-partum use of a calcium channel blocker. Clin Exp Dermatol 1998;23:19–21.
3. Ahn HK, Nava-Ocampo AA, Han JY, Choi JS, Chung JH, Yang JY, Koong MK, Park CT. Exposure to amlodipine in the first trimester of pregnancy and during breastfeeding. Hypertens Pregnancy 2007;26:179–87.
4. Nahapetian A, Oudiz RJ. Serial hemodynamics and complications of pregnancy in severe pulmonary arterial hypertension. Cardiology 2008;109: 237–40.
5. Committee on Drugs, American Academy of Pediatrics. The transfer of drugs and other chemicals into human milk. Pediatrics 2001;108: 776–89.

AMMONIUM CHLORIDE

Respiratory Drug (Expectorant), Urinary Acidifier

PREGNANCY RECOMMENDATION: Compatible
BREASTFEEDING RECOMMENDATION: No Human Data—Probably Compatible

PREGNANCY SUMMARY

Although the data are limited and there are no animal reproduction data, there is no evidence suggesting that usual doses of ammonium chloride present an embryo or fetal risk.

FETAL RISK SUMMARY

The Collaborative Perinatal Project monitored 50,282 mother–child pairs, 365 of whom had 1st trimester exposure to ammonium chloride as an expectorant in cough medications (1, pp. 378–381). For use anytime during pregnancy, 3401 exposures were recorded (1, p. 442). In neither group was evidence found to suggest a relationship to large categories of major or minor malformations. Three possible associations with individual malformations were found but independent confirmation is required to determine the actual risk: inguinal hernia (1st trimester only) (11 cases); cataract (6 cases); and any benign tumor (17 cases) (1, pp. 478, 496)

When consumed in large quantities near term, ammonium chloride may cause acidosis in the mother and the fetus (2,3). In some cases, the decreased pH and pCO_2, increased lactic acid, and reduced oxygen saturation were as severe as those seen with fatal apnea neonatorum. However, the newborns did not appear in distress.

BREASTFEEDING SUMMARY

No reports describing the use of ammonium chloride during lactation have been located.

References

1. Heinonen OP, Slone D, Shapiro S. *Birth Defects and Drugs in Pregnancy*. Littleton, MA: Publishing Sciences Group, 1977.
2. Goodlin RC, Kaiser IH. The effect of ammonium chloride induced maternal acidosis on the human fetus at term. I. pH, hemoglobin, blood gases. Am J Med Sci 1957;233:666–74.
3. Kaiser IH, Goodlin RC. The effect of ammonium chloride induced maternal acidosis on the human fetus at term. II. Electrolytes. Am J Med Sci 1958;235:549–54.

AMOBARBITAL

Sedative/Hypnotic

PREGNANCY RECOMMENDATION: Limited Human Data—No Relevant Animal Data
BREASTFEEDING RECOMMENDATION: No Human Data—Potential Toxicity

PREGNANCY SUMMARY

Although the data are limited, there is evidence of structural anomalies in newborns exposed to amobarbital during organogenesis. The absolute risk is unknown but may be low. The drug also is eliminated slowly in newborns. If possible, the drug should be avoided during organogenesis and near delivery.

FETAL RISK SUMMARY

Amobarbital is a member of the barbiturate class. The drug crosses the placenta, achieving levels in the cord serum similar to those in the maternal serum (1,2). Single or continuous dosing of the mother near term does not induce amobarbital hydroxylation in the fetus as demonstrated by the prolonged elimination of the drug in the newborn (half-life 2.5 times maternal). An increase in the incidence of congenital defects in infants exposed in utero to amobarbital has been reported (3,4, pp. 336, 344). In one survey of 1369 patients exposed to multiple drugs, 273 received amobarbital during the 1st trimester (3). Ninety-five of the exposed mothers delivered infants with major or minor abnormalities. Malformations associated with barbiturates, in general, were as follows:

Anencephaly	Congenital dislocation of the hip
Congenital heart disease	Soft-tissue deformity of the neck
Severe limb deformities	Hypospadias
Cleft lip and palate	Accessory auricle
Intersex	Polydactyly
Papilloma of the forehead	Nevus
Hydrocele.	

The Collaborative Perinatal Project monitored 50,282 mother–child pairs, 298 of whom had 1st trimester exposure to amobarbital (4, pp. 336, 344). For use anytime during pregnancy, 867 exposures were recorded (4, p. 438). A possible association was found between the use of the drug in the 1st trimester and the following: cardiovascular malformations (7 cases), polydactyly in blacks (2 cases in 29 blacks), genitourinary malformations other than hypospadias (3 cases), inguinal hernia (9 cases), and clubfoot (4 cases).

In contrast to the above reports, a 1964 survey of 187 pregnant patients who had received various neuroleptics, including amobarbital, found a 3.1% incidence of malformations in the offspring (5). This is approximately the expected incidence of abnormalities in a nonexposed population. Arthrogryposis and multiple defects were reported in an infant exposed to amobarbital during the 1st trimester (6). The defects were attributed to immobilization of the limbs at the time of joint formation, multiple drug use, and active tetanus.

BREASTFEEDING SUMMARY

No reports describing the use of amobarbital during lactation have been located. Similar to other barbiturates, the drug probably is excreted into breast milk. The effects of this exposure are unknown, but toxicity is possible (e.g., see Phenobarbital).

References

1. Kraver B, Draffan GH, Williams FM, Calre RA, Dollery CT, Hawkins DF. Elimination kinetics of amobarbital in mothers and newborn infants. Clin Pharmacol Ther 1973;14:442–7.
2. Draffan GH, Dollery CT, Davies DS, Krauer B, Williams FM, Clare RA, Trudinger BJ, Darling M, Sertel H, Hawkins DF. Maternal and neonatal elimination of amobarbital after treatment of the mother with barbiturates during late pregnancy. Clin Pharmacol Ther 1976;19:271–5.
3. Nelson MM, Forfar JO. Associations between drugs administered during pregnancy and congenital abnormalities of the fetus. Br Med J 1971;1:523–7.
4. Heinonen OP, Slone D, Shapiro S. *Birth Defects and Drugs in Pregnancy*. Littleton, MA: Publishing Sciences Group, 1977.
5. Favre-Tissot M. An original clinical study of the pharmacologic-teratogenic relationship. Ann Med Psychol (Paris) 1964;1:389.
6. Jago RH. Arthrogryposis following treatment of maternal tetanus with muscle relaxants. Arch Dis Child 1970;45:277–9.

AMOXAPINE

Antidepressant

PREGNANCY RECOMMENDATION: Limited Human Data—Animal Data Suggest Risk
BREASTFEEDING RECOMMENDATION: Limited Human Data—Potential Toxicity

PREGNANCY SUMMARY

The animal data suggest risk, but the human pregnancy experience is too limited to assess the embryo–fetal risk. Until such data are available, the safest course may be to avoid amoxapine during organogenesis.

FETAL RISK SUMMARY

No published reports linking the use of amoxapine with congenital defects have been located. Reproductive studies in mice, rats, and rabbits have found no teratogenicity, but embryotoxicity was observed in rats and rabbits given oral doses approximating the human dose (1). Intrauterine death, stillbirths, decreased weight, and decreased neonatal survival (days 0–4) were seen with oral doses at 3–10 times the human dose.

In a surveillance study of Michigan Medicaid recipients involving 229,101 completed pregnancies conducted between 1985 and 1992, 19 newborns had been exposed to amoxapine during the 1st trimester (F. Rosa, personal communication, FDA, 1993). Three (15.8%) major birth defects were observed (one expected). Data on the specific types of defects were not available, but no cases of cardiovascular defects, oral clefts, spina bifida, polydactyly, limb reduction defects, and hypospadias were observed. Although the total incidence of anomalies is high, the number of exposures is too small to draw a conclusion.

BREASTFEEDING SUMMARY

Amoxapine and its metabolite are excreted into breast milk. A 29-year-old woman suffering from depression was treated with approximately 250 mg/day of amoxapine (2). She developed galactorrhea and oligomenorrhea. Milk samples were collected after 10 and 11 months of therapy and analyzed for amoxapine and the active metabolite, 8-hydroxyamoxapine. The levels of the parent compound at the sample collection times were both <20 ng/mL, but the metabolite was present in both samples, 45 minutes after the last dose at 10 months and 11.5 hours after the last dose at 11 months. Levels of the active metabolite at these times were 113 and 168 ng/mL, respectively. A venous blood specimen obtained simultaneously with the first milk sample had concentrations of amoxapine and 8-hydroxyamoxapine of 97 and 375 ng/mL, respectively. The American Academy of Pediatrics classifies amoxapine as a drug whose effect on the nursing infant is unknown but may be of concern (3).

References

1. Product information. Asendin. Lederle Laboratories, 1997.
2. Gelenberg AJ. Amoxapine, a new antidepressant, appears in human milk. J Nerv Ment Dis 1979;167:635–6.
3. Committee on Drugs, American Academy of Pediatrics. The transfer of drugs and other chemicals into human milk. Pediatrics 2001;108:776–89.

AMOXICILLIN

Antibiotic (Penicillin)

PREGNANCY RECOMMENDATION: **Human Data Suggest Risk in 1st and 3rd Trimesters**
BREASTFEEDING RECOMMENDATION: **Compatible**

PREGNANCY SUMMARY

Penicillins are generally considered low risk at any stage of pregnancy. This assessment may have to be modified for the aminopenicillins (ampicillin and amoxicillin) because there is some evidence that exposure to these two antibiotics during organogenesis is associated with oral clefts (see also Ampicillin). However, even if the association is causal, the absolute risk is very low. In addition, one study reported an association between amoxicillin–clavulanic acid and necrotizing enterocolitis (NEC) when the antibiotic combination was used near preterm birth. Both of these associations require confirmation.

FETAL RISK SUMMARY

Amoxicillin is an aminopenicillin antibiotic similar to ampicillin. The antibiotic is known to cross the placenta.

Reproduction studies have been conducted in mice and rats at doses up to 10 times the human dose. No effect on fertility or fetal harm was observed at this dose (1).

The Collaborative Perinatal Project monitored 50,282 mother–child pairs, 3546 of whom had 1st trimester exposure to penicillin derivatives (2, pp. 297–313). For use anytime during pregnancy, 7171 exposures were recorded (2, p. 435). In neither group was evidence found to suggest a relationship to large categories of major or minor malformations or to individual defects. Amoxicillin has been used as a single 3-g dose to treat bacteriuria in pregnancy without causing fetal harm (3,4).

In a surveillance study of Michigan Medicaid recipients involving 229,101 completed pregnancies conducted between 1985 and 1992, 8538 newborns had been exposed to amoxicillin during the 1st trimester (F. Rosa, personal communication, FDA, 1993). A total of 317 (3.7%) major birth defects were observed (363 expected). Specific data were available for six defect categories, including (observed/expected) 76/85 cardiovascular defects, 16/14 oral clefts, 6/7 spina bifida, 17/24 polydactyly, 9/16 limb reduction defects, and 22/22 hypospadias. These data do not support an association between the drug and the defects.

Several reports have described the use of amoxicillin in pregnancy, either for preterm pre-labor rupture of membranes (5,6) or for the treatment of prenatal *Chlamydia* infection (7–10). The latter reference is of particular interest because of the potential for fetal–newborn harm when amoxicillin–clavulanic acid (ACA) was used. A 2001 randomized study (ORACLE 1) was conducted in patients with preterm, pre-labor rupture of fetal membranes to determine neonatal health benefits of three antibiotic regimens (10). The regimens, compared with a placebo group (N = 1225) were erythromycin (250 mg) (N = 1197), amoxicillin (250 mg)–clavulanic acid (125 mg) (N = 1212), or both (N = 1192) four times daily for 10 days or until delivery. The primary outcome measures were specific outcomes or a composite of neonatal death, chronic lung disease, or major cerebral abnormality. For these neonatal outcomes, the two groups with ACA had no benefit over placebo, whereas erythromycin use resulted in significantly better outcomes (both composite and specific). When any-ACA exposure was compared with no-ACA for outcomes with suspected or proven NEC, the results were 92 (3.8%) and 58 (2.4%) (p = 0.004). The authors thought that a possible mechanism for this outcome was that the ACA combination selected for *Clostridium difficile* and that abnormal colonization of the neonatal intestinal tract was one possible mechanism for NEC (10).

A population based from Denmark examined the association between amoxicillin use in pregnancy and birth weight, preterm birth, congenital anomalies, perinatal death, and spontaneous abortion (SAB) (11). During the study period (1991–2000), 401 primiparous women obtained a prescription for the antibiotic. The control group consisted of 10,237 primiparous women who did not redeem any prescriptions from 3 months before pregnancy until the end of pregnancy. The mean birth weight of subjects was 57 g (95% confidence interval [CI] 9–105) higher than controls. The odds ratio and 95% CI for the other outcomes were as follows: low birth weight (0.63, 0.26–1.53); preterm birth (0.77, 0.49–1.21); congenital anomalies (1.16, 0.54–2.50); and SAB (0.89, 0.66–1.18) (11).

In a 2004 study, 191 women treated with ACA (subjects) in the 1st trimester were matched with 191 controls exposed to amoxicillin only (12). Maternal age, birth weight, gestational age at birth, and rates of live births and abortions were comparable between the two groups. The rates of major malformations in subjects (3/158, 1.9%) and controls (5/163, 3%) (p = 0.49; relative risk 0.62, 95% CI 0.15–2.55) were within the expected baseline risk for the general population. There were no cases of oral clefts (12).

A retrospective cohort study using data from Tennessee Medicaid included 30,049 infants born in 1985–2000 was published in 2009 (13). Infants with fetal exposures in the 1st trimester to four antibiotics recommended for potential bioterrorism attacks (amoxicillin, ciprofloxacin, azithromycin, and doxycycline) were compared to infants with no fetal exposure to any antibiotic. Erythromycin was included as a positive control. In the 7216 infants exposed to amoxicillin and no other antibiotics, the number of cases, risk ratios, and 95% CI were as follows: any malformation (232, 1.09, 0.55–1.37), cardiac (89, 1.15, 0.79–1.68); musculoskeletal (52, 1.05, 0.66–1.69); genitourinary (52, 1.38, 0.78–2.43); gastrointestinal (26, 0.63, 0.35–1.16); CNS (23, 1.08, 0.50–2.32); and orofacial (15, 1.67, 0.56–5.04). The authors concluded that the four antibiotics should not result in a greater incidence of overall major malformations (see also Azithromycin, Ciprofloxacin, and Doxycycline) (13).

A 2012 study used data from the Slone Epidemiology Center Birth Defects Study (1994–2008) to identify 877 infants with cleft lip with/without cleft palate and 471 with cleft palate alone (14). Controls included 6952 infants without defects, 2.1% of whom were exposed to amoxicillin. The adjusted odds ratio (OR) for cleft lip with/without cleft palate for exposure in the 1st trimester was 2.0 (95% CI 1.0–4.1). For third gestational month exposure, the results were OR 4.3 (95% CI 1.4–13.0). For cleft palate, the results for the two exposure periods were OR 1.0 (95% CI 0.4–2.3) and OR 7.1 (95% CI 1.4–36). No elevated risks were observed for other penicillins or cephalosporins, but the risk for ampicillin could not be evaluated because there were fewer than five exposed subjects. Because the risk for oral clefts among penicillins appeared to be related only to the aminopenicillins (ampicillin and amoxicillin), the authors speculated that the aminobenzyl group has a role in the development of oral clefts. Even so, the background risk for oral clefts is about 1–2 per 1000 and a twofold risk would increase the risk to only 2–4 per 1000 (14).

BREASTFEEDING SUMMARY

Amoxicillin is excreted into breast milk in low concentrations. Following a 1-g oral dose given to six mothers, peak milk levels occurred at 4–5 hours, averaging 0.9 mcg/mL (range 0.68–1.3 mcg/mL) (15). Mean milk:plasma ratios at 1, 2, and 3 hours were 0.014, 0.013, and 0.043, respectively. Although no adverse effects have been observed, three potential problems exist for the nursing infant: modification of bowel flora, direct effects on the infant (e.g., allergy or sensitization), and interference with the interpretation of culture results if a fever workup is required.

In a 1993 cohort study, diarrhea was reported in 32 (19.3%) nursing infants of 166 breastfeeding mothers who were taking antibiotics (16). For the 25 women taking amoxicillin, diarrhea was observed in 3 (12%) infants. The diarrhea was considered minor because it did not require medical attention (16).

The American Academy of Pediatrics classifies amoxicillin as compatible with breastfeeding (17).

References

1. Product information. Amoxil. SmithKline Beecham Pharmaceuticals, 2000.
2. Heinonen OP, Slone D, Shapiro S. *Birth Defects and Drugs in Pregnancy*. Littleton, MA: Publishing Sciences Group, 1977.
3. Masterton RG, Evans DC, Strike PW. Single-dose amoxycillin in the treatment of bacteriuria in pregnancy and the puerperium—a controlled clinical trial. Br J Obstet Gynaecol 1985;92:498–505.
4. Jakobi P, Neiger R, Merzbach D, Paldi E. Single-dose antimicrobial therapy in the treatment of asymptomatic bacteriuria in pregnancy. Am J Obstet Gynecol 1987;156:1148–52.
5. Almeida L, Schmauch A, Bergstrom S. A randomised study on the impact of peroral amoxicillin in women with prelabour rupture of membranes preterm. Gynecol Obstet Invest 1996;41:82–4.
6. Magwali TL, Chipato T, Majoko F, Rusakaniko S, Mujaji C. Prophylactic augmentin in prelabor preterm rupture of the membranes. Int J Gynecol Obstet 1999;65:261–5.
7. Magat AH, Alger LS, Nagey DA, Hatch V, Lovchik JC. Double-blind randomized study comparing amoxicillin and erythromycin for the treatment of *Chlamydia trachomatis* in pregnancy. Obstet Gynecol 1993:81:745–9.
8. Alary M, Joly J-M, Mondor M, Boucher M, Fortier A, Pinault J-J, Paris G, Carrier S, Chamberland H, Bernatchez H, Paradis J-F. Randomised comparison of amoxycillin and erythromycin in treatment of genital chlamydia infection in pregnancy. Lancet 1994;344:1461–5.
9. Turrentin MA, Newton ER. Amoxicillin or erythromycin for the treatment of antenatal chlamydial infection: a meta-analysis. Obstet Gynecol 1995;86:1021–5.
10. Kenyon SL, Taylor DJ, Tarnow-Mordi W, for the ORACLE Collaborative Group. Broad-spectrum antibiotics for preterm, prelabour rupture of fetal membranes: the ORACLE I randomised trial. Lancet 2001;357:979–88.
11. Jepsen P, Skriver MV, Floyd A, Lipworth L, Schønheyder HC, Sørensen HT. A population-based study of maternal use of amoxicillin and pregnancy outcome in Denmark. Br J Clin Pharmacol 2003;55:216–21.
12. Berkovitch M, Diav-Citrin O, Greenberg R, Cohen M, Bulkowstein M, Shechtman S, Bortnik O, Arnon J. Ornoy A. First-trimester exposure to amoxycillin/clavulanic acid: a prospective, controlled study. Br J Clin Pharmacol 2004;58:298–302.
13. Cooper WO, Hernandez-Diaz S, Arbogast PG, Dudley JA, Dyer SM, Gideon PS, Hall KS, Kaltenbach LA, Ray WA. Antibiotics potentially used in response to bioterrorism and the risk of major congenital malformations. Paediatr Perinat Epidemiol 2009;23:18–28.
14. Lin KJ, Mitchell AA, Yau W-P, Louik C, Hernandez-Diaz S. Maternal exposure to amoxicillin and the risk of oral clefts. Epidemiology 2012;23:699–705.
15. Kafetzis D, Siafas C, Georgakopoulos P, Papadatos C. Passage of cephalosporins and amoxicillin into the breast milk. Acta Paediatr Scand 1981;70:285–8.
16. Ito S, Blajchman A, Stephenson M, Eliopoulos C, Koren G. Prospective follow-up of adverse reactions in breast-fed infants exposed to maternal medication. Am J Obstet Gynecol 1993;168:1393–9.
17. Committee on Drugs, American Academy of Pediatrics. The transfer of drugs and other chemicals into human milk. Pediatrics 2001;108:776–89.

AMPHETAMINE

Central Stimulant

PREGNANCY RECOMMENDATION: Human and Animal Data Suggest Risk
BREASTFEEDING RECOMMENDATION: Limited Human Data—Potential Toxicity Contraindicated (Nonmedical Use)

PREGNANCY SUMMARY

Although medicinal use of amphetamines appears to be low risk for embryo–fetal harm, abuse of the agent is associated with significant toxicity for the embryo, fetus, and newborn. Such use is contraindicated in pregnancy.

FETAL RISK SUMMARY

The amphetamines are a group of sympathomimetic drugs that are used to stimulate the central nervous system. Members of this group include amphetamine, dextroamphetamine, and methamphetamine. A number of studies have examined the possible relationship between amphetamines and adverse fetal outcome. Women were using these drugs for appetite suppression, narcolepsy, or illicit abuse purposes.

In near-term pregnant sheep administered IV doses at or below what is commonly regarded as abuse, methamphetamine rapidly crossed the placenta and accumulated in the fetus (1). Fetal blood pressure was increased 20%–37% with a decrease in fetal oxyhemoglobin saturation and arterial pH. Approximately similar results were reported in a 1993 abstract that also used pregnant sheep (2). Fetal concentrations of the drug were approximately the same as maternal levels during a 6-hour interval.

The question as to whether amphetamines are teratogenic in humans has been examined in a number of studies and single-patient case histories. Cardiac malformations and other defects were produced in mice injected with very large doses (about 200 times the usual human dose) of dextroamphetamine (3). These same investigators then retrospectively and prospectively examined human infants whose mothers had ingested the drug (4). In the retrospective portion of the study, 219 infants and children under 2 years of age with congenital heart disease were compared with 153 similar-age infants and children without heart defects. Neither maternal exposure to dextroamphetamine during pregnancy nor exposure during the vulnerable period differed statistically between the groups. However, a positive family history of congenital heart disease occurred in 31.1% of the infants with the defects compared with only 5.9% of the control group ($p = 0.001$). The prospective study compared 52 mothers with a documented exposure to dextroamphetamine during the vulnerable period with 50 nonexposed mothers. Neither group produced an infant with congenital heart disease, and the numbers of other congenital abnormalities were similar (nine vs. seven). Thus, this study found no evidence for an association between congenital heart defects and dextroamphetamine. However, in a follow-up study published 3 years later, the investigators reported a significant relationship between dextroamphetamine exposure and heart defects (5). Comparing 184 infants under 1 year of age with congenital heart disease with 108 control infants, significant differences were found for maternal exposure to dextroamphetamine (18% vs. 8%, $p < 0.05$), exposure during the vulnerable period (11% vs. 3%, $p = 0.025$), and positive family history of congenital heart disease (27% vs. 6%, $p < 0.001$). Infants who were both exposed during the vulnerable period and had a positive family history were statistically similar for the groups (5% vs. 1%).

In a fourth study by the above investigative group, 240 women were followed prospectively during their pregnancies to determine exposure to medicinal agents, radiation, and other potential teratogens (6). Thirty-one (13%) women consumed an appetite suppressant (usually dextroamphetamine) during the 1st trimester and an additional 34 (14%) were exposed later in pregnancy. Eight (3.3%) babies had a major congenital defect noted at birth, which is approximately the expected incidence in the United States. Three of the affected infants had been exposed during the 1st trimester to an appetite suppressant. Although the authors identified a wide range of maternal drug consumption during the 1st trimester, no conclusions as to the cause of the defects can be drawn from the data.

Four other reports have related various defects with amphetamine exposure (7–10). An infant with a bifid exencephalia was delivered from a mother who took 20–30 mg of dextroamphetamine daily throughout pregnancy (7). The infant died after an attempt was made at surgical correction. A second case involved a mother who ingested dextroamphetamine daily for appetite suppression and who delivered a full-term infant. The infant died 6 days later as a result of a congenital heart defect (8). Drug histories were obtained from mothers of 11 infants with biliary atresia and compared with the histories of 50 control mothers (9). Amphetamine exposure occurred in five women in the study group and in three of the controls. A 1966 report described a mother with two infants with microcephaly, mental retardation, and motor dysfunction (10). The mother had taken an appetite suppressant containing methamphetamine and phenobarbital during the 1st and 2nd trimesters of both pregnancies (pregnancy numbers 1 and 3). A spontaneous abortion occurred in pregnancy number 2, but no details were given of the mother's drug intake. Her fourth pregnancy, in which she did not take the appetite suppressant, resulted in the delivery of a normal child. There was no family history of developmental disorders, congenital defects, mental retardation, cerebral palsy, or epilepsy.

Fetal structural defects have been associated with maternal abuse of drugs in a large volume of literature (see also Ethanol, Cocaine, Heroin, Lysergic Acid Diethylamide [LSD], Marijuana, and Methadone). For example, in a 1972 case, multiple brain and eye anomalies were observed in an infant exposed in utero to amphetamines, LSD, meprobamate, and marijuana (11). In this and similar cases, the cause of the structural abnormalities is probably multifactorial, involving drug use, life-styles, infections, poor maternal health, and other factors.

In a retrospective study, 458 mothers who delivered infants with major (N = 175) or minor (N = 283) abnormalities were compared with 911 matched controls (12). Appetite suppressants were consumed during pregnancy by significantly more mothers of infants with anomalies than by controls (3.9% vs. 1.1%, $p < 0.01$). Dextroamphetamine consumption accounted for 13 of the 18 maternal exposures in the anomaly group. During the first 56 days of pregnancy, dextroamphetamine-containing compounds were used by 10 mothers in the anomaly group compared with only 5 of the controls (2.2% vs. 0.5%; $p < 0.05$). The abnormalities (3major and 7 minor) observed in the 10 infants were urogenital system defects (4 cases), and 1 case each of congenital heart disease, cleft lip, severe limb deformity, accessory auricles, congenital dislocation of hip, and pilonidal sinus. Although statistically significant results were found in this study, the results must be interpreted cautiously due to the retrospective collection of drug histories and the lack of information pertaining to past and present maternal medical and obstetric histories.

A prospective study of 1824 white mothers who took anorectic drugs (primarily amphetamines) during pregnancy compared with 8989 white mothers who did not take such drugs measured rates of severe congenital defects of 3.7% and 3.4%, respectively, in infants with a gestational age of at least 37 weeks (13). When children of all known gestational ages were included, amphetamine usage occurred in 85% (1694 of 1992) of the group consuming anorectic drugs. The incidence of severe congenital defects in the amphetamine group was 3.4%. Fourteen infants were exposed in the first 84 days after the last menstrual period, and except for three infants with cleft lip and/or palate, no pattern of malformations was observed.

The effects of amphetamine abuse on fetal outcome and subsequent development were described in a series of reports from Sweden (14–18). Twenty-three women who ingested amphetamine during the 1st trimester were divided into two groups: 6 who claimed that they stopped use of the drug after they became aware of their pregnancy or after the 1st trimester, and 17 who continued use of the drug throughout gestation (14). Two of the infants (group not specified) had congenital defects: a stillborn infant had myelomeningocele, and one had extensive telangiectasis (considered to be an inherited disorder). The outcome of the infants exposed throughout gestation included six preterm (<37 weeks), three small-for-gestational-age (all with poor prenatal care), one of whom had a seizure on the first day, and two full-term but extremely drowsy infants. In a later report, 66 infants born to amphetamine-addicted mothers were followed during their first year of life (16). Except for temporary drowsiness in the first few months, all children had normal somatic and psychomotor development at 12 months of age. In the final report from these investigators, the fetal outcome of 69 amphetamine-addicted women who delivered 71 children (1 delivered twice and 1 delivered twins) was described (17). Seventeen of the women claimed to have stopped amphetamine ingestion as previously described, and 52 continued use of amphetamines throughout pregnancy. Three women in the first group and 17 in the second group were alcoholics (18). Four infants had congenital defects: intestinal atresia (two cases—both died and one also had hydrocephalus), congenital heart defect (one case), and epidermolysis bullosa without known heredity (one case). In one of the four cases, the mother was an alcoholic, but the particular case was not specified. Drowsiness was observed in 8 infants and jitteriness in 11 infants; 4 full-term infants required tube feedings. The four studies (14–17) were combined into a single article published in 1980 (18).

The Collaborative Perinatal Project monitored 50,282 mother–child pairs, 671 of whom had 1st trimester exposure to amphetamines (19, pp. 346–347). For use anytime during pregnancy, 1898 exposures were recorded (19, p. 439). In neither group was evidence found to suggest a relationship to large categories of major or minor malformations. Two case reports failed to observe any neonatal effects from the treatment of narcolepsy with large doses of amphetamine (20,21). A 1988 report described a mother who had used amphetamines, barbiturates, cocaine, LSD, alcohol, and marijuana during pregnancy who delivered a female infant with bilateral cerebrovascular accident and resulting porencephaly (22). The infant expired at 2.5 months of age. The fetal injury was thought to be caused by cocaine (see also Cocaine).

A 1992 case report described the use of dextroamphetamine and lovastatin in a human pregnancy (23). A woman was treated for 5 weeks with the combination, starting approximately 6 weeks from her last menstrual period, for progressive weight gain and hypercholesterolemia. Therapy was discontinued when her pregnancy was diagnosed at 11 weeks' gestation. A female infant was delivered by cesarean section at 39 weeks' gestation. Gestational age was confirmed by an ultrasound examination at 21 weeks' gestation and the Dubowitz score at birth. The infant had a constellation of malformations termed the VATER association (vertebral anomalies, anal atresia, tracheoesophageal fistula with esophageal atresia, renal and radial dysplasias). Specific anomalies included an asymmetric chest, thoracic scoliosis, absent left thumb, foreshortened left forearm, left elbow contracture, fusion of the ribs on the left, butterfly vertebrae in the thoracic and lumbar spine, left radial aplasia, and a lower esophageal stricture. Chromosomal analysis was normal, and the family history was noncontributory (23).

The effects of IV methamphetamine abuse on the fetus were evaluated in a 1988 report (24). Maternal use of the drug was identified by self-reporting before delivery in 52 women, and an equal number of controls were selected for comparison. Although self-reporting of illegal drug use is prone to underreporting, the drug histories were validated by social worker interviews and were thought to represent actual drug use in the study population. Other drugs used in the study and control groups were tobacco (24 vs. 6), marijuana (20 vs. 1), cocaine (14 vs. 0), and one each in the study group for alcohol, lorazepam, dextroamphetamine, heroin, opium, LSD, and diazepam. No statistical differences were measured between the groups in the rate of obstetric complications (12% vs. 27%) or neonatal complications (21% vs. 17%). The latter category included meconium (10% vs. 12%), fetal heart rate decelerations (4% vs. 0) and tachycardia (2% vs. 0%), tachypnea (4% vs. 2%), and withdrawal symptoms (2% vs. 0%). Mean birth weight, length, and head circumference were all lower in the study infants compared with controls ($p = 0.001$). Six (12%) of the infants in the study group had a congenital defect compared with seven (14%) of the controls. Statistically, however, the investigators could only conclude that methamphetamine abuse does not cause a ≥12-fold increase in congenital anomalies (24).

A 1992 abstract described the effects of methamphetamine abuse in 48 newborns in comparison to 519 controls (25). Offspring of women positive for opiates, cocaine, alcohol, and toluene were excluded from both groups. Except for a significantly lower birth weight, 3173 vs. 3327 g ($p = 0.03$), all other parameters studied were similar, including birth length, head circumference, Apgar scores, gestational age at delivery, and the incidence of both major and minor malformations.

Intrauterine death occurred at 34 weeks' gestation in the fetus of a 29-year-old amphetamine addict who had injected 500 mg of amphetamine (26). The mother was exhibiting toxic signs and symptoms of amphetamine overdose when she was brought to the hospital. An initial fetal bradycardia of 90–100 beats/minute worsened over the next 50 minutes when the heart sounds became inaudible. Approximately 24 hours later, a 3000-g female stillborn infant without congenital abnormalities was delivered.

Amphetamine withdrawal has been described in newborns whose mothers were addicted to amphetamines during pregnancy (27–29). In a report of four mothers using methamphetamine, symptoms consisting of shrill cries, irritability, jerking, and sneezing were observed in two infants (27). One of the infants was evaluated at 4 months of age and appeared normal except for small size (weight 3rd percentile, head circumference 10th percentile). The author speculated that the symptoms in the newborns may have been caused by hidden narcotic addiction (27). Another report of four women with methamphetamine dependence described one newborn with marked drowsiness lasting for 4 days (28). The mother had not been taking narcotics. The third report of neonatal withdrawal involved an infant delivered from a mother who was a known amphetamine addict (29). Beginning 6 hours after birth, the female infant had diaphoresis, agitation alternating with periods of lassitude, apnea with feedings, a seizure on the 6th day, vomiting, miotic pupils, and a glassy-eyed stare. Her first 3 months were marked by slow development, but at 2.5 years of age, there was no evidence of neurologic disability and intelligence was considered above normal.

Methamphetamine withdrawal characterized by abnormal sleep patterns, poor feeding, tremors, and hypertonia was reported in a 1987 study (30). Infants exposed to methamphetamine or cocaine, either alone or in combination, were combined into a single group ($N = 46$) because of similar maternal and neonatal medical factors. Mothers in the drug group had a significantly greater incidence of prematurity compared with drug-free controls (28% vs. 9%), and a significantly greater incidence of placental hemorrhage and anemia compared with narcotic-using mothers and controls (13% vs. 2% vs. 2.2%, and 13% vs. 2% vs. 0%). Maternal methamphetamine abuse was significantly associated with lower gestational age, birth weight, length, and occipitofrontal circumference (30).

Echoencephalography (ECHO) was performed within 3 days of birth on 74 term (>37 weeks) infants who had tested positive for cocaine or methamphetamine, but who otherwise had uncomplicated perinatal courses (31). The infants had no other known risk factors for cerebral injury. The 74 newborns were classified into three groups: 24 (32%) exposed to methamphetamine, 32 (43%) exposed to cocaine, and 18 (24%) exposed to cocaine plus heroin or methadone, or both. Two comparison groups were formed: a group of 87 term, drug-free infants studied by ECHO because of clinical concerns for hypoxic–ischemic encephalopathy, and a normal group of 19 drug-free term newborns. Both groups of comparison infants were also studied by ECHO within 3 days of birth. Only one structural anomaly, consisting of an absent septum pellucidum, was observed in the infants examined. The affected newborn, exposed to methamphetamine, was also found to have bilateral optic nerve atrophy and diffuse attenuation of the white matter. Twenty-six (35.1%) of the drug-exposed infants had cranial abnormalities detected by ultrasonography, which was similar to the 27.6% (24 of 87) incidence in the group suspected of encephalopathy ($p = 0.7$). The normal controls had an incidence of 5.3% (1 of 19) ($p < 0.01$ in comparison to both of the other groups). The lesions observed in the drug-exposed infants were intraventricular hemorrhage, echodensities known to be associated with necrosis, and cavitary lesions. Lesions were concentrated in the basal ganglion, frontal lobes, and posterior fossa (31). The ECHO abnormalities were not predicted by standard neonatal clinical assessment and were believed to be consistent with those observed in adult abusers of amphetamines and cocaine (31).

Amphetamines do not appear to be human teratogens (32–34). Mild withdrawal symptoms may be observed in the newborns, but the few studies of infant follow-up have not shown long-term sequelae, although more studies of this nature are needed. Illicit maternal use of amphetamines, on the other hand, presents significant risks to the fetus and newborn, including intrauterine growth restriction, premature delivery, and the potential for increased maternal, fetal, and neonatal morbidity. These poor outcomes probably reflect several factors, including multiple drug use, lifestyles, and poor maternal health. However, cerebral injuries occurring in newborns exposed in utero appear to be directly related to the vasoconstrictive properties of amphetamines (31).

BREASTFEEDING SUMMARY

Amphetamine, the racemic mixture of levo—and dextroamphetamine, is concentrated in breast milk (21). After continuous daily dosing of 20 mg, milk concentrations ranged from 55 to 138 ng/mL with milk:plasma ratios varying between 2.8 and 7.5. Amphetamine was found in the urine of the nursing infant. No adverse effects of this exposure were observed over a 24-month period. In a second study, no neonatal insomnia or stimulation was observed in 103 nursing infants whose mothers were taking various amounts of amphetamine (35). The American Academy of Pediatrics classifies amphetamines as contraindicated during breastfeeding because of irritability and poor sleeping pattern (36).

References

1. Burchfield DJ, Lucas VW, Abrams RM, Miller RL, DeVane CL. Disposition and pharmacodynamics of methamphetamine in pregnant sheep. JAMA 1991;265:1968–73.
2. Stek A, Fisher B, Clark KE. Maternal and fetal cardiovascular responses to methamphetamine (abstract). Am J Obstet Gynecol 1993;168:333.

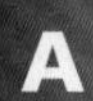

3. Nora JJ, Trasler DG, Fraser FC. Malformations in mice induced by dexamphetamine sulphate. Lancet 1965;2:1021–2.
4. Nora JJ, McNamara DG, Fraser FC. Dextroamphetamine sulphate and human malformations. Lancet 1967;1:570–1.
5. Nora JJ, Vargo T, Nora A, Love KE, McNamara DG. Dextroamphetamine: a possible environmental trigger in cardiovascular malformations. Lancet 1970;1:1290–1.
6. Nora JJ, Nora AH, Sommerville RJ, Hill RM, McNamara DG. Maternal exposure to potential teratogens. JAMA 1967;202:1065–9.
7. Matera RF, Zabala H, Jimenez AP. Bifid exencephalia: teratogen action of amphetamine. Int Surg 1968;50:79–85.
8. Gilbert EF, Khoury GH. Dextroamphetamine and congenital cardiac malformations. J Pediatr 1970;76:638.
9. Levin JN. Amphetamine ingestion with biliary atresia. J Pediatr 1971;79:130–1.
10. McIntire MS. Possible adverse drug reaction. JAMA 1966;197:62–3.
11. Bogdanoff B, Rorke LB, Yanoff M, Warren WS. Brain and eye abnormalities: possible sequelae to prenatal use of multiple drugs including LSD. Am J Dis Child 1972;123:145–8.
12. Nelson MM, Forfar JO. Associations between drugs administered during pregnancy and congenital abnormalities of the fetus. Br Med J 1971;1:523–7.
13. Milkovich L, van den Berg BJ. Effects of antenatal exposure to anorectic drugs. Am J Obstet Gynecol 1977;129:637–42.
14. Eriksson M, Larsson G, Winbladh B, Zetterstrom R. The influence of amphetamine addiction on pregnancy and the newborn infant. Acta Paediatr Scand 1978;67:95–9.
15. Larsson G, Eriksson M, Zetterstrom R. Amphetamine addiction and pregnancy: psycho-social and medical aspects. Acta Psychiatr Scand 1979;60:334–45.
16. Billing L, Eriksson M, Larsson G, Zetterstrom R. Amphetamine addiction and pregnancy. III. One year follow-up of the children: psychosocial and pediatric aspects. Acta Paediatr Scand 1980;69:675–80.
17. Eriksson M, Larsson G, Zetterstrom R. Amphetamine addiction and pregnancy. II. Pregnancy, delivery and the neonatal period: socio-medical aspects. Acta Obstet Gynecol Scand 1981;60:253–9.
18. Larsson G. The amphetamine addicted mother and her child. Acta Paediatr Scand Suppl 1980;278:7–24.
19. Heinonen OP, Slone D, Shapiro S. *Birth Defects and Drugs in Pregnancy.* Littleton, MA: Publishing Sciences Group, 1977.
20. Briggs GG, Samson JH, Crawford DJ. Lack of abnormalities in a newborn exposed to amphetamine during gestation. Am J Dis Child 1975;129:249–50.
21. Steiner E, Villen T, Hallberg M, Rane A. Amphetamine secretion in breast milk. Eur J Clin Pharmacol 1984;27:123–4.
22. Tenorio GM, Nazvi M, Bickers GH, Hubbird RH. Intrauterine stroke and maternal polydrug abuse: case report. Clin Pediatr 1988;27:565–7.
23. Ghidini A, Sicherer S, Willner J. Congenital abnormalities (VATER) in baby born to mother using lovastatin. Lancet 1992;339:1416–7.
24. Little BB, Snell LM, Gilstrap LC III. Methamphetamine abuse during pregnancy: outcome and fetal effects. Obstet Gynecol 1988;72:541–4.
25. Ramin SM, Little BB, Trimmer KJ, Standard DI, Blakely CA, Snell LM. Methamphetamine use during pregnancy in a large urban population (abstract). Am J Obstet Gynecol 1992;166:353.
26. Dearlove JC, Betteridge T. Stillbirth due to intravenous amphetamine. BMJ 1992;304:548.
27. Sussman S. Narcotic and methamphetamine use during pregnancy: effect on newborn infants. Am J Dis Child 1963;106:325–30.
28. Neuberg R. Drug dependence and pregnancy: a review of the problems and their management. J Obstet Gynaecol Br Commonw 1970;66:1117–22.
29. Ramer CM. The case history of an infant born to an amphetamine-addicted mother. Clin Pediatr 1974;13:596–7.
30. Oro AS, Dixon SD. Perinatal cocaine and methamphetamine exposure: maternal and neonatal correlates. J Pediatr 1987;111:571–8.
31. Dixon SD, Bejar R. Echoencephalographic findings in neonates associated with maternal cocaine and methamphetamine use: incidence and clinical correlates. J Pediatr 1989;115:770–8.
32. Chernoff GF, Jones KL. Fetal preventive medicine: teratogens and the unborn baby. Pediatr Ann 1981;10:210–7.
33. Kalter H, Warkany J. Congenital malformations (second of two parts). N Engl J Med 1983;308:491–7.
34. Zierler S. Maternal drugs and congenital heart disease. Obstet Gynecol 1985;65:155–65.
35. Ayd FJ Jr. Excretion of psychotropic drugs in human breast milk. Int Drug Ther News Bull 1973;8:33–40.
36. Committee on Drugs, American Academy of Pediatrics. The transfer of drugs and other chemicals into human milk. Pediatrics 2001;108:776–89.

AMPHOTERICIN B

Antifungal Antibiotic

PREGNANCY RECOMMENDATION: Compatible
BREASTFEEDING RECOMMENDATION: No Human Data—Probably Compatible

PREGNANCY SUMMARY

Although animal reproduction data suggest risk, no adverse effects have been reported in exposed human embryos and fetuses. The drug crosses the human placenta with cord blood concentrations up to those measured in the mother.

FETAL RISK SUMMARY

No reports linking the use of amphotericin B with congenital defects have been located. Reproduction studies of amphotericin B liposome were conducted with maternal nontoxic doses in rats (0.16–0.8 times the recommended human clinical dose range of 1–5 mg/kg based on BSA [RHCD]) and rabbits (0.2–1 times the RHCD) (1). Rabbits administered doses 0.5–2 times the RHCD had a higher rate of spontaneous abortions than did controls (1). No fetal harm was observed in reproduction studies of amphotericin B lipid complex in rats and rabbits at doses up to 0.64 times the human dose (2).

The antibiotic crosses the placenta to the fetus with cord blood:maternal serum ratios ranging from 0.38 to 1.0 (3–5). In a term (42 weeks) infant whose mother was treated with amphotericin B 0.6 mg/kg every other day, cord and maternal blood levels at delivery were both 2.6 mcg/mL, with a cord blood:maternal serum ratio of 1.0 (3). Amniotic fluid concentration was 0.08 mcg/mL at delivery. The time interval between the last dose and delivery was not specified. Concentrations in the cord blood and maternal serum of a woman treated with 16 mg of amphotericin B just before delivery (one-fifth of a planned total dose of 80 mg had infused when delivery occurred) were 0.12 and 0.32 mcg/mL, respectively, a ratio of 0.38 (4). The woman's last dose before this time was 7 days previously when she had received 80 mg. In a third case, a mother was receiving 20 mg IV every other day (0.5 mg/kg) (5). The cord and maternal serum concentrations were 1.3 and 1.9 mcg/mL, respectively, a ratio of 0.68. The levels were determined 26 hours after her last dose.

The Collaborative Perinatal Project monitored 50,282 mother–child pairs, 9 of whom had 1st trimester exposure to amphotericin B (6). Numerous other reports have also described the use of amphotericin B during various stages of pregnancy, including the 1st trimester (4–22). No evidence of adverse fetal effects was found by these studies. Amphotericin B can be used during pregnancy in those patients who will clearly benefit from the drug.

BREASTFEEDING SUMMARY

No reports describing the use of amphotericin B during human lactation have been located. The drug probably is excreted into breast milk, but the risk, if any exists, to a nursing infant is unknown.

References

1. Product information. Ambisome. Fujisawa Healthcare, 2000.
2. Product information. Abelcet. Liposome, 2000.
3. McCoy MJ, Ellenberg JF, Killam AP. Coccidioidomycosis complicating pregnancy. Am J Obstet Gynecol 1980;137:739–40.
4. Ismail MA, Lerner SA. Disseminated blastomycosis in a pregnant woman. Review of amphotericin B usage during pregnancy. Am Rev Respir Dis 1982;126:350–3.
5. Hager H, Welt SI, Cardasis JP, Alvarez S. Disseminated blastomycosis in a pregnant woman successfully treated with amphotericin-B: a case report. J Reprod Med 1988;33:485–8.
6. Heinonen OP, Slone D, Shapiro S. *Birth Defects and Drugs in Pregnancy*. Littleton, MA: Publishing Sciences Group, 1977:297.
7. Neiberg AD, Maruomatis F, Dyke J, Fayyad A. Blastomyces dermatitidis treated during pregnancy. Am J Obstet Gynecol 1977;128:911–2.
8. Philpot CR, Lo D. Cryptococcal meningitis in pregnancy. Med J Aust 1972;2:1005–7.
9. Aitken GWE, Symonds EM. Cryptococcal meningitis in pregnancy treated with amphotericin. A case report. Br J Obstet Gynaecol 1962;69:677–9.
10. Feldman R. Cryptococcosis (torulosis) of the central nervous system treated with amphotericin B during pregnancy. South Med J 1959;52:1415–7.
11. Kuo D. A case of torulosis of the central nervous system during pregnancy. Med J Aust 1962;1:558–60.
12. Crotty JM. Systemic mycotic infections in Northern Territory aborigines. Med J Aust 1965;1:184.
13. Littman ML. Cryptococcosis (torulosis). Current concepts and therapy. Am J Med 1959;27:976–8.
14. Mick R, Muller-Tyl E, Neufeld T. Comparison of the effectiveness of nystatin and amphotericin B in the therapy of female genital mycoses. Wien Med Wochenschr 1975:125:131–5.
15. Silberfarb PM, Sarois GA, Tosh FE. Cryptococcosis and pregnancy. Am J Obstet Gynecol 1972;112:714–20.
16. Curole DN. Cryptococcal meningitis in pregnancy. J Reprod Med 1981;26:317–9.
17. Sanford WG, Rasch JR, Stonehill RB. A therapeutic dilemma: the treatment of disseminated coccidioidomycosis with amphotericin B. Ann Intern Med 1962;56:553–63.
18. Harris RE. Coccidioidomycosis complicating pregnancy. Report of 3 cases and review of the literature. Obstet Gynecol 1966;28:401–5.
19. Smale LE, Waechter KG. Dissemination of coccidioidomycosis in pregnancy. Am J Obstet Gynecol 1970;107:356–9.
20. Hadsall FJ, Acquarelli MJ. Disseminated coccidioidomycosis presenting as facial granulomas in pregnancy: a report of two cases and a review of the literature. Laryngoscope 1973;83:51–8.
21. Daniel L, Salit IE. Blastomycosis during pregnancy. Can Med Assoc J 1984;131:759–61.
22. Peterson CW, Johnson SL, Kelly JV, Kelly PC. Coccidioidal meningitis and pregnancy: a case report. Obstet Gynecol 1989;73:835–6.

AMPICILLIN

Antibiotic (Penicillin)

PREGNANCY RECOMMENDATION: Human Data Suggest Risk in 1st Trimester
BREASTFEEDING RECOMMENDATION: Compatible

PREGNANCY SUMMARY

Penicillins are considered low risk at any stage of pregnancy. This assessment may have to be modified for the aminopenicillins (ampicillin and amoxicillin) because there is some evidence that exposure to these two antibiotics during organogenesis is associated with oral clefts (see also Amoxicillin). However, even if the association is causal, the absolute risk is very low. The association requires confirmation.

FETAL RISK SUMMARY

Ampicillin is an aminopenicillin antibiotic (see also Amoxicillin). The drug rapidly crosses the placenta into the fetal circulation and amniotic fluid (1–6). Fetal serum levels can be detected within 30 minutes and equilibrate with maternal serum in 1 hour. Amniotic fluid levels can be detected in 90 minutes, reaching 20% of the maternal serum peak in about 8 hours. The pharmacokinetics of ampicillin during pregnancy have been reported (7,8).

Ampicillin depresses both plasma-bound and urinary-excreted estriol by inhibiting steroid conjugate hydrolysis in the gut (9–13). Urinary estriol was formerly used to assess the condition of the fetoplacental unit, with depressed levels being associated with fetal distress. This assessment is now made by measuring plasma unconjugated estriol, which is not usually affected by ampicillin. An interaction between ampicillin and oral contraceptives resulting in pregnancy has been suspected (14,15). Two studies, however, failed to confirm this interaction and concluded that alternate contraceptive methods were not necessary during ampicillin therapy (16,17).

The use of ampicillin in early pregnancy was associated with a prevalence ratio estimate of 3.3 (90% confidence interval [CI] 1.3–8.1, $p = 0.02$) for congenital heart disease in a retrospective study (18). A specific defect, transposition of the great arteries, had a risk of 7.7 (90% CI 1.3–38) based on exposure in 2 of the 29 infants with the anomaly. The investigators did note, however, that the results had to be viewed cautiously because the data were subject to recall bias (drug histories were taken by questionnaire or telephone up to a year after presumed exposure) and the study could not distinguish between the fetal effects of the drug versus those of the infectious agent(s) for which the drugs were used. Others have also shared this concern (19). Other reports linking the use of ampicillin with congenital defects have not been located.

The Collaborative Perinatal Project monitored 50,282 mother–child pairs, 3546 of whom had 1st trimester exposure to penicillin derivatives (20, pp. 297–313). For use anytime during pregnancy, 7171 exposures were recorded (20, p. 435). In neither group was evidence found to suggest a relationship to large categories of major or minor malformations or to individual defects. Based on these data, it is unlikely that ampicillin is teratogenic.

In a surveillance study of Michigan Medicaid recipients involving 229,101 completed pregnancies conducted between 1985 and 1992, 10,011 newborns had been exposed to ampicillin during the 1st trimester (F. Rosa, personal communication, FDA, 1993). A total of 441 (4.4%) major birth defects were observed (426 expected). Specific data were available for six defect categories, including (observed/expected) 116/100 cardiovascular defects, 13/16 oral clefts, 6/8 spina bifida, 36/29 polydactyly, 9/17 limb reduction defects, and 27/24 hypospadias. These data do not support an association between the drug and the defects.

Ampicillin is often used in the last half of pregnancies in which either the woman or her fetus is at risk for infections because of premature rupture of the membranes or other risk factors (21–23). In one report, a mother with ruptured membranes at 40 weeks' gestation had an anaphylactic reaction to ampicillin (24). A markedly distressed infant was delivered with severe metabolic acidosis (arterial cord blood pH 6.71). Multifocal clonic seizures and brain edema occurred during the neonatal period, and pronounced neurologic abnormalities were evident at 6 months of age.

A 2001 study from Hungary evaluated the association between ampicillin and birth defects (25). Of 38,151 controls (no defects), 2632 (6.9%) had been treated with ampicillin. In 22,865 cases (with defects), 1643 (7.2%) had been treated with ampicillin. For ampicillin use in the second and third months of gestation, the only significant difference was for cleft palate (odds ratio 4.2, 95% confidence interval 1.4–16.3). However, the authors concluded that the lack of evidence for the association in other studies and in animals suggested that the apparent risk was not real and instead a chance association (25).

BREASTFEEDING SUMMARY

Ampicillin is excreted into breast milk in low concentrations. Milk:plasma ratios have been reported up to 0.2 (26,27). Candidiasis and diarrhea were observed in one infant whose mother was receiving ampicillin (28).

In a 1993 cohort study, diarrhea was reported in 32 (19.3%) nursing infants of 166 breastfeeding mothers who were taking antibiotics (29). For the five women taking ampicillin, diarrhea was observed in one (20%) infant. The diarrhea was considered minor because it did not require medical attention (29).

Although adverse effects are apparently rare, three potential problems exist for the nursing infant: modification of bowel flora, direct effects on the infant (e.g., allergic response or sensitization), and interference with the interpretation of culture results if a fever workup is required.

References

1. Bray R, Boc R, Johnson W. Transfer of ampicillin into fetus and amniotic fluid from maternal plasma in late pregnancy. Am J Obstet Gynecol 1966;96:938–42.
2. MacAulay M, Abou-Sabe M, Charles D. Placental transfer of ampicillin. Am J Obstet Gynecol 1966;96:943–50.
3. Biro L, Ivan E, Elek E, Arr M. Data on the tissue concentration of antibiotics in man. Tissue concentrations of semi-synthetic penicillins in the fetus. Int Z Klin Pharmakol Ther Toxikol 1970;4:321–4.
4. Elek E, Ivan E, Arr M. Passage of penicillins from mother to foetus in humans. Int J Clin Pharmacol Ther Toxicol 1972;6:223–8.
5. Kraybill EN, Chaney NE, McCarthy LR. Transplacental ampicillin: inhibitory concentrations in neonatal serum. Am J Obstet Gynecol 1980;138:793–6.
6. Jordheim O, Hagen AG. Study of ampicillin levels in maternal serum, umbilical cord serum and amniotic fluid following administration of pivampicillin. Acta Obstet Gynecol Scand 1980;59:315–7.
7. Philipson A. Pharmacokinetics of ampicillin during pregnancy. J Infect Dis 1977;136:370–6.
8. Noschel VH, Peiker G, Schroder S, Meinhold P, Muller B. Untersuchungen zur pharmakokinetik von antibiotika und sulfanilamiden in der schwangerschaft und unter der geburt. Zentralbl Gynakol 1982;104:1514–8.
9. Willman K, Pulkkinen M. Reduced maternal plasma and urinary estriol during ampicillin treatment. Am J Obstet Gynecol 1971;109:893–6.
10. Boehn F, DiPietro D, Goss D. The effect of ampicillin administration on urinary estriol and serum estradiol in the normal pregnant patient. Am J Obstet Gynecol 1974;119:98–101.
11. Sybulski S, Maughan G. Effect of ampicillin administration on estradiol, estriol and cortisol levels in maternal plasma and on estriol levels in urine. Am J Obstet Gynecol 1976;124:379–81.
12. Aldercreutz H, Martin F, Lehtinen T, Tikkanen M, Pulkkinen M. Effect of ampicillin administration on plasma conjugated and unconjugated estrogen and progesterone levels in pregnancy. Am J Obstet Gynecol 1977;128: 266–71.
13. Van Look PFA, Top-Huisman M, Gnodde HP. Effect of ampicillin or amoxycillin administration on plasma and urinary estrogen levels during normal pregnancy. Eur J Obstet Gynecol Reprod Biol 1981;12:225–33.
14. Dossetor J. Drug interactions with oral contraceptives. Br Med J 1975;4: 467–8.
15. DeSano EA Jr, Hurley SC. Possible interactions of antihistamines and antibiotics with oral contraceptive effectiveness. Fertil Steril 1982;37:853–4.
16. Friedman CI, Huneke AL, Kim MH, Powell J. The effect of ampicillin on oral contraceptive effectiveness. Obstet Gynecol 1980;55:33–7.
17. Back DJ, Breckenridge AM, MacIver M, Orme M, Rowe PH, Staiger C, Thomas E, Tjia J. The effects of ampicillin on oral contraceptive steroids in women. Br J Clin Pharmacol 1982;14:43–8.
18. Rothman KJ, Fyler DC, Goldblatt A, Kreidberg MB. Exogenous hormones and other drug exposures of children with congenital heart disease. Am J Epidemiol 1979;109:433–9.
19. Zierler S. Maternal drugs and congenital heart disease. Obstet Gynecol 1985;65:155–65.
20. Heinonen OP, Slone D, Shapiro S. *Birth Defects and Drugs in Pregnancy*. Littleton, MA: Publishing Sciences Group, 1977.
21. Boyer KM, Gotoff SP. Prevention of early-onset neonatal group B streptococcal disease with selective intrapartum chemoprophylaxis. N Engl J Med 1986;314:1665–9.
22. Amon E, Lewis SV, Sibai BM, Villar MA, Arheart KL. Ampicillin prophylaxis in preterm premature rupture of the membranes: a prospective randomized study. Am J Obstet Gynecol 1988;159:539–43.
23. Morales WJ, Angel JL, O'Brien WF, Knuppel RA. Use of ampicillin and corticosteroids in premature rupture of membranes: a randomized study. Obstet Gynecol 1989;73:721–6.
24. Heim K, Alge A, Marth C. Anaphylactic reaction to ampicillin and severe complication in the fetus. Lancet 1991;337:859.
25. Czeizel AE, Rockenbauer M, Sorensen HT, Olsen J. A population-based case-control teratologic study of ampicillin treatment during pregnancy. Am J Obstet Gynecol 2001;185:140–7.

26. Wilson J, Brown R, Cherek D, Dailey JW, Hilman B, Jobe PC, Manno BR, Manno JE, Redetzki HM, Stewart JJ. Drug excretion in human breast milk: principles, pharmacokinetics and projected consequences. Clin Pharmacokinet 1980;5:1–66.
27. Knowles J. Excretion of drugs in milk—a review. J Pediatr 1965;66:1068–82.
28. Williams M. Excretion of drugs in milk. Pharm J 1976;217:219.
29. Ito S, Blajchman A, Stephenson M, Eliopoulos C, Koren G. Prospective follow-up of adverse reactions in breast-fed infants exposed to maternal medication. Am J Obstet Gynecol 1993;168:1393–9.

AMPRENAVIR

Antiviral

PREGNANCY RECOMMENDATION: Compatible—Maternal Benefit >> Embryo–Fetal Risk
BREASTFEEDING RECOMMENDATION: Contraindicated

PREGNANCY SUMMARY

The limited human data do not allow a prediction as to the risk of amprenavir during pregnancy. The developmental toxicity observed in animals at doses less than the human clinical dose is a potential concern for human pregnancies. However, if indicated, the drug should not be withheld because of pregnancy.

FETAL RISK SUMMARY

Amprenavir is an inhibitor of HIV type 1 (HIV-1) protease. Protease is an enzyme that is required for the cleavage of viral polyprotein precursors into active functional proteins found in infectious HIV. Amprenavir, in combination with other antiretroviral agents, is indicated for the treatment of HIV-1 infections.

In reproduction studies with amprenavir, doses two times the human clinical exposure based on AUC comparisons (HCE) in male and female rats had no effect on fertility or mating (1). During embryo and fetal development, doses 1/2 the HCE produced thymic elongation and incomplete ossification of bones. When administered from day 7 of gestation to day 22 of lactation, a dose two times the HCE was associated with reduced body weights. However, subsequent development of the offspring, including fertility and reproductive performance, was not affected (1). In rabbits, doses up to 1/20th the HCE were associated with abortions and minor skeletal variations resulting from deficient ossification of the femur, humerus trochlea, and humerus (1).

Amprenavir is transferred across rat and rabbit placentas to the fetus (1). In an ex vivo human placental model, the antiviral agent also readily crossed to the fetus but with a clearance index less than abacavir. No accumulation of the drug was measured (2). The placental transfer is consistent with the molecular weight of amprenavir (about 506).

The Antiretroviral Pregnancy Registry reported, for the period January 1989 through July 2009, prospective data (reported before the outcomes were known) involving 4702 live births that had been exposed during the 1st trimester to one or more antiretroviral agents (3). Congenital defects were noted in 134, a prevalence of 2.8% (95% confidence interval [CI] 2.4–3.4). In the 6100 live births with earliest exposure in the 2nd/3rd trimesters, there were 153 infants with defects (2.5%, 95% CI 2.1–2.9). The prevalence rates for the two periods did not differ significantly. There were 288 infants with birth defects among 10,803 live births with exposure anytime during pregnancy (2.7%, 95% CI 2.4–3.0). The prevalence rate did not differ significantly from the rate expected in a nonexposed population. There were 38 outcomes exposed to amprenavir (28 in the 1st trimester and 10 in the 2nd/3rd trimesters) in combination with other antiretroviral agents. There was one birth defect among those exposed in the 1st trimester and none in those exposed in the 2nd/3rd trimesters. In reviewing the birth defects of prospective and retrospective (pregnancies reported after the outcomes were known) registered cases, the Registry concluded that, except for isolated cases of neural tube defects with efavirenz exposure in retrospective reports, there was no other pattern of anomalies (isolated or syndromic) (3). (See Lamivudine for required statement.)

A public health advisory was issued by the FDA on the association between protease inhibitors and diabetes mellitus (4). Because pregnancy is a risk factor for hyperglycemia, there was concern that these antiviral agents would exacerbate this risk. An abstract published in 2000 described the results of a study involving 34 pregnant women treated with protease inhibitors (none with amprenavir) compared with 41 controls that evaluated the association with diabetes (5). No association between protease inhibitors and an increased incidence of gestational diabetes was found.

Two reviews, one in 1996 and the other in 1997, concluded that all women currently receiving antiretroviral therapy should continue to receive therapy during pregnancy and that treatment of the mother with monotherapy should be considered inadequate therapy (6,7). The same conclusion was reached in a 2003 review with the added admonishment that therapy must be continuous to prevent emergence of resistant viral strains (8). In 2009, the updated U.S. Department of Health and Human Services guidelines for the use of antiretroviral agents in HIV-1-infected patients continued the recommendation that the therapy, with the exception of efavirenz, should be continued during pregnancy (9). If indicated, therefore, protease inhibitors, including amprenavir, should not be withheld in pregnancy because the expected benefit to the HIV-positive mother outweighs the unknown risk to the fetus. Pregnant women taking protease inhibitors should be monitored for hyperglycemia. The updated guidelines for the use of antiretroviral drugs

to reduce perinatal HIV-1 transmission also were released in 2010 (10). Women receiving antiretroviral therapy during pregnancy should continue the therapy but, regardless of the regimen, zidovudine administration is recommended during the intrapartum period to prevent vertical transmission of HIV to the newborn (10).

BREASTFEEDING SUMMARY

No reports describing the use of amprenavir during human lactation have been located. The antiviral agent is excreted into the milk of lactating rats (1). In addition, the molecular weight (about 506) is low enough that excretion into human breast milk should be expected.

Reports on the use of amprenavir during human lactation are unlikely because the antiviral agent is used in the treatment of HIV infections. HIV-1 is transmitted in milk, and in developed countries, breastfeeding is not recommended (6,7,9,11–13). In developing countries, breastfeeding is undertaken, despite the risk, because there are no affordable milk substitutes available. Until 1999, no studies had been published that examined the effect of any antiretroviral therapy on HIV-1 transmission in milk. In that year, a study involving zidovudine was published that measured a 38% reduction in vertical transmission of HIV-1 infection in spite of breastfeeding when compared with controls (see Zidovudine).

References

1. Product information. Agenerase. Glaxo Wellcome, 2000.
2. Bawdon RE. The *ex vivo* human placental transfer of the anti-HIV nucleoside inhibitor abacavir and the protease inhibitor amprenavir. Infect Dis Obstet Gynecol 1998;6:244–6.
3. Antiretroviral Pregnancy Registry Steering Committee. *Antiretroviral Pregnancy Registry International Interim Report for 1 January 1989 through 31 July 2009*. Wilmington, NC: Registry Coordinating Center; 2009. Available at www.apregistry.com. Accessed May 29, 2010.
4. CDC. Public Health Service Task Force recommendations for the use of antiretroviral drugs in pregnant women infected with HIV-1 for maternal health and for reducing perinatal HIV-1 transmission in the United States. MMWR 1998;47:No. RR-2.
5. Fassett M, Kramer F, Stek A. Treatment with protease inhibitors in pregnancy is not associated with an increased incidence of gestational diabetes (abstract). Am J Obstet Gynecol 2000;182:S97.
6. Carpenter CCJ, Fischi MA, Hammer SM, Hirsch MS, Jacobsen DM, Katzenstein DA, Montaner JSG, Richman DD, Saag MS, Schooley RT, Thompson MA, Vella S, Yeni PG, Volberding PA. Antiretroviral therapy for HIV infection in 1996. JAMA 1996;276;146–54.
7. Minkoff H, Augenbraun M. Antiretroviral therapy for pregnant women. Am J Obstet Gynecol 1997;176:478–89.
8. Minkoff H. Human immunodeficiency virus infection in pregnancy. Obstet Gynecol 2003;101:797–810.
9. Panel on Antiretroviral Guidelines for Adults and Adolescents. *Guidelines for the Use of Antiretroviral Agents in HIV-1-Infected Adults and Adolescents*. Department of Health and Human Services. December 1, 2009:1–161. Available at http://www.aidsinfo.nih.gov/ContentFiles/AdultandAdolescentGL.pdf. Accessed September 17, 2010:60, 96–8.
10. Panel on Treatment of HIV-Infected Pregnant Women and Prevention of Perinatal Transmission. *Recommendations for Use of Antiretroviral Drugs in Pregnant HIV-1-Infected Women for Maternal Health and Interventions to Reduce Perinatal HIV Transmission in the United States*. May 24, 2010:1–117. Available at http://aidsinfo.nih.gov/ContentFiles/PerinatalGL.pdf. Accessed September 17, 2010:30 (Table 5).
11. Brown ZA, Watts DH. Antiviral therapy in pregnancy. Clin Obstet Gynecol 1990;33:276–89.
12. De Martino M, Tovo P-A, Pezzotti P, Galli L, Massironi E, Ruga E, Floreea F, Plebani A, Gabiano C, Zuccotti GV. HIV-1 transmission through breast-milk: appraisal of risk according to duration of feeding. AIDS 1992;6:991–7.
13. Van de Perre P. Postnatal transmission of human immunodeficiency virus type 1: the breast feeding dilemma. Am J Obstet Gynecol 1995;173:483–7.

AMRINONE

Cardiac Agent

PREGNANCY RECOMMENDATION: Limited Human Data—Animal Data Suggest Low Risk
BREASTFEEDING RECOMMENDATION: No Human Data—Probably Compatible

PREGNANCY SUMMARY

The data are too limited to assess the risk to the embryo–fetus. The drug probably crosses the placenta. If the maternal condition requires amrinone, it should not be withheld because of pregnancy.

FETAL RISK SUMMARY

Amrinone is a cardiac inotropic agent that also has a vasodilatory effect (1). The drug is unrelated to cardiac glycosides or catecholamines. The principal indication for amrinone is the short-term management of congestive heart failure.

Amrinone is teratogenic in some animal species, producing skeletal and gross external malformations in one type of rabbits but not in other types, and having no effect on fetal rats (1). In pregnant baboons, amrinone infusion did not significantly affect uterine artery blood flow (2).

A single case report has described the use of amrinone in a human pregnancy (3). A 34-year-old woman at 18 weeks' gestation was treated with an amrinone IV infusion (0.5 mg/kg loading dose followed by 2 mcg/kg/minute) for refractory congestive heart failure secondary to bacterial endocarditis. A higher dose was not used because of premature ventricular contractions. Although no fetal adverse effects attributable to the drug were noted, fetal death occurred 11 days after discontinuance of amrinone because of the deteriorating medical condition of the mother (3).

BREASTFEEDING SUMMARY

No reports describing the use of amrinone during lactation have been located. The molecular weight of amrinone (about 187) is low enough, however, that passage into milk should be expected.

References

1. Product information, Inocor. Sanofi Winthrop Pharmaceuticals, 1997.
2. Fishburne JI Jr, Dormer KJ, Payne GG, Gill PS, Ashrafzadeh AR, Rossavik IK. Effects of amrinone and dopamine on uterine blood flow and vascular responses in the gravid baboon. Am J Obstet Gynecol 1988;158:829–37.
3. Jelsema RD, Bhatia RK, Ganguly S. Use of intravenous amrinone in the short-term management of refractory heart failure in pregnancy. Obstet Gynecol 1991;78:935–6.

AMYL NITRITE

Vasodilator

PREGNANCY RECOMMENDATION: Limited Human Data—No Relevant Animal Data
BREASTFEEDING RECOMMENDATION: No Human Data—Probably Compatible

PREGNANCY SUMMARY

The absence of specific human pregnancy experience prevents an assessment of the embryo–fetal risk. However, another vasodilator has limited data and does not appear to cause developmental toxicity (see Nitroglycerin). Transient decreases in maternal blood pressure may occur.

FETAL RISK SUMMARY

Amyl nitrite is a rapid-acting, short-duration vasodilator used primarily for the treatment of angina pectoris. Because of the nature of its indication, experience in pregnancy is limited. The Collaborative Perinatal Project recorded seven 1st trimester exposures to amyl nitrite and nitroglycerin, as well as eight other patients exposed to other vasodilators (1). From this small group of 15 patients, four malformed children were observed. It was not stated whether amyl nitrite was taken by any of the mothers of the affected infants. The number of cases is too small to assess the risk of amyl nitrite in pregnancy.

BREASTFEEDING SUMMARY

No reports describing the use of amyl nitrite during lactation have been located. It is doubtful if maternal use would represent any risk to a nursing infant.

Reference

1. Heinonen OP, Slone D, Shapiro S. *Birth Defects and Drugs in Pregnancy*. Littleton, MA: Publishing Sciences Group, 1977:371–3.

ANAGRELIDE

Hematologic Agent (Antiplatelet)

PREGNANCY RECOMMENDATION: Limited Human Data—Animal Data Suggest Low Risk
BREASTFEEDING RECOMMENDATION: No Human Data—Potential Toxicity

PREGNANCY SUMMARY

Human pregnancy experience with anagrelide is limited. Except for one spontaneous abortion (SAB), all other outcomes were normal babies. Moreover, the animal data suggest low risk. The manufacturer recommends that women should not become pregnant while taking anagrelide, but the benefits of therapy must be weighed against the unknown risks on a case-by-case basis.

FETAL RISK SUMMARY

Anagrelide, an antiplatelet agent, is indicated for the reduction of elevated platelet counts and resulting risk of thrombosis in patients with thrombocythemia.

An animal teratology study observed no congenital abnormalities in pregnant rats given oral doses up to 730 times the maximum recommended human dose based on BSA (MRHD) or in pregnant rabbits administered doses up to 32 times the MRHD (1). In a fertility and reproductive performance study of female rats, however, doses 49 times the MRHD or higher disrupted implantation and produced an adverse effect on embryo–fetal survival (1). The same dosage in a perinatal and postnatal study with pregnant rats caused a delay in parturition, deaths of undelivered dams and their fetuses, and increased mortality in pups that were born (1).

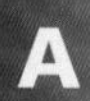

No reports describing the placental transfer of anagrelide in animals or humans have been located. The molecular weight of the drug (about 275 for the free base) is low enough that passage to the embryo and/or fetus should be expected.

The first reported human pregnancy exposure to anagrelide appears to be that described by the manufacturer in its product information (1). Five women became pregnant while receiving the drug at doses of 1–4 mg/day. Therapy was stopped when the pregnancies were diagnosed (timing not specified), and all the women delivered normal, healthy babies.

A 2001 report described 43 pregnancies in 20 women with essential thrombocythemia (ET) (2). Only one pregnancy involved exposure to anagrelide and that one ended in a 1st trimester SAB.

A 2004 case report described the outcome of a pregnancy in which anagrelide was used throughout (3). A 25-year-old woman had been diagnosed with essential thrombocythemia (ET) several years before conception and, because she did not tolerate interferon-α, she was maintained on anagrelide 4 mg/day. She was a heterozygous carrier of the factor V Leiden mutation. When pregnancy was recognized, her dose was reduced to 1 mg/day and low molecular weight heparin was started. Because preeclampsia developed at 32 weeks', an elective cesarean section was performed to deliver a 1400-g baby (no other data given). The infant had normal blood count parameters (3).

A 2005 report described two women with ET who became pregnant while receiving anagrelide (4). A 32-year-old woman was maintained on 1–4 mg/day, the dose adjusted to maintain a normal platelet count. She conceived against medical advice and eventually gave birth to a healthy 2.87-kg baby girl with no congenital defects and a normal full blood count. The second patient was a 28-year-old woman who was maintained on anagrelide 1.5–2.0 mg/day. Her pregnancy was discovered at 12 weeks' gestation. The drug was discontinued and she was maintained on low-molecular-weight heparin until she gave birth to a healthy full-term, 2.1-kg male baby with no congenital defects and a normal blood count (4).

A 32-year-old woman positive for the JAK2V617F mutation ET became pregnant while receiving anagrelide (5). The drug was discontinued in the third week and she was treated with aspirin for the remainder of pregnancy. At 39 4/7 weeks, a normal, healthy 2.8-kg baby girl was born with Apgar scores of 9 and 10. The infant's blood count was normal (5).

BREASTFEEDING SUMMARY

No reports describing the use of anagrelide during lactation have been located. The molecular weight of the compound (about 275 for the free base) is low enough that excretion into milk should be expected. The effect of this exposure on a nursing infant is unknown.

References

1. Product information. Agrylin. Roberts Pharmaceutical, 2000.
2. Wright CA, Tefferi A. A single institutional experience with 43 pregnancies in essential thrombocythemia. Eur J Hematol 2001;66:152–9.
3. Doubek M, Brychtova Y, Doubek R, Janku P, Mayer J. Anagrelide therapy in pregnancy: report of a case of essential thrombocythemia. Ann Hematol 2004;83:726–7.
4. Alkindi S, Dennison D, Pathare A. Successful outcome with anagrelide in pregnancy. Ann Hematol 2005;84:758–9.
5. Sobas MA, Perez Encinas MM, Rabunal Martinez MJ, Quinteiro Garcia C, Bello Lopez JL. Anagrelide treatment in early pregnancy in a patient with JAK2V617F-positive essential thrombocythemia: case report and literature review. Acta Haematol 2009;122:221–2.

ANAKINRA

Immunologic Agent (Immunomodulator)

PREGNANCY RECOMMENDATION: Limited Human Data—Animal Data Suggest Low Risk
BREASTFEEDING RECOMMENDATION: Limited Human Data—Probably Compatible

PREGNANCY SUMMARY

One report has described the use of anakinra throughout pregnancy. The infant was severely growth-restricted, probably due to the mother's disease. No other developmental toxicity was noted. The animal data do not suggest a risk of structural defects, but the agent prevented embryo implantation in one study. Although the near absence of data prevents an assessment of the risk for the human embryo–fetus, interleukin-1 receptor antagonist (IL-1ra) is a natural occurring cytokine that appears to have a role in the protection of the placenta/embryo–fetus from the maternal immune response mechanisms. Therefore, it is doubtful if recommended doses of recombinant IL-1ra will cause direct toxicity to the embryo or fetus. Until human pregnancy data are available, however, the safest course is to avoid anakinra during gestation. Planned or inadvertent pregnancy exposure appears to represent a low risk for the embryo and fetus. If anakinra is used in pregnancy for the treatment of rheumatoid arthritis, health care professionals are encouraged to call the toll-free number (877-311-8972) for information about patient enrollment in the Organization of Teratology Information Specialists (OTIS) Rheumatoid Arthritis Study.

FETAL RISK SUMMARY

Anakinra is a nonglycosylated form of the human cytokine IL-1ra produced by recombinant DNA technology. Anakinra (recombinant IL-1ra) is indicated for the reduction in signs and symptoms of moderate to severe rheumatoid arthritis. By binding to interleukin-1 receptors, IL-1ra competitively inhibits interleukin-1 activity, such as the stimulation of several inflammatory mediators. The terminal elimination half-life ranges from 4 to 6 hours (1).

Native IL-1ra is a normal constituent in the maternal, fetal, and amniotic fluid compartments (2,3). Endogenous IL-1ra has been measured in amniotic fluid and newborn urine. Fetal urine is a major source of the cytokine and is gender-dependent with the highest levels found in females. The investigators of one study concluded that the higher concentrations contributed to the better resistance of female fetuses against preterm birth and perinatal infections (3). Conversely, IL-1ra also has been shown to have partial agonist properties because it increases the prostaglandin E_2 (PGE_2) production of interleukin-1β in fetal membranes that is involved in the initiation of parturition at term (4).

Reproduction studies have been conducted in rats and rabbits. No evidence of impaired fertility or fetal harm was observed in either species at doses up to 100 times the human dose (*assumed to be based on weight*). Animal carcinogenic studies have not been conducted with anakinra, but it was not mutagenic with in vitro and in vivo tests (1).

In contrast to the above animal data, recombinant IL-1ra has been shown in mice to impair embryonic implantation by a direct inhibitory effect on transformation of the epithelial plasma membrane (5,6). Further, the embryos were morphologically normal and were viable when transferred to pseudopregnant mice (6).

In a 1992 mouse study, interleukin-1-induced preterm delivery was blocked by IL-1ra (7). However, IL-1ra did not prevent preterm delivery or prolong pregnancy in mice with endotoxin-induced preterm labor (8).

A 2001 Australian study found evidence that polymorphisms in the gene encoding for endogenous IL-1ra were associated with recurrent miscarriage (three or more consecutive pregnancy losses before 20 weeks' gestation) (9). The study investigated 105 women with idiopathic recurrent miscarriage compared with 91 controls with a history of normal pregnancies and no pregnancy losses. Three alleles of IL-1ra polymorphisms were measured. Study subjects had a significantly higher level of polymorphic allele 2, suggesting that this was a genetic determinant of idiopathic recurrent miscarriage and that IL-1ra acted as a physiologic mediator. The study could not determine the degree of genetic IL-1ra deficiency that was associated with idiopathic recurrent miscarriage (9). In contrast, a 2003 Finnish study found that significantly higher levels of polymorphic allele 3 were associated with recurrent spontaneous abortion, suggesting that the allele frequencies varied considerably in different ethnic groups (10).

Anakinra crosses the rabbit placenta. The cervixes of pregnant rabbits were inoculated with *Escherichia coli* and then the rabbits were given a 5-hour infusion of anakinra (10 mg/kg) (11). Although the treatment did not affect clinical or microbiological outcomes or amniotic fluid levels of tumor necrosis factor-alpha or prostaglandins (PGE_2), amniotic fluid concentrations of anakinra were markedly elevated compared with controls (14.8 ng/mL vs. none detected) (11).

An in vitro study was conducted using term human placentas obtained at cesarean section from uncomplicated pregnancies to determine if recombinant IL-1ra crossed the placenta (12). Both maternal-to-fetal and fetal-to-maternal directions were studied. Minimal transfer occurred in either direction. The findings appear to be consistent with the high molecular weight (17,300) of the 153-amino acid protein.

A 2009 case report described a 33-year-old woman with adult-onset Still disease who was treated with anakinra 100 mg/day throughout pregnancy (13). She gave birth at term to a severely growth-restricted (5th percentile), otherwise-normal 2700-g female infant with Apgar scores of 7, 8, and 9. Intrauterine growth restriction is a known complication of Still disease (see also Breastfeeding Summary) (13).

BREASTFEEDING SUMMARY

A 2009 report (see above) described the use of anakinra 100 mg/day during breastfeeding (13). The mother was treated throughout gestation and continued the therapy while breastfeeding. The small-for-gestational-age infant had appropriate growth (10th to 25th percentile) and normal psychomotor development (13).

Even though the molecular weight of the 153-amino acid cytokine is high (17,300), endogenous IL-1ra is excreted into colostrum and mature milk. In a 1996 study, concentrations of IL-1ra in colostrum were higher than those in milk (14). Both colostrum and milk had significantly higher concentrations than did maternal serum or plasma. The measurements of another 1996 study mirrored these findings of IL-1ra in colostrum, transitional milk, and mature milk (15). In the first study, the high milk concentrations persisted over a sequential collection period of 2–6 months (14). It was thought that the presence of natural IL-1ra contributed to the known anti-inflammatory properties of breast milk. Indeed, in a 2001 study, milk levels of IL-1ra in eight lactating women with acute mastitis were markedly increased (16). Because of the presence of native IL-1ra in milk, there appears to be no risk to a nursing infant from maternal administration of anakinra.

References

1. Product information. Kineret. Amgen, 2004.
2. Romero R, Gomez R, Galasso M, Mazor M, Berry SM, Quintero RA, Cotton DB. The natural interleukin-1 receptor antagonist in the fetal, maternal, and amniotic fluid compartments: the effect of gestational age, fetal gender, and intrauterine infection. Am J Obstet Gynecol 1994;171:912–21.
3. Bry K, Lappalainen U, Waffarn F, Teramo K, Hallman M. Influence of fetal gender on the concentration of interleukin-1 receptor antagonist in amniotic fluid and in newborn urine. Pediatr Res 1994;35:130–4.
4. Brown NL, Alvi SA, Elder MG, Bennett PR, Sullivan MHF. Regulation of prostaglandin production in intact fetal membranes by interleukin-1 and its receptor antagonist. J Endocrinol 1998;159:519–26.
5. Simon C, Frances A, Piquette GN, El Danasouri I, Zurawski G, Dang W, Polan LM. Embryonic implantation in mice is blocked by interleukin-1 receptor antagonist. Endocrinology 1994;134:521–8.
6. Simon C, Valbuena D, Krussel J, Bernal A, Murphy CR, Shaw T, Pellicer A, Polan LM. Interleukin-1 receptor antagonist prevents embryonic implantation by a direct effect on the endometrial epithelium. Fertil Steril 1998;70:896–906.
7. Romero R, Tartakovsky B. The natural interleukin-1 receptor antagonist prevents interleukin-1-induced preterm delivery in mice. Am J Obstet Gynecol 1992;167:1041–5.

8. Fidel PL Jr, Romero R, Cutright J, Wolf N, Gomez R, Araneda H, Ramirez M, Yoon BH. Treatment with interleukin-1 receptor antagonist and soluble tumor necrosis factor receptor Fc fusion protein does not prevent endotoxin-induced preterm parturition in mice. J Soc Gynecol Invest 1997;4:22–6.
9. Unfried G, Tempfer C, Schneeberger C, Widmar B, Nagele F, Huber JC. Interleukin 1 receptor antagonist polymorphism in women with idiopathic recurrent miscarriage. Fertil Steril 2001;75:683–7.
10. Karhukorpi J, Laitinen T, Kivela H, Tiilikainen A, Hurme M. IL-1 receptor antagonist gene polymorphism in recurrent spontaneous abortion. J Reprod Immunol 2003;58:61–7.
11. McDuffie RS Jr, Davies JK, Leslie KK, Lee S, Sherman MP, Gibbs RS. A randomized controlled trial of interleukin-1 receptor antagonist in a rabbit model of ascending infection in pregnancy. Infect Dis Obstet Gynecol 2001;9:233–7.
12. Zaretsky MV, Alexander JM, Byrd W, Bawdon RE. Transfer of inflammatory cytokines across the placenta. Obstet Gynecol 2004;103:546–50.
13. Berger CT, Recher M, Steiner U, Hauser TM. A patient's wish: anakinra in pregnancy. Ann Rheum Dis 2009;68:1794–5.
14. Buescher ES, Malinowska I. Soluble receptors and cytokine antagonists in human milk. Pediatr Res 1996;40:839–44.
15. Srivastave MD, Srivastava A, Brouhard B, Saneto R, Groh-Wargo S, Kubit J. Cytokines in human milk. Res Commun Mol Pathol Pharmacol 1996;93:263–87.
16. Buescher ES, Hair PS. Human milk anti-inflammatory component contents during acute mastitis. Cell Immunol 2001;210:87–95.

ANIDULAFUNGIN

Antifungal

PREGNANCY RECOMMENDATION: No Human Data—Animal Data Suggest Low Risk
BREASTFEEDING RECOMMENDATION: No Human Data—Potential Toxicity

PREGNANCY SUMMARY

No reports describing the use of anidulafungin in human pregnancy have been located. The animal reproduction data suggest low risk, but the absence of human pregnancy experience prevents a complete assessment of embryo–fetal risk. Moreover, there are no reports of human pregnancy experience with caspofungin and micafungin, the other agents in the class. Thus, the best course is to avoid anidulafungin in pregnancy, however, if the woman's condition requires it, the benefit probably outweighs the unknown risk. The lowest possible dose should be used.

FETAL RISK SUMMARY

Anidulafungin is a semisynthetic lipopeptide antifungal agent administered by IV infusion. It is an echinocandin, a class of antifungal agents that also includes caspofungin and micafungin. Anidulafungin is indicated for the treatment of candidemia and other forms of *Candida* infections. Although it does not undergo hepatic metabolism, anidulafungin does undergo chemical degradation at physiologic temperature and pH to inactive peptidic compounds that are subsequently degraded and eliminated. The in vitro degradation half-life of the drug under physiologic conditions is about 24 hours. The terminal elimination half-life is 40–50 hours, with excretion primarily in the feces. Plasma protein binding of anidulafungin is moderate (84%) (1).

Reproduction studies have been conducted in rats and rabbits. In pregnant rats given a dose up two times the recommended human dose based on BSA (RHD), skeletal changes in rat fetuses were observed that included incomplete ossification of various bones and wavy, misaligned, or misshapen ribs. These effects, however, were not dose-related and were within the range of the laboratory's historical control database. In pregnant rabbits, doses four times the RHD (the highest dose) were associated with slightly reduced fetal weights, but maternal toxicity was also noted (1).

Anidulafungin was not genotoxic in several tests. Carcinogenicity studies have not been conducted. There were no adverse effects on fertility from the drug in male and female rats given IV doses that were two times the RHD (1).

It is not known if anidulafungin can cross the human placenta. The molecular weight (about 1140) is high, but the long degradation half-life and moderate plasma protein binding suggest that transfer to the embryo and/or fetus might occur. Moreover, the recommended course of therapy involves daily IV doses for at least 14 days. Anidulafungin does cross the rat placenta and has been detected in fetal plasma (1).

BREASTFEEDING SUMMARY

No reports describing the use of anidulafungin during human lactation have been located.

The molecular weight (about 1140) is high, but the long degradation half-life and moderate plasma protein binding suggest that excretion into breast milk might occur. Moreover, the recommended course of therapy involves daily IV doses for at least 14 days. The effect on a nursing infant from potential exposure to the drug in milk is unknown. Dose-related histamine-mediated symptoms (rash, urticaria, flushing, pruritus, dyspnea, and hypotension) have been observed in adults receiving IV anidulafungin.

Reference

1. Product information. Eraxis. Pfizer, 2007.

ANILERIDINE

[Withdrawn from the market. See 9th edition.]

ANISINDIONE

[Withdrawn from the market. See 9th edition.]

ANISOTROPINE

[Withdrawn from the market. See 9th edition.]

ANTAZOLINE

[Withdrawn from the market. See 9th edition.]

ANTHRALIN

Dermatologic Agent (Anti-Psoriatic)

PREGNANCY RECOMMENDATION: No Human Data—Probably Compatible
BREASTFEEDING RECOMMENDATION: No Human Data—Probably Compatible

PREGNANCY SUMMARY

No reports describing the use of anthralin in human pregnancy have been located. The lack of animal reproduction data and human pregnancy experience prevents an assessment of the embryo–fetal risk. However, a 2002 review of psoriasis in pregnancy stated that there was no evidence of systemic absorption or toxicity with topical anthralin (1). Thus, the embryo–fetal risk probably is nil.

FETAL RISK SUMMARY

Anthralin (dithranol) is a synthetic product used in creams and ointments for the topical treatment of psoriasis. It has been used in the treatment of psoriasis since 1916 (1). Reproduction studies in animals have not been conducted (2).

Either there is no systemic absorption of anthralin or the plasma concentrations are too low to detect. In either case, exposure of the embryo–fetus to clinically significant amounts of anthralin appears to be nil, despite the low molecular weight (about 226).

A case of contact dermatitis to dithranol (anthralin) in a woman at 7 months gestation was reported in 2003 (3). The dermatitis, due to inadvertent exposure, cleared rapidly after exposure was eliminated. No information on the pregnancy outcome was given.

BREASTFEEDING SUMMARY

No reports describing the use of anthralin during human lactation have been located. The molecular weight (about 226) is low enough for excretion into breast milk. However, either there is no systemic absorption of anthralin or the plasma concentrations are too low to detect. In either case, exposure of the nursing infant to clinically significant amounts of anthralin appears to be nil.

References

1. Tauscher AE, Fleischer AB Jr, Phelps KC, Feldman SR. Psoriasis and pregnancy. J Cutan Med Surg 2002;6:561–70.
2. Product information. Psoriatec. Sirius Laboratories, 2004.
3. Strauss RM, Bate J, Pring D. Connubial contact dermatitis: an unusual pregnancy dermatoses. Acta Derm Venereol 2003;83:316.

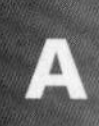

ANTIPYRINE

Analgesic/Antipyretic

PREGNANCY RECOMMENDATION: Limited Human Data—No Relevant Animal Data
BREASTFEEDING RECOMMENDATION: No Human Data—Potential Toxicity

PREGNANCY SUMMARY

The absence of relevant animal reproduction data and the limited human pregnancy experience prevent an assessment of the embryo–fetal risk. The drug is best avoided in pregnancy because of its known toxicity in adults.

FETAL RISK SUMMARY

Because of its rare association with hemolytic anemia and agranulocytosis (1), antipyrine (phenazone), a prostaglandin synthesis inhibitor, is no longer available as a single agent. However, the drug is still available in some topical ear drops and in the prodrug, dichloralphenazone (see also Dichloralphenazone). This latter agent, a combination of chloral hydrate and antipyrine, is a component, along with isometheptene and acetaminophen, of several proprietary mixtures commonly used for tension and vascular (migraine) headaches (see also Isometheptene and Acetaminophen).

Although animal reproductive studies involving antipyrine have not been located, the drug has been used extensively in investigations of fetal metabolism in pregnant sheep as reviewed in a 1993 reference (2). That investigation found that antipyrine did not affect umbilical metabolism but did alter metabolism and blood flow distribution in the fetal lamb (2).

Eight cases of antipyrine exposure (presumably oral), among 27 women using a miscellaneous group of non-narcotic analgesics during the 1st trimester, were reported by the Collaborative Perinatal Project (3). From the 27 mother–child pairs, one infant had a congenital malformation (standard relative risk 0.46), but the specific agent the mother had taken was not identified.

In a double-blind, randomized study of neonatal jaundice prophylaxis, either antipyrine ($N = 24$), 300 mg/day or placebo ($N = 24$) was given from the 38th week of gestation until delivery (4). The average duration of treatment in both groups was 15.5 days. The mean bilirubin concentration in the infants 4 days after birth was 62.6 μmol/L in those exposed to antipyrine compared with 111.5 μmol/L in the placebo group ($p < 0.005$). The authors attributed the decrease in bilirubin to the induction of glucuronyltransferase in the fetal liver, a known effect of antipyrine (4). No adverse effects in the newborns were observed.

BREASTFEEDING SUMMARY

Antipyrine (phenazone), a nonelectrolyte with a molecular weight <200, freely diffuses into the aqueous phase of milk with a milk:plasma ratio of approximately 1.0 (5,6). No reports of its use during lactation have been located.

References

1. Swanson M, Cook R. *Drugs Chemicals and Blood Dyscrasias*. Hamilton, IL: Drug Intelligence Publications, 1977:88–9.
2. Gull I, Charlton V. Effects of antipyrine on umbilical and regional metabolism in late gestation in the fetal lamb. Am J Obstet Gynecol 1993;168:706–13.
3. Heinonen OP, Slone D, Shapiro S. *Birth Defects and Drugs in Pregnancy*. Littleton, MA: Publishing Sciences Group, 1977:287.
4. Lewis PJ, Friedman LA. Prophylaxis of neonatal jaundice with maternal antipyrine treatment. Lancet 1979;1:300–2.
5. Hawkins DF. *Drugs and Pregnancy. Human Teratogenesis and Related Problems*. 2nd ed. New York, NY: Churchill Livingstone, 1987:312.
6. McNamara PJ, Burgio D, Yoo SD. Pharmacokinetics of acetaminophen, antipyrine, and salicylic acid in the lactating and nursing rabbit, with model predictions of milk to serum concentration ratios and neonatal dose. Toxicol Appl Pharmacol 1991;109:149–60.

ANTITHROMBIN III (HUMAN)

Hematologic Agent (Thrombin Inhibitor)

PREGNANCY RECOMMENDATION: Limited Human Data—Animal Data Suggest Low Risk
BREASTFEEDING RECOMMENDATION: No Human Data—Probably Compatible

PREGNANCY SUMMARY

Antithrombin III (human) has been used in the 2nd and 3rd trimesters for the treatment of preeclampsia. Preliminary evidence suggests that this treatment may be beneficial, but further studies are needed to confirm these outcomes. Although the limited animal data are reassuring, there is no human 1st trimester experience with this agent.

FETAL RISK SUMMARY

This product is prepared from pooled units of human plasma from screened normal plasma donors. Although the risk of transmitting infectious agents, such as viruses, has been reduced by measures taken during production, there is still a potential for transmitting disease (1). Antithrombin III is an α_2-glycoprotein that normally is present in human plasma at a concentration of approximately 12.5 mg/dL (1). It is the major plasma inhibitor of thrombin.

Reproduction studies have been conducted with antithrombin III in pregnant rats and rabbits. No evidence of impaired fertility or fetal harm was observed with doses up to four times the human dose (1).

It is not known whether there are physiologic processes that can carry maternal antithrombin to the embryo or fetus. The molecular weight of the protein, about 58,000, should prevent passive diffusion.

Two reports have described the use of antithrombin III in the treatment of preeclampsia (2,3). In both cases, the beneficial effects of antithrombin III were theorized to be related to the inhibition of thrombin, resulting in a reduction in maternal hypertension and an increase in placental circulation (2,3). In a nonrandomized study, women with severe early-onset preeclampsia (mean gestational age at onset 28–29 weeks) with intrauterine growth restriction were treated for 7 days with antithrombin III 1500 IU/day and heparin 5000 U/day (N = 14) or heparin 5000 U/day alone (N = 15) (2). None of the women received antihypertensive agents. The mean gestational age at the beginning of treatment was 30–31 weeks with delivery in both groups occurring at about 32 weeks' gestation. There was no difference in the mean birth weights (1280 vs. 1135 g), but the estimated fetal weight gain (g/day) was higher in the antithrombin group (29.5 vs. 15.3 g, $p < 0.05$). No information was provided on the status of the newborns, but there were no differences between the groups in the fetal biochemical profile score (2).

A total of 133 women with severe preeclampsia (24–35 weeks' gestation) were enrolled in a randomized, double-blind, placebo-controlled trial (3). The patients received either antithrombin III 3000 units once daily for 7 days (N = 66) or albumin once daily for 7 days (N = 67). The mean gestational age at the start of treatment was about 32 weeks in both groups. Treatment was interrupted in 23 and 29 patients in the antithrombin III and placebo groups, respectively, because of worsening of maternal and fetal findings. Patients in each group received antihypertensive agents and/or magnesium sulfate when indicated. There were no significant differences between the groups in the fetal biochemical profile score, but the antithrombin III group had a greater estimated fetal gain (p = 0.029). Pregnancy outcomes all favored the treatment group: gestational age at delivery (34.1 vs. 33.0 weeks, p = 0.007), birth weight (1749 vs. 1409 g, p = 0.004), and number of small-for-gestational-age newborns (65.6% vs. 83.3%, p = 0.020). No adverse effects in the newborns were observed (3).

BREASTFEEDING SUMMARY

No reports describing the use of antithrombin III during lactation have been located. The high molecular weight of the protein (about 58,000) suggests that it will not be excreted into breast milk. However, even if small amounts did enter the milk they likely would be digested in the infant's stomach. Therefore, the risk to a nursing infant from this agent appears to be nil.

References

1. Product information. Thrombate III. Bayer Corporation, Pharmaceutical Division, Biological Products, 2003.
2. Nakabayashi M, Asami M, Nakatani A. Efficacy of antithrombin replacement therapy in severe early-onset preeclampsia. Semin Thromb Hemost 1999;25:463–6.
3. Maki M, Kobayashi T, Terao T, Ikenoue T, Satoh K, Nakabayashi M, Sagara Y, Kajiwara Y, Urata M. Antithrombin therapy for severe preeclampsia. Results of a double-blind, randomized, placebo-controlled trial. Thromb Haemost 2000;84:583–90.

APIXABAN

Anticoagulant

PREGNANCY RECOMMENDATION: **No Human Data—Animal Data Suggest Low Risk**
BREASTFEEDING RECOMMENDATION: **No Human Data—Potential Toxicity**

PREGNANCY SUMMARY

No reports describing the use of apixaban in human pregnancy have been located. The animal reproduction data suggest low risk, but the absence of human pregnancy experience prevents a complete assessment of the embryo–fetal risk. Maternal bleeding during pregnancy and at delivery, as well as fetal or newborn bleeding, is a risk because there is no established way to reverse the anticoagulant effect that may persist for about 24 hours. The treatment of deep venous thrombosis or pulmonary embolism is not an approved indication, and apixaban should not be used as heparin is the treatment of choice for these indications (1). However, if apixaban is the treatment of choice for its approved indication, it should not be withheld because of pregnancy.

FETAL RISK SUMMARY

Apixaban is an oral, reversible, selective active site inhibitor of factor Xa in the same pharmacologic class as rivaroxaban. It is indicated to reduce the risk of stroke and systemic embolism in patients with nonvalvular atrial fibrillation. The agent is partially metabolized (about 25%) to inactive metabolites. Plasma protein binding is about 87%. The half-life is about 6 hours but, because of prolonged absorption, repeated dosing results in an effective half-life of about 12 hours (2).

Reproduction studies have been conducted in mice, rats, and rabbits. In these species that were given apixaban from implantation to the end of gestation, fetal exposures occurred but were not associated with an increased risk of fetal malformations or toxicity, or maternal or fetal deaths due to bleeding. However, an increased incidence of maternal bleeding in mice, rats, and rabbits was observed at maternal exposures that were 19, 4, and 1 times, respectively, the human exposure of unbound drug based on AUC at the maximum human dose of 5 mg twice daily (MHD) (2).

Two-year studies in mice and rats observed no carcinogenicity. Various assays for mutagenic and clastogenic effects also were negative. No effect on fertility was observed in male or female rats given doses up to 3 and 4 times, respectively, the MHD. In rats given doses up to 5 times the MHD from implantation through the end of lactation, no adverse findings were observed in male offspring. Adverse effects in female offspring were decreased mating and fertility indices (2).

It is not known if apixaban crosses the human placenta. The molecular weight (about 460), partial metabolism, moderate plasma protein binding, and long effective half-life suggest that the drug will cross to the embryo–fetus. The drug does cross the rat placenta and distributes in fetal blood, liver, and kidney (3).

BREASTFEEDING SUMMARY

No reports describing the use of apixaban during human lactation have been located. The molecular weight (about 460), partial metabolism, moderate plasma protein binding (about 87%), and long effective half-life (about 12 hours) suggest that the drug will be excreted into breast milk. The effect of this exposure on a nursing infant is unknown. However, bleeding (e.g., gastrointestinal, intracranial, intraocular) has been reported in adults and is potentially fatal. Therefore, the safest course is to not breastfeed if apixaban is taken.

References

1. Greer IA. Thrombosis in pregnancy: updates in diagnosis and management. Hematol Am Soc Hematol Educ Program 2012;203–7. doi:10.1182/asheducation-2012.1.203.
2. Product information. Eliquis. Bristol-Myers Squibb, 2012.
3. Wang L, He K, Maxwell B, Grossman SJ, Tremaine LM, Humphreys WG, Zhang D. Tissue distribution and elimination of [^{14}C]apixaban in rats. Drug Metab Dispos 2011;39:256–64.

APREPITANT

Antiemetic

PREGNANCY RECOMMENDATION: **No Human Data—Animal Data Suggest Low Risk**
BREASTFEEDING RECOMMENDATION: **No Human Data—Potential Toxicity**

PREGNANCY SUMMARY

No reports describing the use of aprepitant in human pregnancy have been located. The animal data suggest low risk, even though low doses relative to the human dose were studied. Use of higher doses was not possible because of saturation of absorption in the animals. The absence of human pregnancy experience prevents a full assessment of the risk. Until additional data are available, the use of aprepitant, if indicated, should be restricted to the 2nd and 3rd trimesters. However, if inadvertent exposure does occur during organogenesis, the embryo–fetal risk appears to be low.

FETAL RISK SUMMARY

Aprepitant is an oral antiemetic indicated, in combination with other antiemetic agents, for the prevention of acute and delayed nausea and vomiting associated with highly emetogenic cancer chemotherapy, such as cisplatin. It is a selective high-affinity antagonist of human substance P/neurokinin 1 (NK_1). Protein binding to plasma protein is >95%. Aprepitant is extensively metabolized to relatively inactive compounds by cytochrome P450 isoenzymes (primarily CYP3A4). The elimination half-life ranges from 9 to 13 hours (1).

Reproduction studies have been conducted in rats and rabbits. In rats, oral doses up to about 1.6 times the human exposure in nonpregnant patients at the recommended dose based on $AUC_{0-24\,h}$ (HERD) revealed no evidence of impaired fertility or fetal harm. Similar results were observed in rabbits at doses up to about 1.4 times the HERD. Higher doses were not used because of saturation of absorption. In 2-year carcinogenicity studies, oral doses up to 0.4–1.4 times the HERD were carcinogenic in male and female rats. Oral doses up to 2.2–2.7 times the HERD were carcinogenic in male mice. No mutagenicity was observed in various assays (1).

It is not known if aprepitant crosses the human placenta. The drug crosses the placenta in rats and rabbits and crosses the blood–brain barrier in humans (1). Although protein binding is high, the molecular weight (about 534) and elimination half-life suggest that the drug will cross the human placenta to the embryo and/or fetus.

BREASTFEEDING SUMMARY

No reports describing the use of aprepitant during human lactation have been located. The molecular weight (about 534) and elimination half-life (9–13 hours) suggest that the drug will be excreted into breast milk. However, the high plasma protein binding (>95%) should attenuate the amount excreted. The potential effect of this exposure on a nursing infant is unknown, but consideration should be given, especially if the exposure is prolonged, to the carcinogenic effects observed in animal studies.

Reference

1. Product information. Emend. Merck, 2005.

APROBARBITAL

[Withdrawn from the market. See 8th edition.]

APROTININ

Hemostatic

PREGNANCY RECOMMENDATION: Limited Human Data—Animal Data Suggest Low Risk
BREASTFEEDING RECOMMENDATION: No Human Data—Probably Compatible

PREGNANCY SUMMARY

No reports linking the use of aprotinin and congenital defects have been located. The drug crosses the placenta and decreases fibrinolytic activity in the newborn (1). The drug has been used safely in severe accidental hemorrhage with coagulation when labor was not established (2).

FETAL RISK SUMMARY

Aprotinin, a polypeptide, is a natural, broad-spectrum protease inhibitor obtained from bovine lung that is indicated for the prophylaxis of perioperative blood loss during cardiopulmonary bypass surgery. After IV administration, aprotinin undergoes rapid distribution into the total extracellular space and the plasma half-life, after the distribution phase, is about 150 minutes. The terminal half-life is about 10 hours (3).

Reproduction studies were conducted in rats with daily IV doses for 11 days up to 2.4 times the human dose based on body weight (HD-BW) or 0.37 times the human dose based on BSA (HD-BSA). Rabbits were given daily IV doses for 13 days up to 1.2 times the HD-BW or 0.36 times the HD-BSA. No effects on fertility or fetal harm were observed in either species (3).

BREASTFEEDING SUMMARY

No reports have been located describing the use of aprotinin during lactation. Because of the indication for this drug, the opportunity for breastfeeding following its use is probably nil. The oral absorption of this polypeptide is unknown, but most likely poor.

References

1. Hoffhauer H, Dobbeck P. Untersuchungen uber die plactapassage des kallikrein-inhibitors. Klin Wochenschr 1970;48:183–4.
2. Sher G. Trasylol in cases of accidental hemorrhage with coagulation disorder and associated uterine inertia. S Afr Med J 1974;48:1452–5.
3. Product information. Trasylol. Bayer, 2000.

ARFORMOTEROL

Respiratory Drug (Bronchodilator)

PREGNANCY RECOMMENDATION: No Human Data—Probably Compatible
BREASTFEEDING RECOMMENDATION: No Human Data—Probably Compatible

PREGNANCY SUMMARY

No reports describing the use of arformoterol in human pregnancy have been located. The animal data suggest low risk, but the absence of human data prevents a complete assessment of the embryo–fetal risk. Although other β-adrenergic agonists are known to interfere with uterine contractions (e.g., see Terbutaline), such an effect from arformoterol is unlikely because of the very low systemic levels obtained from oral inhalation.

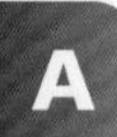

FETAL RISK SUMMARY

Arformoterol is a selective long-acting β_2-adrenergic receptor agonist that acts as a bronchodilator. It is the (*R*,*R*)-enantiomer of formoterol and has twice the potency of racemic formoterol. (See also Formoterol.) Arformoterol is formulated as a solution that is administered by nebulization. Systemic bioavailability of arformoterol is very low with concentrations in the low pg/mL range in nonpregnant patients. The drug is extensively metabolized to inactive metabolites. Plasma protein binding (52%–65%) is moderate, but the mean terminal half-life (26 hours) is prolonged (1).

Reproduction studies have been conducted in rats and rabbits. In pregnant rats, oral doses that resulted in exposures about 370 times the adult exposure (AUC) at the maximum recommended daily inhalation dose (MRDID) caused omphalocele (umbilical hernia). At exposures of about 1100 times the MRDID, increased pup loss at birth and during lactation and decreased pup weights were observed. Delays in development were evident at about 2400 times the MRDID (1).

In pregnant rabbits, fetal malpositioned right kidney was noted at doses producing exposures that were about 8400 times the MRDID. Doses that were about ≥22,000 times the MRDID based on BSA (MRDID-BSA) caused brachydactyly, bulbous aorta, liver cysts, adactyly, lobular dysgenesis of the lung, and interventricular septal defect. At the highest dose (about 43,000 times the MRDID-BSA), embryolethality was observed. Decreased pup weights were noted at doses that were about 22,000 times the MRDID-BSA. There were no teratogenic findings at exposures of about ≤4900 times the MRDID (1).

Two-year studies for carcinogenicity have been conducted in mice (oral) and rats (inhalation). In female mice, there was a dose-related increase in the incidence of uterine and cervical endometrial stromal polyps and stromal cell sarcoma at exposures (AUC) of about 70 times the MRDID. In female rats, exposures that were about 130 times the MRDID caused an increased incidence of thyroid gland C-cell adenoma and carcinoma. No tumor findings occurred with exposures of about 55 times the MRDID. Arformoterol was not mutagenic or clastogenic in multiple assays. There were no effects on fertility or reproductive performance in rats given oral doses up to about 2700 times the MRDID-BSA (1).

It is not known if arformoterol crosses the human placenta. The molecular weight (about 345 for the free base), moderate plasma protein binding, and prolonged terminal half-life suggest that the drug will cross the placenta. However, because of the minimal amounts in the systemic circulation, this exposure appears to be clinically insignificant.

BREASTFEEDING SUMMARY

No reports describing the use of arformoterol during human lactation have been located. The molecular weight (about 345 for the free base), moderate plasma protein binding, and prolonged terminal half-life suggest that the drug will be excreted into breast milk. However, because of the minimal amounts in the systemic circulation, this exposure appears to represent no risk to a nursing infant.

Reference

1. Product information. Brovana. Sepracor, 2007.

ARGATROBAN

Hematologic Agent (Thrombin Inhibitor)

PREGNANCY RECOMMENDATION: Compatible—Maternal Benefit >> Embryo–Fetal Risk
BREASTFEEDING RECOMMENDATION: No Human Data—Potential Toxicity

PREGNANCY SUMMARY

Animal reproductive studies have not shown developmental toxicity, but the doses used were a small fraction of the human dose. The human pregnancy experience is limited to three case reports where argatroban was used in the 2nd and 3rd trimesters. No drug-induced toxicity, such as hemorrhage, was observed in the three exposed infants. Although there are no reports describing the use of argatroban in the 1st trimester, the lack of teratogenicity in animals and another agent in this subclass (see Lepirudin) is encouraging. Thus, if a pregnant woman requires argatroban therapy the benefits to her appear to outweigh the theoretical risks to the embryo or fetus.

FETAL RISK SUMMARY

Argatroban is a synthetic reversible direct thrombin inhibitor derived from L-arginine. It is in the same anticoagulant subclass as bivalirudin, desirudin, and lepirudin. Argatroban is indicated as an anticoagulant for prophylaxis or treatment of thrombosis in patients with heparin-induced thrombocytopenia (HIT). It is also indicated as an anticoagulant in patients with or at risk for HIT undergoing percutaneous coronary intervention. The drug is administered as a continuous IV infusion and undergoes partial metabolism in the liver. Total serum protein binding is 54%, with 20% bound to albumin and 34% to α_1-acid glycoprotein. The terminal elimination half-life is 39–51 minutes (1).

Reproduction studies with IV argatroban have been conducted in pregnant rats and rabbits at doses up to 0.3 and 0.2 times, respectively, the maximum recommended human dose based on BSA. No evidence of impaired fertility or fetal harm was observed in either species (1).

It is not known if argatroban crosses the human placenta. The molecular weight (about 527 for the hydrated form), low metabolism, and moderate serum protein binding suggest that exposure of the embryo–fetus should be expected, especially since the drug is given as a continuous infusion.

The use of argatroban in the 2nd trimester was reported in 2008 (2). A 35-year-old woman with anemia secondary to myelodysplastic syndrome developed a deep vein thrombosis (location and extent not specified) in the 18th week of pregnancy and was treated with unfractionated heparin. Severe thrombocytopenia developed, which was subsequently shown to be caused by bone-marrow dysplasia and not heparin (HIT antibody was negative), and therapy was changed to daily IV doses of danaparoid. In the 22nd week of gestation, pulmonary embolism occurred after a leg massage. An emergency pulmonary embolectomy was performed under cardiopulmonary bypass to remove emboli from the right main pulmonary artery. Anticoagulation during surgery was maintained with argatroban. The woman recovered and eventually delivered a healthy infant by cesarean section at 29 weeks' gestation. No details on the infant were provided (2).

A second 2008 report described the use of argatroban in the 3rd trimester (3). A 26-year-old woman with a nonocclusive portal vein thrombosis and thrombocytopenia secondary to idiopathic thrombocytopenic purpura was treated with enoxaparin at 31 weeks' gestation. Two weeks later, because of worsening thrombocytopenia that initially was thought to be HIT but was later found not to be, treatment was changed to a continuous infusion of argatroban. Dexamethasone was given for 4 days before a scheduled cesarean section to increase the platelet count so that epidural anesthesia could be used. Argatroban was discontinued 7 hours before epidural anesthesia was successfully placed. A 3092-g male infant with Apgar scores of 8 and 9 at 1 and 5 minutes, respectively, was delivered. Examination of the infant revealed a small muscular ventricular septal defect with a patent foramen ovale; neither was due to argatroban. The infant had a normal platelet count at birth. At 6 months of age, the ventricular septal defect had resolved but he still had a patent foramen ovale (3).

Argatroban was used in a 38-year-old woman with an upper extremity deep vein thrombosis who had developed HIT late in the 2nd trimester (4). As the thrombus resolved, her therapy was changed to SC fondaparinux 7.5 mg/day, and this agent was continued until the day before scheduled induction. During labor she was given an IV infusion of argatroban and then discontinued several hours before combined spinal–epidural analgesia. She gave birth to a healthy, 3.8-kg male infant with Apgar scores of 8 and 8 at 1 and 5 minutes, respectively. No bleeding complications were reported in the infant (4).

A 31-year-old woman in her 12th week of pregnancy completely loss her vision in her right eye for 2 minutes (5). After an extensive workup, she was diagnosed with hypereosinophilic syndrome and started on heparin and prednisone. HIT developed and her anticoagulant therapy was changed to argatroban (dose not specified). The thrombocytopenia resolved and, after 15 days, she was discharged home on fondaparinux (75 mg/day) and a tapering dose of prednisone. About 6–7 months later she gave birth to a healthy female infant (no further infant details provided) (5).

In a 2012 case report, a 33-year-old woman, with a history of hereditary antithrombin deficiency, presented at 7 weeks' gestation with a deep venous thrombosis in her left leg due to the deficiency (6). She was treated with urokinase (24,000 units/day), heparin (20,000 units/day), and antithrombin concentrate (3000 units/day). Ten days later, at 9 weeks', HIT was diagnosed; heparin was discontinued and a continuous infusion of argatroban (2.5 mcg/kg/min) was started. At 21 weeks', argatroban was stopped and fondaparinux (2.5 mg/day) was started at 24 weeks'. Argatroban (2.5–3.5 mcg/kg/min) was restarted during labor induction at 37 weeks'. The patient gave birth to a 2800-g male infant with Apgar scores of 9 and 10 at 1 and 5 minutes, respectively. The newborn had 14% of antithrombin activity. The mother and her newborn were discharged home 15 days later (6).

BREASTFEEDING SUMMARY

No studies describing the use argatroban during human lactation have been located. The molecular weight (about 527 for the hydrated form), low metabolism, and moderate serum protein binding suggest that the drug will be excreted into breast milk, especially as it is given as a continuous infusion. Both the effect of this exposure on a nursing infant and the potential for oral absorption are unknown. Severe adverse effects have been observed in adults, such as hypotension, fever, nausea/vomiting, and diarrhea (1). Thus, until human data are available, the safest course is to not breastfeed while receiving argatroban.

References

1. Product information. Argatroban. GlaxoSmithKline, 2009.
2. Taniguchi S, Fukuda I, Minakawa M, Watanabe K, Daitoku K, Suzuki Y. Emergency pulmonary embolectomy during the second trimester of pregnancy: report of a case. Surg Today 2008;38:59–61.
3. Young SK, Al-Mondhiry HA, Vaida SJ, Ambrose A, Botti JJ. Successful use of argatroban during the third trimester of pregnancy: case report and review of the literature. Pharmacotherapy 2008;28:1531–6.
4. Ekbatani A, Asaro LR, Malinow AM. Anticoagulation with argatroban in a parturient with heparin-induced thrombocytopenia. Int J Obstet Anesth 2010;19:82–117.
5. Darki A, Kodali PP, McPheters JP, Virk H, Patel MR, Jacobs W. Hypereosinophilic syndrome with cardiac involvement. Tex Heart Inst J 2011;38:163–5.
6. Tanimura K, Ebina Y, Sonoyama A, Morita H, Miyata S, Yamada H. Argatroban therapy for heparin-induced thrombocytopenia during pregnancy in a woman with hereditary antithrombin deficiency. J Obstet Gynaecol Res 2012;38:749–52.

ARIPIPRAZOLE

Antipsychotic

PREGNANCY RECOMMENDATION: Limited Human Data—Animal Data Suggest Risk
BREASTFEEDING RECOMMENDATION: Limited Human Data—Potential Toxicity

PREGNANCY SUMMARY

Several case reports have described the use of aripiprazole in human pregnancy. No developmental toxicity was observed in these cases. The animal data suggest a risk of developmental toxicity and possibly teratogenicity, but the very limited human pregnancy experience prevents a complete assessment of the embryo–fetal risk. Until such data are available, the safest course is to avoid the drug in pregnancy. However, if the mother's condition requires treatment with aripiprazole, the lowest effective dose, avoiding the 1st trimester if possible, should be used. In addition, long-term evaluation of the infant is warranted.

FETAL RISK SUMMARY

Aripiprazole is an antipsychotic used in the treatment of schizophrenia. Activity is due to both the parent drug and its active metabolite. Both are extensively (>99%) bound to serum proteins, primarily albumin. The mean elimination half-lives of aripiprazole and the active metabolite are about 75 and 94 hours, respectively (1,2). The drug is in the quinolinone subclass of antipsychotics that has no other members.

Reproduction studies have been conducted in rats and rabbits. Female rats were treated for 2 weeks before mating through day 7 of gestation with doses up to six times the maximum recommended human dose based on BSA (MRHD). Fertility was not impaired but increased pre-implantation loss was seen at a dose twice the MRHD or greater and decreased fetal weight was noted at six times the MRHD. In pregnant rats, a dose 10 times the MRHD given during organogenesis caused a slightly prolonged gestation, and a slight delay in fetal development, as evidenced by decreased fetal weight, undescended testes, and delayed skeletal ossification. The latter effect was also seen at three times the MRHD. Some maternal toxicity was observed at 10 times the MRHD, but there was no evidence that the observed adverse effects were secondary to maternal toxicity (1,2). There were no effects on embryo, fetal, or pup survival, but offspring had decreased bodyweights (at 3 and 10 times the MRHD), and increased incidences of hepatodiaphragmatic nodules and diaphragmatic hernia (at 10 times the MRHD). Adverse effects in female offspring exposed in utero at 10 times the MRHD included delayed vaginal opening and impaired reproductive performance (decreased fertility rate, corpora lutea, implants, and live fetuses, and increased post-implantation loss). In perinatal and postnatal rat studies, a dose 10 times the MRHD given from day 17 of gestation through postpartum day 21 resulted in slight maternal toxicity and prolongation of gestation, increases in stillbirths, and decreases in pup weight (persisting into adulthood) and survival. Disturbances in spermatogenesis and prostate atrophy, but not impaired fertility, were observed in male rats given doses 13–19 times the MRHD from 9 weeks before mating through mating (1,2).

In rabbits, a dose 11 times the human exposure at the maximum recommended human dose based on AUC (HE) (up to 65 times the MRHD) during organogenesis resulted in decreased maternal food consumption and increased abortions. Other adverse effects noted were increased fetal mortality (at 11 times the HE), decreased fetal weight (at 3 and 11 times the HE), and increased incidences of skeletal abnormalities (fused sternebrae at 3 and 11 times the HE) and minor skeletal variations (at 11 times the HE) (1,2).

It is not known if aripiprazole or its active metabolite crosses the human placenta early in gestation. However, consistent with the molecular weight of the parent compound (about 448), combined with the prolonged elimination half-lives of aripiprazole and the active metabolite, both cross the placenta to the fetus at term (see case report below).

A 2006 case report described the use of aripiprazole in a 22-year-old woman with a 3-year history of paranoid schizophrenia (3). She had been treated with a variety of antipsychotics, including aripiprazole, but had stopped all therapy 1 year before conception. When her disease relapsed at 29 weeks' gestation, the woman was restarted on aripiprazole 10 mg/day and subsequently increased to 15 mg/day. After 85 days of therapy, the drug was stopped 6 days before spontaneous delivery at the end of week 37 of gestation. The normal, 2.6-kg male infant had Apgar scores of 9 and 10 at 1 and 5 minutes, respectively. He remained healthy at 6 months of age (3).

A second 2006 case report described a 27-year-old woman with schizophrenia who conceived while taking aripiprazole 15 mg/day (4). The woman stopped the drug during the 8th week of gestation. After a relapse during the 20th week of gestation, she restarted aripiprazole 10 mg/day and continued this dose throughout the remainder of her pregnancy. Fetal distress, including tachycardia, was noted at term and a healthy, 3.25-kg infant (sex not specified) was delivered by cesarean section. The infant was doing well at 6 months of age (4).

In a 2008 case report, a 24-year-old woman with schizoaffective disorder took aripiprazole 20 mg/day up to the time of conception and then discontinued the drug because she did not want to expose her fetus (5). She also had stopped her intermittent use of marijuana about 2 weeks before conception. At about 8 weeks', she experienced a severe relapse and aripiprazole was restarted and continued throughout pregnancy. At 40 weeks', she gave birth to a healthy, 3.24-kg male infant with Apgar scores of 9 and 9. The infant was doing well at 12 months of age (5).

Five other reports, similar to those above, have described the use of aripiprazole in six pregnancies (6–10). No adverse effects of the drug therapy were observed in the newborns. In one case, a woman taking aripiprazole 10 mg/day had an elective cesarean section at 39 weeks' gestation (9). At birth, samples were obtained from cord blood 8.6 hours after the last dose. The cord serum concentrations of aripiprazole and the active metabolite were 17 and 8 mcg/L, respectively, while the concentrations in the mother, taken 9.6 hours after dose, were 70 and 45 mcg/L, respectively. The cord:maternal ratios were 0.64 and 0.47, respectively (9).

BREASTFEEDING SUMMARY

In a case mentioned above, a woman taking aripiprazole 15 mg/day breastfed her newborn infant (6). Breast milk samples were collected on postpartum day 3 but the analysis for the drug was unsuccessful. On day 27, milk samples were collected 24 hours after the last dose (30 minutes before the next dose) and 4 and 10 hours after a dose. On day 28, the mother's serum concentrations of the parent drug and metabolite were 207 and 42 ng/mL, respectively. Neither aripiprazole nor its metabolite was detected in any of the three milk specimens. Based on a detection limit of 10 ng/mL, the milk:plasma ratios were <0.04. The estimated relative infant dose based on the mother's weight-adjusted dose was <0.7%. At 3 months of age, the infant was growing normally (6).

Although the above case was unable to find detectable milk concentrations of aripiprazole and its metabolite, confirmation of these results is warranted. Until such data are available, if a woman taking the drug chooses to breastfeed, the infant should be closely monitored for adverse effects. Recommendations for counseling breastfeeding mothers who are taking an antipsychotic drug were listed in a 2013 reference (11). Moreover, long-term evaluation of exposed infants is warranted.

References

1. Product information. Abilify. Bristol-Myers Squibb, 2004.
2. Product information. Abilify. Otsuka America Pharmaceutical, 2004.
3. Mendhekar DN, Sharma JB, Srilakshmi P. Use of aripiprazole during late pregnancy in a woman with psychotic illness. Ann Pharmacother 2006;40:575.
4. Mendhekar DN, Sunder K, Andrade C. Aripiprazole use in a pregnant schizoaffective woman. Bipolar Disord 2006;8:299–300.
5. Mervak B, Collins J, Valenstein M. Case report of aripiprazole usage during pregnancy. Arch Women's Ment Health 2008;11:249–50.
6. Lutz UC, Hiemke C, Wiatr G, Farger G, Arand J, Wildgruber D. Aripiprazole in pregnancy and lactation. A case report. J Clin Psychopharmacol 2010;30:204–5.
7. Watanabe N, Kasahara M, Sugibayashi R, Nakajima K, Watanabe O, Murashima A. Perinatal use of aripiprazole. A case report. J Clin Psychopharmacol 2011;31:377–9.
8. Gentile S, Tofani S, Bellantuono C. Aripiprazole and pregnancy. A case report and literature review. J Clin Psychopharmacol 2011;31:531–2.
9. Nguyen T, Teoh S, Hackett P, Ilett K. Placental transfer of aripiprazole. Aust N Z J Psychiatry 2011;45:500–1.
10. Widschwendter CG, Hofer A. Aripiprazole use in early pregnancy: a case report. Pharmacopsychiatry 2012;45:299–300.
11. Klinger G, Stahl B, Fusar-Poli P, Merlob P. Antipsychotic drugs and breastfeeding. Pediatr Endocrinol 2013;10:308–17.

ARMODAFINIL

Central Stimulant

PREGNANCY RECOMMENDATION: Limited Human Data—Animal Data Suggest Risk
BREASTFEEDING RECOMMENDATION: No Human Data—Potential Toxicity

PREGNANCY SUMMARY

Other than the three cases reported by the manufacturer, no reports describing the use of armodafinil in human pregnancy have been located. Developmental toxicity was observed in two animal species at systemic exposures that were equal to or less than human plasma exposures. The near absence of human pregnancy experience prevents a better assessment of the embryo–fetal risk. Avoiding armodafinil during pregnancy is the best course. Inadvertent exposure does not appear to represent a major risk of embryo–fetal harm but, because of the two cases of intrauterine growth restriction, closer attention than usual to fetal growth might be appropriate.

FETAL RISK SUMMARY

Armodafinil is the R-enantiomer of modafinil which is a mixture of the *R*- and *S*-enantiomers (see also Modafinil). It is indicated to improve wakefulness in patients with excessive sleepiness associated with obstructive sleep apnea/hypopnea syndrome, narcolepsy, and shift-work sleep disorder. Armodafinil is a lipophilic agent that is extensively metabolized to apparently inactive metabolites. The drug is moderately bound (about 60%) to plasma proteins, primarily albumin, and the terminal half-life is about 15 hours (1).

Reproduction studies with armodafinil have been conducted in rats and, with modafinil, in rats and rabbits. In rats, daily oral doses of armodafinil given throughout the period of organogenesis resulted in increased incidences of fetal visceral and skeletal variations and decreased fetal body weights. The no-effect dose for rat embryo–fetal developmental toxicity was associated with a plasma exposure (AUC) that was about 0.03 times the AUC in humans at the maximum recommended daily dose of 250 mg (MRDD) (1).

Daily oral doses of modafinil given to rats throughout organogenesis caused an increase in resorptions and increased incidences of visceral and skeletal variations. The no-effect dose for embryo–fetal developmental toxicity was associated with a plasma exposure (AUC) that was about 0.5 times the AUC in humans at the recommended daily dose of 200 mg (RHD). In another study, no developmental toxicity was observed at plasma modafinil exposure about 2 times the AUC at the RHD. However, when modafinil was given to rats throughout gestation and lactation, decreased viability in the offspring occurred with plasma exposures that were about 0.1 times the AUC at the RHD. No effects on postnatal developmental and neurobehavioral parameters were observed in surviving offspring (1).

In rabbits, daily oral doses of modafinil given throughout organogenesis caused increased incidences of fetal structural alterations and embryo–fetal death at the highest dose. The highest no-effect dose for developmental toxicity was associated with a plasma modafinil exposure that was about equal to the AUC at the RHD (1).

Carcinogenicity studies conducted with modafinil in mice and rats were negative. No evidence of mutagenic or clastogenic potential was found in multiple assays with armodafinil. Fertility studies in male and female rats with modafinil observed an increase in time to mate at the highest dose. The no-effect dose resulted in a plasma exposure that was about equal to the AUC in humans at the RHD (1).

It is not known if armodafinil crosses the human placenta. The molecular weight (about 273), lipophilic nature, moderate plasma protein binding, and long terminal half-life suggest that the drug will cross to the embryo–fetus.

The manufacturer mentioned two cases of intrauterine growth restriction, and one spontaneous abortion had been reported in association with armodafinil and modafinil, but it was not known if the outcomes were drug-related (1). (See also Modafinil.)

BREASTFEEDING SUMMARY

No reports describing the use of armodafinil during human lactation have been located. The molecular weight (about 273), lipophilic nature, moderate plasma protein binding (about 60%), and long terminal half-life (about 15 hours) suggest that the drug will be excreted into breast milk. The effect of this exposure on a nursing infant is unknown. If a lactating woman uses armodafinil, her infant should be closely observed for adverse effects that are commonly seen in adults (i.e., headache, nausea, dizziness, anxiety, and insomnia).

Reference

1. Product information. Nuvigil. Cephalon, 2010.

ARNICA

Herb

PREGNANCY RECOMMENDATION: Contraindicated
BREASTFEEDING RECOMMENDATION: Contraindicated

PREGNANCY SUMMARY

No reports describing the use of arnica in human pregnancy have been located. The herb should not be used in pregnancy as it is a uterine stimulant that has been used traditionally as an abortifacient (1).

FETAL RISK SUMMARY

Arnica is a perennial plant that has bright yellow, daisy-like flowers that, when dried, are the primary parts used, but the roots and rhizomes also are used. The herb has been used medicinally for hundreds of years, especially in Europe. The herb and its extracts have been used as a topical treatment for skin conditions and wounds and are often used in cosmetic formulations. However, clinical evidence to support its use as an anti-inflammatory or analgesic is lacking. The FDA has classified arnica as an unsafe herb when used orally, in which case it is considered a poison, or applied to broken skin where absorption could occur. It is possibly safe when used in amounts commonly found in foods. A large number of chemicals are found in arnica, including flavonoids glycosides, isomeric alcohols, terpenoids (including sesquiterpene lactones), amines, coumarins, carbohydrates, volatile oils, fatty acids, and other compounds. The active ingredients are the sesquiterpene lactones (1–3).

No carcinogenicity, reproductive, or developmental toxicity data are available (3).

In homoeopathic formulations, arnica has been promoted for use before and during labor as helpful for internal and external bruising of both the mother and newborn infant (4). In a survey of 1044 Italian women, 491 (47%) reported that they had taken or were taking one or more herbals in the last year, sometimes during pregnancy (5). Arnica was among the top 10 herbs taken by the women.

BREASTFEEDING SUMMARY

Although it has not been studied, an abstract describing toxicity in a nursing infant suggests that some of the chemicals in arnica are excreted into human milk. A 9-day-old term male infant who was exclusively breastfed presented with a 1-day history of lethargy, decreased milk intake, anemia, and jaundice (6). The mother, who was asymptomatic, had started drinking a tea made from arnica flowers 48 hours before the onset of symptoms. No reason for the infant's jaundice was found on workup. A screening test in the infant for glucose-6-phosphate dehydrogenase (G6PD) was normal. Exchange transfusions were used to lower the bilirubin and correct the infant's anemia. The mother stopped drinking the tea and resumed breastfeeding, and no further hemolysis or other problems were noted in the infant (6).

References

1. Arnica. *The Review of Natural Products*. St. Louis, MO: Wolters Kluwer Health, 2010.
2. Arnica. *Natural Medicines Comprehensive Database*. 10th ed. Stockton, CA: Therapeutic Research Faculty, 2008:83–5.
3. Anonymous. Final report on the safety assessment of arnica montana extract and arnica montana. Int J Toxicol 2001;20(Suppl 2):1–11.
4. Kaplan B. Homoeopathy: 2. In pregnancy and for the under-fives. Prof Care Mother Child 1994;4:185–7.
5. Zaffani S, Cuzzolin L, Benoni G. Herbal products: behaviors and beliefs among Italian women. Pharmacoepidemiol Drug Saf 2006;15:354–9.
6. Miller AD, Ly BT, Clark RF. Neonatal hemolysis associated with nursing mother ingestion of arnica tea (abstract). Clin Toxicol 2009;47:726.

ASENAPINE

Antipsychotic

PREGNANCY RECOMMENDATION: No Human Data—Animal Data Suggest Risk
BREASTFEEDING RECOMMENDATION: No Human Data—Potential Toxicity

PREGNANCY SUMMARY

No reports describing the use of asenapine in human pregnancy have been located. There is no evidence of embryo–fetal harm with other agents in this subclass. However, because of the very limited human pregnancy experience with atypical antipsychotics, the American College of Obstetricians and Gynecologists does not recommend the routine use of these agents in pregnancy, but a risk benefit assessment may indicate that such use is appropriate (1). Until human data are available, the use of other antipsychotics in pregnancy should be considered. Nevertheless, asenapine is indicated for severe debilitating mental disease and the benefits to the mother will probably outweigh the unknown embryo–fetal risk. A 1996 review on the management of psychiatric illness concluded that patients with histories of chronic psychosis represent a high-risk group (for both the mother and the fetus) and should be maintained on pharmacologic therapy before and during pregnancy (2). Folic acid 4 mg/day has been recommended for women taking atypical antipsychotics because they may have a higher risk of neural tube defects due to inadequate folate intake and obesity (3).

FETAL RISK SUMMARY

Asenapine is an atypical antipsychotic agent that is available for sublingual administration. It is indicated for the acute treatment of schizophrenia in adults. Asenapine belongs to the antipsychotic subclass of dibenzapine derivatives that includes clozapine, loxapine, olanzapine, and quetiapine. It is metabolized and eliminated as inactive metabolites. The mean terminal half-life is about 24 hours. Asenapine is highly bound (95%) to plasma proteins, including albumin and α1-acid glycoprotein (4).

Animal reproduction studies have been conducted in rats and rabbits. In these species, asenapine was not teratogenic at IV doses up to 0.7 and 0.4 times, respectively, the maximum recommended human dose of 10 mg twice daily given sublingually based on BSA (MRHD). In rabbits, the highest dose produced plasma levels (AUC) that were twice the human levels resulting from the MRHD. Increases in post-implantation loss and early pup deaths were observed in rats given daily IV doses that were 0.15–0.7 times the MRHD from gestation day 6 through postpartum day 21. Decreases in pup survival and weight gain were seen at IV doses that were 0.4 and 0.7 times the MRHD. Oral dosing had the same effects. The decreases in pup survival were largely due to prenatal drug effects (4).

Lifetime carcinogenicity studies have been conducted in mice and rats. In female mice given SC doses resulting in plasma levels (AUC) that were about 5 times the human levels resulting from the MRHD, an increased incidence of malignant lymphomas was observed. However, the mouse strain used had a high and variable incidence of this cancer, and the significance of this finding to humans is unknown. The no-effect dose was about 1.5 times the human levels resulting from the MRHD. No tumors were observed in male mice or in rats. No evidence of genotoxic potential was found in several tests. In rats, doses up to 10 times the MRHD had no effect on fertility (4).

It is not known if asenapine crosses the human placenta. The molecular weight (about 286 for the free base) and the long terminal elimination half-life suggest that the drug will cross to the embryo–fetus, even though the high plasma protein binding may limit the exposure.

BREASTFEEDING SUMMARY

No reports describing the use of asenapine during human lactation have been located. The molecular weight (about 286 for the free base) and the long terminal elimination half-life (about 24 hours) suggest that the drug will be excreted into breast milk, even though the high (95%) plasma protein binding might limit the exposure. The effect of this exposure on a nursing infant is unknown, but they should be monitored for the most common adverse reactions observed in adults (somnolence, dizziness, akathisia, and oral hypoesthesia).

The manufacturer recommends women receiving asenapine should not breastfeed (4). Moreover, the American Academy of Pediatrics classifies other atypical antipsychotics (e.g., see Clozapine) as drugs whose effect on the nursing infant is unknown but may be of concern (5).

Because of the very limited human experience with atypical antipsychotics, the American College of Obstetricians and Gynecologists does not recommend the routine use of these agents during lactation, but a risk–benefit assessment may indicate that such use is appropriate (1).

References

1. American College of Obstetricians and Gynecologists. Use of psychiatric medications during pregnancy and lactation. *ACOG Practice Bulletin*. Number 92, April 2008. Obstet Gynecol 2008;111:1001–19.
2. Althuler LL, Cohen L, Szuba MP, Burt VK, Gitlin M, Mintz J. Pharmacologic management of psychiatric illness during pregnancy: dilemmas and guidelines. Am J Psychiatry 1996;153:592–606.
3. Koren G, Cohn T, Chitayat D, Kapur B, Remington G, Myles-Reid D, Zipursky RB. Use of atypical antipsychotics during pregnancy and the risk of neural tube defects in infants. Am J Psychiatry 2002;159:136–7.
4. Product information. Saphris. Organon Pharmaceuticals USA, 2013.
5. Committee on Drugs, American Academy of Pediatrics. The transfer of drugs and other chemicals into human milk. Pediatrics 2001;108:776–89.

ASPARAGINASE

Antineoplastic

PREGNANCY RECOMMENDATION: Human and Animal Data Suggest Risk
BREASTFEEDING RECOMMENDATION: No Human Data—Potential Toxicity

PREGNANCY SUMMARY

Based on limited reports in humans, the use of asparaginase, in combination with other antineoplastics, does not seem to pose a major risk to the fetus when used in the 2nd and 3rd trimesters, or when exposure occurs before conception in either women or men. No reports describing the use of only asparaginase in pregnancy have been located. Because of the teratogenicity observed in animals and the lack of human data after 1st trimester exposure, asparaginase should be used cautiously during this period, if at all.

FETAL RISK SUMMARY

The antineoplastic agent asparaginase, which is used in the treatment of certain types of cancers, contains the enzyme, L-asparagine amidohydrolase, type EC-2, derived from *Escherichia coli* (1).

The drug is teratogenic in rabbits, rats, and mice (1–3). In pregnant rabbits given 50 IU/kg (5% of the human dose), asparaginase crossed the placenta and produced malformations of the lung, kidney, and skeleton; spina bifida; abdominal extrusion; and missing tail (2). Doses of 1000 IU/kg (equal to the human dose) or more in rats and mice produced exencephaly and skeletal anomalies (3). Maternal and fetal growth restriction have also been observed in pregnant rats and mice treated with 1000 IU/kg (1).

The reported use of asparaginase during human pregnancy is limited to six pregnancies, all in the 2nd trimester, resulting in the birth of seven infants (one set of twins) (4–9). In each case, multiple other chemotherapeutic agents were used with asparaginase for treatment of the acute leukemias. Therapy with asparaginase was initiated between 16.5 and 22 weeks of pregnancy. No congenital abnormalities were observed in any of the newborn infants, although two newborns had transient, drug-induced bone marrow hypoplasia (4,5). One 34-year-old mother, with acute lymphoblastic leukemia, was treated for 18 weeks, commencing at 22 weeks' gestation, with various combinations of asparaginase, daunorubicin, vincristine, cytarabine, cyclophosphamide, mercaptopurine, and methotrexate (9). Asparaginase, 5000 U/m^2/day, was administered on days 15–28 of therapy. She gave birth to a normal female infant after 40 weeks' gestation. The newborn had a normal karyotype (46,XX) but with gaps and a ring chromosome. The clinical significance of these findings is unknown, but because these abnormalities may persist for several years, the potential exists for an increased risk of cancer as well as for a risk of genetic damage in the next generation (9).

A number of reports have evaluated the reproductive histories of men and women who were exposed to asparaginase and multiple other antineoplastic agents before conception (10–15). Of the 13 men described, 9 fathered 15 children (10–13), including 1 who fathered a child while receiving therapy (10). Two congenital anomalies were observed; one infant had a birthmark (13), and one newborn had multiple anomalies (11). In the latter case, the man, who had been off therapy for at least 3.5 years, also fathered a normal child (11). No relationship between these outcomes and the fathers' exposure to either asparaginase or the other chemotherapeutic agents can be inferred from the two cases.

In 57 women treated with asparaginase and other agents 2 months to 15 years before conception, a total of 83 pregnancies occurred, resulting in 5 spontaneous abortions, 5 elective abortions, 2 stillbirths, and 71 liveborn infants (10,12–15). Among the liveborn infants, four were delivered prematurely, one was growth-restricted, and seven had congenital defects, four minor and three major. The minor abnormalities were an epidermal nevus (13), dark hair patch (14), ear tag (14), and congenital hip dysplasia (15). Infants with major defects were the offspring of women who had been treated 15–24 months before conception with asparaginase, chlorambucil, mercaptopurine, methotrexate, procarbazine, thioguanine, vinblastine, vincristine, and prednisone (14). The defects were hydrocephalus, tracheomalacia, and pelvic asymmetry. The authors concluded that the latter defect was most likely a deformation, resulting from the mother's scoliosis or from uterine scarring caused by radiation, rather than a mutagenic effect of drug therapy (14). Causes for the other two defects were not proposed, but they were not thought to be the result of germ cell damage.

BREASTFEEDING SUMMARY

No reports describing the use of asparaginase during human lactation have been located. Toxicity in a nursing infant is a potential complication if a mother receiving this drug chooses to breastfeed.

References

1. Product information. Elspar. Merck Sharpe & Dohme, 1993.
2. Adamson RH, Fabro S, Hahn MA, Creech CE, Whang-Peng J. Evaluation of the embryotoxic activity of L-asparaginase. Arch Int Pharmacodyn Ther 1970;186:310–20. As cited in Shepard TH. *Catalog of Teratogenic Agents*. 6th ed. Baltimore, MD: Johns Hopkins University Press, 1989:58–9.
3. Ohguro Y, Imamura S, Koyama K, Hara T, Miyagawa A, Hatano M, Kanda K. Toxicological studies on L-asparaginase. Yamaguchi Igaku 1969;18:271–92. As cited in Shepard TH. *Catalog of Teratogenic Agents*. 6th ed. Baltimore, MD: Johns Hopkins University Press, 1989:58–9.
4. Okun DB, Groncy PK, Sieger L, Tanaka KR. Acute leukemia in pregnancy: transient neonatal myelosuppression after combination chemotherapy in the mother. Med Pediatr Oncol 1979;7:315–9.
5. Khurshid M, Saleem M. Acute leukaemia in pregnancy. Lancet 1978;2:534–5.

6. Karp GI, Von Oeyen P, Valone F, Khetarpal VK, Israel M, Mayer RJ, Frigoletto FD, Garnick MB. Doxorubicin in pregnancy: possible transplacental passage. Cancer Treat Rep 1983;67:773–7.
7. Awidi AS, Tarawneh MS, Shubair KS, Issa AA, Dajani YF. Acute leukemia in pregnancy: report of five cases treated with a combination which included a low dose of Adriamycin. Eur J Cancer Clin Oncol 1983;19:881–4.
8. Turchi JJ, Villasis C. Anthracyclines in the treatment of malignancy in pregnancy. Cancer 1988;61:435–40.
9. Schleuning M, Clemm C. Chromosomal aberrations in a newborn whose mother received cytotoxic treatment during pregnancy. N Engl J Med 1987;317:1666–7.
10. Blatt J, Mulvihill JJ, Ziegler JL, Young RC, Poplack DG. Pregnancy outcome following cancer chemotherapy. Am J Med 1980;69:828–32.
11. Evenson DP, Arlin Z, Welt S, Claps ML, Melamed MR. Male reproductive capacity may recover following drug treatment with the L-10 protocol for acute lymphocytic leukemia. Cancer 1984;53:30–6.
12. Green DM, Hall B, Zevon MA. Pregnancy outcome after treatment for acute lymphoblastic leukemia during childhood or adolescence. Cancer 1989;64:2335–9.
13. Green DM, Zevon MA, Lowrie G, Seigelstein N, Hall B. Congenital anomalies in children of patients who received chemotherapy for cancer in childhood and adolescence. N Engl J Med 1991;325:141–6.
14. Mulvihill JJ, McKeen EA, Rosner F, Zarrabi MH. Pregnancy outcome in cancer patients: experience in a large cooperative group. Cancer 1987;60:1143–50.
15. Pajor A, Zimonyi I, Koos R, Lehoczky D, Ambrus C. Pregnancies and offspring in survivors of acute lymphoid leukemia and lymphoma. Eur J Obstet Gynecol Reprod Biol 1991;40:1–5.

ASPARTAME

Artificial Sweetener

PREGNANCY RECOMMENDATION: Compatible
BREASTFEEDING RECOMMENDATION: Compatible (Excluding Those with Phenylketonuria)

PREGNANCY SUMMARY

Ingestion of aspartame-sweetened products during pregnancy does not represent a risk to the fetuses of normal mothers, or of mothers either heterozygous for or who have phenylketonuria (PKU). Elevated plasma levels of phenylalanine, an amino acid that is concentrated in the fetus, are associated with fetal toxicity. Whether a toxic threshold exists for neural toxicity or the toxicity is linear with phenylalanine plasma levels is not known. Women with PKU need to control their consumption of any phenylalanine-containing product. Because aspartame is a source of phenylalanine, although a minor source, this should be considered by these women in their dietary planning. The other components of aspartame—methanol and aspartic acid—and the various degradation products have no toxicity in doses that can be ingested by humans.

FETAL RISK SUMMARY

Aspartame is a nutritive sweetening agent used in foods and beverages. It contains 4 kcal/g and is about 180–200 times as sweet as sucrose. The product was discovered in 1965 and obtained final approval by the FDA as a food additive in certain dry foods in 1981 and in carbonated beverages in 1983 (1). Aspartame is probably the most extensively studied food additive ever approved by the FDA (2,3). Chemically, the compound is *N*-L-α-aspartyl-L-phenylalanine, 1-methyl ester (i.e., the methyl ester of the amino acids L-phenylalanine and L-aspartic acid).

Aspartame is broken down in the lumen of the gut to methanol, aspartate, and phenylalanine (1–4). The major decomposition product when the parent compound is exposed to high temperatures or in liquids is aspartyl-phenylalanine diketopiperazine (DKP), a product formed by many dipeptides (3–5). The rate of conversion of aspartame to degradation products depends on pH and temperature (3). In addition to methanol, the two amino acids, and DKP, other degradation products are L,L-β-aspartame (aspartame is commercially available as the L,L-α isomer), three dipeptides (α-Asp-Phe, β-Asp-Phe, and Phe-Asp), and phenylalanine methyl ester (3). The dipeptide compounds are hydrolyzed to the individual amino acids in the gut, and these, along with methanol, will be evaluated in later sections. None of the other degradation products have shown toxic effects after extensive study (3). Moreover, the DKP compound and the β-isomer of aspartame are essentially inactive biologically (3).

The projected maximum ingestion of aspartame has been estimated to be 22–34 mg/kg/day. The higher dose is calculated as the 99th percentile of projected daily ingestion (2). The 22–34 mg/kg dose range is equivalent to 2.4–3.7 mg/kg/day of methanol, 9.8 mg/kg/day of aspartate, and 12–19 mg/kg/day of phenylalanine (2). The FDA has set the allowable or acceptable daily intake (ADI) of aspartame at 50 mg/kg (1.5 times the 99th percentile of projected daily ingestion) (1,3). In Europe and Canada, the ADI is 40 mg/kg (3). The ADI is defined as an average daily ingestion that is considered harmless, even if continued indefinitely, but does not imply that amounts above this value are harmful (3).

The toxic effects of methanol ingestion are the result of its metabolism to formaldehyde and then to formic acid. Accumulation of this latter product is responsible for the acidosis and ocular toxicity attributable to methanol (1–3). The dose of methanol estimated to cause significant toxicity is estimated to be 200–500 mg/kg (4). Theoretically, since about 10% of aspartame is methanol, the toxic dose of aspartame, in terms only of methanol, would be about 2000 mg/kg, a dose considered far in excess of any possible ingestion (4). In 12 normal subjects, methanol plasma levels were below the level of detection (0.4 mg/dL) after ingestion of aspartame, 34 mg/kg (3). When abuse doses (100, 150, and 200 mg/kg) of aspartame were administered, statistically significant increases in methanol blood concentrations were measured with peak levels of 1.27, 2.14, and 2.58 mg/dL, respectively (3). Methanol was undetectable at 8 hours after the 100-mg/kg dose, but was still present after the higher aspartame doses. Blood and urine formate concentrations were measured after ingestion of 200 mg/kg of aspartame in six healthy subjects (3). No significant increases in blood formate levels were measured, but urinary formate excretion did increase significantly. This indicated that the rate of formate synthesis did not exceed the rate of formate metabolism and excretion (3). No ocular changes or toxicity were observed in the test subjects (3). Moreover, the amount of methanol (approximately 55 mg/L) derived from aspartame-sweetened beverages, containing approximately 555 mg/L of aspartame, is much less than the average methanol content of fruit juices (140 mg/L) (2). Based on the above data, the risk to the fetus from the methanol component of aspartame is nil.

Aspartate is one of two dicarboxylic amino acids (glutamate is the other) that have caused hypothalamic neuronal necrosis in neonatal rodents fed large doses of either the individual amino acids or aspartame (2,5). In neonatal mice, plasma concentrations of aspartate and glutamate must exceed 110 and 75 micro-mol/dL, respectively, before brain lesions are produced (2). Concerns were raised that this toxicity could occur in humans, especially because glutamate is widespread in the food supply (e.g., monosodium glutamate [MSG]) (6). In addition, some aspartate is transaminated to glutamate, and the neural toxicity of the two amino acids is additive (6). However, brain lesions were not produced in nonhuman primates fed large doses of aspartame, aspartate, or MSG (2).

In normal humans, ingestion of aspartame, 34 mg/kg, or equimolar amounts of aspartate, 13 mg/kg, did not increase plasma aspartate levels (7). Adults heterozygous for PKU also metabolized aspartate normally as evidenced by insignificant increases in plasma aspartate concentrations and unchanged levels of those amino acids that could be derived from aspartate, such as glutamate, asparagine, and glutamine (8). When the dose of aspartame was increased to 50 mg/kg, again no increase in plasma aspartate levels was measured (9). When an abuse dose of aspartame, 100 mg/kg, was administered to adults heterozygous for PKU, plasma aspartate levels increased from a baseline of 0.49–0.80 micro-mol/dL (10). The increase was well within the range of normal postprandial levels. In normal adults given a higher abuse dose of aspartame (200 mg/kg), plasma levels of aspartate plus glutamate were increased from a baseline of 2.7–7 micro-mol/dL, still far below the estimated toxic human plasma level of 100 micro-mol/dL for aspartate and glutamate (7). Plasma aspartate levels at 2 hours after the 200-mg/kg dose were less than normal postprandial aspartate levels after a meal containing protein (1). Based on these data, subjects heterozygous for PKU metabolize aspartate normally (2). Moreover, neither aspartate nor glutamate is concentrated in the fetus, unlike most other amino acids (1,2,5,11,12). Human placentas perfused in vitro showed a fetal:maternal ratio of 0.13 for aspartic acid and 0.14 for glutamic acid (11). In pregnant monkeys infused with sodium aspartate, 100 mg/kg/hour, maternal plasma aspartate levels increased from 0.36 to 80.2 micro-mol/dL, whereas fetal levels changed from 0.42 to 0.98 micro-mol/dL (12). Thus, there is no evidence of a risk of fetal aspartate toxicity resulting from maternal ingestion of aspartame, either alone or in combination with glutamate.

High plasma levels of phenylalanine, such as those occurring in PKU, are known to affect the fetus adversely. Phenylalanine, unlike aspartate, is concentrated on the fetal side of the placenta with a fetal:maternal gradient of 1.2:1–1.3:1 (13). The fetus of a mother with PKU may either be heterozygous for PKU (i.e., those who only inherit one autosomal recessive gene and who are nonphenylketonuric) or homozygous for PKU (i.e., those who inherit two autosomal recessive genes and who are phenylketonuric). The incidence of PKU is approximately 1/15,000 persons (5). In contrast, individuals heterozygous for PKU are much more common, with an estimated incidence of 1/50–1/70 persons (8). In the former case, the fetus has virtually no (≤0.3%) phenylalanine hydroxylase activity and is unable to metabolize phenylalanine to tyrosine, thus allowing phenylalanine to accumulate to toxic levels (14). The heterozygous fetus does possess phenylalanine hydroxylase, although only about 10% of normal, with activity of the enzyme detected in the fetal liver as early as 8 weeks' gestation (13,14). Unfortunately, possession of some phenylalanine hydroxylase activity does not reduce the amount of phenylalanine transferred from the mother to the fetus (13). In a study of four families, evidence was found that the heterozygous fetus either did not metabolize the phenylalanine received from the mother or metabolism was minimal (13). This supported previous observations that the degree of mental impairment from exposure to high, continuous maternal levels of phenylalanine is often similar for both the nonphenylketonuric and phenylketonuric fetuses (13). Moreover, the exact mechanism of mental impairment induced by elevated phenylalanine plasma levels has not been determined (4,15,16).

Offspring of women with PKU often are afflicted with mental retardation, microcephaly, congenital heart disease, and low birth weight (16). Pregnancies of these women are also prone to spontaneously abort (16). In one study, maternal phenylalanine plasma levels >120 micro-mol/dL (classic PKU) were consistently associated with microcephaly, although true mental retardation was observed only when plasma levels exceeded 110 micro-mol/dL (16). However, research has not excluded the possibility that lower concentrations may be associated with less severe reductions in intelligence (16–18). For example, in the study cited above, maternal phenylalanine levels <60 μmol/dL (mild hyperphenylalaninemia without urine phenylketones) were associated with normal intelligence in the infants (16). When maternal levels were in the range of 60–100 micro-mol/dL (atypical PKU), most of the infants also had normal intelligence, but their mean IQ was lower than that of the infants of mothers with mild hyperphenylalaninemia. Others have interpreted these and additional data as indicating a 10.5 point reduction in IQ for each 25.0 micro-mol/dL rise in maternal phenylalanine plasma concentration (19,20). A recent study, however, examined the nonhyperphenylalaninemic offspring of 12 mothers with untreated hyperphenylalaninemia (21). The results supported the contention that a maternal plasma phenylalanine threshold of 60 micro-mol/dL existed for an adverse effect on the intelligence of the offspring (21). The investigators, however, were unable to exclude the possibility that nonintellectual dysfunction, such as hyperactivity or attention deficit disorder, may occur at concentrations below the alleged threshold (21). Thus, although this latest study is evidence for a threshold effect, additional studies are needed before the concept of a linear relationship between offspring intelligence and maternal phenylalanine levels can be set aside (19,20,22–24).

In normal subjects, fasting and postprandial (after a meal containing protein) phenylalanine levels are approximately

6 and 12 micro-mol/dL, respectively (2,8). When normal adults were administered either a 34- or 50-mg/kg aspartame dose, the mean maximum phenylalanine concentrations were 9–12 and 16 micro-mol/dL, respectively, with levels returning to baseline 4 hours after ingestion (2,7–9). Single doses of 100–200 mg/kg, representing abuse ingestions of aspartame, resulted in peak phenylalanine plasma levels ranging from 20 to 49 micro-mol/dL (2,25). These elevated levels returned to near baseline values within 8 hours. Normal adults were also dosed with an aspartame-sweetened beverage, providing a 10-mg/kg dose of aspartame, at 2-hour intervals for three successive doses (2,26). Plasma levels of phenylalanine rose slightly after each dose, indicating that the phenylalanine load from the previous dose had not been totally eliminated. However, the increases were not statistically significant, and plasma phenylalanine levels never exceeded normal postprandial limits at any time (26). The results of the above studies suggest that even large doses of aspartame do not pose a fetal risk in the normal subject.

Humans heterozygous for the PKU allele metabolize phenylalanine slower than normal persons because of a decreased amount of liver phenylalanine hydroxylase (2). The conversion of phenylalanine to tyrosine is thus impaired, and potentially toxic levels of phenylalanine may accumulate. When adults with this genetic trait were administered aspartame, 34 mg/kg, the mean peak phenylalanine concentration was 15–16 micro-mol/dL, approximately 36%-45% higher than that measured in normal adults (11 micro-mol/dL) (2,8,27). To determine the effects of abuse doses, a dose of 100 mg/kg was administered, resulting in a mean peak plasma level of 42 micro-mol/dL, approximately 100% higher than that observed in normal individuals (20 micro-mol/dL) (2,10). In both cases, phenylalanine plasma levels were well below presumed toxic levels and returned to baseline values within 8 hours.

A 1986 study examined the effects of a 10-mg/kg dose of aspartame obtained from a commercial product on the basal concentrations of several amino acids, including phenylalanine, in four types of patients: normal, PKU, hyperphenylalaninemic, and PKU carriers (28). One hour after ingestion, mean phenylalanine levels had increased 1.35 micro-mol/dL (+30%) in normal subjects and 1.35 micro-mol/dL (+20%) in PKU carriers, decreased 4.58 micro-mol/dL (-3%) in subjects with PKU, and remained unchanged in hyperphenylalaninemic individuals. The 10-mg/kg dose was selected because it represented, for a 60-kg adult, the dose received from three cans of an aspartame-sweetened soft drink or from approximately 1 quart of aspartame-sweetened Kool-Aid (28).

BREASTFEEDING SUMMARY

Ingestion of aspartame, 50 mg/kg, by normal lactating women results in a small, but statistically significant, rise in overall aspartate and phenylalanine milk concentrations (9). Milk aspartate levels rose from 2.3 to 4.8 micro-mol/dL during a 4-hour fasting interval after the aspartame dose. The rise in phenylalanine milk levels during the same interval was approximately 0.5–2.3 micro-mol/dL. The investigators of this study concluded that these changes, even if spread over an entire 24-hour period, would have no effect on a nursing infant's phenylalanine intake (9). However, because mothers or infants with PKU need to carefully monitor their intake of phenylalanine, the American Academy of Pediatrics classifies aspartame as an agent to be used with caution during breastfeeding if the mother or the infant has PKU (29).

References

1. Sturtevant FM. Use of aspartame in pregnancy. Int J Fertil1985;30:85–7.
2. Stegink LD. The aspartame story: a model for the clinical testing of a food additive. Am J Clin Nutr 1987;46:204–15.
3. Stegink LD, Brummel MC, McMartin K, Martin-Amat G, Filer LJ Jr, Baker GL, Tephly TR. Blood methanol concentrations in normal adult subjects administered abuse doses of aspartame. J Toxicol Environ Health 1981;7:281–90.
4. Dews PB. Summary report of an international aspartame workshop. Food Chem Toxicol 1987;25:549–52.
5. London RS. Saccharin and aspartame: are they safe to consume during pregnancy? J Reprod Med 1988;33:17–21.
6. Council on Scientific Affairs, American Medical Association. Aspartame:review of safety issues. JAMA 1985;254:400–2.
7. Stegink LD, Filer LJ Jr, Baker GL. Effect of aspartame and aspartate loading upon plasma and erythrocyte free amino acid levels in normal adult volunteers. J Nutr 1977;107:1837–45.
8. Stegink LD, Koch R, Blaskovics ME, Filer LJ Jr, Baker GL, McDonnell JE. Plasma phenylalanine levels in phenylketonuric heterozygous and normal adults administered aspartame at 34 mg/kg body weight. Toxicology 1981;20:81–90.
9. Stegink LD, Filer LJ Jr, Baker GL. Plasma, erythrocyte and human milk levels of free amino acids in lactating women administered aspartame or lactose. J Nutr 1979;109:2173–81.
10. Stegink LD, Filer LJ Jr, Baker GL, McDonnell JE. Effect of an abuse dose of aspartame upon plasma and erythrocyte levels of amino acids in phenylketonuric heterozygous and normal adults. J Nutr 1980;110:2216–24.
11. Schneider H, Mohlen KH, Challier JC, Dancis J. Transfer of glutamic acid across the human placenta perfused in vitro. Br J Obstet Gynaecol 1979;86:299–306.
12. Stegink LD, Pitkin RM, Reynolds WA, Brummel MC, Filer LJ Jr. Placental transfer of aspartate and its metabolites in the primate. Metabolism 1979;28:669–76.
13. Levy HL, Lenke RR, Koch R. Lack of fetal effect on blood phenylalanine concentration in maternal phenylketonuria. J Pediatr 1984;104:245–7.
14. Hilton MA, Sharpe JN, Hicks LG, Andrews BF. A simple method for detection of heterozygous carriers of the gene for classic phenylketonuria. J Pediatr 1986;109:601–4.
15. Perry TL, Hansen S, Tischler B, Bunting R, Diamond S. Glutamine depletion in phenylketonuria: a possible cause of the mental defect. N Engl J Med 1970;282:761–6.
16. Levy HL, Waisbren SE. Effects of untreated maternal phenylketonuria and hyperphenylalaninemia on the fetus. N Engl J Med 1983;309:1269–74.
17. Buist NRM, Tuerck J, Lis E, Penn R. Effects of untreated maternal phenylketonuria and hyperphenylalaninemia on the fetus. N Engl J Med 1984;311:52–3.
18. Levy HL, Waisbren SE. Effects of untreated maternal phenylketonuria and hyperphenylalaninemia on the fetus. N Engl J Med 1984;311:53.
19. Pardridge WM. The safety of aspartame. JAMA 1986;256:2678.
20. Pardridge WM. The safety of aspartame. JAMA 1987;258:206.
21. Waisbren SE, Levy HL. Effects of untreated maternal hyperphenylalaninemia on the fetus: further study of families identified by routine cord blood screening. J Pediatr 1990;116:926–9.
22. Levy HL, Waisbren SE. The safety of aspartame. JAMA 1987;258:205.
23. Stegink LD, Krause WL. The safety of aspartame. JAMA 1987;258:205–6.
24. Hilton MA. Consumption of aspartame by heterozygotes for phenylketonuria. J Pediatr 1987;110:662–3.
25. Stegink LD, Filer LJ Jr, Baker GL. Plasma and erythrocyte concentrations of free amino acids in adult humans administered abuse doses of aspartame. J Toxicol Environ Health 1981;7:291–305.
26. Stegink LD, Filer LJ Jr, Baker GL. Effect of repeated ingestion of aspartame-sweetened beverages upon plasma aminograms in normal adults (abstract). Am J Clin Nutr 1983;37:704.
27. Stegink LD, Filer LJ Jr, Baker GL, McDonnell JE. Effect of aspartame loading upon plasma and erythrocyte amino acid levels in phenylketonuric heterozygotes and normal adult subjects. J Nutr 1979;109:708–17.
28. Caballero B, Mahon BE, Rohr FJ, Levy HL, Wurtman RJ. Plasma amino acid levels after single-dose aspartame consumption in phenylketonuria, mild hyperphenylalaninemia, and heterozygous state for phenylketonuria. J Pediatr 1986;109:668–71.
29. Committee on Drugs, American Academy of Pediatrics. The transfer of drugs and other chemicals into human milk. Pediatrics 2001;108:776–89.

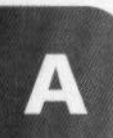

ASPIRIN

Nonsteroidal Anti-inflammatory

PREGNANCY RECOMMENDATION: Compatible (Low-Dose)
Human Data Suggest Risk in 1st and 3rd Trimesters (Full-Dose)
BREASTFEEDING RECOMMENDATION: Limited Human Data—Potential Toxicity

PREGNANCY SUMMARY

The use of aspirin during pregnancy, especially of chronic or intermittent high doses, should be avoided. The drug may affect maternal and newborn hemostasis mechanisms, leading to an increased risk of hemorrhage. High doses may be related to increased perinatal mortality, intrauterine growth restriction (IUGR), and teratogenic effects. Low doses, such as 80 mg/day, appear to have beneficial effects in pregnancies complicated by systemic lupus erythematosus with antiphospholipid antibodies. In pregnancies at risk for the development of gestational hypertension and preeclampsia, and in fetuses with IUGR, low-dose aspirin (40–150 mg/day) may be beneficial, but more studies are required to assess accurately the risk:benefit ratio of such therapy. Near term, aspirin may prolong gestation and labor. Although aspirin has been used as a tocolytic agent, serious bleeding complications may occur in the newborn. Premature closure of the ductus arteriosus may occur in the latter part of pregnancy as a result of maternal consumption of full-dose aspirin. Persistent pulmonary hypertension of the newborn (PPHN) is a potential complication of the closure. If an analgesic or antipyretic is needed, acetaminophen should be considered.

FETAL RISK SUMMARY

Aspirin, a nonsteroidal anti-inflammatory drug (NSAID), is the most frequently ingested drug in pregnancy either as a single agent or in combination with other drugs (1). The terms "aspirin" and "salicylate" are used interchangeably in this monograph unless specifically separated. In eight surveys totaling more than 54,000 patients, aspirin was consumed sometime during gestation by slightly more than 33,000 (61%) (2–9). The true incidence is probably much higher than this because many patients either do not remember taking aspirin or consume drug products without realizing that they contain large amounts of salicylates (2,4,8). Evaluation of the effects of aspirin on the fetus is thus difficult because of this common, and often hidden, exposure. However, some toxic effects on the mother and the fetus from large doses of salicylates have been known since 1893 (10).

Aspirin consumption during pregnancy may produce adverse effects in the mother: anemia, antepartum or postpartum hemorrhage, prolonged gestation, and prolonged labor (5,11–14). The increased length of labor and frequency of postmaturity result from the inhibition of prostaglandin synthesis by aspirin. Aspirin has been shown to significantly delay the induced abortion time in nulliparous (but not multiparous) patients by this same mechanism (15). In an Australian study, regular aspirin ingestion was also found to increase the number of complicated deliveries (cesarean sections, breech, and forceps) (5). Small doses of aspirin may decrease urinary estriol excretion (16).

Aspirin, either alone or in combination with β-mimetics, has been used to treat premature labor (17–19). Although adverse effects in the newborn were infrequent, maternal complications in one study included non–dose-related prolonged bleeding times and dose-related vertigo, tinnitus, headache, and hyperventilation (19).

Failure of intrauterine devices (IUDs) to prevent conception has been described in two patients who consumed frequent doses of aspirin (20). The anti-inflammatory action of aspirin was proposed as the mechanism of the failure.

Low-dose aspirin (about 85 mg/day) was used to treat maternal thrombocytopenia (platelet counts <60,000/mm^3) in 19 patients with either IUGR or toxemia (21). In five women who had a definite response to the aspirin, no improvement in plasma volume or fetal welfare was demonstrated.

In women with systemic lupus erythematosus complicated with either lupus anticoagulant or anticardiolipin antibody (i.e., antiphospholipid antibodies), low-dose aspirin (e.g., 80 mg/day) has been used in combination with prednisone to reduce the incidence of pregnancy loss (22–25) (see reference 22 for a review of this topic). This therapy has not been associated with drug-induced fetal or neonatal complications.

Several studies have investigated the effect of low-dose aspirin (e.g., 40–150 mg/day) on the prevention of gestational hypertension, preeclampsia, and eclampsia, and the associated fetal risks of IUGR and mortality (26–38) (see reference 36 for a review of this topic). Low-dose aspirin exerts its beneficial effects in these disorders by irreversible inactivation of platelet cyclooxygenase, resulting in a greater inhibition of thromboxane A_2 synthesis than that of prostacyclin production. This inhibition restores the ratio of the two substances to a more normal value. Aspirin-induced fetal and neonatal toxicity has not been observed after the chronic use of low-dose aspirin for these indications. The lack of toxicity may be partially explained by the findings of a study published in 1989 (34). In that study, 60–80 mg of aspirin/day, starting 3 weeks before delivery and continuing until birth, inhibited maternal platelet cyclooxygenase, but not that of the newborn. These results were in agreement with other studies using 60–150 mg/day (34). Other toxicities associated with the use of full-dose aspirin near term, such as hemorrhage, premature closure of the ductus arteriosus, pulmonary hypertension, prolonged gestation, and prolonged labor, were not observed with low-dose aspirin therapy (34). Although these results are reassuring, in the opinion of some, too few studies have been reported to allow a true estimate of the fetal risk (36). However, other recent reports have observed no serious neonatal adverse effects, including hemorrhagic complications, in their series (39,40). In one of these studies, 33 women judged to be at risk for gestational hypertension were randomly assigned to either an aspirin (N = 17) or a placebo (N = 16) group during the 12th week of gestation in a single-blind study (39). Patients in the aspirin group, treated with 60 mg/day from enrollment to delivery, had a longer duration of pregnancy (39 vs. 35 weeks) and delivered heavier infants (2922 vs. 2264 g). None of the aspirin-treated women developed gestational hypertension, whereas three of the placebo group did develop the complication. In a double blind study, 65 women with increased blood pressure during the rollover test administered during the 28th or 29th week of pregnancy were randomly divided into two groups: one group was treated with 100 mg/day of aspirin (N = 34) and the other with placebo (N = 31) (40). Four women (11.8%) of the aspirin-treated group developed gestational hypertension compared with 11 (35.5%) of the placebo group.

Fetal and newborn effects, other than congenital defects, from aspirin exposure in utero, may include increased perinatal mortality, IUGR, congenital salicylate intoxication, and depressed albumin-binding capacity (2,5,12,41–43). For the latter effect, no increase in the incidence of jaundice was observed (2). Perinatal mortality in the Australian study was a result of stillbirths more often than neonatal deaths (5, 41). Some of the stillbirths were associated with antepartum hemorrhage and others may have been caused by closure of the ductus arteriosus in utero (44). Closure of the ductus has been shown in animals to be a result of aspirin inhibition of prostaglandin synthetase. In some early cases, in utero premature closure of the ductus arteriosus was probably caused by aspirin but not suspected (45). However, a large prospective American study involving 41,337 patients, 64% of whom used aspirin sometime during gestation, failed to show that aspirin was a cause of stillbirths, neonatal deaths, or reduced birth weight (46). The difference between these findings probably relates to the chronic or intermittent use of higher doses by the patients in the Australian study (44). Excessive use of aspirin was blamed for the stillbirth of a fetus in whom salicylate levels in the fetal blood and liver were 25–30 and 12 mg/dL, respectively (47). Congenital salicylate intoxication was found in two newborns exposed to high aspirin doses before delivery (42,43). Although both infants survived, one infant exhibited withdrawal symptoms beginning on the second neonatal day consisting of hypertonia, agitation, a shrill piercing cry, and increased reflex irritability (41). The serum salicylate level was 31 mg/dL. Most of the symptoms gradually subsided over 6 weeks, but some mild hypertonia may have persisted.

A 1996 case–control study investigated the relationship between aspirin and other NSAIDs and PPHN (48). Case infants (N = 103) weighed at least 2500 g at birth and had no major congenital defects, whereas controls (N = 298) were full-term infants without congenital defects. Aspirin or other NSAIDs were used by mothers of 26 cases. Because 34% of the cases and all of the controls were born at one hospital (inborn), the investigators conducted two analyses, one for inborn infants and one for the total group. For the total group, the odds ratio and 95% confidence interval (CI) for the exposures and PPHN were aspirin 4.9 (1.6–15.3) and other NSAIDs 6.2 (1.8–21.8). For inborn cases, the findings were aspirin 9.6 (2.4–39.0) and other NSAIDs 17.5 (4.3–71.6). The timing of the exposures was earlier than expected, a median 3 months for aspirin and 1 month for NSAIDs. This result led to three potential conclusions: (a) the drugs caused early structural remodeling or functional alterations of the pulmonary vasculature, (b) the agents were also used in the 3rd trimester, or (c) there was another, unidentified primary cause of PPHN. Exposure in the 3rd trimester was the most likely conclusion because it would have been consistent with the presumed mechanism of in utero premature closure of the ductus arteriosus and resulting increased risk of PPHN. However, the investigators could not determine which of the choices was correct (48). A 2001 report also found the association between aspirin and PPHN (49).

Aspirin given in doses of 325–650 mg during the week before delivery may affect the clotting ability of the newborn (50–56). In the initial study by Bleyer and Breckenridge (50), 3 of 14 newborns exposed to aspirin within 1 week of delivery had minor hemorrhagic phenomena vs. only 1 of 17 nonexposed controls. Collagen-induced platelet aggregation was absent in the aspirin group and, although of less clinical significance, factor XII activity was markedly depressed. A direct correlation was found between factor XII activity and the interval between the last dose of aspirin and birth. Neonatal purpuric rash with depressed platelet function has also been observed after maternal use of aspirin close to term (56). The use of salicylates other than aspirin may not be a problem because the acetyl moiety is apparently required to depress platelet function (57–59). In a 1982 study, 10 mothers consuming less than 1 g of aspirin within 5 days of delivery had excessive intrapartum or postpartum blood loss, resulting in hemoglobulin levels that were markedly lower than those of controls (13,14). One mother required a transfusion. Bleeding complications seen in 9 of the 10 infants included numerous petechiae over the presenting part, hematuria, a cephalohematoma, subconjunctival hemorrhage, and bleeding from a circumcision. No life-threatening hemorrhage, effect on Apgar scores, or increased hospital stay was found, nor was bleeding observed in seven mother–infant pairs when aspirin consumption occurred 6–10 days before delivery (13,14).

An increased incidence of intracranial hemorrhage (ICH) in premature or low-birth-weight infants may occur after maternal aspirin use near birth (60). Computed tomographic screening for ICH was conducted on 108 infants 3–7 days after delivery. All of the infants were either ≤34 weeks in gestation or ≤1500 g in birth weight. A total of 53 infants (49%) developed ICH, including 12 (71%) of the 17 aspirin-exposed newborns. This incidence was statistically significant when compared with the 41 (45%) non–aspirin-exposed infants who developed ICH. The conclusions of this study have been challenged and defended (61,62). In view of the potentially serious outcome, however, full doses of aspirin should be used with extreme caution by patients in danger of premature delivery.

Aspirin readily crosses the placenta (10). When given near term, higher concentrations are found in the neonate than in the mother (63). The kinetics of salicylate elimination in the newborn have been studied (63–65).

A 2003 population-based cohort study involving 1055 pregnant women investigated the prenatal use of aspirin, other NSAIDs, and acetaminophen (66). Fifty-three women

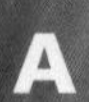

(5%) reported used of NSAIDs around the time of conception or during pregnancy, 13 of whom had a spontaneous abortion (SAB). After adjustment, an 80% increased risk of SAB was found for other NSAIDs (adjusted hazard ratio 1.8, 95% CI 1.0–3.2). Moreover, the association was stronger if the initial use of drugs was around conception or if they were used longer than 1 week. A similar association was found with aspirin, but it was weaker because there were only 22 exposures (5 SABs). No association was observed with acetaminophen (66).

The relationship between aspirin and congenital defects is controversial. Several studies have examined this question with findings either supporting or denying a relationship. In two large retrospective studies, mothers of 1291 malformed infants were found to have consumed aspirin during pregnancy more frequently than mothers of normal infants (67,68). In a retrospective survey of 599 children with oral clefts, use of salicylates in the 1st trimester was almost three times more frequent in the mothers of children with this defect (69). A reviewer of these studies noted several biases, including the fact that they were retrospective, that could account for the results (46). Three other reports of aspirin teratogenicity involving a total of 10 infants have been located (70–72). In each of these cases, other drugs and factors were present.

A 1985 study found a possible association between the use of aspirin in early pregnancy and congenital heart disease (73). The risk for defects in septation of the truncus arteriosus was increased about twofold over nonexposed controls. In an earlier retrospective case–control comparison of the relationship between maternal drug intake and congenital heart disease, aspirin was used by 80 of 390 mothers of infants with defects vs. 203 of 1254 mothers of control infants (74). Twelve of the exposed infants had transposition of the great arteries and six had tetralogy of Fallot, but the association between the drug and these defects was weak. The study could not distinguish between the effects of the drug and the underlying condition for which the drug was used (74). A brief review of this and other investigations that have examined the relationship between aspirin and congenital heart disease was published in 1985 (75). The review concluded that too few data existed to associate aspirin with cardiac defects.

A study published in 1989, however, concluded that 1st trimester use of aspirin did not increase the risk of congenital heart defects in relation to other structural anomalies (76). The interval examined encompassed the time of major cardiac development (i.e., from the 5th week after the onset of the last menstrual period to the 9th week of gestation). The data, from the Slone Epidemiology Unit Birth Defects Study, involved 1381 infants with any structural cardiac defect and five subgroups with selected cardiac defects (subgroups were not mutually exclusive): aortic stenosis (N = 43), coarctation of the aorta (N = 123), hypoplastic left ventricle (N = 98), transposition of the great arteries (N = 210), and conotruncal defects (N = 791). A control group of 6966 infants with other malformations was used for comparison. Infants with syndromes that included cardiac defects, such as Down's syndrome or Holt-Oram syndrome, were excluded from the data, as were mothers who were uncertain about 1st trimester aspirin use or its frequency. After adjustment for potentially confounding factors, the relative risks for the defects among aspirin users in comparison to controls were as follows: 0.9 (95% CI 0.8–1.1) for any cardiac defect, 1.2 (95% CI 0.6–2.3) for aortic stenosis, 1.0 (95% CI 0.6–1.4) for coarctation of the aorta, 0.9 (95% CI 0.6–1.4) for hypoplastic left ventricle, 0.9 (95% CI 0.6–1.2) for transposition of the great arteries, and 1.0 (95% CI 0.8–1.2) for conotruncal defects. No dose–effect relationship was observed (76).

A 2003 case–control study was conducted to identify drug use in early pregnancy that was associated with cardiac defects (77). Cases (cardiovascular defects without known chromosome anomalies) were drawn from three Swedish health registers (N = 5015). Controls were all infants born in Sweden in 1995–2001 (N = 577,730). Associations were identified for several drugs, some of which were probably due to confounding from the underlying disease or complaint or multiple testing, but some were thought to be true drug effects. The total exposed, number of cases, and odds ratio (OR, 95% CI) for NSAIDs and aspirin were 7698, 80 cases, 1.24 (0.99–1.55) and 5920, 52 cases, 1.01 (0.76–1.33), respectively. These results demonstrated no association with cardiac defects (77).

In an FDA surveillance study of Michigan Medicaid recipients involving 229,101 completed pregnancies conducted between 1985 and 1992, 1709 newborns had been exposed to aspirin during the 1st trimester (F. Rosa, personal communication, FDA, 1993). A total of 83 (4.9%) major birth defects were observed (73 expected). Specific data were available for six defect categories, including (observed/expected) 19/17 cardiovascular defects, 2/3 oral clefts, 0/1 spina bifida, 3/5 polydactyly, 1/3 limb reduction defects, and 6/4 hypospadias. These data do not support an association between the drug and the defects.

The Collaborative Perinatal Project monitored 50,282 mother–child pairs, 14,864 of whom used aspirin during the 1st trimester (6). For use anytime during pregnancy, 32,164 (64%) aspirin exposures were recorded. This prospective study did not find evidence of a teratogenic effect with aspirin. However, the data did not exclude the possibility that grossly excessive doses of aspirin may be teratogenic. An Australian study of 144 infants of mothers who took aspirin regularly in pregnancy also failed to find an association between salicylates and malformations (41). Based on these studies and the fact that aspirin usage in pregnancy is so common, it is not possible to determine the teratogenic risk of salicylates, if indeed it exists.

A 1996 case–control study of gastroschisis found a significantly elevated risk with ibuprofen (see Ibuprofen) and other medications and exposures (78). A significant association also was found for aspirin (N = 7, OR 4.67, 95% CI 1.21–18.05). The data supported a vascular hypothesis for the pathogenesis of gastroschisis (78).

Full-dose aspirin has been reported to affect adversely the IQ of children exposed in utero during the first half of pregnancy (79). In a longitudinal prospective study of the effects of prenatal alcohol exposure on child health and development conducted between 1974 and 1975, drug histories were obtained from 1529 women during the 5th month of pregnancy. At birth, 421 children were selected for later follow-up based on a system of prebirth criteria. Of these, 192 (45.6%) had been exposed to aspirin during the first half of pregnancy. A significant and negative association was discovered between aspirin and child IQ and the children's attentional decrements when they were examined at 4 years of age. The association was not changed after adjustment for a wide variety of potentially confounding covariates. Of interest, the data indicated that girls were significantly more affected than boys. The physical growth parameters, height, weight, and head circumference at 4 years of age, were not significantly related to maternal use of aspirin (79).

In a similar study, data were collected in 19,226 pregnancies by the Collaborative Perinatal Project; aspirin exposure during the first half of pregnancy was reported by 10,159 (52.8%) (80). In contrast to the earlier report, the mean child IQs at 4 years of age in the exposed and nonexposed groups were 98.3 and 96.1, respectively. Adjustment for multiple confounders reduced the difference between the groups to less than one point. No relationship between the amount of aspirin consumed and child IQ was found. The investigators concluded that an adverse effect of in utero aspirin exposure on child IQ was unlikely (80).

Women attempting to conceive should not use any NSAID, including aspirin, because of the findings in a variety of animal models that indicate these agents block blastocyst implantation (81,82). Moreover, as noted above, NSAIDs have been associated with SABs in humans (see Ibuprofen for additional studies).

A 2012 report from the National Birth Defects Prevention Study found associations between exposures to NSAIDs (aspirin, ibuprofen, and naproxen) and several birth defects (83). The data for this case–control study came from approximately 20,470 women with expected due dates in 1997–2004. Among this group, 3173 women (15.5%) were exposed to NSAIDs in the 1st trimester. Although the results suggested that NSAIDs are not a major cause of birth defects, the study did find several small-to-moderate but statistically significant increases in nine defects. The drug, adjusted OR and 95% CI for each defect were: anencephaly/craniorachischisis—aspirin (2.1; 1.1–4.3); spina bifida—ibuprofen (1.6; 1.2–2.1); encephalocele—naproxen (3.5; 1.2–10); anophthalmia/microphthalmia—aspirin (3.0; 1.3–7.3), ibuprofen 1.9; 1.1–3.3, and naproxen 2.8; 1.1–7.3); cleft lip ± cleft palate—ibuprofen (1.3; 1.1–1.6) and naproxen (1.7; 1.1–2.5); cleft palate—aspirin (1.8; 1.1–2.9); transverse limb deficiency—naproxen (2.0; 1.0–3.8); amniotic bands/limb body wall—aspirin (2.5; 1.1–5.6) and ibuprofen (2.2; 1.4–3.5); and a heart defect (isolated pulmonary valve stenosis)—naproxen (2.4; 1.3–4.5). The analysis of the latter defect was limited to term births only. The authors acknowledged that further studies were needed because most of these associations had not been reported from other databases (83).

BREASTFEEDING SUMMARY

Aspirin and other salicylates are excreted into breast milk in low concentrations. Sodium salicylate was first demonstrated in human milk in 1935 (84). In one study of a mother taking 4 g daily, no detectable salicylate in her milk or in her infant's serum was found, but the test sensitivity was only 50 mcg/mL (85). Reported milk concentrations are much lower than this level. Following single or repeated oral doses, peak milk levels occurred at around 3 hours and ranged from 1.1 to 10 mcg/mL (86,87). This represented a milk:plasma ratio of 0.03–0.08 at 3 hours. Because salicylates are eliminated more slowly from milk than from plasma, the ratio increased to 0.34 at 12 hours (86). Peak levels have also been reported to occur at 9 hours (88). Only one report has attributed infant toxicity to salicylates obtained in mother's milk (89). A 16-day-old female infant developed severe salicylate intoxication with a serum salicylate level of 24 mg/dL on the third hospital day. Milk and maternal serum aspirin levels were not obtained, but the mother was taking 650 mg every 4 hours. Although the parents denied giving the baby aspirin or other salicylates, it is unlikely, based on the above reports, that she could have received the drug from the milk in the quantities found (89).

Adverse effects on platelet function in the nursing infant exposed to aspirin via the milk have not been reported but are a potential risk. The American Academy of Pediatrics recommends that aspirin should be used cautiously by the mother during lactation because of potential adverse effects in the nursing infant (90).

References

1. Corby DG. Aspirin in pregnancy: maternal and fetal effects. Pediatrics 1978;62(Suppl):930–7.
2. Palmisano PA, Cassady G. Salicylate exposure in the perinate. JAMA 1969;209:556–8.
3. Forfar JO, Nelson MM. Epidemiology of drugs taken by pregnant women: drugs that may affect the fetus adversely. Clin Pharmacol Ther 1973;14:632–42.
4. Finnigan D, Burry AF, Smith IDB. Analgesic consumption in an antenatal clinic survey. Med J Aust 1974;1:761–2.
5. Collins E, Turner G. Maternal effects of regular salicylate ingestion in pregnancy. Lancet 1975;2:335–7.
6. Slone D, Heinonen OP, Kaufman DW, Siskind V, Monson RR, Shapiro S. Aspirin and congenital malformations. Lancet 1976;1:1373–5.
7. Hill RM, Craig JP, Chaney MD, Tennyson LM, McCulley LB. Utilization of over-the-counter drugs during pregnancy. Clin Obstet Gynecol 1977;20:381–94.
8. Harrison K, Thomas I, Smith I. Analgesic use during pregnancy. Med J Aust 1978;2:161.
9. Bodendorfer TW, Briggs GG, Gunning JE. Obtaining drug exposure histories during pregnancy. Am J Obstet Gynecol 1979;135:490–4.
10. Jackson AV. Toxic effects of salicylate on the foetus and mother. J Pathol Bacteriol 1948;60:587–93.
11. Lewis RN, Schulman JD. Influence of acetylsalicylic acid, an inhibitor of prostaglandin synthesis, on the duration of human gestation and labour. Lancet 1973;2:1159–61.
12. Rudolph AM. Effects of aspirin and acetaminophen in pregnancy and in the newborn. Arch Intern Med 1981;141:358–63.
13. Stuart MJ, Gross SJ, Elrad H, Graeber JE. Effects of acetylsalicylic-acid ingestion on maternal and neonatal hemostasis. N Engl J Med 1982;307:909–12.
14. Stuart MJ. Aspirin and maternal or neonatal hemostasis. N Engl J Med 1983;308:281.
15. Niebyl JR, Blake DA, Burnett LS, King TM. The influence of aspirin on the course of induced midtrimester abortion. Am J Obstet Gynecol 1976;124:607–10.
16. Castellanos JM, Aranda M, Cararach J, Cararach V. Effect of aspirin on oestriol excretion in pregnancy. Lancet 1975;1:859.
17. Babenerd VJ, Kyriakidis K. Acetylsalicylic acid in the prevention of premature delivery. Fortschr Med 1979;97:463–6.
18. Wolff F, Bolte A, Berg R. Does an additional administration of acetylsalicylic acid reduce the requirement of betamimetics in tocolytic treatment? Geburtshilfe Frauenheilkd 1981;41:293–6.
19. Wolff F, Berg R, Bolte A. Clinical study of the labour inhibiting effects and side effects of acetylsalicylic acid (ASA). Geburtshilfe Frauenheilkd 1981;41:96–100.
20. Buhler M, Papiernik E. Successive pregnancies in women fitted with intrauterine devices who take antiinflammatory drugs. Lancet 1983;1:483.
21. Goodlin RC. Correction of pregnancy-related thrombocytopenia with aspirin without improvement in fetal outcome. Am J Obstet Gynecol 1983;146:862–4.
22. Gant NF. Lupus erythematosus, the lupus anticoagulant, and the anti-cardiolipid antibody. Supplement No. 6, May/June 1986, to Pritchard JA, MacDonald PC, Gant NF. *Williams Obstetrics*. 17th ed. Norwalk, CT: Appleton-Century-Crofts, 1985.

23. Branch DW, Scott JR, Kochenour NK, Hershgold E. Obstetric complications associated with the lupus anticoagulant. N Engl J Med 1985;313:1322–6.
24. Elder MG, DeSwiet M, Robertson A, Elder MA, Flloyd E, Hawkins DF. Low-dose aspirin in pregnancy. Lancet 1988;1:410.
25. Lockshin MD, Druzin ML, Qamar T. Prednisone does not prevent recurrent fetal death in women with antiphospholipid antibody. Am J Obstet Gynecol 1989;160:439–43.
26. Beaufils M, Uzan S, Donsimoni R, Colau JC. Prevention of pre-eclampsia by early antiplatelet therapy. Lancet 1985;1:840–2.
27. Beaufils M, Uzan S, Donsimoni R, Colau JC. Prospective controlled study of early antiplatelet therapy in prevention of preeclampsia. Adv Nephrol 1986;15:87–94.
28. Ylikorkala O, Makila U-M, Kaapa P, Viinikka L. Maternal ingestion of acetylsalicylic acid inhibits fetal and neonatal prostacyclin and thromboxane in humans. Am J Obstet Gynecol 1986;155:345–9.
29. Spitz B, Magness RR, Cox SM, Brown CEL, Rosenfeld CR, Gant NF. Low-dose aspirin. I. Effect on angiotensin II pressor responses and blood prostaglandin concentrations in pregnant women sensitive to angiotensin II. Am J Obstet Gynecol 1988;159:1035–43.
30. Wallenburg HCS, Rotmans N. Prevention of recurrent idiopathic fetal growth retardation by low-dose aspirin and dipyridamole. Am J Obstet Gynecol 1987;157:1230–5.
31. Wallenburg HCS, Rotmans N. Prophylactic low-dose aspirin and dipyridamole in pregnancy. Lancet 1988;1:939.
32. Uzan S, Beaufils M, Bazin B, Danays T. Idiopathic recurrent fetal growth retardation and aspirin-dipyridamole therapy. Am J Obstet Gynecol 1989;160:763.
33. Wallenburg HCS, Rotmans N. Idiopathic recurrent fetal growth retardation and aspirin-dipyridamole therapy. Reply. Am J Obstet Gynecol 1989;160:763–4.
34. Sibai BM, Mirro R, Chesney CM, Leffler C. Low-dose aspirin in pregnancy. Obstet Gynecol 1989;74:551–7.
35. Trudinger B, Cook CM, Thompson R, Giles W, Connelly A. Low-dose aspirin improves fetal weight in umbilical placental insufficiency. Lancet 1988;2:214–5.
36. Romero R, Lockwood C, Oyarzun E, Hobbins JC. Toxemia: new concepts in an old disease. Semin Perinatol 1988;12:302–23.
37. Lubbe WF. Low-dose aspirin in prevention of toxaemia of pregnancy. Does it have a place? Drugs 1987;34:515–8.
38. Wallenburg HCS, Dekker GA, Makovitz JW, Rotmans P. Low-dose aspirin prevents pregnancy-induced hypertension and pre-eclampsia in angiotensin-sensitive primigravidae. Lancet 1986;1:1–3.
39. Benigni A, Gregorini G, Frusca T, Chiabrando C, Ballerini S, Valcamonico A, Orisio S, Piccinelli A, Pinciroli V, Fanelli R, Gastaldi A, Remuzzi G. Effect of low-dose aspirin on fetal and maternal generation of thromboxane by platelets in women at risk for pregnancy-induced hypertension. N Engl J Med 1989;321:357–62.
40. Schiff E, Peleg E, Goldenberg M, Rosenthal T, Ruppin E, Tamarkin M, Barkai G, Ben-Baruch G, Yahal I, Blankstein J, Goldman B, Mashiach S. The use of aspirin to prevent pregnancy-induced hypertension and lower the ratio of thromboxane A_2 to prostacyclin in relatively high risk pregnancies. N Engl J Med 1989;321:351–6.
41. Turner G, Collins E. Fetal effects of regular salicylate ingestion in pregnancy. Lancet 1975;2:338–9.
42. Earle R Jr. Congenital salicylate intoxication-report of a case. N Engl J Med 1961;265:1003–4.
43. Lynd PA, Andreasen AC, Wyatt RJ. Intrauterine salicylate intoxication in a newborn. A case report. Clin Pediatr (Phila) 1976;15:912–3.
44. Shapiro S, Monson RR, Kaufman DW, Siskind V, Heinonen OP, Slone D. Perinatal mortality and birth-weight in relation to aspirin taken during pregnancy. Lancet 1976;1:1375–6.
45. Arcilla RA, Thilenius OG, Ranniger K. Congestive heart failure from suspected ductal closure in utero. J Pediatr 1969;75:74–8.
46. Collins E. Maternal and fetal effects of acetaminophen and salicylates in pregnancy. Obstet Gynecol 1981;58(Suppl):57S–62S.
47. Aterman K, Holzbecker M, Ellenberger HA. Salicylate levels in a stillborn infant born to a drug-addicted mother, with comments on pathology and analytical methodology. Clin Toxicol 1980;16:263–8.
48. Van Marter LJ, Leviton A, Allred EN, Pagano M, Sullivan KF, Cohen A, Epstein MF. Persistent pulmonary hypertension of the newborn and smoking and aspirin and nonsteroidal antiinflammatory drug consumption during pregnancy. Pediatrics 1996;97:658–63.
49. Alano MA, Ngougmna E, Ostrea EM Jr, Konduri GG. Analysis of nonsteroidal antiinflammatory drugs in meconium and its relation to persistent pulmonary hypertension of the newborn. Pediatrics 2001; 107:519–23.
50. Bleyer WA, Breckenridge RJ. Studies on the detection of adverse drug reactions in the newborn. II. The effects of prenatal aspirin on newborn hemostasis. JAMA 1970;213:2049–53.
51. Corby DG, Schulman I. The effects of antenatal drug administration on aggregation of platelets of newborn infants. J Pediatr 1971;79:307–13.
52. Casteels-Van Daele M, Eggermont E, de Gaetano G, Vermijlen J. More on the effects of antenatally administered aspirin on aggregation of platelets of neonates. J Pediatr 1972;80:685–6.
53. Haslam RR, Ekert H, Gillam GL. Hemorrhage in a neonate possible due to maternal ingestion of salicylate. J Pediatr 1974;84:556–7.
54. Ekert H, Haslam RR. Maternal ingested salicylate as a cause of neonatal hemorrhage. Reply. J Pediatr 1974;85:738.
55. Pearson H. Comparative effects of aspirin and acetaminophen on hemostasis. Pediatrics 1978;62(Suppl):926–9.
56. Haslam RR. Neonatal purpura secondary to maternal salicylism. J Pediatr 1975;86:653.
57. O'Brien JR. Effects of salicylates on human platelets. Lancet 1968;1: 779–83.
58. Weiss HJ, Aledort ML, Shaul I. The effect of salicylates on the haemostatic properties of platelets in man. J Clin Invest 1968;47:2169–80.
59. Bleyer WA. Maternal ingested salicylates as a cause of neonatal hemorrhage. J Pediatr 1974;85:736–7.
60. Rumack CM, Guggenheim MA, Rumack BH, Peterson RG, Johnson ML, Braithwaite WR. Neonatal intracranial hemorrhage and maternal use of aspirin. Obstet Gynecol 1981;58(Suppl):52S–6S.
61. Soller RW, Stander H. Maternal drug exposure and perinatal intracranial hemorrhage. Obstet Gynecol 1981;58:735–7.
62. Corby DG. Editorial comment. Obstet Gynecol 1981;58:737–40.
63. Levy G, Procknal JA, Garrettson LK. Distribution of salicylate between neonatal and maternal serum at diffusion equilibrium. Clin Pharmacol Ther 1975;18:210–4.
64. Levy G, Garrettson LK. Kinetics of salicylate elimination by newborn infants of mothers who ingested aspirin before delivery. Pediatrics 1974;53: 201–10.
65. Garrettson LK, Procknal JA, Levy G. Fetal acquisition and neonatal elimination of a large amount of salicylate. Study of a neonate whose mother regularly took therapeutic doses of aspirin during pregnancy. Clin Pharmacol Ther 1975;17:98–103.
66. Li DK, Liu L, Odouli R. Exposure to non-steroidal anti-inflammatory drugs during pregnancy and risk of miscarriage: population based cohort study. BMJ 2003;327:368–71.
67. Richards ID. Congenital malformations and environmental influences in pregnancy. Br J Prev Soc Med 1969;23:218–25.
68. Nelson MM, Forfar JO. Associations between drugs administered during pregnancy and congenital abnormalities of the fetus. Br Med J 1971;1:523–7.
69. Saxen I. Associations between oral clefts and drugs during pregnancy. Int J Epidemiol 1975;4:37–44.
70. Benawra R, Mangurten HH, Duffell DR. Cyclopia and other anomalies following maternal ingestion of salicylates. J Pediatr 1980;96:1069–71.
71. McNiel JR. The possible effect of salicylates on the developing fetus. Brief summaries of eight suggestive cases. Clin Pediatr (Phila) 1973;12: 347–50.
72. Sayli BS, Asmaz A, Yemisci B. Consanguinity, aspirin, and phocomelia. Lancet 1966;1:876.
73. Zierler S, Rothman KJ. Congenital heart disease in relation to maternal use of Bendectin and other drugs in early pregnancy. N Engl J Med 1985;313:347–52.
74. Rothman KJ, Fyler DC, Goldblatt A, Kreidberg MB. Exogenous hormones and other drug exposures of children with congenital heart disease. Am J Epidemiol 1979;109:433–9.
75. Zierler S. Maternal drugs and congenital heart disease. Obstet Gynecol 1985;65:155–65.
76. Werler MM, Mitchell AA, Shapiro S. The relation of aspirin use during the first trimester of pregnancy to congenital cardiac defects. N Engl J Med 1989;321:1639–42.
77. Kallen BAJ, Olausson PO. Maternal drug use in early pregnancy and infant cardiovascular defect. Reprod Toxicol 2003;17:255–61.
78. Torfs CP, Katz EA, Bateson TF, Lam PK, Curry CJR. Maternal medications and environmental exposures as risk factors for gastroschisis. Teratology 1996;54:84–92.
79. Streissguth AP, Treder RP, Barr HM, Shepard TH, Bleyer WA, Sampson PD, Martin DC. Aspirin and acetaminophen use by pregnant women and subsequent child IQ and attention decrements. Teratology 1987;35:211–9.
80. Klebanoff MA, Berendes HW. Aspirin exposure during the first 20 weeks of gestation and IQ at four years of age. Teratology 1988;37:249–55.

81. Matt DW, Borzelleca JF. Toxic effects on the female reproductive system during pregnancy, parturition, and lactation. In: Witorsch RJ, ed. *Reproductive Toxicology*. 2nd ed. New York, NY: Raven Press, 1995:175–93.
82. Daewood MY. Nonsteroidal antiinflammatory drugs and reproduction. Am J Obstet Gynecol 1993;169:1255–65.
83. Hernandez RK, Werler MM, Romitti P, Sun L, Anderka M; National Birth Defects Prevention Study. Nonsteroidal antiinflammatory drug use among women and the risk of birth defects. Am J Obstet Gynecol 2012;206: 228.e1–8.
84. Kwit NT, Hatcher RA. Excretion of drugs in milk. Am J Dis Child 1935;49: 900–4.
85. Erickson SH, Oppenheim GL. Aspirin in breast milk. J Fam Pract 1979;8: 189–90.
86. Weibert RT, Bailey DN. *Salicylate Excretion in Human Breast Milk (Abstract No. 7)*. Presented at the 1979 Seminar of the California Society of Hospital Pharmacists, Los Angeles, October 13, 1979.
87. Findlay JWA, DeAngelis RL, Kearney MF, Welch RM, Findley JM. Analgesic drugs in breast milk and plasma. Clin Pharmacol Ther 1981;29: 625–33.
88. Anderson PO. Drugs and breast feeding—a review. Drug Intell Clin Pharm 1977;11:208–23.
89. Clark JH, Wilson WG. A 16-day-old breast-fed infant with metabolic acidosis caused by salicylate. Clin Pediatr (Phila) 1981;20:53–4.
90. Committee on Drugs, American Academy of Pediatrics. The transfer of drugs and other chemicals into human milk. Pediatrics 2001;108: 776–89.

ASTEMIZOLE

[Withdrawn from the market. See 9th edition.]

ATAZANAVIR

Antiviral

PREGNANCY RECOMMENDATION: Compatible—Maternal Benefit >> Embryo–Fetal Risk
BREASTFEEDING RECOMMENDATION: Contraindicated

PREGNANCY SUMMARY

Although the limited human data prevent an assessment of the risk of atazanavir during pregnancy, the animal data suggest low risk to the developing fetus. Of note, the systemic exposures in two animal species were very close to those obtained clinically. However, if indicated, the drug should not be withheld because of pregnancy.

FETAL RISK SUMMARY

Atazanavir is an azapeptide HIV type 1 (HIV-1) protease inhibitor. The agent selectively inhibits the virus-specific processing of viral Gag and Gag-Pol polyproteins in HIV-1-infected cells, thereby preventing formation of mature virions (1). The hepatic metabolites of atazanavir are inactive. Plasma protein binding is 86% with about equal amounts bound to albumin and α_1-glycoprotein. The mean elimination half-life is about 7 hours (1).

Reproduction studies have been conducted in rats and rabbits. In rats, doses producing systemic drug exposures that were two times the human exposure from the clinical dose of 400 mg once daily (HE) had no adverse effect on mating or fertility and were not teratogenic or embryotoxic. However, in pre- and postnatal rat development studies, the dose resulted in body weight loss or decreased weight gain in offspring and maternal toxicity. No effects on offspring were observed when the maternal exposure was equivalent to the HE. No teratogenic effects were observed in rabbits at doses producing maternal exposures equal to the HE (1).

It is not known if atazanavir crosses the human placenta. The molecular weight (about 705 for the free base) and moderately long elimination half-life suggest that passage to the embryo and fetus might occur.

The Antiretroviral Pregnancy Registry reported, for the period January 1989 through July 2009, prospective data (reported before the outcomes were known) involving 4702 live births that had been exposed during the 1st trimester to one or more antiretroviral agents (2). Congenital defects were noted in 134, a prevalence of 2.8% (95% confidence interval [CI] 2.4–3.4). In the 6100 live births with earliest exposure in the 2nd/3rd trimesters, there were 153 infants with defects (2.5%, 95% CI 2.1–2.9). The prevalence rates for the two periods did not differ significantly. There were 288 infants with birth defects among 10,803 live births with exposure anytime during pregnancy (2.7%, 95% CI 2.4–3.0). The prevalence rate did not differ significantly from the rate expected in a nonexposed population. There were 528 outcomes exposed to atazanavir (343 in the 1st trimester and 185 in the 2nd/3rd trimesters) in combination with other antiretroviral agents. There were 12 birth defects (9 in the 1st trimester and 3 in the 2nd/3rd trimesters). In reviewing the birth defects of prospective and retrospective (pregnancies reported after the outcomes were known) registered cases, the Registry concluded that, except for isolated cases of neural tube defects with efavirenz exposure in retrospective reports, there was no other pattern of anomalies (isolated or syndromic) (2). (See Lamivudine for required statement.)

Hyperbilirubinemia is a common adverse effect with atazanavir, but it is not known if this will worsen physiologic hyperbilirubinemia in the newborn or young infant and lead to kernicterus. In the prepartum period, additional monitoring and alternative therapy to atazanavir should be considered (1).

A public health advisory was issued by the FDA on the association between protease inhibitors and diabetes mellitus (3). Because pregnancy is a risk factor for hyperglycemia, there was concern that these antiviral agents would exacerbate this risk. An abstract published in 2000 described the results of a study involving 34 pregnant women treated with protease inhibitors (none with amprenavir) compared with 41 controls that evaluated the association with diabetes (4). No association between protease inhibitors and an increased incidence of gestational diabetes was found.

Two reviews, one in 1996 and the other in 1997, concluded that all women currently receiving antiretroviral therapy should continue to receive therapy during pregnancy and that treatment of the mother with monotherapy should be considered inadequate therapy (5,6). The same conclusion was reached in a 2003 review with the added admonishment that therapy must be continuous to prevent emergence of resistant viral strains (7). In 2009, the updated U.S. Department of Health and Human Services guidelines for the use of antiretroviral agents in HIV-1-infected patients continued the recommendation that the therapy, with the exception of efavirenz, should be continued during pregnancy (8). If indicated, therefore, protease inhibitors, including atazanavir, should not be withheld in pregnancy because the expected benefit to the HIV-positive mother outweighs the unknown risk to the fetus. Pregnant women taking protease inhibitors should be monitored for hyperglycemia. Updated guidelines for the use of antiretroviral drugs to reduce perinatal HIV-1 transmission also were released in 2010 (9). Women receiving antiretroviral therapy during pregnancy should continue the therapy but, regardless of the regimen, zidovudine administration is recommended during the intrapartum period to prevent vertical transmission of HIV to the newborn (9).

BREASTFEEDING SUMMARY

No reports describing the use of atazanavir during human lactation have been located. The molecular weight (about 705 for the free base) and the moderately long elimination half-life (about 7 hours) suggest that the drug will be excreted into breast milk. The effect on a nursing infant from this exposure is unknown.

However, reports on the use of atazanavir during lactation are unlikely because of the potential toxicity, especially hyperbilirubinemia, and because the drug is indicated in the treatment of patients with HIV. HIV-1 is transmitted in milk, and in developed countries, breastfeeding is not recommended (5,6,8,10–12). In developing countries, breastfeeding is undertaken, despite the risk, because there are no affordable milk substitutes available.

References

1. Product information. Reyataz. Bristol-Myers Squibb, 2004.
2. Antiretroviral Pregnancy Registry Steering Committee. *Antiretroviral Pregnancy Registry International Interim Report for 1 January 1989 through 31 July 2009*. Wilmington, NC: Registry Coordinating Center; 2009. Available at www.apregistry.com. Accessed May 29, 2010.
3. Centers for Disease Control. Public Health Service Task Force recommendations for the use of antiretroviral drugs in pregnant women infected with HIV-1 for maternal health and for reducing perinatal HIV-1 transmission in the United States. MMWR 1998;47:No. RR-2.
4. Fassett M, Kramer F, Stek A. Treatment with protease inhibitors in pregnancy is not associated with an increased incidence of gestational diabetes (abstract). Am J Obstet Gynecol 2000;182:S97.
5. Carpenter CCJ, Fischi MA, Hammer SM, Hirsch MS, Jacobsen DM, Katzenstein DA, Montaner JSG, Richman DD, Saag MS, Schooley RT, Thompson MA, Vella S, Yeni PG, Volberding PA. Antiretroviral therapy for HIV infection in 1996. JAMA 1996;276;146–54.
6. Minkoff H, Augenbraun M. Antiretroviral therapy for pregnant women. Am J Obstet Gynecol 1997;176:478–89.
7. Minkoff H. Human immunodeficiency virus infection in pregnancy. Obstet Gynecol 2003;101:797–810.
8. Panel on Antiretroviral Guidelines for Adults and Adolescents. *Guidelines for the Use of Antiretroviral Agents in HIV-1-Infected Adults and Adolescents*. Department of Health and Human Services. December 1, 2009;1–161. Available at http://www.aidsinfo.nih.gov/ContentFiles/AdultandAdolescentGL.pdf. Accessed September 17, 2010:60, 96–8.
9. Panel on Treatment of HIV-Infected Pregnant Women and Prevention of Perinatal Transmission. *Recommendations for Use of Antiretroviral Drugs in Pregnant HIV-1-Infected Women for Maternal Health and Interventions to Reduce Perinatal HIV Transmission in the United States*. May 24, 2010; 1–117. Available at http://aidsinfo.nih.gov/ContentFiles/PerinatalGL.pdf. Accessed September 17, 2010:30 (Table 5).
10. Brown ZA, Watts DH. Antiviral therapy in pregnancy. Clin Obstet Gynecol 1990;33:276–89.
11. De Martino M, Tovo P-A, Pezzotti P, Galli L, Massironi E, Ruga E, Floreea F, Plebani A, Gabiano C, Zuccotti GV. HIV-1 transmission through breast-milk: appraisal of risk according to duration of feeding. AIDS 1992;6:991–7.
12. Van de Perre P. Postnatal transmission of human immunodeficiency virus type 1: the breast feeding dilemma. Am J Obstet Gynecol 1995;173:483–7.

ATENOLOL

Sympatholytic (Antihypertensive)

PREGNANCY RECOMMENDATION: Human Data Suggest Risk in 2nd and 3rd Trimesters
BREASTFEEDING RECOMMENDATION: Limited Human Data—Potential Toxicity

PREGNANCY SUMMARY

Atenolol may cause growth restriction and reduced placental weight. The drug does not possess ISA (i.e., partial agonist). The reduced fetal growth appears to be related to increased vascular resistance in both the mother and the fetus and is a function of the length of drug exposure. Treatment starting early in the 2nd trimester is associated with the greatest decrease in fetal and placental weights, whereas treatment restricted to the 3rd trimester primarily affects only placental weight. Although growth restriction is a serious concern, the benefits of maternal therapy with β-blockers, in some cases, might outweigh the risks to the fetus and must be judged on a case-by-case basis. Because only one case has been reported, an association between atenolol and fetal retroperitoneal fibromatosis requires confirmation. Newborns exposed to atenolol near delivery should be closely observed during the first 24–48 hours for signs and symptoms of β-blockade. The long-term effects of prolonged in utero exposure to this class of drugs have not been studied but warrant evaluation.

FETAL RISK SUMMARY

Atenolol is a cardioselective β_1-adrenergic blocking agent used for the treatment of hypertension. The drug did not cause structural anomalies in pregnant rats and rabbits, but a dose-related increase in embryo and fetal resorptions in rats was observed at doses ≥25 times the maximum recommended human antihypertensive dose based on 100 mg/day in a 50-kg patient (MRHD). This effect was not seen in rabbits at doses up to 12.5 times the MRHD (1).

In contrast with propranolol and sotalol, atenolol exposure during gestation did not increase the motor activity or cause poor performance in rat offspring (2). The adverse effects observed with propranolol and sotalol, but not atenolol, were attributed to the β_2-blocking activity of propranolol and sotalol.

A 2002 abstract, reviewing both published and nonpublished sources to assess atenolol developmental toxicity, found that fetal growth restriction occurred in both animals and humans (3). The animal–human concordance was thought to result from the reduced placental and fetal circulation induced by atenolol.

Atenolol readily crosses the placenta to the fetus producing steady-state fetal levels approximately equal to those in the maternal serum (4–11). When 11 pregnant patients were treated with 100 mg/day, the serum half-life (8.1 hours) and the 24-hour urinary excretion (52 mg) were similar to those values in nonpregnant women (8). In nine women treated with atenolol for cardiac disease, the average maternal and cord drug concentrations at delivery were 133 and 126 ng/mL, respectively (11). No evidence of altered atenolol pharmacokinetics during pregnancy was found. Atenolol transfer was one-third to one-fourth the transfer of the more lipid-soluble β-blockers propranolol, timolol, and labetalol in an in vitro experiment using perfused human placentas (12).

In a surveillance study of Michigan Medicaid recipients involving 229,101 completed pregnancies conducted between 1985 and 1992, 105 newborns had been exposed to atenolol during the 1st trimester (F. Rosa, personal communication, FDA, 1993). A total of 12 (11.4%) major birth defects were observed (4 expected). Specific data were available for six defect categories, including (observed/expected) 3/1 cardiovascular defects, 1/0 oral clefts, 0/0 spina bifida, 0/0 polydactyly, 1/0 limb reduction defects, and 4/0 hypospadias. Only with the latter defect is there a suggestion of a possible association, but other factors, including the mother's disease, concurrent drug use, and chance, may be involved.

A 1997 abstract (13) and later full report (14) described a case of retroperitoneal fibromatosis in a fetus exposed in utero to atenolol from the second month of gestation through delivery at 37 weeks. The obese (134 kg at term), 25-year-old mother, in her third pregnancy, was treated for hypertension with 100-mg atenolol daily until giving birth to the 3790-g male infant. Other drug therapy included magnesium supplements and occasional metoclopramide. The mother had no familial history of cancer and both of her other children were normal. Treatment of the tumor with chemotherapy during the first 3 months of life was successful, but a severe scoliosis was present in the child at 4 years of age. The authors attributed the rare tumor to the drug because, among other reasons, the location of the mass was similar to that of fibroses reported in adults exposed to atenolol (13,14).

The use of atenolol for the treatment of hypertension in pregnant women has been described frequently (7,10,15–28). No fetal malformations attributable to atenolol have been reported in these trials, but in most cases, the treatment with atenolol did not occur during the 1st trimester.

In a 1981 study, 13 women—11 in the 3rd trimester and 2 in the 2nd trimester—were treated for gestational hypertension with atenolol 100 mg/day until delivery (15). The birth weights of 12 of the 13 newborns were less than the 50th percentile (3 were less than the 10th percentile), but the authors thought they were consistent with severe preeclampsia. The pharmacokinetic profiles of atenolol in the pregnant subjects were similar to those measured in nonpregnant women (15).

A 1982 study described the pregnancy outcomes of 10 women with chronic hypertension who were treated with atenolol 100–200 mg/day beginning at 11–32 weeks (16). One woman delivered a stillborn infant at 41+ weeks' gestation, but the remaining nine women delivered at a median of 39 weeks. The median birth weight was 82% of the gestational mean with placental weights ranging from 235 to 795 g.

A 1983 retrospective study examined the effects of atenolol (N = 87) and metoprolol (N = 2), either alone or in combination with other antihypertensives, for the treatment of hypertension (chronic or preeclampsia) in pregnancy (17). Birth weights were not given. There were three stillbirths, but the maternal therapy in these cases was not specified.

A randomized, double-blind study published in 1983 compared atenolol (N = 46) with placebo (N = 39) for the treatment of mild-to-moderate gestational hypertension (18). Treatment was started at a mean 34 weeks' gestation in both groups. The mean gestational ages at delivery were 38 weeks (placebo) and 39 weeks (atenolol) ($p < 0.05$). No differences in the incidence of hypoglycemia, respiratory distress syndrome, or hyperbilirubinemia were observed between the groups. Although not statistically significant, both the mean birth weights (2961 vs. 3017 g) and placental weights (549 vs. 608 g) were lower in those treated with atenolol. However, significantly more atenolol-exposed newborns had bradycardia, 39% (18 of 46) vs. 10% (4 of 39) ($p < 0.01$). None of the infants required treatment for the lowered heart rate. Three intrauterine deaths occurred, two in the placebo group and one in the atenolol group (18). In the same year, the authors of this study and a previous report (16) commented briefly on the benefits of β-blockers in the management of hypertension during pregnancy (19).

A 1992 study evaluated the effectiveness of atenolol in three groups of pregnant women having chronic hypertension (N = 12), gestational hypertension without proteinuria

($N = 52$), or preeclampsia ($N = 6$) (20). The mean doses in the three groups were 62.5, 70.0, and 100.0 mg, respectively. The drug was started at a mean gestational age of 24.5, 29.8, and 31.0 weeks, respectively. The mean birth weights observed were approximately 2902, 3059, and 2431 g, respectively.

The effect of β-blockers in pregnancy was reviewed in a 1988 article. Citing only three reports, the authors concluded that atenolol was safe and effective therapy during pregnancy (21).

Antihypertensive therapy with atenolol has been associated with fetal growth restriction in a number of studies (7,10,22–27). A nonrandomized 1983 study compared atenolol ($N = 28$; enrolled before May 1981) with labetalol ($N = 28$; enrolled after May 1981) in the treatment of chronic ($N = 6$) or gestational hypertension ($N = 50$) (7). The average daily doses were 144.6 mg (atenolol) and 614 mg (labetalol). Newborn weights were significantly higher in those exposed to labetalol, 3280 vs. 2750 g, respectively ($p < 0.001$). Two newborns were premature (<37 weeks) in the atenolol group compared with one in the labetalol group. In addition, two mothers treated with atenolol delivered stillborn infants at 29 and 38 weeks, respectively (7).

A 1984 case report described the pregnancy outcome of a woman treated with atenolol (50 mg/day increased to 100 mg/day at 33 weeks') throughout a 36-week gestation (10). Intrauterine growth restriction (IUGR) was diagnosed by ultrasound and a small (weight not given) but otherwise-normal baby girl was delivered with Apgar scores of 5, 7, and 9 at 1, 5, and 10 minutes, respectively. The maternal plasma and cord blood atenolol concentrations were 510 and 380 ng/mL, respectively. Other than a transient decrease in heart rate to 100 beats/minute at 16 hours of age, the infant had no complications (10).

A 1980 report described 60 pregnancy outcomes from 59 women treated with β-blockers for hypertension (22). The agents used were atenolol ($N = 10$; daily dose 100–200 mg), acebutolol ($N = 28$; daily dose 200–600 mg), pindolol ($N = 21$; daily dose 10–20 mg), and propranolol ($N = 1$; daily dose 40 mg). Although the birth weights were not differentiated by drug, 9 newborns weighed <2500 g, 11 were 2500–2800 g, and 40 were >2800 g (21). Two years later, this research group compared atenolol ($N = 31$), acebutolol ($N = 56$), and pindolol ($N = 38$) in a nonrandomized study for the treatment of hypertension during pregnancy (23). One year later, the researchers increased the number of atenolol cases to 37 (24). The mean birth weights of the three groups were 2.82, 3.16, and 3.38 kg, respectively (23,24).

In a prospective, randomized, double-blind study, women with mild essential hypertension were given either atenolol (50–200 mg/day) or placebo starting at a mean gestational age of 15.9 weeks (25). The 15 newborns in the treated group had a significantly lower birth weight than the 14 untreated controls (2620 vs. 3530 g; $p < 0.001$). In the treated group, 5 of the newborns had weights below the 5th percentile and 10 were below the 10th percentile, compared with 1 newborn below the 25th percentile in controls. In addition, the atenolol group had significantly smaller placentas (442 vs. 635 g; $p < 0.002$) (25).

A 1992 report described the outcomes of 29 women with pregnancy-induced hypertension in the 3rd trimester (26). The women were randomized to receive either atenolol ($N = 13$) or pindolol ($N = 16$). The decrease in mean maternal arterial blood pressure in the two groups was similar. In comparing the women's status before and after therapy, several significant changes were measured in fetal hemodynamics with atenolol but, except for fetal heart rate, no significant changes were measured with pindolol. The atenolol-induced changes included a decrease in fetal heart rate; increases in the pulsatility indices (and thus the peripheral vascular resistance) of the fetal thoracic descending aorta, the abdominal aorta, and the umbilical artery; and a decrease in the umbilical venous blood flow (26). Although no difference in birth weights was observed in the two groups, the placental weight in atenolol-treated pregnancies was significantly less, 529 vs. 653 g ($p = 0.03$).

A 1997 report described an open, retrospective survey on the use of antihypertensives in 398 consecutive pregnant women who attended an antenatal hypertension clinic from 1980 to 1995 (27). The 76 women who used atenolol were compared with those using calcium channel blockers ($N = 22$), diuretics ($N = 26$), methyldopa ($N = 17$), other β-blockers ($N = 12$), or no drug therapy ($N = 235$). The mean birth weights/placental weights in the groups were atenolol 2.19 kg/390 g ($p < 0.001$); other β-blockers 2.36 kg/450 g; calcium channel blockers 2.50 kg/385 g ($p = 0.001$); diuretics 2.53 kg/500 g; methyldopa 2.70 kg/500 g; and no drug treatment 2.78 kg/535 g. The ponderal index ($kg/m^3 \times 10^4$), an indirect measure of impaired placental function in some forms of IUGR, also was calculated for each group: 2.21 ($p < 0.001$), 2.44, 2.22, 2.33, 2.67, and 2.39, respectively. The authors concluded that atenolol was associated with IUGR and reduced placental weights and should be avoided in women who are trying to conceive or are in the early stages of gestation (27).

A 1999 retrospective cohort study reported the outcomes of 312 pregnancies in 223 women treated for gestational hypertension ($N = 80$), preeclampsia ($N = 19$), chronic hypertension ($N = 179$), or superimposed preeclampsia on chronic hypertension ($N = 34$) (28). The women were treated with atenolol monotherapy ($N = 78$), other monotherapy ($N = 53$), combination therapy ($N = 90$; atenolol in 57), or no treatment ($N = 91$). The atenolol outcomes were statistically significant when compared with other monotherapy or with no treatment. (Combination therapy implied more severe disease and consistently had the worst outcomes.) Birth weights were as follows: atenolol 2372 g vs. other monotherapy 2756 g or no treatment 3068 g ($p < 0.05$), and combination therapy 2220 g; birth lengths were as follows: atenolol 47.9 cm vs. other monotherapy 48.3 cm, no treatment 50.4 cm, ($p < 0.05$), and combination therapy 46.3 cm. There were two nonsignificant trends: higher prevalence of preterm delivery (<37 weeks) atenolol 33% vs. other monotherapy 26%, no treatment 15%, and combination therapy 46%; and higher prevalence of small-for-gestational-age (<10th percentile) atenolol 49% vs. other monotherapy 34%, no treatment 21%, and combination therapy 52%. The adverse fetal effects of atenolol were more pronounced when the therapy was started early in pregnancy and were duration-dependent (28).

A prospective randomized study compared 24 atenolol-treated women with 27 pindolol-treated women (29). No differences between the groups were found in gestational length, birth weight, Apgar scores, rates of cesarean section, or umbilical cord blood glucose levels. Treatment in both groups started at about 33 weeks' gestation. Placentas in the atenolol group weighed less than those from pindolol-treated women, 440 vs. 533 g, $p < 0.02$.

A 1987 study used Doppler ultrasound to evaluate maternal and fetal circulation during atenolol therapy in 14 women (9 nulliparous) with pregnancy-induced hypertension at a mean gestational age of 35 weeks (range 33–38 weeks) (30). The studies were conducted before and during the first and third days of treatment. During treatment, the volume of blood flow remained unchanged in the fetal descending aorta and the umbilical vein. In contrast, the pulsatility index increased in the fetal descending aorta and the maternal arcuate artery, suggesting that peripheral vascular resistance had increased on both the maternal and fetal sides of the placenta. No effect on placental or fetal weight occurred because of the short treatment period (delivery occurred a mean 18 days after the start of the study) (30). The study design and techniques were criticized based on concerns for reproducibility, including day-to-day variability in Doppler measurements, the lack of controls, and the uncertainty of the clinical significance of velocity waveform measurements (31).

A 1995 randomized study examined the short-term effects of IV 15- to 20-minute infusions of atenolol or pindolol in 24 women with gestational hypertension (32). Comparisons were made for uterine and umbilicoplacental vascular impedance, fetal hemodynamics, and cardiac function. Both drugs significantly decreased maternal blood pressure and maternal heart rate immediately after infusion, but the effect of atenolol still was evident 30 minutes after the end of the infusion. Pindolol produced no changes in uteroplacental or umbilicoplacental vascular impedance, whereas atenolol increased vascular impedance in the nonplacental uterine artery. The umbilical artery pulsatility indices, an indication of increased vascular resistance, were higher after atenolol than after pindolol. Pindolol had no effects on fetal hemodynamics whereas atenolol decreased pulsatility indices in the fetal renal artery. In addition, atenolol significantly decreased peak systolic velocity in the fetal pulmonary trunk. The investigators concluded that both drugs were equally effective in lowering maternal blood pressure, that atenolol increased uteroplacental vascular impedance, and that atenolol had direct effects on fetal hemodynamics. Based on these findings, pindolol was the preferred agent (32).

A 1995 review of vasoactive drugs in pregnancy stated that pregnancy-induced hypertension (now known as gestational hypertension) was associated with increased vascular resistance that could reduce uteroplacental blood flow by 40%–70% (33). In addition, atenolol treatment was associated with increased resistance in uterine arteries and decreased peak velocity in the fetal pulmonary trunk, but that pindolol lacked these effects (32). They concluded that the use of vasoconstricting β-blockers during pregnancy should be reconsidered (33).

Normotensive women at risk for preeclampsia (cardiac output > 7.4 L/minute before 24 weeks' gestation) were enrolled in a 1999 double-blind, randomized, controlled trial to determine if atenolol could reduce this risk (34). The treatment groups were nulliparous: atenolol ($N = 21$) or placebo ($N = 19$); diabetics: atenolol ($N = 7$) or placebo ($N = 9$); and controls: no treatment ($N = 18$). A significant decrease ($p = 0.04$) in the incidence of preeclampsia was noted in the atenolol-treated women, but their offspring had a birth weight of 440 g less than that of placebo infants ($p = 0.02$). However, no increase in the rate of small-for-gestational-age fetuses was observed. Previous research by these investigators had suggested that in women with hypertension, fetal growth restriction occurred primarily when increased vascular resistance was present but not when hypertension was mediated by increased cardiac output (34). They concluded that a change in therapy was indicated if the maternal cardiac output was less than the mean for gestational age or if peripheral resistance was greater than 1150 dyne second/cm^5. If these guidelines had been followed, atenolol therapy would have been changed in seven subjects, including four cases involving the smallest infants (34).

A 2001 retrospective review of pregnancies ($N = 235$) at risk for preeclampsia that were treated with atenolol (25–100 mg/day) early in gestation was reported by the same authors as those of the above study (35). The goals of therapy were to reduce cardiac output to 1 standard deviation above the mean for gestational age and to lower mean arterial pressure to <90 mmHg. To maintain fetal growth, this was modified to maintaining cardiac output above the mean for gestational age and maintaining peripheral vascular resistance at <1150 dyne second/cm^5. Low birth weight was associated with (a) prior pregnancy with IUGR ($p = 0.001$); (b) failure to adjust the dose properly for cardiac output and peripheral vascular resistance ($p < 0.001$); and (c) a pregnancy in an earlier year of the investigator's experience ($p < 0.001$). In the study population, the birth weight increased from the 20th percentile at the beginning of the study period (1991) to the 40th percentile by the end (1999) ($p = 0.002$) (35).

In a group of pregnant women with symptomatic mitral valve stenosis, 11 were treated with atenolol and 14 with propranolol (36). The mean birth weight of the 25 infants was 2.8 kg (range 2.1–3.5 kg). Atenolol, 25 mg twice daily, was administered from 18 weeks' gestation to term in a normotensive woman who had suffered a myocardial infarction (37). She delivered a 2720-g infant with normal Apgar scores and blood gases.

Intrauterine fetal deaths have been observed in women with severe hypertension treated with atenolol, but this also has occurred with other β-blockers and in hypertensive women not treated with drugs (7,16–18,38). Four cases of fetal death (at 18, 29, and 33 weeks) or neonatal death (at 6.5 days) have been reported when the mothers were treated with atenolol combined with either angiotensin-converting enzyme inhibitors (39–41) or a selective angiotensin II receptor antagonist (42).

In eight women treated with atenolol or pindolol, a decrease in the basal fetal heart rate was noted only in atenolol-exposed fetuses (43). Before and during treatment, fetal heart rates in the atenolol patients were 136 and 120 beats/minute, respectively, whereas the rates for the pindolol group were 128 and 132 beats/minute, respectively. In 60 patients treated with atenolol for pregnancy-induced hypertension, no effect on fetal heart rate pattern in response to uterine contractions was observed (44). Accelerations, variables, and late decelerations all were easily distinguishable.

Persistent β-blockade was observed in a newborn whose mother was treated with atenolol, 100 mg/day, for

hypertension (5). At 15 hours of age, the otherwise normal infant developed bradycardia at rest and when crying, and hypotension. The serum atenolol concentration was 0.24 mcg/mL. Urinary excretion of the drug during the first 7 days ranged from 0.085 to 0.196 mcg/mL.

A 1992 case report described a pregnant woman who was diagnosed with a pheochromocytoma at 28 weeks' gestation (45). She was treated with atenolol (100 mg/day) and phenoxybenzamine (30 mg/day) to control her blood pressure. An elective cesarean section was performed at 37 weeks to deliver a normal female infant (birth weight not given).

A woman with a renal transplant was treated with cyclosporine, prednisolone, and atenolol (50 mg/day) throughout a normotensive pregnancy without proteinuria (46). An 820-g (below the 3rd percentile) male infant was delivered at 30 weeks' gestation because of severe IUGR. The authors attributed the growth restriction to cyclosporine, but atenolol and prednisolone probably contributed to the condition.

A review published in 2002 examined the pharmacokinetic and pharmacodynamic issues relevant to the toxic effects of atenolol exposure during pregnancy (47). The authors concluded that (a) maternal hypertension can potentiate the adverse effects of atenolol on placental and fetal circulation, resulting in decreased placental and birth weight; (b) decreased placental weight has been significantly associated with IUGR and lower birth weight independent of gestational age; (c) the effects of atenolol are duration-dependent; and (d) several other agents have a more favorable effect on birth weight, including labetalol, pindolol, acebutolol, and calcium channel blockers (47).

The duration of treatment, rather than the dose used, appears to be a critical factor in causing atenolol-induced fetal growth restriction (48). At one center, adjustment of the dose for maternal cardiac output and peripheral vascular resistance reduced these toxic effects. Infant behavior is apparently not affected by atenolol exposure, as no differences were noted in the development at 1 year of age of offspring from mothers treated during the 3rd trimester for mild-to-moderate pregnancy-induced hypertension with either bed rest alone or rest combined with atenolol (49). The mean duration of therapy in the atenolol-treated patients was 5 weeks.

BREASTFEEDING SUMMARY

Atenolol is excreted into breast milk (6,8,10,47,50–54). The drug is a weak base, and when used during lactation, accumulation in the milk will occur with concentrations significantly greater than corresponding plasma levels (6,8,47,50–53). Peak milk concentrations after single-dose (50 mg) and continuous-dosing (25–100 mg/day) regimens were 3.6 and 2.9 times greater, respectively, than simultaneous plasma levels (52). Atenolol has been found in the serum and urine of breastfed infants in some studies (6,8,10,50). Other studies have been unable to detect the drug in the infant serum (test limit 10 ng/mL) (51,52).

Symptoms consistent with β-adrenergic blockade were observed in a breastfed, 5-day-old, full-term female infant, including cyanosis, hypothermia (35.5°C rectal), and bradycardia (80 beats/minute) (54). Blood pressure was 80/40 mmHg. Except for these findings, physical examination was normal and bacterial cultures from various sites were negative. The mother had been treated orally with atenolol, 50 mg every 12 hours, for postpartum hypertension. Breastfeeding was stopped 3 days after onset of the symptoms and 6 hours later, the infant's symptoms had resolved. A milk sample, collected 10 days postpartum and 1.5 hours after a 50-mg dose, contained 469 ng/mL of atenolol. Concentrations in the infant's serum, 48 and 72 hours after breastfeeding, were 2010 and 140 ng/mL, respectively. The calculated serum half-life in the infant was 6.4 hours. By extrapolation, the minimum daily dose absorbed by the infant was estimated to be 8.97 mg, approximately 9% of the mother's daily dose (54). (These calculations have been questioned and defended [55,56].)

Except for the single case cited above, adverse reactions in infants have not been reported. However, because milk accumulation occurs with atenolol, nursing infants must be closely monitored for bradycardia and other signs and symptoms of β-blockade. Moreover, one author has recommended that water-soluble, low-protein-bound, renally excreted β-blockers, such as atenolol, should not be used during lactation (57). Because of the availability of safer alternatives, this seems to be good advice. Long-term effects on infants exposed to β-blockers from breast milk have not been studied but warrant evaluation.

The American Academy of Pediatrics classifies atenolol as a drug that has been associated with significant effects in nursing infants (cyanosis and bradycardia) and should be used by nursing mothers with caution (58).

References

1. Product information. Tenormin. Zeneca Pharmaceuticals, 2003.
2. Speiser Z, Gordon I, Rehavi M, Gitter S. Behavioral and biochemical studies in rats following prenatal treatment with β-adrenoceptor antagonists. Eur J Pharmacol 1991;195:75–83.
3. Tabacova SA, Kimmel CA, Wall K, McCloskey CA. Animal-human concordance in the developmental toxicity of two antihypertensive agents (abstract). Teratology 2002;65:304.
4. Melander A, Niklasson B, Ingemarsson I, Liedholm H, Schersten B, Sjoberg NO. Transplacental passage of atenolol in man. Eur J Clin Pharmacol 1978;14:93–4.
5. Woods DL, Morrell DF. Atenolol: side effects in a newborn infant. Br Med J 1982;285:691–2.
6. Liedholm H. Transplacental passage and breast milk accumulation of atenolol in humans. Drugs 1983;25(Suppl 2):217–8.
7. Lardoux H, Gerard J, Blazquez G, Chouty F, Flouvat B. Hypertension in pregnancy: evaluation of two beta blockers atenolol and labetalol. Eur Heart J 1983;4(Suppl G):35–40.
8. Thorley KJ. Pharmacokinetics of atenolol in pregnancy and lactation. Drugs 1983;25(Suppl 2):216–7.
9. Boutroy MJ. Fetal and neonatal effects of the beta-adrenoceptor blocking agents. Dev Pharmacol Ther 1987;10:224–31.
10. Fowler MB, Brudenell M, Jackson G, Holt DW. Essential hypertension and pregnancy: successful outcome with atenolol. Br J Clin Pract 1984;38:73–4.
11. Hurst AK, Shotan A, Hoffman K, Johnson J, Goodwin TM, Koda R, Elkayam U. Pharmacokinetic and pharmacodynamic evaluation of atenolol during and after pregnancy. Pharmacotherapy 1998;18:840–6.
12. Schneider H, Proegler M. Placental transfer of B-adrenergic antagonists studied in an in vitro perfusion system of human placental tissue. Am J Obstet Gynecol 1988;159:42–7.
13. Satge D, Sasco AJ, Col JY, Lemonnier PG, Hemet J, Robert E. Antenatal exposure to atenolol and retroperitoneal fibromatosis (abstract). Teratology 1997;55:103.
14. Satge D, Sasco AJ, Col J-Y, Lemonnier PG, Hemet J, Robert E. Antenatal exposure to atenolol and retroperitoneal fibromatosis. Reprod Toxicol 1997;11:539–41.
15. Thorley KJ, McAinsh J, Cruickshank JM. Atenolol in the treatment of pregnancy-induced hypertension. Br J Clin Pharmacol 1981;12:725–30.

16. Rubin PC, Butters L, Low RA, Reid JL. Atenolol in the treatment of essential hypertension during pregnancy. Br J Clin Pharmacol 1982;14:279–81.
17. Liedholm H. Atenolol in the treatment of hypertension of pregnancy. Drugs 1983;25(Suppl 2):206–11.
18. Rubin PC, Butters L, Clark DM, Reynolds B, Sumner DJ, Steedman D, Low RA, Reid JL. Placebo-controlled trial of atenolol in treatment of pregnancy-associated hypertension. Lancet 1983;1:431–4.
19. Rubin PC, Butters L, Low RA, Clark DC, Reid JL. Atenolol in the management of hypertension during pregnancy. Drugs 1983;25(Suppl 2):212–4.
20. Fabregues G, Alvarez L, Varas Juri P, Drisaldi S, Cerrato C, Moschettoni C, Pituelo D, Baglivo HP, Esper RJ. Effectiveness of atenolol in the treatment of hypertension during pregnancy. Hypertension 1992;19(Suppl II):II129–31.
21. Frishman WH, Chesner M. Beta-adrenergic blockers in pregnancy. Am Heart J 1988;115:147–52.
22. Dubois D, Petitcolas J, Temperville B, Klepper A. Beta blockers and high-risk pregnancies. Int J Biol Res Pregnancy 1980;1:141–5.
23. Dubois D, Petitcolas J, Temperville B, Klepper A, Catherine P. Treatment of hypertension in pregnancy with β-adrenoceptor antagonists. Br J Clin Pharmacol 1982;13(Suppl):375S–8S.
24. Dubois D, Peticolas J, Temperville B, Klepper A. Treatment with atenolol of hypertension in pregnancy. Drugs 1983;25(Suppl 2):215–8.
25. Butters L, Kennedy S, Rubin PC. Atenolol in essential hypertension during pregnancy. BMJ 1990;301:587–9.
26. Montan S, Ingemarsson I, Marsal K, Sjoberg N-O. Randomized controlled trial of atenolol and pindolol in human pregnancy: effects on fetal haemodynamics. BMJ 1992;304:946–9.
27. Lip GYH, Beevers M, Churchill D, Shaffer LM, Beevers DG. Effect of atenolol on birth weight. Am J Cardiol 1997;79:1436–8.
28. Lydakis C, Lip GYH, Beevers M, Beevers DG. Atenolol and fetal growth in pregnancies complicated by hypertension. Am J Hypertens 1999;12:541–7.
29. Tuimala R, Hartikainen-Sorri A-L. Randomized comparison of atenolol and pindolol for treatment of hypertension in pregnancy. Curr Ther Res 1988;44:579–84.
30. Montan S, Liedholm H, Lingman G, Marsal K, Sjoberg N-O, Solum T. Fetal and uteroplacental haemodynamics during short-term atenolol treatment of hypertension in pregnancy. Br J Obstet Gynaecol 1987;94:312–7.
31. Rubin PC. Beta blockers in pregnancy. Br J Obstet Gynaecol 1987;94:292–3.
32. Rasanen J, Jouppila P. Uterine and fetal hemodynamics and fetal cardiac function after atenolol and pindolol infusion. A randomized study. Eur J Obstet Gynecol Reprod Biol 1995;62:195–201.
33. Jouppila P, Rasanen J, Alahuhta S, Jouppila R. Vasoactive drugs in obstetrics: a review of data obtained by Doppler and color Doppler methods. Hypertens Pregnancy 1995;14:261–75.
34. Easterling TR, Brateng D, Schmucker B, Brown Z, Millard SP. Prevention of preeclampsia: a randomized trial of atenolol in hyperdynamic patients before onset of hypertension. Obstet Gynecol 1999;93:725–33.
35. Easterling TR, Carr DB, Brateng D, Diederichs C, Schmucker B. Treatment of hypertension in pregnancy: effect of atenolol on maternal disease, preterm delivery, and fetal growth. Obstet Gynecol 2001;98:427–33.
36. Al Kasab SM, Sabag T, Al Zaibag M, Awaad M, Al Bitar I, Halim MA, Abdullah MA, Shahed M, Rajendran V, Sawyer W. β-Adrenergic receptor blockade in the management of pregnant women with mitral stenosis. Am J Obstet Gynecol 1990;163:37–40.
37. Soderlin MK, Purhonen S, Haring P, Hietakorpi S, Koski E, Nuutinen LS. Myocardial infarction in a parturient. Anaesthesia 1994;49:870–2.
38. Lubbe WF. More on beta-blockers in pregnancy. N Engl J Med 1982; 307:753.
39. Knott PD, Thorpe SS, Lamont CA. Congenital renal dysgenesis possibly due to Captopril. Lancet 1989;1:451.
40. Mehta N, Modi N. ACE inhibitors in pregnancy. Lancet 1989;2:96.
41. Smith AM. Are ACE inhibitors safe in pregnancy? Lancet 1989;2:750–1.
42. Briggs GG, Nageotte MP. Fatal fetal outcome with the combined use of valsartan and atenolol. Ann Pharmacother 2001;35:859–61.
43. Ingemarsson I, Liedholm H, Montan S, Westgren M, Melander A. Fetal heart rate during treatment of maternal hypertension with beta-adrenergic antagonists. Acta Obstet Gynecol Scand 1984;118(Suppl):95–7.
44. Rubin PC, Butters L, Clark D, Sumner D, Belfield A, Pledger D, Low RAL, Reid JL. Obstetric aspects of the use in pregnancy-associated hypertension of the B-adrenoceptor antagonist atenolol. Am J Obstet Gynecol 1984;150:389–92.
45. Bakri YN, Ingemansson SE, Ali A, Parikh S. Pheochromocytoma and pregnancy: report of three cases. Acta Obstet Gynecol Scand 1992;71:301–4.
46. Pickrell MD, Sawers R, Michael J. Pregnancy after renal transplantation: severe intrauterine growth retardation during treatment with cyclosporin A. BMJ 1988;296:825.
47. Tabacova SA, Kimmel CA. Atenolol: pharmacokinetic/dynamic aspects of comparative developmental toxicity. Reprod Toxicol 2002;16:1–7.
48. Sibai BM. Chronic hypertension in pregnancy. In reply. Obstet Gynecol 2002;100:1358–9.
49. Reynolds B, Butters L, Evans J, Adams T, Rubin PC. First year of life after the use of atenolol in pregnancy associated hypertension. Arch Dis Child 1984;59:1061–3.
50. Liedholm H, Melander A, Bitzen PO, Helm G, Lonnerholm G, Mattiasson I, Nilsson B, Wahlin-Boll E. Accumulation of atenolol and metoprolol in human breast milk. Eur J Clin Pharmacol 1981;20:229–31.
51. Kulas J, Lunell NO, Rosing U, Steen B, Rane A. Atenolol and metoprolol. A comparison of their excretion into human breast milk. Acta Obstet Gynecol Scand 1984;118(Suppl):65–9.
52. White WB, Andreoli JW, Wong SH, Cohn RD. Atenolol in human plasma and breast milk. Obstet Gynecol 1984;63:42S–4S.
53. White WB. Management of hypertension during lactation. Hypertension 1984;6:297–300.
54. Schmimmel MS, Eidelman AJ, Wilschanski MA, Shaw D Jr, Ogilvie RJ, Koren G. Toxic effects of atenolol consumed during breast feeding. J Pediatr 1989;114:476–8.
55. Diamond JM. Toxic effects of atenolol consumed during breast feeding. J Pediatr 1989;115:336.
56. Koren G. Toxic effects of atenolol consumed during breast feeding. J Pediatr 1989;115:336–7.
57. Anderson PO. Drugs and breast milk. Pediatrics 1995;95:957.
58. Committee on Drugs, American Academy of Pediatrics. The transfer of drugs and other chemicals into human milk. Pediatrics 2001;108:776–89.

ATOMOXETINE

Psychotherapeutic (Miscellaneous)

PREGNANCY RECOMMENDATION: Limited Human Data—Animal Data Suggest Risk
BREASTFEEDING RECOMMENDATION: No Human Data—Potential Toxicity

PREGNANCY SUMMARY

Although the animal data suggest risk, the absence of detailed human pregnancy experience prevents an assessment of the embryo–fetal risk. Until such data are available, the safest course is to avoid the drug in pregnancy. If the mother's condition requires atomoxetine, the lowest effective dose, avoiding the 1st trimester if possible, should be used. However, inadvertent exposure in the 1st trimester does not appear to represent a major risk. Long-term follow-up of exposed offspring may be warranted.

FETAL RISK SUMMARY

Atomoxetine is used for the treatment of attention deficit/hyperactivity disorder (ADHD). Atomoxetine has an equipotent active metabolite, but the plasma concentration is only 1% (in normal metabolizers) of the parent drug. A second active metabolite has much less activity and its plasma levels are 5% (in normal metabolizers) of the parent drug. The plasma elimination half-life in normal (extensive) metabolizers is about 5 hours. In persons who are "poor metabolizers" (7% of whites and 2% of blacks), the drug plasma levels are much higher and the plasma elimination half-life is 24 hours. The plasma protein binding is 98%, primarily to albumin (1).

Reproduction studies have been conducted in rats and rabbits. No effects on rat fertility were observed at doses up to about 6 times the maximum human dose based on BSA (MHD). In one of two studies in which rats were treated in the diet for 2 weeks prior to mating through organogenesis and lactation with doses up to about 6 times the MHD, a decrease in pup weight (female only) and pup survival (also seen at 3 times the MHD) was observed. The no-effect dose for pup survival was about 2 times the MHD. A diet dose about 5 times the MHD given throughout the period of organogenesis resulted in a decrease in fetal weight and an increase in the incidence of incomplete ossification of the vertebral arch in fetuses. The no-effect dose for these effects was about 2.5 times the MHD. No adverse fetal effects were observed when rats were gavage fed with doses up to 17 times the MHD throughout organogenesis (1).

In pregnant rabbits given atomoxetine by gavage, a dose about 23 times the MHD resulted in an increase in early absorptions and a decrease in live fetuses in one of three studies. In addition, slight increases in the incidences of atypical origin of carotid artery and absent subclavian artery were observed, as was slight maternal toxicity. The no-effect dose was about 7 times the MHD. The high dose produced plasma levels (AUC) in rabbits that were about 3.3 times (normal metabolizers) or 0.4 times (poor metabolizers) those in humans receiving the MHD. The no-effect dose for these effects was about 7 times the MHD (1).

It is not known if atomoxetine or its active metabolites cross the human placenta. The molecular weight for the parent drug (about 256 for the free base) combined with elimination half-life suggests that atomoxetine will cross to the embryo and/or fetus. The extensive protein binding, however, will limit the amount available for transfer.

In a brief correspondence, representatives of the manufacturer and others stated that there had been three pregnancies in adult clinical trials with atomoxetine (2). Two resulted in healthy newborns, but the third pregnancy was lost to follow up. No other details were provided.

BREASTFEEDING SUMMARY

No reports describing the use of atomoxetine during human lactation have been located. The molecular weight of the parent drug (about 256 for the free base) and the relatively long elimination half-life (5 hours for normal metabolizers; 24 hours for poor metabolizers) suggest that the drug and/or its metabolites will be excreted into breast milk. The effect of this exposure on a nursing infant is unknown. If a mother chooses to breastfeed while taking atomoxetine, the infant should be monitored for potential toxicity (such as upper abdominal pain, constipation, and dyspepsia).

References

1. Product information. Strattera. Eli Lilly, 2004.
2. Heiligenstein J, Michelson D, Wernicke J, Milton D, Kratochvil CJ, Spencer TJ, Newcorn JH. Atomoxetine and pregnancy. J Am Acad Child Adolesc Psychiatry 2003;42:884–5.

ATORVASTATIN

Antilipemic Agent

PREGNANCY RECOMMENDATION: Contraindicated
BREASTFEEDING RECOMMENDATION: Contraindicated

PREGNANCY SUMMARY

The interruption of cholesterol-lowering therapy during pregnancy should have no effect on long-term treatment of hyperlipidemia. Moreover, because cholesterol and products synthesized by cholesterol are important during fetal development, the use of atorvastatin is contraindicated during pregnancy. However, the absolute embryo risk from inadvertent exposure in the 1st trimester appears to be low.

FETAL RISK SUMMARY

Atorvastatin, a lipophilic 3-hydroxy-3-methylglutaryl-coenzyme A (HMG-CoA) reductase inhibitor (statin), is indicated as an adjunct to diet to reduce total cholesterol, low-density lipoprotein cholesterol, apolipoprotein B, and triglyceride levels in patients with primary hypercholesterolemia and mixed dyslipidemia. It has the same mechanism of action as other available drugs in this class, fluvastatin, lovastatin, pitavastatin, pravastatin, rosuvastatin, and simvastatin (cerivastatin was withdrawn from the market in 2001). Atorvastatin is extensively metabolized and some of the metabolites are as pharmacologically active as the parent compound. Atorvastatin is highly bound (≥98%) to plasma proteins and it has a mean plasma elimination of about 14 hours. However, because of the active metabolites, the half-life of inhibitory activity for HMG-CoA reductase is 20–30 hours (1,2).

In reproduction studies with pregnant rats and rabbits, doses that were about 30 and 20 times, respectively, the human exposure (HE) based on BSA, were not teratogenic. With maternal dosing in rats from gestation day 7 through lactation day 21 (weaning), at a dose 22 times the HE based on AUC, there was decreased pup survival at birth, during the neonatal period, at weaning, and at maturity, and decreased pup weight at birth, during nursing, and at maturity. In addition, pup development was inhibited at this dose (1–3). A 1994 report described developmental toxicity of atorvastatin at maternally toxic doses in pregnant rats and rabbits (4). There was no evidence, however, of teratogenicity in either species (4).

It is not known if atorvastatin or its active metabolites cross the human placenta. The relatively high molecular weight (about 1161 for the nonhydrated form) and extensive protein binding suggest that transfer across the placenta will be inhibited. In pregnant rats, however, fetal liver levels of atorvastatin were equivalent to maternal concentrations (1–3).

A 2002 report described the use of atorvastatin in early pregnancy (5). A 35-year-old woman with several diseases (hypertension, diabetes mellitus, hypercholesterolemia, anxiety disorder, epilepsia, and morbid obesity) conceived while being treated with multiple drugs: atorvastatin (40 mg/day), rosiglitazone, gliclazide (a sulfonylurea), acarbose, spironolactone, hydrochlorothiazide, carbamazepine, thioridazine, amitriptyline, chlordiazepoxide, and pipenzolate bromide (an antispasmodic). Her pregnancy was diagnosed in the 8th week of gestation and all medications were stopped. She was treated with methyldopa and insulin for the remainder of her pregnancy. At 36 weeks' gestation, a healthy, 3.5-kg female infant was delivered by cesarean section. Apgar scores were 7 and 8 at 1 and 5 minutes, respectively. The infant was developing normally after 4 months (5).

A 2004 report described the outcomes of pregnancy that had been exposed to statins and reported to the FDA (see Lovastatin).

A 2005 abstract reported 19 pregnancies exposed to a statin in the 1st trimester, 7 of which involved atorvastatin (6). The pregnancy outcomes included one healthy newborn, two spontaneous abortions (one with trisomy 18), one elective abortion, one newborn with jaundice, and two infants with congenital defects (VACTERL association, also exposed to trandolapril and insulin) and unilateral dilated renal pelvis (also exposed to enalapril) (6).

A 2008 prospective, observational cohort study compared the pregnancy outcomes of 64 women who had taken a statin in the 1st trimester with 64 matched controls without exposure to known teratogens (7). The statin exposures were atorvastatin ($N = 46$), simvastatin ($N = 9$), pravastatin ($N = 6$), and rosuvastatin ($N = 3$). Sixty-one women discontinued the drug in the 1st trimester, but three continued taking a statin into the 2nd trimester. Twenty-one (33%) women in the exposed group had other medical conditions, in addition to hyperlipidemia, and seven had more than one chronic condition. The rates of major malformations in the two groups were 2.2% (1/46 live births) and 1.9% (1/52 live births) ($p = 0.93$), respectively. There were also no statistical differences in the other outcomes: live births (71.9% vs. 81.2%), spontaneous abortions (21.9% vs. 17.2%), elective abortions (4.7% vs. 0%), and stillbirths (1.5% vs. 1.6%). Gestational age at birth (38.4 vs. 39.3 weeks) and birth weight (3.14 vs. 3.45 kg) were significantly lower in the exposed group (7).

BREASTFEEDING SUMMARY

No reports describing the use of atorvastatin in human lactation have been located. The relatively high molecular weight (about 1161 for the nonhydrated form) suggests that excretion into milk would be inhibited, but some excretion should be expected. Because of the potential for adverse effects in a nursing infant, women who are taking atorvastatin should not breastfeed.

References

1. Product information. Lipitor. Parke-Davis, 2004.
2. Product information. Lipitor. Pfizer, 2004.
3. Henck JW, Craft WR, Black A, Colgin J, Anderson JA. Pre- and postnatal toxicity of the HMG-CoA reductase inhibitor atorvastatin in rats. Toxicol Sci 1998;41:88–99.
4. Dostal LA, Schardein JL, Anderson JA. Developmental toxicity of the HMG-CoA reductase inhibitor, atorvastatin, in rats and rabbits. Teratology 1994;50:387–94.
5. Yaris F, Yaris E, Kadioglu M, Ulku C, Kesim M, Kalyoncu NI. Normal pregnancy outcome following inadvertent exposure to rosiglitazone, gliclazide, and atorvastatin in a diabetic and hypertensive woman. Reprod Toxicol 2004;18:619–21.
6. McElhatton P. Preliminary data on exposure to statins during pregnancy (abstract). Reprod Toxicol 2005;20:471–2.
7. Taguchi N, Rubin ET, Hosokawa A, Choi J, Ying AY, Moretti M, Koren G, Ito S. Prenatal exposure to HMG-CoA reductase inhibitors: effects on fetal and neonatal outcomes. Reprod Toxicol 2008;26:175–7.

ATOVAQUONE

Antiprotozoal

PREGNANCY RECOMMENDATION: Compatible—Maternal Benefit >> Embryo–Fetal Risk
BREASTFEEDING RECOMMENDATION: No Human Data—Potential Toxicity

PREGNANCY SUMMARY

The use of atovaquone, usually combined with proguanil (see also Proguanil), during human pregnancy does not appear to increase the risk of major birth defects. The lack of toxicity in animals with doses close to those used in humans is reassuring. Two reviews, one in 2004 (1) and the other in 2011 (2), concluded that the drug could be used in pregnancy. Because the maternal benefit appears to exceed the unknown embryo–fetal risk, the agent should not be withheld because of pregnancy.

FETAL RISK SUMMARY

Atovaquone is an analog of ubiquinone that is indicated for the prevention and treatment of *Pneumocystis carinii* pneumonia in patients intolerant of trimethoprim–sulfamethoxazole (3). The agent, when combined with proguanil, is also indicated for the prevention and treatment of malaria due to *Plasmodium falciparum* (2,4). Unlabeled uses include the treatment of babesiosis (in combination with quinine and/or clindamycin and/or azithromycin) and toxoplasmosis (in combination with pyrimethamine) (5). The drug undergoes little, if any, metabolism and is extensively bound (99.9%) to plasma proteins. The elimination half-life is long, ranging from about 67–78 hours (3).

Reproduction studies have been conducted in rats and rabbits (3,4). In rats, no teratogenicity or reproductive toxicity was observed at plasma concentrations 2–3 times the estimated human exposure (HE) for *P. carinii* (3) or 5–6.5 times the HE for malaria (4). In rabbits, plasma concentrations about 0.5 times the HE for *P. carinii* (3) and 0.6–1.3 times the HE for malaria (4) were maternally toxic. At these exposures, mean fetal body weights and lengths were decreased, and there were higher numbers of early resorption and post-implantation losses. These effects may have been due to the maternal toxicity (3,4). The combination of atovaquone and proguanil was not teratogenic in rats (1.7 and 0.10 times the HE for malaria, respectively) or rabbits (0.34 and 0.82 times the HE for malaria, respectively). There was also no embryotoxicity in rabbits at these exposures (4).

Atovaquone was not carcinogenic in rats, but hepatocellular adenoma and carcinoma were observed with all doses tested in mice (1.4–3.6 times the average plasma concentrations in humans). In other tests, there was no evidence of atovaquone-induced mutagenicity or genotoxicity (3).

It is not known if atovaquone crosses the human placenta. The molecular weight (about 367), absence of metabolism, and long elimination half-life suggest that atovaquone will cross the human placenta to the embryo–fetus. However, the extensive plasma protein binding might limit the amount that crosses.

In an antenatal clinic in Thailand, 24 pregnant women who had tested positive for malaria were treated with a triple combination of atovaquone (20 mg/kg/day), proguanil (8 mg/kg/day), and artesunate (4 mg/kg/day) for 3 days (5). The study was conducted to determine the pharmacokinetic properties of the drugs in pregnancy. The median estimated gestational age at the start of treatment was 28.5 weeks (range 19.1–35.9 weeks). No adverse effects of the therapy were observed in the fetuses or newborns (5).

Some of the same authors in the above report used the identical regimen to treat 27 pregnant women with multidrug-resistant malaria (6). The treatment occurred at a mean gestational age of 28.2 weeks. They found no evidence of toxicity in the mothers or the fetuses (6).

The 3-day triple anti-infective regimen described above was compared with a 7-day supervised trial of quinine for the treatment of uncomplicated falciparum malaria (7). There were 39 pregnant women in the three-drug group and 42 in the one-drug group. All of the women were in the 2nd or 3rd trimesters. The three-drug regimen was significantly better and had a much lower failure rate. There were no significant differences in pregnancy duration, birth weight, congenital anomalies, or in growth and development of infants monitored for 1 year (7).

A combination tablet containing atovaquone 250 mg and proguanil 100 mg was used to treat 26 women (gestational age 24–34 weeks) with acute uncomplicated *P. falciparum* malaria (8). The study was designed to determine the pharmacokinetics of the two drugs and cycloguanil, the active metabolite of proguanil. No serious toxicities were observed and the newborns had no physical anomalies (8).

A large nationwide cohort study from Denmark, covering the period 2000–2008, compared the pregnancy outcomes (live births) of women exposed to atovaquone–proguanil during the 1st trimester with those not exposed (9). In weeks 3–8 after conception, 93 were exposed (1 major birth defect, 1.1%) compared with 570,784 unexposed (13,994 major birth defects, 2.5%). The adjusted prevalence odds ratio (POR) was 0.43 and 95% confidence interval (CI) 0.06–3.11. For exposure anytime in the 1st trimester, 149 were exposed (2 major birth defects, 1.3%) compared with 570,728 unexposed (13,993 major birth defects, 2.5%), POR 0.55, and 95% CI 0.14–2.21. The birth defects were those observed in the first year of life (9).

BREASTFEEDING SUMMARY

No reports describing the use of atovaquone during lactation have been located. The molecular weight (about 367), absence of metabolism, and long elimination half-life (about 67–78 hours) suggest that the drug will be excreted into breast milk. However, the extensive plasma protein binding (99.9%) should limit the amount in milk. The effect of this exposure on a nursing infant is unknown. The severity of the mother's illness, such as infection with HIV, may preclude breastfeeding. In addition, the potential for severe adverse effects in a nursing infant, such as gastrointestinal symptoms, rash, fever, headache, hepatic toxicity, and carcinogenicity, suggests that even HIV-negative women should not breastfeed if they are taking this drug.

References

1. Rosenblatt JE. Antiparasitic agents. Mayo Clin Proc 1999;74:1161–75.
2. Irvine MH, Einarson A, Bozzo P. Prophylactic use of antimalarials during pregnancy. Can Fam Physician 2011;57:1279–81.
3. Product information. Mepron. GlaxoSmithKline, 2004.
4. Product information. Malarone. GlaxoSmithKline, 2004.
5. McGready R, Stepniewska K, Edstein MD, Cho T, Gilveray G, Looareesuwan S, White NJ, Nosten F. The pharmacokinetics of atovaquone and proguanil in pregnant women with acute falciparum malaria. Eur J Clin Pharmacol 2003;59:545–52.
6. McGready R, Keo NK, Villegas L, White NJ, Looareesuwan S, Nosten F. Artesunate-atovaquone-proguanil rescue treatment of multidrug-resistant *Plasmodium falciparum* malaria in pregnancy: a preliminary report. Trans R Soc Trop Med Hyg 2003;97:592–4.
7. McGready R, Ashley EA, Moo E, Cho T, Barends M, Hutagalung R, Looareesuwan S, White NJ, Nosten F. A randomized comparison of artesunate-atovaquone-proguanil versus quinine in treatment of uncomplicated falciparum malaria during pregnancy. J Infect Dis 2005;192:846–53.
8. Na-Bangchang K, Manyando C, Ruengweerayut R, Kioy D, Mulenga M, Miller GB, Konsil J. The pharmacokinetics and pharmacodynamics of atovaquone and proguanil for the treatment of uncomplicated falciparum malaria in third-trimester pregnant women. Eur J Clin Pharmacol 2005;61:573–82.
9. Pasternak B, Hviid A. Atovaquone-proguanil use in early pregnancy and the risk of birth defects. Arch Intern Med 2011;171:259–60.

ATRACURIUM

Skeletal Muscle Relaxant

PREGNANCY RECOMMENDATION: Limited Human Data—Probably Compatible
BREASTFEEDING RECOMMENDATION: No Human Data—Probably Compatible

PREGNANCY SUMMARY

No adverse effects in the fetus or newborn attributable to in utero atracurium exposure have been reported. Because of the drug's high molecular weight and ionization at physiologic pH, only small amounts cross the human placenta, thus limiting the exposure of the embryo or fetus. Moreover, direct administration to the fetus in the latter part of pregnancy has not been associated with fetal harm. Human fetal exposures early in pregnancy, however, have not been reported. Animal reproduction studies have only been conducted in rabbits, and although the drug may be a potential teratogen in this species, further studies are required to determine the magnitude of this potential. Based on the data below, the use of atracurium during the latter portion of human pregnancy appears to represent little, if any, risk.

FETAL RISK SUMMARY

The competitive (nondepolarizing) neuromuscular blocking agent, atracurium besylate, provides muscle relaxation during surgery or mechanical ventilation. The drug undergoes rapid, nonenzymatic, spontaneous degradation in the plasma (Hofmann elimination) that is independent of hepatic or renal mechanisms (1,2).

In reproduction studies in rabbits with SC doses of 0.15 mg/kg once daily or 0.10 mg/kg twice daily (human IV bolus doses vary from 0.08 to 0.5 mg/kg), an increased incidence of spontaneously occurring visceral or skeletal anomalies was observed in both treatment groups when compared with nontreated controls (3). Moreover, in comparison to controls, a lower percentage of male fetuses (41% vs. 51%) and a higher percentage of post-implantation losses (15% vs. 8%) were observed in the 0.15 mg/kg-once-daily group (3).

In a study conducted by the manufacturer published in 1983, SC doses of atracurium, identical to those above, were injected into rabbits on days 6–18 of pregnancy (4). Rabbits, and cats in the perinatal study below, were used because the pharmacokinetics of atracurium in these species are similar to those in humans, whereas the kinetics in rats is markedly different from humans. No teratogenicity or adverse effects were observed in the rabbit fetuses (4).

Theoretically, the relatively high molecular weight (about 1244) of atracurium besylate and its high degree of ionization at physiologic pH should inhibit the placental passage of atracurium. In the perinatal portion of the study cited above, six pregnant cats, 1–3 days before term, were given a single dose of atracurium, 0.6 mg/kg IV (4). No atracurium was detected in fetal blood, leading to the conclusion that the drug did not cross the placenta (4). Moreover, no depression of respiratory activity was observed when a dose of 0.6 mg/kg was injected directly into the fetuses. A brief 1985 report described the failure to detect placental transfer of atracurium during a 60-minute interval after a 0.5-mg/kg IV dose in five pregnant sheep (5). Small amounts of laudanosine, the major metabolite, crossed the placenta and were detected in some of the fetuses. The metabolite, however, is considered to be inactive at the doses of parent drug used clinically (1).

In contrast to the above animal data, human placental transfer of atracurium has been documented (6,7). In five women, from a total group of 26 undergoing cesarean section, average venous concentrations of the drug, following a 0.3-mg/kg IV dose, ranged from 3.34 mcg/mL at 3 minutes to 0.7 mcg/mL at 10 minutes (6). Venous cord blood concentrations of atracurium ranged from undetectable to 0.23 mcg/mL, suggesting that the cord:maternal ratio varied from 5% to 20% (6). In the second report by these authors, 53 women, delivered by cesarean section, received atracurium 0.3 mg/kg IV followed by increments of 0.1–0.2 mg/kg IV as necessary to maintain surgical relaxation (7). Concentrations of the drug in 16 women at delivery ranged from 0.54 to 3.34 mcg/mL. Only one patient received a second IV dose (0.2 mg/kg). Venous cord concentrations in seven newborns were undetectable (<0.1 mcg/mL in two and <0.05 mcg/mL in five), one cord blood sample was contaminated, and in eight newborns, concentrations ranged from 0.05 to 0.23 mcg/mL. The cord:maternal blood ratio varied from 0.03 to 0.33 (mean 0.12). Newborn neuromuscular activity was reported as normal in all newborns. Further, no adverse effects on Apgar scores or on the time to sustained respiration attributable to atracurium were observed in these two studies (6,7) or in an earlier report by the same authors (8).

A number of reports have described the safe use of atracurium during human pregnancy (9–13). A woman scheduled for a cesarean section had a low plasma concentration of cholinesterase activity. Atracurium, which does not depend on plasma cholinesterase for its metabolism, was successfully used for neuromuscular blockade in a dose of 0.4 mg/kg IV bolus (9). A healthy newborn with Apgar scores of 8 and 10 at 1 and 5 minutes, respectively, was delivered 10 minutes after the IV bolus. In another case, an IV infusion of atracurium was used during a 16-hour interval to maintain maternal muscle paralysis in a patient with pneumococcal pneumonia who required mechanical ventilation (10). In addition to other anesthetic agents, the woman received 520 mg of atracurium over 16 hours or an average of 32.5 mg/hour until vaginal delivery of a 1800-g female infant. No neuromuscular blockade was observed in the newborn that had Apgar scores of 7, 10, and 10 at 1, 5, and 10 minutes, respectively. Neuromuscular blockade with atracurium was used in a pregnant woman at 24 weeks' gestation that underwent resection of a pheochromocytoma (11). She eventually delivered a healthy, 2977-g male infant at 39 weeks' gestation. Normal newborns were also described in two other reports following the use of atracurium prior to cesarean section (12,13). Moreover, a 1986 review on obstetrical anesthesia concluded that atracurium was safe to use in obstetric patients (14).

Three studies have described the direct human fetal administration of atracurium to achieve neuromuscular blockade (15–17). In one study, atracurium (0.4 mg/kg) was used in 11 fetuses during 18 intrauterine transfusions and compared with pancuronium (0.1 mg/kg, 12 fetuses, 19 transfusions) (gestational ages not specified in either group) (15). The two agents were similar in onset of neuromuscular blockade. Atracurium, however, was statistically superior to pancuronium in terms of return of fetal movements (22 vs. 67 minutes), more fetal movements, fetal movements/minute, and more heart accelerations than pancuronium after transfusion (15). The authors concluded that atracurium was the preferred drug if fetal paralysis was required. A 1988 reference also used a 0.4-mg/kg IV fetal dose after determining that a 0.2-mg/kg dose was inadequate to arrest fetal activity during intrauterine transfusions (16). Atracurium was used in 6 women undergoing 12 transfusion procedures for fetal Rh isoimmunization. Onset of paralysis occurred within 1–5 minutes and fetal activity returned between 20 and 130 minutes. One fetus developed bradycardia and died 1 hour after transfusion of severe erythroblastosis fetalis and rupture of the spleen.

Atracurium, 1.0 mg/kg IM (fetal gluteal muscle), was used in five fetuses for various intrauterine procedures conducted between 32 and 38 weeks' gestation (17). In comparison to five fetuses treated with pancuronium, 0.15 mg/kg IM, neuromuscular blockade was achieved slightly faster (mean 4.7 vs. 5.8 minutes) and fetal movements returned sooner (mean 36 vs. 92 minutes) with atracurium. One fetus with peritonitis given pancuronium was stillborn, one fetus with peritonitis given atracurium was born alive with a gastrointestinal perforation, and one fetus given atracurium for ascites drainage and albumin transfusion died after birth. Although the authors did not discuss these outcomes, they do not appear to be related to the neuromuscular blocking agents. No evidence of soft tissue, nerve, or muscle damage at the sites of injection was observed in the newborns.

BREASTFEEDING SUMMARY

No reports describing the use of atracurium during human lactation have been located. Atracurium undergoes rapid, spontaneous degradation in plasma (Hofmann elimination) with an elimination half-life of approximately 20 minutes. The metabolites are not biologically active. In addition, the drug has a relatively high molecular weight (about 1244) and is highly ionized at physiologic pH, both of which are factors that would markedly reduce transfer into milk. Although usage in a lactating woman is possible, at least several hours (and most likely much more time) would pass after use of atracurium before lactation was resumed. The rapid breakdown of atracurium that occurs in plasma would also be expected in milk, even though the latter medium is slightly more acidic than plasma. Thus, any amounts that were transferred into milk would most likely be rapidly degraded. Based on these data, nursing can probably be safely resumed, especially after single-dose use, following recovery from atracurium-induced neuromuscular blockade. A 1994 review of anesthetic agents also concluded that nursing could be allowed as soon as feasible after surgery (18).

References

1. Drenck NE, Viby-Mogensen J, Ostergaard D, Seraj M. Atracurium (tracrium). Middle East J Anesthesiol 1988;9:457–65.
2. Anonymous. Atracurium. Lancet 1983;1:394–5.
3. Product information. Tracrium. Glaxo Wellcome, 1998.
4. Skarpa M, Dayan AD, Follenfant M, James DA, Moore WB, Thomson PM, Lucke JN, Morgan M, Lovell R, Medd R. Toxicity testing of atracurium. Br J Anaesth 1983;55:27S–9S.
5. Mandel MB, Stiller RL, Kennedy RL, Tyler IL, Edelmann CA, Cook DR. Placental transfer of atracurium and laudanosine in the pregnant ewe (abstract). Anesthesiology 1985;63:A429.
6. Frank M, Flynn PJ, Hughes R. Atracurium in obstetric anaesthesia. A preliminary report. Br J Anaesth 1983;55:113S–4S.
7. Flynn PJ, Frank M, Hughes R. Use of atracurium in caesarean section. Br J Anaesth 1984;56:599–604.
8. Flynn PJ, Frank M, Hughes R. Evaluation of atracurium in caesarian section using train-of-four responses (abstract). Anesthesiology 1982;57:A286.
9. Baraka A, Jaude CA. Atracurium in a parturient with atypical cholinesterase. Br J Anaesth 1984;56:930–1.
10. Thomas D, Windsor JPW. Prolonged sedation and paralysis in a pregnant patient. Delivery of an infant with a normal Apgar score. Anaesthesia 1985;40:465–7.
11. Mitchell SZ, Freilich JD, Brant D, Flynn M. Anesthetic management of pheochromocytoma resection during pregnancy. Anesth Analg 1987;66: 478–80.
12. Hardy PAJ. Atracurium and bradycardia. Anaesthesia 1985;40:504–5.
13. Stuart JC, Kan AF, Rowbottom SJ, Yau G, Gin T. Acid aspiration prophylaxis for emergency caesarean section. Anaesthesia 1996;51:415–21.
14. Biehl D, Palahniuk RJ. Update on obstetrical anaesthesia. Can Anaesth Soc J 1986;33:238–45.
15. Mouw RJC, Hermans J, Brandenburg HCR, Kanhai HHH. Effects of pancuronium or atracurium on the anemic fetus during and directly after intrauterine transfusion (IUT): a double blind randomized study (abstract). Am J Obstet Gynecol 1997;176:S18.
16. Bernstein HH, Chitkara U, Plosker H, Gettes M, Berkowitz RL. Use of atracurium besylate to arrest fetal activity during intrauterine intravascular transfusions. Obstet Gynecol 1988;72:813–6.
17. Fan SZ, Huang FY, Lin SY, Wang YP, Hsieh FJ. Intrauterine neuromuscular blockade in fetus. Acta Anaesth Sin 1990;28:31–4.
18. Spigset O. Anaesthetic agents and excretion in breast milk. Acta Anaesthesiol Scand 1994;38:94–103.

ATROPINE

Parasympatholytic

PREGNANCY RECOMMENDATION: Human Data Suggest Low Risk
BREASTFEEDING RECOMMENDATION: Limited Human Data—Probably Compatible

PREGNANCY SUMMARY

Although the human data describing pregnancy outcomes are limited, there is no evidence of embryo or fetal harm.

FETAL RISK SUMMARY

Atropine, an anticholinergic, rapidly crosses the placenta (1–4). Atropine exposure in the 1st, 2nd, and 3rd trimesters was estimated in one study to be 11.3, 6.7, and 6.3/1000 women, respectively (5). The drug has been used to test placental function in high-risk obstetric patients by producing fetal vagal blockade and subsequent tachycardia (6).

IV atropine (0.5 mg) caused a decrease of 10%–100% in fetal breathing in 13 of 15 fetuses, an increase of 300% in 1 fetus, and no effect in another (7). The decrease in fetal breathing occurred approximately 2 minutes after administration of the drug and lasted 5–10 minutes. No fetal hypoxia was observed, nor was there an effect on fetal heart rate or beat-to-beat variability.

The Collaborative Perinatal Project monitored 50,282 mother–child pairs, 401 of whom used atropine in the 1st trimester (8, pp. 346–353). For use anytime during pregnancy, 1198 exposures were recorded (8, p. 439). In neither group was evidence found for an association with malformations. However, when the group of parasympatholytics were taken as a whole (2323 exposures), a possible association with minor malformations was found (8, pp. 346–353).

In a surveillance study of Michigan Medicaid recipients involving 229,101 completed pregnancies conducted between 1985 and 1992, 381 newborns had been exposed to atropine during the 1st trimester (F. Rosa, personal communication, FDA, 1993). A total of 18 (4.7%) major birth defects were observed (16 expected). Specific data were available for six defect categories, including (observed/expected) 4/4 cardiovascular defects, 0/0.5 oral clefts, 1/0 spina bifida, 2/0 polydactyly, 1/1 hypospadias, and 2/0 limb reduction defects. Only with the latter defect is there a suggestion of a possible association, but other factors such as the mother's disease, concurrent drug use, and chance may be involved.

Atropine has been used to reduce gastric secretions before cesarean section without producing fetal or neonatal effects (9,10). In a study comparing atropine and glycopyrrolate, 10 women in labor received 0.01 mg/kg of IV atropine (11). No statistically significant changes were noted in fetal heart rate or variability nor was there any effect on uterine activity.

A single case of a female infant born at 36 weeks' gestation with multiple defects, including Ebstein anomaly, was described in a 1989 report (12). In addition to the cardiac defect, other abnormalities noted were hypertelorism, epicanthal folds, low-set posteriorly rotated ears, a cleft uvula, medially rotated hands, deafness, and blindness. The mother had taken Lomotil (diphenoxylate and atropine) for diarrhea during the 10th week of gestation. Because exposure was beyond the susceptible stages of development for these defects, the drug combination was not considered causative. However, a possible viremia in the mother as a cause of the diarrhea could not be excluded as playing a role in the infant's anomalies.

BREASTFEEDING SUMMARY

The passage of atropine into breast milk is controversial (13). It has not been adequately documented whether measurable amounts are excreted or, if excretion does occur, whether it may affect the nursing infant. Although neonates are particularly sensitive to anticholinergic agents, no adverse effects have been reported in nursing infants whose mothers were taking atropine. The American Academy of Pediatrics classifies the agent as compatible with breastfeeding (14).

References

1. Nishimura H, Tanimura T. *Clinical Aspects of The Teratogenicity of Drugs*. New York, NY: American Elsevier, 1976:63.
2. Kivalo I, Saarikoski S. Placental transmission of atropine at full-term pregnancy. Br J Anaesth 1977;49:1017–21.
3. Kanto J, Virtanen R, Iisalo E, Maenpaa K, Liukko P. Placental transfer and pharmacokinetics of atropine after a single maternal intravenous and intramuscular administration. Acta Anaesth Scand 1981;25:85–8.
4. Onnen I, Barrier G, d'Athis PH, Sureau C, Olive G. Placental transfer of atropine at the end of pregnancy. Eur J Clin Pharmacol 1979;15:443–6.
5. Piper JM, Baum C, Kennedy DL, Price P. Maternal use of prescribed drugs associated with recognized fetal adverse drug reactions. Am J Obstet Gynecol 1988;159:1173–7.
6. Hellman LM, Fillisti LP. Analysis of the atropine test for placental transfer in gravidas with toxemia and diabetes. Am J Obstet Gynecol 1965;91: 797–805.
7. Roodenburg PJ, Wladimiroff JW, Van Weering HK. Effect of maternal intravenous administration of atropine (0.5 mg) on fetal breathing and heart pattern. Contrib Gynecol Obstet 1979;6:92–7.
8. Heinonen OP, Slone D, Shapiro S. *Birth Defects and Drugs in Pregnancy*. Littleton, MA: Publishing Sciences Group, 1977.
9. Diaz DM, Diaz SF, Marx GF. Cardiovascular effects of glycopyrrolate and belladonna derivatives in obstetric patients. Bull NY Acad Med 1980;56: 245–8.
10. Roper RE, Salem MG. Effects of glycopyrrolate and atropine combined with antacid on gastric acidity. Br J Anaesth 1981;53:1277–80.
11. Abboud T, Raya J, Sadri S, Grobler N, Stine L, Miller F. Fetal and maternal cardiovascular effects of atropine and glycopyrrolate. Anesth Analg 1983;62:426–30.
12. Siebert JR, Barr M Jr, Jackson JG, Benjamin DR. Ebstein's anomaly and extracardiac defects. Am J Dis Child 1989;143:570–2.
13. Stewart JJ. Gastrointestinal drugs. In: Wilson JT, ed. *Drugs in Breast Milk*. Balgowlah, Australia: ADIS Press, 1981:65–71.
14. Committee on Drugs, American Academy of Pediatrics. The transfer of drugs and other chemicals into human milk. Pediatrics 2001;108:776–89.

AURANOFIN

Immunologic Agent (Antirheumatic)

PREGNANCY RECOMMENDATION: No Human Data—Animal Data Suggest Low Risk
BREASTFEEDING RECOMMENDATION: No Human Data—Probably Compatible

PREGNANCY SUMMARY

No reports describing the use of auranofin in human pregnancy have been located. Although there was evidence of embryo–fetal toxicity and/or teratogenicity in animals, the doses used caused maternal toxicity and the comparisons to the human dose (HD) were based on body weight. Doses that were not maternally toxic did not cause these effects. Based on experience with other gold compounds (see Gold Sodium Thiomalate), gold does not appear to pose a major risk to the fetus. However, long-term follow-up studies of exposed fetuses have not been reported. If auranofin is indicated in a pregnant woman she should be informed of this information.

FETAL RISK SUMMARY

Auranofin is an oral disease-modifying antirheumatic drug (DMARD) containing 29% gold. It is indicated in the management of adults with active classical or definite rheumatoid arthritis who have had an insufficient therapeutic response to, or are intolerant of, an adequate trial of full dose of one or more nonsteroidal anti-inflammatory drugs. Auranofin is rapidly metabolized and intact auranofin is undetectable in blood. Approximately 25% of the gold in auranofin is absorbed. The gold in auranofin is moderately bound (60%) to plasma proteins. The mean terminal plasma half-life of auranofin gold at steady state is 26 days (range 21–31 days), whereas the mean terminal body half-life at steady state is 80 days (range 42–128 days) (1).

Reproduction studies have been conducted in rabbits, rats, and mice. In rabbits, maternal toxic (impaired food intake) doses about 4–50 times the HD resulted in decreased fetal weights, increased incidence or resorptions and abortions, and an increased incidence of congenital abnormalities, mainly abdominal defects such as gastroschisis and umbilical hernia. No teratogenicity was noted in rats given a maternal toxic dose 42 times the HD, but there was an increase in the incidence of resorptions and a decrease in litter size and weight. A dose 21 times the HD that was not maternally toxic did not cause these effects or teratogenicity. In mice, a dose 42 times the HD was not teratogenic or maternal toxic (1).

In a 24-month carcinogenicity study in rats, doses that were 3–21 times the HD resulted in renal tumors. In a 12-month study in rats, a dose 192 times the HD caused renal tumors, whereas a dose 30 times the HD did not. In an 18-month study in mice, doses that were 8–72 times the HD were not associated with a significant increase in tumors. Auranofin was mutagenic in one assay but not in other assays (1). The effects of the drug animal fertility were apparently not studied.

Intact auranofin is not available to cross to the embryo or fetus because the agent has not been detected in blood. However, gold, released from auranofin, will cross the placenta (see Gold Sodium Thiomalate).

BREASTFEEDING SUMMARY

No reports describing the use of auranofin during human lactation have been located. Intact auranofin has not been detected in blood and, thus, would not be excreted into breast milk. However, gold, released from auranofin, will be excreted into milk (see Gold Sodium Thiomalate). Based solely on that information, breastfeeding when the mother is being treated with auranofin is probably compatible.

Reference

1. Product information. Ridaura. Prometheus Laboratories, 2007.

AUROTHIOGLUCOSE

[Withdrawn from the market. See 9th edition.]

AVANAFIL

Impotence Agent

PREGNANCY RECOMMENDATION: No Human Data—Animal Data Suggest Low Risk
BREASTFEEDING RECOMMENDATION: No Human Data—Potential Toxicity

PREGNANCY SUMMARY

No reports describing the use of avanafil in human pregnancy have been located. Animal data suggest low risk, but the absence of human pregnancy experience prevents a more complete assessment of embryo–fetal risk. Such reports are unlikely because of the indication. However, the drug is a vasodilator and could be used for other indications (e.g., see Sildenafil).

FETAL RISK SUMMARY

Avanafil, a vasodilator, is a phosphodiesterase inhibitor that enhances the effect of nitric oxide. It is in the same pharmacologic class as sildenafil and yohimbine. Avanafil is indicated for the treatment of erectile dysfunction. It undergoes partial hepatic metabolism. Plasma protein binding is about 99% and terminal elimination half-life is about 5 hours (1).

Reproduction studies have been conducted in rats and rabbits. In rats given the drug during gestation days 6–17, no evidence of teratogenicity, or embryo or fetal toxicity was observed at exposures up to about 8 times the exposure at the maximum recommended human dose of 200 mg based on AUC for total avanafil (protein bound plus free drug) (MRHD). At the maternally toxic dose producing exposures about 30 times the MRHD, decreased fetal body weight with no signs of structural anomalies was noted. When the drug was given from gestation day 6 through lactation day 20, maternal exposures that were ≥17 times the human exposure caused reduced offspring growth and maturation. There was no observed effect on reproductive performance of maternal rats or offspring, or on the behavior of offspring at the highest dose. In rabbits given the drug during gestation days 6–18, no evidence of teratogenicity was observed at exposures about 6 times the exposure at the MRHD. At a maternally toxic (reduced body weights) dose, increased post-implantation loss was observed consistent with increased late resorptions (1).

Studies for carcinogenicity in mice and rats were negative, as were various assays for mutagenic and clastogenic effects. In fertility impairment studies in male and female rats, a decrease in fertility, altered estrous cycles, no or reduced sperm motility, and an increased percentage of abnormal sperm occurred at exposures that were about 11 times the MRHD (1).

It is not known if avanafil crosses the human placenta. The molecular weight (about 484) and moderately long termination half-life suggest that the drug will cross to the embryo–fetus. However, the high plasma protein binding should limit the amount available to cross.

BREASTFEEDING SUMMARY

No reports describing the use of avanafil during human lactation have been located. Such reports are unlikely given its indication. However, the drug is a vasodilator and could be used for other indications (e.g., see Sildenafil). The molecular weight (about 484) and moderately long termination half-life (about 5 hours) suggest that the drug will be excreted into breast milk. However, the high plasma protein binding (about 99%) should limit the amount excreted. The most common (≥2%) adverse effects observed in adults were headache, flushing, nasal congestion, nasopharyngitis, and back pain (1). Although use of the drug during breastfeeding is unlikely, nursing infants of mothers receiving the drug should be monitored for these effects.

Reference

1. Product information. Stendra. VIVUS, 2013.

AXITINIB

Antineoplastic (Tyrosine Kinase Inhibitor)

PREGNANCY RECOMMENDATION: Contraindicated
BREASTFEEDING RECOMMENDATION: Contraindicated

PREGNANCY SUMMARY

No reports describing the use of axitinib during human pregnancy have been located. In one animal species, the drug was teratogenic, embryotoxic, and fetotoxic at maternal exposures that were lower than human exposures. Moreover, axitinib impairs fertility in both female and male animals. Although the human risk is unknown, women taking this drug should be informed of the potential risk to their embryo–fetus if they become pregnant.

FETAL RISK SUMMARY

Axitinib, available as oral tablets, is an inhibitor of receptor tyrosine kinases including vascular endothelial growth factor receptors that are implicated in pathologic angiogenesis, tumor growth, and cancer progression. There are several other agents in this subclass (see Appendix). It is indicated for the treatment of advanced renal cell carcinoma after failure of one prior systemic therapy. The drug is metabolized to relatively inactive metabolites and is highly bound (>99%) to plasma proteins with preferential binding to albumin and moderate binding to a_1-acid glycoprotein. The plasma half-life is 2.5–6.1 hours (1).

Reproduction studies have been conducted in mice. An increase in post-implantation loss was observed when mice were given twice-daily doses up to about 10 times the systemic exposure (AUC) from the recommended human starting dose (RHSD) before mating and through the first week of pregnancy. In mice given twice-daily doses during organogenesis, embryo–fetal toxicities were observed, in the absence of maternal toxicity, that included cleft palate and variation in skeletal ossification at about 0.5 and 0.15 times, respectively, the exposure from the RHSD (1).

Carcinogenicity studies have not been conducted with axitinib. The drug was not mutagenic or clastogenic in two in vitro assays, but was genotoxic in an in vivo assay. In fertility studies with male mice and dogs, testes/epididymis toxicity was observed that included decreased organ weight, atrophy or degeneration, decreased numbers of germinal cells, hypospermia or abnormal sperm forms, and reduced sperm

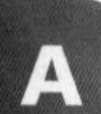

density and count. Findings in the female reproductive tracts of these species included delayed sexual maturity, reduced or absent corpora lutea, decreased uterine weights, and uterine atrophy (1).

It is not known if axitinib crosses the human placenta. The molecular weight (about 387) and plasma half-life suggest that the agent will cross to the embryo–fetus, but the high plasma protein binding might limit the amount crossing.

BREASTFEEDING SUMMARY

No reports describing the use of axitinib during human lactation have been located. The molecular weight (about 387) and plasma half-life (2.5–6.1 hours) suggest that the agent will be excreted into breast milk, but the high plasma protein binding (>99%) might limit the amount in milk. However, the drug is given orally and, if excreted into milk, it could be absorbed into the systemic circulation by a nursing infant. The effect of this exposure on a nursing infant is unknown, but severe toxicity is a potential concern. Consequently, mothers taking this drug should not breastfeed.

Reference

1. Product information. Inlyta. Pfizer Laboratories, 2012.

AZACITIDINE

Antineoplastic

PREGNANCY RECOMMENDATION: No Human Data—Animal Data Suggest Risk
BREASTFEEDING RECOMMENDATION: Contraindicated

PREGNANCY SUMMARY

No reports describing the use of azacitidine in human pregnancy have been located. The animal reproduction data at a small fraction of the human dose suggest risk, but the absence of human pregnancy experience prevents a more complete assessment. Pregnant women should not be given this drug, especially in the 1st trimester. If an inadvertent pregnancy occurs, the woman should be advised of the potential risk for severe adverse effects in the embryo and fetus. In addition, because of the animal fertility studies, men should be advised not to father a child while receiving azacitidine (1), and for several months after treatment.

FETAL RISK SUMMARY

Azacitidine, a pyrimidine nucleoside analog of cytidine, inhibits methylation of DNA. It is the same antineoplastic subclass as decitabine and nelarabine. Azacitidine is given by injection. It is indicated for the treatment of patients with the following myelodysplastic syndrome (MDS) subtypes: refractory anemia or ringed refractory anemia with ringed sideroblasts (if accompanied by neutropenia or thrombocytopenia or requiring transfusions), refractory anemia with excess blasts, refractory anemia with excess blasts in transformation, and chronic myelomonocytic leukemia (1). The metabolites are apparently inactive. The mean elimination half-lives of azacitidine and its metabolites are about 4 hours (1).

Reproduction studies have been conducted in mice and rats. In pregnant mice, a single intraperitoneal (IP) dose, which was 8% of the recommended human daily dose based on BSA (RHDD), on gestation day 10 caused a 44% frequency of embryo death (resorption). IP doses that were about 4%–16% of the RHDD given on or before gestation day 15 were associated with developmental abnormalities in the brain. In pregnant rats, embryotoxicity was evident when an IP dose (about 8% of the RHDD) was given on gestation days 4–8 (post-implantation). No embryotoxicity was observed when the drug was given on gestation days 1–3 (pre-implantation). Fetal deaths were observed when a single IP dose was given on gestation days 9 or 10; on day 9, the average number of live animals per liter was reduced to 9% of controls. In addition, single IP doses on gestation days 9, 10, 11, or 12 were associated with CNS anomalies (exencephaly/encephalocele), limb defects (micromelia, club foot, and syndactyly), micrognathia, gastroschisis, edema, and rib abnormalities (1).

Azacitidine was carcinogenic in long-term studies in mice and rats. Tumors of the hematopoietic system were seen in female mice given IP doses that were about 8% of the RHDD 3 times weekly for 52 weeks. A similar dose given once per week in mice for 50 weeks caused an increased incidence of tumors in the lymphoreticular system, lung, mammary gland, and skin. A study in male rats dosed twice weekly with about 20%–80% of the RHDD revealed an increased incidence of testicular tumors. Azacitidine was mutagenic and clastogenic in multiple tests (1).

In fertility studies, daily doses that were about 9% of the RHDD given to male mice for 3 days before mating with untreated females were associated with reduced fertility and loss of offspring during subsequent embryonic and postnatal development. When male rats were dosed 3 times weekly for 11 or 16 weeks at about 20%–40% of the RHDD, decreased weight of the testes and epididymides and decreased sperm counts accompanied by decreased pregnancy rates and increased loss of embryos in mated females were observed (1).

It is not known if azacitidine crosses the human placenta. The molecular weight (244) and elimination half-life suggest that the drug will cross to the embryo and/or fetus.

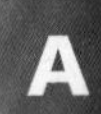

BREASTFEEDING SUMMARY

No reports describing the use of azacitidine during human lactation have been located. The molecular weight (244) and the elimination half-life (about 4 hours) suggest that the drug will be excreted into breast milk. The potential effects of this exposure on a nursing infant are unknown, but the effects may be severe. In adults, the most common adverse effects are nausea, anemia, thrombocytopenia, vomiting, pyrexia, leukopenia, diarrhea, fatigue, constipation, neutropenia, and ecchymosis (1).

Reference

1. Product information. Vidaza. Pharmion, 2007.

AZATADINE

[Withdrawn from the market. See 9th edition.]

AZATHIOPRINE

Immunologic Agent (Immunosuppressant)

PREGNANCY RECOMMENDATION: Human Data Suggest Risk in 3rd Trimester
BREASTFEEDING RECOMMENDATION: Limited Human Data—Probably Compatible

PREGNANCY SUMMARY

Although teratogenic in two animal species, azathioprine does not appear to cause structural anomalies in humans when used during organogenesis. Exposure in the 3rd trimester has been linked to immunosuppression. In addition, bone marrow suppression of the newborn has been reported, but modification of the dose in the 3rd trimester appears to reduce the risk of this toxicity. Intrauterine growth restriction also has been reported, but this effect may have been a consequence of multiple factors, one of which was azathioprine, working in combination. Taken in sum, however, the evidence suggests that the maternal benefit of treatment outweighs the potential risk to the fetus and newborn. If azathioprine is used in pregnancy for Crohn's disease, health-care professionals are encouraged to call the toll-free number (877-311-8972) for information about patient enrollment in an Organization of Teratology Information Specialists (OTIS) study.

FETAL RISK SUMMARY

Azathioprine is used primarily in patients with organ transplants or in those with inflammatory bowel disease as an immunosuppressant. Prednisone is commonly combined with azathioprine in these patients. The drug readily crosses the placenta, and trace amounts of its metabolite, 6-mercaptopurine (6-MP), have been found in fetal blood (see also Mercaptopurine) (1). 6-MP is converted intracellularly to active nucleotides (2), also called thioguanine nucleotides (TGNs); (see references 45 and 46).

Azathioprine is teratogenic in rabbits, producing limb reduction defects after small doses, but not in mice and rats (3). The manufacturer, however, has reproduction data on file indicating that azathioprine, in doses equivalent to the human dose (5 mg/kg/day), was teratogenic in both mice and rabbits (4). Malformations included skeletal defects and visceral anomalies.

In a surveillance study of Michigan Medicaid recipients involving 229,101 completed pregnancies conducted between 1985 and 1992, 7 newborns had been exposed to azathioprine during the 1st trimester (F. Rosa, personal communication, FDA, 1993). One (14.3%) major birth defect was observed (none expected), but information on the type of malformation is not available. No cases were observed in six defect categories, including cardiovascular defects, oral clefts, spina bifida, polydactyly, limb reduction defects, and hypospadias.

Most investigators have found azathioprine to be relatively safe in pregnancy (5–26). Several references have described the use of azathioprine during pregnancy in women who have received renal transplants (23,26–30), liver transplants (31–33), or a heart transplant (34). The drug has not been associated with congenital defects in these reports.

Sporadic anomalies have been reported, but these are not believed to be related to the drug therapy (23,27). Defects observed include pulmonary valvular stenosis (35); preaxial polydactyly (thumb polydactyly type) (36); hypothyroidism and atrial septal defect (azathioprine therapy started in 2nd trimester) (37); hypospadias (mother also had severe diabetes mellitus) (20); and plagiocephaly with neurologic damage, congenital heart disease (mild mitral regurgitation), bilateral pes equinovarus, cerebral palsy (frontal hemangioma) and cerebral hemorrhage (died at 2 days of age) in twins, hypospadias, and congenital cytomegalovirus infection (14). The latter infection had also been reported in another infant whose mother was taking azathioprine (11). Chromosomal aberrations were noted in three infants after in utero exposure to the drug, but the relationship to azathioprine and the clinical significance of the findings are questionable (14,38).

Immunosuppression of the newborn was observed in one infant whose mother received 150 mg of azathioprine and 30 mg of prednisone daily throughout pregnancy (11). The suppression was characterized by lymphopenia, decreased survival of lymphocytes in culture, absence of immunoglobulin M, and reduced levels of immunoglobulin G. Recovery occurred at about 15 weeks of age. An infant exposed to 125 mg of azathioprine plus 12.5 mg of prednisone daily during pregnancy was born with pancytopenia and severe combined immune deficiency (39). The infant died at 28 days of complications brought on by irreversible bone marrow and lymphoid hypoplasia. To avoid neonatal leukopenia and thrombocytopenia, maternal doses of azathioprine were reduced during the 3rd trimester in a 1985 study (40). A significant correlation was found between maternal leukocyte counts at 32 weeks' gestation and at delivery and cord blood leukocyte count. If the mother's count was ≤1 SD for normal pregnancy, her dose of azathioprine was halved. Before this technique was used, several newborns had leukopenia and thrombocytopenia, but no low levels were measured after institution of the new procedure (40).

Intrauterine growth restriction may be related to the use of azathioprine in pregnancy. Based on animal experiments and analysis of human exposures, one investigator concluded that growth restriction was associated with the drug (41). Reports that are more recent have also supported this association (42). The incidence of small-for-gestational-age infants from women who have undergone renal transplants and who are maintained on azathioprine and corticosteroids is approximately 20% (21,23), but some centers have rates as high as 40% (42). However, the effects of the underlying disease, including hypertension, vascular disease, and renal impairment, as well as the use of multiple medications other than azathioprine, cannot be excluded as major or sole contributors to the growth restriction.

Azathioprine has been reported to interfere with the effectiveness of intrauterine devices (IUDs) (23,43). Two renal transplant patients, maintained on azathioprine and prednisone, received a copper IUD (Cu7) and both became pregnant with the IUD in place (43). At another institution, 6 of 20 renal transplant patients became pregnant with an IUD in place (23). Because of these failures, additional or other methods of contraception should be considered in sexually active women receiving azathioprine and prednisone.

BREASTFEEDING SUMMARY

A study of four women, two with systemic lupus erythematosus (SLE) and two after liver transplant, who were taking azathioprine (50–100 mg/day) while nursing was reported in 2006 (44). Serial milk samples in two of the women with SLE (both taking 100 mg/day) were analyzed for 6-MP, the active metabolite of azathioprine. 6-MP was not detected in any sample (limit of detection 5 ng/mL). The absolute theoretical infant dose was <0.09% of the mother's weight-adjusted dose. Milk samples were collected from the other two mothers but were not analyzed. No adverse effects were observed in the four infants and all were doing well at follow-up (44). In a letter correspondence (45) and subsequent reply (46), it was pointed out that the active metabolites of azathioprine are actually toxic TGNs that are converted from 6-MP intracellularly. Six mother–infant pairs were sampled to determine if TGNs were detectable in the serum of lactating women taking azathioprine and their infants (45). Neither TGNs nor other potentially toxic metabolites were detected. These additional data combined with the absence of detectable 6-MP in milk suggested that the nursing infant would not be exposed to the toxic metabolites of azathioprine (45,46).

References

1. Sarrikoski S, Seppala M. Immunosuppression during pregnancy. Transmission of azathioprine and its metabolites from the mother to the fetus. Am J Obstet Gynecol 1973;115:1100–6.
2. Mercaptopurine. In: Sweetman SC, ed. *Martindale. The Complete Drug Reference*. 34th ed. London, UK: Pharmaceutical Press, 2005:567–8.
3. Tuchmann-Duplessis H, Mercier-Parot L. Foetopathes therapeutiques: production experimentale de malformations des membres. Union Med Can 1968;97:283–8. As cited in Shepard TH. *Catalog of Teratogenic Agents*. 6th ed. Baltimore, MD: Johns Hopkins University Press, 1989:63.
4. Product information. Imuran. FARO Pharmaceuticals, 2000.
5. Gillibrand PN. Systemic lupus erythematosus in pregnancy treated with azathioprine. Proc R Soc Med 1966;59:834.
6. Board JA, Lee HM, Draper DA, Hume DM. Pregnancy following kidney homotransplantation from a non-twin: report of a case with concurrent administration of azathioprine and prednisone. Obstet Gynecol 1967;29:318–23.
7. Kaufmann JJ, Dignam W, Goodwin WE, Martin DC, Goldman R, Maxwell MH. Successful, normal childbirth after kidney homotransplantation. JAMA 1967;200:338–41.
8. Anonymous. Eleventh annual report of human renal transplant registry. JAMA 1973;216:1197.
9. Nolan GH, Sweet RL, Laros RK, Roure CA. Renal cadaver transplantation followed by successful pregnancies. Obstet Gynecol 1974;43:732–8.
10. Sharon E, Jones J, Diamond H, Kaplan D. Pregnancy and azathioprine in systemic lupus erythematosus. Am J Obstet Gynecol 1974;118:25–7.
11. Cote CJ, Meuwissen HJ, Pickering RJ. Effects on the neonate of prednisone and azathioprine administered to the mother during pregnancy. J Pediatr 1974;85:324–8.
12. Erkman J, Blythe JG. Azathioprine therapy complicated by pregnancy. Obstet Gynecol 1972;40:708–9.
13. Price HV, Salaman JR, Laurence KM, Langmaid H. Immunosuppressive drugs and the foetus. Transplantation 1976;21:294–8.
14. The Registration Committee of the European Dialysis and Transplant Association. Successful pregnancies in women treated by dialysis and kidney transplantation. Br J Obstet Gynaecol 1980;87:839–45.
15. Golby M. Fertility after renal transplantation. Transplantation 1930;10:201–7.
16. Rabau-Friedman E, Mashiach S, Cantor E, Jacob ET. Association of hypoparathyroidism and successful pregnancy in kidney transplant recipient. Obstet Gynecol 1982;59:126–8.
17. Myers RL, Schmid R, Newton JJ. Childbirth after liver transplantation. Transplantation 1980;29:432.
18. Williams PF, Johnstone M. Normal pregnancy in renal transplant recipient with history of eclampsia and intrauterine death. Br Med J 1982;285:1535.
19. Westney LS, Callender CO, Stevens J, Bhagwanani SG, George JPA, Mims OL. Successful pregnancy with sickle cell disease and renal transplantation. Obstet Gynecol 1984;63:752–5.
20. Ogburn PL Jr, Kitzmiller JL, Hare JW, Phillippe M, Gabbe SG, Miodovnik M, Tagatz GE, Nagel TC, Williams PP, Goetz FC, Barbosa JJ, Sutherland DE. Pregnancy following renal transplantation in class T diabetes mellitus. JAMA 1986;255:911–5.
21. Marushak A, Weber T, Bock J, Birkeland SA, Hansen HE, Klebe J, Kristoffersen K, Rasmussen K, Olgaard K. Pregnancy following kidney transplantation. Acta Obstet Gynecol Scand 1986;65:557–9.
22. Key TC, Resnik R, Dittrich HC, Reisner LS. Successful pregnancy after cardiac transplantation. Am J Obstet Gynecol 1989;160:367–71.
23. Davison JM, Lindheimer MD. Pregnancy in renal transplant recipients. J Reprod Med 1982;27:613–21.
24. Symington GR, Mackay IR, Lambert RP. Cancer and teratogenesis: infrequent occurrence after medical use of immunosuppressive drugs. Aust NZ J Med 1977;7:368–72.
25. Alstead EM, Ritchie JK, Lennard-Jones JE, Farthing MJG, Clark ML. Safety of azathioprine in pregnancy in inflammatory bowel disease. Gastroenterology 1990;99:443–6.
26. Haugen G, Fauchald P, Sødal G, Halvorsen S, Oldereid N, Moe N. Pregnancy outcome in renal allograft recipients: influence of ciclosporin A. Eur J Obstet Gynecol Reprod Biol 1991;39:25–9.

27. Kossoy LR, Herbert CM III, Wentz AC. Management of heart transplant recipients: guidelines for the obstetrician-gynecologist. Am J Obstet Gynecol 1988;159:490–9.
28. Cararach V, Carmona F, Monleón FJ, Andreu J. Pregnancy after renal transplantation: 25 years experience in Spain. Br J Obstet Gynaecol 1993;100:122–5.
29. Sturgiss SN, Davison JM. Perinatal outcome in renal allograft recipients: prognostic significance of hypertension and renal function before and during pregnancy. Obstet Gynecol 1991;78:573–7.
30. Sturgiss SN, Davison JM. Effect of pregnancy on long-term function of renal allografts. Am J Kidney Dis 1992;19:167–72.
31. Laifer SA, Darby MJ, Scantlebury VP, Harger JH, Caritis SN. Pregnancy and liver transplantation. Obstet Gynecol 1990;76:1083–8.
32. Zaballos J, Perez-Cerda F, Riao D, Davila P, Martinez P, Sevillano A, Garcia I, de Andres A, Moreno E. Anesthetic management of liver transplantation in a pregnant patient with fulminant hepatitis. Transplant Proc 1991;23:1994–5.
33. Ville Y, Fernandez H, Samuel D, Bismuth H, Frydman R. Pregnancy in liver transplant recipients: course and outcome in 19 cases. Am J Obstet Gynecol 1993;168:896–902.
34. Kirk EP. Organ transplantation and pregnancy. A case report and review. Am J Obstet Gynecol 1991;164:1629–34.
35. Nishimura H, Tanimura T. *Clinical Aspects of the Teratogenicity of Drugs*. New York, NY: American Elsevier, 1976:106–7.
36. Williamson RA, Karp LE. Azathioprine teratogenicity: review of the literature and case report. Obstet Gynecol 1981;58:247–50.
37. Burleson RL, Sunderji SG, Aubry RH, Clark DA, Marbarger P, Cohen RS, Scruggs BF, Lagraff S. Renal allotransplantation during pregnancy. Successful outcome for mother, child, and kidney. Transplantation 1983; 36:334.
38. Leb DE, Weisskopf B, Kanovitz BS. Chromosome aberrations in the child of a kidney transplant recipient. Arch Intern Med 1971;128:441–4.
39. DeWitte DB, Buick MK, Cyran SE, Maisels MJ. Neonatal pancytopenia and severe combined immunodeficiency associated with antenatal administration of azathioprine and prednisone. J Pediatr 1984;105:625–8.
40. Davison JM, Dellagrammatikas H, Parkin JM. Maternal azathioprine therapy and depressed haemopoiesis in the babies of renal allograft patients. Br J Obstet Gynaecol 1985;92:233–9.
41. Scott JR. Fetal growth retardation associated with maternal administration of immunosuppressive drugs. Am J Obstet Gynecol 1977;128:668–76.
42. Pirson Y, Van Lierde M, Ghysen J, Squifflet JP, Alexandre GPJ, van Ypersele De Strihou C. Retardation of fetal growth in patients receiving immunosuppressive therapy. N Engl J Med 1985;313:328.
43. Zerner J, Doil KL, Drewry J, Leeber DA. Intrauterine contraceptive device failures in renal transplant patients. J Reprod Med 1981;26:99–102.
44. Moretti ME, Verjee Z, Ito S, Koren G. Breast-feeding during maternal use of azathioprine. Ann Pharmacother 2006;40:2269–72.
45. Gardiner SJ, Gearry RB, Roberts RI, Zhang M, Barclay ML, Begg EJ. Comment: breast-feeding during maternal use of azathioprine. Ann Pharmacother 2007;41:719–20.
46. Moretti ME, Verjee Z, Ito S, Koren G. Reply. Comment: breast-feeding during maternal use of azathioprine. Ann Pharmacother 2007;41:720.

AZELASTINE

Antihistamine

PREGNANCY RECOMMENDATION: No Human Data—Animal Data Suggest Low Risk
BREASTFEEDING RECOMMENDATION: No Human Data—Probably Compatible

PREGNANCY SUMMARY

No reports describing the use of azelastine in human pregnancy have been located. The animal data suggest that the risk to the embryo–fetus is low. Moreover, the systemic bioavailability of the antihistamine after intranasal administration is only 40% and it is much lower after ocular administration. Nevertheless, the complete absence of human pregnancy experience prevents a full assessment of the risk. A 2000 review of the use of newer asthma and allergy medications in pregnancy stated that, based on the animal studies, there were better choices available than azelastine (1).

FETAL RISK SUMMARY

The antihistamine azelastine is formulated for intranasal and ophthalmic administration. It is a phthalazinone derivative that has histamine H_1-receptor antagonist activity. Azelastine nasal spray is indicated for the treatment of the symptoms of seasonal allergic rhinitis such as rhinorrhea, sneezing, and nasal pruritus and for the treatment of the symptoms of vasomotor rhinitis, such as rhinorrhea, nasal congestion, and postnasal drip (2). The ophthalmic preparation is indicated for the treatment of itching of the eye associated with allergic conjunctivitis (3).

The systemic bioavailability, after nasal administration, is 40% with peak plasma concentrations obtained in 2–3 hours (2). In contrast, very small amounts are absorbed after ophthalmic administration (3). The plasma concentrations of the major active metabolite desmethylazelastine range from 20% to 50% of the parent drug concentrations (2). The elimination half-lives of azelastine and the active metabolite are 22 and 54 hours, respectively.

Reproduction studies have been conducted in mice, rats, and rabbits. In pregnant mice, an oral dose about 280 times the maximum recommended daily intranasal dose in adults based on BSA (MRDID) caused embryo–fetal death, malformations (cleft palate; short or absent tail; fused, absent, or branched ribs), delayed ossification, and decreased fetal weight. However, the dose also was maternally toxic (decreased weight). Neither maternal nor fetal toxicity was noted at a dose 10 times the MRDID (2). In rats, a dose about 240 times the MRDID was not maternally toxic but did cause fetal malformations (oligo- and brachydactylia), and delayed and skeletal variations. A maternal toxic dose (560 times the MRDID) resulted in embryo–fetal death and decreased fetal weight. A dose 25 times the MRDID caused no toxicity in the mother or fetus (2,4). In rabbits, doses greater than 500 times the MRDID caused severe maternal toxicity and resulted in abortions, delayed ossification, and reduced fetal weight. Neither maternal nor fetal adverse effects were observed with a dose 5 times the MRDID (2,4). In peri- and postnatal studies with rats, doses 25–240 times the MRDID were not associated with toxicity in the pups in terms of physical growth, reflexive behavior, activity, motor coordination, and learning and reproductive performance (4).

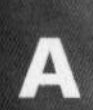

No carcinogenic effects in mice and rats were observed in 2-year studies at doses 100 and 240 times the MRDID, respectively. In addition, studies with azelastine for genotoxicity were also negative, as were fertility tests in rats at 240 times the MRDID (2).

It is not known if azelastine crosses the human placenta. The molecular weight (about 382 for the free base) and prolonged elimination half-life suggest that the drug could cross to the embryo and fetus. However, the low systemic concentrations of the parent drug and major active metabolite suggest that the amount available at the maternal:fetal interface will be clinically insignificant.

BREASTFEEDING SUMMARY

No reports describing the use of azelastine during human lactation have been located. The relatively low molecular weight (about 382 for the free base) and the prolonged elimination half-lives of the parent drug and major active metabolite suggest that the drugs will be excreted into breast milk. However, the systemic bioavailability after intranasal administration is only 40% and is much lower after ocular administration. Therefore, it is doubtful if clinically significant amounts will be excreted into milk.

References

1. Joint Committee of the American College of Obstetricians and Gynecologists (ACOG) and the American College of Allergy, Asthma and Immunology (ACAAI). The use of newer asthma and allergy medications during pregnancy. Ann Allergy Asthma Immunol 2000;84:475–80.
2. Product information. Astelin. MedPointe Pharmaceuticals, 2004.
3. Product information. Optivar. MedPointe Pharmaceuticals, 2004.
4. Suzuki Y, Okada F, Mikami T, Goto M, Hasegawa H, Chiba T. Teratology and reproduction studies of azelastine, a novel antiallergic agent, in rats and rabbits. Arzneimittelforschung 1981;31:1225–30.

AZFICEL-T

Dermatologic Agent

PREGNANCY RECOMMENDATION: No Human Data—Probably Compatible
BREASTFEEDING RECOMMENDATION: No Human Data—Probably Compatible

PREGNANCY SUMMARY

No reports describing the use of azficel-T in human pregnancy have been located.

Because it is an autologous product that is obtained from the patient by skin biopsy, reproduction studies in animals have not been conducted. The risk to an embryo or fetus appears to be nil.

FETAL RISK SUMMARY

Azficel-T is an autologous cellular product composed of dermal fibroblasts suspended in a sterile medium. The fibroblasts are obtained from postauricular skin biopsy tissue and sent to the manufacturer for aseptic expansion using standard tissue culture procedures. The cells are shipped back to the clinic when sufficient cells for three doses have been obtained and when patient administration has been scheduled. The product is given as three intradermal injections at 3- to 6-week intervals. Azficel-T is indicated for improvement of the appearance of moderate-to-severe nasolabial fold wrinkles in adults (1). Information on metabolism, plasma protein binding, and half-life is not relevant.

Studies in animals or by other means have not been conducted for reproduction, carcinogenicity, mutagenicity, and fertility.

Because the cells are injected intradermal they should not be in the systemic circulation. Moreover, intact cells should not cross the placenta.

BREASTFEEDING SUMMARY

No reports describing the use of azficel-T during human lactation have been located. Because the cells are injected intradermal they should not be in the systemic circulation and would not be present in breast milk. Moreover, the product is made from the patient's own cells and would not be expected to harm a nursing infant.

Reference

1. Product information. Laviv. Fibrocell Technologies, 2011.

AZILSARTAN

Antihypertensive

PREGNANCY RECOMMENDATION: Human Data Suggest Risk in 2nd and 3rd Trimesters
BREASTFEEDING RECOMMENDATION: No Human Data—Probably Compatible

PREGNANCY SUMMARY

No reports describing the use of azilsartan in human pregnancy have been located. The limited 1st-trimester experience with other agents in this class does not suggest a risk of major anomalies. The antihypertensive mechanisms of action of azilsartan and angiotensin converting enzyme (ACE) inhibitors are very close. That is, the former selectively blocks the binding of angiotensin II to AT_1 receptors, whereas the latter prevents the formation of angiotensin II itself. Therefore, use of this drug during the 2nd and 3rd trimesters may cause teratogenicity and severe fetal and neonatal toxicity identical to that seen with ACE inhibitors (e.g., see Captopril or Enalapril). Fetal toxic effects may include anuria, oligohydramnios, fetal hypocalvaria, intrauterine growth restriction, prematurity, and patent ductus arteriosus. Anuria-associated anhydramnios/oligohydramnios may produce fetal limb contractures, craniofacial deformation, and pulmonary hypoplasia. Severe anuria and hypotension, resistant to both pressor agents and volume expansion, may occur in the newborn following in utero exposure to valsartan. Newborn renal function and blood pressure should be closely monitored.

FETAL RISK SUMMARY

Azilsartan, an angiotensin II receptor blocker (ARB) given orally, is the active form of the commercially available prodrug azilsartan medoxomil. It is indicated, either alone or with other agents, for the treatment of hypertension. Azilsartan is in the same class of angiotensin II receptor blockers as candesartan, eprosartan, irbesartan, losartan, olmesartan, telmisartan, and valsartan. It is metabolized to inactive metabolites. Plasma protein binding, primarily to albumin, is high (>99%) and the elimination half-life is about 11 hours (1).

Animal reproduction studies have not been conducted with azilsartan. Long-term studies for carcinogenic potential in mice and rats were negative. Assays for mutagenicity have shown both positive and negative effects. The drug had no effect on the fertility of male and female rats (1).

It is not known if azilsartan crosses the human placenta. The molecular weight (about 607) and the elimination half-life suggest that the drug will cross to the embryo–fetus, even though the high plasma protein binding should limit the exposure. However, other agents in this class are known to cross the placenta and the same should be expected for azilsartan.

A 2012 review of the use of ACE inhibitors and ARBs in the 1st trimester concluded that there may be an elevated teratogenic risk, but the risk appeared to be related to other factors (2). The factors that typically coexist with hypertension in pregnancy included diabetes, advanced maternal age, and obesity.

BREASTFEEDING SUMMARY

No reports describing the use of azilsartan during human lactation have been located. The molecular weight (about 607) and the elimination half-life (about 11 hours) suggest that the drug will be excreted into breast milk, but the high plasma protein binding should limit the amount excreted. The effect of this exposure on a nursing infant is unknown. Diarrhea was the most common (2%) adverse reaction in adults (1). The American Academy of Pediatrics classifies ACE inhibitors, a closely related group of antihypertensive agents, as compatible with breastfeeding (see Captopril or Enalapril).

References

1. Product information. Edarbi. Takeda Pharmaceuticals America, 2011.
2. Polifka JE. Is there an embryopathy associated with first-trimester exposure to angiotensin-converting enzyme inhibitors and angiotensin receptor antagonists? A critical review of the evidence. Birth Defects Res (Part A) 2012;94:576–98.

AZITHROMYCIN

Antibiotic

PREGNANCY RECOMMENDATION: Compatible
BREASTFEEDING RECOMMENDATION: Compatible

PREGNANCY SUMMARY

The human pregnancy data do not suggest an embryo–fetal risk of developmental toxicity from azithromycin. The antibiotic has not been associated with an increased risk of pyloric stenosis.

FETAL RISK SUMMARY

Azithromycin, an azalide antibiotic, is derived from erythromycin. It is in the macrolide anti-infective class that includes clarithromycin and erythromycin.

Animal studies using rats and mice treated with daily doses up to maternal toxic levels revealed no impairment of fertility or harm to the fetus. These daily doses were about 1 and 0.5 times, respectively, the human dose of 2 g/day based on BSA (HD) (1).

Long-term studies for carcinogenic effects have not been conducted, but tests for mutagenic and clastogenic effects were negative. No evidence of impaired fertility was found in rats given daily doses up to about 0.05 times the HD (1).

Azithromycin crosses the human placenta at term (2,3). In 20 women scheduled for elective cesarean section, a single 1-g oral dose of azithromycin was given 6 (N = 2), 12 (N = 7), 24 (N = 5), 72 (N = 5), or 168 (N = 1) hours before delivery. The mean maternal concentrations at delivery for the five groups were 311, 144, 63, 60, and <10 ng/mL, respectively, whereas the corresponding mean cord serum levels were 19, 26, 27, 19, and <10 ng/mL, respectively. Cerebrospinal fluid levels in the mothers (all had spinal anesthesia) were undetectable (<16 ng/mL) in each group.

In an ex vivo experiment with term human placentas utilizing a single placental cotyledon model, the mean transplacental transfer of three macrolide antibiotics (azithromycin, erythromycin, and roxithromycin) were 2.6%, 3.0%, and 4.3%, respectively (3). The percentages were calculated as the ratio between the steady-state level in fetal venous and maternal arterial sides (3).

A number of reports (4–22) have described the use of azithromycin in human pregnancy. A 1994 abstract reported that 16 pregnant patients with cervicitis caused by *Chlamydia* had been treated with a single 1-g oral dose of the antibiotic in a comparison trial with erythromycin (4). Fifteen of the women had negative tests for *Chlamydia* after treatment. No data were given on gestational age at the time of treatment or on the pregnancy outcomes. In a second, similar report, also comparing efficacy with erythromycin, 15 pregnant women with chlamydial cervicitis were treated with a single 1-g oral dose (5). All of the women had negative cervical swabs for *Chlamydia* as analyzed by direct DNA assay 14 days after the dose. Three more recent reports have also documented the efficacy of azithromycin in the treatment of pregnant women with *Chlamydia* (6–8). Of the five reports, only the last study (8) indicated the gestational age at treatment (about 24 weeks), but none provided information on fetal outcome. In contrast to the effectiveness of azithromycin for *Chlamydia* infections, a single 1-g oral dose of the antibiotic was ineffective in reducing lower genital colonization with ureaplasma in pregnant women between 22 and 34 weeks' gestation with ruptured membranes or preterm labor (9). Two women with scrub typhus (tsutsugamushi disease) in the 2nd trimester were treated successfully with 3-day courses of azithromycin (10). Both delivered healthy infants.

A 1998 noninterventional observational cohort study described the outcomes of pregnancies in women who had been prescribed ≥1 of 34 newly marketed drugs by general practitioners in England (11). Data were obtained by questionnaires sent to the prescribing physicians 1 month after the expected or possible date of delivery. In 831 (78%) of the pregnancies, a newly marketed drug was thought to have been taken during the 1st trimester with birth defects noted in 14 (2.5%) singleton births of the 557 newborns (10 sets of twins). In addition, two birth defects were observed in aborted fetuses. However, few of the aborted fetuses were examined. Azithromycin was taken during the 1st trimester in 11 pregnancies. The outcomes of these pregnancies were 1 elective abortion and 10 normal, term babies (11).

In a 2005 abstract, 145 pregnant women were exposed to a new macrolide (38 azithromycin, 53 clarithromycin, and 54 roxithromycin), of which 103 were exposed in the 1st trimester (12). The rates of congenital anomalies compared with 928 exposed to a nonteratogen were similar (4.0% vs. 3.75%, p = 0.156). In a 2006 study, comparisons were made between three groups each containing 123 pregnancies: azithromycin (88 exposed in 1st trimester), nonteratogenic antibiotics, and nonteratogenic agents (13). The rates of congenital anomalies were not significantly different, 3.4%, 2.3%, and 3.4%, respectively. The authors concluded that azithromycin was relatively safe during pregnancy (13).

A retrospective cohort study using data from Tennessee Medicaid included 30,049 infants born in 1985–2000 was published in 2009 (14). Infants with fetal exposures in the 1st trimester to four antibiotics recommended for potential bioterrorism attacks (azithromycin, amoxicillin, ciprofloxacin, and doxycycline) were compared with infants with no fetal exposure to any antibiotic. Erythromycin was included as a positive control. In the 559 infants exposed to azithromycin and no other antibiotics, the number of cases, risk ratios, and 95% CI were as follows: any malformation (23, 1.37, 0.85–2.22), cardiac (7, 1.13, 0.50–2.55), musculoskeletal (8, 1.58, 0.61–4.10), genitourinary (4, 1.34, 0.44–4.03), gastrointestinal (4, 1.57, 0.52–4.75), CNS (1, 0.81–6.27), and orofacial (2, 4.85, 0.88–26.60). The authors concluded that the four antibiotics should not result in a greater incidence of overall major malformations (see also Amoxicillin, Ciprofloxacin, and Doxycycline) (14).

A 2009 case report described the use of azithromycin (500 mg/day for 6 days) for the treatment of Q fever in the 9th week of pregnancy (15). A healthy 3500-g infant was born at 40 weeks'.

A study evaluating the effects of mass treatment (cefixime, azithromycin, and metronidazole) for AIDS prevention in Uganda was published in 1999 (16). Compared with controls, the prevalences of trichomoniasis, bacterial vaginosis, gonorrhea, and *Chlamydia* infection were significantly lower, but no difference was observed in the incidence of HIV infection. A second study using this same group of patients found, in addition to the lower rates of infection, reduced rates of neonatal death, low birth weight, and preterm delivery (17). However, in a third study involving the same Uganda women as above, children of 94 women with *Trichomonas vaginalis* who had been treated during pregnancy with the three-drug combination had increased low birth weight (<2500 g) and preterm birth rate compared with untreated controls (18). The authors concluded that treatment of the condition during pregnancy was harmful and that it was most likely due to metronidazole.

A prospective multicenter study published in 2008 compared pregnant women exposed to a new macrolide (azithromycin, clarithromycin, or roxithromycin) with two comparison groups (19). Of 161 women exposed to a macrolide, 118 were exposed in the 1st trimester. The rate of major malformations in the study group was 4.1% compared with 2.1% of those exposed to other antibiotics (OR = 1.41, 95% CI 0.47–4.23). The authors concluded that the use of the new macrolides did not represent an increased risk of congenital defects strong enough for an elective abortion (19).

A prospective, multicenter observational 2012 study was conducted by teratogen information services in Italy, Israel, Czech Republic, the Netherlands, and Germany (20). Of the 608 women exposed to macrolides, 511 were exposed in the 1st trimester. The study group was compared with 773 women exposed to nonteratogens in the 1st trimester. The rate of major congenital defects were similar in the groups (3.4% vs. 2.4%, $p = 0.36$; OR 1.42, 95% CI 0.70–2.88) or in the rate of cardiovascular defects (1.6% vs. 0.9%). The rates for azithromycin ($N = 134$) were 5.2% vs. 2.4% ($p = 0.09$; OR 2.23, 95% CI 0.91–5.5) and 3% vs. 0.9% ($p = 0.06$; OR 3.59, 95% CI 0.99–12.88) (20).

Two reports, one an abstract, have examined the potential of azithromycin in the prevention of premature birth (21,22). In the abstract, azithromycin combined with metronidazole was compared with placebo in three different periods: <32 weeks', <35 weeks', and <37 weeks' (21). The combination did not decrease the incidence of preterm birth. In the other report, azithromycin was compared with placebo. The results provided no evidence that the use of the antibiotic could prevent preterm birth (22).

In a 2003 Danish study, 188 women received a macrolide (see Breastfeeding Summary) within 30 days of birth and none of their infants had infantile hypertrophic pyloric stenosis (23).

BREASTFEEDING SUMMARY

Azithromycin accumulates in breast milk. A woman, in the 1st week after a term vaginal delivery, was treated with a single 1-g oral dose of azithromycin for a wound infection following a bilateral tubal ligation and then, because of worsening symptoms, was given 48 hours of IV gentamicin and clindamycin (24). She was discharged from the hospital on a 5-day course of azithromycin, 500 mg daily, but only took three doses because she wanted to resume breastfeeding that had been stopped during azithromycin therapy. The patient continued pumping her breasts during this time to maintain milk flow and resumed breastfeeding 24 hours after the third dose of the antibiotic. Drug doses and approximate time from the first dose were 1 g (0 hours), 500 mg (59 hours), 500 mg (83 hours), and 500 mg (107 hours). Milk concentrations of azithromycin and times from the first dose were 0.64 mcg/mL (48 hours), 1.3 mcg/mL (60 hours), and 2.8 mcg/mL (137 hours) (maternal serum concentrations were not determined). The authors attributed the antibiotic's milk accumulation to its lipid solubility and ion trapping of a weak base (24).

A 2003 study investigated the association between maternal use of macrolides and infantile hypertrophic pyloric stenosis (23). The Danish population-based cohort study comprised 1166 women who had been a prescribed macrolide (azithromycin, clarithromycin, erythromycin, spiramycin, or roxithromycin) from birth to 90 days postnatally compared with up to 41,778 controls. The odds ratios (ORs) for stenosis were 2.3–3.0, depending on the postnatal period of exposure (42, 56, 70, or 90 days), but none were significant. When stratified by gender, the ORs for males were 1.8–3.1 and again were not statistically significant. For females, the ORs at 70 and 90 days post-birth were 10.3 and 7.5, respectively, but only the former was significant (95% CI 1.2–92.3) (23).

Investigators from Israel examined the possible association between macrolide (azithromycin, clarithromycin, erythromycin, or roxithromycin) exposure in milk and infantile hypertrophic pyloric stenosis in a 2009 study (25). They compared 55 infants exposed to a macrolide antibiotic with 36 infants exposed to amoxicillin. In the macrolide group, seven (12.7%) had an adverse reaction (rash, diarrhea, loss of appetite, or somnolence), whereas three infants (8.3%) in the amoxicillin group had an adverse reaction (rashes or somnolence). The rates of adverse reactions were comparable. No cases of infantile hypertrophic pyloric stenosis were observed (25).

References

1. Product information. Zithromax. Pfizer Labs, 1994.
2. Ramsey PS, Vaules MB, Vasdev GM, Andrews WW, Ramin KD. Maternal and transplacental pharmacokinetics of azithromycin. Am J Obstet Gynecol 2003;188:714–8.
3. Heikkinen T, Laine K, Neuvonen PJ, Ekblad U. The transplacental transfer of the macrolide antibiotics erythromycin, roxithromycin and azithromycin. Br J Obstet Gynaecol 2000;107:770–5.
4. Edwards M, Rainwater K, Carter S, Williamson F, Newman R. Comparison of azithromycin and erythromycin for Chlamydia cervicitis in pregnancy (abstract). Am J Obstet Gynecol 1994;170:419.
5. Bush MR, Rosa C. Azithromycin and erythromycin in the treatment of cervical chlamydial infection during pregnancy. Obstet Gynecol 1994;84:61–3.
6. Rosenn M, Macones GA, Silverman N. A randomized trial of erythromycin and azithromycin for the treatment of chlamydia infection in pregnancy (abstract). Am J Obstet Gynecol 1996;174:410.
7. Wehbeh H, Ruggiero R, Ali Y, Lopez G, Shahem S, Zarou D. A randomized clinical trial of a single dose of azithromycin in the treatment of chlamydia among pregnant women (abstract). Am J Obstet Gynecol 1996;174:361.
8. Wehbeh HA, Ruggeirio RM, Shahem S, Lopez G, Ali Y. Single-dose azithromycin for chlamydia in pregnant women. J Reprod Med 1998;43:509–14.
9. Ogasawara KK, Goodwin TM. Efficacy of azithromycin in reducing lower genital ureaplasma colonization in women at risk for preterm delivery (abstract). Am J Obstet Gynecol 1997;176:S57.
10. Choi EK, Pai H. Azithromycin therapy for scrub typhus during pregnancy. Clin Infect Dis 1998;27:1538–9.
11. Wilton LV, Pearce GL, Martin RM, Mackay FJ, Mann RD. The outcomes of pregnancy in women exposed to newly marketed drugs in general practice in England. Br J Obstet Gynaecol 1998;105:882–9.
12. Tellem R, Shechtman S, Arnon J, Diav-Citrin O, Bar-Oz B, Berkovitch M, Ornoy A. Pregnancy outcome after gestational exposure to the new macrolides: a prospective controlled cohort study (abstract). Reprod Toxicol 2005;20:484.
13. Sarkar M, Woodland C, Koren G, Einarson A. Pregnancy outcome following gestational exposure to azithromycin. BMC Pregnancy Childbirth 2006;6:18. [Epub 2006 May 30].
14. Cooper WO, Hernandez-Diaz S, Arbogast PG, Dudley JA, Dyer SM, Gideon PS, Hall KS, Kaltenbach LA, Ray WA. Antibiotics potentially used in response to bioterrorism and the risk of major congenital malformations. Paediatr Perinat Epidemiol 2009;23:18–28.
15. Cerar D, Karner P, Avsic-Zupanc T, Strle F. Azithromycin for acute Q fever in pregnancy. Wien Klin Wochenschr 2009;121:469–72.
16. Wawer MJ, Sewankambo NK, Serwadda D, Quinn TC, Paxton LA, Kiwanuka N, Wabwire-Mangen F, Li C, Lutalo T, Nalugoda F, Gaydos CA, Moulton LH, Meehan MO, Ahmed S, the Rakai Project Study Group, Gray RH. Control of sexually transmitted disease for AIDS prevention in Uganda: a randomised community trial. Lancet 1999;353:525–35.
17. Gray RH, Wabwire-Mangen F, Kigozi G, Sewankambo NK, Serwadda D, Moulton LH, Quinn TC, O'Brien KL, Meehan M, Abramowsky C, Robb M, Wawer MJ. Randomized trial of presumptive sexually transmitted disease therapy during pregnancy in Rakai, Uganda. Am J Obstet Gynecol 2001;185:1209–17.
18. Kigozi GG, Brahmbhatt H, Wabwire-Mangen F, Wawer MJ, Serwadda D, Sewankambo N, Gray RH. Treatment of *Trichomonas* in pregnancy and adverse outcomes of pregnancy: a subanalysis of a randomized trial in Rakai, Uganda. Am J Obstet Gynecol 2003;189:1398–400.
19. Bar-Oz B, Diav-Citrin O, Shechtman S, Tellem R, Arnon J, Francetic I, Berkovitch M, Ornoy A. Pregnancy outcome after gestational exposure to the new macrolides: a prospective multi-center observational study. Eur J Obstet Gynecol Reprod Biol 2008;141:31–4.
20. Bar-Oz B, Weber-Schoendorfer C, Berlin M, Clementi M, Di Gianantonio D, de Vries L, De Saints M, Merlob P, Stahl B, Eleftheriou G, Manakova E, Hubickova-Heringova L, Youngster I, Berkovitch M. The outcomes of pregnancy in women exposed to the new macrolides in the first trimester: a prospective, multicentre, observations study. Drug Saf 2012;35:589–98.

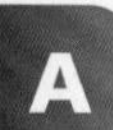

21. Hauth JC, Cliver S. Hodgkins P, Andrews WW, Schwebke JR, Hook EW, Goldenberg RL. Mid-trimester metronidazole and azithromycin did not prevent preterm birth in women at increased risk: a double-blind trial. Am J Obstet Gynecol 2001;185(6 Suppl):S86.
22. van den Broek NR, White SA, Goodall M, Ntonya C, Kayira E, Kafulafula G, Neilson JP. The APPLe study: a randomized, community-based, placebo-controlled trial of azithromycin for the prevention of preterm birth, with meta analysis. PloS Med 2009;6:e100091.
23. Sorensen HT, Skriver MV, Pedersen L, Larsen H, Ebbesen F, Schonheyder HC. Risk of infantile hypertrophic pyloric stenosis after maternal postnatal use of macrolides. Scand J Infect Dis 2003;35:104–6.
24. Kelsey JJ, Moser LR, Jennings JC, Munger MA. Presence of azithromycin breast milk concentrations: a case report. Am J Obstet Gynecol 1994;170:1375–6.
25. Goldstein LH, Berlin M, Tsur L, Bortnik O, Binyamini L, Berkovitch M. The safety of macrolides during lactation. Breastfeed Med 2009;4:157–200.

AZTREONAM

Antibiotic

PREGNANCY RECOMMENDATION: No Human Data—Animal Data Suggest Low Risk
BREASTFEEDING RECOMMENDATION: Compatible

PREGNANCY SUMMARY

No reports describing the therapeutic use of aztreonam in human pregnancy have been located. However, several studies have found that the drug crosses the human placenta and have described the pharmacokinetics in pregnancy. The animal reproduction data suggest low risk, but the absence of therapeutic experience in pregnancy prevents a more complete assessment of the embryo–fetal risk. Nevertheless, if the drug is indicated, it should not be withheld because of pregnancy.

FETAL RISK SUMMARY

Aztreonam is a synthetic, monocyclic β-lactam antibiotic that is structurally different from other β-lactam antibiotics, such as the penicillins and cephalosporins. Administration of high IV doses of the drug to pregnant rats (15 times the maximum recommended human dose [MRHD]) and rabbits (5 times the MRHD) did not produce embryotoxic, fetotoxic, or teratogenic effects (1–5).

Single 1-g IV doses of aztreonam administered 2–8 hours before elective termination produced detectable concentrations of the antibiotic in fetal serum and amniotic fluid (6). In other studies, the drug was rapidly distributed into cord serum and amniotic fluid (7–11). Six studies have described the pharmacokinetics of aztreonam in pregnancy (7–12). No maternal or fetal adverse effects were reported in these studies.

BREASTFEEDING SUMMARY

Aztreonam is excreted into breast milk (7,11,13). In one study, peak milk concentrations 6 hours after a single 1-g IV dose were <0.4–1.0 mcg/mL (7). In an earlier study, 12 lactating women received a single 1-g dose of the antibiotic either by IM injection ($N = 6$) or by the IV route ($N = 6$) (13). Infants were not allowed to breastfeed during the study. Milk and serum samples were collected at scheduled intervals for 8 hours after the dose. In the IM group, the mean peak milk concentration was estimated to be 0.3 mcg/mL, corresponding to a milk:serum ratio of 0.007. Similar calculations for the IV group yielded a peak value of 0.2 mcg/mL and a ratio of 0.002. The low milk concentrations measured in the study were compatible with the acidic nature of the drug and its very low lipid solubility. In another study, the milk concentration was 0.1–0.4 mcg/mL (11).

These data, combined with the poor oral absorption of the antibiotic, indicate that direct systemic effects from the antibiotic in nursing infants are unlikely (13).

The American Academy of Pediatrics classifies aztreonam as compatible with breastfeeding (14).

References

1. Furuhashi T, Kato I, Igarashi Y, Nakayoshi H. Toxicity study of azthreonam: fertility study in rats. Chemotherapy 1985;33:190–202. As cited in Shepard TH. *Catalog of Teratogenic Agents*. 6th ed. Baltimore, MD: Johns Hopkins University Press, 1989:66.
2. Furuhashi T, Ushida K, Sato K, Nakayoshi H. Toxicity study on azthreonam: teratology study in rats. Chemotherapy 1985;33:203–18. As cited in Shepard TH. *Catalog of Teratogenic Agents*. 6th ed. Baltimore, MD: Johns Hopkins University Press, 1989:66.
3. Furuhashi T, Ushida K, Kakei A, Nakayoshi H. Toxicity study on azthreonam: perinatal and postnatal study in rats. Chemotherapy 1985;33:219–31. As cited in Shepard TH. *Catalog of Teratogenic Agents*. 6th ed. Baltimore, MD: Johns Hopkins University Press, 1989:66.
4. Singhvi SM, Ita CE, Shaw JM, Keim GR, Migdalof BH. Distribution of aztreonam into fetuses and milk of rats. Antimicrob Agents Chemother 1984;26:132–5.
5. Product information. Azactam. E. R. Squibb & Sons, 1994.
6. Hayashi R, Devlin RG, Frantz M, Stern M. Concentration of aztreonam in body fluids in mid-pregnancy (abstract). Clin Pharmacol Ther 1984;35:246.
7. Ito K, Hirose R, Tamaya T, Yamada Y, Izumi K. Pharmacokinetic and clinical studies on aztreonam in the perinatal period. Jpn J Antibiot 1990;43:719–26.
8. Matsuda S, Oh K, Hirayama H. Transplacental transfer and clinical application of aztreonam. Jpn J Antibiot 1990;43:700–5.
9. Obata I, Yamato T, Hayashi S, Imakawa N, Hayashi S. Pharmacokinetic study of aztreonam transfer from mother to fetus. Jpn J Antibiot 1990;43:70–80.
10. Cho N, Fukunaga K, Kunii K, Kobayashi I. Studies on aztreonam in the perinatal period. Jpn J Antibiot 1990;43:706–18.
11. Nau H. Clinical pharmacokinetics in pregnancy and perinatology. II. Penicillins. Dev Pharmacol Ther 1987;10:174–98.
12. Cook V, Allen S, Summersgill J, Gall S. The pharmacokinetics of aztreonam during pregnancy (abstract). Am J Obstet Gynecol 1994;170:420.
13. Fleiss PM, Richwald GA, Gordon J, Stern M, Frantz M, Devlin RG. Aztreonam in human serum and breast milk. Br J Clin Pharmacol 1985;19:509–11.
14. Committee on Drugs, American Academy of Pediatrics. The transfer of drugs and other chemicals into human milk. Pediatrics 2001;108:776–89.

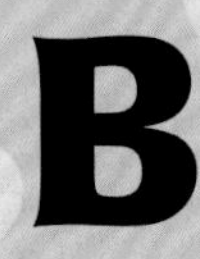

B

BACAMPICILLIN

[Withdrawn from the market. See 9th edition.]

BACITRACIN

Antibiotic

PREGNANCY RECOMMENDATION: Compatible (Topical)
BREASTFEEDING RECOMMENDATION: Compatible (Topical)

PREGNANCY SUMMARY

The pregnancy information is very limited, but the risk from topical use probably is nil. The IM formulation is not approved for use in adults and should not be used in pregnancy.

FETAL RISK SUMMARY

No reports linking the use of bacitracin with congenital defects have been located. The drug is primarily used topically, although the injectable form is available. One study listed 18 patients exposed to the drug in the 1st trimester (1). The route of administration was not specified. No association with malformations was found.

BREASTFEEDING SUMMARY

No reports describing the use of bacitracin during human lactation have been located. Such reports are unlikely because the drug is not approved for use in adults.

Reference

1. Heinonen OP, Slone D, Shapiro S. *Birth Defects and Drugs in Pregnancy*. Littleton, MA: Publishing Sciences Group, 1977:297, 301.

BACLOFEN

Muscle Relaxant

PREGNANCY RECOMMENDATION: Limited Human Data—Animal Data Suggest Low Risk
BREASTFEEDING RECOMMENDATION: Limited Human Data—Probably Compatible

PREGNANCY SUMMARY

The human pregnancy experience with baclofen is limited to 10 cases, 7 of which involved intrathecal administration. This method results in plasma concentrations 100 times less than those achieved with oral administration (1). Late onset neonatal seizures were observed in one case in which the mother was taking 80 mg/day, the maximum recommended daily oral dose. No signs of toxicity were observed in the other two pregnancies in which the mothers were taking lower oral doses. This appears to be consistent with a dose–effect relationship, because the chemical and pharmacokinetic characteristics of baclofen suggest that it will cross the placenta. Although the human data are very limited, there is no evidence of developmental toxicity from other agents in the same pharmacologic class. The animal reproduction data have reduced relevance because, in one study, the teratogenic dose also caused maternal toxicity and, in another, a comparison with the human dose was not made. However, three other studies observed no teratogenicity in mice, rats, and rabbits, so the risk appears to be low. Taken in sum, more human data are required to assess the risk to the embryo and/or fetus adequately. However, the intrathecal route is probably low risk because of the expected very low systemic exposure. If a woman requires oral baclofen, it should not be withheld because of pregnancy, but the lowest dose possible should be used and offspring should be monitored for late-onset seizures.

B

FETAL RISK SUMMARY

Baclofen, an analog of γ-aminobutyric acid, is a centrally acting skeletal muscle relaxant. Although their specific mechanisms of action may differ, baclofen is in the same class of centrally acting skeletal muscle relaxants as carisoprodol, chlorzoxazone, cyclobenzaprine, metaxalone, methocarbamol, orphenadrine, and tizanidine. Plasma protein binding is only about 30%, and 70%–80% of the drug is excreted unchanged in the urine. The plasma elimination half-life is 3–4 hours, whereas the elimination half-life in the cerebrospinal fluid is 1–5 hours. The maximum recommended daily oral dose is 80 mg (1,2). Because of its specialized indication to control spasticity secondary to multiple sclerosis and other spinal cord diseases and injuries, its use in pregnancy is anticipated to be limited.

Reproduction studies have been conducted in pregnant rats, mice, and rabbits. In rats, a maternal toxic (decreased food intake and weight gain) dose approximately 3 times the maximum recommended human dose based on BSA was associated with an increased incidence of omphalocele (ventral hernias) in fetuses. This defect was not observed in mice and rabbits (1). Shepard reviewed three studies involving rats, mice, and rabbits in which the drug was administered during organogenesis and all reported negative teratogenic findings (3). In contrast, in a 1995 study of pregnant rats that administered 30- or 60-mg/kg doses, vertebral arch widening was observed on day 10 of gestation at the lower dose, similar to that produced by valproic acid in rats (4). The author concluded that baclofen could produce spina bifida or other neural tube defects in rats. Interestingly, the 60-mg/kg dose did not produce this effect, causing speculation that the dose caused a greater severity of neural tube defects, and thus a greater number of unrecorded early fetal deaths (4).

It is not known if baclofen crosses the human placenta. The molecular weight (about 214), low plasma protein binding and metabolism, and the plasma elimination half-life suggest that the drug will cross to the embryo and fetus.

Six reports involving seven pregnancies have been published in which a continuous intrathecal infusion of baclofen was administered via an implanted pump in six and intrathecal bolus dose in one (5–10). The first case involved a 29-year-old woman with quadriplegia who was treated with 1000 mcg/day for 15 months to control her intractable spasticity (5). Conception occurred after ovulation stimulation with clomiphene. The baclofen dose was gradually increased to 1200 mcg/day to maintain control of her spasticity as the pregnancy progressed. Because of severe symptoms of autonomic dysfunction and loss of spasticity control (even at 1400 mcg/day), a cesarean section was performed under epidural bupivacaine anesthesia during the 35th week of gestation. A 2.04-kg healthy female infant was delivered with Apgar scores of 9 and 10, presumably at 1 and 5 minutes, respectively (5).

The second and third cases, both involving the same woman, were published in 2000 (6). A 38-year-old woman became pregnant after approximately 3.5 years of continuous intrathecal baclofen infusion to control severe spasticity resulting from a complete 5th cervical vertebra (C5)–level medullar injury. Good control of her spasticity was obtained with 140 mcg/day throughout her pregnancy. A healthy, 2.155-kg male infant was delivered by cesarean section at 36 weeks' gestation with Apgar scores of 9 and 10 at 1 and 5 minutes, respectively. The birth weight, length (47 cm), and head circumference (33 cm) were appropriate for gestational age. No major or minor malformations were noted on physical and ultrasonography examinations, and the child was developing normally at 24 months of age (6). Three months after delivery of her first infant, the woman became pregnant a second time while receiving 140 mcg/day throughout gestation. A cesarean section was performed at 34 weeks with delivery of a healthy, 2.24-kg male infant with Apgar scores of 8 and 10 at 1 and 5 minutes, respectively. The weight, length (46 cm), and head circumference (32 cm) were appropriate for gestational age. No abnormalities were noted in the infant, and he was developing normally at 12 months of age (6).

A 17-year-old woman, 27 weeks pregnant, presented with clinical symptoms and signs of severe tetanus (7). She was treated with intrathecal bolus doses of baclofen for 21 days to control her muscular contractures and paroxysms. The mean daily dose was 1350 mcg (range 250–1500 mcg).

She also received a continuous IV infusion of diazepam 20–200 mg/day. Diazepam was stopped at about 32 weeks' gestation, 3 days before the onset of spontaneous labor. A healthy 1.50-kg male infant was delivered with an Apgar score of 10 at 5 minutes. The infant had no muscular weakness or evidence of respiratory or neurologic distress. The infant was discharged home with his mother at 9 days of age (7).

A 23-year-old paraplegic woman at 30 weeks' gestation was started on intrathecal baclofen for increasing spasticity and spasticity-related pain (8). An infusion pump was implanted under general anesthesia with an initial dose of 150 mcg/day. Over the following 6 weeks, the infusion dose required to control her spasms increased to 375 mcg/day. Labor was induced at 37 weeks' gestation, and she gave birth to a healthy 2.81-kg female infant. The child was developing normally at 2 years of age (8).

A 2008 report described a 38-year-old woman with multiple sclerosis complicated by spasticity (9). The spasticity was treated with intrathecal baclofen 202.6 mcg/day throughout gestation. Because of spontaneous rupture of the membranes and a transverse lie at 36 5/7 weeks, a healthy 2.68-kg male infant was delivered by cesarean section. Apgar scores were 9 and 10, presumably at 1 and 5 minutes, respectively. No follow-up of the infant was reported (9). In a similar case, but in which intrathecal baclofen (dose not reported) was used throughout gestation to control spasticity secondary to cerebral palsy, a 28-year-old woman gave birth at 38 weeks to a healthy 3.30-kg infant (sex not specified) (10). Apgar scores were 9 and 10 at 1 and 5 minutes, respectively. At 1-year follow-up, the infant was doing well.

A 2001 case report described a paraplegic woman who had used baclofen 80 mg/day (*the maximum recommended daily oral dose*), oxybutynin 9 mg/day, and trimethoprim 100 mg/day throughout an uneventful pregnancy (11). The fetus developed tachycardia at an unspecified gestational age and an apparently healthy female infant was delivered (birth weight not given). Apgar scores were 10 at 1 and 5 minutes. At 7 days of age, the infant was admitted to the hospital for generalized seizures, but the mother had noted abnormal movements 2 days after birth. All diagnostic test results were negative and the seizures did not respond to phenytoin, phenobarbital, clonazepam, lidocaine, or pyridoxine. Because seizures had been reported in adults after abrupt withdrawal of baclofen, a dose of 1 mg/kg divided into four daily doses was started and the seizures stopped 30 minutes after the first dose. Baclofen was slowly tapered and then discontinued after 2 weeks. Magnetic resonance imaging of the infant's brain on day 17 suggested a short hypoxic ischemic insult that was thought to have been secondary to the seizures (11).

A 41-year-old woman with stiff-limb syndrome was treated with oral baclofen and diazepam throughout an uncomplicated pregnancy (12). The dose of baclofen during the 1st trimester was 100 mg/day (i.e., >maximum recommended dose), whereas the diazepam dose was 60 mg/day. She was able to reduce the dose of the two drugs to 25 and 15 mg/day, respectively, from the 2nd trimester onward. Despite a birth complicated by fetal distress requiring assisted forceps delivery, the apparently healthy female infant had no evidence of sedation or withdrawal and remained well during breastfeeding. No other details regarding the infant were provided (12).

A 27-year-old woman was diagnosed about 2 months before pregnancy with stiff person syndrome (Moersche-Woltman syndrome) (13). She was treated with gabapentin (2700 mg/day), diazepam (30 mg/day), and a prednisone taper. When pregnancy was diagnosed, diazepam was discontinued but, without the drug, her muscle spasms increased and baclofen (30 mg/day) was started. The patient was able to wean down her medications in the 2nd and 3rd trimesters (specific details not provided). Labor commenced at about 40 weeks while still on gabapentin and baclofen. A cesarean section was conducted because of fetal repetitive late decelerations to deliver a 3230-g female infant with Apgar scores of 5 and 8 at 1 and 5 minutes, respectively. The infant, discharged home on day 4, was doing well (age assumed to be 6 weeks) (13).

A 2004 report described the pregnancy outcome of a 38-year-old woman with reflex sympathetic dystrophy who was treated throughout gestation with baclofen 20 mg/day, clonazepam 2 mg/day, and oxycodone 50 mg/day in divided doses (14). A 3.71-kg female infant was delivered by cesarean section at 39 2/7 weeks' gestation because of breech presentation and maternal health considerations. The baclofen concentration in cord blood was below the level of quantitation (0.08 mcg/mL), but the interval between the last dose and birth was not specified. The infant developed transient respiratory distress shortly after birth that was attributed to retained lung fluid. Oral baclofen 0.5 mg/kg/day in four divided doses was started shortly after birth and tapered over 9 days. Although no seizure activity was observed, phenobarbital was started on day 2 because of narcotic withdrawal symptoms. On day 16 of life, the infant was discharged home on low-dose phenobarbital. Neurologic examination results were normal at discharge and at 6 weeks (14).

BREASTFEEDING SUMMARY

In an animal study, the γ-aminobutyric acid agonist, baclofen, was a potent inhibitor of suckling-induced prolactin release from the anterior pituitary (15). The drug had no effect on milk ejection. Because prolactin release is required to maintain lactation, the potential for decreased milk production with chronic use may exist. However, no human studies on this topic have been located.

Small amounts of baclofen are excreted into human milk after oral administration. A 20-year-old woman with spastic paraplegia, who was 14 days postpartum, was given a single 20-mg (94 microM) oral dose of baclofen (16). No mention was made as to whether her infant was nursing. Serum samples were drawn at 1, 3, 6, and 20 hours after the dose, and milk samples were obtained at 2, 4, 8, 14, 20, and 26 hours. The highest serum concentration measured, 1.419 microM/L, occurred at 3 hours, whereas the highest milk level, 0.608 microM/L, was obtained at 4 hours. The total amount of drug recovered from the milk during the 26-hour sampling period was 22 mcg (0.10 microM), or about 0.1% of the mother's dose. The authors speculated that this amount would not lead to toxic levels in a nursing infant (16).

The American Academy of Pediatrics classifies baclofen as compatible with breastfeeding (17).

References

1. Product information. Lioresal Intrathecal. Medtronic, 2002.
2. Baclofen. In: Sweetman SC, ed. *Martindale: The Complete Drug Reference*. 34th ed. London, UK: Pharmaceutical Press, 2005:1386–8.
3. Shepard TH. *Catalog of Teratogenic Agents*. 6th ed. Baltimore, MD: Johns Hopkins University Press, 1989:66.
4. Briner W. Muscimol- and baclofen-induced spina bifida in the rat. Med Sci Res 1995;24:639–40.
5. Delhaas EM, Verhagen J. Pregnancy in a quadriplegic patient treated with continuous intrathecal baclofen infusion to manage her severe spasticity. Case report. Paraplegia 1992;30:527–8.
6. Munoz FC, Marco DG, Perez AV, Camacho MM. Pregnancy outcome in a woman exposed to continuous intrathecal baclofen infusion. Ann Pharmacother 2000;34:956.
7. Engrand N, Van de Perre P, Vilain G, Benhamou D. Intrathecal baclofen for severe tetanus in a pregnant woman. Eur J Anaesthesiol 2001;18:261–3.
8. Roberts AG, Graves CR, Konrad PE, Groomes TE, Pfister AA, Damian MM, Charles PD. Intrathecal baclofen pump implantation during pregnancy. Neurology 2003;61:1156–7.
9. Dalton CM, Keenan E, Jarrett L, Buckley L, Stevenson VL. The safety of baclofen in pregnancy: intrathecal therapy in multiple sclerosis. Mult Scler 2008;14:571–2.
10. Ali Sakr Esa W, Toma I, Tetzlaff JE, Barsoum S. Epidural analgesia in labor for a woman with an intrathecal baclofen pump. Int J Obstet Anesth 2009;18:64–6.
11. Ratnayaka BDM, Dhaliwal H, Watkin S. Neonatal convulsions after withdrawal of baclofen. BMJ 2001;323:85.
12. Weatherby SJM, Woolner P, Clarke CE. Pregnancy in stiff-limb syndrome. Mov Disord 2004;19:852–4.
13. Goldkamp J, Blaskiewicz R, Myles T. Stiff person syndrome and pregnancy. Obstet Gynecol 2011;118:454–7.
14. Moran LR, Almeida PG, Worden S, Huttner KM. Intrauterine baclofen exposure: a multidisciplinary approach. Pediatrics 2004;114:e267–9.
15. Lux VA, Somoza GM, Libertun C. Beta-(-4 chlorophenyl) GABA (baclofen) inhibits prolactin and thyrotropin release by acting on the rat brain. Proc Soc Exp Biol Med 1986;183:358–62.
16. Eriksson G, Swahn C-G. Concentrations of baclofen in serum and breast milk from a lactating woman. Scand J Clin Lab Invest 1981;41:185–7.
17. Committee on Drugs, American Academy of Pediatrics. The transfer of drugs and other chemicals into human milk. Pediatrics 2001;108:776–89.

B

BALSALAZIDE

Anti-inflammatory Bowel Disease Agent

PREGNANCY RECOMMENDATION: No Human Data—Animal Data Suggest Low Risk
BREASTFEEDING RECOMMENDATION: No Human Data—Potential Toxicity

PREGNANCY SUMMARY

No reports describing the use of balsalazide in human pregnancy have been located. Balsalazide is a prodrug that is converted in the bowel to mesalamine (see Mesalamine). A 2002 review concluded that mesalamine is safe to use during pregnancy (1). Therefore, the maternal benefits of balsalazide appear to outweigh the unknown risks to the fetus.

FETAL RISK SUMMARY

The oral prodrug balsalazide is enzymatically cleaved in the colon to produce mesalamine (5-aminosalicylic acid) (see also Mesalamine). It is indicated for the treatment of mildly to moderately active ulcerative colitis. A very small portion of a balsalazide dose is absorbed intact into the systemic circulation where it is extensively (≥99%) protein bound (2).

Reproduction studies have been conducted in rats and rabbits. In pregnant rats and rabbits, doses up to 2.4 and 4.7 times the recommended human dose based on BSA, respectively, revealed no evidence of impaired fertility or fetal harm. In addition, studies with mesalamine in these species did not observe fetal toxicity or teratogenicity (see Mesalamine) (2).

It is not known if balsalazide crosses the human placenta. The molecular weight (about 437) is low enough but the very small amounts in the plasma and extensive plasma protein binding suggest that little if any drug crosses to the embryo–fetus. Moreover, only small amounts of mesalamine are absorbed into the systemic circulation and then are rapidly excreted in the urine.

BREASTFEEDING SUMMARY

No reports describing the use of the prodrug balsalazide during human lactation have been located. Only small amounts of balsalazide and its active metabolite mesalamine are absorbed into the systemic circulation. Moreover, the parent drug is extensively (≥99%) bound to plasma proteins. A 2002 review concluded that mesalamine was safe to use by nursing mothers (1). However, a possible allergic reaction (diarrhea) was observed in a nursing infant whose mother was using mesalamine rectal suppositories. Because of this adverse effect, nursing infants should be closely observed for changes in bowel function if the mother is taking balsalazide.

References

1. Schroeder KW. Role of mesalazine in acute and long-term treatment of ulcerative colitis and its complications. Scand J Gastroentrol Suppl 2002;236:42–7.
2. Product information. Colazal. Salix Pharmaceuticals, 2004.

BASILIXIMAB

Immunologic Agent (Immunosuppressant)

PREGNANCY RECOMMENDATION: Compatible—Maternal Benefit >> Embryo–Fetal Risk
BREASTFEEDING RECOMMENDATION: No Human Data—Probably Compatible

PREGNANCY SUMMARY

No reports describing the use of basiliximab in human pregnancy have been located. The animal data suggest low risk, but the absence of human pregnancy experience prevents a full assessment of the embryo–fetal risk. A 2004 review concluded that immunosuppressive antibodies, such as basiliximab, have little implication for pregnancy because they are used either for induction immunosuppression or to prevent an acute rejection episode (1). If exposure does occur during pregnancy, the risk for developmental toxicity appears to be low, but long-term studies of exposed offspring for functional abnormalities and other developmental toxicity are warranted. The manufacturer recommends that women of childbearing potential use effective contraception before and during therapy, and for 4 months afterward (2).

FETAL RISK SUMMARY

Basiliximab, an interleukin-2 (IL-2) receptor antagonist, is a chimeric (murine/human) monoclonal antibody (IgG_{1k}) indicated for the prophylaxis of acute organ rejection in patients receiving renal transplantation (2). Basiliximab is classified as a nondepleting (i.e., does not destroy T- or B-lymphocytes) protein immunosuppressant (3). It binds only to IL-2 receptor sites expressed on the surface of activated T-lymphocytes.

This binding inhibits IL-2-mediated activation of lymphocytes. Basiliximab is used with immunosuppressive regimens that include cyclosporine and corticosteroids. The elimination half-life is about 7 days (2).

Reproduction studies have been conducted in monkeys. No maternal toxicity, embryotoxicity, or teratogenicity was observed when doses producing blood concentrations 13 times higher than those observed in humans were given during organogenesis. However, immunologic toxicity studies were not performed in the offspring (2).

It is not known if basiliximab crosses the human placenta. The molecular weight of the glycoprotein (about 144,000) may prevent transfer. However, the prolonged elimination half-life and the fact that immunoglobulin G molecules are known to cross the placenta, at least in the 3rd trimester, suggest that some exposure of the embryo and/or fetus will occur.

IL-2 receptors may have an important role in the development of the immune system, but the potential effect of basiliximab on this development was not evaluated in monkey offspring. Moreover, while in the circulation, basiliximab impairs the response of the immune system to antigenic challenges. It is unknown if the ability to respond to these challenges returns to normal after clearance of basiliximab (2).

BREASTFEEDING SUMMARY

No reports describing the use of basiliximab during human lactation have been located. Because immunoglobulins and other large molecules are excreted into colostrum in the first 2–3 days after birth, basiliximab is also probably excreted during this time. It may not be possible to avoid exposure during this early period of lactation because of the prolonged elimination half-life (about 7 days). Excretion into mature milk also is possible. Although partial digestion of the antibody in the gastrointestinal tract is probable, the effects, if any, on a nursing infant from this exposure are unknown.

References

1. Danesi R, Del Tacca M. Teratogenesis and immunosuppressive treatment. Transplant Proc 2004;36:705–7.
2. Product information. Simulect. Novartis Pharmaceuticals, 2005.
3. Halloran PF. Immunosuppressive drugs for kidney transplantation. N Engl J Med 2004;351:2715–29.

BECLOMETHASONE

Respiratory Drug (Corticosteroid)

PREGNANCY RECOMMENDATION: Compatible
BREASTFEEDING RECOMMENDATION: Limited Human Data—Probably Compatible

PREGNANCY SUMMARY

In a position statement from a joint committee of the American College of Obstetricians and Gynecologists (ACOG) and the American College of Allergy, Asthma, and Immunology (ACAAI) published in 2000, either beclomethasone or budesonide were considered the inhaled steroids of choice for use during pregnancy (1).

FETAL RISK SUMMARY

Beclomethasone dipropionate is given by inhalation for the chronic treatment of bronchial asthma in patients requiring corticosteroid therapy for the control of symptoms. It is also available for intranasal use and, outside of the United States, for topical application.

Beclomethasone was embryocidal (increased fetal resorption) and teratogenic when administered by SC injection to mice and rabbits at approximately 10 times the human dose (HD) (2,3). Congenital malformations observed included cleft palate, agnathia, microstomia, absence of the tongue, delayed ossification, and agenesis of the thymus. Similar toxic effects in both species were observed with SC injections that were approximately one-half the maximum recommended adult daily inhalation dose based on BSA (4). In the rat, no embryo or fetal harm was found with inhaled (at 10 times the HD) or oral (at 1000 times the HD) beclomethasone (2,3).

No human reports associating the use of beclomethasone with human congenital anomalies have been found. A 1975 report briefly mentioned seven healthy babies born from mothers who had used beclomethasone aerosol for >6 months (5). In another report, beclomethasone was used during 45 pregnancies in 40 women (6). Dosage ranged between 4 and 16 inhalations/day (mean 9.5), with each inhalation delivering 42 mcg of drug. Three of the 33 prospectively studied pregnancies ended in abortion that was not thought to be caused by the maternal asthma. Forty-three living infants resulted from the remaining 42 pregnancies. Six infants had low birth weights, including two of the three premature newborns (<37 weeks' gestation). There was no evidence of neonatal adrenal insufficiency. One full-term infant had cardiac malformations (double ventricular septal defect, patent ductus arteriosus, and subaortic stenosis). However, the mother's asthma was also treated with prednisone, theophylline, and epinephrine. In addition, she had schizophrenia and diabetes mellitus for which she took fluphenazine and insulin (6). Cardiac malformations are known to occur with diabetes mellitus (see Insulin).

In a surveillance study of Michigan Medicaid recipients involving 229,101 completed pregnancies conducted between 1985 and 1992, 395 newborns had been exposed to beclomethasone during the 1st trimester (F. Rosa, personal communication, FDA, 1993). A total of 16 (4.1%) major birth defects were observed (16 expected). Specific information was not available on the defects, but no anomalies were

B

observed in six categories (cardiovascular defects, oral clefts, spina bifida, polydactyly, limb reduction defects, and hypospadias). These data do not support an association between the drug and congenital defects.

A 2004 prospective, double-blind, double placebo-controlled, randomized study compared inhaled beclomethasone (194 women) with theophylline (191 women) for the treatment of moderate asthma during pregnancy (7). The mean gestational age at randomization was about 20 weeks in both groups. There was no significant difference in the rate of asthma exacerbations between the groups, but significantly fewer discontinued beclomethasone because of adverse effects. There also were no differences in maternal or perinatal outcomes (7).

A 2004 study examined the effect of inhaled corticosteroids on low birth weight, preterm births, and congenital malformations in pregnant asthmatic patients (8). The inhaled steroids with the number of patients were beclomethasone (*N* = 277), fluticasone (*N* = 132), triamcinolone (*N* = 81), budesonide (*N* = 43), and flunisolide (*N* = 25). Compared with the general population, the study found no increased incidence of small-for-gestational-age infants (<10th percentile for gestational age), low birth weight (<2500 g), preterm births, and congenital malformations (8).

A 2006 meta-analysis on the use of inhaled corticosteroids during pregnancy was published in 2006 (9). The analysis included five agents: beclomethasone, budesonide, flunisolide, fluticasone, and triamcinolone. The results showed that these agents do not increase the risk of major congenital defects, preterm delivery, low birth weight, and pregnancy-induced hypertension. Thus, they could be used during pregnancy (9).

A 2007 report described the use of inhaled beclomethasone in 29 pregnant women (10). No effects on fetal growth or pregnancy outcomes were observed. Beclomethasone was metabolized by placental enzymes (10).

BREASTFEEDING SUMMARY

It is not known whether beclomethasone is excreted into breast milk. Other corticosteroids are excreted into milk in low concentrations (see Prednisone), and the passage of beclomethasone into milk should be expected. One report mentioned three cases of maternal beclomethasone use during breastfeeding (5). Effects on the nursing infants were not mentioned.

References

1. Joint Committee of the American College of Obstetricians and Gynecologists (ACOG) and the American College of Allergy, Asthma, and Immunology (ACAAI). Position statement. The use of newer asthma and allergy medications during pregnancy. Ann Allergy Asthma Immunol 2000;84:475–80.
2. Product information. Beconase. Glaxo Wellcome, 2000.
3. Product information. Vancenase; Vanceril. Schering, 2000.
4. Product information. Beclovent. Glaxo Wellcome, 2000.
5. Brown HM, Storey G. Treatment of allergy of the respiratory tract with beclomethasone dipropionate steroid aerosol. Postgrad Med J 1975;51(Suppl 4):59–64.
6. Greenberger PA, Patterson R. Beclomethasone dipropionate for severe asthma during pregnancy. Ann Intern Med 1983;98:478–80.
7. Dombrowski MP, Schatz M, Wise R, Thom EA, Landon M, Mabie W, Newman RB, McNellis D, Hauth JC, Lindheimer M, Caritis SN, Leveno KJ, Meis P, Miodovnik M, Wapner RJ, Varner MW, O'Sullivan MJ, Conway DL, for the National Institute of Child Health and Human Development Maternal-Fetal Medicine Units Network, and the National Heart, Lung, and Blood Institute. Randomized trial of inhaled beclomethasone dipropionate versus theophylline for moderate asthma during pregnancy. Am J Obstet Gynecol 2004;190:737–44.
8. Namazy J, Schatz M, Long L, Lipkowitz M, Lillie M, Voss M, Deitz RJ, Petitti D. Use of inhaled steroids by pregnant asthmatic women does not reduce intrauterine growth. J Allergy Clin Immunol 2004;113:427–32.
9. Rahimi R, Nikfar S, Abdollahi M. Meta-analysis finds use of inhaled corticosteroids during pregnancy safe: a systematic meta-analysis review. Hum Exp Toxicol 2006;25:447–52.
10. Murphy VE, Fittock RJ, Zarzycki PK, Delahunty MM, Smith R, Clifton VL. Metabolism of synthetic steroids by the human placenta. Placenta 2007;28:39–46.

BEDAQUILINE

Antituberculosis

PREGNANCY RECOMMENDATION: No Human Data—Animal Data Suggest Low Risk
BREASTFEEDING RECOMMENDATION: No Human Data—Potential Toxicity

PREGNANCY SUMMARY

No reports describing the use of bedaquiline in human pregnancy have been located. The animal data suggest low risk but the absence of human pregnancy experience prevents a full assessment of embryo–fetal risk. Nevertheless, tuberculosis is a severe infection and, if indicated, bedaquiline should not be withheld because of pregnancy.

FETAL RISK SUMMARY

Bedaquiline fumarate is an oral diarylquinoline antimycobacterial drug. It is indicated as part of combination therapy in adults (≥18 years) with pulmonary multidrug-resistant tuberculosis. It is metabolized to an inactive metabolite (M2). Plasma protein binding of bedaquiline is >99.9%. The mean terminal elimination half-life of both bedaquiline and M2 is about 5.5 months, thought to reflect the slow release from peripheral tissues (1).

Reproduction studies have been conducted in rats and rabbits. In these studies, no evidence of fetal harm was found. The plasma exposure in rats was twofold higher (lower in rabbits) than the human plasma exposure (1).

Bedaquiline was not mutagenic or clastogenic in several assays. The drug had no effects on fertility in male and female rats (1).

It is not known if bedaquiline or M2 cross the human placenta. The molecular weight of bedaquiline (about 556) and the very long elimination half-lives of the parent compound and M2 suggest that both may cross to the embryo–fetus. However, the high plasma protein binding might reduce the amount available to cross the placenta.

BREASTFEEDING SUMMARY

No reports describing the use of bedaquiline during breastfeeding have been located. The molecular weight of bedaquiline (about 556) and the very long elimination half-lives (about 5.5 months) of the parent compound and M2 suggest that both may be excreted into breast milk, but the high plasma protein binding might reduce the amount excreted. However, bedaquiline is concentrated in the milk of rats with concentrations 6–12 times the maximum maternal plasma level. If a mother chooses to nurse while receiving the drug, her infant should be observed for nausea, arthralgia, headache, hemoptysis, and chest pain, the most common (≥10%) adverse reactions observed in patients.

Reference

1. Product information. Sirturo. Janssen Therapeutics, 2012.

BELATACEPT

Immunologic Agent (Immunosuppressant)

PREGNANCY RECOMMENDATION: **No Human Data—Animal Data Suggest Low Risk Contraindicated—1st Trimester (If Combined with Mycophenolate)**

BREASTFEEDING RECOMMENDATION: **No Human Data—Probably Compatible Contraindicated (If Combined with Mycophenolate)**

PREGNANCY SUMMARY

No reports describing the use of belatacept in human pregnancy have been located. The animal data suggest low risk but the absence of human pregnancy experience prevents a better assessment. However, belatacept is used in combination with basiliximab induction, mycophenolate, and corticosteroids, and the latter two agents are known human teratogens (see Mycophenolate and Prednisone). Nevertheless, rejection of a transplanted organ has serious consequences for the mother and her pregnancy. Therefore, if indicated, the drug should not be withheld because of pregnancy but the woman should be informed of the potential risk to her embryo–fetus. In addition, physicians are encouraged to register pregnant patients in the National Transplant Pregnancy Registry by calling 1-877-955-6877.

FETAL RISK SUMMARY

Belatacept, a selective T-cell costimulation blocker given as an IV infusion, is a protein that is fused to a portion of human immunoglobulin G1 antibody. The parent molecule, abatacept, differs from belatacept by two amino acids. Belatacept is indicated for prophylaxis of organ rejection in adult patients receiving a kidney transplant and is used in combination with basiliximab induction, mycophenolate mofetil, and corticosteroids. Although information on the metabolism of belatacept was not provided by the manufacturer, the terminal half-life was about 8–10 days depending on the dose (1).

Reproduction studies have been conducted in rats and rabbits. In these species, no teratogenicity was observed at exposures that were 16 and 19 times the maximum recommended human dose during the first month of treatment based on AUC (MRHD). In rats, daily belatacept during gestation and throughout the lactation period was associated with maternal toxicity (infections) in a small percentage of dams at doses that were ≥3 times the MRHD. This toxicity resulted in increased pup mortality (up to 100% in some dams), but there were no abnormalities or malformations in surviving pups. The in vitro data indicate that belatacept has lower potency in rodents than in humans, but the in vivo difference in potency is unknown. Thus, the relevance of the rat toxicities to humans and the significance of the magnitude of the relative exposures to humans are unknown (1).

Carcinogenicity studies have not been conducted with belatacept but have been with abatacept, the more active analog in rodents. Weekly SC injections of abatacept in mice were associated with increases in the incidences of malignant lymphomas and mammary gland tumors (in females). The clinical significance of these findings is unknown because the mice were infected with endogenous murine leukemia and mouse mammary tumor viruses which are associated with an increased incidence of lymphomas and mammary gland tumors, respectively. However, cases of posttransplant lymphoproliferative disorder (a premalignant or malignant proliferation of B lymphocytes) have been reported in clinical trials. Genotoxicity studies have not been conducted with belatacept because they are not required for protein therapeutics. No effects on male or female fertility were observed (1).

It is not known if belatacept crosses the human placenta. The protein is known to cross the placenta of animals. The molecular weight (about 90,000) suggests that transfer of the agent across the placenta will be limited, but the elimination half-life will place it at the maternal–fetal interface for a prolonged period. Moreover, the parent molecule, abatacept

B

crosses the placenta. In addition, immunoglobulin G crosses the placenta, especially in the latter portion of pregnancy and belatacept is an immunoglobulin G antibody. Therefore, exposure of the embryo and/or fetus should be expected.

BREASTFEEDING SUMMARY

No reports describing the use of belatacept during human lactation have been located. The molecular weight (about 90,000) suggests that excretion of the agent into breast milk will be limited, but the terminal half-life is very long (8–10 days). Immunoglobulin G is excreted into colostrum and belatacept is an immunoglobulin G antibody. Moreover, belatacept is used in combination with basiliximab induction, mycophenolate mofetil, and corticosteroids. Basiliximab and corticosteroids appear to be compatible with breastfeeding (see Basiliximab and Prednisone), but mycophenolate is contraindicated (see Mycophenolate). Thus, although belatacept alone is probably compatible, if taken with mycophenolate breastfeeding should be avoided.

Reference

1. Product information. Nulojix. Bristol-Myers Squibb, 2011.

BELIMUMAB

Immunologic Agent (Immunomodulator)

PREGNANCY RECOMMENDATION: No Human Data—Probably Compatible
BREASTFEEDING RECOMMENDATION: No Human Data—Probably Compatible

PREGNANCY SUMMARY

No reports describing the use of belimumab in human pregnancy have been located. Teratogenicity was not observed in cynomolgus monkeys. This species was chosen because belimumab binds cynomolgus monkey and human B-lymphocyte stimulator protein with equal affinity. Compared with controls, an increased risk of fetal death was observed at the lowest but not the highest dose. An increased risk of infant death compared with controls also was observed with both doses. A dose relationship was not apparent in either outcome and the rates were consistent with historical control data for macaques. No other forms of developmental toxicity were observed in the offspring. If belimumab is used in pregnancy, patients should be informed of the lack of human pregnancy experience.

FETAL RISK SUMMARY

Belimumab is a human immune globulin G1 lambda (IgG1λ) monoclonal antibody that is a specific inhibitor of soluble human B-lymphocyte stimulator protein. It is indicated for the treatment of adult patients with active, autoantibody-positive, systemic lupus erythematosus who are receiving standard therapy. The terminal half-life is 19.4 days (1).

Reproduction studies have been conducted in pregnant cynomolgus monkeys with IV infusion doses of 0 (controls), 5, and 150 mg/kg (the highest dose was about 9 times the anticipated maximum human exposure based on AUC) given every 2 weeks from gestation day 20 to 150. The antibody was not associated with direct or indirect teratogenicity. Skeletal and cardiac variations were observed but the rates were within historical control rates. Fetal deaths were observed in 14%, 24%, and 15%, respectively, and infant deaths were observed in 0%, 8%, and 5%, respectively. The cause of the deaths was not known, but the incidences were considered incidental as they were comparable with historical control data for macaques. After cessation of treatment, B-cell numbers recovered about 1 year postpartum in adult monkeys and by 3 months of age in offspring (1,2).

Neither the carcinogenic potential nor the mutagenic potential has been evaluated. The effects on male and female fertility in animals have not been studied (1).

Although the molecular weight is high (about 147,000), belimumab crossed the placenta late in gestation in cynomolgus monkeys as expected for an immune globulin antibody (2). Because the human and monkey placentas are similar, exposure of the human fetus probably occurs.

BREASTFEEDING SUMMARY

No reports describing the use belimumab during human lactation have been located. Although the molecular weight is high (about 147,000), belimumab was excreted into the milk of cynomolgus monkeys (1). In addition, because maternal antibodies are excreted into breast milk, the presence of belimumab in milk should be expected. The effect of this exposure on a nursing infant is unknown.

References

1. Product information. Benlysta. Human Genome Sciences, 2011.
2. Auyeung-Kim DJ, Devalaraja MN, Migone TS, Cai W, Chellman GJ. Developmental and peri-postnatal study in cynomolgus monkeys with belimumab, a monoclonal antibody directed against B-lymphocyte stimulator. Reprod Toxicol 2009;28:443–55.

B

BELLADONNA

Parasympatholytic

PREGNANCY RECOMMENDATION: Limited Human Data—No Relevant Animal Data
BREASTFEEDING RECOMMENDATION: No Human Data—Probably Compatible

PREGNANCY SUMMARY

The limited pregnancy experience showing teratogenicity requires confirmation. In general, however, anticholinergics appear to be low risk in pregnancy. (See Atropine.)

FETAL RISK SUMMARY

Belladonna is an anticholinergic agent. The Collaborative Perinatal Project monitored 50,282 mother–child pairs, 554 of whom used belladonna in the 1st trimester (1, pp. 346–353). Belladonna was found to be associated with malformations in general and with minor malformations. Specifically, increased risks (standardized relative risk >1.5) were observed for respiratory tract anomalies, hypospadias, and eye and ear malformations. The association between belladonna and eye and ear malformations was statistically significant. Interpretation of these data is difficult, however, because the authors of the study emphasized that even though some agents had elevated risks and significant associations did occur, a cause-and-effect relationship could not be inferred. For use anytime during pregnancy, 1355 exposures were recorded (1, p. 439). No association was found in this group.

A 1994 case report described the use of belladonna alkaloid (4 times daily for 5 days) in two women with hyperemesis and excessive salivation (2). A phenothiazine (specific agent not mentioned) antiemetic also was given. One woman gave birth to a normal female infant at term, whereas the other gave birth to twins at 30 weeks. All three infants had normal examinations (2).

BREASTFEEDING SUMMARY

No reports describing the use of belladonna during lactation have been located. In general, however, agents in this class are probably compatible with breastfeeding. (See Atropine.)

References

1. Heinonen OP, Slone D, Shapiro S. *Birth Defects and Drugs in Pregnancy*. Littleton, MA: Publishing Sciences Group, 1977.
2. Freeman JJ, Altieri RH, Baptiste HJ, Kuo T, Crittenden S, Fogarty K, Moultrie M, Coney E, Kanegis K. Evaluation and management of sialorrhea of pregnancy with concomitant hyperemesis. J Natl Med Assoc 1994;86:704–8.

BENAZEPRIL

Antihypertensive

PREGNANCY RECOMMENDATION: Human Data Suggest Risk in 2nd and 3rd Trimesters
BREASTFEEDING RECOMMENDATION: No Human Data—Probably Compatible

PREGNANCY SUMMARY

The fetal toxicity of benazepril in the 2nd and 3rd trimesters is similar to other angiotensin-converting enzyme (ACE) inhibitors. The use of this drug during the 2nd and 3rd trimesters may cause teratogenicity and severe fetal and neonatal toxicity. Fetal toxic effects may include anuria, oligohydramnios, fetal hypocalvaria, intrauterine growth restriction (IUGR), prematurity, and patent ductus arteriosus. Stillbirth or neonatal death may occur. Anuria-associated oligohydramnios may produce fetal limb contractures, craniofacial deformation, and pulmonary hypoplasia. Severe anuria and hypotension, which is resistant to both pressor agents and volume expansion, may occur in the newborn following in utero exposure. Newborn renal function and blood pressure should be closely monitored.

FETAL RISK SUMMARY

Benazepril is an ACE inhibitor. It is indicated for the treatment of hypertension. It is metabolized to benazeprilat, a more potent active metabolite. The effective half-life of accumulation of benazeprilat is 10–11 hours (1).

Reproduction studies have been conducted in mice, rats, and rabbits. No teratogenic effects were observed at doses that were 9, 60, and >0.8 times, respectively, the maximum recommended human dose based on BSA (assuming a 50-kg woman) (1).

Benazepril crosses the human placenta (1). This is consistent with the molecular weight (about 425 for the free base of the parent drug) and suggests that its active metabolite also will cross.

A 1997 report described the use of benazepril (40 mg/day) in a 35-year-old woman with chronic hypertension (2). Treatment began several years before conception. Anhydramnios was noted at 27 weeks' gestation and the drug was discontinued. Twelve days later, complete resolution of the severe oligohydramnios was documented and the woman eventually delivered a healthy 2600-g (10th percentile) male infant at 38 weeks' gestation. No signs or symptoms of impaired renal function were observed in the healthy infant (2).

A retrospective study using pharmacy-based data from the Tennessee Medicaid program identified 209 infants born between 1985 and 2000 who had 1st trimester exposure to ACE inhibitors (3). Infants of mothers with evidence of diabetes, either before or during pregnancy, were excluded, as were those exposed to angiotensin-receptor antagonists (ARBs), ACE inhibitors, or other antihypertensives beyond the 1st trimester, and known teratogens. The subject group (*N*=209) was compared with two groups, other antihypertensives (*N*=202) and no antihypertensives (*N*=29,096). The number of major birth defects in each of the three groups was 18 (8.6%), 4 (2%), and 834 (2.9%), respectively. Compared with the no antihypertensives group, exposure to ACE inhibitors was associated with a significantly increased risk of major defects (relative risk [RR] 2.71, 95% confidence interval [CI] 1.72–4.27). When the analysis was conducted by the type of defect, the highest rates were with cardiovascular defects, 9, 2, and 294, respectively, RR 3.72, 95% CI 1.89–7.30, and with CNS defects, 3, 0, and 80, respectively, RR 4.39, 95% CI 1.37–14.02. The major defects observed in the subject group were atrial septal defect (*N* = 6) (includes three with pulmonic stenosis and/or three with patent ductus arteriosus [PDA]), renal dysplasia (*N* = 2), PDA alone (*N* = 2), and one each of ventricular septal defect, spina bifida, microcephaly with eye anomaly, coloboma, hypospadias, intestinal and choanal atresia, Hirschsprung disease, and diaphragmatic hernia (3). In an accompanying editorial, it was noted that neither previous reports of 1st trimester exposure to ACE inhibitors nor the animal studies had observed an increased risk of birth defects (4). It also was noted that no mechanism for ACE inhibitor-induced teratogenicity was known. A subsequent communication raising concerns about the validity of the study in terms of adequate exclusion of diabetes, charting and coding errors in busy medical practices, and the effects of maternal obesity (5) was addressed by the investigators (6).

Benazepril and other ACE inhibitors are human teratogens when used in the 2nd and 3rd trimesters, producing fetal hypocalvaria and renal defects. The cause of the defects and other toxicity is probably related to fetal hypotension and decreased renal blood flow. The compromise of the fetal renal system may result in severe, and at times fatal, anuria, both in the fetus and in the newborn. Anuria-associated oligohydramnios may produce pulmonary hypoplasia, limb contractures, persistent PDA, craniofacial deformation, and neonatal death (7,8). IUGR, prematurity, and severe neonatal hypotension may also be observed.

Two reviews of fetal and newborn renal function indicated that both renal perfusion and glomerular plasma flow are low during gestation and that high levels of angiotensin II may be physiologically necessary to maintain glomerular filtration at low perfusion pressures (9,10). Benazepril prevents the conversion of angiotensin I to angiotensin II and, thus, may lead to in utero renal failure. Since the primary means of removal of the drug is renal, the impairment of this system in the newborn prevents elimination of the drug resulting in prolonged hypotension. Newborn renal function and blood pressure should be closely monitored. If oligohydramnios occurs, stopping benazepril may resolve the problem but may not improve infant outcome because of irreversible fetal damage (7).

In those cases in which benazepril must be used to treat the mother's disease, the lowest possible dose should be used combined with close monitoring of amniotic fluid levels and fetal well-being. Guidelines for counseling exposed pregnant patients have been published and should be of benefit to health professionals faced with this task (7,11). However, the observation in Tennessee Medicaid data of an increased risk of major congenital defects after 1st trimester exposure to ACE inhibitors raises concerns about teratogenicity that have not been seen in other studies (4). Medicaid data are a valuable tool for identifying early signals of teratogenicity, but are subject to a number of shortcomings and their findings must be considered hypotheses until confirmed by independent studies.

In a 2002 case report, a woman with chronic hypertension presented at about 24 weeks' gestation with severe oligohydramnios (amniotic fluid index <2) (12). Her medications included benazepril, carvedilol, amiodarone, and furosemide. The fetus had a misshapen cranium with overlapping sutures, pericardial effusion, small bladder, echogenic focus in the heart, echogenic bowel, and normal-appearing kidneys. All the drugs except carvedilol were discontinued. An examination 18 days later revealed normal amniotic fluid volume and normal cranial anatomy. At about 37 weeks, she gave birth to a 2060-g (<3rd percentile) female infant with Apgar scores of 7 and 9 at 1 and 5 minutes, respectively. The infant's initial physical examination was normal. Except for bilious vomiting on day 1, that resolved by day 2, the infant's hospital course was normal. At 1 year of age, the infant was healthy and weighed 18 lb (5th percentile) (12).

A 2012 review of the use of ACE inhibitors and ARBs in the 1st trimester concluded that there may be an elevated teratogenic risk, but the risk appeared to be related to other factors (13). The factors, that typically coexist with hypertension in pregnancy, included diabetes, advanced maternal age, and obesity.

BREASTFEEDING SUMMARY

Benazepril and benazeprilat are excreted into human breast milk (14). Nine women were given benazepril 20 mg/day for 3 days. At 1 hour after a dose, peak milk concentrations of benazepril were 0.9 mcg/L, whereas the peak level of benazeprilat was 2 mcg/L at 1.5 hours postdose. The estimated infant dose as a percentage of the mother's weight-adjusted dose was <0.14% (14). These results are consistent with the data from other ACE inhibitors (see Captopril and Enalapril) that have found low amounts in milk and no adverse effects in nursing infants.

References

1. Product information. Benazepril Hydrochloride. Andrx Pharmaceuticals, 2005.
2. Chisholm CA, Chescheir NC, Kennedy M. Reversible oligohydramnios in a pregnancy with angiotensin-converting enzyme inhibitor exposure. Am J Perinatol 1997;14:511–3.
3. Cooper WO, Hernandez-Diaz S, Arbogast PG, Dudley JA, Dyer S, Gideon PS, Hall K, Ray WA. Major congenital malformations after first-trimester exposure to ACE inhibitors. N Engl J Med 2006;354:2443–51.
4. Friedman JM. ACE inhibitors and congenital anomalies. N Engl J Med 2006;354:2498–500.
5. Scialli AR, Lione A. ACE inhibitors and major congenital malformations. N Engl J Med 2006;355:1280.
6. Cooper WO, Ray WA. Reply—ACE inhibitors and major congenital malformations. N Engl J Med 2006;355:1281.
7. Barr M Jr. Teratogen update: angiotensin-converting enzyme inhibitors. Teratology 1994;50:399–409.
8. Shotan A, Widerhorn J, Hurst A, Elkayam U. Risks of angiotensin-converting enzyme inhibition during pregnancy: experimental and clinical evidence, potential mechanisms, and recommendations for use. Am J Med 1994;96:451–6.
9. Robillard JE, Nakamura KT, Matherne GP, Jose PA. Renal hemodynamics and functional adjustments to postnatal life. Semin Perinatol 1988;12: 143–50.
10. Guignard J-P, Gouyon J-B. Adverse effects of drugs on the immature kidney. Biol Neonate 1988;53:243–52.
11. Brent RL, Beckman DA. Angiotensin-converting enzyme inhibitors, an embryopathic class of drugs with unique properties: information for clinical teratology counselors. Teratology 1991;43:543–6.
12. Muller PR, James A. Pregnancy with prolonged fetal exposure to an angiotensin-converting enzyme inhibitor. J Perinatol 2002;22:582–4.
13. Polifka JE. Is there an embryopathy associated with first-trimester exposure to angiotensin-converting enzyme inhibitors and angiotensin receptor antagonists? A critical review of the evidence. Birth Defects Res (Part A) 2012;94:576–98.
14. Kaiser G, Ackerman R, Dieterle W, Fleiss PM. Benazepril and benazeprilat in human plasma and breast milk (abstract). Eur J Clin Pharmacol 1989;36(Suppl):A303. As cited by National Library of Medicine LactMed database, September 7, 2013.

BENDAMUSTINE

Antineoplastic (Alkylating Agent)

PREGNANCY RECOMMENDATION: Contraindicated—1st Trimester
BREASTFEEDING RECOMMENDATION: Contraindicated

PREGNANCY SUMMARY

No reports describing the use of the alkylating antineoplastic agent bendamustine in human pregnancy have been located. Other agents in this class (see below) are known to cause human teratogenicity and, combined with the animal data strongly suggest that bendamustine should not be given in the 1st trimester. If a woman is inadvertently exposed to the drug during the 1st trimester, she should be informed of the potential risk.

FETAL RISK SUMMARY

Bendamustine is an alkylating antineoplastic agent that is a bifunctional mechlorethamine derivative given by IV infusion. It is in the same subclass of antineoplastics as busulfan, chlorambucil, cyclophosphamide, carmustine, dacarbazine, ifosfamide, mechlorethamine, melphalan, and streptozocin. Bendamustine is indicated for the treatment of patients with chronic lymphocytic leukemia. It also is indicated for indolent B-cell non-Hodgkin's lymphoma that has progressed during or within 6 months of treatment with rituximab or a rituximab-containing regimen. Bendamustine is metabolized to two minor active metabolites (M3 and M4) that have low plasma concentrations (10% and 1% of the parent compound concentrations, respectively). Plasma protein binding of bendamustine is 94%–96%. The elimination half-lives of the parent compound and the two active metabolites are about 40 minutes, 3 hours, and 30 minutes, respectively (1).

Reproduction studies have been conducted in mice and rats. In mice, an intraperitoneal dose about 2.1 times the recommended human dose based on BSA (RHD) given during organogenesis caused an increase in resorptions, decreased fetal body weights, and skeletal and visceral malformations (exencephaly, cleft palates, accessory rib, and spinal deformities). The dose did not cause apparent maternal toxicity. Repeat intraperitoneal dosing on gestational days 7–11 resulted in increased resorptions and similar malformations. In rats, intraperitoneal doses about 1.2 times the RHD given 5 times during gestational days 4–13 caused embryo and fetal death. A significant increase also was observed in external (effect on tail, head, and herniation of external organs [exomphalos]) and internal (hydronephrosis and hydrocephalus) malformations (1).

Bendamustine was carcinogenic in mice, producing peritoneal sarcomas in females after 4 days of intraperitoneal injections and mammary carcinomas and pulmonary adenomas after 4 days of oral dosing. The drug also was mutagenic and clastogenic in several assays. In human males, impaired spermatogenesis, azoospermia, and total germinal aplasia have been reported after treatment with other alkylating agents and might occur with bendamustine (1).

Although it is apparent that bendamustine crosses the placenta in animals, it is not known if it or the active metabolites cross the human placenta. The molecular weight of the parent compound (about 359 for the free base) is low enough for passage, but the short elimination half-life combined with high plasma protein binding should reduce the amount transferred to the embryo or fetus. A similar conclusion can be reached for M4, which has a shorter half-life and a serum concentration that is only 1% of the parent compound's concentration. M3 has a longer half-life and its serum concentration is 10% of the parent compound's concentration.

Occupational exposure of the mother to antineoplastic agents during pregnancy may present a risk to the fetus.

A position statement from the National Study Commission on Cytotoxic Exposure and a research article involving some antineoplastic agents are presented in the monograph for cyclophosphamide. (See Cyclophosphamide.)

BREASTFEEDING SUMMARY

No reports describing the use of bendamustine during human lactation have been located. The molecular weight of the parent compound (about 359 for the free base) and the presence of two active metabolites suggest that excretion into breast milk will occur. Because of the potential for serious toxicity in a nursing infant, breastfeeding should be discontinued while the mother is receiving therapy. Pumping and discarding the milk for at least 24 hours after a dose should prevent exposure of the nursling.

Reference

1. Product information. Treanda. Cephalon, 2008–2009.

BENDROFLUMETHIAZIDE

Diuretic

PREGNANCY RECOMMENDATION: Limited Human Data—Probably Compatible
BREASTFEEDING RECOMMENDATION: No Human Data—Probably Compatible

PREGNANCY SUMMARY

The available pregnancy experience with bendroflumethiazide is limited. Nevertheless, the published experience with 1st trimester use of thiazides and related diuretics does not indicate these agents are teratogenic. One large study (the Collaborative Perinatal Project) did find an increased risk of defects when diuretics were used during the 1st trimester in women with cardiovascular disorders, but causal relationships cannot be inferred from these data without independent confirmation. (See Chlorothiazide.) Diuretics are not recommended for the treatment of gestational hypertension because of the maternal hypovolemia characteristic of this disease. Other risks to the fetus or newborn include hypoglycemia, thrombocytopenia, hyponatremia, hypokalemia, and death from maternal complications. Moreover, thiazide diuretics may have a direct effect on smooth muscle and inhibit labor.

FETAL RISK SUMMARY

Bendroflumethiazide is a thiazide diuretic. Animal reproduction studies during the period of organogenesis have not been conducted with this agent.

In a study reported in 1964, 1011 women received bendroflumethiazide, 5 mg/day, from 30 weeks' gestation until delivery in an attempt to prevent preeclampsia and eclampsia (1). No fetal adverse effects were noted.

See Chlorothiazide for other reports of the clinical use of thiazide diuretics in pregnancy and the potential fetal and newborn toxicity of these agents.

BREASTFEEDING SUMMARY

Bendroflumethiazide has been used to suppress lactation (see Chlorothiazide) (2). The American Academy of Pediatrics classifies bendroflumethiazide as compatible with breastfeeding (3).

References

1. Cuadros A, Tatum HJ. The prophylactic and therapeutic use of bendroflumethiazide in pregnancy. Am J Obstet Gynecol 1964;89:891–7.
2. Healy M. Suppressing lactation with oral diuretics. Lancet 1961;1:1353–4.
3. Committee on Drugs, American Academy of Pediatrics. The transfer of drugs and other chemicals into human milk. Pediatrics 2001;108:776–89.

BENZOCAINE

Local Anesthetic

PREGNANCY RECOMMENDATION: Limited Human Data—Probably Compatible
BREASTFEEDING RECOMMENDATION: No Human Data—Probably Compatible

PREGNANCY SUMMARY

Only one source has described the use of benzocaine in human pregnancy and there are no animal reproduction studies. Systemic absorption may occur from mucous membranes or from damaged skin with the amount absorbed dependent on the administered dose. There are about 50 over-the-counter (OTC) products that contain benzocaine, a number suggesting wide use of this anesthetic. There is no evidence that topical use of this drug class is associated with any aspect of developmental toxicity. Nevertheless, the best course is to avoid use of benzocaine on mucous membranes or damaged skin during pregnancy.

B

FETAL RISK SUMMARY

Benzocaine (ethyl aminobenzoate) is a topical local anesthetic that is indicated for various purposes such as pruritic dermatoses, pruritus, minor burns, insect bites, toothache, and minor sore throat pain. Systemic absorption is poor from intact skin but it is well absorbed from mucous membranes and traumatized skin. It is metabolized, primarily by cholinesterase in plasma, to inactive metabolites. The agent is available OTC in formulations for oral and topical sprays, solutions, lozenges, creams, and gels (1).

Reproduction studies in animals have not been conducted.

It is not known if benzocaine crosses the human placenta. The molecular weight (about 165) is low enough that exposure of the embryo or fetus, if absorption has occurred, should be expected. However, appropriate clinical use should minimize any exposure.

The Collaborative Perinatal Project monitored 50,282 mother–child pairs, 47 of whom had exposure to benzocaine during the 1st trimester (2, pp. 357–363). No evidence of an association with large classes of malformations was found. For use anytime during pregnancy, 238 exposures were recorded (2, p. 440). From these data, no evidence of an association with large categories of major or minor malformations or to individual defects was found. These results were also cited in a 1988 review of anesthetic agents (3).

BREASTFEEDING SUMMARY

No reports describing the use of benzocaine during breastfeeding have been located. Although the molecular weight (about 165) is low enough for excretion into breast milk, systemic absorption is poor from intact skin. However, the anesthetic is well absorbed from mucous membranes and traumatized skin and use of agent on these surfaces should be avoided or kept to minimum during breastfeeding.

References

1. Product information. Benzocaine. Merck Manual Professional, 2007. Available at http://www.merck.com/mmpe/print/lexicomp/benzocaine.html. Accessed January 27, 2011.
2. Heinonen OP, Slone D, Shapiro S. *Birth Defects and Drugs in Pregnancy*. Littleton, MA: Publishing Sciences Group, 1977.
3. Friedman JM. Teratogen update: anesthetic agents. Teratology 1988;37: 69–77.

BENZPHETAMINE

Anorexiant

PREGNANCY RECOMMENDATION: Contraindicated
BREASTFEEDING RECOMMENDATION: Contraindicated

PREGNANCY SUMMARY

No reports describing the use of benzphetamine in human pregnancy have been located. There are no animal reproductive data, but because of its close relationship to amphetamines, the manufacturer classes the drug as contraindicated during pregnancy. Although this drug should not be used in pregnancy, inadvertent exposure to benzphetamine does not appear to represent a significant risk to the embryo or fetus (see Amphetamines).

FETAL RISK SUMMARY

The sympathomimetic amine, benzphetamine, is chemically and pharmacologically related to the amphetamines. The primary pharmacologic actions include CNS stimulation and elevation of blood pressure. The drug is contraindicated in patients with moderate to severe hypertension and several other conditions. Benzphetamine is indicated in the management of obesity in combination with a regimen of weight reduction based on caloric restriction. As with all agents in this class, tolerance and tachyphylaxis may develop. Animal reproduction studies have not been conducted (1).

It is not known if benzphetamine crosses the human placenta to the fetus. The relatively low molecular weight (about 276), however, suggests that exposure of the embryo–fetus will occur.

BREASTFEEDING SUMMARY

No reports describing the use of benzphetamine during lactation have been located. The relatively low molecular weight (about 276) suggests that the drug will be excreted in breast milk. The effects on a nursing infant from exposure via the milk are unknown, but there is potential for severe toxicity. Benzphetamine is chemically and pharmacologically related to the amphetamines. As such, it is contraindicated during nursing. (See Amphetamines.)

Reference

1. Product information. Didrex. Pharmacia, 2000.

BENZTHIAZIDE

Diuretic

See Chlorothiazide.

B

BENZTROPINE

Parasympatholytic

PREGNANCY RECOMMENDATION: Limited Human Data—Probably Compatible
BREASTFEEDING RECOMMENDATION: No Human Data—Probably Compatible

PREGNANCY SUMMARY

One surveillance study found a possible association between benztropine and cardiovascular defects, but confirmation is required. Exposure near term has been associated with paralytic ileus in the newborn.

FETAL RISK SUMMARY

Benztropine is an anticholinergic agent structurally related to atropine (see also Atropine). It also has antihistaminic activity. In a large prospective study, 2323 patients were exposed to this class of drugs during the 1st trimester, 4 of whom took benztropine (1). A possible association was found in the total group with minor, but not major, malformations.

In a surveillance study of Michigan Medicaid recipients involving 229,101 completed pregnancies conducted between 1985 and 1992, 84 newborns had been exposed to benztropine during the 1st trimester (F. Rosa, personal communication, FDA, 1993). Four (4.8%) major birth defects were observed (three expected), three of which were cardiovascular defects (one expected). No anomalies were observed in five other categories of defects (oral clefts, spina bifida, polydactyly, limb reduction defects, and hypospadias) for which specific data were available. Based on a small number of exposures, a possible association is suggested with cardiovascular defects.

Paralytic ileus has been observed in two newborns exposed to chlorpromazine and benztropine at term (2). In one of these infants, other anticholinergic drugs may have contributed to the effect (see Doxepin). The small left colon syndrome was characterized by decreased intestinal motility, abdominal distention, vomiting, and failure to pass meconium. The condition cleared rapidly in both infants after a Gastrografin enema.

A 2008 case report described a 25-year-old pregnant woman who was under treatment for bipolar disorder with lithium carbonate (500 mg twice daily), haloperidol (5 mg twice daily), and benzotropine (2 mg twice daily) (3). Her pregnancy was normal until the last 2 weeks when she began to lose weight and developed hypertension. At 39 weeks, a cesarean section delivered a 2.500-kg male infant with Apgar scores of 9 and 10 at 1 and 5 minutes, respectively. Both the infant and placental weights were below the mean for the population. In addition, the maternal plasma concentrations of phosphatidylcholine and free choline were also below the population means in the 3rd trimester. Because these nutrients are important in pregnancy, the authors speculated that one of her drugs, most likely lithium, was the cause of the low birth and placenta weights (3).

BREASTFEEDING SUMMARY

No reports describing the use of benztropine during human lactation have been located. In general, however, agents in this class are probably compatible with breastfeeding. (See Atropine.)

References

1. Heinonen OP, Slone D, Shapiro S. *Birth Defects and Drugs in Pregnancy*. Littleton, MA: Publishing Sciences Group, 1977:346–53.
2. Falterman CG, Richardson CJ. Small left colon syndrome associated with maternal ingestion of psychotropic drugs. J Pediatr 1980;97:308–10.
3. Gossell-Williams M, Fletcher H, Zeisel SH. Unexpected depletion in plasma choline and phosphatidylcholine concentrations in a pregnant woman with bipolar affective disorder being treated with lithium, haloperidol and benzotropine: a case report. J Med Case Rep 2008;2:55. doi:10.1186/1752-1947-2-55.

BENZYL ALCOHOL

Pediculicide/Anti-infective

PREGNANCY RECOMMENDATION: Limited Human Data—Probably Compatible (Topical) Contraindicated (Injectable)
BREASTFEEDING RECOMMENDATION: No Human Data—Probably Compatible (Topical) Contraindicated (Injectable)

PREGNANCY SUMMARY

Benzyl alcohol is used topically for head lice and as a bacteriostatic preservative in injectable solutions and other drug formulations. The animal reproduction data suggest low risk, but there is only one report describing its use as a preservative in a drug during human pregnancy and none as a pediculicide. Although a dose–response relationship has not been established, it is doubtful if sufficient benzyl alcohol would be absorbed from topical application to cause embryo–fetal toxicity. Thus, the embryo–fetal risk from topical use appears to be low, if it exists at all. The embryo–fetal risk from benzyl alcohol-preserved injectable products given to a pregnant woman is unknown. However, the plasma concentrations of the agent will be much higher than that obtained from topical use, so the safest course is to avoid injectable products, especially IV fluids, containing benzyl alcohol during pregnancy.

FETAL RISK SUMMARY

Benzyl alcohol is a pediculicide that is available as a 5% lotion. It is also used as a preservative in some injectable fluids and in multidose vials. As a lotion, it is indicated for the topical treatment of head lice infestation in patients 6 months of age and older. Treatment is repeated in 7 days. Small amounts of the drug were absorbed in 4 of 19 subjects when an exaggerated exposure period (3 times the normal exposure period) was used. Plasma concentrations in three subjects (6 months–3 years age group) at 0.5 hour posttreatment were 1.97–2.99 mcg/mL, whereas one subject in the 4–11 year age group 1 hour after treatment had a concentration of 1.63 mcg/mL (1). Benzyl alcohol is rapidly oxidized to benzoic acid and then conjugated in the liver with glycine to form hippuric acid (2). No information on the plasma protein binding, pK_a, or elimination half-life has been located.

Comparisons between animal and human exposures could not be conducted because of the low systemic exposures in humans. Consequently, SC injections were given to pregnant rats and rabbits in doses that were 100–500 and 100–400 mg/kg, respectively. No teratogenic effects were noted in either species, but maternal toxicity was observed at the highest doses.

The carcinogenic potential of the lotion in animals has not been evaluated. However, no evidence of carcinogenic activity was observed in oral 2-year high dose studies in rats and mice. Mutagenic studies have revealed positive and negative findings. Fertility studies have not been conducted (1).

It is not known if benzyl alcohol crosses the human placenta. The molecular weight (about 108) is low enough, but the plasma concentrations are very low even after a higher than normal exposure period with the lotion.

A 1977 report described a postpartum woman with severe flaccid paraplegia that was thought to be due to benzyl alcohol. One hour after delivery, normal saline (40 mL) containing 1.5% benzyl alcohol as a preservative had been inadvertently injected into an epidural catheter. The neurologic symptoms gradually improved over the next 16 months (3).

Beginning in pregnancy, a 22-year-old woman who was homozygous for factor V Leiden was treated with dalteparin injections from a multidose vial that contained benzyl alcohol (4). In the fifth month of pregnancy, the physician became aware of the exposure and changed to a dalteparin formulation without the preservative. No toxicity was observed and 4 months later the woman gave birth to a healthy infant (no other details provided) (4).

BREASTFEEDING SUMMARY

No reports describing exposure to benzyl alcohol during lactation have been located. The molecular weight (about 108) is low enough for excretion into milk, but the plasma concentrations after topical use of the lotion are very low, if at all. Higher plasma concentrations should be expected if the mother has an IV catheter requiring flushes with benzyl alcohol preserved fluids or is receiving injections from multidose vials containing the preservative. Premature infants and term neonates typically have immature liver function and may not be able to conjugate benzoic acid, the initial metabolite, to hippuric acid, resulting in metabolic acidosis (2). However, although a dose–response relationship has not been determined, it appears unlikely that a nursing infant's exposure to benzyl alcohol from breast milk would be high enough to cause toxicity.

References

1. Product information. Ulesfia. Shionogi Pharma, 2010.
2. Centers for Disease Control and Prevention. Neonatal deaths associated with use of benzyl alcohol—United States. MMWR 1982;31:290–1.
3. Craig DB, Habib GG. Flaccid paraparesis following obstetrical epidural anesthesia: possible role of benzyl alcohol. Anesth Analg 1977;56:219–21.
4. Moll S. A low-molecular-weight heparin preparation contraindicated during pregnancy. Am J Obstet Gynecol 2001;184:1046.

BEPOTASTINE

Ophthalmic (Antihistamine)

PREGNANCY RECOMMENDATION: No Human Data—Probably Compatible
BREASTFEEDING RECOMMENDATION: No Human Data—Probably Compatible

PREGNANCY SUMMARY

No reports describing the use of bepotastine in human pregnancy have been located. The animal data suggest low risk. The systemic bioavailability is very low from ocular use; in addition, H_1-receptor antihistamines are considered low risk in pregnancy. Although human pregnancy experience is needed, the drug probably is compatible in pregnancy.

B

FETAL RISK SUMMARY

Bepotastine is a histamine H_1-receptor antagonist and inhibitor of the release of histamine from mast cells. It is indicated for the treatment of itching associated with allergic conjunctivitis. The product is available as a 1.5% solution with each milliliter containing 15 mg of bepotastine besilate (equivalent to 10.7 mg of bepotastine). The systemic absorption is minimal. In healthy adults, one drop of solution in both eyes 4 times daily for 7 days produced a peak plasma concentration of 7.3 ng/mL 1–2 hours after instillation. The elimination half-life apparently has not been determined, but plasma levels were below the quantifiable limit (2 ng/mL) at 24 hours. Metabolism also is minimal as about 75%–90% is excreted unchanged in the urine. Plasma protein binding is moderate (about 55%) (1).

Reproduction studies have been conducted with oral doses in rats and rabbits. During organogenesis and fetal development in rats, doses up to about 3300 times the systemic concentrations anticipated for topical ocular use in humans (SCH) were not teratogenic. At a dose 5 times higher, there was potential for causing skeletal abnormalities. When this higher dose was given during the perinatal and lactation periods, an increase in stillbirths and decreased growth and development were observed in rat pups. The no-observed-effect level was about 1650 times the SCH. In rabbits during organogenesis and fetal development, doses >13,000 times the human dose based on body weight were not teratogenic (1).

Bepotastine did not significantly induce neoplasms in mice or rats in long-term studies. There also was no evidence of genotoxicity in multiple assays. There was a slight reduction in fertility index and surviving fetuses when a dose much higher than 3300 times the SCH was given to male and female rats. Infertility was not seen when the dose was lowered to 3300 times the SCH (1).

It is not known if bepotastine crosses the human placenta. The molecular weight (about 389 for free acid) and moderate plasma protein binding suggest that the drug will cross to the embryo–fetus. However, the minimal systemic bioavailability suggests that the exposure will be clinically insignificant.

BREASTFEEDING SUMMARY

No reports describing the use of bepotastine during human lactation have been located. The molecular weight (about 389 for free acid) and moderate plasma protein binding suggest that the drug will be excreted into breast milk. However, the minimal systemic bioavailability suggests that any exposure of a nursing infant will be clinically insignificant.

Reference

1. Product information. Bepreve. ISTA Pharmaceuticals, 2009.

BEPRIDIL

[Withdrawn from the market. See 9th edition.]

BESIFLOXACIN

Ophthalmic (Anti-infective)

PREGNANCY RECOMMENDATION: No Human Data—Animal Data Suggest Low Risk
BREASTFEEDING RECOMMENDATION: No Human Data—Probably Compatible

PREGNANCY SUMMARY

No reports describing the use of besifloxacin in human pregnancy have been located. The animal data suggest low risk. Because the systemic bioavailability of the antibiotic is very low, the risk to the embryo or fetus also appears to be low.

FETAL RISK SUMMARY

Besifloxacin ophthalmic suspension is a quinolone antimicrobial that is indicated for the treatment of bacterial conjunctivitis caused by susceptible bacteria. Besifloxacin is in the same subclass of ophthalmic antibiotics as ciprofloxacin, gatifloxacin, levofloxacin, moxifloxacin, norfloxacin, and ofloxacin. Systemic absorption is minimal. Maximum plasma concentrations after bilateral dosing 3 times daily for 16 doses were <1.3 ng/mL (mean 0.43 ng/mL). The average elimination half-life in plasma was about 7 hours (1).

Reproduction studies using oral besifloxacin have been conducted in rats. No skeletal or visceral malformations were observed in fetuses with doses producing maternal plasma concentrations that were >45,000 times the mean plasma concentrations measured in humans (PCH). Increased post-implantation loss, decreased fetal weights, and decreased fetal ossification were noted, but these doses also produced maternal toxicity (reduced body weight gain and food consumption) and mortality. The no-observed-effect level (NOEL) was >11,000 times the PCH. The NOEL also was the same in a prenatal and postnatal development study in rats (1).

B

Long-term studies in animals for carcinogenicity have not been conducted. The drug was not mutagenic in one test but, similar to other quinolones, was mutagenic in another test. The drug also induced chromosomal aberrations. No impairment of fertility in male and female rats was observed with oral doses that were >10,000 times the daily human ophthalmic dose (1).

It is not known if besifloxacin crosses the human placenta. The molecular weight (about 394 for the free base) and long plasma elimination half-life suggest that the drug will cross to the embryo–fetus. However, the minimal plasma concentrations suggest that the exposure will not be clinically significant.

BREASTFEEDING SUMMARY

No reports describing the use of besifloxacin during human lactation have been located. The molecular weight (about 394 for the free base) and long plasma elimination half-life (7 hours) suggest the drug will be excreted into breast milk. However, the maximum plasma concentrations (<1.3 ng/mL) suggest that exposure of a nursing infant will be clinically insignificant.

Reference

1. Product information. Besivance. Bausch & Lomb, 2009.

β-CAROTENE

Vitamin

PREGNANCY RECOMMENDATION: Compatible
BREASTFEEDING RECOMMENDATION: Compatible

PREGNANCY SUMMARY

There is no known embryo–fetal risk from the use of this vitamin in pregnancy.

FETAL RISK SUMMARY

β-Carotene, a natural precursor to vitamin A found in green and yellow vegetables as well as being commercially available, is partially converted in the small intestine to vitamin A (1). Even with therapeutic doses of the drug, serum levels of vitamin A do not rise above normal. Studies in animals have failed to show a teratogenic effect (see also Vitamin A) (2).

A single case describing the therapeutic use of this vitamin in human pregnancy has been located. A 35-year-old woman at 6.5 weeks' gestation was seen because of her daily intake of 180 mg (300,000 IU) of β-carotene for the past year for the treatment of skin lesions of porphyria (3). She had stopped taking the vitamin at 4.5 weeks' gestation because of the pregnancy, but her skin still had a yellow-orange tinge. Serum levels of β-carotene and retinol (vitamin A) were determined 2 weeks after her last dose. The β-carotene level was markedly elevated (0.403 mg/dL; normal 0.05–0.2 mg/dL) whereas the retinol concentration was low normal (0.069 mg/dL; normal 0.05–0.2 mg/dL) (3). At 18 weeks' gestation, her β-carotene level had fallen to 0.22 mg/dL. She delivered a healthy, normal-appearing, 3910-g male infant without skin discoloration at term. The infant was developing normally at 6 weeks of age.

BREASTFEEDING SUMMARY

Although there are no reports describing the use of β-carotene during human lactation, this vitamin is considered to be compatible with breastfeeding (see also Vitamin A).

References

1. American Hospital Formulary Service. *Drug Information 1997*. Bethesda, MD: American Society of Health-System Pharmacists, 1997:2806–7.
2. Nishimura H, Tanimura T. *Clinical Aspects of the Teratogenicity of Drugs*. New York, NY: American Elsevier, 1978:252.
3. Polifka JE, Dolan CR, Donlan MA, Friedman JM. Clinical teratology counseling and consultation report: high dose β-carotene use during early pregnancy. Teratology 1996;54:103–7.

BETAMETHASONE

Corticosteroid

PREGNANCY RECOMMENDATION: Compatible—Maternal Benefit >> Embryo–Fetal Risk
BREASTFEEDING RECOMMENDATION: No Human Data—Probably Compatible

PREGNANCY SUMMARY

Although no reports linking the use of betamethasone with birth defects have been located, four large epidemiologic studies have associated the use of corticosteroids during the 1st trimester with orofacial clefts. Betamethasone was not specifically identified in these studies, but only one study listed the corticosteroids used (see Hydrocortisone for details).

B

FETAL RISK SUMMARY

Betamethasone is often used in patients with premature labor at about 26–34 weeks' gestation to stimulate fetal lung maturation (1–15). The benefits of this therapy are as follows:

- Reduction in incidence of respiratory distress syndrome (RDS)
- Decreased severity of RDS if it occurs
- Decreased incidence of, and mortality from, intracranial hemorrhage
- Increased survival of premature infants

Betamethasone crosses the placenta to the fetus (16). The drug is partially metabolized (47%) by the perfused placenta to its inactive 11-ketosteroid derivative but less so than other corticosteroids, although the differences are not statistically significant (17).

In patients with premature rupture of the membranes (PROM), administration of betamethasone to the mother does not always reduce the frequency of RDS or perinatal mortality (18–22). An increased risk of maternal infection has also been observed in patients with PROM treated with corticosteroids (19,20). In a study comparing betamethasone therapy with nonsteroidal management of women with PROM, neonatal sepsis was observed in 23% (5 of 22) of steroid-exposed newborns vs. only 2% (1 of 46) of the non–steroid-exposed group (21). A 1985 study also found increased neonatal sepsis in exposed newborns who were delivered >48 hours after PROM, 18.6% (14 of 75) vs. 7.4% (4 of 54) of nonexposed controls (22). In addition, moderate to severe respiratory morbidity was increased over that in controls, 21.3% vs. 11.1%, as well as overall mortality, 8% vs. 1.8% (22). Other reports, however, have noted beneficial effects of betamethasone administration to patients with PROM with no increase in infectious morbidity (15,23,24). In women colonized with group B streptococci, the combined use of betamethasone and ampicillin improved the outcome of preterm pregnancies with PROM (25).

Betamethasone therapy is less effective in decreasing the incidence of RDS in male infants than in female infants (23,26,27). The reasons for this difference have not been discovered. Slower lung maturation in male fetuses has been cited as a major contributing factor to the sex differential noted in neonatal mortality (28). Therapy is also less effective in multiple pregnancies (27,29), even when doses have been doubled (27). In twins, only the first-born seems to benefit from antenatal steroid therapy (27).

An increased incidence of hypoglycemia in newborns exposed in utero to betamethasone has been reported (30). Although other investigators have not observed this effect, maternal betamethasone-induced hyperglycemia is a possible explanation if the drug was given shortly before delivery.

In the initial study examining the effect of betamethasone on RDS, investigators reported an increased risk of fetal death in patients with severe preeclampsia (1). They proposed that the corticosteroid had an adverse effect on placentas already damaged by vascular disease. A second study did not confirm these findings (7).

A case of suspected betamethasone-induced leukemoid reaction was observed in an 880-g female infant at 30 weeks' gestation whose mother received 12 mg of betamethasone 4 hours prior to delivery (31). A second case, in a female infant born at 25–26 weeks 71 hours after betamethasone, was published in 1997 (32). Within about 7–10 days, the white blood cell count had returned to normal in both infants. A 1984 study examined the effect of betamethasone on leukocyte counts in mothers with PROM or premature labor (33). No effect, as compared with untreated controls, was found in either group.

A case of acute, life-threatening exacerbation of muscular weakness requiring intubation and mechanical ventilation was reported in a 24-year-old woman who was treated with betamethasone, 12 mg IM, to enhance fetal lung maturity at 32 weeks' gestation (34). The onset of symptoms occurred 30 minutes after the corticosteroid dose. The authors attributed the crisis to betamethasone (adrenocorticosteroids are known to aggravate myasthenia) after other potential causes were ruled out. The infant was delivered by emergency cesarean section and, except for the typical problems related to prematurity, he had a normal hospital course.

Hypertensive crisis associated with the use of ritodrine and betamethasone has been reported (35). Systolic blood pressure was >300 mmHg with a diastolic pressure of 120 mmHg. Although the hypertension was probably caused by ritodrine, it is not known whether the corticosteroid was a contributing factor.

The effect of betamethasone administration on patent ductus arteriosus (PDA) was investigated in premature infants with a birth weight <2000 g (36). Infants of nontreated mothers had a PDA incidence of 44% vs. 6.5% for infants of treated mothers ($p < 0.01$). This reduction in the incidence of PDA after betamethasone therapy has also been observed in other studies (25). A study published in 1989 indicated that betamethasone caused transient, mild constriction of the ductus arteriosus (37). Eleven women with placenta previa with a mean gestational age of 31.7 weeks (range 27.3–37.3 weeks) were given two 12-mg IM doses of the drug, 24 hours apart, to promote fetal lung maturation. Fetal Doppler echocardiography of the ductus arteriosus was conducted just before the first dose then at 5 and 30 hours after the dose. Two of the fetuses showed mild constriction of the ductus 4–5 hours after the first injection, but the tests were normal when performed at 30 hours. No evidence of tricuspid regurgitation was observed (37). The authors concluded that the changes were probably not clinically significant.

A 1984 article discussed the potential benefits of combining thyroid hormones with corticosteroids to produce an additive or synergistic effect on fetal lung phosphatidylcholine synthesis (38). The therapy may offer advantages over corticosteroid therapy alone, but it is presently not possible because of the lack of commercially available thyroid stimulators that cross the placenta. The thyroid hormones, T4 and T3, are poorly transported across the placenta and thus would not be effective.

Five premature infants (three males and two females), exposed in utero to two 8-mg IM doses of betamethasone administered to the mother 48 and 24 hours before birth, were evaluated to determine the effect of the drug on endogenous progesterone, mineralocorticoid, and glucocorticoid activity (39). Plasma levels of the mineralocorticoids, aldosterone and 11-deoxycorticosterone, were not significantly decreased in the newborns at birth or during the next few days. Glucocorticoid activity in the newborns, as measured by levels of corticosterone, cortisol, cortisone, and 11-deoxycortisol, was significantly depressed at birth but rebounded above normal values when the subjects were 2 hours of age, then returned to normal ranges shortly after this time. Progesterone and 17-hydroxyprogesterone levels in the fetuses and neonates were not affected by betamethasone.

A 1994 case report described a pregnancy in which seven weekly courses (two 12.5-mg IM doses every 12 hours) of betamethasone were given between 24 weeks' gestation and delivery at 34.5 weeks (40). The 2625-g male infant had a "moon facies" appearance and a "buffalo hump" of apparent excess adipose deposition in the upper back. Tests in the mother and infant shortly after delivery were consistent with hypothalamic–pituitary–adrenal axis suppression with low basal serum cortisol levels (40). At 10 months of age, the infant's motor development and cognitive function were normal for age, length and head circumference were at the 20th percentile, and weight was slightly less than the 5th percentile. The cushingoid features had completely resolved (40). Two more recent reports have also described adrenal suppression in women secondary to multiple antenatal betamethasone courses (41,42), and in newborns exposed to ≥3 courses (43). A 1999 study, however, did not observe adrenal suppression in nine infants whose mothers had received a mean of 4.8 treatment courses of betamethasone (44).

Although human studies have usually shown a benefit, the use of corticosteroids in animals has been associated with several toxic effects (45,46):

- Reduced fetal head circumference
- Reduced fetal adrenal weight
- Increased fetal liver weight
- Reduced fetal thymus weight
- Reduced placental weight

None of these effects has been observed in human investigations with single courses of betamethasone. However, multiple courses of betamethasone have been associated with lower birth weights and reduced head circumference at birth (43,47,48).

In children born of mothers treated with betamethasone for premature labor, studies conducted at 4 and 6 years of age have found no differences from controls in cognitive and psychosocial development (49,50). Two studies published in 1990 evaluated children at 10–12 years of age who had been exposed in utero to betamethasone in a randomized, double-blind, placebo-controlled trial of the effects of the corticosteroid on fetal lung maturity (51,52). No differences were found between the exposed and placebo groups in terms of intellectual and motor development, school achievement, and social-emotional functioning (51). Concerning physical development, no differences between the groups were measured in terms of physical growth, neurologic and ophthalmologic development, and lung function (52). However, during the first few years of life the corticoid-exposed group had significantly more hospital admissions relating to infections than did those in the placebo group (52).

Studies conducted on very-low-birth-weight infants (500–1500 g) at 2 years of age indicated that, compared with nonexposed controls, exposed infants received antenatal betamethasone therapy that was associated with a significant improvement in survival, improved growth, and a decrease in early respiratory morbidity (53). Further study of the children at 5 years of age, but limited to those with birth weights of 500–999 g, found significantly improved survival but without significantly improved growth or decrease in early respiratory morbidity (54).

A study published in 1999 (55), with an accompanying editorial (54), reported a decrease in the incidence of cystic periventricular leukomalacia (PL) with prenatal betamethasone, but not with dexamethasone. Among 883 liveborn infants, with gestational ages ranging from 24 to 31 weeks, the rates of cystic PL in infants of mothers given betamethasone (N = 361), dexamethasone (N = 165), or no prenatal corticosteroids (N = 357) were 4.4%, 11.0%, and 8.4%, respectively. Cystic PL (necrosis of the white matter adjacent to the lateral ventricles resulting in the formation of cysts (56)) is the most frequent cause of cerebral palsy in premature infants (55).

A 1999 study reported a modest reduction in the risk of cerebral white matter damage (echolucency) and intraventricular hemorrhage (IVH) but a significant reduction in ventriculomegaly in premature infants weighing 500 to 1500 g (57). Significant reductions in the risk for echolucency and ventriculomegaly were seen in the gestationally youngest infants and in those with IVH, hypothyroxinemia, or vasculitis of the umbilical cord or chorionic plate of the placenta (57). In addition to this study, three other reports have also shown that the risk of IVH is reduced in preterm infants by the administration of antenatal betamethasone (58–60).

Another study on the reduction of PL with betamethasone appeared in 2001 (61). In 1161 neonates born at gestational ages of 24–34 weeks, 400 were exposed to antenatal betamethasone and 761 were not exposed (controls). The effects of antenatal betamethasone compared with controls were PL or IVH 23% vs. 31%, $p = 0.005$; PL with IVH 5% vs. 11%, $p = 0.001$; and isolated PL 3% vs. 7%, $p = 0.009$. The investigators concluded that antenatal betamethasone therapy was associated with a greater than 50% decrease in PL in preterm infants (61).

Among miscellaneous effects of antenatal betamethasone, decreased fetal heart rate variability has been demonstrated (62,63). In addition, a 1999 report described three newborns who developed various degrees of transient hypertrophic cardiomyopathy after multiple courses of antenatal betamethasone (64).

BREASTFEEDING SUMMARY

No reports describing the use of betamethasone during human lactation have been located. However, the molecular weights (about 435 for the acetate salt and about 517 for the sodium phosphate salt) are low enough that excretion into milk should be expected.

References

1. Liggins GC, Howie RN. A controlled trial of antepartum glucocorticoid treatment for prevention of the respiratory distress syndrome in premature infants. Pediatrics 1972;50:515–25.
2. Gluck L. Administration of corticosteroids to induce maturation of fetal lung. Am J Dis Child 1976;130:976–8.
3. Ballard RA, Ballard PL. Use of prenatal glucocorticoid therapy to prevent respiratory distress syndrome: a supporting view. Am J Dis Child 1976;130:982–7.

B

4. Mead PB, Clapp JF III. The use of betamethasone and timed delivery in management of premature rupture of the membranes in the preterm pregnancy. J Reprod Med 1977;19:3–7.
5. Block MF, Kling OR, Crosby WM. Antenatal glucocorticoid therapy for the prevention of respiratory distress syndrome in the premature infant. Obstet Gynecol 1977;50:186–90.
6. Ballard RA, Ballard PL, Granberg JP, Sniderman S. Prenatal administration of betamethasone for prevention of respiratory distress syndrome. J Pediatr 1979;94:97–101.
7. Nochimson DJ, Petrie RH. Glucocorticoid therapy for the induction of pulmonary maturity in severely hypertensive gravid women. Am J Obstet Gynecol 1979;133:449–51.
8. Eggers TR, Doyle LW, Pepperell RJ. Premature labour. Med J Aust 1979;1:213–6.
9. Doran TA, Swyer P, MacMurray B, Mahon W, Enhorning G, Bernstein A, Falk M, Wood MM. Results of a double-blind controlled study on the use of betamethasone in the prevention of respiratory distress syndrome. Am J Obstet Gynecol 1980;136:313–20.
10. Schutte MF, Treffers PE, Koppe JG, Breur W. The influence of betamethasone and orciprenaline on the incidence of respiratory distress syndrome in the newborn after preterm labour. Br J Obstet Gynaecol 1980;87:127–31.
11. Dillon WP, Egan EA. Aggressive obstetric management in late second-trimester deliveries. Obstet Gynecol 1981;58:685–90.
12. Johnson DE, Munson DP, Thompson TR. Effect of antenatal administration of betamethasone on hospital costs and survival of premature infants. Pediatrics 1981;68:633–7.
13. Bishop EH. Acceleration of fetal pulmonary maturity. Obstet Gynecol 1981;58(Suppl):48S–51S.
14. Ballard PL, Ballard RA. Corticosteroids and respiratory distress syndrome: status 1979. Pediatrics 1979;63:163–5.
15. Gamsu HR, Mullinger BM, Donnai P, Dash CH. Antenatal administration of betamethasone to prevent respiratory distress syndrome in preterm infants: report of a UK multicentre trial. Br J Obstet Gynaecol 1989;96:401–10.
16. Ballard PL, Granberg P, Ballard RA. Glucocorticoid levels in maternal and cord serum after prenatal betamethasone therapy to prevent respiratory distress syndrome. J Clin Invest 1975;56:1548–54.
17. Levitz M, Jansen V, Dancis J. The transfer and metabolism of corticosteroids in the perfused human placenta. Am J Obstet Gynecol 1978;132:363–6.
18. Eggers TR, Doyle LW, Pepperell RJ. Premature rupture of the membranes. Med J Aust 1979;1:209–13.
19. Garite TJ, Freeman RK, Linzey EM, Braly PS, Dorchester WL. Prospective randomized study of corticosteroids in the management of premature rupture of the membranes and the premature gestation. Am J Obstet Gynecol 1981;141:508–15.
20. Garite TJ. Premature rupture of the membranes: the enigma of the obstetrician. Am J Obstet Gynecol 1985;151:1001–5.
21. Nelson LH, Meis PJ, Hatjis CG, Ernest JM, Dillard R, Schey HM. Premature rupture of membranes: a prospective, randomized evaluation of steroids, latent phase, and expectant management. Obstet Gynecol 1985;66:55–8.
22. Simpson GF, Harbert GM Jr. Use of β-methasone in management of preterm gestation with premature rupture of membranes. Obstet Gynecol 1985;66:168–75.
23. Kuhn RJP, Speirs AL, Pepperell RJ, Eggers TR, Doyle LW, Hutchison A. Betamethasone, albuterol, and threatened premature delivery: benefits and risks. Obstet Gynecol 1982;60:403–8.
24. Schmidt PL, Sims ME, Strassner HT, Paul RH, Mueller E, McCart D. Effect of antepartum glucocorticoid administration upon neonatal respiratory distress syndrome and perinatal infection. Am J Obstet Gynecol 1984;148:178–86.
25. Morales WJ, Angel JL, O'Brien WF, Knuppel RA. Use of ampicillin and corticosteroids in premature rupture of membranes: a randomized study. Obstet Gynecol 1989;73:721–6.
26. Ballard PL, Ballard RA, Granberg JP, Sniderman S, Gluckman PD, Kaplan SL, Grumbach MM. Fetal sex and prenatal betamethasone therapy. J Pediatr 1980;97:451–4.
27. Avery ME, Aylward G, Creasy R, Little AB, Stripp B. Update on prenatal steroid for prevention of respiratory distress: report of a conference—September 26–28, 1985. Am J Obstet Gynecol 1986;155:2–5.
28. Khoury MJ, Marks JS, McCarthy BJ, Zaro SM. Factors affecting the sex differential in neonatal mortality: the role of respiratory distress syndrome. Am J Obstet Gynecol 1985;151:777–82.
29. Turrentine MA, Dupras-Wilson P, Wilkins IA. A retrospective analysis of the effect of antenatal steroid administration on the incidence of respiratory distress syndrome in preterm twin pregnancies. Am J Perinatol 1996;13:351–4.
30. Papageorgiou AN, Desgranges MF, Masson M, Colle E, Shatz R, Gelfand MM. The antenatal use of betamethasone in the prevention of respiratory distress syndrome: a controlled double-blind study. Pediatrics 1979;63:73–9.
31. Bielawski D, Hiatt IM, Hegyi T. Betamethasone-induced leukaemoid reaction in pre-term infant. Lancet 1978;1:218–9.
32. Hoff DS, Mammel MC. Suspected betamethasone-induced leukemoid reaction in a premature infant. Pharmacotherapy 1997;17:1031–4.
33. Ferguson JE, Hensleigh PA, Gill P. Effects of betamethasone on white blood cells in patients with premature rupture of the membranes and preterm labor. Am J Obstet Gynecol 1984;150:439–41.
34. Catanzarite VA, McHargue AM, Sandberg EC, Dyson DC. Respiratory arrest during therapy for premature labor in a patient with myasthenia gravis. Obstet Gynecol 1984;64:819–22.
35. Gonen R, Samberg I, Sharf M. Hypertensive crisis associated with ritodrine infusion and betamethasone administration in premature labor. Eur J Obstet Gynecol Reprod Biol 1982;13:129–32.
36. Waffarn F, Siassi B, Cabal LA, Schmidt PL. Effect of antenatal glucocorticoids on clinical closure of the ductus arteriosus. Am J Dis Child 1983;137:336–8.
37. Wasserstrum N, Huhta JC, Mari G, Sharif DS, Willis R, Neal NK. Betamethasone and the human fetal ductus arteriosus. Obstet Gynecol 1989;74:897–900.
38. Ballard PL. Combined hormonal treatment and lung maturation. Semin Perinatol 1984;8:283–92.
39. Dorr HG, Versmold HT, Sippell WG, Bidlingmaier F, Knorr D. Antenatal betamethasone therapy: effects on maternal, fetal, and neonatal mineralocorticoids, glucocorticoids, and progestins. J Pediatr 1986;108:990–3.
40. Bradley BS, Kumar SP, Mehta PN, Ezhuthachan SG. Neonatal cushingoid syndrome resulting from serial courses of antenatal betamethasone. Obstet Gynecol 1994;83:869–72.
41. McKenna DS, Wittber GM, Nagaraja HN, Samuels P. The effects of repeated doses of antenatal corticosteroids on maternal adrenal function. Am J Obstet Gynecol 2000;183:669–73.
42. Helal KJ, Gordon MC, Lightner CR, Barth WH Jr. Adrenal suppression induced by betamethasone in women at risk for premature delivery. Obstet Gynecol 2000;96:287–90.
43. Banks BA, Cnaan A, Morgan MA, Parer JT, Merrill JD, Ballard PL, Ballard RA, and the North American Thyrotropin-Releasing Hormone Study Group. Multiple courses of antenatal corticosteroids and outcome of premature neonates. Am J Obstet Gynecol 1999;181:709–17.
44. Terrone DA, Rinehart BK, Rhodes PG, Roberts WE, Miller RC, Martin JN Jr. Multiple courses of betamethasone to enhance fetal lung maturation do not suppress neonatal adrenal response. Am J Obstet Gynecol 1999;180:1349–53.
45. Taeusch HW Jr. Glucocorticoid prophylaxis for respiratory distress syndrome: a review of potential toxicity. J Pediatr 1975;87:617–23.
46. Johnson JWC, Mitzner W, London WT, Palmer AE, Scott R. Betamethasone and the rhesus fetus: multisystemic effects. Am J Obstet Gynecol 1979;133:677–84.
47. French NP, Hagan R, Evans SF, Godfrey M, Newnham JP. Repeated antenatal corticosteroids: size at birth and subsequent development. Am J Obstet Gynecol 1999;180:114–21.
48. Abbasi S, Hirsch D, Davis J, Tolosa J, Stouffer N, Debbs R, Gerdes JS. Effect of single versus multiple courses of antenatal corticosteroids on maternal and neonatal outcome. Am J Obstet Gynecol 2000;182:1243–9.
49. MacArthur BA, Howie RN, Dezoete JA, Elkins J. Cognitive and psychosocial development of 4-year-old children whose mothers were treated antenatally with betamethasone. Pediatrics 1981;68:638–43.
50. MacArthur BA, Howie RN, Dezoete JA, Elkins J. School progress and cognitive development of 6-year-old children whose mothers were treated antenatally with betamethasone. Pediatrics 1982;70:99–105.
51. Schmand B, Neuvel J, Smolders-de Haas H, Hoeks J, Treffers PE, Koppe JG. Psychological development of children who were treated antenatally with corticosteroids to prevent respiratory distress syndrome. Pediatrics 1990;86:58–64.
52. Smolders-de Haas H, Neuvel J, Schmand B, Treffers PE, Koppe JG, Hoeks J. Physical development and medical history of children who were treated antenatally with corticosteroids to prevent respiratory distress syndrome: a 10- to 12-year follow-up. Pediatrics 1990;85:65–70.
53. Doyle LW, Kitchen WH, Ford GW, Rickards AL, Lissenden JV, Ryan MM. Effects of antenatal steroid therapy on mortality and morbidity in very low birth weight infants. J Pediatr 1986;108:287–92.
54. Doyle LW, Kitchen WH, Ford GW, Rickards AL, Kelly EA. Antenatal steroid therapy and 5-year outcome of extremely low birth weight infants. Obstet Gynecol 1989;73:743–6.

55. Baud O, Foix-L'Helias L, Kaminski M, Audibert F, Jarreau PH, Papiernik E, Huon C, Leperco J, Dehan M, Lacaze-Masmonteil T. Antenatal glucocorticoid treatment and cystic periventricular leukomalacia in very premature infants. N Engl J Med 1999;341:1190–6.
56. Fanaroff AA, Hack M. Periventricular leukomalacia—prospects for prevention. N Engl J Med 1999;341:1229–31.
57. Leviton A, Dammann O, Allred EN, Kuban K, Pagano M, Van Marter L, Paneth N, Reuss ML, Susser M, for The Developmental Epidemiology Network Investigators. Antenatal corticosteroids and cranial ultrasonographic abnormalities. Am J Obstet Gynecol 1999;181:1007–17.
58. Ment LR, Oh W, Ehrenkranz RA, Philip AGS, Duncan CC, Makuch RW. Antenatal steroids, delicry mode, and intraventricular hemorrhage in preterm infants. Am J Obstet Gynecol 1995;172:795–800.
59. Garland JS, Buck R, Leviton A. Effect of maternal glucocorticoid exposure on risk of severe intraventricular hemorrhage in surfactant-treated preterm infants. J Pediatr 1995;126:272–9.
60. Chen B, Basil JB, Schefft GL, Cole FS, Sadovsky Y. Antenatal steroids and intraventricular hemorrhage after premature rupture of membranes at 24–28 weeks' gestation. Am J Perinatol 1997;14:171–6.
61. Canterino JC, Verma U, Visintainer PF, Elimian A, Klein SA, Tejani N. Antenatal steroids and neonatal periventricular leukomalacia. Obstet Gynecol 2001;97:135–9.
62. Ville Y, Vincent Y, Tordjman N, Hue MV, Fernandez H, Frydman R. Effect of betamethasone on the fetal heart rate pattern assessed by computerized cardiotocography in normal twin pregnancies. Fetal Diagn Ther 1995;10:301–6.
63. Senat MV, Minoui S, Multon O, Fernandez H, Frydman R, Ville Y. Effect of dexamethasone and betamethasone on fetal heart rate variability in preterm labour: a randomised study. Br J Obstet Gynaecol 1998;105:749–55.
64. Yunis KA, Bitar FF, Hayek P, Mroueh SM, Mikati M. Transient hypertrophic cardiomyopathy in the newborn following multiple doses of antenatal corticosteroids. Am J Perinatol 1999;16:17–21.

BETAXOLOL

Sympatholytic (Antihypertensive)

PREGNANCY RECOMMENDATION: Human Data Suggest Risk in 2nd and 3rd Trimesters
BREASTFEEDING RECOMMENDATION: Limited Human Data—Potential Toxicity

PREGNANCY SUMMARY

In one study, betaxolol was started in the 3rd trimester and no fetal harm was observed. Some β-blockers may cause intrauterine growth restriction (IUGR) and reduced placental weight, especially those lacking intrinsic sympathomimetic activity (ISA) (i.e., partial agonist). Treatment beginning early in the 2nd trimester results in the greatest weight reductions, whereas treatment restricted to the 3rd trimester primarily affects only placental weight. Betaxolol does not possess ISA. However, IUGR and reduced placental weight may potentially occur with all agents within this class. Although growth restriction is a serious concern, the benefits of maternal therapy with β-blockers, in some cases, might outweigh the risks to the fetus and must be judged on a case-by-case basis. If used near delivery, the newborn infant should be closely monitored for 24–48 hours for signs and symptoms of β-blockade. Long-term effects of in utero exposure to β-blockers have not been studied but warrant evaluation.

FETAL RISK SUMMARY

Betaxolol is a cardioselective β_1-adrenergic blocking agent used in the treatment of hypertension and topically in the therapy of glaucoma. Betaxolol is teratogenic in rats producing skeletal and visceral anomalies at maternally toxic doses (600 times the maximum recommended human dose [MRHD]) (1). At this dose, postimplantation loss and reduced litter size and weight were also noted. At doses 6 and 60 times the MRHD, a possible increased incidence of incomplete descent of testes and sternebral reductions were observed (1). No teratogenic effects were observed in rabbits, but an increase in postimplantation loss occurred at the highest dose tested (54 times the MRHD) (1).

Betaxolol rapidly crosses the human placenta (2–4). The mean fetal:maternal ratio at birth was 0.93. The half-life in newborns was 14.8–38.5 hours compared with that in the mothers of 15.6–22.1 hours (mean 19 hours) (2,3).

A 1990 report from France described the pregnancy outcomes of 22 women treated with betaxolol (10–40 mg/day) for mild to moderate hypertension (4). Treatment was begun at a mean of 30.7 weeks. The mean gestational age at birth was 37.2 weeks and the mean birth weight of the 23 neonates (1 set of twins) was 2.6 kg. One of the newborns was growth restricted (onset before betaxolol therapy) and five were premature. All were doing well at 9 months (4).

BREASTFEEDING SUMMARY

Betaxolol is excreted into human milk in quantities sufficient to produce β-blockade in a nursing infant (1). Although no reports have been located that describe the use of this agent during nursing, one study measured betaxolol concentrations in the milk of three mothers who had been treated with drug during pregnancy in the first 3 postpartum days (3). The last maternal dose had been taken 3–26 hours before delivery. The milk concentrations ranged from 3 to 48 ng/mL and the milk:plasma ratios ranged from 2.0 to 11.6, with the highest ratios occurring in one mother 48 and 72 hours after delivery. No mention was made if the mothers breastfed their infants

If betaxolol is used during nursing, the infant should be closely observed for hypotension, bradycardia, and other signs or symptoms of β-blockade. Long-term effects of exposure to β-blockers from milk have not been studied but warrant evaluation.

B

References

1. Product information. Kerlone. G.D. Searle & Co., 1997.
2. Morselli PL, Boutroy MJ, Bianchetti G, Thenot JP. Pharmacokinetics of antihypertensive drugs in the neonatal period. Dev Pharmacol Ther 1989;13:190–8.
3. Morselli PL, Boutroy MJ, Bianchetti G, Zipfel A, Boutroy JL, Vert P. Placental transfer and perinatal pharmacokinetics of betaxolol. Eur J Clin Pharmacol 1990;38:477–83.
4. Boutroy MJ, Morselli PL, Bianchetti G, Boutroy JL, Pepin L, Zipfel A. Betaxolol: a pilot study of its pharmacological and therapeutic properties in pregnancy. Eur J Clin Pharmacol 1990;38:535–9.

BETHANECHOL

Parasympathomimetic (Cholinergic)

PREGNANCY RECOMMENDATION: Limited Human Data—No Relevant Animal Data
BREASTFEEDING RECOMMENDATION: Limited Human Data—Potential Toxicity

PREGNANCY SUMMARY

Human pregnancy experience is too limited to assess the embryo–fetal risk.

FETAL RISK SUMMARY

Bethanechol is indicated for the treatment of nonobstructive urinary retention and neurogenic atony of the urinary bladder with retention. Reproduction studies in animals have not been conducted (1).

The use of bethanechol in human pregnancy has been reported, but too little data are available to analyze (2).

BREASTFEEDING SUMMARY

Specific data on the excretion of bethanechol into breast milk are lacking. The molecular weight (about 197) is low enough, however, that excretion into milk should be expected. One author cautioned that mothers receiving regular therapy with this drug should not breastfeed (3). Abdominal pain and diarrhea have been reported in a nursing infant exposed to bethanechol in milk (4).

References

1. Product information. Urecholine. Merck, 2000.
2. Heinonen OP, Slone D, Shapiro S. *Birth Defects and Drugs in Pregnancy*. Littleton, MA: Publishing Sciences Group, 1977:345–56.
3. Platzker ACD, Lew CD, Stewart D. Drug "administration" via breast milk. Hosp Pract 1980;15:111–22.
4. Shore MF. Drugs can be dangerous during pregnancy and lactations. Can Pharmaceut J 1970;103:358. As cited in: Committee on Drugs, American Academy of Pediatrics. The transfer of drugs and other chemicals into human breast milk. Pediatrics 1983;72:375–83.

BEVACIZUMAB

Antineoplastic

PREGNANCY RECOMMENDATION: Limited Human Data—Animal Data Suggest Moderate Risk
BREASTFEEDING RECOMMENDATION: No Human Data—Potential Toxicity

PREGNANCY SUMMARY

Six reports describing the use of bevacizumab in human pregnancy have been located. All of these reports involved intravitreal injections. Three of the exposures involved unknown pregnancies. The outcomes of the pregnancies were two spontaneous abortions and seven healthy, term infants. The animal reproduction data, although involving only one species, suggest risk. Angiogenesis is critical to fetal development (1), so the drug is best avoided in pregnancy (2). Because of the very long elimination half-life, it could take as long as 100 days (range 55–250 days) to eliminate 97% of the drug from the plasma. If a pregnant woman requires treatment with bevacizumab, she should be advised of the potential risks to the embryo–fetus that include growth restriction, structural anomalies, and death.

FETAL RISK SUMMARY

Bevacizumab is a recombinant humanized monoclonal IgG1 antibody. It is indicated, in combination with IV 5-fluorouracil-based chemotherapy, as first- or second-line treatment of patients with metastatic carcinoma of the colon or rectum. Bevacizumab binds and inhibits the histologic activity of human vascular endothelial growth factor (VEGF). This effect prevents the formation of new blood vessels (angiogenesis). The drug is given as an IV infusion every 2 weeks. The estimated elimination half-life is about 20 days (range 11–50 days) (1). No information is available on metabolism.

B

Reproduction studies have been conducted in rabbits. Doses that approximated the human dose based on body weight were associated with developmental toxicity, including reduced maternal and fetal body weights, an increased number of fetal resorptions, and an increased incidence of specific gross and fetal skeletal alterations. Adverse fetal outcomes were observed at all doses tested (1).

Carcinogenic and mutagenic studies have not been conducted with bevacizumab. Bevacizumab may impair fertility. Female cynomolgus monkeys were given doses that were equal to or 5 times the human 10 mg/kg dose for 13 or 26 weeks. Following recovery, dose-related decreases in ovarian and uterine weights, endometrial proliferation, number of menstrual cycles, and arrested follicular development or absent corpora lutea were observed (1).

It is not known if bevacizumab crosses the human placenta. Although antibodies are large molecules, the molecular weight of bevacizumab is about 149,000, some immune globulins are transported across the placenta to the embryo–fetus (e.g., see Immune Globulin Intravenous).

A brief 2009 report described the use of bevacizumab and verteporfin in a pregnant woman treated for choroidal neovascularization (CNV) secondary to punctate inner choroidopathy (3). She received photodynamic therapy with IV verteporfin about 1–2 weeks postconception. At 3-months postconception, she underwent intravitreal injection of 1.25 mg bevacizumab. The patient delivered a healthy infant at term with no evidence of congenital anomalies at birth or at 3-months of age (3).

A 2009 report described the use of intravitreal 1.25 mg bevacizumab in two early pregnancies, one at about 4 weeks in a 29-year-old and the other at about 3 weeks in a 25-year-old (4). Both pregnancies were spontaneously aborted 7 and 10 days, respectively, after the intravitreal injection. The authors cited a website stating that a 1.25-mg bevacizumab intravitreal injection achieves high systemic concentrations (100's ng/mL) and that blood levels have been detected for up to a month after injection (5). The authors speculated that the abortions resulted from the VEGF action of the drug (4).

In a 2010 case report, a woman with CNV received bevacizumab 1.25-mg intravitreal injection in both eyes, performed 1 week apart, and 6 weeks later, received a second 1.25-mg dose in the left eye (total dose 3.75 mg) (6). Three weeks later, she was diagnosed with a 5-week pregnancy. After an uneventful pregnancy, she gave birth at term to a healthy 3.17-kg female infant. No developmental abnormalities were observed in the infant who was doing well at 12 months of age (6).

Four pregnant women were treated with bevacizumab for CNV in a 2010 report (7). The women received a mean 2.6 injections (range 1–6) during pregnancy. All delivered healthy full-term infants who remained healthy with normal growth and development during infancy (7).

A 2012 report described the pregnancy outcome of a 35-year-old woman with CNV who was treated with bevacizumab (dose not specified) in her 7th gestational week (8). She delivered vaginally a healthy 3.75-kg male infant at term with Apgar scores of 10 and 10. The infant had no congenital anomalies and had normal visual behavior. His growth and development were normal in his first 12 months (8).

BREASTFEEDING SUMMARY

No reports describing the use of bevacizumab during human lactation have been located. Although antibodies are large molecules (the molecular weight of bevacizumab is about 149,000), some immune globulins are excreted into breast milk. Of importance, human IgG is excreted into milk (1). Therefore, the excretion into milk of the closely related bevacizumab should be expected. The effects of this exposure on a nursing infant are unknown, but the toxicity could be severe. Thus, the best course is to not breastfeed if the woman is receiving bevacizumab therapy.

References

1. Product information. Avastin. Genentech, 2007.
2. Kumar N, Sebastian R, Harding S, Pearce I. Bevacizumab: a word of caution. Can J Ophthalmol 2007;42:760–1.
3. Rosen E, Rubowitz A, Ferencz JR. Exposure to verteporfin and bevacizumab therapy for choroidal neovascularization secondary to punctate inner choroidopathy during pregnancy. Eye (Lond) 2009;23:1479.
4. Petrou P, Georgalas I, Giavaras G, Anastasiou E, Ntana Z, Petrou C. Early loss of pregnancy after intravitreal bevacizumab injection. Acta Ophthalmol 2010;88:e136.
5. Cousins SW. Safety surveillance in the anti-VEGF era: myths and misconceptions. Available at http://www.osnsupersite.com/view.aspx?rid=19510. Accessed May 9, 2010.
6. Wu Z, Huang J, Sadda S. Inadvertent use of bevacizumab to treat choroidal neovascularization during pregnancy: a case report. Ann Acad Med Singapore 2010;39:143–5.
7. Tarantola RM, Folk JC, Boldt HC, Mahajan VB. Intravitreal bevacizumab during pregnancy. Retina 2010;30:1405–11.
8. Introini U, Casalino G, Cardani A, Scotti F, Finardi A, Candiani M, Bandello F. Intravitreal bevacizumab for a subfoveal myopic choroidal neovascularization in the first trimester of pregnancy. J Ocul Pharmacol Ther 2012;28:553–5.

BEXAROTENE

Antineoplastic

PREGNANCY RECOMMENDATION: Contraindicated
BREASTFEEDING RECOMMENDATION: No Human Data—Potential Toxicity

PREGNANCY SUMMARY

Bexarotene is contraindicated in pregnancy. No reports describing its use during human pregnancy have been located. Pregnancy should be excluded and the use of effective contraception (two reliable forms used simultaneously) confirmed before bexarotene therapy is started in women of childbearing age. If these criteria are met, therapy should be initiated on

B

the 2nd or 3rd day of a normal menstrual cycle. The contraceptive methods should be used for 1 month before therapy, during therapy, and for 1 month after stopping therapy. The manufacturer also recommends that pregnancy tests be repeated monthly during treatment (1). In addition, male patients with sexual partners who are pregnant, possibly pregnant, or who could become pregnant, should use condoms during sexual intercourse during therapy and for 1 month after therapy has been stopped (1).

FETAL RISK SUMMARY

Bexarotene is a member of a subclass of retinoids that selectively binds and activates retinoid X receptor subtypes (RXRα, RXRβ, and RXRγ). These subtypes then interact with various receptor partners to function as transcription factors that regulate the expression of genes that control cellular differentiation and proliferation. Bexarotene is indicated for the treatment of refractory cutaneous manifestations of cutaneous T-cell lymphoma. Four active metabolites have been identified (1).

In reproduction studies with pregnant rats during organogenesis, an oral dose approximately one-third of the AUC in humans at the recommended dose (RHD) caused incomplete ossification (1). When a dose about 1.33 times the RHD was given, cleft palate, depressed eye bulge/microphthalmia, and small ears were observed. Doses higher than about 0.8 times the RHD caused embryo and fetal death. The no-effect dose was one-sixth the RHD (1). Studies on fertility and carcinogenicity have not been conducted, but tests for mutagenicity or clastogenicity were negative (1).

It is not known if bexarotene crosses the human placenta. The molecular weight (about 348) is low enough that transfer to the fetus should be expected.

BREASTFEEDING SUMMARY

No reports describing the use of bexarotene in human lactation have been located. The molecular weight (about 348) is low enough that excretion into breast milk should be expected. Because of the unknown amounts present in milk and the potential for serious adverse effects in a nursing infant, women receiving bexarotene should probably not breastfeed.

Reference

1. Product information. Targretin. Ligand Pharmaceuticals, 2001.

BIMATOPROST

Ophthalmic (Prostaglandin Agonist)

PREGNANCY RECOMMENDATION: No Human Data—Probably Compatible
BREASTFEEDING RECOMMENDATION: No Human Data—Probably Compatible

PREGNANCY SUMMARY

No reports describing the use of bimatoprost in human pregnancy have been located. The animal data suggest low risk, but the absence of human pregnancy experience prevents a more complete assessment of the embryo–fetal risk. However, clinically significant exposure of the embryo–fetus is unlikely and use of the drug in pregnancy is probably compatible.

FETAL RISK SUMMARY

Bimatoprost is a synthetic structural analog of prostaglandin with ocular hypotensive activity. It is given as one drop in the affected eye(s) once daily. It is in the same class of prostaglandin agonists as latanoprost, tafluprost, and travoprost. Bimatoprost is indicated for the reduction of elevated intraocular pressure in patients with open angle glaucoma or ocular hypertension. In healthy adults given one drop daily in each eye for 2 weeks, blood concentrations peaked (mean 0.08–0.09 ng/mL) at 10 minutes and were below the limit of detection (0.025 ng/mL) in most subjects at 1.5 hours after dosing. The drug is metabolized to apparently inactive metabolites. Plasma protein binding is about 88% and the elimination half-life, after an IV dose, was about 45 minutes (1). A similar elimination half-life appears to reflect the blood levels after ocular administration.

Reproduction studies have been conducted in mice and rats. In these species, abortion occurred at oral doses that were about 33 or 97 times, respectively, the maximum intended human exposure based on blood AUC (MIHE). At doses at least 41 times the MIHE, the gestation length was reduced, and the incidence of dead fetuses, late resorptions, perinatal and postnatal pup mortality was increased. In addition, pup body weights were decreased (1).

Carcinogenicity studies were negative in mice or rats given oral doses of bimatoprost. The drug was not mutagenic or clastogenic in multiple assays. No impairment of fertility was observed in male and female rats given oral doses up to about 103 times MIHE (1).

It is not known if bimatoprost crosses the human placenta. The molecular weight (about 416) and moderate plasma protein binding suggest that the drug will cross to the embryo–fetus. However, the short elimination half-life and the very low blood concentrations probably indicate that any exposure will not be clinically significant.

Prostaglandin F2a has been used for pregnancy termination in humans via intrauterine extra-amniotic infusion to treat missed abortion or intrauterine death. However, there is no evidence that at doses given to reduce elevated ophthalmic pressure, an increased risk for uterine contractions would be seen (see Latanoprost).

BREASTFEEDING SUMMARY

No reports describing the use of bimatoprost during human lactation have been located. The molecular weight (about 416) and moderate plasma protein binding (about 88%) suggest that the drug will be excreted into breast milk. However, the short elimination half-life (about 45 minutes) and the very low blood concentrations suggest that clinically significant exposure will not occur.

Reference

1. Product information. Lumigan. Allergan, 2012.

BIPERIDEN

[Withdrawn from the market. See 9th edition.]

BISACODYL

Gastrointestinal Agent (Laxative)

PREGNANCY RECOMMENDATION: No Human Data—Probably Compatible
BREASTFEEDING RECOMMENDATION: No Human Data—Probably Compatible

PREGNANCY SUMMARY

No reports describing the use of bisacodyl in animal or human pregnancy have been located. A 1984 reference found no reports of adverse effects in pregnancy (1). In addition, a 1985 review considered stimulant laxatives, such as bisacodyl, to be safe in pregnancy, but regular or chronic use should be avoided (2). Because only small amounts are in the systemic circulation, the direct embryo–fetal risk probably is nil.

FETAL RISK SUMMARY

Bisacodyl is a diphenylmethane stimulant laxative that is indicated for the treatment of constipation and for the evacuation of the bowel before diagnostic procedures or surgery (3). It is structurally and pharmacologically related to phenolphthalein (4). (See also Phenolphthalein.) Bisacodyl is available as oral tablets and suppositories. Bisacodyl is converted to its active metabolite in the gastrointestinal tract and acts primarily in the large intestine (3). Only minimal amounts (about 5%) are absorbed into the systemic circulation (3,4).

Animal reproduction studies with bisacodyl have not been located.

It is not known if bisacodyl crosses the human placenta. The molecular weight (about 361) is low enough for passive diffusion across the placenta, but the minimal amounts in the circulation suggest that neither the embryo nor fetus will have clinically significant exposure to the drug.

BREASTFEEDING SUMMARY

No reports describing the use of bisacodyl during human lactation have been located. Although the molecular weight (about 361) is low enough for excretion into milk, only minimal amounts (about 5%) are absorbed into the maternal circulation. The effects of this exposure on a nursing infant are unknown but appear to be negligible. Others have previously arrived at the same conclusion (5,6).

References

1. Onnis A, Grella P. *The Biochemical Effects of Drugs in Pregnancy*. Volume 2. Chichester, UK: Ellis Horwood Limited, 1984:48–9.
2. Lewis JH, Weingold AB, and The Committee on FDA-Related Matters, American College of Gastroenterology. The use of gastrointestinal drugs during pregnancy and lactation. Am J Gastroenterol 1985;80:912–23.
3. Parfitt K, ed. *Martindale. The Complete Drug Reference*. 32nd ed. London, UK: Pharmaceutical Press, 1999:1179.
4. Gattuso JM, Kamm MA. Adverse effects of drugs used in the management of constipation and diarrhoea. Drug Saf 1994;10:47–65.
5. Vorherr H. Drug excretion in breast milk. Postgrad Med 1974;56:97–104.
6. Anderson PO. Drug use during breast-feeding. Clin Pharm 1991;10:594–624.

BISMUTH SUBSALICYLATE

Antidiarrheal

PREGNANCY RECOMMENDATION: Human Data Suggest Low Risk
BREASTFEEDING RECOMMENDATION: No Human Data—Potential Toxicity

B

PREGNANCY SUMMARY

Inorganic bismuth salts, formed from metabolism of bismuth subsalicylate in the gastrointestinal tract, apparently present little or no risk to the fetus from normal therapeutic doses, but the data available for bismuth in pregnancy are poor and the actual fetal risk cannot be determined (1). On the other hand, the potential actions of salicylates on the fetus are complex. Although the risk for toxicity may be small, significant fetal adverse effects have resulted from chronic exposure to salicylates. Because of this, the use of bismuth subsalicylate during gestation should be restricted to the first half of pregnancy, and then only in amounts that do not exceed the recommended doses.

FETAL RISK SUMMARY

Bismuth subsalicylate (bismuth salicylate) is hydrolyzed in the gastrointestinal tract to bismuth salts and sodium salicylate (2,3). Two tablets or 30 mL suspension of the compound yields 204 mg and 258 mg, respectively, of salicylate. Inorganic bismuth salts, in contrast to organic complexes of bismuth, are relatively water-insoluble and poorly absorbed systemically, but significant absorption of salicylate does occur (2,3). A brief 1992 study found minimal absorption of bismuth (exact serum concentrations not specified) from bismuth subsalicylate in 12 healthy subjects as opposed to a peak serum level of 0.050 mcg/mL after a dose of 216 mg of colloidal bismuth subcitrate in a single patient (4). Some bismuth absorption was documented across the normal gastric mucosa, but the primary absorption occurred from the duodenum. Others believe, however, that the design of the study produced the observed results, and that bismuth absorption occurs only in the gastric antrum, not in the gastric body or duodenum (5).

Although absorption of inorganic bismuth salts is negligible, in a study of chronic administration of bismuth tartrate, 5 mg/kg/day, one of four lambs born of treated ewes was stunted, hairless, and exophthalmic, and a second was aborted (6). Moreover, in one case report, the use of an extemporaneously compounded antidiarrheal mixture containing bismuth subsalicylate was associated with bismuth encephalopathy in a 60-year-old man who took an unknown amount of the preparation for a period of 1 month (7). Encephalopathy was diagnosed by an electroencephalogram characteristic of bismuth toxicity and a blood bismuth level of 72 ng/mL (upper limit of normal is 5 ng/mL).

No reports of adverse fetal outcome after the use of commercially available bismuth subsalicylate have been located for humans. The Collaborative Perinatal Project recorded 15 1st trimester exposures to bismuth salts (bismuth subgallate $N = 13$, bismuth subcarbonate $N = 1$, and milk of bismuth $N = 1$), but none to bismuth subsalicylate (8, pp. 384–387). These numbers are small, but no evidence was found to suggest any association with congenital abnormalities. For use anytime during pregnancy, 144 mother–child pairs were exposed to bismuth subgallate and 5 of the in utero–exposed infants had inguinal hernia, a hospital standardized relative risk of 2.6 (8, pp. 442, 497). A causal relationship, however, cannot be determined from these data.

In contrast to bismuth, salicylate is rapidly absorbed with >90% of the dose recovered in the urine. Data on the use of salicylates in human pregnancy, primarily acetylsalicylic acid (aspirin), are extensive. The main concerns from exposure to this drug during pregnancy include congenital defects, increased perinatal mortality from premature closure of the ductus arteriosus in utero, intrauterine growth restriction, and salicylate intoxication (see Aspirin). An increased risk of intracranial hemorrhage in premature or low-birth-weight infants is a potential complication of aspirin exposure near delivery, but other salicylates, including sodium salicylate, probably do not present a risk because the presence of the acetyl moiety seems to be required to suppress platelet function (9–11).

BREASTFEEDING SUMMARY

The excretion of significant amounts of bismuth obtained from bismuth subsalicylate into breast milk is not expected because of the poor absorption of bismuth into the systemic circulation. Salicylates, however, are excreted in milk and are eliminated more slowly from milk than from plasma with milk:plasma ratios rising from 0.03 to 0.08 at 3 hours to 0.34 at 12 hours (12). Because of the potential for adverse effects in the nursing infant, the American Academy of Pediatrics recommends that salicylates should be used cautiously during breastfeeding (13). A review stated that bismuth subsalicylate should be avoided during lactation because of systemic salicylate absorption (14).

References

1. Friedman JM, Little BB, Brent RL, Cordero JF, Hanson JW, Shepard TH. Potential human teratogenicity of frequently prescribed drugs. Obstet Gynecol 1990;75:594–9.
2. Pickering LK, Feldman S, Ericsson CD, Cleary TG. Absorption of salicylate and bismuth from a bismuth subsalicylate-containing compound (Pepto-Bismol). J Pediatr 1981;99:654–6.
3. Feldman S, Chen S-L, Pickering LK, Cleary TG, Ericsson CD, Hulse M. Salicylate absorption from a bismuth subsalicylate preparation. Clin Pharmacol Ther 1981;29:788–92.
4. Menge H, Brosius B, Lang A, Gregor M. Bismuth absorption from the stomach and small intestine. Gastroenterology 1992;102:2192.
5. Nwokolo CU, Pounder RE. Bismuth absorption from the stomach and small intestine. Reply. Gastroenterology 1992;102:2192–3.
6. James LF, Lazar VA, Binns W. Effects of sublethal doses of certain minerals on pregnant ewes and fetal development. Am J Vet Res 1966;27:132–5.
7. Hasking GJ, Duggan JM. Encephalopathy from bismuth subsalicylate. Med J Aust 1982;2:167.
8. Heinonen OP, Slone D, Shapiro S. *Birth Defects and Drugs in Pregnancy*. Littleton, MA: Publishing Sciences Group, 1977.
9. O'Brien JR. Effects of salicylates on human platelets. Lancet 1968;1:779–83.
10. Weiss HJ, Aledort ML, Shaul I. The effect of salicylates on the haemostatic properties of platelets in man. J Clin Invest 1968;47:2169–80.
11. Bleyer WA. Maternal ingested salicylates as a cause of neonatal hemorrhage. J Pediatr 1974;85:736–7.
12. Findlay JWA, DeAngelis RL, Kearney MF, Welch RM, Findley JM. Analgesic drugs in breast milk and plasma. Clin Pharmacol Ther 1981;29:625–33.
13. Committee on Drugs, American Academy of Pediatrics. The transfer of drugs and other chemicals into human milk. Pediatrics 2001;108:776–89.
14. Anderson PO. Drug use during breast feeding. Clin Pharm 1991;10:594–624.

B

BISOPROLOL

Sympatholytic (Antihypertensive)

PREGNANCY RECOMMENDATION: Human Data Suggest Risk in 2nd and 3rd Trimesters
BREASTFEEDING RECOMMENDATION: No Human Data—Potential Toxicity

PREGNANCY SUMMARY

Some β-blockers may cause intrauterine growth restriction (IUGR) and reduced placental weight, especially those lacking intrinsic sympathomimetic activity (ISA) (i.e., partial agonist). Treatment beginning early in the 2nd trimester results in the greatest weight reductions, whereas treatment restricted to the 3rd trimester primarily affects only placental weight. However, IUGR and reduced placental weight may potentially occur with all agents within this class. Although growth restriction is a serious concern, the benefits of maternal therapy with β-blockers, in some cases, might outweigh the risks to the fetus and must be judged on a case-by-case basis.

Newborn infants of mothers consuming the drug near delivery should be closely observed for 24–48 hours for signs and symptoms of β-blockade. Long-term effects of in utero exposure to β-blockers have not been studied but warrant evaluation.

FETAL RISK SUMMARY

Bisoprolol is a cardioselective β_1-adrenergic blocking agent used in the management of hypertension. In animal reproduction studies, bisoprolol was not teratogenic in rats at doses up to 375 and 77 times the maximum recommended human dose (MRHD) based on weight and BSA, respectively, but fetotoxicity (increased late resorptions) was observed (1). No teratogenic effects were observed in rabbits at doses up to 31 and 12 times the MRHD based on body weight and BSA, respectively (1). Embryo lethality (increased early resorptions) was observed in rabbits.

A 2004 case report described a 24-year-old woman who took bisoprolol (5 mg/day), naproxen (550 mg about twice a week), and sumatriptan (100 mg about once a week) for migraine headaches during the first 5 weeks of pregnancy (2). An elective cesarean section was performed at 37 weeks for breech presentation to deliver a 3125-g male infant. The infant had a wide bilateral cleft lip/palate, marked hypertelorism, a broad nose, and bilateral but asymmetric toe abnormalities (missing and hypoplastic phalanges) (2).

BREASTFEEDING SUMMARY

No reports describing the use of bisoprolol in lactating women have been located. Nursing infants of mothers consuming bisoprolol should be closely observed for hypotension, bradycardia, and other signs or symptoms of β-blockade. Long-term effects of exposure to β-blockers from milk have not been studied but warrant evaluation.

References

1. Product information. Zebeta. Lederle Laboratories, 1997.
2. Kajantie E, Somer M. Bilateral cleft lip and palate, hypertelorism and hypoplastic toes. Clin Dysmorphol 2004;13:195–6.

BIVALIRUDIN

Thrombin Inhibitor

PREGNANCY RECOMMENDATION: Compatible—Maternal Benefit >> Embryo–Fetal Risk
BREASTFEEDING RECOMMENDATION: No Human Data—Probably Compatible

PREGNANCY SUMMARY

No reports describing the use of bivalirudin in human pregnancy have been located. The animal data suggest low risk. The absence of human data prevents an assessment of the embryo–fetal risk. However, the manufacturer recommends that bivalirudin should always be used with aspirin (300–325 mg/day) and aspirin may cause developmental toxicity (see Aspirin). In addition, maternal bleeding secondary to both agents is a potential complication, especially in the 3rd trimester, and in the newborn if exposure has occurred within a week of delivery. If indicated, however, the maternal benefit appears to outweigh the potential, but unknown embryo–fetal risk.

FETAL RISK SUMMARY

The reversible direct thrombin inhibitor bivalirudin is a synthetic 20-amino acid peptide. It is indicated, in combination with aspirin, for use as an IV anticoagulant in patients undergoing percutaneous transluminal coronary angioplasty. In patients with normal renal function, bivalirudin has a very short half-life (25 minutes) but may be as long as 3.5 hours for dialysis-dependent patients. Bivalirudin is not bound to plasma proteins (other than thrombin) or to red blood cells (1).

Reproduction studies have been conducted in rats and rabbits. In rats, SC doses up to 1.6 times the maximum recommended

B

human dose based on BSA (MRHD) revealed no evidence of impaired fertility or fetal harm. Similar findings were observed in rabbits with SC doses up to 3.2 times the MRHD (1).

It is not known if bivalirudin crosses the human placenta. The molecular weight (about 2180 for the anhydrous free base) and the very short elimination half-life in patients with normal renal function suggest that little, if any, of the peptide will cross the placenta.

BREASTFEEDING SUMMARY

No reports describing the use of bivalirudin during human lactation have been located. The molecular weight (about 2180 for the anhydrous free base) and short elimination half-life (25 minutes in patients with normal renal function) suggest that little, if any, drug will be excreted into milk. The indication for the drug suggests that women should not breastfeed while receiving bivalirudin. Waiting 3 hours or longer for patients with impaired renal function after the last dose would assure that the exposure of a nursing infant was minimal or nil. In addition, bivalirudin is a peptide that should be digested in the nursing infant's gastrointestinal tract.

Reference

1. Product information. Angiomax. The Medicines Company, 2004.

BLACK SEED/KALANJI

Herb

PREGNANCY RECOMMENDATION: No Human Data—No Relevant Animal Data
BREASTFEEDING RECOMMENDATION: No Human Data—Probably Compatible

PREGNANCY SUMMARY

There are no animal or human pregnancy data for the seeds of *Nigella sativa* (black seed/kalanji) or its active ingredients. However, one animal study did show a protective effect of thymoquinone in pregnant diabetic mice. Hepatotoxicity has been observed in some animal tests and the oil can cause contact dermatitis. Because of its use since antiquity, it is unlikely that black seed/kalanji causes teratogenicity. However, its use to stimulate menstruation and its potential contraceptive properties suggests that the product should be avoided in pregnancy.

FETAL RISK SUMMARY

The seeds of the annual plant *N. sativa*, commonly known as black seed or kalanji, have been used as a medicine and food or spice for several thousand years in the Middle East, Europe, Africa, and India. The seeds contain a large number of compounds, including fixed oils, proteins, alkaloids, saponin, fatty acids, vitamin C, minerals, and essential oil. The main active constituents are thymoquinone, dithymoquinone, thymohydroquinone, and thymol (1,2).

The seeds and/or their active constituents have been used for numerous diseases and conditions and are thought to have beneficial effects on the respiratory, immune, and gastrointestinal systems. They also are claimed to have anticancer effects and have been used for their antioxidant, antidiabetic, anti-inflammatory, analgesic, antihypertensive, broad-spectrum antimicrobial, and anthelmintic properties. However, there are few clinical studies of these uses, and information on the doses taken is lacking. In women, the seeds have been used to stimulate menstruation and increase milk flow (1,2).

Animal reproduction tests with the seeds or its active compounds have not been conducted. However, in a study of pregnant mice with streptozotocin-induced diabetes, thymoquinone (10 mg/kg/day) was shown to reduce the rate of malformations (3). Moreover, studies in rats and guinea pigs with the volatile oil of *N. sativa* have shown anti-oxytocic potential by inhibiting spontaneous uterine contractions and to have a potential contraceptive effect (1,2,4).

It is not known if any of the active constituents or other compounds found in the seeds of *N. sativa* cross the placenta.

BREASTFEEDING SUMMARY

No reports describing the use of black seed/kalanji during breastfeeding have been located. The seeds of *N. sativa* have been used for thousands of years and it is unlikely that they cause significant toxicity in a nursing infant. The product has been used to increase milk flow but, apparently, there are no clinical studies to support this claim (1,2).

References

1. Kalanji. In *The Review of Natural Medicines*. St. Louis, MO: Wolters Kluwer Health, 2008.
2. Black Seed. *Natural Medicines Comprehensive Database*. 10th ed. Stockton, CA: Therapeutic Research Faculty, 2008:191–2.
3. Al-Enazi MM. Effect of thymoquinone on malformations and oxidative stress-induced diabetic mice. Pakistan J Biological Sci 2007;10:3115–9.
4. Aqel M, Shaheen R. Effects of the volatile oil of *Nigella sativa* seeds on the uterine smooth muscle of rat and guinea pig. J Ethnopharmacol 1996;52:23–6.

BLACK WIDOW SPIDER ANTIVENIN

Antidote

PREGNANCY RECOMMENDATION: Limited Human Data—Probably Compatible
BREASTFEEDING RECOMMENDATION: No Human Data—Probably Compatible

B

PREGNANCY SUMMARY

Only three reports describing the use of black widow spider antivenin in pregnancy have been located. In each case, the maternal symptoms did not respond to other therapies but did within 1 hour to the antivenin. No fetal harm was observed in these cases. Although there is a risk of immediate hypersensitivity reaction, the risk can be reduced by sensitivity testing before administration (1). Because the maternal symptoms can be severe and do not always respond to other therapies, the antivenin should not be withheld because of pregnancy if the test for sensitivity is negative (2).

FETAL RISK SUMMARY

Black widow spider antivenin is used to treat patients with symptoms due to bites by the black widow spider (*Latrodectus mactans*). It is a sterile, nonpyrogenic preparation of specific venom-neutralizing globulins obtained from the blood serum of healthy horses immunized against the venom, a neurotoxin, of black widow spiders. It is given either IM or IV. A skin or conjunctival test should be preformed before administration of the antivenin to rule out sensitivity to horse serum (3).

Reproduction studies in animals have not been conducted, nor have studies for carcinogenesis, mutagenesis, and impairment of fertility (3).

It is not known if the globulins cross the human placenta. However, globulins are a family of proteins with high molecular weight. As such, it is doubtful if clinically significant amounts will cross to the embryo–fetus, although exposure in the 3rd trimester might occur.

The first published case of a black widow spider bite in pregnancy was in 1979 (4). A 20-year-old woman in her 16th week of pregnancy was bitten below the right breast. She experienced severe pain accompanied by abdominal and generalized muscle cramps. There was no cervical dilation, vaginal bleeding, or evidence of active labor. Fetal heart tones were 144 beats/minute. After skin testing, she was given an IV dose of antivenin and within 20 minutes was almost asymptomatic. She was discharged home the next day. About 18 weeks later, she gave birth by cesarean section to a healthy 3.7-kg male infant (4).

A 1994 case report described the pregnancy outcome of a 36-year-old woman at 22 weeks' gestation who was bitten by a black widow spider (5). There was no vaginal bleeding and her cervix was long and closed. She experienced restlessness, pain, and muscle cramping and was treated with calcium gluconate, diazepam, and morphine. She had some relief but her symptoms soon returned. After a negative skin test, one 2.5-mL vial of the antivenin was administered IV over 15 minutes. Within 1 hour her symptoms resolved and she was discharged home the following day. No further details on her pregnancy were provided (5).

In a 2000 case report, a 27-year-old woman at 38 1/7 weeks was bitten by a black widow spider (6). Her symptoms included anxiety and severe abdominal, chest, and back pain. She had irregular uterine contractions and her cervix was dilated 1 cm, 50% effaced. She was initially treated with calcium gluconate, morphine, diazepam, and midazolam, but these agents were not effective in relieving her symptoms. After a negative conjunctival test, she was given the antivenin (dose and route not specified) and within 1 hour her symptoms had markedly decreased. She still had uterine contractions and her cervix was now 2 cm, 75% effaced. However, she was discharged home the next day after her contractions stopped and with no further changes in her cervix. One week later, she had a spontaneous vaginal birth of a healthy male infant (6).

BREASTFEEDING SUMMARY

No reports describing the use of black widow spider antivenin during breastfeeding have been located. It is doubtful if such reports will appear because the symptoms of the bites can be quite severe and would probably hinder any attempt to breastfeed. In addition, the antivenin is composed of globulins (i.e., proteins). Even if they were excreted into breast milk, they would probably be digested in the nursing infant's gut. Thus, the limited data suggest that administration of the antivenin to the mother is compatible with breastfeeding.

References

1. Miller JR. Treatment of black widow spider bite. J Am Board Fam Pract 1994;7:183–4.
2. Bailey B. Are there teratogenic risks associated with antidotes used in the acute management of poisoned pregnant women? Birth Defects Res A Clin Mol Teratol 2003;67:133–40.
3. Product information. Antivenin—*Latrodectus mactans*. Merck Sharp & Dohme, 2010.
4. Russell FE, Marcus P, Streng JA. Black widow envenomation during pregnancy. Report of a case. Toxicon 1979;17:188–9.
5. Handel CC, Izquierdo LA, Curet LB. Black widow spider (*Latrodectus mactans*) bite during pregnancy. West J Med 1994;160:261–2.
6. Sherman RP, Groll JM, Gonzalez DI, Aerts MA. Black widow spider (*Latrodectus mactans*) envenomation in a term pregnancy. Curr Surg 2000;57:346–8.

BLEOMYCIN

Antineoplastic

PREGNANCY RECOMMENDATION: Human and Animal Data Suggest Risk
BREASTFEEDING RECOMMENDATION: No Human Data—Potential Toxicity

B

PREGNANCY SUMMARY

Bleomycin caused developmental toxicity (teratogenicity or death) in two animal species, but there are no reports describing the use of the drug during the 1st trimester in humans. When the drug was used later in pregnancy, it was combined with other antineoplastic agents. Although no reports of toxicity in offspring that were attributable to bleomycin were observed, the most frequent adverse effects in adults involve the skin and mucous membranes.

FETAL RISK SUMMARY

Bleomycin is an antineoplastic agent whose mechanism of action is thought to be inhibition of DNA synthesis and lesser inhibition of RNA and protein synthesis. It is in the same antineoplastic subclass of antibiotics as dactinomycin and mitomycin.

The drug is teratogenic in rats. Skeletal malformations, shortened innominate artery, and hydroureter were observed at an intraperitoneal dose about 1.6 times the recommended human dose based on BSA (RHD) given on days 6–15 of gestation. An IV dose about 2.4 times the RHD administered to rabbits on gestational days 6–18 resulted in abortions, but there were no teratogenic effects (1).

No reports linking the use of bleomycin with congenital defects in humans have been located. Chromosomal aberrations in human marrow cells have been reported, but the significance to the fetus is unknown (2). Two separate cases of non-Hodgkin's lymphoma in pregnancy were treated during the 2nd and 3rd trimesters with bleomycin and other antineoplastic agents (3,4). Normal infants without anomalies or chromosomal changes were delivered. In another case, a 21-year-old woman with a Ewing's sarcoma of the pelvis was treated with bleomycin and four other antineoplastic agents at approximately 25 weeks' gestation (5). Nine weeks later, recurrence of tumor growth necessitated delivery of the normal infant by cesarean section to allow for more definitive treatment of the tumor. The child was reported to be developing normally at 4 years of age.

A 1989 case report described the effect of maternal chemotherapy on a premature newborn delivered at approximately 27 weeks' gestation (6). The mother was treated with bleomycin (30 mg), etoposide (165 mg), and cisplatin (55 mg) (all given daily for 3 days), 1 week before delivery, for an unknown primary cancer with metastases to the eye and liver. The mother developed profound neutropenia just before delivery. On the 3rd day after delivery, the 1190-g female infant also developed a profound leukopenia with neutropenia, 10 days after in utero exposure to the antineoplastic agents. The condition resolved after 10 days. At 10 days of age, the infant began losing her scalp hair and experienced a rapid loss of lanugo. Etoposide was thought to be the most likely cause of the neutropenia and the alopecia. By 12 weeks of age, substantial hair regrowth had occurred, and at 1 year follow-up, the child was developing normally except for moderate bilateral hearing loss. The investigators could not determine whether the sensorineural deafness was caused by the maternal and/or neonatal gentamicin therapy, or by the maternal cisplatin chemotherapy (6).

A 25-year-old woman underwent surgery at 25 weeks' gestation for an endodermal sinus tumor of the ovary (7). A chemotherapy cycle consisting of bleomycin (50 mg), cisplatin (75 mg/m^2), and vinblastine (0.25 mg/kg) was started 9 days later. Approximately 3 weeks later she received a second cycle of therapy. A normal, healthy 1900-g male infant was delivered by scheduled cesarean section at 32 weeks' gestation. The infant was alive and growing normally at the time of the report (7).

Combination chemotherapy with bleomycin was used for teratoma of the testis in two men (8). In both cases, recovery of spermatogenesis with apparently successful fertilization occurred but the possibility of alternate paternity could not be excluded.

The long-term effects of combination chemotherapy on menstrual and reproductive function were described in a 1988 report (9). Only 7 of 40 women treated for malignant ovarian germ cell tumors received bleomycin. The results of this study are discussed in the monograph for cyclophosphamide (see Cyclophosphamide).

Occupational exposure of the mother to antineoplastic agents during pregnancy may present a risk to the fetus. A position statement from the National Study Commission on Cytotoxic Exposure and a research article involving some antineoplastic agents are presented in the monograph for cyclophosphamide (see Cyclophosphamide).

BREASTFEEDING SUMMARY

No reports describing the use of bleomycin during human lactation have been located. It is not known if the drug is excreted into breast milk. Because of the risk of serious toxicity to a nursing infant, the safest course is to not breastfeed if the antineoplastic is being administered.

References

1. Product information. Blenoxane. Bristol-Myers Squibb Oncology/Immunology Division, 2000.
2. Bornstein RS, Hungerford DA, Haller G, Engstrom PF, Yarbro JW. Cytogenic effects of bleomycin therapy in man. Cancer Res 1971;31:2004–7.
3. Ortega J. Multiple agent chemotherapy including bleomycin of non-Hodgkin's lymphoma during pregnancy. Cancer 1977;40:2829–35.
4. Falkson HC, Simson IW, Falkson G. Non-Hodgkin's lymphoma in pregnancy. Cancer 1980;45:1679–82.
5. Haerr RW, Pratt AT. Multiagent chemotherapy for sarcoma diagnosed during pregnancy. Cancer 1985;56:1028–33.
6. Raffles A, Williams J, Costeloe K, Clark P. Transplacental effects of maternal cancer chemotherapy: case report. Br J Obstet Gynaecol 1989;96:1099–1100.
7. Malone JM, Gershenson DM, Creasy RK, Kavanagh JJ, Silva EG, Stringer CA. Endodermal sinus tumor of the ovary associated with pregnancy. Obstet Gynecol 1986;68(Suppl):86S–9S.
8. Rubery ED. Return of fertility after curative chemotherapy for disseminated teratoma of testis. Lancet 1983;1:186.
9. Gershenson DM. Menstrual and reproductive function after treatment with combination chemotherapy for malignant ovarian germ cell tumors. J Clin Oncol 1988;6:270–5.

B

BLUE COHOSH

Herb

PREGNANCY RECOMMENDATION: Human and Animal Data Suggest Risk
BREASTFEEDING RECOMMENDATION: No Human Data—Potential Toxicity

PREGNANCY SUMMARY

Blue cohosh is an herbal product that has uterine stimulant properties. Some of its constituents have been shown to be teratogenic and toxic in various animal species. The herb should be avoided in the 1st trimester because of the animal teratogenicity data and its estrogenic effect demonstrated in humans (1). It is used in human pregnancy to induce labor, but the potential fetal and newborn toxicity appears to outweigh any medical benefit (2,3). In addition, preparations of blue cohosh are not standardized as to content or purity.

FETAL RISK SUMMARY

Blue cohosh (*Caulophyllum thalictroides* Michx.; family Berberidaceae [barberries]) is found throughout damp woodlands of the eastern part of North America, especially in the Allegheny Mountains (1,2). It is an early spring, leafy perennial herb with yellowish-green flowers that mature into bitter, bright blue seeds. The medicinal parts, collected in the autumn, are the matted, knotty rootstock (rhizomes) (1,2). *Caulophyllum robustum* Maxim, a species found in Asia, is also used for medicine (2).

Blue cohosh is often used to stimulate labor. In a survey of nurse-midwives, blue cohosh was the most frequently used herbal preparation for this purpose (65% of respondents), usually administered prior to or instead of oxytocin (4). Native Americans used blue cohosh for menstrual cramps and suppression of profuse menstruation (2). It has also been used as an emmenagogue, antispasmodic, antirheumatic, laxative, or for colic, sore throat, hiccups, epilepsy, hysterics, and uterine inflammation (2,3). The roasted seeds have been used as a coffee substitute (3).

The chemical composition of blue cohosh has been investigated since 1863 (5). Because early Native Americans used the herb to facilitate childbirth, researchers in 1954 described a technique to isolate a crystalline glycoside from blue cohosh rhizome and roots that demonstrated marked activity as a smooth muscle stimulant. Increased tone and rate of contraction were observed in rat, rabbit, and guinea pig uteruses, as well as in other smooth muscle preparations (5).

A number of chemical constituents have been isolated from blue cohosh rhizomes. These include anagyrine, baptifoline, 5,6-dehydro-α-islupanine, α-isolupanine, lupanine, sparteine, and *N*-methylcytisine (all are quinolizidine alkaloids), magnoflorine and taspine (aporphine alkaloids), caulophyllosaponin (also known as caulosaponin, a triterpene saponin), and caulosapogenin (1,2,6). In addition, a novel alkaloid, thalictroidine, has been recently found (6). *N*-Methylcytisine (also known as caulophylline) is a nicotinic agonist in animals (1,2).

Citing previously published data, a 1999 study listed the concentrations of the quinolizidine alkaloids found in some blue-cohosh-containing dietary supplements: *N*-methylcytisine 5–850 ppm, anagyrine 2–390 ppm, and baptifoline 9–900 ppm (the lower concentrations were found in liquid-extract products) (6). In contrast, the level of magnoflorine in the *C. thalictroides* rhizomes was 11,000 ppm (6).

N-Methylcytisine was teratogenic in a rat embryo culture, but thalictroidine, anagyrine, and α-isolupanine were not teratogenic in this system at the concentrations tested (6). Marked embryo toxicity, without evidence of teratogenicity, was shown for taspine (6).

In an animal reproduction test, pregnant rats were administered either a low or high potency of *Caulophyllum* extract (homeopathic concentrations) on days 1–5 of pregnancy (7). The lower potency prevented implantation by disrupting the site of implantation. In contrast, the high-potency preparation caused no adverse effect compared with controls, but did increase the average number of young per litter (8 vs. 5 for controls) (7).

Anagyrine is teratogenic in ruminants, such as cattle, causing "crooked calf syndrome" (8–13). The severity of the malformations has been shown to be dose-related (11,12). Malformations include bowed or twisted limbs, spinal or neck curvature, and cleft palate. The defects may result from decreased normal fetal movements, which are required for normal skeletal development, secondary to the action of the alkaloid on fetal muscarinic and nicotinic receptors.

In an experiment with rats, a low-potency extract of blue cohosh (homeopathic concentration) administered between estrus cycles, immediately before estrus, and during estrus was shown to be an effective inhibitor of ovulation and also inhibited physiologic changes in the uterus (14). A high-potency extract (also homeopathic concentration) had no effect on ovulation or uterine changes.

No studies describing the placental crossing of any constituent of blue cohosh have been located. Based on the animal studies above, however, some or all of the alkaloids and other chemicals isolated from the herb probably cross the placenta.

A brief 1996 case report described an adverse newborn outcome after a woman with an uneventful pregnancy was given a combination of black and blue cohosh (dosage not specified) for labor induction (15). After a normal labor, a 3840-g female infant was born with Apgar scores of 1, 4, and 5 at 1, 5, and 10 minutes, respectively. No spontaneous breathing was observed, but resuscitation efforts were successful with the onset of breathing noted at 30 minutes. Mechanical ventilation was required during the hospital course, which was complicated by seizures and acute tubular necrosis. Computed tomography revealed basal ganglia and parasagittal hypoxic injury. Lower limb spasticity was apparent at 3 months of age, and the infant required nasogastric tube feeding. Although the cause of the neurologic toxicity in the newborn was unknown, the authors could not rule out a possible role for the herbal preparation. Citing published data, they speculated that black cohosh may have caused peripheral vasodilation and hypotension, whereas blue cohosh may have caused increased uterine activity. The combination of these actions may have led to a reduction of placental perfusion and caused hypoxia in the infant (15). The accuracy of this assessment has been challenged (16), but the case report below lends credibility to the concept that the use of blue cohosh in pregnancy may cause toxicity (17,18).

A 1998 case report described profound neonatal congestive heart failure in a newborn that was thought to have been caused by the mother's use of blue cohosh to promote uterine contractions (19). The 36-year-old woman had hypothyroidism but was euthyroid on replacement therapy. Except for this one condition, she had an uncomplicated pregnancy. One month before term, she was instructed by a midwife to take one tablet prepared from blue cohosh daily. Instead, for the next 5 weeks, the woman took one tablet 3 times daily. During this period, she reported increased uterine contractions and a decrease in fetal movements. A precipitous delivery occurred 1 hour after the onset of spontaneous labor, 15 minutes after spontaneous rupture of membranes. There was slight meconium-stained amniotic fluid. The 3.66-kg male infant had Apgar scores of 6 and 9 presumably at 1 and 5 minutes, respectively, but cyanosis and poor perfusion developed within minutes of birth that required intubation and mechanical ventilation. At 1 hour of age, on 100% oxygen, umbilical arterial blood pH was 7.07, P_{CO_2} 40 mmHg, and P_{O_2} 38 mmHg. A chest X-ray revealed cardiomegaly and pulmonary edema and an electrocardiogram showed acute myocardial infarction. Hepatomegaly was present in addition to the cardiac abnormalities. The infant's condition gradually improved and he was discharged home after 31 days. At 2 years of age, the child was progressing well with normal growth and development and good exercise tolerance, but continued to receive digoxin therapy. There was persistent cardiomegaly and his left ventricular function remained mildly reduced. The authors attributed the toxicity to blue cohosh because it contains vasoactive glycosides and it is known to cause toxic effects on the heart of animals (19).

A 2004 case report described a stroke in a female, full-term infant (birth weight 3860 g) 26 hours after birth (20). The mother, on advice of her physician, had consumed a tea made from blue cohosh to induce labor. A cesarean section was performed because of a failed attempt at vaginal delivery. Focal motor seizures of the right arm began at 26 hours of age. At 2 days of age, a computed tomographic scan revealed an evolving infarct in the distribution of the left middle cerebral artery. Laboratory tests in the infant for thrombophilia were normal and a family history for clotting disorders was negative. A cocaine metabolite, benzoylecgonine, was detected in the urine, meconium, the mother's bottle of blue cohosh, and the contents of a sealed bottle of a different preparation of the herb. Although cocaine contamination of the products could not be excluded, a blue cohosh preparation (Inca Tea) contains coca leaves and can cause a positive test for cocaine exposure (20). In addition, among the natural constituents of blue cohosh, caulophyllosaponin can cause uterine contraction and coronary-artery constriction in animals (20), and methylcytisine is a nicotine agonist. In subsequent correspondence regarding the presence of benzoylecgonine, a chemical not related to blue cohosh, there was speculation that the mother may have taken cocaine or, more likely, it involved detection of a cross-reacting substance by an insensitive assay (21–23).

BREASTFEEDING SUMMARY

No reports describing the use of blue cohosh during lactation have been located. It is not known if the constituents of the herb are excreted into breast milk. Depending on the maternal serum concentration of the various chemicals, however, some excretion should be expected. The effects of this exposure on a nursing infant are unknown, but the potential toxicity and estrogenic effects are substantial reasons to avoid blue cohosh ingestion during breastfeeding. At least one source states that its use during this period is likely unsafe (3).

References

1. Blue Cohosh. In *PDR for Herbal Medicines*. 2nd ed. Montvale, NJ: Medical Economics, 2000:109–10.
2. Blue Cohosh. In *The Review of Natural Products*. St. Louis, MO: Facts and Comparisons, 2000.
3. Blue Cohosh. In *Natural Medicines Comprehensive Database*. Stockton, CA: Therapeutic Research Faculty, 1999:160–1.
4. McFarlin BL, Gibson MH, O'Rear J, Harman P. A national survey of herbal preparation use by nurse-midwives for labor stimulation. Review of the literature and recommendations for practice. J Nurse-Midwifery 1999;44:205–16.
5. Ferguson HC, Edwards LD. A pharmacological study of a crystalline glycoside of *Caulophyllum thalictroides*. J Am Pharm Assoc 1954;43:16–21.
6. Kennelly EJ, Flynn TJ, Mazzola EP, Roach JA, McClud TG, Danford DE, Betz JM. Detecting potential teratogenic alkaloids from blue cohosh rhizomes using an in vitro rat embryo culture. J Nat Prod 1999;62:1385–9.
7. Chandrasekhar K, Rao Vishwanath C. Studies on the effect of *Caulophyllum* on implantation in rats (abstract). J Reprod Fertil 1974;38:245–6.
8. Shupe JL, Binns W, James LF, Keeler RF. Lupine, a cause of crooked calf disease. J Am Vet Med Assoc 1967;151:198–203.
9. Keeler RF. Lupin alkaloids from teratogenic and nonteratogenic lupins. I. Correlation of crooked calf disease incidence with alkaloid distribution determined by gas chromatography. Teratology 1973;7:23–30.
10. Keeler RF. Lupin alkaloids from teratogenic and nonteratogenic lupins. II. Identification of the major alkaloids by tandem gas chromatography-mass spectrometry in plants producing crooked calf disease. Teratology 1973;7:31–35.
11. Keeler RF. Lupin alkaloids from teratogenic and nonteratogenic lupins. III. Identification of anagyrine as the probable teratogen by feeding trials. J Toxicol Environ Health 1976;1:887–98.
12. Keeler RF, Cronin EH. Lupin alkaloids from teratogenic and nonteratogenic lupins. IV. Concentration of total alkaloids, individual major alkaloids, and the teratogen anagyrine as a function of plant part and stage of growth and their relationship to crooked calf disease. J Toxicol Environ Health 1976;1:899–908.
13. Keeler RF. Teratogens in plants. J Animal Sci 1984;58:1029–39.
14. Chandrasekhar K, Sarma GHR. Observations on the effect of low and high doses of *Caulophyllum* on the ovaries and the consequential changes in the uterus and thyroid in rats (abstract). J Reprod Fertil 1974;38:236–7.
15. Gunn TR, Wright IMR. The use of black and blue cohosh in labour. Lancet 1996;109:410–1.
16. Baillie N, Rasmussen P. Black and blue cohosh in labour. Lancet 1997; 110:20–1.
17. Wright IMR. Neonatal effects of maternal consumption of blue cohosh. J Pediatr 1999;134:384.

18. Jones TK. Neonatal effects of maternal consumption of blue cohosh. Reply. J Pediatr 1999;134:384–5.
19. Jones TK, Lawson BM. Profound neonatal congestive heart failure caused by maternal consumption of blue cohosh herbal medication. J Pediatr 1998;132:550–2.
20. Finkel RS, Zarlengo KM. Blue cohosh and perinatal stroke. N Engl J Med 2004;351:302–3.
21. Potterton D. More on blue cohosh and perinatal stroke. N Engl J Med 2004;351:2239–40.
22. Chan GM, Nelson LS. More on blue cohosh and perinatal stroke. N Engl J Med 2004;351:2240.
23. Finkel RS, Zarlengo KM. Reply: more on blue cohosh and perinatal stroke. N Engl J Med 2004;351:2240–1.

BOCEPREVIR

Antiviral Agent

PREGNANCY RECOMMENDATION: No Human Data—Animal Data Suggest Low Risk (Contraindicated 3-Drug Combination)
BREASTFEEDING RECOMMENDATION: No Human Data—Potential Toxicity (3-Drug Combination)

PREGNANCY SUMMARY

No reports describing the use of boceprevir in human pregnancy have been located. The animal data suggest low risk. However, the indication for boceprevir involves the combined use with ribavirin and peginterferon alfa. Although peginterferon alfa is probably compatible with pregnancy (see Interferon Alfa), ribavirin is contraindicated because it has caused developmental toxicity in all animal species tested (see Ribavirin). The three-drug combination should be avoided in pregnancy.

FETAL RISK SUMMARY

Boceprevir, a mixture of two diastereomers administered orally, is an inhibitor of the hepatitis C virus protein serine protease. It is indicated, in combination with peginterferon alfa and ribavirin, for the treatment of chronic hepatitis C genotype 1 infection in adults with compensated liver disease, including cirrhosis, who are previously untreated or who have failed previous interferon and ribavirin therapy. It is metabolized by the liver to inactive metabolites. Plasma protein binding is about 75% and the mean elimination plasma half-life is about 3.4 hours (1).

Reproduction studies with boceprevir alone have been conducted in rats and rabbits. AUC exposures in these species that were 11.8 and 2.0 times, respectively, the human exposure at the recommended dose of 800 mg 3 times daily produced no effects on fetal development. However, ribavirin causes dose-related teratogenicity or embryolethality in animals (see Ribavirin) and peginterferon alfa causes dose-related abortions in animals (see Interferon Alfa) (1).

Two-year carcinogenicity studies in rats and mice with boceprevir were negative. Similar studies in these species with ribavirin also were negative. Boceprevir was not genotoxic, but ribavirin was, in multiple assays. Ribavirin induced reversible testicular toxicity in animals and interferon alfa impaired fertility in females. Boceprevir caused reversible effects on fertility and early embryonic development in female rats, as well as dose-related testicular degeneration in male rats. This latter effect was not observed in mice and monkeys, and limited clinical monitoring has revealed no evidence of testicular toxicity in humans (1).

It is not known if boceprevir crosses the human placenta. The molecular weight (about 520), moderate plasma protein binding and elimination half-life suggest that the agent will cross to the embryo–fetus.

BREASTFEEDING SUMMARY

Studies describing the use of boceprevir during human lactation have not been located. The molecular weight (about 520), moderate plasma protein binding (about 75%) and elimination half-life suggest that the agent will be excreted into breast milk. The effects of this exposure on a nursing infant are unknown. However, boceprevir is always combined with ribavirin and peginterferon alfa (see Ribavirin and Interferon Alfa). The latter agent is known to be excreted into breast milk and ribavirin is probably excreted. If a woman taking this therapy is breastfeeding, her nursing infant could be exposed to all three agents. Thus, the best course of action is to not breastfeed.

Reference

1. Product information. Victrelis. Schering Corporation, 2012.

BORTEZOMIB

Antineoplastic (Proteasome Inhibitor)

PREGNANCY RECOMMENDATION: Contraindicated
BREASTFEEDING RECOMMENDATION: Contraindicated

PREGNANCY SUMMARY

No reports describing the use of bortezomib in human pregnancy have been located. The drug caused developmental toxicity (growth restriction and death) at a dose one-half of the human clinical dose of 1.3 mg/m^2 based on body surface area (HCD) in one of two species. Because the recommended dose is given over several weeks, use during pregnancy could result in multiple exposures of the embryo and/or fetus to a cytotoxic agent. The manufacturer recommends that women should be advised to use effective contraceptive measures to prevent pregnancy (1). Until human pregnancy data are available, the best course is to avoid the drug during pregnancy. However, if treatment is required during gestation, the decision to use bortezomib should be made on a case-by-case basis, but the woman should be advised of the potential risk to her embryo–fetus.

FETAL RISK SUMMARY

Bortezomib is a cytotoxic antineoplastic that is given as an IV bolus injection. It is the same class as carfilzomib. Bortezomib is indicated for the treatment of multiple myeloma patients who have received at least one prior therapy. The mean elimination half-life after first dose has ranged 9–15 hours, but has not been fully characterized in multiple myeloma patients. Plasma protein binding is moderate (about 83%). Bortezomib undergoes some metabolism to inactive metabolites, but plasma levels of metabolites at 10 and 30 minutes after a dose were low compared with the parent compound (1).

Reproductive studies have been conducted in rats and rabbits. No teratogenicity was observed at the highest doses tested during organogenesis in rats and rabbits that were about 0.5 times the HCD. However, in rabbits given the highest dose during organogenesis, there was significant postimplantation loss and decreased number of live fetuses, as well as significant decreases in the weight of live fetuses (1).

Carcinogenic studies have not been conducted with bortezomib. The agent was not genotoxic in various tests, but did demonstrate clastogenic activity in one test. Although fertility studies have not been conducted, 6-month studies conducted for general toxicity in rats revealed degenerative changes in the ovaries and testes at doses that were approximately one-fourth and equivalent, respectively, to the HCD (1).

It is not known if bortezomib crosses the human placenta. The molecular weight (about 384), the long elimination half-life, the moderate plasma protein binding, and lack of rapid metabolism all suggest that the drug will cross to the embryo and/or fetus.

BREASTFEEDING SUMMARY

No reports describing the use of bortezomib during human lactation have been located. It is not known if bortezomib is excreted into breast milk. The molecular weight (about 384), the long elimination half-life, the moderate plasma protein binding, and lack of rapid metabolism all suggest that the drug will be excreted in milk. Bortezomib is given as IV bolus injections over several weeks. The effects of this exposure on a nursing infant are unknown, as is the oral bioavailability. However, because the drug is cytotoxic, the best course is to not breastfeed during treatment.

Reference

1. Product information. Velcade. Millennium Pharmaceuticals, 2007.

BOSENTAN

Vasodilator

PREGNANCY RECOMMENDATION: Limited Human Data—Animal Data Suggest Moderate Risk
BREASTFEEDING RECOMMENDATION: Limited Human Data—Potential Toxicity

PREGNANCY SUMMARY

Three reports have described the use of bosentan in human pregnancy. No embryo–fetal harm was observed. Based only on the animal data, the manufacturer states that pregnancy must be excluded and that reliable contraceptive methods should be used before the drug is prescribed. It also recommends monthly pregnancy tests during treatment (1). Pregnant women should not take this drug unless the severity of pulmonary arterial hypertension warrants the risk.

FETAL RISK SUMMARY

The endothelin receptor antagonist bosentan is indicated for the treatment of pulmonary arterial hypertension. It is a neurohormone that binds specifically to endothelin receptor types ET_A and ET_B. After oral administration, bosentan has one active (contributes 10%–20% of the total activity) and two inactive metabolites. Bosentan is highly (98%) bound to plasma albumin (1). It has an elimination half-life of about 5 hours (1,2).

Reproduction studies have been conducted in rats and rabbits. In rats, daily doses equal to or greater than 2 times the maximum recommended human daily dose based on BSA (MRHDD) showed dose-related teratogenicity (defects of the head, mouth, face, and large blood vessels). Increased stillbirths and pup mortality were observed at doses 2 times the MRHDD or higher. Birth defects were not observed in rabbits given doses up to 1500 mg/kg/day (relationship to MRHDD not specified), but plasma concentrations were lower than those obtained in rats. The malformations observed in rats were similar to those observed in animals with other endothelin receptor antagonists and were thought to represent a class effect of these drugs (1).

Bosentan showed dose-related carcinogenicity in mice and rats given the agent over a 2-year period but no mutagenic or clastogenic activity. Short-duration studies showed no effect on fertility in male or female rats (1).

In near-term rats, closure of the fetal ductus arteriosus by indomethacin, N-nitro-L-arginine monomethyl ester (L-name), or dexamethasone was prevented by the simultaneous administration of bosentan (3). An investigational selective endothelin receptor (ET_A) blocker (CI-1020) also was effective in preventing ductus closure (3).

The effects of bosentan on uteroplacental and maternal renal blood flow in pregnant rats were described in a 2002 report (4). On gestational day 19 (term 23 days), bosentan increased uteroplacental blood flow significantly higher than the normal physiologic increase but had no effect on renal blood flow. On gestational days 20–21, bosentan had no effect on uteroplacental blood flow but decreased renal blood flow by 20% (4).

It is not known if bosentan or its active metabolite crosses the human placenta. The molecular weight (about 570) and long elimination half-life suggest that the drug, and possibly the active metabolite, will cross the placenta, but the high plasma protein binding should limit the exposure of the embryo–fetus.

A 2005 case report described the use of bosentan throughout pregnancy in a woman with Eisenmenger's syndrome due to pulmonary hypertension (5). Sildenafil was added at 27 weeks' gestation. At 30 weeks, a planned cesarean section gave birth to a 1.41-kg healthy female infant. Postoperatively, the mother was treated with bosentan, sildenafil, and warfarin. Her infant was nursed in the hospital for 11 weeks without problems, but died at 26 weeks of age from a respiratory infection (5).

A second 2005 report described a woman with pulmonary arterial hypertension who received bosentan and warfarin until 8 weeks when her therapy was changed to inhaled iloprost (6). The woman suffered a cardiorespiratory arrest at about 25 weeks but was successful resuscitated after about 1 minute and was converted to IV iloprost for 5 days. At that time, a cesarean section delivered a 0.65-kg male infant with Apgar scores of 8 and 9. No congenital anomalies were observed in the infant. The child was progressing well at 16 months of age (6).

Bosentan (250/day), sildenafil (150 mg/day), hydroxychloroquine (200 mg/day), azathioprine (100 mg/day), and phenprocoumon were used up to 5 weeks' gestation in a 29-year-old woman with systemic lupus erythematosus-associated pulmonary arterial hypertension (7). At that time, bosentan and phenprocoumon were discontinued and the other three agents were continued along with low-molecular-weight heparin. At 35 weeks, inhaled iloprost was added. At 37 weeks, a planned cesarean section gave birth to a healthy 2.760-kg female infant with Apgar scores of 8, 9, and 10 at 1, 5, and 10 minutes, respectively. Breastfeeding was declined. At the time of the report, the child was doing well (7).

Bosentan is an isoenzymes-inducer and is metabolized by the isoenzymes CYP2C9 and CYP3A4. Because many hormonal contraceptives are metabolized by CYP3A4, treatment with bosentan could cause decreased plasma concentrations and failure of these agents. Therefore, women should not rely on hormonal contraceptives alone (oral, injectable, or implantable) for contraception (1,2).

BREASTFEEDING SUMMARY

One report described the use of bosentan during breastfeeding (see reference 5), but milk concentrations were not determined. The molecular weight (about 570) and long elimination half-life (about 5 hours) suggest that the drug, and possibly the active metabolite, will be excreted into breast milk. However, the high plasma protein binding (98%) should limit the amount of drug in milk. Although the effect of this exposure on a nursing infant is unknown, no adverse effects were mentioned in the above case, but there is a potential for toxicity.

References

1. Cheng JWM. Bosentan. Heart Dis 2003;5:161–9.
2. Product information. Tracleer. Actelion Pharmaceuticals, 2004.
3. Momma K, Nakanishi T, Imamura S. Inhibition of *in vivo* constriction of fetal ductus arteriosus by endothelin receptor blockage in rats. Pediatr Res 2003;53:479–85.
4. Ajne G, Nisell H, Wolff K, Jansson T. The role of endogenous endothelin in the regulation of uteroplacental and renal blood flow during pregnancy in conscious rats. Placenta 2003;24:813–8.
5. Molelekwa V, Akhter P, McKenna P, Bowen M, Walsh K. Eisenmenger's syndrome in a 27 week pregnancy—management with bosentan and sildenafil. Ir Med J 2005;98:87–8.
6. Elliot CA, Stewart P, Webster VJ, Mills GH, Hutchinson SP, Howarth ES, Bu'lock FA, Lawson RA, Armstrong IJ, Kiely DG. The use of iloprost in early pregnancy in patients with pulmonary hypertension. Eur Respir J 2005;26:168–73.
7. Streit M, Speich R, Fischler M, Ulrich S. Successful pregnancy in pulmonary arterial hypertension associated with systemic lupus erythematosus: a case report. J Med Case Rep 2009;3:7255.

BOSUTINIB

Antineoplastic (Tyrosine Kinase Inhibitor)

PREGNANCY RECOMMENDATION: Contraindicated
BREASTFEEDING RECOMMENDATION: Contraindicated

B

PREGNANCY SUMMARY

No reports describing the use of bosutinib in pregnancy have been located. The animal data cannot be interpreted because in one species inadequate doses were used and, in the other, fetal toxicity occurred with maternal toxic doses. Nevertheless, the manufacturer warns that the drug can cause fetal harm based on the drug's mechanism of action (1). Thus, use of bosutinib should be avoided in pregnancy, especially during the 1st trimester.

FETAL RISK SUMMARY

Bosutinib is an oral tyrosine kinase inhibitor. There are several other agents in this subclass (see Appendix). Bosutinib is indicated for the treatment of adult patients with chronic, accelerated, or blast phase Philadelphia chromosome-positive chronic myelogenous leukemia with resistance or intolerance of prior therapy. It is metabolized to inactive metabolites and is highly (96%) bound to plasma protein. The mean terminal phase elimination half-life is 22.5 hours (1).

Reproduction studies have been conducted in rats and rabbits. Rats were given daily oral doses during organogenesis that resulted in exposures that were about <3 times the human exposure at 500 mg/day based on AUC (HE). However, the study did not expose the rats to sufficient drug to fully evaluate adverse outcomes. In rabbits given daily doses during organogenesis, a maternal toxic dose that resulted in exposures that were about 4 times the HE, fetal anomalies (fused sternebrae and various visceral anomalies), and an approximate 6% decrease in fetal body weight were observed (1).

A 2-year carcinogenicity study in male and female rats was negative, as were tests and assays for mutagenic and clastogenic effects. Reduced fertility was observed in male rats given high doses of the drug that resulted in exposures about equal to the HE. Although fertility (number of pregnancies) was not affected in female rats, doses resulting in exposures less than the HE were associated with increased resorptions and decreased implantations and number of viable embryos (1).

It is not known if bosutinib crosses the human placenta. The molecular weight (about 530 for the anhydrous form) and long elimination half-life suggest that the drug will cross to the embryo–fetus. However, the high plasma protein binding might limit the exposure.

BREASTFEEDING SUMMARY

No reports describing the use of bosutinib during human lactation have been located. The molecular weight (about 530 for the anhydrous form) and long elimination half-life (22.5 hours) suggest that the drug will be excreted into breast milk, but the high plasma protein binding (96%) might limit the amount in milk. The effect on a nursing infant from this exposure is unknown. If a woman receiving the drug chooses to nurse, her infant should be closely monitored for the most common adverse effects observed in adults (diarrhea, nausea, vomiting, thrombocytopenia, abdominal pain, rash, anemia, pyrexia, and fatigue).

Reference

1. Product information. Bosulif. Pfizer, 2012.

BOTULINUM TOXIN TYPE A

Central Nervous System Agent (Physical Adjunct)

PREGNANCY RECOMMENDATION: Limited Human Data—Animal Data Suggest Low Risk
BREASTFEEDING RECOMMENDATION: No Human Data—Probably Compatible

PREGNANCY SUMMARY

No reports describing the use of commercially prepared botulinum toxin type A in human pregnancy have been located. The animal data are suggestive of low risk, but the absence of human pregnancy experience prevents a full assessment of the embryo–fetal risk. However, the commercially prepared and wild toxins should be identical. Moreover, the case reports above suggest that the wild toxins do not cross the human placenta in the last half of pregnancy. In addition, the appearance in the systemic circulation of botulinum toxin type A is not expected after IM injections. Therefore, although the safety of use of the commercial toxin in pregnancy is unknown (1,2), the risk of embryo or fetal harm appears to very low or nonexistent.

FETAL RISK SUMMARY

Botulinum toxin type A is produced by fermentation of the anaerobic bacterium *Clostridium botulinum* type A. One unit (U) of the commercial preparation corresponds to the calculated median intraperitoneal lethal dose (LD_{50}) in mice. Botulinum toxin type A causes paralysis by binding to acceptor sites on motor nerve terminals, entering the nerve terminals, and inhibiting the release of acetylcholine (3). The toxin is not expected to enter the systemic circulation following IM injection. Botox is indicated for the treatment of cervical dystonia to decrease the severity of abnormal head position and neck associated with the disorder. It is also indicated for the treatment of strabismus and blepharospasm associated with dystonia, including benign essential blepharospasm or seventh nerve disorders (3). Botox Cosmetic is indicated for the temporary improvement in the appearance of moderate to severe glabellar lines associated with corrugator or procerus muscle activity (4).

Reproduction studies have been conducted in mice, rats, and rabbits. In mice and rats given IM injections during organogenesis, the developmental no-observed-effect level (NOEL) was 4 U/kg. Doses of 8 or 16 U/kg were associated with decreased fetal body weights and/or delayed ossification. Doses >8 U/kg impaired fertility in female rats by altering the estrous cycle. In rabbits, IM doses of 0.125 U/kg/day (gestational days 6–18) or 2 U/kg/day (gestational days 6 and 13) resulted in severe maternal toxicity, abortions, and fetal malformations. Higher doses caused maternal death (3). Interestingly, a 1965 study provided indirect evidence that botulinum toxin type A crossed the placentas of pregnant mice, even though the toxin has a very high molecular weight (5).

It is not known if botulinum toxin type A crosses the human placenta. It is a large protein with a very high molecular weight. In addition, it is not expected to enter the systemic circulation and, therefore, would not be present at the maternal–fetal interface. Moreover, the case reports below provide indirect evidence that botulinum toxins do not cross to the fetus in clinically significant amounts.

The first reported case of botulism in a pregnant woman appeared in 1975 (6). The case report involved a 32-year-old woman at 34 weeks' gestation who developed botulism and required assisted ventilation. Botulinum toxin type A was detected in her serum and she was treated with trivalent botulism antitoxin, but with limited success. Fetal heart tones were 140–160 beats per minute. On the 5th day of illness, she precipitously delivered a 1538-g male infant who was cyanotic with shallow respirations. No botulinum toxin was detected in the infant's serum obtained within 4 hours of birth. The infant's hospital 42-day course included aspiration pneumonia, anemia, seizures, and a probable intraventricular hemorrhage. The infant developed hydrocephalus several months after discharge but the condition resolved spontaneously. At 20 months of age, he was nearly totally blind (probable optic atrophy) and developmentally slow. The infant's condition was attributed to hypoxia, a precipitous delivery, and intraventricular hemorrhage (6).

A 30-year-old woman at about 27 weeks' gestation was admitted to a hospital with signs and symptoms of botulism (7). She had been "skin popping" black tar heroin and had developed multiple abscesses on her left leg. Because botulism was suspected, she received two vials of antitoxin. The abscesses were excised and culture revealed *C. botulinum* type A. Ten days before she was discharged from the hospital, at 34 weeks' gestation, her baby was delivered by cesarean section. No details regarding the infant were provided other than the fact that the infant remained in intensive care at 24 days of age (7).

A 1996 case report described a 37-year-old woman at 23 weeks' gestation who developed botulism from home-produced green beans (8). She eventually required assisted ventilation because of near-complete paralysis. At the peak of the disease, fetal movement was the visible motion. Although she was treated with botulism antitoxin, she required tracheotomy and ventilation for 2 months. Throughout the woman's 3-month hospitalization, repeated surveillance revealed normal fetal development. Four months after the onset of the poisoning, a normal infant was delivered spontaneously (sex and other details of the infant not provided) (8).

A second 1996 case report involved a 24-year-old Alaskan native at 16 weeks' gestation that was poisoned by consumption of fermented whitefish (9). Both *C. botulinum* types A and E were cultured from her stool and type E organisms and toxin were detected in the whitefish. Ultrasonography revealed a fetus with normal breathing and movements. The woman was treated with trivalent botulinum antitoxin and rapidly recovered. At 42 weeks' gestation, she spontaneously delivered a healthy 4300-g male infant. The child's growth and development during the 1st year were normal (9).

In an in vitro study, botulinum toxin type A has been demonstrated to inhibit or completely arrest myometrial activity (10). The investigators thought that the toxin might eventually have application in the prevention of preterm labor after fetal surgery. Moreover, the effects were potentially reversible (10).

BREASTFEEDING SUMMARY

No reports describing the use of botulinum toxin type A during human lactation have been located. Because the toxin is not expected to appear in the systemic circulation, it would not be available for excretion into breast milk. Therefore, the risk to a nursing infant is probably nil.

References

1. Anonymous. Botulinum toxin. Consensus Statement 1990;8:1–20.
2. Tsui JKC. Botulinum toxin as a therapeutic agent. Pharmacol Ther 1996;72;13–24.
3. Product information. Botox. Allergan, 2004.
4. Product information. Botox Cosmetic. Allergan, 2002. As cited by *Facts and Comparisons*. St. Louis, MO: Wolters Kluwer Health, 2002:1997–8a.
5. Hart LG, Dixon RL, Long JP, Mackay B. Studies using *Clostridium botulinum* toxin—type A. Toxicol Appl Pharmacol 1965;7:84–9.
6. St. Clair EH, DiLiberti JH, O'Brien ML. Observations of an infant born to a mother with botulism. J Pediatr 1975;87:658.
7. CDC. Wound botulism—California 1995. MMWR 1995;44:889–92.
8. Polo JM, Martin J, Berciano J. Botulism and pregnancy. Lancet 1996;348:195.
9. Robin L, Herman D, Redett R. Botulism in a pregnant woman. N Engl J Med 1996;335:823–4.
10. Garza JJ, Downard CD, Clayton N, Maher TJ, Fauza DO. *Clostridium botulinum* toxin inhibits myometrial activity in vitro: possible application on the prevention of preterm labor after fetal surgery. J Pediatr Surg 2003;38: 511–3.

BRENTUXIMAB VEDOTIN

Antineoplastic

PREGNANCY RECOMMENDATION: No Human Data—Animal Data Suggest Moderate Risk
BREASTFEEDING RECOMMENDATION: No Human Data—Probably Compatible

B

PREGNANCY SUMMARY

No reports describing the use of brentuximab in human pregnancy have been located. The animal data in the only species studied suggest risk. Moreover, the mechanism of action suggests that the drug can cause fetal harm. If the drug must be used in pregnancy, avoiding the 1st trimester should be considered. In addition, the patient should be informed of the potential risk to her fetus.

FETAL RISK SUMMARY

Brentuximab is an IgG1 antibody specific for human CD30 combined with a microtubule disrupting agent (MMAE) and a protease-cleavable linker. It is given as an IV infusion every 3 weeks. Brentuximab is indicated for the treatment of patients with Hodgkin lymphoma after failure of autologous stem cell transplant (ASCT) or after failure of at least two prior multiagent chemotherapy regimens in patients who are not ASCT candidates. It also is indicated for treatment of patients with systemic anaplastic large cell lymphoma after failure of at least one prior multiagent chemotherapy regimen. The antibody–drug conjugate undergoes minimal metabolism and the terminal half-life is about 4–6 days (1).

Reproduction studies have been conducted in rats. During organogenesis, embryo–fetal toxicities were observed in rats given IV doses of brentuximab that resulted in systemic exposures that were approximately the same as the human exposure. The drug-induced toxicities were increased early resorption (≥99%), postimplantation loss (≥99%), decreased number of live fetuses, and external malformations (umbilical hernias and malrotated hind limbs) (1).

Carcinogenicity studies with brentuximab have not been conducted. Consistent with its mechanism of action, MMAE was genotoxic in the rat bone marrow micronucleus study, but it was not mutagenic in two assays. Fertility studies have not been conducted. However, impairment of male reproductive function and fertility was observed in repeat-dose toxicity studies in rats (1).

It is not known if brentuximab crosses the human placenta. The molecular weight (about 153,000) and minimal metabolism suggest that exposure of the embryo–fetus will be limited. However, immune globulin crosses the placenta, especially late in gestation (see Immune Globulin Intravenous) and the animal data (see above) suggest that the agent crosses the placenta in rats.

BREASTFEEDING SUMMARY

No reports describing the use of brentuximab during human lactation have been located. The molecular weight (about 153,000) and minimal metabolism suggest that exposure of a nursing infant will be limited, if it occurs at all. However, immune globulin is excreted into colostrum during the first few days after birth and brentuximab is an IgG1 antibody-drug conjugate. Nevertheless, the amount of the drug in colostrum or breast milk should be low and the potential for harm of a nursing infant appears to be low.

Reference

1. Product information. Adcetris. Seattle Genetics, 2012.

BRETYLIUM

[Withdrawn from the market. See 9th edition.]

BROMFENAC

Ophthalmic

PREGNANCY RECOMMENDATION: No Human Data—Probably Compatible
BREASTFEEDING RECOMMENDATION: No Human Data—Probably Compatible

PREGNANCY SUMMARY

No reports describing the use of bromfenac in human pregnancy have been located. The animal reproduction data suggest low risk. Although the lack of human pregnancy experience does not allow a more complete assessment, the very small amounts, if any, of the drug in the systemic circulation suggest that it represents no risk to the embryo or fetus.

FETAL RISK SUMMARY

Bromfenac is a nonsteroidal anti-inflammatory drug (NSAID) that is used topically as a 0.09% solution on the eye. It is indicated for the treatment of postoperative inflammation and the reduction of ocular pain in patients who have undergone cataract extraction. The maximum recommended dose is one drop (0.09 mg) in each eye 2 times daily. It is not known if the drug is absorbed into the systemic circulation, but based on the dose, the amount in the systemic circulation is estimated to be below the limit of quantification (50 ng/mL) (1).

Reproduction studies have been conducted in rats and rabbits. In pregnant rats and rabbits, oral doses up to 540 and 4500 times, respectively, the recommended human ophthalmic dose revealed no evidence of teratogenicity. However, the highest dose in rats was associated with embryo, fetal, and neonatal death, and reduced postnatal growth. The highest dose in rabbits caused increased postimplantation loss (1).

It is not known if bromfenac crosses the human placenta. The molecular weight (about 254 for the nonhydrated free acid) is low enough, but only very small amounts, if any, are present in the systemic circulation. Thus, clinically significant exposure of the embryo or fetus is unlikely.

BREASTFEEDING SUMMARY

No reports describing the use of bromfenac during human lactation have been located. The molecular weight (about 254 for the nonhydrated free acid) is low enough for excretion into breast milk, but only very small amounts, if any, are present in the systemic circulation. Moreover, other NSAIDs are compatible with breastfeeding, even when given orally (e.g., see Ibuprofen). Therefore, the use bromfenac should also be compatible.

Reference

1. Product information. Xibrom. ISTA Pharmaceuticals, 2006.

BROMIDES

Anticonvulsant/Sedative

PREGNANCY RECOMMENDATION: Human and Animal Data Suggest Risk
BREASTFEEDING RECOMMENDATION: Limited Human Data—Potential Toxicity

PREGNANCY SUMMARY

Chronic ingestion of drugs containing bromides is a risk for development toxicity. Exposure near delivery has been reported to cause neonatal bromism.

FETAL RISK SUMMARY

The Collaborative Perinatal Project monitored 50,282 mother–child pairs, 986 of whom had 1st trimester exposure to bromides (1, pp. 402–406). For use anytime during pregnancy, 2610 exposures were recorded (1, p. 444). In neither group was evidence found to suggest a relationship to large categories of major or minor malformations. Four possible associations with individual malformations were found, but independent confirmation is required: polydactyly (14 cases), gastrointestinal anomalies (10 cases), clubfoot (7 cases), and congenital dislocation of hip (use anytime) (92 cases).

Two infants with intrauterine growth restriction from a mother who chronically ingested a proprietary product containing bromides (Bromo-Seltzer) have been described (2). Both male infants were microcephalic (one at the 2nd percentile and one at less than the 2nd percentile) and one had congenital heart disease (atrial septal defect with possible pulmonary insufficiency). The mother did not use the product in three other pregnancies, two before and one after the affected children, and all three of these children were of normal height. In a similar case, a woman chronically ingested tablets containing bromides throughout gestation and eventually gave birth to a female infant who was growth restricted (all parameters below the 10th percentile) (3). Follow-up of the infant at 2.5 years of age indicated persistent developmental delay.

Neonatal bromide intoxication from transplacental accumulation has been described in four infants (4–7). In each case, the mother had either taken bromide-containing medications (three cases) or was exposed from employment in a photographic laboratory (one case). Bromide concentrations in three of the four infants were 3650, 2000, and 2420 mcg/mL on days 6, 5, and 5, respectively (4–6). In the fourth case, a serum sample, not obtained until 18 days after birth, contained 150 mcg/mL (7). All four infants exhibited symptoms of neonatal bromism consisting of poor suck, weak cry, diminished Moro reflex, lethargy, and hypotonia. One of the infants also had cyanosis and a large head with dysmorphic face (7). Subsequent examinations of three of the above infants revealed normal growth and development after several months (4–6). One infant, however, had mild residual hypotonia of the neck muscles persisting at 6 and 9.5 months (7).

Cord serum bromide levels were determined on 1267 newborn infants born in Rochester, New York, during the first half of 1984 (8). Mean bromide concentrations were 8.6 mcg/mL (range 3.1–28.5 mcg/mL), which is well below the serum bromide level (>720 mcg/mL) that is considered toxic (8). The measured concentrations were not related to Apgar scores, neonatal condition, or congenital abnormalities. None of the mothers was taking bromide-containing drugs (most of which have been removed from the market), and the concentrations in cord blood were thought to have resulted from occupational exposure to photographic chemicals or from the low levels encountered in food and water.

BREASTFEEDING SUMMARY

The excretion of bromides into breast milk has been known since at least 1907 (9). A 1938 report reviewed this topic and demonstrated the presence of bromides in milk in an additional 10 mothers (9). A 1935 report measured milk concentrations of 1666 mcg/mL in two patients treated with 5 g daily for 1 month (10). Rash and sedation of varying degrees

B

in several nursing infants have been reported as a result of maternal consumption of bromides during lactation (9–11). Although bromide-containing medications are no longer available in the United States, these drugs may be available in other countries. In addition, high maternal serum levels may be obtained from close, frequent exposure to chemicals used in photographic developing. Women who are breastfeeding and are exposed to such chemicals should be alert for symptoms of sedation or drowsiness and unexplained rashes in their infants. Monitoring of bromide levels in these women may be beneficial. Nursing is not recommended for women receiving bromide-containing medications, although the American Academy of Pediatrics classifies bromides as compatible with breastfeeding (12).

References

1. Heinonen OP, Slone D, Shapiro S. *Birth Defects and Drugs in Pregnancy*. Littleton, MA: Publishing Sciences Group, 1977.
2. Opitz JM, Grosse RF, Haneberg B. Congenital effects of bromism? Lancet 1972;1:91–2.
3. Rossiter EJR, Rendel-Short TJ. Congenital effects of bromism? Lancet 1972;2:705.
4. Finken RL, Robertson WO. Transplacental bromism. Am J Dis Child 1963;106:224–6.
5. Mangurten HH, Ban R. Neonatal hypotonia secondary to transplacental bromism. J Pediatr 1974;85:426–8.
6. Pleasure JR, Blackburn MG. Neonatal bromide intoxication: prenatal ingestion of a large quantity of bromides with transplacental accumulation in the fetus. Pediatrics 1975;55:503–6.
7. Mangurten HH, Kaye CI. Neonatal bromism secondary to maternal exposure in a photographic laboratory. J Pediatr 1982;100:596–8.
8. Miller ME, Cosgriff JM, Roghmann KJ. Cord serum bromide concentration: variation and lack of association with pregnancy outcome. Am J Obstet Gynecol 1987;157:826–30.
9. Tyson RM, Shrader EA, Perlman HH. Drugs transmitted through breast milk. III. Bromides. J Pediatr 1938;13:91–3.
10. Kwit NT, Hatcher RA. Excretion of drugs in milk. Am J Dis Child 1935;49:900–4.
11. Van der Bogert F. Bromin poisoning through mother's milk. Am J Dis Child 1921;21:167.
12. Committee on Drugs, American Academy of Pediatrics. The transfer of drugs and other chemicals into human milk. Pediatrics 2001;108:776–89.

BROMOCRIPTINE

Endocrine/Metabolic Agent (Miscellaneous)

PREGNANCY RECOMMENDATION: Compatible
BREASTFEEDING RECOMMENDATION: Contraindicated

PREGNANCY SUMMARY

Bromocriptine apparently does not pose a significant risk to the fetus. The pattern and incidence of anomalies are similar to those expected in a nonexposed population.

FETAL RISK SUMMARY

Bromocriptine has been used during all stages of pregnancy. In 1982, Turkalj et al. (1) reviewed the results of 1410 pregnancies in 1335 women exposed to bromocriptine during gestation. The drug, used for the treatment of infertility as a result of hyperprolactinemia or pituitary tumors including acromegaly, was usually discontinued as soon as pregnancy was diagnosed. The mean duration of exposure after conception was 21 days. The review included all reported cases from 1973 (the year bromocriptine was introduced) through 1980. Since then, 11 other studies have reported the results of treatment in 121 women with 145 pregnancies (2–12). The results of the pregnancies in the combined studies are as follows:

Total patients/pregnancies 1456/1555
Liveborn infants 1369 (88%)
Stillborn infants 5 (0.3%)
Multiple pregnancies (30 twins/3 triplets) 33*(2.1%)
Spontaneous abortions 66 (10.7%)
Elective abortions 26 (1.7%)
Extrauterine pregnancies 12 (0.8%)
Hydatidiform moles (2 patients) 3 (0.2%)
Pregnant at time of report-outcome unknown 10

*Two women with twins were also treated with clomiphene or gonadotropin.

A total of 48 (3.5%) of the 1374 liveborn and stillborn infants had detectable anomalies at birth (1–12). This incidence is similar to the expected rate of congenital defects found in the general population. In the review by Turkalj et al. (1), the mean duration of fetal exposure to bromocriptine was similar between children with congenital abnormalities and normal children. No distinguishable pattern of anomalies was found. The malformations detected at birth are shown below (number of infants indicated in parentheses):

Down's syndrome (2)
Hydrocephalus and multiple atresia of esophagus and intestine (1)
Microcephalus/encephalopathy (1)
Omphalocele/talipes (1)
Pulmonary artery atresia (1)
Reduction deformities (4)
Renal agenesis (1)
Pierre Robin syndrome (1)
Bat ear and plagiocephalous (1)
Cleft palate (1)
Ear lobe deformity (1)
Head posture constrained (1)
Hip dislocation (aplasia of cup) (9)
Hydrocele (3)
Hydrocele/omphalocele (1)
Hypospadias (1)

Inguinal hernia (2)
Skull soft and open fontanella (1)
Single palmar crease (1)
Single umbilical artery (1)
Syndactyly (2)
Talipes (5)
Umbilical hernia (1)
Cutaneous hemangioma (4)
Testicular ectopia (1) (spontaneous correction at age 7 months)

Long-term studies on 213 children followed up to 6 years of age have shown normal mental and physical development (1,2).

In a surveillance study of Michigan Medicaid recipients involving 229,101 completed pregnancies conducted between 1985 and 1992, 50 newborns had been exposed to bromocriptine during the 1st trimester (F. Rosa, personal communication, FDA, 1993). Three (6%) major birth defects were observed (two expected). Specific information was not available on the malformations, but no anomalies were observed in six categories of defects (cardiovascular defects, oral clefts, spina bifida, polydactyly, limb reduction defects, and hypospadias) for which data were available. Based on a small number of exposures, the data do not support an association between the drug and congenital defects.

BREASTFEEDING SUMMARY

Since bromocriptine is indicated for the prevention of physiologic lactation, breastfeeding is not possible during therapy (13,14). However, in one report, a mother taking 5 mg/day for a pituitary tumor was able to breastfeed her infant successfully (3). No effects on the infant were mentioned. Because bromocriptine suppresses lactation, the American Academy of Pediatrics classifies bromocriptine as a drug that should be given to nursing women with caution (15).

References

1. Turkalj I, Braun P, Krupp P. Surveillance of bromocriptine in pregnancy. JAMA 1982;247:1589–91.
2. Konopka P, Raymond JP, Merceron RE, Seneze J. Continuous administration of bromocriptine in the prevention of neurological complications in pregnant women with prolactinomas. Am J Obstet Gynecol 1983;146:935–8.
3. Canales ES, Garcia IC, Ruiz JE, Zarate A. Bromocriptine as prophylactic therapy in prolactinoma during pregnancy. Fertil Steril 1981;36:524–6.
4. Bergh T, Nillius SJ, Larsson SG, Wide L. Effects of bromocriptine-induced pregnancy on prolactin-secreting pituitary tumors. Acta Endocrinol 1981;98:333.
5. Yuen BH, Cannon W, Sy L, Booth J, Burch P. Regression of pituitary microadenoma during and following bromocriptine therapy: persistent defect in prolactin regulation before and throughout pregnancy. Am J Obstet Gynecol 1982;142:634–9.
6. Maeda T, Ushiroyama T, Okuda K, Fujimoto A, Ueki M, Sugimoto O. Effective bromocriptine treatment of a pituitary macroadenoma during pregnancy. Obstet Gynecol 1983;61:117–21.
7. Hammond CB, Haney AF, Land MR, van der Merwe JV, Ory SJ, Wiebe RH. The outcome of pregnancy in patients with treated and untreated prolactin-secreting pituitary tumors. Am J Obstet Gynecol 1983;147:148–57.
8. Cundy T, Grundy EN, Melville H, Sheldon J. Bromocriptine treatment of acromegaly following spontaneous conception. Fertil Steril 1984;42:134–6.
9. Randall S, Laing I, Chapman AJ, Shalet SM, Beardwell CG, Kelly WF, Davies D. Pregnancies in women with hyperprolactinaemia: obstetric and endocrinological management of 50 pregnancies in 37 women. Br J Obstet Gynaecol 1982;89:20–33.
10. Andersen AN, Starup J, Tabor A, Jensen HK, Westergaard JG. The possible prognostic value of serum prolactin increment during pregnancy in hyperprolactinaemic patients. Acta Endocrinol 1983;102:1–5.
11. Van Roon E, van der Vijver JCM, Gerretsen G, Hekster REM, Wattendorff RA. Rapid regression of a suprasellar extending prolactinoma after bromocriptine treatment during pregnancy. Fertil Steril 1981;36:173–77.
12. Crosignani P, Ferrari C, Mattei AM. Visual field defects and reduced visual acuity during pregnancy in two patients with prolactinoma: rapid regression of symptoms under bromocriptine. Case reports. Br J Obstet Gynaecol 1984;91:821–3.
13. Product information. Parlodel. Sandoz Pharmaceuticals, 1985.
14. Thorbert G, Akerlund M. Inhibition of lactation by cyclofenil and bromocriptine. Br J Obstet Gynaecol 1983;90:739–42.
15. Committee on Drugs, American Academy of Pediatrics. The transfer of drugs and other chemicals into human milk. Pediatrics 2001;108:776–89.

BROMODIPHENHYDRAMINE

[Withdrawn from the market. See 9th edition.]

BROMPHENIRAMINE

Antihistamine

PREGNANCY RECOMMENDATION: Limited Human Data—No Relevant Animal Data
BREASTFEEDING RECOMMENDATION: Limited Human Data—Probably Compatible

PREGNANCY SUMMARY

In general, antihistamines are considered low risk in pregnancy. However, exposure near birth of premature infants has been associated with an increased risk of retrolental fibroplasia.

FETAL RISK SUMMARY

The Collaborative Perinatal Project monitored 50,282 mother–child pairs, 65 of whom had 1st trimester exposure to brompheniramine (1, pp. 322–325). Based on 10 malformed infants, a statistically significant association ($p < 0.01$) was found between this drug and congenital defects. This relationship was not found with other antihistamines. For use anytime during pregnancy, 412 exposures were recorded (1, p. 437).

B

In this group, no evidence was found for an association with malformations.

The use of antihistamines in general (specific agents and dose not given) during the last 2 weeks of pregnancy has been associated with an increased risk of retrolental fibroplasia in premature infants (2). Infants weighing <1750 g, who had no detectable congenital anomalies and who survived for at least 24 hours after birth, were enrolled in the multicenter National Collaborative Study on Patent Ductus Arteriosus in Premature Infants conducted between 1979 and 1981 (2). After exclusions, 3026 infants were available for study. Exposures to antihistamines and other drugs were determined by interview and maternal record review. The incidence of retrolental fibroplasia in infants exposed to antihistamines during the last 2 weeks of gestation was 22% (19 of 86) vs. 11% (324 of 2940) in infants not exposed during this interval. Adjustment for severity of disease did not change the estimated rate ratio.

BREASTFEEDING SUMMARY

A single case report has been located describing adverse effects in a 3-month-old nursing infant of a mother consuming a long-acting preparation containing 6 mg of dexbrompheniramine and 120 mg of *d*-isoephedrine (3). The mother began taking the preparation on a twice-daily schedule about 1 or 2 days before the onset of symptoms in the infant. Symptoms consisted of irritability, excessive crying, and disturbed sleeping patterns, which resolved spontaneously within 12 hours when breastfeeding was stopped. One manufacturer considers the drug to be contraindicated for nursing mothers (4). The American Academy of Pediatrics noted the above adverse effects observed with dexbrompheniramine plus *d*-isoephedrine, but classified the combination as usually compatible with breastfeeding (5).

References

1. Heinonen OP, Slone D, Shapiro S. *Birth Defects and Drugs in Pregnancy*. Littleton, MA: Publishing Sciences Group, 1977.
2. Zierler S, Purohit D. Prenatal antihistamine exposure and retrolental fibroplasia. Am J Epidemiol 1986;123:192–6.
3. Mortimer EA Jr. Drug toxicity from breast milk? Pediatrics 1977;60:780–1.
4. Product information. Dimetane. AH Robins Company, 1990.
5. Committee on Drugs, American Academy of Pediatrics. The transfer of drugs and other chemicals into human milk. Pediatrics 2001;108:776–89.

BUCLIZINE

[Withdrawn from the market. See 9th edition.]

BUDESONIDE

Respiratory Drug (Corticosteroid)

PREGNANCY RECOMMENDATION: Compatible (Inhaled/Nasal), No Human Data—Animal Data Suggest Risk (Oral)
BREASTFEEDING RECOMMENDATION: Limited Human Data—Probably Compatible

PREGNANCY SUMMARY

Inhaled budesonide does not appear to represent a significant risk for congenital defects in humans, but a small risk may exist between nasal budesonide and cardiac defects. A small, but statistically significant, increased risk for cleft lip with or without cleft palate has been reported for corticosteroids (see Hydrocortisone). A similar risk for orofacial clefts was observed with inhaled budesonide, but the number of exposed infants was too small for statistical significance. The data from the manufacturer's postmarketing surveillance do not show a clustering of defects and thus, in themselves, cannot be used as evidence of an increased risk for birth defects. Surveillance reports of this type are important for detecting early signals of major teratogens, but they have several difficulties. The primary problems with these voluntary reports are their retrospective nature (reported after the outcome is known), their selection bias (mainly adverse outcomes are reported), and their lack of sufficient details on the mother, her family history, her disease, and her pregnancy. Moreover, these data cannot be used to determine true rates of outcomes.

During pregnancy, the benefits of treating allergic rhinitis with any product, including budesonide, must be carefully weighed against the potential risks of therapy. Consideration should be given to limiting corticosteroid exposure, especially during the 1st trimester. In contrast, poorly controlled asthma may result in adverse maternal, fetal, and neonatal outcomes (1). Maternal complications include an increased risk of preeclampsia, pregnancy-induced hypertension, hyperemesis gravidarum, vaginal hemorrhage, and induced and difficult labors. Fetal and neonatal adverse effects may be an increased risk of perinatal mortality, intrauterine growth restriction (IUGR), prematurity, lower birth weight, and neonatal hypoxia. Because controlling maternal asthma can ameliorate or prevent all of these complications (1), the benefits of therapy outweigh the potential risks of drug-induced teratogenicity or toxicity. Therefore, pregnant women who require an inhaled corticosteroid, such as budesonide, for control of their asthma should be counseled as to the risks and benefits of therapy, but treatment should not be withheld because of their pregnancy.

FETAL RISK SUMMARY

Budesonide is an anti-inflammatory corticosteroid used in the maintenance treatment of asthma as prophylactic therapy (Pulmicort Turbuhaler) or for the management of symptoms of allergic rhinitis (Rhinocort Nasal Inhaler). Pulmicort Turbuhaler delivers approximately 160 mcg of micronized budesonide per actuation, whereas Rhinocort Nasal Inhaler delivers approximately 32 mcg of micronized budesonide per actuation (2,3). The latter dose is suspended in a mixture of propellants (dichlorodifluoromethane, trichloromonofluoromethane, and dichlorotetrafluoroethane) and sorbitan trioleate.

Budesonide has potent glucocorticoid but weak mineralocorticoid activity. Compared with hydrocortisone (cortisol), budesonide is 40 times more potent when administered SC and 25 times more potent when given orally. Approximately 34% of the delivered dose of Pulmicort and 21% of Rhinocort are absorbed systemically (2,3).

Similar to other glucocorticoid agents, budesonide is administered to pregnant rabbits at a SC dose about 0.33 times the maximum recommended human daily inhalation dose based on BSA (MRHD) produced fetal loss, IUGR, and skeletal anomalies (mostly delayed ossification of the vertebra and skull) (2–4). In pregnant rats, a SC dose about 3 times the MRHD resulted in similar outcomes. No teratogenic or embryocidal effects were observed in pregnant rats administered inhalation doses up to about 2 times the MRHD (2,3).

No reports describing the placental transfer of budesonide have been located. The relatively low molecular weight (about 431 for the butyraldehyde formulation) and high lipid solubility suggest substantial placental transfer. The actual amount of active budesonide reaching the fetus, however, may be small because of the low systemic bioavailability after inhaled or nasal administration (see above).

Data from the Swedish Medical Birth Registry involving 2014 infants whose mothers had inhaled budesonide for asthma during early pregnancy were reported in 1999 (5). Drug exposures were identified prospectively, before the pregnancy outcomes were known. Among the mothers of the 2014 infants, 1675 also used β_2-adrenergic agonists, 16 used other inhaled corticosteroids in addition to budesonide, and 316 used no other antiasthmatic drug. A total of 76 infants (3.8%) in the exposed group had a congenital malformation, compared with 3.5% for all infants born in 1995–1997. Major structural defects were observed in 41 of the infants, whereas 35 infants had minor and/or variable conditions. Five of the major defects were chromosomal anomalies. It is unlikely that these were due to drug therapy (4). Four (expected 3.3) of the major anomaly group had an orofacial cleft (median cleft palate [*N* = 2], unilateral cleft lip [*N* = 1], and unilateral cleft lip and palate [*N* = 1]) (relative risk 1.2, 95% confidence interval [CI] 0.3–3.1) (4). Among the major and minor defects, 18 (expected 17–18) involved the heart, including 2 premature infants with patent ductus arteriosus (both categorized as minor defects). The other cardiac malformations were as follows: ventricular septal defects (VSD) with or without other anomalies (*N* = 11); atrial septal defects with or without other anomalies (*N* = 4); and unspecified cardiac defect (*N* = 1). Only two of the cases with VSD, one with transposition of the great vessels and another with tricuspidal atresia (both successfully repaired), were reported to the Swedish Child Cardiology Registry (expected number 5.6). Because the other 16 cases were not reported, the authors concluded that the defects were mild and of little clinical significance (5).

The above Registry was updated in 2003 (6). There were now 2968 mothers who had used inhaled budesonide in early pregnancy and gave birth to infants with normal gestational age, birth weight, and length. There also was no increase in rate of stillbirths. The study was not designed to detect birth defects (6).

Twenty-one pregnancies in which the woman received an active drug were reported to the manufacturer during clinical trials of Pulmicort Turbuhaler (A. Marants, personal communication, Astra Pharmaceuticals, 1999). Two of the pregnancies were terminated voluntarily, 1 woman had a miscarriage, 3 had unknown outcomes, 13 delivered normal infants, and 2 delivered infants with congenital malformations. In one case, the 27-year-old mother was receiving budesonide 1600 mcg/day at conception. She was also taking prednisone 10 mg/day and a combination oral contraceptive (levonorgestrel + ethinyl estradiol). Although the reason for early delivery was not specified, a female infant with coarctation of the aorta was delivered by cesarean section at 30 weeks' gestation. The infant was scheduled for surgical repair of the defect. In the second case, a 41-year-old mother used budesonide inhaler for 22 days (dosage unknown) before discontinuing it because of her pregnancy. Seven months later, she delivered a female infant with double-sided maxillary clefts, double digits of the left hand, and persistent fetal circulation (i.e., patent ductus arteriosus). The infant died at 8 days of age.

The infant outcomes of five asthmatic women who used budesonide during pregnancy were described in retrospective postmarketing reports to the manufacturer (A. Marants, personal communication, Astra Pharmaceuticals, 1999). Only limited data were available for each pregnancy. The first case involved a 36-year-old woman, treated with an unknown dose of budesonide combined with a β_2-adrenergic agonist (albuterol), who delivered an anencephalic infant. In the second case, a 32-year-old woman administering budesonide 1600 mcg/day gave birth to a healthy 2.65-kg baby. A 33-year-old woman was treated with four antiasthmatic agents during gestation, including budesonide 1600 mcg/day, an oral corticosteroid (name not specified), a β_2-adrenergic agonist (not specified), and theophylline. She gave birth to a female infant with agenesis of the left foot who was otherwise healthy. Another 33-year-old woman being treated with budesonide 1600 mcg/day, phenobarbital, and terbutaline (a β_2-adrenergic agonist) delivered an infant with cleft palate, an unspecified cardiac defect, and hydrocephalus. Finally, IUGR and oligohydramnios were noted in a pregnancy of a 36-year-old woman who was being treated with budesonide 400 mcg/day, salmeterol (an inhaled β_2-adrenergic agonist), and terfenadine (an antihistamine). She gave birth to a growth-restricted infant (2.0 kg) who had multiple malformations, including a diaphragmatic hernia, renal hypoplasia, and a VSD. The infant died on the day of birth.

A 2003 case–control study, using data from three Swedish health registers, was conducted to identify drug use in early pregnancy that was associated with cardiac defects (7). Cases of cardiovascular defects without known chromosome anomalies (*N* = 5015) were compared with controls consisting of all infants born in Sweden (1995–2001) (*N* = 577,730).

Associations were identified for several drugs, some of which were probably due to confounding from the underlying disease or complaint or multiple testing, but some were thought to be true drug effects. For all inhaled corticosteroids, there were 66 cases in 7404 exposures (odds ratio [OR] 1.05, 95% CI 0.82–1.34). For inhaled budesonide, there were 16 cases in 6557 exposures (OR 1.12, 95% CI 0.87–1.44). For all nasal corticosteroids, there were 31 cases among 2872 exposures (1.24, 95% CI 0.87–1.78), but 28 of the cases involved nasal budesonide (2230 exposures) (1.45, 95% CI 0.99–2.10). Restricting the analysis of nasal budesonide to less severe defects increased the probability of an association (OR 1.58, 95% CI 1.02–2.46), as also was seen with unspecified cardiovascular defects (OR 2.39, 95% CI 0.96–4.92). The risk for ventricular and atrial septum defects were 1.67 (95% CI 0.99–2.81) and 2.18 (95% CI 0.71–5.08), respectively (7).

A 2004 study examined the effect of inhaled corticosteroids on low birth weight, preterm births, and congenital malformations in pregnant asthmatic patients (8). The inhaled steroids and the number of patients were beclomethasone (*N* = 277), fluticasone (*N* = 132), triamcinolone (*N* = 81), budesonide (*N* = 43), and flunisolide (*N* = 25). Compared with the general population, the study found no increased incidence of small-for-gestational-age infants (<10th percentile for gestational age), low birth weight (<2500 g), preterm births, and congenital malformations (8).

A 2006 meta-analysis on the use of inhaled corticosteroids during pregnancy was published in 2006 (9). The analysis included five agents: beclomethasone, budesonide, flunisolide, fluticasone, and triamcinolone. The results showed that these agents do not increase the risk of major congenital defects, preterm delivery, low birth weight, and pregnancy-induced hypertension. Thus, they could be used during pregnancy (9).

A 2007 report described the use of inhaled budesonide in 42 pregnant women (10). No effects on fetal growth or pregnancy outcomes were observed in these patients. Although most synthetic corticosteroids are partially metabolized by placental enzymes, budesonide was not (10).

BREASTFEEDING SUMMARY

The relatively low molecular weight (about 431 for the butyraldehyde formulation) and the high lipid solubility predict excretion of systemic budesonide into milk. However, the systemic bioavailability of budesonide following inhalation therapy is relatively low (see section above), thus, the actual amount in milk also may be low. The results of the below study are consistent with this assessment.

In a 2007 study, milk and plasma budesonide concentrations were measured in eight mothers receiving maintenance treatment with Pulmicort Turbuhaler (200 or 400 mcg twice daily) (11). Plasma concentrations also were measured in their breastfeeding infants. The mean milk:plasma ratio was 0.46. For both dose levels, the estimated daily infant dose was 0.3% of the daily maternal dose. The average plasma concentrations in nursing infants was estimated to be 1/600th of the maternal concentration (all infant levels were less than the limit of quantification), assuming 100% bioavailability in the infants. The authors concluded that their data supported continued use of inhaled budesonide during breastfeeding (11).

References

1. Quick reference from the Working Group on Managing Asthma during Pregnancy: Recommendations for Pharmacologic Treatment—Update 2004, National Institutes of Health (NIH Publication No. 05-3279). Available at http://www.nhibi.nih.gov/health/prof/lung/asthma/astpreg.htm. Accessed September 2013.
2. Product information. Pulmicort Turbuhaler. AstraZeneca, 2000.
3. Product information. Rhinocort. AstraZeneca, 2000.
4. Kihlstrom I, Lundberg C. Teratogenicity study of the new glucocorticosteroid budesonide in rabbits. Arzneimittelforschung 1987;37:43–6.
5. Kallen B, Rydhstroem H, Aberg A. Congenital malformations after the use of inhaled budesonide in early pregnancy. Obstet Gynecol 1999;93:392–5.
6. Norjavaara E, Gerhardsson de Verdier M. Normal pregnancy outcomes in a population-based study including 2968 pregnant women exposed to budesonide. J Allergy Clin Immunol 2003;111:736–42.
7. Kallen BAJ, Olausson PO. Maternal drug use in early pregnancy and infant cardiovascular defect. Reprod Toxicol 2003;17:255–61.
8. Namazy J, Schatz M, Long L, Lipkowitz M, Lillie M, Voss M, Deitz RJ, Petitti D. Use of inhaled steroids by pregnant asthmatic women does not reduce intrauterine growth. J Allergy Clin Immunol 2004;113:427–32.
9. Rahimi R, Nikfar S, Abdollahi M. Meta-analysis finds use of inhaled corticosteroids during pregnancy safe: a systematic meta-analysis review. Hum Exp Toxicol 2006;25:447–52.
10. Murphy VE, Fittock RJ, Zarzycki PK, Delahunty MM, Smith R, Clifton VL. Metabolism of synthetic steroids by the human placenta. Placenta 2007;28:39–46.
11. Falt A, Bengtsson T, Kennedy BM, Gyllenberg A, Lindberg B, Thorsson L, Strandgarden K. Exposure of infants to budesonide through breast milk of asthmatic mothers. J Allergy Clin Immunol 2007;120:798–802.

BUMETANIDE

Diuretic

PREGNANCY RECOMMENDATION: Limited Human Data—Animal Data Suggest Low Risk
BREASTFEEDING RECOMMENDATION: No Human Data—Probably Compatible

PREGNANCY SUMMARY

No published reports on the use of bumetanide in human pregnancy have been located, but the diuretic has been recommended for the treatment of the nephrotic syndrome occurring during pregnancy (1). Diuretics are not recommended for the treatment of gestational hypertension because of the maternal hypovolemia characteristic of this disease.

B

FETAL RISK SUMMARY

Bumetanide is a potent loop diuretic that is similar in action to furosemide; it shares the same indications and precautions for use during gestation as this latter diuretic (see also Furosemide).

The drug is not teratogenic in rats, mice, hamsters, or rabbits (2,3). In rats, doses 3400 times the maximum therapeutic human dose (MTHD) had a slight embryocidal effect, produced fetal growth restriction, and increased the incidence of delayed ossification of sternebrae (3). In rabbits, which are more sensitive to the effects of bumetanide than other test species, doses 3.4 times the MTHD were slightly embryocidal. At doses 10 times the MTHD, an increased embryocidal effect was observed, as well as an increased incidence of delayed ossification of sternebrae (3).

In a surveillance study of Michigan Medicaid recipients involving 229,101 completed pregnancies conducted between 1985 and 1992, 44 newborns had been exposed to bumetanide during the 1st trimester (F. Rosa, personal communication, FDA, 1993). Two (4.5%) major birth defects were observed (two expected), both of which were cardiovascular defects (0.4 expected).

BREASTFEEDING SUMMARY

No reports describing the use of bumetanide during human lactation have been located. Bumetanide probably is compatible with breastfeeding but, in general, diuretics should be used cautiously during nursing because they may suppress lactation.

References

1. Wood SM, Blainey JD. Hypertension and renal disease. In: Wood SM, Beeley L, eds. *Prescribing in Pregnancy*. Clin Obstet Gynaecol 1981;8:439–53.
2. McClain RM, Dammers KD. Toxicologic evaluation of bumetanide, a potent diuretic agent. J Clin Pharmacol 1981;21:543–54. As cited in Shepard TH. *Catalog of Teratogenic Agents*. 6th ed. Baltimore, MD: Johns Hopkins University Press, 1989:92.
3. Product information. Bumex. Roche Laboratories, 1993.

BUPRENORPHINE

Narcotic Agonist-Antagonist Analgesic

PREGNANCY RECOMMENDATION: Limited Human Data—Animal Data Suggest Low Risk
BREASTFEEDING RECOMMENDATION: Limited Human Data—Potential Toxicity

PREGNANCY SUMMARY

Buprenorphine is a potent narcotic agonist and antagonist that has been used during human pregnancy for analgesia immediately prior to delivery in a small number of cases. One pregnancy case has been located in which the drug was given as a narcotic substitute for heroin dependency. Neonatal withdrawal was observed, but the symptoms were less than that expected with methadone. Animal studies have demonstrated dose-related maternal, embryo, and fetal toxicity and dose-related behavioral changes in offspring, but no congenital malformations. Although the lack of congenital anomalies is reassuring, the behavioral changes in animals combined with the absence of published early human pregnancy experience prevent an assessment of the risk that this drug presents to the embryo or fetus. Because there is substantially more published human pregnancy experience for other narcotic analgesics, they are preferred to buprenorphine, especially during early gestation. Buprenorphine may have a role as substitution therapy for maternal heroin addiction, but additional reports are needed to define its pregnancy safety profile before this use can be recommended.

FETAL RISK SUMMARY

Buprenorphine, an analgesic that possesses both narcotic agonist and antagonist activity, is approximately 33 times more potent than morphine (0.3-mg buprenorphine is equivalent to 10-mg morphine in analgesic and respiratory depressant effects). Although a sublingual formulation is available in other countries, only parenteral buprenorphine has been approved for general use in the United States. The human adult dose is 0.3–0.6 mg IM or IV repeated up to every 6 hours (0.017–0.034 mg/kg/day for a 70-kg person).

Buprenorphine is currently under investigation as an alternative to methadone maintenance treatment of narcotic dependence (1–3). The drug has also been studied as an alternative to cocaine, but it is apparently not effective for this use (2). Although these trials have not yet included pregnant women, the advantages of buprenorphine over methadone during gestation may include less respiratory depression at high doses, less toxicity from overdose, less severe withdrawal after abrupt discontinuance of the drug, and potentially less abuse liability (1,2). Of interest, however, abuse of buprenorphine, often concurrently with opiates, has been reported outside of the United States (4,5). One of these latter citations reported frequent abuse of buprenorphine by pregnant women but provided no outcome data (4).

Reproduction studies in rats and rabbits have been conducted (6–12). No fetal adverse effects were observed in rats and rabbits when their mothers were administered doses up to 5 mg/kg IM during organogenesis (6). Shepard (7) cited a study in which fetal growth restriction, but not congenital defects, was observed in rats exposed to maternal doses of >0.05–5 mg/kg/day (about 3–300 times the recommended human dose [RHD]) given after implantation through delivery. Rat fetuses exposed to 5 mg/kg/day in the last week of pregnancy had a reduced survival rate after delivery (7). As reported by the manufacturer, no major congenital malformations were observed in rats given doses of 10–1000 times (SC or IM) or 160 times (IV) the RHD, but significant increases in postimplantation losses and early fetal deaths were noted with IM doses of 10 and 100 times the RHD (8). A slight increase in postimplantation losses was also observed with IV doses of 40 and 160 times the RHD. In rabbits, IM doses produced a dose-related increase in extra rib formation that was statistically significant at 1000 times the RHD (8). Rats pups exposed in utero throughout gestation to maternal doses of buprenorphine, 1 and 2 mg/kg/day SC, had reduced survival. Minimal effects were observed on the endogenous opioid system, however, as determined by a comparison of the brain enkephalin levels of buprenorphine-exposed pups to those in methadone-exposed pups (9).

In a study involving pregnant rats, buprenorphine was administered by a continuous infusion in doses of 0.3, 1.0, and 3.0 mg/kg/day from day 8 of gestation through parturition (10). At these doses, no evidence of significant maternal toxicity was observed, nor were there any significant effects on the offspring in terms of morbidity and mortality, birth weight, and postnatal growth (up to 60 days) (10). In a second publication by these researchers, using the same drug-administration technique and animal type described above, no disruption in the rest–activity cycle was observed in the exposed offspring at 22 and 30 days of age (11).

The long-term effects on sexual differentiation in rats exposed in utero to maternal injections of buprenorphine, 0.3 or 0.6 mg/kg every 48 hours from day 6 to day 20 of gestation, were described in a study published in 1997 (12). Compared with controls and the lower-dose group, spontaneous parental behavior (at 23–28 days of age) and the expected sex difference in the consumption of a 0.25% saccharin solution (at 42–55 days of age) were impaired in the 0.6-mg/kg-exposed offspring. The authors concluded that the higher dose of buprenorphine produced long-term adverse effects on behavior (12).

As suggested by the molecular weight of the free base (about 468), buprenorphine crosses the placenta to the fetus. In a 1997 case report, a 24-year-old woman was treated with buprenorphine 4 mg/day for heroin addiction, starting in the 4th month of pregnancy (13). Frequent tests during the remainder of the pregnancy and at delivery confirmed her rapid withdrawal from heroin. Except for buprenorphine, all tests were negative for opiates, cocaine, cannabis, and amphetamines. An apparently normal female infant (birth weight not specified) was delivered at 39 weeks' gestation. Apgar scores were 10 and 10 at 1 and 10 minutes, respectively. High levels of buprenorphine and its metabolite were measured in the newborn approximately 20 hours after birth. Maternal trough serum concentrations of buprenorphine and the metabolite, norbuprenorphine, obtained a few days before delivery were 0.3 and 2.3 ng/mL, respectively. Parent drug and metabolite concentrations in the meconium were 107 and 295 ng/g, respectively. Levels of drug and metabolite were, respectively, 1.9 and 1.7 ng/mL in the newborn's serum and 36.8 and 61.1 ng/mL in the newborn's urine. The estimated cord:maternal serum ratio was 6.3, whereas the ratio for the metabolite was 0.7. A weak withdrawal syndrome was observed at 48 hours of age with an adapted Finnegan score (used to evaluate the intensity of withdrawal syndromes; range 0–40) of 12 (13). Symptoms, which resolved without therapy, consisted of agitation, sleep disturbance, tremor, yawning, noisy breathing, and a slight fever (13). The Finnegan score fell to 8 at 3 days of age and was normal by 6 days of age.

The effect of epidural buprenorphine combined with bupivacaine has been compared with epidural combinations of bupivacaine and morphine, fentanyl, sufentanil, and oxymorphone for analgesia during and after cesarean section (14–17). The analgesic effects of the narcotic agents were similar, but buprenorphine caused a significant increase in maternal vomiting (14–16). No adverse neonatal effects were observed in the two studies that used buprenorphine before delivery (14,17).

The use of sublingual buprenorphine for labor pain in 34 primigravida women was described in a 1992 report (18). Each patient received a single 6-mcg/kg dose during the first stage of labor. No effects were observed on the progression of labor and none of the women had nausea or vomiting. Similarly, no changes in fetal heart rate (range 138–150 beats/minute) were observed. Buprenorphine produced no neonatal depression as evidenced by the average Apgar scores (range not specified) at 1 and 5 minutes of 9.71 and 9.94, respectively.

BREASTFEEDING SUMMARY

Buprenorphine is excreted into human milk. In a 1997 case report (see above), a 24-year-old former heroin addict on buprenorphine maintenance therapy (4 mg/day) gave birth to an apparently normal female infant at 39 weeks' gestation (13). She continued taking buprenorphine while nursing her infant. At 4 weeks of age, buprenorphine and its metabolite, norbuprenorphine, were determined in her milk at each feeding over a 24-hour period. The volume of milk drunk was estimated by weighing the infant before and after the feedings. Although the specific milk concentrations were not provided, the authors estimated that the total doses of drug and metabolite ingested by the infant over the 24-hour period were 3.28 and 0.33 mcg, respectively. No withdrawal symptoms in the infant were observed when lactation was abruptly interrupted at 8 weeks of age.

A study published in 1997 described the effects of continuous extradural bupivacaine and buprenorphine on analgesia and breastfeeding in 20 healthy women who had undergone a cesarean section at term (19). The study group ($N = 10$) received a 5-mL bolus of bupivacaine 0.25% with 200 mcg of buprenorphine extradurally at cord clamping, followed by a continuous extradural infusion of bupivacaine (0.25%) and buprenorphine (12 mcg/mL) infused at 0.7 mL/hour for 3 days. The control group ($N = 10$) received the same bolus and continuous infusion, but without the buprenorphine. There were no significant differences in visual analog pain scores between the groups at 2 hours, 1 day, and 2 days, but the controls received significantly more supplemental diclofenac (a nonsteroidal anti-inflammatory agent) during the 2-day period (mean 25 vs. 5 mg, $p < 0.05$). The weight of breast milk ingested at each feeding was estimated by weighing the infant before and after each feeding. Compared with the control group, the buprenorphine group ingested significantly less milk each day (starting at day 3), and the infant's daily weight as a percentage of birth weight was significantly less starting at day 7. In both effects, the significant differences

B

continued up to 11 days, near the time of discharge from the hospital. The investigators speculated that the differences between the two groups might be due to CNS depression in the mother and infant. Although one author thought the stress of the prolonged hospital stay may have depressed the breastfeeding (20), the investigators responded that long hospital stays are normal in Japan and, if stress is a factor, would have affected both groups similarly (19).

Because buprenorphine is excreted into milk and because depression of the nursing infant resulting in lower weight gain is a possibility, mothers receiving buprenorphine should probably not breastfeed. If breastfeeding is undertaken, the mother should be advised of the potential risk to her infant.

References

1. Vocci F, Chiang CN, Cummings L, Hawks R. Overview: medications development for the treatment of drug abuse. NIDA Res Monogr 1995;149: 4–15.
2. Schottenfeld RS. Clinical trials of pharmacologic treatments in pregnant women—methodologic considerations. NIDA Res Monogr 1995;149: 201–23.
3. O'Connor PG, Oliveto AH, Shi JM, Triffleman EG, Carroll KM, Kosten TR, Rounsaville BJ, Pakes JA, Schottenfeld RS. A randomized trial of buprenorphine maintenance for heroin dependence in a primary care clinic for substance users versus a methadone clinic. Am J Med 1998;105:100–5.
4. Stewart MJ. Effect of scheduling of buprenorphine (Temgesic) on drug abuse patterns in Glasgow. BMJ 1991;302:969.
5. Strang J. Abuse of buprenorphine (Temgesic) by snorting. BMJ 1991;302:969.
6. Heel RC, Brogden RN, Speight TM, Avery GS. Buprenorphine: a review of its pharmacological properties and therapeutic efficacy. Drugs 1979;17: 81–110.
7. Mori N, Sakanoue M, Kamata S, Takeuchi M, Shimpo K, Tamagawa M. Toxicological studies of buprenorphine teratogenicity, perinatal and postnatal studies in the rat. Iyaku Kenkyu 1982;13:509–44. As cited in Shepard TH. *Catalog of Teratogenic Agents*. 8th ed. Baltimore, MD: Johns Hopkins University Press, 1995:58–9.
8. Product information. Buprenex. Reckitt & Colman Pharmaceuticals, 1998.
9. Tiong GK, Olley JE. Effects of exposure in utero to methadone and buprenorphine on enkephalin levels in the developing rat brain. Neurosci Lett 1988;93:101–6.
10. Hutchings DE, Zmitrovich AC, Hamowy AS, Liu P-YR. Prenatal administration of buprenorphine using the osmotic minipump: a preliminary study of maternal and offspring toxicity and growth in the rat. Neurotoxicol Teratol 1995;17:419–23.
11. Hutchings DE, Hamowy AS, Williams EM, Zmitrovich AC. Prenatal administration of buprenorphine in the rat: effects on the rest-activity cycle at 22 and 30 days of age. Pharmacol Biochem Behav 1996;55:607–13.
12. Barron S, Chung VM. Prenatal buprenorphine exposure and sexually dimorphic nonreproductive behaviors in rats. Pharmacol Biochem Behav 1997;58:337–43.
13. Marquet P, Chevrel J, Lavignasse P, Merle L, Lachatre G. Buprenorphine withdrawal syndrome in a newborn. Clin Pharmacol Ther 1997;62:569–71.
14. Celleno D, Costantino P, Emanuelli M, Capogna G, Muratori F, Sebastiani M, Cipriani G. Epidural analgesia during and after cesarean delivery. Comparison of five opioids. Reg Anesth 1991;16:79–83.
15. Cohen S, Amar D, Pantuck CB, Pantuck EJ, Weissman AM, Landa S, Singer N. Epidural patient-controlled analgesia after cesarean section: buprenorphine-0.015% bupivacaine with epinephrine versus fentanyl-0.015% bupivacaine with and without epinephrine. Anesth Analg 1992;74:226–30.
16. Cohen S, Amar D, Pantuck CB, Pantuck EJ, Weissman AB. Adverse effects of epidural 0.03% bupivacaine during analgesia after cesarean section. Anesth Analg 1992;75:753–6.
17. Lehmann KA, Stern S, Breuker KH. Obstetrical peridural anesthesia with bupivacaine and buprenorphine. A randomized double-blind study in comparison with untreated controls. Anaesthesist 1992;41:414–22.
18. Roy S, Basu RK. Role of sublingual administration of tablet buprenorphine hydrochloride on relief of labour pain. J Indian Med Assoc 1992;90:151–3.
19. Hirose M, Hosokawa T, Tanaka Y. Extradural buprenorphine suppresses breast feeding after caesarean section. Br J Anaesth 1997;79:120–1.
20. Celebioglu B. Extradural buprenorphine and breast feeding after caesarean section. Br J Anaesth 1998;80:271.

BUPROPION

Antidepressant

PREGNANCY RECOMMENDATION: Limited Human Data Suggest Low Risk
BREASTFEEDING RECOMMENDATION: Limited Human Data—Potential Toxicity

PREGNANCY SUMMARY

The animal and most of the human data suggest low risk. Although increased rates of heart defects were reported in two studies, this outcome has not been confirmed by other studies. One study found a strong association between bupropion use in pregnancy and attention deficit/hyperactivity disorder (ADHD) in offspring, but cigarette smoking was a potential confounder. Additional research is required to clarify this risk. If a woman requires bupropion, she should be informed of the potential risks, but the drug should not be withheld because of pregnancy.

FETAL RISK SUMMARY

Bupropion is a unique antidepressant of the aminoketone class that differs from other antidepressants in that it does not inhibit monoamine oxidase and does not alter the reuptake of norepinephrine or serotonin. Anticholinergic effects are much less frequent and less severe than those observed with other antidepressants. The drug is extensively metabolized with three active metabolites, but the antidepressant activity has not been fully characterized. Plasma protein binding of bupropion and one metabolite is 84%, whereas the binding of a second active metabolite is about half that of bupropion. The elimination half-lives of the three active metabolites range from 20 to 37 hours (1).

Reproduction studies in rats and rabbits at doses up to about 7–11 times the maximum recommended human dose based on BSA (MRHD) revealed no clear evidence of impaired fertility or fetal harm. However, in rabbits, a slight increase in the incidence of fetal malformations and a reduction in fetal weight was observed at doses ≥MRHD (2).

Bupropion caused an increase in nodular proliferative lesions of the liver in rats, but not mice, in lifetime carcinogenicity studies. No increase in malignant tumors of the liver or other organs was observed in either species. Bupropion was mutagenic in one test. In rats, a dose about 11 times the MRHD caused chromosomal aberrations (2).

Consistent with its molecular weight (about 240 for the free base), bupropion crosses the human placenta. In a 2010 report, healthy term placentas were used to determine the transplacental transfer and metabolism of bupropion (3). Following a 4-hour infusion, the amounts of bupropion in the maternal and fetal circulations and in the placenta were 32%, 20%, and 48%, respectively. The amount retained by the placenta was metabolized to threohydrobupropion, one of the active metabolites. The ratio of metabolite to parent compound in the three sites was 0.08, 0.07, and 0.06, respectively (3). In a second report from these investigators, it was found that the placenta metabolized bupropion to all three active metabolites (4). Human placental 11β-hydroxysteroid dehydrogenase was the primary enzyme involved, but CYP2B6 also had activity. Significantly higher amounts of the three active metabolites were measured in the placentas of women who smoked ≥20 cigarettes/day compared with those who smoked ≤10 cigarettes/day and nonsmokers (4).

In a surveillance study of Michigan Medicaid recipients involving 229,101 completed pregnancies conducted between 1985 and 1992, three newborns had been exposed to bupropion during the 1st trimester (F. Rosa, personal communication, FDA, 1993). No major birth defects were observed (none expected).

A prospective comparative study in 136 women exposed to bupropion (for depression or smoking cessation) was published in 2005 (5). The pregnancy outcomes of 105 live births included no major malformations, mean birth weight of 3450 g, mean gestational age of 40 weeks, 20 spontaneous abortions (SABs), 10 elective abortions (EABs), and 1 stillbirth. There also was one neonatal death after delivery at 22 weeks because of abruptio placenta. Compared with nonteratogen-exposed controls, only the number of SABs (14.7% vs. 4.5%; $p = 0.009$) and EABs (7.4% vs. 0.75%; $p = 0.015$) were significantly increased. In a subanalysis, there were no significant differences when women taking bupropion for depression ($N = 91$) were compared with a group using other antidepressants and a nonteratogen exposed group (5).

A 2005 meta-analysis of seven prospective comparative cohort studies involving 1774 patients was conducted to quantify the relationship between seven newer antidepressants and major malformations (6). The antidepressants were bupropion, fluoxetine, fluvoxamine, nefazodone, paroxetine, sertraline, and trazodone. There was no statistical increase in the risk of major birth defects above the baseline of 1%–3% in the general population for the individual or combined studies (6).

The final report of the Bupropion Pregnancy Registry, covering the period September 1, 1997, through March 31, 2008, was issued in August 2008 (7). The Registry was closed to new enrollments on November 1, 2007. The Registry prospectively (before the pregnancy outcome was known) enrolled 1597 pregnancies exposed to bupropion. Among these cases, 31 were still pregnant, 572 were lost to follow-up, and there were 1005 known outcomes (includes 9 sets of twins and 1 set of triplets). The number of outcomes involving earliest exposure in the 1st, 2nd, or 3rd trimester were 806, 147, and 52, respectively. The outcomes of those with earliest exposure in the 1st trimester included 651 live births without defects, 96 SABs, 33 EABs, and 2 fetal deaths, and outcomes with defects included 18 live births, 5 EABs, and 1 fetal death. For earliest exposure in the 2nd trimester, outcomes without reported defects were 142 live births, 1 SAB, and 1 EAB, and outcomes with defects 3 live births. Among exposures in the 3rd trimester, there were no defects in 51 live births and 1 fetal death. After excluding EABs and fetal deaths without known defects and all SABs, the proportion of birth defects with earliest exposure in the 1st trimester was 3.6% (95% confidence interval [CI] 2.3–5.3). The proportion of birth defects with earliest exposure in the 2nd trimester was 2.1% (95% CI 0.5–6.4) (7).

There were 28 outcomes, 25 with earliest exposure in the 1st trimester, with birth defects reported retrospectively (after the pregnancy outcome was known) (7). Although retrospective reports are usually biased, reporting adverse outcomes and not normal infants, nine of the defects involved the heart and great vessels. The Registry has noted the increased number of cardiac defects in the prospective and retrospective groups. However, the relatively small sample size, the potential bias from the large percentage of cases lost to follow-up, and the incomplete descriptions of the defects prevented determining if the data reflect a potential drug effect on the developing cardiovascular system (7).

> ***Required statement:*** *Committee consensus. After reviewing the 1005 prospectively reported pregnancy outcomes, the Bupropion Pregnancy Registry Advisory Committee concludes the Registry has successfully met its primary purpose which was to exclude a major teratogenic effect in pregnancies inadvertently or intentionally exposed to any formulation of bupropion. The Registry was not designed to exclude an increase in the risk of specific defects* (5).

A study published in 2007 was conducted to determine if bupropion exposure in the 1st trimester was associated with congenital malformations (8). Using data collected in 1995–2004, the prevalence of structural defects in 1213 infants exposed to bupropion in the 1st trimester was compared with 4743 infants exposed to other antidepressants and to 1049 infants exposed to bupropion after the 1st trimester. For all congenital anomalies, the prevalence in the 1st trimester bupropion group was 23.1/1000 infants, adjusted odds ratio (AOR) 0.95 (95% CI 0.62–1.45) and 1.00 (95% CI 0.57–1.73) in comparison to other antidepressants (prevalence 23.2/1000) and bupropion exposure after the 1st trimester (prevalence 21.9/1000), respectively. For cardiovascular anomalies, the prevalence for 1st trimester bupropion exposure was 10.7/1000, AOR 0.97 (95% CI 0.52–1.80) and 1.07 (95% CI 0.48–2.40) compared with other antidepressants (prevalence 10.8/1000) and bupropion exposure after the 1st trimester (prevalence 9.5/1000), respectively. The results did not support a hypothesis of a teratogenic effect of 1st trimester exposure to bupropion (8).

A prospective cohort study evaluated a large group of pregnancies exposed to antidepressants in the 1st trimester to determine if there was an association with major malformations (9). The patient population came from the Motherisk database and involved 928 cases that met their criteria. The 928 matched (for age, smoking, and alcohol use) controls were pregnancies not exposed to antidepressants or known teratogens. In addition to the 113 bupropion cases, the other cases were 184 citalopram, 21 escitalopram, 61 fluoxetine, 52 fluvoxamine, 68 mirtazapine, 39 nefazodone, 148 paroxetine, 61 sertraline, 17 trazodone, and 154 venlafaxine. In the antidepressant group, there were 24 (2.5%) major defects compared with 25 (2.6%) in controls (odds ratio [OR] 0.9, 95% CI 0.5–1.61). There were no major defects in the pregnancies exposed to bupropion, escitalopram, or trazodone (9).

A National Birth Defects Prevention Study to determine if bupropion was associated with congenital heart defects was published in 2010 (10). The retrospective case–control study compared 6853 infants with major heart defects with 5869 control infants. Bupropion exposure was defined as any reported use between 1 month before and 3 months after conception. Case infants were more likely to have left outflow tract defects than control infants (OR 2.6, 95% CI 1.2–5.7). The authors noted that additional studies were required to confirm their results (10).

Another study published in 2010 found a significant association between bupropion use in pregnancy and ADHD in offspring (11). A claims-based dataset was used to identify 431 (1.13%) children, from 38,074 families, who had a diagnosis or treatment for ADHD at or before 5 years of age. The average maternal age at delivery was 31 years. Maternal age was not associated with ADHD in offspring, but male children were more likely to have ADHD (OR 2.79, $p < 0.001$). Significant associations were found between the presence of ADHD in children and a diagnosis of ADHD in the mother (OR 4.15, $p < 0.001$) or father (OR 3.54, $p < 0.001$). This finding was consistent with the known strong inheritance of the disorder. Significant associations with ADHD in offspring were also found for the mother, but not the father, for diagnosis of bipolar disorder (OR 5.08, $p < 0.001$), psychotic disorder (OR 4.05, $p = 0.02$), or depression (OR 2.58, $p < 0.001$). Exposure to bupropion, especially in the 2nd trimester (OR 14.66, $p < 0.001$) was associated with ADHD in children, but selective serotonin reuptake inhibitors (SSRIs) were not (OR 0.91, $p = 0.74$). Because cigarette smoking during pregnancy has been related to ADHD (see also Cigarette Smoking) and bupropion is used in smoking cessation programs, the author noted that this was a potential confounder. Women taking bupropion before or after pregnancy did not have a higher risk for having children with ADHD (11).

BREASTFEEDING SUMMARY

Bupropion is excreted into breast milk. A 37-year-old lactating woman was treated with 100 mg of bupropion 3 times daily (12). She was nursing her 14-month-old infant twice daily at times corresponding to 9.5 and 7.5 hours after a dose. Peak milk concentrations of bupropion occurred 2 hours after a 100-mg dose with a value of 0.189 mcg/mL, but the peak plasma level measured, 0.072 mcg/mL, occurred at 1 hour. The milk:plasma (M:P) ratios at 0, 1, 2, 4, and 6 hours after a dose were 7.37, 2.49, 4.31, 8.72, and 6.24, respectively. Two metabolites, hydroxybupropion and threohydrobupropion, were also measured with peak concentrations of both occurring at 2 hours in milk and plasma. The milk concentration ranges for the two metabolites were milk levels 0.093–0.132 and 0.366–0.443 mcg/mL, respectively, whereas the M:P ratios were 0.09–0.11 and 1.23–1.57, respectively. The levels of a third metabolite, erythrohydrobupropion, were too low to be measured in breast milk (test sensitivity 0.02 mcg/mL). No adverse effects were observed in the infant nor was any drug or metabolite found in his plasma, an indication that accumulation had not occurred (12).

Two breastfeeding mothers, one at 15 weeks after birth and the other at 29 weeks, were being treated with bupropion, 75 mg twice daily and sustained release (SR) 150 mg daily, respectively (13). The drug was at steady state in both mothers. Neither bupropion nor its metabolite (hydroxybupropion) was detectable in the infants. No adverse effects were observed in the infants (13).

A 2004 report described the excretion of bupropion and its three active metabolites into breast milk in 10 mothers an average 12.5 months after birth (14). The average weight of the mothers was 59.4 kg. All had stopped breastfeeding and none had taken bupropion before the study. The dose during the study was SR 150 mg/day for 3 days, then SR 300 mg/day for 4 days, and samples were collected on day 7. Milk samples were collected with an electric breast pump. The calculated average bupropion dose in milk, based on 150 mL/kg/day, was 6.75 mcg/kg/day or 0.14% of the mother's weight-adjusted dose. The average M:P ratios of bupropion and the three active metabolites (hydroxybupropion, erythrohydrobupropion, and threohydrobupropion) were 2.8, 0.1, 0.9, and 1.2, respectively. The estimated daily infant doses of the metabolites were 15.75, 10.80, and 68.85 mcg/kg/day, respectively (14).

Seizures were reported in a 6-month-old breastfeeding infant whose mother had just started SR bupropion 150 mg/day (15). The 31-year-old mother, a pediatrician, had taken the agent for depression before pregnancy but had discontinued it before conception. She continued off the drug throughout pregnancy and while nursing her female infant. At 6 months postpartum, she restarted bupropion because of increasing depression. She had taken two doses, about 36 hours apart, when about 72 hours after the first dose she observed the infant arching her back, rolling her eyes, and smacking her lips for about 10–15 seconds. The mother thought the infant was having a seizure. Following this event, the mother observed a 5–10 minute postictal state that included staring and nonresponsiveness. Later examination of the infant at a specialty pediatric seizure clinic revealed a normal physical examination and laboratory tests, as well as an unremarkable electroencephalogram. Neither infant nor maternal bupropion levels were obtained. The mother stopped the drug and continued to nurse with no further seizure activity noted over the next 6 weeks. Because rare seizures have occurred in adults taking the antidepressant, the seizures were attributed to the drug (15).

A 2009 report described bupropion concentrations, but not of metabolites, in the breast milk, serum, and urine of four nursing mothers taking SR 150–300 mg/day at steady state (16). The samples were collected a mean 13 days after birth. The mean peak and trough milk concentrations were 64.1 and 9.2 ng/mL, respectively, whereas the mean M:P ratio was 1.3. Infant serum levels were not checked. In two infants, urine levels of bupropion were not detected (<10 ng/mL) but, in a third infant, born 5.5 weeks prematurely, the bupropion concentration was 41.0 ng/mL. The mean infant dose as a percentage of the mother's weight-adjusted dose was 5.7% (16).

B

The elevated (>1) M:P ratios for bupropion in the three studies above are consistent with the accumulation in milk observed with weak bases (i.e., ion-trapping). A 1996 review of antidepressant treatment during breastfeeding found no information that bupropion exposure during nursing resulted in quantifiable amounts in an infant or that the exposure caused adverse effects (17). The case above that observed seizures may or may not have been related to bupropion. The reported experience in breastfeeding mothers taking bupropion is too limited to determine the relationship. Nevertheless, nursing mothers and their caregivers should be aware of this possible complication. The American Academy of Pediatrics classifies bupropion as a drug whose effect on the nursing infant is unknown but may be of concern (18).

References

1. Weintraub M, Evan P. Bupropion: a chemically and pharmacologically unique antidepressant. Hosp Form 1989;24:254–9.
2. Product information. Wellbutrin. GlaxoSmithKline, 2010.
3. Earhart AD, Patrikeeva S, Wang X, Abdelrahman DR, Hankins GDV, Ahmed MS, Nanovskaya T. Transplacental transfer and metabolism of bupropion. J Matern Fetal Neonatal Med 2010;23:409–16.
4. Wang X, Abdelrahman DR, Zharikova OL, Patrikeeva SL, Hankins CDV, Ahmed MS, Nanovskaya TN. Bupropion metabolism by human placenta. Biochem Pharmacol 2010;79:1684–90.
5. Chun-Fai-Chan B, Koren G, Fayez I, Kalra S, Voyer-Lavigne S, Boshier A, Shakir S, Einarson A. Pregnancy outcome of women exposed to bupropion during pregnancy: a prospective comparative study. Am J Obstet Gynecol 2005;192:932–6.
6. Einarson TR, Einarson A. Newer antidepressants in pregnancy and rates of major malformations: a meta-analysis of prospective comparative studies. Pharmacoepidemiol Drug Saf 2005;14:823–7.
7. The Bupropion Pregnancy Registry. Final Report, 1 September 1997 through 31 March 2008. GlaxoSmithKline, August 2008.
8. Cole JA, Modell JG, Haight BR, Cosmatos IS, Stoler JM, Walker AM. Bupropion in pregnancy and the prevalence of congenital malformations. Pharmacoepidemiol Drug Saf 2007;16:474–84.
9. Einarson A, Choi J, Einarson TR, Koren G. Incidence of major malformations in infants following antidepressant exposure in pregnancy: results of a large prospective cohort study. Can J Psychiatry 2009;54:242–6.
10. Alwan S, Reefhuis J, Botto LD, Rasmussen SA, Correa A, Friedman JM, and the National Birth Defects Prevention Study. Maternal use of bupropion and risk for congenital heart defects. Am J Obstet Gynecol 2010;203:52.e1–6.
11. Figueroa R. Use of antidepressants during pregnancy and risk of attention-deficit/hyperactivity disorder in the offspring. J Dev Behav Pediatr 2010;31:641–8.
12. Briggs GG, Samson JH, Ambrose PJ, Schroeder DH. Excretion of bupropion in breast milk. Ann Pharmacother 1993;27:431–3.
13. Baab S, Peindl K, Piontek C, Wisner K. Serum bupropion levels in 2 breastfeeding mother–infant pairs. J Clin Psychiatry 2002;63:910–1.
14. Haas JS, Kaplan CP, Barenboim DJ 3rd, Benowitz NL. Bupropion in breast milk: an exposure assessment for potential treatment to prevent postpartum tobacco use. Tob Control 2004;13:52–6.
15. Chaudron LH, Schoenecker CJ. Bupropion and breastfeeding: a case of a possible infant seizure. J Clin Psychiatry 2004;65:881–2.
16. Davis MF, Miller HS, Nolan PE Jr. Bupropion levels in breast milk for 4 mother–infant pairs: more answers to lingering questions. J Clin Psychiatry 2009;70:297–8.
17. Wisner KL, Perel JM, Findling RL. Antidepressant treatment during breastfeeding. Am J Psychiatry 1996;153:1132–7.
18. Committee on Drugs, American Academy of Pediatrics. The transfer of drugs and other chemicals into human milk. Pediatrics 2001;108:776–89.

BUSPIRONE

Sedative

PREGNANCY RECOMMENDATION: Limited Human Data—Animal Data Suggest Low Risk
BREASTFEEDING RECOMMENDATION: Limited Human Data—Potential Toxicity

PREGNANCY SUMMARY

Although no drug-induced congenital malformations have been observed after 1st trimester exposure to buspirone, the data are too limited to assess the safety of the drug in human pregnancy. The cause of the intrauterine death cited below is unknown. Moreover, that study lacked the sensitivity to identify minor anomalies because of the absence of standardized examinations. Late-appearing major defects, including neurobehavior effects, may also have been missed due to the timing of the questionnaires.

FETAL RISK SUMMARY

Buspirone is an antianxiety agent that is unrelated chemically and pharmacologically to other sedative and anxiolytic drugs. Reproduction studies in rats and rabbits at doses approximately 30 times the maximum recommended human dose revealed no fertility impairment or fetal adverse effects (1).

A 1993 report described the use of buspirone, in combination with four other agents, all started before conception, in a pregnant woman with major depression, a coexisting panic disorder, and migraine headaches (2). The pregnancy was electively terminated after 12 weeks, resulting in the delivery of a male fetus with normal organ formation and a normal placenta. No dysmorphology was observed during the complete macroscopic and microscopic examination, including a normal 46,XY karyotype.

In a surveillance study of Michigan Medicaid recipients involving 229,101 completed pregnancies conducted between 1985 and 1992, 42 newborns had been exposed to buspirone during the 1st trimester (F. Rosa, personal communication, FDA, 1993). One (2.4%) major birth defect was observed (two expected). The anomaly was not included in six defect categories for which specific data were available (cardiovascular defects, oral clefts, spina bifida, polydactyly, limb reduction defects, and hypospadias).

A 1998 non-interventional observational cohort study described the outcomes of pregnancies in women who had been prescribed ≥1 of 34 newly marketed drugs by general practitioners in England (3). Data were obtained by questionnaires sent to the prescribing physicians 1 month after the expected or possible date of delivery. In 831 (78%) of the pregnancies, a newly marketed drug was thought to have been taken during the 1st trimester with birth defects noted in 14 (2.5%) singleton births of the 557 newborns (10 sets of twins). In addition, two birth defects were observed in aborted fetuses. However, few of the aborted fetuses were examined. Buspirone was taken during the 1st trimester in 16 pregnancies. The outcomes of these pregnancies included 2 elective abortions, 1 intrauterine death, 12 normal term babies, and 1 newborn with a genetic defect (cystic fibrosis) (3).

In a 1998 case report, a 32-year-old woman with bipolar disorder took buspirone, fluoxetine, and carbamazepine (see Breastfeeding Summary for doses and further details) throughout gestation (4). At 42 weeks' gestation she gave birth to a healthy, normally developed 3940-g female infant. The mother continued her medications for 3 weeks while exclusively breastfeeding the infant. She reported seizure-like activity in her infant at 3 weeks, 4 months, and 5.5 months of age (4).

BREASTFEEDING SUMMARY

One report has investigated the excretion of buspirone into human milk. In this 1998 case report, a 32-year-old woman with bipolar disorder took buspirone (45 mg/day), fluoxetine (20 mg/day), and carbamazepine (600 mg/day) throughout pregnancy and during the first 3 weeks postpartum (4). She reported seizure-like activity in the infant at 3 weeks, 4 months, and 5.5 months of age. Breast milk, maternal serum, and infant serum were evaluated for buspirone on postpartum day 13, but the drug was not detected in any of the samples (test sensitivity not reported). Similar evaluations were conducted for fluoxetine, norfluoxetine, and carbamazepine on days 13 and 21 postpartum (see Fluoxetine and Carbamazepine for results). A neurologic examination of the infant, which included electroencephalography, was within normal limits. The authors were unable to determine the cause of the seizure-like activity, if it had indeed occurred (none of the episodes had been observed by medical personnel) (4).

Although buspirone was not detected in breast milk or maternal and infant serum in the above case, the timing of the samples in relation to the mother's ingestion of the drug and the test sensitivity were not specified. Therefore, because other agents in this pharmacologic class are excreted into milk (e.g., see Diazepam), the excretion of buspirone, at least to some degree, should still be expected.

Because of the potential for CNS impairment in a nursing infant, maternal use of the drug, especially for prolonged periods, should be undertaken cautiously, if at all. The American Academy of Pediatrics classifies other antianxiety agents as drugs whose effects on the nursing infant are unknown, but may be of concern because effects on the developing brain may not be apparent until later in life (5).

References

1. Product information. Buspar. Mead Johnson Pharmaceuticals, 1994.
2. Seifritz E, Holsboer-Trachsler E, Haberthur F, Hemmeter U, Pöldinger W. Unrecognized pregnancy during citalopram treatment. Am J Psychiatry 1993;150:1428–9.
3. Wilton LV, Pearce GL, Martin RM, Mackay FJ, Mann RD. The outcomes of pregnancy in women exposed to newly marketed drugs in general practice in England. Br J Obstet Gynaecol 1998;105:882–9.
4. Brent NB, Wisner KL. Fluoxetine and carbamazepine concentrations in a nursing mother/infant pair. Clin Pediatr 1998;37:41–4.
5. Committee on Drugs, American Academy of Pediatrics. The transfer of drugs and other chemicals into human milk. Pediatrics 2001;108:776–89.

BUSULFAN

Antineoplastic

PREGNANCY RECOMMENDATION: Contraindicated—1st Trimester
BREASTFEEDING RECOMMENDATION: Contraindicated

PREGNANCY SUMMARY

Busulfan is a human teratogen when used during organogenesis.

FETAL RISK SUMMARY

Busulfan is an alkylating antineoplastic agent. Reproductive studies in pregnant rats revealed that the drug produced sterility in both male and female offspring due to the absence of germinal cells in testes and ovaries (1).

The use of busulfan has been reported in at least 49 human pregnancies, of which 31 were treated in the 1st trimester (2–10). One of these references reviewed eight earlier cases that are included in the above totals (9). Malformations in six infants were: unspecified malformations, aborted at 20 weeks; anomalous deviation of left lobe liver, bilobar spleen, pulmonary atelectasis; pyloric stenosis; cleft palate, microphthalmia, cytomegaly, hypoplasia of ovaries and thyroid gland, corneal opacity, intrauterine growth restriction (IUGR); myeloschisis, aborted at 6 weeks; IUGR, left hydronephrosis and hydroureter, absent right kidney and ureter, hepatic subcapsular calcifications (2,4–6).

Data from one review indicated that 40% of the infants exposed to anticancer drugs were of low birth weight (2). This finding was not related to the timing of the exposure. One mother with chronic granulocytic leukemia was treated

B

with busulfan and allopurinol beginning at 20 weeks' gestation (8). A growth-restricted infant was delivered at 39 weeks with absence of the right kidney, hydronephrosis of the left kidney, and hepatic subcapsular calcifications. The kidney and liver defects predated the onset of drug therapy, but their cause was unknown. The growth restriction, however, was thought to be caused by busulfan.

Long-term studies of growth and mental development in offspring exposed to busulfan during the 2nd trimester, the period of neuroblast multiplication, have not been conducted (11). However, a few infants have been studied for periods of up to 10 years without evidence of adverse outcome (3,9,10). Moreover, a 1994 review concluded that although there were insufficient data to assess the fetal risk from busulfan, use after the 1st trimester would reduce the risk of birth defects (12).

Chromosomal damage has been associated with busulfan therapy, but the clinical significance of this to the fetus is unknown (13). Irregular menses and amenorrhea, with the latter at times permanent, have been reported in women receiving busulfan (14,15). Reversible ovarian failure with delivery of a normal infant has also been reported after busulfan therapy (16).

Occupational exposure of the mother to antineoplastic agents during pregnancy may present a risk to the fetus. A position statement from the National Study Commission on Cytotoxic Exposure and a research article involving some antineoplastic agents are presented in the monograph for cyclophosphamide (see Cyclophosphamide).

BREASTFEEDING SUMMARY

No studies describing the use of busulfan during human lactation or measuring the amount, if any, excreted into milk have been located. Because of the potential for serious toxicity in a nursing infant, the use of the drug during lactation should be considered contraindicated.

References

1. Product information. Myleran. Glaxo Wellcome Oncology/HIV, 1997.
2. Nicholson HO. Cytotoxic drugs in pregnancy: review of reported cases. J Obstet Gynaecol Br Commonw 1968;75:307–12.
3. Lee RA, Johnson CE, Hanlon DG. Leukemia during pregnancy. Am J Obstet Gynecol 1962;84:455–8.
4. Diamond I, Anderson MM, McCreadie SR. Transplacental transmission of busulfan (Myleran) in a mother with leukemia: production of fetal malformation and cytomegaly. Pediatrics 1960;25:85–90.
5. Abramovici A, Shaklai M, Pinkhas J. Myeloschisis in a six weeks embryo of a leukemic woman treated by busulfan. Teratology 1978;18:241–6.
6. Gililand J, Weinstein L. The effects of cancer chemotherapeutic agents on the developing fetus. Obstet Gynecol Surv 1983;38:6–13.
7. Ozumba BC, Obi GO. Successful pregnancy in a patient with chronic myeloid leukemia following therapy with cytotoxic drugs. Int J Gynecol Obstet 1992;38:49–53.
8. Boros SJ, Reynolds JW. Intrauterine growth retardation following third-trimester exposure to busulfan. Am J Obstet Gynecol 1977;129:111–2.
9. Dugdale M, Fort AT. Busulfan treatment of leukemia during pregnancy. JAMA 1967;199:131–3.
10. Zuazu J, Julia A, Sierra J, Valentin MG, Coma A, Sanz MA, Batlle J, Flores A. Pregnancy outcome in hematologic malignancies. Cancer 1991;67:703–9.
11. Dobbing J. Pregnancy and leukaemia. Lancet 1977;1:1155.
12. Wiebe VJ, Sipila PEH. Pharmacology of antineoplastic agents in pregnancy. Crit Rev Oncol Hematol 1994;16:75–112.
13. Gebhart E, Schwanitz G, Hartwich G. Chromosomal aberrations during busulphan therapy. Dtsch Med Wochenschr 1974;99:52–6.
14. Galton DAG, Till M, Wiltshaw E. Busulfan: summary of clinical results. Ann NY Acad Sci 1958;68:967–73.
15. Schilsky RL, Lewis BJ, Sherins RJ, Young RC. Gonadal dysfunction in patients receiving chemotherapy for cancer. Ann Intern Med 1980;93:109–14.
16. Shalev O, Rahav G, Milwidsky A. Reversible busulfan-induced ovarian failure. Eur J Obstet Gynecol Reprod Biol 1987;26:239–42.

BUTALBITAL

Sedative

PREGNANCY RECOMMENDATION: Limited Human Data—No Relevant Animal Data
BREASTFEEDING RECOMMENDATION: No Human Data—Potential Toxicity

PREGNANCY SUMMARY

The limited evidence suggests that butalbital is not a major human teratogen. However, similar to all barbiturates, chronic exposure in the second half of gestation or high doses near term can cause neonatal withdrawal.

FETAL RISK SUMMARY

Butalbital is a short-acting barbiturate that is contained in a number of analgesic mixtures. In a large prospective study, 112 patients were exposed to this drug during the 1st trimester (1). No association with malformations was found. Severe neonatal withdrawal was described in a male infant whose mother took 150 mg of butalbital daily during the last 2 months of pregnancy in the form of a proprietary headache mixture (Esgic-butalbital 50 mg, caffeine 40 mg, and acetaminophen 325 mg/dose) (2). The infant was also exposed to oxycodone, pentazocine, and acetaminophen during the 1st trimester, but apparently these had been discontinued before the start of the butalbital product. Onset of withdrawal occurred within 2 days of birth.

In a surveillance study of Michigan Medicaid recipients involving 229,101 completed pregnancies conducted between 1985 and 1992, 1124 newborns had been exposed to butalbital during the 1st trimester (F. Rosa, personal communication, FDA, 1993). A total of 53 (4.7%) major birth defects were observed (45 expected). Specific data were available for six defect categories, including (observed/expected) 10/11 cardiovascular defects, 1/2 oral clefts, 0/0.5 spina bifida, 1/3 polydactyly, 2/2 limb reduction defects, and 2/3 hypospadias. These data do not support an association between the drug and congenital defects.

BREASTFEEDING SUMMARY

No reports describing the use of butalbital during human lactation have been located. The drug probably is excreted into breast milk and sedation of a nursing infant is a potential effect.

References

1. Heinonen OP, Slone D, Shapiro S. *Birth Defects and Drugs in Pregnancy*. Littleton, MA: Publishing Sciences Group, 1977:336–7.
2. Ostrea EM. Neonatal withdrawal from intrauterine exposure to butalbital. Am J Obstet Gynecol 1982;143:597–9.

BUTAPERAZINE

[Withdrawn from the market. See 9th edition.]

BUTENAFINE

Antifungal (Topical)

PREGNANCY RECOMMENDATION: No Human Data—Animal Data Suggest Low Risk
BREASTFEEDING RECOMMENDATION: No Human Data—Probably Compatible

PREGNANCY SUMMARY

No reports describing the use of butenafine in human pregnancy have been located. The animal data suggest low risk, as does the very low systemic concentrations. Although a more complete assessment of the embryo–fetal risk cannot be made, the topical use of this agent appears to low risk in human pregnancy.

FETAL RISK SUMMARY

Butenafine, a synthetic antifungal, is a benzylamine derivative with a mechanism of action similar to the allylamine class of antifungal agents. The agent is available as a cream to be applied to the skin. Butenafine is indicated for the topical treatment of the dermatologic infection, tinea (pityriasis) versicolor due to *Malassezia furfur* (formerly *Pityrosporum orbiculare*). Small amounts of butenafine are absorbed into the systemic circulation. After the application 6 and 20 g/day for 14 days, the mean peak plasma concentrations were 1.4 and 5.0 ng/mL, respectively. The biphasic plasma elimination half-lives were estimated to be 35 and >150 hours, respectively. The antifungal agent is metabolized (1).

Reproduction studies have been conducted in rats and rabbits. In rats during organogenesis, daily SC doses up to 0.5 times the maximum recommended human dose for tinea versicolor based on BSA (MRHD) were not teratogenic. In a peri- and postnatal study with rats, daily oral doses up to 2.5 times the MRHD caused no treatment-related effects on postnatal survival, development of the F1 generation, or their subsequent maturation and fertility. In rabbits during organogenesis, daily oral doses up to 16 times the MRHD revealed no evidence of treatment-related fetal harm (1).

Studies for carcinogenic effects have not been conducted with butenafine, but assays for mutagenic and clastogenic effects were negative. No adverse effects on male and female rat fertility were observed with daily SC doses up to 0.5 times the MRHD (1).

It is not known if butenafine crosses the placenta. The molecular weight (about 318 for the free base) and long plasma elimination half-life suggest that the drug will cross to the embryo and fetus, but the very small amounts in the systemic circulation suggest that the exposure will be clinically insignificant.

BREASTFEEDING SUMMARY

No reports describing the use of butenafine during human lactation have been located. The molecular weight (about 318 for the free base) and long plasma elimination half-life suggest that the drug will be excreted into breast milk, but the very small amounts in the systemic circulation suggest that the effects on a nursing infant from this exposure will be clinically insignificant.

Reference

1. Product information. Mentax. Mylan Pharmaceuticals, 2007.

BUTOCONAZOLE

Antifungal

PREGNANCY RECOMMENDATION: Limited Human Data—Probably Compatible
BREASTFEEDING RECOMMENDATION: No Human Data—Probably Compatible

B

PREGNANCY SUMMARY

The limited human pregnancy experience suggests that butoconazole is low risk.

FETAL RISK SUMMARY

Butoconazole is available as a topical cream for the treatment of vaginal fungal infections. It is in the same antifungal class of imidazole derivatives as clotrimazole, econazole, ketoconazole, miconazole, oxiconazole, sertaconazole, sulconazole, and tioconazole.

Butoconazole is teratogenic in some animal species, but only when large oral doses are administered (1).

An average 5.5% of a vaginal dose is absorbed systemically with peak plasma levels appearing at about 24 hours (1). No data are available on the placental transfer of this agent, but the low molecular weight (about 475) indicates that transfer to the fetus probably occurs.

No published reports of butoconazole use in the 1st trimester have been located. However, butoconazole is one of several agents that have been approved for 2nd and 3rd trimester use in the treatment of vulvovaginal mycotic infections (2–4). Therapy for 6 days is recommended if this antifungal is used.

In a surveillance study of Michigan Medicaid recipients involving 229,101 completed pregnancies conducted between 1985 and 1992, 444 newborns had been exposed to vaginal butoconazole during the 1st trimester (F. Rosa, personal communication, FDA, 1993). A total of 16 (3.6%) major birth defects were observed (17 expected). Specific data were available for six defect categories, including (observed/expected) 4/4 cardiovascular defects, 0/1 oral clefts, 1/0 spina bifida, 0/0.5 polydactyly, 0/1 limb reduction defects, and 0/1 hypospadias. These data do not support an association between the vaginal use of the drug and congenital defects.

BREASTFEEDING SUMMARY

No reports describing the use of butoconazole during human lactation have been located. The low systemic bioavailability from topical application suggests that there is little risk to a nursing infant.

References

1. Product information. Femstat. Syntex, 1993.
2. Weisberg M. Treatment of vaginal candidiasis in pregnant women. Clin Ther 1986;8:563–7.
3. Hagler L, Brett L. Treatment of vaginal candidiasis in pregnant women. Clin Ther 1987;9:559–60.
4. Weisberg M. Treatment of vaginal candidiasis in pregnant women. Clin Ther 1987;9:561.

BUTORPHANOL

Narcotic Agonist-Antagonist Analgesic

PREGNANCY RECOMMENDATION: Human Data Suggest Risk in 3rd Trimester
BREASTFEEDING RECOMMENDATION: Limited Human Data—Probably Compatible

PREGNANCY SUMMARY

Although the human pregnancy experience is very limited, and there is no data during the 1st trimester, agents in this class appear to be low risk. Use during labor, however, may cause a sinusoidal fetal heart rate pattern and transient neonatal depression.

FETAL RISK SUMMARY

No reports linking the use of butorphanol with congenital defects have been located. Because it has both narcotic agonist and antagonist properties, prolonged use during gestation may result in fetal addiction with subsequent withdrawal in the newborn (see also Pentazocine). The drug is commercially available as injection and nasal spray formulations.

No teratogenic effects were observed in reproduction studies in rats and rabbits administered butorphanol during organogenesis (1). An increased frequency of stillbirth was observed in rats given 1 mg/kg (5.9 mg/m^2) SC and in rabbits dosed orally with 30 mg/kg (360 mg/m^2) and 60 mg/kg (720 mg/m^2).

At term, butorphanol rapidly crosses the placenta, producing cord serum levels averaging 84% of maternal concentrations (2,3). Depressant effects on the newborn from in utero exposure during labor are similar to those seen with meperidine (2–4).

The use of 1 mg of butorphanol combined with 25 mg of promethazine administered IV to a woman in active labor was associated with a sinusoidal fetal heart rate pattern (5). Onset of the pattern occurred 6 minutes after drug injection and persisted for approximately 58 minutes. The newborn infant showed no effects from the abnormal heart pattern. A subsequent study to determine the incidence of sinusoidal fetal heart rate pattern after butorphanol administration was published in 1986 (6). Fifty-one women in labor who received butorphanol, 1 mg IV, were compared with a control group of 55 women who did not receive narcotic analgesia. A sinusoidal fetal heart rate pattern was observed in 75% (38 of 51) of the treated women vs. 13% (7 of 55) of controls

B

(p <0.001). The mean time of onset of the abnormal tracing was 12.74 minutes after butorphanol with a duration of 31.26 minutes. This duration was significantly longer than that observed in the nontreated controls (13.86 minutes; p <0.02). Because no short-term maternal or neonatal adverse effects were observed, the investigators concluded that, in the absence of other signs, the abnormal heart rate pattern was not indicative of fetal hypoxia (6).

A study comparing the effects of maternal analgesics on neonatal neurobehavior was conducted in 135 patients during their 1st day of life (7). Maternal analgesia consisted of 1 mg of butorphanol (N = 68) or 40 mg of meperidine (N = 67). No difference between the drugs was observed.

BREASTFEEDING SUMMARY

Butorphanol passes into breast milk in concentrations paralleling levels in maternal serum (3). Milk:plasma ratios after IM (12 mg) or oral (8 mg) doses were 0.7 and 1.9, respectively. Using 2 mg IM or 8 mg orally 4 times per day would result in 4 mcg excreted in the full daily milk output (1000 mL). Although it has not been studied, this amount is probably insignificant. The American Academy of Pediatrics classifies butorphanol as compatible with breastfeeding (8).

References

1. Product information. Stadol NS. Bristol-Myers Squibb, 2000.
2. Maduska AL, Hajghassemali M. A double-blind comparison of butorphanol and meperidine in labour: maternal pain relief and effect on the newborn. Can Anaesth Soc J 1978;25:398–404.
3. Pittman KA, Smyth RD, Losada M, Zighelboim I, Maduska AL, Sunshine A. Human perinatal distribution of butorphanol. Am J Obstet Gynecol 1980;138:797–800.
4. Quilligan EJ, Keegan KA, Donahue MJ. Double-blind comparison of intravenously injected butorphanol and meperidine in parturients. Int J Gynaecol Obstet 1980;18:363–7.
5. Angel JL, Knuppel RA, Lake M. Sinusoidal fetal heart rate pattern associated with intravenous butorphanol administration: a case report. Am J Obstet Gynecol 1984;149:465–7.
6. Hatjis CG, Meis PJ. Sinusoidal fetal heart rate pattern associated with butorphanol administration. Obstet Gynecol 1986;67:377–80.
7. Hodgkinson R, Huff RW, Hayashi RH, Husain FJ. Double-blind comparison of maternal analgesia and neonatal neurobehaviour following intravenous butorphanol and meperidine. J Int Med Res 1979;7:224–30.
8. Committee on Drugs, American Academy of Pediatrics. The transfer of drugs and other chemicals into human milk. Pediatrics 2001;108:776–89.

BUTRIPTYLINE

[Withdrawn from the market. See 9th edition.]

C

CABAZITAXEL

Antineoplastic (Antimitotic Taxoid)

PREGNANCY RECOMMENDATION: No Human Data—Animal Data Suggest Risk
BREASTFEEDING RECOMMENDATION: No Human Data—Potential Toxicity

PREGNANCY SUMMARY

No reports describing the use of cabazitaxel in human pregnancy have been located. Animal data in two species suggest risk at exposures much less than human exposures, but the absence of human pregnancy experience prevents a better assessment of the embryo–fetal risk. Such experience is unlikely because the drug is indicated for the treatment of prostate cancer. However, it might be used off-label for other neoplasms.

FETAL RISK SUMMARY

Cabazitaxel, given as 1-hour IV infusion every 3 weeks, is an antimitotic agent that is in the same subclass of taxoids as docetaxel and paclitaxel. It is indicated in combination with prednisone for treatment of patients with hormone-refractory metastatic prostate cancer previously treated with a docetaxel-containing treatment regimen. Cabazitaxel is prepared by semi-synthesis with a precursor extracted from yew needles. The drug is extensively metabolized to about 20 metabolites, 3 of which are active. Human serum binding is 89%–92%, most of which is to albumin (82%) and lipoproteins. It is equally distributed between blood and plasma. The elimination half-life is 95 hours (1).

Reproduction studies have been conducted in rats and rabbits. In rats, a once-daily dose during organogenesis that was about 0.02–0.06 times the peak concentration in patients with cancer at the recommended human dose (RHD) caused embryo–fetal toxicity consisting of postimplantation loss, embryo and fetal deaths. Decreased mean fetal birth weight associated with delays in skeletal ossification was observed at about 0.02 times the RHD. Fetal abnormalities were not observed in rats or rabbits at exposure levels significantly lower than the expected human exposures. Although specific details were not provided, similar effects (embryo and fetal toxicity and abortions) were observed in pregnant rabbits (1).

Long-term animal studies for carcinogenic effects have not been conducted. The drug was clastogenic in one assay and both positive and negative is other mutagenicity assays. Although cabazitaxel had no effect on mating behavior or the ability to become pregnant in female rats, the agent did cause an increase in preimplantation loss and early resorptions. Multi-cycle studies caused atrophy of the uterus and necrosis of the corpora lutea in female rats. In male rats, no effect on mating performance or fertility were observed, but, in higher dose multi-cycle studies, degeneration of seminal vesicle and seminiferous tubule atrophy in the testis were observed. In dogs, minimal testicular degeneration (minimal epithelial single cell necrosis in epididymis) was observed (1).

It is not known if cabazitaxel or its active metabolites cross the human placenta. The molecular weight (about 836 for the solvent-free form), moderate serum binding, and long elimination half-life suggest that the drug will cross to the embryo–fetus.

BREASTFEEDING SUMMARY

No reports describing the use of cabazitaxel during human lactation have been located. The molecular weight (about 836 for the solvent-free form), moderate serum binding (89%–92%), and long elimination half-life (95 hours) suggest that the drug will be excreted into breast milk. The effect of this exposure on a nursing infant is unknown. In adults, the agent can cause severe toxicity that affects many body systems. Although cabazitaxel is indicated for the treatment of prostate cancer, it might be used off-label for other neoplasms. Thus, if a woman is given this drug, the safest course is to not breastfeed.

Reference

1. Product information. Jevtana. Sanofi-Aventis, 2010.

CABERGOLINE

Endocrine/Metabolic Agent (Miscellaneous)

PREGNANCY RECOMMENDATION: Human Data Suggest Low Risk
BREASTFEEDING RECOMMENDATION: Contraindicated

C

PREGNANCY SUMMARY

Cabergoline does not exhibit direct embryo or fetal toxicity or teratogenicity in animals. Because it inhibits prolactin release, the agent can prevent or abort pregnancies in mice and rats, but this has no human relevance because human egg nidation is not regulated by prolactin. A 2002 review stated that cabergoline was the current treatment of choice for most patients with hyperprolactinemia (1). In addition, the review recommended that once ovulatory cycles were established, women should stop treatment 1 month before they intended to conceive. Hyperprolactinemia is a frequent cause of infertility (2). In many of these women, the partial or complete resolution of this condition will result in conception (2). When pregnancy is diagnosed, cabergoline should be discontinued. However, no evidence indicates that exposure to cabergoline in pregnancy is harmful.

FETAL RISK SUMMARY

Cabergoline is a synthetic ergot derivative that is a long-acting dopamine receptor (D_2) agonist with low affinity for other dopamine (D_1), adrenergic (α_1 and α_2), and serotonin (5-HT_1 and 5-HT_2) receptors. The drug has a direct inhibitory effect on prolactin secretion from the anterior pituitary gland. Cabergoline is indicated for the treatment of hyperprolactinemic disorders, either idiopathic or due to pituitary adenomas (3).

Animal reproduction studies have been conducted in mice, rats, and rabbits with daily oral doses (comparisons to human doses are made with the total weekly animal dose and the maximum recommended weekly human dose for a 50-kg human [MRHD], both based on BSA). In mice, doses up to about 55 times the MRHD caused maternal toxicity but no teratogenic effects in the offspring. In rats, a dose about 1/7th the MRHD caused an increase in postimplantation embryo and fetal losses, an effect that was thought to be due to the prolactin inhibitory effects of cabergoline. Conception in female rats was inhibited at a dose 1/28th the MRHD given 2 weeks before mating and throughout the mating period. A similar dose given to pregnant rats from 6 days before delivery throughout the lactation period caused growth restriction and death in offspring because of decreased milk secretion. In rabbits, a dose approximately 19 times the MRHD during organogenesis caused maternal toxicity (decreased food consumption and weight loss). An increased occurrence of various malformations was observed in one rabbit study using a dose 150 times the MRHD, but no increase in defects was observed in a second study at 300 times the MRHD (3).

A 1996 reproduction study in mice, rats, and rabbits concluded that cabergoline did not impair male rat fertility, was not teratogenic in mice and rabbits, had no effects on the latter phase of gestation or parturition in rats, and caused no toxicity in neonatal rats (4). The study also found that cabergoline could inhibit egg nidation in mice and rats and prevent conception. However, this effect has no relevance to humans because egg nidation in these species, but not in humans, is regulated by prolactin through a luteotrophic effect. A 1997 study in rats demonstrated that cabergoline-inhibited prolactin release resulted in the inhibition of ovarian progesterone biosynthesis, thereby preventing implantation and terminating pregnancy (5).

No reports describing the placental crossing of cabergoline in humans have been located. The molecular weight (about 452) is low enough; however, that exposure of the embryo and/or fetus should be expected.

In a group of 56 women with amenorrhea secondary to hyperprolactinemia (serum prolactin levels >20 mcg/L), 17 (81% of pregnancy-seeking women) became pregnant while under treatment with cabergoline (6). Women were instructed to discontinue cabergoline immediately after a positive pregnancy test. Of the 17 pregnancies, there was 1 spontaneous abortion, 10 normal-term outcomes, and 6 outcomes pending. All 10 children have had normal physical and mental development (6).

A 1994 case report described the outcome of a pregnancy exposed to cabergoline (7). A 38-year-old woman with a microadenoma of the pituitary gland was treated for hyperprolactinemia with a stable cabergoline dose of 0.5 mg twice weekly. She had a 17-year history of infertility and was intolerant to bromocriptine therapy. The prolactin level 2 days after a dose was 1133 mU/L (normal range 60–550 mU/L). After return of her menstrual cycles, she became pregnant but had a spontaneous abortion at 17 weeks' gestation (not mentioned if cabergoline was stopped when pregnancy was diagnosed). Approximately 5 months later (2 months after restarting cabergoline), she again became pregnant and cabergoline was stopped (gestational age not specified). Labor was induced at 38 weeks' gestation for intrauterine growth restriction. A 2.26-kg male infant without malformations was delivered with Apgar scores of 3 and 8 at 1 and 5 minutes, respectively. The placenta weight was 370 g. He was discharged home with his mother at 6 days of age (7).

A multinational French study published in 1996 described the outcomes of 226 pregnancies (all singletons) in 205 women who had been receiving cabergoline treatment (0.125–4.0 mg/week) before gestation (2). The women were from a group of 1650 premenopausal hyperprolactinemic women who had been treated with the drug. In seven cases, pregnancy occurred during the first cycle after discontinuation of cabergoline. The time of exposure could not be determined in 18 other cases. In the remaining 201 pregnancies, embryo–fetal exposure to cabergoline was thought to have ranged between 1 and 144 days. The 226 outcomes included early pregnancy loss (*N* = 56), live births (*N* = 148), ongoing pregnancies (*N* = 16), and lost to follow-up (*N* = 6). Among the 56 early pregnancy losses, there were 28 elective abortions (EABs), 23 spontaneous abortions (SABs), 1 intrauterine death (a cord accident at 25 weeks), 1 tubal pregnancy, and 3 EABs for major anomalies (dose and time of exposure shown in parentheses): Down's syndrome, maternal age 42 years, woman later conceived on another cycle and gave birth to a normal infant (0.5 mg/week; exposure for 2 weeks after conception); limb-body wall defect—large abdominal wall defect, deformed left leg, and proximal phocomelia of right lower limb (0.5 mg/week; exposure for 2 weeks

C

after conception); and hydrocephalus, cerebral atrophy, and facial dysmorphic (0.5 mg/week; exposure for 7 weeks after conception) (2).

Among the 148 live births, 17 were preterm, and 2 cases had an unknown length of gestation (2). Birth weights ranged from 1600 to 4350 g, with 10 infants below 2500 g (6.8%, 95% confidence intervals [CI] 3%–12%). In addition to the three cases above, seven infants had birth defects, but only two of them were major defects. The major defects were (dose and exposure times not specified) left megaureter as well as craniosynostosis and scaphocephaly. Thus, there were 5 infants with major malformations among 151 outcomes (3.3%, 95% CI 1.0%–7.6%). The postnatal development of 148 infants was known for various periods after birth, of which 107 were followed up for 1 to 72 months. All the infants showed normal physical and mental development (2).

In a 1997 report, 9 women became pregnant (from a group of 47) against medical advice after a mean of 12.4 months (range 1–37 months) of cabergoline therapy for hyperprolactinemia (8). The doses ranged from 0.25 to 3.5 mg/week. Cabergoline was discontinued as soon as pregnancy was diagnosed. One pregnancy aborted spontaneously, and one woman underwent elective abortion at 8 weeks' gestation. In the remaining cases, all the pregnancies were brought to term without complication. The infants were healthy at birth and all had normal development during long-term follow-up (8 years) that was still ongoing (8).

A 2002 study reported the outcomes of 61 pregnancies in 50 women who had been treated with cabergoline for hyperprolactinemia (9). Pregnancy began during treatment in 60 cases and immediately after stopping treatment in 1 case. The median duration of treatment before pregnancy was 42.5 weeks (range 1–236 weeks) and the mean dose was 1.1 mg/week (range 0.25–7.0 mg/week). The pregnancy outcomes were 5 EABs (1 for a suspected malformation; specific details not available), 6 SABs, 1 hydatidiform mole, and 49 livebirths. Among the livebirths, there was one minor defect and one major defect (trisomy 18) (9).

In a 2005 report, a woman with Parkinson's disease took levodopa/carbidopa 330 mg/day and cabergoline 1 mg/day throughout an uncomplicated pregnancy and gave birth at term to a healthy baby girl (10). A few years later, now at age 34 and receiving levodopa/carbidopa 625 mg/day and cabergoline 4 mg/day, she became pregnant again. At 32 weeks, she underwent a cesarean section because of placenta abruption. The baby girl was doing well (10).

A 2010 review cited evidence from nearly 600 pregnancies that cabergoline exposure during gestation does not cause teratogenic effects (11). The review included three reports published in 2008–2010 that found no increased risk for SABs, stillbirths, low birth weight, or congenital malformations (12–14).

A 2013 case report described a 29-year-old woman with Cushing disease and noncurative transsphenoidal pituitary surgery who was treated with cabergoline throughout pregnancy (15). The woman had received the drug for about 1 year before she conceived. The cumulative dose during pregnancy was 300 mg. Spontaneous labor occurred at 38 weeks and she gave birth to a healthy, 3350-g female infant with Apgar scores of 7 and 9 at 1 and 5 minutes, respectively. The infant had no signs of congenital defects or hypoglycemia and was doing well at 6 weeks of age. Breastfeeding was unsuccessful because the drug (4.5 mg twice weekly) caused poor milk production (15).

BREASTFEEDING SUMMARY

Although it is not an approved indication, cabergoline suppresses lactation because of its inhibition of prolactin release from the anterior pituitary gland. This action is similar to that of bromocriptine, another prolactin-inhibiting agent. A number of studies have examined this effect (16–21). The oral doses ranged from 0.4 mg to 1 mg, usually given as a single dose within 24 hours of delivery, but sometimes given as a divided dose over 2 days. The 1-mg dose appeared to be the most effective for long-term suppression of lactation.

The manufacturer states that cabergoline should not be used to suppress physiologic lactation because of the known toxicities associated with bromocriptine, when used for this purpose (3). These toxicities include hypertension, stroke, and seizures.

References

1. Colao A, di Sarno A, Pivonello R, di Somma C, Lombardi G. Dopamine receptor agonists for treating prolactinomas. Expert Opin Investig Drugs 2002;11:787–800.
2. Robert E, Musatti L, Piscitelli G, Ferrari CI. Pregnancy outcome after treatment with the ergot derivative, cabergoline. Reprod Toxicol 1996;10:333–7.
3. Product information. Dostinex. Pharmacia & Upjohn, 2001.
4. Beltrame D, Longo M, Mazue G. Reproductive toxicity of cabergoline in mice, rats, and rabbits. Reprod Toxicol 1996;10:471–83.
5. Negishi H, Koide SS. Prevention and termination of pregnancy in rats by cabergoline, a dopamine agonist. J Reprod Fertil 1997;109:103–7.
6. Ferrari C, Paracchi A, Mattei AM, de Vincentiis S, D'Alberton A, Grosignani PG. Cabergoline in the long-term therapy of hyperprolactinemic disorders. Acta Endocrinologica 1992;126:489–94.
7. Jones TH, Fraser RB. Cabergoline treated hyperprolactinaemia results in pregnancy in a bromocriptine intolerant patient after seventeen years of infertility. Br J Obstet Gynaecol 1994;101:349–50.
8. Ciccarelli E, Grottoli S, Razzore P, Gaia D, Bertagna A, Cirillo S, Cammarota T, Camanni M, Camanni F. Long-term treatment with cabergoline, a new long-lasting ergoline derivative, in idiopathic or tumorous hyperprolactinaemia and outcome of drug-induced pregnancy. J Endocrinol Invest 1997;20:547–51.
9. Ricci E, Parazzini F, Motta T, Ferrari CI, Colao A, Clavenna A, Rocchi F, Gangi E, Paracchi S, Gasperi M, Lavezzari M, Nicolosi AE, Ferrero S, Landi ML, Beck-Peccoz P, Bonati M. Pregnancy outcome after cabergoline treatment in early weeks of gestation. Reprod Toxicol 2002;16:791–3.
10. Scott M, Chowdhury M. Pregnancy in Parkinson's disease: unique case report and review of the literature. Mov Disord 2005;20:1078–9.
11. Schlechte JA. Update in pituitary 2010. J Clin Endocrinol Metab 2011;96:1–8.
12. Colao A, Abs R, Barcena DG, Chanson P, Paulus W, Kleinberg DL. Pregnancy outcomes following cabergoline treatment: extended results from a 12 year observational study. Clin Endocrinol (Oxf) 2008;68:66–71.
13. Ono M, Miki N, Amano K, Kawamata T, Seki T, Makino R, Tekano K, Izumi S, Okada Y, Hori T. Individualized high dose cabergoline therapy for hyperprolactinemic infertility in women with micro- and macroprolactinomas. J Clin Endocrinol Metab 2010;95:2672–9.
14. Lebbe M, Hubinont C, Bernard P, Maiter D. Outcome of 100 pregnancies initiated under treatment with cabergoline in hyperprolactinaemic women. Clin Endocrinol (Oxf) 2010;73:236–42.
15. Woo I, Ehsanipoor RM, Cabergoline therapy for Cushing disease throughout pregnancy. Obstet Gynecol 2013;122:485–7.
16. Melis GB, Gambacciani M, Paoletti AM, Beneventi F, Mais V, Baroldi P, Fioretti P. Dose-related prolactin inhibitory effect of the new long-acting dopamine receptor agonist cabergoline in normal cycling, puerperal, and hyperprolactinemic women. J Clin Endocrinol Metab 1987;65:541–5.
17. Melis GB, Mais V, Paoletti AM, Beneventi F, Gambacciani M, Fioretti P. Prevention of puerperal lactation by a single oral administration of the new prolactin-inhibiting drug, cabergoline. Obstet Gynecol 1988;71:311–4.

18. Giorda G, de Vincentiis S, Motta T, Casazza S, Fadin M, D'Alberton A. Cabergoline versus bromocriptine in suppression of lactation after cesarean delivery. Gynecol Obstet Invest 1991;31:93–6.
19. Rolland R, Piscitelli G, Ferrari C, Petroccione A, and the European Multicentre Study Group for Cabergoline in Lactation Inhibition. Single dose cabergoline versus bromocriptine in inhibition of puerperal lactation: randomised, double blind, multicentre study. Br Med J 1991;302:1367–71.
20. Caballero-Gordo A, Lopez-Nazareno N, Calderay M, Caballero JL, Mancheno E, Sghedoni D. Oral cabergoline. Single-dose inhibition of puerperal lactation. J Reprod Med 1991;36:717–21.
21. Ferrari C, Piscitelli G, Grosignani PG. Cabergoline: a new drug for the treatment of hyperprolactinaemia. Hum Reprod 1995;10:1647–52.

C

CABOZANTINIB

Antineoplastic (Tyrosine Kinase Inhibitor)

PREGNANCY RECOMMENDATION: Contraindicated
BREASTFEEDING RECOMMENDATION: Contraindicated

PREGNANCY SUMMARY

No reports describing the use of cabozantinib during human pregnancy have been located. The animal data suggest risk, but the absence of human pregnancy experience prevents a more complete assessment of the embryo–fetal risk. However, based on the mechanism of action, embryo–fetal harm may occur. If a woman is pregnant or conceives during treatment, she should be informed of the potential risk to her embryo and/or fetus.

FETAL RISK SUMMARY

Cabozantinib, a substrate of CYP3A4 in vitro, is an oral inhibitor of tyrosine kinase activity. There are several other agents in this subclass (see Appendix). Cabozantinib is indicated for the treatment of patients with progressive, metastatic medullary thyroid cancer. The drug is metabolized to apparently inactive metabolites. Plasma protein binding is high (>99.7%) and the effective half-life is about 55 hours (1).

Reproduction studies have been conducted in rats and rabbits. In rats that were given the drug daily during organogenesis, embryo–fetal death was observed at doses that were <1% of the human exposure by AUC at the recommended dose (HE). The findings included delayed ossifications and skeletal variations at doses that were about ≥0.03% of the HE. In rabbits administered the drug daily during organogenesis, visceral malformations and variations including reduced spleen size and missing lung lobe were observed at a dose that was about 11% of the HE (1).

Studies evaluating the carcinogenic potential of cabozantinib have not been conducted. The drug was not mutagenic or clastogenic in various assays. Fertility was impaired in male rats (decrease in sperm counts and reproductive organ weights) and female rats (decrease in live embryos and increase in pre- and postimplantation losses, and ovarian necrosis). Impairment of fertility also was observed in male (hypospermia) and female (absence of corpora lutea) dogs (1).

It is not known if cabozantinib crosses the human placenta. The molecular weight (about 636 for the malate salt) and the long effective half-life suggest that the drug will cross to the embryo–fetus, but the high plasma protein binding might limit the exposure.

BREASTFEEDING SUMMARY

No reports describing the use of cabozantinib during human lactation have been located. The molecular weight (about 636 for the malate salt) and the long effective half-life (about 55 hours) suggest that the drug will be excreted into breast milk, but the high plasma protein binding (≥99.7%) might limit the exposure. The effect of this exposure on a nursing infant is unknown. However, because the drug commonly (≥25%) causes toxicity in adults, such as diarrhea, stomatitis, decreased appetite and weight, nausea, fatigue, and oral and abdominal pain, the best course is to not use cabozantinib during breastfeeding.

Reference

1. Product information. Cometriq. Exelixis, 2012.

CAFFEINE

Central Stimulant

PREGNANCY RECOMMENDATION: Compatible
BREASTFEEDING RECOMMENDATION: Compatible

C

PREGNANCY SUMMARY

Although the amount of caffeine in commonly used beverages varies widely, caffeine consumption in pregnancy in moderate amounts apparently does not pose a measurable risk to the fetus. When used in moderation, no association with congenital malformations, spontaneous abortions (SABs), preterm birth, and low birth weight has been proved.

FETAL RISK SUMMARY

Caffeine is one of the most popular drugs in the world (1). It is frequently used in combination products containing aspirin, phenacetin, and codeine and is present in a number of commonly consumed beverages, such as coffee, teas, and colas, as well as many food items. The mean caffeine content in the usual servings of some common beverages was reported as caffeinated coffee (66–146 mg), nonherbal tea (20–46 mg), and caffeinated soft drinks (47 mg) (2), but these amounts may vary widely. (For example, see also reference 26 in which it is reported that the average caffeine content in two cups of regular coffee totaled 454 mg, and the average content in a similar amount of decaffeinated coffee totaled 12 mg.)

Caffeine crosses the placenta, and fetal blood and tissue levels similar to maternal concentrations are achieved (1,3–5). Cord blood levels of 1–1.6 mcg/mL have been measured (3). Caffeine has also been found in newborns exposed to theophylline in utero (6).

The mutagenicity and carcinogenicity of caffeine have been evaluated in more than 50 studies involving laboratory animals, human and animal cell tissue cultures, and human lymphocytes in vivo (1,3). The significance of mutagenic and carcinogenic effects found in nonmammalian systems has not been established in man. The drug is an animal teratogen only when doses high enough to cause toxicity in the mother have been given (1).

The Collaborative Perinatal Project (CPP) monitored 50,282 mother–child pairs, 5378 of whom had 1st trimester exposure to caffeine (7, pp. 366–370). No evidence of a relationship to congenital defects was found. For use anytime during pregnancy, 12,696 exposures were recorded (7, pp. 493–494). In this group, slightly increased relative risks were found for musculoskeletal defects, hydronephrosis, adrenal anomalies, and hemangiomas or granulomas, but the results are not interpretable without independent confirmation (7, pp. 493–494). A follow-up analysis by the CPP on 2030 malformed infants and maternal use of caffeine-containing beverages did not support caffeine as a teratogen (8). Other reports have also found no association between the use of caffeine during pregnancy and congenital malformations (9–12).

Several authors have associated high caffeine consumption (six to eight cups of coffee/day) with decreased fertility, increased incidence of SAB, and low birth weights (3,13–17). However, a few of these studies have isolated the effects of caffeine from cigarette or alcohol use, both of which are positively associated with caffeine consumption (3). One German study has observed that high coffee use alone is associated with low birth weights (18). In an American study of more than 12,400 women, low birth weights and short gestations occurred more often among offspring of women who drank four or more cups of coffee/day and who smoked (12). No relationship between low birth weights or short gestation and caffeine was found after controlling for smoking, alcohol intake, and demographic characteristics. However, other investigators have questioned whether this study has accurately assessed the total caffeine intake of the women (19,20). A Canadian study retrospectively investigated 913 newborn infants for the effects of caffeine and cigarette smoking on birth weight and placental weight (21). Significant caffeine–cigarette interactions were found when daily consumption of caffeine was ≥300 mg. Compared with nonsmokers, cigarette smoking significantly lowered mean birth weight. When caffeine use was considered, daily consumption of ≥300 mg combined with smoking ≥15 cigarettes caused an additional significant reduction in weight. Head circumference and body length were not affected by any level of caffeine consumption. Placental weight, which normally increases with cigarette smoking, an effect hypothesized to be due to compensatory hypertrophy induced by chronic fetal hypoxia, was found to decrease significantly in women smoking ≥15 cigarettes/day and ingesting ≥300 mg of caffeine/day (21).

A prospective cohort study examined the relationship between caffeine intake and the incidence of late SAB in 3135 predominantly white, educated, professional women (22). A total of 2483 (79%) of this population used caffeine during pregnancy. Caffeine consumption was calculated based on the intake of coffee (107 mg/serving), tea (34 mg/serving), colas (47 mg/serving), and drugs. Moderate-to-heavy consumption, defined as ≥151 mg of caffeine/day, occurred in 28% (879) and was associated with a twofold increased risk of late 1st and 2nd trimester SAB (relative risk 1.95, $p = 0.07$). Consumption of >200 mg/day did not increase this risk. In women who had an SAB in their last pregnancy, light use of caffeine (0–150 mg/day) was associated with a fourfold increase in late pregnancy loss (relative risk 4.18, $p = 0.04$). The data were adjusted for factors such as demographic characteristics, obstetric and medical histories, contraceptive use, smoking, and alcohol exposure. The investigators cautioned, however, that other independent epidemiologic studies were required to confirm their findings because SAB is of multifactorial etiology (22,23).

No increased risk for SAB, intrauterine growth restriction, or microcephaly was found in a study that was able to identify all abortions that occurred 21 or more days after conception (24). The mean 1st trimester caffeine consumption was statistically similar in those who aborted compared with those who delivered liveborn infants, 125.9 vs. 111.6 mg. After adjustment for other risk factors, notably smoking, the adjusted odds ratios for growth restriction and microcephaly were 1.11 (95% confidence interval [CI] 0.88–1.40) and 1.09 (95% CI 0.86–1.37), respectively (24).

A publication, evaluating studies published between 1981 and 1986, reviewed the effects of caffeine consumption on human pregnancies in terms of congenital malformations, low birth weight, preterm birth, SABs, and behavior

C

in in utero exposed children (25). Based on this evaluation of the literature, the author concluded that moderate intake of caffeine was not related to any adverse pregnancy outcome. A second article (120 references) reviewed the effect of caffeine on pregnancy outcome in both animals and humans (26). This author also concluded that modest amounts of caffeine present no proven risk to the fetus, but that limitation of daily amounts to <300 mg/day may lessen the possibility of growth restriction.

Research on the effects of caffeine consumption on human fecundability (i.e., the probability of becoming clinically pregnant in a given menstrual cycle) was reported in 1988 (27). Drawing from women they had enrolled in a study of very early pregnancy loss, the investigators chose 104 women who had not become pregnant in the first 3 months. Data were recorded daily by the women on menstrual bleeding, intercourse, and caffeine and other substance exposures. Caffeine consumption was calculated by assuming that brewed coffee contained 100 mg, instant coffee 65 mg, tea 50 mg, and soft drinks 40 mg. The subjects were primarily white, college educated, and in their late 20s or early 30s. Caffeinated beverages were consumed by 93% (97 of 104) of the women. The women were grouped into lower caffeine consumers (<3150 mg/month, or about one cup of brewed coffee/day) and higher consumers (>3150 mg/month). Based on this division, the higher consumers were consistently less likely to become pregnant than the lower consumers, with a weighted mean of fecundability ratios across 13 menstrual cycles of 0.59. (The fecundability ratio was determined in each cycle by dividing the number of women who became pregnant by the total number of woman cycles at risk and then by dividing the fraction obtained in the higher caffeine consumption group by the fraction obtained for the lower consumption group.) The ratio was less than 1.0 in every cycle. For cycles occurring after 6 months, the ratio was 0.53, indicating a slightly stronger association between higher caffeine consumption and the inability to become pregnant (27). Statistical adjustment of the data for age, frequency of intercourse, age at menarche, cigarette smoking, vitamin and analgesic intake, alcohol and marijuana use, and the mother's weight and height did not significantly change these findings. Moreover, when caffeine consumption was further subdivided, a partial dose–response relationship was observed, with a ratio of 0.26 for women consuming >7000 mg/month (i.e., >70 cups of coffee/month). Unadjusted data on infertility (defined as women who failed to achieve pregnancy after 1 year) indicated that only 6% of the lower consumption group met this definition compared with 28% of the higher consumption group, an estimated relative risk of 4.7 (p <0.005) (27). Evidence was also found to suggest that the effects of caffeine on fertility were short acting because recent consumption was far more important than previous consumption. Although the study attempted to include all related factors, the investigators cautioned that they could not exclude the possibility that some unknown factor or condition might have accounted for these results and that independent confirmation was required (27,28). Partial confirmation of this study was reported in 1989 (29). In a retrospective analysis of data collected from 1959 to 1967 on 6303 pregnancies, a dose–response relationship was found between caffeine consumption and difficulty in becoming pregnant. Using data adjusted for ethnicity (white, black), parity (0,1), and smoking, the relative risk of decreased fertility for <1 cup of coffee/day was 1.00, 1-3 cups/day 1.20, 4-6 cups/day 1.88, and >7 cups/day 1.96 (29).

Some investigators have expressed concern over the altering of catecholamine levels in the fetus by caffeine (30). Two cups of regular coffee containing a total of 454 mg of caffeine have been shown to increase maternal epinephrine levels significantly but not norepinephrine or dopamine concentrations (31). Decaffeinated coffee (12 mg of caffeine in two cups) did not affect these catecholamine levels.

A 1989 single-blind, crossover study of eight women at 32–36 weeks of gestation investigated the effects of 2 cups of caffeinated (regular) or decaffeinated coffee on fetal breathing movements and heart rate (31). Administration of the test beverages, containing a total of 454 mg and 12 mg of caffeine, respectively, were separated by 1 week, and in each case, were consumed over a 15-minute period. Fetal breathing movements increased significantly during the 3rd hour after regular coffee, rising from 144 breaths/hour to 614 breaths/hour (p <0.01). Fetal heart rate fell 9% (p <0.05) at 1–1.5 hours after the regular coffee and then slowly rose toward control levels at 2 and 4 hours. However, the mean number, amplitude, and duration of fetal heart rate accelerations did not differ statistically from the control period. Decaffeinated coffee also caused a significant increase in fetal breathing movements, rising to 505 breaths/hour during the 2nd hour, but this beverage caused only a slight, nonsignificant lowering of the fetal heart rate. In an earlier study using 200-mg tablets of caffeine, no increase in fetal breathing rates was observed (32). The differences between the two studies may have been related to the lower dose and/or the dosage form of caffeine.

Cardiac arrhythmias and other symptoms in newborn infants were associated with maternal caffeine consumption of >500 mg/day (N = 16) in comparison with the offspring of women who used less than 250 mg/day (N = 56) of caffeine (33). The percentages of observed symptoms in the infants of the high and low caffeine groups were tachyarrhythmias (supraventricular tachycardia and atrial flutter) 25% vs. 1.7% (p <0.01), premature atrial contraction 12.5% vs. 0 (p <0.01), fine tremors 100% vs. 10.7% (p <0.001), and tachypnea (resting respiratory rate >60 respirations/minute) 25% vs. 3.5% (p <0.01), respectively. The authors attributed the symptoms to caffeine withdrawal after birth (33).

Two reports have described adverse fetal outcomes, including teratogenic effects, in the offspring of two mothers taking migraine preparations consisting of ergotamine and caffeine (34,35). Complete details of these cases are provided under Ergotamine.

A 1993 reference compared the effects of maternal caffeine consumption greater than 500 mg/day with those of less than 200 mg/day on fetal behavior in the 3rd trimester (36). Long-term consumption of high amounts of caffeine apparently modulated fetal behavior in terms of quiet sleep (infrequent body movements, regular breathing patterns, and little variability in fetal heart rate [FHR]), active sleep (rapid eye movements [REM], increased body activity, irregular breathing, and increased FHR variability), and arousal (REM, frequent body movements, highly irregular FHR baseline, and breathing activity). Fetuses of mothers in the high caffeine group spent less mean time in active sleep, similar mean time

C

in quiet sleep, and much greater mean time in arousal than did low caffeine-exposed fetuses. It could not be determined if the modulation of behavior had any clinical significance to the newborn or in later life (36).

A 2001 review concluded that, in those who do not smoke or drink alcohol, moderate caffeine consumption (<5–6 mg/kg/day spread throughout the day) did not increase any reproductive risks (37). Use of high doses may be associated with SABs, difficulty in becoming pregnant, and infertility. A dose–response relationship may exist for the latter two problems. However, confirmation of these findings is needed before any firm conclusions can be drawn. The consumption of high caffeine doses with cigarette smoking may increase the risk for delivery of infants with lower birth weight than that induced by smoking alone. Moreover, consumption of large amounts of caffeine may be associated with becoming a smoker and excessive alcohol drinking (37).

BREASTFEEDING SUMMARY

Caffeine is excreted into breast milk (38–45). Milk:plasma ratios of 0.5 and 0.76 have been reported (39,40). Following ingestion of coffee or tea containing known amounts of caffeine (36–335 mg), peak milk levels of 2.09–7.17 mcg/mL occurred within 1 hour (41). An infant consuming 90 mL of milk every 3 hours would ingest 0.01–1.64 mg of caffeine over 24 hours after the mother drank a single cup of caffeinated beverage (41). In another study, peak milk levels after a 100-mg dose were 3.0 mcg/mL at 1 hour (40). In this and an earlier study, the authors estimated a nursing infant would receive 1.5–3.1 mg of caffeine after a single cup of coffee (39,40).

Nine breastfeeding mothers consumed a measured amount of caffeine (750 mg/day) added to decaffeinated coffee for 5 days, then abstained from all caffeine ingestion for the next 4 days (44). In six women, 24-hour pooled aliquots of milk samples from each feeding were collected on days 5 and 9. In another mother, pooled aliquots were collected daily for 9 days. The average milk caffeine concentrations from these seven mothers on day 5 were 4.3 mcg/mL (range <0.25–15.7 mcg/mL). Caffeine was not detected (i.e., <0.25 mcg/mL) in any of the seven samples on day 9. Serum levels in the infants of these seven mothers on day 5 averaged 1.4 mcg/mL (range 0.8–2.8 mcg/mL in five infants, not detectable in two). On day 9, caffeine was detectable in the sera of only two infants, decreasing from 0.8 mcg/mL on day 5 to 0.6 mcg/mL on day 9 in one, and decreasing from 2.8 to 2.4 mcg/mL in the other. The remaining two mothers collected milk samples with each feeding for the entire 9 days of the study but did not pool the samples. These mothers were breastfeeding infants aged 79 and 127 days, and their mean daily milk caffeine levels on days 1–5 ranged from 4.0 to 28.6 mcg/mL. Caffeine could not be detected in any of the milk samples after 5 days. The two infants' sera contained <0.25 mcg/mL (mother's milk 13.4 mcg/mL) and 3.2 mcg/mL (mother's milk 28.6 mcg/mL) on day 5, and both were <0.25 mcg/mL on day 9. The wide variance in milk concentrations of caffeine was attributed to the mother's ability to metabolize caffeine (44). Based on the average level of 4.3 mcg/mL, and assuming an infant consumed 150–180 mL/kg/day, the author calculated the infant would receive 0.6–0.8 mg/kg/day of caffeine (44).

In an extension of the above study, the effect of 500 mg of caffeine consumption/day on infant heart rate and sleep time was evaluated in 11 mother–infant pairs (45). Mothers consumed decaffeinated coffee daily for 5 days and then decaffeinated coffee with added caffeine for another 5-day period. Milk caffeine levels on the last day of the caffeine period ranged from 1.6 to 6.2 mcg/mL, providing an estimated 0.3–1.0 mg/kg/day of caffeine to the infants. No significant difference in 24-hour heart rate or sleep time was observed between the two phases of the study.

The elimination half-life of caffeine is approximately 80 hours in term newborns and 97.5 hours in premature babies (42). A 1987 study investigated the metabolism of caffeine in breast- and formula-fed infants given oral doses of caffeine citrate (46). The serum half-lives of caffeine were greater than three times as long in the breast-fed infants as compared with the formula-fed infants (76 vs. 21 hours at 47–50 weeks postconceptional age; 54 vs. 16 hours at 51–54 weeks postconceptional age). The investigators attributed the findings to inhibition or suppression of caffeine metabolism by the hepatic cytochrome P450 system by some element of breast milk (46).

The amounts of caffeine in breast milk after maternal ingestion of caffeinated beverages are probably too low to be clinically significant. However, accumulation may occur in infants when mothers consume moderate-to-heavy amounts of caffeinated beverages. Irritability and poor sleeping patterns have been observed in nursing infants during periods of heavy maternal use of caffeine (43). The American Academy of Pediatrics classifies usual amounts of caffeinated beverages as compatible with breastfeeding (47).

References

1. Soyka LF. Effects of methylxanthines on the fetus. Clin Perinatol 1979;6:37–51.
2. Bunker ML, McWilliams M. Caffeine content of common beverages. J Am Diet Assoc 1979;74:28–32.
3. Soyka LF. Caffeine ingestion during pregnancy: in utero exposure and possible effects. Semin Perinatol 1981;5:305–9.
4. Goldstein A, Warren R. Passage of caffeine into human gonadal and fetal tissue. Biochem Pharmacol 1962;17:166–8.
5. Parsons WD, Aranda JV, Neims AH. Elimination of transplacentally acquired caffeine in full term neonates. Pediatr Res 1976;10:333.
6. Brazier JL, Salle B. Conversion of theophylline to caffeine by the human fetus. Semin Perinatol 1981;5:315–20.
7. Heinonen OP, Slone D, Shapiro S. *Birth Defects and Drugs in Pregnancy*. Littleton, MA: Publishing Sciences Group, 1977.
8. Rosenberg L, Mitchell AA, Shapiro S, Slone D. Selected birth defects in relation to caffeine-containing beverages. JAMA 1982;247:1429–32.
9. Van't Hoff W. Caffeine in pregnancy. Lancet 1982;1:1020.
10. Kurppa K, Holmberg PC, Kuosma E, Saxen L. Coffee consumption during pregnancy. N Engl J Med 1982;306:1548.
11. Curatolo PW, Robertson D. The health consequences of caffeine. Ann Intern Med 1983;98(Part 1):641–53.
12. Linn S, Schoenbaum SC, Monson RR, Rosner B, Stubblefield PG, Ryan KJ. No association between coffee consumption and adverse outcomes of pregnancy. N Engl J Med 1982;306:141–5.
13. Weathersbee PS, Olsen LK, Lodge JR. Caffeine and pregnancy. Postgrad Med 1977;62:64–9.
14. Anonymous. Caffeine and birth defects—another negative study. Pediatr Alert 1982;7:23–4.
15. Hogue CJ. Coffee in pregnancy. Lancet 1981;2:554.
16. Weathersbee PS, Lodge JR, Caffeine: its direct and indirect influence on reproduction. J Reprod Med 1977;19:55–63.
17. Lechat MF, Borlee I, Bouckaert A, Misson C. Caffeine study. Science 1980;207:1296–7.

18. Mau G, Netter P. Kaffee- und alkoholkonsum-riskofaktoren in der schwangerschaft? Geburtshilfe Frauenheilkd 1974;34:1018–22.
19. Bracken MB, Bryce-Buchanan C, Silten R, Srisuphan W. Coffee consumption during pregnancy. N Engl J Med 1982;306:1548–9.
20. Luke B. Coffee consumption during pregnancy. N Engl J Med 1982; 306:1549.
21. Beaulac-Baillargeon L, Desrosiers C. Caffeine–cigarette interaction on fetal growth. Am J Obstet Gynecol 1987;157:1236–40.
22. Srisuphan W, Bracken MB. Caffeine consumption during pregnancy and association with late spontaneous abortion. Am J Obstet Gynecol 1986;154:14–20.
23. Bracken MB. Caffeine consumption during pregnancy and association with late spontaneous abortion: reply. Am J Obstet Gynecol 1986;155:1147.
24. Mills JL, Holmes LB, Aarons JH, Simpson JL, Brown ZA, Jovanovic-Peterson LG, Conley MR, Graubard BI, Knopp RH, Metzger BE. Moderate caffeine use and the risk of spontaneous abortion and intrauterine growth retardation. JAMA 1993;269:593–7.
25. Leviton A. Caffeine consumption and the risk of reproductive hazards. J Reprod Med 1988;33:175–8.
26. Berger A. Effects of caffeine consumption on pregnancy outcome: a review. J Reprod Med 1988;33:945–56.
27. Wilcox A, Weinberg C, Baird D. Caffeinated beverages and decreased fertility. Lancet 1988;2:1453–6.
28. Wilcox AJ. Caffeinated beverages and decreased fertility. Lancet 1989;1:840.
29. Christianson RE, Oechsli FW, van den Berg BJ. Caffeinated beverages and decreased fertility. Lancet 1989;1:378.
30. Bellet S, Roman L, DeCastro O, Kim KE, Kershbaum A. Effect of coffee ingestion on catecholamine release. Metabolism 1969;18:288–91.
31. Salvador HS, Koos BJ. Effects of regular and decaffeinated coffee on fetal breathing and heart rate. Am J Obstet Gynecol 1989;160:1043–7.
32. McGowan J, Devoe LD, Searle N, Altman R. The effects of long- and short-term maternal caffeine ingestion on human fetal breathing and body movements in term gestations. Am J Obstet Gynecol 1987;157:726–9.
33. Hadeed A, Siegel S. Newborn cardiac arrhythmias associated with maternal caffeine use during pregnancy. Clin Pediatr 1993;32:45–7.
34. Graham JM Jr, Marin-Padilla M, Hoefnagel D. Jejunal atresia associated with Cafergot® ingestion during pregnancy. Clin Pediatr 1983;22:226–8.
35. Hughes HE, Goldstein DA. Birth defects following maternal exposure to ergotamine, beta blockers, and caffeine. J Med Genet 1988;25:396–9.
36. Devoe LD, Murray C, Youssif A, Arnaud M. Maternal caffeine consumption and fetal behavior in normal third-trimester pregnancy. Am J Obstet Gynecol 1993;168:1105–12.
37. Christian MS, Brent RL. Teratogen update: evaluation of the reproductive and developmental risks of caffeine. Teratology 2001;64:51–78.
38. Jobe PC. Psychoactive substances and antiepileptic drugs. In: Wilson JT, ed. *Drugs in Breast Milk*. Balgowlah, Australia: ADIS Press, 1981:40.
39. Tyrala EE, Dodson WE. Caffeine secretion into breast milk. Arch Dis Child 1979;54:787–800.
40. Sargraves R, Bradley JM, Delgado MJM, Wagner D, Sharpe GL, Stavchansky S. Pharmacokinetics of caffeine in human breast milk after a single oral dose of caffeine (abstract). Drug Intell Clin Pharm 1984;18:507.
41. Berlin CM Jr, Denson HM, Daniel CH, Ward RM. Disposition of dietary caffeine in milk, saliva, and plasma of lactating women. Pediatrics 1984;73:59–63.
42. Berlin CM Jr. Excretion of the methylxanthines in human milk. Semin Perinatol 1981;5:389–94.
43. Hill RM, Craig JP, Chaney MD, Tennyson LM, McCulley LB. Utilization of over-the-counter drugs during pregnancy. Clin Obstet Gynecol 1977;20:381–94.
44. Ryu JE. Caffeine in human milk and in serum of breast-fed infants. Dev Pharmacol Ther 1985;8:329–37.
45. Ryu JE. Effect of maternal caffeine consumption on heart rate and sleep time of breast-fed infants. Dev Pharmacol Ther 1985;8:355–63.
46. Le Guennec J-C, Billon B. Delay in caffeine elimination in breast-fed infants. Pediatrics 1987;79:264–8.
47. Committee on Drugs, American Academy of Pediatrics. The transfer of drugs and other chemicals into human milk. Pediatrics 2001;108:776–89.

CALCIFEDIOL

Vitamin

PREGNANCY RECOMMENDATION: Compatible
BREASTFEEDING RECOMMENDATION: Compatible

FETAL RISK SUMMARY

Calcifediol is converted in the kidneys to calcitriol, one of the active forms of vitamin D. See Vitamin D.

BREASTFEEDING SUMMARY

See Vitamin D.

CALCIPOTRIENE

Dermatologic Agent (Anti-Psoriatic)

PREGNANCY RECOMMENDATION: No Human Data—Probably Compatible
BREASTFEEDING RECOMMENDATION: No Human Data—Probably Compatible

PREGNANCY SUMMARY

No reports describing the use of calcipotriene in human pregnancy have been located. The animal data suggest moderate risk, but there is no evidence that vitamin D derivatives cause human developmental toxicity. Only low amounts of the drug are absorbed into the systemic circulation and the embryo–fetal risk is probably similar to calcitriol, a vitamin considered

C

compatible with pregnancy (see Calcitriol). Two reviews discussing the treatment of psoriasis, one in 2002 (1) and the other in 2005 (2), considered the topical use of calcipotriene to be safe in pregnancy. Mild hypercalcemia has been observed in a newborn exposed in utero to calcitriol and is a potential complication with calcipotriene.

FETAL RISK SUMMARY

Calcipotriene, a synthetic derivative of vitamin D_3 (calcitriol), is available in cream, ointment, and solution preparations. It is indicated for the treatment of plaque psoriasis in adults. Clinical studies with the ointment found that about 6% and 5% of the applied dose is absorbed systemically when applied to psoriasis plaques and normal skin, respectively. Much of the absorbed drug is converted to inactive metabolites within 24 hours of application. Metabolism is thought to be similar to calcitriol (3,4). Systemic absorption of the cream or solution has not been studied (3).

Reproduction studies have been conducted in rats and rabbits with oral calcipotriene where the expected bioavailability of the dose was about 40%–60%. The maternal and fetal calculated no-effect exposures in the rat and rabbit studies were about equal to the expected human systemic exposure level from dermal application based on BSA (HSEL). In rats, oral doses about 7.4 times the HSEL resulted in a significantly higher incidence of skeletal abnormalities consisting primarily of enlarged fontanelles (thought to be due to the drug's effect on calcium metabolism) and extra ribs. In rabbits, increased maternal and fetal toxicity was noted at about 7.5 times the HSEL. Doses that were about 17.5 times the HSEL resulted in fetuses with a significant increase in the incidences of pubic bones, forelimb phalanges, and incomplete bone ossification (3,4).

Long-term carcinogenesis studies in mice with topical calcipotriene, without exposure to ultraviolet radiation (UVR), caused no significant changes in tumor incidence. However, when mice also were exposed to UVR, the results suggested that the drug enhanced the effect of UVR to induce skin tumors. Calcipotriene was not mutagenic in multiple assays and, at oral doses up to about 7.5 times the HSEL, did not impair the fertility or reproductive performance in rats (3,4).

It is not known if calcipotriene crosses the human placenta. However, the systemic disposition of calcipotriene is expected to be similar to that of the naturally occurring calcitriol that does enter the fetal circulation (4).

BREASTFEEDING SUMMARY

No reports describing the use of calcipotriene during human lactation have been located. Only small amounts are absorbed into the systemic circulation and probably are excreted into breast milk. However, calcipotriene is a synthetic derivative of calcitriol, an active form of vitamin D. Vitamin D is compatible with breastfeeding (see Vitamin D), and the topical use of calcipotriene probably can be classified similarly.

References

1. Tauscher AE, Fleischer AB Jr, Phelps KC, Feldman SR. Psoriasis and pregnancy. J Cutan Med Surg 2002;6:561–70.
2. Lebwohl M. A clinician's paradigm in the treatment of psoriasis. J Am Acad Dermatol 2005;53:S59–69.
3. Product information. Dovonex cream. LEO Pharma, 2010.
4. Product information. Dovonex ointment. Bristol-Myers Squibb, 2010.

CALCITONIN-SALMON

Calcium Regulation Hormone

PREGNANCY RECOMMENDATION: Limited Human Data—Probably Compatible
BREASTFEEDING RECOMMENDATION: No Human Data—Probably Compatible

PREGNANCY SUMMARY

No reports linking the use of calcitonin-salmon with congenital defects have been located. Marked increases of calcitonin concentrations in fetal serum greater than maternal levels have been demonstrated at term (1). The significance of this finding is unknown.

FETAL RISK SUMMARY

Calcitonin-salmon is a synthetic polypeptide of 32 amino acids in the same linear sequence that is found in the hormone from salmon. The hormone does not cross the placenta (2).

A decrease in fetal birth weights in rabbits has been observed when calcitonin-salmon was administered in doses 14–56 times the recommended human dose. The fetal weight reduction may have been due to metabolic effects on the mother (2).

In a 1990 case, a 28-year-old woman at 30 weeks with a history of a renal transplant was treated for 3 weeks with an IV infusion of calcitonin-salmon for hypercalcemia (3). A cesarean section was performed at 33 weeks for preeclampsia to deliver a normal 1600 g female infant.

BREASTFEEDING SUMMARY

No reports describing the use of calcitonin-salmon during lactation have been located. Because it is a polypeptide, excretion into milk would not be expected. Moreover, calcitonin-salmon has been shown to inhibit lactation in animals (4). Mothers wishing to breastfeed should be informed of this potential complication (2).

References

1. Kovarik J, Woloszczuk W, Linkesch W, Pavelka R. Calcitonin in pregnancy. Lancet 1980;1:199–200.
2. Product information. Miacalcin. Novartis Pharmaceuticals, 2000.
3. Fromm GA, Labarrere CA, Ramirez J, Mautalen CA, Plantalech L, Althabe O, Casco C, Ferraris J. Hypercalcaemia in pregnancy in a renal transplant recipient with secondary hyperparathyroidism—case report. Br J Obstet Gynaecol 1990;97:1049–53.
4. Tohei A, VandeGarde B, Arbogast LA, Voogt JL. Calcitonin inhibition of prolactin secretion in lactating rats: mechanism of action. Neuroendocrinology 2000;71:327–32.

CALCITRIOL

Vitamin

PREGNANCY RECOMMENDATION: Compatible
BREASTFEEDING RECOMMENDATION: Compatible

PREGNANCY SUMMARY

The near absence of human pregnancy experience prevents a complete assessment of the risk for the embryo and fetus. However, there is no evidence that recommended doses of vitamin D during pregnancy are harmful.

FETAL RISK SUMMARY

Calcitriol is one of three physiologically active forms of vitamin D (see Vitamin D). Calcitriol is teratogenic in rabbits given daily doses that were about two and six times the maximum recommended human dose based on BSA (MRHD) (1). Defects observed included external and skeletal malformations. The high dose given on gestation days 7–18 also increased maternal mortality, decreased mean fetal body weight, and reduced the number of newborn surviving to 24 hours. No teratogenic effects were observed in rats treated with daily doses up to about five times the MRHD (1). However, hypercalcemia was measured in the offspring of rats given doses that were about one and three times the MRHD (1).

The manufacturer cites a case of mild hypercalcemia during the first 2 days of life in an infant who was exposed to a maternal dose of 17–36 mcg/day (approximately 17–36 times the maximum recommended dose) during pregnancy (1). The hypercalcemia resolved by the third day.

BREASTFEEDING SUMMARY

See Vitamin D.

Reference

1. Product information. Rocaltrol. Roche Laboratories, 2000.

CALCIUM CARBONATE

Nutrient/Antacid

PREGNANCY RECOMMENDATION: Compatible
BREASTFEEDING RECOMMENDATION: Compatible

PREGNANCY SUMMARY

Sufficient maternal calcium intake is important to ensure adequate mineralization of the fetal skeleton (1). The recommended dietary allowance (RDA) for calcium during pregnancy is based on age: 1300 mg/day for 14–18 years and 1000 mg/day for 19–50 years (2). The primary source of calcium in pregnancy is diet, but antacids and supplements containing calcium carbonate, and prenatal vitamins, also contribute. Recommended doses of calcium carbonate for heartburn relief are safe in pregnancy, but very high doses have caused milk-alkali syndrome and other toxicity. Calcium supplements, such as 1000–2000 mg/day of calcium carbonate, offer few if any benefits for pregnant women if they have adequate dietary calcium intake. However, there may be some benefits for women with low (<600 mg/day) dietary calcium intake.

C

FETAL RISK SUMMARY

Calcium carbonate is commonly used as a source of calcium either alone or as a component of vitamins products. It also is used as an antacid, either alone or in combination with other antacids, to neutralize stomach acid.

Calcium crosses the human placenta by active transport. The fetal concentration of calcium is related to fetal weight so that most accumulation of calcium takes place in the 3rd trimester (3).

A number of studies have evaluated calcium supplementation with calcium carbonate to prevent or reduce the risk of hypertensive disorders in pregnancy (gestational hypertension and preeclampsia), preterm birth, maternal hemodynamic dysfunction, and long-term effects on the blood pressure of offspring (4–15). Although many of these studies reported a reduction in hypertensive disorders, a large 1997 study conducted by the National Institutes of Health (NIH) did not find this outcome (16). In this study, 4589 healthy nulliparous women at 13–21 weeks' gestation were randomized to receive daily treatment throughout their pregnancy with either 2 g of calcium carbonate or placebo. In the calcium group (N = 2295), preeclampsia occurred in 158 (6.9%), whereas in the placebo group (N = 2294), 168 (7.3%) developed preeclampsia (relative risk 0.94, 95% confidence interval 0.76–1.16). There also was no significant difference between the groups for pregnancy-associated hypertension without preeclampsia (15.3% vs. 17.3%) or all hypertensive disorders (22.2% vs. 24.6%). The mean systolic and diastolic blood pressures during pregnancy were similar in the groups. Moreover, calcium supplementation did not reduce the number of preterm births (<37 weeks; 10.8% vs. 10.0%), small-for-gestational-age infants (5.8% vs. 4.9%), or fetal and neonatal deaths (27 vs. 25 cases). In addition, calcium supplementation did not increase urolithiasis (3 vs. 4 cases) (16).

In an editorial accompanying the aforementioned NIH study, the author pointed out that whereas the investigators involved diet in the NIH study, this may not have been done in previous studies and might account for the different outcomes (17). The author also cautioned that although the NIH study clearly demonstrates that supplemental calcium 2 g/day offers no benefit for low-risk women if the desired outcome is reduced preeclampsia or improved fetal or neonatal outcome, it did not indicate that adequate or extra dietary calcium was not important (17).

A 1999 randomized, double-blind, placebo-controlled study examined the effect of calcium carbonate supplementation (≥2 g/day) during the 2nd and 3rd trimesters on fetal bone mineralization (18). A total of 256 infants (128 per group) were studied. The supplementation did increase fetal bone mineralization in women with low dietary calcium intake (<600 mg/day) compared with placebo, but in women with adequate dietary calcium intake, supplementation did not result in major improvement in this outcome (18).

The results of a multicenter, randomized, placebo-controlled, double-blind trial of calcium supplementation in low-calcium-intake pregnant women were published in 2006 (19). The trial found that calcium carbonate supplementation (1.5 g/day) did not prevent preeclampsia but did reduce its severity. Also noted was a slight, nonsignificant lowering of preterm (<37 weeks) birth (9.8% vs. 10.8%) and a significant decrease in early (<32 weeks) preterm birth (2.6% vs. 3.2%). Maternal morbidity and mortality and neonatal mortality were reduced by supplementation, but two other outcomes, low birth weight in term pregnancies and admission to intensive care units, were similar between the two groups (19).

Using data collected for the aforementioned trial, a 2010 study in Argentina evaluated the effect of calcium supplements on fetal growth in pregnant women with low calcium intake (average calcium intake <600 mg/day) (20). The women, at about 13 weeks' gestation, were randomized to either calcium carbonate 1500 mg/day (N = 231) or placebo (N = 230). No differences between the two groups were found in serial fetal biometric measurements taken five times from 20 to 36 weeks' gestation. Moreover, neonatal characteristics and anthropometric measurements at birth were comparable in both groups. The investigators concluded that calcium supplementation of 1500 mg/day in pregnant women with low calcium intake did not improve fetal somatic or skeletal growth (20).

Excessive consumption of calcium carbonate throughout pregnancy was suspected to be the cause of neonatal hypocalcemia, resulting in seizures (21). The mother, a healthy 24-year-old, had heartburn, which she treated with 10 to 14 extra-strength Tums daily (750 mg calcium carbonate/tablet) starting midway through the 1st trimester and continuing until the onset of labor at 39 weeks. The normal-appearing infant weighed about 3.5 kg at birth and was sent home on the second day. Generalized seizures developed at 8 days of age. Laboratory tests were normal, except for a total calcium level of 6.3 mg/dL that decreased to 6.1 mg/dL the next day (normal: 8.5–11.0 mg/dL) and a high phosphorus level (8.2 mg/dL; normal 4.0–7.0 mg/dL). The infant was treated with phenobarbital and IV calcium gluconate, and at 12 days of age, the total calcium was within the normal range, but the phosphorus level did not return to a normal range until 29 days of age. One possible mechanism proposed by the author was that the excessive maternal calcium intake had suppressed fetal parathyroid function. At 3 months of age, the infant was healthy and doing well (21).

Ingestion of calcium carbonate has been associated with three published cases of milk-alkali syndrome in pregnancy (22–24). The first case involved a 34-year-old woman in her second pregnancy (22). She had excessive vomiting and took large quantities (amount not specified) of calcium carbonate, milk, and cheese. She was admitted to the hospital at 23 weeks' gestation with dehydration and a 3-day history of abdominal pain, nausea, vomiting, and diarrhea. Laboratory tests revealed hypercalcemia (14.3 mg/dL), and acute renal insufficiency (serum creatinine 2.1 mg/dL; blood urea nitrogen 52 mg/dL). The hypercalcemia was caused by the milk-alkali syndrome and resulted in pancreatitis and azotemia. Aggressive IV hydration, 5 L of isotonic saline over 12 hours, resulted in a normal calcium level and renal function and her abdominal pain resolved in 4 days. She was discharged home in good health. At 37 weeks, she gave birth to a stillborn fetus. The fetus had short limbs and low-set ears but a normal chromosome analysis. An autopsy revealed no evidence of tissue calcification (22).

A 31-year-old woman at 36 weeks' gestation presented with a 3-day history of disorientation, ataxia, nausea, and vomiting (23). Over the previous 2 weeks she had daily ingested 5 glasses of milk and about 30 antacid tablets, each containing 500 mg calcium carbonate. Her total calcium level was 22.5 mg/mL. Because acute severe hypercalcemia (≥15 mg/dL) can be life-threatening and may result in intractable nausea, vomiting, polyuria, dehydration, coma, cardiac arrhythmias, and circulatory arrest, she was aggressively treated with IV therapy and furosemide, followed by hemodialysis. The fetal condition was normal with external monitoring. An ultrasound examination revealed normal amniotic fluid volume but no fetal breathing, body motion, or tone. Four weeks later, the woman gave birth to a 2950-g normal male infant who was doing well at 1 year of age (23).

A third case of the milk-alkali syndrome in pregnancy secondary to excessive ingestion of calcium carbonate was reported in 2004 (24). A 32-year-old woman at 16 weeks' gestation, who had taken an antacid (Tums; 6–10 tablets/day) for gastroesophageal reflux, presented with severe hypercalcemia (total and ionized calcium 22 mg/dL and 12.16 mg/ dL, respectively), alkalosis, and acute renal insufficiency. The normal ranges for total and ionized calcium were 8.5–10.5 and 4.65–5.20 mg/dL, respectively. At admission, she was treated with IV isotonic saline, furosemide, and a 600-mg dose of IV etidronate. On day 5, symptoms of bisphosphonate-induced hypocalcemia were noted (tingling of the extremities and a positive Chvostek sign). Her symptoms were relieved with IV calcium gluconate and she was started on calcium carbonate. Her low concentrations of total and ionized calcium (7.4–8.0 and 4.00–4.56 mg/dL, respectively) normalized in about 2 weeks. No information was provided on the eventual pregnancy outcome (24).

BREASTFEEDING SUMMARY

The RDA for calcium during lactation is based on age: 1300 mg/day for 14–18 years and 1000 mg/day for 19–50 years (2).

In a small 1994 study, the calcium needed for milk production appeared to be met by decreased urinary excretion and increased bone resorption and not by increased absorption (25). A 1995 study found that calcium carbonate supplements (1000 mg) 5 days each week in Gambian women consuming a low-calcium diet had no effect on breast milk calcium concentration or on maternal bone mineral content. The investigators concluded that physiologic mechanisms worked to furnish calcium for breast milk production (26).

In a 2006 study, pregnant women in Gambia were randomized to calcium carbonate supplementation (1500 mg/day) (N = 61) or placebo (N = 62) from 20 weeks' gestation to delivery (27). Breast milk levels of calcium were analyzed at 2, 13, and 52 weeks after delivery. No differences between subjects and controls in the calcium or phosphorus concentrations in breast milk were noted. Moreover, calcium supplementation had no effect on infant birth weight, growth, or bone mineral status (27).

In Mexican lactating women with high lead levels (mean blood lead 8.5 mcg/mL), a 2003 study measured the effect of calcium carbonate supplementation (1200 mg/day) compared with placebo (28). The supplements resulted in a small decline (0.29 mcg/dL) of blood lead levels. A greater reduction (1.16 mcg/dL) was observed in women who were compliant with supplement use and had high bone lead levels (patella bone lead ≥5 mcg/g bone) (28).

A 1997 study evaluated the effect of calcium carbonate supplementation (1 g/day) compared with placebo on the bone density of the maternal lumbar spine (29). In lactating women, the lumbar spine bone density decreased by 4.2% in the supplement group compared with a 4.9% decrease in the placebo group. In nonlactating women, calcium supplements increased lumbar spine bone density by 2.2% vs. 0.4% with placebo. There was no effect of lactation or supplementation on bone density in the forearm and supplementation did not increase the calcium concentration in breast milk (29). An accompanying editorial supported the findings of the study. The author noted that nursing mothers provide an average of 200–250 mg/day of calcium to their infants and recommended that they increase their calcium intake by 400–800 mg/day (30).

References

1. Thomas M, Weisman SM. Calcium supplementation during pregnancy and lactation: effects on the mother and fetus. Am J Obstet Gynecol 2006;194:937–45.
2. Dietary Supplement Fact Sheet: Calcium. Available at http://ods.od.nih.gov/factsheets/Calcium-HealthProfessional. Accessed February 25, 2013.
3. Care AD. The placental transfer of calcium. J Dev Physiol 1991;15:253–7.
4. Belizan JM, Villar J, Zalazar A, Rojas L, Chan D, Bryce GF. Preliminary evidence of the effect of calcium supplementation on blood pressure in normal pregnant women. Am J Obstet Gynecol 1983;146:175–80.
5. Villar J, Repke J, Belizan JM, Pareja G. Calcium supplementation reduces blood pressure during pregnancy: results of a randomized controlled clinical trial. Obstet Gynecol 1987;70:317–22.
6. Repke JT, Villar J, Anderson C, Pareja G, Dubin N, Belizan JM. Biochemical changes associated with blood pressure reduction induced by calcium supplementation during pregnancy. Am J Obstet Gynecol 1989;160:684–90.
7. Villar J, Repke JT. Calcium supplementation during pregnancy may reduce preterm delivery in high-risk patients. Am J Obstet Gynecol 1990;163:1124–31.
8. Belizan JM, Villar J, Gonzalez L, Campodonico L, Bergel E. Calcium supplementation to prevent hypertensive disorders of pregnancy. N Engl J Med 1991;325:1399–405.
9. Sanchez-Ramos L, Briones DK, Kaunitz AM, Delvalle GO, Gaudier FL, Walker CD. Prevention of pregnancy-induced hypertension by calcium supplementation in angiotensin II-sensitive patients. Obstet Gynecol 1994;84:349–53.
10. Carroli G, Duley L, Belizan JM, Villar J. Calcium supplementation during pregnancy: a systematic review of randomised controlled trials. Br J Obstet Gynaecol 1994;101:753–8.
11. Sanchez-Ramos L, Adair CD, Kaunitz AM, Briones DK, Del Valle GO, Delke I. Calcium supplementation in mild preeclampsia remote from term: a randomized double-blind clinical trial. Obstet Gynecol 1995;85:915–8.
12. Bucher HC, Guyatt GH, Cook RJ, Hatala R, Cook DJ, Lang JD, Hunt D. Effect of calcium supplementation on pregnancy-induced hypertension and preeclampsia—a meta-analysis of randomized controlled trials. JAMA 1996;275:1113–7.
13. Lopez-Jaramillo P, Delgado F, Jacome P, Teran E, Ruano C, Rivera J. Calcium supplementation and risk of preeclampsia in Ecuadorian pregnant teenagers. Obstet Gynecol 1997;90:162–7.
14. Boggess KA, Samuel L, Schmucker BC, Waters J, Easterling TR. A randomized controlled trial of the effect of third-trimester calcium supplementation on maternal hemodynamic function. Obstet Gynecol 1997;90:157–61.
15. Belizan JM, Villar J, Bergel E, del Pino A, Di Fulvio S, Galliano SV, Kattan C. Long term effect of calcium supplementation during pregnancy on the blood pressure of offspring: follow up of a randomised controlled trial. BMJ 1997;313;281–5.
16. Levine RJ, Hauth JC, Curet LB, Sibai BM, Catalano PM, Morris CD, DerSimonian R, Esterlitz JR, Raymond EG, Bild DE, Clemens JD, Cutler JA. Trial of calcium to prevent preeclampsia. N Engl J Med 1997;337:69–76.
17. Roberts JM. Prevention or early treatment of preeclampsia. N Engl J Med 1997;337:124–5.
18. Koo WW, Walters JC, Esterlitz J, Levine RJ, Bush AJ, Sibai B. Maternal calcium supplementation and fetal bone mineralization. Obstet Gynecol 1999;94:577–82.
19. Villar J, Abdel-Aleem H, Merialdi M, Mathai M, Ali MM, Zavaleta N, Purwar M, Hofmeyr J, Ngoc NTN, Campodonico L, Landoulsi S, Carroli G, Lindheimer M, on behalf of the World Organization Calcium Supplementation for the Prevention for Preeclampsia Trial Group. World

Health Organization randomized trial of calcium supplementation among low calcium intake pregnant women. Am J Obstet Gynecol 2006;194:639–49.
20. Abalos E, Merialdi M, Wojdyla D, Carroli G, Campodonico L, Yao SE, Gonzalez R, Deter R, Villar J, Van Look P. Effects of calcium supplementation on fetal growth in mothers with deficient calcium intake: a randomised controlled trial. Paediat Perinat Epidemiol 2010;24:53–62.
21. Robertson WC Jr. Calcium carbonate consumption during pregnancy: an unusual cause of neonatal hypocalcemia. J Child Neurol 2002;17:853–5.
22. Ullian ME, Linas SL. The milk-alkali syndrome in pregnancy—case report. Miner Electrolyte Metab 1988;14:208–10.
23. Kleinman GE, Rodriquez H, Good MC, Caudle MR. Hypercalcemic crisis in pregnancy associated with excessive ingestion of calcium carbonate antacid (milk-alkali syndrome): successful treatment with hemodialysis. Obstet Gynecol 1991;78:496–9.
24. Picolos MK, Sims CR, Mastrobattista JM, Carroll MA, Lavis VR. Milk-alkali syndrome in pregnancy. Obstet Gynecol 2004;104:1201–4.
25. Specker BL, Vieira NE, O'Brien KO, Ho ML, Heubi JE, Abrams SA, Yergey AL. Calcium kinetics in lactating women with low and high calcium intakes. Am J Clin Nutr 1994;59:593–9.
26. Prentice A, Jarjou LMA, Cole TJ, Stirling DM, Dibba B, Fairweather-Tait S. Calcium requirements of lactating Gambian mothers: effects of calcium supplement on breast-milk calcium concentration, maternal bone mineral content, and urinary calcium excretion. Am J Clin Nutr 1995;62:58–67.
27. Jarjou LM, Prentice A, Sawo Y, Laskey MA, Bennett J, Goldberg GR, Cole TJ. Randomized, placebo-controlled, calcium supplementation study in pregnant Gambian women: effects on breast-milk calcium concentrations and infant birth weight, growth, and bone mineral accretion in the first year of life. Am J Clin Nutr 2006;83:657–66.
28. Hernandez-Avila M, Gonzalez-Cossio T, Hernandez-Avila JE, Romieu I, Peterson KE, Aro A, Palazuelos E, Hu H. Dietary calcium supplements to lower blood lead levels in lactating women: a randomized placebo-controlled trial. Epidemiology 2003;14:206–12.
29. Kalkwarf HJ, Specker BL, Bianchi DC, Ranz J, Ho M. The effect of calcium supplementation on bone density during lactation and after weaning. N Engl J Med 1997;337:523–8.
30. Prentice A. Calcium supplementation during breast-feeding. N Engl J Med 1997;337:558–9.

CAMPHOR

Antipruritic/Local Anesthetic

PREGNANCY RECOMMENDATION: Compatible (Topical)
BREASTFEEDING RECOMMENDATION: No Human Data—Probably Compatible

PREGNANCY SUMMARY

Limited data suggest that the topical use of camphor during gestation is of low risk.

FETAL RISK SUMMARY

Camphor is a natural product obtained from the subtropical tree *Cinnamomum camphora* in the form of D-camphor; it is also produced synthetically in the optically inactive racemic form. In reproductive studies in rats and rabbits with oral doses, no evidence of embryotoxicity or teratogenicity was observed even at maternally toxic doses (1).

No reports linking the use of topically applied camphor with congenital defects have been located. Camphor is toxic and potentially a fatal poison if taken orally in sufficient quantities. Four cases of fetal exposure after accidental ingestion, including a case of fetal death and neonatal respiratory failure, have been reported (2–5). The drug crosses the placenta (3). A 1997 case report described a 16-year-old girl at 6 weeks' gestation who ingested 30 g of camphor dissolved in 250 mL of wine in an unsuccessful attempt to induce abortion (6). After successful treatment of the symptoms of camphor poisoning, her pregnancy was electively terminated a few weeks later. An autopsy of the embryo was not done.

The Collaborative Perinatal Project monitored 50,282 mother–child pairs, 168 of whom had 1st trimester exposure to topical camphor (7, pp. 410–412). No association was found with congenital malformations. For use anytime during pregnancy, 763 exposures were recorded and, again, no relationship to defects was noted (7, pp. 444, 499).

BREASTFEEDING SUMMARY

Although there are no reports describing the use of topical camphor during lactation, its use probably is harmless for a nursing infant.

References

1. Leuschner J. Reproductive toxicity studies of D-Camphor in rats and rabbits. Arzneim-Forsch/Drug Res 1997;47:124–8.
2. Figgs J, Hamilton R, Homel S, McCabe J. Camphorated oil intoxication in pregnancy. Report of a case. Obstet Gynecol 1965;25:255–8.
3. Weiss J, Catalano P. Camphorated oil intoxication during pregnancy. Pediatrics 1973;52:713–4.
4. Blackman WB, Curry HB. Camphor poisoning: report of case occurring during pregnancy. J Fla Med Assoc 1957;43:99.
5. Jacobziner H, Raybin HW. Camphor poisoning. Arch Pediatr 1962;79:28.
6. Rabl W, Katzgraber F, Steinlechner M. Camphor ingestion for abortion (case report). Forensic Sci Int 1997;89:137–40.
7. Heinonen OP, Slone D, Shapiro S. *Birth Defects and Drugs in Pregnancy*. Littleton, MA: Publishing Sciences Group, 1977.

CANAKINUMAB

Immunologic Agent (Immunomodulator)

PREGNANCY RECOMMENDATION: No Human Data—Animal Data Suggest Low Risk
BREASTFEEDING RECOMMENDATION: No Human Data—Potential Toxicity

C

PREGNANCY SUMMARY

No reports describing the use of canakinumab in human pregnancy have been located. The animal data in two species suggest low risk, but a no-observed-effect-level (NOEL) for the incomplete fetal skeletal development observed in the species was not reported. The absence of human pregnancy experience prevents an assessment of this and other risks for the human embryo–fetus. If treatment with this antibody is required in pregnancy, the woman should be informed of the absence of human pregnancy data and potential risk.

FETAL RISK SUMMARY

Canakinumab is a recombinant human antihuman interleukin-1 beta (IL-1β) monoclonal antibody that belongs to the IgG1/k isotype subclass. Canakinumab is indicated for the treatment of cryopyrin-associated periodic syndrome, in adults and children 4 years of age and older, including familial cold autoinflammatory syndrome and Muckle–Wells syndrome. The immunomodulator binds to serum IL-1β. The mean terminal half-life is 26 days (1).

Reproduction studies have been conducted in monkeys and mice. In monkeys, SC doses, given twice weekly during gestation days 23–109 that were 23–230 times the human dose based on plasma AUC comparison at the maximum recommended human dose (MRHD-AUC) revealed no evidence of embryotoxicity or fetal malformations. However, increases in the incidence of incomplete fetal skeletal development were observed at all dose levels. Because canakinumab does not cross-react with mouse IL-1, mice were given SC doses of a murine analog of canakinumab on gestation days 6, 11, and 17. A comparison with the human exposure was not given, but the three doses used were identical on a body-weight basis to those given to monkeys. Incomplete fetal skeletal development was increased in a dose-dependent manner at all dose levels tested (1). The NOEL was not reported in either species.

Studies for carcinogenic or mutagenic potential have not been conducted. Fertility studies, using a murine analog of canakinumab, were conducted in male and female mice. SC doses of the analog, identical on a body-weight basis to those given to monkeys, were given before and after mating and had no effect on male or female fertility parameters (1).

It is not known if canakinumab crosses the human placenta. The molecular weight (145,157) suggests that passive transfer will not occur, but the long circulation half-life will place the protein at the maternal: fetal interface for a prolonged period. Moreover, other proteins (e.g., see Immune Globulin Intravenous) cross the placenta. If the delayed skeletal development observed in the two animal species were direct effects (i.e., effects on the embryo and/or fetus and not caused by maternal effects), this would be evidence that the antibody can cross hemochorial placentas.

BREASTFEEDING SUMMARY

No reports describing the use of canakinumab during human lactation have been located. The high molecular weight of this antibody (145,157) and the long circulation half-life (26 days) suggest that excretion into mature breast milk will be inhibited. Because immunoglobulins and other high-molecular-weight substances are excreted into colostrum, exposure of the nursing infant to canakinumab might occur during the first few days after birth. The effect, if any, of this exposure on a nursing infant is unknown. However, an increase in serious infections is a potential complication due to interference with the immune response. Other adverse effects observed in patients treated with this drug include nasopharyngitis, diarrhea, rhinitis, nausea, headache, bronchitis, and gastroenteritis (1). Nursing infants of women receiving the drug should be closely monitored for these effects.

Reference

1. Product information. Ilaris. Novartis Pharmaceuticals, 2009.

CANDESARTAN CILEXETIL

Antihypertensive

PREGNANCY RECOMMENDATION: Human Data Suggest Risk in 2nd and 3rd Trimesters
BREASTFEEDING RECOMMENDATION: No Human Data—Probably Compatible

PREGNANCY SUMMARY

The antihypertensive mechanisms of action of candesartan and angiotensin-converting enzyme (ACE) inhibitors are very close. That is, the former selectively blocks the binding of angiotensin II to AT_1 receptors, whereas the latter prevents the formation of angiotensin II itself. Therefore, use of this drug during the 2nd and 3rd trimesters may cause teratogenicity and severe fetal and neonatal toxicity that is identical to that seen with ACE inhibitors (e.g., see Captopril or Enalapril). Fetal toxic effects may include anuria, oligohydramnios, fetal hypocalvaria, intrauterine growth restriction, prematurity, and patent ductus arteriosus. Stillbirth or neonatal death may occur. Anuria-associated oligohydramnios may produce fetal limb contractures, craniofacial deformation, and pulmonary hypoplasia. Severe anuria and hypotension, which is resistant to both pressor agents and volume expansion, may occur in the newborn following in utero exposure to candesartan cilexetil. Newborn renal function and blood pressure should be closely monitored.

C

FETAL RISK SUMMARY

The prodrug, candesartan cilexetil, is hydrolyzed to the active drug, candesartan, during absorption from the gastrointestinal tract. Candesartan is a selective angiotensin II receptor blocker (ARB) that is used, either alone or in combination with other antihypertensive agents, for the treatment of hypertension. It blocks the vasoconstrictor and aldosterone-secreting effects of angiotensin II by preventing angiotensin II from binding to AT_1 receptors (1).

Reproduction studies have been conducted with candesartan cilexetil in mice, rats, and rabbits at oral doses up to approximately 138, 2.8, and 1.7 times the maximum recommended human dose of 32 mg based on BSA (MRHD), respectively (1). Rat offspring, exposed to the drug during late gestation and through lactation, had decreased survival and an increased incidence of hydronephrosis, whereas no maternal toxicity or fetal harm was observed in pregnant mice. In pregnant rabbits, maternal toxicity (decreased body weight and death) was noted, but, in the offspring of surviving dams, no adverse effects were seen on fetal survival, fetal weight, or on external, visceral, or skeletal development (1). No effects on fertility or reproductive performance were observed in male and female rats given oral doses up to 83 times the MRHD (1).

It is not known if candesartan crosses the human placenta to the fetus. The molecular weight of candesartan (about 440 after hydrolysis of the prodrug, candesartan cilexetil) is low enough such that passage to the fetus should be expected.

In a 2001 case report, candesartan (7 mg/day) was used for mild hypertension throughout gestation (2). Amniotic fluid was reduced at term. The female infant (birth weight not given) had left-sided facial palsy, plexus paresis, and was anuric. On ultrasound, the kidneys were hyperechogenic with poor corticomedullary differentiation. Urine production started at 5 days of age and the sonographic appearance of the kidneys normalized during the following month. At 8 months of age, the infant was developing normally and only a discrete facial and plexus palsy remained (2).

A 41-year-old woman was treated with candesartan throughout a 32-week gestation (3). Because of anhydramnios, she was delivered of a 1120-g (0.4th percentile) male infant in poor condition. The infant had defective ossification of the roof of the calvarium, joint contractures, mild hypospadias, rocker bottom feet, a large abdominal left kidney and absent right kidney. He developed intractable hypotension, unresponsive to hydration, and remained anuric until he died (3).

In a 2003 report, the outcomes of 42 pregnancies exposed to ARAs were described (4). The outcomes of 37 pregnancies (1 set of twins) exposed in the 1st trimester were 3 spontaneous abortions (drugs not specified), 4 elective abortions (one for exencephaly; candesartan until 4 3/7 weeks, carbimazole, hydrochlorothiazide, maternal obesity), 1 stillbirth (no anomalies; valsartan until week 4, cigarette smoking, other antihypertensives), 1 minor malformation (undescended testicles; drug not specified), and 28 healthy newborns. There was one major malformation (cleft palate, patent ductus arteriosus, modest coarctation of the aorta, growth restriction; valsartan until week 13, hydrochlorothiazide, metoprolol, cigarette smoking). Five cases involved late exposure to ARAs and their outcomes involved one or more of the following: oligohydramnios/anhydramnios, anuria, hypoplastic skull bones, limb contractions, lung hypoplasia, and neonatal death (4).

A 2005 article reviewed the mechanism of ARA-induced fetal toxicity (5). This toxicity, observed in 15 case reports, was similar to that observed with angiotensin-converting enzyme (ACE) inhibitors. The primary effect is suppression of the fetal renin–angiotensin system that results in disruption of the fetal vascular perfusion and renal dysfunction (5).

A 38-year-old pregnant woman with chronic hypertension was treated with candesartan (16 mg/day) and propranolol (160 mg/day) (6). Oligohydramnios was diagnosed at 23 weeks and candesartan was stopped and methyldopa was started. At 26 weeks, no amniotic fluid was noted, the fetal kidneys were small and the bladder was empty. An elective abortion delivered a 860-g male fetus with deformities of the extremities and face due to oligohydramnios. The kidneys had severe tubular dysgenesis with a reduced number and poor differentiation of proximal tubules (6).

A 2007 review cited 64 published cases of pregnancies exposed to ARAs, 42.2% of which had unfavorable outcomes (7). The duration of ARA exposure was longer in the cases with poor outcomes compared with those with good outcomes, 26.3 ± 10.5 vs. 17.3 ± 11.6 weeks.

A 2010 case report described the outcome of an unplanned pregnancy that was exposed to aspirin 75 mg/day, metoprolol 25 mg/day, and candesartan 4 mg/day in the first 22 weeks (8). At that time, ultrasound revealed edematous fetal kidneys and reduced levels of amniotic fluid, and candesartan was discontinued. Five weeks later, normal amniotic fluid and a visible fetal bladder were noted, but the kidneys remained enlarged. At 31 weeks, she gave birth to a 2200-g male infant with Apgar scores of 9 and 9. Renal function studies in the 1-day-old infant were within normal limits. However, at 1 and 2 weeks, ultrasound of the kidneys showed bilateral marked calices, small cysts, and parenchymal increased echogenety. There was complete sonographic normalization of the kidneys at 6 weeks of age. At 6 months of age, a urine analysis was normal. The infant had a systolic murmur related to a patent ductus arteriosus. Based on experimental evidence, concern was expressed for renal dysfunction and arterial hypertension in adulthood (8).

A 2012 review of the use of ACE inhibitors and ARBs in the 1st trimester concluded that there may be an elevated teratogenic risk, but the risk appeared to be related to other factors (9). The factors that typically coexist with hypertension in pregnancy, included diabetes, advanced maternal age, and obesity.

BREASTFEEDING SUMMARY

No reports describing the use of candesartan cilexetil during human lactation have been located. Because the molecular weight of the active drug, candesartan, is about 440, excretion into human breast milk should be expected. The effects of this exposure on a nursing infant are unknown. The American Academy of Pediatrics, however, classifies ACE inhibitors, a closely related group of antihypertensive agents, as compatible with breastfeeding (see Captopril or Enalapril).

References

1. Product information. Atacand. AstraZeneca LP, 2000.
2. Hinsberger A, Wingen AM, Hoyer PF. Angiotensin-II-receptor inhibitors in pregnancy. Lancet 2001;357:1620.
3. Cox RM, Anerson JM, Cox P. Defective embryogenesis with angiotensin II receptor antagonists in pregnancy. Br J Obstet Gynaecol 2003;110:1038–40.
4. Schaefer C. Angiotensin II-receptor-antagonists: further evidence of fetotoxicity but not teratogenicity. Birth Defects Res (Part A) 2003;67:591–4.
5. Alwan S, Polifka JE, Friedman JM. Angiotensin II receptor antagonist treatment during pregnancy. Birth Defects Res (Page A) 2005;73:123–30.
6. Vendemmia M, Garcia-Meric P, Rizzotti A, Boubred F, Lacroze V, Liprandi A, Simeoni U. Fetal and neonatal consequences of antenatal exposure to type 1 angiotensin II receptor-antagonists. J Matern Fetal Neonatal Med 2005;19:137–40.
7. Velazquez-Armenta EY, Han JY, Choi JS, Yang KM, Nava-Ocampo AA. Angiotensin II receptor blockers in pregnancy: a case report and systematic review of the literature. Hypertens Pregnancy 2007;26:51–66.
8. Munk PS, von Brandis P, Larsen AI. Reversible fetal renal failure after maternal treatment with candesartan: a case report. Reprod Toxicol 2010;29:381–2.
9. Polifka JE. Is there an embryopathy associated with first-trimester exposure to angiotensin-converting enzyme inhibitors and angiotensin receptor antagonists? A critical review of the evidence. Birth Defects Res (Part A) 2012;94:576–98.

CAPECITABINE

Antineoplastic

PREGNANCY RECOMMENDATION: No Human Data—Animal Data Suggest Risk
BREASTFEEDING RECOMMENDATION: Contraindicated

PREGNANCY SUMMARY

No reports describing the use of capecitabine during human pregnancy have been located. Studies have observed developmental toxicity in mice (structural anomalies and death) and rabbits (death) at systemic exposures less than those observed with the maximum recommended dose in humans. The drug is converted intracellularly to the active metabolite 5-FU. Although there are no human pregnancy data, capecitabine should be avoided in pregnancy. If it must be used for the mother's benefit, consideration should be given to avoiding the period of organogenesis.

FETAL RISK SUMMARY

Capecitabine, a fluoropyrimidine carbamate, is an oral prodrug that, upon absorption from the gut, is converted in the liver to a precursor (5′-DFUR) of 5-fluorouracil (5-FU). The final metabolic step to 5-FU, the active agent, occurs in tumor and normal cells. (See also Fluorouracil.) Capecitabine is classified as an antimetabolite in the subclass of pyrimidine analogs. In addition to fluorouracil, other antineoplastic agents in the subclass are cytarabine, floxuridine, and gemcitabine. Capecitabine is indicated for adjuvant treatment in patients with Dukes' C colon cancer who have undergone complete resection of the primary tumor, as first-line treatment of patients with metastatic colorectal carcinoma, and, either alone or in combination (see Ixabepilone) in some cases of breast cancer. Plasma protein binding of capecitabine and its metabolites is low (<60%). The elimination half-life of capecitabine and 5-FU is very short (about 0.75 hours) (1).

Reproduction studies have been conducted in mice and monkeys. During organogenesis in mice, a dose that resulted in systemic exposures of 5′-DFUR AUC that were about 0.2 times the human exposure from the recommended daily dose (HERDD) produced cleft palate, anophthalmia, microphthalmia, oligodactyly, polydactyly, syndactyly, kinky tail, and dilation of cerebral ventricles. In monkeys, during organogenesis, a dose that resulted in systemic exposures of 5′-DFUR AUC that were about 0.6 times HERDD caused fetal death (1).

The carcinogenic potential of capecitabine has not been evaluated. The drug was not mutagenic in two assays but was clastogenic in one test. However, 5-FU causes mutations in bacteria and yeast and chromosomal abnormalities in mice. In mice, a capecitabine dose resulting in exposures that were about 0.7 times the HERDD caused a reversible decrease in fertility in females and degenerative changes in the testes of males. No fetuses survived this dose in mice that became pregnant (1).

It is not known if capecitabine or the precursor 5′-DFUR crosses the human placenta. The molecular weight of capecitabine (about 359) and the low plasma protein binding suggest that the drug will cross to the embryo–fetus, but the very short elimination half-life should limit the exposure. The molecular weight of 5′-DFUR was not specified, but if it or the parent drug were to cross the placenta, intracellular metabolism in normal tissues could expose the embryo–fetus to 5-FU.

BREASTFEEDING SUMMARY

No reports describing the use of capecitabine during human lactation have been located. The molecular weight of capecitabine (about 359) and the low plasma protein binding (<60%) of capecitabine and 5′-DFUR (molecular weight not specified) suggest that the drugs will be excreted into breast milk, but the very short elimination half-life of capecitabine (about 0.75 hours; unspecified for 5′-DFUR) should limit the exposure. The effects of this exposure on a nursing infant are unknown. However, metabolism of the parent drug and the precursor would expose the infant to 5-FU. The mother should not breastfeed if she is being treated.

Reference

1. Product information. Xeloda. Roche Laboratories, 2006.

CAPREOMYCIN

Antibiotic (Antituberculosis)

PREGNANCY RECOMMENDATION: Limited Human Data—No Relevant Animal Data
BREASTFEEDING RECOMMENDATION: No Human Data—Probably Compatible

PREGNANCY SUMMARY

No reports describing the use of capreomycin during human pregnancy have been located. A 1992 review of tuberculosis and pregnancy stated that the safety of capreomycin in pregnancy was not established, but cited no references of its use (1). Two other sources, one published in 1995 and the other in 1996, concluded that capreomycin should be avoided, if possible, because of the potential for ototoxicity and deafness (2,3). Neither source cited pregnancy data involving capreomycin.

FETAL RISK SUMMARY

Capreomycin is a polypeptide antibiotic isolated from *Streptomyces capreolus*. The antibiotic is a mixture of four active components consisting of capreomycin IA and IB (a combined total of at least 90% of the product) and capreomycin IIA and IIB. Capreomycin is given by IM injection. Less than 1% is absorbed orally. It is indicated, in combination with other antituberculosis agents, as an alternate drug when the primary agents are ineffective or cannot be used because of toxicity. Because the toxicity of capreomycin is similar to aminoglycosides (e.g., cranial nerve VIII and renal), it should not be used with these agents (4).

Capreomycin caused a low incidence of wavy ribs in rats given doses 3.5 times the human dose (1). No studies have been conducted on the effects of the antibiotic on fertility, carcinogenicity, or mutagenicity (4).

It is not known if capreomycin crosses the human placenta. The molecular weight (about 653–669) suggests that the drug will cross to the embryo–fetus.

A 2003 report described the use of capreomycin in a pregnant woman with multidrug-resistant tuberculosis (5). A 22-year-old woman was diagnosed with the infection at 23 weeks' gestation and daily treatment was initiated with rifampin (600 mg), isoniazid (300 mg), and ethambutol (700 mg). Because of lack of response, her therapy was changed after 3 weeks to capreomycin (IV 1000 mg 5 days/week), cycloserine (750 mg/day), levofloxacin (1000 mg/day), *para*-aminosalicylic acid (12 g/day), and pyrazinamide (1500 mg/day). After spontaneous rupture of the membrane, she gave birth at 35 weeks' gestation to a healthy, 2003-g infant. The results of a tuberculin skin test and three nasogastric aspiration cultures were negative, as were a neurologic examination and electrophysiology hearing studies. The infant was kept separated from the mother (5).

A 2003 study reported the outcomes of seven pregnancies treated for multidrug-resistant tuberculosis (6). The seven women received multiple anti-infective agents. Three patients (one throughout, one in 1st trimester, and one postpartum) were treated with IV capreomycin. In 2005, the same group reported the long-term follow-up of six of the offspring; a seventh child, not exposed to capreomycin, was lost to follow-up (7). The average age of the children was 3.7 years and each underwent a comprehensive clinical evaluation. None had hearing loss and all had normal vision and neurologic analysis. Of the three exposed to capreomycin (current age and time of exposure), one had mild speech delay (4.6 years; throughout and postpartum), one was hyperactive (5.1 years; postpartum only), and one had no abnormalities (1.25 years; 1st trimester only). All three were breastfed (7). Neither of the two conditions appears to be related to capreomycin.

BREASTFEEDING SUMMARY

No studies reporting the excretion of capreomycin into breast milk have been located. One report mentioned that two infants whose mothers were receiving IV capreomycin and other antituberculosis agents were breastfed (7). No other details were available, but the long-term follow-up revealed no evidence of capreomycin-induced toxicity (see above).

The molecular weight (about 653–669) suggests that the drug will be excreted into breast milk.

The effect on a nursing infant from this exposure is unknown. Although the systemic absorption of capreomycin in a neonate has not been studied, <1% of an oral dose is absorbed by adults, so the risk, if any, to a nursing infant appears to be minimal.

References

1. Hamadeh MA, Glassroth J. Tuberculosis and pregnancy. Chest 1992;101:1114–20.
2. Davidson PT. Managing tuberculosis during pregnancy. Lancet 1995;346:199–200.
3. Robinson CA, Rose NC. Tuberculosis: current implications and management in obstetrics. Obstet Gynecol Surv 1996;51:115–24.
4. Product information. Capastat. 1990.
5. Klaus-Dieter KLL, Qarah S. Multidrug-resistant tuberculosis in pregnancy—case report and review of the literature. Chest 2003;123:953–6.
6. Shin S, Guerra D, Rich M, Seung K, Mukherjee J, Joseph K, Hurtado R, Alcantara F, Bayona J, Bonilla C, Farmer P, Furin J. Treatment of multidrug-resistant tuberculosis during pregnancy: a report of 7 cases. Clin Infect Dis 2003;36:996–1003.
7. Drobac PC, Castillo HD, Sweetland A, Anca G, Joseph JK, Furin J, Shin S. Treatment of multidrug-resistant tuberculosis during pregnancy: long-term follow-up of 6 children with intrauterine exposure to second-line agents. Clin Infect Dis 2005;40:1689–92.

for neonatal hypotension and renal failure (29). Of interest, a 1991 review concluded that fetal and neonatal renal dysfunction was more common after maternal use of enalapril than with captopril (28).

A 1991 report presented two cases of fetopathy and hypocalvaria in newborns exposed in utero to ACE inhibitors, including one case in which captopril, prednisone, atenolol, and furosemide were used throughout pregnancy (same case as described in reference 24) and one case caused by lisinopril (30). Twelve other cases of hypocalvaria or acalvaria were reviewed, three of which were thought to be caused by captopril (*N* = 2) or enalapril (*N* = 1) and nine others with causes that were either not drug-related or unknown. The authors speculated that the underlying pathogenetic mechanism in these cases was fetal hypotension (30).

In a 1991 article examining the teratogenesis of ACE inhibitors, the authors cited evidence linking fetal calvarial hypoplasia with the use of these agents after the 1st trimester (31). They speculated that the mechanism was related to drug-induced oligohydramnios that allowed the uterine musculature to exert direct pressure on the fetal skull. This mechanical insult, combined with drug-induced fetal hypotension, could inhibit peripheral perfusion and ossification of the calvaria (31).

Investigators in a study published in 1992 examined microscopically the kidneys of nine fetuses exposed to ACE inhibitors, one of which was enalapril (32). The researchers concluded that the renal defects associated with ACE inhibitors were caused by decreased renal perfusion and are similar to the defects seen in other conditions related to reduced fetal renal blood flow (32).

In a retrospective 2000 study, the outcomes of 10 pregnant women treated with low-dose captopril (12.5–25 mg/day) for severe, unresponsive vasoconstricted hypertension were reviewed (33). Maternal hemodynamics improved without fetal or neonatal complications. Assuming an expected complication rate of 5%–10%, however, the number of exposed pregnancies may have been too small to identify adverse effects (33).

A retrospective study using pharmacy-based data from the Tennessee Medicaid program identified 209 infants, born between 1985 and 2000, who had 1st trimester exposure to ACE inhibitors (34). Infants of mothers with evidence of diabetes, either before or during pregnancy, were excluded, as were those exposed to angiotensin-receptor antagonists (ARBs), ACE inhibitors, or other antihypertensives beyond the 1st trimester, and exposure to known teratogens. Two comparison groups, other antihypertensives (*N* = 202) and no antihypertensives (*N* = 29,096), were formed. The number of major birth defects in each of the three groups was 18 (8.6%), 4 (2%), and 834 (2.9%), respectively. Compared with the no antihypertensives group, exposure to ACE inhibitors was associated with a significantly increased risk of major defects (relative risk [RR] 2.71, 95% confidence interval [CI] 1.72–4.27). When the analysis was conducted by the type of defect, the highest rates were with cardiovascular defects, 9, 2, and 294, respectively (RR 3.72, 95% CI 1.89–7.30), and with central nervous system defects, 3, 0, and 80, respectively (RR 4.39, 95% CI 1.37–14.02). The major defects observed in the subject group were as follows: atrial septal defect (*N* = 6) (includes three with pulmonic stenosis and/or three with patent ductus arteriosus (PDA)), renal dysplasia (*N* = 2), PDA alone (*N* = 2), and one each of ventricular septal defect, spina bifida, microcephaly with eye anomaly, coloboma, hypospadias, intestinal and choanal atresia, Hirschsprung disease, and diaphragmatic hernia (34). In an accompanying editorial, it was noted that neither previous reports of 1st trimester exposure to ACE inhibitors nor the animal studies had observed an increased risk of birth defects (35). It also was noted that no mechanism for ACE inhibitor–induced teratogenicity was known. A subsequent communication raising concerns about the validity of the study in terms of adequate exclusion of diabetes, charting and coding errors in busy medical practices, and the effects of maternal obesity (36) was addressed by the investigators (37).

Captopril and other ACE inhibitors are human teratogens when used in the 2nd and 3rd trimesters, producing fetal hypocalvaria and renal defects. The cause of the defects and other toxicity is probably related to fetal hypotension and decreased renal blood flow. The compromise of the fetal renal system may result in severe, and at times fatal, anuria, both in the fetus and in the newborn. Anuria-associated oligohydramnios may produce pulmonary hypoplasia, limb contractures, persistent patent ductus arteriosus, craniofacial deformation, and neonatal death (38,39). IUGR, prematurity, and severe neonatal hypotension may also be observed. Two reviews of fetal and newborn renal function indicated that both renal perfusion and glomerular plasma flow are low during gestation and that high levels of angiotensin II may be physiologically necessary to maintain glomerular filtration at low perfusion pressures (40,41). Captopril prevents the conversion of angiotensin I to angiotensin II and, thus, may lead to in utero renal failure. Newborn renal function and blood pressure should be closely monitored. If oligohydramnios occurs, stopping captopril may resolve the problem but may not improve infant outcome because of irreversible fetal damage (38). In those cases in which captopril must be used to treat the mother's disease, the lowest possible dose should be used combined with close monitoring of amniotic fluid levels and fetal well-being. Guidelines for counseling exposed pregnant patients have been published and should be of benefit to health professionals faced with this task (31,38).

The observation in Tennessee Medicaid data of an increased risk of major congenital defects after 1st trimester exposure to ACE inhibitors raises concerns about teratogenicity that have not been seen in other studies (35). Medicaid data are a valuable tool for identifying early signals of teratogenicity, but are subject to a number of shortcomings, and their findings must be considered hypotheses until confirmed by independent studies.

A 2012 review of the use of ACE inhibitors and ARBs in the 1st trimester concluded that there may be an elevated teratogenic risk, but the risk appeared to be related to other factors (42). The factors, which typically coexist with hypertension in pregnancy, included diabetes, advanced maternal age, and obesity.

BREASTFEEDING SUMMARY

Captopril is excreted into breast milk in low concentrations. In 12 mothers given 100 mg three times/day, average peak milk levels were 4.7 ng/mL at 3.8 hours after their last dose (43,44). This represented an average milk:plasma ratio of 0.012. No differences were found in captopril levels in milk before and after the drug. No effects on the nursing infants were observed. The American Academy of Pediatrics classifies captopril as compatible with breastfeeding (45).

C

References

1. Broughton Pipkin F, Turner SR, Symonds EM. Possible risk with captopril in pregnancy: some animal data. Lancet 1980;1:1256.
2. Broughton Pipkin F, Symonds EM, Turner SR. The effect of captopril (SQ14,225) upon mother and fetus in the chronically cannulated ewe and in the pregnant rabbit. J Physiol 1982;323:415–22.
3. Keith IM, Will JA, Weir EK. Captopril: association with fetal death and pulmonary vascular changes in the rabbit (41446). Proc Soc Exp Biol Med 1982;170:378–83.
4. Lumbers ER, Kingsford NM, Menzies RI, Stevens AD. Acute effects of captopril, an angiotensin-converting enzyme inhibitor, on the pregnant ewe and fetus. Am J Physiol 1992;262 (Regul Integrative Comp Physiol 31):R754–60.
5. Binder ND, Faber JJ. Effects of captopril on blood pressure, placental blood flow and uterine oxygen consumption in pregnant rabbits. J Pharmacol Exp Ther 1992;260:294–9.
6. Anonymous. The 1984 report of the Joint National Committee on Detection, Evaluation, and Treatment of High Blood Pressure. Arch Intern Med 1984;144:1045–6.
7. Lindheimer MD, Katz AI. Current concepts. Hypertension in pregnancy. N Engl J Med 1985;313:675–80.
8. Lip GYH, Churchill D, Beevers M, Auckett A, Beevers DG. Angiotensin-converting-enzyme inhibitors in early pregnancy. Lancet 1997;350:1446–7.
9. Duminy PC, Burger PT. Fetal abnormality associated with the use of captopril during pregnancy. S Afr Med J 1981;60:805.
10. Broude AM. Fetal abnormality associated with captopril during pregnancy. S Afr Med J 1982;61:68.
11. Kaler SG, Patrinos ME, Lambert GH, Myers TF, Karlman R, Anderson CL. Hypertrichosis and congenital anomalies associated with maternal use of minoxidil. Pediatrics 1987;79:434–6.
12. Owen J, Hauth JC. Polyarteritis nodosa in pregnancy: a case report and brief literature review. Am J Obstet Gynecol 1989;160:606–7.
13. Guignard JP, Burgener F, Calame A. Persistent anuria in a neonate: a side effect of captopril? (abstract). Int J Pediatr Nephrol 1981;2:133.
14. Millar JA, Wilson PD, Morrison N. Management of severe hypertension in pregnancy by a combined drug regimen including captopril: case report. NZ Med J 1983;96:796–8.
15. Boutroy MJ, Vert P, Hurault de Ligny B, Miton A. Captopril administration in pregnancy impairs fetal angiotensin-converting enzyme activity and neonatal adaptation. Lancet 1984;2:935–6.
16. Rothberg AD, Lorenz R. Can captopril cause fetal and neonatal renal failure? Pediatr Pharmacol 1984;4:189–92.
17. Coen G, Cugini P, Gerlini G, Finistauri D, Cinotti GA. Successful treatment of long-lasting severe hypertension with captopril during a twin pregnancy. Nephron 1985;40:498–500.
18. Knott PD, Thorpe SS, Lamont CAR. Congenital renal dysgenesis possibly due to captopril. Lancet 1989;1:451.
19. Smith AM. Are ACE inhibitors safe in pregnancy? Lancet 1989;2:750–1.
20. Fiocchi R, Lijnen P, Fagard R, Staessen J, Amery A, Van Assche F, Spitz B, Rademaker M. Captopril during pregnancy. Lancet 1984;2:1153.
21. Caraman PL, Miton A, Hurault de Ligny B, Kessler M, Boutroy MJ, Schweitzer M, Brocard O, Ragage JP, Netter P. Grossesses sous captopril. Therapie 1984;39:59–63.
22. Plouin PF, Tchobroutsky C. Angiotensin-converting-enzyme inhibition during human pregnancy: fifteen cases. Presse Méd 1985;14:2175–8.
23. Ducret F, Pointet PH, Lauvergeon B, Jacoulet C, Gagnaire J. Grossesse sous inhibiteur de l'enzyme de conversion. Presse Méd 1985;14:897.
24. Barr M. Fetal effects of angiotensin converting enzyme inhibitor (abstract). Teratology 1990;41:536.
25. Pryde PG, Nugent CE, Sedman AB, Barr M Jr. ACE inhibitor fetopathy (abstract). Am J Obstet Gynecol 1992;166:348.
26. Kreft-Jais C, Plouin PF, Tchobroutsky C, Boutroy J. Angiotensin-converting enzyme inhibitors during pregnancy: a survey of 22 patients given captopril and nine given enalapril. Br J Obstet Gynaecol 1988;95:420–2.
27. Piper JM, Ray WA, Rosa FW. Pregnancy outcome following exposure to angiotensin-converting enzyme inhibitors. Obstet Gynecol 1992;80:429–32.
28. Hanssens M, Keirse MJNC, Vankelecom F, Van Assche FA. Fetal and neonatal effects of treatment with angiotensin-converting enzyme inhibitors in pregnancy. Obstet Gynecol 1991;78:128–35.
29. Rosa FW, Bosco LA, Graham CF, Milstien JB, Dreis M, Creamer J. Neonatal anuria with maternal angiotensin-converting enzyme inhibition. Obstet Gynecol 1989;74:371–4.
30. Barr M Jr, Cohen MM Jr. ACE inhibitor fetopathy and hypocalvaria: the kidney–skull connection. Teratology 1991;44:485–95.
31. Brent RL, Beckman DA. Angiotensin-converting enzyme inhibitors, an embryopathic class of drugs with unique properties: information for clinical teratology counselors. Teratology 1991;43:543–6.
32. Martin RA, Jones KL, Mendoza A, Barr M Jr, Benirschke K. Effect of ACE inhibition on the fetal kidney: decreased renal blood flow. Teratology 1992;46:317–21.
33. Easterling TR, Carr DB, Davis C, Diederichs C, Brateng DA, Schmucker B. Low-dose, short-acting, angiotensin-converting enzyme inhibitors as rescue therapy in pregnancy. Obstet Gynecol 2000;96:956–61.
34. Cooper WO, Hernandez-Diaz S, Arbogast PG, Dudley JA, Dyer S, Gideon PS, Hall K, Ray WA. Major congenital malformations after first-trimester exposure to ACE inhibitors. N Engl J Med 2006;354:2443–51.
35. Friedman JM. ACE inhibitors and congenital anomalies. N Engl J Med 2006;354:2498–500.
36. Scialli AR, Lione A. ACE inhibitors and major congenital malformations. N Engl J Med 2006;355:1280.
37. Cooper WO, Ray WA. Reply—ACE inhibitors and major congenital malformations. N Engl J Med 2006;355:1281.
38. Barr M Jr. Teratogen update: angiotensin-converting enzyme inhibitors. Teratology 1994;50:399–409.
39. Shotan A, Widerhorn J, Hurst A, Elkayam U. Risks of angiotensin-converting enzyme inhibition during pregnancy: experimental and clinical evidence, potential mechanisms, and recommendations for use. Am J Med 1994;96:451–6.
40. Robillard JE, Nakamura KT, Matherne GP, Jose PA. Renal hemodynamics and functional adjustments to postnatal life. Semin Perinatol 1988;12: 143–50.
41. Guignard JP, Gouyon JB. Adverse effects of drugs on the immature kidney. Biol Neonate 1988;53:243–52.
42. Polifka JE. Is there an embryopathy associated with first-trimester exposure to angiotensin-converting enzyme inhibitors and angiotensin receptor antagonists? A critical review of the evidence. Birth Defects Res (Part A) 2012;94:576–98.
43. Devlin RG, Fleiss PM. Selective resistance to the passage of captopril into human milk. Clin Pharmacol Ther 1980;27:250.
44. Devlin RG, Fleiss PM. Captopril in human blood and breast milk. J Clin Pharmacol 1981;21:110–3.
45. Committee on Drugs, American Academy of Pediatrics. The transfer of drugs and other chemicals into human milk. Pediatrics 2001;108:776–89.

CARBACHOL

Parasympathomimetic (Cholinergic)

PREGNANCY RECOMMENDATION: No Human Data—Probably Compatible
BREASTFEEDING RECOMMENDATION: No Human Data—Probably Compatible

PREGNANCY SUMMARY

Although there are no human reports, carbachol probably is compatible in pregnancy.

FETAL RISK SUMMARY

Carbachol is used in the eye. No reports of its use in pregnancy have been located. As a quaternary ammonium compound, it is ionized at physiologic pH and transplacental passage in significant amounts would not be expected.

BREASTFEEDING SUMMARY

No reports describing the use of carbachol during human lactation have been located. Because clinical significant concentrations are unlikely, the drug should be compatible with breastfeeding.

CARBAMAZEPINE

Anticonvulsant

PREGNANCY RECOMMENDATION: Compatible—Maternal Benefit >> Embryo–Fetal Risk
BREASTFEEDING RECOMMENDATION: Compatible

PREGNANCY SUMMARY

Carbamazepine use in pregnancy is associated with an increased incidence of major and minor malformations, including neural tube defects (NTDs), cardiovascular and urinary tract defects, and cleft palate. A fetal carbamazepine syndrome has been proposed, consisting of minor craniofacial defects, fingernail hypoplasia, and developmental delay. The latter abnormality, however, is controversial; some studies have found mild mental retardation and some have not. Although pregnant women should be advised of these potential adverse outcomes, if the drug is required during pregnancy it should not be withheld because the benefits of preventing seizures outweigh the potential fetal harm.

FETAL RISK SUMMARY

Carbamazepine, a tricyclic anticonvulsant, has been in clinical use since 1962. The drug is teratogenic in rats at doses 10–25 times the maximum human daily dose [MHDD] of 1200 mg/day or 1.5–4 times the MHDD based on BSA (1). Anomalies observed included kinked ribs, cleft palate, talipes, and anophthalmos.

The drug crosses the placenta, with highest concentrations found in fetal liver and kidneys (2–4). Fetal levels are approximately 50%–80% of maternal serum levels (4).

Placental function in women taking carbamazepine has been evaluated (5). No effect was detected from carbamazepine as measured by serum human placental lactogen, 24-hour urinary total estriol excretion, placental weight, and birth weight.

In a surveillance study of Michigan Medicaid recipients involving 229,101 completed pregnancies conducted between 1985 and 1992, 172 newborns had been exposed to carbamazepine during the 1st trimester (F. Rosa, personal communication, FDA, 1993). A total of 13 (7.6%) major birth defects were observed (7 expected), including 4 cardiovascular defects (2 expected), and 1 spina bifida (none expected). No anomalies were observed in four other categories of defects (oral clefts, polydactyly, limb reduction defects, and hypospadias) for which specific data were available. Although the above data have not yet been analyzed to distinguish between combination and monotherapy (F. Rosa, personal communication, FDA, 1993), the total number of malformations suggests an association between the drug and congenital defects (see also discussion of reference 25 below).

Additional reports to the FDA involved five cases of holoprosencephaly in which carbamazepine was used either alone (two cases) or in combination with valproic acid and phenytoin (one case), phenytoin and primidone (one case), or gabapentin (one case) (6). Because of the lack of family histories, an association with familial holoprosencephaly or maternal neurologic problems could not be excluded (6).

A number of reports have described the use of carbamazepine during the 1st trimester (5,7,23,27,33–40). Multiple anomalies were found in one stillborn infant in whom carbamazepine was the only anticonvulsant used by the mother (15). These included closely set eyes, flat nose with single nasopharynx, polydactylia, atrial septal defect, patent ductus arteriosus, absent gallbladder and thyroid, and collapsed fontanel. Individual defects observed in this and other cases include talipes, meningomyelocele, anal atresia, ambiguous genitalia, congenital heart disease, hypertelorism, hypoplasia of the nose, cleft lip, congenital hip dislocation, inguinal hernia, hypoplasia of the nails, and torticollis (7–18). One infant, also exposed to lithium during the 1st trimester, had hydrocephalus and meningomyelocele (18). Decreased head circumference (7 mm less than controls) has been observed in infants exposed only to carbamazepine during gestation (19). The head size was still small by 18 months of age with no catch-up growth evident. Dysmorphic facial features, combined with physical and mental retardation, were described in an infant girl exposed during gestation to 500–1700 mg/day of carbamazepine monotherapy (23). Maternal carbamazepine serum levels had been monitored frequently during gestation and all were reported to be in the therapeutic range (23).

In a 1982 review, Janz stated that nearly all possible malformations had been observed in epileptic patients (24). Minor malformations, such as those seen in the fetal hydantoin syndrome (FHS) (see Phenytoin), have also been observed with carbamazepine monotherapy, causing Janz to conclude that the term FHS was misleading (24). Because carbamazepine was thought to present a lower risk to the fetus, the drug has been recommended as the treatment of choice for women who may become pregnant and who require anticonvulsant therapy for the first time (25). However, a 1989 report has indicated that carbamazepine is also probably a human teratogen (22).

Eight children were identified retrospectively after in utero exposure to carbamazepine either alone (*N* = 4), or in combination with other anticonvulsants (phenobarbital *N* = 2, primidone *N* = 1, or phenobarbital and clonazepam *N* = 1) (22). In six mothers, daily carbamazepine doses ranged from 600 to 1600 mg (dosage unknown in two). The following defects were noted in the children: intrauterine growth restriction (two cases), poor neonatal performance (three cases), postnatal growth deficiency (three cases, not determined in four), developmental delay (three cases, not determined in four), microcephaly (three cases, not determined in four), upslanting palpebral fissures (two cases), short nose with long philtrum (two cases), hypoplastic nails (four cases), and cardiac defect (two cases).

Concurrently with the above evaluations, a prospective study involving 72 women treated with carbamazepine in early pregnancy was conducted (22). Fifty-four liveborn children were evaluated from the 72 mothers, with the remaining 18 excluded for various reasons (seven spontaneous abortions, five therapeutic abortions, and six lost to follow-up before delivery). A control group of 73 pregnant women was prospectively selected for comparison. Anticonvulsant drug therapy in the study group consisted of carbamazepine either alone (*N* = 50) or in combination with phenobarbital (*N* = 12), phenobarbital and valproic acid (*N* = 4), primidone (*N* = 3), valproic acid (*N* = 1), ethosuximide (*N* = 1), and primidone and ethosuximide (*N* = 1). Carbamazepine dosage varied from 200 to 1200 mg/day. Seizures occurred at least once during pregnancy in 59% of the women, but they did not correlate with either malformations or developmental delay in the offspring (22). Of the 54 liveborn children, 48 were examined by the study investigators. Five (10%) of these children had major anomalies consisting of lumbosacral meningomyelocele (*N* = 1), multiple ventricular septal defects (*N* = 1), indirect inguinal hernia (*N* = 1) (all three exposed to carbamazepine alone), and cleft uvula (*N* = 2) (exposed to carbamazepine and phenobarbital). Five (7%) of the control infants also had major anomalies. The incidence of children with two minor malformations was statistically similar for the study and control groups, 23% (11 of 48) vs. 13% (9 of 70), respectively. Those presenting with three or more minor anomalies, however, were more frequent in the exposed group (38%, 18 of 48) than in controls (6%, 4 of 70) ($p = 0.001$). Based on the combined results from the retrospective and prospective studies, the investigators concluded that carbamazepine exposure was associated with a pattern of congenital malformations whose principal features consisted of minor craniofacial defects, fingernail hypoplasia, and developmental delay. Because these defects were similar to those observed with the fetal hydantoin syndrome, and because both carbamazepine and phenytoin are metabolized through the arene oxide pathway, a mechanism was proposed that attributed the teratogenicity to the epoxide intermediates rather than to the specific drugs themselves (22).

In a later correspondence concerning the above study, the investigators cited unofficial data obtained from the FDA involving 1307 pregnancies in which the maternal use of carbamazepine was not confounded by the concomitant use of valproic acid (26). Eight infants with spina bifida were identified in the offspring of these mothers. The incidence of 0.6% (1 in 163) represented a ninefold relative risk for the neural tube defect (26).

A 1991 report cited data accumulated by the FDA on 237 infants with spina bifida born to women taking antiepileptic drugs during gestation (27). Carbamazepine was part of the anticonvulsant regimen in at least 64 of the women, 36 without valproic acid and 28 with valproic acid. The author noted that substantial underreporting was likely in these data, and an accurate assessment of the risk of spina bifida with carbamazepine could not be determined from voluntarily reported cases (27). To overcome these and other biases, the pregnancy outcomes of all Medicaid recipients in Michigan who gave birth in the period from 1980 through 1988, and who took anticonvulsants during the 1st trimester, were examined. Four cases of spina bifida were identified from 1490 women, including 107 who had taken carbamazepine. Three of the infants with spina bifida had been exposed to carbamazepine in utero, one of whom was also exposed to valproic acid, and two of whom were also exposed to phenytoin, barbiturates, or primidone alone or in combination. Combined with other published studies, the author concluded that in utero exposure to carbamazepine during the 1st trimester, without concurrent exposure to valproic acid, results in a 1% risk of spina bifida (27). The relative risk (RR) was estimated to be about 13.7 (95% confidence interval [CI], 5.6–33.7) times the expected rate.

The above study generated several published comments involving the risk of spina bifida after 1st -trimester exposure to carbamazepine (28–32). The last reference described an infant with closed spina bifida resulting from a pregnancy in which the mother took 600 mg of carbamazepine alone throughout gestation (32). The 3400-g female infant, delivered at 36 weeks' gestation, had a lumbosacral myelomeningocele covered with skin and no sensory loss. The authors of this report commented on four other cases of spina bifida after exposure to carbamazepine, either alone or in combination with valproic acid (32).

The effects of exposure (at any time during the 2nd or 3rd month after the last menstrual period) to folic acid antagonists on embryo–fetal development were evaluated in a large, multicenter, case–control surveillance study published in 2000 (33). The report was based on data collected between 1976 and 1998 from 80 maternity or tertiary care hospitals. Mothers were interviewed within 6 months of delivery about their use of drugs during pregnancy. Folic acid antagonists were categorized into two groups: group 1—dihydrofolate reductase inhibitors (aminopterin, methotrexate, sulfasalazine, pyrimethamine, triamterene, and trimethoprim); group 2—agents that affect other enzymes in folate metabolism, impair the absorption of folate, or increase the metabolic breakdown of folate (carbamazepine, phenytoin, primidone, and phenobarbital). The case subjects were 3870 infants with cardiovascular defects, 1962 with oral clefts, and 1100 with urinary tract malformations. Infants with defects associated with a syndrome were excluded as were infants with coexisting NTDs; known to be reduced by maternal folic acid supplementation. Too few infants with limb-reduction defects were identified to be analyzed. Controls (*N* = 8387) were infants with malformations other than oral clefts and cardiovascular, urinary tract, limb reduction, and NTDs, but included infants with chromosomal and genetic defects. The risk of malformations in control infants would not have been reduced by vitamin supplementation, and none of the controls used folic acid antagonists. For group 1 cases, the RRs of cardiovascular defects and oral clefts were 3.4 (95% CI 1.8–6.4) and 2.6 (95% CI 1.1–6.1), respectively. For group II cases, the RRs of cardiovascular, urinary tract defects, and oral clefts were 2.2 (95% CI 1.4–3.5), 2.5 (95% CI 1.2–5.0), and 2.5 (95% CI 1.5–4.2), respectively. Maternal use of multivitamin supplements with folic acid (typically 0.4 mg) reduced the risks in group 1 cases, but not in group 2 cases (33).

A 2001 case–control study, using the same database as in the above study, compared 1242 infants with NTDs (spina bifida, anencephaly, and encephalocele) with a control group of 6660 infants with congenital defects not related to vitamin supplements (34). Based on six exposed cases, the adjusted odds ratio (OR) for carbamazepine was 6.9%, 95% CI 1.9–25.7. For all folic acid antagonists (carbamazepine, phenobarbital, phenytoin, primidone, sulfasalazine, triamterene, and trimethoprim), based on 27 cases, the adjusted OR was 2.9, 95% CI 1.7–4.6 (34).

A 1996 study described typical dysmorphic facial features in 6 of 47 children (aged 6 months to 6 years) who had been exposed to carbamazepine monotherapy during pregnancy (35). Moreover, the average cognitive score for the 47 children was significantly lower than a control group. The authors concluded that the facial features and mild mental retardation were consistent with a carbamazepine syndrome that had been described earlier (see references 22 and 35).

In a 2000 study, a group of 100 Swedish children who had been exposed to antiepileptic drugs (carbamazepine most frequently) in utero was compared with 100 matched controls at 9 months of age (36). Exposed children had a significant increase in the number of minor anomalies, 31 vs. 18, and, after carbamazepine exposure, an increased number of facial anomalies, 11 vs. 6. A blinded assessment of psychomotor development using Griffiths' test (gross motor function, personal and social behavior, hearing and speech, eye and hand coordination, and performance), however, found that antiepileptic drug exposure did not influence the results (36).

The effect of in utero exposure to antiepileptic drugs on fetal growth was described for 977 newborns in another 2000 Swedish study (37). Birth data were collected from 1973 to 1997, during which time the frequency of antiepileptic monotherapy increased from 46% to 88%. As expected, the most marked effects on body weight, length, and head circumference were found with polytherapy. For monotherapy, however, only carbamazepine had a negative influence on these measurements (37).

A 1997 study, using the General Practice Research Database in the United Kingdom, reported an increased prevalence of major malformations in infants of epileptic mothers treated with antiepileptic drugs (3.4%, 10 of 297) compared with matched controls (1.0%, 6 of 594), RR 3.3, 95% CI 1.2–9.2 (38). Eight of the ten congenital anomalies involved carbamazepine (seven with monotherapy): ventricular septal defect; pulmonary stenosis; cleft palate, hare lip; Pierre Robin syndrome with cleft palate (also alcohol abuse); sensorineural deafness; congenital megaureter, hydronephrosis syndrome; vesicoureteric reflux; and Marcus Gunn ptosis (combined with sodium valproate) (38).

A 2000 study, using data from the MADRE (an acronym for MAlformation and DRug Exposure) surveillance project, assessed the human teratogenicity of anticonvulsants (39). Among 8005 malformed infants, cases were defined as infants with a specific malformation, whereas controls were infants with other anomalies. Of the total group, 299 were exposed in the 1st trimester to anticonvulsants. Among these, exposure to monotherapy occurred in the following: phenobarbital (*N* = 65), methobarbital (*N* = 10), carbamazepine (*N* = 46), valproic acid (*N* = 80), phenytoin (*N* = 24), and other agents (*N* = 16). A statistically significant association was found between carbamazepine monotherapy and spina bifida (*N* = 4). When all 1st trimester exposures (mono- and polytherapy) were evaluated, a significant association was found between carbamazepine and hypertelorism with localized skull defects (*N* = 3). Although the study confirmed some previously known associations, several new associations with anticonvulsants were discovered and require independent confirmation (see Mephobarbital, Phenobarbital, Phenytoin, and Valproic Acid) (39).

A prospective study published in 1999 described the outcomes of 517 pregnancies of epileptic mothers identified at one Italian center from 1977 (40). Excluding genetic and chromosomal defects, malformations were classified as severe structural defects, mild structural defects, and deformations. Minor anomalies were not considered. Spontaneous (*N* = 38) and early (*N* = 20) voluntary abortions were excluded from the analysis, as were seven pregnancies that delivered at other hospitals. Of the remaining 452 outcomes, 427 were exposed to anticonvulsants; of which 313 involved monotherapy: carbamazepine (*N* = 113), phenobarbital (*N* = 83), valproate (*N* = 44), primidone (*N* = 35), phenytoin (*N* = 31), clonazepam (*N* = 6), and other (*N* = 1). There were no defects in the 25 pregnancies not exposed to anticonvulsants. Of the 42 (9.3%) outcomes with malformations, 24 (5.3%) were severe, 10 (2.2%) were mild, and 8 (1.8%) were deformities. There were 12 malformations with carbamazepine monotherapy: 7 (6.2%) were severe (spina bifida, hydrocephalus, diaphragmatic hernia, esophagus atresia, pyloric stenosis, omphalocele, renal dysplasia, and hydronephrosis), 1 (0.9%) was mild (inguinal hernia and valgus/varus foot), and 4 (3.5%) were deformations (club foot and hip dislocation). The investigators concluded that the anticonvulsants were the primary risk factor for an increased incidence of congenital malformations (see Clonazepam, Phenobarbital, Phenytoin, Primidone, and Valproic Acid) (40).

A 2001 prospective cohort study, conducted from 1986 to 1993 at five maternity hospitals, was designed to determine if anticonvulsant agents or other factors (e.g., genetic) were responsible for the constellation of abnormalities seen in infants of mothers treated with anticonvulsants during pregnancy (41). A total of 128,049 pregnant women were screened at delivery for exposure to anticonvulsant drugs. Three groups of singleton infants were identified: (a) exposed to anticonvulsant drugs, (b) not exposed to anticonvulsant drugs but with a maternal history of seizures, and (c) not exposed to anticonvulsant drugs and with no maternal history of seizures (control group). After applying exclusion criteria, including exposure to other teratogens, 316, 98, and 508 infants, respectively, were analyzed. Anticonvulsant monotherapy occurred in 223 women: phenytoin (*N* = 87), phenobarbital (*N* = 64), carbamazepine (*N* = 58), and too few cases for analysis with valproic acid, clonazepam, diazepam, and lorazepam. Ninety-three infants were exposed to two or more anticonvulsant drugs. All infants were examined systematically (blinded as to group in 93% of the cases) for embryopathy associated with anticonvulsant exposure (major

C

malformations, hypoplasia of the midface and fingers, microcephaly, and intrauterine growth restriction). Compared with controls, significant associations between anticonvulsants and anticonvulsant embryopathy were phenytoin monotherapy 20.7% (18/87), phenobarbital monotherapy 26.6% (17/64), any monotherapy 20.6% (46/223), exposure to two or more anticonvulsants 28.0% (26/93), and all infants exposed to anticonvulsants (mono- and polytherapy) 22.8% (72/316). Nonsignificant associations were found for carbamazepine monotherapy 13.8% (8/58), nonexposed infants with a maternal history of seizures 6.1% (6/98), and controls 8.5% (43/508). The investigators concluded that the distinctive pattern of physical abnormalities observed in infants exposed to anticonvulsants during gestation was due to the drugs, rather than to epilepsy itself (41).

A study published in 2009 examined the effect of AEDs on the head circumference in newborns (42). Significant reductions in mean birth-weight-adjusted mean head circumference (bw-adj-HC) was noted for monotherapy with carbamazepine and valproic acid. No effect on bw-adj-HC was observed with gabapentin, phenytoin, clonazepam, and lamotrigine. A significant increase in the occurrence of microcephaly (bw-adj-HC smaller than 2 standard deviations below the mean) was noted after any AED polytherapy but not after any monotherapy, including carbamazepine and valproic acid (42).

In a study designed to evaluate the effect of in utero exposure to anticonvulsants on intelligence, 148 Finnish children of epileptic mothers were compared with 105 controls (22). Previous studies had shown intellectual impairment from either this exposure or no effect. Of the 148 children of epileptic mothers, 129 were exposed to anticonvulsant therapy during the first 20 weeks of pregnancy, 2 were only exposed after 20 weeks, and 17 were not exposed. In those mothers treated during pregnancy, 42 received carbamazepine (monotherapy in 9 cases) during the first 20 weeks, and 1 received the drug after 20 weeks. The children were evaluated at 5.5 years of age for both verbal and nonverbal measures of intelligence. A child was considered mentally deficient if the results of both tests were less than 71. Two of the 148 children of epileptic mothers were diagnosed as mentally deficient and 2 others had borderline intelligence (the mother of one of these latter children had not been treated with anticonvulsant medication). None of the controls was considered mentally deficient. One child with profound mental retardation had been exposed in utero to carbamazepine monotherapy, but the condition was compatible with dominant inheritance and was not thought to be caused by drug exposure. Both verbal and nonverbal intelligence scores were significantly lower in the study group children than in controls. In both groups, intelligence scores were significantly lower when seven or more minor anomalies were present. However, the presence of hypertelorism and digital hypoplasia, two minor anomalies considered typical of exposure to some anticonvulsants (e.g., phenytoin), was not predictive of low intelligence (21).

A prospective, controlled, blinded, observational 1994 study compared the global IQ and language development of children exposed in utero with either carbamazepine ($N = 34$) or phenytoin ($N = 36$) monotherapy to their respective matched controls (43). The cognitive tests were administered to the children between the ages of 18 and 36 months. The maternal IQ scores and socioeconomic status in the carbamazepine subjects and their controls were similar, 96.5 vs. 96.0, and 44.7 vs. 46.1, respectively, as they were in the phenytoin subjects and controls, 90.0 vs. 93.9, and 40.8 vs. 40.9, respectively. Compared with controls, no significant differences were measured in either IQ or language development scores between carbamazepine-exposed children and their matched controls. In contrast, phenytoin-exposed children had both lower mean global IQ and language development scores than their matched controls (see Phenytoin). No correlation between the daily dose (mg/kg) of either anticonvulsant and global IQ was found. Major malformations were observed in two carbamazepine-exposed children (missing last joint of right index finger and nail hypoplasia; hypospadias), one carbamazepine control (pulmonary atresia), and two phenytoin-exposed children (42). In subsequent correspondence relating to the above study (44,45), various perceived problems were cited and were addressed in a reply (46).

A 2013 study reported dose-dependent associations with reduced cognitive abilities across a range of domains at 6 years of age after fetal valproate exposure (47). Analysis showed that IQ was significantly lower for valproate (mean 97, 95% CI 94–101) than to carbamazepine (mean 105, 95% CI 102–108; $p = 0.0015$), lamotrigine (mean 108, 95% CI 105–110; $p = 0.0003$), or phenytoin (mean 108, 95% CI 104–112; $p = 0.0006$). Mean IQs were higher in children whose mother's had taken folic acid (mean 108, 95% CI 106–111) compared with children whose mothers had not taken the vitamin (mean 101, 95% CI 98–104; $p = 0.0009$) (47).

A 2001 prospective study compared the outcomes of 210 pregnancies exposed to carbamazepine in the 1st trimester with controls (48). The rate of major defects in exposed subjects was significantly increased compared with controls, RR 2.24, 95% CI 1.1–4.56. There was no specific pattern of defects (48).

A 2002 meta-analysis evaluated pooled data from 21 prospective studies involving 1255 offspring to determine the teratogenic risk of exposure to carbamazepine (49). Of infants, 85 (6.7%) had major defects compared with 88 (2.34%) of 3756 controls ($p < 0.05$). Among 182 untreated women with epilepsy, 5 (2.75%) had major defects. The defects with the greatest increased rate were NTDs, cardiovascular and urinary tract defects, and cleft palate. The drug also may cause a significant, but very small (0.18 weeks) reduction in the mean gestational age at delivery. Combination therapy was more teratogenic than monotherapy (49).

A possible teratogenic mechanism for carbamazepine in combination with other anticonvulsants was proposed in 1984 to account for the higher than expected adverse pregnancy outcome that is observed with combination therapy (50). Accumulation of the toxic oxidative metabolite, carbamazepine-10,11-epoxide, was shown when the drug was combined with other antiepileptic agents, such as phenobarbital, valproic acid, and phenytoin. These last two agents are also known to produce toxic epoxide metabolites that can bind covalently to macromolecules and may produce mutagenic or teratogenic effects (see Phenytoin) (50). However, a 2002 reference pointed out that carbamazepine-10,11-epoxide, while detected in high concentrations in the serum, is stable and nonreactive and is a potent anticonvulsant itself. Moreover, the metabolite was not embryotoxic in animals (51).

A case of attempted suicide with carbamazepine, possibly resulting in a neural tube defect, has been reported (52). A 44-year-old nonepileptic woman at 3–4 weeks after conception (i.e., during the period of neural tube closure) ingested approximately 4.8 g of the drug as a single dose. Her serum carbamazepine levels for 2 days after the ingestion were more than twice the recommended maximum therapeutic level. Subsequently, a large thoracolumbar spinal defect was observed on sonographic examination and her pregnancy was terminated at 20 weeks' gestation. Fetal autopsy of the male infant revealed an open myeloschisis and a hypoplastic left cerebral hemisphere, the latter defect thought to be the result of focal necrosis (52).

The Lamotrigine Pregnancy Registry, an ongoing project conducted by the manufacturer, was first published in January 1997 (53). The final report was published in July 2010. The Registry is now closed. Among 183 prospectively enrolled pregnancies exposed to carbamazepine and lamotrigine, with or without other anticonvulsants, 180 were exposed in the 1st trimester resulting in 157 live births without defects, 10 SABs, 9 EABs, 1 fetal death, and 3 birth defects. There were three exposures in the 2nd/3rd trimesters resulting in live births without defects (53).

A case of neuroblastoma was described in a developmentally normal 2.5-year-old male infant who had been exposed throughout gestation to carbamazepine and phenytoin (54). The tumor was attributed to phenytoin exposure.

The effect of carbamazepine on maternal and fetal vitamin D metabolism was examined in a 1984 study (55). In comparison with normal controls, several significant differences were found in the level of various vitamin D compounds and in serum calcium, but the values were still within normal limits. No alterations were found in alkaline phosphatase and phosphate concentrations. The observed differences were not thought to be of major clinical significance (55).

BREASTFEEDING SUMMARY

Carbamazepine is excreted into breast milk, producing milk:plasma ratios of 0.24–0.69 (2,4,9,14,56–58). The amount of carbamazepine measured in infant serum is low, with typical levels around 0.4 mcg/mL, but levels may be as high as 0.5–1.8 mcg/mL (2,57). In one case, infant serum levels were 15% and 20% of the maternal total and free carbamazepine concentrations, respectively (56). Accumulation does not seem to occur.

In a 1998 case report, seizures were reported by the mother in a nursing infant (58). The mother had bipolar disorder that was being treated with fluoxetine (20 mg/day), buspirone (45 mg/day), and carbamazepine (600 mg/day) (see Fluoxetine and Buspirone). Carbamazepine was detected in breast milk and the infant's serum (both 0.5 ng/mL). A neurologic examination of the infant, which included electroencephalography, was within normal limits. The cause of the seizure-like activity could not be determined, if indeed it had occurred (none of the episodes had been observed by medical personnel) (58).

In a 2010 study, 199 children who had been breastfed while their mothers were taking a single antiepileptic drug (carbamazepine, lamotrigine, phenytoin, or valproate) were evaluated at 3 years of age cognitive outcome (59). Mean adjusted IQ scores for exposed children were 99 (95% CI 96–103), whereas the mean adjusted IQ scores of non-breastfed infants were 98 (95% CI 95–101).

The American Academy of Pediatrics classifies carbamazepine as compatible with breastfeeding (60).

References

1. Product information. Tegretol. Novartis Pharmaceuticals, 2000.
2. Pynnonen S, Kanto J, Sillanpae M, Erkkola R. Carbamazepine: placental transport, tissue concentrations in the foetus and newborns, and level in milk. Acta Pharmacol Toxicol 1977;41:244–53.
3. Rane A, Bertilsson L, Palmer L. Disposition of placentally transferred carbamazepine (Tegretol) in the newborn. Eur J Clin Pharmacol 1975;8:283–4.
4. Nau H, Kuhnz W, Egger HJ, Rating D, Helge H. Anticonvulsants during pregnancy and lactation: transplacental, maternal and neonatal pharmacokinetics. Clin Pharmacokinet 1982;7:508–43.
5. Hiilesmaa VK. Evaluation of placental function in women on antiepileptic drugs. J Perinat Med 1983;11:187–92.
6. Rosa F. Holoprosencephaly and antiepileptic exposures. Teratology 1995;51:230.
7. Geigy Pharmaceuticals. Tegretol in epilepsy. In: *Monograph 319-80950*, Ciba-Geigy, Ardsley, 1978:18–19.
8. McMullin GP. Teratogenic effects of anticonvulsants. Br Med J 1971;4:430.
9. Pynnonen S, Sillanpae M. Carbamazepine and mothers milk. Lancet 1975;2:563.
10. Lander CM, Edwards VE, Endie MJ, Tyrer JH. Plasma anticonvulsant concentrations during pregnancy. Neurology 1977;27:128–31.
11. Nakane Y, Okuma T, Takahashi R, Sato Y, Wada T, Sato T, Fukushima Y, Kumashiro H, Ono T, Takahashi T, Aoki Y, Kazamatsuri H, Inami M, Komai S, Seino M, Miyakoshi M, Tanimura T, Hazama H, Kawahara R, Otsuki S, Hosokawa K, Inanaga K, Nakazawa Y, Yamamoto K. Multi-institutional study on the teratogenicity and fetal toxicity to antiepileptic drugs: a report of a collaborative study group in Japan. Epilepsia 1980;21:633–80.
12. Janz D. The teratogenic risk of antiepileptic drugs. Epilepsia 1975;16: 159–69.
13. Meyer JG. Teratogenic risk of anticonvulsants and the effects on pregnancy and birth. Eur Neurol 1979;10:179–90.
14. Niebyl JR, Blake DA, Freeman JM, Luff RD. Carbamazepine levels in pregnancy and lactation. Obstet Gynecol 1979;53:139–40.
15. Hicks EP. Carbamazepine in two pregnancies. Clin Exp Neurol 1979;16: 269–75.
16. Thomas D, Buchanan N. Teratogenic effects of anticonvulsants. J Pediatr 1981;99:163.
17. Niesen M, Froscher W. Finger- and toenail hypoplasia after carbamazepine monotherapy in late pregnancy. Neuropediatrics 1985;16:167–8.
18. Jacobson SJ, Jones K, Johnson K, Ceolin L, Kaur P, Sahn D, Donnenfeld AE, Rieder M, Santelli R, Smythe J, Pastuszak A, Einarson T, Koren G. Prospective multicentre study of pregnancy outcome after lithium exposure during first trimester. Lancet 1992;339:530–3.
19. Hiilesmaa VK, Teramo K, Granstrom ML, Bardy AH. Fetal head growth retardation associated with maternal antiepileptic drugs. Lancet 1981;2:165–7.
20. Hiilesmaa VK, Bardy A, Teramo K. Obstetric outcome in women with epilepsy. Am J Obstet Gynecol 1985;152:499–504.
21. Gaily E, Kantola-Sorsa E, Granstrom M-L. Intelligence of children of epileptic mothers. J Pediatr 1988;113:677–84.
22. Jones KL, Lacro RV, Johnson KA, Adams J. Pattern of malformations in the children of women treated with carbamazepine during pregnancy. N Engl J Med 1989;320:1661–6.
23. Vestermark V, Vestermark S. Teratogenic effect of carbamazepine. Arch Dis Child 1991;66:641–2.
24. Janz D. Antiepileptic drugs and pregnancy: altered utilization patterns and teratogenesis. Epilepsia 1982;23(Suppl 1):S53–63.
25. Paulson GW, Paulson RB. Teratogenic effects of anticonvulsants. Arch Neurol 1981;38:140–3.
26. Jones KL, Johnson KA, Adams J, Lacro RV. Teratogenic effects of carbamazepine. N Engl J Med 1989;321:1481.
27. Rosa FW. Spina bifida in infants of women treated with carbamazepine during pregnancy. N Engl J Med 1991;324:674–7.
28. Anonymous. Teratogenesis with carbamazepine. Lancet 1991;337:1316–7.
29. Hughes RL. Spina bifida in infants of women taking carbamazepine. N Engl J Med 1991;325:664.
30. Hesdorffer DC, Hauser WA. Spina bifida in infants of women taking carbamazepine. N Engl J Med 1991;325:664.
31. Rosa F. Spina bifida in infants of women taking carbamazepine. N Engl J Med 1991;325:664–5.

C

32. Oakeshott P, Hunt GM. Carbamazepine and spina bifida. Br Med J 1991;303:651.
33. Hernandez-Diaz S, Werler MM, Walker AM, Mitchell AA. Folic acid antagonists during pregnancy and the risk of birth defects. N Engl J Med 2000;343:1608–14.
34. Hernandez-Diaz S, Werler MM, Walker AM, Mitchell AA. Neural tube defects in relation to use of folic acid antagonists during pregnancy. Am J Epidemiol 2001;153:981–8.
35. Ornoy A, Cohen E. Outcome of children born to epileptic mothers treated with carbamazepine during pregnancy. Arch Dis Child 1996;75:517–20.
36. Wide K, Winbladh B, Tomson T, Sars-Zimmer K, Berggren E. Psychomotor development and minor anomalies in children exposed to antiepileptic drugs in utero: a prospective population-based study. Dev Med Child Neurol 2000;42:87–92.
37. Wide K, Winbladh B, Tomson T, Kallen B. Body dimensions of infants exposed to antiepileptic drugs in utero: observations spanning 25 years. Epilepsia 2000;41:854–61.
38. Jick SS, Terris BZ. Anticonvulsants and congenital malformations. Pharmacotherapy 1997;17:561–4.
39. Arpino C, Brescianini S, Robert E, Castilla EE, Cocchi G, Cornel MC, de Vigan C, Lancaster PAL, Merlob P, Sumiyoshi Y, Zampino G, Renzi C, Rosano A, Mastroiacovo P. Teratogenic effects of antiepileptic drugs: use of an international database on malformations and drug exposure (MADRE). Epilepsia 2000;41:1436–43.
40. Canger R, Battino D, Canevini MP, Fumarola C, Guidolin L, Vignoli A, Mamoli D, Palmieri C, Molteni F, Granata T, Hassibi P, Zamperini P, Pardi G, Avanzini G. Malformations in offspring of women with epilepsy: a prospective study. Epilepsia 1999;40:1231–6.
41. Holmes LB, Harvey EA, Coull BA, Huntington KB, Khoshbin S, Hayes AM, Ryan LM. The teratogenicity of anticonvulsant drugs. N Engl J Med 2001;344:1132–8.
42. Almgren M, Kallen B, Lavebratt C. Population-based study of antiepileptic drug exposure in utero—influence on head circumference in newborns. Seizure 2009;18:672–5.
43. Scolnik D, Nulman I, Rovet J, Gladstone D, Czuchta D, Gardner HA, Gladstone R, Ashby P, Weksberg R, Einarson T, Koren G. Neurodevelopment of children exposed in utero to phenytoin and carbamazepine monotherapy. JAMA 1994;271:767–70.
44. Jeret JS. Neurodevelopment after in utero exposure to phenytoin and carbamazepine. JAMA 1994;272:850.
45. Loring DW, Meador KJ, Thompson WO. Neurodevelopment of children exposed in utero to phenytoin and carbamazepine. JAMA 1994;272:850–1.
46. Koren G. Neurodevelopment of children exposed in utero to phenytoin and carbamazepine. JAMA 1994;272:851.
47. Meador KJ, Baker GA, Browning N, Cohen MJ, Bromley RL, Clayton-Smith J, Kalayjian LA, Kanner A, Liporace JD, Pennell PB, Privitera M, Loring DW, for the NEAD Study Group. Fetal antiepileptic drug exposure and cognitive outcomes at age 6 years (NEAD study): a prospective observational study. Lancet Neurol 2013;12:244–52.
48. Diav-Citrin O, Shechtman S, Arnon J, Ornoy A. Is carbamazepine teratogenic? A prospective controlled study of 210 pregnancies. Neurology 2001;57:321–4.
49. Matalon S, Shechtman S, Goldzweig G, Ornoy A. The teratogenic effect of carbamazepine: a meta-analysis of 1255 exposures. Reprod Toxicol 2002;16:9–17.
50. Lindhout D, Höppener RJEA, Meinardi H. Teratogenicity of antiepileptic drug combinations with special emphasis on epoxidation (of carbamazepine). Epilepsia 1984;25:77–83.
51. Koren G. Comment on antiepileptics and antipsychotics. Teratology 2002;66:273.
52. Little BB, Santos-Ramos R, Newell JF, Maberry MC. Megadose carbamazepine during the period of neural tube closure. Obstet Gynecol 1993;82:705–8.
53. The Lamotrigine Pregnancy Registry. Final Report. 1 September 1992 through 31 March 2010. GlaxcoSmithKline, July 2010.
54. Al-Shammri S, Guberman A, Hsu E. Neuroblastoma and fetal exposure to phenytoin in a child without dysmorphic features. Can J Neurol Sci 1992;19:243–5.
55. Markestad T, Ulstein M, Strandjord RE, Aksnes L, Aarskog D. Anticonvulsant drug therapy in human pregnancy: effects on serum concentrations of vitamin D metabolites in maternal and cord blood. Am J Obstet Gynecol 1984;150:254–8.
56. Kok THHG, Taitz LS, Bennett MJ, Holt DW. Drowsiness due to clemastine transmitted in breast milk. Lancet 1982;1:914–5.
57. Wisner KL, Perel JM. Serum levels of valproate and carbamazepine in breastfeeding mother–infant pairs. J Clin Psychopharmacol 1998;18:167–9.
58. Brent NB, Wisner KL. Fluoxetine and carbamazepine concentrations in a nursing mother/infant pair. Clin Pediatr 1998;37:41–4.
59. Meador KJ, Baker GA, Browning N, Clayton-Smith J, Combs-Cantrell DT, Cohen M, Kalayjian LA, Kanner A, Liporace JD, Pennell PB, Privitera M, Loring DW, for the NEAD Study Group. Effects of breastfeeding in children of women taking antiepileptic drugs. Neurology 2010;75:1954–60.
60. Committee on Drugs, American Academy of Pediatrics. The transfer of drugs and other chemicals into human milk. Pediatrics 2001;108:776–89.

CARBARSONE

[Withdrawn from the market. See 8th edition.]

CARBENICILLIN

Antibiotic (Penicillin)

PREGNANCY RECOMMENDATION: Compatible
BREASTFEEDING RECOMMENDATION: Compatible

PREGNANCY SUMMARY

Although the reported pregnancy experience with carbenicillin is limited, all penicillins are considered low risk in pregnancy.

FETAL RISK SUMMARY

Carbenicillin is a penicillin antibiotic (see also Penicillin G). Reproduction studies conducted in mice (200 mg/kg), rats (500 or 1000 mg/kg), and monkeys (500 mg/kg) observed no fetal harm (1).

The drug crosses the placenta and distributes to most fetal tissues (2,3). After a 4-g IM dose, mean peak concentrations in cord and maternal serums at 2 hours were similar. Amniotic fluid levels averaged 7%–11% of maternal peak concentrations.

No published reports linking the use of carbenicillin with congenital defects have been located. The Collaborative Perinatal

Project monitored 50,282 mother–child pairs, 3546 of whom had documented 1st trimester exposure to penicillin derivatives (4, pp. 297–313). For use anytime during pregnancy, 7171 exposures were recorded (4, p. 435). In neither group was evidence found to suggest a relationship to large categories of major or minor malformations or to individual defects.

In a surveillance study of Michigan Medicaid recipients involving 229,101 completed pregnancies conducted between 1985 and 1992, 31 newborns had been exposed to carbenicillin during the 1st trimester (F. Rosa, personal communication, FDA, 1993). A total of five (16.1%) major birth defects were observed (one expected), one of which was a cardiovascular defect (0.5 expected). No anomalies were observed in five other categories of defects (oral clefts, spina bifida, polydactyly, limb reduction defects, and hypospadias) for which specific data were available. The number of exposures is too small to draw any conclusions.

BREASTFEEDING SUMMARY

No reports describing the use of carbenicillin during lactation have been located. Low amounts of the drug were measured in a 1984 study (5). At 5–7 days postpartum in 70 women, the highest mean concentration after a single 1000-mg IM dose was 0.24 mcg/mL at 4 hours. Although adverse effects from other penicillins in breast milk are rare, three potential problems exist for the nursing infant: modification of bowel flora, direct effects on the infant (e.g., allergic response), and interference with the interpretation of culture results if a fever workup is required.

C

References

1. Product information. Geocillin. Pfizer, 2000.
2. Biro L, Ivan E, Elek E, Arr M. Data on the tissue concentration of antibiotics in man. Tissue concentrations of semi-synthetic penicillins in the fetus. Int Z Pharmakol Ther Toxikol 1970;4:321–4.
3. Elek E, Ivan E, Arr M. Passage of penicillins from mother to foetus in humans. Int J Clin Pharmacol Ther Toxicol 1972;6:223–8.
4. Heinonen OP, Slone D, Shapiro S. *Birth Defects and Drugs in Pregnancy*. Littleton, MA: Publishing Sciences Group, 1977.
5. Matsuda S. Transfer of antibiotics into maternal milk. Biol Res Pregnancy 1984;5:57–60.

CARBIDOPA

Antiparkinson Agent

PREGNANCY RECOMMENDATION: Limited Human Data—Animal Data Suggest Risk
BREASTFEEDING RECOMMENDATION: No Human Data—Probably Compatible

PREGNANCY SUMMARY

As expected, a limited number of reports describe the use of carbidopa (in combination with levodopa) during human pregnancy. The indication for this drug in women of childbearing age is relatively rare. Limited studies have not found teratogenicity in animals with carbidopa, except when combined with levodopa, an outcome that may have been related to the latter drug. However, carbidopa did cause fetal deaths in one animal species. The cause of the two miscarriages described above is unknown, but requires further study. Brown fat hemorrhage observed in newborn rats treated during the 1st week of gestation was dose-related, and the toxicity has not been reported in humans. Moreover, the placental passage of carbidopa in animals and humans is limited. Based on the above data and the fact that lower doses of levodopa can be used if carbidopa is added to the mother's regimen, therapy with carbidopa, if indicated, should not be withheld because of pregnancy.

FETAL RISK SUMMARY

This antiparkinson agent has no pharmacologic effect when given alone and is almost always used in conjunction with levodopa (see also Levodopa). Carbidopa (α-methyldopa hydrazine; MK-486) inhibits decarboxylation of extracerebral levodopa. When used in combination with this latter agent, lower doses of levodopa can be administered, resulting in fewer adverse effects, and more levodopa is available for passage to the brain and eventual conversion in that organ to the active metabolite, dopamine.

Combinations of carbidopa and levodopa, as well as levodopa alone, have caused visceral and skeletal malformations in rabbits (1,2). The carbidopa doses were 10–20 times the maximum recommended human dose (MRHD) (2). A dose about two times the MRHD caused a decrease in the number of live pups delivered by rats (2). Carbidopa, 10 or 100 mg/kg/day given orally to rats from day 1 through day 21 of gestation, did not have a teratogenic effect but did cause a significant dose-related increase in brown fat (interscapular brown adipose tissue) hemorrhage and vasodilation in the newborn pups (3). The hemorrhage, 4.6% and 12.1%, respectively, for the two doses, was thought to be related to dopamine. Combining carbidopa and levodopa resulted in a lower incidence of hemorrhage. No teratogenic effects were observed in mice given carbidopa doses up to 10 times the MRHD (2).

A study published in 1978 examined the effect of carbidopa (20 mg/kg SC every 12 hours for 7 days) and levodopa plus carbidopa (200/20 mg/kg SC every 12 hours for 7 days) on the length of gestation in pregnant rats (4). Only the combination had a statistically significant effect on pregnancy duration, causing a delay in parturition of 12 hours. The results were thought to be consistent with dopamine inhibition of oxytocin release (4).

In pregnant rats, small amounts of carbidopa cross the placenta and can be detected in amniotic fluid and fetal tissue (5). Carbidopa concentrations were measured at 1, 2, and 4 hours after a 20-mg/kg IV dose administered near the end of gestation (19th day). The highest levels in the maternal plasma, placenta, amniotic fluid, and fetus (time of maximum concentration shown in parentheses) were 9.9 mcg/mL (1 hour), 2.35 mcg/g (1 hour), 0.32 mcg/mL (2 and 4 hours), and 0.65 mcg/g (2 hours), respectively (5).

Human placental transfer of carbidopa, although the amounts were very small, was documented in a study published in 1995 (6). A 34-year-old woman with juvenile Parkinson's disease was treated with carbidopa/levodopa (200/800 mg/day) during two pregnancies (see also Levodopa). Both pregnancies were electively terminated, one at 8 weeks' gestation and the other at 10 weeks. Mean concentrations of carbidopa (expressed as ng/mg protein) in the maternal serum, placental tissue (including umbilical cord), fetal peripheral organs (heart, kidney, muscle), and fetal neural tissue (brain and spinal cord) were 2.05, 8.0, 0.14, and <0.15, respectively. The low concentrations of carbidopa in the fetus, compared with those in the mother and placenta, were interpreted as evidence for an effective placental barrier to the transport of carbidopa (6).

Because Parkinson's disease is relatively uncommon in women of childbearing age, only a few reports have been located that describes the use of carbidopa, always in combination with levodopa, in human pregnancy (7–11). A woman with at least a 7-year history of parkinsonism conceived while being treated with carbidopa/levodopa (five 25/250-mg tablets/day) and amantadine (100 mg twice/day) (7). She had delivered a normal male infant approximately 6 years earlier, but no medical treatment had been given during that pregnancy. Amantadine was immediately discontinued when the current pregnancy was diagnosed. Other than slight vaginal bleeding in the 1st trimester, there were no maternal or fetal complications. She gave birth to a normal-term infant (sex and weight not specified) who was doing well at 1.5 years of age (7).

A 1987 retrospective report described the use of carbidopa/levodopa, starting before conception in five women during seven pregnancies, one of which was electively terminated during the 1st trimester (8). All of the other pregnancies went to term (newborn weights and sexes not specified). Maternal complications in three pregnancies included slight 1st trimester vaginal bleeding, nausea and vomiting during the 8th and 9th months (only one patient reported nausea and vomiting after the 1st trimester), and depression that resolved postpartum, and preeclampsia. One infant, whose mother took amantadine and carbidopa/levodopa and whose pregnancy was complicated by preeclampsia, had an inguinal hernia. No adverse effects or congenital anomalies were noted in the other five newborns, and all remained healthy at follow-up (approximately 1–5 years of age) (8).

A 27-year-old woman with a history of chemotherapy and radiotherapy for non-Hodgkin's lymphoma occurring approximately 4 years earlier had developed a progressive parkinsonism syndrome that was treated with a proprietary preparation of carbidopa/levodopa (co-careldopa; Sinemet Plus; 375 mg/day) (9). She conceived 5 months after treatment began and eventually delivered a healthy, 3540-g male infant at term. Apgar scores were 9 at both 1 and 10 minutes, respectively. Co-careldopa was continued throughout her pregnancy (9).

A brief case report, published in 1997, described a normal outcome in the third pregnancy of a woman with levodopa-responsive dystonia (Segawa disease) who was treated throughout gestation with 500 mg/day of levodopa alone (10). The male infant weighed 2350 g at birth and was developing normally at the time of the report. Two previous pregnancies had occurred while the woman was being treated with daily doses of levodopa (100 mg) and carbidopa (10 mg). Spontaneous abortions had occurred in both pregnancies: one at 6 weeks and the other at 12 weeks. An investigation failed to find any cause for the miscarriages (10).

A successful pregnancy in a 27-year-old woman with Segawa disease was reported in 2009 (11). The woman was treated throughout gestation with levodopa (1250 mg/day) and, at 36 weeks' gestation, gave birth to a healthy, 2298-g male infant with an Apgar score of 9 at 5 minutes. The infant was doing well at 6 months of age. The authors cited eight other cases of the disease in five pregnant women. Five of the pregnancies were treated with levodopa monotherapy and ended in healthy newborns. In one of those patients, her first two pregnancies were treated with carbidopa/levodopa and both ended in abortions (see reference 10 above). The ninth pregnancy was not treated with any agent and the severely asphyxiated newborn died after birth (11).

A woman with a 12-year history of Parkinson's disease was treated throughout gestation with levodopa, carbidopa, entacapone, and bromocriptine (12). She gave birth at term to a 3175-g female infant, without deformities, with Apgar scores of 9, 10, and 10. Generalized seizures occurred in the infant 1 hour after birth followed by repeated episodes of shivering throughout the first day that responded to diazepam. Slowly improving hypotonia also was observed during the first week. Pneumonia was diagnosed but an extensive workup for the cause of seizures was negative. The child was developing normally at 1 year of age and has not had any other seizures (12).

BREASTFEEDING SUMMARY

No reports describing the use of carbidopa during human lactation have been located. The molecular weight (about 244) suggests that the drug probably will be excreted into breast milk, but the amounts should be low. In at least two cases, breastfeeding was held because of concerns with other drug therapy (levodopa or amantadine) that the mother was taking with carbidopa (7,9). Small amounts are excreted in the milk of lactating rats (5).

References

1. Product information. Sinemet. DuPont Pharma, 2000.
2. Product information. Stalevo. Novartis Pharmaceuticals, 2007.
3. Kitchin KT, DiStefano V. L-Dopa and brown fat hemorrhage in the rat pup. Toxicol Appl Pharmacol 1976;38:251–63.
4. Seybold VS, Miller JW, Lewis PR. Investigation of a dopaminergic mechanism for regulating oxytocin release. J Pharmacol Exp Ther 1978;207:605–10.
5. Vickers S, Stuart EK, Bianchine JR, Hucker HB, Jaffe ME, Rhodes RE, Vandenheuvel WJA. Metabolism of carbidopa [L-(-)-α-hydrazino-3,4-dihydroxy-α-methylhydrocinnamic acid monohydrate], an aromatic amino acid decarboxylase inhibitor, in the rat, dog, rhesus monkey, and man. Drug Metab Dispos 1974;2:9–22.

6. Merchant CA, Cohen G, Mytilineou C, DiRocco A, Moros D, Molinari S, Yahr MD. Human transplacental transfer of carbidopa/levodopa. J Neural Transm Park Dis Dement Sect 1995;9:239–42.
7. Cook DG, Klawans HL. Levodopa during pregnancy. Clin Neuropharmacol 1985;8:93–5.
8. Golbe LI. Parkinson's disease and pregnancy. Neurology 1987;37: 1245–9.
9. Ball MC, Sagar HJ. Levodopa in pregnancy. Mov Disord 1995;10:115.
10. Nomoto M, Kaseda S, Iwata S, Osame M, Fukuda T. Levodopa in pregnancy. Mov Disord 1997;12:261.
11. Watanabe T, Matsubara S, Baba Y, Tanaka H, Suzuki T, Suzuki M. Successful management of pregnancy in a patient with Segawa disease: case report and literature review. J Obstet Gynaecol Res 2009; 35:562–4.
12. Lindh J. Short episode of seizures in a newborn of mother treated with levodopa/carbidopa/entacapone and bromocriptine. Mod Disord 2007;22:1515.

C

CARBIMAZOLE

Antithyroid

Carbimazole is converted in vivo to methimazole. See Methimazole.

CARBINOXAMINE

Antihistamine

PREGNANCY RECOMMENDATION: No Human Data—Probably Compatible
BREASTFEEDING RECOMMENDATION: No Human Data—Probably Compatible

PREGNANCY SUMMARY

No reports describing the use of carbinoxamine in human pregnancy have been located. The antihistamine is in the same subclass of ethanolamines such as clemastine and diphenhydramine. As such, it is probably compatible in pregnancy. However, these agents have marked sedative effects that should be considered if consumed by a pregnant woman.

FETAL RISK SUMMARY

Carbinoxamine is a first-generation (H_1) antihistamine with anticholinergic and sedative properties. Animal reproduction studies have not been conducted with carbinoxamine. Long-term studies for carcinogenesis, mutagenesis, and fertility also have not been conducted (1).

It is not known if carbinoxamine crosses the human placenta. The molecular weight of carbinoxamine maleate (about 407) suggests that the drug will cross to the embryo–fetus.

BREASTFEEDING SUMMARY

No reports describing the use of carbinoxamine during human lactation have been located. The molecular weigh of carbinoxamine maleate (about 407) suggests that the drug will be excreted into breast milk. If the drug is used by a mother while nursing, the infant should be monitored for sedation. Although there are no data, the manufacturer considers the drug contraindicated in nursing mothers (1). The reason given for this is the increased sensitivity of newborn or premature infants to antihistamines.

Reference

1. Product information. Arbinoxa. Hawthorn Pharmaceuticals, 2012.

CARBOPLATIN

Antineoplastic

PREGNANCY RECOMMENDATION: Contraindicated—1st Trimester
BREASTFEEDING RECOMMENDATION: Contraindicated

PREGNANCY SUMMARY

Carboplatin exhibits dose-related embryo toxicity and teratogenicity in one animal species. Treatment during human gestation has been reported in a number of cases, all of which were treated well after organogenesis. Moreover, there also are a large number of women who were treated with carboplatin several years before pregnancy. In both of these time

C

periods, no fetal or neonatal toxicity due to carboplatin was noted. However, the absence of human exposures during organogenesis prevents an assessment of the actual teratogenic risk but, based on the animal data and the pharmacology of the drug, the risk appears to be high. Therefore, pregnant women should not be treated with this agent during the 1st trimester. Moreover, carboplatin is mutagenic and probably carcinogenic in experimental systems, but these effects have not been studied in human pregnancy.

FETAL RISK SUMMARY

The antineoplastic agent, carboplatin, is indicated for the treatment of ovarian cancer. It is closely related to cisplatin, another cancer chemotherapeutic agent. Carboplatin and cisplatin share the same cell-cycle nonspecific mechanism of action, producing inter-strand DNA cross-links. Carboplatin is not protein bound (1).

Carboplatin is mutagenic both in vitro and in vivo. Its carcinogenic potential has not been studied, but drugs with similar mechanisms of action are carcinogenic. Carboplatin is embryotoxic and teratogenic in rats given the drug during organogenesis (dose not specified) (1).

A 1989 study reported dose-related embryolethality and teratogenicity in rats treated in the early phase of organogenesis (2). Previous work by these researchers had found no teratogenicity at a dose of 4 mg/kg/day (relationship to human dose not stated). In their current study, however, a dose of 6 mg/kg/day produced a significant increase in embryo deaths and multiple malformations (e.g., gastroschisis, dilation of cerebral ventricles, cleft sternum, fused ribs, and malformed thoracic vertebrae) (2).

It is not known if carboplatin crosses the placenta early in pregnancy. The molecular weight (about 371) is low enough that passage to the fetal compartment should be expected. A 2002 review of cancer chemotherapy stated that carboplatin was widely distributed throughout all body tissues, including, presumably, the amniotic fluid (3).

A number of reports have described the use of carboplatin in human pregnancy (4–18). In a 1994 study, a 41-year-old primigravid woman at 14 weeks' gestation had surgery for ovarian cancer (4). Beginning at 22 weeks, she received carboplatin every 4 weeks for three cycles. Nine weeks after the last dose, a cesarean section at 37 weeks gave birth to a normal-appearing 3245-g male infant with Apgar scores of 9 and 9. The neonate had normal renal function and no evidence of myelosuppression. Platinum–DNA adducts were found in maternal and cord blood lymphocytes, indicating that the drug crossed the placenta (4).

A 40-year-old woman was treated for ovarian cancer at 20 weeks' gestation with cisplatin and cyclophosphamide (5). A second course of these agents was given a few weeks later. Further cisplatin doses were discontinued because the woman developed ototoxicity. At 30 weeks' gestation carboplatin and cyclophosphamide were given. A normal-appearing 3600-g male infant was delivered by cesarean section 7 weeks later. Apgar scores were 9 and 9 at 1 and 5 minutes, respectively. The infant was developing normally, including normal audiograms and neurologic findings, at 12 months of age (5).

In a follow-up report to the above case, researchers used a modified cisplatin–DNA enzyme-linked immunosorbent assay (ELISA) test to determine if platinum–DNA adducts could be detected in amniotic fluid obtained at 36 weeks or in cord blood at 37 weeks (6). Platinum–DNA adducts were not detected in either sample, but insufficient DNA was extracted from the samples to assay at the limit of ELISA sensitivity. A less-sensitive assay (atomic absorbance spectrometry [AAS]) also failed to detect platinum drug binding to DNA in amniotic fluid or cord blood. In contrast, DNA from the placenta was positive for platinum–DNA adducts in both the ELISA and AAS assays (6).

A 2003 report described the pregnancy outcome of a 30-year-old woman treated with carboplatin and paclitaxel during the 2nd and 3rd trimesters (7). She was diagnosed with an advanced stage of serous papillary adenocarcinoma of the ovary in the 1st trimester. The woman underwent an exploratory laparotomy at 7.5 weeks' gestation and then consented to chemotherapy beginning at 16–17 weeks. She received six cycles of carboplatin and paclitaxel, and was delivered by cesarean hysterectomy 3 weeks after the last cycle at 35.5 weeks. The newborn (sex not specified) had Apgar scores of 9, 9, and 9 at 1, 5, and 10 minutes, respectively. Birth weight was 2500 g (44th percentile), and the physical examination and laboratory tests were normal. In addition, the placenta appeared grossly normal. The infant was doing well at 15 months of age with no evidence of neurologic, renal, growth, or hematologic effects from the exposure (7).

A 28-year-old woman delivered a normal 3.88-kg male infant 4 years after treatment of a bilateral ovarian dysgerminoma (8). Treatment consisted of a laparotomy to remove the right tube and ovary and carboplatin (dose 735 mg). A 29-year-old woman conceived with the assistance of a donated ovum that had been fertilized in vitro, followed by embryo transfer (9). Five years earlier, both ovaries had been removed for stage III borderline ovarian adenocarcinoma. Her last course of carboplatin chemotherapy was given approximately 4 years before the pregnancy (9). In a retrospective study, the postsurgical reproductive histories of 50 women with ovarian cancer treated with unilateral oophorectomy from 1965 to 2000 were analyzed (10). Twenty-four women had attempted pregnancy and 17 (71%) had conceived 32 pregnancies. Six of the 17 had received prior chemotherapy (carboplatin or cisplatin plus paclitaxel in three; cisplatin plus cyclophosphamide in two; melphalan in one). The pregnancy outcomes were 1 on-going pregnancy, 5 spontaneous abortions (SABs), and 26 term gestations. There were no congenital anomalies in any of the offspring (10).

A large cohort study published in 2000 compared the pregnancy outcomes in survivors of various childhood cancers based on the type of treatment received (11). Among the total group of women, 340 had 594 pregnancies. The pregnancies were divided into five groups: 165 (nonsterilizing surgery or no treatment), 113 (chemotherapy with various agents, including an unknown number treated with carboplatin and cisplatin), 97 (abdominal–pelvic radiation), 53 (chemotherapy plus abdominal–pelvic radiation), and 166 (other treatments). The incidence of SABs and perinatal deaths did not differ among the groups. The proportion of live births with low birth weight (excluding preterm births) or congenital anomalies was highest in those treated only with radiation (16.0%) and those treated only with surgery only (9.5%), respectively. The rates of low birth weight (excluding preterm births) and congenital defects in the two chemotherapy groups were 2.3% and 2.3% (chemotherapy only) and 7.1% and 2.4% (chemotherapy plus radiation) (11).

In a novel case report, a 21-year-old woman was diagnosed with metastatic ovarian cancer that was initially treated with surgery that left her uterus, right fallopian tube, and ovary *in situ* (12). She then was enrolled into a phase I transplant protocol and received three cycles of carboplatin and paclitaxel. Subsequent high-dose chemotherapy was then given (carboplatin, paclitaxel, and/or cyclophosphamide). After her chemotherapy, the woman received a successful transplant of autologous peripheral blood stem cells. Approximately 16 months after the transplant she conceived but had a 1st trimester miscarriage. She conceived again several months later and eventually delivered a healthy full-term, 3000-g female infant. The child was developing normally at 17 months of age (12).

In a 2008 case report, a 34-year-old woman became pregnant after 12 years of infertility (13). Gestational diabetes was diagnosed at 5 weeks' gestation (HbA1c 6.9%) and she was treated with insulin. At 16 weeks, bilateral ovarian cancer was diagnosed and, 2 weeks later, she underwent bilateral salpingo-oophorectomy. Four courses of carboplatin were given from 21 to 33 weeks' gestation. At 33 weeks, a cesarean section was conducted to deliver a 2222-g normal male infant with Apgar scores of 9 and 10 at 1 and 5 minutes, respectively. After birth, the mother received five more courses of carboplatin. One year after the completion of therapy, the mother had no evidence of disease and her infant son was normal (13).

A 2008 review described data on seven patients who had received carboplatin during pregnancy (14). Three patients received carboplatin alone, three in combination with other antineoplastics (paclitaxel or cyclophosphamide) and one had received both carboplatin and cisplatin. All of the exposures occurred in the 2nd and 3rd trimesters. No fetal or neonatal toxicity was observed in the seven fetuses, although one neonate (exposed to both carboplatin and cisplatin) had anemia. The offspring were normal at a median follow-up of 13.5 months (range 9–20 months) (14).

Lung cancer with metastasis to the brain was diagnosed in a 33-year-old nonsmoking woman in the 19th week of pregnancy (15). The patient was treated with weekly paclitaxel and carboplatin every 3 weeks. In the 6th week of therapy, progressive disease in the brain was found with only partial response in the lungs. High-dose corticosteroids were given to induce fetal lung maturation and reduce cerebral edema. At 30 weeks, a cesarean section delivered a healthy baby boy (*no other details provided*). The mother died 4 weeks later. The infant was developing normally at 5 months of age (15).

A 32-year-old woman at about 29 weeks' was treated with one cycle of carboplatin and paclitaxel for cervical cancer (16). Because she refused further chemotherapy, a cesarean section at about 33 weeks' delivered a 2190-g male neonate with no signs of drug-induced toxicity. At 4 years of age, the child was developing normally (16).

A 38-year-old woman with breast cancer was treated with weekly trastuzumab in addition to carboplatin and docetaxel beginning at 15 weeks' (17). Fetal renal insufficiency with anhydramnios and missing visualization of the fetal bladder occurred at 21 weeks. The condition reversed after trastuzumab was discontined and three instillations of amniotic fluid. The amount of amniotic stabilized after 24 weeks. Because of fetal growth restriction, a cesarean section was performed at 33 weeks to deliver a male infant with birth weight <3rd percentile. The neonate had normal renal function with normal urinalysis (17).

In a 2013 case report, a 36-year-old primigravid woman at 12 weeks was diagnosed with ovarian cancer (18). She underwent left salpingo-oophorectomy and fertility-sparing staging surgery. At 14 weeks, she was started on intraperitoneal carboplatin given on day 1 and IV paclitaxel given on days 1, 8, and 15 of a 28-day cycle. Mild preeclampsia developed at 32 weeks after four of the planned six cycles had been given. Chemotherapy was held because of persistent thrombocytopenia. At 37 weeks, she underwent a planned cesarean section to give birth to a viable 2126-g male neonate with Apgar scores of 8 and 9 at 1 and 5 minutes, respectively. The infant had congenital bilateral talipes equinovarus (*clubfoot*), but one parent had a family history of this defect. A complete blood count was normal. The infant was doing well at 7 months of age (18).

BREASTFEEDING SUMMARY

Consistent with its molecular weight (about 371), carboplatin is excreted into breast milk. In a 2012 case report, a 40-year-old woman at about 4 months postpartum was exclusively breastfeeding when she began treatment with 6 weekly doses of IV carboplatin and paclitaxel for recurrent papillary thyroid cancer (19). Her infant was fed donor milk during treatment. After the 6th dose, milk samples were collected at 0, 4, 28, 172, and 316 hours. For carboplatin, the relative infant dose was 2.0%, whereas the relative infant dose for paclitaxel was 16.7%. Carboplatin remained detectable (0.16 mg/L) at 316 hours. For paclitaxel, the level at 172 hours was 0.97 mg/L but was undetectable at 316 hours. The authors concluded that although these levels were probably too low to cause toxicity, potential toxicity could include myelosuppression (especially neutropenia and thrombocytopenia), severe hypersensitivity reactions, nephrotoxicity, and neurotoxicity (19). Because of the potential toxicity, women receiving these agents should not nurse.

References

1. Product information. Paraplatin. Bristol-Myers Squibb, 2004.
2. Kai S, Kohmura H, Ishikawa K, Makihara Y, Ohta S, Kawano S, Takahashi N. Teratogenic effects of carboplatin, an oncostatic drug, administered during the early organogenetic period in rats. J Toxicol Sci 1989;14:115–30.
3. Leslie KK. Chemotherapy and pregnancy. Clin Obstet Gynecol 2002;45:153–64.
4. Koc ON, McFee M, Reed E, Gerson SL. Detection of platinum–DNA adducts in cord blood lymphocytes following in utero platinum exposure. Eur J Cancer 1994;30A:716–7.
5. Henderson CE, Elia G, Garfinkel D, Poirier MC, Shamkhani H, Runowicz CD. Platinum chemotherapy during pregnancy for serous cystadenocarcinoma of the ovary. Gynecol Oncol 1993;49:92–4.
6. Shamkhani H, Anderson LM, Henderson CE, Moskal TJ, Runowicz CD, Dove LF, Jones AB, Chaney SG, Rice JM, Poirier MC. DNA adducts in human and patas monkey maternal and fetal tissues induced by platinum drug chemotherapy. Reprod Toxicol 1994;8:207–16.
7. Méndez LE, Mueller A, Salom E, González-Quintero VH. Paclitaxel and carboplatin chemotherapy administered during pregnancy for advanced epithelial ovarian cancer. Obstet Gynecol 2003;102:1200–2.

C

8. Hudson CN, Slevin ML, Tebbutt H. Successful pregnancy after treatment of stage III bilateral ovarian dysgerminoma. Br J Obstet Gynaecol 1995;102:1015–6.
9. Lawal AH, Lynch CB. Borderline ovarian cancer, bilateral surgical castration, chemotherapy and a normal delivery after ovum donation and in vitro fertilisation-embryo transfer. Br J Obstet Gynaecol 1996;103:931–2.
10. Schilder JM, Thompson AM, DePriest PD, Ueland FR, Cibull ML, Kryscio RJ, Modesitt SC, Lu KH, Geisler JP, Higgins RV, Magtibay PM, Cohn DE, Powell MA, Chu C, Stehman FB, van Nagell J. Outcome of reproductive age women with stage 1A or 1C invasive epithelial ovarian cancer treated with fertility-sparing therapy. Gynecol Oncol 2002;87:1–7.
11. Chiarelli AM, Marrett LD, Darlington GA. Pregnancy outcomes in females after treatment for childhood cancer. Epidemiology 2000;11:161–6.
12. Seiden MV, Spitzer TR, McAfee S, Fuller AF. Successful pregnancy after high-dose cyclophosphamide, carboplatinum, and Taxol with peripheral blood stem cell transplant in a young woman with ovarian cancer. Gynecol Oncol 2001;83:412–4.
13. Tabata T, Nishiura K, Tanida K, Kondo E, Okugawa Y, Sagawa N. Carboplatin chemotherapy in a pregnant patient with undifferentiated ovarian carcinoma: case report and review of the literature. Int J Gynecol Cancer 2008;18:181–4.
14. Mir O, Berveiller P, Ropert S, Goffinet F, Goidwasser F. Use of platinum derivatives during pregnancy. Cancer 2008;1133069–74.
15. Azim HA Jr, Scarfone G, Peccatori FA. Carboplatin and weekly paclitaxel for the treatment of advanced non-small cell lung cancer (NSCLC) during pregnancy. J Thorac Oncol 2009;4:559–60.
16. Chun KC, Kim DY, Kim JH, Kim YM, Kim YT, Nam JH. Neoadjuvant chemotherapy with paclitaxel plus platinum followed by radical surgery in early cervical cancer during pregnancy: three case reports. Jpn J Clin Oncol 2010;40:694–8.
17. Gottschalk I, Berg C, Harbeck N, Stressiq R, Kozlowski P. Fetal renal insufficiency following trastuzumab treatment for breast cancer in pregnancy: case report and review of the current literature. Breast Cancer (Basel) 2011;6:475–8.
18. Smith ER, Borowsky ME, Jain VD. Intraperitoneal chemotherapy in a pregnant woman with ovarian cancer. Obstet Gynecol 2013;122:481–3.
19. Griffin SJ, Milla M, Baker TE, Liu T, Wang H, Hale TW. Transfer of carboplatin and paclitaxel into breast milk. J Hum Lact 2012;28:457–9.

CARBOPROST

Endocrine/Metabolic Agent (Prostaglandin)

PREGNANCY RECOMMENDATION: Contraindicated (Unless for Termination/Evacuation of Pregnancy)
BREASTFEEDING RECOMMENDATION: No Human Data—Probably Compatible

PREGNANCY SUMMARY

No reports describing the outcomes of human pregnancies following the use of carboprost in failed medical abortions have been located. Carboprost exposure in animals has resulted in embryotoxicity, but the doses were based on body weight and not compared to the human dose. However, another prostaglandin analog, misoprostol, when used unsuccessfully in the 1st trimester as an abortifacient, has been associated with cranial nerve defects in the fetus.

FETAL RISK SUMMARY

Carboprost tromethamine is a synthetic prostaglandin F2α analog that is given IM to stimulate myometrial contractions in the gravid uterus, leading to evacuation of the products of conception. Carboprost is approved for induced abortion between 13 and 20 weeks' gestation. It also is indicated for postpartum uterine bleeding. In pregnant women in the 2nd trimester who were administered carboprost by continuous IV infusion, the elimination half-life of the drug was approximately 30–45 minutes, with similar findings when carboprost was given by IM injection (1).

Reproductive studies have been conducted with carboprost in rats and rabbits. Rabbits were given doses ranging between 0.0025 and 0.5/mg/kg on 3 consecutive days during organogenesis. Doses above 0.025 mg/kg interfered with implantation, were embryolethal, or induced abortion, but no teratogenic effects were seen. In rats, doses ranging from 0.001 to 1.0 mg/kg were given beginning on gestational day 15. Doses larger than 0.025/mg/kg caused abortions. At doses as low as 0.003 mg/kg, abortions or early deliveries occurred and most pups did not survive. There were no effects on structural development of the pups noted (1).

Studies for carcinogenicity have not been conducted with carboprost. No evidence of mutagenicity was observed in various assays. There was no effect on fertility in male and female rats treated with SC injections of 0.25–1.0 mg/kg for 3 or 6 days before breeding (1).

It is not known if carboprost crosses the placenta. The molecular weight (about 489) suggests that the drug will cross the placenta, but the relatively short elimination half-life should limit passage (1).

No reports describing the outcomes of human pregnancies following the use of carboprost in failed medical abortions have been located. Although a failed attempted abortion would typically be followed by completion of the procedure by some other means; in rare cases a woman may wish to maintain the pregnancy. Isolated case reports suggest that the failed procedure(s) themselves may result in damage to the placenta and therefore damage to the fetus (2). First-trimester exposure to another prostaglandin, misoprostol, in failed induced abortion, has been associated with an increased risk for 6th and 7th cranial nerve damage, leading to Möbius syndrome (3). However, in the case of carboprost, if used as indicated, exposure to the product would typically occur after the first trimester.

BREASTFEEDING SUMMARY

No reports describing the use of carboprost during human lactation have been located. The molecular weight of carboprost (about 489) suggests that the agent might cross into breast milk. Based on the elimination half-life, the manufacturer suggests that breastfeeding be avoided for a minimum of 6 hours after the last dose of carboprost (1).

References

1. Product information. Hemabate. Pfizer, 2004, 2006.
2. Arnon J, Ornoy A. Clinical teratology counseling and consultation case report: outcome of pregnancy after failure of early induced abortions. Teratology 1995;52:126–7.
3. Pastuszak AL, Schuler L, Speck-Martins CE, Coehlo KE, Cordello SM, Vargas F, Brunoni D, Schwarz IV, Larrandaburu M, Safattle H, Meloni VF, Koren G. Use of misprostol during pregnancy and Möbius syndrome in infants. N Engl J Med 1998;338:1881–5.

C

CARFILZOMIB

Antineoplastic (Proteasome Inhibitor)

PREGNANCY RECOMMENDATION: Contraindicated
BREASTFEEDING RECOMMENDATION: Contraindicated

PREGNANCY SUMMARY

No reports describing the use of carfilzomib in human pregnancy have been located. The animal data suggest moderate risk, but the absence of human pregnancy experience prevents a more complete assessment of the embryo–fetal risk. The manufacturer states that the drug can cause fetal harm based on its mechanism of action and findings in animals.

FETAL RISK SUMMARY

Carfilzomib is an antineoplastic agent that is given IV on 2 consecutive days each week for 3 weeks, followed by a 12-day rest period before subsequent cycles are given. It is a proteasome inhibitor in the same class as bortezomib. Carfilzomib is indicated for the treatment of patients with multiple myeloma who have received at least two prior therapies, including bortezomib and an immunomodulatory agent, and have demonstrated disease progression on or within 60 days of completion of the last therapy. The drug is rapidly and extensively metabolized to inactive metabolites. Plasma protein binding averaged 97% and the parent drug is cleared from the systemic circulation with a half-life of ≤1 hour (1).

Reproduction studies have been conducted in rats and rabbits. No teratogenicity was observed in rats given doses of 0.5–2 mg/kg/day (comparison to the human dose not specified) during organogenesis. In pregnant rabbits, doses that were ≥20% of the recommended human dose of 27 mg/m^2 based on BSA (RHD) caused an increase in preimplantation loss. At a maternal toxic dose (40% of the RHD), an increase in early resorptions and postimplantation loss and a decrease in fetal weight was observed (1).

Carcinogenicity studies have not been conducted with carfilzomib. The drug was not mutagenic in one assay, but clastogenic effects were observed in one of two assays. Although fertility studies have not been conducted, no effects on reproductive tissues were noted during 28-day repeat-dose toxicity studies in rats and monkeys or in 6-month rat and 9-month monkey chronic toxicity studies (1).

It is not known if carfilzomib crosses the human placenta. The molecular weight (about 720) suggests that the drug will cross the placenta. However, the rapid metabolism to inactive metabolites, high plasma protein binding, and short half-life in the systemic circulation suggest that exposure of the embryo–fetus will be limited.

BREASTFEEDING SUMMARY

No reports describing the use of carfilzomib during human lactation have been located. The molecular weight (about 720) suggests that the drug will be excreted into breast milk. However, the rapid metabolism to inactive metabolites, high plasma protein binding (97%), and short systemic circulation half-life (≤1 hour) in the systemic circulation suggest that exposure of a nursing infant will be limited. The effects of this potential exposure on a nursing infant are unknown. The most common (≥30%) adverse reactions in adults are fatigue, anemia, nausea, thrombocytopenia, dyspnea, diarrhea, and pyrexia. If a woman receiving this drug is nursing, her infant should be closely monitored for these effects.

Reference

1. Product information. Kyprolis. Onyx Pharmaceuticals, 2012.

CARGLUMIC ACID

Endocrine/Metabolic Agent (Hyperammonemia)

PREGNANCY RECOMMENDATION: No Human Data—Animal Data Suggest Moderate Risk
BREASTFEEDING RECOMMENDATION: No Human Data—Potential Toxicity

C

PREGNANCY SUMMARY

No reports describing the use of carglumic acid in human pregnancy have been located. Although the animal data suggested risk when the drug was used from organogenesis through postpartum day 21, a portion of the risk may have reflected exposure during nursing (see Breastfeeding Summary). Women with *N*-acetylglutamate synthase (NAGS) deficiency must remain on treatment throughout pregnancy to prevent irreversible neurologic damage and death. If a pregnant woman does require this therapy, she should be informed of the absence of human pregnancy experience.

FETAL RISK SUMMARY

Carglumic acid is a structural analog of *N*-acetylglutamate available as oral tablets. It is indicated as adjunctive therapy for the treatment of acute and chronic hyperammonemia due to the deficiency of the hepatic co-enzyme NAGS. The agent is partially metabolized in the gut before absorption. Plasma protein binding has not been determined. The median terminal half-life is 5.6 hours (1).

Reproduction studies have been conducted in rats and rabbits. In these species, oral doses up to 1.3 times the maximum recommended human starting dose based on BSA (MRHSD) resulted in maternal toxicity, but no effects on embryo–fetal development were observed. When female rats received doses up to 1.3 times the MRHSD from organogenesis through day 21 postpartum, a reduction in offspring survival was seen at the highest dose and a reduction in offspring growth was seen at all doses (1).

Carcinogenicity studies have not been conducted with carglumic acid, but the drug was not mutagenic in multiple assays. No effects on fertility or reproductive performance were noted in female rats at doses up to 1.3 times the MRHSD, or mating or fertility in male rats at doses up to 0.6 times the MRHSD (1).

It is not known if carglumic acid crosses the human placenta. The molecular weight (about 190) and moderately long terminal half-life suggest that the drug will cross to the embryo–fetus. However, ionization at physiologic pH could limit the exposure.

BREASTFEEDING SUMMARY

No reports describing the use of carglumic acid during human lactation have been located. The molecular weight (about 190) and moderately long terminal half-life (5.6 hours) suggest that the drug will be excreted into breast milk, but ionization at physiologic pH could limit the exposure. The effect of the exposure on a nursing infant is unknown. However, the drug is excreted into rat milk, resulting in increased mortality and impaired body weight gain (1).

Reference

1. Product information. Carbaglu. Accredo Health Group, 2010.

CARISOPRODOL

Muscle Relaxant

PREGNANCY RECOMMENDATION: Limited Human Data—No Relevant Animal Data
BREASTFEEDING RECOMMENDATION: Limited Human Data—Probably Compatible

PREGNANCY SUMMARY

The limited human pregnancy experience with carisoprodol does not suggest a major risk of embryo or fetal harm. The FDA data do raise a hypothesis of an association with oral clefts, but the risk, if it exists, appears to be low. There have been some reports of congenital defects with meprobamate, the active metabolite of carisoprodol, but two large surveillance studies did not support an association between meprobamate and malformations (see Meprobamate). Although the data do not support a significant risk with carisoprodol, the best course would be to avoid this agent, if possible, during the 1st trimester.

FETAL RISK SUMMARY

Carisoprodol is a centrally acting muscle relaxant. It is metabolized by the liver to meprobamate, the active metabolite. The reproductive effects of this drug in animals have not been studied.

It is not known if carisoprodol crosses the human placenta. The molecular weight (about 260) suggests that it will cross to the embryo and fetus. Moreover, the active metabolite, meprobamate, does cross the placenta (see Meprobamate).

The Collaborative Perinatal Project monitored 50,282 mother–child pairs, 14 of whom were exposed in the 1st trimester to carisoprodol (1). No association of the drug with large classes of malformations or to individual defects was found.

In a surveillance study of Michigan Medicaid recipients involving 229,101 completed pregnancies conducted between 1985 and 1992, 326 newborns had been exposed to carisoprodol during the 1st trimester (F. Rosa, personal communication, FDA, 1993). Twenty (6.1%) major birth defects were observed (14 expected), including (observed/expected) 3/3 cardiovascular defects, 2/0.5 oral clefts, and 1/1 hypospadias. No anomalies were observed in three other categories of defects (spina bifida, polydactyly, and limb-reduction defects) for which data were available. Only with the two cases of oral clefts is there a suggestion of a possible association, but other factors, including the mother's disease, concurrent drug use, and chance, may be involved.

A 2001 case report described the pregnancy outcome of a 27-year-old woman who had taken carisoprodol (700 mg), propoxyphene (70 mg), and acetaminophen (900 mg) three times daily throughout gestation and during the first 6 months of breastfeeding (2). The 2635-g infant (sex not specified), delivered 2 weeks preterm by cesarean section, showed no signs or symptoms of withdrawal after birth. No mention was made of birth defects, and the infant was developing normally at 6 months of age (2).

A similar case was observed in 2006 (3). The woman took carisoprodol (700 mg) four times daily before and throughout gestation for severe back muscle spasm. A healthy female infant was delivered at term. The mother continued treatment while breastfeeding during the first postpartum month. No signs or symptoms of withdrawal were noted in the newborn or in the infant when breastfeeding was stopped about 1 month after birth (3).

BREASTFEEDING SUMMARY

Carisoprodol and its active metabolite, meprobamate, are excreted into breast milk at concentrations two to four times those in the maternal plasma (4). While unique, the two cases below confirm that the drug and its metabolite are present in milk and that the concentrations of meprobamate exceed those in the maternal plasma.

A 2001 case report described the use of carisoprodol (700 mg), propoxyphene (70 mg), and acetaminophen (900 mg) three times daily throughout gestation and during the first 6 months of breastfeeding (2). Levels of carisoprodol and meprobamate were measured in breast milk on 4 consecutive days. The average milk concentrations of the two agents were 0.9 mcg/mL and 11.6 mcg/mL, respectively. Neither the timing of the samples in relationship to the maternal dose nor the maternal plasma levels were specified. Based on an estimated milk intake of 150 mL/kg/day, the absolute and relative doses of carisoprodol plus meprobamate that would have been ingested by an exclusively breastfed infant were 1.9 mg/kg/day and 4.1%, respectively. No signs or symptoms of withdrawal were noted in the infant who had normal psychomotor development at 6 months of age. However, the infant was partially fed formula because of insufficient maternal milk production (2).

In a similar case, a woman took carisoprodol (700 mg) four times daily before and throughout gestation, and during the first postpartum month for severe back muscle spasm (3). The healthy female infant was delivered at term and was exclusively breastfed. The mother also took an analgesic combination (hydrocodone plus acetaminophen) for a short period after delivery. Blood and milk samples were obtained from the mother about a week after delivery. Peak carisoprodol and meprobamate blood concentrations, obtained 2 hours post-dose, were 3 and 9 mcg/mL, respectively, whereas the milk concentrations, obtained at the same time, were 1.4 and 10.9 mcg/mL, respectively. The corresponding milk plasma ratios were 0.3 and 1.4, respectively. Trough blood concentrations, obtained about 4 hours postdose, were <2 and <4 mcg/mL, respectively, whereas the milk values were 0.8 and 17.1 mcg/mL, respectively. The corresponding milk:plasma ratios were ≥ 0.4 and ≥ 4.3, respectively. A blood sample from the infant, obtained 2 hours after breastfeeding that was started 1.5 hours after a maternal dose, revealed undetectable levels of carisoprodol (<2 mcg/mL) and meprobamate (<4 mcg/mL). Nursing was stopped at about 1 month of age. No signs or symptoms of withdrawal or other adverse effects were noted in the newborn or when breastfeeding was stopped about 1 month later (3).

Although the human data are very limited, both cases involved mothers taking carisoprodol doses that were much higher than the recommended dose of 1050–1400 mg/day. The lack of detectable adverse effects in both infants suggests that the risk of toxicity is low, at least in infants that also were exposed during pregnancy. Starting carisoprodol treatment during breastfeeding may have different results in a nursing infant. The American Academy of Pediatrics classifies another centrally acting skeletal muscle relaxant as compatible with breastfeeding (see Baclofen). However, until additional data are available, women taking this drug and who elect to nurse should closely monitor their infants for sedation and other changes in behavior or functions.

References

1. Heinonen OP, Slone D, Shapiro S. *Birth Defects and Drugs in Pregnancy*. Littleton, MA: Publishing Sciences Group, 1977:357–65.
2. Nordeng H, Zahlsen K, Spigset O. Transfer of carisoprodol to breast milk. Ther Drug Monit 2001;23:298–300.
3. Briggs GG, Ambrose PJ, Nageotte MP, Padilla G. High-dose carisoprodol during pregnancy and lactation. Ann Pharmacother 2008:42:898–901.
4. Product information. Soma. Wallace Laboratories, 1994.

CARMUSTINE

Antineoplastic

PREGNANCY RECOMMENDATION: Human and Animal Data Suggest Risk
BREASTFEEDING RECOMMENDATION: Contraindicated

C

PREGNANCY SUMMARY

Typical of many chemotherapeutic agents, carmustine is carcinogenic, mutagenic, clastogenic, embryotoxic, and teratogenic in experimental animals. However, only two reports have described the use of carmustine in human pregnancy. In one of these, a woman was treated with carmustine before and during the first two trimesters. She gave birth to a normal infant. In the other case, a woman who was not treated until late in the 2nd trimester was electively delivered prematurely because of her disease. Her infant was growth restricted 17 months after birth but had apparently normal mental and motor development. As with other cancer chemotherapeutic agents, treatment after the 1st trimester does not appear to result in newborn toxicity, although bone marrow suppression has been reported when multiple agents were used close to delivery (e.g., see Cyclophosphamide). Several alkylating agents are thought to be human teratogens (e.g., busulfan, chlorambucil, and cyclophosphamide), but few infants have been exposed to these drugs in the 1st trimester. Until proven otherwise, carmustine should be considered a potential teratogen if used during the period of organogenesis. Therefore, a woman whose condition requires treatment during organogenesis, or who conceives while under treatment, should be informed of the potential risk to her embryo.

FETAL RISK SUMMARY

Carmustine (BCNU) is an alkylating agent that is chemically classified as a nitrosourea. Other antineoplastics in this group include lomustine (CCNU) and streptozocin. Carmustine is indicated for the palliative therapy of certain brain tumors, multiple myeloma, Hodgkin's disease, and non-Hodgkin's lymphoma. The drug alkylates deoxyribonucleic acid (DNA) and ribonucleic acid (RNA), in addition to inhibiting some enzymes by carbamoylation of amino acids in proteins. Carmustine undergoes rapid degradation in the plasma with a terminal half-life of 22 minutes after an IV dose. The antineoplastic and toxic properties of carmustine are thought to be secondary to metabolites. The most severe toxicities are delayed bone marrow suppression and pulmonary toxicity (1,2).

Carmustine is carcinogenic in mice and rats at doses less than the recommended human dose based on BSA (RHD). The agent was mutagenic in in vitro assays and clastogenic in both in vivo and in vitro tests (2). Reproduction studies have been conducted with carmustine in pregnant rats and rabbits (1,2). A dose about 0.17 times the RHD in rats caused embryotoxicity and fetal malformations (anophthalmia, micrognathia, and omphalocele). In rabbits, increased embryolethality was observed at approximately 1.2 times the RHD (1,2). In another animal study, pregnant rats were given an intraperitoneal dose of 20 mg/kg on embryonic day 15 (3). (*Note: This dose is approximately 3.4 times the RHD.*) Exposed offspring had histologic alterations suggestive of cortical dysplasia (laminar disorganization, cytomegalic neurons, and neuronal heterotopias). Of interest, cortical dysplasia is associated with epilepsy in children and adults (3).

It is not known if carmustine or its metabolites crosses the placenta. The molecular weight (about 214) is low enough that exposure of the embryo or fetus should be expected. Two characteristics of carmustine, its high lipid solubility and its relatively lack of ionization at physiologic pH, will promote transfer of the drug across the placenta. The very short plasma half-life may lessen the transfer of the parent drug, but the pharmacology and pharmacokinetics of the active metabolites have not been fully elucidated.

A 1984 report described a 21-year-old woman with diffuse histiocytic lymphoma who received carmustine and procarbazine for 5 months before conception and throughout the first 24 weeks of pregnancy (4). A second nitrosourea agent, streptozocin, replaced carmustine and procarbazine in the 2nd trimester. Before pregnancy, the patient had received multiple courses of chemotherapy, including cyclophosphamide, doxorubicin, vincristine, bleomycin, methotrexate, cytarabine, and etoposide, in addition to radiation therapy to the neck. Because of the failure of the previous therapy, she was started on carmustine 110 mg IV on day 1 and procarbazine 100 mg orally for 10 days every 4 weeks. She conceived after five monthly cycles of this latter therapy. The woman refused pregnancy termination and received five more cycles of therapy at 4-week intervals starting at 4 weeks' gestation. Three courses of streptozocin, 800 mg IV for 3 days every 4 weeks, were started at 24 weeks' gestation because of disease progression. She received the last dose of streptozocin 2 weeks before delivery at 35 weeks' gestation. The woman's normal- appearing male infant weighed 2.34 kg with a head circumference of 32.5 cm and a length of 51.5 cm. The Apgar scores were 7 and 9 at 1 and 5 minutes, respectively. The initial blood test revealed a normal hemoglobin, white blood cell and platelet counts. All other clinical tests were within normal limits, including electrolytes, multiple chemistry, urinalysis, renal ultrasound, and chromosome studies (4).

In a second case report, a 27-year-old woman with a history of malignant melanoma was admitted to the hospital at 14 weeks' gestation for progressive weight loss and persistent headache (5). Approximately 9 months earlier an enlarged nevus had been removed from her left shoulder and the pathology had revealed the melanoma. The work-up for metastatic disease was negative and she was discharged home. Two months later, the woman was readmitted for severe back pain, which was attributed to diffuse metastatic disease of the spine. At 23 weeks' gestation, she was started on chemotherapy consisting of carmustine 150 mg/m^2 IV on day 1, tamoxifen 80 mg orally twice daily for 7 days, cisplatin 25 mg/m^2 IV on days 1 to 3, and dacarbazine 220 mg/m^2 on days 1 to 3. Approximately 3 weeks later, she received a second course of these agents. Corticosteroids were administered for fetal lung maturity and as an antiemetic for chemotherapy. Because the woman continued to deteriorate, a 1520-g female infant was delivered by cesarean section at 30 weeks' gestation. The 325-g placenta had malignant melanoma in the intervillous space and melanin pigment granules in villous Hofbauer cells and syncytial trophoblasts. The mother died 1 month later. At 17 months of age the child's weight was 6.6 kg (5th percentile), length 74.5 cm

(<5th percentile), and head circumference 47 cm (10th percentile). Examination revealed age-appropriate evaluations for mental age, motor age, and language scores (5).

A number of reports have described pregnancy outcomes after the use of carmustine before conception (6–11). In four studies, the outcomes of 16 pregnancies (12 women) were 14 normal newborns, one stillbirth (twins), and one elective abortion (6–9). In one case, a man treated earlier with carmustine fathered a normal infant (7). A 2000 study analyzed the pregnancy outcomes of 340 cancer survivors who had one or more pregnancies after treatment with carmustine and 11 other alkylating agents (10). The cases were divided into five mutually exclusive treatment groups: nonsterilizing surgery, chemotherapy with alkylating agents, abdominal–pelvic radiation, alkylating agents plus abdominal–pelvic radiation, and all other treatments. The study found no evidence of an increased risk of birth defects or spontaneous abortions (10). In a 2002 study, 1915 women had 4029 pregnancies after chemotherapy with or without radiation (11). No statistical differences in pregnancy outcomes (live births and spontaneous abortions) by treatment group were found, including the 126 pregnancies in women treated with carmustine.

BREASTFEEDING SUMMARY

No reports describing the use of carmustine during lactation have been located. The low molecular weight (about 214), high lipid solubility, and relative lack of ionization at physiologic pH suggest that carmustine will be excreted into breast milk. The short elimination half-life in the plasma may limit the amount of parent drug in milk, but the pharmacology and pharmacokinetics of the active metabolites have not been adequately characterized. Because there is substantial risk of harm for a nursing infant, women who are being treated with carmustine should not nurse.

References

1. Product information. BiCNU. Bristol-Myers Squibb, 1998.
2. Product information. Gliadel Wafer. Guilford Pharmaceuticals, 2003.
3. Benardete EA, Kriegstein AR. Increase excitability and decreased sensitivity to GABA in an animal model of dysplastic cortex. Epilepsia 2002;43:970–82.
4. Schapira DV, Chudley AE. Successful pregnancy following continuous treatment with combination chemotherapy before conception and throughout pregnancy. Cancer 1984;54:800–3.
5. DiPaola RS, Goodin S, Ratzell M, Florczyk M, Karp G, Ravikumar TS. Chemotherapy for metastatic melanoma during pregnancy. Gynecol Oncol 1997;66:526–30.
6. Blatt J, Mulvihill JJ, Ziegler JL, Young RC, Poplack DG. Pregnancy outcome following cancer chemotherapy. Am J Med 1980;69:828–32.
7. Green DM, Zevon MA, Lowrie G, Seigelstein N, Hall B. Congenital anomalies in children of patients who received chemotherapy for cancer in childhood and adolescence. N Engl J Med 1991;325:141–6.
8. Bierman PJ, Bagin RG, Jagannath S, Vose JM, Spitzer G, Kessinger A, Dicke KA, Armitage JO. High dose chemotherapy followed by autologous hematopoietic rescue in Hodgkin's disease: long-term follow-up in 128 patients. Ann Oncol 1993;4:767–73.
9. Brice P, Pautier P, Marolleau JP, Castaigne S, Gisselbrecht C. Pregnancy after autologous bone marrow transplantation for malignant lymphomas. Nouv Rev Fr Hematol 1994;36:387–8.
10. Chiarelli AM, Marrett LD, Darlington GA. Pregnancy outcomes in females after treatment for childhood cancer. Epidemiology 2000;11:161–6.
11. Green DM, Whitton JA, Stovall M, Mertens AC, Donaldson SS, Ruymann FB, Pendergrass TW, Robison LL. Pregnancy outcome of female survivors of childhood cancer: a report from the Childhood Cancer Survivor study. Am J Obstet Gynecol 2002;187:1070–80.

CARPHENAZINE

[Withdrawn from the market. See 8th edition.]

CARTEOLOL

Sympatholytic (Antihypertensive)

PREGNANCY RECOMMENDATION: Human Data Suggest Risk in 2nd and 3rd Trimesters
BREASTFEEDING RECOMMENDATION: No Human Data—Potential Toxicity

PREGNANCY SUMMARY

No studies describing the use of carteolol in human pregnancies have been located. If used near delivery, the newborn infant should be closely observed for 24–48 hours for signs and symptoms of β-blockade. Long-term effects of in utero exposure to β-blockers have not been studied but warrant evaluation. Some β-blockers may cause intrauterine growth restriction (IUGR) and reduced placental weight, especially those lacking intrinsic sympathomimetic activity (ISA) (i.e., partial agonist). Treatment beginning early in the 2nd trimester results in the greatest weight reductions, whereas treatment restricted to the 3rd trimester primarily affects only placental weight. Carteolol does possess ISA. However, IUGR and reduced placental weight may potentially occur with all agents within this class. Although growth restriction is a serious concern, the benefits of maternal therapy with β-blockers, in some cases, might outweigh the risks to the fetus and must be judged on a case-by-case basis.

C

FETAL RISK SUMMARY

Carteolol is a nonselective β_1/β_2-adrenergic blocking agent used in the treatment of hypertension and topically in the therapy of glaucoma. No teratogenic effects were observed in pregnant mice and rabbits treated with doses much higher than the maximum recommended human dose (1–3). A dose-related increase in the incidence of wavy ribs was noted in fetal rats whose mothers were given doses 212 times the maximum recommended human dose (MRHD) (3). Fetotoxicity (increased resorptions and decreased fetal weight) was observed in rats and rabbits at doses up to 5264 and 1052 times the MRHD (3). These effects were not noted in mice at doses up to 1052 times the MRHD (3).

BREASTFEEDING SUMMARY

No reports describing the use of carteolol during human lactation have been located. If carteolol is used during nursing, the infant should be closely observed for hypotension, bradycardia, and other signs or symptoms of β-blockade. Long-term effects of exposure to β-blockers from milk have not been studied but warrant evaluation.

References

1. Tanaka N, Shingai F, Tamagawa M, Nakatsu I. Reproductive study of carteolol hydrochloride in mice, part 1. Fertility and reproductive performance. J Toxicol Sci 1979;4:47–58. As cited in Shepard TH. *Catalog of Teratogenic Agents*. 6th ed. Baltimore, MD: Johns Hopkins University Press, 1989:119.
2. Tamagawa, M, Namoto T, Tanaka N, Hishino H. Reproduction study of carteolol hydrochloride in mice, part 2. Perinatal and postnatal toxicity. J Toxicol Sci 1979;4:59–78. As cited in Shepard TH. *Catalog of Teratogenic Agents*. 6th ed. Baltimore, MD: Johns Hopkins University Press, 1989:119.
3. Product information. Cartrol. Abbott Laboratories, 1997.

CARVEDILOL

Sympatholytic (Antihypertensive)

PREGNANCY RECOMMENDATION: Human Data Suggest Risk in 2nd and 3rd Trimesters
BREASTFEEDING RECOMMENDATION: No Human Data—Probably Compatible

PREGNANCY SUMMARY

Only one report describing the use of carvedilol in human pregnancy has been located. The animal data and the experience with other, similar agents, suggest that the risk of teratogenicity is low. Intrauterine growth restriction (IUGR), however, has been reported in the case below and is known to occur with other α/β-blockers (see Labetalol). Moreover, some β-blockers have caused IUGR and reduced placental weight, especially those lacking intrinsic sympathomimetic activity (ISA) (i.e., partial agonist). Treatment beginning early in the 2nd trimester results in the greatest weight reductions, whereas treatment restricted to the 3rd trimester primarily affects only placental weight. Carvedilol does not possess ISA. IUGR and reduced placental weight may potentially occur with all agents within this class. Although growth restriction is a serious concern, the benefits of maternal therapy with carvedilol (or other α/β-blockers), in some cases, might outweigh the risks to the fetus and must be judged on a case-by-case basis.

FETAL RISK SUMMARY

Carvedilol is a combined α/β-adrenergic blocking agent that is used for the treatment of hypertension and mild-to-moderate heart failure. The α_1-adrenoreceptor blocking activity has been associated with vasodilation and a reduction in peripheral vascular resistance. Carvedilol is extensively metabolized and some of the metabolites are weakly active. Plasma protein binding, primarily to albumin, is >98% and the mean terminal elimination half-life of the parent compound is 7–10 hours (1).

Reproduction studies in rats and rabbits at 50 and 25 times the maximum recommended human dose based on BSA (MRHD), respectively, revealed postimplantation loss in both species. The dose in rats, which was maternal toxic, was also associated with a decrease in fetal weight and an increase in frequency of fetuses with delayed skeletal development (missing or stunted 13th rib). Increased pup mortality at 1 week postpartum was observed when pregnant rats were treated with carvedilol at ≥10 times the MRHD during the last trimester and continued through day 22 of lactation. The no-observed-effect-level (NOEL) for developmental toxicity was 10 times the MRHD for rats and 5 times the MRHD for rabbits. Toxicity (sedation, reduced weight gain) and impaired fertility were observed in adult rats at ≥32 times the MRHD, including a reduced number of successful matings, prolonged mating time, fewer implants per dam, and complete resorption of 18% of the litters. The drug and/or its metabolites cross the rat placenta (1).

It is not known if carvedilol crosses the human placenta. The molecular weight (about 407) and long terminal elimination half-life suggest that exposure of the embryo–fetus probably occurs. However, the high plasma protein binding should limit the amount crossing the placenta.

In a 2002 case report, a woman with chronic hypertension presented at about 24 weeks' gestation with severe oligohydramnios (amniotic fluid index <2) (2). Her medications included benazepril, carvedilol, amiodarone, and furosemide. The fetus had a misshapen cranium with overlapping sutures, pericardial effusion, small bladder, echogenic focus in the heart, echogenic bowel, and normal-appearing kidneys. All the drugs except carvedilol were discontinued. An examination 18 days later revealed normal amniotic fluid volume and normal cranial anatomy. At about 37 weeks' gestation, she gave birth to a 2060 g (<3rd percentile) female infant with Apgar scores of 7 and 9 at 1 and 5 minutes, respectively. The infant's initial physical examination was normal. Except for bilious vomiting on day 1, which resolved by day 2, the infant's hospital course was normal. At 1 year of age, the infant was healthy and weighed 18 lbs (5th percentile) (2).

BREASTFEEDING SUMMARY

No reports describing the use of carvedilol during human lactation have been located. The molecular weight (about 407) and long terminal elimination half-life (7–10 hours) suggest that the drug will be excreted into breast milk, but the high plasma protein binding (>98%) should limit the amount. The potential effects of this exposure on a nursing infant include bradycardia, hypotension, and other symptoms of α/β-blockade. However, a similar agent is classified by the American Academy of Pediatrics as compatible with breastfeeding (see Labetalol).

References

1. Product information. Coreg. GlaxoSmithKline, 2009.
2. Muller PR, James A. Pregnancy with prolonged fetal exposure to an angiotensin-converting enzyme inhibitor. J Perinatol 2002;22:582–4.

CASANTHRANOL

Purgative

PREGNANCY RECOMMENDATION: Compatible
BREASTFEEDING RECOMMENDATION: No Human Data—Probably Compatible

PREGNANCY SUMMARY

Casanthranol is an anthraquinone purgative. Although the data are limited, there is no evidence that drugs in this class pose a risk to the embryo–fetus.

FETAL RISK SUMMARY

In a large prospective study, 109 patients were exposed to this agent during pregnancy, 21 in the 1st trimester (1). No evidence of an increased risk for malformations was found (see also Cascara Sagrada).

In a surveillance study of Michigan Medicaid recipients involving 229,101 completed pregnancies conducted between 1985 and 1992, 96 newborns had been exposed to casanthranol during the 1st trimester (F. Rosa, personal communication, FDA, 1993). Four (4.2%) (four expected) major birth defects were observed. Specific data were available for six defect categories, including (observed/expected) 2/1 cardiovascular defects, 1/0 spina bifida, and 1/0.5 polydactyly. No anomalies were observed in the other three categories (oral clefts, limb-reduction defects, and hypospadias. These data do not support an association between the drug and congenital defects.

BREASTFEEDING SUMMARY

No reports describing the use of casanthranol during human lactation have been located. Although diarrhea in a nursing infant is a potential effect, the drug is probably compatible with breastfeeding. (See also Cascara Sagrada.)

Reference

1. Heinonen OP, Slone D, Shapiro S. *Birth Defects and Drugs in Pregnancy*. Littleton, MA: Publishing Sciences Group, 1977:384–7, 442.

CASCARA SAGRADA

Purgative

PREGNANCY RECOMMENDATION: Limited Human Data—Probably Compatible
BREASTFEEDING RECOMMENDATION: Limited Human Data—Probably Compatible

PREGNANCY SUMMARY

Cascara sagrada is an anthraquinone purgative. Although the data are limited, there is no evidence that drugs in this class pose a risk to the embryo–fetus.

C

FETAL RISK SUMMARY

In a large prospective study, 53 mother–child pairs were exposed to cascara sagrada during the 1st trimester (1, pp. 384–387). Although the numbers are small, no evidence for an increased risk of malformations was found. For anytime use during pregnancy, 188 exposures were recorded (1, pp. 438, 442, 497). The relative risk for benign tumors was higher than expected, but independent confirmation is required (1, pp. 438, 442, 497).

A 1977 study found that more than 50% of the women taking laxatives during pregnancy had taken a laxative of the anthraquinone type (2). Danthron (1:8 dihydroxyanthraquinone) was administered to nine women shortly before induction of labor. Presence of the laxative and/or its metabolite was documented in the amniotic fluid and in the urine of the newborns. No fetal adverse effects were noted (2).

BREASTFEEDING SUMMARY

Most reviewers acknowledge the presence of anthraquinones (e.g., cascara and danthron) in breast milk and warn of the consequences for the nursing infant (3–5). A comprehensive review described the excretion of laxatives into human milk, but little is known about the presence of these agents in breast milk (6). Two reports suggest an increased incidence of diarrhea in infants when nursing mothers are given cascara sagrada or senna for postpartum constipation (7,8). However, the American Academy of Pediatrics classifies cascara and danthron as compatible with breastfeeding (9).

References

1. Heinonen OP, Slone D, Shapiro S. *Birth Defects and Drugs in Pregnancy*. Littleton, MA: Publishing Sciences Group, 1977.
2. Blair AW, Burdon M, Powell J, Gerrard M, Smith R. Fetal exposure to 1:8 dihydroxyanthraquinone. Biol Neonate 1977;31:289–93.
3. Knowles JA. Breast milk: a source of more than nutrition for the neonate. Clin Toxicol 1974;7:69–82.
4. O'Brien TE. Excretion of drugs in human milk. Am J Hosp Pharm 1974;31:844–54.
5. Edwards A. Drugs in breast milk—a review of the recent literature. Aust J Hosp Pharm 1981;11:27–39.
6. Stewart JJ. Gastrointestinal drugs. In: Wilson JT, ed. *Drugs in Breast Milk*. Balgowlah, Australia: ADIS Press, 1981:65–71.
7. Tyson RM, Shrader EA, Perlman HH. Drugs transmitted through breast milk. Part I. Laxatives. J Pediatr 1937;11:824–32.
8. Greenleaf JO, Leonard HSD. Laxatives in the treatment of constipation in pregnant and breast-feeding mothers. Practitioner 1973;210:259–63.
9. Committee on Drugs, American Academy of Pediatrics. The transfer of drugs and other chemicals into human milk. Pediatrics 2001;108:776–89.

CASPOFUNGIN

Antifungal

PREGNANCY RECOMMENDATION: No Human Data—Animal Data Suggest Risk
BREASTFEEDING RECOMMENDATION: No Human Data—Probably Compatible

PREGNANCY SUMMARY

No reports describing the use of caspofungin in human pregnancy have been located. A 2003 review of antifungal agents was also unable to find such reports (1). The animal data are suggestive of human risk, especially if exposure occurs in the 1st trimester. However, the absence of human pregnancy experience prevents an assessment of the embryo–fetal risk. If indicated, maternal treatment should be avoided in the 1st trimester, if possible.

FETAL RISK SUMMARY

Caspofungin inhibits the synthesis of glucan, an integral component of the fungal cell wall, and is the first antifungal agent in this class. It is a semisynthetic lipopeptide (echinocandin) compound that is synthesized from a fermentation product of the fungus *Glarea lozoyenis*. Caspofungin is approved for the treatment of *Candida* infections and for invasive aspergillosis in patients who cannot be treated with other antifungals. Caspofungin is extensively bound to albumin (about 97%). Plasma clearance of caspofungin is primarily from distribution, rather than by excretion or by metabolism. The γ-phase half-life is 40–50 hours (2).

Reproduction studies have been conducted in rats and rabbits. In rats, doses producing exposures similar to those obtained in humans treated with a 70-mg dose (HE) were embryotoxic, resulting in increased resorptions and peri-implantation losses. Other effects included incomplete ossification of the skull and torso and an increased incidence of cervical ribs. The agent was also embryotoxic in rabbits, causing increased resorptions at doses similar to the HE. In addition, incomplete ossifications of the talus/calcaneus were observed in rabbits (2).

Caspofungin crosses the placenta in rats and rabbits (gestational age not specified) and the drug could be detected in fetal plasma (2). It is not known if the agent crosses the human placenta. The molecular weight (about 1213 for the acetate salt) and extensive plasma protein binding should limit the amount crossing the placenta, but the long β-phase half-life should provide substantial amounts of the drug available for transfer.

BREASTFEEDING SUMMARY

No reports describing the use of caspofungin during human lactation have been located. The high molecular weight (about 1213 for the acetate salt) and extensive plasma protein binding (about 97%) should limit the amount of drug excreted in breast milk, but the long γ-phase half-life may allow for some drug in the milk. The effect of this exposure on a nursing infant is unknown. However, other drugs from different classes of antifungal agents, such as fluconazole and ketoconazole, are classified as compatible with breastfeeding by the American Academy of Pediatrics (see Fluconazole and Ketoconazole). The risk of harm from exposure to caspofungin also appears to be low, and women being treated with caspofungin should be allowed to breastfeed. Their infants should be monitored for signs and symptoms of histamine release (e.g., rash, facial swelling, and pruritus) and gastrointestinal complaints.

References

1. Moudgal VV, Sobel JD. Antifungal drugs in pregnancy: a review. Expert Opin Drug Saf 2003;2:475–83.
2. Product information. Cancidas. Merck, 2004.

CASTOR OIL

Laxative/Oxytocic

PREGNANCY RECOMMENDATION: Human Data Suggest Risk
BREASTFEEDING RECOMMENDATION: No Human Data—Potential Toxicity

PREGNANCY SUMMARY

Castor oil has been used since ancient times to induce labor. Nevertheless, neither the efficacy for this indication nor the fetal/newborn safety has been documented. One study found that the drug had no value to labor induction (1). Castor oil can cause severe maternal morbidity and possibly mortality, but this toxicity appears to be rare. However, maternal nausea and diarrhea appear to be very common, although underreported. The mechanism of castor oil's oxytocic effect is unknown, but might be due to systemically absorbed ricinoleic acid stimulating uterine contractions. In recent times, the use of castor oil as an oxytocic agent has declined, probably because of the availability of safer and more physiologic agents, such as oxytocin and the two prostaglandins: dinoprostone and misoprostol. Although the report of multiple congenital defects attributed to castor beans early in gestation requires confirmation, castor beans should be avoided in pregnancy. As for castor oil, the limited human data offer no documented benefits for the mother or fetus. Uterine bleeding and abortion are potential toxicities. Thus, the use of castor oil as a laxative or for other purposes before term pregnancy should be avoided. Use at term should only be on the advice of a healthcare provider.

FETAL RISK SUMMARY

Castor, *Ricinus communis*, is an ornamental plant native to the West Indies, but now grows in the United States and Hawaii (2). Castor oil is cold expressed from castor beans (i.e., seeds) and contains a mixture of triglycerides. The principal compound is ricinoleic acid with smaller amounts of linoleic, oleic, pamitic, and stearic acids. The oil also contains toxins, such as ricin and ricinine, that are removed with further processing (2). Upon ingestion, castor oil is hydrolyzed in the duodenum by pancreatic lipase to release glycerol and the active ingredient, ricinoleic acid (3,4). Castor seeds contain ricin and can cause poisoning (3). Castor oil has been used for the induction of labor, and as a cathartic, contraceptive cream, lubricant, and skin emollient (2,3). It also has been combined with quinine to induce labor at term and topically as a contraceptive and abortifacient (3).

A 1983 report described an infant with growth restriction, convulsions, craniofacial dysmorphia, absent deformity of limbs, and vertebral segmentation defect that was born from a 20-year-old mother (5). The mother had taken a castor oilseed, once per month, as a contraceptive for 3 months before conception and during the first 2 months of gestation. No other drugs were taken during pregnancy. Because ricin is a potent toxin, the authors attributed the defects to the castor oilseeds (4). Of interest, a 2002 review stated (without specific reference) that castor bean had emmenagogue and abortifacient effects (6).

Castor oil has been used since ancient Egypt to induce labor (1,2,7–15). A 1958 study evaluated the efficacy of castor oil for the induction of labor (1). In the first part of the study, the investigator polled obstetric department heads of 50 medical schools. Of the 32 who responded, 16 never used castor oil for labor induction, whereas 16 used it some times. A retrospective review of 114 consecutive inductions (1952–1954) was conducted at the investigator's institution. All of the inductions involved rupture of membranes and oxytocin. The group was divided into four subgroups: rupture of membranes and oxytocin ($N = 24$), added enema ($N = 27$), added castor oil ($N = 31$), and added castor oil and enema ($N = 32$). The average induction times for the four groups were 4, 2, 4, and 4 hours, respectively. The 18 induction failures were nearly equal in the groups: 5, 5, 3, and 5, respectively. These results convinced the investigator that castor oil had no value in the induction of labor (1).

The uterine activity effect of castor oil, soap enema, hot bath, or a combination of all three was described in 60 women at 38–41 weeks' gestation in a 1959 study (7). Castor oil plus soap enema had the most marked effect, but most of the increased activity was due to castor oil. A hot bath had little effect. The effects on delivery times, induction failure, and pregnancy outcomes were not provided. Nevertheless, based solely on uterine activity, the investigators concluded that labor induction with castor oil, with or without soap enema, was useful (7).

C

A 1999 survey found that among 90 nurse-midwives who used herbal products for labor induction, castor oil (93%) was most the common (8). The doses used ranged from 5 to 120 mL. The mechanism of the oxytocic effect is unknown, but various authors have stated that it is secondary to intestinal peristalsis or an increase in the concentrations of prostaglandin E (9,10,12). However, a brief 2002 report stated that the oxytocic effect was due to systemically absorbed ricinoleic acid that caused contractions of the uterine musculature (13). Nausea is a very common adverse effect, as is diarrhea after delivery. The use of castor oil does not appear to directly affect the fetus or the Apgar scores at birth, but most reports fail to mention the condition of the newborn. Two reviews concluded that there is insufficient evidence to support the use of castor oil as an induction agent (14,15).

A 1987 study reported an increase in meconium staining of the amniotic fluid in women given castor oil for labor induction compared with controls (16). Meconium staining occurred in 4 (2.3%) of 174 women given castor oil compared with 0 of the 304 controls ($p < 0.1$). Although the authors deemed the result significant, the difference might not have been if the standard p value of < 0.05 has been used. In another report, 10.4% of women receiving castor oil had meconium-stained amniotic fluid compared with 11.5% of controls (*ns*) (12).

A case report describing amniotic fluid embolism associated temporally with castor oil was published in 1988 (17). A 33-year-old woman at 40 weeks' gestation with an uncomplicated pregnancy and unremarkable medical history ingested 30 mL castor oil for labor induction. About 60 minutes later, spontaneous rupture of membranes occurred, followed by cardiorespiratory arrest. A dead fetus, with no observable abnormalities, was delivered, along with a normal placenta, in the intensive care unit. Maternal blood contained fetal squamous cells and amniotic fluid debris. The clinical course was complicated by seizures and findings consistent with disseminated intravascular coagulation. EEG findings were consistent with anoxic encephalopathy. At the time of the report, the woman remained in a persistent vegetative state (17).

A 2003 case report described uterine rupture in a 39-year-old woman at 39 weeks' gestation (18). The woman experienced a brief bowel movement, followed by severe abdominal pain and rupture of membranes shortly after ingesting castor oil 5 mL for labor induction. A repeat cesarean section, performed for fetal distress and a closed, long cervix, revealed a portion of the umbilical cord protruding from a 2-cm rupture of the lower transverse scar. A female 2724-g female infant was delivered with Apgar scores of 9 at 1 and 5 minutes (18).

An unusual use of castor oil in pregnancy was briefly reported in 1967 (19). Castor oil was applied to the cervical os to facilitate vaginal delivery. The author noted that the use of oil to lubricate the vagina and os during labor was common among midwives in his region.

BREASTFEEDING SUMMARY

No reports describing the use of castor oil during lactation have been located. Castor oil has been used orally to promote the flow of breast milk (2). Evidence for this effect has not been located. The principal active ingredient, ricinoleic acid, is absorbed systemically and could be excreted into milk. Diarrhea in the nursing infant is a potential complication. In a rural region of India, newborn infants are sometimes given castor oil for its laxative properties in the belief that it will clean the intestine of meconium (20). However, this practice has been discouraged because it can be dangerous for the infant, at times causing paralytic ileus and aspiration pneumonia (20).

References

1. Nabors GG. Castor oil as an adjunct to induction of labor: critical re-evaluation. Am J Obstet Gynecol 1958;75:36–8.
2. Castor. *The Review of Natural Products. Facts and Comparisons*. St. Louis, MO: Wolters Kluwer Health, 2007.
3. Castor Oil. Castor Seed. *Natural Medicines Comprehensive Database*. 5th ed. Stockton, CA: Therapeutic Research Faculty, 2003:296–7, 298–9.
4. Gattuso JM, Kamm MA. Adverse effects of drugs used in the management of constipation and diarrhoea. Drug Saf 1994;10:47–65.
5. Mauhoub ME, Khalifa MM, Jaswal OB, Garrah MS. "Ricin syndrome." A possible new teratogenic syndrome associated with ingestion of castor oil seed in early pregnancy: a case report. Ann Trop Paediatr 1983;3: 57–61.
6. Ernst E. Herbal medicinal products during pregnancy: are they safe? Br J Obstet Gynaecol 2002;109:227–35.
7. Mathie JG, Dawson BH. Effect of castor oil, soap enema, and hot bath on the pregnant human uterus near term: a tocographic study. Br Med J 1959;1:1162–5.
8. McFarlin BL, Gibson MH, O'Rear J, Harman P. A national survey of herbal preparation use by nurse-midwives for labor stimulation. J Nurse-Midwifery 1999;44:205–16.
9. Davis L. The use of castor oil to stimulate labor in patients with premature rupture of membranes. J Nurse Midwifery 1984;29:366–70.
10. Harris M, Nye M. Self-administration of castor oil. Mod Midwife 1994;4: 29–30.
11. Summers L. Methods of cervical ripening and labor induction. J Nurse Midwifery 1997;42:71–85.
12. Garry D, Figueroa R, Guillaume J, Cucco V. Use of castor oil in pregnancies at term. Altern Ther Health Med 2000;6:77–9.
13. Lippert TH, Mueck AO. Labour induction with alternative drugs? J Obstet Gynaecol 2002;22:343.
14. Kelly AJ, Kavanagh J, Thomas J. Castor oil, bath and/or enema for cervical priming and induction of labour. Cochrane Database Syst Rev 2002;(2):Art. No: CD003099. doi:10.1002/14651858.CD003099.
15. Tenore JL. Methods for cervical ripening and induction of labor. Am Fam Physician 2003;67:2123–8.
16. Mitri F, Hofmeyr GJ, Van Gelderen CJ. Meconium during labor—self-medication and other associations. S Afr Med J 1987;71:431–3.
17. Steingrub JS, Lopez T, Teres D, Steingart R. Amniotic fluid embolism associated with castor oil ingestion. Crit Care Med 1988;16:642–3.
18. Sicuranza GB, Figueroa R. Uterine rupture associated with castor oil ingestion. J Matern Fetal Neonatal Med 2003;13:133–4.
19. Tendulkar S. Local lubrication in labour. Indian Med J 1967;61:176.
20. Benakappa DG, Shivananda MR, Benakappa AD. Breast-feeding practices in rural Karnataka (India) with special reference to lactation failure. Acta Peadiatr Jpn 1989;31:391–8.

CEFACLOR

Antibiotic (Cephalosporin)

PREGNANCY RECOMMENDATION: Compatible
BREASTFEEDING RECOMMENDATION: Compatible

PREGNANCY SUMMARY

No detectable teratogenic risk with cefaclor and other cephalosporin antibiotics was found in a large 2001 study (see Cephalexin).

C

FETAL RISK SUMMARY

Cefaclor is an oral, semisynthetic cephalosporin antibiotic. Reproduction studies in mice, rats, and ferrets found no evidence of impaired fertility or fetal harm at doses up to 12, 12, and 3 times, respectively, the human dose (1). Cephalosporins are usually considered safe to use during pregnancy (see other cephalosporins for published human experience).

In a surveillance study of Michigan Medicaid recipients involving 229,101 completed pregnancies conducted between 1985 and 1992, 1325 newborns had been exposed to the antibiotic during the 1st trimester (F. Rosa, personal communication, FDA, 1993). A total of 75 (5.7%) major birth defects were observed (56 expected). Specific data were available for six defect categories, including (observed/expected) 19/13 cardiovascular defects, 8/2 oral clefts, 1/0.7 spina bifida, 1/4 polydactyly, 2/2 limb reduction defects, and 3/3 hypospadias. The data for all defects, cardiovascular defects, and oral clefts are suggestive of an association between cefaclor and congenital defects, but other factors, such as the mother's disease, may be involved. However, similar findings were measured for another cephalosporin antibiotic with more than a thousand exposures (see Cephalexin). Positive results were also suggested for cephradine (339 exposures) but not for cefadroxil (722 exposures) (see Cephradine and Cefadroxil). In contrast, other anti-infectives with large cohorts (see Ampicillin, Amoxicillin, Penicillin G, Erythromycin, and Tetracycline) were not associated with congenital defects.

BREASTFEEDING SUMMARY

Cefaclor is excreted into breast milk in low concentrations. Following a single 500-mg oral dose, average milk levels ranged from 0.16 to 0.21 mcg/mL during a 5-hour period (2). Only trace amounts of the antibiotic could be measured at 1 and 6 hours. Even though these levels are low, three potential problems exist for the nursing infant: modification of bowel flora, direct effects on the infant, and interference with the interpretation of culture results if a fever workup is required.

In a 1993 cohort study, diarrhea was reported in 32 (19.3%) nursing infants of 166 breastfeeding mothers who were taking antibiotics (3). For the five women taking cefaclor, diarrhea was observed in 1 (20%) infants. The diarrhea was considered minor because it did not require medical attention (3).

Although not specifically listing cefaclor, the American Academy of Pediatrics classifies other cephalosporin antibiotics as compatible with breastfeeding (e.g., see Cefadroxil and Cefazolin).

References

1. Product information. Ceclor. Eli Lilly and Company, 1997.
2. Takase Z, Shirafuji H, Uchida M. Clinical and laboratory studies of cefaclor in the field of obstetrics and gynecology. Chemotherapy (Tokyo) 1979;27(Suppl):666–72.
3. Ito S, Blajchman A, Stephenson M, Eliopoulos C, Koren G. Prospective follow-up of adverse reactions in breast-fed infants exposed to maternal medication. Am J Obstet Gynecol 1993;168:1393–9.

CEFADROXIL

Antibiotic (Cephalosporin)

PREGNANCY RECOMMENDATION: Compatible
BREASTFEEDING RECOMMENDATION: Compatible

PREGNANCY SUMMARY

No detectable teratogenic risk with cephalosporin antibiotics was found in a large 2001 study (see Cephalexin).

FETAL RISK SUMMARY

Cefadroxil is an oral, semisynthetic cephalosporin antibiotic. Reproduction studies in mice and rats found no evidence of impaired fertility or fetal harm at doses up to 11 times the human dose (1). Cephalosporins are usually considered safe to use during pregnancy (see other cephalosporins for published human experience).

At term, a 500-mg oral dose produced an average peak cord serum level of 4.6 mcg/mL at 2.5 hours (about 40% of maternal serum) (2). Amniotic fluid levels achieved a peak of 4.4 mcg/mL at 10 hours. No infant data were given.

In a surveillance study of Michigan Medicaid recipients involving 229,101 completed pregnancies conducted between 1985 and 1992, 722 newborns had been exposed to cefadroxil during the 1st trimester (F. Rosa, personal communication, FDA, 1993). A total of 27 (3.7%) major birth defects were observed (30 expected). Specific data were available for six defect categories, including (observed/expected) 1/1 cardiovascular defects, 0/1 oral clefts, 0/0.5 spina bifida, 2/2 polydactyly, 2/1 limb reduction defects, and 1/2 hypospadias. These data do not support an association between the drug and congenital defects (see also Cefaclor, Cephalexin, and Cephradine for contrasting results).

C

Cefadroxil, 500 mg twice daily for 10 days following an IV dose of ceftazidime, was used in 12 women for the treatment of asymptomatic bacteriuria during the 1st trimester (see also Ceftazidime) (3). No adverse effects of the treatment were observed.

BREASTFEEDING SUMMARY

Cefadroxil is excreted into breast milk in low concentrations. Following a single 500-mg oral dose, peak milk levels of about 0.6–0.7 mcg/mL occurred at 5–6 hours (2). A 1-g oral dose given to six mothers produced peak milk levels averaging 1.83 mcg/mL (range 1.2–2.4 mcg/mL) at 6–7 hours (4). In this latter group, milk:plasma ratios at 1, 2, and 3 hours were 0.009, 0.011, and 0.019, respectively. Although these levels are low, three potential problems exist for the nursing infant: modification of bowel flora, direct effects on the infant, and interference with the interpretation of culture results if a fever workup is required. The American Academy of Pediatrics classifies cefadroxil as compatible with breastfeeding (5).

References

1. Product information. Duricef. Bristol-Myers Squibb Company, 1997.
2. Takase Z, Shirafuji H, Uchida M. Experimental and clinical studies of cefadroxil in the treatment of infections in the field of obstetrics and gynecology. Chemotherapy (Tokyo) 1980;28(Suppl 2):424–31.
3. Nathorst-Boos J, Philipson A, Hedman A, Arvisson A. Renal elimination of ceftazidime during pregnancy. Am J Obstet Gynecol 1995;172:163–6.
4. Kafetzi DA, Siafas CA, Georgakopoulos PA, Papdatos CJ. Passage of cephalosporins and amoxicillin into the breast milk. Acta Paediatr Scand 1981;70:285–8.
5. Committee on Drugs, American Academy of Pediatrics. The transfer of drugs and other chemicals into human milk. Pediatrics 2001;108:776–89.

CEFAMANDOLE

[Withdrawn from the market. See 9th edition.]

CEFATRIZINE

[Withdrawn from the market. See 9th edition.]

CEFAZOLIN

Antibiotic (Cephalosporin)

PREGNANCY RECOMMENDATION: Compatible
BREASTFEEDING RECOMMENDATION: Compatible

PREGNANCY SUMMARY

No detectable teratogenic risk with cephalosporin antibiotics was found in a large 2001 study (see Cephalexin).

FETAL RISK SUMMARY

Cefazolin is a parenteral, semisynthetic cephalosporin antibiotic. Reproduction studies in mice, rats, and rabbits found no evidence of impaired fertility or fetal harm at doses up to 25 times the human dose (1).

Cefazolin crosses the placenta into the cord serum and amniotic fluid (2–6). In early pregnancy, distribution is limited to the body fluids and these concentrations are considerably lower than those found in the 2nd and 3rd trimesters (3). At term, 15–70 minutes after a 500-mg dose, cord serum levels range from 35% to 69% of the maternal serum (4). The maximum concentration in amniotic fluid after 500-mg dose was 8 mcg/mL at 2.5 hours (5). No data on the newborns were given. Following a 2-g IV dose given to seven women between 23 and 32 weeks' gestation, the mean serum concentration of cefazolin in hydropic and nonhydropic fetuses was 18.04 and 21.02 mcg/mL, respectively, providing evidence that the presence of hydrops did not significantly impair the transfer of the antibiotic (6).

Cefazolin, 2 g IV every 8 hours, has been used in the treatment of pyelonephritis occurring in the second half of pregnancy (7). No adverse fetal outcomes attributable to the drug were observed.

BREASTFEEDING SUMMARY

Cefazolin is excreted into breast milk in low concentrations. Following a 2-g IV dose, the average milk levels ranged from 1.2 to 1.5 mcg/mL over 4 hours (milk:plasma ratio 0.02) (8). When cefazolin was given as a 500-mg IM dose, one to three times daily, the drug was not detectable (5). Although these levels are low, three potential problems exist for the nursing infant: modification of bowel flora, direct effects on the infant, and interference with the interpretation of culture results if a fever workup is required. The American Academy of Pediatrics classifies cefazolin as compatible with breastfeeding (9).

References

1. Product information. Ancef. SmithKline Beecham Pharmaceuticals, 1997.
2. Dekel A, Elian I, Gibor Y, Goldman JA. Transplacental passage of cefazolin in the first trimester of pregnancy. Eur J Obstet Gynecol Reprod Biol 1980;10:303–7.
3. Bernard B, Barton L, Abate M, Ballard CA. Maternal-fetal transfer of cefazolin in the first twenty weeks of pregnancy. J Infect Dis 1977;136:377–82.
4. Cho N, Ito T, Saito T, et al. Clinical studies on cefazolin in the field of obstetrics and gynecology. Chemotherapy (Tokyo) 1970;18:770–7.
5. von Kobyletzki D, Reither K, Gellen J, Kanyo A, Glocke M. Pharmacokinetic studies with cefazolin in obstetrics and gynecology. Infection 1974;2(Suppl):60–7.
6. Brown CEL, Christmas JT, Bawdon RE. Placental transfer of cefazolin and piperacillin in pregnancies remote from term complicated by Rh isoimmunization. Am J Obstet Gynecol 1990;163:938–43.
7. Sanchez-Ramos L, McAlpine KJ, Adair CD, Kaunitz AM, Delke I, Briones DK. Pyelonephritis in pregnancy: once-a-day ceftriaxone versus multiple doses of cefazolin. Am J Obstet Gynecol 1995;172:129–33.
8. Yoshioka H, Cho K, Takimoto M, Maruyama S, Shimizu T. Transfer of cefazolin into human milk. J Pediatr 1979;94:151–2.
9. Committee on Drugs, American Academy of Pediatrics. The transfer of drugs and other chemicals into human milk. Pediatrics 2001;108:776–89.

CEFDINIR

Antibiotic (Cephalosporin)

PREGNANCY RECOMMENDATION: Compatible
BREASTFEEDING RECOMMENDATION: Compatible

PREGNANCY SUMMARY

No detectable teratogenic risk with cephalosporin antibiotics was found in a large 2001 study (see Cephalexin).

FETAL RISK SUMMARY

Cefdinir is an oral, semisynththetic, third-generation cephalosporin antibiotic. No reports describing its use in pregnancy have been located. The molecular weight (about 395) is low enough that passage to the fetus should be expected.

Reproduction studies have been conducted in pregnant rats and rabbits (1). In pregnant rats, oral doses up to 11 times the human dose based on BSA (HD) were not teratogenic, but decreased fetal weight occurred at doses ≥1.1 times the HD. No effects were seen on maternal reproductive performance or offspring survival, behavior, development, or reproductive function. In rabbits, oral doses up to 0.23 times the HD were not teratogenic, but maternal toxicity (decreased body weight) was noted at the highest dose. No adverse effects on offspring were observed (1).

BREASTFEEDING SUMMARY

No published reports describing the use of cefdinir in human lactation have been located. The molecular weight (about 395) is low enough that excretion into breast milk should be expected. However, the drug was not detected in breast milk after a single, 600-mg oral dose (1). Multiple dosing during lactation has apparently not been studied. If excretion does occur, three potential problems exist for the nursing infant: modification of bowel flora, direct effects on the infant, and interference with the interpretation of culture results if a fever workup is required. The American Academy of Pediatrics classifies other cephalosporins as compatible with breastfeeding (e.g., see Cefadroxil and Cefazolin).

Reference

1. Product information. Omnicef. Abbott Laboratories, 2001.

CEFDITOREN

Antibiotic (Cephalosporin)

PREGNANCY RECOMMENDATION: Compatible
BREASTFEEDING RECOMMENDATION: Compatible

PREGNANCY SUMMARY

No detectable teratogenic risk with cephalosporin antibiotics was found in a large 2001 study (see Cephalexin).

C

FETAL RISK SUMMARY

No reports describing the use of cefditoren in human pregnancy have been located. Cefditoren pivosil is a prodrug that is hydrolyzed during absorption to the active drug, cefditoren. It is an oral, semisynthetic cephalosporin antibiotic similar to other agents in this class. Cefditoren probably crosses the placenta, similar to other cephalosporins.

Reproduction studies have been conducted with cefditoren pivosil in rats and rabbits. In pregnant rats and rabbits, doses up to about 24 and 4 times, respectively, the human dose of 200 mg twice daily based on BSA (HD) were not teratogenic. In addition, rat fertility and reproduction were not affected by the highest dose. However, in rabbits, the highest dose caused severe maternal toxicity resulting in fetal toxicity and abortions. In a postnatal study in rats, a dose 18 times the HD produced no adverse effects on postnatal survival, physical and behavioral development, learning abilities, and reproductive capability at sexual maturity (1).

BREASTFEEDING SUMMARY

No reports describing the use of cefditoren in human lactation have been located. Small amounts of antibiotic have been found in breast milk for all cephalosporins that have been studied, so the presence of cefditoren in milk should be expected. In most cases, the effects of this exposure will be insignificant. However, three potential problems exist for the nursing infant exposed to cefditoren in milk: modification of bowel flora, direct effects on the infant, and interference with the interpretation of culture results if a fever workup is required. The American Academy of Pediatrics classifies other cephalosporins as compatible with breastfeeding (for example, see Cefadroxil and Cefazolin).

Reference

1. Product information. Spectracef. Purdue Pharmaceutical Products, 2004.

CEFEPIME

Antibiotic (Cephalosporin)

PREGNANCY RECOMMENDATION: Compatible
BREASTFEEDING RECOMMENDATION: Compatible

PREGNANCY SUMMARY

No detectable teratogenic risk with cephalosporin antibiotics was found in a large 2001 study (see Cephalexin).

FETAL RISK SUMMARY

No reports describing the use of cefepime in human pregnancy have been located. It is a parenteral, semisynthetic cephalosporin antibiotic. Serum protein binding is about 20% (1).

No adverse effects on fertility or reproduction, including embryo toxicity and teratogenicity, were observed in mice, rats, and rabbits dosed at one to four times the recommended maximum human daily dose based on BSA (1).

Consistent with the molecular weight (about 481 for the free base), cefepime crosses the human placenta. In a 2010 study, nine women scheduled for a cesarean section were given IV cefepime 1 g over 60 minutes (2). The transplacental passage rate calculated as a percentage of fetal venous concentration to maternal blood concentration was about 23%, whereas the transfetal passage rate calculated as a percentage of fetal arterial drug concentration to fetal venous concentration was about 79% (2).

BREASTFEEDING SUMMARY

Cefepime is excreted in human milk. The manufacturer reports that a nursing infant consuming about 1000 mL of human milk per day would received about 0.5 mg of cefepime per day (1). In spite of this low dose, three potential problems exist for the nursing infant exposed to cefepime in milk: modification of bowel flora, direct effects on the infant, and interference with the interpretation of culture results if a fever workup is required. Although not specifically listing cefepime, the American Academy of Pediatrics classifies other cephalosporin antibiotics as compatible with breastfeeding (for example, see Cefadroxil and Cefazolin).

References

1. Product information. Maxipime. Bristol-Myers Squibb Company, 2013.
2. Ozyuncu O, Nemutlu E, Katlan D, Kir S, Beksac MS. Maternal and fetal blood levels of moxifloxacin, levofloxacin, cefepime and cefoperazone. Int J Antimicrob Agents 2010;36:175–8.

CEFIXIME

Antibiotic (Cephalosporin)

PREGNANCY RECOMMENDATION: Compatible
BREASTFEEDING RECOMMENDATION: Compatible

PREGNANCY SUMMARY

The limited human pregnancy data do not suggest embryo–fetal risk. In addition, no detectable teratogenic risk with cephalosporin antibiotics was found in a large 2001 study (see Cephalexin).

C

FETAL RISK SUMMARY

Cefixime is an oral, semisynthetic cephalosporin antibiotic. Serum protein binding is about 65% and the elimination half-life is about 3.5 hours (1).

Reproduction studies found no evidence in rats of impaired fertility or reproductive performance at doses up to 125 times the adult therapeutic dose or, in mice and rats, of teratogenicity at doses up to 400 times the human dose (1).

Consistent with the molecular weight (about 453), cefixime crosses the human placenta.

A 2010 study measured cefixime amniotic fluid concentrations in six women given a 400 mg oral dose about 2 hours before amniocentesis (2). The study was conducted between the 16th and 20th gestational weeks. The mean concentrations of cefixime in maternal blood and amniotic fluid were 2.59 mcg/mL and 0.85 mcg/mL, respectvely, and amniotic fluid passage rate of about 38% (2).

A 1998 noninterventional observational cohort study described the outcomes of pregnancies in women who had been prescribed one or more of 34 newly marketed drugs by general practitioners in England (3). Data were obtained by questionnaires sent to the prescribing physicians one month after the expected or possible date of delivery. In 831 (78%) of the pregnancies, a newly marketed drug was thought to have been taken during the 1st trimester, with birth defects noted in 14 (2.5%) singleton births of the 557 newborns (10 sets of twins). In addition, two birth defects were observed in aborted fetuses. However, few of the aborted fetuses were examined. Cefixime was taken during the 1st trimester in 11 pregnancies. The outcomes of these pregnancies included two spontaneous abortions, one elective abortion, seven normal newborns (one premature), and one unknown outcome (3).

A 2003 study evaluated 95 pregnant women with gonorrhea who were treated with either cefixime ($N = 52$) or ceftriaxone ($N = 43$) (4). Treatment in both groups occurred at about 21 weeks' gestation. Both antibiotics were equally effective, with 91 patients cured of the infection. Hyperbilirubinemia occurred more often in infants from mothers treated with ceftriaxone, but the difference was not significant (4).

A study evaluating the effects of mass treatment (cefixime, azithromycin, metronidazole) for AIDS prevention in Uganda was published in 1999 (5). Compared with controls, the prevalences of trichomoniasis, bacterial vaginosis, gonorrhea, and chlamydia infection were significantly lower, but no difference was observed in the incidence of HIV infection. A second study using this same group of patients found, in addition to the lower rates of infection, reduced rates of neonatal death, low birth weight, and preterm delivery (6). However, in a third study involving the same Uganda women as above, children of 94 women with *Trichomonas vaginalis* who had been treated during pregnancy with the 3-drug combination had increased low birth weight (<2500 g) and preterm birth rate compared with untreated controls (7). The authors concluded that treatment of the condition during pregnancy was harmful and that it was most likely due to metronidazole.

BREASTFEEDING SUMMARY

No reports describing the use of cefixime during human lactation have been located. Low concentrations of other cephalosporins have been measured, however, and the presence of cefixime in milk should be expected. Three potential problems exist for the nursing infant exposed to cefixime in milk: modification of bowel flora, direct effects on the infant, and interference with the interpretation of culture results if a fever workup is required. The American Academy of Pediatrics classifies other cephalosporin antibiotics as compatible with breastfeeding (for example, see Cefadroxil and Cefazolin).

References

1. Product information. Suprax. Lupin Pharma, 2013.
2. Ozyuncu O, Beksac MS, Nemutlu E, Katlan D, Kir S. Maternal blood and amniotic fluid levels of moxifloxacin, levofloxacin and cefixime. J Obstet Gynecol 2010;36:484–7.
3. Wilton LV, Pearce GL, Martin RM, Mackay FJ, Mann RD. The outcomes of pregnancy in women exposed to newly marketed drugs in general practice in England. Br J Obstet Gynaecol 1998;105:882–9.
4. Ramus RM, Sheffield JS, Mayfield JA, Wendel GD Jr. A randomized trial that compared oral cefixime and intramuscular ceftriaxone for the treatment of gonorrhea in pregnancy. Am J Obstet Gynecol 2001;185;629–32.
5. Wawer MJ, Sewankambo NK, Serwadda D, Quinn TC, Paxton LA, Kiwanuka N, Wabwire-Mangen F, Li C, Lutalo T, Nalugoda F, Gaydos CA, Moulton LH, Meehan MO, Ahmed S, the Rakai Project Study Group, Gray RH. Control of sexually transmitted disease for AIDS prevention in Uganda: a randomised community trial. Lancet 1999;353:525–35.
6. Gray RH, Wabwire-Mangen F, Kigozi G, Sewankambo NK, Serwadda D, Moulton LH, Quinn TC, O'Brien KL, Meehan M, Abramowsky C, Robb M, Wawer MJ. Randomized trial of presumptive sexually transmitted disease therapy during pregnancy in Rakai, Uganda. Am J Obstet Gynecol 2001;185:1209–17.
7. Kigozi GG, Brahmbhatt H, Wabwire-Mangen F, Wawer MJ, Serwadda D, Sewankambo N, Gray RH. Treatment of *Trichomonas* in pregnancy and adverse outcomes of pregnancy: a subanalysis of a randomized trial in Rakai, Uganda. Am J Obstet Gynecol 2003;189:1398–400.

CEFMETAZOLE

[Withdrawn from the market. See 9th edition.]

C

CEFONICID

[Withdrawn from the market. See 9th edition.]

CEFOPERAZONE

[Withdrawn from the market. See 9th edition.]

CEFORANIDE

[Withdrawn from the market. See 9th edition.]

CEFOTAXIME

Antibiotic (Cephalosporin)

PREGNANCY RECOMMENDATION: Compatible
BREASTFEEDING RECOMMENDATION: Compatible

PREGNANCY SUMMARY

No detectable teratogenic risk with cephalosporin antibiotics was found in a large 2001 study (see Cephalexin).

FETAL RISK SUMMARY

Cefotaxime is a parenteral, semisynthetic cephalosporin antibiotic. Reproduction studies in mice and rats have found no evidence of impaired fertility or fetal harm at doses up to 20 times the human dose (1). Cephalosporins are usually considered safe to use during pregnancy.

During the 2nd trimester, the drug readily crosses the placenta (2). The half-life of cefotaxime in fetal serum and in amniotic fluid was 2.3 and 2.8 hours, respectively. Five women with chorioamnionitis and in labor received cefotaxime (dose not specified) (3). The maternal and cord blood concentrations were nearly equivalent at 8.90 and 8.60 mcg/mL, respectively, but the placental tissue:maternal blood ratio was 0.2 (dose to delivery interval not specified).

BREASTFEEDING SUMMARY

Cefotaxime is excreted into breast milk in low concentrations. Following a 1-g IV dose, mean peak milk levels of 0.33 mcg/mL were measured at 2–3 hours (2,4). The half-life in milk ranged from 2.36 to 3.89 hours (mean 2.93 hours). The milk:plasma ratios at 1, 2, and 3 hours were 0.027, 0.09, and 0.16, respectively. Although these levels are low, three potential problems exist for the nursing infant: modification of bowel flora, direct effects on the infant, and interference with the interpretation of culture results if a fever workup is required. The American Academy of Pediatrics classifies cefotaxime as compatible with breastfeeding (5).

References

1. Product information. Claforan. Hoechst Marion Roussel, 1997.
2. Kafetzis DA, Lazarides CV, Siafas CA, Georgakopoulos PA, Papadatos CJ. Transfer of cefotaxime in human milk and from mother to foetus. J Antimicrob Chemother 1980;6(Suppl A):135–41.
3. Maberry MC, Trimmer KJ, Bawdon RE, Sobhi S, Dax JB, Gilstrap LC III. Antibiotic concentration in maternal blood, cord blood and placental tissue in women with chorioamnionitis. Gynecol Obstet Invest 1992;33:185–6.
4. Kafetzis DA, Siafas CA, Georgakopoulos PA, Papadatos CJ. Passage of cephalosporins and amoxicillin into the breast milk. Acta Paediatr Scand 1981;70:285–8.
5. Committee on Drugs, American Academy of Pediatrics. The transfer of drugs and other chemicals into human milk. Pediatrics 2001;108:776–89.

CEFOTETAN

Antibiotic (Cephalosporin)

PREGNANCY RECOMMENDATION: Compatible
BREASTFEEDING RECOMMENDATION: Compatible

PREGNANCY SUMMARY

No detectable teratogenic risk with cephalosporin antibiotics was found in a large 2001 study (see Cephalexin).

C

FETAL RISK SUMMARY

Cefotetan is a parenteral, semisynthetic cephalosporin antibiotic. Reproduction studies in rats and monkeys found no evidence of impaired fertility or fetal harm at doses up to 20 times the human dose (1). Cephalosporins are usually considered safe to use during pregnancy.

A 1985 study measured the placental passage of the drug when administered just prior to cesarean section (2). Twenty women received a single, 1-g IV bolus dose of the antibiotic at intervals of 1–4 hours before surgery. The peak maternal plasma level obtained was 28 mcg/mL. Cord blood concentrations progressively increased depending on the length of time after a mother received a dose and were highest (12.5 mcg/mL) when she received the drug 4 hours prior to surgery. Similarly, a progressive increase in amniotic fluid concentrations was observed with values of 5.1, 7.5, and 8.1 mcg/mL measured at 2, 3, and 4 hours, respectively. The increases in the level of antibiotic in the amniotic fluid paralleled those in the cord blood.

Three Japanese studies reported placental passage of cefotetan (3–5). Cord blood levels almost double those measured above, 24.7 mcg/mL, were reported 1 hour after a 1-g IV dose (3). This value was 15.4% of the peak maternal serum level, indicating that the peak maternal level was about 160 mcg/mL. The amniotic fluid concentration was 12.3% of the mother's level, or approximately 20 mcg/mL. A confirming study also found high cord blood levels after a single 1-g IV dose with the highest value of 29.0 mcg/mL measured 3.6 hours after the maternal dose (4). The highest amniotic fluid level, however, was 8.6 mcg/mL, which was also observed at 3.6 hours. The third study measured cord serum concentrations of 15, 31.4, and 3.5 mcg/mL at 0.85, 3.75, and 16 hours, respectively, after a 1-g IV dose (5). Amniotic fluid concentrations ranged from 1.18 to 13.6 mcg/mL up to 16 hours after a dose.

BREASTFEEDING SUMMARY

Small amounts of cefotetan are excreted into human breast milk (5,6). A 1982 reference reported milk levels ranging from 0.22 to 0.34 mcg/mL 1–6 hours after a 1-g IV dose (5). In six women treated with cefotetan 1 g IM every 12 hours, mean milk levels 4–10 hours after a dose varied from 0.29 to 0.59 mcg/mL (6). No accumulation in the milk was observed, as evidenced by a steady milk:plasma ratio. The mean ratio 10 hours after the first dose was 0.05 compared with 0.07, 10 hours after the fifth dose.

Even though the amounts of antibiotic are very small, and no reports of adverse effects in a nursing infant have been located, three potential problems exist for the infant exposed to cefotetan in milk: modification of bowel flora, direct effects on the infant, and interference with the interpretation of culture results if a fever workup is required. Although not specifically listing cefotetan, the American Academy of Pediatrics classifies other cephalosporin antibiotics as compatible with breastfeeding (for example, see Cefadroxil and Cefazolin).

References

1. Product information. Cefotan. Zeneca Pharmaceuticals, 1997.
2. Bergogne-Berezin E, Berthelot O, Ravina JH, Yernant D. *Study of Placental Transfer of Cefotetan (Abstract)*. Program and Abstracts of the 25th Interscience Conference on Antimicrobial Agents and Chemotherapy, Minneapolis, MN, September 29–October 2, 1985:144.
3. Takase Z, Fujiwara M, Kawamoto Y, Seto M, Shirafuji H, Uchida M. Laboratory and clinical studies of cefotetan (YM09330) in the field of obstetrics and gynecology (English abstract). Chemotherapy (Tokyo) 1982;30(Suppl 1):869–81.
4. Motomura R, Teramoto C, Souda Y, Fujita A, Chiyoda R, Mori H, Yamabe T. Fundamental and clinical study of cefotetan (YM09330) in the field of obstetrics and gynecology (English abstract). Chemotherapy (Tokyo) 1982;30(Suppl 1):882–7.
5. Cho N, Fukunaga K, Kunii K. Fundamental and clinical studies on cefotetan (YM09330) in the field of obstetrics and gynecology (English abstract). Chemotherapy (Tokyo) 1982;30(Suppl 1):832–42.
6. Novelli A, Mazzei T, Ciuffi M, Nicoletti P, Buzzoni P, Reali EF, Periti P. The penetration of intramuscular cefotetan disodium into human extra-vascular fluid and maternal milk secretion. Chemioterapia 1983;2:337–42.

CEFOXITIN

Antibiotic (Cephalosporin)

PREGNANCY RECOMMENDATION: Compatible
BREASTFEEDING RECOMMENDATION: Compatible

PREGNANCY SUMMARY

No detectable teratogenic risk with cephalosporin antibiotics was found in a large 2001 study (see Cephalexin).

C

FETAL RISK SUMMARY

Cefoxitin is a parenteral, semisynthetic cephalosporin antibiotic. Reproduction studies found no evidence in rats of impaired fertility or reproductive performance at doses three times the maximum recommended human dose (MRHD) or, in mice and rats, fetal harm (other than a slight decrease in fetal weight) or teratogenesis at doses up to approximately 7.5 times the MRHD (1).

Multiple reports have described the transplacental passage of cefoxitin (2–14). Two patients were given 1 g IV just prior to therapeutic abortion at 9 and 10 weeks' gestation (10). At 55 minutes, the serum level in one woman was 10.5 mcg/mL while none was found in the fetal tissues. In the second patient, at 4.25 hours the maternal serum was "nil," while the fetal tissue level was 35.7 mcg/mL.

At term, following IM or rapid IV doses of 1 or 2 g, cord serum levels up to 22 mcg/mL (11%–90%) of maternal levels have been measured (7–10). Amniotic fluid concentrations peaked at 2–3 hours in the 3–15 mcg/mL range (7,8,10,11,14). No apparent adverse effects were noted in any of the newborns.

BREASTFEEDING SUMMARY

Cefoxitin is excreted into breast milk in low concentrations (6,10,12,13,15). Up to 2 mcg/mL has been detected in the milk of women receiving therapeutic doses (J.J. Whalen, personal communication, Merck, Sharpe & Dohme, May 13, 1981). No data on the infants were given. Following prophylactic administration of 2–4 g of cefoxitin to 18 women during and following cesarean section, milk samples were collected a mean 25 hours (range 9–56 hours) after the last dose of antibiotic (15). Only one sample, collected 19 hours after the last dose, contained measurable concentrations of cefoxitin (0.9 mcg/mL). Although these levels are low, three potential problems exist for the nursing infant: modification of bowel flora, direct effects on the infant, and interference with the interpretation of culture results if a fever workup is required. The American Academy of Pediatrics classifies cefoxitin as compatible with breastfeeding (16).

References

1. Product information. Mefoxin. Merck & Company, 1997.
2. Bergone-Berezin B, Kafe H, Berthelot G, Morel O, Benard Y. Pharmacokinetic study of cefoxitin in bronchial secretions. In: *Current Chemotherapy: Proceedings of The 10th International Congress of Chemotherapy, Zurich, Switzerland, September 18–23, 1977*. Washington, DC: American Society for Microbiology, 1978.
3. Aokawa H, Minagawa M, Yamamiohi K, Sugiyama A. Studies on cefoxitin. Chemotherapy (Tokyo) 1977;(Suppl):394.
4. Matsuda S, Tanno M, Kashiwakura S, Furuya H. Basic and clinical studies on cefoxitin. Chemotherapy (Tokyo) 1977;(Suppl):396.
5. Berthelot G, Bergogne-Berezin B, Morel O, Kafe H, Benard Y. *Cefoxitin: Pharmacokinetic Study in Bronchial Secretions-Transplacental Diffusion (Abstract No. 80)*. Paper Presented at 10th International Congress of Chemotherapy, Zurich, Switzerland, September 18–23, 1977.
6. Mashimo K, Mihashi S, Fukaya I, Okubo B, Ohgob M, Saito A. New drug symposium IV. Cefoxitin. Chemotherapy (Tokyo) 1978;26:114–9.
7. Matsuda S, Tanno M, Kashiwakura T, Furuya H. Laboratory and clinical studies on cefoxitin in the field of obstetrics and gynecology. Chemotherapy (Tokyo) 1978;26(Suppl 1):460–7.
8. Cho N, Ubhara K, Suigizaki K, Sed B, Miyagami J, Saito H, Nakayama T. Clinical studies of cefoxitin in the field of obstetrics and gynecology. Chemotherapy (Tokyo) 1978;26(Suppl 1):468–75.
9. Seiga K, Minagawa M, Yamaji K, Sugiyama Y. Study on cefoxitin. Chemotherapy (Tokyo) 1978;26(Suppl 1):491–501.
10. Takase Z, Shirafuji H, Uchida M. Clinical and laboratory studies on cefoxitin in the field of obstetrics and gynecology. Chemotherapy (Tokyo) 1978;26(Suppl 1):502–5.
11. Bergogne-Berezin B, Lambert-Zeohovsky N, Rouvillois JL. *Placental Transfer of Cefoxitin (Abstract No. 314)*. Paper Presented at the 18th Interscience Conference on Antimicrobial Agents and Chemotherapy, Atlanta, Georgia, October 1–4, 1978.
12. Brogden RN, Heel RC, Speight TM, Avery GS. Cefoxitin: a review of its antibacterial activity, pharmacological properties and therapeutic use. Drugs 1979;17:1–37.
13. Dubois M, Delapierre D, Demonty J, Lambotte R, Dresse A. *Transplacental and Mammary Transfer of Cefoxitin (Abstract No. 118)*. Paper Presented at 11th International Congress of Chemotherapy and 19th Interscience Conference on Antimicrobial Agents and Chemotherapy, Boston, MA, October 1–5, 1979.
14. Bergogne-Berezin B, Morel O, Kafe H, Berthelot G, Benard Y, Lambert-Zechevsky N, Rouvillots JL. Pharmacokinetic study of cefoxitin in man: diffusion into the bronchi and transfer across the placenta. Therapie 1979;34:345–54.
15. Roex AJM, van Loenen AC, Puyenbroek JI, Arts NFT. Secretion of cefoxitin in breast milk following short-term prophylactic administration in caesarean section. Eur J Obstet Gynecol Reprod Biol 1987;25:299–302.
16. Committee on Drugs, American Academy of Pediatrics. The transfer of drugs and other chemicals into human milk. Pediatrics 2001;108:776–89.

CEFPODOXIME

Antibiotic (Cephalosporin)

PREGNANCY RECOMMENDATION: Compatible
BREASTFEEDING RECOMMENDATION: Compatible

PREGNANCY SUMMARY

No detectable teratogenic risk with cephalosporin antibiotics was found in a large 2001 study (see Cephalexin).

FETAL RISK SUMMARY

No reports describing the use of cefpodoxime in human pregnancy have been located. It is an oral, semisynthetic cephalosporin antibiotic. Reproduction studies found no evidence in rats of impaired fertility or reproductive performance or, in rats and rabbits, of embryo toxicity or teratogenicity, at doses up to two times the human dose based on BSA (1).

BREASTFEEDING SUMMARY

According to the manufacturer, low concentrations of cefpodoxime are excreted into human milk (1). Following 200-mg oral doses administered to three women, milk concentrations, as a percentage of concomitant serum levels, 4 hours after the dose were 0%, 2%, and 6%, respectively, and at 6 hours, 0%, 9%, and 16%, respectively. Although not specifically stated for these three women, mean serum concentrations in fasted adults after a 200-mg dose were 2.2 mcg/mL at 2 and 3 hours (peak levels), 1.8 mcg/mL at 4 hours, and 1.2 mcg/mL at 6 hours (1).

In spite of these low levels, three potential problems exist for the nursing infant exposed to cefpodoxime in milk: modification of bowel flora, direct effects on the infant, and interference with the interpretation of culture results if a fever workup is required. Although not specifically listing cefpodoxime, the American Academy of Pediatrics classifies other cephalosporin antibiotics as compatible with breastfeeding (for example, see Cefadroxil and Cefazolin).

Reference

1. Product information. Vantin. Pharmacia & Upjohn Company, 1997.

CEFPROZIL

Antibiotic (Cephalosporin)

PREGNANCY RECOMMENDATION: Compatible
BREASTFEEDING RECOMMENDATION: Compatible

PREGNANCY SUMMARY

No detectable teratogenic risk with cephalosporin antibiotics was found in a large 2001 study (see Cephalexin).

FETAL RISK SUMMARY

No reports describing the use of cefprozil in human pregnancy have been located. It is an oral, semisynthetic cephalosporin antibiotic. Reproduction studies found no evidence in animals of impaired fertility or, in mice, rats, and rabbits, of fetal harm at doses of 8.5, 18.5, and 0.8 times, respectively, the maximum human daily dose based on BSA (1).

BREASTFEEDING SUMMARY

Low concentrations of cefprozil are excreted in human milk. In a study published in 1992, nine healthy, lactating women were given a single 1000-mg oral dose of cefprozil consisting of *cis* and *trans* isomers in an approximately 90:10 ratio (2). The mean peak plasma concentrations of the *cis* and *trans* isomers were 14.8 and 1.9 mcg/mL, respectively. For the *cis* isomer, the mean milk concentration over a 24-hour period ranged from 0.25 to 3.36 mcg/mL, whereas the average maximum concentration in milk of the *trans* isomer was <0.26 mcg/mL. Less than 0.3% of the maternal dose was excreted into milk for the two isomers. The investigators estimated that an infant receiving 800 mL/day of milk would ingest a maximum of 3 mg of cefprozil, an amount they assessed as clinically insignificant.

Three potential problems exist for the nursing infant exposed to cefprozil in milk: modification of bowel flora, direct effects on the infant, and interference with the interpretation of culture results if a fever workup is required. The American Academy of Pediatrics classifies cefprozil as compatible with breastfeeding (3).

References

1. Product information. Cefzil. Bristol-Myers Squibb Company, 2000.
2. Shyu WC, Shah VR, Campbell DA, Venitz J, Jaganathan V, Pittman KA, Wilber RB, Barbhaiya RH. Excretion of cefprozil into human breast milk. Antimicrob Agents Chemother 1992;36:938–41.
3. Committee on Drugs, American Academy of Pediatrics. The transfer of drugs and other chemicals into human milk. Pediatrics 2001;108: 776–89.

CEFTAROLINE FOSAMIL

Antibiotic (Cephalosporin)

PREGNANCY RECOMMENDATION: Compatible
BREASTFEEDING RECOMMENDATION: Compatible

PREGNANCY SUMMARY

No reports describing the use of ceftaroline fosamil in human pregnancy have been located. Animal data suggest low risk. Although there is no human pregnancy experience, in general, cephalosporins are considered compatible in pregnancy.

C

FETAL RISK SUMMARY

Ceftaroline fosamil is a cephalosporin antibiotic that is converted to the bioactive ceftaroline after IV administration. It is indicated for the treatment of acute bacterial skin and skin structure infections and community-acquired bacterial pneumonia. Plasma protein binding is about 20% and the elimination half-life after multiple doses is about 2.7 hours (1).

Reproduction studies have been conducted in rats and rabbits. In rats, doses that produced exposures that were about 8 times the human exposure from 600 mg every 12 hours based on AUC (HE) did not cause maternal toxicity or fetal harm. Moreover, a higher dose in rats revealed no evidence of an effect on postnatal development or reproductive performance in offspring. In rabbits, doses that were about 0.8 times the HE or higher were maternal toxic but did not cause malformations (1).

Ceftaroline fosamil was not mutagenic in multiple assays but was clastogenic in an in vitro assay. The latter effect was not observed after metabolic activation. No evidence of impaired fertility was observed in male and female rats at doses up to about 4 times the maximum recommended human dose based on BSA (1).

It is not known if ceftaroline fosamil or ceftaroline crosses the human placenta. The molecular weight of the prodrug (about 685) and lower molecular weight of the active agent, and the elimination half-life and low plasma protein binding, suggest that ceftaroline will cross to the embryo–fetus.

BREASTFEEDING SUMMARY

No reports describing the use of ceftaroline fosamil during human lactation have been located. The molecular weight of the prodrug (about 685) and lower molecular weight of the active agent, and the elimination half-life (about 2.7 hours) and low plasma protein binding (about 20%), suggest that both the prodrug and active agent will be excreted into breast milk. Moreover, low concentrations of other cephalosporins are excreted into milk and the presence in milk of this antibiotic should be expected. Three potential problems exist for the nursing infant: modification of bowel flora, direct effects on the infant, and interference with the interpretation of culture results if a fever workup is required. The American Academy of Pediatrics classifies other cephalosporin antibiotics as compatible with breastfeeding (for example, see Cefadroxil and Cefazolin).

Reference

1. Product information. Teflaro. Forest Pharmaceuticals, 2011.

CEFTAZIDIME

Antibiotic (Cephalosporin)

PREGNANCY RECOMMENDATION: Compatible
BREASTFEEDING RECOMMENDATION: Compatible

PREGNANCY SUMMARY

No detectable teratogenic risk with cephalosporin antibiotics was found in a large 2001 study (see Cephalexin).

FETAL RISK SUMMARY

Ceftazidime is a parenteral, semisynthetic cephalosporin antibiotic. Reproduction studies in mice and rats found no evidence of impaired fertility or fetal harm at doses up to 40 times the human dose (1). Cephalosporins are usually considered safe to use during pregnancy.

Ceftazidime administered at various stages of gestation, including the 1st trimester, crosses the placenta to the fetus and appears in the amniotic fluid (2–4). A brief English abstract of a 1983 Japanese report stated that levels in the cord blood and amniotic fluid following a 1-g IV dose exceeded the minimum inhibitory concentrations for most causative organisms but did not give specific values (2).

Nine women, undergoing abortion for fetuses affected by β-thalassemia major between 19 and 21 weeks' gestation, were given ceftazidime 1 g IM three times a day (3). At least three doses of the antibiotic were administered prior to abortion. The average concentrations of the drug in maternal serum at 2 and 4 hours after the last dose were 19.5 mcg/mL (range 14–25 mcg/mL) and 1.5 mcg/mL (range 1.4–1.6 mcg/mL), respectively. The simultaneous levels in amniotic fluid were 2.7 mcg/mL (range 1.3–4 mcg/mL) and 3.1 mcg/mL (range 2.2–3.9 mcg/mL), respectively, corresponding to approximately 14% and 207% of the maternal concentrations, respectively.

In a 1987 report, 30 women received a single 2-g IV bolus dose over 3 minutes of ceftazidime between 1 and 4 hours prior to undergoing abortion of a fetus at a mean gestational age of 10 weeks (range 7–12 weeks) (4). Antibiotic concentrations were determined in maternal plasma, placental tissue, and amniotic fluid. In maternal plasma, mean levels ranged from 76 mcg/mL at 1 hour to 16.5 mcg/mL at 4 hours. Placental tissue concentrations were constant over this time interval, 12 mg/kg at 1 hour and 13 mg/kg at 4 hours, whereas the amniotic fluid concentration increased from 0.5 to 2.8 mcg/mL, respectively.

Increased renal elimination of ceftazidime was found in 12 women with asymptomatic bacteriuria treated with a 400-mg bolus dose, followed by a continuous infusion of 1 g for 4 hours (5). The initial treatment occurred during the 1st trimester, followed by treatments approximately 2 weeks before delivery at term and after cessation of breastfeeding. The mean renal clearances of the antibiotic during the three administrations were 143, 170, and 103 mL/minute, respectively.

BREASTFEEDING SUMMARY

Low concentrations of ceftazidime are excreted into breast milk (6). Eleven women were treated with 2 g of ceftazidime IV every 8 hours for endometritis following cesarean section. No mention was made as to whether the women were breastfeeding during treatment. Plasma and milk samples were collected between 2 and 4 days of therapy (total number of doses received averaged 12.6). The mean maternal plasma levels of the antibiotic just prior to a dose and 1 hour after a dose were 7.6 and 71.8 mcg/mL, respectively. The mean concentrations in breast milk before a dose and at 1 and 3 hours after a dose were 3.8, 5.2, and 4.5 mcg/mL, respectively. No accumulation of the antibiotic in milk was observed.

Three potential problems exist for the nursing infant exposed to ceftazidime in milk: modification of bowel flora, direct effects on the infant, and interference with the interpretation of culture results if a fever workup is required. The American Academy of Pediatrics classifies ceftazidime as compatible with breastfeeding (7).

References

1. Product information. Fortaz. Glaxo Wellcome, 1997.
2. Cho N, Suzuki H, Mitsukawa M, Tamura T, Yamaguchi Y, Maruyama M, Aoki K, Fukunaga K, Kuni K. Fundamental and clinical evaluation of ceftazidime in the field of obstetrics and gynecology (English abstract). Chemotherapy (Tokyo) 1983;31(Suppl 3):772–82.
3. Giamarellou H, Gazis J, Petrikkos G, Antsaklis A, Aravantinos D, Daikos GK. A study of cefoxitin, moxalactam, and ceftazidime kinetics in pregnancy. Am J Obstet Gynecol 1983;147:914–9.
4. Jørgensen NP, Walstad RA, Molne K. The concentrations of ceftazidime and thiopental in maternal plasma, placental tissue and amniotic fluid in early pregnancy. Acta Obstet Gynecol Scand 1987;66:29–33.
5. Nathorst-Boos J, Philipson A, Hedman A, Arvisson A. Renal elimination of ceftazidime during pregnancy. Am J Obstet Gynecol 1995;172:163–6.
6. Blanco JD, Jorgensen JH, Castaneda YS, Crawford SA. Ceftazidime levels in human breast milk. Antimicrob Agents Chemother 1983;23:479–80.
7. Committee on Drugs, American Academy of Pediatrics. The transfer of drugs and other chemicals into human milk. Pediatrics 2001;108:776–89.

CEFTIBUTEN

Antibiotic (Cephalosporin)

PREGNANCY RECOMMENDATION: Compatible
BREASTFEEDING RECOMMENDATION: Compatible

PREGNANCY SUMMARY

No detectable teratogenic risk with cephalosporin antibiotics was found in a large 2001 study (see Cephalexin).

FETAL RISK SUMMARY

No reports describing the use of ceftibuten in human pregnancy have been located. It is an oral, semisynthetic cephalosporin antibiotic. Reproduction studies in rats found no evidence of impaired fertility at doses up to approximately 43 times the human dose based on BSA (HD). No teratogenesis or fetal harm was found in studies with rats and rabbits at doses up to approximately 8.6 and 1.5 times, respectively, the HD (1).

BREASTFEEDING SUMMARY

No reports describing the use of ceftibuten during human lactation have been located. Low concentrations of other cephalosporins are excreted into milk, however, and the presence of ceftibuten in milk should be expected. Three potential problems exist for the nursing infant exposed to ceftibuten in milk: modification of bowel flora, direct effects on the infant, and interference with the interpretation of culture results if a fever workup is required. The American Academy of Pediatrics classifies other cephalosporin antibiotics as compatible with breastfeeding (for example, see Cefadroxil and Cefazolin).

Reference

1. Product information. Cedax. Schering Corporation, 1997.

CEFTIZOXIME

Antibiotic (Cephalosporin)

PREGNANCY RECOMMENDATION: Compatible
BREASTFEEDING RECOMMENDATION: Compatible

C

PREGNANCY SUMMARY

No fetal or newborn adverse effects following exposure to ceftizoxime during pregnancy have been reported. In addition, no detectable teratogenic risk with cephalosporin antibiotics was found in a large 2001 study (see Cephalexin).

FETAL RISK SUMMARY

Ceftizoxime is a parenteral, semisynthetic cephalosporin antibiotic. Reproduction studies in rats found no evidence of impaired fertility at doses up to approximately two times the maximum human daily dose based on BSA or, in rats and rabbits, of fetal harm (1).

The placental transfer of ceftizoxime and cefoperazone were studied in an in vitro perfused human placental system (2). The mean clearance indices for the two antibiotics were 0.126 and 0.037, respectively. The steady-state fetal concentrations of the two agents were 4–5 and 4 mcg/mL, respectively.

Following 1- or 2-g IV doses administered to women at term, peak cord blood levels occurred at 1–2 hours with concentrations ranging between 12 and 30 mcg/mL (3–7). Amniotic fluid concentrations were lower with peak levels of 10–20 mcg/mL at 2–3 hours. The mean fetal:maternal ratio reported in one group of patients after a 2-g IV dose was 0.28 (7). In a different study, maternal, fetal, and amniotic concentrations were measured in women who had received at least three doses of ceftizoxime 2 g at 8-hour intervals (8). Mean levels at delivery in the various compartments were 11.96, 24.54, and 43.45 mcg/mL, respectively. Cord blood levels averaged 1.6 times higher than maternal levels with average amniotic fluid concentrations 2.9 times those in the maternal serum (8). No adverse fetal or newborn effects were noted in any of the trials.

A 1993 report found that protein binding of ceftizoxime was significantly less in fetal blood than in maternal blood (9). The mean binding to fetal proteins was 21.9% compared with maternal protein binding of 57.8%.

An abstract of a multicenter, double-blind, randomized study published in 1993 found no difference between ceftizoxime (2 g IV every 8 hours) ($N = 154$) and placebo ($N = 152$) in the percentage of women with preterm premature rupture of the membranes who were undelivered at 7 days (10). Only noninfected women who were not in labor were enrolled in the study. A prospective, double-blind, placebo-controlled study published in 1995 found that ceftizoxime (2 g IV every 8 hours) had no effect on the interval to delivery or duration of pregnancy in women, with intact membranes and without chorioamnionitis, who were in preterm (<37 weeks' gestation) labor (11).

BREASTFEEDING SUMMARY

Ceftizoxime is excreted into breast milk in low concentrations (7,12). Mean levels following single doses of 1 and 2 g were less than 0.5 mcg/mL. Even though these levels are low, three potential problems exist for the nursing infant: modification of bowel flora, direct effects on the infant, and interference with the interpretation of culture results if a fever workup is required. Although not specifically listing ceftizoxime, the American Academy of Pediatrics classifies other cephalosporin antibiotics as compatible with breastfeeding (for example, see Cefadroxil and Cefazolin).

References

1. Product information. Cefizox. Fujisawa USA, 1997.
2. Fortunato SJ, Bawdon RE, Maberry MC, Swan KF. Transfer of ceftizoxime surpasses that of cefoperazone by the isolated human placental perfused in vitro. Obstet Gynecol 1990;75:830–3.
3. Cho N, Fukunaga K, Kunii K. Studies on ceftizoxime (CZX) in the field of obstetrics and gynecology. Chemotherapy (Tokyo) 1980;28(Suppl 5): 821–30.
4. Matsuda S, Seida A. Clinical use of ceftizoxime in obstetrics and gynecology. Chemotherapy (Tokyo) 1980;28(Suppl 5):812–20.
5. Okada E, Kawada A, Shirakawa N. Clinical studies on transplacental diffusion of ceftizoxime into fetal blood and treatment of infections in obstetrics and gynecology. Chemotherapy (Tokyo) 1980;28(Suppl 5):874–87.
6. Seiga K, Minagawa M, Egawa J, Yamaji K, Sugiyama Y. Clinical and laboratory studies on ceftizoxime (CZX) in the field of obstetrics and gynecology. Chemotherapy (Tokyo) 1980;28(Suppl 5):845–62.
7. Motomura R, Kohno M, Mori H, Yamabe T. Basic and clinical studies of ceftizoxime in obstetrics and gynecology. Chemotherapy (Tokyo) 1980;28(Suppl 5):888–99.
8. Fortunato SJ, Bawdon RE, Welt SI, Swan KF. Steady-state cord and amniotic fluid ceftizoxime levels continuously surpass maternal levels. Am J Obstet Gynecol 1988;159:570–3.
9. Fortunato SJ, Welt SI, Stewart JT. Differential protein binding of ceftizoxime in cord versus maternal serum. Am J Obstet Gynecol 1993;168:914–5.
10. Blanco J, Iams J, Artal R, Baker D, Hibbard J, McGregor J, Cetrulo C. Multicenter double-blind prospective random trial of ceftizoxime vs. placebo in women with preterm premature ruptured membranes (PPROM). Am J Obstet Gynecol 1993;168:378.
11. Gordon M, Samuels P, Shubert P, Johnson F, Gebauer C, Iams J. A randomized, prospective study of adjunctive ceftizoxime in preterm labor. Am J Obstet Gynecol 1995;172:1546–52.
12. Gerding DN, Peterson LR. Comparative tissue and extravascular fluid concentrations of ceftizoxime. J Antimicrob Chemother 1982;10(Suppl C):105–16.

CEFTRIAXONE

Antibiotic (Cephalosporin)

PREGNANCY RECOMMENDATION: Compatible
BREASTFEEDING RECOMMENDATION: Compatible

PREGNANCY SUMMARY

No detectable teratogenic risk with cephalosporin antibiotics was found in a large 2001 study (see Cephalexin).

FETAL RISK SUMMARY

Ceftriaxone is a parenteral, semisynthetic cephalosporin antibiotic. Reproduction studies in rats found no evidence of impaired fertility or reproduction performance at a dose approximately 20 times the recommended human dose or, in mice, rats, and nonhuman primates, of embryotoxicity, fetotoxicity, or teratogenicity at doses approximately 20, 20, and 3 times, respectively, the recommended human dose (1).

A 1993 report described the pharmacokinetics of ceftriaxone, 2 g IV once daily for about 10 days, in nine women at 28 to 40 weeks' gestation who were being treated for chorioamnionitis or pyelonephritis (2). No accumulation of the antibiotic was noted and the pharmacokinetic profile was similar to healthy, nonpregnant adults. No adverse effects in fetuses or newborns were observed.

Peak levels in cord blood following 1- or 2-g IV doses occurred at 4 hours, with concentrations varying between 19.6 and 40.6 mcg/mL (1–8 hours) (3–5). Amniotic fluid levels over 24 hours ranged from 2.2 to 23.4 mcg/mL with peak levels occurring at 6 hours (3–5). Ceftriaxone concentrations in the first voided newborn urine were highly variable, ranging from 6 to 92 mcg/mL. Elimination half-lives from cord blood (7 hours), amniotic fluid (6.8 hours), and placenta (5.4 hours) were nearly identical to maternal serum (3,4,6). No adverse effects in the newborns were mentioned.

In a surveillance study of Michigan Medicaid recipients involving 229,101 completed pregnancies conducted between 1985 and 1992, 60 newborns had been exposed to ceftriaxone during the 1st trimester (F. Rosa, personal communication, FDA, 1993). Four (6.7%) major birth defects were observed (three expected), including three cardiovascular defects (one expected). No anomalies were observed in five other categories of defects (oral clefts, spina bifida, polydactyly, limb reduction defects, and hypospadias) for which specific data were available. A possible association between ceftriaxone and cardiovascular defects is suggested, but other factors, such as the mother's disease, concurrent drug use, and chance, may be involved. However, other cephalosporin antibiotics from this study have shown possible associations with congenital malformations (see also Cefaclor, Cephalexin, and Cephradine).

Ceftriaxone, 1 g IV daily, has been used in the treatment of pyelonephritis occurring in the second half of pregnancy (7). No adverse fetal outcomes attributable to the drug were observed.

Ceftriaxone 1 g IV has been used for preoperative prophylaxis prior to emergency cesarean section (8). Amniotic fluid and fetal serum levels ranged from 0.016 to 0.25 mcg/mL (mean 0.085 mcg/mL) and from 0.66 to 18.4 mcg/mL (mean 4.6 mcg/mL), respectively.

Gonorrhea infecting 114 pregnant women in the 2nd trimester was treated with a single, 250-mg IM dose of ceftriaxone in a study published in 1993 (9). The treatment was compared with approximately similar numbers of pregnant women treated with spectinomycin or amoxicillin with probenecid. Ceftriaxone and spectinomycin were similar in efficacy and both were superior to the amoxicillin/probenecid regimen. A 20-year-old woman with endocarditis due to *Neisseria sicca* was treated for 4 weeks with ceftriaxone, 2 g IV every 12 hours, late in the 3rd trimester (10). She eventually delivered a term, small-for-gestational-age female infant, whose low weight was attributed to the mother's chronic disease state.

BREASTFEEDING SUMMARY

Ceftriaxone is excreted into breast milk in low concentrations. Following either 1- or 2-g IV or IM doses, peak levels of 0.5–0.7 mcg/mL occurred at 5 hours, approximately 3%–4% of maternal serum (3,4). High protein binding in maternal serum probably limited transfer to the milk (3,4). The antibiotic was still detectable in milk at 24 hours (3). Elimination half-lives after IV and IM doses were 12.8 and 17.3 hours, respectively (3). Chronic dosing would eventually produce calculated steady-state levels in 1.5–3 days in the 3–4 mcg/mL range (4). Although these levels are low, three potential problems exist for the nursing infant: modification of bowel flora, direct effects on the infant, and interference with the interpretation of culture results if a fever workup is required. The American Academy of Pediatrics classifies ceftriaxone as compatible with breastfeeding (11).

References

1. Product information. Rocephin. Roche Laboratories, 1997.
2. Bourget P, Fernandez H, Quinquis V, Delouis C. Pharmacokinetics and protein binding of ceftriaxone during pregnancy. Antimicrob Agents Chemother 1993;37:54–9.
3. Kafetzis DA, Brater DC, Fanourgakis JE, Voyatzis J, Georgakopoulos P. Placental and breast-milk transfer of ceftriaxone (C). In: *Proceedings of the 22nd Interscience Conference on Antimicrobial Agents in Chemotherapy, Miami, FL*, October 4–6, 1982. New York, NY: Academic Press, 1983:155.
4. Kafetzis DA, Brater DC, Fanourgakis JE, Voyatzis J, Georgakopoulos P. Ceftriaxone distribution between maternal blood and fetal blood and tissues at parturition and between blood and milk postpartum. Antimicrob Agents Chemother 1983;23:870–3.
5. Cho N, Kunii K, Fukunago K, Komoriyama Y. Antimicrobial activity, pharmacokinetics and clinical studies of ceftriaxone in obstetrics and gynecology. In: *Proceedings of the 13th International Congress on Chemotherapy, Vienna, Austria, August 28–September 2, 1983*. Princeton, NJ: Excerpta Medica, 1984:100/64–6.
6. Graber H, Magyar T. Pharmacokinetics of ceftriaxone in pregnancy. Am J Med 1984;77:117–8.
7. Sanchez-Ramos L, McAlpine KJ, Adair CD, Kaunitz AM, Delke I, Briones DK. Pyelonephritis in pregnancy: once-a-day ceftriaxone versus multiple doses of cefazolin. Am J Obstet Gynecol 1995;172:129–33.
8. Lang R, Shalit I, Segal J, Arbel Y, Markov S, Hass H, Fejgin M. Maternal and fetal and tissue levels of ceftriaxone following preoperative prophylaxis in emergency cesarean section. Chemotherapy 1993;39:77–81.
9. Cavenee MR, Farris JR, Spalding TR, Barnes DL, Castaneda YS, Wendel GD Jr. Treatment of gonorrhea in pregnancy. Obstet Gynecol 1993;81:33–8.
10. Deger R, Ludmir J. Neisseria sicca endocarditis complicating pregnancy. A case report. J Reprod Med 1992;37:473–5.
11. Committee on Drugs, American Academy of Pediatrics. The transfer of drugs and other chemicals into human milk. Pediatrics 2001;108:776–89.

CEFUROXIME

C

Antibiotic (Cephalosporin)

PREGNANCY RECOMMENDATION: Compatible
BREASTFEEDING RECOMMENDATION: Compatible

PREGNANCY SUMMARY

No detectable teratogenic risk with cefuroxime or other cephalosporin antibiotics was found in a large 2001 study (see Cephalexin).

FETAL RISK SUMMARY

Cefuroxime is an oral and parenteral, semisynthetic cephalosporin antibiotic. Reproduction studies in rats have found no evidence of impaired fertility at doses up to 9 times the maximum recommended human dose based on BSA (MRHD) or, mice and rats, of fetal harm at doses up to 23 times the MRHD (1).

Cefuroxime readily crosses the placenta in late pregnancy and labor, achieving therapeutic concentrations in fetal serum and amniotic fluid (2–7). Therapeutic antibiotic levels in infants can be demonstrated up to 6 hours after birth with measurable concentrations persisting for 26 hours. The pharmacokinetics of cefuroxime in pregnancy have been reported (8). The antibiotic has been used for the treatment of pyelonephritis in pregnancy (9). Adverse effects in the newborn after in utero exposure have not been observed.

In women at 15–35 weeks' gestation, a single 750-mg IV dose produced mean serum concentrations in mothers, hydropic fetuses, and fetuses with oligohydramnios of 7.4, 6.2, and 4.9 mcg/mL, respectively (10). The concentrations did not correlate with gestational age. Nine women with premature rupture of the membranes at 27–33 weeks' gestation received 1.5 g IV of cefuroxime three times daily (11). The mean concentrations of the antibiotic in the mothers (1 hour after a dose), umbilical cord plasma, placenta, and membranes were 35.0 mcg/mL, 3.0 mcg/mL, 11.2 mcg/g, and 35.6 mcg/g, respectively.

In a surveillance study of Michigan Medicaid recipients involving 229,101 completed pregnancies conducted between 1985 and 1992, 143 newborns had been exposed to cefuroxime during the 1st trimester (F. Rosa, personal communication, FDA, 1993). Three (2.1%) major birth defects were observed (six expected), but no anomalies were observed in six categories of defects for which specific data were available (cardiovascular defects, oral clefts, spina bifida, polydactyly, limb-reduction defects, and hypospadias). These data do not support an association between the drug and congenital defects (see also Cefaclor, Cephalexin, and Cephradine for contrasting results).

The pregnancy outcomes of 106 women exposed in the 1st trimester to cefuroxime were described in a 2000 study (12). Compared with 106 matched controls, there was no difference in pregnancy outcomes in terms of live births, spontaneous abortions, gestational age at birth, prematurity, birth weight, fetal distress, method of delivery, and major or minor malformations. Induced abortions, however, occurred in significantly more cefuroxime-exposed women than in controls, possibly due to misinformation and misperception of the risk the antibiotic posed to a pregnancy (12).

BREASTFEEDING SUMMARY

Cefuroxime is excreted into breast milk in low concentrations (1). Even though the levels are low, three potential problems exist for the nursing infant exposed to cefuroxime in milk: modification of bowel flora, direct effects on the infant, and interference with the interpretation of culture results if a fever workup is required. Although not specifically listing cefuroxime, the American Academy of Pediatrics classifies other cephalosporin antibiotics as compatible with breastfeeding (for example, see Cefadroxil and Cefazolin).

References

1. Product information. Ceftin. Glaxo Wellcome, 1997.
2. Craft I, Mullinger BM, Kennedy MRK. Placental transfer of cefuroxime. Br J Obstet Gynaecol 1981;88:141–5.
3. Bousfield P, Browning AK, Mullinger BM, Elstein M. Cefuroxime: potential use in pregnant women at term. Br J Obstet Gynaecol 1981;88:146–9.
4. Bergogne-Berezin E, Pierre J, Even P, Rouvillois JL, Dumez Y. Study of penetration of cefuroxime into bronchial secretions and of its placental transfer. Therapie 1980;35:677–84.
5. Tzingounis V, Makris N, Zolotas J, Michalas S, Aravantinos D. Cefuroxime prophylaxis in caesarean section. Pharmatherapeutica 1982;3:140–2.
6. Coppi G, Berti MA, Chehade A, Franchi I, Magro B. A study of the transplacental transfer of cefuroxime in humans. Curr Ther Res 1982;32:712–6.
7. Bousefield PF. Use of cefuroxime in pregnant women at term. Res Clin Forums 1984;6:53–8.
8. Philipson A, Stiernstedt G. Pharmacokinetics of cefuroxime in pregnancy. Am J Obstet Gynecol 1982;142:823–8.
9. Faro S, Pastorek JG II, Plauche WC, Korndorffer FA, Aldridge KE. Short-course parenteral antibiotic therapy for pyelonephritis in pregnancy. S Med J 1984;77:455–7.
10. Holt DE, Fisk NM, Spencer JAD, de Louvlis J, Hurley R, Harvey D. Transplacental transfer of cefuroxime in uncomplicated pregnancies and those complicated by hydrops or changes in amniotic fluid volume. Arch Dis Child 1993;68:54–7.
11. De Leeuw JW, Roumen FJME, Bouckaert PXJM, Cremers HMHG, Vree TB. Achievement of therapeutic concentrations of cefuroxime in early preterm gestations with premature rupture of the membranes. Obstet Gynecol 1993;81:255–60.
12. Berkovitch M, Segal-Socher I, Greenberg R, Bulkowshtein M, Arnon J, Perlob P, Or-Noy A. First trimester exposure to cefuroxime: a prospective cohort study. Br J Clin Pharmacol 2000;50:161–5.

CELECOXIB

Nonsteroidal Anti-inflammatory

PREGNANCY RECOMMENDATION: Human Data Suggest Risk in 1st and 3rd Trimesters
BREASTFEEDING RECOMMENDATION: Limited Human Data—Probably Compatible

C

PREGNANCY SUMMARY

Celecoxib has been used in human pregnancy as a tocolytic. The animal data are suggestive of a low risk for congenital malformations. Moreover, a brief 2003 editorial on the potential for nonsteroidal anti-inflammatory drug (NSAID)-induced developmental toxicity concluded that NSAIDs, and specifically those with greater COX-2 affinity, had a lower risk of this toxicity in humans than aspirin (1). The use of first-generation NSAIDs during the latter half of pregnancy has been associated with oligohydramnios and premature closure of the ductus arteriosus (e.g., see Indomethacin) (2). Persistent pulmonary hypertension of the newborn may occur if NSAIDs are used in the 3rd trimester close to delivery (2,3). These drugs also have been shown to inhibit labor and prolong pregnancy, both in humans (4) and in animals (5). Similar effects should be expected if celecoxib is used during the 3rd trimester or close to delivery. Women attempting to conceive should not use any prostaglandin synthesis inhibitor, including celecoxib, because of the findings in a variety of animal models that indicate these agents block blastocyst implantation (6,7). Moreover, as noted above, NSAIDs have been associated with spontaneous abortions (SABs) and congenital malformations. The absolute risk for these defects, however, appears to be low. If celecoxib is used in pregnancy for the treatment of rheumatoid arthritis, healthcare professionals are encouraged to call the toll-free number (877-311-8972) for information about patient enrollment in the OTIS Rheumatoid Arthritis study.

FETAL RISK SUMMARY

Celecoxib is a second-generation NSAID that inhibits prostaglandin synthesis via the inhibition of cyclooxygenase-2 (COX-2). It is in the same NSAID subclass (COX-2 inhibitors) as rofecoxib and valdecoxib. In therapeutic concentrations, it does not inhibit, as do first-generation NSAIDs, the cyclooxygenase-1 (COX-1) isoenzyme. Celecoxib is indicated for the relief of the signs and symptoms of osteoarthritis and rheumatoid arthritis (8).

Celecoxib was not mutagenic or clastogenic in Chinese hamster ovary cells or clastogenic in an in vivo micronucleus test in rat bone marrow. Administration to female rats of oral doses that were about six times the maximum recommended human dose based on AUC at 200 mg twice a day (MRHD) resulted in preimplantation and postimplantation losses and reduced embryo–fetal survival, a natural consequence of its inhibition of prostaglandin synthesis (8).

Reproduction studies have been conducted in rats and rabbits. In pregnant rats, a dose-related increase in diaphragmatic hernias was observed in one of two studies at doses about six times the MRHD. No teratogenic effects occurred in pregnant rabbits at doses equal to the MRHD, but at doses about two times the MRHD, an increased incidence of fetal alterations (fused ribs and fused, misshapen sternebrae) was observed. No evidence of delayed labor or parturition at doses up to about seven times the MRHD was observed in rats (8).

Two studies in pregnant rabbits were designed to test the hypothesis that celecoxib was effective in preventing preterm delivery and did not adversely affect fetal ductus arteriosus patency (9,10). In the first study, the rabbits received a daily dose that was about 0.5 times the MRHD for differing periods starting at day 13 of gestation (9). Concentrations of prostanoids, cytokines, and nitric oxide were altered by the treatment, resulting in decrease in the incidence compared with controls of preterm parturition. In the second study, no adverse effect on the fetal ductus arteriosus was observed (10).

No reports describing the placental transfer of celecoxib have been located. The molecular weight (about 381) is low enough that passage to the fetus should be expected. Celecoxib metabolism is mediated by the cytochrome P450 2C9 enzyme, resulting in at least three inactive metabolites (8). Women, in whom metabolism by this enzyme is known or suspected to be deficient, may have abnormally high plasma levels of celecoxib and, thus, more of the drug will be available for placental transfer.

A combined 2001 population-based observational cohort study and a case–control study estimated the risk of adverse pregnancy outcome from the use of NSAIDs (11). The use of NSAIDs during pregnancy was not associated with congenital malformations, preterm delivery, or low birth weight, but a positive association was discovered with SABs. A similar study, also published in 2001, failed to find a relationship, in general, between NSAIDs and congenital malformations, but did find a significant association with cardiac defects and orofacial clefts (12). In addition, a 2003 study found a significant association between exposure to NSAIDs in early pregnancy and SABs (13). (See Ibuprofen for details on these three studies.)

A 2006 case–control study found a significant association between congenital anomalies, specifically cardiac septal defects, and the use of NSAIDs in the 1st trimester (14). A population-based pregnancy registry (N = 36,387) was developed by linking three databases in Quebec. (See Naprosyn for other study details.) Case infants were those with any congenital anomaly diagnosed in the first year of life and were compared with matched controls. There were 93 infants (8.8%) with congenital defects from 1056 mothers who had filled prescriptions for NSAIDs in the 1st trimester. In controls, there were 2478 infants (7%) with anomalies from 35,331 mothers who had not filled such a prescription. The adjusted odds ratio (OR) was 2.21 (95% CI 1.72–2.85). The adjusted OR for cardiac septal closure was 3.34 (95% CI 1.87–5.98). There also was a significant association with anomalies of the respiratory system 9.55 (95% CI 3.08–29.63), but this association disappeared when cases coded as "unspecified anomaly of the respiratory system" were excluded. For the cases involving septal closure, 61% were atrial septal defects and 31% were ventricular septal defects. There were no significant associations for oral clefts or defects involving other major organ systems. The five most common NSAIDs were naproxen (35%), ibuprofen (26%), rofecoxib (15%), diclofenac (9%), and celecoxib (9%). Among these agents, the only significant association was for ibuprofen prescriptions in the 1st trimester and congenital defects ($p < 0.01$) (14).

An in vitro study demonstrated that celecoxib had significant uterine relaxant effects (15). Celecoxib was more potent, in this regard, than nimesulide or meloxicam. A 2002 randomized, double-blind, placebo-controlled study compared the tocolytic effects of celecoxib (100 mg orally every 12 hours for 4 doses) and indomethacin (100 mg rectally, then 50 mg orally every 6 hours for 7 doses) (16). The subjects, 12 in each group, were in preterm labor at 24 to 34 weeks' gestation. Partial premature constriction of the fetal ductus arteriosus occurred in the indomethacin group, but not in the celecoxib group. A transient decrease in amniotic fluid volume was observed in both groups, but more so with indomethacin. Both drugs were equally effective in the maintenance of tocolysis, but the authors concluded that the safety of celecoxib was superior to that of indomethacin (16).

A randomized trial in 2007 compared the tocolytic effects of celecoxib (200 mg/day) and IV magnesium sulfate, each given for 48 hours (17). Gestational ages were 24–34 weeks and each group had 52 women. No statistical difference (81% vs. 87%) in the arrest of labor was found and there were no severe maternal or neonatal complications (17).

BREASTFEEDING SUMMARY

Celecoxib is excreted into human breastmilk (18–20). A 40-year-old woman who was breastfeeding her 5-month-old daughter was admitted to the hospital for surgery. In the postoperative period, she received four doses of celecoxib (100 mg twice/day) in addition to other medications. Starting about 5 hours after her last dose, four milk samples were obtained by hand expression over a 24-hour interval. The elimination half-life range was 4.0–6.5 hours. These data suggest that celecoxib would be eliminated from breast milk about 24 hours after the last dose. Although maternal plasma was not obtained, the estimated milk:plasma ratios (based on reported adult plasma levels) were 0.27–0.59. The infant did not resume breastfeeding until 48 hours after the last dose. If she had nursed, the estimated maximum infant dose would have been about 40 mcg/kg/day (18).

A 2004 study of five breastfeeding women taking celecoxib, three at steady state (200 mg once daily) and two after a single 200-mg dose, measured a mean milk concentration of 66 mcg/L and a mean milk:plasma ratio of 0.23 (19). The mean absolute infant dose was 9.8 mcg/kg/day and the relative infant dose was 0.30% of the mother's weight-adjusted dose. Plasma concentrations in two infants at 17 and 22 months of age, who were nursing every 3–4 hours during the day and once at night, were below the limit of detection (10 mcg/L) (19).

Six lactating women, who stopped nursing after taking celecoxib, were included in a 2005 report (20). After a single 200-mg dose, the median absolute infant dose was 13 mcg/kg/day and the relative infant dose was 0.23% of the mother's weight-adjusted dose.

Several first-generation NSAIDs are considered low risk during nursing (e.g., see Diclofenac, Fenoprofen, Flurbiprofen, Ibuprofen, Ketoprofen, Ketorolac, and Tolmetin) and, based on the available data, celecoxib, at the doses studied, can be similarly classified. Although only 3 of the 12 patients studied were breastfeeding when taking celecoxib, the authors of the studies concluded that celecoxib was unlikely to pose a risk to a nursing infant.

References

1. Tassinari MS, Cook JC, Hunt ME. NSAIDs and development toxicity. Birth Defects Res (Part B) 2003;68:3–4.
2. Levin DL. Effects of inhibition of prostaglandin synthesis on fetal development, oxygenation, and the fetal circulation. Semin Perinatol 1980;4:35–44.
3. Van Marter LJ, Leviton A, Allred EN, Pagano M, Sullivan KF, Cohen A, Epstein MF. Persistent pulmonary hypertension of the newborn and smoking and aspirin and nonsteroidal antiinflammatory drug consumption during pregnancy. Pediatrics 1996;97:658–63.
4. Fuchs F. Prevention of prematurity. Am J Obstet Gynecol 1976;126:809–20.
5. Powell JG, Cochrane RL. The effects of a number of non-steroidal anti-inflammatory compounds on parturition in the rat. Prostaglandins 1982;23:469–88.
6. Matt DW, Borzelleca JF. Toxic effects on the female reproductive system during pregnancy, parturition, and lactation. In: Witorsch RJ, ed. *Reproductive Toxicology*. 2nd ed. New York, NY: Raven Press, 1995:175–93.
7. Dawood MY. Nonsteroidal antiinflammatory drugs and reproduction. Am J Obstet Gynecol 1993;169:1255–65.
8. Product information. Celebrex. G.D. Searle, 1999.
9. Hausman N, Beharry KD, Nishihara KC, Akmal Y, Asrat T. Effect of the antenatal administration of celecoxib during the second and third trimesters of pregnancy on prostaglandin, cytokine, and nitric oxide levels in rabbits. Am J Obstet Gynecol 2003;189:1737–43.
10. Hausman N, Beharry K, Nishihara K, Akmal V, Stavitsky Y, Asrat T. Response of fetal prostanoids, nitric oxide, and ductus arteriosus to the short- and long-term antenatal administration of celecoxib, a selective cyclo-oxygenase-2 inhibitor, in the pregnant rabbit. Am J Obstet Gynecol 2003;189:1744–50.
11. Nielsen GL, Sorensen HT, Larsen H, Pedersen L. Risk of adverse birth outcome and miscarriage in pregnant users of non-steroidal anti-inflammatory drugs: population based observational study and case-control study. Br Med J 2001;322:266–70.
12. Ericson A, Kallen BAJ. Nonsteroidal anti-inflammatory drugs in early pregnancy. Reprod Toxicol 2001;15:371–3.
13. Li DK, Liu L, Odouli R. Exposure to non-steroidal anti-inflammatory drugs during pregnancy and risk of miscarriage: population based cohort study. Br Med J 2003;327:368–71.
14. Ofori B, Oraichi D, Blais L, Rey E, Bérard A. Risk of congenital anomalies in pregnant users of non-steroidal anti-inflammatory drugs: a nested case-control study. Birth Defects Res (Part B) 2006;77:268–79.
15. Slattery MM, Friel AM, Healy DG, Morrison JJ. Uterine relaxant effects of cyclooxygenase-2 inhibitors in vitro. Obstet Gynecol 2001;98:563–9.
16. Stika CS, Gross GA, Leguizamon G, Gerber S, Levy R, Mathur A, Bernhard LM, Nelson DM, Sadovsky Y. A prospective randomized safety trial of celecoxib for treatment of preterm labor. Am J Obstet Gynecol 2002;187:653–60.
17. Borna S, Saeidi FM. Celecoxib versus magnesium sulfate to arrest preterm labor: randomized trial. J Obstet Gynaecol Res 2007;33:631–4.
18. Knoppert DC, Stempak D, Baruchel S, Koren G. Celecoxib in human milk: a case report. Pharmacotherapy 2003;23:97–100.
19. Hale TW, McDonald R, Boger J. Transfer of celecoxib into human milk. J Hum Lact 2004;20:397–403.
20. Gardiner SJ, Doogue MP, Zhang M, Begg EJ. Quantification of infant exposure to celecoxib through breast milk. Br J Clin Pharmacol 2005;61:101–4.

CELIPROLOL

[Withdrawn from the market. See 9th edition.]

CENTRUROIDES (SCORPION) IMMUNE F(ab′)$_2$ (EQUINE)

Antidote

PREGNANCY RECOMMENDATION: Maternal Benefit >> Embryo–Fetal Risk
BREASTFEEDING RECOMMENDATION: No Human Data—Probably Compatible

PREGNANCY SUMMARY

No reports describing the use of *Centruroides* antivenom in pregnancy have been located. Animal reproduction studies have not been conducted, and the absence of human pregnancy experience prevents any assessment of the embryo–fetal risk. It appears, however, that the maternal benefit outweighs the unknown embryo–fetal risk. Therefore, if indicated, the antivenom should not be withheld because of pregnancy.

FETAL RISK SUMMARY

Centruroides antivenom is prepared from horse plasma immunized to venom from five different species of scorpions. It is given IV to bind and neutralize venom toxins, facilitating redistribution away from target tissues and elimination from the body. The antivenom is indicated for the treatment of clinical signs of scorpion envenomation. The half-life is 159 ± 57 hours (1).

Reproduction studies in animals have not been conducted. Moreover, studies for carcinogenic and mutagenic potential have not been conducted, nor have been fertility impairment studies (1).

It is not known if the antivenom crosses the human placenta. The molecular weight of the antivenom was not given by the manufacturer. The molecular weight is probably very high, because the product is a polyvalent preparation of equine immune globulin F(ab′)$_2$ fragments. Exposure of the fetus, at least in early pregnancy, might be clinically insignificant. However, the long elimination half-life will allow the antivenom to be at the maternal–fetal interface for a several days.

BREASTFEEDING SUMMARY

No reports describing the use of *Centruroides* antivenom during human lactation have been located. The molecular weight of the antivenom was not given by the manufacturer. The molecular weight probably is very high, because the product is a polyvalent preparation of equine immune globulin F(ab′)$_2$ fragments. Moreover, the antivenom has a long elimination half-life (159 ± 57 hours) and, if it was given shortly before birth, this might allow excretion of small amounts during the colostral phase. Although the effect of any exposure on nursing is unknown, the antivenom would most likely be digested in the infant's gut.

Reference

1. Product information. Anascorp. Accredo Health Group, 2011.

CEPHALEXIN

Antibiotic (Cephalosporin)

PREGNANCY RECOMMENDATION: Compatible
BREASTFEEDING RECOMMENDATION: Compatible

PREGNANCY SUMMARY

Although some data suggest an association with congenital malformations, most studies have found that cephalosporin antibiotics, in general, are safe to use in pregnancy.

C

FETAL RISK SUMMARY

Cephalexin is an oral, semisynthetic cephalosporin antibiotic. Reproduction studies found no evidence in rats, at doses up to 500 mg/kg, of impaired fertility or reproductive performance or, in mice and rats, of fetal harm (1).

Several published reports have described the administration of cephalexin to pregnant patients in various stages of gestation (2–12). None of these has linked the use of cephalexin with congenital defects or toxicity in the newborn. However, even though cephalosporins are usually considered safe to use during pregnancy, a surveillance study described below found results contrasting to the published data.

In a surveillance study of Michigan Medicaid recipients involving 229,101 completed pregnancies conducted between 1985 and 1992, 3613 newborns had been exposed to cephalexin during the 1st trimester (F. Rosa, personal communication, FDA, 1993). A total of 176 (4.9%) major birth defects were observed (154 expected). Specific data were available for six defect categories, including (observed/expected) 44/36 cardiovascular defects, 11/5 oral clefts, 3/2 spina bifida, 3/10 polydactyly, 1/6 limb reduction defects, and 8/9 hypospadias. The data for total defects, cardiovascular defects, and oral clefts are suggestive of an association between cephalexin and congenital defects, but other factors, such as the mother's disease, concurrent drug use, and chance, may be involved. However, similar findings were measured for another cephalosporin antibiotic with more than a thousand exposures (see Cefaclor). Positive results were also suggested for cephradine (339 exposures) but not for cefadroxil (722 exposures) (see Cephradine and Cefadroxil). In contrast, other anti-infectives with large cohorts (see Ampicillin, Amoxicillin, Penicillin G, Erythromycin, and Tetracycline) had negative findings.

Transplacental passage of cephalexin has been demonstrated only near term (2,3). Following a 1-g oral dose, peak concentrations for maternal serum, cord serum, and amniotic fluid were about 34 (1 hour), 11 (4 hours), and 13 mcg/mL (6 hours), respectively (3). Patients in whom labor was induced were observed to have falling concentrations of cephalexin in all samples when labor was prolonged beyond 18 hours (4). In one report, all fetal blood samples gave a negative Coombs' reaction (2).

The effect of postcoital prophylaxis with a single oral dose of either cephalexin (250 mg) or nitrofurantoin macrocrystals (50 mg) starting before or during pregnancy in 33 women (39 pregnancies) with a history of recurrent urinary tract infections was described in a 1992 reference (11). A significant decrease in the number of infections was documented without fetal toxicity.

The manufacturer has unpublished information on 46 patients treated with cephalexin during pregnancy (C.L. Lynch, personal communication, Dista Products, 1981). Two of these patients received the drug from 1to 2 months prior to conception to term. No effects on the fetus attributable to the antibiotic were observed. Follow-up examination on one infant at 2 months was normal.

A 2001 study used the Hungarian Case-Control Surveillance of Congenital Abnormalities (1980–1996) database to examine the association between cephalosporins (cephalexin, cefaclor, cefamandole, cefoperazone, cefotaxime, ceftibuten, and cefuroxime) and birth defects (12). Cases were drawn from 22,865 pregnant women who had fetuses or newborn infants with congenital abnormalities. Matched controls were obtained from pregnant women who had infants without defects. Most of the 308 case women were treated with cephalexin. No detectable teratogenic risk was found.

BREASTFEEDING SUMMARY

Cephalexin is excreted into breast milk in low concentrations (13,14). A 1-g oral dose given to six mothers produced peak milk levels at 4–5 hours averaging 0.51 mcg/mL (range 0.24–0.85 mcg/mL) (13). Mean milk:plasma ratios at 1, 2, and 3 hours were 0.008, 0.021, and 0.14, respectively.

A 30-year-old, penicillin-allergic, breastfeeding woman developed erysipelas/cellulitis in her breasts 9 days after a cesarean section (14). She was treated with IV cephalothin, 1 g every 6 hours for 3 days, then oral cephalexin and probenecid (both 500 mg four times daily). Severe diarrhea, discomfort, and crying were observed in the nursing infant during IV therapy and continued with oral therapy, but at a decreased level. The symptoms had nearly resolved after partial replacement of breast milk with goat's milk for 7 days. Sixteen days after initiation of oral therapy, the woman collected 12 milk samples (6 pairs of fore- and hind-milk) by manual expression over a 16-hour interval. The average concentrations of cephalexin and probenecid and cephalexin were 0.745 and 0.964 mcg/mL, respectively. The concentrations of the two substances in fore- and hind-milk were not significantly different. The infant doses, based on the milk AUC and an estimated intake of 150 mL/kg/day, of cephalexin and probenecid were 0.5% and 0.7%, respectively, of the mother's weight-adjusted dose. Although these doses were thought to be low enough to exclude systemic effects, it was concluded that cephalexin was the most likely cause of the diarrhea (14).

The above two studies are not comparable because of the dosage and duration. However, they do suggest that probenecid markedly increases the milk concentration of cephalexin. In the absence of any data, it is not known if a lower milk concentration would also have caused the diarrhea observed in the infant. Nevertheless, three potential problems exist for a nursing infant exposed to antibiotics in milk: modification of bowel flora, direct effects on the infant, and interference with the interpretation of culture results if a fever workup is required. Although not specifically listing cephalexin, the American Academy of Pediatrics classifies other cephalosporin antibiotics as compatible with breastfeeding (for example, see Cefadroxil and Cefazolin).

References

1. Product information. Keflex. Dista Products, 1997.
2. Paterson ML, Henderson A, Lunan CB, McGurk S. Transplacental transfer of cephalexin. Clin Med 1972;79:22–4.
3. Creatsas G, Pavlatos M, Lolis D, Kaskarelis D. A study of the kinetics of cephapirin and cephalexin in pregnancy. Curr Med Res Opin 1980;7:43–6.
4. Hirsch HA. Behandlung von harnwegsinfektionen in gynakologic und geburtshilfe mit cephalexin. Int J Clin Pharmacol 1969;2(Suppl):121–3.
5. Brumfitt W, Pursell R. Double-blind trial to compare ampicillin, cephalexin, co-trimoxazole, and trimethoprim in treatment of urinary infection. Br Med J 1972;2:673–6.
6. Mizuno S, Metsuda S, Mori S. Clinical evaluation of cephalexin in obstetrics and gynaecology. In: *Proceedings of a Symposium on the Clinical Evaluation of Cephalexin*, Royal Society of Medicine, London, June 2 and 3, 1969.

7. Guttman D. Cephalexin in urinary tract infections—preliminary results. In: *Proceedings of a Symposium on the Clinical Evaluation of Cephalexin*, Royal Society of Medicine, London, June 2 and 3, 1969.
8. Soto RF, Fesbre F, Cordido A, et al. Ensayo con cefalexina en el tratamiento de infecciones urinarias en pacientes embarazadas. Rev Obstet Ginecol Venez 1972;32:637–41.
9. Campbell-Brown M, McFadyen IR. Bacteriuria in pregnancy treated with a single dose of cephalexin. Br J Obstet Gynaecol 1983;90:1054–9.
10. Jakobi P, Neiger R, Merzbach D, Paldi E. Single-dose antimicrobial therapy in the treatment of asymptomatic bacteriuria in pregnancy. Am J Obstet Gynecol 1987;156:1148–52.
11. Pfau A, Sacks TG. Effective prophylaxis for recurrent urinary tract infections during pregnancy. Clin Infect Dis 1992;14:810–4.
12. Czeizel AE, Rockenbauer M, Sorensen HT, Olsen J. Use of cephalosporins during pregnancy and in the presence of congenital abnormalities: a population-based, case-control study. Am J Obstet Gynecol 2001;184:1289–96.
13. Kafetzis D, Siafas C, Georgakopoulos P, Papadatos CJ. Passage of cephalosporins and amoxicillin into the breast milk. Acta Paediatr Scand 1981;70:285–8.
14. Ilett KF, Hackett LP, Ingle B, Bretz PJ. Transfer of probenecid and cephalexin into breast milk. Ann Pharmacother 2006;40:986–9.

C

CEPHALOTHIN

[Withdrawn from the market. See 9th edition.]

CEPHAPIRIN

[Withdrawn from the market. See 9th edition.]

CEPHRADINE

[Withdrawn from the market. See 9th edition.]

CERIVASTATIN

[Withdrawn from the market. See 8th edition.]

CERTOLIZUMAB PEGOL

Immunologic Agent (Immunomodulator)

PREGNANCY RECOMMENDATION: Limited Human Data—Probably Compatible
BREASTFEEDING RECOMMENDATION: Limited Human Data—Probably Compatible

PREGNANCY SUMMARY

The limited human pregnancy experience suggests that certolizumab pegol is low risk for embryo–fetal harm. In 2011, the World Congress of Gastroenterology stated, "Certolizumab pegol in pregnancy is considered to be low risk and compatible with use during conception and pregnancy in women" (1). Animal reproduction studies could not be conducted because the antibody is human specific. However, studies in rats with a rodent-specific antibody similar to certolizumab pegol found no evidence of fetal harm. There is some similarity between the action of immunomodulators with anti-TNFα activity and the human teratogen thalidomide, a drug that also decreases the activity of TNFα. (See Infliximab and Thalidomide.) However, decreased production of TNFα may not be a primary cause of the teratogenicity of thalidomide. Theoretically, TNFα antagonists could interfere with implantation and ovulation, but this has not been shown clinically (2).

FETAL RISK SUMMARY

Certolizumab pegol is a recombinant, humanized antibody Fab′ fragment that blocks human tumor necrosis factor alpha (TNFα). TNFα is a pro-inflammatory cytokine with a central role in inflammatory processes. Certolizumab is in the same subclass of immunomodulators (blockers of TNFα activity) as adalimumab, golimumab, and infliximab. It is conjugated with polyethylene glycol (PEG) to decrease the renal clearance and metabolism of the antibody. The agent is given by

C

SC injection. Certolizumab pegol is indicated for reducing the signs and symptoms of Crohn's disease and maintaining clinical response in adult patients with moderately to severely active disease that have had an inadequate response to conventional therapy. The terminal elimination half-life is about 14 days (3).

Reproduction studies in animals have not been conducted with certolizumab pegol because it does not cross-react with mouse or rat TNFα. However, studies were conducted in rats using a rodent anti-murine TNFα pegylated Fab′ fragment similar to certolizumab pegol. Doses up to 100 mg/kg revealed no evidence of impaired fertility or fetal harm (3). Although a comparison to the human dose was not specified, the maximum dose was about 17 times the human dose of 5.7 mg/kg from a 400-mg dose given to a 70-kg patient.

Long-term studies to evaluate the carcinogenic potential of certolizumab pegol have not been conducted, but the agent was not genotoxic in multiple assays. The rodent anti-murine TNFα pegylated Fab′ fragment had no effect on the fertility and reproductive performance of male or female rats (3).

Although the molecular weight is very high (about 91,000), certolizumab (but not PEG) crosses the human placenta to the fetus in late gestation (4). In 12 newborns (2 sets of twins) at a mean gestational age of 37.8 weeks (range 36–40 weeks), the median (range) of certolizumab concentrations in cord blood as a percentage of maternal concentration was 3.9% (1.5%–24%). The concentrations in cord blood and in the infant were all ≤1.65 mcg/mL and were undectable in four cord blood samples and three infants (lower limit of quantification <0.41 mcg/mL). PEG was not detected in any cord blood or infant. No birth defects or neonatal intensive care unit stays occurred in any infant (4).

BREASTFEEDING SUMMARY

Certolizumab was not detected in several milk samples from a mother who was breastfeeding her infant (4). The mother was receiving 400 mg every 4 weeks and had received a dose 1 week before delivery and 3 weeks after delivery. At birth, the levels in the cord blood level and infant were 0.94 mcg/mL and 1.02 mcg/mL, respectively. At 4 weeks post-birth, the levels in the mother and infant were 22.93 mcg/mL and 0.84 mcg/mL (3.7%), respectively. Breast milk samples were obtained at 1 and 2 weeks post-birth and at 4 hours, 3 days, and 6 days after the dose at 3 weeks. Concentrations in each of the five milk samples were undectable. PEG was not detected in the infant (4).

References

1. Mahadevan U, Cucchiara S, Hyams JS, Steinwurz F, Nuti F, Travis SPL, Sandborn WJ, Colombel IH. The London position statement of the World Congress of Gastroenterology on biological therapy for IBD with the European Crohn's and Colitis Organization: pregnancy and pediatrics. Am J Gastroenterol 2011;106:214–23.
2. Khanna D, McMahon M, Furst DE. Safety of tumor necrosis factor-α antagonists. Drug Saf 2004;27:307–24.
3. Product information. Cimzia. UCB, 2008.
4. Mahadevan U, Wolf DC, Dubinsky M, Cortot A, Lee SD, Siegel CA, Ullman T, Glover S, Valentine JF, Rubin DT, Miller J, Abreu MT. Placental transfer of anti-tumor necrosis factor agents in pregnant patients with inflammatory bowel disease. Clin Gastroenterol Hepatol 2013;11:286–92.

CETIRIZINE

Antihistamine

PREGNANCY RECOMMENDATION: Limited Human Data—Animal Data Suggest Low Risk
BREASTFEEDING RECOMMENDATION: No Human Data—Probably Compatible

PREGNANCY SUMMARY

Cetirizine is not an animal teratogen, and there is no evidence in human pregnancy that the antihistamine presents a significant risk to the fetus. However, the number of human pregnancy exposures is too few to adequately assess the potential risk. Although cetirizine appears unlikely to be a major human teratogen, an oral first-generation agent, such as chlorpheniramine or tripelennamine, should be considered if antihistamine therapy during pregnancy (especially in the 1st trimester) is required. Cetirizine and loratadine were considered acceptable alternatives, except during the 1st trimester, if a first-generation agent was not tolerated (1–3). The use of cetirizine as an antiemetic needs further study.

FETAL RISK SUMMARY

The antihistamine, cetirizine, is a second-generation, orally active, selective peripheral H_1-receptor antagonist. It is indicated for the relief of seasonal and perennial allergic rhinitis and for the treatment of chronic urticaria. The agent is a human metabolite of hydroxyzine.

Reproduction studies in mice, rats, and rabbits at oral doses up to 40, 180, and 220 times the maximum recommended human daily dose based on BSA (MRHD), respectively, revealed no teratogenic effects (4).

It is not known if cetirizine crosses the human placenta to the fetus. The molecular weight (about 462 for the dihydrochloride salt) is low enough that transfer to the fetus should be expected.

A prospective controlled study published in 1997 evaluated the teratogenic risk of cetirizine and hydroxyzine (see also Hydroxyzine) in human pregnancy (5). A total of 120 pregnancies (2 sets of twins) exposed to either cetirizine (*N* = 39) or hydroxyzine (*N* = 81) during pregnancy were identified and compared with 110 controls. The control group was matched for maternal age, smoking, and alcohol use.

The drugs were taken during the 1st trimester in 37 (95%) of the cetirizine exposures and in 53 (65%) of the hydroxyzine cases for a variety of indications (e.g., rhinitis, urticaria, pruritic urticarial papules and plaques of pregnancy, sedation, and other nonspecified reasons). Fourteen spontaneous abortions (cetirizine 6, hydroxyzine 3, controls 5) and 11 induced abortions (hydroxyzine 6, controls 5) occurred in the three groups. Among the live births, there were no statistical differences among the groups in birth weight, gestational age at delivery, rate of cesarean section, or neonatal distress. Two minor anomalies were observed in liveborn infants exposed to cetirizine during organogenesis; one had an ectopic kidney and one had undescended testes. No major abnormalities were seen in this group. In the hydroxyzine group, two of the live births had major malformations; one had a ventricular septal defect and one a complex congenital heart defect (also exposed to carbamazepine). A third infant, exposed after organogenesis, also had a ventricular septal defect. Minor abnormalities were observed in four hydroxyzine-exposed infants: one case each of hydrocele, inguinal hernia, hypothyroidism (mother also taking propylthiouracil), and strabismus. In the control group, no major malformations were observed, but five infants had minor defects (dislocated hip, growth hormone deficiency, short lingual frenulum, and two unspecified defects). Statistically, there were no differences between the groups in outcome (5).

A recent review compared the published pregnancy outcomes in terms of congenital malformations of various first- and second-generation antihistamines (6). Based on the one study above, the authors calculated a relative risk for cetirizine of 1.2 (95% confidence interval 0.1–11.7). They concluded that in pregnancy, chlorpheniramine is the oral antihistamine of choice and that diphenhydramine should be used if a parenteral antihistamine is required (6).

A 1998 noninterventional observational cohort study described the outcomes of pregnancies in women who had been prescribed one or more of 34 newly marketed drugs by general practitioners in England (7). Data were obtained by questionnaires sent to the prescribing physicians one month after the expected or possible date of delivery. In 831 (78%) of the pregnancies, a newly marketed drug was thought to have been taken during the 1st trimester with birth defects noted in 14 (2.5%) singleton births of the 557 newborns (10 sets of twins). In addition, two birth defects were observed in aborted fetuses. However, few of the aborted fetuses were examined. Cetirizine was taken during the 1st trimester in 20 pregnancies. The outcomes of these pregnancies included 4 spontaneous abortions, 1 elective abortion, and 16 normal- term infants (1 set of twins) (7). Although this study found no major birth defects, it lacked the sensitivity to identify minor anomalies because of the absence of standardized examinations. Further, late-appearing major defects may also have been missed because of the timing of the questionnaires.

A 2000 publication reported the antiemetic effects of cetirizine in 60 women who were using the antihistamine (10 mg/day) for the treatment of allergies during pregnancy (8). A control group of pregnant women, matched for the use of pyridoxine (vitamin B6) but who were not taking an antihistamine, was used for comparison. The cetirizine group had a significantly lower rate of nausea and vomiting (7% vs. 37%, $p = 0.0001$) (8). No pregnancy outcome data were provided.

The safety of cetirizine during pregnancy was evaluated in a 2008 prospective observational cohort study (9). A total of 196 pregnant women who were exposed to cetirizine in the 1st trimester were compared with 1686 control women not exposed to the antihistamine. No significant differences were observed in four outcomes (odds ratio; confidence interval): major birth defects (1.07; 0.21–3.59), spontaneous abortions (0.97; 0.54–1.65), preterm births (0.76; 0.35–1.5), and mean birth weight of term infants ($p = 0.13$) (9).

BREASTFEEDING SUMMARY

No published reports describing the use of cetirizine during human lactation have been located, but the manufacturer states that the antihistamine is excreted into human milk. This would be consistent with the relatively low molecular weight (about 462 for the dihydrochloride salt). The effect of this exposure on a nursing infant is unknown, but sedation is a possibility.

References

1. Mazzotta P, Loebstein R, Koren G. Treating allergic rhinitis in pregnancy. Safety considerations. Drug Saf 1999;20:361–75.
2. Horak F, Stubner UP. Comparative tolerability of second generation antihistamines. Drug Saf 1999;20:385–401.
3. Position Statement of a Joint Committee of the American College of Obstetricians and Gynecologists and the American College of Allergy, Asthma and Immunology. The use of newer asthma and allergy medications during pregnancy. Ann Allergy Asthma Immunol 2000;84:475–80.
4. Product information. Zyrtec. Pfizer, 2001.
5. Einarson A, Bailey B, Jung G, Spizzirri D, Baillie M, Koren G. Prospective controlled study of hydroxyzine and cetirizine in pregnancy. Ann Allergy Asthma Immunol 1997;78:183–6.
6. Schatz M, Petitti D. Antihistamines and pregnancy. Ann Allergy Asthma Immunol 1997;78:157–9.
7. Wilton LV, Pearce GL, Martin RM, Mackay FJ, Mann RD. The outcomes of pregnancy in women exposed to newly marketed drugs in general practice in England. Br J Obstet Gynaecol 1998;105:882–9.
8. Einarson A, Levichek Z, Einarson TR, Koren G. The antiemetic effect of cetirizine during pregnancy. Ann Pharmacol 2000;34:1486–7.
9. Weber-Schoendorfer C, Schaefer C. The safety of cetirizine during pregnancy—a prospective observational cohort study. Reprod Toxicol 2008;26:19–23.

CETUXIMAB

Antineoplastic

PREGNANCY RECOMMENDATION: No Human Data—No Relevant Animal Data
BREASTFEEDING RECOMMENDATION: No Human Data—Potential Toxicity

C

PREGNANCY SUMMARY

No reports describing the use of cetuximab in human or animal pregnancies have been located. It also is not known if the antibody crosses the placenta, but if it does it could disrupt normal embryo–fetal development. Cetuximab binds to epidermal growth factor receptor (EGFR) that is involved in the control of prenatal development and may be essential for normal organogenesis, proliferation, and differentiation in the embryo (1). Because of the potential for embryo and fetal harm, the antibody should not be used in pregnancy. In addition, based on the very long half-life, a woman should not conceive for about 60 days after the last dose. However, head and neck and colorectal cancers can be fatal, so if a woman requires cetuximab and informed consent is obtained, treatment should not be withheld because of pregnancy. If an inadvertent pregnancy occurs, the woman should be advised of the potential risk for severe adverse effects in the embryo and fetus.

FETAL RISK SUMMARY

Cetuximab is a recombinant, human/mouse chimeric monoclonal antibody that is given as a once-weekly IV infusion. It specifically binds to EGFR and competitively inhibits the binding of EGF and other ligands. Cetuximab, in combination with radiation therapy, is indicated for the treatment of locally or regionally advanced squamous cell carcinoma of the head and neck. As a single agent, it is indicated for the treatment of patients with recurrent or metastatic squamous cell carcinoma of the head and neck for which prior platinum-based therapy has failed. It also is indicated, either alone or in combination with irinotecan, for the treatment of EGFR-expressing, metastatic colorectal carcinoma in patients who are refractory or intolerant of irinotecan-based chemotherapy. The mean half-life is about 112 hours (range 63–230 hours).

Cetuximab may cause severe, infusion-related toxicity, including hypotension and other adverse effects. Premedication with an antihistamine (e.g., 50 mg diphenhydramine IV) is recommended (1). Hypotension in a pregnant woman could have deleterious effects on placental perfusion, resulting in embryo and fetal harm.

Animal reproduction studies have not been conducted with cetuximab. Neither have long-term studies for carcinogenicity. However, no mutagenic or clastogenic effects were noted in tests. In a 39-week toxicity study in female cynomolgus monkeys receiving 0.4–4 times the human dose based on BSA, a tendency for impairment of menstrual cycling was observed, as revealed by increased incidences of irregular or absence of cycles compared with controls. These effects began at week 25 and were continued through the 6-week recovery period. No effects on fertility were noted in male monkeys (1).

It is not known if cetuximab crosses the human placenta. The high molecular weight (about 152,000) suggests that it will not cross. However, human immunoglobulin (IgG) does cross and, therefore, cetuximab may also cross (1).

BREASTFEEDING SUMMARY

No reports describing the use of cetuximab during lactation have been located. The very high molecular weight (about 152,000) suggests that it will not be excreted into breast milk. However, human immunoglobulin (IgG) is excreted into milk and, therefore, cetuximab may also be excreted (1). The effect of this potential exposure on a nursing infant is unknown, but immunosuppression and other severe adverse effects are potential complications.

Reference

1. Product information. Erbitux. Bristol-Myers Squibb, 2007.

CEVIMELINE

Parasympathomimetic (Cholinergic)

PREGNANCY RECOMMENDATION: No Human Data—No Relevant Animal Data
BREASTFEEDING RECOMMENDATION: No Human Data—Potential Toxicity

PREGNANCY SUMMARY

No studies describing the use of cevimeline during human pregnancy have been located. The very limited animal data that did not include exposure during organogenesis, and the lack of any reported human pregnancy experience, prevents an assessment of the risk that this drug presents to a fetus.

FETAL RISK SUMMARY

Cevimeline is an oral cholinergic agonist indicated for the treatment of dry mouth in patients with Sjögren's syndrome.

In reproduction studies with rats, a dose, approximately five times the recommended human dose for a 60-kg person based on BSA, given from 14 days before mating through day 7 of gestation caused a reduction in the mean number of implantations. This effect may have been due to maternal toxicity (1).

No studies examining the placental transfer of cevimeline have been located. The molecular weight (about 245 for the hydrated salt form) is low enough, however, that passage to the fetus should be expected.

BREASTFEEDING SUMMARY

No reports describing the use of cevimeline in human lactation have been located. The molecular weight (about 245 for the hydrated salt form) suggests that excretion into breast milk should be expected. Because the effect of this exposure on a nursing infant is unknown, combined with the lack of data on the amount of drug that may be in milk, women who are taking cevimeline should probably not breastfeed.

Reference

1. Product information. Evoxaca. Daiichi Pharmaceutical, 2001.

C

CHAMOMILE

Herb

PREGNANCY RECOMMENDATION: Limited Human Data—No Relevant Animal Data
BREASTFEEDING RECOMMENDATION: No Human Data—Probably Compatible

PREGNANCY SUMMARY

The only reports describing the use of chamomile in human pregnancy involve its use for morning sickness. Some sources recommend avoiding excessive use of oral chamomile in pregnancy because the herb is thought to have uterine stimulant, emmenagogue, and abortifacient properties (1–4). Neither the period of pregnancy when these effects occurred nor the doses producing them have been stated or quantified. There is no information describing these effects after external use of chamomile. Because of the very limited reporting of human pregnancy experience and the absence of relevant animal reproduction data, the best course is to avoid oral chamomile during pregnancy. However, the risk from consumption of the herb, especially from occasional use, must be very rare because chamomile has been used for thousands of years.

FETAL RISK SUMMARY

Chamomile may refer to the German (*Matricaria chamomilla or M. recutita)* or Roman (*Anthemis nobilis or Chamaemelum nobile*) chamomiles. Both plants have been called "true chamomile" (1,5). The fragrant flower heads of the plants are dried and used as teas and extracts. Although the plants are different, the main chemicals in the flower heads are the same: chamazulene, apigenin, bisabolol, and angelic acid (1). Regardless of the source, chamomile and its teas have been used for thousands of years for their astringent, antispasmodic, sedative, anxiolytic, and antibacterial properties (1–3,5,6). There are numerous indications based on the properties, but few have been studied or have proven efficacy (7,8).

Animal reproduction studies have not been conducted with chamomile. However, a study in pregnant rats and rabbits using bisabolol found no evidence of teratogenicity or developmental toxicity after chronic administration of 1 mL/kg (1,4,6). However, in mice, high doses (3 mg/kg) of bisabolol were associated with resorptions of fetuses and reduced birth weight (4,6).

Nurse-midwives frequently prescribe chamomile teas for the treatment of morning sickness (9,10). However, many of these healthcare professionals thought that the use of chamomile teas were unsafe in pregnancy (10).

Both plant sources of chamomile contain coumarin compounds: umbelliferone (in German chamomile) and scopoletin-7-glucoside (in Roman chamomile) (6). Because of the presence of the coumarins, one review cautioned that the use of both chamomiles was a concern for pregnant women with coagulation disorders (11).

BREASTFEEDING SUMMARY

No reports describing the use of chamomile during lactation have been located. However, chamomile-containing teas have been used to treat colic in very young infants and children (6,12,13). Both German and Roman chamomiles have been used for thousands of years. The absence of reported exposures suggests that there is little or no risk from consumption of chamomile during breastfeeding.

References

1. Chamomile. *The Review of Natural Products*. St. Louis, MO: Wolters Kluwer Health, 2007.
2. Roman Chamomile. *Natural Medicines Comprehensive Database*. 5th ed. Stockton, CA: Therapeutic Research Faculty, 2003:1129–31.
3. Chamomile (*Matricaria recutita, Chamaemelum nobile*). Natural Standard Monograph. Available at http://www.naturalstandard.com. Accessed November 25, 2006.
4. Gallo M, Koren G, Smith MJ, Boon H. The use of herbal medicine in pregnancy and lactation. In: Koren G, ed. *Maternal-Fetal Toxicology. A Clinician's Guide*. 3rd ed. New York, NY: Marcel Dekker, 2001:569–601.
5. German Chamomile. *Natural Medicines Comprehensive Database*. 5th ed. Stockton, CA: Therapeutic Research Faculty, 2003:599–601.
6. Gardiner P. Chamomile (*Matricaria recutita, Anthemis nobilis*). The Longwood Herbal Task Force. Available at http://www.mcp.edu/herbal/default.htm and The Center for Holistic Pediatric Education and Research. Available at http://www.childenshospital.org/holistic/. Revised December 30, 1999. Accessed November 29, 2006.

7. Chamomile Flower, German. Blumenthal M, senior ed. *The Complete German Commission E Monographs. Therapeutic Guide to Herbal Medicines.* Austin, TX: American Botanical Council, 1998:107.
8. Chamomile Flower, Roman. Blumenthal M, Senior Editor. *The Complete German Commission E Monographs. Therapeutic Guide to Herbal Medicines.* Austin, TX: American Botanical Council, 1998:320.
9. Allaire AD, Moos MK, Wells SR. Complementary and alternative medicine in pregnancy: a survey of North Carolina certified nurse-midwives. Obstet Gynecol 2000;95:19–23.
10. Wilkinson JM. What do we know about herbal morning sickness treatments? A literature survey. Midwifery 2000;16:224–8.
11. Johns T, Sibeko L. Pregnancy outcomes in women using herbal therapies. Birth Defects Res (Part B) 2003;68:501–4.
12. Kemper KJ. Seven herbs every pediatrician should know. Contemp Pediatrics 1996;13:79–91.
13. Weizman Z, Alkrinawi S, Goldfarb D, Bitran C. Efficacy of herbal tea preparation in infantile colic. J Pediatr 1993;122:650–2.

CHENODIOL

Gastrointestinal Agent (Gallstone Solubilizing Agent)

PREGNANCY RECOMMENDATION: Contraindicated
BREASTFEEDING RECOMMENDATION: No Human Data—Potential Toxicity

PREGNANCY SUMMARY

Based on the observed hepatotoxicity of this agent, the use of chenodiol is contraindicated during pregnancy.

FETAL RISK SUMMARY

Chenodiol (chenodeoxycholic acid) is a naturally occurring bile acid used orally to dissolve gallstones. No reports on the use of this drug during human pregnancy have been located.

Chenodiol is not teratogenic in animals, but fetotoxicity has occurred in some species. Studies with pregnant rats, mice, and baboons did not observe congenital malformations after in utero exposure to the agent during organogenesis (1–3). In one study using three dosage levels, dose-related hepatotoxicity was observed in dams but not in newborn rats (4). No fetal hepatotoxicity was observed in a study of rats in which the drug composed 0.25% of the maternal diet during pregnancy (5). Hepatotoxicity was observed, however, in newborn baboons and rhesus monkeys exposed to chenodiol during gestation (3,6). Extensive hemorrhagic necrosis of the adrenal glands and interstitial hemorrhage of the kidneys were also noted in the newborn rhesus monkeys (6). Theoretically, the main hepatotoxic property of chenodiol in animals is due to its principal bacterial metabolite, lithocholic acid (7). In contrast to humans who readily metabolize lithocholic acid to poorly absorbed, nontoxic compounds, animals such as rabbits, rhesus monkeys, and baboons are unable to fully form sulfate conjugates to detoxify the metabolite, and thus are susceptible to liver damage (7).

One study concluded that dihydroxy bile acids, such as chenodiol, are transferred, at least in rats, from the mother to the fetus (5).

BREASTFEEDING SUMMARY

No reports describing the use of chenodiol during lactation have been located.

References

1. Kitao T, Kamishita S, Yoshikawa H, Sakaguchi M. Teratogenicity studies of chenodeoxycholic acid in rats. Yakuri to Chiryo 1982;10:3887–901 as cited in Shepard TH. *Catalog of Teratogenic Agents.* 6th ed. Baltimore, MD: Johns Hopkins University Press, 1989:127.
2. Takahashi H, Miyashita T, Tozuka K. Effects of chenodeoxycholic acid, administered in the organogenetic period, on the pre- and post-natal development of rat's and mouse's offspring. Oyo Yakuri (Pharmacometrics) 1978;15:1047–55.
3. McSherry CK, Morrissey KP, Swarm RL, May PS, Niemann WH, Glenn F. Chenodeoxycholic acid induced liver injury in pregnant and neonatal baboons. Ann Surg 1976;184:490–9.
4. Celle G, Cavanna M, Bocchini R, Robbiano L. Chenodeoxycholic acid (CDCA) versus ursodeoxycholic acid (UDCA): a comparison of their effects in pregnant rats. Arch Int Pharmacodyn Ther 1980;246:149–58.
5. Sprinkle DJ, Hassan AS, Subbiah MTR. Effect of chenodeoxycholic acid feeding during gestation in the rat on bile acid metabolism and liver morphology. Proc Soc Exp Biol Med 1984;175:386–97.
6. Heywood R, Palmer AK, Foll CV, Lee MR. Pathological changes in fetal rhesus monkey induced by oral chenodeoxycholic acid. Lancet 1973; 2:1021.
7. Allan RN, Thistle JL, Hofmann AF, Carter JA. Lithocholate metabolism during chemotherapy for gallstone dissolution. 1. Serum levels of sulphated and unsulphated lithocholates. Gut 1976;17:405–12.

CHLORAL HYDRATE

Sedative/Hypnotic

PREGNANCY RECOMMENDATION: Limited Human Data—No Relevant Animal Data
BREASTFEEDING RECOMMENDATION: Limited Human Data—Probably Compatible

C

PREGNANCY SUMMARY

The limited human pregnancy experience and the absence of relevant animal data prevent a complete assessment of the embryo–fetal risk.

FETAL RISK SUMMARY

No reports linking the use of chloral hydrate with congenital defects have been located. The drug has been given in labor and demonstrated to be in cord blood at concentrations similar to maternal levels (1). Sedative effects on the neonate have not been studied.

The Collaborative Perinatal Project recorded 71 1st trimester exposures to chloral hydrate (2, pp. 336–44). From this group, 8 infants with congenital defects were observed (standardized relative risk [SRR] 1.68). When only malformations with uniform rates by hospital were examined, the SRR was 2.19. Neither of these relative risks reached statistical significance. Moreover, when chloral hydrate was combined with all tranquilizers and nonbarbiturate sedatives, no association with congenital malformations was found (SRR 1.13; 95% confidence interval [CI] 0.88–1.44). For use anytime during pregnancy, 358 exposures to chloral hydrate were discovered (2, p. 438). The nine infants with anomalies yielded an SRR of 0.98 (95% CI 0.45–1.84).

BREASTFEEDING SUMMARY

Chloral hydrate and its active metabolite are excreted into breast milk. Peak concentrations of about 8 mcg/mL were obtained about 45 minutes after a 1.3-g rectal dose (3). Only trace amounts are detectable after 10 hours.

Mild drowsiness was observed in the nursing infant of a mother taking 1300 mg of dichloralphenazone every evening (4). The mother was also consuming chlorpromazine 100 mg three times daily. Dichloralphenazone is metabolized to trichloroethanol, the same active metabolite of chloral hydrate. Milk levels of trichloroethanol were 60%–80% of the maternal serum. Infant growth and development remained normal during the exposure and at follow-up 3 months after the drug was stopped. The American Academy of Pediatrics classifies the drug as compatible with breastfeeding (5).

References

1. Bernstine JB, Meyer AE, Hayman HB. Maternal and fetal blood estimation following the administration of chloral hydrate during labor. J Obstet Gynecol Br Emp 1954;61:683–5.
2. Heinonen OP, Slone D, Shapiro S. *Birth Defects and Drugs in Pregnancy*. Littleton, MA: Publishing Sciences Group, 1977.
3. Bernstine JB, Meyer AE, Bernstine RL. Maternal blood and breast milk estimation following the administration of chloral hydrate during the puerperium. J Obstet Gynecol Br Emp 1956;63:228–31.
4. Lacey JH. Dichloralphenazone and breast milk. Br Med J 1971;4:684.
5. Committee on Drugs, American Academy of Pediatrics. The transfer of drugs and other chemicals into human milk. Pediatrics 2001;108:776–89.

CHLORAMBUCIL

Antineoplastic

PREGNANCY RECOMMENDATION: Contraindicated—1st Trimester
BREASTFEEDING RECOMMENDATION: Contraindicated

PREGNANCY SUMMARY

The limited data suggest that chlorambucil is a human teratogen.

FETAL RISK SUMMARY

The use of the alkylating agent, chlorambucil, during pregnancy has resulted in both normal and deformed infants (1–7). Two reports observed unilateral agenesis of the left kidney and ureter in male fetuses following 1st trimester exposure to chlorambucil (3,4). Similar defects have been found in animals exposed to the drug (8). In a third case, a pregnant patient was treated with chlorambucil at the 10th week of gestation (5). A full-term infant was delivered, but died 3 days later of multiple cardiovascular anomalies. The fourth case involved a woman treated with 24 mg/day during weeks 3–4 (6). She aborted in the 1st trimester a fetus with a retinal defect. In a 2012 report, a woman with chronic lymphocytic leukemia was treated with chlorambucil 2 mg/day 3 times per week during the first 20 weeks of pregnancy (7). Because of preeclampsia, she had a cesarean section at 36 weeks' gestation to give birth to a healthy 2235-g male infant who had normal growth and development at 3 months of age.

Chlorambucil is mutagenic as well as carcinogenic (9–13). These effects have not been reported in newborns following in utero exposure. Data from one review indicated that 40% of the infants exposed to anticancer drugs were of low birth weight (14). Long-term studies of growth and mental development in offspring exposed to chlorambucil during the 2nd trimester, the period of neuroblast multiplication, have not been conducted (15).

Amenorrhea and reversible azoospermia with high doses have been reported (16–20). Long-term follow-up of menstrual and reproductive function in women treated with various antineoplastic agents was reported in 1988 (20). Only two of the 40 women studied, however, may have been exposed to chlorambucil (see Cyclophosphamide).

Occupational exposure of the mother to antineoplastic agents during pregnancy may present a risk to the fetus. A position statement from the National Study Commission on Cytotoxic Exposure and a research article involving some antineoplastic agents are presented in the monograph for cyclophosphamide (see Cyclophosphamide).

BREASTFEEDING SUMMARY

No reports describing the use of chlorambucil during lactation have been located. Because of the potential for severe adverse effects in a nursing infant, women receiving this alkylating agent should not breastfeed.

References

1. Sokal JE, Lessmann EM. Effects of cancer chemotherapeutic agents on the human fetus. JAMA 1960;172:1765–71.
2. Jacobs C, Donaldson SS, Rosenberg SA, Kaplan HS. Management of the pregnant patient with Hodgkin's disease. Ann Intern Med 1981;95:669–75.
3. Shotton D, Monie IW. Possible teratogenic effect of chlorambucil on a human fetus. JAMA 1963;186:74–5.
4. Steege JF, Caldwell DS. Renal agenesis after first trimester exposure to chlorambucil. South Med J 1980;73:1414–5.
5. Thompson J, Conklin KA. Anesthetic management of a pregnant patient with scleroderma. Anesthesiology 1983;59:69–71.
6. Rugh R, Skaredoff L. Radiation and radiomimetic chlorambucil and the fetal retina. Arch Ophthalmol 1965;74:382–93. As cited by Schardein JL. *Chemically Induced Birth Defects*. 3rd ed. New York, NY: Marcel Dekker, 2000:581–2.
7. Ali R, Kimya Y, Koksal N, Ozkocaman V, Yorulmaz H, Eroglu A, Ozcelik T, Tunali A. Pregnancy in chronic lymphocytic leukemia: experience with fetal exposure to chlorambucil. Leuk Res 2009;33:567–9.
8. Monie IW. Chlorambucil-induced abnormalities of urogenital system of rat fetuses. Anat Rec 1961;139:145.
9. Lawler SD, Lele KP. Chromosomal damage induced by chlorambucil and chronic lymphocytic leukemia. Scand J Haematol 1972;9:603–12.
10. Westin J. Chromosome abnormalities after chlorambucil therapy of polycythemia vera. Scand J Haematol 1976;17:197–204.
11. Catovsky D, Galton DAG. Myelomonocytic leukaemia supervening on chronic lymphocytic leukaemia. Lancet 1971;1:478–9.
12. Rosner R. Acute leukemia as a delayed consequence of cancer chemotherapy. Cancer 1976;37:1033–6.
13. Reimer RR, Hover R, Fraumeni JF, Young RC. Acute leukemia after alkylating-agent therapy of ovarian cancer. N Engl J Med 1977;297:177–81.
14. Nicholson HO. Cytotoxic drugs in pregnancy: review of reported cases. J Obstet Gynaecol Br Commonw 1968;75:307–12.
15. Dobbing J. Pregnancy and leukaemia. Lancet 1977;1:1155.
16. Freckman HA, Fry HL, Mendex FL, Maurer ER. Chlorambucil-prednisolone therapy for disseminated breast carcinoma. JAMA 1964;189:111–4.
17. Richter P, Calamera JC, Morganfeld MC, Kierszenbaum AL, Lavieri JC, Mancinni RE. Effect of chlorambucil on spermatogenesis in the human malignant lymphoma. Cancer 1970;25:1026–30.
18. Morgenfeld MC, Goldberg V, Parisier H, Bugnard SC, Bur GE. Ovarian lesions due to cytostatic agents during the treatment of Hodgkin's disease. Surg Gynecol Obstet 1972;134:826–8.
19. Schilsky RL, Lewis BJ, Sherins RJ, Young RC. Gonadal dysfunction in patients receiving chemotherapy for cancer. Ann Intern Med 1980;93:109–14.
20. Gershenson DM. Menstrual and reproductive function after treatment with combination chemotherapy for malignant ovarian germ cell tumors. J Clin Oncol 1988;6:270–5.

CHLORAMPHENICOL

Antibiotic

PREGNANCY RECOMMENDATION: Compatible
BREASTFEEDING RECOMMENDATION: Limited Human Data—Potential Toxicity

PREGNANCY SUMMARY

Although apparently nontoxic to the fetus, chloramphenicol should be used with caution at term. Specific details were not provided, but one report claimed that cardiovascular collapse (gray syndrome) developed in babies delivered from mothers treated with chloramphenicol during the final stage of pregnancy (1). Additional reports of this severe adverse effect have not been located. It is well known that newborns exposed directly to high doses of chloramphenicol may develop the gray syndrome (2,3). Because of this risk, some authors consider the drug to be contraindicated during pregnancy (4).

FETAL RISK SUMMARY

No reports linking the use of chloramphenicol with congenital defects have been located. The drug crosses the placenta at term producing cord serum concentrations 30%–106% of maternal levels (5,6).

The Collaborative Perinatal Project monitored 50,282 mother–child pairs, 98 of whom had 1st trimester exposure to chloramphenicol (7, pp. 297–301). For use anytime in pregnancy, 348 exposures were recorded (7, p. 435). In neither group was evidence found to suggest a relationship to large categories of major or minor malformations or to individual defects. A 1977 case report described a 14-day course of IV chloramphenicol, 2 g daily, given to a patient with typhoid fever in the 2nd trimester (8). A normal infant was delivered at term. Twenty-two patients, in various stages of gestation, were treated with chloramphenicol for acute pyelonephritis (9). No difficulties in the newborn could be associated with the antibiotic. In a controlled study, 110 patients received one to three antibiotics during the 1st trimester for a total of 589 weeks (10). Chloramphenicol was given for a total of 205 weeks. The incidence of birth defects was similar to that in controls.

A 1998 report described the use of chloramphenicol for the treatment of Rocky Mountain spotted fever in a woman at 28 weeks' gestation (11). She was treated with IV chloramphenicol (3 g/day) and ceftriaxone (2 g/day) for 1 week and then for 3 weeks with oral amoxicillin. She eventually delivered a full-term, healthy 3916-g infant.

C

BREASTFEEDING SUMMARY

Chloramphenicol is excreted into breast milk. Two milk samples, separated by 24 hours in the same patient, were reported as 16 and 25 mcg/mL, representing milk:plasma ratios of 0.51 and 0.61, respectively (12). Both active drug and inactive metabolite were measured. No effect on the infant was mentioned. No infant toxicity was mentioned in a 1964 report that found peak levels occurring in milk 1–3 hours after a single 1-g oral dose (13). In a similar study, continuous excretion of chloramphenicol into breast milk was established after the 1st day of therapy (14). Minimum and maximum milk concentrations were determined for five patients receiving 250 mg orally every 6 hours (0.54 and 2.84 mcg/mL) and for five patients receiving 500 mg orally every 6 hours (1.75 and 6.10 mcg/mL). No infant data were given.

The safety of maternal chloramphenicol consumption and breastfeeding is unknown. The American Academy of Pediatrics classifies the antibiotic as an agent whose effect on the nursing infant is unknown but may be of concern because of the potential for idiosyncratic bone marrow suppression (15). Another publication recommended that chloramphenicol not be used in the lactating patient (16). Milk levels of this antibiotic are too low to precipitate the gray syndrome, but a theoretical risk does exist for bone marrow depression. Two other potential problems of lesser concern involve the modification of bowel flora and possible interference with the interpretation of culture results if a fever workup is required. Several adverse effects were reported in 50 breastfed infants whose mothers were being treated with chloramphenicol, including refusal of the breast, falling asleep during feeding, intestinal gas, and heavy vomiting after feeding (17).

References

1. Oberheuser F. Praktische Erfahrungen mit Medikamenten in der Schwangerschaft. Therapiewoche 1971;31:2200. As reported in Manten A. Antibiotic drugs. In: Dukes MNG, ed. *Meyler's Side Effects of Drugs*. Volume VIII. New York, NY: American Elsevier, 1975:604.
2. Sutherland JM. Fatal cardiovascular collapse of infants receiving large amounts of chloramphenicol. J Dis Child 1959;97:761–7.
3. Weiss CV, Glazko AJ, Weston JK. Chloramphenicol in the newborn infant. A physiologic explanation of its toxicity when given in excessive doses. N Engl J Med 1960;262:787–94.
4. Schwarz RH, Crombleholme WR. Antibiotics in pregnancy. South Med J 1979;72:1315–8.
5. Scott WC, Warner RF. Placental transfer of chloramphenicol (Chloromycetin). JAMA 1950;142:1331–2.
6. Ross S, Burke RG, Sites J, Rice EC, Washington JA. Placental transmission of chloramphenicol (Chloromycetin). JAMA 1950;142:1361.
7. Heinonen OP, Slone D, Shapiro S. *Birth Defects and Drugs in Pregnancy*. Littleton, MA: Publishing Sciences Group, 1977.
8. Schiffman P, Samet CM, Fox L, Neimand KM, Rosenberg ST. Typhoid fever in pregnancy—with probable typhoid hepatitis. NY State J Med 1977;77:1778–9.
9. Cunningham FG, Morris GB, Mickal A. Acute pyelonephritis of pregnancy: a clinical review. Obstet Gynecol 1973;42:112–7.
10. Ravid R, Roaff R. On the possible teratogenicity of antibiotic drugs administered during pregnancy. In: Klingberg MA, Abramovici H, Chemke J, eds. *Drugs and Fetal Development*. New York, NY: Plenum Press, 1972:505–10.
11. Markley KC, Levine AB, Chan Y. Rocky Mountain spotted fever in pregnancy. Obstet Gynecol 1998;91:860.
12. Smadel JE, Woodward TE, Ley HL Jr, Lewthwaite R. Chloramphenicol (Chloromycetin) in the treatment of Tsutsugamushi disease (scrub typhus). J Clin Invest 1949;28:1196–215.
13. Prochazka J, Havelka J, Hejzlar M. Excretion of chloramphenicol by human milk. Cas Lek Cesk 1964;103:378–80.
14. Havelka J, Hejzlar M, Popov V, Viktorinova D, Prochazka J. Excretion of chloramphenicol in human milk. Chemotherapy 1968;13:204–11.
15. Committee on Drugs, American Academy of Pediatrics. The transfer of drugs and other chemicals into human milk. Pediatrics 2001;108:776–89.
16. Anonymous. Update: drugs in breast milk. Med Lett Drugs Ther 1979;21:21–4.
17. Havelka J, Frankova A. Contribution to the question of side effects of chloramphenicol therapy in newborns. Cesk Pediatr 1972;21:31–3.

CHLORCYCLIZINE

Antihistamine

No data are available. See Meclizine for representative agent in this class.

CHLORDIAZEPOXIDE

Sedative

PREGNANCY RECOMMENDATION: Human Data Suggest Risk in 1st and 3rd Trimesters
BREASTFEEDING RECOMMENDATION: No Human Data—Potential Toxicity

PREGNANCY SUMMARY

The effects of benzodiazepines, including chlordiazepoxide, on the human embryo and fetus are controversial. Although some studies have reported an association with various types of congenital defects, other studies have not found such associations. Maternal denial of exposure and concurrent exposure to other toxic drugs and substances (e.g., alcohol and smoking) may be confounding factors. If the drug does cause birth defects, the risk appears to be low. Continuous use during gestation has resulted in neonatal withdrawal, and depression of the newborn may occur if chlordiazepoxide is used close to birth. Consequently, if the maternal condition requires the use of the drug during pregnancy, the lowest possible dose should be taken. Moreover, abrupt discontinuance of chlordiazepoxide should be avoided. Severe withdrawal symptoms (physical and psychological) may occur in the mother and could result in the substitution of other substances (e.g., alcohol) to treat the symptoms. Fetal withdrawal, such as that observed with narcotics, has not been reported, but should be considered.

C

FETAL RISK SUMMARY

Chlordiazepoxide is a benzodiazepine (see also Diazepam). The drug has antianxiety, sedative, appetite-stimulating, and weak analgesic actions (1).

No teratogenic effects were observed in rats given doses of 10–80 mg/kg/day through one or two matings (1). At 100 mg/kg/day, maternal toxicity (decreased interest in mating and nursing) and marked decreases in offspring viability and body weight were attributed to sedative effects of the drug (1). Moreover, at this dose, one newborn in each of two matings had major skeletal abnormalities.

In a study evaluating 19,044 live births, the use of chlordiazepoxide was associated with a greater than fourfold increase in severe congenital anomalies (2). In 172 patients exposed to the drug during the first 42 days of gestation, the following defects were observed: mental deficiency, spastic diplegia and deafness, microcephaly and retardation, duodenal atresia, and Meckel's diverticulum (2). Although not statistically significant, an increased fetal death rate was also found with maternal chlordiazepoxide ingestion (2). A survey of 390 infants with congenital heart disease matched with 1254 normal infants found a higher rate of exposure to several drugs, including chlordiazepoxide, in the offspring with defects (3).

In contrast, other studies have not confirmed a relationship with increased defects or mortality (4–8). The Collaborative Perinatal Project monitored 50,282 mother–child pairs, 257 of whom were exposed in the 1st trimester to chlordiazepoxide (5,8). No association with large classes of malformations or to individual defects was found.

In a surveillance study of Michigan Medicaid recipients involving 229,101 completed pregnancies conducted between 1985 and 1992, 788 newborns had been exposed to chlordiazepoxide during the 1st trimester (F. Rosa, personal communication, FDA, 1993). A total of 44 (5.6%) major birth defects were observed (34 expected). Specific data were available for six defect categories, including (observed/expected) 10/7 cardiovascular defects, 2/1 oral clefts, 0/0.5 spina bifida, 3/2 polydactyly, 1/1 limb-reduction defects, and 2/2 hypospadias. These data do not support an association between the drug and congenital defects.

A 1992 study reported on heavy benzodiazepine exposure during pregnancy from Michigan Medicaid data collected during 1980 to 1983 (9). Of the 2048 women, from a total sample of 104,339, who had received benzodiazepines, 80 had received 10 or more prescriptions for these agents. The records of these 80 women indicated frequent alcohol and substance abuse. Their pregnancy outcomes were 3 intrauterine deaths, 2 neonatal deaths in infants with congenital malformations, and 64 survivors. The outcome for 11 infants was unknown. Six of the surviving infants had diagnoses consistent with congenital defects (9). The investigators concluded that the high rate of congenital anomalies was suggestive of multiple alcohol and substance abuse and may not have been related to benzodiazepine exposure (9).

Neonatal withdrawal consisting of severe tremulousness and irritability has been attributed to maternal use of chlordiazepoxide (10). The onset of withdrawal symptoms occurred on the 26th day of life. Chlordiazepoxide readily crosses the placenta at term in an approximate 1:1 ratio (11–13). The drug has been used to reduce pain during labor, but the maternal benefit was not significant (14,15). Marked depression was observed in three infants whose mothers received chlordiazepoxide within a few hours of delivery (13). The infants were unresponsive, hypotonic, hypothermic, and fed poorly. Hypotonicity persisted for up to a week. Other studies have not seen depression (11,12).

BREASTFEEDING SUMMARY

No reports describing the use of chlordiazepoxide during human lactation have been located. The molecular weight (about 300) is low enough, however, that passage into milk should be expected. Moreover, other benzodiazepines are excreted into milk and have produced adverse effects in nursing infants (see Diazepam). Because of the potential for drug accumulation and toxicity in nursing infants, chlordiazepoxide should be avoided during breastfeeding.

References

1. Product information. Librium. ICN Pharmaceuticals, 2000.
2. Milkovich L, van den Berg BJ. Effects of prenatal meprobamate and chlordiazepoxide hydrochloride on human embryonic and fetal development. N Engl J Med 1974;291:1268–71.
3. Rothman KJ, Fyler DC, Golblatt A, Kreidberg MB. Exogenous hormones and other drug exposures of children with congenital heart disease. Am J Epidemiol 1979;109:433–9.
4. Crombie DL, Pinsent RJ, Fleming DM, Rumeau-Rouguette C, Goujard J, Huel G. Fetal effects of tranquilizers in pregnancy. N Engl J Med 1975;293:198–9.
5. Hartz SC, Heinonen OP, Shapiro S, Siskind V, Slone D. Antenatal exposure to meprobamate and chlordiazepoxide in relation to malformations, mental development, and childhood mortality. N Engl J Med 1975;292:726–8.
6. Bracken MB, Holford TR. Exposure to prescribed drugs in pregnancy and association with congenital malformations. Obstet Gynecol 1981;58:336–44.
7. Committee on Drugs, American Academy of Pediatrics. Psychotropic drugs in pregnancy and lactation. Pediatrics 1982;69:241–4.
8. Heinonen OP, Slone D, Shapiro S. *Birth Defects and Drugs in Pregnancy*. Littleton, MA: Publishing Sciences Group, 1977:336–7.
9. Bergman U, Rosa FW, Baum C, Wiholm B-E, Faich GA. Effects of exposure to benzodiazepine during fetal life. Lancet 1992;340:694–6.
10. Athinarayanan P, Pierog SH, Nigam SK, Glass L. Chlordiazepoxide withdrawal in the neonate. Am J Obstet Gynecol 1976;124:212–3.
11. Decancq HG Jr, Bosco JR, Townsend EH Jr. Chlordiazepoxide in labour: its effect on the newborn infant. J Pediatr 1965;67:836–40.
12. Mark PM, Hamel J. Librium for patients in labor. Obstet Gynecol 1968;32:188–94.
13. Stirrat GM, Edington PT, Berry DJ. Transplacental passage of chlordiazepoxide. Br Med J 1974;2:729.
14. Duckman S, Spina T, Attardi M, Meyer A. Double-blind study of chlordiazepoxide in obstetrics. Obstet Gynecol 1964;24:601–5.
15. Kanto JH. Use of benzodiazepines during pregnancy, labour and lactation, with particular reference to pharmacokinetic considerations. Drugs 1982;23:354–80.

CHLORHEXIDINE

Anti-infective

PREGNANCY RECOMMENDATION: Compatible
BREASTFEEDING RECOMMENDATION: No Human Data—Probably Compatible

C

PREGNANCY SUMMARY

No reports of adverse effects in newborns have been reported even though chlorhexidine is used commonly during labor and in the neonate. Moreover, only very small amounts of disinfectant reach the maternal circulation and, presumably, the fetus. Although the agent is an effective disinfectant, single vaginal applications of chlorhexidine solutions do not appear to offer any advantage over sterile water or saline in the prevention of maternal infections during labor or in the postpartum period.

FETAL RISK SUMMARY

Chlorhexidine, a bisbiguanide antiseptic and disinfectant, is effective against most bacteria, and some fungi and viruses (including HIV). In addition to its topical use on the skin and intravaginally, it has been used for gingivitis and the prevention of dental plaque. Chlorhexidine has also been used as a spermicide (1). No adverse fetal effects were observed in pregnant rats administered chlorhexidine by gastric intubation on days 6 through 15 of gestation (2).

A number of studies have documented the safety and possible effectiveness of vaginal disinfection with chlorhexidine prior to delivery, primarily to prevent colonization of newborns with group B streptococci (3–15). Application to the groin and perineum, to the abdomen prior to cesarean section, and whole body washing has also been effective in preventing fetal and maternal infection (3,16–19). However, two double-blinded, placebo-controlled, randomized studies published in 1997, one utilizing a single intravaginal wash with 20 mL of a 0.4% chlorhexidine solution (20) and the other a 200-mL vaginal irrigation with a 0.2% solution (21), both groups in active labor, did not find a significant reduction in maternal infection rates compared with sterile water or saline. No adverse effects in the newborns were observed.

One author, hypothesizing an etiological connection between sudden infant death syndrome (SIDS) and toxigenic *Escherichia coli* or *Chlamydia* species, has suggested that decontamination of the birth canal with chlorhexidine during labor might reduce infant mortality from this disease (22), but a temporal relationship is speculative. In contrast to the real and theoretical benefits realized by the newborn from maternal chlorhexidine use, a single vaginal washing with a 0.4% chlorhexidine solution was not effective in decreasing the incidence of intra-amniotic infection or endometritis (23).

In one study involving nonpregnant women, swabbing of the entire vagina for 1 minute with gauze sponges soaked in 4% chlorhexidine gluconate did not result in detectable blood concentrations (sensitivity 0.1 mcg/mL) of the agent (24). A second study, utilizing a method ten times more sensitive (sensitivity 0.01 mcg/mL), was able to detect chlorhexidine in maternal blood from 34 of 96 women following vaginal washing with a 0.2% solution (25). Mean blood chlorhexidine concentrations obtained using two different methods of washing were 0.0146 and 0.0104 mcg/mL, respectively (range 0.01–0.083 mcg/mL). No accumulation of chlorhexidine in maternal blood was observed after a second vaginal washing at 6 hours in 14 patients or after a third washing, 6 hours later, in 3. The disinfectant was not detected in 62 of the women.

One writer has cautioned that the potential long-term effects (not specified) in the newborn from exposure to respiratory and other epithelial surfaces following vaginal use of chlorhexidine during labor have not been investigated (26).

BREASTFEEDING SUMMARY

No reports describing the excretion of chlorhexidine into milk have been located. The presence of the drug in breast milk is probably clinically insignificant because of the very small amounts absorbed into the maternal circulation following vaginal washing. As a general precaution, the mother's nipples should be rinsed thoroughly with water if chlorhexidine is used on them as a disinfectant, even though absorption of the agent from the gastrointestinal tract is poor.

References

1. Editorial. Multipurpose spermicides. Lancet 1992;340:211–3.
2. Gilman MR, De Salva SJ. Teratology studies of benzethonium chloride, cetyl pyridinium chloride and chlorhexidine in rats (Abstract). Toxicol Appl Pharmacol 1979;48:A35.
3. Vorherr H, Ulrich JA, Messer RH, Hurwitz EB. Antimicrobial effect of chlorhexidine on bacteria of groin, perineum and vagina. J Reprod Med 1980;24:153–7.
4. Christensen KK, Christensen P, Dykes AK, Kahlmeter G, Kurl DN, Linden V. Chlorhexidine for prevention of neonatal colonization with group B streptococci. I. In vitro effect of chlorhexidine on group B streptococci. Eur J Obstet Gynecol Reprod Biol 1983;16:157–65.
5. Dykes AK, Christensen KK, Christensen P, Kahlmeter G. Chlorhexidine for prevention of neonatal colonization with group B streptococci. II. Chlorhexidine concentrations and recovery of group B streptococci following vaginal washing in pregnant women. Eur J Obstet Gynecol Reprod Biol 1983;16:167–72.
6. Christensen KK, Christensen P. Chlorhexidine for prevention of neonatal colonization with GBS. Antibiot Chemother 1985;35:296–302.
7. Christensen KK, Christensen P, Dykes AK, Kahlmeter G. Chlorhexidine for prevention of neonatal colonization with group B streptococci. III. Effect of vaginal washing with chlorhexidine before rupture of the membranes. Eur J Obstet Gynecol Reprod Biol 1985;19:231–6.
8. Christensen KK, Dykes AK, Christensen P. Reduced colonization of newborns with group B streptococci following washing of the birth canal with chlorhexidine. J Perinat Med 1985;13:239–43.
9. Easmon CSF. Group B streptococcus. Infect Control 1986;7(Suppl 2):135–7.

10. Dykes AK, Christensen KK, Christensen P. Chlorhexidine for prevention of neonatal colonization with group B streptococci. IV. Depressed puerperal carriage following vaginal washing with chlorhexidine during labour. Eur J Obstet Gynecol Reprod Biol 1987;24:293–7.
11. Burman LG, Christensen P, Christensen K, Fryklund B, Helgesson AM, Svenningsen NW, Tullus K, and the Swedish Chlorhexidene Study Group. Prevention of excess neonatal morbidity associated with group B streptococci by vaginal chlorhexidine disinfection during labour. Lancet 1992;340:65–9.
12. Burman LG, Tullus K. Vaginal chlorhexidine disinfection during labour. Lancet 1992;340:791–2.
13. Lindemann R, Henrichsen T, Svenningsen L, Hjelle K. Vaginal chlorhexidine disinfection during labour. Lancet 1992;340:792.
14. Henrichsen T, Lindemann R, Svenningsen L, Hjelle K. Prevention of neonatal infections by vaginal chlorhexidine disinfection during labour. Acta Paediatr 1994;83:923–6.
15. Kollée LAA, Speyer I, van Kuijck MAP, Koopman R, Dony JM, Bakker JH, Wintermans RGF. Prevention of group B streptococci transmission during delivery by vaginal application of chlorhexidine gel. Eur J Obstet Gynecol Reprod Biol 1989;31:47–51.
16. Vorherr H, Vorherr UF, Moss JC. Comparative effectiveness of chlorhexidine, povidone-iodine, and hexachlorophene on the bacteria of the perineum and groin of pregnant women. Am J Infect Control 1988;16:178–81.
17. Brown TR, Ehrlich CE, Stehman FB, Golichowski AM, Madura JA, Eitzen HE. A clinical evaluation of chlorhexidine gluconate spray as compared with iodophor scrub for preoperative skin preparation. Surg Gynecol Obstet 1984;158:363–6.
18. Sanderson PJ, Haji TC. Transfer of group B streptococci from mothers to neonates: effect of whole body washing of mothers with chlorhexidine. J Hosp Infect 1985;6:257–64.
19. Frost L, Pedersen M, Seiersen E. Changes in hygienic procedures reduce infection following caesarean section. J Hosp Infect 1989;13:143–8.
20. Sweeten KM, Ericksen NL, Blanco JD. Chlorhexidine versus sterile water vaginal wash during labor to prevent peripartum infection. Am J Obstet Gynecol 1997;176:426–30.
21. Rouse DJ, Hauth JC, Andrews WW, Mills BB, Maher JE. Chlorhexidine vaginal irrigation for the prevention of peripartal infection: a placebo-controlled randomized clinical trial. Am J Obstet Gynecol 1997;176:617–22.
22. Elfast RA. Chlorhexidine prophylaxis at labor. Prevention of sudden infant death? Lakartidningen 1993;90:3771–2.
23. Eriksen NL, Blanco JD. Chlorhexidine versus sterile water vaginal wash during labor to prevent peripartum infection (Abstract). Am J Obstet Gynecol 1995;172:304.
24. Vorherr H, Vorherr UF, Mehta P, Ulrich JA, Messer RH. Antimicrobial effect of chlorhexidine and povidone-iodine on vaginal bacteria. J Infect 1984;8:195–9.
25. Nilsson G, Larsson L, Christensen KK, Christensen P, Dykes AK. Chlorhexidine for prevention of neonatal colonization with group B streptococci. V. Chlorhexidine concentrations in blood following vaginal washing during delivery. Eur J Obstet Gynecol Reprod Biol 1989;31:221–6.
26. Feldman R, van Oppen C, Noorduyn A. Vaginal chlorhexidine disinfection during labour. Lancet 1992;340:791.

CHLOROQUINE

Antimalarial/Amebicide

PREGNANCY RECOMMENDATION: Compatible—Maternal Benefit >> Embryo–Fetal Risk
BREASTFEEDING RECOMMENDATION: Compatible

PREGNANCY SUMMARY

Although some studies have suggested a low risk of congenital malformations, the lack of a pattern in the defects suggests that a causative association is unlikely. In any event, the maternal and fetal benefit of preventing and treating malaria far outweighs the risk, if any, to the embryo–fetus.

FETAL RISK SUMMARY

Chloroquine is the drug of choice for the prophylaxis and treatment of sensitive malaria species during pregnancy (1–4). The drug is also indicated for the treatment of extraintestinal invasion by the protozoan parasite, *Entamoeba histolytica* (5). Chloroquine is generally considered safe for these purposes by most authorities (1–7). However, the antimalarial is embryotoxic and teratogenic in rats given a 1000-mg/kg dose, causing embryonic death in 27% and producing anophthalmia and microphthalmia in 47% of the surviving fetuses (8).

Chloroquine crosses the placenta to the fetus, with fetal concentrations approximating those in the mother (9). In seven mothers at term in the second stage of labor, chloroquine, 5 mg/kg IM, produced mean levels in maternal blood, cord venous blood, and cord arterial blood that were all about 0.7 mcg/mL. The time interval from administration to sampling averaged 5.3 hours (range 2.4–10.5 hours). In a pregnant monkey, an ^{125}I-labeled chloroquine analog crossed the placenta and concentrated in the fetal adrenal cortex and retina (10). Chloroquine rapidly crosses the placenta in pregnant mice and selectively accumulates in the melanin structures of the fetal eyes (11). The drug was retained in the ocular structures for 5 months after elimination from the rest of the body.

The risks of complications from malarial infection occurring during pregnancy are increased, especially in women not living in endemic areas (i.e., nonimmune women) (12–14). Infection is associated with a number of severe maternal and fetal outcomes: anemia, abortion, stillbirths, prematurity, low birth weight, fetal distress, and congenital malaria (12–14). However, it is not yet clear if all of these are related to malarial infection (13). For example, prevention of low birth weight and the resulting risk of infant mortality by antimalarial chemoprophylaxis has not yet been proven (13). Increased maternal morbidity and mortality includes adult respiratory distress syndrome, massive hemolysis, disseminated intravascular coagulation, acute renal failure, and hypoglycemia, with the latter symptom occurring in up to 50% of women in whom quinine is used (14). Severe *Plasmodium falciparum* malaria in pregnant nonimmune women has a poor prognosis and may be associated with asymptomatic uterine contractions, intrauterine growth restriction, fetal tachycardia, fetal distress, hypoglycemia, and placental insufficiency because of intense parasitization (13). Because of the severity of this disease in pregnancy, chemoprophylaxis is recommended for women of childbearing age traveling in areas where malaria is present (12–14).

Congenital malaria may occur in up to 10% of infants born to mothers not living in endemic areas (14). In most cases, clinical malaria manifests 3–8 weeks after birth, probably as a result of exchange of infected maternal erythrocytes at birth, and is characterized by fever, hepatosplenomegaly, jaundice, and thrombocytopenia (14). In areas of hyperendemicity, transplacental passage of maternal IgG may protect the newborn against development of clinical malaria (14).

Congenital defects have been reported in three infants delivered from one mother who was treated during pregnancy with 250–500 mg/day of chloroquine for discoid lupus erythematosus (15). In addition, this woman also had two normal infants, who had not been exposed to chloroquine during gestation, and one normal infant who had been exposed. Anomalies in the three infants were Wilms' tumor at age 4 years, left-sided hemihypertrophy (one infant), and cochleovestibular paresis (two infants).

A 1985 report summarized the results of 169 infants exposed in utero to 300 mg of chloroquine base once weekly throughout pregnancy (16). The control group consisted of 454 nonexposed infants. Two infants (1.2%) in the study group had anomalies (tetralogy of Fallot and congenital hypothyroidism) compared with four control infants who had defects (0.9%). Based on these data, the authors concluded that chloroquine is not a major teratogen, but a small increase in birth defects could not be excluded (16).

BREASTFEEDING SUMMARY

Chloroquine is excreted into breast milk (9,17). When chloroquine, 5 mg/kg IM, was administered to six nursing mothers 17 days postpartum, mean milk and serum concentrations 2 hours later were 0.227 mcg/mL (range 0.163–0.319 mcg/mL) and 0.648 mcg/mL (range 0.46–0.95 mcg/mL), respectively. The mean milk:blood ratio was 0.358 (range 0.268–0.462). Based on an average consumption of 500 mL of milk/day, an infant would have received about 114 mcg/day of chloroquine, an amount considered safe by the investigators (9). In an earlier study, three women were given a single dose of 600 mg of chloroquine 2–5 days postpartum (17). Serum and milk samples were collected up to 227 hours after administration. The milk:plasma ratios (AUC) for chloroquine and the principal metabolite, desethylchloroquine, ranged from 1.96 to 4.26 and from 0.54 to 3.89, respectively. Based on a daily milk intake of 1000 mL, the nursing infants would have ingested between 2.2% and 4.2% of the maternal doses over a 9-day period (17).

Although the amounts of chloroquine excreted into milk are not considered to be harmful to a nursing infant, they are insufficient to provide adequate protection against malaria (12). The American Academy of Pediatrics classifies chloroquine as compatible with breastfeeding (18).

References

1. Gilles HM, Lawson JB, Sibelas M, Voller A, Allan N. Malaria, anaemia and pregnancy. Ann Trop Med Parasitol 1969;63:245–63.
2. Diro M, Beydoun SN. Malaria in pregnancy. South Med J 1982;75:959–62.
3. Anonymous. Malaria in pregnancy. Lancet 1983;2:84–5.
4. Strang A, Lachman E, Pitsoe SB, Marszalek A, Philpott RH. Malaria in pregnancy with fatal complications: case report. Br J Obstet Gynaecol 1984;91:399–403.
5. D'Alauro F, Lee RV, Pao-In K, Khairallah M. Intestinal parasites and pregnancy. Obstet Gynecol 1985;66:639–43.
6. Ross JB, Garatsos S. Absence of chloroquine induced ototoxicity in a fetus. Arch Dermatol 1974;109:573.
7. Lewis R, Lauresen NJ, Birnbaum S. Malaria associated with pregnancy. Obstet Gynecol 1973;42:698–700.
8. Udalova LD. The effect of chloroquine on the embryonal development of rats. Pharmacol Toxicol (Russian) 1967;2:226–8. As cited in Shepard TH. *Catalog of Teratogenic Agents*. 6th ed. Baltimore, MD: Johns Hopkins University Press, 1989;140–1.
9. Akintonwa A, Gbajumo SA, Biola Mabadeje AF. Placental and milk transfer of chloroquine in humans. Ther Drug Monit 1988;10:147–9.
10. Dencker L, Lindquist NG, Ulberg S. Distribution of an I-125 labeled chloroquine analogue in a pregnant Macaca monkey. Toxicology 1975;5:255–64. As cited in Shepard TH. *Catalog of Teratogenic Agents*. 6th ed. Baltimore, MD: Johns Hopkins University Press, 1989;140–1.
11. Product information. Aralen. Sanofi Pharmaceuticals, 2000.
12. CDC. Recommendations for the prevention of malaria among travelers. MMWR 1990;39:1–10.
13. World Health Organization. Practical chemotherapy of malaria. WHO Tech Rep Ser 1990;805:1–141.
14. Subramanian D, Moise KJ Jr, White AC Jr. Imported malaria in pregnancy: report of four cases and review of management. Clin Infect Dis 1992;15:408–13.
15. Hart CW, Naunton RF. The ototoxicity of chloroquine phosphate. Arch Otolaryngol 1964;80:407–12.
16. Wolfe MS, Cordero JF. Safety of chloroquine in chemosuppression of malaria during pregnancy. Br Med J 1985;290:1466–7.
17. Edstein MD, Veenendaal JR, Newman K, Hyslop R. Excretion of chloroquine, dapsone and pyrimethamine in human milk. Br J Clin Pharmacol 1986;22:733–5.
18. Committee on Drugs, American Academy of Pediatrics. The transfer of drugs and other chemicals into human milk. Pediatrics 2001;108:776–89.

CHLOROTHIAZIDE

Diuretic

PREGNANCY RECOMMENDATION: Compatible
BREASTFEEDING RECOMMENDATION: Compatible

PREGNANCY SUMMARY

The published experience with 1st trimester use of thiazides and related diuretics does not indicate these agents are teratogenic. One large study (the Collaborative Perinatal Project) did find an increased risk of defects when diuretics were used during the 1st trimester in women with cardiovascular disorders, but causal relationships cannot be inferred from these

C

data without independent confirmation. Diuretics are not recommended for the treatment of gestational hypertension or preeclampsia because of the maternal hypovolemia characteristic of this disease. Other risks to the fetus or newborn include hypoglycemia, thrombocytopenia, hyponatremia, hypokalemia, and death from maternal complications. Moreover, thiazide diuretics may have a direct effect on smooth muscle and may inhibit labor.

FETAL RISK SUMMARY

Chlorothiazide is a member of the thiazide group of diuretics. The information in this monograph applies to all members of the group, including the pharmacologically and structurally related diuretics, chlorthalidone, indapamide, metolazone, and quinethazone.

Reproduction studies in mice (500 mg/kg/day), rats (60 mg/kg/day), and rabbits (50 mg/kg/day) revealed no external malformations or growth impairment, and no effect on fetal survival (1). However, these studies did not include a thorough examination for visceral anomalies and skeletal defects (1).

Data from published reports indicate that thiazide and related diuretics are infrequently administered during the 1st trimester. In the past, when these drugs were routinely given to prevent or treat toxemia, therapy was usually begun in the 2nd or 3rd trimester and adverse effects in the fetus were rare (2–11). No increases in the incidence of congenital defects were discovered, and thiazides were considered nonteratogenic (12–15).

In contrast, the Collaborative Perinatal Project monitored 50,282 mother–child pairs, 233 of whom were exposed in the 1st trimester to thiazide or related diuretics (16, pp. 371–373). All of the mothers had cardiovascular disorders, which makes interpretation of the data difficult. However, an increased risk for malformations was found for chlorthalidone (20 patients) and miscellaneous thiazide diuretics (35 patients, excluding chlorothiazide and hydrochlorothiazide). For use anytime during pregnancy, 17,492 exposures were recorded and only polythiazide showed a slight increase in risk (16, p. 441). The statistical significance of these findings is unknown and independent confirmation is required.

In a surveillance study of Michigan Medicaid recipients involving 229,101 completed pregnancies conducted between 1985 and 1992, a number of newborns had been exposed to this class of diuretics during the 1st trimester: 20 (chlorothiazide), 48 (chlorthalidone), and 567 (hydrochlorothiazide) (F. Rosa, personal communication, FDA, 1993). The number of major birth defects observed, the number expected, and the incidence for each drug were: 2/1/10.0%, 2/2/4.2%, and 24/22/4.2%, respectively. Specific data were available for six defect categories (observed/expected): cardiovascular defects 0/0, 1/0.5, and 7/6; oral clefts 0/0, 0/0, and 0/1; spina bifida, 0/0, 0/0, and 0/0.5; polydactyly, 0/0, 0/0, and 1/2; limb-reduction defects 0/0, 0/0, and 0/1; and hypospadias 1/0, 0/0, and 1/1, respectively. Although the number of exposures is small for two of the diuretics, these data do not support an association between the drug and congenital defects.

Many investigators consider diuretics contraindicated in pregnancy, except for patients with heart disease or chronic hypertension, because they do not prevent or alter the course of toxemia and they may decrease placental perfusion (8,17–21). A 1984 study determined that the use of diuretics for hypertension in pregnancy prevented normal plasma volume expansion and did not change perinatal outcome (22). In 4035 patients treated for edema in the last half of the 3rd trimester (hypertensive patients were excluded), higher rates were found for induction of labor, stimulation of labor, uterine inertia, meconium staining, and perinatal mortality (20). All except perinatal mortality were statistically significant compared with 13,103 controls. In another study, a decrease in the endocrine function of the placenta, as measured by placental clearance of estradiol, was found in three patients treated with hydrochlorothiazide (23).

Chlorothiazide readily crosses the placenta at term, and fetal serum levels may equal those of the mother (24). In 10 women, following 2 weeks of hydrochlorothiazide, 50 mg/day, the cord:maternal plasma ratio determined 2–13 hours after the last dose ranged from 0.10 to 0.80 (25). Chlorthalidone also crosses the placenta (26). Other diuretics probably cross to the fetus in similar amounts, although specific data are lacking.

Thiazides are considered mildly diabetogenic because they can induce hyperglycemia (18). Several investigators have noted this effect in pregnant patients treated with thiazides (27–30). Other studies have failed to show maternal hyperglycemia (31,32). Although apparently a low risk, newborns exposed to thiazide diuretics near term should be observed closely for symptoms of hypoglycemia resulting from maternal hyperglycemia (30).

Neonatal thrombocytopenia has been reported following the use near term of chlorothiazide, hydrochlorothiazide, and methyclothiazide (15,27,33–38). Other studies have not found a relationship between thiazide diuretics and platelet counts (39,40). The positive reports involve only 11 patients; however, although the numbers are small, 2 of the affected infants died (27,34). The mechanism of the thrombocytopenia is unknown, but the transfer of antiplatelet antibody from the mother to the fetus has been demonstrated (38). Thiazide-induced hemolytic anemia in 2 newborns was described in 1964 following the use of chlorothiazide and bendroflumethiazide at term (33). Thiazide diuretics may induce severe electrolyte imbalances in the mother's serum, in amniotic fluid, and in the newborn (41–43). In one case, a stillborn fetus was attributed to electrolyte imbalance and/or maternal hypotension (41). Two hypotonic newborns were discovered to be hyponatremic, a condition believed to have resulted from maternal diuretic therapy (42). Fetal bradycardia, 65–70 beats/minute, was shown to be secondary to chlorothiazide-induced maternal hypokalemia (43). In a 1963 study, no relationship was found between neonatal jaundice and chlorothiazide (44). Maternal and fetal deaths in two cases of acute hemorrhagic pancreatitis were attributed to the use of chlorothiazide in the 2nd and 3rd trimesters (45).

BREASTFEEDING SUMMARY

Chlorothiazide is excreted into breast milk in low concentrations (46). Following a single 500-mg oral dose, milk levels were <1 mcg/mL at 1, 2, and 3 hours. The authors speculated that the risks of pharmacologic effects in nursing infants would be remote. However, it has been stated that thrombocytopenia can occur in the nursing infant if the mother is taking chlorothiazide (47). Documentation of this is needed (48). Chlorthalidone has a very low milk:plasma ratio of 0.05 (26).

In one mother taking 50 mg of hydrochlorothiazide (HCTZ) daily, peak milk levels of the drug occurred 5–10 hours after a dose and were about 25% of maternal blood concentrations (49). The mean milk concentration of HCTZ was about 80 ng/mL. An infant consuming 600 mL of milk/day would thus ingest about 50 mcg of the drug, probably an insignificant amount (49). The diuretic could not be detected in the serum of the nursing 1-month-old infant, and the measurements of serum electrolytes, blood glucose, and blood urea nitrogen were all normal.

Thiazide diuretics have been used to suppress lactation (50,51). However, the American Academy of Pediatrics classifies bendroflumethiazide, chlorothiazide, chlorthalidone, and hydrochlorothiazide as compatible with breastfeeding (52).

References

1. Product information. Diuril. Merck, 2000.
2. Finnerty FA Jr, Buchholz JH, Tuckman J. Evaluation of chlorothiazide (Diuril) in the toxemias of pregnancy. Analysis of 144 patients. JAMA 1958;166:141–4.
3. Zuspan FP, Bell JD, Barnes AC. Balance-ward and double-blind diuretic studies during pregnancy. Obstet Gynecol 1960;16:543–9.
4. Sears RT. Oral diuretics in pregnancy toxaemia. Br Med J 1960;2:148.
5. Assoli NS. Renal effects of hydrochlorothiazide in normal and toxemic pregnancy. Clin Pharmacol Ther 1960;1:48–52.
6. Tatum H, Waterman EA. The prophylactic and therapeutic use of the thiazides in pregnancy. GP 1961;24:101–5.
7. Flowers CE, Grizzle JE, Easterling WE, Bonner OB. Chlorothiazide as a prophylaxis against toxemia of pregnancy. Am J Obstet Gynecol 1962;84: 919–29.
8. Weseley AC, Douglas GW. Continuous use of chlorothiazide for prevention of toxemia of pregnancy. Obstet Gynecol 1962;19:355–8.
9. Finnerty FA Jr. How to treat toxemia of pregnancy. GP 1963;27:116–21.
10. Fallis NE, Plauche WC, Mosey LM, Langford HG. Thiazide versus placebo in prophylaxis of toxemia of pregnancy in primigravid patients. Am J Obstet Gynecol 1964;88:502–4.
11. Landesman R, Aguero O, Wilson K, LaRussa R, Campbell W, Penaloza O. The prophylactic use of chlorthalidone, a sulfonamide diuretic, in pregnancy. J Obstet Gynaecol Br Commonw 1965;72:1004–10.
12. Cuadros A, Tatum H. The prophylactic and therapeutic use of bendroflumethiazide in pregnancy. Am J Obstet Gynecol 1964;89:891–7.
13. Finnerty FA Jr, Bepko FJ Jr. Lowering the perinatal mortality and the prematurity rate. The value of prophylactic thiazides in juveniles. JAMA 1966;195:429–32.
14. Kraus GW, Marchese JR, Yen SSC. Prophylactic use of hydrochlorothiazide in pregnancy. JAMA 1966;198:1150–4.
15. Gray MJ. Use and abuse of thiazides in pregnancy. Clin Obstet Gynecol 1968;11:568–78.
16. Heinonen OP, Slone D, Shapiro S. *Birth Defects and Drugs in Pregnancy*. Littleton, MA: Publishing Sciences Group, 1977.
17. Watt JD, Philipp EE. Oral diuretics in pregnancy toxemia. Br Med J 1960;1:1807.
18. Pitkin RM, Kaminetzky HA, Newton M, Pritchard JA. Maternal nutrition: a selective review of clinical topics. Obstet Gynecol 1972;40:773–85.
19. Lindheimer MD, Katz AI. Sodium and diuretics in pregnancy. N Engl J Med 1973;288:891–4.
20. Christianson R, Page EW. Diuretic drugs and pregnancy. Obstet Gynecol 1976;48:647–52.
21. Lammintausta R, Erkkola R, Eronen M. Effect of chlorothiazide treatment of renin–aldosterone system during pregnancy. Acta Obstet Gynecol Scand 1978;57:389–92.
22. Sibai BM, Grossman RA, Grossman HG. Effects of diuretics on plasma volume in pregnancies with long-term hypertension. Am J Obstet Gynecol 1984;150:831–5.
23. Shoemaker ES, Grant NF, Madden JD, MacDonald PC. The effect of thiazide diuretics on placental function. Tex Med 1973;69:109–15.
24. Garnet J. Placental transfer of chlorothiazide. Obstet Gynecol 1963;21: 123–5.
25. Beermann B, Fahraeus L, Groschinsky-Grind M, Lindstrom B. Placental transfer of hydrochlorothiazide. Gynecol Obstet Invest 1980;11:45–8.
26. Mulley BA, Parr GD, Pau WK, Rye RM, Mould JJ, Siddle NC. Placental transfer of chlorthalidone and its elimination in maternal milk. Eur J Clin Pharmacol 1978;13:129–31.
27. Menzies DN. Controlled trial of chlorothiazide in treatment of early pre-eclampsia. Br Med J 1964;1:739–42.
28. Ladner CN, Pearson JW, Herrick CN, Harrison HE. The effect of chlorothiazide on blood glucose in the third trimester of pregnancy. Obstet Gynecol 1964;23:555–60.
29. Goldman JA, Neri A, Ovadia J, Eckerling B, DeVries A. Effect of chlorothiazide on intravenous glucose tolerance in pregnancy. Am J Obstet Gynecol 1969;105:556–60.
30. Senior B, Slone D, Shapiro S, Mitchell AA, Heinonen OP. Benzothiadiazides and neonatal hypoglycaemia. Lancet 1976;2:377.
31. Lakin N, Zeytinoglu J, Younger M, White P. Effect of chlorothiazide on insulin requirements of pregnant diabetic women. JAMA 1960;173: 353–4.
32. Esbenshade JH Jr, Smith RT. Thiazides and pregnancy: a study of carbohydrate tolerance. Am J Obstet Gynecol 1965;92:270–1.
33. Harley JD, Robin H, Robertson SEJ. Thiazide-induced neonatal haemolysis? Br Med J 1964;1:696–7.
34. Rodriguez SU, Leikin SL, Hiller MC. Neonatal thrombocytopenia associated with ante-partum administration of thiazide drugs. N Engl J Med 1964;270:881–4.
35. Leikin SL. Thiazide and neonatal thrombocytopenia. N Engl J Med 1964;271:161.
36. Prescott LF. Neonatal thrombocytopenia and thiazide drugs. Br Med J 1964;1:1438.
37. Jones JE, Reed JF Jr. Renal vein thrombosis and thrombocytopenia in the newborn infant. J Pediatr 1965;67:681–2.
38. Karpatkin S, Strick N, Karpatkin MB, Siskind GW. Cumulative experience in the detection of antiplatelet antibody in 234 patients with idiopathic thrombocytopenic purpura, systemic lupus erythematosus and other clinical disorders. Am J Med 1972;52:776–85.
39. Finnerty FA Jr, Assoli NS. Thiazide and neonatal thrombocytopenia. N Engl J Med 1964;271:160–1.
40. Jerkner K, Kutti J, Victoria L. Platelet counts in mothers and their newborn infants with respect to antepartum administration of oral diuretics. Acta Med Scand 1973;194:473–5.
41. Pritchard JA, Walley PJ. Severe hypokalemia due to prolonged administration of chlorothiazide during pregnancy. Am J Obstet Gynecol 1961;81:1241–4.
42. Alstatt LB. Transplacental hyponatremia in the newborn infant. J Pediatr 1965;66:985–8.
43. Anderson GG, Hanson TM. Chronic fetal bradycardia: possible association with hypokalemia. Obstet Gynecol 1974;44:896–8.
44. Crosland D, Flowers C. Chlorothiazide and its relationship to neonatal jaundice. Obstet Gynecol 1963;22:500–4.
45. Minkowitz S, Soloway HB, Hall JE, Yermakov V. Fatal hemorrhagic pancreatitis following chlorothiazide administration in pregnancy. Obstet Gynecol 1964;24:337–42.
46. Werthmann MW Jr, Krees SV. Excretion of chlorothiazide in human breast milk. J Pediatr 1972;81:781–3.
47. Anonymous. Drugs in breast milk. Med Lett Drugs Ther 1976;16:25–7.
48. Dailey JW. Anticoagulant and cardiovascular drugs. In: Wilson JT, ed. *Drugs in Breast Milk*. Balgowlah, Australia: ADIS Press, 1981:61–4.
49. Miller ME, Cohn RD, Burghart PH. Hydrochlorothiazide disposition in a mother and her breast-fed infant. J Pediatr 1982;101:789–91.
50. Healy M. Suppressing lactation with oral diuretics. Lancet 1961;1:1353–4.
51. Catz CS, Giacoia GP. Drugs and breast milk. Pediatr Clin North Am 1972;19:151–66.
52. Committee on Drugs, American Academy of Pediatrics. The transfer of drugs and other chemicals into human milk. Pediatrics 2001;108:776–89.

CHLOROTRIANISENE

C

[Withdrawn from the market. See 9th edition.]

CHLORPHENIRAMINE

Antihistamine

PREGNANCY RECOMMENDATION: Compatible
BREASTFEEDING RECOMMENDATION: No Human Data—Probably Compatible

PREGNANCY SUMMARY

Use of antihistamines, including chlorpheniramine, is low risk in gestation. However, a possible association with retrolental fibroplasia in premature infants has been reported.

FETAL RISK SUMMARY

The Collaborative Perinatal Project monitored 50,282 mother–child pairs, 1070 of whom had 1st trimester exposure to chlorpheniramine (1, pp. 322–34). For use anytime during pregnancy, 3931 exposures were recorded (1, pp. 437, 488). In neither group was evidence found to suggest a relationship to large categories of major or minor malformations. Several possible associations with individual malformations were found, but independent confirmation is required to determine the actual risk.

Polydactyly in blacks (7 cases in 272 blacks)
Gastrointestinal defects (13 cases)
Eye and ear defects (7 cases)
Inguinal hernia (22 cases)
Hydrocephaly (8 cases)
Congenital dislocation of the hip (16 cases)
Malformations of the female genitalia (6 cases)

A 1971 study found that significantly fewer infants with malformations were exposed to antihistamines in the 1st trimester as compared with controls (2). Chlorpheniramine was the sixth most commonly used antihistamine.

In a surveillance study of Michigan Medicaid recipients involving 229,101 completed pregnancies conducted between 1985 and 1992, 61 newborns had been exposed to chlorpheniramine during the 1st trimester (F. Rosa, personal communication, FDA, 1993). Most of the exposures involved decongestant combinations including adrenergics. Two (3.3%) major birth defects were observed (three expected), including one case of polydactyly (none expected). No anomalies were observed in five other categories of defects (cardiovascular defects, oral clefts, spina bifida, limb-reduction defects, and hypospadias) for which specific data were available. These data do not support an association between the drug and congenital defects.

A case of infantile malignant osteopetrosis was described in a 4-month-old boy exposed in utero on several occasions to Contac (chlorpheniramine, phenylpropanolamine, and belladonna alkaloids) but this is a known genetic defect (3). The boy also had a continual "stuffy" nose.

An association between exposure during the last 2 weeks of pregnancy to antihistamines in general and retrolental fibroplasia in premature infants has been reported. (See Brompheniramine for details.)

BREASTFEEDING SUMMARY

No reports describing the use of chlorpheniramine during human lactation have been reported. As with other antihistamines, the drug probably is compatible with breastfeeding.

References

1. Heinonen OP, Slone D, Shapiro S. *Birth Defects and Drugs in Pregnancy*. Littleton, MA: Publishing Sciences Group, 1977.
2. Nelson MM, Forfar JO. Associations between drugs administered during pregnancy and congenital abnormalities of the fetus. Br Med J 1971;1:523–7.
3. Golbus MS, Koerper MA, Hall BD. Failure to diagnose osteopetrosis in utero. Lancet 1976;2:1246.

CHLORPROMAZINE

Antipsychotic

PREGNANCY RECOMMENDATION: Compatible
BREASTFEEDING RECOMMENDATION: Limited Human Data—Potential Toxicity

PREGNANCY SUMMARY

Although one survey found an increased incidence of defects and a report of ectromelia exists, most studies have found chlorpromazine to be safe for both mother and embryo–fetus if used occasionally in low doses. However, use near term should be avoided due to the danger of maternal hypotension and adverse effects in the newborn.

C

FETAL RISK SUMMARY

Chlorpromazine is a propylamino phenothiazine. The drug readily crosses the placenta (1–4). Reproductive studies in rodents have shown a potential for embryotoxicity, increased neonatal mortality, and decreased offspring performance (5). In animals, selective accumulation and retention occur in the fetal pigment epithelium (6). Although delayed ocular damage from high prolonged doses in pregnancy has not been reported in humans, concern has been expressed for this potential toxicity (6,7).

Chlorpromazine has been used for the treatment of nausea and vomiting of pregnancy during all stages of gestation, including labor, since the mid-1950s (8–10). The drug seems to be safe and effective for this indication. Its use in labor to promote analgesia and amnesia is usually safe, but some patients, up to 18% in one series, have a marked unpredictable fall in blood pressure that could be dangerous to the mother and the fetus (11–15). Use of chlorpromazine during labor should be discouraged because of this adverse effect.

One psychiatric patient, who consumed 8000 mg of chlorpromazine in the last 10 days of pregnancy, delivered a hypotonic, lethargic infant with depressed reflexes and jaundice (4). The adverse effects resolved within 3 weeks.

An extrapyramidal syndrome, which may persist for months, has been observed in some infants whose mothers received chlorpromazine near term (16–20). This reaction is characterized by tremors, increased muscle tone with spasticity, and hyperactive deep tendon reflexes. Hypotonicity has been observed in one newborn and paralytic ileus in two after exposure at term to chlorpromazine (4,21). However, most reports describing the use of chlorpromazine in pregnancy have concluded that it does not adversely affect the fetus or the newborn (22–27).

The Collaborative Perinatal Project (CPP) monitored 50,282 mother–child pairs, 142 of whom had 1st trimester exposure to chlorpromazine (28). For use anytime during pregnancy, 284 exposures were recorded. No evidence was found in either group to suggest a relationship to malformations or an effect on perinatal mortality rate, birth weight, or intelligence quotient scores at 4 years of age. Opposite results were found in a prospective French study that compared 315 mothers exposed to phenothiazines during the 1st trimester with 11,099 nonexposed controls (29). Malformations were observed in 11 exposed infants (3.5%) and in 178 controls (1.6%) ($p < 0.01$). In the phenothiazine group, 57 women took chlorpromazine and four infants had malformations: syndactyly; microcephaly, clubfoot/hand, muscular abdominal aplasia (also exposed to acetylpromazine); endocardial fibroelastosis, brachymesophalangy, clinodactyly (also exposed to pipamazine); and microcephaly (also exposed to promethazine).

The case of microcephaly, although listed as a possible drug-induced malformation, was considered by the authors to be more likely a genetic defect since the mother had already delivered two previous children with microcephaly (29). However, even after exclusion of this case, the association between phenothiazines and malformations remained significant (29). In another report, a stillborn fetus delivered at 28 weeks with ectromelia and omphalocele was attributed to the combined use of chlorpromazine and meclizine in the 1st trimester (30).

In a surveillance study of Michigan Medicaid recipients involving 229,101 completed pregnancies conducted between 1985 and 1992, 36 newborns had been exposed to chlorpromazine during the 1st trimester (F. Rosa, personal communication, FDA, 1993). No major birth defects were observed (two expected).

In an in vitro study, chlorpromazine was shown to be a potent inhibitor of sperm motility (31). A concentration of 53 μmol/L produced a 50% reduction in motility.

Using data from the CPP, researchers discovered that offspring of psychotic/neurotic mothers who had consumed chlorpromazine or other neuroleptics for more than 2 months during gestation, whether or not they were breastfed, were significantly taller than nonexposed controls at 4 months, 1 year, and 7 years of age (32). At 7 years of age, the difference between the exposed and nonexposed groups was approximately 3 cm. The mechanisms behind these effects were not clear, but may have been related to the dopamine receptor-blocking action of the drugs.

Reviewers have concluded that the phenothiazines are not teratogenic (26,33,34) and, because of its extensive clinical experience, chlorpromazine should be included among the treatments of choice if antipsychotic therapy was required during pregnancy (34).

BREASTFEEDING SUMMARY

Chlorpromazine is excreted into breast milk in very small concentrations. Following a 1200 mg oral dose (20 mg/kg), peak milk levels of 0.29 mcg/mL were measured at 2 hours (35). This represented a milk:plasma ratio of less than 0.5. The drug could not be detected following a 600-mg oral dose. In a study of four lactating mothers consuming unspecified amounts of the neuroleptic, milk concentrations of chlorpromazine ranged from 7 to 98 ng/mL, with maternal serum levels ranging from 16 to 52 ng/mL (36). In two mothers, more of the drug was found in the milk than in the plasma. Only two of the mothers breastfed their infants. One infant, consuming milk with a level of 7 ng/mL, showed no ill effects, but the second took milk containing 92 ng/mL and became drowsy and lethargic.

With the one exception described above, there have been no reported adverse effects in breastfed babies whose mothers were ingesting chlorpromazine (26). Based on this report, however, nursing infants exposed to the agent in milk should be observed for sedation. The American Academy of

Pediatrics classifies chlorpromazine as an agent whose effect on the nursing infant is unknown but may be of concern because of the drowsiness and lethargy observed in the infant described above, and because of the galactorrhea induced in adults (37).

References

1. Franchi G, Gianni AM. Chlorpromazine distribution in maternal and fetal tissues and biological fluids. Acta Anaesthesiol (Padava) 1957;8:197–207.
2. Moya F, Thorndike V. Passage of drugs across the placenta. Am J Obstet Gynecol 1962;84:1778–98.
3. O'Donoghue SEF. Distribution of pethidine and chlorpromazine in maternal, foetal and neonatal biological fluids. Nature 1971;229:124–5.
4. Hammond JE, Toseland PA. Placental transfer of chlorpromazine. Arch Dis Child 1970;45:139–40.
5. Product information. Thorazine. SmithKline Beecham Pharmaceuticals, 2000.
6. Ullberg S, Lindquist NG, Sjostrand SE. Accumulation of chorio-retinotoxic drugs in the foetal eye. Nature 1970;227:1257–8.
7. Anonymous. Drugs and the fetal eye. Lancet 1971;1:122.
8. Karp M, Lamb VE, Benaron HBW. The use of chlorpromazine in the obstetric patient: a preliminary report. Am J Obstet Gynecol 1955;69:780–5.
9. Benaron HBW, Dorr EM, Roddick WJ, Johnson RP, Gossack L, Tucker BE. The use of chlorpromazine in the obstetric patient: a preliminary report I. In the treatment of nausea and vomiting of pregnancy. Am J Obstet Gynecol 1955;69:776–9.
10. Sullivan CL. Treatment of nausea and vomiting of pregnancy with chlorpromazine. A report of 100 cases. Postgrad Med 1957;22:429–32.
11. Harer WB. Chlorpromazine in normal labor. Obstet Gynecol 1956;8:1–9.
12. Lindley JE, Rogers SF, Moyer JH. Analgesic-potentiation effect of chlorpromazine during labor; a study of 2093 patients. Obstet Gynecol 1957;10:582–6.
13. Bryans CI Jr, Mulherin CM. The use of chlorpromazine in obstetrical analgesia. Am J Obstet Gynecol 1959;77:406–11.
14. Christhilf SM Jr, Monias MB, Riley RA Jr, Sheehan JC. Chlorpromazine in obstetric analgesia. Obstet Gynecol 1960;15:625–9.
15. Rodgers CD, Wickard CP, McCaskill MR. Labor and delivery without terminal anesthesia. A report of the use of chlorpromazine. Obstet Gynecol 1961;17:92–5.
16. Hill RM, Desmond MM, Kay JL. Extrapyramidal dysfunction in an infant of a schizophrenic mother. J Pediatr 1966;69:589–95.
17. Ayd FJ Jr, ed. Phenothiazine therapy during pregnancy-effects on the newborn infant. Int Drug Ther Newslett 1968;3:39–40.
18. Tamer A, McKay R, Arias D, Worley L, Fogel BJ. Phenothiazine-induced extrapyramidal dysfunction in the neonate. J Pediatr 1969;75:479–80.
19. Levy W, Wisniewski K. Chlorpromazine causing extrapyramidal dysfunction in newborn infant of psychotic mother. NY State J Med 1974;74:684–5.
20. O'Connor M, Johnson GH, James DI. Intrauterine effect of phenothiazines. Med J Aust 1981;1:416–7.
21. Falterman CG, Richardson J. Small left colon syndrome associated with maternal ingestion of psychotropic drugs. J Pediatr 1980;97:308–10.
22. Kris EB, Carmichael DM. Chlorpromazine maintenance therapy during pregnancy and confinement. Psychiatr Q 1957;31:690–5.
23. Kris EB. Children born to mothers maintained on pharmacotherapy during pregnancy and postpartum. Recent Adv Biol Psychiatry 1962;4:180–7.
24. Kris EB. Children of mothers maintained on pharmacotherapy during pregnancy and postpartum. Curr Ther Res 1965;7:785–9.
25. Sobel DE. Fetal damage due to ECT, insulin coma, chlorpromazine, or reserpine. Arch Gen Psychiatry 1960;2:606–11.
26. Ayd FJ Jr. Children born of mothers treated with chlorpromazine during pregnancy. Clin Med 1964;71:1758–63.
27. Loke KH, Salleh R. Electroconvulsive therapy for the acutely psychotic pregnant patient: a review of 3 cases. Med J Malaysia 1983;38:131–3.
28. Slone D, Siskind V, Heinonen OP, Monson RR, Kaufman DW, Shapiro S. Antenatal exposure to the phenothiazines in relation to congenital malformations, perinatal mortality rate, birth weight, and intelligence quotient score. Am J Obstet Gynecol 1977;128:486–8.
29. Rumeau-Rouquette C, Goujard J, Huel G. Possible teratogenic effect of phenothiazines in human beings. Teratology 1976;15:57–64.
30. O'Leary JL, O'Leary JA. Nonthalidomide ectromelia; report of a case. Obstet Gynecol 1964;23:17–20.
31. Levin RM, Amsterdam JD, Winokur A, Wein AJ. Effects of psychotropic drugs on human sperm motility. Fertil Steril 1981;36:503–6.
32. Platt JE, Friedhoff AJ, Broman SH, Bond RN, Laska E, Lin SP. Effects of prenatal exposure to neuroleptic drugs on children's growth. Neuropsychopharmacology 1988;1:205–12.
33. Ananth J. Congenital malformations with psychopharmacologic agents. Compr Psychiatry 1975;16:437–45.
34. Elia J, Katz IR, Simpson GM. Teratogenicity of psychotherapeutic medications. Psychopharmacol Bull 1987;23:531–86.
35. Blacker KH, Weinstein BJ, Ellman GL. Mother's milk and chlorpromazine. Am J Psychol 1962;114:178–9.
36. Wiles DH, Orr MW, Kolakowska T. Chlorpromazine levels in plasma and milk of nursing mothers. Br J Clin Pharmacol 1978;5:272–3.
37. Committee on Drugs, American Academy of Pediatrics. The transfer of drugs and other chemicals into human milk. Pediatrics 2001;108:776–89.

CHLORPROPAMIDE

Antidiabetic Agent

PREGNANCY RECOMMENDATION: Human Data Suggest Risk in 3rd Trimester
BREASTFEEDING RECOMMENDATION: Limited Human Data—Potential Toxicity

PREGNANCY SUMMARY

Although the use of chlorpropamide during human gestation does not appear to be related to structural anomalies, insulin is still the treatment of choice for this disease. Oral hypoglycemics might not be indicated for the pregnant diabetic. Moreover, insulin, unlike chlorpropamide, does not cross the placenta and, thus, eliminates the additional concern that the drug therapy itself is adversely affecting the fetus. Carefully prescribed insulin therapy will provide better control of the mother's blood glucose, thereby preventing the fetal and neonatal complications that occur with this disease. High maternal glucose levels, as may occur in diabetes mellitus, are closely associated with a number of maternal and fetal adverse effects, including fetal structural anomalies if the hyperglycemia occurs early in gestation. To prevent this toxicity, the American College of Obstetricians and Gynecologists recommends that insulin be used for types I and II diabetes occurring during pregnancy and, if diet therapy alone is not successful, for gestational diabetes (1,2). If chlorpropamide is used during pregnancy, therapy should be changed to insulin and chlorpropamide discontinued before delivery (the exact time before delivery is unknown) to lessen the possibility of prolonged hypoglycemia in the newborn.

FETAL RISK SUMMARY

Chlorpropamide is a sulfonylurea used for the treatment of adult-onset diabetes mellitus. It is not the treatment of choice for the pregnant diabetic patient.

In a study using neurulating mouse embryos in whole embryo culture, chlorpropamide produced malformations and growth restriction at concentrations similar to therapeutic levels in humans (3). The defects were not a result of hypoglycemia or of chlorpropamide metabolites.

When administered near term, chlorpropamide crosses the placenta and may persist in the neonatal serum for several days (4–6). One mother, who took 500 mg/day throughout pregnancy, delivered an infant whose serum level was 15.4 mg/dL at 77 hours of life (4). Infants of three other mothers, who were consuming 100–250 mg/day at term, had serum levels varying between 1.8 and 2.8 mg/dL 8–35 hours after delivery (5). All four infants had prolonged symptomatic hypoglycemia secondary to hyperinsulinism lasting for 4–6 days. Another newborn, whose mother had been taking chlorpropamide, had severe, prolonged hypoglycemia and seizures (6). In other reports, totaling 69 pregnancies, chlorpropamide in doses of 100–200 mg or more/day either gave no evidence of neonatal hypoglycemia and hyperinsulinism or no constant relationship between daily maternal dosage and neonatal complications (7,8).

In an abstract (9), and later in a full report (10), the in vitro placental transfer, using a single-cotyledon human placenta, of four oral hypoglycemics agents was described. As expected, molecular weight was the most significant factor for drug transfer, with dissociation constant (pKa) and lipid solubility providing significant additive effects. The cumulative percent placental transfer at 3 hours of the four agents and their approximate molecular weights (shown in parenthesis) were tolbutamide (270) 21.5%, chlorpropamide (277) 11.0%, glipizide (446) 6.6%, and glyburide (494) 3.9% (10).

Although teratogenic in animals, an increased incidence of congenital defects, other than that expected in diabetes mellitus, was not found with chlorpropamide in several studies (11–20). Four malformed infants have been attributed to chlorpropamide but the relationship is unclear: hand and finger anomalies (11); stricture of lower ileum, death (11); preauricular sinus (11); and microcephaly and spastic quadriplegia (14).

In a surveillance study of Michigan Medicaid recipients involving 229,101 completed pregnancies conducted between 1985 and 1992, 18 newborns had been exposed to chlorpropamide during the 1st trimester (F. Rosa, personal communication, FDA, 1993). No major birth defects were observed (one expected).

A 1991 report described the outcomes of pregnancies in 21 non-insulin-dependent diabetic women who were treated with oral hypoglycemic agents (17 sulfonylureas, 3 biguanides, and 1 unknown type) during the 1st trimester (21). The duration of exposure ranged from 3 to 28 weeks, but all patients were changed to insulin therapy at the first prenatal visit. Forty non-insulin-dependent diabetic women matched for age, race, parity, and glycemic control served as a control group. Eleven (52%) of the exposed infants had major or minor congenital malformations compared with six (15%) of the controls. Moreover, ear defects, a malformation that is observed, but uncommonly, in diabetic embryopathy, occurred in six of the exposed infants and in none of the controls. Six of the 11 infants with defects had been exposed in utero to chlorpropamide (length of exposure during pregnancy in weeks): severe microtia right ear, multiple tags left ear (22 weeks); bilateral auricular tags (8 weeks); single umbilical artery (14 weeks); ear tag (10 weeks); facial, auricular, and vertebral defects, deafness, ventricular septal defect (15 weeks); and multiple vertebral anomalies, ventricular septal defect, severe aortic coarctation; bilateral ear tags and posterior rotated ears (14 weeks) (21).

Sixteen livebirths occurred in the exposed group compared with 36 in controls (21). The groups did not differ in the incidence of hypoglycemia at birth (53% vs. 53%), but three of the exposed newborns had severe hypoglycemia lasting 2, 4, and 7 days, even though the mothers had not used oral hypoglycemics (two women had used chlorpropamide) close to delivery. The authors attributed this to irreversible β-cell hyperplasia that may have been increased by exposure to oral hypoglycemics. Hyperbilirubinemia was noted in 10 (67%) of 15 exposed newborns compared with 13 (36%) of controls ($p < 0.04$), and polycythemia and hyperviscosity requiring partial exchange transfusions were observed in 4 (27%) of 15 exposed vs. 1 (3.0%) control ($p < 0.03$) (one exposed infant not included in these data because presented after completion of study) (21).

A study published in 1995 assessed the risk of congenital malformations in infants of mothers with non-insulin-dependent diabetes during a 6-year period (22). Women were included in the study if, during the first 8 weeks of pregnancy, they had not participated in a preconception care program and then had been treated either with diet alone (group 1), diet and oral hypoglycemic agents (predominantly chlorpropamide, glyburide, or glipizide) (group 2), or diet and exogenous insulin (group 3). The 302 women eligible for analysis gave birth to 332 infants (five sets of twins and 16 with two or three separate singleton pregnancies during the study period). A total of 56 (16.9%) of the infants had one or more congenital malformations, 39 (11.7%) of which were classified as major anomalies (defined as those that were either lethal, caused significant morbidity, or required surgical repair). The major anomalies were divided among those involving the central nervous system, face, heart and great vessels, gastrointestinal, genitourinary, and skeletal (includes caudal regression syndrome) systems. Minor anomalies included all of these, except those of the central nervous system, and a miscellaneous group composed of sacral skin tags, cutis aplasia of the scalp, and hydroceles. The number of infants in each group and the number of major and minor anomalies observed were group 1—125 infants, 18 (14.4%) major, 6 (4.8%) minor; group 2—147 infants, 14 (9.5%) major, 9 (6.1%) minor; group 3—60 infants, 7 (11.7%) major, 2 (3.3%) minor. There were no statistical differences among the groups. Six (4.1%) of the infants exposed in utero to oral hypoglycemic agents and four other infants in the other two groups had ear anomalies (included among those with face defects). Other than the incidence of major anomalies, two other important findings of this study were the independent associations between the risk of major anomalies (but not minor defects) and poor glycemic control in early pregnancy, and a younger maternal age at the onset of diabetes. Moreover, the study did not find an association between the use of oral hypoglycemics during organogenesis and congenital malformations because the observed anomalies appeared to be related to poor maternal glycemic control (22).

C

BREASTFEEDING SUMMARY

Chlorpropamide is excreted into breast milk. Following a 500-mg oral dose, the milk concentration in a composite of two samples obtained at 5 hours was 5 mcg/mL (G.G. D'Ambrosio, personal communication, Pfizer Laboratories, 1982). The effects on a nursing infant from this amount of drug are unknown, but hypoglycemia is a potential toxicity.

References

1. American College of Obstetricians and Gynecologists. Pregestational diabetes mellitus. *ACOG Practice Bulletin*. No. 60. March 2005. Obstet Gynecol 2005;105:675–85.
2. American College of Obstetricians and Gynecologists. Gestational diabetes. *ACOG Practice Bulletin*. No. 30. September 2001. Obstet Gynecol 2001;98:525–38.
3. Smoak IW. Embryopathic effects of the oral hypoglycemic agent chlorpropamide in cultured mouse embryos. Am J Obstet Gynecol 1993;169:409–14.
4. Zucker P, Simon G. Prolonged symptomatic neonatal hypoglycemia associated with maternal chlorpropamide therapy. Pediatrics 1968;42:824–5.
5. Kemball ML, McIver C, Milnar RDG, Nourse CH, Schiff D, Tiernan JR. Neonatal hypoglycaemia in infants of diabetic mothers given sulphonylurea drugs in pregnancy. Arch Dis Child 1970;45:696–701.
6. Harris EL. Adverse reactions to oral antidiabetic agents. Br Med J 1971;3:29–30.
7. Sutherland HW, Stowers JM, Cormack JD, Bewsher PD. Evaluation of chlorpropamide in chemical diabetes diagnosed during pregnancy. Br Med J 1973;3:9–13.
8. Sutherland HW, Bewsher PD, Cormack JD, Hughes CRT, Reid A, Russell G, Stowers JM. Effect of moderate dosage of chlorpropamide in pregnancy on fetal outcome. Arch Dis Child 1974;49:283–91.
9. Elliott B, Schenker S, Langer O, Johnson R, Prihoda T. Oral hypoglycemic agents: profound variation exists in their rate of human placental transfer. Society of Perinatal Obstetricians Abstract. Am J Obstet Gynecol 1992;166:368.
10. Elliott BD, Schenker S, Langer O, Johnson R, Prihoda T. Comparative placental transport of oral hypoglycemic agents in humans: a model of human placental drug transfer. Am J Obstet Gynecol 1994;171:653–60.
11. Soler NG, Walsh CH, Malins JM. Congenital malformations in infants of diabetic mothers. Q J Med 1976;45:303–13.
12. Adam PAJ, Schwartz R. Diagnosis and treatment: should oral hypoglycemic agents be used in pediatric and pregnant patients? Pediatrics 1968;42:819–23.
13. Dignan PSJ. Teratogenic risk and counseling in diabetes. Clin Obstet Gynecol 1981;24:149–59.
14. Campbell GD. Chlorpropamide and foetal damage. Br Med J 1963;1:59–60.
15. Jackson WPU, Campbell GD, Notelovitz M, Blumsohn D. Tolbutamide and chlorpropamide during pregnancy in human diabetes. Diabetes 1962;11(Suppl):98–101.
16. Jackson WPU, Campbell GD. Chlorpropamide and perinatal mortality. Br Med J 1963;2:1652.
17. Macphail I. Chlorpropamide and foetal damage. Br Med J 1963;1:192.
18. Malins JM, Cooke AM, Pyke DA, Fitzgerald MG. Sulphonylurea drugs in pregnancy. Br Med J 1964;2:187.
19. Moss JM, Connor EJ. Pregnancy complicated by diabetes. Report of 102 pregnancies including eleven treated with oral hypoglycemic drugs. Med Ann DC 1965;34;253–60.
20. Douglas CP, Richards R. Use of chlorpropamide in the treatment of diabetes in pregnancy. Diabetes 1967;16:60–1.
21. Piacquadio K, Hollingsworth DR, Murphy H. Effects of in-utero exposure to oral hypoglycaemic drugs. Lancet 1991;338:866–9.
22. Towner D, Kjos SL, Leung B, Montoro MM, Xiang A, Mestman JH, Buchanan TA. Congenital malformations in pregnancies complicated by NIDDM. Diabetes Care 1995;18:1446–51.

CHLORPROTHIXENE

[Withdrawn from the market. See 9th edition.]

CHLORTETRACYCLINE

Antibiotic (Tetracycline)

PREGNANCY RECOMMENDATION: Contraindicated in 2nd and 3rd Trimesters
BREASTFEEDING RECOMMENDATION: Compatible

PREGNANCY SUMMARY

Tetracyclines are known human teratogens. See Tetracycline.

BREASTFEEDING SUMMARY

Chlortetracycline is excreted into breast milk. Eight patients were given 2–3 g orally/day for 3–4 days (1). Average maternal and milk concentrations were 4.1 and 1.25 mcg/mL, respectively, producing a milk:plasma ratio of 0.4. Infant data were not given.

Theoretically, dental staining and inhibition of bone growth could occur in breastfed infants whose mothers were consuming chlortetracycline. However, this theoretical possibility seems remote because in infants exposed to a closely related antibiotic, tetracycline, serum levels were undetectable (<0.05 mcg/mL) (2). The American Academy of Pediatrics classifies tetracycline as compatible with breastfeeding (3). Three potential problems may exist for the nursing infant, even though there are no reports in this regard: modification of bowel flora, direct effects on the infant, and interference with the interpretation of culture results if a fever workup is required.

References

1. Guilbeau JA, Schoenbach EB, Schuab IG, Latham DV. Aureomycin in obstetrics; therapy and prophylaxis. JAMA 1950;143:520–6.
2. Posner AC, Prigot A, Konicoff NG. Further observations on the use of tetracycline hydrochloride in prophylaxis and treatment of obstetric infections. In: *Antibiotics Annual 1954-55*. New York, NY: Medical Encyclopedia, 1955:594–8.
3. Committee on Drugs, American Academy of Pediatrics. The transfer of drugs and other chemicals into human milk. Pediatrics 2001;108:776–89.

CHLORTHALIDONE

Diuretic

PREGNANCY RECOMMENDATION: Compatible
BREASTFEEDING RECOMMENDATION: Compatible

C

PREGNANCY SUMMARY

Chlorthalidone is structurally related to the thiazide diuretics (see Chlorothiazide). In general, diuretics are not recommended for the treatment of gestational hypertension because of the maternal hypovolemia characteristic of this disease.

FETAL RISK SUMMARY

Reproduction studies in rats and rabbits at doses up to 420 times the human dose have observed no evidence of fetal harm (1).

BREASTFEEDING SUMMARY

See Chlorothiazide.

Reference

1. Product information. Thalitone. Monarch Pharmaceuticals, 2000.

CHLORZOXAZONE

Muscle Relaxant

PREGNANCY RECOMMENDATION: Limited Human Data—No Relevant Animal Data
BREASTFEEDING RECOMMENDATION: No Human Data—Probably Compatible

PREGNANCY SUMMARY

The available human pregnancy experience does not suggest a risk of teratogenicity.

FETAL RISK SUMMARY

The reproductive effects of the centrally acting muscle relaxant, chlorzoxazone, have not been studied in animals. Moreover, no published reports of its use in human pregnancy have been located. The relatively low molecular weight (about 170) suggests that the drug will cross the placenta.

In a surveillance study of Michigan Medicaid recipients involving 229,101 completed pregnancies conducted between 1985 and 1992, 42 newborns had been exposed to chlorzoxazone during the 1st trimester (F. Rosa, personal communication, FDA, 1993). One (2.4%) major birth defect was observed (two expected), a cardiovascular defect (0.5 expected). Earlier data, obtained from the same source between 1980 and 1983, totaled 264 1st trimester exposures with 17 defects observed (17 expected). These combined data do not support an association between the drug and congenital defects.

BREASTFEEDING SUMMARY

No reports describing the use of chlorzoxazone during lactation have been located. The molecular weight (about 170) is low enough that excretion into breast milk should be expected. The effect of this potential exposure on a nursing infant is unknown. However, other muscle relaxants are excreted in milk and do not appear to harm a nursing infant (e.g., see Baclofen and Carisoprodol).

CHOLECALCIFEROL

Vitamin

PREGNANCY RECOMMENDATION: Compatible
BREASTFEEDING RECOMMENDATION: Compatible

C

PREGNANCY SUMMARY

Cholecalciferol (vitamin D_3) is converted in the liver to calcifediol, which in turn is converted in the kidneys to calcitriol, one of the active forms of vitamin D (see Calcitriol and Vitamin D).

BREASTFEEDING SUMMARY

See Vitamin D.

CHOLESTYRAMINE

Antilipemic

PREGNANCY RECOMMENDATION: Compatible
BREASTFEEDING RECOMMENDATION: No Human Data—Probably Compatible

PREGNANCY SUMMARY

Except for a single case involving maternal and fetal vitamin K deficiency, the use of this drug in pregnancy appears to be low risk.

FETAL RISK SUMMARY

Cholestyramine is a resin used to bind bile acids in a nonabsorbable complex. In a reproductive study involving rats and rabbits, the resin was given in doses up to 2 g/kg/day without evidence of fertility impairment or adverse fetal effects (1). In a comparison between pregnant and nonpregnant rats, administration of cholestyramine failed to lower the plasma cholesterol concentration or to increase bile acid synthesis (2). The drug therapy had no effect, in comparison to control animals, on maternal weight gain, number of fetuses, and fetal weight.

Cholestyramine has been used for the treatment of cholestasis of pregnancy (3–7). Except for the case described below, no adverse fetal effects were observed in these studies. One review recommended the resin as first-line therapy for the pruritus that accompanies intrahepatic cholestasis of pregnancy (6). Cholestyramine also binds fat-soluble vitamins, and long-term use could result in deficiencies of these agents in either the mother or the fetus (8). In one study, treatment with 9 g daily up to a maximum duration of 12 weeks was not associated with fetal or maternal complications (3).

A 31-year-old woman in her third pregnancy was treated with cholestyramine (8 g/day) beginning at 19 weeks' gestation for intrahepatic cholestasis of pregnancy (7). At 22 weeks' gestation, the dose was increased to 16 g/day. Four weeks later, she was clinically jaundiced and at 29 weeks' gestation, she was admitted to the hospital for reduced fetal movements. Fetal ultrasound scans over the next week revealed expanding bilateral subdural hematomas with hydrocephalus, an enlarged liver, and bilateral pleural effusions (7). The mother's prothrombin ratio was markedly elevated but responded to two doses of IV vitamin K. One week later, following labor induction for fetal distress, a 1660-g infant was delivered who died at 15 minutes of age. It was thought that the fetal subdural hematomas were the result of vitamin K deficiency caused by the cholestyramine, cholestasis, or both (7).

A 1989 report described the use of cholestyramine and other agents in the treatment of inflammatory bowel disease during pregnancy (9). Seven patients were treated during gestation with the resin. One of the seven delivered prematurely (<37 weeks' gestation) and one of the newborns was small for gestational age (<10th percentile for gestational age). Both of these outcomes were probably related to the mother's disease, rather than to the therapy.

In a surveillance study of Michigan Medicaid recipients involving 229,101 completed pregnancies conducted between 1985 and 1992, 4 newborns had been exposed to cholestyramine during the 1st trimester (10). Thirty-three other newborns were exposed after the 1st trimester. None of the infants had congenital malformations.

BREASTFEEDING SUMMARY

Cholestyramine is a nonabsorbable resin. No reports describing its use during lactation have been located. Because it binds fat-soluble vitamins, prolonged use may result in deficiencies of these vitamins in the mother and her nursing infant.

References

1. Koda S, Anabuki K, Miki T, Kahi S, Takahashi N. Reproductive studies on cholestyramine. Kiso to Rinsho 1982;16:2040–94. As cited in Shepard TH. *Catalog of Teratogenic Agents*. 7th ed. Baltimore, MD: Johns Hopkins University Press, 1992:90.
2. Innis SM. Effect of cholestyramine administration during pregnancy in the rat. Am J Obstet Gynecol 1983;146:13–6.
3. Lutz EE, Margolis AJ. Obstetric hepatosis: treatment with cholestyramine and interim response to steroids. Obstet Gynecol 1969;33:64–71.
4. Heikkinen J, Maentausta O, Ylostalo P, Janne O. Serum bile acid levels in intrahepatic cholestasis of pregnancy during treatment with phenobarbital or cholestyramine. Eur J Obstet Gynecol Reprod Biol 1982;14:153–62.
5. Shaw D, Frohlich J, Wittmann BAK, Willms M. A prospective study of 18 patients with cholestasis of pregnancy. Am J Obstet Gynecol 1982;142:621–5.

6. Schorr-Lesnick B, Lebovics E, Dworkin B, Rosenthal WS. Liver disease unique to pregnancy. Am J Gastroenterol 1991;86:659–70.
7. Sadler LC, Lane M, North R. Severe fetal intracranial haemorrhage during treatment with cholestyramine for intrahepatic cholestasis of pregnancy. Br J Obstet Gynaecol 1995;102:169–70.
8. American Hospital Formulary Service. *Drug Information 1997*. Bethesda, MD: American Society of Health-System Pharmacists, 1997:1330–4.
9. Fedorkow DM, Persaud D, Nimrod CA. Inflammatory bowel disease: a controlled study of late pregnancy outcome. Am J Obstet Gynecol 1989;160:998–1001.
10. Rosa F. *Anti-cholesterol Agent Pregnancy Exposure Outcomes*. Presented at the 7th International Organization for Teratogen Information Services, Woods Hole, MA, April 1994.

C

CHONDROITIN

Dietary Supplement

PREGNANCY RECOMMENDATION: No Human Data—Probably Compatible
BREASTFEEDING RECOMMENDATION: No Human Data—Probably Compatible

PREGNANCY SUMMARY

No reports describing the use of chondroitin in human pregnancy have been located. The animal data suggest low risk, but the absence of reported human pregnancy experience prevents an assessment of the risk to the embryo–fetus. Moreover, the lack of standardization prevents knowledge of the exact dose taken. The oral bioavailability depends on the molecular weight of the product used, and this may not be known from the product's package insert or label. However, chondroitin is an endogenous substance widely found in human tissues, so the embryo–fetus must synthesize it during development. Therefore, the planned or inadvertent use of chondroitin during gestation does not appear to represent a clinically significant risk of embryo–fetal harm.

FETAL RISK SUMMARY

Chondroitin is a mucopolysaccharide that belongs to a class of very large molecules called glycosaminoglycans (1,2). It is isolated from natural sources, such as shark and bovine cartilage. There are no official standards to regulate its production in the United States, so the actual dose taken cannot be accurately determined. Endogenous chondroitin acts as the flexible connecting matrix (substrate) between protein filaments in cartilage that is found in most mammals. The substance can be found in human cartilage, bone, cornea, skin, and the arterial wall (3). Oral chondroitin, frequently in combination with glucosamine or manganese, is used in the treatment of osteoarthritis, ischemic heart disease, osteoporosis, hyperlipidemia, and other conditions. An IM formulation (not available in the United States) is used for osteoarthritis and topical chondroitin is used for dry eyes and as an adjunct to ocular surgery. With the possible exceptions of its use for osteoarthritis and dry eyes, studies are needed to confirm the efficacy of chondroitin. The oral bioavailability of oral chondroitin has been reported to be minimal, in the range of 0%–13% (1), but is thought to depend on the molecular weight of the chondroitin product studied (3).

Animal reproduction studies have been conducted in mice and rats, but the doses used were not related to the human daily dose in terms of BSA or AUC. Injection of 1 mL (20 mg) of a 2% solution of chondroitin sulfate into mice during organogenesis resulted in cleft palates or kinky tails (4). No adverse effects were observed with oral doses up to 5000 mg/kg of chondroitin polysulfate given to rats and mice during organogenesis (5).

It is not known if chondroitin crosses the animal or human placenta. The molecular weight (5000–50,000) and probable very low blood concentrations suggest that minimal amounts, if any, will cross to the embryo or fetus.

BREASTFEEDING SUMMARY

No reports describing the use of chondroitin during lactation have been located. Depending on the source, the molecular weight (5000–50,000) and probable very low blood concentrations suggest that little, if any, of the drug will be excreted into breast milk. Therefore, the use of chondroitin during lactation is probably compatible.

References

1. Chondroitin. *The Review of Natural Products*. St. Louis, MO: Wolters Kluwer Health, 2004.
2. Chondroitin Sulfate. *Natural Medicines Comprehensive Database*. Stockton, CA: Therapeutic Research Faculty, 2003:345–7.
3. Chondroitin. PDR Health. Available at http://www.pdrhealth.com/drug_info/nmdrugprofiles/nutsupdrugs/cho_0071.shtml. Accessed March 20, 2006.
4. Kamei T. The teratogenic effect of excessive chondroitin sulfate in the DDN strain of mice. Med Biol 1961;60:126–9. As cited in Shepard TH. *Catalog of Teratogenic Agents*. 10th ed. Baltimore, MD: The Johns Hopkins University Press, 2001:107–8.
5. Hamada Y. Studies on anti-atherosclerotic agents. IX. Teratological studies of sodium chondroitin polysulfate. Oyo Yakuri 1972;6:589–94. As cited in Shepard TH. *Catalog of Teratogenic Agents*. 10th ed. Baltimore, MD: The Johns Hopkins University Press, 2001:107.

CICLESONIDE

Respiratory Drug (Corticosteroid)

PREGNANCY RECOMMENDATION: Compatible—Maternal Benefit >> Embryo–Fetal Risk
BREASTFEEDING RECOMMENDATION: No Human Data—Probably Compatible

C

PREGNANCY SUMMARY

No reports describing the use of ciclesonide in human pregnancy have been located. Poorly controlled asthma may result in adverse maternal, fetal, and neonatal outcomes (4,5). Maternal complications include an increased risk of preeclampsia, gestational hypertension, hyperemesis gravidarum, vaginal hemorrhage, and induced and difficult labor. Fetal and neonatal adverse effects may be an increased risk of perinatal mortality, intrauterine growth restriction (IUGR), prematurity, lower birth weight, and neonatal hypoxia (1). Moreover, a recent study reported that asthma exacerbations during the 1st trimester significantly increased the risk of congenital malformations (2). Because controlling maternal asthma can ameliorate or prevent all of these complications, the benefits of therapy outweigh the potential risks of drug-induced teratogenicity or toxicity. Pregnant women who require an inhaled corticosteroid, such as ciclesonide, for control of their asthma should be counseled as to the risks and benefits of therapy, but treatment should not be withheld because of their pregnancy.

FETAL RISK SUMMARY

Ciclesonide is a nonhalogenated glucocorticoid that is available as an inhaled aerosol and intranasal spray. It is a prodrug that is enzymatically hydrolyzed to the active drug des-ciclesonide (RM1). The oral bioavailability of ciclesonide and RM1 is negligible. RM1 has anti-inflammatory activity with an affinity for glucocorticoid receptors that is 120 times greater than that of ciclesonide and 12 times greater than that of dexamethasone. The inhaled aerosol is indicated for the maintenance treatment of asthma as a prophylactic therapy, whereas the intranasal spray is indicated for the treatment of nasal symptoms associated with perennial or seasonal allergic rhinitis (3,4). Compared with an IV 800-mcg dose, the absolute bioavailability of ciclesonide after an oral inhalation 1280-mcg dose (four times the recommended dose) was 22% and the relative systemic exposure of RM1 was 63%. Plasma protein binding for ciclesonide and RM1 was ≥99%. Following IV administration, the mean half-lives of ciclesonide and RM1 were 0.71 and 6–7 hours, respectively (1), but a review cited mean values of 0.38 and 3.5 hours, respectively (5). Only RM1 was detected in the serum after use of the intranasal spray, and then only with daily doses ≥400 mcg (4).

Reproduction studies have been conducted in rats and rabbits. There was no teratogenicity or other fetal effects in rats given oral doses that were about 10 times the maximum human daily inhalation dose based on BSA (MHDID) (3). Similarly, no adverse fetal effects were observed when rats were given doses up to about 35 times the maximum human daily intranasal dose based on BSA (MHDND) (4). When rabbits were given a SC dose that was less than either maximum human dose, fetal toxicity consisting of death, reduced weight, cleft palate, skeletal abnormalities including incomplete ossifications, and skin effects were observed (3,4). No adverse effects were observed with a dose that was one-fifth of the toxic dose.

No carcinogenicity was observed in 2-year studies in mice and rats. Ciclesonide was not mutagenic in two assays, but was clastogenic in one of three tests. Similar findings were observed with dexamethasone, the concurrent reference corticosteroid. In addition, there was no evidence of impaired fertility in male and female rats given oral doses up to about 10 times the MHDID or about 35 times the MHDND (3,4).

It is not known if ciclesonide or RM1 crosses the human placenta. The molecular weight of ciclesonide (about 541) is low enough, but the high plasma protein binding and very short half-life suggests that minimal amounts will cross the placenta. In contrast, the half-life of RM1 suggests that exposure of the embryo–fetus to amounts greater than that from ciclesonide is likely.

BREASTFEEDING SUMMARY

No reports describing the use of ciclesonide during human lactation have been located. The molecular weight of the prodrug ciclesonide (about 541) is low enough, but the high plasma protein binding and very short half-life suggests that minimal amounts will be excreted into breast milk. In contrast, the half-life of the active drug des-ciclesonide (RM1; molecular weight not specified) suggests that exposure of the nursing infant will be greater than that from ciclesonide. Although the prodrug and its active metabolite have negligible oral bioavailability (both <1%), the relatively anti-inflammatory activity of RM1 is 12 times that of dexamethasone. The effects of this exposure on a nursing infant are unknown, but, like all corticosteroids, suppression of the hypothalamic–pituitary–adrenal function is a potential complication.

References

1. Report of the Working Group on Asthma and Pregnancy, National Institutes of Health. *Management of Asthma During Pregnancy*. NIH Publication No. 93-3279, September 1993.
2. Blais L, Forget A. Asthma exacerbations during the first trimester of pregnancy and the risk of congenital malformations among asthmatic women. J Allergy Clin Immunol 2008;121:1379–84.
3. Product information. Alvesco. Nycomed US, 2007.
4. Product information. Omnaris. Sepracor, 2007.
5. Derendorf H. Pharmacokinetic and pharmacodynamic properties of inhaled ciclesonide. J Clin Pharmacol 2007;47:782–9.

CICLOPIROX

Antifungal

PREGNANCY RECOMMENDATION: No Human Data—Probably Compatible
BREASTFEEDING RECOMMENDATION: No Human Data—Probably Compatible

PREGNANCY SUMMARY

Although there is no published human pregnancy data, the low systemic bioavailability and the absence of developmental toxicity in four animal species suggest that the use of ciclopirox is low risk for the embryo–fetus.

FETAL RISK SUMMARY

Ciclopirox is a synthetic anti-infective agent used topically for its antifungal properties. Very small amounts (1.3% of the dose with occlusive dressings) are absorbed systemically from the skin (1).

There was no evidence of teratogenic effects or other fetal harm in animals (mice, rats, rabbits, and monkeys) given doses of 10 times or more the topical human dose by various routes of administration (1).

No reports of its use in human pregnancy have been located. The manufacturer has no reports of congenital abnormalities occurring after use of ciclopirox (C.K. Whitmore, personal communication, Hoechst-Roussel Pharmaceuticals, Inc., 1987).

BREASTFEEDING SUMMARY

No reports describing the use of ciclopirox during lactation have been located. The very small amounts (1.3%) absorbed systemically with occlusive dressings probably indicates that infant exposure via the milk is negligible, if it occurs at all.

Reference

1. Product information. Loprox. MEDICIS, The Dermatology Company, 2000.

CIDOFOVIR

Antiviral

PREGNANCY RECOMMENDATION: Compatible—Maternal Benefit >> Embryo–Fetal Risk
BREASTFEEDING RECOMMENDATION: Contraindicated

PREGNANCY SUMMARY

No reports describing the use of cidofovir during human pregnancy have been located. It is not known whether the drug crosses the placenta to the fetus, but because of its relatively low molecular weight (approximately 315) passage to the fetus should be expected. Because of the lack of human data, the risk to the human embryo and fetus cannot be assessed. Some risk may exist because of the adverse effects observed at very low doses in the limited animal studies. Despite this risk, the use of cidofovir after the 1st trimester in a pregnant HIV-positive woman with sight-threatening cytomegalovirus (CMV) retinitis may be a rational decision.

FETAL RISK SUMMARY

Cidofovir (HPMPC) is used in the treatment of CMV retinitis in patients with AIDS. The antiviral agent is converted to the active metabolite, cidofovir diphosphate, by intracellular enzymes. In animals, cidofovir is carcinogenic, embryotoxic, and teratogenic.

Cidofovir was carcinogenic in female rats, producing mammary adenocarcinoma at doses as low as about 0.04 times the recommended human dose based on AUC (RHD). Reproductive studies with cidofovir have been conducted with rats and rabbits (1). Both maternal toxicity and embryotoxicity (reduced fetal body weights) were observed at daily IV doses in rats and rabbits that were about 0.12 and 0.24 times the RHD, respectively, administered during organogenesis. The no-observable-effect doses for embryotoxicity in rats and rabbits were about 0.04 and 0.05 times the RHD, respectively. Teratogenic effects, consisting of external, soft tissue, and skeletal malformations (meningocele, short snout, and short maxillary bones), were observed in the fetuses of rabbits given a dose that was about 0.24 times the RHD during organogenesis.

Pregnant mice inoculated intranasally with equine herpesvirus 1 in the 2nd or 3rd week of gestation were treated with a single dose of cidofovir 50 mg/kg SC 1 day prior to inoculation (2). A noninfected, control group of pregnant mice was also treated at a similar gestational time with the same dose of cidofovir. In the infected group, cidofovir significantly reduced the incidence of virus transfer to the fetus and subsequent abortion, a predictable effect of the virus. No obvious toxic effects were observed in either group.

BREASTFEEDING SUMMARY

No reports describing the use of cidofovir during lactation have been located. This antiviral agent should not be used during breastfeeding because of the potential severe toxicity in a nursing infant. Moreover, although no studies have been reported in lactating humans, cidofovir has induced mammary cancer with very low doses in female rats.

In addition, the mother's clinical status will usually preclude the use of cidofovir during breastfeeding. The only approved indication for this drug is for the treatment of CMV retinitis in patients infected with HIV type 1 (HIV-1). Because HIV-1 is transmitted in milk, breastfeeding is not recommended in developed countries where there are available affordable milk substitutes (3–5).

C

References

1. Product information. Vistide. Gilead Sciences, 1997.
2. Awan AR, Field HJ. Effects of phosphonylmethoxyalkyl derivatives studied with a murine model for abortion induced by equine herpesvirus 1. Antimicrob Agents Chemother 1993;37:2478–82.
3. Brown ZA, Watts DH. Antiviral therapy in pregnancy. Clin Obstet Gynecol 1990;33:276–89.
4. de Martino M, Tovo P-A, Pezzotti P, Galli L, Massironi E, Ruga E, Floreea F, Plebani A, Gabiano C, Zuccotti GV. HIV-1 transmission through breast-milk: appraisal of risk according to duration of feeding. AIDS 1992;6: 991–7.
5. Van de Perre P. Postnatal transmission of human immunodeficiency virus type 1: the breast-feeding dilemma. Am J Obstet Gynecol 1995;173: 483–7.

CIGARETTE SMOKING

Stimulant

PREGNANCY RECOMMENDATION: Contraindicated
BREASTFEEDING RECOMMENDATION: Contraindicated

PREGNANCY SUMMARY

Maternal and paternal cigarette smoking before pregnancy is associated with reduced fertility and ectopic tubal pregnancies. During pregnancy, maternal smoking is related to increased risks for spontaneous abortions (SABs), premature delivery, placental abruption, placenta previa, and premature rupture of membranes (PROM). Symmetric and asymmetric fetal growth restriction that involves weight, length, and head, chest, and shoulder circumference is a consistent finding of numerous studies. Up to 30% of low-birth-weight infants may be due to maternal smoking. A major consequence of smoking-induced toxicity is a significantly increased perinatal mortality rate, in addition to the losses from SABs. Maternal smoking is also a risk for increased neonatal, infant, and adolescent complications. These include increased admissions to a neonatal intensive care unit (NICU), abnormal neurobehavior development, sudden infant death syndrome (SIDS), and childhood diseases such as asthma, respiratory infections, and obesity. Vascular retinal abnormalities in infants are another complication. Although reversible, the abnormalities might be a harbinger of later vascular disease.

Cigarette smoking appears to be associated with small increases (usually less than twofold) in major birth defects and possible deformations. The defects with positive associations involve the heart and great vessels, limbs, skull, genitourinary system, feet, abdominal wall, small bowel, and muscles. Dose-dependent relationships, gene–smoking interactions, and synergistic combinations with some medications have been noted. However, the prevalence and frequency of maternal cigarette smoking are based on self-reports that typically underestimate the actual amount of smoking. This and the failure to adjust for other confounders may have biased the results of some studies. Biochemical validation should be, but rarely is, a component of studies on the effects of smoking during pregnancy.

FETAL RISK SUMMARY

Cigarette smoking during pregnancy is a significant health hazard to the mother, embryo, fetus, infant, and adolescent. Cigarette smoke contains more than 3000 different compounds, including nicotine, carbon monoxide, ammonia, polycyclic aromatic hydrocarbons, hydrogen cyanide, and vinyl chloride (1–5). Although these and other chemical constituents of cigarette smoke represent a risk to the pregnancy, the principal concerns relate to nicotine and carbon monoxide. Nicotine has a plasma half-life of about 40 minutes, whereas its primary inactive metabolite, cotinine, has a half-life of 15–30 hours (4). Nicotine releases epinephrine that results in a marked reduction in uterine blood flow and an increase in uterine vascular resistance (1–4).

Although the frequency of cigarette smoking during pregnancy is declining, the self-reported overall prevalence ranges from about 13% to 20% (3,4,6,7). The prevalence is dependent on a number of factors, primarily ethnic group, age, and education. The highest frequency is among American Indian or Alaskan Native women (20.2%) and white women (16.2%), whereas it is lower in Black (9.6%), Hispanic (4%) and Asian or Pacific Islander women (3.1%) (5). The highest prevalence of smoking during pregnancy is among women age 18–24 years (5,7) and more women with 12 years of education or less (11.7% to 25.5%) smoke than do women with 13–15 years (9.6%) or ≥16 years (2.2%) of education (5). However, these self-reported rates, whether based on questionnaires, interviews, or birth certificate data, probably underestimate the actual frequency of smoking (5,6,8). The high rates of nondisclosure have led some to recommend that biochemical validation of smoking status should be a part of all studies involving pregnant women (6).

Nicotine and carbon monoxide rapidly cross the placenta (1–5). Nicotine and carboxyhemoglobin fetal concentrations are about 10%–15% higher than those in the mother.

Cigarette smoking before and during pregnancy is associated with a number of adverse reproductive effects. These toxic effects can be classified as follows:

- Subfertility and ectopic pregnancy
- Pregnancy Complications
  - Spontaneous abortions
  - Premature delivery
  - Placental abruption/placenta previa
  - Placental previa
  - Premature rupture of membranes
- Embryo–Fetal Complications
  - Growth restriction

Perinatal mortality
Congenital malformations
Neonatal Complications
Neonatal Intensive Care Unit admissions
Retinal abnormalities
Adolescent Complications
Neurodevelopment
Sudden infant death syndrome
Childhood morbidity

Subfertility and Ectopic Pregnancy

Cigarette smoking adversely effects female fertility (4,9, 10–12). A 1986 review explored this topic in depth and concluded that cigarette smoking adversely affects the ability to conceive during a given menstrual cycle (i.e., reduced fecundity) (11). One of the mechanisms of smoking-induced reduced fecundity might be related to altered uterine tubal function (increased utero-tubal amplitude and tonus). This could also explain the higher incidence of ectopic tubal pregnancies in women who smoke (11). Other potential contributing mechanisms are affects on the preimplantation embryo, implantation, gamete maturation and function, and adverse effects on sperm density, motility, and morphology induced by paternal smoking (11).

Pregnancy Complications

SPONTANEOUS ABORTIONS Cigarette smoking is associated with an increased risk of SABs of fetuses with normal karyotype (1–5,8–11,13,14). Compared with nonsmokers, the risk of abortion may be increased by as much as 20%–80% (2–4,9). An estimated 19,000–141,000 SABs annually may be caused by tobacco (5). However, adjustment for confounding factors, such as a previous history of SAB and alcohol consumption, may reduce the association (9). The mechanism of smoking-induced SAB is unknown but may be due to interference with placentation or implantation (11).

PREMATURE DELIVERY Preterm delivery is increased in women who smoke (1,4,5,7,9,10,14,15). Smoking may be responsible for 14%–15% of all premature births (5,10). The effect of smoking is most pronounced in infants born at less than 33 weeks' gestation (7). The risk increases with the number of cigarettes smoked (9).

PLACENTAL ABRUPTION/PLACENTA PREVIA An increased risk of vaginal bleeding secondary to placental abruption or previa has been shown with smoking (2–4,6,9,10,12–14,16). There is a dose-dependent association with these complications (2,3,10,13). The risk of abruption and previa in those smoking less than one-pack/day was 23% and 25%, respectively, greater than that of nonsmokers, whereas the risk in those smoking one pack/day or more was increased 86% and 92%, respectively (3). Moreover, a smoking history of more than 6 years was associated with an increased incidence of placenta previa of 14.3% and of placental abruption of 72% (4). The estimated annual number of infant deaths from these two complications is 1900–4800 (5).

PREMATURE RUPTURE OF MEMBRANES PROM is an adverse effect of maternal smoking (1,2,4,5,9). Similar to other complications, a dose-dependent relationship has been found (2,4). One cited study found that the incidence of PROM was 1.4% in women smoking 20 or more cigarettes/day, 0.6% in those smoking 1–5 cigarettes/day, and 0.3% in nonsmokers (4).

Embryo–Fetal Complications

GROWTH RESTRICTION IUGR at any gestational age is a well-known complication of cigarette smoking during pregnancy (1–7,10–16). Growth restriction is typically symmetrical IUGR, but aspects of asymmetrical IUGR may be present in the last trimester (7). The negative effects of smoking on fetal growth include weight, length, and head, chest, and shoulder circumference, and involve a dose-dependent relationship. In comparison to infants of women who do not smoke, the infants of smokers, on average, weigh 200 g less (2–4). Moreover, compared with nonsmokers, the risk of having an infant weighing less than 2500 g was 52% greater in those smoking less than one pack/day and 130% greater in those smoking one-pack/day or more (3). Overall, the relative risk (smokers vs. nonsmokers) of giving birth to an infant weighing less than 2500 g is approximately 2.0 (13). In 1993, it was estimated that smoking was responsible for 40,000 low-birth-weight (LBW) infants (4). Smoking during pregnancy may account for 20%–30% of LBW infants (5). Quitting smoking before or during pregnancy decreases the risk of delivering an LBW infant to that of nonsmokers (5,7,13). The primary cause of the growth restriction is thought to be chronic fetal hypoxia secondary to nicotine and carbon monoxide (1,5,10,12). Nicotine-induced vasoconstriction causes reduced placental blood flow. Carbon monoxide binds to hemoglobin, both maternal and fetal, with an affinity that is more than 200 times that of oxygen (5).

PERINATAL MORTALITY An increase in perinatal deaths (fetal deaths after 20 weeks' gestation and infant deaths within 28 days of birth) has been frequently associated with cigarette smoking during pregnancy (1–3,5, 8–11,13,14,16). Increased rates of perinatal death have been reported, with the highest risk found in smoking women who had had multiple pregnancies, were of low socioeconomic class, and were anemic (2,3). A dose-dependent relationship between maternal smoking and perinatal mortality is evident. The increased perinatal mortality is secondary to stillbirths, prematurity, respiratory distress syndrome, pneumonia, placental abruption, and placenta previa. The risk of perinatal mortality from cigarette smoking is about 10% and most deaths occur in infants with IUGR (9). Of interest, heavy tobacco chewing has been associated with decreased birth weight (100–200 g; primarily due to prematurity) and a threefold increase in the stillbirth rate (2,17).

CONGENITAL MALFORMATIONS The relationship between cigarette smoking during pregnancy and structural malformations is controversial (2–5,9,11,14,15). Several reports have found low associations between smoking and various birth defects, but the studies relied on self-reported smoking prevalence. A 2003 statement from the Teratology Society on the benefits of smoking cessation during pregnancy concluded that smoking was not associated with major congenital malformations (5).

CARDIOVASCULAR DEFECTS (In addition to the references cited in this section, see reference 24.)

In a brief 1971 correspondence using data from the 1958 British Perinatal Mortality Survey, a statistically significant association was found for congenital heart disease between smokers (at least one cigarette/day after the fourth month of pregnancy) and nonsmokers (18). Congenital heart disease was determined by medical examination or autopsy.

The incidence of congenital heart disease per 1000 births in smokers and nonsmokers was 7.3 and 4.7, respectively. After adjustment, the smoking effect was independent of maternal age, parity, and social class (18).

A 1978 case–control study found a significant increase in congenital defects in women that smoked 21 or more cigarettes/day (19). There were 1370 cases (41% smoked) and 2968 controls (39% smoked). There was a significant increase in the estimated relative risk (RR) for congenital defects in smokers compared with nonsmokers, 1.6 vs. 1.0, respectively. Defects with RR estimates of 2.0 or higher were heart valves (2.0), inguinal hernia (2.8), pyloric stenosis (3.3), and defects of the digestive system (2.9) (19). A 1978 study, using data from a previous study on the effects of exposure to trace anesthetic agents on the health of healthcare professionals, discovered a significant association between smoking and an increase in the risk of SABs and congenital defects (20). Compared with nonsmokers, there was an increase for cardiovascular, gastrointestinal, and urogenital malformations. For all defects, smokers had a risk as high as 2.3 times that of nonsmokers (20).

A case–control study conducted in California involved 207 cases with conotruncal heart defects, 246 with neural tube defects (NTDs), 178 with limb deficiencies, and 481 controls delivered during 1987–1988 (21). The confirmed heart defects in infants included tetralogy of Fallot, d-transposition of the great arteries, truncus arteriosus communis, double-outlet right ventricle, pulmonary valve atresia with ventricular septal defect (VSD), subaortic VSD type 1, and aortico-pulmonary window (21). Confirmed cases of NTDs and limb deficiencies in infants and fetuses (spontaneous and elective abortions) included anencephaly, spina bifida cystica, craniorrhachischisis, and iniencephaly, and longitudinal, transverse, or amniotic band limb-deficiency defects of the upper and/or lower limbs (21). Moderately elevated associations, but only when both parents smoked, were found for conotruncal heart defects odds ratio (OR) 1.9 (95% CI 1.2–3.1) and limb deficiencies OR 1.7 (95% CI 0.96–2.9), but parenteral smoking was not associated with increased risks for NTDs (21).

Data relating to risk factors for *l*-transposition of the great arteries obtained from the Baltimore-Washington Infant Study (1981–1989), a population-based case–control study, were published in 2003 (22). *L*-transposition of the great arteries is an uncommon congenital cardiovascular malformation. Among 3377 cases of congenital cardiovascular malformations, 36 (1.1%) had the targeted defect. The majority of the cases had multiple cardiovascular anomalies and 47% had a single ventricle. Seventy-five percent of the cases came from two regions (clusters) within the study's boundaries that were characterized by the release of toxic chemicals into the air and hazardous waste sites (22). For the two clusters, the case–control OR of the targeted defect was 13.4, 95% CI 4.7–37.8. Three other possible associations with *l*-transposition of the great arteries were identified: maternal smoking (OR 1.6, 95% CI 1.1–2.4), maternal use of hair dye (OR 3.0, 95% CI 0.9–9.7), and paternal exposure to laboratory chemicals (OR 8.2, 95% CI 1.7–40.1) (22).

NEURAL TUBE DEFECTS (NTDs) (In addition to the references cited in this section, see references 21 and 37.)

A 1979 case–control study examined the effects of cigarette smoking on closure defects of the central nervous system (CNS) (anencephaly, myelomeningocele, and encephalocele) (66 cases) and oral clefts (cleft lip or cleft palate) (66 cases) (23). Smoking frequency was determined from hospital records. Although significantly more case women smoked than did control women (83% vs. 39%), there was no association between smoking and CNS closure defects (33% vs. 39%) (23). Another 1979 study found no association, compared with nonsmokers, between smoking and congenital malformations (2.8% vs. 2.8%) (24). Similarly, no associations with specific defects (cardiovascular, gastrointestinal, genitourinary, musculoskeletal, or oral clefts) were found. After adjustment for socioeconomic class, a possible dose-dependent association with NTDs (anencephaly and spina bifida) was found. However, even if smoking was causal, it was thought to have only modest importance in the etiology of NTDs (24). In addition, women might have understated the number of cigarettes smoked because they were aware of medical opposition to smoking, especially during pregnancy. Information was more likely to be accurate for nonsmokers and heavy smokers (24).

A 1998 Swedish study found a protective effect of maternal smoking on the incidence of NTDs: total NTDs OR 0.75 (95% CI 0.61–0.91); anencephaly OR 0.49 (95% CI 0.28–0.85); and spina bifida OR 0.76 (95% CI 0.61–0.95) (25). Although the exact cause for this unexpected finding was unknown, one logical reason could have been an excess in early losses of embryos with NTDs (25).

LIMB DEFECTS (In addition to the references cited in this section, see reference 21.)

A 1994 case–control study used the Hungarian Congenital Abnormality Registry (1975–1984) and three other sources of ascertainment (1,575,904 births) to examine the association between smoking and isolated congenital limb deficiencies (six types) (26). After adjustment, the relative odds (RO) 1.48 (95% CI 0.98–2.23) were higher among smoking mothers of cases of terminal transverse limb deficiencies (but not five other types of limb deficiencies). A causal relationship could not be proven because of unadjusted potential confounders. However, the data did support the hypothesis of vascular disruption as a cause of the defects (26). A 1997 study used data from Swedish Health registries to identify 610 cases of limb reduction defects among 1,109,299 infants born between 1983 and 1993 (27). The OR for an association between any maternal smoking and all cases of limb reductions was 1.2, 95% CI 1.06–1.50. Of the various types of defects, only transverse limb reductions had an OR and 95% CI above unity (27).

CRANIOSYNOSTOSIS An increased risk of craniosynostosis (premature ossification of the skull and obliteration of the sutures resulting in a misshapen head) in mothers who smoked was reported in 1994 (28). In the Colorado Craniosynostosis Registry (1986–1989), 212 cases confirmed by an independent radiologist were identified and participated in the study. Cases and controls were interviewed between 1989 and 1991. The types of craniosynostosis were lambdoid ($N = 86$), sagittal ($N = 69$), coronal ($N = 25$), metopic ($N = 18$), and multiple suture synostosis ($N = 14$). Smoking was associated with craniosynostosis OR 1.7 (95% CI 1.2–2.6). For mothers who smoked more than one pack/day, the association for all types of craniosynostosis combined was OR 3.5 (95% CI 1.5–8.4) and for coronal synostosis

OR 5.6 (95% CI 2.1–15.3). No significant association was noted for drinking alcohol (28). A 1999 study found a significant association between isolated craniosynostosis and smoking (29). For any smoking, the adjusted OR was 1.67 (95% CI 1.27–2.19), but a dose-dependent association also was found: OR 1.45 (95% CI 1.04–2.02) for <10 cigarettes/day and OR 2.12 (95% CI 1.50–2.99) for ≥10 cigarettes/day. Among the different types of craniosynostosis, only premature closure of the sagittal suture OR 1.48 (95% CI 1.02–2.14) reached statistical significance. Male gender had the strongest association with the defects (29). A 2000 study reported evidence that supported the conclusion of the above studies that smoking was associated with craniosynostosis (30). Using data gathered by the Centers for Disease Control and Prevention's (CDC) population-based surveillance system (1968–1980), 61 mothers of infants with craniosynostosis and 3029 mothers of normal infants were interviewed. After exclusions, 44 cases of isolated craniosynostosis remained, 27 of which were sagittal synostosis. The association between maternal smoking and isolated craniosynostosis was OR 1.92 (95% CI 1.01–3.66) and for sagittal craniosynostosis OR 1.71 (95% CI 0.75–3.89). As with previous studies, male infants were predominantly affected. A limitation of this study was that smoking exposure was only identified for the first 3 months of pregnancy. Smoking frequency may have changed in the last part of pregnancy, which is the most critical period for the development of craniosynostosis (30).

ORAL CLEFTS (In addition to the references cited in this section, see references 23 and 24.)

Several studies and one review have examined the relationship between smoking and isolated oral clefts. In a 1983 Finish study that appeared to be well controlled for many potential confounders, no significant associations between smoking (≥5 cigarettes/day) and oral clefts, CNS defects, or musculoskeletal anomalies were found (31). Using data from the Atlanta Birth Defects Case-Control Study (1968–1980), 238 cases of cleft lip and/or cleft palate and 107 cases of cleft palate were compared with 2809 match controls (32). Smoking was ascertained by structured questionnaire and exposure was defined as maternal smoking during the period 3 months before conception to 3 months after pregnancy began. After adjustment, significant associations were found between smoking and offspring with isolated cleft lip and/or palate OR 1.55 (95% CI 1.10–2.18), and isolated cleft palate OR 1.96 (95% CI 1.10–3.50) (32).

A 1999 case–control study used data from the Slone Epidemiology Unit Births Defect Study (1976–1992) to examine the relationship between smoking in the first 13 weeks of pregnancy and isolated cleft lip and palate (33). Four control groups, all with other malformations, were selected from the database. The OR and 95% CI was nearly identical in the four groups: 1.5–1.6 (95% CI 1.1–1.3, 1.8–2.7). The investigators concluded that infants with malformations other than the defect of interest were suitable controls (33). Using the same database, the investigators examined the relationship between smoking and oral clefts (34). Cases were isolated oral clefts (cleft lip alone [*N* = 334], cleft lip and palate [*N* = 494], or cleft palate [*N* = 244]), and oral clefts with other malformations (cleft lip [*N* = 58], cleft lip and palate [*N* = 140], or cleft palate [*N* = 209]). Controls had other malformations, but not oral clefts or defects possibly associated with smoking. There were no associations between smoking and any oral cleft group. However, a positive dose response was found in infants with cleft lip and palate and other malformations: 1–14 cigarettes/day OR 1.09 (95% CI 0.6–1.9), 15–24 cigarettes/day OR 1.84 (95% CI 1.2–2.9), and >24 cigarettes/day OR 1.85 (95% CI 1.0–3.5). This finding might have been related to the presence of malformations associated with smoking (34). The authors also reviewed 16 other published studies on the association between smoking and oral clefts.

A 1999 study was conducted in Denmark to determine the relationship between smoking and infant transforming growth factor alpha (TGFA) locus mutations and isolated cleft lip and/or palate (35). A second objective was to determine if there was a synergistic effect of these two risk factors. Smoking was associated with a slightly increased risk of cleft lip and/or palate, OR 1.40 (95% CI 0.88–2.00), but not with isolated cleft palate. The TGFA allele is elevated in the Danish population, occurring in 25% of both cases and controls. It was not associated with either type of oral cleft and no synergistic effect with smoking was observed (35).

The 1996 U.S. Natality database involving 3,891,494 live births was used in a 2000 case–control study (36). Four states were excluded because they did not collect smoking data. A total of 2207 live births with cleft lip and palate were compared with 4414 normal controls. After adjustment for maternal age, race, education levels, and maternal conditions (diabetes and gestational hypertension), a significant association was found between smoking and the defect, OR 1.34 (95% CI 1.16–1.54). Moreover, compared with no smoking, a dose response was found as follows: 1–10 cigarettes/day OR 1.50 (95% CI 1.28–1.76), 11–20 cigarettes/day OR 1.55 (95% CI 1.23–1.95), and 21 or more cigarettes/day OR 1.78 (95% CI 1.22–2.59) (36).

A 2002 case–control study examined the status of a biotransformation enzyme *N*-acetyltransferase 2 (NAT2) in 45 cases of mothers who had had a child with an oral cleft, 39 case mothers who had had a child with spina bifida, and 73 control mothers (37). NAT2 is involved in the inactivation of toxic compounds in cigarette smoke and a few drugs. The maternal phenotype, either slow or fast NAT2 acetylators, was determined for case and control mothers. Compared with fast NAT2 acetylators, slow acetylators had no increased risk for oral clefts OR 1.0 (95% CI 0.4–2.3) or spina bifida OR 0.7 (95% CI 0.3–1.7). In the oral cleft group, significantly more mothers smoked and used medications than did controls (36% vs. 18% and 38% vs. 19%, respectively). In the spina bifida group, case mothers were similar to controls for smoking, but significantly more used medications during pregnancy (23% vs. 18% and 44% vs. 19%) (37).

A 1996 review examined the relationship between potentially teratogenic environmental exposures and nonsyndromic oral clefts (38). The origin of oral clefts is multifactorial and involves both genetic and environmental factors, one of which is believed to be cigarette smoking. Several studies, some of which are discussed above, were reviewed, which found negative and positive associations between smoking and oral clefts. Although not arriving at any conclusions as to the specific causes of isolated oral clefts (none were possible), the review did identify common misclassifications and confounding bias that could distort a study's findings (38).

GENITOURINARY DEFECTS (In addition to the references cited in this section, see references 20 and 24.)

A 1996 case–control study assessed the association between smoking and urinary tract anomalies (39). There were 112 cases and 354 controls. After adjustment, a significant association between smoking and urinary tract defects was found, OR 2.3 (95% CI 1.2–4.5). Significant associations also were found for mothers who smoked 1–1000 cigarettes (light smoking) during the entire pregnancy, OR 3.7 (95% CI 1.7–8.6) or during the 1st trimester OR 2.9 (95% CI 1.4–6.7). When analyzed by infant sex, the associations were significant for females OR 6.1 (95% CI 2.0–18.4) and OR 5.7 (95% CI 2.0–16.5), respectively, but not for males OR 2.5 (95% CI 0.8–7.6) and OR 1.7 (95% CI 0.7–4.5), respectively. No significant associations were found for heavy smoking (>1000 cigarettes) either in the entire pregnancy or in the 1st trimester. The authors hypothesized that the lack of a dose response might have been due to a greater prevalence of fetal loss from SAB or stillbirth and that these fetuses may have had major congenital defects that involved the urinary tract (39). A 1997 study used Swedish health registries to identify 483 infants with kidney malformations and 719 infants with other urinary organ malformations with no involvement of the kidneys from 1,117,021 infants born in 1983–1993 with known smoking exposure in early pregnancy (40). A moderate significant association with kidney malformations (agenesis/hypoplasia, dysplasia, or unspecified cystic disease) was found OR 1.22 (95% CI 1.00–1.48), but there was no dose response (<10 cigarettes/day vs. ≥10 cigarettes/day). No association with other urinary organ malformations was observed (40).

A negative association was found between cigarette smoking and hypospadias in a 2002 case–control study (41). Data from the Swedish health registries provided 3262 cases among 1,413,811 infants born in 1983–1996. The association between any smoking (N = 715) and the defect was OR 0.83 (95% CI 0.76–0.90). The results were similar for those <10 cigarettes/day (N = 450) or ?10/day (N = 265). Because the negative association was only found in those cases where the mother's parity was 1 or >4, confounding was suspected (41).

FOOT DEFECTS Several studies have discovered positive associations between maternal smoking and foot deformities. A brief 1998 report described an association between maternal smoking and foot defects, adjusted OR 1.21 (95% CI 1.14–1.29) (42). The authors also cited six other studies examining the relationship between foot defects and smoking, four of which had OR ranging from 1.0 to 2.6 with 95% CI above 1.0 (42). In a 2000 study, 346 infants with isolated clubfoot were identified from the Atlanta Birth Defects Case–Control (1968–1980) database (43). Case infants and normal controls (N = 3029) were born in 1968–1980 and the mothers were interviewed in 1982–1983. The adjusted OR and 95% CI were smoking only 1.34 (1.04–1.72), family history only 6.52 (2.95–14.41), and smoking and family history 20.30 (7.90–52.17). The findings suggested a potentially important gene–environmental factor interaction (43). A 2002 report compared 239 cases of congenital idiopathic clubfoot (talipes equinovarus) to 365 unmatched controls in a population-based study of the relationship between maternal smoking and the foot anomaly (44). The OR for smoking and talipes equinovarus was 2.2 (95% CI 1.5–3.3). A dose-dependent response was seen and, in addition, female infants had a higher risk than males, OR 2.8 vs. 1.8. For isolated clubfoot, the OR for smoking was 2.4 (95% CI 1.6–3.6) (44).

POLAND SYNDROME A 1999 case–control study examined data from the Hungarian Congenital Abnormality Registry (HCAR) (population-based) and the Spanish Collaborative Study of Congenital Malformations (ECEMC) (hospital-based, case–control) to determine if there was an association between maternal cigarette smoking and isolated Poland sequence (45). Poland syndrome or sequence is thought to be caused by interruption of the early embryonic blood supply in the subclavian arteries and is characterized by pectoral muscle defect and ipsilateral hand deficiencies of various types and severity (45). In the HCAR database, 20 cases were identified from 1,575,904 births (prevalence 0.13 per 10,000 births), whereas in the ECEMC database, there were 32 cases among 1,405,392 births (prevalence 0.23 per 10,000 births). Logistic regression analyses (after controlling for maternal age, birth weight, gestational age, and pregnancy order) revealed that maternal smoking was associated with an increased risk of Poland sequence in both databases: HCAR (OR 2.72) and ECEMC (OR 2.61). When combined, the OR was 1.83. The investigators concluded that the results suggested a twofold increase in the risk of Poland sequence from in utero exposure to cigarette smoking. Although the number of cases were small, the results were similar in the two programs with different methodologies and possibly different uncontrolled confounding factors. However, confirmation of the findings is required (45).

GASTROSCHISIS The cause of gastroschisis is unknown, but vascular disruption during early embryonic development has been suggested. No association between cigarette smoking and the abdominal wall defect was found in two studies published in the 1990s (46,47). A 2000 review cited 10 case–control studies that reported various associations with gastroschisis, two of which associated the defect with cigarette smoking, in addition to other factors (48). In one of the studies, smoking ascertainment was obtained from birth certificates, a source known to underestimate maternal smoking, so the significant OR 4.1 (95% CI 1.4–12) is suspect. In the second study, the source was a 2nd trimester interview and the result was OR 2.1 (95% CI 0.9–4.8) (48).

A 2002 abstract examined gastroschisis and small intestine atresia, two defects believed to arise from vascular disruption (49). Maternal smoking and use of vasoconstrictive drugs (pseudoephedrine, phenylpropanolamine, ephedrine, and ecstasy [methylenedioxymethamphetamine]) was ascertained by retrospective interview. The number of cases and controls were 205 gastroschisis, 127 small intestine atresia, 381 malformed controls, and 416 normal controls. In the four groups, the reported use of a vasoconstrictive drug in the first 2 months of pregnancy was 20%, 21%, 13%, and 12%, respectively, whereas maternal smoking was present in 48%, 24%, 34%, and 34%, respectively. The OR for vasoconstrictive drug use or smoking were gastroschisis, 1.7 (95% CI 1.0–2.8) and 1.5 (95% CI 1.1–2.2); small intestine atresia, 2.0 (95% CI 1.0–3.7) and 1.0 (95% CI 0.6–1.7). Combined exposure to the drugs and smoking increased the gastroschisis risk 2.1-fold and the small intestine atresia risk 2.8-fold. Vasoconstrictive drug use and smoking 20 or more cigarettes/day increased the risks 3.6-fold and 4.2-fold, respectively (49).

Neonatal Complications

NEONATAL INTENSIVE CARE UNIT ADMISSIONS Infants of smoking mothers have an increased risk of admission to an NICU (5). Approximately 14,000 to 26,000 admissions annually may be attributable to smoking.

RETINAL ABNORMALITIES A 2000 study investigated the relationship between maternal cigarette smoking and retinal abnormalities in neonates (50). The infants, both cases and controls (162 each), were grouped by birth weight: small for gestational age (SGA), appropriate for gestational age (AGA), and large for gestational age (LGA). All infants were delivered at term, had clear amniotic fluid, Apgar scores of 7 or higher, and were healthy with no signs of fetal distress either at birth or during the first 3 days after birth. Smoking was determined by maternal interview. Infants of mothers who had stopped smoking during pregnancy were excluded. Eye examinations were conducted on the 2nd or 3rd day of life by one ophthalmologist who was blinded to the maternal smoking history. Compared with infants of nonsmoking mothers, a highly significant increase in the incidence of retinal arterial narrowing and straightening (RANS) was observed in the eyes of infants of smoking mothers, 52 vs. 10 eyes, respectively. Significant increases in the incidences of RANS also were observed when the results where analyzed by birth weight: SGA 22 vs. 2, AGA 26 vs. 8, and LGA 4 vs. 0 eyes, respectively. In addition, eyes of infants in the smoking exposure group had a significant increase in the incidence of retinal venous dilatation and tortuosity (RVDT), 100 vs. 36, respectively. The results for RVDT were significant in SGA (38 vs. 10 eyes) and AGA (56 vs. 24 eyes) infants, but not in LGA infants (6 vs. 2 eyes). The hematocrit of the infants was significantly higher in the total smoking group and in each birth weight subgroup. Intraretinal hemorrhage (IH), in association with elevated hematocrit and RVDT, was found in the total smoking group, 61 vs. 31 eyes, respectively. When analyzed by birth weight, only the incidence in AGA infants was significantly increased, 39 vs. 18 eyes, respectively. No IH was observed when RANS was present. The IH resolved within 3 months and the other retinal abnormalities (RANS, RVDT) resolved by 6 months of age. The rapid resolution of the IH and other considerations suggested that it would not lead to amblyopia. However, concern was expressed that the vascular retinal abnormalities could be a sign that the exposed infants were predisposed to vascular disease early in adult life (50).

Infant/Adolescent Complications

NEURODEVELOPMENT Smoking during pregnancy may have long-term effects on the cognitive performance, emotional development, perceptual motor abilities, and behavior of offspring (1–3,5,8,10–13,14,16,51–53). Similar findings have been found in experimental animal studies (5,14). Negative effects on learning, such as reading, mathematics, and general ability, have been detected in children as old as 11 years (2,11,13,51). In addition, behavior problems and attention deficit hyperactivity disorder (ADHD) have been observed (3,8,13,51,52). Mean decreases in IQ of 5 points for each 100-g weight decrement have been reported (3). A 1996 study of 10-year-olds with idiopathic mental retardation (most had mild retardation with an IQ between 50 and 70) found, after adjustment for multiple factors including LBW and alcohol, that maternal smoking was associated with a 44% increase in the prevalence of mental retardation (52). When mothers smoked at least 1 pack/day, the increase was 70% after adjustment. Some of the adverse neurodevelopment outcomes cannot be completely separated from potential confounding factors such as the actual amount of smoking, socioeconomic status, education, and passive smoking (11), but the experimental animal studies support the findings. Moreover, more recent studies have controlled for social and family history factors and have found consistent patterns of deficits (15). For example, a 1996 study and subsequent correspondence found, after adjustment for socioeconomic status, parental IQ and ADHD status, and alcohol, a significant association between maternal smoking and ADHD as well as a nearly significant association with decreased IQ (53–55).

SUDDEN INFANT DEATH SYNDROME An increased risk of SIDS has been associated with maternal cigarette smoking (3–5,7–9,12,13,14,16). Approximately 24% (1200 to 2200 cases) of SIDS/year may be due to smoking (5). Prenatal and postnatal smoking doubles the risk of SIDS from a baseline of 2.3 per 1000 births in nonsmokers to 4.6 per 1000 births in smokers (4). The greatest risk appears to be for infants exposed both prenatally and postnatally (9). The risk is also dose-dependent, increasing with the number of cigarettes smoked per day (4,13).

CHILDHOOD MORBIDITY An increased risk of other diseases and complications has been associated with prenatal and postnatal exposure to cigarette smoke. Separating the effects of these exposure periods on childhood morbidity is very difficult because most infants exposed during gestation will also be exposed postnatally. For example, data from 1988 estimated that only 1.2% of children in the United States exposed to cigarette smoking in utero were not exposed after birth (9). Exposed infants have increased incidences of pneumonia and bronchitis (2,5), childhood asthma (5,12), other respiratory illnesses (7,12), childhood obesity (5), and otitis media (7). Not surprisingly, they also have more hospital admissions for pneumonia and bronchitis (5,12).

Smoking Cessation

See Nicotine Replacement Products.

BREASTFEEDING SUMMARY

Nicotine is excreted into breast milk. Nursing infants of mothers who smoke will be exposed to nicotine by inhalation and orally (13,56). Cigarette smoking may also decrease the volume of milk (56). In addition, smoking decreases the duration of breastfeeding. A 1998 review cited data from an earlier survey that found that the duration of breastfeeding was significantly decreased in women who smoked compared with those who did not smoke (57). In nonsmokers, the duration was 145.0 days, whereas the duration of breastfeeding in those who smoked ≤1 pack/day or >1 pack/day was 99.5 and 77.9 days, respectively. Women who are breastfeeding should be urged to quit because cigarette smoking is a significant risk to their health and to their infant's health (see the above sections on Neonatal Complications and Infant/Adolescent Complications). If a woman cannot stop smoking, at least she should try not to smoke in the same room with the infant or during nursing. The American Academy of Pediatrics encourages smoking cessation during lactation, but makes no recommendation for or against nicotine replacement products because of insufficient data (58).

C

References

1. Longo LD. Environmental pollution and pregnancy: risks and uncertainties for the fetus and infant. Am J Obstet Gynecol 1980;137:162–73.
2. Report of Committee Appointed by Action on Smoking and Health. Mothers who smoke and their children. Practitioner 1980;224:735–9.
3. Longo LD. Some health consequences of maternal smoking: issues without answers. Birth Defects Orig Artic Ser 1982;18:13-31.
4. Lee MJ. Marihuana and tobacco use in pregnancy. Obstet Gynecol Clin North Am 1998;25:65–83.
5. Adams J. Statement of the Public Affairs Committee of the Teratology Society on the importance of smoking cessation during pregnancy. Birth Defects Res (Part A) 2003;67:895–9.
6. Kendrick JS, Merritt RK. Women and smoking: an update for the 1990s. Am J Obstet Gynecol 1996;175:528–35.
7. Floyd RL, Rimer BK, Giovino GA, Mullen PD, Sullivan SE. A review of smoking in pregnancy: effects on pregnancy outcomes and cessation efforts. Annu Rev Publ Health 1993;14:379–411.
8. Slotkin TA. Fetal nicotine or cocaine exposure: which one is worse? J Pharmacol Exp Ther 1998;285:931–45.
9. Werler MM. Teratogen update: smoking and reproductive outcomes. Teratology 1997;55:382–8.
10. Merritt TA. Smoking mothers affect little lives. Am J Dis Child 1981;135: 501–2.
11. Stillman RJ, Rosenberg MJ, Sachs BP. Smoking and reproduction. Fert Steril 1986;46:545–66.
12. Mercelina-Roumans PEAM, Ubachs JMH, van Wersch JWJ. Smoking and pregnancy. Eur J Obstet Gynecol Reprod Biol 1997;75:113–4.
13. King JC, Fabro S. Alcohol consumption and cigarette smoking: effect on pregnancy. Clin Obstet Gynecol 1983;26:437–48.
14. Landesman-Dwyer S, Emanuel I. Smoking during pregnancy. Teratology 1979;19:119–26.
15. Hill RM, Craig JP, Chaney MD, Tennyson LM, McCulley LB. Utilization of over-the-counter drugs during pregnancy. Clin Obstet Gynecol 1977;20:381–94.
16. Niebury P, Marks JS, McLaren NM, Remington PL. The fetal tobacco syndrome. JAMA 1985;253:2998–9.
17. Krishna K. Tobacco chewing in pregnancy. Br J Obstet Gynaecol 1978;85:726–8.
18. Fedrick J, Alberman ED, Goldstein H. Possible teratogenic effect of cigarette smoking. Nature (London) 1971;231:529–30.
19. Kelsey JL, Dwyer T, Holford TR, Bracken MB. Maternal smoking and congenital malformations: an epidemiological study. J Epidemiol Comm Health 1978;32:102–7.
20. Himmelberger DU, Brown BW Jr, Cohen EN. Cigarette smoking during pregnancy and the occurrence of spontaneous abortion and congenital abnormality. Am J Epidemiol 1978;108;470–9.
21. Wasserman CR, Shaw GM, O'Malley CD, Tolarova MM, Lammer EJ. Parental cigarette smoking and risk for congenital anomalies of the heart, neural tube, or limb. Teratology 1996;53:261–7.
22. Kuehl KS, Loffredo CA. Population-based study of l-transposition of the great arteries: possible associations with environmental factors. Birth Defects Res (Part A) 2003;67:162–7.
23. Ericson A, Kallen B, Westerholm P. Cigarette smoking as an etiologic factor in cleft lip and palate. Am J Obstet Gynecol 1979;135:348–51.
24. Evans DR, Newcombe RG, Campbell H. Maternal smoking habits and congenital malformations: a population study. Br Med J 1979;2:171–3.
25. Kallen K. Maternal smoking, body mass index, and neural tube defects. Am J Epidemiol 1998;147:1103–11.
26. Czeizel AE, Kodaj I, Lenz W. Smoking during pregnancy and congenital limb deficiency. Br Med J 1994;308:1473–6.
27. Kallen K. Maternal smoking during pregnancy and limb reduction malformations in Sweden. Am J Public Health 1997;87:29–32.
28. Alderman BW, Bradley CM, Greene C, Fernbach SK, Baron AE. Increase risk of craniosynostosis with maternal cigarette smoking during pregnancy. Teratology 1994;50:13–8.
29. Kallen K. Maternal smoking and craniosynostosis. Teratology 1999;60: 146–50.
30. Honein MA, Rasmussen SA. Further evidence for an association between maternal smoking and craniosynostosis. Teratology 2000;62:145–6.
31. Hemminki K, Mutanen P, Saloniemi I. Smoking and the occurrence of congenital malformations and spontaneous abortions: multivariate analysis. Am J Obstet Gynecol 1983;145:61–6.
32. Khoury MJ, Gomez-Farias M, Mulinare J. Does maternal cigarette smoking during pregnancy cause cleft lip and palate in offspring? Am J Dis Child 1989;143:333–7.
33. Lieff S, Olshan AF, Werler M, Savitz DA, Mitchell AA. Selection bias and the use of controls with malformations in case-control studies of birth defects. Epidemiology 1999;10:238–41.
34. Lieff S, Olshan AF, Werler M, Strauss RP, Smith J, Mitchell A. Maternal cigarette smoking during pregnancy and risk of oral clefts in newborns. Am J Epidemiol 1999;150:683–94.
35. Christensen K, Olsen J, Norgaard-Pedersen B, Basso O, Stovring H, Milhollin-Johnson L, Murray JC. Oral clefts, transforming growth factor alpha gene variants, and maternal smoking: a population-based case-control study in Denmark, 1991–1994. Am J Epidemiol 1999;149:248–55.
36. Chung KC, Kowalski CP, Kim HM, Buchman SR. Maternal cigarette smoking during pregnancy and the risk of having a child with cleft lip/palate. Plast Reconstr Surg 2000;105:485–91.
37. van Rooij IALM, Groenen PMW, van Drongelen M, Te Morsche RHM, Peters WHM, Steegers-Theunissen RPM. Orofacial clefts and spina bifida: *N*-acetyltransferase phenotype, maternal smoking, and medication use. Teratology 2002;66:260–6.
38. Wyszynski DF, Beaty TH. Review of the role of potential teratogens in the origin of human nonsyndromic oral clefts. Teratology 1996;53:309–17.
39. Li DK, Mueller BA, Hickok DE, Daling JR, Fantel AG, Checkoway H, Weiss NS. Maternal smoking during pregnancy and the risk of congenital urinary tract anomalies. Am J Public Health 1996;86:249–53.
40. Kallen K. Maternal smoking and urinary organ malformations. Int J Epidemiol 1997;26:571–4.
41. Kallen K. Role of maternal smoking and maternal reproductive history in the etiology of hypospadias in the offspring. Teratology 2002;66:185–91.
42. Reefhuis J, de Walle HEK, Cornel MC, EUROCAT Working Group. Maternal smoking and deformities of the foot: results of the EUROCAT study. Am J Public Health 1998;88:1554–5.
43. Honein MA, Paulozzi LJ, Moore CA. Family history, maternal smoking, and clubfoot: an indication of a gene–environment interaction. Am J Epidemiol 2000;152:658–65.
44. Skelly AC, Holt VL, Mosca VS, Alderman BW. Talipes equinovarus and maternal smoking: a population-based case-control study in Washington State. Teratology 2002;66:91–100.
45. Martinez-Frias ML, Czeizel AE, Rodriguez-Pinilla E, Bermejo E. Smoking during pregnancy and Poland sequence: results of a population-based registry and a case-control registry. Teratology 1999;59:35–8.
46. Torfs CP, Velie EM, Oechsli FW, Bateson TF, Curry CJR. A population-based study of gastroschisis: demographic, pregnancy, and lifestyle risk factors. Teratology 1994;50:44–53.
47. Penman DG, Fisher RM, Noblett HR, Soothill PW. Increase in incidence of gastroschisis in the south west of England in 1995. Br J Obstet Gynaecol 1998;105:328–31.
48. Curry JI, McKinney P, Thornton JG, Stringer MD. The aetiology of gastroschisis. Br J Obstet Gynaecol 2000;107:1339–46.
49. Werler MM, Mitchell AA. Case-control study of vasoconstrictive exposures and risks of gastroschisis and small intestinal atresia (abstract). Teratology 2002;65:298.
50. Beratis NG, Varvarigou A, Katsibris J, Gartaganis SP. Vascular retinal abnormalities in neonates of mothers who smoked during pregnancy. J Pediatr 2000;136:760–6.
51. Tong S, McMichael AJ. Maternal smoking and neuropsychological development in childhood: a review of the evidence. Dev Med Child Neurol 1992;34:191–7.
52. Drews CD, Murphy CC, Yeargin-Allsopp M, Decoufle P. The relationship between idiopathic mental retardation and maternal smoking during pregnancy. Pediatrics 1996;97:547–53.
53. Milberger S, Biederman J, Faraone SV, Chen L, Jones J. Is maternal smoking during pregnancy a risk factor for attention deficit hyperactivity disorder in children? Am J Psychiatry 1996;153:1138–42.
54. Chabrol H, Peresson G. ADHD and maternal smoking during pregnancy. Am J Psychiatry 1997;154:1177.
55. Milberger S, Biederman J, Faraone SV. ADHD and maternal smoking during pregnancy. Reply. Am J Psychiatry 1997;154:1177–8.
56. U.S. Department of Health and Human Services. *HHS Blueprint for Action on Breastfeeding*. Washington, DC: Office on Women's Health, 2000.
57. Howard CR, Lawrence RA. Breast-feeding and drug exposure. Obstet Gynecol Clin North Am 1998;25:195–217.
58. American Academy of Pediatrics. The transfer of drugs and other chemicals into human milk. Pediatrics 2001;108:776–89.

CIGUATOXIN

Toxin

PREGNANCY RECOMMENDATION: Human Data Suggest Risk
BREASTFEEDING RECOMMENDATION: Contraindicated

PREGNANCY SUMMARY

Of the cases described, none of the liveborn infants appeared to have had lasting sequelae from exposure to the toxin. However, long-term adverse effects could not be completely excluded in the one infant exposed shortly before birth. The timing of the exposure in relation to delivery may have been a factor in this case. The association between the toxin and the abortion cannot be determined from the available data. Transplacental passage of the toxin has not been studied, but its high molecular weight (1112) presumably limits its crossing the placenta.

FETAL RISK SUMMARY

Ciguatoxin is a marine toxin produced by the blue-green algae, *Gambierdiscus toxicus*, that is concentrated in the fish food chain (1). The toxin is stable to cooking, freezing, drying, or salting and results in ciguatera poisoning when infected tropical fish are ingested (1). Other toxins that may be present with ciguatoxin include scaritoxin and maitotoxin (2,3).

Eight cases of ciguatera poisoning during pregnancy have been published (1–4). An Australian woman at term developed symptoms of poisoning within 4 hours of ingesting the toxin from a reef fish (1). Fetal symptoms of poisoning, beginning simultaneously with the mother's symptoms, consisted of "tumultuous fetal movements, and an intermittent peculiar fetal shivering" (1). The unusual fetal movements continued for 18 hours, then gradually subsided over the next 24 hours. A cesarean section performed 2 days later delivered a 3800-g male infant with meconium aspiration and left-sided facial palsy. At 1 day of age, possible myotonia of the muscles of the hands was noted. Pulmonary signs and symptoms of the meconium aspiration resolved with time. At 6 weeks of age, the baby had not yet smiled, but he was otherwise normal (1). The mother was unable to breast feed due to excruciating hyperesthesia of the nipples.

Six cases of ciguatera poisoning during pregnancy (gestational ages not provided) were described by researchers from the San Francisco Bay area in an abstract published in 1991 (2). The women had neurologic, neuromuscular, and cardiovascular signs and symptoms of poisoning, and all experienced increased fetal activity in conjunction with their symptoms. One fetus was aborted during the acute phase of the poisoning (2). The other five women were delivered, at or near term, of apparently normal infants without sequelae from the exposure. The exposure–delivery intervals for the latter five cases were not specified.

In another case from California, a woman in her 16th week of gestation developed ciguatera poisoning 4 hours after eating a meal of cooked barracuda (4). This case may have been briefly mentioned in another reference (3). Increased fetal movements persisted only for a few hours. A cesarean section, performed 19 days past term, delivered a normal, 3630-g male infant who was developing normally at 10 months of age.

BREASTFEEDING SUMMARY

Ciguatoxin is apparently excreted in breast milk. A 4-month-old infant was breastfed 1 hour and 3 hours after his mother consumed a portion of a presumed ciguatera-infected fish (5). The mother's symptoms of poisoning developed within a few hours of ingesting the fish meal and resolved by 3 weeks. She continued to nurse her infant throughout the entire course of her illness. Approximately 10 hours after the first nursing following the mother's fish meal, the baby became colicky, irritable, and developed diarrhea lasting 48 hours, followed by a fine maculopapular rash. The signs and symptoms in the infant, which were considered compatible with ciguatera toxicity by the authors, completely resolved within 2 weeks (5).

Ciguatoxin was thought to be the cause of green stools in a nursing 3-month-old infant who was breastfed 12 hours after the mother had developed symptoms of ciguatera poisoning (6). The infant was changed to formula and then rechallenged with breast milk a few days later, resulting in the reappearance of the green stools. Prompt cessation of breastfeeding again resolved the problem. No other symptoms were observed in the infant.

References

1. Pearn J, Harvey P, De Ambrosis W, Lewis R, McKay R. Ciguatera and pregnancy. Med J Austr 1982;1:57–8.
2. Rivera-Alsina ME, Payne C, Pou A, Payne S. Ciguatera poisoning in pregnancy (Abstract). Am J Obstet Gynecol 1991;164:397.
3. Geller RJ, Olson KR, Senecal PE. Ciguatera fish poisoning in San Francisco, California, caused by imported barracuda. Western J Med 1991;155:639–42.
4. Senecal PE, Osterloh JD. Normal fetal outcome after maternal ciguateric toxin exposure in the second trimester. J Toxicol Clin Toxicol 1991;29:473–8.
5. Blythe DG, de Sylva DP. Mother's milk turns toxic following fish feast. JAMA 1990;264:2074.
6. Thoman M. Letters to the editor. Vet Hum Toxicol 1989;31:71.

CILOSTAZOL

Hematological Agent (Antiplatelet)

C

PREGNANCY RECOMMENDATION: No Human Data—Animal Data Suggest Risk
BREASTFEEDING RECOMMENDATION: No Human Data—Potential Toxicity

PREGNANCY SUMMARY

No reports describing the use of cilostazol during human pregnancy have been located. The drug is teratogenic and toxic in two animal species, but the complete lack of human data prevents any assessment of the risk that cilostazol presents to a human fetus.

FETAL RISK SUMMARY

Cilostazol, an antiplatelet agent, is an inhibitor of cellular phosphodiesterase III. It is indicated for the reduction of symptoms of intermittent claudication. The drug undergoes extensive hepatic metabolism. Two of the metabolites are active.

Reproduction studies have been conducted with cilostazol in rats and rabbits (1). No effects on fertility or mating performance were observed in male and female rats at oral doses up to 1000 mg/kg/day. The highest dose produced systemic exposures less than 1.5 times in males, and about 5 times in females, the human systemic exposure based on AUC of unbound cilostazol at the maximum recommended human dose. In pregnant rats, the 1000-mg/kg/day dose resulted in decreased fetal weights and an increased incidence of congenital malformations in the cardiovascular (ventricular septal, aortic arch, and subclavian artery defects), renal (renal pelvic dilation), and skeletal (14th rib; retarded ossification) systems. Increased incidences of ventricular septal defects and retarded ossification were also observed at 150 mg/kg/day. This same dose administered to rats in late pregnancy was associated with stillbirths and decreased birth weight. In pregnant rabbits, a dose of 150 mg/kg/day was associated with an increased incidence of retarded ossification of the sternum (1).

It is not known if cilostazol crosses the human placenta to the fetus. The molecular weight (about 369) is low enough that transfer to the fetus should be expected. Moreover, transfer of the two active metabolites may also occur.

BREASTFEEDING SUMMARY

No reports describing the use of cilostazol during human lactation have been located. The molecular weight (about 369) suggests that the drug will be excreted into breast milk. The effect on a nursing infant from exposure to cilostazol in milk is unknown. Because of the potential for severe adverse effects, breastfeeding is not recommended.

Reference

1. Product information. Pletal. Otsuka America Pharma, 2000.

CIMETIDINE

Gastrointestinal Agent (Antisecretory)

PREGNANCY RECOMMENDATION: Compatible
BREASTFEEDING RECOMMENDATION: Compatible

PREGNANCY SUMMARY

No increased risk of congenital malformations attributable to cimetidine in humans has been reported. Feminization of the fetus has not been reported, but warrants study.

FETAL RISK SUMMARY

Cimetidine is a histamine 2-receptor antagonist (H2 blocker) that inhibits gastric acid secretion. In pregnancy, the antihistamine is primarily used for the treatment of peptic ulcer disease and for the prevention of gastric acid aspiration (Mendelson's syndrome) prior to delivery.

In studies with multiple animal species, no evidence of impaired fertility or teratogenesis was observed with doses up to 40 times higher than the usual human dose (1). Cimetidine does have weak antiandrogenic effects in animals, as evidenced by a reduction in the size of testes, prostatic glands, and seminal vesicles (2,3), and in humans, by reports of decreased libido and impotence (4). Conflicting reports on the antiandrogenic activity in animals exposed in utero to cimetidine have been published (5–9).

Three references, all from the same research group, described the effects on male rats of exposure to cimetidine from gestation up to the time of weaning (5–7). The rats had decreased weights of testicles, prostate gland, and seminal vesicles at 55 and 110 days of age as compared with nonexposed controls. Exposed animals also had reduced testosterone serum levels, lack of sexual motivation, and decreased sexual performance, but normal luteinizing hormone levels. The observed demasculinization effects were still present 35 days after discontinuation of the drug, indicating that exposure may have modified both central and end-organ androgen receptor activity or responsiveness (5–7). In contrast, researchers from the manufacturer treated rats similarly to the rats in the above reports and found no effect on any of the parameters described previously (8). Another group found no effect of cimetidine exposure during gestation and lactation on masculine sexual development, except for an insensitivity of the pituitary gland to androgen regulation, and no effect at all on female pups (9). These authors concluded that cimetidine was not an animal teratogen.

Cimetidine crosses the placenta to the fetus by simple diffusion (10–14). In an in vitro study, the placental transfer of cimetidine across human and baboon placentas was similar (10). Cimetidine is not metabolized by the placenta (11). At term, cimetidine crosses the placenta, resulting in a peak mean fetal:maternal ratio of 0.84 at 1.5–2 hours (12). In an earlier study, 20 women were administered a single, 200-mg bolus injection of cimetidine prior to delivery (19 vaginal, 1 cesarean section) (13). The drug was detected in all but two cord blood samples with levels of 0.05–1.22 mcg/mL. The injection-to-delivery intervals in the two patients with no cimetidine in cord blood were prolonged, 435 and 780 minutes. A 1983 study measured a peak mean fetal:maternal ratio of about 0.5 at 2.5 hours (14).

The manufacturer has received a number of reports of women who took the drug during pregnancy, including throughout gestation (B. Dickson, personal communication, Smith Kline & French Laboratories, 1986). They were aware of three isolated incidences of congenital defects, apparently unrelated to cimetidine therapy, including congenital heart disease, mental retardation detected later in life, and clubfoot.

Cimetidine was used throughout pregnancy in a case ending in intrauterine fetal death, but the adverse outcome was believed to be due to severe maternal disease and captopril therapy (see Captopril) (15). Three pregnant women with gastric hemorrhage secondary to peptic ulcer disease were described in a 1982 report (16). The women, at 16, 12, and 31 weeks' gestation, were treated for various lengths of time with cimetidine and other standard therapy and all delivered healthy newborns without congenital defects or metabolic disturbances. In another report, transient liver impairment was described in a newborn exposed to cimetidine at term (17). However, other reports have not confirmed this toxicity (13,18–35).

In a surveillance study of Michigan Medicaid recipients involving 229,101 completed pregnancies conducted between 1985 and 1992, 460 newborns had been exposed to cimetidine during the 1st trimester (F. Rosa, personal communication, FDA, 1993). A total of 20 (4.3%) major birth defects were observed (20 expected). Specific data were available for six defect categories, including (observed/expected) 8/5 cardiovascular defects, 0/1 oral clefts, 0/0 spina bifida, 1/1 polydactyly, 0/1 limb reduction defects, and 1/1 hypospadias. These data do not support an association between the drug and congenital defects.

Cimetidine has been used at term either with or without other antacids to prevent maternal gastric acid aspiration pneumonitis (Mendelson's syndrome) (13,14,19–35). No neonatal adverse effects were noted in these studies.

In a 1991 report, 23 women were exposed in the 1st trimester to cimetidine ($N = 9$), ranitidine ($N = 13$), or both ($N = 1$) (36). The pregnancy outcomes were spontaneous abortions (SABs) 2, elective abortions (EABs) 2, normal births 18, and 1 infant with a large hemangioma of the upper eye lid (removed without incidence). The outcomes suggested that the agents were not teratogenic (36).

A 1996 prospective cohort study compared the pregnancy outcomes of 178 women who were exposed during pregnancy to H2 blockers with 178 controls matched for maternal age, smoking, and heavy alcohol consumption (37). All of the women had contacted a teratology information service concerning gestational exposure to H2 blockers (subjects) or nonteratogenic or nonfetotoxic agents (controls). Among subjects (mean daily dose in parentheses), 71% took ranitidine (258 mg), 16% cimetidine (487 mg), 8% famotidine (32 mg), and 5% nizatidine (283 mg). There were no significant differences between the outcomes of subjects and controls in terms of live births, SABs and EABs, gestational age at birth, delivery method, birth weight, infants small for gestational age, or major malformations. Among subjects, there were 3 birth defects (2.1%) among the 142 exposed to H2 blockers in the 1st trimester: one each of atrial septal defect, ventricular septal defect, and tetralogy of Fallot. There were 5 birth defects (3.0%) among the 165 exposed anytime during pregnancy. For controls, the rates of defects were 3.5% (1st trimester) and 3.1% (anytime). There were also no differences between the groups in neonatal health problems and developmental milestones, but two children (one subject and one control) were diagnosed as developmentally delayed. The investigators concluded that 1st trimester exposure to histamine H2 blockers did not represent a major teratogenic risk (37).

Data from the Swedish Medical Birth Registry were presented in 1998 (38). A total of 553 infants (6 sets of twins) were delivered from 547 women who had used acid-suppressing drugs early in pregnancy. The odds ratio (OR) for malformations after H2 blockers was 0.86, 95% confidence interval (CI) 0.33–2.23. Of the 19 infants with birth defects, 9 had been exposed to H2 blockers, 1 of whom was also exposed to omeprazole. Cimetidine was the only acid-suppressing drug exposure in 35 infants. Three other offspring were exposed in utero to cimetidine combined either with famotidine (one infant) or with omeprazole (two infants). Two infants with birth defects were exposed to cimetidine: an encephalocele and an unstable hip (see Omeprazole for additional details of this study) (38).

Two databases, one from England and the other from Italy, were combined for a study published in 1999 that was designed to assess the incidence of congenital malformations in women who had received a prescription during the 1st trimester for an acid-suppressing drug (cimetidine, ranitidine, and omeprazole) (39). Nonexposed women were selected from the same databases to form a control group. SABs and EABs (except two cases for anomalies that were grouped with stillbirths) were excluded from the analysis. Stillbirths were defined as any pregnancy loss occurring at 28 weeks'

C

gestation or later. Cimetidine was taken in 233 pregnancies, resulting in 234 live births (14 [6.0%] premature), 3 stillbirths, and 1 neonatal death. Eleven (4.7%) of the newborns had a congenital malformation (shown by system): craniofacial (cleft lip and palate), musculoskeletal (dysplastic hip/dislocation/clicking hip *N* = 3; polydactyly), genital and urinary (hypospadias *N* = 2; congenital hydrocele/inguinal hernia, ovarian cyst, renal defects/hydronephrosis), and gastrointestinal (pyloric stenosis). In addition, two newborns had a small head circumference for gestational age. In comparison, the outcomes of 1547 nonexposed pregnancies included 1560 live births (115 [7.4%] premature), 15 stillbirths (includes 2 elective abortions for anomalies), and 10 neonatal deaths. Of the newborns, 64 (4.1%) had malformations involving the following: CNS (*N* = 2), head/face (*N* = 13), eye (*N* = 2), heart (*N* = 7), muscle/skeletal (*N* = 13), genital/urinary (*N* = 18), gastrointestinal (*N* = 2), and those of polyformation (*N* = 3) or known genetic defects (*N* = 4). There were 21 newborns that were small for gestational age and 78 had a small head circumference for gestational age. The relative risk of malformation (adjusted for mother's age and prematurity) associated with cimetidine was 1.3 (95% CI 0.7–2.6), with omeprazole 0.9 (95% CI 0.4–2.4), and with ranitidine 1.5 (95% CI 0.9–2.6) (39).

A population-based observational cohort study formed by linking data from three Swedish national healthcare registers over a 10-year period (1995–2004) was reported in 2009 (40). The main outcome measures were a diagnosis of allergic disease or a prescription for asthma or allergy medications. The drug types included in the study were gastric acid suppressors, including H2 blockers, prostaglandins, proton pump inhibitors, combinations for eradication of *Helicobacter pylori*, and drugs for peptic ulcer and gastro-esophageal reflux disease. Of 585,716 children, 29,490 (5.0%) met the diagnosis and 5645 (1%) had been exposed to gastric acid suppression therapy in pregnancy. Of these children, 405 (0.07%) were treated for allergic disease. For developing allergy, the odds ratio (OR) was 1.43, 98% CI 1.29–1.59, irrespective of the drug, time of exposure during pregnancy, and maternal history of allergy. For developing childhood asthma, but not other allergic diseases, the OR was 1.51, 95% CI 1.35–1.69, irrespective of the type of acid-suppressive drug and the time of exposure in pregnancy. The authors proposed three possible mechanisms for their findings: (a) exposure to increased amounts of allergens could cause sensitization to digestion labile antigens in the fetus; (b) maternal Th2 cytokine pattern could promote an allergy-prone phenotype in the fetus; and (c) maternal allergen-specific IgE could cross the placenta and sensitize fetal immune cells to food and airborne allergens. Several limitations of the study that might have affected their findings were identified, including a general increase in childhood asthma but not necessarily an increase in allergic asthma (40). The study requires confirmation.

A 2005 study evaluated the outcomes of 553 pregnancies after exposure to H2 blockers, 501 (91%) in the 1st trimester (41). The data were collected by the European Network of Teratology Information Services (ENTIS), The agents and number of cases were cimetidine 113, famotidine 75, nizatidine 15, ranitidine 335, and roxatidine 15. No increase in the number of major malformations were noted (41).

One group of reviewers has recommended that cimetidine not be used during pregnancy because of the possibility for feminization, as observed in some animals and in nonpregnant humans. This effect from in utero exposure to cimetidine has not been studied (42). However, as additional human pregnancy data accumulated, more reviews on the treatment of GERD have concluded that H2 blockers, with the possible exception of nizatidine, could be used in pregnancy with relative safety (43–46).

A 2009 meta-analysis of published studies was conducted to assess the safety of H2 blockers that were used in 2398 pregnancies (47). Compared with 119,892 nonexposed pregnancies, the OR for congenital malformations was 1.14 (95% CI 0.89–1.45), whereas the ORs and 95% CIs for SABs, preterm birth, and small for gestational age were 0.62 [0.36–1.05], 1.17 [0.94–1.147], and 0.28 [0.06–1.22], respectively. The authors concluded that H2 blockers could be used safely in pregnancy (47).

A 2010 study from Israel identified 1148 infants exposed in the 1st trimester to H2 blockers (48). No association with congenital malformations was found (OR 1.03, 95% CI 0.80–1.32). Moreover, no association was found with EABs, perinatal mortality, premature delivery, low birth weight, or low Apgar scores (48).

BREASTFEEDING SUMMARY

Cimetidine is excreted into breast milk and may accumulate in concentrations greater than that found in maternal plasma (49). Following a single 400-mg oral dose, theoretical milk:plasma ratio of 1.6 has been calculated. Multiple oral doses of 200 and 400 mg result in milk:plasma ratios of 4.6 to 7.44, respectively. An estimated 6 mg of cimetidine per liter of milk could be ingested by the nursing infant. The results of a study published in 1995 suggested that cimetidine was actively transported into milk (50). Using single oral doses of 100, 600, or 1200 mg in healthy lactating volunteers, the average of the mean milk:serum ratios for the three doses was 5.77 (range 5.65–5.84), much higher than that predicted by diffusion.

The clinical significance of an infant ingesting cimetidine from milk is unknown. Theoretically, the drug could adversely affect the nursing infant's gastric acidity, inhibit drug metabolism, and produce central nervous system stimulation, but these effects have not been reported. The American Academy of Pediatrics classifies cimetidine as compatible with breastfeeding (51).

References

1. Product information. Tagamet. SmithKline Beecham Pharmaceuticals, 2000.
2. Finkelstein W, Isselbacher KJ. Cimetidine. N Engl J Med 1978;299:992–6.
3. Pinelli F, Trivulzio S, Colombo R, Cocchi D, Faravelli R, Caviezel F, Galmozzi G, Cavallaro R. Antiprostatic effect of cimetidine in rats. Agents Actions 1987;22:197–201.
4. Sawyer D, Conner CS, Scalley R. Cimetidine: adverse reactions and acute toxicity. Am J Hosp Pharm 1981;38:188–97.
5. Anand S, Van Thiel DH. Prenatal and neonatal exposure to cimetidine results in gonadal and sexual dysfunction in adult males. Science 1982;21:493–4.
6. Parker S, Udani M, Gavaler JS, Van Thiel DH. Pre- and neonatal exposure to cimetidine but not ranitidine adversely affects adult sexual functioning of male rats. Neurobehav Toxicol Teratol 1984;6:313–8.
7. Parker S, Schade RR, Pohl CR, Gavaler JS, Van Thiel DH. Prenatal and neonatal exposure of male rat pups to cimetidine but not ranitidine adversely affects subsequent adult sexual functioning. Gastroenterology 1984;86:675–80.
8. Walker TF, Bott JH, Bond BC. Cimetidine does not demasculinize male rat offspring exposed in utero. Fundam Appl Toxicol 1987;8:188–97.

9. Shapiro BH, Hirst SA, Babalola GO, Bitar MS. Prospective study on the sexual development of male and female rats perinatally exposed to maternally administered cimetidine. Toxicol Lett 1988;44:315–29.
10. Dicke JM, Johnson RF, Henderson GI, Kuehl TJ, Schenker S. A comparative evaluation of the transport of H_2-receptor antagonists by the human and baboon placenta. Am J Med Sci 1988;295:198–206.
11. Schenker S, Dicke J, Johnson RF, Mor LL, Henderson GI. Human placental transport of cimetidine. J Clin Invest 1987;80:1428–34.
12. Howe JP, McGowan WAW, Moore J, McCaughey W, Dundee JW. The placental transfer of cimetidine. Anaesthesia 1981;36:371–5.
13. McGowan WAW. Safety of cimetidine in obstetric patients. J R Soc Med 1979;72:902–7.
14. Johnston JR, Moore J, McCaughey W, Dundee JW, Howard PJ, Toner W, McClean E. Use of cimetidine as an oral antacid in obstetric anesthesia. Anesth Analg 1983;62:720–6.
15. Knott PD, Thorpe SS, Lamont CAR. Congenital renal dysgenesis possibly due to captopril. Lancet 1989;1:451.
16. Corazza GR, Gasbarrini G, Di Nisio Q, Zulli P. Cimetidine (Tagamet) in peptic ulcer therapy during pregnancy: a report of three cases. Clin Trials J 1982;19:91–3.
17. Glade G, Saccar CL, Pereira GR. Cimetidine in pregnancy: apparent transient liver impairment in the newborn. Am J Dis Child 1980;134:87–8.
18. Zulli P, DiNisio Q. Cimetidine treatment during pregnancy. Lancet 1978;2:945–6.
19. Husemeyer RP, Davenport HT. Prophylaxis for Mendelson's syndrome before elective caesarean sections. A comparison of cimetidine and magnesium trisilicate mixture regimens. Br J Obstet Gynaecol 1980;87:565–70.
20. Pickering BG, Palahniuk RJ, Cumming M. Cimetidine premedication in elective caesarean section. Can Anaesth Soc J 1980;27:33–5.
21. Dundee JW, Moore J, Johnston JR, McCaughey W. Cimetidine and obstetric anaesthesia. Lancet 1981;2:252.
22. McCaughey W, Howe JP, Moore J, Dundee JW. Cimetidine in elective caesarean section. Effect on gastric acidity. Anaesthesia 1981;36:167–72.
23. Crawford JS. Cimetidine in elective caesarean section. Anaesthesia 1981;36:641–2.
24. McCaughey W, Howe JP, Moore J, Dundee JW. Cimetidine in elective caesarean section. Anaesthesia 1981;36:642.
25. Hodgkinson R, Glassenberg R, Joyce TH III, Coombs DW, Ostheimer GW, Gibbs CP. Safety and efficacy of cimetidine and antacid in reducing gastric acidity before elective cesarean section. Anesthesiology 1982;57:A408.
26. Ostheimer GW, Morrison JA, Lavoie C, Sepkoski C, Hoffman J, Datta S. The effect of cimetidine on mother, newborn and neonatal neurobehavior. Anesthesiology 1982;57:A405.
27. Hodgkinson R, Glassenberg R, Joyce TH III, Coombs DW, Ostheimer GW, Gibbs CP. Comparison of cimetidine (Tagamet) with antacid for safety and effectiveness in reducing gastric acidity before elective cesarean section. Anesthesiology 1983;59:86–90.
28. Qvist N, Storm K. Cimethidine pre-anesthetic: a prophylactic method against Mendelson's syndrome in cesarean section. Acta Obstet Gynecol Scand 1983;62:157–9.
29. Okasha AS, Motaweh MM, Bali A. Cimetidine-antacid combination as premedication for elective caesarean section. Can Anaesth Soc J 1983;30: 593–7.
30. Frank M, Evans M, Flynn P, Aun C. Comparison of the prophylactic use of magnesium trisilicate mixture B.P.C., sodium citrate mixture or cimetidine in obstetrics. Br J Anaesth 1984;56:355–62.
31. McAuley DM, Halliday HL, Johnston JR, Moore J, Dundee JW. Cimetidine in labour: absence of adverse effect on the high-risk fetus. Br J Obstet Gynaecol 1985;92:350–5.
32. Johnston JR, McCaughey W, Moore J, Dundee JW. Cimetidine as an oral antacid before elective caesarean section. Anaesthesia 1982;37:26–32.
33. Johnston JR, McCaughey W, Moore J, Dundee JW. A field trial of cimetidine as the sole oral antacid in obstetric anaesthesia. Anaesthesia 1982;37:33–8.
34. Thorburn J, Moir DD. Antacid therapy for emergency caesarean section. Anaesthesia 1987;42:352–5.
35. Howe JP, Dundee JW, Moore J, McCaughey W. Cimetidine: Has it a place in obstetric anaesthesia? Anaesthesia 1980;35:421–2.
36. Koren G, Zemlickis DM. Outcome of pregnancy after first trimester exposure to H2 receptor antagonists. Am J Perinatol 1991;8:37–8.
37. Magee LA, Inocencion G, Kamboj L, Rosetti F, Koren G. Safety of first trimester exposure to histamine H_2 blockers. A prospective cohort study. Dig Dis Sci 1996;41:1145–9.
38. Kallen B. Delivery outcome after the use of acid-suppressing drugs in early pregnancy with special reference to omeprazole. Br J Obstet Gynaecol 1998;105:877–81.
39. Ruigomez A, Rodriguez LAG, Cattaruzzi C, Troncon MG, Agostinis L, Wallander MA, Johansson S. Use of cimetidine, omeprazole, and ranitidine in pregnant women and pregnancy outcomes. Am J Epidemiol 1999;150:476–81.
40. Dehlink E, Yen E, Leichtner AM, Hait EJ, Fiebiger E. First evidence of a possible association between gastric acid suppression during pregnancy and childhood asthma: a population-based register study. Clin Exp Allergy 2009;39:246–53.
41. Garbis H, Elefant E, Diav-Citrin O, Mastroiacovo P, Schaefer C, Vial T, Clementi M, Valti E, McElhatton P, Smorlesij C, Rodriguez EP, Robert-Gnansia E, Merlob P, Peiker G, Pexieder T, Schueler L, Ritvanen A, Mathieu-Nolf M. Pregnancy outcome after exposure to ranitidine and other H2-blockers—a collaborative study of the European Network of Teratology Information Services. Reprod Toxicol 2005;453–8.
42. Smallwood RA, Berlin RG, Castagnoli N, Festen HPM, Hawkey CJ, Lam SK, Langman MJS, Lundborg P, Parkinson A. Safety of acid-suppressing drugs. Dig Dis Sci 1995;40(Suppl):63S–80S.
43. Broussard CN, Richter JE. Treating gasto-oesophageal reflux disease during pregnancy and lactation. What are the safest therapy options? Drug Saf 1998;19:325–37.
44. Katz PO, Castell DO. Gastroesophageal reflux disease during pregnancy. Gastroenterol Clin North Am 1998;27:153–67.
45. Richter JE. Gastroesophageal reflux disease during pregnancy. Gastroenterol Clin North Am 2003;32:235–61.
46. Richter JE. Review article: the management of heartburn in pregnancy. Aliment Pharmacol Ther 2005;22:749–57.
47. Gill SK, O'Brien L, Koren G. The safety of histamine 2 (H2) blockers in pregnancy: a meta-analysis. Dig Dis Sci 2009;54:1835–8.
48. Matok I, Gorodischer R, Koren G, Sheiner E, Wiznitzer A, Uziel E, Levy A. The safety of H_2-blockers use during pregnancy. J. Clin Pharmacol 2010;50:81–7.
49. Somogyi A, Gugler R. Cimetidine excretion into breast milk. Br J Clin Pharmacol 1979;7:627–9.
50. Oo CY, Kuhn RJ, Desai N, McNamara PJ. Active transport of cimetidine into human milk. Clin Pharmacol Ther 1995;58:548–55.
51. Committee on Drugs, American Academy of Pediatrics. The transfer of drugs and other chemicals into human milk. Pediatrics 2001;108:776–89.

CINACALCET

Calcium Receptor Agonist

PREGNANCY RECOMMENDATION: Limited Human Data—Animal Data Suggest Low Risk
BREASTFEEDING RECOMMENDATION: No Human Data—Potential Toxicity

PREGNANCY SUMMARY

Two reports described the use of cinacalcet late in the 3rd trimester, but information on the newborn condition was provided only in one case. Cinacalcet is the first member of a new drug class, so there are no other comparable agents. Moreover, therapy in most patients will be prolonged (months). Animal data do show developmental toxicity (growth restriction) but maternal toxicity also was evident. The near absence of human pregnancy experience prevents a more complete assessment of the embryo–fetal risk. Nevertheless, if a woman's condition requires cinacalcet, it should not be withheld because of pregnancy.

FETAL RISK SUMMARY

Cinacalcet increases the sensitivity of the calcium-sensing receptor to activation by extracellular calcium. It is indicated for the treatment of secondary hyperparathyroidism in patients with chronic kidney disease on dialysis. It also is indicated for the treatment of hypercalcemia in patients with parathyroid carcinoma. Cinacalcet is rapidly and extensively metabolized to inactive metabolites. The terminal half-life is 30–40 hours and plasma protein binding is 93%–97% (1).

Reproduction studies have been conducted in rats and rabbits. In pregnant rats, no teratogenicity was observed with daily oral doses that produced exposures up to four times those resulting with a human dose of 180 mg/day based on AUC (HE). Decreased fetal weights were observed with daily doses producing exposures that were less than one to four times the HE, but maternal toxicity (decreased food consumption and body weight gain) also was noted. Daily doses that produced exposures less than the HE given during gestation through lactation revealed no evidence of adverse fetal or pup (postweaning) effects. When higher doses were given (two to three times the HE), maternal signs of hypocalcemia (periparturient mortality and early postnatal pup death) and reductions in postnatal maternal and pup weight were noted. In pregnant rabbits, daily oral doses that produced exposures less than the HE revealed no evidence of fetal harm, but maternal toxicity (reduced food consumption and body weight gain) was observed (1).

No evidence of carcinogenic effects was observed in long-term studies in mice and rats.

Assays for mutagenicity were negative. In fertility studies in male and female rats, only daily doses producing exposures greater than four times the HE were associated with slight toxicity (decreases in food consumption and body weight) (1).

It is not known if cinacalcet crosses the human placenta. The drug crosses the rabbit placenta (1). The molecular weight (about 358 for the free base) and long terminal half-life suggest that the drug will cross to the embryo and fetus. However, the extensive metabolism and high plasma protein binding should decrease the exposure to the parent drug.

A 2009 case report described a pregnant 40-year-old woman with severe primary hyperparathyroidism (2). She presented at 32 weeks' gestation with hypertension and hypercalcemia. Treatment with cinacalcet (240 mg/day) and calcitonin (100 mcg SC every other day) decreased the serum calcium. A planned cesarean section delivery was conducted at 34 weeks. No information on the newborn was provided, except that the cord blood had elevated calcium as compared to the mother's blood, indicating that the physiological calcium gradient between the mother and the child had not been disrupted by cinacalcet (2).

In a 2013 report, a 21-year-old woman with primary hyperparathyroidism attributable to parathyromatosis presented with markedly elevated total calcium and ionized calcium levels at 14 weeks' gestation (3). She underwent surgery at 22 weeks to remove hypercellular parathyroid tissue. Because of persistent hypercalcemia that was increasing, cinacalcet (30 mg/day) was started at 33 weeks' gestation and was successful in decreasing the calcium levels. At 38 weeks, a cesarean section delivered a healthy male infant. Other than that he was doing well at 6 weeks of age; no other details about the infant were provided (3).

BREASTFEEDING SUMMARY

No reports describing the use of cinacalcet during human lactation have been located. The molecular weight (about 358 for the free base) and long terminal half-life (30–40 hours) suggest that the drug will be excreted into breast milk. However, the extensive metabolism and high plasma protein binding (93%–97%) should decrease the amount of parent drug in milk. The effect of this exposure on a nursing infant is unknown, but nausea/vomiting, the most common toxicity observed in adults, and hypocalcemia are potential adverse effects. The latter toxicity is particularly worrisome because of an infant's high requirements for calcium during bone accretion.

References

1. Product information. Sensipar. Amgen, 2007.
2. Horjus C, Groot I, Telting D, van Setten P, van Sorge A, Kovacs CS, Hermus A, de Boer H. Cincacalcet for hyperparathyroidism in pregnancy and puerperium. J Pediatr Endocrinol Metab 2009;22:741–9.
3. Edling KL, Korenman SG, Janzen C, Sohsman MY, Apple SK, Bhuta S, Yeh MW. A pregnant dilemma: primary hyperthyroidism due to parathyromatosis in pregnancy. Endo Pract 2013;6:1–15.

CINNARIZINE

[Withdrawn from the market. See 9th edition.]

CINOXACIN

Urinary Germicide (Quinolone)

PREGNANCY RECOMMENDATION: No Human Data—Animal Data Suggest Low Risk
BREASTFEEDING RECOMMENDATION: No Human Data—Probably Compatible

C

PREGNANCY SUMMARY

No reports describing the use of cinoxacin during human pregnancy have been located. Because of the potential for cinoxacin-induced arthropathy in the fetus and the newborn, the manufacturer recommends that it should not be used in pregnancy (1).

FETAL RISK SUMMARY

Cinoxacin is a synthetic, oral quinolone antibacterial agent indicated for the treatment of urinary tract infections. Its actions and uses are similar to nalidixic acid. No evidence of impaired fertility or fetal harm was observed in reproduction studies in rats and rabbits at doses up to 10 times the daily human dose (1).

It is not known if cinoxacin crosses the placenta. The molecular weight (about 262) is low enough that transfer to the fetus should be expected.

BREASTFEEDING SUMMARY

No reports describing the use of cinoxacin during human lactation have been located. Because of the potential for arthropathy in a nursing infant, the manufacturer recommends that it should not be used in lactating women (1).

Reference

1. Product information. Cinobac. Oclassen Pharmaceuticals, 1998.

CIPROFLOXACIN

Anti-infective (Quinolone)

PREGNANCY RECOMMENDATION: Human Data Suggest Low Risk
BREASTFEEDING RECOMMENDATION: Limited Human Data—Potential Toxicity

PREGNANCY SUMMARY

The use of ciprofloxacin during human gestation does not appear to be associated with an increased risk of major congenital malformations. Although a number of birth defects have occurred in the offspring of women who had taken this drug during pregnancy, the lack of a pattern among the anomalies is reassuring. However, a causal relationship with some of the birth defects cannot be excluded. Because of this and the available animal data, the use of ciprofloxacin during pregnancy, especially during the 1st trimester, should be used with caution, but the overall risk appears to be low. A 1993 review on the safety of fluoroquinolones concluded that these antibacterials should be avoided during pregnancy because of the difficulty in extrapolating animal mutagenicity results to humans and because interpretation of this toxicity is still controversial (1). The authors of this review were not convinced that fluoroquinolone-induced fetal cartilage damage and subsequent arthropathies were a major concern, even though this effect had been demonstrated in several animal species after administration to both pregnant and immature animals and in occasional human case reports involving children (1). Others have also concluded that fluoroquinolones should be considered contraindicated in pregnancy, because safer alternatives are usually available (2).

FETAL RISK SUMMARY

Ciprofloxacin is a synthetic, broad-spectrum antibacterial agent. As a fluoroquinolone, it is in the same class as enoxacin, levofloxacin, lomefloxacin, norfloxacin, ofloxacin, and sparfloxacin. Nalidixic acid and cinoxacin are also quinolone drugs.

Ciprofloxacin did not impair fertility and was not embryotoxic or teratogenic in mice and rats at doses up to 6 times the usual human daily dose. A similar lack of embryo and fetal toxicity was observed in rabbits. As with other quinolones, multiple doses of ciprofloxacin produced permanent lesions and erosion of cartilage in weight-bearing joints, leading to lameness in immature rats and dogs (3).

A 2005 study measured the amount of three fluoroquinolones (ciprofloxacin, ofloxacin, levofloxacin) that crossed the perfused human placenta (4). All three agents crossed the placenta from the maternal to the fetal compartment, but the amounts crossing were small: 3.2%, 3.7%, and 3.9%, respectively.

A number of reports have described the use of ciprofloxacin during human gestation (2,5–16). In a 1993 reference, data on 103 pregnancies exposed to the drug were released by the manufacturer (5). Of these cases, there were 63 normal, live newborns (52 exposed during 1st trimester, 7 during the 2nd or 3rd trimesters, and 4 in which the exposure time was unknown), 18 terminations, 10 spontaneous abortions (SABs) (all 1st trimester), 4 fetal deaths (3 during 1st trimester, 1 in 3rd trimester), and 8 infants with congenital defects (7 exposed between 2 and 12 weeks postmenstruation and 1 on a single day of her last menstrual period) (these defects are included among those shown in reference 11 below).

No congenital malformations were observed in the infants of 38 women who received either ciprofloxacin (*N* = 10) or

C

norfloxacin ($N = 28$) during pregnancy (35 in the 1st trimester) (6). Most ($N = 35$) received the drugs for the treatment of urinary tract infections. Matched to a control group, the fluoroquinolone-exposed pregnancies had a significantly higher rate of cesarean section for fetal distress and their infants were significantly heavier. No differences were found between the groups in infant development or in the musculoskeletal system (6).

A 1995 letter described seven pregnant women with multidrug-resistant typhoid fever who were treated with ciprofloxacin during the 2nd and 3rd trimesters (7). All delivered healthy infants who were doing well at 5 years of age without evidence of cartilage damage. The authors also described the healthy outcome of another pregnant woman treated with ciprofloxacin during the 1st trimester. That infant was doing well at 6 months of age. A subsequent letter, also in women with typhoid fever, described three pregnant women in the 2nd and 3rd trimesters who were treated with ciprofloxacin (8). A normal outcome occurred in one patient and the pregnancies of the other two were progressing satisfactory.

A surveillance study on the use of fluoroquinolones during pregnancy was conducted by the Toronto Motherisk Program among members of the Organization of Teratology Information Services (OTIS) and briefly reported in 1995 (9). Pregnancy outcome data were available for 134 cases, of which 68 involved ciprofloxacin, 61 were exposed to norfloxacin, and 5 were exposed to both the drugs. Most (90%) were exposed during the first 13 weeks postconception. Fluoroquinolone-exposed pregnancies were compared to matched controls and there were no differences in live births (87% vs. 86%), terminations (3% vs. 5%), miscarriages (10% vs. 9%), abnormal outcomes (7% vs. 4%), cesarean section rate (12% vs. 22%), fetal distress (15% vs. 15%), and pregnancy weight gain (15 vs. 16 kg). The mean birth weight of the exposed infants was 162 g higher than those in the control group and their gestations were a mean 1 week longer (9).

A 16-year-old became pregnant about 1.5 years after a combined liver–kidney transplant for type 1 primary hyperoxaluria (10). She was treated with immunosuppressive agents (prednisone 10 mg/day, cyclosporine 200 mg/day, and azathioprine 75 mg/day) and penicillin 500 mg/day and ciprofloxacin 250 mg/day throughout pregnancy. A healthy 2860-g female infant was delivered by cesarean section at 38 weeks' gestation. Apgar scores were 4 and 9 at 1 and 5 minutes, respectively (10).

An abstract, published in 1996, described six pregnancies exposed to ciprofloxacin during the 1st trimester (11). Five healthy babies (one set of twins) had been born and two pregnancies were progressing normally. In another 1996 reference, no congenital anomalies were reported in 32 pregnancies exposed to a fluoroquinolone (9 ciprofloxacin, 13 norfloxacin, 10 ofloxacin) (12). In a 1997 reference, a pregnant woman with Q fever (*Coxiella burnetii*) at 28 weeks' gestation was treated with ciprofloxacin for 3 weeks (13). Because her symptoms did not resolve, a cesarean section was performed at 32 weeks' gestation with delivery of a healthy, female infant. No evidence of transplacental spread of the infection, which is known to cause stillbirth and abortion in animals and humans, was found (13).

A prospective follow-up study conducted by the European Network of Teratology Information Services (ENTIS) analyzed 549 pregnancies exposed to fluoroquinolones (70 to ciprofloxacin) (2). Data on another 116 prospective and 25 retrospective pregnancy exposures to the antibiotics were also included. From the 549 follow-up cases, 509 were treated during the 1st trimester, 22 after the 1st trimester, and in 18 cases the exposure occurred at an unknown gestational time. The liveborn infants were delivered at a mean gestational age of 39.4 weeks and had a mean birth weight of 3302 g, length of 50.3 cm, and head circumference of 34.9 cm. Of the 549 pregnancies, there were 415 liveborn infants (390 exposed during the 1st trimester), 356 of which were normal-term deliveries (including one set of twins), 15 were premature, 6 were small-for-gestational age (IUGR, <10th percentile), 20 had congenital anomalies (19 from mothers exposed during the 1st trimester; 4.9%), and 18 had postnatal disorders unrelated to either prematurity, low birth weight, or malformations (11). Of the remaining 135 pregnancies, there were 56 spontaneous abortions or fetal deaths (none late) (1 malformed fetus), and 79 elective abortions (4 malformed fetuses). A total of 116 (all involving ciprofloxacin) prospective cases were obtained from the manufacturer's registry. Among these, there were 91 liveborn infants, 6 of whom had malformations. Of the remaining 25 pregnancies, 15 were terminated (no malformations reported), and 10 aborted spontaneously (one embryo with acardia, no data available on a possible twin). Thus, of the 666 cases with known outcomes, 32 (4.8%) of the embryos, fetusess or newborns had congenital malformations. Based on previous epidemiologic data, the authors concluded that the 4.8% frequency of malformations did not exceed the background rate. Finally, 25 retrospective reports of infants with anomalies, who had been exposed in utero to fluoroquinolones, were analyzed, but no specific patterns of major congenital malformations were detected (2).

The defects observed in the 10 infants followed prospectively and in the 8 infants reported retrospectively, all with 1st trimester ciprofloxacin exposure, were (2) as follows:

Source: Prospective ENTIS
- Angioma right lower leg
- Hip dysplasia left side
- Trisomy, unspecified (pregnancy terminated)

Source: Prospective Manufacturer's Registry
- Hypospadias
- Auricle indentation, hip dysplasia
- Cerebellum hypoplasia, oculomotor palsy, development retardation
- Hooded foreskin
- Amputation right forearm
- Hypospadias, bilateral hernia inguinalis
- Acardia (spontaneous abortion)

Source: Retrospective Reports
- Teeth discoloration
- Hypoplastic auricle, absence external auditory canal
- Rubinstein–Taybi syndrome
- Femur aplasia
- Femur–fibula–ulna complex
- Ectrodactyly
- Defects of heart, trachea, esophagus, urethra, anus, gallbladder, skeleton, heterotopic gastric mucosa, mucosa
- Heart defect

The authors of the above study concluded that pregnancy exposure to quinolones was not an indication for termination, but that this class of antibacterials should still be considered contraindicated in pregnant women because safer alternatives are usually available (2). Because of their own and previously published findings, they further recommended that the focus of future studies should be on malformations involving the abdominal wall and urogenital system, and limb reduction defects. Moreover, this study did not address the issue of cartilage damage from quinolone exposure and the authors recognized the need for follow-up studies of this potential toxicity in children exposed in utero.

In a surveillance study of Michigan Medicaid recipients involving 229,101 completed pregnancies conducted between 1985 and 1992, 132 newborns had been exposed to ciprofloxacin during the 1st trimester (F. Rosa, personal communication, FDA, 1993). Three (2.3%) major birth defects were observed (six expected), one of which was a case of spina bifida (none expected). No anomalies were observed in five other categories of defects (cardiovascular defects, oral clefts, polydactyly, limb reduction defects, and hypospadias) for which specific data were available. These data do not support an association between the drug and congenital defects.

A 1998 prospective multicenter study reported the pregnancy outcomes of 200 women exposed to fluoroquinolones compared with 200 matched controls (14). Subjects were pregnant women who had called one of four teratogen information services concerning their exposure to fluoroquinolones. The agents, number of subjects, and daily doses were ciprofloxacin ($N = 105$; 500–1000 mg), norfloxacin ($N = 93$; 400–800 mg), and ofloxacin ($N = 2$; 200–400 mg). The most common infections involved the urinary tract (69.4%) or the respiratory tract (24%). The fewer live births in the fluoroquinolone group (173 vs. 188, $p = 0.02$) was attributable to the greater number of spontaneous abortions (18 vs. 10, *ns*) and induced abortions (9 vs. 2, *ns*). There were no differences between the groups in terms of premature birth, fetal distress, method of delivery, low birth weight (<2500 g), or birth weight. Among the liveborn infants exposed during organogenesis, major malformations were observed in 3 of 133 subjects and 5 of 188 controls (*ns*). The defects in subject infants were two cases of ventricular septal defect and one case of patent ductus arteriosus, whereas those in controls were two cases of ventricular septal defect, one case of atrial septal defect with pulmonic valve stenosis, one case of hypospadias, and one case of displaced hip. There were also no differences between the children of the groups in gross motor development milestone achievements (musculoskeletal functions: lifting, sitting, crawling, standing, or walking) as measured by the Denver Developmental Scale (14).

A database cohort study from Denmark evaluated the pregnancy outcomes in two groups of women who had redeemed a fluoroquinolone prescription during pregnancy; those who had at any time in pregnancy and those who had during the 1st trimester or 30 days before conception (15). Among 87 women in the first group, the prevalence ratio of preterm birth was 1.4 (95% confidence interval [CI] 0.6–3.2), one woman had a stillbirth, and no infants died during the perinatal period. Among the 130 women in the second group, the prevalence ratio of congenital anomalies was 0.7 (95% CI 0.3–2.0) and the ratio of bone malformations was 2.2 (95% CI 0.7–6.7). Among the four infants with congenital anomalies, three had bone malformations: unsymmetrical closure of the cranial sutures (ofloxacin), extra toe (fleroxacin), and clubfoot (ciprofloxacin). Although a causal link between the bone defects and fluoroquinolones could not be determined, the authors suggested that future studies should look for this association (15).

A retrospective cohort study using data from Tennessee Medicaid included 30,049 infants born in 1985–2000 was published in 2009 (16). Infants with fetal exposures in the 1st trimester to four antibiotics recommended for potential bioterrorism attacks (ciprofloxacin, amoxicillin, azithromycin, and doxycycline) were compared to infants with no fetal exposure to any antibiotic. Erythromycin was included as a positive control. In the 439 infants exposed to ciprofloxacin and no other antibiotics, the number of cases, risk ratios, and 95% CI were as follows: any malformation (8, 0.64. 0.31–1.30), cardiac (3, 0.70, 0.22–2.26); musculoskeletal (0); genitourinary (2, 0.80, 0.19–3.40); gastrointestinal (2, 0.78, 0.18–3.48); CNS (0); and orofacial (1, 1.72, 0.18–1′, replace:=wdreplaceall, forward:=true, matchwildcards:=false, matchcase:=true6.55). The authors concluded that the four antibiotics should not result in a greater incidence of overall major malformations (see also Amoxicillin, Azithromycin, and Doxycycline) (16).

In a study investigating the pharmacokinetics of ciprofloxacin, 20 pregnant women, between 19 and 25 weeks' gestation (mean 21.16 weeks), were scheduled for pregnancy termination because the fetuses were affected with β-thalassemia major (17). Two doses of ciprofloxacin, 200 mg IV every 12 hours, were given prior to abortion. Serum and amniotic fluid concentrations were drawn concomitantly at 4, 8, and 12 hours after dosing. Mean maternal serum concentrations at these times were 0.28, 0.09, and 0.01 mcg/mL, respectively, compared with mean amniotic fluid levels of 0.12, 0.13, and 0.10 mcg/mL, respectively. The amniotic fluid:maternal serum ratios were 0.43, 1.44, and 10.0, respectively (17).

BREASTFEEDING SUMMARY

When first marketed, the administration of ciprofloxacin during breastfeeding was not recommended because of the potential for arthropathy (based on animal data) and other serious toxicity in the nursing infant (3). Phototoxicity has been observed with some members of the quinolone class of drugs when exposure to excessive sunlight (i.e., ultraviolet light) has occurred. Well-differentiated squamous cell carcinomas of the skin have been produced in mice who were exposed chronically to some quinolones and periodic ultraviolet light (e.g., see Lomefloxacin), but studies to evaluate the carcinogenicity of ciprofloxacin in this manner have not been conducted.

Ciprofloxacin is excreted into human milk (17–19). Ten lactating women were given three oral doses of ciprofloxacin, 750 mg each (17). Six simultaneous serum and milk samples were drawn between 2 and 24 hours after the third dose of the antibacterial. The mean peak serum level (2.06 mcg/mL) occurred at 2 hours, then steadily fell to 0.02 mcg/mL at 24 hours. Milk concentrations exhibited a similar pattern with a mean peak level measured at 2 hours, 3.79 mcg/mL, and the lowest amount at 24 hours, 0.02 mcg/mL. The mean milk:serum ratio varied from 0.85 to 2.14 with the highest ratio occurring 4 hours after the last dose (17).

A 24-year-old woman, 17 days postpartum, was given a single 500-mg dose of the antibacterial to treat a urinary tract infection (18). She was also suffering from acute renal failure and had undergone her final hemodialysis treatment 7 days prior to administration of ciprofloxacin. Her serum creatinine and blood urea nitrogen at the time of the dose were 740 mmol/L and 26.8 mmol/L, respectively. Milk samples were collected at 4, 8, 12, and 16 hours. Concentrations of ciprofloxacin at these times were 9.1, 9.1, 9.1, and 6.0 μmol/L, respectively. (*Note: 9.1 and 6.0 μmol/L are approximately 3.0 and 2.0 mcg/mL, respectively.*) Based on the volume of milk and concentrations, the potential cumulative dose for the infant, who was not allowed to breastfeed, was 1.331 μmol/L (18).

In a 1992 case report, a 4-month-old female infant was being exclusively breastfed six times/day (19). The mother had taken a single night-time dose (500 mg) of the antibacterial for 10 days prior to the collection of simultaneous samples of milk, maternal serum, and infant serum, approximately 11 hours after a dose. On the day of sampling, breastfeeding occurred 8 hours after the mother's dose. Maternal serum, milk, and infant serum ciprofloxacin concentrations were 0.21, 0.98, and $<$0.03 mcg/mL (undetectable), respectively. The authors estimated the infant was consuming 0.92 mg/day (0.15 mg/kg/day) of ciprofloxacin. No adverse effects were observed in the infant (19).

In a second 1992 case report, a 2-month-old breastfed female infant presented with a 1-day history of anorexia, fever, and foul-smelling green diarrhea (20). She was admitted to the hospital with a diagnosis of pseudomembranous colitis. The infant had been hospitalized during the first 14 days of life with a history of necrotizing entercolitis but had been doing well at home for the past month. *Clostridium difficile* toxin was found in the infant's stool. Following a left colectomy and 7 days of oral vancomycin, the infant was thriving at home. Upon inquiry, it was discovered that the infant's mother had self-administered ciprofloxacin (dose not specified) for 6 days before her infant's admission to the hospital. The cause of the pseudomembranous colitis was thought to be ciprofloxacin obtained from breast milk (20).

In unpublished studies available to the manufacturer, peak milk levels occurred approximately 4 hours after a ciprofloxacin dose and were about the same as serum levels (personal communication, Miles Pharmaceutical, June 1990). Levels of the antibacterial were undetectable 36–48 hours after a dose. Based on these data, the manufacturer recommends that 48 hours elapse after the last dose of ciprofloxacin before breastfeeding is resumed (personal communication, Miles Pharmaceutical, June 1990).

In an unusual report, follow-up of infants who had been treated as neonates with ciprofloxacin for severe *Klebsiella pneumoniae* revealed two of five infants with greenish-colored teeth on eruption (21). The teeth were stained uniformly with dyscalcification at the cervical part. The investigators could not determine the cause of the condition. Other reports of this condition have not been located and the clinical significance of this to a nursing infant exposed to fluoroquinolones via the milk is unknown.

Although there is a report of toxicity in a nursing infant that was thought to have been caused by ciprofloxacin, the contribution of the infant's medical history, as well as the mother's unknown ciprofloxacin dose, are confounding factors. Data are limited, but the amount of ciprofloxacin in breast milk does not appear to represent a significant risk to an infant, especially if nursing is held for several hours after a dose. Short courses of maternal therapy are probably compatible with nursing. The American Academy of Pediatrics, without citing the above case report of potential drug-induced toxicity, classified ciprofloxacin as compatible with breastfeeding (22).

References

1. Norrby SR, Lietman PS. Safety and tolerability of fluoroquinolones. Drugs 1993;45(Suppl 3):59–64.
2. Schaefer C, Amoura-Elefant E, Vial T, Ornoy A, Garbis H, Robert E, Rodriguez-Pinilla E, Pexieder T, Prapas N, Merlob P. Pregnancy outcome after prenatal quinolone exposure. Evaluation of a case registry of the European Network of Teratology Information Services (ENTIS). Eur J Obstet Gynecol Reprod Biol 1996;69:83–9.
3. Product information. Cipro. Miles Pharmaceutical, 1993.
4. Polachek H, Holcberg G, Sapir G, Tsadkin-Tamir M, Polacheck J, Katz M, Ben-Zvi Z. Transfer of ciprofloxacin, ofloxacin and levofloxacin across the perfused human placenta in vitro. Eur J Obstet Gynecol Reprod Biol 2005;122:61–5.
5. Bomford JAL, Ledger JC, O'Keeffe BJ, Reiter CH. Ciprofloxacin use during pregnancy. Drugs 1993;45(Suppl 3):461–2.
6. Berkovitch M, Pastuszak A, Gazarian M, Lewis M, Koren G. Safety of the new quinolones in pregnancy. Obstet Gynecol 1994;84:535–8.
7. Koul PA, Wani JI, Wahid A. Ciprofloxacin for multiresistant enteric fever in pregnancy. Lancet 1995;346:307–8.
8. Leung D, Venkatesan P, Boswell T, Innes JA, Wood MJ. Treatment of typhoid in pregnancy. Lancet 1995;346:648.
9. Pastuszak A, Andreou R, Schick B, Sage S, Cook L, Donnenfeld A, Koren G. New postmarketing surveillance data supports a lack of association between quinolone use in pregnancy and fetal and neonatal complications. Reprod Toxicol 1995;9:584.
10. Skannal DG, Dungy-Poythress LJ, Miodovnik M, First MR. Pregnancy in a combined liver and kidney transplant recipient with type 1 primary hyperoxaluria. Obstet Gynecol 1995;86:641–3.
11. Baroncini A, Calzolari E, Calabrese O, Zanetti A. First-trimester exposure to ciprofloxacin (abstract). Teratology 1996;53:24A.
12. Wilton LV, Pearce GI, Mann RD. A comparison of ciprofloxacin, norfloxacin, ofloxacin, azithromycin, and cefixime examined by observational cohort studies. Br J Clin Pharmacol 1996;41:277–84.
13. Ludlam H, Wreghitt TG, Thornton S, Thomson BJ, Bishop NJ, Coomber S, Cunniffe J. Q fever in pregnancy. J Infect 1997;34:75–8.
14. Loebstein R, Addis A, Ho E, Andreou R, Sage S, Donnenfeld AE, Schick B, Bonati M, Mortetti M, Lalkin A, Pastuszak A, Koren G. Pregnancy outcome following gestational exposure to fluoroquinolones: a multicenter prospective controlled study. Antimicrob Ag Chemother 1998;42:1336–9.
15. Wogelius P, Norgaard M, Gislum M, Pedersen L, Schonheyder HC, Sorensen HT. Further analysis of the risk of adverse birth outcome after maternal use of fluoroquinolones. Int J Antimicrob Agents 2005;26:323–6.
16. Cooper WO, Hernandez-Diaz S, Arbogast PG, Dudley JA, Dyer SM, Gideon PS, Hall KS, Kaltenbach LA, Ray WA. Antibiotics potentially used in response to bioterrorism and the risk of major congenital malformations. Paediatr Perinat Epidemiol 2009;23:18–28.
17. Giamarellou H, Kolokythas E, Petrikkos G, Gazis J, Aravantinos D, Sfikakis P. Pharmacokinetics of three newer quinolones in pregnant and lactating women. Am J Med 1989;87(Suppl 5A):49S–51S.
18. Cover DL, Mueller BA. Ciprofloxacin penetration into human breast milk: a case report. Ann Pharmacother 1990;24:703–4.
19. Gardner DK, Gabbe SG, Harter C. Simultaneous concentrations of ciprofloxacin in breast milk and in serum in mother and breast-fed infant. Clin Pharm 1992;11:352–4.
20. Harmon T, Burkhart G, Applebaum H. Perforated pseudomembranous colitis in the breast-fed infant. J Pediatr Surg 1992;27:744–6.
21. Lumbiganon P, Pengsaa K, Sookpranee T. Ciprofloxacin in neonates and its possible effect on the teeth. Pediatr Infect Dis J 1991;10:619–20.
22. Committee on Drugs, American Academy of Pediatrics. The transfer of drugs and other chemicals into human milk. Pediatrics 2001;108: 776–89.

CISAPRIDE

[Withdrawn from the market. See 9th edition.]

C

CISPLATIN

Antineoplastic

PREGNANCY RECOMMENDATION: Contraindicated—1st Trimester
BREASTFEEDING RECOMMENDATION: Contraindicated

PREGNANCY SUMMARY

Exposure to cisplatin in the 1st trimester is limited to two cases. The drug is teratogenic and embryotoxic in two animal species. Because of the potential for embryo toxicity, the drug should be avoided during the 1st trimester. The reported use in the 2nd and 3rd trimesters and long-term follow-up of the offspring are too limited to assess for toxicity appearing later in life.

[*See Carboplatin for additional data.*]

FETAL RISK SUMMARY

Cisplatin is an antineoplastic used in the treatment of various cancers. This agent is mutagenic in bacteria, produces chromosomal aberrations in animal cells in tissue culture, and is teratogenic and embryotoxic in mice (1). Cisplatin is also a transplacental carcinogen in rats, producing tumors in the liver, lung, nervous system, and kidneys of adult offspring (2). The mechanism for the production of these tumors is probably the result of DNA damage in fetal rat tissues (3). A 1994 review also reviewed the animal teratogenicity of cisplatin (4).

Only nine cases of cisplatin usage during pregnancy have been located (5–13). In one case, the mother, in her 10th week of gestation, received a single intravenous dose of 50 mg/kg for carcinoma of the uterine cervix (5). Two weeks later, a radical hysterectomy was performed. The male fetus was morphologically normal for its developmental age.

A 25-year-old woman underwent surgery at 25 weeks' gestation for an endodermal sinus tumor of the ovary (6). The chemotherapy cycle consisting of cisplatin (75 mg/m^2), vinblastine (0.25 mg/kg), and bleomycin (50 mg) was started 9 days later. Approximately 3 weeks later she received a second cycle of therapy. A normal, healthy 1900-g male infant was delivered by scheduled cesarean section at 32 weeks' gestation. The infant was alive and growing normally at the time of the report.

A 1989 case report described the effect of maternal chemotherapy on a premature newborn delivered at approximately 27 weeks' gestation (7). The mother had been treated with cisplatin (55 mg), bleomycin (30 mg), and etoposide (165 mg) (all given daily for 3 days), 1 week prior to delivery, for an unknown primary cancer with metastases to the eye and liver. The mother developed profound neutropenia just prior to delivery. On the 3rd day after birth, the 1190-g female infant also developed a profound leukopenia with neutropenia, 10 days after in utero exposure to the antineoplastic agents. The condition resolved after 10 days. At 10 days of age, the infant began losing her scalp hair along with a rapid loss of lanugo. Etoposide was thought to be the most likely cause of the neutropenia and the alopecia (7). By 12 weeks of age, substantial hair regrowth had occurred, and at 1-year follow-up, the child was developing normally except for moderate bilateral hearing loss. The investigators could not determine whether the sensorineural deafness was due to the maternal and/or neonatal gentamicin therapy or to the maternal cisplatin chemotherapy (7).

A third case of cisplatin usage during pregnancy involved a 28-year-old woman with advanced epithelial ovarian carcinoma (8). Following surgical treatment at 16 weeks' gestation, the patient was treated with cisplatin, 50 mg/m^2, and cyclophosphamide, 750 mg/m^2, every 21 days for seven cycles. Labor was induced at 37–38 weeks' gestation, resulting in the delivery of a healthy, 3275-g male infant. Height, weight, and head circumference were in the 75th–90th percentile. No abnormalities of the kidneys, liver, bone marrow, or auditory-evoked potential were found at birth, and the infant's physical and neurologic growth was normal at 19 months of age.

In a report similar to that above, a 24-year-old woman was treated during the 2nd trimester of pregnancy for epithelial ovarian carcinoma (9). Surgery was performed at 15.5 weeks' gestation, followed by five courses of chemotherapy consisting of cisplatin (100 mg/m^2) and cyclophosphamide (600 mg/m^2 $\times$ 2, 1000 mg/m^2 $\times$ 3). Spontaneous rupture of membranes occurred just prior to the sixth course of chemotherapy at 36.5 weeks' gestation, and she delivered a normal-appearing, 3060-g male infant, who, except for initial mild respiratory distress, has developed normally as of 28 months of age.

A 21-year-old woman with a dysgerminoma was treated surgically at 26 weeks' gestation, followed approximately 1 week later with cisplatin, 20 mg/m^2, and etoposide, 100 mg/m^2, daily for 5 days at 3- to 4-week intervals (10). A healthy, 2320-g female infant was delivered at 38 weeks. The infant is developing normally at 9 months of age.

Three treatments of cisplatin (75 mg/m^2; total dose 330 mg) were administered at 22, 25, and 28 weeks' gestation to a 34-year-old woman with a rapidly progressing cervical cancer (11). A cesarean section was performed at 32 weeks' gestation with delivery of a normal, 2120-g male infant, who was doing well at 12 months of age.

A 35-year-old woman with metastatic non-small-cell lung cancer was treated in the 1st and 2nd trimesters with chemotherapy of an unknown pregnancy (12). After undergoing a craniotomy to remove the metastatic tumor and whole brain irradiation early in pregnancy, she was treated with docetaxel and cisplatin on days 1 and 8 every 21 days for four cycles (gestational weeks 9–18). Because of lack of response, treatment was changed to two cycles of gemcitabine and cisplatin (gestational weeks 19 and 22). About 2 months after the last dose her pregnancy was diagnosed. At 33 weeks'gestation, a cesarean section delivered a normal 1490-g female infant (normal karyotype 46,XX) with Apgar scores of 8, 9, and 10 at 1, 5, and 10 minutes, respectively, and normal blood counts. An extensive examination of the infant failed to find any abnormalities. The infant was developing normally at 10 months of age (12).

A 32-year-old woman underwent surgery at 20 weeks' gestation (from in vitro fertilization) for a ruptured ovarian cyst (13). Ovarian cancer was diagnosed and she was given four cycles of docetaxel and cisplatin before a cesarean section at 34 weeks. The 2245-g female infant had Apgar scores of 3 and 6 at 1 and 10 minutes, respectively. The infant died at 5 days of age from multiple congenital anomalies that had been diagnosed before starting chemotherapy (13).

The long-term effects of cisplatin and other antineoplastic agents on menstrual function in females and reproductive function in females and males after treatment of various cancers have been described (14–16). Of the 76 women studied, cisplatin was used in 9 and in 25 men, cisplatin had been given to 4. The results of one of these studies (14) have been discussed in the monograph for cyclophosphamide (see Cyclophosphamide). In the second report, a normal-term infant was delivered from a woman treated with cisplatin, etoposide, dactinomycin, and intrathecal methotrexate 2 years prior to conception for choriocarcinoma (15). Similarly, no congenital malformations were observed in seven liveborn offspring of four males and two females treated with cisplatin during childhood or adolescence (16).

A 1996 report described successful pregnancy outcomes in 14 women who had been treated prior to conception for ovarian germ cell tumors with a chemotherapy regimen (POMB/ACE) consisting of cisplatin (120 mg/m^2), vincristine, methotrexate, bleomycin, dactinomycin, cyclophosphamide, and etoposide (17). No congenital malformations were observed.

Reversible azoospermia occurred in a male treated for teratoma of the testis with cisplatin, vinblastine, bleomycin, surgery, and radiation (18). Fifteen months after the end of therapy, the sperm count was <50,000 sperm/micro-L with 70% motile and a high percentage of abnormal forms. Three months later, the patient and his wife reported a pregnancy, which was terminated on their request.

A significant reduction in reproductive organ weights, sperm counts, sperm motility, fertility, and levels of testosterone, luteinizing hormone and follicle-stimulating hormone occurred in male rats treated with cisplatin 1 week prior to mating (19). After mating, a significant preimplantation loss and lower fetal weights in comparison with controls were observed.

Occupational exposure of the mother to antineoplastic agents during pregnancy may present a risk to the fetus. A position statement from the National Study Commission on Cytotoxic Exposure and a research article involving some antineoplastic agents are presented in the monograph for cyclophosphamide (see Cyclophosphamide).

BREASTFEEDING SUMMARY

Three studies, two with opposite results from the third, have examined the excretion of cisplatin into human milk. In a 1985 study, a 31-year-old woman, 7 months postpartum with ovarian cancer, was treated with doxorubicin and cisplatin (20). Doxorubicin (90 mg) was given IV over 15 minutes followed by IV cisplatin (130 mg, 100 mg/m^2) infused over 26 hours. Blood and milk samples were collected frequently for cisplatin determination from 0.25 to 71.25 hours after the start of the infusion. Peak plasma concentrations of platinum reached 2.99 mcg/mL, but platinum was undetectable (sensitivity 0.1 mcg/mL) in the milk.

Opposite results were obtained in a 1989 study (21). A 24-year-old woman with an entodermal sinus tumor of the left ovary was treated with cisplatin, 30 mg/m^2 IV for 4 hours daily, for 5 consecutive days. Etoposide and bleomycin were also administered during this time. On the 3rd day of therapy, milk and serum samples were collected 30 minutes before the cisplatin dose was administered. Cisplatin concentrations in the milk and plasma were 0.9 and 0.8 mcg/mL, respectively, a milk:plasma ratio of 1.1. The infant was not allowed to breastfeed.

In the third study, cisplatin measured in breast milk was in the range of 0.1–0.15 mcg/mL (over 2 hours), with a milk:plasma ratio of about 0.1 over an 18-hour sampling period (22). The woman, who was still lactating 2 years after her last delivery, was treated with six courses of cisplatin (100 mg/course) and cyclophosphamide (1600 mg/course) for ovarian cancer.

The American Academy of Pediatrics did not cite either of these latter two studies and classifies cisplatin as compatible with breastfeeding (23). However, based on the two reports, breastfeeding during cisplatin therapy should be considered contraindicated.

References

1. Product information. Platinol. Bristol-Myers Squibb Oncology/Immunology Division, 1997.
2. Diwan BA, Anderson LM, Ward JM, Henneman JR, Rice JM. Transplacental carcinogenesis by cisplatin in F344/NCr rats: promotion of kidney tumors by postnatal administration of sodium barbital. Toxicol Appl Pharmacol 1995;132:115–21.
3. Giurgiovich AJ, Diwan BA, Lee KB, Anderson LM, Rice JM, Poirier MC. Cisplatin-DNA adduct formation in maternal and fetal rat tissues after transplacental cisplatin exposure. Carcinogenesis 1996;17:1665–9.
4. Wiebe VJ, Sipila PEH. Pharmacology of antineoplastic agents in pregnancy. Crit Rev Oncol Hematol 1994;16:75–112.
5. Jacobs AJ, Marchevsky A, Gordon RE, Deppe G, Cohen CJ. Oat cell carcinoma of the uterine cervix in a pregnant woman treated with cis-diamminedichloroplatinum. Gynecol Oncol 1980;9:405–10.
6. Malone JM, Gershenson DM, Creasy RK, Kavanagh JJ, Silva EG, Stringer CA. Endodermal sinus tumor of the ovary associated with pregnancy. Obstet Gynecol 1986;68(Suppl):86S–9S.

7. Raffles A, Williams J, Costeloe K, Clark P. Transplacental effects of maternal cancer chemotherapy: case report. Br J Obstet Gynaecol 1989;96:1099–100.
8. Malfetano JH, Goldkrand JW. Cis-platinum combination chemotherapy during pregnancy for advanced epithelial ovarian carcinoma. Obstet Gynecol 1990;75:545–7.
9. King LA, Nevin PC, Williams PP, Carson LF. Treatment of advanced epithelial ovarian carcinoma in pregnancy with cisplatin-based chemotherapy. Gynecol Oncol 1991;41:78–80.
10. Buller RE, Darrow V, Manetta A, Porto M, DiSaia PJ. Conservative surgical management of dysgerminoma concomitant with pregnancy. Obstet Gynecol 1992;79:887–90.
11. Giacalone P-L, Laffargue F, Benos P, Rousseau O, Hedon B. Cis-platinum neoadjuvant chemotherapy in a pregnant woman with invasive carcinoma of the uterine cervix. Br J Obstet Gynaecol 1996;103:932–4.
12. Kim JH, Kim HS, Sung CW, Kim KJ, Kim CH, Lee KY. Docetaxel, gemcitabine, and cisplatin administered for non-small cell lung cancer during the first and second trimester of an unrecognized pregnancy. Lung Cancer 2008;59:270–3.
13. Rouzi AA, Sahly NN, Sahly NF, Alahwal MS. Cisplatinum and docetaxel for ovarian cancer in pregnancy. Arch Gynecol Obstet 2009;280:823–5.
14. Gershenson DM. Menstrual and reproductive function after treatment with combination chemotherapy for malignant ovarian germ cell tumors. J Clin Oncol 1988;6:270–5.
15. Bakri Y, Pedersen P, Nassar M. Normal pregnancy after curative multiagent chemotherapy for choriocarcinoma with brain metastases. Acta Obstet Gynecol Scand 1991;70:611–3.
16. Green DM, Zevon MA, Lowrie G, Seigelstein N, Hall B. Congenital anomalies in children of patients who received chemotherapy for cancer in childhood and adolescence. N Engl J Med 1991;325:141–6.
17. Bower, M, Fife K, Holden L, Paradinas FJ, Rustin GJS, Newlands ES. Chemotherapy for ovarian germ cell tumours. Eur J Cancer 1996;32A: 593–7.
18. Rubery ED. Return of fertility after curative chemotherapy for disseminated teratoma of testis. Lancet 1983;1:186.
19. Kinkead T, Flores C, Carboni AA, Menon M, Seethalakshmi L. Short term effects of cis-platinum on male reproduction, fertility and pregnancy outcome. J Urol 1992;147:201–6.
20. Egan PC, Costanza ME, Dodion P, Egorin MJ, Bachur NR. Doxorubicin and cisplatin excretion into human milk. Cancer Treat Rep 1985;69:1387–9.
21. De Vries EGE, Van Der Zee AGJ, Uges DRA, Sleijfer DTH. Excretion of platinum into breast milk. Lancet 1989;1:497.
22. Ben-Baruch G, Menczer J, Goshen R, Kaufman B, Gorodetsky R. Cisplatin excretion in human milk. J Natl Cancer Inst 1992;84:451–2.
23. Committee on Drugs, American Academy of Pediatrics. The transfer of drugs and other chemicals into human milk. Pediatrics 2001;198: 776–89.

C

CITALOPRAM

Antidepressant

PREGNANCY RECOMMENDATION: Human Data Suggest Risk in 3rd Trimester
BREASTFEEDING RECOMMENDATION: Limited Human Data—Potential Toxicity

PREGNANCY SUMMARY

Citalopram does not appear to be a major human teratogen. Only one of the studies below observed an increase in defects or pattern of major anomalies over that expected in a nonexposed population. (See Paroxetine.) However, selective serotonin reuptake inhibitor (SSRI) antidepressants, including citalopram, have been associated with several developmental toxicities, including spontaneous abortions (SABs), low birth weight, prematurity, neonatal serotonin syndrome, neonatal behavioral syndrome (withdrawal), possibly sustained abnormal neurobehavior beyond the neonatal period, respiratory distress, and persistent pulmonary hypertension of the newborn (PPHN).

FETAL RISK SUMMARY

The antidepressant, citalopram, is an SSRI that has a chemical structure unrelated to those of other antidepressants (1). All the antidepressant agents in this class (citalopram, escitalopram, fluoxetine, fluvoxamine, paroxetine, and sertraline) share a similar mechanism of action, although they have different chemical structures. These differences could be construed as evidence against any conclusion that they share similar effects on the embryo, fetus, or newborn. In the mouse embryo, however, craniofacial morphogenesis appears to be regulated, at least in part, by serotonin. Interference with serotonin regulation by chemically different inhibitors produces similar craniofacial defects (2). Regardless of the structural differences, therefore, some of the potential adverse effects on the pregnancy may also be similar.

Both mating and fertility were reduced in male and female rats at oral doses approximately five times the maximum recommended human daily dose of 60 mg/day based on BSA (MRHD). The duration of gestation was increased at approximately eight times the MRHD. Citalopram demonstrated dose-related embryo and fetal growth restriction, reduced survival, and teratogenicity in rats dosed during organogenesis at about 18 times the MRHD (1). Fetal malformations included cardiovascular and skeletal defects, but the dose was maternal toxic (clinical signs, decreased weight gain). The developmental no-effect dose was about nine times the MRHD. In contrast, no developmental adverse effects were observed in the offspring of pregnant rabbits given doses up to about five times the MRHD (1).

Increased offspring mortality during the first 4 days after birth and persistent growth restriction were observed when pregnant rats were dosed at about five times the MRHD throughout gestation and early lactation. Similar effects were observed with doses about four times the MRHD in late gestation through weaning. The no-effect dose in this group was about twice the MRHD (1).

In an in vitro experiment using a single placental cotyledon, both citalopram and its metabolite desmethylcitalopram crossed to the fetal side (3). The mean steady-state placental transfer for the two compounds was 9.1% and 5.6%, respectively. A 2003 study of the placental transfer of antidepressants found cord blood:maternal serum ratios for citalopram and its metabolite that were 0.17–1.42 and

C

0.50–1.00, respectively (4). The dose-to-delivery interval was 14–48 hours, with the highest ratio for the parent drug and metabolite occurring at 48 hours.

In a 2002 study, 11 women took citalopram (20–40 mg/day) during pregnancy; 10 throughout gestation and 1 starting at 20 weeks' gestation (5). The mean ratio of two metabolites was significantly higher during pregnancy than at 2 months postdelivery, indicating induction of the CYP2D6 isoenzyme (5). The trough plasma concentrations of citalopram, desmethylcitalopram, and didesmethylcitalopram in the normal newborns were 64%, 66%, and 68% of the maternal concentrations, respectively. The neurodevelopment of the infants up to the age of 1 year was normal (5). All infants were breastfed (see Breastfeeding Summary).

Citalopram is at least eight times more potent in the inhibition of serotonin reuptake than its four metabolites (1). It has an elimination half-life of approximately 35 hours. This is in the same general range as the other SSRI agents with weakly active or inactive metabolites (elimination half-lives of parent compounds in parentheses): fluvoxamine (15.6 hours), paroxetine (21 hours), and sertraline (26 hours). All have much shorter elimination half-lives than fluoxetine (4–6 days) or fluoxetine's active metabolite (4–16 days).

A brief 1993 case report described a woman who was treated with citalopram for major depression during the first 6 weeks of an undiagnosed pregnancy (6). She received 40 mg/day during the first 3 weeks, and then the dose was increased to 60 mg/day. She also took several other drugs for coexisting panic disorder and migraine headaches. All medication was stopped in the sixth week of gestation when the pregnancy was diagnosed. Because of her deteriorating mental status and anxiety concerning fetal development, she requested an abortion, which was performed at 12 weeks' gestation. At autopsy, a thorough macroscopic and microscopic evaluation, including a detailed neuropathological examination, found no evidence of malformation (6).

Five male infants exposed to citalopram (30 mg/day), paroxetine (10–40 mg/day), or fluoxetine (20 mg/day) during gestation exhibited withdrawal symptoms at or within a few days of birth and lasting up to 1 month (7). Symptoms included irritability, constant crying, shivering, increased tonus, eating and sleeping problems, and convulsions.

A 2004 prospective study examined the effect of four SSRIs (citalopram, fluoxetine, paroxetine, and sertraline) on newborn neurobehavior, including behavioral state, sleep organization, motor activity, heart rate variability, tremulousness, and startles (8). Seventeen SSRI-exposed, healthy, full-birth-weight newborns and 17 nonexposed, matched controls were studied. A wide range of disrupted neurobehavioral outcomes were shown in the subject infants. After adjustment for gestational age, the exposed infants were found to differ significantly from controls in terms of tremulousness, behavioral states, and sleep organization. The effects observed on motor activity, startles, and heart rate variability were not significant after adjustment (8).

A 2003 prospective study evaluated the pregnancy outcomes of 138 women treated with SSRIantidepressants during gestation (9). Women using each agent were 73 fluoxetine, 36 sertraline, 19 paroxetine, 7 citalopram, and 3 fluvoxamine. Most (62%) took an SSRI throughout pregnancy and 95% were taking an SSRI at delivery. Birth complications were observed in 28 infants, including preterm birth (9 cases), meconium aspiration, nuchal cord, floppy at birth, and low birth weight. Four infants (2.9%) had low birth weight, all exposed to fluoxetine (40–80 mg/day) throughout pregnancy, including two of the three infants of mothers taking 80 mg/day. One infant had Hirschsprung disease, a major defect, and another had cavum septi pellucidi (neither the size of the cavum nor the SSRI agents were specified) (9). The clinical significance of the cavum septi pellucidi is doubtful as it is nearly always present at birth but resolves in the first several months (10).

The database of the World Health Organization (WHO) was used in a 2005 report on neonatal SSRI withdrawal syndrome (11). In this database, 93 suspected cases with either neonatal convulsions or withdrawal syndrome were identified in the WHO database. The agents were 63 paroxetine, 13 fluoxetine, 1 paroxetine plus fluoxetine, 9 sertraline, and 7 citalopram. The analysis suggested that paroxetine might have an increased risk of convulsions or withdrawal compared with other SSRIs (11).

Evidence for the neonatal behavioral syndrome that is associated with in utero exposure to SSRIs and serotonin and norepinephrine reuptake inhibitors (SNRIs) (collectively called serotonin reuptake inhibitors [SRIs]) in late pregnancy was reviewed in a 2005 reference (12). The report followed a recent agreement by the FDA and manufacturers for a class labeling change about the neonatal syndrome. Analysis of case reports, case series, and cohort studies revealed that late exposure to SRIs carried an overall risk ratio of 3.0 (95% confidence interval [CI] 2.0–4.4) for the syndrome compared with early exposure. The case reports (N = 18) and case series (N = 131) involved 97 cases of paroxetine, 18 fluoxetine, 16 sertraline, 12 citalopram, 4 venlafaxine, and 2 fluvoxamine. There were nine cohort studies analyzed. The typical neonatal syndrome consisted of central nervous system, motor, respiratory, and gastrointestinal signs that were mild and usually resolved within 2 weeks. Only one of 313 quantifiable cases involved a severe syndrome consisting of seizures, dehydration, excessive weight loss, hyperpyrexia, and intubation. There were no neonatal deaths attributable to the syndrome (12).

A significant increase in the risk of low birth weight (<10th percentile) and respiratory distress after prenatal exposure to SSRIs was reported in 2006 (13). The population-based study, representing all live births (N = 119,547) during a 39-month period in British Columbia, Canada, compared pregnancy outcomes of depressed mothers treated with SSRIs with outcomes in depressed mothers not treated with medication and in nonexposed controls. The severity of depression in the depressed groups was accounted for by propensity score matching (13).

A 30% incidence of SSRI-induced neonatal abstinence syndrome was found in a 2006 cohort study (14). Sixty neonates with prolonged in utero exposure to SSRIs were compared to nonexposed controls. The agents used were paroxetine (62%), fluoxetine (20%), citalopram (13%), venlafaxine (3%), and sertraline (2%). Assessment was conducted by the Finnegan score. Ten of the infants had mild and eight had severe symptoms of the syndrome. The maximum mean score in infants with severe symptoms occurred within 2 days of birth, but some occurred as long as 4 days after birth.

Because of the small numbers, a dose–response could only be conducted with paroxetine. Infants exposed to mean maternal doses that were <19 mg/day had no symptoms, <23 mg/day had mild symptoms, and 27 mg/day had severe symptoms (14).

A 2005 prospective comparative study of citalopram in pregnancy was reported in 2005 (15). Three groups, citalopram, disease, and nonteratogen, each containing 132 pregnant women were closely matched. In the citalopram group, 125 (95%) took the drug at least in the 1st trimester and 71 (54%) continued the drug throughout gestation. The outcomes in the citalopram-exposed pregnancies were 114 live births, 14 SABs, 2 elective abortions, and 2 stillbirths. One male infant, exposed during organogenesis, had a major anomaly (umbilical and scrotal hernia). There were no statistical differences among the three groups in terms of mean birth weight, structural defects, gestational age at birth, and fetal survival. However, for infants exposed in the 3rd trimester, there were increased risks for complications in general (relative risk [RR] 1.5, 95% CI 1.0–2.4) and for neonatal intensive care unit (NICU) admissions (RR 4.2, 95% CI 1.7–10.3) (i.e., poor neonatal adaptation syndrome) (15).

A meta-analysis of clinical trials (1990–2005) with SSRIs was reported in 2006 (16). The SSRI agents included were citalopram, fluoxetine, fluvoxamine, paroxetine, and sertraline. The specific outcomes analyzed were major, minor, and cardiac malformations, and SABs. The odd ratio [OR] with 95% CI for the four outcomes were 1.394 (0.906–2.145), 0.97 (0.13–6.93), 1.193 (0.531–2.677), and 1.70 (1.28–2.25), respectively. Only the risk of SABs was significantly increased (16).

A brief 2005 report described significant associations between the use of SSRIs in the 1st trimester and congenital defects (17). The data were collected by the CDC-sponsored National Birth Defects Prevention Study in an on-going case–control study of birth defect risk factors. Case infants (N = 5357) with major birth defects were compared with 3366 normal controls. A positive association was found with omphalocele (N = 161; OR 3.0, 95% CI 1.4–6.1). Paroxetine, which accounted for 36% of all SSRI exposures, had the strongest association with the defect (OR 6.3, 95% CI 2.0–19.6). The study also found a significant association between the use of any SSRI and craniosynostosis (N = 372; OR 1.8, 95% CI 1.0–3.2) (17). An expanded report from this group was published in 2007 (see reference 25 below).

In 1999, the Swedish Medical Birth Registry compared the use of antidepressants in early pregnancy and delivery outcome for the years 1995–1997 (18). There were no significant differences for birth defects, infant survival, or risk of low birth weight (<2500 g) among singletons between those exposed to any depressant, SSRIs only, and non-SSRIs only, but a shorter gestational duration (<37 weeks) was observed for any antidepressant exposure (OR 1.43, 95% CI 1.14–1.80). Fifteen (4.0%) of the citalopram-exposed infants had anomalies, but one was a trisomy 13 syndrome and five were classified as uncertain anomalies (18). A second Registry report, published in 2006 covering the years 1995–2003, analyzed the relationship between antidepressants and major malformations and cardiac defects (19). There was no significant increase in the risk of major malformations with any antidepressant. The strongest effect among cardiac anomalies was with ventricular or atrial septum defects (VSDs-ASDs). Significant increases were found with paroxetine (OR 2.22, 95% CI 1.39–3.55) and clomipramine (OR 1.87, 95% CI 1.16–2.99 (19). In 2007, the analysis was expanded to include the years 1995–2004 (20). There were 6481 women (6555 infants) who had reported the use of SSRIs in early pregnancy. The number of women using a single SSRI during the 1st trimester was 2579 citalopram, 1807 sertraline, 908 paroxetine, 860 fluoxetine, 66 escitalopram, and 36 fluvoxamine. After adjustment, only paroxetine was significantly associated with an increased risk of cardiac defects (N = 13, RR 2.62, 95% CI 1.40–4.50) or VSDs-ASDs (N = 8, RR 3.07, 95% CI 1.32–6.04). Analysis of the combined SSRI group, excluding paroxetine, revealed no associations with cardiac defects or VSDs-ASDs. The study also found no association with omphalocele or craniostenosis (20).

A 2007 study evaluated the association between 1st-trimester exposure to paroxetine and cardiac defects by quantifying the dose–response relationship (21). A population-based pregnancy registry was used by linking three administrative databases so that it included all pregnancies in Quebec between 1997 and 2003. There were 101 infants with major congenital defects, 24 involving the heart, among the 1403 women using only one type of antidepressant during the 1st trimester. The use of paroxetine or other SSRIs did not significantly increase the risk of major defects or cardiac defects compared with non-SSRI antidepressants. However, a paroxetine dose >25 mg/day during the 1st trimester was significantly associated with an increased risk of major defects (OR 2.23, 95% CI 1.19–4.17) and of cardiac defects (OR 3.07, 95% CI 1.00–9.42) (21).

A 2007 retrospective cohort study examined the effects of exposure to SSRIs or venlafaxine in the 3rd trimester on 21 premature and 55 term newborns (22). The randomly selected unexposed control group consisted of 90 neonates of mothers not taking antidepressants, psychotropic agents, or benzodiazepines at the time of delivery. There were significantly more premature infants among the subjects (27.6%) than in controls (8.9%), but the groups were not matched. The antidepressants, number of subjects, and daily doses in the exposed group were paroxetine (46; 5—40 mg), fluoxetine (10; 10–40 mg), venlafaxine (9; 74–150 mg), citalopram (6; 10–30 mg), sertraline (3; 125–150 mg), and fluvoxamine (2; 50–150 mg). The behavioral signs that were significantly increased in exposed compared with nonexposed infants were central nervous system (CNS) —abnormal movements, shaking, spasms, agitation, hypotonia, hypertonia, irritability, and insomnia; respiratory system—indrawing, apnea/bradycardia, and tachypnea; and other—vomiting, tachycardia, and jaundice. In exposed infants, CNS (63.2%) and respiratory system (40.8%) signs were most common, appearing during the first day of life and lasting for a median duration of 3 days. All of the exposed premature infants exhibited behavioral signs compared with 69.1% of exposed term infants. The duration of hospitalization was significantly longer in exposed premature compared with nonexposed premature infants, 14.5 days vs. 3.7 days, respectively. In 75% of the term and premature infants, the signs resolved within 3 and 5 days, respectively. There were six infants in each group with congenital malformations, but the drugs involved were not specified (22).

A 2007 review conducted a literature search to determine the risk of major congenital malformations after 1st trimester exposure to SSRIs and SNRIs (23). Fifteen controlled studies were analyzed. The data were adequate to suggest that citalopram, fluoxetine, sertraline, and venlafaxine were not associated with an increased risk of congenital defects. In contrast, the analysis did suggest an increased risk with paroxetine. The data were inadequate to determine the risk for the other SSRIs and SNRIs (23).

A case–control study, published in 2006, was conducted to test the hypothesis that exposure to SSRIs in late pregnancy was associated with persistent pulmonary hypertension of the newborn (24). A total of 1213 women were enrolled in the study, 377 cases whose infants had PPHN and 836 matched controls and their infants. Mothers were interviewed by nurses who were blinded to the hypothesis. Fourteen case infants had been exposed to an SSRI after the 20th week of gestation compared with six control infants (adjusted odds ratio 6.1, 95% CI 2.2–16.8). The numbers were too small to analyze the effects of dosage, SSRI used, or reduction of the length of exposure before delivery. No increased risk of PPHN was found with the use of SSRIs before the 20th week or with the use of non-SSRI antidepressants at any time in pregnancy. If the relationship was causal, the absolute risk was estimated to be about 1% (24).

Two large case–control studies assessing associations between SSRIs and major birth defects were published in 2007 (25,26). The findings related to SSRIs as a group, as well as to four specific agents: citalopram, fluoxetine, paroxetine, and sertraline. One of the studies did find a significant association between citalopram and a group of defects (anencephaly, craniosynostosis, and omphalocele) (25). An accompanying editorial discussed the findings and limitations of these and other related studies (27). Details of the studies and the editorial are described in the paroxetine review (see Paroxetine).

A prospective cohort study evaluated a large group of pregnancies exposed to antidepressants in the 1st trimester to determine if there was an association with major malformations (28). The patient population came from the Motherisk database and involved 928 cases that met their criteria. The 928 matched (for age, smoking, and alcohol use) controls were pregnancies not exposed to antidepressants or known teratogens. In addition to the 184 citalopram cases, the other cases were 113 bupropion, 21 escitalopram, 61 fluoxetine, 52 fluvoxamine, 68 mirtazapine, 39 nefazodone, 148 paroxetine, 61 sertraline, 17 trazodone, and 154 venlafaxine. In the antidepressant group, there were 24 (2.5%) major defects compared with 25 (2.6%) in controls (odds ratio 0.9, 95% CI 0.5–1.61). There were eight major anomalies in the citalopram group: umbilical hernia, duplex kidney, club foot, pyloric stenosis, neural tube defect, atrial septal defect, congenital pneumothorax, and hypospadias. There were no major defects in the pregnancies exposed to bupropion, escitalopram, or trazodone (28).

BREASTFEEDING SUMMARY

Citalopram is excreted into human milk. A 1997 report described breast milk concentrations of the antidepressant in two lactating women under treatment for depression and one healthy lactating volunteer (29). All three subjects were extensive metabolizers of citalopram with respect to the liver enzymes (CYP2C19 and CYP2D6) involved in the metabolism of the drug. The two women with depression were being treated with 20 mg/day and 40 mg/day at 2 and 4 months postpartum, respectively. The healthy volunteer was given a single dose of 40 mg at 10 months postpartum. The milk:serum ratio in the two women ranged from 1.16 to 1.88, whereas in the volunteer, the ratio was 1.00, based on the AUC. The dose ingested by an infant was calculated to range from 4.3 to 17.6 mcg/kg/day (0.7%–5.9% of the weight-adjusted maternal dose) in the two women on chronic therapy, and 11.2 mcg/kg/day (1.8% of the weight-adjusted maternal dose based on AUC) in the volunteer. The two mothers on chronic therapy observed no adverse effects in their nursing infants. Compared with other SSRI antidepressants, the relative dose to the infant from citalopram (0.7%–5.9%) was comparable to fluoxetine and its active metabolite (1.2%–6.5%) but higher than that for fluvoxamine (0.5%), sertraline (0.45%), and paroxetine (0.34%). Based on these data, the authors recommended that caution should be used with the administration of citalopram during lactation (29).

In a second 1997 report, a 21-year-old mother developed severe depression 2 months after delivery of a female infant and was begun on citalopram (30). Blood and milk samples were collected after 8 days of a continuous 20 mg/day dose. The mean milk:serum ratio over a 24-hour period was approximately 3 for both citalopram and its inactive metabolite. The estimated citalopram weight-adjusted infant dose was 4.8% of the mother's dose. After 3 weeks of therapy, the citalopram serum concentration in the infant was about 1/15th of the mother's trough level; the metabolite was undetectable. The levels indicated that no accumulation of citalopram or the metabolite occurred in the infant. No adverse effects or unusual behavior were observed in the infant (30).

A 2000 report measured citalopram concentrations in the milk and plasma of seven women who were nursing their infants (mean age 4.1 months) (31). The median citalopram dose was 0.36 mg/kg/day. The mean milk:plasma ratios of citalopram and the metabolite, desmethylcitalopram, were 1.8 (range 1.2–3) and 1.8 (range 1.0–2.5), respectively. Citalopram was detected in the plasma of three infants (2.0–2.3 ng/mL), two of which also had detectable levels of the metabolite (2.2 ng/mL). The mean combined dose of citalopram and metabolite (expressed as a percentage of the maternal weight-normalized dose) was 4.4%–5.1%. No adverse effects were observed in the infants and all had normal Denver developmental quotients (31).

A 29-year-old woman, 4 weeks after delivery, was started on citalopram (40 mg/day) for postpartum depression (32). Eight days later, single samples of milk and maternal serum (time from last dose not specified) yielded concentrations of 205 ng/mL and 98.9 ng/mL, respectively. Uneasy sleep was noted in the breastfed infant starting about 2–3 days after initiation of drug therapy. The citalopram concentration in the infant's serum after 16 days of maternal therapy was 12.7 ng/mL. Reducing the dose to 20 mg/day and substituting two breastfeedings with artificial nutrition normalized the infant's sleeping. One week later, the serum concentrations of citalopram in the mother and infant were 49.0 ng/mL and 4.5 ng/mL, respectively (32).

C

In their product information, the manufacturer describes two infants with excessive somnolence, decreased feeding, and weight loss associated with nursing from mothers receiving citalopram (1). Both cases involved reports to the manufacturer that apparently were not published. Although the information is incomplete, the manufacturer was able to obtain partial details of these cases (G. Fagen, personal communication, Forrest Pharmaceuticals, 2000). One full-term infant was born to a Danish woman who had been started on citalopram, 40 mg/day, shortly before delivery. The infant was presumably breastfed. When the adverse effects were noted 3–4 days after birth, the mother stopped the drug. The infant made a full recovery. The second case involved an 8-day-old Swedish baby who developed tiredness, weight loss, and decreased suckling. The mother had started taking citalopram, 20 mg/day, approximately 1 year earlier. She was also taking an antihistamine. Five days before the onset of the adverse symptoms, without medical advice, she increased her dose to 30 mg/day. A single milk sample (timing in relationship to the dose not specified) yielded a drug concentration of 377 nmol/L (about 0.122 mcg/mL) (1 mol of citalopram = 324.4 g (23)). The concentration of the metabolite was 111 nmol/L. These amounts are very close to those reported in the above published cases. No other details of the case were available, although it is known that the infant was doing well at 4 years of age.

Nine women treated with citalopram during pregnancy (see Fetal Risk Summary) continued to use the antidepressant while nursing their infants (5). Maternal plasma concentrations of the parent compound and metabolites demonstrated a tendency to rise at 2 weeks and 2 months postpartum. The milk:plasma ratios for citalopram, desmethylcitalopram, and didesmethylcitalopram ranged from 1.2 to 3.3, 1.3 to 4.1, and 1.1 to 4.6, respectively. In contrast, the infant plasma concentrations of the parent compound and two metabolites at various intervals up to 2 months of age all declined from those measured at birth. The weight and neurodevelopment of the infants up to 1 year of age were normal (5).

A prospective, observational cohort study designed to determine the frequency of adverse effects in nursing infants exposed to citalopram in milk was published in 2004 (33). Three groups of nursing women were formed: 31 women who were depressed and taking citalopram; 12 women who were depressed but who were taking other SSRI antidepressants; and 31 healthy women matched to the first group by maternal age and parity. There was no statistically significant difference in the rate of adverse events among the nursing infants in the three groups (3/31 events, 0/12 events, and 1/31 events, respectively). In the citalopram group, two of the events were colic and decreased feeding, but both were considered nonspecific and insignificant and did not require intervention. The third event involved irritability and restlessness that were observed in the infant when the mother started citalopram at 2 months postpartum. Breastfeeding was stopped after 2 weeks and the symptoms resolved (33).

A 2004 study was conducted in 25 women (nursing 26 infants) to quantify the concentration of the SSRI or SNRI in their breast milk (34). The antidepressants taken by the women were citalopram (nine mothers/10 infants), paroxetine (six), sertraline (six), fluoxetine (one), and venlafaxine (three). The maternal mean dose of citalopram was 24 mg/day (20–50 mg/day). The mean milk concentration was 389 nmol/L (157–725 nmol/L, resulting in a theoretical maximum infant dose that was 5.2% of the mother's weight-adjusted dose. Citalopram was detected in six of the infants serum (mean 1.9 nmol/L, range 0–8 nmol/L). There was no evidence of adverse effects in the breastfeeding infants (34).

A 2010 study using human and animal models found that drugs that disturb serotonin balance such as SSRIs and SNRIs can impair lactation (35). The authors concluded that mothers taking these drugs may need additional support to achieve breastfeeding goals.

A 1999 review of SSRI agents concluded that if there were compelling reasons to treat a mother for postpartum depression, a condition in which a rapid antidepressant effect is important, the benefits of therapy with SSRIs would most likely outweigh the risks (36). Nevertheless, nursing women receiving citalopram, in particular those taking doses >20 mg/day or concurrently with other sedative agents, should be warned of the potential for toxicity in their infants. Moreover, the long-term consequences of exposure to SSRI antidepressants in breast milk on the infant's neurobehavior development are unknown (no such adverse effects have been reported to date, but additional research is needed). Avoiding nursing around the time of peak maternal concentrations (about 4 hours after a dose) may limit infant exposure. However, the long elimination half-lives of all SSRIs and their weakly basic properties, which are conducive to ion trapping in the relatively acidic milk, probably will lessen the effectiveness of this strategy. The American Academy of Pediatrics classifies other SSRIs as drugs whose effect on the nursing infant is unknown but may be of concern (see Fluoxetine, Fluvoxamine, Paroxetine, and Sertraline).

References

1. Product information. Celexa. Forest Pharmaceuticals, 2000.
2. Shuey DL, Sadler TW, Lauder JM. Serotonin as a regulator of craniofacial morphogenesis: site specific malformations following exposure to serotonin uptake inhibitors. Teratology 1992;46:367–78.
3. Heikkinen T, Ekblad U, Laine K. Transplacental transfer of citalopram, fluoxetine and their primary demethylated metabolites in isolated perfused human placenta. BJOG 2002;109:1003–8.
4. Hendrick V, Stowe ZN, Altshuler LL, Hwang S, Lee E, Haynes D. Placental passage of antidepressant medications. Am J Psychiatry 2003;160:993–6.
5. Heikkinen T, Ekblad U, Kero P, Ekblad S, Laine K. Citalopram in pregnancy and lactation. Clin Pharmacol Ther 2002;72:184–91.
6. Seifritz E, Holsboer-Trachsler E, Haberthur F, Hemmeter U, Poldinger W. Unrecognized pregnancy during citalopram treatment. Am J Psychiatry 1993;150:1428–9.
7. Nordeng H, Lindemann R, Perminov KV, Reikvam A. Neonatal withdrawal syndrome after in utero exposure to selective serotonin reuptake inhibitors. Acta Paediatr 2001;90:288–91.
8. Zeskind PS, Stephens LE. Maternal selective serotonin reuptake inhibitor use during pregnancy and newborn neurobehavior. Pediatrics 2004;113: 368–75.
9. Hendrick V, Smith LM, Suri R, Hwang S, Haynes D, Altshuler L. Birth outcomes after prenatal exposure to antidepressant medication. Am J Obstet Gynecol 2003;188:812–5.
10. DeMyer W. Brain, midline caves. In: Buyse ML, Editor-in-Chief. *Birth Defects Encyclopedia*. Cambridge, MA: Blackwell Scientific Publications, 1990:238.
11. Sanz EJ, De-las-Cuevas C, Kiuru A, Edwards R. Selective serotonin reuptake inhibitors in pregnant women and neonatal withdrawal syndrome: a database analysis. Lancet 2005;365:482–7.
12. Moses-Kolko EL, Bogen D, Perel J, Bregar A, Uhl K, Levin B, Wisner KL. Neonatal signs after late in utero exposure to serotonin reuptake inhibitors. JAMA 2005;293:2372–83.
13. Oberlander TF, Warburton W, Misri S, Aghajanian J, Hertzman C. Neonatal outcomes after prenatal exposure to selective serotonin reuptake inhibitor antidepressants and maternal depression using population-based linked health data. Arch Gen Psychiatry 2006;63:898–906.

14. Levinson-Castiel R, Merlob P, Linder N, Sirota L, Klinger G. Neonatal abstinence syndrome after in utero exposure to selective serotonin reuptake inhibitors in term infants. Arch Pediatr Adoles Med 2006;160:173–6.
15. Sivojelezova A, Shuhaiber S, Sarkissian L, Einarson A, Koren G. Citalopram use in pegnancy: prospective comparative evaluation of pregnancy and fetal outcome. Am J Obstet Gynecol 2005;193:2004–9.
16. Rahimi R, Nikfar S, Abdollahi M. Pregnancy outcomes following exposure to serotonin reuptake inhibitors: a meta-analysis of clinical trials. Reprod Toxicol 2006;22:571–5.
17. Alwan S, Reefhuis J, Rasmussen S, Olney R, Friedman JM. Maternal use of selective serotonin reuptake inhibitors and risk for birth defects (abstract). Birth Defects Res (Part A) 2005;73:291.
18. Ericson A, Kallen B, Wiholm BE. Delivery outcome after the use of antidepressants in early pregnancy. Eur J Clin Pharmacol 1999;55:503–8.
19. Kallen B, Olausson PO. Antidepressant drugs during pregnancy and infant congenital heart defect. Reprod Toxicol 2006;21:221–2.
20. Kallen BAJ, Olausson PO. Maternal use of selective serotonin re-uptake inhibitors in early pregnancy and infant congenital malformations. Birth Defects Res (Part A) 2007;79:301–8.
21. Berard A, Ramos E, Rey E, Blais L, St Andre M, Oraichi D. First trimester exposure to paroxetine and risk of cardiac malformations in infants: the importance of dosage. Birth Defects Res (Part B) 2007;80:18–27.
22. Ferreira E, Carceller AM, Agogue C, Martin BZ, St-Andre M, Francoeur D, Berard A. Effects of selective serotonin reuptake inhibitors and venlafaxine during pregnancy in term and preterm neonates. Pediatrics 2007;119:52–9.
23. Bellantuono C, Migliarese G, Gentile S. Serotonin reuptake inhibitors in pregnancy and the risk of major malformations: a systematic review. Hum Psychopharmacol Clin Exp 2007;22:121–8.
24. Chambers CD, Hernandez-Diaz S, Van Marter LJ, Werler MM, Louik C, Jones KL, Mitchell AA. Selective serotonin-reuptake inhibitors and risk of persistent pulmonary hypertension of the newborn. N Engl J Med 2006;354:579–87.
25. Alwan S, Reefhuis J, Rasmussen SA, Olney RS, Friedman JM, for the National Birth Defects Prevention Study. Use of selective serotonin-reuptake inhibitors in pregnancy and the risk of birth defects. N Engl J Med 2007;356:2684–92.
26. Louik C, Lin AE, Werler MM, Hernandez-Diaz S, Mitchell AA. First-trimester use of selective serotonin-reuptake inhibitors and the risk of birth defects. N Engl J Med 2007;356:2675–83.
27. Greene MF. Teratogenicity of SSRIs—serious concern or much ado about little? N Engl J Med 2007;356:2732–3.
28. Einarson A, Choi J, Einarson TR, Koren G. Incidence of major malformations in infants following antidepressant exposure in pregnancy: results of a large prospective cohort study. Can J Psychiatry 2009;54:242–6.
29. Spigset O, Carleborg L, Ohman R, Norstrom A. Excretion of citalopram in breast milk. Br J Clin Pharmacol 1997;44:295–8.
30. Jensen PN, Olesen OV, Bertelsen A, Linnet K. Citalopram and desmethylcitalopram concentrations in breast milk and in serum of mother and infant. Therap Drug Monitor 1997;19:236–9.
31. Rampono J, Kristensen JH, Hackett LP, Paech M, Kohan R, Ilett KF. Citalopram and demethylcitalopram in human milk; distribution, excretion and effects in breast fed infants. Br J Clin Pharmacol 2000;50:263–8.
32. Schmidt K, Olesen OV, Jensen PN. Citalopram and breast-feeding: serum concentration and side effects in the infant. Biol Psychiatry 2000;47: 164–5.
33. Lee A, Woo J, Ito S. Frequency of infant adverse events that are associated with citalopram use during breast-feeding. Am J Obstet Gynecol 2004;190:218–21.
34. Berle JO, Steen VM, Aamo TO, Breilid H, Zahlsen K, Spigset O. Breastfeeding during maternal antidepressant treatment with serotonin reuptake inhibitors: infant exposure, clinical symptoms, and cytochrome P450 genotypes. J Clin Psychiatry 2004;65:1228–34.
35. Marshall AM, Nommsen-Rivers LA, Hernandez LI, Dewey KG, Chantry CJ, Gregerson KA, Horseman ND. Serotonin transport and metabolism in the mammary gland modulates secretory activation and involution. J Clin Endocrin Metab 2010;95:837–46.
36. Edwards JG, Anderson I. Systematic review and guide to selection of selective serotonin reuptake inhibitors. Drugs 1999;57:507–33.

CLADRIBINE

Antineoplastic

PREGNANCY RECOMMENDATION: Contraindicated
BREASTFEEDING RECOMMENDATION: Contraindicated

PREGNANCY SUMMARY

No reports describing the use of cladribine in human pregnancy have been located. However, other drugs that inhibit DNA synthesis (e.g., methotrexate and aminopterin) are known human teratogens. If possible, the drug should be avoided in pregnancy, especially during the 1st trimester. Because hairy cell leukemia usually has an indolent disease course, deferring treatment until after delivery may be appropriate (1).

FETAL RISK SUMMARY

The prodrug cladribine is a synthetic antineoplastic agent that is administered as a single course given by continuous IV infusion for 7 consecutive days. It is indicated for the treatment of active hairy cell leukemia as defined by clinically significant anemia, neutropenia, thrombocytopenia or disease-related symptoms. The drug is classified as an antimetabolite in the same subclass of purine analogs and related agents as clofarabine, fludarabine, mercaptopurine, pentostatin, and thioguanine. Cladribine undergoes intracellular metabolism to its active metabolite. About 20% is bound to plasma proteins and the mean terminal half-life is 5.4 hours (2).

Reproduction studies have been conducted in mice and rabbits (routes not specified but assumed to be oral). In mice, a significant increase in fetal variations was observed with a daily dose that was about 17 times the human dose based on body weight. The drug was embryotoxic in mice when given at doses equivalent to the human dose. When the daily dose was doubled, increased resorptions, reduced litter size, and fetal malformations were observed. Fetal death and malformations were observed in rabbits given a daily dose that was about 33 times the human dose based on body weight. The no-observed-effect-dose (NOEL) in these species was about 6 and 11 times the human dose, respectively (2).

Carcinogenic studies have not been conducted with cladribine. The drug was not mutagenic in various assays but was clastogenic. When given IV to monkeys, the drug caused suppression of rapidly generating cells, including testicular cells. The effect on human fertility is unknown (2).

It is not known if cladribine crosses the human placenta. The molecular weight (about 286), low plasma protein binding, terminal half-life, and long infusion time suggest that the drug will cross to the embryo–fetus.

In a letter correspondence, a woman at 10 week's gestation was diagnosed with hairy cell leukemia (3). Because she wished to continue her pregnancy, treatment was deferred until after delivery. At 16 weeks' gestation, during an otherwise normal pregnancy, she underwent a splenectomy for an enlarged spleen that was causing abdominal discomfort. She gave birth at term to a healthy female infant. Treatment was again deferred for 6 months while she breastfed her infant. Six weeks after treatment, a repeat bone marrow biopsy specimen and aspirate were normal (3).

A 37-year-old woman with hairy cell leukemia was treated with a 7-day infusion of cladribine and obtained a complete remission (4). Eleven months after completion of therapy, she became pregnant. Her pregnancy was uncomplicated and she gave birth to a term, healthy, female infant whose birth weight (actual birth weight not specified) was appropriate for gestational age. At 9 months of age, the infant was developing normally and meeting all developmental milestones (4).

BREASTFEEDING SUMMARY

No reports describing the use of cladribine during human lactation have been located. The molecular weight (about 286), low plasma protein binding (about 20%), terminal half-life (5.4 hours), and long infusion time (7 consecutive days) suggest that the drug will be excreted into breast milk. The effect of this exposure on a nursing infant is unknown. However, because of the risk for significant toxicity in a nursing infant, women receiving this antineoplastic agent should not breastfeed. Hairy cell leukemia usually has an indolent disease course and deferring treatment until breastfeeding is stopped appears to be an option (see above case report).

C

References

1. Robak T. Current treatment options in hairy cell leukemia and hairy cell leukemia variant. Cancer Treat Rev 2006;32:365–76.
2. Product information. Leustatin. Centocor Ortho Biotech, 2007.
3. Alothman A, Sparling TG. Managing hairy cell leukemia in pregnancy. Ann Intern Med 1994;120:1048–9.
4. Orlowski RZ. Successful pregnancy after cladribine therapy for hairy cell leukemia. Leuk Lymphoma 2004;45:187–8.

CLARITHROMYCIN

Antibiotic

PREGNANCY RECOMMENDATION: Compatible
BREASTFEEDING RECOMMENDATION: Compatible

PREGNANCY SUMMARY

The animal reproduction data suggest high risk, but the available human pregnancy experience suggests that the risk, if it exists, is low. The antibiotic has not been associated with an increased risk of pyloric stenosis.

FETAL RISK SUMMARY

Clarithromycin, a semisynthetic antibiotic structurally related to erythromycin, belongs to the same macrolide class of anti-infectives as azithromycin, dirithromycin, erythromycin, and troleandomycin.

The effects of clarithromycin on fertility and reproduction in rats, mice, rabbits, and monkeys have been reported by the manufacturer. Doses up to 1.3 times the recommended maximum human dose based on BSA (MRHD) (serum levels approximately 2 times the levels in humans) in male and female rats produced no adverse effects on the estrous cycle, fertility, parturition, or fetal outcome. No teratogenic effects were observed in four studies involving one rat strain using oral and IV doses up to 1.3 times the MRHD, but a low incidence of cardiovascular anomalies was seen in two studies, with a second rat strain at an oral dose about 1.2 times the MRHD. A variable incidence of cleft palate occurred in mice given oral doses about 2–4 times the MRHD (1).

In rabbits, IV doses 17 times less than the MRHD resulted in fetal death, but teratogenic effects were not observed with various oral or IV doses (1). Embryonic loss attributed to maternal toxicity occurred in monkeys administered oral doses 2.4 times the MRHD (serum levels three times the levels in humans). In monkeys, an oral dose approximately equal to the MRHD (serum levels about twice those obtained in humans) caused fetal growth restriction.

Clarithromycin crosses the human placenta (2). In an in vitro experiment using perfused term placentas, the mean transplacental transfer of clarithromycin was 6.1%.

At a 1996 meeting, a teratogen information service (TIS) reported the outcomes of 34 exposures to clarithromycin during pregnancy (3). All of the exposures occurred during the 1st and early 2nd trimesters for the treatment of upper respiratory infections. Among the 29 known pregnancy outcomes (5 were pending), there were 8 (28%) abortions (4 spontaneous/4 voluntary), 20 (69%) normal newborns, and 1 (3%) infant with a 0.5-cm brown mark on the temple. One of the normal newborns, delivered at 26 weeks, died from complications of prematurity. Although follow-up of the remaining newborns had not been sufficiently long to exclude completely the presence of congenital malformations, these outcomes do not appear to be different from those expected in a nonexposed population.

Case reports of clarithromycin and congenital anomalies available to the FDA through June 1996 were limited to six diverse birth defects: cystic head, pregnancy terminated; craniofacial anomalies, absent clavicles, bilateral hip deformities, and underdeveloped left heart; spina bifida; cleft lip; pulmonary hypoplasia, anomalous infradiaphragmatic venous return; and CHARGE syndrome (F. Rosa, personal communication, FDA, 1996). By definition, infants having CHARGE association or syndrome must have two or more of the following: coloboma of the eye or eye defects, heart disease, choanal atresia, restricted growth and development with or without CNS anomalies, genital hypoplasia, and ear anomalies with or without deafness (4). The diversity of the malformations lessens the probability of an association with clarithromycin and any or all of these outcomes may have occurred by chance.

A 1998 prospective controlled multicenter study compared the outcomes of 157 pregnancies exposed to clarithromycin with an equal number of matched controls (5). All of the women had called a TIS. The most common indications for use of the antibiotic were respiratory infections. Of the subjects, 122 (78%) were exposed during the 1st trimester. The outcomes of subjects and controls were spontaneous abortions (SABs) (22 vs. 11, $p = 0.04$), elective abortions (EABs) (11 vs. 3, $p = 0.04$), live births (123 vs. 143, $p = 0.003$), stillbirths (1 vs. 0, *ns*), major malformations (3 vs. 2, *ns*), and minor malformations (7 vs. 7, *ns*). The major anomalies (exposure occurred in the 3rd trimester in one case) in the study group were hydrocephalus, Turner's syndrome, and stenosis uteropelvic junction and cranial synostosis. The minor malformations were a large birth mark, a reflux valve problem, an enlarged right ventricle (brain), a minor ventricular septal defect, undescended testes, a blocked tear ducts defect, and excess breast tissue on the right. The types of malformations in controls were comparable, with no pattern of defects apparent in either group. Although the increased number of SABs in exposed women was within the expected background rate and may have been affected by confounding factors, the investigators concluded that it warranted further study (5).

A prospective, multicenter study published in 2008 compared pregnant women exposed to a new macrolide (azithromycin, clarithromycin, or roxithromycin) with two comparison groups (6). Of the 161 women exposed to a macrolide, 118 were exposed in the 1st trimester. The rate of major malformations in the study group was 4.1% compared with 2.1% of those exposed to other antibiotics (OR = 1.41, 95% confidence interval (CI) 0.47–4.23). The authors concluded that the use of the new macrolides did not represent an increased risk of congenital defects strong enough for an EAB (6).

A 2012 prospective, multicenter observational study was conducted by TISs in Italy, Israel, Czech Republic, the Netherlands, and Germany (7). Of the 608 women exposed to macrolides, 511 were exposed in the 1st trimester. The study group was compared with 773 women exposed to nonteratogens in the 1st trimester. The rate of major congenital defects were similar in the groups (3.4% vs. 2.4%, $p = 0.36$; OR 1.42, 95% CI 0.70–2.88) or in the rate of cardiovascular defects (1.6% vs. 0.9%). The rates for clarithromycin ($N = 218$) were 1.8% vs. 2.4%, $p = 0.80$; OR 0.76, 95% CI 0.25–2.27 and 0.5% vs. 0.9%, $p = 0.99$; OR 0.54, 95% CI 0.06–4.48 (7).

A register-based, nationwide cohort study conducted in Denmark, covering the period 1997–2007, was published in 2013 (8). The study identified 931,504 pregnancies (705,837 live birth, 77,553 SABs, and 148,114 EABs), 401 of whom were exposed to clarithromycin in the 1st trimester. The hazard ratio (HR) of having an SAB after exposure to clarithromycin was 1.56, 95% CI 1.14–2.13. A significant HR was not found with 1st trimester exposure to three other antibiotics and proton pump inhibitors (PPIs) (HR and 95% CI): amoxicillin ($N = 4584$, 0.92, 0.82–1.04); erythromycin ($N = 6492$, 1.03, 0.94–1.13); Penicillin V ($N = 33,469$, 1.00, 0.96–1.04); and PPIs ($N = 3577$, 1.03, 0.91–1.18). Among the 253 exposed offspring diagnosed with a major malformation, 9 (3.6%) were exposed to clarithromycin (odds ratio [OR] 1.03, 95% CI 0.53–2.00). The authors concluded that further research was required to examine the possible effects of treatment indications on the above association (8).

Three pregnant women with documented *Helicobacter pylori* infections, persistent nausea and vomiting, and epigastric pain were treated in the 2nd trimester with a 2-week course of clarithromycin combined with amoxicillin and with famotidine, omeprazole, or ranitidine (9). The therapy was effective in eliminating the conditions. No adverse effects on the pregnancy outcomes were noted.

In a 2005 abstract, 145 pregnant women were exposed to a new macrolide (38 azithromycin, 53 clarithromycin, 54 roxithromycin), of which 103 were exposed in the 1st trimester (10). The rates of congenital anomalies compared with 928 exposed to a nonteratogen were similar (4.0% vs. 3.75%, $p = 0.156$). In a 2003 Danish study, 188 women received a macrolide (see Breastfeeding Summary) within 30 days of birth and none of their infants had infantile hypertrophic pyloric stenosis (11).

BREASTFEEDING SUMMARY

Clarithromycin is excreted into breast milk. In a 1993 study, 12 mothers were given clarithromycin 250 mg twice daily (12). Both the parent drug and metabolite were excreted into milk, with peaks levels measured at 2.2 and 2.8 hours, respectively, The half-lives of the drug and metabolite were 4.3 and 9 hours, respectively. The combined exposure for an exclusively breastfed infant was about 2% of the mother's weight-adjusted dose (12).

A 2003 study investigated the association between maternal use of macrolides and infantile hypertrophic pyloric stenosis (11). The Danish population-based cohort study comprised 1166 women who had a prescribed macrolide (azithromycin, clarithromycin, erythromycin, spiramycin, or roxithromycin) from birth to 90 days postnatally compared with up to 41,778 controls. The OR for stenosis was 2.3–3.0, depending on the postnatal period of exposure (42, 56, 70, or 90 days), but none of the ORs was significant. When stratified by gender, the ORs for males were 1.8–3.1 and again were not statistically significant. For females, the ORs at 70 and 90 days postbirth were 10.3 and 7.5, but only the former was significant (95% CI 1.2–92.3) (11).

Investigators from Israel examined the possible association between macrolide (azithromycin, clarithromycin, erythromycin, or roxithromycin) exposure in milk and infantile hypertrophic pyloric stenosis in a 2009 study (13). They compared 55 infants exposed to a macrolide antibiotic to 36 infants exposed to amoxicillin. In the macrolide group, 7 (12.7%) had an adverse reaction (rash, diarrhea, loss of appetite, somnolence), whereas 3 infants (8.3%) in the amoxicillin group had an adverse reaction (rashes, somnolence). The rates of adverse reactions were comparable. No cases of infantile hypertrophic pyloric stenosis were observed (13).

References

1. Product information. Biaxin. Abbott Laboratories, 1996.
2. Witt A, Sommer EM, Cichna M, Postlbauer K, Widhalm A, Gregor H, Reisenberger K. Placental transfer of clarithromycin surpasses other macrolide antibiotics. Am J Obstet Gynecol 2003;188:816–9.
3. Schick B, Hom M, Librizzi R, Donnenfeld A. Pregnancy outcome following exposure to clarithromycin (abstract). Abstracts of the Ninth International Conference of the Organization of Teratology Information Services, May 2–4, 1996, Salt Lake City, Utah. Reprod Toxicol 1996;10:162.
4. Escobar LF, Weaver DD. Charge association. In: Buyse ML, ed. *Birth Defects Encyclopedia*. Vol. 1. Dover, MA: Center for Birth Defects Information Services, 1990:308–9.
5. Einarson A, Phillips E, Mawji F, D'Alimonte D, Schick B, Addis A, Mastroiacova P, Mazzone T, Matsui D, Koren G. A prospective controlled multicentre study of clarithromycin in pregnancy. Am J Perinatol 1998;15:523–5.
6. Bar-Oz B, Diav-Citrin O, Shechtman S, Tellem R, Arnon J, Francetic I, Berkovitch M, Ornoy A. Pregnancy outcome after gestational exposure to the new macrolides: a prospective multi-center observational study. Eur J Obstet Gynecol Reprod Biol 2008;141:31–4.
7. Bar-Oz B, Weber-Schoendorfer C, Berlin M, Clementi M, Di Gianantonio D, de Vries L, De Saints M, Merlob P, Stahl B, Eleftheriou G, Manakova E, Hubickova-Heringova L, Youngster I, Berkovitch M. The outcomes of pregnancy in women exposed to the new macrolides in the first trimester: a prospective, multicentre, observations study. Drug Saf 2012;35:589–98.
8. Andersen JT, Petersen M, Jimenez-Solem E, Broedbaek K, Andersen NL, Torp-Pedersen C, Keiding N, Poulsen HE. Clarithromycin in early pregnancy and the risk of miscarriage and malformation: a register-based nationwide cohort study. PLoS One 2013;8:e53327. doi:10.1371/journal.pone.0053327. Epub 2013 Jan 2.
9. Jacoby EB, Porter KB. *Helicobacter pylori* infection and persistent hyperemesis gravidarum. Am J Perinatol 1999;16:85–8.
10. Tellem R, Shechtman S, Arnon J, Diav-Citrin O, Bar-Oz B, Berkovitch M, Ornoy A. Pregnancy outcome after gestational exposure to the new macrolides: a prospective controlled cohort study (abstract). Reprod Toxicol 2005;20:484.
11. Sorensen HT, Skriver MV, Pedersen L, Larsen H, Ebbesen F, Schonheyder HC. Risk of infantile hypertrophic pyloric stenosis after maternal postnatal use of macrolides. Scand J Infect Dis 2003;35:104–6.
12. Sedimayr TH, Peters F, Raasch W, Kees F. Clarithromycin, a new macrolide antibiotic: effectiveness in puerperal infections and pharmacokinetics in breast milk. Geburtshilfe Frauenheilkd 1993;53:488–91.
13. Goldstein LH, Berlin M, Tsur L, Bortnik O, Binyamini L, Berkovitch M. The safety of macrolides during lactation. Breastfeed Med 2009;4:157–200.

CLAVULANATE, POTASSIUM

Anti-infective

PREGNANCY RECOMMENDATION: Compatible
BREASTFEEDING RECOMMENDATION: No Human Data—Probably Compatible

PREGNANCY SUMMARY

Several studies have described the use of amoxicillin and potassium clavulanate for various infections in pregnant women. Most studies have observed no adverse effects in the fetus or newborn attributable to the combination (see Amoxicillin and Ticarcillin). However, one study did report an association with necrotizing enterocolitis (NEC) in newborns.

FETAL RISK SUMMARY

Clavulanic acid is a β-lactamase inhibitor produced by *Streptomyces clavuligerus* that is combined, as the potassium salt, with the penicillin antibiotics, amoxicillin or ticarcillin, to broaden their antibacterial spectrum of activity. No adverse fetal effects were observed in mice, rats, and pigs administered potassium clavulanate in combination with amoxicillin or ticarcillin during gestation (1–5).

Following a single oral dose of amoxicillin (250 mg) and potassium clavulanate (125 mg) in humans, both agents crossed the placenta to the fetus (6,7). Cord blood levels were found 1 hour after the dose, with peak levels occurring at 2–3 hours. In one study, the mean peak maternal serum and umbilical cord blood levels occurred at 2 hours with values of 2.20 and 1.23 mcg/mL, respectively (fetal:maternal ratio 0.56) (7). Both amoxicillin and potassium clavulanate have been demonstrated in the amniotic fluid (6–8), with peak concentrations of clavulanate (0.44 mcg/mL) measured 5.5 hours after administration (7). A study using in vitro perfused human placentas demonstrated the transfer of potassium clavulanate when concentrations on the maternal side were 10–13 mcg/mL, but not at 2–6 mcg/mL (8). A fetal/maternal gradient of 1:1 was obtained at the higher concentrations.

In addition to the above, several studies have described the use of amoxicillin–clavulanic acid (ACA) for various infections in pregnant women either without causing fetal or newborn harm (9–11) or causing newborn harm (12).

A 2001 randomized study (ORACLE 1) was conducted in patients with preterm, prelabor rupture of fetal membranes to determine neonatal health benefits of three antibiotic regimens (12). The regimens, compared with a placebo group ($N = 1225$) were erythromycin (250 mg) ($N = 1197$), amoxicillin (250 mg)–clavulanic acid (125 mg) ($N = 1212$), or both ($N = 1192$) four times daily for 10 days or until delivery. The primary outcome measures were specific outcomes or a composite of neonatal death, chronic lung disease, or major cerebral abnormality. For these neonatal outcomes, the two groups with ACA had no benefit over placebo, whereas erythromycin use resulted in significantly better outcomes (both composite and specific). When any-ACA exposure was compared with no-ACA for outcomes with suspected or proven NEC, the results were 92 (3.8%) and 58 (2.4%) ($p = 0.004$). The authors thought that a possible mechanism for this outcome was that the ACA combination selected for *Clostridium difficile* and that abnormal colonization of the neonatal intestinal tract was one possible mechanism for NEC (12).

In a surveillance study of Michigan Medicaid recipients involving 229,101 completed pregnancies conducted between 1985 and 1992, 556 newborns had been exposed to clavulanic acid (presumably in combination with penicillins) during the 1st trimester (F. Rosa, personal communication,

C

FDA, 1993). A total of 24 (4.3%) major birth defects were observed (24 expected). Specific data were available for six defect categories, including (observed/expected) 5/6 cardiovascular defects, 2/1 oral clefts, 1/2 polydactyly, 0/1 limb-reduction defects, 1/1 hypospadias, and 2/0.3 spina bifida. Only with the latter defect is there a suggestion of a possible association, but other factors, including the mother's disease, concurrent drug use, and chance, may be involved.

In a 1997 prospective, double-blind, randomized, controlled study, two antibiotic regimens (ampicillin–sulbactam for 72 hours followed by amoxicillin–clavulanate or ampicillin for 72 hours followed by amoxicillin) were effective for prophylaxis in women with preterm premature rupture of the membranes who had received antenatal corticosteroids alone (13). Although both combinations reduced the frequency of neonatal mortality, sepsis, and respiratory distress syndrome and increased birth weight compared with corticosteroids alone, statistical significance was reached only with the ampicillin–sulbactam/amoxicillin–clavulanate combination (26.3% vs. 48.6%; $p \leq 0.05$).

In a 2004 study, 191 women treated with amoxicillin–clavulanic acid (subjects) in the 1st trimester were matched with 191 controls exposed to amoxicillin only (14). Maternal age, birth weight, gestational age at birth, and rates of live births and abortions were comparable between the two groups. The rates of major malformations in subjects (3/158, 1.9%) and controls (5/163, 3%) ($p = 0.49$; relative risk 0.62, 95% confidence interval 0.15–2.55) were within the expected baseline risk for the general population (14).

BREASTFEEDING SUMMARY

Both amoxicillin and ticarcillin are excreted into breast milk (see Amoxicillin and Ticarcillin), but data pertaining to potassium clavulanate have not been located. Excretion probably occurs because of the low molecular weight (about 237). The effects of the β-lactamase inhibitor on the nursing infant are unknown.

References

1. Baldwin JA, Schardein JL, Koshima Y. Reproduction studies of BRL14151K and BRL25000. I. Teratology studies in rats. Chemotherapy (Tokyo) 1983;31(Suppl 2):238–51.
2. Baldwin JA, Schardein JL, Koshima Y. Reproduction studies of BRL14151K and BRL25000. II. Peri- and post-natal studies in rats. Chemotherapy (Tokyo) 1983;31(Suppl 2):252–62.
3. Hirakawa T, Suzuki T, Sano Y, Tamura K, Koshima Y, Hiura KI, Fujita K, Hardy TL. Reproduction studies of BRL14151K and BRL25000. III. Fertility studies in rats. Chemotherapy (Tokyo) 1983;31(Suppl 2):263–72.
4. James PA, Hardy TL, Koshima Y. Reproduction studies of BRL 25000. IV. Teratology in pig. Chemotherapy (Tokyo) 1983;31(Suppl 2):274–9.
5. Tasker TCG, Cockburn A, Jackson D, Mellows G, White D. Safety of ticarcillin/potassium clavulanate. J Antimicrob Chemother 1986;17:225–32.
6. Matsuda S, Tanno M, Kashiwagura T, Seida A. Fundamental and clinical studies on BRL25000 (clavulanic acid–amoxicillin) in the field of obstetrics and gynecology. Chemotherapy (Tokyo) 1982;30(Suppl 2):538–47.
7. Takase Z, Shirafuji H, Uchida M. Clinical and laboratory studies on BRL25000 (clavulanic acid–amoxicillin) in the field of obstetrics and gynecology. Chemotherapy (Tokyo) 1982;30(Suppl 2):579–86.
8. Fortunato SJ, Bawdon RE, Swan KF, Bryant EC, Sobhi S. Transfer of Timentin (ticarcillin and clavulanic acid) across the in vitro perfused human placenta: comparison with other agents. Am J Obstet Gynecol 1992;167:1595–9.
9. Matsuda S. Augmentin treatment in obstetrics and gynaecology. In: Leigh DA, Robinson OPW, eds. *Augmentin: Proceedings of an International Symposium*, Montreux, Switzerland, July 1981. Excerpta Medica 1982: 179–91.
10. Mayer HO, Jeschek H, Kowatsch A. Augmentin in the treatment of urinary tract infection in pregnant women and pelvic inflammatory disease. In: *Proceedings of the European Symposium on Augmentin*, Scheveningen, June 1982, 1983:207–17.
11. Pedler SJ, Bint AJ. Comparative study of amoxicillin–clavulanic acid and cephalexin in the treatment of bacteriuria during pregnancy. Antimicrob Agents Chemother 1985;27:508–10.
12. Kenyon SL, Taylor DJ, Tarnow-Mordi W, for the ORACLE Collaborative Group. Broad-spectrum antibiotics for preterm, prelabour rupture of fetal membranes: the ORACLE I randomised trial. Lancet 2001;357:979–88.
13. Lovett SM, Weiss JD, Diogo MJ, Williams PT, Garite TJ. A prospective, double-blind, randomized, controlled clinical trial of ampicillin-sulbactam for preterm premature rupture of membranes in women receiving antenatal corticosteroid therapy. Am J Obstet Gynecol 1997;176:1030–8.
14. Berkovitch M, Diav-Citrin O, Greenberg R, Cohen M, Bulkowstein M, Shechtman S, Bortnik O, Arnon J. Ornoy A. First-trimester exposure to amoxycillin/clavulanic acid: a prospective, controlled study. Br J Clin Pharmacol 2004;58:298–302.

CLEMASTINE

Antihistamine

PREGNANCY RECOMMENDATION: Compatible
BREASTFEEDING RECOMMENDATION: Limited Human Data—Potential Toxicity

PREGNANCY SUMMARY

In general, antihistamines are considered compatible with pregnancy. However, a possible association with retrolental fibroplasia in premature infants has been reported.

FETAL RISK SUMMARY

Reproductive studies with the antihistamine, clemastine, in rats and rabbits have revealed no evidence of teratogenic effects (1). No published reports describing the use of clemastine in human pregnancy have been located.

In a surveillance study of Michigan Medicaid recipients involving 229,101 completed pregnancies conducted between 1985 and 1992, 1617 newborns had been exposed to clemastine during the 1st trimester (F. Rosa, personal communication, FDA, 1993). A total of 71 (4.4%) major birth defects were observed (68 expected). Specific data were available for six defect categories, including (observed/expected) 13/16 cardiovascular defects, 3/3 oral clefts, 3/1 spina bifida, 4/5 polydactyly, 4/4 hypospadias, and 5/1.9 limb-reduction defects. Only with the latter defect is there a suggestion of a possible association, but other factors, including the mother's disease, concurrent drug use, and chance, may be involved.

A 2002 study found no increased risk of teratogenicity or other pregnancy or newborn complications for antihistamines when used in early pregnancy for the treatment of nausea and vomiting ($N = 12,394$) and allergy ($N = 5041$) (2). Clemastine was used by 1230 women.

An association between exposure to antihistamines during the last 2 weeks of pregnancy and retrolental fibroplasia in premature infants has been reported. See Brompheniramine for details.

BREASTFEEDING SUMMARY

Clemastine is excreted into breast milk (3). A 10-week-old girl developed drowsiness, irritability, refusal to feed, neck stiffness, and a high-pitched cry 12 hours after the mother began taking the antihistamine, 1 mg twice daily. The mother also was also taking phenytoin and carbamazepine. Twenty hours after the last dose, clemastine levels in maternal plasma and milk were 20 and 5–10 ng/mL, respectively, a milk:plasma ratio of 0.25–0.5. The drug could not be detected in the infant's plasma. Symptoms in the baby resolved within 24 hours after the drug was stopped, although breastfeeding was continued. Examination 3 weeks later was also normal. Owing to the above case report, the American Academy of Pediatrics states that the drug should be used with caution during breastfeeding (4).

References

1. Product information. Tavist. Sandoz Pharmaceuticals, 1993.
2. Kallen B. Use of antihistamine drugs in early pregnancy and delivery outcome. J Matern Fetal Neonatal Med 2002;11:146–52.
3. Kok THHG, Taitz LS, Bennett MJ, Holt DW. Drowsiness due to clemastine transmitted in breast milk. Lancet 1982;1:914–5.
4. Committee on Drugs, American Academy of Pediatrics. The transfer of drugs and other chemicals into human milk. Pediatrics 2001;108:776–89.

CLEVIDIPINE

Calcium Channel Blocker

PREGNANCY RECOMMENDATION: No Human Data—Animal Data Suggest Risk
BREASTFEEDING RECOMMENDATION: No Human Data—Probably Compatible

PREGNANCY SUMMARY

No reports describing the use of clevidipine in human pregnancy have been located. The animal reproduction data suggest risk, but the absence of human pregnancy experience prevents a complete assessment of the embryo–fetal risk. However, other calcium channel blockers have been used extensively in human pregnancy as antihypertensives and tocolytics without evidence of developmental toxicity (e.g., see Nicardipine, Nifedipine, and Verapamil). Nevertheless, until human pregnancy data are available, other agents, such as IV labetalol, are probably preferred to treat severe hypertension in pregnancy if IV therapy is required.

FETAL RISK SUMMARY

Clevidipine is a calcium channel blocker that is given by IV infusion. It is indicated for the reduction of blood pressure when oral therapy is not feasible or desirable. Clevidipine is rapidly metabolized to inactive metabolites. One of the metabolites is formaldehyde. Plasma protein binding is high (>99.5%) and the terminal half-life is very short (about 15 minutes) (1).

Reproduction studies have been conducted in rats and rabbits. In these species, during organogenesis, doses that were 0.7 and 2 times, respectively, the maximum recommended human dose based on BSA (MRHD) decreased fetal survival. Clevidipine crosses the rat placenta. In rats dosed during late gestation and lactation, there were dose-related increases in maternal mortality, length of gestation, and prolonged parturition at doses that were about ≥ 0.17 times the MRHD. When mated, offspring of these dams had a lower conception rate than controls (1).

Long-term animal carcinogenicity studies have not been conducted with clevidipine because of the intended short-term use in humans. Clevidipine was genotoxic in three in vitro assays but not in an in vivo test. The positive in vitro tests were thought likely to be due to the metabolite formaldehyde.

Fertility and mating performance was not affected in male and female rats at doses about equivalent to the MRHD, but female rats demonstrated pseudopregnancy and changes in estrus cycle at doses as low as one-fourth the MRHD.

It is not known if clevidipine crosses the human placenta. The molecular weight (about 456) is low enough, but the rapid metabolism, high plasma protein binding, and a very short terminal half-life suggests that little active drug will cross to the embryo or fetus.

BREASTFEEDING SUMMARY

No reports describing the use of clevidipine during human lactation have been located. The molecular weight (about 456) is low enough, but the rapid metabolism, high plasma protein binding, and a very short terminal half-life suggests that little of the active drug will be excreted into breast milk. Moreover, the drug is given as an IV infusion for hypertension when oral medication is not feasible or desirable. In such cases, it is doubtful if the mother would be nursing a child.

Reference

1. Product information. Cleviprex. The Medicines Company, 2008.

C

CLIDINIUM

Parasympatholytic

PREGNANCY RECOMMENDATION: Limited Human Data—No Relevant Animal Data
BREASTFEEDING RECOMMENDATION: No Human Data—Probably Compatible

PREGNANCY SUMMARY

The limited human pregnancy experience and absence of relevant animal data prevent a complete assessment of the embryo–fetal risk.

FETAL RISK SUMMARY

Clidinium is an anticholinergic quaternary ammonium bromide. In a large prospective study, 2323 patients were exposed to this class of drugs during the 1st trimester, 4 of whom took clidinium (1). A possible association was found between the total group and minor malformations.

BREASTFEEDING SUMMARY

No reports describing the use of clidinium during human lactation have been located (see also Atropine).

Reference

1. Heinonen OP, Slone D, Shapiro S. *Birth Defects and Drugs in Pregnancy.* Littleton, MA: Publishing Sciences Group, 1977:346–53.

CLINDAMYCIN

Antibiotic

PREGNANCY RECOMMENDATION: Compatible
BREASTFEEDING RECOMMENDATION: Compatible

PREGNANCY SUMMARY

No reports linking the use of clindamycin with congenital defects have been located.

FETAL RISK SUMMARY

Reproduction studies in mice and rats with oral doses up to about 1.1 and 2.1 times the maximum recommended human adult dose based on BSA (MRHD), respectively, revealed no evidence of teratogenicity. In addition, SC doses in the two species up to 0.5 and 0.9 times the MRHD, respectively, failed to show teratogenicity (1).

The drug crosses the placenta, achieving maximum cord serum levels of approximately 50% of the maternal serum (2,3). Levels in the fetus were considered therapeutic for susceptible pathogens. A study published in 1988 measured a mean cord:maternal ratio of 0.15 in three women given an unknown amount of clindamycin in labor for the treatment of chorioamnionitis (4). At the time of sampling, mean maternal blood, cord blood, and placental membrane concentrations of the antibiotic were 1.67 mcg/mL, 0.26 mcg/mL, and 1.86 mcg/g, respectively (placenta:maternal ratio 1.11). Fetal tissue levels increase following multiple dosing with the drug concentrating in the fetal liver (2). Maternal serum levels after dosing at various stages of pregnancy were similar to those of nonpregnant patients (3,5). Clindamycin has been used for prophylactic therapy prior to cesarean section (6).

In a surveillance study of Michigan Medicaid recipients involving 229,101 completed pregnancies conducted between 1985 and 1992, 647 newborns had been exposed to clindamycin during the 1st trimester (includes both maternal systemic and nonsystemic administration) (F. Rosa, personal communication, FDA, 1993). A total of 31 (4.8%) major birth defects were observed (28 expected). Specific data were available for six defect categories, including (observed/expected) 5/6 cardiovascular defects, 0/1 oral clefts, 1/0.5 spina bifida, 1/2 polydactyly, 0/1 limb-reduction defects, and 3/2 hypospadias. These data do not support an association between the drug and congenital defects.

BREASTFEEDING SUMMARY

Clindamycin is excreted into breast milk. In two patients receiving 600 mg IV every 6 hours, milk levels varied from 2.1 to 3.8 mcg/mL (0.2–3.5 hours after drug) (7). When the patients were changed to 300 mg orally every 6 hours, levels varied from 0.7 to 1.8 mcg/mL (2–7 hours after drug). Maternal serum levels were not given.

Two grossly bloody stools were observed in a nursing infant whose mother was receiving clindamycin and gentamicin (8). No relationship to either drug could be established. However, the condition cleared rapidly when breastfeeding was stopped. Except for this one case, no other adverse effects in nursing infants have been reported.

Three potential problems that may exist for the nursing infant are modification of bowel flora, direct effects on the infant, and interference with the interpretation of culture results if a fever workup is required. The American Academy of Pediatrics classifies clindamycin as compatible with breastfeeding (9).

References

1. Product information. Cleocin. Pharmacia & Upjohn, 2000.
2. Philipson A, Sabath LD, Charles D. Transplacental passage of erythromycin and clindamycin. N Engl J Med 1973;288:1219–21.
3. Weinstein AJ, Gibbs RS, Gallagher M. Placental transfer of clindamycin and gentamicin in term pregnancy. Am J Obstet Gynecol 1976;124:688–91.
4. Gilstrap LC III, Bawdon RE, Burris J. Antibiotic concentration in maternal blood, cord blood, and placental membranes in chorioamnionitis. Obstet Gynecol 1988;72:124–5.
5. Philipson A, Sabath LD, Charles D. Erythromycin and clindamycin absorption and elimination in pregnant women. Clin Pharmacol Ther 1976;19:68–77.
6. Rehu M, Jahkola M. Prophylactic antibiotics in caesarean section: effect of a short preoperative course of benzyl penicillin or clindamycin plus gentamicin on postoperative infectious morbidity. Ann Clin Res 1980;12:45–8.
7. Smith JA, Morgan JR, Rachlis AR, Papsin FR. Clindamycin in human breast milk. Can Med Assoc J 1975;112:806.
8. Mann CF. Clindamycin and breast-feeding. Pediatrics 1980;66:1030–1.
9. Committee on Drugs, American Academy of Pediatrics. The transfer of drugs and other chemicals into human milk. Pediatrics 2001;108:776–89.

CLOBAZAM

Anticonvulsant

PREGNANCY RECOMMENDATION: Limited Human Data—Potential Toxicity
BREASTFEEDING RECOMMENDATION: Limited Human Data—Potential Toxicity

PREGNANCY SUMMARY

There is limited information on the effects of clobazam in human pregnancy, but the animal data suggest risk. Clobazam, a benzodiazepine, is usually used in combination with other anticonvulsants. It is well known that antiepileptic polytherapy increases the risk to the embryo and/or fetus. Although the risk of structural anomalies appears to be low with agents in this class, benzodiazepines can cause clinically significant neonatal toxicity when used close to birth. These toxicities have been described with diazepam (see Diazepam) and include the floppy infant syndrome and a withdrawal syndrome. Folic acid 5 mg/day is recommended before and during pregnancy for women taking clobazam (1). Pregnant women taking clobazam are encouraged to enroll in the North American Antiepileptic Drug Pregnancy Registry by calling the toll-free number 1-800-233-2334.

FETAL RISK SUMMARY

Clobazam is an antiepileptic drug available as oral tablets. It is in the same class of benzodiazepine agents as alprazolam, chlordiazepoxide, clonazepam, diazepam, flunitrazepam, lorazepam, midazolam, oxazepam, quazepam, temazepam, and triazolam. Although it is approved as an anticonvulsant, clobazam causes somnolence or sedation similar to that caused by all drugs in this class. Clobazam is indicated for the adjunctive treatment of seizures associated with Lennox-Gastaut syndrome in patients 2 years of age or older. The drug undergoes extensive hepatic metabolism to an active metabolite. The relative potency of the active metabolite compared to clobazam ranges from 20% to equal potency. Plasma protein binding of the parent drug and active metabolite are about 80%–90% and 70%, respectively, whereas the mean elimination half-lives are about 36–42 and 71–82 hours, respectively (2).

A 1979 reproduction study in rats and mice conducted by the manufacturer found no teratogenic or fertility-disturbing effects from administration of clobazam in food (3). In contrast, the current product information states that animal data suggest developmental toxicity, including an increased incidence of fetal abnormalities following oral administration of doses similar to those used in humans (2). However, the animal species and specific doses were not reported.

Rats were used in a 2005 report on the central nervous system (CNS) effects of clobazam (4). Pregnant rats were given clobazam 125 mg/kg daily (comparison to human dose not specified) during the first 7 days of gestation and fetuses were examined on day 20 of gestation. Although there were no gross abnormalities, histologic examination revealed extensive teratogenic effects that included necrosis and hypoplasia of the brain (4).

The manufacturer states that the carcinogenic potential has not been adequately studied, but a 2-year limited study in rats found an increased incidence of thyroid follicular cell adenomas in males at the highest dose (100 mg/kg) of clobazam tested. The drug and the active metabolite were not mutagenic in multiple assays. There are no studies on the effect of the drug on fertility (2).

Clobazam and its active metabolite cross the human placenta at term. In a 1982 study, women at term were given a single 20 mg dose of the drug before giving birth (5). Clobazam was detectable in the umbilical blood in 16 of 19 newborns at birth and in the blood in 9 of 14 infants at 5 days of age. The maternal vein and umbilical vein concentrations were nearly the same. In an in vitro test using human placentas, both the parent drug and its active metabolite crossed the placenta (5). The above results are compatible with the molecular weight (about 301) of clobazam, lipophilic nature, moderate plasma protein binding, and prolonged elimination half-life. These characteristics suggest that the drug will cross the placenta throughout gestation.

A 1984 study described the effect of clobazam on seizure control in 14 women (6). Two of the women had been taking the drug for 12–15 months but only around the time of menstruation. The drug was discontinued when they became pregnant. Pregnancy outcome was not described in either case (6).

In a 2011 study, there were 109,344 pregnant women in the Quebec Pregnancy Registry of whom 349 (0.32%) were epileptic (7). Of these, 42 used no antiepileptic drugs (non-use), 217 used monotherapy, and 90 took polytherapy. During pregnancy, the three most prevalent antiepileptic agents used were carbamazepine (29.9%), valproic acid (19.7%), and phenytoin (11.5%). For polytherapy, the most common drug combinations were carbamazepine combined with clobazam (2.5%), phenytoin (1.6%), or valproic acid (1.6%). Although pregnancy outcomes were provided for non-use, monotherapy, and polytherapy, specific agents associated with the outcomes were not identified. The outcomes in the non-use, monotherapy, and polytherapy groups, respectively, were as follows: planned abortions—45.2%, 40.5%, 44.4%; spontaneous abortions—0%, 2.8%, 4.4%; stillbirths—2.4%, 0%, 2.4%; live births—95.0%, 100%, 51.1%; major defects—10.5%, 9.9%, 19.0%; low birth weight—10.5%, 8.2%, 7.1%; small for gestational age—5.3%, 18.2%, 11.9%; and prematurity (<37 weeks)—15.8%, 10.0%, 9.5%. Because the number of outcomes analyzed in each group declined depending on the specificity of the analysis, none of the differences was statistical significant (7).

The Lamotrigine Pregnancy Registry, an ongoing project conducted by the manufacturer, was first published in January 1997 (8). The final report was published in July 2010. The Registry is now closed. Among 13 prospectively enrolled pregnancies exposed to clobazam and lamotrigine in the 1st trimester, with or without other anticonvulsants, there were 12 live births without defects, and 1 induced abortion with a birth defect. The woman in the birth defect case was taking lamotrigine and clobazam before and during gestation. The fetus had a lumbar neural tube defect with early evidence of ventriculomegaly and a derangement of the posterior fossa (8).

Retrospective cases (reported after the pregnancy outcome was known) are often biased (only adverse outcomes are reported), but they are useful in identifying specific patterns of anomalies suggestive of a common cause (8). There were nine pregnancies with birth defects exposed to clobazam with other antiepileptics reported retrospectively to the Registry, five involving earliest exposure to clobazam in the 1st trimester, two in the 2nd and 3rd trimesters, and one in the 3rd trimester of exposure. No specific pattern was observed (8).

BREASTFEEDING SUMMARY

Clobazam is excreted into breast milk. This is consistent with the molecular weight (about 301), lipophilic nature, moderate plasma protein binding (80%–90%), and prolonged elimination half-life (36–42 hours). Its active metabolite is also present in milk because of its characteristics (plasma protein binding about 70% and mean elimination half-life about 71–82 hours).

Neonatal withdrawal due to clobazam in milk was described in a 2000 review (9). Both clobazam and its metabolite were excreted into milk with an a milk:plasma (parent drug plus metabolite) after 2 days of treatment of 0.13–0.36. After 5 days, the M:P declined to 0.13 possibly because of accumulation of the metabolite in the maternal plasma. The average infant weight-adjusted dose was estimated to be 4.6%, with a maximum dose of 7.5%. The authors of the review thought that breastfeeding should be allowed but the infant should be monitored for sedation and poor sucking (9).

Another 2000 review concluded that the use of clobazam would be safe during breastfeeding if the maternal dose was low and if the exposure was short (10). The authors estimated that the maximum infant exposure would be 10% of the usual therapeutic pediatric dose that was used in the treatment of seizures. However, long-term maternal use could result in infant toxicity and the same monitoring, as described above, was recommended (10).

References

1. Brodie MJ, Dichter MA. Established antiepileptic drugs. Seizure 1997;6:159–74.
2. Product information. Onfi. Lundbeck, 2011.
3. Schütz E. Toxicology of clobazam. Br J Clin Pharmacol 1979;7:33S–5S.
4. Pundey SK, Gupta S. Neuroembryopathic effect of clobazam in rat: a histological study. Nepal Med Coll J 2005;7:10–2.
5. Nandakumaran M, Rey E, Helou A, Challier JC, de Lauture D, Francoual C, Guerre-Millo M, Chavinie J, Olive G. Materno-fetal placental transfer of clobazam and norclobazam in late gestation. Dev Pharmacol Ther 1982;4 (Suppl 1):135–43.
6. Feely M, Gibson J. Intermittent clobazam for catamenial epilepsy: tolerance avoided. J Neurol Neurosurg Psychiatry 1984;47:1279–82.
7. Kulaga S, Sheehy O, Zargarzadeh AH, Moussally K, Bérard A. Antiepileptic drug use during pregnancy: perinatal outcomes. Seizure 2011;20:667–72.
8. The Lamotrigine Pregnancy Registry. Final Report. 1 September 1992 through 31 March 2010. GlaxcoSmithKline, July 2010.
9. Bar-Oz B, Nulman I, Koren G, Ito S. Anticonvulsants and breast feeding—a clinical review. Paediatr Drugs 2000;2:113–26.
10. Hägg S, Spigset O. Anticonvulsant use during lactation. Drug Saf 2000;22:425–40.

CLOFARABINE

Antineoplastic

PREGNANCY RECOMMENDATION: No Human Data—Animal Data Suggest Risk
BREASTFEEDING RECOMMENDATION: No Human Data—Potential Toxicity

PREGNANCY SUMMARY

No reports describing the use of clofarabine in human pregnancy have been located. The animal pregnancy data suggest risk, as does the potential for impaired fertility. The absence of human pregnancy experience prevents a complete assessment of the embryo–fetal risk. Women of reproductive age should use effective contraceptive methods to prevent pregnancy while receiving this drug (1). However, lymphoblastic leukemia is a potential fatal disease. Thus, if a woman does conceive and informed consent is obtained, clofarabine should not be withheld because of pregnancy.

C

FETAL RISK SUMMARY

Clofarabine is a purine nucleoside antimetabolite antineoplastic that is sequentially metabolized intracellularly to the active 5′-triphosphate metabolite that inhibits DNA synthesis. The drug is classified as an antimetabolite in the same subclass of purine analogs and related agents as cladribine, fludarabine, pentostatin, mercaptopurine, and thioguanine. Clofarabine is indicated for the treatment of pediatric patients (1–21 years of age) with relapsed or refractory acute lymphoblastic leukemia after at least two prior regimens. Plasma protein binding, primarily to albumin, is 47%. The terminal half-life is about 5.2 hours with 49%–60% of the drug excreted unchanged in the urine within 24 hours (1).

Reproduction studies have been conducted in rats and rabbits. In pregnant rats and rabbits, doses that were about equal to and 0.23 times, respectively, the recommended human clinical dose based on BSA (RHCD) resulted in increased incidences of malformations and variations (gross external, soft tissue, skeletal and retarded ossification) and developmental toxicity (reduced fetal body weight and increased postimplantation loss) (1).

Studies for carcinogenicity have not been conducted with clofarabine. Although not mutagenic in one assay, the drug was clastogenic in two assays. Fertility studies have been conducted in mice, rats, and dogs. Toxicity was observed in male reproductive organs in these species at doses that were about 0.17, 3, and 0.14 times, respectively, the RHCD. In female mice, a dose 4 times the RHCD resulted in ovarian atrophy or degeneration and uterine mucosal apoptosis (1).

It is not known if clofarabine crosses the human placenta. The molecular weight (about 304), plasma protein binding, and elimination half-life suggest that exposure of the embryo and fetus will occur.

BREASTFEEDING SUMMARY

No reports describing the use of clofarabine during human lactation have been located. The molecular weight (about 304), plasma protein binding (47%), and elimination half-life (5.2 hours) suggest that the drug will be excreted into breast milk. The effects of this exposure on a nursing infant are unknown, but severe toxicity potentially involving multiple systems throughout the body is a concern. Thus, the best course is to not breastfeed while receiving clofarabine therapy.

Reference

1. Product information. Clolar. Genzyme, 2007.

CLOFAZIMINE

Anti-infective (Leprostatic)

PREGNANCY RECOMMENDATION: Limited Human Data—Animal Data Suggest Low Risk
BREASTFEEDING RECOMMENDATION: Limited Human Data—Potential Toxicity

PREGNANCY SUMMARY

Limited human pregnancy experience and the animal data suggest that the risk of developmental toxicity is low, if it exists at all. Pigmentation of the newborn's skin is a potential complication.

FETAL RISK SUMMARY

Clofazimine, a bright-red dye with antibacterial properties against *Mycobacterium leprae*, is used for the treatment of lepromatous leprosy. Animal studies involving mice and rats with doses up to 50 mg/kg/day, and rabbits, 15 mg/kg/day, found no evidence of teratogenicity (1). Fetotoxicity in mice at doses 12–25 times the human dose, however, included retardation of fetal skull ossification, increased incidence of abortions and stillbirths, and decreased neonatal survival (2).

A number of studies have reported the use of clofazimine throughout human pregnancies (3–9). In 13 pregnancies, three exposed newborns died shortly after birth, but none of the outcomes could be attributed to clofazimine. The causes of death were unspecified (died 3 hours after birth), prematurity and antemortem hemorrhage, and gastroenteritis (5,7). The mother of the newborn who died at 3 hours was steroid dependent, but she had stopped her prednisolone 4 weeks before delivery (5). No congenital anomalies were observed in any of the 13 infants, although some of the infants were pigmented at birth. In at least 3 infants (data not provided in 10 infants), the pigmentation gradually resolved over a 1-year period (8).

A 1982 case report described the effects of clofazimine exposure during pregnancy on two newborns (10). The first case involved a woman with erythema nodosum leprosum who was treated throughout gestation with clofazimine, 300 mg/day, and prednisone. Rifampin was also used early in pregnancy. Oligohydramnios developed just prior to delivery after a gestation of uncertain dates. Thick, foul-smelling, meconium-stained fluid was present, and the placenta showed signs of acute severe amnionitis. A 2575-g male infant was delivered vaginally, who appeared normal except for his skin, which was "not excessively pigmented." Bilateral hydrocele and iron deficiency anemia were diagnosed at 14 days of age with fever of unknown origin occurring then and again at 5 months of age. The infant was doing well at 12 months of age. In the second case, a woman was treated throughout pregnancy with clofazimine, 300 mg/day, for tuberculoid leprosy. A normal, healthy 3070-g female infant was delivered vaginally at an unspecified gestational age, and she is growing and developing normally at 3 years of age. Skin pigmentation was not mentioned.

A 1984 reference examined the results of 79 pregnancies from 76 women with lepromatous leprosy, of whom 4 (5 pregnancies) were treated with clofazimine (300 mg/week) (11). No information was given on the outcome of these pregnancies, although the authors stated that clofazimine was the best drug available, if given after the 1st trimester, to prevent transient relapses and to prevent or treat erythema nodosum leprosy (11).

BREASTFEEDING SUMMARY

Clofazimine is excreted into breast milk, and pigmentation of the nursing infant may result. In one case, a mother was ingesting clofazimine, between 100 and 300 mg/day (exact dose not specified), 6 days/week, for a 6-month period (3). Her nursing infant became "ruddy and then slightly hypermelanotic." The baby's skin returned to a normal color 5 months after the mother's medication was stopped.

The American Academy of Pediatrics classifies clofazimine as a drug whose effect on the nursing infant is unknown (other than the skin pigmentation) but may be of concern (12).

References

1. Stenger EG, Aeppli L, Peheim E, Thomann PE. Zur toxikologie des leprostaticums 3-(*p*-chloranilino)-10-(*p*-chlorophenyl)-2-10-dihydro 2(isopropylamino)phenazin (G-30320). Arzneimittelforschung 1970;20:794–9. As cited in Shepard TH. *Catalog of Teratogenic Agents*. 6th ed. Baltimore, MD: Johns Hopkins University Press, 1989:157.
2. Product information. Lamprene. Ciba-Geigy Corp, 1992.
3. Browne SG, Hogerzeil LM. "B 663" in the treatment of leprosy. Preliminary report of a pilot trial. Lepr Rev 1962;33:6–10.
4. Imkamp FMJH. A treatment of corticosteroid-dependent lepromatous patients in persistent erythema nodosum leprosum. A clinical evaluation of G.30320 (B663). Lepr Rev 1968;39:119–25.
5. Plock H, Leiker DL. A long-term trial with clofazimine in reactive lepromatous leprosy. Lepr Rev 1976;47:25–34.
6. De las Aguas JT. Treatment of leprosy with Lampren (B.663 Geigy). Int J Lepr Other Mycobact Dis 1971;39:493–503.
7. Schulz EJ. Forty-four months' experience in the treatment of leprosy with clofazimine (Lamprene (Geigy)). Lepr Rev 1972;42:178–87.
8. Karat AB. Long-term follow-up of clofazimine (Lamprene) in the management of reactive phases of leprosy. Lepr Rev 1975;46(Suppl):105–9.
9. Waters MFR. Symposium on B.663 (Lamprene, Geigy) in the treatment of leprosy and leprosy reactions. Int J Lepr 1968;36:560–1.
10. Farb H, West DP, Pedvis-Leftick A. Clofazimine in pregnancy complicated by leprosy. Obstet Gynecol 1982;59:122–3.
11. Duncan ME, Pearson JMH. The association of pregnancy and leprosy. III. Erythema nodosum leprosum in pregnancy and lactation. Lepr Rev 1984;55:129–42.
12. Committee on Drugs, American Academy of Pediatrics. The transfer of drugs and other chemicals into human milk. Pediatrics 2001;108:776–89.

CLOFIBRATE

[Withdrawn from the market. See 9th edition.]

CLOMIPHENE

Fertility Agent (Nonhormonal)

PREGNANCY RECOMMENDATION: Contraindicated
BREASTFEEDING RECOMMENDATION: No Human Data—Potential Toxicity

PREGNANCY SUMMARY

Patients requiring the use of clomiphene should be cautioned that each new course of the drug should be started only after pregnancy has been excluded.

FETAL RISK SUMMARY

Clomiphene is used to induce ovulation and is contraindicated after conception has occurred. Multiple pregnancies, most often twins, may be a complication of ovulation induction with clomiphene (1).

Shepard reviewed five animal reproduction studies involving the use of clomiphene in mice, rats, and monkeys (2). Hydramnios, cataracts, dose-related fetal mortality, and multiple abnormalities of the genital tract were observed in fetal mice and rats, but no congenital anomalies resulted

C

after exposure of monkeys during the embryonic period. In mice, preovulatory administration of clomiphene produced a decrease in implantation rates, and growth restriction and an increased incidence of exencephaly in surviving fetuses (3). The decreased rate of implantation and growth restriction, which were most pronounced when the drug was given immediately before ovulation, apparently were caused by impairment of uterine function, rather than by a direct effect on the embryo itself (3).

Several case reports of neural tube defects have been reported after stimulating ovulation with clomiphene (4–8). However, an association between the drug and these defects has not been established (9–17). In one review, the percentage of congenital anomalies after clomiphene use was no greater than in the normal population (9). Similarly, another study involving 1034 pregnancies after clomiphene-induced ovulation found no association with the incidence or type of malformation (18). Recent studies have also failed to find an association between ovulation induction with clomiphene and neural tube defects (19–25) or any defects (19,23). Congenital malformations reported in patients who received clomiphene before conception include the following (8,9,26–40):

- Hydatidiform mole
- Retinal aplasia
- Syndactyly
- Clubfoot
- Pigmentation defects
- Microcephaly
- Congenital heart defects
- Cleft lip/palate
- Down's syndrome
- Ovarian dysplasia
- Hypospadias
- Polydactyly
- Hemangioma
- Anencephaly
- Persistent hyperplastic primary vitreous

A 1996 prospective study examined the possible relationship between clomiphene and spontaneous abortions (41). The outcomes of 1744 clomiphene-induced pregnancies were compared with the outcomes of 3245 spontaneous pregnancies. The incidence of spontaneous abortion (clinical and preclinical) was higher in clomiphene-induced pregnancies than in spontaneous pregnancies (23.7% vs. 20.4%, $p < 0.01$).

Acardius acephalus in a monozygotic twin was observed in a pregnancy occurring after ovulation induced with clomiphene (42). Because monozygotic twining is associated with an increased incidence of congenital defects, and because clomiphene-induced ovulation increases the incidence of multiple gestation and possibly of monozygotic twins, the investigators thought that the drug may have had a causative role, either directly or indirectly, in the defect. Another case of acardius acephalus similar to the one above was published in 1995 (43). The authors also mentioned a third case that had been published in 1990 (44). However, they concluded that there was insufficient evidence to establish a relationship between clomiphene and acardiac twinning (43).

A single case of hepatoblastoma in a 15-month-old female was thought to be caused by the use of clomiphene and follicle-stimulating/luteinizing hormone prior to conception (45).

Inadvertent use of clomiphene early in the 1st trimester has been reported in two patients (32,38). A ruptured lumbosacral meningomyelocele was observed in one infant exposed during the 4th week of gestation (32). There was no evidence of neurologic defect in the lower limbs or of hydrocephalus. The second infant was delivered with esophageal atresia with fistula, congenital heart defects, hypospadias, and absent left kidney (38). The mother also took methyldopa throughout pregnancy for mild hypertension.

In a surveillance study of Michigan Medicaid recipients involving 229,101 completed pregnancies conducted between 1985 and 1992, 41 newborns may have been exposed to clomiphene during the 1st trimester (F. Rosa, personal communication, FDA, 1993). Three (7.3%) (two expected) major birth defects were observed, one of which was a cardiovascular defect (0.5 expected). No anomalies were observed in five other categories of defects (oral clefts, spina bifida, polydactyly, limb-reduction defects, and hypospadias) for which specific data were available. Although the number of exposures is small, these data do not support an association between the drug and congenital defects.

BREASTFEEDING SUMMARY

No reports describing the use of clomiphene during lactation have been located. The drug may reduce lactation in some patients (46).

References

1. Product information. Serophene. Serono Laboratories, 1993.
2. Shepard TH. *Catalog of Teratogenic Agents*. 6th ed. Baltimore, MD: Johns Hopkins University Press, 1989:158–9.
3. Dziadek M. Preovulatory administration of clomiphene citrate to mice causes fetal growth retardation and neural tube defects (exencephaly) by an indirect maternal effect. Teratology 1993;47:263–73.
4. Barrett C, Hakim C. Anencephaly, ovulation stimulation, subfertility, and illegitimacy. Lancet 1973;2:916–7.
5. Dyson JL, Kohler HG, Anencephaly and ovulation stimulation. Lancet 1973;1:1256–7.
6. Field B, Kerr C. Ovulation stimulation and defects of neural tube closure. Lancet 1974;2:1511.
7. Sandler B. Anencephaly and ovulation stimulation. Lancet 1973;2:379.
8. Biale Y, Leventhal H, Altaras M, Ben-Aderet N. Anencephaly and clomiphene-induced pregnancy. Acta Obstet Gynecol Scand 1978;57:483–4.
9. Asch RH, Greenblatt RB. Update on the safety and efficacy of clomiphene citrate as a therapeutic agent. J Reprod Med 1976;17:175–180.
10. Harlap S. Ovulation induction and congenital malformations. Lancet 1976;2:961.
11. James WH, Clomiphene, anencephaly, and spina bifida. Lancet 1977;1:603.
12. Ahlgren M, Kallen B, Rannevik G. Outcome of pregnancy after clomiphene therapy. Acta Obstet Gynecol Scand 1976;55:371–5.
13. Elwood JM. Clomiphene and anencephalic births. Lancet 1974;1:31.
14. Czeizel A. Ovulation induction and neural tube defects. Lancet 1989;2:167.
15. Cuckle H, Wald N. Ovulation induction and neural tube defects. Lancet 1989;2:1281.
16. Cornel MC, Ten Kate LP, Graham Dukes MN, De Jong-V D Berg LTW, Meyboom RHB, Garbis H, Peters PWJ. Ovulation induction and neural tube defects. Lancet 1989;1:1386.
17. Cornel MC, Ten Kate LP, Te Meerman GJ. Ovulation induction, in-vitro fertilisation, and neural tube defects. Lancet 1989;2:1530.
18. Kurachi K, Aono T, Minagawa J, Miyake A. Congenital malformations of newborn infants after clomiphene-induced ovulation. Fertil Steril 1983;40:187–9.
19. Mills JL, Simpson JL, Rhoads GG, Graubard BI, Hoffman H, Conley MR, Lassman M, Cunningham G. Risk of neural tube defects in relation to maternal fertility and fertility drug use. Lancet 1990;336:103–4.
20. Rosa F. Ovulation induction and neural tube defects. Lancet 1990;336:1327.
21. Mills JL. Clomiphene and neural-tube defects. Lancet 1991;337:853.

22. Van Loon K, Besseghir K, Eshkol A. Neural tube defects after infertility treatment: a review. Fertil Steril 1992;58:875–84.
23. Shoham Z, Zosmer A, Insler V. Early miscarriage and fetal malformations after induction of ovulation (by clomiphene citrate and/or human menotropins), in vitro fertilization, and gamete intrafallopian transfer. Fertil Steril 1991;55:1–11.
24. Werler MM, Louik C, Shapiro S, Mitchell AA. Ovulation induction and risk of neural tube defects. Lancet 1994;344:445–6.
25. Greenland S, Ackerman DL. Clomiphene citrate and neural tube defects: a pooled analysis of controlled epidemiologic studies and recommendations for future studies. Fertil Steril 1995;64:936–41.
26. Miles PA, Taylor HB, Hill WC. Hydatidiform mole in a clomiphene related pregnancy: a case report. Obstet Gynecol 1971;37:358–9.
27. Schneiderman CI, Waxman B. Clomid therapy and subsequent hydatidiform mole formation: a case report. Obstet Gynecol 1972;39:787–8.
28. Wajntraub G, Kamar R, Pardo Y. Hydatidiform mole after treatment with clomiphene. Fertil Steril 1974;25:904–5.
29. Berman P. Congenital abnormalities associated with maternal clomiphene ingestion. Lancet 1975;2:878.
30. Drew AL. Letter to the editor. Dev Med Child Neurol 1974;16:276.
31. Hack M, Brish M, Serr DM, Insler V, Salomy M, Lunenfeld B. Outcome of pregnancy after induced ovulation. Follow-up of pregnancies and children born after clomiphene therapy. JAMA 1972;220:1329–33.
32. Ylikorkala O. Congenital anomalies and clomiphene. Lancet 1975;2:1262–3.
33. Laing IA, Steer CR, Dudgeon J, Brown JK. Clomiphene and congenital retinopathy. Lancet 1981;2:1107–8.
34. Ford WDA, Little KET. Fetal ovarian dysplasia possibly associated with clomiphene. Lancet 1981;2:1107.
35. Kistner RW. Induction of ovulation with clomiphene citrate. Obstet Gynecol Surv 1965;20:873–99.
36. Goldfarb AF, Morales A, Rakoff AE, Protos P. Critical review of 160 clomiphene-related pregnancies. Obstet Gynecol 1968;31:342–5.
37. Oakely GP, Flynt IW. Increased prevalence of Down's syndrome (mongolism) among the offspring of women treated with ovulation-inducing agents. Teratology 1972;5:264.
38. Singhi M, Singhi S. Possible relationship between clomiphene and neural tube defects. J Pediatr 1978;93:152.
39. Mor-Joseph S, Anteby SO, Granat M, Brzezinsky A, Evron S. Recurrent molar pregnancies associated with clomiphene citrate and human gonadotropins. Am J Obstet Gynecol 1985;151:1085–6.
40. Bishai R, Arbour L, Lyons C, Koren G. Intrauterine exposure to clomiphene and neonatal persistent hyperplastic primary vitreous. Teratology 1999;60:143–5.
41. Dickey RP, Taylor SN, Curole DN, Rye PH, Pyrzak R. Incidence of spontaneous abortion in clomiphene pregnancies. Hum Reprod 1996;11:2623–8.
42. Haring DAJP, Cornel MC, Van Der Linden JC, Van Vugt JMG, Kwee ML. Acardius acephalus after induced ovulation: a case report. Teratology 1993;47:257–62.
43. Martinez-Roman S, Torres PJ, Puerto B. Acardius acephalus after ovulation induction by clomiphene. Teratology 1995;51:231–2.
44. Sceusa DK, Klein PE. Ultrasound diagnosis of an acardius acephalic monster in a quintuplet pregnancy. JDMS 1990;2:109–12. As cited by Martinez-Roman S, Torres PJ, Puerto B. Acardius acephalus after ovulation induction by clomiphene. Teratology 1995;51:231–2.
45. Melamed I, Bujanover Y, Hammer J, Spirer Z. Hepatoblastoma in an infant born to a mother after hormonal treatment for sterility. N Engl J Med 1982;307:820.
46. Product information. Clomid. Hoechst Marion Roussel, 2000.

CLOMIPRAMINE

Antidepressant

PREGNANCY RECOMMENDATION: Human Data Suggest Risk in 1st and 3rd Trimesters
BREASTFEEDING RECOMMENDATION: Limited Human Data—Potential Toxicity

PREGNANCY SUMMARY

Clomipramine was not teratogenic in animals, but a statistically significant association between clomipramine and cardiac defects was found in a human study. These results require confirmation. In addition, newborn toxicity may occur due to apparent drug withdrawal. In two cases, in utero exposure to a benzodiazepine sedative may have contributed to the observed symptoms. Although the data are very limited, no long-term effects of in utero exposure to clomipramine have been observed.

FETAL RISK SUMMARY

Clomipramine is a tricyclic antidepressant in the same class as amitriptyline, doxepin, imipramine, and trimipramine. No teratogenic effects were observed after dosing with clomipramine via the oral (mice and rats), SC (mice and rats), and IV (mice and rabbits) routes (1). Congenital malformations (2,3) and toxic symptoms (caused by apparent drug withdrawal) (4–10) have been reported in human fetuses exposed to clomipramine.

In a 1996 descriptive large case series, the European Network of the Teratology Information Services (ENTIS) prospectively examined the outcomes of 689 pregnancies exposed to antidepressants (2). Multiple drug therapy occurred in about two-thirds of the mothers. Clomipramine (134 exposures) was the most commonly used tricyclic antidepressant. The outcomes of these pregnancies were 20 elective abortions, 22 spontaneous abortions, 4 stillbirths, 76 normal newborns (includes 2 premature infants), 9 normal infants with neonatal disorder (primarily withdrawal symptoms), and 3 infants with congenital defects. The defects (all exposed in the 1st trimester or longer) were Down's syndrome, bilateral talipes (also exposed to prazepam), and Harlequin syndrome with multiple anomalies (exposed to multiple other agents).

A 2003 case–control study, using data from three Swedish health registers, was conducted to identify drug use in early pregnancy that was associated with cardiac defects (3). Cases (cardiovascular defects without known chromosome anomalies) (N = 5015) were compared with controls consisting of all infants born in Sweden (1995–2001) (N = 577,730). Associations were identified for several drugs, some of which were probably due to confounding from the underlying disease or complaint or multiple testing, but some were thought to be true drug effects (2). For all antidepressants, there were 40 cases in 4068 exposures (odds ratio [OR] 1.14, 95% confidence interval [CI] 0.83–1.56). There was an increased OR for the tricyclic/tetracyclic antidepressants (16 cases, 1018 exposures; OR 1.77, 95% CI 1.07–2.91), but the association was due to clomipramine (15 cases, 838 exposures; OR 2.03, 95% CI 1.22–3.40). The lack of an association with other antidepressants suggested to the investigators that it was unlikely that the underlying disease itself caused the association with clomipramine (3).

A mother took clomipramine 25 mg three times daily throughout a normal pregnancy (4). Twelve hours after birth, the 3140-g male infant became dusky and was hypothermic (rectal temperature 35.4°C). Hypothermia persisted for 4 days and was aggravated by feeding and handling. Jitteriness, attributed to drug withdrawal, developed on the 2nd day and persisted for 48 hours. The symptoms were controlled with phenobarbital. Plasma levels of clomipramine and its metabolite, chlordesipramine, were <20 and 116 ng/mL, respectively, at 1 day of age, and <20 and 96 ng/mL, respectively, at age 3 days. Recovery was uneventful and normal development was noted at 3 and 6 months of age (4).

Drug withdrawal was observed in two newborns exposed throughout gestation to clomipramine (5). A 3550-g infant, exposed to 200 mg/day, appeared normal at birth but became lethargic, cyanotic, and tachypneic with moderate respiratory acidosis within a few hours. Oxygen therapy corrected the cyanosis and respiratory acidosis. Jitteriness and tremors developed by the end of the 1st day, followed by intermittent hypertonia and hypotonia, tachypnea, and feeding problems. Phenobarbital was used to control the symptoms, which resolved completely in 1 week. A 4020-g newborn, whose mother had taken 100 mg/day of clomipramine, had symptoms similar to those observed in the first infant. Oxygen and phenobarbital therapy were used, and although the neurologic symptoms had resolved within a few days, tachypnea and feeding difficulties persisted for 16 days. Both infants were developing normally at 5 months of age (5).

Neonatal convulsions were observed in two male infants after in utero exposure to clomipramine (maternal doses not specified) (6). The onset of seizures occurred at 8 and 7 hours. The first infant, a 3420-g newborn whose mother had been treated with clomipramine during the last 7 weeks of gestation, had persistent intermittent convulsions, despite treatment with phenobarbital and paraldehyde, until 53 hours of age, after which he remained hypertonic and jittery with ankle clonus until the 11th day. The second infant, exposed throughout gestation to clomipramine and flurazepam (dose not specified), delivered at 33 weeks' gestation with a birth weight of 2360 g, had convulsions that were unresponsive to phenobarbital. At 24 hours of age, 0.4 mg of clomipramine was given intravenously over 2 hours, resulting in complete cessation of the symptoms for 11 hours. Upon their recurrence, a dose of 0.5 mg over 2 hours was given, followed by a continuous tapering infusion until age 12 days when oral therapy was started (doses not given). No additional convulsions were observed, but he remained jittery. All therapy was stopped at age 17 days without adverse effect. No follow-up of either infant was mentioned. The combined concentrations of drug and metabolite in the mothers were 610 and 549 ng/mL, respectively, both higher than the suggested therapeutic range of 200–500 ng/mL. Although the exact values could not be obtained from the graphs used in the reference, the initial combined serum levels of clomipramine and metabolite in the infants appear to be in the range of 250–400 ng/mL. The authors attributed the convulsions to the initial steep decline in serum drug levels, with clomipramine therapy in the second infant permitting a more gradual decline in concentrations and, thus, control of the infant's symptoms. Neurologic symptoms in the infants did not resolve completely until the concentration of clomipramine was <10 ng/mL (6).

Six cases of fetal exposure to clomipramine were described in a 1991 report (7). One infant, with meconium-stained fluid in the trachea, had mild respiratory distress with acidosis, mild hypotonia, and a tremor at birth. At 12 hours of age, the newborn developed jitteriness that resolved spontaneously, along with the other symptoms, by 6 days of age. At birth, clomipramine concentrations were 474.4 ng/mL in the maternal serum and 266.6 ng/mL in the neonatal plasma (ratio 1.8). Levels of the metabolite were not determined. The mother's dose at this time was 125 mg/day. The elimination half-life of clomipramine in the infant during the first week, when the male infant was not breastfeeding, was 92.8 hours. Among the other five cases, one woman had a therapeutic abortion at 9 weeks' gestation, one stopped clomipramine therapy when she realized she was pregnant, and the remaining three continued therapy with daily doses between 75 and 250 mg throughout gestation. Mild hypotonia, persisting for several weeks, was observed in one of the four liveborn infants, and transient tachypnea requiring oxygen therapy was observed in another. No other symptoms or signs of toxicity were noted (7).

Three additional cases of drug withdrawal to clomipramine have been reported (8–10). A short 1990 case report described symptoms of drug withdrawal in a newborn exposed during the last 8–9 weeks of gestation to daily doses of 125 mg of clomipramine and 3 mg of lorazepam (8). The 3900-g infant was normal until 8 hours of age, when tachypnea, with a respiratory rate of 100–120 breaths/minute, and recessions developed. Other symptoms noted in the infant over the next 10 days were intermittent hypertonia and marked diaphoresis. Treatment consisted of intravenous fluids, oxygen, and empiric antibiotic therapy. No follow-up of the infant was reported (8). In the second case, a 33-year-old woman with an obsessive-compulsive disorder was treated with clomipramine, 100–150 mg/day, from the 12th week of gestation through the 32nd week (9). At that time, the mother decided on her own to discontinue the drug and, 4 days later, she presented in premature labor and imminent delivery, and a 2.7-kg infant was delivered by cesarean section. Repetitive seizures, rigidity, irritability, and decerebrate-like posturing, which was unresponsive to phenobarbital and phenytoin, occurred 10 minutes after birth. After 3 days of convulsions, 0.5 mg of clomipramine was given via gastric tube with resolution of the seizures within 30 minutes. When the seizures recurred 10 hours later, clomipramine, 0.5 mg three times daily, was started and the phenobarbital discontinued. The clomipramine was gradually tapered over the next 20 days. An EEG shortly after birth showed a left temporal epileptogenic focus, but was normal after 20 days of clomipramine therapy. The infant was discharged home at the age of 1 month with no signs or symptoms of neurological damage (9). The third case involved a term male infant who

C

had been exposed throughout gestation to 100 mg/day (10). Generalized, stimulate sensitive, status myoclonus developed at age 2 days (clomipramine serum level <10 ng/mL) that were successfully treated with 0.5 mg clomipramine. Previous treatment with clonazepam and phenobarbital was unsuccessful. At 3 weeks of age, only mild jitteriness in response to touch was noted (10).

A 2002 prospective study compared two groups of mother–child pairs exposed to antidepressants throughout gestation (46 exposed to tricyclics—7 to clomipramine; 40 to fluoxetine) to 36 nonexposed, not depressed controls (11). Offspring were studied between the ages 15 and 71 months for effects of antidepressant exposure in terms of IQ, language, behavior, and temperament. Exposure to antidepressants did not adversely affect the measured parameters, but IQ was significantly and negatively associated with the duration of depression, and language was negatively associated with the number of depression episodes after delivery (11).

BREASTFEEDING SUMMARY

Clomipramine is excreted into human milk (7). A woman taking 125 mg/day of the antidepressant had milk and plasma concentrations determined on the 4th and 6th postpartum days. Her infant was not breastfeeding during this time. Milk levels were 342.7 and 215.8 ng/mL, respectively, compared with plasma levels of 211.0 and 208.4 ng/mL, respectively. The milk:plasma ratios on the 4th and 6th days were 1.62 and 1.04, respectively. Neonatal plasma concentrations of clomipramine, from drug obtained in utero, declined from 266.6 ng/mL at birth to 94.8 ng/mL on the 6th day. The baby was allowed to breastfeed commencing at 7 days of age; at the same time, the mother's dose was increased to 150 mg/day. Repeat determinations of milk and plasma clomipramine concentrations were made between 10 and 14 hours after the daily dose on the 10th, 14th, and 35th days after delivery. Milk levels ranged from 269.8 to 624.2 ng/mL compared with plasma concentrations of 355.0–509.8 ng/mL, corresponding to milk:plasma ratios of 0.76–1.22. The highest concentrations for both the milk and the plasma occurred on the 35th day, but neonatal drug levels continued to decline from 45.4 ng/mL on the 10th day to 9.8 ng/mL on the 35th day. No adverse effects were noted in the infant during breastfeeding (7).

A 1996 review of antidepressant treatment during breastfeeding found no information that clomipramine exposure during nursing resulted in quantifiable amounts in an infant or that the exposure caused adverse effects (12).

Ten nursing infants of mothers taking antidepressants (two with clomipramine 75–125 mg/day) were compared with 15 bottle-fed infants of mothers with depression who did not breastfeed (13). Concentrations of clomipramine in fore-milk and hind-milk ranged from 32 to 212 ng/mL and 32 to 436 ng/mL, respectively. The milk:maternal plasma ratios were 0.4–1.2 and 0.4–3.0, respectively. One infant had plasma levels of 3.2 ng/mL when the mother was taking 75 mg/day and 5.5 ng/mL when the dose was increased to 125 mg/day. No toxic effects or delays in development were observed in the infants. The estimated daily dose consumed by the infants was about 1% of the mother's weight-adjusted dose (13).

The American Academy of Pediatrics classifies clomipramine as a drug whose effect on the nursing infant is unknown but may be of concern (14).

References

1. Watanabe N, Nakai T, Iwanami K, Fujii T. Toxicological studies of clomipramine hydrochloride. Kiso to Rinsho 1970;4:2105–24. As cited in Shepard TH. *Catalog of Teratogenic Agents*. 6th ed. Baltimore, MD: Johns Hopkins University Press, 1989:159–60.
2. McElhatton PR, Garbis HM, Elefant E, Vial T, Bellemin B, Mastroiacovo P, Arnon J, Rodriguez-Pinilla E, Schaefer C, Pexieder T, Merlob P, Dal Verme S. The outcome of pregnancy in 689 women exposed to therapeutic doses of antidepressants. A collaborative study of the European Network of Teratology Information Services (ENTIS). Reprod Toxicol 1996;10:285–94.
3. Kallen BAJ, Olausson PO. Maternal drug use in early pregnancy and infant cardiovascular defect. Reprod Toxicol 2003;17:255–61.
4. Ben Muza A, Smith CS. Neonatal effects of maternal clomipramine therapy. Arch Dis Child 1979;54:405.
5. Ostergaard GZ, Pedersen SE. Neonatal effects of maternal clomipramine treatment. Pediatrics 1982;69:233–4.
6. Cowe L, Lloyd DJ, Dawling S. Neonatal convulsions caused by withdrawal from maternal clomipramine. Br Med J 1982;284:1837–8.
7. Schimmell MS, Katz EZ, Shaag Y, Pastuszak A, Koren G. Toxic neonatal effects following maternal clomipramine therapy. J Toxicol Clin Toxicol 1991;29:479–84.
8. Singh S, Gulati S, Narang A, Bhakoo ON. Non-narcotic withdrawal syndrome in a neonate due to maternal clomipramine therapy. J Pediatr Child Health 1990;26:110.
9. Bromiker R, Kaplan M. Apparent intrauterine fetal withdrawal from clomipramine hydrochloride. JAMA 1994;272:1722–3.
10. Bloem BR, Lammers GJ, Roofthooft DWE, De Beaufort AJ, Brouwer OF. Clomipramine withdrawal in newborns. Arch Dis Child Fetal Neonatal Ed 1999;81:F77.
11. Nulman I, Rovet J, Stewart DE, Wolpin J, Pace-Asciak P, Shuhaiber S, Koren G. Child development following exposure to tricyclic antidepressants or fluoxetine throughout fetal life: a prospective, controlled study. Am J Psychiatry 2002;159:1889–95.
12. Wisner KL, Perel JM, Findling RL. Antidepressant treatment during breast-feeding. Am J Psychiatry 1996;153:1132–7.
13. Yoshida K, Smith B, Craggs M, Kumar RC. Investigation of pharmacokinetics and of possible adverse effects in infants exposed to tricyclic antidepressants in breast-milk. J Affect Disord 1997;43:225–37.
14. Committee on Drugs, American Academy of Pediatrics. The transfer of drugs and other chemicals into human milk. Pediatrics 2001;108:776–89.

CLOMOCYCLINE

Antibiotic (Tetracycline)

See Tetracycline.

C

CLONAZEPAM

Anticonvulsant

PREGNANCY RECOMMENDATION: Human Data Suggest Low Risk
BREASTFEEDING RECOMMENDATION: Compatible*

PREGNANCY SUMMARY

Clonazepam was teratogenic in one animal species but not in another. Published human pregnancy experience in the 1st trimester is limited to 71 cases. In these exposures, one major congenital defect was observed. Fetal and neonatal toxicity also has been reported. Although the true incidence of teratogenicity and toxicity cannot be determined, the risk of adverse pregnancy outcome appears to be low, but additional study is needed. Until such data are available, the safest course is to avoid the drug during the 1st trimester. However, if clonazepam is indicated, it should not be withheld because of pregnancy.

FETAL RISK SUMMARY

Clonazepam is a benzodiazepine anticonvulsant that is chemically and structurally similar to diazepam (1). The drug is used either alone or in combination with other anticonvulsants.

Reproduction studies in mice and rats during organogensis at doses up to 4 and 20 times, respectively, the maximum recommended human dose of 20 mg/day for seizures [MRHD-S], and 20 and 100 times, respectively, the maximum recommended human dose of 4 mg/day for panic disorders [MRHD-P], based on BSA, revealed no evidence of embryo or fetal effects (2). In rabbits administered doses that were 0.2–10 times the MRHD-S and 1–50 times the MRHD-P, a low, non-dose-related incidence of a similar pattern of malformations (cleft palate, open eyelid, fused sternebrae, and limb defects) was observed in all dosage groups (2). At the highest dose (twice the dose that produced reductions in maternal weight gain), intrauterine growth restriction was also observed.

In a small series of patients (N = 150) matched with nonepileptic controls, anticonvulsant therapy, including five women using clonazepam, had no effect on the incidence of gestational hypertension, albuminuria, premature contractions, premature labor, bleeding in pregnancy, duration of labor, blood loss at delivery, cesarean sections, and vacuum extractions (3).

In a surveillance study of Michigan Medicaid recipients involving 229,101 completed pregnancies conducted between 1985 and 1992, 19 newborns had been exposed to clonazepam during the 1st trimester (F. Rosa, personal communication, FDA, 1993). Three (15.8%) major birth defects were observed (one expected), two of which were cardiovascular defects (0.2 expected). No anomalies were observed in five other categories of defects (oral clefts, spina bifida, polydactyly, limb-reduction defects, and hypospadias) for which specific data were available.

A prospective study published in 1999 described the outcomes of 517 pregnancies of epileptic mothers identified at one Italian center from 1977 (4). Excluding genetic and chromosomal defects, malformations were classified as severe structural defects, mild structural defects, and deformations. Minor anomalies were not considered. Spontaneous (N = 38) and elective (N = 20) abortions were excluded from the analysis, as were 7 pregnancies that delivered at other hospitals. Of the remaining 452 outcomes, 427 were exposed to anticonvulsants; of which, 313 involved monotherapy: clonazepam (N = 6), carbamazepine (N = 113), phenobarbital (N = 83), valproate (N = 44), primidone (N = 35), phenytoin (N = 31), and other (N = 1). There were no defects in the 25 pregnancies not exposed to anticonvulsants. Of the 42 (9.3%) outcomes with malformations, 24 (5.3%) were severe, 10 (2.2%) were mild, and 8 (1.8%) were deformities. There were no malformations with clonazepam monotherapy. The investigators concluded that the anticonvulsants were the primary risk factor for an increased incidence of congenital malformations (see also Carbamazepine, Phenobarbital, Phenytoin, Primidone, and Valproic Acid) (4).

A 2001 report described the pregnancy outcomes of 38 women treated during gestation with clonazepam for panic disorder (5). Twenty-nine of the women were taking clonazepam at the time of conception and 27 were taking the drug at delivery. The Apgar scores were within normal limits. Hospital records were available for 27 infants, 17 of whom were exposed to the agent at delivery. In the 27 infants, there was no evidence of neonatal withdrawal or congenital anomalies, but 2 infants had minor defects: hydrocele; two-vessel umbilical cord. One infant had cardiac disease (no specific details) but was not exposed to clonazepam in the 1st trimester (5).

The database of the Hungarian Case–Control Surveillance of Congenital Abnormalities (1980–1996) was used in a 2002 report that evaluated the teratogenicity of five benzodiazepines: clonazepam, alprazolam, medazepam, nitrazepam, and tofisopam (6). There were 22,865 women who delivered infants with congenital abnormalities, 57 (0.25%) of whom used one of the benzodiazepines in pregnancy. Clonazepam was used throughout gestation in four cases (cleft lip and/or palate, cardiovascular defect, hypospadias, and multiple defects). Although the data were limited, no teratogenic risk was found for clonazepam or the other agents (6).

*Potential toxicity if combined with other CNS depressants.

In a 2004 report, the medical records of 28,565 infants were surveyed to identify cases exposed to anticonvulsants (7). Of 166 cases, 52 had been exposed to clonazepam, 43 as monotherapy. Thirty-three of the monotherapy cases had been exposed in the 1st trimester. Congenital defects were noted in one (3.0%) infant: dysmorphic facial features (small eyes, ptosis, and external auditory canal stenosis), tetralogy of Fallot, 11 pair of ribs, and growth restriction (length and head circumference <5th percentile). As with other case series, the data are limited but no increase in congenital malformations was observed (7).

The Lamotrigine Pregnancy Registry, an ongoing project conducted by the manufacturer, was first published in January 1997 (8). The final report was published in July 2010. The Registry is now closed. Among 103 prospectively enrolled pregnancies exposed to clonazepam and lamotrigine, with or without other anticonvulsants, 98 were exposed in the 1st trimester, resulting in 88 live births without defects, 5 spontaneous abortions, 2 elective abortions, and 3 birth defects. There were five exposures in the 2nd/3rd trimesters resulting in three live births, one fetal death, and one birth defect (8).

Toxicity in the newborn, apparently related to clonazepam, has been reported. Apnea, cyanosis, lethargy, and hypotonia developed at 6 hours of age in an infant of 36 weeks' gestational age exposed throughout pregnancy to an unspecified amount of clonazepam (9). There was no evidence of congenital defects in the 2750-g newborn. Cord and maternal serum levels of clonazepam were 19 and 32 ng/mL, respectively, a ratio of 0.59. Both levels were within the therapeutic range (5–70 ng/mL). At 18 hours of age, the clonazepam level in the infant's serum measured 4.4 ng/mL. Five episodes of prolonged apnea (16–43 seconds/occurrence) were measured by pneumogram over the next 12 hours. Hypotonia and lethargy resolved within 5 days, but overt clinical apnea persisted for 10 days. Follow-up pneumograms demonstrated apnea spells until 10 weeks of age, but the presence of the drug in breast milk may have contributed to the condition (see Breastfeeding Summary). The authors concluded that apnea due to prematurity was not a significant factor. Neurologic development was normal at 5 months (9).

A 1995 case report described paralytic ileus of the small bowel in a fetus at 32 weeks' gestation associated with polyhydramnios (10). The fetal stomach was enlarged (more than 2 standard deviations above the mean). The mother had been treated with clonazepam (4 mg/day) and carbamazepine (1800 mg/day) for epilepsy throughout gestation. A 2420-g male infant was delivered by cesarean section at 36 weeks' gestation. Normal bowel movements started after three gastrographin enemas. No evidence of cystic fibrosis or Hirschsprung disease was found and the child was developing normally at 20 months of age. The ileus was attributed to clonazepam (10).

A study published in 2009 examined the effect of AEDs on the head circumference in newborns (11). Significant reductions in mean birth-weight-adjusted mean head circumference (bw-adj-HC) was noted for monotherapy with carbamazepine and valproic acid. No effect on bw-adj-HC was observed with gabapentin, phenytoin, clonazepam, and lamotrigine. A significant increase in the occurrence of microcephaly (bw-adj-HC smaller than 2 standard deviations below the mean) was noted after any AED polytherapy but not after any monotherapy, including carbamazepine and valproic acid. The potential effects of these findings on child development warrant study (11).

BREASTFEEDING SUMMARY

Clonazepam is excreted into breast milk. In a woman treated with an unspecified amount of the anticonvulsant, milk concentrations remained constant between 11 and 13 ng/mL (9). The milk:maternal serum ratio was approximately 0.33. After 7 days of nursing, the infant, described above, had a serum concentration of 2.9 ng/mL. A major portion of this probably resulted from in utero exposure because the elimination half-life of clonazepam in neonates is thought to be prolonged. No evidence of drug accumulation after breastfeeding was found. Persistent apneic spells, lasting until 10 weeks of age, were observed, but it was not known whether breastfeeding contributed to the condition. Based on this case, the authors recommended that infants exposed in utero or during breastfeeding to clonazepam should have serum levels of the drug determined and be closely monitored for central nervous system depression or apnea (9).

A 1988 report described a woman who was treated with clonazepam (4 mg/day) and phenytoin (400 mg/day) throughout gestation and during nursing (12). The healthy, 3930-g infant was delivered at term. Maternal serum and milk samples were collected several times over postpartum days 2–4 at 0–11 hours after a dose. The concentrations of clonazepam in the serum ranged from 51to 104 nmol/L (about 16–33 ng/mL), whereas those in the milk ranged from <10 to 34 nmol/L (about 3–11 ng/mL). The infant's serum level of clonazepam in the pooled sample from days 2 to 4 was 15 nmol/L (about 5 ng/mL). The study could not determine the proportions of the infant drug level that resulted from placental transfer and ingestion from milk. No effects on the infant were mentioned (12).

A 2006 report described six women taking quetiapine and other psychotropic agents during breastfeeding (13). Milk samples in one woman at 17.5 weeks postpartum were obtained after doses of clonazepam (0.5 mg), quetiapine (25 mg), and paroxetine (60 mg) (timing of samples and daily doses were not specified). None of the drugs was detected in the milk (<30 nmol/L). The estimated infant daily dose for all three drugs was <0.01 mg/kg/day. In addition, the infant's behavior was assessed with the Bayley Scales of Infant Development, Second Edition. The results suggested normal development (13).

The effects of exposure to benzodiazepines during breastfeeding were reported in a 2012 study (14). In a 15-month period spanning 2010–2011, 296 women called the Motherisk Program in Toronto, Ontario, seeking advice on the use of these drugs during lactation and 124 consented to the study. The most commonly used benzodiazepines were lorazepam (52%), clonazepam (18%), and midazolam (15%). Neonatal sedation was reported in only two infants. Clonazepam was not taken by either mother. There was no significant difference between the characteristics of these 2 and the 122 that reported no sedation in terms of maternal age, gestational age at birth, daily amount of time nursing, amount of time infant slept each day, and the benzodiazepine dose (mg/kg/day). The only difference was in the number of CNS depressants that the mothers were taking: 3.5 vs. 1.7 ($p = 0.0056$). In one of the two infants with sedation, the mother reported using clonazepam (0.25 mg twice daily), flurazepam (1 mg/day), bupropion (1 mg/day), and risperidone (0.75 mg/day). The infant also was exposed in utero. The investigators concluded that their results supported the recommendation that the use benzodiazepines was not a reason to avoid breastfeeding (14).

C

References

1. Reith H, Schafer H. Antiepileptic drugs during pregnancy and the lactation period. Pharmacokinetic data. Dtsch Med Wochenschr 1979;104:818–23.
2. Product information. Klonopin. Roche Laboratories, 2000.
3. Hiilesmaa VK, Bardy A, Teramo K. Obstetric outcome in women with epilepsy. Am J Obstet Gynecol 1985;152:499–504.
4. Canger R, Battino D, Canevini MP, Fumarola C, Guidolin L, Vignoli A, Mamoli D, Palmieri C, Molteni F, Granata T, Hassibi P, Zamperini P, Pardi G, Avanzini G. Malformations in offspring of women with epilepsy: a prospective study. Epilepsia 1999;40:1231–6.
5. Weinstock L, Cohen LS, Bailey JW, Blatman R, Rosenbaum JF. Obstetrical and neonatal outcome following clonazepam use during pregnancy: a case series. Psychother Psychosom 2001;70:158–62.
6. Eros E, Czeizel AE, Rockenbauer M, Sorensen HT, Olsen J. A population-based case–control teratology study of nitrazepam, medazepam, tofisopam, alprazolam, and clonazepam treatment during pregnancy. Eur J Obstet Gynecol Reprod Biol 2002;101:147–54.
7. Lin AE, Peller AJ, Westgate MN, Houde K, Franz A, Holmes LB. Clonazepam use in pregnancy and the risk of malformations. Birth Defects Res (Part A) 2004;70:534–6.
8. The Lamotrigine Pregnancy Registry. Final Report. 1 September 1992 through 31 March 2010. GlaxoSmithKline, July 2010.
9. Fisher JB, Edgren BE, Mammel MC, Coleman JM. Neonatal apnea associated with maternal clonazepam therapy: a case report. Obstet Gynecol 1985;66(Suppl):34S–5S.
10. Haeusler MC, Hoellwarth ME, Holzer P. Paralytic ileus in a fetus-neonate after maternal intake of benzodiazepine. Prenat Diagn 1995;15:1165–7.
11. Almgren M, Kallen B, Lavebratt C. Population-based study of antiepileptic drug exposure in utero—influence on head circumference in newborns. Seizure 2009;18:672–5.
12. Soderman P, Matheson I. Clonazepam in breast milk. Eur J Pediatrics 1988;147:212–3.
13. Misri S, Corral M, Wardrop AA, Kendrick K. Quetiapine augmentation in lactation. A series of case reports. J Clin Psychopharm 2006;26:508–11.
14. Kelly LE, Poon S, Madadi P, Koren G. Neonatal benzodiazepines exposure during breastfeeding. J Pediatr 2012;161:448–51.

CLONIDINE

Antihypertensive/Central Analgesic

PREGNANCY RECOMMENDATION: Limited Human Data—Animal Data Suggest Risk
BREASTFEEDING RECOMMENDATION: Limited Human Data—Probably Compatible

PREGNANCY SUMMARY

No reports linking the use of clonidine with congenital defects have been located. The drug has been used during all trimesters, but experience during the 1st trimester is very limited. Adverse fetal effects attributable to clonidine have not been observed (1–8).

FETAL RISK SUMMARY

Reproduction studies in rats at doses as low as 1/3 the oral maximum recommended daily human dose MRDHD-W (based on weight) or 1/15 times the MRDHD-BSA (based on BSA), started before gestation, resulted in increased resorptions (9). Decreased embryo–fetal survival was not observed when these doses were used on gestation days 6–15, but did occur in both mice and rats at doses 40 times the MRDHD-W or 4 to 8 times the MRDHD-BSA. No embryo or fetal toxicity or teratogenicity was observed in rabbits given doses up to 3 times the MRDHD-W (9).

In a surveillance study of Michigan Medicaid recipients involving 229,101 completed pregnancies conducted between 1985 and 1992, 59 newborns had been exposed to clonidine during the 1st trimester (F. Rosa, personal communication, FDA, 1993). Three (5.1%) major birth defects were observed (three expected), two of which were cardiovascular defects (0.6 expected). No anomalies were observed in five other categories of defects (oral clefts, spina bifida, polydactyly, limb-reduction defects, and hypospadias) for which specific data were available. The number of exposures is too small to draw any conclusions.

The pharmacokinetics of clonidine during pregnancy have been reported (10). The mean maternal and cord serum concentrations in 10 women were 0.46 and 0.41 ng/mL, respectively, corresponding to a cord:maternal ratio of 0.89. The mean amniotic fluid concentration was 1.50 ng/mL. The mean maternal dose was 330 mcg/day. Results of neurologic examinations and limited blood chemistry tests in the exposed infants were similar to those in untreated controls. No neonatal hypotension was observed.

BREASTFEEDING SUMMARY

Clonidine is secreted into breast milk (8,10). Following a 150-mcg oral dose, milk concentrations of 1.5 ng/mL may be achieved (milk:plasma ratio 1.5) (P.A. Bowers, personal communication, Boehringer Ingelheim, Ltd., 1981). In a study of nine nursing women taking mean daily doses of 391.7 mcg (postpartum days 1–5), 309.4 mcg (postpartum days 10–14), and 241.7 mcg (postpartum days 45–60), milk concentrations were approximately twice those in maternal serum (10). Mean milk levels were close to 2 ng/mL or higher during the three sampling periods. Hypotension was not observed in the nursing infants, although clonidine was found in the serum of the infants (mean levels less than maternal). The long-term significance of this exposure is not known.

C

References

1. Turnbull AC, Ahmed S. Catapres in the treatment of hypertension in pregnancy, a preliminary study. In: *Catapres in Hypertension*. Symposium of the Royal College of Surgeons. London, 1970:237–45.
2. Johnston CI, Aickin DR. The control of high blood pressure during labour with clonidine. Med J Aust 1971;2:132.
3. Raftos J, Bauer GE, Lewis RG, Stokes GS, Mitchell AS, Young AA, Maclachlan I. Clonidine in the treatment of severe hypertension. Med J Aust 1973;1:786–93.
4. Horvath JS, Phippard A, Korda A, Henderson-Smart DJ, Child A, Tiller DJ. Clonidine hydrochloride—a safe and effective antihypertensive agent in pregnancy. Obstet Gynecol 1985;66:634–8.
5. Horvath JS, Korda A, Child A, Henderson-Smart D, Phippard A, Duggin GC, Hall BM, Tiller DJ. Hypertension in pregnancy: a study of 142 women presenting before 32 weeks' gestation. Med J Aust 1985;143:19–21.
6. Ng Wing Tin L, Frelon JH, Beaute Y, Pellerin M, Guillaumin JP. Clonidine et traitement de l'hypertension arterielle de la femme enceinte. Cahiers d'Anesthésiologie 1986;34:389–93.
7. Ng-Wing Tin L, Frelon JH, Beaute Y, Pellerin M, Guillaumin JP, Bazin C. Clonidine et traitement de l'hypertension arterielle de la femme enceinte. Rev fr Gynécol Obstét 1986;81:563–6.
8. Ng Wing-Tin L, Frelon JH, Hardy F, Bazin C. Clonidine et traitement des urgences hypertensives de la femme enceinte. Rev fr Gynécol Obstét 1987;82:519–22.
9. Product information. Catapres. Boehringer Ingelheim Pharmaceuticals, 2000.
10. Hartikainen-Sorri A-L, Heikkinen JE, Koivisto M. Pharmacokinetics of clonidine during pregnancy and nursing. Obstet Gynecol 1987;69:598–600.

CLOPIDOGREL

Hematologic Agent (Antiplatelet)

PREGNANCY RECOMMENDATION: Limited Human Data—Probably Compatible
BREASTFEEDING RECOMMENDATION: No Human Data—Probably Compatible

PREGNANCY SUMMARY

Clopidogrel is not teratogenic in two animal species, but the limited human pregnancy experience prevents a more complete assessment of the embryo–fetal risk. However, the known benefits to a woman appear to far outweigh the unknown embryo–fetal risks. If a patient's condition requires clopidogrel, the treatment should not be withheld because of pregnancy.

FETAL RISK SUMMARY

Clopidogrel is a direct inhibitor of adenosine diphosphate (ADP)-induced platelet aggregation. It is a prodrug that must be biotransformed to an active metabolite to inhibit platelet aggregation. Neither clopidogrel nor its main circulating metabolite has platelet-inhibiting activity. The active metabolite, which has not been identified, acts by irreversibly inhibiting ADP binding to its receptor and the subsequent ADP-mediated activation of the glycoprotein GPIIb/IIIa complex. Clopidogrel is indicated for the reduction of atherosclerotic events (myocardial infarction, stroke, and vascular death) in patients with atherosclerosis documented by recent occurrences of myocardial infarction, stroke, or established peripheral arterial disease (1).

Reproduction studies have been conducted in pregnant rats and rabbits at doses up to 65 and 78 times, respectively, the recommended daily human dose based on BSA (1). No evidence of impaired fertility or fetotoxicity was seen in either species.

It is not known if clopidogrel, or its active and inactive metabolites, cross the human placenta. The molecular weight of the inactive parent drug (about 420 for the bisulfate) is low enough that some drug probably crosses to the embryo or fetus. The identity and characteristics of the active metabolite, however, have not been determined.

A woman with a history of essential thrombocythemia and myocardial infarction received treatment with chemotherapy (details not specified) to normalize her platelet count and then cardiac bypass surgery (2). After surgery, she conceived while taking aspirin (300 mg/day) and ticlopidine (500 mg/day) but aborted the pregnancy in the 2nd trimester (6 months after surgery). Her treatment was then changed to clopidogrel (150 mg/day) combined with intermittent low-molecular-weight heparin (dalteparin), which she took throughout a second pregnancy. Clopidogrel was discontinued 10 days before vaginal delivery of a healthy, 3170-g female infant. The Apgar scores were 9, 10, 10, and 10 at 1, 5, 10, and 60 minutes, respectively. The mother had no unusual bleeding at delivery and the repair of a mediolateral episiotomy was uneventful. There was no evidence of infarcts or areas of fibrin deposits in the normal placenta. The bottle-fed infant was discharged home with her mother 5 days after delivery (2).

A 43-year-old woman, with a history of diabetes and hypertension, was in her sixth pregnancy when she had an acute myocardial infarction (AMI) at 20 weeks' gestation (3). She was treated with aspirin, nitroglycerin, and then tirofiban with heparin for percutaneous transluminal coronary angioplasty and intracoronary stenting. She was discharged home, 5 days after the procedure, on aspirin, clopidogrel, and metoprolol (doses not specified). The mother and fetus were apparently doing well with appropriate follow-up (3).

A 44-year-old woman at 8 weeks' gestation presented with an AMI (4). She was treated with intracoronary stent placement and clopidogrel (600 mg), heparin, and a 24-hour IV infusion of eptifibatide. The next day, she was started on clopidogrel, aspirin, and propranolol and discharged home on these agents. At 36 weeks' gestation, she underwent a planned cesarean section for a healthy infant (no further details on the newborn were provided) (4).

A 38-year-old woman with severe coronary artery disease and hypertension was started on clopidogrel 75 mg/day, aspirin 75 mg/day, labetalol 200 mg/day, and enoxaparin at about 27 weeks' gestation (5). One week later, she underwent percutaneous coronary intervention to place a sirolimus-eluting stent. At 35 weeks' gestation, a cesarean section under general anesthesia delivered a 2.03-kg male infant with Apgar scores of 5 and 8 at 1 and 5 minutes, respectively. No further information on the newborn was provided (5).

A 43-year-old woman, with a history of diabetes and hypertension, was in her sixth pregnancy when she had an AMI at 20 weeks' gestation (6). She was treated with aspirin, nitroglycerin, and then tirofiban with heparin for intracoronary stenting. She was discharged home, 5 days after the procedure, on clopidogrel, aspirin, and metoprolol (doses not specified). The pregnancy was ongoing at the time of the report (6).

In another case similar to those above, a 43-year-old woman at 21 weeks' gestation had an AMI and underwent stent placement (7). She was then treated with clopidogrel 75 mg/day and aspirin 100 mg/day for 2 weeks. The aspirin was continued until 1 week before a planned cesarean section at 32 weeks' gestation and heparin therapy was started. A healthy, 1.967-kg infant with an Apgar of 9 was delivered. Both mother and infant were discharged 8 days later (7).

A brief 2009 case report described a 39-year-old woman at 6 weeks' gestation who developed an AMI and was started on clopidogrel, aspirin, and heparin (8). Following placement of a stent, the woman again experienced chest pain, and thrombus was discovered in three coronary arteries that were removed under coverage of abciximab and intracoronary adenosine. She was maintained on clopidogrel and aspirin throughout pregnancy. At 41 weeks, she was given platelet concentrates and a cesarean section delivered a female infant with appropriate weight (not specified). Defects in the infant included a patent foramen ovale, a muscular ventricular septal defect, and moderate mitral regurgitation. The authors considered the anomalies relatively common with a benign prognosis (8).

Five other case reports have described the use of clopidogrel in pregnancy, two throughout gestation (9,10) and the others starting at 10, 25, and 31 weeks' gestation (11–13). No congenital anomalies were observed in the five newborns.

BREASTFEEDING SUMMARY

No reports describing the use of clopidogrel during human lactation have been located. The molecular weight of the inactive parent drug (about 420 for the bisulfate) suggests that it will be excreted into breast milk. The effect of this possible exposure on a nursing infant is unknown.

References

1. Product information. Plavix, Bristol-Myers Squibb, 2002.
2. Klinzing P, Markert UR, Liesaus K, Peiker G. Case report: successful pregnancy and delivery after myocardial infarction and essential thrombocythemia treated with clopidogrel. Clin Exp Obstet Gynecol 2001;28:215–6.
3. Boztosun B, Olcay A, Avci A, Kirma C. Treatment of acute myocardial infarction in pregnancy with coronary artery balloon angioplasty and stenting: use of tirofiban and clopidogrel. Int J Cardiol 2008;127:413–6.
4. Al-Aqeedi RF, Al-Nabti AD. Drug-eluting stent implantation for acute myocardial infarction during pregnancy with use of glycoprotein IIb/IIIa inhibitor. J Invasive Cardiol 2008;20:E146–9.
5. Cuthill JA, Young S, Greer IA, Oldroyd K. Anaesthetic considerations in a parturient with critical coronary artery disease and a drug-eluting stent presenting for caesarean section. Int J Obstet Anesth 2005;14:167–71.
6. Boztosun B, Olcay A, Avci A, Kirma C. Treatment of acute myocardial infarction in pregnancy with coronary artery balloon angioplasty and stenting: use of tirofiban and clopidogrel. Int J Cardiol 2008;127:413–6.
7. Arimura T, Mitsutake R, Miura S, Nishikawa H, Kawamura A, Saku K. Acute myocardial infarction associated with pregnancy successfully treated with percutaneous coronary intervention. Inter Med 2009;48:1383–6.
8. Santiago-Diaz P, Arrebola-Moreno AL, Ramirez-Hernandez JA, Melgares-Moreno R. Use of antiplatelet drugs during pregnancy. Rev Exp Cardiol 2009;62:1197–8.
9. De Santis M, De Luca C, Mappa I, Cesari E, Mazza A, Quattrocchi T, Caruso A. Clopidogrel treatment during pregnancy: a case report and a review of the literature. Intern Med 2011;50:1769–73.
10. Myers GR, Hoffman MK, Marshall ES. Clopidogrel use throughout pregnancy in a patient with a drug-eluting coronary stent. Obstet Gynecol 2011;118:32–3.
11. Babic Z, Gabric ID, Pintaric H. Successful primary percutaneous coronary intervention in the first trimester of pregnancy. Catheter Cardiovasc Inter 2011;77:522–5.
12. Jaiswal A, Rashid M, Balek M, Park C. Acute myocardial infarction during pregnancy: a clinical checkmate. Indian Heart J 2013;65:464–8.
13. Duarte FP, O'Neill P, Centeno MJ, Ribeiro I, Moreira J. Myocardial infarction in the 31st week of pregnancy—case report. Rev Bras Anestesiol 2011;61:225–31.

CLORAZEPATE

Sedative/Anticonvulsant

PREGNANCY RECOMMENDATION: Human Data Suggest Risk
BREASTFEEDING RECOMMENDATION: No Human Data—Potential Toxicity

PREGNANCY SUMMARY

The effects of benzodiazepines on the human embryo and fetus are controversial. Although some studies have reported an association with various types of congenital defects, other studies have not found such associations (see also Chlordiazepoxide or Diazepam). Maternal denial of exposure and concurrent exposure to other toxic drugs and substances (e.g., alcohol and smoking) may be confounding factors. If the maternal condition requires use of the drug during pregnancy, the lowest possible dose should be taken.

C

FETAL RISK SUMMARY

Clorazepate is a member of the benzodiazepine class of agents. The drug undergoes rapid metabolism to an active metabolite, nordiazepam, so there is essentially no circulating parent drug. Plasma protein binding of nordiazepam and its elimination half-life is about 40–50 hours. No teratogenic effects were observed in rats and rabbits fed large doses of the drug during gestation (1). The pharmacokinetics of clorazepate have been determined in pregnant women (2,3).

Consistent with the molecular weight (about 409) of the parent drug, the active metabolite, nordiazepam, crosses the human placenta and has been measured in amniotic fluid at 13 to 40 weeks' gestation, umbilical cord blood (both arterial and venous), and in milk (2).

One report described multiple anomalies in an infant exposed to clorazepate during the 1st trimester (4). Exposure may have commenced as early as the 3rd week of gestation (5th week after the last menstrual period). The woman reportedly consumed 23 doses of the drug during the 1st trimester. Deformities present in the infant at birth were distended abdomen, oval mass in the suprapubic area, skin tag at site of penis without a urethral opening, absent scrotum and anus, marked shortening of the right thigh, bifid distal part of left foot, left great toe abnormality, right foot with four toes and an abnormal great toe, short digit attached to right finger in place of the thumb on left hand, deformities of the sacrum and fourth and fifth lumbar vertebrae with a narrowed pelvis, underdeveloped right femur, absent right fibula, absence of two left metacarpal bones, hypoplasia of first right metacarpal bone, patent ductus arteriosus, absence of right lung lobe, cecum, rectum, and right kidney, and the presence of several supernumerary spleens. The infant died 24 hours after birth (4).

In an unconfirmed, retrospective report of oral contraceptive drug interactions, one woman became pregnant while taking a combination tablet of ethinyl estradiol 80 mcg/norethindrone 1 mg (5). The only other medications consumed immediately prior to the pregnancy were clorazepate and an unidentified cold tablet. The authors speculated that a possible interaction may have occurred between the antihistamine in the cold tablet and the contraceptive. Although the woman claimed she did not miss any doses of the oral contraceptive, there was no confirmation of compliance (5). Interpretation of this interaction, if it exists, is not possible.

The Lamotrigine Pregnancy Registry, an ongoing project conducted by the manufacturer, was first published in January 1997 (6). The final report was published in July 2010. The Registry is now closed. In two prospectively enrolled pregnancies exposed in the 1st trimester to clorazepate and lamotrigine, with or without other anticonvulsants, there was one fetal death and one spontaneous abortion (6).

BREASTFEEDING SUMMARY

No reports describing the use of clorazepate during human lactation have been located.

However, following a single 20-mg clorazepate dose administered IM to seven women during labor, low concentrations of nordiazepam, the active metabolite, were found in milk at 2 days postdose (average 10.0 ng/mL, range 7.5–15.5 ng/mL) and at 4 days (average 9.4 ng/mL, range 6–12 ng/mL). The milk:maternal blood ratios were 0.18 and 0.23, respectively. In infant blood at 2 days, only trace amounts were measured in five with 4 ng/mL and 7.5 ng/mL levels in the other two. In five infants at 4 days, the average concentration was 5.7 ng/mL (range 4–8.5 ng/mL). In the other two infants, one had trace amounts and the other had a coagulated sample. In absolute terms, the amounts were considered negligible (2).

Other benzodiazepines accumulate in human milk, and adverse effects in the nursing infant have been reported (see Diazepam). The American Academy of Pediatrics classifies other benzodiazepines as drugs whose effect on the nursing infant is unknown but may be of concern (e.g., see Diazepam).

References

1. Product information. Clorazepate Dipotassium. Mylan Pharmaceuticals, 2010.
2. Rey E, Giraux P, d'Athis PH, Turquais JM, Chavinie J, Olive G. Pharmacokinetics of the placental transfer and distribution of clorazepate and its metabolite nordiazepam in the feto-placental unit and in the neonate. Eur J Clin Pharmacol 1979;15:181–5.
3. Rey E, d'Athis PH, Giraux P, de Lauture D, Turquais JM, Chavinie J, Olive G. Pharmacokinetics of clorazepate in pregnant and non-pregnant women. Eur J Clin Pharmacol 1979;15:175–80.
4. Patel DA, Patel AR. Clorazepate and congenital malformations. JAMA 1980;244:135–6.
5. DeSano EA Jr, Hurley SC. Possible interactions of antihistamines and antibiotics with oral contraceptive effectiveness. Fertil Steril 1982;37:853–4.
6. The Lamotrigine Pregnancy Registry. Final Report. 1 September 1992 through 31 March 2010. GlaxoSmithKline, July 2010.

CLOTRIMAZOLE

Antifungal

PREGNANCY RECOMMENDATION: Compatible
BREASTFEEDING RECOMMENDATION: Compatible

PREGNANCY SUMMARY

The absorption of clotrimazole from the skin and vagina is minimal. Three large surveillance studies found no association between clotrimazole and birth defects. However, one study did find a significant increase in the risk of spontaneous abortions (SABs) with 1st trimester vaginitis treatment. A later study speculated that this effect might have been due to inhibition of the critical enzyme aromatase. Until there are more data regarding this possible association, the best course is to avoid the use of clotrimazole for vaginitis treatment in the 1st trimester or the application of the antifungal to large areas of skin at any time in pregnancy.

FETAL RISK SUMMARY

Clotrimazole is in the same antifungal class of imidazole derivatives as butoconazole, econazole, ketoconazole, miconazole, oxiconazole, sertaconazole, sulconazole, and tioconazole. No reports linking the use of clotrimazole with congenital defects have been located. The topical use of the drug in pregnancy has been studied (1–4). No adverse effects attributable to clotrimazole were observed. Absorption of the agent from the skin and vagina is minimal (5).

Suspected birth defect diagnoses occurred in 6564 offspring of 104,339 women in a retrospective analysis of women who had delivered in Michigan hospitals during 1980–1983 (6). First-trimester vaginitis treatment with clotrimazole occurred in 74 of the 6564 deliveries linked to birth defect diagnoses and in 1012 of the 97,775 cases not linked to such diagnoses. The estimated relative risk of birth defects when clotrimazole was used was 1.09 (95% confidence interval [CI] 0.9–1.4). An estimated relative risk for SABs of 1.36 (95% CI 1.1–1.6) was calculated based on 112 clotrimazole exposures among 4264 abortions compared with 1086 1st trimester exposures among 55,736 deliveries. Although an increased relative risk for birth defects was not found, this study could not exclude the possibility of an association with a specific birth defect (6).

In a surveillance study of Michigan Medicaid recipients involving 229,101 completed pregnancies conducted between 1985 and 1992, 2624 newborns had been exposed to clotrimazole (maternal vaginal use) during the 1st trimester (F. Rosa, personal communication, FDA, 1993). A total of 118 (4.5%) major birth defects were observed (112 expected). Specific data were available for 6 defect categories, including (observed/expected) 27/26 cardiovascular defects, 4/4 oral clefts, 3/1 spina bifida, 9/7 polydactyly, 1/4 limb-reduction defects, and 6/6 hypospadias. These data do not support an association between vaginal use of clotrimazole and congenital defects.

Data from the Hungarian Case-Control Surveillance of Congenital Abnormalities (1980–1992) were used to examine the potential teratogenic effects of vaginal and/or topical use of clotrimazole (7). Although clotrimazole use was not associated with an increase in the prevalence of any birth defect (fetal and live births), there was a suggestion that it was associated with a decrease in the prevalence of undescended testis (prevalence odds ratio 0.72, 95% CI 0.54–0.95) (7).

A 2002 study evaluated azole antifungals commonly used in pregnancy for their potential to inhibit placental aromatase, an enzyme that is critical for the production of estrogen and for the maintenance of pregnancy (8). The authors speculated that the embryotoxicity observed in animals and humans (see also Miconazole and Sulconazole) might be explained by inhibition of aromatase. They found that the most potent inhibitors of aromatase were (shown in order of decreasing potency) econazole, bifonazole (not available in United States), sulconazole, clotrimazole, and miconazole. However, an earlier study reported a pregnancy that was maintained even when there was severe fetal and placental aromatase deficiency (<0.3% of that of controls) caused by a rare genetic defect (9). In this case, both the fetus and mother were virilized because of diminished conversion of androgens to estrogen. Because the pregnancy was maintained and the virilization, the case suggested that the main function of placental aromatase was to protect the mother and fetus from exposure to adrenal androgens (9).

BREASTFEEDING SUMMARY

The absorption of clotrimazole from the skin and vagina is minimal (5). Therefore, it is doubtful if measurable amounts of the antifungal agent appear in milk.

References

1. Tan CG, Good CS, Milne LJR, Loudon JDO. A comparative trial of six-day therapy with clotrimazole and nystatin in pregnant patients with vaginal candidiasis. Postgrad Med 1974;50(Suppl 1):102–5.
2. Frerich W, Gad A. The frequency of Candida infections in pregnancy and their treatment with clotrimazole. Curr Med Res Opin 1977;4:640–4.
3. Haram K, Digranes A. Vulvovaginal candidiasis in pregnancy treated with clotrimazole. Acta Obstet Gynecol Scand 1978;57:453–5.
4. Svendsen E, Lie S, Gunderson TH, Lyngstad-Vik I, Skuland J. Comparative evaluation of miconazole, clotrimazole and nystatin in the treatment of candidal vulvo-vaginitis. Curr Ther Res 1978;23:666–72.
5. Product information. Lotrimin. Schering, 2000.
6. Rosa FW, Baum C, Shaw M. Pregnancy outcomes after first-trimester vaginitis drug therapy. Obstet Gynecol 1987;69:751–5.
7. Czeizel AE, Toth M, Rockenbauer M. No teratogenic effect after clotrimazole therapy during pregnancy. Epidemiology 1999;10:437–40.
8. Kragie L, Turner SD, Patten CJ, Crespi CL, Stresser DM. Assessing pregnancy risks of azole antifungals using a high throughput aromatase inhibition assay. Endocr Res 2002;28:129–40.
9. Harada N. Genetic analysis of human placental aromatase deficiency. J Steroid Biochem Mol Bi ol 1993;44:331–40.

CLOXACILLIN

[Withdrawn from the market. See 9th edition.]

CLOZAPINE

Antipsychotic

PREGNANCY RECOMMENDATION: Compatible—Maternal Benefit >> Embryo–Fetal Risk
BREASTFEEDING RECOMMENDATION: Limited Human Data—Potential Toxicity

PREGNANCY SUMMARY

No reports have linked clozapine with congenital malformations, but the data are limited. There is no evidence of embryo or fetal harm with other agents in this subclass. Because clozapine is indicated for severe debilitating mental disease, the benefits to the mother appear to outweigh the unknown embryo–fetal risk. However, there is a risk of extrapyramidal and/or withdrawal symptoms in the newborn if the drug is used in the 3rd trimester. Moreover, clozapine may cause agranulocytosis and other adverse reactions, so it is available only through a restricted program (1). Because of the limited human pregnancy experience with atypical antipsychotics, the American College of Obstetricians and Gynecologists does not recommend the routine use of these agents in pregnancy, but a risk–benefit assessment may indicate that such use is appropriate (2). A 1996 review on the management of psychiatric illness concluded that patients with histories of chronic psychosis represent a high-risk group (for both the mother and the fetus) and should be maintained on pharmacologic therapy before and during pregnancy (3). Folic acid, 4 mg/day, has been recommended for women taking atypical antipsychotics because they may have a higher risk of neural tube defects due to inadequate folate intake and obesity (4).

FETAL RISK SUMMARY

Clozapine is an atypical antipsychotic indicated for treatment-resistant schizophrenia. It belongs to the antipsychotic subclass of dibenzapine derivatives that includes asenapine, loxapine, olanzapine, and quetiapine. Clozapine is almost completely metabolized to weakly active and inactive metabolites. Plasma protein binding is about 97% and the dose-dependent mean elimination half-life is about 12 hours at steady state (1).

Reproduction studies in rats and rabbits at doses up to 0.4 and 0.9 times, respectively, the maximum recommended human dose based on BSA found no evidence of impaired fertility or fetal harm (1).

A brief 1993 report described a woman who was treated prior to and throughout gestation with clozapine (dose not given) for treatment-resistant chronic undifferentiated schizophrenia (5). An apparently healthy, about 3689-g male infant was delivered at term. The authors cited information on 14 other women who had taken clozapine during gestation apparently without fetal adverse effects (6).

Consistent with the molecular weight (about 327), clozapine crosses the placenta, at least at term. A 1994 report described a woman who was maintained on 100 mg/day before and during the first 32 weeks of gestation (7). The dose was then lowered to 50 mg/day until she delivered at term a normal female infant. No psychomotor abnormalities were observed in the infant up to 6 months of age. Clozapine plasma levels, measured in the mother throughout her pregnancy, ranged from 38–55 ng/mL (100 mg/day) to 14.1–15.4 ng/mL (50 mg/day). At birth, the cord blood concentration was 27 ng/mL (maternal 14.1 ng/mL), representing a ratio of approximately 2. The amniotic fluid concentration was 11.6 ng/mL (7).

Nine diverse case reports of adverse pregnancy outcomes involving the use of clozapine during pregnancy have been reported to the FDA (F. Rosa, personal communication, FDA, 1995). In the absence of a cohort denominator, the cases do not suggest a fetal risk and may have been caused by chance. The cases were neonatal hypocalcemia, convulsions; asymmetry of buttock crease; Turner's syndrome (chromosomal abnormality); spontaneous abortion (SAB), hydropic villous degeneration (chromosomal abnormality); SAB 8th week (abnormal gestational sac); multiple congenital defects (unspecified) (pregnancy terminated); congenital blindness; clinodactyly thumbs and big toes; and neonatal cerebral hemorrhage.

A case report in 1996 described an otherwise healthy male infant, exposed throughout gestation to clozapine (200–300 mg/day) and lorazepam (7.5–12.5 mg/day), who developed transient, mild floppy infant syndrome after delivery at 37 weeks' gestation (8). The mother had taken the combination therapy for the treatment of schizophrenia. The hypotonia, attributed to lorazepam because of the absence of such reports in pregnancies exposed to clozapine alone, resolved 5 days after birth (8).

A 2005 study, involving women from Canada, Israeli, and England, described 151 pregnancy outcomes in women using atypical antipsychotic drugs (9). The exposed group was matched with a comparison group (N = 151) who had not been exposed to these agents. The drugs and number of pregnancies were olanzapine (N = 60), risperidone (N = 49), quetiapine (N = 36), and clozapine (N = 6). In those exposed, there were 110 live births (72.8%), 22 SABs (14.6%), 15 elective abortions (9.9%), and 4 stillbirths (2.6%). Among the live births, one infant exposed in utero to olanzapine had multiple anomalies, including midline defects (cleft lip, encephalocele, and aqueductal stenosis). The mean birth weight was 3341 g. There were no statically significant differences, including rates of neonatal complications, between the cases and controls, with the exceptions of low birth weight (10% vs. 2%, p = 0.05) and elective abortions (9.9% vs. 1.3%, p = 0.003). The low birth weight may have been caused by the increased rate of cigarette smoking (38% vs. 13%, $p \leq 0.001$) and heavy/binge alcohol use (5 vs. 1) in the exposed group (9).

BREASTFEEDING SUMMARY

Clozapine is concentrated in breast milk (7). While taking clozapine 50 mg/day, a mother (described above) on her first postpartum day had a plasma concentration of 14.7 ng/mL and a concentration of 63.5 ng/mL from the first portion of her breast milk (milk:plasma ratio [M:P] 4.3). One week postpartum, 4 days after the dose was increased to 100 mg/day, the two concentrations were 41.4 and 115.6 ng/mL (M:P ratio 2.8), respectively. The infant was not allowed to breastfeed (7).

In a 1995 report, four mothers taking clozapine were breastfeeding their infants, one of whom had drowsiness and another developed agranulocytosis that was possibly due to clozapine. No further details were provided (10).

A 2007 report described a case in which the mother took clozapine 100 mg/day throughout pregnancy and breastfeeding (11). She gave birth to a healthy female infant who was breastfed up to 1 year of age. The infant's development was normal except for her speech that was delayed. She did not achieve normal, fluent speech until 5 years of age. The cause of the developmental delay could not be determined (11).

The American Academy of Pediatrics classifies clozapine as a drug whose effect on the nursing infant is unknown but may be of concern (12).

References

1. Product information. Clozaril. Novartis Pharmaceuticals, 2013.
2. American College of Obstetricians and Gynecologists. Use of psychiatric medications during pregnancy and lactation. *ACOG Practice Bulletin*. Number 92, April 2008. Obstet Gynecol 2008;111:1001–19.
3. Althuler LL, Cohen L, Szuba MP, Burt VK, Gitlin M, Mintz J. Pharmacologic management of psychiatric illness during pregnancy: dilemmas and guidelines. Am J Psychiatry 1996;153:592–606.
4. Koren G, Cohn T, Chitayat D, Kapur B, Remington G, Myles-Reid D, Zipursky RB. Use of atypical antipsychotics during pregnancy and the risk of neural tube defects in infants. Am J Psychiatry 2002;159:136–7.
5. Walderman MD, Safferman AZ. Pregnancy and clozapine. Am J Psychiatry 1993;150:168–9.
6. Lieberman J, Safferman AZ. Clinical profile of clozapine: adverse reactions and agranulocytosis. In: Lapierre Y, Jones B, eds. *Clozapine in Treatment Resistant Schizophrenia: A Scientific Update*. London: Royal Society of Medicine, 1992. As cited in Walderman MD, Safferman AZ. Pregnancy and clozapine. Am J Psychiatry 1993;150:168–9.
7. Barnas C, Bergant A, Hummer M, Saria A, Fleischhacker WW. Clozapine concentrations in maternal and fetal plasma, amniotic fluid, and breast milk. Am J Psychiatry 1994;151:945.
8. Di Michele V, Ramenghi LA, Sabatino G. Clozapine and lorazepam administration in pregnancy. Eur Psychiatry 1996;11:214.
9. McKenna K, Koren G, Tetelbaum M, Wilton L, Shakir S, Diav-Citrin O, Levinson A, Zipursky RB, Einarson A. Pregnancy outcome of women using atypical antipsychotic drugs: a prospective comparative study. J Clin Psychiatry 2005;66:444–9.
10. Dev VJ, Krupp P. Adverse event profile and safety of clozapine. Rev Contemp Pharmacother 1995;6:197–208. As cited in Clozapine, National Library of Medicine LactMed database, 2013.
11. Mendhekar D. Possible delayed speech acquisition with clozapine therapy during pregnancy and lactation. J Neuropsychiatry Clin Neurosci 2007;19:196–7.
12. Committee on Drugs, American Academy of Pediatrics. The transfer of drugs and other chemicals into human milk. Pediatrics 2001;108:776–89.

COCAINE

Sympathomimetic

PREGNANCY RECOMMENDATION: Contraindicated (Systemic) Compatible (Topical)
BREASTFEEDING RECOMMENDATION: Contraindicated (Systemic) Compatible (Topical)

PREGNANCY SUMMARY

The widespread abuse of cocaine has resulted in major toxicity in the mother, the fetus, and the newborn. The use of cocaine is often significantly correlated with the heavy use of other abuse drugs. Many of the studies reviewed here were unable completely to separate this usage in their patient populations or were unable to verify self-reported usage of cocaine, thus resulting in the possible misclassification of patients into the various groups. Whether the reported consequences of maternal cocaine exposure are due to these biases, to cocaine itself, to other drugs acting independently or in conjunction with cocaine, to poor lifestyles, or to other maternal characteristics are not presently clear. It is clear, however, that women who use cocaine during pregnancy are at significant risk for shorter gestations, premature delivery, spontaneous abortions, abruptio placentae, and death. The drug decreases uterine blood flow and induces uterine contractions. An increased risk may exist for premature rupture of the membranes but apparently not for placenta previa. The unborn children of these women may be growth restricted or severely distressed, and they are at risk for increased mortality. In utero cerebrovascular accidents with profound morbidity and mortality may occur. Congenital abnormalities involving the genitourinary tract, heart, limbs, and face may occur, and cocaine abuse should be considered teratogenic. Bowel atresias have also been observed in newborn infants, which may be due to intrauterine bowel infarctions. The exact mechanism of cocaine-induced malformations is presently uncertain, but it may be related to the placental vasoconstriction and fetal hypoxia produced by the drug, with the resulting intermittent vascular disruptions and ischemia actually causing the fetal damage. Interactions with other drugs, however, may play a role. In addition to the above toxicities, the newborn child exposed to cocaine during gestation is at risk for severe neurobehavior and neurophysiologic abnormalities that may persist for months. An increased incidence of sudden infant death syndrome in the first few months after birth may also be a consequence of maternal cocaine abuse in conjunction with other factors. Long-term studies of cocaine-exposed children need to be completed before a true assessment of the damage caused by this drug can be determined.

FETAL RISK SUMMARY

Cocaine, a naturally occurring alkaloid, is legally available in the United States as a topical anesthetic, but its illegal use as a central nervous system stimulant far exceeds any medicinal market for the drug. Cocaine is a sympathomimetic, producing hypertension and vasoconstriction as a result of its direct cardiovascular activity. The increasing popularity of cocaine is due to its potent ability to produce euphoria, an effect that is counterbalanced by the strong addictive properties of the drug (1). As of 1985, an estimated 30 million Americans had used cocaine and 5 million were believed to be using it regularly (1). Although the exact figures are unknown, current usage probably exceeds these estimates. Preliminary results of a study conducted between July 1984 and June 1987 in the Boston area indicated that 117 (17%) of 679 urban women used cocaine at least once during pregnancy as determined by prenatal and postpartum interviews and urine assays for cocaine metabolites (2). Final results from this study, now involving a total of 1226 mothers, found that 216 (18%) used cocaine during pregnancy, but that only 165 (76%) of these women would have been detected by history alone (3). Fifty-one women who had denied use of cocaine had positive urine assays for cocaine metabolites. Other investigators have reported similar findings (4). Of 138 women who had positive urine screens for cocaine at delivery, only 59 (43%) would have been identified by drug history alone. In this same study, the increasing prevalence of maternal cocaine abuse was demonstrated (4). Over a 24-month period (September 1986–August 1988), the incidence of positive urine screens for cocaine in women at delivery rose steadily, starting at 4% in the first 6-month quarter and increasing to 12% in the final quarter. The total number of women (1776) was approximately equally divided among the four quarters.

Illicitly obtained cocaine varies greatly in purity, and it is commonly adulterated with substances such as lactose, mannitol, lidocaine, and procaine (5). Cocaine is detoxified by liver and plasma cholinesterases (1,5). Activity of the latter enzyme system is much lower in the fetus and in infants and is decreased in pregnant women, resulting in slower metabolism and elimination of the drug (1,5). Moreover, most studies have found a correlation between cocaine use and the use of other drugs of abuse such as heroin, methadone, methamphetamine, marijuana, tobacco, and alcohol. Compared with drug-free women, this correlation was highly significant ($p < 0.0001$) and, further, users were significantly more likely to be heavy abusers of these substances ($p < 0.0001$) (2).

Research on the effects of maternal and fetal cocaine exposure has focused on several different areas. It reflects the wide-ranging concerns for fetal safety this drug produces:

- Placental transfer of cocaine
- Pregnancy complications
- Placental receptor function
- Premature labor and delivery
- Spontaneous abortions
- Premature rupture of membranes (PROM)
- Placenta previa
- Gestational hypertension
- Abruptio placentae
- Ruptured ectopic pregnancy
- Maternal mortality
- Fetal complications
- Growth restriction
- Fetal distress
- Cerebrovascular accidents
- Congenital anomalies
- Infant complications
- Neurobehavior
- Mortality
- Hospitalizations

Placental Transfer

Although the placental transfer of cocaine has not been quantified in humans, cocaine metabolites are frequently found in the urine of in utero-exposed newborns. Because cocaine has high water and lipid solubility, low molecular weight (about 340), and low ionization at physiologic pH, it should freely cross to the fetus (5). In pregnant sheep given IV cocaine, 0.5 mg/kg, to produce plasma levels similar to those observed in humans, fetal plasma levels at 5 minutes were 46.8 ng/mL compared with simultaneous maternal levels of 405 ng/mL (fetus 12% of mother) (6). At 30 minutes, the levels for fetal and maternal plasma had decreased to 11.8 and 83 ng/mL, respectively (fetus 14% of mother). Uterine blood flow was decreased in a dose-dependent manner by 36% after the above dose (6). Decreases in uterine blood flow of similar magnitude have also been observed in other studies with pregnant sheep (7,8). In one report, the reduction was accompanied by fetal hypoxemia, hypertension, and tachycardia, which were more severe than when cocaine was administered directly to the fetus (8).

Pregnancy Complications

PLACENTAL RECEPTOR FUNCTION In a study examining the effects of prenatal cocaine exposure on human placental tissue, significant decreases, as compared with nonexposed controls, were found for the total number of β-adrenergic receptor-binding sites (202 vs. 313 fmol/mg, $p < 0.01$), μ-opiate receptor-binding sites (77 vs. 105 fmol/mg, $p < 0.05$), and δ-opiate receptor-binding sites (77 vs. 119 fmol/mg, $p < 0.01$) (9). These effects were interpreted as a true down-regulation of the receptor population and may be associated with increased levels of adrenergic compounds (9,10). The authors speculated that if a similar down-regulation of the fetal adrenergic receptor-binding sites also occurred, it could result in disruption of synaptic development of the fetal nervous system. However, the clinical significance of these findings has not yet been determined (9).

PREMATURE LABOR/DELIVERY The effect of maternal cocaine use on the duration of gestation has been included in several research papers (3,4,11–25). When compared with non-drug-using controls, in utero cocaine exposure invariably resulted in significantly shortened mean gestational periods ranging up to 2 weeks. A statistically significant mean shorter (1.9 weeks) gestational period was also observed when cocaine–polydrug users (20% used heroin) were compared with noncocaine–polydrug users (26% used heroin) (13). Two other studies, comparing cocaine/amphetamine (18) or cocaine/methadone (17) consumption with noncocaine heroin/methadone-abusing women, found nonsignificant shorter gestational lengths, 37.9 vs. 38.3 weeks and 37.2 vs. 38.1 weeks, respectively. A third study classified some of their subjects into two subgroups: cocaine only ($N = 24$) and cocaine plus polyabuse drugs ($N = 46$) (20). No statistical differences were measured for gestational age at delivery (36.6 vs. 37.4 weeks) or for the incidence of preterm (<37 weeks) delivery (25.0% vs. 23.9%). When included as part of the research format, the incidence of premature labor and delivery was significantly increased in comparison to that in drug-free women (4,11,18–25). When comparisons were made with noncocaine opiate abusers, the incidences were higher but not significant. One investigation also found that cocaine use significantly increased the incidence of precipitous labor (11). Although objective data were not provided, a 1985 report mentioned that several cocaine-exposed women had noted uterine contractions and increased fetal activity within minutes of using cocaine (26). This same group reported in 1989 that infants who had been exposed to cocaine throughout pregnancy ($N = 52$) (average maternal dose/use = 0.5 g) had a significantly shorter mean gestational age than infants of drug-free women ($N = 40$), 38.0 weeks vs. 39.8 weeks ($p < 0.001$), respectively (24). The gestational period of those who used cocaine only during the 1st trimester was a mean 38.9 weeks, which was not significantly different from that of either of the other two groups. The incidence of preterm delivery (defined as <38 weeks) in the three groups was 17% (4 of 23; 1st trimester use only), 31% (16 of 52; cocaine use throughout pregnancy), and 3% (1 of 40; drug-free controls) (24). Only the difference between the latter two groups was statistically significant ($p < 0.003$). In another 1989 study, bivariate comparisons of 114 cocaine users (as determined by positive urine assays) with 1010 nonusers (as determined by interview and negative urine assays) indicated the difference in gestational length to be statistically significant (38.8 weeks vs. 39.3 weeks, $p < 0.05$) (3). However, multivariate analyses to control the effect of other substances and maternal characteristics known to affect pregnancy outcome adversely resulted in a loss of significance, thus demonstrating that, in this population, cocaine exposure alone did not affect the duration of gestation (3).

SPONTANEOUS ABORTIONS A 1985 report found an increased rate of spontaneous abortions (SABs) in previous pregnancies of women using cocaine either alone or with narcotics compared with women using only narcotics and women not abusing drugs (26). These data were based on patient recall, so the authors were unable to determine whether a causal relationship existed. In a subsequent report on this patient population, the incidence of previous abortions (not differentiated between elective and spontaneous) was significantly greater in women who predominantly used cocaine either alone or with opiates when compared with those who used only opiates or with non-drug-using controls (25). A statistically significant ($p < 0.05$) higher incidence of one or more SABs was found in 117 users (30%) compared with 562 nonusers (21%) (2). Other studies, examining cocaine consumption in current pregnancies, found no correlation between the drug and SABs (5,15–17,22).

PREMATURE RUPTURE OF MEMBRANES Premature rupture of membranes (PROM) was observed in 2% of 46 women using cocaine and/or methamphetamine vs. 10% of 49 women using narcotics vs. 4.4% of 45 drug-free controls (differences not significant) (18). Similarly, no difference in PROM rates was noted between two groups of women admitted in labor without previous prenatal care (cocaine group $N = 124$, noncocaine group $N = 218$) (23). However, a 1989 report found a statistically significant increase in the incidence of PROM in women with a positive urine screen for cocaine (29 of 138, 21%) in comparison with non-cocaine-using controls (3 of 88, 3%) ($p < 0.0005$) (4). Although not statistically significant, the risk of PROM was higher in women who predominantly used cocaine either alone (10%, 6 of 63) or with opiates (14%, 4 of 28) than in drug-free controls (2%, 3 of 123) (26). The incidence of placenta previa was also not increased by cocaine use in this study (22). In contrast, 33% of 50 "crack" (alkaloidal cocaine that is smoked) users had PROM compared with 18% of non-drug-using controls ($p = 0.05$) (21). Drug abuse patterns in both groups were determined by interview, which may have introduced classification error into the results, but the authors reasoned that any error would have underestimated the actual effect of the cocaine exposure (21).

GESTATIONAL HYPERTENSION Two studies have measured the incidence of gestational hypertension in their patients (22,23). In one, the rate of this complication in cocaine-exposed and nonexposed women was too low to report (22). In the second, 25% (13 of 53) of cocaine-exposed women vs. 4% (4 of 100) of nonexposed controls had the disorder ($p < 0.05$) (23). Other factors such as maternal age, race, use of multiple abuse drugs, small numbers, and self-reported cocaine exposure may have accounted for this difference.

ABRUPTIO PLACENTAE Two cases of abruptio placentae after IV and intranasal cocaine use were reported in 1983 (27). Since this initial observation, a number of similar cases of this complication have been described (1,4,5,11,14,18,19,21,24–26,28–30), although some investigators either did not observe any cases (31) or the number of cases in the studied patients was too low to report (22). The findings of one study indicated that abruptio placentae-induced stillbirths in cocaine users ($N = 50$), multiple drug users (some of whom used cocaine) ($N = 110$), and drug-free controls ($N = 340$) were 8%, 4.5%, and 0.8%, respectively (5). The difference between the cocaine-only group and the controls was significant ($p < 0.001$). The four mothers in the cocaine group suffered placental abruption after IV and intranasal administration (one each) and smoking (two cases). Two of the five mothers in the multiple drug use group suffered the complication after injection of a "speed ball" (heroin plus cocaine) (5). Thus, 6 of the 12 cases were associated with cocaine use. Onset of labor with abruptio placentae was observed in 4 of 23 women after the use of IV cocaine (25). Additional information was provided by these investigators in a series of papers extending into 1989 (11,14,20,24,25). The latest data indicated that in women who had used cocaine during pregnancy ($N = 75$; 23 of whom used cocaine only during the 1st trimester), 10 (13.3%) had suffered abruptio placentae compared with none of the 40 drug-free controls ($p < 0.05$) (24). Retroplacental hemorrhages, including placental abruption, were significantly increased in a cocaine and/or methamphetamine group (13% of 46) in comparison with either opiate users (2% of 49) or drug-free controls (2.2% of 45) ($p < 0.05$) (18). Two cases of abruptio placentae were observed in 55 women using "crack" (none in 55 drug-free controls) (21) and one case in a woman using cocaine in 102 consecutive deliveries at a Texas hospital (28). Three additional cases of sonographically diagnosed abruption probably related to cocaine use were described in a 1988 report (29). Although the exact mechanism of cocaine-induced abruptio placentae is still unknown, the pharmacologic effects of the drug offer a reasonable explanation. Cocaine prevents norepinephrine reuptake at nerve terminals, producing peripheral and placental vasoconstriction, reflex tachycardia with acute hypertension, and uterine contractions. The net effect of these actions in some cases may be abruptio placentae (1,5,11,18,24,26,27,32).

RUPTURED ECTOPIC PREGNANCY Two cases of rupture of ectopic pregnancies were reported in 1989 (33). In both incidences, the women described severe abdominal pain immediately after consuming cocaine (smoking in one, nasally in the other). While the authors of this report could not totally exclude spontaneous rupture of the tubal pregnancies, they concluded that the short time interval between cocaine ingestion and the onset of symptoms made the association appear likely (33).

Maternal Mortality

Fatalities following adult cocaine use have been reported frequently, but only two cases have been located that involve pregnant women (34,35). A 24-year-old woman, who smoked "crack" daily, presented at 34 weeks' gestation with acute onset of severe headache and photophobia (34). Her symptoms were determined to be due to subarachnoid hemorrhage resulting from a ruptured aneurysm. Following surgery to relieve intracranial pressure and an unsuccessful attempt to isolate the aneurysm, the patient gave birth to a normal 2400-g male infant. Her condition subsequently worsened on postpartum day 21 and she died 4 days later from recurrent intracranial hemorrhage. The second case involved a 21-year-old in approximately her 16th week of pregnancy (35). She was admitted to the hospital in a comatose condition after about 1.5 g of cocaine had been placed in her vagina. She was maintained on life support systems and eventually delivered, by cesarean section, a female infant at 33 weeks' gestation with severe brain abnormalities. The infant died at 10 days of age, and the mother died approximately 4 months later.

Fetal Complications

GROWTH RESTRICTION Fetal complications reported after exposure to cocaine include growth restriction, fetal distress, cerebrovascular accidents, and congenital anomalies. A large number of studies have examined the effect of in utero cocaine exposure on fetal growth parameters (birth weight, length, and head circumference) (2–5,11–26,36–39). Most of these studies found, after correcting for confounding variables, that cocaine exposure, when compared with non-drug-abuse populations, was associated with reduced fetal growth. This reduction was comparable, in most cases, with that observed in fetuses exposed to opiates, such as heroin or methadone. A survey of 117 users compared to 562 nonusers discovered that 14% of the former had given birth to a low-birth-weight infant vs. 8% of the nonexposed women ($p < 0.05$) (2). In one investigation, when maternal drug use included both cocaine (or amphetamines) and narcotics, the infants ($N = 9$) had a significant reduction in birth weight, length, and head circumference compared to either stimulant or narcotic use alone (18). In an earlier report, no significant differences were observed in fetal growth parameters between groups of women consuming cocaine ($N = 12$), cocaine plus methadone ($N = 11$), methadone ($N = 15$), and noncocaine/nonmethadone controls ($N = 15$) (26). However, in a subsequent publication from these researchers, women who used cocaine throughout gestation (as opposed to those who only used it during the 1st trimester) were significantly more likely than drug-free controls to deliver low-birth-weight infants; 25% (13 of 52) vs. 5% (2 of 40) ($p < 0.003$), respectively (24). Fetal growth parameters (birth weight, length, and head circumference) were also significantly ($p < 0.001$) depressed compared with those of controls if the woman used cocaine throughout pregnancy (24). Exposure during the 1st trimester only resulted in reduced growth, but the difference was not significant. Some investigators have suggested that the decrease in fetal growth in two studies may have been due to poor nutrition or to alcohol intake (40,41). In both instances, however, women abusing alcohol either had been excluded or their exclusion would not have changed the findings (42,43). In one study that found no statistical difference in birth weights between infants of cocaine users and noncocaine users, only 10 cocaine-exposed newborns were involved (28). The cocaine group had been identified from obstetric records of 102 consecutively delivered women. However, the sample size is very small and the character of cocaine use (e.g., dose, frequency, etc.) could not always be determined. In addition, recent research has shown that self-reporting of cocaine use probably underestimates the actual usage (3,4).

A single case of oligohydramnios at 17 weeks' gestation with two increased serum α-fetoprotein levels (125 and 168 mcg/L) has been described, but any relationship between these events and the mother's history of cocaine abuse is unknown (44). Intrauterine growth restriction was diagnosed at 26 weeks' gestation followed shortly thereafter by fetal death in utero. Analysis of fetal whole blood showed a cocaine level of 1 mcg/mL, within the range associated with fatalities in adults (44).

In a prospective 1989 study involving 1226 mothers, 18% used cocaine as determined by interview or urine assay (3). After controlling for potentially confounding variables and other substance abuse, infants of women with positive urine assay for cocaine, compared with infants of nonusers, had lower birth weights (93 g less, $p = 0.07$), lengths (0.7 cm less, $p = 0.01$), and head circumferences (0.43 cm less, $p = 0.01$). The effect of cocaine on birth weight was even greater if prepregnancy weight and pregnancy weight gain were not considered. The mean reduction in infant birth weight was now 137 g vs. 93 g when these factors were considered ($p < 0.01$). In those cases where the history of cocaine use was positive but the urine assay was negative, no significant differences were found by multivariate analyses. The authors concluded not only that cocaine impaired fetal growth but also that urine assays (or another biologic marker) were important to show the association (3).

Multiple ultrasound examinations (two to four) were used to evaluate fetal growth in a series of 43 women with primary addiction to cocaine (45). An additional 24 women were studied, but their ultrasound examinations were incomplete in one aspect or another and they were not included in the analysis. Careful attention was given to establishing gestational age. Complete ultrasonic parameters included biparietal diameter, femur length, and head and abdominal circumferences. The number of addicted infants with birth weight, head circumference, and femur length at ≤50th,

≤25th, and ≤10th percentile ranks did not differ significantly from expected standard growth charts. However, the number of examinations yielding values for biparietal diameter and abdominal circumference at the ≤50th and ≤25th percentile ranks was significantly more than expected ($p = 0.001$). Because biparietal diameter and head circumference are not independent parameters, each being an indicator of fetal head size, the authors speculated that the most logical explanation for their findings was late-onset dolichocephalia (45). Based on these findings, the study concluded that maternal cocaine use had adversely affected fetal growth. If only birth weight had been used as a criterion, this effect may have been missed (45).

FETAL DISTRESS Several studies have included measurements of fetal distress in their research findings (11,15–21,23,26,31,37,39). In some reports, perinatal distress was significantly ($p < 0.05$) increased in cocaine abusers over women using heroin/methadone (11,12) and drug-free controls (19). Perinatal distress was also noted more frequently in other studies comparing cocaine users with drug-free controls (10% vs. 5.7% and 11.1% vs. 3.7%, respectively), but the differences were not significant (20,21). Compared with non-drug users, higher rates of fetal tachycardia (2% vs. 0%) and bradycardia (17% vs. 6%) have been observed, but, again, the differences were not significant (18). One-minute Apgar scores were lower after in utero cocaine exposure in several studies (4,15–17,20,23,37) but only statistically significant in some (15–17,23) and no different in another (25). In contrast, only two studies, one a series of three reports on the same group of patients, found a significant lowering of the 5-minute Apgar score (15–17,25). Other studies observed no difference in this value (4,20,23,26,31,37,39). Significantly more ($p < 0.05$) meconium-stained infants were observed in studies comparing cocaine users with methadone-maintained women (25% vs. 8.2%) (10) and with noncocaine/other drug-exposed subjects (25% vs. 4%) (23). Three other studies observed nonsignificant increased rates of meconium staining or passage (22% vs. 17%, 29% vs. 23%, and 73% vs. 58%) (18,20,25), and a fourth reported a lower incidence (22% vs. 27%), compared with non-drug-using controls (21).

CEREBROVASCULAR ACCIDENTS Eight reports have described perinatal or newborn cerebrovascular accidents and resulting brain damage in infants exposed in utero to cocaine (11,14,18,46–50). The first report of this condition was published in 1986 (46). A mother who had used an unknown amount of cocaine intranasally during the first 5 weeks of pregnancy and approximately 5 g during the 3 days before delivery, gave birth to a full-term, 3660-g male infant. The last dose of approximately 1 g had been consumed 15 hours before delivery. Fetal monitoring during the 12 hours before delivery showed tachycardia (180–200 beats/minute) and multiple variable decelerations. At birth, the infant was limp, he had a heart rate of 80 beats/minute, and thick meconium staining (without aspiration) was noted. Apnea, cyanosis, multiple focal seizures, intermittent tachycardia (up to 180 beats/minute), hypertension (up to 140 mmHg by palpation), abnormalities in tone (both increased and decreased depending on the body part), and miotic pupils were noted beginning at 16 hours of age. Noncontrast computed tomographic scan at 24 hours of age showed an acute infarction in the distribution of the left middle cerebral artery. Repeat scans showed a persistent left-sided infarct with increased gyral density (age 7 days) and a persistent area of focal encephalomalacia at the site of the infarction (age 2.5 months). One other infant with perinatal cerebral infarction associated with maternal cocaine use in the 48–72 hours prior to delivery has been mentioned by these investigators (11,14,24). A separate report described a mother who had used cocaine and multiple other abuse drugs during gestation had delivered a female infant (gestational age not specified) with bilateral cerebrovascular accident and resulting porencephaly (47). The infant died at 2.5 months of age. In another study of 55 infants exposed to cocaine (with or without opiates), one infant with perinatal asphyxia had a cerebral infarction (18). A severely depressed male infant delivered at 38 weeks' gestation had an electroencephalogram and cranial ultrasound suggestive of hemorrhagic infarction (48). Follow-up during the neonatal period indicated mild-to-moderate neurodevelopmental abnormalities. Brain lesions were described in 39% (11 of 28) of infants with a positive urine assay for cocaine and in 33% (5 of 15) of newborns with a positive assay for methamphetamine (49). The brain injuries, which were not differentiated by drug type, were hemorrhagic infarction in the deep brain (six cases; three around the internal capsule/basal ganglion), cystic lesions in the deep brain (four cases), large posterior fossa hemorrhage (three cases), absent septum pellucidum with atrophy (one case), diffuse atrophy (one case), and brain edema (one case) (49). In a control group of 20 term infants with severe asphyxia, only one had a similar brain lesion. A second report also described brain lesions in infants exposed in utero to cocaine (50). The 11 infants all had major CNS anomalies, and 10 of the infants also had craniofacial defects (described later). The CNS defects were hydranencephaly (one case), porencephaly (two cases), hypoplastic corpus callosum with unilateral parietal lobe cleft and heterotopias (one case), intraparenchymal hemorrhage (five cases), unilateral three-vessel hemispheric infarction (one case), and encephalomalacia (one case). In addition, three infants had arthrogryposis multiplex congenita of central origin (50). Four of the infants died, and the other seven had serious neurodevelopmental disabilities (50).

Echoencephalography (ECHO) was performed within 3 days of birth on 74 term (>37 weeks) infants who had tested positive for cocaine or methamphetamine but who otherwise had uncomplicated perinatal courses (51). The infants had no other known risk factors for cerebral injury. The 74 newborns were classified into three groups: 32 (43%) cocaine exposed, 24 (32%) methamphetamine exposed, and 18 (24%) exposed to cocaine plus heroin or methadone, or both. Two comparison groups were formed: a group of 87 term, drug-free infants studied by ECHO because of clinical concerns for hypoxic–ischemic encephalopathy and a normal group of 19 drug-free term newborns. Both groups of comparison infants were also studied by ECHO within 3 days of birth. Only one structural anomaly, consisting of an absent septum pellucidum, was observed in the infants examined. The affected newborn, exposed to methamphetamine, was also found to have bilateral optic nerve atrophy and diffuse attenuation of the white matter. Twenty-six (35.1%) of the drug-exposed infants had cranial abnormalities detected by ultrasonography, which was similar to the 27.6% (24 of 87) incidence in the

C

comparison group with possible hypoxic–ischemic encephalopathy ($p = 0.7$). The normal controls had an incidence of 5.3% (1 of 19) ($p < 0.01$ in comparison to both of the other groups). The lesions observed in the drug-exposed infants were intraventricular hemorrhage, echodensities known to be associated with necrosis, and cavitary lesions. Lesions were concentrated in the basal ganglion, frontal lobes, and posterior fossa (51). Cerebral infarction was found in two cocaine-exposed infants. The ECHO abnormalities that were not predicted by standard neonatal clinical assessment were believed to be consistent with those observed in adult abusers of cocaine and amphetamines (51).

CONGENITAL ANOMALIES Maternal cocaine abuse has been associated with numerous other congenital malformations. In a series of publications extending from 1985 to 1989, a group of investigators described the onset of ileal atresia (with bowel infarction in one) within the first 24 hours after birth in two infants and genitourinary tract malformations in nine infants (11,13,20,24,26). The abnormalities in the nine infants were prune belly syndrome with urethral obstruction, bilateral cryptorchidism (one also had absence of third and fourth digits on the left hand and a second-degree hypospadias) (two males), female pseudohermaphroditism (one case) (defects included hydronephrosis, ambiguous genitalia with absent uterus and ovaries, anal atresia, absence of third and fourth on the left hand, and clubfoot), secondary hypospadias (two cases), hydronephrosis (three cases), and unilateral hydronephrosis with renal infarction of the opposite kidney (one case). Data from the metropolitan Atlanta Birth Defects Case–Control study, involving 4929 liveborn and stillborn infants with major defects compared with 3029 randomly selected controls, showed a statistically significant association between cocaine use and urinary tract malformations (adjusted odds ratio 4.81, 95% CI 1.15–20.14) (52,53). The adjusted risk for anomalies of the genitalia was 2.27 (*ns*). Cocaine exposure for this analysis was based on self-reported use any time from 1 month before conception through the first 3 months of pregnancy (52,53).

The rates of major congenital malformations in a study involving 50 cocaine-only users, 110 cocaine plus polydrug users, and 340 drug-free controls were 10% (five cases), 4.5% (five cases), and 2% (seven cases), respectively (4). The groups were classified by history and infant urine assays; chronic alcohol abusers were excluded. The difference between the first and last groups was significant ($p < 0.01$). The incidence of minor abnormalities (e.g., hypertelorism, epicanthal folds, and micrognathia) was similar among the groups (5). Congenital heart defects were observed in all three groups as follows: cocaine-only, transposition of the great arteries (one case) and hypoplastic right heart syndrome (one case); cocaine plus polydrug, ventricular septal defects (three cases); controls, ventricular septal defect (one case), patent ductus arteriosus (one case), and pulmonary stenosis (one case). Skull defects were observed in three infants in the cocaine-only group: exencephaly (stillborn), interparietal encephalocele, and parietal bone defects without herniation of meninges or cerebral tissue. One infant in the cocaine plus polydrug group had microcephalia. Significantly more major and minor malformations were seen in a group of cocaine-exposed infants ($N = 53$) (five major/four minor) than in a matched, nonexposed sample ($N = 100$) (two major/four minor) ($p < 0.05$) (23). Congenital heart defects occurred in four of the cocaine-exposed infants: atrial septal defect (one case), ventricular septal defects (two cases), and cardiomegaly (one case). None of the infants born from controls had heart defects ($p < 0.01$). The authors noted, however, that their findings were weakened by the self-reported nature of the drug histories (23).

A 1989 report of 138 women at delivery with positive urine cocaine tests found 10 (7%) infants with congenital anomalies: ventricular septal defect (two), atrial septal defect (one), complete heart block (one), inguinal hernia (two), esophageal atresia (one), hypospadias (one), cleft lip and palate with trisomy 13 (one), and polydactyly (one) (4). Only two (2%) infants of 88 non-cocaine-using controls had congenital defects, but the difference between the two groups was not significant. When the cocaine group was divided into cocaine only (114 women) and cocaine plus other abuse drugs (24 women), five infants in each group were found to have a malformation. The difference between these subgroups was highly significant ($p < 0.005$).

Necrotizing enterocolitis has been described in two infants after in utero cocaine exposure (48). One of the infants was also exposed to heroin and methamphetamine. The proposed mechanism for the injuries was cocaine-induced ischemia of the fetal bowel, followed by invasion of anaerobic bacteria (48). In another report, three newborns (two may have been described immediately above) presented with intestinal defects: one each with midcolonic atresia, ileal atresia, and widespread infarction of the bowel distal to the duodenum (54). Five other infants plus one of those with intestinal disruption had congenital limb-reduction defects: unilateral terminal transverse defect (three), Poland sequence (one) (i.e., unilateral defect of pectoralis muscle and syndactyly of hand (55)), bilateral upper limb anomalies including ulnar ray deficiencies (one), and bilateral radial ray defects (two) (54). The defects were thought to be caused by cocaine-induced vascular disruption or hypoperfusion (54).

Facial defects seen in 10 of 11 infants exposed either to cocaine alone (6 of 11) or to cocaine plus other abuse drugs (5 of 11) included blepharophimosis (two), ptosis and facial diplegia (one), unilateral oro-orbital cleft (one), Pierre Robin anomaly (one), cleft palate (one), cleft lip and palate (one), skin tags (two), and cutis aplasia (one) (50). All of the infants had major brain abnormalities, which have been described above.

Ocular defects consisting of persistent hyperplastic primary vitreous in one eye and changes similar to those observed in retinopathy of prematurity in the other eye were described in a case report of an infant exposed throughout gestation to cocaine and multiple other abuse drugs (56). The association of the two defects was thought to be coincidental and not likely due to cocaine (56). Thirteen newborns with cocaine toxicity (each infant with multiple symptoms and positive urine assay) had a complete ophthalmic examination; six were discovered to have marked dilation and tortuosity of the iris vasculature (57). The five infants who were most severely affected were followed for at least 3 months and all showed a gradual resolution of the defects without apparent visual impairment. Transient iris vasculature defects have also been found in infants of diabetic mothers (both gestational and insulin-dependent) (58) and in non-cocaine-exposed controls

(57,59). However, the vascular changes have not yet been observed in infants of mothers abusing methadone, heroin, amphetamines, marijuana, or a combination of these drugs (specific data on the number of infants examined in these categories were not given) (58).

Two mothers who had used cocaine during the 1st trimester produced infants with unusual abnormalities (60,61). Both mothers used other abuse drugs, heroin in one case and marijuana and methaqualone in the other. The anomalies observed were chromosomal aneuploidy 45,X, bilaterally absent fifth toes, and features consistent with Turner's syndrome in one (60) and multiple defects including hypothalamic hamartoblastoma in the other (61). Hydrocephaly was noted in one infant (from a group of 10) exposed in utero to cocaine, marijuana, and amphetamines (28). No major anomalies were seen in 8 infants exposed to cocaine (all had positive urine assays for cocaine) and other abuse drugs, but two infants had minor defects consisting of a sacral exostosis and capillary hemangioma in one and a capillary hemangioma in the other (37). In the latter case, the mother claimed to have used cocaine only during the month preceding delivery. Cocaine was not considered a causative agent in any of these cases (28,37,60,61).

In contrast to the above reports, no congenital abnormalities were observed in several series of cocaine-exposed women totaling 55 (21), 39 (31), 56 (39), and 38 (62) subjects. A prospective 1989 study mentioned previously found cocaine metabolites in the urine assays from 114 (9.3%) of 1226 women (3). After controlling for the effects of other substances and maternal characteristics known to affect pregnancy outcome adversely, no significant association was found between cocaine and one or more minor anomalies, a constellation of three minor anomalies, or one major anomaly (3). An association with the latter two, however, was suggested by the data ($p = 0.10$) (3). Although animal data cannot be directly extrapolated to humans, administration of cocaine to pregnant rats and mice did not increase the incidence of congenital abnormalities (63).

Infant Complications

NEUROBEHAVIOR Newborn infants who have been exposed in utero to cocaine may have significant neurobehavior impairment in the neonatal period. An increased degree of irritability, tremulousness, and muscular rigidity has been observed by a number of researchers (4,11,15–19, 21,23,26,62,64). Gastrointestinal symptoms (vomiting, diarrhea) have also been observed (4,21). The onset of these symptoms usually occurs 1–2 days after birth with peak severity of symptoms occurring on days 2 and 3 (19,21,62,64). Seizures, which may have been related to withdrawal, have been observed (14,23). The overall incidence of severe withdrawal symptoms, however, is apparently not increased over that expected in opiate-addicted newborns (15–17). In one report that identified 138 infants whose mothers tested positive for cocaine, 24 (17%) of the mothers also tested positive for other abuse substances, usually opiates (4). The incidence of withdrawal in infants of the cocaine-only group was 25% (28 of 114) vs. 54% (13 of 24) in infants of the multiple abuse drug group ($p < 0.005$).

The Neonatal Behavior Assessment Scale (NBAS) has been used in several studies to quantify the observed symptoms (11,24,26,64). In a blinded study comparing infants of methadone-maintained women with those of cocaine-exposed women, the latter group had a significantly increased degree of irritability, tremulousness, and state lability ($p < 0.03$) (11). Expansion of this study to include drug-free controls and cluster analysis of the NBAS revealed that the cocaine group had significant impairment in state organization compared with either the opiate group infants or controls (24,26). The NBAS was used to evaluate 16 term newborn infants with cocaine-positive urine assays (65). All demonstrated no to very poor visual attention and tracking, abnormal state regulation, and mild-to-moderate hypertonicity with decreased spontaneous movement (65). Flash-evoked visual potentials were abnormal in 11 of 12 infants studied, and the disturbances remained in six infants studied at 4–6 months (65).

Ultrasound was used in a study published in 1989 to evaluate the behavior of 20 fetuses exposed to cocaine as a predictor of neonatal outcome (66). All fetuses were exposed to cocaine during the 1st trimester; 4 during the 1st trimester only, 7 during the 1st and 2nd trimesters, and 9 throughout gestation. The investigators were able to document that fetal state organization was predictive of newborn neurobehavioral well-being and state organization. In this study, the most frequent indicators of neurobehavioral well-being were excessive tremulousness of the extremities, unexplained tachypnea, or both (66). Abnormal state organization was shown by hyperresponsiveness and difficulty in arousal (66).

Electroencephalographic (EEG) abnormalities indicative of cerebral irritation have been documented in cocaine-exposed neonates (31,64, 65). Normalization of the EEG abnormalities may require up to 12 months (31,64).

MORTALITY Increased perinatal mortality was observed in a study published in 1989, although in comparison to controls, the higher incidence was not significant (4). Seven (5%) of 140 infants (138 mothers, two sets of twins) whose mothers tested positive for cocaine at delivery died compared with none of 88 infants whose mothers did not test positive for cocaine at delivery. The seven cases included three intrauterine fetal deaths and four neonatal deaths.

An increased risk of sudden infant death syndrome (SIDS) has been suggested by three studies (11,17,67). Two infants, from a group of 50 exposed in utero to cocaine and methadone, died of SIDS, one at 1 month of age and the other at 3 months (17). It could not be determined whether a relationship existed between the deaths and maternal cocaine use (17). In one study, 10 of 66 infants (15%) exposed to cocaine in utero died of SIDS over a 9- to 180-day interval (mean 46 days) following birth (11). This incidence was estimated to be approximately 30 times that observed in the general population and almost 4 times that seen in the infants of opiate-abusing women (11). Based on this experience, a prospective study was commenced and the results were reported in 1989 (67). Of cocaine-using mothers, 32 infants were compared with 18 infants of heroin/methadone-addicted mothers. Eight of the mothers in the cocaine group also used heroin/methadone. The mothers of both groups received similar prenatal care, and they used similar amounts of alcohol, cigarettes, and marijuana. Infants in both groups were delivered at a gestational age of 38 weeks or more, and mean birth weight, length, and head circumference were identical. Cardiorespiratory recordings (pneumograms), conducted in

C

most cases at 8–14 days of age, were abnormal in 13 infants, 12 cocaine exposed and 1 opiate exposed ($p < 0.05$). Five of the cocaine-exposed infants had an episode of life-threatening apnea of infancy requiring home resuscitation before the pneumograms could be performed. The 13 infants were treated with theophylline until age 6 months, or longer if the pneumogram had not yet normalized. No cases of SIDS were observed in any of the 50 infants. In an earlier study, pneumograms were used to quantify abnormal sleeping ventilatory patterns in infants of substance-abusing mothers (68). Of three cocaine-exposed infants, one had an abnormal pneumogram. Apnea and/or abnormal pneumograms were observed in 20 (14%) of 138 infants whose mothers tested positive for cocaine at delivery (4). None of the 88 control infants whose mothers tested negative for cocaine at delivery had apnea or abnormal pneumograms ($p < 0.0005$). In a large study examining the relationship between SIDS and cocaine exposure, 1 of 175 infants exposed to cocaine died of SIDS compared with 4 of 821 infants who were not exposed (36). The risks per 1000 in the two groups were similar, 5.6 and 4.9, respectively, corresponding to a relative risk for SIDS among infants of cocaine-abusing women of 1.17 (95% CI 0.13–10.43) (36). Based on these data, the study concluded that the increased rates reported previously probably reflected other risk factors that were independently associated with SIDS (36). However, because the study relied on self-reported cocaine use and urine screens (only detects recent exposure), some of the women may have been misclassified as nonusers (69). Analysis of the hair, where the drug accumulates for months, has been advocated as a technique to ensure accurate assessment of past exposure (69).

HOSPITALIZATION Increased neonatal hospitalization in infants whose mothers tested positive for cocaine at delivery has been reported (4). In 137 infants (138 mothers, 2 sets of twins, 3 fetal deaths excluded), the mean number of days hospitalized was 19.2 compared with 5.1 for 88 infants of mothers who tested negative for cocaine at delivery ($p < 0.0001$). Moreover, the incidences of neonatal hospitalization for longer than 3 and 10 days were both significantly greater for the cocaine group (80% vs. 24%, respectively, $p < 0.00001$; 35% vs. 10%, respectively, $p < 0.0005$). The implications of these findings on the limited resources available to hospitals are, obviously, very important.

BREASTFEEDING SUMMARY

Milk:plasma ratios of cocaine in breast milk have not been determined. In one case, the urine of a normal, breastfed, 6-week-old boy was positive for a cocaine metabolite (70). The mother was using an unspecified amount of cocaine. In another patient, a milk sample 12 hours after the last dose of approximately 0.5 g taken intranasally over 4 hours contained measurable levels (specific data not given) of cocaine and the metabolite, benzoylecgonine, that persisted until 36 hours after the dose (71). The 14-day-old infant was breastfed five times over the 4-hour period during which the mother ingested the cocaine. Approximately 3 hours after the first dose, the child became markedly irritable with onset of vomiting and diarrhea. Other symptoms observed upon examination were tremulousness, increased startle response, hyperactive Moro reaction, increased symmetrical deep tendon reflexes with bilateral ankle clonus, and marked lability of mood (71). The irritability and tremulousness steadily improved over the next 48 hours. Large amounts of cocaine and the metabolite were found in the infant's urine 12 hours after the mother's last dose, which persisted until 60 hours postdose. On discharge (time not specified), the physical and neurologic examinations were normal. Additional follow-up of the infant was not reported.

In an unusual case report, a mother applied cocaine powder to her nipples to relieve soreness shortly before breastfeeding her 11-day-old infant (72). Although a breast shield was used, the unsheathed nipple protruded to allow feeding. Three hours after feeding, the infant was found gasping, choking, and blue. Seizures, which occurred with other symptoms of acute cocaine ingestion, stopped 2 hours after admission to the hospital. The mother's milk was negative for cocaine and metabolites but the infant's urine was positive. Physical and neurologic examinations were normal on discharge 5 days later and again at 6 months. Computed tomography (CT) scan during hospitalization showed a small area of lucency in the left frontal lobe and an EEG at this time was abnormal. A repeat CT scan and EEG were normal at 2 months of age.

Based on the toxicity exhibited in the infant after exposure via the milk, maternal cocaine use during breastfeeding should be strongly discouraged and considered contraindicated. Obviously, mothers should also be warned against using the drug topically for nipple soreness. The American Academy of Pediatrics classifies the use of cocaine as contraindicated during breastfeeding (73).

References

1. Cregler LL, Mark H. Special report: medical complications of cocaine abuse. N Engl J Med 1986;315:1495–500.
2. Frank DA, Zuckerman BS, Amaro H, Aboagye K, Bauchner H, Cabral H, Fried L, Hingson R, Kayne H, Levenson SM, Parker S, Reece H, Vinci R. Cocaine use during pregnancy: prevalence and correlates. Pediatrics 1988;82:888–95.
3. Zuckerman B, Frank DA, Hingson R, Amaro H, Levenson SM, Kayne H, Parker S, Vinci R, Aboagye K, Fried LE, Cabral H, Timperi R, Bauchner H. Effects of maternal marijuana and cocaine use on fetal growth. N Engl J Med 1989;320:762–8.
4. Neerhof MG, MacGregor SN, Retzky SS, Sullivan TP. Cocaine abuse during pregnancy: peripartum prevalence and perinatal outcome. Am J Obstet Gynecol 1989;161:633–8.
5. Bingol N, Fuchs M, Diaz V, Stone RK, Gromisch DS. Teratogenicity of cocaine in humans. J Pediatr 1987;110:93–6.
6. Moore TR, Sorg J, Miller L, Key TC, Resnik R. Hemodynamic effects of intravenous cocaine on the pregnant ewe and fetus. Am J Obstet Gynecol 1986;155:883–8.
7. Foutz SE, Kotelko DM, Shnider SM, Thigpen JW, Rosen MA, Brookshire GL, Koike M, Levinson G, Elias-Baker B. Placental transfer and effects of cocaine on uterine blood flow and the fetus (Abstract). Anesthesiology 1983;59:A422.
8. Woods JR Jr, Plessinger MA, Clark KE. Effect of cocaine on uterine blood flow and fetal oxygenation. JAMA 1987;257:957–61.
9. Wang CH, Schnoll SH. Prenatal cocaine use associated with down regulation of receptors in human placenta. Neurotoxicol Teratol 1987;9:301–4.
10. Wang CH, Schnoll SH. Prenatatal cocaine use associated with down regulation of receptors in human placenta. Natl Inst Drug Abuse Res Monogr Ser 1987;76:277.
11. Chasnoff IJ, Burns KA, Burns WJ. Cocaine use in pregnancy: perinatal morbidity and mortality. Neurotoxicol Teratol 1987;9:291–3.
12. Chasnoff IJ. Cocaine- and methadone-exposed infants: a comparison. Natl Inst Drug Abuse Res Monogr Ser 1987;76:278.
13. Chasnoff IJ, Chisum GM, Kaplan WE. Maternal cocaine use and genitourinary tract malformations. Teratology 1988;37:201–4.

14. Chasnoff I, MacGregor S. Maternal cocaine use and neonatal morbidity (Abstract). Pediatr Res 1987;21:356A.
15. Ryan L, Ehrlich S, Finnegan L. Outcome of infants born to cocaine using drug-dependent women (Abstract). Pediatr Res 1986;20:209A.
16. Ryan L, Ehrlich S, Finnegan LP. Cocaine abuse in pregnancy: effects on the fetus and newborn. Natl Inst Drug Abuse Res Monogr Ser 1987;76:280.
17. Ryan L, Ehrlich S, Finnegan L. Cocaine abuse in pregnancy: effects on the fetus and newborn. Neurotoxicol Teratol 1987;9:295–9.
18. Oro AS, Dixon SD. Perinatal cocaine and methamphetamine exposure: maternal and neonatal correlates. J Pediatr 1987;111:571–8.
19. Dixon SD, Oro A. Cocaine and amphetamine exposure in neonates: perinatal consequences (Abstract). Pediatr Res 1987;21:359A.
20. MacGregor SN, Keith LG, Chasnoff IJ, Rosner MA, Chisum GM, Shaw P, Minogue JP. Cocaine use during pregnancy: adverse perinatal outcome. Am J Obstet Gynecol 1987;157:686–90.
21. Cherukuri R, Minkoff H, Feldman J, Parekh A, Glass L. A cohort study of alkaloidal cocaine ("crack") in pregnancy. Obstet Gynecol 1988;72: 147–51.
22. Chouteau M, Namerow PB, Leppert P. The effect of cocaine abuse on birth weight and gestational age. Obstet Gynecol 1988;72:351–4.
23. Little BB, Snell LM, Klein VR, Gilstrap LC III. Cocaine abuse during pregnancy: maternal and fetal implications. Obstet Gynecol 1989;73:157–60.
24. Chasnoff IJ, Griffith DR, MacGregor S, Dirkes K, Burns KA. Temporal patterns of cocaine use in pregnancy: perinatal outcome. JAMA 1989;261:1741–4.
25. Keith LG, MacGregor S, Friedell S, Rosner M, Chasnoff IJ, Sciarra JJ. Substance abuse in pregnant women: recent experience at the Perinatal Center for Chemical Dependence of Northwestern Memorial Hospital. Obstet Gynecol 1989;73:715–20.
26. Chasnoff IJ, Burns WJ, Schnoll SH, Burns KA. Cocaine use in pregnancy. N Engl J Med 1985;313:666–9.
27. Acker D, Sachs BP, Tracey KJ, Wise WE. Abruptio placentae associated with cocaine use. Am J Obstet Gynecol 1983;146:220–1.
28. Little BB, Snell LM, Palmore MK, Gilstrap LC III. Cocaine use in pregnant women in a large public hospital. Am J Perinatol 1988;5:206–7.
29. Townsend RR, Laing FC, Jeffrey RB Jr. Placental abruption associated with cocaine abuse. AJR 1988;150:1339–40.
30. Collins E, Hardwick RJ, Jeffery H. Perinatal cocaine intoxication. Med J Aust 1989;150:331–4.
31. Doberczak TM, Shanzer S, Senie RT, Kandall SR. Neonatal neurologic and electroencephalographic effects of intrauterine cocaine exposure. J Pediatr 1988;113:354–8.
32. Finnegan L. The dilemma of cocaine exposure in the perinatal period. Natl Inst Drug Abuse Res Monogr Ser 1988;81:379.
33. Thatcher SS, Corfman R, Grosso J, Silverman DG, DeCherney AH. Cocaine use and acute rupture of ectopic pregnancies. Obstet Gynecol 1989;74:478–9.
34. Henderson CE, Torbey M. Rupture of intracranial aneurysm associated with cocaine use during pregnancy. Am J Perinatol 1988;5:142–3.
35. Greenland VC, Delke I, Minkoff HL. Vaginally administered cocaine overdose in a pregnant woman. Obstet Gynecol 1989;74:476–7.
36. Bauchner H, Zuckerman B, McClain M, Frank D, Fried LE, Kayne H. Risk of sudden infant death syndrome among infants with in utero exposure to cocaine. J Pediatr 1988;113:831–4.
37. Madden JD, Payne TF, Miller S. Maternal cocaine abuse and effect on the newborn. Pediatrics 1986;77:209–11.
38. Fulroth R, Phillips B, Durand DJ. Perinatal outcome of infants exposed to cocaine and/or heroin in utero. Am J Dis Child 1989;143:905–10.
39. Hadeed AJ, Siegel SR. Maternal cocaine use during pregnancy: effect on the newborn infant. Pediatrics 1989;84:205–10.
40. Bauchner H, Zuckerman B, Amaro H, Frank DA, Parker S. Teratogenicity of cocaine. J Pediatr 1987;111:160–1.
41. Donvito MT. Cocaine use during pregnancy: adverse perinatal outcome. Am J Obstet Gynecol 1988;159:785–6.
42. Bingol N, Fuchs M, Diaz V, Stone RK, Gromisch DS. Teratogenicity of cocaine (reply). J Pediatr 1987;111:161.
43. MacGregor SN. Cocaine use during pregnancy: adverse perinatal outcome (reply). Am J Obstet Gynecol 1988;159:786.
44. Critchley HOD, Woods SM, Barson AJ, Richardson T, Lieberman BA. Fetal death in utero and cocaine abuse: case report. Br J Obstet Gynaecol 1988;95:195–6.
45. Mitchell M, Sabbagha RE, Keith L, MacGregor S, Mota JM, Minoque J. Ultrasonic growth parameters in fetuses of mothers with primary addiction to cocaine. Am J Obstet Gynecol 1988;159:1104–9.
46. Chasnoff IJ, Bussey ME, Savich R, Stack CM. Perinatal cerebral infarction and maternal cocaine use. J Pediatr 1986;108:456–9.
47. Tenorio GM, Nazvi M, Bickers GH, Hubbird RH. Intrauterine stroke and maternal polydrug abuse. Clin Pediatr 1988;27:565–7.
48. Telsey AM, Merrit TA, Dixon SD. Cocaine exposure in a term neonate: necrotizing enterocolitis as a complication. Clin Pediatr 1988;27: 547–50.
49. Dixon SD, Bejar R. Brain lesions in cocaine and methamphetamine exposed neonates (Abstract). Pediatr Res 1988;23:405A.
50. Kobori JA, Ferriero DM, Golabi M. CNS and craniofacial anomalies in infants born to cocaine abusing mothers (Abstrasct). Clin Res 1989;37:196A.
51. Dixon SD, Bejar R. Echoencephalographic findings in neonates associated with maternal cocaine and methamphetamine use: incidence and clinical correlates. J Pediatr 1989;115:770–8.
52. Chavez GF, Mulinare J, Cordero JF. Maternal cocaine use and the risk for genitourinary tract defects: an epidemiologic approach (Abstract). Am J Hum Genet 1988;43(Suppl):A43.
53. Chavez GF, Mulinare J, Cordero JF. Maternal cocaine use during early pregnancy as a risk factor for congenital urogenital anomalies. JAMA 1989;262:795–8.
54. Hoyme HE, Jones KL, Dixon SD, Jewett T, Hanson JW, Robinson LK, Msall ME, Allanson J. Maternal cocaine use and fetal vascular disruption (Abstract). Am J Hum Genet 1988;43(Suppl):A56.
55. Smith DW, Jones KL. *Recognizable Patterns of Human Malformations.* 3rd ed. Philadelphia, PA: WB Saunders, 1982:224.
56. Teske MP, Trese MT. Retinopathy of prematurity-like fundus and persistent hyperplastic primary vitreous associated with maternal cocaine use. Am J Ophthalmol 1987;103:719–20.
57. Isenberg SJ, Spierer A, Inkelis SH. Ocular signs of cocaine intoxication in neonates. Am J Ophthalmol 1987;103:211–4.
58. Ricci B, Molle F. Ocular signs of cocaine intoxication in neonates. Am J Ophthalmol 1987;104:550–1.
59. Isenberg SJ, Inkelis SH, Spierer A. Ocular signs of cocaine intoxication in neonates (reply). Am J Ophthalmol 1987;104:551.
60. Kushnick T, Robinson M, Tsao C. 45,X chromosome abnormality in the offspring of a narcotic addict. Am J Dis Child 1972;124:772–3.
61. Huff DS, Fernandes M. Two cases of congenital hypothalamic hamartoblastoma, polydactyly, and other congenital anomalies (Pallister-Hall syndrome). N Engl J Med 1982;306:430–1.
62. LeBlanc PE, Parekh AJ, Naso B, Glass L. Effects of intrauterine exposure to alkaloidal cocaine ("crack"). Am J Dis Child 1987;141:937–8.
63. Fantel AG, MacPhail BJ. The teratogenicity of cocaine. Teratology 1982;26:17–9.
64. Doberczak TM, Shanzer S, Kandall SR. Neonatal effects of cocaine abuse in pregnancy (Abstract). Pediatr Res 1987;21:359A.
65. Dixon SD, Coen RW, Crutchfield S. Visual dysfunction in cocaine-exposed infants (Abstract). Pediatr Res 1987;21:359A.
66. Hume RF Jr, O'Donnell KJ, Staner CL, Killam AP, Gingras JL. In utero cocaine exposure: observations of fetal behavioral state may predict neonatal outcome. Am J Obstet Gynecol 1989;161:685–90.
67. Chasnoff IJ, Hunt CE, Kletter R, Kaplan D. Prenatal cocaine exposure is associated with respiratory pattern abnormalities. Am J Dis Child 1989;143:583–7.
68. Davidson Ward SL, Schuetz S, Krishna V, Bean X, Wingert W, Wachsman L, Keens TG. Abnormal sleeping ventilatory pattern in infants of substance-abusing mothers. Am J Dis Child 1986;140:1015–20.
69. Graham K, Koren G. Maternal cocaine use and risk of sudden infant death. J Pediatr 1989;115:333.
70. Shannon M, Lacouture PG, Roa J, Woolf A. Cocaine exposure among children seen at a pediatric hospital. Pediatrics 1989;83:337–42.
71. Chasnoff IJ, Lewis DE, Squires L. Cocaine intoxication in a breast-fed infant. Pediatrics 1987;80:836–8.
72. Chaney NE, Franke J, Wadlington WB. Cocaine convulsions in a breast-feeding baby. J Pediatr 1988;112:134–5.
73. Committee on Drugs, American Academy of Pediatrics. The transfer of drugs and other chemicals into human milk. Pediatrics 2001;108: 776–89.

CODEINE

C

Narcotic Agonist Analgesic, Respiratory Drug (Antitussive)

PREGNANCY RECOMMENDATION: Human Data Suggest Risk
BREASTFEEDING RECOMMENDATION: Human Data Suggest Potential Toxicity

PREGNANCY SUMMARY

Various reports have described associations between 1st-trimester exposure to opioid analgesics, including codeine, and congenital defects. Although the studies contained some unavoidable confounders that could have affected the results, such as the doses used, the reasons for use (e.g., maternal diseases and addiction), and exposures to other drugs, some data do suggest a small absolute risk of congenital birth defects if exposure occurs during organogenesis. Moreover, there is evidence of fetal and newborn toxicity if the mother is addicted to codeine or other opioids, or consumes high doses of these agents during the later half of pregnancy or close to delivery. Consequently, if possible, these agents should be avoided in pregnancy, especially in the 1st and 3rd trimesters.

FETAL RISK SUMMARY

Codeine is an opioid analgesic that is indicated for the control of pain. It is often combined with other agents, such as acetaminophen. In addition, an unproved indication for codeine is suppression of cough. Codeine is metabolized by the liver to morphine, hydrocodone, norcodeine, normorphine, and other metabolites (1). The analgesic effects appear to be primarily due to morphine and unmetabolized codeine. Codeine and its metabolites are excreted almost entirely by the kidneys, with a plasma elimination half-life of 3–4 hours (1).

Reproduction studies have been conducted in mice, rats, hamsters, and rabbits. In hamsters, high SC doses ranging from 73 to 360 mg/kg resulted in an incidence of 6%–8% of cranioschisis; no dose response was found (2). In another hamster study, maternal-toxic oral doses of 150 mg/kg resulted in increased resorptions, reduced fetal weight, and a small increase in meningoencephaloceles (2,3). SC doses in mice caused skeletal abnormalities, but no teratogenicity was observed with oral doses (3). Further, codeine was not teratogenic in rats and rabbits (3).

The Collaborative Perinatal Project monitored 50,282 mother–child pairs, 563 of whom had 1st trimester exposure to codeine (4, pp. 287–295). No evidence was found to suggest a relationship to large categories of major or minor malformations. Associations were found with six individual defects (4, pp. 287–295, 471) (independent confirmation is required for all associations found in this study): respiratory (8 cases); genitourinary (other than hypospadias) (7 cases); Down's syndrome (1 case); tumors (4 cases); umbilical hernia (3 cases); and inguinal hernia (12 cases). For use anytime during pregnancy, 2522 exposures were recorded (4, p. 434). With the same qualifications, possible associations with four individual defects were found (4, p. 484): hydrocephaly (7 cases); pyloric stenosis (8 cases); umbilical hernia (7 cases); and inguinal hernia (51 cases).

In an investigation comparing 1427 malformed newborns with 3001 controls, 1st trimester use of narcotic analgesics (most commonly codeine) was associated with inguinal hernias, cardiac and circulatory system defects, cleft lip and palate, dislocated hip and other musculoskeletal defects. Second-trimester use was associated with alimentary tract defects (5). In a large retrospective Finnish study, the use of opiates (mainly codeine) during the 1st trimester was associated with an increased risk of cleft lip and palate (6,7). Finally, a survey of 390 infants with congenital heart disease matched with 1254 normal infants found a higher rate of exposure to several drugs, including codeine, in the offspring with defects (8).

In a surveillance study of Michigan Medicaid recipients involving 229,101 completed pregnancies conducted between 1985 and 1992, 7640 newborns had been exposed to codeine during the 1st trimester (F. Rosa, personal communication, FDA, 1993). A total of 375 (4.9%) major birth defects were observed (325 expected). Specific data were available for six defect categories, including (observed/expected) 74/76 cardiovascular defects, 14/13 oral clefts, 4/4 spina bifida, 25/22 polydactyly, 15/13 limb-reduction defects, and 14/18 hypospadias. Only with the total number of defects is there a suggestion of an association between codeine and congenital defects, but other factors, including the mother's disease, concurrent drug use, and chance, may be involved.

Results of a National Birth Defects Prevention Study (1997–2005) were published in 2011 (9). This population-based case–control study examined the association between maternal use of opioid analgesics and >30 types of major structural birth defects. In 17,449 case mothers, therapeutic opioid use was reported by 454 (2.6%) compared with 134 (2.0%) of 6701 control mothers. Indications for use of opioid analgesics were surgical procedures (41%), infections (34%), chronic diseases (20%), and injuries (18%). Dose, duration, or frequency were not evaluated. The exposure period evaluated was from 1 month before to 3 months after conception. Limiting the exposure period to the first 2 months after conception produced similar results. Infants with >1 defect were included in multiple birth defect categories. The following opioids were included (number of cases for each agent not specified): codeine, hydrocodone, hydromorphone, fentanyl, meperidine, methadone, morphine, oxycodone, pentazocine, propoxyphene, and tramadol. The birth defect, total number, number exposed, and the adjusted odds ratio (aOR) with 95% confidence interval (CI) were as follows:

Birth Defect	Total	Cases	aOR (95% CI)
Spina bifida	718	26	2.0 (1.3–3.2)
Any heart defect (20 types)	7724	211	1.4 (1.1–1.7)
Atrioventricular septal defect	175	9	2.4 (1.2–4.8)
Teratology of Fallot	672	21	1.7 (1.1–2.8)
Conotruncal defect	1481	41	1.5 (1.0–2.1)
Conoventricular septal defect	110	6	2.7 (1.1–6.3)
Left ventricular outflow tract obstruction defect	1195	36	1.5 (1.0–2.2)
Hypoplastic left heart syndrome	357	17	2.4 (1.4–4.1)
Right ventricular outflow tract obstruction defect	1175	40	1.6 (1.1–2.3)
Pulmonary valve stenosis	867	34	1.7 (1.2–2.6)
Atrial septal defect (ASD)	511	17	2.0 (1.2–3.6)
Ventricular septal defect + ASD	528	17	1.7 (1.0–2.9)
Hydrocephaly	301	11	2.0 (1.0–3.7)
Glaucoma/anterior chamber defects	103	5	2.6 (1.0–6.6)
Gastroschisis	726	26	1.8 (1.1–2.9)

The authors speculated that the activity of opioids and their receptors as growth regulators during the development of the embryo might be a mechanism to explain the above findings. The exposure data were obtained by retrospective maternal self-report; the authors acknowledged that recall bias and misclassification might have affected their results. They concluded that the absolute risk was a modest absolute increase above the baseline risk for birth defects (9).

A large Norwegian population-based cohort study, also published in 2011, reported results for codeine that were the opposite of the above study (10). In this report, 2666 women who used codeine during pregnancy were compared with 65,316 women who used no opioids during pregnancy. There was no statistical difference in the congenital malformation rate (aOR 0.9, 95% CI 0.8–1.1) between codeine-exposed and unexposed infants. There also was no difference in the infant survival rate (aOR 0.9, 95% CI 0.6–1.5) (10).

A 2003 report described an association between opiate-dependent mothers and strabismus in their infants (11). In an 18-month period from 1998 to 2000, 72 infants born to opiate-dependent mothers, 50 of whom had been treated for neonatal abstinence syndrome, were identified. During pregnancy, 57% of the mothers took methadone alone, 30% methadone and heroin, 8% heroin alone, and 4% morphine or codeine. Benzodiazepines and amphetamines were also used in some cases. The investigators were able to contact the mothers of 49 infants, 29 of whom had a full ophthalmological examination. The remaining 20 cases completed a telephone interview. The age of the 49 children ranged from 6 to 39 months. Strabismus was found in seven (14%) of the infants and another 14% had a history of strabismus. The mean age at which the eye abnormality was noted in the 14 cases was 8.5 months. The incidence of strabismus was at least 10 times that in the general population (11).

Use of codeine during labor produces neonatal respiratory depression to the same degree as other opioid analgesics (12). The first-known case of neonatal codeine addiction was described in 1965 (13). The mother had taken analgesic tablets containing 360–480 mg of codeine/day for 8 weeks before delivery.

A second report described neonatal codeine withdrawal in two infants of nonaddicted mothers (14). The mother of one infant began consuming a codeine cough medication 3 weeks before delivery. Approximately 2 weeks before delivery, analgesic tablets with codeine were taken at a frequency of up to six tablets/day (48 mg of codeine/day). The second mother was treated with a codeine cough medication consuming 90–120 mg of codeine/day for the last 10 days of pregnancy. Apgar scores of both infants were 8–10 at 1 and 5 minutes. Typical symptoms of narcotic withdrawal were noted in the infants shortly after birth but not in the mothers (14).

A 25-year-old woman with well-controlled insulin-dependent diabetes underwent a cesarean section at 34 weeks' gestation because of spontaneous rupture of the membranes (15). The 2.5-kg (75th centile) male infant had Apgar scores of 9, 10, and 10 at 1, 5, and 10 minutes, respectively. He was admitted to the neonatal unit because of hypoglycemia. Between 24 and 48 hours of age, he developed a tremor and became restless and irritable with a strong cry and with other symptoms of drug withdrawal. A brief seizure occurred at 36 hours of age and he became hypertonic with loose stools at 48 hours of age. The mother was interviewed and admitted taking a drug containing codeine and acetaminophen for severe headache and lower back pain throughout the last 2 months of pregnancy. The estimated daily dose of codeine was 90 mg. The infant recovered but specific details were not provided (15).

In Washington State, neonatal abstinence syndrome rates increased significantly between 2000 and 2008 and, in 2008, were higher than the national figures (3.3 compared with 2.8 per 1000 births $p < 0.05$) (16). The broad categories of drug exposures associated with the syndrome were opioids and related narcotics, cocaine, and other psychotropic agents. The proportion of neonates exposed prenatally to opioids increased from 26.4% in 2000 to 41.7% in 2008 ($p < 0.05$) (16).

BREASTFEEDING SUMMARY

Codeine, and its metabolite morphine, pass into breast milk in very small amounts that are usually considered insignificant (17–20). However, three reports provide evidence that this low-risk classification requires reassessment (21–23).

In a 1993 study, concentrations of codeine and morphine were determined in the breastmilk of 7 mothers and in the plasma of 11 healthy, term neonates at 1–5 days of age (20). Milk samples were not obtained from four mothers for various reasons. The mean birth weight was 3.3 kg. The mothers were treated with codeine 60 mg every 6 hours and milk samples were collected 16–54 hours postpartum. In milk, codeine and morphine levels were 33.8–314 ng/mL and 1.9–20.5 ng/mL, respectively, 20–240 minutes after a 60-mg codeine dose. Neonatal plasma samples were collected 1–4 hours after breastfeeding that had been completed 1 hour after a dose. The mean number of codeine doses taken by the mothers before neonatal sampling was 4.1 (range 1–12). Neonatal codeine and morphine plasma concentrations were <0.8–4.5 ng/mL and <0.5–2.2 ng/mL, respectively. Because no toxicity was observed in the neonates, the authors concluded that short-term use of codeine (up to four 60-mg doses) was safe for healthy, full-term infants in the first days of life (20).

C

A 2006 case report described the death of a nursing infant secondary to maternal codeine use (21). On the first postpartum day, the mother took an oral analgesic product containing codeine 30 mg and acetaminophen 500 mg, 2 tablets every 12 hours, for episiotomy pain. The mother reduced the dose by one-half on day 2 because of sedation and constipation, and continued this dose for 2 weeks. On day 7, the healthy, full-term, male infant was lethargic and had difficulty feeding but, by day 11, had regained his birth weight. On day 12, his skin was gray and his milk intake had fallen. He was found dead on day 13. At postmortem, his blood morphine concentration was 70 ng/mL. Because of the infant's decreased milk intake, the mother had stored milk on day 10. Analysis of this milk yielded a morphine concentration of 87 ng/mL. An analysis for cytochrome P450 2D6 (CYP2D6), the enzyme responsible for metabolizing codeine to morphine, was conducted on family members and the infant. The mother was heterozygous for a CYP2D6*2A allele with CYP2D6*2×2 gene duplication, classified as an ultrarapid metabolizer, thus converting codeine to morphine at an increased rate. The sedation and constipation she experienced were consistent with this genotype. The maternal grandmother was also an ultrarapid metabolizer, whereas the father, maternal grandfather, and infant had two functional CYP2D6 alleles (CYP2D6*1/*2 genotypes) and were classified as extensive metabolizers. The authors considered the polymorphism to be clinically important because of the frequency of CYP2D6 ultrarapid metabolizers (CYP2D6UMs): 1% in Finland and Denmark; 10% in Greece and Portugal; and 29% in Ethiopia (21).

The pharmacogenetics of neonatal opioid toxicity was examined in a 2009 report (22). Among 72 mother–child pairs who had contacted the Motherisk Program in Toronto, 17 (24%) breastfed infants exhibited central nervous system (CNS) depression when their mothers took codeine. In each case, there was observable sedation in the infant while feeding and a marked improvement after codeine or breastfeeding was stopped. There also was concordance between maternal and infant CNS depression as 12 (71%) of the 17 mothers also showed signs of toxicity. As expected, a dose–effect relationship was found as the 17 mothers of symptomatic infants took a higher codeine dose than the 55 mothers of asymptomatic infants, 1.62 vs. 1.02 mg/kg/day. Two mothers whose infants had severe toxicity (one of whom is described in reference 21) were CYP2D6UMs and of the UGT2B7*2/*2 genotype. The investigators concluded that nursing infants of mothers who are CYP2D6UMs combined with the genotype were at risk of life-threatening CNS depression (22).

A 2009 report searched the medical literature to find other reports of CNS depression from exposure to codeine in breast milk (23). In addition to the 17 cases described in references 21 and 22, the authors found reports of toxicity in 18 other breastfeeding infants (total 35). The ages of the infants ranged from 3 days to 4 months. The adverse drug reactions reported included apnea, poor breathing, bradycardia, CNS depression, cyanosis, drowsiness, sedation, and constipation (23).

In 2007, the FDA released a statement regarding use of codeine by nursing mothers (24). Although codeine is considered to be the safest choice among narcotic pain relievers, some mothers may be CYP2D6UMs and could put their nursing infants at risk. If a physician prescribes a codeine-containing product, the lowest dose needed for the shortest amount of time should be prescribed (24).

A 2009 study used coupled physiologically based pharmacokinetic models for the mother and child to estimate the risk of maternal consumption of codeine products during breastfeeding (25). The investigators considered combinations of genotype, assuming typical breastfeeding schedules and maternal doses of ≤2.5 mg/kg/day. Their stimulations showed that potentially toxic morphine plasma concentrations in the neonate could be reached within 4 days after repeated codeine dosing to the mother (25).

Based on the above, long-term consumption of codeine-containing products should be avoided during breastfeeding. Short-term therapy, such as 1–2 days, and close monitoring of the infant should be standard (21,23). If the mother or infant demonstrates symptoms of opioid toxicity, such as sedation, lethargy, or poor milk intake, breastfeeding should be stopped. A trial of naloxone, a narcotic antagonist, could be diagnostic. Guidelines developed by Motherisk in Canada for the safe use of codeine-containing drugs during breastfeeding were published in 2009 (26).

References

1. Codeine sulfate. In: Sweetman SC, ed. *Martindale: The Complete Drug Reference*. 34th ed. London: Pharmaceutical Press, 2005:27.
2. Shepard TH. *Catalog of Teratogenic Agents*. 10th ed. Baltimore, MD: The Johns Hopkins University Press, 2001:127.
3. Schardein JL. *Chemically Induced Birth Defects*. 3rd ed. New York, NY: Marcel Dekker, 2000:140.
4. Heinonen OP, Slone D, Shapiro S. *Birth Defects and Drugs in Pregnancy*. Littleton, MA: Publishing Sciences Group, 1977.
5. Bracken MB, Holford TR. Exposure to prescribed drugs in pregnancy and association with congenital malformations. Obstet Gynecol 1981;58:336–44.
6. Saxen I. Associations between oral clefts and drugs taken during pregnancy. Int J Epidemiol 1975;4;37–44.
7. Saxen I. Epidemiology of cleft lip and palate: an attempt to rule out chance correlations. Br J Prev Soc Med 1975;29:103–10.
8. Rothman KJ, Fyler DC, Goldblatt A, Kreidberg MB. Exogenous hormones and other drug exposures of children with congenital heart disease. Am J Epidemiol 1979;109:433–9.
9. Broussard CS, Rasmussen SA, Reefhuis J, Friedman JM, Jann MW, Riehle-Colarusso T, Honein MA, for the National Birth Defects Prevention Study. Maternal treatment with opioid analgesics and risk for birth defects. Am J Obstet Gynecol 2011;204:314–7.
10. Nezvalova-Henriksen K, Spigset O, Nordeng H. Effects of codeine on pregnancy outcome: results from a large population-based cohort study. Eur J Clin Pharmacol 2011;67:1253–61.
11. Gill AC, Oei J, Lewis NL, Younan N, Kennedy I, Lui K. Strabismus in infants of opiate-dependent mothers. Acta Paediatr 2003;92:379–85.
12. Bonica JJ. *Principles and Practice of Obstetric Analgesia and Anesthesia*. Philadelphia, PA: FA Davis, 1967:245.
13. Van Leeuwen G, Guthrie R, Stange F. Narcotic withdrawal reaction in a newborn infant due to codeine. Pediatrics 1965;36;635–6.
14. Mangurten HH, Benawra R. Neonatal codeine withdrawal in infants of nonaddicted mothers. Pediatrics 1980;65:159–60.
15. Khan K, Chang J. Neonatal abstinence syndrome due to codeine. Arch Dis Child 1997;76:F59–60.
16. Creanga AA, Sabel JC, Ko JY, Wasserman CR, Shapiro-Mendoza CK, Taylor P, Barfield W, Cawthon L, Paulozzi LJ. Maternal drug use and its effect on neonates—a population-based study in Washington state. Obstet Gynecol 2012;119:924–33.
17. Kwit NT, Hatcher RA. Excretion of drugs in milk. Am J Dis Child 1935;49:900–4.
18. Horning MG, Stillwell WG, Nowlin J, Lertratanangkoon K, Stillwell RN, Hill RM. Identification and quantification of drugs and drug metabolites in human breast milk using GC-MS-COM methods. Mod Probl Paediatr 1975;15:73–9.
19. Anonymous. Drugs in breast milk. Med Lett Drugs Ther 1974;16:25–7.

20. Meny RG, Naumburg EG, Alger LS, Brill-Miller JL, Brown S. Codeine and the breastfed neonate. J Hum Lact 1993;9:237–40.
21. Koren G, Cairns J, Chitayat D, Gaedigk A, Leeder SJ. Pharmacogenetics of morphine poisoning in a breastfed neonate of a codeine-prescribed mother. Lancet 2006;368:704.
22. Madadi P, Ross CJD, Hayden MR, Carleton BC, Gaedigk A, Leeder JS, Koren G. Pharmacogenetics of neonatal opioid toxicity following maternal use of codeine during breastfeeding: a case-control study. Clin Pharmacol Ther 2009;85:31–5.
23. Madadi P, Shirazi F, Walter FG, Koren G. Establishing causality of CNS depression in breastfed infants following maternal codeine use. Paediatr Drugs 2008;10:399–404.
24. US Food and Drug Administration. Public Health Advisory. Use of codeine products in nursing mothers. August 17, 2007. http://www.fda.gov/Drugs/DrugSafety/PostmarketDrugSafetyInformationforPatientsandProviders/DrugSafetyInformationforHeathcareProfessionals/PublicHealthAdvisories/ucm054717.htm. Accessed September 17, 2013.
25. Willmann S, Edginton AN, Coboeken K, Ahr G, Lippert J. Risk to the breast-fed neonate from codeine treatment to the mother: a quantitative mechanistic modeling study. Clin Pharmacol Ther 2009;86:634–43.
26. Madadi P, Moretti M, Djokanovic N, Bozzo P, Nulman I, Ito S, Koren G. Guidelines for maternal codeine use during breastfeeding. Can Fam Physician 2009;55:1077–8.

COLCHICINE

Antigout

PREGNANCY RECOMMENDATION: Compatible
BREASTFEEDING RECOMMENDATION: Limited Human Data—Probably Compatible

PREGNANCY SUMMARY

Although colchicine is teratogenic in animals, the human pregnancy experience suggests that the risk to the embryo–fetus is low, if it exists at all. The use of colchicine by the father before conception does not appear to represent a significant reproductive risk, but azoospermia may be a rare complication. Because some reports suggested a risk of chromosome abnormalities, routine amniocentesis was recommended in cases of familial Mediterranean fever (FMF) treated with colchicine (1). However, more recent data suggest that routine amniocentesis is not justified (2,3).

FETAL RISK SUMMARY

Colchicine is used in the treatment of gout and FMF. Seven animal studies, reviewed by Shepard (4), indicated that colchicine, or its derivative, demecolcine (desacetylmethylcolchicine), were teratogenic in mice and rabbits at low doses and embryocidal in mice, rats, and rabbits at higher doses. Mutagenic effects were also observed in rabbit blastocysts. No adverse fetal effects were observed in limited studies with pregnant monkeys (4).

A number of reports have described the use of colchicine or demecolcine in human pregnancy (2,3,5–23). In these reports, no evidence of teratogenicity or other forms of developmental toxicity was found when these agents were used at recommended doses. In a woman treated throughout pregnancy with colchicine 1 mg/day, drug concentrations in the mother and cord blood at 38 weeks' gestation were 3.15 ng/mL and 0.47 ng/mL, respectively (23).

A 2011 case report described a successful 15 course of colchicine 1 mg/day, prednisolone 15 mg/day, and azathioprine 100 mg/day in a woman at 28 weeks' gestation with idiopathic granulomatous mastitis (24). No information on the pregnancy outcome was provided.

The mutagenic effects of colchicine and the possible relationship of this drug to sperm abnormalities and congenital malformations were the subjects of several publications (25–32). A 1965 report described three pregnancies occurring in a woman between the ages of 24 and 27 years, two of which ended abnormally (25). Her first pregnancy resulted in an SAB of a macerated fetus at 4.5 months, her second in the delivery of a normal girl, and her third in the delivery of a male with atypical Down's syndrome (trisomy 21), who died 24 hours after birth. The infant had palmar transverse folds on the hands, inner epicanthic folds, unspecified cardiac malformations, trigger thumbs, syndactyly in the second and third toes, hypognathous, cleft palate, low-set ears, and an incompletely developed scapha helix. The father was 27–30 years of age during these pregnancies and was being treated for gout on an intermittent basis with 1–2 mg/day of colchicine. Cultures of leukocytes obtained from him demonstrated mutagenic changes when exposed to colchicine, but blood and sperm samples, collected 3 months after the end of colchicine therapy, were normal. The investigators theorized that the colchicine therapy may have caused diploid spermatozoa that resulted in the production of triploid children (25).

A brief report, from the same laboratory as the reference above, described the analysis of lymphocyte cultures from three male patients being treated with colchicine (26). Compared with controls, a significant increase in the number of cells with abnormal numbers of chromosomes was found in the colchicine-exposed men. The investigators proposed that this finding indicated that these men were at higher risk of producing trisomic offspring than were nonexposed men. Of 54 children with Down's syndrome in their clinic, two had been fathered by men being treated with colchicine (26). The validity of this proposed association between colchicine and Down's syndrome was the subject of several references (27–30). One of the arguments against the association included the high possibility of Down's syndrome and colchicine therapy occurring at the same time in an older population (28). Moreover, several references have described healthy children fathered by men who were being treated with colchicine (6–8,31,32).

A 2005 study analyzed the reproductive histories of 326 couples in which at least one of the partners had FMF (236 women—628 pregnancies; 90 men—273 pregnancies) (1).

C

Among the 901 pregnancies, there were 891 singletons and 10 sets of twins. After excluding abortions and fetal deaths, there were 777 viable pregnancies to determine if colchicine was teratogenic. Amniocentesis to detect chromosomal abnormalities was conducted in 558 of the viable pregnancies. Seven numerical chromosomal abnormalities were found (4.99 expected, *ns*), six of which were unbalanced structural abnormalities (3.22 expected; *ns*). There were seven major malformations, also lower than expected. Although not significant, the authors concluded that the higher number of chromosomal abnormalities justified continuing the policy of routine amniocentesis in this patient population (1). However, two reports concluded that amniocentesis was not justified (2,3).

The effect of colchicine on sperm production is controversial. Hamsters and mice treated chronically with SC injections of demecolcine developed extensive damage to the germinal epithelium, resulting in azoospermia within 35–45 days (33). One study observed azoospermia in a 36-year-old patient induced by 1.2 mg/day of colchicine, but not with 0.6 mg/day (34). A second study, however, using 1.8–2.4 mg/day in seven healthy men 20–25 years old, measured no effect on sperm production or on serum levels of testosterone, luteinizing hormone, or follicle-stimulating hormone (35). The authors of this second report, however, could not exclude the fact that some men may be unusually sensitive to the drug, resulting in testicular toxicity (35). A 1998 review concluded that colchicine by itself may not have a significant direct adverse effect on sperm production or function (36).

BREASTFEEDING SUMMARY

Colchicine is excreted into breast milk (9–11). A 31-year-old woman, receiving long-term therapy with colchicine (0.6 mg twice daily) for FMF, was treated throughout a normal pregnancy, labor, and delivery (9). Milk, urine, and serum samples were obtained from her between 16 and 21 days after delivery. Colchicine was detected in three of five milk samples collected on days 16–20 with levels ranging from 1.2 to 2.5 ng/mL (test sensitivity 0.5 ng/mL). However, the authors could not determine whether their analysis was recovering all of the drug in the milk because of the high lipid content of the samples. Two serum samples collected on days 19 and 21 measured 0.7 and 1.0 ng/mL of the drug, indicating that the milk:plasma ratio exceeded 1.0. Daily urine colchicine concentrations (days 16–20) ranged from 70 to 390 ng/mL. No apparent effects were observed in the nursing infant over the first 6 months of life (9).

In four lactating women on long-term colchicine therapy (1–1.5 mg/day for at least 7 years) for FMF, serum and milk samples were drawn before a dose and at 1, 3, and 6 hours after a dose (10). Maximum breast milk drug concentrations ranged between 1.9 and 8.6 ng/mL, whereas maximum serum concentrations ranged from 3.6 to 6.46 ng/mL. The peak concentrations in milk and serum both occurred at 1 hour and the colchicine concentration time curves for milk and serum were parallel. No apparent effects in the nursing infants were observed over a 10-month period. The authors concluded that nursing was safe for women taking colchicine, but that waiting 12 hours after a dose to breastfeed would minimize exposure of the nursing infant (10).

Much higher colchicine milk concentrations were measured in a second study. A 21-year-old woman had taken colchicine (1 mg/day) throughout gestation and continued while breastfeeding her normal infant (11). On postpartum days 5 and 15, colchicine concentrations in the mother's 24-hour urine sample were 276,000 and 123,000 ng/24 hours, respectively, while none was detected (test sensitivity 5 ng/mL) in the infant's 12-hour urine collection. Milk samples were collected four times each on day 5 (2, 4, 15, and 21 hours after a dose) and day 15 (0, 4, 7, and 11 hours after a dose). Colchicine concentrations in the 2-hour and 4-hour samples on day 5 were 31 and 24 ng/mL, respectively, and below the level of detection at 15 and 21 hours. On day 15, levels at 0 and 11 hours were below detection, while those at 4 and 7 hours were 27 and 10 ng/mL, respectively. Assuming 100% of the dose in milk was absorbed, the infant's estimated dose during the 8-hour period after a dose was 10% of the mother's weight-adjusted dose. Although no adverse effects were observed in the infant, the authors recommended that a mother could minimize drug exposure from her milk by taking her dose at bedtime and waiting 8 hours to breastfeed (11).

Because of the absence of infant toxicity observed during nursing in one of the above cases (9), the American Academy of Pediatrics classified colchicine as compatible with breastfeeding (37).

References

1. Berenstadt M, Welsz B, Cuckle H, Di-Castro M, Guetta E, Barkai G. Chromosomal abnormalities and birth defects among couples with colchicine treated familial Mediterranean fever. Am J Obstet Gynecol 2005;193:1513–6.
2. Diav-Citrin O, Shechtman S, Schwartz V, Avgil-Tsadok M, Finkel-Pekarsky V, Wajnberg R, Arnon J, Berkovitch M, Ornoy A. Pregnancy outcome after in utero exposure to colchicine. Am J Obstet Gynecol 2010;203:144.e1–8.
3. Ben-Chetrit E, Ben-Chetrit A, Berkun Y, Ben-Chetrit E. Pregnancy outcomes in women with familial Mediterranean fever receiving colchicine: is amniocentesis justified? Arthritis Care Res 2010;62:143–8.
4. Shepard TH. *Catalog of Teratogenic Agents*. 6th ed. Baltimore, MD: Johns Hopkins University Press, 1989:164–6.
5. Sokal JE, Lessmann EM. Effects of cancer chemotherapeutic agents on the human fetus. JAMA 1960;172:1765–72.
6. Cohen MM, Levy M, Eliakim M. A cytogenetic evaluation of long-term colchicine therapy in the treatment of familial Mediterranean fever (FMF). Am J Med Sci 1977;274:147–52.
7. Levy M, Yaffe C. Testicular function in patients with familial Mediterranean fever on long-term colchicine treatment. Fertil Steril 1978;29:667–8.
8. Zemer D, Pras M, Sohar E, Gafni J. Colchicine in familial Mediterranean fever. N Engl J Med 1976;294:170–1.
9. Milunsky JM, Milunsky A. Breast-feeding during colchicine therapy for familial Mediterranean fever. J Pediatr 1991;119:164.
10. Ben-Chetrit E, Scherrmann JM, Levy M. Colchicine in breast milk of patients with familial Mediterranean fever. Arthritis Rheum 1996;39:1213–7.
11. Guillonneau M, Aigrain EJ, Galliot M, Binet M-H, Darbois Y. Colchicine is excreted at high concentrations in human breast milk. Eur J Obstet Gynecol Reprod Biol 1995;61:177–8.
12. Ehrenfeld M, Brzezinski A, Levy M, Eliakim M. Fertility and obstetric history in patients with familial Mediterranean fever on long-term colchicine therapy. Br J Obstet Gynaecol 1987;94:1186–91.
13. Shimoni Y, Shalev E. Pregnancy and complicated familial Mediterranean fever. Int J Gynaecol Obstet 1990;33:165–9.
14. Rabinovitch O, Zemer D, Kukia E, Sohar E, Mashlach S. Colchicine treatment in conception and pregnancy: two hundred thirty-one pregnancies in patients with familial Mediterranean fever. Am J Reprod Immunol 1992;28:245–6.
15. Mordel N, Birkenfeld A, Rubinger D, Schenker JG, Sadovsky E. Successful full-term pregnancy in familial Mediterranean fever complicated with amyloidosis: case report and review of the literature. Fetal Diagn Ther 1993;8:129–34.
16. Ditkoff EC, Sauer MV. Successful pregnancy in familial Mediterranean fever patient following assisted reproduction. J Assist Reprod Genet 1996;13:684–5.

17. Michael O, Goldman RD, Koren G, and Motherisk Team. Safety of colchicine during pregnancy. Can Fam Physician 2003;49:967–9.
18. Ben-Chetrit E, Berkun Y, Ben-Chetrit E, Ben-Chetrit A. The outcome of pregnancy in the wives of men with familial Mediterranean fever treated with colchicine. Semin Arthritis Rheum 2004;34:549–52.
19. Cerquaglia C, Diaco M, Nucera G, La Regina M, Montalto M, Manna R. Pharmacological and clinical basis of treatment of familial Mediterranean fever (FMF) with colchicine or analogues: an update. Curr Drug Targets Inflamm Allergy 2005;4:117–24.
20. Tutuncu L, Atasoyu EM, Evrenkaya R, Mungen E. Familial Mediterranean fever-related nephrotic syndrome and successful full-term pregnancy. Arch Med Res 2006;37:178–80.
21. Ofir D, Levy A, Wiznitzer A, Mazor M, Sheiner E. Familial Mediterranean fever during pregnancy: an independent risk factor for preterm delivery. Eur J Obstet Gynecol Reprod Biol 2008;141:115–8.
22. Cerquaglia C, Verrecchia E, Fonnesu C, Giovinale G, Marinaro A, De Socio G, Manna R. Female reproductive dysfunction in familial Mediterranean fever patients with and without colchicine treatment. Clin Exp Rheumatol 2010;28 (4 Suppl 60):S101. Epub 2010 Sep 24.
23. Amoura Z, Schermann JM, Weclisler B, Zerah X, Goodeau P. Transplacental passage of colchicine in familial Mediterranean fever. J Rheumatol 1944;21:383.
24. Salesi M, Karimifar M, Salimi F, Mahzouni P. A case of granulomatous mastitis with erythema nodosum and arthritis. Rheumatol Int 2011;31:1093–5.
25. Cestari AN, Botelho Vieira Filho JP, Yonenaga Y, Magnelli N, Imada J. A case of human reproductive abnormalities possibly induced by colchicine treatment. Rev Bras Biol 1965;25:253–6.
26. Ferreira NR, Buoniconti A. Trisomy after colchicine therapy. Lancet 1968;2:1304.
27. Walker FA. Trisomy after colchicine therapy. Lancet 1969;1:257–8.
28. Timson J. Trisomy after colchicine therapy. Lancet 1969;1:370.
29. Hoefnagel D. Trisomy after colchicine therapy. Lancet 1969;1:1160.
30. Ferreira NR, Frota-Pessoa O. Trisomy after colchicine therapy. Lancet 1969;1:1160–1.
31. Yu TF, Gutman AB. Efficacy of colchicine prophylaxis in gout. Prevention of recurrent gouty arthritis over a mean period of five years in 208 gouty subjects. Ann Intern Med 1961;55:179–92.
32. Goldfinger SE. Colchicine for familial Mediterranean fever: possible adverse effects. N Engl J Med 1974;290:56.
33. Poffenbarger PL, Brinkley BR. Colchicine for familial Mediterranean fever: possible adverse effects. N Engl J Med 1974;290:56.
34. Merlin HE. Azoospermia caused by colchicine—a case report. Fertil Steril 1972;23:180–1.
35. Bremer WJ, Paulsen CA. Colchicine and testicular function in man. N Engl J Med 1976;294:1384–5.
36. Haimov-Kochman R, Ben-Chetrit E. The effect of colchicine treatment on sperm production and function: a review. Hum Reprod 1998;13:360–2.
37. Committee on Drugs, American Academy of Pediatrics. The transfer of drugs and other chemicals into human milk. Pediatrics 2001;108:776–89.

COLESEVELAM

Antilipemic Agent

PREGNANCY RECOMMENDATION: Limited Human Data—Probably Compatible
BREASTFEEDING RECOMMENDATION: No Human Data—Probably Compatible

PREGNANCY SUMMARY

The effect of colesevelam on the absorption of vitamins and other nutrients from the gastrointestinal tract in pregnant women has not been studied (1). Fat-soluble vitamin deficiency, especially vitamin K, is a potential complication if this agent is used during pregnancy.

FETAL RISK SUMMARY

This nonabsorbed, polymeric, lipid-lowering agent binds bile acids to prevent their absorption. Because cholesterol is the sole precursor of bile acids, this action eventually results in the lowering of low-density lipoprotein (LDL) cholesterol levels in the blood. It is indicated, either alone or in combination with an HMG-CoA reductase inhibitor (atorvastatin, cerivastatin, fluvastatin, lovastatin, pravastatin, or simvastatin), as adjunctive therapy to diet and exercise for the reduction of elevated LDL cholesterol in patients with primary hypercholesterolemia (1). Because the drug is not absorbed, no direct embryo or fetal exposure will occur.

Reproduction studies have been conducted in pregnant rats and rabbits (1). Doses that were about 50 and 17 times, respectively, the maximum human dose based on body weight (MHD) revealed no evidence of fetal harm. In addition, no effect on rat fertility was seen at 50 times the MHD (1). In rats, doses >30 times the MHD caused vitamin K deficiency and hemorrhage, but the absorption of fat-soluble (A, D, E, and K) vitamins was not significantly impaired (1).

A 2012 report described five cases of familial hypercholesterolemia in pregnancy that occurred between 2004 and 2010 (2). Colesevelam (625 mg twice daily) was started before pregnancy. Two women stopped the therapy less than 4 weeks into their pregnancies, but the other three continued the drug throughout gestation. All five women had uncomplicated pregnancies and gave birth to healthy infants at term (2).

BREASTFEEDING SUMMARY

No reports describing the use of colesevelam in lactation have been located. The drug is not absorbed after oral administration so the nursing infant will not be exposed to the drug via breast milk. However, maternal deficiency of fat-soluble vitamins, especially vitamin K (see above), is a potential complication. This may result in lower fat-soluble vitamin concentrations in milk because these vitamins are natural constituents of breast milk.

References

1. Product information. Welchol. Sankyo Pharma, 2001.
2. Eapen DJ, Valiani K, Reddy S, Sperling L. Management of familial hypercholesterolemia during pregnancy: case series and discussion. J Clin Lipidol 2012;61:88–91.

COLESTIPOL

Antilipemic Agent

PREGNANCY RECOMMENDATION: No Human Data—Probably Compatible
BREASTFEEDING RECOMMENDATION: No Human Data—Probably Compatible

PREGNANCY SUMMARY

The actions of colestipol are similar to those of cholestyramine, another exchange resin (see also Cholestyramine). It is not absorbed into the systemic circulation, so it should have no direct effect on the fetus. However, as with cholestyramine, prolonged use of colestipol may result in reduced intestinal absorption of the fat-soluble vitamins, A, D, E, and K. Because the interruption of cholesterol-lowering therapy during pregnancy should have no effect on the long-term treatment of hyperlipidemia, the use of colestipol should probably be halted during gestation.

FETAL RISK SUMMARY

The anion exchange resin, colestipol, is used to bind bile acids in the intestine into a nonabsorbable complex that is excreted in the feces. The prevention of the systemic reabsorption of the bile acids lowers the total amount of cholesterol in the patient. Because less than 0.17% of a dose is absorbed systemically, it is not expected to cause fetal harm when administered during pregnancy in recommended doses (1).

In a reproductive study with rats and rabbits, doses up to 1000 mg/kg/day produced no adverse effects on the fetuses (2). No published or unpublished cases involving the use of colestipol during human pregnancy have been located. Rosa also reported finding no recipients of this drug in his 1994 presentation on the outcome of pregnancies following exposure to anticholesterol agents (3).

BREASTFEEDING SUMMARY

Because colestipol is poorly absorbed (less than 0.17% of a dose) into the systemic circulation, its use by the lactating woman should have no direct effect on the nursing infant. Prolonged use of the exchange resin, however, may result in decreased maternal absorption of the fat-soluble vitamins, A, D, E, and K. The resulting deficiencies in the mother would lessen the amounts of these vitamins in her milk.

References

1. Product information. Colestid. Pharmacia & Upjohn, 2000.
2. Webster HD, Bollert JA. Toxicologic, reproductive and teratologic studies of colestipol hydrochloride: a new bile acid sequestrant. Toxicol Appl Pharmacol 1974;28:57–65. As cited in Shepard TH. *Catalog of Teratogenic Agents*. 7th ed. Baltimore, MD: Johns Hopkins University Press, 1992:105.
3. Rosa F. *Anti-cholesterol Agent Pregnant Exposure Outcomes*. Presented at the 7th International Organization for Teratogen Information Services, Woods Hole, MA, April 1994.

COLISTIMETHATE

Antibiotic

PREGNANCY RECOMMENDATION: Limited Human Data—Animal Data Suggest Moderate Risk
BREASTFEEDING RECOMMENDATION: Limited Human Data—Probably Compatible

PREGNANCY SUMMARY

No reports linking the use of colistimethate with congenital defects have been located. The drug crosses the placenta at term (1).

FETAL RISK SUMMARY

Colistimethate was not teratogenic in rats at IM doses about 0.13 and 0.30 times the maximum recommended human dose based on BSA (MRHD) (2). The same weight doses in rabbits (about 0.25 and 0.55 times the MRHD) resulted in talipes varus in 2.6% and 2.9% of the fetuses, respectively. Increased resorption of rabbit embryos occurred at the highest dose.

BREASTFEEDING SUMMARY

Colistimethate is excreted into breast milk. The milk:plasma ratio is 0.17–0.18 (3). Although this level is low, three potential problems exist for the nursing infant: modification of bowel flora, direct effects on the infant, and interference with the interpretation of culture results if a fever workup is required.

References

1. MacAulay MA, Charles D. Placental transmission of colistimethate. Clin Pharmacol Ther 1967;8:578–86.
2. Product information. Coly-Mycin. Monarch Pharmaceuticals, 2000.
3. Wilson JT. Milk/plasma ratios and contraindicated drugs. In: Wilson JT, ed. *Drugs in Breast Milk*. Balgowlah, Australia: ADIS Press, 1981:78–9.

COLLAGENASE *CLOSTRIDIUM HISTOLYTICUM*

Dermatologic Agent

PREGNANCY RECOMMENDATION: No Human Data—Probably Compatible
BREASTFEEDING RECOMMENDATION: No Human Data—Probably Compatible

PREGNANCY SUMMARY

No reports describing the use of collagenase *Clostridium histolycticum* in human pregnancy have been located. Reproduction studies in rats revealed no evidence of harm to the fetus, but the comparison to the human dose was based on body weight and may not be interpretable. However, in humans, quantifiable levels of the drug did not occur in the systemic circulation after injection into a Dupuytren cord. Almost all patients treated with collagenase *C. histolyticum* develop antiproduct antibodies after treatment. The clinical significance of antiproduct antibody formation on a developing fetus is not known.

FETAL RISK SUMMARY

Collagenase *Clostridium histolyticum* is a polypeptide consisting of two microbial collagenases (proteinases), collagenase AUX-I and collagenase AUX-II, isolated from the fermentation of *C. histolyticum* bacteria. It is indicated for the treatment of adult patients with Dupyutren contracture with a palpable cord. The drug is given by local injection into the hand. After injection into a Dupuytren cord, neither of the collagenases had quantifiable levels in the systemic circulation (the lower limit of quantification for AUX I and AUX II in human plasma is 5 and 25 ng/mL, respectively).

Reproduction studies have been performed in rats. No evidence of fetal harm was observed in pregnant rats given IV doses up to about 45 times the IV human dose based on body weight (HD) (1).

Carcinogenicity studies with collagenase *C. histolyticum* have not been conducted. Various assays for mutagenic and clastogenic effects were negative. The polypeptide did not impair fertility or early embryonic development when administered IV to rats at doses up to about 45 times the HD (1).

It is not known if the two collagenases cross the human placenta. The molecular weights of collagenase AUX-1 and collagenase AUX-II are 114,000 and 113,000, respectively, and nonquantifiable systemic levels suggest that clinically significant exposure of the embryo or fetus is unlikely.

BREASTFEEDING SUMMARY

No reports on the use of collagenase *C. histolyticum* during lactation have been located. The molecular weights of collagenase AUX-1 and collagenase AUX-II are 114,000 and 113,000, respectively, and, combined with the nonquantifiable systemic levels, suggest that the presence in milk of clinically significant amounts is unlikely.

Reference

1. Product information. Xiaflex. Auxilium Pharmaceuticals, 2010.

CONIVAPTAN

Vasopressin Receptor Antagonist

PREGNANCY RECOMMENDATION: No Human Data—Animal Data Suggest Moderate Risk
BREASTFEEDING RECOMMENDATION: No Human Data—Potential Toxicity

PREGNANCY SUMMARY

No reports describing the use of conivaptan during human pregnancy have been located. Developmental toxicity (death) was observed in one of two animal species. Because of the administration method, exposure of the embryo and fetus will probably occur. The absence of human pregnancy experience prevents a more complete assessment of the embryo–fetal risk. If a pregnant woman requires conivaptan therapy, she should be advised of the potential risk (abortion or fetal/neonatal death).

C

FETAL RISK SUMMARY

Conivaptan is a nonpeptide, dual antagonist of arginine vasopressin receptors. It is indicated for the treatment of euvolemic hyponatremia (e.g., the syndrome of inappropriate secretion of antidiuretic hormone, or in the setting of hypothyroidism, adrenal insufficiency, pulmonary disorders, etc) in hospitalized patients. It is given as a continuous IV infusion over several days. The mean terminal elimination half-life after conivaptan infusion is 5 hours. The drug is extensively bound to plasma proteins (99%). Some of the metabolites have activity equivalent to the parent compound but, overall, the activity of the metabolites was only 7% that of conivaptan (1).

Reproduction studies have been conducted in rats and rabbits. When female rats were given daily IV bolus doses that resulted in systemic exposures that were less than the human therapeutic exposure based on AUC (HTE) before mating and during the first 7 days of pregnancy, prolonged diestrus, decreased fertility, and increased pre- and postnatal implantation loss occurred. No effects were observed with these doses on male fertility. No significant maternal or fetal effects were observed at daily doses resulting in systemic exposures that were less than the HTE during organogenesis (days 7–17). When dosing was continued through lactation day 20 (weaning), no maternal toxicity was observed, but pups showed decreased neonatal viability, weaning indices, delayed growth and physical development (including sexual maturation), and delayed reflex development. No pup adverse effects were observed when the daily dose was reduced by one-half or more. In pregnant rabbits given daily IV doses resulting in systemic exposures less than the HTE during organogenesis, there were no fetal adverse effects, but maternal toxicity was evident at all doses tested (1).

During labor, daily doses given orally to rats that resulted in systemic exposures equivalent to the HTE delayed delivery. Daily IV doses that resulted in systemic exposures less than the HTE caused increased peripartum pup mortality. These effects may have been secondary to conivaptan activity on oxytocin receptors in rats (1).

No carcinogenicity was observed in mice and rats given daily doses by gavage for 2 years that resulted in systemic exposures that were up to six and two times, respectively, the HTE. Conivaptan was not mutagenic or clastogenic, with or without metabolic activation, in several tests (1).

Conivaptan crosses the rat placenta with fetal tissue concentrations <10% of maternal plasma levels, but placental levels were 2.2 times higher than maternal plasma levels. Moreover, conivaptan was slowly cleared from fetal tissues, suggesting that fetal accumulation may occur (1). It is not known if conivaptan crosses the human placenta. The molecular weight (about 499 for the free base) and the administration of a continuous intravenous infusion over several days suggest that the drug will cross to the human embryo and fetus.

BREASTFEEDING SUMMARY

No reports describing the use of conivaptan during human lactation have been located. It is not known if conivaptan is excreted into breast milk. The molecular weight (about 499 for the free base) and the administration of a continuous intravenous infusion over several days suggest that the drug will be excreted into milk. Although the effects on a nursing infant are unknown, there is a potential for severe toxicity in several organ systems as observed in adults receiving IV infusions. Moreover, as a weak base, ion trapping in the relatively acidic milk will allow conivaptan to accumulate in milk. Therefore, until data relating to milk concentrations are available, women receiving conivaptan should probably not breastfeed.

Reference

1. Product information. Vaprisol. Astellas Pharma US, 2007.

CORTICOTROPIN/COSYNTROPIN

Corticosteroid Stimulating Hormone

PREGNANCY RECOMMENDATION: Limited Human Data—No Relevant Animal Data
BREASTFEEDING RECOMMENDATION: No Human Data—Probably Compatible

PREGNANCY SUMMARY

Studies reporting the use of corticotropin in pregnancy have not demonstrated adverse fetal effects (1–4). However, corticosteroids have been suspected of causing malformations (see Hydrocortisone). Because corticotropin stimulates the release of endogenous corticosteroids, this relationship should be considered when prescribing the drug to women in their reproductive years.

BREASTFEEDING SUMMARY

No reports describing the use of corticotropin during human lactation have been located. The use of this agent during breastfeeding probably is compatible.

References

1. Johnstone FD, Campbell S. Adrenal response in pregnancy to long-acting tetracosactin. J Obstet Gynaecol Br Commonw 1974;81:363–7.
2. Simmer HH, Tulchinsky D, Gold EM, Frankland M, Greipel M, Gold AS. On the regulation of estrogen production by cortisol and ACTH in human pregnancy at term. Am J Obstet Gynecol 1974;119:283–96.
3. Aral K, Kuwabara Y, Okinaga S. The effect of adrenocorticotropic hormone and dexamethasone, administered to the fetus in utero, upon maternal and fetal estrogens. Am J Obstet Gynecol 1972;113:316–22.
4. Potert AJ. Pregnancy and adrenalcortical hormones. Br Med J 1962;2:967–72.

C

CORTISONE

Corticosteroid

PREGNANCY RECOMMENDATION: Human Data Suggest Risk
BREASTFEEDING RECOMMENDATION: No Human Data—Probably Compatible

PREGNANCY SUMMARY

Cortisone (Compound E) is an inactive corticosteroid precursor that is secreted by the adrenal cortex. It is converted by reduction to hydrocortisone, primarily in the liver. See Hydrocortisone.

BREASTFEEDING SUMMARY

See Hydrocortisone.

COUMARIN DERIVATIVES

Anticoagulant

PREGNANCY RECOMMENDATION: Contraindicated—1st Trimester
BREASTFEEDING RECOMMENDATION: Compatible; Contraindicated (Phenindione)

PREGNANCY SUMMARY

The use of coumarin derivatives during the 1st trimester carries with it a significant risk to the fetus. For all cases, only about 70% of pregnancies are expected to result in a normal infant. Exposure in the 6th–9th weeks of gestation may produce a pattern of defects termed the fetal warfarin syndrome with an incidence up to 25% or greater in some series. Infants exposed before and after this period have had other congenital anomalies, but the relationship between warfarin and these defects is unknown. Infrequent central nervous system defects, which have greater clinical significance to the infant than the defects of the fetal warfarin syndrome, may be deformations related to hemorrhage and scarring, with subsequent impaired growth of brain tissue. Spontaneous abortions, stillbirths, and neonatal deaths may also occur. If the mother's condition requires anticoagulation, the use of heparin from the start of the 6th gestational week through the end of the 12th gestational week, and again at term, may lessen the risk to the fetus of adverse outcome.

FETAL RISK SUMMARY

Coumarin derivatives (dicumarol, ethyl biscoumacetate, and warfarin) are oral anticoagulants, as are the indandione derivatives (anisindione and phenindione). Use of any of these agents during pregnancy may result in significant problems for the fetus and newborn. Since the first case of fetal coumarin embryopathy described by DiSaia in 1966 (1), a large volume of literature has accumulated. Hall and coworkers (2) reviewed this subject in 1980 (167 references). In the 3 years following this review, a number of other reports have appeared (3–12). The principal problems confronting the fetus and newborn are as follows:

- Embryopathy (fetal warfarin syndrome)
- Central nervous system defects
- Spontaneous abortion
- Stillbirth
- Prematurity
- Hemorrhage

First-trimester use of coumarin derivatives may result in the fetal warfarin syndrome (FWS) (1–4). The common characteristics of the FWS are nasal hypoplasia because of failure of development of the nasal septum and stippled epiphyses. The bridge of the nose is depressed, resulting in a flattened, upturned appearance. Neonatal respiratory distress occurs frequently because of upper airway obstruction. Other features that may be present are as follows:

- Birth weight <10th percentile for gestational age
- Eye defects (blindness, optic atrophy, microphthalmia) when drug also used in 2nd and 3rd trimesters
- Hypoplasia of the extremities (ranging from severe rhizomelic dwarfing to dystrophic nails and shortened fingers)
- Developmental retardation
- Seizures
- Scoliosis
- Deafness/hearing loss
- Congenital heart disease
- Death

The critical period of exposure, based on the work of Hall and coworkers (2), seems to be the 6th–9th weeks of gestation. All of the known cases of FWS were exposed during at least a portion of these weeks. Exposure after the 1st trimester carries the risk of central nervous system (CNS) defects. No constant grouping of abnormalities was observed, nor were there an apparent correlation between time of exposure and the defects, except that all fetuses were exposed in the 2nd and/or 3rd trimesters. After elimination of those cases that were probably caused by late fetal or neonatal hemorrhage, the CNS defects in 13 infants were thought to represent deformations that occurred as a result of abnormal growth arising from an earlier fetal hemorrhage and subsequent scarring (2). Two patterns were recognized: (a) dorsal midline dysplasia characterized by agenesis of corpus callosum, Dandy-Walker malformations, and midline cerebellar atrophy (encephaloceles may be present); and (b) ventral midline dysplasia characterized by optic atrophy (eye anomalies).

Other features of CNS damage in the 13 infants were (number of infants shown in parenthesis):

- Mental retardation (13)
- Blindness (7)
- Spasticity (4)
- Seizures (3)
- Deafness (1)
- Scoliosis (1)
- Growth failure (1)
- Death (3)

Long-term effects in the children with CNS defects were more significant and debilitating than those from the fetal warfarin syndrome (2).

Fetal outcomes for the 471 cases of in utero exposure to coumarin derivatives reported through 1983 are summarized below (2–12):

1ST TRIMESTER EXPOSURE (263):
- Normal infants—167 (63%)
- Spontaneous abortions—41 (16%)
- Stillborn/neonatal death—17 (6%)
- FWS—27 (10%)
- CNS/other defects—11 (4%)

2ND TRIMESTER EXPOSURE (208):
- Normal infants—175 (84%)
- Spontaneous abortions—4 (2%)
- Stillborn/neonatal death—19 (9%)
- CNS/other defects—10 (5%)

TOTAL INFANTS EXPOSED (471):
- Normal infants—342 (73%)
- Spontaneous abortions—45 (10%)
- Stillborn/neonatal death—36 (8%)
- FWS/CNS/other defects—48 (10%)

Hemorrhage was observed in 11 (3%) of the normal newborns (premature and term). Two of the patients in the 2nd- and 3rd trimester groups were treated with the coumarin derivatives, phenprocoumon and nicoumalone. Both infants were normal.

Congenital abnormalities that did not fit the pattern of the FWS or CNS defects were reported in 10 infants (2,9). These were thought to be incidental malformations that were probably not related to the use of coumarin derivatives (see also three other cases, in which the relationship to coumarin derivatives is unknown, described in the text below, references 16,20,22).

- Asplenia, two-chambered heart, agenesis of pulmonary artery
- Anencephaly, spina bifida, congenital absence of clavicles
- Congenital heart disease, death
- Fetal distress, focal motor seizures
- Bilateral polydactyly
- Congenital corneal leukoma
- Nonspecified multiple defects
- Asplenia, congenital heart disease, incomplete rotation of gut, short broad phalanges, hypoplastic nails
- Single kidney, toe defects, other anomalies, death
- Cleft palate

A 1984 study examined 22 children, with a mean age of 4.0 years, who were exposed in utero to warfarin (13). Physical and mental development of the children was comparable to that of matched controls.

Since publication of the above data, a number of additional reports and studies have appeared, describing the outcomes of pregnancies treated at various times with coumarin derivatives (13–25). The largest series involved 156 women with cardiac valve prostheses who had 223 pregnancies (14). During a period of 19 years, the women were grouped based on evolving treatment regimens: group I—68 pregnancies treated with acenocoumarol until the diagnosis of pregnancy was made, and then treated with dipyridamole or aspirin, or both; group II—128 pregnancies treated with acenocoumarol throughout gestation; group III—12 pregnancies treated with acenocoumarol, except when heparin was substituted from pregnancy diagnosis to the 13th week of gestation, and again from the 38th week until delivery; and group IV—15 pregnancies in women with biologic prostheses who were not treated with anticoagulant therapy. The fetal outcomes in the four groups were as follows: spontaneous abortions, 10.3% vs. 28.1% vs. 0% vs. 0% ($p < 0.0005$); stillbirths, 7.4% vs. 7.1% vs. 0% vs. 6.7%; and neonatal deaths, 0% vs. 2.3% vs. 0% vs. 0%. (See reference for maternal outcomes in the various groups.) Of the 38 children examined in group II, 3 (7.9%) had features of the FWS.

In a subsequent report from these investigators, the outcomes of 72 pregnancies studied prospectively were described in 1986 (15). The pregnancies were categorized into three groups according to the anticoagulant therapy: group I—23 pregnancies treated with acenocoumarol except for heparin from the 6th to 12th week of gestation; group II—12 pregnancies treated the same as group I except that heparin treatment was started after the 7th week; and group III—37 pregnancies treated with acenocoumarol throughout gestation (pregnancies in this group were not detected until after the 1st trimester). In most patients, heparin was substituted for the coumarin derivative after the 38th week of gestation. The fetal outcomes in the three groups were spontaneous abortions, 8.7% vs. 25% vs. 16.2%; and stillbirths, 0% vs. 8.3% vs. 0%. Not all of the infants born to the mothers were examined, but of those that were, the FWS was observed in 0% of group I (0 of 19), 25.0% of group II (2 of 8), and 29.6% of group III (8 of 27). Thus, 10 (28.6%) of the 35 infants examined who were exposed at least during the first 7 weeks of gestation had warfarin embryopathy.

A 1983 report described 14 pregnancies in 13 women with a prosthetic heart valve who were treated throughout pregnancy with warfarin (16). Two patients had spontaneous abortions, two delivered premature stillborn infants (one infant had anencephaly), and two newborns died during the neonatal period. The total fetal and neonatal mortality in this series was 43%. Other defects noted were corneal changes in two, bradydactyly and dysplastic nails in two, and nasal hypoplasia in one.

In 18 pregnancies of 16 women with an artificial heart valve, heparin was substituted for warfarin when pregnancy was diagnosed (between 6 and 8 weeks after the last menstrual period) and continued until the 13th week of gestation (17). Nine of the 18 pregnancies aborted, but none of the nine liveborn infants had congenital anomalies or other complications.

Three reports described the pregnancy outcomes in mothers with prosthetic heart valves and who were treated with anticoagulants (18–20). A study published in 1991 described the outcomes of 64 pregnancies in 40 women with cardiac valve replacement, 34 of whom had mechanical valves (18). Warfarin was used in 47 pregnancies (23 women), heparin in 11 pregnancies (11 women), and no anticoagulation was given in 6 pregnancies (6 women). Fetal wastage (spontaneous abortions, neonatal death after preterm delivery, and stillbirths) occurred in 25 (53%) of the warfarin group, 4 (36%) of those treated with heparin, and 1 (17%) of those not treated. Two infants, both exposed to warfarin, had congenital malformations: single kidney and toe, and finger defects in one; cleft lip and palate in the other.

Two groups of pregnant patients with prosthetic heart valves were compared in a study published in 1992 (19). In group 1 ($N = 40$), all treated with coumarin-like drugs until near term when therapy was changed to heparin, 34 (85%) had mechanical valves, whereas none of those in group 2 ($N = 20$) were treated with anticoagulation and all had biological valves. The pregnancy outcomes of the two groups were as follows: spontaneous abortions 7 and 0, prematurity 14 and 2 ($p < 0.05$), low birth weight 15 and 2 ($p < 0.05$), stillbirth 1 and 0, neonatal mortality 5 and 0, and birth defects 4 and 0. The 4 infants from group 1 with birth defects included 3 with typical features of FWS (1 with low birth weight and upper airway obstruction) and 1 with left ventricular hypoplasia and aortic atresia (died in neonatal period). The other 4 neonatal deaths involved 3 from respiratory distress syndrome and 1 from a cerebral hemorrhage.

A 1994 reference compared retrospectively two groups of pregnant women: Group 1 (56 pregnancies in 31 women) with mechanical valve replacements, all of whom were treated with warfarin; and group 2 (95 pregnancies in 57 women) with porcine tissue valves, none of whom received anticoagulation (20). Twenty women in group 1 either continued the warfarin throughout delivery ($N = 12$) or discontinued the drug ($N = 8$) 1–2 days before delivery. The pregnancy outcomes of the two groups were as follows: induced abortion 9 and 22, fetal loss before 20 weeks' gestation 7 and 8, fetal loss after 20 weeks' gestation 6 and 1 ($p < 0.01$), total fetal loss 13 and 9 ($p < 0.05$), and live births 34 and 64 ($p < 0.05$). Two infants, both in group 1 had birth defects—a ventricular septal defect in 1 and a hypoplastic nose in the other (20).

Five reports have described single cases of exposure to warfarin during pregnancy (21–25). A woman with Marfan's syndrome had replacement of her aortic arch and valve combined with coronary artery bypass performed during the 1st week of her pregnancy (1–8 days after conception) (21). She was treated with warfarin throughout gestation. A normal female infant was delivered by elective cesarean section at 34 weeks' gestation. Warfarin was used to treat a deep vein thrombosis during the 3rd trimester in a 34-year-old woman because of heparin-induced maternal thrombocytopenia (22). A normal infant was delivered at term. In another case involving a woman with a deep vein thrombosis that had occurred before the present pregnancy, warfarin therapy was continued through the first 14 weeks of gestation (23). At term, a 3660-g infant was delivered, who did not breathe and who died after 35 minutes. At autopsy, an almost total agenesis of the left diaphragm and hypoplasia of both lungs were noted. The relationship between warfarin and the defect is unknown.

The use of warfarin to treat a deep vein thrombosis associated with circulating lupus anticoagulant during pregnancy has been described (24). Therapy was started after the ninth week of gestation. Because of severe pregnancy-induced hypertension, a 1830-g female infant was delivered by cesarean section at 31 weeks. No information was provided about the condition of the infant.

A woman with a mitral valve replacement 8 months before pregnancy was treated continuously with warfarin until 6 weeks after her last menstrual period (25). Warfarin was then stopped and except for cigarette smoking, no other drugs were taken during the pregnancy. A growth-restricted (2340 g, 3rd percentile; 50 cm length, 50th percentile; 35 cm head circumference, 50th percentile) female infant was delivered at term. Congenital abnormalities noted in the infant were triangular face with broad forehead, micrognathia, microglossia, hypoplastic fingernails and toenails, and hypoplasia of the distal phalanges. No epiphyseal stippling was seen on a skeletal survey. A normal female karyotype, 46,XX, was found on chromosomal analysis. Psychomotor development was normal at 1 year of age, but physical growth remained restricted (3rd percentile). The authors concluded that the pattern of defects represented the earliest teratogenic effects of warfarin, but they could not exclude a chance association with the drug.

In a surveillance study of Michigan Medicaid recipients involving 229,101 completed pregnancies conducted between 1985 and 1992, 22 newborns had been exposed to warfarin during the 1st trimester (F. Rosa, personal communication, FDA, 1993). One (4.5%) major birth defect was observed (one expected), a cardiovascular defect (0.2 expected).

A report published in 1994 assessed the neurological, cognitive, and behavioral development of 21 children (8–10 years of age) who had been exposed in utero to coumarin derivatives (26). A control group of 17 children was used for comparison. Following examination, 32 of the children were classified as normal (18 exposed and 14 control children), 5 had minor neurological dysfunction (2 exposed and 3 control children), and 1 child had severe neurological abnormalities, which were thought to be due to oral anticoagulants. Although no significant differences were measured between the groups, the children with the lowest neurological assessments and the lowest IQ scores had been exposed to coumarin derivatives (26).

In a 2013 report, a 19-year-old primigravid woman at 32 weeks' gestation was admitted to the hospital with coagulopathy (27). She had spontaneous bleeding from the oral mucosa and from nicks on her legs from shaving and frank hematuria. Her international normalized ratio (INR) was >9. The fetus showed evidence of acidosis. Fresh-frozen plasma was given and bleeding stopped after about 1 hour. A 2180-g female infant was delivered by emergent cesarean section with Apgar scores of 0, 2, and 3 at 1, 5, and 10 minutes, respectively. The infant's INR was >9. She died on day 4 of life. Further history was obtained from the mother and it was learned that she had ingested brodifacoum, a second-generation rodenticidal anticoagulant. The agent was identified in maternal serum and cord blood. Because brodifacoum is lipophilic and has a very long half-life (up to several months), the mother required IV vitamin K (35 mg over several days) and high oral doses (up to 60 mg/day). Thirty days after presentation, her INR had decreased to 1.8 (27).

BREASTFEEDING SUMMARY

Excretion of coumarin (dicumarol, ethyl biscoumacetate, and warfarin) and indandione (anisindione and phenindione) derivatives into breast milk is dependent on the agent used. Three reports on warfarin have been located, totaling 15 lactating women (28–30). Doses ranged between 2 and 12 mg/day in 13 patients (7 nursing, 6 not nursing) with serum levels varying from 1.6 to 8.5 μmol/L (28,29). Warfarin was not detected in the milk of any of the 13 patients or in the plasma of the 7 nursing infants. No anticoagulant effect was found in the plasma of the three infants tested. In another report, the warfarin doses in two breastfeeding women were not specified nor were maternal plasma drug levels determined (30). However, no spectrophotometric evidence for the drug was found in the milk of one mother and no anticoagulant effect was measured in either nursing infant.

Exposure to ethyl biscoumacetate in milk resulted in bleeding in 5 of 42 exposed infants in one report (31). The maternal dosage was not given. An unidentified metabolite was found in the milk that may have led to the high complication rate. A 1959 study measured ethyl biscoumacetate levels in 38 milk specimens obtained from four women taking 600–1200 mg/day (32). The drug was detected in only 13 samples with levels varying from 0.09 to 1.69 mcg/mL. No correlation could be found between the milk concentrations and the dosage or time of administration. Twenty-two infants were breastfed from these and other mothers receiving ethyl biscoumacetate. No adverse effects were observed in the infants, but coagulation tests were not conducted (32).

More than 1600 postpartum women were treated with dicumarol to prevent thromboembolic complications in a 1950 study (33). Doses were titrated to adjust the prothrombin clotting time to 40%–50% of normal. No adverse effects or any change in prothrombin times were noted in any of the nursing infants.

Phenindione use in a lactating woman resulted in a massive scrotal hematoma and wound oozing in a 1.5-month-old breastfed infant shortly after a herniotomy was performed (34). The mother was taking 50 mg every morning and alternating between 50 and 25 mg every night for suspected pulmonary embolism that developed postpartum. Milk levels varying from 1 to 5 mcg/mL have been reported after 50- or 75-mg single doses of phenindione (35). When the dose was 25 mg, only 18 of 68 samples contained detectable amounts of the anticoagulant.

Maternal warfarin consumption apparently does not pose a significant risk to normal, full-term, breastfed infants. Other oral anticoagulants should be avoided by the lactating woman. The American Academy of Pediatrics classifies phenindione (which is not used in the United States) as contraindicated during breastfeeding because of the risk of hemorrhage in the infant (36). Both warfarin and dicumarol (bishydroxycoumarin) are classified by the Academy as compatible with breastfeeding.

References

1. DiSaia PJ. Pregnancy and delivery of a patient with a Starr-Edwards mitral valve prosthesis. Obstet Gynecol 1966;28:469–71.
2. Hall JG, Pauli RM, Wilson KM. Maternal and fetal sequelae of anticoagulation during pregnancy. Am J Med 1980;68:122–40.
3. Baillie M, Allen ED, Elkington AR. The congenital warfarin syndrome: a case report. Br J Ophthalmol 1980;64:633–5.
4. Harrod MJE, Sherrod PS. Warfarin embryopathy in siblings. Obstet Gynecol 1981;57:673–6.
5. Russo R, Bortolotti U, Schivazappa L, Girolami A. Warfarin treatment during pregnancy: a clinical note. Haemostasis 1979;8:96–8.
6. Biale Y, Cantor A, Lewenthal H, Gueron M. The course of pregnancy in patients with artificial heart valves treated with dipyridamole. Int J Gynaecol Obstet 1980;18:128–32.
7. Moe N. Anticoagulant therapy in the prevention of placental infarction and perinatal death. Obstet Gynecol 1982;59:481–3.
8. Kaplan LC, Anderson GG, Ring BA. Congenital hydrocephalus and Dandy-Walker malformation associated with warfarin use during pregnancy. Birth Defects 1982;18:79–83.
9. Chen WWC, Chan CS, Lee PK, Wang RYC, Wong VCW. Pregnancy in patients with prosthetic heart valves: an experience with 45 pregnancies. Q J Med 1982;51:358–65.
10. Vellenga E, Van Imhoff GW, Aarnoudse JG. Effective prophylaxis with oral anticoagulants and low-dose heparin during pregnancy in an antithrombin III deficient woman. Lancet 1983;2:224.
11. Michiels JJ, Stibbe J, Vellenga E, Van Vliet HHDM. Prophylaxis of thrombosis in antithrombin III-deficient women during pregnancy and delivery. Eur J Obstet Gynecol Reprod Biol 1984;18:149–53.
12. Oakley C. Pregnancy in patients with prosthetic heart valves. Br Med J 1983;286:1680–3.
13. Chong MKB, Harvey D, De Swiet M. Follow-up study of children whose mothers were treated with warfarin during pregnancy. Br J Obstet Gynaecol 1984;91:1070–3.
14. Salazar E, Zajarias A, Gutierrez N, Iturbe I. The problem of cardiac valve prostheses, anticoagulants, and pregnancy. Circulation 1984;70(Suppl 1):I169–77.
15. Iturbe-Alessio I, Fonseca MDC, Mutchinik O, Santos MA, Zajarias A, Salazar E. Risks of anticoagulant therapy in pregnant women with artificial heart valves. N Engl J Med 1986;315:1390–3.
16. Sheikhzadeh A, Ghabusi P, Hakim S, Wendler G, Sarram M, Tarbiat S. Congestive heart failure in valvular heart disease in pregnancies with and without valvular prostheses and anticoagulant therapy. Clin Cardiol 1983;6:465–70.
17. Lee P-K, Wang RYC, Chow JSF, Cheung K-L, Wong VCW, Chan T-K. Combined use of warfarin and adjusted subcutaneous heparin during pregnancy in patients with an artificial heart valve. J Am Coll Cardiol 1986;8:221–4.
18. Ayhan A, Yapar EG, Yuce K, Kisnisci HA, Nazli N, Ozmen F. Pregnancy and its complications after cardiac valve replacement. Int J Gynecol Obstet 1991;35:117–22.
19. Born D, Martinez EE, Almeida PAM, Santos DV, Carvalho ACC, Moron AF, Miyasaki CH, Moraes SD, Ambrose JA. Pregnancy in patients with prosthetic heart valves: the effects of anticoagulation on mother, fetus, and neonate. Am Heart J 1992;124:413–7.
20. Lee C-N, Wu C-C, Lin P-Y, Hsieh F-J, Chen H-Y. Pregnancy following cardiac prosthetic valve replacement. Obstet Gynecol 1994;83:353–60.
21. Cola LM, Lavin JP Jr. Pregnancy complicated by Marfan's syndrome with aortic arch dissection, subsequent aortic arch replacement and triple coronary artery bypass grafts. J Reprod Med 1985;30:685–8.
22. Copplestone A, Oscier DG. Heparin-induced thrombocytopenia in pregnancy. Br J Haematol 1987;65:248.

23. Normann EK, Stray-Pedersen B. Warfarin-induced fetal diaphragmatic hernia: case report. Br J Obstet Gynaecol 1989;96:729–30.
24. Campbell JM, Tate G, Scott JS. The use of warfarin in pregnancy complicated by circulating lupus anticoagulant; a technique for monitoring. Eur J Obstet Gynecol Reprod Biol 1988;29:27–32.
25. Ruthnum P, Tolmie JL. Atypical malformations in an infant exposed to warfarin during the first trimester of pregnancy. Teratology 1987;36:299–301.
26. Olthof E, De Vries TW, Touwen BCL, Smrkovsky M, Geven-Boere LM, Heijmans HSA, Van der Veer E. Late neurological, cognitive and behavioural sequelae of prenatal exposure to coumarins: a pilot study. Ear Hum Develop 1994;38:97–109.
27. Mehlhaff KM, Baxter CC, Rudinsky K, McKenna DS. Lethal neonatal coagulopathy after maternal ingestion of a superwarfarin. Obstet Gynecol 2013;122:500–2.
28. Orme ML, Lewis PJ, De Swiet M, Serlin MJ, Sibeon R, Baty JD, Breckenridge AM. May mothers given warfarin breast-feed their infants? Br Med J 1977;1:1564–5.
29. De Swiet M, Lewis PJ. Excretion of anticoagulants in human milk. N Engl J Med 1977;297:1471.
30. McKenna R, Cole ER, Vasan U. Is warfarin sodium contraindicated in the lactating mother? J Pediatr 1983;103:325–7.
31. Gostof, Momolka, Zilenka. Les substances derivees du tromexane dans le lait maternal et leurs actions paradoxales sur la prothrombine. Schweiz Med Wochenschr 1952;30:764–5. As cited in Daily JW. Anticoagulant and cardiovascular drugs. In: Wilson JT, ed. *Drugs in Breast Milk*. Balgowlah, Australia: ADIS Press, 1981:63.
32. Illingworth RS, Finch E. Ethyl biscoumacetate (Tromexan) in human milk. J Obstet Gynaecol Br Commonw 1959;66:487–8.
33. Brambel CE, Hunter RE. Effect of dicumarol on the nursing infant. Am J Obstet Gynecol 1950;59:1153–9.
34. Eckstein HB, Jack B. Breast-feeding and anticoagulant therapy. Lancet 1970;1:672–3.
35. Goguel M, Noel G, Gillet JY. Therapeutique anticoagulante et allaitement: etude du passage de la phenyl-2-dioxo,1,3 indane dans le lait maternal. Rev Fr Gynecol Obstet 1970;65:409–12. As cited in Anderson PO. Drugs and breast feeding—a review. Drug Intell Clin Pharm 1977;11:208–23.
36. Committee on Drugs, American Academy of Pediatrics. The transfer of drugs and other chemicals into human milk. Pediatrics 2001;108:776–89.

CRIZOTINIB

Antineoplastic (Tyrosine Kinase Inhibitor)

PREGNANCY RECOMMENDATION: Contraindicated
BREASTFEEDING RECOMMENDATION: Contraindicated

PREGNANCY SUMMARY

No reports describing the use of crizotinib during human pregnancy have been located. Developmental toxicity was observed in two animal species at doses close to the human dose. Based on the drug's mechanism of action, crizotinib should be avoided in pregnancy.

FETAL RISK SUMMARY

Crizotinib is an oral receptor tyrosine kinase inhibitor that is indicated for the treatment of patients with locally advanced or metastatic non-small cell lung cancer that is anaplastic lymphoma kinase (ALK)-positive as detected by an FDA-approved test. The drug is administered orally in 250 mg doses given twice daily. Crizotinib is metabolized to inactive metabolites and plasma protein binding is moderately high (91%). The mean terminal half-life is 42 hours following a single dose but may be lengthened by multiple dosing (1).

In rats treated during organogenesis, postimplantation loss was increased at doses that were about 1.2 times the recommended human dose (RHD) based on AUC (RHD-AUC). No increase in structural anomalies was observed in rats at doses up to the maternally toxic dose that was about 5 times the RHD-AUC or in rabbits at doses of up to about 3 times the RHD-AUC. However, fetal body weights were reduced at these doses (1).

Carcinogenicity studies with crizotinib have not been conducted. Crizotinib was genotoxic in multiple assays but not mutagenic in one assay. No studies have been conducted in animals to evaluate the effect on fertility. However, in toxicity studies in rats, males exhibited testicular pachytene spermatocyte degeneration when given doses that were greater than 3 times the RHD-AUC for 28 days. In female rats, single-cell necrosis of ovarian follicles occurred at doses that were about 10 times the RHD based on BSA given for 3 days (1).

It is not known if crizotinib crosses the human placenta. The molecular weight (about 450) and the long elimination half-life suggest that it will cross to the embryo–fetus. However, the amount crossing may be limited by the moderately high plasma protein binding.

BREASTFEEDING SUMMARY

No reports describing the use of crizotinib during human lactation have been located. The molecular weight (about 450) and the long elimination half-life (42 hours after a single dose) suggest that the drug will be excreted into breast milk, but the amount excreted may be limited by the moderately high (91%) plasma protein binding. Until additional data on the amount in breast milk are available, the safest course is to not breastfeed when taking this drug.

Reference

1. Product Information. Xalkori. Pfizer Labs, 2011.

CROFELEMER

Gastrointestinal Agent (Antidiarrheal)

PREGNANCY RECOMMENDATION: No Human Data—Probably Compatible
BREASTFEEDING RECOMMENDATION: No Human Data—Probably Compatible

PREGNANCY SUMMARY

No reports describing the use of crofelemer in human pregnancy have been located. Doses used in animal reproduction studies were compared with the human dose based on body weight and, in one species, maternal toxicity occurred, so the results are not interpretable. Nevertheless, the botanical drug is minimally absorbed, so clinically significant exposure of the embryo–fetus probably does not occur.

FETAL RISK SUMMARY

Crofelemer, a botanical drug substance, is an oral inhibitor of two functions of intestinal epithelial cells that regulate fluid secretion, thus preventing high-volume water loss in diarrhea. It is indicated for symptomatic relief of noninfectious diarrhea in patients with HIV/AIDS on anti-retroviral therapy. The drug is minimally absorbed and concentrations of crofelemer in plasma are below the level of quantitation (50 ng/mL). No metabolites have been identified (1).

Reproduction studies have been conducted in rats and rabbits. In rats, oral doses up to 177 times the recommended daily human dose of 4.2 mg/kg (RHD) revealed no evidence of fetal harm. There also was no evidence of adverse prenatal or postnatal effects in offspring. In rabbits, a dose that was about 96 times the RHD caused abortions and resorptions of fetuses, but maternal toxicity also was evident.

Long-term studies of carcinogenicity have not been conducted, but three assays for mutagenicity were negative. At doses up to 177 times the RHD, crofelemer had no effects on fertility or reproductive performance of male and female rats (1).

It is not known if crofelemer crosses the human placenta. Although high, the molecular weight of the botanical drug cannot be determined because of extensive polymerization. Moreover, systemic concentrations of the drug are minimal, so exposure of an embryo or fetus probably appears to be nil.

BREASTFEEDING SUMMARY

No reports describing the use of crofelemer during human lactation have been located. Because the drug is minimally absorbed, clinically significant amounts of crofelemer in milk probably do not occur.

Reference

1. Product information. Fulyzaq. Salix Pharmaceuticals, 2013.

CROMOLYN SODIUM

Respiratory Drug (Anti-inflammatory)

PREGNANCY RECOMMENDATION: Compatible
BREASTFEEDING RECOMMENDATION: No Human Data—Probably Compatible

PREGNANCY SUMMARY

Neither the human nor the animal reproduction data suggest a risk of structural anomalies.

FETAL RISK SUMMARY

Cromolyn sodium is an inhaled anti-inflammatory agent used for the prevention of bronchial asthma. The drug is generally considered safe for use during pregnancy (1–6). Although small amounts are absorbed systemically from the lungs, it is not known whether the drug crosses the placenta to the fetus (6).

Reproductive studies using SC doses of cromolyn in mice, rats, and both SC and IV in rabbits have not revealed teratogenicity (7,8). In one source, the doses used in the three animal species were 27, 16, and 98 times the maximum recommended human dose based on BSA, respectively (8). Increased resorptions and decreased fetal weight were observed only with high parenteral doses that were associated with maternal toxicity (8).

A 1984 study, cited by Shepard, reported over 300 pregnancies in which cromolyn was used in combination with other drugs, most often with isoproterenol, without a link with congenital defects (9).

Congenital malformations were noted in four (1.35%) newborns in a 1982 study of 296 women treated throughout gestation with cromolyn sodium (10). This incidence is less than the expected rate of 2%–3% in a nonexposed population. The defects observed were patent ductus arteriosus, clubfoot, nonfused septum, and harelip alone. The author concluded that there was no association between the defects and cromolyn sodium (10).

As of 1983, the manufacturer had reports of 185 women treated during all or parts of pregnancy, but the small number probably reflects underreporting of the actual usage (personal communication, Fisons Corporation, 1983). From these cases, 10 infants had been born with congenital defects, at least 3 of which appeared to be genetic in origin. Multiple drug exposure was common. In none of the 10 cases was there evidence to link the defects with cromolyn sodium.

In a surveillance study of Michigan Medicaid recipients involving 229,101 completed pregnancies conducted between 1985 and 1992, 191 newborns had been exposed to cromolyn during the 1st trimester (F. Rosa, personal communication, FDA, 1993). Seven (3.7%) major birth defects were observed (eight expected). Specific data were available for six defect categories, including (observed/expected) 1/2 cardiovascular defects, 1/0.5 oral clefts, 0/0 spina bifida, 1/0.5 polydactyly, 0/0.5 limb-reduction defects, and 0/0.5 hypospadias. These data do not support an association between the drug and congenital defects.

BREASTFEEDING SUMMARY

No reports describing the use of cromolyn sodium during lactation have been located.

References

1. Dykes MHM. Evaluation of an antiasthmatic agent cromolyn sodium (Aarane, Intal). JAMA 1974;227:1061–2.
2. Greenberger P, Patterson R. Safety of therapy for allergic symptoms during pregnancy. Ann Intern Med 1978;89:234–7.
3. Weinstein AM, Dubin BD, Podleski WK, Spector SL, Farr RS. Asthma and pregnancy. JAMA 1979;241:1161–5.
4. Pratt WR. Allergic diseases in pregnancy and breast feeding. Ann Allergy 1981;47:355–60.
5. Mawhinney H, Spector SL. Optimum management of asthma in pregnancy. Drugs 1986;32:178–87.
6. Niebyl JR. *Drug Use in Pregnancy*. Philadelphia, PA: Lea & Febiger, 1982:53.
7. Cox JSG, Beach JE, Blair AMJN, Clarke AJ. Disodium cromoglycate (Intal). Adv Drug Res 1970;5:135–6. As cited in Shepard TH. *Catalog of Teratogenic Agents*. 6th ed. Baltimore, MD: Johns Hopkins University Press, 1989:174.
8. Product information. Intal. Rhone-Poulenc Rorer Pharmaceuticals, 2000.
9. Shepard TH. *Catalog of Teratogenic Agents*. 6th ed. Baltimore, MD: Johns Hopkins University Press, 1989:174.
10. Wilson J. Use of sodium cromoglycate during pregnancy: results on 296 asthmatic women. Acta Therap 1982;8(Suppl):45–51.

CYCLACILLIN

[Withdrawn from the market. See 9th edition.]

CYCLAMATE

Artificial Sweetener

PREGNANCY RECOMMENDATION: Limited Human Data—Probably Compatible
BREASTFEEDING RECOMMENDATION: No Human Data—Probably Compatible

PREGNANCY SUMMARY

The very limited human pregnancy data does not suggest a major risk of structural anomalies.

FETAL RISK SUMMARY

Cyclamate crosses the placenta to produce fetal blood levels of about 25% of maternal serum (1). The drug has been suspected of having cytogenetic effects in human lymphocytes (2). One group of investigators attempted to associate these effects with an increased incidence of malformations and behavioral problems, but a causal relationship could not be established (3).

BREASTFEEDING SUMMARY

No reports describing the use of cyclamate during human lactation have been located.

References

1. Pitkin RM, Reynolds WA, Filer LJ. Placental transmission and fetal distribution of cyclamate in early human pregnancy. Am J Obstet Gynecol 1970;108:1043–50.
2. Bauchinger M. Cytogenetic effect of cyclamate on human peripheral lymphocytes in vivo. Dtsch Med Wochenschr 1970;95:2220–3.
3. Stone D, Matalka E, Pulaski B. Do artificial sweeteners ingested in pregnancy affect the offspring? Nature 1971;231:53.

CYCLANDELATE

C

[Withdrawn from the market. See 9th edition.]

CYCLAZOCINE

[Withdrawn from the market. See 8th edition.]

CYCLIZINE

Antihistamine/Antiemetic

PREGNANCY RECOMMENDATION: Compatible
BREASTFEEDING RECOMMENDATION: No Human Data—Probably Compatible

PREGNANCY SUMMARY

In general, antihistamines are considered low risk in pregnancy. However, exposure near birth of premature infants has been associated with an increased risk of retrolental fibroplasia.

FETAL RISK SUMMARY

Cyclizine is a piperazine antihistamine that is used as an antiemetic (see Buclizine and Meclizine for closely related drugs). The drug is teratogenic in animals but apparently not in humans. In 111 patients given cyclizine during the 1st trimester, no increased malformation rate was observed (1). Similarly, the Collaborative Perinatal Project found no association between 1st trimester cyclizine use and congenital defects, although the number of exposed patients ($N = 15$) was small compared with the total sample (2). The Food and Drug Administration's OTC Laxative Panel acting on this data concluded that cyclizine is not teratogenic (3). In 1974, investigators searching for an association between antihistamines and oral clefts found no relationship between this defect and the cyclizine group (4). Finally, a retrospective study in 1971 found that significantly fewer infants with malformations were exposed to antihistamines/antiemetics in the 1st trimester as compared with controls (5). Cyclizine was the fifth most commonly used antiemetic.

An association between exposure during the last 2 weeks of pregnancy to antihistamines in general and retrolental fibroplasia in premature infants has been reported. See Brompheniramine for details.

BREASTFEEDING SUMMARY

No reports describing the use of cyclizine during human lactation have been located.

References

1. Milkovich L, Van den Berg BJ. An evaluation of the teratogenicity of certain antinauseant drugs. Am J Obstet Gynecol 1976;125:244–8.
2. Heinonen OP, Slone D, Shapiro S. *Birth Defects and Drugs in Pregnancy*. Littleton, MA: Publishing Sciences Group, 1977:323.
3. Anonymous. Meclizine; cyclizine not teratogenic. Pink Sheets. FDC Rep 1974:T&G-2.
4. Saxen I. Cleft palate and maternal diphenhydramine intake. Lancet 1974;1:407–8.
5. Nelson MM, Forfar JO. Associations between drugs administered during pregnancy and congenital abnormalities of the fetus. Br Med J 1971;1:523–7.

CYCLOBENZAPRINE

Skeletal Muscle Relaxant

PREGNANCY RECOMMENDATION: Limited Human Data—Animal Data Suggest Low Risk
BREASTFEEDING RECOMMENDATION: No Human Data—Potential Toxicity

PREGNANCY SUMMARY

The animal reproduction data and human pregnancy experience suggest that the use of cyclobenzaprine in pregnancy is low risk.

C

FETAL RISK SUMMARY

Cyclobenzaprine is a centrally acting skeletal muscle relaxant that is closely related to the tricyclic antidepressants (e.g., imipramine). The agent is not teratogenic or embryotoxic in mice, rats, and rabbits given doses up to 20 times the human dose (1). No published reports of its use in human pregnancy have been located.

It is not known if cyclobenzaprine crosses the human placenta. The molecular weight (about 276 for the free base) is low enough that exposure of the embryo or fetus probably occurs.

In a surveillance study of Michigan Medicaid recipients involving 229,101 completed pregnancies conducted between 1985 and 1992, 545 newborns had been exposed to cyclobenzaprine during the 1st trimester (F. Rosa, personal communication, FDA, 1993). A total of 24 (4.4%) major birth defects were observed (23 expected), including (observed/expected) 5/5 cardiovascular defects, 1/1 oral clefts, and 2/2 polydactyly. No anomalies were observed in three other categories of defects (spina bifida, limb-reduction defects, and hypospadias) for which data were available. Earlier data, obtained from the same source between 1980 and 1983, totaled 168 1st-trimester exposures with 12 defects observed (10 expected). These combined data do not support an association between the drug and congenital defects.

BREASTFEEDING SUMMARY

No reports have been located on the excretion of cyclobenzaprine into milk. The molecular weight (about 276 for the free base) is low enough that excretion into milk should be expected. In addition, the closely related tricyclic antidepressants (e.g., see Imipramine) are excreted into milk and this should be considered before cyclobenzaprine is used during lactation.

Reference

1. Product information. Flexeril. Merck Sharpe & Dohme, 1993.

CYCLOPENTHIAZIDE

[Withdrawn from the market. See 9th edition.]

CYCLOPHOSPHAMIDE

Antineoplastic

PREGNANCY RECOMMENDATION: Contraindicated—1st Trimester
BREASTFEEDING RECOMMENDATION: Contraindicated

PREGNANCY SUMMARY

Cyclophosphamide is known to cause congenital defects when exposure occurs during organogenesis. Fetal bone marrow suppression is a potential toxicity when exposure occurs later in pregnancy. [*See Rituximab for additional data.*]

FETAL RISK SUMMARY

Cyclophosphamide is an alkylating antineoplastic agent. Both normal and malformed newborns have been reported following the use of cyclophosphamide in pregnancy (1–33). Ten malformed infants have resulted from 1st trimester exposure (1–8). Radiation therapy was given to most of the mothers, and at least one patient was treated with other antineoplastics (1,2,4). Defects observed in four of the infants are shown in the list below, and three other infants are described in the text that follows:

- Flattened nasal bridge, palate defect, skin tag, four toes each foot, hypoplastic middle phalanx fifth finger, bilateral inguinal hernia sacs
- Toes missing, single coronary artery
- Hemangioma, umbilical hernia
- Imperforate anus, rectovaginal fistula, growth restricted

A newborn exposed in utero to cyclophosphamide during the 1st trimester presented with multiple anomalies (6). The mother, who was being treated for a severe exacerbation of systemic lupus erythematosus, received two IV doses of 200 mg each between 15 and 46 days' gestation. Except for prednisone, 20 mg daily, no other medication was given during the pregnancy. The 3150-g female infant was delivered at 39 weeks' gestational age with multiple abnormalities, including dysmorphic facies: multiple eye defects including bilateral blepharophimosis with left microphthalmos; abnormally shaped, low-set ears; cleft palate, bilaterally absent thumbs, and dystrophic nails. Borderline microcephaly, hypotonia, and possible developmental delay were observed at 10 months of age.

A 1993 publication reported a 29-year-old woman with twins who was treated for acute lymphocytic leukemia throughout gestation with cyclophosphamide (200 mg/day) and intermittent prednisone (7). Therapy was stopped at 33 weeks' gestation and she delivered 4 weeks later. Both infants recovered from their severe respiratory distress syndromes. The 1250-g female twin has developed normally

C

and is now 22 years of age. Except for strabismus repair at age 9, she has not required any further hospitalizations (7). In contrast, the 1190-g male twin required hospitalization until 10 months of age due to multiple congenital anomalies: dyschondrosteosis (Madelung's deformity) of the right arm, esophageal atresia, abnormal inferior vena cava, abnormal renal collecting system later diagnosed as cross-renal atopia, and a rudimentary left testicle (found later) (7). Chromosomal analysis of the child revealed a normal karyotype (46, XY). Developmental and neurologic problems were diagnosed at about 8 years of age and an IQ test performed at 11 years of age was in the low average range (full scale IQ of 81) with even lower verbal skills (7). At 14 years of age, a stage III neuroblastoma arising from the left adrenal gland was diagnosed and was treated with surgery and radiation. At 16 years of age, metastatic papillary thyroid cancer was found and this was treated with surgery. In addition, three courses of radioactive iodine were administered to treat the primary cancer and two recurrences (7). The authors speculated that the different outcomes in the twins might have been due to differences in metabolism, either by the individual placentas or by the hepatic cytochrome P-450 activity of the fetuses (7). In either case, two cyclophosphamide active metabolites, phosphoramide mustard and acrolein, may have actually caused the malformations. Moreover, because of the timing of the two malignancies in the boy, the authors also thought it was possible that they were the result of in utero exposure to cyclophosphamide (7).

A 23-year-old woman with hypertension and lupus nephritis received four IV doses of cyclophosphamide (20 mg/kg/dose), three of which were given before conception and one during the 6th week of gestation (8). She delivered a female, 1705-g (<5th percentile) infant at 37 weeks' gestation with Apgar scores of 5 and 7 at 1 and 5 minutes, respectively. The infant's length was 46 cm (5th–10th percentile) and the head circumference 30.2 cm (<5th percentile). Other medications received throughout gestation were prednisone, nifedipine, atenolol, clonidine, potassium chloride, and aspirin. In addition to respiratory distress syndrome, multiple anomalies were noted, including microbrachycephaly, coronal craniosynostosis, blepharophimosis, shallow orbits, proptosis, hypertelorism, broad, flat nasal bridge, bulbous nasal tip, overfolded small ears, left preauricular pit, microstomia, high-arched palate, micrognathia, hypoplastic thumbs, 5th finger clinodactyly, and absent 4th and 5th toes bilaterally (8). Other malformations were detected in the skeleton and central nervous system during diagnostic workups. Growth delay (<3rd percentile in all growth parameters) and gross motor skills continued to be impaired at age 17.5 months. Based on their comparisons with previous cases of cyclophosphamide-induced congenital defects, the authors concluded that cyclophosphamide was a human teratogen and that a distinct phenotype existed (8).

A case report of a 16-year-old woman with ovarian endodermal sinus tumor presenting in two pregnancies was published in 1979 (19). Conservative surgery, suction curettage to terminate a pregnancy estimated to be at 8–10 weeks' gestation, and chemotherapy with cyclophosphamide, dactinomycin, and vincristine (VAC) produced a complete clinical response for 12 months. The patient then refused further therapy and presented a second time, 6 months later, with tumor recurrence and a pregnancy estimated at 18–20 weeks' gestation. She again refused chemotherapy, but her disease progressed to the point where she allowed VAC chemotherapy to be reinstated 4 weeks later. At 33 weeks' gestation, 2 weeks after her last dose of chemotherapy, she spontaneously delivered a normal 2213-g female infant. The infant was developing normally when last seen at 8 months of age. In a similar case, a woman, treated with surgery and chemotherapy in her 15th week of pregnancy for an ovarian endodermal sinus tumor, delivered a normal 2850-g male infant at 37 weeks' gestation (20). Chemotherapy, begun during the 16th gestational week, included six courses of VAC chemotherapy. The last course was administered 5 days prior to delivery. No information was provided on the subsequent growth and development of the infant.

Following surgical treatment at 16 weeks' gestation, a 28-year-old woman with advanced epithelial ovarian carcinoma was treated with cyclophosphamide, 750 mg/m^2, and cisplatin, 50 mg/m^2, every 21 days for seven cycles (21). Labor was induced at 37–38 weeks' gestation resulting in the delivery of a healthy, 3275-g male infant. Height, weight, and head circumference were in the 75th–90th percentiles. No abnormalities of the kidneys, liver, bone marrow, or audiometry-evoked potential were found at birth, and the infant's physical and neurologic growth was normal at 19 months of age.

Pancytopenia occurred in a 1000-g male infant exposed to cyclophosphamide and five other antineoplastic agents in the 3rd trimester (14). In a similar case, maternal treatment for leukemia was begun at 12.5 weeks' gestation and eventually included cyclophosphamide, five other antineoplastic agents, and whole brain radiation (25). A normally developed, premature female infant was delivered at 31 weeks, who subsequently developed transient severe bone marrow hypoplasia in the neonatal period. The myelosuppression was probably due to mercaptopurine therapy.

In a brief 1997 report, three pregnant women with breast cancer were successfully treated with two or three courses of vinorelbine (20–30 mg/m^2) and fluorouracil (500–750 mg/m^2) at 24, 28, and 29 weeks' gestation, respectively (33). Delivery occurred at 34, 41, and 37 weeks' gestation, respectively. One patient also required six courses of epidoxorubicin and cyclophosphamide. Her infant developed transient anemia at 21 days of age that resolved spontaneously. No adverse effects were observed in the other two newborns. All three infants were developing normally at about 2–3 years of age (33).

A 1999 report from France described the outcomes of pregnancies in 20 women with breast cancer who were treated with antineoplastic agents (34). The first cycle of chemotherapy occurred at a mean gestational age of 26 weeks, with delivery occurring at a mean 34.7 weeks. A total of 38 cycles were administered during pregnancy with a median of two cycles per woman. None of the women received radiation therapy during pregnancy. The pregnancy outcomes included two spontaneous abortions (SABs) (both exposed in the 1st trimester), one intrauterine death (exposed in the 2nd trimester), and 17 live births, one of whom died at 8 days of age without apparent cause. The 16 surviving children were developing normally at a mean follow-up of 42.3 months (34). Cyclophosphamide (C), in combination with various other agents (doxorubicin [D], epirubicin [E], fluorouracil [F], or mitoxantrone [M]), was administered to 13 of the women at a mean dose of 600 mg/m^2 (range 300–1200 mg/m^2). The outcomes were one SAB (CEF; 1st trimester), one stillbirth (one cycle of CE at 23 weeks' gestation), one neonatal death (one cycle of CEF 32 days before birth), and 11 surviving liveborn infants (one CE, six CEF, two CDF, and two CFM; all in the 3rd trimester). One of the infants, exposed to two cycles of CEF with the last at 25 days before birth, had transient leukopenia and another was growth restricted (1460-g, born at 33 weeks' gestation after two cycles of CFM) (34).

Data from one review indicated that 40% of the patients exposed to anticancer drugs during pregnancy delivered low-birth-weight infants (35). This finding was not related to the timing of exposure. Use of cyclophosphamide in the 2nd and 3rd trimesters does not seem to place the fetus at risk for congenital defects. Except in a few individual cases, long-term studies of growth and mental development in offspring exposed to cyclophosphamide during the 2nd trimester, the period of neuroblast multiplication, have not been conducted (36).

Cyclophosphamide is one of the most common causes of chemotherapy-induced menstrual difficulties and azoospermia (37–45). Permanent secondary amenorrhea with evidence of primary ovarian damage has been observed after long-term (20 months) use of cyclophosphamide (45). In contrast, successful pregnancies have been reported following high-dose therapy (39,40,46–50). Moreover, azoospermia appears to be reversible when the drug is stopped (41–44,51).

One report associated paternal use of cyclophosphamide and three other antineoplastics prior to conception with congenital anomalies in an infant (52). Defects in the infant included syndactyly of the first and second digits of the right foot and tetralogy of Fallot. In a group of men treated over a minimum of 3.5 years with multiple chemotherapy for acute lymphocytic leukemia, one man fathered a normal child whereas a second fathered two children, one with multiple anomalies (53). Any relationship between these outcomes and paternal use of cyclophosphamide is doubtful because of the lack of experimental evidence and confirming reports.

Cyclophosphamide-induced chromosomal abnormalities are also of doubtful clinical significance but have been described in some patients after use of the drug. A study published in 1974 reported chromosome abnormalities in patients treated with cyclophosphamide for rheumatoid arthritis and scleroderma (54). In contrast, chromosomal studies were normal in a mother and infant treated during the 2nd and 3rd trimesters in another report (16). In another case, a 34-year-old woman with acute lymphoblastic leukemia was treated with multiple antineoplastic agents from 22 weeks' gestation until delivery of a healthy female infant 18 weeks later (22). Cyclophosphamide was administered three times between the 26th and 30th weeks of gestation. Chromosomal analysis of the newborn revealed a normal karyotype (46,XX) but with gaps and a ring chromosome. The clinical significance of these findings is unknown, but because these abnormalities may persist for several years, the potential existed for an increased risk of cancer as well as for a risk of genetic damage in the next generation (22).

The long-term effects of cyclophosphamide on female and male reproductive function have been reported (55,56). In a 1988 publication, 40 women who had been treated with combination chemotherapy for malignant ovarian germ cell tumors (median age at diagnosis 15 years, range 6–29 years) were evaluated approximately 10 years later (median age 25.5 years, range 14–40 years) (55). Cyclophosphamide had been used in 33 (83%) of the women. Menstrual function in these women after chemotherapy was as follows: premenarchal ($N = 1$), regular menses ($N = 27$), irregular menses ($N = 5$), oligomenorrhea ($N = 2$), amenorrhea ($N = 4$), and premature menopause ($N = 1$). Of the 12 women with menstrual difficulties, only 3 of the difficulties were considered serious or persistent. Evaluation of the reproductive status after chemotherapy revealed that 24 had not attempted to become pregnant, 9 had problem-free conceptions, 3 had initial infertility followed by conceptions, and 4 had chronic infertility. Of the 12 women who had conceived on one or more occasions, 1 had an elective abortion at 10 weeks' gestation, and 11 had delivered 22 healthy infants, although 1 had amelogenesis imperfecta.

A study published in 1985 examined 30 men to determine the effect of cyclophosphamide on male hormone levels and spermatogenesis (56). The men had been treated at a mean age of 9.4 years for a mean duration of 280 days. The mean age of the men at the time of the study was 22 years with a mean interval from end of treatment to evaluation of 12.8 years. Four of the men were azoospermic, 9 were oligospermic, and 17 were normospermic. Compared with normal controls, however, the 17 men classified as normospermic had lower ejaculate volumes (3.1 mL vs. 3.3 mL), lower sperm density (54.5×10^6/mL vs. 79×10^6/mL), decreased sperm motility (42% vs. 61%, $p < 0.05$), and less normal sperm forms (61% vs. 70%, $p < 0.05$). Concentrations of testosterone, dehydroepiandrosterone sulfate, and prolactin were not significantly different between patients and controls. One oligospermic man (sperm density 12×10^6/mL) had fathered a child.

The effect of occupational exposure to antineoplastic agents on pregnancy outcome was examined in a 1985 case–control study involving 124 nurses in 17 Finnish hospitals compared with 321 matched controls (57). The cases involved nurses working in 1979 and 1980 in hospitals that used at least 100 g of cyclophosphamide (the most commonly administered antineoplastic agent in Finland) per year or at least 200 g of all antineoplastic drugs per year. The average total antineoplastic drug use for all hospitals was 1898 g, but a lower total use, 887 g, occurred for intravenous drugs (58). Moreover, the nurses had to be 40 years of age or younger in 1980 and had to work in patient areas where antineoplastic agents were mixed and administered (57). The agents were prepared without the use of vertical-airflow biologic-safety hoods or protective clothing (58). Exposure to these agents during the 1st trimester was significantly associated with early fetal loss (odds ratio [OR] 2.30, 95% confidence interval [CI] 1.20–4.39) ($p = 0.01$) (57). Cyclophosphamide, one of four individual antineoplastic agents to which at least 10 women had been exposed, had an OR for fetal loss of 2.66 (95% CI 1.25–5.71). Other significant associations were found for doxorubicin (OR 3.96, 95% CI 1.31–11.97) and vincristine (OR 2.46, 95% CI 1.13–5.37). The association between fluorouracil and fetal loss (OR 1.70, 95% CI 0.55–5.21) was not significant. Based on the results of their study and data from previous studies, the investigators concluded that nursing personnel should exercise caution in handling these agents (57).

Although there is no current consensus on the danger posed to pregnant women from the handling of antineoplastic agents (e.g., the above study generated several letters that questioned the observed association (59–62)), pharmacy and

C

nursing personnel should take precautions to avoid exposure to these potent agents. The National Study Commission on Cytotoxic Exposure published a position statement on this topic in January 1987 (63). Owing to the importance of this issue, the statement is quoted in its entirety below:

"The Handling of Cytotoxic Agents by Women Who Are Pregnant, Attempting to Conceive, or Breast Feeding"

"There are substantial data regarding the mutagenic, teratogenic and abortifacient properties of certain cytotoxic agents both in animals and humans who have received therapeutic doses of these agents. Additionally the scientific literature suggests a possible association of occupational exposure to certain cytotoxic agents during the first trimester of pregnancy with fetal loss or malformation. These data suggest the need for caution when women who are pregnant or attempting to conceive, handle cytotoxic agents. Incidentally, there is no evidence relating male exposure to cytotoxic agents with adverse fetal outcome.

There are no studies which address the possible risk associated with the occupational exposure to cytotoxic agents and the passage of these agents into breast milk. Nevertheless, it is prudent that women who are breast feeding should exercise caution in handling cytotoxic agents.

If all procedures for safe handling, such as those recommended by the Commission are complied with, the potential for exposure will be minimized.

Personnel should be provided with information to make an individual decision. This information should be provided in written form and it is advisable that a statement of understanding be signed.

It is essential to refer to individual state right-to-know laws to insure compliance."

BREASTFEEDING SUMMARY

Cyclophosphamide is excreted into breast milk (64). Although the concentrations were not specified, the drug was found in milk up to 6 hours after a single 500-mg IV dose. The mother was not nursing. A brief 1977 correspondence from investigators in New Guinea described neutropenia in a breastfed infant whose mother received weekly injections of 800 mg of cyclophosphamide, 2 mg of vincristine, and 30-mg daily oral doses of prednisolone for 6 weeks (65). Absolute neutropenia was present 9 days after breastfeeding had been stopped, which persisted for at least 12 days (65). Serial determinations of the infant's white cell and neutrophil counts were begun 2 days after the last exposure to breast milk. The lowest measured absolute lymphocyte count was 4750/microL. Except for the neutropenia and a brief episode of diarrhea, no other adverse effects were observed in the infant.

A 1979 report involved a case of an 18-year-old woman with Burkitt's lymphoma diagnosed in the 26th week of gestation (66). She was treated with a 7-day course of cyclophosphamide, 10 mg/kg IV, as a single daily dose (total dose 3.5 g). Six weeks after the last chemotherapy dose, she delivered a normal, 2160-g male infant. Analysis of the newborn's blood counts was not conducted. The tumor recurred in the postpartum period and treatment with cyclophosphamide, 6 mg/kg/day IV, was started 20 days after delivery. Although she was advised not to nurse her infant, she continued to do so until her sudden death after the third dose of cyclophosphamide. Blood counts were conducted on both the mother and the infant during therapy. Immediately prior to the first dose, the infant's leukocyte and platelet counts were $4800/mm^3$ (abnormally low for age) and $270,000/mm^3$, respectively. After the third maternal dose, the infant's counts were $3200/mm^3$ and $47,000/mm^3$, respectively. Both counts were interpreted by the investigator as signs of cyclophosphamide-induced toxicity. It was concluded that breastfeeding should be stopped during therapy with the agent (66).

The American Academy of Pediatrics classifies cyclophosphamide as a drug that may interfere with cellular metabolism of the nursing infant (67). Because of the reported cases of neutropenia and thrombocytopenia, and the potential for adverse effects relating to immune suppression, growth, and carcinogenesis, women receiving this drug should not nurse.

References

1. Greenberg LH, Tanaka KR. Congenital anomalies probably induced by cyclophosphamide. JAMA 1964;188:423–6.
2. Toledo TM, Harper RC, Moser RH. Fetal effects during cyclophosphamide and irradiation therapy. Ann Intern Med 1971;74:87–91.
3. Coates A. Cyclophosphamide in pregnancy. Aust N-Z J Obstet Gynaecol 1970;10:33–4.
4. Murray CL, Reichert JA, Anderson J, Twiggs LB. Multimodal cancer therapy for breast cancer in the first trimester of pregnancy. JAMA 1984;252: 2607–8.
5. Sweet DL, Kinzie J. Consequences of radiotherapy and antineoplastic therapy for the fetus. J Reprod Med 1976;17:241–6.
6. Kirshon B, Wasserstrum N, Willis R, Herman GE, McCabe ERB. Teratogenic effects of first-trimester cyclophosphamide therapy. Obstet Gynecol 1988;72:462–4.
7. Zemlickis D, Lishner M, Erlich R, Koren G. Teratogenicity and carcinogenicity in a twin exposed in utero to cyclophosphamide. Teratogenesis Carcinog Mutagen 1993;13:139–43.
8. Enns GM, Roeder E, Chan RT, Catts ZA-K, Cox VA, Golabi M. Apparent cyclophosphamide (Cytoxan) embryopathy: a distinct phenotype? Am J Med Genet 1999;86:237–41.
9. Lasher MJ, Geller W. Cyclophosphamide and vinblastine sulfate in Hodgkin's disease during pregnancy. JAMA 1966;195:486–8.
10. Lergier JE, Jimenez E, Maldonado N, Veray F. Normal pregnancy in multiple myeloma treated with cyclophosphamide. Cancer 1974;34:1018–22.
11. Garcia V, San Miguel J, Borrasca AL. Doxorubicin in the first trimester of pregnancy. Ann Intern Med 1981;94:547.
12. Lowenthal RM, Funnell CF, Hope DM, Stewart IG, Humphrey DC. Normal infant after combination chemotherapy including teniposide for Burkitt's lymphoma in pregnancy. Med Pediatr Oncol 1982;10:165–9.
13. Daly H, McCann SR, Hanratty TD, Temperley IJ. Successful pregnancy during combination chemotherapy for Hodgkin's disease. Acta Haematol (Basel) 1980;64:154–6.
14. Pizzuto J, Aviles A, Noriega L, Niz J, Morales M, Romero F. Treatment of acute leukemia during pregnancy: presentation of nine cases. Cancer Treat Rep 1980;64:679–83.
15. Sears HF, Reid J. Granulocytic sarcoma: local presentation of a systemic disease. Cancer 1976;37:1808–13.
16. Falkson HC, Simson IW, Falkson G. Non-Hodgkin's lymphoma in pregnancy. Cancer 1980;45:1679–82.
17. Webb GA. The use of hyperalimentation and chemotherapy in pregnancy: a case report. Am J Obstet Gynecol 1980;137:263–6.
18. Gililland J, Weinstein L. The effects of cancer chemotherapeutic agents on the developing fetus. Obstet Gynecol Surv 1983;38:6–13.
19. Weed JC Jr, Roh RA, Mendenhall HW. Recurrent endodermal sinus tumor during pregnancy. Obstet Gynecol 1979;54:653–6.
20. Kim DS, Park MI. Maternal and fetal survival following surgery and chemotherapy of endodermal sinus tumor of the ovary during pregnancy: a case report. Obstet Gynecol 1989;73:503–7.
21. Malfetano JH, Goldkrand JW. Cis-platinum combination chemotherapy during pregnancy for advanced epithelial ovarian carcinoma. Obstet Gynecol 1990;75:545–7.
22. Schleuning M, Clemm C. Chromosomal aberrations in a newborn whose mother received cytotoxic treatment during pregnancy. N Engl J Med 1987;317:1666–7.

23. Haerr RW, Pratt AT. Multiagent chemotherapy for sarcoma diagnosed during pregnancy. Cancer 1985;56:1028–33.
24. Turchi JJ, Villasis C. Anthracyclines in the treatment of malignancy in pregnancy. Cancer 1988;61:435–40.
25. Okun DB, Groncy PK, Sieger L, Tanaka KR. Acute leukemia in pregnancy: transient neonatal myelosuppression after combination chemotherapy in the mother. Med Pediatr Oncol 1979;7:315–9.
26. Ortega J. Multiple agent chemotherapy including bleomycin of non-Hodgkin's lymphoma during pregnancy. Cancer 1977;40:2829–35.
27. Hardin JA. Cyclophosphamide treatment of lymphoma during third trimester of pregnancy. Obstet Gynecol 1972;39:850–1.
28. Khurshid M, Saleem M. Acute leukaemia in pregnancy. Lancet 1978;2:534–5.
29. Yankowitz J, Kuller JA, Thomas RL. Pregnancy complicated by Goodpasture syndrome. Obstet Gynecol 1992;79:806–8.
30. Barry C, Davis S, Garrard P, Ferguson IT. Churg-Strauss disease: deterioration in a twin pregnancy. Successful outcome following treatment with corticosteroids and cyclophosphamide. Br J Obstet Gynaecol 1997;104:746–7.
31. Mavrommatis CG, Daskalakis GJ, Papageorgiou IS, Antsaklis AJ, Michalas SK. Non-Hodgkin's lymphoma during pregnancy—case report. Eur J Obstet Gynecol Reprod Biol 1998;79:95–7.
32. Dayoan ES, Dimen LL, Boylen CT. Successful treatment of Wegener's granulomatosis during pregnancy. A case report and review of the medical literature. Chest 1998;113:836–8.
33. Cuvier C, Espie M, Extra JM, Marty M. Vinorelbine in pregnancy. Eur J Cancer 1997;33:168–9.
34. Giacalone PL, Laffargue F, Benos P. Chemotherapy for breast carcinoma during pregnancy. Cancer 1999;86:2266–72.
35. Nicholson HO. Cytotoxic drugs in pregnancy: review of reported cases. J Obstet Gynaecol Br Commonw 1968;75:307–12.
36. Dobbing J. Pregnancy and leukaemia. Lancet 1977;1:1155.
37. Schilsky RL, Lewis BJ, Sherins RJ, Young RC. Gonadal dysfunction in patients receiving chemotherapy for cancer. Ann Intern Med 1980;93:109–14.
38. Stewart BH. Drugs that cause and cure male infertility. Drug Ther 1975;5:42–8.
39. Schwartz PE, Vidone RA. Pregnancy following combination chemotherapy for a mixed germ cell tumor of the ovary. Gynecol Oncol 1981;12:373–8.
40. Bacon C, Kernahan J. Successful pregnancy in acute leukaemia. Lancet 1975;2:515.
41. Qureshji MA, Pennington JH, Goldsmith HJ, Cox PE. Cyclophosphamide therapy and sterility. Lancet 1972;2:1290–1.
42. George CRP, Evans RA. Cyclophosphamide and infertility. Lancet 1972;1:840–1.
43. Sherins RJ, DeVita VT Jr. Effect of drug treatment for lymphoma on male reproductive capacity. Ann Intern Med 1973;79:216–20.
44. Lendon M, Palmer MK, Hann IM, Shalet SM, Jones PHM. Testicular histology after combination chemotherapy in childhood for acute lymphoblastic leukaemia. Lancet 1978;2:439–41.
45. Uldall PR, Feest TG, Morley AR, Tomlinson BE, Kerr DNS. Cyclophosphamide therapy in adults with minimal-change nephrotic syndrome. Lancet 1972;2:1250–3.
46. Card RT, Holmes IH, Sugarman RG, Storb R, Thomas D. Successful pregnancy after high dose chemotherapy and marrow transplantation for treatment of aplastic anemia. Exp Hematol 1980;8:57–60.
47. Deeg HJ, Kennedy MS, Sanders JE, Thomas ED, Storb R. Successful pregnancy after marrow transplantation for severe aplastic anemia and immunosuppression with cyclosporine. JAMA 1983;250:647.
48. Javaheri G, Lifchez A, Valle J. Pregnancy following removal of and long-term chemotherapy for ovarian malignant teratoma. Obstet Gynecol 1983;61:8S–9S.
49. Rustin GJS, Booth M, Dent J, Salt S, Rustin F, Bagshawe KD. Pregnancy after cytotoxic chemotherapy for gestational trophoblastic tumours. Br Med J 1984;288:103–6.
50. Lee RB, Kelly J, Elg SA, Benson WL. Pregnancy following conservative surgery and adjunctive chemotherapy for stage III immature teratoma of the ovary. Obstet Gynecol 1989;73:853–5.
51. Hinkes E, Plotkin D. Reversible drug-induced sterility in a patient with acute leukemia. JAMA 1973;223:1490–1.
52. Russell JA, Powles RL, Oliver RTD. Conception and congenital abnormalities after chemotherapy of acute myelogenous leukaemia in two men. Br Med J 1976;1:1508.
53. Evenson DP, Arlin Z, Welt S, Claps ML, Melamed MR. Male reproductive capacity may recover following drug treatment with the L-10 protocol for acute lymphocytic leukemia. Cancer 1984;53:30–6.
54. Tolchin SF, Winkelstein A, Rodnan GP, Pan SF, Nankin HR. Chromosome abnormalities from cyclophosphamide therapy in rheumatoid arthritis and progressive systemic sclerosis (scleroderma). Arthritis Rheum 1974;17:375–82.
55. Gershenson DM. Menstrual and reproductive function after treatment with combination chemotherapy for malignant ovarian germ cell tumors. J Clin Oncol 1988;6:270–5.
56. Watson AR, Rance CP, Bain J. Long term effects of cyclophosphamide on testicular function. Br Med J 1985;291:1457–60.
57. Selevan SG, Lindbohm M-L, Hornung RW, Hemminki K. A study of occupational exposure to antineoplastic drugs and fetal loss in nurses. N Engl J Med 1985;313:1173–8.
58. Selevan SG, Hornung RW. Antineoplastic drugs and spontaneous abortion in nurses. N Engl J Med 1986;314:1050–1.
59. Kalter H. Antineoplastic drugs and spontaneous abortion in nurses. N Engl J Med 1986;314:1048–9.
60. Mulvihill JJ, Stewart KR. Antineoplastic drugs and spontaneous abortion in nurses. N Engl J Med 1986;314:1049.
61. Chabner BA. Antineoplastic drugs and spontaneous abortion in nurses. N Engl J Med 1986;314:1049–50.
62. Zellmer WA. Antineoplastic drugs and spontaneous abortion in nurses. N Engl J Med 1986;314:1050.
63. Jeffrey LP, Chairman, National Study Commission on Cytotoxic Exposure. Position statement. The handling of cytotoxic agents by women who are pregnant, attempting to conceive, or breast feeding. January 12, 1987.
64. Wiernik PH, Duncan JH. Cyclophosphamide in human milk. Lancet 1971;1:912.
65. Amato D, Niblett JS. Neutropenia from cyclophosphamide in breast milk. Med J Aust 1977;1:383–4.
66. Durodola JI. Administration of cyclophosphamide during late pregnancy and early lactation: a case report. J Natl Med Assoc 1979;71:165–6.
67. Committee on Drugs, American Academy of Pediatrics. The transfer of drugs and other chemicals into human milk. Pediatrics 2001;108:776–89.

CYCLOSERINE

Antituberculosis Agent

PREGNANCY RECOMMENDATION: Limited Human Data—Animal Data Suggest Moderate Risk
BREASTFEEDING RECOMMENDATION: Limited Human Data—Probably Compatible

PREGNANCY SUMMARY

The limited animal and human pregnancy data prevent a complete assessment of the embryo–fetal risk. The best course is to avoid cycloserine during gestation. However, the drug should not be withheld because of pregnancy if the maternal condition requires the antibiotic.

C

FETAL RISK SUMMARY

Cycloserine is a broad-spectrum antibiotic used primarily for active pulmonary and extrapulmonary tuberculosis. No teratogenic effects were observed in rats given doses up to 100 mg/kg/day through two generations (1).

The Collaborative Perinatal Project monitored 50,282 mother–child pairs, 3 of whom had 1st trimester exposure to cycloserine (2). No evidence of adverse fetal effects was suggested by the data. The American Thoracic Society recommends avoidance of cycloserine during pregnancy, if possible, due to the lack of information on the fetal effects of the drug (3).

BREASTFEEDING SUMMARY

Cycloserine is excreted into breast milk. Milk concentrations in four lactating women taking 250-mg of the drug four times daily ranged from 6 to 19 mcg/mL, an average of 72% of serum levels (4). Approximately 0.6% of the mother's daily dose was estimated to be in the milk (5). No adverse effects were observed in the nursing infants (4). The American Academy of Pediatrics classifies cycloserine as compatible with breastfeeding (6).

References

1. Product information. Seromycin. Dura Pharmaceuticals, 2000.
2. Heinonen OP, Slone D, Shapiro S. *Birth Defects and Drugs in Pregnancy*. Littleton, MA: Publishing Sciences Group, 1977:297.
3. American Thoracic Society. Medical Section of the American Lung Association: Treatment of tuberculosis and tuberculosis infection in adults and children. Am Rev Respir Dis 1986;134:355–63.
4. Morton RF, McKenna MH, Charles E. Studies on the absorption, diffusion, and excretion of cycloserine. Antibiot Annu 1955–1956;3:169–72. As cited by Snider DE Jr, Powell KE. Should women taking antituberculosis drugs breast-feed? Arch Intern Med 1984;144:589–90.
5. Vorherr H. Drug excretion in breast milk. Postgrad Med 1974;56:97–104. As cited by Snider DE Jr, Powell KE. Should women taking antituberculosis drugs breast-feed? Arch Intern Med 1984;144:589–90.
6. Committee on Drugs, American Academy of Pediatrics. The transfer of drugs and other chemicals into human milk. Pediatrics 2001;108:776–89.

CYCLOSPORINE

Immunologic Agent (Immunosuppressant)

PREGNANCY RECOMMENDATION: Limited Human Data—Animal Data Suggest Low Risk
BREASTFEEDING RECOMMENDATION: Limited Human Data—Potential Toxicity

PREGNANCY SUMMARY

Based on relatively small numbers, the use of cyclosporine during pregnancy apparently does not pose a major risk to the fetus. Cyclosporine is not an animal teratogen (1,2), and the limited experience in women indicates that it is unlikely to be a human teratogen. No pattern of defects has emerged in the few newborns with anomalies. Skeletal defects, other than the single case of osseous malformation, have not been observed. When used as an immunosuppressant, the disease process itself makes these pregnancies high risk and subject to numerous potential problems, of which the most common is growth restriction. This latter problem is probably related to the mother's disease rather than to her drug therapy, but a contribution from cyclosporine and corticosteroids cannot be excluded. Long-term follow-up studies are warranted, however, to detect latent effects, including those in subsequent generations. If cyclosporine is used in pregnancy for the treatment of rheumatoid arthritis or psoriasis, healthcare professionals are encouraged to call the toll-free number (877-311-8972) for information about patient enrollment in the OTIS Rheumatoid Arthritis study.

FETAL RISK SUMMARY

Cyclosporine (cyclosporin A), an antibiotic produced by certain fungi, is used as an immunosuppressive agent to prevent rejection of kidney, liver, or heart allografts. Other indications for the drug are the treatment of severe, active rheumatoid arthritis and severe (i.e., extensive and/or disabling), recalcitrant, plaque psoriasis (1).

In reproduction studies, cyclosporine produced embryo and fetal toxicity only at maternally toxic dose levels in rats (0.8 times the human transplant dose of 6 mg/kg corrected for BSA) and in rabbits (5.4 times the human dose). Toxic effects included increased pre- and postnatal mortality, and reduced fetal weight and related skeletal restriction. No teratogenic effects were observed (1).

Cyclosporine readily crosses the placenta to the fetus (3–7). In a 1983 study, the cord blood:maternal plasma ratio at delivery was 0.63 (3). In a second study, cord blood and amniotic fluid levels 8 hours after a dose of 325 mg were 57 and 234 ng/mL, respectively (4). Concentrations in the newborn fell to 14 ng/mL at 14 hours and were undetectable (<4 ng/mL) at 7 days. Cord blood:maternal plasma ratios in twins delivered at 35 weeks' gestation were 0.35 and 0.57, respectively (5). A similar ratio of 0.40 was reported in a case delivered at 31 weeks' gestation (6).

Several case reports describing the use of cyclosporine throughout gestation have been published (3–14). Maternal doses ranged between 260 and 550 mg/day (3–5,8,10,11,14). Cases usually involved maternal renal transplantation (3–5, 7–13), but one report described a successful pregnancy in a woman after heart transplantation (6), one involved a combined transplant of a kidney and paratropic segmental pancreas in a diabetic woman (11), and one involved a patient with a liver transplant (14). In addition, a report has described a successful pregnancy in a woman with aplastic anemia who was treated with bone marrow transplantation

(15). In this case, however, cyclosporine therapy had been stopped prior to conception. Guidelines for counseling heart transplant patients who wish to become pregnant have been published (16).

As of October 1987, the manufacturer had knowledge of 34 pregnancies involving cyclosporine (A. Poploski and D. A. Colasante, personal communication, Sandoz Pharmaceuticals Corporation, 1987) (16). Some of these cases are described above. These pregnancies resulted in six abortions (one after early detection of anencephaly, three elective, and two spontaneous abortions, one at 20 weeks' gestation), one pregnancy still ongoing, and 27 live births. One of the newborns died at age 3 days. Autopsy revealed a complete absence of the corpus callosum.

A 1989 case report described an infant with hypoplasia of the right leg and foot after in utero exposure to cyclosporine (12). The right leg was 2 cm shorter than the left. Hypoplasia of the muscles and subcutaneous tissue of the right leg was also present. The authors proposed a possible mechanism for the defect, which involved cyclosporine inhibition of lymphocytic interleukin-2 release and subsequent interference with the differentiation of osteoclasts (12).

Many of the liveborn infants were growth restricted (4,8,10–14). Birth weights of full-term newborns ranged from 2160 to 3200 g (13,14) (A. Poploski and D.A. Colasante, personal communication, 1987). A 1985 review article observed that growth restriction was common in the offspring of renal transplant patients, occurring in 8%–45% of reported pregnancies (17). Although the specific cause of the diminished growth could not be determined, the most likely processes involved were considered to be maternal hypertension, renal function, and immunosuppressive drugs (17).

Follow-up of children exposed in utero to cyclosporine has been conducted in a few cases (5,11) (A. Poploski and D.A. Colasante, personal communication, 1987). In 15 of 27 surviving neonates, early postnatal development was normal except for one infant with slight growth restriction. Postnatal development of 10 children followed from 1 to 13 months revealed normal physical and mental development. No abnormal renal or liver function has been reported in the exposed newborns (5,11) (A. Poploski and D.A. Colasante, personal communication, 1987).

A 2006 report described 71 pregnancies among 45 women after liver transplantation (2). Tacrolimus and cyclosporine were used in 42 and 29 of the pregnancies, respectively. The outcomes of the pregnancies were live births (29 vs. 21), spontaneous abortions (7 vs. 6), elective abortions (5 vs. 1), molar pregnancy (1 vs. 0), and intrauterine death (0 vs. 1) (all *ns*). The median gestation and birth weight were 37.5 vs. 37 weeks, and 2660 vs. 2951 g, respectively (all *ns*). Pregnancies occurring within 1 year of transplantation had the highest incidence of prematurity and lowest birth weight. There were no congenital anomalies observed (2).

Two reviews discussing the treatment of psoriasis, one in 2002 (18) and the other in 2005 (19), considered the use of cyclosporine to be appropriate for the management of severe psoriasis.

BREASTFEEDING SUMMARY

Cyclosporine is excreted into breast milk. In a patient taking 450 mg of cyclosporine/day, milk levels on postpartum days 2, 3, and 4 were 101, 109, and 263 ng/mL, respectively (3). No details were given about the relationship of maternal doses with these levels. In another patient, milk concentrations 22 hours after a dose of 325 mg were 16 ng/mL, whereas maternal blood levels were 52 ng/mL, a milk:plasma ratio of 0.31 (4). A milk:plasma ratio of 0.40 was reported in one study (6) and a ratio of approximately 0.17 was measured in another (7). Breastfeeding was not allowed in any of these studies and has been actively discouraged by most sources because of concerns for potential toxicity in the nursing infant (13,14,16).

A 2001 study reported the use of cyclosporin in a woman who was breastfeeding (20). The woman had a simultaneous kidney–pancreas transplant 13 months before conception. She was treated before, during, and after pregnancy with cyclosporine (300 mg twice daily), azathioprine (100 mg/day), and prednisone (10 mg/day). At 34 weeks' gestation, she delivered an 1800-g male infant with Apgar scores of 5 and 8 at 1 and 5 minutes, respectively. Mild hyperbilirubinemia, treated with phototherapy, was the infant's only complication. The mother's cyclosporine levels during pregnancy were 75–173 ng/mL (therapeutic range 100–125 ng/mL in whole blood) but were not determined at birth. The cord blood cyclosporine concentration was 67 ng/mL. Breastfeeding was initiated 2 hours after birth and continued exclusively for the first 10.5 months of life. Random cyclosporine levels in the infant's serum were <25 ng/mL at approximately 1, 1.5, 2.5, 4, and 10.5 months of age. Maternal serum cyclosporine levels at approximately 1, 1.5, and 2.5 months were 193, 273, and 123 ng/mL, respectively, and breast milk levels were 160, 286, and 79 ng/mL, respectively. No adverse effects from exposure to cyclosporine were observed in the infant. At 12 months of age, his weight and height were at the 46th and 55th percentile, respectively. The mother has subsequently delivered a second child that was also breastfed (20).

Infant cyclosporine exposure was quantified in five mother–infant pairs in a 2003 report (21). The five mothers had taken cyclosporine throughout pregnancy and continued the drug while nursing their infants. In two cases, the milk:maternal blood ratios were 0.45 and 1.4 (not specified in the other three cases). In the latter case, the infant's dose from milk was about 1% of the therapeutic dose (weight basis). The infant's blood levels were as high as 78% of the corresponding maternal trough concentrations that were in the therapeutic range. Cyclosporine was not detected in the blood of three other infants (not tested in one infant). In the five cases, the estimated infant dose from milk, based on a milk consumption of 150 mL/kg/day, ranged from 0.2% to 2.1% of the mother's weight-adjusted dose. No adverse effects in the infants were observed, but specific immunologic effects were not investigated (21).

The American Academy of Pediatrics classifies cyclosporine as a drug that may interfere with cellular metabolism in the nursing infant (22).

References

1. Product information. Neoral, Sandimmune. Novartis Pharmaceuticals, 2005.
2. Christopher V, Al-Chalabi T, Richardson PD, Muiesan P, Rela M, Heaton ND, O'Grady JG, Heneghan MA. Pregnancy outcome after liver transplantation: a single-center experience of 71 pregnancies in 45 recipients. Liver Transpl 2006;12:1138–43.

3. Lewis GJ, Lamont CAR, Lee HA, Slapak M. Successful pregnancy in a renal transplant recipient taking cyclosporin A. Br Med J 1983;286:603.
4. Flechner SM, Katz AR, Rogers AJ, Van Buren C, Kahan BD. The presence of cyclosporine in body tissues and fluids during pregnancy. Am J Kidney Dis 1985;5:60–3.
5. Burrows DA, O'Neil TJ, Sorrells TL. Successful twin pregnancy after renal transplant maintained on cyclosporine A immunosuppression. Obstet Gynecol 1988;72:459–61.
6. Lowenstein BR, Vain NW, Perrone SV, Wright DR, Boullon FJ, Favaloro RG. Successful pregnancy and vaginal delivery after heart transplantation. Am J Obstet Gynecol 1988;158:589–90.
7. Ziegenhagen DJ, Grombach G, Dieckmann M, Zehnter E, Wienand P, Baldamus CA. Pregnancy under cyclosporine administration after renal transplantation. Dtsch Med Wochenschr 1988;113:260–3.
8. Klintmalm G, Althoff P, Appleby G, Segerbrandt E. Renal function in a newborn baby delivered of a renal transplant patient taking cyclosporine. Transplantation 1984;38:198–9.
9. Grischke E, Kaufmann M, Dreikorn K, Linderkamp O, Kubli F. Successful pregnancy after kidney transplantation and cyclosporin A. Geburtshilfe Frauenheilkd 1986;46:176–9.
10. Pikrell MD, Sawers R, Michael J. Pregnancy after renal transplantation: severe intrauterine growth retardation during treatment with cyclosporin A. Br Med J 1988;296:825.
11. Calne RY, Brons IGM, Williams PF, Evans DB, Robinson RE, Dossa M. Successful pregnancy after paratopic segmental pancreas and kidney transplantation. Br Med J 1988;296:1709.
12. Pujals JM, Figueras G, Puig JM, Lloveras J, Aubia J, Masramon J. Osseous malformation in baby born to woman on cyclosporin. Lancet 1989;1:667.
13. Al-Khader AA, Absy M, Al-Hasani MK, Joyce B, Sabbagh T. Successful pregnancy in renal transplant recipients treated with cyclosporine. Transplantation 1988;45:987–8.
14. Sims CJ, Porter KB, Knuppel RA. Successful pregnancy after a liver transplant. Am J Obstet Gynecol 1989;161:532–3.
15. Deeg HJ, Kennedy MS, Sanders JE, Thomas ED, Storb R. Successful pregnancy after marrow transplantation for severe aplastic anemia and immunosuppression with cyclosporine. JAMA 1983;250:647.
16. Kossoy LR, Herbert CM III, Wentz AC. Management of heart transplant recipients: guidelines for the obstetrician—gynecologist. Am J Obstet Gynecol 1988;159:490–9.
17. Lau RJ, Scott JR. Pregnancy following renal transplantation. Clin Obstet Gynecol 1985;28:339–50.
18. Tauscher AE, Fleischer AB Jr, Phelps KC, Feldman SR. Psoriasis and pregnancy. J Cutan Med Surg 2002;6:561–70.
19. Lebwohl M. A clinician's paradigm in the treatment of psoriasis. J Am Acad Dermatol 2005;53:S59–69.
20. Thiagarajan (Munoz-Flores) KD, Easterling T, Davis C, Bond EF. Breastfeeding by a cyclosporin-treated mother. Obstet Gynecol 2001;97:816–8.
21. Moretti ME, Sgro M, Johnson DW, Sauve RS, Woolgar MJ, Taddio A, Verjee Z, Giesbrecht E, Koren G, Ito S. Cyclosporin excretion into breast milk. Transplantation 2003;75:2144–6.
22. Committee on Drugs, American Academy of Pediatrics. The transfer of drugs and other chemicals into human milk. Pediatrics 2001;108:776–89.

CYCLOTHIAZIDE

[Withdrawn from the market. See 9th edition.]

CYCRIMINE

[Withdrawn from the market. See 8th edition.]

CYPROHEPTADINE

Antihistamine/Antiserotonin

PREGNANCY RECOMMENDATION: Limited Human Data—Animal Data Suggest Low Risk
BREASTFEEDING RECOMMENDATION: No Human Data—Probably Compatible

PREGNANCY SUMMARY

The animal reproduction data and limited human pregnancy experience suggest that cyproheptadine is low risk for structural anomalies. Although reporting bias is evident, preterm birth occurred in three women exposed to the drug during pregnancy. Because preterm birth has been associated with other serotonin antagonists (e.g., selective serotonin reuptake inhibitors), there might be a causal association with cyproheptadine.

FETAL RISK SUMMARY

Cyproheptadine has been used as a serotonin antagonist to prevent habitual abortion in patients with increased serotonin production (1,2). No congenital defects were observed when the drug was used for this purpose.

Reproductive studies in mice, rats, and rabbits with oral or SC doses up to 32 times the maximum recommended human dose found no evidence of impaired fertility or fetal harm (3,4). In contrast, Shepard cited a 1982 study that observed dose-related fetotoxicity characterized by skeletal retardation, hydronephrosis, liver and brain toxicity, and increased mortality in fetuses of rats administered 2–50 mg/kg/day intraperitoneally during organogenesis (5).

Two patients, who were being treated with cyproheptadine for Cushing's syndrome, conceived while taking the drug (6,7). Therapy was stopped at 3 months in one patient but continued throughout gestation in the second. Apparently healthy infants were delivered prematurely (33–34 weeks and 36 weeks) from both mothers. Fatal gastroenteritis developed at 4 months of age in the 33- to 34-week gestational infant who was exposed throughout pregnancy to the drug (6). The use of cyproheptadine to treat a pregnant woman with Cushing's syndrome secondary to bilateral adrenal hyperplasia was described in a 1990 reference (8). Specific details were not provided on the case, except that the fetus was delivered prematurely at 33 weeks' gestation. In a separate case, a woman with Cushing's was successfully treated with cyproheptadine; 2 years after stopping the drug, she conceived and eventually delivered a healthy male infant (9).

In a surveillance study of Michigan Medicaid recipients involving 229,101 completed pregnancies conducted between 1985 and 1992, 285 newborns had been exposed to cyproheptadine during the 1st trimester (F. Rosa, personal communication, FDA, 1993). A total of 12 (4.2%) major birth defects were observed (12 expected), including (observed/expected) 2/3 cardiovascular defects, 2/0.6 oral clefts, and 2/0.7 hypospadias. Only with the latter two defects is there a suggestion of an association with this drug, but other factors, including the mother's disease, concurrent drug use, and chance, may be involved. No anomalies were observed in three other categories of anomalies (spina bifida, polydactyly, and limb-reduction defects) for which specific data were available.

A woman at 4 weeks' gestation attempted suicide with cyproheptadine (400 mg), diazepam (200 mg), and trimetozine (12,000 mg) (an antianxiety agent that is no longer available) (10). A 2.65-kg male infant was born at 40 weeks' gestation. No congenital abnormalities were noted in the infant.

BREASTFEEDING SUMMARY

No reports describing the use of cyproheptadine during lactation have been located. Chronic use of cyproheptadine will lower serum prolactin levels and it has been used in the management of galactorrhea (11). No studies have been found, however, that evaluated its potential to interfere with the normal lactation process. Because of the increased sensitivity of newborns to antihistamines and the potential for adverse reactions, the manufacturer considers cyproheptadine to be contraindicated in nursing mothers (3).

References

1. Sadovsky E, Pfeifer Y, Polishuk WZ, Sulman FG. A trial of cyproheptadine in habitual abortion. Isr J Med Sci 1972;8:623–5.
2. Sadovsky E, Pfeifer Y, Sadovsky A, Sulman FG. Prevention of hypothalamic habitual abortion by Periactin. Harefuah 1970;78:332–4. As cited in Anonymous. References and reviews. JAMA 1970;212:1253.
3. Product information. Periactin. Merck & Co., 1997.
4. Pfeifer Y, Sadovsky E, Sulman FG. Prevention of serotonin abortion in pregnant rats by five serotonin antagonists. Obstet Gynecol 1969;33:709–14.
5. Shepard TH. *Catalog of Teratogenic Agents*. 8th ed. Baltimore, MD: Johns Hopkins University Press, 1995:121–2.
6. Kasperlik-Zaluska A, Migdalska B, Hartwig W, Wilczynska J, Marianowski L, Stopinska-Gluszak U, Lozinska D. Two pregnancies in a woman with Cushing's syndrome treated with cyproheptadine. Br J Obstet Gynaecol 1980;87:1171–3.
7. Khir ASM, How J, Bewsher PD. Successful pregnancy after cyproheptadine treatment for Cushing's disease. Eur J Obstet Gynecol Reprod Biol 1982;13:343–7.
8. Aron DC, Schnall AM, Sheeler LR. Cushing's syndrome and pregnancy. Am J Obstet Gynecol 1990;162:244–52.
9. Griffith DN, Ross EJ. Pregnancy after cyproheptadine treatment for Cushing's disease. N Engl J Med 1981;305:893–4.
10. Czeizel AE, Mosonyi A. Monitoring of early human fetal development in women exposed to large doses of chemicals. Environ Mol Mutagen 1997;30:240–4.
11. Wortsman J, Soler NG, Hirschowitz J. Cyproheptadine in the management of the galactorrhea–amenorrhea syndrome. Ann Intern Med 1979;90:923–5.

CYTARABINE

Antineoplastic

PREGNANCY RECOMMENDATION: Human Data Suggest Risk
BREASTFEEDING RECOMMENDATION: Contraindicated

PREGNANCY SUMMARY

The limited human pregnancy experience and the use of combination therapy prevent a complete assessment of the embryo–fetal risk. In addition to the potential for structural anomalies, cytarabine may cause fetal bone marrow suppression.

FETAL RISK SUMMARY

Cytarabine is an antineoplastic agent used in the treatment of various types of leukemia. It is classified as an antimetabolite in the subclass of pyrimidine analogs. Other antineoplastic agents in the subclass are capecitabine, floxuridine, fluorouracil, and gemcitabine.

The drug is teratogenic in the hamster and rat (1). Cytarabine is classified as an antimetabolite in the subclass of pyrimidine analogs. Other antineoplastic agents in the subclass are capecitabine, floxuridine, and gemcitabine.

Normal infants have resulted following in utero exposure to cytarabine during all stages of gestation (2–27). Follow-up of seven infants exposed in utero during the 2nd trimester to cytarabine revealed normal infants at 4–60 months (20,22–26). Two cases of intrauterine fetal death after cytarabine combination treatment have been located (20,23). In one case, maternal treatment for 5 weeks starting at the 15th week of gestation ended in intrauterine death at 20 weeks' gestation of a fetus without abnormalities or leukemic infiltration (20). The second case also involved a woman treated from the 15th week who developed severe

C

pregnancy-induced hypertension at 29 weeks' gestation (23). An apparently normal fetus died 1 week later, most likely as a consequence of the preeclampsia.

Use during the 1st and 2nd trimesters has been associated with congenital and chromosomal abnormalities (21,28–30). One leukemic patient treated during the 2nd trimester elected to have an abortion at 24 weeks' gestation (21). The fetus had trisomy for group C autosomes without mosaicism. A second pregnancy in the same patient with identical therapy ended normally. In another case, a 34-year-old woman with acute lymphoblastic leukemia was treated with multiple antineoplastic agents from 22 weeks' gestation until delivery of a healthy female infant 18 weeks later (28). Cytarabine was administered only during the 27th week of gestation. Chromosomal analysis of the newborn revealed a normal karyotype (46,XX) but with gaps and a ring chromosome. The clinical significance of these findings is unknown, but because these abnormalities may persist for several years, the potential existed for an increased risk of cancer as well as for a risk of genetic damage in the next generation (28). Two women, one treated during the 1st trimester and the other treated throughout pregnancy, delivered infants with the following multiple anomalies:

- Bilateral microtia and atresia of external auditory canals, right hand lobster claw with three digits, bilateral lower limb defects (29)
- Two medial digits of both feet missing, distal phalanges of both thumbs missing with hypoplastic remnant of the right thumb (30)

Congenital anomalies have also been observed after paternal use of cytarabine plus other antineoplastics prior to conception (31). The investigators suggested that the antineoplastic agents may have damaged the sperm without producing infertility in the two fathers. The relationship between use of the chemotherapy in these men and the defects observed is doubtful due to the lack of experimental evidence and confirming reports. The results of these pregnancies were as follows: tetralogy of Fallot, syndactyly of first and second digits of right foot, and a stillborn with anencephaly. Cytarabine may produce reversible azoospermia (32,33). However, male fertility has been demonstrated during maintenance therapy with cytarabine (34).

Pancytopenia was observed in a 1000-g male infant exposed to cytarabine and five other antineoplastic agents during the 3rd trimester (12).

Data from one review indicated that 40% of the mothers exposed to antineoplastic drugs during pregnancy delivered low-birth-weight infants (35). This finding was not related to the timing of exposure. Except for the few cases noted above, long-term studies of growth and mental development in offspring exposed to cytarabine during the 2nd trimester, the period of neuroblast multiplication, have not been conducted (36).

Occupational exposure of the mother to antineoplastic agents during pregnancy may present a risk to the fetus. A position statement from the National Study Commission on Cytotoxic Exposure and a research article involving some antineoplastic agents are presented in the monograph for cyclophosphamide (see Cyclophosphamide).

BREASTFEEDING SUMMARY

No reports describing the use of cytarabine during lactation have been located. Because of the potential for serious adverse effects in nursing infants, women receiving this drug should not breastfeed.

References

1. Product information. Cytosar-U. Pharmacia & Upjohn, 2000.
2. Pawliger DF, McLean FW, Noyes WD. Normal fetus after cytosine arabinoside therapy. Ann Intern Med 1971;74:1012.
3. Au-Yong R, Collins P, Young JA. Acute myeloblastic leukemia during pregnancy. Br Med J 1972;4:493–4.
4. Raich PC, Curet LB. Treatment of acute leukemia during pregnancy. Cancer 1975;36:861–2.
5. Gokal R, Durrant J, Baum JD, Bennett MJ. Successful pregnancy in acute monocytic leukaemia. Br J Cancer 1976;34:299–302.
6. Sears HF, Reid J. Granulocytic sarcoma: local presentation of a systemic disease. Cancer 1976;37:1808–13.
7. Durie BGM, Giles HR. Successful treatment of acute leukemia during pregnancy. Arch Intern Med 1977;137:90–1.
8. Lilleyman JS, Hill AS, Anderton KJ. Consequences of acute myelogenous leukemia in early pregnancy. Cancer 1977;40:1300–3.
9. Moreno H, Castleberry RP, McCann WP. Cytosine arabinoside and 6-thioguanine in the treatment of childhood acute myeloblastic leukemia. Cancer 1977;40:998–1004.
10. Newcomb M, Balducci L, Thigpen JT, Morrison FS. Acute leukemia in pregnancy: successful delivery after cytarabine and doxorubicin. JAMA 1978;239:2691–2.
11. Manoharan A, Leyden MJ. Acute non-lymphocytic leukaemia in the third trimester of pregnancy. Aust N-Z J Med 1979;9:71–4.
12. Pizzuto J, Aviles A, Noriega L, Niz J, Morales M, Romero F. Treatment of acute leukemia during pregnancy: presentation of nine cases. Cancer Treat Rep 1980;64:679–83.
13. Colbert N, Najman A, Gorin NC, Blum F, Treisser A, Lasfargues G, Cloup M, Barrat H, Duhamel G. Acute leukaemia during pregnancy: favourable course of pregnancy in two patients treated with cytosine arabinoside and anthracyclines. Nouv Presse Med 1980;9:175–8.
14. Tobias JS, Bloom HJG. Doxorubicin in pregnancy. Lancet 1980;1:776.
15. Taylor G, Blom J. Acute leukemia during pregnancy. South Med J 1980;73:1314–5.
16. Dara P, Slater LM, Armentrout SA. Successful pregnancy during chemotherapy for acute leukemia. Cancer 1981;47:845–6.
17. Plows CW. Acute myelomonocytic leukemia in pregnancy: report of a case. Am J Obstet Gynecol 1982;143:41–3.
18. De Souza JJL, Bezwoda WR, Jetham D, Sonnendecker EWW. Acute leukaemia in pregnancy: a case report and discussion on modern management. S Afr Med J 1982;62:295–6.
19. Feliu J, Juarez S, Ordonez A, Garcia-Paredes ML, Gonzalez-Baron M, Montero JM. Acute leukemia and pregnancy. Cancer 1988;61:580–4.
20. Volkenandt M, Buchner T, Hiddemann W, Van De Loo J. Acute leukaemia during pregnancy. Lancet 1987;2:1521–2.
21. Maurer LH, Forcier RJ, McIntyre OR, Benirschke K. Fetal group C trisomy after cytosine arabinoside and thioguanine. Ann Intern Med 1971;75:809–10.
22. Lowenthal RM, Marsden KA, Newman NM, Baikie MJ, Campbell SN. Normal infant after treatment of acute myeloid leukaemia in pregnancy with daunorubicin. Aust N-Z J Med 1978;8:431–2.
23. O'Donnell R, Costigan C, O'Donnell LG. Two cases of acute leukaemia in pregnancy. Acta Haematol 1979;61:298–300.
24. Doney KC, Kraemer KG, Shepard TH. Combination chemotherapy for acute myelocytic leukemia during pregnancy: three case reports. Cancer Treat Rep 1979;63:369–71.
25. Cantini E, Yanes B. Acute myelogenous leukemia in pregnancy. South Med J 1984;77:1050–2.
26. Alegre A, Chunchurreta R, Rodrigueq-Alarcon J, Cruz E, Prada M. Successful pregnancy in acute promyelocytic leukemia. Cancer 1982;49:152–3.
27. Hamer JW, Beard MEJ, Duff GB. Pregnancy complicated by acute myeloid leukaemia. N-Z Med J 1979;89:212–3.

28. Schleuning M, Clemm C. Chromosomal aberrations in a newborn whose mother received cytotoxic treatment during pregnancy. N Engl J Med 1987;317:1666–7.
29. Wagner VM, Hill JS, Weaver D, Baehner RL. Congenital abnormalities in baby born to cytarabine treated mother. Lancet 1980;2:98–9.
30. Schafer AI. Teratogenic effects of antileukemic chemotherapy. Arch Intern Med 1981;141:514–5.
31. Russell JA, Powles RL, Oliver RTD. Conception and congenital abnormalities after chemotherapy of acute myelogenous leukaemia in two men. Br Med J 1976;1:1508.
32. Lendon M, Palmer MK, Hann IM, Shalet SM, Jones PHM. Testicular histology after combination chemotherapy in childhood for acute lymphoblastic leukaemia. Lancet 1978;2:439–41.
33. Lilleyman JS. Male fertility after successful chemotherapy for lymphoblastic leukaemia. Lancet 1979;2:1125.
34. Matthews JH, Wood JK. Male fertility during chemotherapy for acute leukemia. N Engl J Med 1980;303:1235.
35. Nicholson HO. Cytotoxic drugs in pregnancy: review of reported cases. J Obstet Gynaecol Br Commonw 1968;75:307–12.
36. Dobbing J. Pregnancy and leukaemia. Lancet 1977;1:1155.

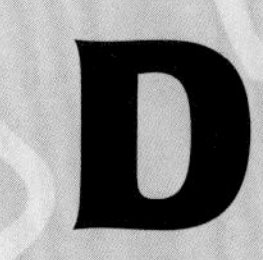

D

DABIGATRAN ETEXILATE

Anticoagulant (Thrombin Inhibitor)

PREGNANCY RECOMMENDATION: No Human Data—Animal Data Suggest Moderate Risk
BREASTFEEDING RECOMMENDATION: No Human Data—Potential Toxicity

PREGNANCY SUMMARY

No reports describing the use of dabigatran etexilate in human pregnancy have been located. The animal data suggest moderate risk, but the absence of human pregnancy experience prevents a more complete assessment of the embryo–fetal risk. Until such data are available, other anticoagulants, such as the low-molecular-weight heparins, appear to be a better choice in pregnancy.

FETAL RISK SUMMARY

Dabigatran etexilate is a direct thrombin inhibitor that is given orally. It is indicated to reduce the risk of stroke and systemic embolism in patients with nonvalvular atrial fibrillation. After oral dosing, dabigatran etexilate is converted to dabigatran, the active agent. Dabigatran is further metabolized to four different acyl glucuronides, all of which have similar activity to dabigatran. Plasma protein binding is about 35% and the half-life is 12–17 hours (1).

Reproduction studies have been conducted in rats and rabbits. In pregnant rats, a dose that was about 2.6–3 times the human exposure from the maximum recommended dose of 300 mg/day based on AUC (MRHD) given after implantation resulted in an increase in dead offspring and caused excess vaginal/uterine bleeding close to parturition. This dose also increased the incidence of delayed or irregular ossification of fetal skull bones and vertebrae. However, the drug did not induce major malformations in the rat or rabbit (dose in rabbits not specified). The number of implantations was decreased when dabigatran was given to male and female rats before mating and up to implantation at the above dose (1).

In 2-year studies, dabigatran was not carcinogenic in mice and rats. The drug was not mutagenic in multiple assays. No adverse effects on male and female rat fertility were observed, but, as noted above, the drug decreased the number of implantations when given up to implantation (gestation day 6) (1).

It is not known if dabigatran etexilate or dabigatran crosses the human placenta. The molecular weights of the parent compound and dabigatran (about 628 and 499 for the free bases), low plasma protein binding, and the long elimination half-life suggest that it will cross to the embryo–fetus. However, without referencing, a 2010 review of new oral anticoagulants stated that dabigatran does not cross the placenta (2).

BREASTFEEDING SUMMARY

No reports describing the use of dabigatran etexilate during human lactation have been located. The molecular weight of the parent compound (about 628 for the free base), low plasma protein binding (about 35%), and the long elimination half-life (12–17 hours) suggest that the drug and its active metabolites will be excreted into breast milk. The effect of the exposure on a nursing infant is unknown, but the drug is absorbed orally. Until such data are available, use of other anticoagulants, such as the low-molecular-weight heparins, should be considered.

References

1. Product information. Pradaxa. Boehringer Ingelheim Pharmaceuticals, 2011.
2. Huisman MV. Further issues with new oral anticoagulants. Curr Pharm Des 2010;16:3487–9.

DACARBAZINE

Antineoplastic

PREGNANCY RECOMMENDATION: Contraindicated—1st Trimester
BREASTFEEDING RECOMMENDATION: No Human Data—Potential Toxicity

D

PREGNANCY SUMMARY

Dacarbazine is an alkylating antineoplastic agent. Other agents in this class (see also Busulfan, Chlorambucil, and Cyclophosphamide) are known to be human teratogens and, combined with the animal data, strongly suggest that dacarbazine should not be given in the 1st trimester.

FETAL RISK SUMMARY

Single intraperitoneal doses of 800 or 1000 mg/kg in pregnant rats produced skeletal reduction defects, cleft palates, and encephaloceles in their offspring (1).

Dacarbazine was used for the treatment of melanoma in the 1st trimester of one pregnancy (2). The pregnancy was electively aborted. In a second case, a woman at 21 weeks', received two cycles of chemotherapy for Hodgkin's disease (3). Each cycle consisted of dacarbazine (375 mg/m^2 IV, days 1 and 14), doxorubicin, bleomycin, and vinblastine. At 29 weeks', a healthy, 2400-g female infant was born, who is alive and well at 10 years of age.

No congenital malformations were observed in four liveborn offspring of one male and another female treated with dacarbazine during childhood or adolescence (4). In a 2002 study, 1915 women had 4029 pregnancies after chemotherapy with or without radiation (5). No statistical differences in pregnancy outcomes (live births and spontaneous abortions) by treatment group were found, including the 170 pregnancies in women treated with dacarbazine.

Occupational exposure of the mother to antineoplastic agents during pregnancy may present a risk to the fetus. A position statement from the National Study Commission on Cytotoxic Exposure and a research article involving some antineoplastic agents are presented in the monograph for cyclophosphamide (see Cyclophosphamide).

BREASTFEEDING SUMMARY

No reports describing the use of dacarbazine during lactation have been located. Because of the potential for severe adverse effects, such as hematopoietic depression in a nursing infant, the drug should not be used during breastfeeding.

References

1. Chaube S. Protective effects of thymidine, and 5-aminoimidazolecarboxamide and riboflavin against fetal abnormalities produced in rats by 5-(3,3-dimethyl-1-triazeno)imidazole-4-carboxamide. Cancer Res 1973;33:2231–40. As cited in Shepard TH. *Catalog of Teratogenic Agents.* 6th ed. Baltimore, MD: Johns Hopkins University Press, 1989:189.
2. Zemlickis D, Lishner M, Degendorfer P, Panzarella T, Sutcliffe SB, Koren G. Fetal outcome after in utero exposure to cancer chemotherapy. Arch Intern Med 1992;152:573–6.
3. Anselmo AP, Cavalier E, Maurizi Enrici R, Pescarmona E, Guerrisi V, Paesano R, Pachi A, Mandelli F. Hodgkin's disease during pregnancy: diagnostic and therapeutic management. Fetal Diagn Ther 1999;14:102–5.
4. Green DM, Zevon MA, Lowries G, Seigelstein N, Hall B. Congenital anomalies in children of patients who received chemotherapy for cancer in childhood and adolescence. N Engl J Med 1991;325:141–6.
5. Green DM, Whitton JA, Stovall M, Mertens AC, Donaldson SS, Ruymann FB, Pendergrass TW, Robison LL. Pregnancy outcome of female survivors of childhood cancer: a report from the Childhood Cancer Survivor study. Am J Obstet Gynecol 2002;187:1070–80.

DACLIZUMAB

Immunologic Agent (Immunosuppressant)

PREGNANCY RECOMMENDATION: Compatible—Maternal Benefit >> Embryo–Fetal Risk
BREASTFEEDING RECOMMENDATION: No Human Data—Probably Compatible

PREGNANCY SUMMARY

No reports describing the use of daclizumab in human pregnancy have been located. The lack of animal and human pregnancy experience prevents an assessment of the embryo–fetal risk. However, basiliximab, an antibody with a similar mechanism of action, did not cause noticeable developmental toxicity in cynomolgus monkeys. (See Basiliximab.) A 2004 review concluded that immunosuppressive antibodies have little implication for pregnancy because they are used either for induction immunosuppression or to prevent an acute rejection episode (1). If exposure does occur during pregnancy, the risk for developmental toxicity is unknown but may be low. Long-term studies of exposed offspring for functional abnormalities and other developmental toxicity are warranted. The manufacturer recommends that women of childbearing potential use effective contraception before and during therapy, and for 4 months afterward (2).

FETAL RISK SUMMARY

Daclizumab, an interleukin-2 (IL-2) receptor antagonist, is an immunosuppressive, humanized (90% human/10% murine) immunoglobulin G1 (IgG1) monoclonal antibody indicated for the prophylaxis of acute organ rejection in patients receiving renal transplants (2). Daclizumab is classified as a nondepleting (i.e., does not destroy T- or B-lymphocytes) protein immunosuppressant (3). It binds only to IL-2 receptor sites expressed on the surface of activated T-lymphocytes.

This binding inhibits IL-2-mediated activation of lymphocytes. Daclizumab is used with immunosuppressive regimens that include cyclosporine and corticosteroids. The elimination half-life is about 20 days (2).

Reproduction studies have not been conducted with daclizumab (2).

D

It is not known if daclizumab crosses the human placenta. The molecular weight of the glycoprotein (about 144,000) may prevent transfer. However, the prolonged elimination half-life and the fact that IgG molecules are known to cross the placenta, at least in the 3rd trimester, suggest that some exposure of the embryo and/or fetus will occur.

IL-2 receptors may have an important role in the development of the immune system, but the potential effect of daclizumab on this development is unknown. While in the circulation, daclizumab impairs the response of the immune system to antigenic challenges. It is unknown if the ability to respond to these challenges returns to normal after clearance of daclizumab (2).

BREASTFEEDING SUMMARY

No reports describing the use of daclizumab during human lactation have been located. Because immunoglobulins and other large molecules are excreted into colostrum in the first 2–3 days after birth, daclizumab is also probably excreted during this time. It may not be possible to avoid exposure during this early period of lactation because of the prolonged elimination half-life (about 20 days). Excretion into mature milk also is possible. Although partial digestion of the antibody in the gastrointestinal tract is probable, the effect on a nursing infant from this exposure is unknown.

References

1. Danesi R, Del Tacca M. Teratogenesis and immunosuppressive treatment. Transplant Proc 2004;36:705–7.
2. Product information. Zenapax. Roche Laboratories, 2005.
3. Halloran PF. Immunosuppressive drugs for kidney transplantation. N Engl J Med 2004;351:2715–29.

DACTINOMYCIN

Antineoplastic

PREGNANCY RECOMMENDATION: Limited Human Data—Animal Data Suggest High Risk
BREASTFEEDING RECOMMENDATION: No Human Data—Potential Toxicity

PREGNANCY SUMMARY

The human pregnancy experience is limited, none of which involved 1st trimester exposure. The animal data suggest high risk. If the drug must be used in pregnancy, exposure during organogenesis during should be avoided.

FETAL RISK SUMMARY

Dactinomycin is an antimitotic antineoplastic agent. It is in the same antineoplastic subclass of antibiotics as bleomycin and mitomycin.

Reproduction studies in the rat, rabbit, and hamster at IV doses 3–7 times the maximum recommended human dose has shown embryo and fetal toxicity and teratogenic effects (1).

Normal pregnancies have followed the use of this drug prior to conception (2–10). However, women were less likely to have a live birth following treatment with this drug than with other antineoplastics (6).

Eight women who were treated with dactinomycin in childhood or adolescence subsequently produced 20 liveborn offspring, 3 (15%) of whom had congenital anomalies (11). This rate was the highest among 14 antineoplastic agents studied. Another report, however, observed no major congenital malformations in 52 offspring born to 11 men and 25 women who had been treated with dactinomycin during childhood or adolescence, suggesting that the results of the initial study occurred by chance (12).

Reports on the use of dactinomycin in six pregnancies have been located (13–18). In these cases, dactinomycin was administered during the 2nd and 3rd trimesters and apparently normal infants were delivered. The infant from one of the pregnancies was continuing to do well 4 years after birth (15). Two of the other pregnancies (16,17) are discussed in more detail in the monograph for cyclophosphamide (see Cyclophosphamide).

Data from one review indicated that 40% of the infants exposed to anticancer drugs were of low birth weight (13). This finding was not related to the timing of exposure. Long-term studies of growth and mental development in offspring exposed to dactinomycin during the 2nd trimester, the period of neuroblast multiplication, have not been conducted (19).

The long-term effects of combination chemotherapy on menstrual and reproductive function have been described in a 1988 report (20). Thirty-two of the 40 women treated for malignant ovarian germ cell tumors received dactinomycin. The results of this study are discussed in the monograph for cyclophosphamide (see Cyclophosphamide).

Occupational exposure of the mother to antineoplastic agents during pregnancy may present a risk to the fetus. A position statement from the National Study Commission on Cytotoxic Exposure and a research article involving some antineoplastic agents are presented in the monograph for cyclophosphamide (see Cyclophosphamide).

BREASTFEEDING SUMMARY

No reports describing the use of dactinomycin during human lactation have been located. Although its relatively high molecular weight (about 1255) should impede the excretion into milk, women receiving this drug should not breastfeed because of the potential risk of severe adverse reactions in the nursing infant.

References

1. Product information. Cosmegen. Merck, 2000.
2. Ross GT. Congenital anomalies among children born of mothers receiving chemotherapy for gestational trophoblastic neoplasms. Cancer 1976;37:1043–7.
3. Walden PAM, Bagshawe KD. Pregnancies after chemotherapy for gestational trophoblastic tumours. Lancet 1979;2:1241.
4. Schwartz PE, Vidone RA. Pregnancy following combination chemotherapy for a mixed germ cell tumor of the ovary. Gynecol Oncol 1981;12: 373–8.
5. Pastorfide GB, Goldstein DP. Pregnancy after hydatidiform mole. Obstet Gynecol 1973;42:67–70.
6. Rustin GJS, Booth M, Dent J, Salt S, Rustin F, Bagshawe KD. Pregnancy after cytotoxic chemotherapy for gestational trophoblastic tumours. Br Med J 1984;288:103–6.
7. Evenson DP, Arlin Z, Welt S, Claps ML, Melamed MR. Male reproductive capacity may recover following drug treatment with the L-10 protocol for acute lymphocytic leukemia. Cancer 1984;53:30–6.
8. Sivanesaratnam V, Sen DK. Normal pregnancy after successful treatment of choriocarcinoma with cerebral metastases: a case report. J Reprod Med 1988;33:402–3.
9. Lee RB, Kelly J, Elg SA, Benson WL. Pregnancy following conservative surgery and adjunctive chemotherapy for stage III immature teratoma of the ovary. Obstet Gynecol 1989;73:853–5.
10. Bakri YN, Pedersen P, Nassar M. Normal pregnancy after curative multiagent chemotherapy for choriocarcinoma with brain metastases. Acta Obstet Gynecol Scand 1991;70:611–3.
11. Green DM, Zevon MA, Lowrie G, Seigelstein N, Hall B. Congenital anomalies in children of patients who received chemotherapy for cancer in childhood and adolescence. N Engl J Med 1991;325:141–6.
12. Byrne J, Nicholson HS, Mulvihill JJ. Absence of birth defects in offspring of women treated with dactinomycin. N Engl J Med 1992;326:137.
13. Nicholson HO. Cytotoxic drugs in pregnancy: review of reported cases. J Obstet Gynaecol Br Commonw 1968;75:307–12.
14. Gililland J, Weinstein L. The effects of cancer chemotherapeutic agents on the developing fetus. Obstet Gynecol Surv 1983;38:6–13.
15. Haerr RW, Pratt AT. Multiagent chemotherapy for sarcoma diagnosed during pregnancy. Cancer 1985;56:1028–33.
16. Weed JC Jr, Roh RA, Mendenhall HW. Recurrent endodermal sinus tumor during pregnancy. Obstet Gynecol 1979;54:653–6.
17. Kim DS, Park MI. Maternal and fetal survival following surgery and chemotherapy of endodermal sinus tumor of the ovary during pregnancy: a case report. Obstet Gynecol 1989;73:503–7.
18. Kim DS, Moon H, Lee JA, Park MI. Anticancer drugs during pregnancy: are we able to discard them? Am J Obstet Gynecol 1992;166:265.
19. Dobbing J. Pregnancy and leukaemia. Lancet 1977;1:1155.
20. Gershenson DM. Menstrual and reproductive function after treatment with combination chemotherapy for malignant ovarian germ cell tumors. J Clin Oncol 1988;6:270–5.

DALFAMPRIDINE

Potassium Channel Blocker

PREGNANCY RECOMMENDATION: No Human Data—Animal Data Suggest Moderate Risk
BREASTFEEDING RECOMMENDATION: No Human Data—Potential Toxicity

PREGNANCY SUMMARY

No reports describing the use of dalfampridine in human pregnancy have been located. Although the animal data suggest risk, the complete absence of human pregnancy experience prevents an assessment of the embryo–fetal risk. If the drug is indicated in a pregnant woman, she should be advised of the absence of data.

FETAL RISK SUMMARY

Dalfampridine is a broad-spectrum potassium channel blocker that is taken as extended-release oral tablets. It is indicated to improve walking in patients with multiple sclerosis. The drug is metabolized to inactive metabolites. Plasma protein binding is very low (1%–3%) and the elimination half-life is 5.2–6.5 hours (1).

Reproduction studies have been conducted in rats and rabbits. In these species, oral doses up to about 5 times the maximum recommended human dose based on BSA (MRHD) revealed no evidence of developmental toxicity. Maternal toxicity was observed at the highest dose. When rats were given oral doses throughout pregnancy and lactation, decreased offspring survival and growth were observed. The no-effect dose for prenatal and postnatal developmental toxicity was about 0.5 times the MRHD (1).

There was no evidence of drug-induced carcinogenesis in 2-year studies in mice. However, a significant increase in uterine polyps was noted in rats at the highest dose tested (about 9 times the MRHD). In vitro and in vivo assays for mutagenesis were negative. The drug had no effect on the fertility of male and female rats (1).

It is not known if dalfampridine crosses the human placenta. The very low molecular (about 94) and plasma protein binding combined with a moderately long elimination half-life suggest that the drug will cross to the embryo–fetus.

BREASTFEEDING SUMMARY

No reports describing the use of dalfampridine during human lactation have been located. The very low molecular weight (about 94) and plasma protein binding (1%–3%) combined with a moderately long elimination half-life (5.2–6.5 hours) suggest that the drug will be excreted into breast milk. The effect of this exposure on a nursing infant is unknown. Exposed infants should be monitored for the most common adverse effects seen in adults, such as insomnia, headache, nausea, dizziness, constipation, and other reactions.

Reference

1. Product information. Ampyra. Acorda Therapeutics, 2010.

DALTEPARIN

Anticoagulant

PREGNANCY RECOMMENDATION: Compatible
BREASTFEEDING RECOMMENDATION: Compatible

D

PREGNANCY SUMMARY

The use of dalteparin during pregnancy appears to present no more fetal or newborn risk than that from standard, unfractionated heparin.

FETAL RISK SUMMARY

Dalteparin is a low-molecular-weight heparin prepared by depolymerization of heparin obtained from porcine intestinal mucosa. The molecular weight of dalteparin varies from <3000 to >8000, but 65%–78% is in the 3000–8000 range (1). Reproduction studies found no evidence of impaired fertility in male and female rats or fetal harm in rats and rabbits (1).

Because of its relatively high molecular weight, dalteparin is not expected to cross the placenta to the fetus (2). Thirty women undergoing elective pregnancy termination in the 2nd trimester (*N* = 15) or 3rd trimester (*N* = 15) for fetal malformations or chromosomal abnormalities were administered a single SC dose of 2500 IU or 5000 IU, respectively, of dalteparin immediately prior to the procedure (3). Heparin activity was not evident in fetal blood, demonstrating the lack of transplacental passage at this stage of gestation.

Dalteparin was administered as a continuous IV infusion at 36 weeks' gestation in a woman being treated for a deep vein thrombosis that had occurred during the 1st trimester (4). During the 1st trimester, she had been treated with IV heparin and then was maintained on SC doses for 4 weeks before developing an allergic reaction. Skin testing revealed immediate-type allergic reactions to heparin and some other derivatives but not to dalteparin. She was changed to warfarin therapy at 14 weeks' gestation, and this therapy was continued until the change to dalteparin at 36 weeks. Following stabilization of the anti-factor Xa plasma levels with a continuous infusion (400 anti-factor Xa U/hour), dalteparin therapy was changed to SC dosing, which was continued until delivery at 38.5 weeks of a healthy, 3010-g female infant. No anti-factor Xa activity was detected in the cord blood.

A 1992 report described the use of dalteparin in seven women at 16–23 weeks' gestation just before undergoing therapeutic termination of pregnancy (5). SC dalteparin was given at 15 and 3 hours before pregnancy termination. Heparin activity (anti-factor Xa) was detected in all mothers but not in any of the fetuses. In the second part of the study, 11 pregnant women with a history of severe thromboembolic tendency, as evidenced by recurrent miscarriages, were treated throughout gestation with SC dalteparin (5). All of the women gave birth to healthy infants without complication. As with heparin, maternal osteoporosis may be a complication resulting from the use of low-molecular-weight heparins, including dalteparin, during pregnancy (see also Heparin and Vitamin D). However, in the 11 patients described above, all had normal mineral mass as determined by bone density scans performed shortly after delivery (5). Moreover, a study published in 1996 compared two groups of pregnant women receiving SC dalteparin, either 5000 IU daily (*N* = 9) or 5000 IU daily in the 1st trimester, then twice daily thereafter (*N* = 8), both starting in the 1st trimester, with a control group (*N* = 8) that did not receive heparin (6). Lumbar spine bone density fell by similar amounts in all pregnancies, and the normal physiological change of pregnancy was not increased by dalteparin.

The use of dalteparin in 184 pregnant women for thromboprophylaxis was reviewed in a brief 1994 report (7). No placental passage of the drug was found in the 9 patients investigated. Congenital malformations were observed in 3.3% of the outcomes, a rate believed to be normal for this population. Another 1994 letter reference described the use of dalteparin in five pregnant women starting between 15 and 18 weeks' gestation (8). Apparently normal infants were delivered.

Dalteparin was used for thromboembolic prophylaxis in 24 pregnant women with a risk of thromboembolic disease (9). The women received total daily doses of 2500 (16 mg) to 10,000 (32 mg) anti-factor Xa IU. Anti-factor Xa activity was demonstrated in the blood samples from the mothers but not in the normal newborns, indicating the lack of placental transfer of the drug.

A 1997 case report described the successful use of dalteparin in the 3rd trimester of a pregnant woman with iliofemoral vein thrombosis who was resistant to use unfractionated heparin (10). She was treated with 7000 IU (100 IU/kg) every 12 hours from 30 weeks' gestation until 24 hours before an uncomplicated vaginal delivery at 38 weeks'.

In a randomized 1999 trial, unfractionated heparin (*N* = 55; mean 20,569 IU/day) and dalteparin (*N* = 50; mean 4631 IU/day) were compared in 105 pregnant women with previous or current thromboembolism (11). There were no recurrences of thromboembolism or cases of thrombocytopenia in either group, but there were more bleeding complications in the patients receiving unfractionated heparin. The pregnancy outcomes in terms of blood loss at delivery, number of cesarean sections, birth weight, and Apgar scores were similar.

In a 2000 trial, a prophylactic dalteparin dose of 5000 IU/day given during pregnancy was adequate for 25 women (mean weight 70.2 kg), but the dose was decreased in 6 women (mean 58.0 kg) and increased in 2 (mean 102.5 kg) after the first anti-Xa activity measurement (12). An adjusted-weight therapeutic dose (100 IU/kg twice daily) was appropriate during pregnancy based on measured anti-Xa activity.

BREASTFEEDING SUMMARY

No reports describing the use of dalteparin during lactation have been located. Dalteparin, a low- molecular-weight heparin, still has a relatively high molecular weight (65%–78% in the range of 3000–8000) and, as such, should not be expected to be excreted into human milk. Because the drug would be inactivated in the gastrointestinal tract, the risk to a nursing infant from ingestion of dalteparin from milk appears to be negligible.

References

1. Product information. Fragmin. Pharmacia & Upjohn Company, 1997.
2. Nelson-Piercy C. Low molecular weight heparin for obstetric thromboprophylaxis. Br J Obstet Gynaecol 1994;101:6–8.
3. Forestier F, Solé Y, Aiach M, Alhenc Gélas M, Daffos F. Absence of transplacental passage of Fragmin (Kabi) during the second and the third trimesters of pregnancy. Thromb Haemost 1992;67:180–1.
4. De Boer K, Heyboer H, ten Cate JW, Borm JJJ, van Ginkel CJW. Low molecular weight heparin treatment in a pregnant woman with allergy to standard heparins and heparinoid. Thromb Haemost 1989;61:148.
5. Melissari E, Parker CJ, Wilson NV, Monte G, Kanthou C, Pemberton KD, Nicolaides KH, Barrett JJ, Kakkar VV. Use of low molecular weight heparin in pregnancy. Thromb Haemost 1992;68:652–6.
6. Shefras J, Farquharson RG. Bone density studies in pregnant women receiving heparin. Eur J Obstet Gynecol Reprod Biol 1996;65:171–4.
7. Wahlberg TB, Kher A. Low molecular weight heparin as thromboprophylaxis in pregnancy. Haemostasis 1994;24:55–6.
8. Manoharan A. Use of low molecular weight heparin during pregnancy. J Clin Pathol 1994;47:94–5.
9. Rasmussen C, Wadt J, Jacobsen B. Thromboembolic prophylaxis with low molecular weight heparin during pregnancy. Int J Gynecol Obstet 1994;47:121–5.
10. Anand SS, Brimble S, Ginsberg JS. Management of iliofemoral thrombosis in a pregnant patient with heparin resistance. Arch Intern Med 1997;157:815–6.
11. Pettila V, Kaaja R, Leinonen P, Ekblad U, Kataja M, Ikkala E. Thromboprophylaxis with low molecular weight heparin (dalteparin) in pregnancy. Thromb Res 1999;96:275–82.
12. Rey E, Rivard GE. Prophylaxis and treatment of thromboembolic diseases during pregnancy with dalteparin. Int J Gynecol Obstet 2000;71:19–24.

DANAPAROID

[Withdrawn from the market. See 9th edition.]

DANAZOL

Androgen

PREGNANCY RECOMMENDATION: Contraindicated
BREASTFEEDING RECOMMENDATION: Contraindicated

PREGNANCY SUMMARY

A number of reports have described the inadvertent use of danazol during human gestation resulting in female pseudohermaphroditism. This teratogenic condition is characterized by a normal XX karyotype and internal female reproductive organs, but ambiguous external genitalia. No adverse effects in male fetuses have been associated with danazol.

FETAL RISK SUMMARY

Danazol is a synthetic androgen derived from ethisterone that is used in the treatment of various conditions, such as endometriosis, fibrocystic breast disease, and hereditary angioedema. No fetal harm was observed in reproduction studies with pregnant rats at doses 7–15 times the human dose, but fetal development was inhibited in rabbits at doses 2–4 times the human dose (1).

Early studies with this agent had examined its potential as an oral contraceptive (2–4). This use was abandoned, however, because low doses (e.g., 50–100 mg/day) were associated with pregnancy rates ≤10% and higher doses were unacceptable to the patient due to adverse effects (2,4).

In experimental animals, danazol crosses the placenta to the fetus, but human data are lacking. The molecular weight (about 338) suggests that it does reach the human embryo and fetus. Because danazol is used to treat endometriosis, frequently in an infertile woman, a barrier (nonhormonal) contraception method is recommended to prevent accidental use during pregnancy.

The first published report of female pseudohermaphroditism appeared in 1981 (5). A woman was treated for endometriosis with a total danazol dose of 81 g divided over 101 days. Subsequent evaluation revealed that the treatment period corresponded to approximately the first 14 weeks of pregnancy. The female infant, whose length and weight were at the 5th percentile, had mild clitoral enlargement and a urogenital sinus evident at birth. Physical findings at 2 years of age were normal except for clitoromegaly, empty, darkened, rugated labia majora, and a complete urogenital sinus formation. Studies indicated the child had a normal vagina, cervix, fallopian tubes, and ovaries. The mother had no evidence of virilization.

A second case reported in 1981 involved a woman with endometriosis who was inadvertently treated with danazol, 800 mg/day, during the first 20 weeks of gestation (6). The mother went into premature labor at 27 weeks and delivered a female infant with a birth weight of 980 g. Ambiguous genitalia were evident at birth, consisting of marked clitoromegaly with fusion of the labia scrotal folds. A urogenital sinus, with well-developed vagina and uterus, was noted on genitogram. Bilateral inguinal hernias with palpable gonads were also present. At 4 days of age, clinical and laboratory findings compatible with a salt-losing congenital adrenal hyperplasia were observed. The infant was successfully treated for this complication, which was thought to be due to a transitory block of the steroid 21- and 11-monooxygenases (6). At 1 year of age, the infant was asymptomatic, and no signs of progressive virilization were observed.

The authors of the above report cited knowledge of 27 other pregnancies in which danazol had been accidentally used (6). Seven of these pregnancies were terminated by abortion. Of the remaining 20 pregnancies, 14 delivered female infants and 5 (36%) of these had evidence of virilization with ambiguous genitalia.

A 1982 case report described female pseudohermaphroditism in an infant exposed to a total danazol dose of 96 g administered over 120 days, corresponding to approximately the first 16 weeks of gestation (7). The infant, weighing 3100 g (5th percentile) with a length of 53.5 cm (25th–50th percentile), had fused labia with coarse rugations, mild clitoromegaly, and a urogenital sinus opening below the clitoris. An 8-cm mass, eventually shown to be a hydrometrocolpos, was surgically drained because of progressive obstructive uropathy. A balanced somatic chromosomal translocation was an incidental finding in this case, most likely inherited from the mother. Growth and development were normal at 6 months of age with no further masculinization.

Two brief 1982 communications described infants exposed in utero to danazol (8,9). In one, a 2400-g term female infant with ambiguous genitalia had been exposed to danazol (dose not specified) during the first 4 months of pregnancy (8). The infant's phallus measured 0.75 cm and complete posterior labial fusion was observed. The second case involved a woman treated with danazol, 200 mg/day, during the first 6 weeks of gestation, who eventually delivered a female infant with normal external genitalia (9). The absence of virilization of the infant's genitalia, as evidenced by a normal clitoris and no labial fusion, indicates the drug was stopped prior to the onset of fetal sensitivity to androgens.

British investigators reported virilization of the external genitalia consisting of clitoromegaly, a fused, scrotalized labia with a prominent median raphe, and a urogenital sinus in a female infant exposed in utero to danazol, 400 mg/day, during the first 18 weeks of pregnancy (10). The mother showed no signs of virilization.

A summary of known cases of danazol exposure during pregnancy was reported in 1984 by Rosa, an investigator from the epidemiology branch of the FDA (11). A total of 44 cases of pregnancy exposure, all to 800 mg/day, were known as of this date, but this number was considered to be understated since normal outcomes were unlikely to be reported (11). Each of the cases of exposure was thought to have occurred after conception had taken place. Of the 44 cases, 7 (16%) aborted and the outcome in 14 others was unknown. Seven males and 15 females resulted from the 22 pregnancies that had been completed. Ten (67%) of the females had virilization and one male infant had multiple congenital abnormalities (details not given). No cases of virilization were observed when the drug was discontinued prior to the 8th week of gestation, the onset of androgen receptor sensitivity (11).

An Australian case of an infant with masculinized external genitalia secondary to danazol was reported in 1985 (12). The mother had been treated with 400 mg/day, without evidence of virilization, until the 19th week of gestation. The infant was developing normally at 6 months of age, except for a minimally enlarged clitoris, rugose and fused labia with a thick median raphe, and a urogenital sinus opening at the base of the phallus.

A 1985 case report described a female fetus exposed in utero to 800 mg/day of danazol until pregnancy was terminated at 20 weeks' gestation (13). A urogenital sinus was identified in the aborted fetus but the external genitalia were normal except for a single opening in the vulva. Citing a personal communication from the manufacturer, the authors noted a total of 74 cases of danazol exposure during pregnancy (13). Among these cases were 29 term females, 9 (31%) of whom had clitoromegaly and labial fusion.

A retrospective review of fetal exposure to danazol included cases gathered from multiple sources, including individual case reports, data from the Australian Drug Reactions Advisory Committee, the FDA, and direct reports to the manufacturers (14). Of the 129 total pregnancies that were exposed to danazol, 23 were electively terminated and 12 miscarried. Among the 94 completed pregnancies, there were 37 normal males, 34 nonvirilized females, and 23 virilized females. All of the virilized female offspring were exposed beyond 8 weeks' gestation. The lowest daily dose that resulted in virilization was 200 mg.

In a surveillance study of Michigan Medicaid recipients involving 229,101 completed pregnancies conducted between 1985 and 1992, 10 newborns had been exposed to danazol during the 1st trimester (F. Rosa, personal communication, FDA, 1993). No major birth defects were observed.

There is no conclusive evidence of fetal harm when conception occurs in a menstrual cycle shortly after cessation of danazol therapy (15–17). A 1978 publication noted 4 intrauterine fetal deaths occurring from a total of 39 pregnancies following danazol treatment, presumably after elimination of the drug from the mother (18). The stillbirths, two each in the 2nd and 3rd trimesters, occurred in women who had conceived within 0–3 cycles of stopping danazol. However, one of the fetal deaths was due to cord torsion and a second death in a twin was due to placental insufficiency, neither of which can be attributed to danazol.

No long-term follow-up studies of children exposed in utero to danazol have been located. A 1982 reference, however, did describe this type of evaluation in 12 young women, aged 16–27 years, who had been exposed to in utero synthetic androgenic progestins resulting in the virilization of the external genitalia in 11 of them (19). Despite possible virilization of early behavior with characterization as "tomboys" (e.g., increased amounts of "rough-and-tumble play" and "an avid interest in high school sports"), all of the women eventually "displayed stereotypically feminine sexual behavior" without any suggestion of behavior abnormalities (19).

BREASTFEEDING SUMMARY

No reports describing the use of danazol during lactation have been located. Because of the potential for severe adverse effects in a nursing infant, women taking this drug should not breastfeed.

References

1. Product information. Danocrine. Sanofi Pharmaceuticals, 2000.
2. Greenblatt RB, Oettinger M, Borenstein R, Bohler CSS. Influence of danazol (100 mg) on conception and contraception. J Reprod Med 1974;13:201–3.
3. Colle ML, Greenblatt RB. Contraceptive properties of danazol. J Reprod Med 1976;17:98–102.
4. Lauersen NH, Wilson KH. Evaluation of danazol as an oral contraceptive. Obstet Gynecol 1977;50:91–6.
5. Duck SC, Katayama KP. Danazol may cause female pseudohermaphroditism. Fertil Steril 1981;35:230–1.
6. Castro-Magana M, Cheruvanky T, Collipp PJ, Ghavami-Maibodi Z, Angulo M, Stewart C. Transient adrenogenital syndrome due to exposure to danazol in utero. Am J Dis Child 1981;135:1032–4.
7. Peress MR, Kreutner AK, Mathur RS, Williamson HO. Female pseudohermaphroditism with somatic chromosomal anomaly in association with in utero exposure to danazol. Am J Obstet Gynecol 1982;142:708–9.
8. Schwartz RP. Ambiguous genitalia in a term female infant due to exposure to danazol in utero. Am J Dis Child 1982;136:474.
9. Wentz AC. Adverse effects of danazol in pregnancy. Ann Intern Med 1982;96:672–3.
10. Shaw RW, Farquhar JW. Female pseudohermaphroditism associated with danazol exposure in utero. Case report. Br J Obstet Gynecol 1984;91:386–9.
11. Rosa FW. Virilization of the female fetus with maternal danazol exposure. Am J Obstet Gynecol 1984;149:99–100.
12. Kingsbury AC. Danazol and fetal masculinization: a warning. Med J Aust 1985;143:410–1.
13. Quagliarello J, Greco MA. Danazol and urogenital sinus formation in pregnancy. Fertil Steril 1985;43:939–42.
14. Brunskill PJ. The effects of fetal exposure to danazol. Br J Obstet Gynaecol 1992;99:212–5.
15. Daniell JF, Christianson C. Combined laparoscopic surgery and danazol therapy for pelvic endometriosis. Fertil Steril 1981;35:521–5.
16. Fayez JA, Collazo LM, Vernon C. Comparison of different modalities of treatment for minimal and mild endometriosis. Am J Obstet Gynecol 1988;159:927–32.
17. Butler L, Wilson E, Belisle S, Gibson M, Albrecht B, Schiff I, Stillman R. Collaborative study of pregnancy rates following danazol therapy of stage I endometriosis. Fertil Steril 1984;41:373–6.
18. Dmowski WP, Cohen MR. Antigonadotropin (danazol) in the treatment of endometriosis. Evaluation of posttreatment fertility and three-year follow-up data. Am J Obstet Gynecol 1978;130:41–8.
19. Money J, Mathews D. Prenatal exposure to virilizing progestins: an adult follow-up study of twelve women. Arch Sex Behav 1982;11:73–83.

D

DANTHRON

[Withdrawn from the market. See 9th edition.]

DANTROLENE

Muscle Relaxant

PREGNANCY RECOMMENDATION: Limited Human Data—No Relevant Animal Data
BREASTFEEDING RECOMMENDATION: Hold Breastfeeding

PREGNANCY SUMMARY

Dantrolene has been used in a limited number of pregnant patients shortly before delivery. No fetal or newborn adverse effects have been observed, but a risk:benefit ratio has not yet been defined. Moreover, published 1st and 2nd trimester experience with this drug is completely lacking.

FETAL RISK SUMMARY

In obstetrics, the only documented use of dantrolene, a hydantoin derivative used as a direct-acting skeletal muscle relaxant, is to prevent or treat malignant hyperthermia. The syndrome of malignant hyperthermia is a potentially lethal complication of anesthesia induced with halogenated anesthetics and depolarizing skeletal muscle relaxants. References describing the use of dantrolene in pregnant patients for chronic spasticity or during the 1st or 2nd trimesters have not been located. The agent is embryocidal in animals and, in some species, produced minor skeletal variations at the highest dose tested (1–3).

Three studies have described the transfer of dantrolene across the human placenta to the fetus with cord:maternal serum ratios of 0.29–0.69 (4–6). Two women, who were considered to be malignant hyperthermia susceptible (MHS), were treated with oral doses of the drug prior to cesarean section (4). One woman received 100 mg twice daily for 3 days prior to elective induction of labor. The second patient received 150 mg on admission in labor and a second dose of 100 mg 6 hours later. Both women were delivered by cesarean section because of failure to progress in labor. Neither was exposed to malignant hyperthermia-triggering agents and neither developed the complication. The cord and maternal blood concentrations in the two cases were 0.40 and 1.38 mcg/mL (ratio 0.29), and 1.39 and 2.70 mcg/mL (ratio 0.51), respectively. The timing of the doses in relationship to delivery was not specified by the author. No adverse effects of the drug exposure were noted in the infants.

A second report described the prophylactic use of dantrolene, administered as a 1-hour IV infusion (2.2 mg/kg) 7.5 hours prior to vaginal delivery, under epidural anesthesia, of a healthy, vigorous infant (5). The mother had been confirmed to be MHS by previous muscle biopsy. At the time of delivery, the cord and maternal blood dantrolene concentrations were 2.1 and 4.3 mcg/mL, respectively, a ratio of 0.48. The mother did not experience malignant hyperthermia. No respiratory depression or muscle weakness was noted in the newborn.

A study published in 1988 treated 20 pregnant women diagnosed as MHS with oral dantrolene, 100 mg/day, for 5 days prior to delivery and for 3 days following delivery (6). Three of the patients were delivered by cesarean section. Known anesthetic malignant hyperthermia-triggering agents were avoided and no cases of the syndrome were observed. All fetuses had reactive nonstress tests and normal biophysical profiles before and after the onset of dantrolene administration. The mean maternal predelivery dantrolene serum concentration was 0.99 mcg/mL compared with a mean cord blood level of 0.68 mcg/mL, a ratio of 0.69. The mean serum half-life of dantrolene in the newborns was 20 hours (6). Extensive neonatal testing up to 3 days after delivery failed to discover any adverse effects of the drug.

Prophylactic dantrolene, 600 mg given as escalating oral doses over 3 days, was administered to a woman with biopsy-proven MHS 3 days prior to a repeat cesarean section (7). The woman had experienced malignant hyperthermia during her first cesarean section but did not during this surgery. No adverse effects were noted in the newborn.

Although no dantrolene-induced complications have been observed in fetuses or newborns exposed to the drug shortly before birth, some investigators do not recommend prophylactic use of the agent because safety in pregnancy has not been sufficiently documented, and the incidence of malignant hyperthermia in the anesthetized patient is very low (8–10). (A recent reference cited incidences of 1/12,000 anesthesias in children and 1/40,000 in adults (11).) They recommend avoidance of those anesthetic agents that might trigger the syndrome, careful monitoring of the patient during delivery, and preparation to treat the complication if it occurs.

BREASTFEEDING SUMMARY

Dantrolene is excreted into human breast milk. A 37-year-old woman undergoing an urgent cesarean section with general anesthesia (succinylcholine, thiopental, nitric oxide, oxygen, and isoflurane) developed tachycardia, respiratory acidosis, and hyperthermia (12). After delivery of the infant and cord clamping, IV dantrolene (160 mg) was administered. Over the next 3 days, she received decreasing total doses of IV dantrolene: 560 mg on day 1320 mg on day 2, and 80 mg on day 3. The infant was not allowed to nurse during this time. Seven breast milk samples were obtained (volume of milk samples and collection method not specified) over an 84-hour interval after the first dose. Milk concentrations of dantrolene ranged from a maximum of 1.2 mcg/mL (day 2; 36 hours after the first dose with a total dose of 720 mg at the time) to 0.05 mcg/mL on day 3 (total dose 1120 mg received at the time). The estimated elimination half-life from milk was 9.02 hours (12). Thus, waiting 2 days after the last dantrolene dose to breastfeed would assure that the exposure of the nursing infant would be negligible.

References

1. Nagaoka T, Osuka F, Hatano M. Reproductive studies of dantrolene. Teratogenicity study in rabbits. Clinical Report 1977;11:2212–17. As cited in Shepard TH. *Catalog of Teratogenic Agents*. 6th ed. Baltimore, MD: Johns Hopkins University Press, 1989:549.
2. Nagaoka T, Osuka F, Shigemura T, Hatano M. Reproductive test of dantrolene. Teratogenicity test on rats. Clinical Report 1977;11:2218–30. As cited in Shepard TH. *Catalog of Teratogenic Agents*. 6th ed. Baltimore, MD: Johns Hopkins University Press, 1989:549.
3. Product information. Dantrium. Norwich Eaton Pharmaceuticals, 1993.
4. Morison DH. Placental transfer of dantrolene. Anesthesiology 1983;59:265.
5. Glassenberg R, Cohen H. Intravenous dantrolene in a pregnant malignant hyperthermia susceptible (MHS) patient (abstract). Anesthesiology 1984;61:A404.
6. Shime J, Gare D, Andrews J, Britt B. Dantrolene in pregnancy: lack of adverse effects on the fetus and newborn infant. Am J Obstet Gynecol 1988;159:831–4.
7. Cupryn JP, Kennedy A, Byrick RJ. Malignant hyperthermia in pregnancy. Am J Obstet Gynecol 1984;150:327–8.
8. Khalil SN, Williams JP, Bourke DL. Management of a malignant hyperthermia susceptible patient in labor with 2-chloroprocaine epidural anesthesia. Anesth Analg 1983;62:119–21.
9. Kaplan RF, Kellner KR. More on malignant hyperthermia during delivery. Am J Obstet Gynecol 1985;152:608–9.
10. Sorosky JI, Ingardia CJ, Botti JJ. Diagnosis and management of susceptibility to malignant hyperthermia in pregnancy. Am J Perinatol 1989;6:46–8.
11. Sessler DI. Malignant hyperthermia. J Pediatr 1986;109:9–14.
12. Fricker RM, Hoerauf KH, Drewe J, Kress HG. Secretion of dantrolene into breast milk after acute therapy of a suspected malignant hyperthermia crisis during cesarean section. Anesthesiology 1998;89:1023–5.

DAPSONE

Leprostatic/Antimalarial

PREGNANCY RECOMMENDATION: Compatible—Maternal Benefit >> Embryo–Fetal Risk
BREASTFEEDING RECOMMENDATION: Limited Human Data—Potential Toxicity

PREGNANCY SUMMARY

The use of dapsone during pregnancy does not appear to present a major risk to the fetus or the newborn. The agent has been used extensively for malarial treatment or chemoprophylaxis and for the treatment of leprosy and certain other dermatologic conditions without producing major fetotoxicity or causing birth defects. If used in combination with pyrimethamine (a folic acid antagonist) for malaria prophylaxis, folic acid supplements or leucovorin should be given.

FETAL RISK SUMMARY

Dapsone (DDS), a sulfone antibacterial agent, is used in the treatment of leprosy and dermatitis herpetiformis, and for various other unlabeled indications, including antimalarial prophylaxis, the treatment of *Pneumocystis carinii* pneumonia, inflammatory bowel disease, rheumatic and connective tissue disorders, and relapsing polychondritis. Because the drug is known to cause blood dyscrasias in adults, some of which have been fatal, close patient monitoring is required during use.

Although reproduction studies in animals have not been conducted (1), a 1980 reference described a study investigating carcinogenicity that was conducted in pregnant and lactating mice and rats (2). A maximum maternally tolerated dose, 100 mg/kg (usual human dose 50–300 mg/day), was administered twice in late gestation and 5 times a week during lactation and then was continued in the offspring after weaning. A small but significant increase in tumors was noted.

A number of studies have described the use of dapsone during all stages of human pregnancy. A few fetal or newborn adverse effects directly attributable to dapsone have been reported, but no congenital anomalies thought to be due to the drug have been observed. The indications for use of dapsone during pregnancy have included dermatologic conditions, leprosy, malaria, and *P. carinii*.

A brief 1968 reference described Heinz-body hemolytic anemia in a mother and her newborn during therapy with dapsone (3). The mother had been diagnosed with herpes gestationis at 22 weeks' gestation, for which she was treated with sulfapyridine for 1 week. At 26 weeks, treatment with dapsone was begun at 400 mg/day for 1 week, 300 mg/day during weeks 2 and 3, 200 mg/day in week 4, 100 mg/day in week 5, then 200 mg/day until delivery of a male infant at 36 weeks' gestation. She developed well-compensated Heinz-body hemolytic anemia 6 days after starting dapsone. The anemia in the infant, who had a normal glucose-6-phosphate dehydrogenase (G6PD) level, completely resolved within 10 days, and he has remained hematologically normal.

In three cases, dapsone was used for the treatment of dermatitis herpetiformis or its variant, herpes gestationis (4,5). In two other reports of herpes gestationis (also referred to as pemphigoid gestationis) occurring during pregnancy, dapsone was not started until after delivery (6,7). A 26-year-old pregnant woman with recurrent herpes gestationis was treated with dapsone and other nonspecific therapy from the 24th week of gestation until delivery of a normal male infant at 38 weeks (4). A 25-year-old woman with dermatitis herpetiformis was treated with dapsone, 100–150 mg/day, during the first 3 months of pregnancy (5). The drug was discontinued briefly during the 4th month of pregnancy because of concerns of teratogenicity, then resumed at 50 mg/day because of worsening of her disease. She eventually gave birth to a full-term, normal infant who developed dapsone-induced hemolytic anemia while breastfeeding (see Breastfeeding Summary below). A 33-year-old woman, treated with dapsone, 25–50 mg/day, throughout pregnancy for dermatitis herpetiformis delivered a healthy full-term infant (8).

A 1978 paper described the clinical courses of 62 pregnancies in 26 women treated for leprosy (Hansen's disease) (9). All of the patients received therapy, with sulfone drugs (specific drugs not mentioned) being used in 58 (94%) of the pregnancies. Two (3.6%) infants (about the expected rate) among the 56 pregnancies with infants who reached an age of viability had congenital anomalies. One infant had a cleft palate, and another had a congenital hip dislocation. A review, published in 1993, discussed the adverse association of leprosy and pregnancy (10). Although dapsone was not thought to cause adverse toxic effects or teratogenicity in the fetus, resistance to dapsone monotherapy has become a problem, and combination therapy, such as dapsone, clofazimine, and rifampin, is recommended for all forms of leprosy (10). Normal pregnancy outcomes of 15 women treated for leprosy were noted in a 1996 letter (N = 13) (11) and in a 1997 report (N = 2) (12). The patients had been treated throughout gestation with dapsone, 100 mg/day, plus rifampin, 600 mg once monthly (11), or with dapsone alone (12). In addition, two had also received clofazimine, and two had taken intermittent prednisolone (11).

Neonatal hyperbilirubinemia, suspected of being due to displacement of bilirubin from albumin-binding sites, has been attributed to the use of dapsone during gestation (13). A 25-year-old woman with leprosy was treated with dapsone, 300 mg/week, until 3 months before delivery. At that time, her dose was decreased to 50 mg/week and then was discontinued 1 week prior to a normal spontaneous vaginal delivery of a 3740-g male infant. The infant, who was not breastfed and had no evidence of ABO incompatibility, developed hyperbilirubinemia that was attributed to dapsone. In a subsequent pregnancy, dapsone therapy was stopped 1 month prior to delivery of a healthy 4070-g male infant who did not develop hyperbilirubinemia.

The combination of dapsone and pyrimethamine (Maloprim) has been frequently used during pregnancy for the chemoprophylaxis of malaria (14–21). Most consider the benefits of this combination in the prevention of maternal malaria to outweigh the risks to the fetus (16–21), but two authors classified the combination as contraindicated in pregnancy (14,15). The adverse effects of the combination were reviewed in a 1993 reference (22). Because of the potential for significant dose-related toxicity, the authors considered the drug combination to be a second-line choice for use in areas where the risk of malaria was high. Folic acid supplements should be given when pyrimethamine is used (21). (See also Pyrimethamine.)

A study published in 1990 compared chlorproguanil plus dapsone (N =44), chloroquine alone (N = 58), and pyrimethamine plus sulfadoxine (N = 54) in a group of pregnant women with falciparum malaria parasitemia (23). A single dose of chlorproguanil plus dapsone during the 3rd trimester cleared the parasitemia in all women within 1 week, compared with 84% and 94%, respectively, in the other two groups. Six weeks after treatment, the proportion of those with parasitemia in each group was 81%, 84%, and 23%, respectively. No adverse effects of the therapy in the fetuses or newborns were mentioned.

An adverse pregnancy outcome in a mother who received malarial chemoprophylaxis with three drugs was the subject of a brief 1983 communication (24). During the 1st month of pregnancy, the 31-year-old woman had taken chloroquine (100 mg/day) and Maloprim (dapsone 100 mg plus pyrimethamine 12.5 mg) on days 10, 20, and 30 after conception. The stillborn male infant was delivered at 26 weeks' gestation with a defect of the abdominal and thoracic wall with exteriorization of most of the abdominal viscera, the heart, and the lungs (a variant of ectopia cordis?) and a missing left arm. The authors concluded that the defects were due to pyrimethamine, but others have questioned this conclusion (see Pyrimethamine).

Dapsone, either alone or in combination with pyrimethamine or trimethoprim, has been suggested as having utility in the prophylaxis of *P. carinii* during pregnancy (25,26).

Although the efficacy of these therapeutic options has not been confirmed, the risks of the disease to the mother far outweigh the risks to the fetus (26).

A 1992 report described an attempted suicide with dapsone and alcohol in a 29-year-old pregnant woman (length of gestation not specified) under treatment for dermatitis herpetiformis (27). The woman had ingested 50 tablets (100 mg each) of dapsone plus six alcoholic drinks. She developed severe methemoglobinemia and hemolytic anemia, treated successfully with methylene blue (total dose about 7 mg/kg) and other therapy, and splenomegaly that resolved spontaneously. No mention was made of the pregnancy outcome.

Folic acid 5 mg/day or leucovorin 5 mg/week should be used if dapsone is combined with pyrimethamine (a folic acid antagonist) for malaria prophylaxis (21,28).

BREASTFEEDING SUMMARY

Dapsone and its primary metabolite, monoacetyldapsone, are excreted into human milk (5,29,30). A 25-year-old woman with dermatitis herpetiformis was treated with dapsone throughout most of her pregnancy and continued this therapy while breastfeeding her infant (5). During the latter two-thirds of her pregnancy and during lactation she took dapsone, 50 mg/day. Approximately 6 weeks after delivery, mild hemolytic anemia was diagnosed in the mother and her infant. Measurements of dapsone and the metabolite were conducted on the mother's serum and milk and on the infant's serum. Dapsone concentrations were 1622, 1092, and 439 ng/mL, respectively, whereas those of the metabolite were 744 ng/mL, none detected, and 204 ng/mL, respectively. The milk:plasma ratio of dapsone was 0.67. The investigators noted that the weak base properties of dapsone, its high lipid solubility, and its long serum half-life (about 20 hours) all favored excretion and entrapment of the drug in milk (5). Moreover, both the mother and her infant appeared to be rapid acetylator phenotypes because of the relatively high ratios of metabolite to parent drug in both (0.459 in the mother, 0.465 in the infant) (5). Neither patient was tested for G6PD deficiency, although persons with this genetic defect are especially susceptible to dapsone-induced hemolytic anemia. Dose-related hemolytic anemia is the most common toxicity reported with dapsone and occurs in patients with or without G6PD deficiency (1).

A 1952 reference studied the excretion into breast milk of dapsone (diaminodiphenylsulfone) and another sulfone antibacterial agent in one and five women, respectively, with leprosy (29). Although stating that dapsone was excreted in the mother's milk and absorbed and excreted in the infant's urine, the investigator did not quantify the amount in the milk.

Three women, 2–5 days postpartum, who were not breastfeeding, were given a single dose of dapsone (100 mg) plus pyrimethamine (12.5 mg; Maloprim) and a single dose of chloroquine (300 mg base) (30). Milk and serum samples for dapsone analysis were collected at intervals up to 52, 102, and 124 hours, yielding milk:plasma ratios, based on AUC, of 0.38, 0.45, and 0.22, respectively. The authors calculated that the amounts of dapsone excreted into milk, based on 1000 mL/day, were 0.31, 0.85, and 0.59 mg, respectively, which are too small to afford malarial chemoprophylaxis to a nursing infant (30).

Although not citing the case of dapsone-induced hemolytic anemia in a nursing infant described above, the American Academy of Pediatrics classifies dapsone as compatible with breastfeeding (31).

References

1. Product information. Dapsone. Jacobus Pharmaceutical, 1997.
2. Griciute L, Tomatis L. Carcinogenicity of dapsone in mice and rats. Int J Cancer 1980;25:123–9.
3. Hocking DR. Neonatal haemolytic disease due to dapsone. Med J Aust 1968;1:1130–1.
4. Diamond WJ. Herpes gestationis. S Afr Med J 1976;50:739–40.
5. Sanders SW, Zone JJ, Foltz RL, Tolman KG, Rollins DE. Hemolytic anemia induced by dapsone transmitted through breast milk. Ann Intern Med 1982;96:465–6.
6. Sills ES, Mabie WC. A refractory case of herpes gestationis. J Tenn Med Assoc 1992;85:559–60.
7. Kirtschig G, Collier PM, Emmerson RW, Wojnarowska F. Severe case of pemphigoid gestationis with unusual target antigen. Br J Dermatol 1994;131:108–11.
8. Tuffanelli DL. Successful pregnancy in a patient with dermatitis herpetiformis treated with low-dose dapsone. Arch Dermatol 1982;118:876.
9. Maurus JN. Hansen's disease in pregnancy. Obstet Gynecol 1978;52:22–5.
10. Duncan ME. An historical and clinical review of the interaction of leprosy and pregnancy: a cycle to be broken. Soc Sci Med 1993;37:457–72.
11. Bhargava P, Kuldeep CM, Mathur NK. Antileprosy drugs, pregnancy and fetal outcome. Int J Lepr Other Mycobact Dis 1996;64:457.
12. Lyde CB. Pregnancy in patients with Hansen disease. Arch Dermatol 1997;133:623–7.
13. Thornton YS, Bowe ET. Neonatal hyperbilirubinemia after treatment of maternal leprosy. South Med J 1989;82:668.
14. Sturchler D. Malaria prophylaxis in travelers: the current position. Experientia 1984;40:1357–62.
15. Brown GV. Chemoprophylaxis of malaria. Med J Aust 1986;144: 696–702.
16. Anonymous. Prevention of malaria in pregnancy and early childhood. Br Med J 1984;289:1296–7.
17. Greenwood AM, Armstrong JRM, Byass P, Snow RW, Greenwood BM. Malaria chemoprophylaxis, birth weight and child survival. Trans R Soc Trop Med Hyg 1992;86:483–5.
18. Greenwood AM, Menendez C, Todd J, Greenwood BM. The distribution of birth weights in Gambian women who received malaria chemoprophylaxis during their first pregnancy and in control women. Trans R Soc Trop Med Hyg 1994;88:311–2.
19. Menendez C, Todd J, Alonso PL, Lulat S, Francis N, Greenwood BM. Malaria chemoprophylaxis, infection of the placenta and birth weight in Gambian primigravidae. J Trop Med Hyg 1994;97:244–8.
20. Kahn G. Dapsone is safe during pregnancy. J Am Acad Dermatol 1985;13:838–9.
21. Spracklen FHN, Monteagudo FSE. Malaria prophylaxis. S Afr Med J 1986;70:316.
22. Luzzi GA, Peto TEA. Adverse effects of antimalarials. An update. Drug Saf 1993;8:295–311.
23. Keuter M, van Eijk A, Hoogstrate M, Raasveld M, van de Ree M, Ngwawe WA, Watkins WM, Were JBO, Brandling-Bennett AD. Comparison of chloroquine, pyrimethamine and sulfadoxine, and chlorproguanil and dapsone as treatment for falciparum malaria in pregnant and non-pregnant women, Kakamega district, Kenya. Br Med J 1990;301:466–70.
24. Harpey J-P, Darbois Y, Lefebvre G. Teratogenicity of pyrimethamine. Lancet 1983;2:399.
25. Connelly RT, Lourwood DL. *Pneumocystis carinii* pneumonia prophylaxis during pregnancy. Pharmacotherapy 1994;14:424–9.
26. American College of Obstetricians and Gynecologists. Human immunodeficiency virus infections in pregnancy. *Educational Bulletin*. No. 232, January 1997.
27. Erstad BL. Dapsone-induced methemoglobinemia and hemolytic anemia. Clin Pharm 1992;11:800–5.
28. Spracklen FHN. Malaria 1984. Part I. Malaria prophylaxis. S Afr Med J 1984;65:1037–41.
29. Dreisbach JA. Sulphone levels in breast milk of mothers on sulphone therapy. Lepr Rev 1952;23:101–6.
30. Edstein MD, Veenendaal JR, Newman K, Hyslop R. Excretion of chloroquine, dapsone and pyrimethamine in human milk. Br J Clin Pharmacol 1986;22:733–5.
31. Committee on Drugs, American Academy of Pediatrics. The transfer of drugs and other chemicals into human milk. Pediatrics 2001;108:776–89.

DAPTOMYCIN

Antibiotic

PREGNANCY RECOMMENDATION: Limited Human Data—Animal Data Suggest Low Risk
BREASTFEEDING RECOMMENDATION: Limited Human Data—Probably Compatible

D

PREGNANCY SUMMARY

Three reports describing the use of daptomycin in the 2nd and 3rd trimesters have been located. The animal reproduction data suggest low risk, but the limited human pregnancy experience prevents a better assessment of the embryo–fetal risk. However, the high molecular weight should limit exposure of the embryo–fetus. Moreover, most antibiotics can be classified as low risk in gestation. Therefore, if the antibiotic is required, it should not be withheld because of pregnancy.

FETAL RISK SUMMARY

Daptomycin is a cyclic lipopeptide derived from the fermentation of *Streptomyces roseosporus*. It is a bactericidal antibiotic that is administered IV for the treatment of skin and skin structure infections caused by susceptible gram-positive bacteria. Daptomycin is about 92% reversibly bound to plasma proteins, primarily albumin. In patients with normal renal function, the mean elimination half-life is about 9 hours with elimination primarily via the urine. Elimination is prolonged in patients with renal impairment. For example, for patients on dialysis, the elimination half-life is about 30 hours (1).

Reproduction studies have been conducted in pregnant rats and rabbits with IV doses up to three and six times, respectively, the human dose based on BSA (HD). No evidence of fetal harm was observed in these studies (1,2). At the highest dose, maternal toxicity (decreased food consumption and weight) was observed. The no-observed-effect level for maternal toxicity was about one-fourth the maximum dose in both species (2). In male and female rats, doses up to nine times the HD had no effect on fertility (1). Carcinogenicity studies have not been conducted with daptomycin, but neither mutagenic nor clastogenic potential were observed in a number of assays (1).

It is not known if daptomycin crosses the human placenta. The high molecular weight (about 1621) should limit passive transfer across the placenta. However, vancomycin, an antibiotic with a similar spectrum and molecular weight (about 1486), is known to cross the human placenta late in the 2nd trimester to produce detectable concentrations in amniotic fluid and cord blood. (See Vancomycin.)

A 2005 report described a woman in the 3rd trimester who was treated with a 6-week course of IV daptomycin (6 mg/kg/day) for tricuspid valve acute bacterial endocarditis (3). Other antibiotics had failed to clear the methicillin-sensitive *Staphylococcus aureus* infection that was secondary to a peripherally inserted central catheter (PICC) line for hyperalimentation. At the time of the report, the woman was still pregnant.

A case similar to the one above was reported in 2010 (4). The woman presented at 14 weeks' gestation with a history of IV drug abuse and tricuspid valve endocarditis caused by methicillin-sensitive *S. aureus*. She was treated with a 6-week course of IV daptomycin 6 mg/kg/day with resolution of the infection. A cesarean section at 37 weeks' delivered a healthy, about 3.068 kg-male infant with Apgar scores of 8 and 9 at 1 and 5 minutes, respectively (4).

Vancomycin-resistant *Enterococcus faecium* pyelonephritis occurred in a woman at 27 weeks' gestation (5). She also had positive cultures for *Ralstonia pickettii*, methicillin-resistant *S. epidermidis*, and *Enterobacter gergoviae* from blood drawn through a PICC line. The woman was successfully treated with a 14-day course of IV daptomycin 4 mg/kg/day and meropenem 1 g every 8 hours. The woman went into premature labor 1 month after completion of the therapy and delivered a baby without evidence of infection or abnormalities (no other details were provided) (5).

BREASTFEEDING SUMMARY

Daptomycin is excreted into breast milk in very low concentrations (6). A woman nursing her infant 5 months after delivery was treated with a 28-day IV course of daptomycin 6.7 mg/kg/day and ertapenem 1 g/day for a complex case of pelvic inflammatory disease (6). Serial milk concentrations were obtained on day 27. The highest measured concentration was 44.7 ng/mL 8 hours after the dose. The estimated milk:plasma ratio was 0.0012. No adverse effects were noted in the breastfeeding infant (6). A 2009 review briefly summarized this and other cases of anti-infectives used for methicillin-resistant *S. aureus* infections during lactation (7).

The very low concentrations of daptomycin in breast milk are consistent with the high molecular weight (about 1621). Confirmation is needed, however, because vancomycin, an antibiotic with a similar spectrum and molecular weight (about 1486), is excreted into breast milk with concentrations nearly identical to the mother's trough serum concentration. (See Vancomycin.) Since daptomycin must be given IV, systemic absorption by the nursing infant is not expected even if the antibiotic is excreted into milk. However, modification of the infant's bowel flora resulting in diarrhea and other gastrointestinal complaints are potential concerns. Therefore, if a lactating woman requires treatment with the antibiotic, her nursing infant should be closely observed for changes in bowel function.

References

1. Product information. Cubicin. Cubist Pharmaceuticals, 2005.
2. Liu SL, Howard LC, Van Lier RBL, Markham JK. Teratology studies with daptomycin administered intravenously (IV) to rats and rabbits (abstract). Teratology 1988;37:475.
3. Cunha BA, Hamid N, Kessler H, Parchuri S. Daptomycin cure after cefazolin treatment failure of methicillin-sensitive *Staphylococcus aureus* (MSSA)

tricuspid valve acute bacterial endocarditis from a peripherally inserted central catheter (PICC) line. Heart Lung 2005;34:442–7.
4. Stroup JS, Wagner J, Badzinski T. Use of daptomycin in a pregnant patient with *Staphylococcus aureus* endocarditis. Ann Pharmacother 2010;44:746–9.
5. Shea K, Hilburger E, Baroco A, Oldfield E. Successful treatment of vancomycin-resistant *Enterococcus faecium* pyelonephritis with daptomycin during pregnancy. Ann Pharmacother 2008;42:722–5.
6. Buitrago MI, Crompton JA, Bertolami S, North DS, Nathan RA. Extremely low excretion of daptomycin into breast milk of a nursing mother with methicillin-resistant *Staphylococcus aureus* pelvic inflammatory disease. Pharmacotherapy 2009;29:347–51.
7. Mitrano JA, Spooner LM, Belliveau P. Excretion of antimicrobials used to treat methicillin-resistant *Staphylococcus aureus* infections during lactation: safety in breastfeeding infants. Pharmacotherapy 2009;29:1103–9.

DARBEPOETIN ALFA

Hematopoietic

PREGNANCY RECOMMENDATION: Compatible—Maternal Benefit >> Embryo–Fetal Risk
BREASTFEEDING RECOMMENDATION: No Human Data—Probably Compatible

PREGNANCY SUMMARY

Several reports have described the use of darbepoetin alfa in human pregnancy, apparently all ending in normal outcomes. The absence of major toxicity in animals and the experience with epoetin alfa (see Epoetin Alfa) suggest that darbepoetin does not represent a significant embryo or fetal risk. Because anemia and the need for frequent blood transfusions present significant risks to the mother and fetus, the benefits derived from darbepoetin probably outweigh the known risks.

FETAL RISK SUMMARY

Darbepoetin is an erythropoiesis 165-amino acid protein produced by recombinant DNA technology in Chinese hamster ovary cells. It is indicated for the treatment of anemia and is closely related to epoetin alfa. The half-life after SC administration is 49 hours (range 27–89 hours) that is reflective of its slow absorption, whereas after IV administration the terminal half-life is 21 hours.

Reproduction studies have been conducted in pregnant rats and rabbits. No evidence of direct embryotoxic, fetotoxic, or teratogenic effects was observed at IV doses up to 20 mcg/kg/day. (*Note: dose is about 300 times the recommended human dose of 0.45 mcg/kg once weekly based on body weight in patients with chronic renal failure [RHD-CRF] or about 60 times the recommended human dose of 2.25 mcg/kg once weekly based on body weight in cancer patients receiving chemotherapy [RHD-C]*). A slight reduction in fetal weight was observed at doses that were ≥1 mcg/kg/day (*≥15 times RHD-CRF; ≥3 times RHD-C*), but this was a maternal toxic dose. In rats, IV doses of ≥2.5 mcg/kg every other day (*about ≥20 times the RHD-CRF or about ≥4 times the RHD-C*) from day 6 of gestation through day 23 of lactation caused decreased body weights and delayed eye opening and preputial separation. Darbepoetin had no adverse effect on uterine implantation in rats or rabbits. However, an increase in postimplantation fetal loss was observed in rats given doses ≥0.5 mcg/kg three times weekly (*about ≥3 times the RHD-CRF; about ≥0.7 times the RHD-C*) (1).

It is not known if darbepoetin alfa crosses the human placenta. The very high molecular weight (about 37,000) of this glycoprotein argues against transfer across the placenta. A closely related drug, epoetin alfa, has a lower molecular weight (about 30,000) and it does not cross to the fetus. (See Epoetin Alfa.)

A 2005 case report described the use of darbepoetin alfa in a 20-year-old woman at 28 weeks' gestation (2). Darbepoetin was given weekly. She had received a kidney transplant about 4 years earlier and had been maintained on rapamycin and iron therapy until 22 weeks' gestation, at which time the rapamycin was discontinued and replaced with cyclosporine. A cesarean section was performed at 37 weeks' because of fetal distress to deliver a healthy 6-pound (about 2.224 kg) female infant with Apgar scores of 7 and 8 at 1 and 5 minutes, respectively (2).

A 2006 report described two pregnancies that were treated with darbepoetin alfa (3). The women, a 33-year-old with chronic renal failure of unknown cause, and a 31-year-old with insulin-dependent diabetes complicated by hypertension and nephropathy, were treated with weekly doses of darbepoetin alfa from the 22nd and 20th week of gestation, respectively. The first mother gave birth at 37 weeks' to a healthy, 2.010-kg infant (sex not specified) with an Apgar score of 10, whereas the second gave birth by cesarean section at 32 weeks' to a 1.730-kg female infant with Apgar scores of 9 and 10. The status of the first infant was not specified, but the second infant was doing well (3).

A 21-year-old woman with nephrotic syndrome was treated with weekly doses of darbepoetin alfa starting at 26 weeks' (4). Because of worsening renal failure, labor was induced and she gave birth at 36 weeks'. No information of the infant was included in the report.

A 27-year-old woman with HbH disease, an intermediate clinical form of alpha thalassemia, was treated with two doses of epoetin at 15 weeks' then darbepoetin alfa 500 IU every 3 weeks from 16 weeks' until delivery by an emergency cesarean section for fetal distress (umbilical cord around the neck of the fetus) at 38 weeks'. The healthy, 3.13-kg male infant had Apgar scores of 8 and 10 (5).

BREASTFEEDING SUMMARY

No reports describing the use of darbepoetin in human lactation have been located. Darbepoetin is a 165-amino acid glycoprotein with a molecular weight of 37,000. Passage into milk is not expected, but in the event that some transfer did occur, digestion in the nursing infant's gastrointestinal tract would occur. Moreover, preterm infants have been treated with epoetin alfa, a closely related agent. (See Epoetin Alfa.) Thus, the risk to a nursing infant from ingestion of the drug via the milk appears to be nonexistent.

References

1. Product information. Aranesp. Amgen, 2004.
2. Goshom J, Youell TD. Darbepoetin alfa treatment for post-renal transplantation anemia during pregnancy. Am J Kidney Dis 2005;46:e81–6.
3. Sobito-Jarek L, Popowska-Drojecka J, Muszytowski M, Wanic-Kossowska M, Kobelski M, Czekalski S. Anemia treatment with darbepoetin alpha in pregnant female with chronic renal failure: report of two cases. Adv Med Sci 2006;51:309–11.
4. Ghosh A, Ayers KJ. Darbepoetin alfa for treatment of anaemia in a case of chronic renal failure during pregnancy—case report. Clin Exp Obstet Gynecol 2007;34:193–4.
5. Maccio A, Madeddu C, Chessa P, Mantovani G, Galanello R. Use of erythropoiesis stimulating agents for the treatment of anaemia and related fatigue in a pregnant woman with HbH disease. Br J Haematol 2009;146:335–7.

D

DARIFENACIN

Urinary Tract Agent (Antispasmodic)

PREGNANCY RECOMMENDATION: No Human Data—Animal Data Suggest Low Risk
BREASTFEEDING RECOMMENDATION: No Human Data—Probably Compatible

PREGNANCY SUMMARY

No reports describing the use of darifenacin in human pregnancy have been located. The animal reproduction data suggest low risk, but the absence of human pregnancy experience prevents an assessment of the embryo–fetal risk. Thus, the use of darifenacin during pregnancy is not recommended. However, inadvertent exposure appears to represent a low risk of embryo–fetal harm.

FETAL RISK SUMMARY

The anticholinergic agent darifenacin is a competitive muscarinic receptor antagonist available in extended-release tablets. It is indicated for the treatment of overactive bladder with symptoms of urge urinary incontinence, urgency and urinary frequency. It is in the same subclass as flavoxate, oxybutynin, solifenacin, tolterodine, and trospium. Darifenacin is extensively metabolized by the liver to inactive metabolites by the cytochrome P450 isoenzymes CYP2D6 and CYP3A4. Protein binding, primarily to α_1-acid-glycoprotein, is about 98% and the elimination half-life is 13–19 hours (1).

Reproduction studies have been conducted in rats and rabbits. In rats, a dose about 59 times the maximum recommended human dose based on AUC (MRHD) resulted in delayed ossification of the sacral and caudal vertebrae. This effect was not observed at about 13 times the MRHD. Dystocia was observed in dams and slight developmental delay occurred in pups at about 17 times the MRHD. The no-effect dose on dams and pups was about five times the MRHD. In rabbits, a dose about 28 times the MRHD caused increased postimplantation loss, but a dose about nine times the MRHD did not. At 28 times the MRHD, dilated ureter and/or kidney pelvis were observed in offspring. There was also one case of this effect, along with urinary bladder dilation, at nine times the MRHD, an effect consistent with the pharmacological action of darifenacin. The no-effect dose in rabbits was 2.8 times the MRHD.

No evidence of carcinogenicity was observed in studies with mice and rats. Darifenacin was neither mutagenic or clastogenic, and there was no evidence of impaired fertility in male or female rats.

It is not known if darifenacin crosses the human placenta. The molecular weight (about 508) and the long elimination half-life suggest that exposure of the embryo and/or fetus should be expected. However, the extensive metabolism and protein binding will decrease the amount of parent drug available for transfer at the maternal:fetal interface.

BREASTFEEDING SUMMARY

No reports describing the use of darifenacin during human lactation have been located. The molecular weight (about 508) and the long elimination half-life suggest that the drug will be excreted into breast milk, but the extensive metabolism and protein binding should decrease the amount of active drug in milk. The effect of exposure on a nursing infant is unknown. If a mother taking darifenacin is breastfeeding, the infant should be monitored for adverse effect, particularly those involving the gastrointestinal tract (e.g., dry mouth, constipation, abdominal pain, and nausea).

Reference

1. Product information. Enablex. Novartis, 2004.

DARUNAVIR

Antiviral

PREGNANCY RECOMMENDATION: Compatible—Maternal Benefit >> Embryo–Fetal Risk
BREASTFEEDING RECOMMENDATION: Contraindicated

PREGNANCY SUMMARY

Several reports have described the use of darunavir in human pregnancy. The animal data suggest low risk, but the obtainable systemic exposures were very low. If indicated, the drug should not be withheld because of pregnancy.

FETAL RISK SUMMARY

Darunavir is an inhibitor of HIV type 1 (HIV-1) protease. Darunavir, coadministered with 100 mg ritonavir, as well as other antiretroviral agents, is indicated for the treatment of HIV infection in antiretroviral-experienced adult patients, such as those with HIV-1 strains resistant to more than one protease inhibitor. Darunavir and ritonavir are combined because darunavir is primarily metabolized by CYP3A and ritonavir inhibits CYP3A, thereby markedly increasing the plasma concentrations of darunavir (lopinavir and tipranavir are combined with ritonavir for the same reason). The metabolites of darunavir are basically inactive, only having about 10% of the activity of darunavir. Plasma protein binding of darunavir is 95%, mainly to α1-acid glycoprotein. The terminal elimination half-life is about 15 hours when combined with ritonavir (1).

Reproduction studies with darunavir have been conducted mice, rats, and rabbits. No embryotoxicity or teratogenicity was observed in these species with doses producing exposures (AUC) that were about 50%, 50%, and 5%, respectively, of the human exposure obtained with the recommended clinical dose boosted with ritonavir based on AUC. The low exposures in the animals resulted from the limited oral bioavailability of darunavir and/or dosing limitations. Long-term carcinogenicity studies in rodents have not been completed. Assays for mutagenicity and chromosomal damage were negative. There was no effect on fertility in rats (1).

Darunavir crosses the human placenta (2–4). The darunavir umbilical cord plasma:maternal plasma ratios at term in two women taking 600/100 mg (darunavir/ritonavir) twice daily during pregnancy were 0.154 and 0.315 (2). The drug also was detected in cord blood at birth in two other women (3,4). The presence of the drug in fetal blood is consistent with the molecular weight (about 594) and prolonged elimination half-life.

Two case reports described the use of darunavir in two pregnancies beginning at 28 and 30 weeks' gestation (5,6). Both pregnancies ended with births of healthy infants.

The Antiretroviral Pregnancy Registry reported, for the period January 1989 through July 2009, prospective data (reported before the outcomes were known) involving 4702 live births that had been exposed during the 1st trimester to one or more antiretroviral agents (7). Congenital defects were noted in 134, a prevalence of 2.8% (95% confidence interval [CI] 2.4–3.4). In the 6100 live births with earliest exposure in the 2nd/3rd trimesters, there were 153 infants with defects (2.5%, 95% CI 2.1–2.9). The prevalence rates for the two periods did not differ significantly. There were 288 infants with birth defects among 10,803 live births with exposure anytime during pregnancy (2.7%, 95% CI 2.4–3.0). The prevalence rate did not differ significantly from the rate expected in a nonexposed population. There were 51 outcomes exposed to darunavir (31 in the 1st trimester and 20 in the 2nd/3rd trimesters) in combination with other antiretroviral agents. There were two birth defects (two in the 1st trimester and none in the 2nd/3rd trimesters). In reviewing the birth defects of prospective and retrospective (pregnancies reported after the outcomes were known) registered cases, the Registry concluded that, except for isolated cases of neural tube defects with efavirenz exposure in retrospective reports, there was no other pattern of anomalies (isolated or syndromic) (7). (See Lamivudine for required statement.)

In 1998, a public health advisory was issued by the FDA on the association between protease inhibitors and diabetes mellitus (8). Because pregnancy is a risk factor for hyperglycemia, there was concern that these antiretroviral agents would exacerbate this risk. The manufacturer's product information also notes the potential risk for new-onset diabetes, exacerbation of preexisting diabetes, and hyperglycemia in HIV-infected patients receiving protease inhibitor therapy (1). An abstract published in 2000 described the results of a study involving 34 pregnant women treated with protease inhibitors compared with 41 controls that evaluated the association with diabetes (9). No association between protease inhibitors and an increased incidence of gestational diabetes was found.

Two reviews, one in 1996 and the other in 1997, concluded that all women currently receiving antiretroviral therapy should continue to receive therapy during pregnancy and that treatment of the mother with monotherapy should be considered inadequate therapy (10,11). The same conclusion was reached in a 2003 review with the added admonishment that therapy must be continuous to prevent emergence of resistant viral strains (12). In 2009, the updated U.S. Department of Health and Human Services guidelines for the use of antiretroviral agents in HIV-1-infected patients continued the recommendation that therapy, with the exception of efavirenz, should be continued during pregnancy (13). If indicated, therefore, protease inhibitors, including darunavir, should not be withheld in pregnancy because the expected benefit to the HIV-positive mother outweighs the unknown risk to the fetus. Pregnant women taking protease inhibitors should be monitored for hyperglycemia. Updated guidelines for the use of antiretroviral drugs to reduce perinatal HIV-1 transmission also were released in 2010 (14). Women receiving antiretroviral therapy during pregnancy should continue the therapy, but, regardless of the regimen, zidovudine administration is recommended during the intrapartum period to prevent vertical transmission of HIV to the newborn (14).

BREASTFEEDING SUMMARY

No reports describing the use of darunavir during lactation have been located. The molecular weight (about 594) and prolonged elimination half-life (about 15 hours) suggest that the drug will be excreted into breast milk. The effect on a nursing infant is unknown.

Reports on the use of darunavir during human lactation are unlikely because the antiviral agent is used in the treatment of HIV infections. HIV-1 is transmitted in milk, and in developed countries, breastfeeding is not recommended (10,11,13,15–17). In developing countries, breastfeeding is undertaken, despite the risk, because there are no affordable milk substitutes available. Until 1999, no studies had been published that examined the effect of any antiretroviral therapy on HIV-1 transmission in milk. In that year, a study involving zidovudine was published that measured a 38% reduction in vertical transmission of HIV-1 infection despite breastfeeding when compared with controls (see Zidovudine).

References

1. Product information. Prezista. Tibotec Therapeutics, 2007.
2. Ripamonti D, Cattaneo D, Cortinovis M, Maggiolo F, Suter F. Transplacental passage of ritonavir-boosted darunavir in two pregnant women. Int J STD Aids 2009;20:215–6.
3. Furco A, Gosrani B, Nicholas S, Williams A, Braithwaite W, Pozniak A, Taylor G, Asboe D, Lyall H, Shaw A, Kapembwa M. Successful use of darunavir, etravirine, enfuvirtide and tenofovir/emtricitabine in pregnant woman with multiclass HIV resistance. AIDS 2009;23:434–5.
4. Pinnetti C, Tamburrini E, Ragazzoni E, De Luca A, Navarra P. Decreased plasma levels of darunavir/ritonavir in a vertically infected pregnant woman carrying multiclass-resistant HIV type-1. Antivir Ther 2010;15:127–9.
5. Sued O, Lattner J, Gun A, Patterson P, Abusamra L, Cesar C, Fink V, Krolewiecki A, Cahn P. Use of darunavir and enfuvirtide in a pregnant woman. Int J STD Aids 2008;19:866–7.
6. Pacanowski J, Bollens D, Poirier JM, Morand-Joubert L, Castaigne V, Girard PM, Meyohas MC. Efficacy of darunavir despite low plasma trough levels during late pregnancy in an HIV-hepatitis C virus-infected patient. AIDS 2009;23:1923–4.
7. Antiretroviral Pregnancy Registry Steering Committee. *Antiretroviral Pregnancy Registry International Interim Report for 1 January 1989 through 31 July 2009*. Wilmington, NC: Registry Coordinating Center, 2009. Available at www.apregistry.com. Accessed May 29, 2010.
8. CDC. Public Health Service Task Force recommendations for the use of antiretroviral drugs in pregnant women infected with HIV-1 for maternal health and for reducing perinatal HIV-1 transmission in the United States. MMWR 1998;47:No. RR-2.
9. Fassett M, Kramer F, Stek A. Treatment with protease inhibitors in pregnancy is not associated with an increased incidence of gestational diabetes (abstract). Am J Obstet Gynecol 2000;182:S97.
10. Carpenter CCJ, Fischi MA, Hammer SM, Hirsch MS, Jacobsen DM, Katzenstein DA, Montaner JSG, Richman DD, Saag MS, Schooley RT, Thompson MA, Vella S, Yeni PG, Volberding PA. Antiretroviral therapy for HIV infection in 1996. JAMA 1996;276;146–54.
11. Minkoff H, Augenbraun M. Antiretroviral therapy for pregnant women. Am J Obstet Gynecol 1997;176:478–89.
12. Minkoff H. Human immunodeficiency virus infection in pregnancy. Obstet Gynecol 2003;101:797–810.
13. Panel on Antiretroviral Guidelines for Adults and Adolescents. *Guidelines for the Use of Antiretroviral Agents in HIV-1-Infected Adults and Adolescents*. Department of Health and Human Services. December 1, 2009:1–161. Available at http://www.aidsinfo.nih.gov/ContentFiles/AdultandAdolescentGL.pdf. Accessed September 17, 2010:60, 96–8.
14. Panel on Treatment of HIV-Infected Pregnant Women and Prevention of Perinatal Transmission. *Recommendations for Use of Antiretroviral Drugs in Pregnant HIV-1-Infected Women for Maternal Health and Interventions to Reduce Perinatal HIV Transmission in the United States*. May 24, 2010:1–117. Available at http://aidsinfo.nih.gov/ContentFiles/PerinatalGL.pdf. Accessed September 17, 2010:30, 39–44 (Table 5).
15. Brown ZA, Watts DH. Antiviral therapy in pregnancy. Clin Obstet Gynecol 1990;33:276–89.
16. De Martino M, Tovo P-A, Pezzotti P, Galli L, Massironi E, Ruga E, Floreea F, Plebani A, Gabiano C, Zuccotti GV. HIV-1 transmission through breast-milk: appraisal of risk according to duration of feeding. AIDS 1992;6:991–7.
17. Van de Perre P. Postnatal transmission of human immunodeficiency virus type 1: the breast feeding dilemma. Am J Obstet Gynecol 1995;173:483–7.

DASATINIB

Antineoplastic (Tyrosine Kinase Inhibitor)

PREGNANCY RECOMMENDATION: Contraindicated
BREASTFEEDING RECOMMENDATION: Contraindicated

PREGNANCY SUMMARY

The limited human experience involves therapy that was started before conception and then discontinued when pregnancy was diagnosed. The data are too limited to assess the embryo–fetal risk. There are human pregnancy data for imatinib, a drug in the same subclass and with the same mechanism of action as dasatinib. (See Imatinib.) Agents in this subclass inhibit angiogenesis, a critical component of embryonic and fetal development. Women of childbearing potential should use adequate contraception to prevent pregnancy. However, leukemia can be fatal, so if a woman requires dasatinib and informed consent is obtained, treatment should not be withheld because of pregnancy. If an inadvertent pregnancy occurs, the woman should be advised of the potential risk for severe adverse effects in the embryo and fetus.

FETAL RISK SUMMARY

Dasatinib is an oral tyrosine kinase inhibitor that inhibits tumor growth, pathologic angiogenesis, and metastatic progression of cancer. There are several other agents in this antineoplastic subclass (see Appendix). Dasatinib is indicated for the treatment of adults with chronic, accelerated, or myeloid or lymphoid blast-phase chronic myeloid leukemia with resistance or intolerance to prior therapy including imatinib. It is extensively metabolized in the liver. One of the metabolites has activity that is equipotent to dasatinib. The exposure of the active metabolite is about 5% of the dasatinib AUC. The mean plasma elimination half-life is 3–5 hours. Elimination is primarily in the feces. The binding of dasatinib and the active metabolite by human plasma proteins is high, about 96% and 93%, respectively (1).

Reproduction studies have been conducted in rats and rabbits. In pregnant rats and rabbits, the lowest doses tested produced maternal AUCs that were 0.3 and 0.1 times, respectively, the human AUC in females at the recommended dose of 70 mg twice daily. At this dose, fetal death was observed in rats. Other embryo–fetal toxicities included skeletal malformations at multiple sites (scapula, humerus, femur, radius, ribs, and clavicle), reduced ossification (sternum; thoracic, lumbar, and sacral vertebrae; forepaw phalanges; pelvis; and hyoid body), edema, and microhepatia (1).

Studies for carcinogenicity and effects on sperm counts, function, and fertility have not been conducted. Dasatinib was not mutagenic or genotoxic in tests, but was clastogenic in one test, with and without metabolic activation (1).

It is not known if dasatinib crosses the human placenta. The molecular weight (about 486 for the nonhydrated form) is low enough, but the short plasma elimination half-life and high plasma protein binding should limit the amount crossing to the embryo–fetus. However, the drug has a very high volume of distribution, suggesting that it is extensively distributed into extravascular space (1).

A 2010 case report described a woman who was being treated with dasatinib (80 mg/day) for chronic myeloid leukemia (2). An unplanned pregnancy occurred and the drug was discontinued about 8 weeks after conception. Treatment was changed to interferon alfa (9 million IU/day). At 33 weeks' gestation, a cesarean section delivered a healthy, 2.1-kg male infant with an Apgar score of 9 at 10 minutes. No malformations were evident and the infant's growth and development were normal through 8 months of age (2).

The authors of the above report also cited a study that had been presented at a scientific meeting (3). Of eight women exposed to dasatinib during early pregnancy, two had spontaneous abortions, three had elective abortions, and three delivered apparently normal infants (3).

BREASTFEEDING SUMMARY

No reports describing the use of dasatinib during human lactation have been located. The molecular weight (about 486 for the nonhydrated form) of the parent compound is low enough, but the short plasma elimination half-lives of dasatinib and its active metabolite and the high plasma protein binding should limit the amounts excreted into breast milk. The risk to a nursing infant is unknown, but there is potential for severe toxicity affecting multiple systems.

References

1. Product information. Sprycel. Bristol-Myers Squibb, 2007.
2. Conchon M, Sanabani SS, Serpa M, Novaes MMY, Nardinelli L, Ferreira PB, Dorliac-Llacer PE, Bendit I. Successful pregnancy and delivery in a patient with chronic myeloid leukemia while on dasatinib therapy. Adv Hematol 2010:136252 [Epub 2010 Mar 7].
3. Cortes J, O'Brien S, Ault P, Borthakur G, Jabbour E, Bradley-Garelik B, Debreczeni K, Yang D, Liu D, Kantarjian H. Pregnancy outcomes among patients with chronic myeloid leukemia treated with dasatinib. Blood 2008;112:Abstract No. 3230. As cited by Conchon M, Sanabani SS, Serpa M, Novaes MMY, Nardinelli L, Ferreira PB, Dorliac-Llacer PE, Bendit I. Successful pregnancy and delivery in a patient with chronic myeloid leukemia while on dasatinib therapy. Adv Hematol 2010:136252 [Epub 2010 Mar 7].

DAUNORUBICIN

Antineoplastic

PREGNANCY RECOMMENDATION: Human and Animal Data Suggest Risk
BREASTFEEDING RECOMMENDATION: Contraindicated

PREGNANCY SUMMARY

Human exposures to daunorubicin during organogenesis are too limited to assess the risk magnitude for congenital defects. Bone marrow suppression, a common toxicity in adults receiving the drug, is a potential fetal complication.

FETAL RISK SUMMARY

Daunorubicin is a cytotoxic antibiotic used as an antineoplastic agent. It is indicated, in combination with other approved anticancer drugs, for remission induction in acute nonlymphocytic leukemia (myelogenous, monocytic, erythroid) of adults and for remission induction in acute lymphocytic leukemia in children and adults. It is in the same antineoplastic subclass of anthracyclines as doxorubicin, epirubicin, idarubicin, and valrubicin (1).

In animal reproduction studies, exposure to daunorubicin during pregnancy produced teratogenic and toxic effects in rabbits, rats, and mice (1). In rabbits, a dose that was about 0.01 times the maximum recommended human dose based on BSA (MRHD) resulted in an increased incidence of abortions and fetal anomalies (parieto-occipital cranioschisis, umbilical hernias, or rachischisis). Malformations in rats administered doses about 0.5 times the MRHD included esophageal, cardiovascular, and urogenital malformations, as well as fused ribs. Restricted fetal and neonatal growth was observed in mice after maternal administration of daunorubicin (1).

The use of daunorubicin during pregnancy has been reported in 29 patients, four during the 1st trimester (2–19). No congenital defects were observed in the 22 (one set of twins) liveborns, but one of these infants was anemic and hypoglycemic and had multiple serum electrolyte abnormalities (8). Two infants had transient neutropenia at 2 months of age (4). Severe, transient, drug-induced bone marrow hypoplasia occurred in one newborn after in utero exposure to daunorubicin and five other antineoplastic agents (18). The myelosuppression may have been secondary to mercaptopurine, but bone marrow suppression also is a toxic effect of daunorubicin. The infant made an uneventful recovery. Results of the remaining pregnancies were three elective abortions (one with enlarged spleen), three intrauterine deaths (one probably due to severe pregnancy-induced hypertension), one stillborn with diffuse myocardial necrosis, and one maternal death (8,9,15,17). Thirteen of the infants (including one set of twins) were studied for periods ranging from 6 months to 9 years and all showed normal growth and development (4,9–11,14,15,17–19).

Data from one review indicated that 40% of the infants exposed to anticancer drugs were of low birth weight (20). This finding was not related to timing of the exposure. Except for the infants noted above, long-term studies of growth and mental development in offspring exposed to daunorubicin during the 2nd trimester, the period of neuroblast multiplication, have not been conducted (21).

In one report, the use of daunorubicin and other antineoplastic drugs in two males was thought to be associated with congenital defects in their offspring (22). The defects observed were tetralogy of Fallot and syndactyly of the first and second digits of the right foot, and an anencephalic stillborn. Although the authors speculated that the drugs damaged the germ cells without producing infertility and thus were responsible for the defects, any relationship to paternal use of daunorubicin is doubtful due to the lack of experimental evidence and other confirming reports. In a third male, fertilization occurred during treatment with daunorubicin and resulted in the birth of a healthy infant (23). Successful pregnancies have also been reported in two women after treatment with daunorubicin (24).

Chromosomal aberrations were observed in the fetus of a 34-year-old woman with acute lymphoblastic leukemia who was treated with multiple antineoplastic agents (12). Daunorubicin was administered for approximately 3 weeks beginning at 22 weeks' gestation. A healthy female infant was delivered 18 weeks after the start of therapy. Chromosomal analysis of the newborn revealed a normal karyotype (46,XX) but with gaps and a ring chromosome. The clinical significance of these findings is unknown, but since these abnormalities may persist for several years, the potential existed for an increased risk of cancer as well as for a risk of genetic damage in the next generation (12).

Occupational exposure of the mother to antineoplastic agents during pregnancy may present a risk to the fetus. A position statement from the National Study Commission on Cytotoxic Exposure and a research article involving some antineoplastic agents are presented in the monograph for cyclophosphamide (see Cyclophosphamide).

BREASTFEEDING SUMMARY

No reports describing the use of daunorubicin during lactation have been located. Because of the potential for severe toxicity in a nursing infant, the use of this agent is contraindicated during breastfeeding.

References

1. Product information. Cerubidine. Bedford Laboratories, 1999.
2. Sears HF, Reid J. Granulocytic sarcoma: local presentation of a systemic disease. Cancer 1976;37:1808–13.
3. Lilleyman JS, Hill AS, Anderton KJ. Consequences of acute myelogenous leukemia in early pregnancy. Cancer 1977;40:1300–3.
4. Colbert N, Najman A, Gorin NC, Blum F. Acute leukaemia during pregnancy: favourable course of pregnancy in two patients treated with cytosine arabinoside and anthracyclines. Nouv Presse Med 1980;9:175–8.
5. Tobias JS, Bloom HJG. Doxorubicin in pregnancy. Lancet 1980;1:776.
6. Sanz MA, Rafecas FJ. Successful pregnancy during chemotherapy for acute promyelocytic leukemia. N Engl J Med 1982;306:939.
7. Alegre A, Chunchurreta R, Rodriguez-Alarcon J, Cruz E, Prada M. Successful pregnancy in acute promyelocytic leukemia. Cancer 1982;49:152–3.
8. Gililand J, Weinstein L. The effects of cancer chemotherapeutic agents on the developing fetus. Obstet Gynecol Surv 1983;38:6–13.
9. Feliu J, Juarez S, Ordonez A, Garcia-Paredes ML, Gonzalez-Baron M, Montero JM. Acute leukemia and pregnancy. Cancer 1988;61:580–4.
10. Volkenandt M, Buchner T, Hiddemann W, Van De Loo J. Acute leukaemia during pregnancy. Lancet 1987;2:1521–2.
11. Turchi JJ, Villasis C. Anthracyclines in the treatment of malignancy in pregnancy. Cancer 1988;61:435–40.
12. Schleuning M, Clemm C. Chromosomal aberrations in a newborn whose mother received cytotoxic treatment during pregnancy. N Engl J Med 1987;317:1666–7.
13. Gokal R, Durrant J, Baum JD, Bennett MJ. Successful pregnancy in acute monocytic leukaemia. Br J Cancer 1976;34:299–302.
14. Lowenthal RM, Marsden KA, Newman NM, Baikie MJ, Campbell SN. Normal infant after treatment of acute myeloid leukaemia in pregnancy with daunorubicin. Aust NZ J Med 1978;8:431–2.
15. O'Donnell R, Costigan C, O'Connell LG. Two cases of acute leukaemia in pregnancy. Acta Haematol 1979;61:298–300.
16. Hamer JW, Beard MEJ, Duff GB. Pregnancy complicated by acute myeloid leukaemia. NZ Med J 1979;89:212–3.
17. Doney KC, Kraemer KG, Shepard TH. Combination chemotherapy for acute myelocytic leukemia during pregnancy: three case reports. Cancer Treat Rep 1979;63:369–71.
18. Okun DB, Groncy PK, Sieger L, Tanaka KR. Acute leukemia in pregnancy: transient neonatal myelosuppression after combination chemotherapy in the mother. Med Pediatr Oncol 1979;7:315–9.
19. Cantini E, Yanes B. Acute myelogenous leukemia in pregnancy. South Med J 1984;77:1050–2.
20. Nicholson HO. Cytotoxic drugs in pregnancy: review of reported cases. J Obstet Gynaecol Br Commonw 1968;75:307–12.
21. Dobbing J. Pregnancy and leukaemia. Lancet 1977;1:1155.
22. Russell JA, Powles RL, Oliver RTD. Conception and congenital abnormalities after chemotherapy of acute myelogenous leukaemia in two men. Br Med J 1976;1:1508.
23. Matthews JH, Wood JK. Male fertility during chemotherapy for acute leukemia. N Engl J Med 1980;303:1235.
24. Estiu M. Successful pregnancy in leukaemia. Lancet 1977;1:433.

DECAMETHONIUM

[Withdrawn from the market. See 8th edition.]

D

DECITABINE

Antineoplastic

PREGNANCY RECOMMENDATION: No Human Data—Animal Data Suggest Risk
BREASTFEEDING RECOMMENDATION: Contraindicated

PREGNANCY SUMMARY

No reports describing the use of decitabine in human pregnancy have been located. The animal reproduction data at a small fraction of the human dose suggest risk, but the absence of human pregnancy experience prevents a more complete assessment of embryo–fetal risk. Pregnant women should not be given this drug, especially in the 1st trimester. If an inadvertent pregnancy occurs, the woman should be advised of the potential risk for severe adverse effects in the embryo and fetus. In addition, because of the animal fertility studies, men should be advised not to father a child while receiving decitabine and for 2 months after treatment (1).

FETAL RISK SUMMARY

Decitabine is an analog of the natural nucleoside 2′-deoxycytidine that is administered by IV infusion every 8 hours for 3 days, and then repeated 6 weeks for at least four cycles. It is in the same antineoplastic subclass as azacitidine and nelarabine. Decitabine is indicated for the treatment of patients with myelodysplastic syndromes (MDS) including previously treated and untreated, de novo and secondary MDS of all French-American-British subtypes (refractory anemia, refractory anemia with ringed sideroblasts, refractory anemia with excess blasts, refractory anemia with excess blasts in transformation, and chronic myelomonocytic leukemia) and Intermediate-1, Intermediate-2, and High-Risk International Prognostic Scoring System groups (1). The metabolic fate of decitabine is not known, but the terminal-phase half-life is about 0.5 hours. Plasma protein binding is <1% (1).

Reproduction studies have been conducted in mice and rats. In pregnant mice, a single intraperitoneal (IP) dose, given on gestational days 8, 9, 10, or 11, that was 2% of the daily recommended clinical dose based on BSA (DRCD) was associated with reduced fetal weight and supernumerary ribs. A dose that was about 7% of the DRCD caused reduced fetal weight, fetal death, and defects (supernumerary ribs, fused vertebrae and ribs, cleft palate, vertebral defects, hindlimb defects, and digital defects of fore- and hindlimbs). Moreover, when the 7% dose was given on gestational day 10, body weights of offspring were significantly reduced at all postnatal time points. Neither the 2% nor 7% doses caused maternal toxicity (1).

In pregnant rats, single IP doses, given on gestational days 9–12, that were about 5%, 8%, or 13% of the DRCD, respectively, were not maternal toxic but did cause developmental toxicity. There were no surviving fetuses with any dose given on day 9. A dose that was ≥8% of the DRCD given on day 10 caused a significant decrease in fetal survival and reduced fetal weight. Dose-related malformations also were observed: Increased incidences of vertebral and rib anomalies (all dose levels); fore-digit defects (doses ≥8% of the DRCD); and exophthalmia, exencephaly, and cleft palate (13% of the DRCD). The highest dose also was associated with reduced size and ossification of the long bones in the limbs (1).

Studies for carcinogenicity have not been conducted with decitabine, but the drug was mutagenic and caused chromosomal rearrangements in larvae of fruit flies. Fertility tests have been conducted in mice. Untreated female mice, when mated with males exposed in utero had decreased fertility. No adverse effects on survival, body weight gain, or hematological measurements were observed in male mice given IP doses that were about 0.3% to 1% of the DRCD 3 times a week for 7 weeks. However, a dose about 0.7% of the DRCD was associated with reduced testes weight, abnormal histology, and significant decreases in sperm count. In female mice mated with these males, pregnancy rates were reduced and postimplantation loss was significantly increased (1).

It is not known if decitabine crosses the human placenta. The molecular weight (about 228) and lack of plasma protein binding suggest that the drug will cross, but the very short terminal phase half-life will limit the amount of drug at the maternal: fetal interface.

BREASTFEEDING SUMMARY

No reports describing the use of decitabine during human lactation have been located.

The molecular weight (about 228) and lack of plasma protein binding suggest that the drug will be excreted into breast milk, but the very short terminal-phase half-life will limit the amount excreted. The effect of this exposure on a nursing infant is unknown, but the potential toxicity may be severe. In adults, the most common adverse effects are neutropenia, thrombocytopenia, anemia, fatigue, pyrexia, nausea, cough, petechiae, constipation, diarrhea, and hyperglycemia (1).

Reference

1. Product information. Dacogen. MGI Pharma, 2007.

DEFERASIROX

Antidote/Chelating Agent

PREGNANCY RECOMMENDATION: Limited Human Data—Animal Data Suggest Low Risk
BREASTFEEDING RECOMMENDATION: No Human Data—Potential Toxicity

PREGNANCY SUMMARY

Three reports describing the use of deferasirox in human pregnancy have been located (1–3). Doses that were very low in comparison with the human dose were used in the animal studies, presumably because higher doses were maternally toxic. The lack of fetal harm in these studies suggests that the risk in human pregnancy is low, but the limited human pregnancy experience prevents a more complete assessment. Another iron-chelating agent, deferoxamine, has been used in pregnancy without any evidence of fetal toxicity (see Deferoxamine).

FETAL RISK SUMMARY

Deferasirox is an oral iron-chelating agent indicated for the treatment of chronic iron overload due to blood transfusions. Although the affinity for zinc and copper is much lower, deferasirox also may lower serum concentrations of these metals. The absolute oral bioavailability is 70%, and the drug accumulates after multiple doses. Protein binding, almost exclusively to albumin, is very high (99%). Elimination of deferasirox and its metabolites is primarily by excretion in the feces, with an elimination half-life of 8–16 hours (4).

Reproduction studies have been conducted in rats and rabbits. No evidence of impaired fertility or fetal harm was observed in these species with oral doses up to about 0.8 times the recommended human dose based on BSA (RHD). No effects on fertility and reproductive performance were observed in male and female rats at doses up to about 0.6 times the RHD. Studies for carcinogenicity and mutagenicity also were negative (4).

It is not known if deferasirox crosses the human placenta. The molecular weight (about 373) and long elimination half-life suggest that exposure of the embryo and/or fetus will occur, but the very high protein binding should limit the exposure.

Three case reports have described the use of deferasirox in pregnant women with thalassemia (1–3). In each case, the drug was started before conception and continued until pregnancy was diagnosed at 22, 20, and 12 weeks'. No abnormalities related to the exposure were observed in the normal newborns (1–3).

BREASTFEEDING SUMMARY

No reports describing the use of deferasirox during human lactation have been located. The molecular weight (about 373) and long elimination half-life (8–16 hours) suggest that the drug will be excreted into breast milk. The amount of oral absorption in an infant is unknown. However, in adults, the absolute oral bioavailability is 70%, and the drug accumulates after multiple doses (4). The recommended therapy with deferasirox is very long (months), and such therapy during breastfeeding might deplete the infant's iron stores. Therefore, if the mother is taking deferasirox, the safest course is not to breastfeed.

References

1. Vini D, Servos P, Drosou M. Normal pregnancy in a patient with β-thalassaemia major receiving iron chelation therapy with deferasirox (Exjade). Eur J Haematol 2011;86:274–5.
2. Anastasi S, Lisi R, Abbate G, Caruso V, Giovannini M, De Sanctis V. Absence of teratogenicity of deferasirox treatment during pregnancy in a thalassaemic patient. Pediatr Endocrinol Rev 2011;8(Suppl 2):345–7.
3. Ricchi P, Costantini S, Spasiano A, Di Matola T, Cinque P, Prossomariti L. A case of well-tolerated and safe deferasirox administration during the first trimester of a spontaneous pregnancy in advanced maternal age thalassemic patient. Acta Haematol 2011;125:222–4.
4. Product information. Exjade. Novartis Pharmaceutical, 2005.

DEFEROXAMINE

Antidote/Chelating Agent

PREGNANCY RECOMMENDATION: Compatible
BREASTFEEDING RECOMMENDATION: No Human Data—Probably Compatible

PREGNANCY SUMMARY

Deferoxamine produces toxicity and teratogenicity in various animal species. Although the number of published human pregnancy exposures to deferoxamine is limited, none of the reports have observed adverse human developmental effects. In one the reports discussed, the authors reviewed over 65 cases of human pregnancy exposure to the agent that occurred during the management of thalassemia or iron overdose (1). No toxic or teratogenic effects were documented. A 1998 review of metal-chelating agents also failed to find any published evidence of human developmental toxicity (2).

D

FETAL RISK SUMMARY

Deferoxamine is used for the treatment of acute iron intoxication and chronic iron overload. Animal reproduction studies have shown delayed ossification in mice and skeletal anomalies in rabbits with daily doses up to 4.5 times the maximum daily human dose. No fetal adverse effects were observed in rats administered similar doses (3).

In another animal reproduction study, pregnant mice were administered intraperitoneal doses of deferoxamine (44, 88, 176, and 352 mg/kg/day) on gestational days 6 through 15. On a weight basis, the lower two doses are comparable to the therapeutic human dose. The no-observed-adverse-effect-level (NOAEL) for maternal toxicity (reduced body weight) was <44 mg/kg/day, whereas the NOAEL for fetal developmental toxicity was 176 mg/kg/day. The only fetal toxic effect was a decrease in the number of live fetuses that was observed at 352 mg/kg/day (4).

A number of reports have described the use of deferoxamine in human pregnancy either for acute iron overdose or for transfusion-dependent thalassemia (1,5–9). A brief mention of three other pregnant patients treated with deferoxamine for acute overdose appeared in an earlier report, but no details were given except that all of the infants were normal (10). The authors have knowledge of a seventh patient treated in the 3rd trimester for overdose with normal outcome (S.M. Lovett, unpublished data, 1985).

In a thalassemia patient, deferoxamine was given by continuous subcutaneous infusion pump, 2 g every 12 hours, for the first 16 weeks of pregnancy (5). A cesarean section was performed at 33 weeks' gestation for vaginal bleeding and premature rupture of the membranes, with delivery of a normal preterm male infant. The neonatal period was complicated by hypoglycemia and prolonged jaundice lasting 6 weeks, but neither problem was thought to be related to deferoxamine. A 1999 report described the use of deferoxamine in an 18-year-old pregnant woman with hemoglobin E beta zero thalassemia, chronic hepatitis C, and iron overload (1). She conceived while receiving an SC dose of 40 mg/kg 4 days/week plus an additional 50-mg/kg IV every month with a transfusion. Therapy was stopped when the pregnancy was diagnosed, but then was restarted at 18 weeks' gestation because of increased iron accumulation. The dose was increased in increments in response to her high ferritin levels, eventually reaching a 50-mg/kg/day IV dose. She delivered an approximately 2298-g, normal male infant at 38 weeks' gestation. The boy was developing normally at 10 months of age and no toxic effects on bone formation, the auditory system, or the ocular system were found (1).

Several pregnant women have received deferoxamine therapy for iron overdose that occurred at 15–38 weeks' gestation (6–9). The women were treated with IM deferoxamine, and one also received the drug nasogastrically. Spontaneous labor with rupture of the membranes occurred 8 hours after iron ingestion in a 34-week gestation patient, resulting in the vaginal delivery 6 hours later of a normal male infant (6). The cord blood iron level was 121 mcg/dL (normal 106–227 mcg/dL) but fell to 21 mcg/dL at 12 hours. The infant's clinical course was normal except for low iron levels requiring iron supplementation. The authors suggested that the low neonatal iron levels were due to chelation of iron by transplacentally transferred deferoxamine. In another case, a normal-term male infant was delivered without evidence of injury from deferoxamine (6). Normal infants were delivered also in the other two cases, both at times distant from the use of deferoxamine (8,9).

BREASTFEEDING SUMMARY

No reports describing the use of deferoxamine in lactation have been located. The molecular weight (about 657) is low enough that some excretion into breast milk probably occurs. The effects, if any, on a nursing infant from this exposure are unknown.

References

1. Singer ST, Vichinsky EP. Deferoxamine treatment during pregnancy: is it harmful? Am J Hematol 1999;60:24–6.
2. Domingo JL. Developmental toxicity of metal chelating agents. Reprod Toxicol 1998;12:499–510.
3. Product information. Desferal. Novartis Pharmaceuticals, 2000.
4. Bosque MA, Domingo JL, Corbella J. Assessment of the developmental toxicity of deferoxamine in mice. Arch Toxicol 1995;69:467–71.
5. Thomas RM, Skalicka AE. Successful pregnancy in transfusion-dependent thalassaemia. Arch Dis Child 1980;55:572–4.
6. Rayburn WF, Donn SM, Wulf ME. Iron overdose during pregnancy: successful therapy with deferoxamine. Am J Obstet Gynecol 1983;147:717–8.
7. Blanc P, Hryhorczuk D, Danel I. Deferoxamine treatment of acute iron intoxication in pregnancy. Obstet Gynecol 1984;64:12S–4S.
8. Van Ameyde KJ, Tenenbein M. Whole bowel irrigation during pregnancy. Am J Obstet Gynecol 1989;160:646–7.
9. Lacoste H, Goyert GL, Goldman LS, Wright DJ, Schwartz DB. Acute iron intoxication in pregnancy: case report and review of the literature. Obstet Gynecol 1992;80:500–1.
10. Strom RL, Schiller P, Seeds AE, Ten Bensel R. Fatal iron poisoning in a pregnant female: case report. Minn Med 1976;59:483–9.

DEHYDROEPIANDROSTERONE

Dietary Supplement

PREGNANCY RECOMMENDATION: Limited Human Data—Animal Data Suggest Risk
BREASTFEEDING RECOMMENDATION: No Human Data—Probably Compatible

PREGNANCY SUMMARY

No reports investigating the potential teratogenic effects from use of dehydroepiandrosterone (DHEA) in human pregnancy have been located. DHEA and its active metabolite (DHEA sulfate; DHEA-S) are weak androgens and intermediates in the biosynthesis of testosterone and estradiol. The animal reproduction data suggest that DHEA and/or DHEA-S may cause virilization of the external genitalia in female fetuses and inhibit implantation or development of the pregnancy when administered shortly after conception. However, the doses used in these studies were not compared with the human dose based on BSA or AUC, so the results might not be interpretable for estimating human risk. Moreover, DHEA-S, and probably also DHEA, crosses the human placenta. Although the intrauterine fluid DHEA-S concentrations were very low, higher levels in the embryos and fetuses may have been present. If the agent is used in pregnancy, the patient should be informed of the animal data and limited human pregnancy experience.

FETAL RISK SUMMARY

Although not approved by the FDA, DHEA is available as an over-the-counter nutritional or dietary supplement. The dose of the drug in individual products is not known. Endogenous DHEA and DHEA-S are secreted by the adrenal cortex. In the systemic circulation, most DHEA is present as DHEA-S. DHEA has been promoted for treatment of systemic lupus erythematosus, fat burn, boosting libido, as an anti-aging treatment, and for other uses, but none of these benefits has been demonstrated in controlled studies. In the plasma, DHEA is weakly bound, whereas DHEA-S is strongly bound to albumin. The half-lives of DHEA and DHEA-S are 1–3 hours and 10–20 hours, respectively (1). The metabolic clearance rate of DHEA-S fluctuates throughout pregnancy (2).

Developmental and reproductive toxicity of DHEA has been studied in three species. In rats, DHEA was associated with failure of implantation (3) and dose-related virilization of female fetuses (increased anogenital distance) and reduced fetal weight (4). Rats exposed to DHEA on gestation days 6–17 demonstrated increased early resorptions (5). In mice, prenatal exposure to DHEA on days 11–17 was associated with increased anogenital distance but did not have a significant effect on behavior of the offspring (6). In another study, maternal weight, number, survival, and weight of pups were affected by DHEA (7). In rabbits, no effects on embryonic or fetal development were seen at various doses of DHEA during gestation days 7–20 (5).

No studies on the carcinogenic or mutagenic potential of DHEA have been located. However, a European case–control study found an association between higher serum concentrations of DHEA-S and breast cancer (8).

DHEA-S, and most likely DHEA, crosses the human placenta. This is consistent with the molecular weights of the two compounds, about 288 and 371, respectively. DHEA-S was found in intrauterine fluids only at the limit of detection in a study of 12 pregnant women at a gestational age of 8–12 weeks (9). The authors postulated that because the concentration of androgens was much lower in the intrauterine fluids compared with maternal serum, that there might be a mechanism for the protection of the embryo from higher concentrations of these hormones. Concentrations in the embryos or fetuses were not measured.

In a study of 25 women with diminished ovarian reserve, patients received 25 mg of DHEA three times daily for 16 weeks between two in vitro fertilization (IVF) cycles (10). Significant increases in fertilized oocytes, normal 3-day embryos, embryos transferred, and average embryo scores per oocyte were observed. A follow-up case–control study with 190 women undergoing IVF treatment due to diminished ovarian function demonstrated that DHEA supplementation resulted in significantly higher cumulative pregnancy rates (11).

BREASTFEEDING SUMMARY

No reports on the use of DHEA during lactation have been located. Estrogens have been associated with decreased milk production and concentrations of nitrogen and protein (see Ethinyl Estradiol). As DHEA is an intermediate in the biosynthesis of estrogen, it could decrease milk production as well (12). Although it has not been studied, this effect should be dose-related. If used during breastfeeding, infant weight gain should be closely monitored.

References

1. Kroboth PD, Salek FS, Pittenger AL, Fabian TJ, Frye RF. DHEA and DHEA-S: a review. J Clin Pharmacol 1999;39:327–48.
2. Cohen H, Cohen M. DHAS half-life in pregnancy, its prognostic value in high risk pregnancies. J Steroid Biochem 1977;8:381–3.
3. Harper MJ. Estrogenic effects of dehydroepiandrosterone and its sulfate in rats. Endocrinology 1969;84:229–35.
4. Goldman AS. Virilization of the external genitalia of the female rat fetus by dehydroepiandrosterone. Endocrinology 1970;87:432–5.
5. Kirchner DL, Mercieca MD, Crowell JA, Levine BS. Developmental toxicity of dehydroepiandrosterone (DHEA) in rats and rabbits. Teratology 1998;57:243.
6. Gandelman R, Simon NG, McDermott NJ. Prenatal exposure to testosterone and its precursors influences morphology and later behavioral responsiveness to testosterone of female mice. Physiol Behav 1979;23:23–6.
7. de Catanzaro D, MacNiven E, Ricciuti F. Comparison of the adverse effects of adrenal and ovarian steroids on early pregnancy in mice. Psychoneuroendocrinology 1991;16:525–36.
8. Kaaks R, Berrino F, Key T, Rinaldi S, Dossus L, Biessy C, Secreto G, Amiano P, Bingham S, Boeing H, Bueno de Mesquita HB, Chang-Claude J, Clavel-Chapelon F, Fournier A, van Gils CH, Gonzalez CA, Gurrea AB, Critselis E, Khaw KT, Krogh V, Lahmann PH, Nagel G, Olsen A, Onland-Moret NC, Overvad K, Palli D, Panico S, Peeters P, Quirós JR, Roddam A, Thiebaut A, Tjønneland A, Chirlaque MD, Trichopoulou A, Trichopoulos D, Tumino R, Vineis P, Norat T, Ferrari P, Slimani N, Riboli E. Serum sex steroids in premenopausal women and breast cancer risk within the European Prospective Investigation into Cancer and Nutrition (EPIC). J Natl Cancer Inst 2005;97:755–65.
9. Atkinson G, Campbell DJ, Cawood ML, Oakey RE. Steroids in human intrauterine fluids of early pregnancy. Clin Endocrinol (Oxf) 1996;44:435–40.
10. Barad D, Gleicher N. Effect of dehydroepiandrosterone on oocyte and embryo yields, embryo grade and cell number in IVF. Hum Reprod 2006;21:2845–9.
11. Barad D, Brill H, Gleicher N. Update on the use of dehydroepiandrosterone supplementation among women with diminished ovarian function. J Assist Reprod Genet 2007;24:629–34.
12. Oladapo OT, Fawole B. Treatments for suppression of lactation. Cochrane Database Syst Rev 2009;(1):CD005937.

DELAVIRDINE

Antiviral

PREGNANCY RECOMMENDATION: Compatible—Maternal Benefit >> Embryo–Fetal Risk
BREASTFEEDING RECOMMENDATION: Contraindicated

D

PREGNANCY SUMMARY

The limited human data do not allow a prediction as to the risk of delavirdine during pregnancy. The animal data indicate that the drug may represent a risk to the developing human fetus. If indicated, the drug should not be withheld because of pregnancy.

FETAL RISK SUMMARY

Delavirdine is a synthetic nonnucleoside reverse transcriptase inhibitor (nnRTI) that is used in the treatment of HIV type 1 (HIV-1). Because resistant viruses emerge rapidly with delavirdine monotherapy, the drug should always be used in combination with other antiretroviral agents (1). Other drugs in this class are efavirenz and nevirapine.

Reproductive studies with delavirdine have been conducted in rats and rabbits. Ventricular septal defects were produced when pregnant rats were administered the agent during organogenesis at doses producing systemic levels equal to or lower than the expected human exposure at the recommended dose (EHE) (1). Reduced pup survival on the day of birth was also noted at this dose. At doses producing 5 times the EHE, marked maternal toxicity, embryo toxicity, fetal developmental delay, and reduced pup survival were observed. Delavirdine administered during organogenesis to rabbits caused maternal toxicity, embryo toxicity, and abortions (1). The lowest dose producing these effects was about six times the EHE. No malformations were observed in the surviving rabbit offspring, but only a few were available for examination (1).

It is not known if delavirdine crosses the human placenta. The molecular weight of the free base (about 457) is low enough that passage to the fetus should be expected.

During premarketing clinical studies, seven unplanned pregnancies occurred, resulting in three ectopic pregnancies, three healthy live births, and one premature infant with a birth defect (1). The infant, exposed early in gestation to about 6 weeks of delavirdine and zidovudine, had a small muscular ventricular septal defect.

The Antiretroviral Pregnancy Registry reported, for January 1989 through July 2009, prospective data (reported before the outcomes were known) involving 4702 live births that had been exposed during the 1st trimester to one or more antiretroviral agents (2). Congenital defects were noted in 134, a prevalence of 2.8% (95% confidence interval [CI] 2.4–3.4). In the 6100 live births with earliest exposure in the 2nd/3rd trimesters, there were 153 infants with defects (2.5%, 95% CI 2.1–2.9). The prevalence rates for the two periods did not differ significantly. There were 288 infants with birth defects among 10,803 live births with exposure anytime during pregnancy (2.7%, 95% CI 2.4–3.0). The prevalence rate did not differ significantly from the rate expected in a nonexposed population. There were 14 outcomes exposed to delavirdine (11 in the 1st trimester and 3 in the 2nd/3rd trimesters) in combination with other antiretroviral agents. There were no birth defects. In reviewing the birth defects of prospective and retrospective (pregnancies reported after the outcomes were known) registered cases, the Registry concluded that, except for isolated cases of neural tube defects with efavirenz exposure in retrospective reports, there was no other pattern of anomalies (isolated or syndromic) (2). (See Lamivudine for required statement.)

Two reviews, one in 1996 and the other in 1997, concluded that all women currently receiving antiretroviral therapy should continue to receive therapy during pregnancy and that treatment of the mother with monotherapy should be considered inadequate therapy (3,4). The same conclusion was reached in a 2003 review with the added admonishment that therapy must be continuous to prevent emergence of resistant viral strains (5). In 2009, the updated U.S. Department of Health and Human Services guidelines for the use of antiretroviral agents in HIV-1-infected patients continued the recommendation that therapy, with the exception of efavirenz, should be continued during pregnancy (6). If indicated, delavirdine should not be withheld in pregnancy because the expected benefit to the HIV-positive mother outweighs the unknown risk to the fetus. Updated guidelines for the use of antiretroviral drugs to reduce perinatal HIV-1 transmission also were released in 2006 (7). Women receiving antiretroviral therapy during pregnancy should continue the therapy but, regardless of the regimen, zidovudine administration is recommended during the intrapartum period to prevent vertical transmission of HIV to the newborn (7).

BREASTFEEDING SUMMARY

No reports describing the use of delavirdine during lactation have been located. The molecular weight of the free base (about 457) is low enough that excretion into breast milk should be expected. The effect on a nursing infant is unknown.

Reports on the use of delavirdine during human lactation are unlikely, however, because the antiviral agent is used in the treatment of HIV infections. HIV-1 is transmitted in milk, and in developed countries, breastfeeding is not recommended (3,4,6,8–10). In developing countries, breastfeeding is undertaken, despite the risk, because there are no affordable milk substitutes available. Until 1999, no studies had been published that examined the effect of any antiretroviral therapy on HIV-1 transmission in milk. In that year, a study involving zidovudine was published that measured a 38% reduction in vertical transmission of HIV-1 infection despite breastfeeding when compared with controls (see Zidovudine).

References

1. Product information. Rescriptor. Pfizer, 2006.
2. Antiretroviral Pregnancy Registry Steering Committee. *Antiretroviral Pregnancy Registry International Interim Report for 1 January 1989 through 31 July 2009*. Wilmington, NC: Registry Coordinating Center, 2009. Available at www.apregistry.com. Accessed May 29, 2010.
3. Carpenter CCJ, Fischi MA, Hammer SM, Hirsch MS, Jacobsen DM, Katzenstein DA, Montaner JSG, Richman DD, Saag MS, Schooley RT, Thompson MA, Vella S, Yeni PG, Volberding PA. Antiretroviral therapy for HIV infection in 1996. JAMA 1996;276;146–54.
4. Minkoff H, Augenbraun M. Antiretroviral therapy for pregnant women. Am J Obstet Gynecol 1997;176:478–89.
5. Minkoff H. Human immunodeficiency virus infection in pregnancy. Obstet Gynecol 2003;101:797–810.
6. Panel on Antiretroviral Guidelines for Adults and Adolescents. *Guidelines for the Use of Antiretroviral Agents in HIV-1-Infected Adults and Adolescents*. Department of Health and Human Services. December 1, 2009:1–161. Available at http://www.aidsinfo.nih.gov/ContentFiles/AdultandAdolescentGL.pdf. Accessed September 17, 2010:60, 96–8.
7. Panel on Treatment of HIV-Infected Pregnant Women and Prevention of Perinatal Transmission. *Recommendations for Use of Antiretroviral Drugs in Pregnant HIV-1-Infected Women for Maternal Health and Interventions to Reduce Perinatal HIV Transmission in the United States*. May 24, 2010:1–117. Available at http://aidsinfo.nih.gov/ContentFiles/PerinatalGL.pdf. Accessed September 17, 2010:30 (Table 5).
8. Brown ZA, Watts DH. Antiviral therapy in pregnancy. Clin Obstet Gynecol 1990;33:276–89.
9. De Martino M, Tovo P-A, Pezzotti P, Galli L, Massironi E, Ruga E, Floreea F, Plebani A, Gabiano C, Zuccotti GV. HIV-1 transmission through breast-milk: appraisal of risk according to duration of feeding. AIDS 1992;6:991–7.
10. Van de Perre P. Postnatal transmission of human immunodeficiency virus type 1: the breast feeding dilemma. Am J Obstet Gynecol 1995;173: 483–7.

D

DEMECARIUM

[Withdrawn from the market. See 9th edition.]

DEMECLOCYCLINE

Antibiotic (Tetracycline)

See Tetracycline.

DENILEUKIN DIFTITOX

Antineoplastic

PREGNANCY RECOMMENDATION: No Human Data—No Relevant Animal Data
BREASTFEEDING RECOMMENDATION: No Human Data—Probably Compatible

PREGNANCY SUMMARY

No reports describing the use of denileukin diftitox in human pregnancy have been located. The absence of both animal and human pregnancy experience prevents an assessment of the embryo–fetal risk. The potential for severe infusion-related toxicity is an important risk factor. Until human pregnancy experience is available, the best course is to avoid use of this agent in pregnancy. However, if a woman requires denileukin diftitox and informed consent is obtained, it should not be withheld because of pregnancy. If an inadvertent pregnancy occurs, the woman should be advised of the unknown risk to her embryo and/or fetus.

FETAL RISK SUMMARY

The biological response modifier, denileukin diftitox, is a recombinant DNA-derived cytotoxic protein composed of amino acid sequences for diphtheria toxin fragments and for interleukin-2. It is in the same antineoplastic subclass as aldesleukin. Denileukin diftitox is indicated for the treatment of patients with persistent or recurrent cutaneous T-cell lymphoma. After an IV infusion, the half-lives of the distribution phase (about 2–5 minutes) and the terminal elimination phase (about 70–80 minutes) are rapid. Denileukin diftitox is metabolized by proteolytic degradation (1).

Denileukin diftitox may cause severe, infusion-related toxicity, including hypotension and other adverse effects. Treatment with IV antihistamines, corticosteroids, and epinephrine may be required (1). Hypotension in a pregnant woman could have deleterious effects on placental perfusion, resulting in embryo and fetal harm. Moreover, the potent α-adrenergic properties of epinephrine also can cause decreased placental perfusion. IV ephedrine might be a better choice to treat maternal hypotension.

Neither animal reproduction studies nor fertility studies have been conducted with denileukin diftitox. Studies for carcinogenicity also have not been conducted, but there was no evidence of mutagenic effects.

It is not known if denileukin diftitox crosses the human placenta. The molecular weight of the protein, about 58,000, suggests that it does not cross. However, other proteins, such as the immunoglobulins, cross the placenta. Moreover, the protein rapidly distributes into tissues (e.g., primarily into the liver and kidneys in rats). The very short distribution and elimination half-lives may limit the amount reaching the embryo and fetus.

BREASTFEEDING SUMMARY

No reports describing the use of denileukin diftitox during human lactation have been located. The molecular weight of the protein , about 58,000, suggests that it will not be excreted into breast milk. However, other proteins, such as the immunoglobulins, are excreted into milk and so may denileukin diftitox. The very short distribution (2–5 minutes) and elimination (70–80 minutes) half-lives may limit the amount in milk. Waiting about 7 hours after a dose to breastfeed should limit the potential exposure of the infant even more. The effect of exposure on a nursing infant is unknown.

Reference

1. Product information. Ontak. Ligand Pharmaceuticals, 2007.

DENOSUMAB

Immunologic Agent (Antiosteoporosis)

PREGNANCY RECOMMENDATION: Contraindicated
BREASTFEEDING RECOMMENDATION: No Human Data—Probably Compatible

PREGNANCY SUMMARY

No reports describing the use of denosumab in human pregnancy have been located. Such reports are unlikely because the monoclonal antibody is indicated only for postmenopausal women. The animal data in monkeys suggest low risk. Although exposure to denosumab during pregnancy might impair mammary gland development and subsequent lactation, the absence of human pregnancy experience prevents an accurate assessment of the maternal and embryo–fetal risk. If a woman becomes pregnant during denosumab therapy, physicians are encouraged to enroll her in the Amgen Pregnancy Surveillance Program by calling 800-77-AMGEN (800-772-6436) (1). Pregnant patients also can enroll themselves by calling the same number.

FETAL RISK SUMMARY

Denosumab is a human IgG2 monoclonal antibody that binds to a protein that is essential for bone resorption, thereby decreasing bone resorption and increasing bone mass. It is indicated for the treatment of postmenopausal women with osteoporosis at high risk for fracture or for patients who have failed or are intolerant to other available osteoporosis therapy. Denosumab is given as an SC injection every 6 months. Because hypocalcemia may occur, all patients should receive calcium (1000 mg/day) and vitamin D (at least 400 IU/day). The mean serum half-life of denosumab is about 25 days (1).

Reproduction studies have been conducted in cynomolgus monkeys. In monkeys, during organogenesis, SC doses up to 13 times the recommended human dose of 60 mg given once every 6 months based on body weight (RHD) revealed no evidence of maternal toxicity or fetal harm. However, fetal lymph nodes were not examined and the toxicity of the antibody in the 2nd and 3rd trimesters, the periods when increasing amounts of monoclonal antibodies are expected to cross the placenta was not studied (1).

In pregnant mice lacking the protein target of denosumab (knockout mice), absence of the target led to fetal lymph node agenesis and postnatal impairment of dentition and bone growth. The mice also had altered maturation of the maternal mammary gland and impaired lactation (1).

Studies of carcinogenicity and mutagenicity have not been conducted. No effects on female fertility or male reproductive organs were observed in monkeys given doses that were 13–50 times the RHD (1).

It is not known if denosumab crosses the human placenta. The molecular weight (about 147,000) suggests that transfer will be inhibited but the long serum half-life will favor transfer. The manufacturer states that monoclonal antibodies are transported across the placenta with the highest amounts in the 3rd trimester (1).

BREASTFEEDING SUMMARY

No reports describing the use of denosumab during human lactation have been located. Such reports are unlikely because the monoclonal antibody is only indicated for postmenopausal women. The molecular weight (about 147,000) suggests that excretion into breast milk will be inhibited but the long serum half-life may favor excretion. If there is excretion, digestion in the infant's gut will probably occur.

Reference

1. Product information. Prolia. Amgen, 2010.

DESFLURANE

General Anesthetic

PREGNANCY RECOMMENDATION: Limited Human Data—Animal Data Suggest Low Risk
BREASTFEEDING RECOMMENDATION: No Human Data—Probably Compatible

PREGNANCY SUMMARY

Desflurane is not teratogenic in two animal species, but there are no reports of its use early in human gestation. The animal data are reassuring, but the absence of human data during organogenesis precludes an estimation of the risk for structural anomalies. In addition, general anesthesia usually involves the use of several pharmacological agents. Although no teratogenicity has been observed with three other halogenated general anesthetic agents (halothane, isoflurane, and methoxyflurane), only halothane has 1st trimester human exposure data (1). The use of desflurane during cesarean section does not appear to affect the newborn any differently from other general anesthetic agents. All such agents can cause depression in the newborn that may last for 24 hours or more. The potential reproductive toxicity (spontaneous abortion and infertility) of occupational exposure to desflurane has not been studied but is a concern based on the exposure concentration found in one study. In addition, occupational exposure to nitrous oxide also was measured in that study, and indicated that the nurses were exposed to both nitrous oxide and volatile anesthetic agents at the same time.

FETAL RISK SUMMARY

Desflurane, a general inhalation anesthetic agent administered via vaporizer, is indicated for the induction and/or maintenance of anesthesia during surgery. It is a nonflammable, volatile liquid that is in the same class of halogenated agents as enflurane, halothane, isoflurane, methoxyflurane, and sevoflurane. Desflurane is closely related chemically to enflurane and isoflurane. The only difference between desflurane and isoflurane is the substitution of fluorine in desflurane for the single chlorine atom in isoflurane. This small change, however, produces marked pharmacokinetic and clinical effects. The potency of desflurane is 20% that of isoflurane, the blood–gas partition coefficient is reduced (i.e., reduced solubility in blood) (0.42 vs. 1.46) as is tissue solubility (brain–blood partition coefficient 1.3 vs. 1.6), and recovery from anesthesia is faster (2).

Three mutagenic tests with desflurane found no evidence of genotoxicity (3). No teratogenic effects were observed in reproduction tests with rats and rabbits at doses of approximately 10 and 13 cumulative minimum alveolar anesthetic concentration (MAC-hour) exposures at 1 MAC-hour/day, respectively, during organogenesis. (*Note: MAC is the concentration that causes immobility in 50% of patients exposed to a noxious stimulus such as a surgical incision; it represents the* ED_{50} [4]). However, an approximately 6% decrease in the body weight of male rat pups delivered prematurely by cesarean section was noted at this dose. No treatment-related behavioral changes or other toxicity (dystocia or decreased body weight) were observed in rat offspring exposed to desflurane 1 MAC-hour/day from gestation day 15–lactation day 21 (3).

The low molecular weight (about 168) and the presence of desflurane in the brain suggest that it will cross the placenta to the fetus. Two reviews have concluded that, in general, inhalational anesthetic agents are freely transferred to fetal tissues (1,5) and, in most cases, the maternal and fetal blood concentrations are approximately equivalent (5). The relatively low human blood–gas partition coefficient and the rapid clearance from the maternal blood also suggest that desflurane will be rapidly cleared from the fetus, thus reducing the potential for neurobehavior depression of the newborn.

A brief 1993 report compared the closely related anesthetic agents, desflurane and enflurane (10 patients in each group), during cesarean delivery (6). Uterine tone increased significantly over time (a potential risk factor for maternal bleeding), but there were no differences between the groups. The mean umbilical vein:maternal artery ratios were 0.69 and 0.51, respectively. No differences between the groups were measured in the Neurological and Adaptive Capacity Scores (NACS) at 2 and 24 hours, 1 and 5 minute Apgar scores (8.0 and 8.9 vs. 7.5 and 9.0, respectively), and cord arterial blood gases or pH (6).

Two end-tidal concentrations of desflurane (3% and 6%) were compared with enflurane (0.6%) for cesarean section delivery in a 1995 study (7). The MACs for the three groups were 0.45, 0.90, and 0.40, respectively, thus representing subanesthetic concentrations. A 50%–50% mixture of nitrous oxide and oxygen was administered with the anesthetic agents (25 patients in each group). Maternal blood loss was similar among the groups. In the newborns, the time-to-sustained-respiration was >90 seconds in one (4%), seven (28%), and five (20%), respectively. The increased incidence in the 6% desflurane group was significantly longer than in the 3% desflurane group. There were no significant differences in the NACS at 2 and 24 hours, but some depression was noted: NACS <35 at 2 hours in four (16%), seven (28%), and six (24%); and at 24 hours—one (4%), one (4%), and none, respectively. Low Apgar scores (<7) were found at 1 minute in three (12%), seven (28%), and six (24%), respectively (*ns*), and at 5 minutes in none, one (4%), and one (4%), respectively (*ns*) (7).

A 1995 study compared desflurane (1.0%–4.5%) and oxygen ($N = 40$) with nitrous oxide (30%–60%) in oxygen (N = 40) for analgesia during vaginal delivery (8). Maternal analgesia scores and blood loss were similar between the groups. Four (10%) of the desflurane group had an NACS < 35 at 2 hours compared with seven (18%) of those exposed to nitrous oxide (*ns*). At 24 hours, none of desflurane group had an NACS <35 compared with three (8%) in the nitrous oxide group (*ns*). Apgar scores <7 at 1 minute occurred in

13% and 8% (*ns*), respectively, but all Apgar scores were ≥7 at 5 minutes. However, nine patients in the desflurane group had amnesia for delivery, a potentially undesirable effect in an obstetrical patient (8).

A study published in 1998 evaluated the exposure of nine nurses in a postanesthesia care unit (PACU) to exhaled desflurane and isoflurane and compared these exposures with the National Institute of Occupational Safety and Health (NIOSH)-recommended exposure limits (9). The NIOSH recommendation for volatile anesthetics (without concomitant nitrous oxide exposure) is a maximum of 2 ppm, but it has not been adopted by the Occupational Safety and Health Administration. Moreover, the recommended limit is controversial and is thought by some to be inappropriately low. However, a potential for reproductive risk (spontaneous abortion and infertility) is thought to exist for some anesthetic agents. The study involved exposure in the PACU to exhaled anesthetic gases from 50 adult patients (desflurane $N = 31$, isoflurane $N = 19$) over an approximate 1-hour recovery time. About half the patients were extubated in the PACU. Exposure was continuously measured from the shoulders (i.e., breathing zone) of the nurses. Breathing-zone anesthetic concentrations of desflurane and isoflurane exceeded the NIOSH limits in 87% and 37% of the cases, respectively. These exposures were above the limit 49% of the time for desflurane and 12% of the time for isoflurane. The investigators listed several limitations to their study and concluded that the results might represent a "worst-case analysis" (9).

A 2004 study found a significant association between maternal occupational exposure to waste anesthetic gases during pregnancy and developmental deficits in their children, including gross and fine motor ability, inattention/hyperactivity, and IQ performance (see Nitrous Oxide).

BREASTFEEDING SUMMARY

Although desflurane has been administered during labor and delivery, the effects of this exposure on the infant that begins nursing immediately after birth have not been described. Desflurane is probably excreted into colostrum and milk as suggested by its presence in the maternal blood and its low molecular weight (about 168), but the toxic potential of this exposure for the infant is unknown. However, the risk to a nursing infant from exposure to desflurane is probably very low (10). Moreover, the concentrations in milk should be less than other halogenated anesthetic agents because of the decreased blood and tissue solubility of desflurane and its rapid washout from the mother's system. The manufacturer states that excretion in milk was not clinically important 24 hours after anesthesia (3). Another halogenated inhalation anesthetic, halothane, is classified as compatible with breastfeeding (see Halothane).

References

1. Friedman JM. Teratogen update: anesthetic agents. Teratology 1988;37:69–77.
2. Eger EI II. Desflurane animal and human pharmacology: aspects of kinetics, safety, and MAC. Anesth Analg 1992;75:S3–9.
3. Product information. Suprane. Baxter Healthcare Corporation, Anesthesia & Critical Care, 2002.
4. Trevor AJ, Miller RD. General anesthetics. In: Katzung BG, ed. *Basic and Clinical Pharmacology*. 8th ed. New York, NY: McGraw-Hill, 2001:426.
5. Kanto J. Risk–benefit assessment of anaesthetic agents in the puerperium. Drug Saf 1991;6:285–301.
6. Wallace DH, Armstrong A, Darras A, Gajraj N, Gambling D, White P. The effect of desflurane or low-dose enflurane on uterine tone at cesarean delivery: placental transfer and recovery (abstract). Anesthesiology 1993;79:A1019.
7. Abboud TK, Zhu J, Richardson M, Peres Da Silva P, Donovan M. Desflurane: a new volatile anesthetic for cesarean section. Maternal and neonatal effects. Acta Anaesthesiol Scand 1995;39:723–6.
8. Abboud TK, Swart F, Zhu J, Donovan MM, Peres Da Silva E, Yakal K. Desflurane analgesia for vaginal delivery. Acta Anaethesiol Scan 1995;39:259–61.
9. Sessler DI, Badgwell JM. Exposure of postoperative nurses to exhaled anesthetic gases. Anesth Analg 1998;87:1083–8.
10. Spigset O. Anaesthetic agents and excretion in breast milk. Acta Anaesthesiol Scand 1994;38:94–103.

DESIPRAMINE

Antidepressant

PREGNANCY RECOMMENDATION: Human Data Suggest Low Risk
BREASTFEEDING RECOMMENDATION: Limited Human Data—Potential Toxicity

PREGNANCY SUMMARY

Although the data are limited, desipramine does not appear to be a major human teratogen.

FETAL RISK SUMMARY

Desipramine, a tricyclic antidepressant, is an active metabolite of imipramine (see also Imipramine). No reports linking the use of desipramine with congenital defects have been located. Neonatal withdrawal symptoms, including cyanosis, tachycardia, diaphoresis, and weight loss, were observed after desipramine was taken throughout pregnancy (1).

In a surveillance study of Michigan Medicaid recipients involving 229,101 completed pregnancies conducted between 1985 and 1992, 31 newborns had been exposed to desipramine during the 1st trimester (F. Rosa, personal communication, FDA, 1993). One (3.2%) major birth defect was observed (one expected). No anomalies were observed in six defect categories (cardiovascular defects, oral clefts, spina bifida, polydactyly, limb reduction defects, and hypospadias) for which specific data were available. The number of exposures is too small for comment.

In a 1996 descriptive case series, the European Network of the Teratology Information Services (ENTIS) prospectively examined the outcomes of 689 pregnancies exposed to antidepressants (2). Multiple drug therapy occurred in about two-thirds of the mothers. Desipramine was used in one pregnancy and the outcome was a spontaneous abortion.

In an in vitro study, desipramine was shown to be a potent inhibitor of sperm motility (3). A concentration of 27 μmol/L produced a 50% reduction in motility.

A 2002 prospective study compared two groups of mother-child pairs: one group exposed to antidepressants throughout gestation (46 exposed to tricyclics - 3 to desipramine; 40 to fluoxetine) and, the other group, 36 nonexposed, not depressed controls (4). Offspring between the ages 15 and 71 months were studied for effects of antidepressant exposure in terms of IQ, language, behavior, and temperament. Exposure to antidepressants did not adversely affect the measured parameters, but IQ was significantly and negatively associated with the duration of depression, and language was negatively associated with the number of depression episodes after delivery (4).

BREASTFEEDING SUMMARY

Desipramine is excreted into breast milk (5–7). No reports of adverse effects have been located. In one patient, milk:plasma ratios of 0.4–0.9 were measured with milk levels ranging between 17 and 35 mcg/mL (5). A 35-year-old mother in her 9th postpartum week took 300 mg of desipramine daily at bedtime for depression (7). One week later, simultaneous milk and serum samples were collected about 9 hours after a dose. Concentrations of desipramine in the milk and serum were 316 and 257 ng/mL (ratio 1.2), respectively, whereas levels of the metabolite, 2-hydroxydesipramine, were 381 and 234 ng/mL (ratio 1.6), respectively. The measurements were repeated 1 week later, 10.33 hours after the dose, and milk levels of the parent drug and metabolite were 328 and 327 ng/mL, respectively. No drug was detected in the infant's serum nor were any clinical signs of toxicity observed in the infant after 3 weeks of maternal treatment (7).

A 1996 review of antidepressant treatment during breastfeeding found no information that desipramine exposure during nursing resulted in quantifiable amounts in an infant or that the exposure caused adverse effects (8). The American Academy of Pediatrics classifies desipramine as a drug whose effect on the nursing infant is unknown but may be of concern (9).

References

1. Webster PA. Withdrawal symptoms in neonates associated with maternal antidepressant therapy. Lancet 1973;2:318–9.
2. McElhatton PR, Garbis HM, Elefant E, Vial T, Bellemin B, Mastroiacovo P, Arnon J, Rodriguez-Pinilla E, Schaefer C, Pexieder T, Merlob P, Dal Verme S. The outcome of pregnancy in 689 women exposed to therapeutic doses of antidepressants. A collaborative study of the European Network of Teratology Information Services (ENTIS). Reprod Toxicol 1996;10:285–94.
3. Levin RM, Amsterdam JD, Winokur A, Wein AJ. Effects of psychotropic drugs on human sperm motility. Fertil Steril 1981;36:503–6.
4. Nulman I, Rovet J, Stewart DE, Wolpin J, Pace-Asciak P, Shuhaiber S, Koren G. Child development following exposure to tricyclic antidepressants or fluoxetine throughout fetal life: a prospective, controlled study. Am J Psychiatry 2002;159:1889–95.
5. Sovner R, Orsulak PJ. Excretion of imipramine and desipramine in human breast milk. Am J Psychiatry 1979;136:451–2.
6. Erickson SH, Smith GH, Heidrich F. Tricyclics and breast-feeding. Am J Psychiatry 1979;136:1483.
7. Stancer HC, Reed KL. Desipramine and 2-hydroxydesipramine in human breast milk and the nursing infant's serum. Am J Psychiatry 1986;143:1597–600.
8. Wisner KL, Perel JM, Findling RL. Antidepressant treatment during breastfeeding. Am J Psychiatry 1996;153:1132–7.
9. Committee on Drugs, American Academy of Pediatrics. The transfer of drugs and other chemicals into human milk. Pediatrics 2001;108:776–89.

DESIRUDIN

Hematological Agent (Thrombin Inhibitor)

PREGNANCY RECOMMENDATION: No Human Data—Animal Data Suggest Risk
BREASTFEEDING RECOMMENDATION: No Human Data—Probably Compatible

PREGNANCY SUMMARY

No reports describing the use of desirudin in human pregnancy have been located. The animal reproductive data suggest risk, but the absence of human pregnancy experience prevents an assessment of the embryo–fetal risk. Desirudin probably does not cross the placenta in clinically significant amounts but this needs study, especially in light of the teratogenicity observed in two animal species. Both unfractionated and low-molecular-weight heparin have been studied in pregnancy and probably are the preferred agents for prophylaxis against deep vein thrombus after surgery in a pregnant patient.

FETAL RISK SUMMARY

Desirudin, a specific inhibitor of human thrombin, is a single polypeptide chain with a protein structure differing slightly from that of hirudin, the anticoagulant present in the peripharyngeal glands of the medicinal leech, *Hirudo medicinalis*. Desirudin is indicated for the prophylaxis of deep vein thrombosis, which may lead to pulmonary embolism, in patients undergoing elective hip replacement surgery. It is administered as an SC injection. Desirudin is metabolized and eliminated by the kidney. The mean terminal elimination half-life is about 2 hours (1).

Reproduction studies have been conducted in rats and rabbits. In pregnant rats, daily SC doses that were 0.3–4 times the maximum recommended human dose based on BSA

(MRHD) were teratogenic. Defects observed were omphalocele, asymmetric and fused sternebrae, shortened hind limbs, and other nonspecified defects. Edema also was observed. In pregnant rabbits, daily SC doses that were 0.3–3 times the MRHD were associated with spina bifida, malrotated hindlimb, hydrocephaly, gastroschisis, and other nonspecified defects (1).

D

Carcinogenic studies have not been performed. Desirudin was not genotoxic in three tests but produced equivocal results in a fourth test. No effect on fertility in male and female rats was observed with doses ≤2.7 times the MRHD (1).

It is not known if desirudin crosses the human placenta. The animal data suggest that the drug had either a direct or an indirect effect on the embryos. However, the molecular weight, about 6964, and short elimination half-life suggest that exposure of embryo or fetus is unlikely.

BREASTFEEDING SUMMARY

No reports describing the use of desirudin during human lactation have been located. The molecular weight of this polypeptide (about 6964), and short elimination half-life (about 2 hours) suggest that excretion into breast milk is unlikely. However, even if the drug were excreted, it probably would be digested in the infant's gut because it is a protein. Thus, the risk to a nursing infant appears to be low, if it exists at all.

Reference

1. Product information. Iprivask. Aventis Pharmaceuticals, 2007.

DESLANOSIDE

Cardiac Glycoside

See Digitalis.

DESLORATADINE

Antihistamine

PREGNANCY RECOMMENDATION: No Human Data—Animal Data Suggest Low Risk
BREASTFEEDING RECOMMENDATION: Limited Human Data—Probably Compatible

PREGNANCY SUMMARY

The animal reproduction data suggest low risk, but the absence of human pregnancy experience prevents a full assessment of the risk. Although there are no reports describing the use of desloratadine in human pregnancy, there are reports for loratadine, the parent compound. (See Loratadine.) The data for loratadine are adequate to demonstrate that it is not a major human teratogen. Because desloratadine is a major metabolite of loratadine, it is reasonable to presume that desloratadine also is not a major teratogen (1). Moreover, antihistamines, in general, are not thought to cause human developmental toxicity at recommended doses. Although subjects classified as slow metabolizers will probably have greater embryo–fetal exposure to desloratadine, and possibly to its active metabolite, there is no reported evidence that such exposure will result in embryo–fetal toxicity. If an oral antihistamine is required during pregnancy, first-generation agents such as chlorpheniramine or tripelennamine should be considered. However, if a woman has taken desloratadine during a known or unknown pregnancy, the absolute embryo–fetal risk appears to be low.

FETAL RISK SUMMARY

Desloratadine is a second-generation, peripherally selective H_1-receptor histamine antagonist that is indicated for the relief of nasal and nonnasal symptoms of allergic rhinitis. It is a major active metabolite of loratadine. (See also Loratadine.) Desloratadine itself is metabolized to an active metabolite by an enzyme that has not been identified. About 7% of the general population has decreased ability (i.e., slow metabolizers) to metabolize desloratadine, but the incidence is about 20% in blacks. The median exposure to desloratadine, based on AUC, was about six-fold greater in subjects classified as slow metabolizers than in those with unaltered metabolism. Protein binding of desloratadine and its active metabolite is in the range of 82%–89%. In patients with unaltered metabolism, the mean elimination half-life of desloratadine is 27 hours, but it exceeds 50 hours in slow metabolizers (2).

Reproduction studies with desloratadine have been conducted in rats and rabbits. There was no evidence of teratogenicity or effect on fertility in rats at desloratadine and active metabolite exposures up to about 210 and 130 times, respectively, the AUC in humans at the recommended daily oral dose (RDOD). However, at about 120 times the RDOD, an increase in preimplantation loss and a decrease in the number of implantations and fetuses were observed. At about 50 times the RDOD, reduced body weight and slow righting reflex were noted. At about 7 times the RDOD, no effect was noted on pup development. In rabbits, there was no evidence of teratogenicity at desloratadine exposure up to about 230 times the RDOD (2).

It is not known if desloratadine (or its active metabolite) crosses the placenta. The molecular weight of desloratadine (about 311) and the prolonged elimination half-life suggest that it will cross to the embryo–fetal compartment. Moreover, patients who are slow metabolizers will have much higher plasma concentrations of desloratadine and an approximate doubling of the elimination time. Both of these properties should increase the amount of drug reaching the embryo–fetus.

BREASTFEEDING SUMMARY

Although there are no reports describing the use of desloratadine during human lactation, the parent compound (loratadine) has been studied. Both loratadine and desloratadine are excreted into human breast milk. The American Academy of Pediatrics classifies loratadine as compatible with breastfeeding. (See Loratadine.)

References

1. Gilbert C, Mazzotta P, Loebstein R, Koren G. Fetal safety of drugs used in the treatment of allergic rhinitis: a critical review. Drug Saf 2005;28:707–19.
2. Product information. Clarinex. Schering Corporation, 2005.

D

DESMOPRESSIN

Pituitary Hormone, Synthetic

PREGNANCY RECOMMENDATION: Limited Human Data—Animal Data Suggest Low Risk
BREASTFEEDING RECOMMENDATION: Compatible

PREGNANCY SUMMARY

Desmopressin is a synthetic polypeptide structurally related to vasopressin. Although the data are limited, no drug-induced toxicity related to its use in pregnancy has been reported. (See also Vasopressin.)

FETAL RISK SUMMARY

Reproduction studies with desmopressin in rats and rabbits at doses up to approximately 0.1 times and 38 times, respectively, the maximum systemic human exposure based on BSA, did not reveal fetal harm (1).

A 1997 report described five women with diabetes insipidus that were treated with desmopressin during six pregnancies (2). No desmopressin-related adverse effects were observed in the eight newborns (two sets of twins). A 1998 review cited 53 cases of desmopressin use during all stages of pregnancy for the management of diabetes insipidus (3). No adverse effects were noted in the cases. In a 1998 case report, diabetes insipidus in a woman with Sheehan's syndrome was managed with intranasal desmopressin in two pregnancies (4). No information on the status of the newborns was provided.

BREASTFEEDING SUMMARY

See Vasopressin.

References

1. Product information. DDAVP. Rhone-Poulenc Rorer Pharmaceuticals, 2000.
2. Hamai Y, Fujii T, Nishina H, Kozuma S, Yoshikawa H, Taketani Y. Differential clinical courses of pregnancies complicated by diabetes insipidus which does, or does not, pre-date the pregnancy. Hum Reprod 1997;12:1816–8.
3. Ray JG. DDAVP use during pregnancy: an analysis of its safety for mother and child. Obstet Gynecol Surv 1998;53:450–5.
4. Briet JW. Diabetes insipidus, Sheehan's syndrome and pregnancy. Eur J Obstet Gynecol 1998;77:201–3.

DESVENLAFAXINE

Antidepressant

PREGNANCY RECOMMENDATION: Human Data Suggest Risk in 3rd Trimester
BREASTFEEDING RECOMMENDATION: Limited Human Data—Potential Toxicity

PREGNANCY SUMMARY

No reports describing the use of desvenlafaxine in human pregnancy have been located. The drug is the major active metabolite of venlafaxine that has some human pregnancy data (see also Venlafaxine). Neither the animal reproduction nor the limited human pregnancy experience with venlafaxine and other serotonin–norepinephrine reuptake inhibitors (SNRIs) suggest a major risk for structural anomalies. However, SNRIs and selective serotonin reuptake inhibitors (SSRIs) have been associated with spontaneous abortions, low birth weight, and prematurity. Exposure in the latter part of pregnancy has been associated with neonatal serotonin syndrome, neonatal behavioral syndrome (withdrawal including seizures), possible sustained abnormal neurobehavior beyond the neonatal period, and respiratory distress. These symptoms are consistent with a direct toxic effect, drug discontinuance syndrome, or a serotonin syndrome. Persistent pulmonary hypertension of the newborn (PPHN) is an additional potential risk, but confirmation is needed.

FETAL RISK SUMMARY

Desvenlafaxine, available as immediate- and extended-release formulations, is in the same antidepressant subclass of SNRIs as duloxetine, milnacipran, and venlafaxine. Desvenlafaxine is indicated for the treatment of major depressive disorder. It undergoes partial metabolism to apparently inactive metabolites. Plasma protein binding is low (30%) and the mean terminal half-life is about 11 hours (1).

Reproduction studies have been conducted in rats and rabbits. When these species were given desvenlafaxine during organogenesis, no evidence of structural anomalies was observed with doses up to 10 and 15 times, respectively, the human dose of 100 mg/day based on BSA (HD). However, fetal weights were decreased in rats, with a no-effect dose 10 times the HD. Exposure of rats throughout gestation and lactation was associated with decreased pup weights and increased pup deaths during the first 4 days of lactation. The cause of the deaths was not known. The no-effect dose for pup mortality was 10 times the HD. Postweaning growth and reproductive performance of the offspring were not affected by maternal treatment at a dose 29 times the HD (1).

Desvenlafaxine was not carcinogenic in 2-year studies in mice and rats. Assays and studies for mutagenic and clastogenic effects also were negative. Reduced fertility was observed in male and female rats given doses about 10 times the HD. There was no effect on fertility with doses that were about 3 times the HD (1).

At term, desvenlafaxine crosses the human placenta (2). This is consistent with the molecular weight (about 381 for the nonhydrated form), low plasma protein binding, moderately long terminal half-life, and the toxicity observed in newborns. Although placental transfer of the drug has not been studied at other times, exposure of the embryo–fetus should be expected throughout gestation.

The use of desvenlafaxine late in the pregnancy may result in functional and behavioral deficits in the newborn infant. The observed toxicities with SNRIs and SSRIs include respiratory distress, cyanosis, apnea, seizures, temperature instability, feeding difficulty, vomiting, hypoglycemia, hypotonia, hypertonia, hyperreflexia, tremor, jitteriness, irritability, and constant crying. The clinical features are consistent with either a direct toxic effect or drug discontinuation syndrome and, occasionally, may resemble a serotonin syndrome. The complications may require prolonged hospitalization, respiratory support, and tube feeding (1). (See Venlafaxine for additional information.)

BREASTFEEDING SUMMARY

Consistent with the molecular weight (about 381 for the nonhydrated form), low plasma protein binding (30%), and moderately long elimination half-life (about 11 hours), desvenlafaxine is excreted into breast milk. (See also Venlafaxine.)

A 1998 study measured the excretion of venlafaxine and its active metabolite desvenlafaxine in the milk of three breastfeeding women (3). The three mothers, started on the antidepressant after delivery, had been taking a stable dose (3.04–8.18 mg/kg/day) for 0.23–5 months. The ages of the infants were 0.37–6 months. The mean milk:plasma (M:P) ratio (in two cases based on AUC and in one on a single point) for the parent drug was 4.14 (range 3.26–5.18), whereas it was 3.06 (range 2.93–3.19) for the metabolite. The mean infant doses for venlafaxine and metabolite were 3.49% and 4.08% of the mother's weight-adjusted dose, respectively. Venlafaxine was not detected in infant plasma, but the median infant metabolite plasma concentration was 100 mcg/L (range 23–225 mcg/L). The mean total infant dose was 7.57% (range 4.74%–9.23%). No adverse effects in the infants were noted. Because of the relatively high infant dose in comparison with other antidepressants, it was recommended that close observation of the infant for short-term adverse effects (e.g., agitation, insomnia, poor feeding, or failure to thrive) was required (3).

A 2002 study determined the milk:plasma (M:P) ratios based on AUC and infant doses of venlafaxine and its metabolite desvenlafaxine in six mothers (mean age 34.5 years and weight 84.3 kg) and their seven nursing infants (mean age 7.0 months and weight 7.3 kg) (4). The median venlafaxine dose was 244 mg/day. The mean M:P ratios for the drug and its metabolite were 2.5 (range 2.0–3.2) and 2.7 (range 2.3–3.2), respectively, whereas the mean maximum milk concentrations were 1161 and 796 mcg/L, respectively. Using an estimated milk production rate of 150 mL/kg/day, the mean infant exposure expressed as a percentage of the weight-adjusted maternal dose was 3.2% (95% confidence interval [CI] 1.7–4.7) for venlafaxine and 3.2% (95% CI 1.9–4.9) for desvenlafaxine. Venlafaxine was detected in the plasma of one infant (5 mcg/L), whereas desvenlafaxine was detected in four infants (range 3–38 mcg/L). All of the infants were healthy (4).

In a 2009 report, 13 women taking venlafaxine (mean dose 194.3 mg/day) and their nursing infants (mean age about 21 weeks) were studied (5). The highest venlafaxine and desvenlafaxine concentrations in milk occurred 8 hours after maternal ingestion. For combined venlafaxine plus desvenlafaxine, the mean M:P ratio was 2.75, and the theoretical infant dose was 0.208 mg/kg/day. The relative infant dose as a percentage of the mother's weight-adjusted dose was 8.1%. The theoretical and relative infant doses for desvenlafaxine were 1.97 and 2.24 times higher than those for venlafaxine. No adverse effects were observed or reported in the infants (5).

A study of a woman taking desvenlafaxine 250 mg/day and amisulpride (an atypical antipsychotic not available in the United States) 100 mg/day for depression and nursing her 5-month-old infant was reported in 2010 (6). The absolute (theoretical) infant doses of the two drugs were 294 and

183 mcg/kg/day, respectively. The relative infant doses as a percentage of the mother's weight-adjusted doses were 7.8% and 6.1%, respectively. The infant was achieving expected developmental progress for age and no adverse effects were noted (6).

In a 2011 study of 10 women taking desvenlafaxine (50–150 mg/day) and their nursing infants (mean age 4.3 months, range 0.9–12.7 months), 8 of whom were exclusively breastfed, no adverse effects were noted in the infants (7). The mean theoretical infant dose was 85 mcg/kg/day and the relative infant dose as a percentage of the mother's weight-adjusted dose was 6.8%.

Maternal plasma concentrations of desvenlafaxine and venlafaxine determine the amount of drug excreted into milk. In this regard, a 2009 study appears to have important implications for choosing which agent to use in a lactating woman (8). The study evaluated the effect of cytochrome P450 2D6 extensive metabolizer (EM) or poor metabolizer (PM) status on the pharmacokinetics of single doses of venlafaxine extended release and desvenlafaxine in healthy adults. The maximum plasma concentrations and AUC of desvenlafaxine were statistically similar in the two groups. In contrast, venlafaxine concentrations and AUC were significantly higher in the PM phenotype compared with the EM phenotype, whereas the desvenlafaxine concentrations and AUC were significantly lower in the PM group (8).

In summary, the available data suggest that exposure to desvenlafaxine from milk does not represent a major risk to a nursing infant. However, nursing preterm and newborn infants were not involved in the above studies and they should be closely observed for excessive sedation and appropriate weight gain if the agent is used by the mother. Additional studies, especially long-term follow-up of exposed infants, are warranted.

References

1. Product information. Pristiq. Wyeth, 2011.
2. Rampono J, Simmer K, Ilett KF, Hackett LP, Doherty DA, Elliot R, Kok CH, Coenen A, Forman T. Placental transfer of SSRI and SNRI antidepressants and effects on the neonate. Pharmacopsychiatry 2009;42:95–100.
3. Ilett KF, Hackett LP, Dusci LJ, Roberts MJ, Kristensen JH, Paech M, Groves A, Yapp P. Distribution and excretion of venlafaxine and *O*-desmethylvenlafaxine in human milk. Br J Clin Pharmacol 1998;45:459–62.
4. Ilett KF, Kristensen JH, Hackett LP, Paech M, Kohan R, Rampono J. Distribution of venlafaxine and its O-desmethyl metabolite in human milk and their effects in breastfed infants. Br J Clin Pharmacol 2002;53: 17–22.
5. Newport DJ, Ritchie JC, Knight BT, Glover BA, Zach EB, Stowe ZN. Venlafaxine in human breast milk and nursing infant plasma: determination of exposure. J Clin Psychiatry 2009;70:1304–10.
6. Ilett KF, Watt F, Hackett LP, Kohan R, Teoh S. Assessment of infant dose through milk in a lactating woman taking amisulpride and desvenlafaxine for treatment-resistant depression. Ther Drug Monit 2010;32:704–7.
7. Rampono J, Teoh S, Hackett LP, Kohan R, Ilett KF. Estimation of desvenlafaxine transfer into milk and infant exposure during its use in lactating women with postnatal depression. Arch Womens Ment Health 2011;14:49–53.
8. Preskorn S, Patroneva A, Silman H, Jiang Q, Isler JA, Burczynski ME, Ahmed S, Paul J, Nichols AI. Comparison of the pharmacokinetics of venlafaxine extended release and desvenlafaxine in extensive and poor cytochrome P450 2D6 metabolizers. J Clin Psychopharmacol 2009;29:39–43.

DEXAMETHASONE

Corticosteroid

FETAL RISK RECOMMENDATION: **Compatible—Maternal Benefit >> Embryo–Fetal Risk**
BREASTFEEDING RECOMMENDATION: **No Human Data—Probably Compatible**

PREGNANCY SUMMARY

Dexamethasone is a corticosteroid with potency similar to betamethasone. Use in the 1st trimester has a small absolute risk of oral clefts. However, depending on the indication, the benefit of therapy may outweigh the risk.

FETAL RISK SUMMARY

Although most sources have not linked the use of dexamethasone with congenital defects, four large epidemiologic studies have found positive associations between systemic corticosteroids and nonsyndromic orofacial clefts. Specific corticosteroids were not identified in three of these studies (see Hydrocortisone for details), but dexamethasone and other agents were listed in a 1999 study discussed below.

In a case–control study, the California Birth Defects Monitoring Program evaluated the association between selected congenital anomalies and the use of corticosteroids 1 month before to 3 months after conception (periconceptional period) (1). Case infants or fetal deaths diagnosed with orofacial clefts, conotruncal defects, neural tubal defects (NTDs), and limb anomalies were identified from a total of 552,601 births that occurred from 1987 through the end of 1989. Controls, without birth defects, were selected from the same database. Following exclusion of known genetic syndromes, mothers of case and control infants were interviewed by telephone, an average of 3.7 years (cases) or 3.8 years (controls) after delivery, to determine various exposures during the periconceptional period. The number of interviews completed were orofacial cleft case mothers ($N = 662$, 85% of eligible), conotruncal case mothers ($N = 207$, 87%), NTD case mothers ($N = 265$, 84%), limb anomaly case mothers ($N = 165$, 82%), and control mothers ($N = 734$, 78%) (1). Orofacial clefts were classified into four phenotypic groups: isolated cleft lip with or without cleft palate (ICLP, $N = 348$), isolated cleft palate (ICP, $N = 141$), multiple cleft lip with or without cleft palate (MCLP, $N = 99$), and multiple cleft palate (MCP, $N = 74$). A total of 13 mothers reported using corticosteroids during the periconceptional period for a wide variety of indications. Six case mothers of ICLP and 3 of ICP used corticosteroids (unspecified corticosteroid $N = 1$, prednisone $N = 2$, cortisone $N = 3$,

D

triamcinolone acetonide $N = 1$, dexamethasone $N = 1$, and cortisone plus prednisone $N = 1$). One case mother of an infant with NTD used cortisone and an injectable unspecified corticosteroid, and three controls used corticosteroids (hydrocortisone $N = 1$ and prednisone $N = 2$). The odds ratio for corticosteroid use and ICLP was 4.3 (95% confidence interval [CI] 1.1–17.2), whereas the odds ratio for ICP and corticosteroid use was 5.3 (95% CI 1.1–26.5). No increased risks were observed for the other anomaly groups. Commenting on their results, the investigators thought that recall bias was unlikely because they did not observe increased risks for other malformations, and it was also unlikely that the mothers would have known of the suspected association between corticosteroids and orofacial clefts (1).

Maternal free estriol and cortisol are significantly depressed after dexamethasone therapy, but the effects of these changes on the fetus have not been studied (2–4).

Dexamethasone has been used in patients with premature labor at about 26–34 weeks' gestation to stimulate fetal lung maturation (5–15). Although this therapy is supported by many clinicians, its use is still controversial since the beneficial effects of steroids are greatest in singleton pregnancies with female fetuses (16–19). These benefits are as follows:

- Reduction in incidence of respiratory distress syndrome (RDS)
- Decreased severity of RDS if it occurs
- Decreased incidence of and mortality from intracranial hemorrhage
- Increased survival of premature infants

Toxicity in the fetus and newborn following the use of dexamethasone is rare.

In studies of women with premature rupture of the membranes (PROM), administration of corticosteroids does not always reduce the frequency of RDS or perinatal mortality (20–22). In addition, an increased risk of maternal infection has been observed in patients with PROM treated with corticosteroids (21,22). A recent report, however, found no difference in the incidence of maternal complications between treated and nontreated patients (23).

Dexamethasone crosses the placenta to the fetus (24,25). The drug is partially metabolized (54%) by the perfused placenta to its inactive 11-ketosteroid derivative, more so than betamethasone, but the difference is not statistically significant (25).

Leukocytosis has been observed in infants exposed antenatally to dexamethasone (26,27). The white blood cell counts returned to normal in about a week.

The use of corticosteroids, including dexamethasone, for the treatment of asthma during pregnancy has not been related to a significantly increased risk of maternal or fetal complications (28). A slight increase in the number of premature births was found, but it could not be determined whether this was an effect of the corticosteroids. An earlier study also recorded a shortening of gestation with chronic corticosteroid use (29).

In Rh-sensitized women, the use of dexamethasone may have prevented intrauterine fetal deterioration and the need for fetal transfusion (30). Five women, in the 2nd and 3rd trimesters, were treated with 24 mg of the steroid weekly for 2–7 weeks resulting, in each case, in a live newborn.

Dexamethasone, 4 mg/day for 15 days, was administered to a woman late in the 3rd trimester for the treatment of autoimmune thrombocytopenic purpura (31). Therapy was given in an unsuccessful attempt to prevent fetal/neonatal thrombocytopenia due to the placental transfer of antiplatelet antibody. Platelet counts in the newborn were 38,000–49,000/mm^3, but the infant made an uneventful recovery.

The use of dexamethasone for the pharmacologic suppression of the fetal adrenal gland has been described in two women with 21-hydroxylase deficiency (32,33). This deficiency results in the overproduction of adrenal androgens and the virilization of female fetuses. Dexamethasone, in divided doses of 1 mg/day, was administered from early in the 1st trimester (5th week and 10th week) to term. Normal female infants resulted from both pregnancies.

Although human studies have usually shown a benefit, the use of corticosteroids in animals has been associated with several toxic effects (34,35):

- Reduced fetal head circumference
- Reduced fetal adrenal weight
- Increased fetal liver weight
- Reduced fetal thymus weight
- Reduced placental weight

Fortunately, none of these effects has been observed in human investigations. Long-term follow-up evaluations of children exposed in utero to dexamethasone have shown no adverse effects from this exposure (36,37).

BREASTFEEDING SUMMARY

No reports describing the use of dexamethasone during lactation have been located. The molecular weight (about 516) is low enough for passage into breast milk. Moreover, trace amounts of other corticosteroids are excreted into milk (e.g., see Hydrocortisone and Prednisone) and the excretion of dexamethasone into milk should be expected.

References

1. Carmichael SL, Shaw GM. Maternal corticosteroid use and risk of selected congenital anomalies. Am J Med Genet 1999;86:242–4.
2. Reck G, Nowostawski, Bredwoldt M. Plasma levels of free estriol and cortisol under ACTH and dexamethasone during late pregnancy. Acta Endocrinol 1977;84:86–7.
3. Kauppilla A. ACTH levels in maternal, fetal and neonatal plasma after short term prenatal dexamethasone therapy. Br J Obstet Gynaecol 1977;84:128–34.
4. Warren JC, Cheatum SG. Maternal urinary estrogen excretion: effect of adrenal suppression. J Clin Endocrinol 1967;27:436–8.
5. Caspi I, Schreyer P, Weinraub Z, Reif R, Levi I, Mundel G. Changes in amniotic fluid lecithin-sphingomyelin ratio following maternal dexamethasone administration. Am J Obstet Gynecol 1975;122:327–31.
6. Spellacy WN, Buhi WC, Riggall FC, Holsinger KL. Human amniotic fluid lecithin/sphingomyelin ratio changes with estrogen or glucocorticoid treatment. Am J Obstet Gynecol 1973;115:216–8.
7. Caspi E, Schreyer P, Weinraub Z, Reif R, Levi I, Mundel G. Prevention of the respiratory distress syndrome in premature infants by antepartum glucocorticoid therapy. Br J Obstet Gynaecol 1976;83:187–93.
8. Ballard RA, Ballard PL. Use of prenatal glucocorticoid therapy to prevent respiratory distress syndrome. Am J Dis Child 1976;130:982–7.
9. Thornfeldt RE, Franklin RW, Pickering NA, Thornfeldt CR, Amell G. The effect of glucocorticoids on the maturation of premature lung membranes: preventing the respiratory distress syndrome by glucocorticoids. Am J Obstet Gynecol 1978;131:143–8.
10. Ballard PL, Ballard RA. Corticosteroids and respiratory distress syndrome: status 1979. Pediatrics 1979;63:163–5.
11. Taeusch HW Jr, Frigoletto F, Kitzmiller J, Avery ME, Hehre A, Fromm B, Lawson E, Neff RK. Risk of respiratory distress syndrome after prenatal dexamethasone treatment. Pediatrics 1979;63:64–72.

12. Caspi E, Schreyer P, Weinraub Z, Lifshitz Y, Goldberg M. Dexamethasone for prevention of respiratory distress syndrome: multiple perinatal factors. Obstet Gynecol 1981;57:41–7.
13. Bishop EH. Acceleration of fetal pulmonary maturity. Obstet Gynecol 1981;58(Suppl):48S–51S.
14. Farrell PM, Engle MJ, Zachman RD, Curet LB, Morrison JC, Rao AV, Poole WK. Amniotic fluid phospholipids after maternal administration of dexamethasone. Am J Obstet Gynecol 1983;145:484–90.
15. Ruvinsky ED, Douvas SG, Roberts WE, Martin JN Jr, Palmer SM, Rhodes PG, Morrison JC. Maternal administration of dexamethasone in severe pregnancy-induced hypertension. Am J Obstet Gynecol 1984;149:722–6.
16. Avery ME. The argument for prenatal administration of dexamethasone to prevent respiratory distress syndrome. J Pediatr 1984;104:240.
17. Sepkowitz S. Prenatal corticosteroid therapy to prevent respiratory distress syndrome. J Pediatr 1984;105:338–9.
18. Avery ME. Prenatal corticosteroid therapy to prevent respiratory distress syndrome (reply). J Pediatr 1984;105:339.
19. Levy DL. Maternal administration of dexamethasone to prevent RDS. J Pediatr 1984;105:339.
20. Eggers TR, Doyle LW, Pepperell RJ. Premature rupture of the membranes. Med J Aust 1979;1:209–13.
21. Garite TJ, Freeman RK, Linzey EM, Braly PS, Dorchester WL. Prospective randomized study of corticosteroids in the management of premature rupture of the membranes and the premature gestation. Am J Obstet Gynecol 1981;141:508–15.
22. Garite TJ. Premature rupture of the membranes: the enigma of the obstetrician. Am J Obstet Gynecol 1985;151:1001–5.
23. Curet LB, Morrison JC, Rao AV. Antenatal therapy with corticosteroids and postpartum complications. Am J Obstet Gynecol 1985;152:83–4.
24. Osathanondh R, Tulchinsky D, Kamali H, Fencl M, Taeusch HW Jr. Dexamethasone levels in treated pregnant women and newborn infants. J Pediatr 1977;90:617–20.
25. Levitz M, Jansen V, Dancis J. The transfer and metabolism of corticosteroids in the perfused human placenta. Am J Obstet Gynecol 1978;132:363–6.
26. Otero L, Conlon C, Reynolds P, Duval-Arnould B, Golden SM. Neonatal leukocytosis associated with prenatal administration of dexamethasone. Pediatrics 1981;68:778–80.
27. Anday EK, Harris MC. Leukemoid reaction associated with antenatal dexamethasone administration. J Pediatr 1982;101:614–6.
28. Schatz M, Patterson R, Zeitz S, O'Rourke J, Melam H. Corticosteroid therapy for the pregnant asthmatic patient. JAMA 1975;233:804–7.
29. Jenssen H, Wright PB. The effect of dexamethasone therapy in prolonged pregnancy. Acta Obstet Gynecol Scand 1977;56:467–73.
30. Navot D, Rozen E, Sadovsky E. Effect of dexamethasone on amniotic fluid absorbance in Rh-sensitized pregnancy. Br J Obstet Gynaecol 1982;89: 456–8.
31. Yin CS, Scott JR. Unsuccessful treatment of fetal immunologic thrombocytopenia with dexamethasone. Am J Obstet Gynecol 1985;152:316–7.
32. David M, Forest MG. Prenatal treatment of congenital adrenal hyperplasia resulting from 21-hydroxylase deficiency. J Pediatr 1984;105:799–803.
33. Evans MI, Chrousos GP, Mann DW, Larsen JW Jr, Green I, McCluskey J, Loriaux L, Fletcher JC, Koons G, Overpeck J, Schulman JD. Pharmacologic suppression of the fetal adrenal gland in utero. JAMA 1985;253: 1015–20.
34. Taeusch HW Jr. Glucocorticoid prophylaxis for respiratory distress syndrome: a review of potential toxicity. J Pediatr 1975;87:617–23.
35. Johnson JWC, Mitzner W, London WT, Palmer AE, Scott R. Betamethasone and the rhesus fetus: multisystemic effects. Am J Obstet Gynecol 1979;133:677–84.
36. Wong YC, Beardsmore CS, Silverman M. Antenatal dexamethasone and subsequent lung growth. Arch Dis Child 1982;57:536–8.
37. Collaborative Group on Antenatal Steroid Therapy. Effects of antenatal dexamethasone administration in the infant: long-term follow-up. J Pediatr 1984;104:259–67.

DEXBROMPHENIRAMINE

Antihistamine

PREGNANCY RECOMMENDATION: No Human Data—Probably Compatible
BREASTFEEDING RECOMMENDATION: Limited Human Data—Probably Compatible

PREGNANCY SUMMARY

Dexbrompheniramine is the *dextro*-isomer of brompheniramine (see Brompheniramine). No reports linking its use with congenital defects have been located. In general, antihistamines are considered low risk in pregnancy. However, exposure near birth of premature infants has been associated with an increased risk of retrolental fibroplasia.

BREASTFEEDING SUMMARY

See Brompheniramine.

DEXCHLORPHENIRAMINE

Antihistamine

PREGNANCY RECOMMENDATION: Compatible
BREASTFEEDING RECOMMENDATION: No Human Data—Probably Compatible

PREGNANCY SUMMARY

In general, antihistamines are considered low risk in pregnancy. However, exposure near birth of premature infants has been associated with an increased risk of retrolental fibroplasia.

FETAL RISK SUMMARY

Dexchlorpheniramine is the *dextro*-isomer of chlorpheniramine (see also Chlorpheniramine). No reports linking its use with congenital defects have been located. One study recorded 14 exposures in the 1st trimester without evidence for an association with malformations (1). Animal studies for chlorpheniramine have not shown a teratogenic effect (2).

In a surveillance study of Michigan Medicaid recipients involving 229,101 completed pregnancies conducted between 1985 and 1992, 1080 newborns had been exposed to dexchlorpheniramine during the 1st trimester (F. Rosa, personal communication, FDA, 1993). A total of 50 (4.6%) major birth defects were observed (43 expected). Specific data were available for six defect categories, including (observed/expected) 10/11 cardiovascular defects, 2/2 oral clefts, 0/0.5 spina bifida, 3/3 polydactyly, 0/2 limb reduction defects, and 4/3 hypospadias. These data do not support an association between the drug and congenital defects.

An association between exposure during the last 2 weeks of pregnancy to antihistamines in general and retrolental fibroplasia in premature infants has been reported. See Brompheniramine for details.

BREASTFEEDING SUMMARY

No reports describing the use of dexchlorpheniramine during human lactation have been located. (See also Chlorpheniramine.)

References

1. Heinonen OP, Slone D, Shapiro S. *Birth Defects and Drugs in Pregnancy*. Littleton, MA: Publishing Sciences Group, 1977:323.
2. Product information. Polaramine. Schering Corporation, 1990.

DEXFENFLURAMINE

[Withdrawn from the market. See 9th edition.]

DEXLANSOPRAZOLE

Gastrointestinal Drug (Antisecretory)

PREGNANCY RECOMMENDATION: **No Human Data—Animal Data Suggest Low Risk**
BREASTFEEDING RECOMMENDATION: **No Human Data—Potential Toxicity**

PREGNANCY SUMMARY

Although there are no human data for dexlansoprazole, there are data for racemic lansoprazole (see Lansoprazole). These data, combined with the data for the other proton pump inhibitors (PPIs), suggest that the risk of developmental toxicity, including structural anomalies, is low. Human pregnancy experience with three other PPIs (see Lansoprazole, Omeprazole, and Pantoprazole) has not shown a causal relationship with congenital malformations. In some cases, malformations may have been missed because of the design and size of the studies. The carcinogenic and mutagenic data for lansoprazole and other PPIs are a potential concern, but the absence of follow-up studies prevents a risk assessment for exposed offspring. A study showing an association between in utero exposure to gastric acid-suppressing drugs and childhood allergy and asthma requires confirmation. As with all drug therapy, avoidance of dexlansoprazole during pregnancy, especially during the 1st trimester, is the safest course. If dexlansoprazole is required or if inadvertent exposure does occur early in gestation, the known risk to the embryo–fetus for congenital defects appears to be low. Long-term follow-up of offspring exposed during gestation is warranted.

FETAL RISK SUMMARY

Dexlansoprazole is a PPI that blocks gastric acid secretion by a direct inhibitory effect on the gastric parietal cell. It is indicated for healing of all grades of erosive esophagitis for up to 8 weeks, the maintenance of healed erosive esophagitis for up to 6 months, and for the treatment of heartburn associated with nonerosive gastroesophageal reflux disease (GERD) for 4 weeks. Dexlansoprazole is the R-enantiomer of racemic lansoprazole. It is in the same drug class as esomeprazole, lansoprazole, omeprazole, pantoprazole, and rabeprazole. The drug is extensively metabolized to inactive metabolites. Plasma protein binding is about 96%–99% and the elimination half-life is about 1–2 hours (1).

Reproduction studies have been conducted in rabbits. At oral doses about 9 times the maximum recommended human dose, no evidence of fetal harm was observed (1). (See also Lansoprazole.)

Studies for carcinogenicity, mutagenicity, and impairment of fertility were conducted for lansoprazole (see Lansoprazole).

It is not known if dexlansoprazole crosses the human placenta. The molecular weight (about 369) and the elimination half-life suggest that the drug will cross to the embryo–fetus, but the high plasma protein binding might limit the exposure.

A meta-analysis of PPIs in pregnancy was reported in 2009 (2). Based on 1530 exposed compared with 133,410 not exposed pregnancies, the OR for major malformations was 1.12, 95% CI 0.86–1.45. There also was no increased risk for spontaneous abortions (OR 1.29, 95% CI 0.84–1.97) or preterm birth (OR 1.13, 95% CI 0.96–1.33) (2).

A population-based, observational, cohort study formed by linking data from three Swedish national healthcare registers over a 10-year period (1995–2004) was reported in 2009 (3). The main outcome measures were a diagnosis of allergic disease or a prescription for asthma or allergy medications. The drug types included in the study were gastric acid suppressors, including H2-receptor antagonists, prostaglandins, PPIs, combinations for eradication of *Helicobacter pylori*, and drugs for peptic ulcer and GERD. Of 585,716 children, 29,490 (5.0%) met the diagnosis and 5645 (1%) had been exposed to gastric acid suppression therapy in pregnancy. Of these children, 405 (0.07%) were treated for allergic disease. For developing allergy, the odds ratio (OR) was 1.43, 98% confidence interval (CI) 1.29–1.59, irrespective of the drug, time of exposure during pregnancy, and maternal history of allergy. For developing childhood asthma, but not other allergic diseases, the OR was 1.51, 95% CI 1.35–1.69, irrespective of the type of acid-suppressive drug and the time of exposure in pregnancy. The authors proposed three possible mechanisms for their findings: (a) exposure to increased amounts of allergens could cause sensitization to digestion of labile antigens in the fetus; (b) maternal Th2 cytokine pattern could promote an allergy-prone phenotype in the fetus; and (c) maternal allergen-specific immunoglobulin E could cross the placenta and sensitize fetal immune cells to food and airborne allergens. Several limitations of the study that might have affected their findings were identified, including a general increase in childhood asthma but not necessarily an increase in allergic asthma (3). The study requires confirmation.

Several reports and reviews describing the use of PPIs during human pregnancy have observed no increased risk of developmental toxicity (see Esomeprazole, Lansoprazole, Omeprazole, Pantoprazole, and Rabeprazole).

D

BREASTFEEDING SUMMARY

No reports describing the use of dexlansoprazole during human lactation have been located. The molecular weight (about 369) and the elimination half-life (about 1–2 hours) suggest that the drug will be excreted into breast milk, but the high plasma protein binding (about 96%–99%) might limit the amount excreted. The effect of this exposure on a nursing infant is unknown. Because of the carcinogenicity observed in animals with lansoprazole, and the potential for suppression of gastric acid secretion in the nursing infant, the use of dexlansoprazole during lactation is best avoided.

References

1. Product information. Kapidex. Takeda Pharmaceuticals America, 2009.
2. Gill SK, O'Brien L, Einarson TR, Koren G. The safety of proton pump inhibitors (PPIs) in pregnancy: a meta-analysis. Am J Gastroenterol 2009;104:1541–5.
3. Dehlink E, Yen E, Leichtner AM, Hait EJ, Fiebiger E. First evidence of a possible association between gastric acid suppression during pregnancy and childhood asthma: a population-based register study. Clin Exp Allergy 2009;39:246–53.

DEXMEDETOMIDINE

Sedative

PREGNANCY RECOMMENDATION: Limited Human Data—Animal Data Suggest Moderate Risk
BREASTFEEDING RECOMMENDATION: No Human Data—Probably Compatible

PREGNANCY SUMMARY

The human pregnancy experience with dexmedetomidine is limited to short-term use immediately before or during delivery in three women. The drug crosses the human placenta at term. A 2009 editorial concluded that off-label use of dexmedetomidine might be beneficial in providing pain relief for laboring women unwilling or unable to receive neuraxial analgesia (1). However, newborn toxicity, such as hypotension and sedation, is a potential concern. Moreover, dexmedetomidine may increase uterine contractions and this property should be considered if the drug is used during pregnancy.

FETAL RISK SUMMARY

Dexmedetomidine, a relatively selective α_2-adrenergic agonist with sedative properties, is given as an IV infusion. It is indicated for sedation of initially intubated and mechanically ventilated patients during treatment in an intensive care setting and for sedation of nonintubated patients before and/or during surgical and other procedures. At recommended doses, dexmedetomidine does not cause respiratory depression. The drug undergoes nearly complete metabolism to inactive metabolites. Plasma protein binding is 94% and the terminal elimination half-life is about 2 hours (2).

Reproduction studies have been conducted in rats and rabbits. In rats, dexmedetomidine crossed the placenta. No teratogenicity was observed in rats given SC doses during organogenesis (gestation day 5–16) up to about the maximum recommended human IV dose (MRHD) based on BSA (MRHD-BSA). However, at the highest dose, postimplantation losses and a reduced number of live pups were observed. The no-observed-effect-level (NOEL) was less than the MRHD-BSA. In another rat study that used SC doses less than the MRHD-BSA from gestation day 16 through weaning, lower offspring weights were observed. Moreover, when offspring were allowed to mate, elevated fetal and embryocidal toxicity and delayed motor development were observed in second-generation offspring. No teratogenicity was noted in rabbits during organogenesis (day 6–18) given IV doses up to about 0.5 times the exposure at the MRHD based on AUC (2).

D

A study using pregnant rats evaluated the effects of chronic vs. acute exposure on fetal development and postnatal behavior (3). The rats were given either daily SC doses (gestation days 7–19) or a single SC dose on day 19. No structural anomalies were observed and there were no differences between the groups in terms of pup postnatal weight gain or behavioral performance (3). Extrapolating from the aforementioned information, all of the doses appeared to be less than the MRHD-BSA.

Studies for carcinogenicity have not been conducted. Assays for mutagenicity were negative but the drug was clastogenic in some tests. Fertility in male and female rats was not affected by SC doses that were less than the MRHD-BSA (2).

The relatively low molecular weight (about 201 for the free base) suggests that dexmedetomidine will cross the human placenta, but the plasma protein binding and short terminal elimination half-life might limit the exposure of the embryo and/or fetus, at least early in gestation. The manufacturer reported that the drug crossed the human placenta in an in vitro study but provided no other details (2). Term placentas were used in a single placental cotyledon study to measure the amount of dexmedetomidine compared with clonidine that crossed to the fetal circulation over a 2-hour period (4). Dexmedetomidine disappeared faster than clonidine from the maternal circulation, but the amount of drug appearing in the fetal circulation at 2 hours was less (12.5% vs. 22.1%). The difference was explained by greater placental retention of dexmedetomidine (48.1% vs. 11.3%). The fetal: maternal concentration ratio at 2 hours was 0.77 (4).

The sedative, analgesic, and hemodynamic controlling properties of dexmedetomidine have been reported in three pregnant women in labor (5–7). A 35-year-old woman with spinal muscular atrophy presented for cesarean section at 35 weeks' gestation (5). She was given an IV infusion of dexmedetomidine with a total dose of 1.84 mcg/kg over 38 minutes, followed by general anesthesia. A male infant (weight not specified) was delivered 68 minutes after discontinuation of the infusion. Apgar scores were 6 and 8 at 1 and 5 minutes, respectively. The initially oxygen saturation in the newborn was 88% but with treatment improved to 95% at 5 minutes. At delivery, the umbilical arterial and maternal venous concentrations were 540 and 710 pg/mL, respectively, a ratio of 0.76. The initial low Apgar score was thought to be secondary to a combination of gestational age and residual inhalational anesthetic. However, a contribution from dexmedetomidine could not be excluded. The healthy infant was discharged home with his mother 1 week later (5).

A 37-year-old woman at 38 weeks' gestation with diabetes and preeclampsia presented in labor (6). Because she refused epidural analgesia, an IV infusion of dexmedetomidine was started. Three hours later, a cesarean section under general anesthesia was conducted because of persistent late decelerations in the fetal heart rate. A healthy, 3.7-kg female infant was delivered with Apgar scores of 8 and 9. The mother and infant were doing well and discharged home after 7 days (6).

In another 2009 report, a morbidly obese 31-year-old woman with spina bifida occulta and a tethered spinal cord at L5-S1 presented at 40 weeks' for elective induction of labor (7). Patient-controlled analgesia with IV fentanyl was started but was unsuccessful in controlling pain from her contractions. An IV infusion of dexmedetomidine was added, which immediately resulted in a marked decrease in her pain. Because of prolonged labor and the diagnosis of chorioamnionitis, a cesarean section was conducted under general anesthesia. The dexmedetomidine infusion was continued during the procedure. A healthy male infant (weight not specified) was delivered with Apgar scores of 7 and 8. The infant did well and was discharged 4 days later (7).

A 2005 in vitro study described the effects of dexmedetomidine on human myometrium (8). At simulated clinical plasma concentrations, the drug enhanced the frequency and amplitude of contractions.

BREASTFEEDING SUMMARY

No reports describing the use of dexmedetomidine during human lactation have been located.

The relatively low molecular weight (about 201 for the free base) suggests that the drug will be excreted into breast milk, but the plasma protein binding (94%) and short terminal elimination half-life (2 hours) should limit the amount in milk. However, as with other weak bases, accumulation in the relatively acidic milk may occur. The oral absorption of the drug is unknown, as is the effect, if any, of exposure in a nursing infant. Nevertheless, the sedative properties of the drug in the mother will limit the opportunities for breastfeeding.

References

1. Sia AT, Sng BL. Editorial. Intravenous dexmedetomidine for obstetric anaesthesia and analgesia: converting a challenge into an opportunity? Int J Obstet Anesth 2009;18:204–6.
2. Product information. Precedex. Hospira, 2010.
3. Tariq M, Cerny V, Elfaki I, Ahmad Khan H. Effects of subchronic versus acute in utero exposure to dexmedetomidine on foetal developments in rats. Basic Clin Pharmacol Toxicol 2008;103:180–5.
4. Ala-Kokko TI, Pienimäki P, Lampela E, Hollmén AI, Pelkonen O, Vahakangas K. Transfer of clonidine and dexmedetomidine across the isolated perfused human placenta. Acta Anaesthesiol Scand 1997;41:313–9.
5. Neumann MM, Davio MB, Macknet MR, Applegate II RL. Dexmedetomidine for awake fiberoptic intubation in a parturient with spinal muscular atrophy type III for cesarean delivery. Int J Obstet Anesth 2009;18:403–7.
6. Abu-Halaweh SA, Al Oweidi AKS, Abu-Malooh H, Zabalawi M, Alkazaleh F, Abu-Ali H, Ramsay MAE. Intravenous dexmedetomidine infusion for labour analgesia in patient with preeclampsia. Eur J Anaesthesiol 2009;26:86–7.
7. Palanisamy A, Klickovich RJ, Ramsay M, Ouyang DW, Tsen LC. Intravenous dexmedetomidine as an adjunct for labor analgesia and cesarean delivery anesthesia in a parturient with a tethered spinal cord. Int J Obstet Anesth 2009;18:258–61.
8. Sia AT, Kwek K, Yeo GS. The in vitro effects of clonidine and dexmedetomidine on human myometrium. Int J Obstet Anesth 2005;14:104–7.

DEXMETHYLPHENIDATE

Central Stimulant

PREGNANCY RECOMMENDATION: No Human Data—Animal Data Suggest Low Risk
BREASTFEEDING RECOMMENDATION: No Human Data—Potential Toxicity

D

PREGNANCY SUMMARY

No reports describing the use of dexmethylphenidate in human pregnancy have been located. No teratogenicity was observed in two animal species, but the maximum maternal systemic exposures obtained were very close to those measured in humans clinically. Reported pregnancy exposures to methylphenidate, a closely related agent, are limited, but have not shown a major risk for embryo–fetal harm (see also Methylphenidate). Until human data are available for dexmethylphenidate, the safest course is to avoid the drug in pregnancy. If the mother's condition requires the drug, the lowest effective dose, avoiding the 1st trimester if possible, should be used. Long-term follow-up of exposed offspring may be warranted.

FETAL RISK SUMMARY

Dexmethylphenidate is a CNS stimulant that is indicated for the treatment of attention deficit/hyperactivity disorder (ADHD). There are no active metabolites. The mean plasma elimination half-life is about 2.2 hours (1).

Reproduction studies have been conducted in rats and rabbits. No evidence of teratogenicity was observed in rats treated during organogenesis with doses resulting in maternal plasma levels (AUC) up to five times the levels (AUC) obtained in adult humans taking the recommended dose of 20 mg/day (RHD). However, at the highest dose, delayed skeletal ossification was seen. When doses resulting in plasma levels up to five times the RHD were given throughout gestation and lactation, the highest dose resulted in decreased postweaning body weight in male offspring. In rabbits, no evidence of teratogenicity was observed at plasma levels up to one time the RHD (1).

It is not known if dexmethylphenidate crosses the human placenta. The molecular weight (about 234 for the free base) suggests that the drug will cross to the embryo and/or the fetus. The relatively short half-life, however, should limit the amount crossing the placenta.

BREASTFEEDING SUMMARY

No reports describing the use dexmethylphenidate during human lactation have been located. The molecular weight (about 234 for the free base) is low enough that excretion into breast milk should be expected. However, the relatively short plasma elimination half-life should limit the amount of the drug in milk. The effect of this exposure on a nursing infant is unknown. If a mother chooses to breastfeed while taking dexmethylphenidate, the infant should be monitored for adverse effects observed in children and adults (e.g., abdominal pain, fever, anorexia, and nausea).

Reference

1. Product information. Focalin. Novartis Pharmaceuticals, 2003.

DEXPANTHENOL

Vitamin/Gastrointestinal Agent (Stimulant)

PREGNANCY RECOMMENDATION: No Human Data—No Relevant Animal Data
BREASTFEEDING RECOMMENDATION: No Human Data—Potential Toxicity

PREGNANCY SUMMARY

No reports describing the use of dexpanthenol in human pregnancy have been located. The absence of animal and human pregnancy experience prevents an assessment of the embryo–fetal risk. The potential dose over a 24-hour period for postoperative adynamic ileus (500—2500 mg) ranges from 50 to 250 times the U.S. recommended daily allowance in pregnancy (10 mg) for pantothenic acid. Although a 1982 review (1) recommended dexpanthenol for functional constipation in pregnant women, without providing any data in pregnancy, the safest course is to avoid the drug in pregnancy and certainly in the 1st trimester. Increased fluid intake and a high fiber diet are still the best way to decrease constipation in pregnancy (2).

FETAL RISK SUMMARY

Dexpanthenol is administered by IM or IV injection to prevent paralytic ileus, for the treatment of intestinal atony causing abdominal distention, and for postoperative or postpartum retention of flatus, or delay in resumption of intestinal motility. It also is used topically for the treatment of minor skin disorders. Dexpanthenol, the alcoholic analogue of *d*-pantothenic acid, is a prodrug that is converted in vivo to pantothenic acid, a B complex vitamin. (See Pantothenic Acid.) The vitamin is a precursor of coenzyme A, the cofactor for enzyme-catalyzed reactions involving the transfer of acetyl groups. The plasma elimination half-life and protein binding have not been reported (3).

Animal reproduction studies have not been conducted with dexpanthenol. Neither have animal studies been performed for carcinogenicity, mutagenicity, or impairment of fertility (3).

Studies describing the placental crossing of dexpanthenol have not been located. The molecular weight (about 205) is low enough that exposure of the embryo and fetus should be expected. Moreover, the active metabolite, pantothenic acid, is required for good health and crosses the placenta to the fetus (see Pantothenic Acid).

BREASTFEEDING SUMMARY

No studies describing the use of dexpanthenol during human lactation have been located. The molecular weight (about 205) is low enough that excretion into breast milk should be expected. The active metabolite, pantothenic acid, is excreted into milk. (See Pantothenic Acid.) The U.S. recommended daily allowance during lactation has not been established for pantothenic acid, but the potential dose of dexpanthenol is very high. (See Pregnancy Summary.). Although most of the dexpanthenol dose should be converted to the B vitamin, excretion of unmetabolized prodrug could potentially cause colic and diarrhea in a nursing infant.

References

1. Hanck AB, Goffin H. Dexpanthenol (Ro 01-4709) in the treatment of constipation. Acta Vitaminol Enzymol 1982;4:87–97.
2. Nolan TE, Schilder JM. Lower gastrointestinal tract disorders. Clinical Updates in Women's Health Care. Am Coll Obstetricians Gynecologists 2006;5(1):5.
3. Product information. Ilopan. Adria Laboratories, 1989.

DEXRAZOXANE

Antineoplastic Cytoprotectant

PREGNANCY RECOMMENDATION: Compatible—Maternal Benefit >> Embryo–Fetal Risk
BREASTFEEDING RECOMMENDATION: No Human Data—Probably Compatible

PREGNANCY SUMMARY

No reports describing the use of dexrazoxane in human pregnancy have been located. Developmental toxicity was observed in two animal species, but the doses studied were greater than the dose causing maternal toxicity. Nevertheless, the absence of human pregnancy experience prevents a more complete assessment of the embryo–fetal risk. However, dexrazoxane is intended to protect the patient from doxorubicin-induced cardiomyopathy. Thus, if a pregnant woman requires dexrazoxane and gives informed consent, the maternal benefit from the drug appears to outweigh the potential embryo–fetal risk. If inadvertent exposure occurs during pregnancy, the woman should be advised of the potential risk for adverse effects in the embryo and fetus.

FETAL RISK SUMMARY

Dexrazoxane, a cyclic derivative of ethylenediaminetetraacetic acid (EDTA) that readily penetrates cell membranes, is given as an IV dose immediately prior to a dose of doxorubicin. It is indicated for reducing the incidence and severity of cardiomyopathy associated with doxorubicin in women with metastatic breast cancer who have received a cumulative doxorubicin dose of 300 mg/m^2 and who will continue to receive doxorubicin therapy to maintain tumor control. Dexrazoxane is partially metabolized to inactive metabolites and is not bound to plasma proteins. The mean dose-related plasma elimination half-lives were 2.1 and 2.5 hours (1).

Reproduction studies have been conducted in rats and rabbits, but the route of administration was not specified in either species. Maternal toxicity was observed in pregnant rats given a dose that was about 0.025 times the human dose based on BSA (HD). When given daily to rats during organogenesis, a dose that was about 0.1 times the HD was embryotoxic and teratogenic. Teratogenic effects were imperforate anus, microphthalmia, and anophthalmia. In rabbits, a daily dose during organogenesis that was about 0.1 times the HD caused maternal toxicity. A higher dose, about 0.5 times the HD, was embryotoxic and teratogenic, including skeletal malformations (short tail, rib, and thoracic defects), soft tissue variations (subcutaneous, eye, and cardiac hemorrhagic areas), and agenesis of the gallbladder and of the intermediate lobe of the lung (1).

Long-term studies for carcinogenic potential have been conducted. Dexrazoxane was not mutagenic in one test but was clastogenic in two other tests. Fertility was impaired in mature male and female rats exposed in utero during organogenesis to doses that were about 0.1 times the HD. Testicular atrophy was observed in rats given a dose that was about 0.33 times the HD for 6 weeks, and in dogs given a dose about equal to the HD for 13 weeks (route of administration not specified) (1).

It is not known if dexrazoxane crosses the human placenta. The molecular weight (about 268), lack of plasma protein binding, and elimination half-life suggest that the drug will cross to the embryo and/or fetus.

BREASTFEEDING SUMMARY

No reports describing the use dexrazoxane during human lactation have been located.

The molecular weight (about 268), lack of plasma protein binding, and elimination half-life (2.1 or 2.5 hours) suggest that the drug will be excreted into breast milk. The effect of this exposure on a nursing infant is unknown. However, because the drug is given as a short IV infusion immediately before doxorubicin, and breastfeeding would be unlikely at this time, the risk of exposing an infant to dexrazoxane when nursing is later resumed appears to be nil.

Reference

1. Product information. Zinecard. Pharmacia & Upjohn, 2007.

D

DEXTROAMPHETAMINE

Central Stimulant

See Amphetamine.

DEXTROMETHORPHAN

Respiratory Drug (Antitussive)

PREGNANCY RECOMMENDATION: Compatible
BREASTFEEDING RECOMMENDATION: Compatible

PREGNANCY SUMMARY

The available human data on the reproductive effects of dextromethorphan do not demonstrate a major teratogenic risk. Except for one study involving chick embryos, there are no published animal reproductive studies. Unpublished pregnant rat and rabbit data have been cited, though, that indicated there was no embryo or fetal harm with the doses used. Extrapolation of the chick embryo data to humans is not possible because of the lethal dose used and the absence of maternal and placental metabolizing systems. Moreover, prior teratology studies have not shown agreement between the chick and mammalian models (1). Fetuses of women with the phenotype for slow dextromethorphan metabolism should have higher concentrations of the drug than fetuses of mothers with normal metabolism, but this may not be clinically significant in the absence of a demonstrated dose–effect. Use of liquid preparations of dextromethorphan that contain ethanol, however, should be avoided during pregnancy because ethanol is a known teratogen.

Many authors consider dextromethorphan to be safe for consumption during pregnancy. This opinion appears to have been based on the low incidence of congenital defects reported in surveillance studies and its wide appeal as a cough suppressant, rather than on evidence derived from human pregnancy research with dextromethorphan or from studies in any animal model. The latest data, however, provide more assurance that dextromethorphan is not a major teratogen.

FETAL RISK SUMMARY

Dextromethorphan, a derivative of the narcotic analgesic levorphanol (see also Levorphanol) that is widely used as a cough suppressant in over-the-counter (OTC) preparations, produces little or no CNS depression. Although it is an antitussive without expectorant, analgesic, or addictive characteristics, abuse of the liquid product, possibly because of the ethanol vehicle used in some proprietary mixtures, is a potential complication (see case below). The agent is available either alone (as capsules, lozenges, or oral solutions) or in combination with a large variety of other compounds used for upper respiratory tract symptoms. Combination products containing ethanol should be avoided during pregnancy (see also Ethanol).

No information is available on the placental transfer of dextromethorphan. The molecular weight (about 271) is low enough that transfer to the fetus should be expected.

Only one published animal reproduction study involving dextromethorphan has been located (see reference 2 for unpublished data). A 1998 report examined the effects of dextromethorphan on chick embryos (3). The authors hypothesized that *N*-methyl-D-aspartate (NMDA) receptor antagonists, such as ethanol and dextromethorphan, induced neural crest (craniofacial and cardiac septal defects) and neural tube defects (NTDs). Dextromethorphan, an NMDA receptor antagonist that acts as a channel blocker at the receptor, was injected into chick embryos in ovo for 3 consecutive days at doses of 0.5, 5, 50, and 500 nmol/embryo/day. The embryos were examined 24 hours after the third dose (none of the embryos were allowed to hatch). Dextromethorphan caused a dose-related increase in embryo mortality with rates of 14.1% with the 50-nmol dose ($p < 0.05$ vs. controls) and 56.7% with the 500-nmol dose ($p < 0.001$ vs. controls). Seven (1.2%) of the 595 control embryos injected only with the vehicle (normal saline) had anomalies (spinal defect [*N* = 1], craniofacial defects [*N* = 4], and multiple defects [*N* = 2]), whereas 30 (8.0%) of all dextromethorphan-treated embryos had anomalies (spinal defect [*N* = 1], craniofacial defects [*N* = 12], multiple defects [*N* = 16], and other defects [*N* = 1]). Only the number of defects (about 15%) in the 500-nmol group, however, was significantly increased ($p < 0.001$) over the number in the control group. The authors cited published evidence that the receptors blocked by dextromethorphan in the chick embryos are analogous to receptors in other animals, including humans, during early development and that the drug would also block these receptors, resulting in similar malformations (3).

Interpretation of the results of the above study have been criticized (1,2,4) and defended (5). The primary concerns raised were the inappropriateness of the chick embryo model for determining human teratogenicity and the design of the study (1,4). Of particular concern, no embryos were allowed to hatch (the doses used were lethal) so it could not be determined if dextromethorphan was actually teratogenic. In addition, one author cited unpublished animal reproduction data from a drug manufacturer showing that in pregnant rats and rabbits, daily doses up to 20 and 100 times the human therapeutic dose on a body weight basis, respectively, caused no embryo or fetal harm in comparison with controls (1).

Metabolism of dextromethorphan has been shown to be primarily a result of O-demethylation to dextrorphan (6). The ability to metabolize many drugs, including O-demethylation of dextromethorphan, is genetically determined in adults. In this study of 155 adult volunteers, 144 (93%) metabolized dextromethorphan rapidly, and 11 (7%) were poor metabolizers, but the poor (slow) drug metabolizer phenotype has been reported in 5%–10% of whites (6). In poor metabolizers, unmetabolized drug was the main excretion product, implying that these individuals had much higher and more prolonged plasma concentrations of dextromethorphan than did those who were extensive metabolizers. Moreover, using microsomal preparations obtained from aborted 10- to 30-week-old human fetuses and live newborn infants, the average activity of O-demethylation was less than 1% of the adult value and did not begin to rise until after birth (6). Thus, accumulation of unmetabolized dextromethorphan in the fetal compartment is a potential result of maternal ingestion of the drug during pregnancy (6).

The Collaborative Perinatal Project monitored 50,282 mother–child pairs, 300 of whom took dextromethorphan during the 1st trimester (7, p. 378). Twenty-four of the infants exposed in utero had a congenital malformation, a standardized relative risk (SRR) of 1.18. When only malformations showing uniform rates by hospital were considered, 17 (SRR 1.21) infants had a congenital defect (7, p. 379). Of these 17, 9 had major defects (SRR 1.10) and 8 had minor defects (SRR 1.30) (7, p. 382). For use anytime during pregnancy, 580 exposures were recorded, 15 of which had a malformation (SRR 1.39) (7, pp. 438, 442). Ten of these defects were inguinal hernias (7, p. 496). The SSRs do not support a relationship between the drug and congenital malformations.

A case report published in 1981 described a woman who consumed 480–840 mL/day of a cough syrup throughout pregnancy (8). The potential maximum daily doses based on 840 mL of syrup were 1.68 g of dextromethorphan, 16.8 g of guaifenesin, 5.0 g of pseudoephedrine, and 79.8 mL of ethanol. The infant had facial features of the fetal alcohol syndrome (bilateral epicanthal folds; short palpebral fissures; short, upturned nose; hypoplastic philtrum and upper lip with thinned vermilion; and a flattened midface [8]). (See also Ethanol.) Other defects noted were an umbilical hernia and labia that appeared hypoplastic. The infant displayed irritability, tremors, and hypertonicity. It is not known if dextromethorphan or the drugs other than ethanol were associated with the adverse effects observed in the infant.

The use of dextromethorphan in four of five cases of a rare and distinct malformation complex was reported in 1984 (9). The complex of defects included absence of external genitalia, urinary, genital, and anal orifices, and persistence of the cloaca (9).

Chromosome analysis in four of the cases was normal and genetics did not appear to be a cause of the defects. Although a causative relationship could not be determined, the authors noted that three of the pregnancies, possibly all five, were exposed to doxylamine during the first 50 days of pregnancy (9). Dextromethorphan, however, was not thought to be related to the outcomes because only four of the mothers had symptoms of respiratory infection or took dextromethorphan during the critical period.

A surveillance study published in 1985 examined the prevalence of certain major birth defects among liveborn infants of 6509 mothers (10). Dextromethorphan was assumed to have been used by 59 of the mothers, only one of whom gave birth to an infant with a major anomaly. This study found no strong association between any of the commonly used drugs and the congenital malformations surveyed (10).

Data from the Spanish Collaborative Study of Congenital Malformations (ECEMC) evaluating prenatal exposure to cough medicines containing dextromethorphan were published in 2001 (11). Using standardized methods, all newborn infants born in more than 77 hospitals throughout Spain were examined during the first 3 days of life for major and/or minor congenital defects. The case–control study was conducted between 1976 and 1998 and included 1,575,388 liveborn infants, 27,864 of whom had congenital defects detected during the first 3 days. Each case infant (those with defects) and its control (the next nonmalformed, same sex-infant born) were obtained from the same hospital. Among the case and control mothers, 0.26% (*N* = 70) and 0.18% (*N* = 48), respectively, had taken cough medicines containing dextromethorphan during the 1st trimester. The data were primarily analyzed for NTD and cardiac defects to test the hypothesis raised in the chick embryo study cited above (reference 3), but about 600 different categories of defects were also examined. Most of these categories, however, had no cases or controls. The adjusted (for maternal age, fever, drugs other than dextromethorphan, flu/cold, first-degree relatives with the same defects) odds ratio and 95% confidence intervals for selected anomalies were NTD 0.67 (0.09–4.94), CNS defects 1.36 (0.39–4.72), hydrocephaly 3.39 (0.38–30.35), congenital heart defects 0.92 (0.13–6.61), oral clefts 4.72 (0.55–40.24), and cleft palate 3.26 (0.35–30.34). When data on the amount consumed were available, the estimated total dextromethorphan dose and duration for cases and controls was about 101 mg/2.69 days and 117 mg/3.96 days, respectively. The investigators concluded that the use of dextromethorphan during the 1st trimester was not associated with an increase in congenital defects (11).

A 1984 review on the effect of OTC drugs on human pregnancy concluded that dextromethorphan was safe to use during this period (12). Other reference sources (13–16) have also concluded that this antitussive does not pose a risk to the human fetus, and a 1998 source states that dextromethorphan is one of the drugs of choice during pregnancy for cough (17). Two of these references recommended a combination of guaifenesin plus dextromethorphan as the preferred antitussive in pregnant asthmatic patients (15,16).

A study published in 2001 described the outcomes of 184 pregnancies exposed to dextromethorphan, 128 of which were exposed in the 1st trimester, compared with 184 matched controls (18). The subjects were women who had called a teratogen information service concerning their use of dextromethorphan during pregnancy. There were six major birth defects (type not specified) in the subject group. One was a chromosomal abnormality and two were born to women who had used the antitussive after the 1st trimester. Among controls, there were five major birth defects (type not specified), one of which was a chromosomal abnormality. There were also no statistical differences between all subjects and controls in other outcomes: live births (172 vs. 174), spontaneous abortions (10 vs. 8), therapeutic abortions (1 vs. 2), stillbirths (1 vs. 0), minor malformations (10 vs. 8), and birth weight (3381 g vs. 3446 g) (18).

BREASTFEEDING SUMMARY

No reports describing the use of dextromethorphan during human lactation or measuring the amount, if any, excreted into milk have been located. The relatively low molecular weight of dextromethorphan (about 271) suggests that passage into milk probably occurs. Many preparations containing dextromethorphan also contain ethanol. These products should be avoided during nursing (see Ethanol). Preparations without ethanol, however, are probably safe to use during breastfeeding.

References

1. Brent RL. Studies of the fetal effects of dextromethorphan in ovo. Teratology 1999;60:57–8. (Originally published as an untitled letter to the editor: Pediatr Res 1998;44:415–6.)
2. Polifka JE, Shepard TH. Studies of the fetal effects of dextromethorphan in ovo. Teratology 1999;60:56–7. (Originally published as an untitled letter to the editor: Pediatr Res 1998;44:415.)
3. Andaloro VJ, Monaghan DT, Rosenquist TH. Dextromethorphan and other *N*-methyl-D-aspartate receptor antagonists are teratogenic in the avian embryo model. Pediatr Res 1998;43:1–7.
4. Brent RL, Shepard TH, Polifka JE. Response to Dr. Rosenquist's comments pertaining to the paper by Andaloro et al. ('98) "Dextromethorphan and other N-methyl-D-aspartate receptor antagonists are teratogenic in the avian embryo model" and letters to the editor by Polifka JE and Shepard TH ('98) and Brent RL ('98). Teratology 1999;60:61–2.
5. Rosenquist TH. Studies of the fetal effects of dextromethorphan in ovo. Teratology 1999;60:56–60. (Originally published as an untitled author's response: Pediatr Res 1998;44:416–7.)
6. Jacqz-Aigrain E, Cresteil T. Cytochrome P450-dependent metabolism of dextromethorphan: fetal and adult studies. Dev Pharmacol Ther 1992;18:161–8.
7. Heinonen OP, Slone D, Shapiro S. *Birth Defects and Drugs in Pregnancy*. Littleton, MA: Publishing Sciences Group, 1977.
8. Chasnoff IJ, Diggs G, Schnoll SH. Fetal alcohol effects and maternal cough syrup abuse. Am J Dis Child 1981;135:968.
9. Robinson HB Jr, Tross K. Agenesis of the cloacal membrane. A probable teratogenic anomaly. Perspect Pediatr Pathol 1984;8:79–96.
10. Aselton P, Jick H, Milunsky A, Hunter JR, Stergachis A. First-trimester drug use and congenital disorders. Obstet Gynecol 1985;65:451–5.
11. Martinez-Frias ML, Rodriguez-Pinilla E. Epidemiologic analysis of prenatal exposure to cough medicines containing dextromethorphan: no evidence of human teratogenicity. Teratology 2001;63:38–41.
12. Rayburn WF. OTC drugs and pregnancy. Perinatol Neonatol 1984;8:21–7.
13. Berglund F, Flodh H, Lundborg P, Prame B, Sannerstedt R. Drug use during pregnancy and breast-feeding. A classification system for drug information. Acta Obstet Gynecol Scand Suppl 1984;126:1–55.
14. Onnis A, Grella P. *The Biochemical Effects of Drugs in Pregnancy*. Vol. 2. West Sussex, England: Ellis Horwood Limited, 1984:62–3.
15. Clark SL. Asthma in Pregnancy. National Asthma Education Program Working Group on Asthma and Pregnancy, National Institutes of Health, National Heart, Lung, and Blood Institute. Obstet Gynecol 1993;82:1036–40.
16. Report of the Working Group on Asthma and Pregnancy. Executive summary: management of asthma during pregnancy. J Allergy Clin Immunol 1994;93:139–62.
17. Koren G, Pastuszak A, Ito S. Drugs in pregnancy. N Engl J Med 1998;338:1128–37.
18. Einarson A, Lyszkiewicz D, Koren G. The safety of dextromethorphan in pregnancy. Results of a controlled study. Chest 2001;119:466–9.

DEXTROTHYROXINE

Antilipemic

PREGNANCY RECOMMENDATION: No Human Data—Probably Compatible
BREASTFEEDING RECOMMENDATION: No Human Data—Probably Compatible

PREGNANCY SUMMARY

Although formerly used to treat hypothyroidism, the drug is now used exclusively for the therapy of hyperlipidemia. Except for the one report below, no mention of its use in human pregnancy has been located.

FETAL RISK SUMMARY

Dextrothyroxine is the *dextro*-isomer of levothyroxine (see also Levothyroxine). In a study of placental passage of dextrothyroxine, approximately 9% of a radiolabeled dose given 2–8 hours before delivery was found in the cord blood (1).

BREASTFEEDING SUMMARY

No reports describing the use of dextrothyroxine during human lactation have been located.

Reference

1. Kearns JE, Hutson W. Tagged isomers and analogues of thyroxine (their transmission across the human placenta and other studies). J Nucl Med 1963;4:453–61.

DIATRIZOATE

Diagnostic

PREGNANCY RECOMMENDATION: Limited Human Data—Probably Compatible
BREASTFEEDING RECOMMENDATION: Limited Human Data—Probably Compatible

PREGNANCY SUMMARY

Diatrizoate is available as diatrizoate sodium for IV use (1) and as diatrizoate meglumine for instillation into the bladder (retrograde cystourethrography) (2). When administered alone, neither form of diatrizoate has been associated with suppression of the fetal thyroid. The guidelines of the Contrast Media Safety Committee of the European Society of Urogenital Radiology recommend that iodinated contrast media may be used in pregnancy if such use is essential. However, neonatal thyroid function should be checked during the 1st week (3).

FETAL RISK SUMMARY

Diatrizoate sodium is a water-soluble organic iodide contrast medium that is given IV. It is indicated for excretory urography, cerebral and peripheral angiography, aortography, intraosseous venography, direct cholangiography, hysterosalpingography, splenoportography, and contrast enhancement of computed tomographic head imaging. It is not metabolized but excreted unchanged in the urine. The alpha and beta half-lives are 30 and 120 minutes, respectively, but, in patients with renal impairment, the beta half-life can be up to several days (1).

Diatrizoate meglumine is a water-soluble contrast medium of organically bound iodine that is instilled directly into the bladder. It is indicated for retrograde cystourethrography.

Studies of reproduction, carcinogenicity, mutagenicity, or fertility have not been conducted with either salt form of diatrizoate.

The use of diatrizoate (both salt forms) for amniography has been described in several studies (4–13). Except for inadvertent injection of the contrast media into the fetus during amniocentesis, the use of diatrizoate was not thought to result in fetal harm. More recent studies have examined the effect of the drug on fetal thyroid function.

All of the various preparations of diatrizoate contain a high concentration of organically bound iodine. Twenty-eight pregnant women received intra-amniotic injections (50 mL) of diatrizoate meglumine for diagnostic indications (14). When compared with nontreated controls, no effect was observed on cord blood levothyroxine (T4) or liothyronine resin uptake values regardless of the time interval between injection and delivery. The authors concluded that the iodine remained organically bound until it was eliminated in 2–4 days from the amniotic fluid (14).

In another report, seven patients within 13 days or less of term were injected intra-amniotically with a mixture of ethiodized oil (12 mL) and diatrizoate meglumine (30 mL) (15). Thyrotropin (TSH) levels were determined in the cord blood of five newborns and in the serum of all seven infants on the 5th day of life. TSH was markedly elevated in three of five cord samples and six of seven neonatal samples. Three of the infants had signs and symptoms of hypothyroidism:

- Elevated TSH/normal T4; apathy and jaundice clearing immediately with thyroid therapy (1 infant)
- Elevated TSH/decreased T4 (1 infant)
- Elevated TSH/decreased T4 with goiter (1 infant)

In contrast to the initial report, the severity of thyroid suppression seemed greater when the time interval between injection and delivery was longer. The explanation offered for these different results was the use of the more sensitive TSH serum test and the use of only water-soluble contrast media in the first study (15).

BREASTFEEDING SUMMARY

Diatrizoate was not detected in breast milk in one study. A woman, 7 weeks postpartum, received the contrast medium (a mixture of sodium and meglumine salts) for urography (16). Nine hours after the dose, no measurable drug was identified by spectrophotometer. Based on this report, the American Academy of Pediatrics classifies diatrizoate as compatible with breastfeeding (17). In addition, a 2005 review concluded that breastfeeding may be continued normally when iodinated agents are given to the mother (3).

References

1. Product information. Hypaque Sodium. Amersham Health, 2006.
2. Product information. Cystografin. Bracco Diagnostics, 2006.
3. Webb JAW, Thomsen HS, Morcos SK. The use of iodinated and gadolinium contrast media during pregnancy and lactation. Eur Radiol 2005;15:1234–40.
4. McLain CR Jr. Amniography studies of the gastrointestinal motility of the human fetus. Am J Obstet Gynecol 1963;86:1079–87.
5. McLain CR Jr. Amniography, a versatile diagnostic procedure in obstetrics. Obstet Gynecol 1964;23:45–50.
6. McLain CR Jr. Amniography for diagnosis and management of fetal death in utero. Obstet Gynecol 1965;26:233–6.
7. Ferris EJ, Shapiro JH, Spira J. Roentgenologic aspects of intrauterine transfusion. JAMA 1966;196:127–8.
8. Wiltchik SG, Schwarz RH, Emich JP Jr. Amniography for placental localization. Obstet Gynecol 1966;28:641–5.
9. Misenhimer HR. Fetal hemorrhage associated with amniocentesis. Am J Obstet Gynecol 1966;94:1133–5.
10. Blumberg ML, Wohl GT, Wiltchik S, Schwarz R, Emich JP. Placental localization by amniography. AJR 1967;100:688–97.
11. Berner HW Jr. Amniography, an accurate way to localize the placenta. Obstet Gynecol 1967;29:200–6.
12. Creasman WT, Lawrence RA, Thiede HA. Fetal complications of amniocentesis. JAMA 1968;204:949–52.
13. Bottorff MK, Fish SA. Amniography. S Med J 1971;64:1203–6.
14. Morrison JC, Boyd M, Friedman BI, Bucovaz ET, Whybrew WD, Koury DN, Wiser WL, Fish SA. The effects of Renografin-60 on the fetal thyroid. Obstet Gynecol 1973;42:99–103.
15. Rodesch F, Camus M, Ermans AM, Dodion J, Delange F. Adverse effect of amniofetography on fetal thyroid function. Am J Obstet Gynecol 1976;126:723–6.
16. FitzJohn TP, Williams DG, Laker MF, Owen JP. Intravenous urography during lactation. Br J Radiol 1982;55:603–5.
17. Committee on Drugs, American Academy of Pediatrics. The transfer of drugs and other chemicals into human milk. Pediatrics 2001;108:776–89.

D

DIAZEPAM

Sedative

PREGNANCY RECOMMENDATION: Human Data Suggest Risk in 1st and 3rd Trimesters
BREASTFEEDING RECOMMENDATION: Limited Human Data—Potential Toxicity

PREGNANCY SUMMARY

The effects of benzodiazepines, including diazepam, on the human embryo and fetus are controversial. Although a number of studies have reported an association with various types of congenital defects, other studies have not found such associations. Maternal denial of exposure, as reported in one study, and the concurrent exposure to other toxic drugs and substances (e.g., alcohol and smoking) may be confounding factors. If the drug does cause birth defects, the risk appears to be low. Continuous use during gestation has resulted in neonatal withdrawal and a dose-related syndrome is apparent if diazepam is used close to delivery. Consequently, if the maternal condition requires the use of diazepam during pregnancy, the lowest possible dose should be taken. Moreover, abrupt discontinuance of diazepam should be avoided.

FETAL RISK SUMMARY

Shepard (1) reviewed six studies of the reproductive effects of the benzodiazepine, diazepam in rats and mice in 1989. Cleft palates in mice and delayed neurobehavioral development and postnatal malignancies in rats were the only adverse effects noted (1).

Diazepam and its metabolite, desmethyldiazepam, freely cross the placenta and accumulate in the fetal circulation with newborn levels about 1–3 times greater than maternal serum levels (2–13). Transfer across the placenta has been demonstrated as early as 6 weeks' gestation (12). Of interest, fetal drug levels were independent of maternal serum concentrations and time from drug administration to sampling. These data suggest that diazepam accumulates in the fetal circulation and tissues during organogenesis (12). At term, equilibrium between mother and fetus occurs in 5–10 minutes after IV administration (11). The maternal and fetal serum binding capacity for diazepam is reduced in pregnancy and is not correlated with albumin (14,15). The plasma half-life in newborns is significantly increased due to a decreased clearance of the drug. Because the transplacental passage is rapid at term, timing of the IV administration with uterine contractions will greatly reduce the amount of drug transferred to the fetus (7).

In a case of gross overdose, a mother who took 580 mg of diazepam as a single dose on about the 43rd day of gestation delivered an infant with cleft lip and palate, craniofacial asymmetry, ocular hypertelorism, and bilateral periauricular tags (16). The authors concluded that the drug ingestion was responsible for the defects. An association between diazepam and an increased risk of cleft lip or palate has been suggested by several studies (17–20). The findings indicated that 1st or 2nd trimester use of diazepam, and selected other drugs, is significantly greater among mothers of children born with oral clefts. However, a review of these studies, published in 1976, concluded that a causal relationship between diazepam and oral clefts had not yet been established, but even if it had, the actual risk was only 0.2% for cleft palate and only 0.4% for cleft lip with or without cleft palate (21). In addition, large retrospective studies showing no association between diazepam and cleft lip/palate have been published (22–25). The results of one of these studies has been criticized and defended (26,27). Although no association was found with cleft lip/palate, a statistically significant association was discovered between diazepam and inguinal hernia (27). This same association, along with others, was found in another investigation (28).

In 1427 malformed newborns compared with 3001 controls, 1st trimester use of tranquilizers (diazepam most common) was associated with inguinal hernia, cardiac defects, and pyloric stenosis (28). Second trimester exposure was associated with hemangiomas and cardiac and circulatory defects. The combination of cigarette smoking and tranquilizer use increased the risk of delivering a malformed infant by 3.7-fold as compared with those who smoked but did not use tranquilizers (28). A survey of 390 infants with congenital heart disease matched with 1254 normal infants found a higher rate of exposure to several drugs, including diazepam, in the offspring with defects (29). Other congenital anomalies reported in infants exposed to diazepam include absence of both thumbs (two cases), spina bifida (one case), and absence of left forearm and syndactyly (one case) (30–32). Any relationship between diazepam and these defects is unknown.

A 1989 report described dysmorphic features, growth restriction, and central nervous system defects in eight infants exposed either to diazepam, 30 mg/day or more, or oxazepam, 75 mg/day or more throughout gestation (33). Three of the mothers denied use of drugs during pregnancy, but diazepam and its metabolite were demonstrated in their plasma in early pregnancy. The mothers did not use alcohol or street drugs, had regular prenatal care, and had no record of criminality or prostitution. The mean birth weight of the infants was 1.2 standard deviations below the Swedish average, only one having a weight above the mean, and one was small for gestational age. Six of the newborns had low Apgar scores primarily due to apnea, five needed resuscitation, all were hypotonic at birth, and all had neonatal drug withdrawal with episodes of opisthotonos and convulsions. Seven of the eight infants had feeding difficulties caused by a lack of rooting and sucking reflexes. Craniofacial defects observed in the infants (number of infants with defect shown in parenthesis) were short nose with low nasal bridge (six), uptilted nose (six), slanted eyes (eight), epicanthic folds (eight), telecanthus (two), long eyelashes (three), highly arched palate (four), cleft hard palate and bifid uvula (two), low-set/abnormal ears (four), webbed neck (three), flat upper lip (five), full lips (four), hypoplastic mandible (five), and microcephaly (two). Other defects present were small, wide-spaced nipples (two), renal defect (one), inguinal hernia (two), and cryptorchidism (two). An infant with severe psychomotor retardation died of possible sudden infant death syndrome at 11 weeks of age. Microscopic examination of the brain demonstrated slight cortical dysplasia and an increased number of single-cell neuronal heterotopias in the white matter. Six other children had varying degrees of mental retardation, some had severely disturbed visual perception, all had gross motor disability, and hyperactivity and attention deficits were common. Extensive special examinations were conducted to identify other possible etiologies, but the only common factor in the eight cases was maternal consumption of benzodiazepines (33). Based on the apparent lack of other causes, the investigators concluded that the clinical characteristics observed in the infants probably represented a teratogenic syndrome due to benzodiazepines.

A 1992 study reported on heavy benzodiazepine exposure during pregnancy from Michigan Medicaid data collected during 1980–1983 (34). Of the 2048 women, from a total sample of 104,339, who had received benzodiazepines, 80 had received 10 or more prescriptions for these agents. The records of these 80 women indicated frequent alcohol and substance abuse. Their pregnancy outcomes were three intrauterine deaths, two neonatal deaths in infants with congenital malformations, and 64 survivors. The outcome for 11 infants was unknown. Six of the 64 surviving infants had diagnoses consistent with congenital defects and neurological abnormalities. No cases of oral clefts were found in 1354 1st trimester benzodiazepine exposures. The investigators concluded that the high rate of congenital anomalies was suggestive of multiple alcohol and substance abuse and may not have been related to benzodiazepine exposure. However, subtle defects, developmental abnormalities, and retardations may not have been included in the records (34).

A 1992 letter correspondence suggested that the Möbius' syndrome observed in a 3-week-old infant was the result of in utero exposure to benzodiazepines (diazepam and oxazepam) (35). The mother had been treated for hypertension starting at 16 weeks' gestation with methyldopa. Diazepam (20 mg/day) was added at 25 weeks', and shortly thereafter, hyoscine butylbromide, oxazepam (20 mg/day), and ritodrine were added. The infant had normal weight, length, and head circumference but was markedly hypotonic at birth. In addition to an expressionless face, malformations observed were epicanthal folds, short palpebral fissures, convergent strabismus, low nasal bridge, short upturned nose, hypertelorism, and high arched palate (35). An electromyogram confirmed bilateral cranial nerve VII palsy. The authors speculated that the Möbius' syndrome and the strabismus were caused by the benzodiazepine therapy based on previous reports. At least one mechanism of Möbius' syndrome (VI and VII nerve palsy), however, was thought to be a result of mechanical trauma induced by uterine contractions early in gestation that results in ischemia in the cranial nuclei VI and VII (see Shepard, 1995, in Misoprostol).

The pregnancy outcomes of five women who had attempted suicide with diazepam combined with other drugs early in gestation were described in a 1997 report (36). The gestational ages when the overdoses occurred were 3–4 weeks and the diazepam doses ranged from 90 mg to 200 mg. All five of the infants were delivered at term and, except for an infant with bilateral undescended testes, were normal. The undescended testes were not thought to have been related to the self-poisoning (36).

A meta-analysis of cohort and case–control studies involving the association of 1st trimester exposure to benzodiazepines and major malformations was published in 1998 (37). Analysis of nine cohort studies (nonepileptic patients) showed no relationship to major malformations (odds ratio [OR] 0.90, 95% confidence interval [CI] 0.61–1.35) or to oral clefts (OR 1.19, 95% CI 0.34–4.15). Two cohort studies involving epileptic patients were also negative. In contrast, pooled data from nine case–control studies showed an association with major defects (OR 3.01, 95% CI 1.32–6.84) or to oral clefts alone (OR 1.79, 95% CI 1.13–2.82) (37). In correspondence concerning this study, objections were raised as to the exclusion of certain studies and to the statistical methods used (38–40).

Another 1998 study described the outcomes of 460 pregnancies (subjects) exposed to benzodiazepines, 98% during the 1st trimester, compared with 424 control pregnancies (41). Subjects and controls had called the Israeli Teratogen Information Service concerning exposure to either benzodiazepines (subjects) or various other nonteratogenic exposures (controls). Diazepam was used by 89 women, but several subjects in the total group used more than one type of benzodiazepine. Subjects were older (31.7 vs. 29.4 years, $p = 0.001$) and called earlier in pregnancy (10.3 vs. 12.9 weeks', $p = 0.001$) than controls. There were also more spontaneous and induced abortions in subjects, 8.7% vs. 5.2% $p = 0.047$ and 14.1% vs. 4.7% $p = 0.001$, respectively. None of the induced abortions involved major congenital defects. The higher rates of spontaneous and induced abortions were thought to be related to the lower gestational ages at calling and to the counseling of the callers, respectively (41). The gestational ages and birth weights of the two groups were similar. Major malformations were observed in 11 of the 355 subject live births (3.1%) and in 10 of 382 control live births (2.6%) (*ns*). The birth defects in infants of subjects were four cases of congenital heart disease (ventricular septal defect, pulmonic stenosis, and two unspecified with one neonatal death; carbamazepine used in two cases), two cases of polydactyly, two cases of hydronephrosis, and one each of esophageal atresia, cerebral palsy, and Down's syndrome (41).

Several investigators have observed that the use of diazepam during labor is not harmful to the mother or her infant (42–49). A dose response is likely as the frequency of newborn complications rises when doses exceed 30–40 mg or when diazepam is taken for extended periods, allowing accumulation to occur (50–56). Two major syndromes of neonatal complications have been observed:

Floppy infant syndrome:
- Hypotonia
- Lethargy
- Sucking difficulties

Withdrawal syndrome:
- Intrauterine growth restriction
- Tremors
- Irritability
- Hypertonicity
- Diarrhea/vomiting
- Vigorous sucking

Under miscellaneous effects, diazepam may alter thermogenesis, cause loss of beat-to-beat variability in the fetal heart rate, and decrease fetal movements (33,57–62).

Abrupt discontinuance of benzodiazepines should be avoided because severe withdrawal symptoms (physical and psychological) may occur in the mother and could result in the substitution of other substances (e.g., alcohol) to treat the symptoms (63). Fetal withdrawal, such as that observed with narcotics, has not been reported, but should be considered.

BREASTFEEDING SUMMARY

Diazepam and its metabolite, *n*-demethyldiazepam, enter breast milk (61,62,64–69). Lethargy and loss of weight have been reported (67,69). Milk:plasma ratios varied between 0.2 and 2.7 (66).

A mother who took 6–10 mg daily throughout pregnancy delivered a full-term, normally developed male infant (69). The infant was breastfed and the mother continued to take her diazepam. Sedation was noted in the infant if nursing occurred less than 8 hours after taking a dose. Paired samples of maternal serum and breast milk were obtained on five occasions between 1 and 4 months after delivery. Milk concentrations of diazepam and desmethyldiazepam varied between 7.5 and 87 ng/mL and 19.2 and 77 ng/mL, respectively. The milk:serum ratios for diazepam varied between 0.14 and 0.21 in four samples but was 1.0 in one sample. The ratio for desmethyldiazepam varied from 0.10 to 0.18 in four samples and was 0.53 in the sample with the high diazepam ratio. A serum level was drawn from the infant on one occasion, revealing levels of diazepam and the metabolite of 0.7 and 46 ng/mL, respectively (69).

Diazepam may accumulate in breastfed infants, and its use in lactating women is not recommended. The American Academy of Pediatrics classifies the effects of diazepam on the nursing infant as unknown but may be of concern (70).

References

1. Shepard TH. *Catalog of Teratogenic Agents*. 6th ed. Baltimore, MD: Johns Hopkins University Press, 1989:203–6.
2. Erkkola R, Kanto J, Sellman R. Diazepam in early human pregnancy. Acta Obstet Gynecol Scand 1974;53:135–8.
3. Kanto J, Erkkola R, Sellman R. Accumulation of diazepam and *n*-demethyldiazepam in the fetal blood during labor. Ann Clin Res 1973;5:375–9.
4. Idanpaan-Heikkila JE, Jouppila PI, Puolakka JO, Vorne MS. Placental transfer and fetal metabolism of diazepam in early human pregnancy. Am J Obstet Gynecol 1971;109:1011–6.
5. Mandelli M, Morselli PL, Nordio S, Pardi G, Principi N, Sereni F, Tognoni G. Placental transfer of diazepam and its disposition in the newborn. Clin Pharmacol Ther 1975;17:564–72.
6. Gamble JAS, Moore J, Lamke H, Howard PJ. A study of plasma diazepam levels in mother and infant. Br J Obstet Gynaecol 1977;84:588–91.
7. Haram K, Bakke DM, Johannessen KH, Lund T. Transplacental passage of diazepam during labor: influence of uterine contractions. Clin Pharmacol Ther 1978;24:590–9.
8. Bakke OM, Haram K, Lygre T, Wallem G. Comparison of the placental transfer of thiopental and diazepam in caesarean section. Eur J Clin Pharmacol 1981;21:221–7.
9. Haram K, Bakke OM. Diazepam as an induction agent for caesarean section: a clinical and pharmacokinetic study of fetal drug exposure. Br J Obstet Gynaecol 1980;87:506–12.
10. Kanto JH. Use of benzodiazepines during pregnancy, labour and lactation, with particular reference to pharmacokinetic considerations. Drugs 1982;23:354–80.
11. Bakke OM, Haram K. Time-course of transplacental passage of diazepam: influence of injection-delivery interval on neonatal drug concentrations. Clin Pharmacokinet 1982;7:353–62.
12. Jauniaux E, Jurkovic D, Lees C, Campbell S, Gulbis B. In-vivo study of diazepam transfer across the first trimester human placenta. Hum Reprod 1996;11:889–92.
13. Jorgensen NP, Thurmann-Nielsen E, Walstad RA. Pharmacokinetics and distribution of diazepam and oxazepam in early pregnancy. Acta Obstet Gynecol Scand 1988;67:493–7.
14. Lee JN, Chen SS, Richens A, Menabawey M, Chard T. Serum protein binding of diazepam in maternal and foetal serum during pregnancy. Br J Clin Pharmacol 1982;14:551–4.
15. Ridd MJ, Brown KF, Nation RL, Collier CB. Differential transplacental binding of diazepam: causes and implications. Eur J Clin Pharmacol 1983;24:595–601.
16. Rivas F, Hernandez A, Cantu JM. Acentric craniofacial cleft in a newborn female prenatally exposed to a high dose of diazepam. Teratology 1984;30:179–80.
17. Safra JM, Oakley GP Jr. Association between cleft lip with or without cleft palate and prenatal exposure to diazepam. Lancet 1975;2:478–80.
18. Saxen I. Epidemiology of cleft lip and palate: an attempt to rule out chance correlations. Br J Prev Soc Med 1975;29:103–10.
19. Saxen I. Associations between oral clefts and drugs taken during pregnancy. Int J Epidemiol 1975;4:37–44.
20. Saxen I, Saxen L. Association between maternal intake of diazepam and oral clefts. Lancet 1975;2:498.
21. Safra MJ, Oakley GP Jr. Valium: an oral cleft teratogen? Cleft Palate J 1976;13:198–200.
22. Czeizel A. Diazepam, phenytoin, and etiology of cleft lip and/or cleft palate. Lancet 1976;1:810.
23. Rosenberg L, Mitchell AA, Parsells JL, Pashayan H, Louik C, Shapiro S. Lack of relation of oral clefts to diazepam use during pregnancy. N Engl J Med 1983;309:1282–5.

24. Shiono PH, Mills JL. Oral clefts and diazepam use during pregnancy. N Engl J Med 1984;311:919–20.
25. Lakos P, Czeizel E. A teratological evaluation of anticonvulsant drugs. Acta Paediatr Acad Sci Hung 1977;18:145–53.
26. Entman SS, Vaughn WK. Lack of relation of oral clefts to diazepam use in pregnancy. N Engl J Med 1984;310:1121–2.
27. Rosenberg L, Mitchell AA. Lack of relation of oral clefts to diazepam use in pregnancy. N Engl J Med 1984;310:1122.
28. Bracken MB, Holford TR. Exposure to prescribed drugs in pregnancy and association with congenital malformations. Obstet Gynecol 1981;58:336–44.
29. Rothman KJ, Fyler DC, Goldblatt A, Kreidberg MB. Exogenous hormones and other drug exposures of children with congenital heart disease. Am J Epidemiol 1979;109:433–9.
30. Istvan EJ. Drug-associated congenital abnormalities. Can Med Assoc J 1970;103:1394.
31. Ringrose CAD. The hazard of neurotrophic drugs in the fertile years. Can Med Assoc J 1972;106:1058.
32. Fourth Annual Report of the New Zealand Committee on Adverse Drug Reactions. NZ Med J 1969;70:118–22.
33. Laegreid L, Olegard R, Walstrom J, Conradi N. Teratogenic effects of benzodiazepine use during pregnancy. J Pediatr 1989;114:126–31.
34. Bergman U, Rosa FW, Baum C, Wiholm B-E, Faich GA. Effects of exposure to benzodiazepine during fetal life. Lancet 1992;340:694–6.
35. Courtens W, Vamos E, Hainaut M, Vergauwen P. Moebius syndrome in an infant exposed in utero to benzodiazepines. J Pediatr 1992;121:833–4.
36. Czeizel AE, Mosonyi A. Monitoring of early human fetal development in women exposed to large doses of chemicals. Environ Mol Mutagen 1997;30:240–4.
37. Dolovich LR, Addis A, Vaillancourt JMR, Power JDB, Koren G, Einarson TR. Benzodiazepine use in pregnancy and major malformations or oral cleft: meta-analysis of cohort and case-controlled studies. Br Med J 1998;317:839–43.
38. Game E, Bergman U. Benzodiazepine use in pregnancy and major malformations or oral clefts. Br Med J 1999;319:918.
39. Cates C. Pooled results are sensitive to zero transformation used. Br Med J 1999;319:918–9.
40. Khan KS, Wukes C, Gee H. Quality of primary studies must influence inferences made from meta-analyses. Br Med J 1999;319:919.
41. Ornoy A, Arnon J, Shechtman S, Moerman L, Lukashova I. Is benzodiazepine use during pregnancy really teratogenic? Reprod Toxicol 1998;12:511–5.
42. Greenblatt DJ, Shader RI. Effect of benzodiazepines in neonates. N Engl J Med 1975;292:649.
43. Modif M, Brinkman CR, Assali NS. Effects of diazepam on uteroplacental and fetal hemodynamics and metabolism. Obstet Gynecol 1973;41:364–8.
44. Toaff ME, Hezroni J, Toaff R. Effect of diazepam on uterine activity during labor. Isr J Med Sci 1977;13:1007–9.
45. Shannon RW, Fraser GP, Aitken RG, Harper JR. Diazepam in preeclamptic toxaemia with special reference to its effect on the newborn infant. Br J Clin Pract 1972;26:271–5.
46. Yeh SY, Paul RIT, Cordero L, Hon EH. A study of diazepam during labor. Obstet Gynecol 1974;43:363–73.
47. Kasturilal D, Shetti RN. Role of diazepam in the management of eclampsia. Curr Ther Res 1975;18:627–30.
48. Eliot BW, Hill JG, Cole AP, Hailey DM. Continuous pethidine/diazepam infusion during labor and its effects on the newborn. Br J Obstet Gynaecol 1975;82:126–31.
49. Lean TH, Retnam SS, Sivasamboo R. Use of benzodiazepines in the management of eclampsia. J Obstet Gynaecol Br Commonw 1968;75:856–62.
50. Scanlon JW. Effect of benzodiazepines in neonates. N Engl J Med 1975;292:649.
51. Gillberg C. "Floppy infant syndrome" and maternal diazepam. Lancet 1977;2:244.
52. Haram K. "Floppy infant syndrome" and maternal diazepam. Lancet 1977;2:612–3.
53. Speight AN. Floppy-infant syndrome and maternal diazepam and/or nitrazepam. Lancet 1977;1:878.
54. Rementeria JL, Bhatt K. Withdrawal symptoms in neonates from intrauterine exposure to diazepam. J Pediatr 1977;90:123–6.
55. Thearle MJ, Dunn PM. Exchange transfusions for diazepam intoxication at birth followed by jejunal stenosis. Proc R Soc Med 1973;66:13–4.
56. Backes CR, Cordero L. Withdrawal symptoms in the neonate from presumptive intrauterine exposure to diazepam: report of case. J Am Osteopath Assoc 1980;79:584–5.
57. Cree JE, Meyer J, Hailey DM. Diazepam in labour: its metabolism and effect on the clinical condition and thermogenesis of the newborn. Br Med J 1973;4:251–5.
58. McAllister CB. Placental transfer and neonatal effects of diazepam when administered to women just before delivery. Br J Anaesth 1980;52:423–7.
59. Owen JR, Irani SF, Blair AW. Effect of diazepam administered to mothers during labour on temperature regulation of neonate. Arch Dis Child 1972;47:107–10.
60. Scher J, Hailey DM, Beard RW. The effects of diazepam on the fetus. J Obstet Gynaecol Br Commonw 1972;79:635–8.
61. Van Geijn HP, Jongsma HW, Doesburg WH, Lemmens WA, deHaan J, Eskes TK. The effect of diazepam administration during pregnancy or labor on the heart rate variability of the newborn infant. Eur J Obstet Gynaecol Reprod Biol 1980;10:187–201.
62. Birger M, Homberg R, Insler V. Clinical evaluation of fetal movements. Int J Gynaecol Obstet 1980;18:377–82.
63. Einarson A, Selby P, Koren G. Abrupt discontinuation of psychotropic drugs during pregnancy: fear of teratogenic risk and impact on counseling. J Psychiatry Neurosci 2001;26:44–8.
64. Van Geijn HP, Kenemans P, Vise T, Vanderkleijn E, Eskes TK. Pharmacokinetics of diazepam and occurrence in breast milk. In: *Proceedings of the Sixth International Congress of Pharmacology*, Helsinki, Finland 1975:514.
65. Hill RM, Nowlin J, Lertratanangkoon K, Stillwell WG, Stillwell RN, Horning MG. The identification and quantification of drugs in human breast milk. Clin Res 1974;22:77A.
66. Cole AP, Hailey DM. Diazepam and active metabolite in breast milk and their transfer to the neonate. Arch Dis Child 1975;50:741–2.
67. Patrick MJ, Tilstone WJ, Reavey P. Diazepam and breast-feeding. Lancet 1972;1:542–3.
68. Catz CS. Diazepam in breast milk. Drug Ther 1973;3:72–3.
69. Wesson DR, Camber S, Harkey M, Smith DE. Diazepam and desmethyldiazepam in breast milk. J Psychoactive Drugs 1985;17:55–6.
70. Committee on Drugs, American Academy of Pediatrics. The transfer of drugs and other chemicals into human milk. Pediatrics 2001;108:776–89.

DIAZOXIDE

Antihypertensive

PREGNANCY RECOMMENDATION: Human Data Suggest Risk in 3rd Trimester
BREASTFEEDING RECOMMENDATION: No Human Data—Potential Toxicity

PREGNANCY SUMMARY

Because other antihypertensive drugs are available for severe maternal hypertension and the long-term effects on the infant have not been evaluated, diazoxide should be used with caution, if at all, during pregnancy. If diazoxide is needed after other therapies have failed, small doses are recommended.

FETAL RISK SUMMARY

Diazoxide readily crosses the placenta and reaches fetal plasma concentrations similar to maternal levels (1). The drug has been used for the treatment of severe hypertension associated with pregnancy (1–12). Daily doses of 30, 21, and 10 mg/kg in rats, rabbits, and dogs, respectively, were associated with reduced fetal and pup survival, and reduced fetal growth (13).

Some investigators have cautioned against the use of diazoxide in pregnancy (14,15). In one study, the decrease in maternal blood pressure was sufficient to produce a state of clinical shock and endanger placental perfusion (14). Transient fetal bradycardia has been reported in other studies following a rapid, marked decrease in maternal blood pressure (7,16). Fatal maternal hypotension has been reported in one patient after diazoxide therapy (17). Recommendations have been made that the infusion technique, rather than rapid IV boluses, is preferred to prevent maternal and fetal complications (18). However, small IV boluses at frequent intervals (30 mg every 1–2 minutes) have successfully controlled maternal hypertension without producing fetal toxicity (19).

Diazoxide is a potent relaxant of uterine smooth muscle and may inhibit uterine contractions if given during labor (2,3,5–7,20–22). The degree and duration of uterine inhibition are dose dependent (21). Augmentation of labor with oxytocin may be required in patients receiving diazoxide.

Hyperglycemia in the newborn (glucose 500–700 mg/dL) secondary to IV diazoxide therapy in a mother just prior to delivery has been observed to persist for up to 3 days (23). In some series, all of the mothers and newborns had hyperglycemia without ketoacidosis (14). The glucose levels returned to near normal within 24 hours.

The use of oral diazoxide for the last 19–69 days of pregnancy has been associated with alopecia, hypertrichosis lanuginosa, and decreased ossification of the wrist (1). However, long-term oral therapy has not caused similar problems in other newborns exposed in utero (4).

BREASTFEEDING SUMMARY

No reports describing the use of diazoxide during lactation have been located. The molecular weight (about 231), however, suggests that the drug will be excreted into breast milk.

References

1. Milner RDG, Chouksey SK. Effects of fetal exposure to diazoxide in man. Arch Dis Child 1972;47:537–43.
2. Finnerty FA Jr, Kakaviatos N, Tuckman J, Magill J. Clinical evaluation of diazoxide: a new treatment for acute hypertension. Circulation 1963;28:203–8.
3. Finnerty FA Jr. Advantages and disadvantages of furosemide in the edematous states of pregnancy. Am J Obstet Gynecol 1969;105:1022–7.
4. Pohl JEF, Thurston H, Davis D, Morgan MY. Successful use of oral diazoxide in the treatment of severe toxaemia of pregnancy. Br Med J 1972;2:568–70.
5. Pennington JC, Picker RH. Diazoxide and the treatment of the acute hypertensive emergency in obstetrics. Med J Aust 1972;2:1051–4.
6. Koch-Weser J. Diazoxide. N Engl J Med 1976;294:1271–4.
7. Morris JA, Arce JJ, Hamilton CJ, Davidson EC, Maidman JE, Clark JH, Bloom RS. The management of severe preeclampsia and eclampsia with intravenous diazoxide. Obstet Gynecol 1977;49:675–80.
8. Keith TA III. Hypertension crisis: recognition and management. JAMA 1977;237:1570–7.
9. MacLean AB, Doig JR, Aickin DR. Hypovolaemia, pre-eclampsia and diuretics. Br J Obstet Gynaecol 1978;85:597–601.
10. Barr PA, Gallery ED. Effect of diazoxide on the antepartum cardiotocograph in severe pregnancy-associated hypertension. Aust NZ J Obstet Gynaecol 1981;21:11–5.
11. MacLean AB, Doig JR, Chatfield WR, Aickin DR. Small-dose diazoxide administration in pregnancy. Aust NZ J Obstet Gynaecol 1981;21:7–10.
12. During VR. Clinical experience obtained from use of diazoxide (Hypertonalum) for treatment of acute intrapartum hypertensive crisis. Zentralbl Gynakol 1982;104:89–93.
13. Product information. Hyperstat. Schering, 2000.
14. Neuman J, Weiss B, Rabello Y, Cabal L, Freeman RK. Diazoxide for the acute control of severe hypertension complicating pregnancy: a pilot study. Obstet Gynecol 1979;53(Suppl):50S–5S.
15. Perkins RP. Treatment of toxemia of pregnancy. JAMA 1977;238:2143–4.
16. Michael CA. Intravenous diazoxide in the treatment of severe preeclamptic toxaemia and eclampsia. Aust NZ J Obstet Gynaecol 1973;13:143–6.
17. Henrich WL, Cronin R, Miller PD, Anderson RJ. Hypotensive sequelae of diazoxide and hydralazine therapy. JAMA 1977;237:264–5.
18. Thien T, Koene RAP, Schijf C, Pieters GFFM, Eskes TKAB, Wijdeveld PGAB. Infusion of diazoxide in severe hypertension during pregnancy. Eur J Obstet Gynaecol Reprod Biol 1980;10:367–74.
19. Dudley DKL. Minibolus diazoxide in the management of severe hypertension in pregnancy. Am J Obstet Gynecol 1985;151:196–200.
20. Barden TP, Keenan WJ. Effects of diazoxide in human labor and the fetus-neonate (abstract). Obstet Gynecol 1971;37:631–2.
21. Landesman R, Adeodato de Souza FJ, Countinho EM, Wilson KH, Bomfim de Sousa FM. The inhibitory effect of diazoxide in normal term labor. Am J Obstet Gynecol 1969;103:430–3.
22. Paulissian R. Diazoxide. Int Anesthesiol Clin 1978;16:201–36.
23. Milsap RL, Auld PAM. Neonatal hyperglycemia following maternal diazoxide administration. JAMA 1980;243:144–5.

DIBENZEPIN

[Withdrawn from the market. See 9th edition.]

DICHLORALPHENAZONE

Sedative

PREGNANCY RECOMMENDATION: Limited Human Data—Probably Compatible
BREASTFEEDING RECOMMENDATION: Limited Human Data—Probably Compatible

PREGNANCY SUMMARY

There is limited information on the use of dichloralphenazone during human pregnancy. The lack of developmental toxicity in one animal species and the absence of human reports describing embryo–fetal toxicity suggest that the risk, if any, is low.

D

FETAL RISK SUMMARY

Dichloralphenazone is a sedative hypnotic composed of two molecules of chloral hydrate (a sedative/hypnotic) (see also Chloral Hydrate) bound together with the analgesic/antipyretic, phenazone (see also Antipyrine) (1). Antipyrine and chloral hydrate are derived from dichloralphenazone and the latter drug is metabolized to the active agent, trichloroethanol. Little information is available on the reproductive effects of antipyrine, chloral hydrate, or the prodrug, dichloralphenazone, a component, along with isometheptene and acetaminophen, of several proprietary mixtures commonly used for tension and vascular (migraine) headaches (see also Isometheptene and Acetaminophen).

Two studies have been located that examined the effect of dichloralphenazone in pregnant rats (1,2). No teratogenic or other adverse fetal effects were observed when doses ranging from 50 to 500 mg/kg/day were fed to rats throughout gestation.

No published reports describing the use of dichloralphenazone in human pregnancy have been located, although one reference commented that the drug has been "widely used" during pregnancy (3). The Collaborative Perinatal Project recorded 71 1st trimester exposures to chloral hydrate (4, pp. 336–344), one of the drugs derived from dichloralphenazone. From this group, eight infants with congenital defects were observed (standardized relative risk (SRR) 1.68). When only malformations with uniform rates by hospital were examined, the SRR was 2.19. Neither of these relative risks reached statistical significance. Moreover, when chloral hydrate was combined with all tranquilizers and nonbarbiturate sedatives, no association with congenital malformations was found (SRR 1.13; 95% confidence interval [CI] 0.88–1.44). For use anytime during pregnancy, 358 exposures to chloral hydrate were discovered (4, p. 438). The nine infants with anomalies yielded an SRR of 0.98 (95% CI 0.45–1.84). (See also Antipyrine for additional information.)

BREASTFEEDING SUMMARY

Dichloralphenazone is a prodrug composed of the sedative/hypnotic, chloral hydrate, bound together with the analgesic/antipyretic, phenazone. Trichlorethanol, an active metabolite of chloral hydrate, is excreted into human breast milk as is phenazone (see Antipyrine).

Mild morning drowsiness was observed in a nursing infant of a woman taking 1300 mg (13 times the dose per capsule in the proprietary headache products mentioned above) of dichloralphenazone at bedtime (5). The mother was also taking chlorpromazine, 100 mg 3 times daily. Milk concentrations of trichloroethanol were 60% to 80% of the maternal serum levels. The metabolite was not detected in the infant's plasma 20 hours after a dose. Infant growth and development remained normal during the exposure and at follow-up 3 months after the drug was stopped. Apparently, no attempt was made in this study to determine the milk concentration of phenazone, the other component of dichloralphenazone. The American Academy of Pediatrics classifies chloral hydrate as compatible with breastfeeding (see Chloral Hydrate).

References

1. McColl JD, Globus M, Robinson S. Effect of some therapeutic agents on the developing rat fetus. Toxicol Appl Pharmacol 1965;7:409–17. As cited in Shepard TH. *Catalog of Teratogenic Agents*. 7th ed. Baltimore, MD: Johns Hopkins University Press, 1992:131.
2. Onnis A, Grella P. *The Biochemical Effects of Drugs in Pregnancy*. Vol. 1. West Sussex, England: Ellis Horwood Limited, 1984:60.
3. Lewis PJ, Friedman LA. Prophylaxis of neonatal jaundice with maternal antipyrine treatment. Lancet 1979;1:300–2.
4. Heinonen OP, Slone D, Shapiro S. *Birth Defects and Drugs in Pregnancy*. Littleton, MA: Publishing Sciences Group, 1977.
5. Lacey JH. Dichloralphenazone and breast milk. Br Med J 1971;4:684.

DICHLORPHENAMIDE

Diuretic (Carbonic Anhydrase Inhibitor)

PREGNANCY RECOMMENDATION: No Human Data—No Relevant Animal Data
BREASTFEEDING RECOMMENDATION: No Human Data—Probably Compatible

PREGNANCY SUMMARY

No reports of human use of dichlorphenamide during pregnancy have been located. The drug is best avoided during organogenesis.

D

FETAL RISK SUMMARY

Dichlorphenamide is a carbonic anhydrase inhibitor used in the treatment of glaucoma. Its mechanism of action is similar to, but much more potent than, acetazolamide or methazolamide (see also Acetazolamide and Methazolamide). The drug is teratogenic in chicks, mice, and rats, producing otolith deficits and forelimb deformities in the fetuses of the latter two species, respectively (1). Skeletal anomalies were observed in rats at a dose 100 times the human dose (2).

It is not known if dichlorphenamide crosses the human placenta. The molecular weight (about 305) is low enough, however, that passage to the embryo or fetus should be expected.

BREASTFEEDING SUMMARY

No reports describing the use of dichlorphenamide during lactation have been located. The molecular weight (about 305) is low enough that excretion into milk should be expected.

References

1. Shepard TH. *Catalog of Teratogenic Agents*. 6th ed. Baltimore, MD: Johns Hopkins University Press, 1989:213.
2. Product information. Daranide. Merck, 2000.

DICLOFENAC

Nonsteroidal Anti-inflammatory

PREGNANCY RECOMMENDATION: Human Data Suggest Risk in 1st and 3rd Trimesters
BREASTFEEDING RECOMMENDATION: No Human Data—Probably Compatible

PREGNANCY SUMMARY

Constriction of the ductus arteriosus in utero is a pharmacologic consequence arising from the use of prostaglandin synthesis inhibitors during pregnancy, as is inhibition of labor, prolongation of pregnancy, and suppression of fetal renal function (see also Indomethacin) (1). As indicated above and published cases with other nonsteroidal anti-inflammatory drugs (NSAIDs), persistent pulmonary hypertension of the newborn may occur if these agents are used in the 3rd trimester close to delivery (1,2). Women attempting to conceive should not use any prostaglandin synthesis inhibitor, including diclofenac, because of the findings in a variety of animal models that indicate these agents block blastocyst implantation (3,4). Moreover, as noted below, NSAIDs have been associated with spontaneous abortions (SABs) and congenital malformations (see also Ibuprofen). The risk for these defects, however, appears to be low.

FETAL RISK SUMMARY

Diclofenac is an NSAID used for the treatment of arthritis, acute and chronic pain, and primary dysmenorrhea. Similar to other agents in this class, it also has antipyretic activity. Diclofenac is in the same subclass (acetic acids) as three other NSAIDs (indomethacin, sulindac, and tolmetin).

In reproduction studies in mice, rats, and rabbits, the drug was not teratogenic with doses up to those that produced maternal and fetal toxicity. Maternal toxic doses, however, were associated with dystocia, prolonged gestation, decreased fetal survival (5), and intrauterine growth restriction (5,6).

A 1990 report described an investigation on the effects of several nonsteroidal anti-inflammatory agents on mouse palatal fusion both in vivo and in vitro (7). The compounds, including diclofenac, were found to induce cleft palate. In the rat, diclofenac, presumably by inhibiting prostaglandin synthesis, has been shown to inhibit implantation and placentation.

The tocolytic effect of diclofenac was demonstrated in a study that used mifepristone (RU 486) to induce preterm labor in rats (8). Diclofenac inhibited preterm delivery but had no effect on mifepristone-induced cervical maturation.

Diclofenac crosses the human placenta. In a 2000 study, 30 women undergoing termination of pregnancy at a mean gestational age of 10.2 weeks (range 8–12 weeks) were given two 50-mg oral doses at a mean 13.5 and 2.5 hours before the procedure (9). Diclofenac was detected in all maternal serum (mean 183.9 ng/mL) and fetal tissue (mean 279.2 ng/mL) samples, producing a mean maternal serum:fetal tissue ratio of 0.95 (range 0.05–4.26). Only 7 of the 30 amniotic fluid samples contained detectable diclofenac (range 0.6–3.5 ng/mL), whereas 17 of 30 coelomic fluid samples contained the drug (range 1.1–33.4 ng/mL) (9).

In a surveillance study of Michigan Medicaid recipients involving 229,101 completed pregnancies conducted between 1985 and 1992, 51 newborns had been exposed to diclofenac during the 1st trimester (F. Rosa, personal communication, FDA, 1993). One unspecified major birth defect was observed (two expected). No anomalies were observed in six defect categories (cardiovascular defects, oral clefts, spina bifida, polydactyly, limb reduction defects, and hypospadias) for which specific data were available. Although the number of exposures is small, these data do not support an association between the drug and congenital defects.

A 29-year-old woman at 33 weeks' gestation was diagnosed by clinical symptoms and ultrasound as having a spontaneous rupture of the right renal pelvis with a small amount of perinephric extravasation of urine (10). She was treated conservatively with diclofenac while hospitalized (50 mg twice daily; duration not specified) and delivered a healthy female infant 5 weeks later. A follow-up examination of her kidney by ultrasonography 5 days postpartum was normal (10).

D

A combined 2001 population-based, observational cohort study and a case–control study estimated the risk of adverse pregnancy outcome from the use of NSAIDs (11). The use of NSAIDs during pregnancy was not associated with congenital malformations, preterm delivery, or low birth weight, but a positive association was discovered with SABs. A similar study, also published in 2001, failed to find a relationship, in general, between NSAIDs and congenital malformations, but did find a significant association with cardiac defects and orofacial clefts (12). In addition, a 2003 study found a significant association between exposure to NSAIDs in early pregnancy and SABs (13). (See Ibuprofen for details on these three studies.)

A brief 2003 editorial on the potential for NSAID-induced developmental toxicity concluded that NSAIDs, and specifically those with greater cyclooxygenase 2 (COX-2) affinity, had a lower risk of this toxicity in humans than aspirin (14).

A 2003 case–control study was conducted to identify drug use in early pregnancy that was associated with cardiac defects (15). Cases (cardiovascular defects without known chromosome anomalies) were drawn from three Swedish health registers (*N* = *5015*) and controls consisting of all infants born in Sweden (1995–2001) (*N* = *577,730*). Among the NSAIDs, only naproxen had a positive association with the defects (see Naproxen). For diclofenac, there were 1362 pregnant women exposed and 15 cases of cardiac defects (odds ratio 1.30, 95% confidence interval [OR] 0.78–2.16) (15).

A 2006 case–control study found a significant association between congenital anomalies, specifically cardiac septal defects, and the use of NSAIDs in the 1st trimester (16). A population-based pregnancy registry (*N* = 36,387) was developed by linking three databases in Quebec. (See Naprosyn for other study details.) Case infants were those with any congenital anomaly diagnosed in the first year of life and were compared with matched controls. There were 93 infants (8.8%) with congenital defects from 1056 mothers who had filled prescriptions for NSAIDs in the 1st trimester. In controls, there were 2478 infants (7%) with anomalies from 35,331 mothers who had not filled such a prescription. The adjusted OR was 2.21 (95% CI 1.72–2.85). The adjusted OR for cardiac septal closure was 3.34 (95% CI 1.87–5.98). There also was a significant association for anomalies of the respiratory system OR 9.55 (95% CI 3.08–29.63), but this association disappeared when cases coded as "unspecified anomaly of the respiratory system" were excluded. For the cases involving septal closure, 61% were atrial septal defects and 31% were ventricular septal defects. There were no significant associations for oral clefts or defects involving other major organ systems. The five most common NSAIDs were naproxen (35%), ibuprofen (26%), rofecoxib (15%), diclofenac (9%), and celecoxib (9%). Among these agents, the only significant association was for ibuprofen prescriptions in the 1st trimester and congenital defects ($p < 0.01$) (16).

Premature closure of the ductus arteriosus in a fetus who was exposed to diclofenac, 50 mg twice daily, for 2 weeks from the 34th week of gestation was reported in 1998 (17). The mother had taken the drug for musculoskeletal back pain and carpal tunnel syndrome. At 41 weeks' gestation, a fetal echocardiogram revealed the ductus defect, enlargement of the right side of the heart, and early cardiac failure. An emergency cesarean section was performed and the baby was successfully resuscitated (17). Another 1998 case described the effects of diclofenac in late gestation (18). The woman, in the 35th week of pregnancy, was treated for thrombophlebitis with a 5-day course of diclofenac (75 mg twice daily) and heparin. Thirteen days after completion of therapy, she delivered a 3200-g female infant with Apgar scores of 6 and 2 at 1 and 5 minutes, respectively. The infant was treated for severe pulmonary hypertension secondary to intrauterine ductal closure. Normal motor and mental development was noted at 2 years of age, but the infant still had cardiac dysfunction (18).

A 1999 report described constriction of the fetal ductus following a single 75-mg IM dose of diclofenac administered at 36 weeks' gestation (19). The constriction resolved within 24 hours and, 32 hours after the dose, the mother delivered 2780-g female infant with an Apgar score of 9 at 1 minute.

In another 1999 case, a woman took diclofenac (50 mg twice daily) for severe arthritis of the hands for 10 days during gestational weeks 34 and 35 (20). She also was occasionally taking Chinese herbs in what was thought to be homeopathic doses. Fetal distress was noted at 41 weeks' gestation and an ultrasound revealed hydrops fetalis with cardiomegaly and right atrial and right ventricular dilatation. An emergency cesarean section delivered a 3980-g female infant with Apgar scores of 6, 7, and 9, at 1, 5, and 10 minutes, respectively. The infant was flaccid with profound bradycardia requiring resuscitation. An echocardiogram within 30 minutes of birth revealed a severely dilated, poorly contractile right ventricle, dilated right atrium, a patent foramen ovale with right to left shunt, moderate tricuspid regurgitation, and a closed ductus arteriosus. The findings were compatible with pulmonary hypertension. The infant markedly improved over the next 4 weeks and was asymptomatic with normal growth and intellectual development at 18 months of age (20).

A 2004 case report described severe pulmonary hypertension in a newborn exposed in utero to diclofenac near delivery (21). The mother, at about 38 weeks' gestation, had been prescribed diclofenac (25 mg three times daily for 3 days) for flu-like symptoms. Immediately after completion of the prescribed course, fetal bradycardia was detected and the mother was delivered of a 3.4-kg male infant by cesarean section. The nonhydropic infant was cyanotic with respiratory distress and required mechanical ventilation. An echocardiogram was consistent with severe neonatal pulmonary hypertension and transient right-sided hypertrophic cardiomyopathy caused by premature closure of the ductus arteriosus. The condition was thought to have resulted from diclofenac. By 40 days of age, the pulmonary hypertension had resolved and the right ventricular hypertrophy had markedly regressed (21).

BREASTFEEDING SUMMARY

No reports describing the use of diclofenac during lactation have been located. The manufacturer states that diclofenac is excreted into the milk of nursing mothers but does not cite quantitative data (5). One reviewer classified diclofenac as one of several low-risk alternatives, because of its short adult serum half-life (1.1 hours) and toxicity profile compared with other similar agents, if an NSAID was required while nursing (22). Other reviewers have also stated that diclofenac can be safely used during breastfeeding (23,24). Another NSAID in the same subclass as diclofenac is classified as compatible with breastfeeding by the American Academy of Pediatrics (see Indomethacin).

References

1. Levin DL. Effects of inhibition of prostaglandin synthesis on fetal development, oxygenation, and the fetal circulation. Semin Perinatol 1980;4:35–44.
2. Van Marter LJ, Leviton A, Allred EN, Pagano M, Sullivan KF, Cohen A, Epstein MF. Persistent pulmonary hypertension of the newborn and smoking and aspirin and nonsteroidal antiinflammatory drug consumption during pregnancy. Pediatrics 1996;97:658–63.
3. Matt DW, Borzelleca JF. Toxic effects on the female reproductive system during pregnancy, parturition, and lactation. In: Witorsch RJ, ed. *Reproductive Toxicology*. 2nd ed. New York, NY: Raven Press, 1995:175–93.
4. Dawood MY. Nonsteroidal antiinflammatory drugs and reproduction. Am J Obstet Gynecol 1993;169:1255–65.
5. Product information. Voltaren. Geigy Pharmaceuticals, 1995.
6. Carp HJA, Fein A, Nebel L. Effect of diclofenac on implantation and embryonic development in the rat. Eur J Obstet Gynecol Reprod Biol 1988;28:273–7.
7. Montenegro MA, Palomino H. Induction of cleft palate in mice by inhibitors of prostaglandin synthesis. J Craniofac Genet Del Biol 1990;10:83–94.
8. Cabrol D, Carbonne B, Bienkiewicz A, Dallot E, Alj AE, Cedard L. Induction of labor and cervical maturation using mifepristone (RU 486) in the late pregnant rat. Influence of a cyclooxygenase inhibitor (diclofenac). Prostaglandins 1991;42:71–9.
9. Siu SSN, Yeung JHK, Lau TK. A study on placental transfer of diclofenac in first trimester of human pregnancy. Hum Reprod 2000;15:2423–5.
10. Royburt M, Peled Y, Kaplan B, Hod M, Friedman S, Ovadia J. Non-traumatic rupture of kidney in pregnancy—case report and review. Acta Obstet Gynecol Scand 1994;73:663–7.
11. Nielsen GL, Sorensen HT, Larsen H, Pedersen L. Risk of adverse birth outcome and miscarriage in pregnant users of non-steroidal anti-inflammatory drugs: population based observational study and case-control study. Br Med J 2001;322:266–70.
12. Ericson A, Kallen BAJ. Nonsteroidal anti-inflammatory drugs in early pregnancy. Reprod Toxicol 2001;15:371–5.
13. Li DK, Liu L, Odouli R. Exposure to non-steroidal anti-inflammatory drugs during pregnancy and risk of miscarriage: population based cohort study. Br Med J 2003;327:368–71.
14. Tassinari MS, Cook JC, Hurtt ME. NSAIDs and developmental toxicity. Birth Defects Res (Part B) 2003;68:3–4.
15. Kallen BAJ, Olausson PO. Maternal drug use in early pregnancy and infant cardiovascular defect. Reprod Toxicol 2003;17:255–61.
16. Ofori B, Oraichi D, Blais L, Rey E, Bérard A. Risk of congenital anomalies in pregnant users of non-steroidal anti-inflammatory drugs: a nested case-control study. Birth Defects Res (Part B) 2006;77:268–79.
17. Adverse Drug Reactions Advisory Committee. Premature closure of the fetal ductus arteriosus after maternal use of non-steroidal anti-inflammatory drugs. Med J Aust 1998;169:270–1.
18. Zenker M, Klinge J, Kruger C, Singer H, Scharf J. Severe pulmonary hypertension in a neonate caused by premature closure of the ductus arteriosus following maternal treatment with diclofenac: a case report. J Perinat Med 1998;26:231–4.
19. Rein AJJT, Nadjari M, Elchalal U, Nir A. Contraction of the fetal ductus arteriosus induced by diclofenac. Fetal Diagn Ther 1999;14:24–5.
20. Mas C, Menahem S. Premature in utero closure of the ductus arteriosus following maternal ingestion of sodium diclofenac. Aust NZ J Obstet Gynaecol 1999;39:106–7.
21. Siu KL, Lee WH. Maternal diclofenac sodium ingestion and severe neonatal pulmonary hypertension. J Paediatr Child Health 2004;40:152–3.
22. Anderson PO. Medication use while breast feeding a neonate. Neonatal Pharmacol Q 1993;2:3–14.
23. Goldsmith DP. Neonatal rheumatic disorders. View of the pediatrician. Rheum Dis Clin North Am 1989;15:287–305.
24. Needs CJ, Brooks PM. Antirheumatic medication during lactation. Br J Rheumatol 1985;24:291–7.

D

DICLOXACILLIN

Antibiotic (Penicillin)

PREGNANCY RECOMMENDATION: Compatible
BREASTFEEDING RECOMMENDATION: Compatible

PREGNANCY SUMMARY

Although the reported pregnancy experience with dicloxacillin is limited, all penicillins are considered low risk in pregnancy.

FETAL RISK SUMMARY

Dicloxacillin is a penicillin antibiotic (see also Penicillin G). The drug crosses the placenta into the fetal circulation and amniotic fluid. Levels are low compared with other penicillins due to the high degree of maternal protein binding (1,2). Following a 500-mg IV dose, the fetal peak serum level of 3.4 mcg/mL occurred at 2 hours (8% of maternal peak) (2). A peak of 1.8 mcg/mL was obtained at 6 hours in the amniotic fluid.

No reports linking the use of dicloxacillin with congenital defects have been located. The Collaborative Perinatal Project monitored 50,282 mother–child pairs, 3546 of whom had 1st trimester exposure to penicillin derivatives (3, pp. 297–313). For use anytime in pregnancy, 7171 exposures were recorded (3, p. 435). In neither case was evidence found to suggest a relationship to large categories of major or minor malformations or to individual defects.

In a surveillance study of Michigan Medicaid recipients involving 229,101 completed pregnancies conducted between 1985 and 1992, 46 newborns had been exposed to dicloxacillin during the 1st trimester (F. Rosa, personal communication, FDA, 1993). One (2.2%) major birth defect was observed (two expected). No anomalies were observed in six defect categories (cardiovascular defects, oral clefts, spina bifida, polydactyly, limb reduction defects, and hypospadias) for which specific data were available. Although the number of exposures is small, these data do not support an association between the drug and congenital defects.

BREASTFEEDING SUMMARY

No reports describing the use of dicloxacillin during lactation have been located. Because other penicillins are excreted into breast milk in low concentrations (e.g., see Ampicillin and Penicillin G) the presence of dicloxacillin should also be expected. Although adverse effects from other penicillins in breast milk are rare, three potential problems exist for the nursing infant: modification of bowel flora, direct effects on the infant (e.g., allergic response), and interference with the interpretation of culture results if a fever workup is required.

References

1. MacAulay M, Berg S, Charles D. Placental transfer of dicloxacillin at term. Am J Obstet Gynecol 1968;102:1162–8.
2. Depp R, Kind A, Kirby W, Johnson W. Transplacental passage of methicillin and dicloxacillin into the fetus and amniotic fluid. Am J Obstet Gynecol 1970;107:1054–7.
3. Heinonen OP, Slone D, Shapiro S. *Birth Defects and Drugs in Pregnancy*. Littleton, MA: Publishing Sciences Group, 1977.

D

DICUMAROL

[Withdrawn from the market. See 9th edition.]

DICYCLOMINE

Parasympatholytic

PREGNANCY RECOMMENDATION: Compatible
BREASTFEEDING RECOMMENDATION: Limited Human Data—Potential Toxicity

PREGNANCY SUMMARY

The use of dicyclomine during human pregnancy does not appear to represent a risk to the fetus or newborn. A 1990 review on the teratogenic risk of commonly used drugs categorized the risk from dicyclomine as "none" (1).

FETAL RISK SUMMARY

This anticholinergic/antispasmodic agent was a component of a proprietary mixture (Bendectin, others) used for the treatment and prevention of pregnancy-induced nausea and vomiting from 1956 until 1976, when the product was reformulated. Dicyclomine was removed at that time because it was discovered that it did not contribute to the effectiveness of the mixture as an antiemetic (see also Doxylamine).

Animal studies conducted with dicyclomine alone, and in combination with doxylamine and pyridoxine (i.e., Bendectin), have found no evidence of impaired fertility or adverse fetal effects (2,3).

In the Collaborative Perinatal Project, 1024 mother–child pairs of the 50,282 studied were exposed to dicyclomine during the 1st trimester (4, pp. 346–356). It was the most common parasympatholytic agent consumed by the women studied. A statistically significant association (standardized relative risk (SRR) 1.46) was discovered for minor malformations with 21 malformed children (4, p. 353). Other defects with an SRR greater than 1.5, and the number of affected newborns, were polydactyly in blacks (SRR 1.89; $N = 6$; 277 black mothers), macrocephaly (SRR 8.8; $N = 3$), diaphragmatic hernia (SRR 12.0; $N = 3$), and clubfoot (SRR 1.8; $N = 7$) (3, pp. 353, 477). For use anytime during pregnancy, 1593 women consumed dicyclomine and an increased SRR was measured for macrocephaly (6.2; $N = 3$) and pectus excavatum (1.8; $N = 9$) (4, p. 492). The authors of this study, however, strongly cautioned that a causal relationship could not be inferred from any of these data, especially when the drug was used after the 1st trimester, and that independent confirmation was required with other studies.

A retrospective study published in 1971, involving more than 1200 mothers, examined the relationship between drugs and congenital malformations (5). This investigation found that significantly fewer mothers of infants with major anomalies, as compared with normal controls, took antiemetics during the first 56 days of pregnancy. Dicyclomine was the fourth most frequently ingested antiemetic.

In a surveillance study of Michigan Medicaid recipients involving 229,101 completed pregnancies conducted between 1985 and 1992, 642 newborns had been exposed to dicyclomine during the 1st trimester (F. Rosa, personal communication, FDA, 1993). A total of 31 (4.8%) major birth defects were observed (27 expected). Specific data were available for six defect categories, including (observed/expected) 5/6 cardiovascular defects, 1/1 oral clefts, 0/0.5 spina bifida, 0/1 limb reduction defects, 0/2 hypospadias, and 3/1 polydactyly. Only with the latter defect is there a suggestion of a possible association, but other factors, including the mother's disease, concurrent drug use, and chance may be involved.

BREASTFEEDING SUMMARY

No published reports on the excretion of dicyclomine into breast milk have been located. The manufacturer has received a case report of apnea in a breastfed 12-day-old infant whose mother was receiving dicyclomine (personal communication, N.G. Dahl, Marion Merrell Dow, Inc., 1992). Following the adverse event, the mother was administered a single, 20-mg dose of the drug and breastfeeding was suspended for 24 hours. Plasma and milk concentrations of dicyclomine 2 hours after the dose were 59 ng/mL and 131 ng/mL (milk:plasma ratio 2.2), respectively. Although a causal relationship between dicyclomine and apnea was not established, similar adverse reactions have occurred when the drug was administered directly to infants (1). Consequently, the safest course is to avoid dicyclomine during nursing.

References

1. Friedman JM, Little BB, Brent RL, Cordero JF, Hanson JW, Shepard TH. Potential human teratogenicity of frequently prescribed drugs. Obstet Gynecol 1990;75:594–9.
2. Product information. Bentyl. Marion Merrell Dow, Inc., 1992.
3. Gibson JP, Staples RE, Larson EJ, Kuhn WL, Holtkamp DE, Newberne JW. Teratology and reproduction studies with an antinauseant. Toxicol Appl Pharmacol 1968;13:439–47.
4. Heinonen OP, Slone D, Shapiro S. *Birth Defects and Drugs in Pregnancy*. Littleton, MA: Publishing Sciences Group, 1977.
5. Nelson MM, Forfar JO. Associations between drugs administered during pregnancy and congenital abnormalities of the fetus. Br Med J 1971;1:523–7.

D

DIDANOSINE

Antiviral

PREGNANCY RECOMMENDATION: Compatible—Maternal Benefit >>Embryo–Fetal Risk
BREASTFEEDING RECOMMENDATION: Contraindicated

PREGNANCY SUMMARY

An increased risk of congenital defects after 1st trimester exposure to didanosine was reported by the Antiretroviral Pregnancy Registry, but the rate has decreased as the number of exposures has increased. Theoretically, exposure to didanosine at the time of implantation could result in impaired fertility due to embryonic cytotoxicity, but this has not been studied in humans. Mitochondrial dysfunction in offspring exposed in utero or postnatally to nucleoside reverse transcriptase inhibitors (NRTIs) has been reported (see Lamivudine and Zidovudine). However, if indicated, the drug should not be withheld because of pregnancy.

FETAL RISK SUMMARY

Didanosine (2′,3′-dideoxyinosine; ddI) inhibits viral reverse transcriptase and DNA synthesis. It is classified as an NRTI used for the treatment of HIV infections. Its mechanism of action is similar to that of five other nucleoside analogues: abacavir, lamivudine, stavudine, zalcitabine, and zidovudine. Didanosine is converted by intracellular enzymes to the active metabolite, dideoxyadenosine triphosphate (ddATP).

No evidence of teratogenicity or toxicity was observed in pregnant rats and rabbits administered doses of didanosine up to 12 and 14.2 times the human dose, respectively (1). In another report, didanosine was given to pregnant mice in doses ranging from 10 to 300 mg/kg/day, through all or part of gestation, without resulting in teratogenic effects or other toxicity (2).

The reproductive toxicity of 2′,3′-dideoxyadenosine (ddA; the unphosphorylated active metabolite of didanosine) in rats was compared in a combined in vitro/in vivo experiment with four other nucleoside analogs (vidarabine phosphate, ganciclovir, zalcitabine, and zidovudine), and these results were then compared with previous data obtained under identical conditions with acyclovir (3). Utilizing various concentrations of the drug in a whole-embryo culture system and direct administration to pregnant females (200 mg/kg subcutaneously every 4 hours for three doses) during organogenesis, in vitro vidarabine showed the highest potential to interfere with embryonic development, whereas in vivo acyclovir had the highest teratogenic potential. In this study, the in vitro reproductive toxicity of ddA was less than that of the other agents, except for zidovudine. The in vivo toxicity was less than that of acyclovir, vidarabine, and ganciclovir, and equal to that observed with zalcitabine and zidovudine.

Antiretroviral nucleosides have been shown to have a direct dose-related cytotoxic effect on preimplantation mouse embryos. A 1994 report compared this toxicity among zidovudine and three newer compounds, didanosine, stavudine, and zalcitabine (4). Whereas significant inhibition of blastocyst formation occurred with a 1 μmol/L concentration of zidovudine, stavudine, and zalcitabine toxicity was not detected until 100 μmol/L, and no toxicity was observed with didanosine up to 100 μmol/L. Moreover, postblastocyst development was severely inhibited in those embryos that did survive exposure to 1 μmol/L zidovudine. As for the other compounds, stavudine, at a concentration of 10 μmol/L (2.24 mcg/mL), inhibited postblastocyst development, but no effect was observed with concentrations up to 100 μmol/L of didanosine or zalcitabine. An earlier study found no cytotoxicity in preimplantation mouse embryos exposed to didanosine concentrations ≤500 μmol/L (2). Although there are no human data, the authors of the 1994 study concluded that the three newer agents may be safer than zidovudine to use in early pregnancy (4).

A 1995 report described the effect of exposure to a relatively high concentration of didanosine (20 μmol/L vs. recommended therapeutic concentrations of 3–5 μmol/L) for prolonged periods (2–11 days) on trophoblasts from term and 1st trimester placentas (5). No significant effects on trophoblast function, as measured by human chorionic gonadotropin (hCG) secretion, protein synthesis, progesterone synthesis, and glucose consumption, were observed.

A 1999 study also investigated the effects of a single 24-hour exposure of zidovudine (AZT) or didanosine on human trophoblast cells using a human choriocarcinoma cell line that exhibited many characteristics of the early placenta (6). Two drug concentrations (7.6 mM or 0.076 mM) were studied for their effects on trophoblast cell proliferation and hormone production (hCG, estradiol (E_2) and progesterone (P_4)). The higher concentrations of AZT or ddI resulted in significant decreases in cell numbers and growth rate (38% and 51% of control values, respectively), but increased production of hCG, E_2, and P_4. The decrease in trophoblast cell proliferation may have been the mechanism for the increased incidence of rodent embryo loss observed with AZT (6). In contrast, the lower concentrations of AZT and ddI did not cause changes in cell numbers, producing only significant increases in E_2 production. Because of these findings, the researchers concluded that high therapeutic doses of either AZT or ddI during early human gestation were potentially embryo toxic (6).

Didanosine crosses the placenta to the fetus in both animals and humans (1,7–13). In pregnant macaques, didanosine was administered by constant infusion at a dose of either 42.5 or 425 mcg/minute/kg (7). The compound crossed the placenta by simple diffusion, resulting in fetal:maternal concentration ratios for both doses of approximately 0.5. In near-term rhesus monkeys, a single IV bolus (2.0 mg/kg) of didanosine resulted in mean fetal concentrations of unmetabolized drug of 33% of the maternal plasma concentrations (8). Concentrations of didanosine were 20% of those in the fetal plasma by 3 hours. However, ddATP was not found in any fetal tissue.

Using a perfused term human placenta, investigators concluded in a 1992 publication that the placental transfer of didanosine was most likely due to passive diffusion (9). Two other studies, again using perfused human placenta, found that only about 50% of the drug would be passively transferred to the fetal circulation (10), and at approximately half the rate of zidovudine (11). In contrast to zidovudine (see Zidovudine), no metabolite was detected in the placenta (10).

Two HIV-positive women, at 21 and 24 weeks' gestation, respectively, were given a single 375-mg oral dose of didanosine immediately prior to pregnancy termination (12). Drug concentrations in the maternal blood, fetal blood, and amniotic fluid at slightly more than 1 hour after the dose were 295, 42, and <5 ng/mL, respectively, in the first patient, and 629, 121, and 135 ng/mL, respectively, in the second woman. The fetal:maternal blood ratios were 0.14 and 0.19, respectively. Although single-drug-level determinations are difficult to interpret, a study published in 1993 found that human placental first-pass metabolism was not the reason for these low fetal and amniotic fluid levels (13).

Three experimental in vitro models using perfused human placentas to predict the placental transfer of NRTIs (didanosine, stavudine, zalcitabine, and zidovudine) were described in a 1999 publication (14). For each drug, the predicted fetal:maternal plasma drug concentration ratios at steady state with each of the three models were close to those actually observed in pregnant macaques. Based on these results, the authors concluded that their models would accurately predict the mechanism, relative rate, and the extent of in vivo human placental transfer of NRTIs (14).

The pharmacokinetics of IV (1.6 mg/kg/hr) and oral (200 mg twice daily) didanosine have been studied in pregnant women with HIV infection at 31 weeks' gestation, during labor, and 6 weeks postpartum (15). This study also described the pharmacokinetics of oral didanosine (60 mg/m^2) in infants at day 1 and at week 6 after birth.

The Antiretroviral Pregnancy Registry reported, for January 1989 through July 2009, prospective data (reported before the outcomes were known) involving 4702 live births that had been exposed during the 1st trimester to one or more antiretroviral agents (16). Congenital defects were noted in 134, a prevalence of 2.8% (95% confidence interval [CI] 2.4–3.4). In the 6100 live births with earliest exposure in the 2nd/3rd trimesters, there were 153 infants with defects (2.5%, 95% CI 2.1–2.9). The prevalence rates for the two periods did not differ significantly. There were 288 infants with birth defects among 10,803 live births with exposure anytime during pregnancy (2.7%, 95% CI 2.4–3.0). The prevalence rate did not differ significantly from the rate expected in a nonexposed population. There were 627 outcomes exposed to didanosine (370 in the 1st trimester and 257 in the 2nd/3rd trimesters) in combination with other antiretroviral agents. There were 22 birth defects (17 in the 1st trimester and 5 in the 2nd/3rd trimesters). In reviewing the birth defects of prospective and retrospective (pregnancies reported after the outcomes were known) registered cases, the Registry concluded that, except for isolated cases of neural tube defects with efavirenz exposure in retrospective reports, there was no other pattern of anomalies (isolated or syndromic) (16). (See Lamivudine for required statement.)

A case of life-threatening anemia following in utero exposure to antiretroviral agents was described in 1998 (17). A 30-year-old woman with HIV infection was treated with zidovudine, didanosine, and trimethoprim/sulfamethoxazole (three times weekly) during the 1st trimester. Vitamin supplementation was also given. Because of an inadequate response, didanosine was discontinued and lamivudine and zalcitabine were started in the 3rd trimester. Two weeks before delivery the HIV viral load was undetectable. At term, a pale, male infant was delivered, who developed respiratory distress shortly after birth. Examination revealed a hyperactive precordium and hepatomegaly without evidence of hydrops. The hematocrit was 11% with a reticulocyte count of zero. An extensive work-up of the mother and infant failed to determine the cause of the anemia. Bacterial and viral infections, including HIV, parvovirus B19, cytomegalovirus, and others, were excluded. The infant received a transfusion and was apparently doing well at 10 weeks of age. Because no other cause of the anemia could be found, the authors attributed the condition to bone morrow suppression, most likely to zidovudine (17). A contribution of the other agents to the condition, however, could not be excluded.

A 2000 case report described the adverse pregnancy outcomes, including NTD, of two pregnant women with HIV infection who were treated with the anti-infective combination, trimethoprim/sulfamethoxazole, for prophylaxis against *Pneumocystsis carinii*, concurrently with antiretroviral agents (18). Exposure to didanosine occurred in one of these cases. A 31-year-old woman presented at 15 weeks' gestation. She was receiving trimethoprim/sulfamethoxazole, didanosine, stavudine, nevirapine, and vitamin B supplements (specific vitamins and dosage not given) that had been started before conception. A fetal ultrasound at 19 weeks' gestation revealed spina bifida and ventriculomegaly. The patient elected to terminate her pregnancy. The fetus did not have HIV infection. Defects observed at autopsy included ventriculomegaly, an Arnold–Chiari malformation, sacral spina bifida, and a lumbosacral meningomyelocele. The authors attributed the NTDs in both cases to the antifolate activity of trimethoprim (18).

No data are available on the advisability of treating pregnant women who have been exposed to HIV via occupational exposure, but one author discourages this use (19).

Two reviews, one in 1996 and the other in 1997, concluded that all women currently receiving antiretroviral therapy should continue to receive therapy during pregnancy and that treatment of the mother with monotherapy should be considered inadequate therapy (20,21). The same conclusion was reached in a 2003 review with the added admonishment that therapy must be continuous to prevent emergence of resistant viral strains (22). In 2009, the updated U.S. Department of Health and Human Services guidelines for the use of antiretroviral agents in HIV type 1 (HIV-1)-infected patients continued the recommendation that therapy, with the exception of efavirenz, should be continued during pregnancy (23). If indicated, didanosine should not be withheld in pregnancy because the expected benefit to the HIV-positive mother outweighs the unknown risk to the fetus. The updated guidelines for the use of antiretroviral drugs to reduce perinatal HIV-1 transmission also were released in 2010 (24). Women receiving antiretroviral therapy during pregnancy should continue the therapy, but, regardless of the regimen, zidovudine administration is recommended during the intrapartum period to prevent vertical transmission of HIV to the newborn (24).

BREASTFEEDING SUMMARY

No reports describing the use of didanosine during lactation have been located. The molecular weight (about 236) is low enough that excretion into milk should be expected. The effect on a nursing infant is unknown.

Reports on the use of didanosine during human lactation are unlikely because the antiviral agent is used in the treatment of HIV infections. HIV-1 is transmitted in milk, and in developed countries, breastfeeding is not recommended (20,21,23,25–27). In developing countries, breastfeeding is undertaken, despite the risk, because there are no affordable milk substitutes available. Until 1999, no studies had been published that examined the effect of any antiretroviral therapy on HIV-1 transmission in milk. In that year, a study involving zidovudine was published that measured a 38% reduction in vertical transmission of HIV-1 infection despite breastfeeding when compared with controls (see Zidovudine).

References

1. Product information. Videx. Bristol-Myers Squibb, 2001.
2. Sieh E, Coluzzi ML, Cusella de Angelis MG, Mezzogiorno A, Floridia M, Canipari R, Cossu G, Vella S. The effects of AZT and DDI on pre- and post-implantation mammalian embryos: an in vivo and in vitro study. AIDS Res Hum Retroviruses 1992;8:639–49.
3. Klug S, Lewandowski C, Merker H-J, Stahlmann R, Wildi L, Neubert D. In vitro and in vivo studies on the prenatal toxicity of five virustatic nucleoside analogues in comparison to aciclovir. Arch Toxicol 1991;65:283–91.
4. Toltzis P, Mourton T, Magnuson T. Comparative embryonic cytotoxicity of antiretroviral nucleosides. J Infect Dis 1994;169:1100–2.
5. Esterman AL, Rosenberg C, Brown T, Dancis J. The effect of zidovudine and 2′3′-dideoxyinosine on human trophoblast in culture. Pharmacol Toxicol 1995;76:89–92.
6. Plessinger MA, Miller RK. Effects of zidovudine (AZT) and dideoxyinosine (ddI) on human trophoblast cells. Reprod Toxicol 1999;13:537–46.
7. Pereira CM, Nosbisch C, Winter HR, Baughman WL, Unadkat JD. Transplacental pharmacokinetics of dideoxyinosine in pigtailed macaques. Antimicrob Agents Chemother 1994;38:781–6.
8. Sandberg JA, Binienda Z, Lipe G, Rose LM, Parker WB, Ali SF, Slikker W Jr. Placental transfer and fetal disposition of 2′3′-dideoxycytidine and 2′3′-dideoxyinosine in the rhesus monkey. Drug Metab Dispos 1995;23:881–4.
9. Bawdon RE, Sobhi S, Dax J. The transfer of anti-human immunodeficiency virus nucleoside compounds by the term human placenta. Am J Obstet Gynecol 1992;167:1570–4.
10. Dancis J, Lee JD, Mendoza S, Liebes L. Transfer and metabolism of dideoxyinosine by the perfused human placenta. J Acquir Immune Defic Syndr 1993;6:2–6.
11. Henderson GI, Perez AB, Yang Y, Hamby RL, Schenken RS, Schenker S. Transfer of dideoxyinosine across the human isolated placenta. Br J Clin Pharmacol 1994;38:237–42.
12. Pons JC, Boubon MC, Taburet AM, Singlas E, Chambrin V, Frydman R, Papiernik E, Delfraissy JF. Fetoplacental passage of 2′,3′-dideoxyinosine. Lancet 1991;337:732.
13. Dalton JT, Au JL-S. 2′3′-Dideoxyinosine is not metabolized in human placenta. Drug Metab Dispos 1993;21:544–6.
14. Tuntland T, Odinecs A, Pereira CM, Nosbisch C, Unadkat JD. In vitro models to predict the in vivo mechanism, rate, and extent of placental transfer of dideoxynucleoside drugs against human immunodeficiency virus. Am J Obstet Gynecol 1999;180:198–206.
15. Wang Y, Livingston E, Patil S, McKinney RE, Bardeguez AD, Gandia J, O'Sullivan MJ, Clax P, Huang S, Unadkat JD. Pharmacokinetics of didanosine in antepartum and postpartum human immunodeficiency virus-infected pregnant women and their neonates: an AIDS Clinical Trials Group study. J Infect Dis 1999;180:1536–41.
16. Antiretroviral Pregnancy Registry Steering Committee. *Antiretroviral Pregnancy Registry International Interim Report for 1 January 1989 through 31 July 2009*. Wilmington, NC: Registry Coordinating Center, 2009. Available at www.apregistry.com. Accessed May 29, 2010.
17. Watson WJ, Stevens TP, Weinberg GA. Profound anemia in a newborn infant of a mother receiving antiretroviral therapy. Pediatr Infect Dis J 1998;17:435–6.
18. Richardson MP, Osrin D, Donaghy S, Brown NA, Hay P, Sharland M. Spinal malformations in the fetuses of HIV infected women receiving combination antiretroviral therapy and co-trimoxazole. Eur J Obstet Gynecol Reprod Biol 2000;93:215–7.
19. Gerberding JL. Management of occupational exposures to blood-borne viruses. N Engl J Med 1995;332:444–51.
20. Carpenter CCJ, Fischi MA, Hammer SM, Hirsch MS, Jacobsen DM, Katzenstein DA, Montaner JSG, Richman DD, Saag MS, Schooley RT, Thompson MA, Vella S, Yeni PG, Volberding PA. Antiretroviral therapy for HIV infection in 1996. JAMA 1996;276;146–54.
21. Minkoff H, Augenbraun M. Antiretroviral therapy for pregnant women. Am J Obstet Gynecol 1997;176:478–89.
22. Minkoff H. Human immunodeficiency virus infection in pregnancy. Obstet Gynecol 2003;101:797–810.
23. Panel on Antiretroviral Guidelines for Adults and Adolescents. *Guidelines for the Use of Antiretroviral Agents in HIV-1-Infected Adults and Adolescents*. Department of Health and Human Services. December 1, 2009:1–161. Available at http://www.aidsinfo.nih.gov/ContentFiles/AdultandAdolescentGL.pdf. Accessed September 17, 2010:60, 96–8.
24. Panel on Treatment of HIV-Infected Pregnant Women and Prevention of Perinatal Transmission. *Recommendations for Use of Antiretroviral Drugs in Pregnant HIV-1-Infected Women for Maternal Health and Interventions to Reduce Perinatal HIV Transmission in the United States*. May 24, 2010:1–117. Available at http://aidsinfo.nih.gov/ContentFiles/PerinatalGL.pdf. Accessed September 17, 2010:30 (Table 5).
25. Brown ZA, Watts DH. Antiviral therapy in pregnancy. Clin Obstet Gynecol 1990;33:276–89.
26. De Martino M, Tovo P-A, Tozzi AE, Pezzotti P, Galli L, Livadiotti S, Caselli D, Massironi E, Ruga E, Fioredda F, Plebani A, Gabiano C, Zuccotti GV. HIV-1 transmission through breast-milk: appraisal of risk according to duration of feeding. AIDS 1992;6:991–7.
27. Van de Perre P. Postnatal transmission of human immunodeficiency virus type 1: the breast-feeding dilemma. Am J Obstet Gynecol 1995;173:483–7.

DIENESTROL

[Withdrawn from the market. See 9th edition.]

D

DIETHYLPROPION

Central Stimulant/Anorexiant

PREGNANCY RECOMMENDATION: Human Data Suggest Low Risk
BREASTFEEDING RECOMMENDATION: Limited Human Data—Probably Compatible

PREGNANCY SUMMARY

No reports, in humans or animals, linking the use of diethylpropion with congenital defects have been located.

FETAL RISK SUMMARY

Diethylpropion has been studied as an appetite suppressant in 28 pregnant patients and, although adverse effects were common in the women, no problems were observed in their offspring (1). A retrospective survey of 1232 patients exposed to diethylpropion during pregnancy found no difference in the incidence of defects (0.9%) when compared with a matched control group (1.1%) (2). No impairment of fertility, teratogenicity, or fetotoxicity was observed in animal studies with doses up to nine times those used in humans (3,4).

BREASTFEEDING SUMMARY

Diethylpropion and its metabolites are excreted into breast milk (4). No reports of adverse effects in a nursing infant have been located.

References

1. Silverman M, Okun R. The use of an appetite suppressant (diethylpropion hydrochloride) during pregnancy. Curr Ther Res 1971;13:648–53.
2. Bunde CA, Leyland HM. A controlled retrospective survey in evaluation of teratogenicity. J New Drugs 1965;5:193–8.
3. Schardein JL. *Drugs as Teratogens*. Cleveland, OH: CRC Press, 1976:73–5.
4. Product information. Tenuate. Marion Merrell Dow, Inc., 1992.

DIETHYLSTILBESTROL

Estrogenic Hormone

PREGNANCY RECOMMENDATION: Contraindicated
BREASTFEEDING RECOMMENDATION: Contraindicated

PREGNANCY SUMMARY

Diethylstilbestrol (DES) is a known human teratogen. It causes developmental toxicity in both female and male offspring. It is contraindicated in pregnancy.

FETAL RISK SUMMARY

Between 1940 and 1971, an estimated 6 million mothers and their fetuses were exposed to DES to prevent reproductive problems such as miscarriage, premature delivery, intrauterine fetal death, and toxemia (1–4). Controlled studies have since proven that DES was not successful in preventing these disorders (5,6). This use has resulted, however, in significant complications of the reproductive system in both female and male offspring (1–12). Two large groups have been established to monitor these complications: the Registry for Research on Hormonal Transplacental Carcinogenesis and the Diethylstilbestrol Adenosis (DESAD) Project (4). The published findings and recommendations of the DESAD project through 1980 plus a number of other studies including the Registry were reviewed in a 1981 National Institutes of Health booklet available from the National Cancer Institute (4). This information was also reprinted in a 1983 journal article (13). The complications identified in female and male children exposed in utero to DES are as follows:

Female
- Lower müllerian tract
- Vaginal adenosis
- Vaginal and cervical clear cell adenocarcinoma
- Cervical and vaginal fornix defects (10)
- Cock's comb (hood, transverse ridge of cervix)
- Collar (rim, hood, transverse ridge of cervix)

Pseudopolyp
Hypoplastic cervix (immature cervix)
Altered fornix of vagina
Vaginal defects (exclusive of fornix) (10)
Incomplete transverse septum
Incomplete longitudinal septum
Upper müllerian tract
Uterine structural defects
Fallopian tube structural defects

Male
Reproductive dysfunction
Altered semen analysis
Infertility

The Registry was established in 1971 to study the epidemiologic, clinical, and pathologic aspects of clear cell adenocarcinoma of the vagina and cervix in DES-exposed women (2). More than 400 cases of clear cell adenocarcinoma have been reported to the Registry. Additional reports continue to appear in the literature (14). The risk of carcinoma is apparently higher when DES treatment was given before the 12th week of gestation and is estimated to be 0.14–1.4/1000 for women younger than 25 years (2,4).

The first-known case of adenosquamous carcinoma of the cervix in an exposed patient was described in 1983 (15). In a second case, a fatal malignant teratoma of the ovary developed in a 12-year-old exposed girl (16). The relationship between these tumors and DES is unknown.

The frequency of dysplasia and carcinoma in situ (CIS) of the cervix and vagina in 3980 DESAD Project patients was significantly increased over controls with an approximately 2- to 4-fold increase in risk (11). These results were different from earlier studies of these same women, which had indicated no increased risk for dysplasia and CIS (17,18). Researchers speculated that the increased incidence now observed was related to the greater amount of squamous metaplasia found in DES-exposed women (11). Scanning electron microscopy of the cervicovaginal transformation zone has indicated that maturation of epithelium is slowed or arrested at the stage of immature squamous epithelium in some DES-exposed women (19). This process may produce greater susceptibility to factors such as herpes and papillomavirus obtained through early coitus with multiple partners and result in the observed increased rates of dysplasia/CIS (11). Of interest in this regard, a 1983 article reported detectable papillomavirus antigen in the cervical–vaginal biopsies of 16 (43%) of 37 DES-exposed women (20).

The incidence of cervical or vaginal structural changes has been reported to occur in up to 85% of exposed women, although most studies place the incidence in the 22%–58% range (2,3,5,7,12,21–24). The structural changes are outlined earlier. The DESAD Project reported an incidence of approximately 25% in 1655 women (10). Selection bias was eliminated by analyzing only those patients identified by record review. Patients referred by physicians and self-referrals had much higher rates of defects, about 49% and 43%, respectively. Almost all of the defects were confined to the cervical–vaginal fornix area, with only 14 patients having vaginal changes exclusive of the fornix and nearly all of these being incomplete transverse septums (10).

Reports linking the use of DES with major congenital anomalies have not been located. The Collaborative Perinatal Project monitored 614 mother–child pairs with 1st trimester exposure to estrogens, including 164 with exposure to DES (25, pp. 389, 391). Evidence for an increase in the expected frequency for cardiovascular defects, eye and ear anomalies, and Down's syndrome was found for estrogens as a group, but not for DES (25, pp. 389, 391, 395). Reevaluation of these data in terms of timing of exposure, vaginal bleeding in early pregnancy, and previous maternal obstetric history, however, failed to support an association between estrogens and cardiac malformations (26). An earlier study also failed to find any relationship with nongenital malformations (27).

Alterations in the body of the uterus have led to concern regarding increased pregnancy wastage and premature births (8,22,28–31). Increased rates of spontaneous abortions, premature births, and ectopic pregnancies are well established by these latter reports, although the relationship to the abnormal changes of the cervix and/or vagina is still unclear (8). Serial observations of vaginal epithelial changes indicate that the frequency of such changes decreases with age (4,17,24).

Spontaneous rupture of a term uterus has been described in a 25-year-old primigravid with DES-type changes in her vagina, cervix, and uterus (32). Other reports of this type have not been located.

In a 1984 study, DES exposure had no effect on the age at menarche, first coitus, pregnancy, or live birth, or on a woman's ability to conceive (33). One group of investigators found that although anomalies in the upper genital tract increased the risk for poor pregnancy outcome, they could not relate specific changes to specific types of outcomes (34).

Hirsutism and irregular menses were found in 72% and 50%, respectively, of 32 DES-exposed women (35). The degree of hirsutism was age related, with the mean ages of severely and mildly hirsute women being 28.8 and 24.7 years, respectively. Based on various hormone level measurements, the authors concluded that in utero DES exposure might result in hypothalamic–pituitary–ovarian dysfunction (35). However, other studies in much larger exposed populations have not observed disturbances of menstruation or excessive hair growth (36).

Data on DES-exposed women who had undergone major gynecologic surgical procedures, excluding cesarean section, were reported in a 1982 study (37). Of 309 exposed women, 33 (11%) had a total of 43 procedures. The authors suggested that DES exposure resulted in an increased incidence of adnexal disease involving adhesions, benign ovarian cysts, and ectopic pregnancies (37). Surgical manipulation of the cervix (cryocautery or conization) in DES-exposed patients results in a high incidence of cervical stenosis and possible development of endometriosis (38,39). Both studies concluded, however, that the causes of infertility in these patients were comparable to those in a non–DES-exposed population.

Adverse effects in male offspring attributable to in utero DES exposure have been reported (1,5,40–46). Abnormalities thought to occur at greater frequencies include the following:

Epididymal cysts
Hypotrophic testis
Microphallus
Varicocele
Capsular induration
Altered semen (decreased count, concentration, motility, and morphology)

D

An increase in problems with passing urine and urogenital tract infections has also been observed (40).

DES exposure has been proposed as a possible cause of infertility in male offspring (1). However, in a controlled in vitro study, no association was found between exposure to DES and reduced sperm penetration of zona-free hamster eggs (46). In addition, a study of 828 exposed males found no increase over controls for risk of genitourinary abnormalities, infertility, or testicular cancer (47). Based on their data, the authors proposed that previous studies showing a positive relationship might have had selection biases, differences in DES use, or both.

Testicular tumors have been reported in three DES-exposed patients (6,48). In one case, a teratoma was discovered in a 23-year-old male (6). Two patients, 27 and 28 years of age, were included in the second report (48). Both had left-sided anaplastic seminomas, and one had epididymal cysts. A male sibling of one of the patients, also exposed to DES, had severe oligospermia, and two exposed sisters had vaginal adenosis and vaginal adenocarcinoma.

Changes in the psychosexual performance of young boys have been attributed to in utero exposure to DES and progesterone (49,50). The mothers received estrogen/progestogen regimens for diabetes. A trend to less heterosexual experience and fewer masculine interests than controls was shown. A 2-fold increase in psychiatric disease, especially depression and anxiety, has been observed in both male and female exposed offspring (6).

BREASTFEEDING SUMMARY

No data are available. Decreased milk volume and nitrogen–protein content may occur if DES is used during lactation (see Mestranol and Ethinyl Estradiol).

References

1. Stenchever MA, Williamson RA, Leonard J, Karp LE, Ley B, Shy K, Smith D. Possible relationship between in utero diethylstilbestrol exposure and male fertility. Am J Obstet Gynecol 1981;140:186–93.
2. Herbst AL. Diethylstilbestrol and other sex hormones during pregnancy. Obstet Gynecol 1981;58(Suppl):35s–40s.
3. Nordquist SAB, Medhat IA, Ng AB. Teratogenic effects of intrauterine exposure to DES in female offspring. Compr Ther 1979;5:69–74.
4. Robboy SJ, Noller KL, Kaufman RH, Barnes AB, Townsend D, Gundersen JH, Nash S. Information for physicians. Prenatal diethylstilbestrol (DES) exposure: recommendations of the Diethylstilbestrol–Adenosis (DESAD) Project for the identification and management of exposed individuals. NIH Publication No. 81-2049, 1981.
5. Stillman RJ. In utero exposure to diethylstilbestrol: adverse effects on the reproductive tract and reproductive performance in male and female offspring. Am J Obstet Gynecol 1982;142:905–21.
6. Vessey MP, Fairweather DVI, Norman-Smith B, Buckley J. A randomized double-blind controlled trial of the value of stilboestrol therapy in pregnancy: long-term follow-up of mothers and their offspring. Br J Obstet Gynaecol 1983;90:1007–17.
7. Prins RP, Morrow P, Townsend DE, Disaia PJ. Vaginal embryogenesis, estrogens, and adenosis. Obstet Gynecol 1976;48:246–50.
8. Sandberg EC, Riffle NL, Higdon JV, Getman CE. Pregnancy outcome in women exposed to diethylstilbestrol in utero. Am J Obstet Gynecol 1981;140:194–205.
9. Noller KL, Townsend DE, Kaufman RH, Barnes AB, Robboy SJ, Fish CR, Jefferies JA, Bergstralh EJ, O'Brien PC, McGorray SP, Scully R. Maturation of vaginal and cervical epithelium in women exposed in utero to diethylstilbestrol (DESAD Project). Am J Obstet Gynecol 1983;146:279–85.
10. Jefferies JA, Robboy SJ, O'Brien PC, Bergstralh EJ, Labarthe DR, Barnes AB, Noller KL, Hatab PA, Kaufman RH, Townsend DE. Structural anomalies of the cervix and vagina in women enrolled in the Diethylstilbestrol Adenosis (DESAD) Project. Am J Obstet Gynecol 1984;148:59–66.
11. Robboy SJ, Noller KL, O'Brien P, Kaufman RH, Townsend D, Barnes AB, Gundersen J, Lawrence WD, Bergstrahl E, McGorray S, Tilley BC, Anton J, Chazen G. Increased incidence of cervical and vaginal dysplasia in 3,980 diethylstilbestrol-exposed young women. Experience of the National Collaborative Diethylstilbestrol Adenosis Project. JAMA 1984;252:2979–83.
12. Chanen W, Pagano R. Diethylstilboestrol (DES) exposure in utero. Med J Aust 1984;141:491–3.
13. NCI DES Summary. Prenatal diethylstilbestrol (DES) exposure. Clin Pediatr 1983;22:139–43.
14. Kaufman RH, Korhonen MO, Strama T, Adam E, Kaplan A. Development of clear cell adenocarcinoma in DES-exposed offspring under observation. Obstet Gynecol 1982;59(Suppl):68S–72S.
15. Vandrie DM, Puri S, Upton RT, Demeester LJ. Adenosquamous carcinoma of the cervix in a woman exposed to diethylstilbestrol in utero. Obstet Gynecol 1983;61(Suppl):84S–7S.
16. Lazarus KH. Maternal diethylstilboestrol and ovarian malignancy in offspring. Lancet 1984;1:53.
17. O'Brien PC, Noller KL, Robboy SJ, Barnes AB, Kaufman RH, Tilley BC, Townsend DE. Vaginal epithelial changes in young women enrolled in the National Cooperative Diethylstilbestrol Adenosis (DESAD) Project. Obstet Gynecol 1979;53:300–8.
18. Robboy SJ, Kaufman RH, Prat J, Welch WR, Gaffey T, Scully RE, Richart R, Fenoglio CM, Virata R, Tilley BC. Pathologic findings in young women enrolled in the National Cooperative Diethylstilbestrol Adenosis (DESAD) Project. Obstet Gynecol 1979;53:309–17.
19. McDonnell JM, Emens JM, Jordan JA. The congenital cervicovaginal transformation zone in young women exposed to diethylstilboestrol in utero. Br J Obstet Gynaecol 1984;91:574–9.
20. Fu YS, Lancaster WD, Richart RM, Reagan JW, Crum CP, Levine RU. Cervical papillomavirus infection in diethylstilbestrol-exposed progeny. Obstet Gynecol 1983;61:59–62.
21. Ben-Baruch G, Menczer J, Mashiach S, Serr DM. Uterine anomalies in diethylstilbestrol-exposed women with fertility disorders. Acta Obstet Gynecol Scand 1981;60:395–7.
22. Pillsbury SG Jr. Reproductive significance of changes in the endometrial cavity associated with exposure in utero in diethylstilbestrol. Am J Obstet Gynecol 1980;137:178–82.
23. Professional and Public Relations Committee of the Diethylstilbestrol and Adenosis Project of the Division of Cancer Control and Rehabilitation. Exposure in utero to diethylstilbestrol and related synthetic hormones. Association with vaginal and cervical cancers and other abnormalities. JAMA 1976;236:1107–9.
24. Burke L, Antonioli D, Friedman EA. Evolution of diethylstilbestrol-associated genital tract lesions. Obstet Gynecol 1981;57:79–84.
25. Heinonen OP, Slone D, Shapiro S. *Birth Defects and Drugs in Pregnancy*. Littleton, MA: Publishing Sciences Group, 1977.
26. Wiseman RA, Dodds-Smith IC. Cardiovascular birth defects and antenatal exposure to female sex hormones: a reevaluation of some base data. Teratology 1984;30:359–70.
27. Wilson JG, Brent RL. Are female sex hormones teratogenic? Am J Obstet Gynecol 1981;141:567–80.
28. Herbst AL, Hubby MM, Blough RR, Azizi F. A comparison of pregnancy experience in DES-exposed daughters. J Reprod Med 1980;24:62–9.
29. Barnes AB, Colton T, Gundersen J, Noller KL, Tilley BC, Strama T, Townsend DE, Hatab P, O'Brien PC. Fertility and outcome of pregnancy in women exposed in utero to diethylstilbestrol. N Engl J Med 1980;302:609–13.
30. Veridiano NP, Dilke I, Rogers J, Tancer ML. Reproductive performance of DES-exposed female progeny. Obstet Gynecol 1981;58:58–61.
31. Mangan CE, Borow L, Burnett-Rubin MM, Egan V, Giuntoli RL, Mikuta JJ. Pregnancy outcome in 98 women exposed to diethylstilbestrol in utero, their mothers, and unexposed siblings. Obstet Gynecol 1982; 59:315–9.
32. Williamson HO, Sowell GA, Smith HE. Spontaneous rupture of gravid uterus in a patient with diethylstilbestrol-type changes. Am J Obstet Gynecol 1984;150:158–60.
33. Barnes AB. Menstrual history and fecundity of women exposed and unexposed in utero to diethylstilbestrol. J Reprod Med 1984;29:651–5.
34. Kaufman RH, Noller K, Adam E, Irwin J, Gray M, Jefferies JA, Hilton J. Upper genital tract abnormalities and pregnancy outcome in diethylstilbestrol-exposed progeny. Am J Obstet Gynecol 1984;148:973–84.
35. Peress MR, Tsai CC, Mathur RS, Williamson HO. Hirsutism and menstrual patterns in women exposed to diethylstilbestrol in utero. Am J Obstet Gynecol 1982;144:135–40.
36. Verkauf BS. Discussion. Am J Obstet Gynecol 1982;144:139–40.
37. Schmidt G, Fowler WC Jr. Gynecologic operative experience in women exposed to DES in utero. South Med J 1982;75:260–3.

38. Haney AF, Hammond MG. Infertility in women exposed to diethylstilbestrol in utero. J Reprod Med 1983;28:851–6.
39. Stillman RJ, Miller LC. Diethylstilbestrol exposure in utero and endometriosis in infertile females. Fertil Steril 1984;41:369–72.
40. Henderson BE, Benton B, Cosgrove M, Baptista J, Aldrich J, Townsend D, Hart W, Mack TM. Urogenital tract abnormalities in sons of women treated with diethylstilbestrol. Pediatrics 1976;58:505–7.
41. Gill WB, Schumacher GFB, Bibbo M. Pathological semen and anatomical abnormalities of the genital tract in human male subjects exposed to diethylstilbestrol in utero. J Urol 1977;117:477–80.
42. Gill WB, Schumacher GFB, Bibbo M, Strous FH, Schoenberh HW. Association of diethylstilbestrol exposure in utero with cryptorchidism, testicular hypoplasia and semen abnormalities. J Urol 1979;122:36–9.
43. Gill WB, Schumacher GFB, Bibbo M. Structural and functional abnormalities in the sex organs of male offspring of mothers treated with diethylstilbestrol (DES). J Reprod Med 1976;16:147–53.
44. Driscoll SG, Taylor SM. Effects of prenatal maternal estrogen on the male urogenital system. Obstet Gynecol 1980;56:537–42.
45. Bibbo M, Gill WB, Azizi F, Blough R, Fang VS, Rosenfield RL, Schaumacher GFB, Sleeper K, Sonek MG, Wied GL. Follow-up study of male and female offspring of DES-exposed mothers. Obstet Gynecol 1977;49:1–8.
46. Shy KK, Stenchever MA, Karp LE, Berger RE, Williamson RA, Leonard J. Genital tract examinations and zona-free hamster egg penetration tests from men exposed in utero to diethylstilbestrol. Fertil Steril 1984;42:772–8.
47. Leary FJ, Resseguie LJ, Kurland LT, O'Brien PC, Emslander RF, Noller KL. Males exposed in utero to diethylstilbestrol. JAMA 1984;252:2984–9.
48. Conley GR, Sant GR, Ucci AA, Mitcheson HD. Seminoma and epididylmal cysts in a young man with known diethylstilbestrol exposure in utero. JAMA 1983;249:1325–6.
49. Yalom ID, Green R, Fisk N. Prenatal exposure to female hormones. Effect on psychosexual development in boys. Arch Gen Psychiatry 1973;28:554–61.
50. Burke L, Apfel RJ, Fischer S, Shaw J. Observations on the psychological impact of diethylstilbestrol exposure and suggestions on management. J Reprod Med 1980;24:99–102.

D

DIFLUNISAL

Nonsteroidal Anti-inflammatory

PREGNANCY RECOMMENDATION: Human Data Suggest Risk in 1st and 3rd Trimesters
BREASTFEEDING RECOMMENDATION: Limited Human Data—Probably Compatible

PREGNANCY SUMMARY

Constriction of the ductus arteriosus in utero is a pharmacologic consequence arising from the use of prostaglandin synthesis inhibitors during pregnancy (see also Indomethacin) (1). Persistent pulmonary hypertension of the newborn may occur if these agents are used in the 3rd trimester close to delivery (1,2). These drugs also have been shown to inhibit labor and prolong pregnancy, both in humans (3) (see also Indomethacin) and in animals (4). Women attempting to conceive should not use any prostaglandin synthesis inhibitor, including diflunisal, because of the findings in a variety of animal models that indicate these agents block blastocyst implantation (5,6). Moreover, nonsteroidal anti-inflammatory drugs (NSAIDs) have been associated with spontaneous abortions (SABs) and congenital malformations. The absolute risk for these defects, however, appears to be low.

FETAL RISK SUMMARY

Diflunisal is an NSAID used in the treatment of mild-to-moderate pain, osteoarthritis, and rheumatoid arthritis. The drug is teratogenic and embryotoxic in rabbits administered 40–60 mg/kg/day, the highest dose equivalent to 2 times the maximum human dose (7). Similar results were not observed in mice and rats treated with 45–100 mg/kg/day (7,8) or in monkeys treated with 80 mg/kg during organogenesis (9). No published reports describing the use of this drug in human pregnancy have been located.

In a surveillance study of Michigan Medicaid recipients involving 229,101 completed pregnancies conducted between 1985 and 1992, 258 newborns had been exposed to diflunisal during the 1st trimester (F. Rosa, personal communication, FDA, 1993). A total of 19 (7.4%) major birth defects were observed (10 expected). Specific data were available for six defect categories, including (observed/expected) 1/3 cardiovascular defects, 1/0.4 oral clefts, 0/0 spina bifida, 1/1 polydactyly, 0/0 limb reduction defects, and 1/1 hypospadias. It remains to be investigated whether an unusual frequency distribution of the other 15 defects is in the overall excess of birth defects.

A combined 2001 population-based, observational cohort study and a case–control study estimated the risk of adverse pregnancy outcome from the use of NSAIDs (10). The use of NSAIDs during pregnancy was not associated with congenital malformations, preterm delivery, or low birth weight, but a positive association was discovered with SABs. A similar study, also published in 2001, failed to find a relationship, in general, between NSAID and congenital malformations, but did find a significant association with cardiac defects and orofacial clefts (11). In addition, a 2003 study found a significant association between exposure to NSAIDs in early pregnancy and SABs (12). (See Ibuprofen for details on these three studies.)

A brief 2003 editorial on the potential for NSAID-induced developmental toxicity concluded that NSAIDs, and specifically those with cyclooxygenase 2 (COX-2) affinity, had a lower risk of this toxicity in humans than aspirin (13).

BREASTFEEDING SUMMARY

Diflunisal is excreted into human milk. Milk concentrations range from 2% to 7% of the levels in the mother's plasma (7). No reports describing the use of this agent during lactation have been located.

References

1. Levin DL. Effects of inhibition of prostaglandin synthesis on fetal development, oxygenation, and the fetal circulation. Semin Perinatol 1980;4:35–44.

2. Van Marter LJ, Leviton A, Allred EN, Pagano M, Sullivan KF, Cohen A, Epstein MF. Persistent pulmonary hypertension of the newborn and smoking and aspirin and nonsteroidal antiinflammatory drug consumption during pregnancy. Pediatrics 1996;97:658–63.
3. Fuchs F. Prevention of prematurity. Am J Obstet Gynecol 1976;126:809–20.
4. Powell JG, Cochrane RL. The effects of a number of non-steroidal anti-inflammatory compounds on parturition in the rat. Prostaglandins 1982;23:469–88.
5. Matt DW, Borzelleca JF. Toxic effects on the female reproductive system during pregnancy, parturition, and lactation. In: Witorsch RJ, ed. *Reproductive Toxicology*. 2nd ed. New York, NY: Raven Press, 1995:175–93.
6. Dawood MY. Nonsteroidal antiinflammatory drugs and reproduction. Am J Obstet Gynecol 1993;169:1255–65.
7. Product information. Dolobid. Merck Sharpe & Dohme, 1993.
8. Nakatsuka T, Fujii T. Comparative teratogenicity study of diflunisal (MK-647) and aspirin in the rat. Oyo Yakuri 1979;17:551–7. As cited in Shepard TH. *Catalog of Teratogenic Agents*. 6th ed. Baltimore, MD: Johns Hopkins University Press, 1989:222.
9. Rowland JM, Robertson RT, Cukierski M, Prahalada S, Tocco D, Hendrickx AG. Evaluation of the teratogenicity and pharmacokinetics of diflunisal in cynomolgus monkeys. Fund Appl Toxicol 1987;8:51–8. As cited in Shepard TH. *Catalog of Teratogenic Agents*. 6th ed. Baltimore, MD: Johns Hopkins University Press, 1989:222.
10. Nielsen GL, Sorensen HT, Larsen H, Pedersen L. Risk of adverse birth outcome and miscarriage in pregnant users of non-steroidal anti-inflammatory drugs: population based observational study and case-control study. Br Med J 2001;322:266–70.
11. Ericson A, Kallen BAJ. Nonsteroidal anti-inflammatory drugs in early pregnancy. Reprod Toxicol 2001;15:371–5.
12. Li DK, Liu L, Odouli R. Exposure to non-steroidal anti-inflammatory drugs during pregnancy and risk of miscarriage: population based cohort study. Br Med J 2003;327:368–71.
13. Tassinari MS, Cook JC, Hurtt ME. NSAIDs and developmental toxicity. Birth Defects Res (Part B) 2003;68:3–4.

DIGITALIS

Cardiac Glycoside

PREGNANCY RECOMMENDATION: Compatible
BREASTFEEDING RECOMMENDATION: Compatible

PREGNANCY SUMMARY

No reports linking digitalis or the various digitalis glycosides with congenital defects have been located. Animal studies have not shown a teratogenic effect (1).

FETAL RISK SUMMARY

Rapid passage to the fetus has been observed after administration of digoxin and digitoxin (2–9). One group of investigators found that the amount of digitoxin recovered from the fetus depended on the length of gestation (2). In the late 1st trimester, only 0.05%–0.10% of the injected dose was recovered from three fetuses. Digitoxin metabolites accounted for 0.18%–0.33%. At 34 weeks' gestation, digitoxin recovery was 0.85% and metabolite recovery was 3.49% from one fetus. Average cord concentrations of digoxin in three reports were 50%, 81%, and 83% of the maternal serum (3,4,9). The highest fetal concentrations of digoxin in the second half of pregnancy were found in the heart (5). The fetal heart has only a limited binding capacity for digoxin in the first half of pregnancy (5). In animals, amniotic fluid acts as a reservoir for digoxin, but no data are available in humans after prolonged treatment (5). The pharmacokinetics of digoxin in pregnant women have been reported (10,11).

Digoxin has been used for both maternal and fetal indications (e.g., congestive heart failure and supraventricular tachycardia) during all stages of gestation without causing fetal harm (12–25). Direct administration of digoxin to the fetus by periodic IM injections has been used to treat supraventricular tachycardia when indirect therapy via the mother failed to control the arrhythmia (26).

In a surveillance study of Michigan Medicaid recipients involving 229,101 completed pregnancies conducted between 1985 and 1992, 34 newborns had been exposed to digoxin during the 1st trimester (F. Rosa, personal communication, FDA, 1993). One (2.9%) major birth defect was observed (one expected), an oral cleft. Although the number of exposures is small, these data are supportive of previous experience for a lack of association between the drug and congenital defects.

Fetal toxicity resulting in neonatal death has been reported after maternal overdose (27). The mother, in her 8th month of pregnancy, took an estimated 8.9 mg of digitoxin as a single dose. Delivery occurred 4 days later. The baby demonstrated digitalis cardiac effects until death at age 3 days from prolonged intrauterine anoxia.

In a series of 22 multiparous patients maintained on digitalis, spontaneous labor occurred more than 1 week earlier than in 64 matched controls (28). The first stage of labor in the treated patients averaged 4.3 hours vs. 8 hours in the control group. In contrast, others found no effect on duration of pregnancy or labor in 122 patients with heart disease (29).

BREASTFEEDING SUMMARY

Digoxin is excreted into breast milk. Data for other cardiac glycosides have not been located. Digoxin milk:plasma ratios have varied from 0.6 to 0.9 (4,7,30,31). Although these amounts seem high, they represent very small amounts of digoxin due to significant maternal protein binding. No adverse effects in the nursing infant have been reported. The American Academy of Pediatrics classifies digoxin as compatible with breastfeeding (32).

References

1. Shepard TH. *Catalog of Teratogenic Agents*. 3rd ed. Baltimore, MD: Johns Hopkins University Press, 1980:116–7.

2. Okita GT, Plotz EF, Davis ME. Placental transfer of radioactive digitoxin in pregnant women and its fetal distribution. Circ Res 1956;4:376–80.
3. Rogers MC, Willserson JT, Goldblatt A, Smith TW. Serum digoxin concentrations in the human fetus, neonate and infant. N Engl J Med 1972;287:1010–3.
4. Chan V, Tse TF, Wong V. Transfer of digoxin across the placenta and into breast milk. Br J Obstet Gynaecol 1978;85:605–9.
5. Saarikoski S. Placental transfer and fetal uptake of ^{3}H-digoxin in humans. Br J Obstet Gynaecol 1976;83:879–84.
6. Allonen H, Kanto J, Lisalo E. The foeto-maternal distribution of digoxin in early human pregnancy. Acta Pharmacol Toxicol 1976;39:477–80.
7. Finley JP, Waxman MB, Wong PY, Lickrish GM. Digoxin excretion in human milk. J Pediatr 1979;94:339–40.
8. Soyka LF. Digoxin: placental transfer, effects on the fetus, and therapeutic use in the newborn. Clin Perinatol 1975;2:23–35.
9. Padeletti L, Porciani MC, Scimone G. Placental transfer of digoxin (beta-methyl-digoxin) in man. Int J Clin Pharmacol Biopharm 1979;17:82–3.
10. Marzo A, Lo Cicero G, Brina A, Zuliani G, Ghirardi P, Pardi G. Preliminary data on the pharmacokinetics of digoxin in pregnancy. Boll Soc Ital Biol Sper 1980;56:219–23.
11. Luxford AME, Kellaway GSM. Pharmacokinetics of digoxin in pregnancy. Eur J Clin Pharmacol 1983;25:117–21.
12. Lingman G, Ohrlander S, Ohlin P. Intrauterine digoxin treatment of fetal paroxysmal tachycardia: case report. Br J Obstet Gynaecol 1980;87:340–2.
13. Kerenyi TD, Gleicher N, Meller J, Brown E, Steinfeld L, Chitkara U, Raucher H. Transplacental cardioversion of intrauterine supraventricular tachycardia with digitalis. Lancet 1980;2:393–4.
14. Harrigan JT, Kangos JJ, Sikka A, Spisso KR, Natarajan N, Rosenfeld D, Leiman S, Korn D. Successful treatment of fetal congestive heart failure secondary to tachycardia. N Engl J Med 1981;304:1527–9.
15. Diro M, Beydoun SN, Jaramillo B, O'Sullivan MJ, Kieval J. Successful pregnancy in a woman with a left ventricular cardiac aneurysm: a case report. J Reprod Med 1983;28:559–63.
16. Heaton FC, Vaughan R. Intrauterine supraventricular tachycardia: cardioversion with maternal digoxin. Obstet Gynecol 1982;60:749–52.
17. Simpson PC, Trudinger BJ, Walker A, Baird PJ. The intrauterine treatment of fetal cardiac failure in a twin pregnancy with an acardiac, acephalic monster. Am J Obstet Gynecol 1983;147:842–4.
18. Spinnato JA, Shaver DC, Flinn GS, Sibai BM, Watson DL, Marin-Garcia J. Fetal supraventricular tachycardia: in utero therapy with digoxin and quinidine. Obstet Gynecol 1984;64:730–5.
19. Bortolotti U, Milano A, Mazzucco A, Valfre C, Russo R, Valente M, Schivazappa L, Thiene G, Gallucci V. Pregnancy in patients with a porcine valve bioprosthesis. Am J Cardiol 1982;50:1051–4.
20. Rotmensch HH, Rotmensch S, Elkayam U. Management of cardiac arrhythmias during pregnancy: current concepts. Drugs 1987;33:623–33.
21. Tamari I, Eldar M, Rabinowitz B, Neufeld HN. Medical treatment of cardiovascular disorders during pregnancy. Am Heart J 1982;104:1357–63.
22. Dumesic DA, Silverman NH, Tobias S, Golbus MS. Transplacental cardioversion of fetal supraventricular tachycardia with procainamide. N Engl J Med 1982;307:1128–31.
23. Gleicher N, Elkayam U. Cardiac problems in pregnancy. II. Fetal aspects: advances in intrauterine diagnosis and therapy. JAMA 1984;252:78–80.
24. Golichowski AM, Caldwell R, Hartsough A, Peleg D. Pharmacologic cardioversion of intrauterine supraventricular tachycardia. A case report. J Reprod Med 1985;30:139–44.
25. Reece EA, Romero R, Santulli T, Kleinman CS, Hobbins JC. In utero diagnosis and management of fetal tachypnea. A case report. J Reprod Med 1985;30:221–4.
26. Weiner CP, Thompson MIB. Direct treatment of fetal supraventricular tachycardia after failed transplacental therapy. Am J Obstet Gynecol 1988;158:570–3.
27. Sherman JL Jr, Locke RV. Transplacental neonatal digitalis intoxication. Am J Cardiol 1960;6:834–7.
28. Weaver JB, Pearson JF. Influence of digitalis on time of onset and duration of labour in women with cardiac disease. Br Med J 1973;3:519–20.
29. Ho PC, Chen TY, Wong V. The effect of maternal cardiac disease and digoxin administration on labour, fetal weight and maturity at birth. Aust NZ J Obstet Gynaecol 1980;20:24–7.
30. Levy M, Granit L, Laufer N. Excretion of drugs in human milk. N Engl J Med 1977;297:789.
31. Loughnan PM. Digoxin excretion in human breast milk. J Pediatr 1978;92:1019–20.
32. Committee on Drugs, American Academy of Pediatrics. The transfer of drugs and other chemicals into human milk. Pediatrics 2001;108:776–89.

DIGITOXIN

Cardiac Glycoside

See Digitalis.

DIGOXIN

Cardiac Glycoside

See Digitalis.

DIGOXIN IMMUNE FAB (OVINE)

Antidote

PREGNANCY RECOMMENDATION: Compatible—Maternal Benefit >> Embryo–Fetal Risk
BREASTFEEDING RECOMMENDATION: Compatible

PREGNANCY SUMMARY

Several reports have described the use of digoxin immune Fab (ovine) in pregnancy, but all involved patients who had preeclampsia. Although no fetal harm related to digoxin immune Fab (ovine) was observed, none of the cases involved exposure during organogenesis. Nevertheless, in cases of digoxin overdose, the maternal benefits of therapy should take priority over the embryo–fetus. Thus, if indicated, therapy with this product should not be withheld because of pregnancy (1).

D

FETAL RISK SUMMARY

Digoxin immune Fab (ovine) is given IV. It is indicated for the treatment of patients with life-threatening or potentially life-threatening digoxin toxicity or overdose. Digoxin immune Fab (ovine) binds digoxin, thereby preventing the cardiac agent from binding to cells. The Fab-digoxin complex is then excreted in the urine. The elimination half-life is approximately 15–20 hours. Reproduction studies in animals have not been conducted (2).

It is not known if digoxin immune Fab (ovine) can cross the human placenta to the embryo–fetus. The antibody fragments probably do not cross, at least early in pregnancy, because of their high molecular weight (about 46,000), but some antibodies are able to cross the placenta in the 3rd trimester (e.g., see Immune Globulin Intravenous).

A 1988 case report described the use of digoxin immune Fab (ovine) in a woman with severe preeclampsia (3). In five additional reports involving 56 women, 13 in the immediate postpartum period (4) and 44 in the 2nd and 3rd trimesters (5–8), the drug was used for the same indication. No drug-induced adverse effects were observed in the fetuses or newborns.

BREASTFEEDING SUMMARY

No reports describing the use of digoxin immune Fab (ovine) during lactation have been located. It is doubtful that clinically significant amounts are excreted into breast milk. Even if some excretion did occur, it would be digested in the nursing infant's stomach. Therefore, the risk to a nursing infant appears to be nil. In addition, the maternal benefits of therapy in cases of digoxin overdose should outweigh the unknown risk to a nursing infant.

References

1. Bailey B. Are there teratogenic risks associated with antidotes used in the acute management of poisoned pregnant women? Birth Defects Res (Part A) 2003;67:133–40.
2. Product information. Digifab. Savage Laboratories, 2008.
3. Goodlin RC. Antidigoxin antibodies in eclampsia. N Engl J Med 1988;318: 518–9.
4. Adair CD, Luper A, Rose JC, Russell G, Veille JC, Buckalew VM. The hemodynamic effects of intravenous digoxin-binding fab immunoglobulin in severe preeclampsia: a double-blind, randomized, clinical trial. J Perinatol 2009;29:284–9.
5. Adair CD, Buckalew V, Taylor K, Ernest JM, Frye AH, Evans C, Veille JC. Elevated endoxin-like factor complicating a multifetal second trimester pregnancy: treatment with digoxin-binding immunoglobulin. Am J Nephrol 1996;16:529–31.
6. Adair CD, Buckalew VM, Kipikasa J, Torres C, Stallings SP, Briery CM. Repeated dosing of digoxin-fragmented antibody in preterm preeclampsia. J Perinatol 2009;29:163–5.
7. Adair CD, Buckalew VM, Graves SW, Lam GK, Johnson DD, Saade G, Lewis DF, Robinson C, Danoff TM, Chauhan N, Hopoate-Sitake M, Porter KB, Humphrey RG, Trofatter KF, Amon E, Ward S, Johnson JA. Digoxin immune fab treatment for severe preeclampsia. Am J Perinatol 2010;27:655–62.
8. Lam GK, Hopoate-Sitake M, Adair CD, Buckalew VM, Johnson DD, Lewis DF, Robinson CJ, Saade GR, Graves SW. Digoxin antibody fragment, antigen binding (Fab), treatment of preeclampsia in women with endogenous digitalis-like factor: a secondary analysis of the DEEP trial. Am J Obstet Gynecol 2013;209:119.e1–6.

DIHYDROCODEINE

Narcotic Agonist Analgesic

PREGNANCY RECOMMENDATION: Human Data Suggest Risk in 3rd Trimester
BREASTFEEDING RECOMMENDATION: No Human Data—Probably Compatible

PREGNANCY SUMMARY

No reports linking the use of dihydrocodeine with congenital defects have been located. Usage in pregnancy is primarily confined to labor. Respiratory depression in the newborn has been reported to be less than that with meperidine, but depression is probably similar when equianalgesic doses are compared (1–4). If dihydrocodeine is used in pregnancy, health-care professionals are encouraged to call the toll-free number (800-670-6126) for information about patient enrollment in the Motherisk study.

BREASTFEEDING SUMMARY

No reports describing the use of dihydrocodeine bitartrate during lactation have been located. Because other opiates are excreted into milk (e.g., see Morphine) and the molecular weight (about 452) of dihydrocodeine bitartrate is low enough, the presence of the narcotic in milk should be expected. The long-term effects on neurobehavior and development in a nursing infant are unknown but warrant study.

References

1. Sliom CM. Analgesia during labour: a comparison between dihydrocodeine and pethidine. S Afr Med J 1970;44:317–9.
2. Ruch WA, Ruch RM. A preliminary report on dihydrocodeine-scopolamine in obstetrics. Am J Obstet Gynecol 1957;74:1125–7.
3. Myers JD. A preliminary clinical evaluation of dihydrocodeine bitartrate in normal parturition. Am J Obstet Gynecol 1958;75:1096–100.
4. Bonica JJ. *Principles and Practice of Obstetric Analgesia and Anaesthesia*. Philadelphia, PA: FA Davis, 1967:245.

DIHYDROERGOTAMINE

Sympatholytic (Antimigraine)

PREGNANCY RECOMMENDATION: Contraindicated
BREASTFEEDING RECOMMENDATION: Contraindicated

PREGNANCY SUMMARY

Dihydroergotamine is a potent semi-synthetic ergot alkaloid that has oxytocic and sympatholytic properties. The animal data suggest a risk of intrauterine growth restriction probably resulting from reduced uteroplacental blood flow and/or increased myometrial tone. Although there is no evidence that it is a teratogen, dihydroergotamine is contraindicated in pregnancy, especially near term. Inadvertent exposure early in gestation, however, does not appear to represent a major risk.

FETAL RISK SUMMARY

Dihydroergotamine is the hydrogenated derivative of ergotamine (see also Ergotamine). It is available only in formulations for injection and nasal spray because oral absorption is poor. Both preparations are indicated for the acute treatment of migraine headaches with or without aura. In addition, the injectable formulation is indicated for the acute treatment of cluster headaches. The mean bioavailability of the nasal spray is 32% relative to the injectable administration. Plasma protein binding is 93% and the elimination half-life is about 9 hours (1,2). Another source, however, states that elimination is biphasic with half-lives of about 1–2 hours and 22–32 hours, respectively (3).

The oxytocic properties of ergotamine have been known since the early 1900s, producing a prolonged and marked increase in uterine tone that may lead to fetal hypoxia (4). The pharmacologic properties of dihydroergotamine are different from ergotamine, as the former is a much more potent sympatholytic (4). In a 1952 study, the oxytocic and toxic effects of dihydroergotamine were demonstrated (5). Twenty women at term were given 1 mg of dihydroergotamine in 500 mL distilled water IV over a period of 2–4 hours to induce labor. Labor induction was successful in eight women (40%), but in six other women the outcomes were four stillborns, one neonatal death 1.25 hours after delivery, and one severely depressed infant that developed seizures 3 days after delivery (progressing satisfactorily at 3 months of age with no abnormal neurological signs). The investigators concluded that dihydroergotamine should not be used to induce labor (5).

Reproduction studies have been conducted in rats and rabbits. In rats, intranasal administration throughout the period of organogenesis at doses producing maternal plasma exposures (AUC) about 0.4–1.2 times the human exposure (AUC) from the maximum recommended daily dose of ≥4 mg (MRDD) resulted in decreased fetal body weights and/or skeletal ossification. Administration of the dose throughout pregnancy and lactation resulted in reduced body weights and impaired reproductive function in the offspring. The no-effect level for rat embryo–fetal toxicity was not established. In rabbits administered the nasal spray during organogenesis, maternal exposures at about 7 times the MRDD also resulted in delayed skeletal ossification. The no-effect dose for rabbit embryo–fetal toxicity was about 2.5 times the MRDD. The embryo–fetal toxic doses in both species did not cause maternal toxicity. The in utero growth restriction in the animal studies was thought to have resulted from reduced uteroplacental blood flow and/or increased myometrial tone (1,2).

A study in guinea pigs quantified the effect of dihydroergotamine on uteroplacental blood flow (6). Pregnant guinea pigs were given the drug (14 mcg/kg/day) from day 30 to 60 of pregnancy (*gestational length for guinea pigs is 64–68 days*). At term, placental blood flow was decreased by 51% and, fetal weight and fetal weight/placental weight ratio were significantly decreased compared with controls (6).

It is not known if dihydroergotamine crosses the human placenta. The molecular weight of the free base (about 584) and long elimination half-life suggest that the drug will cross the placenta, but the extensive protein binding will limit passage.

The Collaborative Perinatal Project monitored 50,282 mother–child pairs, 32 of whom were exposed to ergot derivatives (three to dihydroergotamine) other than ergotamine during the 1st trimester (7). Three malformed children were observed from this group, but the numbers are too small to draw any conclusion.

A brief 1993 report described a 31-year-old woman with depression, panic disorder, and migraine headaches who was exposed to a number of drugs in the first 6 weeks of pregnancy, including dihydroergotamine, citalopram, buspirone, thioridazine, and etilefrine (a sympathomimetic agent) (8). An elective abortion was performed at 12 weeks' gestation. A thorough macroscopic and microscopic examination of the male fetus revealed no evidence of malformation. A detailed neuropathological examination and chromosome analysis (46,XY karyotype) was normal (8).

BREASTFEEDING SUMMARY

No reports describing the use of dihydroergotamine during human lactation have been located. The molecular weight of the free base (about 584) and long elimination half-life (may be as long as 22 hours) suggest that the drug will be excreted into breast milk, but the high protein binding (about 93%) will limit this excretion. The closely related agent ergotamine is excreted into milk (see Ergotamine). An ergot product has been associated with symptoms of ergotism (vomiting, diarrhea, and convulsions) in nursing infants of mothers taking the agent for the treatment of migraine (see Ergotamine). Moreover, dihydroergotamine is a member of the same chemical family as bromocriptine, an agent that is used to suppress lactation. Although no specific information has been located relating to the effects of dihydroergotamine on lactation, ergot alkaloids may hinder lactation by inhibiting maternal pituitary prolactin secretion (9).

D

References

1. Product information. D.H.E. 45. Novartis Pharmaceuticals, 2001.
2. Product information. Migranal. Novartis Pharmaceuticals, 2001.
3. Parfitt K, ed. *Martindale. The Complete Drug Reference*. 32nd ed. London: Pharmaceutical Press, 1999:444–5.
4. Gill RC, Farrar JM. Experiences with di-hydro-ergotamine in the treatment of primary uterine inertia. J Obstet Gynaecol Br Emp 1951;58:79–91.
5. Altman SG, Waltman R, Lubin S, Reynolds SRM. Oxytocic and toxic actions of dihydroergotamine-45. Am J Obstet Gynecol 1952;64:101–9.
6. Hohmann M, Künzel W. Dihydroergotamine causes fetal growth restriction in guinea pigs. Arch Gynecol Obstet 1992;251:187–92.
7. Heinonen OP, Sloan D, Shapiro S. *Birth Defects and Drugs in Pregnancy*. Littleton, MA: Publishing Sciences Group, 1977:358–9.
8. Seifritz E, Holsboer-Trachsler E, Haberthur F, Hemmeter U, Poldinger W. Unrecognized pregnancy during citalopram treatment. Am J Psychiatry 1993;150:1428–9.
9. Vorherr H. Contraindications to breast-feeding. JAMA 1974;227:676.

DIHYDROTACHYSTEROL

Vitamin

PREGNANCY RECOMMENDATION: Compatible
BREASTFEEDING RECOMMENDATION: Compatible

PREGNANCY SUMMARY

Dihydrotachysterol is a synthetic analog of vitamin D. It is converted in the liver to 25-hydroxydihydrotachysterol, an active metabolite. See Vitamin D.

BREASTFEEDING SUMMARY

See Vitamin D.

DILTIAZEM

Calcium Channel Blocker

PREGNANCY RECOMMENDATION: Human Data Suggest Low Risk
BREASTFEEDING RECOMMENDATION: Limited Human Data—Probably Compatible

PREGNANCY SUMMARY

The animal reproductive data suggest high risk, but it is based on body weight comparison, not on BSA or AUC. The limited human pregnancy data suggest that the risk is low, if it exists at all.

FETAL RISK SUMMARY

Diltiazem is a calcium channel inhibitor used for the treatment of angina. Reproductive studies in mice, rats, and rabbits at doses ≤5–10 times (on a body weight basis) the daily recommended human dose found increased mortality in embryos and fetuses. These doses also produced abnormalities of the skeletal system. An increased incidence of stillbirths was observed in perinatal animal studies at ≥20 times the human dose (1). In fetal sheep, diltiazem, like ritodrine and magnesium sulfate, inhibited bladder contractions, resulting in residual urine (2).

A 34-year-old woman, in her 1st month of pregnancy, was treated with diltiazem, 60 mg 4 times/day, and isosorbide dinitrate, 20 mg 4 times/day, for symptomatic myocardial ischemia (3). Both medications were continued throughout the remainder of gestation. Normal twins were delivered by repeat cesarean section at 37 weeks' gestation. Both infants were alive and well at 6 months of age.

In a surveillance study of Michigan Medicaid recipients involving 229,101 completed pregnancies conducted between 1985 and 1992, 27 newborns had been exposed to diltiazem during the 1st trimester (F. Rosa, personal communication, FDA, 1993). Four (14.8%) major birth defects were observed (one expected), two of which were cardiovascular defects (0.3 expected). No anomalies were observed in five other categories of defects (oral clefts, spina bifida, polydactyly, limb reduction defects, and hypospadias) for which data were available. Although the number of exposures is small, the total number of defects and the number of cardiovascular defects are suggestive of an association, but other factors, including the mother's disease, concurrent drug use, and chance may be involved.

A prospective, multicenter cohort study of 78 women (81 outcomes; 3 sets of twins) who had 1st trimester exposure to calcium channel blockers, including 13% to diltiazem, was reported in 1996 (4). Compared with controls, no increase in the risk of major congenital malformations was found.

A 22-year-old woman with Eisenmenger syndrome that was managed with sildenafil 50 mg/day was diagnosed with an atrial septal defect that was closed surgically (5). Eight days after surgery, the patient reported 7 weeks of amenorrhea and a pregnancy test was positive. Sildenafil 150 mg/day and diltiazem 60 mg/day were started. Two weeks later sildenafil was discontinued because of its high cost and the dose of diltiazem was increased to 180 mg/day. Because of worsening pulmonary hypertension at 31 weeks, sildenafil 150 mg/day was restarted and diltiazem was discontinued. The fetal weight was estimated to be in the 15th percentile. At 32 weeks, L-arginine (a nitric oxide donor) 3 g/day was started. During the next 2 weeks, the estimated fetal weight increased to the 35th percentile. Because of superimposed preeclampsia, a cesarean section was performed at 36 weeks to deliver a 2.290-kg male infant with Apgar scores of 9 and 9. No additional information on the infant was provided (5).

Diltiazem has been used as a tocolytic agent (6). In a prospective randomized trial, 22 women treated with the agent were compared with 23 treated with nifedipine. No differences between the groups in outcomes or maternal effects were observed.

BREASTFEEDING SUMMARY

Diltiazem is excreted into human milk (7). A 40-year-old woman, 14 days postpartum, was unsuccessfully treated with diltiazem, 60 mg 4 times/day, for resistant premature ventricular contractions. Her infant was not allowed to breastfeed during the treatment period. Simultaneous serum and milk levels were drawn at several times on the 4th day of therapy. The peak level in milk was approximately 200 ng/mL, almost the same as the peak serum concentration. Milk and serum concentrations were nearly the same during the measurement interval, with changes in the concentrations closely paralleling each other. The data indicated that diltiazem freely diffuses into milk (7). In a separate case described earlier, a mother nursed twins for at least 6 months while being treated with diltiazem and isosorbide dinitrate (3). Milk concentrations were not determined, but both infants were alive and well at 6 months of age. The American Academy of Pediatrics classifies diltiazem as compatible with breastfeeding (8).

References

1. Product information. Cardizem. Hoechst Marion Roussel, 1997.
2. Kogan BA, Iwamoto HS. Lower urinary tract function in the sheep fetus: studies of autonomic control and pharmacologic responses of the fetal bladder. J Urol 1989;141:1019–24.
3. Lubbe WF. Use of diltiazem during pregnancy. NZ Med J 1987;100:121.
4. Magee LA, Schick B, Donnenfeld AE, Sage SR, Conover B, Cook L, McElhatton PR, Schmidt MA, Koren G. The safety of calcium channel blockers in human pregnancy: a prospective, multicenter cohort study. Am J Obstet Gynecol 1996;174:823–8.
5. Lacassie HJ, Germain AM, Valdes G, Fernandez MS, Allamand F, Lopez H. Management of Eisenmenger syndrome in pregnancy with sildenafil and L-arginine. Obstet Gynecol 2004;103:1118–20.
6. El-Sayed Y, Holbrook RH Jr. Diltiazem (D) for the maintenance tocolysis of preterm labor (PTL): a prospective randomized trial (abstract). Am J Obstet Gynecol 1996;174:468.
7. Okada M, Inoue H, Nakamura Y, Kishimoto M, Suzuki T. Excretion of diltiazem in human milk. N Engl J Med 1985;313:992–3.
8. Committee on Drugs, American Academy of Pediatrics. The transfer of drugs and other chemicals into human milk. Pediatrics 2001;108:776–89.

DIMENHYDRINATE

Antihistamine/Antiemetic

PREGNANCY RECOMMENDATION: Compatible
BREASTFEEDING RECOMMENDATION: No Human Data—Probably Compatible

PREGNANCY SUMMARY

In general, antihistamines are considered low risk in pregnancy. However, exposure near birth of premature infants has been associated with an increased risk of retrolental fibroplasia.

FETAL RISK SUMMARY

Dimenhydrinate is the chlorotheophylline salt of the antihistamine diphenhydramine. A prospective study in 1963 compared dimenhydrinate usage in three groups of patients: 266 with malformed infants and two groups of 266 each without malformed infants (1). No difference in usage of the drug was found between the three groups.

The Collaborative Perinatal Project monitored 50,282 mother–child pairs, 319 of whom had 1st trimester exposure to dimenhydrinate (2, pp. 367–370). For use anytime in pregnancy, 697 exposures were recorded (2, p. 440). In neither case was evidence found to suggest a relationship to large categories of major or minor malformations. Two possible associations with individual malformations were found: cardiovascular defects (five cases) and inguinal hernia (eight cases). Independent confirmation is required to determine the actual risk for these anomalies (2, p. 440).

A number of reports have described the oxytocic effect of IV dimenhydrinate (3–13). When used either alone or with oxytocin, most studies found a smoother, shorter labor. However, in one study of 30 patients who received a 100-mg dose during 3.5 minutes, some (at least two, but exact number not specified) also showed evidence of uterine hyperstimulation and fetal distress (e.g., bradycardia and loss of beat-to-beat variability) (13). Owing to these effects, dimenhydrinate should not be used for this purpose.

Dimenhydrinate has been used for the treatment of hyperemesis gravidarum (14). In 64 women presenting with the condition prior to 13 weeks' gestation, all were treated with dimenhydrinate followed by various other antiemetics. Three of the newborns had integumentary abnormalities consisting of one case of webbed toes with an extra finger, and two cases of skin tags (one preauricular and one sacral). The defects were not thought to be related to the drug therapy (14).

An association between exposure during the last 2 weeks of pregnancy to antihistamines in general and retrolental fibroplasia in premature infants has been reported. See Brompheniramine for details.

BREASTFEEDING SUMMARY

No reports describing the use of dimenhydrinate during lactation have been located. The molecular weight (about 470) is low enough that excretion into milk should be expected. For a closely related product, see Diphenhydramine.

References

1. Mellin GW, Katzenstein M. Meclozine and fetal abnormalities. Lancet 1963;1:222–3.
2. Heinonen OP, Slone D, Shapiro S. *Birth Defects and Drugs in Pregnancy*. Littleton, MA: Publishing Sciences Group, 1977.
3. Watt LO. Oxytocic effects of dimenhydrinate in obstetrics. Can Med Assoc J 1961;84:533–4.
4. Rotter CW, Whitaker JL, Yared J. The use of intravenous Dramamine to shorten the time of labor and potentiate analgesia. Am J Obstet Gynecol 1958:75:1101–4.
5. Scott RS, Wallace KH, Badley DN, Watson BH. Use of dimenhydrinate in labor. Am J Obstet Gynecol 1962;83:25–8.
6. Humphreys DW. Safe relief of pain during labor with dimenhydrinate. Clin Med (Winnetka) 1962;69:1165–8.
7. Cooper K. Failure of dimenhydrinate to shorten labor. Am J Obstet Gynecol 1963;86:1041–3.
8. Harkins JL, Van Praagh IG, Irwin NT. A clinical evaluation of intravenous dimenhydrinate in labor. Can Med Assoc J 1964;91:164–6.
9. Scott RS. The use of intravenous dimenhydrinate in labor. New Physician 1964;13:302–7.
10. Klieger JA, Massart JJ. Clinical and laboratory survey into the oxytocic effects of dimenhydrinate in labor. Am J Obstet Gynecol 1965;92:1–10.
11. Hay TB, Wood C. The effect of dimenhydrinate on uterine contractions. Aust NZ J Obstet Gynaecol 1967;1:81–9.
12. Shephard B, Cruz A, Spellacy W. The acute effects of Dramamine on uterine contractibility during labor. J Reprod Med 1976;16:27–8.
13. Hara GS, Carter RP, Krantz KE. Dramamine in labor: potential boon or a possible bomb? J Kans Med Soc 1980;81:134–6, 155.
14. Gross S, Librach C, Cecutti A. Maternal weight loss associated with hyperemesis gravidarum: a predictor of fetal outcome. Am J Obstet Gynecol 1989;160:906–9.

DIMERCAPROL

Antidote

PREGNANCY RECOMMENDATION: Compatible—Maternal Benefit >> Embryo–Fetal Risk
BREASTFEEDING RECOMMENDATION: Contraindicated

PREGNANCY SUMMARY

Although the limited animal data suggest low embryo–fetal risk, there are no reports of dimercaprol use during organogenesis in humans. This absence of data prevents an assessment of the human embryo risk. However, the maternal benefit, and indirect embryo–fetal benefit, appears to far outweigh the unknown embryo–fetal risk. Therefore, if indicated, dimercaprol should not be withheld because of pregnancy (1).

FETAL RISK SUMMARY

Dimercaprol is a chelating agent indicated in the treatment of arsenic, gold, and acute mercury poisoning, and for lead poisoning when used concomitantly with edetate calcium disodium. It is not very effective for chronic mercury poisoning. Dimercaprol is administered by IM injection. The mechanism of action involves dimercaprol sulfhydryl groups forming complexes with certain heavy metals, thereby preventing or reversing the metal from binding sulfhydryl-containing enzymes (2).

A 1998 review cited five studies that evaluated the reproductive toxicity of dimercaprol in animals (3). The antidote was given to pregnant mice in doses of 15–60 mg/kg/day for 4 days to protect against methylmercury-induced developmental toxicity. Similar single or multiple doses given to mice daily did not alleviate arsenate-induced fetal toxicity, but no dimercaprol-induced developmental toxicity was noted. In another study, SC dimercaprol (125 mg/kg/day) in mice on gestational days 9–12 resulted in embryotoxicity (growth restriction, increased mortality) and teratogenicity (digits with abnormal direction and situation, cleft palate, and cerebral hernia) (3). (*Note: the human IM dose, depending on the type of poisoning, varies from 2.5 mg/kg/day to 18 mg/kg/day with up to 13-day courses.*)

It is not known if dimercaprol can cross the human placenta. The low molecular weight (about 124) suggests that the drug does cross to the embryo–fetal compartment.

The first reported case of dimercaprol in a human pregnancy appeared in 1948 (4). An 18-year-old woman at about 26 weeks' gestation was given dimercaprol for arsenical encephalopathy. The woman had received several arsenic-containing injections for vaginal and perineal warts 10 days earlier. She was given a total dose of 5440 mg over 13 days. Labor was induced at about 36 weeks' gestation because of eclampsia, and she delivered a 5.5-lb male infant who required resuscitation but was otherwise healthy. Long-term follow-up of the infant was not reported (4).

A 1969 case report detailed the pregnancy outcome of a 17-year-old patient at 30 weeks' gestation who had ingested approximately 30 mL of arsenic trioxide containing 1.32% of total elemental arsenic (5). About 24 hours after ingestion, she was treated with 150 mg of IM dimercaprol but developed renal failure over the next 72 hours. Spontaneous labor occurred, and she delivered a 1.1-kg female infant with an Apgar score of 4 at 1 minute. A qualitative test for arsenic on the baby's plasma was negative. The infant died 11 hours later of respiratory distress syndrome. At autopsy, toxicologic analysis for arsenic (reported as arsenic trioxide per 100 g of wet tissue) revealed that the metal had crossed the placenta to the fetus with the following concentrations: 0.740 mg (liver), 0.150 mg (kidneys), and 0.0218 mg (brain). The arsenic levels in the infant were all significantly higher than those measured in adult autopsy material. The authors could locate only one other similar case of inorganic arsenic poisoning in pregnancy. In that case, published in 1928 in a French journal, both the mother and infant died. Arsenic levels for the infant were not reported, but the level in the maternal liver was 0.56 g/100 g, less than the level found in the current infant (5).

A 2002 report described the use of IV edetate and IM dimercaprol (dose not specified) in a woman at 30 weeks' gestation with a high blood lead concentration (5.2 μmol/L; goal ≤0.48 μmol/L) (6). Twenty-four hours after initiation of chelation therapy, her lead level was 2.3 μmol/L. Twelve hours later, labor was induced because of uterine hemorrhage and she gave birth to a 1.6-kg (75th percentile) female infant. Lead concentration in the cord blood was 7.6 μmol/L. The Apgar scores were 4 and 6 (presumably at 1 and 5 minutes, respectively). The newborn was flaccid with absent reflexes, no movement to noxious stimuli, and no gag reflex, but she did have spontaneous eye movement. Bilateral diaphragmatic palsy was confirmed by fluoroscopy. During her 7 months of hospitalization, the infant received multiple courses of chelation to treat the intrauterine lead intoxication. In spite of this therapy, she had right sensorineural deafness and neurodevelopment delay at discharge. Oral succimer was continued at home because the blood lead level was still elevated (0.95 μmol/L). The mother's lead source was identified as herbal tablets that had been prescribed for a gastrointestinal complaint. She had taken the tablets periodically over the past 9 years and throughout her pregnancy. Mercury also was present in some of the tablets. The lead intake during pregnancy was estimated to be 50 times the average weekly intake of Western populations (6). In a 2003 case report and review of severe lead poisoning in pregnancy, seven new cases and eight from the literature were identified (7). Ten of the women admitted to intentional ingestion of pica. Among the 15 cases, five underwent chelation while they were pregnant, four with edetate calcium disodium, including one who also received IM dimercaprol, and one who received succimer. No lead-induced congenital defects were noted in the infants, but all received chelation therapy in the neonatal period (7).

D

BREASTFEEDING SUMMARY

No reports describing the use of dimercaprol during human lactation have been located. The molecular weight (about 124) and the typical prolonged therapy (13 days) suggest that the antidote will be excreted into breast milk. The effect, if any, of this exposure on a nursing infant is unknown. Because the use of dimercaprol implies poisoning with arsenic, gold, mercury, or lead, these metals also will be excreted into milk and are toxic to a nursing infant. Therefore, breastfeeding is contraindicated in women receiving dimercaprol.

References

1. Bailey B. Are there teratogenic risks associated with antidotes used in the acute management of poisoned pregnant women? Birth Def Res A Clin Mol Teratol 2003;67:133–40.
2. Product information. BAL in oil. Akorn, 2004.
3. Domingo JL. Developmental toxicity of metal chelating agents. Reprod Toxicol 1998;12:499–510.
4. Kantor HI, Levin PM. Arsenical encephalopathy in pregnancy with recovery. Am J Obstet Gynecol 1948;56:370–4.
5. Lugo G, Cassady G, Palmisano P. Acute maternal arsenic intoxication with neonatal death. Am J Dis Child 1969;117:328–30.
6. Tait PA, Vora A, James S, Fitzgerald DJ, Pester BA. Severe congenital lead poisoning in a preterm infant due to a herbal remedy. Med J Aust 2002;177:193–5.
7. Shannon M. Severe lead poisoning in pregnancy. Ambul Pediatr 2003;3:37-9.

DIMETHINDENE

[Withdrawn from the market. See 9th edition.]

DIMETHOTHIAZINE

[Withdrawn from the market. See 9th edition.]

DINOPROSTONE

Endocrine/Metabolic Agent (Prostaglandin)

PREGNANCY RECOMMENDATION: First 28 Weeks of Pregnancy—Contraindicated Unless for Termination/ Evacuation of Pregnancy Near or At Term—Compatible
BREASTFEEDING RECOMMENDATION: No Human Data—Probably Compatible

D

PREGNANCY SUMMARY

No reports describing human pregnancy outcomes following use of dinoprostone in failed medical abortions have been located. In animals, prostaglandin E2 exposure has resulted in embryotoxicity and an increase in skeletal anomalies. Another prostaglandin analog, misoprostol, when used unsuccessfully in the 1st trimester as an abortifacient, has been associated with cranial nerve defects in the fetus. Use of dinoprostone for cervical ripening near term has not been associated with an excess of adverse outcomes for the infant.

FETAL RISK SUMMARY

Dinoprostone is a naturally occurring prostaglandin E2 that is available in vaginal suppository form and is used for induced abortion between 12 and 20 weeks' gestation, for evacuation of uterine contents in the case of missed abortion or intrauterine death up to 28 weeks' gestation, and in the management of benign hydatidiform mole. Dinoprostone is also available as a controlled-release vaginal insert and in gel form, and is used for cervical ripening in term or near-term pregnancies. Dinoprostone, when given as a vaginal suppository, functions to stimulate the myometrium of the uterus to contract. Dinoprostone has a short half-life of 2.5–5 minutes (1,2).

Reproductive studies have been conducted with prostaglandin E2 in rats and rabbits. In both species given the agent during organogenesis, embryotoxicity and fetal skeletal variations were observed (1,2).

No carcinogenicity or fertility studies have been conducted for dinoprostone. No evidence of mutagenicity was observed in the various assays (1,2).

It is not known if prostaglandin E2 crosses the placenta. The molecular weight (about 352) suggests that exogenous prostaglandin E2 will cross the placenta. However, the indicated uses for the drug and the very short elimination half-life (2.5–5 minutes) suggest that little drug may actually cross to the embryo–fetus (1,2).

No reports describing the outcomes of human pregnancies following the use of dinoprostone in failed medical abortions have been located. Although a failed attempted abortion would typically be followed by completion of the procedure by some other means, in rare cases a woman may wish to maintain the pregnancy. Isolated case reports suggest that the failed procedure(s) themselves may result in damage to the placenta and therefore damage to the fetus (3). First trimester exposure to another prostaglandin, misoprostol, in failed induced abortion, has been associated with an increased risk for 6th and 7th cranial nerve damage leading to Möbius' syndrome (see Misoprostol). However, in the case of dinoprostone, the most common use of the product would be after the first trimester.

BREASTFEEDING SUMMARY

No reports describing the use of dinoprostone during human lactation have been located. The molecular weight of dinoprostone (about 352) suggests that it will be excreted in breast milk. However, the local use of the product and the very short elimination half-life (2.5–5 minutes) suggest that clinically significant amounts will not be present in milk (1,2).

References

1. Product information. Cervidil. Forest Laboratories, 2011.
2. Product information. Prostin E2. Pfizer, 2006.
3. Arnon J, Ornoy A. Clinical teratology counseling and consultation case report: outcome of pregnancy after failure of early induced abortions. Teratology 1995;52:126–7.

DIOXYLINE

[Withdrawn from the market. See 8th edition.]

DIPHEMANIL

[Withdrawn from the market. See 9th edition.]

DIPHENADIONE

[Withdrawn from the market. See 9th edition.]

DIPHENHYDRAMINE

Antihistamine

PREGNANCY RECOMMENDATION: Compatible
BREASTFEEDING RECOMMENDATION: Limited Human Data—Probably Compatible

D

PREGNANCY SUMMARY

Both the animal data and the published human experience suggest that diphenhydramine is safe for use in human pregnancy. The exception is the case–control study discussed below that showed an association with cleft palate. In addition, premature infants exposed within 2 weeks of birth may be at risk for toxicity. At least one review has concluded that diphenhydramine is the drug of choice if parenteral antihistamines are indicated in pregnancy (1).

FETAL RISK SUMMARY

Diphenhydramine is a first-generation antihistamine agent. Reproductive studies with diphenhydramine in rats and rabbits at doses up to 5 times the human dose revealed no evidence of impaired fertility or fetal harm (2). Rapid placental transfer of diphenhydramine has been demonstrated in pregnant sheep with a fetal:maternal ratio of 0.85 (3). Peak fetal concentrations occurred within 5 minutes of a 100-mg IV dose.

The Collaborative Perinatal Project monitored 50,282 mother–child pairs, 595 of whom had 1st trimester exposure to diphenhydramine (4, pp. 323–337). For use anytime during pregnancy, 2948 exposures were recorded (4, p. 437). In neither case was evidence found to suggest a relationship to large categories of major or minor malformations. Several possible associations with individual malformations were found, but independent confirmation is required to determine the actual risk: genitourinary (other than hypospadias) (5 cases); hypospadias (3 cases); eye and ear defects (3 cases); syndromes (other than Down's syndrome) (3 cases); inguinal hernia (13 cases); clubfoot (5 cases); any ventricular septal defect (open or closing) (5 cases); and malformations of diaphragm (3 cases) (4, pp. 323–337, 437, 475).

Cleft palate and diphenhydramine usage in the 1st trimester were statistically associated in a 1974 case–control study (5). A group of 599 children with oral clefts was compared with 590 controls without clefts. In utero exposures to diphenhydramine in the groups were 20 and 6, respectively, a significant difference. However, in a 1971 report significantly fewer infants with malformations were exposed to antihistamines in the 1st trimester as compared with controls (6). Diphenhydramine was the second most commonly used antihistamine. In addition, a 1985 study reported 1st trimester use of diphenhydramine in 270 women from a total group of 6509 (7). No association between the use of the drug and congenital abnormalities was found.

In a surveillance study of Michigan Medicaid recipients involving 229,101 completed pregnancies conducted between 1985 and 1992, 1461 newborns had been exposed to diphenhydramine during the 1st trimester (F. Rosa, personal communication, FDA, 1993). A total of 80 (5.5%) major birth defects were observed (62 expected). Specific data were available for six defect categories, including (observed/expected) 14/14 cardiovascular defects, 3/2 oral clefts, 0/1 spina bifida, 9/4 polydactyly, 1/2 limb reduction defects, and 3/4 hypospadias. Possible associations with congenital defects are suggested for the total number of anomalies and for polydactyly, but other factors, including the mother's disease, concurrent drug use, and chance may be involved.

Diphenhydramine withdrawal was reported in a newborn infant whose mother had taken 150 mg/day during pregnancy (8). Generalized tremulousness and diarrhea began on the 5th day of life. Treatment with phenobarbital resulted in the gradual disappearance of the symptoms.

A stillborn, full-term, 1000-g female infant was exposed during gestation to high doses of diphenhydramine, theophylline, ephedrine, and phenobarbital, all used for maternal asthma (9). Except for a ventricular septal defect, no other macroscopic internal or external anomalies were observed. However, complete triploidy was found in lymphocyte cultures, which is unusual because very few such infants survive until term (9). No relationship between the chromosome abnormality or the congenital defect and the drug therapy can be inferred from this case.

A 1996 report described the use of diphenhydramine, droperidol, metoclopramide, and hydroxyzine in 80 women with hyperemesis gravidarum (10). The mean gestational age at the start of treatment was 10.9 weeks. The patients received 200 mg/day IV of diphenhydramine for 2–3 days and 12 (15%) required a second course of therapy when their symptoms recurred. Three of the mothers (all treated in the 2nd trimester) delivered offspring with congenital defects: Poland's syndrome, fetal alcohol syndrome, and hydrocephalus and hypoplasia of the right cerebral hemisphere. Only the latter anomaly is a potential drug effect, but the most likely cause was thought to be the result of an in utero fetal vascular accident or infection (10).

A 2001 study, using a treatment method similar to the above study, described the use of droperidol and diphenhydramine in 28 women hospitalized for hyperemesis gravidarum (11). Pregnancy outcomes in the study group were compared with a historical control of 54 women who had received conventional antiemetic therapy. Oral metoclopramide and hydroxyzine were used after discharge from the hospital. Therapy was started in the study and control groups at mean gestational ages of 9.9 and 11.1 weeks', respectively. The study group appeared to have more severe disease than controls as suggested by a greater mean loss from the prepregnancy weight, 2.07 vs. 0.81 kg (*ns.*), and a slightly lower serum potassium level, 3.4 vs. 3.5 mmol/L (*ns.*). Compared with controls, the droperidol group had a shorter duration of hospitalization (3.53 vs. 2.82 days, $p = 0.023$), fewer readmissions (38.9% vs. 14.3%, $p = 0.025$), and lower average daily nausea and vomiting scores (both $p < 0.001$). There were no statistical differences ($p > 0.05$) in outcomes (study vs. controls) in terms of spontaneous abortions ($N = 0$ vs. $N = 2$ [4.3%]), elective abortions ($N = 3$ [12.0%] vs. $N = 3$ [6.5%]), Apgar scores at 1, 5, and 10 minutes, age at birth (37.3 vs. 37.9 weeks'), and birth weight (3114 vs. 3347 g). In controls, there was one (2.4%) major malformation of unknown cause, an acardiac fetus in a set of triplets, and one newborn with a genetic defect (Turner's syndrome). There was also one unexplained major birth defect (4.4%) in the droperidol group (bilateral hydronephrosis), and two genetic defects (translocation of chromosomes 3 and 7; tyrosinemia) (11).

A potential drug interaction between diphenhydramine and temazepam resulting in the stillbirth of a term female infant has been reported (12). The mother had taken diphenhydramine 50 mg for mild itching of the skin and approximately 1.5 hours later, had taken 30 mg of temazepam for sleep. Three hours later she awoke with violent intrauterine fetal movements, which lasted several minutes and then abruptly stopped. The stillborn infant was delivered approximately 4 hours later. Autopsy revealed no gross or microscopic anomalies. In an experiment with pregnant rabbits, neither of the drugs alone caused fetal mortality, but when combined, 51 (81%) of 63 fetuses were stillborn or died shortly after birth (12). No definite mechanism could be established for the suggested interaction.

A 1980 report described the oxytocic properties of diphenhydramine when used in labor (13). Fifty women were given 50 mg IV over 3.5 minutes in a study designed to compare its effect with dimenhydrinate (see also Dimenhydrinate). The effects on the uterus were similar to those of dimenhydrinate but not as pronounced. Although no uterine hyperstimulation or fetal distress was observed, the drug should not be used for this purpose due to these potential complications (13).

Regular (every 1–2 minutes with intervening uterine relaxation), painful uterine contractions were observed in a 19-year-old woman at 26 week's gestation, following ingestion of about 35 capsules of diphenhydramine and an unknown amount of acetaminophen in a suicide attempt (14). The uterine contractions responded promptly to IV magnesium sulfate tocolysis and 5 hours later, after treatment with oral activated charcoal for the overdose, no further contractions were observed. The eventual outcome of the pregnancy was not mentioned.

An association between exposure during the last 2 weeks of pregnancy to antihistamines in general and retrolental fibroplasia in premature infants has been reported. See Brompheniramine for details.

BREASTFEEDING SUMMARY

Diphenhydramine is excreted into human breast milk, but levels have not been reported (15). Although the levels are not thought to be sufficiently high to affect the infant after therapeutic doses, the manufacturer considers the drug contraindicated in nursing mothers (2). The reason given for this is the increased sensitivity of newborn or premature infants to antihistamines.

References

1. Schatz M, Petitti D. Antihistamines and pregnancy. Ann Allergy Asthma Immunol 1997;78:157–9.
2. Product information. Benadryl. Parke-Davis, 1997.
3. Yoo GD, Axelson JE, Taylor SM, Rurak DW. Placental transfer of diphenhydramine in chronically instrumented pregnant sheep. J Pharm Sci 1986;75:685–7.
4. Heinonen OP, Sloan D, Shapiro S. *Birth Defects and Drugs in Pregnancy*. Littleton, MA: Publishing Sciences Group, 1977.
5. Saxen I. Cleft palate and maternal diphenhydramine intake. Lancet 1974;1:407–8.
6. Nelson MM, Forfar JO. Associations between drugs administered during pregnancy and congenital abnormalities of the fetus. Br Med J 1971;1:523–7.
7. Aselton P, Jick H, Milunsky A, Hunter JR, Stergachis A. First-trimester drug use and congenital disorders. Obstet Gynecol 1985;65:451–5.
8. Parkin DE. Probable Benadryl withdrawal manifestations in a newborn infant. J Pediatr 1974;85:580.
9. Halbrecht I, Komlos L, Shabtay F, Solomon M, Bock JA. Triploidy 69,XXX in a stillborn girl. Clin Genet 1973;4:210–2.
10. Nageotte MP, Briggs GG, Towers CV, Asrat T. Droperidol and diphenhydramine in the management of hyperemesis gravidarum. Am J Obstet Gynecol 1996;174:1801–6.
11. Turcotte V, Ferreira E, Duperron L. Utilité du dropéridol et de la diphenhydramine dans l'hyperemesis gravidarum. J Soc Obstet Gynaecol Can 2001;23:133–9.
12. Kargas GA, Kargas SA, Bruyere HJ Jr, Gilbert EF, Opitz JM. Perinatal mortality due to interaction of diphenhydramine and temazepam. N Engl J Med 1985;313:1417.
13. Hara GS, Carter RP, Krantz KE. Dramamine in labor: potential boon or a possible bomb? J Kans Med Soc 1980;81:134–6, 155.
14. Brost BC, Scardo JA, Newman RB. Diphenhydramine overdose during pregnancy: lessons from the past. Am J Obstet Gynecol 1996;175:1376–7.
15. O'Brien TE. Excretion of drugs in human milk. Am J Hosp Pharm 1974;31:844–54.

DIPHENOXYLATE

Antidiarrheal

PREGNANCY RECOMMENDATION: Limited Human Data—Animal Data Suggest Low Risk
BREASTFEEDING RECOMMENDATION: Limited Human Data—Potential Toxicity

PREGNANCY SUMMARY

Neither the animal data, although based on body weight, nor the limited human pregnancy data suggest that the combination of diphenoxylate and atropine causes developmental toxicity.

FETAL RISK SUMMARY

Diphenoxylate is a narcotic related to meperidine. It is available only in combination with atropine (to discourage overdosage) for the treatment of diarrhea. Diphenoxylate is rapidly metabolized to diphenoxylic acid (difenoxin), a biologically active metabolite (1).

Reproduction studies have been conducted in mice, rats, and rabbits with oral doses of 0.4–20 mg/kg/day (1). Because of the experimental design and small numbers of litters, embryotoxic, fetotoxic, and teratogenic effects could not be adequately assessed, but examination of the available fetuses did not reveal any evidence of teratogenicity (1).

No reports describing the placental transfer of diphenoxylate to the fetus have been located. The molecular weight of the active, major metabolite difenoxin (425 for the free base) is low enough that the presence of this agent in the fetus should be expected.

In one study, no malformed infants were observed after 1st trimester exposure in seven patients (2). A single case of a female infant born at 36 weeks' gestation with multiple defects, including Ebstein's anomaly, was described in a 1989 report (3). In addition to the cardiac defect, other abnormalities noted were hypertelorism, epicanthal folds, low-set posteriorly rotated ears, a cleft uvula, medially rotated hands, deafness, and blindness. The mother had taken Lomotil (diphenoxylate and atropine) for diarrhea during the 10th week of gestation. Since exposure was beyond the susceptible stages of development for these defects, the drug combination was not considered causative. A possible viremia in the mother as a cause of the diarrhea and the defects could not be excluded.

In a surveillance study of Michigan Medicaid recipients involving 229,101 completed pregnancies conducted between 1985 and 1992, 179 newborns had been exposed to diphenoxylate (presumably combined with atropine) during the 1st trimester (F. Rosa, personal communication, FDA, 1993). Nine (5.0%) major birth defects were observed (seven expected). Specific data were available for six defect categories, including (observed/expected) 3/2 cardiovascular defects, 0/0.3 oral clefts, 1/0 spina bifida, 1/0.5 polydactyly, 1/0.3 limb reduction defects, and 1/0.4 hypospadias. These data do not support an association between the drug and congenital defects.

D

BREASTFEEDING SUMMARY

The manufacturer reports that the active metabolite, diphenoxylic acid (difenoxin), is probably excreted into breast milk, and the effects of that drug and atropine may be evident in the nursing infant (1). One source recommends that the drug should not be used in lactating mothers (4). However, the American Academy of Pediatrics classifies atropine (diphenoxylate was not listed) as compatible with breastfeeding (5).

References

1. Product information. Lomotil. G.D. Searle and Company, 2000.
2. Heinonen OP, Slone D, Shapiro S. *Birth Defects and Drugs in Pregnancy*. Littleton, MA: Publishing Sciences Group, 1977:287.
3. Siebert JR, Barr M Jr, Jackson JC, Benjamin DR. Ebstein's anomaly and extracardiac defects. Am J Dis Child 1989;143:570–2.
4. Stewart JJ. Gastrointestinal drugs. In: Wilson JT, ed. *Drugs in Breast Milk*. Balgowlah, Australia: ADIS Press, 1981:71.
5. Committee on Drugs, American Academy of Pediatrics. The transfer of drugs and other chemicals into human milk. Pediatrics 2001;108:776–89.

DIPHTHERIA/TETANUS TOXOIDS (ADULT)

Toxoid

PREGNANCY RECOMMENDATION: Compatible—Maternal Benefit >> Embryo–Fetal Risk
BREASTFEEDING RECOMMENDATION: No Human Data—Probably Compatible

PREGNANCY SUMMARY

Diphtheria and tetanus produce severe morbidity in the mother with mortality rates of 10% and 30%, respectively (1). In neonates, the tetanus mortality rate is 60%. The risk to the fetus from diphtheria/tetanus toxoids (Td) is unknown, but there is no evidence of teratogenicity (1,2). The CDC and the American College of Obstetricians and Gynecologists (ACOG) recommend Td booster vaccination in pregnancy if ≥10 years have elapsed since a previous Td booster or if booster protection against diphtheria is needed (3,4). If tetanus or diphtheria protection is needed during pregnancy, the diphtheria and reduced tetanus toxoids/acellular pertussis vaccine (Tdap; see Vaccine, Pertussis [Acellular]), instead of Td, may be considered in the 2nd or 3rd trimesters, or earlier if protection is needed urgently. Tdap should only be given once during a lifetime.

FETAL RISK SUMMARY

Diphtheria/tetanus toxoids (Td) for adult use are the specific toxoids of *Corynebacterium diphtheriae* and *Clostridium tetani* adsorbed onto aluminum compounds. Reproduction studies in animals have not been conducted with this product (2).

In a 1999 study using the Hungarian Case-Control Surveillance of Congenital Abnormalities, 1980–1994, database, exposure to tetanus toxoid during pregnancy was examined in 21,563 women who had offspring with congenital defects (5). The control group consisted of 35,727 women who had infants without defects. Exposure to tetanus toxoid occurred in 25 (0.12%) case women (13 in the 1st trimester) compared with 33 (0.09%) control women (17 in the 1st trimester). The difference was not significant (5).

BREASTFEEDING SUMMARY

No reports describing the use of Td during human lactation have been located. The CDC and ACOG recommend Tdap in breastfeeding women who have not received the vaccine previously or 2 years or more have elapsed since the most recent Td administration (3,4).

References

1. Amstey MS. Vaccination in pregnancy. Clin Obstet Gynaecol 1983;10:13–22.

2. Product information. Tetanus and Diphtheria Toxoids Adsorbed (for adult use). Aventis Pasteur, 2001.
3. American College of Obstetricians and Gynecologists. Update on immunization and pregnancy: tetanus, diphtheria, and pertussis vaccination. *Committee Opinion*, Number 438, August 2009.
4. Advisory Committee on Immunization Practices (ACIP). Prevention of pertussis, tetanus, and diphtheria among pregnant and postpartum women and their infants. MMWR 2008;57(RR4):1–51. Available at http://www.cdc.gov/mmwr/PDF/rr/n5704.pdf. Accessed December 28, 2009.
5. Czeizel AE, Rockenbauer M. Tetanus toxoid and congenital abnormalities. Int J Gynecol Obstet 1999;64:253–8.

D

DIPHTHERIA/TETANUS TOXOIDS/ACELLULAR PERTUSSIS VACCINE ADSORBED

Vaccine/Toxoid

See Vaccine, Pertussis (Acellular)

DIPYRIDAMOLE

Hematological Agent (Antiplatelet)

PREGNANCY RECOMMENDATION: Limited Human Data—Animal Data Suggest Low Risk
BREASTFEEDING RECOMMENDATION: Limited Human Data—Probably Compatible

PREGNANCY SUMMARY

Neither the animal nor the limited human pregnancy data suggest that dipyridamole causes developmental toxicity.

FETAL RISK SUMMARY

Dipyridamole is a platelet inhibitor that is indicated as an adjunct to coumarin anticoagulants in the prevention of postoperative thromboembolic complications of cardiac valve replacement. The drug has a terminal elimination half-life of about 10 hours and is highly bound to plasma proteins (1).

Reproduction studies have been conducted in mice, rats, and rabbits at doses up to 1.3, 20, and 1.6 times the maximum recommended daily human dose based on BSA, respectively. No evidence of fetal harm was found in these studies (1).

No reports linking the use of dipyridamole with congenital defects have been located. The drug has been used in pregnancy (2–9). A single IV 30-mg dose of dipyridamole was shown to increase uterine perfusion in the 3rd trimester in 10 patients (10). In one pregnancy, a malformed infant was delivered, but the mother was also taking warfarin (2). The multiple defects in the infant were consistent with the fetal warfarin syndrome (see Coumarin Derivatives).

In a randomized, nonblinded study to prevent preeclampsia, 52 high-risk patients treated from the 13th week of gestation through delivery with daily doses of 300 mg of dipyridamole plus 150 mg of aspirin were compared with 50 high-risk controls (11). Four treated patients were excluded from analysis (spontaneous abortions before 16 weeks) vs. five controls (two lost to follow-up plus three spontaneous abortions). Hypertension occurred in 41 patients—19 treated and 22 controls. The outcome of pregnancy was significantly better in treated patients in three areas: preeclampsia (0 vs. 6), fetal and neonatal loss (0 vs. 5), and severe intrauterine growth restriction (0 vs. 4). No fetal malformations were observed in either group. Other reports and reviews have documented the benefits of this therapy, namely a reduction in the incidence of stillbirth, placental infarction, and intrauterine growth restriction (12–18).

BREASTFEEDING SUMMARY

Dipyridamole is excreted into breast milk (1). The effect of this exposure on a nursing infant is unknown.

References

1. Product information. Persantine. Boehringer Ingelheim Pharmaceuticals, 2004.
2. Tejani N. Anticoagulant therapy with cardiac valve prosthesis during pregnancy. Obstet Gynecol 1973;42:785–93.
3. Del Bosque MR. Dipiridamol and anticoagulants in the management of pregnant women with cardiac valvular prosthesis. Ginecol Obstet Mex 1973;33:191–8.
4. Littler WA, Bonnar J, Redman CWG, Beilin LJ, Lee GD. Reduced pulmonary arterial compliance in hypertensive patients. Lancet 1973;1:1274–8.
5. Biale Y, Lewenthal H, Gueron M, Beu-Aderath N. Caesarean section in patient with mitral-valve prosthesis. Lancet 1977;1:907.
6. Taguchi K. Pregnancy in patients with a prosthetic heart valve. Surg Gynecol Obstet 1977;145:206–8.
7. Ahmad R, Rajah SM, Mearns AJ, Deverall PB. Dipyridamole in successful management of pregnant women with prosthetic heart valve. Lancet 1976;2:1414–5.
8. Biale Y, Cantor A, Lewenthal H, Gueron M. The course of pregnancy in patients with artificial heart valves treated with dipyridamole. Int J Gynaecol Obstet 1980;18:128–32.
9. Salazar E, Zajarias A, Gutierrez N, Iturbe I. The problem of cardiac valve prostheses, anticoagulants, and pregnancy. Circulation 1984;70(Suppl 1):I169–77.

10. Lauchkner W, Schwarz R, Retzke U. Cardiovascular action of dipyridamole in advanced pregnancy. Zentralbl Gynaekol 1981;103:220–7.
11. Beaufils M, Uzan S, Donsimoni R, Colau JC. Prevention of pre-eclampsia by early antiplatelet therapy. Lancet 1985;1:840–2.
12. Beaufils M, Uzan S, Donsimoni R, Colau JC. Prospective controlled study of early antiplatelet therapy in prevention of preeclampsia. Adv Nephrol 1986;15:87–94.
13. Wallenburg HCS, Rotmans N. Prevention of recurrent idiopathic fetal growth retardation by low-dose aspirin and dipyridamole. Am J Obstet Gynecol 1987;157:1230–5.
14. Uzan S, Beaufils M, Bazin B, Danays T. Idiopathic recurrent fetal growth retardation and aspirin-dipyridamole therapy. Am J Obstet Gynecol 1989;160:763.
15. Wallenburg HCS, Rotmans N. Idiopathic recurrent fetal growth retardation and aspirin-dipyridamole therapy. Reply. Am J Obstet Gynecol 1989;160:763–4.
16. Wallenburg HCS, Rotmans N. Prophylactic low-dose aspirin and dipyridamole in pregnancy. Lancet 1988;1:939.
17. Capetta P, Airoldi ML, Tasca A, Bertulessi C, Rossi E, Polvani F. Prevention of pre-eclampsia and placental insufficiency. Lancet 1986;1:919.
18. Romero R, Lockwood C, Oyarzun E, Hobbins JC. Toxemia: new concepts in an old disease. Semin Perinatol 1988;12:302–23.

DIRITHROMYCIN

[Withdrawn from the market. See 9th edition.]

DISOPYRAMIDE

Antiarrhythmic

PREGNANCY RECOMMENDATION: Human Data Suggest Risk in 3rd Trimester
BREASTFEEDING RECOMMENDATION: Limited Human Data—Probably Compatible

PREGNANCY SUMMARY

No reports linking the use of disopyramide with congenital defects in humans or animals have been located. The drug is indicated for the treatment of cardiac arrhythmias. There is evidence that disopyramide has oxytocic effects.

FETAL RISK SUMMARY

Reproduction studies of disopyramide have been conducted in rats and rabbits. Maternal toxicity (decreased food consumption and weight gain), embryotoxicity (decreased number of implantation sites), and fetotoxicity (decreased growth and pup survival) were observed in pregnant rats dosed at ≥20 times the recommended human dose of 12 mg/kg/day, assuming a patient weighing at least 50 kg (RHD) (1). Increased resorption rates occurred in rabbits dosed at doses ≥5 times the RHD, but implantation rates, fetal growth, and offspring survival were not evaluated.

At term, a cord blood level of 0.9 mcg/mL (39% of maternal serum) was measured 6 hours after a maternal 200-mg dose (2). A 27-year-old woman took disopyramide throughout a full-term gestation, 1350 mg/day for the last 16 days, and delivered a healthy, 2920-g female infant (2). Concentrations of disopyramide and the metabolite *N*-monodesalkyl disopyramide in the cord and maternal serum were 0.7 and 0.9 mcg/mL, and 2.7 and 2.1 mcg/mL, respectively. The cord:maternal ratios for the parent drug and metabolite were 0.26 and 0.43, respectively (3). In a separate study, the mean fetal:maternal total plasma ratio was 0.78 when the mother's plasma concentration was within the therapeutic range of 2.0–5.0 mcg/mL (4).

Disopyramide has been used throughout other pregnancies without evidence of congenital abnormalities or growth restriction (2,5,6) (M.S. Anderson, personal communication, G.D. Searle and Company, 1981). Early onset of labor has been reported in one patient (7). The mother, in her 32nd week of gestation, was given 300 mg orally, followed by 100 or 150 mg every 6 hours for posterior mitral leaflet prolapse. Uterine contractions, without vaginal bleeding or cervical changes, and abdominal pain occurred 1–2 hours after each dose. When disopyramide was stopped, symptoms subsided over the next 4 hours. Oxytocin induction 1 week later resulted in the delivery of a healthy infant.

The oxytocic effect of disopyramide was studied in 10 women at term (8). Eight of the 10 women, treated with 150 mg every 6 hours for 48 hours, delivered within 48 hours, compared with none in a placebo group. In one patient, use of 200 mg twice daily during the 18th and 19th weeks of pregnancy was not associated with uterine contractions or other observable adverse effects in the mother or fetus (9). Most reviews of antiarrhythmic drug therapy consider the drug probably safe during pregnancy (5,10), but one does not recommend it for routine therapy (11), and one warns of its oxytocic effects (12).

BREASTFEEDING SUMMARY

Disopyramide is excreted into breast milk (3,6,13,14). In a woman taking 200 mg 3 times daily, samples obtained on the 5th–8th days of treatment revealed a mean milk:plasma ratio of 0.9 for disopyramide and 5.6 for the active metabolite (13). Neither drug was detected in the infant's plasma. In a second case, a mother was taking 450 mg of disopyramide every 8 hours 2 weeks postpartum (3). Milk and serum samples were obtained at 0, 2, 4, and 8 hours after the dose following an overnight fast. Milk concentrations of disopyramide and its metabolite, *N*-monodesalkyl disopyramide, ranged from 2.6 to 4.4 mcg/mL and from 9.6 to 12.3 mcg/mL, respectively. In both cases, the lowest levels occurred at the 8-hour sampling time. The mean milk:plasma ratios for the two were 1.06 and 6.24, respectively. Disopyramide was not detected in the infant's serum (test sensitivity 0.45 mcg/mL), but both disopyramide and the metabolite were found in the infant's urine, 3.3 and 3.7 mcg/mL, respectively. A brief 1985 report described a woman taking 100 mg five times a day throughout pregnancy who delivered a normal female infant (6). On the 2nd postpartum day and 2 hours after a dose, paired milk and serum sample were obtained. The concentrations of disopyramide in the aqueous phase of the milk and the serum were 4.0 and 10.3 μmol/L, respectively, a milk:serum ratio of 0.4. The same ratio was obtained 2 weeks later with samples drawn 3 hours after a dose and levels of 5.0 and 11.5 μmol/L, respectively. No disopyramide was found in the infant's serum (limit of test accuracy 1.5 μmol/L) during the second sampling. A woman taking 200 mg twice daily had milk and serum samples drawn before and 3.5 hours after a dose (14). The concentrations in the serum were 3.7 and 5.5 μmol/L, and those in the milk were 1.7 and 2.9 μmol/L, respectively. The milk:serum ratios were 0.46 before and 0.53 after the dose. No adverse effects were noted in the nursing infants in any of the above cases. The American Academy of Pediatrics classifies disopyramide as compatible with breastfeeding (15).

References

1. Product information. Norpace. G. D. Searle and Company, 2000.
2. Shaxted EJ, Milton PJ. Disopyramide in pregnancy: a case report. Curr Med Res Opin 1979;6:70–2.
3. Ellsworth AJ, Horn JR, Raisys VA, Miyagawa LA, Bell JL. Disopyramide and N-monodesalkyl disopyramide in serum and breast milk. Drug Intell Clin Pharm 1989;23:56–7.
4. Echizen H, Nakura M, Saotome T, Minoura S, Ishizaki T. Plasma protein binding of disopyramide in pregnant and postpartum women, and in neonates and their mothers. Br J Clin Pharmacol 1990;29:423–30.
5. Rotmensch HH, Elkayam U, Frishman W. Antiarrhythmic drug therapy during pregnancy. Ann Intern Med 1983;98:487–97.
6. MacKintosh D, Buchanan N. Excretion of disopyramide in human breast milk. Br J Clin Pharmacol 1985;19:856–7.
7. Leonard RF, Braun TE, Levy AM. Initiation of uterine contractions by disopyramide during pregnancy. N Engl J Med 1978;299:84–5.
8. Tadmor OP, Keren A, Rosenak D, Gal M, Shaia M, Hornstein E, Yaffe H, Graff E, Stern S, Diamant YZ. The effect of disopyramide on uterine contractions during pregnancy. Am J Obstet Gynecol 1990;162:482–6.
9. Stokes IM, Evans J, Stone M. Myocardial infarction and cardiac arrest in the second trimester followed by assisted vaginal delivery under epidural analgesia at 38 weeks gestation. Case report. Br J Obstet Gynaecol 1984;91:197–8.
10. Tamari I, Eldar M, Rabinowitz B, Neufeld HN. Medical treatment of cardiovascular disorders during pregnancy. Am Heart J 1982;104:1357–63.
11. Rotmensch HH, Rotmensch S, Elkayam U. Management of cardiac arrhythmias during pregnancy: current concepts. Drugs 1987;33:623–33.
12. Ward RM. Maternal drug therapy for fetal disorders. Semin Perinatol 1992;16:12–20.
13. Barnett DB, Hudson SA, McBurney A. Disopyramide and its N-monodesalkyl metabolite in breast milk. Br J Clin Pharmacol 1982;14:310–2.
14. Hoppu K, Neuvonen PJ, Korte T. Disopyramide and breast feeding. Br J Clin Pharmacol 1986;21:553.
15. Committee on Drugs, American Academy of Pediatrics. The transfer of drugs and other chemicals into human milk. Pediatrics 2001;108:776–89.

DISULFIRAM

Antialcoholic Agent

PREGNANCY RECOMMENDATION: Limited Human Data—No Relevant Animal Data
BREASTFEEDING RECOMMENDATION: No Human Data—Potential Toxicity

PREGNANCY SUMMARY

The lack of teratogenicity in animals and the absence of a clustering of similar birth defects in human pregnancies exposed to disulfiram suggest that this drug is not a major human teratogen. Obviously, women taking disulfiram should not drink alcohol, but this is occasionally the case because of the findings of fetal alcohol syndrome and defects that are suggestive of fetal alcohol exposure.

FETAL RISK SUMMARY

Disulfiram is used to prevent alcohol consumption in patients with a history of alcohol abuse. In animals, disulfiram is embryotoxic, possibly due to copper chelation, but it is not teratogenic (1).

No reports describing the placental transfer of disulfiram have been located. The molecular weight (about 297) is low enough that transfer to the fetus probably occurs.

Published reports describing the use of disulfiram in gestation involve 36 pregnancies (2–9). Eleven of the 38 exposed fetuses (two sets of twins) had congenital defects, 6 pregnancies were terminated electively, a spontaneous abortion occurred in 1 case, 1 was stillborn, 5 were lost to follow-up, and 14 newborns were normal. No congenital malformations were observed in autopsies conducted on three of the elective terminations (4). The malformations observed, some of which were or may have been related to alcohol exposure or other causes, were as follows:

- Clubfoot (two cases) (2)
- Multiple anomalies with VACTERL syndrome (radial aplasia, vertebral fusion, tracheoesophageal fistula) (twin) (3)
- Phocomelia of lower extremities (one case) (3)
- Microcephaly, mental retardation (possible fetal alcohol syndrome) (one case) (5)
- Pierre–Robin sequence, pulmonary atresia (one case) (6)
- Cleft soft palate, short palpebral fissure (twin) (8)

Limb reduction right forearm (radius and ulna), 2 rudimentary fingers without nails, short palpebral fissure (twin) (8)
Fetal alcohol syndrome (two cases; both mothers continued to drink) (9)
Fetal hydantoin syndrome (mother also took phenytoin) (one case) (9)

In a surveillance study of Michigan Medicaid recipients involving 229,101 completed pregnancies conducted between 1985 and 1992, 25 newborns had been exposed to disulfiram during the 1st trimester (F. Rosa, personal communication, FDA, 1993). One (4.0%) major birth defect was observed (one expected), a cardiovascular defect.

BREASTFEEDING SUMMARY

No reports describing the use of disulfiram during lactation have been located. Because of the relatively low molecular weight (about 297), excretion into milk should be expected. The potential effect of this exposure on a nursing infant is unknown.

References

1. Shepard TH. *Catalog of Teratogenic Agents*. 6th ed. Baltimore, MD: Johns Hopkins University Press, 1989:239–40.
2. Favre-Tissot M, Delatour P. Psychopharmacologie et teratogenese a propos du sulfirame: essal experimental. Annales Medico-psychogiques 1965;1:735–40. As cited in Shepard TH. *Catalog of Teratogenic Agents*. 6th ed. Baltimore, MD: Johns Hopkins University Press, 1989:239–40.
3. Nora AH, Nora JJ, Blu J. Limb-reduction anomalies in infants born to disulfiram-treated alcoholic mothers. Lancet 1977;2:664.
4. Hamon B, Soyez C, Jonville AP, Autret E. Grossesse chez les malades traitées par le disulfirame. Press Med 1991;20:1092.
5. Gardner RJM, Clarkson JE. A malformed child whose previously alcoholic mother had taken disultiram. NZ Med J 1981;93:184–6. As cited in Reitnauer PJ, Callanan NP, Farber RA, Aylsworth AS. Prenatal exposure to disulfiram implicated in the cause of malformations in discordant monozygotic twins. Teratology 1997;56:358–62.
6. Dehaene P, Titran M, Dubois D. Syndrome de Pierre Robin et malformations cardiaques chez un nouveau-ne. Presse Med 1984;13:1394–5. As cited in Reitnauer PJ, Callanan NP, Farber RA, Aylsworth AS. Prenatal exposure to disulfiram implicated in the cause of malformations in discordant monozygotic twins. Teratology 1997;56:358–62.
7. Helmbrecht GD, Hoskins IA. First trimester disulfiram exposure: report of two cases. Am J Perinatol 1993;10:5–7.
8. Reitnauer PJ, Callanan NP, Farber RA, Aylsworth AS. Prenatal exposure to disulfiram implicated in the cause of malformations in discordant monozygotic twins. Teratology 1997;56:358–62.
9. Johnson KA, Jones KL, Chambers CC, Hames C, Emery M. The effect of disulfiram on the unborn baby (abstract). Teratology 1991;43:438.

DOBUTAMINE

Sympathomimetic (Adrenergic)

PREGNANCY RECOMMENDATION: Limited Human Data—Animal Data Suggest Low Risk
BREASTFEEDING RECOMMENDATION: No Human Data—Probably Compatible

PREGNANCY SUMMARY

Although the animal data suggest low risk, the limited human pregnancy experience prevents an assessment of the embryo–fetal risk.

FETAL RISK SUMMARY

Dobutamine, an inotropic agent, is structurally related to dopamine. Reproduction studies in rats (at doses up to the normal human dose of 10 mcg/kg/min for 24 hours for a total daily dose of 14.4 mg/kg [NHD]) and rabbits (at doses up to 2 times the NHD) did not reveal any evidence of fetal harm (1).

No reports describing the placental transfer of dobutamine or studying its effects during human pregnancy have been located (see also Dopamine). The relatively low molecular weight (about 301) suggests that exposure of the embryo and fetus probably occurs. Short-term use in one patient with a myocardial infarction at 18 weeks' gestation was not associated with any known fetal adverse effects (2).

In a 1996 abstract, eight women with severe preeclampsia who required pulmonary artery catheter monitoring were given an IV infusion of dobutamine (3). The drug was effective in improving oxygen delivery in patients with depressed left ventricular function. No mention was made of fetal effects.

A 2009 report described a pregnant woman with dilated cardiomyopathy who was treated with dobutamine starting at 22 weeks' (4). She underwent a cesarean section at 28 weeks' and the 830-g infant was in stable condition.

BREASTFEEDING SUMMARY

No reports describing the use of dobutamine during human lactation have been located. The relatively low molecular weight (about 301) suggests that the drug will be excreted into breast milk. The effect of this exposure on a nursing infant is unknown.

References

1. Product information. Dobutrex. Eli Lilly and Company, 2000.
2. Stokes IM, Evans J, Stone M. Myocardial infarction and cardiac arrest in the second trimester followed by assisted vaginal delivery under epidural analgesia at 38 weeks' gestation. Case report. Br J Obstet Gynaecol 1984;91:197–8.
3. Graves C, Wheeler T, Troiano N. The effect of dobutamine hydrochloride on ventricular function and oxygen transport in patients with severe preeclampsia (abstract). Am J Obstet Gynecol 1996;174:332.
4. Cho FN. Management of pregnant women with cardiac diseases at potential risk of thromboembolism—experience and review. Int J Cardiol 2009;136:229–32.

DOCETAXEL

Antineoplastic

PREGNANCY RECOMMENDATION: Limited Human Data—Animal Data Suggest Risk
BREASTFEEDING RECOMMENDATION: Contraindicated

PREGNANCY SUMMARY

Docetaxel, always in combination with other antineoplastics, has been reported in eight pregnancies, two of which involved the 1st trimester but only one during organogenesis. Both of the 1st trimester exposures had normal infant outcomes. Mild hydrocephalus, which resolved spontaneously, was observed in one fetus exposed in the 2nd and 3rd trimesters; the cause is unknown. In another case, multiple anomalies were identified before chemotherapy was started and the infant died shortly after birth. The animal reproduction data suggest risk at doses that were a small fraction of the human dose, but maternal toxicity also was evident. Based on the very limited human pregnancy experience, docetaxel, if indicated, should not be withheld because of pregnancy, but avoiding organogenesis should be considered.

FETAL RISK SUMMARY

Docetaxel is an antineoplastic with antimitotic activity. It is in the same antineoplastic subgroup of taxoids as cabazitaxel and paclitaxel. Docetaxel is indicated either alone or in combination with other antineoplastics for the treatment of breast cancer, non-small-cell lung cancer, prostate cancer, gastric adenocarcinoma, and head and neck cancer. Plasma protein binding of the highly lipophilic drug is about 94%, mainly to α_1-acid glycoprotein, albumin, and lipoproteins. The terminal half-life is 11.1 hours (1).

Reproduction studies have been conducted in rats and rabbits. In these species, doses given during organogenesis, which were 1/50 and 1/300 the daily maximum recommended human dose based on BSA, were embryotoxic and fetotoxic, manifested as intrauterine death, increased resorption, reduced fetal weight, and fetal ossification delay. These doses also caused maternal toxicity (1).

Long-term studies for carcinogenic potential have not been conducted. The drug was clastogenic in several tests but did not induce mutagenicity in assays. No impairment of fertility was noted in rats, but decreased testicular weights did occur. In a 10-cycle toxicity study (dosing once every 21 days for 6 months) in rats and dogs, testicular atrophy or degeneration was observed (1).

It is not known if docetaxel crosses the human placenta. The molecular weight (about 862), highly lipophilic nature, and the long terminal half-life suggest that the drug will cross to the embryo–fetus. However, the plasma protein binding might limit the transfer.

The first case of docetaxel use in pregnancy was reported in 2000 (2). A 34-year-old woman presented at 15 weeks' gestation with recurrent breast cancer. Approximately 1 year before presentation, she had undergone a modified radical mastectomy followed by chemotherapy for treatment of breast cancer. Chemotherapy at that time had been epirubicin, cyclophosphamide, fluorouracil, and methotrexate. At 19 weeks', vinorelbine was given, but, because of rapid disease progress, that agent was discontinued and docetaxel was given every 3 weeks for 3 cycles. A planned cesarean section was performed at 32 weeks' that delivered a normal, 1620-g female infant with Apgar scores of 8 and 9 presumably at 1 and 5 minutes, respectively. The infant did well and her psychophysical development was normal at 20 months of age.

In a 2006 report, a 35-year-old woman at 13 weeks' gestation with breast cancer was treated with four 21-day cycles of fluorouracil, doxorubicin, and cyclophosphamide (3). No response was noted and at 25 weeks' her therapy was changed to 21-day cycles of docetaxel. She gave birth at 39 weeks to a healthy, 3.09-kg, length 51-cm male infant with normal Apgar scores and blood counts (3). No other information on the infant was provided.

A second 2006 report described two cases of docetaxel exposure in pregnancy (4). In the first case, a 29-year-old woman at 12 weeks' gestation was diagnosed with breast cancer. Treatment with doxorubicin and cyclophosphamide every 2 weeks for four cycles was started at 14 weeks'. At 17 weeks', a fetal ultrasound revealed hydrocephalus (dilated lateral and third ventricle). A modified radical mastectomy and axillary node dissection was conducted at 24 weeks', followed by docetaxel every 2 weeks between 26 and 32 weeks' gestation for four cycles. At 34 weeks', she gave birth to an infant with mild hydrocephalus that regressed spontaneously over several months. The child's development at 28 months was normal (no other details of the infant were provided). The second case involved a 38-year-old woman who was diagnosed with breast cancer at 10 weeks' gestation. At 14 weeks', docetaxel and doxorubicin every 3 weeks for six cycles was started. She developed preeclampsia and a cesarean section was conducted at 35 weeks' to deliver a healthy infant with no detectable malformations. The infant was developing normally at 9 months of age (no additional details were provided) (4).

A brief case report described a 44-year-old woman with advanced-stage breast cancer (5). She was treated with fluorouracil, epirubicin, and cyclophosphamide before undergoing a mastectomy before she became pregnant. During pregnancy, she was treated with five weekly doses of docetaxel because of symptomatic bone metastases starting at about 35 weeks' gestation. She gave birth at 40 weeks to a normal male infant who was doing well and developing normally at 15 months of age (5).

A 2007 case report described a 28-year-old woman with a history of radical mastectomy, chemotherapy, and radiotherapy 1 year before pregnancy (6). Because of metastases, she was treated with docetaxel and trastuzumab at 23 and 26 weeks' gestation, trastuzumab alone at 27 weeks', and docetaxel alone at 30 weeks'. Trastuzumab was omitted at 30 weeks' because an ultrasound revealed anhydramnios and fetal growth at the fifth percentile. The anhydramnios was thought to be due to trastuzumab. At 33 weeks', oligohydramnios was noted. An elective cesarean section was conducted at 36 weeks' to deliver a 2.23-kg male infant with Apgar scores of 7 and 9 at 1 and 5 minutes, respectively. No evidence of positional deformations or respiratory abnormalities from the prolonged low amniotic fluid was noted and the neonatal urine output was normal. The development of the infant also was normal (6).

A 35-year-old woman with metastatic non-small-cell lung cancer was treated in the 1st and 2nd trimesters with chemotherapy of an unknown pregnancy (7). After undergoing a craniotomy to remove the metastatic tumor and whole brain irradiation early in pregnancy, she was treated with docetaxel and cisplatin on days 1 and 8 every 21 days for four cycles (gestational weeks 9–18). Because of lack of response, treatment was changed to two cycles of gemcitabine and cisplatin (gestational weeks 19 and 22). About 2 months after the last dose her pregnancy was diagnosed. At 33 weeks', a cesarean section delivered a normal 1490-g female infant (normal karyotype 46,XX) with Apgar scores of 8, 9, and 10 at 1, 5, and 10 minutes, respectively, and normal blood counts. An extensive examination of the infant failed to find any abnormalities. The infant was developing normally at 10 months of age (7).

A 32-year-old woman underwent surgery at 20 weeks' gestation (from in vitro fertilization) for a ruptured ovarian cyst (8). Ovarian cancer was diagnosed and she was given four cycles of docetaxel and cisplatin before a cesarean section at 34 weeks. The 2245-g female infant had Apgar scores of 3 and 6 at 1 and 10 minutes, respectively. The infant died at 5 days of age from multiple congenital anomalies that had been diagnosed before starting chemotherapy (8).

BREASTFEEDING SUMMARY

No reports describing the use of docetaxel during human lactation have been reported. The molecular weight (about 862), highly lipophilic nature, and the long terminal half-life (11.1 hours) suggest that the drug will be excreted into breast milk, although the plasma protein binding (about 94%) might limit the excretion. The effect of this exposure on a nursing infant is unknown, but serious toxicities (e.g., bone marrow depression, allergic reactions, nausea, vomiting, and diarrhea) have been reported in adults and are a potential complication. If a mother is receiving this drug, she should not breastfeed.

References

1. Product information, Taxotere. Sanofi-Aventis, 2008.
2. De Santis M, Lucchese A, De Carlos S, De Carolis S, Ferrazzani S, Caruso A. Metastatic breast cancer in pregnancy: first case of chemotherapy with docetaxel. Eur J Cancer Care (Engl) 2000;9:235–7.
3. Nieto Y, Santisteban M, Armendia JM, Fernandez-Hidalgo O, Garcia-Manero M, Lopez G. Docetaxel administered during pregnancy for inflammatory breast carcinoma. Clin Breast Cancer 2006;6:533–4.
4. Potluri V, Lewis D, Burton GV. Chemotherapy with taxanes in breast cancer during pregnancy: case report and review of the literature. Clin Breast Cancer 2006;7;167–70.
5. Gainford MC, Clemons M. Breast cancer in pregnancy: are taxanes safe? Clin Oncol (R Coll Radiol) 2006;18:159.
6. Sekar R, Stone PR. Trastuzumab use for metastatic breast cancer in pregnancy. Obstet Gynecol 2007;110:507–10.
7. Kim JH, Kim HS, Sung CW, Kim KJ, Kim CH, Lee KY. Docetaxel, gemcitabine, and cisplatin administered for non-small cell lung cancer during the first and second trimester of an unrecognized pregnancy. Lung Cancer 2008;59:270–3.
8. Rouzi AA, Sahly NN, Sahly NF, Alahwal MS. Cisplatinum and docetaxel for ovarian cancer in pregnancy. Arch Gynecol Obstet 2009;280:823–5.

DOCUSATE CALCIUM

Laxative

See Docusate Sodium.

DOCUSATE POTASSIUM

Laxative

See Docusate Sodium.

DOCUSATE SODIUM

Laxative

PREGNANCY RECOMMENDATION: Compatible
BREASTFEEDING RECOMMENDATION: Compatible

PREGNANCY SUMMARY

No reports linking the use of docusate sodium (DSS) with congenital defects have been located. DSS is a common ingredient in many over-the-counter laxative preparations.

D

FETAL RISK SUMMARY

In a large prospective study, 116 patients were exposed to this drug during pregnancy (1). No evidence for an association with malformations was found. Similarly, no evidence of fetal toxicity was noted in 35 women treated with a combination of docusate sodium and dihydroxyanthraquinone (2).

In a surveillance study of Michigan Medicaid recipients involving 229,101 completed pregnancies conducted between 1985 and 1992, 232 newborns had been exposed to a docusate salt during the 1st trimester (F. Rosa, personal communication, FDA, 1993). Nine (3.9%) major birth defects were observed (nine expected), including one cardiovascular defect (two expected) and one polydactyly (one expected). No anomalies were observed in four other categories of defects (oral clefts, spina bifida, limb reduction defects, and hypospadias) for which specific data were available. These data do not support an association between the drug and congenital defects.

Chronic use of 150–250 mg/day or more of docusate sodium throughout pregnancy was suspected of causing hypomagnesemia in a mother and her newborn (3). At 12 hours of age, the neonate exhibited jitteriness, which resolved spontaneously. Neonatal serum magnesium levels ranged from 0.9 to 1.1 mg/dL between 22 and 48 hours of age with a maternal level of 1.2 mg/dL on the 3rd postpartum day. All other laboratory parameters were normal.

BREASTFEEDING SUMMARY

A combination of docusate sodium and dihydroxyanthraquinone was given to 35 postpartum women in a 1973 study (2). One infant developed diarrhea, but the relationship between the symptom and the laxative is unknown.

References

1. Heinonen OP, Slone D, Shapiro S. *Birth Defects and Drugs in Pregnancy*. Littleton, MA: Publishing Sciences Group, 1977:442.
2. Greenhalf JO, Leonard HSD. Laxatives in the treatment of constipation in pregnant and breast-feeding mothers. Practitioner 1973;210:259–63.
3. Schindler AM. Isolated neonatal hypomagnesaemia associated with maternal overuse of stool softener. Lancet 1984;2:822.

DOFETILIDE

Antiarrhythmic

PREGNANCY RECOMMENDATION: No Human Data—Animal Data Suggest Risk
BREASTFEEDING RECOMMENDATION: No Human Data—Potential Toxicity

PREGNANCY SUMMARY

No reports describing the use of dofetilide during human pregnancy have been located. Although the antiarrhythmic is teratogenic and toxic in animals at exposures slightly above those expected in humans, the lack of human data prevents an assessment of the potential embryo–fetal risk. However, if dofetilide therapy is required in a pregnant woman, the benefits appear to outweigh the unknown risk.

FETAL RISK SUMMARY

Dofetilide is an antiarrhythmic agent with Class III (cardiac action potential duration prolongation) properties that is indicated for the maintenance of normal sinus rhythm in patients with atrial fibrillation/flutter. Only about 20% of the drug is metabolized.

In reproduction studies in mice and rats, oral doses of dofetilide equal to or greater than 4 and 2 times, respectively, the maximum likely human exposure based on AUC (MHE), caused sternebral and vertebral anomalies in both species (1). In addition, an increased incidence of unossified calcaneum was noted in mice. In rats given doses approximately equal to the MHE, an increased incidence of unossified metacarpals and the occurrence of hydroureter and hydronephroses were observed. When the dose was doubled (twice the MHE) in rats, additional defects noted were cleft palate, adactyly, levocardia, and dilation of cerebral ventricles. The no-effect adverse-effect dose in mice was approximately equal to the MHE, whereas in rats it was about half the MHE (1).

Dofetilide had no effect on mating and fertility in rats at doses up to three times the MHE (1). It was also not mutagenic in various assays nor was it carcinogenic in tests with mice and rats. Chronic administration of dofetilide did cause testicular atrophy, decreased testicular weight, and/or epididymal oligospermia in mice, rats, and dogs at doses greater than 3, 4, and 1.3 times, respectively, the MHE (1).

In a 1996 study, the embryo toxicity and teratogenicity of dofetilide in rats were shown to be gestational age related and resulted from dose-dependent bradycardia in in vitro (rat embryo culture) and in vivo (pregnant rat) experiments (2). In the embryo cultures, the minimum effective concentration for significant bradycardia (22 ng/mL) was about six times the human peak plasma concentration achieved after an oral dose of 12 mcg/kg (3.5 ng/mL) (2). An embryo culture dose twice the minimum effective dose caused an almost complete cessation of the heartbeat. In pregnant rats, single oral doses of various concentrations were given on different gestational days. On gestational day (GD) 10, a high incidence of resorptions occurred, but no malformations except one fetus with a short tail. Defects and/or toxicity seen on other days included GD 11 (right-sided cleft lip), GD 12 (small number of defects; 100% lethality at highest dose), and GD 13 (most sensitive day; hindlimb defects; resorptions at higher doses). The defects were preceded by hemorrhage, but the investigators could not determine if the hemorrhage caused the defect or if the hemorrhage and defect were caused by the bradycardia-induced hypoxia (2).

It is not known if dofetilide crosses the human placenta. The molecular weight (about 442) is low enough that transfer to the fetus should be expected.

BREASTFEEDING SUMMARY

No reports describing the use of dofetilide in human lactation have been located. The molecular weight (about 442) is low enough that excretion in breast milk should be expected. The effect of this exposure on a nursing infant is unknown. Until the effects on a nursing infant from exposure to the drug in milk have been clarified, women receiving this agent should probably not breastfeed.

D

References

1. Product information. Tikosyn. Pfizer, 2001.
2. Webster WS, Brown-Woodman PDC, Snow MD, Danielsson BRG. Teratogenic potential of almokalant, dofetilide, and d-sotalol: drugs with potassium channel blocking activity. Teratology 1996;53:168–75.

DOLASETRON

Antiemetic

PREGNANCY RECOMMENDATION: **No Human Data—Animal Data Suggest Low Risk**
BREASTFEEDING RECOMMENDATION: **No Human Data—Probably Compatible**

PREGNANCY SUMMARY

Summary: No reports describing the use of dolasetron during human pregnancy have been located. Among other agents with similar mechanisms of actions and indications (see Granisetron and Ondansetron), only ondansetron has published human pregnancy experience. Based on this experience and the lack of embryo–fetal toxicity in two animal species, dolasetron appears to represent minimal, if any, risk to a human fetus.

FETAL RISK SUMMARY

Dolasetron is a specific and selective serotonin subtype 3 ($5\text{-}HT_3$) receptor antagonist that is used for the treatment and prevention of nausea and vomiting in the postoperative period and after chemotherapy. The drug has no effect on plasma prolactin levels (1).

Dolasetron had no effect on fertility and reproductive performance in female rats at doses up to 8 times the recommended human dose based on BSA (RHD) or in male rats at doses up to 32 times the RHD. No evidence of impaired fertility or fetal harm was observed in pregnant rats and rabbits at oral doses up to 8 and 16 times, respectively, the RHD (1). In 24-month carcinogenicity studies, there was a dose-related significant increase in combined hepatocellular adenomas and carcinomas in male mice, but not in female mice or in male and female rats. No mutagenicity was observed in various tests (1).

It is not known if dolasetron crosses the human placenta. The molecular weight of the free base (about 325 for the free base) is low enough that transfer to the fetus should be expected.

BREASTFEEDING SUMMARY

No reports describing the use of dolasetron in human lactation have been located. The molecular weight (about 325 for the free base) is low enough that excretion into breast milk should be expected. The effect of this exposure on a nursing infant is unknown.

Reference

1. Product information. Anzemet. Aventis Pharmaceuticals, 2001.

DOMPERIDONE

[Withdrawn from the market. See 9th edition.]

D

DONEPEZIL

Cholinesterase Inhibitor (CNS Agent)

PREGNANCY RECOMMENDATION: No Human Data—Animal Data Suggest Low Risk
BREASTFEEDING RECOMMENDATION: No Human Data—Potential Toxicity

PREGNANCY SUMMARY

No reports describing the use of donepezil in human pregnancy have been located. Because of its indication, such reports should be rare. Moreover, the animal data suggest that the risk to the embryo and/or fetus is low. Therefore, inadvertent exposure to donepezil during pregnancy should not be a reason for pregnancy termination.

FETAL RISK SUMMARY

Donepezil (known previously as E2020) is a reversible cholinesterase inhibitor that is indicated for the treatment of mild-to-moderate dementia of the Alzheimer's type. Two metabolites of donepezil are known to be active. The drug is extensively protein bound (about 96%) in the plasma, primarily to albumin (about 75%) and α_1-acid glycoprotein. The plasma elimination half-life is about 70 hours (1,2).

Reproduction studies have been conducted in rats and rabbits. In rats, doses up to about 13 times the maximum recommended human dose based on BSA (MRHD) were not teratogenic. At 8 times the MRHD given from gestational day 17 through postpartum day 20, there was a slight increase in stillbirths and a slight decrease in pup survival through postpartum day 4. Donepezil had no effect on rat fertility at doses up to about 8 times the MRHD. In rabbits, no teratogenic effects were observed at a dose 16 times the MRHD (1,2).

It is not known if donepezil or its active metabolites cross the human placenta. The molecular weight of the parent compound (about 416) and its long plasma elimination half-life suggest that the drug will cross to the embryo–fetus, but the extensive protein binding will limit this transfer.

BREASTFEEDING SUMMARY

No reports describing the use of donepezil during human lactation have been located. Because of its indication, such reports should be rare. Donepezil has two active metabolites. The molecular weight of the parent compound (about 416) and its long plasma elimination half-life (about 70 hours) suggest that donepezil, and possible the active metabolites, will be excreted into breast milk. The extensive protein binding (about 96%), however, should limit this excretion. The effects of this exposure on a nursing infant are unknown.

References

1. Product information. Aricept. Eisai, 2004.
2. Product information. Aricept. Pfizer, 2004.

DOPAMINE

Sympathomimetic (Adrenergic)

PREGNANCY RECOMMENDATION: Compatible—Maternal Benefit >> Embryo-Fetal Risk
BREASTFEEDING RECOMMENDATION: No Human Data—Probably Compatible

PREGNANCY SUMMARY

Experience with dopamine in human pregnancy is limited. No reports of embryo–fetal harm have been located. Since dopamine is indicated only for life-threatening situations, chronic use would not be expected.

FETAL RISK SUMMARY

Animal studies have shown both increases and decreases in uterine blood flow (1,2). In a study in pregnant baboons, dopamine infusion increased uterine vascular resistance and thus impaired uteroplacental perfusion (1). Because of this effect, the investigators concluded that the drug should not be used in patients with severe preeclampsia or eclampsia (1).

However, although human studies on uterine perfusion have not been conducted, the use in women with severe toxemia has not been associated with fetal harm. The drug has been used to prevent or treat renal failure in 10 oliguric or anuric eclamptic patients by reestablishing diuresis (3,4).

In another study of six women with severe preeclampsia and oliguria, low-dose dopamine infusion produced a significant rise in urine and cardiac output (5). No significant changes in blood pressure, central venous pressure, or pulmonary capillary wedge pressure occurred. In another case, low-dose dopamine was successful in treating oliguria due to severe maternal pulmonary hypertension (6).

Dopamine has been used to treat hypotension in 26 patients undergoing cesarean section (2). No adverse effects attributable to dopamine were observed in the fetuses or newborns of the mothers in these studies.

BREASTFEEDING SUMMARY

No reports describing the use of dopamine during lactation have been located. Because it is only indicated for life-threatening situations, it is doubtful if such reports will occur.

References

1. Fishburne JI Jr, Dormer KJ, Payne GG, Gill PS, Ashrafzadeh AR, Rossavik IK. Effects of amrinone and dopamine on uterine blood flow and vascular responses in the gravid baboon. Am J Obstet Gynecol 1988;158:829–37.
2. Clark RB, Brunner JA III. Dopamine for the treatment of spinal hypotension during cesarean section. Anesthesiology 1980;53:514–7.
3. Gerstner G, Grunberger W. Dopamine treatment for prevention of renal failure in patients with severe eclampsia. Clin Exp Obstet Gynecol 1980;7:219–22.
4. Nasu K, Yoshimatsu J, Anai T, Miyakawa I. Lose-dose dopamine in treating acute renal failure caused by preeclampsia. Gynecol Obstet Invest 1996;42:140–1.
5. Kirshon B, Lee W, Mauer MB, Cotton DB. Effects of low-dose dopamine therapy in the oliguric patient with preeclampsia. Am J Obstet Gynecol 1988;159:604–7.
6. Leduc L, Kirshon B, Diaz SF, Cotton DB. Intrathecal morphine analgesia and low-dose dopamine for oliguria in severe maternal pulmonary hypertension—a case report. J Reprod Med 1990;35:727–9.

D

DORIPENEM

Antibiotic

PREGNANCY RECOMMENDATION: No Human Data—Probably Compatible
BREASTFEEDING RECOMMENDATION: No Human Data—Probably Compatible

PREGNANCY SUMMARY

No reports describing the use of doripenem in human pregnancy have been located. In two animal species, the low exposures were not associated with teratogenicity or other developmental toxicity. Moreover, there is no evidence that β-lactam antibiotics (e.g., penicillins and cephalosporins) cause developmental toxicity in humans at therapeutic doses. Therefore, if the maternal condition requires the use of doripenem, the antibiotic should not be withheld because of pregnancy.

FETAL RISK SUMMARY

Doripenem, an antibiotic that is structurally related to β-lactam antibiotics, has activity against aerobic and anaerobic gram-positive and gram-negative bacteria. It is given as an IV infusion. It was approved by the FDA in 2007. Doripenem is classified as a carbapenem in the same class as ertapenem, imipenem–cilastatin, and meropenem. Both plasma protein binding (about 8.1%) and metabolism (about 18%) are low. The mean terminal plasma elimination half-life is about 1 hour (1).

Reproduction studies have been conducted in rats and rabbits. In these species, IV doses producing exposures that were at least 2.4 and 0.8 times, respectively, the human exposure based on AUC from a 500-mg dose every 8 hours (HE) were not teratogenic and did not produce effects on ossification, developmental delays, or fetal weight (1).

It is not known if doripenem crosses the human placenta. The molecular weight (about 421), low metabolism, and minimal plasma protein binding suggest that exposure of the embryo–fetus probably occurs, but the short elimination half-life should limit the amount of exposure.

BREASTFEEDING SUMMARY

No reports describing the use of doripenem during human lactation have been located. It is not known if doripenem is excreted into breast milk. The molecular weight (about 421), low metabolism (18%), and minimal plasma protein binding (about 8.1%) suggest that it will be excreted into milk. However, the short elimination half-life (about 1 hour) should limit the amount of exposure. The effect on a nursing infant from this exposure is unknown but of doubtful clinical significance. Most antibiotics are excreted into breast milk in low concentrations, and adverse effects are rare. Potential problems for the nursing infant are modification of bowel flora, direct effects on the infant (e.g., allergic response), and interference with the interpretation of culture results if a fever workup is required.

Reference

1. Product information. Doribax. Ortho-McNeil Pharmaceutical, 2007.

DORNASE ALFA

Respiratory Agent (Mucolytic)

PREGNANCY RECOMMENDATION: No Human Data—Probably Compatible
BREASTFEEDING RECOMMENDATION: No Human Data—Probably Compatible

PREGNANCY SUMMARY

No reports describing the use of dornase alfa in human pregnancy have been located. The animal data suggest low risk for developmental toxicity. Moreover, inhalation of dornase alfa does not result in higher concentrations of endogenous DNase in the maternal circulation. These data suggest that the risk of using dornase alfa during pregnancy is negligible.

FETAL RISK SUMMARY

Dornase alfa is recombinant human deoxyribonuclease I (rhDNase), an enzyme that selectively cleaves DNA. Dornase alfa is produced from Chinese hamster ovary cells. It is a glycoprotein containing 260 amino acids with a molecular weight of about 37,000. The primary amino acid sequence is identical to that of the native human enzyme. Dornase alfa is administered by inhalation of an aerosol mist to improve pulmonary function in the management of cystic fibrosis patients (1).

Reproduction studies have been conducted in rats and rabbits. There was no evidence of impaired fertility, fetal harm, or effects on development with IV doses that were >600 times the systemic exposures expected with the recommended human dose (1).

It is not known if dornase alfa crosses the human placenta. Cynomolgus monkeys were given IV dornase alfa at term in a study to determine if the enzyme crosses the monkey placenta (2). Consistent with the high molecular weight, dornase alfa was not detected in either the fetus or the amniotic fluid. Native human DNase is an endogenous enzyme in the maternal circulation. In humans, inhaled dornase alfa does not produce serum levels of DNase significantly higher than normal endogenous levels, and no accumulation has been noted after prolonged use (1). Because the monkey and human placentas are similar (both are hemomonochorial), the absence of transfer in the former suggests that the agent is not transferred to the fetal compartment in the latter.

BREASTFEEDING SUMMARY

No reports describing the use of dornase alfa during lactation have been located. Inhaled dornase alfa does not result in a significant increase in the serum concentrations of endogenous DNase. Therefore, it would not be expected in the milk (1). Because the enzyme is a natural constituent of the mother's circulation, the risk to a nursing infant from the mother's use of dornase alfa is negligible.

References

1. Product information. Pulmozyme. Genentech, 2005.
2. Hardy L, McCormick G, Sinicropi D, Baughman S, Osterburg I, Korte R. Placental transfer/secretion in milk of rhDNase in cynomolgus monkeys (abstract). Teratology 1996;53:111–2.

DOTHIEPIN

[Withdrawn from the market. See 9th edition.]

DOXAPRAM

Central Stimulant

PREGNANCY RECOMMENDATION: No Human Data—Animal Data Suggest Low Risk
BREASTFEEDING RECOMMENDATION: No Human Data—Potential Toxicity

PREGNANCY SUMMARY

No reports describing the use of doxapram in human pregnancy have been located. The animal data are limited but do not suggest a major risk for the embryo and/or fetus. Moreover, although the elimination half-life of the drug is unknown, the duration of effect is very short and the agent is extensively metabolized. Thus, the embryo and/or fetal exposure are probably limited except when continuous infusions are administered. The commercial product contains 0.9% benzyl alcohol as a preservative. Since benzyl alcohol can cross the placenta, the use of doxapram near term, especially continuous infusions, should be avoided because of the potential for toxicity in the newborn. However, if indicated, the maternal benefit from single injections of doxapram at any time in pregnancy appears to outweigh the unknown embryo–fetal risk.

FETAL RISK SUMMARY

Doxapram is a short-acting respiratory stimulant. It is administered IV to stimulate respiration in acute situations such as postanesthesia, mild-to-moderate respiratory and central nervous system depression due to drug overdosage, and hypercapnia in patients with chronic obstructive pulmonary disease. The duration of effect varies from 5 to 12 minutes (1). Doxapram is extensively metabolized by the liver after IV injection (2).

Reproduction studies have been conducted in mice and rats. In rats, doses up to 1.6 times the human dose revealed no evidence of impaired fertility or fetal harm. The dose, assumed to be based on weight, was given by the IM and oral routes, but the human dose (either a single dose of 1–2 mg/kg, or an IV infusion of 1–3 mg/kg/hr) are given IV (1). In another study, no teratogenicity was observed in rats (3). In pregnant mice, a dose of 144 mg/kg/day was given intraperitoneal during organogenesis (4). No gross defects were observed, but fetal death and growth restriction were noted. In addition, minor skeletal defects occurred in the fetuses of one pregnancy (4).

Doxapram crosses the sheep placenta and stimulates fetal breathing (5). Doxapram was infused into a maternal vein over 2–5 minutes and peak fetal plasma levels occurred between 0.08 and 0.17 hours after the start of the infusion. The increase in fetal breathing, up to about 41% during the infusion, was dose related (5).

It is not known if doxapram crosses the human placenta. The drug does cross the placenta in dogs (1) and sheep (5). The molecular weight of the free base (about 379) is low enough for transfer, but the very short duration of action suggests that limited amounts will be available at the maternal:fetal interface after single injections. However, continuous infusions of doxapram probably allows for placental passage to the embryo–fetus.

In an in vitro study, doxapram was shown to undergo substantial metabolism by the human fetal liver (6). The fetal livers were obtained from elective abortions conducted at 10–20 weeks' gestation.

BREASTFEEDING SUMMARY

No reports describing the use of doxapram during human lactation have been located. In addition, the indications for the drug suggest that such reports will be rare. However, doxapram has been given to newborns at risk for respiratory depression when narcotic analgesics or general anesthetics were used during delivery (7). No adverse effects attributable to doxapram were observed. The molecular weight of the free base (about 379) suggests that the drug will be excreted into breast milk. The maternal plasma elimination half-life is unknown, but the relatively short duration of effect combined with the extensive hepatic metabolism, probably indicates a short half-life, at least for the parent compound. Of note though, doxapram is a basic drug and accumulation in the relatively acidic breast milk by ion trapping is a potential concern, especially if continuous infusions are used. An additional concern involves benzyl alcohol, the preservative used in the commercial preparation that is known to be toxic in newborns.

References

1. Product information. Dopram. A. H. Robins, 1986.
2. Parfitt K, ed. *Martindale. The Complete Drug Reference*. 32nd ed. London, UK: Pharmaceutical Press, 1999:1480.
3. Imai K. Effect of Doxapram hydrochloride administered to pregnant rats on pre- and post-natal development of their offspring. Oyo Yakuri 1974;8:237–43. As cited by Shepard TH. *Catalog of Teratogenic Agents*. 10th ed. Baltimore, MD: The Johns Hopkins University Press, 2001:186.
4. Imai K. Effect of Doxapram hydrochloride administered to pregnant mice on pre- and post-natal development of their offspring. Oyo Yakuri 1974;8:229–36. As cited by Shepard TH. *Catalog of Teratogenic Agents*. 10th ed. Baltimore, MD: The Johns Hopkins University Press, 2001:186.
5. Hogg MIJ, Golding RH, Rosen M. The effect of doxapram on fetal breathing in the sheep. Br J Obstet Gynaecol 1977;84:48–50.
6. Bairam A, Branchaud C, Beharry K, Rex J, Laudignon N, Papageorgiou A, Aranda JV. Doxapram metabolism in human fetal hepatic organ culture. Clin Pharmacol Ther 1991;50:32–8.
7. Gupta PK, Moore J. The use of doxapram in the newborn. J Obstet Gynaecol Br Commonw 1973;80:1002–6.

DOXAZOSIN

Sympatholytic (Antiadrenergic)

PREGNANCY RECOMMENDATION: Limited Human Data—Animal Data Suggest Moderate Risk
BREASTFEEDING RECOMMENDATION: No Human Data—Potential Toxicity

PREGNANCY SUMMARY

One report describing the use of doxazosin in human pregnancy has been located.

FETAL RISK SUMMARY

Doxazosin is a peripherally acting α_1-adrenergic blocking agent used in the treatment of hypertension.

No adverse fetal effects were observed when pregnant rats and rabbits were given oral doses 4 and 10 times the human serum levels achieved with a 12 mg/day therapeutic dose (HD), respectively. However, reduced fetal survival occurred in rabbits dosed at 20 times the HD and delayed postnatal development was observed in rat pups whose mothers were given doses 8 times the HD during the perinatal and postnatal periods. Doxazosin crosses the placenta in rats (1).

It is not known if doxazosin crosses the human placenta. The molecular weight (about 548) suggests that the drug will cross to the embryo and/or fetus.

In a 2012 report, a 36-year-old pregnant woman developed pheochromocytoma at 26 weeks' (2). She was initially treated with proroxan (an alpha adrenergic blocker not available in the United States) (15 mg three times daily). Eleven days after treatment started, her condition worsened and doxazosin (dose not specified), a calcium channel blocker (name and dose not specified), and an ACE inhibitor (name and dose not specified) were added. The four-drug combination was continued until a cesarean section was performed at 30 4/7 weeks' gestation to deliver a 1.700-kg male infant. A simultaneous laparatomic right-sided adrenalectomy also was performed. Apgar scores were 6 and 8 at 1 and 5 minutes, respectively. No further details on the premature infant were provided. The woman underwent a hysterectomy for placenta increta (2).

D

BREASTFEEDING SUMMARY

No reports describing the use of doxazosin during human lactation have been located.

References

1. Product information. Cardura. Pfizer, 2000.
2. Pirtskhalava N. Pheochromocytoma and pregnancy: complications and solutions (case report). Georgian Med News 2012;208–9:76–82.

DOXEPIN

Antidepressant

PREGNANCY RECOMMENDATION: Human Data Suggest Low Risk
BREASTFEEDING RECOMMENDATION: Limited Human Data—Potential Toxicity

PREGNANCY SUMMARY

Doxepin was not teratogenic in four animal species. One large database reported a possible association with birth defects, but no confirming reports have been located. In general, tricyclic antidepressants are not thought to cause structural anomalies.

FETAL RISK SUMMARY

Doxepin is a tricyclic antidepressant in the same class as amitriptyline, clomipramine, imipramine, and trimipramine. It was not teratogenic in rats, rabbits, monkeys, and dogs (1–3). At the highest doses used, however, an increase in neonatal death was observed in rats and rabbits (1,2). Because of the relatively low molecular weight (280 for the free base), placental transfer of the drug to the fetus should be expected.

In a surveillance study of Michigan Medicaid recipients involving 229,101 completed pregnancies conducted between 1985 and 1992, 118 newborns had been exposed to doxepin during the 1st trimester (F. Rosa, personal communication, FDA, 1993). A total of 12 (10.2%) major birth defects were observed (4.5 expected), including (observed/expected) cardiovascular defects (2/1), oral clefts (2/0.2), and polydactyly (2/0.3). No anomalies were observed in three other categories of malformations (spina bifida, limb reduction defects, and hypospadias) for which specific data were available. The total number of major birth defects and the cases of polydactyly are suggestive of an association, but other factors, including concurrent drug use and chance, may be involved.

In a 1996 descriptive case series, the European Network of the Teratology Information Services (ENTIS) prospectively examined the outcomes of 689 pregnancies exposed to antidepressants (4). Multiple drug therapy occurred in about two-thirds of the mothers. Doxepin was used in 14 pregnancies. The outcomes of these pregnancies were four elective abortions, one spontaneous abortion, one stillbirth, and eight normal newborns.

Paralytic ileus has been observed in an infant exposed to doxepin at term (5). The condition was thought to be primarily due to chlorpromazine, but the authors speculated that the anticholinergic effects of doxepin worked synergistically with the phenothiazine.

A 2002 prospective study compared two groups of mother–child pairs exposed to antidepressants throughout gestation, 46 exposed to tricyclics (2 to doxepin) and 40 exposed to fluoxetine, with 36 nonexposed, nondepressed controls (6). Offspring were studied between the ages 15 and 71 months for effects of antidepressant exposure in terms of IQ, language, behavior, and temperament. Exposure to antidepressants did not adversely affect the measured parameters, but IQ was significantly and negatively associated with the duration of depression, and language was negatively associated with the number of depression episodes after delivery (6).

BREASTFEEDING SUMMARY

Doxepin and its active metabolite, *N*-desmethyldoxepin, are excreted into breast milk (7–9). A 36-year-old woman was treated with doxepin, 10 mg daily, for approximately 5 weeks starting 2 weeks after the birth of her daughter (7). The dose was increased to 25 mg 3 times daily 4 days before the wholly breastfed 8-week-old infant was found pale, limp, and near respiratory arrest. Although drowsiness and shallow respirations continued on admission to the hospital, the baby made a rapid recovery and was normal in 24 hours. A peak milk concentration of doxepin, 29 ng/mL, was measured 4–5 hours after a dose, whereas two levels obtained just prior to a dose (12 hours after the last dose in each case) were 7 and 10 ng/mL, respectively. Milk concentrations of the metabolite ranged from "not detectable" (lower limit of detection 7 ng/mL) to 11 ng/mL. The averages of nine determinations for doxepin and the metabolite in the milk were 18 and 9 ng/mL, respectively. Maternal serum doxepin and *N*-desmethyldoxepin levels ranged from trace to 21 ng/mL (average 15 ng/mL) and 33 to 66 ng/mL (average 57 ng/mL), respectively. The milk:serum ratio for doxepin on two determinations was 0.9, whereas ratios for the metabolite were 0.12 and 0.17. Doxepin was almost undetectable (estimated to be 3 ng/mL) in the infant's serum, but the levels of the metabolite on two occasions were 58 and 66 ng/mL, demonstrating marked accumulation in the infant's serum. The initial infant urine sample contained 39 ng/mL of the metabolite (7).

A 26-year-old woman, 30 days postpartum, was treated with doxepin (150 mg/day) (8). Blood samples were obtained a mean 18 hours after a dose on days 7, 14, 22, 28, 36, 43, 50, and 99 days of treatment. On the same days that blood specimens were drawn, milk samples were collected at the start of feeding (17.2 hours after the last dose) and at the end of feeding (17.7 hours after the last dose). Plasma concentrations of doxepin varied between 35 and 68 ng/mL, with a mean value of 46 ng/mL. Levels for the metabolite, *N*-desmethyldoxepin, ranged from 65 to 131 ng/mL, with a mean of 90 ng/mL. Mean pre- and postfeed milk:plasma ratios for doxepin were 1.08 (range 0.51–1.44) and 1.66 (range 0.79–2.39), respectively, and for the metabolite, 1.02 (range 0.54–1.45) and 1.53 (range 0.85–2.35), respectively. A plasma sample drawn from the infant on day 43 showed no detectable doxepin (sensitivity 5 ng/mL) and 15 ng/mL of the metabolite. No adverse effects of the exposure to doxepin were observed in the infant (8).

Muscle hypotonia, drowsiness, poor sucking and swallowing, and vomiting were reported in a 9-day-old breastfed, 2950-g male baby whose mother was taking doxepin 35 mg/day (9). The mother had started doxepin in the 3rd trimester and continued it postpartum. The normal, full-term, 3030-g infant had Apgar scores of 10 and 10 at 1 and 5 minutes, respectively. Breastfeeding began 8 hours after birth. Hyperbilirubinemia (indirect bilirubin 17 mg/dL) was diagnosed at age 3 days. He was discharged at age 5 days with a bilirubin of 9 mg/dL and a weight of 3100 g. At presentation 9 days after birth, jaundice was again present (indirect bilirubin 18 mg/dL) and was treated with 24 hours of phototherapy. The concentrations of doxepin and metabolite in the infant's serum at 11 days of age, 2 hours after breastfeeding, were about 10 ng/mL and <10 ng/mL, respectively. The milk:plasma ratio, 13–15 hours after the last dose, was estimated to be 1.0–1.7 (doxepin plus metabolite). The calculated infant dose, based on 150–200 mL milk/kg/day, was 10–20 mcg/kg/day, or about 2.5% of the weight-adjusted maternal dose. Breastfeeding was stopped at age 14 days because of persistent drowsiness and vomiting and, about 24 hours later, his symptoms resolved. He was asymptomatic when discharged home 2 days later (9).

D

Adverse effects were observed in two of the three cases cited above and were potentially lethal to one infant. Based on these reports, doxepin should be avoided during lactation. The American Academy of Pediatrics classifies doxepin as an agent whose effect on the nursing infant is unknown but may be of concern (10).

References

1. Owaki Y, Momiyama H, Onodera N. Effects of doxepin hydrochloride administered to pregnant rats upon the fetuses and their postnatal development. Oyo Yakuri 1971;5:913–24. As cited in Shepard TH. *Catalog of Teratogenic Agents*. 6th ed. Baltimore, MD: Johns Hopkins University Press, 1989:243.
2. Owaki Y, Momiyama H, Onodera N. Effects of doxepin hydrochloride administered to pregnant rabbits upon the fetuses. Oyo Yakuri 1971;5:905–12. As cited in Shepard TH. *Catalog of Teratogenic Agents*. 6th ed. Baltimore, MD: Johns Hopkins University Press, 1989:243.
3. Product information. Sinequan. Pfizer, 2000.
4. McElhatton PR, Garbis HM, Elefant E, Vial T, Bellemin B, Mastroiacovo P, Arnon J, Rodriguez-Pinilla E, Schaefer C, Pexieder T, Merlob P, Dal Verme S. The outcome of pregnancy in 689 women exposed to therapeutic doses of antidepressants. A collaborative study of the European Network of Teratology Information Services (ENTIS). Reprod Toxicol 1996;10:285–94.
5. Falterman CG, Richardson CJ. Small left colon syndrome associated with maternal ingestion of psychotropic drugs. J Pediatr 1980;97:308–10.
6. Nulman I, Rovet J, Stewart DE, Wolpin J, Pace-Asciak P, Shuhaiber S, Koren G. Child development following exposure to tricyclic antidepressants or fluoxetine throughout fetal life: a prospective, controlled study. Am J Psychiatry 2002;159:1889–95.
7. Matheson I, Pande H, Alertsen AR. Respiratory depression caused by *N*-desmethyldoxepin in breast milk. Lancet 1985;2:1124.
8. Kemp J, Ilett KF, Booth J, Hackett LP. Excretion of doxepin and *N*-desmethyldoxepin in human milk. Br J Clin Pharmacol 1985;20:497–9.
9. Frey OR, Scheidt P, von Brenndorff AI. Adverse effects in a newborn infant breast-fed by a mother treated with doxepin. Ann Pharmacother 1999;33:690–3.
10. Committee on Drugs, American Academy of Pediatrics. The transfer of drugs and other chemicals into human milk. Pediatrics 2001;108:776–89.

DOXORUBICIN

Antineoplastic

PREGNANCY RECOMMENDATION: Contraindicated—1st Trimester
BREASTFEEDING RECOMMENDATION: Contraindicated

PREGNANCY SUMMARY

Doxorubicin caused structural anomalies and death in two animal species, and has been associated with similar outcomes in humans after exposure during organogenesis. Exposure during the 1st trimester should be avoided. [*See* Rituximab for additional data.]

FETAL RISK SUMMARY

Doxorubicin is an antineoplastic agent used for the treatment of various types of cancer. It is in the same antineoplastic subclass of anthracyclines as daunorubicin, epirubicin, idarubicin, and valrubicin. The drug is embryotoxic and teratogenic in rats and embryotoxic and abortifacient in rabbits (1).

Several reports have described the use of doxorubicin in pregnancy, including three during the 1st trimester (2–21).

D

One of the fetuses exposed during the 1st trimester to doxorubicin, cyclophosphamide, and unshielded radiation was born with an imperforate anus and rectovaginal fistula (15). At about 3 months of age, the infant was small with a head circumference of 46 cm (<5th percentile) but was doing well after two corrective surgeries (15). A 1983 report described the use of doxorubicin and other antineoplastic agents in two pregnancies, one of which ended in fetal death 36 hours after treatment had begun (18). Other than maceration, no other fetal abnormalities were observed. The investigators could not determine the exact cause of the outcome but concluded that the chemotherapy was probably not responsible. The only other complication observed in exposed infants was transient polycythemia and hyperbilirubinemia in one subject. Infants who have been evaluated have shown normal growth and development.

A 1999 report from France described the outcomes of pregnancies in 20 women with breast cancer who were treated with antineoplastic agents (18). The first cycle of chemotherapy occurred at a mean gestational age of 26 weeks with delivery occurring at a mean 34.7 weeks. A total of 38 cycles were administered during pregnancy with a median of two cycles per woman. None of the women received radiation therapy during pregnancy. The pregnancy outcomes included two spontaneous abortions (both exposed in the 1st trimester), one intrauterine death (exposed in the 2nd trimester), and 17 live births, one of whom died at 8 days of age without apparent cause. The 16 surviving children were developing normally at a mean follow-up of 42.3 months (18). Doxorubicin (D), in combination with cyclophosphamide (C), fluorouracil (F), or vincristine (V), was administered to four of the women at a mean dose of 68.7 mg/m^2 (range 50–100 mg/m^2). The outcomes were four surviving liveborn infants (two exposed to DCF and one each to DF and DV in the 2nd or 3rd trimesters).

Three studies have investigated the placental passage of doxorubicin (2,19,20). In one, the drug was not detected in the amniotic fluid at 20 weeks' gestation, which suggested that the drug was not transferred in measurable amounts to the fetus (2). Placental transfer was demonstrated in a 17-week-old aborted fetus, however, using high-performance liquid chromatography (HPLC) (20). High concentrations were found in fetal liver, kidney, and lung. The drug was not detected in amniotic fluid (<1.66 ng/mL), brain, intestine, or gastrocnemius muscle. A third study examined the placental passage of doxorubicin in two pregnancies, one resulting in the birth of a healthy infant at 34 weeks' gestation and one ending with a stillborn fetus at 31 weeks' gestation (19). Using HPLC, doxorubicin was demonstrated in the first case, 48 hours after a 45-mg/m^2 dose (total cumulative dose, 214 mg/m^2), on both sides of the placenta and in the umbilical cord but not in cord blood plasma. In the stillborn, doxorubicin was not detected in any fetal tissue, 36 hours after a single dose of 45 mg/m^2. However, a substance was detected in all fetal tissues analyzed that the investigators concluded may have represented an unknown doxorubicin metabolite (19).

In a 2004 case report, a 17-year-old woman at 22 weeks' gestation was diagnosed with an extraskeletal Ewing's sarcoma (21). She was treated with doxorubicin 50 mg/m^2 by 48-hour continuous infusion and ifosfamide 2 g/m^2 as a single injection, both given at 25, 28, and 30 weeks'. Mild fetal growth restriction was noted from the 29th week of gestation. An elective cesarean section delivered a 1.245-kg male infant with Apgar scores of 7 and 9 at 1 and 5 minutes, respectively. Based on weight and length (38 cm), the infant was small for gestational age. The infant had no congenital anomalies and no respiratory distress syndrome, but did have mild hyperbilirubinemia. He was growing well at 8 months of age (21).

A 2006 case report described the pregnancy outcome of a 21-year-old woman with Burkitt's lymphoma who was treated with intensive chemotherapy (22). Beginning at 26 weeks', she was treated with two cycles of chemotherapy that included ifosfamide, cyclophosphamide, vincristine, doxorubicin, cytarabine, etoposide, cytarabine, and mesna. At 32 weeks', a cesarean section delivered a 1.731-kg male infant with Apgar scores of 8 and 9 at 1 and 5 minutes, respectively. His weight, length, and head circumference were within normal limits for gestational age. No anomalies were noted but respiratory distress was evident. At 9 months of age, his weight was 6.36 kg. He had mild delayed motor skills that were thought to result from his premature birth. Otherwise he was healthy (22).

Long-term studies of growth and mental development of offspring exposed to doxorubicin and other antineoplastic agents in the 2nd trimester, the period of neuroblast multiplication, have not been conducted (23).

Doxorubicin may cause reversible testicular dysfunction (24,25). Similarly, normal pregnancies have occurred in women treated before conception with doxorubicin (26). In 436 long-term survivors treated with chemotherapy for gestational trophoblastic tumors between 1958 and 1978, 33 (8%) received doxorubicin as part of their treatment regimens (26). Of the 33 women, five (15%) had at least one live birth (data given in parentheses refer to mean/maximum doxorubicin dose in milligrams) (100/100), two (6%) had no live births (150/200), one (3%) failed to conceive (100/100), and 25 (76%) did not try to conceive (140/400). Additional details, including congenital anomalies observed, are described in the monograph for methotrexate (see Methotrexate).

The long-term effects of combination chemotherapy on menstrual and reproductive function have been described in a 1988 report (27). Only one of the 40 women treated for malignant ovarian germ cell tumors received doxorubicin. The results of this study are discussed in the monograph for cyclophosphamide (see Cyclophosphamide).

Occupational exposure of the mother to antineoplastic agents during pregnancy may present a risk to the fetus. A position statement from the National Study Commission on Cytotoxic Exposure and a research article involving some antineoplastic agents, including doxorubicin, are presented in the monograph for cyclophosphamide (see Cyclophosphamide).

BREASTFEEDING SUMMARY

Doxorubicin is excreted into human milk. A 31-year-old woman, 7 months postpartum, was given doxorubicin (70 mg/m^2), infused over 15 minutes, for the treatment of ovarian cancer (28). Both doxorubicin and the metabolite, doxorubicinol, were detected in the plasma and the milk. Peak concentrations of the two substances in the plasma occurred at the first sampling time (0.5 hour) and were 805 and 82 ng/mL, respectively. In the milk, the peak concentrations occurred at 24 hours with levels of 128 and 111 ng/mL, respectively. The AUC of the parent compound and metabolite in the plasma were 8.3 and 1.7 μmol/L × hours, respectively, while the AUC

D

in the milk were 9.9 and 16.5 µmol/L × hours, respectively. The highest milk:plasma ratio, 4.43, was measured at 24 hours. Although milk concentrations often exceeded those in the plasma, the total amount of active drug available in the milk was only 0.24 mcg/mL (28). If the infant consumed 150 mL/kg/day, the estimated dose would be 0.036 mg/kg/day

Although the above amounts might be considered negligible, the American Academy of Pediatrics classifies doxorubicin as a drug that may interfere with the cellular metabolism of the nursing infant (29).

References

1. Product information. Adriamycin. Pharmacia & Upjohn, 2000.
2. Roboz J, Gleicher N, Wu K, Kerenyi T, Holland J. Does doxorubicin cross the placenta? Lancet 1979;2:1382–3.
3. Khursid M, Saleem M. Acute leukaemia in pregnancy. Lancet 1978;2: 534–5.
4. Newcomb M, Balducci L, Thigpen JT, Morrison FS. Acute leukemia in pregnancy: successful delivery after cytarabine and doxorubicin. JAMA 1978;239:2691–2.
5. Hassenstein E, Riedel H. Zur teratogenitat von Adriamycin ein fallbericht. Geburtshilfe Frauenheilkd 1978;38:131–3.
6. Cervantes F, Rozman C. Adriamycina y embarazo. Sangre (Barc) 1980;25:627.
7. Pizzuto J, Aviles A, Noriega L, Niz J, Morales M, Romero F. Treatment of acute leukemia during pregnancy: presentation of nine cases. Cancer Treat Rep 1980;64:679–83.
8. Tobias JS, Bloom HJG. Doxorubicin in pregnancy. Lancet 1980;1:776.
9. Garcia V, San Miguel J, Borrasca AL. Doxorubicin in the first trimester of pregnancy. Ann Intern Med 1981;94:547.
10. Garcia V, San Miguel IJ, Borrasca AL. Adriamycin and pregnancy. Sangre (Barc) 1981;26:129.
11. Dara P, Slater LM, Armentrout SA. Successful pregnancy during chemotherapy for acute leukemia. Cancer 1981;47:845–6.
12. Lowenthal RM, Funnell CF, Hope DM, Stewart IG, Humphrey DC. Normal infant after combination chemotherapy including teniposide for Burkitt's lymphoma in pregnancy. Med Pediatr Oncol 1982;10:165–9.
13. Webb GA. The use of hyperalimentation and chemotherapy in pregnancy: a case report. Am J Obstet Gynecol 1980;137:263–6.
14. Gililland J, Weinstein L. The effects of cancer chemotherapeutic agents on the developing fetus. Obstet Gynecol Surv 1983;38:6–13.
15. Murray CL, Reichert JA, Anderson J, Twiggs LB. Multimodal cancer therapy for breast cancer in the first trimester of pregnancy. A case report. JAMA 1984;252:2607–8.
16. Haerr RW, Pratt AT. Multiagent chemotherapy for sarcoma diagnosed during pregnancy. Cancer 1985;56:1028–33.
17. Turchi JJ, Villasis C. Anthracyclines in the treatment of malignancy in pregnancy. Cancer 1988;61:435–40.
18. Giacalone PL, Laffargue F, Benos P. Chemotherapy for breast carcinoma during pregnancy. Cancer 1999;86:2266–72.
19. Karp GI, Von Oeyen P, Valone F, Khetarpal VK, Israel M, Mayer RJ, Frigoletto FD, Garnick MB. Doxorubicin in pregnancy: possible transplacental passage. Cancer Treat Rep 1983;67:773–7.
20. D'Incalci M, Broggini M, Buscaglia M, Pardi G. Transplacental passage of doxorubicin. Lancet 1983;1:75.
21. Nakajima W, Ishida A, Takahashi M, Hirayama M, Washino N, Ogawa M, Takahashi S, Okada K. Good outcome for infant of mother treated with chemotherapy for Ewing sarcoma at 25 to 30 weeks' gestation. J Pediatr Hematol Oncol 2004;26:308–11.
22. Lam MSH. Treatment of Burkitt's lymphoma during pregnancy. Ann Pharmacother 2006;40:2048–52.
23. Dobbing J. Pregnancy and leukaemia. Lancet 1977;1:1155.
24. Lendon M, Palmer MK, Hann IM, Shalet SM, Jones PHM. Testicular histology after combination chemotherapy in childhood for acute lymphoblastic leukaemia. Lancet 1978;2:439–41.
25. Schilsky RL, Lewis BJ, Sherins RJ, Young RC. Gonadal dysfunction in patients receiving chemotherapy for cancer. Ann Intern Med 1980;93:109–14.
26. Rustin GJS, Booth M, Dent J, Salt S, Rustin F, Bagshawe KD. Pregnancy after cytotoxic chemotherapy for gestational trophoblastic tumours. Br Med J 1984;288:103–6.
27. Gershenson DM. Menstrual and reproductive function after treatment with combination chemotherapy for malignant ovarian germ cell tumors. J Clin Oncol 1988;6:270–5.
28. Egan PC, Costanza ME, Dodion P, Egorin MJ, Bachur NR. Doxorubicin and cisplatin excretion into human milk. Cancer Treat Rep 1985;69:1387–9.
29. Committee on Drugs, American Academy of Pediatrics. The transfer of drugs and other chemicals into human milk. Pediatrics 2001;108:776–89.

DOXYCYCLINE

Antibiotic (Tetracycline)

PREGNANCY RECOMMENDATION: Contraindicated in 2nd and 3rd Trimesters
BREASTFEEDING RECOMMENDATION: Compatible

PREGNANCY SUMMARY

See Tetracycline.

BREASTFEEDING SUMMARY

Doxycycline is excreted into breast milk. Oral doxycycline, 200 mg, followed after 24 hours by 100 mg, was given to 15 nursing mothers (1). Milk:plasma ratios determined at 3 and 24 hours after the second dose were 0.3 and 0.4, respectively. Mean milk concentrations were 0.77 and 0.38 mcg/mL.

Theoretically, dental staining and inhibition of bone growth could occur in breastfed infants whose mothers were consuming doxycycline. However, this theoretical possibility seems remote, because in infants exposed to a closely related antibiotic, tetracycline, serum levels were undetectable (less than 0.05 mcg/mL) (2).

The American Academy of Pediatrics classifies tetracycline as compatible with breastfeeding (3). Three potential problems may exist for the nursing infant even though there are no reports in this regard: modification of bowel flora, direct effects on the infant, and interference with the interpretation of culture results if a fever workup is required.

References

1. Morganti G, Ceccarelli G, Ciaffi EG. Comparative concentrations of a tetracycline antibiotic in serum and maternal milk. Antibiotica 1968;6: 216–23.
2. Posner AC, Prigot A, Konicoff NG. Further observations on the use of tetracycline hydrochloride in prophylaxis and treatment of obstetric infections. *Antibiotics Annual 1954–55*. New York, NY: Medical Encyclopedia, 1955:594–8.
3. Committee on Drugs, American Academy of Pediatrics. The transfer of drugs and other chemicals into human milk. Pediatrics 2001;108: 776–89.

D

DOXYLAMINE

Antihistamine/Antiemetic

PREGNANCY RECOMMENDATION: Compatible
BREASTFEEDING RECOMMENDATION: No Human Data—Probably Compatible

PREGNANCY SUMMARY

The preponderance of data supports the assessment that the fixed combination of doxylamine–pyridoxine is safe in human pregnancy, including the 1st trimester. Positive associations with congenital malformations have been observed but probably reflect outcomes that have occurred by chance or are the consequences of nausea and vomiting itself. Moreover, these reports do not consistently describe a specific syndrome or group of malformations. Therefore, pregnant women who request medication for nausea and vomiting can be offered this drug combination, but, as with any treatment during pregnancy, the available evidence should be reviewed with them to obtain their informed consent before initiating therapy.

FETAL RISK SUMMARY

Doxylamine, an antihistamine of the ethanolamine class, is approved for use as a sedative, either alone or in combination with other agents in cough and cold preparations. It is not used in the United States for the symptomatic relief of hypersensitivity reactions, most likely because of its pronounced sedative effects.

The antihistamine was a component of the proprietary product, Bendectin, which contained equal concentrations of doxylamine, pyridoxine (vitamin B6), and dicyclomine (an antispasmodic). Bendectin was marketed in 1956 for the prevention and treatment of nausea and vomiting during pregnancy. The product was reformulated in 1976 to eliminate dicyclomine because that component was not found to contribute to the antiemetic effectiveness. A similar Canadian two-drug formulation (doxylamine and pyridoxine), Diclectin, was marketed in 1978. More than 30 million women have taken this product during pregnancy, making it one of the most heavily prescribed drugs for this condition. The US manufacturer ceased producing the drug combination in 1983 because of litigation and adverse media coverage over its alleged association with congenital limb defects. The fixed two-drug combination, although no longer available in the United States, continues to be produced in Canada and the individual components are marketed worldwide by various manufacturers.

Six studies in rodents and nonhuman primates have not observed teratogenic effects with Bendectin or its components (1–6), but dose-related toxicity was observed in three studies. In a 1968 publication, the reproductive effects of dicyclomine, doxylamine, and Bendectin (the three-drug combination of doxylamine [10 mg], dicyclomine [10 mg], and pyridoxine [10 mg]) in rats and rabbits were reported (1). Dicyclomine and doxylamine were given as pure compounds, whereas Bendectin was administered as pulverized tablets. In rats, dicyclomine and doxylamine (10–100 mg/kg/day) (15–150 times the maximum recommended human dose [four tablets] for a 60-kg human [MRHD]) were given orally for 80 days or more before pregnancy and continued during one (dicyclomine) or two (doxylamine) successive liters. The Bendectin group received 3–60 mg/kg/day (5–90 times the MRHD) orally beginning on the first day of gestation and continued throughout the remainder of the study. First-generation male and female offspring from the control and 60 mg/kg/day groups were then bred (nonsibling matings) and their progeny examined. Compared with nonexposed controls, no increase in congenital malformations or other adverse effects were noted in the pregnancy outcomes of the three drug groups. The one exception appeared to be a small dose-related decrease in fetal weight that was observed in the dicyclomine and doxylamine groups. Pregnant rabbits were administered 10–100 mg/kg/day (15–150 times the MRHD) orally of dicyclomine or doxylamine, or 3–30 mg/kg/day (5–45 times the MRHD) orally of Bendectin on days 9 through 16 of gestation (1). Similar to the study with rats, no adverse effects in pregnancy outcomes were noted when compared with controls except when toxic (100 mg/kg/day) doses were used in the pure drug groups (1).

A 1993 reference studied the effects of three antiemetic histamine H_1 antagonists, doxylamine, chlorcyclizine, and promethazine, on the skeletons of rat fetuses exposed during organogenesis (days 7–13) (2). Doxylamine was given orally at doses of 500 and 750 mg/kg (750 and 1125 times the MRHD). Compared with controls, a dose-dependent loss of skeletal integrity and marked fragility occurred with each antihistamine (2). The investigators concluded that the fragility was due to a defect in joint development rather than to intrauterine growth restriction.

No increase in malformations was observed in rats given Bendectin (two-drug combination) during organogenesis in doses of 0, 200, 500, and 800 mg/kg/day (3). Both maternal and fetal toxicity were evident at the two highest doses. The developmental toxicity observed was reduced prenatal viability (800 mg/kg/day) and reduced fetal body weight/litter (500 and 800 mg/kg/day).

Three of the reproduction studies involved nonhuman primates (4–6). In an unpublished study, rhesus monkeys were given a dose of 7 mg/kg/day (10 times the MRHD) without producing malformations (4). A second study, published in 1985, administered pulverized Bendectin (10 mg doxylamine plus 10 mg pyridoxine) to pregnant cynomolgus monkeys, rhesus monkeys, and baboons (5). A commercial preparation of doxylamine (Decapryn) was used in some baboons to reduce the total amount of drug if they would not take Bendectin.

Nonexposed controls were used in each species. Most animals received the study drugs daily from gestation day 22–50, the major period of organogenesis (5). Cynomolgus and rhesus monkeys were given doses 10–40 times the MRHD, whereas baboons received doses 1–10 times the MRHD of Bendectin or 10 times the MRHD of doxylamine. A few cynomolgus monkeys (short-term exposure group) received Bendectin doses 20 times the MRHD for 4 consecutive days on gestation days 22–25, 26–29, 30–33, 34–37, or 38–41. Some of the long-term exposure monkey groups, all of the short-term exposure groups, and all of the baboon fetuses were removed by hysterotomy prenatally at day 100 of gestation. The remaining monkey fetuses were delivered at term (150–160 days). In the offspring examined prenatally, the incidence of ventricular septal defect (VSD) was 40% (6 of 15) in cynomolgus monkeys, 0% (0 of 8) in cynomolgus monkey short-term exposure groups, 18% (2 of 11) in rhesus monkeys, 23% (3 of 13) in Bendectin-exposed baboons, and 20% (1 of 5) in doxylamine-exposed baboons. The VSD was restricted to the muscular portion of the septum in 91% (11 of 12). No other defects were observed in the monkeys and no dose response was evident among the long-term-treated groups. In addition to the VSD, one baboon fetus (drug group not specified) had exophthalmia, micrognathia, reduction of first and fifth digits on both hands, facial hemangioma, and ambiguous genitalia, and was small for gestational age. The cause of the multiple defects was unknown, but a genetic basis for the anomalies could not be excluded. (Karyotyping was not available at that time.) (5). At term, no cases of VSD were found in nine cynomolgus and four rhesus monkey offspring, but one cynomolgus monkey had a mitral valve defect. Data from the author's laboratory indicated a very low incidence of spontaneous VSD in the three species: 0.3% (1 of 297) cynomolgus monkeys; 0% (0 of 1692) rhesus monkeys; 1.6% (1 of 61) baboons (5). The authors concluded, therefore, that the results suggested a delay in closure of the ventricular septum but that closure would occur before birth (5).

In the second part of the above investigation, daily Bendectin (doxylamine plus pyridoxine) doses 2, 5, and 20 times the MRHD were administered double-blind to cynomolgus monkeys ($N = 69$) from gestational days 22 through 50 (6). A control group ($N = 21$) received placebo tablets containing inert excipients and coatings similar to those in Bendectin. The doses for the four groups (three active, one placebo) were prepared by the manufacturer, and their identity was unknown to the researchers. Delivery occurred at term (approximately 155 days of gestation). No congenital malformations were noted, and no evidence of embryo, fetal, or maternal toxicity was observed.

More than 160 cases of congenital defects have been reported in the literature or to the FDA as either "Bendectin-induced" or associated with use of the drug in the 1st trimester (7–12). Defects observed included skeletal, limb, and cardiac anomalies as well as cleft lip or palate. A 1983 study found an association between Debendox (three-drug formulation) and clefts of the lip, palate, or both, although the authors stated that the association may have been due to chance alone (13).

In a 1989 study, the association between maternal use of marijuana and childhood acute nonlymphoblastic leukemia (ANLL) was investigated (see Marijuana) (14). An incidental finding was that the relative risk (RR) for ANLL in offspring of case mothers who used antinauseant medication was 1.75 (95% confidence interval [CI] 0.98–3.20) ($p = 0.06$). A statistically significant dose–response relationship was observed when the RR increased to 2.81 if the use of antinauseant medication continued for more than 10 weeks. Although not all of the mothers used Bendectin, most of them specifically named the product (14). However, several factors make a causal relationship between Bendectin and ANLL unlikely, including the possibility of recall bias between cases and controls, the absence of biological plausibility, the likelier possibility that the leukemia was induced by other toxins (e.g., marijuana, herbicides, or pesticides), and the lack of other reports of such an association.

D

A possible association between doxylamine–pyridoxine and diaphragmatic hernia was reported in 1983 and was assumed to reflect earlier findings of a large prospective study (12). Authors of the latter study, however, cautioned that their results could not be interpreted, even when apparently strong associations existed, without independent confirmation (15,16). In a large case–control study, infants exposed to the combination in utero had a slightly greater RR of 1.40 for congenital defects (17). The risk was more than doubled (RR 2.91) if the mother also smoked. An increased risk for heart valve anomalies (RR 2.99) was also found. A minimal relationship was found between congenital heart disease and doxylamine (Bendectin) use in early pregnancy in another 1985 report comparing 298 cases with 738 controls (18). The authors went to great efforts to establish that their drug histories were accurate. Their findings provided evidence that if an association existed, it was very small.

In one of the above studies, an association was discovered between Bendectin and pyloric stenosis (RR 4.33–5.24), representing about a 4-fold increase in risk for this anomaly (17). Similarly, the Boston Collaborative Drug Surveillance Programs reported preliminary findings to the FDA indicating a 2.7-fold increase in risk (19). A 1983 case–control study, however, found no association between Bendectin use and the anomaly (20). In evaluating these three reports, the FDA considered them the best available information on the topic but concluded that no definite causal relationship had been shown between Bendectin and pyloric stenosis (19). In addition, the FDA commented that even if there were evidence for an association between the drug and the defect, it did not necessarily constitute evidence of a causal relationship since the nausea and vomiting themselves, or the underlying disease causing the condition, could be responsible for the increased risk (19). A 1984 study, which was not included in the above FDA evaluation, found a possible association with pyloric stenosis but could not eliminate the possibility that it was due to other factors (21). Compared with a control group, the odds ratio (OR) for pyloric stenosis in the offspring of mothers using Bendectin was 2.5 (95% CI 1.2–5.2). However, the authors stated that a conclusion supporting a causal association was not warranted because of the absence of a plausible biologic basis for the defect and conflicting results from other studies (21). Of interest, the *Birth Defects Encyclopedia* describes the etiology of pyloric stenosis (i.e., congenital hypertrophic pyloric stenosis) as probably polygenic and sex-modified, with an occurrence rate of 1/250 births (1200 males; 1/1000 females) (22).

The evidence indicating that doxylamine–pyridoxine is safe in pregnancy is impressive. A number of large studies, many reviewed in a 1983 article (23), have discovered no relationship between the drug combination and birth weight or length, head circumference, gestational age, congenital malformations, or other adverse fetal outcomes (24–40). An editorial accompanying the review article pointed out that Bendectin met none of the criteria for judging that a drug was a teratogen (41). One study was unable to observe chromosomal abnormalities associated with the drug combination, whereas a second study found that use of the drugs was not related to the Poland anomaly (unilateral absence of the pectoralis major muscle with or without ipsilateral hand defect) (42,43).

The Northern California Kaiser Permanente Birth Defects Study, published in 1989, prospectively studied the occurrence of 58 categories of major congenital defects in 31,564 newborns in relation to maternal Bendectin use (44). The OR for any major anomaly and Bendectin was 1.0 (95% CI 0.8–1.4). Three categories of defects were statistically associated with the drug: microcephaly (OR 5.3, 95% CI 1.8–15.6); congenital cataract (OR 5.3, 95% CI 1.2–24.3); and lung malformations (OR 4.6, 95% CI 1.9–10.9). However, this was the exact number of associations that would have been expected by chance alone (44). The authors then reviewed an earlier independent study that did not involve Bendectin and found strong positive associations of microcephaly and congenital cataract with vomiting in pregnancy (44). They concluded, therefore, that Bendectin use during the 1st trimester was not associated with an increase in congenital malformations and that the associations found were unlikely to be causal (44).

A meta-analysis of 17 studies involving the use of Bendectin in pregnancy was published in 1988 (45). The OR 1.01 (95% CI 0.66–1.55) for all studies indicated that Bendectin was not related to congenital defects. The studies were then separated by study type (cohort and case–control studies), and again, no relationship to birth defect outcomes was found (45). Another meta-analysis, published in 1994, examined 16 cohort and 11 case–control studies that had reported birth defects in pregnancies exposed to Bendectin during the 1st trimester (46). The RR of any birth defect in association with exposure to Bendectin was 0.95 (95% CI 0.88–1.04). The RR and 95% CI intervals for specific defects were cardiac (0.90, 0.77–1.05), central nervous system (1.00, 0.83–1.20), neural tube (0.99, 0.76–1.29), limb reduction (1.12, 0.83–1.48), genital tract (0.98, 0.79–1.22), oral clefts (0.81, 0.64–1.03), and pyloric stenosis (1.04, 0.85–1.29). These results indicate that the use of Bendectin during the 1st trimester is unlikely to be associated with congenital malformations (46).

A five-part analysis of the medical literature involving Bendectin and pregnancy outcomes, published in 1995, was used as a demonstration of methodology to determine if a drug presented a human reproductive hazard (47). Some of the legal history surrounding Bendectin's alleged reproductive hazards was also reviewed. The analysis included: (a) analysis of human epidemiologic studies, (b) the relationship between the secular trend of birth defects and the population exposure to drugs, (c) the ability to develop an animal model, (d) analysis of dose–response relationships and pharmacokinetics of the drug in animals and humans, and (e) the biological plausibility for the alleged teratogenicity (47). The author reviewed eight in vitro studies that examined the toxicity, mutagenicity, teratogenicity, and other toxicities of doxylamine. None of these studies found toxicity at serum concentrations obtainable in humans. Moreover, the author emphasized the fact that in vitro studies, by themselves, cannot establish human teratogenicity (47). Based on the total data presented in this analysis, a strong case was made for the contention that Bendectin has no measurable teratogenic effects. In response to this and other publications, however, an intense debate in the scientific literature has developed between some who contend that Bendectin is safe and a proponent of the view that Bendectin induces limb reduction defects (48–53).

Interestingly, a population-based case–control study conducted in 1982–1983 by the Atlanta Birth Defects Case–Control Study and published in 1999 found a protective effect from Bendectin for congenital heart defects (54). The use of antiemetic medication, particularly Bendectin (two- and three-drug combinations), in early moderate to severe nausea during pregnancy was associated with a lower risk for heart defects compared with the absence of nausea (OR 0.67, 95% CI 0.50–0.92), and nausea without medication use (OR 0.70, 95% CI 0.50–0.94). The authors concluded that the results suggested that pregnancy hormones, other factors, or a component of Bendectin (most likely pyridoxine) may be important for normal heart development (54).

In spite of the abundant evidence supporting the safety of doxylamine–pyridoxine in pregnancy, the adverse media publicity and litigation proceedings surrounding Bendectin have affected the use of the combination in other countries. A 1995 article briefly reviewed the history of Bendectin in the United States and compared it with a similar Canadian product, Diclectin (55). Diclectin is the drug of choice for the treatment of emesis in pregnancy as specified by a Canadian Department of Health and Welfare task force, and is labeled for this indication. It is used less frequently, however, than another antihistamine, dimenhydrinate (Gravol; Dramamine in the United States), that is not specifically labeled for pregnancy use. The reason for this appears to be a fear of possible teratogenicity and subsequent litigation (55).

A 2003 ecological analysis of Bendectin found no evidence of a teratogenic effect (56). This study was accompanied by a historical review of the drug and a recommendation that the combination be reintroduced in the American market (57).

A double-blind, placebo-controlled trial published in 2010 was designed to evaluate the effectiveness of a delayed release formulation of doxylamine and pyridoxine (Diclectin), similar to Bendectin, for the treatment of nausea and vomiting of pregnancy (58). Pregnant women were randomized to a 14-day treatment regimen of either the drug combination (N = 131) or placebo (N = 125). The drug combination was significantly better in controlling nausea and vomiting and significantly more women (48.9% vs. 32.8%) wanted to continue the combination at the end of the study (58).

BREASTFEEDING SUMMARY

No reports describing the use of doxylamine or the fixed combination of doxylamine–pyridoxine during human lactation have been located. Both components of the fixed combination, however, are available as single agents. Pyridoxine is excreted into breast milk but presents no risk to a nursing infant (see Pyridoxine). Doxylamine is an antihistamine that is used not only as an antiemetic, but also as a hypnotic and in cough and common cold preparations. The molecular weight of doxylamine succinate, about 389, is low enough that passage into breast milk should be expected. The effect on a nursing infant is unknown, but sedative and other antihistamine actions are a potential concern. The manufacturer of at least one doxylamine preparation states that the drug is contraindicated during nursing (59).

References

1. Gibson JP, Staples RE, Larson EJ, Kuhn WL, Holtkamp DE, Newberne JW. Teratology and reproduction studies with an antinauseant. Toxicol Appl Pharmacol 1968;13:439–47.
2. Sturman G, Freeman P, Bailey AR, Meade HM, Seeley NA. Loss of skeletal integrity in rat fetuses from dams treated with histamine H_1 antagonists. Agents Actions 1993;38:C185–7.
3. Tyl RW, Price CJ, Marr MC, Kimmel CA. Developmental toxicity evaluation of Bendectin in CD rats. Teratology 1988;37:539–52.
4. McClure HM. Research and development studies relative to the experimental induction of oral facial malformation in the Rhesus monkey. No. 1 DE52452 Final report, May 1975–July 1981, August 1982. As cited in Brent RL. Bendectin: review of the medical literature of a comprehensively studied human nonteratogen and the most prevalent tortogen-litigen. Reprod Toxicol 1995;9:337–49.
5. Hendrickx AG, Cukierski M, Prahalada S, Janos G, Rowland J. Evaluation of Bendectin embryotoxicity in nonhuman primates: I. Ventricular septal defects in prenatal macaques and baboon. Teratology 1985;32:179–89.
6. Hendrickx AG, Cukierski M, Prahalada S, Janos G, Booher S, Nyland T. Evaluation of Bendectin embryotoxicity in nonhuman primates: II. Double-blind study in term cynomolgus monkeys. Teratology 1985;32:191–4.
7. Korcok M. The Bendectin debate. Can Med Assoc J 1980;123:922–8.
8. Soverchia G, Perri PF. Two cases of malformations of a limb in infants of mothers treated with an antiemetic in a very early phase of pregnancy. Pediatr Med Chir 1981;3:97–9.
9. Donaldson GL, Bury RG. Multiple congenital abnormalities in a newborn boy associated with maternal use of fluphenazine enanthate and other drugs during pregnancy. Acta Paediatr Scand 1982;71:335–8.
10. Grodofsky MP, Wilmott RW. Possible association of use of Bendectin during early pregnancy and congenital lung hypoplasia. N Engl J Med 1984;311:732.
11. Fisher JE, Nelson SJ, Allen JE, Holsman RS. Congenital cystic adenomatoid malformation of the lung. A unique variant. Am J Dis Child 1982;136:1071–4.
12. Bracken MB, Berg A. Bendectin (Debendox) and congenital diaphragmatic hernia. Lancet 1983;1:586.
13. Golding J, Vivian S, Baldwin JA. Maternal anti-nauseants and clefts of lip and palate. Human Toxicol 1983;2:63–73.
14. Robison LL, Buckley JD, Daigle AE, Wells R, Benjamin D, Arthur DC, Hammond GD. Maternal drug use and risk of childhood nonlymphoblastic leukemia among offspring: an epidemiologic investigation implicating marijuana (a report from the Children's Cancer Study Group). Cancer 1989;63:1904–11.
15. Heinonen OP, Slone D, Shapiro S. *Birth Defects and Drugs in Pregnancy*. Littleton, MA: Publishing Sciences Group, 1977:474–5.
16. Ohga K, Yamanaka R, Kinumaki H, Awa S, Kobayashi N. Bendectin (Debendox) and congenital diaphragmatic hernia. Lancet 1983;1:930.
17. Eskenazi B, Bracken MB. Bendectin (Debendox) as a risk factor for pyloric stenosis. Am J Obstet Gynecol 1982;144:919–24.
18. Zierler S, Rothman KJ. Congenital heart disease in relation to maternal use of Bendectin and other drugs in early pregnancy. N Engl J Med 1985;313:347–52.
19. Bendectin and pyloric stenosis. FDA Drug Bull 1983;13:14–5.
20. Mitchell AA, Schwingl PJ, Rosenberg L, Louik C, Shapiro S. Birth defects in relation to Bendectin use in pregnancy. II. Pyloric stenosis. Am J Obstet Gynecol 1983;147:737–42.
21. Aselton P, Jick H, Chentow SJ, Perera DR, Hunter JR, Rothman KJ. Pyloric stenosis and maternal Bendectin exposure. Am J Epidemiol 1984;120:251–6.
22. Pyloric stenosis. In: Buyse ML, ed. *Birth Defects Encyclopedia*. Vol. II. Cambridge, MA: Blackwell Scientific Publications, 1990:1448.
23. Holmes LB. Teratogen update: Bendectin. Teratology 1983;27:277–81.
24. Aselton P, Jick H, Milunsky A, Hunter JR, Stergachis A. First-trimester drug use and congenital malformations. Obstet Gynecol 1985;65:451–5.
25. Milkovich L, van den Berg BJ. An evaluation of the teratogenicity of certain antinauseant drugs. Am J Obstet Gynecol 1976;125:244–8.
26. Shapiro S, Heinonen OP, Siskind V, Kaufman DW, Monson RR, Slone D. Antenatal exposure to doxylamine succinate and dicyclomine hydrochloride (Bendectin) in relation to congenital malformations, perinatal mortality rate, birth weight, intelligence quotient score. Am J Obstet Gynecol 1977;128:480–5.
27. Rothman KJ, Flyer DC, Goldblatt A, Kreidberg MB. Exogenous hormones and other drug exposures of children with congenital heart disease. Am J Epidemiol 1979;109:433–9.
28. Bunde CA, Bowles DM. A technique for controlled survey of case records. Curr Ther Res 1963;5:245–8.
29. Gibson GT, Collen DP, McMichael AJ, Hartshorne JM. Congenital anomalies in relation to the use of doxylamine/dicyclomine and other antenatal factors. An ongoing prospective study. Med J Aust 1981;1:410–4.
30. Correy JF, Newman NM. Debendox and limb reduction deformities. Med J Aust 1981;1:417–8.
31. Clarke M, Clayton DG. Safety of Debendox. Lancet 1981;2:659–60.
32. Harron DWG, Griffiths K, Shanks RG. Debendox and congenital malformations in Northern Ireland. Br Med J 1980;4:1379–81.
33. Smithells RW, Sheppard S. Teratogenicity testing in humans: a method demonstrating safety of Bendectin. Teratology 1978;17:31–5.
34. Morelock S, Hingson R, Kayne H, Dooling E, Zuckerman B, Day N, Alpert JJ, Flowerdew G. Bendectin and fetal development: a study at Boston City Hospital. Am J Obstet Gynecol 1982;142:209–13.
35. Cordero JF, Oakley GP, Greenberg F, James LM. Is Bendectin a teratogen? JAMA 1981;245:2307–10.
36. Mitchell AA, Rosenberg L, Shapiro S, Slone D. Birth defects related to Bendectin use in pregnancy: I. Oral clefts and cardiac defects. JAMA 1981;245:2311–4.
37. Fleming DM, Knox JDE, Crombie DL. Debendox in early pregnancy and fetal malformation. Br Med J 1981;283:99–101.
38. Greenberg G, Inman WHW, Weatherall JAC, Adelstein AM, Haskey JC. Maternal drug histories and congenital abnormalities. Br Med J 1977;2:853–6.
39. Aselton PJ, Jick H. Additional follow-up of congenital limb disorders in relation to Bendectin use. JAMA 1983;250:33–4.
40. McCredie J, Kricker A, Elliott J, Forrest J. The innocent bystander: doxylamine/dicyclomine/pyridoxine and congenital limb defects. Med J Aust 1984;140:525–7.
41. Brent RR. Editorial. The Bendectin saga: another American tragedy. Teratology 1983;27:283–6.
42. Hughes DT, Cavanagh N. Chromosomal studies on children with phocomelia, exposed to Debendox during early pregnancy. Lancet 1983;2:399.
43. David TJ. Debendox does not cause the Poland anomaly. Arch Dis Child 1982;57:479–80.
44. Shiono PH, Klebanoff MA. Bendectin and human congenital malformations. Teratology 1989;40:151–5.
45. Einarson TR, Leeder JS, Koren G. A method for meta-analysis of epidemiological studies. Drug Intell Clin Pharm 1988;22:813–24.
46. McKeigue PM, Lamm SH, Linn S, Kutcher JS. Bendectin and birth defects: I. A meta-analysis of the epidemiologic studies. Teratology 1994;50:27–37.
47. Brent RL. Bendectin: review of the medical literature of a comprehensively studied human nonteratogen and the most prevalent tortogen-litigen. Reprod Toxicol 1995;9:337–49.
48. Newman SA. Bendectin—birth defects controversy. JAMA 1990;264:569.
49. Skolnick A. Bendectin—birth defects controversy. Reply. JAMA 1990;264:569–70.
50. Scialli AR. Editor's note. Reprod Toxicol 1999;13:239.
51. Newman SA. Dr. Brent and scientific debate. Reprod Toxicol 1999;13:241–4.
52. Brent RL. Response to Dr. Stuart Newman's commentary on an article entitled "Bendectin: review of the medical literature of a comprehensively studied human nonteratogen and the most prevalent tortogen-litigen". Reprod Toxicol 1999;13:245–53.
53. Newman SA. Response to Dr. Brent's commentary on "Dr. Brent and scientific debate". Reprod Toxicol 1999;13:255–60.
54. Boneva RS, Moore CA, Botto L, Wong L-Y, Erickson JD. Nausea during pregnancy and congenital heart defects: a population-based case-control study. Am J Epidemiol 1999;149:717–25.
55. Ornstein M, Einarson A, Koren G. Bendectin/Diclectin for morning sickness: a Canadian follow-up of an American tragedy. Reprod Toxicol 1995;9:1–6.
56. Kutcher JS, Engle A, Firth J, Lamm SH. Bendectin and birth defects II: ecological analyses. Birth Defects Res (Part A) 2003;67:88–97.
57. Brent R. Bendectin and birth defects: hopefully, the final chapter. Birth Defects Res (Part A) 2003;67:79–87.
58. Koren G, Clark S, Hankins GDV, Cartis SN, Miodovnik M, Umans JG, Mattison DR. Effectiveness of delayed-release doxylamine and pyridoxine for nausea and vomiting of pregnancy: a randomized placebo-controlled trial. Am J Obstet Gynecol 2010;203:571.e1–7.
59. Product information. Unisom SleepTabs. Pfizer Inc., 1999.

DRONABINOL

Antiemetic

PREGNANCY RECOMMENDATION: Limited Human Data—Animal Data Suggest Low Risk
BREASTFEEDING RECOMMENDATION: Contraindicated

D

PREGNANCY SUMMARY

Only one report has described the use of dronabinol in human pregnancy. Studies in animals revealed no teratogenicity, but dose-related maternal toxicity resulting in embryo–fetal death was observed. The human data are too limited to assess the risk to the embryo–fetus. Marijuana is contraindicated in pregnancy (see Marijuana) but that product is usually smoked, whereas dronabinol is taken orally. Nevertheless, the use of dronabinol in a pregnant woman should be classified as a "last resort" option.

FETAL RISK SUMMARY

Dronabinol (delta-9-tetrahydrocannabinol [delta-9-THC, THC]) is a synthetic formulation of the naturally occurring component of marijuana. It is indicated for the treatment of anorexia associated with weight loss in patients with AIDS and nausea and vomiting associated with cancer chemotherapy in patients who have failed to respond adequately to conventional antiemetic treatments. Dronabinol undergoes extensive hepatic metabolism to both active and inactive metabolites. Dronabinol and its principal active metabolite, 11-OH-delta-9-THC, are present in approximately equal concentrations in the plasma. Plasma protein binding of dronabinol and its metabolites is about 97% and the terminal elimination half-life is 25–36 hours (1).

Reproduction studies have been conducted in mice and rats. Pregnant mice were given doses that were 0.2–5 times the maximum recommended human dose based on BSA (MRHD) in patients with cancer (MRHD-C) or 1–30 times the MRHD in patients with AIDs (MRHD-A), whereas rats received doses that were 0.8–3 times the MRHD-C or 5–20 times the MRHD-A. No evidence of teratogenicity was observed in these studies. However, dose-dependent maternal toxicity was observed, resulting in decreased maternal weight gain and number of viable pups, and increased fetal mortality and early resorptions (1).

In 2-year carcinogenicity studies, no evidence of carcinogenic effects was observed in rats. In mice, similar studies produced thyroid follicular cell adenoma in males and females but the tumors were not observed at higher doses. Three assays for mutagenicity were negative, whereas one assay produced a weak positive response. Fertility studies were conducted in rats with doses that were 0.3–1.5 times the MRHD-C or 2–10 times the MRHD-A. At these doses, reduced ventral prostate, seminal vesicle, and epididymal weights were observed, as well as decreases in seminal volume, spermatogenesis, number of developing germ cells, and number of Leydig cells in the testis. However, sperm count, mating success, and testosterone concentrations were not affected (1).

THC and one of its metabolites, 9-carboxy-THC, cross the human placenta at term. Data for other periods of gestation and for other metabolites are not available (see Marijuana).

A 2009 case report described the use of dronabinol in pregnancy (2). A 26-year-old woman who had been treated for 2 years with dronabinol (5 mg three times daily) for a complex hyperkinetic movement disorder became pregnant. Because the drug had improved her condition, treatment was continued during pregnancy. No signs of tolerance or need for dose escalation were noted. Her appetite was stimulated and she gained a total of 21 kg weight and her BMI increased to 31. She gave birth vaginally to a healthy baby (additional details not provided) (2).

BREASTFEEDING SUMMARY

No reports describing the use of dronabinol during human lactation have been located. THC is excreted and concentrated in breast milk (see Marijuana).

A 1990 report studied 68 breastfed infants exposed to marijuana in the mother's milk in the first month postpartum and compared their development at 1 year with 68 infants not exposed (3). The exposure appeared to be associated with a decrease in infant motor development at 1 year of age. On the basis of this report, additional research is warranted to confirm or refute these effects. Until such data are available, mothers taking dronabinol should not breastfeed.

References

1. Product information. Marinol. Abbott Laboratories, 2010.
2. Farooq MU, Ducommun E, Goudreau J. Treatment of a hyperkinetic movement disorder during pregnancy with dronabinol. Parkinsonism Relat Disord 2009;15:249–51.
3. Astley SJ, Little RE. Maternal marijuana use during lactation and infant development at one year. Neurotoxicol Teratol 1990;12:161–8.

DRONEDARONE

Antiarrhythmic

PREGNANCY RECOMMENDATION: No Human Data—Animal Data Suggest Risk
BREASTFEEDING RECOMMENDATION: No Human Data—Potential Toxicity

D

PREGNANCY SUMMARY

No reports describing the use of dronedarone in human pregnancy have been located. Major structural anomalies in two animal species and embryo–fetal death in one species were caused by doses equal to or less than the human dose based on BSA. These data strongly suggest that dronedarone should not be used in the 1st trimester of human pregnancy. The manufacturer states that women of childbearing potential must use effective contraception while taking dronedarone (1). The effects of exposure later in pregnancy are completely unknown.

FETAL RISK SUMMARY

Dronedarone is an oral benzofuran derivative that has antiarrhythmic properties belonging to all four Vaughan–Williams classes. It is indicated to reduce the risk of cardiovascular hospitalization in patients with paroxysmal atrial fibrillation (AF) or atrial flutter (AFL), with a recent episode of AF/AFL and associated cardiovascular risk factors (i.e., age >70, hypertension, diabetes, prior cerebrovascular accident, left atrial diameter ≥50 mm, or left ventricular ejection fraction <40%), who are in sinus rhythm or who will be cardioverted. Dronedarone is extensively metabolized to a less potent but active metabolite. Further metabolism results in a large number of inactive metabolites. Plasma protein binding of dronedarone and the active metabolite is >98%. The elimination half-life of the parent compound is 13–19 hours (1).

Reproduction studies have been conducted in rats and rabbits. In pregnant rats, doses equal to or greater than the maximum recommended human dose based on BSA (MRHD) resulted in increased rates of external, visceral, and skeletal malformations (cranioschisis, cleft palate, incomplete evagination of pineal body, brachygnathia, partially fused carotid arteries, truncus arteriosus, abnormal lobation of the liver, partially duplicated inferior vena cava, brachydactyly, ectrodactyly, syndactyly, and anterior and/or posterior club feet). In pregnant rabbits, a dose that was about half the MRHD (the lowest dose tested) caused an increased rate of skeletal abnormalities (anomalous ribcage and vertebrae, pelvic asymmetry) (1).

In 2-year studies for carcinogenicity, an increased incidence of histiocytic sarcomas in male mice, mammary adenocarcinomas in female mice, and hemangiomas in male rats were observed. No genotoxic potential was noted in multiple assays. In fertility studies with female rats, a dose 0.12 times the MRHD given before breeding and implantation caused an increase in irregular estrus cycles and cessation of cycling. Doses that were 1.2 times the MRHD were associated with decreased corpora lutea, implantations, and live fetuses. However, doses up to 1.2 times the MRHD had no effect on the mating behavior or fertility of male rats (1).

It is not known if dronedarone and its active metabolite cross the human placenta. The molecular weight of the parent drug (about 557 for the free base) and long elimination half-life suggest that it will cross to the embryo–fetus, although the high plasma protein binding might limit the exposure.

BREASTFEEDING SUMMARY

No reports describing the use of dronedarone during human lactation have been located. The molecular weight of the parent drug (about 457 for the free base) and long elimination half-life (13–19 hours) suggest that it will cross to the embryo–fetus, although the high plasma protein binding (>98%) of dronedarone and its active metabolite might limit the exposure. The effect of this exposure on a nursing infant is unknown. Adverse reactions that were most common in patients treated with the drug included diarrhea, nausea, abdominal pain, vomiting, dyspeptic signs and symptoms, weakness, and bradycardia (1). If a nursing mother chooses to breastfeed while taking this drug, her infant should be closely observed for these effects.

Reference

1. Product information. Multaq. Sanofi-Aventis, 2009.

DROPERIDOL

Antiemetic/Antipsychotic

PREGNANCY RECOMMENDATION: Compatible
BREASTFEEDING RECOMMENDATION: No Human Data—Potential Toxicity

PREGNANCY SUMMARY

The limited animal and human data suggest that droperidol does not represent a significant risk to the fetus for major anomalies. The drug is a potent antiemetic that is effective for the treatment of severe nausea and vomiting of pregnancy.

D

FETAL RISK SUMMARY

Droperidol is a butyrophenone derivative structurally related to haloperidol (see also Haloperidol). The agent is not teratogenic in animals, but has produced a slight increase in the mortality of newborn rats (1). After IM administration, the increased pup mortality was attributed to CNS depression of the dams resulting in their failure to remove the placentae from the offspring (1).

The relatively low molecular weight of droperidol (about 379) suggests that the drug crosses the placenta to the fetus. In humans, the placental transfer of droperidol is slow (2).

Droperidol promotes analgesia for patients undergoing cesarean section without affecting the respiration of the newborn (2,3). The drug was also administered during labor as a sedative in a study comparing 48 women treated with droperidol with 52 women receiving promethazine (4). These investigators noted eight other reports in which the drug was used in a similar manner. No serious maternal or fetal adverse effects were observed.

Droperidol has been used for the treatment of severe nausea and vomiting occurring during pregnancy (5,6). A 1996 report described the use of droperidol and other drugs (diphenhydramine, metoclopramide, and hydroxyzine) in 80 women with hyperemesis gravidarum (6). The mean gestational age at the start of treatment was 10.9 weeks and the mean total dose received for the approximately 2 days of therapy was 49.6 mg. Twelve (15%) of the women required a second hospitalization and were again treated with the same therapy. Three of the mothers (all treated in the 2nd trimester) delivered offspring with congenital defects: Poland's syndrome, fetal alcohol syndrome, and hydrocephalus and hypoplasia of the right cerebral hemisphere. Only the latter anomaly is a potential drug effect, but the most likely cause was thought to be the result of an in utero fetal vascular accident or infection (6).

A 2001 study, using a treatment method similar to the above study, described the use of droperidol and diphenhydramine in 28 women hospitalized for hyperemesis gravidarum (7). Pregnancy outcomes in the study group were compared with a historical control of 54 women who had received conventional antiemetic therapy. Oral metoclopramide and hydroxyzine were used after discharge from the hospital. Therapy was started in the study and control groups at mean gestational ages of 9.9 and 11.1 weeks', respectively. The study group appeared to have more severe disease than controls, as suggested by a greater mean loss from the prepregnancy weight, 2.07 vs. 0.81 kg (*ns*), and a slightly lower serum potassium level, 3.4 vs. 3.5 mmol/L (*ns*). Compared with controls, the droperidol group had a shorter duration of hospitalization (3.53 vs. 2.82 days, $p = 0.023$), fewer readmissions (38.9% vs. 14.3%, $p = 0.025$), and lower average daily nausea and vomiting scores (both $p < 0.001$). There were no statistical differences ($p > 0.05$) in outcomes (study vs. controls) in terms of spontaneous abortions ($N = 0$ vs. $N = 2$ [4.3%]), elective abortions ($N = 3$ [12.0%] vs. $N = 3$ [6.5%]), Apgar scores at 1, 5, and 10 minutes, age at birth (37.3 vs. 37.9 weeks'), and birth weight (3114 vs. 3347 g) (7). In controls, there was one (2.4%) major malformation of unknown cause, an acardiac fetus in a set of triplets, and one newborn with a genetic defect (Turner's syndrome). There was also one unexplained major birth defect (4.4%) in the droperidol group (bilateral hydronephrosis), and two genetic defects (translocation of chromosomes 3 and 7; tyrosinemia) (7).

In a nonrandomized, prospective study, two doses (0.5 and 1.0 mg/hr) of droperidol plus diphenhydramine for hyperemesis gravidarum were compared with historical controls (8). The number of patients in each group was 34, 67, and 54, respectively. Data were available for major anomalies in 26, 53, and 21 infants, respectively. Major anomalies, excluding those that were obviously not drug-induced (i.e., genetic, chromosomal, or amniotic bands), observed in the study were one (clubfoot—possible genetic defect), one (bilateral hydronephrosis), and none, respectively (8).

BREASTFEEDING SUMMARY

No reports describing the use of droperidol during lactation have been located. The molecular weight (about 379) is low enough that excretion into human milk should be expected. Because the drug is only available as an injectable formulation, the opportunity for exposure of a nursing infant appears to be limited. The effect of exposure on a nursing infant is unknown.

References

1. Product information. Inapsine. Akorn, 1997.
2. Zhdanov GG, Ponomarev GM. The concentration of droperidol in the venous blood of the parturients and in the blood of the umbilical cord of neonates. Anesteziol Reanimatol 1980;4:14–6.
3. Smith AM, McNeil WT. Awareness during anesthesia. Br Med J 1969;1:572–3.
4. Pettit GP, Smith GA, McIlroy WL. Droperidol in obstetrics: a double-blind study. Milit Med 1976;141:316–7.
5. Martynshin MYA, Arkhengel'skii AE. Experience in treating early toxicoses of pregnancy with metoclopramide. Akush Ginekol 1981;57:44–5.
6. Nageotte MP, Briggs GG, Towers CV, Asrat T. Droperidol and diphenhydramine in the management of hyperemesis gravidarum. Am J Obstet Gynecol 1996;174:1801–6.
7. Turcotte V, Ferreira E, Duperron L. Utilité du dropéridol et de la diphenhydramine dans l'hyperemesis gravidarum. J Soc Obstet Gynaecol Can 2001;23:133–9.
8. Ferreira E, Bussieres J-F, Turcotte V, Duperron L, Ouellet G. Case-control study comparing droperidol plus diphenhydramine with conventional treatment in hyperemesis gravidarum. J Pharm Technol 2003;19:349–54.

DROTRECOGIN ALFA (ACTIVATED)

Hematologic Agent (Thrombolytic)

PREGNANCY RECOMMENDATION: Compatible—Maternal Benefit >> Embryo–Fetal Risk
BREASTFEEDING RECOMMENDATION: No Human Data—Probably Compatible

D

PREGNANCY SUMMARY

The lack of animal reproductive studies and the near absence of human pregnancy experience prevent an assessment of the embryo–fetal risk. The drug does not appear to cross the placenta so that a direct risk to the embryo or fetus seems unlikely. However, drotrecogin alfa (activated) has been associated with a nonsignificant trend to more maternal hemorrhage and this would be a major risk to both the mother and fetus (1). Nevertheless, as demonstrated by the two case reports below, if the drug is indicated, it should not be withheld because of pregnancy (2,3).

FETAL RISK SUMMARY

Drotrecogin alfa (activated), a serine protease, is a recombinant (from a human cell line) form of human activated protein C. This glycoprotein is indicated for the reduction of mortality in adult patients with severe sepsis who have a high risk of death. It is administered as a continuous IV infusion because of its very short elimination half-life. The antithrombotic action of drotrecogin alfa (activated) is a result of inhibition of Factors Va and VIIIa. The agent is inactivated by endogenous plasma protease inhibitors. Animal reproduction studies have not been conducted with drotrecogin alfa (activated) (4).

It is not known if drotrecogin alfa (activated) crosses the human placenta to the embryo or fetus, but the molecular weight (about 55,000) of this glycoprotein should inhibit transfer. In addition, because the fetus can synthesize coagulation factors from early in gestation, there are no known physiologic processes in which endogenous maternal activated protein C would be actively transported across the placenta (1). Further, in vitro studies have found no evidence that endogenous protein C crosses the placenta or that it is metabolized by the placenta (1). However, the effect on these processes from high maternal plasma concentrations of activated protein C resulting from infusion of the drug has not been studied.

Drotrecogin alfa (activated) has been recommended for the treatment of preeclampsia because this disease is similar in some ways to severe sepsis: diffuse effects on the maternal vascular endothelium resulting in multiple organ dysfunctions (1,5). A 2002 publication reviewed previous reports on the pathogenesis of preeclampsia to determine whether administration of drotrecogin alfa (activated) could be beneficial in the treatment of this disease (1). The authors of this in-depth assessment concluded that, although the data were limited, there was adequate evidence to support phase II clinical studies in women with early-onset preeclampsia (before 33 weeks' gestation) or severe or worsening postpartum disease (1).

A preliminary report of a phase II study describing the use of human activated protein C for the treatment of disseminated intravascular coagulation (DIC) was published in 1999. A total of 16 women with moderate-to-severe placental abruption were treated over a 2-day period (4). The activated protein C was prepared by extracting protein C from human plasma and activating it with human thrombin. Clinical signs were markedly improved and all coagulation/fibrinolysis parameters, except for the number of platelets, demonstrated significant changes toward normal values. No adverse effects attributable to the treatment were observed (6).

Two case reports described the successful use of drotrecogin alfa (activated) in the 2nd and 3rd trimesters of two women with severe sepsis (2,3). Use of the drug in these cases was indicated because severe sepsis is characterized, among other problems, by dysregulation of coagulation. The women received a continuous infusion of drotrecogin alfa (activated) for 96 hours and their conditions significantly improved. Both eventually gave birth to normal infants (2,3).

BREASTFEEDING SUMMARY

No reports describing the use of drotrecogin alfa (activated) during human lactation have been located. It is doubtful if a nursing infant would have access to the breast milk of a woman treated with this drug because of its indication for severe, life-threatening disease. The very high molecular weight of this glycoprotein (about 55,000) should inhibit excretion into milk, but even if such excretion occurred, the drug would most likely be digested in the infant's gut.

References

1. von Dadelszen P, Magee LA, Lee SK, Stewart SD, Simone C, Koren G, Walley KR, Russell JA. Activated protein C in normal human pregnancy and pregnancies complicated by severe preeclampsia: a therapeutic opportunity? Crit Care Med 2002;30:1883–92.
2. Gupta R, Strickland KM, Mertz HL. Successful treatment of severe sepsis with recombinant activated protein C during the third trimester of pregnancy. Obstet Gynecol 2011;118:492–4.
3. Eppert HD, Goddard KB, King CL. Successful treatment with drotrecogin alfa (activated) in a pregnant women with severe sepsis. Pharmacotherapy 2011;31:333. doi:10.1592/phco.31.3.333.
4. Product information. Xigris. Eli Lilly and Company, 2003.
5. Lapinsky SE, Mehta S. Activated protein C for preeclampsia: tailoring the disease to the therapy. Crit Care Med 2002;30:1929–30.
6. Kobayashi T, Terao T, Maki M, Ikenoue T. Activated protein C is effective for disseminated intravascular coagulation associated with placental abruption. Throm Haemost 1999;82:1363.

DULOXETINE

Antidepressant

PREGNANCY RECOMMENDATION: Human Data Suggest Risk in 3rd Trimester
BREASTFEEDING RECOMMENDATION: Limited Human Data—Potential Toxicity

D

PREGNANCY SUMMARY

Duloxetine causes developmental toxicity in animals (growth restriction in rats and rabbits; behavior deficits and death in rats) at doses <10 times the maximum recommended human dose of 60 mg/day based on BSA (MRHD). No structural anomalies were observed in these species. The human data for duloxetine are limited and incomplete. However, the pharmacologic action of duloxetine is similar to that of venlafaxine and selective serotonin reuptake inhibitors (SSRIs). SSRIs and venlafaxine have been associated with developmental toxicities, including spontaneous abortions, low birth weight, prematurity, neonatal serotonin syndrome, neonatal behavioral syndrome (withdrawal), possible sustained abnormal neurobehavior beyond the neonatal period, respiratory distress, and persistent pulmonary hypertension of the newborn (PPHN). Some of these symptoms are thought to be consistent with a direct toxic effect, drug discontinuance syndrome, or a serotonin syndrome. If duloxetine is used in pregnancy, healthcare professionals are encouraged to call the toll-free number (800-670-6126) for information about patient enrollment in the Motherisk study.

FETAL RISK SUMMARY

Duloxetine is a selective serotonin and norepinephrine reuptake inhibitor (SNRI). It has both antidepressant and central pain inhibitory action. Other drugs in the same class are desvenlafaxine, milnacipran, and venlafaxine. Duloxetine is extensively metabolized to inactive metabolites. The parent compound is highly bound (>90%) to plasma albumin and α_1-acid glycoprotein. The elimination half-life is about 12 hours (range 8–17 hours) (1).

Reproduction studies have been conducted in rats and rabbits. In pregnant rats, there was no evidence of fetal structural defects at doses up to seven times the MRHD administered during organogenesis. However, fetal weights were decreased at this dose. The no-effect dose was twice the MRHD. When duloxetine was administered throughout gestation and lactation, pup survival to 1 day postpartum and pup body weights at birth and during lactation were decreased at a dose five times the MRHD. In addition, pup behavior was adversely affected as shown by increased reactivity (e.g., increased startle response to noise and decreased habituation of locomotor activity). No adverse effects were observed on postweaning growth and reproductive performance. In pregnant rabbits, no evidence of fetal structural defects was observed at doses up to 15 times the MRHD during organogenesis, but fetal growth restriction was noted. The no-effect dose was three times the MRHD (1).

Duloxetine crosses the human placenta, at least at term. In a 2009 case report, the cord blood duloxetine concentration about 14 hours after a 60-mg extended release dose was 65 mcg/L (2). This is consistent with the molecular weight (about 298 for the free base) and the long elimination half-life of the drug.

Approximately 10 women became pregnant in a study of duloxetine in the treatment of depression (3). Treatment was discontinued and no additional information was provided.

A 2007 review conducted a literature search to determine the risk of major congenital malformations after 1st trimester exposure to SSRIs and SNRIs (4). Fifteen controlled studies were analyzed. The data were adequate to suggest that citalopram, fluoxetine, sertraline, and venlafaxine were not associated with an increased risk of congenital defects. In contrast, the analysis did suggest an increased risk with paroxetine. The data were inadequate to determine the risk for the other SSRIs and SNRIs (4).

A case–control study, published in 2006, found that exposure to SSRIs in late pregnancy was associated with persistent pulmonary hypertension of the newborn (PPHN) (5) (see Paroxetine or other SSRIs). Although there were no exposures to duloxetine in this study, the action of duloxetine is similar enough to the SSRIs that it might cause the same effect.

A brief report in 2008 described a case of poor neonatal behavioral syndrome due to duloxetine (6). The 36-year-old mother had been treated with monotherapy duloxetine 90 mg/day during pregnancy. Her female infant was born at 38 weeks' with Apgar scores of 7 and 9 (birth weight not provided). At delivery, the infant was blue, with minimal respiratory effort and oxygen saturation was in the 80s. Laboratory and other tests to determine the cause of the infant's condition were normal. "Jerky rhythmic movements" or "twitchiness" and episodes of shaking began on day 3. The initial electroencephalogram (EEG) showed nonspecific encephalopathy, but a repeat test at 7 days was suggestive of subclinical seizures. The infant was treated with phenobarbital but continued occasional twitching. At 7 weeks, the EEG was normal and phenobarbital was discontinued. At age 2 years, the child is healthy with normal neurobehavioral development (6).

A 2009 report described the use of duloxetine during the second half of pregnancy (2). The 20-year-old woman, treated for depression, was taking 60 mg once daily (868 mcg/kg/day or 34 mg/m^2). She gave birth to a healthy, 2.916-kg female infant at 38 weeks'. The Apgar scores were 8 and 9 at 1 and 5 minutes, respectively. The concentration of duloxetine in the cord blood (see above) was greater than the mother's peak plasma concentration obtained 6 hours after a dose 32 days after birth (see Breastfeeding Summary below). No evidence of developmental toxicity or other toxicity was observed in the infant (2).

Using the Lilly Safety System, a database for the collection, storage, and reporting of adverse events involving Lilly products, investigators identified 400 pregnancies (233 prospective; 167 retrospective) with known outcomes (7). The data collection period was from 2004 (drug approval) through October 2011. Of the prospectively reported cases, 170 (73%) were spontaneous reports, 58 (25%) were from clinical trials, and 5 (2%) involved post-marketing studies. In addition, 176 reports involving duloxetine from the FDA Adverse Events Reporting System through September 2011 were also examined. Analysis of the two data sources suggested that the frequency of abnormal outcomes were generally consistent with historic control rates in the general population (7).

BREASTFEEDING SUMMARY

Duloxetine is excreted into breast milk (2,8). A 2008 study conducted by the manufacturer described the use of duloxetine 40 mg every 12 hours for 3.5 days in six healthy women, at least 12 weeks postpartum, who had stopped nursing when the study was started (8). Seven paired milk and blood samples were collected on day 4 (probably at steady state). The mean milk:plasma ratio was 0.25 (90% confidence interval 0.18–0.35). The theoretical infant dose (TID) was 1.72 mcg/kg/day (range 0.59–3.05) and the mean maternal weight-adjusted dose was 1210 mcg/kg/day, resulting in a relative infant dose (RID) of 0.14% (range 0.068–0.249) (8).

In the case described in the Fetal Risk Summary, the mother exclusively breastfed her infant and, on day 32, milk and plasma samples (peak and trough) and a peak infant plasma sample were obtained (2). The milk:plasma ratios for the peak and trough collections were 1.2 and 1.3, respectively, whereas the drug was not detected in the infant plasma. The TID was 7.1 mcg/kg/day, whereas the mother's weight-adjusted dose was 868 mcg/kg/day. This yielded an RID of 0.82%. No signs of toxicity were noted in the infant at any time (2).

A 2010 study using human and animal models found that drugs that disturb serotonin balance such as SSRIs and SNRIs can impair lactation (9). The authors concluded that mothers taking these drugs may need additional support to achieve breastfeeding goals.

The presence of duloxetine in milk is consistent with the molecular weight (about 298 for the free base) and long elimination half-life (12 hours). Moreover, because milk is relatively acidic compared with blood, the milk:plasma ratio that was >1 also is consistent. Although no toxicity was observed in the above case, the long-term effects of exposure to duloxetine and similar antidepressants have not been adequately studied. The long-term effects on neurobehavior and cognitive development from exposure to potent SNRIs and SSRIs during a period of rapid CNS development have not been adequately studied. Therefore, the best course is to avoid duloxetine, if possible, during nursing. The American Academy of Pediatrics classifies antidepressants as drugs for which the effect on nursing infants is unknown but may be of concern (10).

References

1. Product information. Cymbalta. Eli Lilly, 2006.
2. Briggs GG, Ambrose PJ, Ilett KF, Hackett LP, Nageotte MP, Padilla G. Use of duloxetine in pregnancy and lactation. Ann Pharmacother 2009;43:1898–902.
3. Raskin J, Goldstein DJ, Mallinckrodt CH, Ferguson MB. Duloxetine in the long-term treatment of major depressive disorder. J Clin Psychiatry 2003;64:1237–44.
4. Bellantuono C, Migliarese G, Gentile S. Serotonin reuptake inhibitors in pregnancy and the risk of major malformations: a systematic review. Hum Psychopharmacol Clin Exp 2007;22:121–8.
5. Chambers CD, Hernandez-Diaz S, Van Marter LJ, Werler MM, Louik C, Jones KL, Mitchell AA. Selective serotonin-reuptake inhibitors and risk of persistent pulmonary hypertension of the newborn. N Engl J Med 2006;354:579–87.
6. Eyal R, Yaeger D. Poor neonatal adaptation after in utero exposure to duloxetine. Am J Psychiatry 2008;165:651.
7. Hoog SL, Cheng Y, Elpers J, Dowsett SA. Duloxetine and pregnancy outcomes: safety surveillance findings. Int J Med Sci 2013;10:413–9.
8. Lobo ED, Loghin C, Knadler M, Quinlan T, Zhang L, Chappell J, Lucas R, Bergstrom RF. Pharmacokinetics of duloxetine in breast milk and plasma of healthy postpartum women. Clin Pharmacokinet 2008;47:103–9.
9. Marshall AM, Nommsen-Rivers LA, Hernandez LI, Dewey KG, Chantry CJ, Gregerson KA, Horseman ND. Serotonin transport and metabolism in the mammary gland modulates secretory activation and involution. J Clin Endocrin Metab 2010;95:837–46.
10. Committee on Drugs. American Academy of Pediatrics. The transfer of drugs and other chemicals into human milk. Pediatrics 2001;108:776–89.

DYPHYLLINE

Respiratory Drug (Bronchodilator)

PREGNANCY RECOMMENDATION: Limited Human Data—No Relevant Animal Data
BREASTFEEDING RECOMMENDATION: Limited Human Data—Probably Compatible

PREGNANCY SUMMARY

The absence of animal reproductive data and the very limited human pregnancy experience prevent a complete assessment of the embryo–fetal risk. However, this xanthine derivative is closely related to theophylline, an agent considered compatible in pregnancy. (See also Theophylline.)

FETAL RISK SUMMARY

No published reports describing the use of dyphylline in human pregnancy have been located. In a surveillance study of Michigan Medicaid recipients involving 229,101 completed pregnancies conducted between 1985 and 1992, 97 newborns had been exposed to dyphylline during the 1st trimester (F. Rosa, personal communication, FDA, 1993). Seven (7.2%) major birth defects were observed (four expected), including (observed/expected) cardiovascular defects (3/1), and polydactyly (1/0.3). No anomalies were observed in four other categories of defects (oral clefts, spina bifida, limb reduction defects, and hypospadias) for which specific data were available. Only with cardiovascular defects is there a suggestion of a possible association, but other factors, including the mother's disease, concurrent drug use, and chance may be involved.

BREASTFEEDING SUMMARY

Dyphylline is excreted into breast milk. In 20 normal lactating women, a single 5 mg/kg IM dose produced an average milk:plasma ratio of 2.08 (1). The milk and serum elimination rates were equivalent. Although the drug accumulates in milk, the American Academy of Pediatrics classifies dyphylline as compatible with breastfeeding (2).

References

1. Jarboe CH, Cook LN, Malesic I, Fleischaker J. Dyphylline elimination kinetics in lactating women: blood to milk transfer. J Clin Pharmacol 1981;21:405–10.
2. Committee on Drugs, American Academy of Pediatrics. The transfer of drugs and other chemicals into human milk. Pediatrics 2001;108:776–89.

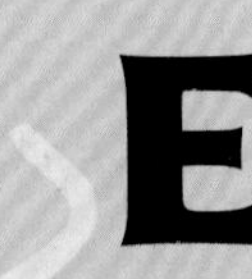

E

ECALLANTIDE

Hematological Agent (Kallikrein Inhibitor)

PREGNANCY RECOMMENDATION: No Human Data—Animal Data Suggest Low Risk
BREASTFEEDING RECOMMENDATION: No Human Data—Probably Compatible

PREGNANCY SUMMARY

No reports describing the use of ecallantide in human pregnancy have been located. The protein caused developmental toxicity (death) in one animal species, but the dose comparison was based on body weight, not BSA or AUC, and maternal toxicity was present. Although a rare genetic disorder, acute episodic attacks of hereditary angioedema can cause localized swelling, inflammation, and pain. If a pregnant woman requires ecallantide, consideration should be given to avoiding early gestation. She should be informed of the lack of human pregnancy experience and the potential risk of embryo death. Moreover, the woman should be informed of the risk of anaphylaxis that has occurred in 3.9% of treated patients (1).

FETAL RISK SUMMARY

Ecallantide, a small protein, is a human plasma kallikrein inhibitor. There are no other agents in this class. It is indicated for the treatment of acute attacks of hereditary angioedema in patients 16 years of age and older. After a single SC dose in healthy subjects, the mean elimination half-life was 2 hours. No information was provided for metabolism and plasma protein binding (1).

Reproduction studies have been conducted in rats and rabbits. In rats, an IV dose that was about 13 times the maximum recommended human dose (MRHD) based on body weight (MRHD-BW) caused increased numbers of early resorptions and percentages of resorbed conceptuses in the presence of mild maternal toxicity. No developmental toxicity was observed with IV doses that were about eight times the MRHD-BW. There were no adverse effects on rat embryo–fetal development with SC doses resulting in exposures up to about 2.4 times the MRHD based on AUC (MRHD-AUC). In rabbits, IV doses resulting in exposures up to about six times the MRHD-AUC were not associated with adverse effects on embryo–fetal development (1).

Studies for carcinogenic or mutagenic potential have not been conducted. SC doses up to about 21 times the MRHD-BW had no effect on fertility and reproductive performance in rats (1).

It is not known if ecallantide crosses the human placenta. The drug is a small protein with a molecular weight of 7054 and a short elimination half-life. These characteristics suggest that clinically significant amounts of the drug will not reach the embryo or fetus.

BREASTFEEDING SUMMARY

No reports describing the use of ecallantide during human lactation have been located. The drug is a small protein with a molecular weight of 7054 and a short 2-hour elimination half-life. These characteristics suggest that clinically significant amounts of the drug will not be excreted into breast milk. The risks to a nursing infant from exposure to the protein appear to be low, if they exist at all.

Reference

1. Product information. Kalbitor. Dyaz, 2009.

ECHINACEA

Herb

PREGNANCY RECOMMENDATION: Limited Human Data—No Relevant Animal Data
BREASTFEEDING RECOMMENDATION: No Human Data—Potential Toxicity

PREGNANCY SUMMARY

Echinacea is an ancient preparation that has recently undergone resurgence in use. Use during pregnancy creates the potential for exposure of the embryo and fetus to multiple chemical compounds that have not undergone reproductive toxicity testing in animals or humans. Moreover, standardization of any herbal product as to its constituents, concentrations, and the presence of contaminants are generally lacking. Two sources recommend that parenteral administration of the herb (a product form not available in the United States) should not be used in pregnancy (1,2). Another source states that echinacea should be avoided during pregnancy because of the lack of information (3). There is only one published report describing human pregnancy exposure. Although this study found no increased risk for major malformations, it was limited by its small sample size, the self-selection of the study group, and the lack of dose standardization (4). Thus, the safety of echinacea products during pregnancy remains to be established and, until such additional evidence is published, pregnant women should be counseled of such.

FETAL RISK SUMMARY

The traditional uses of echinacea are topically to enhance wound healing and systemically as an immunostimulant (5). It was used by the Native Americans before colonization of the continent and was a common medicine in the United States in the late 19th and early 20th centuries (6). The herb is available orally as capsules, as expressed, fresh juice, and as tinctures. In Germany, an intravenous preparation is also available (7). Specific indications for systemic echinacea listed in one publication are prophylaxis and treatment of viral upper respiratory tract infections and combined with conventional anti-infective agents in the treatment of more severe infections (6). Specific topical indications listed are the treatment of eczema, psoriasis, and herpes simplex. Another publication lists antiseptic and antiviral indications (8).

Echinacea angustifolia, the plant most commonly used for medicinal purposes, is a perennial herb of the Compositae family that grows to a height of 3 feet, terminating in a single colorful flower head. The plant is indigenous to the central United States. Related species that have been used in traditional medicine include *E. purpurea* and *E. pallida* (5,9). Because *E. angustifolia* and *E. pallida* closely resemble each other, preparations of echinacea may be mislabeled or contain mixtures of the two species. German authors recommend the use of the above-ground parts (not the roots) of *E. purpurea* or the roots of *E. angustifolia* for medicinal purposes (9).

The principal anti-inflammatory and immunostimulant compounds are found in the hydrophilic and lipophilic fractions of the root, leaves, and flowers (5,6). The specific active ingredients accounting for the medicinal effects of the herb have not been identified. The water-soluble polysaccharides in the roots, however, appear to be a major component of the anti-inflammatory and immune-stimulating properties (6). Essential oil from the root also contains unsaturated alkyl ketones and isobutylamides. Although not all components from the various parts of the plant have been identified, the chemical compounds that have been isolated include echinacoside (a caffeic acid glycoside), a volatile germacrene alcohol (not usually found in dried plant material), echinacein (an isobutylamide responsible for the pungent odor), echinacin B, chicoric acid, cyanrine, chlorogenic acid, caftaric acid, (z)-1,8-pentadecadiene (also known as Z-pentadeca-1,8-diene), and arabinogalactan (5,6).

No animal studies examining the reproductive effects of any of the species of echinacea or their components have been located. One prospective report, however, described the use of this herb in human pregnancies (4). Between 1996 and 1998, 206 women contacted a teratogen information service regarding their exposure to echinacea products (primarily *E. angustifolia* and *E. purpurea*) during gestation. Of these, 112 used echinacea during the 1st trimester. The total cohort was disease matched to 206 women exposed to nonteratogenic agents by maternal age, alcohol, and cigarette use. There were three sets of twins in the study group and none in the control group. Both groups were followed prospectively to determine pregnancy outcomes. No statistically significant differences between the study and control women were found for the following outcomes: live birth (94.7% vs. 96.1%), spontaneous abortion (6.3% vs. 3.4%), induced abortion (0.5% vs. 0.5%), vaginal delivery (83.1% vs. 81.3%), maternal weight gain (15.2 vs. 14.4 kg), gestational age at delivery (39.2 vs. 39.2 weeks), birth weight (3466 vs. 3451 g) (excluding twins), fetal distress (23.6% vs. 21.1%), major malformations (in total group) (3.6% vs. 3.5%), and minor malformations (3.6% vs. 3.5%). Among the 98 newborns exposed during the 1st trimester, there were four (4.1%) major defects: left inguinal hernia requiring surgical repair; bilateral hydronephrosis; syndactyly of the second and third toes; and duplicate left renal pelvis. The authors concluded that there was no increased risk for major anomalies (4).

An in vitro study using *E. purpura* reported adverse effects in human sperm (10). In a sperm penetration assay, zona-free hamster oocytes were incubated for 1 hour with two concentrations of *E. purpura*, 0.8 and 8 mg/mL, dissolved in HEPES-buffered synthetic human tubal fluid (modified HTF). Fresh human donor sperm was suspended in the modified HTF and then mixed with the oocytes for 3 hours. Modified HTF served as the control. At the 0.8 mg/mL concentration, 5 of 9 (56%) of the oocytes were penetrated, whereas at 8 mg/mL, only 1 of 8 (13%) of oocytes was penetrated. The decrease in penetration was not associated with a decrease in sperm motility. In the second part of the study, sperm were incubated with the herbal solutions for 7 days. Both concentrations caused significant sperm DNA denaturation concomitant with decreases in sperm viability compared with controls. Extrapolation of these data to the reproductive risk of echinacea in males is difficult, in part because the concentration of echinacea in semen or sperm has not been studied (10). Moreover, although the doses used in this study are small fractions of the actual recommended human dose, there is no published evidence that the adverse effects observed have occurred in vivo.

BREASTFEEDING SUMMARY

No reports describing the use of echinacea during lactation have been located. For the reasons discussed above, and because of the immaturity of an infant's metabolic and elimination systems, use of this herb should probably be avoided during nursing.

References

1. Blumenthal M, ed. Echinacea purpurea herb. In: *The Complete German Commission E Monographs: Therapeutic Guide to Herbal Medicines*. Austin, TX: American Botanical Council, 1998:122–3.
2. *PDR for Herbal Medicines*. Montvale, NJ: Medical Economics Company, 1998:816–23.
3. *Natural Medicines Comprehensive Database*. 3rd ed. Stockton, CA: Therapeutic Research Faculty, 2000:388–90.
4. Gallo M, Sarkar M, Au W, Pietrzak K, Comas B, Smith M, Jaeger TV, Einarson A, Koren G. Pregnancy outcome following gestational exposure to echinacea. A prospective controlled study. Arch Intern Med 2000;160:3141–3.
5. Echinacea. *The Review of Natural Products*. St. Louis, MO: Facts and Comparisons, 1996.
6. Pepping J. Alternative therapies: Echinacea. Am J Health-Syst Pharm 1999;56:121–2.
7. Zink T, Chaffin J. Herbal 'health' products: what family physicians need to know. Am Fam Physician 1998;58:1133–40.
8. Ernst E. Harmless herbs? A review of the recent literature. Am J Med 1998;104:170–8.
9. Miller LG. Herbal medicinals. Selected clinical considerations focusing on known or potential drug-herb interactions. Arch Intern Med 1998;158:2200–11.
10. Ondrizek RR, Chan PJ, Patton WC, King A. An alternative medicine study of herbal effects on the penetration of zona-free hamster oocytes and the integrity of sperm deoxyribonucleic acid. Fertil Steril 1999;71:517–22.

ECHOTHIOPHATE

Parasympathomimetic (Cholinergic)

PREGNANCY RECOMMENDATION: Limited Human Data—Probably Compatible
BREASTFEEDING RECOMMENDATION: No Human Data—Probably Compatible

PREGNANCY SUMMARY

Echothiophate is a long-acting, relatively irreversible organophosphate that is used in the eye for its anticholinesterase activity. One report of its use in pregnancy has been located.

FETAL RISK SUMMARY

As a quaternary ammonium compound, echothiophate is ionized at physiologic pH and transplacental passage in significant amounts would not be expected (see also Neostigmine). However, 1968 case report suggested otherwise. A 22-year-old woman was treated with echothiophate iodide 0.125% instilled daily into both eyes and acetazolamide 1 g/day (1). She became pregnant shortly after starting this treatment, which was continued until 32 weeks' at which time the therapy was changed to pilocarpine and betamethasone eye drops. Two months later, a normal, full-term female infant was born. Pseudocholinesterase activity was measured in the mother and infant at 10 days, 28 days, and 3 months after birth. Increasing activity with time was shown in both mother and infant. The authors concluded that the drug had crossed the placenta to lower the enzyme activity in the fetus (1).

BREASTFEEDING SUMMARY

No reports describing the use of echothiophate during human lactation have been located.

Reference

1. Birks DA, Prior VJ. Echothiophate iodide treatment of glaucoma in pregnancy. Arch Ophthal 1968;79:283–5.

ECONAZOLE

Antifungal

PREGNANCY RECOMMENDATION: Compatible
BREASTFEEDING RECOMMENDATION: No Human Data—Probably Compatible

PREGNANCY SUMMARY

Topical econazole does not appear to represent a risk to the human fetus. No teratogenic effects were observed in three animal species following oral and SC dosing that produced systemic exposures far greater than those obtained in humans. The very low systemic bioavailability of this antifungal agent after topical or vaginal application prevents clinically significant amounts from reaching the maternal circulation. Although details of the available human pregnancy experience are incomplete, the risk to an embryo or fetus from the maternal use of econazole appears to be nil. However, one study speculated that antifungals that inhibit placental aromatase, such as econazole, have a potential to cause spontaneous abortions. Until additional data are available on this potential association, the best course is to avoid the use of econazole for vaginitis treatment in the 1st trimester or the application of the antifungal to large areas of skin at any time in pregnancy.

E

FETAL RISK SUMMARY

Econazole is available only in a topical cream formulation. Vaginal suppositories, spray powder, lotion, and spray solution are available outside of the United States. Econazole is in the same antifungal class of imidazole derivatives as butoconazole, clotrimazole, ketoconazole, miconazole, oxiconazole, sertaconazole, sulconazole, and tioconazole. It is indicated for the treatment of dermatologic fungal infections including candidiasis. Systemic absorption from the skin or vagina is minimal, with less than 1% of a dose absorbed and recovered in the urine and feces (1–3).

In reproduction studies with oral econazole, no evidence of teratogenicity was observed in mice, rats, or rabbits. Oral doses 10–80 times the human dermal dose, however, did cause embryo and fetal toxicity in some or all members of these species. In addition, prolonged gestation was observed in rats (1). SC doses have also been studied in pregnant mice and rabbits (4). Although no teratogenicity was observed, prolonged gestation and/or fetal death were noted.

It is not known if econazole nitrate crosses the human placenta. The molecular weight (about 445) is low enough, but the amount of drug in the systemic circulation is very low. It is doubtful that clinically significant amounts of the antifungal agent reach the embryo or fetus.

A 1979 report described the use of econazole vaginal suppositories (150 mg at bedtime for 3 days) for the treatment of vaginal candidiasis (5). Some patients required a second course of therapy. Among the patients treated, 24 were pregnant, but the gestational timing of the treatment and pregnancy outcomes were not provided. In a 1981 study, 33 women in various phases of gestation used the same dose and route of administration (6). A second 3-day course of treatment was given to nine of these patients. No details on pregnancy outcomes were reported.

Pregnancy outcome after treatment with a 3-day regimen of econazole vaginal suppositories for vaginal candidiasis was detailed in a 1985 open study (7). Treated were 117 pregnant women with a mean gestational age of 30 weeks (range 10–42 weeks), 44.4% at or after the 36th week of gestation. The number of patients in each trimester was not specified. In 106 pregnancies for which outcome data were available (107 infants, including one set of twins), 13 deliveries were premature. No prolongation of gestation was observed. There were three stillbirths among the 107 infants: one twin; one after intrauterine infection (no fungus recovered); and one death in utero. No congenital defects were observed in the 104 healthy newborns. The mean weight and height were 3301 g and 50.3 cm, respectively. One newborn developed oral thrush, but the mother was still infected at delivery (7).

A 2002 study evaluated azole antifungals commonly used in pregnancy for their potential to inhibit placental aromatase, an enzyme that is critical for the production of estrogen and for the maintenance of pregnancy (8). The authors speculated that the embryotoxicity observed in animals and humans (see also Clotrimazole, Miconazole, and Sulconazole) might be explained by inhibition of aromatase. They found that the most potent inhibitors of aromatase were (shown in order of decreasing potency) econazole, bifonazole (not available in the United States), sulconazole, clotrimazole, and miconazole. However, an earlier study reported a pregnancy that was maintained even when there was severe fetal and placental aromatase deficiency (<0.3% of that of controls) caused by a rare genetic defect (9). In this case, both the fetus and mother were virilized because of diminished conversion of androgens to estrogen. Because the pregnancy was maintained and the virilization, the case suggested that the main function of placental aromatase was to protect the mother and fetus from exposure to adrenal androgens (9).

A population-based case–control study of vaginal econazole in pregnancy was conducted using the Hungarian Case–Control Surveillance of Congenital Abnormalities (10). The study compared 22,843 case women who had newborn infants with a congenital defect with 38,151 controls. Vaginal econazole treatment was used in 68 cases and 122 controls. The crude prevalence odds ratio was 0.9, 95% confidence interval 0.7–1.3 (*ns*). There also was no evidence that econazole use in the 2nd and 3rd month of pregnancy was associated with teratogenicity (10).

BREASTFEEDING SUMMARY

Although no reports describing the use of topical or vaginal econazole during lactation have been located, the very low systemic bioavailability after topical use suggests that little, if any, of this antifungal will be excreted into breast milk. Therefore, the risk of this exposure to a nursing infant appears to be nil.

References

1. Product information. Spectazole. Ortho-McNeil Pharmaceuticals, 2001.
2. Parfitt K, ed. *Martindale. The Complete Drug Reference*. 32nd ed. London, UK: Pharmaceutical Press, 1999:377.
3. Econazole Nitrate. *Drug Facts and Comparisons*. 2000:1612.
4. Maruoka H, Kadota Y, Upshima M, Uesako T, Takemoto Y, Sato H. Toxicological studies on econazole nitrate. 4. Teratological studies in mice and rabbits. Iyakuhin Kenkyu 1978;9:955–70. As cited in Shepard TH. *Catalog of Teratogenic Agents*. 10th ed. Baltimore, MD: The Johns Hopkins University Press, 2001:189.
5. Lecart C, Claerhout F, Franck R, Godts P, Lilien C, Macours L, Schuerwegh, Longree H, Mine M, Strebelle P, Van Gijsegem M, Wesel S. A new treatment of vaginal candidiasis: three-day treatment with econazole. Eur J Obstet Gynecol Reprod Biol 1979;9:125–7.
6. Karoussos K, Carvalho A, Coelho P, Gomes V, Graca L, Carvalho J, Bacelar Autunes A, Andrade C, Filipe G, Helena Pereira M. Gyno-Pevaryl 150: a new drug for the treatment of vaginal candidosis. J Int Med Res 1981;9:165–7.

7. Goormans E, Beck JM, Declercq JA, Loendersloot EW, Roelofs HJM, van Zanten A. Efficacy of econazole ('Gyno-Pevaryl' 150) in vaginal candidosis during pregnancy. Curr Med Res Opin 1985;9:371–7.
8. Kragie L, Turner SD, Patten CJ, Crespi CL, Stresser DM. Assessing pregnancy risks of azole antifungals using a high throughput aromatase inhibition assay. Endocr Res 2002;28:129–40.
9. Harada N. Genetic analysis of human placental aromatase deficiency. J Steroid Biochem Mol Biol 1993;44:331–40.
10. Czeizel AE, Kazy Z, Vargha P. A population-based case-control teratological study of vaginal econazole treatment during pregnancy. Eur J Obstet Gynecol Reprod Biol 2003;111:135–40.

ECSTASY

Central Stimulant

PREGNANCY RECOMMENDATION: **Contraindicated**
BREASTFEEDING RECOMMENDATION: **Contraindicated**

PREGNANCY SUMMARY

The use of amphetamines under controlled conditions, such as 3,4-methylenedioxymethamphetamine (MDMA) in the animal studies above and as amphetamines in the treatment of human disease (see Amphetamine), suggests that these agents are not teratogenic when used alone and do not cause clinically significant fetal toxicity. Other abuse drugs (e.g., lysergic acid diethylamide [LSD] and marijuana) are also not teratogenic (see Lysergic Acid Diethylamide and Marijuana), but alcohol and cocaine are well-known teratogens and/or fetal toxins (see Cocaine and Ethanol). However, ecstasy is not used under controlled conditions. Neither the dosage nor the actual chemical consumed is usually known and, in many cases, the product is taken with other abuse drugs. Because both human studies involved voluntary reporting, a true incidence of major congenital defects cannot be determined, but there does not appear to be a clustering of similar anomalies.

FETAL RISK SUMMARY

In the United States, ecstasy ("Adam"), a central stimulant, is an illicit substance of abuse that is used for its mind-altering properties. It has been associated with dance events known as "raves" (1). Chemically, ecstasy is a member of the amphetamine (3,4-methylenedioxymethamphetamine; MDMA) class of drugs (see also Amphetamine) (1,2).

A brief 2000 publication reported the results of a chemical analysis of 107 pills of ecstasy that were voluntarily and anonymously donated to the authors for analysis after a nationwide solicitation (1). However, because the donors were required to pay a fee for the analysis, the findings may not represent what is actually available. Of the total, only 67 pills (63%) contained some MDMA or a closely related analog (either 3,4-methylenedioxy-ethyl-amphetamine or 3,4-methylenedioxyamphetamine) (1). Forty (37%) contained no MDMA or related amphetamine. Of these, 23 (58%) contained the antitussive dextromethorphan (see also Dextromethorphan) and 9 (23%) contained no identifiable drug. Other substances identified were caffeine, ephedrine, pseudoephedrine, and salicylates (1).

MDMA was not teratogenic in pregnant rats at oral doses of 2.5 or 10 mg/kg/day administered on alternate days from gestational day 6 to day 18 (3). The drug had no effect on gestational duration, litter sizes, or birth weights. Although most pup neurobehavior parameters were unaffected, olfactory discrimination was enhanced in both males and females, and negative geotaxis was delayed in females. However, the density of brain serotonin-uptake sites and levels of brain serotonin and 5-hydroxyindoleacetic acid (5-HIAA; metabolite of serotonin) were not affected. There was a significant reduction of maternal weight and a dose-dependent decrease in maternal brain serotonin (5-HT) (3).

In another study with pregnant rats, MDMA 20 mg/kg SC was administered twice daily on days 14–17 of gestation (4). Marked, long-lasting maternal hyperthermia was observed after the first dose, but the response was attenuated with further doses. The body weight of the dams decreased during treatment and there was a 20% decrease in litter size. There was a slight reduction in pup weights on postnatal day 7, but the difference was not statistically significant compared with controls. In the dams, a significant decrease in the concentration of 5-HT and 5-HIAA in the hippocampus, striatum, and cortex of the brain were measured 1 week after parturition (i.e., nearly 2 weeks after the last dose). In contrast, neither the 5-HT nor 5-HIAA level in the dorsal telencephalon of the pups was different from that of controls. The lack of MDMA-induced toxicity in the fetal brains suggested that either MDMA was not being metabolized to free radical-producing entities or the fetal brains were more efficient than adult brains in eliminating the toxic free radical metabolites (4).

Although there is no information on the placental passage of MDMA, other amphetamines rapidly cross the human placenta (see Amphetamine). Moreover, the relatively low molecular weight of MDMA (about 179, compared with about 135 for amphetamine) suggests that it also rapidly crosses to the fetus.

An abstract published in 1998 described the pregnancy outcomes of 49 women who had called a teratology information service (TIS) in Holland concerning their exposure to pure MDMA or to closely related amphetamines (methylene dioxyamphetamine [MDA]; methylene dioxyethylamphetamine [MDEA]; or other) (5). In 47 cases, the exposure occurred during the 1st trimester; the other 2 were in the 2nd trimester. The mean age of the women was 26 (range 17–44). Other abuse drugs, usually cocaine or marijuana, were taken by

43%, 34% of the women drank alcohol, and 63% of the women smoked cigarettes. Eleven pregnancies were still ongoing. The outcomes of the remaining 38 pregnancies were 2 spontaneous abortions, 2 elective abortions (1 fetus with a defect suggestive of an omphalocele), and 36 liveborn infants (6 premature including one set of triplets). One term newborn, exposed in utero to ecstasy alone, had a congenital heart defect and died a few hours after birth (5).

E

A 1999 report from the United Kingdom National TIS cited 302 inquiries from pregnant women concerning ecstasy from January 1989 to June 1998 (6). Of the total, 31 pregnancies were ongoing and 135 were lost to follow-up. Outcome data were available for 136 pregnancies (1 set of twins). Among this group, 74 women took only ecstasy, and 62 took ecstasy with other drugs, including amphetamines (N = 37), cocaine (N = 20), marijuana (N = 16), alcohol (N = 13), and/or LSD (N = 9). Exposure to ecstasy was limited to the 1st trimester in 127 pregnancies (71 to ecstasy alone, 56 to ecstasy plus other drugs of abuse), to the 1st and 2nd trimesters in 2, to the 2nd trimester in 2, to the 3rd trimester in 1, and throughout gestation in 4. Thus, 133 of the pregnancies (98%) were exposed to ecstasy in the 1st trimester. The outcomes included 11 spontaneous abortions (8%) and 48 elective abortions (35%). One elective abortion occurred at 22 weeks' gestation because of a fetus with absent upper limbs, left scapula, clavicles, and hypoplasticity of the first rib pair. The mother said she had taken only ecstasy during the 1st trimester. No data were available on the other aborted fetuses. There were 12 infants with congenital defects among the 78 born live infants (15.4%, 95% confidence interval [CI] 8.2–25.4). One newborn (without apparent birth defects), who was exposed in utero to ecstasy, heroin, and methadone throughout pregnancy died from an unknown cause. The birth defects and drug exposures (all in the 1st trimester except 1 case) were ecstasy only (6 cases): left 4th toe underlying 3rd toe, right-sided plagiocephaly, 2 with unilateral talipes, bilateral talipes, pyloric stenosis; ecstasy and amphetamine (2 cases): clicking hips, intrauterine growth restriction, ambiguous sex (1 of twins born at 25 weeks'); ecstasy, amphetamine, and gamma hydroxybutyric acid (1 case): ventricular septal defect (VSD) (possibly atrial and ventricular), bilateral hydronephrosis, bilateral clinodactyly; ecstasy and alcohol (3 cases): VSD, pigmentation of the right thigh, ptosis of left eye (exposed in 2nd trimester). There were three female infants with talipes (3.8%, 95% CI 8–109) compared with the expected rate of 0.1% (6). In addition, in Great Britain, there is a 3:1 male predominance of idiopathic talipes equinovarus (6). Neither the sex ratio nor birth weights of term infants (specific data not provided) were adversely affected by the exposures (6).

BREASTFEEDING SUMMARY

No reports describing the use of ecstasy or MDMA during human lactation have been located. The molecular weight (about 179) is low enough, however, that excretion into milk should be expected. The closely related drug amphetamine is concentrated in breast milk with milk:plasma ratios ranging from 2.8 to 7.5 (see Amphetamine). The American Academy of Pediatrics classifies amphetamines as contraindicated during breastfeeding (7).

References

1. Baggott M, Heifets B, Jones RT, Mendelson J, Sferios E, Zehnder J. Chemical analysis of ecstasy pills. JAMA 2000;284:2190.
2. Plessinger MA. Prenatal exposure to amphetamines. Risks and adverse outcomes in pregnancy. Obstet Gynecol Clin North Am 1998;25:119–38.
3. St Omer VEV, Ali SF, Holson RR, Duhart HM, Scalzo FM, Slikker W Jr. Behavioral and neurochemical effects of prenatal methylenedioxymethamphetamine (MDMA) exposure in rats. Neurotoxicol Teratol 1991;13:13–20.
4. Colado MI, O'Shea E, Granados R, Misra A, Murray TK, Green AR. A study of the neurotoxic effect of MDMA ('ecstasy') on 5-HT neurones in the brains of mothers and neonates following administration of the drug during pregnancy. Br J Pharmacol 1997;121:827–33.
5. van Tonningen MR, Garbis H, Reuvers M. Ecstasy exposure during pregnancy (abstract). Teratology 1998;58:33A.
6. McElhatton PR, Bateman DN, Evans C, Pughe KR, Thomas SHL. Congenital anomalies after prenatal ecstasy exposure. Lancet 1999;354:1441–2.
7. Committee on Drugs, American Academy of Pediatrics. The transfer of drugs and other chemicals into human milk. Pediatrics 2001;108:776–89.

ECULIZUMAB

Immunologic Agent (Antihemolysis)

PREGNANCY RECOMMENDATION: Maternal Benefit >> Embryo–Fetal Risk
BREASTFEEDING RECOMMENDATION: No Human Data—Probably Compatible

PREGNANCY SUMMARY

The human pregnancy experience with eculizumab is very limited. The animal data from one species, using a murine version of the antibody, suggest risk. However, eculizumab is indicated for paroxysmal nocturnal hemoglobinuria (PNH), a high-risk complication in pregnancy manifested by hemolytic anemia, bone marrow failure, and thrombosis (1–3). Significant morbidity and mortality have occurred from PNH-induced venous thromboembolism with maternal and perinatal mortality up to 20% and 10%, respectively (1). Supportive therapy (red blood cells and platelet transfusions) and routine prophylactic anticoagulation are recommended. Moreover, there also is a need for additional iron and folic acid supplements because of the hemolysis. In nonpregnant and the limited number of pregnant patients, the use of eculizumab, usually in combination with low-molecular-weight heparin (LMWH), has reduced the need for transfusions and the rate of hemolytic episodes and thrombosis (1–3). Thus, if indicated, the maternal benefit appears to far outweigh the unknown embryo–fetal risk.

FETAL RISK SUMMARY

Eculizumab, an anti-C5 antibody, is a recombinant humanized monoclonal $IgG_{2/4K}$ antibody that contains human constant regions from IgG2 and IgG4 sequences. It is given as an IV infusion once weekly for 5 weeks and then every 2 weeks. The antibody binds to the complement protein C5 to inhibit its cleavage thereby preventing terminal complement mediated intravascular hemolysis. Eculizumab is indicated for the treatment of patients with PNH to reduce hemolysis. Eculizumab increases a patient's susceptibility to serious meningococcal infections (septicemia and/or meningitis), so all patients must be given meningococcal vaccine at least 2 weeks before starting eculizumab therapy and revaccinated according to current medical guidelines. The half-life of the antibody is 272 hours (4).

Reproduction studies have been conducted in mice using a murine anti-C5 antibody. Mice were given doses that were about 2–4 times (low dose) or 4–8 times (high dose) the recommended human dose based on body weight (RHD). When maternal exposure occurred during organogenesis, two cases of retinal dysplasia and one case of umbilical hernia were observed in the high-dose group among 230 offspring. There was no increase in fetal loss or neonatal death. When the antibody was given from implantation through weaning, male offspring had an increased risk of death (1/25 controls, 2/25 low-dose group, and 5/25 high-dose group). Surviving offspring had normal development and reproductive performance (4).

Carcinogenic and mutagenic studies have not been conducted with eculizumab. No effects on reproductive performance or fertility were observed in male and female mice given IV doses of the murine anti-C5 antibody up to 4–8 times the RHD (4).

Although the molecular weight (about 148,000) is very high, the manufacturer states that the antibody is expected to cross the human placenta (4). There are data suggesting that all IgG subtypes can potentially cross the placenta but the IgG2 sequence having the least transfer of the subtypes (3). However, in two newborns (one at term and the other at 28 weeks'), the antibody was not detected in cord blood; in two others (twins at 35 weeks'), low levels within the background level for the assay were found (see reference 8). These cases suggest that the fetus will not be exposed to clinical significant concentrations of eculizumab.

In a 2006 correspondence, brief mention was made of a woman who became pregnant during a study of eculizumab in PNH, even though pregnancy was a study exclusion (5). Eculizumab therapy was discontinued and the woman had a successful full-term birth without complications.

A 34-year-old woman with PNH was treated with eculizumab in a twin pregnancy resulting from in vitro fertilization (6). Her first pregnancy 2 years earlier had ended with a spontaneous abortion (SAB) at 6 weeks' despite anticoagulation with LMWH. Ongoing active hemolysis before and during the current pregnancy was documented and the patient was treated with therapeutic LMWH. At 30 weeks', eculizumab was started with the recommended induction dose of 600 mg weekly for 4 weeks, followed by 900 mg every other week and LMWH was continued. At 35 weeks', thrombocytopenia (60,000/μL) and increasing peripheral edema were observed. One week later, a cesarean section was conducted to deliver a 2919-g male infant and a 2199-g female infant with Apgar scores of 9 and 10 and 8 and 9, respectively. The female twin had an obstructed duplicated kidney that had been diagnosed early in the pregnancy. No additional information was provided on the status of the twins (6).

A 2010 reference described the pregnancy outcomes of seven women exposed to eculizumab for the treatment of PNH (7). All of the patients were initially on the standard maintenance dose of 900 mg every 2 weeks unless specified otherwise. Five of these cases were from the 106 women enrolled in clinical trials of the antibody in PNH. In one case, the woman underwent an elective abortion (EAB) and continued on eculizumab. In three cases, eculizumab was discontinued at 4, 5, and 14 weeks' gestation, respectively. All delivered healthy newborns without any adverse effects. The fifth patient conceived after having been on eculizumab for 5 years. She withdrew from the trial and continued the antibody combined with LMWH throughout pregnancy. Because of breakthrough hemolysis, the eculizumab dosing interval was reduced to 12 days. She gave birth vaginally at term to a healthy, 4-kg male infant. The mother had a therapeutic eculizumab concentration (116.1 mcg/mL; time from last dose not specified) at delivery but the antibody was not detected in cord blood. The sixth patient, with twins, was treated with eculizumab for 2 years before stopping therapy for embryo implantation. She was maintained on therapeutic LMWH. At 27 weeks', eculizumab was restarted with the recommended induction regime (600 mg every week for 4 weeks, then 900 mg every 2 weeks) but, because of continued intravascular hemolysis and hemoglobinuria, the 900 mg maintenance dosing interval was shortened to once weekly. An elective cesarean section at 35 weeks' delivered two healthy infants (sex not specified) weighing 2.4 kg and 2 kg, respectively. At delivery, the mother had a therapeutic antibody concentration (80.5 mcg/mL; time from last dose not specified). The cord blood samples from the twins had subtherapeutic eculizumab concentrations (19.2 and 14.4 mcg/mL) that were within the background level for the assay. Patient number 7 had been receiving eculizumab and warfarin for PNH before conception. She also had chronic hypertension. At 5 weeks' gestation, warfarin was discontinued and replaced with LMWH. At 28 weeks', preeclampsia developed and a cesarean section delivered a 900-g infant (sex not specified). The mother had a therapeutic eculizumab concentration (63.2 mcg/mL; time from last dose not specified) at delivery but the antibody was not detected in cord blood. The mother and baby were doing well (7,8).

Another 2010 report described the pregnancy outcome of a 29-year-old woman with PNH who had been treated with eculizumab for 3 years before conception (9). Although the patient had never had thrombotic complications, LMWH was added when her pregnancy was discovered. Eculizumab and LMWH were continued throughout an uneventful pregnancy. At 38 weeks', she vaginally delivered a healthy 3.43-kg male infant with Apgar scores of 9 and 10 at 1 and 5 minutes, respectively. At 9 months of age, the infant was developing normally (9).

In a 2013 case report, a 26-year-old white woman at 17 weeks' had a recurrence of atypical hemolytic uremic syndrome that was initially controlled with multiple plasma exchanges with fresh-frozen plasma (10). The disease recurred at 26 weeks' and she was treated with IV eculizumab 900 mg every 14 days until a cesarean section at 38 weeks'. The healthy, 3650-g female infant had Apgar scores of 9 and 10 at 1 and 5 minutes, respectively. The infant had normal laboratory values and was discharged home after 1 week (10).

BREASTFEEDING SUMMARY

No reports describing the use of eculizumab during human lactation have been located. In a case described above where the mother received eculizumab (900 mg) at 12-day intervals and had a therapeutic serum concentration (116.1 mcg/mL) at delivery, the antibody was not detected in milk samples obtained on postpartum days 1, 2, 3, 9, and 10 (8). Neither the time of the last dose nor the detection limit of the assay was specified. Nevertheless, the findings are compatible with the high molecular weight (about 148,000) of eculizumab. However, because human IgG is found in milk, additional reports are required to confirm that eculizumab is not excreted in detectable amounts.

The manufacturer states that published data suggest that breast milk antibodies are not systemically absorbed by nursing infants in substantial amounts (4). Consequently, breastfeeding by women receiving eculizumab is probably compatible, but meningococcal infections are a serious potential risk. Moreover, nursing infants should be closely observed for the most common (>10%) adverse effects observed in adults: headache, nasopharyngitis, back pain, nausea, fatigue, and cough.

References

1. Ziakas PD, Poulou LS, Pomoni A. Thrombosis in paroxysmal nocturnal hemoglobinuria at a glance: a clinical review. Curr Vasc Pharmacol 2008;6:347–53.
2. Brodsky RA. How I treat paroxysmal nocturnal hemoglobinuria. Blood 2009;113:6522–7.
3. Danilov AV, Brodsky RA, Craigo S, Smith H, Miller KB. Managing a pregnant patient with paroxysmal nocturnal hemoglobinuria in the era of eculizumab. Leuk Res 2010;34:566–71.
4. Product information. Solaris. Alexion Pharmaceuticals, 2009.
5. Hillmen P. Eculizumab in paroxysmal nocturnal hemoglobinuria. Author reply. N Engl J Med 2006;355:2787–8.
6. Danilov AV, Smith H, Craigo S, Feeney DM, Relias V, Miller KB. Paroxysmal nocturnal hemoglobinuria (PNH) and pregnancy in the era of eculizumab. Leuk Res 2009;33:e4–5.
7. Kelly R, Arnold L, Richards S, Hill A, Bomken C, Hanley J, Loughney A, Beauchamp J, Khursigara G, Rother RP, Chalmers E, Fyfe A, Fitzsimons E, Nakamura R, Gaya A, Rotoli B, Risitano AM, Schubert J, Hillmen P. Successful pregnancy outcome in paroxysmal nocturnal haemoglobinuria on long term eculizumab. Haematologica 2009;94:452 (Abstract).
8. Kelly R, Arnold L, Richards S, Hill A, Bomken C, Hanley J, Loughney A, Beauchamp J, Khursigara G, Rother RP, Chalmers E, Fyfe A, Fitzsimons E, Nakamura R, Gaya A, Risitano AM, Schubert J, Norfolk D, Simpson N, Hillmen P. The management of pregnancy in paroxysmal nocturnal haemoglobinuria on long term eculizumab. Br J Haematol 2010;149: 446–50.
9. Marasca R, Coluccio V, Santachiara R, Leonardi G, Torelli G, Notaro R, Luzzatto L. Pregnancy in PNH: another eculizumab baby. Br J Haematol 2010;150:707–8.
10. Ardissino G, Ossola MW, Baffero GM, Rigotti A, Cugno M. Eculizumab for atypical hemolytic uremic syndrome in pregnancy. Obstet Gynecol 2013;122:487–9.

EDETATE CALCIUM DISODIUM

Antidote

PREGNANCY RECOMMENDATION: Compatible—Maternal Benefit >> Embryo–Fetal Risk
BREASTFEEDING RECOMMENDATION: Contraindicated

PREGNANCY SUMMARY

Only two reports of human pregnancy experience with edetate, both involving a short course in late gestation, have been located. Moreover, interpretation of the rat study is hindered by the presumed oral administration of edetate, a drug that is poorly absorbed from the gastrointestinal (GI) tract. That study did suggest, however, that the observed fetal malformations were induced by zinc deficiency. The human cases and limited animal data are insufficient to assess the risk for the human embryo and fetus. Dietary zinc supplementation might be an option if prolonged treatment with edetate calcium disodium was required during pregnancy, but this has not been studied. In addition, hypotension is a reported adverse effect in adults, and in a pregnant patient, this could jeopardize placental perfusion and the fetus. However, lead is a well-known reproductive toxicant that has significant associations with preterm birth, reduced birth weight and postnatal growth, minor congenital anomalies, and deficits in postnatal neurological or neurobehavioral status (1). Therefore, if indicated, the maternal, and possibly the embryo–fetal, benefit of therapy appear to outweigh any unknown direct or indirect risks (2).

FETAL RISK SUMMARY

The chelating agent edetate calcium disodium (edetate) is the calcium chelate of disodium ethylenediaminetetraacetate. It is indicated for the reduction of blood levels and depot stores of lead in acute or chronic lead poisoning and lead encephalopathy. Edetate also forms stable chelates with other divalent or trivalent metals that can displace calcium, such as cadmium, iron, manganese, mercury, and zinc, but not copper. However, insignificant amounts of iron and manganese are chelated, and mercury is either too tightly bound to be chelated or is stored in inaccessible body compartments. In contrast, the excretion of zinc is significantly increased. Edetate must be given by injection (IM preferred but also by IV) because it is poorly absorbed from the GI tract. The drug is not metabolized and is excreted by the kidneys with an elimination half-life of 20–60 minutes (3).

Reproduction studies have been conducted in pregnant rats. In one study, doses up to 13 times the human dose (presumed to be based on body weight) revealed no evidence of impaired fertility or fetal harm. In a second study, doses up to about 25–40 times the human dose caused fetal malformations, but the anomalies were prevented by simultaneous supplementation of dietary zinc (3).

A 1998 review summarized the developmental toxicity of metal chelating agents, including ethylenediaminetetraacetic acid (EDTA) and its salts (disodium, trisodium, calcium disodium, and tetrasodium edetate) (4). The author cited several animal studies showing teratogenicity that was proven to be secondary to EDTA-induced zinc deficiency. Different incidences of teratogenicity were observed depending on the route of administration (IV, SC, gavage, or diet) and dose. In one study, oral administration of EDTA and its salts, even at maternally toxic doses, had little or no teratogenic effects in rats. The different outcomes were thought to be partially due to poor absorption of the compounds after oral administration (4).

It is not known if edetate crosses the human placenta to the embryo or fetus. The molecular weight (about 374) is low enough for transfer to the fetus. In addition, small amounts of the drug cross the blood–brain barrier as about 5% of the plasma concentration can be found in spinal fluid. However, the very short elimination half-life will limit the amount of drug at the maternal–fetal interface.

The first known case of lead poisoning treated with edetate in a pregnant woman was reported in 1964 (5). A family of six (father, mother, and four male siblings) was diagnosed with lead poisoning caused by using battery cases as fuel in the living room stove for several months. The mother, who was 8 months pregnant, had a blood lead level of 0.24 mg/dL. She was treated with a 7-day course of edetate (75 mg/kg/day). Four weeks later, she delivered an apparently healthy 3.2-kg male infant. The cord blood lead level was undetectable (<0.06 mg/dL). At follow-up, the physical and neurologic examination and developmental assessment were normal at 4.25 years (5).

An unusual case of lead poisoning in a 17-year-old pregnant woman was apparently reported by two different groups of authors from the same New York hospital (6,7). The patient had eaten paint from the walls of her apartment for several months during pregnancy. She was hospitalized at about 38 weeks' gestation because of abdominal pain, paresthesias in her feet, and calf pain. A blood sample yielded a lead level of 86 mcg/mL, whereas the amniotic fluid lead level was 90 mcg/mL. She was treated with IV edetate 1 g twice daily for 3 days. Two days after chelation therapy, her blood level was 41 mcg/mL. Six days later, she delivered a 2665-g female infant spontaneously. The cord blood lead concentration was 60 mcg/mL, whereas the maternal level at discharge was 26 mcg/mL. The small-for-date infant's head circumference was 32 cm (10th percentile), and the length was 45 cm (25th percentile). Radiographs revealed a dense skull with delayed deciduous dental development and abnormal long bones. At about 2 years of age, the girl's growth and development were normal (6,7).

A 2002 report described the use of IV edetate (dose not specified) and IM dimercaprol in a woman at 30 weeks' gestation with a high blood lead concentration (5.2 μmol/L; goal ≤0.48 μmol/L) (8). Twenty-four hours after initiation of chelation therapy, her lead level was 2.3 μmol/L. Twelve hours later, labor was induced because of uterine hemorrhage, and she gave birth to a 1.6-kg (75th percentile) female infant. Lead concentration in the cord blood was 7.6 μmol/L. The Apgar scores were 4 and 6 (presumably at 1 and 5 minutes, respectively). The newborn was flaccid with absent reflexes, no movement to noxious stimuli, and no gag reflex, but she did have spontaneous eye movement. Bilateral diaphragmatic palsy was confirmed by fluoroscopy. During her 7 months of hospitalization, the infant received multiple courses of chelation to treat the intrauterine lead intoxication. In spite of this therapy, she had right sensorineural deafness and neurodevelopment delay at discharge. Oral succimer was continued at home because the blood lead level was still elevated (0.95 μmol/L). The mother's lead source was identified as herbal tablets that had been prescribed for a GI complaint. She had taken the tablets periodically over the last 9 years and throughout pregnancy. Mercury also was present in some of the tablets. The lead intake during pregnancy was estimated to be 50 times the average weekly intake of Western populations (8).

In a 2003 report, four women with severe lead poisoning were treated with IV edetate during the 3rd trimester, including one also treated with dimercaprol. The source of the lead in most cases was the ingestion of pica (soil/clay-based substances). No lead-induced congenital defects were noted in the infants, but all received chelation therapy in the neonatal period (9).

BREASTFEEDING SUMMARY

No reports describing the use of edetate calcium disodium (edetate) during lactation have been located. The molecular weight (about 374) suggests that the drug will be excreted into breast milk, but the very short elimination half-life will limit the amount excreted. Moreover, edetate is poorly absorbed after oral dosing, at least from the adult GI tract. The risk to a nursing infant from exposure to the drug in milk is unknown but appears to be very low or nonexistent. However, because the use of edetate implies poisoning with lead, this metal also will be excreted into milk and is toxic to a nursing infant. Therefore, breastfeeding is contraindicated in women receiving edetate.

References

1. Schardein JL. Metals. *Chemically Induced Birth Defects*. 3rd ed. New York, NY: Marcel Dekker, 2000:879.
2. Bailey B. Are there teratogenic risks associated with antidotes used in the acute management of poisoned pregnant women? Birth Def Res (Part A) 2003;67:133–40.
3. Product information. Calcium Disodium Versenate. Eli Lilly and Company, 2004.
4. Domingo JL. Developmental toxicity of metal chelating agents. Reprod Toxicol 1998;12:499–510.
5. Angle CR, McIntire MS. Lead poisoning during pregnancy. Fetal tolerance of calcium disodium edetate. Am J Dis Child 1964;108:436–9.
6. Timpo AE, Amin JS, Casalino MB, Yuceoglu AM. Congenital lead intoxication. J Pediatr 1979;94:765–7.
7. Pearl M, Boxi LM. Radiographic findings in congenital lead poisoning. Radiology 1980;136:83–4.
8. Tait PA, Vora A, James S, Fitzgerald DJ, Pester BA. Severe congenital lead poisoning in a preterm infant due to a herbal remedy. Med J Aust 2002;177:193–5.
9. Shannon M. Severe lead poisoning in pregnancy. Ambul Pediatr 2003;3:37–9.

EDROPHONIUM

Parasympathomimetic (Cholinergic)

PREGNANCY RECOMMENDATION: Human Data Suggest Risk in 3rd Trimester
BREASTFEEDING RECOMMENDATION: No Human Data—Probably Compatible

E

PREGNANCY SUMMARY

Edrophonium is a short-acting quaternary ammonium chloride with anticholinesterase activity used in the diagnosis of myasthenia gravis. The drug has been used in pregnancy without producing fetal malformations (1–7).

FETAL RISK SUMMARY

Because it is ionized at physiologic pH, significant amounts of edrophonium would not be expected to cross the placenta. The molecular weight (about 202 for edrophonium chloride) is low enough that placental transfer of the nonionized fraction probably occurs.

Caution has been advised against the use during pregnancy of IV anticholinesterases because they may cause premature labor (1,3). This effect on the pregnant uterus increases near term. IM neostigmine has been recommended as an alternative to IV edrophonium if diagnosis of myasthenia gravis is required in a pregnant patient (3). However, vaginal bleeding and abortion have occurred with IM neostigmine and are potential complications (see Neostigmine). In one report, IV edrophonium was given to a woman in the 2nd trimester in an unsuccessful attempt to treat tachycardia secondary to Wolff–Parkinson–White syndrome (6). No effect on the uterus was mentioned and she continued with an uneventful full-term pregnancy.

Transient muscular weakness has been observed in about 20% of newborns of mothers with myasthenia gravis (8). The neonatal myasthenia is caused by transplacental passage of anti-acetylcholine receptor immunoglobulin G antibodies (8).

BREASTFEEDING SUMMARY

No reports describing the use of edrophonium during lactation have been located. Edrophonium is ionized at physiologic pH and is not expected to be excreted into breast milk (9). The molecular weight (about 202 for edrophonium chloride) is low enough that excretion of the nonionized fraction into milk may occur. The effects, if any, on a nursing infant from this exposure are unknown (9).

References

1. Foldes FF, McNall PG. Myasthenia gravis: a guide for anesthesiologists. Anesthesiology 1962;23:837–72.
2. Plauche WG. Myasthenia gravis in pregnancy. Am J Obstet Gynecol 1964;88:404–9.
3. McNall PG, Jafarnia MR. Management of myasthenia gravis in the obstetrical patient. Am J Obstet Gynecol 1965;92:518–25.
4. Hay DM. Myasthenia gravis in pregnancy. J Obstet Gynaecol Br Commonw 1969;76:323–9.
5. Heinonen OP, Slone D, Shapiro S. *Birth Defects and Drugs in Pregnancy*. Littleton, MA: Publishing Sciences Group, 1977:345–56.
6. Gleicher N, Meller J, Sandler RZ, Sullum S. Wolff-Parkinson-White syndrome in pregnancy. Obstet Gynecol 1981;58:748–52.
7. Blackhall MI, Buckley GA, Roberts DV, Roberts JB, Thomas BH, Wilson A. Drug-induced neonatal myasthenia. J Obstet Gynaecol Br Commonw 1969;76:157–62.
8. Plauche WC. Myasthenia gravis in pregnancy: an update. Am J Obstet Gynecol 1979;135:691–7.
9. Wilson JT. Pharmacokinetics of drug excretion. In: Wilson JT, ed. *Drugs in Breast Milk*. Balgowlah, Australia: ADIS Press, 1981:17.

EFALIZUMAB

Immunologic Agent (Immunosuppressant)

PREGNANCY RECOMMENDATION: No Human Data—Animal Data Suggest Low Risk
BREASTFEEDING RECOMMENDATION: No Human Data—Potential Toxicity

PREGNANCY SUMMARY

No reports describing the use of efalizumab in human pregnancy have been located. The animal data suggest that the human embryo and fetal risk are low, but the absence of human pregnancy experience prevents a full assessment of the risk. Because psoriasis is common in women of childbearing potential, the long elimination half-life of efalizumab suggests that exposure of inadvertent pregnancies is highly probable. Based on the animal data, suppression of the antibody response in infants exposed in utero late in gestation is a potential complication.

FETAL RISK SUMMARY

Efalizumab is an immunosuppressant recombinant humanized immunoglobulin (IgG1) kappa isotype monoclonal antibody. It is indicated for the treatment of chronic moderate to severe plaque psoriasis in patients who are candidates for systemic therapy or phototherapy. It is administered by SC injection. After the last steady-state dose, the mean time to eliminate efalizumab was 25 days (range 13–35 days) (1). (*Note: This corresponds to a mean elimination half-life of about 5 days.*)

Animal reproduction studies with efalizumab have not been conducted. However, a study was conducted in mice during organogenesis using an antimouse CD11a antibody with SC doses up to 30 times the equivalent of the recommended clinical dose of efalizumab (ERCD). In this study, no evidence of maternal toxicity, embryotoxicity, or teratogenicity was observed. When doses 3–30 times the ERCD were administered in late gestation and during lactation, no adverse effects on behavior, reproduction, or growth were noted. However, at 11 weeks of age, offspring exhibited a significant reduction in their ability to mount an antibody response. There was evidence at 25 weeks of age that this effect was partially reversible.

The transplacental passage of efalizumab in humans has not been studied. However, immunoglobulin G is known to cross the human placenta. Thus, exposure of the human embryo or fetus should be expected.

BREASTFEEDING SUMMARY

No reports describing the use of efalizumab during human lactation have been located. As an immune globulin, efalizumab is probably excreted into breast milk. Because of the long elimination time (about 25 days), holding breastfeeding after a dose to allow clearance from the mother's system does not appear to be practical. The effect of this exposure on a nursing infant is unknown, but the immune globulin would most likely undergo some degree of digestion in the infant's gut. However, suppression of the infant's antibody response is a potential complication. Until data are available, avoiding nursing during use of efalizumab is the safest course.

Reference

1. Product information. Raptiva. Genentech, 2005.

EFAVIRENZ

Antiviral

PREGNANCY RECOMMENDATION: Compatible—Maternal Benefit >> Embryo–Fetal Risk
BREASTFEEDING RECOMMENDATION: Contraindicated

PREGNANCY SUMMARY

The human data are too limited to allow a prediction as to the risk of efavirenz during pregnancy. The teratogenicity observed in cynomolgus monkeys and the embryo toxicity in rats suggests that there is a potential for risk in the developing human. Exposure of the human embryo–fetus is likely to occur because the agent was found to easily cross the placenta of all animal species tested. Moreover, the case report of a myelomeningocele was considered to be consistent with the toxicity observed in monkeys. Taken in sum, however, the total data do not support the concept that efavirenz is a major teratogen. If indicated, the drug should not be withheld because of pregnancy.

FETAL RISK SUMMARY

Efavirenz is an orally active, nonnucleoside reverse transcriptase inhibitor (nnRTI) that is specific for HIV-1. It is indicated, in combination with other antiretroviral agents, for the treatment of HIV-1 infections. Efavirenz has a terminal half-life of 52–76 hours after a single dose and 40–55 hours after multiple dosing (1). The shorter elimination time after chronic dosing is a result of cytochrome P450 enzyme induction that induces its own metabolism.

In reproduction studies, cynomolgus monkeys were administered oral efavirenz (60 mg/kg/day) throughout pregnancy (postcoital days 20–150). This dose produced plasma drug concentrations similar to those achieved in humans given 600 mg/day. Three of 20 exposed newborns had major congenital malformations, compared with 0 of 20 in nonexposed control monkeys. The defects observed were one case each of anencephaly and unilateral anophthalmia, microphthalmia, and cleft palate. In pregnant rats, doses producing plasma concentrations similar to those in humans resulted in an increase in fetal resorptions. Neither mating nor fertility was impaired in rats at these doses. No teratogenic or toxic effects were observed in rabbits given doses producing plasma concentrations similar to those in humans (1).

It is not known if efavirenz crosses the human placenta to the fetus. The relatively low molecular weight (about 316) suggests that the drug is transferred to the fetus. Placental transfer of efavirenz has been documented in cynomolgus monkeys, rats, and rabbits, with fetal blood concentrations approximately the same as maternal plasma concentrations (1).

A 2002 case report described the pregnancy outcome of a 34-year-old woman with asymptomatic HIV infection (2). The woman was taking zidovudine, stavudine, efavirenz, and folic acid before and during the first 24 weeks of gestation, at which time pregnancy was diagnosed. Therapy was then changed to lamivudine, stavudine, and nelfinavir. At 38 weeks' gestation, a 3450-g male infant was born with length 49 cm and head circumference 34.5 cm. The infant had a large sacral myelomeningocele lesion (10 cm diameter) and a triventricular hydrocephalus. The serologic test for HIV was positive. Surgical repair of the neural tube defect was performed along with ventriculoperitoneal shunting. Because of the reproduction studies in monkeys, the authors attributed the infant's defect to efavirenz (2).

The Antiretroviral Pregnancy Registry reported, for the period January 1989 through July 2009, prospective data (reported before the outcomes were known) involving 4702 liveborn infants who had been exposed during the 1st trimester to one or more antiretroviral agents (3). Congenital defects were noted in 134, a prevalence of 2.8% (95% confidence interval [CI] 2.4–3.4). In the 6100 live births with earliest exposure in the 2nd/3rd trimesters, there were 153 infants with defects (2.5%, 95% CI 2.1–2.9). The prevalence rates for the two periods did not differ significantly. There were 288 infants with birth defects among 10,803 live births with exposure anytime during pregnancy (2.7%, 95% CI 2.4–3.0). The prevalence rate did not differ significantly from the rate expected in a nonexposed population. There were 556 outcomes exposed to efavirenz (501 in the 1st trimester and 55 in the 2nd/3rd trimesters) in combination with other antiretroviral agents. There were 16 birth defects (14 exposures in the 1st trimester and 2 in the 2nd/3rd trimesters). One of the defects from a 1st trimester exposure was a neural tube defect. In reviewing the birth defects of prospective and retrospective (pregnancies reported after the outcomes were known) registered cases, the Registry concluded that, except for isolated cases of neural tube defects with efavirenz exposure in retrospective reports, there was no other pattern of anomalies (isolated or syndromic) (3). (See Lamivudine for required statement.)

Two reviews, one in 1996 and the other in 1997, concluded that all women receiving antiretroviral therapy should continue to receive therapy during pregnancy and that treatment of the mother with monotherapy should be considered inadequate (4,5). The same conclusion was reached in a 2003 review with the added admonishment that therapy must be continuous to prevent emergence of resistant viral strains (6). In 2009, the updated U.S. Department of Health and Human Services guidelines for the use of antiretroviral agents in HIV-1 infected patients continued the recommendation that therapy, with the exception of efavirenz, should be continued during pregnancy (7). The guidelines recommended avoiding efavirenz in pregnancy, particularly during the 1st trimester, because of the teratogenic effects observed in primates and the report of a neural tube defect in a newborn (7). Updated guidelines for the use of antiretroviral drugs to reduce perinatal HIV-1 transmission also were released in 2010 (8). Women receiving antiretroviral therapy during pregnancy should continue the therapy but, regardless of the regimen, zidovudine administration is recommended during the intrapartum period to prevent vertical transmission of HIV to the newborn (8).

BREASTFEEDING SUMMARY

No reports describing the use of efavirenz during human lactation have been located. The molecular weight (about 316) is low enough that excretion into breast milk should be expected. The effect on a nursing infant is unknown.

Reports on the use of efavirenz during human lactation are unlikely because the antiviral agent is used in the treatment of HIV infection. HIV-1 is transmitted in milk, and in developed countries, breastfeeding is not recommended (4,5,7,9–11). In developing countries, breastfeeding is undertaken, despite the risk, because there are no affordable milk substitutes available. Until 1999, no studies had been published that examined the effect of any antiretroviral therapy on HIV-1 transmission in milk. In that year, a study involving zidovudine was published that measured a 38% reduction in vertical transmission of HIV-1 infection despite breastfeeding when compared with controls (see Zidovudine).

References

1. Product information. Sustiva. DuPont Pharma, 2000.
2. Fundaro C, Genovese O, Rendell C, Tamburrini E, Salvaggio E. Myelomeningocele in a child with intrauterine exposure to efavirenz. AIDS 2002;16:299–300.
3. Antiretroviral Pregnancy Registry Steering Committee. *Antiretroviral Pregnancy Registry International Interim Report for 1 January 1989 through 31 July 2009*. Wilmington, NC: Registry Coordinating Center; 2009. Available at www.apregistry.com. Accessed May 29, 2010.
4. Carpenter CCJ, Fischi MA, Hammer SM, Hirsch MS, Jacobsen DM, Katzenstein DA, Montaner JSG, Richman DD, Saag MS, Schooley RT, Thompson MA, Vella S, Yeni PG, Volberding PA. Antiretroviral therapy for HIV infection in 1996. JAMA 1996;276;146–54.
5. Minkoff H, Augenbraun M. Antiretroviral therapy for pregnant women. Am J Obstet Gynecol 1997;176:478–89.
6. Minkoff H. Human immunodeficiency virus infection in pregnancy. Obstet Gynecol 2003;101:797–810.
7. Panel on Antiretroviral Guidelines for Adults and Adolescents. *Guidelines for the Use of Antiretroviral Agents in HIV-1-Infected Adults and Adolescents*. Department of Health and Human Services. December 1, 2009;1–161. Available at http://www.aidsinfo.nih.gov/ContentFiles/AdultandAdolescentGL.pdf. Accessed September 17, 2010:60, 96–8.
8. Panel on Treatment of HIV-Infected Pregnant Women and Prevention of Perinatal Transmission. *Recommendations for Use of Antiretroviral Drugs in Pregnant HIV-1-Infected Women for Maternal Health and Interventions to Reduce Perinatal HIV Transmission in the United States*. May 24, 2010:1–117. Available at http://aidsinfo.nih.gov/ContentFiles/PerinatalGL.pdf. Accessed September 17, 2010:30 (Table 5).
9. Brown ZA, Watts DH. Antiviral therapy in pregnancy. Clin Obstet Gynecol 1990;33:276–89.
10. De Martino M, Tovo P-A, Pezzotti P, Galli L, Massironi E, Ruga E, Floreea F, Plebani A, Gabiano C, Zuccotti GV. HIV-1 transmission through breast-milk: appraisal of risk according to duration of feeding. AIDS 1992;6:991–7.
11. Van de Perre P. Postnatal transmission of human immunodeficiency virus type 1: the breast feeding dilemma. Am J Obstet Gynecol 1995;173:483–7.

ELECTRICITY

Miscellaneous

PREGNANCY RECOMMENDATION: Human Data Suggest Risk
BREASTFEEDING RECOMMENDATION: No Human Data—Potential Toxicity (Mother)

PREGNANCY SUMMARY

Exposure of the pregnant woman to electric current may produce dramatically different fetal outcomes depending on the source and type of current. Based on published reports previous to 1997, otherwise harmless maternal exposure to household alternating current was usually fatal to the fetus. In contrast, a 1997 prospective controlled cohort study cited below described live births in 94% of their cases (1,2); the difference between this report and the previous published experience is most likely due to selective reporting of adverse outcomes, the level of voltage involved (110 vs. 220 V), and whether the current passed through the uterus. Although the new data should lessen a woman's concern for her fetus after electric shock, pregnant women who have experienced this type of injury, even when deemed to be minor, should be advised to consult their health care provider. Oligohydramnios, intrauterine growth restriction, and fetal death may be late effects of exposure to alternating current (3). Lightning strikes of any human are often fatal, but in those rare cases in which the victim is pregnant and survives, about half of the fetuses will also survive. Electroconvulsive therapy (ECT) and direct-current cardioversion do not seem to pose a significant risk to the fetus. The most frequent adverse effect of ECT in the mother was premature contractions and labor, whereas in the fetus it was bradyarrhythmias. Based on one report, the use of a Taser weapon on a pregnant woman may result in spontaneous abortion.

E

FETAL RISK SUMMARY

Published reports have described the exposure of pregnant women to electric currents through five different means: accidental electric injury in the home, lightning strikes, ECT, antiarrhythmic direct-current cardioversion, and from a Taser weapon. Dramatically different fetal outcomes have occurred based on the type of exposure.

Four reports involving 14 women described accidental electric shock with alternating current, either 110 or 220 V, from appliances or wiring in the home (3–6). In each of the cases, the electric current took a presumed hand-to-foot pattern through the body and, thus, probably through the uterus. Gestational ages varied from 12 to 40 weeks. Although none of the mothers was injured or even lost consciousness, in these otherwise harmless events, fetal death occurred in 10 (71%). In at least five of the cases, immediate cessation of fetal movements was noted. One mother, who received the shock at about 28 weeks' gestation, subsequently developed hydramnios and delivered an infant 4 weeks later (4). Burn marks were evident on the newborn, who died 3 days after birth. A second growth-restricted infant was stillborn at 33 weeks' gestation, 12 weeks after the electrical injury (3). In most cases, no specific clinical or pathologic signs could be noted (3). However, oligohydramnios was observed in two cases in which the fetuses survived. The accidents occurred at 20 and 32 weeks' gestation, with injury-to-delivery intervals of 6 and 21 weeks, respectively. The specific cause of fetal damage has not been determined. It may be due to changes in fetal heart conduction resulting in cardiac arrest (4,5) or by lesions in the uteroplacental bed (3).

A 1997 paper described 20 cases from the literature of electric shock during pregnancy with healthy newborn outcomes occurring in only 5 cases (1). An abstract of their preliminary findings was published in 1995 (2). The authors of this report then described the outcomes of 31 women studied prospectively after exposure to home appliances with 110 V ($N = 26$) or 220 V ($N = 2$), or to high voltage (2000 and 8000 V) from electrified fences ($N = 2$), or to a low-voltage (12 V) telephone line ($N = 1$). An additional 16 women who had received electric shocks during pregnancy were either lost to follow-up ($N = 10$) or had not yet given birth ($N = 6$). Of the 31 outcomes, there were 2 spontaneous abortions, one of which may have been caused by the electric shock. In that case, the abortion occurred 2 weeks after the mother had received the shock. One of the live newborns had a ventricular septal defect that eventually closed spontaneously. In comparison to the group of 20 cases from the literature, there were significant differences discovered in the number of live births (94% vs. 25%), voltage involved (77% to 110 V vs. 76% to 220 V), and current crossing the uterus (i.e., hand-to-foot transmission suggesting that the current crossed the uterus) (10% vs. 62%) (1).

Lightning strikes of pregnant women are rare, with only 12 cases described since 1833 (4,7–11). All mothers survived the event, but 6 (50%) of the fetuses died. A 1965 reference reported a lightning strike of a woman in approximately the 11th week of gestation (4). The woman briefly lost consciousness, but other than transient nausea and anxiety that decreased as the pregnancy progressed, she was unhurt. She subsequently delivered a healthy term infant who was developing normally at 5 months of age. This report also described five other cases of lightning strikes of pregnant women that occurred between 1833 and 1959 with two fetal deaths. In one of the latter cases, the electrical injury caused uterine rupture in a mother at 6 months' gestation requiring an immediate cesarean section that was unable to save the fetus. Two cases of lightning strikes in term pregnant women were reported in 1972 (7). Both women were in labor when examined shortly after the events. One infant was delivered 12.5 hours after the maternal injury but died 15.5 hours after birth apparently secondary to congestive heart failure. In the other case, a healthy infant was delivered 14 hours after the lightning strike. A 1979 report described a near-fatal lightning strike in the chest of a 21-year-old woman at 34 weeks' gestation (8). Successful cardiopulmonary resuscitation was performed on the mother, but fetal heart tones were absent on initial examination. A stillborn fetus was delivered 48 hours after admission while the mother was still comatose. No fetal movements were felt by a 12-year-old mother at term after awakening from a lightning strike (9). She went into labor 9 days after the accident and delivered a macerated male fetus. Both the fetus and the placenta appeared grossly normal. A case of a woman in her 7th month of pregnancy who was struck in the right arm by lightning was published in 1982 (10). She apparently did not lose consciousness. Examination revealed minimal maternal injury and normal fetal heart tones. A healthy infant was delivered 10 weeks later who is developing normally at 19 months of age. Finally, the picture and brief description of a 41-year-old woman, in her 26th week of pregnancy, who was struck by lightning, was presented in 1994 (11). The woman, but not the fetus, survived. Interestingly, the direction of the lightning strike in the mother was discussed in later correspondence (12,13).

ECT for depression and psychosis in pregnant patients has been the subject of a large number of references (14–45). The procedure has been used in all trimesters of pregnancy and has been considered safe for the fetus. However, the published data suggest that a better assessment is low risk.

General guidelines for ECT established by the National Institutes of Health (NIH) were published in 1985 (34). The NIH report recommended that ECT, instead of drug therapy, be considered for pregnant patients with severe depression or psychosis in their 1st trimester but did not mention use in the other phases of gestation. Guidelines for the use of ECT in pregnant women were first proposed in 1978 (29) and then later expanded in 1984 (33). The combined guidelines from these two sources are (a) thorough physical examination, including a pelvic examination, if not completed earlier; (b) the presence of an obstetrician; (c) endotracheal intubation; (d) low-voltage, nondominant ECT with EEG monitoring; (e) ECG monitoring of the mother; (f) evaluation of arterial blood gases during and immediately after ECT; (g) Doppler ultrasonography of fetal heart rate (FHR); (h) tocodynamometer recording of uterine tone; (i) administration of glycopyrrolate (see Glycopyrrolate) as the anticholinergic of choice during anesthesia; and (j) weekly nonstress tests.

One report described mental retardation in a 32-month-old child whose mother had received 12 ECT treatments in the 2nd and 3rd trimesters for schizophrenia, but the investigators did not believe the treatments were responsible (37). A 1955 reference examined 16 children who had been exposed in utero to maternal ECT between the 9th and 21st weeks of pregnancy (38). The age of the children at examination ranged from 14 to 81 months and all exhibited normal mental and physical development. Transient (2.5 minutes) fetal heart rate deceleration was observed in a twin pregnancy in which the mother was receiving ECT under general anesthesia (39). A total of eight ECT treatments were given, two before the observed deceleration and five afterwards.

Only one report has been located that described arterial blood gas analyses during ECT in a pregnant patient (28). As observed in previous studies, maternal blood pressure (average systolic blood pressure increase 10 mmHg) and heart rate (average pulse increase 15 beats/minute) rose slightly immediately after the shock, but no maternal hypoxia was measured. A fetal arrhythmia lasting about 15 minutes occurred that was apparently unrelated to oxygen changes in the mother (28).

Transient maternal hypotension after ECT was described in a 1984 case report (32). The adverse effect was attributed to decreased intravascular volume. IV hydration preceded subsequent ECT treatments in the patient, and no further episodes of hypotension were observed (32).

A 1991 report noted mild, bright red vaginal bleeding and uterine contractions after each of seven weekly ECT treatments between 30 and 36 weeks' gestation (35). A cesarean section, performed at 37 weeks' gestation because of bleeding, confirmed a diagnosis of abruptio placentae. The authors attributed the complication to the transient marked hypertension caused by the ECT. Only one other report, however, has described vaginal bleeding after ECT (26). Three women, all in the 8th or 9th month of pregnancy, complained either of severe recurrent abdominal pain ($N = 2$) or vaginal bleeding ($N = 1$) after ECT. Therapy was stopped in these cases, and normal infants were eventually delivered.

A 2007 case report described the pregnancy outcome of woman that had received ECT every 2 weeks throughout pregnancy (40). Labor was induced at 36 weeks' because of preeclampsia to deliver a 2.550-kg male infant with Apgar scores of 4 and 7. The infant had multiple brain infarcts that were attributed to the ECT. An accompanying editorial, however, thought that the infarcts were unlikely to have been caused by the ECT (41). Multiple ECT sessions were associated with premature labor in two reports (42,43).

A 2009 review cited 339 cases of ECT in pregnancy that had been reported over a 65-year interval (1941–2007) (44). Of the 25 fetal or neonatal complications that occurred in these cases, the authors thought that 11, which included 2 deaths, were likely related to ECT. The 11 cases included 8 cases of transient fetal arrhythmias, 1 fetal death due to maternal status epilepticus, 1 miscarriage in the 1st trimester, and 1 case of multiple brain infarcts (same case as reference 40). The review did not cite the above editorial (reference 41). The most frequent adverse effect of ECT in the mother was premature contractions and labor, whereas in the fetus it was bradyarrhythmias (44).

Antiarrhythmic, direct-current cardioversion is considered a safe procedure during gestation (45–48). Cardioversion has been used in the 2nd trimester in a woman with atrial fibrillation after mitral valvulotomy (45), in the 1st trimester in a patient with atrial flutter in 1:1 atrioventricular conduction (46), seven times during three pregnancies in one patient for atrial tachycardia resistant to drug therapy (47), and twice in a single patient in two pregnancies for atrial fibrillation (48). No fetal harm was noted from the procedure in any of these cases. Two review articles on cardiac arrhythmias during pregnancy considered cardioversion (with energies of 10–50 J (49)) to be safe and usually effective in this patient population (49,50).

A 1992 reference described the effect from using a Taser (an electronic immobilization and defense weapon) on a pregnant woman at an estimated 8–10 weeks' gestation (51). The subject, in custody at the time because of drug abuse, was struck by one dart above the uterus and by a second dart in the left thigh, thereby establishing a current path through the uterus. Vaginal spotting began the next day and heavy vaginal bleeding began 7 days after the Taser incident. Uterine curettage performed 7 days later confirmed the presence of an incomplete spontaneous abortion (51).

BREASTFEEDING SUMMARY

No data are available.

References

1. Einarson A, Bailey B, Inocencion G, Ormond K, Koren G. Accidental electric shock in pregnancy: a prospective cohort study. Am J Obstet Gynecol 1997;176:678–81.
2. Einarson A, Innocencion G, Koren G. Accidental electric shock in pregnancy: a prospective cohort study (abstract). Reprod Toxicol 1995;9:581.
3. Leiberman JR, Mazor M, Molcho J, Haiam E, Maor E, Insler V. Electrical accidents during pregnancy. Obstet Gynecol 1986;67:861–3.

4. Rees WD. Pregnant woman struck by lightning. Br Med J 1965;1:103–4.
5. Peppler RD, Labranche FJ, Comeaux JJ. Intrauterine death of a fetus in a mother shocked by an electric current: a case report. J La State Med Soc 1972;124:37–8.
6. Jaffe R, Fejgin M, Aderet NB. Fetal death in early pregnancy due to electric current. Acta Obstet Gynecol Scand 1986;65:283.
7. Chan Y-F, Sivasamboo R. Lightning accidents in pregnancy. J Obstet Gynaecol Br Commonw 1972;79:761–2.
8. Weinstein L. Lightning: a rare cause of intrauterine death with maternal survival. South Med J 1979;72:632–3.
9. Guha-Ray DK. Fetal death at term due to lightning. Am J Obstet Gynecol 1979;134:103–5.
10. Flannery DB, Wiles H. Follow-up of a survivor of intrauterine lightning exposure. Am J Obstet Gynecol 1982;142:238–9.
11. Zehender M. Images in clinical medicine: struck by lightning. N Engl J Med 1994;330:1492.
12. Bourke DL, Harrison CM, Sprung J. Direction of a lightning strike. N Engl J Med 1994;331:953.
13. Zehender M, Wiesinger J. Direction of a lightning strike. N Engl J Med 1994;331:954.
14. Goldstein HH, Weinberg J, Sankstone MI. Shock therapy in psychosis complicating pregnancy: a case report. Am J Psychiatry 1941;98:201–2.
15. Thorpe FT. Shock treatment in psychosis complicating pregnancy. Br Med J 1942;2:281.
16. Polatin P, Hoch P. Electroshock therapy in pregnant mental patients. NY J Med 1945;45:1562–3.
17. Sands DE. Electro-convulsion therapy in 301 patients in a general hospital. Br Med J 1946;2:289–93.
18. Gralnick A. Shock therapy in psychoses complicated by pregnancy; report of two cases. Am J Psychiatry 1946;102:780–2.
19. Turner CC, Wright LD. Shock therapy in psychoses during pregnancy; report of one case. Am J Psychiatry 1947;103:834–6.
20. Moore MT. Electrocerebral shock therapy; a reconsideration of former contraindications. Arch Neurol Psychiatry 1947;57:693–711.
21. Simon JL. Electric shock treatment in advanced pregnancy. J Nerv Ment Dis 1948;107:579–80.
22. Block S. Electric convulsive therapy during pregnancy. Am J Psychiatry 1948;104:579.
23. Charatan FB, Oldham AJ. Electroconvulsive treatment in pregnancy. J Obstet Gynaecol Br Emp 1954;61:665–7.
24. Laird DM. Convulsive therapy in psychoses accompanying pregnancy. N Engl J Med 1955;252:934–6.
25. Smith S. The use of electroplexy (E.C.T.) in psychiatric syndromes complicating pregnancy. J Ment Sci 1956;102:796–800.
26. Sobel DE. Fetal damage due to ECT, insulin coma, chlorpromazine, or reserpine. Arch Gen Psychiatry 1960;2:606–11.
27. Impastato DJ, Gabriel AR, Lardaro HH. Electric and insulin shock therapy during pregnancy. Dis Nerv Syst 1964;25:542–6.
28. Levine R, Frost EAM. Arterial blood-gas analyses during electroconvulsive therapy in a parturient. Anesth Analg 1975;54:203–5.
29. Remick RA, Maurice WL. ECT in pregnancy. Am J Psychiatry 1978;135: 761–2.
30. Fink M. Convulsive and drug therapies of depression. Annu Rev Med 1981;32:405–12.
31. Loke KH, Salleh R. Electroconvulsive therapy for the acutely psychotic pregnant patient: a review of 3 cases. Med J Malaysia 1983;38:131–3.
32. Repke JT, Berger NG. Electroconvulsive therapy in pregnancy. Obstet Gynecol 1984;63(Suppl):39S–41S.
33. Wise mg, Ward SC, Townsend-Parchman W, Gilstrap LC III, Hauth JC. Case report of ECT during high-risk pregnancy. Am J Psychiatry 1984;141:99–101.
34. Office of Medical Applications of Research, National Institutes of Health. Electroconvulsive therapy. JAMA 1985;254:2103–8.
35. Sherer DM, D'Amico ML, Warshal DP, Stern RA, Grunert HF, Abramowicz JS. Recurrent mild abruptio placentae occurring immediately after repeated electroconvulsive therapy in pregnancy. Am J Obstet Gynecol 1991;165:652–3.
36. Yellowlees PM, Page T. Safe use of electroconvulsive therapy in pregnancy. Med J Aust 1990;153:679–80.
37. Yamamoto J, Hammes EM, Hammes EM Jr. Mental deficiency in a child whose mother was given electric convulsive therapy during gestation. A case report. Minn Med 1953;36:1260–1.
38. Forssman H. Follow-up study of sixteen children whose mothers were given electric convulsive therapy during gestation. Acta Psychiatr Neurol Scand 1955;30:437–41.
39. Livingston JC, Johnstone WM Jr, Hadi HA. Electroconvulsive therapy in a twin pregnancy: a case report. Am J Perinatol 1994;11:116–8.
40. Pinette mg, Santarpio C, Wax JR, Blackstone J. Electroconvulsive therapy in pregnancy. Obstet Gynecol 2007;110:465–6.
41. Richards DS. Is electroconvulsive therapy in pregnancy safe? Obstet Gynecol 2007;110:451–2.
42. Kasar M, Saatcioglu O, Kutlar T. Electroconvulsive therapy in pregnancy. J ECT 2007;23:183–4.
43. Pesiridou A, Baquero G, Cristancho P, Wakil L, Altinay M, Kim D, O'Reardon JP. A case of delayed onset of threatened premature labor in association with electroconvulsive therapy in the third trimester of pregnancy. J ECT 2010;26:228–30.
44. Anderson EL, Reti IM. ECT in pregnancy: a review of the literature from 1941 to 2007. Psychosom Med 2009;71:235–42.
45. Vogel JHK, Pryor R, Blount SG Jr. Direct-current defibrillation during pregnancy. JAMA 1965;193:970–1.
46. Sussman HF, Duque D, Lesser ME. Atrial flutter with 1:1 A-V conduction; report of a case in a pregnant woman successfully treated with DC countershock. Dis Chest 1966;49:99–103.
47. Schroeder JS, Harrison DC. Repeated cardioversion during pregnancy; treatment of refractory paroxysmal atrial tachycardia during 3 successive pregnancies. Am J Cardiol 1971;27:445–6.
48. McKenna WJ, Harris L, Rowland E, Whitelaw A, Storey G, Holt D. Amiodarone therapy during pregnancy. Am J Cardiol 1983;51:1231–3.
49. Brown CEL, Wendel GD. Cardiac arrhythmias during pregnancy. Clin Obstet Gynecol 1989;32:89–102.
50. Rotmensch HH, Rotmensch S, Elkayam U. Management of cardiac arrhythmias during pregnancy. Current concepts. Drugs 1987;33:623–33.
51. Mehl LE. Electrical injury from tasering and miscarriage. Acta Obstet Gynecol Scand 1992;71:118–23.

ELETRIPTAN

Antimigraine

PREGNANCY RECOMMENDATION: No Human Data—Animal Data Suggest Moderate Risk
BREASTFEEDING RECOMMENDATION: Compatible

PREGNANCY SUMMARY

No reports describing the use of eletriptan in human pregnancy have been located. The animal data suggest moderate risk, but an assessment of the actual risk cannot be determined until human pregnancy experience is available. Although a 2008 review of triptans in pregnancy found no evidence for teratogenicity, the data did suggest a possible increase in the rate of preterm birth (1).

FETAL RISK SUMMARY

Eletriptan is an oral selective serotonin (5-hydroxytryptamine; $5HT_{1B/1D}$) receptor agonist that has high affinity for $5HT_{1B}$, $5HT_{1D}$, and $5HT_{1F}$ receptors. The drug is closely related to almotriptan, frovatriptan, naratriptan, rizatriptan, sumatriptan, and zolmitriptan. It is indicated for the acute treatment of migraine with or without aura in adults. Protein binding is moderate (about 85%). One active metabolite has been identified. The elimination half-life of eletriptan is about 4 hours, whereas the half-life of the active metabolite is about 13 hours (2).

E

Reproduction studies have been conducted in rats and rabbits. In rats, eletriptan was given during organogenesis at doses ranging from about 1.2 to 12 times the maximum recommended human daily dose of 80 mg based on BSA (MRHDD). At 12 times the MRHDD, fetal weights were decreased and the incidence of vertebral and sternebral variations were increased, but this dose was also maternal toxic (decreased body weight gain). The no-effect-dose for developmental toxicity in rats was about four times the MRHDD. When rabbits were administered doses ranging from about 1.2 to 12 times the MRHDD throughout organogenesis, fetal weights were reduced at the highest dose. All doses were associated with increased incidences of fused sternebrae and vena cava deviations. Maternal toxicity was not observed with the doses used. A no-effect-dose for development toxicity in rabbits was not determined (2).

It is not known if eletriptan or its active metabolite crosses the human placenta to the fetus. The molecular weight of the parent compound (about 382 for the free base) is low enough that passage to the fetus should be expected. In addition, the moderate protein binding and elimination half-life suggest that the drug will be available for transfer at the maternal–fetal interface.

BREASTFEEDING SUMMARY

Eletriptan is excreted into human breast milk. In a study conducted by the manufacturer, eight women were given a single oral dose of 80 mg (2). The mean amount of drug recovered from milk over a 24-hour period was approximately 0.02% of the maternal dose. The mean milk:plasma ratio was 1:4, but there was great variability. At 18–24 hours after the dose, the drug was still present in milk in low concentrations (mean 1.7 ng/mL). The active metabolite was not measured in the milk (2).

The effect of this exposure on a nursing infant is unknown. However, the very low concentrations measured in milk suggest that eletriptan is compatible with breastfeeding.

References

1. Soldin OP, Dahlin J, O'Mara DM. Triptans in pregnancy. Ther Drug Monit 2008;30:5–9.
2. Product information. Relpax. Pfizer, 2004.

ELTROMBOPAG

Hematological Agent (Hematopoietic)

PREGNANCY RECOMMENDATION: **Compatible—Maternal Benefit >> Embryo–Fetal Risk**
BREASTFEEDING RECOMMENDATION: **No Human Data—Potential Toxicity**

PREGNANCY SUMMARY

Eltrombopag is in a pharmacologic class by itself. Only one report describing the use of eltrombopag in human pregnancy has been located. The animal reproduction data suggest low risk, but the doses tested were very low. A more complete assessment of the potential for human embryo–fetal risk cannot be made until human data are available. Nevertheless, if eltrombopag is indicated, the maternal benefit appears to outweigh the unknown embryo–fetal risk, and the drug should not be withheld because of pregnancy. Health care professionals are encouraged to enroll exposed patients in the Promacta Pregnancy Registry by calling 888-825-5249.

FETAL RISK SUMMARY

Eltrombopag is a hematopoietic agent that is in the subclass of thrombopoietin receptor agonists. There are no other agents in the subclass. Because of the risk of hepatotoxicity and other risks, the drug only is available through a restricted distribution program. Eltrombopag is indicated for the treatment of thrombocytopenia in patients with chronic immune (idiopathic) thrombocytopenic purpura (ITP) who have had an insufficient response to corticosteroids, immunoglobulins, or splenectomy. Moreover, it should only be given if the patient's degree of thrombocytopenia and clinical condition increase the risk of bleeding (1). Eltrombopag is extensively metabolized. The drug is highly bound to plasma proteins (>99%). Elimination is primarily via feces with a half-life of 21–32 hours in healthy subjects and 26–35 hours in ITP patients. Systemic concentrations approximately 40% higher in healthy African-American subjects were noted in one clinical study (1).

Reproduction studies have been conducted in rats and rabbits. In pregnant rats, a dose that was seven times the human clinical exposure based on AUC (HCE) was maternal toxic (decreases in body weight gain and food consumption). At this dose, fetal weights were significantly reduced and there was a slight increase in the presence of cervical ribs. No maternal or fetal adverse effects were observed in rats at a dose that was twice the HCE. In pregnant rabbits, no evidence of fetotoxicity, embryolethality, or teratogenicity was observed with doses up to 0.6 times the HCE (1).

Carcinogenicity studies have been conducted in mice and rats. No carcinogenic effect was observed with doses up to 4–5 times the HCE. The drug was not mutagenic or clastogenic in various assays, but was marginally positive (more than threefold increase in mutation frequency) in a mouse lymphoma assay. Eltrombopag had no effect on the fertility of female and male rats at doses that were two and five times the HCE, respectively (1).

It is not known if eltrombopag crosses the human placenta. The molecular weight (about 443 for the free acid) and the long elimination half-life suggest that the drug will cross the placenta, but the high-protein binding should limit the amount crossing the placenta. The drug was detected in the plasma of rat offspring exposed during gestation (1).

A 2012 case report described the pregnancy of a 34-year-old woman at 27 weeks' with systemic lupus erythematosus who developed severe thrombocytopenia (2). She was treated with high-dose corticosteroids, IV immunoglobulin, rituximab (weekly for four doses), one dose of cyclophosphamide, and anti-D immunoglobulin. At about 32 weeks', she received eltrombopag, 50–75 mg/day for about 3 days, but the thrombocytopenia was resistant to all of these agents. Romiplostim (weekly for three doses) was then given and the platelet count rose from 4×10^9/L to 91×10^9/L. Because her platelet count began to fall, she was given the third dose of romiplostim 1 day before induction of labor at 34 weeks'. A healthy normal female baby was born with a normal platelet count (*no additional details were provided*) (2).

BREASTFEEDING SUMMARY

No reports describing the use of eltrombopag during human lactation have been located. The molecular weight (about 443 for the free acid) and the long elimination half-life suggest that the drug will be excreted into breast milk, but the high protein binding should limit the amount excreted. The risk to a nursing infant from exposure to the drug in milk is unknown.

The maximum oral absorption of eltrombopag in adults is approximately 52%, but the absorption in infants is unknown. However, eltrombopag chelates polyvalent cations such as calcium and iron, and, in adults, this interaction can decrease plasma systemic exposure by as much as 70% (1). Thus, chelation by the calcium in milk might prevent clinically significant amounts from being absorbed. Nevertheless, the safest course is not to breastfeed if the mother is taking eltrombopag. If she chooses to do so, the infant should be monitored for the same adverse effects observed in adults: nausea and vomiting, myalgia, dyspepsia, ecchymosis, hepatotoxicity (increases in alanine aminotransferase [ALT], aspartate aminotransferase [AST], and bilirubin), conjunctival hemorrhage, and cataracts.

References

1. Product information. Promacta. GlaxoSmithKline, 2008.
2. Alkaabi J, Alkindi S, Riyami N, Zia F, Balla L, Balla S. Successful treatment of severe thrombocytopenia with romiplostim in a pregnant patient with systemic lupus erythematosus. Lupus 2012;21:1571–4.

EMTRICITABINE

Antiviral

PREGNANCY RECOMMENDATION: Compatible—Maternal Benefit >> Embryo–Fetal Risk
BREASTFEEDING RECOMMENDATION: Contraindicated

PREGNANCY SUMMARY

The animal data suggest low risk, but the limited human pregnancy experience prevents a complete assessment of the embryo–fetal risk. If indicated, the drug should not be withheld because of pregnancy.

FETAL RISK SUMMARY

Emtricitabine is a synthetic nucleoside analog reverse transcriptase inhibitor. It is indicated, in combination with other antiretroviral agents, for the treatment of HIV-1 infections. Emtricitabine is in the same antiviral class as abacavir, didanosine, lamivudine, stavudine, tenofovir, zalcitabine, and zidovudine. Plasma protein binding of emtricitabine is <4% and the plasma elimination half-life is about 10 hours (1).

Reproduction studies have been conducted in mice, rats, and rabbits. In mice and rabbits, no evidence of fetal variations or congenital malformations was observed at systemic exposures (AUC) about 60 and 120 times, respectively, the human exposure at the recommended human daily dose of 200 mg based on AUC (HE). Fertility was normal in mice offspring exposed in utero through sexual maturity at about 60 times the HE. In addition, no effects on fertility were observed in male rats exposed to about 140 times the HE, or in male and female mice exposed to about 60 times the HE (1,2).

Emtricitabine crosses the placenta to the fetus in mice and rabbits. The average fetal plasma:maternal plasma ratio was about 0.40 in mice and 0.50 in rabbits (2). The placental passage is consistent with the relatively low molecular weight (about 247), low plasma protein binding, and long plasma elimination half-life of the antiviral. These factors suggest also that the agent will cross the human placenta.

The Antiretroviral Pregnancy Registry reported, for the period January 1989 through July 2009, prospective data (reported before the outcomes were known) involving 4702 live births that had been exposed during the 1st trimester to one or more antiretroviral agents (3). Congenital defects were noted in 134, a prevalence of 2.8% (95% confidence interval [CI] 2.4–3.4). In the 6100 live births with earliest exposure in the 2nd/3rd trimesters, there were 153 infants with defects (2.5%, 95% CI 2.1–2.9). The prevalence rates for the two periods did not differ significantly. There were 288 infants with birth defects among 10,803 live births with exposure anytime during pregnancy (2.7%, 95% CI 2.4–3.0). The prevalence rate did not differ significantly from the rate expected in a nonexposed population. There were 631 outcomes exposed to emtricitabine (384 exposed in the 1st trimester and 247 exposed in the 2nd/3rd trimesters) in combination with other antiretroviral agents. There were 16 birth defects (11 in the 1st trimester exposure and 5 in the 2nd/3rd trimesters). In reviewing the birth defects of prospective and retrospective (pregnancies reported after the outcomes were known) registered cases, the Registry concluded that, except for isolated cases of neural tube defects with efavirenz exposure in retrospective reports, there was no other pattern of anomalies (isolated or syndromic) (3). (See Lamivudine for required statement.)

Two reviews, one in 1996 and the other in 1997, concluded that all women receiving antiretroviral therapy should continue to receive therapy during pregnancy and that treatment of the mother with monotherapy should be considered inadequate therapy (4,5). The same conclusion was reached in a 2003 review with the added admonishment that therapy must be continuous to prevent emergence of resistant viral strains (6). In 2009, the updated U.S. Department of Health and Human Services guidelines for the use of antiretroviral agents in HIV-1 infected patients continued the recommendation that therapy, with the exception of efavirenz, should be continued during pregnancy (7). If indicated, emtricitabine should not be withheld in pregnancy because the expected benefit to the HIV-positive mother outweighs the unknown risk to the fetus. Updated guidelines for the use of antiretroviral drugs to reduce perinatal HIV-1 transmission also were released in 2010 (8). Women receiving antiretroviral therapy during pregnancy should continue the therapy but, regardless of the regimen, zidovudine administration is recommended during the intrapartum period to prevent vertical transmission of HIV to the newborn (8).

Three studies have reported the pharmacokinetics of emtricitabine in pregnant women with HIV (9–11).

A brief 2009 study reported multi-class HIV resistance in a 38-year-old pregnant woman with twins (12). Starting at 25 weeks', she was successfully treated with a multidrug combination that included emtricitabine. The twins were born at 32 weeks'. Both had negative blood tests for HIV (12).

BREASTFEEDING SUMMARY

Consistent with the molecular weight (about 247), low plasma protein binding (<4%), and long plasma elimination half-life (about 10 hours), emtricitabine is excreted into human breast milk. Five women in Abidjan, Cote d'Ivoire, who were exclusively breastfeeding their infants were given emtricitabine/tenofovir at the start of labor and one tablet daily for 7 days postpartum (13). Maternal blood and milk samples were drawn on days 1, 2, 3, and 7. The median breast milk doses of emtricitabine and tenofovir were 2% and 0.03%, respectively, of the proposed oral infant doses (13).

In developed countries, reports on the use of emtricitabine during lactation are unlikely because the drug is indicated in the treatment of patients with HIV infection. HIV-1 is transmitted in milk, and in developed countries, breastfeeding is not recommended (4,5,7,14–16). In developing countries, breastfeeding is undertaken, despite the risk, because there are no affordable milk substitutes available.

References

1. Product information. Emtriva. Gilead Sciences, 2004.
2. Szczech GM, Wang LH, Walsh JP, Rousseau FS. Reproductive toxicology profile of emtricitabine in mice and rabbits. Reprod Toxicol 2003;17:95–108.
3. Antiretroviral Pregnancy Registry Steering Committee. *Antiretroviral Pregnancy Registry International Interim Report for 1 January 1989 through 31 July 2009*. Wilmington, NC: Registry Coordinating Center; 2009. Available at www.apregistry.com. Accessed May 29, 2010.
4. Carpenter CCJ, Fischi MA, Hammer SM, Hirsch MS, Jacobsen DM, Katzenstein DA, Montaner JSG, Richman DD, Saag MS, Schooley RT, Thompson MA, Vella S, Yeni PG, Volberding PA. Antiretroviral therapy for HIV infection in 1996. JAMA 1996;276:146–54.
5. Minkoff H, Augenbraun M. Antiretroviral therapy for pregnant women. Am J Obstet Gynecol 1997;176:478–89.
6. Minkoff H. Human immunodeficiency virus infection in pregnancy. Obstet Gynecol 2003;101:797–810.
7. Panel on Antiretroviral Guidelines for Adults and Adolescents. *Guidelines for the Use of Antiretroviral Agents in HIV-1-Infected Adults and Adolescents*. Department of Health and Human Services. December 1, 2009:1–161. Available at http://www.aidsinfo.nih.gov/ContentFiles/AdultandAdolescentGL.pdf. Accessed September 17, 2010:60, 96–8.
8. Panel on Treatment of HIV-Infected Pregnant Women and Prevention of Perinatal Transmission. *Recommendations for Use of Antiretroviral Drugs in Pregnant HIV-1-Infected Women for Maternal Health and Interventions to Reduce Perinatal HIV Transmission in the United States*. May 24, 2010:1–117. Available at http://aidsinfo.nih.gov/ContentFiles/PerinatalGL.pdf. Accessed September 17, 2010:30 (Table 5).
9. Hirt D, Urien S, Rey E, Arrive E, Ekouevi DK, Coffie P, Leang SK, Lalsab S, Avit D, Nerrienet E, McIntyre J, Blanche S, Dabis F, Treluyer JM. Population pharmacokinetics of emtricitabine in human immunodeficiency virus type 1-infected pregnant women and their neonates. Antimicrob Agents Chemother 2009;53:1067–73.
10. Stek AM, Best BM, Luo W, Capparelli E, Burchett S, Hu C, Li H, Read JS, Jennings A, Barr E, Smith E, Rossi SS, Mirochnick M. Effect of pregnancy on emtricitabine pharmacokinetics. HIV Med 2012;13:226–35.
11. Colbers APH, Hawkins DA, Gingelmaier A, Kabeya K, Rockstroh JK, Wyen C, Weizsacker K, Sadiq ST, Ivanovic J, Giaquinto C, Taylor GP, Molto J, Burger DM, on behalf of the PANNA network. The pharmacokinetics, safety and efficacy of tenofovir and emtricitabine in HIV-1-infected pregnant women. AIDS 2013;27:739–48.
12. Furco A, Gosrani B, Nicholas S, Williams A, Braithwaite W, Pozniak A, Taylor G, Asboe D, Lyall H, Shaw A, Kapembwa M. Successful use of darunavir, etravirine, enfuvirtide and tenofovir/emtricitabine in pregnant woman with multiclass HIV resistance. AIDS 2009;23:434–5.
13. Benaboud S, Pruvost A, Coffie PA, Ekouevi DK, Urien S, Arrive E, Blanche S, Theodoro F, Avit D, Dabis F, Treluyer JM, Hirt D. Concentrations of tenofovir and emtricitabine in breast milk of HIV-1-infected women in Abidjan, Cote d'Ivoire, in the ANRS 12109 TEmAA study, step 2. Antimicrob Agents Chemother 2011;55:1315–7.
14. Brown ZA, Watts DH. Antiviral therapy in pregnancy. Clin Obstet Gynecol 1990;33:276–89.
15. De Martino M, Tovo P-A, Pezzotti P, Galli L, Massironi E, Ruga E, Floreea F, Plebani A, Gabiano C, Zuccotti GV. HIV-1 transmission through breast-milk: appraisal of risk according to duration of feeding. AIDS 1992;6:991–7.
16. Van de Perre P. Postnatal transmission of human immunodeficiency virus type 1: the breast feeding dilemma. Am J Obstet Gynecol 1995;173:483–7.

ENALAPRIL

Antihypertensive

PREGNANCY RECOMMENDATION: Human Data Suggest Risk in 2nd and 3rd Trimesters
BREASTFEEDING RECOMMENDATION: Limited Human Data—Probably Compatible

E

PREGNANCY SUMMARY

The fetal toxicity of enalapril in the 2nd and 3rd trimesters is similar to other angiotensin-converting enzyme (ACE) inhibitors. The use of this drug during the 2nd and 3rd trimesters may cause teratogenicity and severe fetal and neonatal toxicity. Fetal toxic effects may include anuria, oligohydramnios, fetal hypocalvaria, intrauterine growth restriction (IUGR), prematurity, and patent ductus arteriosus. Anuria-associated anhydramnios/oligohydramnios may produce fetal limb contractures, craniofacial deformation, and pulmonary hypoplasia. Severe anuria and hypotension, resistant to both pressor agents and volume expansion, may occur in the newborn following in utero exposure to valsartan. Newborn renal function and blood pressure should be closely monitored.

FETAL RISK SUMMARY

Enalapril, an ACE inhibitor, is used for the treatment of hypertension. Following oral administration, the prodrug enalapril is bioactivated by hydrolysis to the active agent, enalaprilat. Use of the drug in pregnant rats produced fetal growth restriction and, in two fetuses, incomplete skull ossification (1).

Enalaprilat crosses the human placenta. In an in vitro experiment using a human placental lobe, enalaprilat crossed to the fetal side with a mean transfer of 2.99% (2). The maximum concentration on the fetal side was about 20–48 ng/mL.

A number of references on the use of enalapril during pregnancy have appeared (3–22). A 1991 review summarized the cases of enalapril-exposed pregnancies published prior to January 1, 1990 (23). Use of enalapril limited to the 1st trimester does not appear to present a significant risk to the fetus, but fetal exposure after this time has been associated with teratogenicity and severe toxicity in the fetus and newborn, including death. Of interest, an apparent autosomal recessive syndrome of renal tubular dysplasia with fetal/neonatal anuric renal failure, IUGR, and skull ossification defects, but without exposure to ACE inhibitors, has been described in five infants from two separate kindreds (24).

In a surveillance study of Michigan Medicaid recipients involving 229,101 completed pregnancies conducted between 1985 and 1992, 40 newborns had been exposed to enalapril during the 1st trimester (F. Rosa, personal communication, FDA, 1993). Four (10.0%) major birth defects were observed (two expected), including (observed/expected) 2/0.4 cardiovascular defects and 1/0.1 polydactyly. No anomalies were observed in four other categories of defects (oral clefts, spina bifida, limb reduction defects, and hypospadias) for which specific data were available.

A European survey on the use of ACE inhibitors in pregnancy briefly reviewed the results obtained in nine mother–child pairs (3). Two spontaneous abortions occurred: one at 7 weeks in a 44-year-old woman and one at 11 weeks in a 41-year-old diabetic patient. Enalapril, 20 mg/day, had been used from conception until abortion in the first case and from conception until 6 weeks' gestation in the second. In both cases, factors other than the drug therapy were probably responsible for the pregnancy losses. In a third case, enalapril (30 mg/day) was started at 24 weeks; the patient, with severe glomerulopathy, delivered a stillborn infant 2 weeks later. It is not known whether enalapril therapy was associated with the adverse outcome. The remaining six women were being treated at the time of conception with 10–20 mg/day for essential hypertension or lupus-induced hypertension. Therapy was discontinued by 7 weeks' gestation in four pregnancies, and at 28 weeks in one, and enalapril was continued throughout gestation (40 weeks) in one. Two infants were small for gestational age; one had been exposed only during the first 4 weeks, and one was exposed throughout (40 weeks). No anomalies were mentioned, nor were any other problems in the exposed liveborn infants. The growth restriction was probably due to the severe maternal disease (3).

A 1988 case report described a woman with pregnancy-induced hypertension who was treated with methyldopa and verapamil for 6 weeks with poor control of her blood pressure (4). At 32 weeks' gestation, methyldopa was discontinued and enalapril (20 mg/day) was combined with verapamil (360 mg/day), resulting in good control. An elective cesarean section was performed after 17 days of combination therapy. Oligohydramnios was noted, as was meconium staining. The 2100-g female infant was anuric during the first 2 days, although tests indicated normal kidneys without obstruction. A renal biopsy showed hyperplasia of the juxtaglomerular apparatus. She began producing urine on the 3rd day (2 mL in a period of 24 hours), 12 hours after the onset of peritoneal dialysis. She remained oliguric when dialysis was stopped at age 10 days, producing only 30 mL of urine in a period of 24 hours. By the 19th postnatal day, her urine output had reached 125 mL/24 hours. The plasma enalaprilat concentration was 28 ng/mL before dialysis and then fell to undetectable (<0.16 ng/mL) levels after dialysis. ACE levels (normal 95 nmol/mL-minute) were <1 (days 2 and 3), 2.1 (day 5), 15.6 (day 8), 127 (day 31), and >130 nmol/mL (day 90). Angiotensin II concentrations (normal 182 fmol/mL) were still suppressed (39.8) on day 31; plasma renin activity, active renin, and total renin were all markedly elevated until day 90. By this time, renal function had returned to normal. Clinical follow-up at 1 year of age was normal (4).

A renal transplant patient was treated with enalapril, azathioprine, atenolol, and prednisolone (doses not given) throughout pregnancy (5). Ultrasound at 32 weeks' gestation indicated oligohydramnios and asymmetrical growth restriction. A 1280-g (10th percentile) male infant with a head circumference of 25.7 cm (3rd percentile) was delivered by cesarean section. Severe hypotension (mean 25 mmHg), present at birth, was resistant to volume expansion and pressor agents. The newborn was anuric for 72 hours, then oliguric, passing only 2.5 mL during the next 36 hours. Ultrasonography revealed a normal-sized kidney and a normal urinary tract. Peritoneal dialysis was commenced on day 8, but the infant died 2 days later. Defects secondary to oligohydramnios were squashed facies, contractures of the extremities, and pulmonary hypoplasia. Ossification of the occipital skull was absent. A chromosomal abnormality was excluded based on a normal male karyotype (46,XY). The renal failure and skull hypoplasia were probably caused by enalapril (5).

A 24-year-old woman with malignant hypertension and familial hypophosphatemic rickets was treated from before conception with enalapril (10 mg/day), furosemide (40 mg/day), calciferol, and slow phosphate (6). Blood pressure was normal at 15 weeks' gestation as was fetal growth. However, oligohydramnios developed 2 weeks later; by 20 weeks' gestation, virtually no fluid was present. Fetal growth restriction was also evident at this time. Enalapril and furosemide therapy were slowly replaced by labetalol over the next week, and a steady improvement in amniotic fluid volume was noted by 24 weeks. Volume was normal at 27 weeks' gestation, but shortly thereafter, abruptio placentae occurred, requiring an emergency cesarean section. A 720-g (below 3rd percentile) male infant was delivered who died on day 6. A postmortem examination indicated a normal urogenital tract (6).

An 18-year-old woman with severe chronic hypertension had four pregnancies over an approximately 4-year period, all while taking ACE inhibitors and other antihypertensives (7). During her first pregnancy, she had been maintained on captopril and she delivered a premature, growth-restricted, but otherwise healthy female infant who survived. In the postpartum period, captopril was discontinued and enalapril (10 mg/day) was started while continuing atenolol (100 mg/day) and nifedipine (40 mg/day). She next presented in the 13th week of her second pregnancy with unchanged antihypertensive therapy. Fetal death occurred at 18 weeks' gestation. The 340-g male fetus was macerated but otherwise normal. Her third and fourth pregnancies, again with basically unchanged antihypertensive therapy except for the addition of aspirin (75 mg/day) at the 10th week, resulted in the delivery of an 1170-g female and a 1540-g male, both at 29 weeks (7).

The case of a 27-year-old woman with scleroderma renal disease who was treated with both enalapril and captopril at different times in her pregnancy was published in 1989 (8). Treatment with enalapril (10 mg/day) and nifedipine (60 mg/day) had begun approximately 4 years before the woman presented at an estimated 29 weeks' gestation. Because of concerns for the potential fetal harm induced by the current treatment, therapy was changed to methyldopa. This agent failed to control the woman's hypertension and therapy with captopril (150 mg/day) was initiated at approximately 33 weeks' gestation, 4 weeks prior to delivery of a normal male infant weighing 1740 g. No evidence of renal impairment was observed in the infant (8).

A woman with active systemic lupus erythematosus became severely hypertensive at 22 weeks' gestation (9). Therapy included prednisone, phenytoin (for one episode of tonic-clonic seizure activity), and the antihypertensive agents enalapril, hydralazine (used only briefly), clonidine, nitroprusside, nifedipine, and propranolol. A 600-g male infant with hyaline membrane disease was delivered by cesarean section at 26 weeks' gestation. Severe, persistent hypotension (mean blood pressure during first 24 hours 18–23 mmHg) was observed that was resistant to volume expansion and dopamine. Both kidneys were normal by ultrasonography but no urine was visualized in the bladder. The infant died on the 7th day. Gross and microscopic examination of the kidneys at autopsy revealed no abnormalities. Nephrogenesis was appropriate for gestational age (9).

A 1710-g male infant, delivered by cesarean section for fetal distress at 35 weeks' gestation, had been exposed to enalapril (20 mg/day) and diazepam (5 mg/day) from the 32nd week of pregnancy for the treatment of maternal hypertension (10). Prior to this, treatment had consisted of a 2-week course of methyldopa and amiloride plus hydrochlorothiazide. Except for a few drops, the growth-restricted infant produced no urine, and peritoneal dialysis was started at 86 hours of age. Renal ultrasonography indicated normal kidneys without evidence of obstruction. Renal function slowly improved following dialysis, but some impairment was still present at 18 months of age (10).

Investigators at the FDA reviewed five cases of enalapril-induced neonatal renal failure, one of which had been published previously in a 1989 report (11). Enalapril doses ranged from 10 to 45 mg/day. Two of the mothers were treated throughout gestation, one was treated from 27 to 34 weeks' gestation, and one was treated during the last 3 weeks only. All of the infants required dialysis for anuria. Renal function eventually recovered in two infants, it was still abnormal 1 month after birth in one, and tubular acidosis occurred in the fourth infant 60 days after delivery. Hypotension was reported in three of the four newborns. The authors cautioned that if enalapril was used during pregnancy, then preparations should be made for neonatal hypotension and renal failure (11).

In a 1991 abstract, the FDA investigators updated their previous report on ACE inhibitors and perinatal renal failure by listing a total of 29 cases: 18 were caused by enalapril, 9 by captopril, and 2 by lisinopril (12). Of the 29 cases, 12 (41%) were fatal (another fatal case was listed but it was apparently not caused by renal failure), 9 recovered, and 8 had persistent renal impairment. Only 2 deaths occurred among dialyzed patients. Two cases of oligohydramnios resolved when therapy was stopped before delivery, but one of the infants was stillborn (12).

A 1990 case report suggested that structural kidney defects may be a consequence of enalapril therapy (13). A 22-year-old mother, with systemic lupus erythematosus and severe chronic hypertension, was treated throughout gestation with enalapril (20 mg/day), propranolol (40 mg/day), and hydrochlorothiazide (50 mg/day). Blood pressure was well controlled on this regimen, and no evidence of active lupus occurred during pregnancy. Normal amniotic fluid volume was documented at 16 weeks' gestation followed by severe oligohydramnios at 27 weeks. Although normal fetal growth was observed, the male infant was delivered at

34 weeks' gestation by emergency cesarean section because thick meconium was found on amniocentesis. No meconium was found below the vocal cords. The profound neonatal hypotension induced by enalapril required aggressive treatment with fluids and pressor agents. The newborn had the characteristic features of the oligohydramnios sequence. Both kidneys were morphologically normal by renal ultrasonogram, but no urine output was observed, and no urine was found in the bladder. The infant died at about 25 hours of age. Pulmonary hypoplasia, a condition secondary to oligohydramnios, was found at autopsy. Except for their large size, approximately 1.5 times the expected weight, the kidneys were grossly normal with normal vessels and ureters and a contracted bladder. Microscopic examination revealed a number of kidney abnormalities: irregular corticomedullary junctions; glomerular maldevelopment with a decreased number of lobulations in many of the glomeruli, and some congested glomeruli; a reduced number of tubules in the upper portion of the medulla with increased mesenchymal tissue; and tubular distension in the cortex and medulla. The investigators could not determine whether the renal defects were due to reduced renal blood flow secondary to enalapril, a direct teratogenic effect of the drug, or an effect of the specific drug combination. However, no renal anomalies have been reported after use of the other two drugs (see Hydrochlorothiazide and Propranolol), and similar renal defects have not been reported as a complication of maternal lupus (13).

Three cases of in utero exposure to ACE inhibitors, one of which was enalapril, were reported in a 1992 abstract (14). The infant, delivered at 32 weeks' gestation because of severe oligohydramnios and fetal distress, had growth restriction, hypocalvaria, short limbs, and renal tubular dysplasia. Profound neonatal hypotension and anuria were observed at birth and improved only with dialysis, but the infant died at 9 days of age due to the renal failure (14).

A woman took enalapril (10 mg/day) and furosemide (80 mg/day) throughout gestation for hypertension and delivered a 2.76-kg male infant at 37 weeks' gestation (19). An ultrasound at 20 weeks' had noted oligohydramnios, multicystic kidneys, a small thorax, and no visible bladder. The newborn died a few minutes after birth. Autopsy revealed low set ears, small epicanthic folds, bilateral talipes, a markedly bell-shaped thorax, grossly cystic kidneys, and no apparent normal renal tissue. The karyotype was normal (19).

A 1997 case report described the pregnancy outcome of a woman who was treated with enalapril (20 mg/day) for gestational hypertension from about 28 weeks' gestation to delivery at 36 weeks' (20). Severe oligohydramnios had developed shortly before delivery. The growth-restricted, 2000-g male infant had hypocalvaria, anuria, and profound hypotension. Peritoneal dialysis was started at age 3 days. Before dialysis, the serum ACE level was 7.4 μmol/mL (normal 20–30 μmol/mL). After dialysis, the level was 20.5 μmol/mL, whereas enalaprilat concentrations in the infant's serum and dialysate were 6.92 and 3.3 mcg/mL, respectively. Blood pressure normalized after 4 days of dialysis but chronic renal failure persisted. At 8 months of age, expansion of the calvarial bones with gradual closing of the fontanelles was evident and development, other than growth, was normal. However, the renal failure had worsened and the infant was on the waiting list for a renal transplant (20).

Ten pregnancies treated with enalapril were reported in a 1997 study of 19 pregnancies exposed to ACE inhibitors (21). Enalapril therapy was stopped in the 1st trimester in eight pregnancies and at 14 and 15 weeks', respectively, in the others. No congenital anomalies or renal dysfunction were noted in the 10 neonates (21).

The outcomes of 21 pregnancies exposed to ACE inhibitors between 1991 and 1996 were reported using data from the Danish Birth Registry (22). Exposure to the agents occurred at a median of 8 weeks' gestation (range 5–15 weeks'). No fetal or neonatal complications attributable to the drug therapy were discovered (22).

A 1992 reference described the effects of ACE inhibitors on pregnancy outcome (25). Among 106,813 women enrolled in the Tennessee Medicaid program who delivered either a liveborn or stillborn infant, 19 had taken either enalapril, captopril, or lisinopril during gestation. One newborn, exposed in utero to enalapril, was delivered at 29 weeks' gestation for severe oligohydramnios, IUGR, and fetal distress. Gradual resolution of the infant's renal failure occurred following dialysis (25).

Fourteen cases of fetal hypocalvaria or acalvaria were reviewed in a 1991 reference, one of which was due to enalapril (26). It was speculated that the underlying pathogenetic mechanism in these cases was fetal hypotension.

In an article examining the teratogenesis of ACE inhibitors, evidence was cited linking fetal calvarial hypoplasia with the use of these agents after the 1st trimester (27). The mechanism was thought to be related to drug-induced oligohydramnios that allowed the uterine musculature to exert direct pressure on the fetal skull. This mechanical insult, combined with drug-induced fetal hypotension, could inhibit peripheral perfusion and ossification of the calvaria (27).

A study published in 1992 examined microscopically the kidneys of nine fetuses from chronically hypertensive mothers, one of whom was taking enalapril (28). It was concluded that the renal defects associated with ACE inhibitors were due to decreased renal perfusion and were similar to the defects seen in other conditions related to reduced fetal renal blood flow (28).

Because the fetal toxicity observed in humans in the second half of pregnancy does not have a similar counterpart in experimental animals, a 2001 review compared the pharmacokinetic and pharmacodynamic aspects of enalapril in humans and animals (29). The human fetus is more vulnerable to enalapril-induced toxicity because the specific targets of ACE inhibitors, the kidney and the renin-angiotensin system, are developed before the end of the 1st trimester. This is earlier than the development in animal species, where these specific targets develop near term. In animals, the best concordance in fetal pharmacodynamics to the human is seen with the rhesus monkey, and the least concordance is in rats, which may be partly attributable to pharmacokinetics. Although the placental passage of enalapril in rats has not been studied, the passage of ACE inhibitors with structures similar to enalapril is very low (29).

A retrospective study using pharmacy-based data from the Tennessee Medicaid program identified 209 infants, born between 1985 and 2000, that had 1st trimester exposure to ACE inhibitors (30). Infants of mothers with evidence of diabetes, either before or during pregnancy, were excluded, as were those exposed to angiotensin-receptor antagonists

(ARBs), ACE inhibitors or other antihypertensives beyond the 1st trimester, and exposure to known teratogens. Two comparison groups, other antihypertensives N = 202) and no antihypertensives (N = 29,096), were formed. The number of major birth defects in each of the three groups was 18 (8.6%), 4 (2%), and 834 (2.9%), respectively. Compared with the no-antihypertensives group, exposure to ACE inhibitors was associated with a significantly increased risk of major defects (relative risk [RR] 2.71, 95% confidence interval [CI] 1.72–4.27). When the analysis was conducted by the type of defect, the highest rates were with cardiovascular defects, 9, 2, and 294 respectively, RR 3.72, 95% CI 1.89–7.30, and with central nervous system defects, 3, 0, and 80, respectively, RR 4.39, 95% CI 1.37–14.02. The major defects observed in the subject group were: atrial septal defect (N = 6) (includes three with pulmonic stenosis and/or three with patent ductus arteriosus [PDA]), renal dysplasia (N = 2), PDA alone (N = 2), and one each of ventricular septal defect, spina bifida, microcephaly with eye anomaly, coloboma, hypospadias, intestinal and choanal atresia, Hirschsprung disease, and diaphragmatic hernia (30). In an accompanying editorial, it was noted that neither previous reports of 1st trimester exposure to ACE inhibitors nor the animal studies had observed an increased risk of birth defects (31). It also was noted that no mechanism for ACE inhibitor-induced teratogenicity was known. A subsequent communication raising concerns about the validity of the study in terms of adequate exclusion of diabetes, charting and coding errors in busy medical practices, and the effects of maternal obesity (32) was addressed by the investigators (33).

Enalapril and other ACE inhibitors are human teratogens when used in the 2nd and 3rd trimesters, producing fetal hypocalvaria and renal defects. The cause of the defects and other toxicity is probably related to fetal hypotension and decreased renal blood flow. The compromise of the fetal renal system may result in severe, and at times fatal, anuria, both in the fetus and in the newborn. Anuria-associated oligohydramnios may produce pulmonary hypoplasia, limb contractures, persistent PDA, craniofacial deformation, and neonatal death (34,35). IUGR, prematurity, and severe neonatal hypotension may also be observed. Two reviews of fetal and newborn renal function indicated that both renal perfusion and glomerular plasma flow are low during gestation and that high levels of angiotensin II may be physiologically necessary to maintain glomerular filtration at low perfusion pressures (36,37). Enalapril prevents the conversion of angiotensin I to angiotensin II and, thus, may lead to in utero renal failure. Since the primary means of removal of the drug is renal, the impairment of this system in the newborn prevents elimination of the drug and its active metabolite, enalaprilat, resulting in prolonged hypotension. Newborn renal function and blood pressure should be closely monitored. If oligohydramnios occurs, stopping enalapril may resolve the problem but may not improve infant outcome because of irreversible fetal damage (34). In those cases in which enalapril must be used to treat the mother's disease, the lowest possible dose should be used combined with close monitoring of amniotic fluid levels and fetal well-being. Guidelines for counseling exposed pregnant patients have been published and should be of benefit to health professionals faced with this task (27,34).

The observation in Tennessee Medicaid data of an increased risk of major congenital defects after 1st trimester exposure to ACE inhibitors raises concerns about teratogenicity that have not been seen in other studies. Medicaid data are a valuable tool for identifying early signals of teratogenicity, but are subject to a number of shortcomings, and their findings must be considered hypotheses until confirmed by independent studies.

A 2012 review of the use of ACE inhibitors and ARBs in the 1st trimester concluded that there may be an elevated teratogenic risk, but the risk appeared to be related to other factors (38). The factors, that typically coexist with hypertension in pregnancy, included diabetes, advanced maternal age, and obesity.

BREASTFEEDING SUMMARY

A study published in 1989 was unable to demonstrate the excretion of enalapril and enalaprilat in breast milk (39). Direct concentrations of enalapril, however, were not measured in this study. Three women, 3–45 days postpartum, were treated with enalapril for hypertension. One woman with chronic glomerulonephritis and slightly impaired renal function was treated with 5 mg twice daily for 40 days before the study. The other two women, both with essential hypertension and normal renal function, were treated with 10 mg (duration not specified). ACE activity in the serum of the women was markedly depressed 4 hours after treatment with activity dropping from 18.7–24.0 to 0.4–0.7 U/mL (reference value in controls 28.0 U/mL). ACE activity in milk samples was not affected: 11.7–18.6 U/mL before the dose vs. 12.4–15.4 U/mL 4 hours after the dose (reference value in controls 9.1–22.6 U/mL), indicating that little if any of the drug was excreted into milk. Concentrations of enalaprilat in maternal serum ranged from 23.9 to 48.0 ng/mL in the two women with normal renal function and 179 ng/mL in the woman with renal impairment. Milk levels were all <0.2 ng/mL, the level of sensitivity for the assay (39).

In contrast to the above study, concentrations of both enalapril and enalaprilat were measured in a study published in 1991 (40). A woman, 12 months postpartum, had been treated with enalapril (10 mg/day) for essential hypertension for 11 months. Twenty-four hours after her last dose, she was given 10 mg, and milk samples were drawn at 0, 4, 8.75, and 24 hours. Serum samples were also drawn at various times over the next 24 hours. The total amount of the enalapril and enalaprilat measured in the milk over the 24-hour sample period were 81.9 and 36.1 ng, respectively. These values corresponded to 1.44 and 0.63 ng/mL, respectively. The peak concentration of enalapril, 2.05 ng/mL, occurred in the 4-hour sample, whereas that of enalaprilat, 0.75 ng/mL, occurred in the 8.75-hour sample. When milk levels were compared with serum concentrations at these sampling times, the milk:serum ratios were 0.14 and 0.02, respectively (40).

In a third study, milk and serum concentrations of enalapril and enalaprilat were measured in five women at 0, 4, 6, and 24 hours after a single 20-mg dose (41). The mean maximum milk concentration of enalapril was 1.74 ng/mL, whereas that of enalaprilat was 1.72 ng/mL. No enalapril was measured in the milk of one patient. The milk:serum ratio for the parent compound and the metabolite varied from 0 to 0.043 and from 0.021 to 0.031, respectively (41).

Based on the above data, the amount of enalapril and enalaprilat that could potentially be ingested by a breastfeeding infant appears to be negligible and is probably clinically insignificant. The American Academy of Pediatrics classifies enalapril as compatible with breastfeeding (42).

References

1. Valdés G, Marinovic D, Falcón C, Chuaqui R, Duarte I. Placental alterations, intrauterine growth retardation and teratogenicity associated with enalapril use in pregnant rats. Biol Neonate 1992;61:124–30.
2. Reisenberger K, Egarter C, Sternberger B, Eckenberger P, Eberle E, Weissenbacher ER. Placental passage of angiotensin-converting enzyme inhibitors. Am J Obstet Gynecol 1996;174:1450–5.
3. Kreft-Jais C, Plouin P-F, Tchobroutsky C, Boutroy M-J. Angiotensin-converting enzyme inhibitors during pregnancy: a survey of 22 patients given captopril and nine given enalapril. Br J Obstet Gynaecol 1988;95:420–2.
4. Schubiger G, Flury G, Nussberger J. Enalapril for pregnancy-induced hypertension: acute renal failure in a neonate. Ann Intern Med 1988;108:215–6.
5. Mehta N, Modi N. ACE inhibitors in pregnancy. Lancet 1989;2:96.
6. Broughton Pipkin F, Baker PN, Symonds EM. ACE inhibitors in pregnancy. Lancet 1989;2:96–7.
7. Smith AM. Are ACE inhibitors safe in pregnancy? Lancet 1989;2:750–1.
8. Baethge BA, Wolf RE. Successful pregnancy with scleroderma renal disease and pulmonary hypertension in a patient using angiotensin converting enzyme inhibitors. Ann Rheum Dis 1989;48:776–8.
9. Scott AA, Purohit DM. Neonatal renal failure: a complication of maternal antihypertensive therapy. Am J Obstet Gynecol 1989;160:1223–4.
10. Hulton SA, Thomson PD, Cooper PA, Rothberg AD. Angiotensin-converting enzyme inhibitors in pregnancy may result in neonatal renal failure. S Afr Med J 1990;78:673–6.
11. Rosa FW, Bosco LA, Graham CF, Milstien JB, Dreis M, Creamer J. Neonatal anuria with maternal angiotensin-converting enzyme inhibition. Obstet Gynecol 1989;74:371–4.
12. Rosa FW, Bosco L. Infant renal failure with maternal ACE inhibition (abstract 92). Am J Obstet Gynecol 1991;164:273.
13. Cunniff C, Jones KL, Phillipson J, Benirschke K, Short S, Wujek J. Oligohydramnios sequence and renal tubular malformation associated with maternal enalapril use. Am J Obstet Gynecol 1990;162:187–9.
14. Pryde PG, Nugent CE, Sedman AB, Barr M Jr. ACE inhibitor fetopathy (abstract). Am J Obstet Gynecol 1992;166:348.
15. Neerhof MG, Shlossman PA, Poll DS, Ludomirsky A, Weiner S. Idiopathic aldosteronism in pregnancy. Obstet Gynecol 1991;78:489–91.
16. Boutroy M-J. Fetal effects of maternally administered clonidine and angiotensin-converting enzyme inhibitors. Dev Pharmacol Ther 1989;13: 199–204.
17. Svensson A, Andersch B, Dahlof B. ACE-hammare i samband med graviditet kan medfora risker for fostret. Lakartidningen 1986;83:699–700.
18. Scanferla F, Coli U, Landini S, et al. Treatment of pregnancy-induced hypertension with ACE inhibitor enalapril (abstract). Clin Exp Hypertens Pregn 1987;B6:45.
19. Thorpe-Beeston JG, Armar NA, Dancy M, Cochrane GW, Ryan G, Rodeck CH. Pregnancy and ACE inhibitors. Br J Obstet Gynaecol 1993;100:692–3.
20. Lavoratti G, Seracini D, Fiorini P, Cocchi C, Materassi M, Donzelli G, Pela I. Neonatal anuria by ACE inhibitors during pregnancy. Nephron 1997;76:235–6.
21. Lip GYH, Churchill D, Beevers M, Auckett A, Beevers DG. Angiotensin-converting-enzyme inhibitors in early pregnancy. Lancet 1997;350:1446–7.
22. Steffensen FH, Nielsen GL, Sorensen HT, Olesen C, Olsen J. Pregnancy outcome with ACE-inhibitor use in early pregnancy. Lancet 1998;351:596.
23. Hanssens M, Keirse MJNC, Vankelecom F, Van Assche FA. Fetal and neonatal effects of treatment with angiotensin-converting enzyme inhibitors in pregnancy. Obstet Gynecol 1991;78:128–35.
24. Kumar D, Moss G, Primhak R, Coombs R. Congenital renal tubular dysplasia and skull ossification defects similar to teratogenic effects of angiotensin converting enzyme (ACE) inhibitors. J Med Genet 1997;34:541–5.
25. Piper JM, Ray WA, Rosa FW. Pregnancy outcome following exposure to angiotensin-converting enzyme inhibitors. Obstet Gynecol 1992;80: 429–32.
26. Barr M Jr, Cohen MM Jr. ACE inhibitor fetopathy and hypocalvaria: the kidney-skull connection. Teratology 1991;44:485–95.
27. Brent RL, Beckman DA. Angiotensin-converting enzyme inhibitors, an embryopathic class of drugs with unique properties: information for clinical teratology counselors. Teratology 1991;43:543–6.
28. Martin RA, Jones KL, Mendoza A, Barr M Jr, Benirschke K. Effect of ACE inhibition on the fetal kidney: decreased renal blood flow. Teratology 1992;46:317–21.
29. Tabacova SA, Kimmel CA. Enalapril: pharmacokinetic/dynamic inferences for comparative developmental toxicity. A review. Reprod Toxicol 2001;15:467–78.
30. Cooper WO, Hernandez-Diaz S, Arbogast PG, Dudley JA, Dyer S, Gideon PS, Hall K, Ray WA. Major congenital malformations after first-trimester exposure to ACE inhibitors. N Engl J Med 2006;354:2443–51.
31. Friedman JM. ACE inhibitors and congenital anomalies. N Engl J Med 2006;354:2498–2500.
32. Scialli AR, Lione A. ACE inhibitors and major congenital malformations. N Engl J Med 2006;355:1280.
33. Cooper WO, Ray WA. Reply—ACE inhibitors and major congenital malformations. N Engl J Med 2006;355:1281.
34. Barr M Jr. Teratogen update: angiotensin-converting enzyme inhibitors. Teratology 1994;50:399–409.
35. Shotan A, Widerhorn J, Hurst A, Elkayam U. Risks of angiotensin-converting enzyme inhibition during pregnancy: experimental and clinical evidence, potential mechanisms, and recommendations for use. Am J Med 1994;96:451–6.
36. Robillard JE, Nakamura KT, Matherne GP, Jose PA. Renal hemodynamics and functional adjustments to postnatal life. Semin Perinatol 1988;12: 143–50.
37. Guignard J-P, Gouyon J-B. Adverse effects of drugs on the immature kidney. Biol Neonate 1988;53:243–52.
38. Polifka JE. Is there an embryopathy associated with first-trimester exposure to angiotensin-converting enzyme inhibitors and angiotensin receptor antagonists? A critical review of the evidence. Birth Defects Res (Part A) 2012;94:576–98.
39. Huttunen K, Gronhagen-Riska C, Fyhrquist F. Enalapril treatment of a nursing mother with slightly impaired renal function. Clin Nephrol 1989;31:278.
40. Rush JE, Snyder BA, Barrish A, Hichens M. Comment. Clin Nephrol 1991;35:234.
41. Redman CWG, Kelly JG, Cooper WD. The excretion of enalapril and enalaprilat in human breast milk. Eur J Clin Pharmacol 1990;38:99.
42. Committee on Drugs, American Academy of Pediatrics. The transfer of drugs and other chemicals into human milk. Pediatrics 2001;108: 776–89.

ENCAINIDE

[Withdrawn from the market. See 8th edition.]

ENFLURANE

General Anesthetic

PREGNANCY RECOMMENDATION: Limited Human Data—Animal Data Suggest Low Risk
BREASTFEEDING RECOMMENDATION: No Human Data—Probably Compatible

PREGNANCY SUMMARY

Enflurane is teratogenic in mice but not in rats. No reports of its use early in human gestation have been located. The absence of human experience during organogenesis prevents an assessment of the risk for structural anomalies. In addition, general anesthesia usually involves the use of multiple pharmacological agents. Although no teratogenicity has been observed with other halogenated general anesthetic agents, only halothane has 1st trimester human exposure data (see Halothane). The potential reproductive toxicity (spontaneous abortion and infertility) of occupational exposure to halogenated general anesthetic agents has not been adequately studied.

E

FETAL RISK SUMMARY

Enflurane, a nonflammable general inhalation anesthetic agent administered via vaporizer, is indicated for the induction and/or maintenance of anesthesia during surgery. It also provides analgesia for vaginal delivery and, in low concentrations, is used to supplement other general anesthetic agents during delivery by cesarean section. Enflurane is in the same class of volatile liquid halogenated agents as desflurane, halothane, isoflurane, methoxyflurane, and sevoflurane. It is closely related chemically to desflurane and isoflurane (1). The blood–gas partition coefficient is 1.9 (1). This is higher (i.e., increased solubility in blood) than the value for either isoflurane (1.46) or desflurane (0.42) (see Desflurane or Isoflurane).

Studies in animals have not revealed evidence of carcinogenic or mutagenic effects. Reproduction studies, conducted in rats and rabbits at doses up to four times the human dose, revealed no evidence of impaired fertility or fetal harm (1).

In a 1981 study with mice, chronic exposure to subanesthetic and anesthetic concentrations of enflurane was evaluated. High exposures, about 100 times greater than the level of human occupational exposure in unscavenged operating rooms, were associated with minor developmental variations (lumbar ribs and increased pelvic cavitation) and defects (cleft palate, minor skeletal and visceral anomalies). The effects were greater than those observed with methoxyflurane, but less than those with halothane (2).

In a second study by the authors of the above report, the effects of four general anesthetic agents were compared in pregnant rats (3). The doses and agents used were nitrous oxide (75%; 0.55 MAC), enflurane (1.65%; 0.75 MAC), halothane (0.8%; 0.75 MAC), and isoflurane (1.05%; 0.75 MAC). (*Note: The minimum alveolar anesthetic concentration [MAC] is the concentration that causes immobility in 50% of patients exposed to a noxious stimulus such as a surgical incision; it represents the ED_{50} (4).*) Each agent was administered for 6 hours on each of three consecutive days in one of three gestational periods: pregnancy days 8–10, 11–13, or 14–16. Compared with controls, significantly decreased maternal weight gain was observed in three of the groups (nitrous oxide, isoflurane, and enflurane) after exposure on days 14–16. Exposure on those days resulted in significantly decreased fetal weight in all four groups, and when exposure occurred on days 8–10 in three groups (all except nitrous oxide). Nitrous oxide exposure during days 14–16 resulted in significant increases in total fetal wastage and resorptions (threefold increases). However, no major or minor teratogenic effects were observed in any of the groups (3).

The teratogenic potential of isoflurane, enflurane, and sevoflurane was studied by evaluating the effect of each agent on the proliferation and differentiation of cells exiting from the G1 phase of the cell cycle (5). The theory behind the study was that normal development during embryogenesis, organogenesis, and histogenesis depended upon the proliferation and differentiative processes of cell migration (5). For example, valproate, a known human teratogen, is a potent G1-phase inhibitor of the in vitro proliferation rate at concentrations less than two times the therapeutic plasma concentration. At anesthetic concentrations less than two times the MAC, the antiproliferative potency of the three agents was isoflurane = enflurane >> sevoflurane. However, in the growth-arrested cell population, there was no specific accumulation of any cell-cycle phase and no specific effect on the G1 phase. The investigators concluded that the three agents lacked the specific in vitro characteristics of valproate (5).

In a 1990 study, mice were exposed for 8 hours to sevoflurane and enflurane combined with three different concentrations of oxygen (6). Both anesthetic agents caused cleft palate, but the incidence was lower than that observed with halothane. Increasing the concentrations of oxygen lowered the incidence of the defect (6).

Reviews have concluded that, in general, inhalational anesthetics are freely transferred to fetal tissues (7,8) and, in most cases, the maternal and fetal concentrations are equivalent (8). The low molecular weight (about 185) and the presence of enflurane in the maternal brain support this assertion.

Two reports described the use of enflurane in 100 women for anesthesia for cesarean section (9,10). No increase in newborn adverse effects was observed.

A small 1983 study compared the neonatal outcomes in four groups (10 patients each) of women receiving general anesthesia for cesarean section: 50% nitrous oxide and 50% oxygen either alone, or combined with 0.5% halothane, 1.0% enflurane, or 0.75% isoflurane (11). One newborn had an Apgar score less than 7 at 1 minute (enflurane group), but all newborns in all groups had scores of 7 or greater at 5 minutes. There were no significant differences between the groups in neonatal neurobehavior assessment 2–4 hours after delivery or in maternal or umbilical blood gas analysis at delivery (11).

In a 1977 in vitro study, enflurane was shown to have a statistically significant depressive effect on myometrial strips from nongravid and gravid uteri (12). Three anesthetic agents, isoflurane, enflurane, and halothane, were studied at three concentrations (0.5, 1.0, and 1.5 MAC). The amount of depression was dose-related for each agent and was similar with all agents (12).

In a study to determine if pregnancy decreases the MAC, enflurane and halothane were administered to 16 women (8 with each agent) scheduled for pregnancy termination at 8–13 weeks' gestation (13). A comparison group of 16 nonpregnant women undergoing laparoscopic sterilization received either enflurane or halothane (8 in each group). In pregnant women, the median MAC of 1.15 volume% (range 0.95–1.25) was less than that in nonpregnant women, 1.65% volume% (range 1.45–1.75) ($p = 0.0007$). The percentage decrease (95% confidence interval) for pregnant women was 30% (24%–36%). Similar results were found with halothane (13).

Chronic occupational exposure to anesthetic gases in operating rooms during pregnancy has raised concerns that such exposure could cause birth defects and spontaneous abortions (14). The concentration of enflurane in an operating-room environment was stated to 5–46 parts per million (ppm) near the anesthesiologist and 1–8 ppm near the surgeon. A 1988 review cited a number of studies investigating the possible association between occupational exposure to anesthetic gases and adverse pregnancy outcomes (7). The reviewer concluded that serious methodological weaknesses in these studies precluded arriving at a firm conclusion, but a slightly increased risk of miscarriage was a possibility. However, there was no evidence of an association between occupational exposure and congenital anomalies (7).

In a 1982 study, the infants of mothers who had received analgesia before vaginal delivery consisting of either enflurane, nitrous oxide (both mixed with oxygen), or no inhalation agent were evaluated for neurobehavior during the first 24 hours (15). The infants were tested with the Neurologic and Adaptive Capacity Score at 15 minutes, 2 hours, and 24 hours, and with the Early Neonatal Neurobehavioral Scale at 2 and 24 hours. For all groups, scores were the lowest at 2 hours, but no significant differences were measured between the groups (15).

A 2004 study, however, found a significant association between maternal occupational exposure to waste anesthetic gases during pregnancy and developmental deficits in their children, including gross and fine motor ability, inattention/hyperactivity, and IQ performance (see Nitrous Oxide).

Enflurane has been used immediately prior to delivery for analgesia and anesthesia. This use does not appear to affect the newborn any differently than other general anesthetic agents. The uterine effects of enflurane (relaxation and increased blood loss) also appear to be similar to other agents in this class, but the low concentrations used clinically minimize these actions (16). All anesthetic agents can cause depression in the newborn that may last for 24 hours or more but, again, this is lessened by the low doses.

BREASTFEEDING SUMMARY

Although enflurane has been administered during labor and delivery, the effects of this exposure on the infant that begins nursing immediately after birth have not been described. Enflurane is probably excreted into colostrum and milk as suggested by its presence in the maternal blood and its low molecular weight (about 185), but the toxic potential of this exposure for the infant is unknown. However, the risk to a nursing infant from exposure to enflurane via milk is probably very low (17,18). Another halogenated inhalation anesthetic, halothane, is classified as compatible with breastfeeding by the American Academy of Pediatrics (see Halothane).

E

References

1. Product information. Ethrane. Abbott Laboratories (NZ), 1999.
2. Wharton RS, Mazze RI, Wilson AI. Reproduction and fetal development in mice chronically exposed to enflurane. Anesthesiology 1981;54:505–10.
3. Mazze RI, Fujinaga M, Rice SA, Harris SB, Baden JM. Reproductive and teratogenic effects of nitrous oxide, halothane, isoflurane, and enflurane in Sprague-Dawley rats. Anesthesiology 1986;64:339–44.
4. Trevor AJ, Miller RD. General anesthetics. In: Katzung BG, ed. *Basic and Clinical Pharmacology*. 8th ed. New York, NY: McGraw-Hill, 2001:426.
5. O'Leary G, Bacon CL, Odumeru O, Fagan C, Fitzpatrick T, Gallagher HC, Moriarty DC, Regan CM. Antiproliferative actions of inhalational anesthetics: comparisons to the valproate teratogen. Int J Dev Neurosci 2000;18: 39–45.
6. Natsume N, Miura S, Sugimoto S, Nakamura T, Horiuchi R, Kondo S, Furukawa H, Inagaki S, Kawai T, Yamada M, Arai T, Hosoda R. Teratogenicity caused by halothane, enflurane, and sevoflurane, and changes depending on O_2 concentration (abstract). Teratology 1990;42:30A.
7. Friedman JM. Teratogen update: anesthetic agents. Teratology 1988;37: 69–77.
8. Kanto J. Risk-benefit assessment of anaesthetic agents in the puerperium. Drug Saf 1991;6:285–301.
9. Coleman AJ, Downing JW. Enflurane anesthesia for cesarean section. Anesthesiology 1975;43:354–7.
10. Dick W, Knoche E, Traub E. Clinical investigations concerning the use of Ethrane for cesarean section. J Perinat Med 1979;7:125–33.
11. Warren TM, Datta S, Ostheimer GW, Naulty JS, Weiss JB, Morrison JA. Comparison of the maternal and neonatal effects of halothane, enflurane, and isoflurane for cesarean section. Anesth Analg 1983;62:516–20.
12. Munson ES, Embro WJ. Enflurane, isoflurane, and halothane and isolated human uterine muscle. Anesthesiology 1977;46:11–4.
13. Chan MTV, Mainland P, Gin T. Minimum alveolar concentration of halothane and enflurane are decreased in early pregnancy. Anesthesiology 1996;85:782–6.
14. Corbett TH. Cancer and congenital anomalies associated with anesthetics. Ann NY Acad Sci 1976;271:58–66.
15. Stefani SJ, Hughes SC, Shnider SM, Levinson G, Abboud TK, Henriksen EH, Williams V, Johnson J. Neonatal neurobehavioral effects of inhalation analgesia for vaginal delivery. Anesthesiology 1982;56:351–5.
16. Quail AW. Modern inhalational anaesthetic agents: a review of halothane, isoflurane and enflurane. Med J Aust 1989;150:95–102.
17. Lee JJ, Rubin AP. Breast feeding and anaesthesia. Anaesthesia 1993;48: 616–25.
18. Spigset O. Anaesthetic agents and excretion in breast milk. Acta Anaesthesiol Scand 1994;38:94–103.

ENFUVIRTIDE

Antiviral

PREGNANCY RECOMMENDATION: Compatible—Maternal Benefit >> Embryo–Fetal Risk
BREASTFEEDING RECOMMENDATION: Contraindicated

PREGNANCY SUMMARY

Although the animal data suggest low risk, the limited human pregnancy experience prevents a more complete assessment of embryo–fetal risk. However, enfuvirtide has not been detected in cord blood at delivery or on the fetal side in the ex vivo human placenta perfusion model. If indicated, the drug should not be withheld because of pregnancy.

E

FETAL RISK SUMMARY

Enfuvirtide, a linear 36-amino acid synthetic peptide administered by SC injection, is an inhibitor of the fusion of HIV-1 with CD4+ cells. It is in the same antiviral subclass of entry inhibitors as maraviroc. Enfuvirtide is indicated, in combination with other antiretroviral agents, for the treatment of HIV-1 infection in treatment-experienced patients with evidence of HIV-1 replication despite ongoing antiretroviral therapy. Plasma protein binding of enfuvirtide is about 92%, primarily to albumin and, to a lesser extent, to α_1-acid glycoprotein. The agent is thought to undergo catabolism to the constituent amino acids with subsequent recycling of the amino acids in the body pool. The mean elimination half-life is 3.8 hours (1).

Reproduction studies have been conducted in rats and rabbits. In these species, SC doses up to 27 and 3.2 times, respectively, the human dose based on BSA (HD) revealed no evidence of fetal harm. In male and female rats, SC doses up to 1.6 times the HD had no effect on fertility (1).

Consistent with the high molecular weight (4492) and protein binding, three studies have found that the drug does not cross the human placenta. No transfer to the fetal side was noted in an ex vivo study, even with very high concentrations on the maternal side (2). The mean concentration in the maternal compartment of three term placentas from healthy women was 12,400 ng/mL, 2.5 times the maximum concentration recommended for treated patients, but the drug was not detected (<50 ng/mL) in the fetal venous samples (2). In a clinical study, maternal enfuvirtide (doses not specified) concentrations in two patients immediately before delivery at term were 3647 and 4135 ng/mL, but the drug was undetectable in cord blood (<50 ng/mL) in both cases (3). In a third report, the drug was not detected in the cord blood samples of twins born at 34 weeks from a woman treated with SC enfuvirtide 90 mg twice daily from 25 to 34 weeks (4).

Three reports have described the use of enfuvirtide with other antivirals for multidrug-resistant HIV during the second half of pregnancy. Healthy infants were delivered without evidence of HIV infection at birth or during long-term follow-up (5–7).

The Antiretroviral Pregnancy Registry reported, for the period January 1989 through July 2009, prospective data (reported before the outcomes were known) involving 4702 live births that had been exposed during the 1st trimester to one or more antiretroviral agents (8). Congenital defects were noted in 134, a prevalence of 2.8% (95% confidence interval [CI] 2.4–3.4). In the 6100 live births with earliest exposure in the 2nd/3rd trimesters, there were 153 infants with defects (2.5%, 95% CI 2.1–2.9). The prevalence rates for the two periods did not differ significantly. There were 288 infants with birth defects among 10,803 live births with exposure anytime during pregnancy (2.7%, 95% CI 2.4–3.0). The prevalence rate did not differ significantly from the rate expected in a nonexposed population. There were 31 outcomes exposed to enfuvirtide (19 in the 1st trimester and 12 in the 2nd/3rd trimesters) in combination with other antiretroviral agents. There were no birth defects. In reviewing the birth defects of prospective and retrospective (pregnancies reported after the outcomes were known) registered cases, the Registry concluded that, except for isolated cases of neural tube defects with efavirenz exposure in retrospective reports, there was no other pattern of anomalies (isolated or syndromic) (8). (See Lamivudine for required statement.)

Two reviews, one in 1996 and the other in 1997, concluded that all women currently receiving antiretroviral therapy should continue to receive therapy during pregnancy and that treatment of the mother with monotherapy should be considered inadequate therapy (9,10). The same conclusion was reached in a 2003 review with the added admonishment that therapy must be continuous to prevent emergence of resistant viral strains (11). In 2009, the updated U.S. Department of Health and Human Services guidelines for the use of antiretroviral agents in HIV-1 infected patients continued the recommendation that therapy, with the exception of efavirenz, should be continued during pregnancy (12). If indicated, enfuvirtide should not be withheld in pregnancy because the expected benefit to the HIV-positive mother outweighs the unknown risk to the fetus. Updated guidelines for the use of antiretroviral drugs to reduce perinatal HIV-1 transmission also were released in 2010 (13). Women receiving antiretroviral therapy during pregnancy should continue the therapy but, regardless of the regimen, zidovudine administration is recommended during the intrapartum period to prevent vertical transmission of HIV to the newborn (13).

BREASTFEEDING SUMMARY

No reports describing the use of enfuvirtide during human lactation have been located. The high molecular weight (4492) and protein binding (92%) should inhibit, but may not prevent, excretion into human breast milk. The effect on a nursing infant is unknown. However, enfuvirtide is a 36-amino acid peptide and any amounts that enter milk should be digested by the nursing infant.

Reports on the use of enfuvirtide during lactation are unlikely because the drug is indicated in the treatment of patients with HIV infection. HIV-1 is transmitted in milk, and in developed countries, breastfeeding is not recommended (9,10,12,14–16). In developing countries, breastfeeding is undertaken, despite the risk, because there are no affordable milk substitutes available.

References

1. Product information. Fuzeon. Roche Pharmaceuticals, 2004.
2. Ceccaldi PF, Ferreira C, Gavard L, Gil S, Peytavin G, Mandelbrot L. Placental transfer of enfuvirtide in the ex vivo human placental perfusion model. Am J Obstet Gynecol 2008;198:433.e1–2.

3. Brennan-Benson P, Pakianathan M, Rice P, Bonora S, Chakraborty R, Sharland M, Hay P. Enfuvirtide prevents vertical transmission of multidrug-resistant HIV-1 in pregnancy but does not cross the placenta. AIDS 2006;20:297–9.
4. Furco A, Gosrani B, Nicholas S, Williams A, Braithwaite W, Pozniak A, Taylor G, Asboe D, Lyall H, Shaw A, Kapembwa M. Successful use of darunavir, etravirine, enfuvirtide and tenofovir/emtricitabine in pregnant woman with multiclass HIV resistance. AIDS 2009;23:434–5.
5. Wensing AMJ, Boucher CAB, van Kasteren M, van Dijken PJ, Geelen SP, Juttmann JR. Prevention of mother-to-child transmission of multi-drug resistant HIV-1 using maternal therapy with both enfuvirtide and tipranavir. AIDS 2006;20:1465–7.
6. Madeddu G, Calia GM, Campus ML, Lovigu C, Mannazzu M, Olmeo P, Mela MG, Mura MS. Successful prevention of multidrug resistant HIV mother-to-child transmission with enfuvirtide use in late pregnancy. Int J STD AIDS 2008;19:644–5.
7. Sued O, Lattner J, Patterson P, Abusamra L, Cesar C, Fink V, Krolewiecki A, Cahn P. Use of darunavir and enfuvirtide in a pregnant woman. Int J STD AIDS 2008;19:866–7.
8. Antiretroviral Pregnancy Registry Steering Committee. *Antiretroviral Pregnancy Registry International Interim Report for 1 January 1989 through 31 July 2009*. Wilmington, NC: Registry Coordinating Center; 2009. Available at www.apregistry.com. Accessed May 29, 2010.
9. Carpenter CCJ, Fischi MA, Hammer SM, Hirsch MS, Jacobsen DM, Katzenstein DA, Montaner JSG, Richman DD, Saag MS, Schooley RT, Thompson MA, Vella S, Yeni PG, Volberding PA. Antiretroviral therapy for HIV infection in 1996. JAMA 1996;276:146–54.
10. Minkoff H, Augenbraun M. Antiretroviral therapy for pregnant women. Am J Obstet Gynecol 1997;176:478–89.
11. Minkoff H. Human immunodeficiency virus infection in pregnancy. Obstet Gynecol 2003;101:797–810.
12. Panel on Antiretroviral Guidelines for Adults and Adolescents. *Guidelines for the Use of Antiretroviral Agents in HIV-1-Infected Adults and Adolescents*. Department of Health and Human Services. December 1, 2009:1–161. Available at http://www.aidsinfo.nih.gov/ContentFiles/AdultandAdolescentGL.pdf. Accessed September 17, 2010:60, 96–8.
13. Panel on Treatment of HIV-Infected Pregnant Women and Prevention of Perinatal Transmission. *Recommendations for Use of Antiretroviral Drugs in Pregnant HIV-1-Infected Women for Maternal Health and Interventions to Reduce Perinatal HIV Transmission in the United States*. May 24, 2010:1–117. Available at http://aidsinfo.nih.gov/ContentFiles/PerinatalGL.pdf. Accessed September 17, 2010:30 (Table 5).
14. Brown ZA, Watts DH. Antiviral therapy in pregnancy. Clin Obstet Gynecol 1990;33:276–89.
15. De Martino M, Tovo P-A, Pezzotti P, Galli L, Massironi E, Ruga E, Floreea F, Plebani A, Gabiano C, Zuccotti GV. HIV-1 transmission through breast-milk: appraisal of risk according to duration of feeding. AIDS 1992;6:991–7.
16. Van de Perre P. Postnatal transmission of human immunodeficiency virus type 1: the breast-feeding dilemma. Am J Obstet Gynecol 1995;173:483–7.

E

ENOXACIN

[Withdrawn from the market. See 9th edition.]

ENOXAPARIN

Anticoagulant

PREGNANCY RECOMMENDATION: Compatible
BREASTFEEDING RECOMMENDATION: Compatible

PREGNANCY SUMMARY

The use of enoxaparin during pregnancy appears to present no more fetal and/or newborn risk, and perhaps less, than that from standard, unfractionated heparin or from no therapy.

FETAL RISK SUMMARY

Enoxaparin is a low-molecular-weight-heparin (LMWH) product prepared from porcine intestinal mucosa heparin. The anticoagulant is not teratogenic or embryotoxic in rats and rabbits (1).

Enoxaparin has an average molecular weight of about 4500 (1). Because this is a relatively large molecule, it does not cross the placenta (2,3) and, thus, presents a low risk to the fetus.

Several reports have described the use of enoxaparin during pregnancy without maternal or fetal complications (4–15).

A woman with an extensive lower limb venous thrombosis was treated with unfractionated heparin for 2 weeks starting at 11 weeks' gestation and then changed to enoxaparin (4). She was continued on enoxaparin until delivery of a healthy infant at 34 weeks' gestation.

A 1992 reference described the use enoxaparin in six pregnant women for the treatment and prophylaxis of thromboembolism (5). In two women treated from the 8th or 9th gestational week, one ended with a healthy term infant and the other was progressing normally at 18 weeks (outcome was not available at time of the report). Three other women were treated during the 2nd and/or 3rd trimesters and had normal term deliveries. In the remaining case, a woman with Sjögren's syndrome and a history of deep venous thrombosis (DVT) and pulmonary embolism, developed a DVT at 18 weeks' gestation. She was treated for 10 days with IV heparin and then started on enoxaparin 40 mg twice daily. The DVT recurred at 25 weeks' gestation and she was again treated with a course of IV heparin followed by SC heparin. Due to severe fetal distress after 5 days of SC heparin, an emergency cesarean section was performed. The infant died a few minutes after birth, but permission for an autopsy was refused. An examination of the placenta showed multiple hemorrhages (5).

The use of enoxaparin for the achievement of successful thromboprophylaxis in 16 women during 18 pregnancies was described in a 1994 communication (6). The mean gestational age at the start of therapy was 10 weeks. Eight women had a history of thromboembolism, six had thrombophilia, and two had systemic lupus erythematosus. A 20 mg SC dose once daily was used in the first 11 women, but because of low anti-factor Xa levels, the dose was increased to 40 mg SC once daily in the last 7 pregnancies. From the 18 pregnancies, there were 2 missed abortions and 2 mid-trimester abortions, all in pregnancies of women with anticardiolipin syndrome (6).

E

The thromboprophylaxis of 41 pregnancies (34 women), most with 40 mg enoxaparin SC daily, was described in a 1996 report (7). Some of these cases had been reported earlier in a 1995 abstract (8). Only one thromboembolic event occurred, a hepatic infarction in a woman treated with 20 mg/day SC. No maternal hemorrhages were observed even though the therapy was continued throughout labor, delivery, and the immediate postpartum period. Nineteen of the women underwent 24 surgical procedures while receiving enoxaparin, including cervical cerclage ($N = 2$), amniocentesis ($N = 5$), 2nd trimester terminations ($N = 4$), and cesarean section ($N = 13$). Epidural anesthesia during labor was used in nine women. No abnormal bleeding was observed in any of these cases and there were no reports of intraventricular hemorrhage in the neonates (7).

Enoxaparin, usually 40 mg SC daily starting in the 1st trimester, was used for prophylaxis in 61 women (69 pregnancies) at high risk for thromboembolism in a prospective study published in 1997 (9). Some of these patients ($N = 18$) had been reported earlier (6). Mean steady-state plasma heparin levels, as determined by anti-factor Xa assay, following a 40 mg dose were three times as high as those with 20 mg, 0.09 vs. 0.03 U/mL, respectively, but were not affected by gestational age. No increased bleeding risk during pregnancy was observed and no episodes of thromboembolism in pregnancy occurred, although one patient, treated with 20 mg, had a postpartum pulmonary embolus. Further, no cases of epidural hematomas were observed in the 43 patients receiving regional analgesia or anesthesia. Six pregnancy losses were recorded, four described earlier (6) and two new cases of fetal deaths at 18 and 26 weeks, both in women with lupus anticoagulant and previous fetal loss. Other than seven preterm deliveries, none of which were attributable to drug therapy, the remaining fetal and newborn outcomes were normal. Decreased bone density after delivery (lumbar spine or hip; 1 SD below the mean for nonpregnant age-matched women) was measured in 9 of 26 women after 28 pregnancies. In seven of these cases, unfractionated heparin had been used previously. Based on other published studies, the investigators could not determine whether the low bone density was present before treatment with enoxaparin, or if it was caused by pregnancy and breastfeeding, but a previous study with another LMWH (see Dalteparin) found no effect on bone density (9).

A 1997 case report described the use of enoxaparin (dose not specified) throughout most of the gestation, including labor, in a woman with congenital hypofibrinogenemia and protein S deficiency (10). A male infant with hypofibrinogenemia was delivered by cesarean section at 38 weeks' gestation.

A number of other studies (11–15) and reviews (3,16–22) have described the safe use of enoxaparin and other LMWH agents during pregnancy. Use of LMWH within 2 hours prior to cesarean section, however, was associated with an increase in wound hematoma (23). Also, lower maximum enoxaparin concentrations and anti-factor Xa activity levels occur during pregnancy compared with the nonpregnant state, thus requiring dose adjustments (24).

An opinion of the American College of Obstetricians and Gynecologists (ACOG) states that LMWH is at least as effective in pregnant patients with venous thrombosis, pulmonary embolism, or thrombophilic disorders as unfractionated heparin (25). Moreover, LMWHs have the advantages of ease of administration and less frequent laboratory monitoring. LMWHs may also reduce maternal complications, compared with standard heparin, such as bleeding, osteoporosis, and thrombocytopenia (3). However, there is inadequate information to recommend the use of LMWH in a pregnant woman with a mechanical heart valve (25).

BREASTFEEDING SUMMARY

No reports describing the use of enoxaparin during lactation have been located. However, due to the relatively high molecular weight of this drug, and its inactivation in the gastrointestinal tract if it was ingested orally, its passage into milk and subsequent risk to a nursing infant should be considered negligible.

References

1. Product information. Lovenox. Rhone-Poulenc Rorer, 1993.
2. Nelson-Piercy C. Low molecular weight heparin for obstetric thromboprophylaxis. Br J Obstet Gynaecol 1994;101:6–8.
3. American College of Obstetricians and Gynecologists. Thromboembolism in pregnancy. *ACOG Practice Bulletin*. No. 19, August 2000.
4. Priollet P, Roncato M, Aiach M, Housset E, Poissonnier MH, Chavinie J. Low-molecular-weight heparin in venous thrombosis during pregnancy. Br J Haematol 1986;63:605–6.
5. Gillis S, Shushan A, Eldor A. Use of low molecular weight heparin for prophylaxis and treatment of thromboembolism in pregnancy. Int J Gynecol Obstet 1992;39:297–301.
6. Sturridge F, de Swiet M, Letsky E. The use of low molecular weight heparin for thromboprophylaxis in pregnancy. Br J Obstet Gynaecol 1994;101:69–71.
7. Dulitzki M, Pauzner R, Langevitz P, Pras M, Many A, Schiff E. Low-molecular-weight heparin during pregnancy and delivery: preliminary experience with 41 pregnancies. Obstet Gynecol 1996;87:380–3.
8. Dulitzki M, Seidman DS, Sivan E, Horowitz A, Barkai G, Schiff E. Low-molecular-weight heparin in pregnancy and delivery: experience with 24 cases. Society of Perinatal Obstetricians Abstracts. Am J Obstet Gynecol 1995;172:363.
9. Nelson-Piercy C, Letsky EA, de Swiet M. Low-molecular-weight heparin for obstetric thromboprophylaxis: experience of sixty-nine pregnancies in sixty-one women at high risk. Am J Obstet Gynecol 1997;176:1062–8.
10. Funai EF, Klein SA, Lockwood CJ. Successful pregnancy outcome in a patient with both congenital hypofibrinogenemia and protein S deficiency. Obstet Gynecol 1997;89:858.
11. Casele H, Laifer S. Prospective evaluation of bone density changes in pregnant women on low molecular weight heparin (abstract). Am J Obstet Gynecol 1998;178:S65.
12. Laifer SA, Stiller RJ, Dunston-Boone G, Whetham JCG. Low-molecular weight heparin for treatment of pulmonary embolism in a pregnant woman. Thromb Haemost 1999;82:1361–2.
13. Ellison J, Walker ID, Greer IA. Antenatal use of enoxaparin for prevention and treatment of thromboembolism in pregnancy. Br J Obstet Gynaecol 2000;107:1116–21.
14. Magdelaine A, Verdy E, Coulet F, Berkane N, Girot R, Uzan S, Soubrier F. Deep vein thrombosis during enoxaparin prophylactic treatment in a young pregnant woman homozygous for factor V Leiden and heterozygous

for the G127-A mutation in the thrombomodulin gene. Blood Coagul Fibrinolysis 2000;11:761–5.
15. Younis JS, Ohel G, Brenner B, Haddad S, Lanir N, Ben-Ami M. The effect of thrombophylaxis on pregnancy outcome in patients with recurrent pregnancy loss associated with factor V Leiden mutation. Br J Obstet Gynaecol 2000;107:415–9.
16. Schulman S. Long-term prophylaxis in venous thromboembolism: LMWH or oral anticoagulation? Haemostasis 1998;28(Suppl 3):17–21.
17. Conard J, Horellou MH, Samama MM. Management of pregnancy in women with thrombophilia. Haemostasis 1999;29(Suppl 1):98–104.
18. Bates SM. Optimal management of pregnant women with acute venous thromboembolism. Haemostasis 1999;29(Suppl 1):107–11.
19. Chan WS, Ray JG. Low molecular weight heparin use during pregnancy: issues of safety and practicality. Obstet Gynecol Surv 1999;54:649–54.
20. Robin F, Lecuru F, Desfeux P, Boucaya V, Taurelle R. Anticoagulant therapy in pregnancy. Eur J Obstet Gynecol Reprod Biol 1999;83:171–7.
21. Sanson BJ, Lensing AWA, Prins MH, Ginsberg JS, Barkagan ZS, Lavenne-Pardonge E, Brenner B, Dulitzky M, Nielsen JD, Boda Z, Turi S, MacGillavry MR, Hamulyak K, Theunissen IM, Hunt BJ, Buller HR. Safety of low-molecular-weight heparin in pregnancy: a systematic review. Thromb Haemost 1999;81:668–72.
22. Ensom MHH, Stephenson MD. Low-molecular-weight heparin in pregnancy. Pharmacotherapy 1999;19:1013–25.
23. Wolf H, Piek JMJ, van Wijk FH, Buller HR. Administration of low molecular weight heparin within two hours prior to cesarean section increases the prevalence of wound hematoma (abstract). Am J Obstet Gynecol 2000;182:S158.
24. Casele HL, Laifer SA, Woelkers DA, Venkataramanan R. Changes in the pharmacokinetics of the low-molecular-weight heparin enoxaparin sodium during pregnancy. Am J Obstet Gynecol 1999;181:1113–7.
25. American College of Obstetricians and Gynecologists. Anticoagulation with low-molecular-weight heparin during pregnancy. *Committee Opinion*. No. 211, November 1998.

E

ENTACAPONE

Anti-Parkinson Agent

PREGNANCY RECOMMENDATION: Limited Human Data—Animal Data Suggest Moderate Risk
BREASTFEEDING RECOMMENDATION: No Human Data—Potential Toxicity

PREGNANCY SUMMARY

One report describing the use entacapone in human pregnancy has been located. The drug is teratogenic in rats at plasma exposures close to those observed in humans, but no teratogenicity was seen in rabbits. Entacapone is always used with levodopa/carbidopa and, although the data are very limited, these latter agents do not appear to present a major risk to the human fetus. (See Carbidopa and Levodopa.) Moreover, conditions requiring the use of levodopa/carbidopa during the childbearing years are relatively uncommon and, thus, the use of entacapone should also be uncommon. Although the near absence of human pregnancy experience prevents an assessment of the risk to the embryo–fetus, inadvertent exposure to entacapone during early gestation does not appear to represent a significant risk.

FETAL RISK SUMMARY

Entacapone is indicated as an adjunct to levodopa/carbidopa in patients experiencing end-of-dose "wearing off" effect. The agent is a selective and reversible inhibitor of catechol-O-methyltransferase (COMT), an enzyme involved in the metabolism of levodopa. Inhibition of COMT by entacapone allows for more sustained plasma levels of levodopa resulting in greater beneficial effects on the signs and symptoms of Parkinson's disease. Entacapone is nearly completely metabolized and elimination is biphasic with elimination half-lives of 0.4–0.7 hours (β-phase; serum) and 2.4 hours (γ-phase; tissue) (1).

Entacapone did not impair fertility or general reproductive performance in rats at doses producing systemic exposures up to 28 times the human exposure based on AUC from a maximum recommended daily dose of 1600 mg (HE-MRDD), but did delay mating at the highest dose. In addition, entacapone was mutagenic and clastogenic in one in vitro mouse assay but not in other assays (1).

Reproduction tests have been conducted in rats and rabbits. In pregnant rats treated during organogenesis, systemic exposure 34 times the HE-MRDD, without producing overt maternal toxicity, caused increased incidences of variations in fetal development. There was no evidence of impaired development in the offspring when this dose was given during late gestation and throughout lactation. When doses producing systemic exposures seven times the HE-MRDD or greater were given before mating and during early gestation, an increased incidence of fetal eye anomalies (microphthalmia, anophthalmia) was observed. In pregnant rabbits, systemic exposure 0.4 times the HE-MRDD or greater during organogenesis resulted in increased incidences of abortions, late/total resorptions, and decreased fetal weights. However, these doses were maternal toxic in rabbits. No teratogenic effects were observed in rabbits (1).

Although entacapone is always combined with levodopa/carbidopa, and levodopa is known to cause fetal toxicity and visceral and skeletal malformations in rabbits (see Levodopa), the potential reproductive toxicity and teratogenicity of combined entacapone–levodopa/carbidopa has not been studied in animals (1).

It is not known if entacapone crosses the human placenta to the fetus. The molecular weight (about 305) is low enough that embryo and fetal exposure probably occur, but the short elimination half-life will limit the degree of exposure.

A woman with a 12-year history of Parkinson's disease was treated throughout gestation with levodopa, carbidopa, entacapone, and bromocriptine (2). She gave birth at term to a 3175-g female infant, without deformities, with Apgar scores of 9, 10, and 10. Generalized seizures occurred in the infant 1 hour after birth followed by repeated episodes of shivering throughout the first day that responded to diazepam. Slowly improving hypotonia also was observed during the first week. Pneumonia was diagnosed but an extensive workup for the cause of seizures was negative. The child was developing normally at 1 year of age and has not had any other seizures (2).

BREASTFEEDING SUMMARY

No reports describing the use of entacapone during human lactation have been located. The molecular weight (about 305) is low enough that excretion into milk should be expected, but the relatively short elimination half-life should limit the amount in milk. Entacapone is always given with levodopa/carbidopa. Even though levodopa inhibits prolactin release, normal lactation has been reported while women were being treated with the drug, and levodopa is excreted into breast milk. In addition, the effect of entacapone on levodopa metabolism will increase the amount of plasma levodopa available for transfer into milk. The use of carbidopa during lactation has also been described. (See Carbidopa.) Therefore, a nursing infant will probably be exposed to all three drugs via the milk. The effects of this multiple exposure on a nursing infant are unknown but warrant investigation.

References

1. Product information. Comtan. Novartis Pharmaceuticals, 2003.
2. Lindh J. Short episode of seizures in a newborn of mother treated with levodopa/carbidopa/entacapone and bromocriptine. Mod Disord 2007;22:1515.

ENTECAVIR

Antiviral

PREGNANCY RECOMMENDATION: Compatible—Maternal Benefit >> Embryo–Fetal Risk
BREASTFEEDING RECOMMENDATION: Contraindicated (HIV) No Human Data—Probably Compatible (Hepatitis B)

PREGNANCY SUMMARY

The human pregnancy experience with entecavir is limited. No structural anomalies have been reported. The animal data suggest low risk. If indicated, the drug should not be withheld because of pregnancy.

FETAL RISK SUMMARY

Entecavir is a guanosine nucleoside analog with selective activity against hepatitis B virus (HBV). It is indicated for the treatment of chronic hepatitis B infection in adults with evidence of active viral replication and other evidence of persistent elevations in serum aminotransferases (ALT or AST) or histologically active disease. This indication is based on responses after 1-year of treatment in nucleoside-treatment-naïve and lamivudine-resistant adult patients with HBeAg-positive or HBeAg-negative chronic HBV infection with compensated liver disease and on more limited data in adult patients with HIV/HBV co-infection who have received prior lamivudine therapy. Binding to human serum proteins is low (about 13%) and only minor metabolites have been identified. The terminal elimination half-life is about 128–149 hours (1).

Reproduction studies have been conducted in rats and rabbits. Oral doses in these species resulting in systemic exposures up to about 28 and 212 times the human exposure achieved with the maximum recommended human dose of 1 mg/kg (MRHD), respectively, caused no embryo or maternal toxicity. In rats, doses 3100 times the MRHD caused maternal toxicity, embryo–fetal toxicity (resorptions), lower fetal body weights, tail and vertebral malformations, reduced ossification (vertebrae, sternebrae, and phalanges), and extra lumbar vertebrae and ribs. In rabbits, exposures 883 times the MRHD caused embryo–fetal toxicity (resorptions), reduced ossification (hyoid), and an increased incidence of 13th rib. In a rat peri-postnatal study, systemic exposures greater than 94 times the MRHD revealed no evidence of adverse effects in offspring (1).

Long-term carcinogenicity studies in mice and rats were positive. In mice, exposures from 3 to 42 times the MRHD resulted in various tumors involving the lungs (may have been a species effect), hepatocellular carcinomas, hemangiomas of ovaries and uterus, and hemangiosarcomas of the spleen. In female rats, hepatocellular adenomas, and combined carcinomas and adenomas were observed at 24 times the MRHD, whereas skin fibromas were induced at 4 times the MRHD. In male and female rats, brain gliomas were induced at 35 and 24 times the MRHD, respectively. Entecavir was not mutagenic in various assays, but clastogenicity was observed in human lymphocyte culture (1).

No evidence of impaired fertility was observed in male and female rats given doses resulting in exposures greater than 90 times the MRHD. However, in other studies, exposures greater than 35 times the MRHD resulted in seminiferous tubular degeneration in rodents and dogs, but not in monkeys (1).

It is not known if entecavir crosses the human placenta. The molecular weight (about 277), minimal metabolism, and long elimination half-life suggest that the drug will cross to the embryo and fetus.

The Antiretroviral Pregnancy Registry reported, for the period January 1989 through July 2009, prospective data (reported before the outcomes were known) involving 4702 live births that had been exposed during the 1st trimester to one or more antiretroviral agents (2). Congenital defects were noted in 134, a prevalence of 2.8% (95% confidence interval [CI] 2.4–3.4). In the 6100 live births with earliest exposure in the 2nd/3rd trimesters, there were 153 infants with defects (2.5%, 95% CI 2.1–2.9). The prevalence rates for the two periods did not differ significantly. There were 288 infants with birth defects among 10,803 live births with exposure anytime during pregnancy (2.7%, 95% CI 2.4–3.0). The prevalence rate did not differ significantly from the rate expected in a nonexposed population. There were 10 outcomes exposed to entecavir (9 in the 1st trimester and 1 in the 2nd/3rd trimesters) in combination with other antiretroviral agents. There were no birth defects. In reviewing the birth defects of prospective and retrospective (pregnancies reported after the outcomes were known) registered cases, the Registry concluded that, except for isolated cases of neural tube defects with efavirenz exposure in retrospective reports, there was no other pattern of anomalies (isolated or syndromic) (2). (See Lamivudine for required statement.)

BREASTFEEDING SUMMARY

No reports describing the use of entecavir during human lactation have been located. The molecular weight (about 277), minimal metabolism, and long elimination half-life (128–149 hours) suggest that the drug will be excreted into breast milk. The effect of this exposure on a nursing infant is unknown. Infants of HBsAg-positive or HBeAg-positive mothers should receive hepatitis B immune globulin at birth, followed by the start of the hepatitis B vaccine series soon after birth (3). After the infant receives the first dose of immune globulin, breastfeeding is then permitted (4). However, breastfeeding is contraindicated in women infected with HIV.

References

1. Product information. Baraclude. Bristol-Meyers Squibb, 2007.
2. Antiretroviral Pregnancy Registry Steering Committee. *Antiretroviral Pregnancy Registry International Interim Report for 1 January 1989 through 31 July 2009*. Wilmington, NC: Registry Coordinating Center; 2009. Available at www.apregistry.com. Accessed May 29, 2010.
3. Product information. HyperHeb B S/D. Talecris Biotherapeutics, 2007.
4. Lawrence RA, Lawrence RM. *Breastfeeding. A Guide for the Medical Profession*. 5th ed. St. Louis, MO: Mosby, 1999:225.

ENZALUTAMIDE

Antineoplastic (Antiandrogen)

PREGNANCY RECOMMENDATION: Contraindicated
BREASTFEEDING RECOMMENDATION: Contraindicated

PREGNANCY SUMMARY

No reports describing the use of enzalutamide in human pregnancy have been located. However, such reports are unlikely because of the indication. Animal reproductive studies have not been conducted. If the drug was used in pregnancy, the mechanism of action suggests that it could cause fetal harm. A 2013 study concluded that the androgen receptor was a key regulator for myometrial cell proliferation and disruption of myometrial growth could affect the outcome of pregnancy and labor (1).

FETAL RISK SUMMARY

Enzalutamide is an oral antineoplastic that is given daily (160 mg/day). It is an androgen receptor inhibitor that acts on different steps in the androgen receptor signaling pathway. Enzalutamide is indicated for the treatment of patients with metastatic castration-resistant prostate cancer who have previously received docetaxel. The drug undergoes hepatic metabolism to an active and inactive metabolites. Enzalutamide is 97%–98% bound to plasma proteins, primarily to albumin, whereas the active metabolite is 95% bound to plasma protein. The mean terminal half-life after a single dose in patients is 5.8 days (range 2.8–10.2 days). After a single 160 mg dose in healthy volunteers, the mean terminal half-life for the active metabolite was about 7.8–10.6 days (2).

Reproduction studies in animals have not been conducted (2).

Long-term animal studies to evaluate the potential for carcinogenicity have not been conducted. The drug was not mutagenic in multiple assays. In a long-term study in male rats, atrophy of the prostate and seminal vesicles was observed at dose that was equal to the human exposure based on AUC (HE). In dogs, hypospermatogenesis and atrophy of the prostate and epididymides was observed at a dose that was 0.3 times the HE (2).

It is not known if enzalutamide or its active metabolite cross the human placenta. The molecular weight (about 464) and the long elimination half-life suggest that the drug will cross to the embryo–fetus, although the high plasma protein binding (97%–98%) might limit the amount crossing.

BREASTFEEDING SUMMARY

No reports describing the use of enzalutamide during human lactation have been located. However, such reports are unlikely because of the indication. Nevertheless, if the drug was used during breastfeeding, the molecular weight (about 464) of the parent drug and its long mean elimination half-life (5.8 days; range 2.8–10.2 days) in patients suggest that the drug will be excreted into breast milk, although the high plasma protein binding (97%–98%) might limit the amount excreted.

References

1. Liu L, Li Y, Xie N, Shynlova O, Challis JRG, Slater D, Lye S, Dong X. Proliferative action of the androgen receptor in human uterine myometrial cells—a key regulator for myometrium phenotype programming. J Clin Endocrinol Metab 2013;98:218–27.
2. Product information. Xtandi. Astellas Pharma US, 2012.

EPHEDRINE

Sympathomimetic/Bronchodilator

PREGNANCY RECOMMENDATION: Compatible
BREASTFEEDING RECOMMENDATION: Limited Human Data—Potential Toxicity

E

PREGNANCY SUMMARY

Ephedrine is a sympathomimetic used widely for bronchial asthma, allergic disorders, hypotension, and the alleviation of symptoms caused by upper respiratory infections. It is a common component of proprietary mixtures containing antihistamines, bronchodilators, and other ingredients. Thus, it is difficult to separate the effects of ephedrine on the fetus from other drugs, disease states, and viruses. Ephedrine-like drugs are teratogenic in some animal species, but human teratogenicity has not been suspected (1,2).

FETAL RISK SUMMARY

The Collaborative Perinatal Project monitored 50,282 mother–child pairs, 373 of whom had 1st trimester exposure to ephedrine (3, pp. 345–356). For use anytime during pregnancy, 873 exposures were recorded (3, p. 439). No evidence for a relationship to large categories of major or minor malformations or to individual defects was found. However, an association in the 1st trimester was found between the sympathomimetic class of drugs as a whole and minor malformations (not life-threatening or major cosmetic defects), inguinal hernia, and clubfoot (3, pp. 345–356).

Ephedrine is routinely used to treat or prevent maternal hypotension following spinal anesthesia (4–7). Significant increases in fetal heart rate and beat-to-beat variability may occur, but these effects may have been the result of normal reflexes following hypotension-associated bradycardia. A recent study, however, has demonstrated the placental passage of ephedrine with fetal levels at delivery approximately 70% of the maternal concentration (8). The presence of ephedrine in the fetal circulation is probably a major cause of the fetal heart rate changes.

BREASTFEEDING SUMMARY

A single case report has been located describing adverse effects in a 3-month-old nursing infant of a mother consuming a long-acting preparation containing 120 mg of *d*-isoephedrine and 6 mg of dexbrompheniramine (9). The mother had begun taking the preparation on a twice daily schedule 1 or 2 days prior to onset of the infant's symptoms. The infant exhibited irritability, excessive crying, and disturbed sleeping patterns that resolved spontaneously within 12 hours when breastfeeding was stopped.

References

1. Nishimura H, Tanimura T. *Clinical Aspects of the Teratogenicity of Drugs*. New York, NY: American Elsevier, 1976:231.
2. Shepard TH. *Catalog of Teratogenic Agents*. 3rd ed. Baltimore, MD: The Johns Hopkins University Press, 1980:134–5.
3. Heinonen OP, Slone D, Shapiro S. *Birth Defects and Drugs in Pregnancy*. Littleton, MA: Publishing Sciences Group, 1977.
4. Wright RG, Shnider SM, Levinson G, Rolbin SH, Parer JT. The effect of maternal administration of ephedrine on fetal heart rate and variability. Obstet Gynecol 1981;57:734–8.
5. Antoine C, Young BK. Fetal lactic acidosis with epidural anesthesia. Am J Obstet Gynecol 1982;142:55–9.
6. Datta S, Alper MH, Ostheimer GW, Weiss JB. Method of ephedrine administration and nausea and hypotension during spinal anesthesia for cesarean section. Anesthesiology 1982;56:68–70.
7. Antoine C, Young BK. Fetal lactic acidosis with epidural anesthesia. Am J Obstet Gynecol 1982;142:55–9.
8. Hughes SC, Ward MG, Levinson G, Shnider SM, Wright RG, Gruenke LD, Craig JC. Placental transfer of ephedrine does not affect neonatal outcome. Anesthesiology 1985;63:217–9.
9. Mortimer EA Jr. Drug toxicity from breast milk? Pediatrics 1977;60:780–1.

EPINASTINE

Antihistamine (Ophthalmic)

PREGNANCY RECOMMENDATION: No Human Data—Probably Compatible
BREASTFEEDING RECOMMENDATION: No Human Data—Probably Compatible

PREGNANCY SUMMARY

No reports describing the use of epinastine in human pregnancy have been located. The animal reproduction data, even though the comparison to the human dose was based on body weight, suggest low risk. Although the absence of human pregnancy experience prevents a more complete assessment, the very low systemic bioavailability, and the human experience with other agents in the antihistamine class, suggests that there is little if any embryo or fetal risk from epinastine.

FETAL RISK SUMMARY

Epinastine, a topically active H_1-receptor antagonist and inhibitor of histamine from mast cells, is indicated for the prevention of itching associated with allergic conjunctivitis. It is administered as a 0.05% ophthalmic solution. Systemic bioavailability is low with average maximum plasma concentrations of 0.04 ng/mL measured after one drop in each eye twice daily for 7 days. There was no accumulation in the plasma. Less than 10% of epinastine undergoes metabolism. Binding to plasma proteins (64%) is moderate, but the terminal plasma elimination half-life is prolonged (about 12 hours) (1).

Reproduction studies have been conducted in rats and rabbits. In pregnant rats, maternal toxicity with no embryo or fetal effects was observed with an oral dose that was about 150,000 times the maximum recommended ocular human dose based on body weight (MROHD). However, pup body weight gain was reduced at a dose that was about 90,000 times the MROHD. In pregnant rabbits, resorptions and abortion occurred at an oral dose that was about 55,000 times the MROHD (1).

Carcinogenicity studies in mice and rats were negative at doses up to 30,000 times the MROHD. Epinastine also was negative in multiple studies for mutagenic and clastogenic effects. There was no effect on fertility in male rats, but decreased fertility was noted in female rats at an oral dose of about 90,000 times the MROHD (1).

It is not known if epinastine crosses the human placenta. The molecular weight (about 250 for the free base), low metabolism, moderate plasma protein binding, and prolonged elimination half-life suggest that the antihistamine will cross the placenta. However, the low systemic bioavailability probably prevents clinically significant amounts of the drug from reaching the embryo and fetus.

E

BREASTFEEDING SUMMARY

No reports describing the use epinastine during human lactation have been located. The molecular weight (about 250 for the free base), low metabolism, moderate plasma protein binding (64%), and prolonged elimination half-life (about 12 hours) suggest that the antihistamine will be excreted into human breast milk. However, the low systemic bioavailability probably prevents clinically significant amounts of the drug from appearing in milk. Moreover, in general, antihistamines obtaining therapeutic systemic concentrations are classified as compatible with breastfeeding. Epinastine should be classified similarly.

Reference

1. Product information. Elestat. Inspire Pharmaceuticals, 2007.

EPINEPHRINE

Sympathomimetic/Bronchodilator

PREGNANCY RECOMMENDATION: Human Data Suggest Risk
BREASTFEEDING RECOMMENDATION: No Human Data—Potential Toxicity

PREGNANCY SUMMARY

In situations such as maternal hypotension where a pressor agent is required, use of ephedrine is a better choice than epinephrine.

FETAL RISK SUMMARY

Epinephrine is a sympathomimetic that is widely used for conditions such as shock, glaucoma, allergic reactions, bronchial asthma, and nasal congestion. Because it occurs naturally in all humans, it is difficult to separate the effects of its administration from effects on the fetus induced by endogenous epinephrine, other drugs, disease states, and viruses.

The drug readily crosses the placenta (1). Epinephrine is teratogenic in some animal species, but human teratogenicity has not been suspected (2,3). The Collaborative Perinatal Project monitored 50,282 mother–child pairs, 189 of whom had 1st trimester exposure to epinephrine (4, pp. 345–356). For use anytime during pregnancy, 508 exposures were recorded (4, p. 439). A statistically significant association was found between 1st trimester use of epinephrine and major and minor malformations. An association was also found with inguinal hernia after both 1st trimester and anytime use (4, pp. 477, 492). Although not specified, these data may reflect the potentially severe maternal status for which epinephrine administration is indicated.

In a surveillance study of Michigan Medicaid recipients involving 229,101 completed pregnancies conducted between 1985 and 1992, 35 newborns had been exposed to epinephrine (route not specified) during the 1st trimester (F. Rosa, personal communication, FDA, 1993). No major birth defects were observed (1.5 expected).

Theoretically, epinephrine's α-adrenergic properties might lead to a decreased in uterine blood flow. A large intravenous dose of epinephrine, 1.5 mL of a 1:1000 solution during a 1-hour period to reverse severe hypotension secondary to an allergic reaction, may have contributed to intrauterine anoxic insult to a 28-week-old fetus (5). Decreased fetal movements occurred after treatment and the infant, delivered at 34 weeks' gestation, had evidence of intracranial hemorrhage at birth and died 4 days later.

BREASTFEEDING SUMMARY

No reports describing the use of epinephrine during human lactation have been located.

References

1. Morgan CD, Sandler M, Panigel M. Placental transfer of catecholamines in vitro and in vivo. Am J Obstet Gynecol 1972;112:1068–75.
2. Nishimura H, Tanimura T. *Clinical Aspects of the Teratogenicity of Drugs*. New York, NY: American Elsevier, 1976:231.
3. Shepard TH. *Catalog of Teratogenic Agents*. 3rd ed. Baltimore, MD: The Johns Hopkins University Press, 1980:134–5.
4. Heinonen OP, Slone D, Shapiro S. *Birth Defects and Drugs in Pregnancy*. Littleton, MA: Publishing Sciences Group, 1977.
5. Entman SS, Moise KJ. Anaphylaxis in pregnancy. S Med J 1984;77:402.

E

EPIRUBICIN

Antineoplastic

PREGNANCY RECOMMENDATION: Contraindicated—1st Trimester
BREASTFEEDING RECOMMENDATION: Contraindicated

PREGNANCY SUMMARY

Epirubicin is a cell-cycle phase nonspecific anthracycline in the same antineoplastic class as daunorubicin, doxorubicin, idarubicin, and valrubicin. It is used as adjuvant therapy in patients with breast cancer. The mechanism of action includes the inhibition of nucleic acid (DNA and RNA), protein synthesis, and DNA helicase activity. There are no reports describing the use of this agent during organogenesis.

FETAL RISK SUMMARY

In reproduction studies, epirubicin was embryolethal (increased resorptions and postimplantation loss) in pregnant rats administered an IV dose about 0.04 times the maximum recommended single human dose based on BSA (MRHD) during days 5–15 of gestation (1). Intrauterine growth restriction (IUGR), but not teratogenicity, was also observed with this dose. Doses as low as 0.005 times the MRHD resulted in embryolethality, and IUGR was evident at a dose 0.0015 times the MRHD. At a dose approximately 2.5 times the MRHD given on days 9 and 10 of gestation, fetal deaths, reduced placental weight, and multiple congenital malformations (external: anal atresia, misshapen tail, abnormal genital tubercle; visceral: gastrointestinal, urinary, and cardiovascular systems; skeletal: deformed long bones and girdles, rib abnormalities, irregular spinal ossification) were observed (1). In contrast, a dose 0.02 times the MRHD during days 6–18 of gestation in rabbits was not embryotoxic or teratogenic (1). Administration of maternally toxic doses in rabbits caused abortions and delayed ossification, but no teratogenicity. In fertility studies with male and female rats, mice, rabbits, and dogs, various low doses of epirubicin were associated with atrophy of the testes and epididymis, reduced spermatogenesis, or uterine atrophy (1).

It is not known if epirubicin crosses the placenta. The molecular weight (about 580) is low enough that transfer to the human embryo and fetus should be expected.

The manufacturer's product information describes two human pregnancies in which epirubicin was administered (1). In the first case, a 34-year-old woman at 28 weeks' gestation, who was diagnosed with breast cancer, was treated with epirubicin and cyclophosphamide every 3 weeks for three cycles. The last dose was given at 34 weeks' gestation and she delivered a healthy baby 1 week later. No follow-up of the infant after birth was mentioned. The second case involved a 34-year-old woman with breast cancer metastatic to the liver who was randomized to the FEC-50 regimen (epirubicin, 5-fluorouracil, and cyclophosamide). She was removed from the study because of pregnancy, but the gestational age and number of doses received were not specified. The pregnancy ended with a spontaneous abortion (1).

A 30-year-old woman at about 25 weeks' gestation was treated with four courses of epirubicin (100 mg) and vincristine (2 mg) for non-Hodgkin's lymphoma (2). Prednisolone was also given during each treatment and then tapered. Her disease responded well to the therapy. Labor was induced at 34 weeks' gestation and she gave birth to a normal 2.32-kg, 44.5-cm long female infant with Apgar scores of 8 at 1 and 5 minutes. The mother has remained in complete remission and her child appeared to be doing well at 4 years of age.

A 1996 report described the case of a 39-year-old woman with extensive metastatic breast cancer who had a unilateral mastectomy and axillary dissection at 29 weeks' gestation (3). After surgery, she was started on combination chemotherapy with epirubicin (50 mg/m^2), 5-fluorouracil (600 mg/m^2), and cyclophosphamide (600 mg/m^2). At 35 weeks' gestation, a few days after receiving her second course of therapy, she developed eclamptic tonic-clonic seizures. She subsequently delivered a healthy but growth-restricted (1650-g; <10th percentile) infant. Although hypertension and proteinuria were not detected before the seizures, both were documented in the postpartum period. No follow-up of the infant after delivery was reported.

A 1999 report from France described the outcomes of pregnancies in 20 women with breast cancer who were treated with antineoplastic agents (4). The first cycle of chemotherapy occurred at a mean gestational age of 26 weeks' with delivery occurring at a mean 34.7 weeks. A total of 38 cycles were administered during pregnancy with a median of two cycles per woman. None of the women received radiation therapy during pregnancy. The pregnancy outcomes included two spontaneous abortions (SAB) (both exposed in the 1st trimester), one intrauterine death (exposed in the 2nd trimester), and 17 live births, one of whom died at 8 days of age without apparent cause. The 16 surviving children were developing normally at a mean follow-up of 42.3 months (4). Epirubicin (E), in combination with various other agents (cyclophosphamide [C], fluorouracil [F], methotrexate [M], or vincristine [V]) was administered to 10 of the women at a mean dose of 70 mg/m^2 (range 50–100 mg/m^2). The outcomes were two SAB (ECF, EMV; 1st trimester), one stillbirth (one cycle of EC at 23 weeks'), one neonatal death (one cycle of ECF 32 days before birth), and six surviving liveborn infants (one EC, five ECF; all in the 3rd trimester). One of the infants, exposed to two cycles of ECF with the last at 25 days before birth, had transient leukopenia (4).

Occupational exposure of the mother to antineoplastic agents during pregnancy may present a risk to the fetus. A position statement from the National Study Commission on Cytotoxic Exposure and a research article involving some antineoplastic agents are presented in the monograph for cyclophosphamide (see Cyclophosphamide).

BREASTFEEDING SUMMARY

No reports describing the use of epirubicin during human lactation have been located. The molecular weight (about 580) is low enough that excretion into breast milk should be expected. In addition, another anthracycline (see Doxorubicin) is excreted into human milk. Because of the potential for serious adverse effects, such as immune suppression, carcinogenesis, neutropenia, and unknown effects on growth, women receiving epirubicin should not breastfeed.

E

References

1. Product information. Ellence. Pharmacia & Upjohn, 2001.
2. Goldwasser F, Pico JL, Cerrina J, Fernandez H, Pons JC, Cosset JM, Hayat M. Successful chemotherapy including epirubicin in a pregnant non-Hodgkin's lymphoma patient. Leuk Lymphoma 1995;20:173–6.
3. Muller T, Hofmann J, Steck T. Eclampsia after polychemotherapy for nodal-positive breast cancer during pregnancy. Eur J Obstet Gynecol Reprod Biol 1996;67:197–8.
4. Giacalone PL, Laffargue F, Benos P. Chemotherapy for breast carcinoma during pregnancy. Cancer 1999;86:2266–72.

EPOETIN ALFA

Hematopoietic

PREGNANCY RECOMMENDATION: Compatible—Maternal Benefit >> Embryo–Fetal Risk
BREASTFEEDING RECOMMENDATION: Compatible

PREGNANCY SUMMARY

The use of recombinant human erythropoietin (epoetin alfa) does not seem to present a major risk to the fetus. The glycoprotein does not cross the human placenta to the fetus. The severe maternal hypertension or worsening of renal disease requiring delivery of the fetus that occurred in four pregnancies may be an adverse effect of the drug therapy, a consequence of the preexisting renal disease or current pregnancy, or a combination of these factors. The contribution of epoetin alfa to the case of abruptio placentae in a woman with severe hypertension and chronic renal insufficiency is unknown. No cases of thrombosis were reported in pregnant women treated with epoetin alfa, but this is a potentially serious complication. Because anemia and the need for frequent blood transfusions also present significant risks to the mother and fetus, it appears that the benefits derived from the use of epoetin alfa outweigh the known risks.

FETAL RISK SUMMARY

Recombinant human erythropoietin (epoetin alfa), a 165-amino acid glycoprotein produced by a recombinant DNA method with the same biologic effects as endogenous erythropoietin, is used to stimulate red blood cell production.

Fetal toxicity (decreased growth, delays in appearance of abdominal hair, delayed eyelid opening, delayed ossification, and decreases in the number of caudal vertebrae) was observed in the offspring of pregnant rats dosed with 500 U/kg (five times the human dose) (1). In addition, a trend toward increased fetal wastage occurred in pregnant rats dosed with 100 and 500 U/kg. No fetal adverse effects were seen in rabbits at doses up to 500 U/kg from day 6 to 18 of gestation (1).

Epoetin alfa crosses the placenta in significant amounts to the fetus in pregnant mice (2) but not from the mother to the fetus (3) or from the fetus to the mother in sheep (4). Another study also found no transfer of recombinant epoetin alfa to the fetus in sheep and monkeys, in spite of high maternal concentrations (5). The question of human placental transfer of endogenous erythropoietin and epoetin alfa was examined in a 1993 review (6). Five reasons arguing against transfer were presented: poor correlation between maternal and fetal levels, high correlation between fetal plasma and amniotic fluid levels, high molecular weight, animal studies, and one human in vitro study (6). Since then, several studies have investigated whether or not epoetin alfa is transferred across the human placenta (7–15).

A 1992 study measured an elevated cord erythropoietin level (62 mIU/mL; normal <19) in an infant whose mother was receiving 150 U/kg/week (9000 U/week) of the drug (7). However, because the mother had insulin-dependent diabetes, a disease known to display elevated cord levels of erythropoietin (8–10), the investigators could not determine whether the cord concentrations were due to exogenous or endogenous erythropoietin (7). The lack of correlation between maternal and fetal erythropoietin concentrations, at least between 19 and 28 weeks' gestation, suggests that endogenous maternal erythropoietin does not cross the placenta to the fetus (10). At 7–12 weeks' gestation, however, mean maternal and extraembryonic coelomic fluid concentrations of endogenous erythropoietin were nearly identical, 15.4 mU/mL (range 6.8–32.1 mU/mL) compared with 15.45 mU/mL (range 5.6–29.4 mU/mL), respectively (11). Passage of maternal erythropoietin to the coelomic fluid via the decidualized endometrium was offered as a possible explanation for the identical levels. This latter study also found low amniotic fluid levels of erythropoietin, mean 5.0 mU/mL (range $<$5.0–5.8 mU/mL), at 7–12 weeks' gestation, but their samples may have been contaminated with coelomic fluid (11). An earlier study was unable to find endogenous erythropoietin in amniotic fluid before the 11th week of gestation (12). More recent investigations have demonstrated the lack of placental passage of recombinant epoetin alfa across the human placenta (13–15).

In the fetus, erythropoietin is primarily produced by the fetal liver during most of pregnancy (16). Erythropoietin binding sites have been found in the 1st trimester of pregnancy in the human fetal liver and lung (17) and in cultures of umbilical vein endothelial cells derived at cesarean section (18). A 1994 report compared the levels of endogenous erythropoietin measured in the umbilical serum in normal women at term and in premature labor, and in those with preeclampsia or diabetes (19). Women with preeclampsia had the highest concentrations (95.8 mU/mL), followed by those with diabetes (38.0 mU/mL), women in premature labor (25.2 mU/mL), and normal women (21.1 mU/mL), demonstrating that fetal hypoxia was not the only factor that determines levels of this glycoprotein (19).

The first published report on the use of epoetin alfa in human pregnancy appeared in a 1990 abstract (20). A 28-year-old Japanese woman with chronic glomerulonephritis became pregnant 8 years after the start of dialysis and approximately 22 months after the initiation of weekly doses of epoetin alfa. She had been amenorrheic prior to epoetin alfa therapy; her menses returned 17 months after start of treatment. The duration of her dialysis treatments (in hours per week) was gradually increased throughout gestation. She received 4500–9000 U/week of epoetin alfa from the 20th gestational week (doses prior to this time were not specified) until delivery at 36 weeks' gestation. Her blood pressure was normal throughout pregnancy, as was intrauterine fetal growth. The 2396-g, healthy, male infant was normal at birth with Apgar scores of 9 and 9 at 1 and 5 minutes, respectively. He was discharged with his mother 12 days after birth.

A report published in 1991 described a 32-year-old hypertensive woman with end-stage renal disease of unknown origin, who had been on hemodialysis for 4 years (21). She was started on epoetin alfa early in the 1st trimester and continued until delivery (36 weeks by dates, 34 weeks by ultrasound). No transfusions were required during pregnancy. An emergency cesarean section was performed because of fetal distress secondary to severe maternal hypertension. The 1140-g male infant had Apgar scores of 7 and 8 at 1 and 5 minutes, respectively. No congenital malformations were noted in the infant, who was discharged home at 35 days of age.

A second 1991 publication involved a 37-year-old woman who was treated throughout pregnancy with escalating doses of epoetin alfa (22). The patient had received a renal transplant 9 years before pregnancy because of reflux nephropathy, but the onset of chronic rejection caused progressive renal failure. Due to persistent anemia, she was started on a regimen of epoetin alfa, 4000 U/week, and supplemental iron shortly before conception. The dose was increased at 18 weeks' gestation to 8000 U/week, and then to 12,000 U/week at 27 weeks. Hemodialysis was started during the 25th week of pregnancy because of severe renal failure, polyhydramnios, and fetal intrauterine growth restriction. Her blood pressure was controlled with atenolol and nifedipine. Severe intrauterine growth restriction and fetal distress were diagnosed at 31 weeks and, after betamethasone therapy for fetal lung maturation, a cesarean section was performed to deliver a 780-g female infant. Birth weight was below the 3rd percentile for gestational age. Although the growth restriction was attributed to the mother's renal disease, the use of atenolol was probably a factor (see Atenolol). Except for transient coagulopathy and thrombocytopenia found at birth, both thought to be due to the mother's condition or premature delivery, the infant progressed normally and was discharged home at 66 days of age with a weight of 2140 g.

A 1992 report described the use of epoetin alfa, combined with supplemental oral iron, in three human pregnancies that resulted in the birth of four (one set of twins) infants (7). The birth weights of the newborns were all at approximately the 50th percentile for gestational age (7). Two of the women developed polyhydramnios after starting treatment with epoetin alfa, and all developed preeclampsia or worsening renal impairment, but the authors could not determine whether these were effects of the drug treatment or the underlying disease (7). Hematocrit values were maintained in the targeted 30%–33% range, and no coagulation problems or significant changes in platelet counts were observed. The three pregnancies are described below.

A 30-year-old woman, with onset of renal disease secondary to immunoglobulin A nephropathy and chronic hypertension before pregnancy, was treated with epoetin alfa 50–65 U/kg/week starting in the 20th gestational week (7). Polyhydramnios was noted at 32 weeks' gestation. Because of worsening renal failure, labor induction was initiated at 35 weeks resulting in the delivery of a 2570-g male infant with Apgar scores of 8 and 8 at 1 and 5 minutes, respectively. The newborn had mild hyperbilirubinemia and required oxygen, but no other problems were noted. He was doing well at 3 months.

The second patient, a 33-year-old woman with hypertension, diabetes, and renal impairment, was treated with 150 U/kg/week of epoetin alfa beginning at 26 weeks' gestation (7). Polyhydramnios developed, and labor was induced at 32 weeks because of worsening renal function and superimposed preeclampsia. After maternal betamethasone therapy to accelerate fetal lung maturity, a 2020-g male infant was delivered, with Apgar scores of 4 and 7 at 1 and 5 minutes, respectively. The infant had mild hypoglycemia and hyperbilirubinemia and, initially, required oxygen therapy. He was discharged home at 2 weeks of age.

The third patient was a 26-year-old with renal disease secondary to crescentic segmental necrotizing glomerulonephritis following streptococcal pharyngitis (7). She was treated with azathioprine and prednisone throughout a twin gestation to control her renal disease. Beginning at 14 weeks' gestation, she was treated with epoetin alfa, 85–160 U/kg/week, continuously until 33 weeks' gestation, except for a 4-week period at 23–27 weeks. Therapy was halted during that time because of a low ferritin level, and therapy was discontinued when it recurred at 33 weeks. Labor was induced at 35 weeks for worsening renal function. A cesarean section was required because of failure to descend, resulting in the delivery of a 2220-g female (Apgar scores of 4 and 8, respectively) and a 2410-g male (Apgar scores of 2 and 5, respectively). The infants were developing normally at 7 months of age (7).

The pregnancies of six women who became pregnant while on dialysis for end-stage renal disease and who were treated with epoetin alfa have been described (23,24). No effects on the mothers' blood pressure control were observed in these cases, and in one of the reports, the investigators found no evidence that the drug crossed the placenta to the fetuses (24).

A number of additional studies have been published describing the use of epoetin alfa during human pregnancy (25–32). In most of the studies or reports, the drug was used to treat the maternal anemia associated with severe renal disease (25–29), but in three reports, epoetin alfa was used in women with either heterozygous β thalassemia (30), hypoproliferative anemia and a low serum erythropoietin level (31), or acute promyelocytic leukemia (32). Except for a single complication in which abruptio placentae with resulting fetal death occurred at 23 weeks' gestation and drug therapy could not be excluded as a contributing factor (28), no other fetal and/or newborn adverse effects attributable to epoetin alfa were observed.

BREASTFEEDING SUMMARY

Epoetin is a 165-amino acid glycoprotein produced by recombinant DNA technology that has the same biologic activity as endogenous erythropoietin. No reports describing its use during lactation have been located. Passage into milk is not expected, but in the event that some transfer did occur, digestion in the nursing infant's gastrointestinal system would occur. Moreover, preterm infants have been treated directly with the drug (33). Thus, the risk to a nursing infant from ingestion of the agent via the milk appears to be nonexistent.

References

1. Product information. Epogen. Amgen, 2000.
2. Koury MJ, Bondurant MC, Graber SE, Sawyer ST. Erythropoietin messenger RNA levels in developing mice and transfer of ^{125}I-erythropoietin by the placenta. J Clin Invest 1988;82:154–9.
3. Widness JA, Sawyer ST, Schmidt RL, Chestnut DH. Lack of maternal to fetal transfer of ^{125}I-labelled erythropoietin in sheep. J Dev Physiol 1991;15: 139–43.
4. Widness JA, Malone TA, Mufson RA. Impermeability of the ovine placenta to ^{35}S-recombinant erythropoietin. Pediatr Res 1989;25:649–51.
5. Zanjani ED, Pixley JS, Slotnick N, MacKintosh ER, Ekhterae D, Clemons G. Erythropoietin does not cross the placenta into the fetus. Pathobiology 1993;61:211–5.
6. Huch R, Huch A. Maternal and fetal erythropoietin: physiological aspects and clinical significance. Ann Med 1993;25:289–93.
7. Yankowitz J, Piraino B, Laifer SA, Frassetto L, Gavin L, Kitzmiller JL, Crombleholme W. Erythropoietin in pregnancies complicated by severe anemia of renal failure. Obstet Gynecol 1992;80:485–8.
8. Widness JA, Teramo KA, Clemons GK, Voutilainen P, Stenman UH, McKinlay SM, Schwartz R. Direct relationship of antepartum glucose control and fetal erythropoietin in human type 1 (insulin-dependent) diabetic pregnancy. Diabetologia 1990;33:378–83.
9. Salvesen DR, Brudenell JM, Snijders RJM, Ireland RM, Nicolaides KH. Fetal plasma erythropoietin in pregnancies complicated by maternal diabetes mellitus. Am J Obstet Gynecol 1993;168:88–94.
10. Thomas RM, Canning CE, Cotes PM, Linch DC, Rodeck CH, Rossiter CE, Huehns ER. Erythropoietin and cord blood haemoglobin in the regulation of human fetal erythropoiesis. Br J Obstet Gynaecol 1983;90:795–800.
11. Campbell J, Wathen N, Lewis M, Fingerova H, Chard T. Erythropoietin levels in amniotic fluid and extraembryonic coelomic fluid in the first trimester of pregnancy. Br J Obstet Gynaecol 1992;99:974–6.
12. Zivny J, Kobilkova J, Neuwirt J, Andrasova V. Regulation of erythropoiesis in fetus and mother during normal pregnancy. Obstet Gynecol 1982;60: 77–81.
13. Malek A, Sager R, Eckardt K-U, Bauer C, Schneider H. Lack of transport of erythropoietin across the human placenta as studied by an in vitro perfusion system. Pflügers Arch 1994;427:157–61.
14. Santolaya-Forgas J, Meyer W, Gauthier D, Vengalil S, Duval J, Gottmann D. Transplacental passage of erythropoietin (EPO-Alfa): a case control study. Society of Perinatal Obstetricians Abstract. Am J Obstet Gynecol 1997;176:S83.
15. Reisenberger K, Egarter C, Kapiotis S, Sternberger B, Gregor H, Husslein P. Transfer of erythropoietin across the placenta perfused in vitro. Obstet Gynecol 1997;89:738–42.
16. Finne PH, Halvorsen S. Regulation of erythropoiesis in the fetus and newborn. Arch Dis Child 1972;47:683–7.
17. Pekonen F, Rosenlof K, Rutanen EM, Fyhrquist F. Erythropoietin binding sites in human foetal tissues. Acta Endocrinol 1987;116:561–7.
18. Anagnostou A, Lee ES, Kessimian N, Levinson R, Steiner M. Erythropoietin has a mitogenic and positive chemotactic effect on endothelial cells. Proc Natl Acad Sci USA 1990;87:5978–82.
19. Mamopoulos M, Bili H, Tsantali C, Assimakopoulos E, Mantalenakis S, Farmakides G. Erythropoietin umbilical serum levels during labor in women with preeclampsia, diabetes, and preterm labor. Am J Perinatol 1994;11:427–9.
20. Fujimi S, Hori K, Miijima C, Shigematsu M. Successful pregnancy and delivery in a patient following rHuEPO therapy and on long-term dialysis (abstract). J Am Soc Nephrol 1990;1:391.
21. Barri YM, Al-Furayh O, Qunibi WY, Rahman F. Pregnancy in women on regular hemodialysis. Dial Transplant 1991;20:652–4, 656, 695.
22. McGregor E, Stewart G, Junor BJR, Rodger RSC. Successful use of recombinant human erythropoietin in pregnancy. Nephrol Dial Transplant 1991;6:292–3.
23. Gadallah MF, Ahmad B, Karubian F, Campese VM. Pregnancy in patients with chronic ambulatory peritoneal dialysis. Am J Kidney Dis 1992;20:407–10.
24. Hou S, Orlowski J, Pahl M, Ambrose S, Hussey M, Wong D. Pregnancy in women with end-stage renal disease: treatment of anemia and premature labor. Am J Kidney Dis 1993;21:16–22.
25. Barth W Jr, Lacroix L, Goldberg M, Greene M. Recombinant human erythropoietin (rHEpo) for severe anemia in pregnancies complicated by renal disease. Society of Perinatal Obstetricians Abstract. Am J Obstet Gynecol 1994;170:329.
26. Scott LL, Ramin SM, Richey M, Hanson J, Gilstrap LC III. Erythropoietin use in pregnancy: two cases and review of the literature. Am J Perinatol 1995;12:22–4.
27. Amoedo ML, Fernandez E, Borras M, Pais B, Montoliu J. Successful pregnancy in a hemodialysis patient treated with erythropoietin. Nephron 1995;70:262–3.
28. Braga J, Marques R, Branco A, Goncalves J, Lobato L, Pimentel JP, Flores MM, Goncalves E, Jorge CS. Maternal and perinatal implications of the use of human recombinant erythropoietin. Acta Obstet Gynecol Scand 1996;75:449–53.
29. Pascual J, Liano F, Ortuno J. Pregnancy in an anephric woman. Am J Obstet Gynecol 1995;172:1939.
30. Junca J, Vela D, Orts M, Riutort N, Feliu E. Treating the anaemia of a pregnancy with heterozygous β thalassaemia with recombinant human erythropoietin (r-HuEPO). Eur J Haematol 1995;55:277–8.
31. Harris SA, Payne G Jr, Putman JM. Erythropoietin treatment of erythropoietin-deficient anemia with renal disease during pregnancy. Obstet Gynecol 1996;87:812–4.
32. Lin C-P, Huang M-J, Liu H-J, Chang IY, Tsai C-H. Successful treatment of acute promyelocytic leukemia in a pregnant Jehovah's Witness with all-trans retinoic acid, rhG-CSF, and erythropoietin. Am J Hematol 1996;51:251–2.
33. Emmerson AJB, Coles HJ, Stern CMM, Pearson TC. Double blind trial of recombinant human erythropoietin in preterm infants. Arch Dis Child 1993;68:291–6.

EPOPROSTENOL

Vasodilator

PREGNANCY RECOMMENDATION: Compatible—Maternal Benefit >> Embryo–Fetal Risk
BREASTFEEDING RECOMMENDATION: No Human Data—Probably Compatible

E

PREGNANCY SUMMARY

Epoprostenol is not teratogenic in animals, but the human data are too limited to assess with only three human cases involving exposure early in gestation. The placental transfer of the prostaglandin has not been characterized, but it is unlikely if clinically significant amounts of exogenous epoprostenol reach the fetus. Because the prostaglandin occurs naturally in the fetus, it is also unlikely that maternal administration would produce a direct adverse effect on the embryo or fetus. The adverse fetal outcomes that have been noted (bradycardia, fetal heart rate [FHR] decelerations, and death) were most likely due to severe maternal disease or other factors. Although the maternal benefits obtained from use of epoprostenol for severe preeclampsia have not been well documented, its use for pulmonary hypertension is beneficial and appears to far outweigh any potential risks to the fetus.

FETAL RISK SUMMARY

The naturally occurring prostaglandin, epoprostenol (prostacyclin, PGI_2, PGX), is a metabolite of arachidonic acid. Available in the United States since 1995, it is a potent direct vasodilator of pulmonary and systemic arterial vascular beds and an inhibitor of platelet aggregation. Epoprostenol is indicated for the long-term IV treatment of primary pulmonary hypertension (1).

Reproduction studies have revealed no evidence of impaired fertility or fetal harm in pregnant rats and rabbits at 2.5 and 4.8 times the recommended human dose based on BSA, respectively (1).

In animals, epoprostenol causes dose-related changes on the heart rate: bradycardia at low doses and reflex tachycardia secondary to vasodilation and hypotension at higher doses. Other pharmacologic effects in animals include bronchodilation, inhibition of gastric acid secretion, and decreased gastric emptying (1).

No reports describing the placental transfer of epoprostenol have been located. The molecular weight (about 374) of the drug is low enough for placental transfer, but the clinical significance of this is unknown because the agent is rapidly hydrolyzed and undergoes enzymatic degradation in the plasma. In addition, other factors (e.g., ionization, placental metabolism) may limit transfer to the fetus. Continuous infusions of the prostaglandin, which reach steady-state plasma levels within 15 minutes in animals and are proportional to infusion rates, could potentially provide a reservoir to allow placental transfer. But the in vivo plasma half-life of tritium-labeled epoprostenol in animals is very short (2.7 minutes) (1). In humans, the in vitro half-life in blood is slightly longer, approximately 6 minutes, and the in vivo half-life, although it has not yet been determined, is expected to be no longer than this time (1). Thus, even if placental transfer does occur the amounts reaching the fetus may be clinically insignificant. The effects of adding to the endogenous concentrations of the prostaglandin in the fetus are unknown.

In an in vitro study, prostacyclin was shown to be a potent inhibitor of human fetal and maternal platelet aggregation and more potent than *S*-nitroso-*N*-acetylpenicillamine (a releaser of nitric oxide) (2). Moreover, fetal platelets were more sensitive to both agents than were maternal platelets.

The effects of various drugs on the production of maternal and fetal endogenous prostacyclin have been studied in in vivo and in vitro systems. For ritodrine, one study found an increase in the synthesis of the prostaglandin (3), whereas a second reported no effect (4). Ethanol was shown to decrease prostacyclin synthesis in a dose-related manner (5). No effect on prostacyclin production was shown with aspirin (6–8) or magnesium sulfate (9).

The enzymes involved in the synthesis of prostacyclin (PGI_2) and thromboxane A_2 (TXA_2) were studied in maternal and fetal platelets and venous endothelium in a 1991 publication (10). Three groups of pregnant women were studied: normal controls; mild preeclampsia; and severe preeclampsia. Based on their findings, the authors concluded that the production of both PGI_2 and TXA_2 was equal in mild preeclampsia, but in severe preeclampsia, the rise in TXA_2 exceeded that of PGI_2.

A number of reports have described the use of epoprostenol for the treatment of severe preeclampsia (11–17) or pulmonary hypertension (18–20). In a 1980 case report, a 29-year-old woman at 27 weeks' gestation with hypertension uncontrolled with oral methyldopa (3 g/day) and hydralazine (150 mg/day) was started on a continuous infusion of epoprostenol at 8 ng/kg/minute (11). Diastolic pressure fell from 140 to 80 mmHg and remained at or below 95 mmHg during the next 3 days. Adverse effects in the mother included flushing, tachycardia (95–100 beats/minute [bpm]), and transient, nonspecific chest and abdominal pain. On day 4 of therapy, prolonged (1–2 minutes) fetal bradycardia occurred (60 bpm) and delivery by cesarean section was initiated. During the induction phase of anesthesia, the epoprostenol infusion was stopped for 4 minutes. During this interval, the blood pressure rose to 200/100 mmHg but returned to 130/80 mmHg when the infusion was restarted. More than normal bleeding occurred during the procedure and the infusion was discontinued. The 730-g newborn was alive and making good progress at 3 weeks of age.

A continuous IV infusion of epoprostenol was started at 25 weeks' gestation in a 27-old-woman with preeclampsia only partially responsive to methyldopa, aspirin (300 mg every other day), and hydralazine (12). The woman had a history of two previous pregnancies complicated by pregnancy-induced hypertension, severe intrauterine growth restriction, and fetal death at 27 weeks' gestation. Epoprostenol was chosen because of a rise in her diastolic pressure to 90 mmHg, a slowing of fetal growth, and a falling maternal plasma concentration of 6-oxo-PGF$_{1\alpha}$ (6-keto-prostaglandin F$_{1\alpha}$), the hydrolyzed product of epoprostenol (12). Mild nausea, facial flushing, and headache limited the dose tolerated by the patient to 4 ng/kg/minute. The maternal diastolic blood pressure stabilized at or below 85 mmHg and her pulse rate increased from 69 bpm to 84 bpm, but the FHR remained unchanged. In spite of almost continuous FHR monitoring, the fetus died on the 4th day of the infusion, after which a macerated 430-g female fetus was delivered. The authors speculated that intervention with epoprostenol came too late to save the pregnancy (12).

A study published in 1985 examined the effect of IV infusions of epoprostenol in five women (gestational ages 24–30 weeks) with severe preeclampsia that was unresponsive to various combinations of other antihypertensive therapy (methyldopa, hydralazine, labetalol, and atenolol) (13). The maximum continuous IV infusion doses tolerated by the patients ranged from 1 to 6 ng/kg/minute with durations varying from 5 hours to 11 days. Facial flushing, nausea and vomiting, and headache were dose-limiting adverse effects. Four infants were delivered by cesarean section when the infusions (duration 5 hours to 7 days) were stopped, but one newborn (mother treated for 4 days) died 5 hours after delivery (birth weight 480 g). Another fetus (600 g) was stillborn at 26 weeks' gestation on the 11th day of epoprostenol (2.5 ng/kg/minute). Ultrasound and FHR monitoring did not detect any significant changes in the fetus prior to death. The authors thought that the two deaths were not related to the drug. The blood pressures of the mothers were reduced, but dose-limiting adverse effects prevented satisfactory control in one patient. Epoprostenol had no effect on uterine activity in any of the cases (13).

No significant changes in placental (intervillous) and umbilical vein blood flow were measured in a study of 13 women (gestational ages 28–38 weeks) with either superimposed preeclampsia ($N = 6$) or preeclampsia ($N = 7$) (14). The infusion dose was increased in four increments (1, 2, 4, and 8 ng/kg/minute), each given for 20 minutes. All women experienced facial flushing and two complained of headache. Significant decreases in maternal blood pressure and consistent increases in maternal plasma or urinary 6-keto-prostaglandin F$_{1\alpha}$ levels were measured. In contrast, no changes in maternal or fetal pulse rates or uterine activity were observed. The fetuses were delivered 1–13 days after the study. Except for one 850-g newborn delivered at 30 weeks' gestation who died at age 2 days from respiratory distress syndrome, the other newborns (birth weights 980–2840 g) were well at birth and survived (14).

Two vasodilators, epoprostenol ($N = 22$) or dihydralazine ($N = 25$), were compared in a prospective randomized study of women with proteinuria and acute diastolic blood pressures >110 mmHg immediately before delivery (15). The mean gestational age in both groups was 36 weeks (range 32–40 weeks). The epoprostenol infusion was started at 0.5 ng/kg/minute and was increased to a maximum of 10 ng/kg/minute within 120 minutes, if needed to control the blood pressure. The initial dihydralazine dose was 0.5 mg/kg/minute and increased to a maximum of 1.5 mg/kg/minute, if needed. Both drugs were continued for 24 hours after delivery and during delivery for those requiring cesarean section. Increases in maternal pulse rate occurred in both groups, but the rise in the epoprostenol patients (6 bpm) was significantly less than the rise with dihydralazine (22 bpm) ($p = 0.0024$). Blood pressures were reduced in both groups, but the difference between them was not significant. Cesarean sections were performed in 13 (60%) (11 for FHR decelerations) of the epoprostenol group and in 20 (80%) (14 for FHR decelerations) of those receiving dihydralazine (*ns*). One neonatal death occurred in each group, but neither was related to the drug therapy (15).

A brief 1992 communication reported the treatment of a 35-year-old woman with thrombotic microangiopathy superimposed on preeclampsia at about 26 weeks' gestation (16). Epoprostenol was started at 2 ng/kg/minute and increased to 20 ng/kg/minute over 24 hours with reduction of her blood pressure and a rise in the platelet count. After stabilization, therapy was stopped but restarted later when her condition worsened. Improvement was again achieved, but she was delivered at 28 weeks' because of oligohydramnios and growth restriction. The baby girl died a week later from respiratory arrest. In addition, the authors described, without details, the successful treatment of a 27-year-old patient with HELLP (**h**emolysis, **e**levated **l**iver enzymes, and **l**ow **p**latelets) syndrome (16). Epoprostenol has also been used to treat a severe case of HELLP syndrome in the immediate postpartum period (17).

A 1999 publication described the use of epoprostenol for the treatment of pulmonary hypertension in three women in the 3rd trimester (18). One patient, at 28 weeks' gestation, died from severe disease within hours of the diagnosis. The other two women delivered newborns of 3333 g and 2905 g, respectively, but the condition and status of the newborns was not mentioned.

In another case of primary pulmonary hypertension, a 34-year-old woman became pregnant with twins after 1.5 years of continuous IV infusion of epoprostenol (40 ng/kg/hour) (19). She was also taking warfarin, digoxin, furosemide, spironolactone, and ferrous sulfate. She first presented at 15 weeks' gestation at which time the warfarin was discontinued. A ultrasound examination 2 weeks later revealed the death of twin A and hydrocephalus and bilateral clubfeet in twin B. She refused pregnancy termination. She was treated twice for central catheter-related septicemia with vancomycin and gentamicin. The dose of epoprostenol was increased as pregnancy progressed, eventually reaching a dose of 60 ng/kg/hour. Betamethasone was given for lung maturity. Nitric oxide via nasal cannula was started just prior to cesarean section for breech presentation. A live, 2155-g male infant was delivered with Apgar scores of 7 and 8 at 1 and 5 minutes, respectively. The infant had severe hydrocephalus and facial anomalies consistent with fetal warfarin syndrome (19). He was alive but still hospitalized at the time of the report. The nitric oxide was discontinued after 40 days and the mother was discharged home 43 days after delivery on epoprostenol 77 ng/kg/hour.

A 2004 case report described the use of IV and inhaled epoprostenol for the treatment of severe primary pulmonary hypertension (20). The woman was started on the IV drug at 26 weeks' gestation. Because of concern that systemic administration could inhibit platelet aggregation and place the patient at risk during epidural catheter placement for labor, she was changed to inhaled epoprostenol at 35 weeks' gestation. A healthy, 2250-g male infant was delivered vaginally with Apgar scores of 7 and 9 at 1 and 5 minutes, respectively. The infant was doing well at 6 months of age (20).

Three pregnant women with pulmonary arterial hypertension were treated with epoprostenol during pregnancy in a 2005 report (21). In two patients, epoprostenol and warfarin were begun before pregnancy with warfarin changed to low-molecular-weight heparin early in gestation. The third patient was started on epoprostenol at 16 weeks' gestation. The women were delivered by cesarean section at 32, 32, and 28 weeks', respectively, with birth weights of 1700, 1500, and 795 g, respectively. The latter infant, delivered from a mother with Eisenmenger syndrome, was delivered early because of growth restriction, but all three infants were alive and well (21).

BREASTFEEDING SUMMARY

No reports describing the use of epoprostenol during lactation have been located. There is potential for its use during breastfeeding, such as in postpartum women with pulmonary hypertension on long-term infusions of the drug. However, this situation must be exceedingly rare. Because of its rapid degradation at physiologic pH and probably in the gut, the clinical significance of any transfer into milk to a nursing infant is probably nil. Moreover, the prostaglandin has been given directly by inhalation to a premature neonate with beneficial effects (22).

References

1. Product information. Flolan. Glaxo Wellcome, 2000.
2. Varela AF, Runge A, Ignarro LJ, Chaudhuri G. Nitric oxide and prostacyclin inhibit fetal platelet aggregation: a response similar to that observed in adults. Am J Obstet Gynecol 1992;167:1599–604.
3. Jouppila P, Kirkinen P, Koivula A, Ylikorkala O. Ritodrine infusion during late pregnancy: effects on fetal and placental blood flow, prostacyclin, and thromboxane. Am J Obstet Gynecol 1985;151:1028–32.
4. Ekblad U, Erkkola R, Uotila P, Kanto J, Palo P. Ritodrine infusion at term: effects on maternal and fetal prostacyclin, thomboxane and prostaglandin precursor fatty acids. Gynecol Obstet Invest 1988;25:106–12.
5. Randall CL, Saulnier JL. Effect of ethanol on prostacyclin, thromboxane, and prostaglandin E production in human umbilical veins. Alcohol Clin Exp Res 1995;19:741–6.
6. Martin C, Varner MW, Brance DW, Rodgers G, Mitchell MD. Dose-related effects of low dose aspirin on hemostasis parameters and prostacyclin/thromboxane ratios in late pregnancy. Prostaglandins 1996;51:321–30.
7. Tulppala M, Marttunen M, Soderstrom-Anttila V, Foudila T, Ailus K, Palosuo T, Ylikorkala O. Low-dose aspirin in prevention of miscarriage in women with unexplained or autoimmune related recurrent miscarriage: effect on prostacyclin and thromboxane A_2 production. Hum Reprod 1997;12:1567–72.
8. Vainio M, Maenpaa J, Riutta A, Ylitalo P, Ala-Fossi SL, Tuimala R. In the dose range of 0.5–2.0 mg/kg, acetylsalicylic acid does not affect prostacyclin production in hypertensive pregnancies. Acta Obstet Gynecol Scand 1999;78:82–8.
9. Walsh SW, Romney AD, Wang Y, Walsh MD. Magnesium sulfate attenuates peroxide-induced vasoconstriction in the human placenta. Am J Obstet Gynecol 1998;178:7–12.
10. Satoh K, Seki H, Sakamoto H. Role of prostaglandins in pregnancy-induced hypertension. Am J Kidney Dis 1991;17:133–8.
11. Fidler J, Bennett MJ, De Swift M, Ellis C, Lewis PJ. Treatment of pregnancy hypertension with prostacyclin. Lancet 1980;2:31–2.
12. Lewis PJ, Shepherd GL, Ritter J, Chan SMT, Bolton PJ, Jogee M, Myatt L, Elder MG. Prostacyclin and pre-eclampsia. Lancet 1981;1:559.
13. Belch JJF, Thorburn J, Greer IA, Sarfo S, Prentice CRM. Intravenous prostacyclin in the management of pregnancies complicated by severe hypertension. Clin Exp Hypertens Preg 1985;B4:75–86.
14. Jouppila P, Kirkinen P, Koivula A, Ylikorkala O. Failure of exogenous prostacyclin to change placental and fetal blood flow in preeclampsia. Am J Obstet Gynecol 1985;151:661–5.
15. Moodley J, Gouws E. A comparative study of the use of epoprostenol and dihydralazine in severe hypertension in pregnancy. Br J Obstet Gynaecol 1992;99:727–30.
16. De Belder AJ, Weston MJ. Epoprostenol infusions in thrombotic microangiopathy of pregnancy. Lancet 1992;339:741–2.
17. Huber W, Schweigart U, Classen M. Epoprostenol and plasmapheresis in complicated HELLP syndrome with pancreatitis. Lancet 1994;343:848.
18. Easterling TR, Ralph DD, Schmucker BC. Pulmonary hypertension in pregnancy: treatment with pulmonary vasodilators. Obstet Gynecol 1999;93:494–8.
19. Badalian SS, Silverman RK, Aubry RH, Longo J. Twin pregnancy in a woman on long-term epoprostenol therapy for primary pulmonary hypertension. A case report. J Reprod Med 2000;45:149–52.
20. Bildirici I, Shumway JB. Intravenous and inhaled epoprostenol for primary pulmonary hypertension during pregnancy and delivery. Obstet Gynecol 2004;103:1102–5.
21. Bendayan D, Hod M, Oron G, Sagie A, Eidelman L, Shitrit D, Kramer MR. Pregnancy outcome in patients with pulmonary arterial hypertension receiving prostacyclin therapy. Obstet Gynecol 2005;106:1206–10.
22. Soditt V, Aring C, Groneck P. Improvement of oxygenation induced by aerosolized prostacyclin in a preterm infant with persistent pulmonary hypertension of the newborn. Intensive Care Med 1997;23:1275–8.

EPROSARTAN

Antihypertensive

PREGNANCY RECOMMENDATION: Human Data Suggest Risk in 2nd and 3rd Trimesters
BREASTFEEDING RECOMMENDATION: No Human Data—Probably Compatible

PREGNANCY SUMMARY

No reports describing the use of eprosartan during human pregnancy have been located. The antihypertensive mechanisms of action of eprosartan and angiotensin-converting enzyme (ACE) inhibitors are very close. That is, the former selectively blocks the binding of angiotensin II to AT_1 receptors, whereas the latter blocks the formation of angiotensin II itself. Therefore, use of this drug during the 2nd and 3rd trimesters may cause teratogenicity and severe fetal and neonatal toxicity that is identical to that seen with ACE inhibitors (see Captopril or Enalapril). Fetal toxic effects may include anuria, oligohydramnios, fetal hypocalvaria, intrauterine growth restriction, prematurity, and patent ductus arteriosus. Anuria-associated oligohydramnios may produce fetal limb contractures, craniofacial deformation, and pulmonary hypoplasia. Severe anuria and hypotension, that is resistant to both pressor agents and volume expansion, may occur in the newborn following in utero exposure to eprosartan. Newborn renal function and blood pressure should be closely monitored.

FETAL RISK SUMMARY

Eprosartan is a selective angiotensin II receptor blocker (ARB) that is used, either alone or in combination with other antihypertensive agents, for the treatment of hypertension. Eprosartan blocks the vasoconstrictor and aldosterone-secreting effects of angiotensin II by preventing angiotensin II from binding to AT_1 receptors.

Reproduction studies have been conducted in rats and rabbits (1). No teratogenic effects were observed in either species, but dose-related toxicity occurred in pregnant rabbits. In pregnant rats, no adverse effects on the fetus or on the postnatal development and maturation of offspring were observed at oral doses up to approximately 0.6 times the human exposure based on AUC at the maximum recommended human dose or 800 mg/day (MRHD). Similarly, a dose approximately 0.8 times the MRHD did not result in fetal or maternal toxicity in pregnant rabbits. Increasing the dose to approximately 2.7 times the MRHD in pregnant rabbits, however, caused both maternal (reduced body weight, decreased food consumption, and death) and embryo–fetal (resorptions, abortions, and litter loss) toxicity (1).

It is not known if eprosartan crosses the human placenta. The molecular weight (about 521) is low enough that passage to the fetus should be expected.

A 2012 review of the use of ACE inhibitors and ARBs in the 1st trimester concluded that there may be an elevated teratogenic risk, but the risk appeared to be related to other factors (2). The factors, that typically coexist with hypertension in pregnancy, included diabetes, advanced maternal age, and obesity.

BREASTFEEDING SUMMARY

No reports describing the use of eprosartan during human lactation have been located. The molecular weight (about 521) is low enough that excretion into breast milk should also be expected. The effects of this exposure on a nursing infant are unknown. The American Academy of Pediatrics, however, classifies ACE inhibitors, a closely related group of antihypertensive agents, as compatible with breastfeeding (see Captopril and Enalapril).

References

1. Product information. Teveten. Unimed Pharmaceuticals, 2001.
2. Polifka JE. Is there an embryopathy associated with first-trimester exposure to angiotensin-converting enzyme inhibitors and angiotensin receptor antagonists? A critical review of the evidence. Birth Defects Res (Part A) 2012;94:576–98.

EPTIFIBATIDE

Hematologic Agent (Antiplatelet)

PREGNANCY RECOMMENDATION: **Limited Human Data—Animal Data Suggest Low Risk**
BREASTFEEDING RECOMMENDATION: **Hold Breastfeeding**

PREGNANCY SUMMARY

One report describing the use of eptifibatide in human pregnancy has been located. The animal data are reassuring but more human pregnancy experience is required to assess the risk this agent presents to the embryo–fetus. The primary risk, however, appears to be from maternal hemorrhage during drug administration. If this is adequately controlled, the benefits of the drug to the mother appear to far outweigh the unknown risks to the fetus.

FETAL RISK SUMMARY

The cyclic heptapeptide, eptifibatide, is indicated for the treatment of acute coronary syndrome in patients who will be managed medically or in those undergoing percutaneous coronary intervention. Eptifibatide acts as a reversible inhibitor of platelet aggregation by blocking the GP IIb/IIIa receptor on the platelet surface. It is in the same subclass of antiplatelet agents as abciximab and tirofiban. The drug undergoes some metabolism. Plasma protein binding is about 25% and the plasma elimination half-life is about 2.5 hours (1).

Reproduction studies with eptifibatide have been conducted in rats and rabbits. In pregnant rats and rabbits, continuous daily IV infusions at total daily doses up to about four times the maximum recommended human daily dose based on BSA (MRHDD) revealed no evidence of fetal harm. Although long-term studies in animals for carcinogenicity have not been conducted, no evidence of mutagenicity was found in several tests. Similarly, no evidence of impaired fertility or reproductive performance was observed in rats given daily doses up to about four times the MRHDD (1).

It is not known if eptifibatide crosses the human placenta to the fetus. The molecular weight (about 832), low plasma protein binding, and the elimination half-life suggest that the drug will cross to the embryo–fetus. Moreover, the drug is given as a continuous IV infusion for periods up to 72 hours, thus allowing for prolonged contact at the maternal–fetal interface.

A 44-year-old woman at 8 weeks' gestation presented with an acute myocardial infarction (2). She was treated with intracoronary stent placement and clopidogrel (600 mg), heparin, and a 24-hour IV infusion of eptifibatide. The next day, she was started on clopidogrel, aspirin, and propranolol and discharged home on these agents. At 36 weeks, she underwent a planned cesarean section for a healthy infant (no further details on the newborn were provided) (2).

BREASTFEEDING SUMMARY

No reports describing the use of eptifibatide during lactation have been located. Because of the indications for eptifibatide, it is doubtful if such reports will be forthcoming. The molecular weight (about 832), low plasma protein binding, and the elimination half-life suggest that the drug will be excreted into breast milk. Moreover, the drug is given as a continuous IV infusion for periods up to 72 hours. The effect of this exposure for a nursing infant is unknown, but most likely the risk is very low or nil because the drug should be digested in the infant's gastrointestinal tract. Until data are available, however, the safest course is to hold breastfeeding while the drug is being infused.

References

1. Product information. Integrilin. Schering, 2009.
2. Al-Aqeedi RF, Al-Nabti AD. Drug-eluting stent implantation for acute myocardial infarction during pregnancy with use of glycoprotein IIb/IIIa inhibitor. J Invasive Cardiol 2008;20:E146–9.

ERGOCALCIFEROL

Vitamin

PREGNANCY RECOMMENDATION: Compatible
BREASTFEEDING RECOMMENDATION: Compatible

PREGNANCY SUMMARY

Ergocalciferol (vitamin D_2) is converted in the liver to 25-hydroxyergocalciferol, which in turn is converted in the kidneys to 1,25-dihydroxyergocalciferol, one of the active forms of vitamin D. See Vitamin D.

BREASTFEEDING SUMMARY

See Vitamin D.

ERGOTAMINE

Sympatholytic (Antimigraine)

PREGNANCY RECOMMENDATION: Contraindicated
BREASTFEEDING RECOMMENDATION: Contraindicated

PREGNANCY SUMMARY

Small, infrequent doses of ergotamine used for migraine headaches do not appear to be fetotoxic or teratogenic, but idiosyncratic responses may occur that endanger the fetus. Larger doses or frequent use, however, may cause fetal toxicity or teratogenicity that is probably due to maternal and/or fetal vascular disruption. Based on one report, the combination of ergotamine, caffeine, and propranolol may represent an added risk. Because the risk has not been adequately defined, and also due to the oxytocic properties of the agent, ergotamine should be avoided during pregnancy.

FETAL RISK SUMMARY

Ergotamine is a naturally occurring ergot alkaloid that is used in the prevention or treatment of vascular headaches, such as migraine. The oxytocic properties of ergotamine have been known since the early 1900s, but because it produces a prolonged and marked increase in uterine tone that may lead to fetal hypoxia, it is not used for this purpose (1). A semisynthetic derivative, dihydroergotamine, has also been abandoned as an oxytocic for the same reason (2). (See Dihydroergotamine.) Small amounts of ergotamine have been reported to cross the placenta to the fetus (3).

Ergotamine is not an animal teratogen (4). In pregnant mice, rats, and rabbits, however, doses sufficient to affect maternal weight gain were fetotoxic, producing increased prenatal mortality and growth restriction. The mechanism proposed for these effects was an impairment of blood supply to the uterus and placenta (4). Another study demonstrating fetal death in pregnant rats arrived at the same conclusion (5). Ergotamine (0.25%) fed to pregnant sheep produced severe ergotism, fetal death, and abortions (6).

Most authorities consider ergotamine in pregnancy to be either contraindicated or to be used sparingly and with caution, due to the oxytocic properties of the drug (7–10). Fortunately, the frequency of migraine attacks decreases during pregnancy, thus lessening the need for any medication (8–10).

The Collaborative Perinatal Project monitored 50,282 mother–child pairs, 25 of whom were exposed to ergotamine during the 1st trimester (11). Two malformed children were observed from this group, but the numbers are too small to draw any conclusion.

In a surveillance study of Michigan Medicaid recipients involving 229,101 completed pregnancies conducted between 1985 and 1992, 59 newborns had been exposed to ergotamine during the 1st trimester (F. Rosa, personal communication, FDA, 1993). A total of nine (15.3%) major birth defects were observed (two expected). Specific data were available for six defect categories, including (observed/expected) 1/0.6 cardiovascular defects, 0/0 oral clefts, 0/0 spina bifida, 1/0 polydactyly, 0/0 limb reduction defects, and 1/0 hypospadias. The total number of defects is suggestive of an association, but other factors, such as the mother's disease, concurrent drug use, and chance may be involved.

A retrospective study published in 1978 evaluated the reproductive outcome of women attending a migraine clinic (12). The study group was composed of 777 women enrolling in the clinic for the first time. A control group composed of 182 wives of new male patients at the clinic was formed for comparison. Of the women with migraine, 450 (58%) had been pregnant vs. 136 (75%) of the women without migraine. The difference in the percentage of pregnancies may have been because all of the control women were married while the marriage status of the study women was not known (12). The incidence of at least one spontaneous abortion or stillbirth, 27% vs. 29%, including 1st trimester loss, and the occurrence of toxemia, 18% vs. 18%, were similar for the groups. The total number of pregnancies was 1142 in the study patients and 342 in the controls, with a mean number of pregnancies per patient of 2.54 vs. 2.51, respectively. The migraine group had 924 (81%) live births compared with 277 (81%) for the control women. Congenital defects observed among the live births totaled 31 (3.4%) for the study group vs. 11 (4.0%) for the controls (*ns*). Major abnormalities, found in 20 (2.2%) of the infants from the women with migraine compared with 7 (2.5%) of the infants from controls, were of similar distribution to those found in the geographic area of the clinic (12). Moreover, the incidence of defects was similar to the expected frequency for that location (12). Although the investigators were unable to document reliable and accurate drug histories during the pregnancies because of the retrospective nature of the study, 70.8% of the women with migraine indicated they had used ergotamine in the past. They concluded, therefore, that ergotamine exposure during pregnancy, especially early in gestation, was highly likely, and that this drug and others used for the prevention or treatment of the disease were probably not teratogenic (12).

In contrast to the above study, six case reports have described adverse fetal outcomes attributable to ergotamine (13–18). An infant, who died at 4 weeks of age, was delivered at 24 weeks' gestation with a large rugated, perineal mass, no external genitalia or anal orifice, and a small, polycystic left kidney (13). Two separate sacs made up the mass, one of which resembled a urinary bladder with two ureteral and a vaginal orifice, and the other containing bowel, left ovary, uterus, and right kidney (13). The mother had used an ergotamine inhaler once or twice weekly during the first 8 weeks of pregnancy for migraine headaches. The inhaler delivered 0.36 mg of ergotamine per inhalation and she received two or three inhalations during each headache for a total dose of 0.72–1.08 mg once or twice weekly. The mother also smoked about 10 cigarettes daily.

A female infant with multiple congenital malformations was delivered from a woman who had used a proprietary preparation containing ergotamine, caffeine, belladonna, and pentobarbital during the 2nd month of pregnancy for migraine (14). Two other similar cases in pregnant women who did not receive an ergotamine preparation were included in the report. The birth defects included hydrocephalus, sacral or coccygeal agenesis, digital and muscle hypoplasia, joint contractures, short stature, short perineum, and pilonidal sinus. Because of the similarity of the cases, the authors thought it might be a new syndrome, which they termed cerebroarthrodigital syndrome, in which the primary pathogenetic event is a neural tube-neural crest dysplasia (14). Although they could not determine the cause, they considered an environmental agent, such as ergotamine, or a genetic cause as possibilities (14).

A 1983 report described a 27-year-old woman with migraine headaches who consumed up to 8 tablets/day of a preparation containing 1 mg of ergotamine tartrate and 100 mg of caffeine throughout a total of six pregnancies (15). The 1st pregnancy resulted in the birth of a 2200-g female infant, whose subsequent growth varied between the 3rd and 10th percentiles. She had no medical problems other than enuresis and hay fever. The woman's 2nd, 4th, 5th, and 6th pregnancies all ended in spontaneous abortions. A male infant was delivered in the 3rd pregnancy at 35 weeks' gestation. Birth weight, 1892 g, and length, 43 cm, were at the 20th percentile for gestational age. The infant died at 25 days of age secondary to hyaline membrane disease and after two surgical attempts to correct jejunal atresia. At autopsy, a short small intestine with portions of incomplete or absent muscular coat around the bowel lumen was found. The authors could not exclude a hereditary cause for the anomaly, but they believed the most likely cause was a disruptive vascular mechanism resulting from an interruption of the superior mesenteric arterial supply to the affected organ (15).

In a suicide attempt, a 17-year-old pregnant woman, at 35 weeks' gestation, took a single dose of 10 ergotamine tablets (20 mg) (16). Five hours after ingestion, the fetal heart rate was 165 beats/minute with fetal movement. Uterine contractions were mild but frequent, with little relaxation between contractions. Fetal death occurred approximately 8.5 hours later, about 13.5 hours after ingestion. The most likely mechanism for the fetal death was impairment of placental perfusion by the uterine contractions resulting in fetal hypoxia (16). However, the authors considered two other possible mechanisms: arterial spasm causing decreased uterine arterial perfusion, and altered peripheral resistance and venous return resulting in fetal myocardial ischemia (16).

A 1988 case report described the result of a pregnancy complicated by severe migraine headaches (17). The mother consumed a variety of drugs, including 1–4 rectal suppositories/week during the first 14 weeks of gestation, with each dose containing ergotamine (2 mg), belladonna (0.25 mg), caffeine (100 mg), and phenobarbital (60 mg). Other medications, frequency of ingestion, and gestational weeks of exposure were propranolol (40 mg; 2/day; 0–20 weeks), acetaminophen/codeine (325 mg/8 mg; 6–20/day; 0–16 weeks), and dimenhydrinate (75 mg; 0–3/week; 0–12 weeks). The term, female infant was a breech presentation weighing 2860 g, with a length of 46 cm. The infant was microcephalic and paraplegic with underdeveloped and hypotonic lower limbs. The anal, knee, and ankle reflexes were absent. Sensation was absent to the level of the knees and variably absent on the thighs. This pattern was suggestive of a spinal cord defect in the upper lumbar region (17). Other abnormalities apparent were dislocated hips and marked bilateral talipes equinovarus. Computed tomography of the brain revealed a small organ with lissencephaly, a primitive Sylvian fissure, and ventriculomegaly (17). The above findings were compatible with arrest of cerebral development that occurred after 10–13 weeks (17). The authors concluded that the most likely etiology was a disruptive vascular mechanism, and that the combination of ergotamine, caffeine, and propranolol may have potentiated the vasoconstriction (17).

In response to the case report above, a 1989 letter cited prospective and retrospective data from the Hungarian Case–Control Surveillance of Congenital Anomalies, 1980–1986 system (19). Among controls (normal infants, but including those with Down's syndrome), 0.11% (18 of 16,477) had used ergotamine during pregnancy, whereas 0.14% (13 of 9460) of pregnancies with a birth defect had been exposed to the drug (*ns*). Four of the index cases, however, involved neural tube defects compared with none of the controls ($p < 0.01$), a finding that prompted the author to state that further study was required.

A female infant, the smaller of dizygotic twins, was born at 32 weeks' gestation (18). Paraplegia and arthrogryposis multiplex was present at birth and thought to be due to prenatal cord trauma. The mother had a severe reaction (intractable nausea, vertigo and dizziness requiring bed rest for 3 days) following the use of one rectal suppository containing ergotamine, caffeine, belladonna, and butalbital at 4.5 months' gestation. Because of this reaction, the authors speculated that ergotamine may have caused vascular spasm of a fetal medullary artery that resulted in spinal cord ischemia and neuronal loss (18).

The accidental use at 38 weeks' gestation of a rectal suppository containing ergotamine (2 mg) and caffeine (100 mg) in a woman with nonproteinuric hypertension produced sudden fetal distress that led to an emergency cesarean section (20). A growth-restricted, 2660-g female infant was delivered with Apgar scores of 4 and 8 at 1 and 5 minutes, respectively. The obstetrician, who was unaware of the drug administration, noted the strikingly small amount (100 mL) of blood loss during the procedure. The infant was doing well at 10 years of age.

A 1995 reference reviewed the teratogenicity of ergotamine (21). Because many of the reports of adverse outcomes following the use of the drug during pregnancy are consistent with vascular injury, and because ergotamine toxicity is known to cause vasospasm, the author recommended that the drug should be avoided during all parts of pregnancy (21). The use of the agent in small, appropriate doses, however, was thought to have a low teratogenic potential because ergotamine appeared to be teratogenic only at higher doses, or possibly in those cases involving idiosyncratic susceptibility (21). Recommendations for counseling of exposed women included not only determining the dosage and timing of exposure but also asking questions relating to the presence or absence of signs and symptoms of ergotism, past usage, and possible continuing abuse (21).

BREASTFEEDING SUMMARY

Ergotamine is excreted into breast milk, but data quantifying this excretion have not been located. A 1934 study reported that 90% of nursing infants of mothers using an ergot preparation for migraine therapy had symptoms of ergotism (22). Because of the vomiting, diarrhea, and convulsions observed in this study, the American Academy of Pediatrics classifies ergotamine as a drug that has been associated with significant effects on some nursing infants and should be given to nursing mothers with caution (23). Moreover, ergotamine is a member of the same chemical family as bromocriptine, an agent that is used to suppress lactation. Although no specific information has been located relating to the effects of ergotamine on lactation, ergot alkaloids may hinder lactation by inhibiting maternal pituitary prolactin secretion (24).

References

1. Gill RC, Farrar JM. Experiences with di-hydro-ergotamine in the treatment of primary uterine inertia. J Obstet Gynaecol Br Emp 1951;58:79–91.
2. Altman SG, Waltman R, Lubin S, Reynolds SR. Oxytocic and toxic actions of dihydroergotamine-45. Am J Obstet Gynecol1952;64:101–9.
3. Griffith RW, Grauwiler J, Holdel CH, Leist KH, Matter B. Toxicologic considerations. In: Berde B, Schild HO, eds. *Ergot Alkaloids and Related Compounds. Handbook of Experimental Pharmacology*. Vol. 49. Berlin, Germany: Springer Verlag, 1979:805–51. As cited in Hughes HE, Goldstein DA. Birth defects following maternal exposure to ergotamine, beta-blockers, and caffeine. J Med Genet 1988;25:396–9.
4. Grauwiler J, Schon H. Teratological experiments with ergotamine in mice, rats, and rabbits. Teratology 1973;7:227–36.
5. Schon H, Leist KH, Grauwiler J. Single-day treatment of pregnant rats with ergotamine (abstract). Teratology 1975;11:32A.
6. Greatorex JC, Mantle PG. Effect of rye ergot on the pregnant sheep. J Reprod Fertil 1974;37:33–41.
7. Foster JB. Migraine-traditional uses of ergot compounds. Postgrad Med J 1976;52(Suppl 1):12–4.
8. Massey EW. Migraine during pregnancy. Obstet Gynecol Surv 1977;32: 693–6.
9. Lance JW. The pharmacotherapy of migraine. Med J Aust 1986;144:85–8.
10. Reik L Jr. Headaches in pregnancy. Semin Neurol 1988;8:187–92.
11. Heinonen OP, Sloan D, Shapiro S. *Birth Defects and Drugs in Pregnancy*. Littleton, MA: Publishing Sciences Group, 1977:358–60.
12. Wainscott G, Sullivan FM, Volans GN, Wilkinson M. The outcome of pregnancy in women suffering from migraine. Postgrad Med J 1978;54:98–102.
13. Peeden JN Jr, Wilroy RS Jr, Soper RG. Prune perineum. Teratology 1979;20:233–6.
14. Spranger JW, Schinzel A, Myers T, Ryan J, Giedion A, Opitz JM. Cerebroarthrodigital syndrome: a newly recognized formal genesis syndrome in three patients with apparent arthromyodysplasia and sacral agenesis, brain malformation and digital hypoplasia. Am J Med Genet 1980;5:13–24.

15. Graham JM Jr, Marin-Padilla M, Hoefnagel D. Jejunal atresia associated with Cafergot ingestion during pregnancy. Clin Pediatr 1983;22: 226–8.
16. Au KL, Woo JSK, Wong VCW. Intrauterine death from ergotamine overdosage. Eur J Obstet Gynecol Reprod Biol 1985;19:313–5.
17. Hughes HE, Goldstein DA. Birth defects following maternal exposure to ergotamine, beta blockers, and caffeine. J Med Genet 1988;25: 396–9.
18. Verloes A, Emonts P, Dubois M, Rigo J, Senterre J. Paraplegia and arthrogryposis multiplex of the lower extremities after intrauterine exposure to ergotamine. J Med Genet 1990;27:213–4.
19. Czeizel A. Teratogenicity of ergotamine. J Med Genet 1989;26:69–70.
20. de Groot ANJA, van Dongen PWJ, van Roosmalen J, Eskes TKAB. Ergotamine-induced fetal stress: review of side effects of ergot alkaloids during pregnancy. Eur J Obstet Gynecol Reprod Biol 1993;51:73–7.
21. Raymond GV. Teratogen update: ergot and ergotamine. Teratology 1995;51:344–7.
22. Fomina PI. Untersuchungen uber den Ubergang des aktiven Agens des Mutterkorns in die milch stillender Mutter. Arch Gynaek 1934;157:275. As cited by Knowles JA. Excretion of drugs in milk-a review. J Pediatr 1965;66:1068–82.
23. Committee on Drugs, American Academy of Pediatrics. The transfer of drugs and other chemicals into human milk. Pediatrics 2001;108:776–89.
24. Vorherr H. Contraindications to breast-feeding. JAMA 1974;227:676.

ERIBULIN

Antineoplastic

PREGNANCY RECOMMENDATION: Contraindicated
BREASTFEEDING RECOMMENDATION: Contraindicated

PREGNANCY SUMMARY

No reports describing the use of eribulin in human pregnancy have occurred. Although developmental toxicity occurred in rats at maternal toxic doses, the doses were much less than the recommended human dose. Because of the risk for severe toxicity in an embryo and/or a fetus, eribulin should not be used in pregnancy.

FETAL RISK SUMMARY

Eribulin is a nontaxane microtubule dynamics inhibitor that is given IV on days 1 and 8 of a 21-day cycle. It is indicated for the treatment of patients with metastatic breast cancer who have previously received at least two chemotherapeutic regimens for the treatment of metastatic disease. There are no major metabolites of eribulin. Plasma protein binding is in the range of 49%–65%. The mean elimination half-life is about 40 hours (1).

Reproduction studies have been conducted in rats. In this species, IV doses were given during organogenesis (gestation days 8, 10, and 12) that were about 0.04–0.64 times the recommended human dose based on BSA (RHD). At the highest dose, abortions and severe external or soft-tissue malformations were observed. The malformations included the absence of a lower jaw, tongue, stomach, and spleen. At 0.43 times the RHD, increased embryo–fetal death/resorption, reduced fetal weights, and minor skeletal anomalies consistent with developmental delay were noted. However, at doses ≥0.43 times the RHD, maternal toxicity that included enlarged spleen, reduced maternal weight gain, and decreased food consumption occurred (1).

Studies of carcinogenicity have not been conducted. Eribulin was not mutagenic in bacterial assays but was mutagenic in other assays and was clastogenic in one assay. Although fertility studies have not been conducted, dog and rat toxicology studies have observed testicular toxicity in both species suggesting that the drug may compromise male fertility (1).

It is not known if eribulin crosses the human placenta. The molecular weight (about 730 for the free base), lack of metabolism, moderate protein binding, and long half-life suggest that the drug will cross to the embryo–fetus.

BREASTFEEDING SUMMARY

No reports describing the use of eribulin during human lactation have been located. The molecular weight (about 730 for the free base), lack of metabolism, moderate protein binding, and long half-life suggest that the drug will be excreted into breast milk. Moreover, as a basic drug, higher concentrations of eribulin in milk compared with the plasma may occur. The effect of this exposure on a nursing infant is unknown but there is potential for severe toxicity. Consequently, breastfeeding during therapy with this agent should be considered contraindicated.

Reference

1. Product Information. Halaven. Eisai, 2010.

ERLOTINIB

Antineoplastic (Tyrosine Kinase Inhibitor)

PREGNANCY RECOMMENDATION: Limited Human Data—Animal Data Suggest Moderate Risk
BREASTFEEDING RECOMMENDATION: No Human Data—Potential Toxicity

PREGNANCY SUMMARY

Two reports describing the use of erlotinib in human pregnancy has been located. The animal data suggest risk, but the near absence of human pregnancy experience prevents a complete assessment of the embryo–fetal risk. If a woman receives erlotinib during pregnancy, she should be informed of the unknown risk to her embryo–fetus.

E

FETAL RISK SUMMARY

Erlotinib is an oral antineoplastic agent that is indicated, in combination with gemcitabine, for the first-line treatment of patients with locally advanced, unresectable or metastatic pancreatic cancer. The drug is a human epidermal growth factor type 1/epidermal growth factor receptor tyrosine kinase inhibitor in the same subclass as several other agents (see Appendix). Erlotinib is extensively metabolized by the liver to apparently inactive metabolites. The elimination half-life is about 32 hours. About 93% of erlotinib is bound to the plasma proteins albumin and alpha-1 acid glycoprotein (1,2).

Reproduction studies have been conducted in rats and rabbits. In pregnant rats and rabbits during organogenesis, there was no increased incidence of embryo–fetal lethality, abortion, or teratogenic effects with doses that achieved plasma concentrations that were about equal to those in humans from a 150 mg daily dose based on AUC (HDD). However, when pregnant rabbits were given a dose that produced exposures that were about three times the HDD, maternal toxicity with associated embryo–fetal lethality and abortion occurred. In addition, female rats given daily doses that were about 0.3 or 0.7 times the human dose based on BSA prior to mating, and through the first week of pregnancy had an increase in early resorptions resulting in a decrease in the number of live fetuses (1).

Carcinogenic studies have not been conducted with erlotinib. Multiple tests for genotoxicity were negative, as were the effects on male and female rat fertility (1).

It is not known if erlotinib crosses the human placenta. The molecular weight (about 394 for the free base) and long elimination half-life suggest that the drug will cross. However, the extensive metabolism and moderately high plasma protein binding may limit the amount of active drug reaching the embryo–fetus.

A woman with metastatic nonsmall cell lung cancer was treated with six cycles of cisplatin, gemcitabine, and bisphosphonates that resulted in stable disease (3). No additional therapy was given for 12 months until progressive disease was found and erlotinib 100 mg/day was started. Pregnancy was diagnosed 2 months later. Conception was thought to have occurred at about the same time that erlotinib had been started. The drug was discontinued for the remainder of the pregnancy. At 42 weeks' gestation, a cesarean section delivered a normal, 3490-g female infant. No congenital malformations or other abnormalities were noted in the healthy infant (3).

A 2011 case report described a 38-year-old woman at 26 weeks' gestation who was diagnosed with lung cancer (4). The woman had never smoked. She was initially treated with erlotinib 100 mg/day and then changed about 2 weeks later to gefitinib 250 mg/day. Gefitinib was continued through the remainder of her pregnancy. At 36 weeks', she gave birth to a healthy 2.08-kg infant with an Apgar score of 9 at 1 minute. The baby weighed 2.98 kg 6 weeks later (4).

BREASTFEEDING SUMMARY

No reports describing the use of erlotinib during human lactation have been located. The molecular weight (about 394 for the free base) and long elimination half-life suggest that the drug will be excreted into breast milk. However, the extensive metabolism and moderately high plasma protein binding may limit the amount of active drug reaching the milk. The effects on a nursing infant are unknown, but there is a potential for severe toxicity. Moreover, the systemic bioavailability of erlotinib is markedly increased in adults when the dose is taken with food, and this might also occur in nursing infants. Therefore, until the amount of erlotinib in breast milk has been determined, the safest course is not to breastfeed.

References

1. Product information. Tarceva. Genentech, 2007.
2. Product information. Tarceva. OSI Pharmaceuticals, 2007.
3. Zambelli A, Antonio Da Prada G, Fregoni V, Ponchio L, Sagrada P, Pavesi L. Erlotinib administration for advanced non-small cell lung cancer during the first 2 months of unrecognized pregnancy. Lung Cancer 2008;60:455–7.
4. Lee CH, Liam CK, Pang YK, Chua KT, Lim BK, Lai NL. Successful pregnancy with epidermal growth factor receptor tyrosine kinase inhibitor treatment of metastatic lung adenocarcinoma presenting with respiratory failure. Lung Cancer 2011;74:349–51.

ERTAPENEM

Antibiotic

PREGNANCY RECOMMENDATION: No Human Data—Probably Compatible
BREASTFEEDING RECOMMENDATION: Limited Human Data—Probably Compatible

PREGNANCY SUMMARY

No reports describing the use of ertapenem in human pregnancy have been located. No teratogenicity was observed in two animal species, although mild fetal toxicity was observed in one at a dose very close to that used in humans. Moreover, there is no evidence that any beta-lactam antibiotic (e.g., penicillins and cephalosporins) causes developmental toxicity in humans at therapeutic doses. Therefore, if the maternal condition requires the use of ertapenem, the antibiotic probably is safe at any time during gestation.

FETAL RISK SUMMARY

Ertapenem is a broad-spectrum carbapenem antibiotic that is administered by either IM injection or IV infusion. It is structurally related to the beta-lactam antibiotics and belongs to the same class as imipenem (available as imipenem-cilastatin) and meropenem.

Reproduction studies have been conducted in mice and rats. No evidence of structural teratogenicity was observed at IV doses up to three times the recommended human dose of 1 g based on BSA (mice) and 1.2 times the human exposure at the recommended dose of 1 g based on AUC (rats) (1). However, the maximum dose in mice resulted in decreased fetal weight and decreases in the average number of ossified sacrocaudal vertebrae. The antibiotic had no effect on mating performance, fecundity, fertility, or embryonic survival in either species (1).

Ertapenem crosses the placenta in rats, but this has not been studied in humans. The molecular weight (about 498) is low enough that passage to the fetus should be expected.

BREASTFEEDING SUMMARY

Ertapenem is excreted into breast milk (1). Five women 5–14 days postpartum were treated with 1 g IV daily for 3–10 days. Milk concentrations of the antibiotic were measured at random times for 5 consecutive days after the last dose. Samples obtained within 24 hours of the last dose ranged from <0.13 (lower limit of quantitation) to 0.38 mcg/mL. By day 5, ertapenem could not be detected in the milk of four women and was <0.13 mcg/mL in one woman (1).

The effects on a nursing infant from exposure to ertapenem via milk are unknown but are of doubtful clinical significance. Most antibiotics are excreted into breast milk in low concentrations, and adverse effects are rare. Potential problems for the nursing infant are modification of bowel flora, direct effects on the infant (e.g., allergic response), and interference with the interpretation of culture results if a fever workup is required.

Reference

1. Product information. Invanz. Merck & Company, 2003.

ERYTHRITYL TETRANITRATE

Vasodilator

See Nitroglycerin or Amyl Nitrite.

ERYTHROMYCIN

Antibiotic

PREGNANCY RECOMMENDATION: Compatible (Excludes Estolate Salt)
BREASTFEEDING RECOMMENDATION: Compatible

PREGNANCY SUMMARY

Most reports, including one animal study, have found no evidence of developmental toxicity with erythromycin. Although one report found an association with cardiovascular defects (see reference 17), the investigators could not determine if it was a true drug effect. There also is no evidence that maternal erythromycin treatment late in pregnancy causes infantile hypertrophic pyloric stenosis (IHPS). Because most studies do not indicate a risk, erythromycin can be used in pregnancy if indicated.

E

FETAL RISK SUMMARY

Erythromycin is a macrolide anti-infective that is in the same class as azithromycin, clarithromycin, dirithromycin, and troleadomycin.

The drug was not teratogenic in female rats fed erythromycin (up to 0.25% of the diet) before and during mating, and throughout gestation and weaning (1).

Erythromycin crosses the placenta but in concentrations too low to treat most pathogens (2–4). Fetal tissue levels increase after multiple doses (4). However, a case has been described in which erythromycin was used successfully to treat maternal syphilis but failed to treat the fetus adequately (5). During pregnancy, erythromycin serum concentrations vary greatly as compared with those in normal men and nonpregnant women, which might account for the low levels observed in the fetus (6).

The estolate salt of erythromycin has been observed to induce hepatotoxicity in pregnant patients (7). Approximately 10% of 161 women treated with the estolate form in the 2nd trimester had abnormally elevated levels of serum glutamic-oxaloacetic transaminase, which returned to normal after therapy was discontinued.

The use of erythromycin in the 1st trimester was reported in a mother who delivered an infant with left absence-of-tibia syndrome (8). The mother was also exposed to other drugs, which makes a relationship to the antibiotic unlikely.

The Collaborative Perinatal Project monitored 50,282 mother–child pairs, 79 of whom had 1st trimester exposure to erythromycin (9, pp. 297–313). For use anytime during pregnancy, 230 exposures were recorded (9, p. 435). No evidence was found to suggest a relationship to large categories of major and minor malformations or to individual defects. Erythromycin, like many other antibiotics, lowers urine estriol concentrations (see also Ampicillin for mechanism and significance) (10). The antibiotic has been used during the 3rd trimester to reduce maternal and infant colonization with group B β-hemolytic streptococcus (11,12). Erythromycin has also been used during pregnancy for the treatment of genital mycoplasma (13,14). A reduction in the rates of pregnancy loss and low-birth-weight infants was seen in patients with mycoplasma infection after treatment with erythromycin.

In a surveillance study of Michigan Medicaid recipients involving 229,101 completed pregnancies conducted between 1985 and 1992, 6972 newborns had been exposed to erythromycin during the 1st trimester (F. Rosa, personal communication, FDA, 1993). A total of 320 (4.6%) major birth defects were observed (297 expected). Specific data were available for six defect categories, including (observed/expected) 77/70 cardiovascular defects, 14/11 oral clefts, 1/3 spina bifida, 22/20 polydactyly, 14/12 limb reduction defects, and 11/17 hypospadias. These data do not support an association between the drug and congenital malformations.

Data from the Hungarian Case–Control Surveillance of Congenital Abnormalities, 1980–1996, regarding exposure to erythromycin during organogenesis were published in 1999 (15). Cases (*N* = 22,865) were fetuses or infants with congenital abnormalities, 113 (0.5%) of whom had been exposed to erythromycin. Among controls (*N* = 38,151), newborns without any congenital anomalies, 172 (0.5%) had been exposed to erythromycin. There were 20 cases and 43 controls exposed during the 2nd–3rd months (i.e., organogenesis), odds ratio (OR) 0.8, 95% confidence interval (CI) 0.5–1.4. For exposures during months 4–9, there were 78 cases and 112 controls, OR 1.2, 95% CI 0.9–1.6, and for the entire pregnancy, OR 1.1, 95% CI 0.9–1.5. The study found no detectable teratogenic risk from erythromycin (15).

A 2001 randomized study (ORACLE 1) was conducted in patients with preterm, prelabor rupture of fetal membranes to determine neonatal health benefits of three antibiotic regimens (16). The regimens, compared with a placebo group (*N* = 1225), were erythromycin (250 mg) (*N* = 1197), amoxicillin (250 mg)–clavulanic acid (125 mg) (*N* = 1212), or both (*N* = 1192) four times daily for 10 days or until delivery. The primary outcome measures were specific outcomes or a composite of neonatal death, chronic lung disease, or major cerebral abnormality. For these neonatal outcomes, the two groups with ACA had no benefit over placebo, whereas erythromycin use resulted in significantly better outcomes (both composite and specific). When any-ACA exposure was compared with no-ACA for outcomes with suspected or proven NEC, the results were 92 (3.8%) and 58 (2.4%) (p = 0.004). The authors thought that a possible mechanism for this outcome was that the ACA combination selected for *Clostridium difficile* and that abnormal colonization of the neonatal intestinal tract was one possible mechanism for NEC (16).

A 2003 case–control study, using data from three Swedish health registers, was conducted to identify drug use in early pregnancy that was associated with cardiac defects (17). Cases (cardiovascular defects without known chromosome anomalies) (*N* = 5015) were compared with controls consisting of all infants born in Sweden (1995–2001) (*N* = 577,730). Associations were identified for several drugs, some of which were probably due to confounding from the underlying disease or complaint or multiple testing, but some were thought to be true drug effects. For erythromycin, there were 27 cases in 1588 exposures (OR 1.91, 95% CI 1.30–2.80). The study could not determine if the association was due to confounding, multiple testing, or a true drug effect (17).

Three reports have examined the association between maternal treatment with erythromycin during pregnancy and IHPS in their infants (18–20). The first report evaluated the presence of IHPS in the infants (not treated with erythromycin) of mothers who were prescribed a macrolide antibiotic within three pregnancy time periods (18). The antibiotics were primarily erythromycin, but included azithromycin and clarithromycin and the infants were not treated with erythromycin. For the three time periods, the relative risk for subsequent infant IHPS and 95% CI were: anytime in pregnancy, 1.15, 0.5–2.4; within 10 weeks of delivery, including delivery date 1.76, 0.7–4.2; and within 10 weeks of delivery, excluding delivery date 1.84, 0.8–4.4 (18).

The second report used data collected between 1976 and 1998 as part of an ongoing case–control surveillance program (19). Cases, 1044 infants with IHPS, were compared with two control groups, normal and malformed. Erythromycin exposure in case subjects were identified in three pregnancy time periods: 1–24 weeks, 25–40 weeks, and 33–40 weeks. The number of cases, OR, 95% CI for each time period with normal controls were: 26, 1.0, 0.6–1.6; 10, 0.6, 0.3–1.1; and 6, 0.7, 0.3–1.8, respectively. For malformed controls, the OR and 95% CI for each period was: 1.1, 0.8–1.7; 0.6, 0.3–1.1; and 0.6, 0.3–1.3, respectively. The results indicated no evidence of an increased risk of pyloric stenosis with erythromycin (19).

The third study, published in 2002, used the Tennessee Medicaid/Tenn Care 1985–1997 database (20). Among the 260,799 mother–infant pairs, 13,146 mothers filled prescriptions for erythromycin and 621 filled prescriptions for nonerythromycin macrolides (azithromycin, clarithromycin, clindamycin, dirithromycin) or lincomycin from 32 weeks' gestation through delivery. The number of infant IHPS cases, OR, and 95% CI, in the erythromycin group was 38, 1.17, 0.84–1.64 after 32 weeks' gestation. There were 22,418 mother–infant pairs with erythromycin exposure anytime in pregnancy with 53 cases, 1.15, 0.84–1.56. For nonerythromycin macrolides, the data for the two pregnancy periods were 3 cases, 2.45, 0.78–7.68 and, for anytime in pregnancy, 1287 exposures, 6 cases, 2.77, 1.22–6.30. Although the latter data reached statistical significance, the authors concluded that a causal inference was limited by the small number of infants and for other reasons (20).

In a 2003 Danish study, 188 women received a macrolide (see Breastfeeding Summary) within 30 days of birth and none of their infants had IHPS (21).

Several reports have described the use of erythromycin for the successful treatment of *Chlamydia* infection in the second half of pregnancy (22–27). Although such use is effective, fewer maternal gastrointestinal adverse effects have been observed with amoxicillin (see Amoxicillin) (25–27).

BREASTFEEDING SUMMARY

Erythromycin is excreted into breast milk (28). Following oral doses of 400 mg every 8 hours, milk levels ranged from 0.4 to 1.6 mcg/mL. Oral doses of 2 g/day produced milk concentrations of 1.6–3.2 mcg/mL. The milk:plasma ratio in both groups was 0.5 (28).

In a 1993 cohort study, diarrhea was reported in 32 (19.3%) nursing infants of 166 breastfeeding mothers who were taking antibiotics (29). For the 17 women taking erythromycin, diarrhea was observed in 2 (12%) infants. The diarrhea was considered minor because it did not require medical attention (29).

A 2003 study investigated the association between maternal use of macrolides and infantile hypertrophic pyloric stenosis (21). The Danish population–based cohort study comprised 1166 women who had a prescribed macrolide (azithromycin, clarithromycin, erythromycin, spiramycin, or roxithromycin) from birth to 90 days postnatally compared with up to 41,778 controls. The ORs for stenosis was 2.3–3.0, depending on the postnatal period of exposure (42, 56, 70, or 90 days), but none were significant. When stratified by gender, the ORs for males were 1.8–3.1 and again were not statistically significant. For females, the OR at 70 and 90 days postbirth were 10.3 and 7.5, respectively, but only the former was significant (95% CI 1.2–92.3) (21).

Investigators from Israel examined the possible association between macrolide (azithromycin, clarithromycin, erythromycin, or roxithromycin) exposure in milk and infantile hypertrophic pyloric stenosis in a 2009 study (30). They compared 55 infants exposed to a macrolide antibiotic to 36 infants exposed to amoxicillin. In the macrolide group, 7 (12.7%) had an adverse reaction (rash, diarrhea, loss of appetite, somnolence), whereas 3 infants (8.3%) in the amoxicillin group had an adverse reaction (rashes, somnolence). The rates of adverse reactions were comparable. No cases of infantile hypertrophic pyloric stenosis were observed (30).

The American Academy of Pediatrics classified erythromycin as compatible with breastfeeding in 2001 (31).

References

1. Product information. Ery-Tab. Abbott Laboratories, 2000.
2. Heilman FR, Herrell WE, Wellman WE, Geraci JE. Some laboratory and clinical observations on a new antibiotic, erythromycin (Ilotycin). Proc Staff Meet Mayo Clin 1952;27:285–304.
3. Kiefer L, Rubin A, McCoy JB, Foltz EL. The placental transfer of erythromycin. Am J Obstet Gynecol 1955;69:174–7.
4. Philipson A, Sabath LD, Charles D. Transplacental passage of erythromycin and clindamycin. N Engl J Med 1973;288:1219–20.
5. Fenton LJ, Light IJ. Congenital syphilis after maternal treatment with erythromycin. Obstet Gynecol 1976;47:492–4.
6. Philipson A, Sabath LD, Charles D. Erythromycin and clindamycin absorption and elimination in pregnant women. Clin Pharmacoal Ther 1976;19:68–77.
7. McCormack WM, George H, Donner A, Kodgis LF, Albert S, Lowe EW, Kass EH. Hepatotoxicity of erythromycin estolate during pregnancy. Antimicrob Agents Chemother 1977;12:630–5.
8. Jaffe P, Liberman MM, McFadyen I, Valman HB. Incidence of congenital limb-reduction deformities. Lancet 1975;1:526–7.
9. Heinonen OP, Slone D, Shapiro S. *Birth Defects and Drugs in Pregnancy*. Littleton, MA: Publishing Sciences Group, 1977.
10. Gallagher JC, Ismail MA, Aladjem S. Reduced urinary estriol levels with erythromycin therapy. Obstet Gynecol 1980;56:381–2.
11. Merenstein GB, Todd WA, Brown G, Yost CC, Luzier T. Group B B-hemolytic streptococcus: randomized controlled treatment study at term. Obstet Gynecol 1980;55:315–8.
12. Easmon CSF, Hastings MJG, Deeley J, Bloxham B, Rivers RPA, Marwood R. The effect of intrapartum chemoprophylaxis on the vertical transmission of group B streptococci. Br J Obstet Gynaecol 1983;90:633–5.
13. Quinn PA, Shewchuk AB, Shuber J, Lie KI, Ryan E, Chipman ML, Nocilla DM. Efficacy of antibiotic therapy in preventing spontaneous pregnancy loss among couples colonized with genital mycoplasmas. Am J Obstet Gynecol 1983;145:239–44.
14. Kass EH, McCormack WM. Genital mycoplasma infection and perinatal morbidity. N Engl J Med 1984;311:258.
15. Czeizel AE, Rockenbauer M, Sørensen HT, Olsen J. A population-based case-control teratologic study of oral erythromycin treatment during pregnancy. Repro Toxicol 1999;13:531–6.
16. Kenyon SL, Taylor DJ, Tarnow-Mordi W, for the ORACLE Collaborative Group. Broad-spectrum antibiotics for preterm, prelabour rupture of fetal membranes: the ORACLE I randomised trial. Lancet 2001;357:979–88.
17. Kallen BAJ, Olausson PO. Maternal drug use in early pregnancy and infant cardiovascular defect. Reprod Toxicol 2003;17:255–61.
18. Mahon BE, Rosenman MB, Kleiman MB. Maternal and infant use of erythromycin and other macrolide antibiotics as risk factors for infantile hypertrophic pyloric stenosis. J Pediatr 2001;139;380–4.
19. Louik C, Werler MM, Mitchell AA. Erythromycin use during pregnancy in relation to pyloric stenosis. Am J Obstet Gynecol 2002;186:288–90.
20. Cooper WO, Ray WA, Griffin MR. Prenatal prescription of macrolide antibiotics and infantile hypertrophic pyloric stenosis. Obstet Gynecol 2002;100:101–6.
21. Sorensen HT, Skriver MV, Pedersen L, Larsen H, Ebbesen F, Schonheyder HC. Risk of infantile hypertrophic pyloric stenosis after maternal postnatal use of macrolides. Scand J Infect Dis 2003;35:104–6.
22. FitzSimmons J, Callahan C, Shanahan B, Jungkind D. Chlamydial infections in pregnancy. J Reprod Med 1986;31:19–22.
23. Black-Payne C, Ahrabi MM, Bocchini JA Jr, Ridenour CR, Brouillette RM. Treatment of Chlamydia trachomatis identified with chlamydiazyme during pregnancy: impact on perinatal complications and infants. J Reprod Med 1990;35:362–7.
24. Cohen I, Veille JC, Calkins BM. Improved pregnancy outcome following successful treatment of chlamydial infection. JAMA 1990;263:3160–3.
25. Magat AH, Alger LS, Nagey DA, Hatch V, Lovchik JC. Double-blind randomized study comparing amoxicillin and erythromycin for the treatment of *Chlamydia trachomatis* in pregnancy. Obstet Gynecol 1993:81:745–9.
26. Alary M, Joly J-M, Mondor M, Boucher M, Fortier A, Pinault J-J, Paris G, Carrier S, Chamberland H, Bernatchez H, Paradis J-F. Randomised comparison of amoxycillin and erythromycin in treatment of genital chlamydia infection in pregnancy. Lancet 1994;344:1461–5.
27. Turrentin MA, Newton ER. Amoxicillin or erythromycin for the treatment of antenatal chlamydial infection: a meta-analysis. Obstet Gynecol 1995;86:1021–5.

28. Knowles JA. Drugs in milk. Pediatr Currents 1972;21:28–32.
29. Ito S, Blajchman A, Stephenson M, Eliopoulos C, Koren G. Prospective follow-up of adverse reactions in breast-fed infants exposed to maternal medication. Am J Obstet Gynecol 1993;168:1393–9.
30. Goldstein LH, Berlin M, Tsur L, Bortnik O, Binyamini L, Berkovitch M. The safety of macrolides during lactation. Breastfeed Med 2009;4:157–200.
31. Committee on Drugs, American Academy of Pediatrics. The transfer of drugs and other chemicals into human milk. Pediatrics 2001;108:776–89.

ESCITALOPRAM

E

Antidepressant

PREGNANCY RECOMMENDATION: Human Data Suggest Risk in 3rd Trimester
BREASTFEEDING RECOMMENDATION: Limited Human Data—Potential Toxicity

PREGNANCY SUMMARY

Human pregnancy experience with escitalopram is very limited. The animal data suggest that the risk to an embryo–fetus is low. Two large case–control studies did find increased risks for some birth defects, but the absolute risk appears to be small. However, selective serotonin reuptake inhibitor (SSRI) antidepressants have been associated with several developmental toxicities, including spontaneous abortions, low birth weight, prematurity, neonatal serotonin syndrome, neonatal behavioral syndrome (withdrawal), possibly sustained abnormal neurobehavior beyond the neonatal period, respiratory distress, and persistent pulmonary hypertension of the newborn (PPHN).

FETAL RISK SUMMARY

Escitalopram is the S-enantiomer of racemic citalopram. It is an SSRI that is indicated for the treatment of depression. The metabolites of escitalopram apparently do not contribute to the antidepressant activity. Plasma protein binding is moderate (56%), but the plasma elimination half-life is long (27–32 hours) (1).

All the antidepressant agents in this class (citalopram, escitalopram, fluoxetine, fluvoxamine, paroxetine, and sertraline) share a similar mechanism of action, although only citalopram and escitalopram have similar chemical structures. These differences could be construed as evidence against any conclusion that they share similar effects on the embryo, fetus, or newborn. In the mouse embryo, however, craniofacial morphogenesis appears to be regulated, at least in part, by serotonin. Interference with serotonin regulation by chemically different inhibitors produces similar craniofacial defects (2). Regardless of the structural differences, therefore, some of the potential adverse effects on the pregnancy also may be similar.

Reproduction studies have been conducted in rats. In rats, doses up to ≥56 times the maximum recommended human dose of 20 mg/day based on BSA (MRHD) resulted in decreased fetal body weight and delayed ossification. Mild maternal toxicity (clinical signs and decreased body weight gain and food consumption) was evident at the developmental no-effect dose (28 times the MRHD). No teratogenicity was evident at any dose up to 75 times the MRHD. In rats treated throughout pregnancy and through weaning with doses up to 24 times the MRHD, slightly increased offspring mortality and growth restriction were observed at the highest dose. Mild maternal toxicity (same as noted above) was evident at the highest dose. The no-effect dose was 6 times the MRHD (1). (See also Citalopram for fertility studies in rats and teratology studies in rats and rabbits.)

It is not known if escitalopram crosses the human placenta. The molecular weight (about 324 for the free base), moderate plasma protein binding, and prolonged elimination half-life suggest that escitalopram will cross to the embryo and/or fetus.

A significant increase in the risk of low birth weight (<10th percentile) and respiratory distress after prenatal exposure to SSRIs was reported in 2006 (3). The population-based study, representing all live births (*N* = 119,547) during a 39-month period in British Columbia, Canada, compared pregnancy outcomes of depressed mothers treated with SSRIs with outcomes in depressed mothers not treated with medication and in nonexposed controls. The severity of depression in the depressed groups was accounted for by propensity score matching (3).

A brief 2005 report described significant associations between the use of SSRIs in the 1st trimester and congenital defects (4). The data were collected by the CDC-sponsored National Birth Defects Prevention Study in an ongoing case–control study of birth defect risk factors. Case infants (*N* = 5357) with major birth defects were compared with 3366 normal controls. A positive association was found with omphalocele (*N* = 161; odds ratio [OR] 3.0, 95% confidence interval [CI] 1.4–6.1). Paroxetine, which accounted for 36% of all SSRI exposures, had the strongest association with the defect (OR 6.3, 95% CI 2.0–19.6). The study also found a significant association between the use of any SSRI and craniosynostosis (*N* = 372; OR 1.8, 95% CI 1.0–3.2) (4). An expanded report from this group was published in 2007 (see reference 11).

A 2006 report using the database (1995–2003) of the Swedish Medical Birth Registry examined the relationship between maternal use of antidepressants and major malformations and cardiac defects (5). There was no significant increase in the risk of major malformations with any antidepressant. The strongest effect among cardiac anomalies was with ventricular or atrial septum defects (VSDs-ASDs). Significant increases were found with paroxetine (OR 2.22, 95% CI 1.39–3.55) and clomipramine (OR 1.87, 95% CI 1.16–2.99) (5). In 2007, the analysis of the Registry database was expanded to include the years 1995–2004 (6). There were

6481 women (6555 infants) who had reported the use of SSRIs in early pregnancy. The number using a single SSRI (i.e., no other SSRI or non-SSRI antidepressant) during the 1st trimester was 2579 citalopram, 1807 sertraline, 908 paroxetine, 860 fluoxetine, 66 escitalopram, and 36 fluvoxamine. Only paroxetine was significantly associated with cardiovascular effects (20 cases; OR 1.63, 95% CI 1.05–2.53). Paroxetine also had the strongest association with VSDs-ASDs, but did not reach significance (13 cases; relative risk [RR] 1.81, 95% CI 0.96–3.09). When the analysis was repeated after excluding women with body mass index >26, born outside of Sweden, or with reported subfertility (*N* = 405) , only paroxetine was significantly associated with any cardiac defect (13 cases, RR 2.62, 95% CI 1.40–4.50) and with VSDs-ASDs (8 cases, RR 3.07, 95% CI 1.32–6.04). The RR remained significant after also excluding women who took neuroleptics, sedatives, hypnotics, folic acid, nonsteroidal anti-inflammatory agents, or anticonvulsants (*N* = 340). Analysis of the combined SSRI group, excluding paroxetine, revealed no associations with cardiac defects or VSDs-ASDs. The study also found no association with omphalocele or craniostenosis (6).

A 2006 case report described a pregnancy of a 36-year-old woman who had stopped her treatment of obsessive-compulsive disorder immediately before conception (7). Escitalopram 20 mg/day was restarted at 24 weeks' gestation because of a major depressive episode. She was concerned about the risk for poor neonatal adaptation syndrome, so the escitalopram was gradually tapered during the last month of pregnancy. She delivered a healthy 3.6-kg male infant at term with Apgar scores of 9 and 10 at 1 and 5 minutes, respectively. Escitalopram 20 mg/day was restarted 15 days after delivery while she was breastfeeding. No adverse effects had been reported in the infant who was currently 3 months of age (7).

A 2007 study evaluated the association between 1st trimester exposure to paroxetine and cardiac defects by quantifying the dose–response relationship (8). A population-based pregnancy registry was used by linking three administrative databases so that it included all pregnancies in Quebec between 1997 and 2003. There were 101 infants with major congenital defects, 24 involving the heart, among the 1403 women using only one type of antidepressant during the 1st trimester. The use of paroxetine or other SSRIs did not significantly increase the risk of major defects or cardiac defects compared with non-SSRI antidepressants. However, a paroxetine dose >25 mg/day during the 1st trimester was significantly associated with an increased risk of major defects (OR 2.23, 95% CI 1.19–4.17) and of cardiac defects (OR 3.07, 95% CI 1.00–9.42) (8).

A 2007 review conducted a literature search to determine the risk of major congenital malformations after 1st trimester exposure to SSRIs and selective serotonin and norepinephrine reuptake inhibitors (SNRIs) (9). Fifteen controlled studies were analyzed. The data were adequate to suggest that citalopram, fluoxetine, sertraline, and venlafaxine were not associated with an increased risk of congenital defects. In contrast, the analysis did suggest an increased risk with paroxetine. The data were inadequate to determine the risk for the other SSRIs and SNRIs (9).

A case–control study, published in 2006, was conducted to test the hypothesis that exposure to SSRIs in late pregnancy was associated with PPHN (10). A total of 1213 women were enrolled in the study, 377 cases whose infants had PPHN and 836 matched controls and their infants. Mothers were interviewed by nurses that were blinded to the hypothesis. Fourteen case infants had been exposed to an SSRI after the 20th week of gestation compared with six control infants (adjusted odds ratio 6.1, 95% CI 2.2–16.8). The numbers were too small to analyze the effects of dosage, SSRI used, or reduction of the length of exposure before delivery. No increased risk of PPHN was found with the use of SSRIs before the 20th week or with the use of non-SSRI antidepressants at any time in pregnancy. If the relationship was causal, the absolute risk was estimated to be about 1% (10).

Two large case–control studies assessing associations between SSRIs and major birth defects were published in 2007 (11,12). The findings related to SSRIs as a group, as well as to four specific agents: citalopram, fluoxetine, paroxetine, and sertraline. An accompanying editorial discussed the findings and limitations of these and other related studies (13). Details of the studies and the editorial are described in the paroxetine review (see Paroxetine).

A prospective cohort study evaluated a large group of pregnancies exposed to antidepressants in the 1st trimester to determine if there was an association with major malformations (14). The patient population came from the Motherisk database and involved 928 cases that met their criteria. The 928 matched (for age, smoking, and alcohol use) controls were pregnancies not exposed to antidepressants or known teratogens. In addition to the 21 escitalopram cases, the other cases were 113 bupropion, 184 citalopram, 61 fluoxetine, 52 fluvoxamine, 68 mirtazapine, 39 nefazodone, 148 paroxetine, 61 sertraline, 17 trazodone, and 154 venlafaxine. In the antidepressant group, there were 24 (2.5%) major defects compared with 25 (2.6%) in controls (OR 0.9, 95% CI 0.5–1.61). There were no major defects in the pregnancies exposed to bupropion, escitalopram, or trazodone (14).

Necrotizing enterocolitis was reported in an infant exposed throughout pregnancy and during breastfeeding to escitalopram 20 mg/day (15). A cesarean section had delivered a 3.033-kg female infant at 38 weeks' gestation. She was treated for 2 days for respiratory distress syndrome thought to be related to retained fetal lung fluid. On day 5 after birth, the initial symptoms of necrotizing enterocolitis were lethargy, decreased oral intake, and grossly bloody stools. She was discharged home after 15 days. The authors concluded that exposure to escitalopram was the cause of the necrotizing enterocolitis based on a detailed discussion of the pharmacologic effects of the drug. Because the mother was still taking escitalopram, further breastfeeding was stopped (15).

BREASTFEEDING SUMMARY

Consistent with the molecular weight (about 324 for the free base), moderate plasma protein binding (56%), and prolonged elimination half-life (27–32 hours), escitalopram is excreted into breast milk. In a 2006 study, multiple blood and milk samples were obtained from eight women taking a mean 10 mg/day of the drug for postpartum depression (16). The mean age of the infants was 3.6 months. The mean milk:plasma ratios for escitalopram and its metabolite were 2.2, and the absolute infant doses were 7.6 and 3.0 mcg/kg/day, respectively. The total (parent drug plus metabolite) was 5.3%. All of the infants had normal development and no adverse effects were observed (16).

A 2006 case report described a 32-year-old woman who began taking escitalopram after birth of a healthy 3.560-kg infant (17). Milk and blood samples were collected at 1 and 7 weeks after start of therapy. The mother was taking a 5-mg dose at week 1 and 10-mg dose at week 7. The milk:serum ratios at the two collection periods were 2.49 and 2.03, respectively, whereas the infant's daily doses were 3.74 and 11.4 mcg/kg/day, respectively. The weight-adjusted relative infant doses were 5.1% and 7.7%, respectively. No adverse effects were reported by the mother and the infant was in good health (17).

E

Although no adverse effects in the nursing infants were reported in the above studies, adverse effects have been reported in infants exposed to citalopram (see Citalopram).

Until additional data are available, nursing infants whose mothers are taking escitalopram should be closely monitored for evidence of toxicity. The American Academy of Pediatrics classifies other SSRI antidepressants as drugs for which the effect on nursing infants is unknown but may be of concern (e.g., see Fluoxetine).

A 2010 study using human and animal models found that drugs that disturb serotonin balance such as SSRIs and SNRIs can impair lactation (18). The authors concluded that mothers taking these drugs may need additional support to achieve breastfeeding goals.

A 2012 prospective cohort study appears to have confirmed the above conclusion (19). The breastfeeding rates of 466 women were compared between three groups: (i) those who were taking an SSRI at the time of delivery (N = 167); (ii) those who stopped the SSRI before delivery (N = 117); and (iii) those not exposed (N = 182). The data were collected over a 10-year period by the California Teratogen Information Service Clinical Research Program. The first two groups were significantly less likely to initiate breastfeeding (OR 0.43, 95% CI 0.20–0.94 and OR 0.34, 95% CI 0.16–0.72, respectively) compared with unexposed women (19).

References

1. Product information. Lexapro. Forest Pharmaceuticals, 2004.
2. Shuey DL, Sadler TW, Lauder JM. Serotonin as a regulator of craniofacial morphogenesis: site specific malformations following exposure to serotonin uptake inhibitors. Teratology 1992;46:367–78.
3. Oberlander TF, Warburton W, Misri S, Aghajanian J, Hertzman C. Neonatal outcomes after prenatal exposure to selective serotonin reuptake inhibitor antidepressants and maternal depression using population-based linked health data. Arch Gen Psychiatry 2006;63:898–906.
4. Alwan S, Reefhuis J, Rasmussen S, Olney R, Friedman JM. Maternal use of selective serotonin reuptake inhibitors and risk for birth defects (abstract). Birth Defects Res (Part A) 2005;73:291.
5. Kallen B, Olausson PO. Antidepressant drugs during pregnancy and infant congenital heart defect. Reprod Toxicol 2006;21:221–2.
6. Kallen BAJ, Olausson PO. Maternal use of selective serotonin re-uptake inhibitors in early pregnancy and infant congenital malformations. Birth Defects Res (Part A) 2007;79:301–8.
7. Gentile S. Escitalopram late in pregnancy and while breast-feeding. Ann Pharmacother 2006;40:1696–7.
8. Berard A, Ramos E, Rey E, Blais L, St Andre M, Oraichi D. First trimester exposure to paroxetine and risk of cardiac malformations in infants: the importance of dosage. Birth Defects Res (Part B) 2007;80:18–27.
9. Bellantuono C, Migliarese G, Gentile S. Serotonin reuptake inhibitors in pregnancy and the risk of major malformations: a systematic review. Hum Psychopharmacol Clin Exp 2007;22:121–8.
10. Chambers CD, Hernandez-Diaz S, Van Marter LJ, Werler MM, Louik C, Jones KL, Mitchell AA. Selective serotonin-reuptake inhibitors and risk of persistent pulmonary hypertension of the newborn. N Engl J Med 2006;354:579–87.
11. Alwan S, Reefhuis J, Rasmussen SA, Olney RS, Friedman JM, for the National Birth Defects Prevention Study. Use of selective serotonin-reuptake inhibitors in pregnancy and the risk of birth defects. N Engl J Med 2007;356:2684–92.
12. Louik C, Lin AE, Werler MM, Hernandez-Diaz S, Mitchell AA. First-trimester use of selective serotonin-reuptake inhibitors and the risk of birth defects. N Engl J Med 2007;356:2675–83.
13. Greene MF. Teratogenicity of SSRIs—serious concern or much ado about little? N Engl J Med 2007;356:2732–3.
14. Einarson A, Choi J, Einarson TR, Koren G. Incidence of major malformations in infants following antidepressant exposure in pregnancy: results of a large prospective cohort study. Can J Psychiatry 2009;54:242–6.
15. Potts AL, Young KL, Carter BS, Shenai JP. Necrotizing entercolitis associated with in utero and breast milk exposure to the selective serotonin reuptake inhibitor, escitalopram. J Perinatol 2007;27:120–2.
16. Rampono J, Hackett LP, Kristensen JH, Kohan R, Page-Sharp M, Ilett KF. Transfer of escitalopram and its metabolite demethylescitalopram into breast milk. Br J Clin Pharmacol 2006;62:316–22.
17. Castberg I, Spigset O. Excretion of escitalopram in breast milk. J Clin Psychopharmacol 2006;26:536–8.
18. Marshall AM, Nommsen-Rivers LA, Hernandez LI, Dewey KG, Chantry CJ, Gregerson KA, Horseman ND. Serotonin transport and metabolism in the mammary gland modulates secretory activation and involution. J Clin Endocrin Metab 2010;95:837–46.
19. Gorman JR, Kao K, Chambers CD. Breastfeeding among women exposed to antidepressants during pregnancy. J Hum Lact 2012;28:181–8.

ESMOLOL

Sympatholytic

PREGNANCY RECOMMENDATION: Compatible—Maternal Benefit >> Embryo–Fetal Risk
BREASTFEEDING RECOMMENDATION: No Human Data—Probably Compatible

PREGNANCY SUMMARY

Cardioselective β_1-adrenergic blocking agents are not thought to cause structural anomalies. However, maternal exposure to esmolol has resulted in persistent β-blockade of the fetus and/or newborn.

FETAL RISK SUMMARY

Esmolol is a short-acting cardioselective β_1-adrenergic blocking agent that is structurally related to atenolol and metoprolol. The drug is used for the rapid, temporary treatment of supraventricular tachyarrhythmias (e.g., atrial flutter or fibrillation, sinus tachycardia) and for hypertension occurring during surgery. Because hypotension may occur with its use—up to 50% of patients in some trials—the potential for decreased uterine blood flow and resulting fetal hypoxia should be considered.

Reproduction studies in rats with IV doses up to 10 times the maximum human maintenance dose (MHMD) for 30 minutes daily revealed no evidence of embryo or fetal harm (1). Maternal toxicity and lethality were evident at 33 times the MHMD. Studies in pregnant rabbits with nonmaternal toxic doses also failed to demonstrate embryo or fetal harm (1).

In pregnant sheep, the mean fetal:maternal serum ratio at the end of an infusion of esmolol was 0.08 (2). The drug was not detectable in the fetus 10 minutes after the end of the infusion. However, the hemodynamic effects in the fetal sheep, in terms of decreases in mean arterial pressure and heart rate, were similar to those in the mothers.

A 31-year-old woman at 22 weeks' gestation complicated by a subarachnoid hemorrhage was treated with esmolol prior to induction of anesthesia (3). The estimated weight of her fetus, by ultrasound, was 350 g. She was administered bolus doses of esmolol of up to 2 mg/kg with a continuous infusion of 200 mcg/kg/minute. Fetal heart rate (FHR) decreased from 139–144 to 131–137 beats/minute (bpm) during esmolol treatment. No loss in FHR variability was observed. Administration of the drug was continued during surgery. A healthy, 2880-g boy was delivered at 37 weeks' gestation who was alive and well at 9 months of age.

A 29-year-old woman at 38 weeks' gestation presented with supraventricular tachycardia thought to be due to thyrotoxicosis (4). The FHR was 150–160 bpm. A bolus dose of esmolol, 0.5 mg/kg, followed by a continuous infusion of 50 mcg/kg/minute was given to the mother. Approximately 20 minutes later, the FHR increased to 170–175 bpm, then 4 minutes later fell to 70–80 bpm. The severe bradycardia persisted despite stopping the esmolol and an emergency cesarean section was performed to deliver a 2660-g male infant. The infant's initial pulse was 60 bpm, but increased to 140 bpm within 60 seconds in response to oxygen therapy. The umbilical vein blood pH was 7.09. The mother's arrhythmia was successfully converted after delivery with verapamil. Both mother and infant recovered uneventfully. The authors speculated that the cause of the fetal bradycardia was an esmolol-induced decrease in placental blood flow or interference with fetal compensation for a marginal placental perfusion (4).

A laboring mother at 39 weeks' gestation had a recurrence of tachyarrhythmia (225–235 bpm) that resulted in symptomatic hypotension and fetal bradycardia (5). She was treated with esmolol by IV bolus and continuous infusion (total dose 1060 mg) until delivery of 3390-g female infant with Apgar scores of 7 and 9. Symptoms of β-blockade in the infant included hypotonicity, weak cry, and dusky appearance and apnea with feeding, but except for mild jaundice, other evaluations (calcium, magnesium, and glucose serum levels) were normal. The feeding difficulties had resolved by 48 hours of age and the other symptoms by 60 hours of age.

β-Blockade in the fetus and newborn was described in a case in which the mother was treated with esmolol, 25 mcg/kg/minute, for hypertrophic obstructive cardiomyopathy during labor (6). Within 10 minutes of starting esmolol and receiving IV fentanyl, the fetal heart declined from 160 to 100 bpm with loss of beat-to-beat variability. The newborn had Apgar scores of 8 and 9 at 1 and 5 minutes, respectively, but was hypotensive (mean arterial pressure 34–39 mmHg), mildly hypotonic, hypoglycemic, and fed poorly. All of the symptoms had resolved by 36 hours of age.

A 1994 report described a woman who suffered a myocardial infarction at 26 weeks' gestation who was treated with an infusion of esmolol and other agents (7). She eventually delivered a healthy female infant at 39 weeks.

A 2013 review on the treatment of hypertensive crisis in pregnancy and the postpartum period listed esmolol as one of the preferred agents for this condition (8). Maternal adverse effects included 1st-degree heart block, bradycardia, congestive heart failure, and bronchospasm. Fetal adverse effects included bradycardia and persistent β-blockade (8).

BREASTFEEDING SUMMARY

No reports describing the use of esmolol during lactation have been located. Because of the indications for this drug and the fact that it must be given by injection, the opportunities for use of esmolol while nursing are probably nil.

References

1. Product information. Brevibloc. Baxter Pharmaceutical, 2000.
2. Ostman PL, Chestnut DH, Robillard JE, Weiner CP, Hdez MJ. Transplacental passage and hemodynamic effects of esmolol in the gravid ewe. Anesthesiology 1988;69:738–41.
3. Losasso TJ, Muzzi DA, Cucchiara RF. Response of fetal heart rate to maternal administration of esmolol. Anesthesiology 1991;74:782–4.
4. Ducey JP, Knape KG. Maternal esmolol administration resulting in fetal distress and cesarean section in a term pregnancy. Anesthesiology 1992;77:829–32.
5. Gilson GJ, Knieriem KJ, Smith JF, Izquierdo L, Chatterjee MS, Curet LB. Short-acting beta-adrenergic blockade and the fetus. A case report. J Reprod Med 1992;37:277–9.
6. Fairley CJ, Clarke JT. Use of esmolol in a parturient with hypertrophic obstructive cardiomyopathy. Br J Anaesthesia 1995;75:801–4.
7. Sanchez-Ramos L, Chami YG, Bass TA, DelValle GO, Adair CD. Myocardial infarction during pregnancy: management with transluminal coronary angioplasty and metallic intracoronary stents. Am J Obstet Gynecol 1994;171:1392–3.
8. Too GT, Hill JB. Hypertensive crisis during pregnancy and postpartum period. Semin Perinatol 2013;37:280–7.

ESOMEPRAZOLE

Gastrointestinal Agent (Antisecretory)

PREGNANCY RECOMMENDATION: Limited Human Data—Animal Data Suggest Low Risk
BREASTFEEDING RECOMMENDATION: No Human Data—Potential Toxicity

PREGNANCY SUMMARY

There is very limited human pregnancy data for esomeprazole. A study showing an association between in utero exposure to gastric acid suppressing drugs and childhood allergy and asthma requires confirmation. The animal data and human pregnancy experience with other drugs in this class suggest low risk, but the risk of esomeprazole cannot be fully assessed without additional human data. Until such data are available, if a proton pump inhibitor (PPI) is required, the safest course is to use omeprazole or other drugs in this class that have human data, such as lansoprazole or pantoprazole. (See also Omeprazole, Lansoprazole, and Pantoprazole.) Inadvertent exposure in pregnancy, however, does not appear to represent a clinically significant risk to the embryo or fetus.

FETAL RISK SUMMARY

Esomeprazole, a PPI, is the S-isomer of omeprazole, which is a mixture of the S- and R-isomers. It is in the same drug class as dexlansoprazole, lansoprazole, omeprazole, pantoprazole, and rabeprazole. Esomeprazole is indicated for the short-term (4–8 weeks) treatment and maintenance in the healing and symptomatic resolution of gastrointestinal reflux disease. It is also indicated for the reduction in the occurrence of gastric ulcers in patients receiving continuous nonsteroidal anti-inflammatory therapy and, in combination with amoxicillin and clarithromycin, for the treatment of patients with *Helicobacter pylori* infection and duodenal ulcers. Esomeprazole is extensively metabolized in the liver by cytochrome P450 isoenzymes, primarily CYP2C19, but also by CYP3A4. Approximately 3% of whites and 15%–20% of Asians lack CYP2C19 (i.e., "poor metabolizers"). Plasma concentrations in poor metabolizers are about twice those of subjects with unaltered metabolism. In the plasma, esomeprazole is 97% protein bound with an elimination half-life of about 1–1.5 hours (1).

Reproduction studies have been conducted with esomeprazole in rats and rabbits. In these species, oral doses up to about 57 and 35 times, respectively, the human dose of 20 mg/day based on BSA (HD) revealed no evidence of impaired fertility or fetal harm (1).

Studies with omeprazole, a mixture of the S- and R-isomers, found no evidence of teratogenicity in rats and rabbits at doses up to 56 times the HD in both species. However, in rats given doses ranging about 5.6–56 times the HD, dose-related embryo–fetal toxicity and postnatal developmental toxicity were observed (toxicities not specified). In addition, in rabbits given doses ranging about 5.5–56 times the HD, dose-related increases in embryolethality, fetal resorptions, and pregnancy disruptions were noted (1). The no-adverse-effect levels in these studies were not specified.

The carcinogenic potential of esomeprazole was assessed using omeprazole studies. A significant dose-related occurrence of gastric enterochromaffin-like (ECL) cell carcinoid tumors and ECL cell hyperplasia were observed in male and female rats (1). In a mutagenic study with esomeprazole, the in vitro human lymphocyte chromosome aberration test was positive, but three other mutagenesis assays were negative (1).

Consistent with its molecular weight (about 345 for the anhydrous free base), esomeprazole probably crosses the human placenta. Although this has not been specifically studied with esomeprazole, omeprazole has been shown to cross to the fetus at term. (See Omeprazole.)

A meta-analysis of PPIs in pregnancy was reported in 2009 (2). Based on 1530 exposed compared with 133,410 not-exposed pregnancies, the odds ratio (OR) for major malformations was 1.12 and 95% confidence interval (CI) 0.86–1.45. There also was no increased risk for spontaneous abortions (OR 1.29, 95% CI 0.84–1.97) or preterm birth (OR 1.13, 95% CI 0.96–1.33) (2).

A population-based observational cohort study formed by linking data from three Swedish national health care registers over a 10-year period (1995–2004) was reported in 2009 (3). The main outcome measures were a diagnosis of allergic disease or a prescription for asthma or allergy medications. The drug types included in the study were gastric acid suppressors, including H_2-receptor antagonists, prostaglandins, PPIs, combinations for eradication of *H. pylori*, and drugs for peptic ulcer and gastro-esophageal reflux disease, such as sucralfate. Of 585,716 children, 29,490 (5.0%) met the diagnosis and 5645 (1%) had been exposed to gastric acid suppression therapy in pregnancy. Of these children, 405 (0.07%) were treated for allergic disease. For developing allergy, the OR was 1.43, 98% CI 1.29–1.59, irrespective of the drug, time of exposure during pregnancy, and maternal history of allergy. For developing childhood asthma, but not other allergic diseases, the OR was 1.51, 95% CI 1.35–1.69, irrespective of the type of acid-suppressive drug and the time of exposure in pregnancy. The authors proposed three possible mechanisms for their findings: (i) exposure to increased amounts of allergens could cause sensitization to digestion labile antigens in the fetus; (ii) maternal Th2 cytokine pattern could promote an allergy-prone phenotype in the fetus; and (iii) maternal allergen-specific IgE could cross the placenta and sensitize fetal immune cells to food and airborne allergens. Several limitations of the study that might have affected their findings were identified, including a general increase in childhood asthma but not necessarily an increase in allergic asthma (3). The study requires confirmation.

In a 2010 study from Denmark, covering the period 1996–2008, there were 840,968 live births among whom 5082 were exposed to PPIs between 4 weeks before conception and the end of the 1st trimester (4). In the exposed group, there were 174 (3.4%) major malformations compared with 21,811 (2.6%) not exposed to PPIs (adjusted prevalence odds ratio [aPOR] 1.23, 95 CI 1.05–1.44). When the analysis was limited to exposure in the 1st trimester, there were 118 (3.2%) major malformations among 3651 exposed infants (aPOR 1.10, 95% CI 0.91–1.34). For exposure to esomeprazole in the 1st trimester, there were 23 (3.4%) major birth defects among 668 live births (aPOR 1.19, 95% CI 0.77–1.84) (see Lansoprazole, Omeprazole, Pantoprazole, and Rabeprazole for their data). The data showed that exposure to PPIs in the 1st trimester was not associated with a significantly increased risk of major birth defects (4). An accompanying editorial discussed the strengths and weaknesses of the study (5).

A 2012 case report described the use of esomeprazole (40 mg/day) throughout pregnancy in a woman with an intestinal transplant (6). Other medications used were prednisone (5 mg/day), diphenoxylate-atropine (2 tablets/day), tacrolimus (12 mg/day), ferrous sulfate (650 mg/day), ascorbic acid (1 g/day), prenatal vitamins (1/day), and magnesium supplementation. At 39 3/7 weeks, labor was induced and she had a spontaneous vaginal delivery of a healthy female infant (6).

In a 2012 publication, the National Birth Defects Prevention study, a multi-site population-based case–control study, examined whether nausea/vomiting of pregnancy (NVP) or its treatment were associated with the most common noncardiac defects (nonsyndromic cleft lip with or without cleft palate [CL/P], cleft palate alone [CP], neural tube defects [NTDs], and hypospadias) (7). PPI exposure included esomeprazole. lansoprazole, and omeprazole. There were 4524 cases and 5859 controls. NVP was not associated with cleft palate or NTDs, but modest risk reductions were observed for CL/P and hypospadias. Increased risks were found for PPIs ($N = 7$) and hypospadias (adjusted OR [aOR] 4.36, 95% CI 1.21–15.81), steroids ($N = 10$) and hypospadias (aOR 2.87, 95% CI 1.03–7.97), and ondansetron ($N = 11$) and CP (aOR 2.37, 95% CI 1.18–4.76) (7).

A third 2012 reference, using the Danish nationwide registries, evaluated the risk of hypospadias after exposure to PPIs during the 1st trimester and throughout gestation (8). The study period, 1997–2009, included all liveborn boys that totaled 430,569 of whom 2926 were exposed to maternal PPI use. Hypospadias was diagnosed in 20 (0.7%) exposed boys, whereas 2683 (0.6%) of the nonexposed had hypospadias (adjusted prevalence ratio [aPR] 1.1, 95% CI 0.7–1.7). For the 5227 boys exposed throughout pregnancy, 32 (0.6%) had hypospadias (PR 1.0, 95% CI 0.7–1.4). When the analysis was restricted to mothers with two or more PPI prescriptions, the aPR of overall hypospadias was 1.7 (95% CI 0.9–3.3) and 1.6 (95% CI 0.7–3.9) for omeprazole. The authors concluded that PPIs were not associated with hypospadias (8).

Five reviews on the treatment of gastroesophageal reflux disease (GERD) have concluded that PPIs can be used in pregnancy with relative safety (9–13). Because there is either very limited or no human pregnancy data for the three newest agents in this class (dexlansoprazole, esomeprazole, and rabeprazole), other drugs in the class are preferred.

BREASTFEEDING SUMMARY

No reports describing the use of esomeprazole, the S-isomer of omeprazole, during human lactation have been located. The molecular weight (about 345 for the anhydrous free base) is low enough that excretion into breast milk should be expected. The effect of esomeprazole on a nursing infant is unknown. The potential for toxic effects such as those seen in adults (e.g., headache, diarrhea, and abdominal pain) and the suppression of gastric acid secretion are a concern, as is the potential for the gastric tumors that have been observed in animals after long-term use.

Small amounts of omeprazole, a mixture of the S- and R-isomers, are excreted into milk, but the quantity excreted needs further clarification. (See Omeprazole.) If a lactating woman's condition requires esomeprazole, consideration of the drug's properties might allow her to nurse without significantly exposing her infant. Esomeprazole is dosed once daily because the inhibition of gastric acid secretion is prolonged. In contrast, the plasma elimination half-life is short (about 1–1.5 hours). Thus, waiting 5–7.5 hours after a dose should eliminate up to 97% of the drug from the plasma. Moreover, the mean peak plasma concentration is reported to occur 1.6 hours after the dose (1), and waiting 5–7.5 hours would avoid the period when the greatest amount of drug is available to enter milk. Emptying both breasts near the end of the waiting period and discarding the milk completes the strategy to limit the infant's exposure. This strategy was used in one case involving omeprazole but warrants further study.

References

1. Product information. Nexium. AstraZeneca, 2004.
2. Gill SK, O'Brien L, Einarson TR, Koren G. The safety of proton pump inhibitors (PPIs) in pregnancy: a meta-analysis. Am J Gastroenterol 2009;104:1541–5.
3. Dehlink E, Yen E, Leichtner AM, Hait EJ, Fiebiger E. First evidence of a possible association between gastric acid suppression during pregnancy and childhood asthma: a population-based register study. Clin Exp Allergy 2009;39:246–53.
4. Pasternak B, Hviid A. Use of proton-pump inhibitors in early pregnancy and the risk of birth defects. N Engl J Med 2010;363:2114–23.
5. Mitchell AA. Proton-pump inhibitors and birth defects—some reassurance, but more needed. N Engl J Med 2010;363:2161–3.
6. Gomez-Lobo V, Landy HJ, Matsumoto C, Fishbein TM. Pregnancy in an intestinal transplant recipient. Obstet Gynecol 2012;120:497–500.
7. Anderka M, Mitchell AA, Louik C, Werler MM, Hernandez-Diaz S, Rasmussen SA, and the National Birth Defects Prevention Study. Medications used to treat nausea and vomiting of pregnancy and the risk of selected birth defects. Birth Defects Res A Clin Mol Teratol 2012;94:22–30.
8. Erichsen R, Mikkelsen E, Pedersen L, Sorensen HT. Maternal use of proton pump inhibitors during early pregnancy and the prevalence of hypospadias in male offspring. Am J Ther 2012 Feb 3. [epub ahead of print].
9. Broussard CN, Richter JE. Treating gasto-oesophageal reflux disease during pregnancy and lactation. What are the safest therapy options? Drug Saf 1998;19:325–37.
10. Katz PO, Castell DO. Gastroesophageal reflux disease during pregnancy. Gastroenterol Clin N Am 1998;27:153–67.
11. Ramakrishnan A, Katz PO. Pharmacologic management of gastroesophageal reflux disease. Curr Treat Options Gastroenterol 2002;5:301–10.
12. Richter JE. Gastroesophageal reflux disease during pregnancy. Gastroenterol Clin N Am 2003;32:235–61.
13. Richter JE. Review article: the management of heartburn in pregnancy. Aliment Pharmacol Ther 2005;22:749–57.

ESTAZOLAM

Hypnotic

PREGNANCY RECOMMENDATION: Human Data Suggest Risk in 1st and 3rd Trimesters
BREASTFEEDING RECOMMENDATION: No Human Data—Potential Toxicity

PREGNANCY SUMMARY

No reports describing the use of estazolam in human pregnancy have been located. The effects of this drug on the fetus should be similar to other benzodiazepines (see Diazepam). Maternal use near delivery may potentially cause neonatal motor depression and withdrawal.

E

FETAL RISK SUMMARY

Estazolam is a benzodiazepine hypnotic agent in the same general class as flurazepam, quazepam, temazepam, and triazolam. It is indicated for the short-term management of insomnia. The metabolites have low potencies and concentrations and are not significant contributors to the hypnotic activity of estazolam. Plasma protein binding of estazolam is high (93%) and the range of estimated elimination half-life varies from 10 to 24 hours (1).

Animal reproduction studies have apparently not been conducted with estazolam. The manufacturer considers the drug contraindicated in pregnancy (1).

It is not known if estazolam crosses the human placenta. The molecular weight (about 295) and moderately long elimination half-life suggest that the drug will be transferred to the embryo–fetus. Of note, the benzodiazepine, diazepam, freely crosses the placenta and accumulates in the fetal circulation (see Diazepam).

BREASTFEEDING SUMMARY

No reports describing the use of estazolam during human lactation have been located. The molecular weight (about 295) and moderately long elimination half-life (10–24 hours) suggest that the drug will be excreted into breast milk. Other agents in this class are excreted into milk in low concentrations (e.g., see Quazepam and Temazepam). No toxicity was observed in the nursing infants exposed to these two agents. However, the effects, if any, on an infant's CNS function are unknown. In recognition of this, the American Academy of Pediatrics classified quazepam and temazepam, especially when taken by nursing mothers for long periods, as agents whose effects on an infant are unknown, but may be of concern. Estazolam should be classified similarly.

Reference

1. Product information. ProSom. Abbott Laboratories, 2004.

ESTRADIOL

Estrogenic Hormone

PREGNANCY RECOMMENDATION: Contraindicated
BREASTFEEDING RECOMMENDATION: Compatible

PREGNANCY SUMMARY

Estrogens are contraindicated because there are usually no benefits from their use in pregnancy.

FETAL RISK SUMMARY

Estradiol and its salts (cypionate, valerate) are used for treatment of menopausal symptoms, female hypogonadism, and primary ovarian failure. The more potent synthetic derivative, ethinyl estradiol, has similar indications and is also used in oral contraceptives (see also Oral Contraceptives).

The Collaborative Perinatal Project monitored 614 mother–child pairs with 1st trimester exposure to estrogenic agents (including 48 with exposure to estradiol) (1, pp. 389, 391). An increase in the expected frequency of cardiovascular defects, eye and ear anomalies, and Down's syndrome was found for estrogens as a group but not for estradiol (1, pp. 389, 391, 395). Reevaluation of these data in terms of timing of exposure, vaginal bleeding in early pregnancy, and previous maternal obstetric history, however, failed to support an association between estrogens and cardiac malformations (2). An earlier study also failed to find any relationship with nongenital malformations (3).

In a surveillance study of Michigan Medicaid recipients involving 229,101 completed pregnancies conducted between 1985 and 1992, 29 newborns had been exposed to ethinyl estradiol during the 1st trimester (F. Rosa, personal communication, FDA, 1993). Four (13.8%) major birth defects were observed (one expected), including (observed/expected) 1/0.3 cardiovascular defects and 1/0 hypospadias. No anomalies were observed in four other categories of defects (oral clefts, spina bifida, polydactyly, and limb reduction defects) for which specific data were available. The number of exposures is too small for any conclusion.

Developmental changes in the psychosexual performance of boys have been attributed to in utero exposure to estradiol and progesterone (4). The mothers received an estrogen/progestogen regimen for their diabetes. Hormone-exposed males demonstrated a trend to have less heterosexual experience and fewer masculine interests than controls. Estradiol has been administered to women in labor in an attempt to potentiate the cervical ripening effects of prostaglandins (5). No detectable effect was observed.

BREASTFEEDING SUMMARY

Estradiol has been used to suppress postpartum breast engorgement in patients who did not desire to breastfeed. Following the administration of vaginal suppositories containing 50 or 100 mg of estradiol to six lactating women who wished to stop breastfeeding, less than 10% of the dose appeared in breast milk (6). The American Academy of Pediatrics classifies estradiol as compatible with breastfeeding (7).

References

1. Heinonen OP, Slone D, Shapiro S. *Birth Defects and Drugs in Pregnancy*. Littleton, MA: Publishing Sciences Group, 1977.
2. Wiseman RA, Dodds-Smith IC. Cardiovascular birth defects and antenatal exposure to female sex hormones: a reevaluation of some base data. Teratology 1984;30:359–70.
3. Wilson JG, Brent RL. Are female sex hormones teratogenic? Am J Obstet Gynecol 1981;141:567–80.
4. Yalom ID, Green R, Fisk N. Prenatal exposure to female hormones. Effect of psychosexual development in boys. Arch Gen Psychiatry 1973;28: 554–61.
5. Luther ER, Roux J, Popat R, Gardner A, Gray J, Soubiran E, Korcaz Y. The effect of estrogen priming on induction of labor with prostaglandins. Am J Obstet Gynecol 1980;137:351–7.
6. Nilsson S, Nygren KG, Johansson EDB. Transfer of estradiol to human milk. Am J Obstet Gynecol 1978;132:653–7.
7. Committee on Drugs, American Academy of Pediatrics. The transfer of drugs and other chemicals into human milk. Pediatrics 2001;108:776–89.

E

ESTROGENS, CONJUGATED

Estrogenic Hormone

PREGNANCY RECOMMENDATION: Contraindicated
BREASTFEEDING RECOMMENDATION: No Human Data—Probably Compatible

PREGNANCY SUMMARY

Estrogens are contraindicated because there are usually no benefits from their use in pregnancy.

FETAL RISK SUMMARY

Conjugated estrogens are a mixture of estrogenic substances (primarily estrone). The Collaborative Perinatal Project monitored 13 mother–child pairs who were exposed to conjugated estrogens during the 1st trimester (1, pp. 389, 391). An increased risk for malformations was found, although identification of the malformations was not provided. Estrogenic agents as a group were monitored in 614 mother–child pairs. An increase in the expected frequency of cardiovascular defects, eye and ear anomalies, and Down's syndrome was reported (1, p. 395). Reevaluation of these data in terms of timing of exposure, vaginal bleeding in early pregnancy, and previous maternal obstetric history, however, failed to support an association between estrogens and cardiac malformations (2).

An earlier study also failed to find any relationship with nongenital malformations (3). No adverse effects were observed in one infant exposed during the 1st trimester to conjugated estrogens (4). However, in an infant exposed during the 4th–7th weeks of gestation to conjugated estrogens, multiple anomalies were found: cleft palate, micrognathia, wormian bones, heart defect, dislocated hips, absent tibiae, bowed fibulae, polydactyly, and abnormal dermal patterns (5). Multiple other agents were also taken during this pregnancy, but only conjugated estrogens and prochlorperazine (see also Prochlorperazine) appeared to have been taken during the critical period for the malformations.

Conjugated estrogens have been used to induce ovulation in anovulatory women (6). They have also been used as partially successful contraceptives when given within 72 hours of unprotected, mid-cycle coitus (7). No fetal adverse effects were mentioned in either of these reports.

BREASTFEEDING SUMMARY

No reports of adverse effects from conjugated estrogens in the nursing infant have been located. It is possible that decreased milk volume and decreased nitrogen and protein content could occur (see Mestranol, Ethinyl Estradiol).

References

1. Heinonen OP, Slone D, Shapiro S. *Birth Defects and Drugs in Pregnancy*. Littleton, MA: Publishing Sciences Group, 1977.
2. Wiseman RA, Dodds-Smith IC. Cardiovascular birth defects and antenatal exposure to female sex hormones: a reevaluation of some base data. Teratology 1984;30:359–70.
3. Wilson JG, Brent RL. Are female sex hormones teratogenic? Am J Obstet Gynecol 1981;141:567–80.
4. Hagler S, Schultz A, Hankin H, Kunstadter RH. Fetal effects of steroid therapy during pregnancy. Am J Dis Child 1963;106:586–90.
5. Ho CK, Kaufman RL, McAlister WH. Congenital malformations. Cleft palate, congenital heart disease, absent tibiae, and polydactyly. Am J Dis Child 1975;129:714–6.
6. Price R. Pregnancies using conjugated oestrogen therapy. Med J Aust 1980;2:341–2.
7. Dixon GW, Schlesselman JJ, Ory HW, Blye RP. Ethinyl estradiol and conjugated estrogens as postcoital contraceptives. JAMA 1980;244:1336–9.

ESTRONE

Estrogenic Hormone

See Estrogens, Conjugated.

ESZOPICLONE

Hypnotic

PREGNANCY RECOMMENDATION: No Human Data—Animal Data Suggest Low Risk
BREASTFEEDING RECOMMENDATION: Limited Human Data—Potential Toxicity

E

PREGNANCY SUMMARY

No reports describing the use eszopiclone in human pregnancy have been located. The animal data suggest low risk, but the absence of human pregnancy experience prevents further assessment. However, there is human pregnancy experience with racemic zopiclone. A small 1999 observational study compared the pregnancy outcomes of 40 women exposed in the 1st trimester to zopiclone with those of 40 nonexposed controls (1,2). The outcomes in the two groups were spontaneous abortions 7 vs. 3, respectively; elective abortions 1 vs. 0, respectively; and minor defects 1 vs. 1 (congenital dislocation of the hip in each group), respectively. No difference between the groups in the incidence of major defects was observed: 0/31 (0%) exposed vs. 1/37 (2.7%) controls. Taken in sum, the available data suggest that eszopiclone exposure in pregnancy probably is low risk, but until data are available, the safest course would be use a hypnotic agent with published human pregnancy experience.

FETAL RISK SUMMARY

Eszopiclone is an oral nonbenzodiazepine sedative/hypnotic. It is the active component [(S)-isomer] of racemic zopiclone [(R,S)-zopiclone], a sedative/hypnotic that has been available outside the United States since the 1980s. Eszopiclone is indicated for the treatment of insomnia. It is extensively metabolized to inactive metabolites. Plasma protein binding is low, in the range of 52%–59%, and the terminal elimination half-life is about 6 hours (3).

Reproduction studies with eszopiclone have been conducted in rats and rabbits. In rats, oral doses during organogenesis up to 800 times the maximum recommended human dose based on BSA (MRHD-BSA), a maternal toxic dose, revealed no evidence of structural defects in the fetuses. Slight reductions in fetal weight and evidence of developmental delay were observed with doses about 400 times the MRHD-BSA that also were maternal toxic. These fetal effects were not observed with a nontoxic maternal dose (about 200 times the MRHD-BSA). When eszopiclone was administered throughout pregnancy and lactation at doses ranging from about 200 to 600 times the MRHD-BSA, increased postimplantation loss, decreased postnatal pup weights and survival, and increased pup startle response were seen at all doses. No structural defects were observed in rabbits given oral doses during organogenesis up to 100 times the MRHD-BSA (3).

In female and male rats, the no-effect eszopiclone dose for fertility was 16 times the MRHD-BSA. The no-effect doses for increased preimplantation loss, abnormal estrus cycles, and decreases in sperm number and motility and increases in abnormal sperm were 80, 80, and 16 times, respectively, the MRHD-BSA (3).

Eszopiclone was not carcinogenic in female and male rats given gavage doses resulting in plasma concentrations about 80 and 20 times, respectively, the maximum recommended dose based on AUC (MRHD-AUC) (1). When racemic zopiclone was given in the diet to female and male rats, eszopiclone plasma concentrations were about 150 and 70 times, respectively, the MRHD-AUC. In this study, an increase in mammary gland adenocarcinoma (females) and thyroid gland follicular cell adenomas and carcinomas (males) were observed. Carcinogenicity (pulmonary carcinomas and carcinomas plus adenomas) also was noted in female mice given racemic zopiclone in a diet that resulted in eszopiclone plasma concentrations about eight times the MRHD-AUC. However, an increase in pulmonary tumors was not observed in female mice given gavage doses of eszopiclone resulting in plasma concentrations about 90 times the MRHD-AUC. In tests for mutagenicity or clastogenicity, eszopiclone and one of its metabolites produced mixed results. Results of various assays ranged from positive through equivocal to negative (3).

It is not known if eszopiclone crosses the human placenta. The low molecular weight (about 389), low plasma protein binding, and moderately long elimination half-life suggest that the drug will cross to the embryo and/or fetus. However, the extensive metabolism should limit the degree of embryo–fetal exposure.

BREASTFEEDING SUMMARY

No reports describing the use of eszopiclone [(S)-zopiclone)] during human lactation have been located. However, racemic zopiclone is excreted into breast milk. A 1982/1983 study found a milk:plasma AUC ratio of about 0.60 and 0.80 (both values reported) after a single 7.5-mg oral dose of zopiclone in three nursing mothers (4,5). For eszopiclone, the molecular weight (about 389), low plasma protein binding (52%–59%), and moderately long elimination half-life (about 6 hours) suggest that it also will be excreted into breast milk. The effect of this exposure on a nursing infant is unknown, but sedation is a potential effect. In addition, there is concern for central nervous system toxicity with long-term use.

References

1. Diav-Citrin O, Okotore B, Lucarelli K, Koren G. Pregnancy outcome following first trimester exposure to zopiclone: a prospective controlled cohort study. Am J Perinatol 1999;16:157–60.
2. Diav-Citrin O, Okotore B, Lucarelli K, Koren G. Zopiclone use during pregnancy. Can Fam Physician 2000;46:63–4.
3. Product information. Lunesta. Sepracor, 2005.

4. Gaillot J, Heusse D, Houghton GW, Marc Aurele J, Dreyfus JF. Pharmacokinetics and metabolism of zopiclone. Int Pharmacopsychiatry 1982;17(Suppl 2):76–91.

5. Gaillot J, Heusse D, Houghton GW, Marc Aurele J, Dreyfus JF. Pharmacokinetics and metabolism of zopiclone. Pharmacology 1983;27(Suppl 2): 76–91.

ETANERCEPT

Immunologic Agent (Immunomodulator)

PREGNANCY RECOMMENDATION: Limited Human Data—Animal Data Suggest Low Risk
BREASTFEEDING RECOMMENDATION: Limited Human Data—Probably Compatible

PREGNANCY SUMMARY

Etanercept was not toxic or teratogenic in animal reproduction tests at doses much higher than those used clinically. Although the human pregnancy experience is limited, there is no firm evidence of embryo–fetal harm. However, the human data are too limited for a full assessment of the risk. If etanercept is used in pregnancy for the treatment of rheumatoid arthritis, health care professionals are encouraged to call the toll free number (877-311-8972) for information about patient enrollment in the OTIS Rheumatoid Arthritis Study.

FETAL RISK SUMMARY

Etanercept is a dimeric fusion protein, produced by recombinant DNA technology, consisting of the extracellular ligand-binding portion of the human kilodalton (p75) tumor necrosis factor receptor (TNFR) linked to the Fc portion of human immunoglobulin G1 (IgG1). The protein binds specifically to TNF, a cytokine involved in inflammatory and immune responses, to block its interaction with cell-surface TNFRs (1,2). Etanercept is in the same subclass of immunomodulators that inhibit TNF as adalimumab, certolizumab, golimumab, and infliximab. It is indicated for reducing the signs and symptoms and delaying structural damage in moderate to severe rheumatoid arthritis, including juvenile arthritis. The drug is administered by SC injection.

Reproduction studies in rats and rabbits at doses 60–100 times the human dose revealed no fetal harm (1,2). Animal fertility and carcinogenic studies have not been conducted with etanercept, but it was not mutagenic in in vitro and in vivo tests.

A 32-year-old woman with a 1-year history of rheumatoid arthritis and infertility was treated with SC etanercept (25 mg twice weekly), oral methotrexate (2.5 mg/week), and rofecoxib (25 mg/day) (3). Three months after stopping methotrexate and rofecoxib, and 4 weeks after the last dose of etanercept (total dose 3300 mg over 64 months), she underwent ovulation induction and intrauterine insemination. A successful pregnancy occurred and she delivered a healthy, 2659-g female infant at term. The baby was doing well at 3 months of age (3).

A 37-year-old woman with infertility secondary to antiphospholipid antibodies and elevated natural killer (NK) cells was treated with etanercept (25 mg SC twice weekly), low-dose aspirin (81 mg/day), and low-molecular-weight heparin (enoxaparin 30 mg SC daily) (4). The woman also had a history of chronic leukopenia that was attributed to Epstein-Barr virus. She became pregnant 1 month after the start of therapy. All three agents were discontinued at gestational week 32. At about 38 weeks', she delivered a healthy male (about 2486-g) infant that was doing well at 21 months of age. Although it could not be proven, the authors speculated that etanercept might have played a role in the pregnancy by inhibiting TNF produced by the NK cells in the lining of the woman's uterus (4).

Etanercept was used in a woman who had experienced implantation failure in five previous in vitro fertilization treatments (5). Etanercept 25 mg SC every 4 days was started 4 weeks before ovulation induction and then discontinued upon commencement of gonadotropins. The woman delivered male twins at 34.5 weeks (no additional information provided) (5).

A survey of 600 members of the American College of Rheumatology, partially conducted to determine the outcomes of pregnancies exposed to disease-modifying antirheumatic drugs (DMARD) (etanercept, infliximab, leflunomide, and methotrexate), was published in 2003 (6). From the 175 responders, the outcomes of 15 pregnancies exposed to etanercept were 6 full-term healthy infants, 1 spontaneous abortion (SAB) (also taking methotrexate), 1 elective abortion (EAB), 3 unknown outcomes, and 4 women still pregnant (6).

An early review recommended that pregnancy should be excluded before etanercept was administered to women of childbearing age and that effective contraception should be used during treatment (7). Another review speculated that etanercept could disrupt pregnancy because of its anticytokine activity (8). However, this theoretical concern has not been shown clinically (9).

The preliminary results of an ongoing prospective collaborative study of rheumatoid arthritis medicines in pregnancy conducted by the Organization of Teratology Information Specialists (OTIS) have been reported (10,11). The study covered the period 1999–2004. There were 33 women exposed in the 1st trimester to either etanercept ($N = 29$) or infliximab ($N = 4$). The outcomes of these pregnancies were compared with 77 prospectively ascertained disease-matched controls (did not use anti-TNFα agents) and 50 prospectively ascertained healthy controls. Three controls were lost to follow-up. There was no difference between the groups in the number of SABs and EABs. One malformation (1/33; 3.0%) was reported in the subject group (a chromosomal anomaly, trisomy 18; spontaneously aborted by a woman exposed to etanercept).

Major malformations in the other groups were 4.0% (3/75) in disease-matched controls and 4.1% (2/49) in healthy controls. However, women exposed to etanercept or infliximab and disease-matched controls were significantly more likely to give birth to infants <37 weeks' gestation and to have lower-birth-weight full-term infants than healthy controls. These results suggested that the disease itself was the causal factor (10,11).

A 2006 communication from England described the pregnancy outcomes of 23 women directly exposed to TNFα agents at the time of conception (17 etanercept, 3 adalimumab, and 3 infliximab) (12). Additional therapy included methotrexate in nine women and leflunomide in two. There also were nine patients (4 etanercept, 5 infliximab) that discontinued therapy before conception. The outcomes for the 32 pregnancies were 7 SABs, 3 EABs, and 22 live births. No major anomalies were observed in the live births, including one infant exposed to adalimumab and methotrexate early in gestation (12).

A 2007 case report and literature review described the use of etanercept in two pregnancies (13).

In the first pregnancy, the woman was started on etanercept 25 mg twice weekly before conception. Her pregnancy was diagnosed at about 2 months' gestation. Although ultrasound revealed no abnormalities and normal growth, she elected to terminate the pregnancy. The second case involved a 21-year-old woman who was treated before conception with etanercept 25 mg twice weekly and prednisone 5 mg/ day. She became pregnant about 9 months later with her last dose of etanercept given at about 4 weeks' gestation. At term, she gave birth to a healthy 3.520-kg male infant. During the neonatal period, the infant was treated for a urinary tract infection and jaundice. Adrenal congenital hyperplasia with 21-hydroylase deficiency, known in the father, was detected at 5 days of age and treated with prednisone. At 2 years of age, the child was developing normally (13).

A report using data from the FDA database described 61 congenital anomalies in 41 children born to mothers taking a TNF antagonist (22 etanercept and 19 infliximab) (14). The authors concluded that 24 of the children had one or more of the congenital anomalies that are part of VACTERL association (**v**ertebral anomalies, **a**nal atresia, **c**ardiac defects, **t**racheo**e**sophageal, **r**enal, and **l**imb abnormalities) and the rate was higher than historical controls (14). An accompanying editorial, however, concluded that the evidence for teratogenicity or with the VACTERL association was lacking (15). Many of the anomalies reported occur commonly, such as ventricular septal defects. In addition, such databases have selection bias (only cases with adverse outcomes are reported and emphasis is placed on exposures to new drugs) (15).

A 2009 study from France reported the outcomes of 15 women who took anti-TNF drugs during pregnancy (10 etanercept, 3 infliximab, and 2 adalimumab) (16). The drugs were given in the 1st, 2nd, and 3rd trimesters in 12, 3, and 2 cases, respectively. The outcomes were 2 SABs, 1 EAB, and 12 healthy babies without malformation or neonatal illness. They also reviewed the literature regarding the use of anti-TNF agents in pregnancy and found more than 300 cases. They concluded that, although only 29 were treated throughout gestation, the malformation rate was similar to the general population (16).

A woman with severe rheumatoid arthritis that was well controlled with etanercept was diagnosed with a pregnancy at 6 weeks' gestation (17). Etanercept was discontinued but restarted at 20 weeks' because of worsening arthritis. She was continued throughout the remainder of pregnancy. She gave birth at 39 weeks to 2.740-kg female infant with Apgar scores of 10 and 10. No malformations were observed in the newborn (17).

A 40-year-old woman was treated with SC etanercept 25 mg twice weekly and prednisolone 9 mg/day before and throughout pregnancy (18). Maternal blood concentrations of etanercept were measured in each trimester and at delivery. The concentrations decreased during pregnancy from 3849 ng/mL in the 1st trimester to 2239 ng/mL at delivery. She gave birth at 36 weeks' to a 1.906-kg female infant with Apgar scores of 8 and 9. The cord serum concentration at delivery was 81 ng/ mL, about 4% of the mother's concentration. No abnormalities were observed in the infant (18).

BREASTFEEDING SUMMARY

In the case described above (18), the mother exclusively breastfed her infant while continuing the same dose of etanercept. Maternal blood concentrations at postpartum weeks 1, 3, and 12 were relatively constant (2306–3512 ng/mL), whereas the infant's serum concentrations, 81 ng/mL at birth, decreased from 21 ng/mL at 1 week to not detectable (detection level not stated) at 12 weeks. A breast milk concentration, measured at 12 weeks, was 3.5 ng/mL (18).

A woman 30 days after delivery was started on SC etanercept 25 mg twice weekly for an acute flare of arthritis (19). She did not breastfeed her infant. After the fifth dose, a blood sample (data not shown) was drawn and daily milk samples were obtained on postpartum days 44–49. The peak concentration in milk was 75 ng/mL, 1 day after the dose, and the concentration in the other samples declined from 50 to 25 mcg/mL. The estimated dose a nursing infant would have received was 50–90 mcg/day (19).

There is a marked difference in the milk concentrations in the two studies. The timing of the samples in relationship to the dose was only provided in the first case, and then only in approximate terms. Nevertheless, the milk concentrations are very low and there appeared to be no systemic absorption by the one infant that was breastfed. If confirmed, this would be evidence that the protein is digested in the infants' gastrointestinal tract. Although additional data are required, the limited information suggests that breastfeeding is compatible with maternal use of etanercept.

References

1. Product information. Enbrel. Immunex, 2001.
2. Product information. Enbrel. Wyeth-Ayerst Pharmaceuticals, 2001.
3. Sills ES, Perloe M, Tucker MJ, Kaplan CR, Palermo GD. Successful ovulation induction, conception, and normal delivery after chronic therapy with etanercept: a recombinant fusion anti-cytokine treatment for rheumatoid arthritis. Am J Reprod Immunol 2001;46:366–8.
4. Wallace DJ, Weisman MH. The use of etanercept and other tumor necrosis factor-α blockers in infertility: it's time to get serious. J Rheumatol 2003;30:1897–9.
5. Walsh DJ, Shkrobot LV, Palermo GD, Walsh APH. Clinical experience with intravenous immunoglobulin and TNF-A inhibitor therapies for recurrent pregnancy loss. Ulster Med J 2009;70:57–8.
6. Chakravarty EF, Sanchez-Yamamoto D, Bush TM. The use of disease modifying antirheumatic drugs in women with rheumatoid arthritis of childbearing age: a survey of practice patterns and pregnancy outcomes. J Rheumatol 2003;30:241–6.

7. Janssen NM, Genta MS. The effects of immunosuppressive and anti-inflammatory medications on fertility, pregnancy, and lactation. Arch Intern Med 2000;160:610–9.
8. Jarvis B, Faulds D. Etanercept. A review of its use in rheumatoid arthritis. Drugs 1999;57:945–66.
9. Khanna D, McMahon M, Furst DE. Safety of tumour necrosis factor-α antagonists. Drug Saf 2004;27:307–24.
10. Chambers CD, Johnson DL, Jones KL, The OTIS Collaborative Research Group. Pregnancy outcome in women exposed to anti-TNF-alpha medications: The OTIS Rheumatoid Arthritis in Pregnancy study (abstract). Arthritis Rheum 2004;50:S479.
11. Chambers CD, Johnson DL, Jones KL. Safety of anti-TNF-α medications in pregnancy (abstract). J Am Acad Dermatol 2005;52(Suppl 1):P196.
12. Hyrich KL, Symmons DPM, Watson KD, Silman AJ. Pregnancy outcome in women who were exposed to anti-tumor necrosis factor agents: results from a national population register. Arthritis Rheum 2006;54:2701–2.
13. Roux CH, Brocq O, Breuil V, Albert C, Euller-Ziegler L. Pregnancy in rheumatology patients exposed to anti-tumour necrosis factor (TNF)-α therapy. Rheumatology 2007;46:695–8.
14. Carter JD, Ladhani A, Ricca LR, Valeriano J, Vasey FB. A safety assessment of tumor necrosis factor antagonists during pregnancy: a review of the Food and Drug Administration database. J Rheumatol 2009;36:635–41.
15. Koren G, Inoue M. Do tumor necrosis factor inhibitors cause malformations in humans? J Rheumatol 2009;36:465–6.
16. Berthelot JM, De Bandt M, Goupille P, Solau-Gervais E, Liote F, Goeb V, Azais I, Martin A, Pallot-Prades B, Maugars Y, Mariette X, on behalf of CRI (Club Rhumatismes et Inflammation). Exposition to anti-TNF drugs during pregnancy: outcome of 15 cases and review of the literature. Joint Bone Spine 2009;76:28–34.
17. Umeda N, Ito S, Hayashi T, Goto D, Matsumoto I, Sumida T. A patient with rheumatoid arthritis who had a normal delivery under etanercept treatment. Inter Med 2010;49:187–9.
18. Murashima A, Watanabe N, Ozawa N, Saito H, Yamaguchi K. Etanercept during pregnancy and lactation in a patient with rheumatoid arthritis: drug levels in maternal serum, cod blood, breast milk and the infant's serum. Ann Rheum Dis 2009;68:1793–4.
19. Ostensen M, Eigenmann GO. Etanercept in breast milk. J Rheumatol 2004;31:1017–8.

E

ETHACRYNIC ACID

Diuretic

PREGNANCY RECOMMENDATION: Limited Human Data—Animal Data Suggest Low Risk
BREASTFEEDING RECOMMENDATION: No Human Data—Probably Compatible

PREGNANCY SUMMARY

Although limited 1st trimester human experience has not shown an increased incidence of malformations, ethacrynic acid is not recommended for use in pregnant women (1). Diuretics do not prevent or alter the course of toxemia, but they may decrease placental perfusion (see also Chlorothiazide) (2–4). In general, diuretics are not recommended for the treatment of gestational hypertension because of the maternal hypovolemia characteristic of this disease.

FETAL RISK SUMMARY

Ethacrynic acid is a potent diuretic. It has been used for toxemia, pulmonary edema, and diabetes insipidus during pregnancy (5–14).

Reproduction studies in mice and rabbits at doses up to 50 times the human dose showed no evidence of external malformations (15). Doses of 10 or 2.5 times the human dose in rats and dogs, respectively, did not impair fertility or growth and development of pups. Intrauterine growth restriction was observed in the offspring of rats at a dose 50 times the human dose, but there was no effect on survival or postnatal development (15).

Ototoxicity has been observed in a mother and her newborn following the use of ethacrynic acid and kanamycin during the 3rd trimester (see also Kanamycin) (16).

BREASTFEEDING SUMMARY

No reports describing the use of ethacrynic acid during lactation have been located (see also Chlorothiazide). The manufacturer recommends that ethacrynic acid not be used in nursing mothers (15).

References

1. Wilson AL, Matzke GR. The treatment of hypertension in pregnancy. Drug Intell Clin Pharm 1981;15:21–6.
2. Pitkin RM, Kaminetzky HA, Newton M, Pritchard JA. Maternal nutrition: a selective review of clinical topics. Obstet Gynecol 1972;40:773–85.
3. Lindheimer MD, Katz AI. Sodium and diuretics in pregnancy. N Engl J Med 1973;288:891–4.
4. Christianson R, Page EW. Diuretic drugs and pregnancy. Obstet Gynecol 1976;48:647–52.
5. Delgado Urdapilleta J, Dominguez Robles H, Villalobos Roman M, Perez Diaz A. Ethacrynic acid in the treatment of toxemia of pregnancy. Ginecol Obstet Mex 1968;23:271–80.
6. Felman D, Theoleyre J, Dupoizat H. Investigation of ethacrynic acid in the treatment of excessive gain in weight and pregnancy arterial hypertension. Lyon Med 1967;217:1421–8.
7. Sands RX, Vita F. Ethacrynic acid (a new diuretic), pregnancy, and excessive fluid retention. Am J Obstet Gynecol 1968;101:603–9.
8. Kittaka S, Aizawa M, Tokue I, Shimizu M. Clinical results in Edecril tablet in the treatment of toxemia of late pregnancy. Obstet Gynecol (Jpn) 1968;36:934–7.
9. Mahon R, Dubecq JP, Baudet E, Coqueran J. Use of Edecrin in obstetrics. Bull Fed Soc Gynecol Obstet Lang Fr 1968;20:440–2.
10. Imaizumi S, Suzuoki Y, Torri M, et al. Clinical trial of ethacrynic acid (Edecril) for toxemia of pregnancy. Jpn J Med Consult New Remedies 1969;6:2364–8.
11. Young BK, Haft JI. Treatment of pulmonary edema with ethacrynic acid during labor. Am J Obstet Gynecol 1970;107:330–1.
12. Harrison KA, Ajabor LN, Lawson JB. Ethacrynic acid and packed-blood-cell transfusion in treatment of severe anaemia in pregnancy. Lancet 1971;1:11–4.
13. Fort AT, Morrison JC, Fisk SA. Iatrogenic hypokalemia of pregnancy by furosemide and ethacrynic acid: two case reports. J Reprod Med 1971;6:21–2.
14. Pico I, Greenblatt RB. Endocrinopathies and infertility. IV. Diabetes insipidus and pregnancy. Fertil Steril 1969;20:384–92.
15. Product information. Edecrin. Merck, 2000.
16. Jones HC. Intrauterine ototoxicity: a case report and review of literature. J Natl Med Assoc 1973;65:201–3.

ETHAMBUTOL

Antituberculosis Agent

PREGNANCY RECOMMENDATION: Compatible
BREASTFEEDING RECOMMENDATION: Limited Human Data—Probably Compatible

E

PREGNANCY SUMMARY

The literature supports the safety of ethambutol in combination with isoniazid and rifampin during pregnancy (1–5). One investigator studied 38 patients (42 pregnancies) receiving antitubercular therapy (1). The minor abnormalities noted were within the expected frequency of occurrence. Another researcher observed six aborted fetuses at 5–12 weeks of age (2). Embryonic optic systems were specifically examined and were found to be normal. Most reviewers consider ethambutol, along with isoniazid and rifampin, to be the safest antituberculosis therapy (6,7). However, long-term follow-up examinations for ocular damage have not been reported, causing concern among some clinicians (8).

FETAL RISK SUMMARY

No reports linking the use of ethambutol with congenital defects have been located. The drug crosses the placenta to the fetus (9,10). In a woman who delivered at 38 weeks' gestation, ethambutol concentrations in the cord and maternal blood 30 hours after an 800-mg (15 mg/kg) dose were 4.1 and 5.5 ng/mL, respectively, with a cord:maternal serum ratio of 0.75 (9). The amniotic fluid ethambutol level was 9.5 ng/mL. These levels were within the range (1–5 ng/mL) required to inhibit the growth of *Mycobacterium tuberculosis* (9).

BREASTFEEDING SUMMARY

Ethambutol is excreted into human milk. Milk concentrations in two women (unpublished data) were 1.4 mcg/mL (after an oral dose of 15 mg/kg) and 4.60 mcg/mL (dosage not given) (11). Corresponding maternal serum levels were 1.5 and 4.62 mcg/mL, respectively, indicating milk:serum ratios of approximately 1:1. The American Academy of Pediatrics classifies ethambutol as compatible with breastfeeding (12).

References

1. Bobrowitz ID. Ethambutol in pregnancy. Chest 1974;66:20–4.
2. Lewit T, Nebel L, Terracina S, Karman S. Ethambutol in pregnancy: observations on embryogenesis. Chest 1974;66:25–6.
3. Snider DE, Layde PM, Johnson MW, Lyle MA. Treatment of tuberculosis during pregnancy. Am Rev Respir Dis 1980;122:65–79.
4. Brock PG, Roach M. Antituberculous drugs in pregnancy. Lancet 1981;1:43.
5. Kingdom JCP, Kennedy DH. Tuberculous meningitis in pregnancy. Br J Obstet Gynaecol 1989;96:233–5.
6. American Thoracic Society. Treatment of tuberculosis and tuberculosis infection in adults and children. Am Rev Respir Dis 1986;134:355–63.
7. Medchill MT, Gillum M. Diagnosis and management of tuberculosis during pregnancy. Obstet Gynecol Surv 1989;44:81–4.
8. Wall MA. Treatment of tuberculosis during pregnancy. Am Rev Respir Dis 1980;122:989.
9. Shneerson JM, Francis RS. Ethambutol in pregnancy–foetal exposure. Tubercle 1979;60:167–9.
10. Holdiness MR. Transplacental pharmacokinetics of the antituberculosis drugs. Clin Pharmacokinet 1987;13:125–9.
11. Snider DE Jr, Powell KE. Should women taking antituberculosis drugs breast-feed? Arch Intern Med 1984;144:589–90.
12. Committee on Drugs, American Academy of Pediatrics. The transfer of drugs and other chemicals into human milk. Pediatrics 2001;108:776–89.

ETHANOL

Sedative

PREGNANCY RECOMMENDATION: Contraindicated
BREASTFEEDING RECOMMENDATION: Hold Breastfeeding

PREGNANCY SUMMARY

Ethanol is a teratogen and its use during pregnancy, especially during the first 2 months after conception, is associated with significant risk to the fetus and newborn. Heavy maternal use is related to a spectrum of defects collectively termed the fetal alcohol syndrome. Even moderate use may be related to spontaneous abortions and to developmental and behavioral dysfunction in the infant. A safe dose of alcohol in pregnancy has not been established and a woman should abstain from any intake during pregnancy.

FETAL RISK SUMMARY

The teratogenic effects of ethanol (alcohol) have been recognized since antiquity, but this knowledge gradually fell into disfavor and was actually dismissed as superstition in the 1940s (1). Approximately three decades later, the characteristic pattern of anomalies that came to be known as the fetal alcohol syndrome (FAS) were rediscovered, first in France and then in the United States (2–5). By 1981, over 800 clinical and research papers on the FAS had been published (6).

Mild FAS (low birth weight) has been induced by the daily consumption of as little as two drinks (1 ounce of absolute alcohol or about 30 mL) in early pregnancy, but the complete syndrome is usually seen when maternal consumption is four to five drinks (60–75 mL of absolute alcohol) per day or more. The Council on Scientific Affairs of the American Medical Association and the American Council on Science and Health have each published reports on the consequences of maternal alcohol ingestion during pregnancy (7,8). The incidence of the FAS, depending upon the population studied, is estimated to be between 1/300 and 1/2000 live births with 30%–40% of the offspring of alcoholic mothers expected to show the complete syndrome (7). The true incidence may be even higher because the diagnosis of FAS can be delayed for many years (9) (e.g., see reference 25 below). In addition, the incidence of alcohol abuse seems to be rising. A 1989 report found that alcohol abuse during 1987 in 1032 pregnant women was 1.4% compared with 0.7% of 5602 pregnant women during 1977–1980 (10). The difference in frequency was significant ($p < 0.05$).

Heavy alcohol intake by the father prior to conception has been suspected of producing the FAS (11,12), although this association has been challenged (13). The report by the AMA Council states that growth restriction and some adverse aspects of fetal development may be due to paternal influence but conclusive evidence for the complete FAS is lacking (7).

Evidence supporting an association between "regular drinking" by the father in the month before conception and the infant's birth weight was published in two reports, both by the same authors (14,15). "Regular drinking" was defined as "an average of at least 30 mL of ethanol daily or of 75 mL or more on a single occasion at least once a month" (14). "Occasional drinking" was defined as anything less than this. The mean birth weight, 3465 g, of 174 infants of "regular drinking" fathers was 181 g less than the mean birth weight, 3646 g, of 203 infants of "occasional drinking" fathers, a significant difference ($p < 0.001$). Using regression analysis, a 137-g decrease in birth weight was predicted (15). Statistical significance was also present when the data were categorized by sex (males 3561 vs. 3733 g, females 3364 vs. 3538 g), percentage of infants less than 3000 g (15% vs. 9%), and percentage of infants at or greater than 4000 g (12% vs. 23%). Infant characteristics unrelated to the father's drinking were length, head circumference, gestational age, and Apgar scores (15). Consideration of the mother's drinking, smoking, and marijuana use did not change the statistical significance of the data. Nor could the differences be attributed to any of 20 reproductive and socioeconomic variables that were examined, including paternal smoking and marijuana use. No increases in structural defects were detected in the infants of the "regular drinking" fathers, but the sample size may have been too small to detect such an increase (14). In contrast to these data, other researchers have been unable to find an association between paternal drinking and infant birth weight (16). Thus, additional research is required, especially because the biologic mechanisms for the proposed association have not been determined (15).

The mechanism of ethanol's teratogenic effect is unknown but may be related to acetaldehyde, a metabolic byproduct of ethanol (7). One researcher reported higher blood levels of acetaldehyde in mothers of children with FAS than in alcoholics who delivered normal children (17). However, the analysis techniques used in that study have been questioned, and the high concentrations may have been due to artifactual formation of acetaldehyde (18). At the cellular level, alcohol or one of its metabolites may disrupt protein synthesis, resulting in cellular growth restriction with serious consequences for fetal brain development (19). Other proposed mechanisms that may contribute, as reviewed by Shepard (20), include poor protein intake, vitamin B deficiency, lead contamination of alcohol, and genetic predisposition. Of interest, metronidazole, a commonly used anti-infective agent, has been shown to markedly potentiate the fetotoxicity and teratogenicity of alcohol in mice (21). Human studies of this possible interaction have not been reported.

Complete FAS consists of abnormalities in three areas with a fourth area often involved: (a) craniofacial dysmorphology, (b) prenatal and antenatal growth deficiencies, (c) central nervous system dysfunction, and (d) various other abnormalities (7,8). Problems occurring in the latter area include cardiac and renogenital defects and hemangiomas in about one half of the cases (3–5, 22). Cardiac malformations were described in 43 patients (57%) in a series of 76 children with the FAS evaluated for 0–6 years (age: birth to 18 years) (23). Functional murmurs (12 cases, 16%) and ventricular septal defects (VSD) (20 patients, 26%) accounted for the majority of anomalies. Other cardiac lesions present, in descending order of frequency, were: double outlet right ventricle and pulmonary atresia, dextrocardia (with VSD), patent ductus arteriosus with secondary pulmonary hypertension, and cor pulmonale. Liver abnormalities have also been reported (24, 25). Behavioral problems, including minimal brain dysfunction, are long-term effects of the FAS (1).

Ten-year follow-up of the original 11 children who were first diagnosed as having the FAS was reported in 1985 (25). Of the 11 children, 2 were dead, 1 was lost to follow-up, 4 had borderline intelligence with continued growth deficiency and were dysmorphic, and 4 had severe intelligence deficiency as well as growth deficiency and dysmorphic appearance. Moreover, the degree of growth deficiency and intellectual impairment was directly related to the degree of craniofacial abnormalities (25). In the eight children examined, height, weight, and head circumference were deficient, especially the latter two parameters. The authors concluded that the slow head growth after birth may explain why, in some cases, the FAS is not diagnosed until 9–12 months of age (25). Cardiac malformations originally observed in the infants, atrial septal defect (one), patent ductus arteriosus (one), and ventricular septal defect (six), had either resolved spontaneously or were no longer clinically significant. Three new features of the FAS were observed: dental malalignments, malocclusions, and eustachian tube dysfunction (associated with maxillary hypoplasia and leading to chronic serous otitis media) (25).

Fetal Alcohol Syndrome (2–9,11–13, 22–38)

Craniofacial

Eyes: short palpebral fissures, ptosis, strabismus, epicanthal folds, myopia, microphthalmia, blepharophimosis

Ears: poorly formed concha, posterior rotation, eustachian tube dysfunction

Nose: short, upturned hypoplastic philtrum

Mouth: prominent lateral palatine ridges, thinned upper vermilion, retrognathia in infancy, micrognathia or relative prognathia in adolescence, cleft lip or palate,

small teeth with faulty enamel, Class III malocclusion, poor dental alignment
Maxilla: hypoplastic
Central nervous system
Dysfunction demonstrated by mild to moderate retardation, microcephaly, poor coordination, hypotonia, irritability in infancy, and hyperactivity in childhood
Growth
Prenatal (affecting body length more than weight) and postnatal deficiency (length, weight, and head circumference)
Cardiac
Murmurs, atrial septal defect, ventricular septal defect, great vessel anomalies, tetralogy of Fallot
Renogenital
Labial hypoplasia, hypospadias, renal defects
Cutaneous
Hemangiomas, hirsutism in infancy
Skeletal
Abnormal palmar creases, pectus excavatum, restriction of joint movement, nail hypoplasia, radioulnar synostosis, pectus carinatum, bifid xiphoid, Klippel–Feil anomaly, scoliosis
Muscular
Hernias of diaphragm, umbilicus or groin, diastasis recti

A study published in 1987 found that craniofacial abnormalities were closely related to alcohol consumption in a dose–response manner (39). Although a distinct threshold was not defined, the data indicated that the consumption of more than six drinks (90 mL of ethanol) per day was clearly related to structural defects, with the critical period for alcohol-induced teratogenicity around the time of conception (39). A 1989 study that examined 595 live singleton births found a significant correlation between alcohol use in the first 2 months of pregnancy and intrauterine growth restriction and structural abnormalities (40). Analysis of alcohol use during the other periods of pregnancy did not show a significant association with these outcomes.

A prospective study, conducted between 1974 and 1977 at the Kaiser Permanente health maintenance organization in Northern California, was conducted to determine whether light to moderate drinking during pregnancy was associated with congenital abnormalities (41). A total of 32,870 women met all of the criteria for enrollment in the study. Of the total study population, 15,460 (47%) used alcohol during pregnancy, 17,114 (52%) denied use, and 296 (1%) provided incomplete information on their drinking. Of those drinking, 14,502 (94%) averaged less than one drink/day, 793 (5%) drank one to two drinks/day, 127 (0.8%) consumed three to five drinks/day, and 38 (0.2%) drank six or more drinks/day. The total (major and minor) malformation rates were similar between nondrinkers and light (less than one drink/day) or moderate (one to two drinks/day) drinkers; 78.1/1000, 77.3/1000, and 83.2/1000, respectively. A significant trend ($p = 0.034$) was found with increasing alcohol use and congenital malformations of the sex organs (e.g., absence or hypertrophy of the labia, clitoris, and vagina; defects of the ovaries, fallopian tubes, and uterus; hypoplastic or absent penis or scrotum; intersex and unspecified genital anomalies) (41). Rates per 1000 for defects of the sex organs in nondrinkers and the four drinking groups were 2.8, 2.6, 6.3, 7.9, and 26.3, respectively. Genitourinary malformations (i.e., cryptorchidism, hypospadias, and epispadias) also followed an increasing trend with rates per 1000 women of 27.2, 27.5, 31.5, 47.2, and 78.9 (p value for trend = 0.04), respectively. At the levels of alcohol consumption observed in the study, no increase in the other malformations commonly associated with the FAS was found with increasing alcohol use.

A strong association between moderate drinking (>30 mL of absolute alcohol twice per week) and 2nd trimester (15–27 weeks) spontaneous abortions has been found (27,28). Alcohol consumption at this level may increase the risk of miscarriage by 2–4-fold, apparently by acting as an acute fetal toxin. Consumption of smaller amounts of alcohol, such as one drink (approximately 15 mL of absolute alcohol) per week, was not associated with an increased risk of miscarriage in a 1989 report (42).

Ethanol was once used to treat premature uterine contractions. In a retrospective analysis of women treated for premature labor between 1968 and 1973, 239 singleton pregnancies were identified (43). In 136, the women had received oral and/or IV ethanol, in addition to bed rest and oral β-mimetics. The remaining 103 women had been treated only with bed rest and oral β-mimetics. The alcohol group received an average of 38 g of ethanol/day for 2–34 days. In addition, 73 of these women continued to use oral alcohol at home as needed to arrest uterine contractions. Treatment with ethanol was begun at 12 weeks' gestation or less in 82 (60.3%) of the treated women. The mean birth weights of the alcohol-exposed and nonexposed infants were similar, 3385 vs. 3283 g, respectively. No significant differences were found between the groups in the number of infants who were small for gestational age (weight or length <10th percentile), birth length, fetal and neonatal deaths, and infants with anomalies. No relationship was found between ethanol dose and birth weight, length, or neonatal outcome. None of the exposed infants had features of the typical fetal alcohol syndrome. Psychomotor development (age to sit, walk, speak sentences of a few words, and read) and growth velocity were similar between the two groups. One of the infants whose mother had been treated with IV alcohol was growth restricted from birth to 14 years of age. Eight (6.1%) of 131 alcohol-exposed infants were considered to have problems in school (hyperactivity, carelessness) compared with 2 (2.0%) of 99 controls, but the difference was not significant. Other complications observed were aphasia and impaired hearing in two infants of the treated group and a third infant with blindness in the right eye (this infant was delivered at 27 weeks' gestation and the condition was thought to be due to oxygen therapy). The authors concluded that the alcohol treatment for threatened 1st or 2nd trimester abortions did not cause fetal damage (43). However, an earlier study concluded that adverse effects occurred after even short-term exposure (44). This conclusion was reached in an evaluation of 25 children, 4–7 years of age whose mothers had been treated with alcohol infusions to prevent preterm labor (44). In comparison with matched controls, seven children born during or within 15 hours of termination of the infusion had significant pathology in developmental and personality evaluations.

Two reports have described neural tube defects in six infants exposed to heavy amounts of alcohol during early gestation (45,46). Lumbosacral meningomyelocele was observed in five of the newborns and anencephaly in one. One of the infants also had a dislocated hip and clubfeet (45).

A possible association between maternal drinking and clubfoot was proposed in a short 1985 report (47). Three of 43 infants, delivered from maternal alcoholics, had fetal talipes equinovarus (clubfoot), an incidence significantly greater than expected ($p < 0.00001$).

Gastroschisis has been observed in dizygotic twins delivered from a mother who consumed 150–180 mL of absolute ethanol/day during the first 10 weeks of gestation (48). Although an association could not be proven, the authors speculated that the defects resulted from the heavy alcohol ingestion.

A 1982 report described four offspring of alcoholic mothers with clinical and laboratory features of combined FAS and DiGeorge syndrome (49). Several characteristics of the two syndromes are similar, including craniofacial, cardiac, central nervous system, renal, and immune defects (49). Features not shared are hypoparathyroidism (part of DiGeorge syndrome) and skeletal anomalies (part of FAS). A possible causative relationship was suggested between maternal alcoholism and the DiGeorge syndrome.

An unusual chromosomal anomaly was discovered in a 2-year-old girl whose mother drank heavily during early gestation (50). The infant's karyotype revealed an isochromosome for the long arm of number 9: 46,XX,−9,+i(9q). The infant had several characteristics of the FAS, including growth restriction. The relationship between the chromosomal defect and alcohol is unknown.

Prospective analysis of 31,604 pregnancies found that the percentage of newborns below the 10th percentile of weight for gestational age increased sharply as maternal alcohol intake increased (51). In comparison with nondrinkers, mean birth weight was reduced 14 g in those drinking less than one drink per day and 165 g in those drinking three to five drinks per day. The risk for growth restriction was markedly increased by the ingestion of one to two drinks each day. Other investigators discovered that women drinking more than 100 g of absolute alcohol/week at the time of conception had an increased risk of delivering a growth-restricted infant (52). The risk was twice that of women ingesting less than 50 g/week. Of special significance, the risk for growth restriction was not reduced if drinking was reduced later in pregnancy. However, a 1983 report found that if heavy drinkers reduced their consumption in mid-pregnancy, growth impairment was also reduced, although an increased incidence of congenital defects was still evident (53). Significantly smaller head circumferences have been measured in offspring of mothers who drank more than an average of 20 mL of alcohol/day compared with nondrinkers (54). In this same study, the incidence of major congenital anomalies in drinkers and nondrinkers was 1.2% vs. none (54). These authors concluded that there was no safe level of alcohol consumption in pregnancy.

Alcohol ingestion has been shown to abolish fetal breathing (55). Eleven women, at 37–40 weeks' gestation, were given 0.25 g/kg of ethanol. Within 30 minutes, fetal breathing movements were almost abolished and remained so for 3 hours. No effect on gross fetal body movements or fetal heart rate was observed. However, a 1986 report described four women admitted to a hospital because of marked alcohol intoxication (56). In each case, fetal heart rate tracings revealed no or poor variability and no reactivity to fetal movements or external stimuli. Because of suspected fetal distress, an emergency cesarean section was performed in one patient, but no signs of hypoxia were present in the healthy infant. In the remaining three women, normalization of the fetal heart rate patterns occurred within 11–14 hours when the mothers became sober.

A study of the relationship between maternal alcohol ingestion and the risk of respiratory distress syndrome (RDS) in their infants was published in 1987 (57). Of the 531 infants in the study, 134 were delivered at a gestational age of 28–36 weeks. The 134 mothers of these preterm infants were classified by the amount of alcohol they consumed per occasion into abstainers ($N = 58$) (none), occasional ($N = 21$) (less than 15 mL), social ($N = 15$) (15–30 mL), binge ($N = 12$) (greater than 75 mL), and alcoholic ($N = 28$). The incidence of RDS in the infants from the five groups was 44.8%, 38.1%, 26.7%, 16.7%, and 21.4%, respectively. The difference between abstainers and those frankly alcoholic was significant ($p < 0.05$). Moreover, assuming equal intervals of alcohol intake among the five groups, the decrease in incidence of RDS with increasing alcohol intake was significant ($p < 0.02$). Adjustment of the data for smoking, gestational age, birth weight, Apgar score, and sex of the infant did not change the findings. The authors concluded that chronic alcohol ingestion may have enhanced fetal lung maturation (57).

Neonatal alcohol withdrawal has been demonstrated in offspring of mothers ingesting a mean of 21 ounces (630 mL) of alcohol/week during pregnancy (58). In comparison to infants exposed to an equivalent amount of ethanol only during early gestation or to infants whose mothers never drank, the heavily exposed infants had significantly more withdrawal symptoms. No differences were found between the infants exposed only during early gestation and those never exposed. Electroencephalogram (EEG) testing of infants at 4–6 weeks of age indicated that the irritability and tremors may be due to a specific effect of ethanol on the fetal brain and not to withdrawal or prematurity (59). Persistent EEG hypersynchrony was observed in those infants delivered from mothers who drank more than 60 mL of alcohol/day during pregnancy. The EEG findings were found in the absence of dysmorphology and as a result, the authors suggested that this symptom should be added to the definition of the FAS (59).

Combined fetal alcohol and hydantoin syndromes have been described in several reports (60–63). The infants exhibited numerous similar features from exposure to alcohol and phenytoin. The possibility that the agents are also carcinogenic in utero has been suggested by the finding of ganglioneuroblastoma in a 35-month-old boy and Hodgkin's disease in a 45-month-old girl, both with the combined syndromes (see also Phenytoin) (61–63). Adrenal carcinoma in a 13-year-old girl with FAS has also been reported (64). These findings may be fortuitous, but long-term follow-up of children with the FAS is needed.

An unusual cause of FAS was described in 1981 (65). A woman consumed, throughout pregnancy, 480–840 mL/day of an over-the-counter cough preparation. Since the cough syrup contained 9.5% alcohol, the woman was ingesting 45.6–79.8 mL of ethanol/day. The infant had the typical facial features of the FAS, plus an umbilical hernia and hypoplastic labia. Irritability, tremors, and hypertonicity were also evident.

A safe level of maternal alcohol consumption has not been established (7,8,66). Based on practical considerations, the American Council on Science and Health recommends that pregnant women limit their alcohol consumption to no more than two drinks daily (1 ounce or 30 mL of absolute alcohol) (8). However, the safest course for women who are pregnant, or who are planning to become pregnant, is abstinence (7,66).

BREASTFEEDING SUMMARY

Although alcohol passes freely into breast milk, reaching concentrations approximating maternal serum levels, the effect on the infant has been considered insignificant except in rare cases or at very high concentrations (67). Recent research on the effects of chronic exposure of the nursing infant to alcohol in breast milk, however, should cause a reassessment of this position.

Chronic exposure to alcohol in breast milk was found to have an adverse effect on psychomotor development of breastfeeding infants in a 1989 report (68). In this study, "breastfed" was defined as a breastfeeding child who received no more than 473 mL (16 ounces) of its nourishment in the form of supplemental feedings/day. Statistical methods were used to control for alcohol exposure during gestation. Of the 400 infants studied, 153 were breastfed by mothers who were classified as "heavier" drinkers (i.e., an average daily consumption of 1 ounce of ethanol or about two drinks, or binge drinkers who consumed 2.5 ounces or more of ethanol on a single occasion). The population sampled was primarily white, well-educated, middle-class women who belonged to a health maintenance organization. The investigators measured the mental and psychomotor development of the infants at 1 year of age using the Bayley Scales of Infant Development. Mental development was unrelated to maternal drinking during breastfeeding. In contrast, psychomotor development was adversely affected in a dose–response relation ($p = 0.006$ for linear trend). The mean Psychomotor Development Index (PDI) of infants of mothers who had at least one drink daily was 98, compared with 103 for infants of mothers consuming less alcohol ($p < 0.01$). The decrease in PDI was even greater if only those women not supplementing breastfeeding were considered. Regression analysis predicted that the PDI of totally breastfed infants of mothers who consumed an average of two drinks daily would decrease by 7.5 points. These associations persisted even after more than 100 potentially confounding variables, including maternal tobacco, marijuana, and heavy caffeine exposures, were controlled for during pregnancy and the first 3 months after delivery. The authors cautioned that their findings were only suggestive and should not be extrapolated to other patient populations because of the relative homogeneity of their sample (68). Although the conclusions of this study have been criticized and defended (69,70), judgment on the risks to the nursing infant from alcohol in milk must be withheld until additional research has been completed.

The toxic metabolite of ethanol, acetaldehyde, apparently does not pass into milk even though considerable levels can be measured in the mother's blood (71). One report calculated the amount of alcohol received in a single feeding from a mother with a blood concentration of 100 mg/dL (equivalent to a heavy, habitual drinker) as 164 mg, an insignificant amount (72). Maternal blood alcohol levels have to reach 300 mg/dL before mild sedation might be seen in the baby. However, a 1937 report described a case of alcohol poisoning in an 8-day-old breastfed infant whose mother drank an entire bottle (750 mL) of port wine (73). Symptoms in the child included deep sleep, no response to painful stimuli, abnormal reflexes, and weakly reactive pupils. Alcohol was detected in the infant's blood. The child made an apparently uneventful recovery. Potentiation of severe hypoprothrombic bleeding, a pseudo-Cushing's syndrome, and an effect on the milk-ejecting reflex have been reported in nursing infants of alcoholic mothers (74–76).

Because of the risk of toxicity in a nursing infant, the safest course would be to hold nursing for 1–2 hours for each ounce of alcohol consumed, thereby allowing the alcohol level in milk to decrease. The American Academy of Pediatrics classifies ethanol as compatible with breastfeeding, although it is recognized that adverse effects may occur (77). The Institute of Medicine recommends a maximum daily consumption of 0.5 g/kg ethanol (78).

References

1. Shaywitz BA. Fetal alcohol syndrome: an ancient problem rediscovered. Drug Ther 1978;8:95–108.
2. Lemoine P, Harroussean H, Borteyrn JP. Les enfants de parents alcooliques: anomalies observees. A propos de 127 cas. Quest Med 1968;25: 477–82.
3. Ulleland CN. The offspring of alcoholic mothers. Ann NY Acad Sci 1972;197:167–9.
4. Jones KL, Smith DW, Ulleland CN, Streissguth AP. Pattern of malformation in offspring of chronic alcoholic mothers. Lancet 1973;1:1267–71.
5. Jones KL, Smith DW. Recognition of the fetal alcohol syndrome in early infancy. Lancet 1973;2:999–1001.
6. Abel EL. *Fetal Alcohol Syndrome, Volume 1: An Annotated and Comprehensive Bibliography*. Boca Raton, FL: CRC Press, 1981. As cited in Anonymous. Alcohol and the fetus—is zero the only option? Lancet 1983;1:682–3.
7. Council on Scientific Affairs, American Medical Association. Fetal effects of maternal alcohol use. JAMA 1983;249:2517–21.
8. Alcohol Use during Pregnancy. A report by the American Council on Science and Health. As reprinted in Nutrition Today 1982;17:29–32.
9. Lipson AH, Walsh DA, Webster WS. Fetal alcohol syndrome. A great paediatric imitator. Med J Aust 1983;1:266–9.
10. Little BB, Snell LM, Gilstrap LC III, Gant NF, Rosenfeld CR. Alcohol abuse during pregnancy: changes in frequency in a large urban hospital. Obstet Gynecol 1989;74:547–50.
11. Scheiner AP, Donovan CM, Burtoshesky LE. Fetal alcohol syndrome in child whose parents had stopped drinking. Lancet 1979;1:1077–8.
12. Scheiner AP. Fetal alcohol syndrome in a child whose parents had stopped drinking. Lancet 1979;2:858.
13. Smith DW, Graham JM Jr. Fetal alcohol syndrome in child whose parents had stopped drinking. Lancet 1979;2:527.
14. Little RE, Sing CF. Association of father's drinking and infant's birth weight. N Engl J Med 1986;314:1644–5.
15. Little RE, Sing CF. Father's drinking and infant birth weight: report of an association. Teratology 1987;36:59–65.
16. Rubin DH, Leventhal JM, Krasilnikoff PA, Weile B, Berget A. Fathers' drinking (and smoking) and infants' birth weight. N Engl J Med 1986;315:1551.
17. Veghelyi PV. Fetal abnormality and maternal ethanol metabolism. Lancet 1983;2:53–4.
18. Ryle PR, Thomson AD. Acetaldehyde and the fetal alcohol syndrome. Lancet 1983;2:219–20.
19. Kennedy LA. The pathogenesis of brain abnormalities in the fetal alcohol syndrome: an integrating hypothesis. Teratology 1984;29:363–8.
20. Shepard TH. *Catalog of Teratogenic Agents*. 6th ed. Baltimore, MD: The Johns Hopkins University Press, 1989:54.
21. Damjanov I. Metronidazole and alcohol in pregnancy. JAMA 1986;256:472.
22. FDA Drug Bulletin, *Fetal Alcohol Syndrome*. Vol. 7. National Institute on Alcohol Abuse and Alcoholism, 1977:4.
23. Sandor GGS, Smith DF, MacLeod PM. Cardiac malformations in the fetal alcohol syndrome. J Pediatr 1981;98:771–3.
24. Habbick BF, Casey R, Zaleski WA, Murphy F. Liver abnormalities in three patients with fetal alcohol syndrome. Lancet 1979;1:580–1.

25. Streissguth AP, Clarren SK, Jones KL. Natural history of the fetal alcohol syndrome: a 10-year follow-up of eleven patients. Lancet 1985;2:85–91.
26. Khan A, Bader JL, Hoy GR, Sinks LF. Hepatoblastoma in child with fetal alcohol syndrome. Lancet 1979;1:1403–4.
27. Harlap S, Shiono PH. Alcohol, smoking and incidence of spontaneous abortions in the first and second trimester. Lancet 1980;2:173–6.
28. Kline J, Shrout P, Stein Z, Susser M, Warburton D. Drinking during pregnancy and spontaneous abortion. Lancet 1980;2:176–80.
29. Hanson JW, Jones KL, Smith DW. Fetal alcohol syndrome experience with 41 patients. JAMA 1976;235:1458–60.
30. Goetzman BW, Kagan J, Blankenship WJ. Expansion of the fetal alcohol syndrome. Clin Res 1975;23:100A.
31. DeBeukelaer MM, Randall CL, Stroud DR. Renal anomalies in the fetal alcohol syndrome. J Pediatr 1977;91:759–60.
32. Qazi Q, Masakawa A, Milman D, McGann B, Chua A, Haller J. Renal anomalies in fetal alcohol syndrome. Pediatrics 1979;63:886–9.
33. Steeg CN, Woolf P. Cardiovascular malformations in the fetal alcohol syndrome. Am Heart J 1979;98:636–7.
34. Halliday HL, Reid MM, McClure G. Results of heavy drinking in pregnancy. Br J Obstet Gynaecol 1982;89:892–5.
35. Beattie JO, Day RE, Cockburn F, Garg RA. Alcohol and the fetus in the west of Scotland. Br Med J 1983;287:17–20.
36. Tsukahara M, Kajii T. Severe skeletal dysplasias following intrauterine exposure to ethanol. Teratology 1988;37:79–80.
37. Charness ME, Simon RP, Greenberg DA. Ethanol and the nervous system. N Engl J Med 1989;321:442–54.
38. Golden NL, Sokol RJ, Kuhnert BR, Bottoms S. Maternal alcohol use and infant development. Pediatrics 1982;70:931–4.
39. Ernhart CB, Sokol RJ, Martier S, Moron P, Nadler D, Ager JW, Wolf A. Alcohol teratogenicity in the human: a detailed assessment of specificity, critical period, and threshold. Am J Obstet Gynecol 1987;156:33–9.
40. Day NL, Jasperse D, Richardson G, Robles N, Sambamoorthi U, Taylor P, Scher M, Stoffer D, Cornelius M. Prenatal exposure to alcohol: effect on infant growth and morphologic characteristics. Pediatrics 1989;84:536–41.
41. Mills JL, Graubard BI. Is moderate drinking during pregnancy associated with an increased risk for malformations? Pediatrics 1987;80:309–14.
42. Halmesmaki E, Valimaki M, Roine R, Ylikahri R, Ylikorkala O. Maternal and paternal alcohol consumption and miscarriage. Br J Obstet Gynaecol 1989;96:188–91.
43. Halmesmaki E, Ylikorkala O. A retrospective study on the safety of prenatal ethanol treatment. Obstet Gynecol 1988;72:545–9.
44. Sisenwin FE, Tejani NA, Boxer HS, DiGiuseppe R. Effects of maternal ethanol infusion during pregnancy on the growth and development of children at four to seven years of age. Am J Obstet Gynecol 1983;147:52–6.
45. Friedman JM. Can maternal alcohol ingestion cause neural tube defects? J Pediatr 1982;101:232–4.
46. Castro-Gago M, Rodriguez-Cervilla J, Ugarte J, Novo I, Pombo M. Maternal alcohol ingestion and neural tube defects. J Pediatr 1984;104:796–7.
47. Halmesmaki E, Raivio K, Ylikorkala O. A possible association between maternal drinking and fetal clubfoot. N Engl J Med 1985;312:790.
48. Sarda P, Bard H. Gastroschisis in a case of dizygotic twins: the possible role of maternal alcohol consumption. Pediatrics 1984;74:94–6.
49. Ammann AJ, Wara DW, Cowan MJ, Barrett DJ, Stiehm ER. The DiGeorge syndrome and the fetal alcohol syndrome. Am J Dis Child 1982;136: 906–8.
50. Gardner LI, Mitter N, Coplan J, Kalinowski DP, Sanders KJ. Isochromosome 9q in an infant exposed to ethanol prenatally. N Engl J Med 1985;312:1521.
51. Mills JL, Graubard BI, Harley EE, Rhoads GG, Berendes HW. Maternal alcohol consumption and birth weight. How much drinking during pregnancy is safe? JAMA 1984;252:1875–9.
52. Wright JT, Waterson EJ, Barrison IG, Toplis PJ, Lewis IG, Gordon MG, MacRae KD, Morris NF, Murray-Lyon IM. Alcohol consumption, pregnancy, and low birthweight. Lancet 1983;1:663–5.
53. Rosett HL, Weiner L, Lee A, Zuckerman B, Dooling E, Oppenheimer E. Patterns of alcohol consumption and fetal development. Obstet Gynecol 1983;61:539–46.
54. Davis PJM, Partridge JW, Storrs CN. Alcohol consumption in pregnancy. How much is safe? Arch Dis Child 1982;57:940–3.
55. McLeod W, Brien J, Loomis C, Carmichael L, Probert C, Patrick J. Effect of maternal ethanol ingestion on fetal breathing movements, gross body movements, and heart rate at 37 to 40 weeks' gestational age. Am J Obstet Gynecol 1983;145:251–7.
56. Halmesmaki E, Ylikorkala O. The effect of maternal ethanol intoxication on fetal cardiotocography: a report of four cases. Br J Obstet Gynaecol 1986;93:203–5.
57. Ioffe S, Chernick V. Maternal alcohol ingestion and the incidence of respiratory distress syndrome. Am J Obstet Gynecol 1987;156:1231–5.
58. Coles CD, Smith IE, Fernhoff PM, Falek A. Neonatal ethanol withdrawal: characteristics in clinically normal, nondysmorphic neonates. J Pediatr 1984;105:445–51.
59. Ioffe S, Childiaeva R, Chernick V. Prolonged effects of maternal alcohol ingestion on the neonatal electroencephalogram. Pediatrics 1984;74: 330–5.
60. Wilker R, Nathenson G. Combined fetal alcohol and hydantoin syndromes. Clin Pediatr 1982;21:331–4.
61. Seeler RA, Israel JN, Royal JE, Kaye CI, Rao S, Abulaban M. Ganglioneuroblastoma and fetal hydantoin-alcohol syndromes. Pediatrics 1979;63: 524–7.
62. Ramilo J, Harris VJ. Neuroblastoma in a child with the hydantoin and fetal alcohol syndrome. The radiographic features. Br J Radiol 1979;52:993–5.
63. Bostrom B, Nesbit ME Jr. Hodgkin disease in a child with fetal alcohol-hydantoin syndrome. J Pediatr 1983;103:760–2.
64. Hornstein L, Crowe C, Gruppo R. Adrenal carcinoma in child with history of fetal alcohol syndrome. Lancet 1977;2:1292–3.
65. Chasnoff IJ, Diggs G, Schnoll SH. Fetal alcohol effects and maternal cough syrup abuse. Am J Dis Child 1981;135:968.
66. Anonymous. Alcohol and the fetus—is zero the only option? Lancet 1983;1:682–3.
67. Anonymous. Update: drugs in breast milk. Med Lett Drugs Ther 1979;21:21.
68. Little RE, Anderson KW, Ervin CH, Worthington-Roberts B, Clarren SK. Maternal alcohol use during breast-feeding and infant mental and motor development at one year. N Engl J Med 1989;321:425–30.
69. Lindmark B. Maternal use of alcohol and breast-fed infants. N Engl J Med 1990;322:338–9.
70. Little RE. Maternal use of alcohol and breast-fed infants. N Engl J Med 1990;322:339.
71. Kesaniemi YA. Ethanol and acetaldehyde in the milk and peripheral blood of lactating women after ethanol administration. J Obstet Gynaecol Br Commonw 1974;81:84–6.
72. Wilson JT, Brown RD, Cherek DR, Dailey JW, Hilman B, Jobe PC, Manno BR, Manno JE, Redetzki HM, Stewart JJ. Drug excretion in human breast milk. Principles, pharmacokinetics and projected consequences. Clin Pharmacol 1980;5:1–66.
73. Bisdom CJW. Alcohol and nicotine poisoning in nurslings. Maandschrift voor Kindergeneeskunde, Leyden 1937;6:332. As cited in Anonymous. References. JAMA 1937;109:178.
74. Hoh TK. Severe hypoprothrombinaemic bleeding in the breast-fed young infant. Singapore Med J 1969;10:43–9.
75. Binkiewicz A, Robinson MJ, Senior B. Pseudo-Cushing syndrome caused by alcohol in breast milk. J Pediatr 1978;93:965.
76. Cobo E. Effect of different doses of ethanol on the milk-ejecting reflex in lactating women. Am J Obstet Gynecol 1973;115:817–21.
77. Committee on Drugs, American Academy of Pediatrics. The transfer of drugs and other chemicals into human milk. Pediatrics 2001;108:776–89.
78. Howard CR, Lawrence RA. Breast-feeding and drug exposure. Obstet Gynecol Clin N Am 1998;25:195–217.

ETHCHLORVYNOL

Hypnotic

PREGNANCY RECOMMENDATION: Limited Human Data—Animal Data Suggest Moderate Risk
BREASTFEEDING RECOMMENDATION: No Human Data—Potential Toxicity

PREGNANCY SUMMARY

No reports linking the use of ethchlorvynol with congenital defects have been located.

FETAL RISK SUMMARY

In pregnant rats, a dose of 40 mg/kg/day was associated with an increase in the number of stillbirths and a lower survival rate among the offspring (1).

The Collaborative Perinatal Project reported 68 patients with 1st trimester exposure to miscellaneous tranquilizers and nonbarbiturate sedatives, 12 of which had been exposed to ethchlorvynol (2). For the group as a whole, six infants with malformations were delivered, but details on individual exposures were not given.

Animal data indicate that rapid equilibrium occurs between maternal and fetal blood with maximum fetal blood levels measured within 2 hours of maternal ingestion (3). The authors concluded that following maternal ingestion of a toxic or lethal dose, delivery should be accomplished before equilibrium occurs. Neonatal withdrawal symptoms, consisting of mild hypotonia, poor suck, absent rooting, poor grasp, and delayed-onset jitteriness, have been reported (B.H. Rumack, P.A. Walravens, personal communication, Department of Pediatrics, University. of Colorado Medical Center, 1981). The mother had been taking 500 mg daily during the 3rd trimester.

BREASTFEEDING SUMMARY

No reports describing the use of ethchlorvynol during human lactation have been located. Because the drug rapidly crosses the placenta to the fetus, excretion into milk should be expected. Sedation of the nursing infant is a possible consequence.

References

1. Product information. Placidyl. Abbott Laboratories, 2000.
2. Heinonen OP, Slone D, Shapiro S. *Birth Defects and Drugs in Pregnancy*. Littleton, MA: Publishing Sciences Group, 1977:336–7.
3. Hume AS, Williams JM, Douglas BH. Disposition of ethchlorvynol in maternal blood, fetal blood, amniotic fluid, and chorionic fluid. J Reprod Med 1971;6:54–6.

ETHINAMATE

[Withdrawn from the market. See 8th edition.]

ETHINYL ESTRADIOL

Estrogenic Hormone

PREGNANCY RECOMMENDATION: Contraindicated
BREASTFEEDING RECOMMENDATION: No Human Data—Probably Compatible

PREGNANCY SUMMARY

Estrogens are contraindicated because there are usually no benefits from their use in pregnancy.

FETAL RISK SUMMARY

Ethinyl estradiol is used frequently in combination with progestins for oral contraception (see Oral Contraceptives). The Collaborative Perinatal Project monitored 89 mother–child pairs who were exposed to ethinyl estradiol during the 1st trimester (1, pp. 389, 391). An increased risk for malformations was found, although identification of the malformations was not provided. Estrogenic agents as a group were monitored in 614 mother–child pairs. An increase in the expected frequency of cardiovascular defects, eye and ear anomalies, and Down's syndrome was reported (1, p. 395).

Reevaluation of these data in terms of timing of exposure, vaginal bleeding in early pregnancy, and previous maternal obstetric history, however, failed to support an association between estrogens and cardiac malformations (2). An earlier study also failed to find any relationship with nongenital malformations (3). In a smaller study, 12 mothers were exposed to ethinyl estradiol during the 1st trimester (4). No fetal abnormalities were observed. Ethinyl estradiol has also been used as a contraceptive when given within 72 hours of unprotected midcycle coitus (5). Use of estrogenic hormones during pregnancy is contraindicated.

BREASTFEEDING SUMMARY

Estrogens are frequently used for suppression of postpartum lactation (6, 7). Very small amounts are excreted in milk (7).

When used in oral contraceptives, ethinyl estradiol has been associated with decreased milk production and decreased composition of nitrogen and protein content in human milk (8). Although the magnitude of these changes is low, the differences in milk production and composition may be of nutritional importance to nursing infants of malnourished mothers. If breastfeeding is desired, the lowest dose of oral contraceptives should be chosen. Monitoring of infant weight gain and the possible need for nutritional supplementation should be considered (see Oral Contraceptives).

References

1. Heinonen OP, Slone D, Shapiro S. *Birth Defects and Drugs in Pregnancy*. Littleton, MA: Publishing Sciences Group, 1977.
2. Wiseman RA, Dodds-Smith IC. Cardiovascular birth defects and antenatal exposure to female sex hormones: a reevaluation of some base data. Teratology 1984;30:359–70.
3. Wilson JG, Brent RL. Are female sex hormones teratogenic? Am J Obstet Gynecol 1981;141:567–80.
4. Hagler S, Schultz A, Hankin H, Kunstadler RH. Fetal effects of steroid therapy during pregnancy. Am J Dis Child 1963;106:586–90.
5. Dixon GW, Schlesselman JJ, Ory HW, Blye RP. Ethinyl estradiol and conjugated estrogens as postcoital contraceptives. JAMA 1980;244:1336–9.
6. Gilman AG, Goodman LS, Gilman A, eds. *The Pharmacological Basis of Therapeutics*. 6th ed. New York, NY: MacMillan Publishing, 1980:1431.
7. Klinger G, Claussen C, Schroder S. Excretion of ethinyloestradiol sulfonate in the human milk. Zentralbl Gynaekol 1981;103:91–5.
8. Lonnerdal B, Forsum E, Hambraeus L. Effect of oral contraceptives on composition and volume of breast milk. Am J Clin Nutr 1980;33:816–24.

ETHIODIZED OIL

Diagnostic

PREGNANCY RECOMMENDATION: Human Data Suggest Risk in 2nd and 3rd Trimesters
BREASTFEEDING RECOMMENDATION: No Human Data—Probably Compatible

PREGNANCY SUMMARY

Ethiodized oil contains a high concentration of organically bound iodine. Use of this agent close to term has been associated with neonatal hypothyroidism (see Diatrizoate).

BREASTFEEDING SUMMARY

See Potassium Iodide.

ETHIONAMIDE

Anti-infective (Antituberculosis)

PREGNANCY RECOMMENDATION: Human Data Suggest Low Risk
BREASTFEEDING RECOMMENDATION: Limited Human Data—Probably Compatible

PREGNANCY SUMMARY

Although the animal reproductive suggest risk, the human data suggest that the risk probably is low. If indicated, the drug should not be withheld because of pregnancy.

FETAL RISK SUMMARY

The oral anti-infective agent, ethionamide, is indicated for the treatment of tuberculosis when *Mycobacterium tuberculosis* is resistant to isoniazid or rifampin, or when the patient is intolerant to other drugs. Although it apparently has not been studied, the relatively low molecular weight (about 166) suggests that it is transferred to the fetus.

Ethionamide was teratogenic in rats and rabbits at doses higher than those used in humans (1). Nishimura and Tanimura (2), Shepard (3), and Schardein (4) reviewed nine animal studies involving pregnant mice, rats, and rabbits. All of the studies, except one, showed various developmental anomalies.

Five human studies describing the outcome of pregnancies exposed to ethionamide have been briefly reviewed in three sources (2–4). Only one of the studies found an increased incidence of birth defects, reporting 7 cases, 2 of which were Down's syndrome, from 23 exposed infants (2–4). The other reports found no association with congenital malformations (4).

A 2003 study reported the outcomes of seven pregnancies treated for multidrug-resistant tuberculosis (5). The seven women received multiple anti-infective agents. Two patients (one throughout and one postpartum) were treated with ethionamide. In 2005, the same group reported the long-term follow-up of six of the offspring; a seventh child, not exposed to ethionamide was lost to follow-up (6). The average age of the children was 3.7 years and each underwent a comprehensive clinical evaluation. None had hearing loss and all had normal vision and neurologic analysis. Of the two exposed to ethionamide (current age and time of exposure) one had mild speech delay (4.6 years; throughout and postpartum) and one was hyperactive (5.1 years; postpartum only). Both infants were breastfed (6). Neither of the two conditions appears to be related to ethionamide.

BREASTFEEDING SUMMARY

One report mentioned that two mothers were taking ethionamide and other antitubercular medications while breastfeeding their infants (6). However, no reports have been located that measured the drug in milk. The relatively low molecular weight (about 166) suggests that ethionamide will be excreted into breast milk. The effect of this exposure on a nursing infant is unknown.

References

1. Product information. Trecator. Wyeth-Ayerst Pharmaceuticals, 2001.
2. Nishimura H, Tanimura T. *Clinical Aspects of the Teratogenicity of Drugs*. Amsterdam: Excerta Medica, 1976:139–41.
3. Shepard TH. *Catalog of Teratogenic Agents*. 9th ed. Baltimore, MD: The Johns Hopkins University Press, 1998:188.
4. Schardein JL. *Chemically Induced Birth Defects*. 3rd ed. New York, NY: Marcel Dekker, 2000:393–4.
5. Shin S, Guerra D, Rich M, Seung K, Mukherjee J, Joseph K, Hurtado R, Alcantara F, Bayona J, Bonilla C, Farmer P, Furin J. Treatment of multidrug-resistant tuberculosis during pregnancy: a report of 7 cases. Clin Infect Dis 2003;36:996–1003.
6. Drobac PC, Castillo HD, Sweetland A, Anca G, Joseph JK, Furin J, Shin S. Treatment of multidrug-resistant tuberculosis during pregnancy: long-term follow-up of 6 children with intrauterine exposure to second-line agents. Clin Infect Dis 2005;40:1689–92.

ETHISTERONE

[Withdrawn from the market. See 9th edition.]

ETHOHEPTAZINE

[Withdrawn from the market. See 9th edition.]

ETHOPROPAZINE

[Withdrawn from the market. See 9th edition.]

ETHOSUXIMIDE

Anticonvulsant

PREGNANCY RECOMMENDATION: Human Data Suggest Risk
BREASTFEEDING RECOMMENDATION: Limited Human Data—Probably Compatible

PREGNANCY SUMMARY

Ethosuximide is a succinimide anticonvulsant indicated for the treatment of petit mal epilepsy (1). Ethosuximide has a much lower teratogenic potential than the oxazolidinedione class of anticonvulsants (see also Trimethadione and Paramethadione) (2, 3). However, combination therapy with other anticonvulsants markedly increases the risk of structural anomalies. The succinimide anticonvulsants have been considered the anticonvulsants of choice for the treatment of petit mal epilepsy during the 1st trimester.

FETAL RISK SUMMARY

Ethosuximide has been associated with structural anomalies, but the data are not adequate to prove a definite causal relationship (1). In many of the cases described below, the mother was receiving combination therapy with anticonvulsants known to be human teratogens.

Consistent with its low molecular weight (about 141), the drug crosses the human placenta with many newborns having concentrations within the therapeutic range (1, 4, 5).

In eight pregnancies, the mean maternal and fetal ethosuximide concentrations at birth were 40.15 and 35.82 mcg/mL, respectively, with the time of the last dose ranging from 4.5 to 16 hours before birth. The mean fetal:maternal ratio was 0.97 and the neonatal half-life in three infants was 32–38 hours (4). In another case, the plasma drug concentrations in the mother and cord blood were 240 and 250 μmol/L, respectively, a ratio of 1.0 (5).

In 163 pregnancies exposed to ethosuximide in combination with other anticonvulsants, abnormalities were observed in 10 pregnancies: patent ductus arteriosus (8 cases); cleft lip and/or palate (7 cases); mongoloid facies, short neck, altered palmar crease, and an accessory nipple (1 case); and hydrocephalus (1 case) (2,6–15). Spontaneous hemorrhage in the neonate following in utero exposure to ethosuximide also has been reported (see also Phenytoin and Phenobarbital) (12).

In a surveillance study of Michigan Medicaid recipients involving 229,101 completed pregnancies conducted between 1985 and 1992, 18 newborns had been exposed to ethosuximide during the 1st trimester (F. Rosa, personal communication, FDA, 1993). No major birth defects were observed (one expected).

A 1984 publication described the outcomes of 13 newborns from 10 epileptic mothers compared with pair-matched controls (4). Eleven of the mothers received combination therapy with one or more anticonvulsants (carbamazepine, clonazepam, phenobarbital, phenytoin, primidone, or valproic acid). Two infants had major structural anomalies (hare lip and bilateral clefting) with combination therapy (ethosuximide with phenobarbital or primidone). The mean number of minor anomalies was higher compared with controls (6.2 vs. 2.1), but the number and types did not differ from previous reports of anticonvulsant therapy. Sedation and poor sucking were observed in seven infants, six of whom had been exposed in utero to phenobarbital or primidone. Withdrawal symptoms, characterized by hyperexcitability and other symptoms, lasting for several weeks were observed in five infants, two of whom were exposed to phenobarbital or primidone (4).

The Lamotrigine Pregnancy Registry, an ongoing project conducted by the manufacturer, was first published in January 1997 (16). The final report was published in July 2010. The Registry is now closed. Among nine prospectively enrolled pregnancies exposed to ethosuximide and lamotrigine, with or without other anticonvulsants, eight were exposed in the 1st trimester resulting in seven live births without defects and one spontaneous abortion. There was one exposure in the 2nd/3rd trimesters resulting in a live birth without defects (16).

A 1992 report analyzed pooled data from five prospective European studies involving 1379 children exposed in utero to anticonvulsants (17). There were 13 pregnancies exposed to ethosuximide monotherapy with 1 major defect, and 44 exposed to combination therapy (5 with phenobarbital and 39 with valproic acid) with 5 major defects. These outcomes were not significantly different in comparison with other anticonvulsants (17).

BREASTFEEDING SUMMARY

Ethosuximide freely enters the breast milk in concentrations similar to the maternal serum. Five reports measured milk:plasma ratios of 0.86–1.0 (4,5,18–20). In one case, the infant's plasma concentration of ethosuximide was 120 μmol/L, compared with the mother's level of 370 μmol/L, a ratio of 0.32, but the milk:plasma ratio was 1.0 (5). One fully breastfed infant was sedated at birth with poor sucking and had no weight gain during 4 weeks of breastfeeding (4). Hyperexcitability lasting several weeks has been observed in infants exposed in utero to ethosuximide (4). This condition does not appear to be related to maternal use of the drug during breastfeeding because it also was noted in nonbreastfed infants. No other adverse effects in infants exposed to ethosuximide from milk have been reported. The American Academy of Pediatrics classifies ethosuximide as compatible with breastfeeding (21).

E

References

1. Product information. Ethosuximide. Pliva, 2009.
2. Fabro S, Brown NA. Teratogenic potential of anticonvulsants. N Engl J Med 1979;300:1280–1.
3. The National Institute of Health. Anticonvulsants found to have teratogenic potential. JAMA 1981;241:36.
4. Kuhnz W, Koch S, Jakob S, Hartman A, Helge H, Nau H. Ethosuximide in epileptic women during pregnancy and lactation period. Placental transfer, serum concentrations in nursed infants and clinical status. Br J Clin Pharmacol 1984;18:671–7.
5. Tomson T, Villen T. Ethosuximide enantiomers in pregnancy and lactation. Ther Drug Monit 1994;16:621–3.
6. Speidel BD, Meadow SR. Maternal epilepsy and abnormalities of the fetus and newborn. Lancet 1972;2:839–43.
7. Fedrick J. Epilepsy and pregnancy: a report from the Oxford Record Linkage Study. Br Med J 1973;2:442–8.
8. Lowe CR. Congenital malformations among infants born to epileptic women. Lancet 1973;1:9–10.
9. Starreveld-Zimmerman AAE, van der Kolk WJ, Meinardi H, Elshve J. Are anticonvulsants teratogenic? Lancet 1973;2:48–9.
10. Kuenssberg EV, Knox JDE. Teratogenic effect of anticonvulsants. Lancet 1973;2:198.
11. Speidel BD, Meadow SR. Epilepsy, anticonvulsants and congenital malformations. Drugs 1974;8:354–65.
12. Janz D. The teratogenic risk of antiepileptic drugs. Epilepsia 1975;16: 159–69.
13. Nakane Y, Okuma T, Takahashi R. Multi-institutional study on the teratogenicity and fetal toxicity of antiepileptic drugs: a report of a collaborative study group in Japan. Epilepsia 1980;21:663–80.
14. Heinonen OP, Slone D, Shapiro S. *Birth Defects and Drugs in Pregnancy*. Littleton, MA: Publishing Sciences Group, 1977:358–9.
15. Dansky L, Andermann E, Andermann F. Major congenital malformations on the offspring of epileptic patients: genetic and environment risk factors. In: *Epilepsy, Pregnancy and the Child*. Proceedings of a workshop held in Berlin, September 1980. New York, NY: Raven Press, 1981.
16. The Lamotrigine Pregnancy Registry. Final Report. 1 September 1992 through 31 March 2010. GlaxcoSmithKline, July 2010.
17. Samren EB, van Duijn CM, Koch S, Hiilesmaa VK, Klepel H, Bardy AH, Beck Mannagetta G, Deichl AW, Gaily E, Granstrom ML, Meinardi H, Grobbee DE, Hofman A, Janz D, Lindhout D. Maternal use of antiepileptic drugs and the risk of major congenital malformations: a joint European prospective study of human teratogenesis associated with maternal epilepsy. Epilepsia 1992;38: 981–90.
18. Koup JR, Rose JQ, Cohen ME. Ethosuximide pharmacokinetics in pregnant patient and her newborn. Epilepsia 1978;19:535.
19. Kaneko S, Sato T, Suzuki K. The levels of anticonvulsants in breast milk. Br J Clin Pharmacol 1979;7:624–6.
20. Horning MG, Stillwell WG, Nowlin J, Lertratanangkoon K, Stillwill RN, Hill RM. Identification and quantification of drugs and drug metabolites in human breast milk using GC-MS-COM methods. Mod Probl Paediatr 1975;15:73–9.
21. Committee on Drugs, American Academy of Pediatrics. The transfer of drugs and other chemicals into human milk. Pediatrics 2001;108: 776–89.

ETHOTOIN

Anticonvulsant

PREGNANCY RECOMMENDATION: Compatible—Maternal Benefit >> Embryo–Fetal Risk
BREASTFEEDING RECOMMENDATION: No Human Data—Probably Compatible

E

PREGNANCY SUMMARY

Although the human pregnancy experience is very limited, the embryo–fetal risk is thought to be lower than the more potent phenytoin.

FETAL RISK SUMMARY

Ethotoin is a low-potency hydantoin anticonvulsant (1). The fetal hydantoin syndrome has been associated with the use of the more potent phenytoin (see Phenytoin). Only six reports describing the use of ethotoin during the 1st trimester have been located (2–4). Cleft lip/palate and patent ductus arteriosus were observed in two of the offspring (3,4).

BREASTFEEDING SUMMARY

No reports describing the use of ethotoin during human lactation have been located. However, a more potent hydantoin anticonvulsant (see Phenytoin) is considered compatible with breastfeeding and ethotoin should be classified the same.

References

1. Schmidt RP, Wilder BJ. Epilepsy. In: *Contemporary Neurology Services*. Vol. 2. Philadelphia, PA: FA Davis Co, 1968:154.
2. Heinonen OP, Slone D, Shapiro S. *Birth Defects and Drugs in Pregnancy*. Littleton, MA: Publishing Sciences Group, 1977:358–9.
3. Zablen M, Brand N. Cleft lip and palate with the anticonvulsant ethantoin. N Engl J Med 1978;298:285.
4. Nakane Y, Okuma T, Takahashi R, Sato Y, Wada T, Sato T, Fukushima Y, Kumashiro H, Ono T, Takahashi T, Aoki Y, Kazamatsuri H, Inami M, Komai S, Seino M, Miyakoshi M, Tanimura T, Hazama H, Kawahara R, Otsuki S, Hosokawa K, Inanaga K, Nakazawa Y, -Yamamoto K. Multi-institutional study on the teratogenicity and fetal toxicity of antiepileptic drugs: a report of a collaborative study group in Japan. Epilepsia 1980;21:663–80.

ETHYL BISCOUMACETATE

Anticoagulant

See Coumarin Derivatives.

ETHYNODIOL

Progestogenic Hormone

PREGNANCY RECOMMENDATION: Contraindicated
BREASTFEEDING RECOMMENDATION: No Human Data—Probably Compatible

PREGNANCY SUMMARY

Ethynodiol should not be used in pregnancy because there are no benefits for the mother, embryo, or fetus. The agent is used primarily in oral contraceptives (see Oral Contraceptives).

BREASTFEEDING SUMMARY

See Oral Contraceptives.

ETIDRONATE

Bisphosphonate

PREGNANCY RECOMMENDATION: Limited Human Data—Animal Data Suggest Low Risk
BREASTFEEDING RECOMMENDATION: No Human Data—Probably Compatible

E

PREGNANCY SUMMARY

Although the dose comparisons were based on body weight, etidronate did not cause developmental toxicity in animals at doses that were close to those used in humans. Two reports have described the use of bisphosphonates before or during six human pregnancies. Because the oral bioavailability is low and the plasma clearance is rapid, clinically significant amounts of etidronate may not cross the human placenta. Nonetheless, the drug is slowly released from bone over weeks to years. The amount of drug retained in bone and eventually released back into the systemic circulation is directly related to the dose and duration of treatment. Thus, administration before pregnancy may result in low-level, continuous exposure throughout gestation. The use of etidronate in women who may become pregnant or during pregnancy is not recommended. However, based on the animal and limited human data, inadvertent exposure during early pregnancy does not appear to represent a major risk to the embryo–fetus.

FETAL RISK SUMMARY

Etidronate (EHDP), a hydrophilic bisphosphonate, is a synthetic analog of pyrophosphate that binds to the hydroxyapatite found in bone to inhibit bone resorption. Etidronate is indicated for the treatment of symptomatic Paget's disease of bone and in the prevention and treatment of heterotopic ossification after total hip replacement or because of spinal cord injury. Other agents in this pharmacologic class are alendronate, ibandronate, pamidronate, risedronate, tiludronate, and zoledronic acid. Only about 3% of an oral dose is absorbed into the systemic circulation. Etidronate is not metabolized. The plasma half-life ranges from 1 to 6 hours. About half of the absorbed drug is distributed to bone from which it is slowly released over a prolonged period. Although the elimination half-life from bone is not known with certainty, the clearance from bone in animals is up to 165 days (1).

Reproduction studies have been conducted with etidronate in rats and rabbits. In pregnant rats and rabbits, doses 5–20 times the human clinical dose based on body weight (HCD) did not cause teratogenic or other adverse effects in the offspring. At doses 15–60 times the HCD, etidronate exposure in pregnant rats was associated with skeletal anomalies in the offspring. These defects were thought to be secondary to the action of etidronate on bone. Decreased live births were observed with maternally toxic doses 25–300 times the HCD (1). Shepard reviewed four animal studies in which etidronate was given orally, subcutaneously, or intraperitoneally to mice, rats, and rabbits during gestation (2). Skeletal abnormalities were produced with high doses, but no other developmental toxic effects were observed.

No evidence of carcinogenic effects was observed in long-term studies in rats (1). Studies for mutagenic and clastogenic effects apparently have not been conducted.

It is not known if etidronate crosses the human placenta. The relatively low molecular weight (250), the absence of metabolism, and the prolonged clearance from bone all suggest that exposure of the embryo–fetus will occur. The relatively short plasma half-life, low lipid solubility, and oral bioavailability should limit this exposure.

A 1992 case report described the in utero treatment of a fetus with etidronate early in the 3rd trimester (3). Based on ultrasonography and the mother's obstetric history, a presumptive diagnosis of a rare disorder, idiopathic arterial calcification of infancy (IACI), was made in the fetus at 29 weeks' gestation. The fetus was treated with two courses of etidronate by percutaneous umbilical vein puncture. Fetal distress occurred 1 week later and the 1700-g female infant was delivered by emergency cesarean section with Apgar scores of 2 and 6 at 1 and 5 minutes, respectively. IACI was confirmed in the neonate 1 week after birth. The infant was treated with etidronate over the next several months. Radiographs of her skeleton showed severe growth plate malformations resembling rickets that were thought to be secondary to etidronate. The infant died at 7.5 months of age despite aggressive therapy for prematurity and her disease (3).

A 2008 review described 51 cases of exposure to bisphosphonates before or during pregnancy: alendronate (N = 32), pamidronate (N = 11), etidronate (N = 5), risedronate (N = 2), and zoledronic acid (N = 1) (4). The authors concluded that although these drugs may affect bone modeling and development in the fetus, no such toxicity has yet been reported.

BREASTFEEDING SUMMARY

No reports describing the use of etidronate during lactation have been located. The molecular weight (250) and the lack of metabolism suggest that the drug will be excreted into breast milk, but the low plasma concentrations and relatively short plasma half-life (1–6 hours) suggest that minimal amounts will be excreted into milk. Moreover, the oral bioavailability of etidronate, at least in adults, is only 3%. Although the effect of exposure on a nursing infant is unknown, it appears to be negligible.

References

1. Product information. Didronel. Procter & Gamble Pharmaceuticals, 2006.
2. Shepard TH. *Catalog of Teratogenic Agents*. 10th ed. Baltimore, MD: The Johns Hopkins University Press, 2001:211–2.
3. Bellah RD, Zawodniak L, Librizzi RJ, Harris MC. Idiopathic arterial calcification of infancy: prenatal and postnatal effects of therapy in an infant. J Pediatr 1992;121:930–3.
4. Djokanovic N, Klieger-Grossmann C, Koren G. Does treatment with bisphosphonates endanger the human pregnancy? J Obstet Gynaecol Can 2008;30:1146–8.

ETODOLAC

Nonsteroidal Anti-inflammatory

PREGNANCY RECOMMENDATION: Human Data Suggest Risk in 1st and 3rd Trimesters
BREASTFEEDING RECOMMENDATION: No Human Data—Potential Toxicity

E

PREGNANCY SUMMARY

No reports describing the use of etodolac in human pregnancy have been located. The animal data suggest low risk for congenital malformations. A brief 2003 editorial on the potential for nonsteroidal anti-inflammatory drug (NSAID)–induced developmental toxicity concluded that NSAIDs, and specifically those with greater COX-2 affinity, had a lower risk of this toxicity in humans than aspirin (1).

Constriction of the ductus arteriosus in utero is a pharmacologic consequence arising from the use of prostaglandin synthesis inhibitors during late pregnancy, as is inhibition of labor, prolongation of pregnancy, and suppression of fetal renal function (see also Indomethacin) (2). Persistent pulmonary hypertension of the newborn may occur if these agents are used in the 3rd trimester close to delivery (2,3). Women attempting to conceive should not use any prostaglandin synthesis inhibitor, including etodolac, because of the findings in a variety of animal models that indicate these agents block blastocyst implantation (4,5). Moreover, as noted above, NSAIDs have been associated with spontaneous abortions (SABs) and congenital malformations. The risk for these defects, however, appears to be low.

FETAL RISK SUMMARY

The NSAID etodolac is used in the treatment of arthritis, and acute and chronic pain. Etodolac is in a NSAID subclass (pyranocarboxylic acid) that contains no other members.

In reproduction studies with rats, the drug produced isolated occurrences of alterations in limb development (polydactyly, oligodactyly, syndactyly, and unossified phalanges) at doses close to human clinical doses (2–14 mg/kg/day). These same doses produced oligodactyly and synostosis of metatarsals in rabbits. However, a clear drug or dose–response relationship was not established. Similar to other agents in this class, etodolac increased the incidence of dystocia, prolonged gestation, and decreased pup survival in rats (6).

It is not known if etodolac crosses the human placenta. The molecular weight (about 287) is low enough that passage to the fetus should be expected.

A combined 2001 population-based observational cohort study and a case–control study estimated the risk of adverse pregnancy outcome from the use of NSAIDs (7). The use of NSAIDs during pregnancy was not associated with congenital malformations, preterm delivery, or low birth weight, but a positive association was discovered with SABs. A similar study, also published in 2001, failed to find a relationship, in general, between NSAIDs and congenital malformations, but did find a significant association with cardiac defects and orofacial clefts (8). In addition, a 2003 study found a significant association between exposure to NSAIDs in early pregnancy and SABs (9). (See Ibuprofen for details on these three studies.)

BREASTFEEDING SUMMARY

No reports describing the use of etodolac during lactation have been located. Because of the relatively low molecular weight (about 287), the excretion of etodolac into breast milk should be expected. Moreover, because of its long termination adult plasma half-life (7.3 hours), other agents may be preferred during lactation. One reviewer listed several low-risk alternatives (diclofenac, fenoprofen, flurbiprofen, ibuprofen, ketoprofen, ketorolac, and tolmetin) if a NSAID is required while nursing (10).

References

1. Tassinari MS, Cook JC, Hurtt ME. NSAIDs and developmental toxicity. Birth Defects Res (Part B) 2003;68:3–4.
2. Levin DL. Effects of inhibition of prostaglandin synthesis on fetal development, oxygenation, and the fetal circulation. Semin Perinatol 1980;4:35–44.
3. Van Marter LJ, Leviton A, Allred EN, Pagano M, Sullivan KF, Cohen A, Epstein MF. Persistent pulmonary hypertension of the newborn and smoking and aspirin and nonsteroidal antiinflammatory drug consumption during pregnancy. Pediatrics 1996;97:658–63.
4. Matt DW, Borzelleca JF. Toxic effects on the female reproductive system during pregnancy, parturition, and lactation. In: Witorsch RJ, ed. *Reproductive Toxicology*. 2nd ed. New York, NY: Raven Press, 1995:175–93.
5. Dawood MY. Nonsteroidal antiinflammatory drugs and reproduction. Am J Obstet Gynecol 1993;169:1255–65.
6. Product information. Lodine. Wyeth-Ayerst Laboratories, 2000.
7. Nielsen GL, Sorensen HT, Larsen H, Pedersen L. Risk of adverse birth outcome and miscarriage in pregnant users of non-steroidal anti-inflammatory drugs: population based observational study and case-control study. Br Med J 2001;322:266–70.
8. Ericson A, Kallen BAJ. Nonsteroidal anti-inflammatory drugs in early pregnancy. Reprod Toxicol 2001;15:371–5.
9. Li DK, Liu L, Odouli R. Exposure to non-steroidal anti-inflammatory drugs during pregnancy and risk of miscarriage: population based cohort study. Br Med J 2003;327:368–71.
10. Anderson PO. Medication use while breast feeding a neonate. Neonatal Pharmacol Q 1993;2:3–14.

ETOMIDATE

Hypnotic

PREGNANCY RECOMMENDATION: Limited Human Data—Animal Data Suggest Risk
BREASTFEEDING RECOMMENDATION: Limited Human Data—Probably Compatible

E

PREGNANCY SUMMARY

The human pregnancy experience with etomidate is limited to women undergoing cesarean section. A 1988 review found no reports of congenital malformations in children of women anesthetized with this agent (1). The animal data suggest risk (embryo–fetal death), but the dose was based on body weight and may not be relevant. However, no structural anomalies have been observed in animals. When used immediately before birth, etomidate causes a transient decrease in newborn cortisol concentrations. The clinical significance of this effect is unknown. Although the data are limited, use of etomidate for induction of general anesthesia at or near term does not appear to represent a risk of fetal or newborn harm.

FETAL RISK SUMMARY

Etomidate is a rapid, short-acting hypnotic drug without analgesic activity that is given as an IV injection. Etomidate is indicated for the induction of general anesthesia. The agent is metabolized in the liver to inactive metabolites. Blood concentrations of etomidate decrease rapidly up to 30 minutes after injection and thereafter more slowly with an elimination half-life about 75 minutes (2, 3).

Reproduction studies have been conducted in rats and rabbits. In rats, doses that were ≥1 times the human dose (*based on body weight*) were embryocidal. In rats and rabbits, doses that were 1–16 and 5–15 times the human dose, respectively, resulted in decreased pup survival. The highest doses caused maternal toxicity including death. No teratogenicity has been observed in animals (2, 3).

Studies for carcinogenicity and mutagenicity have not been conducted. No impairment of fertility was noted in male and female rats (2, 3).

It is not known if etomidate crosses the human placenta early in pregnancy but it does at term. A 1988 abstract described seven women undergoing elective cesarean section (4). General anesthesia was induced with a 0.3 mg/kg IV dose of etomidate. The elimination half-life was 132 minutes. At delivery, the fetal:maternal ratio was 0.51. Etomidate was detected in the urine of the newborns up to 16 hours after birth (4). One study reported an umbilical:maternal vein ratio of 0.5 after use of the drug for cesarean section in 20 women (5). Apgar scores were ≥7 and 9/10 at 1 and 5 minutes, respectively. Another study measured an umbilical:maternal ratio of 0.48 in 20 women at cesarean section (6). A 1992 study of 20 women undergoing cesarean section also found that the drug crossed to the fetus (7). All of these results are consistent with the relatively low molecular weight (about 244) of etomidate.

In one of the studies described above, etomidate was associated with a transient reduction in neonatal cortisol concentrations in comparison with a methohexitone group (6). The difference between the two groups was most evident 2 hours after birth. There was no difference at 5 hours. The decrease was thought to be secondary to inhibition of cortisol synthesis in the adrenal cortex, a known effect of etomidate (6). In another study, 11 mothers undergoing elective cesarean sections were given 0.3 mg/kg etomidate for induction of general anesthesia (8). Serum cortisol in the newborns was compared with 11 newborns of mothers who had been given thiopentone for induction. At 1 hour of age, the cortisol concentrations were significantly lower ($p < 0.001$) in the etomidate group (8).

One of the first reports describing the use of etomidate for induction of general anesthesia before cesarean section was published in 1984 (9). Seventy-two women received the agent and no clinical effects were observed in the newborns. Other reports also have described the use of etomidate for this purpose, apparently without harm to the newborns (10–14).

BREASTFEEDING SUMMARY

No reports describing the use of etomidate during human lactation have been located. Such studies are not expected because of the indication for the drug. However, the drug crosses the placenta when given for cesarean section (4–7). In one study involving 20 women who had received a single 0.3 mg/kg IV dose, etomidate was detected in the colostrum (7). Mean colostrum drug concentrations at 30 and 120 minutes after the dose were 79.3 ng/mL (range 0–420 ng/mL) and 16.2 ng/mL (range 0–60 ng/mL), respectively. Etomidate was not detected in any sample 4 hours after the dose. The colostrum:plasma ratio at 30 minutes was 1.2; at 120 minutes, plasma concentrations were undetectable (7). Because of the very small amounts of colostrum that are available at these times, the risk to a nursing infant probably is nil.

References

1. Friedman JM. Teratogen update: anesthetic agents. Teratology 1988;37:69–77.
2. Product information. Etomidate injection. Bedford Laboratories, 2004.
3. Product information. Amidate. Hospira, 2009.
4. Suresh MS, Ahmed AE, Solanki DR, Helms TH, Nguyen S. Etomidate pharmacokinetics during cesarean section (abstract). Anesthesiology 1988;65:A388.
5. Gregory MA, Davidson DG. Plasma etomidate levels in mother and fetus. Anaesthesia 1991;46:716–8.
6. Crozier TA, Flamm C, Speer CP, Rath W, Wuttke W, Kuhn W, Kettler D. Effects of etomidate on the adrenocortical and metabolic adaptation of the neonate. Br J Anaesth 1993;70:47–53.
7. Esener Z, Sarihasan B, Güven H, Üstün E. Thiopentone and etomidate concentrations in maternal and umbilical plasma, and in colostrum. Br J Anaesth 1992;69:586–8.
8. Reddy BK, Pizer B, Bull PT. Neonatal serum cortisol suppression by etomidate compared with thiopentone, for elective caesarean section. Eur J Anaesthesia 1998;5:171–6.

9. Regaert P, Noorduin H. General anesthesia with etomidate, alfentanil and droperidol for caesarean section. Acta Anaethesiol Belg 1984;35:193–200.
10. Tay SM, Ong BC, Tan SA. Cesarean section in a mother with uncorrected congenital coronary to pulmonary artery fistula. Can J Anesth 1999;46:368–71.
11. Orme RMLE, Grange CS, Ainsworth QP, Crebenik CR. General anaesthesia using remifentanil for caesarean section in parturients with critical aortic stenosis: a series of four cases. Int J Obstet Anesth 2004;13:83–7.
12. Bilehjani E, Kianfar AA, Toofan M, Fakhari S. Anesthesia with etomidate and remifentanil for cesarean section in a patient with severe peripartum cardiomyopathy. Middle East J Anesthesiol 2008;19:1141–7.
13. Coskun D, Mahli A, Korkmaz S, Demir FS, Inan GK, Erer D, Ozdogan ME. Anaesthesia for caesarean section in the presence of multivalvular heart disease and severe pulmonary hypertension: a case report. Cases J 2009;2:9383.
14. Duman A, Sarkilar G, Dayioglu M, Özden M, Görmüs N. Use of remifentanil in a patient with Eisenmenger syndrome requiring urgent cesarean section. Middle East J Anesthesiol 2010;20:577–80.

E

ETOPOSIDE

Antineoplastic

PREGNANCY RECOMMENDATION: Human and Animal Data Suggest Risk
BREASTFEEDING RECOMMENDATION: Contraindicated

PREGNANCY SUMMARY

Etoposide is a potent animal teratogen and potentially may be a teratogen in humans, but exposure during organogenesis has not been reported. Five cases of maternal exposure to this agent and other antineoplastics during the 2nd and 3rd trimesters resulted in growth restriction and/or severe myelosuppression in three fetuses–newborns, two of whom were delivered prematurely, and one had reversible alopecia. Successful pregnancies, commencing after etoposide treatment, have also been reported.

FETAL RISK SUMMARY

Etoposide (VP-16, VP-16-213) is a semisynthetic derivative of podophyllotoxin used as an antineoplastic agent. Low doses of the drug, 1/20th–1/2 of the recommended clinical dose based on BSA, are teratogenic and embryocidal in rats and mice (1). A dose-related increase in the occurrence of embryotoxicity and congenital malformations was observed in these animals. Defects included decreased weight, skeletal anomalies, retarded ossification, exencephaly, encephalocele, and anophthalmia. The drug is also mutagenic in mammalian cells and, although not tested in animals, should be considered a potential carcinogen in humans (1).

When etoposide was administered intraperitoneally to pregnant mice during organogenesis, various anomalies were observed, including exencephaly, encephalocele, hydrocephalus, gastroschisis (including abnormal stomach or liver), microphthalmia or anophthalmia, dextrocardia (including missing lung lobe), and axial skeleton defects (2). In whole-embryo rat culture, a concentration of 2 micro-M (no-observed-adverse-effect-level 1.0 micro-M; embryotoxic range 2–5 micro-M) produced growth restriction and brain anomalies (hypoplasia of prosencephalon and edema of rhombencephalon) and microphthalmia (3).

Reported use of etoposide during human pregnancy is limited to five cases (4–8). A 21-year-old woman with a dysgerminoma was treated surgically at 26 weeks' gestation, followed 6 days later with etoposide (100 mg/m^2) and cisplatin (20 mg/m^2), daily for 5 days at 3- to 4-week intervals (4). Four cycles of chemotherapy were given. Because of oligohydramnios and probable intrauterine growth restriction, labor was induced and she delivered a healthy, 2320-g female infant at 38 weeks. The hematologic profile of the newborn was normal, as was her development at 9 months of age.

A 36-year-old woman at 25 weeks' gestation was treated for acute myeloid leukemia with combination chemotherapy consisting of two courses of etoposide (400 mg/m^2/day, days 8–10), cytarabine (1 g/m^2/day, days 1–3), and daunorubicin (45 mg/m^2/day, days 1–3) (5). No fetal growth was observed during serial ultrasound examinations from 30 to 32 weeks. An emergency cesarean section was performed because of fetal distress at 32 weeks' gestation, 11 days after the second course of chemotherapy. The pale, 1460-g (10th percentile) female infant required resuscitation at birth. Analysis of the cord blood revealed anemia and leukopenia, and profound neutropenia and thrombocytopenia were discovered at 30 hours of age. Following successful therapy, the child, at 1 year of age, was no longer receiving any treatment, had normal peripheral blood counts, and was apparently progressing normally.

A 32-year-old woman at 26 weeks' gestation presented with an unknown primary, poorly differentiated adenocarcinoma of the liver and with a mass in the posterior chamber of the right eye (6). She was treated with daily doses of etoposide (165 mg), bleomycin (30 mg), and cisplatin (55 mg), for 3 days. The patient became profoundly neutropenic, developed septicemia, and went into premature labor. A 1190-g female infant was born with Apgar scores of 3 and 8 at 1 and 5 minutes, respectively. Severe respiratory distress was successfully treated over the next 10 days. Although the antineoplastics were chosen because they are highly protein bound (etoposide, 97%; cisplatin, 90% of plasma platinum; bleomycin, no data) and less likely to cross the placenta, marked leukopenia with neutropenia developed in the infant on day 3 (10 days after in utero exposure to the chemotherapy). Scalp hair loss and a rapid loss of lanugo were observed at 10 days of age. By 12 weeks of age, substantial hair regrowth had occurred, and at 1 year follow-up, the child was developing normally, except for moderate bilateral sensorineural hearing loss. The investigators could not determine if the deafness was due to the in utero exposure to cisplatin or to the maternal and/or neonatal aminoglycoside therapy. The alopecia and bone marrow depression in the infant were attributed to etoposide.

Treatment of nonlymphoblastic acute leukemia, diagnosed at 18 weeks' gestation, was described in a brief 1993 report (7). Therapy consisted of two courses of etoposide (100 mg/m^2/day) and daunorubicin (60 mg/m^2/day) on days 1–3, and cytarabine (100 mg/m^2/day) on days 1–7. Follow-up therapy consisted of mitoxantrone, cytarabine, and amsacrine. The patient eventually delivered a term, 2930-g, healthy male infant who was developing normally.

Non-Hodgkin's lymphoma, diagnosed in a 36-year-old woman at 22 weeks' gestation, was treated with a 12-week chemotherapy course consisting of etoposide (125 mg/m^2), vincristine (1.4 mg/m^2), and bleomycin (9 mg/m^2) in weeks 2, 4, 6, 8, 10, and 12, and cyclophosphamide (375 mg/m^2) and doxorubicin (50 mg/m^2) in weeks 1, 3, 5, 7, 9, and 11 (8). Prednisolone was given during the entire 12-week period. A healthy, 3200-g male infant, delivered 3 weeks after the completion of therapy, was alive and well at 21 months of age. At this time also, the mother had just delivered another healthy male infant.

Seven reports, including the one above, have described women who became pregnant following treatment with etoposide (8–14) and one report described the return of normal menstrual function after etoposide therapy (15). One woman delivered a normal term infant following treatment for choriocarcinoma with nine courses of etoposide (100 mg/m^2/day), cisplatin, dactinomycin, and intrathecal methotrexate 2 years prior to conception (9). Pregnancies occurred, about 6–7 years after treatment, in 3 women from a group of 128 who had been previously treated with high-dose chemotherapy for refractory or relapsed Hodgkin's disease (10). The current chemotherapy regimen consisted of etoposide (600–900 mg/m^2), cyclophosphamide, and carmustine, followed by either autologous bone marrow or peripheral progenitor cell transplantation. One of the women conceived after receiving a donated ovum and delivered a healthy child. A second one became pregnant with twins after receiving ovulatory stimulating agents, but aborted both at 5 1/2 months' gestation. The third woman spontaneously conceived and delivered a healthy child.

Two women had normal pregnancies and babies after treatment with high-dose chemotherapy for relapsed Hodgkin's disease and non-Hodgkin's lymphoma, respectively (11). The first patient was treated with etoposide (800 mg/m^2), carmustine, and melphalan, followed by autologous stem cell transplantation (ASCT). She conceived 19 months after completion of treatment. The second woman received etoposide (1000 mg/m^2), cyclophosphamide, and carmustine, followed by ASCT. She became pregnant 33 months later.

Of 33 women (>18 years old) treated with multiple courses of chemotherapy for ovarian germ cell tumors and fertility conserving surgery, 14 (42%) had successful pregnancies (12). No congenital abnormalities in their offspring were observed. The chemotherapy consisted of etoposide (100 mg/m^2 $\times$ 3 days/course), bleomycin, cisplatin, cyclophosphamide, dactinomycin, methotrexate, vincristine, and folinic acid.

A 1993 report described return of ovulation in 25 women under 40 years of age from a group of 34 patients treated with etoposide for gestational trophoblastic disease (13). Nine apparently healthy infants were delivered from the group. In another study, 12 women with methotrexate-resistant gestational trophoblastic disease were treated with etoposide (100 mg/m^2/day $\times$ 5 days every 10 days) (14). Two of the women had successful pregnancies, 3 and 4 years, respectively, after treatment.

Etoposide (200 mg/m^2/day $\times$ 5 days) was successfully used to treat a cervical pregnancy in one woman (15). Her baseline menstrual function returned 60 days after completion of therapy, but it was not stated if she attempted to conceive. A man, who had received etoposide for acute nonlymphoblastic leukemia in a cumulative dose of 3193 mg/m^2, fathered two children, one of whom had a unspecified birthmark (16). There is no evidence that the treatment, that also included irradiation to the brain and lumbar spine, vincristine, thioguanine, doxorubicin, cyclophosphamide, and cytarabine, resulted in the birth defect.

Occupational exposure of the mother to antineoplastic agents during pregnancy may present a risk to the fetus. A position statement from the National Study Commission on Cytotoxic Exposure and a research article involving some antineoplastic agents are presented in the monograph for cyclophosphamide (see Cyclophosphamide).

BREASTFEEDING SUMMARY

Etoposide is excreted into breast milk (17). After delivery of a healthy, 2960-g female at 34 weeks' gestation, a 28-year-old woman with acute promyelocytic leukemia in remission (see Mitoxantrone for details of treatment during gestation) was treated with a second consolidation course of cytarabine and mitoxantrone followed by a third consolidation course consisting of etoposide (80 mg/m^2, days 1–5), mitoxantrone (6 mg/m^2, days 1–3), and cytarabine (170 mg/m^2, days 1–5). She maintained milk secretion by pumping her breasts during the chemotherapy courses. The peak milk concentrations of etoposide measured on days 3, 4, and 5 of therapy were approximately (exact concentrations or times of sample collections were not specified) 0.6, 0.6, and 0.8 mcg/mL, respectively. Milk concentrations of etoposide were undetectable within 24 hours of drug administration on each day. The rapid disappearance of etoposide from the milk is compatible with the lack of plasma accumulation and an elimination half-life of 4–11 hours in adults (1). Against medical advice, the mother began breastfeeding 21 days after drug administration (see Mitoxantrone).

Because of the potential for severe toxicity in a nursing infant, such as bone marrow depression, alopecia, and carcinogenicity, breastfeeding should be stopped for at least 55 hours after the last dose of etoposide to account for the elimination half-life range noted above. However, if other antineoplastic agents have also been administered, breastfeeding should be withheld until all of the agents have been eliminated from the mother's system.

References

1. Product information. VePesid. Bristol-Myers Squibb Oncology, 2000.
2. Sieber SM, Whang-Peng J, Botkin C, Knutsen T. Teratogenic and cytogenic effects of some plant-derived antitumor agents (vincristine, colchicine, maytansine, VP-16-213 and VM-26) in mice. Teratology 1978;18:31–47.

3. Mirkes PE, Zwelling LA. Embryotoxicity of the intercalating agents in m-AMSA and o-AMSA and the epipodophyllotoxin VP-16 in postimplantation rat embryos in vitro. Teratology 1990;41:679–88.
4. Buller RE, Darrow V, Manetta A, Porto M, DiSaia PJ. Conservative surgical management of dysgerminoma concomitant with pregnancy. Obstet Gynecol 1992;79:887–90.
5. Murray NA, Acolet D, Deane M, Price J, Roberts IAG. Fetal marrow suppression after maternal chemotherapy for leukaemia. Arch Dis Child 1994;71:F209–10.
6. Raffles A, Williams J, Costeloe K, Clark P. Transplacental effects of maternal cancer chemotherapy. Case report. Br J Obstet Gynaecol 1989;96:1099–1100.
7. Brunet S, Sureda A, Mateu R, Domingo-Albos A. Full-term pregnancy in a patient diagnosed with acute leukemia treated with a protocol including VP-16. Med Clin (Barc) 1993;100:757–8.
8. Rodriguez JM, Haggag M. VACOP-B chemotherapy for high grade non-Hodgkin's lymphoma in pregnancy. Clin Oncol (R Coll Radiol) 1995;7:319–20.
9. Bakri YN, Pedersen P, Nassar M. Normal pregnancy after curative multiagent chemotherapy for choriocarcinoma with brain metastases. Acta Obstet Gynecol Scand 1991;70:611–3.
10. Bierman PJ, Bagin RG, Jagannath S, Vose JM, Spitzer G, Kessinger A, Dicke KA, Armitage JO. High dose chemotherapy followed by autologous hematopoietic rescue in Hodgkin's disease: long term follow-up in 128 patients. Ann Oncol 1993;4:767–73.
11. Brice P, Pautier P, Marolleau JP, Castaigne S, Gisselbrecht C. Pregnancy after autologous bone marrow transplantation for malignant lymphomas. Nouv Rev Fr Hematol 1994;36:387–8.
12. Bower M, Fife K, Holden L, Paradinas FJ, Rustin GJS, Newlands ES. Chemotherapy for ovarian germ cell tumours. Eur J Cancer 1996;32A: 593–7.
13. Matsui H, Eguchi O, Kimura H, Inaba N, Takamizawa H. The effect of etoposide on ovarian function in patients with gestational trophoblastic disease. Acta Obstet Gynaecol Jpn 1993;45:437–43.
14. Mangili G, Garavaglia E, Frigerio L, Candotti G, Ferrari A. Management of low-risk gestational trophoblastic tumors with etoposide (VP-16) in patients resistant to methotrexate. Gyn Oncol 1996;61:218–20.
15. Segna RA, Mitchell DR, Misas JE. Successful treatment of cervical pregnancy with oral etoposide. Obstet Gynecol 1990;76:945–7.
16. Green DM, Zevon MA, Lowrie G, Seigelstein N, Hall B. Congenital anomalies in children of patients who received chemotherapy for cancer in childhood and adolescence. N Engl J Med 1991;325:141–6.
17. Azuno Y, Kaku K, Fujita N, Okubo M, Kaneko T. Mitoxantrone and etoposide in breast milk. Am J Hematol 1995;48:131–2.

ETRAVIRINE

Antiviral

PREGNANCY RECOMMENDATION: Compatible—Maternal Benefit >>Embryo–Fetal Risk
BREASTFEEDING RECOMMENDATION: Contraindicated

PREGNANCY SUMMARY

There is limited human pregnancy experience with etravirine. No structural defects have been reported. The animal data suggest low risk. If indicated, the drug should not be withheld because of pregnancy.

FETAL RISK SUMMARY

Etravirine is a specific, non-nucleoside reverse transcriptase inhibitor (NNRTI). It is in the same antiviral class as delavirdine, efavirenz, and nevirapine. Etravirine is indicated, in combination with other antiretroviral agents, for the treatment of HIV-1 infection in antiretroviral treatment–experienced adult patients who have evidence of viral replication and HIV-1 strains resistant to an NNRTI and other antiretroviral agents. The drug is metabolized by the liver to metabolites that are at least 90% less active than etravirine. Plasma protein binding of etravirine is 99.6% to albumin and about the same to alpha 1-acid glycoprotein. The elimination half-life is prolonged (41 ± 20 hours) (1).

Animal reproduction studies have been conducted in rats and rabbits. In pregnant rats and rabbits, no evidence of fetal harm was observed at exposures equivalent to the exposure from the recommended human dose of 400 mg/day (1).

Etravirine crosses the human placenta at 34 weeks (2). The etravirine umbilical cord blood concentrations in twins from a mother taking 200 mg twice daily were 577 and 1020 ng/mL. The presence of the drug in fetal blood is consistent with the molecular weight (about 435), prolonged elimination half-life, and lipid solubility.

The Antiretroviral Pregnancy Registry reported, for the period January 1989 through July 2009, prospective data (reported before the outcomes were known) involving 4702 live births that had been exposed during the 1st trimester to one or more antiretroviral agents (3). Congenital defects were noted in 134, a prevalence of 2.8% (95% confidence interval [CI] 2.4–3.4). In the 6100 live births with earliest exposure in the 2nd/3rd trimesters, there were 153 infants with defects (2.5%, 95% CI 2.1–2.9). The prevalence rates for the two periods did not differ significantly. There were 288 infants with birth defects among 10,803 live births with exposure anytime during pregnancy (2.7%, 95% CI 2.4–3.0). The prevalence rate did not differ significantly from the rate expected in a nonexposed population. There were 18 outcomes exposed to etravirine (9 in the 1st trimester and 9 in the 2nd/3rd trimesters) in combination with other antiretroviral agents. There were no birth defects. In reviewing the birth defects of prospective and retrospective (pregnancies reported after the outcomes were known) registered cases, the Registry concluded that, except for isolated cases of neural tube defects with efavirenz exposure, there was no other pattern of anomalies (isolated or syndromic). (See Lamivudine for required statement.)

Two reviews, one in 1996 and the other in 1997, concluded that all women currently receiving antiretroviral therapy should continue to receive the therapy during pregnancy and that treatment of the mother with monotherapy should be considered inadequate (4,5). The same conclusion was reached in a 2003 review with the added admonishment that therapy must be continuous to prevent emergence of resistant viral strains (6). In 2009, the updated U.S. Department of Health and Human Services guidelines for the use of antiretroviral agents in patients infected with HIV-1 continued the recommendation that therapy, with the exception of efavirenz, should be continued during pregnancy (7). If indicated, etravirine should not be withheld in pregnancy because the expected benefit to the HIV-positive mother outweighs the unknown risk to the fetus. Updated guidelines for the use of antiretroviral drugs to reduce perinatal HIV-1 transmission also were released in 2010 (8). Women receiving antiretroviral therapy during pregnancy should continue the therapy but, regardless of the regimen, zidovudine administration is recommended during the intrapartum period to prevent vertical transmission of HIV to the newborn (8). Health care professionals are encouraged to register patients exposed to etravirine during pregnancy in the Antiviral Pregnancy Registry by calling 1-800-258-4263.

BREASTFEEDING SUMMARY

No reports describing the use of etravirine during lactation have been located. The molecular weight (about 435), long elimination half-life (41 ± 20 hours), and lipid solubility suggest that the drug will be excreted into breast milk. However, the high (up to 99.6%) protein binding might limit the amount of exposure. The effect of exposure on a nursing infant is unknown.

Reports on the use of etravirine during human lactation are unlikely, however, because the antiviral agent is used in the treatment of HIV-1 infection. HIV-1 is transmitted in milk, and in developed countries, breastfeeding is not recommended (4,5,7,9–11). In developing countries, breastfeeding is undertaken, despite the risk because no affordable milk substitutes are available. Until 1999, no studies had been published that examined the effect of any antiretroviral therapy on HIV-1 transmission in milk. In that year, a study involving zidovudine was published that measured a 38% reduction in vertical transmission of HIV-1 infection despite breastfeeding when compared with controls (see Zidovudine).

References

1. Product information. Intelence. Tibotec Therapeutics, 2008.
2. Furco A, Gosrani B, Nicholas S, Williams A, Braithwaite W, Pozniak A, Taylor G, Asboe D, Lyall H, Shaw A, Kapembwa M. Successful use of darunavir, etravirine, enfuvirtide and tenofovir/emtricitabine in pregnant woman with multiclass HIV resistance. AIDS 2009;23:434–5.
3. Antiretroviral Pregnancy Registry Steering Committee. *Antiretroviral Pregnancy Registry International Interim Report for 1 January 1989 through 31 July 2009*. Wilmington, NC: Registry Coordinating Center; 2009. Available at www.apregistry.com. Accessed May 29, 2010.
4. Carpenter CCJ, Fischi MA, Hammer SM, Hirsch MS, Jacobsen DM, Katzenstein DA, Montaner JSG, Richman DD, Saag MS, Schooley RT, Thompson MA, Vella S, Yeni PG, Volberding PA. Antiretroviral therapy for HIV infection in 1996. JAMA 1996;276;146–54.
5. Minkoff H, Augenbraun M. Antiretroviral therapy for pregnant women. Am J Obstet Gynecol 1997;176:478–89.
6. Minkoff H. Human immunodeficiency virus infection in pregnancy. Obstet Gynecol 2003;101:797–810.
7. Panel on Antiretroviral Guidelines for Adults and Adolescents. *Guidelines for the Use of Antiretroviral Agents in HIV-1-Infected Adults and Adolescents*. Department of Health and Human Services. December 1, 2009:1–161. Available at http://www.aidsinfo.nih.gov/ContentFiles/AdultandAdolescentGL.pdf. Accessed September 17, 2010:60, 96–8.
8. Panel on Treatment of HIV-Infected Pregnant Women and Prevention of Perinatal Transmission. *Recommendations for Use of Antiretroviral Drugs in Pregnant HIV-1-Infected Women for Maternal Health and Interventions to Reduce Perinatal HIV Transmission in the United States*. May 24, 2010:1–117. Available at http://aidsinfo.nih.gov/ContentFiles/PerinatalGL.pdf. Accessed September 17, 2010:30 (Table 5).
9. Brown ZA, Watts DH. Antiviral therapy in pregnancy. Clin Obstet Gynecol 1990;33:276–89.
10. De Martino M, Tovo P-A, Pezzotti P, Galli L, Massironi E, Ruga E, Floreea F, Plebani A, Gabiano C, Zuccotti GV. HIV-1 transmission through breast-milk: appraisal of risk according to duration of feeding. AIDS 1992;6:991–7.
11. Van de Perre P. Postnatal transmission of human immunodeficiency virus type 1: the breast feeding dilemma. Am J Obstet Gynecol 1995;173:483–7.

ETRETINATE

Vitamin

PREGNANCY RECOMMENDATION: Contraindicated
BREASTFEEDING RECOMMENDATION: No Human Data—Potential Toxicity

PREGNANCY SUMMARY

Etretinate, an orally active synthetic retinoid and vitamin A derivative, is used for the treatment of severe recalcitrant psoriasis. It is contraindicated in pregnant women and in those likely to become pregnant. Following oral administration, etretinate is stored in subcutaneous fat and is slowly released over a prolonged interval (1,2). In some patients after chronic therapy, detectable serum drug levels may occur up to 2.9 years after treatment has been stopped (2,3). Due to this variable excretion pattern, the exact length of time to avoid pregnancy after discontinuing treatment is unknown (2,3).

FETAL RISK SUMMARY

As with other retinoids (see also Isotretinoin and Vitamin A), etretinate is a potent animal teratogen (4). Data accumulated since release of this drug now indicate that it must be considered a human teratogen as well (1–3,5,6).

As of June 1986, a total of 51 pregnancies had occurred during treatment with etretinate (1,7,8). Of these pregnancies, 23 were still ongoing at the time of the reports and were unable to be evaluated (1). In the remaining 28 cases, 17 resulted in normal infants and 3 were normal fetuses after induced abortion. Skeletal anomalies were evident in eight cases: three liveborns, one stillbirth at 5 months, and four induced abortions. In addition, marked cerebral abnormalities, including meningomyeloceles, were observed in the stillborn and in three of the aborted fetuses.

A 1988 correspondence listed 22 documented etretinate exposures during pregnancy in West Germany as of

September 1988 (9). The outcomes of these pregnancies were six induced abortions (no anomalies observed), four spontaneous abortions (no anomalies observed), six normal infants, and six infants with malformations (9).

Fifty-three pregnancies are known to have occurred following discontinuance of etretinate therapy (1,10). Malformations were observed in a fetus and an infant among the 38 pregnancies with known outcomes. In one case, a 22-year-old woman, treated intermittently over 5 years, became pregnant 4 months after etretinate therapy had been stopped (1,11,12). Serum concentrations of etretinate and the metabolite, etretin, were 7 and 8 ng/mL, respectively, during the 8th week of gestation (6 months after the last dose). Following induced abortion at 10 weeks' gestation, the fetus was found to have unilateral skeletal defects of the lower limb consisting of a rudimentary left leg with one toe, missing tibia and fibula, and a hypoplastic femur (11,12). Evaluation of the face, skull, and brain was not possible. The defect was attributed to etretinate.

The second case also involved a 22-year-old woman who conceived 51 weeks after her last dose of etretinate (10). Other than the use of metoclopramide at 8 weeks' gestation for nausea and vomiting, no other drug history was mentioned. A growth-restricted (2850 g, 46 cm long, 3rd percentile) female infant was delivered by cesarean section at 38 weeks' gestation. Multiple congenital anomalies were noted involving the central nervous system, head, face, and heart, which included tetralogy of Fallot, microcephaly, hair whorls, small mandible, asymmetrical nares, protruding ears with malformed antihelices, absent lobules, and enlarged, keyhole-shaped entrances to the external ear canals, strabismus, left peripheral facial nerve paresis, and poor head control. Etretinate was detected in the mother's serum 3.5 months after delivery, but the concentration was below the test's lower limit of accuracy (2 ng/mL). No etretinate was detected in the infant's serum. Etretinate was considered responsible for the defects based partially on the presence of the drug in the mother's serum, and the fact that the pattern of malformation was identical to that observed with isotretinoin, another synthetic retinoid. The author also concluded that women treated with etretinate should avoid conception indefinitely (10).

Some of the defects noted in the above infant are also components of the CHARGE (coloboma, heart defects, choanal atresia, retardation, genital [males only], and ear anomalies) association (13), but in a response, the author of the case immediately above noted that such a relationship does not exclude etretinate as the etiology of the defects (14). Others have questioned whether an indefinite recommendation to avoid pregnancy is practical or necessary (15,16). In West Germany, 2 years of conception avoidance are recommended followed by determination of serum levels of etretinate and its metabolites (16). In six women treated with etretinate from 4 to 78 months, plasma concentrations of the drug were detected after 12 months in three patients (4, 8, and 8 ng/mL) and after 18 months in one patient (10 ng/mL) (16). Two women had no measurable etretinate 12 and 14 months after stopping therapy. The metabolites, acitretin and cis-acitretin, were detectable in two women (at 8 and 18 months) and five women (at 8–18 months).

The range of malformations, as listed by the manufacturer, includes meningomyelocele, meningoencephalocele, multiple synostoses, facial dysmorphia, syndactylies, absence of terminal phalanges, malformations of hip, ankle and forearm, low-set ears, high palate, decreased cranial volume, and alterations of the skull and cervical vertebrae (2).

Pronounced jaundice with elevations of the transaminase enzymes, glutamic-oxaloacetic transaminase and glutamic-pyruvic transaminase, was observed in an otherwise normal male newborn following in utero exposure to etretinate (17). The cause of the liver pathology was unknown. No other abnormalities were observed, and the infant was normal at 5 months of age.

One source has suggested that male patients treated with etretinate should avoid fathering children during treatment; if this does occur, ultrasound of the fetus is indicated (18). Although there is no evidence that etretinate adversely affects sperm, and even if it did, that this could result in birth defects, the authors defended their comment as practicing "defensive" medicine (19, 20).

BREASTFEEDING SUMMARY

It is not known if etretinate is excreted into human milk (2). The closely related retinoid, vitamin A, is excreted (see Vitamin A) and the presence of etretinate in breast milk should be expected. The manufacturer considers use of the drug during lactation to be contraindicated due to the potential for adverse effects (2).

References

1. Orfanos CE, Ehlert R, Gollnick H. The retinoids: a review of their clinical pharmacology and therapeutic use. Drugs 1987;34:459–503.
2. Roche Scientific Summary. *The Clinical Evaluation of Tegison*. Roche Laboratories, Division of Hoffmann-La Roche, Inc, 1986.
3. Anonymous. Etretinate approved. FDA Drug Bull 1986;16:16–7.
4. Kamm JJ. Toxicology, carcinogenicity, and teratogenicity of some orally administered retinoids. J Am Acad Dermatol 1982;6:652–9.
5. Anonymous. Etretinate (Tegison) for skin disease. Drug Ther Bull 1983;21: 9–11.
6. Anonymous. Etretinate for psoriasis. Med Lett Drugs Ther 1987;29:9–10.
7. Happle R, Traupe H, Bounameaux Y, Fisch T. Teratogenicity of etretinate in humans. Dtsch Med Wochenschr 1984;109:1476–80.
8. Rosa FW, Wilk AL, Kelsey FO. Teratogen update: vitamin A congeners. Teratology 1986;33:355–64.
9. Hopf G, Mathias B. Teratogenicity of isotretinoin and etretinate. Lancet 1988;2:1143.
10. Lammer EJ. Embryopathy in infant conceived one year after termination of maternal etretinate. Lancet 1988;2:1080–1.
11. Grote W, Harms D, Janig U, Kietzmann H, Ravens U, Schwarze I. Malformation of fetus conceived 4 months after termination of maternal etretinate treatment. Lancet 1985;1:1276.
12. Kietzmann H, Schwarze I, Grote W, Ravens U, Janig U, Harms D. Fetal malformation after maternal etretinate treatment of Darier's disease. Dtsch Med Wochenschr 1986;111:60–2.
13. Blake KD, Wyse RKH. Embryopathy in infant conceived one year after termination of maternal etretinate: a reappraisal. Lancet 1988;2:1254.
14. Lammer E. Etretinate and pregnancy. Lancet 1989;1:109.
15. Greaves MW. Embryopathy in infant conceived one year after termination of maternal etretinate: a reappraisal. Lancet 1988;2:1254.
16. Rinck G, Gollnick H, Orfanos CE. Duration of contraception after etretinate. Lancet 1989;1:845–6.
17. Jager K, Schiller F, Stech P. Congenital ichthyosiforme erythroderma, pregnancy under aromatic retinoid treatment. Hautarzt 1985;36:150–3.
18. Ellis CN, Voorhees JJ. Etretinate therapy. J Am Acad Dermatol 1987;16: 267–91.
19. Katz R. Etretinate and paternity. J Am Acad Dermatol 1987;17:509.
20. Ellis CN, Voorhees JJ. Etretinate and paternity (reply). J Am Acad Dermatol 1987;17:509.

EVANS BLUE

Dye (Diagnostic)

PREGNANCY RECOMMENDATION: Limited Human Data—Probably Compatible
BREASTFEEDING RECOMMENDATION: No Human Data—Probably Compatible

E

PREGNANCY SUMMARY

No reports linking the use of Evans blue with congenital defects have been located.

FETAL RISK SUMMARY

Evans blue is teratogenic in some animal species (1). The dye has been injected intra-amniotically for diagnosis of ruptured membranes without apparent effect on the fetus except for temporary staining of the skin (2,3). The use of Evans blue during pregnancy for plasma volume determinations has been routine (4–8). No toxicity in the fetus or newborn have been attributed to this use.

BREASTFEEDING SUMMARY

No reports describing the use of Evans blue during lactation have been located.

References

1. Wilson JG. Teratogenic activity of several azo dyes chemically related to trypan blue. Anat Rec 1955;123:313–34.
2. Atley RD, Sutherst JR. Premature rupture of the fetal membranes confirmed by intraamniotic injection of dye (Evans blue T-1824). Am J Obstet Gynecol 1970;108:993–4.
3. Morrison L, Wiseman HJ. Intra-amniotic injection of Evans blue dye. Am J Obstet Gynecol 1972;113:1147.
4. Quinlivan WLG, Brock JA, Sullivan H. Blood volume changes and blood loss associated with labor. I. Correlation of changes in blood volume measured by I^{131}-albumin and Evans blue dye, with measured blood loss. Am J Obstet Gynecol 1970;106:843–9.
5. Sibai BM, Abdella TN, Anderson GD, Dilts PV Jr. Plasma volume findings in pregnant women with mild hypertension: therapeutic considerations. Am J Obstet Gynecol 1983;145:539–44.
6. Goodlin RC, Anderson JC, Gallagher TF. Relationship between amniotic fluid volume and maternal plasma volume expansion. Am J Obstet Gynecol 1983;146:505–11.
7. Hays PM, Cruikshank DP, Dunn LJ. Plasma volume determination in normal and preeclamptic pregnancies. Am J Obstet Gynecol 1985;151: 958–66.
8. Brown MA, Mitar DA, Whitworth JA. Measurement of plasma volume in pregnancy. Clin Sci 1992;83:29–34.

EVENING PRIMROSE OIL

Herb

PREGNANCY RECOMMENDATION: Limited Human Data—Probably Compatible (Labor Induction)
No Human Data—No Relevant Animal Data (Before Term)
BREASTFEEDING RECOMMENDATION: Limited Human Data—Probably Compatible

PREGNANCY SUMMARY

Although there are limited published data, the use of evening primrose oil (EPO) for labor induction is apparently common among nurse-midwives. No adverse effects have been reported in the fetus or newborn. The embryo–fetal risk for other purposes or during other portions of pregnancy is unknown. One source recommended avoiding its use in pregnancy (1).

FETAL RISK SUMMARY

The seeds of evening primrose, a large plant native to North America, contain 14% of oil. It is grown commercially. The oil from the commercial variety of evening primrose contains the fatty acids cis-linoleic acid and gamma-linolenic acid in concentrations of 72% and 9%, respectively. Essential fatty acids are involved in cellular structural elements and as precursors of prostaglandins. Reported uses of EPO in nonpregnant patients include rheumatoid arthritis and diabetic neuropathy. The typical dose used in clinical trials with nonpregnant patients is 6–8 g/day in adults and 2–4 g/day in children (2).

Based on a national survey of nurse-midwifery education programs, EPO was the most frequently mentioned herbal preparation for the induction of labor (3). Twenty-three (64%) of 36 respondents stated that they discussed the use of EPO with their students. The doses prescribed varied widely and included both oral and vaginal doses (3).

A 1999 study examined the effect of EPO on the length of pregnancy (4). Oral doses of EPO from the 37th gestational week until birth did not shorten pregnancy or decrease the overall length of labor, but was associated with an increase in prolonged rupture of membranes, oxytocin augmentation, arrest of descent, and vacuum extraction.

A 2003 review examined the pregnancy outcomes when herbal therapies were used (5). It concluded that EPO was safe for labor induction.

A 2006 randomized, double-blind, placebo controlled trial compared the effects of EPO and placebo on the Bishop score and cervical length in 71 women at term (6). One capsule of EPO (strength not specified) given three times daily for 1 week significantly improved the Bishop score and reduced cervical length compared with placebo. Significantly fewer subjects required cesarean sections compared with placebo. No adverse effects of EPO were observed in fetuses monitored by the biophysical profile and nonstress tests or in the birth weights of newborns (6).

BREASTFEEDING SUMMARY

Fatty acids, such as cis-linoleic and gamma-linolenic, are natural constituents of breast milk (2). In a placebo-controlled trial, 18 subjects were given a total daily dose of 2800-mg linoleic acid and 320 mg of gamma-linoleic acid, whereas 18 controls received placebos (7). The study was conducted for 8 months starting between the 2nd and 6th month of lactation. Not surprisingly, subjects had significantly higher milk concentrations of the fatty acids at the end of the study, whereas controls had decreased levels. No adverse effects were reported in the mothers or infants (7).

References

1. Evening Primrose Oil. *Natural Medicines Comprehensive Database*. 5th ed. Stockton, CA: Therapeutic Research Faculty, 2003:531–3.
2. Evening Primrose Oil. *The Review of Natural Products*. St. Louis, MO: Wolters Kluwer Health, 2006.
3. NcFarlin BL, Gibson MH, O'Rear J, Harman P. A national survey of herbal preparation use by nurse-midwives for labor stimulation. J Nurse-Midwifery 1999;44:205–16.
4. Dove D, Johnson P. Oral primrose oil: its effect on length of pregnancy and selected intrapartum outcomes in low-risk nulliparous women. J Nurse Midwifery 1999;44:320–4.
5. Johns T, Sibeko L. Pregnancy outcomes in women using herbal therapies. Birth Defects Res (Part B) 2003;68:501–4.
6. Ty-Torredes KA. The effect of oral evening primrose oil on Bishop score and cervical length among term gravidas (abstract). Am J Obstet Gynecol 2006;195:S30.
7. Cant A, Shay J, Horrobin DF. The effect of maternal supplementation with linoleic and γ-linolenic acids on the fat composition and content of human milk: a placebo-controlled study. J Nutr Sci Vitaminol 1991;37:573–9.

EVEROLIMUS

Antineoplastic (mTOR Inhibitor)

PREGNANCY RECOMMENDATION: Limited Human Data—Animal Data Suggest Moderate Risk
BREASTFEEDING RECOMMENDATION: Contraindicated

PREGNANCY SUMMARY

Only two reports describing the use of everolimus in human pregnancy have been located and, in both cases, normal infant outcomes occurred. Severe embryo toxicities, in the absence of maternal toxicity, were observed in one animal species at exposures much lower than those occurring in humans taking the recommended dose. The limited human pregnancy experience prevents a full assessment of the embryo–fetal risk. The manufacturer advices women of childbearing potential to use an effective method of contraception during treatment and for up 8 weeks after ending treatment (1). If a woman becomes pregnant while receiving everolimus, she should be advised of the potential for embryo–fetal harm.

FETAL RISK SUMMARY

Everolimus is a mTOR inhibitor (mammalian target of rapamycin) that is available as oral tablets. It is indicated for the treatment of various cancers and for prophylaxis of organ rejection in kidney and liver transplantation. The other agent in this subclass is temsirolimus. After oral absorption, everolimus is metabolized to relatively inactive metabolites. Plasma protein binding is about 74% and the mean elimination half-life is about 30 hours (1, 2). Everolimus is a derivative of sirolimus (see Sirolimus) (3). Reproduction studies have been conducted in rats and rabbits. Oral doses given to rats before mating and through organogenesis resulted in increased resorptions, preimplantation and postimplantation loss decreased number of live fetuses, malformation (e.g., sternal cleft), and retarded skeletal development. The embryo–fetal toxicities occurred at about 4% of the exposure (AUC) in patients receiving the recommended human dose (RHD) of 10 mg/day and in the absence of maternal toxicity. In a prenatal and postnatal study with rats, no adverse effects on delivery or lactation or maternal toxicity were noted at a dose that was about 10% of the RHD based on BSA. However, this dose was associated with a slight reduction in pup body weight and survival, but no drug-related effects on offspring development were observed. In rabbits, embryotoxicity as evident as an increase in resorptions occurred at a dose that was about 1.6 times the RHD based on BSA. However, maternal toxicity also was evident (1).

Two-year studies for carcinogenicity in mice and rats were negative, as were multiple assays for genotoxic and mutagenic effects. Everolimus caused infertility in male rats that was partially reversible when the drug exposure was stopped. In female rats, the increases in preimplantation loss suggested that the drug may reduce female fertility (1).

It is not known if everolimus crosses the human placenta. The molecular weight (about 958), moderate plasma protein binding, and long elimination half-life suggest that the drug will cross to the embryo–fetus.

In a 2011 case report, a woman with a kidney transplant conceived while receiving everolimus (4). The pregnancy was discovered at 12 weeks' gestation. Because of worsening renal function, proteinuria, and severe hypertension during week 30, a cesarean section was performed to deliver a 1.280-kg healthy female infant with an Apgar score of 10. No congenital anomalies were noted. The infant had normal growth without detectable disorders at 12 months of age (4).

A 2012 case report described the pregnancy outcome of a woman who had received a kidney transplant 4 years before conceiving (5). The woman received everolimus, cyclosporine, and corticosteroids throughout pregnancy. At term, she gave birth to a healthy, 3.020-kg infant with an initial Apgar score of 9. The child was in good health at 3 years of age (5).

BREASTFEEDING SUMMARY

No reports describing the use of everolimus during human lactation have been located. The molecular weight (about 958), moderate (about 74%) plasma protein binding, and long (about 30 hours) elimination half-life suggest that the drug will be excreted into breast milk. Based on animal data, the concentration in milk may exceed the maternal plasma concentration. The effect of this exposure on a nursing infant is unknown. However, marked toxicity has been observed in adults, such as gastrointestinal disorders (stomatitis, diarrhea, nausea, vomiting), infections, anorexia, respiratory (cough, dyspnea, epistaxis, pneumonitis), skin and subcutaneous disorders, headache, and other toxicities.

E

References

1. Product information. Afinitor. Novartis Pharmaceuticals, 2012.
2. Product information. Zortress. Novartis Pharmaceuticals, 2013.
3. Halloran PF. Immunosuppressive drugs for kidney transplantation. N Engl J Med 2004;351:2715–29.
4. Veroux M, Corona D, Veroux P. Pregnancy under everolimus-based immunosuppression. Trans Int 2011;24:e115–7.
5. Carta P, Caroti L, Zanazzi M. Pregnancy in a kidney transplant patient treated with everolimus. Am J Kidney Dis 2012;60:329.

EXEMESTANE

Antineoplastic (Hormone)

PREGNANCY RECOMMENDATION: Contraindicated
BREASTFEEDING RECOMMENDATION: Contraindicated

PREGNANCY SUMMARY

No reports describing the use of exemestane in human pregnancy have been located. The animal data suggest moderate risk. The antineoplastic is indicated for postmenopausal women with breast cancer who have been treated with tamoxifen for 2–3 years. The drug prevents the conversion of androgens to estrogen. Because estrogen is required to maintain pregnancy, exemestane is contraindicated in pregnancy.

FETAL RISK SUMMARY

Exemestane is an oral steroidal aromatase inactivator that binds irreversibly to the enzyme, thus preventing conversion of androgens to estrogen both in pre- and postmenopausal women. It is indicated for adjuvant treatment of postmenopausal women with estrogen-receptor positive early breast cancer who have received 2–3 years of tamoxifen and are changed to exemestane for completion of a total of 5 consecutive years of adjuvant hormonal therapy. The drug is extensively metabolized in inactive or minimally active compounds. Plasma protein binding to albumin and α_1-acid glycoprotein is 90%. The mean terminal half-life is about 24 hours (1).

Reproduction studies have been conducted in rats and rabbits. When rats were given a daily dose that was about 1.5 times the recommended human daily dose based on BSA (RHDD) from 14 days before mating to day 15 or 20 of gestation, an increase in placental weight was observed. At doses about ≥8 times the RHDD, prolonged gestation, abnormal or difficult labor, increased resorption, reduced number of live fetuses, decreased fetal weight, and retarded ossification were observed. No malformations were observed with doses that were about 320 times the RHDD. Exemestane and its metabolites crossed the rat placenta at doses about equal to the RHDD resulting in approximately equal concentrations in maternal and fetal blood. In rabbits, daily doses given during organogenesis that were about 70 times the RHDD caused a decrease in placental weight. At about 210 times the RHDD, abortions, an increase in resorptions, and a decrease in fetal body weight occurred but no increase in malformations occurred (1,2).

A 2-year carcinogenicity study in mice resulted in an increased incidence of hepatocellular adenomas and/or carcinomas in both males and females, and an increased incidence of renal tubular adenomas in males. The doses used in male and female mice produced plasma AUC levels that were 34 and 75 times the AUC in postmenopausal patients at the recommended clinical dose. No evidence of carcinogenicity was observed in a separate study with rats. The drug was not mutagenic in two assays and was not clastogenic in an in vivo assay. In fertility studies, untreated female rats showed reduced fertility when mated with male rats given doses of exemestane that were ≥200 times the RHDD (1,2).

It is not known if exemestane or its metabolites cross the human placenta. The molecular weight (about 296) and long elimination half-life suggest that exposure of the embryo and/or fetus to the parent drug and metabolites will occur.

BREASTFEEDING SUMMARY

No reports describing the use exemestane during human lactation have been located. The molecular weight (about 296) and long elimination half-life (about 24 hours) suggest that the drug will be excreted into breast milk. The effect of this exposure on a nursing infant is unknown. However, because the drug prevents conversion of androgens to estrogen, breastfeeding is contraindicated if the woman is receiving exemestane.

References

1. Product information. Aromasin. Pharmacia & Upjohn Company, 2008.
2. Beltrame D, di Salle E, Giavini E, Gunnarsson K, Brughera M. Reproductive toxicity of exemestane, an antitumoral aromatase inactivator, in rats and rabbits. Reprod Toxicol 2001;195–213.

EXENATIDE

Antidiabetic Agent

PREGNANCY RECOMMENDATION: No Human Data—Animal Data Suggest Moderate Risk
BREASTFEEDING RECOMMENDATION: No Human Data—Probably Compatible

PREGNANCY SUMMARY

No reports describing the use of exenatide in human pregnancy have been located. The developmental toxicity (structural anomalies, neonatal death) that was observed in one animal species suggests moderate risk. However, the absence of any human pregnancy experience prevents a more-complete assessment of the embryo–fetal risk. Until such data are available, the best course is to avoid exenatide in pregnancy.

FETAL RISK SUMMARY

Exenatide (also known as exendin-4) enhances glucose-dependent insulin secretion from pancreatic beta cells, suppresses inappropriately elevated glucagon secretion, and slows gastric emptying (1). It is a 39-amino acid peptide amide that is administered SC. Exenatide is indicated as adjunctive therapy to improve glycemic control in patients with type 2 diabetes mellitus who are taking metformin, a sulfonylurea, or a combination of these agents but have not achieved adequate glycemic control. It is eliminated primarily by glomerular filtration with subsequent proteolytic degradation. The mean elimination half-life is 2.4 hours (1).

Reproduction studies with exenatide have been conducted in mice and rabbits. No evidence of fetal harm was observed in mice given SC doses producing systemic exposures up to 390 times the exposure from the maximum recommended human dose based on AUC (MRHD) before and during mating, and through day 7 of gestation. During organogenesis (days 6 through 15), reduced fetal and neonatal growth, cleft palates (some with holes), and irregular skeletal ossification of rib and skull bones were observed at SC doses producing systemic exposures three times the MRHD. An increase in neonatal deaths was noted on postpartum days 2–4 with an SC dose producing a systemic exposure three times the MRHD from day 6 through lactation day 20 (weaning) (1).

In pregnant rabbits, irregular skeletal ossifications were observed with an SC dose producing a systemic exposure 12 times the MRHD during organogenesis (days 6 through 18) (1).

No evidence of carcinogenicity was observed in mice given SC doses resulting in systemic exposures up to 95 times the MRHD over a 2-year period. In a 2-year study in female rats, however, a dose-related increase in benign thyroid C-cell adenomas was observed with systemic exposures that were 5–130 times the MRHD. Exenatide was not mutagenic or clastogenic in various assays and did not impair fertility in mice in a 4-week study with an exposure 390 times the MRHD (1).

A 2003 ex vivo study using single human cotyledons from healthy term placentas investigated whether exenatide crossed the placenta (2). Consistent with the drug's high molecular weight (about 4187) and the short elimination half-life, the fetal:maternal ratio was ≤0.017. Although these results might not be reproducible throughout gestation, it is likely that embryo and/or fetal exposure to exenatide is negligible.

BREASTFEEDING SUMMARY

No reports describing the use of exenatide during human lactation have been located. The high molecular weight (about 4187) and short elimination half-life (2.4 hours) suggest that clinically insignificant amounts will be excreted into breast milk. What little is excreted will probably be digested in the stomach of the nursing infant. Therefore, although the effect of the exposure on a nursing infant is unknown, the risk appears to be negligible. Nevertheless, blood glucose monitoring of the infant should be considered.

References

1. Product information. Byetta. Amylin Pharmaceuticals, 2005.
2. Hiles RA, Bawdon RE, Petrella EM. Ex vivo human placental transfer of the peptides pramlintide and exenatide (synthetic exendin-4). Hum Exp Toxicol 2003;22:623–8.

EZETIMIBE

Antilipemic Agent

PREGNANCY RECOMMENDATION: No Human Data—Animal Data Suggest Moderate Risk
BREASTFEEDING RECOMMENDATION: No Human Data—Potential Toxicity

E

PREGNANCY SUMMARY

No reports describing the use of ezetimibe in human pregnancy have been located. Although the animal data suggest low risk, the lack of human pregnancy experience prevents an assessment of the risk this agent presents to the embryo and fetus. Generally, discontinuing treatment of hypercholesterolemia during pregnancy is not thought to put the mother at risk. If treatment during pregnancy is mandated, ezetimibe appears to be a better choice than treatment with HMG-CoA reductase inhibitors (i.e., "statins" are contraindicated) or the fibric acid derivative fenofibrate.

FETAL RISK SUMMARY

Ezetimibe selectively inhibits the intestinal absorption of cholesterol and related phytosterols. It is indicated, either alone or in combination with HMG-CoA reductase inhibitors, as adjunctive therapy to diet for the reduction of cholesterol and triglycerides in patients with primary hypercholesterolemia. Ezetimibe is extensively metabolized in the small intestine and liver and both the parent compound and the metabolite are pharmacologically active. In addition, both are highly bound (>90%) to plasma proteins and have an elimination half-life of about 22 hours (1,2).

Reproduction studies have been conducted in rats and rabbits. In rats, there was no evidence of impaired fertility or embryolethal effects at doses up to about 10 times the human exposure at 10 mg/day based on AUC for total ezetimibe (HD). At the highest dose, increased incidences of skeletal abnormalities (extra pair of thoracic ribs, unossified cervical vertebral centra, and shortened ribs) were noted. In rabbits, doses up to about 150 times the HD did not cause embryolethal effects, but an increased incidence of extra thoracic ribs was observed (1,2).

No evidence of carcinogenicity was observed in mice and rats administered high doses over a 2-year period. There was also no evidence of mutagenic, clastogenic, or genotoxic effects with various other assays (1,2).

It is not known if ezetimibe or its active metabolite crosses the human placenta. The parent compound does cross the rat and rabbit placentas (1,2). The molecular weight (about 409 for the parent compound) and prolonged elimination half-life suggest that passage to the human embryo and/or fetus will occur, but the high plasma protein binding should limit the transfer.

BREASTFEEDING SUMMARY

No reports describing the use of ezetimibe during human lactation have been located. The molecular weight (about 409 for the parent compound) and the prolonged elimination half-life (about 22 hours) for both ezetimibe and its active metabolite suggest that the drug and/or its metabolite will be excreted into breast milk. However, the high plasma protein binding (>90%) should limit the amount excreted. The effect on a nursing infant from this exposure is unknown. If ezetimibe is taken during lactation, the nursing infant should be closely observed for adverse effects that are commonly seen in adults (e.g., headache, diarrhea, pharyngitis, sinusitis, arthralgia).

References

1. Product information. Zetia. Merck/Schering-Plough Pharmaceuticals, 2004.
2. Product information. Zetia. Schering, 2004.

EZOGABINE

Anticonvulsant

PREGNANCY RECOMMENDATION: No Human Data—Animal Data Suggest Risk
BREASTFEEDING RECOMMENDATION: No Human Data—Potential Toxicity

PREGNANCY SUMMARY

No reports describing the use of ezogabine in human pregnancy have been located. The animal data in two species suggest risk but the absence of human pregnancy experience prevents a better assessment. If a woman becomes pregnant while taking the drug or is prescribed the drug during pregnancy, she should be advised of the absence of human data and the potential risk to her embryo and/or fetus. Pregnant women taking ezogabine are encouraged to enroll in the North American Antiepileptic Drug Pregnancy Registry by calling the toll-free number 1-800-233-2334.

E

FETAL RISK SUMMARY

Ezogabine is a potassium channel opener that is available as oral tablets. It is indicated as adjunctive treatment of partial-onset seizures in patients aged 18 years and older. Ezogabine is metabolized to an *N*-acetyl metabolite (NAMR) that has antiepileptic activity but less than the parent drug, as well as inactive metabolites. Plasma protein binding of ezogabine and NAMR are about 80% and 45%, respectively, whereas the elimination half-lives are 7–11 hours for both molecules (1).

Reproductive studies have been conducted in rats and rabbits. In rats given ezogabine during organogenesis, fetal skeletal variations were observed. When the drug was given throughout pregnancy and lactation, increased prenatal and postnatal mortality, decreased body weight gain, and delayed reflex development in the offspring were observed. The no-effect dose for embryo–fetal toxicity in both of these periods produced maternal plasma exposures (AUC) of ezogabine and NAMR that were less than those in humans at the maximum recommended human dose (MRHD). In rabbits, exposure throughout organogenesis resulted in decreased fetal body weights and increased incidences of fetal skeletal variations. The no-effect dose for embryo–fetal toxicity was associated with plasma levels of ezogabine and NAMR that were less than those in humans at the MRHD. In both rats and rabbits, the maximum doses evaluated were by maternal toxicity (acute neurotoxicity) (1).

In a 1-year study, a dose-related increased in the frequency of lung neoplasms was noted in male mice. No evidence of carcinogenicity was observed in a 2-year study in rats. In studies for mutagenicity with ezogabine, three assays were negative and one was positive. For assays with NAMR, one was negative and one was positive. In male and female rats, ezogabine had no effect on fertility, reproductive performance, or early embryonic development at doses producing a plasma ezogabine exposure (AUC) less than that in humans at the MRHD (1).

It is not known if ezogabine or its active metabolite NAMR crosses the placenta. The molecular weight of ezogabine (about 303), and the moderate plasma protein binding and long elimination half-lives of the parent drug and active metabolite suggest that both will cross to the embryo–fetus.

BREASTFEEDING SUMMARY

No reports describing the use of ezogabine during human lactation have been located. The molecular weight of ezogabine (about 303) and the moderate plasma protein binding (80% for ezogabine; 45% for the active metabolite [NAMR]) and long elimination half-lives (7–11 hours for both) suggest that ezogabine and NAMR will be excreted into breast milk. Although the systemic absorption in infants is unknown, the parent drug is well absorbed in adults. The drug is best avoided during breastfeeding because of the concern for clinically significant toxicity in a nursing infant.

Reference

1. Product information. Potiga. GlaxoSmithKline, 2012.

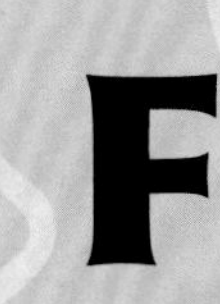

FACTOR XIII CONCENTRATE (HUMAN)

Hematologic Agent (Antihemophilic)

PREGNANCY RECOMMENDATION: Compatible
BREASTFEEDING RECOMMENDATION: Compatible

PREGNANCY SUMMARY

Factor XIII concentrate (human) (FXIII) is a necessary therapy for patients with congenital deficiency of FXIII. In women without such therapy, severe bleeding will occur, as well as abortions if they become pregnant.

FETAL RISK SUMMARY

FXIII is a heat-treated, lyophilized coagulation factor XIII concentrate made from pooled human plasma. It is an endogenous plasma glycoprotein consisting of two A-subunits and two B-subunits that circulates in blood and is present in platelets, monocytes, and macrophages. FXIII is indicated for routine IV prophylactic treatment of congenital FXIII deficiency. The effectiveness of the product is based on maintaining a trough FXIII activity of about 5%–20%. The half-life of FXIII is about 6.6 days (1).

Reproduction studies in animal have not been conducted.

Congenital FXIII deficiency is associated with severe bleeding, impaired wound healing and, in pregnancy, a high risk of spontaneous abortions (2–4). Several sources have described the use of FXIII throughout pregnancy to prevent these complications (5–11). Because FXIII is an endogenous substance, no adverse effects were expected or reported in the offspring of exposed pregnancies.

BREASTFEEDING SUMMARY

No reports describing the use of FXIII during human lactation have been located. However, congenital FXIII deficiency is a life-threatening disorder. FXIII is an endogenous glycoprotein and excretion into breast milk should not occur. However, even if small amounts were excreted during the colostral phase, it should be digested in the infant's gut and have no effect on a nursing infant. Consequently, if a mother with this condition chooses to breastfeed her infant, FXIII should not be withheld.

References

1. Product information. Corifact. CSL Behring, 2012.
2. Asahina T, Kobayashi T, Okada Y, Itoh M, Yamashita M, Inamoto Y, Terao T. Studies on the role of adhesive proteins in maintaining pregnancy. Horm Res 19988;50(Suppl 2):37–45.
3. Hsiseh L, Nugent D. Factor XIII deficiency. Haemophilia 2008;14:1190–1200.
4. Karimi M, Bereczky Z, Cohan N, Muszbek L. Factor XIII deficiency. Semin Thromb Hemost 2009;35:426–38.
5. Rodeghiero F, Castaman GC, Di Bona E, Ruggeri M, Dini E. Successful pregnancy in a woman with congenital factor XIII deficiency treat with substitutive therapy. Blut 1987;55:45–8.
6. Kobayashi T, Terao T, Kojima T, Takamatsu J, Kamiya T, Saito H. Congenital factor XIII deficiency with treatment of factor XIII concentrate and normal vaginal delivery. Gynecol Obstet Invest 1990;29:235–8.
7. Burrows RF, Ray JG, Burrows EA. Bleeding risk and reproductive capacity among patients with factor XIII deficiency: a case presentation and review of the literature. Obstet Gynecol Surv 2000;55:103–8.
8. Asahina T, Kobayashi T, Okada Y, Goto J, Terao T. Maternal blood coagulation factor XIII is associated with the development of cytotrophoblastic shell. Placenta 2000;21:388–93.
9. Ichinose A, Asahina T, Kobayashi T. Congenital blood coagulation factor XIII deficiency and perinatal management. Curr Drug Targets 2005;6:541–9.
10. Asahina T, Kobayashi T, Takeuchi K, Kanayama N. Congenital blood coagulation factor XIII deficiency and successful deliveries: a review of the literature. Obstet Gynecol Surv 2007;62:255–60.
11. Takahashi T, Hatao K, Suzukawa M, Oji T. Congenital factor XIII deficiency required high-dose factor XIII concentrate in late pregnancy. Rinsho Ketsueki 2007;48:418–20.

FAMCICLOVIR

Antiviral

PREGNANCY RECOMMENDATION: Limited Human Data—Animal Data Suggest Low Risk
BREASTFEEDING RECOMMENDATION: No Human Data—Potential Toxicity

PREGNANCY SUMMARY

The limited human pregnancy experience and the animal reproductive data suggest that the risk for the embryo–fetus is low. The manufacturer (Novartis Pharmaceuticals) maintains a pregnancy registry to monitor the maternal–fetal outcomes of women exposed to famciclovir during pregnancy (1). Patients can be registered by calling (888) 669-6682.

FETAL RISK SUMMARY

Famciclovir is a prodrug administered orally for the treatment of infections involving herpes simplex virus types 1 and 2, or varicella zoster virus. After administration, the drug undergoes rapid biotransformation to penciclovir, the active antiviral compound. Specific indications are the treatment of recurrent episodes of genital herpes and the management of acute herpes zoster (shingles) (1).

Carcinogenic, but not embryotoxic or teratogenic, effects were observed in animal studies with famciclovir. A significant increase in the incidence of mammary adenocarcinoma was seen in female rats administered famciclovir 600 mg/kg/day, 1.5–9.0 times the levels achieved with the recommended human doses based on AUC comparisons for penciclovir. At this dose in female rats and at doses ≤2.4 times the human dose (AUC comparison) in male mice, marginal increases in the incidence of SC tissue fibrosarcomas and squamous cell carcinomas of the skin were observed. The tumors, however, were not observed in male rats and female mice. The reason for these gender differences is apparently unknown (1).

Both famciclovir and the active metabolite, penciclovir, were tested for teratogenicity in pregnant rats and rabbits. Based on the penciclovir levels achieved with the recommended human doses (AUC comparison), oral doses of famciclovir 2.7–10.8 times (rats) and 1.4–5.4 times (rabbits) those concentrations had no effect on embryo and fetal development. IV famciclovir also had no effect on embryo and fetal development in either the rat or the rabbit at doses up to 1.5–6 and 1.1–4.5 times, respectively, the human dose, based on BSA (HD). A similar lack of toxicity was observed with IV penciclovir at doses in pregnant rats and rabbits 0.3–1.3 and 0.5–2.1 times, respectively, the HD (1).

It is not known whether famciclovir or its active metabolite, penciclovir, crosses the placenta to the fetus. Because of the molecular weight of famciclovir (about 321), passage to the fetus should be expected.

A 1998 noninterventional observational cohort study described the outcomes of pregnancies in women who had been prescribed one or more of 34 newly marketed drugs by general practitioners in England (2). Data were obtained by questionnaires sent to the prescribing physicians one month after the expected or possible date of delivery. Of 1067 exposed pregnancies, famciclovir was taken during the 1st trimester in 7 pregnancies. The outcomes of these pregnancies included one ectopic pregnancy; two missed abortions; and four normal, full-term infants.

A 2010 review on the safety of famciclovir in all types of patients stated that the drug should be avoided in pregnant and lactating women because of the lack of data (3).

BREASTFEEDING SUMMARY

No studies describing the use of famciclovir during breastfeeding have been located. The drug is probably excreted into human milk and there is a potential for toxicity. Until human data are available, women taking famciclovir should not breastfeed (3).

References

1. Product information. Famvir. Novartis Pharmaceuticals, 2007.
2. Wilton LV, Pearce GL, Martin RM, Mackay FJ, Mann RD. The outcomes of pregnancy in women exposed to newly marketed drugs in general practice in England. Br J Obstet Gynaecol 1998;105:882–9.
3. Mubareka S, Leung V, Aoki FY, Vinh DC. Famciclovir: a focus on efficacy and safety. Expert Opin Drug Saf 2010;9:643–58.

FAMOTIDINE

Gastrointestinal Agent (Antisecretory)

PREGNANCY RECOMMENDATION: Compatible
BREASTFEEDING RECOMMENDATION: Limited Human Data—Probably Compatible

PREGNANCY SUMMARY

The animal reproductive data suggest low risk, but the human pregnancy experience is limited. Nevertheless, there is no evidence that histamine H_2-receptor antagonists pose a clinically significant risk to the embryo or fetus. A study showing an association between in utero exposure to gastric acid suppressors and childhood allergy and asthma requires confirmation.

FETAL RISK SUMMARY

Famotidine, a reversible competitive inhibitor of histamine H_2-receptors (H2 blockers), is more potent than either cimetidine or ranitidine. It is indicated for the treatment of gastric and duodenal ulcers, in the treatment of gastroesophageal reflux disease (GERD), and in the therapy of pathologic hypersecretory conditions, such as Zollinger-Ellison syndrome. The drug undergoes minimal first-pass metabolism. Plasma protein binding is low (15%–20%) and the elimination half-life is 2.5–3.5 hours (1).

Reproduction studies have been conducted in rats and rabbits. No significant evidence of impaired fertility or harm to the fetus at oral doses up to 2000 and 500 mg/kg/day (comparison to the human dose not stated), respectively, or IV doses up to 200 mg/kg/day in both species were observed. Sporadic abortions were observed in rabbits given maternal toxic (decreased food intake) oral doses that were 250 times the usual human dose (1). In published studies in rats and rabbits, using oral doses ≤2000 mg/kg/day and IV doses of 100–200 mg/kg/day, found no evidence of impaired fertility, fetotoxic effects, teratogenicity, or changes in postnatal behavior attributable to famotidine (2,3).

Famotidine is known to cross the term human placenta based on in vitro studies (4). This is consistent with the molecular weight (about 337), low plasma protein binding, and the elimination half-life.

In a surveillance study of Michigan Medicaid recipients involving 229,101 completed pregnancies conducted between 1985 and 1992, 33 newborns had been exposed to famotidine during the 1st trimester (F. Rosa, personal communication, FDA, 1993). Two (6.1%) major birth defects were observed (one expected). No anomalies were observed in six defect categories (cardiovascular defects, oral clefts, spina bifida, polydactyly, limb reduction defects, and hypospadias) for which specific data were available. The number of exposures is too small to draw any conclusions.

A 1996 prospective cohort study compared the pregnancy outcomes of 178 women who were exposed during pregnancy to H2 blockers with 178 controls matched for maternal age, smoking, and heavy alcohol consumption (5). All of the women had contacted a teratology information service concerning gestational exposure to H2 blockers (subjects) or nonteratogenic or nonfetotoxic agents (controls). Among subjects (mean daily dose in parentheses), 71% took ranitidine (258 mg), 16% cimetidine (487 mg), 8% famotidine (32 mg), and 5% nizatidine (283 mg). There were no significant differences between the outcomes of subjects and controls in terms of live births, spontaneous abortions (SABs) and elective abortions (EABs), gestational age at birth, delivery method, birth weight, infants small for gestational age, or major malformations. Among subjects, there were 3 birth defects (2.1%) among the 142 exposed to H2 blockers in the 1st trimester: one each of atrial septal defect, ventricular septal defect, and tetralogy of Fallot. There were 5 birth defects (3.0%) among the 165 exposed anytime during pregnancy. For controls, the rates of defects were 3.5% (1st trimester) and 3.1% (anytime). There were also no differences between the groups in neonatal health problems and developmental milestones, but two children (one subject and one control) were diagnosed as developmentally delayed. The investigators concluded that 1st trimester exposure to H2 blockers did not represent a major teratogenic risk (5).

Data from the Swedish Medical Birth Registry were presented in 1998 (6). A total of 553 infants (6 sets of twins) were delivered from 547 women who had used acid-suppressing drugs early in pregnancy. Famotidine was the only acid-suppressing drug exposure in 58 infants. Three other offspring were exposed in utero to famotidine combined either with cimetidine (one infant) or with ranitidine (two infants). The odds ratio (OR) for malformations after H2 blockers was 0.86, 95% confidence interval (CI) 0.33–2.23. Of the 19 infants with birth defects, 9 had been exposed to H2 blockers, 1 of whom had also been exposed to omeprazole. No birth defects were observed in those exposed to famotidine (see Omeprazole for additional details of this study) (6).

A population-based observational cohort study formed by linking data from three Swedish national healthcare registers over a 10-year period (1995–2004) was reported in 2009 (7). The main outcome measures were a diagnosis of allergic disease or a prescription for asthma or allergy medications. The drug types included in the study were gastric acid suppressors, including H2 blockers, prostaglandins, proton pump inhibitors, combinations for eradication of *Helicobacter pylori*, and drugs for peptic ulcer and gastroesophageal reflux disease. Of 585,716 children, 29,490 (5.0%) met the diagnosis and 5645 (1%) had been exposed to gastric acid suppression therapy in pregnancy. Of these children, 405 (0.07%) were treated for allergic disease. For developing allergy, the OR was 1.43, 98% CI 1.29–1.59, irrespective of the drug, time of exposure during pregnancy, and maternal history of allergy. For developing childhood asthma, but not other allergic diseases, the OR was 1.51, 95% CI 1.35–1.69, irrespective of the type of acid-suppressive drug and the time of exposure in pregnancy. The authors proposed three possible mechanisms for their findings: (i) exposure to increased amounts of allergens could cause sensitization to digestion labile antigens in the fetus; (ii) maternal Th2 cytokine pattern could promote an allergy-prone phenotype in the fetus; and (iii) maternal allergen-specific IgE could cross the placenta and sensitize fetal immune cells to food and airborne allergens. Several limitations of the study that might have affected their findings were identified, including a general increase in childhood asthma but not necessarily an increase in allergic asthma (7). The study requires confirmation.

A 2005 study evaluated the outcomes of 553 pregnancies after exposure to H2 blockers, 501 (91%) in the 1st trimester (8). The data were collected by the European Network of Teratology Information Services (ENTIS). The agents and number of cases were famotidine 75, cimetidine 113, nizatidine 15, ranitidine 335, and roxatidine 15. No increase in the number of major malformations were noted (8).

A 2009 meta-analysis of published studies was conducted to assess the safety of H2 blockers that were used in 2398 pregnancies (9). Compared with 119,892 nonexposed pregnancies, the OR for congenital malformations was 1.14 (95% CI 0.89–1.45), whereas the ORs and 95% CIs for SABs, preterm birth, and small for gestational age were 0.62 (0.36–1.05), 1.17 (0.94–1.147), and 0.28 (0.06–1.22), respectively. The authors concluded that H2 blockers could be used safely in pregnancy (9).

F

Four reviews on the treatment of GERD have concluded that H2 blockers, with the possible exception of nizatidine, could be used in pregnancy with relative safety (10–13).

A 2010 study from Israel identified 1148 infants exposed in the 1st trimester to H2 blockers (13). No association with congenital malformations was found (OR 1.03, 95% CI 0.80–1.32). Moreover, no association was found with EABs, perinatal mortality, premature delivery, low birth weight, or low Apgar scores (14).

F

BREASTFEEDING SUMMARY

Famotidine is concentrated in breast milk, but to a lesser degree than either cimetidine or ranitidine (15). Following a single 40-mg dose administered to eight postpartum women who were not breastfeeding, the mean milk:plasma ratios at 2, 6, and 24 hours were 0.41, 1.78, and 1.33, respectively. The mean peak milk concentration, 72 ng/mL, occurred at 6 hours compared with 2 hours for plasma (mean 75 ng/mL). Exposure of the nursing infant to famotidine via milk has not been reported. Although a potential risk may exist for adverse effects, the American Academy of Pediatrics classifies a similar drug (cimetidine) as compatible with breastfeeding. A 1991 reference source suggested that because famotidine and two other H2 blockers, nizatidine and roxatidine, are less concentrated in milk, they might be preferred in the nursing woman in place of cimetidine or ranitidine (16).

References

1. Product information. Pepcid. Merck Sharp & Dohme, 1996.
2. Burek JD, Majka JA, Bokelman DL. Famotidine: summary of preclinical safety assessment. Digestion 1985;32(Suppl 1):7–14.
3. Shibata M, Kawano K, Shiobara Y, Yoshinaga T, Fujiwara M, Uchida T, Odani Y. Reproductive studies on famotidine (YM 11170) in rats and rabbits. Oyo Yakuri 1983;26:489–97, 543–78, 831–40. As cited in Shepard TH. *Catalog of Teratogenic Agents*. 6th ed. Baltimore, MD: The Johns Hopkins University Press, 1989:273.
4. Dicke JM, Johnson RF, Henderson GI, Kuehl TJ, Schenker S. A comparative evaluation of the transport of H2-receptor antagonists by the human and baboon placenta. Am J Med Sci 1988;295:198–206.
5. Magee LA, Inocencion G, Kamboj L, Rosetti F, Koren G. Safety of first trimester exposure to histamine H_2 blockers. A prospective cohort study. Dig Dis Sci 1996;41:1145–9.
6. Kallen B. Delivery outcome after the use of acid-suppressing drugs in early pregnancy with special reference to omeprazole. Br J Obstet Gynaecol 1998;105:877–81.
7. Dehlink E, Yen E, Leichtner AM, Hait EJ, Fiebiger E. First evidence of a possible association between gastric acid suppression during pregnancy and childhood asthma: a population-based register study. Clin Exp Allergy 2009;39:246–53.
8. Garbis H, Elefant E, Diav-Citrin O, Mastroiacovo P, Schaefer C, Vial T, Clementi M, Valti E, McElhatton P, Smorlesij C, Rodriguez EP, Robert-Gnansia E, Merlob P, Peiker G, Pexieder T, Schueler L, Ritvanen A, Mathieu-Nolf M. Pregnancy outcome after exposure to ranitidine and other H2-blockers—a collaborative study of the European Network of Teratology Information Services. Reprod Toxicol 2005;453–8.
9. Gill SK, O'Brien L, Koren G. The safety of histamine 2 (H2) blockers in pregnancy: a meta-analysis. Dig Dis Sci 2009;54:1835–8.
10. Broussard CN, Richter JE. Treating gasto-oesophageal reflux disease during pregnancy and lactation. What are the safest therapy options? Drug Saf 1998;19:325–37.
11. Katz PO, Castell DO. Gastroesophageal reflux disease during pregnancy. Gastroenterol Clin North Am 1998;27:153–67.
12. Richter JE. Gastroesophageal reflux disease during pregnancy. Gastroenterol Clin N Am 2003;32:235–61.
13. Richter JE. Review article: the management of heartburn in pregnancy. Aliment Pharmacol Ther 2005;22:749–57.
14. Matok I, Gorodischer R, Koren G, Sheiner E, Wiznitzer A, Uziel E, Levy A. The safety of H_2-blockers use during pregnancy. J Clin Pharmacol 2010;50:81–7.
15. Courtney TP, Shaw RW, Cedar E, Mann SG, Kelly JG. Excretion of famotidine in breast milk. Br J Clin Pharmacol 1988;26:639P.
16. Anderson PO. Drug use during breast-feeding. Clin Pharm 1991;10:594–624.

FEBUXOSTAT

Antigout (Uricosuric)

PREGNANCY RECOMMENDATION: No Human Data—Animal Data Suggest Low Risk
BREASTFEEDING RECOMMENDATION: No Human Data—Potential Toxicity

PREGNANCY SUMMARY

No reports describing the use of febuxostat in human pregnancy have been located. The animal reproduction data suggest low risk, but the absence of human pregnancy experience prevents a complete assessment of the embryo–fetal risk. Because this agent will be taken for long periods, the best course would be to consider other uricosurics with pregnancy experience, such as probenecid.

FETAL RISK SUMMARY

Febuxostat is a xanthine oxidase inhibitor that acts by decreasing serum uric acid. It is in the same class of uricosurics as allopurinol, probenecid, and sulfinpyrazone. Febuxostat is indicated for the chronic management of hyperuricemia in patients with gout. It is metabolized to four pharmacologically active metabolites, all of which occur in human plasma at a much lower concentration than the parent drug. Febuxostat, taken once daily, is highly bound to plasma protein (about 99%) and the mean terminal elimination half-life is about 5–8 hours (1).

Reproduction studies have been conducted in rats and rabbits. No teratogenicity was observed in these species with oral doses up to 40 and 51 times, respectively, the human plasma exposure at 80 mg/day for equal BSA (HPE) during organogenesis. In rats, doses up to 40 times the HPE during organogenesis and through the lactation period were associated with an increase in neonatal mortality and a reduction in neonatal body weight gain (1). However, a no-observed-effect-level was not established.

In 2-year studies for carcinogenic effects conducted in rats and mice, increased transitional cell papilloma and carcinoma of the urinary bladder were observed. The urinary bladder neoplasms were secondary to calculus formation in the kidney and bladder. Febuxostat was mutagenic in one assay but was negative in other assays. No effect on fertility or reproductive performance was observed in male and female rats given doses up to 35 times the HPE (1).

It is not known if febuxostat or any of the active metabolites cross the human placenta. The molecular weight (about 316) and long elimination half-life suggest that the drug will cross to the embryo–fetus. The extensive plasma protein binding may limit the exposure.

BREASTFEEDING SUMMARY

No reports describing the use of febuxostat during human lactation have been located. The molecular weight (about 316) and long elimination half-life (about 5–8 hours) suggest that the drug will be excreted into breast milk. The extensive plasma protein binding (about 99%) may limit the exposure. The effect of this exposure on a nursing infant is unknown. If the mother does decide to nurse, the infant should be observed for the most common adverse effects reported in adults: liver function abnormalities, nausea, arthralgia, and rash. However, because the drug will be taken for long periods, the best course might be to avoid it during breastfeeding.

Reference

1. Product information. Uloric. Takeda Pharmaceuticals America, 2009.

F

FELBAMATE

Anticonvulsant

PREGNANCY RECOMMENDATION: Limited Human Data—Animal Data Suggest Moderate Risk
BREASTFEEDING RECOMMENDATION: Limited Human Data—Potential Toxicity

PREGNANCY SUMMARY

There is limited information on the effects of felbamate in human pregnancy. The drug is structurally similar to meprobamate. Serious adult toxicity, including fatal cases of aplastic anemia and acute liver failure, was reported to the manufacturer in July and September 1994. One adverse pregnancy outcome, an infant with mental retardation whose mother was on monotherapy, has been reported to the FDA (F. Rosa, personal communication, FDA, 1994), but the relationship to the drug is unknown.

FETAL RISK SUMMARY

Citing information obtained from the manufacturer, one review stated that 10 women had become pregnant while enrolled in clinical trials of the drug and were subsequently dropped from the studies (1). Two of these women underwent elective termination of their pregnancies. A third patient was changed to phenytoin at 4 weeks' gestation and had a spontaneous abortion at 9.5 weeks. The remaining seven women eventually gave birth without any problems, but details on these pregnancies, whether felbamate or other anticonvulsants were continued throughout gestation, and the status of the newborns were not provided.

Felbamate was not teratogenic in rats and rabbits at doses up to 13.9 times and 4.2 times, respectively, the human daily dose based on body weight, or 3 times and <2 times, respectively, the human dose based on BSA (2). In rats, however, there was a decrease in pup weight and an increase in pup deaths during lactation. The cause of the deaths was not known. The no-effect dose in rats was 6.9 times the human dose based on body weight (1.5 times based on BSA) (2).

The drug crosses the placenta without accumulation in pregnant rats (2,3). Transplacental passage apparently has not been described in humans but should occur because of the low molecular weight (about 238).

The Lamotrigine Pregnancy Registry, an ongoing project conducted by the manufacturer, was first published in January 1997 (4). The final report was published in July 2010. The Registry is now closed. There were two prospectively enrolled pregnancies exposed in the 1st trimester to felbamate and lamotrigine, with and without other anticonvulsants, resulting in a live birth without defects and an induced abortion (4).

BREASTFEEDING SUMMARY

Felbamate is excreted into human breast milk (2). No reports have been located that describe the effects, if any, of exposure to this anticonvulsant via breast milk in human infants. Because of the potential for serious toxicity (e.g., aplastic anemia and acute liver failure) in a nursing infant, felbamate probably should not be used during breastfeeding.

References

1. Wagner ML. Felbamate: a new antiepileptic drug. Am J Hosp Pharm 1994;51:1657–66.
2. Product information. Felbatol. Wallace Laboratories, 2000.
3. Adusumalli VE, Yang JT, Wong KK, Kucharczyk N, Sofia RD. Felbamate pharmacokinetics in the rat, rabbit, and dog. Drug Metab Dispos Biol Fate Chem 1991;19:1116–25.
4. The Lamotrigine Pregnancy Registry. Final Report. 1 September 1992 through 31 March 2010. GlaxoSmithKline, July 2010.

FELODIPINE

Calcium Channel Blocker

PREGNANCY RECOMMENDATION: Limited Human Data—Animal Data Suggest Risk
BREASTFEEDING RECOMMENDATION: No Human Data—Probably Compatible

F

PREGNANCY SUMMARY

Although the animal data suggest risk, the very limited human pregnancy experience prevents a complete assessment of the embryo–fetal risk. However, there is no evidence that drugs in this class are teratogenic.

FETAL RISK SUMMARY

Felodipine is a calcium channel-blocking agent used in the treatment of hypertension. The drug is teratogenic in rabbits, producing digital anomalies consisting of a reduction in size and degree of ossification of the terminal phalanges (1). The frequency and severity of the defects appeared to be dose-related over a range of 0.4–4 times the maximum recommended human dose based on BSA (MRHD). The defects may have been related to decreased uterine blood flow (1). Similar effects were not observed in rats or monkeys. In the latter species, however, an abnormal position of the distal phalanges was observed in about 40% of the fetuses. At doses four times the MRHD, delayed parturition with difficult labor, an increased incidence of stillbirths, and a decreased incidence of postnatal survival were noted in rats (1).

A prospective, multicenter cohort study of 78 women (81 outcomes, 3 sets of twins) who had 1st trimester exposure to calcium channel blockers, including 1% to felodipine, was reported in 1996 (2). Compared with controls, no increase in the risk of major congenital malformations was found. A 1997 report described three pregnant women treated with felodipine for chronic essential hypertension (3). Therapy was started before or during the 1st trimester in each case. One woman, treated with felodipine and atenolol throughout gestation, delivered a growth-restricted, 2020-g (<5th percentile) female infant at 37 weeks' with Apgar scores of 8 and 9 at 1 and 5 minutes, respectively. The intrauterine growth restriction was most likely due to atenolol and hypertension. The birth weights of the other two infants were in the 10th and 15th percentile. Although a contribution from felodipine cannot be excluded, the low weights were probably secondary to maternal hypertension.

BREASTFEEDING SUMMARY

No reports describing the use of felodipine during human lactation have been located. Because of its relatively low molecular weight (about 384), however, excretion into human milk should be expected. The effect of this exposure on a nursing infant is unknown.

References

1. Product information. Plendil. Merck Sharp & Dohme, 2000.
2. Magee LA, Schick B, Donnenfeld AE, Sage SR, Conover B, Cook L, McElhatton PR, Schmidt MA, Koren G. The safety of calcium channel blockers in human pregnancy: a prospective, multicenter cohort study. Am J Obstet Gynecol 1996;174:823–8.
3. Casele HL, Windley KC, Prieto JA, Gratton R, Laifer SA. Felodipine use in pregnancy. Report of three cases. J Reprod Med 1997;42:378–81.

FENFLURAMINE

[Withdrawn from the market. See 9th edition.]

FENOFIBRATE

Antilipemic

PREGNANCY RECOMMENDATION: Limited Human Data—Animal Data Suggest Risk
BREASTFEEDING RECOMMENDATION: No Human Data—Potential Toxicity

PREGNANCY SUMMARY

Only two reports describing the use of fenofibrate in human pregnancy has been located. Although the near absence of human pregnancy experience prevents an assessment of the risk, the combined animal data are reason for concern if this drug is used for prolonged periods in pregnancy. As with other antilipemic agents, there is apparently no benefit in otherwise healthy women from the use of fenofibrate during gestation. However, fenofibrate may be of benefit to treat or prevent hyperlipidemia-associated pancreatitis. If used during pregnancy, the woman should be informed of the limited human data.

FETAL RISK SUMMARY

Fenofibrate is a prodrug that is rapidly hydrolyzed by esterases after oral administration to the active metabolite, fenofibric acid. The active metabolite is further metabolized to inactive metabolites. Fenofibric acid is indicated as adjunctive therapy to diet for the treatment of primary hypercholesterolemia or mixed dyslipidemia, and for hypertriglyceridemia. Fenofibric acid is extensively bound to serum protein (about 99%) and has an elimination half-life of 20 hours (1,2).

Reproduction studies have been conducted in pregnant rats and rabbits (1,2). The drug was embryocidal and teratogenic in pregnant rats given 7–10 times the maximum recommended human dose based on BSA (MRHD). At 9 times the MRHD given before and throughout gestation to rats, reproductive toxicity included delayed parturition in 100% of the dams, a 60% increase in postimplantation loss with a decrease in litter size, reduced birth weight, an increase in spina bifida, and decreased pup survival (40% at birth, 4% during neonatal period, and 0% to weaning). Similar findings were observed at seven times the MRHD given from day 15 of gestation through weaning. When pregnant rats were dosed at 10 times the MRHD during organogenesis, an increased incidence of congenital malformations was observed, including domed head/hunched shoulders/rounded body/abnormal chest, kyphosis, stunted fetuses, elongated sternal ribs, malformed sternebrae, extra foramen in palatine, misshapen vertebrae, and supernumerary ribs (1). Embryocidal effects were also observed in rabbits. Doses 9 and 18 times the MRHD caused abortions in 10% and 25% of the dams, respectively. At 18 times the MRHD, 7% of the fetuses died (1,2).

Fenofibrate had no mutagenic potential in four different tests, but the drug was carcinogenic in rats, significantly increasing the incidence of liver carcinoma, pancreatic carcinoma and adenomas, and benign testicular interstitial cell tumors in a dose-related manner (1,2). Some of these tumors (pancreatic acinar adenomas and testicular interstitial cell tumors) were also seen in a second strain of rats at lower doses (1,2).

It is not known if fenofibrate or fenofibric acid crosses the human placenta. Fenofibrate is rapidly metabolized and is not detected in the plasma (1,2). The molecular weight of the metabolite, fenofibric acid (about 319), and the prolonged elimination half-life suggest that the drug will cross, but the high serum protein binding should limit the amount available for transfer to the embryo or fetus.

A 2011 case report described the use of fenofibrate in the 3rd trimester (3). A 30-year-old G4P1SAB2 woman with adequately treated hypothyroidism presented at 32 weeks' gestation with hypertriglyceridemia-associated pancreatitis. Diet alone did not control her dyslipidemia and she was started on an unspecified dose of fenofibrate. Recurrence of pancreatitis was prevented and at 35 weeks' gestation she gave birth spontaneously to a healthy, 2452-g male infant with Apgar scores of 8 and 9, presumably at 1 and 5 minutes (3).

A 30-year-old woman with high triglyceride levels was started on fenofibrate 267 mg/day (4). One year later, an unplanned pregnancy was diagnosed at 8 weeks' gestation and the drug was stopped. At 36 weeks, a cesarean section delivered a healthy 3200-g (75th percentile) male infant with Apgar scores of 7, 9, and 10 at 1, 5, and 10 minutes, respectively. No congenital anomalies were found and the infant was healthy at 1 year of age (4).

BREASTFEEDING SUMMARY

No reports describing the use of fenofibrate in human lactation have been located. The relative low molecular weight of the active metabolite (about 319) suggests that it is excreted into breast milk. Although the effect of this exposure on a nursing infant is unknown, women taking fenofibrate should probably not breastfeed because of potential toxicity in a nursing infant.

References

1. Product information. Tricor. Abbott Laboratories, 2001.
2. Product information. Lofibra. GATE Pharmaceuticals, 2004.
3. Whitten AE, Lorenz RP, Smith JM. Hyperlipidemia-associated pancreatitis in pregnancy managed with fenofibrate. Obstet Gynecol 2011;117:517–9.
4. Sunman H, Canpolat U, Sahiner L, Aytemir K. Use of fenofibrate during the first trimester of an unplanned pregnancy in a patient with hypertriglyceridemia. Ann Pharmacother 2012;46:e5. doi:10.1345/aph.1Q626.

FENOLDOPAM

Antihypertensive

PREGNANCY RECOMMENDATION: **No Human Data—Animal Data Suggest Low Risk**
BREASTFEEDING RECOMMENDATION: **No Human Data—Probably Compatible**

PREGNANCY SUMMARY

The absence of human pregnancy experience prevents an assessment of the fetal risk from exposure to fenoldopam mesylate, but the animal data are reassuring. Because it is used for the emergency reduction of severe hypertension, the maternal benefit probably outweighs the unknown fetal risk. However, rapid reduction of maternal blood pressure may compromise the placental perfusion, resulting in fetal hypoxia and subsequent bradycardia. Fetal death is a potential consequence of this effect. Fetal heart rate monitoring, therefore, is recommended during IV infusions of fenoldopam.

F

FETAL RISK SUMMARY

An IV infusion of fenoldopam mesylate, a dopamine D_1-like receptor agonist, is indicated for the short-term (up to 48 hours), rapid-onset, management of severe hypertension. It is a vasodilator, affecting coronary, renal, mesenteric, and peripheral arteries in animals.

Reproduction studies have been conducted in rats and rabbits with oral doses up to 200 mg/kg/day and 25 mg/kg/day, respectively (1). Although maternal toxicity was evident at the highest doses, no evidence of impaired fertility or fetal harm was observed.

It is not known if fenoldopam mesylate crosses the human placenta. The molecular weight (about 402) is low enough that transfer to the fetus should be expected.

BREASTFEEDING SUMMARY

No reports describing the use of fenoldopam mesylate in human lactation have been located. The molecular weight (about 402) suggests that excretion into breast milk probably occurs. The effect of this exposure on a nursing infant is unknown. Because of the nature of the indication, opportunities for use of this drug during breastfeeding are probably very rare.

Reference

1. Product information. Corlopam. Abbott Laboratories, 2001.

FENOPROFEN

Nonsteroidal Anti-inflammatory

PREGNANCY RECOMMENDATION: Human Data Suggest Risk in 1st and 3rd Trimesters
BREASTFEEDING RECOMMENDATION: Limited Human Data—Probably Compatible

PREGNANCY SUMMARY

Prostaglandin synthesis inhibitors can cause constriction of the ductus arteriosus in utero (see also Indomethacin) (1). Persistent pulmonary hypertension of the newborn may occur if these agents are used in the 3rd trimester close to delivery (1,2). These drugs also have been shown to inhibit labor and prolong pregnancy, both in humans (3) (see also Indomethacin), and in animals (4). Women attempting to conceive should not use any prostaglandin synthesis inhibitor, including fenoprofen, because of the findings in various animal models that indicate these agents block blastocyst implantation (5,6). Moreover, nonsteroid anti-inflammatory drugs (NSAIDs) have been associated with spontaneous abortions (SABs) and congenital malformations. The absolute risk for these defects, however, appears to be low.

FETAL RISK SUMMARY

Fenoprofen is an NSAID in the same subclass (propionic acids) as five other agents (flurbiprofen, ibuprofen, ketoprofen, naproxen, and oxaprozin). It is indicated for the relief of the signs and symptoms of rheumatoid arthritis and osteoarthritis (7).

Fenoprofen given to rats during pregnancy and continued until labor resulted in prolonged parturition (7).

It is not known if fenoprofen crosses the human placenta. The molecular weight (about 559) is low enough that passage to the fetus should be expected. However, in one study, the drug was used during labor (8). No data were given except that the drug could not be detected in cord blood or amniotic fluid.

In a surveillance study of Michigan Medicaid recipients involving 229,101 completed pregnancies conducted between 1985 and 1992, 191 newborns had been exposed to fenoprofen during the 1st trimester (F. Rosa, personal communication, FDA, 1993). A total of six (3.1%) major birth defects were observed (eight expected), including (observed/expected) 1/2 cardiovascular defects and 1/1 polydactyly. No anomalies were observed in four other categories of defects (oral clefts, spina bifida, limb reduction defects, and hypospadias) for which specific data were available. These data do not support an association between the drug and congenital defects.

A combined 2001 population-based observational cohort study and a case–control study estimated the risk of adverse pregnancy outcome from the use of NSAIDs (9). The use of

NSAIDs during pregnancy was not associated with congenital malformations, preterm delivery, or low birth weight, but a positive association was discovered with SABs. A similar study, also published in 2001, failed to find a relationship, in general, between NSAIDs and congenital malformations, but did find a significant association with cardiac defects and orofacial clefts (10). In addition, a 2003 study found a significant association between exposure to NSAIDs in early pregnancy and SABs (11) (see Ibuprofen for details on these three studies).

A brief 2003 editorial on the potential for NSAID-induced developmental toxicity concluded that NSAIDs, and specifically those with greater cyclooxygenase-2 (COX-2) affinity, had a lower risk of this toxicity in humans than aspirin (12).

BREASTFEEDING SUMMARY

Fenoprofen passes into breast milk in very small quantities. The milk:plasma ratio in nursing mothers given 600 mg every 6 hours for 4 days was approximately 0.017 (8). Although the clinical significance of this amount is unknown, another NSAID in the same subclass is classified as compatible with breastfeeding by the American Academy of Pediatrics (see Ibuprofen).

References

1. Levin DL. Effects of inhibition of prostaglandin synthesis on fetal development, oxygenation, and the fetal circulation. Semin Perinatol 1980;4: 35–44.
2. Van Marter LJ, Leviton A, Allred EN, Pagano M, Sullivan KF, Cohen A, Epstein MF. Persistent pulmonary hypertension of the newborn and smoking and aspirin and nonsteroidal antiinflammatory drug consumption during pregnancy. Pediatrics 1996;97:658–63.
3. Fuchs F. Prevention of prematurity. Am J Obstet Gynecol 1976;126: 809–20.
4. Powell JG, Cochrane RL. The effects of a number of non-steroidal anti-inflammatory compounds on parturition in the rat. Prostaglandins 1982;23:469–88.
5. Matt DW, Borzelleca JF. Toxic effects on the female reproductive system during pregnancy, parturition, and lactation. In: Witorsch RJ, ed. *Reproductive Toxicology*. 2nd ed. New York, NY: Raven Press, 1995: 175–93.
6. Dawood MY. Nonsteroidal antiinflammatory drugs and reproduction. Am J Obstet Gynecol 1993;169:1255–65.
7. Product information. Nalfon. Dista Products, 2001.
8. Rubin A, Chernish SM, Crabtree R, Gruber CM Jr, Helleberg L, Rodda BE, Warrick P, Wolen RL, Ridolfo AS. A profile of the physiological disposition and gastro-intestinal effects of fenoprofen in man. Curr Med Res Opin 1974;2:529–44.
9. Nielsen GL, Sorensen HT, Larsen H, Pedersen L. Risk of adverse birth outcome and miscarriage in pregnant users of non-steroidal anti-inflammatory drugs: population based observational study and case-control study. Br Med J 2001;322:266–70.
10. Ericson A, Kallen BAJ. Nonsteroidal anti-inflammatory drugs in early pregnancy. Reprod Toxicol 2001;15:371–5.
11. Li DK, Liu L, Odouli R. Exposure to non-steroidal anti-inflammatory drugs during pregnancy and risk of miscarriage: population based cohort study. Br Med J 2003;327:368–71.
12. Tassinari MS, Cook JC, Hurtt ME. NSAIDs and developmental toxicity. Birth Defects Res B Dev Reprod Toxicol 2003;68:3–4.

FENOTEROL

[Withdrawn from the market. See 9th edition.]

FENTANYL

Narcotic Agonist Analgesic

PREGNANCY RECOMMENDATION: Human Data Suggest Risk
BREASTFEEDING RECOMMENDATION: Compatible

PREGNANCY SUMMARY

The National Birth Defects Prevention Study discussed below found evidence that opioid use during organogenesis is associated with a low absolute risk of congenital birth defects.

Respiratory depression in the newborn is a potential complication if fentanyl is used close to delivery. As with all opioids, neonatal withdrawal may occur after chronic, long-term exposure during pregnancy.

FETAL RISK SUMMARY

Fentanyl is an opioid analgesic. When given by IV injection, the terminal elimination half-life is 219 minutes. Although not teratogenic in rats, fentanyl impaired fertility and was embryotoxic at IV doses 0.3 times the upper human dose given for a period of 12 days (1).

The placental transfer of fentanyl has been documented in the 1st and 2nd trimesters (2) and at term (3–7). A study published in 1998 measured fentanyl concentrations in fetal fluids (amniotic and/or chorionic cavities), fetal blood (after 12 weeks' gestation), and maternal serum 5–22 minutes after an IV bolus (1.5 mcg/kg) in 42 healthy women scheduled for pregnancy termination (between 6 and 16 weeks) under general anesthesia (2). Fentanyl was detected in amniotic fluid at less than 12 weeks', but not later, and in fetal blood. None of the samples of chorionic fluid, however, contained detectable fentanyl (2).

In a study comparing women in labor who received 50 or 100 mcg of fentanyl IV every hour as needed ($N = 137$) (mean dose 140 mcg, range 50–600 mcg) to those not requiring analgesia (epidural or narcotic) ($N = 112$), no statistical differences were found in newborn outcome in terms of the incidence of depressed respirations, Apgar scores, and the need for naloxone (3). In blinded measurements taken at 2–4 and 24 hours, no differences were observed between the two groups of infants in respiratory rate, heart rate, blood pressure, adaptive capacity, neurologic evaluation, and overall assessment. The last dose of fentanyl was given at a mean of 112 minutes before delivery. Cord blood levels of the narcotic were always significantly lower than maternal serum levels (cord:maternal ratios were approximately 0.5 but exact data were not given) ($p < 0.03$). Doses used were considered equianalgesic to 5–10 mg of morphine or 37.5–75 mg of meperidine (3).

Respiratory depression has been observed in one infant whose mother received epidural fentanyl during labor (4). Fentanyl may produce loss of fetal heart rate (FHR) variability without causing fetal hypoxia (3,5). However, no effect on FHR variability or accelerations was observed when epidural fentanyl was given to women receiving adequate epidural lidocaine analgesia (6). The narcotic has been combined with bupivacaine for spinal anesthesia during labor (7,8). In four studies, the addition of fentanyl to bupivacaine had no effect on neonatal respiration (9,10–12) and, in two, did not adversely affect neurobehavioral scores (9,12). Placental transfer of fentanyl was documented in one study with cord:maternal venous plasma ratios of 1.12 for total drug and 1.20 for free drug (9). A study of a continuous epidural infusion of fentanyl and bupivacaine found no accumulation of either drug over a 1- to 15-hour interval in 21 laboring women and observed no adverse fetal effects (13). The mean cord:maternal venous fentanyl concentration was 0.94.

In 15 women undergoing elective cesarean section, fentanyl 1 mcg/kg given IV within 10 minutes of delivery produced an average cord blood:maternal blood ratio over 10 minutes of 0.31 (range 0.06–0.43) (14). No respiratory depression was observed, and all neurobehavioral scores were normal at 4 and 24 hours.

A 1998 case report described respiratory muscle rigidity in a newborn that was attributed to fentanyl (15). Because of severe maternal disease (pulmonary valve stenosis with congestive heart failure and pregnancy-induced hypertension) and Doppler measurements showing periodically absent diastolic flow in the umbilical cord, a cesarean section under general anesthesia was performed at 31 weeks' gestation to deliver a 1440-g male infant. Betamethasone had been given to the mother for fetal lung maturation before delivery. The mother was premedicated with morphine (7.5 mg) and scopolamine (0.3 mg), followed by fentanyl (300 mcg; *note: reference states "mg" but assumed to be "mcg"*), diazepam (7.5 mg), ketamine (300 mg), and vecuronium (7 mg). The newborn had no respiratory movements and had a heart rate of about 100 beats/minute (Apgar score 3 at 1 minute). Attempts to ventilate the infant by mask and then by intubation with positive pressure produced no chest movements until 8 minutes after delivery. A chest X-ray showed normal lungs with no sign of hyaline membrane disease. After treatment of severe respiratory alkalosis at 1 hour of age, the infant made an uneventful recovery and was developing normally at 1 year of age. The author attributed the chest wall rigidity to fentanyl because this is a common adverse effect in adults administered the agent during anesthesia (15).

A 31-year-old woman was treated with transdermal fentanyl patches (125 mcg/hr) throughout gestation for severe cervical and lumbar spinal injuries sustained in a road traffic accident before conception (16). An elective cesarean section was performed at 38 weeks' gestation to deliver a healthy, 3.13-kg female infant with Apgar scores of 9 at 1 and 5 minutes, respectively. The infant's head circumference was 35.4 cm (50th percentile). Blood concentrations of fentanyl were as follows: mother (predelivery) 3.56 ng/mL, infant 1.23 ng/mL (at birth), 0.31 ng/mL (day 1), and <0.25 ng/mL) (day 2). At 24 hours of age, the bottle-fed baby was noted to be jittery, fisting, and irritable with a high-pitched cry. The mean Finnegan scores (an assessment of acute opioid withdrawal in newborns based on nursing observations) on days 1 and 2 were 4.5 ("mild" is 0–7) with a single peak of 11 ("abstinence" is 8–11) at 72 hours of age. Finnegan scores were consistently less than 4 by day 4 and, at 96 hours of age the infant had no signs of opioid withdrawal. No drug therapy of the withdrawal was required at any time. The infant was developing normally at follow-up (16).

Results of a National Birth Defects Prevention Study (1997–2005) were published in 2011 (17). This population-based case–control study examined the association between maternal use of opioid analgesics and >30 types of major structural birth defects. In 17,449 case mothers, therapeutic opioid use was reported by 454 (2.6%) compared with 134 (2.0%) of 6701 control mothers. Indications for use of opioid analgesics were surgical procedures (41%), infections (34%), chronic diseases (20%), and injuries (18%). Dose, duration, or frequency was not evaluated. The exposure period evaluated was from 1 month before to 3 months after conception. Limiting the exposure period to the first 2 months after conception produced similar results. Infants with >1 defect were included in multiple birth defect categories. The following opioids were included (number of cases for each agent not specified): codeine, hydrocodone, hydromorphone, fentanyl, meperidine, methadone, morphine, oxycodone, pentazocine, propoxyphene, and tramadol. The birth defect, total number, number exposed, and the adjusted odds ratio (aOR) with 95% confidence interval (CI) were as follows (see below table):

Birth Defect	Total	Cases	aOR (95% CI)
Spina bifida	718	26	2.0 (1.3–3.2)
Any heart defect (20 types)	7724	211	1.4 (1.1–1.7)
Atrioventricular septal defect	175	9	2.4 (1.2–4.8)
Teratology of Fallot	672	21	1.7 (1.1–2.8)
Conotruncal defect	1481	41	1.5 (1.0–2.1)
Conoventricular septal defect	110	6	2.7 (1.1–6.3)
Left ventricular outflow tract obstruction defect	1195	36	1.5 (1.0–2.2)
Hypoplastic left heart syndrome	357	17	2.4 (1.4–4.1)
Right ventricular outflow tract obstruction defect	1175	40	1.6 (1.1–2.3)
Pulmonary valve stenosis	867	34	1.7 (1.2–2.6)
Atrial septal defect (ASD)	511	17	2.0 (1.2–3.6)
Ventricular septal defect + ASD	528	17	1.7 (1.0–2.9)
Hydrocephaly	301	11	2.0 (1.0–3.7)
Glaucoma/anterior chamber defects	103	5	2.6 (1.0–6.6)
Gastroschisis	726	26	1.8 (1.1–2.9)

The authors speculated that the activity of opioids and their receptors as growth regulators during development of the embryo might be a mechanism to explain the above findings. The exposure data were obtained by retrospective maternal self-report; the authors acknowledged that recall bias and misclassification might have affected their results. They concluded that the absolute risk was a modest absolute increase above the baseline risk for birth defects (17).

BREASTFEEDING SUMMARY

Fentanyl is excreted into milk. A study published in 1992 measured fentanyl colostrum concentrations in 13 healthy women who had received fentanyl (2 mcg/kg) during cesarean section or postpartum tubal ligation (18). Serum and colostrum samples were collected at six intervals up to 10 hours after drug administration. The peak serum and colostrum fentanyl levels occurred at 0.75 hours, with mean values of 0.19 and 0.40 ng/mL, respectively, falling to undectable and 0.05 ng/mL, respectively, at 10 hours. Colostrum fentanyl concentrations were always greater than serum levels at every measurement. It was concluded that breastfeeding was safe because of the low colostrum concentrations and the low oral bioavailability of fentanyl (18).

The American Academy of Pediatrics classifies fentanyl as compatible with breastfeeding (19).

References

1. Product information. Duragesic. Janssen Pharmaceutica, 2000.
2. Shannon C, Jauniaux E, Gulbis B, Thiry P, Sitham M, Bromley L. Placental transfer of fentanyl in early human pregnancy. Hum Reprod 1998;13:2317–20.
3. Rayburn W, Rathke A, Leuschen MP, Chleborad J, Weidner W. Fentanyl citrate analgesia during labor. Am J Obstet Gynecol 1989;161:202–6.
4. Carrie LES, O'Sullivan GM, Seegobin R. Epidural fentanyl in labour. Anaesthesia 1981;36:965–9.
5. Johnson ES, Colley PS. Effects of nitrous oxide and fentanyl anesthesia on fetal heart-rate variability intra- and postoperatively. Anesthesiology 1980;52:429–30.
6. Viscomi CM, Hood DD, Melone PJ, Eisenach JC. Fetal heart rate variability after epidural fentanyl during labor. Anesth Analg 1990;71:679–83.
7. Justins DM, Francis D, Houlton PG, Reynolds F. A controlled trial of extradural fentanyl in labour. Br J Anaesth 1982;54:409–13.
8. Milon D, Bentue-Ferrer D, Noury D, Reymann JM, Sauvage J, Allain H, Saint-Marc C, van den Driessche J. Peridural anesthesia for cesarean section employing a bupivacaine–fentanyl combination. Ann Fr Anesth Reanim 1983;2:273–9.
9. Fernando R, Bonello E, Gill P, Urquhart J, Reynolds F, Morgan B. Neonatal welfare and placental transfer of fentanyl and bupivacaine during ambulatory combined spinal epidural analgesia for labour. Anaesthesia 1997;52:517–24.
10. Benlabed M, Dreizzen E, Ecoffey C, Escourrou P, Migdal M, Gaultier C. Neonatal patterns of breathing after cesarean section with or without epidural fentanyl. Anesthesiology 1990;73:1110–3.
11. Halonen PM, Paatero H, Hovorka J, Haasio J, Korttila K. Comparison of two fentanyl doses to improve epidural anaesthesia with 0.5% bupivacaine for cesarean section. Acta Anaesthesiol Scand 1993;37:774–9.
12. Porter J, Bonello E, Reynolds F. Effect of epidural fentanyl on neonatal respiration. Anesthesiology 1998;89:79–85.
13. Bader AM, Fragneto R, Terui K, Arthur GR, Loferski B, Datta S. Maternal and neonatal fentanyl and bupivacaine concentrations after epidural infusion during labor. Anesth Analg 1995;81:829–32.
14. Eisele JH, Wright R, Rogge P. Newborn and maternal fentanyl levels at cesarean section (abstract). Anesth Anal 1982;61:179–80.
15. Lindemann R. Respiratory muscle rigidity in a preterm infant after use of fentanyl during cesarean section. Eur J Pediatr 1998;157:1012–3.
16. Regan J, Chambers F, Gorman W, MacSullivan R. Neonatal abstinence syndrome due to prolonged administration of fentanyl in pregnancy. Br J Obstet Gynaecol 2000;107:570–2.
17. Broussard CS, Rasmussen SA, Reefhuis J, Friedman JM, Jann MW, Riehle-Colarusso T, Honein MA, for the National Birth Defects Prevention Study. Maternal treatment with opioid analgesics and risk for birth defects. Am J Obstet Gynecol 2011;204:314–7.
18. Steer PL, Biddle CJ, Marley WS, Lantz RK, Sulik PL. Concentration of fentanyl in colostrum after an analgesic dose. Can J Anaesth 1992;39:231–5.
19. Committee on Drugs, American Academy of Pediatrics. The transfer of drugs and other chemicals into human milk. Pediatrics 2001;108:776–89.

FESOTERODINE

Urinary Tract Agent (Antispasmodic)

PREGNANCY RECOMMENDATION: No Human Data—Animal Data Suggest Low Risk
BREASTFEEDING RECOMMENDATION: No Human Data—Probably Compatible

PREGNANCY SUMMARY

No reports describing the use of fesoterodine in human pregnancy have been located. Reproduction studies in animals observed developmental toxicity but only at levels causing maternal toxicity. There was no evidence of drug-induced malformations or developmental delay in surviving offspring. Although the absence of human pregnancy experience prevents a full assessment of the embryo–fetal risk, there is no evidence that other anticholinergics (e.g., see Atropine) cause developmental toxicity. Until human experience is available, the safest course is to avoid fesoterodine in pregnancy. However, if inadvertent exposure in pregnancy does occur, the embryo–fetal risk probably is low.

F

FETAL RISK SUMMARY

The prodrug fesoterodine is a competitive muscarinic receptor antagonist (anticholinergic) that inhibits urinary bladder smooth muscle. After oral administration, fesoterodine is converted to the active metabolite, 5-hydroxymethyl tolterodine (5-HT), the same metabolite responsible for the action of tolterodine (see also Tolterodine). 5-HT undergoes hepatic metabolism to inactive compounds. Because of the rapid and extensive metabolism, fesoterodine cannot be detected in the plasma. Fesoterodine is indicated for the treatment of overactive bladder with symptoms of urge urinary incontinence, urgency, and frequency. It is the same subclass as darifenacin, flavoxate, oxybutynin, solifenacin, tolterodine, and trospium. Plasma protein binding of 5-HT is about 50%, primarily to albumin and α_1-acid glycoprotein, and the terminal half-life is about 6–9 hours (range about 4–20 hours) (1,2).

Reproduction studies have been conducted in mice and rabbits. In mice, oral doses resulting in exposures 6–27 times the expected human exposure (AUC) from the maximum recommended human dose of 8 mg (MRHD) caused no dose-related teratogenicity. One case of cleft palate was observed at each dose tested, but the incidence was within the background historical range. However, increased resorptions and decreased live fetuses were observed. In a prenatal and postnatal development study in mice with an oral dose that was 40% of the dose used in the teratogenicity study, maternal toxicity (decreased body weight) and delayed ear opening of the pups was observed (1).

In rabbits, oral doses producing exposures that were 3–11 times the MRHD were associated with retardation of bone development in the fetuses. No dose-related teratogenicity was observed in rabbits given SC doses up to 9–11 times the exposure from the MRHD, but maternal toxicity and retarded bone development in fetuses (incidence within the background historical range) were observed. Maternal toxicity was observed at exposures three times the MRHD in the absence of any fetal effects (1).

Fesoterodine was not carcinogenic in a 2-year study with oral doses in mice and rats. The drug was not mutagenic nor genotoxic in multiple assays. In mice, fesoterodine had no effect on reproductive function, fertility, or early embryonic development at maternally nontoxic doses (1).

It is not known if 5-HT crosses the human placenta. The molecular weight (about 342), low plasma protein binding, and prolonged terminal half-life suggest that it will cross to the embryo–fetus.

BREASTFEEDING SUMMARY

No reports describing the use of fesoterodine during human lactation have been located.

The molecular weight of the active metabolite 5-HT (about 342), its low plasma protein binding (about 50%), and its long terminal half-life (about 6–9 hours with a range of about 4–20 hours) suggest that it will be excreted into breast milk. The effect of this exposure on a nursing infant is unknown. Although neonates are particular sensitive to anticholinergic agents, atropine is classified as compatible with breastfeeding by the American Academy of Pediatrics (see Atropine).

References

1. Product information. Toviaz. Pfizer, 2008.
2. Malhotra B, Guan Z, Wood N, Gandelman K. Pharmacokinetic profile of fesoterodine. Int J Clin Pharmacol Therapeutics 2008;46:556–63.

FEVERFEW

Herb

PREGNANCY RECOMMENDATION: Contraindicated
BREASTFEEDING RECOMMENDATION: No Human Data—Potential Toxicity

PREGNANCY SUMMARY

No reports describing the use of feverfew in human pregnancy have been located. The only animal reproduction study used a dose, based on weight, that was much higher than a typical human dose. This dose comparison cannot be assessed because doses should be compared based on BSA or AUC. Although embryolethality was suggested by the study, this outcome did not reach statistical significance. Moreover, no structural anomalies were observed in the study. The herb has been used in traditional and folk medicine for approximately 2500 years, so it is doubtful if consumption of the herb is associated with major birth defects. Feverfew does have emmenagogue activity and might cause abortion but, apparently, the doses used for this purpose have not been quantified. Its reported use for morning sickness, again without specifying a dose, suggests that a dose–effect relationship exists. Because the toxic dose is unknown, feverfew should not be used in pregnancy.

FETAL RISK SUMMARY

Feverfew is a plant that grows wild throughout the world, including North America. It is a short, bushy plant with a height up to 1 m (about 3.3 feet) and yellow flowers that bloom from July to October. The herb has been used in traditional and folk medicine for approximately 2500 years. The name feverfew comes from its antipyretic properties. It has been known as "medieval aspirin." Feverfew has been used for a long list of medical conditions, including migraine. It also has been used to treat labor, menstrual disorders, potential miscarriage, morning sickness, and as an abortifacient. Because of the risk of abortion, it is considered contraindicated in pregnancy (1–3).

A large number of chemicals have been identified in feverfew. The major biologically active constituents are thought to be the sesquiterpene lactones, 85% of which are parthenolide. Other chemicals found in the plant are flavonoids, volatile oils, and miscellaneous other substances (1).

Because of the absence of animal reproduction studies, a 2006 study was conducted to screen pregnant rats to determine if a full reproductive study was warranted (3). The daily feverfew dose used was 839 mg/kg, which was 58.7 times the recommended human dose of 1 g/day (assumed to be in a 70-kg adult). Rats were treated daily on either gestational days (GDs) 1–8 to establish if the herb affects implantation and early development, or GDs 8–15 to detect if feverfew affects major organ development. In the GD1–8 group, an increase in preimplantation loss was observed, but the increase was not statistically significant. However, the number of liveborn pups was significantly fewer in the GD1–8 group compared with the GD8–15 group. There was also some indication that fetuses had lower weights than controls in the GD8–15 group, but this may have been due to the increased number of runts (defined as two standard deviations less than the mean litter weight of the controls) in the feverfew-exposed group. None of the treated fetuses had gross internal or external structural anomalies. Based on the overall results, the investigators concluded that a full reproductive study was warranted (3).

It is not known if feverfew crosses the human placenta. The dried leaf powder is standardized to contain at least 0.2% of parthenolide that has a molecular weight of about 248 (4). The molecular weight alone suggests that it will cross to the embryo and/or fetus.

BREASTFEEDING SUMMARY

No reports describing the use of feverfew during lactation have been located. The dried leaf powder is standardized to contain at least 0.2% of parthenolide that has a molecular weight of about 248 (4). The molecular weight alone suggests that it will be excreted into breast milk. Because of the potential risk of toxicity for a nursing infant, women consuming feverfew should not breastfeed (1,2).

References

1. Feverfew. *The Review of Natural Products*. St. Louis, MO: Facts and Comparisons, 2006.
2. Feverfew. *Natural Medicines Comprehensive Database*. 10th ed. Stockton, CA: Therapeutic Research Faculty, 2008:584–5.
3. Yao M, Ritchie HE, Brown-Woodman PD. A reproductive screening test of feverfew: is a full reproductive study warranted? Reprod Toxicol 2006;22:688–93.
4. Feverfew. In: Sweetman SC, ed. *Martindate: The Complete Drug Reference*. 34th ed. London, UK: Pharmaceutical Press, 2005:469.

FEXOFENADINE

Antihistamine

PREGNANCY RECOMMENDATION: No Human Data—Animal Data Suggest Moderate Risk
BREASTFEEDING RECOMMENDATION: Limited Human Data—Probably Compatible

PREGNANCY SUMMARY

No reports describing the use of fexofenadine during human pregnancy have been located. However, studies in rats found dose-related embryo and fetal toxicity, but the risk to a human fetus cannot be assessed at this time. Because of the extensive human data available, several reviews have recommended that oral first-generation antihistamines (e.g., chlorpheniramine or tripelennamine) should be considered if antihistamine therapy during pregnancy (especially in the 1st trimester) is required (1–3). The second-generation agents, cetirizine or loratadine, were considered acceptable alternatives, except during the 1st trimester, if a first-generation antihistamine was not tolerated.

FETAL RISK SUMMARY

Fexofenadine is a second-generation (peripherally selective), histamine H_1-receptor antagonist that is used for the relief of symptoms associated with seasonal allergic rhinitis (4). It is a metabolite of another second-generation antihistamine, terfenadine (no longer available). As a group, second- generation antihistamines are less sedating than first-generation agents.

Fertility studies in rats and reproduction studies in rats and rabbits have been conducted with fexofenadine. In rats, doses producing systemic exposures that were ≥3 times the human exposure obtained with a 60-mg twice-daily dose (HTD) were associated with a dose-related decrease in the number of implantations and an increase in the number of postimplantation losses. No evidence of teratogenicity was noted in pregnant rats and rabbits at oral doses up to 4 and 47 times the HTD, respectively. However, dose-related decreases in pup weight gain and survival were observed in rats at three times the HTD (4).

It is not known if fexofenadine crosses the human placenta to the fetus. The molecular weight (about 502 for the free base) is low enough that transfer to the fetus should be expected.

BREASTFEEDING SUMMARY

Consistent with the molecular weight (about 502 for the free base), fexofenadine is excreted into breast milk. Four lactating women were given terfenadine (60 mg every 12 hours for four doses), and then milk and plasma samples were collected after the last dose at various times for 30 hours (5). None of the parent compound was detected in the milk or plasma. The maximum concentrations of the active metabolite fexofenadine were 309 and 41 ng/mL, respectively—both occurring approximately 4 hours after the last dose. Based on the 12-hour excretion, the mean milk:plasma ratio was 0.21. The maximum estimated exposure of a nursing infant was 0.45% of the recommended maternal weight-corrected dose (5).

The above estimated exposure of a nursing infant may not be applicable when the mother is actually taking fexofenadine. Moreover, the effect of this exposure on a nursing infant is unknown because the four women did not nurse their infants during the study. However, the American Academy of Pediatrics classifies fexofenadine as compatible with breastfeeding (6).

References

1. Mazzotta P, Loebstein R, Koren G. Treating allergic rhinitis in pregnancy. Safety considerations. Drug Saf 1999;20:361–75.
2. Horak F, Stubner UP. Comparative tolerability of second generation antihistamines. Drug Saf 1999;20:385–401.
3. Joint committee of the American College of Obstetricians and Gynecologists (ACOG) and the American College of Allergy, Asthma and Immunology (ACAAI). Position statement. The use of newer asthma and allergy medications during pregnancy. Ann Allergy Asthma Immunol 2000;84:475–80.
4. Product information. Allegra. Hoechst Marion Roussel, 2000.
5. Lucas BD, Purdy CY, Scarim SK, Benjamin S, Abel SR, Hilleman DE. Terfenadine pharmacokinetics in breast milk in lactating women. Clin Pharmacol Ther 1995;57:398–402.
6. Committee on Drugs, American Academy of Pediatrics. The transfer of drugs and other chemicals into human milk. Pediatrics 2001;108:776–89.

FIDAXOMICIN

Antibiotic

PREGNANCY RECOMMENDATION: No Human Data—Animal Data Suggest Low Risk
BREASTFEEDING RECOMMENDATION: No Human Data—Probably Compatible

PREGNANCY SUMMARY

No reports describing the use of fidaxomicin in human pregnancy have been located. The animal reproduction data suggest low risk. Because only minimal amounts (in the ng/mL range) of fidaxomicin are detected in the systemic circulation, the drug is probably compatible in pregnancy.

FETAL RISK SUMMARY

Fidaxomicin is an oral macrolide antibacterial agent. It is indicated in adults (≥18 years of age) for the treatment of *Clostridium difficile*–associated diarrhea. The drug is in the same macrolide antibacterial class as azithromycin, clarithromycin, dirithromycin, erythromycin, and troleandomycin. Fidaxomicin acts in the gastrointestinal tract. Systemic absorption is minimal with plasma concentrations in the ng/mL range. It is metabolized to an active metabolite (OP-1118) in the gut and both the parent drug and metabolite are excreted in the feces with elimination half-lives of 9 and 10 hours, respectively (1).

Reproduction studies have been conducted in rats and rabbits. In these species, IV doses producing plasma exposures that were about 200 and 66 times, respectively, the human exposure based on AUC (HE) revealed no evidence of fetal harm (1).

Long-term carcinogenicity studies have not been conducted with fidaxomicin. Neither the parent drug nor OP-1118 was mutagenic in two assays, but fidaxomicin was clastogenic in one test. No effects on fertility in male and female rats were observed with systemic exposures that were about 100 times the HE (1).

It is not known if fidaxomicin crosses the human placenta. Minimal concentrations of other macrolide antibacterials cross the placenta (e.g., azithromycin and erythromycin) and fidaxomicin might also cross. However, fidaxomicin plasma concentrations are minimal and any exposure of the embryo–fetus should be clinically insignificant.

BREASTFEEDING SUMMARY

No reports describing the use of fidaxomicin during human lactation have been located. Because plasma concentrations of the antibacterial are minimal (ng/mL range), adverse effects in a nursing infant are not expected.

Reference

1. Product information. Optimer Pharmaceuticals, 2011.

FILGRASTIM

Hematopoietic

PREGNANCY RECOMMENDATION: Compatible—Maternal Benefit >> Embryo–Fetal Risk
BREASTFEEDING RECOMMENDATION: No Human Data—Probably Compatible

PREGNANCY SUMMARY

Neither the animal nor the human pregnancy data suggest a major risk for the human embryo or fetus from maternal filgrastim therapy. Although the human pregnancy experience is limited, no congenital malformations or other toxicities attributable to filgrastim have been observed. The cases submitted to the manufacturer suggest selective reporting (i.e., preferentially reporting of abnormal outcomes). Amounts sufficient to produce a biological effect in the fetus apparently cross the human placenta, at least in the 2nd and 3rd trimesters. Additional study is warranted, but filgrastim treatment should not be withheld because of pregnancy.

FETAL RISK SUMMARY

The human granulocyte colony-stimulating factor (G-CSF) filgrastim is a 175-amino acid glycoprotein produced by recombinant DNA technology. Filgrastim is indicated to decrease the incidence of infection, as manifested by febrile neutropenia, in patients with nonmyeloid malignancies receiving myelosuppressive chemotherapy associated with a significant incidence of severe neutropenia with fever. The agent is administered either SC or IV. The elimination half-life is approximately 3.5 hours (1).

Reproduction studies with filgrastim have been conducted in rats and rabbits. No effects on fertility were observed in male and female rats at doses ≤500 mcg/kg. (*Note: The human dose is 5–10 mcg/kg/day.*) In pregnant rats treated during organogenesis, IV injections ≤575 mcg/kg/day were not associated with fetal death, teratogenicity, or behavioral effects. In offspring of pregnant rats treated with doses >20 mcg/kg/day, a delay of external differentiation (detachment of auricles and descent of testes) and slight growth restriction were observed. These effects may have been due to lower maternal body weight during rearing and nursing. At 100 mcg/kg/day, newborn pups had decreased body weights and a slightly decreased 4-day survival rate. Treating pregnant rabbits during organogenesis with doses of 80 mcg/kg/day resulted in increased resorptions and embryolethality but not external defects. This dose, however, was maternally toxic (genitourinary bleeding and decreased body weight and food consumption) (1).

Filgrastim crosses the rat placenta late in gestation (2). In a rat study, filgrastim (50 mcg/kg) was given twice daily for 2, 4, and 6 days before delivery. Filgrastim crossed the placenta within 30 minutes, reaching peak fetal serum levels 4 hours after the dose. Peak serum levels in the fetuses were 1000-fold lower than levels measured in the dams, but the agent still induced bone marrow and spleen myelopoiesis in the fetus and neonate (2). In a continuation of this study, the investigators demonstrated that the 6-day course of filgrastim administered before delivery significantly increased the survival of pups that were infected at birth with Group B β-hemolytic *Streptococcus* (3).

Although it has a very high molecular weight (18,800), filgrastim also crosses the human placenta, at least in the 2nd and 3rd trimesters. A single IV dose of filgrastim (25 mcg/kg) was given to 11 women (1 set of twins) with an imminent delivery at ≤30 weeks' gestation (4). Ten infants were delivered within 30 hours of the dose (mean 10.8 hours) ("early delivery"), and two infants were delivered at 54 and 108 hours ("late delivery"). Three of 10 cord blood samples in the "early delivery" group had G-CSF levels higher than those of 10 untreated controls, but there was no difference in cord blood neutrophil concentrations. Cord blood from the two infants in the "late delivery" group had G-CSF levels similar to those of controls but much higher neutrophil levels that remained elevated for 1 week. The investigators concluded that filgrastim crossed the placenta in amounts sufficient to produce a biologic effect in the fetus, and that this effect was most noticeable in cases where delivery was delayed at least 30 hours after a dose (4).

A 1998 study by the same investigators as above evaluated the effects of filgrastim therapy in women in preterm labor (5). Of the 26 women enrolled in the study, 16 (eight G-CSF subjects and eight controls) delivered within 3 weeks of the dose and were eligible for evaluation. G-CSF cases received a single 25 mcg/kg dose administered as an IV infusion over 4 hours, whereas controls received an IV infusion without the drug. No adverse effects on pregnancy duration or maternal discomfort were noted. Neutrophil production was assessed by bone marrow aspiration in neonates 24 hours after delivery. The mean time between G-CSF or placebo administration and delivery was 3.9 and 6.3 days, respectively. Compared with controls, the neonates of case mothers had a significantly greater marrow proliferative pool and a significant improvement in Scores for Neonatal Acute Physiologic State (5).

A 27-year-old patient at 26 weeks' gestation was diagnosed with acute myeloid leukemia (6). Because she was otherwise well, she decided to hold chemotherapy to allow the fetus to mature. The woman became neutropenic and, at 27 weeks' gestation, developed fever secondary to a systemic infection. In addition to antibiotics, a 12-day course of filgrastim (dose not specified) was given to allow further time for fetal maturation. A cesarean section was performed at 32 weeks' gestation to deliver a healthy baby boy (weight and other details not provided). The infant was doing well at 5 months of age (6).

A brief 1996 report described the use of filgrastim in a pregnant woman with acute promyelocytic leukemia (7). In addition to other treatment, filgrastim (75 mcg/day SC) was given for 7 days early in the 2nd trimester. She eventually delivered a healthy female infant at term (7).

A number of other studies have reported the use of filgrastim in human pregnancy (8–12). In four studies, the outcomes of 15 pregnancies were (period of exposure shown in parentheses) as follows: one normal infant (3rd trimester) (8); two normal infants (throughout); one with bilateral hydronephrosis (throughout); two with cyclic neutropenia (throughout and 3rd trimester; mothers also had the disorder); one normal infant (1st trimester); three elective abortions (EABs) (1st trimester; one fetus with "abnormal embryogenesis"); and one infant with cardiac septal defects (3rd trimester) (9); one normal infant (2–3 weeks' gestation); one normal infant and one spontaneous abortion (SAB) (treatment before pregnancy in both) (10); and one normal infant (3rd trimester) (11).

Two reports from the Severe Chronic Neutropenia International Registry (SCNIR), one in 2002 (12) and the other in 2003 (13), discussed the outcomes of 23 pregnancies in women who were treated with filgrastim. Three women became pregnant during clinical trials and, although they were excluded from the study, continued to receive commercially available filgrastim (12). Two of the women with cyclic neutropenia had normal infants (one with cyclic neutropenia; one electively aborted her first pregnancy, then carried a second pregnancy to term). The third woman had idiopathic neutropenia and she had an EAB because of abnormal bleeding but subsequently died (12). The Registry also collected data on 20 pregnancies in women who had been exposed to filgrastim and 105 pregnancies in women who were not exposed to the agent (historical controls) (13). The outcomes of the exposed group, treated for an average of two trimesters (range one to three), were 13 normal infants, 3 SABs, and 4 EABs (nonmedical). Among the 105 historical controls, there were 75 live births (includes two sets of twins and five infants with medical conditions—primarily respiratory), 24 SABs, and 8 EABs (12,13).

The SCNIR also reported the outcomes of nine pregnancies based on information submitted to the manufacturer (12). Of the nine cases, there were four normal infants, one SAB, and four infants with congenital renal and/or cardiac malformations (12).

BREASTFEEDING SUMMARY

No reports describing the use of filgrastim during human lactation have been located. Filgrastim is a glycoprotein and, although it may be excreted into breast milk, it would probably be digested in a nursing infant's stomach. The risk to a nursing infant is unknown but appears to be low to nonexistent. Therefore, treatment with filgrastim should not be held because of breastfeeding.

References

1. Product information. Neupogen. Amgen, 2004.
2. Medlock ES, Kaplan DL, Cecchini M, Ulich TR, del Castillo J, Andresen J. Granulocyte colony-stimulating factor crosses the placenta and stimulates fetal rat granulopoiesis. Blood 1993;81:916–22.
3. Novales JS, Salva AM, Mondanlou HD, Kaplan DL, del Castillo J, Andresen J, Medlock ES. Maternal administration of granulocyte colony-stimulating factor improves neonatal rat survival after a lethal group B streptococcal infection. Blood 1993;81:923–7.
4. Calhoun DA, Ross C, Christensen RD. Transplacental passage of recombinant human granulocyte colony-stimulating factor in women with an imminent preterm delivery. Am J Obstet Gynecol 1996;174:1306–11.
5. Calhoun DA, Christensen RD. A randomized pilot trial of administration of granulocyte colony-stimulating factor to women before preterm delivery. Am J Obstet Gynecol 1998;179:766–71.
6. Cavenagh JD, Richardson DS, Cahill MR, Bernard T, Kelsey SM, Newland AC. Treatment of acute myeloid leukaemia in pregnancy. Lancet 1995;346:441–2.
7. Lin C-P, Huang M-J, Liu H-J, Chang IY, Tsai C-H. Successful treatment of acute promyelocytic leukemia in a pregnant Jehovah's Witness with all-trans-retinoic acid, rhG-CSF, and erythropoietin. Am J Hematol 1996;51:251–2.
8. Arango HA, Kalter CS, Decesare SL, Fiorica JV, Lyman GH, Spellacy WN. Management of chemotherapy in a pregnancy complicated by a large neuroblastoma. Obstet Gynecol 1994;84:665–8.
9. Welter K, Boxer LA. Severe chronic neutropenia: pathophysiology and therapy. Semin Hematol 1997;34:267–78.
10. Cavallaro AM, Lilleby K, Majolino I, Storb R, Appelbaum FR, Rowley SD, Bensinger WI. Three- to six-year follow-up of normal donors who received recombinant human granulocyte colony-stimulating factor. Bone Marrow Transplant 2000;25:85–9.
11. Sangalli MR, Peek M, McDonald A. Prophylactic granulocyte colony-stimulating factor treatment for acquired chronic severe neutropenia in pregnancy. Aust N Z J Obstet Gynaecol 2001;41:470–1.
12. Cottle TE, Fier CJ, Donadieu J, Kinsey SE. Risk and benefit of treatment of severe chronic neutropenia with granulocyte colony-stimulating factor. Semin Hematol 2002;39:134–40.
13. Dale DC, Cottle TE, Fier CJ, Bolyard AA, Bonilla MA, Boxer LA, Cham B, Freedman MH, Kannourakis G, Kinsey SE, Davis R, Scarlata D, Schwinzer B, Zeidler C, Welte K. Severe chronic neutropenia: treatment and follow-up of patients in the Severe Chronic Neutropenia International Registry. Am J Hematol 2003;72:82–93.

FINGOLIMOD

Immunologic Agent (Immunomodulator)

PREGNANCY RECOMMENDATION: No Human Data—Contraindicated
BREASTFEEDING RECOMMENDATION: No Human Data—Probably Compatible

PREGNANCY SUMMARY

No reports describing the use of fingolimod in human pregnancy have been located. The receptor affected by fingolimod is involved in angiogenesis and vascular formation during embryogenesis. An increase in malformations has been noted in rats given doses similar to the recommended human dose based on BSA (RHD). Reduced pre- and postnatal survival and an increase in learning deficits have also been seen. In rabbits, an increase in embryo–fetal death and growth restriction has been noted, with the no-effect-dose-level approximately 20 times the RHD. On the basis of the termination half-life of the drug, the manufacturer suggests that fingolimod be discontinued at least 2 months before attempting conception.

F

FETAL RISK SUMMARY

Fingolimod is an orally administered drug that modulates sphingosine 1-phosphate receptors. Its active metabolite, fingolimod-phosphate, binds with high affinity to sphingosine 1-phosphate receptors and blocks capacity of lymphocytes to egress from the lymph nodes. It is indicated for the treatment of patients with relapsing forms of multiple sclerosis to delay the frequency of clinical exacerbations and to delay the accumulation of physical disability. Both fingolimod and its active metabolite are highly (99.7%) plasma protein bound. The terminal elimination half-life for both is 6–9 days. The receptor affected by fingolimod affects angiogenesis and is known to be involved in vascular formation during embryogenesis (1,2).

Reproduction studies have been conducted in rats and rabbits. In rats, at oral doses of 0.03–10 mg/kg/day, increased incidences of malformations and embryo–fetal deaths were observed at all but the lowest dose. The lowest end of the dosing range in these studies is less than the RHD. The most common malformations reported in rats were persistent truncus arteriosus and ventricular septal defects. In addition, in rats administered fingolimod during pregnancy and lactation at 0.05–0.5 mg/kg/day, pup survival was decreased at all doses and learning deficits were seen at the highest dose. The lowest dose administered is similar to the RHD. In rabbits, increased incidences of embryo–fetal mortality and growth restriction were seen at doses of 1.5 and 5 mg/kg/day. The no-effect dose in rabbits was about 20 times the RHD (1).

The carcinogenic potential of fingolimod was evaluated in mice and rats. In mice at oral doses of 0.025–2.5 mg/kg/day for up to 2 years, the incidence of malignant lymphoma was increased at the mid and high doses. However, in rats at doses up to 50 times the RHD, no increase in tumors was seen. Both in vitro and in vivo assays for fingolimod were negative for mutagenicity.

No effects on male and female fertility in rats were noted at the highest dose tested, which is approximately 200 times the RHD (1).

It is not known if fingolimod or its active metabolite crosses the human placenta. The relatively low molecular weight (about 307) and the long terminal half-life suggest that the drug will cross, but the high plasma protein binding may limit the exposure of the embryo–fetus (1,3).

BREASTFEEDING SUMMARY

No reports describing the use of fingolimod during human lactation have been located. The molecular weight (about 307) and the long terminal half-life (6–9 days) suggest that the drug and its active metabolite will be excreted into breast milk, but the high plasma protein binding (99.7%) may limit the amount (1,3). The effect of this exposure on a nursing infant is unknown.

References

1. Product information. Gilenya. Novartis, 2011.
2. Schmid G, Guba M, Ischenko I, Papyan A, Joka M, Schrepfer S, Bruns CJ, Jauch KW, Heeschen C, Graeb C. The immunosuppressant FTY720 inhibits tumor angiogenesis via the sphingosine 1-phosphate receptor 1. J Cell Biochem 2007;101:259–70.
3. Chun J, Hartung H-P. Mechanism of action of oral fingolimod (FTY720) in multiple sclerosis. Clin Neuropharmacol 2010;33:91–101.

FLAVOXATE

Urinary Tract Agent (Antispasmodic)

PREGNANCY RECOMMENDATION: Limited Human Data—Animal Data Suggest Low Risk
BREASTFEEDING RECOMMENDATION: No Human Data—Probably Compatible

PREGNANCY SUMMARY

The available human pregnancy data available for flavoxate are very limited and are completely lacking for 1st trimester exposure. Moreover, most of the treated women apparently received short-term therapy (i.e., no more than a few doses), and none involved the oral route with tablets, the only available form of the drug in the United States. The limitations also include a lack of information on the growth and development of the exposed infants. Although these uncertainties markedly limit the validity of any fetal safety assessment, the absence of reported toxicity in the fetus and newborn coupled with the lack of fetal toxicity in animals appears to indicate that the use of flavoxate during the second half of pregnancy presents a small, if any, risk to the fetus. The potential fetal effects of flavoxate exposure in the first half of pregnancy are unknown.

FETAL RISK SUMMARY

Flavoxate is a tertiary amine that is a direct inhibitor of smooth muscle spasm of the urinary tract. The drug also possesses some antimuscarinic (i.e., atropine-like) activity. It is used for the symptomatic relief of urinary tract discomfort resulting from inflammatory conditions. Flavoxate is in the same subclass as darifenacin, oxybutynin, solifenacin, tolterodine, and trospium.

Reproduction studies in mice, rats, and rabbits at doses up to 34 times the human therapeutic dose found no evidence of impaired fertility or fetal harm (1–3). At doses approximately 40 times the therapeutic dose, cleft palate (not thought to be drug-induced) and fetal resorption occurred in mice, and intrauterine growth restriction was observed in fetal mice and rabbits (3).

No reports on the placental transfer of flavoxate have been located. The molecular weight (about 392 for the free base) is low enough that passage to the fetus should be expected.

One presentation at a 1975 conference in Yugoslavia described the use of flavoxate during human pregnancy (4). Although specific obstetric data were not provided, IV flavoxate, often as a single dose in combination with antibiotics, was routinely used in pregnant women for the treatment of pyelonephritis. In addition, the effect of flavoxate on uterine contractions, using total IV doses ranging from 100 to 600 mg, was studied in 30 women at term and in 5 women with premature labor at 7–8 months. Uterine contractions were not modified in any of these patients and no fetal or newborn adverse effects were observed.

A 1984 source cited a 1972 study in which IM flavoxate, 100 mg 3 times daily followed by 400 mg/day by suppository, was used as a tocolytic in 66 women with premature labor (3). The 1984 source cited a second study that involved a reduction in the duration of labor in 120 women with a 100-mg IV dose of flavoxate (3). In neither of the cited studies were adverse effects noted in the mothers or fetuses.

BREASTFEEDING SUMMARY

No reports describing the use of flavoxate during lactation have been located. The molecular weight of the drug (about 392 for the free base) is low enough that excretion into milk should be expected. The effect of this exposure on a nursing infant is unknown.

References

1. Product information. Urispas. SmithKline Beecham Pharmaceuticals, 1998.
2. Schardein JL. *Chemically Induced Birth Defects*. 2nd ed. New York, NY: Marcel Dekker, 1993:447.
3. Onnis A, Grella P. *The Biochemical Effects of Drugs in Pregnancy*. Vol. 1. West Sussex, England: Ellis Norwood Limited, 1984:221–2.
4. Esposito A. *Preliminary Studies on the Use of Flavoxate in Obstetrics and Gynaecology*. International Round Table Discussion on Flavoxate, Opatija, Yugoslavia, March 30, 1975:66–73 (translation provided by BA Wallin, Smith Kline & French Laboratories, 1987).

FLECAINIDE

Antiarrhythmic

PREGNANCY RECOMMENDATION: Limited Human Data—Animal Data Suggest Moderate Risk
BREASTFEEDING RECOMMENDATION: Limited Human Data—Probably Compatible

PREGNANCY SUMMARY

The limited human pregnancy experience includes only one case in which flecainide was used in the 1st trimester. Although the animal data suggest moderate risk, the human data are too limited to allow a complete assessment of risk to the embryo. However, the fetal risk from treatment of refractory fetal arrhythmias appears to be low.

FETAL RISK SUMMARY

Flecainide is an antiarrhythmic agent that is structurally related to encainide and procainamide. In one breed of rabbits, flecainide produced dose-related teratogenicity and embryotoxicity at approximately four times the usual human dose (1). Structural defects observed were club paws, sternebrae and vertebrae abnormalities, and pale hearts with contracted ventricular septum. Similar toxic effects and malformations were not observed in a second breed of rabbits, or in mice and rats, but dose-related delayed sternebral and vertebral ossification was observed in rat fetuses (1).

Two 1988 reports of human use of flecainide during pregnancy may have described a single incidence of exposure to the drug (2,3). IV flecainide was given to a pregnant woman at 30 weeks' gestation for persistent fetal supraventricular tachycardia resistant to digoxin (2,3). The fetal heart rate pattern quickly converted to a sinus rhythm and the mother was maintained on oral flecainide, 100 mg 3 times daily, until delivery was induced at 38 weeks' gestation. The 3450-g female infant had no cardiac problems during the 10 days of observation. Flecainide concentrations in the cord blood and maternal serum at delivery 5 hours after the last dose were 533 and 833 ng/mL, respectively, a ratio of 0.63 (2).

Flecainide 100 mg twice daily, combined with the β-blocker sotalol, was used throughout gestation in one woman for the treatment of ventricular tachycardia and polymorphous ventricular premature complexes associated with an aneurysm of the left ventricle (4). A cesarean section was performed at approximately 37 weeks' gestation. Flecainide concentrations in umbilical cord and plasma samples at delivery, 11 hours after the last dose, were 0.394

and 0.455 mcg/mL, respectively, a ratio of 0.86. No adverse effects, including bradycardia, were observed in the fetus or newborn, who was growing normally at 1 year of age.

A 22-year-old woman at approximately 31 weeks' gestation was treated with flecainide, 100 mg every 8 hours, for fetal arrhythmia associated with fetal hydrops unresponsive to therapeutic levels of digoxin (5). Therapeutic levels of flecainide were measured in the mother over the next 4 days, during which time the fetal heart rate (FHR) converted to a normal sinus rhythm of 120 beats/minute. Approximately 2 days later, a nonreactive nonstress test was documented and flecainide and digoxin were discontinued, but the FHR returned to pretreatment levels within 36 hours. Flecainide was restarted at 150 mg every 12 hours, and within 30 minutes of the first dose, the FHR converted to normal. This dose was continued for 4 days, during which time the FHR remained normal at 120 beats/minute, but with a nonreactive nonstress test. Gradual reduction of the dose to 50 mg every 12 hours maintained a normal FHR with return of a reactive nonstress test and normal beat-to-beat variability. Fetal ascites was completely resolved after 10 days of therapy. A normal 3480-g infant, Apgar scores of 9 and 10 at 1 and 5 minutes, respectively, was delivered vaginally at 41 weeks' gestation. Maternal and fetal serum trough levels at delivery were 0.2 and 0.1 mcg/mL, respectively (5). A postnatal echocardiogram performed on the newborn was normal.

A 1991 report described the experimental use of flecainide, 300–400 mg/day orally, in 14 women at a mean gestational age of 31 weeks (range 23–36 weeks) to treat fetal hydrops and ascites secondary to supraventricular tachycardias or atrial flutter (6). The duration of treatment ranged from 2 days to 5 weeks. Although specific data were not given, the cord:maternal plasma ratio at birth was approximately 0.80, and all fetuses had flecainide concentrations within the usual therapeutic range (400–800 mcg/L). Twelve of the fourteen newborns were alive and well at the time of the report, and one infant, not under treatment at the time, died of sudden infant death syndrome at 4.5 months of age. One intrauterine death occurred after 3 days of therapy and may have been caused by either a flecainide-induced arrhythmia or fetal blood sampling (6).

A woman in the 3rd trimester was initially treated with flecainide 100 mg orally twice daily, then decreased to 50 mg twice daily, for fetal tachycardia that resolved within 4 days (7). The fetal ascites and polyhydramnios also resolved around this time. Approximately 6 weeks after treatment was begun, she gave birth to a 3320-g, male infant. The cord blood:maternal serum ratio of the drug was 0.97 (235.4/241.2 ng/mL), but the flecainide concentration in the amniotic fluid was 6426.5 ng/mL, about 27 times the level in the fetus.

Other publications have described the successful use of flecainide for the treatment of fetal tachycardia (8–14), and in one of these, flecainide and digoxin were considered the drugs of choice for this condition (8). However, flecainide is superior to digoxin for the treatment of tachycardia in hydropic fetuses (9,10).

The loss of FHR variability and accelerations was described in a case of supraventricular tachycardia treated with 300 mg/day of flecainide during the 3rd trimester (11). The heart rate of the 3690-g male infant returned to a reactive pattern 5 days after delivery. One day later, the infant's serum concentration of flecainide was below the detection level. A general review of drug therapy used for the treatment of fetal arrhythmias was published in 1994 (12). Flecainide has also been used to treat new-onset maternal ventricular tachycardia presenting during the 3rd trimester (15).

Conjugated hyperbilirubinemia thought to be caused by flecainide was described in a 1995 reference (16). Flecainide, 150 mg twice daily, was started at about 28 weeks' gestation for the treatment of fetal supraventricular tachycardia after a trial of digoxin and adenosine had failed to halt the arrhythmia. Other fetal complications, in addition to the arrhythmia, were polyhydramnios, ascites, pericardial effusion, cardiomegaly, and tricuspid and mitral valve regurgitation. Successful conversion to a sinus rhythm occurred within 24 hours. The mother discontinued the therapy 1 week later, and a second course of flecainide was started when the fetal tachycardia and ascites reoccurred. The 2843-g, male infant, delivered vaginally at 36 weeks, developed transient conjugated hyperbilirubinemia within a few days of birth. The authors attributed the hyperbilirubinemia to flecainide because no other cause of the toxicity could be found and the drug is known to produce a similar condition in adults. Follow-up of the infant at 2 months of age revealed that the liver toxicity had resolved and, at 28 months of age, the child was continuing to do well (16).

BREASTFEEDING SUMMARY

Flecainide is concentrated in breast milk (4,17), but no reports of infant exposure to the drug from nursing have been located. A woman was treated throughout gestation and in the postpartum period with flecainide, 100 mg twice daily, and sotalol (see Sotalol) (4). Simultaneous samples of milk and plasma were drawn 3 hours after the second daily dose on the 5th and 7th days postpartum. Flecainide concentrations on day 5 were 0.891 and 0.567 mcg/mL, respectively, and 1.093 and 0.500 mcg/mL, respectively, on day 7. Milk:plasma ratios were 1.57 and 2.18, respectively. The infant was not breastfed (4).

Eleven healthy women volunteers who intended not to breastfeed were given flecainide 100 mg orally every 12 hours for 5.5 days starting on postpartum day 1 (17). The breasts were emptied by a mechanical breast suction pump every 3–4 hours during the study. Peak milk levels of the drug occurred at 3–6 hours after a dose with a mean half-life of elimination of 14.7 hours. The highest daily average concentration of the drug ranged from 270 to 1529 ng/mL, with milk:plasma ratios on days 2, 3, 4, and 5 of 3.7, 3.2, 3.5, and 2.6, respectively. An estimated maximum steady-state concentration of flecainide in an infant consuming approximately 700 mL of milk per day (assumed to be the total milk production) was 62 ng/mL, an apparently nontoxic level. Based on this, the investigators concluded that the risk of adverse effects in a nursing infant whose mother was consuming flecainide was minimal (17). The American Academy of Pediatrics classifies flecainide as compatible with breastfeeding (18).

References

1. Product information, Tambocor. 3M Pharmaceuticals, 1993.
2. Wren C, Hunter S. Maternal administration of flecainide to terminate and suppress fetal tachycardia. Br Med J 1988;296:249.

3. Macphail S, Walkinshaw SA. Fetal supraventricular tachycardia: detection by routine auscultation and successful in-utero management: case report. Br J Obstet Gynaecol 1988;95:1073–6.
4. Wagner X, Jouglard J, Moulin M, Miller AM, Petitjean J, Pisapia A. Coadministration of flecainide acetate and sotalol during pregnancy: lack of teratogenic effects, passage across the placenta, and excretion in human breast milk. Am Heart J 1990;119:700–2.
5. Kofinas AD, Simon NV, Sagel H, Lyttle E, Smith N, King K. Treatment of fetal supraventricular tachycardia with flecainide acetate after digoxin failure. Am J Obstet Gynecol 1991;165:630–1.
6. Allan LD, Chita SK, Sharland GK, Maxwell D, Priestley K. Flecainide in the treatment of fetal tachycardias. Br Heart J 1991;65:46–8.
7. Bourget P, Pons J-C, Delouis C, Fermont L, Frydman R. Flecainide distribution, transplacental passage, and accumulation in the amniotic fluid during the third trimester of pregnancy. Ann Pharmacother 1994;28:1031–4.
8. van Engelen AD, Weijtens O, Brenner JI, Kleinman CS, Copel JA, Stoutenbeek P, Meijboom EJ. Management outcome and follow-up of fetal tachycardia. J Am Coll Cardiol 1994;24:1371–5.
9. Simpson JM, Sharland GK. Fetal tachycardias: management and outcome of 127 consecutive cases. Heart 1998;79:576–81.
10. Wren C. Mechanisms of fetal tachycardia. Heart 1998;79:536–7.
11. van Gelder-Hasker MR, de Jong CLD, de Vries JIP, van Geijn HP. The effect of flecainide acetate on fetal heart rate variability: a case report. Obstet Gynecol 1995;86:667–9.
12. Ito S, Magee L, Smallhorn J. Drug therapy for fetal arrhythmias. Clin Perinatol 1994;21:543–72.
13. Amano K, Harada Y, Shoda T, Nishijima M, Hiraishi S. Successful treatment of supraventricular tachycardia with flecainide acetate: a case report. Fetal Diagn Ther 1997;12:328–31.
14. Jaeggi E, Fouron JC, Drblik SP. Fetal atrial flutter: diagnosis, clinical features, treatment, and outcome. J Pediatr 1998;132:335–9.
15. Connaughton M, Jenkins BS. Successful use of flecainide to treat new-onset maternal ventricular tachycardia in pregnancy. Br Heart J 1994;72:297.
16. Vanderhal AL, Cocjin J, Santulli TV, Carlson DE, Rosenthal P. Conjugated hyperbilirubinemia in a newborn infant after maternal (transplacental) treatment with flecainide acetate for fetal tachycardia and fetal hydrops. J Pediatr 1995;126:988–90.
17. McQuinn RL, Pisani A, Wafa S, Chang SF, Miller AM, Frappell JM, Chamberlain GVP, Camm AJ. Flecainide excretion in human breast milk. Clin Pharmacol Ther 1990;48:262–7.
18. Committee on Drugs, American Academy of Pediatrics. The transfer of drugs and other chemicals into human milk. Pediatrics 2001;108:776–89.

FLOSEQUINAN

[Withdrawn from the market. See 9th edition.]

FLOXURIDINE

Antineoplastic (Antimetabolite)

PREGNANCY RECOMMENDATION: Contraindicated—1st Trimester
BREASTFEEDING RECOMMENDATION: Contraindicated

PREGNANCY SUMMARY

No reports describing the use of floxuridine in human pregnancy have been located. The drug has caused some form of developmental toxicity (structural anomalies, functional deficits, and death) in several animal species. Although the magnitude of human risk is unknown, floxuridine is best avoided in pregnancy, especially in the 1st trimester, because it interferes with DNA, RNA, and protein synthesis.

FETAL RISK SUMMARY

Floxuridine, a fluorinated pyrimidine, is a prodrug antineoplastic antimetabolite that is given by intra-arterial infusion. It is rapidly metabolized to one of two active agents, 5-fluorouracil or floxuridine-monophosphate, and several inactive metabolites (see also Fluorouracil). It is classified as an antimetabolite in the subclass of pyrimidine analogs. In addition to fluorouracil, other antineoplastic agents in the subclass are capecitabine and gemcitabine. Floxuridine is indicated for the palliative management of gastrointestinal adenocarcinoma metastatic to the liver. Pharmacokinetic data are not available (1,2).

Reproduction studies have been conducted in the chick embryo, mice, and rats. The drug was teratogenic in the three species at doses that were 4.2–125 times the recommended human therapeutic dose. Malformations included cleft palates, skeletal defects and deformed appendages, paws, and tails (2). In addition, a 1998 study concluded that the postpubertal reproduction dysfunction observed in male mice that had been exposed to floxuridine as embryos resulted from excessive cell death in the developing brain (3).

Long-term carcinogenicity studies have not been conducted with floxuridine. Floxuridine and its active metabolite, fluorouracil, are known to be mutagenic. With the exception of the above study, reproductive performance and fertility studies have not been conducted with floxuridine. However, fluorouracil is known to cause chromosomal aberrations and changes in chromosome organization of spermatogonia, as well as transient infertility in rats. In female rats, intraperitoneal doses of fluorouracil administered in the preovulatory phase of oogenesis significantly reduced the number of fertile matings, delayed the development of embryos, increased the incidence of preimplantation lethality, and induced chromosomal anomalies in the embryos (2).

It is not known if floxuridine or its active metabolites cross the human placenta. The molecular weight of the parent compound (about 246) suggests that the drug will cross to the embryo–fetus.

BREASTFEEDING SUMMARY

No reports describing the use of floxuridine during human lactation have been located. The antineoplastic agent is converted into two active metabolites, 5-fluorouracil and floxuridine-monophosphate (see also Fluorouracil). The molecular weight of the parent compound (about 246) suggests that the drug will be excreted into breast milk. If a nursing woman is treated with floxuridine, breastfeeding should be avoided because the drug interferes with DNA, RNA, and protein synthesis.

References

1. Product information. FUDR. Roche Laboratories, 1987.
2. Product information. Floxuridine. Bedford Laboratories, 2000.
3. Nagao T, Kuwagata M, Saito Y. Effects of prenatal exposure to 5-fluoro-2′-deoxyuridine on developing central nervous system and reproductive function in male offspring of mice. Teratog Carcinog Mutagen 1998;18:73–92.

F

FLUCONAZOLE

Antifungal

PREGNANCY RECOMMENDATION: Human Data Suggest Risk (≥400 mg/day)
BREASTFEEDING RECOMMENDATION: Compatible

PREGNANCY SUMMARY

Although the data are very limited, the use of fluconazole during the 1st trimester appears to be teratogenic with continuous daily doses of 400 mg/day or more. The malformations may resemble those observed in the Antley-Bixler syndrome. The published experience with the use of smaller doses, such as those prescribed for vaginal fungal infections, suggests that the risk for adverse outcomes is low, if it exists at all. In those instances in which continuous, high-dose fluconazole is the only therapeutic choice during the 1st trimester, the patient should be informed of the potential risk to her fetus.

FETAL RISK SUMMARY

Fluconazole is a triazole antifungal agent in the same class as itraconazole, posaconazole, terconazole, and voriconazole.

In studies with pregnant rabbits, abortions were noted at a dose 20–60 times the recommended human dose (RHD) but no fetal anomalies (1). In pregnant rats, doses <20–60 times the RHD produced increases in fetal anatomical variants (supernumerary ribs, renal pelvis dilation, and delays in ossification). At doses 20 to ≥60 times the RHD, embryo deaths were observed as well as structural abnormalities consisting of wavy ribs, cleft palate, and abnormal craniofacial ossification (1). These effects were thought to be consistent with inhibition of estrogen synthesis (1).

One hypothesis for the teratogenic effects of phenytoin involves the production of toxic intermediates, such as an epoxide (arene oxide) (2). Because fluconazole inhibits the cytochrome P450 pathway responsible for phenytoin metabolism, authors of a 1999 study reasoned that the drug combination could provide a test of the hypothesis. The theory was not supported, however, when pretreatment with a nonembryotoxic fluconazole dose doubled (from 6.2% to 13.3%) the incidence of phenytoin-induced cleft palate in mice. Administering both drugs closely together significantly increased the incidence of resorptions ($p < 0.05$) but not malformations. This lack of effect on malformations may have been related to the increased embryolethality of the combination (2). The mechanism for the teratological interaction between the drugs was unknown.

It is not known if fluconazole crosses the human placenta. The molecular weight (about 306) is low enough that passage to the fetus should be expected.

A case published in 1992 described the pregnancy outcome in a 22-year-old black woman who was treated before and throughout gestation with fluconazole, 400 mg/day orally, for disseminated coccidioidomycosis (3). Premature rupture of the membranes occurred at 27 weeks' gestation; 1 week later, a cesarean section was performed because of chorioamnionitis. A 1145-g female infant with grossly dysmorphic features and with Apgar scores of 0 and 6 at 1 and 5 minutes, respectively, was delivered. The infant died shortly after birth. Anatomic abnormalities included cranioschisis of the frontal bones, craniostenosis of the sagittal suture, hypoplasia of the nasal bones, cleft palate, humeral–radial fusion, bowed tibia and femur, bilateral femoral fractures, contractures of both upper and lower extremities, an incompletely formed right thumb, medial deviation of both feet with a short left first toe, and short right first, fourth, and fifth toes (3). No evidence of coccidioidomycosis was found on microscopic examination.

A 1996 publication described three infants (one of whom is described above) with congenital malformations who had been exposed to fluconazole in utero during the 1st trimester or beyond (4). One woman with *Coccidioides immitis* meningitis took 800 mg/day of fluconazole through the first 7 weeks of pregnancy, then resumed the therapy during the 9th week of gestation and continued until delivery by cesarean section at 38 weeks' gestation. The male infant was small for gestational age (1878 g), was cyanotic, and had a poor tone. He suffered a femur fracture when his limbs were straightened for measurement shortly after birth. Multiple malformations were observed, involving the head and face: brachycephaly, maxillary hypoplasia, small ear helices, exotropia, craniofacial disproportion, large anterior fontanelle, trigonocephaly, supraorbital ridge hypoplasia, and micrognathia; the skeleton: femoral bowing, femoral fracture, thin clavicles, ribs, and long bones, and diffuse osteopenia; and the heart: tetralogy of Fallot, pulmonary artery hypoplasia, patent foramen ovale, and patent ductus arteriosus.

The pregnancy outcome of a woman (her second pregnancy), first described by Lee et al. in 1992 (3), was also reviewed in the above 1996 reference. In her next pregnancy (her third), she delivered a healthy male infant (4). Although she had been told to take fluconazole 400 mg/day, nontherapeutic serum levels documented that the patient was not compliant with these instructions. After this, the woman conceived a fourth time, and therapeutic serum fluconazole concentrations were documented while she was taking 400 mg/day. Therapy was discontinued when her pregnancy was diagnosed at 4 months' gestation. The full-term female infant (weight not specified) had multiple malformations involving the head and face: cleft palate, low ears, tracheomalacia, rudimentary epiglottis, and proptosis; the skeleton: femoral bowing, clavicular fracture, thin wavy ribs, absent distal phalanx (toe), and arachnodactyly; and the heart: ventricular septal defect and pulmonary artery hypoplasia. The infant died at age 3 months from complications related to her tracheomalacia.

The anomalies noted in the 1992 case report were at first thought to be consistent with an autosomal recessive genetic disorder known as the Antley-Bixler syndrome (3). However, because of the second case in the same mother and the third infant, the defects were now thought to represent the teratogenic effect of fluconazole (4). Moreover, several of the defects observed were similar to those described in fetal rats exposed to fluconazole.

The FDA in January 1996 received a report of congenital defects in an infant exposed to 800 mg/day of fluconazole during the 1st trimester (F. Rosa, personal communication, FDA, 1996). Similar to the case described by Lee et al. (3), the infant had craniostenosis of the sagittal suture and a rare bilateral humeral–radial fusion anomaly. Other malformations were rocker-bottom feet and orbital hypoplasia. Additional individual adverse reports involving fluconazole that were received by the FDA included three cases of cleft palate, one case each of miscarriage with severe shortening of all limbs and of syndactyly, both after a single 150-mg dose in the 1st trimester, and single cases of hydrocephalus, omphalocele, and deafness.

A 1997 case report described a 27-year-old woman with chronic *C. immitis* meningitis who was treated with fluconazole (400 mg/day through the fourth or fifth week, then 800 mg/day) during the first 9 weeks of an unknown pregnancy (5). Fluconazole was stopped when the pregnancy was diagnosed and amphotericin B therapy was initiated. At 22 weeks' gestation, amphotericin B was discontinued and fluconazole was restarted at 1200 mg/day. Spontaneous rupture of the membranes occurred at 31 weeks and a 1300-g male infant was delivered by cesarean section. Craniofacial anomalies noted in the newborn included a soft calvarium, widely separated sutures, prominent forehead, mild exorbitism, a large pear-shaped nose, and small ears with overfolded helices (5). Other malformations included immobile elbows, hypoplastic nails, subluxed hips, rocker-bottom feet, and bilateral radialhumeral synostosis. Because of the similarity to the other reported cases, the authors concluded that fluconazole produces an Antley-Bixler-like syndrome (5). *(Note: The malformations observed in this infant are very similar to those described by Rosa above, and may have been the same case.)*

In contrast to the above adverse outcomes, a retrospective review of 289 pregnancies was reported in which the mothers received either a single 150-mg dose (N = 275), multiple 50-mg doses (N = 3), or multiple 150-mg doses (N = 11) of fluconazole (6). All of the women were treated during (gestational age of exposure not specified) or shortly before pregnancy for vaginal candidiasis, even though the authors noted that fluconazole was contraindicated for the treatment of this condition in pregnancy. The outcomes of the 289 pregnancies included 178 infants (5 sets of twins), 39 (13.5%) spontaneous abortions, 38 elective abortions, 2 ectopic pregnancies, and 37 unknown outcomes. Four infants with anomalies were observed, but in each case the mother had taken fluconazole before conception (1 week to >26 weeks before the last monthly menstrual period).

A prospective study published in 1996 compared the pregnancy outcomes of 226 women exposed to fluconazole during the 1st trimester with 452 women exposed to nonteratogenic agents (7). The dosage taken by the exposed group consisted of a single, 150 mg dose (N = 105, 47%), multiple doses of 150 mg (N = 81, 36%), 50-mg single dose (N = 3, 1%), 50-mg multiple doses (N = 23, 10%), 100-mg single dose (N = 5, 2%), or 100-mg multiple doses (N = 9, 4%). Most women (90.7%) were treated for vaginal candidiasis. There were no differences between the two groups in the number of miscarriages, stillbirths, congenital malformations, prematurity, low birth weight, cesarean section, or prolonged hospital stay. Seven (4.0% of live births) of the exposed women delivered infants with anomalies compared with 17 (4.2% of live births) of controls. There was no pattern among the congenital anomalies in the exposed group except for two cases of trisomy 21.

A brief 1996 case report described a normal pregnancy outcome in a 24-year-old woman treated with 21 days of fluconazole (600 mg/day) (because of intolerance to amphotericin B) for *Torulopsis glabrata* fungemia beginning at 14 weeks' gestation (8). Although the patient's course was complicated by shock and intracerebral hemorrhage, she eventually delivered at term a healthy 2.95-kg infant (sex not specified) who was doing well at 18 months of age.

In another 1996 case report, a 24-year-old woman at about 19 weeks' gestation had chorioretinitis, candidiasis, fever, pneumonia, and low body weight attributed to *Candida albicans* sepsis (9). Because of massive nausea and vomiting after a test dose of amphotericin B, she was treated with IV fluconazole (10 mg/kg/day or about 400 mg/day) for 16 days and then the same dosage orally for another 34 days. She responded well to the antifungal therapy and gave birth at 39 weeks to a healthy 2.834-kg female infant with Apgar scores of 8 and 9 at 1 and 5 minutes, respectively. The infant had normal growth and mental development at 2 years of age (9).

A regional drug information center reported the pregnancy outcomes of 16 women (17 outcomes, 1 set of twins) who had called to inquire about the effect of fluconazole on their pregnancies (10). The median fluconazole dose was 300 mg (range 150–1000 mg) starting at a mean 4 weeks' gestation (range 1–26 weeks). The twins were stillborn (no malformations), but the other 15 newborns were normal.

A 1998 noninterventional observational cohort study described the outcomes of pregnancies in women who had been prescribed one or more of 34 newly marketed drugs by general practitioners in England (11). Data were obtained by questionnaires sent to the prescribing physicians one month after the expected or possible date of delivery. In 831 (78%) of the pregnancies, a newly marketed drug was thought to have been taken during the 1st trimester with birth defects noted in 14 (2.5%) singleton births of the 557 newborns (10 sets of twins). In addition, two birth defects were observed in aborted fetuses. However, few of the aborted fetuses were examined. Fluconazole was taken during the 1st trimester in 48 pregnancies, but the dose and duration of therapy were not specified. The outcomes of these pregnancies included 4 spontaneous abortions, 5 elective abortions, 4 pregnancies lost to follow-up, and 37 normal newborns (3 premature; 2 sets of full-term twins) (11). Although no congenital malformations were observed, the study lacked the sensitivity to identify minor anomalies because of the absence of standardized examinations. Late-appearing major defects may also have been missed due to the timing of the questionnaires.

A short 1998 report described the pregnancy outcome of a 38-year-old woman who had been treated with a single 150-mg oral dose of fluconazole about the date of conception (12). Chorionic villus sampling was conducted at 12 weeks' gestation finding a normal karyotype (46,XY). The male infant, delivered by cesarean section at 39 weeks', had an encephalocele. Echocardiography revealed dextrocardia and that both the pulmonary artery and the aorta emerged from the right ventricle (12). He died at 7 days of age. The cause of the anomalies was unknown, but it could not have been secondary to fluconazole because of the timing of the exposure.

A 42-year-old woman with achalasia at 31 weeks' gestation was diagnosed with *Candida* esophagitis (13). IV fluconazole, 150 mg/day, was given for 14 days with resolution of the vomiting and lessening of her nausea. She was treated before and after fluconazole with parenteral hyperalimentation. An apparently healthy 2.438-kg female infant, Apgar scores of 9 and 9 at 1 and 5 minutes, respectively, was delivered at 38 weeks' gestation.

In a 1999 report, fluconazole exposures and pregnancy outcomes were examined using the Danish Jutland Pharmaco-Epidemiological Prescription Database (14). A total of 165 women who had received a single, oral 150-mg dose of fluconazole for vaginal candidiasis just before or during pregnancy from 1991 to 1996 were identified. Of these, 121 had been exposed during the 1st trimester. The outcomes of exposed women were compared with the outcomes of 13,327 women who had not received any prescription medication during their pregnancies (controls). In the comparison of exposed newborns with controls, no elevated risk for preterm delivery (odds ratio [OR] 1.17, 95% confidence interval [CI] 0.63–2.17) or low birth weight (OR 1.19, 95% CI 0.37–3.79) was discovered. Similarly, the prevalence of congenital malformations was 3.3% (4 of 121) in exposed compared with 5.2% (697 of 13,327) in controls (OR 0.65, 95% CI 0.24–1.77) (14).

In a 2005 case, a woman with HIV infection was treated with multiple drugs, including fluconazole 400 mg/day, during pregnancy (15). The infant, delivered at 37 weeks', was noted to have seizures secondary to withdrawal from methadone and multiple malformations. Examination at 9 months of age revealed craniosynostosis, shallow orbital region, hypoplastic supraorbital ridges, hypertelorism, mild ptosis, radioulinar synostosis, and metacarpophalangeal–proximal interphalangeal symphalangism of D2–D5 bilaterally. Antley-Bixler and other syndromes were excluded. Compared with four previous cases, the findings in the present case of craniosynostosis, multiple symphalangism, and long-bone abnormalities were similar and suggested a clearly identifiable phenotype (15).

A 1998 review concluded that the risk of embryo–fetal harm was low when small doses were used, such as those for vaginal fungal infections (16).

In a 2013 case report, a woman at 21 3/7 weeks' gestation had a cervical cerclage for early labor (17). A culture of the amniotic fluid taken before the cerclage placement was positive for *C. albicans*. Because she refused removal of the cerclage, she was treated with an 800-mg IV dose of fluconazole, followed by 400 mg/day orally. After a 14-day course of fluconazole, a repeat amniotic fluid culture remained positive for the fungus. The woman still refused removal of the cerclage. A 40-mg dose of fluconazole was then instilled into the amniotic fluid, followed by another 800 mg IV loading dose and 400 mg/day. A terconazole 80-mg vaginal suppository was given nightly. Intra-amniotic fluconazole was given weekly, with the next two doses being 100 mg and 80 mg. Four weeks later, at 27 2/7 weeks, an emergent cesarean section for placental abruption delivered a viable female infant with Apgar scores of 5 and 7. The infant was discharged home after a 67-day stay in the neonatal intensive care unit. A second case very similar to that above also was reported. This patient presented at 23 1/7 weeks and was treated similar to the first case until she underwent cesarean delivery for presumed placental abruption at 31 5/7 weeks. The 1.62-kg female infant had Apgar scores of 7 and 8 and, after a 39-day stay, was discharged home without sequelae (17).

A registry-based cohort of liveborn infants in Denmark that examined 1st trimester exposure to fluconazole was published in 2013 (18). No increased risk of birth defects with oral doses of 150 mg or 300 mg was found in the 7352 exposed pregnancies (prevalence 2.86%) compared with 968,236 unexposed pregnancies (prevalence 2.60%) (OR 1.06, 95% CI 0.92–1.21). However, a significantly increased risk for tetralogy of Fallot was found (7 cases vs. 287 cases; prevalence 0.10% vs. 0.03%; OR 3.13, 95% CI 1.49–6.71). As noted by the authors, the absolute risk for tetralogy of Fallot was small and requires confirmation from other studies (18).

BREASTFEEDING SUMMARY

Fluconazole is excreted into human milk (19,20). A 42-year-old lactating 54.5-kg woman was taking fluconazole 200 mg once daily (19). On her 18th day of therapy (8 days postpartum), milk samples were obtained at 0.5 hour before a dose and at 2, 4, and 10 hours after a dose. Serum samples were drawn 0.5 hour before the dose and 4 hours after the dose. On her last day of therapy (20 days postpartum), milk samples were again collected at 12, 24, 36, and 48 hours after the dose. Peak milk concentrations of fluconazole, up to 4.1 mcg/mL, were measured 2 hours after the mother's dose. The milk:plasma ratios at 0.5 hour before dose and 4 hours after dose were both 0.90. The elimination half-lives in the milk and serum were 26.9 hours and 18.6 hours, respectively. No mention was made of the nursing infant (19).

A 29-year-old woman who was nursing her 12-week-old infant developed a vaginal fungal infection (20). Breastfeeding was halted at the patient's request and she was given 150 mg of fluconazole orally. Fluconazole concentrations were determined in milk (pooled from both breasts) and plasma samples obtained at 2, 5, 24, and 48 hours after the dose. Milk concentrations were 2.93, 2.66, 1.76, and 0.98 mcg/mL, respectively, while plasma concentrations were 6.42, 2.79, 2.52, and 1.19 mcg/mL, respectively. The milk:plasma ratios were 0.46, 0.85, 0.85, and 0.83, respectively, with half-lives of 30 and 35 hours, respectively, in the milk and plasma. The author estimated that after three plasma half-lives, 87.5% of the dose would have been eliminated from a woman with normal renal function, thereby greatly reducing the amount of drug a nursing infant would ingest (20).

Although the risk to a nursing infant from exposure to fluconazole in breast milk is unknown, the safe use of this antifungal agent in neonates has been reported (21–23). A brief 1989 report described a 48-day-old infant, born at 36 weeks' gestation, who was treated with IV fluconazole, 6 mg/kg/day, for disseminated *C. albicans* (21). The dosage was reduced to 3 mg/kg/day when a slight, transient increase in serum transaminase values was measured. The infant was discharged home at 80 days of age in good condition. In the second case, IV fluconazole 6 mg/kg/day was administered for 20 days to an approximately 6-week-old, premature infant (born at 28 weeks' gestation) with a disseminated *C. albicans* infection (22). Results of follow-up studies of the infant during the next 4 months were apparently normal. In a similar case, a 1-month-old premature infant was treated with IV fluconazole (5 mg/kg for 1 hour daily) for 21 days and orally for 8 days for meningitis caused by a *Candida* species (23). He was doing well at 9 months of age.

A mother, breastfeeding her third infant, experienced severe pain from cracked nipples associated with a fungal infection (24). She had successfully breastfed her two previous infants for 1–2 years. The fungal infection was successfully treated with fluconazole (200 mg loading dose, then 100 mg/day for 15 days, and then 200 mg/day for 15 days) (24).

The safety of fluconazole during breastfeeding cannot be completely extrapolated from these cases, but the dose administered to these infants far exceeds the amount they would have received via breast milk. Since no drug-induced toxicity was encountered in the infants, fluconazole is probably safe to use during breast feeding. The American Academy of Pediatrics classifies fluconazole as compatible with breastfeeding (25).

References

1. Product information. Diflucan. Pfizer, 2001.
2. Tiboni GM, Iammarrone E, Giampietro F, Lamonaca D, Bellati U, Di Ilio C. Teratological interaction between the bis-triazole antifungal agent fluconazole and the anticonvulsant drug phenytoin. Teratology 1999;59:81–7.
3. Lee BE, Feinberg M, Abraham JJ, Murthy AR. Congenital malformations in an infant born to a woman treated with fluconazole. Pediatr Infect Dis J 1992;11:1062–4.
4. Pursley TJ, Blomquist IK, Abraham J, Andersen HF, Bartley JA. Fluconazole-induced congenital anomalies in three infants. Clin Infect Dis 1996;22:336–40.
5. Aleck KA, Bartley DL. Multiple malformation syndrome following fluconazole use in pregnancy: report of an additional patient. Am J Med Genet 1997;72:253–6.
6. Inman W, Pearce G, Wilton L. Safety of fluconazole in the treatment of vaginal candidiasis. A prescription-event monitoring study, with special reference to the outcome of pregnancy. Eur J Clin Pharmacol 1994;46:115–8.
7. Mastroiacovo P, Mazzone T, Botto LD, Serafini MA, Finardi A, Caramelli L, Fusco D. Prospective assessment of pregnancy outcomes after first-trimester exposure to fluconazole. Am J Obstet Gynecol 1996;175:1645–50.
8. Kremery V Jr, Huttova M, Masar O. Teratogenicity of fluconazole. Pediatr Infect Dis 1996;15:841.
9. Wiesinger EC, Mayerhofer S, Wenisch C, Breyer S, Graninger W. Fluconazole in *Candida albicans* sepsis during pregnancy: case report and review of the literature. Infection 1996;24:263–6.
10. Campomori A, Bonati M. Fluconazole treatment for vulvovaginal candidiasis during pregnancy. Ann Pharmacother 1997;118–9.
11. Wilton LV, Pearce GL, Martin RM, Mackay FJ, Mann RD. The outcomes of pregnancy in women exposed to newly marketed drugs in general practice in England. Br J Obstet Gynaecol 1998;105:882–9.
12. Sanchez JM, Moya G. Fluconazole teratogenicity. Prenat Diagn 1998;18:862–3.
13. Kalish RB, Garry D, Figueroa R. Achalasia with Candida esophagitis during pregnancy. Obstet Gynecol 1999;94:850.
14. Sorensen HT, Nielsen GL, Olesen C, Larsen H, Steffensen FH, Schonheyder HC, Olsen J, Czeizel AE. Risk of malformations and other outcomes in children exposed to fluconazole in utero. Br J Clin Pharmacol 1999;48:234–8.
15. Lopez-Rangel E, Van Allen MI. Prenatal exposure to fluconazole: an identifiable dysmorphic phenotype. Birth Defects Res A Clin Mol Teratol 2005;73:919–23.
16. King CT, Rogers PD, Cleary JD, Chapman SW. Antifungal therapy during pregnancy. Clin Infect Dis 1998;27:1151–60.
17. Bean LM, Jackson JR, Dobak WJ, Beiswenger TR, Thorp JA. Intra-amniotic fluconazole therapy for *Candida albicans* intra-amniotic infection. Obstet Gynecol 2013;121:452–4.
18. Molgaard-Nielsen D, Pasternak B, Hviid A. Use of oral fluconazole during pregnancy and the risk of birth defects. N Engl J Med 2013;369:830–9.
19. Schilling CG, Seay RE, Larson TA, Meier KR. Excretion of fluconazole in human breast milk (abstract no. 130). Pharmacotherapy 1993;13:287.
20. Force RW. Fluconazole concentrations in breast milk. Pediatr Infect Dis J 1995;14:235–6.
21. Viscoli C, Castagnola E, Corsini M, Gastaldi R, Soliani M, Terragna A. Fluconazole therapy in an underweight infant. Eur J Clin Microbiol Infect Dis 1989;8:925–6.
22. Wiest DB, Fowler SL, Garner SS, Simons DR. Fluconazole in neonatal disseminated candidiasis. Arch Dis Child 1991;66:1002.
23. Gurses N, Kalayci AG. Fluconazole monotherapy for Candidal meningitis in a premature infant. Clin Infect Dis 1996;23:645–6.
24. Bodley V, Powers D. Long-term treatment of a breastfeeding mother with fluconazole-resolved nipple pain caused by yeast: a case study. J Hum Lact 1997;13:307–11.
25. Committee on Drugs, American Academy of Pediatrics. The transfer of drugs and other chemical into human milk. Pediatrics 2001;108:776–89.

FLUCYTOSINE

Antifungal

PREGNANCY RECOMMENDATION: Contraindicated—1st Trimester
BREASTFEEDING RECOMMENDATION: No Human Data—Potential Toxicity

PREGNANCY SUMMARY

A major concern with flucytosine exposure in the 1st trimester is that it is partially metabolized to 5-fluorouracil, a known human teratogen (see below). Thus, if possible, avoiding the 1st trimester is the best course.

FETAL RISK SUMMARY

Flucytosine is indicated only in the treatment of serious infections caused by susceptible strains of Candida and/or Cryptococcus. The drug is partially metabolized and binding to serum proteins is low. The mean half-life is about 4 hours (1).

Reproduction studies have been conducted in rats, mice, and rabbits. Flucytosine was teratogenic in rats at doses 0.27–4.7 times the maximum recommended human dose (MRHD), producing vertebral fusions, cleft lip and palate, and micrognathia. In mice, a dose 2.7 times the MRHD was associated with a low, nonsignificant, incidence of cleft palate. Flucytosine was not teratogenic in rabbits at 0.68 times the MRHD (1).

Consistent with its molecular weight (about 129), low metabolism and serum protein binding, and moderate half-life, flucytosine crosses the human placenta. A woman at 21 weeks' gestation with cryptococcal meningitis was treated with flucytosine and amphotericin B for 1 week before elective termination (2). Both agents were found in the amniotic fluid and cord blood.

Following oral administration, about 4% of flucytosine is metabolized within the gut or by fungal organisms to 5-fluorouracil, an antineoplastic agent (1,3). Fluorouracil is suspected of producing congenital defects in humans (see Fluorouracil).

Several case reports of pregnant patients treated with flucytosine, usually in combination with amphotericin B, in the 2nd and 3rd trimesters have been located (4–8). No defects were observed in the newborns.

BREASTFEEDING SUMMARY

No reports describing the use of flucytosine during lactation have been located. Because of the potential for serious adverse effects in a nursing infant, breastfeeding is not recommended when taking flucytosine.

References

1. Product information. Ancobon. ICN Pharmaceuticals, 2000.
2. Stafford CR, Fisher JF, Fadel HE, Espinel-Ingroff AV, Shadomy S, Hamby M. Cryptococcal meningitis in pregnancy. Obstet Gynecol 1983;62(3 Suppl): 35s–7s.
3. Diasio RB, Lakings DE, Bennett JE. Evidence for conversion of 5-fluorocytosine to 5-fluorouracil in humans: possible factor in 5-fluorocytosine clinical toxicity. Antimicrob Agents Chemother 1978;14:903–8.
4. Philpot CR, Lo D. Cryptococcal meningitis in pregnancy. Med J Aust 1972;2:1005–7.
5. Schonebeck J, Segerbrand E. Candida albicans septicaemia during first half of pregnancy successfully treated with 5-fluorocytosine. Br Med J 1973;4:337–8.
6. Curole DN. Cryptococcal meningitis in pregnancy. J Reprod Med 1981;26:317–9.
7. Chotmongkol V, Siricharoensang S. Cryptococcal meningitis in pregnancy: a case report. J Med Assoc Thai 1991;74:421–2.
8. Chen CP, Wang KG. Cryptococcal meningitis in pregnancy. Am J Perinatol 1996;13:35–6.

FLUDARABINE PHOSPHATE

Antineoplastic

PREGNANCY RECOMMENDATION: Limited Human Data—Animal Data Suggest Risk
BREASTFEEDING RECOMMENDATION: Contraindicated

PREGNANCY SUMMARY

Only one report describing the use of fludarabine in human pregnancy has been located. In that report, exposure occurred in the 2nd trimester and no fludarabine-induced toxicity was thought to have occurred. However, the animal reproduction data suggest risk if the drug is used during organogenesis. Thus, if indicated, avoiding exposure during the 1st trimester would be the best course. The manufacturer states that women of childbearing potential and fertile males must take contraceptive measures during and at least for 6 months after the cessation of therapy (1,2).

FETAL RISK SUMMARY

Fludarabine phosphate, available in oral and IV formulations, is a synthetic purine antimetabolite that is rapidly dephosphorylated in the plasma to an active metabolite. It is a fluorinated nucleotide analog of vidarabine. Fludarabine is in the same antineoplastic subclass of purine analogs and related agents as cladribine, clofarabine, mercaptopurine, pentostatin, and thioguanine. It is indicated as a single agent for the treatment of adult patients with B-cell chronic lymphocytic leukemia whose disease has not responded to or has progressed during or after treatment with at least one standard alkylating-agent containing regimen. Plasma protein binding of the active metabolite is about 19%–29% and the terminal half-life is about 20 hours (1,2).

Reproduction studies have been conducted in rats and rabbits. In rats during organogenesis, repeated IV doses that were 1.5 and 4.5 times the recommended human oral dose based on BSA (RHOD) caused an increase in resorptions, skeletal and visceral malformations (cleft palate, exencephaly, and vertebrae deformities), and decreased body weights. The highest dose was maternal toxic (slight body weight decreases). In rabbits, repeated IV doses that were ≥0.3 times the RHOD were associated with a significant increase in malformations, including cleft palate, hydrocephaly, adactyly, brachydactyly, fusion of the digits, diaphragmatic hernia, heart and great vessel defects, and vertebrae and rib anomalies. At 2.4 times the RHOD, increases in embryo (increased resorptions) and fetal (decreased live fetuses) lethality were observed (1,2).

Studies for carcinogenesis have not been conducted. Both the parent drug and the active metabolite were clastogenic but not mutagenic. Fertility studies in mice, rats, and dogs have shown dose-related adverse effects on the male reproductive system that included decreases in testicular weights and degeneration and necrosis of spermatogenic epithelium in the testes (1,2).

It is not known if fludarabine crosses the human placenta. The molecular weights of the parent drug and active metabolite, 365 and 269, respectively, the low plasma protein binding, and the elimination half-life suggest that both compounds will cross to the embryo–fetus.

In a 2009 case report, a woman with relapse of acute myeloid leukemia at 22 weeks' gestation was treated with fludarabine, cytarabine, mitoxantrone, idarubicin, and gemtuzumab ozogamicin (3). The fetus developed signs of idarubicin-induced cardiomyopathy, transient cerebral ventriculomegaly, anemia, and intrauterine growth restriction. The newborn, delivered at 33 weeks by cesarean section, showed no congenital malformations.

A 20-year-old woman with Fanconi anemia became pregnant 93 months after allogeneic stem cell transplantation from an unrelated donor (4). The preparative regimen for the transplantation consisted of fludarabine, cyclophosphamide, methotrexate, tacrolimus, and antithymocyte globulin. She gave birth at 38 weeks' gestation to a normal, 2828-g male infant after an uncomplicated pregnancy.

BREASTFEEDING SUMMARY

No reports describing the use of fludarabine during human lactation have been located. The molecular weights of the parent drug and active metabolite, 365 and 269, respectively, the low plasma protein binding (19%–29%), and the elimination half-life (20 hours) suggest that both compounds will be excreted into breast milk. The effect of this exposure on a nursing infant is unknown. However, in patients treated with the drug, clinically significant toxicities were observed that involved the hematopoietic, nervous, pulmonary, gastrointestinal, cardiovascular, and genitourinary systems, as well as the skin. Taken in sum, the potential risks suggest that if a woman is receiving fludarabine, she should not breastfeed her infant.

References

1. Product information. Oforta. Sanofi-Aventis, 2009.
2. Product information. Fludarabine Phosphate. Antisoma Research Limited, 2009.
3. Baumgartner AK, Oberhoffer R, Jacobs VR, Ostermayer E, Menzel H, Voigt M, Schneider KT, Pildner von Steinburg S. Reversible foetal cerebral ventriculomegaly and cardiomyopathy under chemotherapy for maternal AML. Onkologie 2009;32:40–3.
4. Yabe H, Koike T, Shimizu T, Ishiguro H, Morimoto T, Hyodo H, Akiba T, Kato S, Yabe M. Natural pregnancy and delivery after unrelated bone marrow transplantation using fludarabine-based regimen in a Fanconi anemia patient. Int J Hematol 2010;91:350–1.

FLUMAZENIL

Antidote

PREGNANCY RECOMMENDATION: Compatible—Maternal Benefit >> Embryo–Fetal Risk
BREASTFEEDING RECOMMENDATION: No Human Data—Probably Compatible

PREGNANCY SUMMARY

No reports describing the use of flumazenil during the 1st trimester in humans have been located. Two cases, however, have reported use of the agent in the 3rd trimester. In addition, a second case report (1) was cited in a 2003 review (2). Although an assessment of the teratogenic risk in humans cannot be made, the animal data suggest the risk is low. Moreover, the indication for flumazenil is such that the maternal benefit should far outweigh the unknown embryo–fetal risk. Therefore, if indicated, flumazenil should not be withheld during pregnancy (3).

FETAL RISK SUMMARY

Flumazenil, a benzodiazepine receptor antagonist, rapidly inhibits the actions of benzodiazepines on the CNS. It is indicated for the complete or partial reversal of the sedative effects of benzodiazepines following therapeutic use or for the management of benzodiazepine overdose. Although it has weak partial agonist activity in some animals, flumazenil has little or no agonist action in humans. After IV administration, flumazenil has a mean terminal half-life of 54 minutes (range 41–79 minutes). Approximately 50% of the agent is protein bound in the plasma and the metabolites are inactive (4).

Reproduction studies have been conducted in rats and rabbits. No evidence of impaired fertility was observed in male and female rats at oral doses up to 120 times the human exposure based on AUC obtained with the maximum recommended IV dose of 5 mg (HEMRD). In rats and rabbits, no teratogenicity was observed when flumazenil was given during organogenesis at oral doses up to 120–600 times the HEMRD. However, embryocidal effects (increased pre- and postimplantation losses) were noted in rabbits at 200 times the HEMRD. The no-effect dose was 60 times the HEMRD. In rats, oral doses 120 times the HEMRD during lactation resulted in decreased pup survival and increased pup liver weight at weaning. Other adverse effects noted were delayed incisor eruption and ear opening. The no-effect level was 24 times the HEMRD (4).

It is not known if flumazenil crosses the human placenta to the embryo/fetus. The molecular weight (about 303) and moderate plasma protein binding suggest that transfer may occur, but the very short elimination half-life will limit the embryo–fetal exposure.

A 1993 case report described the use of flumazenil in a 22-year-old woman at 36 weeks' gestation (5). The woman was somnolent but was able to respond appropriately to questions. She had taken 50–60 5-mg tablets of diazepam. After initial emergency treatment, serum levels approximately 7 hours after ingestion of diazepam and two metabolites (oxazepam and *N*-desmethyldiazepam) were 1.9, 0.8, and 0.9 μmol/L, respectively. The fetal heart rate was 130–160 beats/minute with decreased variability, absence of accelerations, and occasional decelerations. Flumazenil, 0.3 mg IV, was given to distinguish between fetal asphyxia and an influence of benzodiazepines. Shortly afterward, the patient awakened and the fetal heart rate was noted to have accelerations and increased variability. Approximately 24 hours later, the maternal and fetal symptoms recurred and a second 0.3 mg dose of IV flumazenil was given. Both the mother and the fetus responded as before and no further doses were required. Two weeks later, she delivered a healthy 3620-g (head circumference 33 cm) male infant with Apgar scores of 7, 10, and 10 at 1, 5, and 10 minutes, respectively. No adverse effects of the overdose were observed in the infant who was discharged home with his mother at 5 days of age (5).

BREASTFEEDING SUMMARY

No reports describing the use of flumazenil during human lactation have been located.

The molecular weight (about 303) and moderate plasma protein binding suggest that transfer into breast milk may occur, but the very short elimination half-life (mean 54 minutes) will mitigate this transfer. IV flumazenil has been given directly to neonates to reverse the sedative effects of diazepam administered to the mother immediately before delivery (6,7). If indicated, flumazenil should not be withheld during lactation. However, because of the potential for adverse effects in a nursing infant that may be similar to those observed in treated adults (such as fatigue, nausea/vomiting, agitation, and cutaneous vasodilation), holding breastfeeding for a few hours after the last dose to allow drug elimination from the mother should be considered.

References

1. Shibata T, Kubota N, Yokoyama H. A pregnant woman with convulsion treated with diazepam, which was reversed with flumazenil just prior to cesarean section [Japanese]. Masui 1994;43:572. As cited by Bailey B. Are there teratogenic risks associated with antidotes used in the acute management of poisoned pregnant women? Birth Defects Res A Clin Mol Teratol 2003;67:133–40.
2. Bailey B. Are there teratogenic risks associated with antidotes used in the acute management of poisoned pregnant women? Birth Defects Res A Clin Mol Teratol 2003;67:133–40.
3. Weinbroum AA, Flaishon R, Sorkine P, Szold O, Rudick V. A risk–benefit assessment of flumazenil in the management of benzodiazepine overdose. Drug Saf 1997;17:181–96.
4. Product information. Romazicon. Roche Pharmaceuticals, 2004.
5. Stahl MMS, Saldeen P, Vinge E. Reversal of fetal benzodiazepine intoxication using flumazenil. Br J Obstet Gynaecol 1993;100:185–8.
6. Richard P, Autret E, Bardol J, Soyez C, Barbier P, Jonville AP, Ramponi N. The use of flumazenil in a neonate. J Toxicol Clin Toxicol 1991;29:137–40.
7. Dixon JC, Speidel BD, Dixon JJ. Neonatal flumazenil therapy reverses maternal diazepam. Acta Paediatr 1998;87:225–6.

FLUNISOLIDE

Respiratory Agent (Corticosteroid)

PREGNANCY RECOMMENDATION: Compatible
BREASTFEEDING RECOMMENDATION: No Human Data—Probably Compatible

PREGNANCY SUMMARY

The animal data suggest risk, but the limited human pregnancy experience prevents a complete assessment of the embryo–fetal risk. Moreover, human pregnancy data exist only for inhaled flunisolide. Inhaled corticosteroids play an important role in preventing acute exacerbations of asthma. In a position statement from a joint committee of the American College of Obstetricians and Gynecologists (ACOG) and the American College of Allergy, Asthma, and Immunology (ACAAI) published in 2000, either beclomethasone or budesonide were considered the inhaled steroids of choice for use during pregnancy (1).

FETAL RISK SUMMARY

The oral inhaled formulation of the corticosteroid flunisolide is indicated for the maintenance treatment of asthma as prophylactic therapy (2). The nasal spray product is indicated for the management of the nasal symptoms of seasonal or perennial rhinitis (3). Flunisolide has potent anti-inflammatory and antiallergic activity, but it is not a bronchodilator and is not indicated for the relief of bronchospasm. Total systemic bioavailability of inhaled flunisolide is 40%. The agent is rapidly metabolized by the liver to low potency or inactive metabolites; the plasma half-life of flunisolide is about 1.8 hours. Plasma accumulation has not been observed after 2 weeks of therapy with 2 mg/day (2). After use of the nasal spray, 50% of the dose reaches the systemic circulation as unmetabolized flunisolide with a plasma half-life of 1–3 hours (3).

Reproduction studies have been conducted with oral flunisolide in rats and rabbits. As with other corticosteroids, flunisolide was teratogenic and fetotoxic at daily oral doses of 1180 mcg/m^2 and 480 mcg/m^2, respectively (2,3). A reproduction study in pregnant mice observed dose-related teratogenicity (cleft palate) and reduced fetal weight, but the SC doses also caused maternal toxicity (reduced body weight) (4). Another study used pregnant rats and observed dose-related growth restriction, multiple congenital defects, and increased mortality (5).

The maximum recommended daily human dose (MRDHD) for the inhaled and nasal formulations are 2000 mcg and 464 mcg, respectively (2,3). If the systemic bioavailability of the two formulations are 40% (800 mcg) and 50% (232 mcg), respectively, and if a typical patient has a BSA of about 1.8 m^2, then the systemic bioavailable doses are about 444 and 129 mcg/m^2, respectively. Thus, based on systemic bioavailability, the dose in rats causing developmental toxicity was about 3 and 9 times the MRDHD, respectively, and in rabbits, about 1 and 4 times the MRDHD, respectively.

It is not known if flunisolide crosses the human placenta. The molecular weights of the formulations (about 434 and 444) are low enough to cross the placenta, but the short elimination half-lives and extensive metabolism should limit the amount reaching the embryo or fetus.

A 2004 study examined the effect of inhaled corticosteroids on low birth weight, preterm births, and congenital malformations in pregnant asthmatic patients (6). The inhaled steroids and the number of patients were beclomethasone (N = 277), fluticasone (N = 132), triamcinolone (N = 81), budesonide (N = 43), and flunisolide (N = 25). Compared with the general population, the study found no increased incidence of small-for-gestational-age infants (less than 10th percentile for gestational age), low birth weight (<2500 g), preterm births, and congenital malformations (6).

In another 2004 study, 722 asthmatic women used inhaled corticosteroids during pregnancy (7). Although the number of subjects using flunisolide was not mentioned, there were no significant relationships between the inhaled steroid users and low birth weight, small for gestational age, major malformations, gestational hypertension, or preterm birth (7).

The two studies cited above suggest that the embryo–fetal risk is low. However, the one study (7) examining perinatal outcomes was too small to have identified an association with oral clefts, if it had existed. Systemic corticosteroids are known to be associated with a low risk for isolated, nonsyndromic oral clefts (cleft lip and/or palate) when used in the 1st trimester, as well as fetal growth restriction when used for long periods later in gestation. (See Hydrocortisone.).

A 2006 meta-analysis on the use of inhaled corticosteroids during pregnancy was published in 2006 (8). The analysis included five agents: beclomethasone, budesonide, flunisolide, fluticasone, and triamcinolone. The results showed that these agents do not increase the risk of major congenital defects, preterm delivery, low birth weight, and pregnancy-induced hypertension. Thus, they could be used during pregnancy (8).

BREASTFEEDING SUMMARY

No reports describing the use of flunisolide during human lactation have been located. The molecular weights of the inhaled and nasal spray formulations (about 434 and 444) are low enough for excretion into breast milk, but the short elimination half-lives and extensive metabolism should limit the amount. Other corticosteroids are excreted into milk in low concentrations (see Prednisone), and the passage of flunisolide into milk should be expected. The effects of this exposure on a nursing infant are unknown, but the amounts excreted into milk should be low. Therefore, use of flunisolide during breastfeeding probably is compatible.

References

1. Joint Committee of the American College of Obstetricians and Gynecologists (ACOG) and the American College of Allergy, Asthma, and Immunology (ACAAI). Position statement. The use of newer asthma and allergy medications during pregnancy. Ann Allergy Asthma Immunol 2000;84:475–80.
2. Product information. Aerobid. Forest Pharmaceuticals, 2006.
3. Product information. Nasarel. IVAX Laboratories, 2006.
4. Tamagawa M, Hatori M, Ooi A, Nishioeda R, Tanaka N. Comparative teratological study of flunisolide in mice. Oyo Yakuri (Pharmacometrics) 1982;24:741–50.
5. Itabashi M, Inoue T, Yokota M, Takehara K, Tajima M. Reproductive studies on flunisolide in rats: oral administration during the period of organogenesis. Oyo Yakuri (Pharmacometrics) 1982;24:643–59.
6. Namazy J, Schatz M, Long L, Lipkowitz M, Lillie MA, Voss M, Deitz RJ, Petitti D. Use of inhaled steroids by pregnant asthmatic women does not reduce intrauterine growth. J Allergy Clin Immunol 2004;113:427–32.
7. Schatz M, Dombrowski M, Wise R, Momirova V, Landon M, Mabie W, Newman RB, Hauth JC, Lindheimer M, Caritis SN, Leveno KJ, Meis P, Miodovnik M, Wapner RJ, Paul RH, Varner MW, O'Sullivan MJ, Thurnau GR, Conway DL, for The National Institute of Child Health and Development Maternal-Fetal Medicine Units Network and The National Heart, Lung, and Blood Institute. The relationship of asthma medication use to perinatal outcomes. J Allergy Clin Immunol 2004;113:1040–5.
8. Rahimi R, Nikfar S, Abdollahi M. Meta-analysis finds use of inhaled corticosteroids during pregnancy safe: a systematic meta-analysis review. Hum Exp Toxicol 2006;25:447–52.

FLUNITRAZEPAM

[Withdrawn from the market. See 9th edition.]

FLUOCINOLONE

Corticosteroid (Topical/Ophthalmic Implant)

PREGNANCY RECOMMENDATION: Limited Human Data—Animal Data Suggest Risk
BREASTFEEDING RECOMMENDATION: No Human Data—Potential Toxicity

PREGNANCY SUMMARY

Systemic corticosteroids are known to cause dose-related developmental toxicity (i.e., growth restriction and structural anomalies) in animals and humans. The limited pregnancy experience with fluocinolone does not appear to represent a risk, probably because the systemic amounts were insufficient to cause embryo or fetal toxicity. Although the amount of topical fluocinolone reaching the systemic circulation is uncertain, suppression of the hypothalamic–pituitary–adrenal (HPA) axis has been observed when other topically fluorinated corticosteroids were used for long periods in nonpregnant patients (see Fluocinonide). Use of occlusive dressings will increase the amount absorbed. Because the amounts absorbed systemically from topical fluocinolone are unknown and probably highly variable, a less-potent agent should be considered for pregnant women requiring long-term topical corticosteroid therapy. Fluocinolone is not absorbed systemically in detectable amounts from the ocular implant, so the embryo–fetal risks from this therapy appear to be negligible.

FETAL RISK SUMMARY

Fluocinolone is a potent, synthetic, fluorinated corticosteroid that has anti-inflammatory, antipyretic, and vasoconstrictive properties. It is available in various topical formulations as a cream, ointment, solution, shampoo, and oil in concentrations ranging from 0.01% to 0.2%. It also is available as an ocular implant (0.59 mg) that is indicated for the treatment of chronic noninfectious uveitis affecting the posterior segment of the eye (3). Topical fluocinolone is indicated for the relief of the inflammatory and pruritic manifestations of corticosteroid-responsive dermatoses (1,2). Systemic absorption of detectable amounts has not been observed after administration of the ocular implant (3). However, systemic absorption probably occurs with topical use. The degree of absorption is affected by inflammation, integrity of the epidermal barrier, and the use of occlusive dressings. Suppression of the HPA axis is a potential complication after topical use (1,2) and has occurred with other fluorinated corticosteroids (see Fluocinonide).

A number of animal reproduction studies have demonstrated that corticosteroids cause developmental toxicity (growth restriction, structural anomalies, and death) (see Hydrocortisone). Potent topical corticosteroids also can cause structural anomalies after dermal application (2,3).

It is not known if fluocinolone crosses the human placenta. The molecular weight (about 453 as the acetonide) is low enough that exposure of the embryo and fetus should be expected from the amounts absorbed systemically. The placenta does contain an enzyme that degrades corticosteroids (e.g., see Betamethasone, Dexamethason, Hydrocortisone, and Prednisolone), although active drug still crosses.

The use of fluocinolone for the treatment of pruritus vulvae in 17 pregnant women was described in a 1967 reference (4). Typically, the treatment was given five to seven times over a 24-hour period before voluntarily discontinuance after two or three days. No information was given about the pregnancy outcomes.

A large 1997 case–control study of the teratogenic potential of oral and topical corticosteroids involving 1,923,413 total births from 1980 to 1994 was conducted with the Hungarian Case–Control Surveillance of Congenital Abnormalities (5). Among the 20,830 malformed case infants, 73 (0.35%) used a topical corticosteroid during the 1st trimester compared with 118 (0.33%) of the 35,727 normal control infants ($p = 0.69$). The number of cases and controls that used topical fluocinolone cream was 16 and 47, respectively (5).

A 2003 review stated that a topical product containing fluocinolone, hydroquinone, and tretinoin (Tri-Luma®) was effective for the treatment of melasma, a localized facial hyperpigmentation also known as the "mask of pregnancy" (6). Tretinoin, when given systemically, is a known human teratogen (see Tretinoin [Systemic]) and, although the systemic bioavailability is poor, concerns have been raised with topical tretinoin (see Tretinoin [Topical]). Thus, the safest course is to avoid use of the combination in pregnancy, at least during the 1st trimester.

BREASTFEEDING SUMMARY

No reports describing the use of fluocinolone during human lactation have been located.

If fluocinolone reaches the systemic circulation, the molecular weight (about 453 as the acetonide) is low enough that excretion into breast milk should be expected. The amount of topically applied fluocinolone reaching the systemic circulation is uncertain, but suppression of the HPA axis has been observed with other topically applied fluorinated corticosteroids (see Fluocinonide) in nonpregnant patients. Because of this uncertainty, if a nursing woman requires long-term topical therapy, consideration should be given to a less-potent corticosteroid.

References

1. Product information. Synalar Cream 0.025%. MEDICIS, The Dermatology Company, 2007.
2. Product information. Synalar Solution 0.01%. MEDICIS, The Dermatology Company, 2007.
3. Product information. Retisert. Bausch & Lomb, 2005.

4. Godat J. Effective treatment of pruritus vulvae due to Candida. J La State Med Soc 1967;119:203–4.
5. Czeizel AE, Rockenbauer M. Population-based case-control study of teratogenic potential of corticosteroids. Teratology 1997;56:335–40.
6. Stulberg DI, Clark N, Tovey D. Common hyperpigmentation disorders in adults: part II. Melanoma, seborrheic keratoses, acanthosis nigricans, melasma, diabetic dermopathy, tinea versicolor, and postinflammatory hyperpigmentation. Am Fam Physician 2003;68:1963–8.

FLUOCINONIDE

Corticosteroid (Topical)

PREGNANCY RECOMMENDATION: Limited Human Data—Animal Data Suggest Risk
BREASTFEEDING RECOMMENDATION: No Human Data—Potential Toxicity

PREGNANCY SUMMARY

The only report describing the use of fluocinonide in human pregnancy involved a woman in the 3rd trimester. The amount of topically applied fluocinonide reaching the systemic circulation is uncertain, but suppression of the hypothalamic–pituitary–adrenal (HPA) axis has been observed in nonpregnant patients. Use of occlusive dressings will increase the amount absorbed. Moreover, it is not known if the amounts absorbed can cause the congenital defects and growth restriction observed in humans with systemic corticosteroids. One manufacturer recommends treatment for no more than 2 weeks with a total dosage not exceeding 60 g/week (1). If a pregnant woman requires long-term topical corticosteroid therapy, the use of a less-potent agent should be considered.

FETAL RISK SUMMARY

Fluocinonide is a potent, synthetic, fluorinated corticosteroid that has anti-inflammatory, antipruritic, and vasoconstrictive properties. It is available in various topical formulations, such as creams, ointments, gels, and solutions in concentrations of 0.05% or 0.1%. Fluocinonide is indicated for the relief of the inflammation and pruritic manifestations of corticosteroid-responsive dermatoses (1). Systemic absorption does occur with topical use with the amount of absorption affected by inflammation, the integrity of the epidermal barrier, and the use of occlusive dressings. Suppression of the HPA axis is a potential complication. Application of a 0.1% cream twice daily in pediatric and adult patients has been associated with suppression of the HPA axis (1).

A number of animal reproduction studies have demonstrated that corticosteroids cause developmental toxicity (growth restriction, structural anomalies, and death) (see Hydrocortisone). Potent topical corticosteroids also can cause structural anomalies after dermal application (1).

It is not known if fluocinonide crosses the human placenta. The molecular weight (about 495) is low enough that exposure of the embryo and fetus should be expected. The placenta does contain an enzyme that degrades corticosteroids (e.g., see Betamethasone, Dexamethason, Hydrocortisone, and Prednisolone), although some active drug still crosses. The amount of fluocinonide reaching the systemic circulation apparently has not been measured, but amounts sufficient to suppress the HPA axis has been shown clinically, as indicated above.

A 2006 case report described a 21-year-old woman in the 3rd trimester with a diagnosis of food-induced acute generalized exanthematous pustulosis (2). She was successively treated with fluocinonide cream 0.05% and tapering doses of systemic methylprednisolone (doses and durations not specified). She eventually gave birth at 40 weeks' gestation to a healthy male infant (2).

BREASTFEEDING SUMMARY

No reports describing the use of fluocinonide during human lactation have been located.

If fluocinonide reaches the systemic circulation, the molecular weight (about 495) is low enough that excretion into breast milk should be expected. The amount of topically applied fluocinonide reaching the systemic circulation is uncertain, but suppression of the HPA axis has been observed in nonpregnant patients. Because of this uncertainty, if a nursing woman requires long-term topical corticosteroid therapy, consideration should be given to a less-potent corticosteroid.

References

1. Product information. Vanos. MEDICIS, The Dermatology Company, 2007.
2. Valkova S. Food-induced acute generalized exanthematous pustulosis in a pregnant woman. Skinmed 2006;5:199–201.

FLUORESCEIN SODIUM

Diagnostic Agent

PREGNANCY RECOMMENDATION: Limited Human Data—Animal Data Suggest Low Risk
BREASTFEEDING RECOMMENDATION: Limited Human Data—Potential Toxicity (IV)
Limited Human Data—Probably Compatible (Topical)

PREGNANCY SUMMARY

One report has described the use of fluorescein sodium in human pregnancy. Use of the topical solution in the eye (as well as IV injection) produces measurable concentrations of the dye in the systemic circulation (see references 5 and 6) and passage to the fetus should be expected.

FETAL RISK SUMMARY

The diagnostic agent, fluorescein sodium (dye and coloring Yellow No. 8), is available as a topical solution, dye-impregnated paper strips, and as a solution for IV injection.

No adverse fetal effects were observed in the offspring of pregnant albino rats administered IV sodium fluorescein (10%) at a dose of 5 mL/kg (1). The agent crossed the placenta and distributed throughout the fetuses within 15 minutes. Using phenobarbital in mature rats exposed in utero to multiple maternal IV doses of 10% sodium fluorescein, the investigators determined that in utero exposure to the dye had no effect on their drug detoxification systems later in life (1). No adverse effects on fetal development were observed when pregnant rats and rabbits were treated by gavage with multiple high doses (up to 1500 mg/kg in rats and up to 250 mg/kg in rabbits) of sodium fluorescein during organogenesis (2). Similarly, no adverse fetal outcomes occurred when pregnant rabbits were administered multiple 1.4-mL IV doses of 10% sodium fluorescein during the first two-thirds of gestation (3).

A 2009 report described a 45-year-old woman with choroidal neovascularization and an unknown pregnancy, who received fluorescein angiography at 9 weeks and verteporfin at 12 weeks (4). Pregnancy was diagnosed at about 25 weeks. At about 37 weeks, she gave birth spontaneously to a healthy, 2410-g female infant without congenital anomalies and with Apgar scores of 9 and 10. The normal infant was doing well at 16 months of age (4).

BREASTFEEDING SUMMARY

Fluorescein sodium is excreted into breast milk (5,6). A 29-year-old woman, who suffered acute central vision loss shortly after prematurely delivery of twins, was administered a 5-mL IV dose of 10% fluorescein sodium for diagnostic angiography (5). Her hospitalized infants were not fed her milk because of concern that the fluorescein in the milk could cause a phototoxic reaction if consumed (a severe bullous skin eruption was observed in a premature infant receiving phototherapy for hyperbilirubinemia shortly after administration of IV fluorescein angiography [7]). Milk concentrations of the dye were measured in seven samples collected between 6 and 76 hours after fluorescein administration. The highest and lowest concentrations, 372 ng/mL and 170 ng/mL, were measured at 6 and 76 hours, respectively. The elimination half-life of fluorescein in the woman's milk was approximately 62 hours (5).

In a second case, a 28-year-old woman at 3 months postpartum was administered a topical 2% solution in both eyes (6). Her infant was not allowed to breastfeed on the day of instillation. Absorption into the systemic circulation was documented with plasma fluorescein concentrations of 36 and 40 ng/mL at 45 and 75 minutes, respectively, after the dose. Milk concentrations at 30, 60, and 90 minutes were 20, 22, and 15 ng/mL, respectively. Because of these data, the authors recommended that mothers should not breastfeed for 8–12 hours after fluorescein topical administration (6).

The two mothers in the above cases either did not breastfeed or temporarily withheld nursing to allow the dye to clear from their milk because of concerns for a fluorescein-induced phototoxic reaction in their infants. Although the American Academy of Pediatrics classifies fluorescein as compatible with breastfeeding (8), the much higher milk concentrations obtained following IV fluorescein indicate that a risk may exist, especially in those infants undergoing phototherapy, and feeding should be temporarily withheld (9).

References

1. Salem H, Loux JJ, Smith S, Nichols CW. Evaluation of the toxicologic and teratogenic potentials of sodium fluorescein in the rat. Toxicology 1979;12:143–50.
2. Burnett CM, Goldenthal EI. The teratogenic potential in rats and rabbits of D and C Yellow no. 8. Food Chem Toxicol 1986;24:819–23.
3. McEnerney JK, Wong WP, Peyman GA. Evaluation of the teratogenicity of fluorescein sodium. Am J Ophthalmol 1977;84:847–50.
4. Rodrigues M, Meira D, Batista S, Carrilho MM. Accidental pregnancy exposure to verteporfin: obstetrical and neonatal outcomes: a case report. Aust NZ J Obstet Gynaecol 2009;49:236–7.
5. Maguire AM, Bennett J. Fluorescein elimination in human breast milk. Arch Ophthalmol 1986;106:718–9.
6. Mattern J, Mayer PR. Excretion of fluorescein into breast milk. Am J Ophthalmol 1990;109:598–9.
7. Kearns GL, Williams BJ, Timmons OD. Fluorescein phototoxicity in a premature infant. J Pediatr 1985;107:796–8.
8. Committee on Drugs, American Academy of Pediatrics. The transfer of drugs and other chemicals into human milk. Pediatrics 2001;108:776–89.
9. Anderson PO. Medication use while breast feeding a neonate. Neonatal Pharmacol Q 1993;2:3–14.

FLUOROURACIL

Antineoplastic

PREGNANCY RECOMMENDATION: Contraindicated—1st Trimester
BREASTFEEDING RECOMMENDATION: Contraindicated

PREGNANCY SUMMARY

Fluorouracil is classified as an antimetabolite in the subclass of pyrimidine analogs. Other antineoplastic agents in the subclass are capecitabine, cytarabine, floxuridine, and gemcitabine. It is frequently used in combination with other antineoplastics. Structural anomalies are a potential complication if this agent is given systemically during the 1st trimester.

FETAL RISK SUMMARY

Fluorouracil was embryotoxic and teratogenic in mice, rats, and hamsters given parenteral doses equivalent to the human dose (1). Although not teratogenic in monkeys, divided doses above 40 mg/kg resulted in abortions. Animal reproduction studies with topical fluorouracil have not been conducted (1).

When applied topically in patients with actinic keratoses, the amount of fluorouracil absorbed systemically is approximately 6% (1). The amount absorbed from mucous membranes is unknown. One manufacturer reported an infant with cleft lip and palate from a woman who appropriately used topical fluorouracil and a second infant with a ventricular septal defect from a woman who used the drug topically on mucous membranes (1). In addition, spontaneous abortions (SAB) have been reported following use on mucous membrane areas (1). It is not known if there is a causative relationship between the topically applied drug and these outcomes.

Following systemic therapy in the 1st trimester (also with exposure to 5 rad of irradiation), multiple defects were observed in an aborted fetus: radial aplasia; absent thumbs and three fingers; hypoplasia of lungs, aorta, thymus, and bile duct; aplasia of esophagus, duodenum, and ureters; single umbilical artery; absent appendix; imperforate anus; and a cloaca (2).

A 33-year-old woman with metastatic breast cancer was treated with a modified radical mastectomy during her 3rd month of pregnancy, followed by oophorectomy at 13 weeks' gestation (3). Chemotherapy, consisting of 5-fluorouracil, cyclophosphamide, and doxorubicin, was started at approximately 11 weeks' gestation and continued for six 3-week cyclic courses. Methotrexate was substituted for doxorubicin at this time and the new three-drug regimen was continued until delivery by cesarean section at 35 weeks of a 2260-g female infant. No abnormalities were noted at birth, and continued follow-up at 24 months of age revealed normal growth and development. Toxicity consisting of cyanosis and jerking extremities has been reported in a newborn exposed to fluorouracil in the 3rd trimester (4).

In a surveillance study of Michigan Medicaid recipients involving 229,101 completed pregnancies conducted between 1985 and 1992, 14 newborns had been exposed to fluorouracil (includes nonsystemic administration) during the 1st trimester (F. Rosa, personal communication, FDA, 1993). One (7.1%) major birth defect was observed (one expected). No anomalies were observed in six defect categories (cardiovascular defects, oral clefts, spina bifida, polydactyly, limb reduction defects, and hypospadias) for which specific data were available.

In a brief 1997 report, three pregnant women with breast cancer were successfully treated with two or three courses of vinorelbine (20–30 mg/m^2) and fluorouracil (500–750 mg/m^2) at 24, 28, and 29 weeks' gestation, respectively (5). Delivery occurred at 34, 41, and 37 weeks' gestation, respectively. One patient also required six courses of epidoxorubicin and cyclophosphamide. Her infant developed transient anemia at 21 days of age that resolved spontaneously. No adverse effects were observed in the other two newborns. All three infants were developing normally at about 2–3 years of age (5).

A 1999 report from France described the outcomes of pregnancies in 20 women with breast cancer who were treated with antineoplastic agents (6). The first cycle of chemotherapy occurred at a mean gestational age of 26 weeks, with delivery occurring at a mean 34.7 weeks. A total of 38 cycles were administered during pregnancy with a median of two cycles per woman. None of the women received radiation therapy during pregnancy. The pregnancy outcomes included two SAB (both exposed in the 1st trimester), one intrauterine death (exposed in the 2nd trimester), and 17 live births, one of whom died at 8 days of age without apparent cause. The 16 surviving children were developing normally at a mean follow-up of 42.3 months (6). Fluorouracil (F), in combination with various other agents (cyclophosphamide [C], doxorubicin [D], epirubicin [E], mitoxantrone [M], or vinorelbine [V]) was administered to 16 of the women at a mean dose of 535 mg/m^2 (range 300–750 mg/m^2). The outcomes were one SAB (FCE; 1st trimester), one neonatal death (one cycle of FCE 32 days before birth), and 14 surviving liveborn infants (five FEC, four FV, two FDC, two FCM, and one FD in the 2nd or 3rd trimester). One of the infants, exposed to two cycles of FCE with the last at 25 days before birth, had transient leukopenia and another was growth restricted (1460-g, born at 33 weeks' gestation after two cycles of FCM) (6).

Amenorrhea has been observed in women treated with fluorouracil for breast cancer, but this was probably caused by concurrent administration of melphalan (7,8) (see also Melphalan). The long-term effects of combination chemotherapy on menstrual and reproductive function have been described in two 1988 reports (9,10). In one report, only 2 of the 40 women treated for malignant ovarian germ cell tumors received fluorouracil (9). The results of this study are discussed in the monograph for cyclophosphamide (see Cyclophosphamide). The other report described the reproductive results of 265 women who had been treated from 1959 to 1980 for gestational trophoblastic disease (10). Single-agent chemotherapy was administered to 91 women, including 54 cases in which fluorouracil was the only agent used; sequential (single agent) and combination therapies were administered to 67 and 107 women, respectively. Of the total group, 241 were exposed to pregnancy and 205 (85%) of these women conceived, with a total of 355 pregnancies. The time interval between recovery and pregnancy was 1 year or less (8.5%), 1–2 years (32.1%), 2–4 years (32.4%), 4–6 years (15.5%), 6–8 years (7.3%), 8–10 years (1.4%), and more than 10 years (2.8%). A total of 303 (4 sets of twins) liveborn infants resulted from the 355 pregnancies, 3 of whom had congenital malformations: anencephaly, hydrocephalus, and congenital heart disease (one in each case). No gross developmental abnormalities were observed in the dead fetuses. Cytogenetic studies were conducted on the peripheral lymphocytes of 94 children, and no significant chromosomal abnormalities were noted. Moreover, follow-up of the children, more than 80% of the group older than 5 years of age (the oldest was 25 years old), revealed normal development. The reproductive histories and pregnancy outcomes of the treated women were comparable to those of the normal population (10).

Occupational exposure of the mother to antineoplastic agents during pregnancy may present a risk to the fetus. A position statement from the National Study Commission on Cytotoxic Exposure and a research article involving some antineoplastic agents are presented in the monograph for cyclophosphamide (see Cyclophosphamide).

BREASTFEEDING SUMMARY

No reports describing the use of fluorouracil during lactation have been located. The low molecular weight (about 130) probably indicates that the drug is excreted into milk. Because of the potential for severe toxicity in a nursing infant, women should not nurse while receiving fluorouracil.

References

1. Product information. Efudex. ICN Pharmaceuticals, 2000.
2. Stephens JD, Golbus MS, Miller TR, Wilber RR, Epstein CJ. Multiple congenital anomalies in a fetus exposed to 5-fluorouracil during the first trimester. Am J Obstet Gynecol 1980;137:747–9.
3. Turchi JJ, Villasis C. Anthracyclines in the treatment of malignancy in pregnancy. Cancer 1988;61:435–440.
4. Stadler HE, Knowles J. Fluorouracil in pregnancy: effect on the neonate. JAMA 1971;217:214–5.
5. Cuvier C, Espie M, Extra JM, Marty M. Vinorelbine in pregnancy. Eur J Cancer 1997;33:168–9.
6. Giacalone PL, Laffargue F, Benos P. Chemotherapy for breast carcinoma during pregnancy. Cancer 1999;86:2266–72.
7. Fisher B, Sherman B, Rockette H, Redmond C, Margolese K, Fisher ER. L-Phenylalanine (L-PAM) in the management of premenopausal patients with primary breast cancer. Cancer 1979;44:847–57.
8. Schilsky RL, Lewis BJ, Sherins RJ, Young RC. Gonadal dysfunction in patients receiving chemotherapy for cancer. Ann Intern Med 1980;93:109–14.
9. Gershenson DM. Menstrual and reproductive function after treatment with combination chemotherapy for malignant ovarian germ cell tumors. J Clin Oncol 1988;6:270–5.
10. Song H, Wu P, Wang Y, Yang X, Dong S. Pregnancy outcomes after successful chemotherapy for choriocarcinoma and invasive mole: long-term follow-up. Am J Obstet Gynecol 1988;158:538–45.

FLUOXETINE

Antidepressant

PREGNANCY RECOMMENDATION: Human Data Suggest Risk in 3rd Trimester
BREASTFEEDING RECOMMENDATION: Limited Human Data—Potential Toxicity

PREGNANCY SUMMARY

The available animal and human experience indicates that fluoxetine is not a major teratogen. However, one animal study has shown that fluoxetine can produce changes, perhaps permanently, in the fetal brain. Moreover, the increased rate of three or minor anomalies found in one investigation may be evidence that the drug does adversely affect embryonic development. The other studies cited above lacked the sensitivity to identify minor anomalies because of the absence of standardized examinations. Two large case–control studies did find increased risks for some birth defects, but the absolute risk appears to be small. However, selective serotonin reuptake inhibitor (SSRI) antidepressants, including fluoxetine, have been associated with several developmental toxicities, including spontaneous abortions (SABs), low birth weight, prematurity, neonatal serotonin syndrome, neonatal behavioral syndrome (withdrawal), possibly sustained abnormal neurobehavior beyond the neonatal period, respiratory distress, and persistent pulmonary hypertension of the newborn (PPHN).

FETAL RISK SUMMARY

Fluoxetine, an SSRI, is used for the treatment of depression. The chemical structure of fluoxetine is unrelated to other antidepressant agents.

All of the antidepressant agents in the SSRI class (citalopram, escitalopram, fluoxetine, fluvoxamine, paroxetine, and sertraline) share a similar mechanism of action, although they have different chemical structures. These differences could be construed as evidence against any conclusion that they share similar effects on the embryo, fetus, or newborn. In the mouse embryo, however, craniofacial morphogenesis appears to be regulated, at least in part, by serotonin. Interference with serotonin regulation by chemically different inhibitors produces similar craniofacial defects (1). Regardless of the structural differences, therefore, some of the potential adverse effects on pregnancy outcome may also be similar.

Reproduction studies in rats and rabbits revealed no evidence of teratogenicity when using up to 1.5 and 3.6 times the maximum recommended human daily dose based on BSA (MRHDD), respectively, throughout organogenesis (2,3). In rats, however, doses of 1.5 times the MRHDD during gestation or 0.9 times the MRHDD during gestation and lactation were associated with an increase in stillbirths, a decrease in pup weight, and a decrease in pup survival during the first 7 days postpartum (2). The no-effect dose for pup mortality was 0.6 times the MRHDD (2). There was no evidence of developmental neurotoxicity in the surviving pups exposed to 1.5 times the MRHDD during gestation (2).

Using uterine rings from midterm (gestation day 14) and term pregnant rats, fluoxetine, and two other antidepressants (imipramine and nortriptyline), were shown to attenuate the activity of serotonin-induced spontaneous uterine contractions (4). Although a direct myometrial role could not be demonstrated for these monoamine reuptake inhibitors, the investigators discussed several other possible pathways that fluoxetine could induce preterm delivery (4).

Administration of fluoxetine to pregnant rats produced a down-regulation of fetal cortical ^{3}H-imipramine binding sites that was still evident 90 days after birth (5). The clinical significance of this finding to the development of the human fetal brain is unknown.

In a study to determine if fluoxetine increased the bleeding risk in neonates, pregnant rats were administered fluoxetine (5.62 mg/kg/day) from day 7 of gestation until the delivery (6). The dose was approximately five times the maximum recommended human dose. Compared with controls, fluoxetine-exposed pups had a significantly higher frequency of skin hematomas. The mechanism was thought to be related to the inhibition of serotonin uptake by platelets (6).

Both fluoxetine and the active metabolite, norfluoxetine, cross the placenta and distribute within the embryo or fetus in rats (7). Consistent with the relatively low molecular weight (about 310 for the free base), fluoxetine and the metabolite desmethylfluoxetine (norfluoxetine) cross the human term placenta. In an in vitro experiment using a single placental cotyledon, the mean steady-state placental transfer for the two compounds was 8.7% and 9.1%, respectively (8). A 2003 study of the placental transfer of antidepressants found cord blood:maternal serum ratios for fluoxetine and its metabolite that ranged from 0.32 to 1.36 and 0.12 to 1.58, respectively (9). The dose-to-delivery interval was 9–37 hours, with the highest ratio for the parent drug and metabolite occurring at 26 hours. Moreover, two studies (cited below as references 19 and 20), have documented the human placental transfer of the antidepressant and its active metabolite at term.

During clinical trials with fluoxetine, a total of 17 pregnancies occurred during treatment, even though the women were required to use birth control, suggesting lack of compliance (3). No pregnancy complications or adverse fetal outcomes were observed.

A prospective evaluation of 128 women treated with a mean daily dose of 25.8 mg of fluoxetine during the 1st trimester was reported in 1993 (10). Two matched control groups were selected: one with exposure to tricyclic antidepressants (TCAs) and the other with exposure only to nonteratogens. No differences were found in the rates of major birth defects (2, 0, and 2, respectively) among the groups. An increased risk was observed, although not statistically significant, in the rate of SAB when the fluoxetine group was compared with those in the nonteratogen group, 14.8% vs. 7.8% (relative risk 1.9; 95% confidence interval [CI] 0.92–3.92). Because only 74 TCA 1st trimester exposures were available for matching, comparisons between the three groups were based on 74 women in each group. The rates of SAB from this analysis were 13.5% (fluoxetine), 12.2% (TCAs), and 6.8% (nonteratogens), again without reaching statistical significance (10).

A 1992 prospective multicenter study evaluated the effects of lithium exposure during the 1st trimester in 148 women (11). One of the pregnancies was terminated at 16 weeks' gestation because of a fetus with a rare congenital heart defect—Ebstein's anomaly. The fetus had been exposed to lithium, fluoxetine, trazodone, and L-thyroxine during the 1st trimester. The defect was probably caused by lithium exposure.

In a surveillance study of Michigan Medicaid recipients involving 229,101 completed pregnancies conducted between 1985 and 1992, 142 newborns had been exposed to fluoxetine, 109 during the 1st trimester (F. Rosa, personal communication, FDA, 1994). Two (1.8%) major birth defects were observed (five expected), but details of the abnormalities were not available. No anomalies were observed in eight defect categories (cardiovascular defects, oral clefts, spina bifida, polydactyly, limb reduction defects, hypospadias, brain defects, and eye defects) for which specific data were available. These data do not support an association between the drug and congenital defects.

A 1993 letter to the editor from representatives of the manufacturer summarized the postmarketing database for the antidepressant (12). Of the 1103 prospectively reported exposed pregnancies, 761 of which had potentially reached term, data were available for 544 (71%) outcomes, including 91 elective terminations. Among the remaining 453 pregnancies, there were 72 (15.9%) SABs; 2 (0.4%) stillbirths; and 20 (4.4%) infants with major malformations, 7 of which were identified in the postperinatal period. Details of the aborted fetuses and stillbirths were not given. The malformations observed in the perinatal period were abdominal wall defect (in one twin), atrial septal defect, constricted band syndrome, hepatoblastoma, bilateral hydroceles, gastrointestinal anomaly, intestinal blockage, macrostomia, stubbed and missing digits, trisomy 18, trisomy 21, and ureteral disorder (2 cases). The postperinatal cases included an arrhythmia, pyloric stenosis (2 cases), tracheal malacia (3 cases), and volvulus. Additional 28 cases of major malformations reported retrospectively to the manufacturer were mentioned, but no details were given other than the fact that the malformations lacked similarity and were not indicative of a pattern of anomalies (12).

A review that appeared in 1996 (before reference 14) examined the published data relating to the safety of fluoxetine use during gestation and lactation in both experimental animals and humans (13). Using previously published criteria for identifying human teratogens, the authors concluded that the use of fluoxetine during pregnancy did not result in an increased frequency of birth defects or effects on neurobehavior (13).

A prospective study published in 1996 compared the pregnancy outcomes of 228 women who took fluoxetine with 254 nonexposed controls (14). The rates of spontaneous abortion in the two groups were 10% (exposed) and 8.5% (controls), but 13.6% (23 of 169) among those who were enrolled in the study during the 1st trimester and who had 1st trimester exposure. No significant difference in the rates of major defects among liveborn infants from subjects and controls was observed and no anomaly patterns were evident in either group. A total of 250 infants (97 study and 153 controls) were examined (by a physician who was unaware of the infant's drug exposure [15]) for minor anomalies and among those with three or more anomalies, 15 (15.5%) were exposed and 10 (6.5%) were not exposed ($p = 0.03$). In comparison with those infants who were exposed to fluoxetine during the 1st trimester or not exposed at all, late-exposed infants had a significant increase in perinatal complications, including prematurity (after excluding twins), rate of admission to special-care nurseries (after excluding preterm infants), poor neonatal adaptation, lower mean birth weight and shorter length in full-term infants, and a higher proportion of full-term infants with birth weights at ≤10th percentile. Moreover, two (2.7%) of the full-term infants who were exposed late had PPHN, a complication that is estimated to occur in the general population at a rate of 0.07%–0.10%. Although the authors concluded that the number of major structural anomalies and the rate of SABs were not significantly increased by fluoxetine exposure in this study, the increased rate of three or more minor anomalies, an unusual finding, is indicative that the drug does affect embryonic development and raises the concern of occult malformations, such as those involving brain development (14).

A 1993 case report described possible fluoxetine-induced toxicity in a term 3580-g male newborn (15). The infant's 17-year-old mother had taken the antidepressant (20 mg/day) throughout most of her pregnancy for severe depression and suicidal ideation. The infant was initially alert and active with mild hypoglycemia (33 mg/dL). At 4 hours of age, marked acrocyanosis was noted and the infant became jittery. Tachypnea developed with a respiratory rate of 70. His condition continued to worsen with symptoms peaking at 36 hours. The symptoms included continuous crying, irritability, moderate to marked tremors, increased muscle tone, a hyperactive Moro reflex, and emesis. An extensive diagnostic workup, including a drug screen, was negative. The cord blood fluoxetine and norfluoxetine levels were 26 ng/mL and 54 ng/mL, respectively, both within a nontoxic range for adults. The infant was asymptomatic at 96 hours of age at which time the serum levels of the parent drug and metabolite were <25 ng/mL and 55 ng/mL, respectively. The toxicity was attributed to fluoxetine (15).

A case report in 1997 described a 3020-g male newborn who was delivered at term from a 34-year-old woman with obsessive-compulsive disorder treated with fluoxetine 60 mg/day (16). Apgar scores were 7 and 8 at 1 and 5 minutes, respectively. The newborn was jittery and hypertonic with mild grunting, flaring, and retracting. Scattered petechiae on the face and trunk and a cephalohematoma were noted. A right, nondisplaced clavicular fracture was noted on chest X-ray. On the 2nd day of life, the serum fluoxetine and norfluoxetine concentrations were 129 ng/mL and 227 ng/mL, respectively, both in the normal adult range. The mother did not breastfeed the infant. Marked improvement in the jitteriness was observed by 2 weeks of age and by 5 months of age, the infant was considered normal. The symptoms, including the bruising and bleeding, were thought to have been caused by the antidepressant (16).

In a 1996 descriptive case series, the European Network of the Teratology Information Services (ENTIS) prospectively examined the outcomes of 689 pregnancies exposed to antidepressants (17). Multiple drug therapy occurred in about two-thirds of the mothers. Fluoxetine was used in 96 pregnancies. The outcomes of these pregnancies were 15 elective abortions, 13 SABs, 1 stillbirth, 60 normal newborns (includes 6 premature infants), 3 normal infants with neonatal disorder (asphyxia and bradycardia, periventricular bleeding; gastroesophageal regurgitation and bradycardia; and withdrawal symptoms), 2 infants with minor defects (angioma right eyebrow and pilonidal sinus), and 2 infants with congenital defects. The defects (all exposed in the 1st trimester or longer) were ventricular septal defect; and hypospadias (exposed to multiple other agents) (17).

Using data from the manufacturer's prospective pregnancy registry, postnatal complications that had been reported in 112 pregnancies (115 infants) exposed to fluoxetine during the 3rd trimester were tabulated in a 1995 reference (18). Maternal doses were 10–80 mg/day, but were not reported in 20 pregnancies. Postnatal complications, unrelated to congenital malformations, were noted in 15 singleton term infants, including 2 infants with jitteriness and 3 with irritability. Irritability was also observed in one premature infant (gestational age not given). Except in one infant, the complications were considered mild and transitory. No relationship to the maternal dose was observed, but plasma drug levels were not measured in any of the infants (18).

A study published in 1997 described the outcomes among 796 pregnancies with confirmed 1st trimester exposure to fluoxetine that had been reported prospectively to the manufacturer's worldwide fluoxetine pregnancy registry (19) (this is an update of the data presented in reference 12). Of the total number, 37 pregnancies were identified during clinical trials and 759 from spontaneous reports. SABs occurred in 110 (13.8%) cases and, for the remaining 686 pregnancies, malformations, deformations, and disruptions occurred in 34 (5.0%). No consistent pattern of defects was observed and only one minor malformation was reported. Moreover, no recurring patterns of malformations, increase in unusual defects, or adverse outcomes were observed in 89 infants from 426 retrospectively reported pregnancies. Based on these data, the authors concluded that it was unlikely that the drug was related to an increased risk of malformations (19).

The neurodevelopment of children ages 16–86 months, who had been exposed in utero for varying lengths of duration to fluoxetine (N = 55) or TCAs (N = 80), were described in 1997 (20). A control group (N = 84) of children not exposed to any agent known to adversely affect the fetus was used for comparison. Assessments of neurodevelopment were based on tests for global IQ and language development and were conducted in a blinded manner. No statistically significant differences were found between the three groups in terms of gestational age at birth, birth weight, and weight, height or head circumference at testing. The mean global IQ scores in the fluoxetine, tricyclic, and control groups were 117, 118, and 115, respectively (*ns*). Moreover, there were no significant differences in the language scores, or assessment of temperament, mood, arousability, activity level, distractibility, or behavior problems. In addition, no significant differences between the three groups were found with analysis of the data by comparing those exposed only during the 1st trimester to those exposed throughout pregnancy (20).

A 1998 noninterventional observational cohort study described the outcomes of pregnancies in women who had been prescribed ≥1 of 34 newly marketed drugs by general practitioners in England (21). Data were obtained by questionnaires sent to the prescribing physicians 1 month after the expected or possible date of delivery. In 831 (78%) of the pregnancies, a newly marketed drug was thought to have been taken during the 1st trimester with birth defects noted in 14 (2.5%) singleton births of the 557 newborns (10 sets of twins). In addition, two birth defects were observed in aborted fetuses. However, few of the aborted fetuses were examined. Fluoxetine was taken during the 1st trimester in 52 pregnancies. The outcomes of these pregnancies included 2 ectopic pregnancies, 6 SABs, 6 elective abortions, 11 cases lost to follow-up, 25 normal newborns (1 premature), and 2 infants with major malformations. The birth defects were spina bifida with hydrocephalus (the mother also took dothiepin, sodium valproate, and carbamazepine) and congenital hypothyroidism. In addition, one newborn with a normal chromosome pattern had a minor congenital anomaly (single palmar creases) (21).

Two reviews published in 1998 (22,23) and a meta-analytical review published in 2000 (24) concluded that fluoxetine was not associated with human teratogenicity.

In a 1998 case report, a 32-year-old woman with bipolar disorder took fluoxetine, buspirone, and carbamazepine (see Breastfeeding Summary for doses and further details) throughout gestation (25). At 42 weeks' gestation she gave birth to a healthy 3940-g female infant. The mother continued her medications for 3 weeks while exclusively breastfeeding the infant. She reported seizure-like activity in her infant at 3 weeks, 4 months, and 5.5 months of age (25).

Five male infants exposed to citalopram (30 mg/day), paroxetine (10–40 mg/day), or fluoxetine (20 mg/day) during gestation exhibited withdrawal symptoms at or within a few days of birth and lasting up to 1 month (26). Symptoms included irritability, constant crying, shivering, increased tonus, eating and sleeping problems, and convulsions.

A 2002 prospective study compared two groups of mother–child pairs exposed to antidepressants throughout gestation (40 exposed to fluoxetine and 46 to tricyclics) with 36 nonexposed, not depressed controls (27). Offspring were studied between the ages of 15 and 71 months for effects of antidepressant exposure in terms of IQ, language, behavior, and temperament. Exposure to antidepressants did not adversely affect the measured parameters, but IQ was significantly and negatively associated with the duration of depression, and language was negatively associated with the number of depression episodes after delivery (27).

The effect of SSRIs on birth outcomes and postnatal neurodevelopment of children exposed prenatally was reported in 2003 (28). Thirty-one children (mean age 12.9 months) exposed during pregnancy to SSRIs (15 sertraline, 8 paroxetine, 7 fluoxetine, and 1 fluvoxamine) were compared with 13 children (mean age 17.7 months) of mothers with depression who elected not to take medications during pregnancy. All of the mothers had healthy lifestyles. The timing of the exposures was 71% in the 1st trimester, 74% in the 3rd trimester, and 45% throughout. The average duration of breastfeeding in the subjects and controls was 6.4 and 8.5 months. Twenty-eight (90%) subjects nursed their infants, 17 of who took SSRIs (10 sertraline, 4 paroxetine, and 3 fluoxetine) compared with 11 (85%) controls, 3 of who took sertraline. There were no significant differences between the groups in terms of gestational age at birth, premature births, birth weight, and length or, at follow-up, in sex distribution or gain in weight and length (expressed at percentage). Seven (23%) of the exposed infants were admitted to a neonatal intensive care unit (six respiratory distress, four meconium aspiration, and one cardiac murmur) compared with none of the controls (*ns*). Follow-up examinations were conducted by a pediatric neurologist, psychologist, and a dysmorphologist who were blinded as to the mother's mediations status. The mean Apgar scores at 1 and 5 minutes were lower in the exposed group than in controls (7.0 vs. 8.2, and 8.4 vs. 9.0, respectively). There was one major defect in each group: small asymptomatic ventricular septal defect (exposed); bilateral lacrimal duct stenosis that required surgery (control). The test outcomes for mental development were similar in the groups, but significant differences in the subjects included a slight delay in psychomotor development and lower behavior motor quality (tremulousness and fine motor movements) (28).

A 2004 prospective study examined the effect of four SSRIs (citalopram, fluoxetine, paroxetine, and sertraline) on newborn neurobehavior, including behavioral state, sleep organization, motor activity, heart rate variability, tremulousness, and startles (29). Seventeen SSRI-exposed, healthy, full-birth-weight newborns and 17 nonexposed, matched controls were studied. A wide range of disrupted neurobehavioral outcomes were shown in the subject infants. After adjustment for gestational age, the exposed infants were found to differ significantly from controls in terms of tremulousness, behavioral states, and sleep organization. The effects observed on motor activity, startles, and heart rate variability were not significant after adjustment (29).

A 2003 prospective study evaluated the pregnancy outcomes of 138 women treated with SSRI antidepressants during gestation (30). Women using each agent were 73 fluoxetine, 36 sertraline, 19 paroxetine, 7 citalopram, and 3 fluvoxamine. Most (62%) took an SSRI throughout pregnancy and 95% were taking an SSRI at delivery. Birth complications were observed in 28 infants, including preterm birth (9 cases), meconium aspiration, nuchal cord, floppy at birth, and low birth weight. Four infants (2.9%) had low birth weight, all exposed to fluoxetine (40–80 mg/day) throughout pregnancy, including two of the three infants of mothers taking 80 mg/day. One infant had Hirschsprung disease, a major defect, and another had cavum septi pellucidi (neither the size of the cavum nor the SSRI agents were specified) (30). The clinical significance of the cavum septi pellucidi is doubtful as it is nearly always present at birth but resolves in the first several months (31).

In 2004, an expert panel of the National Toxicology Program (NTP) Center for the Evaluation of Risks to Human Reproduction (CEHR) evaluated the developmental toxicity of fluoxetine (32). The panel concluded that fluoxetine, especially when used late in pregnancy, caused developmental toxicity that was characterized by an increased rate of poor neonatal adaptation, such as jitteriness, tachypnea, hypoglycemia, hypothermia, poor tone, respiratory distress, weak or absent cry, diminished pain reactivity, or desaturation with feeding (32). Other toxicities included low birth weight and decreased duration of gestation. The panel also concluded that fluoxetine can impair human fertility as demonstrated by reversible, impaired sexual function, specifically orgasm. The mechanism of these effects was unknown but could be related to the drug, disease, or to the pharmacological action of the drug (32).

A 2005 meta-analysis of seven prospective comparative cohort studies involving 1774 patients was conducted to quantify the relationship between seven newer antidepressants and major malformations (33). The antidepressants were bupropion, fluoxetine, fluvoxamine, nefazodone, paroxetine, sertraline, and trazodone. There was no statistical increase in the risk of major birth defects above the baseline of 1%–3% in the general population for the individual or combined studies (33).

The database of the World Health Organization (WHO) was used in a 2005 report on neonatal SSRI withdrawal syndrome (34). Ninety-three suspected cases with either neonatal convulsions or withdrawal syndrome were identified in the WHO database. The agents were 64 paroxetine, 14 fluoxetine, 9 sertraline, and 7 citalopram. The analysis suggested that paroxetine might have an increased risk of convulsions or withdrawal compared with other SSRIs (34).

Evidence for the neonatal behavioral syndrome that is associated with in utero exposure to SSRIs and serotonin and norepinephrine reuptake inhibitors (SNRIs) (collectively called *serotonin reuptake inhibitors* [SRIs]) in late pregnancy was reviewed in a 2005 reference (35). The report followed a recent agreement by the FDA and manufacturers for a class labeling change about the neonatal syndrome. Analysis of case reports, case series, and cohort studies revealed that late exposure to SRIs carried an overall risk ratio of 3.0 (95% CI 2.0–4.4) for the syndrome compared with early exposure. The case reports (*N* = 18) and case series (*N* = 131) involved 97 cases of paroxetine, 18 fluoxetine, 16 sertraline, 12 citalopram, 4 venlafaxine, and 2 fluvoxamine. There were nine cohort studies analyzed. The typical neonatal syndrome consisted of CNS, motor, respiratory, and gastrointestinal signs that were mild and usually resolved within 2 weeks. Only 1 of 313 quantifiable cases involved a severe syndrome consisting of seizures, dehydration, excessive weight loss, hyperpyrexia, and intubation. There were no neonatal deaths attributable to the syndrome (35).

Possible sustained neurobehavioral outcomes beyond the neonatal period were reported in 2005 (36). Based on the previous findings that prenatally exposed newborns had reduced pain responses, biobehavioral responses to acute pain (heel lance) were prospectively studied in 2-month-old infants. The responses included facial action (Neonatal Facial Coding System) and cardiac autonomic reactivity (derived from respiratory activity and heart rate variability). Three groups of infants were formed: 11 infants with prenatal SSRI exposure alone (2 fluoxetine and 9 paroxetine), 30 infants with prenatal and postnatal (from breast milk) SSRI exposure (6 fluoxetine, 20 paroxetine, and 4 sertraline), and 22 nonexposed controls (mothers not depressed). The exposure during breastfeeding was considered to be very low. Heel lance-induced facial action increased in all three groups but was significantly lowered (blunted) in the first group. Heart rate was significantly lower in the exposed infants during recovery. Moreover, exposed infants had a greater return of parasympathetic cardiac modulation, whereas controls had a sustained sympathetic response. The findings were consistent with the patterns of pain reactivity observed in exposed newborns and suggested sustained neurobehavioral outcomes (36).

A significant increase in the risk of low birth weight (<10th percentile) and respiratory distress after prenatal exposure to SSRIs was reported in 2006 (37). The population-based study, representing all live births (*N* = 119,547) during a 39-month period in British Columbia, Canada, compared pregnancy outcomes of depressed mothers treated with SSRIs with outcomes in depressed mothers not treated with medication and in nonexposed controls. The severity of depression in the depressed groups was accounted for by propensity score matching (37).

A 30% incidence of SSRI-induced neonatal abstinence syndrome was found in a 2006 cohort study (38). Sixty neonates with prolonged in utero exposure to SSRIs were compared with nonexposed controls. The agents used were paroxetine (62%), fluoxetine (20%), citalopram (13%), venlafaxine (3%), and sertraline (2%). Assessment was conducted by the Finnegan score. Ten of the infants had mild and eight had severe symptoms of the syndrome. The maximum mean score in infants with severe symptoms occurred within 2 days of birth, but some occurred as long as 4 days after birth. Because of the small numbers, a dose response could only be conducted with paroxetine. Infants exposed to mean maternal doses that were <19 mg/day had no symptoms, <23 mg/day had mild symptoms, and 27 mg/day had severe symptoms (38).

A meta-analysis of clinical trials (1990–2005) with SSRIs was reported in 2006 (39). The SSRI agents included were citalopram, fluoxetine, fluvoxamine, paroxetine, and sertraline. The specific outcomes analyzed were major, minor, and cardiac malformations and SABs. The odds ratio (OR) with 95% CI for the four outcomes were 1.394 (0.906–2.145), 0.97 (0.13–6.93), 1.193 (0.531–2.677), and 1.70 (1.28–2.25), respectively. Only the risk of SABs was significantly increased (39).

A brief 2005 report described significant associations between the use of SSRIs in the 1st trimester and congenital defects (40). The data were collected by the CDC-sponsored National Birth Defects Prevention Study in an ongoing case–control study of birth defect risk factors. Case infants (*N* = 5357) with major birth defects were compared with 3366 normal controls. A positive association was found with omphalocele (*N* = 161; OR 3.0, 95% CI 1.4–6.1). Paroxetine, which accounted for 36% of all SSRI exposures, had the strongest association with the defect (OR 6.3, 95% CI 2.0–19.6). The study also found a significant association between the use of any SSRI and craniosynostosis (*N* = 372; OR 1.8, 95% CI 1.0–3.2) (40). An expanded report from this group was published in 2007 (see reference 49 below).

In a multicenter, prospective controlled study, the pregnancy outcomes of three groups of women were evaluated: (a) paroxetine 330 (286 in the 1st trimester), (b) fluoxetine 230 (206 in the 1st trimester), and (c) 1141 exposures not known to cause birth defects (41). Compared with controls, there was a higher rate of congenital defects among those exposed to paroxetine in the 1st trimester, 5.1% vs. 2.6%, relative risk (RR) 1.92, 95% CI 1.01–3.65. There also was a higher rate for cardiovascular anomalies, 1.9% vs. 0.6%, RR 3.46, 95% CI 1.06–11.42. In addition, perinatal complications were more prevalent in both SSRI groups than in controls (41).

In 1999, the Swedish Medical Birth Registry compared the use of antidepressants in early pregnancy and delivery outcomes for the years 1995–1997 (42). There were no significant differences for birth defects, infant survival, or risk of low birth weight (<2500 g) among singletons between those exposed to any depressant, SSRIs only, or non-SSRIs only, but a shorter gestational duration (<37 weeks) was observed for any antidepressant exposure (OR 1.43, 95% CI 1.14–1.80) (42). A second Registry report, published in 2006 and covering the years 1995–2003, analyzed the relationship between antidepressants and major malformations or cardiac defects (43). There was no significant increase in the risk of major malformations with any antidepressant. The strongest effect among cardiac defects was with ventricular or atrial septum defects (VSDs-ASDs). Significant increases were found with paroxetine (OR 2.22, 95% CI 1.39–3.55) and clomipramine (OR 1.87, 95% CI 1.16–2.99 (44). In 2007, the analysis was expanded to include the years 1995–2004 (44). There were 6481 women (6555 infants) who had reported the use of SSRIs in early pregnancy. The number of women using a single SSRI during the 1st trimester was 2579 citalopram, 1807 sertraline, 908 paroxetine, 860 fluoxetine, 66 escitalopram, and 36 fluvoxamine. After adjustment, only paroxetine was significantly associated with an increased risk of cardiac defects (N = 13, RR 2.62, 95% CI 1.40–4.50) or VSDs-ASDs (N = 8, RR 3.07, 95% CI 1.32–6.04). Analysis of the combined SSRI group, excluding paroxetine, revealed no associations with these defects. The study found no association with omphalocele or craniostenosis (44).

A 2007 study evaluated the association between 1st trimester exposure to paroxetine and cardiac defects by quantifying the dose–response relationship (45). A population-based pregnancy registry was used by linking three administrative databases so that it included all pregnancies in Quebec between 1997 and 2003. There were 101 infants with major congenital defects, 24 involving the heart, among the 1403 women using only one type of antidepressant during the 1st trimester. The use of paroxetine or other SSRIs did not significantly increase the risk of major defects or cardiac defects compared with non-SSRI antidepressants. However, a paroxetine dose >25 mg/day during the 1st trimester was significantly associated with an increased risk of major defects (OR 2.23, 95% CI 1.19–4.17) and of cardiac defects (OR 3.07, 95% CI 1.00–9.42) (45).

A 2007 retrospective cohort study examined the effects of exposure to SSRIs or venlafaxine in the 3rd trimester on 21 premature and 55 term newborns (46). The randomly selected unexposed control group consisted of 90 neonates of mothers not taking antidepressants, psychotropic agents, or benzodiazepines at the time of delivery. There were significantly more premature infants among the subjects (27.6%) than in controls (8.9%), but the groups were not matched. The antidepressants, as well as the number of subjects, and daily doses (in parentheses) in the exposed group were paroxetine (46; 5–40 mg), fluoxetine (10; 10–40 mg), venlafaxine (9; 74–150 mg), citalopram (6; 10–30 mg), sertraline (3; 125–150 mg), and fluvoxamine (2; 50–150 mg). The behavioral signs that were significantly increased in exposed compared with nonexposed infants were as follows: CNS: abnormal movements, shaking, spasms, agitation, hypotonia, hypertonia, irritability, and insomnia; respiratory system: indrawing, apnea/bradycardia, and tachypnea; and other: vomiting, tachycardia, and jaundice. In exposed infants, CNS (63.2%) and respiratory system (40.8%) signs were most common, appearing during the 1st day of life and lasting for a median duration of 3 days. All of the exposed premature infants exhibited behavioral signs compared with 69.1% of exposed term infants. The duration of hospitalization was significantly longer in exposed premature compared with nonexposed premature infants (14.5 days vs. 3.7 days, respectively). In 75% of the term and premature infants, the signs resolved within 3 and 5 days, respectively. There were six infants in each group with congenital malformations, but the drugs involved were not specified (46).

A 2007 review conducted a literature search to determine the risk of major congenital malformations after 1st trimester exposure to SSRIs and SNRIs (47). Fifteen controlled studies were analyzed. The data were adequate to suggest that citalopram, fluoxetine, sertraline, and venlafaxine were not associated with an increased risk of congenital defects. In contrast, the analysis did suggest an increased risk with paroxetine. The data were inadequate to determine the risk for the other SSRIs and SNRIs (47).

A case–control study, published in 2006, was conducted to test the hypothesis that exposure to SSRIs in late pregnancy was associated with PPHN (48). The study concept evolved from a 1996 study (see above) in which two (2.7%) newborns exposed to fluoxetine late in pregnancy had PPHN (14). A total of 1213 women were enrolled in the study, consisting of 377 cases whose infants had PPHN and 836 matched controls and their infants. Mothers were interviewed by nurses who were blinded to the hypothesis. Fourteen case infants had been exposed to an SSRI after the 20th week of gestation compared with six control infants (adjusted OR 6.1, 95% CI 2.2–16.8). The numbers were too small to analyze the effects of dosage, SSRI used, or reduction of the length of exposure before delivery. No increased risk of PPHN was found with the use of SSRIs before the 20th week or with the use of non-SSRI antidepressants at any time in pregnancy. If the relationship was causal, the absolute risk was estimated to be about 1% (48).

Two large case–control studies assessing associations between SSRIs and major birth defects were published in 2007 (49,50). The findings related to SSRIs as a group as well as to four specific agents: citalopram, fluoxetine, paroxetine, and sertraline. An accompanying editorial discussed the findings and limitations of these and other related studies (51). Details of the studies and the editorial are described in the paroxetine review (see Paroxetine).

A 16-year-old primigravida with narcolepsy, cataplexy, and glutaric aciduria type II (an autosomal recessive disorder) was treated throughout pregnancy with modafinil 200 mg/day, fluoxetine 20 mg/day, L-carnitine, and riboflavin (52). Because the episodes of narcolepsy and cataplexy increased in frequency, a cesarean section was conducted at 38 weeks' to deliver a 2.360-kg infant (sex not specified) with Apgar scores of 7, 8, and 9. No signs of withdrawal or abnormalities in vital signs or behavior were noted in the infant, who was discharged home with the mother after 3 days (52).

A prospective cohort study evaluated a large group of pregnancies exposed to antidepressants in the 1st trimester to determine if there was an association with major malformations (53). The patient population came from the Motherisk database and involved 928 cases that met their criteria. The 928 matched (for age, smoking, and alcohol use) controls were pregnancies not exposed to antidepressants or known teratogens. In addition to the 61 fluoxetine cases, the other cases were 113 bupropion, 184 citalopram, 21 escitalopram, 52 fluvoxamine, 68 mirtazapine, 39 nefazodone, 148 paroxetine, 61 sertraline, 17 trazodone, and 154 venlafaxine. In the antidepressant group, there were 24 (2.5%) major defects compared with 25 (2.6%) in controls (odds ratio 0.9, 95% CI 0.5–1.61). There were three major anomalies in the fluoxetine group: pulmonary valve stenosis, hypospadias, and ventricular septal defect. There were no major defects in the pregnancies exposed to bupropion, escitalopram, or trazodone (53).

BREASTFEEDING SUMMARY

Fluoxetine is excreted into breast milk. A 1990 case report described a woman, 3 months postpartum, who was started on fluoxetine, 20 mg every morning, for depression (54). No drug-related adverse effects were noted in the infant by the mother or the infant's pediatrician. However, the woman's husband, also a pediatrician, thought that the nursing infant showed increased irritability during the first 2 weeks of therapy. Two months after treatment had begun, plasma and milk samples were obtained from the mother (time in relationship to the dose was not specified). Plasma concentrations of the antidepressant and its active metabolite, norfluoxetine, were 100.5 and 194.5 ng/mL, respectively. Similar measurements in the milk were 28.8 and 41.6 ng/mL, respectively. The milk:plasma ratios for the parent compound and the metabolite were 0.29 and 0.21, respectively (54).

A 1992 report described a woman treated for postpartum depression with fluoxetine, 20 mg at bedtime, 10 weeks after delivery (55). The dosing time was chosen just before the infant's longest period of sleep to lessen his exposure to the drug. After 53 days of therapy, milk and serum samples were collected 8 hours after the usual dose and 4 hours after a subsequent dose administered to approximate peak concentrations of fluoxetine. Serum concentrations of fluoxetine and the active metabolite at 4 hours were 135 and 149 ng/mL, respectively, and at 8 hours were 124 and 141 ng/mL, respectively. The variation in the milk samples was greater, with values at 4 hours of 67 and 52 ng/mL (hand-expressed foremilk), respectively, and at 8 hours of 17 and 13 ng/mL (hand-expressed hindmilk obtained after nursing), respectively. Assuming that the milk contained a steady concentration of 120 ng/mL of fluoxetine and norfluoxetine, and the infant was ingesting 150 mL/kg/day of milk, the maximum theoretical infant dose was 15–20 mcg/kg/day. No adverse effects were observed in the nursing infant's behavior, feeding patterns, or growth during the treatment period (55).

A 1993 case study described colicky symptoms consisting of increased crying, irritability, decreased sleep, vomiting, and watery stools in a breastfed infant whose mother was taking fluoxetine, 20 mg/day (56). The mother had begun breastfeeding the infant immediately after birth and began taking fluoxetine 3 days later. The baby began to show symptoms at 6 days of age. The mother was enrolled in a study of infant crying at 3 weeks postpartum and, at 6 weeks, the infant was switched to a commercial formula for 3 weeks. The mother continued to pump her breasts during this time. She noted a marked change in the infant's behavior shortly after the change to formula feeding. The milk concentrations of fluoxetine and norfluoxetine were 69 ng/mL and 90 ng/mL, respectively. After 3 weeks of bottle-feeding, feeding with the mother's milk from a bottle was resumed; within 24 hours, the colic returned and she restarted feeding with the commercial formula. Drugs levels of fluoxetine and metabolite, determined by a commercial laboratory, in the infant's serum on the 2nd day after the return to mother's milk were 340 ng/mL and 208 ng/mL, respectively. The authors associated the symptoms of colic with the presence of fluoxetine in the mother's milk (56).

The very high infant serum levels of fluoxetine and metabolite, similar to therapeutic range in adults, are difficult to explain based on the mother's low dose. A 1996 review suggested that one possible explanation was laboratory error (57).

The presence of fluoxetine and its active metabolite, norfluoxetine, was measured in the breast milk of 10 women and in serum or urine of some of the 11 (one set of twins) nursing infants (median age 185 days) (58). The women had been taking fluoxetine at an unchanged dose for 7–14 days. The mean maternal dose of fluoxetine was 0.39 mg/kg/day (range 0.17–0.85 mg/kg/day). Milk concentrations of fluoxetine, over a 24-hour interval, were 17.4–293 ng/mL, whereas those for norfluoxetine were 23.4–379.1 ng/mL. In three women, the mean milk:plasma ratios for the two agents were 0.88 (range 0.52–1.51) and 0.82 (range 0.60–1.15), respectively. Peak milk concentrations of fluoxetine occurred within 6 hours in 8 women, more than 12 hours in 2, and undetermined in 1. A plasma sample obtained from one infant contained no measurable drug or metabolite (limit of detection for both <1 ng/mL). Fluoxetine was detected in four of five infant urine samples (1.7–17.4 ng/mL) and norfluoxetine was measured in two of the five samples (10.5 and 13.3 ng/mL). Based on an ingestion of 1000 mL of milk per day, the mean infant doses of fluoxetine and norfluoxetine were 0.077 mg/day and 0.084 mg/day, respectively, or about 10.8% of the weight-adjusted maternal dose. No adverse effects in the nursing infants, including alterations in sleeping, eating, or behavior patterns, were reported by the mothers (58).

In a 1998 case report, a 32-year-old woman with bipolar disorder took fluoxetine (20 mg/day), buspirone (45 mg/day), and carbamazepine (600 mg/day) throughout pregnancy and during the first 3 weeks postpartum (25). She reported seizure-like activity in the infant at 3 weeks, 4 months, and 5.5 months of age. Breast milk and infant serum were evaluated for the presence of fluoxetine and metabolite on postpartum days 13 and 21. On day 13, fluoxetine concentrations in breast milk were 45 ng/mL and 68 ng/mL (right and left breasts), whereas norfluoxetine levels were 68 and 57 ng/mL (right and left breasts). On day 21, the milk concentrations of the drug and metabolite were 38 and 28 ng/mL (mixed milk), respectively. The infant's serum had no detectable fluoxetine on day 13, but the level was 61 ng/mL on day 21. Norfluoxetine concentrations in infant serum on day 13 and 21 were 58 and 57 ng/mL, respectively. Maternal serum samples were not obtained for fluoxetine analysis. Similar analyses were conducted for buspirone and carbamazepine

F

(see Buspirone and Carbamazepine for results). A neurologic examination of the infant, which included electroencephalography, was within normal limits. The authors were unable to determine the cause of the seizure-like activity, if indeed it had occurred (none of the episodes had been observed by medical personnel) (25).

Serum and milk concentrations of fluoxetine (maternal dose 20–40 mg/day) and norfluoxetine in four breastfeeding women were reported in a 1998 study (59). Maternal fluoxetine serum concentrations ranged from 71 to 250 ng/mL, whereas the levels for the metabolite were 67–177 ng/mL. Hindmilk levels of fluoxetine and norfluoxetine (always higher than foremilk) were 37–132 ng/mL and 11–74 ng/mL, respectively. Neither the parent drug nor metabolite could be detected in the serum or urine samples from the nursing infants. No neurological abnormalities were detected in the infants and all had normal mental and psychomotor performance development up to 12–13 months of age, as assessed by the Bayley Scales of Infant Development (59).

In 14 breastfeeding women receiving a mean fluoxetine dose of 0.51 mg/kg/day, the mean milk:plasma ratios for the parent drug and metabolite were 0.68 and 0.56, respectively (60). The mean total infant dose (fluoxetine plus active metabolite) was estimated to be 6.81% (range 2.15%–12%) of the weight-adjusted maternal dose. In nine infants for which plasma samples were obtained, fluoxetine was detected in five (range 20–252 ng/mL) and norfluoxetine in seven (range 17–187 ng/mL). In eight cases, the antidepressant had also been taken during pregnancy and three of these infants had the highest plasma concentrations of fluoxetine. Two infants had colic, which had resolved in one infant before the study. Two other infants, with the highest plasma levels of fluoxetine, norfluoxetine, or both, exhibited symptoms of withdrawal consisting of uncontrollable crying, irritability, and poor feeding. In one case, however, maternal methadone use may have contributed to the symptoms (60).

An abstract of a study published in 1999 examined the effect of maternal fluoxetine therapy on the weight gain of nursing infants (61). A total of 64 women took the antidepressant during pregnancy and 26 continued the drug during breastfeeding. The other 38 women, who also breastfed their infants but who had discontinued the drug, were used as controls. Fluoxetine-exposed nursing infants had a growth curve significantly below the controls, averaging a deficit in weight gain of 392 g (95% CI −5, −780) in measurements taken between 2 weeks and 6 months of age. Although no adverse effects in the exposed nursing infants were reported by the mothers, the reduced growth was thought to be of possible clinical significance if infant weight gain was already of concern (61).

A 2001 case report described a woman who had been taking fluoxetine (40 mg/day) for 8 years, including throughout pregnancy (62). The infant was delivered at 37 weeks' gestation with a birth weight of about 2.76 kg. The infant was drowsy in the immediate postpartum period but was able to nurse. On day 3 of life, the infant was difficult to arouse, stopped rooting, closed her mouth, nursed only for a few minutes, and began to moan and grunt. On day 11, signs and symptoms included fever (102°F) and continuous moaning with an expiratory grunt; in addition, the infant was drowsy and difficult to arouse and hypotonic. An examination for sepsis was negative. Breastfeeding was stopped. The mother's serum fluoxetine and norfluoxetine levels were 453 and 422 ng/mL, respectively, whereas her milk levels were 114 and 124 ng/mL, respectively. The infant's serum levels of fluoxetine and metabolite were <40 ng/mL and 142 ng/mL, respectively. Eight days after nursing was stopped, the infant's serum levels were <40 ng/mL and 86 ng/mL, respectively. The infant recovered over the next 3 weeks (62).

A 2010 study using human and animal models found that drugs disturbing serotonin balance such as SSRIs and SNRIs can impair lactation (63). The authors concluded that mothers taking these drugs may need additional support to achieve breastfeeding goals.

Although some of the above reports described toxicity, the long-term effects on neurobehavior and development from exposure to this potent serotonin reuptake blocker during a period of rapid CNS development have not been adequately studied. Further, the reduced weight gain identified in one study may have clinical significance in some situations. As reported by the FDA, the manufacturer was advised to revise the labeling of fluoxetine to contain a recommendation against its use by nursing mothers (64). The current labeling contains this revision (2). In contrast, the authors of a 1996 review stated that they encouraged women to continue breastfeeding while taking the drug (13). Similarly, a 1999 review of SSRI agents concluded that if there were compelling reasons to treat a mother for postpartum depression, a condition in which a rapid antidepressant effect is important, the benefits of therapy with SSRIs would most likely outweigh the risks (65). The American Academy of Pediatrics classifies the effects of fluoxetine on the nursing infant to be unknown but may be of concern (66).

References

1. Shuey DL, Sadler TW, Lauder JM. Serotonin as a regulator of craniofacial morphogenesis: site-specific malformations following exposure to serotonin uptake inhibitors. Teratology 1992;46:367–78.
2. Product information. Prozac. Dista Products, 2000.
3. Cooper GL. The safety of fluoxetine—an update. Br J Psychiatry 1988;153(Suppl 3):77–86.
4. Vedernikov Y, Bolanos S, Bytautiene E, Fulep E, Saade GR, Garfield RE. Effect of fluoxetine on contractile activity of pregnant rat uterine rings. Am J Obstet Gynecol 2000;182:296–9.
5. Montero D, de Ceballos ML, Del Rio J. Down-regulation of 3H-imipramine binding sites in rat cerebral cortex after prenatal exposure to antidepressants. Life Sci 1990;46:1619–26.
6. Stanford MS, Patton JH. In utero exposure to fluoxetine HCl increases hematoma frequency at birth. Pharmacol Biochem Behav 1993;45:959–62.
7. Pohland RC, Byrd TK, Hamilton M, Koons JR. Placental transfer and fetal distribution of fluoxetine in the rat. Toxicol Appl Pharmacol 1989;98: 198–205.
8. Heikkinen T, Ekblad U, Laine K. Transplacental transfer of citalopram, fluoxetine, and their primary demethylated metabolites in isolated perfused human placenta. BJOG 2002;109:1003–8.
9. Hendrick V, Stowe ZN, Altshuler LL, Hwang S, Lee E, Haynes D. Placental passage of antidepressant medications. Am J Psychiatry 2003;160:993–6.
10. Pastuszak A, Schick-Boschetto B, Zuber C, Feldkamp M, Pinelli M, Sihn S, Donnenfeld A, McCormack M, Leen-Mitchell M, Woodland C, Gardner A, Hom M, Koren G. Pregnancy outcome following first-trimester exposure to fluoxetine (Prozac). JAMA 1993;269:2246–8.
11. Jacobson SJ, Jones K, Johnson K, Ceolin L, Kaur P, Sahn D, Donnenfeld AE, Rieder M, Santelli R, Smythe J, Pastuszak A, Einarson T, Koren G. Prospective multicentre study of pregnancy outcome after lithium exposure during first trimester. Lancet 1992;339:530–3.
12. Goldstein DJ, Marvel DE. Psychotropic medications during pregnancy: risk to the fetus. JAMA 1993;270:2177.
13. Nulman I, Koren G. The safety of fluoxetine during pregnancy and lactation. Teratology 1996;53:304–8.
14. Chambers CD, Johnson KA, Dick LM, Felix RJ, Jones KL. Birth outcomes in pregnant women taking fluoxetine. N Engl J Med 1996;335:1010–5.

15. Spencer MJ. Fluoxetine hydrochloride (Prozac) toxicity in a neonate. Pediatrics 1993;92:721–2.
16. Mhanna MJ, Bennet JB II, Izatt SD. Potential fluoxetine chloride (Prozac) toxicity in a newborn. Pediatrics 1997;100:158–9.
17. McElhatton PR, Garbis HM, Elefant E, Vial T, Bellemin B, Mastroiacovo P, Arnon J, Rodriguez-Pinilla E, Schaefer C, Pexieder T, Merlob P, Dal Verme S. The outcome of pregnancy in 689 women exposed to therapeutic doses of antidepressants. A collaborative study of the European Network of Teratology Information Services (ENTIS). Reprod Toxicol 1996;10:285–94.
18. Goldstein DJ. Effects of third trimester fluoxetine exposure on the newborn. J Clin Psychopharmacol 1995;15:417–20.
19. Goldstein DJ, Corbin LA, Sundell KL. Effects of first-trimester fluoxetine exposure on the newborn. Obstet Gynecol 1997;89:713–8.
20. Nulman I, Rovet J, Stewart DE, Wolpin J, Gardner HA, Theis JGW, Kulin N, Koren G. Neurodevelopment of children exposed in utero to antidepressant drugs. N Engl J Med 1997;336:258–62.
21. Wilton LV, Pearce GL, Martin RM, Mackay FJ, Mann RD. The outcomes of pregnancy in women exposed to newly marketed drugs in general practice in England. Br J Obstet Gynaecol 1998;105:882–9.
22. Gupta S, Masand PS, Rangwani S. Selective serotonin reuptake inhibitors in pregnancy and lactation. Obstet Gynecol Surv 1998;53:733–6.
23. Austin MPV, Mitchell PB. Psychotropic medications in pregnant women: treatment dilemmas. Med J Aust 1998;169:428–31.
24. Addis A, Koren G. Safety of fluoxetine during the first trimester of pregnancy: a meta-analytical review of epidemiological studies. Psychologic Med 2000;30:89–94.
25. Brent NB, Wisner KL. Fluoxetine and carbamazepine concentrations in a nursing mother/infant pair. Clin Pediatr 1998;37:41–4.
26. Nordeng H, Lindemann R, Perminov KV, Reikvam A. Neonatal withdrawal syndrome after in utero exposure to selective serotonin reuptake inhibitors. Acta Paediatr 2001;90:288–91.
27. Nulman I, Rovet J, Stewart DE, Wolpin J, Pace-Asciak P, Shuhaiber S, Koren G. Child development following exposure to tricyclic antidepressants or fluoxetine throughout fetal life: a prospective, controlled study. Am J Psychiatry 2002;159:1889–95.
28. Casper RC, Fleisher BE, Lee-Ancajas JC, Gilles A, Gaylor E, DeBattista A, Hoyme HE. Follow-up of children of depressed mothers exposed or not exposed to antidepressant drugs during pregnancy. J Pediatr 2003;142: 402–8.
29. Zeskind PS, Stephens LE. Maternal selective serotonin reuptake inhibitor use during pregnancy and newborn neurobehavior. Pediatrics 2004;113: 368–75.
30. Hendrick V, Smith LM, Suri R, Hwang S, Haynes D, Altshuler L. Birth outcomes after prenatal exposure to antidepressant medication. Am J Obstet Gynecol 2003;188:812–5.
31. DeMyer W. Brain, midline caves. In: Buyse ML, editor-in-chief. *Birth Defects Encyclopedia*. Cambridge, MA: Blackwell Scientific Publications, 1990:238.
32. Hines RN, Adams J, Buck GM, Faber W, Holson JF, Jacobson SW, Keszler M, McMartin K, Segraves RT, Singer LT, Sipes IG, Williams PL, NTP-CERHR expert panel report on the reproductive and developmental toxicity of fluoxetine. Birth Defects Res B Dev Reprod Toxicol 2004;71:193–280.
33. Einarson TR, Einarson A. Newer antidepressants in pregnancy and rates of major malformations: a meta-analysis of prospective comparative studies. Pharmacoepidemiol Drug Saf 2005;14:823–7.
34. Sanz EJ, De-las-Cuevas C, Kiuru A, Edwards R. Selective serotonin reuptake inhibitors in pregnant women and neonatal withdrawal syndrome: a database analysis. Lancet 2005;365:482–7.
35. Moses-Kolko EL, Bogen D, Perel J, Bregar A, Uhl K, Levin B, Wisner KL. Neonatal signs after late in utero exposure to serotonin reuptake inhibitors. JAMA 2005;293:2372–83.
36. Oberlander TF, Grunau RE, Fitzgerald C, Papsdorf M, Rurak D, Riggs W. Pain reactivity in 2-month-old infants after prenatal and postnatal selective serotonin reuptake inhibitor medication exposure. Pediatrics 2005;115:411–25.
37. Oberlander TF, Warburton W, Misri S, Aghajanian J, Hertzman C. Neonatal outcomes after prenatal exposure to selective serotonin reuptake inhibitor antidepressants and maternal depression using population-based linked health data. Arch Gen Psychiatry 2006;63:898–906.
38. Levinson-Castiel R, Merlob P, Linder N, Sirota L, Klinger G. Neonatal abstinence syndrome after in utero exposure to selective serotonin reuptake inhibitors in term infants. Arch Pediatr Adoles Med 2006;160:173–6.
39. Rahimi R, Nikfar S, Abdollahi M. Pregnancy outcomes following exposure to serotonin reuptake inhibitors: a meta-analysis of clinical trials. Reprod Toxicol 2006;22:571–5.
40. Alwan S, Reefhuis J, Rasmussen S, Olney R, Friedman JM. Maternal use of selective serotonin reuptake inhibitors and risk for birth defects (abstract). Birth Defects Res A Clin Mol Teratol 2005;73:291.
41. Diav-Citrin O, Shechtman S, Weinbaum D, Arnon J, Gianantonio ED, Clementi M, Ornoy A. Paroxetine and fluoxetine in pregnancy: a multicenter, prospective, controlled study (abstract). Reprod Toxicol 2005;20:459.
42. Ericson A, Kallen B, Wiholm BE. Delivery outcome after the use of antidepressants in early pregnancy. Eur J Clin Pharmacol 1999;55:503–8.
43. Kallen B, Olausson PO. Antidepressant drugs during pregnancy and infant congenital heart defect. Reprod Toxicol 2006;21:221–2.
44. Kallen BAJ, Olausson PO. Maternal use of selective serotonin re-uptake inhibitors in early pregnancy and infant congenital malformations. Birth Defects Res A Clin Mol Teratol 2007;79:301–8.
45. Berard A, Ramos E, Rey E, Blais L, St-Andre M, Oraichi D. First trimester exposure to paroxetine and risk of cardiac malformations in infants: the importance of dosage. Birth Defects Res B Dev Reprod Toxicol 2007;80: 18–27.
46. Ferreira E, Carceller AM, Agogue C, Martin BZ, St-Andre M, Francoeur D, Berard A. Effects of selective serotonin reuptake inhibitors and venlafaxine during pregnancy in term and preterm neonates. Pediatrics 2007;119: 52–9.
47. Bellantuono C, Migliarese G, Gentile S. Serotonin reuptake inhibitors in pregnancy and the risk of major malformations: a systematic review. Hum Psychopharmacol Clin Exp 2007;22:121–8.
48. Chambers CD, Hernandez-Diaz S, Van Marter LJ, Werler MM, Louik C, Jones KL, Mitchell AA. Selective serotonin-reuptake inhibitors and risk of persistent pulmonary hypertension of the newborn. N Engl J Med 2006;354:579–87.
49. Alwan S, Reefhuis J, Rasmussen SA, Olney RS, Friedman JM, for the National Birth Defects Prevention Study. Use of selective serotonin-reuptake inhibitors in pregnancy and the risk of birth defects. N Engl J Med 2007;356:2684–92.
50. Louik C, Lin AE, Werler MM, Hernandez-Diaz S, Mitchell AA. First-trimester use of selective serotonin-reuptake inhibitors and the risk of birth defects. N Engl J Med 2007;356:2675–83.
51. Greene MF. Teratogenicity of SSRIs—serious concern or much ado about little? N Engl J Med 2007;356:2732–3.
52. Williams SF, Alvarez JR, Pedro HF, Apuzzio JJ. Glutaric aciduria type II and narcolepsy in pregnancy. Obstet Gynecol 2008;111:522–4.
53. Einarson A, Choi J, Einarson TR, Koren G. Incidence of major malformations in infants following antidepressant exposure in pregnancy: results of a large prospective cohort study. Can J Psychiatry 2009;54:242–6.
54. Isenberg KE. Excretion of fluoxetine in human breast milk. J Clin Psychiatry 1990;51:169.
55. Burch KJ, Wells BG. Fluoxetine/norfluoxetine concentrations in human milk. Pediatrics 1992;89:676–7.
56. Lester BM, Cucca J, Andreozzi L, Flanagan P, Oh W. Possible association between fluoxetine hydrochloride and colic in an infant. J Am Acad Child Adolesc Psychiatr 1993;32:1253–5.
57. Wisner KL, Perel JM, Findling RL. Antidepressant treatment during breast feeding. Am J Psychiatry 1996;153:1132–7.
58. Taddio A, Ito S, Koren G. Excretion of fluoxetine and its metabolite, norfluoxetine, in human breast milk. J Clin Pharmacol 1996;36:42–7.
59. Yoshida K, Smith B, Craggs M, Channi Kumar R. Fluoxetine in breast-milk and developmental outcome of breast-fed infants. Br J Psychiatry 1998;172:175–9.
60. Kristensen JH, Ilett KF, Hackett LP, Yapp P, Paech M, Begg EJ. Distribution and excretion of fluoxetine and norfluoxetine in human milk. Br J Clin Pharmacol 1999;48:521–7.
61. Chambers CD, Anderson PO, Thomas RG, Dick LM, Felix RJ, Johnson KA, Jones KL. Weight gain in infants breastfed by mothers who take fluoxetine (abstract). Pediatrics 1999;104:1120–1.
62. Hale TW, Shum S, Grossberg M. Fluoxetine toxicity in a breastfed infant. Clin Pediatr 2001;40:681–4.
63. Marshall AM, Nommsen-Rivers LA, Hernandez LI, Dewey KG, Chantry CJ, Gregerson KA, Horseman ND. Serotonin transport and metabolism in the mammary gland modulates secretory activation and involution. J Clin Endocrin Metab 2010;95:837–46.
64. Nightingale SL. Fluoxetine labeling revised to identify phenytoin interaction and to recommend against use in nursing mothers. JAMA 1994; 271:1067.
65. Edwards JG, Anerson I. Systematic review and guide to selection of selective serotonin reuptake inhibitors. Drugs 1999;57:507–33.
66. Committee on Drugs, American Academy of Pediatrics. The transfer of drugs and other chemicals into human milk. Pediatrics 2001;108:776–89.

FLUOXYMESTERONE

Androgenic Hormone

PREGNANCY RECOMMENDATION: Contraindicated
BREASTFEEDING RECOMMENDATION: Contraindicated

F

PREGNANCY SUMMARY

Only one report describing the use of fluoxymesterone in human pregnancy has been located. Fluoxymesterone is contraindicated in pregnancy because of the risk for nonadrenal female pseudohermaphroditism (see Testosterone).

FETAL RISK SUMMARY

The androgenic hormone fluoxymesterone is indicated as replacement therapy in conditions associated with symptoms of deficiency or absence of endogenous testosterone. It is also indicated for the palliation of androgen-responsive recurrent mammary cancer. Fluoxymesterone inhibits the release of testosterone by inhibition of pituitary luteinizing hormone. Large doses may also suppress spermatogenesis by inhibiting follicle-stimulating hormone (1). The relatively low molecular weight (about 336) suggests that the drug will cross the placenta.

Fluoxymesterone (10 mg/day) was given to a 31-year-old woman in the third month of pregnancy for gigantomastia (2). "Several weeks" of therapy had no effect on the size of the breasts nor did diuretic therapy with chlorothiazide (6000 mg/day). The woman was eventually hospitalized at 6 months' gestation because of breast tissue necrosis and hemorrhage. A single IM dose of testosterone and estradiol (Deladumone) had no effect and both breasts continued to enlarge. An 8-day course of combination oral contraceptives was discontinued because of superficial thrombophlebitis in the right thigh. When the breast ulcer became infected, a bilateral simple mastectomy was performed. She eventually delivered a normal healthy, 3.8-kg male infant (2).

BREASTFEEDING SUMMARY

No reports describing the use of fluoxymesterone during human lactation have been located. Because testosterone and its derivatives inhibit lactation (see Testosterone), fluoxymesterone is contraindicated in women who are breastfeeding.

References

1. Product information. Halotestin. Upjohn, 1995.
2. Moss WH. Gigantomastia with pregnancy. A case report with review of the literature. Arch Surg 1968;96:27–37.

FLUPENTHIXOL

[Withdrawn from the market. See 9th edition.]

FLUPHENAZINE

Antipsychotic

PREGNANCY RECOMMENDATION: Human Data Suggest Risk in 3rd Trimester
BREASTFEEDING RECOMMENDATION: No Human Data—Potential Toxicity

PREGNANCY SUMMARY

Extrapyramidal and/or withdrawal have been reported when fluphenazine was used during gestation. Although one case report described multiple anomalies, most evidence suggests that phenothiazines are relatively low risk during pregnancy (see also Prochlorperazine).

FETAL RISK SUMMARY

Fluphenazine is a piperazine phenothiazine in the same group as prochlorperazine. Phenothiazines readily cross the placenta (1).

Shepard reviewed two studies, in which fluphenazine was given to pregnant rats at doses up to 100 mg/kg orally without producing adverse fetal effects (2). Pregnant mice were given fluphenazine (1 mg/kg) or diphenylhydantoin (50 mg/kg), or both, by gavage during organogenesis (3).

As compared with controls, a significant reduction in fetal weight and length was observed in all treatment groups. The combination produced a significant increase in the incidence of skeletal defects (incomplete ossification of sternebrae and skull bones) and in the incidence of dilated cerebral ventricles (already increased in the fluphenazine-alone group) (3).

An apparently normal pregnancy outcome was described in a woman receiving psychotherapy and being treated with fluphenazine decanoate (2 mL IM every 3 weeks) (4). In addition, she also smoked cigarettes (up to 4 packs/day) and drank four or five cocktails each evening. She eventually delivered a 1-week postterm 3.38-kg, male infant, who developed minor extrapyramidal symptoms (or withdrawal) 4 weeks after delivery. The symptoms readily responded to oral diphenhydramine. At 2 months of age, the infant was healthy and weighed 4.66 kg. The infant boy was reported by the mother to be doing well at 20 months of age.

A 22-year-old woman with schizophrenia was treated with chlorpromazine (up to 1200 mg/day) throughout gestation, fluphenazine decanoate (50 mg IM every 2 weeks) from the 14th week of gestation, and electroconvulsive therapy at 18 weeks (5). The fluphenazine dose was increased to 100 mg IM every 2 weeks at 24 weeks' gestation. In addition, she smoked 3–4 packs of cigarettes per day. An apparently normal, 3.53-kg male infant was delivered by cesarean section at 39 weeks, who did well during the first 3 weeks. At that time (6 weeks after the mother's last fluphenazine dose), the infant developed excessive irritability, choreiform and dystonic movements mostly in the upper limbs, jittery behavior, and hypertonicity. Two doses of diphenhydramine given on the 24th and 25th days failed to resolve the condition. Over the next few weeks, the symptoms subsided only to return on the 58th day with the same earlier intensity (5). Diphenhydramine (62.5 mg) was restarted every 6 hours with slow improvement in his condition. At 15 weeks of age, the infant's progress appeared normal. At 6 months of age, the diphenhydramine was gradually withdrawn. Follow-up at 15 months of age was normal. The authors attributed the infant's condition to fluphenazine withdrawal (5).

An infant with multiple anomalies was born to a mother treated with fluphenazine enanthate injections throughout pregnancy (6). The mother also took Debendox (see Doxylamine) during the 1st trimester. Anomalies included: ocular hypertelorism with telecanthus; cleft lip and palate; imperforate anus; hypospadias of penoscrotal type; jerky, roving eye movements; episodic rapid nystagmoid movements; rectourethral fistula; and poor ossification of frontal skull bone.

In a surveillance study of Michigan Medicaid recipients involving 229,101 completed pregnancies conducted between 1985 and 1992, 13 newborns had been exposed to fluphenazine during the 1st trimester (F. Rosa, personal communication, FDA, 1993). One (7.7%) major birth defect was observed (0.6 expected), a cardiovascular defect (0 expected). The number of exposures is too small for comment.

A 35-year-old woman with schizophrenia was treated throughout gestation with fluphenazine, 10 mg orally twice daily, then decreased to 5 mg orally twice daily during the 3rd trimester (7). The fluphenazine concentration in cord blood was <1.0 ng/mL. She delivered a normal, 2855-g, female infant at 39 weeks' gestation, who developed severe rhinorrhea and upper respiratory distress at 8 hours of age. Oral feedings were poor and complicated by periodic episodes of vomiting, course choreoathetoid movements of the arms and legs, and intermittent arching of the body (7). Marked improvement in her symptoms occurred following a single dose of pseudoephedrine solution (0.75 mg) that was repeated once the next day. Although the infant had no further extrapyramidal symptoms, the rhinorrhea and nasal congestion persisted for 3 months.

BREASTFEEDING SUMMARY

No reports describing the use of fluphenazine during human lactation have been located. Because other phenothiazines are excreted into milk (see also Prochlorperazine), passage of fluphenazine into milk should be expected. The American Academy of Pediatrics classifies the effects of other antipsychotic phenothiazine agents (e.g., see Chlorpromazine) on the nursing infant to be unknown but may be of concern.

References

1. Moya F, Thorndike V. Passage of drugs across the placenta. Am J Obstet Gynecol 1962;84:1778–98.
2. Shepard TH. *Catalog of Teratogenic Effects*. 8th ed. Baltimore, MD: The Johns Hopkins University Press, 1995:190–1.
3. Abdel-Hamid HA, Abdel-Rahman MS, Abdel-Rahman SA. Teratogenic effect of diphenylhydantoin and/or fluphenazine in mice. J Appl Toxicol 1996;16:221–5.
4. Cleary MF. Fluphenazine decanoate during pregnancy. Am J Psychiatry 1977;134:815–6.
5. O'Connor M, Johnson GH, James DI. Intrauterine effect of phenothiazines. Med J Aust 1981;1:416–7.
6. Donaldson GL, Bury RG. Multiple congenital abnormalities in a newborn boy associated with maternal use of fluphenazine enanthate and other drugs during pregnancy. Acta Paediatr Scand 1982;71:335–8.
7. Nath SP, Miller DA, Muraskas JK. Severe rhinorrhea and respiratory distress in a neonate exposed to fluphenazine hydrochloride prenatally. Ann Pharmacother 1996;30:35–7.

FLURAZEPAM

Hypnotic

PREGNANCY RECOMMENDATION: Limited Human Data—Animal Data Suggest Low Risk
BREASTFEEDING RECOMMENDATION: Limited Human Data—Probably Compatible*

*Potential toxicity if combined with other CNS depressants

PREGNANCY SUMMARY

Limited reports describing the use of flurazepam in human pregnancy have been located. The effects of this drug on the fetus should be similar to other benzodiazepines (see Diazepam). Maternal use near delivery may potentially cause neonatal motor depression and withdrawal.

FETAL RISK SUMMARY

Flurazepam is a benzodiazepine used to induce sleep. No teratogenic or other adverse fetal or postnatal effects were observed in studies using rats and rabbits administered 80 mg/kg and 20 mg/kg, respectively, during various stages of gestation (1). Similarly, no reports of congenital abnormalities attributable to human exposure with flurazepam have been located. One group of investigators classified the risk to the fetus from exposure to flurazepam as "none–minimal," but the quality of the data was judged to be "poor" (2). Studies involving other members of this class, however, have found evidence that some of these agents may cause fetal abnormalities (see Chlordiazepoxide and Diazepam).

Although published data are lacking, the molecular weight of flurazepam (about 461) suggests it is transferred to the fetus. Data from the manufacturer indicate that an active metabolite of flurazepam crosses the human placenta and may adversely affect the newborn (3). In a case cited in their product information, a woman ingested flurazepam, 30 mg nightly, for 10 days immediately preceding delivery. The newborn appeared sleepy and lethargic during the first 4 days of life. The effect was thought to be due to a long-acting metabolite, N_1-desalkylflurazepam, found in the newborn's serum.

In a surveillance study of Michigan Medicaid recipients involving 229,101 completed pregnancies conducted between 1985 and 1992, 73 newborns had been exposed to flurazepam during the 1st trimester (F. Rosa, personal communication, FDA, 1993). Four (5.5%) (three expected) major birth defects were observed, including (observed/expected) 2/1 cardiovascular defects, 1/0 oral clefts, and 1/0 polydactyly. These data do not support an association between the drug and congenital defects.

A brief 1982 case report described convulsions attributable to clomipramine in a newborn who was exposed to that drug and flurazepam throughout gestation (4). The 2360-g male infant was delivered vaginally at 33 weeks' gestation (the reason for the premature delivery was not stated) and had Apgar scores of 9 and 9 at 1 and 5 minutes, respectively. Convulsions, consisting of myoclonic jerks that were unresponsive to phenobarbital, started at 7 hours of age and were eventually successfully treated with IV and oral clomipramine, although the infant remained jittery. The contribution of flurazepam, which is known to cause convulsions after abrupt withdrawal following prolonged use in adults, to the seizures observed in the newborn is unknown. However, a correlation between declining serum levels of clomipramine and its active metabolite and the condition of the infant probably indicates that the seizures were not due to flurazepam.

BREASTFEEDING SUMMARY

Studies measuring the amount of flurazepam excreted into breast milk have not been located. However, the passage of this agent and its active, long-acting metabolite into milk should be expected (see also Diazepam).

The effects of exposure to benzodiazepines during breastfeeding were reported in a 2012 study (5). In a 15-month period spanning 2010–2011, 296 women called the Motherisk Program in Toronto, Ontario, seeking advice on the use of these drugs during lactation, and 124 consented to the study. The most commonly used benzodiazepines were lorazepam (52%), clonazepam (18%), and midazolam (15%). Neonatal sedation was reported in only two infants. There was no significant difference between the characteristics of these 2 and the 122 that reported no sedation in terms of maternal age, gestational age at birth, daily amount of time nursing, amount of time infant slept each day, and the benzodiazepine dose (mg/kg/day). The only difference was in the number of CNS depressants that the mothers were taking: 3.5 vs. 1.7 (p = 0.0056). In the two infants with sedation, one mother reported using alprazolam (two doses of 0.25 mg), sertraline (50 mg/day), and zopiclone (about 2.5 mg every 3 days), whereas the other mother took clonazepam (0.25 mg twice daily), flurazepam (1 mg/day), bupropion (1 mg/day), and risperidone (0.75 mg/day). The infant in this latter case also was exposed in utero. The investigators concluded that their results supported the recommendation that the use benzodiazepines was not a reason to avoid breastfeeding (5).

The American Academy of Pediatrics classifies the effects of lorazepam on the nursing infant as unknown but may be of concern if exposure is prolonged (6).

References

1. Hoffmann-LaRoche Company, Personal Communication, 1979. As cited by Shepard TH. *Catalog of Teratogenic Agents*. 6th ed. Baltimore, MD: The Johns Hopkins University Press, 1989:285.
2. Friedman JM, Little BB, Brent RL, Cordero JF, Hanson JW, Shepard TH. Potential human teratogenicity of frequently prescribed drugs. Obstet Gynecol 1990;75:594–9.
3. Product information. Dalmane. Roche Laboratories, 1993.
4. Cowe L, Lloyd DJ, Dawling S. Neonatal convulsions caused by withdrawal from maternal clomipramine. Br Med J 1982;284:1837–8.
5. Kelly LE, Poon S, Madadi P, Koren G. Neonatal benzodiazepines exposure during breastfeeding. J Pediatr 2012;161:448–51.
6. Committee on Drugs, American Academy of Pediatrics. The transfer of drugs and other chemicals into human milk. Pediatrics 2001;108:776–89.

FLURBIPROFEN

Nonsteroidal Anti-inflammatory

PREGNANCY RECOMMENDATION: Human Data Suggest Risk in 1st and 3rd Trimesters
BREASTFEEDING RECOMMENDATION: Compatible

PREGNANCY SUMMARY

No reports describing the use of flurbiprofen during human pregnancy have been located. Constriction of the ductus arteriosus in utero is a pharmacologic consequence arising from the use of prostaglandin synthesis inhibitors during pregnancy, as is inhibition of labor, prolongation of pregnancy, and suppression of fetal renal function (see also Indomethacin) (1). Persistent pulmonary hypertension of the newborn may occur if these agents are used in the 3rd trimester close to delivery (1,2). Women attempting to conceive should not use any prostaglandin synthetase inhibitor, including flurbiprofen, because of the findings in various animal models that indicate these agents block blastocyst implantation (3,4). Moreover, as noted below, nonsteroidal anti-inflammatory drugs (NSAIDs) have been associated with spontaneous abortions (SABs) and congenital malformations. The absolute risk for these defects, however, appears to be low.

FETAL RISK SUMMARY

Flurbiprofen is an NSAID that shares the same precautions for human pregnancy use as other NSAIDs. It is in the same subclass (propionic acids) as five other agents (fenoprofen, ibuprofen, ketoprofen, naproxen, and oxaprozin). Flurbiprofen is used in the treatment of arthritis and is available in an ocular formulation for inhibition of intraoperative miosis. No teratogenic effects were observed in mice, rats, and rabbits administered this drug during gestation (5).

Like other NSAIDs, systemic use of flurbiprofen in rats has been associated with prolonged gestation, fetal growth restriction, and decreased fetal survival (6). In one study of pregnant rats, flurbiprofen inhibition of parturition appeared to be dose-related (7).

A combined 2001 population-based, observational cohort study and a case–control study estimated the risk of adverse pregnancy outcome from the use of NSAIDs (8). The use of NSAIDs during pregnancy was not associated with congenital malformations, preterm delivery, or low birth weight, but a positive association was discovered with SABs. (A similar study, also published in 2001, failed to find a relationship, in general, between NSAIDs and congenital malformations, but did find a significant association with cardiac defects and orofacial clefts (9), In addition, a 2003 study found a significant association between exposure to NSAIDs in early pregnancy and SABs (10) (see Ibuprofen for details on these three studies).

A brief 2003 editorial on the potential for NSAID-induced developmental toxicity concluded that NSAIDs, and specifically those with greater cyclooxygenase 2 (COX-2) affinity, had a lower risk of this toxicity in humans than aspirin (11). Two reviews, both on antirheumatic drug therapy in pregnancy, recommended that if an NSAID was needed, agents with short elimination adult half-lives should be used at the maximum tolerated dosage interval, using the smallest effective dose, and that therapy should be stopped within 8 weeks of the expected delivery date (12,13). Flurbiprofen has a short plasma elimination half-life (5.7 hours), but other factors, such as its toxicity profile, need to be considered.

BREASTFEEDING SUMMARY

Very small amounts of flurbiprofen are excreted into breast milk (14,15). In 10 nursing mothers, at least 1 month postpartum, a single 100-mg oral dose of flurbiprofen was administered and milk and blood samples were obtained over a 48-hour period (14). The average peak plasma concentration (14.7 mcg/mL) occurred at 1.5 hours with a mean half-life of 5.8 hours. The average peak milk concentration was 0.09 mcg/mL with an average of 0.05% (range 0.03%–0.07%) of the maternal dose recovered in breast milk. Breastfeeding was discontinued during and after the study.

In a multiple dosing study, 12 lactating women, 3–5 days after delivery, were administered nine doses of flurbiprofen over a 3-day period (50 mg 4 times daily) (15). Paired milk and plasma samples were obtained at several times during the period and after the last dose. The mean maternal plasma half-life of the drug was 4.8 hours. Flurbiprofen milk concentrations were less than 0.05 mcg/mL in 10 of the mothers. In the remaining two mothers, only three of their milk samples contained flurbiprofen: 0.06, 0.07, and 0.08 mcg/mL. The authors concluded that these small amounts were safe for a nursing infant. The mothers did not breastfeed their infants (15).

The small amounts of flurbiprofen recovered from transitional and mature breast milk seem to indicate that the risk posed by flurbiprofen to a nursing infant is slight, if it exists at all. One reviewer classified flurbiprofen as one of several low-risk alternatives, because of its short adult serum half-life and toxicity profile compared with other similar agents, if an NSAID was required while nursing (16). Other reviewers have also stated that flurbiprofen can be safely used during breastfeeding (17,18). Ibuprofen, another NSAID in the same subclass as flurbiprofen, is considered compatible with breastfeeding by the American Academy of Pediatrics (see Ibuprofen).

References

1. Levin DL. Effects of inhibition of prostaglandin synthesis on fetal development, oxygenation, and the fetal circulation. Semin Perinatol 1980;4:35–44.

2. Van Marter LJ, Leviton A, Allred EN, Pagano M, Sullivan KF, Cohen A, Epstein MF. Persistent pulmonary hypertension of the newborn and smoking and aspirin and nonsteroidal antiinflammatory drug consumption during pregnancy. Pediatrics 1996;97:658–63.
3. Matt DW, Borzelleca JF. Toxic effects on the female reproductive system during pregnancy, parturition, and lactation. In: Witorsch RJ, ed. *Reproductive Toxicology*. 2nd ed. New York, NY: Raven Press, 1995:175–93.
4. Dawood MY. Nonsteroidal antiinflammatory drugs and reproduction. Am J Obstet Gynecol 1993;169:1255–65.
5. Product information. Ansaid. The Upjohn Company, 1995.
6. Product information. Ocufen. Allergan America, 1987.
7. Powell JG Jr, Cochrane RL. The effects of a number of non-steroidal anti-inflammatory compounds on parturition in the rat. Prostaglandins 1982;23:469–88.
8. Nielsen GL, Sorensen HT, Larsen H, Pedersen L. Risk of adverse birth outcome and miscarriage in pregnant users of non-steroidal anti-inflammatory drugs: population based observational study and case-control study. Br Med J 2001;322:266–70.
9. Ericson A, Kallen BAJ. Nonsteroidal anti-inflammatory drugs in early pregnancy. Reprod Toxicol 2001;15:371–5.
10. Li DK, Liu L, Odouli R. Exposure to non-steroidal anti-inflammatory drugs during pregnancy and risk of miscarriage: population based cohort study. Br Med J 2003;327:368–71.
11. Tassinari MS, Cook JC, Hurtt ME. NSAIDs and developmental toxicity. Birth Defects Res B Dev Reprod Toxicol 2003;68:3–4.
12. Needs CJ, Brooks PM. Antirheumatic medication in pregnancy. Br J Rheumatol 1985;24:282–90.
13. Ostesen M. Optimisation of antirheumatic drug treatment in pregnancy. Clin Pharmacokinet 1994;27:486–503.
14. Cox SR, Forbes KK. Excretion of flurbiprofen into breast milk. Pharmacotherapy 1987;7:211–5.
15. Smith IJ, Hinson JL, Johnson VA, Brown RD, Cook SM, Whitt RT, Wilson JT. Flurbiprofen in post-partum women: plasma and breast milk disposition. J Clin Pharmacol 1989;29:174–84.
16. Anderson PO. Medication use while breast feeding a neonate. Neonatal Pharmacol Q 1993;2:3–14.
17. Goldsmith DP. Neonatal rheumatic disorders. View of the pediatrician. Rheum Dis Clin North Am 1989;15:287–305.
18. Needs CJ, Brooks PM. Antirheumatic medication during lactation. Br J Rheumatol 1985;24:291–7.

FLUTICASONE

Respiratory Drug (Corticosteroid)

PREGNANCY RECOMMENDATION: Compatible
BREASTFEEDING RECOMMENDATION: No Human Data—Probably Compatible

PREGNANCY SUMMARY

Four reports totaling 201 women have described the use of fluticasone during pregnancy. No increase in the rates of embryo, fetal, or newborn toxicity were observed. Although the animal data suggest high risk, SC doses were used, resulting in much higher systemic concentrations than those obtained in humans after inhalation. Because of the initial absence of human pregnancy experience, two reviews concluded that either beclomethasone or budesonide were the inhaled corticosteroids of choice if such therapy is initiated in pregnancy (1,2). However, the new data suggest that if a nonpregnant woman has shown a good response to fluticasone, or if the agent is indicated in a pregnant woman, the drug is compatible with pregnancy.

FETAL RISK SUMMARY

Fluticasone, a synthetic trifluorinated glucocorticoid, is indicated for the maintenance treatment of asthma as a prophylactic therapy. In human lung preparations, the affinity of fluticasone for the glucocorticoid receptor is almost twice that of the active metabolite of betamethasone, and more than 3 and 18 times greater that of budesonide and dexamethasone, respectively. Although the oral bioavailability of fluticasone is negligible (<1%), the systemic bioavailability after inhalation is high (about 30% of the dose). Peak plasma levels after an 880-mcg inhaled dose were in the range of 0.1–1.0 ng/mL. The only metabolite that has been identified in humans is relativity inactive (about 2000 times less affinity than the parent drug for the glucocorticoid receptor). Plasma protein binding of the parent compound is about 91%. Excretion is mostly in the feces with a terminal plasma elimination half-life of about 7.8 hours (3).

Reproduction studies have been conducted with SC doses in mice, rats, and rabbits. In mice and rats, SC doses approximately 0.1 and 0.5 times the maximum human daily inhalation dose based on BSA (MRHID), respectively, revealed embryonic growth restriction, omphalocele, cleft palate, and retarded cranial ossification. This toxicity was considered characteristic of potent glucocorticoid compounds as rodents may be more prone to teratogenic effects from these agents than humans (3). In male and female rats, no evidence of impaired fertility was observed with SC doses up to about 0.25 times the MRHID, but prostate weight was significantly reduced. Fluticasone was not tumorigenic in long-term studies in mice and rats, nor was it mutagenic or clastogenic in various in vitro assays. In pregnant rabbits, SC doses approximately 0.04 times the MRHID were associated with fetal weight reduction and cleft palate. Oral doses approximately 3 times the MRHID did not cause maternal toxicity or increase the incidence of external, visceral, or skeletal fetal defects. After oral doses in rats and rabbits that were about 0.5 and 3 times the MRHID, respectively, less than 0.008% of the dose crossed the placenta. However, consistent with its poor oral absorption, fluticasone was not detected in the maternal rabbit plasma (3). Although not stated, poor absorption in the rat probably also occurred.

It is not known if fluticasone can cross the human placenta. As noted above, the systemic concentrations of fluticasone after inhalation are very low. Moreover, the placenta is a rich source of enzymes that can metabolize corticosteroids (e.g., see Betamethasone, Dexamethasone, Hydrocortisone, and Prednisolone). These factors suggest that clinically significant exposure of the embryo or fetus is unlikely.

A 2004 study examined the effect of inhaled corticosteroids on low birth weight, preterm births, and congenital malformations in pregnant asthmatic patients (4). The inhaled steroids and the number of patients were beclomethasone (*N* = 277), fluticasone (*N* = 132), triamcinolone (*N* = 81), budesonide (*N* = 43), and flunisolide (*N* = 25). Compared with the general population, the study found no increased incidence of small-for-gestational-age infants (less than 10th percentile for gestational age), low birth weight (<2500 g), preterm births, and congenital malformations (4).

Three reports described the use of fluticasone nasal spray in 69 pregnant women, sometimes compared with placebo controls (5–7). No effects on fetal growth or pregnancy outcomes were observed in these patients. Although most synthetic corticosteroids are partially metabolized by the placental enzymes, budesonide and fluticasone were not (6).

A 2006 meta-analysis on the use of inhaled corticosteroids during pregnancy was published in 2006 (8). The analysis included five agents: beclomethasone, budesonide, flunisolide, fluticasone, and triamcinolone. The results showed that these agents do not increase the risk of major congenital defects, preterm delivery, low birth weight, and pregnancy-induced hypertension. Thus, they could be used during pregnancy (8).

BREASTFEEDING SUMMARY

No reports describing the use of fluticasone during human lactation have been located. Because of the low systemic concentrations obtained with fluticasone inhalation, and the drug's poor oral bioavailability, it is doubtful if clinically significant amounts would be ingested by a nursing infant.

References

1. Tan KS, Thomson NC. Asthma in pregnancy. Am J Med 2000;109:727–33.
2. Joint Committee of the American College of Obstetrics and Gynecologists (ACOG) and the American College of Allergy, Asthma and Immunology (ACAAI). Position statement. The use of newer asthma and allergy medications during pregnancy. Ann Allergy Asthma Immunol 2000;84:475–80.
3. Product information. Flovent. GlaxoSmithKline, 2005.
4. Namazy J, Schatz M, Long L, Lipkowitz M, Lillie M, Voss M, Deitz RJ, Petitti D. Use of inhaled steroids by pregnant asthmatic women does not reduce intrauterine growth. J Allergy Clin Immunol 2004;113:427–32.
5. Ellegard EK, Hellgren M, Karlsson NG. Fluticasone propionate aqueous nasal spray in pregnancy rhinitis. Clin Otolaryngol 2001;26:394–400.
6. Murphy VE, Fittock RJ, Zarzycki PK, Delahunty MM, Smith R, Clifton VL. Metabolism of synthetic steroids by the human placenta. Placenta 2007;28:39–46.
7. Choi JS, Han JY, Kim MY, Velazquez-Armenta EY, Nava-Ocampo AA. Pregnancy outcomes in women using inhaled fluticasone during pregnancy: a case series. Allergol Immunopathol (Madr) 2007;35:239–42.
8. Rahimi R, Nikfar S, Abdollahi M. Meta-analysis finds use of inhaled corticosteroids during pregnancy safe: a systematic meta-analysis review. Hum Exp Toxicol 2006;25:447–52.

FLUVASTATIN

Antilipemic Agent

PREGNANCY RECOMMENDATION: **Contraindicated**
BREASTFEEDING RECOMMENDATION: **Contraindicated**

PREGNANCY SUMMARY

Because the interruption of cholesterol-lowering therapy during pregnancy should have no effect on the long-term treatment of hyperlipidemia, and because cholesterol and other products synthesized from cholesterol are required for fetal development, the use of fluvastatin is contraindicated during pregnancy.

FETAL RISK SUMMARY

The cholesterol-lowering, hydrophilic agent fluvastatin (a "statin") has the same mechanism of action (i.e., inhibition of hepatic 3-hydroxy-3-methylglutaryl-coenzyme A [HMG-CoA] reductase) as other available agents in this class, atorvastatin, lovastatin, pitavastatin, pravastatin, rosuvastatin, and simvastatin (cerivastatin was withdrawn from the market in 2001).

Fluvastatin was not teratogenic in rats and rabbits at doses up to 36 and 10 mg/kg/day, respectively (1,2). Moreover, at the highest doses tested in rats for effects on fertility and reproductive performance, 20 mg/kg/day in males and 6 mg/kg/day in females, no adverse effects were observed (2). Significant maternal body weight loss and an increase in stillborns, neonatal morbidity, and maternal morbidity, however, were observed with fluvastatin doses of either 12 or 24 mg/kg/day administered to pregnant rats from the 15th day after coitus through weaning (2). The maternal morbidity was attributed to the occurrence of cardiomyopathy in the affected animals. The adverse effects of fluvastatin were lessened or prevented by the co-administration of mevalonic acid, a product produced by the enzyme HMG-CoA reductase, indicating that the toxicity was a result of inhibition of this enzyme.

Rosa (3) reported finding no recipients of this drug in his 1994 presentation on the outcome of pregnancies following exposure to anticholesterol agents. However, a 1999 case report described the pregnancy outcome of a 28-year-old woman who had taken fluvastatin (20 mg/day) for 18 months before conception and during the first 9 weeks of pregnancy (4). The patient, who had a kidney transplantation 6 years before pregnancy, took prednisone, cyclosporine, azathioprine, cephalexin, and ranitidine throughout gestation. She delivered a healthy, 2901-g female infant at term with

Apgar scores of 4 and 9 at 1 and 5 minutes, respectively. Except for transient tachypnea, no other complications were noted. At age 19 months, the infant's growth (weight, height, and head circumference all at the 50th percentile or higher) and development were normal (4).

A 2004 report described the outcomes of pregnancy that had been exposed to statins and reported to the FDA (see Lovastatin).

Among 19 cases followed by a teratology information service in England, one involved 1st trimester exposure to fluvastatin (5). The pregnancy outcome was a newborn with bradycardia and intrauterine growth restriction.

BREASTFEEDING SUMMARY

No published reports describing the use of fluvastatin during lactation have been located. The manufacturer reports that fluvastatin is present in breast milk at a milk:plasma ratio of 2 (1). Because of the potential for adverse effects in the nursing infant, the drug should not be used during lactation.

References

1. Product information. Lescol. Sandoz Pharmaceuticals, 1995.
2. Hrab RV, Hartman HA, Cox RH Jr. Prevention of fluvastatin-induced toxicity, mortality, and cardiac myopathy in pregnant rats by mevalonic acid supplementation. Teratology 1994;50:19–26.
3. Rosa F. *Anti-cholesterol Agent Pregnancy Exposure Outcomes*. Presented at the 7th International Organization for Teratogen Information Services, Woods Hole, MA, April 1994.
4. Seguin J, Samuels P. Fluvastatin exposure during pregnancy. Obstet Gynecol 1999;93:847.
5. McElhatton P. Preliminary data on exposure to statins during pregnancy (abstract). Reprod Toxicol 2005;20:471–2.

FLUVOXAMINE

Antidepressant

PREGNANCY RECOMMENDATION: Human Data Suggest Risk in 3rd Trimester
BREASTFEEDING RECOMMENDATION: Limited Human Data—Potential Toxicity

PREGNANCY SUMMARY

The limited animal and human data do not suggest a major teratogenic risk from the use of fluvoxamine. However, the above studies lack the sensitivity to identify minor anomalies because of the absence of standardized examinations. Late-appearing major defects may also have been missed because of the timing of the questionnaires. Selective serotonin reuptake inhibitor (SSRI) antidepressants, including fluvoxamine, have been associated with several developmental toxicities, including spontaneous abortions (SABs), low birth weight, prematurity, neonatal serotonin syndrome, neonatal behavioral syndrome (withdrawal), possible sustained abnormal neurobehavior beyond the neonatal period, respiratory distress, and persistent pulmonary hypertension of the newborn (PPHN).

FETAL RISK SUMMARY

Fluvoxamine is an antidepressant used in the treatment of obsessive-compulsive disorder. The mechanism of action is unknown, but the drug is an SSRI resulting in the potentiation of serotonin activity in the brain. The chemical structure of fluvoxamine is unrelated to other antidepressants.

All the antidepressant agents in the SSRI class (citalopram, escitalopram, fluoxetine, fluvoxamine, paroxetine, and sertraline) share a similar mechanism of action, although they have different chemical structures. These differences could be construed as evidence against any conclusion that they share similar effects on the embryo, fetus, or newborn. In the mouse embryo, however, craniofacial morphogenesis appears to be regulated, at least in part, by serotonin. Interference with serotonin regulation by chemically different inhibitors produces similar craniofacial defects (1). Regardless of the structural differences, therefore, some of the potential adverse effects on pregnancy outcome may also be similar.

No evidence of teratogenicity was observed in reproductive studies with rats and rabbits administered oral doses approximately twice the maximum human daily dose based on BSA (MHDD) (2). Increased pup mortality at birth and decreased postnatal pup weight were seen, however, when rats were dosed at 2 and 4 times the MHDD, respectively, throughout pregnancy and weaning. These effects may have been partially due to maternal toxicity, but a direct toxic effect on the fetuses and pups could not be excluded (2).

No reports describing the transfer across the human placenta have been located. The molecular weight (about 434 for the maleate salt) is low enough that passage to the fetus should be expected.

In a 1996 descriptive case series, the European Network of the Teratology Information Services (ENTIS) prospectively examined the outcomes of 689 pregnancies exposed to antidepressants (3). Multiple drug therapy occurred in about two-thirds of the mothers. Fluvoxamine was used in 67 pregnancies. The outcomes of these pregnancies were 9 elective abortions (EABs) (1 with defect—see below), 6 SABs, 2 stillbirths, 47 normal newborns (includes 2 premature infants), 2 infants with neonatal disorders (withdrawal, cyanosis), and 2 infants with congenital defects. The three cases of defects (all exposed in the 1st trimester or longer and to multiple agents) were multicystic left kidney, right megaureter with neonatal renal insufficiency; and hydrocephaly; right diaphragmatic hernia; and agenesis of the corpus callosum (EAB) (3).

A 1998 noninterventional ,observational cohort study described the outcomes of pregnancies in women who had been prescribed one or more of 34 newly marketed drugs by general practitioners in England (4). Data were obtained by questionnaires sent to the prescribing physicians one month after the expected or possible date of delivery. In 831 (78%) of the pregnancies, a newly marketed drug was thought to have been taken during the 1st trimester, with birth defects noted in 14 (2.5%) singleton births of the 557 newborns (10 sets of twins). In addition, two birth defects were observed in aborted fetuses. However, few of the aborted fetuses were examined. Fluvoxamine was taken during the 1st trimester in 21 pregnancies. The outcomes of these pregnancies included one ectopic pregnancy, five SABs, two EABs, nine normal full-term newborns, one premature delivery (twins), and three lost to follow-up. One of the EABs was for a genetic abnormality (47,XXX) (4).

A prospective, multicenter, controlled cohort study published in 1998 evaluated the pregnancy outcomes of 267 women exposed to one or more of three SSRI antidepressants during the 1st trimester: fluvoxamine ($N = 26$); paroxetine ($N = 97$); and sertraline ($N = 147$) (5). The women were combined into a study group without differentiation as to the drug they had consumed. A randomly selected control group ($N = 267$) was formed from women who had exposures to nonteratogenic agents. The pregnancy outcomes were determined, in most cases, 6–9 months after delivery. No significant differences were measured in the number of live births, SABs or EABs, stillbirths, major malformations, birth weight, or gestational age at birth. Nine major malformations were observed in each group. The relative risk for major anomalies was 1.06 (95% confidence interval [CI] 0.43–2.62). No clustering of defects was apparent. The outcomes of women who took an antidepressant throughout gestation were similar to those who took an antidepressant only during the 1st trimester (5). All of the 267 women in the study group had taken an antidepressant during embryogenesis (6).

The effect of SSRIs on birth outcomes and postnatal neurodevelopment of children exposed prenatally was reported in 2003 (7). Thirty-one children (mean age 12.9 months) exposed during pregnancy to SSRIs (15 sertraline, 8 paroxetine, 7 fluoxetine, and 1 fluvoxamine) were compared with 13 children (mean age 17.7 months) of mothers with depression who elected not to take medications during pregnancy. All of the mothers had healthy lifestyles. The timing of the exposures was 71% in the 1st trimester, 74% in the 3rd trimester, and 45% throughout. The average duration of breastfeeding in the subjects and controls was 6.4 and 8.5 months, respectively. Twenty-eight (90%) subjects nursed their infants, 17 of who took SSRIs (10 sertraline, 4 paroxetine, and 3 fluoxetine) compared with 11 (85%) controls, three of whom took sertraline. There were no significant differences between the groups in terms of gestational age at birth, premature births, birth weight and length or, at follow-up, in sex distribution or gain in weight and length (expressed at percentage). Seven (23%) of the exposed infants were admitted to a neonatal intensive care unit (six respiratory distress, four meconium aspiration, and one cardiac murmur) compared with none of the controls (*ns*). Follow-up examinations were conducted by a pediatric neurologist, psychologist, and a dysmorphologist who were blinded as to the mother's mediations status. The mean Apgar scores at 1 and 5 minutes were lower in the exposed group than in controls, 7.0 vs. 8.2, and 8.4 vs. 9.0, respectively. There was one major defect in each group: small asymptomatic ventricular septal defect (exposed); bilateral lacrimal duct stenosis that required surgery (control). The test outcomes for mental development were similar in the groups, but significant differences in the subjects included a slight delay in psychomotor development and lower behavior motor quality (tremulousness and fine motor movements) (7).

A 2005 meta-analysis of seven prospective comparative cohort studies involving 1774 patients was conducted to quantify the relationship between seven newer antidepressants and major malformations (8). The antidepressants were bupropion, fluoxetine, fluvoxamine, nefazodone, paroxetine, sertraline, and trazodone. There was no statistical increase in the risk of major birth defects above the baseline of 1%–3% in the general population for any of the individual or combined studies (8).

In a 2006 report, a 33-year-old woman with severe psychotic depression was treated with fluvoxamine 200 mg/day and quetiapine 400 mg/day (9). After appropriate counseling, she continued this therapy and conceived and, after a normal pregnancy, delivered a healthy 2600-g, 49-cm-long female infant with Apgar scores of 9 and 10 at 1 and 5 minutes, respectively. The infant was developing normally at 3 months (9).

A 2003 prospective study evaluated the pregnancy outcomes of 138 women treated with SSRI antidepressants during gestation (10). Women using each agent were 73 fluoxetine, 36 sertraline, 19 paroxetine, 7 citalopram, and 3 fluvoxamine. Most (62%) took an SSRI throughout pregnancy and 95% were taking an SSRI at delivery. Birth complications were observed in 28 infants, including preterm birth (9 cases), meconium aspiration, nuchal cord, floppy at birth, and low birth weight. Four infants (2.9%) had low birth weight, all exposed to fluoxetine (40–80 mg/day) throughout pregnancy, including two of the three infants of mothers taking 80 mg/day. One infant had Hirschsprung disease, a major defect, and another had cavum septi pellucidi (neither the size of the cavum nor the SSRI agents was specified) (10). The clinical significance of the cavum septi pellucidi is doubtful as it is nearly always present at birth but resolves in the first several months (11).

Evidence for the neonatal behavioral syndrome that is associated with in utero exposure to SSRIs and serotonin and norepinephrine reuptake inhibitors (SNRIs) (collectively called serotonin reuptake inhibitors [SRIs]) in late pregnancy was reviewed in a 2005 reference (12). The report followed a recent agreement by the FDA and manufacturers for a class labeling change about the neonatal syndrome. Analysis of case reports, case series, and cohort studies revealed that late exposure to SRIs carried an overall risk ratio of 3.0 (95% CI 2.0–4.4) for the syndrome compared with early exposure. The case reports ($N = 18$) and case series ($N = 131$) involved 97 cases of paroxetine, 18 fluoxetine, 16 sertraline, 12 citalopram, 4 venlafaxine, and 2 fluvoxamine. There were nine cohort studies analyzed. The typical neonatal syndrome consisted of CNS, motor, respiratory, and gastrointestinal signs that were mild and usually resolved within 2 weeks. Only one of 313 quantifiable cases involved a severe syndrome consisting of seizures, dehydration, excessive weight loss, hyperpyrexia, and intubation. There were no neonatal deaths attributable to the syndrome (12).

A significant increase in the risk of low birth weight (<10th percentile) and respiratory distress after prenatal exposure to SSRIs was reported in 2006 (13). The population-based study, representing all live births (*N* = 119,547) during a 39-month period in British Columbia, Canada, compared pregnancy outcomes of depressed mothers treated with SSRIs with outcomes in depressed mothers not treated with medication and in nonexposed controls. The severity of depression in the depressed groups was accounted for by propensity score matching (13).

A meta-analysis of clinical trials (1990–2005) with SSRIs was reported in 2006 (14). The SSRI agents included were citalopram, fluoxetine, fluvoxamine, paroxetine, and sertraline. The specific outcomes analyzed were major, minor, and cardiac malformations, and SABs. The odds ratios (ORs) with 95% CI for the four outcomes were 1.394 (0.906–2.145), 0.97 (0.13–6.93), 1.193 (0.531–2.677), and 1.70 (1.28–2.25), respectively. Only the risk of SABs was significantly increased (14).

A brief 2005 report described significant associations between the use of SSRIs in the 1st trimester and congenital defects (15). The data were collected by the CDC-sponsored National Birth Defects Prevention Study in an on-going case–control study of birth defect risk factors. Case infants (*N* = 5357) with major birth defects were compared with 3366 normal controls. A positive association was found with omphalocele (*N* = 161; OR 3.0, 95% CI 1.4–6.1). Paroxetine, which accounted for 36% of all SSRI exposures, had the strongest association with the defect (OR 6.3, 95% CI 2.0–19.6). The study also found a significant association between the use of any SSRI and craniosynostosis (*N* = 372; OR 1.8, 95% CI 1.0–3.2) (15). An expanded report from this group was published in 2007 (see reference 22 below).

A 2006 report using the database (1995–2003) of the Swedish Medical Birth Registry examined the relationship between maternal use of antidepressants and major malformations and cardiac defects (16). There was no significant increase in the risk of major malformations with any antidepressant. The strongest effect among cardiac anomalies was with ventricular or atrial septum defects (VSDs-ASDs). Significant increases were found with paroxetine (OR 2.22, 95% CI 1.39–3.55) and clomipramine (OR 1.87, 95% CI 1.16–2.99 (16). In 2007, the analysis of the Registry database was expanded to include the years 1995–2004 (17). There were 6481 women (6555 infants) who had reported the use of SSRIs in early pregnancy. The number using a single SSRI (i.e., no other SSRI or non-SSRI antidepressant) during the 1st trimester was 2579 citalopram, 1807 sertraline, 908 paroxetine, 860 fluoxetine, 66 escitalopram, and 36 fluvoxamine. Only paroxetine was significantly associated with cardiovascular effects (20 cases; OR 1.63, 95% CI 1.05–2.53). Paroxetine also had the strongest association with VSDs-ASDs, but did not reach significance (13 cases; relative risk [RR] 1.81, 95% CI 0.96–3.09). When the analysis was repeated after excluding women with body mass index >26, born outside of Sweden, or with reported subfertility (*N* = 405) , only paroxetine was significantly associated with any cardiac defect (13 cases, RR 2.62, 95% CI 1.40–4.50) and with VSDs-ASDs (8 cases, RR 3.07, 95% CI 1.32–6.04). The RR remained significant after also excluding women who took neuroleptics, sedatives, hypnotics, folic acid, nonsteroidal anti-inflammatory agents, or anticonvulsants (*N* = 340). Analysis of the combined SSRI group, excluding paroxetine, revealed no associations with cardiac defects or VSDs-ASDs. The study also found no association with omphalocele or craniostenosis (17).

A 2007 study evaluated the association between 1st trimester exposure to paroxetine and cardiac defects by quantifying the dose–response relationship (18). A population-based pregnancy registry was used by linking three administrative databases so that it included all pregnancies in Quebec between 1997 and 2003. There were 101 infants with major congenital defects, 24 involving the heart, among the 1403 women using only one type of antidepressant during the 1st trimester. The use of paroxetine or other SSRIs did not significantly increase the risk of major defects or cardiac defects compared with non-SSRI antidepressants. However, a paroxetine dose >25 mg/day during the 1st trimester was significantly associated with an increased risk of major defects (OR 2.23, 95% CI 1.19–4.17) and of cardiac defects (OR 3.07, 95% CI 1.00–9.42) (18).

A 2007 retrospective cohort study examined the effects of exposure to SSRIs or venlafaxine in the 3rd trimester on 21 premature and 55 term newborns (19). The randomly selected unexposed control group consisted of 90 neonates of mothers not taking antidepressants, psychotropic agents, or benzodiazepines at the time of delivery. There were significantly more premature infants among the subjects (27.6%) than in controls (8.9%), but the groups were not matched. The antidepressants, as well as the number of subjects and daily doses (shown in parentheses) in the exposed group were paroxetine (46; 5–40 mg), fluoxetine (10; 10–40 mg), venlafaxine (9; 74–150 mg), citalopram (6; 10–30 mg), sertraline (3; 125–150 mg), and fluvoxamine (2; 50–150 mg). The behavioral signs that were significantly increased in exposed than in nonexposed infants were as follows: CNS—abnormal movements, shaking, spasms, agitation, hypotonia, hypertonia, irritability, and insomnia; respiratory system—indrawing, apnea/bradycardia, and tachypnea; and other—vomiting, tachycardia, and jaundice. In exposed infants, CNS (63.2%) and respiratory system (40.8%) signs were most common, appearing during the first day of life and lasting for a median duration of 3 days. All of the exposed premature infants exhibited behavioral signs compared with 69.1% of exposed term infants. The duration of hospitalization was significantly longer in exposed premature than in nonexposed premature infants, 14.5 days vs. 3.7 days, respectively. In 75% of the term and premature infants, the signs resolved within 3 and 5 days, respectively. There were six infants in each group with congenital malformations, but the drugs involved were not specified (19).

A 2007 review conducted a literature search to determine the risk of major congenital malformations after 1st trimester exposure to SSRIs and SNRIs (20). Fifteen controlled studies were analyzed. The data were adequate to suggest that citalopram, fluoxetine, sertraline, and venlafaxine were not associated with an increased risk of congenital defects. In contrast, the analysis did suggest an increased risk with paroxetine. The data were inadequate to determine the risk for the other SSRIs and SNRIs (20).

A case–control study, published in 2006, was conducted to test the hypothesis that exposure to SSRIs in late pregnancy was associated with PPHN (21). A total of 1213 women were enrolled in the study, 377 cases whose infants had PPHN and 836 matched controls and their infants. Mothers were interviewed by nurses who were blinded to the hypothesis. Fourteen case infants had been exposed to an SSRI after the 20th week of gestation compared with six control infants (adjusted OR 6.1, 95% CI 2.2–16.8). The numbers were too small to analyze the effects of dosage, SSRI used, or reduction of the length of exposure before delivery. No increased risk of PPHN was found with the use of SSRIs before the 20th week or with the use of non-SSRI antidepressants at any time in pregnancy. If the relationship was causal, the absolute risk was estimated to be about 1% (21).

Two large case–control studies assessing associations between SSRIs and major birth defects were published in 2007 (22,23). The findings related to SSRIs as a group, as well as to four specific agents: citalopram, fluoxetine, paroxetine, and sertraline. The studies found increased risks for some birth defects, but the absolute risk appeared to be small. An accompanying editorial discussed the findings and limitations of these and other related studies (24). Details of the studies and the editorial are described in the paroxetine review (see Paroxetine).

A prospective cohort study evaluated a large group of pregnancies exposed to antidepressants in the 1st trimester to determine if there was an association with major malformations (25). The patient population came from the Motherisk database and involved 928 cases that met their criteria. The 928 matched (for age, smoking, and alcohol use) controls were pregnancies not exposed to antidepressants or known teratogens. In addition to the 52 fluvoxamine cases, the other cases were 113 bupropion, 184 citalopram, 21 escitalopram, 61 fluoxetine, 68 mirtazapine, 39 nefazodone, 148 paroxetine, 61 sertraline, 17 trazodone, and 154 venlafaxine. In the antidepressant group, there were 24 (2.5%) major defects compared with 25 (2.6%) in controls (OR 0.9, 95% CI 0.5–1.61). There were two major anomalies in the fluvoxamine group: atrial septal defect and an umbilical hernia. There were no major defects in the pregnancies exposed to bupropion, escitalopram, or trazodone (25).

BREASTFEEDING SUMMARY

Fluvoxamine is excreted into human milk. A 23-year-old, 70-kg woman in her 12th postpartum week was treated for postnatal depression with fluvoxamine, 100 mg twice daily (2.86 mg/kg/day) (26). Two weeks after the start of therapy, single milk and plasma samples were obtained 5 hours after a dose and concentrations of 0.09 and 0.31 mcg/mL, respectively, were measured. It was estimated that the infant was ingesting about 0.5% of the mother's daily dose (26).

In a brief 1997 communication, plasma and breast milk samples were obtained from a breastfeeding mother 3 hours after her morning fluvoxamine dose (100 mg/day; 1.43 mg/kg/day) (27). The concentrations in the plasma and milk were 0.17 and 0.05 mcg/mL, respectively, a milk:plasma ratio of 0.29. The estimated infant dose was slightly less than 0.0075 mg/kg/day (0.5% of the mother's daily dose). The nursing infant had been exposed to the drug in milk for about 3–4 weeks when breastfeeding was discontinued. No adverse effects from the exposure were noted on infant assessments conducted up to 21 months of age (27).

A 2000 case report described a 31-year-old breastfeeding woman, 3 months postpartum, on a stable dose (100 mg twice daily) of fluvoxamine (28). Serum and foremilk samples were collected every hour for 12 hours after a dose. The mean milk:serum ratio was 1.32. The estimated dose ingested by the nursing infant was 48 mcg/kg/day or 1.58% of the weight-adjusted maternal dose. No adverse effects or unusual behavior was noted in the nursing infant (28). Foremilk samples in women ingesting SSRI agents have been shown to contain much less drug than hindmilk because of the higher fat content of hindmilk and the lipid solubility of these drugs (see Paroxetine and Sertraline). Therefore, because only foremilk was collected from each breast, the milk:serum ratio and the actual dose ingested by the infant were probably higher.

In a second 2000 communication, a 26-year-old woman was started on fluvoxamine for severe obsessive-compulsive disorder symptoms at 19 days postpartum (29). About 8 weeks later, while on a dose of 25 mg three times daily, six breast milk (2–4 ounces) samples were collected (before each dose and before each feeding) over a 24-hour period. Blood samples were obtained from the mother and infant at the same time; 10 hours after a dose and 2–3 hours after the last feeding, respectively. Milk concentrations of fluvoxamine were 24–40 ng/mL over the collection period. Maternal and infant serum concentrations were 20 ng/mL and 9 ng/mL, respectively. The authors speculated that the atypically high infant serum concentration (45% of the mother's level) may have been related to the infant's hepatic function. The estimated maximum dose ingested by the nursing infant was 6 mcg/kg/day, or about 0.62% of the weight-adjusted maternal dose. No adverse effects or interference with normal developmental milestones up to 4 months of age was observed in the nursing infant (29).

In a 2006 case described in the Fetal Summary, a woman took fluvoxamine 200 mg/day and quetiapine 400 mg/day throughout a normal pregnancy (9). She continued this therapy while attempting to breastfeed her healthy female infant. Because of insufficient milk production, formula supplementation was required. The infant was developing normally and meeting all milestones at 3 months of age (9).

A 1999 review of SSRI agents concluded that if there were compelling reasons to treat a mother for postpartum depression, a condition in which a rapid antidepressant effect is important, the benefits of therapy with SSRIs would most likely outweigh the risks (30). However, because the long-term effects of exposure to SSRI antidepressants in breast milk on the infant's neurobehavioral development are unknown, stopping or reducing the frequency of breastfeeding should be considered if therapy with these agents is required. Avoiding nursing around the time of peak maternal concentration (about 4 hours after a dose) may limit infant exposure. However, the long elimination half-lives of all SSRIs and their weakly basic properties, which are conducive to ion trapping in the relatively acidic milk, probably will lessen the effectiveness of this strategy. The American Academy of Pediatrics classifies fluvoxamine as a drug whose effect on a nursing infant is unknown, but may be of concern (31).

References

1. Shuey DL, Sadler TW, Lauder JM. Serotonin as a regulator of craniofacial morphogenesis: site-specific malformations following exposure to serotonin uptake inhibitors. Teratology 1992;46:367–78.
2. Product information. Luvox. Solvay Pharmaceuticals, 1996.
3. McElhatton PR, Garbis HM, Elefant E, Vial T, Bellemin B, Mastroiacovo P, Arnon J, Rodriguez-Pinilla E, Schaefer C, Pexieder T, Merlob P, Dal Verme S. The outcome of pregnancy in 689 women exposed to therapeutic doses of antidepressants. A collaborative study of the European Network of Teratology Information Services (ENTIS). Reprod Toxicol 1996;10:285–94.
4. Wilton LV, Pearce GL, Martin RM, Mackay FJ, Mann RD. The outcomes of pregnancy in women exposed to newly marketed drugs in general practice in England. Br J Obstet Gynaecol 1998;105:882–9.
5. Kulin NA, Pastuszak A, Sage SR, Schick-Boschetto B, Spivey G, Feldkamp M, Ormond K, Matsui D, Stein-Schechman AK, Cook L, Brochu J, Rieder M, Koren G. Pregnancy outcome following maternal use of the new selective serotonin reuptake inhibitors. A prospective controlled multicenter study. JAMA 1998;279:609–10.
6. Koren G. In reply. Risk of fetal anomalies with exposure to selective serotonin reuptake inhibitors. JAMA 1998;279:1873–4.
7. Casper RC, Fleisher BE, Lee-Ancajas JC, Gilles A, Gaylor E, DeBattista A, Hoyme HE. Follow-up of children of depressed mothers exposed or not exposed to antidepressant drugs during pregnancy. J Pediatr 2003;142:402–8.
8. Einarson TR, Einarson A. Newer antidepressants in pregnancy and rates of major malformations: a meta-analysis of prospective comparative studies. Pharmacoepidemiol Drug Saf 2005;14:823–7.
9. Gentile S. Quetiapine-fluvoxamine combination during pregnancy and while breastfeeding. Arch Womens Ment Health 2006;9:158–9.
10. Hendrick V, Smith LM, Suri R, Hwang S, Haynes D, Altshuler L. Birth outcomes after prenatal exposure to antidepressant medication. Am J Obstet Gynecol 2003;188:812–5.
11. DeMyer W. Brain, midline caves. In: Buyse ML, ed. *Birth Defects Encyclopedia*. Cambridge, MA: Blackwell Scientific Publications, 1990:238.
12. Moses-Kolko EL, Bogen D, Perel J, Bregar A, Uhl K, Levin B, Wisner KL. Neonatal signs after late in utero exposure to serotonin reuptake inhibitors. JAMA 2005;293:2372–83.
13. Oberlander TF, Warburton W, Misri S, Aghajanian J, Hertzman C. Neonatal outcomes after prenatal exposure to selective serotonin reuptake inhibitor antidepressants and maternal depression using population-based linked health data. Arch Gen Psychiatry 2006;63:898–906.
14. Rahimi R, Nikfar S, Abdollahi M. Pregnancy outcomes following exposure to serotonin reuptake inhibitors: a meta-analysis of clinical trials. Reprod Toxicol 2006;22:571–5.
15. Alwan S, Reefhuis J, Rasmussen S, Olney R, Friedman JM. Maternal use of selective serotonin reuptake inhibitors and risk for birth defects (abstract). Birth Defects Res A Clin Mol Teratol 2005;73:291.
16. Kallen B, Olausson PO. Antidepressant drugs during pregnancy and infant congenital heart defect. Reprod Toxicol 2006;21:221–2.
17. Kallen BAJ, Olausson PO. Maternal use of selective serotonin re-uptake inhibitors in early pregnancy and infant congenital malformations. Birth Defects Res A Clin Mol Teratol 2007;79:301–8.
18. Berard A, Ramos E, Rey E, Blais L, St-Andre M, Oraichi D. First trimester exposure to paroxetine and risk of cardiac malformations in infants: the importance of dosage. Birth Defects Res B Dev Reprod Toxicol 2007;80:18–27.
19. Ferreira E, Carceller AM, Agogue C, Martin BZ, St-Andre M, Francoeur D, Berard A. Effects of selective serotonin reuptake inhibitors and venlafaxine during pregnancy in term and preterm neonates. Pediatrics 2007;119:52–9.
20. Bellantuono C, Migliarese G, Gentile S. Serotonin reuptake inhibitors in pregnancy and the risk of major malformations: a systematic review. Hum Psychopharmacol Clin Exp 2007;22:121–8.
21. Chambers CD, Hernandez-Diaz S, Van Marter LJ, Werler MM, Louik C, Jones KL, Mitchell AA. Selective serotonin-reuptake inhibitors and risk of persistent pulmonary hypertension of the newborn. N Engl J Med 2006;354:579–87.
22. Alwan S, Reefhuis J, Rasmussen SA, Olney RS, Friedman JM, for the National Birth Defects Prevention Study. Use of selective serotonin-reuptake inhibitors in pregnancy and the risk of birth defects. N Engl J Med 2007;356:2684–92.
23. Louik C, Lin AE, Werler MM, Hernandez-Diaz S, Mitchell AA. First-trimester use of selective serotonin-reuptake inhibitors and the risk of birth defects. N Engl J Med 2007;356:2675–83.
24. Greene MF. Teratogenicity of SSRIs—serious concern or much ado about little? N Engl J Med 2007;356:2732–3.
25. Einarson A, Choi J, Einarson TR, Koren G. Incidence of major malformations in infants following antidepressant exposure in pregnancy: results of a large prospective cohort study. Can J Psychiatry 2009;54:242–6.
26. Wright S, Dawling S, Ashford JJ. Excretion of fluvoxamine in breast milk. Br J Clin Pharmacol 1991;31:209.
27. Yoshida K, Smith B, Channi Kumar R. Fluvoxamine in breast-milk and infant development. Br J Clin Pharmacol 1997;44:209–13.
28. Hagg S, Granberg K, Carleborg L. Excretion of fluvoxamine into breast milk. Br J Clin Pharmacol 2000;49:286–8.
29. Arnold LM, Suckow RF, Lichtenstein PK. Fluvoxamine concentrations in breast milk and in maternal and infant sera. J Clin Psychopharmacol 2000;20:491–3.
30. Edwards JG, Anerson I. Systematic review and guide to selection of selective serotonin reuptake inhibitors. Drugs 1999;57:507–33.
31. Committee on Drugs, American Academy of Pediatrics. The transfer of drugs and other chemicals into human milk. Pediatrics 2001;108:776–89.

FOLIC ACID

Vitamin

PREGNANCY RECOMMENDATION: Compatible
BREASTFEEDING RECOMMENDATION: Compatible

PREGNANCY SUMMARY

Folic acid deficiency during pregnancy is a common problem in undernourished women and in women not receiving supplements. The relationship between folic acid levels and various maternal or fetal complications is complex. Evidence has accumulated that interference with folic acid metabolism or folate deficiency induced by drugs such as anticonvulsants and some antineoplastics early in pregnancy results in congenital anomalies. Moreover, a substantial body of evidence is now available that non-drug-induced folic acid deficiency, or abnormal folate metabolism, is related to the occurrence of birth defects and some neural tube defects (NTDs). Lack of the vitamin or its metabolites may also be responsible for some cases of spontaneous abortion and intrauterine growth restriction. For other complications, it is probable that a number of factors, of which folic acid deficiency may be one, contribute to poor pregnancy outcome. To ensure good maternal and fetal health, all pregnant women should receive sufficient dietary or supplementary folic acid to maintain normal maternal folate levels.

FETAL RISK SUMMARY

Folic acid, a water-soluble B complex vitamin, is essential for nucleoprotein synthesis and the maintenance of normal erythropoiesis (1). The National Academy of Sciences' recommended dietary allowance (RDA) for folic acid in pregnancy is 0.4 mg (1). However, a recommended dietary intake of 0.5 mg/day has been proposed that would meet the needs of women with poor folate stores, those with essentially no other dietary folate, and those with multiple pregnancies (2).

Rapid transfer of folic acid to the fetus occurs in pregnancy (3–5). One investigation found that the placenta stores folic acid and transfer occurs only after placental tissue vitamin receptors are saturated (6). Results compatible with this hypothesis were measured in a 1975 study using radiolabeled folate in women undergoing 2nd trimester abortions (7).

Folic acid deficiency is common during pregnancy (8–11). If not supplemented, maternal serum and red blood cell (RBC) folate values decline during pregnancy (8,12–16). Even with vitamin supplements, however, maternal folate hypovitaminemia may result (8). This depletion is thought to result from preferential uptake of folic acid by the fetal circulation such that at birth, newborn levels are significantly higher than maternal levels (8,15–18). At term, mean serum folate in 174 mothers was 5.6 ng/mL (range 1.5–7.6 ng/mL), whereas in their newborns, it was 18 ng/mL (range 5.5–66.0 ng/mL) (8). In an earlier study, similar serum values were measured with RBC folate decreasing from 157 ng/mL at 15 weeks' gestation to 118 ng/mL at 38 weeks (12). Folic acid supplementation prevented the decrease in both serum and RBC folate. Although supplementation is common during pregnancy in some countries, not all authorities believe this is necessary for the entire population (19,20). The main controversy is whether all women should receive supplements because of the cost involved in identifying those at risk (19), or whether supplements should be given only to those in whom a clear indication has been established (20).

The most common complication of maternal folic acid deficiency is megaloblastic anemia (9,21–30). Pancytopenia secondary to folate deficiency has also been reported during pregnancy (31). The three main factors involved in the pathogenesis of megaloblastic anemia of pregnancy are depletion of maternal folic acid stores by the fetus, inadequate maternal intake of the vitamin, and faulty absorption (27). Multiple pregnancy, hemorrhage, and hemolytic anemia hasten the decline of maternal levels (13,27). A 1969 study used 1-mg daily supplements to produce a uniformly satisfactory hematologic response in these conditions (29). In anemia associated with β-thalassemia minor, 5 mg/day of folic acid was significantly better than 0.25 mg/day in increasing predelivery hemoglobin concentrations in both nulliparous and multiparous Chinese women (32). Patients with iron deficiency, chronic blood loss, and parasitic infestation were excluded.

The proposed effects on the mother and fetus resulting from folate deficiency, not all of which appear to be related to the vitamin, can be summarized as follows:

Fetal anomalies (NTDs; other defects)
Placental abruption
Gestational hypertension (GHTN)
Abortions
Placenta previa
Premature delivery
Low birth weight

Fetal Anomalies (Neural Tube Defects; Other Defects)

Several investigations have suggested a relationship between folic acid deficiency and neural tube defects (NTDs). (Studies conducted with multiple vitamin products and not specifically with folic acid are described under Vitamins, Multiple.) In a randomized, double-blind trial to prevent recurrences of NTDs, 44 women took 4 mg/day of folic acid from before conception through early pregnancy (33). There were no recurrences in this group. A placebo group of 51 women plus 16 noncompliant patients from the treated group had four and two recurrences, respectively. The difference between the supplemented and nonsupplemented patients was significant ($p = 0.04$). Other researchers reported significantly lower RBC folate levels in mothers of infants with NTDs than in mothers of normal infants, but not all of the affected group had low serum folate (34). In a subsequent report by these investigators, very low vitamin B_{12} concentrations were found, suggesting that the primary deficiency may have been due to this latter vitamin with resulting depletion of RBC and tissue folate (35). A large retrospective study found a protective effect with folate administration during pregnancy, leading to a conclusion that deficiency of this vitamin may be teratogenic (36).

Evidence was published in 1989 that low dietary intake of folic acid is related to the occurrence of NTDs (37). In this Australian population-based case–control study, 77 mothers whose pregnancies involved an isolated NTD were compared with 77 mothers of infants with other defects (control group 1) and 154 mothers of normal infants (control group 2). Free folate intake was classified into four levels (in mcg/day): 8.0–79.8, 79.9–115.4, 115.5–180.5, and 180.6–1678.0. After adjustment for potential confounding variables, a statistically significant trend for protection against an NTD outcome was observed with increasing free folate intake in comparison to both control groups: $p = 0.02$ for control group 1, and $p < 0.001$ for control group 2. The odds ratios (ORs) for the highest intake compared with the control groups were 0.31 and 0.16, respectively. When total folate intake was examined, the trends were less: $p = 0.10$ for control group 1 and $p = 0.03$ for control group 2. In an accompanying editorial comment, criticism of the above study focused on the authors' estimation of dietary folate intake (38). The commentary cited evidence that nutrition tables are unreliable for the estimation of folate content, and that the only conclusion the study could claim was that dietary factors, but not necessarily folate, had a role in the etiology of NTDs.

A 1989 study conducted in California and Illinois examined three groups of patients to determine whether multivitamins had a protective effect against NTDs (39). The groups were composed of women who had a conceptus with an NTD ($N = 571$) and two control groups: those who had a stillbirth or an infant with another defect ($N = 546$) and women who had delivered a normal child ($N = 573$). In this study, NTDs included anencephaly, meningocele, myelomeningocele, encephalocele, rachischisis, iniencephaly, and lipomeningocele. The periconceptional use of multivitamins, both in

F

terms of vitamin supplements only and when combined with fortified cereals, was then evaluated for each of the groups. The outcome of this study, after appropriate adjustment for potential confounding factors, revealed an OR of 0.95 for NTD-supplemented mothers (i.e., those who received the RDA of vitamins or more) compared with unsupplemented mothers of abnormal infants, and an OR of 1.00 when the NTD group was compared with unsupplemented mothers of normal infants. Only slight differences from these values occurred when the data were evaluated by considering vitamin supplements only (no fortified cereals) or vitamin supplements of any amount (i.e., less than the RDA). Similarly, examination of the data for an effect of folate supplementation on the occurrence of NTDs did not change the results. Thus, this study could not show that the use of either multivitamin or folate supplements reduced the frequency of NTDs. However, the investigators cautioned that their results could not exclude the possibility that vitamins might be of benefit in a high-risk population. Several reasons were proposed by the authors to explain why their results differed from those obtained in other studies: (a) recall bias, (b) a declining incidence of NTDs, (c) geographic differences such that a subset of vitamin-preventable NTDs did not occur in the areas of the current study, and (d) others had not considered the vitamins contained in fortified cereals (39). However, other researchers concluded that this study led to a null result because (a) the vitamin consumption history was obtained after delivery, (b) the history was obtained after the defect was identified, or (c) the study excluded those women taking vitamins after they knew they were pregnant (40).

In contrast to the above report, a Boston study published in 1989 found a significant effect of folic acid–containing multivitamins on the occurrence of NTDs (40). The study population comprised 22,715 women for whom complete information on vitamin consumption and pregnancy outcomes was available. Women were interviewed at the time of a maternal serum α-fetoprotein screen or an amniocentesis. Thus, in most cases, the interview was conducted before the results of the tests were known to either the patient or the interviewer. A total of 49 women had an NTD outcome (2.2/1000). Among these, three cases occurred in 107 women with a history of previous NTDs (28.0/1000), and two were in 489 women with a family history of NTDs in someone other than an offspring (4.1/1000). After excluding the 87 women whose family history of NTDs was unknown, the incidence of NTDs in the remaining women was 44 cases in 22,093 (2.0/1000). Among the 3157 women who did not use a folic acid–containing multivitamin, 11 cases of NTDs occurred, a prevalence of 3.5/1000. For those using the preparation during the first 6 weeks of pregnancy, 10 cases occurred from a total of 10,713 women (prevalence 0.9/1000). Among mothers who, during the first 6 weeks, used vitamins that did not contain folic acid, the prevalence was three cases in 926, a ratio of 3.2/1000. When vitamin use was started in the 7th week of gestation, there were 25 cases of NTD from 7795 mothers using the folic acid–multivitamin supplements (3.2/1000; prevalence ratio 0.92) and no cases in the 66 women who started consuming multivitamins without folate. This study, then, observed a markedly reduced risk of NTDs when folic acid–containing multivitamin preparations were consumed in the first 6 weeks of gestation.

A 1989 preliminary report of a Hungarian, controlled, double-blind study evaluated the effect on congenital defects and first occurrence of NTDs of periconceptional supplementation with a multivitamin combination containing 0.8 mg folic acid compared with a trace-element supplement (controls) (41). Women were randomized to the vitamin formulation or control 1 month before through 3 months after the last menstrual period. The differences in outcome between the groups (number of subjects $N = 1302$) were not significant. Statistical significance was obtained, however, in the final report, published in 1992 (42) with an accompanying editorial (43), where pregnancy outcome was known in 2104 vitamin-supplemented cases and 2052 controls. Significantly more congenital malformations occurred in the control group (22.9/1000 vs. 13.3/1000, $p = 0.02$), including six cases of NTDs in controls compared with none in those taking vitamins ($p = 0.029$) (42). The rate of NTD occurrence in the control group corresponded to the expected rate in Hungary (41).

In 1991, the results of an 8-year study to examine the effects of folic acid supplementation, with or without other vitamins, on the recurrence rate of NTDs was published (44). This randomized, double-blind study conducted by the British Medical Research Council (MRC) was carried out at 33 medical centers in the United Kingdom, Australia, Canada, France, Hungary, Israel, and Russia. A total of 1817 women, all of whom had a previous pregnancy affected by an NTD (anencephaly, spina bifida cystica, or encephalocele), were enrolled in the study prior to conception and randomized to one of four treatment groups: folic acid (4 mg/day) ($N = 449$), folic acid (4 mg/day) plus other vitamins ($N = 461$), other vitamins (A, D, B_1, B_2, B_6, C, and nicotinamide) ($N = 453$), and no vitamins (placebo capsules containing ferrous sulfate and dicalcium phosphate) ($N = 454$). Women with epilepsy were excluded, as were those with infants whose NTD was associated with genetic factors. Women who conceived were continued in the study until the 12th week of gestation. The study was terminated after 1195 women had a completed pregnancy where the outcome could be classified as either NTD or no NTD, because the preventive effect of folic acid was clear. Six NTDs were observed in the two folic acid groups (6/593; 10/1000) and 21 were observed in the nonfolic acid groups (21/602; 35/1000). Analysis of the data indicated that folic acid had prevented 72% of the NTD recurrences compared with other vitamins, which gave no protective effect. The benefit of folic acid was the same for anencephaly as for spina bifida and encephalocele. The study found no evidence that any other vitamin had a protective effect, nor did other vitamins enhance the effect of folic acid. Based on the results of the study, the MRC recommended that all women who have had a previous pregnancy outcome with an NTD should take folic acid supplements. The study could not determine, however, whether 4 mg/day of folic acid was required or whether a smaller dose, such as 0.36 mg, would have been equally efficacious. They speculated, however, that even small doses should have some preventive effect.

The CDC published interim recommendations for folic acid supplementation based on the MRC study, pending further research to determine the required dose, for women who have had an infant or fetus with an NTD (spina bifida, anencephaly, or encephalocele) (45): 4 mg/day of folic acid at least 4 weeks before conception through the first 3 months of pregnancy. This supplementation was not recommended for (a) women who have never had an infant or fetus with an NTD, (b) relatives of women who have had an infant or fetus with an NTD, (c) women who themselves have spina bifida, and (d) women who take valproic acid (45). Approximately 1 year later, the CDC, in conjunction with other American health agencies, published the recommendation that all women of childbearing age should consume 0.4 mg of folic acid per day either from the diet or from supplements (46). This recommendation included women who had an NTD-affected pregnancy, unless they were planning to become pregnant. In that case, the CDC suggested that the 4-mg/day dose was still appropriate. Although the 0.4-mg dose may be as effective, the higher dose was based on a study designed to prevent NTDs, and the risks of an NTD-affected infant may be greater than the maternal risks from 4 mg/day of folic acid.

Several unanswered questions have been raised by the findings of the MRC trial, in addition to the one involving dosage, including the following: (a) How long before conception is supplementation needed (47)?, (b) What are the risks from supplementation (47–49)?, (c) If there are risks, are they the same for 4 mg and 0.4 mg (47–49)?, (d) Will the benefits of supplementation be the same for all ethnic groups, even in those with much lower prevalence rates of NTDs (47)?, (e) Will the benefits be as great for women who are not at an increased risk for producing a child with an NTD (47)?, (f) Can the required folic acid be obtained from food (47)?, (g) Is one mechanism of folic acid's action in preventing NTDs related to the correction of genetic defects, such as inborn errors of homocysteine metabolism (50)?, and (h) Is folic acid itself or its metabolite, 5-methyltetrahydrofolate (5-MTHF), the active form of the vitamin (48,49)?

Two uncontrolled trials conducted in the United Kingdom during the MRC study described above provided additional evidence that folic acid supplementation is beneficial in preventing recurrences of NTDs (51,52). Women at high-risk for recurrence, but who refused to be enrolled in the MRC trial, primarily out of fear of being placed in the placebo group, were treated with 4 mg/day of folic acid at least 1 month prior to conception through the 12th week of gestation (51). Of the 255 women supplemented, 234 achieved a pregnancy with 235 fetuses/infants (one set of twins). Two cases of NTDs were observed (spina bifida; encephalocele), a recurrence risk of 8.5/1000, approximately one-third the expected incidence of 30/1000 and nearly identical to the results in the MRC study. In the second trial, 208 high-risk women were treated similarly, but with a multivitamin preparation containing 0.36 mg of folic acid (52). Of the 194 who had delivered (14 were still pregnant), only one NTD was observed (an incidence of 5.2/1000), and that mother admitted poor compliance in taking the vitamins.

The results of three other studies, one conducted in 12 Irish hospitals beginning in 1981 (53), one in Spain between 1974 and 1990 (54), and one in the United States and Canada from 1988 through 1991 (55,56), indicated that folic acid may be protective at a much lower dosage (e.g., ≥0.3 mg/day) than that used in the MRC trial. In the American/Canadian study, folic acid (the most commonly used daily dose was 0.4 mg) consumed 28 days before through 28 days after the last menstrual period decreased the risk for first occurrence of NTDs by approximately 60% (55). The investigators also found evidence that a relatively high dietary intake of folate reduced the risk of NTDs (55).

In a search for a possible mechanism of folic acid prevention of NTDs, several studies have compared the concentrations of folic acid in mothers who have produced a child with an NTD with control mothers with no history of NTDs in their infants (57–60). A brief 1991 report found no relation between NTDs and low folate levels in fetal blood, fetal red cells, or maternal blood, thus eliminating poor placental transfer of folic acid as a possible mechanism (57).

A study conducted in Dublin found no difference in serum folate or vitamin B_{12} levels in mothers whose pregnancies ended with an NTD infant or fetus when compared with 395 normal controls (58). The serum samples were obtained during a routine screening program for rubella antibody conducted in three Dublin hospitals. After testing, the samples were frozen and then later used for this study. During the study period, 116 cases of NTDs were identified, but serum was available for only 32 of the cases: 16 with anencephalus, 15 with spina bifida, and 1 with encephalocele. In half of the cases, serum was obtained between 9 week's and 13 weeks' gestation. The mean serum folate concentrations in the cases and controls were both 3.4 ng/mL, and levels of vitamin B_{12} were 297 and 277 pg/mL, respectively.

Another trial found significantly lower RBC folate levels in pregnancies ending with an NTD (59). This Scottish study measured vitamin levels in 20 women younger than 35 years of age who had a history of two or more NTD pregnancies. A control group of 20 women with no pregnancies ending in NTDs, but matched for age, obstetric history, and social class, was used for comparison. No significant differences between the two groups were found in assays for plasma or serum vitamin A, thiamine, riboflavin, pyridoxine, vitamin B_{12}, folate, vitamin C, vitamin E, total protein, albumin, transferrin, copper, magnesium, zinc, and white cell vitamin C. RBC folate, however, was significantly lower in the case mothers than in controls, 178 vs. 268 ng/mL ($p = 0.005$), respectively, although both were within the normal range (106–614 ng/mL). Moreover, a linear relationship was found between RBC folate and the number of NTD pregnancies. Women who had three or four such pregnancies also had the lowest concentrations of RBC folate (59). The dietary intake of folic acid was lower in the case mothers than in controls, but the difference was not statistically significant. Because the lower RBC folate levels could not be attributed entirely to dietary intake of folic acid, the authors speculated that one factor predisposing to the occurrence of NTDs may be an inherited disorder of folate metabolism (59).

A study conducted in Finland, published in 1992, was similar in design and findings to the Dublin study described above (60). Serum samples from women who had delivered an infant with an NTD were analyzed and compared with samples from 178 matched controls. Cases of NTDs with known or suspected causes unrelated to vitamins were excluded. Maternal serum had been drawn during the first or second prenatal care appointment for reasons not related to the study, all within 8 weeks of neural tube closure, and kept frozen in a central laboratory. No statistical differences were found between case mothers and controls in serum levels of folate, vitamin B_{12}, and retinol. After adjustment, the ORs for being a case mother were

F

1.00 for folate, 1.05 for vitamin B_{12}, and 0.99 for retinol. Several possible explanations have been offered as to why this study was unable to find differences between case and control mothers (61): (a) Serum samples may not have been obtained early enough in pregnancy, (b) maternal serum vitamin concentrations may not be a good test of the folic acid deficiency necessary to cause NTDs, and (c), most likely, the group tested may not have been at risk to have a vitamin-sensitive NTD since the normal incidence of NTDs in the studied population is very low.

At least three publications have commented on the potential risks of high-dose folic acid supplementation (45,62,63). Megaloblastic anemia resulting from vitamin B_{12} deficiency may be masked by folic acid doses of 4 mg/day but still allow the neurologic damage of the deficiency to progress (45,62). Responding to this, a Canadian editorial recommended that a woman's vitamin B_{12} status be checked prior to commencing high-dose folic acid supplementation (62). A second risk identified concerned the inhibition of dihydropteridine reductase (DHPR), a key enzyme in the maintenance of tetrahydrobiopterin levels, by folic acid but not by 5-MTHF (63). Children with an inherited deficiency of this enzyme have lowered levels of dopamine, noradrenaline, serotonin, and folates in the CNS, which results in gross neurologic damage and death if untreated, thus raising the potential that high-dose folic acid could cause damage to embryonic neural tissue.

Folic acid deficiency is a known experimental animal teratogen (64). In humans, the relationship between fetal defects other than NTDs and folate deficiency is less clear. Several reports have claimed an increase in congenital malformations associated with low levels of this vitamin (9,24–26,33,36,65,66), and one study observed a significant decrease in birth defects when a multivitamin–folic acid preparation was used before and during early gestation (42) (see details above). Other investigators have stated that maternal deficiency does not result in fetal anomalies (22,23,67–73). One study found the folate status of mothers giving birth to severely malformed fetuses to be no different from that of the general obstetric population and much better than that of mothers with overt megaloblastic anemia (67). Similar results were found in other series (71–73).

The strongest evidence for an association between folic acid and fetal defects comes from cases treated with drugs that either are folic acid antagonists or induce folic acid deficiency, although agreement with the latter is not universal (70,74,75). The folic acid antagonists, aminopterin and methotrexate, are known teratogens (see Aminopterin and Methotrexate). A very high incidence of defects resulted when aminopterin was used as an unsuccessful abortifacient in the 1st trimester. These antineoplastic agents may cause fetal injury by blocking the conversion of folic acid to tetrahydrofolic acid in both the fetus and the mother.

In contrast, certain anticonvulsants, such as phenytoin and phenobarbital, induce maternal folic acid deficiency, possibly by impairing gastrointestinal absorption or increasing hepatic metabolism of the vitamin (70,74,75). Whether these agents also induce folic acid deficiency in the fetus is less certain, because the fetus seems to be efficient in drawing on available maternal stores of folic acid. Low maternal folate levels, however, have been proposed as a mechanism for the increased incidence of defects observed in infants exposed in utero to some anticonvulsants. In a 1984 article, investigators reported research on the relationship among folic acid, anticonvulsants, and fetal defects (74). In the retrospective part of this study, a group of 24 women who were treated with phenytoin and other anticonvulsants produced 66 infants, of whom 10 (15%) had major anomalies. Two of the mothers with affected infants had markedly low RBC folate concentrations. A second group of 22 epileptic women was then given supplements of daily folic acid, 2.5–5.0 mg, starting before conception in 26 pregnancies and within the first 40 days in 6 pregnancies. This group produced 33 newborns (32 pregnancies, one set of twins) with no defects, a significant difference from the group not receiving supplementation. Negative associations between anticonvulsant-induced folate deficiency and birth defects have also been reported (70,75). Investigators studied a group of epileptic women taking anticonvulsants and observed only two defects (2.9%) in pregnancies producing a live baby, which is a rate similar to that expected in a healthy population (70). Although folate levels were not measured in this retrospective survey, maternal folate deficiency was predicted by the authors, based on their current research with folic acid in patients taking anticonvulsants. Another group of researchers observed 20 infants (15%) with defects from 133 women taking anticonvulsants (75). No NTDs were found, but this defect is rare in Finland and an increase in the anomaly could have been missed (75). All of the women were given folate supplements of 0.1–1.0 mg/day (average 0.5 mg/day) from the 6th to 16th weeks of gestation until delivery. Folate levels were usually within the normal range (normal considered to be serum >1.8 ng/mL, RBC >203 ng/mL).

Whole embryo cultures of rats have been tested with valproic acid and folinic acid, a folic acid derivative (76). The anticonvulsant produced a dose-related increase in the incidence of NTDs that was not prevented by the addition of the vitamin. Experiments in embryonic mice, however, indicated that valproic acid-induced NTDs were related to interference with embryonic folate metabolism (77). Teratogenic doses of valproic acid caused a significant reduction in embryonic levels of formylated tetrahydrofolates and increased the levels of tetrahydrofolate by inhibition of the enzyme glutamate formyltransferase. The result of this inhibition would have serious consequences on embryonic development, including neural tube closure (77).

A review of teratogenic mechanisms involving folic acid and antiepileptic therapy was published in 1992 (78). Several studies conducted by the authors and others demonstrated that phenytoin, phenobarbital, and primidone, but not carbamazepine or valproic acid, significantly reduced serum and RBC levels of folate, and that polytherapy decreased these levels significantly more than monotherapy. Animal studies cited indicated that valproic acid disrupts folic acid metabolism, possibly by inhibiting key enzymes, rather than by lowering concentrations of the vitamin, whereas phenytoin may act on folic acid by both mechanisms (78). Data from a study conducted by the authors indicated that a significant association existed between low serum and RBC folate levels, especially <4 ng/mL, before or early in pregnancy in epileptic women and spontaneous abortions and the occurrence of congenital malformations (78). The reviewers concluded that folic acid supplementation may be effective in preventing some poor pregnancy outcomes in epileptic women.

Another 1992 report, based on the results of a 1990 workshop addressing the use of antiepileptic drugs during pregnancy, offered guidelines to counsel women with epilepsy who plan pregnancy or who are pregnant (79). Included among the guidelines was the recommendation that adequate folic acid be consumed daily, either from the diet or from supplements, to maintain normal serum and RBC levels of folate before and during the first months of pregnancy (i.e., during organogenesis). A specific folic acid dose was not recommended.

In a 2013 case–control study from Japan covering the period 2001–2012, 360 women who had given birth to spina bifida-affected offspring were compared with 2333 women who had given birth to offspring without spina bifida (80). Four variables were significantly associated with the risk of having a newborn with spina bifida: not taking folic acid supplements (OR 2.5, 95% confidence interval [CI] 1.72–3.64, presence of spina bifida patients within third-degree relatives (OR 4.26, 95% CI 1.12–16.19), taking anticonvulsants without taking folic acid (OR 20.20, 95% CI 2.06–198.17), and low birth weight ≤2500 g (OR 4.21, 95% 3.18–5.59). In 2000, the Japanese government recommended that women planning a pregnancy should take 0.4 mg/day of folic acid. Because the prevalence rate of spina bifida, 5–6 per 10,000 total births, had not changed in 11 years, the authors recommended that mandatory food fortification with folic acid should be implemented (80).

Placental Abruption

Several articles have proposed that maternal folic acid status is associated with placental abruption (25,26,28,66,81). In a review and analysis of 506 consecutive cases of abruptio placentae, defective folate metabolism was found as a predisposing factor in 97.5%. The authors theorized that folic acid deficiency early in pregnancy caused irreversible damage to the fetus, chorion, and decidua, leading to abruption, abortion, premature delivery, low birth weight, and fetal malformations. Other studies have discovered that 60% of their patients with abruption were folate deficient, but their numbers were too small for statistical analysis (82). In other series, no correlation was found between low levels of folic acid and this complication (16,69,83).

Gestational Hypertension

A relationship between folate deficiency and GHTN is doubtful. In a study of women with megaloblastic anemia, 14% had GHTN compared with the predicted incidence of 6% for that population (22). In another report, 22 (61%) of 36 GHTN patients had folate deficiency, but the authors were unable to conclude that the association was causative (66,82). Other investigators have also failed to find a relationship between low levels of the vitamin and GHTN (23,27). In one of these studies, the incidence of GHTN in megaloblastic anemia was 12.2% compared with 14.0% in normoblastic anemia (27). A second group of investigators studied folate levels in 101 preeclamptic and 17 eclamptic women and compared them with 52 normal controls and 29 women with overt megaloblastic anemia (84). No correlation was found between levels of folic acid and the complications.

Abortions and Placenta Previa

Several papers have associated folic acid deficiency with abortion (25,26,66,78,81,85–87). The cause of some abortions, as proposed by some, is faulty folate metabolism in early pregnancy, producing irreversible injury to the fetus and placenta (81). Others have been unable to detect any significant relationship between serum and RBC folate levels and abortion (12,68,88). In a series of 66 patients with early spontaneous abortions, the incidence of folate deficiency was the same as in those with uncomplicated pregnancies (88). These researchers did find a relationship between low folic acid levels and placenta previa. However, others found no evidence of an association between folate deficiency and either abortion or antepartum hemorrhage (12).

F

Premature Birth and Low Birth Weight

The relationship among prematurity, low birth weight, and folic acid levels has been investigated. In one study, significantly lower folate levels were measured in the blood of low-birth-weight neonates than in that of normal-weight infants (18). The incidences of both premature delivery and infants with birth weight <2500 g were increased in folate-deficient mothers in a 1960 report (22). These patients all had severe megaloblastic anemia and a poor standard of nutrition. In a later study of 510 infants from folate-deficient mothers, 276 (54%) weighed ≤2500 g compared with a predicted incidence of 8.6% (81). A study of women with uterine bleeding during pregnancy found a significant association between serum folate and low birth weight (86). Similarly, another study reported a significant relationship between folate levels at the end of the 2nd trimester and newborn birth weight (89). A 1992 report described the effects of supplementation with ferrous sulfate (325 mg/day) and folic acid (1 mg/day), beginning at the first prenatal visit, on infant birth weight (90). A significant association between low serum folate levels at 30 weeks' gestation and fetal growth restriction (defined as below the 15th percentile for gestational age) was discovered. Adjustment for psychosocial status, maternal race, body mass index, smoking history, history of a low-birth-weight infant, and infant gender did not change the results. In contrast, others have found no association between folic acid deficiency and prematurity (27,69,91,92) or between serum folate and birth weight (12,69,93,94).

Two reports have alluded to problems with high folic acid levels in the mother during pregnancy (95,96). An isolated case report described an anencephalic fetus whose mother was under psychiatric care (95). She had been treated with very high doses of folic acid and vitamins B_1, B_6, and C. The relationship between the vitamins and the defect is questionable. A 1984 study examined the effect of folic acid, zinc, and other nutrients on pregnancy outcome (96). Total complications of pregnancy (infection, bleeding, fetal distress, prematurity or death, pregnancy-induced hypertension, and tissue fragility) were associated with high serum folate and low serum zinc levels. The explanation offered for these surprising findings was that folate inhibits intestinal absorption of zinc, which, they proposed, was responsible for the complications. This study also found an association between low folate and abortion.

The CDC and other U.S. health agencies recommend a daily consumption of 0.4 mg of folic acid, from either the diet or supplements or both, for all women of childbearing age before the onset of pregnancy (46,97). An increased risk of adverse fetal outcome can be lowered by folic acid supplementation in at least two groups of women. Women with a history of a fetus or infant with an NTD should receive supplementation with 4 mg/day of folic acid beginning 1 month (3 months has been recommended in England [98]) before conception and continuing through the 12th week of gestation (45,98,99). Also, women receiving antiepileptic medications should receive sufficient folic acid from either the diet or supplementation or both to maintain normal serum and RBC levels of the vitamin beginning before conception and continuing through the period of organogenesis. A specific dosage recommendation has not been located for women receiving anticonvulsants, but 4 or 5 mg/day has been used.

F

BREASTFEEDING SUMMARY

Folic acid is actively excreted into breast milk (100–109). Accumulation of folate in milk takes precedence over maternal folate needs (100). Levels of folic acid are relatively low in colostrum but as lactation proceeds, concentrations of the vitamin rise (101–103). Folate levels in newborns and breastfed infants are consistently higher than those in mothers and normal adults (104,105). In Japanese mothers, mean breast milk folate concentrations were 141.4 ng/mL, resulting in a total intake by the infant of 14–25 mcg/kg/day (105). Much lower mean levels were measured in pooled human milk in an English study examining preterm (26 mothers, at 29–34 weeks) and term (35 mothers, at ≥39 weeks) patients (103). Preterm milk folate concentrations rose from 10.6 ng/mL (colostrum) to 30.5 ng/mL (16–196 days), whereas term milk folate concentrations increased during the same period from 17.6 to 42.3 ng/mL.

Supplementation with folic acid is apparently not needed in mothers with good nutritional habits (103–107). Folic acid deficiency and megaloblastic anemia did not develop in women not receiving supplements even when lactation exceeded 1 year (103,104). In another study, maternal serum and RBC folate levels increased significantly after 1 mg of folic acid/day for 4 weeks, but milk folate levels remained unchanged (105). Investigators gave well-nourished lactating women a multivitamin preparation containing 0.8 mg of folic acid (106). At 6 months postpartum, milk concentrations of folate did not differ significantly from those of controls who were not receiving supplements. Other investigators measured more-than-adequate blood folate levels in American breastfed infants during the 1st year of life (107). The mean milk concentration of folate consumed by these infants was 85 ng/mL.

In patients with poor nutrition, lactation may lead to severe maternal folic acid deficiency and megaloblastic anemia (100). For these patients, there is evidence that low folate levels, as part of the total nutritional status of the mother, are related to the length of the lactation period (103). In one study, lactating mothers with megaloblastic anemia were treated with 5 mg/day of folic acid for 3 days (102). Breast milk folate rose from 7–9 ng/mL to 15–40 ng/mL 1 day after treatment began. The elevated levels were maintained for 3 weeks without further treatment. Nine lower-socioeconomic-status women were treated with multivitamins containing 0.8 mg of folic acid and were compared with seven untreated controls (108). Breast milk folate was significantly higher in the treated women. In another study of lactating women with low nutritional status, supplementation with folic acid, 0.2–10.0 mg/day, resulted in mean milk concentrations of 2.3–5.6 ng/mL (109). Milk concentrations were directly proportional to dietary intake.

Folic acid concentrations were determined in preterm and term milk in a study to determine the effect of storage time and temperature (110). Storage of milk in a freezer resulted in progressive decreases over 3 months such that the RDA of folate for infants could not be provided from milk stored for this length of time. Storage in a refrigerator for 24 hours did not affect folate levels.

The National Academy of Sciences' RDA for folic acid during lactation is 0.280 mg (1). If the lactating woman's diet adequately supplies this amount, maternal supplementation with folic acid is not needed. Maternal supplementation with the RDA for folic acid is recommended for those patients with inadequate nutritional intake. The American Academy of Pediatrics considers maternal consumption of folic acid to be compatible with breastfeeding (111).

References

1. American Hospital Formulary Service. *Drug Information 1997*. Bethesda, MD: American Society of Health-System Pharmacists, 1997:2809–11.
2. Herbert V. Recommended dietary intakes (RDI) of folate in humans. Am J Clin Nutr 1987;45:661–70.
3. Frank O, Walbroehl G, Thomson A, Kaminetzky H, Kubes Z, Baker H. Placental transfer: fetal retention of some vitamins. Am J Clin Nutr 1970;23:662–3.
4. Kaminetzky HA, Baker H, Frank O, Langer A. The effects of intravenously administered water-soluble vitamins during labor in normovitaminemic and hypovitaminemic gravidas on maternal and neonatal blood vitamin levels at delivery. Am J Obstet Gynecol 1974;120:697–703.
5. Hill EP, Longo LD. Dynamics of maternal–fetal nutrient transfer. Fed Proc 1980;39:239–44.
6. Baker H, Frank O, Deangelis B, Feingold S, Kaminetzky HA. Role of placenta in maternal–fetal vitamin transfer in humans. Am J Obstet Gynecol 1981;141:792–6.
7. Landon MJ, Eyre DH, Hytten FE. Transfer of folate to the fetus. Br J Obstet Gynaecol 1975;82:12–9.
8. Baker H, Frank O, Thomason AD, Langer A, Munves ED, De Angelis B, Kaminetzky HA. Vitamin profile of 174 mothers and newborns at parturition. Am J Clin Nutr 1975;28:59–65.
9. Kaminetzky HA, Baker H. Micronutrients in pregnancy. Clin Obstet Gynecol 1977;20:263–80.
10. Dostalova L. Correlation of the vitamin status between mother and newborn during delivery. Dev Pharmacol Ther 1982;4(Suppl 1):45–57.
11. Bruinse HW, Berg HVD, Haspels AA. Maternal serum folacin levels during and after normal pregnancy. Eur J Obstet Gynecol Reprod Biol 1985;20:153–8.
12. Chanarin I, Rothman D, Ward A, Perry J. Folate status and requirement in pregnancy. Br Med J 1968;2:390–4.
13. Ball EW, Giles C. Folic acid and vitamin B_{12} levels in pregnancy and their relation to megaloblastic anemia. J Clin Pathol 1964;17:165–74.
14. Ek J, Magnus EM. Plasma and red blood cell folate during normal pregnancies. Acta Obstet Gynecol Scand 1981;60:247–51.
15. Baker H, Ziffer H, Pasher I, Sobotka H. A Comparison of maternal and foetal folic acid and vitamin B_{12} at parturition. Br Med J 1958;1:978–9.
16. Avery B, Ledger WJ. Folic acid metabolism in well-nourished pregnant women. Obstet Gynecol 1970;35:616–24.
17. Ek J. Plasma and red cell folate values in newborn infants and their mothers in relation to gestational age. J Pediatr 1980;97:288–92.
18. Baker H, Thind IS, Frank O, DeAngelis B, Caterini H, Liquria DB. Vitamin levels in low-birth-weight newborn infants and their mothers. Am J Obstet Gynecol 1977;129:521–4.
19. Horn E. Iron and folate supplements during pregnancy: supplementing everyone treats those at risk and is cost effective. Br Med J 1988;297:1325,1327.

20. Hibbard BM. Iron and folate supplements during pregnancy: supplementation is valuable only in selected patients. Br Med J 1988;297:1324,1326.
21. Chanarin I, MacGibbon BM, O'Sullivan WJ, Mollin DL. Folic-acid deficiency in pregnancy: the pathogenesis of megaloblastic anaemia of pregnancy. Lancet 1959;2:634–9.
22. Gatenby PBB, Lillie EW. Clinical analysis of 100 cases of severe megaloblastic anaemia of pregnancy. Br Med J 1960;2:1111–4.
23. Pritchard JA, Mason RA, Wright MR. Megaloblastic anemia during pregnancy and the puerperium. Am J Obstet Gynecol 1962;83:1004–20.
24. Fraser JL, Watt HJ. Megaloblastic anemia in pregnancy and the puerperium. Am J Obstet Gynecol 1964;89:532–4.
25. Hibbard BM. The role of folic acid in pregnancy: with particular reference to anaemia, abruption and abortion. J Obstet Gynaecol Br Commonw 1964;71:529–42.
26. Hibbard BM, Hibbard ED, Jeffcoate TNA. Folic acid and reproduction. Acta Obstet Gynecol Scand 1965;44:375–400.
27. Giles C. An account of 335 cases of megaloblastic anaemia of pregnancy and the puerperium. J Clin Pathol 1966;19:1–11.
28. Streiff RR, Little AB. Folic acid deficiency in pregnancy. N Engl J Med 1967;276:776–9.
29. Pritchard JA, Scott DE, Whalley PJ. Folic acid requirements in pregnancy-induced megaloblastic anemia. JAMA 1969;208:1163–7.
30. Rothman D. Folic acid in pregnancy. Am J Obstet Gynecol 1970;108:149–75.
31. Solano FX Jr, Councell RB. Folate deficiency presenting as pancytopenia in pregnancy. Am J Obstet Gynecol 1986;154:1117–8.
32. Leung CF, Lao TT, Chang AMZ. Effect of folate supplement on pregnant women with beta-thalassaemia minor. Eur J Obstet Gynecol Reprod Biol 1989;33:209–13.
33. Laurence KM, James N, Miller MH, Tennant GB, Campbell H. Double-blind randomised controlled trial of folate treatment before conception to prevent recurrence of neural-tube defects. Br Med J 1981;282:1509–11.
34. Smithells RW, Sheppard S, Schorah CJ. Vitamin deficiencies and neural tube defects. Arch Dis Child 1976;51:944–50.
35. Schorah CJ, Smithells RW, Scott J. Vitamin B_{12} and anencephaly. Lancet 1980;1:880.
36. Nelson MM, Forfar JO. Associations between drugs administered during pregnancy and congenital abnormalities of the fetus. Br Med J 1971;1: 523–7.
37. Bower C, Stanley FJ. Dietary folate as a risk factor for neural-tube defects: evidence from a case–control study in Western Australia. Med J Aust 1989;150:613–9.
38. Mann J. Dietary folate and neural-tube defects. Med J Aust 1989;150:609.
39. Mills JL, Rhoads GG, Simpson JL, Cunningham GC, Conley MR, Lassman MR, Walden ME, Depp OR, Hoffman HJ. The absence of a relation between the periconceptional use of vitamins and neural-tube defects. N Engl J Med 1989;321:430–5.
40. Milunsky A, Jick H, Jick SS, Bruell CL, MacLaughlin DS, Rothman KJ, Willett W. Multivitamin/folic acid supplementation in early pregnancy reduces the prevalence of neural tube defects. JAMA 1989;262:2847–52.
41. Czeizel A, Fritz G. Letter to the editor. JAMA 1989;262:1634.
42. Czeizel AE, Dudás I. Prevention of the first occurrence of neural-tube defects by periconceptional vitamin supplementation. N Engl J Med 1992;327:1832–5.
43. Rosenberg IH. Editorial. Folic acid and neural-tube defects—time for action? N Engl J Med 1992;327:1875–7.
44. MRC Vitamin Study Research Group. Prevention of neural tube defects: results of the Medical Research Council vitamin study. Lancet 1991;338:131–7.
45. CDC. Use of folic acid for prevention of spina bifida and other neural tube defects—1983–1991. MMWR 1991;40:513–6.
46. CDC. Recommendations for the use of folic acid to reduce the number of cases of spina bifida and other neural tube defects. MMWR 1992; 41(RR-14):1–7.
47. Anonymous. Folic acid and neural tube defects. Lancet 1991;338:153–4.
48. Scott JM, Kirke P, O'Broin S, Weir DG. Folic acid to prevent neural tube defects. Lancet 1991;338:505.
49. Lucock MD, Wild J, Hartley R, Levene MI, Schorah CJ. Vitamins to prevent neural tube defects. Lancet 1991;338:894–5.
50. Steegers-Theunissen RPM, Boers GHJ, Trijbels FJM, Eskes TKAB. Neural-tube defects and derangement of homocysteine metabolism. N Engl J Med 1991;324:199–200.
51. Laurence KM. Folic acid to prevent neural tube defects. Lancet 1991;338:379.
52. Super M, Summers EM, Meylan B. Preventing neural tube defects. Lancet 1991;338:755–6.
53. Kirke PN, Daly LE, Elwood JH for the Irish Vitamin Study Group. A randomised trial of low dose folic acid to prevent neural tube defects. Arch Dis Child 1992;67:1442–6.
54. Martinez-Frias M-L, Rodriguez-Pinilla E. Folic acid supplementation and neural tube defects. Lancet 1992;340:620.
55. Werler MM, Shapiro S, Mitchell AA. Periconceptional folic acid exposure and risk of occurrent neural tube defects. JAMA 1993;269:1257–61.
56. Oakley GP Jr. Folic acid—preventable spina bifida and anencephaly (editorial). JAMA 1993;269:1292–3.
57. Holzgreve W, Tercanli S, Pietrzik K. Vitamins to prevent neural tube defects. Lancet 1991;338:639–40.
58. Molloy AM, Kirke P, Hillary I, Weir DG, Scott JM. Maternal serum folate and vitamin B_{12} concentrations in pregnancies associated with neural tube defects. Arch Dis Child 1985;60:660–5.
59. Yates JRW, Ferguson-Smith MA, Shenkin A, Guzman–Rodriguez R, White M, Clark BJ. Is disordered folate metabolism the basis for the genetic predisposition to neural tube defects? Clin Genet 1987;31:279–87.
60. Mills JL, Tuomilehto J, Yu KF, Colman N, Blaner WS, Koskela P, Rundle WE, Forman M, Tolvanen L, Rhoads GG. Maternal vitamin levels during pregnancies producing infants with neural tube defects. J Pediatr 1992;120:863–71.
61. Holmes LB. Prevention of neural tube defects (editorial). J Pediatr 1992;120:918–9.
62. Glanville NT, Cook HW. Folic acid and prevention of neural tube defects. Can Med Assoc J 1992;146:39.
63. Leeming RJ, Blair JA, Brown SE. Vitamins to prevent neural tube defects. Lancet 1991;338:895.
64. Shepard TH. *Catalog of Teratogenic Agents*. 6th ed. Baltimore, MD: The Johns Hopkins University Press, 1989:285–8.
65. Hibbard ED, Smithells RW. Folic acid metabolism and human embryopathy. Lancet 1965;1:1254.
66. Stone ML. Effects on the fetus of folic acid deficiency in pregnancy. Clin Obstet Gynecol 1968;11:1143–53.
67. Scott DE, Whalley PJ, Pritchard JA. Maternal folate deficiency and pregnancy wastage. II. Fetal malformation. Obstet Gynecol 1970;36:26–8.
68. Pritchard JA, Scott DE, Whalley PJ, Haling RF Jr. Infants of mothers with megaloblastic anemia due to folate deficiency. JAMA 1970;211:1982–4.
69. Kitay DZ, Hogan WJ, Eberle B, Mynt T. Neutrophil hypersegmentation and folic acid deficiency in pregnancy. Am J Obstet Gynecol 1969;104: 1163–73.
70. Pritchard JA, Scott DE, Whalley PJ. Maternal folate deficiency and pregnancy wastage. IV. Effects of folic acid supplements, anticonvulsants, and oral contraceptives. Am J Obstet Gynecol 1971;109:341–6.
71. Emery AEH, Timson J, Watson-Williams, EJ. Pathogenesis of spina bifida. Lancet 1969;2:909–10.
72. Hall MH. Folates and the fetus. Lancet 1977;1:648–9.
73. Emery AEH. Folates and fetal central nervous system malformations. Lancet 1977;1:703.
74. Biale Y, Lewenthal H. Effect of folic acid supplementation on congenital malformations due to anticonvulsive drugs. Eur J Obstet Gynecol Reprod Biol 1984;18:211–6.
75. Hiilesmaa VK, Teramo K, Granstrom M-L, Bardy AH. Serum folate concentrations during pregnancy in women with epilepsy: relation to antiepileptic drug concentrations, number of seizures, and fetal outcome. Br Med J 1983;287:577–9.
76. Hansen DK, Grafton TF. Lack of attenuation of valproic acid-induced effects by folinic acid in rat embryos in vitro. Teratology 1991;43:575–82.
77. Wegner C, Nau H. Alteration of embryonic folate metabolism by valproic acid during organogenesis: implications for mechanism of teratogenesis. Neurology 1992;42(Suppl 5):17–24.
78. Dansky LV, Rosenblatt DS, Andermann E. Mechanisms of teratogenesis: folic acid and antiepileptic therapy. Neurology 1992;42(Suppl 5):32–42.
79. Delgado-Escueta AV, Janz D. Consensus guidelines: preconception counseling, management, and care of the pregnant woman with epilepsy. Neurology 1992;42(Suppl 5):149–60.
80. Kondo A, Morota N, Ihara S, Saisu T, Inoue K, Shimokawa S, Fujimaki H, Matsuo K, Shimosuka Y, Watanabe T. Risk factors for the occurrence of spina bifida (a case-control study) and the prevalence rate of spina bifida in Japan. Birth Defects Res (Part A) 2013;97:610–5.
81. Hibbard BM, Jeffcoate TNA. Abruptio placentae. Obstet Gynecol 1966;27:155–67.
82. Stone ML, Luhby AL, Feldman R, Gordon M, Cooperman JM. Folic acid metabolism in pregnancy. Am J Obstet Gynecol 1967;99:638–48.
83. Whalley PJ, Scott DE, Pritchard JA. Maternal folate deficiency and pregnancy wastage. I. Placental abruption. Am J Obstet Gynecol 1969;105:670–8.

84. Whalley PJ, Scott DE, Pritchard JA. Maternal folate deficiency and pregnancy wastage. III. Pregnancy-induced hypertension. Obstet Gynecol 1970;36:29–31.
85. Martin JD, Davis RE. Serum folic acid activity and vaginal bleeding in early pregnancy. J Obstet Gynaecol Br Commonw 1964;71:400–3.
86. Martin RH, Harper TA, Kelso W. Serum-folic-acid in recurrent abortions. Lancet 1965;1:670–2.
87. Martin JD, Davis RE, Stenhouse N. Serum folate and vitamin B12 levels in pregnancy with particular reference to uterine bleeding and bacteriuria. J Obstet Gynaecol Br Commonw 1967;74:697–701.
88. Streiff RR, Little B. Folic acid deficiency as a cause of uterine hemorrhage in pregnancy. J Clin Invest 1965;44:1102.
89. Whiteside MG, Ungar B, Cowling DC. Iron, folic acid and vitamin B_{12} levels in normal pregnancy, and their influence on birth-weight and the duration of pregnancy. Med J Aust 1968;1:338–42.
90. Goldenberg RL, Tamura T, Cliver SP, Cutter GR, Hoffman HJ, Copper RL. Serum folate and fetal growth retardation: a matter of compliance? Obstet Gynecol 1992;79:719–22.
91. Husain OAN, Rothman D, Ellis L. Folic acid deficiency in pregnancy. J Obstet Gynaecol Br Commonw 1963;70:821–7.
92. Abramowicz M, Kass EH. Pathogenesis and prognosis of prematurity (continued). N Engl J Med 1966;275:938–43.
93. Scott KE, Usher R. Fetal malnutrition: its incidence, causes, and effects. Am J Obstet Gynecol 1966;94:951–63.
94. Varadi S, Abbott D, Elwis A. Correlation of peripheral white cell and bone marrow changes with folate levels in pregnancy and their clinical significance. J Clin Pathol 1966;19:33–6.
95. Averback P. Anencephaly associated with megavitamin therapy. Can Med Assoc J 1976;114:995.
96. Mukherjee MD, Sandstead HH, Ratnaparkhi MV, Johnson LK, Milne DB, Stelling HP. Maternal zinc, iron, folic acid, and protein nutriture and outcome of human pregnancy. Am J Clin Nutr 1984;40:496–507.
97. CDC. Recommendations for use of folic acid to reduce number of spina bifida cases and other neural tube defects. MMWR 1992;41(RR-14):1–7. As cited in Anonymous. From the Centers for Disease Control and Prevention. JAMA 1993;269:1233,1236,1238.
98. Hibbard BM. Folates and fetal development. Br J Obstet Gynaecol 1993;100:307–9.
99. Committee on Obstetrics: Maternal and Fetal Medicine. American College of Obstetrics and Gynecology. Folic acid for the prevention of recurrent neural tube defects. No. 120. March 1993.
100. Metz J. Folate deficiency conditioned by lactation. Am J Clin Nutr 1970;23:843–7.
101. Cooperman JM, Dweck HS, Newman LJ, Garbarino C, Lopez R. The folate in human milk. Am J Clin Nutr 1982;36:576–80.
102. Ford JE, Zechalko A, Murphy J, Brooke OG. Comparison of the B vitamin composition of milk from mothers of preterm and term babies. Arch Dis Child 1983;58:367–72.
103. Ek J. Plasma, red cell, and breast milk folacin concentrations in lactating women. Am J Clin Nutr 1983;38:929–35.
104. Ek J, Magnus EM. Plasma and red blood cell folate in breastfed infants. Acta Paediatr Scand 1979;68:239–43.
105. Tamura T, Yoshimura Y, Arakawa T. Human milk folate and folate status in lactating mothers and their infants. Am J Clin Nutr 1980;33:193–7.
106. Thomas MR, Sneed SM, Wei C, Nail PA, Wilson M, Sprinkle EE III. The effects of vitamin C, vitamin B_6, vitamin B_{12}, folic acid, riboflavin, and thiamine on the breast milk and maternal status of well-nourished women at 6 months postpartum. Am J Clin Nutr 1980;33:2151–6.
107. Smith AM, Picciano MF, Deering RH. Folate intake and blood concentrations of term infants. Am J Clin Nutr 1985;41:590–8.
108. Sneed SM, Zane C, Thomas MR. The effects of ascorbic acid, vitamin B_6, vitamin B_{12}, and folic acid supplementation on the breast milk and maternal nutritional status of low socioeconomic lactating women. Am J Clin Nutr 1981;34:1338–46.
109. Deodhar AD, Rajalakshmi R, Ramakrishnan CV. Studies on human lactation. Part III. Effect of dietary vitamin supplementation on vitamin contents of breast milk. Acta Paediatr (Stockholm) 1964;53:42–8.
110. Bank MR, Kirksey A, West K, Giacoia G. Effect of storage time and temperature on folacin and vitamin C levels in term and preterm human milk. Am J Clin Nutr 1985;41:235–42.
111. Committee on Drugs, American Academy of Pediatrics. The transfer of drugs and other chemicals into human milk. Pediatrics 2001;108:776–89.

FOMEPIZOLE

Antidote

PREGNANCY RECOMMENDATION: Compatible—Maternal Benefit >> Embryo–Fetal Risk
BREASTFEEDING RECOMMENDATION: Hold Breastfeeding

PREGNANCY SUMMARY

Other than one case, no other human pregnancy experience is available. Although an assessment of the risk that this agent presents to a human embryo or fetus cannot be made, the maternal benefits should far outweigh the unknown fetal risks. Therefore, the drug should not be withheld because of pregnancy (1).

FETAL RISK SUMMARY

Fomepizole, given IV every 12 hours for ≥48 hours, is a competitive inhibitor of alcohol dehydrogenase, an enzyme that catalyzes the oxidation of alcohol to acetaldehyde. The enzyme also catalyzes the initial steps in the metabolism of ethylene glycol and methanol to their toxic metabolites. Fomepizole is indicated as an antidote for ethylene glycol (such as antifreeze or coolants) or methanol ingestion. It undergoes extensive metabolism to inactive metabolites. The elimination half-life has not been determined (2).

According to the manufacturer, animal reproduction studies have not been conducted with fomepizole. One source cited a 1982 abstract, however, that reported that the drug was not teratogenic in mice (3).

It is not known if fomepizole crosses the human placenta to the embryo or fetus. The very low molecular weight (about 82) suggests that the drug will cross the placenta.

Only one report describing the use of fomepizole in human pregnancy has been located. A 21-year-old woman at 11 weeks' gestation in her second pregnancy was treated with fomepizole (two doses of 15 mg IV over 30 minutes, approximately 8 hours apart) for inhalation of carburetor cleaner (4). The cleaner contained a mixture of methanol, toluene, methylene chloride, and carbon dioxide. Her history included chronic abuse of toluene and inhalants. After release from the hospital, she was again admitted for the same problem about 6 weeks later and was treated with one dose of fomepizole. Attempts to contact the patient after discharge were unsuccessful and the eventual outcome of the pregnancy was unknown (4).

BREASTFEEDING SUMMARY

No reports describing the use of fomepizole during human lactation have been located. The very low molecular weight (about 82) suggests that the drug will be excreted into breast milk. The effects of this exposure on a nursing infant are unknown (the most common adverse effects in patients and normal volunteers were headache, nausea, dizziness, and bad taste/metallic taste [2]). Since the maternal benefits of therapy are great, breastfeeding should be temporarily discontinued, at least until the therapy is completed and the drug eliminated from the maternal system. The time required to eliminate the drug is unknown, but waiting for 24 hours would allow for nearly complete elimination if the half-life was ≥5 hours. Moreover, fomepizole is extensively metabolized to inactive metabolites and this will serve to lessen infant exposure. Furthermore, fomepizole is indicated as an antidote for ethylene glycol (such as antifreeze or coolants) or methanol ingestion, and these substances could be toxic to a nursing infant if they were excreted into milk.

References

1. Bailey B. Are there teratogenic risks associated with antidotes used in the acute management of poisoned pregnant women? Birth Def Res A Clin Mol Teratol 2003;67:133–40.
2. Product information. Antizol. Orphan Medical, 2000.
3. Giknis MLA, Damjanov I. The effects of pyrazole and its derivatives on the transplacental embryotoxicity of ethanol. Teratology 1982;25:43A–4A. As cited by Schardein JL. *Chemically Induced Birth Defects*. 3rd ed. New York, NY: Marcel Dekker, 2000:633.
4. Velez LI, Kulstad E, Shepherd G, Roth B. Inhalational methanol toxicity in pregnancy treated twice with fomepizole. Vet Hum Toxicol 2003;45: 28–30.

F

FONDAPARINUX

Anticoagulant

PREGNANCY RECOMMENDATION: Limited Human Data—Probably Compatible
BREASTFEEDING RECOMMENDATION: No Human Data—Probably Compatible

PREGNANCY SUMMARY

Although the human pregnancy experience with fondaparinux is limited, no reports of embryo–fetal harm have been located. Several reviews have stated that the agent is safe in pregnancy. Thus, if indicated it should not be withheld because of pregnancy.

FETAL RISK SUMMARY

Fondaparinux is a synthetic selective inhibitor of activated factor X (Xa) that is administered by SC injection. The drug is indicated for the prophylaxis of deep vein thrombosis in patients undergoing hip fracture, hip replacement, or knee replacement surgery. Distribution to extravascular fluid is characterized as minor. The drug is extensively (at least 94%) and specifically bound to antithrombin III but not to other plasma proteins or red blood cells. The binding to antithrombin III significantly potentiates the neutralization of factor Xa by antithrombin III. Fondaparinux has no effect on thrombin or platelet function. The metabolism of fondaparinux has not been investigated, but most of a dose is excreted unchanged in the urine. The drug is contraindicated in patients weighing <50 kg because total clearance in this group is reduced by approximately 30% (1).

Reproduction studies in pregnant rats and rabbits at SC doses up to 32 and 65 times the recommended human dose based on BSA, respectively, revealed no evidence of impaired fertility or fetal harm (1).

Fondaparinux did not cross the placenta in an in vitro human dually perfused, cotyledon model using placentas from six healthy white women approximately 31 years of age (2,3). The dose tested corresponded to the therapeutic plasma concentrations observed with the recommended human dose. The result is consistent with the high molecular weight (about 1728) and minimal extravascular distribution of fondaparinux. However, in a 2004 study of five women treated near delivery, the concentrations of fondaparinux in cord plasma were <5–40 ng/mL (4). The patient with undetectable drug had received only one dose, whereas the other four patients were at steady state with plasma levels of 255–340 ng/mL. The fetal concentrations were about 10% of the maternal levels (4).

A 31-year-old woman in her 12th week of pregnancy completely loss her vision in her right eye for 2 minutes (5). After an extensive work-up, she was diagnosed with hypereosinophilic syndrome and started on heparin and prednisone. HIT developed and her anticoagulant therapy was changed to argatroban (dose not specified). The thrombocytopenia resolved and, after 15 days, she was discharged home on fondaparinux (75 mg/day) and a tapering dose of prednisone. About 6–7 months later, she gave birth to a healthy female infant (no further details on the infant was provided) (5).

In a 2012 case report, a 33-year-old woman, with a history of hereditary antithrombin deficiency, presented at 7 weeks' gestation with a deep venous thrombosis in her left leg due to the deficiency (6). She was treated with urokinase (24,000 units/day), heparin (20,000 units/day), and antithrombin concentrate (3000 units/day). Ten days later, at 9 weeks, HIT was diagnosed; heparin was discontinued and a continuous infusion of argatroban (2.5 mcg/kg/min) was started. At 21 weeks, argatroban was stopped and fondaparinux (2.5 mg/day) was started at 24 weeks'. Argatroban (2.5–3.5 mcg/kg/min) was restarted during labor induction at 37 weeks. The patient gave birth to 2800-g male infant with Apgar scores of 9 and 10 at 1 and 5 minutes, respectively. The newborn had

14% of antithrombin activity. The mother and her newborn were discharged home 15 days later (6).

In addition to the above two reports, four other reports have described the use of fondaparinux during human pregnancy without causing embryo or fetal harm (7–10). In addition, four reviews have stated that the drug can be used safely in pregnancy (11–14).

BREASTFEEDING SUMMARY

No reports describing the use of fondaparinux during human lactation have been located. Despite the high molecular weight (about 1728), the drug may be excreted into milk. The potential effects of this exposure on a nursing infant are unknown but are probably not clinically significant.

F

References

1. Product information. Arixtra. Sanofi-Synthelabo, 2003.
2. Lagrange F, Brun J-L, Vergnes MC, Paolucci F, Nadal T, Leng J-J, Saux MC, Bannwarth B. Fondaparinux sodium does not cross the placental barrier. Study using the in-vitro human dually perfused cotyledon model. Clin Pharmacokinet 2002;41(Suppl 2):47–9.
3. Lagrange F, Vergnes C, Brun JL, Paolucci F, Nadal T, Leng JJ, Saux MC, Banwarth B. Absence of placental transfer of pentasaccharide (Fondaparinux, Arixtra®) in the dually perfused human cotyledon in vitro. Thromb Haemost 2002;87:831–5.
4. Dempfle C-EH. Minor transplacental passage of fondaparinux in vivo. N Engl J Med 2004;350:1914–5.
5. Darki A, Kodali PP, McPheters JP, Virk H, Patel MR, Jacobs W. Hypereosinophilic syndrome with cardiac involvement. Tex Heart Inst J 2011;38:163–5.
6. Tanimura K, Ebina Y, Sonoyama A, Morita H, Miyata S, Yamada H. Argatroban therapy for heparin-induced thrombocytopenia during pregnancy in a woman with hereditary antithrombin deficiency. J Obstet Gynaecol Res 2012;38:749–52.
7. Wijesiriwardana A, Lees DAR, Lush C. Fondaparinux as anticoagulant in a pregnant woman with heparin allergy. Blood Coagul Fibrinolysis 2006;17:147–8.
8. Mazzolai L, Hohlfeld P, Spertini F, Hayoz D, Schapira M, Duchosal MA. Fondaparinux is a safe alternative in case of heparin intolerance during pregnancy. Blood 2006;108:1569–70.
9. Harenberg J. Treatment of a woman with lupus and thromboembolism and cutaneous intolerance to heparins using fondaparinux during pregnancy. Thromb Res 2007;119:385–8.
10. Gerhardt A, Zotz RB, Stockschlaeder M, Scharf RE. Fondaparinux is an effective alternative anticoagulant in pregnant women with high risk of venous thromboembolism and intolerance to low-molecular-weight heparins and heparinoids. Thromb Haemost 2007;97:496–7.
11. Hawkins D, Evans J. Minimising the risk of heparin-induced osteoporosis during pregnancy. Expert Opin Drug Saf 2005;4:583–90.
12. James AH. Prevention and management of venous thromboembolism in pregnancy. Am J Med 2007;120(10 Suppl 2):S26–34.
13. Deruelle P, Coulon C. The use of low-molecular-weight heparins in pregnancy—how safe are they? Curr Opin Obstet Gynecol 2007;19:573–7.
14. Desai P, Suk M. Orthopedic trauma in pregnancy. Am J Orthop 2007;36:E160–6.

FORMOTEROL

Respiratory Drug (Bronchodilator)

PREGNANCY RECOMMENDATION: **Limited Human Data—Probably Compatible**
BREASTFEEDING RECOMMENDATION: **No Human Data—Probably Compatible**

PREGNANCY SUMMARY

The animal data suggest low risk, but the limited human pregnancy experience prevents a more complete assessment of the embryo–fetal risk. However, there is no published evidence that drugs in this class cause developmental toxicity (growth restriction, structural defects, functional/behavior defects, or death). β-Adrenergic agonists (e.g., see Albuterol and Terbutaline) have been used as tocolytics and inhibition of uterine contractions and labor is a potential complication. Although SC formoterol has potent tocolytic activity in rodents, this effect has not been studied in humans. Moreover, the systemic bioavailability of the drug after inhalation is probably too low to inhibit uterine activity. Of note, among the five premature births in the surveillance study, four of the women were using inhaled formoterol at the time. Other potential toxic effects of formoterol are maternal hyperglycemia (especially in diabetics) resulting in newborn hypoglycemia, and maternal pulmonary edema (especially when used with corticosteroids). Although published studies of these potential adverse effects from inhaled formoterol have not been located, the reported plasma drug concentrations appear to be too low to cause these toxicities. Because of the availability of extensive human pregnancy experience, either albuterol or salmeterol would be a better choice if a pregnant woman required an inhaled β-adrenergic bronchodilator. However, if a nonpregnant woman had a good response to inhaled formoterol, it would be reasonable to continue her on this drug during pregnancy. If formoterol is used in pregnancy, healthcare professionals are encouraged to call the toll-free number (877-311-8972) for information about patient enrollment in an Organization of Teratology Information Specialists (OTIS) study.

FETAL RISK SUMMARY

Formoterol is a potent, long-acting, selective β_2-adrenergic agonist that acts as a bronchodilator. It is formulated as a dry powder into capsules intended for oral inhalation using the Aerolizer inhaler. Formoterol is indicated for the long-term maintenance treatment of asthma and in the prevention of bronchospasm. It also is indicated for the long-term maintenance treatment of bronchoconstriction in patients with chronic obstructive pulmonary disease (COPD), including chronic bronchitis and emphysema, and for the acute prevention of exercise-induced bronchospasm. Plasma protein binding in vitro was 61%–64% (31%–38% to albumin) over a wide range of drug concentrations. The mean plasma terminal elimination half-life after a single inhaled dose was 10 hours (1).

Reproduction studies have been conducted with formoterol in rats and rabbits. In pregnant rats, oral doses about 2000 times the maximum recommended daily inhalation dose in humans based on BSA (MRDID-BSA) or higher in late pregnancy resulted in stillbirth and neonatal mortality. These effects were not produced at doses about 70 times the MRDID-BSA. Oral doses about 70 times the MRDID-BSA or greater during organogenesis caused delayed ossification and, at 2000 times the MRDID-BSA or greater, reduced fetal weight. Oral dosing in pregnant rats and rabbits did not cause congenital malformations (1).

In long-term, high-dose studies, formoterol was carcinogenic in mice and rats. In these species, the doses used were about 25 and 45 times the human exposure based on AUC at the MRDID or higher, respectively. Formoterol was not mutagenic or clastogenic in multiple assays and did not impair fertility in rats (1).

In studies, both in vitro and in vivo, conducted in mice and rats, formoterol was a potent inhibitor of uterine contractions. The tocolytic activity of formoterol was about 1000 times that of ritodrine (2,3).

It is not known if formoterol crosses the human placenta. The molecular weight of the dihydrate fumarate salt (about 841), low protein binding, and prolonged elimination half-life suggest that the drug will pass to the embryo and/or fetus. However, the mean steady-state plasma concentrations of the drug after twice-daily dosing ranged from 4.0 to 8.8 pg/mL. Thus, very low drug concentrations will be available for placental transfer at the maternal–fetal interface.

A 2002 postmarketing surveillance study in England reported the outcomes of 34 pregnancies (33 women) exposed to formoterol (4). Most exposures ($N = 31$) occurred in the 1st trimester. Of these, there were 20 term live births, 5 premature births (31–36 weeks' gestation), 3 spontaneous abortions (SABs), and 3 elective pregnancy terminations. One of the premature infants had a fetal heart rate anomaly (no other information provided), and a term infant had pyloric stenosis. Formoterol treatment was ongoing in 16 of the 25 cases at the time of birth, including four of the premature births. Three women started treatment in the 2nd or 3rd trimester, and all had live term births. Exposure was uncertain in an additional pregnancy that ended in an SAB (4).

BREASTFEEDING SUMMARY

No reports describing the use of formoterol during human lactation have been located. The molecular weight of the dihydrate fumarate salt (about 841), low protein binding, and prolonged elimination half-life suggest that the drug will be excreted into breast milk. However, the very low plasma drug concentrations (4.0–8.8 pg/mL) suggest that the amount in milk will be clinically insignificant. Terbutaline, another β-adrenergic agonist, is classified by the American Academy of Pediatrics as compatible with breastfeeding (5). Thus, maternal inhalation of formoterol probably is compatible with nursing.

References

1. Product information. Foradil Aerolizer. Schering, 2005.
2. Shinkai N, Takasuna K, Takayama S. Tocolytic activity of formoterol against premature delivery in mice. J Pharm Pharmacol 2002;54:1637–43.
3. Shinkai N, Takasuna K, Takayama S. Inhibitory effects of formoterol on lipopolysaccharide-induced premature delivery through modulation of proinflammatory cytokine production in mice. Reproduction 2003;125:199–203.
4. Wilton LV, Shakir SA. A post-marketing surveillance study of formoterol (Foradil): its use in general practice in England. Drug Saf 2002;25:213–23.
5. Committee on Drugs. American Academy of Pediatrics. The transfer of drugs and other chemicals into human milk. Pediatrics 2001;108:776–89.

FOSAMPRENAVIR

Antiviral

PREGNANCY RECOMMENDATION: Compatible—Maternal Benefit >> Embryo–Fetal Risk
BREASTFEEDING RECOMMENDATION: Contraindicated

PREGNANCY SUMMARY

Although the limited human data does not allow a prediction as to the risk of fosamprenavir during pregnancy, the animal data indicate that the drug may represent a risk to the developing fetus. However, if indicated, the drug should not be withheld because of pregnancy.

FETAL RISK SUMMARY

Fosamprenavir is a prodrug of amprenavir, an inhibitor of HIV protease. After in vivo conversion in the gut during absorption, amprenavir binds to the active site of HIV type 1 (HIV-1) protease to prevent the processing of viral Gag and Gag-Pol polyprotein precursors, resulting in the formation of immature, noninfectious viral particles. Fosamprenavir is indicated, in combination with other antiretroviral agents, for the treatment of HIV infection (1).

Fosamprenavir was not mutagenic or genotoxic in assays conducted in vitro and in vivo. The agent did not impair fertility or general reproductive performance in male and female rats treated with doses producing systemic exposures of three (males) or four (females) times the systemic exposure obtained with the maximum recommended human dose when given alone (MRHD), or similar to the systemic exposure obtained with the maximum recommended human dose when given in combination with ritonavir (MRHD-RIT) (1).

Reproduction studies have been conducted in pregnant rats and rabbits. In rats given fosamprenavir from gestational days 6–17, no major effects on embryo–fetal development were observed at doses 0.7 and 2 times the MRHD-RIT and MRHD, respectively. Dosing of female rats before and during mating, throughout gestation, and during the first six postpartum days was associated with a reduction in pup survival and body weights. An increased incidence of abortion was observed in pregnant rabbits given fosamprenavir from gestational days 7–20 at doses 0.3 and 0.8 times the MRHD-RIT and MRHD, respectively. In contrast, amprenavir was associated with abortions and an increase in the incidence of minor skeletal variations (deficient ossification of the femur, humerus, and trochlea) in rabbits at a dose about 1/20th the human exposure obtained from the recommended dose (1).

Consistent with its molecular weight (about 506), amprenavir crosses the rat and rabbit placentas to the fetus. Amprenavir also has been shown to readily cross the ex vivo human placenta (see Amprenavir).

The Antiretroviral Pregnancy Registry reported, for the period January 1989 through July 2009, prospective data (reported before the outcomes were known) involving 4702 live births that had been exposed during the 1st trimester to one or more antiretroviral agents (2). Congenital defects were noted in 134, a prevalence of 2.8% (95% confidence interval [CI] 2.4–3.4). In the 6100 live births with earliest exposure in the 2nd/3rd trimester, there were 153 infants with defects (2.5%, 95% CI 2.1–2.9). The prevalence rates for the two periods did not differ significantly. There were 288 infants with birth defects among 10,803 live births, with exposure anytime during pregnancy (2.7%, 95% CI 2.4–3.0). The prevalence rate did not differ significantly from the rate expected in a nonexposed population. There were 98 outcomes exposed to fosamprenavir (70 in the 1st trimester and 28 in the 2nd/3rd trimesters) in combination with other antiretroviral agents. There were two birth defects (one in the 1st trimester and one in the 2nd/3rd trimester). In reviewing the birth defects of prospective and retrospective (pregnancies reported after the outcomes were known) registered cases, the Registry concluded that, except for isolated cases of neural tube defects with efavirenz exposure in retrospective reports, there was no other pattern of anomalies (isolated or syndromic) (2) (see Lamivudine for required statement).

The FDA issued a public health advisory on the association between protease inhibitors and diabetes mellitus (3). Because pregnancy is a risk factor for hyperglycemia, there was concern that these antiviral agents would exacerbate this risk. An abstract published in 2000 described the results of a study involving 34 pregnant women treated with protease inhibitors (none with fosamprenavir or amprenavir) compared with 41 controls that evaluated the association with diabetes (4). No association between protease inhibitors and an increased incidence of gestational diabetes was found.

Two reviews, one in 1996 and the other in 1997, concluded that all women currently receiving antiretroviral therapy should continue to receive therapy during pregnancy and that treatment of the mother with monotherapy should be considered inadequate therapy (5,6). The same conclusion was reached in a 2003 review with the added admonishment that therapy must be continuous to prevent emergence of resistant viral strains (7). In 2009, the updated U.S. Department of Health and Human Services guidelines for the use of antiretroviral agents in HIV-1-infected patients continued the recommendation that therapy, with the exception of efavirenz, should be continued during pregnancy (8). If indicated, therefore, protease inhibitors, including fosamprenavir, should not be withheld in pregnancy because the expected benefit to the HIV-positive mother outweighs the unknown risk to the fetus. Pregnant women taking protease inhibitors should be monitored for hyperglycemia. The updated guidelines for the use of antiretroviral drugs to reduce perinatal HIV-1 transmission also were released in 2010 (9). Women receiving antiretroviral therapy during pregnancy should continue the therapy but, regardless of the regimen, zidovudine administration is recommended during the intrapartum period to prevent vertical transmission of HIV to the newborn (9).

BREASTFEEDING SUMMARY

No reports describing the use of fosamprenavir during lactation have been located. Amprenavir is excreted into the milk of lactating rats. In addition, the molecular weight of amprenavir (about 506) is low enough that excretion into breast milk should be expected (see Amprenavir).

Reports on the use of fosamprenavir during human lactation are unlikely because the antiviral agent is used in the treatment of HIV infection. HIV-1 is transmitted in milk, and, in developed countries, breastfeeding is not recommended (5,6,8,10–12). In developing countries, breastfeeding is undertaken, despite the risk, because there are no affordable milk substitutes available. Until 1999, no studies had been published that examined the effect of any antiretroviral therapy on HIV-1 transmission in milk. In that year, a study involving zidovudine was published that measured a 38% reduction in vertical transmission of HIV-1 infection despite breastfeeding when compared with controls (see Zidovudine).

References

1. Product information. Lexiva. GlaxoSmithKline, 2003.
2. Antiretroviral Pregnancy Registry Steering Committee. *Antiretroviral Pregnancy Registry International Interim Report for 1 January 1989 through 31 July 2009*. Wilmington, NC: Registry Coordinating Center; 2009. Available at www.apregistry.com. Accessed May 29, 2010.
3. CDC. Public Health Service Task Force recommendations for the use of antiretroviral drugs in pregnant women infected with HIV-1 for maternal health and for reducing perinatal HIV-1 transmission in the United States. MMWR 1998;47:No. RR-2.
4. Fassett M, Kramer F, Stek A. Treatment with protease inhibitors in pregnancy is not associated with an increased incidence of gestational diabetes (abstract). Am J Obstet Gynecol 2000;182:S97.
5. Carpenter CCJ, Fischi MA, Hammer SM, Hirsch MS, Jacobsen DM, Katzenstein DA, Montaner JSG, Richman DD, Saag MS, Schooley RT, Thompson MA, Vella S, Yeni PG, Volberding PA. Antiretroviral therapy for HIV infection in 1996. JAMA 1996;276;146–54.
6. Minkoff H, Augenbraun M. Antiretroviral therapy for pregnant women. Am J Obstet Gynecol 1997;176:478–89.
7. Minkoff H. Human immunodeficiency virus infection in pregnancy. Obstet Gynecol 2003;101:797–810.
8. Panel on Antiretroviral Guidelines for Adults and Adolescents. *Guidelines for the Use of Antiretroviral Agents in HIV-1-Infected Adults and Adolescents*. Department of Health and Human Services. December 1, 2009:1–161. Available at http://www.aidsinfo.nih.gov/ContentFiles/AdultandAdolescentGL.pdf. Accessed September 17, 2010:60, 96–8.
9. Panel on Treatment of HIV-Infected Pregnant Women and Prevention of Perinatal Transmission. *Recommendations for Use of Antiretroviral Drugs in Pregnant HIV-1-Infected Women for Maternal Health and Interventions*

to Reduce Perinatal HIV Transmission in the United States. May 24, 2010:1–117. Available at http://aidsinfo.nih.gov/ContentFiles/PerinatalGL.pdf. Accessed September 17, 2010:30 (Table 5).
10. Brown ZA, Watts DH. Antiviral therapy in pregnancy. Clin Obstet Gynecol 1990;33:276–89.
11. De Martino M, Tovo P-A, Pezzotti P, Galli L, Massironi E, Ruga E, Floreea F, Plebani A, Gabiano C, Zuccotti GV. HIV-1 transmission through breast-milk: appraisal of risk according to duration of feeding. AIDS 1992;6:991–7.
12. Van de Perre P. Postnatal transmission of human immunodeficiency virus type 1: the breast feeding dilemma. Am J Obstet Gynecol 1995;173:483–7.

FOSCARNET

Antiviral

PREGNANCY RECOMMENDATION: Compatible—Maternal Benefit >> Embryo–Fetal Risk
BREASTFEEDING RECOMMENDATION: Contraindicated

PREGNANCY SUMMARY

One 1992 review suggested that foscarnet would be a first-line agent for pregnant HIV-positive patients with sight-threatening cytomegalovirus (CMV) retinitis (1). Because of the frequent occurrence of renal toxicity experienced with foscarnet in adults, however, the reviewer recommended frequent antepartum testing of the fetus and close monitoring of the amniotic fluid volume to observe for fetal renal toxicity.

FETAL RISK SUMMARY

Foscarnet has antiviral in vitro activity against all known herpes viruses, including CMV, herpes simplex virus (HSV) types 1 and 2, human herpesvirus 6, Epstein–Barr virus, and varicella–zoster virus (2). The drug is also active in vitro against HIV (3). It is used in patients with AIDS who have CMV retinitis or in immunocompromised patients with mucocutaneous acyclovir-resistant HSV infections.

Reproductive studies in pregnant rats with SC doses of 150 mg/kg/day, approximately one-eighth the estimated maximum daily human exposure based on AUC comparison, caused an increase in the frequency of skeletal malformations or variations. Administration to pregnant rabbits with 75 mg/kg/day, approximately one-third the human dose (AUC comparison), produced similar skeletal defects or variations. In addition, dose-related genotoxic effects were seen in two in vitro tests and in one in vivo test in mice (2).

It is not known if foscarnet crosses the human placenta. The molecular weight (about 300 for the sodium salt) is low enough that passage to the fetus should be expected.

Only one report describing the use of foscarnet during human pregnancy has been located. A 21-year-old woman at 18 weeks' gestation was treated with an 8-day course of IV foscarnet (total dose 43.8 g) for severe, genital acyclovir-resistant HSV type 2 (3). The patient also had a 3-year history of HIV disease that was being treated with saquinavir, lamivudine, and zidovudine. After discharge from the hospital, repeat cultures yielded HSV type 2 sensitive to acyclovir and she was treated with oral doses of this antiviral agent for the remainder of her pregnancy. She underwent a cesarean section at term to deliver a healthy, HIV-negative, female infant who was developing normally at 1 year of age. The authors, citing information received from the manufacturer, briefly reviewed two other cases of IV foscarnet therapy. In one case, a HIV-negative woman with acyclovir-resistant HSV encephalitis and retinitis had been treated with foscarnet (60 mg/kg IV every 8 hours) for 17 days starting at 32 weeks' gestation. She eventually delivered a healthy infant at term. The second case involved a HIV-positive patient who was treated with foscarnet (40 mg/kg IV every 8 hours) for genital HSV type 2 beginning at 29 weeks' gestation. No further information was available on this case (3).

BREASTFEEDING SUMMARY

No reports describing the use of foscarnet during human lactation have been located. Because excretion into human milk most likely occurs, and because of the potentially severe toxicity that might occur in a nursing infant, women receiving foscarnet should not breastfeed.

References

1. Watts DH. Antiviral agents. Obstet Gynecol Clin North Am 1992;19:563–85.
2. Product information. Foscavir. AstraZeneca, 2001.
3. Alvarez-McLeod A, Havlik J, Drew KE. Foscarnet treatment of genital infection due to acyclovir-resistant herpes simplex virus type 2 in a pregnant patient with AIDS: case report. Clin Infect Dis 1999;29:937–8.

FOSFOMYCIN

Antibiotic

PREGNANCY RECOMMENDATION: Compatible
BREASTFEEDING RECOMMENDATION: Limited Human Data—Probably Compatible

PREGNANCY SUMMARY

The lack of teratogenicity in animals and the apparently safe use of fosfomycin during human pregnancy appear to indicate that the drug presents a low risk, if any, to the fetus.

FETAL RISK SUMMARY

F

Fosfomycin is a synthetic, broad-spectrum, bactericidal phosphonic acid antibiotic given as a single 3-g oral dose of the trometamol salt for the treatment of uncomplicated urinary tract infections (acute cystitis) in women (1). Outside of the United States, other salt forms (calcium salt for oral administration, disodium salt for IM or IV dosing) are also available. Following absorption, fosfomycin tromethamine is rapidly converted to the free acid, fosfomycin.

Studies in male and female rats found no effect on fertility or impairment of reproductive performance (1). No teratogenic effects were observed in pregnant rats administered doses up to 1000 mg/kg/day, about 9 and 1.4 times the human dose based on body weight and BSA (HD), respectively (1). In pregnant rabbits, fetotoxicity was observed at doses up to 1000 mg/kg/day, about 9 and 2.7 times the HD, respectively, a maternally toxic dose in the rabbit.

The placental transfer of fosfomycin, following a single 1-g IM dose (14–20 mg/kg), was studied in a group of women at term in active labor (2). Samples of maternal and fetal blood were obtained before delivery at 30, 90, and 120–210 minutes after the dose in 7, 8, and 7 women, respectively. Mean maternal blood concentrations of fosfomycin at the three time intervals were 14.24, 23.32, and 15.86 mcg/mL, respectively, whereas those in the fetal blood were 1.58, 5.35, and 11.5 mcg/mL, respectively. Another report found that the drug crossed the placenta, resulting in detectable concentrations in amniotic fluid and cord blood in three women (3).

Although the above studies were conducted with IM dosing, the results appear to be comparable with those expected after oral dosing. The mean maximum maternal serum concentration of fosfomycin, after a single 3-g oral dose of fosfomycin tromethamine under fasting conditions, was 26.1 mcg/mL within 2 hours (1). As should be expected because of the normal physiologic changes that occur during gestation, pregnant women will have lower peak levels. In four pregnant women at 28–32 weeks' gestation after a single 3-g oral dose, the mean peak serum level at 2 hours was 20.5 mcg/mL (4).

A number of reports have described the use of fosfomycin during human pregnancy. Although appropriate precautions had been taken to exclude and prevent pregnancies during clinical trials, three women conceived shortly after enrolling and all received a single 3-g oral dose of fosfomycin (H.A. Schneier, personal communication, Forest Laboratories, 1997). The dose was apparently consumed about 3 days before conception in one case, 8 days after the last menstrual period (probably before conception) in a second, and 14 days after the last menstrual period (assumed to be around the time of conception) in a third. The first woman was lost to follow-up and the other two delivered healthy male newborns who were developing normally at 3 years of age.

In a case of stillbirth reported by the manufacturer to the FDA, the mother was hospitalized following a car accident and approximately 10 days later received a single 3-g oral dose of fosfomycin for a urinary tract infection (H.A. Schneier, personal communication, Forest Laboratories, 1997). About 5 days later, ultrasound demonstrated no fetal heartbeat and an induced abortion was performed. The cause of death was thought to be caused by progressive multiple placental infarctions and fetal hypotrophy.

Several published reports have studied the efficacy and safety of oral fosfomycin during pregnancy (4–15). The drug has been used in all trimesters of pregnancy without apparent harm to the fetus or newborn.

A 1998 noninterventional observational cohort study described the outcomes of pregnancies in women who had been prescribed ≥1 of 34 newly marketed drugs by general practitioners in England (16). Of 1067 exposed pregnancies, fosfomycin was taken during the 1st trimester in two, both concluding with normal, full-term infants.

BREASTFEEDING SUMMARY

No reports describing the use of fosfomycin during human lactation have been located. However, consistent with the molecular weight (about 259), the drug is excreted into colostrum and breast milk (3). In two women, the average colostrum and milk concentrations were 4.8 and 3.6 mcg/mL, respectively (colostrum:plasma and milk:plasma ratios 0.07). The risk to a nursing infant from this exposure is unknown, but modification of the infant's bowel flora may occur.

References

1. Product information. Monurol. Forest Laboratories, 2001.
2. Ferreres L, Paz M, Martin G, Gobernado M. New studies on placental transfer of fosfomycin. Chemotherapy 1977;23(Suppl 1):175–9.
3. Kirby WMM. Pharmacokinetics of fosfomycin. Chemotherapy 1977;23 (Suppl 1):141–51.
4. De Cecco L, Ragni N. Urinary tract infections in pregnancy: Monuril single-dose treatment versus traditional therapy. Eur Urol 1987;13(Suppl 1): 108–13.
5. Ragni N. *Fosfomycin Trometamol Single Dose versus Pipemidic Acid 7 Days in the Treatment of Bacteriuria in Pregnancy*. Clinical Report, 29 November 1990. Data on file, Forest Laboratories.
6. Reeves DS. Treatment of bacteriuria in pregnancy with single dose fosfomycin trometamol: a review. Infection 1992;20(Suppl 4):S313–6.
7. Moroni M. *Monuril Effectiveness and Tolerability in the Treatment and Prevention of Urinary Tract Infections*. Clinical Report. Data on file, Forest Laboratories.
8. Paladini A, Paladini AA, Balbi C, Carati L. *Efficacy and Safety of Fosfomycin Trometamol in the Treatment of Bacteriuria in Pregnancy*. Clinical Report. Data on file, Forest Laboratories.
9. Ragni N, Pivetta C, Paccagnella F, Foglia G, Del Bono GP, Fontana P. Urinary tract infections in pregnancy. In: Neu HC, Williams JD, eds. *New Trends in Urinary Tract Infections. International Symposium Rome 1987*. Basel, Switzerland: Karger, 1988:197–206.
10. Zinner S. Fosfomycin trometamol versus pipemidic acid in the treatment of bacteriuria in pregnancy. Chemotherapy 1990;36(Suppl 1):50–2.
11. Marone P, Concia E, Catinella M, Andreoni M, Guaschino S, Marino L, Grossi F, Cellani F. Fosfomycin trometamol in the treatment of urinary tract infections during pregnancy. A multicenter study. In: *3rd International Congress, Infections in Obstetrics and Gynecology*, Pavia, Italy, 1988.

12. Thoumsin H, Aghayan M, Lambotte R. Fosfomycin trometamol versus nitrofurantoin in multiple dose in pregnant women. Preliminary results. Infection 1990;18(Suppl 2):S94–7.
13. Moroni M. Monurol in lower uncomplicated urinary tract infections in adults. Eur Urol 1987;13(Suppl 1):101–4.
14. De Andrade J, Mendes Carvalho Lopes C, Carneiro daSilva D, Champi Ribeiro MG, Souza JEMR. Fosfomycin trometamol single-dose in the treatment of uncomplicated urinary tract infections in cardiac pregnant or nonpregnant women. A controlled study. J Bras Ginec 1994;104: 345–51.
15. Gobernado M, Perez de Leon A, Santos M, Mateo C, Ferreres L. Fosfomycin in the treatment of gynecological infections. Chemotherapy 1977;23(Suppl 1): 287–92.
16. Wilton LV, Pearce GL, Martin RM, Mackay FJ, Mann RD. The outcomes of pregnancy in women exposed to newly marketed drugs in general practice in England. Br J Obstet Gynaecol 1998;105:882–9.

FOSINOPRIL

Antihypertensive

PREGNANCY RECOMMENDATION: Human Data Suggest Risk in 2nd and 3rd Trimesters
BREASTFEEDING RECOMMENDATION: No Human Data—Probably Compatible

PREGNANCY SUMMARY

No reports describing the use of fosinopril in human pregnancy have been located. The 1st trimester experience with other angiotensin-converting enzyme (ACE) inhibitors does not suggest a risk of major anomalies. The use of this drug during the 2nd and 3rd trimesters may cause teratogenicity and severe fetal and neonatal toxicity. Fetal toxic effects may include anuria, oligohydramnios, fetal hypocalvaria, intrauterine growth restriction (IUGR), prematurity, and patent ductus arteriosus. Anuria-associated anhydramnios/oligohydramnios may produce fetal limb contractures, craniofacial deformation, and pulmonary hypoplasia. Severe anuria and hypotension, resistant to both pressor agents and volume expansion, may occur in the newborn following in utero exposure to valsartan. Newborn renal function and blood pressure should be closely monitored.

FETAL RISK SUMMARY

Fosinopril is an ACE inhibitor. In reproduction studies in rats at doses about 80–250 times the maximum recommended human dose based on body weight (MRHD), three similar orofacial malformations and one fetus with situs inversus were observed (1). No teratogenic effects were observed in rabbits at a dose up to 25 times the MRHD (1).

A retrospective study using pharmacy-based data from the Tennessee Medicaid program identified 209 infants, born between 1985 and 2000, who had 1st trimester exposure to ACE inhibitors (2). Infants of mothers with evidence of diabetes, either before or during pregnancy, were excluded, as were those exposed to angiotensin-receptor antagonists (ARBs), ACE inhibitors, or other antihypertensives beyond the 1st trimester, and those exposed to known teratogens. Two comparison groups, those taking other antihypertensives (N = 202) and those taking no antihypertensives (N = 29,096), were formed. The number of major birth defects in each of the three groups was 18 (8.6%), 4 (2%), and 834 (2.9%), respectively. Compared with the no antihypertensives group, exposure to ACE inhibitors was associated with a significantly increased risk of major defects (relative risk [RR] 2.71, 95% confidence interval [CI] 1.72–4.27). When the analysis was conducted by the type of defect, the highest rates were with cardiovascular defects, 9, 2, and 294 respectively, RR 3.72, 95% CI 1.89–7.30, and with CNS defects, 3, 0, and 80, respectively, RR 4.39, 95% CI 1.37–14.02. The major defects observed in the subject group were as follows: atrial septal defect (N = 6) (includes three with pulmonic stenosis and/or three with patent ductus arteriosus (PDA), renal dysplasia (N = 2), PDA alone (N = 2), and one each of ventricular septal defect, spina bifida, microcephaly with eye anomaly, coloboma, hypospadias, intestinal and choanal atresia, Hirschsprung disease, and diaphragmatic hernia (2). In an accompanying editorial, it was noted that neither previous reports of 1st trimester exposure to ACE inhibitors nor the animal studies had observed an increased risk of birth defects (3). It also was noted that no mechanism for ACE inhibitor-induced teratogenicity was known. A subsequent communication raising concerns about the validity of the study in terms of adequate exclusion of diabetes, charting and coding errors in busy medical practices, and the effects of maternal obesity (4) was addressed by the investigators (5).

ACE inhibitors are human teratogens when used in the 2nd and 3rd trimesters, producing fetal hypocalvaria and renal defects. The cause of the defects and other toxicity is thought to be related to fetal hypotension and decreased renal blood flow. The compromise of the fetal renal system may result in severe, and at times fatal, anuria, both in the fetus and in the newborn. Anuria-associated oligohydramnios may produce pulmonary hypoplasia, limb contractures, PDA, craniofacial deformation, and neonatal death (6,7). Prematurity, IUGR, and severe neonatal hypotension may also be observed. Two reviews of fetal and newborn renal function indicated that both renal perfusion and glomerular plasma flow are low during gestation and that high levels of angiotensin II may be physiologically necessary to maintain glomerular filtration at low perfusion pressures (8,9). Fosinopril prevents the conversion of angiotensin I to angiotensin II and, thus, may lead to in utero renal failure. Since the primary means of removal of the drug is renal, the impairment of this system in the newborn prevents elimination of the drug, resulting in prolonged hypotension. Newborn renal function and blood pressure should be closely monitored. If oligohydramnios occurs, stopping fosinopril may resolve the problem but may not improve infant outcome because of irreversible fetal damage (6). In those cases in which fosinopril must be used to treat the mother's disease, the lowest possible dose should be used, combined with close monitoring of amniotic fluid levels and fetal well-being. Guidelines for counseling exposed pregnant patients have been published and should be of benefit to health professionals faced with this task (6,10).

A 2012 review of the use of ACE inhibitors and ARBs in the 1st trimester concluded that there may be an elevated teratogenic risk, but the risk appeared to be related to other factors (11). The factors that typically coexist with hypertension in pregnancy included diabetes, advanced maternal age, and obesity.

BREASTFEEDING SUMMARY

No published reports describing the use of fosinopril during lactation have been located. The manufacturer states that the drug can be detected in milk after a daily dose of 20 mg given for 3 days (1). Although the effects of this exposure on a nursing infant are unknown, the American Academy of Pediatrics classifies two other similar agents (see Captopril and Enalapril) as compatible with breastfeeding.

References

1. Product information. Monopril. Bristol-Myers Squibb, 2000.
2. Cooper WO, Hernandez-Diaz S, Arbogast PG, Dudley JA, Dyer S, Gideon PS, Hall K, Ray WA. Major congenital malformations after first-trimester exposure to ACE inhibitors. N Engl J Med 2006;354:2443–51.
3. Friedman JM. ACE inhibitors and congenital anomalies. N Engl J Med 2006;354:2498–500.
4. Scialli AR, Lione A. ACE inhibitors and major congenital malformations. N Engl J Med 2006;355:1280.
5. Cooper WO, Ray WA. Reply—ACE inhibitors and major congenital malformations. N Engl J Med 2006;355:1281.
6. Barr M Jr. Teratogen update: angiotensin-converting enzyme inhibitors. Teratology 1994;50:399–409.
7. Shotan A, Widerhorn J, Hurst A, Elkayam U. Risks of angiotensin-converting enzyme inhibition during pregnancy: experimental and clinical evidence, potential mechanisms, and recommendations for use. Am J Med 1994;96:451–6.
8. Robillard JE, Nakamura KT, Matherne GP, Jose PA. Renal hemodynamics and functional adjustments to postnatal life. Semin Perinatol 1988;12:143–50.
9. Guignard J-P, Gouyon J-B. Adverse effects of drugs on the immature kidney. Biol Neonate 1988;53:243–52.
10. Brent RL, Beckman DA. Angiotensin-converting enzyme inhibitors, an embryopathic class of drugs with unique properties: information for clinical teratology counselors. Teratology 1991;43:543–6.
11. Polifka JE. Is there an embryopathy associated with first-trimester exposure to angiotensin-converting enzyme inhibitors and angiotensin receptor antagonists? A critical review of the evidence. Birth Defects Res (Part A) 2012;94:576–98.

FOSPROPOFOL

Hypnotic

PREGNANCY RECOMMENDATION: No Human Data—Animal Data Suggest Low Risk
BREASTFEEDING RECOMMENDATION: No Human Data—Probably Compatible

PREGNANCY SUMMARY

No reports describing the use of fospropofol in human pregnancy have been located. The agent is converted to its active metabolite propofol for which there is limited human pregnancy experience but not in the first half of gestation. Although the animal data suggest low risk, human data are required for a complete assessment of the embryo–fetal risk. As with propofol, use of the prodrug near birth may cause transient depression of the newborn (see Propofol).

FETAL RISK SUMMARY

Fospropofol is a prodrug that is metabolized by alkaline phosphatases to propofol, which undergoes further metabolism. It is indicated for monitored anesthesia care sedation in adult patients undergoing diagnostic or therapeutic procedures. The mean elimination half-life of fospropofol is 0.88 hours, whereas the mean elimination half-life of propofol from fospropofol is 1.13 hours. Both fospropofol and its active metabolite propofol are highly plasma protein bound (about 98%) primarily to albumin (1).

Reproduction studies have been conducted in rats and rabbits. In these species, doses up to 0.6 and 1.7 times, respectively, the anticipated human dose for a 16-minute procedure based on BSA (HD) revealed no evidence of embryo–fetal harm or impaired fertility. In rats, the highest doses caused significant maternal toxicity, whereas in rabbits all doses caused significant maternal toxicity. When rats were given doses up to 0.2 times the HD from gestation day 7 through lactation day 20, no clear treatment-related effects on growth, development, behavior (passive avoidance and water maze), or fertility and mating capacity of the offspring were noted (1).

Long-term studies for carcinogenicity have not been conducted with fospropofol. The drug was not genotoxic in two assays, with or without metabolic activation. However, in a third assay, fospropofol was mutagenic in the presence of metabolic activation but the finding was thought to have been an artifact of the culture conditions (1).

It is not known if fospropofol crosses the human placenta. The molecular weight (about 332 for the disodium salt form) is low enough, but the extensive plasma protein binding and relatively short elimination half-life suggest that transfer will be limited. However, the active metabolite propofol does cross, with an umbilical vein:maternal vein ratio of 0.7 (see Propofol).

BREASTFEEDING SUMMARY

No reports describing the use of fospropofol during human lactation have been located. The molecular weight (about 332 for the disodium salt form) is low enough for excretion, but the extensive plasma protein binding and relatively short elimination half-life should limit the amount in milk. Small amounts of the active metabolite propofol are excreted into colostrum and milk following use of the agent for the induction and maintenance of maternal anesthesia during cesarean delivery (see Propofol).

Reference

1. Product information. Lusedra. Eisai, 2009.

FROVATRIPTAN

Antimigraine

PREGNANCY RECOMMENDATION: No Human Data—Animal Data Suggest Low Risk
BREASTFEEDING RECOMMENDATION: No Human Data—Probably Compatible

PREGNANCY SUMMARY

No reports describing the use of frovatriptan in human pregnancy have been located. The animal data suggest low risk, but an assessment of the actual risk cannot be determined until human pregnancy experience is available. Although a 2008 review of triptans in pregnancy found no evidence for teratogenicity, the data did suggest a possible increase in the rate of preterm birth (1).

FETAL RISK SUMMARY

Frovatriptan is an oral selective serotonin (5-hydroxytryptamine [5-HT]) receptor agonist that has high affinity for 5-HT_{1B} and 5-HT_{1D} receptors. The drug is closely related to almotriptan, eletriptan, naratriptan, rizatriptan, sumatriptan, and zolmitriptan. It is indicated for the acute treatment of migraine with or without aura in adults. Protein binding is minimal (about 15%). Several metabolites have been identified, but only one has affinity, lower than frovatriptan, for the 5-$HT_{1B/1D}$ receptors. The mean terminal elimination half-life of frovatriptan is about 26 hours (2).

Reproduction studies have been conducted in rats and rabbits. In rats, frovatriptan was given during organogenesis at oral doses ranging from 130 to 1300 times the maximum recommended human dose based on BSA (MRHD). Dose-related increases were found in the incidences of dilated ureters, unilateral and bilateral pelvic cavitation, hydronephrosis, and hydroureters. The renal effects were thought to be consistent with a slight delay in fetal maturation. A no-effect dose for this toxicity was not established. Skeletal variations (incomplete ossification of the sternebrae, skull, and nasal bones) were observed at all doses. In pregnant rabbits, oral doses up to 210 times the MRHD during organogenesis revealed no effects on fetal development (2).

It is not known if frovatriptan or its less active metabolite crosses the human placenta to the fetus. The molecular weight of the parent compound (about 243 for the free base) is low enough that passage to the fetus should be expected. In addition, the minimal protein binding and prolonged elimination half-life suggest that the drug will be available for transfer at the maternal:fetal interface.

BREASTFEEDING SUMMARY

No reports describing the use of frovatriptan during human lactation have been located. The molecular weight (about 243 for the free base), low plasma protein binding (about 15%), and prolonged elimination half-life (about 26 hours) suggest that the drug will be excreted into breast milk. The effect of this exposure on a nursing infant is unknown, but using an antimigraine agent with a shorter half-life should be considered.

References

1. Soldin OP, Dahlin J, O'Mara DM. Triptans in pregnancy. Ther Drug Monit 2008;30:5–9.
2. Product information. Frova. Elan Biopharmaceuticals, 2004.

FURAZOLIDONE

Anti-infective

PREGNANCY RECOMMENDATION: Limited Human Data—No Relevant Animal Data
BREASTFEEDING RECOMMENDATION: No Human Data—Potential Toxicity

PREGNANCY SUMMARY

No reports linking the use of furazolidone with congenital defects have been located.

FETAL RISK SUMMARY

The Collaborative Perinatal Project monitored 50,282 mother–child pairs, 132 of whom had 1st trimester exposure to furazolidone (1). No association with malformations was found. Theoretically, furazolidone could produce hemolytic anemia in a glucose-6-phosphate dehydrogenase-deficient newborn if given at term. Placental passage of the drug has not been reported.

F

BREASTFEEDING SUMMARY

No reports describing the use of furazolidone during human lactation have been located.

Reference

1. Heinonen OP, Slone D, Shapiro S. *Birth Defects and Drugs in Pregnancy*. Littleton, MA: Publishing Sciences Group, 1977:299–302.

FUROSEMIDE

Diuretic

PREGNANCY RECOMMENDATION: Human Data Suggest Low Risk
BREASTFEEDING RECOMMENDATION: Limited Human Data—Probably Compatible

PREGNANCY SUMMARY

Administration of furosemide during pregnancy does not significantly alter amniotic fluid volume (1). Serum uric acid levels, which are increased in toxemia, are further elevated by furosemide (2). No association was found in a 1973 study between furosemide and low platelet counts in the neonate (3). Unlike the thiazide diuretics, neonatal thrombocytopenia has not been reported for furosemide.

FETAL RISK SUMMARY

Furosemide is a potent diuretic. The drug has caused maternal deaths and abortions in rabbits at doses 2, 4, and 8 times the maximum recommended human dose of 600 mg/day (4).

An increase in the incidence and severity of hydronephrosis (distention of the renal pelvis and in some cases of the ureters) has also been observed in the offspring of mice and rabbits (4). Wavy ribs and some skeletal defects have been observed in the offspring of rats given furosemide during organogenesis (5). These effects appeared to be caused directly or indirectly by the diuretic action of the drug.

Cardiovascular disorders, such as pulmonary edema, severe hypertension, or congestive heart failure, are probably the only valid indications for this drug in pregnancy. Furosemide crosses the placenta (6). Following oral doses of 25–40 mg, peak concentrations in cord serum of 330 ng/mL were recorded at 9 hours. Maternal and cord levels were equal at 8 hours. Increased fetal urine production after maternal furosemide therapy has been observed (7,8). Administration of furosemide to the mother has been used to assess fetal kidney function by provoking urine production, which is then visualized by ultrasonic techniques (9,10). Diuresis was found more often in newborns exposed to furosemide shortly before birth than in controls (11). Urinary sodium and potassium levels in the treated newborns were significantly greater than in the nonexposed controls.

In a surveillance study of Michigan Medicaid recipients involving 229,101 completed pregnancies conducted between 1985 and 1992, 350 newborns had been exposed to furosemide during the 1st trimester (F. Rosa, personal communication, FDA, 1993). A total of 18 (5.1%) major birth defects were observed (15 expected). Specific data were available for six defect categories, including (observed/expected) 2/4 cardiovascular defects, 1/1 oral clefts, 0/0 spina bifida, 1/1 polydactyly, 1/1 limb reduction defects, and 3/1 hypospadias. Only with the latter defect is there a suggestion of an association, but other factors, including the mother's disease, concurrent drug use, and chance, may be involved.

In the 2nd and 3rd trimesters, furosemide has been used for edema, hypertension, and toxemia of pregnancy without causing fetal or newborn adverse effects (1,12–33). One case report described the use of oral furosemide throughout gestation for the treatment of Gordon's syndrome (short stature, defective dentition, hyperkalemic hyperchloremic acidosis, and chronic hypertension) (34). A cesarean section at 32 weeks' gestation gave birth to an 1100-g female infant with Apgar scores of 8 and 9. Except for respiratory distress due to prematurity and hyperkalemia that required treatment, the infant did well.

Many investigators now consider diuretics contraindicated in pregnancy, except for patients with cardiovascular disorders, since they do not prevent or alter the course of toxemia and they may decrease placental perfusion (35–38). A 1984 study determined that the use of diuretics for hypertension in pregnancy prevented normal plasma volume expansion and did not change perinatal outcome (39). Thus, diuretics are not recommended for the treatment of gestational hypertension and/or preeclampsia because of the maternal hypovolemia characteristic of these conditions.

BREASTFEEDING SUMMARY

Furosemide is excreted into breast milk (4,40). No reports of adverse effects in nursing infants have been found. Thiazide diuretics have been used to suppress lactation (see Chlorothiazide).

References

1. Votta RA, Parada OH, Windgrad RH, Alvarez OH, Tomassinni TL, Patori AA. Furosemide action on the creatinine concentration of amniotic fluid. Am J Obstet Gynecol 1975;123:621–4.
2. Carswell W, Semple PF. The effect of furosemide on uric acid levels in maternal blood, fetal blood and amniotic fluid. J Obstet Gynaecol Br Commonw 1974;81:472–4.
3. Jerkner K, Kutti J, Victorin L. Platelet counts in mothers and their newborn infants with respect to antepartum administration of oral diuretics. Acta Med Scand 1973;194:473–5.
4. Product information. Furosemide. Mylan Pharmaceuticals, 2000.
5. Shepard TH. *Catalog of Teratogen Agents*. 9th ed. Baltimore, MD: The Johns Hopkins University Press, 1998:215.
6. Beermann B, Groschinsky-Grind M, Fahraeus L, Lindstroem B. Placental transfer of furosemide. Clin Pharmacol Ther 1978;24:560–2.
7. Wladimiroff JW. Effect of furosemide on fetal urine production. Br J Obstet Gynaecol 1975;82:221–4.
8. Stein WW, Halberstadt E, Gerner R, Roemer E. Effect of furosemide on fetal kidney function. Arch Gynekol 1977;224:114–5.
9. Barrett RJ, Rayburn WF, Barr M Jr. Furosemide (Lasix) challenge test in assessing bilateral fetal hydronephrosis. Am J Obstet Gynecol 1983;147:846–7.
10. Harman CR. Maternal furosemide may not provoke urine production in the compromised fetus. Am J Obstet Gynecol 1984;150:322–3.
11. Pecorari D, Ragni N, Autera C. Administration of furosemide to women during confinement, and its action on newborn infants. Acta Biomed (Italy) 1969;40:2–11.
12. Pulle C. Diuretic therapy in monosymptomatic edema of pregnancy. Minerva Med 1965;56:1622–3.
13. DeCecco L. Furosemide in the treatment of edema in pregnancy. Minerva Med 1965;56:1586–91.
14. Bocci A, Pupita F, Revelli E, Bartoli E, Molaschi M, Massobrio A. The water–salt metabolism in obstetrics and gynecology. Minerva Ginecol 1965;17:103–10.
15. Sideri L. Furosemide in the treatment of oedema in gynaecology and obstetrics. Clin Ter 1966;39:339–46.
16. Wu CC, Lee TT, Kao SC. Evaluation of new diuretic (furosemide) on pregnant women. A pilot study. J Obstet Gynecol Republ China 1966;5:318–20.
17. Loch EG. Treatment of gestosis with diuretics. Med Klin 1966;61:1512–5.
18. Buchheit H, Nicolai KH. Influence of furosemide (Lasix) on gestational edemas. Med Klin 1966;61:1515–8.
19. Tanaka T. Studies on the clinical effect of Lasix in edema of pregnancy and toxemia of pregnancy. Sanka To Fujinka 1966;41:914–20.
20. Merger R, Cohen J, Sadut R. Study of the therapeutic effects of furosemide in obstetrics. Rev Fr Gynecol 1967;62:259–65.
21. Nascimento R, Fernandes R, Cunha A. Furosemide as an accessory in the therapy of the toxemia of pregnancy. Hospital (Portugal) 1967;71:137–40.
22. Finnerty FA Jr. Advantages and disadvantages of furosemide in the edematous states of pregnancy. Am J Obstet Gynecol 1969;105:1022–7.
23. Das Gupta S. Frusemide in blood transfusion for severe anemia in pregnancy. J Obstet Gynaecol India 1970;20:521–5.
24. Kawathekar P, Anusuya SR, Sriniwas P, Lagali S. Diazepam (Calmpose) in eclampsia: a preliminary report of 16 cases. Curr Ther Res 1973;15:845–55.
25. Pianetti F. Our results in the treatment of parturient patients with oedema during the five years 1966–1970. Atti Accad Med Lomb 1973;27:137–40.
26. Azcarte Sanchez S, Quesada Rocha T, Rosas Arced J. Evaluation of a plan of treatment in eclampsia (first report). Ginecol Obstet Mex 1973;34:171–86.
27. Bravo Sandoval J. Management of preeclampsia–eclampsia in the third gyneco-obstetrical hospital. Cir Cirjjands 1973;41:487–94.
28. Franck H, Gruhl M. Therapeutic experience with nortensin in the treatment of toxemia of pregnancy. Munch Med Wochenschr 1974;116:521–4.
29. Cornu P, Laffay J, Ertel M, Lemiere J. Resuscitation in eclampsia. Rev Prat 1975;25:809–30.
30. Finnerty FA Jr. Management of hypertension in toxemia of pregnancy. Hosp Med 1975;11:52–65.
31. Saldana-Garcia RH. Eclampsia: maternal and fetal mortality. Comparative study of 80 cases. In VIII World Congress of Gynecology and Obstetrics. Int Cong Ser 1976;396:58–9.
32. Palot M, Jakob L, Decaux J, Brundis JP, Quereux C, Wahl P. Arterial hypertensions of labor and the postpartum period. Rev Fr Gynecol Obstet 1979;74:173–6.
33. Clark AD, Sevitt LH, Hawkins DF. Use of furosemide in severe toxaemia of pregnancy. Lancet 1972;1:35–6.
34. Kirshon B, Edwards J, Cotton DB. Gordon's syndrome in pregnancy. Am J Obstet Gynecol 1987;156:1110–1.
35. Pitkin RM, Kaminetzky HA, Newton M, Pritchard JA. Maternal nutrition: a selective review of clinical topics. Obstet Gynecol 1972;40:773–85.
36. Lindheimer MD, Katz AI. Sodium and diuretics in pregnancy. N Engl J Med 1973;288:891–4.
37. Christianson R, Page EW. Diuretic drugs and pregnancy. Obstet Gynecol 1976;48:647–52.
38. Gant NF, Madden JD, Shteri PK, MacDonald PC. The metabolic clearance rate of dehydroisoandrosterone sulfate. IV. Acute effects of induced hypertension, hypotension, and natriuresis in normal and hypertensive pregnancies. Am J Obstet Gynecol 1976;124:143–8.
39. Sibai BM, Grossman RA, Grossman HG. Effects of diuretics on plasma volume in pregnancies with long-term hypertension. Am J Obstet Gynecol 1984;150:831–5.
40. Product information. Lasix. Hoechst–Roussel Pharmaceuticals, 1990.

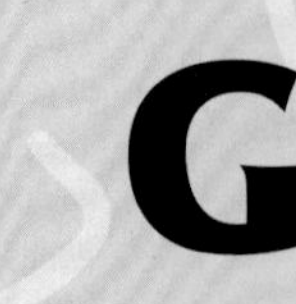

GABAPENTIN

Anticonvulsant

PREGNANCY RECOMMENDATION: Limited Human Data—Animal Data Suggest Risk
BREASTFEEDING RECOMMENDATION: Limited Human Data—Probably Compatible

PREGNANCY SUMMARY

A 2005 report of gabapentin monotherapy raises concerns of drug-induced developmental toxicity (1). Although limited, other studies involving monotherapy have not confirmed these findings. Moreover, a 2012 review concluded that the available data were not sufficient to determine whether or not exposure to gabapentin was harmful to the fetus (2). Because the agent is often combined with other anticonvulsants, the actual cause of a defect may be obscured. If a woman's condition requires gabapentin, the benefits of therapy to her appear to outweigh the potential risks to her embryo and/or fetus. A 2009 review on the treatment of cluster headache in pregnancy and lactation concluded that, if indicated, gabapentin was the drug of choice (3).

FETAL RISK SUMMARY

Gabapentin (Neurontin) is an anticonvulsant used as adjunctive therapy for the treatment of partial seizures in patients with epilepsy (4,5). The drug also is indicated for the management of postherpetic neuralgia in adults (5). Gabapentin enacarbil (Horizant) is a prodrug that is undergoes extensive first-pass hydrolysis by enterocytes and to a lesser extent in the liver to form gabapentin so that blood levels are low and transient (≤2% of gabapentin plasma levels) (6). The prodrug is indicated for the treatment of moderate-to-severe restless legs syndrome (6). Gabapentin has been used off-label for multiple other conditions, including migraine and chronic headache, bipolar disorder, peripheral neuropathy, diabetic neuropathy, complex regional pain syndrome, attention deficit disorder, trigeminal neuralgia, periodic limb movement disorder of sleep, and alcohol withdrawal syndrome (7).

Fetotoxicity in mice exposed during organogenesis to maternal oral doses of about 1–4 times the maximum recommended human dose based on BSA (MRHD) was characterized by delayed ossification of bones in the skull, vertebrae, forelimbs, and hindlimbs. The no-effect dose in mice was about half of the MRHD. Delayed ossification was also observed in rats exposed in utero to 1–5 times the MRHD. Hydroureter or hydronephrosis was observed in rat pups exposed in utero during organogenesis and during the perinatal and postnatal periods after similar doses. The causes of the urinary tract anomalies were unclear. The no-effect dose in rats during organogenesis was approximately equal to the MRHD in the teratogenicity study. When compared with controls, exposure to gabapentin during organogenesis did not increase congenital malformations, other than hydroureter or hydronephrosis in rats, in mice, rats, and rabbits at 4, 5, or 8 times, respectively, the MRHD. In rabbits, doses less than about ¼ to 8 times the MRHD caused an increased incidence of postimplantation fetal loss (5).

Animal reproduction studies have been conducted with gabapentin enacarbil (6). In rats and rabbits given the drug throughout organogenesis, increased embryo–fetal mortality and decreased fetal body weights were observed. The no-effect dose in rats and rabbits was about 3 and 16 times, respectively, the recommended human dose of 600 mg/day based on BSA (RHD). When rats were dosed throughout pregnancy and lactation, decreased growth and survival were noted. The no-effect dose was about three times the RHD (6).

Both gabapentin and gabapentin enacarbil were carcinogenic (pancreatic acinar cell adenomas and carcinomas) in rats, but assays for mutagenicity were negative. No adverse effects on fertility were observed with either agent (5,6).

Consistent with its low molecular weight (about 171), absence of metabolism and plasma protein binding, gabapentin crosses the placenta. In a 2005 study involving six women, the mean cord:maternal plasma concentration ratio was 1.7 (range 1.3–2.1) (8). The drug declined in the neonates with an estimated half-life of 14 hours.

No cases of fetal or newborn adverse outcomes were reported to the FDA through 1996 (F. Rosa, personal communication, FDA, 1996).

A 2005 abstract reported 62 pregnancy outcomes after exposure to gabapentin, lamotrigine, or topiramate (1). The study included a blinded dysmorphology examination. Thirty women used gabapentin, one of whom delivered an infant with a major malformation: pyloric stenosis with bilateral fifth finger clinodactyly and prominent epicanthal folds (mother treated for seizures with monotherapy). Two of the 13 infants that were examined by a dysmorphologist had anticonvulsant facies (one monotherapy and the other combined with carbamazepine). In addition, two had neurologic abnormalities:

failure to gaze up (sunsetting), opisthotonus, frontal bossing, medial flare of the eyebrows, and small for gestational age (mother treated for depression with gabapentin, doxepin, clonazepam, nefazodone, and zolpidem); sunsetting and metopic ridge (mother treated for chronic fatigue and fibromyalgia with gabapentin, lorazepam, and fluoxetine). Although they were not conclusive, the findings suggested reason for concern with gabapentin, as well as the same phenotype that has been observed with older anticonvulsants (1).

In a brief 1995 communication, a newborn exposed to gabapentin and carbamazepine during pregnancy had a cyclops holoprosencephaly (no nose and one eye) (9). Of the seven suspected cases of holoprosencephaly described in this report, five involved the use of carbamazepine (two cases of monotherapy and three of combined therapy). Because of the lack of family histories, an association with familial holoprosencephaly or maternal neurologic problems could not be excluded (9).

The Lamotrigine Pregnancy Registry, an ongoing project conducted by the manufacturer, was first published in January 1997 (10). The final report was published in July 2010. The Registry is now closed. Among 32 prospectively enrolled pregnancies exposed to gabapentin and lamotrigine, with or without other anticonvulsants, 27 were exposed in the 1st trimester, resulting in 25 live births without defects, 1 spontaneous abortion (SAB), and 1 birth defect. There were five exposures in the 2nd/3rd trimester resulting in live births without defects (10).

A 1998 noninterventional observational cohort study described the outcomes of pregnancies in women who had been prescribed ≥1 of 34 newly marketed drugs by general practitioners in England (11). Data were obtained by questionnaires sent to the prescribing physicians 1 month after the expected or possible date of delivery. In 831 (78%) of the pregnancies, a newly marketed drug was thought to have been taken during the 1st trimester with birth defects noted in 14 (2.5%) singleton births of the 557 newborns (10 sets of twins). In addition, two birth defects were observed in aborted fetuses. However, few of the aborted fetuses were examined. Gabapentin was taken during the 1st trimester in 17 pregnancies. The outcomes of these pregnancies included 2 SABs, 4 elective abortions (EABs), and 11 normal newborns (1 premature) (11). Although no congenital malformations were observed, the study lacked the sensitivity to identify minor anomalies. Late-appearing major defects may also have been missed due to the timing of the questionnaires.

A 1996 review reported 16 pregnancies exposed to gabapentin from preclinical trials and postmarketing surveillance (12). The outcomes of these pregnancies included five EABs, one ongoing pregnancy, seven normal infants, and three infants with birth defects. No specific information was provided on the defects other than that there was no pattern of malformation and all had been exposed to polytherapy for epilepsy (12).

A 2002 review concluded that gabapentin could be used for chronic headache during early pregnancy but not later because of concerns about delaying fetal bony growth plate development (13). The reason for this concern was not stated, but the animal data above may have influenced the conclusion. In a 2002 report of a postmarketing surveillance study in England, there were no congenital anomalies in the 11 infants of women who used gabapentin in the 1st trimester (14).

Results from the Neurontin Pregnancy Registry were reported in 2003 (15). There were 51 fetuses, including 3 sets of twins, from 39 women with epilepsy and other disorders. At conception, 17 were taking gabapentin alone, 30 were taking it with other antiepileptic drugs, and 4 were not receiving gabapentin. At delivery, the numbers were 19, 21, and 4, respectively. There were six SABs and one EAB. Among the 44 live births, there were 2 (4.5%) major anomalies: hypospadia (gabapentin plus valproate) and single kidney (gabapentin alone, changed to phenobarbital at 16 weeks'). There also was one (2.3%) minor defect (defect of left external ear canal and two small skin tags on the jaw). The outcomes were comparable to the risk of major (4%–8%) defects in infants of epileptic mothers and the risk of minor (3%–10%) defects in the general population (15).

The United Kingdom Epilepsy and Pregnancy Register prospective study reported the malformation risks of antiepileptic drugs (AEDs) (16). Among the 3607 cases, there were 31 pregnancies (excludes an unspecified number of pregnancy losses with no major defects) exposed to gabapentin monotherapy. There was one major anomaly (type not specified). Compared to no exposure to AED, the adjusted odds ratio was 1.76, 95% confidence interval 0.22–14.49 ($p = 0.596$) (16).

A brief report described the use of gabapentin in seven women with hyperemesis gravidarum (17). Therapy was started at a mean gestational age of 8 weeks and discontinued at a median gestational age of 21 weeks (range 10–25 weeks). The mean dose was 1843 mg (range 1200–3000 mg). Two birth defects were observed: hydronephrosis and tethered spinal cord. The latter defect occurred in an infant conceived by in vitro fertilization, a process known to increase the risk of congenital defects (17).

A study published in 2009 examined the effect of AEDs on the head circumference in newborns (18). Significant reductions in mean birth-weight-adjusted mean head circumference (bw-adj-HC) was noted for monotherapy with carbamazepine and valproic acid. No effect on bw-adj-HC was observed with gabapentin, phenytoin, clonazepam, and lamotrigine. A significant increase in the occurrence of microcephaly (bw-adj-HC smaller than 2 standard deviations below the mean) was noted after any AED polytherapy but not after any monotherapy, including carbamazepine and valproic acid. The potential effects of these findings on child development warrant study (18).

A 2013 prospective cohort study compared the outcomes of 223 pregnancies exposed to gabapentin (average dose 1000 mg/day, range 100–4800 mg/day combined with other drugs) with 223 pregnancies not exposed to gabapentin or known teratogens (19). Indications for use of gabapentin were known in 207 cases: epilepsy (34%), pain (90%), and psychiatric conditions (22%). In the two groups, there was no statistical difference in the number of major malformations 7 (4.1%) vs. 5 (2.5%), SABs 22 (9.8%) vs. 17 (7.6%), stillbirths 2 (1.1%) vs. 0, or IUGR 6 (3.5%) vs. 4 (1.9%). Statistically significant outcomes were found for live births (76.2% vs. 90%), EABs (13% vs. 2.2%), preterm birth (10.5% vs. 3.9%), and low (<2500 g) birth weight (10.5% vs. 4.4%). The seven infants with major malformations were exposed to gabapentin and other drugs in the 1st trimester. The defects were ventricular septal defect (2 infants); anencephaly; macrocephaly, microtrognathism, and cutis marmorata; pyloric stenosis; bilateral varus clubfoot; and cryptorchidism. Although the authors noted the small size of their study, and the absence of a comparative group with other antiepileptic drugs, they concluded that gabapentin did not appear to increase the risk for major malformations (19).

A 27-year-old woman was diagnosed about 2 months before pregnancy with stiff person syndrome (Moersche-Woltman syndrome) (20). She was treated with gabapentin (2700 mg/day), diazepam (30 mg/day), and a prednisone taper. When pregnancy was diagnosed, diazepam was discontinued but, without the drug, her muscle spasms increased and baclofen (30 mg/day) was started. The patient was able to wean down her medications in the 2nd and 3rd trimesters (specific details not provided). Labor commenced at about 40 weeks' while still on gabapentin and baclofen. A cesarean section was conducted because of fetal repetitive late decelerations to deliver a 3230-g female infant with Apgar scores of 5 and 8 at 1 and 5 minutes, respectively. The infant, discharged home on day 4, was doing well (age assumed to be 6 weeks) (20).

BREASTFEEDING SUMMARY

Consistent with its low molecular weight (about 171) and lack of plasma protein binding, gabapentin is excreted breast milk. A 2005 study described the use of gabapentin during pregnancy in five women, three of whom breastfed their infants (7). One infant was born at 33 weeks', but all five had normal Apgar scores. No congenital defects were noted in the five infants. In the three women who breastfed, their doses were 600, 1800, and 2100 mg/day, respectively. Milk and plasma sampling occurred on postpartum days 21, 16, and 97, respectively. Infant plasma levels of gabapentin after completion of nursing were 1.3, 1.5, and 1.9 μM, respectively, and the milk:plasma ratios were 1.0, 1.3, and 0.8, respectively. The estimated infant dose as a percentage of the mother's weight-adjusted dose was 1.3%–3.8% (not specified by infant) (7).

In a 2006 case report, a 34-year-old mother had been taking gabapentin 600 mg three times daily (36.7 mg/kg/day) and amitriptyline 2.5 mg/day for 6 weeks while nursing her male infant (21). On the date the milk samples were obtained, her infant was 1.6 months old and weighed 3.1 kg. The milk:plasma ratio was 0.86 and the relative infant was 2.34% of the mother's weight-adjusted dose. The plasma concentration in the infant (0.4 mg/L) was about 6% of the mother's plasma concentration. No adverse effects were noted in the infant, who was doing well (21).

References

1. Chambers CD, Kao KK, Felix RJ, Alvarado S, Chavez C, Ye N, Dick LM, Jones KL. Pregnancy outcome in infants prenatally exposed to newer anticonvulsants (abstract). Birth Defects Res (Part A) 2005;73:316.
2. Holmes LB, Hernandez-Diaz S. Newer anticonvulsants: lamotrigine, topiramate, and gabapentin. Birth Defects Res A Clin Mol Teratol 2012;94:599–606.
3. Jurgens TP, Schaefer C, May A. Treatment of cluster headache in pregnancy and lactation. Cephalalgia 2009;29:391–400.
4. Dichter MA, Brodie MJ. New antiepileptic drugs. N Engl J Med 1996;334:1583–90.
5. Product information. Neurontin. Parke-Davis, 2012.
6. Product information. Horizant. GlaxoSmithKline, 2012.
7. Mack A. Examination of the evidence for off-label use of gabapentin. J Managed Care Pharm 2003;9:559–68.
8. Ohman I, Vitols S, Tomson T. Pharmacokinetics of gabapentin during delivery, in the neonatal period, and lactation: does a fetal accumulation occur during pregnancy? Epilepsia 2005;46:1621–4.
9. Rosa F. Holoprosencephaly and antiepileptic exposures. Teratology 1995;51:230.
10. The Lamotrigine Pregnancy Registry. Final Report. 1 September 1992 through 31 March 2010. GlaxcoSmithKline, July 2010.
11. Wilton LV, Pearce GL, Martin RM, Mackay FJ, Mann RD. The outcomes of pregnancy in women exposed to newly marketed drugs in general practice in England. Br J Obstet Gynaecol 1998;105:882–9.
12. Morrell MJ. The new antiepileptic drugs and women: efficacy, reproductive health, pregnancy, and fetal outcome. Epilepsia 1996;37(Suppl 6):S34–44.
13. Marcus DA. Pregnancy and chronic headache. Expert Opin Pharmacother 2002;3:389–93.
14. Wilton LV, Shakir S. A postmarketing surveillance study of gabapentin as add-on therapy for 3100 patients in England. Epilepsia 2002;43:983–92.
15. Montouris G. Gabapentin exposure in human pregnancy: results from the gabapentin pregnancy registry. Epilepsy Bevav 2003;4:310–7.
16. Morrow J, Russell A, Guthrie E, Parsons L, Robertson I, Waddell R, Irwin B, McGivern RC, Morrison PJ, Craig J. Malformation risks of antiepileptic drugs in pregnancy: a prospective study from the UK Epilepsy and Pregnancy Register. J Neurol Neurosurg Psychiatry 2006;77:193–8.
17. Guttuso T Jr, Robinson LK, Amankwah KS. Gabapentin use in hyperemesis gravidarum: a pilot study. Early Hum Dev 2010;86:65–6.
18. Almgren M, Kallen B, Lavebratt C. Population-based study of antiepileptic drug exposure in utero—influence on head circumference in newborns. Seizure 2009;18:672–5.
19. Fujii H, Goel A, Bernard N, Pistelli A, Yates LM, Stephens S, Han JY, Matsui D, Erwell F, Einarson R, Koren G, Einarson A. Pregnancy outcomes following gabapentin use: results of a prospective comparative cohort study. Neurology 2013;80:1–6.
20. Goldkamp J, Blaskiewicz R, Myles T. Stiff person syndrome and pregnancy. Obstet Gynecol 2011;118:454–7.
21. Kristensen JH, Ilett KF, Hackett LP, Kohan R. Gabapentin and breastfeeding: a case report. J Hum Lact 2006;22:426–8.

GADOBENATE DIMEGLUMINE

Diagnostic Agent

PREGNANCY RECOMMENDATION: Limited Human Data—Animal Data Suggest Moderate Risk
BREASTFEEDING RECOMMENDATION: Limited Human Data—Probably Compatible

PREGNANCY SUMMARY

Gadolinium-based contrast agents are complexes with chelating agents that lower the potential toxicity in patients receiving the agents by preventing the cellular uptake of free gadolinium. The complexes cross the placenta to the fetus and are excreted by the fetal kidneys into the amniotic fluid, where they remain for long periods. The complexes themselves are relatively nontoxic, but dissociation may occur to release free gadolinium into the amniotic fluid where it could expose fetal lungs and gut. Presently, the risk of gadolinium-induced toxicity in the fetus is unknown but may be harmful (1–3). A concern has been raised for a risk of gadolinium-induced nephrogenic systemic fibrosis (3). The American College of Radiology recommends that these agents should not be routinely used in pregnancy and, if such use is indicated, a written informed consent be obtained from the patient (1). The guidelines of the Contrast Media Safety Committee of the European Society of Urogenital Radiology and a review article recommend that gadolinium-based contrast media may be used in pregnancy if such use is important to the mother's health (4,5).

FETAL RISK SUMMARY

Gadobenate dimeglumine, a paramagnetic agent, is a complex formed between a chelating agent and a paramagnetic ion, gadolinium. It is in the same subclass of gadolinium-based contrast agents as gadodiamide, gadofosveset trisodium, gadopentetate dimeglumine, gadoteridol, and gadoversetamide. Gadobenate dimeglumine is given IV for magnetic resonance imaging (MRI) of the central nervous system in adults. Neither metabolism nor plasma protein binding of the agent has been detected. The mean elimination half-life is about 1–2 hours (6).

Reproduction studies have been conducted in rats and rabbits. In rats, no evidence of teratogenicity, other developmental toxicities (i.e., birth, survival, growth, development, and fertility of the next generation), or maternal toxicity at a daily IV dose that was three times the human dose based on BSA (HD). Teratogenicity (microphthalmia/small eye and/or focal retinal fold in three fetuses from three litters) was observed in rabbits given a daily IV dose during organogenesis that was six times the HD. A dose that was 10 times the HD resulted in increased intrauterine deaths (6).

Long-term studies to evaluate the potential for carcinogenicity have not been conducted. Assays for mutagenicity and chromosome aberrations assay were negative. No effect on male and female rat fertility was observed with daily IV doses up to three times the HD. A dose five times the HD caused irreversible toxicity in male rat reproductive organs. These effects were not observed in dog and monkey studies with doses up to about 11 and 10 times, respectively, the HD (6).

BREASTFEEDING SUMMARY

Although no reports describing the administration of gadobenate dimeglumine during human lactation have been located, reviewers consider gadolinium contrast media to be compatible with breastfeeding because of the very small amounts excreted into milk and potentially being absorbed by a nursing infant (2–4). The American Academy of Pediatrics classifies gadopentetate dimeglumine as compatible with breastfeeding (7) (see Gadopentetate Dimeglumine).

References

1. Kanal E, Barkovich AJ, Bell C, Borgstede JP, Bradley WG Jr, Froelich JW, Gilk T, Gimbel JR, Gosbee J, Kuhni-Kaminski E, Lester JW Jr, Nyenhuis J, Parag Y, Schaefer DJ, Sebek-Scoumis EA, Weinreb J, Zaremba LA, Wilcox P, Lucey L, Sass N, for the ACR Blue Ribbon Panel on MR Safety. ACR guidance document for safe MR practices: 2007. AJR Am J Roentgenol 2007;188:1447–74.
2. Lin SP, Brown JJ. MR contrast agents: physical and pharmacologic basics. J Magn Reson Imaging 2007;25:884–99.
3. Chen MM, Coakley FV, Kaimal A, Laros RK Jr. Guidelines for computed tomography and magnetic resonance imaging use during pregnancy and lactation. Obstet Gynecol 2008;112:333–40.
4. Webb JAW, Thomsen HS, Morcos SK, and members of Contrast Media Safety Committee of European Society of Urogenital Radiology (ESUR). The use of iodinated and gadolinium contrast media during pregnancy and lactation. Eur Radiol 2005;15:1234–40.
5. Garcia-Bournissen F, Shrim A, Koren G. Safety of gadolinium during pregnancy. Can Fam Physician 2006;52:309–10.
6. Product information. Multihance. Bracco Diagnostics, 2007.
7. Committee on Drugs, American Academy of Pediatrics. The transfer of drugs and other chemicals into human milk. Pediatrics 2001;106:776–89.

GADOBUTROL

Diagnostic (Radiopaque Agent)

PREGNANCY RECOMMENDATION: No Human Data—Animal Data Suggest Moderate Risk
BREASTFEEDING RECOMMENDATION: No Human Data—Probably Compatible

PREGNANCY SUMMARY

No reports describing the use a gadobutrol in human pregnancy have been located. Gadolinium-based contrast agents are complexes with chelating agents that lower the potential toxicity in patients receiving the agents by preventing the cellular uptake of free gadolinium. The complexes cross the placenta to the fetus and are excreted by the fetal kidneys into the amniotic fluid, where they remain for long periods. The complexes themselves are relatively nontoxic, but dissociation may occur to release free gadolinium into the amniotic fluid, where it could expose fetal lungs and gut. Presently, the risk of gadolinium-induced toxicity in the fetus is unknown but may be harmful (1–3). A concern has been raised for a risk of gadolinium-induced nephrogenic systemic fibrosis (3). The American College of Radiology recommends that these agents should not be routinely used in pregnancy and, if such use is indicated, a written informed consent be obtained from the patient (1). The guidelines of the Contrast Media Safety Committee of the European Society of Urogenital Radiology and a review article recommend that gadolinium-based contrast media may be used in pregnancy if such use is important to the mother's health (4,5).

FETAL RISK SUMMARY

Gadobutrol, a gadolinium-based contrast agent, is a paramagnetic macrocyclic administered for magnetic resonance imaging (MRI). It is indicated for IV use in diagnostic MRI in adults and children 2 years of age or older to detect and visualize areas with disrupted blood–brain barrier and/or abnormal vascularity of the central nervous system. The agent does not display any particular protein binding and is not metabolized. The mean terminal half-life is 1.81 hours (6).

Reproduction studies have been conducted in rats, rabbits, and monkeys. In rats, maternally toxic doses that were 12 times the human equivalent dose based on BSA (HED) caused retardation of the embryo development and embryolethality. Similar toxicity, but without evidence of maternal toxicity, occurred in rabbits at doses that were 8 times the HED. In rabbits, the toxicity occurred despite minimal placental transfer (0.01% of the dose detected in the fetuses). In monkeys, gadobutrol was not teratogenic but was embryolethal when given IV during organogenesis in doses up to 8 times the recommended single human dose based on BSA. However, pregnant animals received repeated daily doses so their exposure was much higher than that obtained with the standard single dose in humans (6).

Studies for carcinogenicity have not been conducted. Multiple assays for mutagenicity were negative. No effect on fertility and general reproductive performance was observed in male and female rats (6).

It is not known if gadobutrol crosses the human placenta, However, other gadolinium-based contrast agents cross (see Gadobenate Dimeglumine and other agents in this subclass) and exposure of the embryo–fetus should be expected with gadobutrol. The molecular weight (about 605) and the terminal half-life are consistent with placenta transfer.

BREASTFEEDING SUMMARY

No reports describing the use of gadobutrol during human lactation have been located. However, the molecular weight (about 605) and terminal half-life (1.81 hours) suggest that the drug will be excreted into breast milk. Although there are no reports, reviewers consider gadolinium contrast media to be compatible with breastfeeding because of the very small amounts excreted into milk and potentially being absorbed by a nursing infant (2–4). The American Academy of Pediatrics classifies gadopentetate dimeglumine as compatible with breastfeeding (7) (see Gadopentetate Dimeglumine).

References

1. Kanal E, Barkovich AJ, Bell C, Borgstede JP, Bradley WG Jr, Froelich JW, Gilk T, Gimbel JR, Gosbee J, Kuhni-Kaminski E, Lester JW Jr, Nyenhuis J, Parag Y, Schaefer DJ, Sebek-Scoumis EA, Weinreb J, Zaremba LA, Wilcox P, Lucey L, Sass N, for the ACR Blue Ribbon Panel on MR Safety. ACR guidance document for safe MR practices: 2007. AJR Am J Roentgenol 2007;188:1447–74.
2. Lin SP, Brown JJ. MR contrast agents: physical and pharmacologic basics. J Magn Reson Imaging 2007;25:884–99.
3. Chen MM, Coakley FV, Kaimal A, Laros RK Jr. Guidelines for computed tomography and magnetic resonance imaging use during pregnancy and lactation. Obstet Gynecol 2008;112:333–40.
4. Webb JAW, Thomsen HS, Morcos SK, and members of Contrast Media Safety Committee of European Society of Urogenital Radiology (ESUR). The use of iodinated and gadolinium contrast media during pregnancy and lactation. Eur Radiol 2005;15:1234–40.
5. Garcia-Bournissen F, Shrim A, Koren G. Safety of gadolinium during pregnancy. Can Fam Physician 2006;52:309–10.
6. Product information. Gadavist. Bayer HealthCare Pharmaceuticals, 2011.
7. Committee on Drugs, American Academy of Pediatrics. The transfer of drugs and other chemicals into human milk. Pediatrics 2001;106:776–89.

GADODIAMIDE

Diagnostic Agent

PREGNANCY RECOMMENDATION: Limited Human Data—Animal Data Suggest Moderate Risk
BREASTFEEDING RECOMMENDATION: Limited Human Data—Probably Compatible

PREGNANCY SUMMARY

Available gadolinium-based contrast agents are complexes with chelating agents that lower the potential toxicity in patients receiving the agents by preventing the cellular uptake of free gadolinium. The complexes cross the placenta to the fetus and are excreted by the fetal kidneys into the amniotic fluid, where they remain for long periods. The complexes themselves are relatively nontoxic, but dissociation may occur to release free gadolinium into the amniotic fluid, where it could expose fetal lungs and gut. Presently, the risk of gadolinium-induced toxicity in the fetus is unknown but may be harmful (1–3). A concern has been raised for a risk of gadolinium-induced nephrogenic systemic fibrosis (3). The American College of Radiology recommends that these agents should not be routinely used in pregnancy and, if such use is indicated, a written informed consent be obtained from the patient (1). In addition, the guidelines of the Contrast Media Safety Committee of the European Society of Urogenital Radiology and a review article recommend that gadolinium-based contrast media may be used in pregnancy if such use is important to the mother's health (4,5).

FETAL RISK SUMMARY

Gadodiamide, a paramagnetic agent, is a complex formed between a chelating agent and a paramagnetic ion, gadolinium. It is in the same subclass of gadolinium-based contrast agents as gadobenate dimeglumine, gadofosveset trisodium, gadopentetate dimeglumine, gadoteridol, and gadoversetamide. Gadodiamide is indicated for IV use in magnetic resonance imaging (MRI) to visualize lesions with abnormal vascularity (or those thought to cause abnormalities in the blood–brain barrier) in the brain (intracranial lesions), spine, and associated tissues. It is also indicated for IV administration to facilitate the visualization of lesions with abnormal vascularity within the thoracic (noncardiac), abdominal, and pelvic cavities, and the retroperitoneal space. Neither metabolism nor plasma protein binding has been detected. The elimination half-life is about 78 minutes (6).

Reproduction studies have been conducted in rats and rabbits. Increased incidences of flexed appendages and skeletal malformations were observed in rabbits given a daily IV dose for 13 days during gestation that was about 0.6 times the human dose (HD) based on mmol/m^2. The skeletal malformations may have due to maternal toxicity (reduced body weight). Neither fetal abnormalities nor maternal toxicity were observed in rats at a daily IV dose given for 10 days during gestation that was 1.3 times the HD based on mg/m^2 (6).

Long-term studies to evaluate the potential for carcinogenicity have not been conducted. Assays for mutagenicity and chromosome aberrations assay were negative. No effect on male and female rat fertility was observed with a low IV dose given three times weekly (6).

BREASTFEEDING SUMMARY

Although no reports describing the administration of gadodiamide during human lactation have been located, reviewers consider gadolinium contrast media to be compatible with breastfeeding because of the very small amounts excreted into milk and potentially being absorbed by a nursing infant (2–4). The American Academy of Pediatrics classifies gadopentetate dimeglumine as compatible with breastfeeding (7) (see Gadopentetate Dimeglumine).

References

1. Kanal E, Barkovich AJ, Bell C, Borgstede JP, Bradley WG Jr, Froelich JW, Gilk T, Gimbel JR, Gosbee J, Kuhni-Kaminski E, Lester JW Jr, Nyenhuis J, Parag Y, Schaefer DJ, Sebek-Scoumis EA, Weinreb J, Zaremba LA, Wilcox P, Lucey L, Sass N, for the ACR Blue Ribbon Panel on MR Safety. ACR guidance document for safe MR practices: 2007. AJR Am J Roentgenol 2007;188:1447–74.
2. Lin SP, Brown JJ. MR contrast agents: physical and pharmacologic basics. J Magn Reson Imaging 2007;25:884–99.
3. Chen MM, Coakley FV, Kaimal A, Laros RK Jr. Guidelines for computed tomography and magnetic resonance imaging use during pregnancy and lactation. Obstet Gynecol 2008;112:333–40.
4. Webb JAW, Thomsen HS, Morcos SK, and members of Contrast Media Safety Committee of European Society of Urogenital Radiology (ESUR). The use of iodinated and gadolinium contrast media during pregnancy and lactation. Eur Radiol 2005;15:1234–40.
5. Garcia-Bournissen F, Shrim A, Koren G. Safety of gadolinium during pregnancy. Can Fam Physician 2006;52:309–10.
6. Product information. Omniscan. GE Healthcare, 2005.
7. Committee on Drugs, American Academy of Pediatrics. The transfer of drugs and other chemicals into human milk. Pediatrics 2001;106:776–89.

GADOFOSVESET

Diagnostic Agent

PREGNANCY RECOMMENDATION: Limited Human Data—Animal Data Suggest Moderate Risk
BREASTFEEDING RECOMMENDATION: No Human Data—Potential Toxicity

PREGNANCY SUMMARY

Available gadolinium-based contrast agents are complexes with chelating agents that lower the potential toxicity in patients receiving the agents by preventing the cellular uptake of free gadolinium. The complexes cross the placenta to the fetus and are excreted by the fetal kidneys into the amniotic fluid, where they remain for long periods. The complexes themselves are relatively nontoxic, but dissociation may occur to release free gadolinium into the amniotic fluid, where it could expose fetal lungs and gut. Presently, the risk of gadolinium-induced toxicity in the fetus is unknown but may be harmful (1–3). A concern has been raised for a risk of gadolinium-induced nephrogenic systemic fibrosis (3). The American College of Radiology recommends that these agents should not be routinely used in pregnancy and, if such use is indicated, a written informed consent be obtained from the patient (1). In addition, the guidelines of the Contrast Media Safety Committee of the European Society of Urogenital Radiology and a review article recommend that gadolinium-based contrast media may be used in pregnancy if such use is important to the mother's health (4,5).

FETAL RISK SUMMARY

Gadofosveset, a paramagnetic agent, is a complex formed between a chelating agent and a paramagnetic ion, gadolinium. It is in the same subclass of gadolinium-based contrast agents as gadobenate dimeglumine, gadodiamide, gadopentetate dimeglumine, gadoteridol, and gadoversetamide. Gadofosveset trisodium is indicated for use as a contrast agent in magnetic resonance angiography (MRA) to evaluate aortoiliac occlusive disease in adults with known or suspected peripheral vascular disease. It binds reversibly to serum albumin, resulting in longer time in the vascular system than non-protein-binding contrast agents. Metabolism has not been detected and the mean elimination half-life is about 16 hours (6).

Reproduction studies have been conducted in rats and rabbits. In rats and rabbits, daily doses up to about 11 and 21.5 times, respectively, the human dose based on BSA (HD) did not cause fetal anomalies. In both species, the highest dose caused maternal toxicity. In rabbits, a daily dose 3 times the HD caused increased postimplantation loss, resorptions, and dead fetuses (6).

Long-term studies to evaluate the potential for carcinogenicity have not been conducted. Assays for mutagenicity and chromosome aberrations assay were negative. Male and female rat fertility was not impaired with daily doses up to 8.3 times the HD given for 4 and 2 weeks, respectively (6).

BREASTFEEDING SUMMARY

Although no reports describing the administration of gadofosveset during human lactation have been located, reviewers consider other gadolinium-based contrast media to be compatible with breastfeeding because of the very small amounts excreted into milk and potentially being absorbed by a nursing infant (2–4). The American Academy of Pediatrics classifies gadopentetate dimeglumine as compatible with breastfeeding (7) (see Gadopentetate Dimeglumine). However, gadofosveset has a much longer elimination half-life (16 hours) than other gadolinium-based contrast agents and, even though the agent is bound to albumin, the binding is reversible. Until human data are available, withholding breastfeeding for 24 hours or longer should lessen the amount available for excretion into breast milk.

G

References

1. Kanal E, Barkovich AJ, Bell C, Borgstede JP, Bradley WG Jr, Froelich JW, Gilk T, Gimbel JR, Gosbee J, Kuhni-Kaminski E, Lester JW Jr, Nyenhuis J, Parag Y, Schaefer DJ, Sebek-Scoumis EA, Weinreb J, Zaremba LA, Wilcox P, Lucey L, Sass N, for the ACR Blue Ribbon Panel on MR Safety. ACR guidance document for safe MR practices: 2007. AJR Am J Roentgenol 2007;188:1447–74.
2. Lin SP, Brown JJ. MR contrast agents: physical and pharmacologic basics. J Magn Reson Imaging 2007;25:884–99.
3. Chen MM, Coakley FV, Kaimal A, Laros RK Jr. Guidelines for computed tomography and magnetic resonance imaging use during pregnancy and lactation. Obstet Gynecol 2008;112:333–40.
4. Webb JAW, Thomsen HS, Morcos SK, and members of Contrast Media Safety Committee of European Society of Urogenital Radiology (ESUR). The use of iodinated and gadolinium contrast media during pregnancy and lactation. Eur Radiol 2005;15:1234–40.
5. Garcia-Bournissen F, Shrim A, Koren G. Safety of gadolinium during pregnancy. Can Fam Physician 2006;52:309–10.
6. Product information. Ablavar. Lantheus Medical Imaging, 2009.
7. Committee on Drugs, American Academy of Pediatrics. The transfer of drugs and other chemicals into human milk. Pediatrics 2001;106:776–89.

GADOPENTETATE DIMEGLUMINE

Diagnostic Agent

PREGNANCY RECOMMENDATION: Limited Human Data—Animal Data Suggest Risk
BREASTFEEDING RECOMMENDATION: Compatible

PREGNANCY SUMMARY

Available gadolinium-based contrast agents are complexes with chelating agents that lower the potential toxicity in patients receiving the agents by preventing the cellular uptake of free gadolinium. The complexes cross the placenta to the fetus and are excreted by the fetal kidneys into the amniotic fluid, where they remain for long periods. The complexes themselves are relatively nontoxic, but dissociation may occur to release free gadolinium into the amniotic fluid, where it could expose fetal lungs and gut. Presently, the risk of gadolinium-induced toxicity in the fetus is unknown but may be harmful (1–3). A concern has been raised for a risk of gadolinium-induced nephrogenic systemic fibrosis (3). The American College of Radiology recommends that these agents should not be routinely used in pregnancy and, if such use is indicated, a written informed consent be obtained from the patient (1). In addition, the guidelines of the Contrast Media Safety Committee of the European Society of Urogenital Radiology and a review article recommend that gadolinium-based contrast media may be used in pregnancy if such use is important to the mother's health (4,5).

FETAL RISK SUMMARY

Gadopentetate dimeglumine, a paramagnetic agent, is a complex formed between a chelating agent and a paramagnetic ion, gadolinium. It is in the same subclass of gadolinium-based contrast agents as gadobenate dimeglumine, gadodiamide, gadoversetamide, and gadoteridol. Gadopentetate dimeglumine is indicated for use with magnetic resonance imaging (MRI) in adults, and pediatric patients (2 years of age and older) to visualize lesions with abnormal vascularity in the brain (intracranial lesions), spine, and associated tissues. It also is indicated for use with MRI in adults and pediatric patients (2 years of age and older) to facilitate the visualization of lesions with abnormal vascularity in the head, neck, and body (excluding the heart). Neither metabolism nor plasma protein binding has been detected. The mean elimination half-life is 1.6 hours (6).

Reproduction studies have been conducted in rats and rabbits. Although no congenital malformations were observed, daily IV doses in these species that were 7.5–12.5 times the human dose based on body weight (HD) resulted in slight retardation of development. Doses that were 2.5 times the HD did not cause this effect (6). The contrast agent crosses the placenta to the fetus in rabbits (7).

Long-term studies for carcinogenicity potential have not been conducted. The drug was not mutagenic or clastogenic in several assays. High doses impaired fertility in male and female rats, including dose-related irreversible toxicity of male rat reproductive organs (6).

In a 1997 report, 11 women at 16–37 weeks' gestation underwent gadolinium-enhanced MRI for suspected uterine or placental abnormalities (8). The placentas were rapidly and intensely enhanced immediately after administration of the contrast agent. Three patients were in the 2nd trimester and eight were in the 3rd trimester. All infants were healthy at birth (8).

A 1992 case report described the inadvertent IV bolus administration of gadopentetate dimeglumine (0.2 mmol/kg) to a woman with multiple sclerosis shortly after conception (9). Her last menstrual period had occurred 23 days before the MRI procedure, thus giving her an estimated gestational length of 9 days. Because this was before the period of organogenesis, the authors of the report concluded that the most likely adverse effect would have been an early spontaneous abortion, rather than congenital malformations. A normal pregnancy occurred, however, terminating in the delivery of a healthy baby girl at 39 weeks' gestation. The infant was developing normally at 3 months of age (9).

A 1993 report described two women at 3 and 5 months' gestation, respectively, who were given the contrast agent for MRI diagnosis of Crohn's disease (10). Both patients delivered healthy infants at term.

Eleven women with symptomatic hydronephrosis at 19–34 weeks' underwent gadolinium-enhanced (gadopentetate dimeglumine) MRI excretory urography (11). There were no adverse effects of the procedure in the pregnancies. All of the infants had good Apgar scores, none had a birth weight below the third centile adjusted for gestational age and sex, and one had an umbilical hernia.

A prospective cohort study, conducted by a teratology information service in Italy, described the outcomes of 26 women who had an MRI with gadopentetate dimeglumine immediately before or after conception (12). Two cases were exposed preconceptional (4 and 12 days after the last menstrual period) and 24 were exposed at about a mean 30 days after the last menstrual period. Because of the short half-life of the agent, all of the exposures occurred before organogenesis. The outcomes were two spontaneous abortions (SABs), one elective abortion (mother taking valproic acid), two infants with low birth weight, and one infant with a congenital anomaly (hemangiomas; mother exposed at 31 days). No information was available on the two SABs. The 23 live births were all at term (12).

BREASTFEEDING SUMMARY

Gadopentetate dimeglumine is excreted into breast milk. A woman breastfeeding her infant was given the contrast agent 13 weeks after birth (13). Small amounts of the drug were found in her milk at 2, 11, 17, and 24 hours with a cumulative amount of 1.60 mcg-mols (0.023% of the administered dose).

A 2000 study described the excretion of gadopentetate dimeglumine into the breast milk of 19 women (14). One woman who was undergoing MRI received 0.2 mmol/kg IV (15 mmol), but the other 18 women received 0.1 mmol/kg (mean 5.9 mmol). Breastfeeding was stopped for at least 24 hours. The cumulative amount of drug excreted into milk over 24 hours was 0.57 μmol (range 0.05–3.0 μmol). This amount was a mean 0.009% (range 0.001% to 0.04%) of the mother's dose. Because the amount excreted into milk would be far less than the recommended IV dose for neonates (200 μmol/kg), and because very little of orally administered gadopentetate dimeglumine is absorbed systemically, the authors concluded that waiting 24 hours to resume breastfeeding was not warranted (14). An editorial also concluded that waiting 24 hours was not required because of the small amounts in milk and the safety profile of the contrast agent in infants and children (15). The American Academy of Pediatrics classifies gadopentetate dimeglumine as compatible with breastfeeding (16), as do other reviewers (2–4).

References

1. Kanal E, Barkovich AJ, Bell C, Borgstede JP, Bradley WG Jr, Froelich JW, Gilk T, Gimbel JR, Gosbee J, Kuhni-Kaminski E, Lester JW Jr, Nyenhuis J, Parag Y, Schaefer DJ, Sebek-Scoumis EA, Weinreb J, Zaremba LA, Wilcox P, Lucey L, Sass N, for the ACR Blue Ribbon Panel on MR Safety. ACR guidance document for safe MR practices: 2007. AJR Am J Roentgenol 2007;188:1447–74.
2. Lin SP, Brown JJ. MR contrast agents: physical and pharmacologic basics. J Magn Reson Imaging 2007;25:884–99.
3. Chen MM, Coakley FV, Kaimal A, Laros RK Jr. Guidelines for computed tomography and magnetic resonance imaging use during pregnancy and lactation. Obstet Gynecol 2008;112:333–40.
4. Webb JAW, Thomsen HS, Morcos SK, and members of Contrast Media Safety Committee of European Society of Urogenital Radiology (ESUR). The use of iodinated and gadolinium contrast media during pregnancy and lactation. Eur Radiol 2005;15:1234–40.
5. Garcia-Bournissen F, Shrim A, Koren G. Safety of gadolinium during pregnancy. Can Fam Physician 2006;52:309–10.
6. Product information. Magnevist. Bayer HealthCare Pharmaceuticals, 2009.
7. Novak Z, Thurmond AS, Ross PL, Jones MK, Thornburg KL, Katzberg RW. Gadolinium-DTPA transplacental transfer and distribution in fetal tissue in rabbits. Invest Radiol 1993;28:828–30.
8. Marcos HB, Semelka RC, Worawattanakul S. Normal placenta: gadolinium-enhanced dynamic MR imaging. Radiology 1997;205:493–6.
9. Barkhof F, Heijboer RJJ, Algra PR. Inadvertent IV administration of gadopentetate dimeglumine during early pregnancy. AJR Am J Roentgenol 1992;158:1171.
10. Shoenut JP, Semelka RC, Silverman R, Yaffe CS, Micflikier AB. MRI in the diagnosis of Crohn's disease in two pregnant women. J Clin Gastroenterol 1993;17:244–7.
11. Spencer JA, Tomlinson AJ, Weston MJ, Lloyd SN. Early report: comparison of breath-hold MR excretory urography, Doppler ultrasound and isotope renography in evaluation of symptomatic hydronephrosis in pregnancy. Clin Radiol 2000;55:446–53.
12. De Santis M, Straface G, Cavaliere AF, Carducci B, Caruso A. Gadolinium periconceptional exposure: pregnancy and neonatal outcome. Acta Obstet Gynecol 2007;86:99–101.
13. Rofsky NM, Weinreb JC, Litt AW. Quantitative analysis of gadopentetate dimeglumine excreted in breast milk. J Magn Reson Imaging 1993;3:131–2.
14. Kubik-Huch RA, Gottstein-Aalame NM, Frenzel T, Seifert B, Puchert E, Wittek S, Debatin JF. Gadopentetate dimeglumine excretion into human breast milk during lactation. Radiology 2000;216:555–8.
15. Hylton NM. Suspension of breast-feeding following gadopentetate dimeglumine administration. Radiology 2000;216:325–6.
16. Committee on Drugs, American Academy of Pediatrics. The transfer of drugs and other chemicals into human milk. Pediatrics 2001;106:776–89.

G

GADOTERIDOL

Diagnostic Agent

PREGNANCY RECOMMENDATION: Limited Human Data—Animal Data Suggest Risk
BREASTFEEDING RECOMMENDATION: Limited Human Data—Probably Compatible

PREGNANCY SUMMARY

Available gadolinium-based contrast agents are complexes with chelating agents that lower the potential toxicity in patients receiving the agents by preventing the cellular uptake of free gadolinium. The complexes cross the placenta to the fetus and are excreted by the fetal kidneys into the amniotic fluid, where they remain for long periods. The complexes themselves are relatively nontoxic, but dissociation may occur to release free gadolinium into the amniotic fluid, where it could expose fetal lungs and gut. Presently, the risk of gadolinium-induced toxicity in the fetus is unknown but may be harmful (1–3). A concern has been raised for a risk of gadolinium-induced nephrogenic systemic fibrosis (3). The American College of Radiology recommends that these agents should not be routinely used in pregnancy and, if such use is indicated, a written informed consent be obtained from the patient (1). In addition, the guidelines of the Contrast Media Safety Committee of the European Society of Urogenital Radiology and a review article recommend that gadolinium-based contrast media may be used in pregnancy if such use is important to the mother's health (4,5).

FETAL RISK SUMMARY

Gadoteridol, a paramagnetic agent, is a nonionic complex formed between a chelating agent and a paramagnetic ion, gadolinium. It is in the same subclass of gadolinium-based contrast agents as gadobenate dimeglumine, gadodiamide, gadofosveset trisodium, gadopentetate dimeglumine, and gadoversetamide. Gadoteridol is indicated for use in MRI in adults and children over 2 years of age to visualize lesions with abnormal vascularity in the brain (intracranial lesions), spine, and associated tissues. It also is indicated for use in MRI in adults to visualize lesions in the head and neck. It is not known if gadoteridol is metabolized or if it binds to plasma proteins. The elimination half-life is about 1.57 hours (6).

Reproduction studies have been conducted in rats and rabbits. In rats, a daily IV dose given for 12 days during gestation that was six times the human dose based on mmol/m^2 (HD) doubled the incidence of postimplantation loss. This dose and a daily dose that was 40% lower given for 12 days caused an increase in spontaneous locomotor activity in rat offspring. In rabbits, an increase in the incidence of spontaneous abortions and early delivery was noted at a dose that was seven times the HD (6).

Studies to evaluate the potential for carcinogenicity or potential effects on fertility have not been conducted. Assays for mutagenicity and chromosome aberrations assay were negative. No effect on male and female rat fertility was observed with a low IV dose given three times weekly (6).

BREASTFEEDING SUMMARY

Although no reports describing the administration of gadoteridol during human lactation have been located, reviewers consider gadolinium contrast media to be compatible with breastfeeding because of the very small amounts excreted into milk and potentially being absorbed by a nursing infant (2–4). The American Academy of Pediatrics classifies gadopentetate dimeglumine as compatible with breastfeeding (7) (see Gadopentetate Dimeglumine).

References

1. Kanal E, Barkovich AJ, Bell C, Borgstede JP, Bradley WG Jr, Froelich JW, Gilk T, Gimbel JR, Gosbee J, Kuhni-Kaminski E, Lester JW Jr, Nyenhuis J, Parag Y, Schaefer DJ, Sebek-Scoumis EA, Weinreb J, Zaremba LA, Wilcox P, Lucey L, Sass N, for the ACR Blue Ribbon Panel on MR Safety. ACR guidance document for safe MR practices: 2007. AJR Am J Roentgenol 2007;188:1447–74.
2. Lin SP, Brown JJ. MR contrast agents: physical and pharmacologic basics. J Magn Reson Imaging 2007;25:884–99.
3. Chen MM, Coakley FV, Kaimal A, Laros RK Jr. Guidelines for computed tomography and magnetic resonance imaging use during pregnancy and lactation. Obstet Gynecol 2008;112:333–40.
4. Webb JAW, Thomsen HS, Morcos SK, and members of Contrast Media Safety Committee of European Society of Urogenital Radiology (ESUR). The use of iodinated and gadolinium contrast media during pregnancy and lactation. Eur Radiol 2005;15:1234–40.
5. Garcia-Bournissen F, Shrim A, Koren G. Safety of gadolinium during pregnancy. Can Fam Physician 2006;52:309–10.
6. Product information. Prohance. Bracco Diagnostics, 2007.
7. Committee on Drugs, American Academy of Pediatrics. The transfer of drugs and other chemicals into human milk. Pediatrics 2001;106:776–89.

GADOVERSETAMIDE

Diagnostic Agent

PREGNANCY RECOMMENDATION: Limited Human Data—Animal Data Suggest Risk
BREASTFEEDING RECOMMENDATION: Limited Human Data—Probably Compatible

PREGNANCY SUMMARY

Available gadolinium-based contrast agents are complexes with chelating agents that lower the potential toxicity in patients receiving the agents by preventing the cellular uptake of free gadolinium. The complexes cross the placenta to the fetus and are excreted by the fetal kidneys into the amniotic fluid, where they remain for long periods. The complexes themselves are relatively nontoxic, but dissociation may occur to release free gadolinium into the amniotic fluid, where it could expose fetal lungs and gut. Presently, the risk of gadolinium-induced toxicity in the fetus is unknown but may be harmful (1–3).

A concern has been raised for a risk of gadolinium-induced nephrogenic systemic fibrosis (3). The American College of Radiology recommends that these agents should not be routinely used in pregnancy and, if such use is indicated, a written informed consent be obtained from the patient (1). In addition, the guidelines of the Contrast Media Safety Committee of the European Society of Urogenital Radiology and a review article recommend that gadolinium-based contrast media may be used in pregnancy if such use is important to the mother's health (4,5).

FETAL RISK SUMMARY

Gadoversetamide, a paramagnetic agent, is a complex formed between a chelating agent (versetamide) and a paramagnetic ion (gadolinium). It is in the same subclass of gadolinium-based contrast agents as gadobenate dimeglumine, gadodiamide, gadofosveset trisodium, gadopentetate dimeglumine, and gadoteridol. Gadoversetamide is indicated for use with magnetic resonance imaging (MRI) in patients with abnormal blood–brain barrier or abnormal vascularity of the brain, spine, and associated tissues. The agent also is indicated for use with MRI to provide contrast enhancement and facilitate visualization of lesions with abnormal vascularity in the liver in patients who are highly suspect for structural abnormalities of liver on computed tomography. Neither metabolites nor plasma protein binding has been detected. The mean elimination half-life is about 104 ± 20 minutes (6).

Reproduction studies have been conducted in rats and rabbits. In rats, daily IV doses given for 5 weeks (including gestation) that were equal to the human dose based on BSA (HD) reduced neonatal weights from birth through weaning. A dose 0.2 times the HD did not cause the effect. Neither dose was maternal toxic. A daily IV dose given on gestational days 7–17 that was 10 times the HD did cause maternal toxicity, as well as reduced mean fetal weight, abnormal liver lobation, delayed ossification of sternebrae, and delayed behavioral development (startle reflex and air rights reflex). These effects were not observed with doses that were equal to the HD. In rabbits, daily IV doses given during gestational days 6–18 that were 1 and 4 times the HD caused forelimb flexures and cardiovascular changes (malformed thoracic arteries, a septal defect, and abnormal ventricle) in fetuses. These effects were not observed at doses that were 0.3 times the HD. Maternal toxicity was not observed at any dose (6).

Long-term studies to evaluate the potential for carcinogenicity have not been conducted. Genotoxicity assays were negative but a chromosome aberration assay was positive. In fertility studies, daily IV doses given for 4 and 7 weeks that were 6 and 4 times the HD, respectively, caused irreversible toxicity in male rat reproductive organs and impaired fertility. These effects were not observed with a dose equal to the HD, nor were they observed in similar studies conducted in dogs. In a rat single-dose study, no adverse effects were seen on the male reproductive system 24 hours and 14 days after doses that were 1–25 times the HD (6).

BREASTFEEDING SUMMARY

Although no reports describing the administration of gadoversetamide during human lactation have been located, reviewers consider gadolinium contrast media to be compatible with breastfeeding because of the very small amounts excreted into milk and potentially being absorbed by a nursing infant (2–4). The American Academy of Pediatrics classifies gadopentetate dimeglumine as compatible with breastfeeding (7) (see Gadopentetate Dimeglumine).

References

1. Kanal E, Barkovich AJ, Bell C, Borgstede JP, Bradley WG Jr, Froelich JW, Gilk T, Gimbel JR, Gosbee J, Kuhni-Kaminski E, Lester JW Jr, Nyenhuis J, Parag Y, Schaefer DJ, Sebek-Scoumis EA, Weinreb J, Zaremba LA, Wilcox P, Lucey L, Sass N, for the ACR Blue Ribbon Panel on MR Safety. ACR guidance document for safe MR practices: 2007. AJR Am J Roentgenol 2007;188:1447–74.
2. Lin SP, Brown JJ. MR contrast agents: physical and pharmacologic basics. J Magn Reson Imaging 2007;25:884–99.
3. Chen MM, Coakley FV, Kaimal A, Laros RK Jr. Guidelines for computed tomography and magnetic resonance imaging use during pregnancy and lactation. Obstet Gynecol 2008;112:333–40.
4. Webb JAW, Thomsen HS, Morcos SK, and members of Contrast Media Safety Committee of European Society of Urogenital Radiology (ESUR). The use of iodinated and gadolinium contrast media during pregnancy and lactation. Eur Radiol 2005;15:1234–40.
5. Garcia-Bournissen F, Shrim A, Koren G. Safety of gadolinium during pregnancy. Can Fam Physician 2006;52:309–10.
6. Product information. OptiMARK. Mallinckrodt, 2009.
7. Committee on Drugs, American Academy of Pediatrics. The transfer of drugs and other chemicals into human milk. Pediatrics 2001;106:776–89.

GALANTAMINE

Cholinesterase Inhibitor (CNS Agent)

PREGNANCY RECOMMENDATION: No Human Data—Animal Data Suggest Low Risk
BREASTFEEDING RECOMMENDATION: No Human Data—Potential Toxicity

PREGNANCY SUMMARY

No reports describing the use of galantamine in human pregnancy have been located. Because of its indication, such reports should be rare. Moreover, the animal data suggest that the risk to the embryo and/or fetus is low. Therefore, inadvertent exposure to galantamine during pregnancy should not be a reason for pregnancy termination.

FETAL RISK SUMMARY

Galantamine is a reversible cholinesterase inhibitor that is indicated for the treatment of mild-to-moderate dementia of the Alzheimer's type. The metabolites are apparently inactive. Plasma protein binding is low (18%) and the plasma elimination half-life is about 7 hours (1).

Reproduction studies have been conducted in rats and rabbits. In rats, a dose three times the maximum recommended human dose based on BSA (MRHD) given for 14 days before mating through organogenesis caused a slight increase in skeletal variations. No major malformations were observed with a dose seven times the MRHD. When rats were given doses three and seven times the MRHD from the beginning of organogenesis through postpartum day 21, pup weights were decreased. However, no other adverse effects on postnatal development were observed. The above doses also caused slight maternal toxicity. No impairment of fertility was observed in female rats given doses up to seven times the MRHD for 14 days or in male rats for 60 days before mating. In rabbits, doses up to 32 times the MRHD during organogenesis revealed no evidence of teratogenicity (1).

It is not known if galantamine crosses the human placenta. The molecular weight (about 287 for the free base), low plasma protein binding, and the moderately long plasma elimination half-life suggest that the drug will cross to the embryo and/or fetus.

BREASTFEEDING SUMMARY

No reports describing the use of galantamine during human lactation have been located. Because of its indication, such reports should be rare. The molecular weight (about 287 for the free base), its low plasma protein binding (18%), and moderately long plasma elimination half-life (about 7 hours) suggest that galantamine will be excreted into breast milk. The effects of this exposure on a nursing infant are unknown.

Reference

1. Product information. Razadyne. Janssen Pharmaceutica Products, 2004.

GALSULFASE

Endocrine/Metabolic Agent (Enzyme)

PREGNANCY RECOMMENDATION: No Human Data—Animal Data Suggest Low Risk
BREASTFEEDING RECOMMENDATION: No Human Data —Probably Compatible

PREGNANCY SUMMARY

No reports describing the use of galsulfase in human pregnancy have been located. The animal data in two species suggest low risk. Because Maroteaux-Lamy syndrome is a debilitating chronic disease, the drug should not be withheld because of pregnancy.

FETAL RISK SUMMARY

Galsulfase is a purified human enzyme that is produced by DNA technology. It is a glycoprotein that is given as weekly IV infusions. Galsulfase is indicated for patients with mucopolysaccharidosis VI (MPS V1; Maroteaux-Lamy syndrome) to improve walking and stair-climbing capacity. In 13 patients with MPS VI the medium half-life at weeks 1 and 24 were 9 and 26 minutes, respectively (1).

Reproduction studies have been conducted in rats and rabbits. In these species, IV doses up to about 0.5 and 0.97 times, respectively, the recommended human dose of 1 mg/kg based on BSA (RHD) revealed no evidence of impaired fertility or harm to the fetus (1).

Long-term studies in animals for carcinogenicity and mutagenicity have not been conducted. In male and female rats, an IV dose that was about 0.5 times the RHD had no effect on fertility and reproductive performance (1).

It is not known if galsulfase crosses the human placenta. The molecular weight (about 56,000) and brief half-life suggest that exposure of the embryo or fetus will be minimal, if it occurs at all.

Pregnant women treated with this agent are encouraged to enroll in the MPS VI Clinical Surveillance Program by calling 800-983-4587 (1).

BREASTFEEDING SUMMARY

No reports describing the use of galsulfase during lactation have been located. The molecular weight (about 56,000) and brief half-life (9–26 minutes) suggest that excretion into breast milk will be minimal, if it occurs at all. Moreover, as a glycoprotein, the agent would most likely be digested in the infant's gut.

Reference

1. Product information. Naglazyme. BioMarin Pharmaceutical, 2011.

GANCICLOVIR

Antiviral

PREGNANCY RECOMMENDATION: Compatible—Maternal Benefit >> Embryo–Fetal Risk
BREASTFEEDING RECOMMENDATION: No Human Data—Potential Toxicity

PREGNANCY SUMMARY

Cytomegalovirus (CMV) is the most common cause of congenital viral infection in the United States, infecting 0.2%–2.2% of all liveborn infants (1). Approximately 40% of primary CMV infections occurring during pregnancy will result in transplacental passage of the virus to the fetus. A relatively small percentage of these infants, however, will exhibit structural damage, such as symmetric growth restriction, hepatosplenomegaly, chorioretinitis, microphthalmia, cerebral calcification, hydrocephaly, and microcephaly. Some infants infected in utero will develop later toxicity as evidenced by deafness (CMV is the leading cause of congenital hearing loss), mental retardation, and impaired psychomotor development (1). The effectiveness of ganciclovir in preventing or ameliorating these effects is unknown. Only six cases of its use in human pregnancy are known. No adverse effects attributable to ganciclovir were apparent in the five cases with outcome details, although one infant had a positive CMV urine culture without signs or symptoms of infection. Long-term evaluation of three of the four exposed infants for late-appearing toxicity has not been reported. The fourth infant was developing normally at 3 years of age (2). Because of the potential for fetal toxicity and the known toxic effects in animals, some investigators have recommended that ganciclovir should only be used during pregnancy for life-threatening disease or in immunocompromised patients with major CMV infections, such as retinitis (3–5). The only approved indications for ganciclovir are for the treatment of CMV retinitis or prevention of CMV disease in immunocompromised patients or in solid organ transplant recipients (3). However, based on the above cases and avoiding the 1st trimester, if possible, the use of ganciclovir to prevent or treat fetal infection might be reasonable.

FETAL RISK SUMMARY

Ganciclovir, a synthetic nucleoside analog that inhibits replication of herpes viruses, is used in the treatment of CMV retinitis and other viral infections.

The drug is embryotoxic in mice and rabbits, causing fetal resorption in at least 85% of animals exposed to two times the human dose based on AUC (HD). Month-old male offspring of female mice administered 1.7 times HD before and during gestation and during lactation had hypoplastic testes and seminal vesicles and pathologic changes in the nonglandular region of the stomach. In pregnant rabbits given doses two times the HD, fetal effects included growth restriction and teratogenicity (cleft palate, anophthalmia/microphthalmia, aplastic kidneys and pancreas, hydrocephaly, and brachygnathia) (3).

Ganciclovir is both carcinogenic and mutagenic in mice (3). Moreover, inhibition of spermatogenesis has been observed in mice and dogs. One study using cultured fetal rat hepatocytes, however, found little or no toxic effects, in terms of cell growth and cell membrane permeability, of high concentrations (0.5–30 mcg/mL) of ganciclovir (6).

Passage of ganciclovir across the perfused human placenta has been reported (4,6). In a 1993 report, ganciclovir was found initially to concentrate on the maternal placental surface and then to cross passively, without metabolism, to the fetus (6). In a second study, ganciclovir and acyclovir were discovered to cross the placenta in approximately similar amounts by simple diffusion (4).

Six reports (three unpublished) have described the use of ganciclovir during human pregnancy (2,7,8). In the first case, a 31-year-old woman received a renal transplant approximately 3 weeks after her last menstrual period (LMP) (8 and 10 days after unprotected intercourse) (7). Medications related to maintaining the transplant included methylprednisolone tapered to prednisone, azathioprine, and cyclosporine. Other drugs added shortly after surgery were trimethoprim, nifedipine, and acyclovir. Her worsening hypertension was controlled with nifedipine. Six weeks after surgery (9 weeks after her LMP), she developed CMV infection that was treated with IV ganciclovir (2.5 mg/kg twice daily) for 2 weeks and a single dose of IV CMV hyperimmune globulin. CMV cultures were negative after treatment and remained so throughout the remainder of the pregnancy. A normal 2640-g male infant was born at 38 weeks' gestation with Apgar scores of 9 and 9 at 1 and 5 minutes, respectively. Placental villitis consistent with CMV was noted and the infant had a positive CMV urine culture, but he remained healthy and was developing normally at 18 months of age (7).

The second case involved a 29-year-old who was a CMV-negative woman and who had received a CMV-positive liver transplant (8). She became pregnant 5 months after the transplant. She received oral ganciclovir (3 g/day), tacrolimus, and prednisone before conception and throughout the 1st trimester. Ganciclovir was discontinued when pregnancy was diagnosed at 3 months' gestation. Steroid-induced hyperglycemia was not observed, but worsening preeclampsia and fetal distress resulted in delivery at 30 weeks' gestation of a 790-g female infant with Apgar scores of 4 and 7 at 1 and 5 minutes, respectively. No malformations were observed and, except for her small size and mild respiratory problems, she did well and was discharged home on day 50 of life. The author also mentioned three other, unpublished, ganciclovir-treated pregnancies that had been reported to the manufacturer. One patient had been lost to follow-up, one had been treated with IV ganciclovir during the last 4 weeks of pregnancy, and one had been treated with oral ganciclovir at 14–18 weeks' gestation. The two pregnancies with known outcomes resulted in normal infants (8).

A 2005 report described the use of ganciclovir to treat CMV infection in a fetus at 22 weeks' gestation (2). The mother had received a renal transplant before pregnancy and had been treated for CMV infection subsequent to a blood transfusion. Although the mother had no signs or symptoms of infection, an amniocentesis at 21–4/7 weeks' gestation suggested fetal CMV infection. Oral ganciclovir 3 g/day was started at 22 weeks'. At 25 weeks, a repeat amniocentesis revealed that the CMV–DNA level had decreased to within the negative range. The minimum inhibitory concentration for CMV was 3 μM, whereas the amniotic fluid concentration of ganciclovir was 14.5 μM. A cesarean section at 36 weeks' delivered a healthy female infant with no signs or symptoms of CMV infection. At 3 years of age, the child had no signs of neurological, ophthalmological, or developmental abnormalities (2).

BREASTFEEDING SUMMARY

No reports describing the use of ganciclovir during lactation have been located. Because of the potential for serious toxicity in a nursing infant, mothers taking ganciclovir should probably not breastfeed. However, the drug has been used in newborns. The pharmacokinetics of ganciclovir in newborns with congenital cytomegalovirus infections has been reported (9).

References

1. American College of Obstetricians and Gynecologists. Perinatal viral and parasitic infections. *ACOG Practice Bulletin*. No. 20, September 2000.
2. Puliyanda DP, Silverman NS, Lehman D, Vo A, Bunnapradist S, Radha RK, Toyoda M, Jordan SC. Successful use of oral ganciclovir for the treatment of intrauterine cytomegalovirus infection in a renal allograft recipient. Transpl Infect Dis 2005;7:71–4.
3. Product information. Cytovene. Roche Laboratories, 2001.
4. Gilstrap LC, Bawdon RE, Roberts SW, Sobhi S. The transfer of the nucleoside analog ganciclovir across the perfused human placenta. Am J Obstet Gynecol 1994;170:967–73.
5. DeArmond B. Safety considerations in the use of ganciclovir in immunocompromised patients. Transplant Proc 1991;23(Suppl 1):26–9.
6. Henderson GI, Hu ZQ, Yang Y, Perez TB, Devi BG, Frosto TA, Schenker S. Ganciclovir transfer by human placenta and its effects on rat fetal cells. Am J Med Sci 1993;306:151–6.
7. Miller BW, Howard TK, Goss JA, Mostello DJ, Holcomb WL Jr, Brennan DC. Renal transplantation one week after conception. Transplantation 1995;60:1353–4.
8. Pescovitz MD. Absence of teratogenicity of oral ganciclovir used during early pregnancy in a liver transplant recipient. Transplantation 1999;67:758–9.
9. Trang JM, Kidd L, Gruber W, Storch G, Demmler G, Jacobs R, Dankner W, Starr S, Pass R, Stagno S, Alford C, Soong S-J, Whitley RJ, Sommadossi J-P, and the NIAID Collaborative Antiviral Study Group. Linear single-dose pharmacokinetics of ganciclovir in newborns with congenital cytomegalovirus infections. Clin Pharmacol Ther 1993;53:15–21.

GARLIC

Herb

PREGNANCY RECOMMENDATION: Compatible
BREASTFEEDING RECOMMENDATION: Compatible

PREGNANCY SUMMARY

Ingestion of garlic as a food flavoring appears to be safe during pregnancy. The herb has been used since ancient times and its use is so common that it is doubtful that it presents any risk to the embryo or fetus. Some components of garlic do cross the placenta to the fetus, as shown by detection of a garlic odor in the amniotic fluid and on the newborn's breath. The use of high-dose garlic during gestation is not common and apparently has not been reported. Moreover, the lack of standardization of therapeutic garlic preparations would make any such study suspect unless analysis of the chemical constituents of the actual product used in the study was also reported. The complete lack of data on the outcome of animal or human pregnancies after high-dose garlic does not allow any assessment of its fetal risk. At least one source considers the use of large amounts of garlic during pregnancy to be contraindicated because of the potential for inducing menstruation or uterine contractions (1).

FETAL RISK SUMMARY

Allium sativum L. (Family, Alliaceae), better known as garlic, is a perennial bulb used as a food flavoring. In much higher doses, the herb has been used for medicinal purposes since ancient times. The medicinal parts of garlic are the whole fresh bulb, the dried bulb, and the oil. Studies have demonstrated antibacterial, antimycotic, lipid-lowering, and platelet aggregation inhibition properties. Garlic may prolong bleeding and clotting time and enhance fibrinolytic activity. The average daily doses for medicinal indications are 4 g of fresh garlic, 8 mg of essential oil, and one or two fresh garlic cloves (1–5).

The primary chemical constituents of garlic are the alliins (alkylcysteine sulfoxides), in particular the odorless, colorless amino acid, alliin (S-allyl-L-cysteine sulfoxide). This amino acid, which has no pharmacologic activity, is converted by the enzyme, allinase (released from neighboring vascular bundle sheath cells by cutting or crushing the bulb) to allicin (diallyl-disulfide-mono-S-oxide, but also known as diallyl thiosulfinate responsible for the pungent characteristic garlic odor), a sulfur-containing volatile oil. The unstable allicin then undergoes further changes to two major products, diallyldisulfide (a predominant compound in garlic breath) and diallytrisulfide, and several minor products, cycloalliin, vinyl dithiins, ajoene (4,5,9, trithiadodeca-1,6,11-triene 9-oxide), and methylallyltrisulfide (2–5).

Depending on the method of preparation, commercial garlic products may vary widely in their content of allicin, especially those in oil (4). In some cases, no detectable levels of allicin were found. A 1992 study that evaluated 18 garlic preparations of the approximate 70 that were commercially available in Germany found that only five had an allicin content equivalent to 4 g of fresh garlic, the average daily dose required for therapeutic effects. The other 13 products were considered "expensive placebos" because they had no pharmacologic activity (4).

Korean garlic juice was administered to rats to investigate whether it would protect against embryotoxicity induced by maternal ingestion of methylmercuric chloride (6). Analysis of Korean garlic juice indicated that it contained several types of free amino acids, including (numbers in parentheses is the number of amino acids for each type) neutral ($N = 7$), sulfur-containing ($N = 3$), acidic ($N = 2$), basic ($N = 2$), imino acid ($N = 1$), and aromatic acid ($N = 3$) with a total content of approximately 55 mg/mL. The pregnant rats were given 20 mg of methylmercuric chloride on gestational day 7 and then treated with either 0.5 or 1.0 g/kg Korean garlic juice or saline. A fourth group of rats was not treated with mercury or garlic juice. Korean garlic juice was effective, in a dose-related manner, in preventing or reversing the toxicity of organic mercury in terms of increasing maternal and fetal body weights, increasing fetal survival, and decreasing mercury levels in the organs and blood of dams and fetuses. The investigators concluded that the effects of Korean garlic juice were most likely due to the thiol groups found on several of the amino acids that resulted in chelation of the mercury, thereby protecting essential maternal and fetal enzyme systems (6).

Some of the chemical components apparently cross the placenta of animals and humans. In fetal sheep, the taste system develops between 50 and 100 days after conception (7). To determine if garlic crosses the sheep placenta, sheep were administered 6 mL of Egyptian garlic oil by gavage on approximately day 110 of gestation. A sensory panel of 16 judges, selected because of demonstrated ability to detect dilute concentrations of garlic in water, was used to determine if the odor was present in allantoic and amniotic fluid, fetal blood, and maternal blood. Samples were drawn at 0, 50, 100, and 150 minutes after the maternal dose. Paired samples (treated and untreated) were presented to each judge. Garlic odor was detected in amniotic fluid at 100 and 150 minutes and in allantoic fluid, fetal blood, and maternal blood at 50, 100, and 150 minutes (7). In a brief letter, one correspondent said the odor of garlic had been noted on the breath of some human newborns (8). In a 1995 study, a sensory panel of 13 judges, screened for normal olfactory function, smelled paired samples of amniotic fluid from 10 women (9). At 48 minutes before amniocentesis in the 2nd trimester, five of the women received capsules containing the essential oil of garlic and five received placebo capsules containing lactose. The odor of garlic was judged stronger in four of the five women who had ingested the capsules with garlic. Therefore, this study demonstrated that components of garlic were transferred across the placenta and altered the odor of amniotic fluid (9). Although the specific components of garlic in the amniotic fluid were not identified, allicin (diallyl thiosulfinate) and at least one of its degradation products (diallyldisulfide) were most likely present because these are responsible for the characteristic odor of garlic (see above).

Two brief reports by a group of investigators in London stated that garlic might have benefits in preventing preeclampsia and intrauterine growth restriction (IUGR) (10,11). In an in vitro experiment, the investigators added increasing concentrations of garlic extract to a homogenate of human placental villous tissue to demonstrate a dose-related increase in nitric oxide synthase (enzyme that produces nitric oxide) activity (10). Because both calcium-dependent and calcium-independent nitric oxide synthase activities are decreased in preeclampsia and IUGR, the researchers speculated that garlic might be beneficial in these vascular conditions. In the second study, also using human placental villous tissue, both garlic extract and perchloric acid-treated garlic extract (allicin-negative) were shown to have cyclooxygenase inhibitor activity similar to that of aspirin (11).

G

BREASTFEEDING SUMMARY

Garlic ingestion by a lactating woman may impart garlic odor to her milk. The clinical significance of occasional garlic odor in milk appears to relate only to the amount of time the infant will be attached to the breast and this effect will disappear if the mother ingests the herb frequently.

At least some garlic constituents are excreted into breast milk. A 1994 study in lactating mice evaluated the effects on xenobiotic metabolizing enzymes in mouse pups from garlic administered to the mother (12). The lactating mice received either 200 or 400 mg/kg of crushed fresh garlic diluted in a volume of 0.1 mL of water for 14 or 21 days postpartum. Significant hepatic enzyme changes were measured in both the dams and pups, but the clinical significance of the changes is unknown.

Eight women, all exclusively breastfeeding their 3- to 4-month old infants, were the subject of a study published in 1991 examining the effect of garlic on the odor of breast milk and the nursling's behavior (13). None of the women was a regular user of garlic and their consumption of other sulfur-containing foods was limited before and during the study. In addition to breastfeeding, milk samples were also collected from the women every hour for 4 hours. They were given either placebo or garlic (1.5 g of garlic extract) capsules on alternate days. A sensory panel of 11 judges, all screened for normal olfactory function, were able consistently to detect the odor of garlic from paired samples of expressed milk (treated and untreated) with a peak effect at 2 hours. It also appeared that the nursing infants detected the garlic odor because when the mother had ingested garlic capsules, the infants attached to the breast for significantly longer periods and sucked more. Although not significant, the infants also tended to consume more milk, but consumption may have been limited by the amount of milk available to the infant (13). A subsequent study confirmed that infants remained attached to the breast longer than usual when their mothers started taking garlic but that this effect disappeared with continued garlic ingestion (14).

The clinical significance of the above investigations is unknown. A review on the effect of various flavors in milk concluded that it was not known whether flavors such as garlic in milk had any effect on the subsequent development of food habits or willingness to accept new foods at weaning or later in life (15).

References

1. Garlic. *Natural Medicines Comprehensive Database*. Stockton, CA: Therapeutic Research Faculty, 1999:366–8.
2. Allium Sativum. Garlic. *PDR for Herbal Medicines*, Montvale, NJ: Medical Economics, 1998:626–8.
3. Garlic. Blumenthal M, ed. *The Complete German Commission E Monographs. Therapeutic Guide to Herbal Medicines*. Austin, TX: American Botanical Council, 1998:134.
4. Robbers JE, Tyler VE. *Tyler's Herbs of Choice. The Therapeutic Use of Phytomedicinals*. Binghamton, NY: Haworth Press, 2000:132–7.
5. Garlic. *The Lawrence Review of Natural Products*. St. Louis, MO: Facts and Comparisons, 1994.
6. Lee JH, Kang HS, Roh J. Protective effects of garlic juice against embryotoxicity of methylmercuric chloride administered to pregnant Fischer 344 rats. Yonsei Med J 1999;40:483–9.
7. Nolte DL, Provenza FD, Callan R, Panter KE. Garlic in the ovine fetal environment. Physiol Behav 1992;52:1091–3.
8. Snell SB. Garlic on the baby's breath. Lancet 1973;2:43.
9. Mennella JA, Johnson A, Beauchamp GK. Garlic ingestion by pregnant women alters the odor of amniotic fluid. Chem Senses 1995;20:207–9.
10. Das I, Khan NS, Sooranna SR. Nitric oxide synthase activation is a unique mechanism of garlic action. Biochem Soc Trans 1995;23:136S.
11. Das I, Patel S, Sooranna SR. Effects of aspirin and garlic on cyclooxygenase-induced chemiluminescence in human term placenta. Biochem Soc Trans 1997;25:99S.
12. Chhabra SK, Rao AR. Transmammary exposure of mouse pups to allium sativum (garlic) and its effect on the neonatal hepatic xenobiotic metabolizing enzymes of mice. Nutrition Res 1994;14:195–210.
13. Mennella JA, Beauchamp GK. Maternal diet alters the sensory qualities of human milk and the nursling's behavior. Pediatrics 1991;88:737–44.
14. Mennella JA, Beauchamp GK. The effects of repeated exposure to garlic-flavored milk on the nursling's behavior. Pediatr Res 1993;34:805–8.
15. Mennella JA. Mother's milk: a medium for early flavor experiences. J Hum Lact 1995;11:39–45.

G

GATIFLOXACIN

Ophthalmic (Anti-infective)

PREGNANCY RECOMMENDATION: **No Human Data—Probably Compatible**
BREASTFEEDING RECOMMENDATION: **No Human Data—Probably Compatible**

PREGNANCY SUMMARY

No reports describing the use of ophthalmic gatifloxacin during human pregnancy have been located. The risk to an embryo or fetus appears to be nil because serum concentrations after ophthalmic use were below the lower limit of quantification. The oral and IV formulations have been withdrawn and only the ophthalmic preparation is available.

FETAL RISK SUMMARY

Gatifloxacin is a synthetic, broad-spectrum, fluoroquinolone antibacterial agent. It is in the same anti-infective class as ciprofloxacin, enoxacin, gemifloxacin, levofloxacin, lomefloxacin, moxifloxacin, norfloxacin, ofloxacin, sparfloxacin, and trovafloxacin. In an escalated dosing regimen up to 2 drops 8 times daily for 3 days, serum gatifloxacin concentrations were below the lower limit of quantification (5 ng/mL) (1).

In reproduction studies with rats and rabbits, oral doses up to about 1000 times the maximum recommended ophthalmic dose (MROD) were not teratogenic. In rats, skeletal/craniofacial anomalies or delayed ossification, atrial enlargement, and reduced fetal weight were observed in fetuses at about 3000 times the MROD. In a perinatal/postnatal study, increased postimplantation loss and neonatal/perinatal death were observed at a dose that was about 4000 times the MROD (1).

It is not known if gatifloxacin crosses the human placenta. Although the molecular weight of the hydrate (about 402) is low enough, serum concentrations are below the lower limit of quantification. Thus, clinically significant exposure of the embryo and/or fetus should not occur.

BREASTFEEDING SUMMARY

No reports describing the use of gatifloxacin in human lactation have been located. Because serum concentrations are below the lower limit of quantification (5 ng/mL), clinically significant amounts of gatifloxacin are not expected in breast milk.

Reference

1. Product information. Zymaxid. Allergan, 2012.

GEFITINIB

Antineoplastic (Tyrosine Kinase Inhibitor)

PREGNANCY RECOMMENDATION: **Limited Human Data—Animal Data Suggest Risk**
BREASTFEEDING RECOMMENDATION: **No Human Data—Potential Toxicity**

PREGNANCY SUMMARY

One report describing the use of gefitinib in the 2nd and 3rd trimesters has been located. There was developmental toxicity (growth restriction and death) in two animal species, but the very limited human pregnancy experience prevents a more complete assessment of the embryo–fetal risk.

FETAL RISK SUMMARY

Gefitinib is an oral epidermal growth factor receptor tyrosine kinase inhibitor. It is in the same subclass as several other agents (see Appendix). It is indicated as monotherapy for the continued treatment of patients with locally advanced or metastatic non-small-cell cancer after failure of other chemotherapies. Gefitinib is extensively metabolized and one of the metabolites is partially active. The elimination half-life of gefitinib is about 48 hours. Plasma protein binding to albumin and α-1 glycoprotein is 90% (1).

Reproduction studies have been conducted in rats and rabbits. Pregnant rats were treated from the beginning of organogenesis to the end of weaning with daily doses (5 mg/kg) that were about one-fifth the recommended human dose based on BSA (RHD), there was a decrease in the number of pups born alive. When the dose was increased to 20 mg/kg, the effect was more severe with more pups dying soon after birth. The no-effect dose was 1 mg/kg. In pregnant rabbits, a dose about twice the RHD caused reduced fetal weight (1). No mention of maternal toxicity was made in any of the animal studies.

Carcinogenicity studies have not been conducted with gefitinib. Genotoxicity studies in several tests were negative (1).

It is not known if gefitinib crosses the human placenta. After a single dose of 5 mg/kg (about one-fifth the RHD), gefitinib crossed the rat placenta (1). The molecular weight (about 447) and long elimination half-life suggest that gefitinib also will cross the human placenta.

A 2011 case report described a 38-year-old woman at 26 weeks' gestation who was diagnosed with lung cancer (2). The woman had never smoked. She was initially treated with erlotinib 100 mg/day and then changed about 2 weeks later to gefitinib 250 mg/day. Gefitinib was continued through the remainder of her pregnancy. At 36 weeks', she gave birth to a healthy 2.08-kg infant with an Apgar score of 9 at 1 minute. The baby weighed 2.98 kg 6 weeks later (2).

BREASTFEEDING SUMMARY

No reports describing the use gefitinib during human lactation have been located. The molecular weight (about 447) and long elimination half-life suggest that gefitinib will be excreted into breast milk. The effect of this exposure on a nursing infant is unknown, but could be serious. In adults, the most common adverse effects were diarrhea, rash, acne, dry skin, nausea, and vomiting. Until human data are available, the safest course is to not breastfeed while taking gefitinib.

References

1. Product information. Iressa. AstraZeneca Pharmaceuticals, 2007.
2. Lee CH, Liam CK, Pang YK, Chua KT, Lim BK, Lai NL. Successful pregnancy with epidermal growth factor receptor tyrosine kinase inhibitor treatment of metastatic lung adenocarcinoma presenting with respiratory failure. Lung Cancer 2011;74:349–51.

GEMCITABINE

Antineoplastic (Antimetabolite)

PREGNANCY RECOMMENDATION: **Contraindicated—1st Trimester**
BREASTFEEDING RECOMMENDATION: **Contraindicated**

PREGNANCY SUMMARY

Two case reports have described the use of gemcitabine in the 2nd trimester. One of the reports speculated that two unusual complications (chronic lung disease and excessive lung excretions) might have been related to the therapy. The animal data suggest risk. Gemcitabine is indicated for the treatment of cancers with a high mortality, often in combination with other antineoplastics. Nevertheless, the maternal benefit appears to outweigh the unknown fetal risk, but avoiding organogenesis is a reasonable option.

FETAL RISK SUMMARY

Gemcitabine is a nucleoside analog antineoplastic. It is classified as an antimetabolite in the subclass of pyrimidine analogs. Other antineoplastic agents in the subclass are capecitabine, cytarabine, floxuridine, and fluorouracil. Gemcitabine is indicated in combination with carboplatin for ovarian cancer, with paclitaxel for breast cancer, and with cisplatin for non-small-cell lung cancer. It also is indicated for locally advanced or metastatic adenocarcinoma of the pancreas. Gemcitabine is metabolized intracellularly to the active diphosphate and triphosphate nucleosides. Gemcitabine triphosphate can be extracted from peripheral blood mononuclear cells and has a half-life of the terminal phase from these cells of 1.7–19.4 hours. An inactive metabolite is found in the plasma. The half-lives of gemcitabine in women 29 and 45 years of age were 49 and 57 minutes, respectively. Plasma protein binding is negligible (1).

Reproduction studies have been conducted in mice and rabbits. In mice, gemcitabine was embryotoxic, causing cleft palate and incomplete ossification at doses about 1/200th of the recommended human dose based on BSA (RHD). This dose was also maternally toxic. Fetotoxicity or embryolethality was observed at about 1/1300th of the RHD (1). A 1993 study in mice that was conducted by the manufacturer expanded on the maternal and developmental toxicities noted above (2). In rabbits, embryotoxicity (decreased fetal viability, reduced live litter sizes, and developmental delays) and fetotoxicity (fused pulmonary artery and absence of the gall bladder) at doses about 1/600th of the RHD (1).

Carcinogenesis studies have not been conducted with gemcitabine. The drug was associated with mutagenic and clastogenic effects in some assays. Effects on the fertility of male mice were noted at a dose 1/700th of the RHD, consisting of hypospermatogenesis, decreased fertility, and decreased implantations. The fertility of female mice was not affected at doses up to about 1/200th of the RHD (1).

It is not known if gemcitabine crosses the human placenta. The molecular weight (about 264 for the free base) and negligible plasma protein binding suggest that the drug will cross the placenta. However, the very short plasma elimination half-life of the drug should reduce the amount reaching the embryo–fetus.

A 2008 report described the use of gemcitabine, docetaxel, and cisplatin in a woman who had lung cancer with brain metastases and an unrecognized pregnancy (3). Very early in gestation, she underwent craniotomy with tumor removal, followed by whole brain irradiation. Starting at 9 weeks' gestation, she was treated with four cycles of docetaxel and cisplatin (days 1 and 8) every 3 weeks. At 19 weeks', therapy was changed to gemcitabine and cisplatin (days 1 and 8) at 3-week intervals for two cycles. About 2 months after the last dose, her pregnancy was diagnosed. A cesarean section was performed at 33 weeks to deliver a normal, 1490-g female infant (normal karyotype 46, XX) with Apgar scores of 8, 9, and 10 at 1, 5, and 10 minutes, respectively, and normal blood counts. An extensive examination of the infant failed to find any abnormalities. She was developing normally at 10 months of age (3).

In a second case, a 38-year-old woman was treated for lung cancer at 25 weeks' gestation with gemcitabine (1000 mg/m^2 on day 1 and 8) and carboplatin AUC 5 (day 1) (4). She gave birth by an elective cesarean section at 28 4/7 weeks to a baby girl with Apgar scores of 7 and 9 at 1 and 5 minutes, respectively. The infant had multiple complications secondary to prematurity. The authors speculated that two unusual features, chronic lung disease and excessive secretions from her lungs, might have been related to either the chemotherapy or an effect of the malignancy itself. At 8 months of age, the infant had been weaned off of oxygen therapy and her neurodevelopment was age-appropriate (4).

Occupational exposure of the mother to antineoplastic agents during pregnancy may present a risk to the fetus. A position statement from the National Study Commission on Cytotoxic Exposure and a research article involving some antineoplastic agents are presented in the monograph for cyclophosphamide (see Cyclophosphamide).

BREASTFEEDING SUMMARY

It is not known if gemcitabine is excreted into human breast milk. The molecular weight (about 264 for the free base) and negligible plasma protein binding suggest that the drug will be excreted into milk, but the very short elimination half-life (49–57 minutes) should mitigate the amount entering milk. However, the cytotoxicity of the drug and its use in combination with other antineoplastics strongly suggests that women being treated with gemcitabine should not breastfeed.

References

1. Product information. Gemzar. Eli Lilly, 2007.
2. Eudaly JA, Tizzano JP, Higdon GL, Todd GC. Developmental toxicity of gemcitabine, an antimetabolite oncolytic, administered during gestation to CD-1 mice. Teratology 1993;48:365–81.
3. Kim JH, Kim HS, Sung CW, Kim KJ, Kim CH, Lee KY. Docetaxel, gemcitabine, and cisplatin administered for non-small cell lung cancer during the first and second trimester of an unrecognized pregnancy. Lung Cancer 2008;59:270–3.
4. Gurumurthy M, Koh P, Singh R, Bhide A, Satodia P, Hocking M, Anbarasu A, Wood LEP. Metastatic non-small-cell lung cancer and the use of gemcitabine during pregnancy. J Perinatol 2009;29:63–5.

GEMFIBROZIL

Antilipemic Agent

PREGNANCY RECOMMENDATION: Limited Human Data—Animal Data Suggest Risk
BREASTFEEDING RECOMMENDATION: No Human Data—Potential Toxicity

PREGNANCY SUMMARY

The animal data suggest risk, but the limited human pregnancy experience prevents a more complete assessment of the embryo–fetal risk. Teratogenic effects secondary to the drug have not been observed in the few case reports. Because the drug is used for a severe maternal condition, it should not be withheld, if indicated, because of pregnancy, but starting therapy after the 1st trimester should be considered.

FETAL RISK SUMMARY

Gemfibrozil is a lipid-regulating agent. It is indicated as adjunctive therapy to diet for treatment of adult patients with very high serum triglyceride levels who present a risk of pancreatitis and who do not respond adequately to a determined dietary effort. The drug is extensively metabolized to multiple metabolites, one of which may be active (see reference 9). Gemfibrozil is highly bound to plasma proteins but may be displaced by other drugs. The plasma half-life is 1.5 hours following multiple doses (1).

Reproductive tests have been conducted in rats and rabbits. In male and female rats, gemfibrozil was tumorigenic (benign liver nodules, liver carcinoma, and benign Leydig cell tumors) at 0.2 and 1.3 times the human exposure based on AUC. Treatment of female rats before and during gestation with 0.6 and 2 times the human dose based on BSA (HD) produced dose-related decreases in the conception rate, birth weight, and pup growth during lactation, and increased skeletal variations. Anophthalmia was observed rarely. The highest dose also resulted in an increased rate of stillbirths. Pregnant rabbits given 1 and 3 times the HD during organogenesis had a decreased litter size and, at the highest dose, an increased incidence of parietal bone variations (1). Two other studies have found no evidence of reproductive or teratogenic effects in rats and rabbits (2, 3).

It is not known if gemfibrozil crosses the human placenta during early pregnancy. The molecular weight (about 250) suggests that the drug will cross to the embryo–fetus. Although the extensive metabolism, high plasma protein binding, and short half-life should limit the exposure, the drug and an active metabolite cross near term (see reference 9).

In a surveillance study of Michigan Medicaid recipients involving 229,101 completed pregnancies conducted between 1985 and 1992, 8 newborns had been exposed to gemfibrozil during the 1st trimester and 7 in the 2nd or 3rd trimester (4). One defect, a structural brain anomaly, was observed in an infant delivered from a mother who took the agent after the 1st trimester. In a separate case included in this report, an infant with Pierre Robin syndrome, suspected of being associated with 1st trimester exposure to gemfibrozil, was reported retrospectively to the FDA. The syndrome (cleft palate–micrognathia–glossoptosis) was most likely due to autosomal recessive inheritance (4).

A 1992 report described the use of gemfibrozil starting at 20 weeks' gestation in a 33-year-old woman with eruptive xanthomas (5). The patient had a similar condition in her first pregnancy that included hypertriglyceridemia, fulminant pancreatitis, and acute respiratory distress syndrome (5). A dose of 600 mg 4 times daily for 2 months lowered the triglyceride level from 7530 to 4575 mg/dL, and the total cholesterol level from 1515 to 1325 mg/dL, but the xanthomas persisted throughout her pregnancy. A healthy, term infant (birth weight and sex not specified) was eventually delivered (5).

A 1999 case report described the use of gemfibrozil 600 mg twice daily in a 22-year-old woman for severe acute pancreatitis due to hypertriglyceridemia throughout pregnancy (except for gestational week 11) (6). After treatment in the hospital, she did well during the remainder of her pregnancy without a recurrence of her pancreatitis or other complications. She gave birth to a full-term, healthy, male infant (no other details on the infant were given) (6).

A 29-year-old woman with lipoatrophic diabetes mellitus was treated throughout gestation with gemfibrozil 600 mg twice daily (7). The lipoatrophic diabetes was thought to be consistent with congenital partial lipodystrophy (Kobberling-Dunnigan syndrome). At 37 weeks' gestation, labor was induced and she gave birth to a 2800-g female infant with Apgar scores of 7 and 8. No other information about the infant was provided (7).

A 18-year-old woman with familial chylomicronemia syndrome had lipoprotein lipase deficiency and hypertriglyceridemia since birth (8). During pregnancy, she was managed with a very-low-fat diet and, in the 3rd trimester, with gemfibrozil. Because of a risk for pancreatitis, labor was induced at 38 weeks' and she gave birth to a healthy 2.77-kg male infant. No details on the infant were given (8).

A 23-year-old woman with primary lipoprotein lipase deficiency was managed with a low-fat diet throughout gestation (9). In week 29, gemfibrozil 600 mg/day was started and increased to 900 mg/day a week later. A second episode of pancreatitis prompted labor induction at 35 weeks and a female infant (about 2355 g) with a 5-minute Apgar of 9 was delivered vaginally. Analysis of the cord blood revealed similar concentrations of gemfibrozil and its active metabolite in both umbilical vein and artery at levels within the normal reference for adults. The infant was intubated for 48 hours for respiratory distress. The mother and her daughter were both healthy and doing well 11 years later (9).

BREASTFEEDING SUMMARY

No reports describing the use of gemfibrozil during lactation have been located. The molecular weight (about 250) suggests that the drug will be excreted into milk. However, the extensive metabolism, high plasma protein binding, and short half-life (1.5 hours) should limit the exposure. Nevertheless, there is a potential for severe toxicity in a nursing infant and the drug should probably not be used during breastfeeding.

References

1. Product information. Gemfibrozil. Watson Laboratories, 2004.
2. Kurtz SM, Fitzgerald JE, Fisken RA, Schardein JL, Reutner TF, Lucas JA. Toxicological studies on gemfibrozil. Proc R Soc Med 1976;69(Suppl 2): 15–23. As cited in Schardein JL. *Chemically Induced Birth Defects*. 2nd ed. New York, NY: Marcel Dekker, 1993:81.
3. Fitzgerald JE, Petrere JA, De La Iglesia FA. Experimental studies on reproduction with the lipid-regulating agent gemfibrozil. Fund Appl Toxicol 1987;8:454–64. As cited in Shepard TH. *Catalog of Teratogenic Agents*. 7th ed. Baltimore, MD: The Johns Hopkins University Press, 1992:188.
4. Rosa F. *Anti-cholesterol Agent Pregnancy Exposure Outcomes*. Presented at the 7th International Organization for Teratogen Information Services, Woods Hole, MA, April 1994.
5. Jaber PW, Wilson BB, Johns DW, Cooper PH, Ferguson JE II. Eruptive xanthomas during pregnancy. J Am Acad Dermatol 1992;27:300–2.
6. Saadi HF, Kurlander DJ, Erkins JM, Hoogwerf BJ. Severe hypertriglyceridemia and acute pancreatitis during pregnancy: treatment with gemfibrozil. Endocr Pract 1999;5:33–6.
7. Morse AN, Whitaker MD. Successful pregnancy in a woman with lipoatrophic diabetes mellitus: a case report. J Reprod Med 2000;45:850–2.
8. Al-Shali K, Wang J, Fellows F, Huff MW, Wolfe BM, Hegele RA. Successful pregnancy outcome in a patient with severe chylomicronemia due to compound heterozygosity for mutant lipoprotein lipase. Clin Biochem 2002;35:125–30.
9. Tsai E, Brown JA, Veldee MY, Anderson GJ, Chait A, Brunzell JD. Potential of essential fatty acid deficiency with extremely low fat diet in lipoprotein lipase deficiency during pregnancy: a case report. BMC Pregnancy Childbirth 2004;4:27.

GEMIFLOXACIN

Anti-infective (Quinolone)

PREGNANCY RECOMMENDATION: Human Data Suggest Low Risk
BREASTFEEDING RECOMMENDATION: No Human Data—Probably Compatible

PREGNANCY SUMMARY

No reports describing the use of gemifloxacin during human pregnancy have been located. The animal toxicity (fetal growth restriction) observed at exposures close to those obtained in humans should be considered before this agent is used in pregnant women. Moreover, some reviewers have concluded that all fluoroquinolones should be considered contraindicated in pregnancy (e.g., see Ciprofloxacin and Norfloxacin) because safer alternatives are usually available.

FETAL RISK SUMMARY

Gemifloxacin is a synthetic, broad-spectrum, fluoroquinolone antibacterial agent. It is in the same anti-infective class as ciprofloxacin, enoxacin, gatifloxacin, levofloxacin, lomefloxacin, moxifloxacin, norfloxacin, ofloxacin, sparfloxacin, and trovafloxacin. Gemifloxacin is available in an oral formulation. Gemifloxacin and its metabolites are primarily eliminated in the feces (about 61%), with the remainder excreted in the urine (about 36%). Plasma protein binding ranges from 55% to 73% and the elimination half-life is about 7 hours (range 4–12 hours) (1).

Reproduction studies have been conducted with gemifloxacin in mice, rats, and rabbits. Fetal growth restriction was observed in all three species given doses resulting in exposures, based on AUC, that were two-, four-, and three-fold greater, respectively, than those obtained in women given oral doses of 325 mg (HD). The growth restriction appeared to be reversible in rats, but this was not studied in mice and rabbits. In rats, a dose eight times the HD not only caused fetal brain and ocular malformations but also caused maternal toxicity. The no-observed-effect-level (NOEL) in pregnant animals was about 0.8–3 times the HD (1).

It is not known if gemifloxacin crosses the human placenta. The molecular weight of the mesylate salt (about 485), plasma protein binding (55%–73%), and elimination half-life (about 7 hours) suggest that passage to the fetus should be expected.

BREASTFEEDING SUMMARY

No reports describing the use of gemifloxacin in lactating humans have been located. The molecular weight (about 485), plasma protein binding (55%–73%), and elimination half-life (about 7 hours) suggest that the drug will be excreted into breast milk. The effect of this exposure on a nursing infant is unknown. However, other fluoroquinolones are classified by the American Academy of Pediatrics as compatible with breastfeeding (see Ciprofloxacin).

Reference

1. Product information. Factive. GeneSoft Pharmaceuticals, 2004.

GEMTUZUMAB OZOGAMICIN

[Withdrawn from the marker. See 9th edition.]

GENTAMICIN

Antibiotic (Aminoglycoside)

PREGNANCY RECOMMENDATION: Human Data Suggest Low Risk
BREASTFEEDING RECOMMENDATION: Compatible

PREGNANCY SUMMARY

Gentamicin is used frequently in pregnancy to treat maternal infections. Developmental toxicity has not been associated with this agent.

FETAL RISK SUMMARY

Gentamicin is an aminoglycoside antibiotic. The antibiotic did not impair fertility or cause fetal harm in rats and rabbits (1). Not surprisingly, gentamicin produces dose-related nephrotoxicity in fetal rats (2–4). High doses (110 mg/kg/day SC) of gentamicin during gestation have also been shown to produce significant and persistent increases in the blood pressure, as well as nephrotoxicity, in exposed rat offspring (5).

Gentamicin rapidly crosses the placenta into the fetal circulation and amniotic fluid (6–15). Following 40- to 80-mg IM doses given to patients in labor, peak cord serum levels averaging 34%–44% of maternal levels were obtained at 1–2 hours (6,9,13,14). Following a single 80-mg IM injection before delivery, mean peak amniotic fluid concentrations (5.17 mcg/mL) occurred at 8 hours (14). No toxicity attributable to gentamicin was seen in any of the newborns. Patients undergoing 1st and 2nd trimester abortions were given 1 mg/kg IM (10). Gentamicin could not be detected in their cord serum before 2 hours. Amniotic fluid levels were undetectable at this dose up to 9 hours after injection. Doubling the dose to 2 mg/kg allowed detectable levels in the fluid in one of two samples 5 hours after injection.

The pharmacokinetics of gentamicin in 23 women with pyelonephritis at a mean gestational age of 21.8 weeks was described in 1994 (16). Similar to that observed in postpartum women, standard weight-adjusted doses of gentamicin produced low, subtherapeutic serum levels in most of the women.

A brief study published in 2000 compared gentamicin serum levels in infants of women who had received the antibiotic IV (240-mg single daily dose vs. 80 mg 3 times daily) during labor (17). In the single daily dose group ($N = 11$), all of the mothers had received one dose a mean 5.12 hours before delivery, whereas in the divided-dose group ($N = 10$), 9 of 10 mothers received one dose a mean 4.72 hours before delivery. The mean serum levels in the newborn infants were 1.94 and 0.98 mcg/mL, respectively ($p = 0.01$). There was no correlation between the infant's serum level and the time interval from the mother's dose (17). Based on their analysis, the authors concluded that the divided-dose regimen was best for women in labor (17).

In an abstract published in 1997, women undergoing midtrimester terminations received gentamicin either as a 10-mg intra-amniotic infusion ($N = 16$) or a single 80-mg IV dose (18). Low median gentamicin plasma levels were measured in the mothers and fetuses after the intra-amniotic dose: 0.28 mcg/mL in the mothers and 0.4 mcg/mL in the fetuses. In contrast, the median amniotic fluid concentration, 46 mcg/mL, was sustained for >24 hours. After IV dosing, amniotic fluid concentrations were low throughout the study (median 0.35 mcg/mL). The authors concluded that intra-amniotic infusions of gentamicin were a safe method to administer the antibiotic without reaching toxic levels in the mother or the fetus (18).

Intra-amniotic instillations of gentamicin were given to 11 patients with premature rupture of the membranes (19). Ten patients received 25 mg every 12 hours and one received 25 mg every 8 hours, for a total of 1–19 doses per patient. Maternal gentamicin serum levels ranged from 0.063 to 6 mcg/mL (all but one were <0.6 mcg/mL and that one was believed to be caused by error). Cord serum levels varied from 0.063 to 2 mcg/mL (all but two were <0.6 mcg/mL). No harmful effects were seen in the newborns after prolonged exposure to high local concentrations of gentamicin.

Only one report linking the use of gentamicin to congenital defects has been located. A 34-year-old woman, who was not known to be pregnant at the time, received a 10-day course of gentamicin (300 mg/day) in gestational week 7 (20). The appropriateness of this dose cannot be determined because the mother's height and weight and renal function were not given. The mother was also treated with prednisolone (50 mg/day for 5 days) for an "allergic reaction" to the antibiotic. She delivered an apparently healthy, 2950-g (6 pounds 8 ounces) male infant at 37 weeks' gestation. His growth after birth was less than the 5th percentile and, at 4.5 years of age, the child was evaluated for short stature (<5th percentile). At this time, he was noted to have impaired renal function. Ultrasound examination revealed small kidneys, both <5th percentile for age, with increased echotexture, markedly decreased corticomedullary differentiation, and small bilateral cysts. Although the exact cause of the renal cystic dysplasia was unknown, and a potential genetic defect could not be excluded, the authors speculated, on the basis of animal studies, that the combination of gentamicin and prednisolone had induced the abnormal nephrogenesis.

Gentamicin, in combination with ampicillin ($N = 62$), was compared with two groups of women treated with cefazolin ($N = 58$) or ceftriaxone ($N = 59$) in a randomized trial of the treatment of acute pyelonephritis in pregnancy (21). The mean gestational age at the start of therapy was 14 to 15 weeks. There were no significant differences among the three groups in clinical or pregnancy outcomes. The pregnancy outcomes included gestational age at delivery, preterm delivery, birth weight, neonatal intensive care admission, and length of stay in the neonatal intensive care if admitted (21).

The population-based dataset of the Hungarian Case-Control Surveillance of Congenital Abnormalities, covering the period of 1980–1996, was used to evaluate the teratogenicity of aminoglycoside antibiotics (parenteral gentamicin, streptomycin, tobramycin, and oral neomycin) in a study published in 2000 (22). A case group of 22,865 women who had fetuses or newborns with congenital malformations were compared with 38,151 women who had no newborns with structural defects. A total of 38 cases and 42 controls were treated with aminoglycosides. There were 19 women in the case and control groups, 0.08% and 0.05%, respectively, treated with gentamicin (odds ratio 1.7, 95% confidence interval 0.9–3.2). A case–control pair analysis for the 2nd and 3rd months of gestation also failed to show a risk for teratogenicity. The investigators concluded that there was no detectable teratogenic risk for structural defects for any of the aminoglycoside antibiotics (22). Although it was not investigated in this study, they also concluded that the risk of deafness after in utero aminoglycoside exposure was small.

Ototoxicity, which is known to occur after gentamicin therapy, has not been reported as an effect of in utero exposure. However, eighth-cranial nerve toxicity in the fetus is well known following exposure to other aminoglycosides (see Kanamycin and Streptomycin) and may potentially occur with gentamicin. Gentamicin and vancomycin, both of which can cause ototoxicity and nephrotoxicity, have been used together during pregnancy without apparent harm to the fetus or newborn (see Vancomycin).

Potentiation of $MgSO_4$-induced neuromuscular weakness has been reported in a neonate exposed during the last 32 hours of pregnancy to 24 g of $MgSO_4$ (23). The depressed infant was treated with gentamicin for sepsis at 12 hours of age. After the second dose, the infant's condition worsened with rapid onset of respiratory arrest. Emergency treatment was successful, and no lasting effects of the toxic interaction were noted.

BREASTFEEDING SUMMARY

Small amounts of gentamicin are excreted into breast milk and absorbed by the nursing infant. In a reference published in 1994, 10 women, who had just delivered term infants, were administered antibiotic prophylaxis with gentamicin (80 mg IM 3 times daily) (24). On the 4th day of a 5-day therapy course, milk and serum samples were obtained. The mean maternal serum levels of gentamicin at 1 and 7 hours after a dose were 3.94 and 1.02 mcg/mL, respectively. Mean milk levels at 1, 3, 5, and 7 hours after a dose were 0.42, 0.48, 0.49, and 0.41 mcg/mL, respectively, providing mean milk:plasma ratios at 1 and 7 hours of 0.11 and 0.44, respectively. The infants were allowed to breastfeed 1 hour after a dose and serum samples were collected 1 hour later. Five of the 10 infants had detectable (>0.27 mcg/mL) gentamicin serum levels with a mean level of 0.41 mcg/mL.

In a case report, a nursing infant developed two grossly bloody stools while his mother was receiving gentamicin and clindamycin (25). The condition cleared rapidly when breastfeeding was discontinued. Although both antibiotics are known to be excreted into milk, the cause of the infant's diarrhea cannot be determined with certainty. The American Academy of Pediatrics classifies gentamicin as compatible with breastfeeding (26).

References

1. Product information. Garamycin. Schering, 1997.
2. Mallie JP, Coulon G, Billerey C, Faucourt A, Morin JP. In utero aminoglycosides-induced nephrotoxicity in rat neonates. Kidney Int 1988;33:36–44.
3. Smaoui H, Mallie J-P, Schaeverbeke M, Robert A, Schaeverbeke J. Gentamicin administered during gestation alters glomerular basement membrane development. Antimicrob Agents Chemother 1993;37:1510–7.
4. Lelievre-Pegorier M, Euzet S, Merlet-Benichou C. Effect of fetal exposure to gentamicin on phosphate transport in young rat kidney. Am J Physiol 1993;265:F807–12.
5. Stahlmann R, Chahoud I, Thiel R, Klug S, Forster C. The developmental toxicity of three antimicrobial agents observed only in nonroutine animal studies. Reprod Toxicol 1997;11:1–7.
6. Percetto G, Baratta A, Menozzi M. Observations on the use of gentamicin in gynecology and obstetrics. Minerva Ginecol 1969;21:1–10.
7. von Kobyletzki D. *Experimental Studies on the Transplacental Passage of Gentamicin.* Presented at Fifth International Congress on Chemotherapy, Vienna, 1967.
8. von Koblyetzki D, Wahlig H, Gebhardt F. *Pharmacokinetics of Gentamicin during Delivery. Antimicrobial Anticancer Chemotherapy.* Proceedings of the Sixth International Congress on Chemotherapy, Tokyo, 1969;1: 650–2.
9. Yoshioka H, Monma T, Matsuda S. Placental transfer of gentamicin. J Pediatr 1972;80:121–3.
10. Garcia S, Ballard C, Martin C, Ivler D, Mathies A, Bernard B. Perinatal pharmacology of gentamicin. Clin Res 1972;20:252.
11. Daubenfeld O, Modde H, Hirsch H. Transfer of gentamicin to the foetus and the amniotic fluid during a steady state in the mother. Arch Gynecol 1974;217:233–40.
12. Kauffman R, Morris J, Azarnoff D. Placental transfer and fetal urinary excretion of gentamicin during constant rate maternal infusion. Pediatr Res 1975;9:104–7.
13. Weinstein A, Gibbs R, Gallagher M. Placental transfer of clindamycin and gentamicin in term pregnancy. Am J Obstet Gynecol 1976;124:688–91.
14. Creatsas G, Pavlatos M, Lolis D, Kaskarelis D. Ampicillin and gentamicin in the treatment of fetal intrauterine infections. J Perinat Med 1980;8:13–8.
15. Gilstrap LC III, Bawdon RE, Burris J. Antibiotic concentration in maternal blood, cord blood, and placental membranes in chorioamnionitis. Obstet Gynecol 1988;72:124–5.
16. Graham JM, Blanco JD, Oshiro BT, Magee KP. Gentamicin levels in pregnant women with pyelonephritis. Am J Perinatol 1994;11:40–41.
17. Regev RH, Litmanowitz I, Arnon S, Shiff J, Dolfin T. Gentamicin serum concentrations in neonates born to gentamicin-treated mothers. Pediatr Infect Dis J 2000;19:890–1.
18. Barak J, Mankuta D, Pak I, Glezerman M, Katz M, Danon A. Transabdominal amnioinfusion of gentamicin: a pharmacokinetic study of maternal plasma and intraamniotic levels (abstract). Am J Obstet Gynecol 1997;176:S59.
19. Freeman D, Matsen J, Arnold N. Amniotic fluid and maternal and cord serum levels of gentamicin after intra-amniotic instillation in patients with premature rupture of the membranes. Am J Obstet Gynecol 1972;113:1138–41.
20. Hulton S-A, Kaplan BS. Renal dysplasia associated with in utero exposure to gentamicin and corticosteroids. Am J Med Genet 1995;58:91–3.
21. Wing DA, Hendershott CM, Debuque L, Millar LK. A randomized trial of three antibiotic regimens for the treatment of pyelonephritis in pregnancy. Obstet Gynecol 1998;92:249–53.
22. Czeizel AE, Rockenbauer M, Olsen J, Sorensen HT. A teratological study of aminoglycoside antibiotic treatment during pregnancy. Scand J Infect Dis 2000;32:309–13.
23. L'Hommedieu CS, Nicholas D, Armes DA, Jones P, Nelson T, Pickering LK. Potentiation of magnesium sulfate-induced neuromuscular weakness by gentamicin, tobramycin, and amikacin. J Pediatr 1983;102:629–31.
24. Celiloglu M, Celiker S, Guven H, Tuncok Y, Demir N, Erten O. Gentamicin excretion and uptake from breast milk by nursing infants. Obstet Gynecol 1994;84:263–5.
25. Mann CF. Clindamycin and breast-feeding. Pediatrics 1980;66:1030–1.
26. Committee on Drugs, American Academy of Pediatrics. The transfer of drugs and other chemicals into human milk. Pediatrics 2001;108: 776–89.

GENTIAN VIOLET

Disinfectant/Anthelmintic

PREGNANCY RECOMMENDATION: Limited Human Data—No Relevant Animal Data
BREASTFEEDING RECOMMENDATION: No Human Data—Potential Toxicity

PREGNANCY SUMMARY

The Collaborative Perinatal Project monitored 50,282 mother–child pairs, 40 of whom had 1st trimester exposure to gentian violet (1). Evidence was found to suggest a relationship to malformations based on defects in 4 patients. Independent confirmation is required to determine the actual risk.

BREASTFEEDING SUMMARY

No reports describing the use of gentian violet during human lactation have been located.

Reference

1. Heinonen OP, Slone D, Shapiro S. *Birth Defects and Drugs in Pregnancy*. Littleton, MA: Publishing Sciences Group, 1977:302.

GINGER

Herb

PREGNANCY RECOMMENDATION: Compatible
BREASTFEEDING RECOMMENDATION: No Human Data—Probably Compatible

G

PREGNANCY SUMMARY

There is no evidence of ginger-induced developmental toxicity. The herb has been used safely as an antiemetic for nausea and vomiting of pregnancy.

FETAL RISK SUMMARY

The rhizome of the perennial plant, ginger (*Zingiber officinale*), is used as a dried powdered spice in foods and as a natural medicine for its alleged carminative, cardiotonic, antithrombotic, antibacterial, antioxidant, antitussive, antiemetic, stimulant, antihepatotoxic, anti-inflammatory, antimutagenic, diaphoretic, diuretic, spasmolytic, immunostimulant, and cholagogue actions (1). The active ingredients in ginger are thought to be primarily a class of structurally cardiotonic compounds called gingerols. Other pharmacologically active compounds that have been identified in ginger include shogaol, dehydrogingerdiones, gingerdiones, and zingerone. Some of these ingredients inhibit prostaglandin synthetase (cyclooxygenase) but, in some cases, this activity may be confined only to fresh ginger (1).

In a reproduction study, ginger tea (20 or 50 g/L) was given to rats during organogenesis (days 6–15) via their drinking water (2). The lower concentration (20 g/L) was equivalent to the ginger tea consumed by humans (2). No maternal toxicity or teratogenicity was seen, but early embryonic loss was double that of the controls ($p < 0.05$) at both doses. In addition, surviving fetuses, especially females, were significantly heavier than controls and had more advanced skeletal growth (2). Another rat study used a patented standardized ethanol extract of *Z. officinale* (EV.EXT 33) to administer doses up to 1000 mg/kg/day during organogenesis (3). Compared with a control group, no embryo toxicity, teratogenicity, or treatment-related adverse effects were observed in the pregnant rats or their offspring.

Several authors have commented on or reported, with mixed results, studies examining the antiemetic properties of ginger in nonpregnant patients (4–10), and a review of this topic was published in 2000 (11). The oral dose in the studies varied from 1 to 2 g/day of the powdered root or rhizome. Although the exact mechanism of action is unknown, it appears to be a local effect in the gastrointestinal tract rather than a central action (7,10). The effect may be mediated by antagonism of gastrointestinal 5-hydroxytryptamine (serotonin) to prevent stimulation of the vagus nerve and, thus, the vomiting center (8,10). One author commented that ginger has been long used in Chinese herbal or folk medicine for the treatment of pregnancy-induced nausea and vomiting (5).

The efficacy of ginger as an antiemetic in pregnancy was studied in a double-blind, randomized, cross-over trial involving women with hyperemesis gravidarum (12). All the subjects had been admitted to a hospital with hyperemesis and if their symptoms persisted for more than 2 days, they were enrolled in the study after giving informed consent. A total of 27 women at a mean gestational age of about 11 weeks completed the study. The women were administered either powdered root of ginger (1 g/day) or placebo for 4 days, then nothing for 2 days, then given the alternate agent for 4 days. More patients stated a preference for ($p = 0.003$), and had greater relief from their symptoms ($p = 0.035$), with ginger than with placebo. No maternal adverse effects were observed. The pregnancy outcomes were one spontaneous abortion in the 12th week of gestation, one elective abortion for reasons other than nausea and vomiting, and 25 normal living infants. The mean gestational age at delivery was 39.9 weeks (range 36–41 weeks) with a mean birth weight of 3585 g (range 2450–5150 g). All had Apgar scores of 9–10 at 5 minutes, and none had a congenital abnormality (12).

In a comment relating to the above study, one author urged caution in the use of ginger during pregnancy, citing ginger's action as a thromboxane synthetase inhibitor, which, theoretically, could affect testosterone-receptor binding and result in adverse sex-steroid differentiation of the fetal brain (13). Although the author's research failed to find evidence of toxicity due to ginger, he recommended that it not be used in pregnancy until this effect was studied. No published reports to refute or support this alleged effect, however, have been located.

A 2001 randomized, double-masked study also evaluated the effect on ginger on nausea and vomiting of pregnancy (14). Ginger 1 g/day was compared with placebo for 4 days starting at a mean gestational age of about 10 weeks. Ginger resulted in a significant decrease in the severity of nausea and vomiting. No adverse effects on pregnancy outcome were detected (14).

The result of a prospective study of women consuming ginger in the 1st trimester for nausea and vomiting was reported in 2003 (15). The pregnancy outcomes of the exposed women were compared with a control group who were exposed to nonteratogenic drugs that were not antiemetics. The outcomes in the 187 ginger-exposed subjects were 3 spontaneous abortions, 1 elective abortion (Down's syndrome), 2 stillbirths, and 181 live births. Three liveborn infants had birth defects: ventricular septal defect, right lung abnormality, and a kidney abnormality (pelviectasis). In addition, a female child was later diagnosed with idiopathic central precocious puberty at 2 years of age. The mean birth weight was 3542 g and the mean gestational age at birth was 39 weeks. Except for the fact that more control infants weighed <2500 g, the outcomes between the groups did not differ significantly. Sixty-six women rated the effectiveness of ginger in controlling nausea and vomiting. On a 10-point scale (0 being no effect and 10 the best effect), the mean score was 3.3 (within the "mild effect" range) (15).

A 2004 randomized, controlled trial was conducted in women <16 weeks' gestation (16). Women were treated for 3 weeks with either ginger (*N* = 146) (1.05 g/day) or vitamin B6 (*N* = 145) (75 mg/day) and the efficacy of the treatments was measured at 7, 14, and 21 days. The median gestational age at the start of the study in the two groups was 8.5 and 8.6 weeks, respectively. There was no difference between the groups, averaged over time, in reducing nausea, retching, or vomiting. There also was no difference in the pregnancy outcomes, except that the ginger group had slightly more live births (16).

BREASTFEEDING SUMMARY

No studies describing the use of ginger during lactation have been located. It is unlikely, however, that small doses of ginger, such as those used as a spice, would affect a nursing infant. The effects, if any, of the higher doses used as an antiemetic are also unknown, but they are probably of little consequence to the infant. The oral bioavailability of ginger and its active ingredients, however, has not been studied in animals or humans.

References

1. Ginger. *The Review of Natural Products*. St Louis, MO: Facts and Comparisons, 2000.
2. Wilkinson JM. Effect of ginger tea on the fetal development of Sprague-Dawley rats. Reprod Toxicol 2000;14:507–12.
3. Weidner MS, Sigwart K. Investigation of the teratogenic potential of a *Zingiber officinale* extract in the rat. Reprod Toxicol 2001;15:75–80.
4. Mowrey DB, Clayson DE. Motion sickness, ginger, and psychophysics. Lancet 1982;1:655–7.
5. Liu WHD. Ginger root, a new antiemetic. Anaesthesia 1990;45:1085.
6. Bone ME, Wilkinson DJ, Young JR, McNeil J, Charlton S. Ginger root—a new antiemetic. The effect of ginger root on postoperative nausea and vomiting after major gynaecological surgery. Anaesthesia 1990;45:669–71.
7. Phillips S, Ruggier R, Hutchinson SE. *Zingiber officinale* (Ginger)—an antiemetic for day case surgery. Anaesthesia 1993;48:715–7.
8. Lumb AB. Mechanism of antiemetic effect of ginger. Anaesthesia 1993;48:1118.
9. Arfeen Z, Owen H, Plummer JL, Ilsley AH, Sorby-Adams RAC, Doecke CJ. A double-blind randomized controlled trial of ginger for the prevention of postoperative nausea and vomiting. Anaesth Intens Care 1995;23:449–52.
10. Visalyaputra S, Petchpaisit N, Somcharoen K, Choavaratana R. The efficacy of ginger root in the prevention of postoperative nausea and vomiting after outpatient gynaecological laparoscopy. Anaesthesia 1998;53:486–510.
11. Ernst E, Pittler MH. Efficacy of ginger for nausea and vomiting: a systematic review of randomized clinical trials. Br J Anaesth 2000;84:367–71.
12. Fischer-Rasmussen W, Kjaer SK, Dahl C, Asping U. Ginger treatment of hyperemesis gravidarum. Eur J Obstet Gynecol Rep Biol 1990;38:19–24.
13. Backon J. Ginger in preventing nausea and vomiting of pregnancy: a caveat due to its thromboxane synthetase activity and effect on testosterone binding. Eur J Obstet Gynecol Rep Biol 1991;42:163.
14. Vutyavanich T, Kraisarin T, Ruangsri RA. Ginger for nausea and vomiting in pregnancy: randomized, double-masked, placebo-controlled trial. Obstet Gynecol 2001;97:577–82.
15. Portnoi G, Chng LA, Karimi-Tabesh L, Koren G, Tan MP, Einarson A. Prospective comparative study of the safety and effectiveness of ginger for the treatment of nausea and vomiting in pregnancy. Am J Obstet Gynecol 2003;189:1374–7.
16. Smith C, Crowther C, Willson K, Hotham N, McMillian V. A randomized controlled trial of ginger to treat nausea and vomiting of pregnancy. Obstet Gynecol 2004;103:639–45.

GINKGO BILOBA

Herb

PREGNANCY RECOMMENDATION: No Human Data—Animal Data Suggest Low Risk
BREASTFEEDING RECOMMENDATION: No Human Data—Potential Toxicity

PREGNANCY SUMMARY

No reports describing the use of ginkgo biloba during human pregnancy have been located. No mutagenicity in animals or human sperm was observed and no teratogenicity occurred in one animal species, but the data and details of the animal studies are very limited. Moreover, a large number of chemicals have been identified from this herb and none has undergone rigorous reproductive testing. However, because ginkgo is an ancient herb and its use is widespread, it is doubtful that a major teratogenic effect or other significant reproductive toxicity would have escaped notice. More subtle or low-incidence effects, however, including structural and behavioral teratogenicity, the induction of abortions, and infertility may have escaped detection, and further study is required before human reproductive risk or safety can be assessed.

Because of the uncertainties described above, various sources can be found that either state there are no restrictions against it use in pregnancy (1) or that the herb is contraindicated during gestation (2–4). The safest course is to avoid ginkgo products during pregnancy.

FETAL RISK SUMMARY

Ginkgo biloba (scientific name) is a popular herbal preparation. The dioecious ginkgo tree may live as long as several 100–1000 years. It is the sole survivor of the family *Ginkgoaceae*, which dates back >200 million years. The tree, which may grow to a height of 30–40 m (approximately 98–131 feet), has fan-shaped leaves and is indigenous to China, Japan, and Korea (2,3,5). Commercial plantations of ginkgo trees in the United States, however, are pruned to shrub height to allow mechanical picking of the leaves (6).

The medicinal parts of ginkgo are the fresh and dried leaves, and the seeds separated from their fleshy outer layer (5). Ginkgo leaf extract, however, is the most commonly used form of this herb (3). Numerous uses have been recommended for the various IV (not available in United States) and oral preparations of ginkgo leaf extract, some of which are symptomatic relief of organic brain syndrome (e.g., cerebral insufficiency, anxiety and stress, memory impairment, headache, and dementias), intermittent claudication and other circulatory disorders, asthma, and vertigo and tinnitus of vascular origin (1–3,5,6).

Ginkgo seed, although not commercially available in the United States, is used orally as an antitussive and expectorant, as an aid for digestion, to prevent drunkenness, in asthma and bronchitis, and for genitourinary complaints. Topical uses include scabies and skin sores. Roasted seeds with the pulp removed are eaten for food in Japan and China (3).

The content of active compounds in ginkgo leaves may vary widely depending on the season (2,7). Seasonal and other factors, such as location and method of harvest, may result in variance as much as 300% in the concentrations of active compounds (7). Ginkgo leaf extract is prepared using an acetone–water extraction process and subsequent purification steps without adding concentrates or isolated ingredients (1,3,5,6). A number of chemical constituents have been identified in the extract (percentages refer to German Commission E standards): 22%–27% flavanone glycosides (flavonoids consisting of monosides, biosides, and triosides of quercetin, kaempferol, isorhamnetins, and 3′-O-methylmyristicins); 5%–7% terpene lactones (terpenoids) (2.8%–3.4% ginkgolides A, B, C, and M [trilactonic diterpenes], 2.6%–3.2% bilobalide [trilactone sesquiterpene]); and <5 ppm of ginkgolic acids (1–3,5,6). Other chemical constituents found in the leaf before processing, in addition to those identified in the extract, include amino acid 6-hydroxykynurenic acid, bioflavonoids (dimeric bioflavones: amentoflavone, bilobetin, ginkgetin, isoginkgetin, 5-methoxybilobetin, sciadopitysin) (about 40 different bioflavonoids have been identified), terpene lactone (ginkgolide J), steroids (sitosterol, stigmasterol), polyprenols, organic acids (shikimic, vanillic, ascorbic, p-coumaric), benzoic acid derivatives, carbohydrates, straight-chain hydrocarbons, alcohol, ketones, and 2-hexenol (2). A 1993 reference detailed the chemical structures of the active ingredients (flavonoids and terpene lactones) (8).

The seed contains 38% carbohydrate, 4% protein, and <2% fat (2). This part of the tree is not marketed in the United States, but may contaminate other ginkgo products (9). Chemicals found in the seed are alkaloids (e.g., ginkgotoxin), amino acids, cyanogenetic glycosides, and long-chain phenols (e.g., anacaric acid, bilobol, and cardanol) (2).

Reproduction studies in animals have revealed no mutagenic or teratogenic effects. No teratogenicity was observed in pregnant rats given oral doses up to 1600 mg/kg/day (2).

In a sperm penetration assay, zona-free hamster oocytes were incubated for 1 hour with two concentrations of ginkgo, 0.1 and 1.0 mg/mL, dissolved in HEPES-buffered synthetic human tubal fluid (modified HTF) (10). Fresh human donor sperms was suspended in the modified HTF and then mixed with the oocytes for 3 hours. Modified HTF served as the control. At the 0.1 mg/mL concentration, three of nine oocytes were penetrated, whereas at 1.0 mg/mL, zero (0 of 8) penetration occurred. The decrease in penetration was not associated with a decrease in sperm motility. In the second part of the study, sperms were incubated with the herbal solutions for 7 days. Neither concentration caused significant sperm DNA denaturation or mutation of a selected sperm sentinel gene (BRCA1 exon 11 gene), but the higher concentration reduced sperm viability compared with controls. Extrapolation of these data to the reproductive risk of ginkgo in males is difficult, in part because the concentration of the herb in semen or sperm has not been studied (10). Moreover, although the doses used in this study are small fractions of the actual recommended human dose, usually expressed in milligrams of ginkgo, no published evidence indicates that the adverse effects observed have occurred in vivo.

Although some ginkgo preparations may be standardized, the standardization of any herbal product as to its constituents, concentrations, and the presence of contaminants is generally lacking. Consumption of these products during pregnancy may result in fetal exposure to unintended chemicals and doses.

BREASTFEEDING SUMMARY

No reports describing the use of ginkgo biloba during lactation have been located. Although one source states that there are no restrictions to its use during lactation (1), other sources consider the use of the herb during lactation to be contraindicated (2–4). The latter course is the safest because of the large number of chemical compounds in the herb and the absence of information on the effects of exposure to these substances in a nursing infant.

References

1. Ginkgo Biloba Leaf Extract. Blumenthal M, ed. *The Complete German Commission E Monographs. Therapeutic Guide to Herbal Medicines*. Austin, TX: American Botanical Council, 1998:136–8.
2. Ginkgo. *The Review of Natural Products*. St. Louis, MO: Facts and Comparisons, 1998.
3. Ginkgo Leaf, Ginkgo Leaf Extract, Ginkgo Seed. *Natural Medicines Comprehensive Database*. Stockton, CA: Therapeutic Research Faculty, 1999:377–81.
4. Wong AHC, Smith M, Boon HS. Herbal remedies in psychiatric practice. Arch Gen Psychiatry 1998;55:1033–44.
5. Ginkgo Biloba. *PDR for Herbal Medicines*. Montvale, NJ: Medical Economics, 1998:871–3.
6. Robbers JE, Tyler VE. *Tyler's Herbs of Choice: The Therapeutic Use of Phytomedicinals*. Binghamton, NY: Haworth Press, 2000:141–6.
7. Product information. BioGinkgo 27/7. Pharmanex, 1998.
8. Sticher O. Quality of ginkgo preparations. Planta Medica 1993;59:2–11.
9. Boullata JI, Nace AM. Safety issues with herbal medicine. Pharmacotherapy 2000;20:257–69.
10. Ondrizek RR, Chan PJ, Patton WC, King A. An alternative medicine study of herbal effects on the penetration of zona-free hamster oocytes and the integrity of sperm deoxyribonucleic acid. Fertil Steril 1999;71:517–22.

G

GINSENG

Herb

PREGNANCY RECOMMENDATION: Limited Human Data—Animal Data Suggest Low Risk
BREASTFEEDING RECOMMENDATION: No Human Data—Potential Toxicity

G

PREGNANCY SUMMARY

Ginseng is an ancient popular herb that is used extensively throughout the world. The reproductive effects of the herb in pregnant animals, except in one case, have not been studied. Similarly, only one small study has investigated its effect in human pregnancy, but the study did not mention if birth defects were observed. As with most herbal preparations, there appears to be little or no quality control in the production of commercial products, and mislabeling of these products is probably common. Ginseng is known to act on multiple organ systems. Depending on the product ingested and the dose and duration of use, the herb can produce clinically significant adverse reactions in nonpregnant patients. Hypertension and hypoglycemia have been reported with ginseng (1). These effects could complicate pregnancies with hypertensive disorders or diabetes. However, because ginseng has been used in medicine for more than 2000 years and its current use is widespread, it is doubtful if it causes major birth defects or other clinically significant developmental toxicity. More subtle or low-incidence effects, however, including structural and behavioral teratogenicity, the induction of abortions, and infertility, may have escaped detection. Further study using products identified by chemical analysis is required before human reproductive risk or safety can be assessed.

FETAL RISK SUMMARY

Ginseng is a plant that is found throughout the world. The root is considered the most important part of the plant because it contains the pharmacologically active ginsenosides. Ginseng has been used in medicine for >2000 years. The herb is promoted as having multiple pharmacologic effects, including adaptogenic, CNS, cardiovascular, endocrine, ergogenic, antineoplastic, and immunomodulatory effects. It is available as fresh or dried roots, extracts, solutions, tablets, sodas, teas, chewing gum, cigarettes, and candy (1–3).

Although the name ginseng (common names, if given, shown in parentheses) commonly refers to *Panax quinquefollus* L. (American or Canadian ginseng) or *P. ginseng* C.A. Meyer (Asian, Chinese, Korean, or Oriental ginseng; red ginseng [steamed]), one source listed seven other recognized medicinal ginsengs (1). They are *P. japonicus* var *bipinnatifidus*, *P. japonicus* C.A. Meyer (Japanese, Chikusetsu, or zhu je ginseng), *P. japonicus* var *major*, *P. notoginseng* (Western or Five-fingers ginseng; Sang; San-chi; Tien-chan or tienqi ginseng), *P. pseudoginseng* subsp. *himalaicus* (Himalayan ginseng), *P. pseudoginseng* var *major* (Zhuzishen), and *P. vietnamensis* Ha et Grushv. (Vietnamese ginseng) (1).

A 1994 letter stated that there were eight species and three varieties of genus *Panax* in the Northern Hemisphere (4). The eight species were *ginseng*, *quinquefolium*, *notoginseng*, *pseudoginseng*, *zingigerensis*, *trifolus*, *stipuleanatus*, and *japonicus*. The varieties of *P. japonicus* were identified as var *major*, var *angustifolius*, and var *bipinnatifidus*.

Ginseng products are commercially available as food flavorings and herbal medicines. Although the minor constituents of ginseng listed below might have some role, the principal pharmacologically active ingredients of ginseng appear to be a group of steroid-like compounds linked to sugars, called saponins (ginsenosides) (1). At least 13 major saponins, as well as numerous minor glycosides, have been identified. Minor constituents include volatile oils, β-elemine, sterols, acetylenes, polysaccharides, starch, flavonoids, peptides, various B-complex vitamins, minerals, enzymes, and choline (1). Xanthines (e.g., caffeine, theophylline, and theobromine), produced by the plant, may also be present in various concentrations and may contribute to the pharmacologic action of the product (1).

The actual amount of ginsenosides in commercial preparations varies widely. This variance partially reflects poor quality control, but may also depend on the species, age of the root, location, season of harvest, and preservation or curing method (1). In addition, products sold as ginseng may actually contain no ginsenosides (2,5). For example, other herbal species that do not contain ginsenosides are also called "ginseng," such as Siberian ginseng (*Eleutherococcus senticosus*; active constituents are eleutherosides) and Brazilian ginseng (*Pfaffia paniculata*) (6). In addition, Chinese silk vine (*Periploca sepium*), an herb that contains cardiac glycosides but no ginsenosides, is a common substitute for Siberian ginseng (7).

A reproduction study with rats was conducted with an extract (G115) of Oriental ginseng (*P. ginseng*) (8). Two generations of rats, male and female, were fed a diet supplemented with ginseng extract at doses of 1.5, 5, or 15 mg/kg/day or a control diet. No differences in treatment-related effects were observed between the groups in terms of body weights, food consumption, hematologic and clinical chemical data. In addition, no differences were noted in ophthalmic, gross and histopathologic examinations, or in autopsies (8).

Ginseng (*P. ginseng*) was used as a fetal protectant in a study involving rats given hexavalent chromium throughout gestation (9). Hexavalent chromium, the most toxic form of chromium for the embryo and fetus, was fed to two groups of female rats in their drinking water. In one of the groups, ginseng (20 mg/kg/day) was also given. A third group received ginseng only, whereas a control group received neither agent. The rats receiving chromium plus ginseng had significantly better pregnancy outcomes than those receiving only chromium in terms of increased maternal weight gain, fewer pre- and postimplantation losses, resorptions, and stillbirths, and lower rates of visceral and skeletal anomalies (9).

The effects of American ginseng (*P. quinquefolium*) on male copulatory behavior have been studied in rats (10). Doses of 10–100 mg/kg/day given for 28 days significantly stimulated copulatory behavior. In comparison with controls, no effects were noted on plasma luteinizing hormone or testosterone levels, or on sex organs, but plasma prolactin concentrations were significantly decreased in ginseng-treated animals (10).

Three brief reports have described an estrogen-like effect (11) and vaginal bleeding (12,13) in three postmenopausal women taking ginseng (*P. ginseng* in two; unknown source in one).

A 30-year-old woman took an herbal preparation alleged to be pure Siberian ginseng (1300 mg/day—twice the manufacturer's recommended dose) throughout pregnancy and during the first 2 weeks of breastfeeding (14). In late pregnancy, she had repeated occurrences of premature uterine contractions. She also thought that the hair growth on her head, face, and pubic region had increased and was thicker. The term, 3.3-kg male infant had thick black hair in the pubic region and over the entire forehead, and swollen, red nipples (14). The mother stopped breastfeeding 2 weeks postpartum on medical advice because she did not want to stop taking the herb. At 7.5 weeks of age, the infant's weight (5.8 kg) and length (60.6 cm) were above the 97th percentile, but the pubic and forehead hair, which had begun to fallout at 2 weeks, was scant. A physical examination revealed testes that were enlarged (volume = 3 mL) but were otherwise normal. In addition, there was no evidence of adrenogenital syndrome because the serum concentrations of 17-hydroxyprogesterone, testosterone, and cortisol were within normal ranges. The investigators noted that ginseng increases testosterone levels in male rats and testes growth in rabbits, and could significantly increase corticotropin and corticosteroid levels. Therefore, they concluded that the product she was taking might have caused the hirsutism in the mother and infant and the infant's excessive weight gain (14).

In response to the above case, a representative for a government agency argued that the cited animal studies involving ginseng had no relevance because the active constituents of Siberian ginseng were eleutherosides that are completely different from ginsenosides (15). In reply, one of the investigators stated that they had recently given the woman doses either of her Siberian ginseng or placebo in a double-blind manner. Her testosterone levels were undetectable when she was taking the herb and normal when she received placebo. The investigator hypothesized that the product she was taking contained a compound that suppressed, but acted like, endogenous testosterone (16). In the last correspondence on this case, three bulk lots of powder supposedly containing Siberian ginseng were obtained from the manufacturer of the product taken by the woman. The lot dates overlapped the period of her pregnancy. Chemical analysis revealed that the powder was actually Chinese silk vine (*P. sepium*), the bark of which contains cardioactive glycosides (17). Inadvertent substitution of Chinese silk vine for Siberian ginseng had occurred previously and may have resulted because of confusion surrounding the Chinese names of the herbs (17).

A brief 1991 correspondence compared the outcomes of 88 Asian women who had taken ginseng during pregnancy with 88 matched controls who had not taken the herb (18). No statistically significant differences were found in the mode of delivery, birth weight, low birth weight (<2500 g), preterm delivery (<37 weeks), low Apgar scores (<7), and stillbirths or neonatal deaths. Regarding pregnancy complications, there were no differences in the incidence of gestational diabetes, or antepartum or postpartum hemorrhage, but significantly more controls than subjects had preeclampsia (1 vs. 8; $p < 0.02$). No mention was made of congenital malformations in either group (18).

BREASTFEEDING SUMMARY

No studies describing the use of ginseng during human lactation have been located. Confusion has arisen over the actual identity of commercial products (see above) and without chemical analysis, the actual herb ingested is uncertain. Ginseng can affect multiple organ systems in users and, potentially, could adversely affect a nursing infant if the ginsenosides (active constituents) were excreted into breast milk. However, it is doubtful if ginseng has caused clinically significant effects in nursing infants because of its ancient and widespread use. Although more subtle effects on a nursing infant could have been missed, the proven benefits of breastfeeding may outweigh the unknown risk from exposure to the active and inactive constituents of ginseng. Women taking this herb and nursing should be informed of this uncertainty.

References

1. Ginseng, Panax. *The Review of Natural Products*. St. Louis, MO: Facts and Comparisons, 2001.
2. Robbers JE, Tyler VE. *Tyler's Herbs of Choice*. Binghamton, NY: Haworth Herbal Press, 1999:238.
3. Attele AS, Wu JA, Yuan CS. Ginseng pharmacology. Multiple constituents and multiple actions. Biochem Pharmacol 1999;58:1685–93.
4. Vigano C, Ceppi E. What is in ginseng? Lancet 1994;344:619.
5. Cui J, Garle M, Eneroth P, Bjōrkem I. What do commercial ginseng preparations contain? Lancet 1994;344:134.
6. Walker AF. What is in ginseng? Lancet 1994;344:619.
7. Wong HCG. Probable false authentication of herbal plants: ginseng. Arch Intern Med 1999;159:1142.
8. Hess FG Jr, Parent RA, Cox GE, Stevens KR, Becci PJ. Reproduction study in rats of ginseng extract G115. Food Chem Toxicol 1982;20:189–92.
9. Elsaleed EM, Nada SA. Teratogenicity of hexavalent chromium in rats and the beneficial role of ginseng. Bull Environ Contam Toxicol 2002;68:361–8.
10. Murphy LL, Cadena RS, Chavez D, Ferraro JS. Effect of American ginseng (*Panax quinquefolium*) on male copulatory behavior in the rat. Physiol Behav 1998;64:445–50.
11. Punnonen R, Lukola A. Oestrogen-like effect of ginseng. Br Med J 1980; 281:1110.
12. Greenspan EM. Ginseng and vaginal bleeding. JAMA 1983;249:2018.
13. Palop-Larrea V, Gonzálvez-Perales JL, Catalán-Oliver C, Belenguer-Varea A, Martínez-Mir I. Metrorrhagia and ginseng. Ann Pharmacother 2000;34:1347–8.
14. Koren G, Randor S, Martin S, Danneman D. Maternal ginseng use associated with neonatal androgenization. JAMA 1990;264:2866.
15. Awang DVC. Maternal use of ginseng and neonatal androgenization. JAMA 1991;265:1828.
16. Koren G. Maternal use of ginseng and neonatal androgenization. JAMA 1991;265:1828.
17. Awang DVC. Maternal use of ginseng and neonatal androgenization. JAMA 1991;266:363.
18. Chin RKH. Ginseng and common pregnancy disorders. Asia Oceania J Obstet Gynaecol 1991;17:379–80.

GITALIN

[Withdrawn from the market. See 8th edition.]

GLATIRAMER

Immunologic Agent (Immunosuppressive)

PREGNANCY RECOMMENDATION: Compatible—Maternal Benefit >> Embryo–Fetal Risk
BREASTFEEDING RECOMMENDATION: Limited Human Data—Probably Compatible

PREGNANCY SUMMARY

The use of glatiramer during pregnancy appears to be low risk. In addition, the benefits of the drug in reducing the number of relapses of multiple sclerosis appear to outweigh the potential, but unknown risks to the embryo–fetus. If indicated, glatiramer should not be withheld because of pregnancy.

FETAL RISK SUMMARY

Glatiramer (copolymer-1) is an immunosuppressant agent given by SC injection to reduce the frequency of relapses in patients with relapsing–remitting multiple sclerosis, including patients who experienced a first clinical episode and have features consistent with multiple sclerosis. It is the acetate salts of synthetic polypeptides containing four naturally occurring amino acids: L-glutamic acid, L-alanine, L-lysine, and L-tyrosine. Chemically, glatiramer is a designated L-glutamic acid polymer with L-alanine, L-lysine, and L-tyrosine, acetate (salt).

A substantial fraction of the dose is hydrolyzed locally, but some may enter the systemic circulation intact (1).

Reproduction studies during organogenesis have been conducted in rats and rabbits at SC doses up to 18 and 36 times the human dose of 20 mg based on BSA (HD), respectively. No adverse fetal effects were observed in either species. Pregnant rats were also given glatiramer at doses up to about 18 times the HD from gestational day 15 and throughout lactation. No significant effects were observed on delivery or pup growth or development.

Long-term studies for carcinogenesis in mice and rats were negative, as were assays for mutagenesis or clastogenic effects. In fertility and reproductive performance studies in rats at SC doses up to 18 times the HD, no adverse effects were observed on reproductive or developmental parameters (1).

It is not known if glatiramer crosses the human placenta to the fetus. The average molecular weight of glatiramer acetate is 5000–9000, suggesting that it does not cross by simple diffusion.

A prospective observational cohort study from a Teratology Information Service in Berlin compared the pregnancy outcomes of four groups: exposure to glatiramer (*N* = 31) or interferon (*N* = 69) (either beta-1a (*N* = 48) or beta-1b (*N* = 21), women with multiple sclerosis not exposed to these agents (*N* = 64), and a healthy comparative group (*N* = 1556) (2). Spontaneous abortions (SABs), all within the expected range, in the four groups were 3.9%, 11.7%, 9.8%, and 9.1%, respectively. The higher rate in the interferon group was due to a 27.8% rate in the beta-1b subgroup. Major birth defects occurred in two exposed to glatiramer, none in the interferon group, three in the multiple sclerosis group, and 23 of the healthy controls. In the glatiramer-exposed group, club feet occurred in a term infant who was exposed until gestational week 6. The second defect in the glatiramer group was a complex heart defect diagnosed by ultrasound. The mother in this case had received the drug until gestational week 13. She also had received moxifloxacin for 1 day and levofloxacin for 5 days in week 6, as well as IV glucocorticoids for 3 days for relapse. Her pregnancy was electively terminated. The male fetus had a complete atrioventricular canal (grade III) with a normal karyotype. In all groups, the mean birth weights were within the normal range (>3200 g) but were significantly lower in the interferon group. The birth weights also were significantly lower in mothers who had relapsed. The authors concluded that neither glatiramer or interferon was a major risk for developmental toxicity (2).

A 2010 study reported the pregnancy outcomes of 13 women (14 newborns—one set of twins) with multiple sclerosis (3). Glatiramer was used throughout gestation in nine cases, discontinued early (weeks 4 or 5) in gestation in three cases, and discontinued at 19 weeks in one case. There were no birth defects in the 14 newborns (3).

A brief 2011 report described three women with multiple sclerosis who received glatiramer throughout gestation (4). The pregnancy outcomes were compared with seven women with more complicated (increased relapses) multiple sclerosis who were treated with interferon beta-1a throughout gestation. Birth weight was lower in the glatiramer group, 3142 g vs. 3444 g, but the glatiramer group was born earlier (38.3 vs. 39.7 weeks). In the glatiramer group, a male infant had hypospadias that required surgical correction. In the interferon group, a male infant had a valvular stenosis of the pulmonary artery (4).

In a 2012 study from Germany, pregnancy outcomes in women with multiple sclerosis were compared in three groups: glatiramer (*N* = 41), interferon beta (*N* = 78), and pregnancies not exposed to these agents (*N* = 216) (5). There were no differences between the groups in terms of birth weight, body length, gestational age at birth, and preterm birth. Congenital anomalies were observed in two infants in the glatiramer group (defect of urinary bladder and hip dysplasia), three in the interferon group (ventricular septal defect [VSD], valvular stenosis of the pulmonary artery, and hip dysplasia), and seven in the control group (5).

A 2012 study from Italy evaluated the pregnancy outcomes in 423 cases where the mother had multiple sclerosis (6). In the prospective observational multicenter study, 17 were exposed to glatiramer, 88 to interferon beta, and 318 nonexposed. Glatiramer was not associated with a higher frequency of SAB or other negative pregnancy and fetal outcomes (6).

BREASTFEEDING SUMMARY

Because of the high molecular weight (about 5000–9000), it is doubtful if unmetabolized glatiramer is excreted into breast milk. In a 2010 report described above, 8 of 13 mothers receiving glatiramer chose to breastfeed their infants (3). The duration of nursing was 1 day to 6 months, but only two breastfed for a significant period (2 and 6 months). No other information was provided.

Three mothers who taken glatiramer throughout pregnancy continued the therapy during exclusive breastfeeding for 6 months (4). None of the infants had noticeable problems.

In the above study from Germany, 170 of 335 women throughout all three groups breastfed exclusively (5). Significantly reduced relapse rates of multiple sclerosis during the first 3 months occurred compared with nonexclusive breastfeeding or nonbreastfeeding women ($p < 0.0001$).

References

1. Product information. Copaxone. Teva Neuroscience, 2012.
2. Weber-Schoendorfer C, Schaefer C. Multiple sclerosis, immunomodulators, and pregnancy outcome: a prospective observational study. Mult Scler 2009;15:1037–42.
3. Salminen HJ, Leggett H, Boggild M. Glatiramer acetate exposure in pregnancy: preliminary safety and birth outcomes. J Neurol 2010;257: 2020–23.
4. Hellwig K, Gold R. Glatiramer acetate and interferon-beta throughout gestation and postpartum in women with multiple sclerosis. J Neurol 2011;258:502–3.
5. Hellwig K, Haghikia A, Gold R. Multiple sclerosis and pregnancy: experience from a nationwide database in Germany. Ther Adv Neurol Disord 2012;5:247–53.
6. Giannini M, Portaccio E, Ghezzi A, Hakiki B, Pasto L, Razzolini L, Piscolla E, De Giglio L, Pozzilli C, Paolicelli D, Trojano M, Marrosu MG, Patti F, La Mantia L, Mancardia G, Solaro C, Totaro R, TolaMR, De Luca G, Lugaresi A, Moiola L, Martinelli V, Comi MP, Amato MP. Pregnancy and fetal outcomes after glatiramer acetate exposure in patients with multiple sclerosis: a prospective observational multicentric study. BMC Neurol 2012;12:124. doi:10.1186/1471-2377-12-124.

GLIMEPIRIDE

Antidiabetic Agent

PREGNANCY RECOMMENDATION: Limited Human Data—Animal Data Suggest Low Risk
BREASTFEEDING RECOMMENDATION: No Human Data—Probably Compatible

PREGNANCY SUMMARY

One report describing the use of glimepiride during human pregnancy has been located. Insulin is the treatment of choice for pregnant diabetic patients because, in general, other hypoglycemic agents do not provide adequate glycemic control. Moreover, insulin, unlike most oral agents, does not cross the placenta to the fetus, thus eliminating the additional concern that the drug therapy itself will adversely affect the fetus. Carefully prescribed insulin therapy provides better control of the mother's glucose, thereby preventing the fetal and neonatal complications that occur with this disease. High maternal glucose levels, as may occur in diabetes mellitus, are closely associated with a number of maternal and fetal adverse effects, including fetal structural anomalies if the hyperglycemia occurs early in gestation. To prevent this toxicity, the American College of Obstetricians and Gynecologists recommends that insulin be used for types 1 and 2 diabetes occurring during pregnancy and, if diet therapy alone is not successful, for gestational diabetes (1,2).

FETAL RISK SUMMARY

Glimepiride is a second-generation sulfonylurea in the same class as glipizide and glyburide (see also Glipizide and Glyburide). It is used as an adjunct to diet and exercise, either alone or in combination with other oral agents, in the treatment of type 2 diabetes (non-insulin-dependent diabetes mellitus). It has also been used in combination with insulin when diet, exercise, and an oral hypoglycemic have not controlled hyperglycemia.

Reproduction studies in animals have been conducted with glimepiride. No teratogenic effects were observed in rats and rabbits given doses up to approximately 4000 and 60 times, respectively, the maximum recommended human dose based on BSA (MRHD). However, in some studies, rat pups, nursing from mothers given high doses of glimepiride during pregnancy and lactation, developed skeletal deformities consisting of shortening, thickening, and bending of the humerus during the postnatal period. Moreover, fetotoxicity (intrauterine death) occurred in both rats and rabbits at 50 and 0.1 times, respectively, the MRHD. The fetotoxicity, which has also been observed with other sulfonylureas, occurred only at doses that produced maternal hypoglycemia and was thought to be due to that effect. No effect on the fertility of male and female rats was noted at doses up to 4000 times the MRHD (3).

It is not known if glimepiride crosses the placenta, but the molecular weight (about 491) is low enough that transfer to the fetus should be expected. Hypoglycemia in the newborn may occur if glimepiride is taken close to delivery.

A 2005 case report described the pregnancy outcome of a 33-year-old woman treated with glimepiride for type 2 diabetes mellitus in the first 8 weeks of an unplanned pregnancy (4). Other diseases in the patient were hypertension, hypercholesterolemia, and morbid obesity that were treated with orlistat, ramipril, thiocolchicoside (a muscle relaxant), simvastatin, metformin, ciprofloxacin, and aspirin. When pregnancy was diagnosed at 8 weeks, all medications were stopped, and she was started on methyldopa and insulin. She gave birth at 38 weeks to a 3.470-kg female infant with Apgar scores of 5 and 7 at 1 and 5 minutes, respectively. No minor or major malformations were observed in the infant (4).

BREASTFEEDING SUMMARY

No reports describing the use of glimepiride during human lactation have been located. The relatively low molecular weight (about 491) suggests that the drug will be excreted into breast milk. Because neonatal hypoglycemia is a potential effect, women taking glimepiride should consider changing to insulin therapy while nursing.

References

1. American College of Obstetricians and Gynecologists. Pregestational diabetes mellitus. *ACOG Practice Bulletin*. No. 60. March 2005. Obstet Gynecol 2005;105:675–85.
2. American College of Obstetricians and Gynecologists. Gestational diabetes. *ACOG Practice Bulletin*. No. 30. September 2001. Obstet Gynecol 2001;98:525–38.
3. Product information. Amaryl. Hoechst Marion Roussel, 2000.
4. Kalyoncu NI, Yaris F, Kadioglu M, Kesim M, Ulku C, Yaris E, Unsal M, Dikici M. Pregnancy outcome following exposure to orlistat, ramipril, glimepiride in a woman with metabolic syndrome. Saudi Med J 2005;26:497–9.

GLIPIZIDE

Antidiabetic Agent

PREGNANCY RECOMMENDATION: Limited Human Data—Animal Data Suggest Low Risk
BREASTFEEDING RECOMMENDATION: Limited Human Data—Probably Compatible

PREGNANCY SUMMARY

Although the use of glipizide may be beneficial for decreasing the incidence of fetal and newborn morbidity and mortality in developing countries where the proper use of insulin is problematic, insulin is still the treatment of choice for this disease during pregnancy. Moreover, insulin, unlike glipizide, does not cross the placenta, which eliminates the additional concern that the drug therapy itself is adversely affecting the fetus. Carefully prescribed insulin therapy will provide better control of the mother's blood glucose, thereby preventing the fetal and neonatal complications that occur with this disease. High maternal glucose levels, as may occur in diabetes mellitus, are associated with a number of maternal and fetal adverse effects, including fetal structural anomalies if the hyperglycemia occurs early in gestation. To prevent this toxicity, the American College of Obstetricians and Gynecologists recommends that insulin be used for types 1 and 2 diabetes occurring during pregnancy and, if diet therapy alone is not successful, for gestational diabetes (1,2). If glipizide is used during pregnancy, therapy should be changed to insulin. If glipizide is continued, it should be stopped before delivery (the exact time before delivery is unknown) to lessen the possibility of prolonged hypoglycemia in the newborn.

FETAL RISK SUMMARY

Glipizide is an oral sulfonylurea agent, structurally similar to glyburide that is used for the treatment of adult-onset diabetes mellitus. It is not the treatment of choice for the pregnant diabetic patient.

Reproductive studies in male and female rats showed no effect on fertility. Mild fetotoxicity (type not specified) was observed at all doses tested in rats and was thought to be caused by the hypoglycemic action of glipizide. No teratogenic effects were observed in rats or rabbits (3).

A 1994 report described the in vitro placental transfer, using a single cotyledon human placenta, of four oral hypoglycemic agents (4). As expected, molecular weight was the most significant factor for drug transfer, with dissociation constant (pK_a) and lipid solubility providing significant additive effect. The cumulative percentage placental transfer at 3 hours of the four agents and their approximate molecular weights (shown in parentheses) were tolbutamide (270) 21.5%, chlorpropamide (277) 11.0%, glipizide (446) 6.6%, and glyburide (494) 3.9% (4).

A 1984 source cited a study that described the use of glipizide in four diabetic patients from the 32nd week of gestation through delivery (5). No adverse effects in the fetuses were observed.

A study published in 1995 assessed the risk of congenital malformations in infants of mothers with non-insulin-dependent diabetes during a 6-year period (6). Women were included in the study if, during the first 8 weeks of pregnancy, they had not participated in a preconception care program and then had been treated either with diet alone (group 1), diet and oral hypoglycemic agents (predominantly chlorpropamide, glyburide, or glipizide) (group 2), or diet and exogenous insulin (group 3). The 302 women eligible for analysis gave birth to 332 infants (5 sets of twins and 16 with two or three separate singleton pregnancies during the study period). A total of 56 (16.9%) infants had one or more congenital malformations, 39 (11.7%) of which were classified as major anomalies (defined as those that were either lethal, caused significant morbidity, or required surgical repair). The major anomalies were divided among those involving the CNS, face, heart and great vessels, gastrointestinal, genitourinary, and skeletal (includes caudal regression syndrome) systems. Minor anomalies included all of these, except those of the CNS, and a miscellaneous group composed of sacral skin tags, cutis aplasia of the scalp, and hydroceles. The number of infants in each group and the number of major and minor anomalies observed were group 1—125 infants, 18 (14.4%) major, 6 (4.8%) minor; group 2—147 infants, 14 (9.5%) major, 9 (6.1%) minor; and group 3—60 infants, 7 (11.7%) major, 2 (3.3%) minor. There were no statistical differences among the groups. Six (4.1%) of the infants exposed in utero to oral hypoglycemic agents and four other infants in the other two groups had ear anomalies (included among those with face defects). Other than the incidence of major anomalies, two other important findings of this study were (1) the independent associations between the risk of major anomalies (but not minor defects) and poor glycemic control in early pregnancy and (2) a younger maternal age at the onset of diabetes. Moreover, the study did not find an association between the use of oral hypoglycemics during organogenesis and congenital malformations, in that the observed anomalies appeared to be related to poor maternal glycemic control (6).

BREASTFEEDING SUMMARY

Nondetectable levels of glipizide were reported in three of four milk samples from two women nursing their infants (7). The two women were on a steady-state dose of glipizide (5-mg immediate-release tablet every morning for 6 and 15 days). In one woman, the peak milk concentration (3 hours after dose) was 0.20 mcg/mL and the trough level was nondetectable (detection limit 0.08 mcg/mL). In the second woman, both the peak and trough samples had nondetectable glipizide levels. Blood glucose levels were normal in both of the exclusively breastfed infants (7).

References

1. American College of Obstetricians and Gynecologists. Pregestational diabetes mellitus. *ACOG Practice Bulletin*. No. 60. March 2005. Obstet Gynecol 2005;105:675–85.
2. American College of Obstetricians and Gynecologists. Gestational diabetes. *ACOG Practice Bulletin*. No. 30. September 2001. Obstet Gynecol 2001;98:525–38.
3. Product information. Glucotrol. Pfizer Inc., 1997.
4. Elliott BD, Schenker S, Langer O, Johnson R, Prihoda T. Comparative placental transport of oral hypoglycemic agents in humans: a model of human placental drug transfer. Am J Obstet Gynecol 1994;171:653–60.
5. Onnis A, Grella P. *The Biochemical Effects of Drugs in Pregnancy*. Vol 2. West Sussex, England: Ellis Horwood Limited, 1984:174–5.
6. Towner D, Kjos SL, Leung B, Montoro MM, Xiang A, Mestman JH, Buchanan TA. Congenital malformations in pregnancies complicated by NIDDM. Diabetes Care 1995;18:1446–51.
7. Feig DS, Briggs GG, Kraemer JM, Ambrose PJ, Moskovitz DN, Nageotte MP, Donat DJ, Padilla G, Wan S, Klein J, Koren G. Transfer of glyburide and glipizide into breast milk. Diabetes Care 2005;28:1851–5.

GLUCAGON

Antidote

PREGNANCY RECOMMENDATION: Compatible—Maternal Benefit >> Embryo–Fetal Risk
BREASTFEEDING RECOMMENDATION: Compatible

PREGNANCY SUMMARY

The limited animal and human pregnancy data suggest that the embryo and/or fetal risks from glucagon are very low or negligible. Apparently, the drug does not cross the placenta.

As with all antidotes, maternal treatment usually is paramount. Thus, in cases of severe hypoglycemia, when IV glucose cannot be administered, glucagon should not be withheld because of concern for embryo–fetal safety. The maternal consequences of withholding treatment might place the pregnancy at far greater risk than the undocumented risk from the drug.

FETAL RISK SUMMARY

Glucagon is a single-chain polypeptide hormone produced by recombinant DNA technology that is identical to human glucagon. Glucagon increases blood glucose by stimulating hepatic glycogenolysis and relaxes smooth muscle of the gastrointestinal tract. It also is used as an antidote for β-blocker overdose. Glucagon must be given parenterally because it is destroyed in the gastrointestinal tract and is not active when taken orally. The polypeptide contains 29 amino acid residues with a molecular weight of 3483. Glucagon treats severe hypoglycemia by the conversion of liver glycogen to glucose. It is also indicated as a diagnostic aid in the radiologic examination of the gastrointestinal tract when diminished intestinal motility is advantageous. The hormone is extensively metabolized in the liver, kidney, and plasma and has a very short elimination half-life (range 8–18 minutes) (1).

Reproduction studies have not been conducted with recombinant glucagon, but have been performed with animal-source glucagon. In rats, doses up to 40 times the human dose based on BSA revealed no evidence of impaired fertility or fetal harm (1).

An in vitro mouse study examined the effect of glucagon and other metabolic factors (insulin, β-hydroxybutyrate, and acetoacetate) on the preimplantation development of mouse embryos (2). Glucagon, as well as the other factors, demonstrated a statistically significant dose-related inhibition of blastocyst development when cultured over 72 hours. However, the relationship of the observed embryotoxicity to a typical human clinical exposure is doubtful.

The metabolic response to glucagon injections (1 mcg/kg to 1 mg/kg) was studied in chronically catheterized fetal lambs near term (3). A significant hyperglycemia occurred within 15–30 minutes but, in contrast to neonatal lambs, did not induce a significant ketogenesis.

In a 1992 study, no effects on renal function were observed in near-term fetal sheep administered pharmacologic doses of glucagon (0.5 mcg/kg/min) for 1.5 hours (4). However, a significant increase in fetal heart rate, without changes in arterial pressure, was noted.

Glucagon does not cross the placenta in sheep or humans (5–8). In an experiment with pregnant sheep at term, no transfer of radioiodine-labeled glucagon was detected either from the mother to the fetus or from the fetus to the mother (5). A 1972 human study failed to find evidence of glucagon placental transfer in three mothers at term (6). Similarly, in an in vitro study using human chorion, no transfer of glucagon to the fetal side was detected (7). In a 1976 study, 15 women received a 1-mg IV dose of glucagon within 40 minutes of delivery (8). Compared with 47 control subjects, no change in glucagon concentrations in umbilical cord blood was observed, suggesting a lack of significant placental transfer.

A 1987 study reported the outcomes of seven pregnant women who had received glucagon for severe hypoglycemia on 12 occasions during pregnancy (9). In each case, a single 1-mg dose was given SC or IM by a spouse or other family member, resulting in glucose levels of 100–200 mg/dL within 30 minutes in 11 cases. In one case, the woman did not respond and required IV glucose in the emergency room. Although the gestational timing of the glucagon doses was not given, all of the infants survived and had normal Apgar scores at birth (9).

Glucagon was used as an antidote in a pregnant woman who had taken a massive overdose (15.2 g) of the β-blocker, metoprolol (10). At 20 weeks' gestation, the woman ingested 152 100-mg tablets in a suicide attempt. She suffered cardiac arrest in the hospital. Despite prolonged, but successful, cardiopulmonary resuscitation, she remained in severe cardiogenic shock with low systolic blood pressure. When the nature of the ingestion was learned, the woman was given glucagon 1-mg IV. Her condition markedly improved after the glucagon, but intrauterine fetal death had occurred and an induced abortion was performed 10 days later (10).

A 2003 review on the effects of antidotes in pregnancy concluded that there was probably no teratogenic risk because of the endogenous nature of glucagon (11). However, doses >1 mg in human pregnancy have not been reported.

BREASTFEEDING SUMMARY

No reports describing the use of glucagon during lactation have been located. It is doubtful if such reports would be forthcoming because of the nature of its indications (severe hypoglycemia; antidote; diagnostic agent) and its very short elimination half-life (8–18 minutes). Moreover, even if the high molecular weight (3483) polypeptide hormone were excreted into milk, it would be broken down to its constituent amino acids or fragments thereof in the infant's digestive tract. Thus, the risk to a nursing infant appears to be negligible.

References

1. Product information. Glucagon. Eli Lilly, 2001.
2. Zusman I, Yaffe P, Ornoy A. Effects of metabolic factors in the diabetic state on the in vitro development of preimplantation mouse embryos. Teratology 1987;35:77–85.
3. Philipps AF, Dubin JW, Matty PJ, Raye JR. Influence of exogenous glucagon on fetal glucose metabolism and ketone production. Pediatr Res 1983;17:51–6.
4. Moore RS, Lumbers ER. Renal and metabolic effects of glucagon in the fetus. J Dev Physiol 1992;17:47–9.
5. Sperling MA, Erenberg A, Fiser RH, Oh W, Fisher DA. Placental transfer of glucagon in sheep. Endocrinology 1973;93:1435–8.
6. Johnston DI, Bloom SR, Greene KR, Beard RW. Failure of the human placenta to transfer pancreatic glucagon. Biol Neonate 1972;21:375–80.
7. Moore WMO, Ward BS, Gordon C. Human placental transfer of glucagon. Clin Sci Mol Med 1974;46:125–9.
8. Spellacy WN, Buhi WC. Glucagon, insulin and glucose levels in maternal and umbilical cord plasma with studies of placental transfer. Obstet Gynecol 1976;47:291–4.
9. Rayburn W, Piehl E, Sanfield J, Compton A. Reversing severe hypoglycemia during pregnancy with glucagon therapy. Am J Perinatol 1987;4:259–61.
10. Tai YT, Lo CW, Chow WH, Cheng CH. Successful resuscitation and survival following massive overdose of metoprolol. Br J Clin Pract 1990;44:746–7.
11. Bailey B. Are there teratogenic risks associated with antidotes used in the acute management of poisoned pregnant women? Birth Defects Res A Clin Mol Teratol 2003;67:133–40.

GLUCARPIDASE

Antidote

PREGNANCY RECOMMENDATION: No Human Data—Probably Compatible
BREASTFEEDING RECOMMENDATION: No Human Data—Probably Compatible

PREGNANCY SUMMARY

No reports describing the use of glucarpidase in human or animal pregnancy have been located, but such reports are unlikely because of the drug's indication. The use of methotrexate in pregnancy is contraindicated (see Methotrexate). However, if the drug was used because a pregnant woman inadvertently received methotrexate, the benefit–risk ratio might favor glucarpidase.

FETAL RISK SUMMARY

Glucarpidase is a carboxypeptidase produced by recombinant DNA technology. The enzyme is a homodimer protein that converts methotrexate to its inactive metabolites. It is indicated for the treatment of toxic plasma methotrexate concentrations (>1 μmol/L) in patients with delayed methotrexate clearance due to impaired renal function. The metabolism and plasma protein binding data were not specified, but the elimination half-life is 9 hours (1).

Reproduction studies in animals have not been conducted. Neither have studies been conducted for carcinogenic and mutagenic potential, and studies for impairment of fertility.

It is not known if glucarpidase crosses the human placenta. The molecular weight (83,000) suggests that the protein will not cross to the embryo–fetus, at least early in gestation.

BREASTFEEDING SUMMARY

No reports describing the use of glucarpidase during human lactation have been located. The molecular weight (83,000) suggests that the protein will not be excreted into mature milk, but might be excreted during the colostral phase. However, reports of its use during breastfeeding are unlikely because of its indication. Methotrexate is contraindicated during breastfeeding (see Methotrexate).

Reference

1. Product information. Voraxaze. BTG International, 2012.

G

GLUCOSAMINE

Dietary Supplement

PREGNANCY RECOMMENDATION: Limited Human Data—Probably Compatible
BREASTFEEDING RECOMMENDATION: No Human Data—Probably Compatible

PREGNANCY SUMMARY

Except for the one study, no reports describing the use of glucosamine in human pregnancy have been located. The very limited animal data suggest low risk, but the human data are too limited to determine the risk of glucosamine in pregnancy. However, glucosamine is an endogenous substance widely found in human tissues, so the embryo–fetus must synthesize it during development. Moreover, the availability of free glucosamine to cross the placenta also is apparently very limited. Therefore, the planned or inadvertent use of glucosamine during gestation does not appear to represent a clinically significant risk of embryo–fetal harm.

FETAL RISK SUMMARY

Glucosamine, an amino-sugar, is an endogenous substance found in chitin, glycoproteins, and glycosaminoglycans (formerly known as mucopolysaccharides). It not only is derived from marine exoskeletons but also is prepared synthetically. Endogenous glucosamine is involved in the process of cartilage tissue formation and is present in tendons and ligaments. Commercial formulations of glucosamine, sometimes in combination with chondroitin or manganese, are used to treat osteoarthritis and other inflammatory conditions (1–4). The drug is available in oral, injectable (intra-articular, IM, and IV), and topical formulations, but only the oral form is available in the United States (2,3,5). Oral bioavailability (26%) is limited by hepatic metabolism, whereas IM bioavailability is 96%. After absorption, glucosamine is incorporated into plasma proteins, and the elimination half-life is 57–70 hours (5). No official standards regulate glucosamine production in the United States, so the actual dose taken cannot be accurately determined.

In a 1956 study, no teratogenicity was observed in mice and rabbits (6). However, glucosamine has been suspected of inhibiting protein, RNA, and DNA synthesis (1). The clinical significance of this is unknown.

It is not known if glucosamine crosses the animal or human placenta. The molecular weight (about 179) and prolonged plasma protein elimination half-life suggest that the drug will cross to the embryo–fetus. However, unbound glucosamine is concentrated in articular cartilage and free drug is undectable in the plasma (3). Therefore, it appears that free drug at the maternal:fetal interface is very limited and that little, if any, glucosamine would be available to cross the placenta.

A 2005 abstract cited data from an ongoing study involving the exposure of pregnant patients to glucosamine (7). Of the 55 women in the study, outcome data were available for 34 pregnancies (20 pregnancies ongoing; 1 case no data provided): 33 livebirths (2 sets of twins) and 3 spontaneous abortions. A male infant had a scrotal hernia, which was repaired surgically (7). The timing of the exposures, doses, and other information were not provided in this brief abstract.

Concern has been expressed that glucosamine might alter glucose metabolism (1–5). A 2006 review, however, concluded that the agent could be used in some patients without affecting glucose control, but data in diabetic patients were limited (8). Because pregnancy is a state of insulin resistance, pregnant women with diabetes should be monitored closely for changes in glucose control.

BREASTFEEDING SUMMARY

No reports describing the use of glucosamine during human lactation have been located. The molecular weight (about 179) and prolonged plasma protein elimination half-life suggest that the drug could be excreted in breast milk. However, unbound glucosamine is undetectable in the plasma (3).

Therefore, it appears that little, if any, drug will be excreted into milk, and its use during lactation probably is compatible.

References

1. Glucosamine. *The Review of Natural Products.* St. Louis, MO: Wolters Kluwer Health, 2004.
2. Glucosamine hydrochloride. *Natural Medicines Comprehensive Database.* Stockton, CA: Therapeutic Research Faculty, 2003:626–8.
3. Glucosamine Sulfate. *Natural Medicines Comprehensive Database.* Stockton, CA: Therapeutic Research Faculty, 2003:628–31.
4. Glucosamine. PDR Health. Available at http://www.pdrhealth.com/drug_info/nmdrugprofiles/nutsupdrugs/glu_0122.shtml. Accessed March 20, 2006.
5. Glucosamine. Micromedex (R) Healthcare Series. Available at http://126.0.10.223/mdxcgi/display.exe?CTL=D:\Root \MMDX\MDX\MDXCGI\MEGAT. Accessed March 24, 2006.
6. Didock KA, Jackson D, Robson JM. The action of some nucleotoxic substances in pregnancy. Br J Pharmacol 1956;11:437–41. As cited in Schardein JL. *Chemically Induced Birth Defects.* 3rd ed. New York, NY: Marcel Dekker, 2000:699.
7. Sivojelezova A, Einarson A, Koren G. A prospective cohort study evaluating pregnancy outcomes and risk perceptions of pregnant women following glucosamine use during pregnancy (abstract). Birth Defects Res (Part A) 2005;73:395.
8. Stumpf JL, Lin SW. Drug information rounds: effect of glucosamine on glucose control. Ann Pharmacother 2006;40:694–8.

G

GLYBURIDE

Antidiabetic Agent

PREGNANCY RECOMMENDATION: Human Data Suggest Low Risk
BREASTFEEDING RECOMMENDATION: Limited Human Data—Probably Compatible

PREGNANCY SUMMARY

The evidence suggests that glyburide may be an acceptable alternative to insulin in gestational diabetes, but the risk factors for failure need to be considered in the decision to use the oral agent. Glyburide also may be beneficial for decreasing the incidence of fetal and newborn morbidity and mortality in developing countries and in some populations where the proper use of insulin is problematic. Moreover, either the agent does not cross the placenta in detectable amounts or is actively transported back to the mother. In either case, neonatal hypoglycemia secondary to glyburide appears to be a low risk. Insulin is the treatment of choice for diabetic types 1 and 2. For non-insulin-dependent diabetics (type 2), close control of the mother's blood glucose with insulin, preferably starting before conception, will help to prevent the fetal and neonatal complications that occur with this disease. High maternal glucose levels, as may occur in diabetes mellitus, are associated with a number of maternal and fetal adverse effects, including fetal structural anomalies if the hyperglycemia occurs early in gestation. To prevent this toxicity, the American College of Obstetricians and Gynecologists recommends that insulin be used for types 1 and 2 diabetes occurring during pregnancy and, if diet therapy alone is not successful, for gestational diabetes (1,2).

FETAL RISK SUMMARY

Glyburide is a second-generation, oral sulfonylurea agent, structurally similar to acetohexamide and glipizide that is used for the treatment of adult-onset diabetes mellitus. It is not the treatment of choice for the pregnant diabetic patient. Glyburide is metabolized to inactive metabolites. The decrease in glyburide serum levels is biphasic with a terminal half-life of about 10 hours (3).

No fetotoxicity or teratogenicity was observed in pregnant mice, rats, and rabbits fed large doses of the agent (4). In pregnant rats, glyburide crossed the placenta to the fetus (fetal:maternal ratio 0.541) in amounts similar to diazepam (fetal:maternal ratio 0.641) (5).

In studies using in vitro techniques with human placentas, only relatively small amounts of glyburide were observed to transfer from the maternal to the fetal circulation (6–11), and the use of placentas from diabetic patients (7) or with high glucose concentrations (8) did not change the amounts transferred. Concentrations used on the maternal side of the perfused placenta model were approximately 800 ng/mL, much higher than the average peak serum level of 140–350 ng/mL obtained after a single 5-mg oral dose (9). Transport of the drug to the fetal side of the placenta was 0.62% at 2 hours.

The in vitro placental transfer, using a single cotyledon human placenta, of four oral hypoglycemic agents has been described (10). As expected, molecular weight was the most significant factor for drug transfer, with the dissociation constant (pK_a) and lipid solubility providing a significant additive effect. The cumulative percentage placental transfer at 3 hours of the four agents and their approximate molecular weights (shown in parentheses) were tolbutamide (270) 21.5%, chlorpropamide (277) 11.0%, glipizide (446) 6.6%, and glyburide (494) 3.9% (10). In a study using similar in vitro techniques with human placentas, glyburide did not increase glucose transfer to the fetus or affect the placental uptake of glucose (11).

A commentary in 2001 considered several factors (pK_a, molecular weight, lipid solubility, elimination half-life, and protein binding) that could limit glyburide from crossing the placenta (12). The short elimination half-life (4 hours) and extensive protein binding (99.8%) were thought to be the major determinants limiting transplacental transfer (12).

A 2006 study using an in vitro perfused human placental cotyledon reported evidence of active glyburide transport from the fetal to the maternal side (13). The transfer was against a concentration gradient, as the initial fetal:maternal concentration ratio was 0.92 and then decreased over 3 hours to 0.31. The investigators concluded that this was the first direct evidence of active transport from the fetus to the mother of any medicinal drug used during pregnancy (13).

A 1991 report described the outcomes of pregnancies in 21 non-insulin-dependent diabetic women who were treated with oral hypoglycemic agents (17 sulfonylureas, 3 biguanides, and 1 unknown type) during the 1st trimester (14). The duration of exposure was 3–28 weeks, but all patients were changed to insulin therapy at the first prenatal visit. Forty non-insulin-dependent diabetic matched women served as a control group. Eleven (52%) of the exposed infants had major or minor congenital malformations compared with 6 (15%) of the controls. Moreover, ear defects, a malformation that is observed, but uncommonly, in diabetic embryopathy, occurred in six of the exposed infants and in none of the controls. Two of the infants with defects (anencephaly; ventricular septal defect) were exposed in utero to glyburide during the first 10 and 23 weeks of gestation, respectively, but these and the other malformations observed, with the possible exception of the ear defects, were thought to be related to poor blood glucose control during organogenesis. The cluster of ear defects, however, suggested a drug effect or synergism between the drug and lack of metabolic control in the mother. Sixteen live births occurred in the exposed group compared with 36 in the control group. The groups did not differ in the incidence of hypoglycemia at birth (53% vs. 53%), but 3 of the exposed newborns (not exposed to glyburide) had severe hypoglycemia lasting 2, 4, and 7 days, even though the mothers had not used oral hypoglycemics close to delivery. This was attributed to irreversible β-cell hyperplasia that may have been increased by exposure to oral hypoglycemics. Hyperbilirubinemia was noted in 10 (67%) of 15 exposed newborns compared to 13 (36%) of controls ($p < 0.04$), and polycythemia and hyperviscosity requiring partial exchange transfusions were observed in 4 (27%) of 15 exposed vs. 1 (3.0%) control ($p < 0.03$) (1 exposed infant was not included in these data because of delivery after completion of study) (14).

The use of glyburide in all phases of human gestation has been reported in other studies (15–19). In these studies, glyburide (glibenclamide) was either used alone or combined with the oral antihyperglycemic agent, metformin (see Metformin). Neonatal hypoglycemia (blood glucose <25 mg/dL) was present in 4 of 15 (27%) newborns who were exposed to glyburide during gestation (16,17). This adverse effect was 3.5 times that observed in a group of newborns whose mothers were treated with insulin. Moreover, in one newborn, the hypoglycemia persisted for more than 48 hours (16).

A study published in 1995 assessed the risk of congenital malformations in infants of mothers with non-insulin-dependent diabetes (NIDDM) over a 6-year period (20). Women were included in the study if, during the first 8 weeks of pregnancy, they had not participated in a preconception care program and then had been treated either with diet alone (group 1), diet and oral hypoglycemic agents (predominantly chlorpropamide, glyburide, or glipizide) (group 2), or diet and exogenous insulin (group 3). The 302 women eligible for analysis gave birth to 332 infants (5 sets of twins and 16 with two or three separate singleton pregnancies during the study period). A total of 56 (16.9%) of the infants had one or more congenital malformations, 39 (11.7%) of which were classified as major anomalies (defined as those that were either lethal, caused significant morbidity, or required surgical repair). The major anomalies were divided among those involving the central nervous system, face, heart and great vessels, gastrointestinal, genitourinary, and skeletal (includes caudal regression syndrome) systems. Minor anomalies included all of these, except those of the central nervous system, and a miscellaneous group composed of sacral skin tags, cutis aplasia of the scalp, and hydroceles. The number of infants in each group and the number of major and minor anomalies observed were group 1—125 infants, 18 (14.4%) major, 6 (4.8%) minor; group 2—147 infants, 14 (9.5%) major, 9 (6.1%) minor; and group 3—60 infants, 7 (11.7%) major, 2 (3.3%) minor. There were no statistical differences among the groups. Six (4.1%) of the infants exposed in utero to oral hypoglycemic agents and four other infants in the other two groups had ear anomalies (included among those with face defects). Another important finding of this study was the independent association between the risk of major anomalies and poor glycemic control in early pregnancy. The study did not find an association between the use of oral hypoglycemics during organogenesis and congenital malformations because the observed anomalies appeared to be related to poor maternal glycemic control (20).

In a surveillance study of Michigan Medicaid recipients involving 229,101 completed pregnancies conducted between 1985 and 1992, 37 newborns had been exposed to glyburide during the 1st trimester (F. Rosa, personal communication, FDA, 1993). One (2.7%) major birth defect was observed (two expected), which was a cardiovascular defect (0.4 expected). No anomalies were observed in five other categories of defects (oral clefts, spina bifida, polydactyly, limb reduction defects, and hypospadias) for which specific data were available.

A study published in 2000 compared the pregnancy outcomes in gestational diabetic women with singleton pregnancies who were randomly assigned to treatment with glyburide or insulin (21). A majority of the women (83%) were Hispanic, mostly Mexican American. The study was not blinded. The goals of treatment were the achievement of a mean glucose concentration of 90–105 mg% and fasting, preprandial, and postprandial glucose levels of 60–90, 80–95, and <120 mg%, respectively. A total of 404 women were enrolled, 201 in the glyburide group and 203 in the insulin group. The mean pretreatment glucose concentrations, fasting, preprandial, and postprandial concentrations, and the glycosylated hemoglobin's in the glyburide and insulin groups were 114 vs. 116 mg%, 104 vs. 108 mg%, 104 vs. 107 mg%, 130 vs. 129 mg%, and 5.7% vs. 5.6%, respectively. These results are indicative of mild hyperglycemia. There were no significant differences between the groups in terms of any characteristic, including the gestational age at start of therapy and at delivery. The mean doses of glyburide and insulin were 9 mg/day and 85 units/day, respectively. Eight (4%) of the women randomized to glyburide failed to achieve good glycemic control and were changed to insulin. During treatment, the mean blood glucose concentrations and the mean fasting, preprandial, and postprandial values did not differ significantly between the glyburide and insulin groups. Nor was there a difference in the mean glycosylated hemoglobin values, 5.5% vs. 5.4%, respectively, measured late in the 3rd trimester. In 12 randomly selected women a mean 8 hours after the last dose, the glyburide maternal serum concentrations ranged from 50 to 150 ng/mL, whereas glyburide was undetectable in cord serum. No significant differences were measured between the groups in terms of neonatal features, metabolic outcomes, or perinatal mortality (21). An accompanying editorial explored the strengths and limitations of the study (22).

Several reports and an editorial have studied (23–27) or discussed (28) the use of glyburide for the treatment of gestational diabetes not controlled by diet. The studies reported favorable control of glucose levels with relatively few patients requiring a change to insulin therapy. However, in one study, glyburide-treated women had an increased risk of preeclampsia and their infants were more likely to require phototherapy for hyperbilirubinemia (25). Several risk factors have been identified that were predictors of glyburide failure: higher mean glucose values on glucose challenge test and more likely to have a test value ≥200 mg/dL (26); and diagnoses of diabetes earlier in gestation (23 vs. 28 weeks') of older age (34 vs. 29 years) and multiparity, and with higher fasting glucoses (>110 mg/dL) (27).

G

BREASTFEEDING SUMMARY

Nondetectable levels of glyburide in breast milk were reported in a 2005 study involving 11 lactating women, 3 of whom were nursing infants (29). The analysis of glyburide in milk was conducted at two different laboratories. Of eight nonbreastfeeding subjects, six received a single 5- mg dose and two received a single 10-mg dose. Glyburide was not detected in the milk of these cases (detection limit 0.005 mcg/mL). Three breastfeeding women on a steady-state dose of glyburide (5 mg every morning for 4–7 days) also had nondetectable peak (4 hours post-dose) and trough glyburide levels in their milk (detection limit 0.080 mcg/mL). Blood glucose levels were normal in two of the breastfed infants (not determined in the third infant because supplements were being given) (29).

References

1. American College of Obstetricians and Gynecologists. Pregestational diabetes mellitus. *ACOG Practice Bulletin*. No. 60. March 2005. Obstet Gynecol 2005;105:675–85.
2. American College of Obstetricians and Gynecologists. Gestational diabetes. *ACOG Practice Bulletin*. No. 30. September 2001. Obstet Gynecol 2001;98:525–38.
3. Product information. Diaβeta. Aventis Pharmaceuticals, 2004.
4. Shepard TH. *Catalog of Teratogenic Agents*. 8th ed. Baltimore, MD: The Johns Hopkins University Press, 1995:202.
5. Sivan E, Feldman B, Dolitzki M, Nevo N, Dekel N, Karasik A. Glyburide crosses the placenta in vivo in pregnant rats. Diabetologia 1995;38:753–6.
6. Elliott BD, Langer O, Schenker S, Johnson RF. Insignificant transfer of glyburide occurs across the human placenta. Am J Obstet Gynecol 1991;165:807–12.
7. Elliott BD, Bynum D, Langer O. Glyburide does not cross the diabetic placenta in significant amounts. Society of Perinatal Obstetricians Abstracts. Am J Obstet Gynecol 1993;168:360.
8. Elliott BD, Bynum D, Langer O. Maternal hyperglycemia does not alter in-vitro placental transfer of the oral hypoglycemic agent glyburide. Society of Perinatal Obstetricians Abstracts. Am J Obstet Gynecol 1993;168:360.
9. Elliott B, Langer O, Schenker S, Johnson R. Glyburide is insignificantly transported to the fetal circulation by the human placenta in vitro (abstract). Am J Obstet Gynecol 1991;164:247.
10. Elliott BD, Schenker S, Langer O, Johnson R, Prihoda T. Comparative placental transport of oral hypoglycemic agents in humans: a model of human placental drug transfer. Am J Obstet Gynecol 1994;171:653–60.
11. Elliott BD, Crosby-Schmidt C, Langer O. Human placental glucose uptake and transport are not altered by pharmacologic levels of the oral hypoglycemic agent, glyburide. Society of Perinatal Obstetricians Abstracts. Am J Obstet Gynecol 1994;170:321.
12. Koren G. Glyburide and fetal safety; transplacental pharmacokinetic considerations. Reprod Toxicol 2001;15:227–9.
13. Kraemer J, Klein J, Lubetsky A, Koren G. Perfusion studies of glyburide transfer across the human placenta: implications for fetal safety. Am J Obstet Gynecol 2006;195:270–4.
14. Piacquadio K, Hollingsworth DR, Murphy H. Effects of in-utero exposure to oral hypoglycaemic drugs. Lancet 1991;338:866–9.
15. Coetzee EJ, Jackson WPU. Diabetes newly diagnosed during pregnancy. A 4-year study at Groote Schuur Hospital. S Afr Med J 1979;56:467–75.
16. Coetzee EJ, Jackson WPU. Pregnancy in established non-insulin-dependent diabetics: a five-and-a-half year study at Groote Schuur Hospital. S Afr Med J 1980;58:795–802.
17. Coetzee EJ, Jackson WPU. Oral hypoglycaemics in the first trimester and fetal outcome. S Afr Med J 1984;65:635–7.
18. Coetzee EJ, Jackson WPU. The management of non-insulin-dependent diabetes during pregnancy. Diabetes Res Clin Pract 1986;5:281–7.
19. Ravina A. Insulin-dependent diabetes of pregnancy treated with the combination of sulfonylurea and insulin. Isr J Med Sci 1995;31:623–5.
20. Towner D, Kjos SL, Leung B, Montoro MM, Xiang A, Mestman JH, Buchanan TA. Congenital malformations in pregnancies complicated by NIDDM. Diabetes Care 1995;18:1446–51.
21. Langer O, Conway DL, Berkus MD, Xenakis EMJ, Gonzales O. A comparison of glyburide and insulin in women with gestational diabetes mellitus. N Engl J Med 2000;343:1134–8.
22. Greene MF. Oral hypoglycemic drugs for gestational diabetes. N Engl J Med 2000;343:1178–9.
23. Velazquez MD, Bolnick J, Cloakey D, Gonzalez JL, Curet LB. The use of glyburide in the management of gestational diabetes. Obstet Gynecol 2003;101(Suppl):88S.
24. Kremer CJ, Duff P. Glyburide for the treatment of gestational diabetes. Am J Obstet Gynecol 2004;190:1438–9.
25. Jacobson GF, Ramos GA, Ching JV, Kirby RS, Ferrara A, Field DR. Comparison of glyburide and insulin for the management of gestational diabetes in a large managed care organization. Am J Obstet Gynecol 2005;193:118–24.
26. Rochon M, Rand L, Roth L, Gaddipati S. Glyburide for the management of gestational diabetes: risk factors predictive of failure and associated pregnancy outcomes. Am J Obstet Gynecol 2006;195:1090–4.
27. Kahn BF, Davies JK, Lynch AM, Reynolds RM, Barbour LA. Predictors of glyburide failure in the treatment of gestational diabetes. Obstet Gynecol 2006;107:1303–9.
28. Durnwald C, Landon MB. Glyburide: the new alternative for treating gestational diabetes? Am J Obstet Gynecol 2005;193:1–2.
29. Feig DS, Briggs GG, Kraemer JM, Ambrose PJ, Moskovitz DN, Nageotte MP, Donat DJ, Padilla G, Wan S, Klein J, Koren G. Transfer of glyburide and glipizide into breast milk. Diabetes Care 2005;28:1851–5.

GLYCERIN

Laxative

PREGNANCY RECOMMENDATION: Limited Human Data—Probably Compatible
BREASTFEEDING RECOMMENDATION: No Human Data—Probably Compatible

PREGNANCY SUMMARY

Only one report describing the use of glycerin in human pregnancy has been located. The near absence of human pregnancy experience prevents a full assessment of the embryo–fetal risk.

FETAL RISK SUMMARY

In a 2013 case report, a 24-year-old woman at 22 weeks' gestation was treated with 6 weeks of meropenem (3 g/day) and cefotaxime (2 g/day) for a brain abscess (1). Glycerin (20 g/day) was given to reduce intracranial pressure. She responded well to the therapy. At term, she gave birth to a normal 2890-g female infant (1).

BREASTFEEDING SUMMARY

No data are available.

Reference

1. Yoshida M, Matsuda H, Furuya K. Successful prognosis of brain abscess during pregnancy. J Reprod Infertil 2013;14:152–5.

G

GLYCOPYRROLATE

Parasympatholytic (Anticholinergic)

PREGNANCY RECOMMENDATION: Limited Human Data—No Relevant Animal Data
BREASTFEEDING RECOMMENDATION: No Human Data—Probably Compatible

PREGNANCY SUMMARY

Glycopyrrolate is an anticholinergic agent. Although the data are very limited, there is no evidence that drugs in this class cause developmental toxicity.

FETAL RISK SUMMARY

In pregnant sheep, the transfer of glycopyrrolate (0.025 mg/kg) across the placenta was significantly less than that of atropine (0.05 mg/kg) (1). No change in maternal or fetal arterial pressure, fetal heart rate, or beat-to-beat variability was observed. In pregnant dogs, the placental passage of glycopyrrolate was again significantly less than that of atropine (2).

In a large prospective study, 2323 patients were exposed to this class of drugs during the 1st trimester, only 4 of whom took glycopyrrolate (3). A possible association was found between the total group and minor malformations.

Glycopyrrolate has been used before cesarean section to decrease gastric secretions (4–7). Maternal heart rate, but not blood pressure, was increased. Uterine activity increased as expected for normal labor. Fetal heart rate and variability were not changed significantly, confirming the limited placental transfer of this quaternary ammonium compound. No effects in the newborns were observed.

In a 1999 double-blind, randomized, controlled study, women were treated with either glycopyrrolate ($N = 24$) or placebo ($N = 25$) immediately before induction of subarachnoid anesthesia for elective cesarean section to determine if the drug reduced the incidence and severity of nausea (8). Glycopyrrolate reduced the frequency ($p = 0.02$) and severity ($p = 0.03$) of nausea. It also reduced the severity of hypotension as evidenced by reduced ephedrine requirements ($p = 0.02$). There was no difference in Apgar scores between the two groups (8).

A 2011 study was conducted to determine if glycopyrrolate prevents bradycardia in women receiving spinal anesthesia for cesarean section (9). In the double-blind, placebo-controlled study, 34 patients received glycopyrrolate and 35 received saline. Bradycardia (heart rate <60/min) occurred in none of the glycopyrrolate patients and in six of the placebo group ($p = 0.02$) (9).

Glycopyrrolate has been recommended as the anticholinergic of choice during anesthesia for electroconvulsive therapy in pregnant patients (10).

BREASTFEEDING SUMMARY

No reports describing the use of glycopyrrolate during human lactation have been located (see also Atropine).

References

1. Murad SHN, Conklin KA, Tabsh KMA, Brinkman CR III, Erkkola R, Nuwayhid B. Atropine and glycopyrrolate: hemodynamic effects and placental transfer in the pregnant ewe. Anesth Analg 1981;60:710–4.
2. Proakis AG, Harris GB. Comparative penetration of glycopyrrolate and atropine across the blood–brain and placental barriers in anesthetized dogs. Anesthesiology 1978;48:339–44.
3. Heinonen OP, Slone D, Shapiro S. *Birth Defects and Drugs in Pregnancy*. Littleton, MA: Publishing Sciences Group, 1977:346–53.
4. Diaz DM, Diaz SF, Marx GF. Cardiovascular effects of glycopyrrolate and belladonna derivatives in obstetric patients. Bull NY Acad Med 1980;56:245–8.
5. Abboud TK, Read J, Miller F, Chen T, Valle R, Henriksen EH. Use of glycopyrrolate in the parturient: effect on the maternal and fetal heart and uterine activity. Obstet Gynecol 1981;57:224–7.
6. Roper RE, Salem MG. Effects of glycopyrrolate and atropine combined with antacid on gastric acidity. Br J Anaesth 1981;53:1277–80.
7. Abboud T, Raya J, Sadri S, Grobler N, Stine L, Miller F. Fetal and maternal cardiovascular effects of atropine and glycopyrrolate. Anesth Analg 1983;62:426–30.

8. Ure D, James KS, McNeill M, Booth JV. Glycopyrrolate reduces nausea during spinal anaesthesia for cesarean section without affecting neonatal outcome. Br J Anaesthesia 1999;82:277–9.
9. Chamchad D, Horrow JC, Nakhamchik L, Sauter J, Roberts N, Aronzon B, Gerson A, Medved M. Prophylactic glycopyrrolate prevents bradycardia after spinal anesthesia for cesarean section: a randomized, double-blind, placebo-controlled prospective trial with heart rate variability correlation. J Clin Anesth 2011;23:361–6.
10. Wise MG, Ward SC, Townsend-Parchman W, Gilstrap LC III, Hauth JC. Case report of ECT during high-risk pregnancy. Am J Psychiatry 1984;141:99–101.

GOLDENSEAL

Herb

PREGNANCY RECOMMENDATION: Contraindicated
BREASTFEEDING RECOMMENDATION: No Human Data—Potential Toxicity (High or Frequent Doses)

G

PREGNANCY SUMMARY

Goldenseal and its active isoquinoline alkaloids, hydrastine and berberine, should be avoided in pregnancy because they can stimulate uterine contractions and induce labor. Although dosage information and clinical reports are lacking, goldenseal has been used traditionally as an abortifacient. Nevertheless, goldenseal preparations have been available for centuries, and the absence of reports describing human pregnancy toxicity suggests low risk, at least from usual doses. However, the safest course is to avoid this herb in pregnancy, especially high doses and/or frequent use.

FETAL RISK SUMMARY

The perennial herb, goldenseal is found in the woods of the Ohio River valley and other locations in the northeastern United States. It also is grown commercially in Washington State, New York, North Carolina, and Canada (1). Goldenseal has been used for hundreds of years and is one of the five top-selling herbal products in the United States (2). The principal active components, found in the roots, include the isoquinoline alkaloids (range of concentrations) hydrastine (1.5%–4%) and berberine (0.5%–6%). Other alkaloids with apparently less activity include canadine (tetrahydroberberine), palmatine, and berberastine. For goldenseal, the typical daily doses for tablets and capsules is 0.75–3.4 g/day, 0.9–3 mL of fluid extract, 6–12 mL of tincture, and 1.5–3 g of dried root as a decoction (1,2).

Goldenseal is a component of many over-the-counter products, such as dietary supplements, digestive aids, eardrops, cold/flu and allergy remedies, and laxatives. The herb or individual alkaloids have been used for their antimicrobial, antidiarrheal, anti-inflammatory, antiproliferative, cardiovascular, ophthalmic, immunostimulant, and other effects, but controlled trials are lacking. Moreover, the alkaloids are poorly absorbed when taken orally (1,2).

Reproduction studies have been conducted in rats and mice (3–8). In pregnant rats, a daily oral dose that was 65 times the human dose based on body weight was given on gestation days 1–8 or 8–15 (3). Compared with controls, there was no increase in pre- or postimplantation losses, no change in fetal weight, and no difference in the incidence of external or internal malformations. In a separate study, rat embryos were explanted on gestation day 10.5 and cultured with increasing concentrations (0.5–6 μL/mL) of goldenseal extract for 26 hours in rat serum. Compared with nonexposed embryos, growth restriction and embryotoxicity were observed in a dose-dependent manner beginning at 1 μL/mL. The different results observed were thought to be due to the poor oral absorption of goldenseal. Because goldenseal is unlikely to be absorbed to the same extent as the concentrations used in the in vitro study, the authors thought that the herb, at the prescribed human dose, would not cause human embryo toxicity (3).

In a series of studies conducted by the National Toxicology Program, no developmental toxicity was observed in pregnant rats and mice at doses that were less than the maternal toxic dose (4–9).

It is not known if the active isoquinoline alkaloids of goldenseal cross the human placenta. The molecular weights of two alkaloids, berberine (about 353) and canadine (about 339), are low enough to cross. However, the poor systemic bioavailability after recommended oral doses suggests that little will reach the maternal circulation and be available to expose the embryo–fetus. Higher doses, however, may result in greater bioavailability and, consequently, greater embryo–fetal exposure.

Hydrastine and berberine are known to be uterine stimulants (1,2). Although published clinical trials are lacking, herbs containing these constituents have been used traditionally as abortifacients (2). The dose required for this effect has not been published.

BREASTFEEDING SUMMARY

No reports describing the use of goldenseal or its active constituents during lactation have been located. Systemic absorption is poor after ingestion of recommended doses, so the amount of alkaloids in milk is most likely very low. High or frequent doses, however, might result in systemic concentrations and excretion into breast milk. Berberine, one of the active isoquinoline alkaloids of goldenseal, is known to displace bilirubin from albumin in animal studies, resulting in increased serum total and direct bilirubin concentrations (2). The risk of this for a nursing infant is unknown but probably low if the mother is ingesting low, infrequent doses of goldenseal. However, high doses or frequent use of goldenseal, or use of the specific alkaloids, could place the infant at risk of icterus or jaundice. Until human data are available, the safest course is to avoid goldenseal or its active alkaloids while breastfeeding (10).

References

1. Goldenseal. *The Review of Natural Products*. St. Louis, MO: Facts and Comparisons, 2008.
2. Goldenseal (Hydrastis canadensis). Natural Standard Monograph. Available at www.naturalstandard.com. Accessed March 3, 2009.
3. Yao M, Ritchie HE, Brown-Woodman D. A reproductive screening test for goldenseal. Birth Defects Res B Dev Reprod Toxicol 2005;74:399–404.
4. NTP Study TER98007. *Developmental Toxicity Evaluation for Goldenseal Root Powder (Hydrastis canadensis) Administered in the Feed to Sprague-Dawley (CD®) Rats on Gestational Days 6 to 20*. National Toxicology Program. Springfield, VA: National Technical Information Services, 2002.
5. NTP Study TER98008. *Developmental Toxicity Evaluation for Berberine Chloride Dihydrate (CAS no. 5956-60-5) Administered in the Feed to Sprague-Dawley (CD®) Rats on Gestational Days 6 to 20*. National Toxicology Program. Springfield, VA: National Technical Information Services, 2003.
6. NTP Study TER99002. *Developmental Toxicity Evaluation for Berberine Chloride Dihydrate (CAS no. 5956-60-5) Administered in the Feed to Swiss (CD-1®) Mice on Gestational Days 6 to 17*. National Toxicology Program. Springfield, VA: National Technical Information Services, 2003.
7. NTP Study TER99004. *Developmental Toxicity Evaluation for Goldenseal (Hydrastis canadensis) Root Powder Administered in the Feed to Swiss (CD-1®) Mice on Gestational Days 6-17*. National Toxicology Program. Springfield, VA: National Technical Information Services, 2002.
8. NTP Study TER20102. *Developmental Toxicity Research Evaluation for Berberine Chloride Dihydrate (CAS no. 5956-60-5) Administered by Gavage to Sprague-Dawley (CD®) Rats on Gestational Days 6 Through 19*. National Toxicology Program. Springfield, VA: National Technical Information Services, 2002.
9. NTP Study TER20103. *Developmental Toxicity Research Evaluation for Berberine Chloride Dihydrate (CAS no. 5956-60-5) Administered by Gavage to Swiss (CD-1®) Mice on Gestational Days 6 Through 16*. National Toxicology Program. Springfield, VA: National Technical Information Services, 2003.
10. National Center for Complementary and Alternative Medicine. Goldenseal. *Herbs at A Glance*. National Institutes of Health, U.S. Department of Health and Human Services, 2008. Available at http://nccam.nih.gov/health/goldenseal. Accessed August 3, 2009.

GOLD SODIUM THIOMALATE

Immunologic Agent (Antirheumatic)

PREGNANCY RECOMMENDATION: Limited Human Data—Animal Data Suggest Low Risk
BREASTFEEDING RECOMMENDATION: Limited Human Data—Probably Compatible

PREGNANCY SUMMARY

Although gold compounds apparently do not pose a major risk to the fetus, the clinical experience is limited and long-term follow-up studies of exposed fetuses have not been reported.

FETAL RISK SUMMARY

Gold sodium thiomalate is indicated in the treatment of active rheumatoid arthritis. Teratogenic effects were observed in rats and rabbits given SC doses 140 and 175 times the usual human dose, respectively, during organogenesis (1). In rats, the defects were hydrocephaly and microphthalmia, whereas those in rabbits were limb malformations and gastroschisis.

Gold compounds have been used for the treatment of maternal rheumatoid arthritis and other conditions in a small number of pregnancies (2–7). One review noted that several pregnant patients had been treated with gold salts without harmful effects observed in the newborns (2). In a Japanese report, 119 patients were treated during the 1st trimester with gold, 26 of whom received the drug throughout pregnancy (3). Two anomalies were observed in the newborns—a dislocated hip in one infant and a flattened acetabulum in another—but the association with the therapy is unknown. A German case history involved a woman who received her last injection of gold for chronic polyarthritis in the 3rd week of pregnancy (4). A growth-restricted, 1750-g female infant was delivered at 40 weeks' gestation. Other than the low birth weight, no other abnormalities were noted in the infant, whose development during the next 2 years was normal. In another case, a woman had been treated with gold sodium thiomalate (sodium aurothiomalate) for 2 years immediately prior to pregnancy, receiving her last dose when several weeks pregnant (5). No adverse effects in the newborn were mentioned.

Gold compounds cross the placenta. A patient who had received a total dose of 570 mg of gold sodium thiomalate from before conception through the 20th week of gestation elected to terminate her pregnancy (6). No obvious fetal abnormalities were observed, but gold deposits were found in the fetal liver and kidneys. A second patient received monthly 100-mg injections of gold throughout pregnancy (7). The last dose, given 3 days prior to delivery, produced a cord serum concentration of 2.25 mcg/mL, 57% of the simultaneous maternal serum level. No anomalies were observed in the infant.

BREASTFEEDING SUMMARY

Gold is excreted in milk (5,8–10). A woman received a total aurothioglucose dose of 135 mg in the postpartum period (8). Gold levels in two milk samples collected a week apart were 8.64 and 9.97 mcg/mL, respectively. The validity of these figures has been challenged on a mathematical basis, so the exact amount excreted is open to question (9). In addition, the timing of the samples in relation to the dose was not given. Of interest, however, was the demonstration of gold levels in the infant's red blood cells (0.354 mcg/mL) and serum (0.712 mcg/mL) obtained on the same date as the second milk sample. The author speculated that this unexpected oral absorption may have been the cause of various unexplained adverse reactions noted in nursing infants of mothers receiving gold injections, such as rashes, nephritis, hepatitis, and hematologic abnormalities (8).

Another report described a lactating woman who was treated with 50 mg of gold sodium thiomalate weekly for 7 weeks after an initial 20-mg dose (total dose 370 mg) (10). Milk and infant urine samples collected 66 hours after the last dose yielded gold levels of 22 and 0.4 ng/mL, respectively. Repeat samples collected 7 days after an additional 25-mg dose produced milk and urine levels of 40 and <0.4 ng/mL, respectively. Three months after cessation of therapy, transient facial edema was observed in the nursing infant, but it was not known whether this was related to the maternal gold administration (10).

In a 1986 report, two women were given IM injections of gold sodium thiomalate (5). One patient received 20 mg on day 1 followed by 50 mg on day 3. Milk concentrations rose from a low of 17 ng/mL (1.4% of simultaneous maternal serum) 10 hours after the first dose to a peak of 153 ng/mL (approximately 4.6% of maternal serum) 22 hours after the second dose. The second patient received three doses of the gold salt consisting of 10 mg on day 1, 20 mg on day 8, and 20 mg on day 12. The peak milk concentration, 185 ng/mL (10.4% of maternal serum), occurred 3 hours after the third dose. The levels of gold in the milk of both patients increased steadily over the sampling periods. The investigators estimated that the nursing infant would receive about 20% of the maternal dose (5).

Three studies have described the excretion of gold into breast milk, with milk concentrations in two of the studies similar in magnitude. Gold absorption by the nursing infant has been documented. Although adverse effects have been suggested, a direct cause-and-effect relationship has not been proven. At least one set of investigators cautioned that, due to the prolonged maternal elimination time after gold administration and the potential for toxicity in the infant, nursing should be avoided (5). However, the American Academy of Pediatrics classifies gold salts as compatible with breastfeeding (11).

References

1. Product information. Myochrysine. Merck, 2000.
2. Freyberg RH, Ziff M, Baum J. Gold therapy for rheumatoid arthritis. In: Hollander JL, McCarty DJ Jr, eds. *Arthritis and Allied Conditions*. 8th ed. Philadelphia, PA: Lea & Febiger, 1972:479.
3. Miyamoto T, Miyaji S, Horiuchi Y, Hara M, Ishihara K. Gold therapy in bronchial asthma—special emphasis upon blood level of gold and its teratogenicity. J Jpn Soc Intern Med 1974;63:1190–7.
4. Fuchs U, Lippert TH. Gold therapy and pregnancy. Dtsch Med Wochenschr 1986;111:31–4.
5. Ostensen M, Skavdal K, Myklebust G, Tomassen Y, Aarbakke J. Excretion of gold into human breast milk. Eur J Clin Pharmacol 1986;31:251–2.
6. Rocker I, Henderson WJ. Transfer of gold from mother to fetus. Lancet 1976;2:1246.
7. Cohen DL, Orzel J, Taylor A. Infants of mothers receiving gold therapy. Arthritis Rheum 1981;24:104–5.
8. Blau SP. Metabolism of gold during lactation. Arthritis Rheum 1973;16: 777–8.
9. Gottlieb NL. Suggested errata. Arthritis Rheum 1974;17:1057.
10. Bell RAF, Dale IM. Gold secretion in maternal milk. Arthritis Rheum 1976;19:1374.
11. Committee on Drugs, American Academy of Pediatrics. The transfer of drugs and other chemicals into human milk. Pediatrics 2001;108: 776–89.

GOLIMUMAB

Immunologic Agent (Immunomodulator)

PREGNANCY RECOMMENDATION: No Human Data—Animal Data Suggest Low Risk
Contraindicated (if combined with methotrexate)
BREASTFEEDING RECOMMENDATION: No Human Data—Probably Compatible
Contraindicated (if combined with methotrexate)

PREGNANCY SUMMARY

No reports describing the use of golimumab in human pregnancy have been located. The animal data from one species suggest that the embryo–fetal risk is low. However, the lack of human pregnancy experience prevents a full assessment of the risk. There is some similarity between the action of immunomodulators with antitumor necrosis factor alpha (TNFα) activity and the human teratogen thalidomide, a drug that also decreases the activity of TNFα (see Thalidomide). However, decreased production of TNFα may not be a primary cause of the teratogenicity of thalidomide. Theoretically, TNFα antagonists could interfere with implantation and ovulation, but this has not been shown clinically (1). If golimumab is indicated in a pregnant woman, she should be informed of the absence of human pregnancy data. Moreover, until adequate human data are available, the safest course is to avoid the drug during organogenesis (20–55 days after conception or 34–69 days from the first day of the last menstrual period).

FETAL RISK SUMMARY

Golimumab is a human IgG1k monoclonal antibody that blocks human TNFα. TNFα is a pro-inflammatory cytokine with a central role in inflammatory processes. Golimumab is in the same subclass of immunomodulators as adalimumab, certolizumab pegol, etanercept, and infliximab that block TNF. It is indicated, in combination with methotrexate, for the treatment of adult patients with moderately to severely active rheumatoid arthritis. Golimumab also is indicated, either alone or with methotrexate, for the treatment of adult patients with active psoriatic arthritis and, alone for the treatment of adult patients with active ankylosing spondylitis. The median terminal half-life is about 2 weeks (2).

Reproduction studies have been conducted in monkeys. Pregnant monkeys were given twice-weekly SC doses during the 1st trimester that were up to 300 times the maximum recommended human dose based on weight. No evidence of maternal or fetal harm or developmental defects was observed. The drug crossed the placenta as indicated by its presence in umbilical cord blood obtained at the end of the 2nd trimester. When monkeys were given twice-weekly SC doses during the 2nd and 3rd trimesters, no evidence of maternal or neonatal harm was noted. The doses produced maternal and neonatal exposures that were 860 and 310 times, respectively, the maximal steady state human blood levels. This exposure during pregnancy and lactation had no effect on the development and maturation of the immune system in offspring (2,3).

Studies for neither carcinogenicity nor mutagenicity have been conducted with golimumab. A study in mice using an analogous anti-mouse TNFα antibody showed no impairment of fertility (2).

It is not known if golimumab crosses the human placenta. The molecular weight (about 150,000–151,000) is high, but immunoglobulin G crosses the placenta late in pregnancy (see Immune Globulin Intravenous). Placental transfer of IgG was a function of dose, as well as gestational age. Moreover, golimumab crossed to the fetus in monkeys and, because the placentas in monkeys are similar to those in humans, the antibody should be expected to cross to the human fetus.

BREASTFEEDING SUMMARY

No reports describing the use of golimumab during human lactation have been located. It is not known if the antibody is excreted into breast milk. The molecular weight (about 150,000–151,000) is high, but the terminal half-life is very long (about 2 weeks). Because immunoglobulins are excreted into milk, exposure of a nursing infant should be expected. The effect of this exposure is unknown, but serious infections have been observed in human adults treated with golimumab. However, exposure during lactation had no effect on the development and maturation of the immune system in monkey offspring (3). Nevertheless, if a woman elects to nurse her infant while receiving this agent, close observation of the infant for signs and symptoms of infection should be considered.

References

1. Khanna D, McMahon M, Furst DE. Safety of tumor necrosis factor-α antagonists. Drug Saf 2004;27:307–24.
2. Product information. Simponi. Centocor Ortho Biotech, 2009.
3. Martin PL, Oneda S, Treacy G. Effects of an anti-TNF-α monoclonal antibody, administered throughout pregnancy and lactation, on the development of the macaque immune system. Am J Reprod Immunol 2007;58:138–49.

GRANISETRON

Antiemetic

PREGNANCY RECOMMENDATION: Limited Human Data—Animal Data Suggest Low Risk
BREASTFEEDING RECOMMENDATION: No Human Data—Probably Compatible

PREGNANCY SUMMARY

Three reports describing the use of granisetron during human gestation have been located. Because of the indication for this drug, the opportunity for fetal exposure appears to be minimal.

FETAL RISK SUMMARY

Granisetron is an antiemetic used for the prevention of nausea and vomiting in patients receiving cancer chemotherapy. The drug is a selective 5-hydroxytryptamine$_3$ (5-HT$_3$)-receptor antagonist with little or no affinity for other serotonin receptors (1). No evidence of an effect on plasma prolactin concentrations has been found in clinical studies.

Reproductive studies at doses up to 146 and 96 times, respectively, the recommended human dose based on BSA in pregnant rats and rabbits found no evidence of impaired fertility or harm to the fetus (1). Shepard reviewed three studies conducted in rats and rabbits before and after conception or in the perinatal and postnatal periods that found no adverse fetal effects or drug-related effects on behavior (2).

It is not known whether granisetron crosses the placenta to the fetus. The molecular weight (about 349) is low enough that passage to the fetus should be expected.

Granisetron has been used to prevent vomiting during cesarean section (3) and with chemotherapy in the 3rd trimester (4,5). No fetal or newborn complications related to the antiemetic were reported.

BREASTFEEDING SUMMARY

No reports describing the use of granisetron during lactation have been located. The indication for granisetron therapy, however, suggests that the opportunities for use of the drug during lactation are minimal. Because of its low molecular weight (about 349), transfer into breast milk should be expected.

References

1. Product information. Kytril. SmithKline Beecham Pharmaceuticals, 1997.
2. Shepard TH. *Catalog of Teratogenic Agents*. 8th ed. Baltimore, MD: The Johns Hopkins University Press, 1995:204–5.
3. Fujii Y. Prevention of emetic episodes during cesarean delivery performed under regional anesthesia in parturients. Curr Drug Saf 2007;2: 25–32.
4. Merimsky O, Le Cesne A. Soft tissue and bone sarcomas in association with pregnancy. Acta Oncol 1998;37:721–7.
5. Merimsky O, Le Chevalier T, Missenard G, Lepechoux C, Cojean-Zelek I, Mesurolle B, Le Cesne A. Management of cancer in pregnancy: a case of Ewing's sarcoma of the pelvis in the third trimester. Ann Oncol 1999;10: 345–50.

G

GRISEOFULVIN

Antifungal

PREGNANCY RECOMMENDATION: Limited Human Data—Probably Compatible
BREASTFEEDING RECOMMENDATION: No Human Data—Potential Toxicity

PREGNANCY SUMMARY

Although the animal reproductive data suggest risk, the human pregnancy experience is too limited for a complete assessment of the embryo–fetal risk. However, griseofulvin is best avoided during organogenesis because the use of an antifungal agent is seldom essential during this time.

G

FETAL RISK SUMMARY

Griseofulvin is a fungistatic antibiotic derived from a species of *Penicillium*. The drug is tumorigenic, embryotoxic, and teratogenic in some species of animals. Chronic oral exposure to griseofulvin in several strains of mice has induced hepatic and thyroid tumors (1). Hepatic tumors were also induced by relatively low weekly SC doses in mice during the first 3 weeks of life (1). Multiple malformations, including defects of the eye, skeleton, urogenital tract, and the central nervous system, were observed in fetuses of pregnant rats injected with 50–500 mg/kg on days 11–14 of gestation (2). Daily doses of 1250–1500 mg/kg (about 60–75 times the usual human dose) on days 6 through 15 of gestation in rats produced tail defects and occasional exencephaly (2). Because of the animal toxicity, at least one publication suggested that it not be given during pregnancy (3).

Human placental transfer of griseofulvin has been demonstrated at term (4).

In a surveillance study of Michigan Medicaid recipients involving 229,101 completed pregnancies conducted between 1985 and 1992, 34 newborns had been exposed to griseofulvin during the 1st trimester (F. Rosa, personal communication, FDA, 1993). One (2.9%) major birth defect was observed (one expected). No anomalies were observed in six defect categories (cardiovascular defects, oral clefts, spina bifida, polydactyly, limb reduction defects, and hypospadias) for which specific data were available. The number of exposures is too small to draw any conclusions.

A possible interaction between oral contraceptives and griseofulvin has been reported in 22 women (5). The study described transient intermenstrual bleeding in 15 women, amenorrhea in 5, and unintended pregnancies in 2.

In a report from the FDA, two sets of conjoined twins were observed in a sample of >20,000 birth defect cases with 1st trimester drug exposure (6). The first case involved female twins conjoined at the head and chest (craniothoracopagus syncephalus), and the second involved male dicephalic twins joined in the thorax and lumbar areas with a single seven-chamber heart. In both cases, the mothers had taken griseofulvin during early pregnancy. Fission with twinning is normally completed by the 20th day after ovulation, and thus, the cause of conjoined twinning would have to be present prior to this time (6). In both cases, maternal griseofulvin use was the only drug exposure (of those drugs under surveillance by the FDA). Because the incidence of conjoined twins is rare (approximately 1 in 50,000 births) and thoracopagus is even less common (1 in 250,000), the authors concluded that the cases provided evidence for an association with griseofulvin (6). The FDA investigators also examined other data on 1st trimester griseofulvin exposure involving 55,736 deliveries from one geographic area between 1980 and 1983 (6). Of these cases, griseofulvin was taken during the first 3 months by 37 mothers, two of whom delivered infants with birth defects: one with a congenital heart defect and the other with an unknown defect. The incidence of 5.4% (2 of 37) was approximately the incidence in the total sample. However, in 4264 women with spontaneous or threatened abortion diagnoses, 7 had been prescribed the drug during the preceding 3 months, a relative risk of 2.5 (95% confidence interval 1.01–6.1) (6).

Prompted by the above report, investigators in two other countries reported data from their respective congenital anomaly registries (7,8). One of these, from Hungary, found 39 sets of conjoined twins in a sample of more than 100,000 cases of congenital anomalies observed between 1970 and 1986 (griseofulvin was marketed in Hungary in 1970) (7). None of the mothers of the 39 conjoined twins took griseofulvin. The prevalence of conjoined twins in Hungary is approximately 1 in 60,000 births (7). The investigators also reported data from their case–control surveillance system for the period 1980–1984 (7). Of 6786 congenital anomaly cases, 2 were exposed to griseofulvin–one infant with a heart defect was exposed during the 2nd and 3rd months, and one infant with pyloric stenosis was exposed during the 1st month. Three exposures occurred in the 10,962 matched controls, all in the late 2nd and 3rd trimesters.

The second report involved data from the International Clearinghouse for Birth Defects Monitoring Systems (8). None of the 47 sets of conjoined twins in more than 3 million births had been exposed to griseofulvin. Thus, neither of these reports was able to support the FDA report of an association between griseofulvin and the rare defect.

A 2003 review concluded that griseofulvin was contraindicated in pregnancy because of a high risk of teratogenicity and the availability of safer alternatives (9). In contrast, a 2004 report of a population-based case–control study did not detect a teratogenic risk of oral griseofulvin treatment during pregnancy (10). The data for this study came from the Hungarian Case-Control Surveillance of Congenital Anomalies in 1980–1996 and the Hungarian Congenital Abnormalities Registry for 1970–2002. The control group was composed of 38,151 pregnant women who gave birth to normal infants compared with 22,843 case women who had fetuses or newborns with birth defects. Griseofulvin was used in 7 (0.03%) of the cases and 24 (0.06%) of the controls. No teratogenic potential was found by a comparison of the expected and observe number of different congenital anomalies. In addition, there were 55 conjoined twins and none had been exposed to griseofulvin (10).

BREASTFEEDING SUMMARY

No reports describing the use of griseofulvin during lactation have been located. Because of the potential for toxicity in a nursing infant, the use of griseofulvin during breastfeeding does not appear to be warranted.

References

1. Product information. Fulvicin. Schering, 2000.
2. Shepard TH. *Catalog of Teratogenic Agents*. 9th ed. Baltimore, MD: The Johns Hopkins University Press, 1998:224–5.
3. Anonymous. Griseofulvin: a new formulation and some old concerns. Med Lett Drugs Ther 1976;18:17.
4. Rubin A, Dvornik D. Placental transfer of griseofulvin. Am J Obstet Gynecol 1965;92:882–3.
5. van Dijke CPH, Weber JCP. Interaction between oral contraceptives and griseofulvin. Br Med J 1984;288:1125–6.
6. Rosa FW, Hernandez C, Carlo WA. Griseofulvin teratology, including two thoracopagus conjoined twins. Lancet 1987;1:171.
7. Metneki J, Czeizel A. Griseofulvin teratology. Lancet 1987;1:1042.
8. Knudsen LB. No association between griseofulvin and conjoined twinning. Lancet 1987;2:1097.
9. Moudgal VV, Sobel JD. Antifungal drugs in pregnancy: a review. Expert Opin Drug Saf 2003;2:475–83.
10. Czeizel AE, Metneki J, Kazy Z, Puho E. A population-based case–control study of oral griseofulvin treatment during pregnancy. Acta Obstet Gynecol 2004;83:827–31.

GUAIFENESIN

Respiratory Drug (Expectorant)

PREGNANCY RECOMMENDATION: Compatible
BREASTFEEDING RECOMMENDATION: No Human Data—Probably Compatible

PREGNANCY SUMMARY

The available pregnancy data do not support an association between guaifenesin and developmental toxicity.

FETAL RISK SUMMARY

The Collaborative Perinatal Project monitored 197 mother–child pairs with 1st trimester exposure to guaifenesin (1, p. 478). An increase in the expected frequency of inguinal hernias was found. For use anytime during pregnancy, 1336 exposures were recorded (1, p. 442). In this latter case, no evidence for an association with malformations was found. In another large study in which 241 women were exposed to the drug during pregnancy, no strong association was found between guaifenesin and congenital defects (2).

A 1981 report described a woman who consumed, throughout pregnancy, 480–840 mL/day of a cough syrup (3). The potential maximum daily doses based on 840 mL of syrup were 16.8 g of guaifenesin, 5.0 g of pseudoephedrine, 1.68 g of dextromethorphan, and 79.8 mL of ethanol. The infant had features of the fetal alcohol syndrome (see Ethanol) and displayed irritability, tremors, and hypertonicity. It is not known whether guaifenesin or the other drugs, other than ethanol, were associated with the adverse effects observed in the infant.

In a surveillance study of Michigan Medicaid recipients involving 229,101 completed pregnancies conducted between 1985 and 1992, 141 newborns had been exposed to guaifenesin during the 1st trimester (F. Rosa, personal communication, FDA, 1993). Nine (6.4%) major birth defects were observed (6 expected), including two cardiovascular defects (1.4 expected). No anomalies were observed in five other categories of defects (oral clefts, spina bifida, polydactyly, limb reduction defects, and hypospadias) for which specific data were available. An additional 1338 newborns were exposed to the general class of expectorants during the 1st trimester with 63 (4.7%) major birth defects observed (57 expected). Specific malformations were (observed/expected) 9/13 cardiovascular defects, 0/2 oral clefts, 1/1 spina bifida, 7/4 polydactyly, 1/2 limb reduction defects, and 3/3 hypospadias. These data do not support an association between either guaifenesin or the general class of expectorants and congenital defects.

BREASTFEEDING SUMMARY

No reports describing the use of guaifenesin during lactation have been located.

References

1. Heinonen OP, Slone D, Shapiro S. Birth Defects and Drugs in Pregnancy. Littleton, MA:Publishing Sciences Group, 1977.
2. Aselton P, Jick H, Milunsky A, Hunter JR, Stergachis A. First-trimester drug use and congenital disorders. Obstet Gynecol 1985;65:451–5.
3. Chasnoff IJ, Diggs G, Schnoll SH. Fetal alcohol effects and maternal cough syrup abuse. Am J Dis Child 1981;135:968.

GUANABENZ

[Withdrawn from the marker. See 9th edition.]

GUANADREL

[Withdrawn from the marker. See 9th edition.]

GUANETHIDINE

Sympatholytic (Antihypertensive)

PREGNANCY RECOMMENDATION: Limited Human Data—Animal Data Suggest Low Risk
BREASTFEEDING RECOMMENDATION: Limited Human Data—Potential Toxicity

PREGNANCY SUMMARY

Although most reports of guanethidine have not been associated with drug-induced adverse fetal or newborn outcome, only three cases of 1st trimester exposure have been described. Two of these were reported in a surveillance study, in which one malformed infant was delivered from a group of 13 women who took miscellaneous antihypertensives. Thus, the data are too limited to assess the safety of the drug during early human pregnancy. Moreover, the use of this potent antihypertensive has been supplanted by the use of safer, more effective agents for pregnant women. Because of this, it probably should be considered as a drug of last choice during pregnancy (1).

FETAL RISK SUMMARY

Guanethidine is a peripherally acting, antiadrenergic agent used in the treatment of hypertension. In nonpregnant adults, the drug is often combined with diuretics. Because orthostatic hypotension resulting from adrenergic inhibition and unopposed parasympathetic function is a common problem with this agent, its usefulness in the pregnant patient is markedly reduced (1–4).

In a reproduction study in pregnant rats, guanethidine 10 mg/kg/day (average human dose <1.0 mg/kg/day) produced no adverse effects in the offspring (5). Guanethidine was listed in a later reference as a drug that causes maternal death before any effect on the fetus is observed (6). Without citing details, another publication cited guanethidine as a drug capable of producing embryopathy (i.e., death or malformation or both) in laboratory animals (7).

Guanethidine neurotoxicity has been observed in newborn rats and mice that were given the drug early in postnatal life (8,9). In one study, newborn rats were given guanethidine (50 mg/kg SC) once daily for 5 days starting on postnatal day 2 (8). In contrast to adult rats, a possible drug-induced delay in cellular proliferation resulting in initially low brain weights occurred that was thought to be related to passage of guanethidine into the brain because of immature function of the neonatal blood–brain barrier (8). An earlier study found a dysfunctional blood–brain barrier in newborn mice, but not in adult mice, when administration of guanethidine caused a long-lasting reduction in brain catecholamine (norepinephrine and dopamine) levels (9). It is not known if these neurotoxicities would have occurred in the animal fetuses from exposure to the much smaller amounts of drug that would have presumably resulted after placental transfer.

No studies relating to the placental transfer of guanethidine in animals or humans have been located. The commercially available form of the drug, guanethidine monosulfate, has a molecular weight of about 296, which is low enough that passage to the embryo and fetus in measurable amounts should occur.

Several reports have described the use of guanethidine during all phases of human pregnancy (10–16). The Collaborative Perinatal Project monitored 50,282 mother–child pairs, 13 of whom had 1st trimester exposure to a miscellaneous group of antihypertensives, 2 of which were exposed to guanethidine (10). There was 1 infant with a malformation from the total group of 13.

Three references described the use of guanethidine during the 3rd trimester for the treatment of preeclampsia (11–13). Although the outcomes of many of these pregnancies were poor, including fetal death, they appeared to be related to the severity of the mother's disease rather than to the drug therapy. In a fourth reference, the use of guanethidine, tolazoline, phentolamine, and methyldopa for severe hypertension of pregnancy was curtailed over a 3-year period in favor of reserpine and phenoxybenzamine because the authors concluded that the latter two agents gave better control of hypertension, improvement of renal function, and greater predictability of results (14). No fetal or newborn adverse effects were mentioned. A fifth reference also concluded that guanethidine was not an effective antihypertensive, in comparison to other available agents, for the treatment of severe hypertension presenting late in pregnancy (15).

A 1977 report described a 29-year-old woman who was treated with guanethidine (10 mg/day) and hydrochlorothiazide (50 mg twice daily) for hypertension during the first 12 weeks of pregnancy (16). This therapy was stopped, and she was eventually diagnosed with pheochromocytoma that was resected during delivery of a healthy, full-term, 5400-g female infant. The infant was alive and well at 8 years of age.

BREASTFEEDING SUMMARY

The manufacturer states that very small amounts of guanethidine are excreted into milk (17), but published reports describing the use of guanethidine during lactation have not been located. The molecular weight (about 296) of the commercially available form guanethidine monosulfate suggests that the drug will be excreted into breast milk. The effect of this exposure on a nursing infant is unknown.

References

1. Sullivan JM. Blood pressure elevation in pregnancy. Prog Cardiovasc Dis 1974;16:375–94.
2. Finnerty FA Jr. Hypertension in pregnancy. Clin Obstet Gynecol 1975;18:145–54.
3. Kelly JV. Drugs used in the management of toxemia of pregnancy. Clin Obstet Gynecol 1977;20:395–409.
4. Berkowitz RL. Anti-hypertensive drugs in the pregnant patient. Obstet Gynecol Surv 1980;35:191–204.
5. West GB. Drugs and rat pregnancy. J Pharm Pharmacol 1962;14:828–30.
6. West GB. Pregnancy tests using new drugs (abstract). Biochem Pharmacol 1963;12(Suppl):246–7.
7. Woollam DHM. Principles of teratogenesis: mode of action of thalidomide. Proc R Soc Med 1965;58:497–501.
8. Bartolome J, Bartolome M, Seidler FJ, Anderson TR, Slotkin TA. Effects of early postnatal guanethidine administration on adrenal medulla and brain of developing rats. Biochem Pharmacol 1976;25:2387–90.
9. Liuzzi A, Foppen FH, Angeletti PU. Adrenaline, noradrenaline and dopamine levels in brain and heart after administration of 6-hydroxydopamine and guanethidine to newborn mice. Biochem Pharmacol 1974;23:1041–4.
10. Heinonen OP, Sloan D, Shapiro S. *Birth Defects and Drugs in Pregnancy*. Littleton, MA: Publishing Sciences Group, 1977:372–3.
11. Coyle MG, Greig M, Walker J. Blood-progesterone and urinary pregnanediol and oestrogens in foetal death from severe pre-eclampsia. Lancet 1962;2:275–7.
12. Daftary SN, Desa Souza JM, Kumar A, Mandrekar SS, Lotlikar KD, Sheth UK. A controlled clinical trial of guanethidine in toxemia of pregnancy. Indian J Med Sci 1963;17:812–8.
13. Wallace SJ, Michie EA. A follow-up study of infants born to mothers with low oestriol excretion during pregnancy. Lancet 1966;2:560–3.
14. Maughan GB, Shabanah EH, Toth A. Experiments with pharmacologic sympatholysis in the gravid. Am J Obstet Gynecol 1967;97:764–76.
15. Ratnam SS, Lean TH, Sivasamboo R. A comparison of hypotensive drugs in patients with hypertensive disorders in late pregnancy. Aust N-Z J Obstet Gynaecol 1971;11:78–84.
16. Leak D, Carroll JJ, Robinson DC, Ashworth EJ. Management of pheochromocytoma during pregnancy. Can Med Assoc J 1977;116:371–5.
17. Product information. Ismelin. Ciba Pharmaceutical, 1995.

GUANFACINE

Sympatholytic (Antihypertensive)

PREGNANCY RECOMMENDATION: Limited Human Data—Animal Data Suggest Low Risk
BREASTFEEDING RECOMMENDATION: No Human Data—Potential Toxicity

PREGNANCY SUMMARY

Although the limited human pregnancy data for guanfacine have not shown developmental toxicity, if an antihypertensive is indicated, agents with greater pregnancy experience should be used.

FETAL RISK SUMMARY

Guanfacine is a centrally acting antihypertensive agent. The drug did not produce reproductive dysfunction or adverse fetal effects in rats and rabbits given doses 70 and 20 times the maximum recommended human dose (MRHD). At doses 200 and 100 times the MRHD, respectively, increased fetal mortality and maternal toxicity were observed (1).

Although guanfacine crosses the placenta in animals (1,2), this has not been studied in humans. The molecular weight (about 247 for the free base) is low enough that exposure of the embryo and fetus should be expected.

The manufacturer is aware of two unreported cases of exposure during pregnancy that resulted in the birth of healthy infants (A.H. Robins Company, personal communication, 1987). A third patient, who was participating in a clinical trial of the drug for the treatment of hypertension, became pregnant during treatment (3). Guanfacine therapy was discontinued at approximately 8 weeks of gestation. She subsequently delivered a healthy male infant.

Guanfacine is not approved for the treatment of preeclampsia, but one study has been located that describes the use of the agent for this purpose. A 1980 German report summarized the use of guanfacine for the treatment of hypertension secondary to preeclampsia in 30 women (4). The gestational ages of the women at the time of treatment were not specified. Therapy was administered for 16–68 days with doses ranging from 1 to 4 mg/day (mean dose approximately 2 mg/day). Mean systolic blood pressures (supine/standing) before treatment were about 160/164 mmHg compared with 136/139 mmHg just before parturition. Mean diastolic pressures (supine/standing) before treatment and just before delivery were 105/106 and 88/92 mmHg, respectively. No significant changes in fetal heart rate were observed during the trial. Six infants were growth restricted, but this was probably secondary to the maternal hypertension. No drug-induced adverse effects were observed in any of the infants, and all were developing normally on follow-up (duration of follow-up not specified).

BREASTFEEDING SUMMARY

No reports describing the use of guanfacine during human lactation have been located. The molecular weight (about 247 for the free base) is low enough that excretion into human milk should be expected. The effect of this exposure on a nursing infant is unknown. Guanfacine reduces serum prolactin concentrations in some patients and, theoretically, could cause inhibition of milk secretion.

References

1. Product information. Tenex. A.H. Robins Company, 2000.
2. Sorkin EM, Heel RC. Guanfacine. A review of its pharmacodynamic and pharmacokinetic properties, and therapeutic efficacy in the treatment of hypertension. Drugs 1986;31:301–36.
3. Karesoja M, Takkunen H. Guanfacine, a new centrally acting antihypertensive agent in long-term therapy. Curr Ther Res 1981;29:60–5.
4. Philipp E. Guanfacine in the treatment of hypertension due to pre-eclamptic toxaemia in thirty women. Br J Clin Pharmacol 1980;10(Suppl 1):137S–40S.

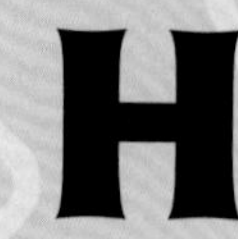

HALOPERIDOL

Antipsychotic

PREGNANCY RECOMMENDATION: Limited Human Data—Animal Data Suggest Moderate Risk
BREASTFEEDING RECOMMENDATION: Limited Human Data—Potential Toxicity

PREGNANCY SUMMARY

Although the animal data suggest moderate risk, the limited human pregnancy experience with haloperidol prevents a more complete assessment of embryo–fetal risk. Neonatal tardive dyskinesia may be an uncommon complication of exposure throughout gestation. There does not appear to be an increased risk of major congenital defects, but there were three cases of limb defects after 1st trimester haloperidol exposure and a fourth case after exposure to a drug in the same class (penfluridol). This potential association requires further study. Until such data are available, avoiding 1st trimester exposure, if possible, should be considered.

FETAL RISK SUMMARY

Haloperidol, a butyrophenone, is indicated for the management of manifestations of psychotic disorders (e.g., schizophrenia) and Tourette's disorder. It is available in both oral and IM formulations (1).

Animal reproductive studies with haloperidol in mice, rats, rabbits, and dogs have not revealed a teratogenic effect attributable to this tranquilizer. In rodents, doses 2–20 times the usual maximum human dose (oral or parenteral) were associated with an increased incidence of resorption, reduced fertility, delayed delivery, and pup mortality (1,2). With single injections up to maternal toxic levels in hamsters, haloperidol was associated with fetal mortality and dose-related anomalies (3). Exposure of male rats in utero to haloperidol throughout most of gestation had no effect on typical parameters of adult sexual activity other than subtle changes involving ultrasonic vocalization (4).

Consistent with the molecular weight (about 376), haloperidol crosses the human placenta. In a 2007 study, 13 women taking a staple dose (mean 2.2 mg/day) of haloperidol for a mean 22 weeks before delivery had maternal and cord concentrations of the drug determined at birth (5). The cord blood concentration was 65.5% of the maternal concentration. The mean Apgar scores were 7.4 and 8.9 at 1 and 5 minutes, respectively. There were four neonatal complications (two cardiovascular, 1 respiratory, and 1 hypotonia; complications were not further described). No infants were admitted to the neonatal intensive care unit (5).

A 31-year-old woman with atypical psychosis was treated with oral haloperidol 3 mg/day and biperiden 3 mg/day at 36 weeks' (6). As her condition worsened, her doses were increased to IM 5 mg twice daily for each drug. At about 38 weeks', 3.5 hours after a dose of both drugs, she gave birth to a healthy 3260-g male infant with Apgar scores of 9 and 9. At delivery, maternal plasma concentrations of haloperidol and biperiden were 10.2 and 4.4 ng/mL, whereas in the newborn they were 4.6 ng/mL and not detectable, respectively (6).

Three reports have described limb defects in three infants after 1st trimester exposure to haloperidol (7–9). In one of these cases, high doses (15 mg/day) were used (8). Defects were observed in two infants: ectromelia (phocomelia) in one infant (7), and multiple upper- and lower-limb defects and an aortic valve defect in the other (8). The infant in the latter case died.

The third case was identified in a 2005 international prospective cohort study that compared 215 pregnancies exposed to either haloperidol ($N = 188$) or penfluridol ($N = 27$) (a butyrophenone antipsychotic not available in the United States) with 631 controls (9). The pregnancy outcomes were determined by telephone interviews and/or mailed questionnaires. In 161 pregnancies, exposure occurred in the 1st trimester, 136 to haloperidol and 25 to penfluridol. The median doses for haloperidol were oral 5 mg/day (2.25–10 mg) or parenteral 100 mg/4 weeks. There were no statistical differences between the butyrophenone and control groups in terms of spontaneous abortions (8.8% vs. 5.5%), ectopic pregnancies (0.5% vs. 0.2%), stillbirths (0 vs. 0.2%), or major malformations (3.4% vs. 3.8%). Significant differences were observed in the rates of elective terminations (8.8% vs. 3.8%), preterm births (13.9% vs. 6.9%), birthweight (3155 vs. 3370 g), birthweight of full-term infants (3250 vs. 3415 g), and cesarean section delivery (25.5% vs. 16.3%). There were three major defects in pregnancies exposed to haloperidol in the 1st trimester: absent left fourth finger, common wrist (carpal) of left first and second fingers; carbamazepine syndrome, developmental delay, congenital heart defect (also exposed to carbamazepine); and ventricular septal defect (also exposed to perphenazine). The haloperidol doses in the three cases were 12.5 mg IM every 4 weeks, 150 mg IM every month, and 10 mg/day orally. There was one major defect with 1st trimester exposure to penfluridol (oral 20 mg/ week): upper limb reduction defect and foot deformity. The small size of the study prevented excluding a possible association between butyrophenones and limb defects (9). Of interest, though, other studies have not observed limb defects in haloperidol-exposed pregnancies (10–14).

In 98 of 100 patients treated with haloperidol for hyperemesis gravidarum in the 1st trimester, no effects were produced on birth weight, duration of pregnancy, sex ratio, or fetal or neonatal mortality, and no malformations were found in abortuses, stillborn, or liveborn infants (10). Two of the patients were lost to follow-up. In 31 infants with severe reduction deformities born over a 4-year period, none of the mothers remembered taking haloperidol (11). Haloperidol has been used for the control of chorea gravidarum and manic-depressive illness during the 2nd and 3rd trimesters (15,16). During labor, the drug has been administered to the mother without causing neonatal depression or other effects in the newborn (12).

In a surveillance study of Michigan Medicaid recipients involving 229,101 completed pregnancies conducted between 1985 and 1992, 56 newborns had been exposed to haloperidol during the 1st trimester (F. Rosa, personal communication, FDA, 1993). Three (5.4%) (two expected) major birth defects were observed, two of which were cardiovascular defects (0.6 expected). No anomalies were observed in five other defect categories (oral clefts, spina bifida, polydactyly, limb reduction defects, and hypospadias) for which specific data were available.

A 1989 report described a case of withdrawal emergent syndrome, a subtype of tardive dyskinesia, in a newborn infant who had been exposed to oral haloperidol (2–6 mg/day) throughout gestation (17). The mother had been treated with haloperidol for schizophrenia, but she stopped the drug 2 weeks before delivery at 38 weeks' gestation. The male infant (weight not given except as "appropriate for gestational age") had Apgar scores of 8 and 9 at 1 and 5 minutes, respectively. One hour after delivery, he became irritable and developed continuous tongue thrust. In addition, poor suck resulting in difficult feeding, vomiting, abdominal posturing of the hands, and tremors of the trunk and extremities were noted. By 8 days of age, all of the signs had resolved except for the tongue thrusting. This symptom continued to persist at 6 months of age, but otherwise, his development and examination were normal (17). A second, similar case of tardive dyskinesia was described in a 2003 case report (18). The mother had been treated for schizophrenia with haloperidol 200 mg IM every 2 weeks throughout gestation. She received her last dose 3 weeks before delivery of an infant (sex and weight not given) with Apgar scores of 9 and 9 at 1 and 5 minutes, respectively. The newborn was noted to be jittery and developed diarrhea and metabolic acidosis. Irritability increased over the next 8 days when tonic-clonic movements in all extremities were noted (seizures were excluded by an electroencephalogram) as well as tongue thrusting and torticollis. Treatment with clonazepam resolved the condition and the infant was discharged home at 21 days of age (18).

Premature labor, loss of fetal cardiac variability and acceleration, an unusual fetal heart rate pattern (double phase baseline), and depression at birth (Apgar scores of 4 and 7 at 1 and 5 minutes, respectively) were observed in a comatose mother and her infant after an acute overdose of an unknown amount of haloperidol and lithium at 31 weeks' gestation (19). Because of progressive premature labor, the 1526-g female infant was delivered about 3 days after the overdose. The lithium concentrations of the maternal plasma, amniotic fluid, and cord vein plasma were all >4 mmol/L (severe toxic effect >2.5 mmol/L), whereas the maternal level of haloperidol at delivery was about 1.6 ng/mL. The effects observed in the fetus and newborn were attributed to cardiac and cerebral manifestations of lithium intoxication. No follow-up on the infant was reported (19).

BREASTFEEDING SUMMARY

Haloperidol is excreted into breast milk. In a patient receiving an average of 29.2 mg/day, a milk level of 5 ng/mL was detected (20). When the dose was decreased to 12 mg, a level of 2 ng/mL was measured. In a second patient taking 10 mg daily, milk levels up to 23.5 ng/mL were found (21). A milk:plasma ratio of 0.6–0.7 was calculated. No adverse effects were noted in the nursing infant.

In a 1985 report, the haloperidol milk concentration was 1.7 ng/mL 3 hours after an unspecified dose (total daily dose 6 mg but the number of doses per day not specified) and 12 days after birth (6). However, the mother had not been breastfeeding and attempts had been made to halt milk production.

A 1992 reference measured haloperidol in the breast milk of three women receiving chronic therapy (22). The maternal doses were 3, 4, and 6 mg/day, and the corresponding haloperidol concentrations in their milk were 32, 17, and 4.7 ng/mL, respectively. The patient receiving 6 mg/day, but with the lowest milk concentration, was thought to be noncompliant with her therapy. No mention of nursing infants was made (22).

A study published in 1998 described 12 mothers who breastfed their infants while taking haloperidol, chlorpromazine, or trifluoperazine for bipolar depression (3 cases), manic disorder (1 case), schizo-affective disorder (5 cases), or schizophrenia (3 cases) (23). Haloperidol doses were 1–40 mg/day. The ages of the nursing infants at the start of therapy were 1–18 weeks. Using an enzyme immunoassay technique, the range of concentrations in fore-milk and hind-milk were <10–988 and 23–140 ng/mL, respectively, whereas the range of ratios of fore-milk and hind-milk to maternal plasma were 0.8–5.2 and 1.7–8.0, respectively. Plasma concentrations of haloperidol in the four nursing infants who were tested were 0.8, 1.2 and 2.1, 6.8, and 8.0 ng/mL, respectively. Two of the samples (6.8 and 8.0 ng/ mL) were in the adult range. In addition, the urine of all seven infants tested contained haloperidol (1.6–7.9 ng/mL). The maximum infant dose ingested was 3% of the weight-adjusted maternal dose. As assessed using the Bayley Scales of Infant Development, all three of the infants whose mothers were taking both haloperidol (20–40 mg/day) and chlorpromazine (200–600 mg/day) showed a decline in mental and psychomotor development from the first (at 1–4 months of age) to the second assessment (at 12–18 months of age). Because of this decline, the investigators concluded that breastfeeding might not be best if a breastfeeding mother is taking neuroleptics, either alone or in combination, at the upper end of their recommended dose ranges (23).

The American Academy of Pediatrics classifies haloperidol as an agent whose effect on the nursing infant is unknown but may be of concern (24).

References

1. Product information. Haloperidol. Major Pharmaceuticals, 2012.
2. Tuchmann-Duplessis H, Mercier-Parot L. Influence of neuroleptics on prenatal development in mammals. In: Tuchmann-Duplessis H, Fanconi G, Burgio GR, eds. *Malformations, Tumors and Mental Defects, Pathogenetic Correlations*. Milan, Italy: Carlo Erba Foundation, 1971. As cited in Shepard TH. *Catalog of Teratogenic Agents*. 6th ed. Baltimore, MD: The Johns Hopkins University Press, 1989:308–9.
3. Gill TS, Guram MS, Geber WF. Haloperidol teratogenicity in the fetal hamster. Dev Pharmacol Ther 1982;4:1–5. As cited in Elia J, Katz IR, Simpson GM. Teratogenicity of psychotherapeutic medications. Psychopharmacol Bull 1987;23:531–86.
4. Bignami G, Laviola G, Alleva E, Cagiano R, Lacomba C, Cuomo V. Developmental aspects of neurobehavioural toxicity. Toxicol Ltrs 1992;64/65:231–7.
5. Newport DJ, Calamaras MR, DeVane CL, Donovan J, Beach AJ, Winn S, Knight BT, Gibson BB, Viguera AC, Owens MJ, Nemeroff CB, Stowe ZN. Atypical antipsychotic administration during late pregnancy: placental passage and obstetrical outcomes. Am J Psychiatry 2007;164:1214–20.
6. Kuniyoshi M, Inanaga K. Haloperidol and biperiden plasma levels in a pregnant atypical psychotic woman and a neonate—a case report. Kurume Med J 1985;32:199–202.
7. Dieulangard P, Coignet J, Vidal JC. Sur un cas d'ectro-phocomelie peut-etre d'origine medicamenteuse. Bull Fed Gynecol Obstet 1966;18:85–7.
8. Kopelman AE, McCullar FW, Heggeness L. Limb malformations following maternal use of haloperidol. JAMA 1975;231:62–4.
9. Diav-Citrin O, Shechtman S, Ornoy S, Arnon J, Schaefer C, Garbis H, Clementi M, Ornoy A. Safety of haloperidol and penfluridol in pregnancy: a multicenter, prospective, controlled study. J Clin Psychiatry 2005;66:317–22.
10. Van Waes A, Van de Velde E. Safety evaluation of haloperidol in the treatment of hyperemesis gravidarum. J Clin Pharmacol 1969;9:224–7.
11. Hanson JW, Oakley GP. Haloperidol and limb deformity. JAMA 1975;231:26.
12. Ayd FJ Jr. Haloperidol: fifteen years of clinical experience. Dis Nerv Syst 1972;33:459–69.
13. Magnier P. On hyperemesis gravidarum; a therapeutical study of R 1625. Gynecol Prat 1964;15:17–23.
14. Loke KH, Salleh R. Electroconvulsive therapy for the acutely psychotic pregnant patient: a review of 3 cases. Med J Malaysia 1983;38:131–3.
15. Donaldson JO. Control of chorea gravidarum with haloperidol. Obstet Gynecol 1982;59:381–2.
16. Nurnberg HG. Treatment of mania in the last six months of pregnancy. Hosp Community Psychiatry 1980;31:122–6.
17. Sexon WR, Barak Y. Withdrawal emergent syndrome in an infant associated with maternal haloperidol therapy. J Perinatol 1989;9:170–2.
18. Collins KO, Comer JB. Maternal haloperidol therapy associated with dyskinesia in a newborn. Am J Health-Syst Pharm 2003;60:2253–5.
19. Nishiwaki T, Tanaka K, Sekiya S. Acute lithium intoxication in pregnancy. Int J Gynecol Obstet 1996;52:191–2.
20. Stewart RB, Karas B, Springer PK. Haloperidol excretion in human milk. Am J Psychiatry 1980;137:849–50.
21. Whalley LJ, Blain PG, Prime JK. Haloperidol secreted in breast milk. Br Med J 1981;282:1746–7.
22. Ohkubo T, Shimoyama R, Sugawara K. Measurement of haloperidol in human breast milk by high-performance liquid chromatography. J Pharm Sci 1992;81:947–9.
23. Yoshida K, Smith B, Craggs M, Kumar R. Neuroleptic drugs in breast milk: a study of pharmacokinetics and of possible adverse effects in breast-fed infants. Psychol Med 1998;28:81–91.
24. Committee on Drugs, American Academy of Pediatrics. The transfer of drugs and other chemicals into human milk. Pediatrics 2001;108:776–89.

HALOTHANE

General Anesthetic

PREGNANCY RECOMMENDATION: Limited Human Data—Animal Data Suggest Low Risk
BREASTFEEDING RECOMMENDATION: Limited Human Data—Probably Compatible

PREGNANCY SUMMARY

Halothane has demonstrated teratogenicity and toxicity in some animal studies, but this may have occurred at maternally toxic doses. The potential for long-term behavioral teratogenicity in animals or humans has not been adequately studied but such studies are needed. The anesthetic does not appear to cause human structural anomalies nor does it appear to be related to embryotoxicity (e.g., abortions), but this is based on limited 1st trimester experience. Others also have reached this same conclusion (1). In addition, general anesthesia usually involves the use of multiple pharmacologic agents which complicates attempts at fetal risk assessment. In the past, halothane frequently was used during delivery for analgesia and anesthesia. This use does not appear to affect the newborn any differently than use of other general anesthetic agents does. The uterine effects of halothane (relaxation and increased blood loss) also appear to be similar to those of other agents in this class. All anesthetic agents can cause depression in the newborn that may last for 24 hours or more. The potential reproductive toxicity (spontaneous abortion and infertility) of occupational exposure to halothane has not been adequately studied.

FETAL RISK SUMMARY

Halothane, a nonflammable, volatile liquid administered via vaporizer, is indicated for the induction and/or maintenance of anesthesia during surgery. It is a fluorinated inhalation anesthetic agent that was the first such agent in a class that now includes desflurane, enflurane, isoflurane, methoxyflurane, and sevoflurane. Halothane has a high blood–gas partition coefficient (2.5) compared with other anesthetics in this class (2). The agent has been used in obstetric anesthesia since the 1950s.

In a 1968 reproduction study, pregnant rats were administered a subanesthetic mixture of 0.8% halothane in 25% oxygen–nitrogen for 12 hours at different stages of gestation (3). Higher incidences of lumbar ribs, vertebral anomalies, and fetal resorptions were observed. An abstract published the same year described the effects on pregnant mice exposed to either 1% or 1.5% halothane for 3 hours during organogenesis (4). An increased incidence of cleft palate, limb hematomas, and ossification defects in the limbs was observed.

An increased incidence of resorptions, as well as decreased fetal weight and length, was observed in pregnant hamsters exposed on the 9th, 10th, or 11th day of gestation to a mixture of 0.6% halothane and 60% nitrous oxide (5). In contrast, subanesthetic concentrations of halothane (50–3200 ppm) administered to rats on days 8–12 of pregnancy did not increase fetal death and resorption rates, growth restriction, or frequency of skeletal anomalies (6). Skeletal variations and ossification defects were observed in all groups but were not dose-related.

In a 1978 study, male and female mice were exposed to subanesthetic and anesthetic concentrations of halothane before mating (5–7 days/week for 9 weeks), then the females were exposed daily throughout gestation (7). Halothane exposures ranged from 0.025 to 4.0 minimum alveolar anesthetic concentration (MAC) hours/day. (*Note: MAC is the concentration that causes immobility in 50% of patients exposed to a noxious stimulus such as a surgical incision; it represents the* ED_{50} *(8).*) Maternal (decreased weight gain), fetal (decreased weight and length), and neonatal (decreased early postnatal weight gain) toxicity were observed at ≥0.4 MAC hours/day. At 1.2 MAC hours/day, the pregnancy rate, implantation rate, and number of live fetuses per litter were all significantly decreased, but the percentage of resorptions and postnatal offspring survival were not altered. The smallest dose at which toxicity was observed was estimated to be 40 times greater than the level of occupational exposure in unscavenged operating rooms (7). Two studies of similar design using subanesthetic mixtures of halothane and nitrous oxide found a decrease in ovulation and implantation and a slight decrease in fetal growth (9,10). No increase in resorptions or major defects was observed in either study. However, cytogenetic damage to bone marrow and spermatogonial cells were noted after prolonged exposure (9,10).

High subanesthetic concentrations of halothane or halot hane plus nitrous oxide resulted in fetal growth restriction in pregnant rats, but did not increase fetal death or congenital malformations (11). Another study in rats also found no minor or major congenital defects using 0.75 MAC of halothane (0.8%) for 6 hours/day for 3 consecutive days at different intervals during gestation (12).

A 1999 study examined the effects on mice exposed to 1.2 MAC of halothane (1.5%) before and during gestation (13). The dose was equivalent to that used clinically. Treatment before gestation had no effect on fertility or the number of live young delivered. Compared with controls, there were an increased number of offspring deaths before weaning, and the immune response of the offspring was impaired. The clinical significance of the impairment was unknown (13).

The effects of halothane on growing neural tips (growth cones) in the forebrains of neonatal rat pups were described in a 1993 report (14). The pups were exposed to three concentrations of halothane (0.5%, 0.75%, and 1.0%) over a 6-hour period on postnatal day 1. A dose–response chart on the activity of a growth cone enzyme (protein kinase C [PKC]) was found, with the lowest concentration having no effect on the enzyme. The 1.0% concentration, however, reduced the activity to about 71%. The 0.75% dose also reduced the PKC activity but to a lesser degree. The authors thought that the reduced enzyme activity could be related to long-term morphologic or behavioral neuroabnormalities in the pups (14).

The molecular weight (about 197) suggests that halothane will cross the placenta to the embryo and fetus. In agreement, research has demonstrated the rapid uptake of halothane by the fetus (15). Two reviews have concluded that, in general, inhalational anesthetic agents are freely transferred to fetal tissues (1,16), and in most cases, the maternal and fetal blood concentrations are approximately equivalent (16). Lower levels were reported in a 1977 study in which 15 women undergoing cesarean section received 0.65% halothane combined with 50% nitrous oxide in oxygen (17). The umbilical vein:maternal artery ratio at delivery was 0.35. The ratio in a second group of 15 women who received the anesthetic mixture with 0.2% halothane was 0.51. The time from start of halothane to delivery was about 10.5 minutes in both groups.

Pregnant women, at least in early gestation, require less halothane for anesthesia than nonpregnant women. A 1996 study compared eight women scheduled for pregnancy termination at 8–13 weeks' gestation with eight nonpregnant women undergoing laparoscopic sterilization (18). In pregnant women the median MAC of 0.58 volume% (range 0.53–0.58) was less than that in nonpregnant women, 0.75 volume% (range 0.70–0.78; $p = 0.0005$). The percentage decrease (95% confidence interval) for pregnant women was 27% (20%–27%). Similar results were found with enflurane (18).

Halothane and similar anesthetic agents (e.g., isoflurane and enflurane) have a relaxant effect on the pregnant uterus (2,19–24). This effect has been known since the 1950s and was considered one reason to avoid using halothane during routine, uncomplicated obstetric procedures (2,19). A 1970 study using low concentrations (0.5% or 0.8%) found no increase in blood loss at cesarean section (23). However, it was recognized that decreasing uterine tone could result in increased postpartum hemorrhage. Indeed, a 1989 review concluded that halothane, isoflurane, and enflurane all increased blood loss through a dose-related depression of uterine activity (24). In agreement with the dose-related uterine effects, a 1991 reviewer thought that low halothane concentrations (≤0.5%) were not associated with an increased risk of uterine hemorrhage (25). In the 1970 study cited above, the 0.8% concentration of halothane was associated with an increased incidence of maternal hypotension, most likely secondary to compression of the inferior vena cava by the uterus and vasodilatation (23). However, uterine blood flow is maintained during maternal hypotension because of uterine artery dilation (24). In addition, low concentrations of halothane (0.25%–0.5%) did not depress the neonatal cardiac or respiratory systems (24).

Halothane was once frequently prescribed for both vaginal and cesarean deliveries (17,20,26,27). For example, one hospital conducted 2500 vaginal deliveries over a 6-year period with a combination of halothane, nitrous oxide, and oxygen (20). The decline in obstetric use was probably due to the availability of agents with reduced solubility in blood (e.g., see Desflurane and Isoflurane) and the recognition that general anesthesia can cause depression in the newborn.

Several studies have documented decreased initial Apgar scores in newborns following cesarean section under general anesthesia (17,23,26–28). Because the halothane concentrations often were subanesthetic and combined with nitrous oxide, it was not always clear whether the depression was secondary to a specific agent or the combination. In one study, reducing the amount of nitrous oxide from 75% to 50% and adding 0.5% halothane substantially improved the Apgar scores at 2 minutes (23). In an earlier study that combined halothane anesthesia with succinylcholine, reducing the halothane dose markedly improved the condition of the newborns as measured by Apgar scores (26). Another study found no difference in Apgar scores between groups given 0.3%–0.5% halothane combined with either 40% or 25% nitrous oxide (27). In a direct comparison between 0.5% halothane and 0.75% isoflurane, both combined with 50% nitrous oxide, the isoflurane group required significantly less succinylcholine, recovered faster from anesthesia, and had less uterine relaxation and bleeding (28). The mean Apgar scores were significantly higher at 1 minute in the isoflurane group (7.4 vs. 6.7) but were similar at 5 minutes (8.9 vs. 8.8).

A 1989 study compared 0.5% halothane, 0.5% isoflurane, and 1.0% isoflurane (*N* = 20 in each group) during cesarean section delivery (29). No differences among the groups were observed in the incidence of low 1-minute Apgar scores or in the Neurologic and Adaptive Capacity Scores (NACS) at 15 minutes, 2 hours, and 24 hours. The percentage of infants who scored 35–40 on the NACS was similar in the three groups (29). A small 1983 study compared the neonatal outcomes in four groups (10 patients each) of women receiving general anesthesia for cesarean section: 50% nitrous oxide and 50% oxygen either alone or combined with 0.5% halothane, 1.0% enflurane, or 0.75% isoflurane (30). There were no differences among the groups in low Apgar scores at 1 and 5 minutes, neonatal neurobehavioral assessment 2–4 hours after delivery, or maternal or umbilical blood–gas analysis at delivery. A randomized study examined the effects of halothane (*N* = 32) and isoflurane (*N* = 34) (both at 0.7 MAC) on newborn Apgar scores and acid–base status after anesthesia for emergency cesarean section (31). There were no statistically significant differences in the percentage of infants with low Apgar scores (<7) at 1 and 5 minutes. Similarly, there were no significant differences in the hydrogen ion concentration, partial pressure of carbon dioxide, partial pressure of oxygen, or base deficit in blood samples from umbilical arteries and veins (31).

The Collaborative Perinatal Project monitored 50,282 mother–child pairs, 25 of whom had 1st trimester exposure to halothane (32). Two children had unspecified malformations, but there was no evidence of an association between halothane and the defects (32). A 1965 report on fetal hazards of surgery during pregnancy described the outcomes of 20 women who were administered general anesthesia (halothane plus nitrous oxide) during pregnancy (7, 9, and 4 women in the 1st, 2nd, and 3rd trimesters, respectively) (33). One unspecified birth defect was observed (timing of exposure not specified).

A possible association between surgery in the 1st trimester and neural tube defects (NTD) was published in 1990 (34). Using data from Swedish health care registries, investigators studied 2252 infants whose mothers had surgery during the 1st trimester. Six of the infants had NTD (expected 2.5), one of whom was thought to have Meckel's syndrome. An additional infant had a diagnosis of hydranencephaly, but the autopsy report indicated that the diagnosis was uncertain and it may have been a very large encephalocele. In the total group, 572 had operations during the period of neural tube closure (gestational weeks 4 and 5). Mothers of five of the six infants with NTD (expected 0.6) had surgery during this period, but only one had been exposed to halothane (in combination with nitrous oxide). The mother of the hydranencephaly case had surgery in gestational week 8 and was exposed to halothane in combination with thiopental and succinylcholine. The authors could not determine whether the findings represented a causal association with surgery or just a random occurrence (34).

Chronic occupational exposure to anesthetic gases in operating rooms during pregnancy has raised concerns that such exposure could cause spontaneous abortions (35,36). The principal concern relates to unscavenged environments in which high concentrations of halothane (0.001% or 10 ppm) and nitrous oxide (0.03% or 300 ppm) had been measured (35). Lower concentrations of halothane also have been reported near the anesthesiologist (1–26 ppm) and the surgeon (1–2 ppm) (37). A 1988 review cited a number of studies investigating the possible association between occupational exposure to anesthetic gases and adverse pregnancy outcomes (15). The reviewer concluded that serious methodological weaknesses in these studies precluded arriving at a firm conclusion, but a slightly increased risk of miscarriage was a possibility. However, there was no evidence of an association between occupational exposure and congenital anomalies (15).

A review published in 1991 briefly evaluated the possibility that some drugs and environmental agents could cause behavioral teratogenicity (38). Anesthetics (e.g., halothane) were listed as "suspected" human behavioral teratogens apparently based solely on animal studies. However, specific data for any anesthetic agent, including halothane, were not cited.

A 2004 study, however, found a significant association between maternal occupational exposure to waste anesthetic gases during pregnancy and developmental deficits in their children, including gross and fine motor ability, inattention/hyperactivity, and IQ performance (see Nitrous Oxide).

A 1993 study evaluated the effect of halothane anesthesia for fetal surgery in pregnant ewes (39). Compared with ketamine, halothane decreased fetal cardiac output and placental blood flow. An increase in total vascular resistance, highest in the placenta, resulted in the shunting of blood away from the placenta (39). The combination of these effects resulted in depressed respiratory gas exchange. The investigators concluded that halothane was a poor anesthetic for fetal surgery (39).

BREASTFEEDING SUMMARY

Halothane is excreted into breast milk (40–42). Breast milk samples were collected on 2 days from a lactating anesthesiologist while she was working (40). The milk concentrations of 2 ppm were consistent with the concentrations at the anesthesiologist's face in the operating room. Because respiratory excretion of halothane by operating room personnel continues for ≤72 hours, the authors thought that the trace milk concentrations would be detectable for a similar period of time (40).

No reports measuring the amount of halothane excreted in milk of patients who have received halothane anesthesia have been located. Of interest, a 1993 reference stated that respiratory excretion of halothane in patients may occur for ≤20 days after exposure and that trace amounts of halothane should be expected in milk during that interval (41). One review considered the potential amounts in milk after halothane anesthesia, when nursing was feasible, to be negligible (42). The American Academy of Pediatrics classifies halothane as a drug that usually is compatible with breastfeeding (43).

References

1. Friedman JM. Teratogen update: anesthetic agents. Teratology 1988;37:69–77.
2. Product information. Halothane. Abbott Laboratories, 1975.
3. Basford AB, Fink BR. The teratogenicity of halothane in the rat. Anesthesiology 1968;29:1167–73.
4. Smith BE, Usubliaga LE, Lehrer SB. Cleft palate induced by halothane anesthesia in C-57 black mice (abstract). Teratology 1971;4:242.
5. Bussard DA, Stoelting RK, Peterson C, Ishaq M. Fetal changes in hamsters anesthetized with nitrous oxide and halothane. Anesthesiology 1974;41:275–8.
6. Lansdown ABG, Pope WDB, Halsey MJ, Bateman PE. Analysis of fetal development in rats following maternal exposure to subanesthetic concentrations of halothane. Teratology 1976;13:299–304.
7. Wharton RS, Mazze RI, Baden JM, Hitt BA, Dooley JR. Fertility, reproduction and postnatal survival in mice chronically exposed to halothane. Anesthesiology 1978;48:167–74.
8. Trevor AJ, Miller RD. General anesthetics. In: Katzung BG, ed. *Basic and Clinical Pharmacology*. 8th ed. New York, NY: McGraw-Hill, 2001:426.
9. Coate WB, Kapp RW Jr, Lewis TR. Chronic exposure to low concentrations of halothane–nitrous oxide: reproductive and cytogenetic effects in the rat. Anesthesiology 1979;50:310–8.
10. Coate WB, Kapp RW Jr, Ulland BM. Toxicity of low concentration long-term exposure to an airborne mixture of nitrous oxide and halothane. J Environ Pathol Toxicol 1979;2:209–31.
11. Pope WDB, Halsey MJ, Lansdown ABG, Simmonds A, Bateman PE. Fetotoxicity in rats following chronic exposure to halothane, nitrous oxide, or methoxyflurane. Anesthesiology 1978;48:11–6.
12. Mazze RI, Fujinaga M, Rice SA, Harris SB, Baden JM. Reproductive and teratogenic effects of nitrous oxide, halothane, isoflurane, and enflurane in Sprague-Dawley rats. Anesthesiology 1986;64:339–44.
13. Puig NR, Amerio N, Piaggio E, Barragan J, Comba JO, Elena GA. Effects of halothane reexposure in female mice and their offspring. Reprod Toxicol 1999;13:361–7.
14. Saito S, Fujita T, Igarashi M. Effects of inhalational anesthetics on biochemical events in growing neuronal tips. Anesthesiology 1993;79:1338–47.
15. Dwyer R, Fee JPH, Moore J. Uptake of halothane and isoflurane by mother and baby during caesarean section. Br J Anaesth 1995;74:379–83.
16. Kanto J. Risk-benefit assessment of anaesthetic agents in the puerperium. Drug Saf 1991;6:285–301.
17. Latto IP, Waldron BA. Anaesthesia for caesarean section. Br J Anaesth 1977;49:371–8.
18. Chan MTV, Mainland P, Gin T. Minimum alveolar concentration of halothane and enflurane are decreased in early pregnancy. Anesthesiology 1996;85:782–6.
19. Crawford JS. The place of halothane in obstetrics. Br J Anaesth 1962;34:386–90.
20. Stoelting VK. Fluothane in obstetric anesthesia. Anesth Analg 1964;43:243–6.
21. Munson ES, Embro WJ. Enflurane, isoflurane, and halothane and isolated human uterine muscle. Anesthesiology 1977;46:11–4.
22. Naftalin NJ, McKay DM, Phear WPC, Goldberg AH. The effects of halothane on pregnant and nonpregnant human myometrium. Anesthesiology 1977;46:15–9.
23. Moir DD. Anaesthesia for caesarean section. Br J Anaesth 1970;42:136–42.
24. Quail AW. Modern inhalational anaesthetic agents. A review of halothane, isoflurane and enflurane. Med J Aust 1989;150:95–102.
25. Nandi PR, Morrison PF, Morgan BM. Effects of general anaesthesia on the fetus during caesarean section. Anaesth Rev 1991;8:103–22.
26. Johnstone M, Breen PJ. Halothane in obstetrics: elective caesarean section. Br J Anaesth 1966;38:386–93.
27. Galbert MW, Gardner AE. Use of halothane in a balanced technic for cesarean section. Anesth Analg 1972;51:701–4.
28. Ghaly RG, Flynn RJ, Moore J. Isoflurane as an alternative to halothane for caesarean section. Anaesthesia 1988;43:5–7.
29. Abboud TK, D'Onofrio I, Reyes A, Mosaad P, Zhu J, Mantilla M, Gangolly J, Crowell D, Cheung M, Afrasiabi A, Khoo N, Davidson J, Steffens Z, Zaki N. Isoflurane or halothane for cesarean section: comparative maternal and neonatal effects. Acta Anaesthesiol Scand 1989;33:578–81.
30. Warren TM, Datta S, Ostheimer GW, Naulty JS, Weiss JB, Morrison JA. Comparison of the maternal and neonatal effects of halothane, enflurane, and isoflurane for cesarean delivery. Anesth Analg 1983;62:516–20.
31. Mokriski BK, Malinow AM. Neonatal acid-base status following general anesthesia for emergency abdominal delivery with halothane or isoflurane. J Clin Anest 1992;4:97–100.
32. Heinonen OP, Slone D, Shapiro S. *Birth Defects and Drugs in Pregnancy*. Littleton, MA: Publishing Sciences Group, 1977:358–60.
33. Shnider SM, Webster GM. Maternal and fetal hazards of surgery during pregnancy. Am J Obstet Gynecol 1965;92:891–900.
34. Kallen B, Mazze RI. Neural tube defects and first trimester operations. Teratology 1990;41:717–20.
35. Corbett TH. Anesthetics as a cause of abortion. Fert Steril 1972;23:866–9.
36. Brodsky JB. Anesthesia and surgery during early pregnancy and fetal outcome. Clin Obstet Gynecol 1983;26:449–57.
37. Corbett TH. Cancer and congenital anomalies associated with anesthetics. Ann NY Acad Sci 1976;271:58–66.
38. Nelson BK. Evidence for behavioral teratogenicity in humans. J Appl Toxicol 1991;11:33–7.
39. Sabik JF, Assad RS, Hanley FL. Halothane as an anesthetic for fetal surgery. J Pediatr Surg 1993;28:542–7.
40. Cote CJ, Kenepp NB, Reed SB, Strobel GE. Trace concentrations of halothane in human breast milk. Br J Anaesth 1976;48:541–3.
41. Lee JJ, Rubin AP. Breast feeding and anaesthesia. Anaesthesia 1993;48:616–25.
42. Spigset O. Anaesthetic agents and excretion in breast milk. Acta Anaesthesiol Scand 1994;38:94–103.
43. Committee on Drugs, American Academy of Pediatrics. The transfer of drugs and other chemicals into human milk. Pediatrics 2001;108:776–89.

HEMIN

Hematopoietic

PREGNANCY RECOMMENDATION: Limited Human Data—No Relevant Animal Data
BREASTFEEDING RECOMMENDATION: No Human Data—Probably Compatible

PREGNANCY SUMMARY

Animal reproduction studies have not been conducted with hemin and there is only one report on its use in human pregnancy. The citations below, however, suggest that hemin has been used more frequently in pregnant women. The primary embryo or fetal risk from hemin appears to be from the transmission of viruses or other agents from a hemin-induced maternal infection or from a hemin-induced maternal adverse reaction (e.g., thrombocytopenia or coagulopathy). Therefore, the drug should not be withheld because of pregnancy.

FETAL RISK SUMMARY

The enzyme inhibitor hemin (previously known as hematin) limits the hepatic and/or marrow synthesis of porphyrin. It is indicated for the amelioration of recurrent attacks of acute intermittent porphyria that are temporally related to the menstrual cycle (1). Hemin is an iron molecule derived from human red blood cells. Although multiple steps have been taken to lessen the chance of blood-borne infection, a risk still exists for the transmission of infectious agents, such as viruses, and for the agent that causes Creutzfeldt-Jacob disease (1).

Reproduction studies in animals have not been conducted. It is not known if hemin can cross the human placenta to the fetus. As a natural constituent of human blood, it is unlikely that clinically significant amounts would cross to the fetal compartment.

A 1989 review summarized the prevalence, genetics, biochemistry, classification, and the treatment of acute intermittent porphyria (2). The authors also cited evidence that female hormones affect the onset and expression of the disease. Before an understanding of the disease and improved prenatal care were achieved, porphyria was associated with significant maternal mortality and poor pregnancy outcome (2). Although the authors did not specifically state that hemin treatment was indicated during pregnancy, they did state that patients with acute attacks should be hospitalized for symptomatic treatment. They also noted that treatment with hemin could shorten the duration of the attack and reduce its severity (2).

Earlier, a brief response to a question concerning porphyria and pregnancy hinted at the potential severity of this disease. The author, although noting the lack of information relating to the potential to cause adverse pregnancy outcomes, still recommended hematin therapy for an acute porphyric attack before considering termination of pregnancy (3). Responding to this recommendation, another author suggested that glucose infusions were safer and expressed concern that the anticoagulant effect of hemin could jeopardize a pregnancy (4). However, hemin was not thought to have a clinically significant anticoagulant effect at low doses and was indicated in pregnancy if glucose infusions were not effective in reversing the disease process (5).

A 34-year-old woman, in the 1st or 2nd month of pregnancy, was treated with hematin, 3 mg/kg/day administered as an IV infusion for 5 days, for an exacerbation of acute intermittent porphyria (6). A second IV infusion course, 1.5 mg/kg/day for 2 weeks, was started 41 days after the first course. No adverse fetal effects of the exposure were noted and the woman eventually delivered a healthy, 2570-g male infant at 39 weeks' gestation. At follow-up, no evidence of porphyria was noted in the 5-year-old child (6).

A 1984 study investigated the effect of hematin on bilirubin binding (7). Cord blood of newborn infants with ABO hemolytic disease was thought to contain endogenous hematin, which could increase the risk of kernicterus. In an in vitro experiment, hematin was added to bilirubin-enriched cord blood and was found to have a significant adverse effect on bilirubin binding. However, the high concentrations required were not physiologic and, thus, were not thought to have clinical significance for infants with ABO-isoimmune hemolysis (7).

A 2010 review of the treatment of acute intermittent porphyria in pregnancy concluded that although the available information was limited, hemin could be safely given in pregnancy (8).

BREASTFEEDING SUMMARY

No reports describing the use of hemin during lactation have been located. Hemin is an enzyme inhibitor that is derived from human red blood cells. It is doubtful if hemin is excreted in milk but even if small amounts were excreted, they would be digested in the infant's gut.

References

1. Product information. Panhematin. Ovation Pharmaceuticals, 2004.
2. Kanaan C, Veille JC, Lakin M. Pregnancy and acute intermittent porphyria. Obstet Gynecol Surv 1989;44:244–9.
3. Bissell DM. Acute intermittent porphyria and pregnancy. JAMA 1985; 252:1457.
4. Loftin EB III. Hematin therapy in acute porphyria. JAMA 1985;254:613.
5. Bissell DM. In reply: hematin therapy in acute porphyria. JAMA 1985;254:1457.
6. Wenger S, Meisinger V, Brücke T, Deecke L. Acute porphyric neuropathy during pregnancy—effect of haematin therapy. Eur Neurol 1998;39:187–8.
7. Kirk JJ, Ritter DA, Kenny JD. The effect of hematin on bilirubin binding in bilirubin-enriched neonatal cord serum. Biol Neonate 1984;45:53–7.
8. Farfaras A, Zagouri F, Zografos G, Kostopoulou A, Sergentanis N, Antoniou S. Acute intermittent porphyria in pregnancy: a common misdiagnosis. Clin Exp Obstet Gynecol 2010;37:256–60.

HEPARIN

Anticoagulant

PREGNANCY RECOMMENDATION: Compatible
BREASTFEEDING RECOMMENDATION: Compatible

PREGNANCY SUMMARY

No reports linking the use of heparin during gestation with developmental toxicity have been located. Because heparin probably does not cross the placenta, other fetal complications are related to the severe maternal disease necessitating anticoagulant therapy.

FETAL RISK SUMMARY

Hall et al. (1) reviewed the use of heparin and other anticoagulants during pregnancy (167 references) (see also Coumarin Derivatives). They concluded from the published cases in which heparin was used without other anticoagulants that significant risks existed for the mother and fetus and that heparin was not a clearly superior form of anticoagulation during pregnancy. Nageotte and coworkers (2) analyzed the same data to arrive at a different conclusion.

	Hall	Nageotte
Total number of cases	135	120
Term liveborn—no complications	86	86
Premature—survived without complications	19	19
Liveborn—complications (not specified)	1	1
Premature—expired		
Heparin therapy appropriate[a]	10	5
Heparin therapy not appropriate[a]		4[b]
Severe maternal disease making successful outcome of pregnancy unlikely		1[c]
Spontaneous abortions		
Unknown cause	2	1
Maternal death due to pulmonary embolism		1
Stillbirths		
Heparin therapy appropriate[a]	17	8
Heparin therapy not appropriate[a]		7[d]
Heparin and Coumadin used		2

[a]Appropriateness as determined by current standards.
[b]Hypertension of pregnancy (4).
[c]Tricuspid atresia (1).
[d]Hypertension of pregnancy (6); proliferative glomerulonephritis (1).

By eliminating the 15 cases in which maternal disease or other drugs were the most likely cause of the fetal problem, the analysis of Nageotte and coworkers results in a 13% (15 of 120) unfavorable outcome vs. the 22% (30 of 135) of Hall and associates. This new value appears to be significantly better than the 31% (133 of 426) abnormal outcome reported for coumarin derivatives (see Coumarin Derivatives). Furthermore, in contrast to coumarin derivatives in which a definite drug-induced pattern of malformations has been observed (fetal warfarin syndrome), heparin has not been related to congenital defects nor does it cross the placenta (3–5). Consequently, the mechanism of heparin's adverse effect on the fetus, if it exists, must be indirect. Hall and coworkers theorized that fetal effects may be caused by calcium (or other cation) chelation resulting in the deficiency of that ion(s) in the fetus. A more likely explanation, in light of the report of the Nageotte group, is severe maternal disease that could be relatively independent of heparin. Thus, heparin appears to have major advantages over oral anticoagulants as the treatment of choice during pregnancy (6–13).

A retrospective study, published in 1989, lends support to the argument that heparin therapy is safe for the mother and fetus (14). A total of 77 women were treated with heparin during 100 pregnancies. In 98 pregnancies, therapy was administered for the prevention or treatment of venous thromboembolism; in 2 pregnancies treatment was because of prosthetic heart valves. In comparison with normal pregnancies, no difference was seen in the treated mothers in terms of prematurity, spontaneous abortions, stillbirths, neonatal deaths, or congenital malformations (6). Two bleeding episodes occurred, but there were no symptomatic thrombolic events.

In a surveillance study of Michigan Medicaid recipients involving 229,101 completed pregnancies conducted between 1985 and 1992, 65 newborns had been exposed to heparin during the 1st trimester (F. Rosa, personal communication, FDA, 1993). Seven (10.8%) major birth defects were observed (three expected). Specific data were available for six defect categories, including (observed/expected) 4/0.6 cardiovascular defects, 0/0 oral clefts, 0/0 spina bifida, 1/0 polydactyly, 0/0 limb reduction defects, and 1/0 hypospadias. The data for total malformations and for cardiovascular defects are suggestive of possible associations, but other factors, most likely the mother's disease, but also possibly concurrent drug therapy and chance, are probably involved.

Long-term heparin therapy during pregnancy has been associated with maternal osteopenia (15–19). Both low-dose (10,000 U/day) and high-dose heparin have been implicated, but the latter is more often related to this complication. One study found bone demineralization to be dose related, with more severe changes occurring after long-term therapy (>25 weeks) and in patients who had also received heparin in a previous pregnancy (18). The significant decrease in 1,25-dihydroxyvitamin D levels measured in heparin-treated pregnant patients may be related to the pathogenesis of this adverse effect (16,17). Similar problems have not been reported in newborns.

BREASTFEEDING SUMMARY

Heparin is not excreted into breast milk because of its high molecular weight (15,000) (20). Moreover, it is not absorbed after oral administration.

References

1. Hall JG, Pauli RM, Wilson KM. Maternal and fetal sequelae of anticoagulation during pregnancy. Am J Med 1980;68:122–40.
2. Nageotte MP, Freeman RK, Garite TJ, Block RA. Anticoagulation in pregnancy. Am J Obstet Gynecol 1981;141:472.
3. Flessa HC, Kapstrom AB, Glueck HI, Will JJ, Miller MA, Brinker B. Placental transport of heparin. Am J Obstet Gynecol 1965;93:570–3.
4. Russo R, Bortolotti U, Schivazappa L, Girolami A. Warfarin treatment during pregnancy: a clinical note. Haemostasis 1979;8:96–8.
5. Moe N. Anticoagulant-therapy in the prevention of placental infarction and perinatal death. Obstet Gynecol 1982;59:481–3.
6. Hellgren M, Nygards EB. Long-term therapy with subcutaneous heparin during pregnancy. Gynecol Obstet Invest 1982;13:76–89.
7. Cohen AW, Gabbe SG, Mennuti MT. Adjusted-dose heparin therapy by continuous intravenous infusion for recurrent pulmonary embolism during pregnancy. Am J Obstet Gynecol 1983;146:463–4.

8. Howell R, Fidler J, Letsky E. The risks of antenatal subcutaneous heparin prophylaxis: a controlled trial. Br J Obstet Gynaecol 1983;90:1124–8.
9. Vellenga E, van Imhoff GW, Aarnoudse JG. Effective prophylaxis with oral anticoagulants and low-dose heparin during pregnancy in an antithrombin III deficient woman. Lancet 1983;2:224.
10. Bergqvist A, Bergqvist D, Hallbook T. Deep vein thrombosis during pregnancy. Acta Obstet Gynecol Scand 1983;62:443–8.
11. Michiels JJ, Stibbe J, Vellenga E, van Vliet HHDM. Prophylaxis of thrombosis in antithrombin III-deficient women during pregnancy and delivery. Eur J Obstet Gynecol Reprod Biol 1984;18:149–53.
12. Nelson DM, Stempel LE, Fabri PJ, Talbert M. Hickman catheter use in a pregnant patient requiring therapeutic heparin anticoagulation. Am J Obstet Gynecol 1984;149:461–2.
13. Romero R, Duffy TP, Berkowitz RL, Chang E, Hobbins JC. Prolongation of a preterm pregnancy complicated by death of a single twin in utero and disseminated intravascular coagulation: effects of treatment with heparin. N Engl J Med 1984;310:772–4.
14. Ginsberg JS, Kowalchuk G, Hirsh J, Brill-Edwards P, Burrows R. Heparin therapy during pregnancy: risks to the fetus and mother. Arch Intern Med 1989;149:2233–6.
15. Wise PH, Hall AJ. Heparin-induced osteopenia in pregnancy. Br Med J 1980;281:110–1.
16. Aarskog D, Aksnes L, Lehmann V. Low 1,25-dihydroxyvitamin D in heparin-induced osteopenia. Lancet 1980;2:650–1.
17. Aarskog D, Aksnes L, Markestad T, Ulstein M, Sagen N. Heparin-induced inhibition of 1,25-dihydroxyvitamin D formation. Am J Obstet Gynecol 1984;148:1141–2.
18. De Swiet M, Dorrington Ward P, Fidler J, Horsman A, Katz D, Letsky E, Peacock M, Wise PH. Prolonged heparin therapy in pregnancy causes bone demineralization. Br J Obstet Gynaecol 1983;90:1129–34.
19. Griffiths HT, Liu DTY. Severe heparin osteoporosis in pregnancy. Postgrad Med J 1984;60:424–5.
20. O'Reilly RA. Anticoagulant, antithrombotic, and thrombolytic drugs. In: Gilman AG, Goodman LS, Gilman A, eds. *The Pharmacological Basis of Therapeutics*. 6th ed. New York, NY: MacMillan, 1980:1350.

HEROIN

Narcotic Agonist Analgesic

PREGNANCY RECOMMENDATION: Human Data Suggest Risk
BREASTFEEDING RECOMMENDATION: Contraindicated

PREGNANCY SUMMARY

In the United States, heroin exposure during pregnancy is confined to illicit use as opposed to in other countries, such as Great Britain, where the drug is commercially available. The documented fetal toxicity of heroin derives from the illicit use and resulting maternal–fetal addiction. In the form available to the addict, heroin is adulterated with various substances (such as lactose, glucose, mannitol, starch, quinine, amphetamines, strychnine, procaine, or lidocaine) or contaminated with bacteria, viruses, or fungi (1,2). Maternal use of other drugs, abuse and nonabuse, is likely. It is, therefore, difficult to separate entirely the effects of heroin on the fetus from the possible effects of other chemical agents, multiple diseases with addiction, and life-style. However, there are data that morphine, which is closely related to heroin, and other opioids are human teratogens (see Morphine).

FETAL RISK SUMMARY

Heroin rapidly crosses the placenta, entering fetal tissues within 1 hour of administration. Withdrawal of the drug from the mother causes the fetus to undergo simultaneous withdrawal. Intrauterine death may occur from meconium aspiration (3,4).

Assessment of fetal maturity and status is often difficult because of uncertain dates and an accelerated appearance of mature lecithin:sphingomyelin ratios (5).

Until recently, the incidence of congenital anomalies was not thought to be increased (6–8). Current data, however, suggest that a significant increase in major anomalies can occur (9). In a group of 830 heroin-addicted mothers, the incidence of infants with congenital abnormalities was significantly greater than in a group of 400 controls (9). Higher rates of jaundice, respiratory distress syndrome, and low Apgar scores were also found. Malformations reported with heroin are multiple and varied with no discernible patterns of defects (6–13). In addition, all of the mothers in the studies reporting malformed infants were consuming numerous other drugs, including drugs of abuse.

Characteristics of the infant delivered from a heroin-addicted mother may include the following (14):

- Accelerated liver maturity with a lower incidence of jaundice (8,15)
- Lower incidence of hyaline membrane disease after 32 weeks' gestation (5,16)
- Normal Apgar scores (6)
- (*Note*: *The findings of Ostrea and Chavez (9) are in disagreement with the above statements.*)
- Low birth weight; up to 50% weigh less than 2500 g
- Small size for gestational age
- Narcotic withdrawal in about 85% (58%–91%): symptoms (hyperactivity, respiratory distress, fever, diarrhea, mucus secretion, sweating, convulsions, yawning, and face scratching) apparent usually within the first 48 hours, with some delaying up to 6 days; incidence is directly related to daily dose and length of maternal addiction (7,8)
- Meconium staining of amniotic fluid
- Elevated serum magnesium levels when withdrawal signs are present (up to twice normal)
- Increased perinatal mortality; rates up to 37% in some series (13)

Random chromosomal damage was significantly higher when Apgar scores were 6 or less (12,17). However, only one case has appeared relating chromosomal abnormalities to congenital anomalies (12). The clinical significance of this is doubtful. The lower incidence of hyaline membrane disease may be caused by elevated prolactin blood levels in fetuses of addicted mothers (18).

Long-term effects on growth and behavior have been reported (19). As compared with controls, children aged 3–6 years delivered from addicted mothers were found to have lower weights, lower heights, and impaired behavioral, perceptual, and organizational abilities.

BREASTFEEDING SUMMARY

Heroin crosses into breast milk in sufficient quantities to cause addiction in the infant (20). A milk:plasma ratio has not been reported. Previous investigators have considered breastfeeding as one method for treating the addicted newborn (21). However, the American Academy of Pediatrics classifies heroin abuse as a contraindication to breastfeeding (22).

References

1. Anonymous. Diagnosis and management of reactions to drug abuse. Med Lett Drugs Ther 1980;22:74.
2. Thomas L. Notes of a biology-watcher. N Engl J Med 1972;286:531–3.
3. Chappel JN. Treatment of morphine-type dependence. JAMA 1972; 221:1516.
4. Rementeria JL, Nunag NN. Narcotic withdrawal in pregnancy: stillbirth incidence with a case report. Am J Obstet Gynecol 1973;116:1152–6.
5. Gluck L, Kulovich MV. Lecithin/sphingomyelin ratios in amniotic fluid in normal and abnormal pregnancy. Am J Obstet Gynecol 1973;115:539–46.
6. Reddy AM, Harper RG, Stern G. Observations on heroin and methadone withdrawal in the newborn. Pediatrics 1971;48:353–8.
7. Stone ML, Salerno LJ, Green M, Zelson C. Narcotic addiction in pregnancy. Am J Obstet Gynecol 1971;109:716–23.
8. Zelson C, Rubio E, Wasserman E. Neonatal narcotic addiction: 10 year observation. Pediatrics 1971;48:178–89.
9. Ostrea EM, Chavez CJ. Perinatal problems (excluding neonatal withdrawal) in maternal drug addiction: a study of 830 cases. J Pediatr 1979;94:292–5.
10. Perlmutter JF. Drug addiction in pregnant women. Am J Obstet Gynecol 1967;99:569–72.
11. Krause SO, Murray PM, Holmes JB, Burch RE. Heroin addiction among pregnant women and their newborn babies. Am J Obstet Gynecol 1958;75:754–8.
12. Kushnick T, Robinson M, Tsao C. 45,X chromosome abnormality in the offspring of a narcotic addict. Am J Dis Child 1972;124:772–3.
13. Naeye RL, Blanc W, Leblanc W, Khatamee MA. Fetal complications of maternal heroin addiction: abnormal growth, infections and episodes of stress. J Pediatr 1973;83:1055–61.
14. Perlmutter JF. Heroin addiction and pregnancy. Obstet Gynecol Surv 1974;29:439–46.
15. Nathenson G, Cohen MI, Liff IF, McNamara H. The effect of maternal heroin addiction on neonatal jaundice. J Pediatr 1972;81:899–903.
16. Glass L, Rajegowda BK, Evans HE. Absence of respiratory distress syndrome in premature infants of heroin-addicted mothers. Lancet 1971;2:685–6.
17. Amarose AP, Norusis MJ. Cytogenetics of methadone-managed and heroin-addicted pregnant women and their newborn infants. Am J Obstet Gynecol 1976;124:635–40.
18. Parekh A, Mukherjee TK, Jhaveri R, Rosenfeld W, Glass L. Intrauterine exposure to narcotics and cord blood prolactin concentrations. Obstet Gynecol 1981;57:447–9.
19. Wilson GS, McCreary R, Kean J, Baxter JC. The development of preschool children of heroin-addicted mothers: a controlled study. Pediatrics 1979;63:135–41.
20. Lichtenstein PM. Infant drug addiction. NY Med J 1915;102:905. As cited in Cobrinik RW, Hood TH Jr, Chusid E. The effect of maternal narcotic addiction on the newborn infant: review of literature and report of 22 cases. Pediatrics 1959;24:288–304.
21. Cobrinik RW, Hood RT Jr, Chusid E. The effect of maternal narcotic addiction on the newborn infant: review of literature and report of 22 cases. Pediatrics 1959;24:288–304.
22. Committee on Drugs, American Academy of Pediatrics. The transfer of drugs and other chemicals into human milk. Pediatrics 2001;108:776–89.

H

HETACILLIN

[Withdrawn from the market. See 8th edition.]

HEXACHLOROPHENE

Anti-infective

PREGNANCY RECOMMENDATION: Compatible (Topical; Excludes Mucous Membranes)
BREASTFEEDING RECOMMENDATION: Compatible

PREGNANCY SUMMARY

One report has suggested that heavy use of hexachlorophene during the 1st trimester may cause birth defects in exposed offspring, but several criticisms have been directed at this study on methodological grounds. Moreover, in nonprimate animal species, only very high levels (i.e., that approached maternal toxicity) of hexachlorophene are teratogenic. These considerations, coupled with the absence of confirming reports in humans, suggest a lack of an association between routine handwashing with hexachlorophene and human congenital malformations. Because of other toxicities, use of the antiseptic on mucous membranes, such as in the vagina, or on injured skin should be avoided.

FETAL RISK SUMMARY

Hexachlorophene, a polychlorinated biphenol compound, is a topical antiseptic used primarily as a surgical hand scrub and as a bacteriostatic skin cleanser. Although no longer recommended, hexachlorophene has also been used as a douching agent and in feminine hygiene sprays. The drug is rapidly absorbed systemically following topical administration to injured skin, but percutaneous absorption also occurs across intact skin (1–3). Because of very rapid absorption, hexachlorophene should not be used on mucous membranes or injured skin (1,2).

Blood concentrations of the anti-infective have been documented in premature and full-term newborns who were bathed with hexachlorophene and in adults after chronic handwashing (3). CNS toxicity has been observed following the topical use of hexachlorophene in burn patients and after intravaginal application (3).

Hexachlorophene crosses the human placenta (4,5). Newborn whole cord blood concentrations in one study ranged from 0.003 to 0.182 mcg/g with a mean of 0.022 mcg/g (1 mcg/g = 1 ppm) (4). The source of the drug was thought to be from vaginal sprays used by the mothers and from preparation of the skin immediately before delivery. In a second study, a commercially available 3% emulsion of hexachlorophene was used as antiseptic lubricant for vaginal examinations during labor (5). At delivery, detectable maternal serum concentrations of the drug occurred in 12 of 28 women (range 0.142–0.942 mcg/mL) and in the whole cord blood of 9 of 28 newborns (range 0.177–0.617 mcg/mL). Because of the potential for toxicity, the authors recommended the use of alternative lubricants.

A number of studies have examined the reproductive toxicity of hexachlorophene in various animal species (6–14). A marked reduction in the sperm count was observed in male rats administered a single oral dose of 125 mg/kg (6). In pregnant rats, dose-related teratogenicity was demonstrated following acute and chronic oral dosing (6–9). No malformations resulted with relatively low doses (6–8), but high maternal doses were associated with cleft palate (8) and with microphthalmia, anophthalmia, and rib anomalies (9). Intravaginal administration of hexachlorophene in pregnant rats resulted in frequent microphthalmia, anophthalmia, wavy ribs, and less frequently, cleft palate in the offspring (10,11). Blood concentrations were 6–10 times higher after vaginal or oral administration than after dermal application (11). Oral doses of 6 mg/kg/day in pregnant rabbits produced defects of the ribs in a small percentage of exposed fetuses, indicating a minimal teratogenic response (9).

Three studies have described the distribution of hexachlorophene in the fetuses of pregnant mice, rats, and monkeys (12–14). In fetal mice, the drug selectively accumulated in the brain, optic vesicles, and neural tube in early gestation (12). During late gestation, high fetal concentrations were measured in the blood, liver, and intestine. A similar pattern of distribution during gestation was described in fetal monkeys (13). In both mice and monkeys, a partial blood–brain barrier was demonstrated to hexachlorophene in term fetuses (12,13). Hexachlorophene crossed the placenta in pregnant rats after both oral and dermal administration with concentrations detected in the placenta, amniotic fluid, and fetus (14).

Only one study has associated the routine use of hexachlorophene with human teratogenicity (15). The results of the investigation were summarized as a news item in a medical journal approximately a year before publication of the original study (16). In a retrospective analysis of the pregnancy outcomes among nurses who had washed their hands with hexachlorophene during the 1st trimester, 25 severe malformations were observed in 460 neonates (15). No major congenital defects were observed among 233 newborns delivered from similarly employed mothers who did not use hexachlorophene. The exposed nurses had worked at one of six Swedish hospitals between 1969 and 1975 and had washed their hands 10–60 times per day with either a 0.5% or 3% hexachlorophene liquid soap. Three of the hospitals also used a 0.3% or 0.5% hexachlorophene hand cream. Among the exposed group, 46 newborns, in addition to the 25 with major defects, had minor malformations for a total of 71 affected infants (15.4%). The major malformations included cleft lip and/or palate, microphthalmia, anal atresia and hypospadias, cystic kidneys, esophageal atresia and kidney defects, limb reductions, diaphragmatic hernia, neural tube defects, pulmonary stenosis, and cardiac defects. Minor malformations included dislocations of the hip, undescended testes, polydactyly, various foot anomalies, and mild cardiac defects. Eight (3.4%) minor malformations were observed in the control group.

Criticisms of this study on methodological grounds have been published (17,18). Most of the hexachlorophene-exposed nurses were selected because of an infant malformation, not on the basis of exposure to the drug, thus leading to a higher rate of malformations in the exposed group. The selection of the control group was also criticized and was considered, at least on statistical grounds, not to be representative of random selection (17). Concern was expressed over the identification of the minor defects and how diligently these defects were searched for at the various hospitals (18). Furthermore, another study evaluated delivery data on women working in Swedish hospitals from 1973 to 1975 and compared them with births in the general Swedish population during the same period (19). A cluster of malformed infants was found during 1973–1974 that was similar to that observed in the report associating defects with hexachlorophene. However, the rates of perinatal deaths and congenital malformations did not differ between 3007 infants born to women heavily exposed to hexachlorophene in 31 hospitals and 1653 infants born to women working in 18 hospitals where the antiseptic was not used at all or was used only sporadically (19).

BREASTFEEDING SUMMARY

Hexachlorophene has been measured in breast milk following the presumed use of the antiseptic as a nipple wash between nursings (20). The specific history of hexachlorophene use by the women was not available. Six samples of milk were found to have a range of hexachlorophene levels from trace (<2 ppb) to 9.0 ppb (1 ng/g = 1 ppb). The authors concluded that the low milk concentrations of hexachlorophene found in their study were not a risk to a nursing infant. The American Academy of Pediatrics has not found any reports describing signs or symptoms in a nursing infant or effect on lactation after use of the drug but notes that nipple washing with hexachlorophene may contaminate the milk (21).

References

1. American Hospital Formulary Service. *Drug Information 1997*. Bethesda, MD: American Society of Health-System Pharmacists, 1997:2716–8.
2. Product information. pHisoHex. Sanofi Winthrop Pharmaceuticals, 1993.
3. Lockhart JD. How toxic is hexachlorophene? Pediatrics 1972;50:220–35.
4. Curley A, Hawk RE, Kimbrough RD, Nathenson G, Finberg L. Dermal absorption of hexachlorophene in infants. Lancet 1971;2:296–7.
5. Strickland DM, Leonard RG, Stavchansky S, Benoit T, Wilson RT. Vaginal absorption of hexachlorophene during labor. Am J Obstet Gynecol 1983;147:769–72.
6. Thorpe E. Some pathological effects of hexachlorophene in the rat. J Comp Pathol 1967;77:137–42.
7. Gaines TB, Kimbrough RD. The oral and dermal toxicity of hexachlorophene in rats. Toxicol Appl Pharmacol 1971;19:375–6.
8. Oakley GP, Shepard TH. Possible teratogenicity of hexachlorophene in rats (abstract). Teratology 1972;5:264.
9. Kennedy GL Jr, Smith SH, Keplinger ML, Calandra JC. Evaluation of the teratological potential of hexachlorophene in rabbits and rats. Teratology 1975;12:83–8.
10. Kimmel CA, Moore W Jr, Stara JF. Hexachlorophene teratogenicity in rats. Lancet 1972;2:765.
11. Kimmel CA, Moore W Jr, Hysell DK, Stara JF. Teratogenicity of hexachlorophene in rats. Comparison of uptake following various routes of administration. Arch Environ Health 1974;28:43–8.
12. Brandt I, Dencker L, Larsson Y. Transplacental passage and embryonic-fetal accumulation of hexachlorophene in mice. Toxicol Appl Pharmacol 1979;49:393–401.
13. Brandt I, Dencker L, Larsson KS, Siddall RA. Placental transfer of hexachlorophene (HCP) in the marmoset monkey (*Callithrix jacchus*). Acta Pharmacol Toxicol 1983;52:310–3.
14. Kennedy GL Jr, Dressler IA, Keplinger ML, Calandra JC. Placental and milk transfer of hexachlorophene in the rat. Toxicol Appl Pharmacol 1977;40:571–6.
15. Halling H. Suspected link between exposure to hexachlorophene and malformed infants. Ann NY Acad Sci 1979;320:426–35.
16. Check W. New study shows hexachlorophene is teratogenic in humans. JAMA 1978;240:513–4.
17. Källen B. Hexachlorophene teratogenicity in humans disputed. JAMA 1978;240:1585–6.
18. Janerich DT. Environmental causes of birth defects: the hexachlorophene issue. JAMA 1979;241:830–1.
19. Baltzar B, Ericson A, Källen B. Pregnancy outcome among women working in Swedish hospitals. N Engl J Med 1979;300:627–8.
20. West RW, Wilson DJ, Schaffner W. Hexachlorophene concentrations in human milk. Bull Environ Contam Toxicol 1975;13:167–9.
21. Committee on Drugs, American Academy of Pediatrics. The transfer of drugs and other chemicals into human milk. Pediatrics 2001;108:776–89.

H

HEXAMETHONIUM

[Withdrawn from the market. See 8th edition.]

HEXOCYCLIUM

[Withdrawn from the market. See 8th edition.]

HEXOPRENALINE

[Withdrawn from the market. See 9th edition.]

HOMATROPINE

Parasympatholytic (Anticholinergic)

PREGNANCY RECOMMENDATION: Limited Human Data—No Relevant Animal Data
BREASTFEEDING RECOMMENDATION: No Human Data—Probably Compatible

PREGNANCY SUMMARY

The limited human experience and absence of animal reproductive data prevent an assessment of the embryo–fetal risk. In general, however, anticholinergics are not thought to present a clinically significant risk of developmental toxicity (see also Atropine).

FETAL RISK SUMMARY

Homatropine is an anticholinergic agent. The Collaborative Perinatal Project monitored 50,282 mother–child pairs, 26 of whom used homatropine in the 1st trimester (1, pp. 346–353). For use anytime during pregnancy, 86 exposures were recorded (1, p. 439). Only for anytime use was a possible association with congenital defects discovered. In addition, when the group of parasympatholytics was taken as a whole (2323 exposures), a possible association with minor malformations was found (1, pp. 346–353).

BREASTFEEDING SUMMARY

No reports describing the use of homatropine during human lactation have been located (see also Atropine).

Reference

1. Heinonen OP, Slone D, Shapiro S. *Birth Defects and Drugs in Pregnancy*. Littleton, MA: Publishing Sciences Group, 1977.

HORMONAL PREGNANT TEST TABLETS

H

[Withdrawn from the market. See 8th edition.]

HYDRALAZINE

Antihypertensive

PREGNANCY RECOMMENDATION: Human Data Suggest Risk in 3rd Trimester
BREASTFEEDING RECOMMENDATION: Limited Human Data—Probably Compatible

PREGNANCY SUMMARY

No reports linking the use of hydralazine with congenital defects have been located. However, fetal toxicity has been associated with use of the drug in the 3rd trimester.

FETAL RISK SUMMARY

In England, hydralazine is the most commonly used antihypertensive agent in pregnant women (1). Neonatal thrombocytopenia and bleeding secondary to maternal ingestion of hydralazine have been reported in three infants (2). In each case, the mother had consumed the drug daily throughout the 3rd trimester. This complication has also been reported in series examining severe maternal hypertension and may be related to the disease rather than to the drug (3,4).

Hydralazine readily crosses the placenta to the fetus (5). Serum concentrations in the fetus are equal to or greater than those in the mother.

The Collaborative Perinatal Project monitored 50,282 mother–child pairs, 8 of whom had 1st trimester exposure to hydralazine (6, p. 372). For use anytime during pregnancy, 136 cases were recorded (6, p. 441). No defects were observed with 1st trimester use. There were eight infants born with defects who were exposed in the 2nd or 3rd trimester. This incidence (5.9%) is greater than the expected frequency of occurrence, but the severe maternal disease necessitating the use of hydralazine is probably responsible. Patients with preeclampsia are at risk for a marked increase in fetal mortality (7–10).

In a surveillance study of Michigan Medicaid recipients involving 229,101 completed pregnancies conducted between 1985 and 1992, 40 newborns had been exposed to hydralazine during the 1st trimester (F. Rosa, personal communication, FDA, 1993). One (2.5%) major birth defect was observed (two expected), a hypospadias (none expected).

A number of studies involving the use of hydralazine either alone or in combination with other antihypertensives have found the drug to be relatively safe for the fetus (4,7–17). Fatal maternal hypotension has been reported in one patient after combined therapy with hydralazine and diazoxide (18).

In a woman with chronic hypertension maintained on methyldopa, an increase in blood pressure at about 35 weeks' gestation prompted the addition of hydralazine, 25 mg twice daily, to the treatment regimen (19). Fetal premature atrial contractions were diagnosed 1 week later, but tachyarrhythmias, which can be initiated by premature atrial contractions, were not observed (19). Hospitalization with bed rest allowed the patient's blood pressure to decline enough to discontinue hydralazine therapy. Within 24 hours of stopping hydralazine, the fetal arrhythmia resolved. The infant was delivered at 38 weeks and cardiac evaluation after discharge at 3 days indicated a regular heart rate.

A syndrome resembling lupus erythematosus was diagnosed in a 29-year-old woman treated with IV hydralazine during the 28th week of pregnancy (20). The patient received 425 mg during a 6-day period for the treatment of hypertension. IV methyldopa was administered on the 6th day of therapy. Labor was induced for fetal distress and a 780-g growth-restricted male infant was delivered vaginally. The infant expired at 36 hours of age secondary to cardiac tamponade induced by 7 mL of clear sterile transudate in the pericardial space. Lupus-like symptoms consisting of macular rash, arthralgia, and bilateral pleural effusion developed in the mother on the 5th day of hydralazine therapy and gradually resolved after discontinuance of the drug and delivery. The findings of pericardial effusion and cardiac tamponade in the infant were also thought to represent clinical evidence of a lupus-like syndrome (20). The symptoms in both the mother and fetus were attributed to hydralazine sensitivity resulting in the induction of a lupus-like syndrome.

BREASTFEEDING SUMMARY

Hydralazine is excreted into breast milk (5). In one patient treated with 50 mg 3 times daily, the milk:plasma ratio 2 hours after a dose was 1.4. This value is in close agreement with the predicted ratio calculated from the pK_a (21). The available dose of hydralazine in 75 mL of milk was estimated to be 13 mcg (5). No adverse effects were noted in the nursing infant from this small concentration. The American Academy of Pediatrics classifies hydralazine as compatible with breastfeeding (22).

References

1. De Swiet M. Antihypertensive drugs in pregnancy. Br Med J 1985;291:365–6.
2. Widerlov E, Karlman I, Storsater J. Hydralazine-induced neonatal thrombocytopenia. N Engl J Med 1980;303:1235.
3. Brazy JE, Grimm JK, Little VA. Neonatal manifestations of severe maternal hypertension occurring before the thirty-sixth week of pregnancy. J Pediatr 1982;100:265–71.
4. Sibai BM, Anderson GD. Pregnancy outcome of intensive therapy in severe hypertension in first trimester. Obstet Gynecol 1986;67:517–22.
5. Liedholm H, Wahlin-Boll E, Ingemarsson I, Melander A. Transplacental passage and breast milk concentrations of hydralazine. Eur J Clin Pharmacol 1982;21:417–9.
6. Heinonen OP, Slone D, Shapiro S. *Birth Defects and Drugs in Pregnancy*. Littleton, MA: Publishing Sciences Group, 1977.
7. Bott-Kanner G, Schweitzer A, Schoenfeld A, Joel-Cohen J, Rosenfeld JB. Treatment with propranolol and hydralazine throughout pregnancy in a hypertensive patient. Isr J Med Sci 1978;14:466–8.
8. Pritchard JA, Pritchard SA. Standardized treatment of 154 consecutive cases of eclampsia. Am J Obstet Gynecol 1975;123:543–52.
9. Chapman ER, Strozier WE, Magee RA. The clinical use of Apresoline in the toxemias of pregnancy. Am J Obstet Gynecol 1954;68:1109–17.
10. Johnson GT, Thompson RB. A clinical trial of intravenous Apresoline in the management of toxemia of late pregnancy. J Obstet Gynecol 1958;65:360–6.
11. Kuzniar J, Skret A, Piela A, Szmigiel Z, Zaczek T. Hemodynamic effects of intravenous hydralazine in pregnant women with severe hypertension. Obstet Gynecol 1985;66:453–8.
12. Hogstedt S, Lindeberg S, Axelsson O, Lindmark G, Rane A, Sandstrom B, Lindberg BS. A prospective controlled trial of metoprolol-hydralazine treatment in hypertension during pregnancy. Acta Obstet Scand 1985;64:505–10.
13. Gallery EDM, Ross MR, Gyory AZ. Antihypertensive treatment in pregnancy: analysis of different responses to oxprenolol and methyldopa. Br Med J 1985;291:563–6.
14. Horvath JS, Korda A, Child A, Henderson-Smart D, Phippard A, Duggin GG, Hall BM, Tiller DJ. Hypertension in pregnancy: a study of 142 women presenting before 32 weeks' gestation. Med J Aust 1985;143:19–21.
15. Rosenfeld J, Bott-Kanner G, Boner G, Nissenkorn A, Friedman S, Ovadia J, Merlob P, Reisner S, Paran E, Zmora E, Biale Y, Insler V. Treatment of hypertension during pregnancy with hydralazine monotherapy or with combined therapy with hydralazine and pindolol. Eur J Obstet Gynecol Reprod Biol 1986;22:197–204.
16. Mabie WC, Gonzalez AR, Sibai BM, Amon E. A comparative trial of labetalol and hydralazine in the acute management of severe hypertension complicating pregnancy. Obstet Gynecol 1987;70:328–33.
17. Owen J, Hauth JC. Polyarteritis nodosa in pregnancy: a case report and brief literature review. Am J Obstet Gynecol 1989;160:606–7.
18. Henrich WL, Cronin R, Miller PD, Anderson RJ. Hypotensive sequelae of diazoxide and hydralazine therapy. JAMA 1977;237:264–5.
19. Lodeiro JG, Feinstein SJ, Lodeiro SB. Fetal premature atrial contractions associated with hydralazine. Am J Obstet Gynecol 1989;160:105–7.
20. Yemini M, Shoham (Schwartz) Z, Dgani R, Lancet M, Mogilner BM, Nissim F, Bar-Khayim Y. Lupus-like syndrome in a mother and newborn following administration of hydralazine: a case report. Eur J Obstet Gynecol Reprod Biol 1989;30:193–7.
21. Daily JW. Anticoagulant and cardiovascular drugs. In: Wilson JT, ed. *Drugs in Breast Milk*. Balgowlah, Australia: ADIS Press, 1981:61–4.
22. Committee on Drugs, American Academy of Pediatrics. The transfer of drugs and other chemicals into human milk. Pediatrics 2001;108:776–89.

HYDRIODIC ACID

[Withdrawn from the market. See 8th edition.]

HYDROCHLOROTHIAZIDE

Diuretic

See Chlorothiazide.

HYDROCODONE

Narcotic Agonist Analgesic, Respiratory Drug (Antitussive)

PREGNANCY RECOMMENDATION: **Human Data Suggest Risk**
BREASTFEEDING RECOMMENDATION: **Limited Human Data—Potential Toxicity**

PREGNANCY SUMMARY

The National Birth Defects Prevention Study discussed below found evidence that opioid use during organogenesis is associated with a low absolute risk of congenital birth defects. Interestingly, this supports the FDA data also presented below. Similar to other opioid analgesics, the use of hydrocodone late in pregnancy has the potential to cause respiratory depression and withdrawal in the newborn (see also Codeine).

FETAL RISK SUMMARY

Hydrocodone is a centrally acting narcotic agent that is related to codeine. It is combined with other drugs for use as an analgesic or as an antitussive. In a reproductive study in hamsters, a single SC injection (102 mg/kg) during the critical period of CNS organogenesis produced malformations (cranioschisis and various other lesions) in 3.4% of the offspring (1). Because of its narcotic properties, withdrawal could theoretically occur in infants exposed in utero to prolonged maternal ingestion of hydrocodone.

In a surveillance study of Michigan Medicaid recipients involving 229,101 completed pregnancies conducted between 1985 and 1992, 332 newborns had been exposed to hydrocodone during the 1st trimester (F. Rosa, personal communication, FDA, 1993). A total of 24 (7.2%) major birth defects were observed (14 expected), 5 of which were cardiovascular defects (3 expected). No anomalies were observed in five other defect categories (oral clefts, spina bifida, polydactyly, limb reduction defects, and hypospadias) for which specific data were available. The total number of malformations is suggestive of a possible association but other factors, including the mother's disease, concurrent drug use, and chance, may be involved.

At a 1996 meeting, data on 118 women using hydrocodone ($N = 40$) or oxycodone ($N = 78$) during the 1st trimester for postoperative pain, general pain, or upper respiratory infection were matched with a similar group using codeine for these purposes (2). Six (5.1%) of the infants exposed to hydrocodone or oxycodone had malformations, an odds ratio of 2.61 (95% confidence interval 0.6–11.5) ($p = 0.13$). There was no pattern evident among the six malformations (2).

Results of a National Birth Defects Prevention Study (1997–2005) were published in 2011 (3). This population-based case–control study examined the association between maternal use of opioid analgesics and >30 types of major structural birth defects. In 17,449 case mothers, therapeutic opioid use was reported by 454 (2.6%) compared with 134 (2.0%) of 6701 control mothers. Indications for use of opioid analgesics were surgical procedures (41%), infections (34%), chronic diseases (20%), and injuries (18%). Dose, duration, and frequency were not evaluated. The exposure period evaluated was from 1 month before to 3 months after conception. Limiting the exposure period to the first 2 months after conception produced similar results. Infants with >1 defect were included in multiple birth defect categories. The following opioids were included (number of cases for each agent not specified): codeine, hydrocodone, hydromorphone, fentanyl, meperidine, methadone, morphine, oxycodone, pentazocine, propoxyphene, and tramadol. The birth defect, total number, number exposed, and the adjusted odds ratio (aOR) with 95% confidence interval (CI) were as follows:

Birth Defect	Total	Cases	aOR (95% CI)
Spina bifida	718	26	2.0 (1.3–3.2)
Any heart defect (20 types)	7724	211	1.4 (1.1–1.7)
Atrioventricular septal defect	175	9	2.4 (1.2–4.8)
Teratology of Fallot	672	21	1.7 (1.1–2.8)
Conotruncal defect	1481	41	1.5 (1.0–2.1)
Conoventricular septal defect	110	6	2.7 (1.1–6.3)
Left ventricular outflow tract obstruction defect	1195	36	1.5 (1.0–2.2)
Hypoplastic left heart syndrome	357	17	2.4 (1.4–4.1)
Right ventricular outflow tract obstruction defect	1175	40	1.6 (1.1–2.3)
Pulmonary valve stenosis	867	34	1.7 (1.2–2.6)
Atrial septal defect (ASD)	511	17	2.0 (1.2–3.6)
Ventricular septal defect + ASD	528	17	1.7 (1.0–2.9)
Hydrocephaly	301	11	2.0 (1.0–3.7)
Glaucoma/anterior chamber defects	103	5	2.6 (1.0–6.6)
Gastroschisis	726	26	1.8 (1.1–2.9)

The authors speculated that the activity of opioids and their receptors as growth regulators during development of the embryo might be a mechanism to explain the above findings. The exposure data were obtained by retrospective maternal self-report; the authors acknowledged that recall bias and misclassification might have affected their results. They concluded that the absolute risk was a modest absolute increase above the baseline risk for birth defects (3).

BREASTFEEDING SUMMARY

A mother, breastfeeding her third infant, experienced severe pain from cracked nipples associated with a fungal infection (4). She had successfully breastfed her two previous infants for 1–2 years. At about 3 weeks postpartum, because acetaminophen alone or combined with codeine had not been successful in controlling her pain, she was started on hydrocodone/acetaminophen (10/650 mg/tablet) two tablets every 4 hours. Good analgesia was obtained, but both the mother and infant were "groggy and sleepy most of the day." After 24 hours, the mother decreased the dose to 1 tablet every 3–5 hours alleviating the symptoms in her and the infant. She eventually discontinued the drug combination completely after 3 weeks. The fungal infection was successfully treated with long-term (30 days) oral fluconazole (4). Although hydrocodone milk concentrations were not measured, it is obvious that sufficient amounts were excreted into milk to cause marked sedation in the infant. Such excretion is consistent with the molecular weight (about 381) of hydrocodone.

Severe apnea, requiring mouth-to-mouth resuscitation, intubation, and IV naloxone, developed in a 5-week old, 3.8-kg breastfed infant (5). The mother had been prescribed methadone and hydrocodone/acetaminophen (doses not specified) for migraine headaches and had taken these agents before breastfeeding the infant. The infant's urine drug screen was positive for opioids. It could not be determined if the infant toxicity was due to methadone, hydrocodone, or a combination of the two agents (5).

A 2007 study reported milk concentrations of hydrocodone in two women (6). In the first case, a 22-year-old, 63.6-kg woman was treated during the 3rd trimester with hydrocodone/acetaminophen two tablets every 3–4 hours to control headaches caused by left-sided temporal schwannoma (skull-based tumor). She continued the analgesic combination after delivery at 35 weeks' gestation. On postpartum day 7, the patient underwent a craniotomy to remove the tumor and was continued on 5 mg of hydrocodone/acetaminophen one to two tablets every 4 hours as needed. She received 105 mg hydrocodone over 81 hours. During that time, an electric pump was used to obtain breast milk for her infant. The milk hydrocodone concentrations were 8.6–127.3 mcg/L with the levels dependent upon the mother's dose and the time interval from the last dose. The average milk concentration, based on AUC, was 57.2 mcg/L. The infant dose, if exclusively breastfed, was 8.58 mcg/kg/day, or 3.1% of the mother's weight-adjusted dose. In the second case, a 22-year-old, 73.5-kg woman at 16 days postpartum was admitted to the hospital for treatment of mastitis and urosepsis. In addition to antibiotics, she received hydrocodone/acetaminophen (5/500 mg) every 6 hours, but only took three doses (15 mg hydrocodone) over a 24-hour period. Milk was obtained as in the first case. Milk concentrations of the opioid were 5.2–47.2 mcg/L depending on the time from the last dose. The average milk concentration, based on AUC, was 20.4 mcg/L. The infant dose, if exclusively breastfed, was 3.07 mcg/kg/day, or 3.7% of the mother's weight-adjusted dose (6).

In their comments, the authors noted that although the infant doses relative to their mother's weight-adjusted dose were nearly the same (3.1% vs. 3.7%), the absolute infant doses were much different (8.58 vs. 3.07 mcg/kg/day) (6). Because the infants were not hospitalized, the authors could not determine if either infant experienced an adverse reaction. However, toxicity would have been more likely in the first infant because of the higher dose.

In a 2011 study, 30 postpartum women received hydrocodone–acetaminophen for pain while fully breastfeeding their infants (7). The study period averaged 55.3 hours (range 16.9–84.1 hours). The average milk concentration of hydrocodone was 14.2 mcg/L. The infant dose as a percentage of the mother's weight-adjusted dose was 1.6% (range 0.2%–9%). Hydromorphone, a metabolite of hydrocodone, was detected in 12 of the 30 women. The total median opiate dosage from breast milk was 0.7% (range 0.1%–9.9%) of the therapeutic dose for older infants. The infants were not followed for evidence of adverse effects (7).

Occasional doses of hydrocodone probably represent a minimal risk for a nursing infant, but higher or frequent maternal dosing may cause toxicity. Regardless, mothers taking hydrocodone products while breastfeeding should observe their infants for breathing difficulty, sedation, excessive sleepiness, gastrointestinal effects, and changes in feeding patterns.

References

1. Geber WF, Schramm LC. Congenital malformations of the central nervous system produced by narcotic analgesics in the hamster. Am J Obstet Gynecol 1975;123:705–13.
2. Schick B, Hom M, Tolosa J, Librizzi R, Donnfeld A. *Preliminary Analysis of First Trimester Exposure to Oxycodone and Hydrocodone (Abstract).* Presented at the Ninth International Conference of the Organization of Teratology Information Services, Salt Lake City, Utah, May 2–4, 1996. Reprod Toxicol 1996;10:162.
3. Broussard CS, Rasmussen SA, Reefhuis J, Friedman JM, Jann MW, Riehle-Colarusso T, Honein MA, for the National Birth Defects Prevention Study. Maternal treatment with opioid analgesics and risk for birth defects. Am J Obstet Gynecol 2011;204:314–7.
4. Bodley V, Powers D. Long-term treatment of a breastfeeding mother with fluconazole-resolved nipple pain caused by yeast: a case study. J Hum Lact 1997;13:307–11.
5. Meyer D, Tobias JD. Adverse effects following the inadvertent administration of opioids to infants and children. Clin Pediatr (Phil) 2005;44:499–503.
6. Anderson PO, Sauberan JB, Lane JR, Rossi SS. Hydrocodone excretion into breast milk: the first two reported cases. Breastfeed Med 2007;2:10–14.
7. Sauberan JB, Anderson PO, Lane JR, Rafie S, Nguyen N, Rossi SS, Stellwagen LM. Breast milk hydrocodone and hydromorphone levels in mothers using hydrocodone for postpartum pain. Obstet Gynecol 2011;117:611–7.

HYDROCORTISONE

Corticosteroid

PREGNANCY RECOMMENDATION: Human Data Suggest Risk
BREASTFEEDING RECOMMENDATION: Limited Human Data—Probably Compatible

PREGNANCY SUMMARY

Hydrocortisone and its inactive precursor, cortisone, appear to present a small risk to the human fetus. These corticosteroids produce dose-related teratogenic and toxic effects in genetically susceptible experimental animals consisting of cleft palate, cataracts, spontaneous abortion, intrauterine growth restriction (IUGR), and polycystic kidney disease. Although the large amount data do not support these effects in the great majority of human pregnancies, adverse outcomes have been observed and may have been caused by corticosteroids. Moreover, the decrease in birth weight and a small increase in the incidence of cleft lip with or without cleft palate is supported by large epidemiologic studies. In addition, cataracts, resulting from a toxicity observed in humans administered the drug directly, have been reported in human offspring exposed in utero, but a causal relationship to maternal corticosteroid use is less certain. Because the benefits of corticosteroids appear to far outweigh the fetal risks, these agents should not be withheld if the mother's condition requires their use. The mother, however, should be informed of the risks so that she can actively participate in the decision on whether to use these agents during her pregnancy.

FETAL RISK SUMMARY

Hydrocortisone (Cortisol; Compound F) is a corticosteroid secreted by the adrenal cortex. An inactive precursor, cortisone (Compound E), is also secreted by the adrenal cortex and is converted by reduction, primarily by the liver, to hydrocortisone (1). Hydrocortisone is used for various indications. Physiologic doses are used to treat adrenal hormone deficiency, and higher, pharmacologic amounts for the anti-inflammatory and immunosuppressant properties and other effects.

Multiple studies have described the effects of hydrocortisone or cortisone on the pregnancy outcomes of experimental animals (2–14). In five different strains of pregnant mice administered a daily IM dose of cortisone ranging from 0.625 to 10.0 mg for 4–5 days, a dose-related and strain-related incidence of cleft palate and resorption were observed (2). Depending on the day of gestation that treatment started, the percentage of young with cleft palate ranged from 2.9% to 79.1%. (Pups with cleft lip and palate similar to the spontaneous defects that sometimes occur in untreated pups were excluded (2).) In contrast, no cases of cleft palate were observed in the young from control mice injected with an inert cortisone-free vehicle. Other anomalies observed in the offspring of treated groups included marked IUGR, shortening of the head and mandible, and spina bifida.

In a continuation of the above work, this same research group studied the effects on pregnant mice of a daily 2.5-mg IM cortisone dose given for 4 consecutive days beginning on gestational days 7 through 18 (3). The maximum percentage of litters resorbed occurred on day 7 (88%) and declined thereafter as the gestational age increased at the first dose. Depending on the mother's genotype, the 4-day cortisone treatment beginning on gestational day 11 resulted in an incidence of cleft palate in the offspring varying from 4% to 100%. Much of this and earlier experiments were reviewed by these investigators in a 1957 paper (4).

Hydrocortisone was shown to produce an incidence of cleft palate in mice offspring similar to cortisone (95%) in genetically susceptible pregnant mice treated with 2.5 mg/day IM for 4 days starting on the 10th or 11th gestational day (5). No other gross external malformations were observed in the offspring.

The effect of cortisone treatment in mice on litter size, birth weight, cleft palate, gestation length, and spontaneous cleft lip (with or without palate) has been investigated (6). Litter size was reduced only if treatment was begun before the 12th gestational day, whereas birth weight was primarily reduced (mean reduction 31.2%) by treatment after this time. Cortisone administration had no effect on mean gestation length or on the frequency of spontaneous cleft lip but did induce cleft palate in some offspring. A 1998 correspondence reiterated the negative effect of cortisone on intrauterine growth that was found in this study (7).

The teratogenic potency of three corticosteroids to produce cleft palate in mice was the subject of a study published in 1965 (8). Therapeutically equivalent IM doses of hydrocortisone (4 mg), prednisolone (1 mg), or dexamethasone (0.15 mg) were administered to pregnant mice (weight 20 to 25 g) on gestational days 11 through 14. After exclusion of offspring with spontaneous cleft lip and palate, the frequency of cleft palate with the three agents was 18%, 77%, and 100%, respectively (8). In another study, cleft palate (palatoschisis) and cataract were frequently observed in the offspring of pregnant mice (weight 20 g) administered 1 mg of hydrocortisone SC for 2–4 days between gestational days 9 and 16 (9). Resorption of part or all of the litters was common.

One study investigated the effect of IM cortisone, 1–5.7 mg/kg/day administered for 1–33 days, on reproduction in rabbits (10). Gross congenital anomalies were not seen in offspring that survived, but IUGR was evident in some. Further, a marked increase in fetal and neonatal death was observed. In a later study, pregnant rabbits received IM cortisone, 25 or 30 mg (approximately 7–8 mg/kg/day), for 4 days beginning on gestational day 14 or 15 (11). (Total gestation time in rabbits is 31–34 days (12)) Seventeen of the 35 embryos had a cleft palate, including 9 of the 12 born dead. Embryos with cleft palate, living or stillborn, usually weighed less than their siblings. In addition, two of the seven exposed litters were completely resorbed. All 36 offspring from nonexposed controls were born alive without cleft palate.

Reduced lung and body weights were observed in rabbit fetuses given a 2-mg IM injection of hydrocortisone on gestational day 24 (13). Treated fetuses also had fewer lung cells as indicated by decreased DNA per lung. The deficiencies in the number of lung cells and the weights of lung and body recovered within 30 days of birth. In a 1979 study, hydrocortisone, 57 mg/kg/day intraperitoneal on day 12 or 15 of gestation, had no effect on the development of brain monoamine cell bodies or the arrival of axon terminals in the regions where the synapses form (14).

A study published in 1991 demonstrated that a single 250 mg/kg SC dose of hydrocortisone in pregnant mice on gestational days 11 through 17 could induce polycystic kidney disease in the fetus (15). (Total gestation time in mice is 18–20 days (12).) The highest incidence of the defect occurred after exposure on gestational day 12, corresponding to the expected onset of metanephric renal differentiation in the fetal mouse (15).

Hydrocortisone and cortisone cross the human placenta to the fetus (16–19). Six pregnant women, immediately before an elective cesarean section at term, received a continuous IV infusion of a mixture of radioactive-labeled hydrocortisone and cortisone (16). By measurement of the hormones in the mothers and newborns, the investigators demonstrated that most (about 75%) of the hydrocortisone in the fetus was endogenous, whereas most of the cortisone was from the mother. Two other studies described low transfer of hydrocortisone to the fetus because of placental metabolism (17,18). The placenta is a rich source of the enzyme 11β-ol-dehydrogenase which can convert hydrocortisone to cortisone, the biologically inactive 11-ketosteroid (17,18). In an in vivo experiment, radioactive-labeled IV hydrocortisone was administered to five women immediately before an elective abortion at 13–18 weeks' gestation (17). The concentrations of hydrocortisone and cortisone in umbilical cord serum and the placenta exhibited similar patterns: about 15% for hydrocortisone and 85% for cortisone, indicating that most of hydrocortisone crossing the placenta had been converted to cortisone (17). Using a perfused human placenta, one investigation discovered that the percentage of hydrocortisone converted to cortisone in three different perfusion mediums was 73% (buffer), 85% (1% human serum albumin), and 78% (washed calf red blood cells) (18).

In a 1982 report, researchers measured the concentration of hydrocortisone in the cord blood of 71 premature infants (mean gestational age 32.5 weeks) after administration of the drug in an attempt to prevent respiratory distress syndrome (RDS) (19). The mothers received an IV dose of 100 mg, followed by 100 mg IM every 8 hours up to a total of 400 mg. The infants were delivered between 6 minutes and 85 hours after the first dose. The peak cord blood concentration (32 mcg/100 mL) occurred approximately 1 hour after a dose, representing a 3.8-fold increase over endogenous levels (8.5 mcg/100 mL). Nearly all of the exogenous hydrocortisone was cleared between doses as indicated by the elimination half-life of about 2 hours (19).

Hydrocortisone is frequently prescribed during human pregnancy and case reports and other references have described the use of this agent or its precursor, cortisone, during pregnancies that produced an infant with a congenital malformation. In most cases, however, a relationship between the drug and the outcome cannot be determined.

The Collaborative Perinatal Project monitored 50,282 mother–child pairs, of whom 21 and 34 infants, respectively, were exposed in the 1st trimester to hydrocortisone and cortisone (20, pp. 388–400). Three of the infants exposed in utero to hydrocortisone had a major malformation (relative risk [RR] 2.79), whereas one infant had a defect following exposure to cortisone (RR 0.46) (type of defect not specified). There were 74 exposures to hydrocortisone anytime during pregnancy with three malformed infants (RR 1.70) (20, p. 443). Although the number of exposures is limited, no evidence of an association with congenital malformations was found with these data (20, p. 398).

Several case reports have described congenital anomalies in newborns exposed to corticosteroids with and without other drug exposures (21–25). Some of these cases are included in the review discussed below (26). A brief 1953 correspondence describes four infants with defects (club foot, coarctation of the aorta, cataract, and hypospadias) who were delivered to mothers treated during the 1st trimester with cortisone for nausea and vomiting (21). Microcephaly was noted in a newborn whose mother was treated with two 100-mg IV doses of hydrocortisone and a single IM dose of procaine penicillin at about the 8th week of gestation (22). A male cyclops with a single orbit containing one eyeball with two corneas and two irides was described in a 1973 publication (23). The mother had been treated with "high doses" (specifics not given) of cortisone, procaine penicillin, and sodium salicylate at about 4 weeks fetal age for symptoms of diarrhea, fever, and a maculopapular rash. The infant died 5 minutes after birth. In addition to the cyclops, the nose was absent and the ears were low set, and at autopsy, the brain was found to be small and severely malformed. Although the mother had a positive rubella titer, a definite diagnosis of rubella could not be made (23). Moreover, the defects noted in the infant were not consistent with those required for a diagnosis of congenital rubella syndrome (see Vaccine, Rubella). Two malformed infants, one with gastroschisis and the other with hydrocephalus, were briefly noted in a 1965 reference (24). The mothers had used cortisone (doses not specified) throughout their pregnancies for ulcerative colitis and severe asthma, respectively. Bilateral nuclear cataract was diagnosed in a male infant who had been exposed to prednisone (15–60 mg/day) throughout gestation for maternal Crohn's disease (25). In addition, "high-dose" (amount not specified) cortisone had been given during the 6th month of gestation.

A brief 1995 article reviewed the available literature to assess whether the use of corticosteroids (hydrocortisone, cortisone, prednisone, prednisolone, or dexamethasone) during the first 70 days after human conception was teratogenic (26). The disorders treated were mainly systemic lupus erythematosus, asthma, and infertility. From 18 case reports, the researchers identified 26 exposed pregnancies of which 7 (27%) ended with malformed offspring. Four (57%) of the anomalies were cleft palate (three of these cases are described below in references 27–29) and the other three were bilateral nuclear cataract, gastroschisis, and hydrocephalus. Although the number of infants with congenital defects is much higher than expected, the authors thought it likely that they represented reporting bias. In addition, they reviewed 17 reported series of 457 mothers exposed to the corticosteroids during the 1st trimester. In this group, 16 (3.5%) of the offsprings, an incidence close to that expected, had malformations. Of these, two had cleft palate (0.2 expected based on population frequency). The other defects were anencephaly (*N* = 2), clubfoot (*N* = 3), dislocated hip (*N* = 1), coarctation of the aorta (*N* = 2; 1 with a positive family history), transposition of the great vessels (*N* = 1; with a positive family history), cataract (*N* = 2; 1 with a positive family history), hypospadias (*N* = 2), and undescended testis (*N* = 1). Other adverse effects including stillbirth, neonatal death, prematurity, and low birth weight accounted for 21% of the outcomes, but the authors were unable to separate the effect of the drug treatment from the disease process itself. They concluded that there was little teratogenic risk, if any, from the use of corticosteroids in human pregnancy (26).

The first reported case of cleft palate in an infant delivered from a woman treated with cortisone was published in 1956 (27). A 30-year-old woman with idiopathic steatorrhea was administered oral cortisone, 100 mg 3 times daily, beginning on the 38th day of pregnancy. Therapy was gradually tapered and then discontinued about 9 weeks later when pregnancy was diagnosed. The woman eventually delivered a term stillborn male child with a cleft palate. The cause of death was thought to be intrauterine anoxia. A second case was also reported in 1956 (28). A woman with disseminated lupus erythematosus was treated throughout her pregnancy with oral cortisone (100 mg/day) and tolazoline (400 mg/day). She delivered a premature, growth-restricted 2 pound 11 ounce (about 1.22 kg) male infant between 35 and 36 weeks' gestation. The infant, who died of pneumonia 14 days after birth, had a cleft palate but no other malformations were observed at autopsy. A 1962 paper mentioned an infant with a cleft palate whose mother had taken 62.5 mg/day of cortisone during the first 6 months of pregnancy (29).

A 1960 reference cited pregnancy outcome data from 31 reports totaling 260 pregnancies exposed to pharmacologic doses of cortisone or its analogs (30). The outcomes included 8 stillborn, 1 abortion, 15 premature infants, and 7 newborns with various disorders, 1 of which involved transient adrenocortical failure. (Disorders in the other six were not specified.) The authors did not attempt to list the type or frequency of congenital defects, stating only that most "... showed no malformations." They did, however, mention four cases of cleft palate (two from their series and two from unpublished data) in infants exposed to large doses of corticosteroids during the 1st trimester (30).

Data from the MADRE (Malformation Drug Exposure Surveillance) project were published in 1994 (31). This large surveillance study, a part of the International Clearinghouse for Birth Defects Monitoring Systems, compared congenital malformations with 1st trimester drug exposures from six countries (Australia, France, Israel, Italy, Japan, and South America) during a 2-year period (1990–1991) (31). A total of 1448 infants with birth defects were studied. Most of the programs, however, did not report abortions. Moreover, individual drugs were not identified but were grouped into 45 pharmacologic classes. The maternal drug exposure history was determined by interview in the postpartum period. Of interest, seven infants with facial clefts (cleft lip $N = 5$, cleft lip and palate $N = 2$) were exposed to systemic corticosteroids (odds ratio [OR] 3.16; 95% confidence interval [CI] 1.08–7.91; $p = 0.04$). The authors noted that the association may have occurred by chance (31).

The MADRE database again was used in a 2003 case–control study (32). The time interval for data collection was 13 years (1990–2002) and included 11,150 reported congenital malformations (included live births, stillbirths, and induced abortion) with 1st trimester drug exposure. For the present study, cases were defined as infants with cleft lip and/or palate and exposure to systemic corticosteroids during the 1st trimester. Controls were defined as infants with any other birth defect. There were nine cases of cleft lip or cleft palate (OR 2.10, 95% CI 1.03–4.26). Two of the cases were cleft palate only (OR 1.17, 95% CI 0.28–4.92) and seven were cleft lip with or without cleft palate (OR 2.59, 95% CI 1.18–5.67). Because of a decreasing trend of the number of cases per year and animal data, the results were thought to suggest a possible interaction with environmental pesticides (32).

The case–control study, Spanish Collaborative Study of Congenital Malformations, surveying more than 1.2 million infants born live from 1976 to 1995 was published in 1995 (33). The study's purpose was to determine if the occurrence of nonsyndromic cleft lip (with or without cleft palate) was related to 1st trimester exposure to systemic corticosteroids. Three control groups were used: (a) paired controls, (b) controls born at the same hospital ±45 days of the case's birth date, and (c) malformed infants without oral clefts. Statistical analysis was employed to control for four potential confounding factors: (a) maternal smoking; (b) maternal hyperthermia; (c) first-degree malformed relatives with cleft lip with or without cleft palate; and (d) 1st trimester drug exposure to anticonvulsants, benzodiazepines, metronidazole, or sex hormones. A total of 1184 case infants were identified with nonsyndromic oral clefts, 5 (0.42%) of whom were exposed during the 1st trimester to corticosteroids. Among the 31,752 control infants, 36 (0.11%) had been exposed to corticosteroids during the 1st trimester. None of the 5 case infants had been exposed to known teratogens or known risk factors for oral clefts during the 1st trimester. Based on four cases (a case of cleft soft palate was excluded), there was an increased risk of cleft lip (with or without cleft palate) following 1st trimester exposure to systemic corticosteroids (OR 6.55; 95% CI 1.44–29.76; $p = 0.015$) (32). Control of the four confounding factors made the association slightly stronger (OR 6.64; 95% CI 1.46–30.18; $p = 0.014$). The corticosteroids identified in these four cases were hydrocortisone ($N = 1$; 40 mg/day throughout pregnancy), prednisone ($N = 2$; 15–30 mg/day during 1st trimester), and triamcinolone ($N = 1$; 8 mg/day during 2nd month) (33).

Another large case–control study of the teratogenic potential of oral and topical corticosteroids involving 1,923,413 total births from 1980 to 1994 was conducted with the Hungarian Case–Control Surveillance of Congenital Abnormalities and published in 1997 (34). Among the 20,830 malformed case infants, 322 (1.55%) were exposed to systemic corticosteroids (all oral except for 4 who received parenteral doses) during the 1st trimester compared with 503 (1.41%) (all oral except for 3 who received parenteral doses) of the 35,727 normal control infants ($p = 0.19$). A corticosteroid ointment was used in 73 (0.35%) of the cases and in 118 (0.33%) of the controls ($p = 0.69$). A corticosteroid spray was used by 8 case mothers (0.04%) and 11 controls (0.03%) ($p = 0.63$), but the offspring from those mothers were excluded from the detailed analysis because of the small numbers. The indications for systemic corticosteroids during the 1st trimester were primarily for asthma, hay fever, rheumatoid disorders, and subfertility, whereas the ointments were used for skin diseases. Most of the systemic exposures in both cases and controls were to dexamethasone and prednisolone. None of the patients in either group received systemic hydrocortisone and only 15 cases and 22 controls received systemic cortisone. Hydrocortisone ointment was used by 24 case mothers and 32 controls. No association between the rate of different abnormalities and the use of corticosteroids (oral and ointment) in the 2nd and 3rd months of gestation or during the 1st trimester was found based on the analysis of the case–control pairs. In the 1st gestational month, three cases with cleft lip (with or without cleft palate) (OR 5.88, 95% CI 1.70–20.32) and multiple defects (OR 4.88, 95% CI 1.41–16.88) were observed. However, exposures that occurred only during the 1st gestational month (the 1st half of this month is before conception and the other half involves the processes of preimplantation and implantation) cannot cause defects because this time is before the critical period for induction of congenital malformations (34).

In a case–control study published in 1999, the California Birth Defects Monitoring Program evaluated the association between selected congenital anomalies and the use of corticosteroids 1 month before to 3 months after conception (periconceptional period) (35). Case infants or fetal deaths diagnosed with orofacial clefts, conotruncal defects, neural tubal defects (NTD), and limb anomalies were identified from a total of 552,601 births that occurred from 1987 through the end of 1989. Controls, without birth defects, were selected from the same database. Following exclusion of known genetic syndromes, mothers of case and control infants were interviewed by telephone, an average of 3.7 years (cases) or 3.8 years (controls) after delivery, to determine various exposures during the periconceptional period. The number of interviews completed were orofacial cleft case mothers (N = 662, 85% of eligible), conotruncal case mothers (N = 207, 87%), NTD case mothers (N = 265, 84%), limb anomaly case mothers (N = 165, 82%), and control mothers (N = 734, 78%) (34). Orofacial clefts were classified into four phenotypic groups: isolated cleft lip with or without cleft palate (ICLP, N = 348), isolated cleft palate (ICP, N = 141), multiple cleft lip with or without cleft palate (MCLP, N = 99), and multiple cleft palate (MCP, N = 74). A total of 13 mothers reported using corticosteroids during the periconceptional period for a wide variety of indications. Six case mothers of ICLP and 3 of ICP used corticosteroids (unspecified corticosteroid, N = 1; prednisone, N = 2; cortisone, N = 3; triamcinolone acetonide, N = 1; dexamethasone, N = 1; and cortisone plus prednisone, N = 1). One case mother of an infant with NTD used cortisone and an injectable unspecified corticosteroid, and three controls used corticosteroids (hydrocortisone, N = 1; and prednisone, N = 2). The OR for corticosteroid use and ICLP was 4.3 (95% CI 1.1–17.2), whereas the OR for ICP and corticosteroid use was 5.3 (95% CI 1.1–26.5). No increased risks were observed for the other anomaly groups. Commenting on their results, the investigators thought that recall bias was unlikely because they did not observe increased risks for other malformations, and it was unlikely that the mothers would have known of the suspected association between corticosteroids and orofacial clefts (35).

A 2002 study, using data from a Danish prescription database and a birth registry, examined the relationship between topical corticosteroids and low birth weight, malformations, and preterm delivery (36). The pregnancy outcomes of 363 women, who had received prescriptions for the drugs 30 days before conception and/or during pregnancy, were compared with 9263 controls, who had received no prescriptions at all. The incidence of birth defects in 170 pregnancies with 1st trimester exposure was 1.8% (3 of 170) and in controls was 3.6%. The defects in the exposed group were clubfoot, flat foot, and metatarsus varus. For use anytime in pregnancy, no associations were found with low birth weight and preterm delivery. Stratification by corticosteroid strength (weak to very strong) did not change any of the results (36).

In a 2004 report, the Israeli Teratogen Information Service prospectively collected and followed 311 pregnancies exposed to systemic corticosteroids (37). The pregnancy outcomes, in terms of major congenital defects, of exposed and 790 controls did not differ significantly (4.6% vs. 2.6%). There were no cases of oral clefts in the exposed group. However, significant differences were observed in the rates of spontaneous abortion (11.5% vs. 7.0%) and preterm births (22.7% vs. 10.8%). Moreover, exposed infants had a lower median birth weight (3080 vs. 3290 g) and were born at an earlier median gestational age (39 vs. 40 weeks). The study had a power to find a 2.5-fold increase in the overall rate of major congenital defects (37).

Hydrocortisone was only partly successful in an attempt to prevent in utero virilization by adrenal suppression of a female fetus with congenital adrenal hyperplasia (21-hydroxylase deficiency) (38). A daily oral dose of 40 mg was started at 9.4 weeks' gestation and increased to 50 mg/day during mid-pregnancy. At delivery, low amniotic fluids of estriol suggested only partial suppression of the fetal adrenal glands. The infant had moderate virilization as indicated by clitoral hypertrophy and slight posterior fusion. In contrast, dexamethasone was used successfully in a second mother (see Dexamethasone). The failure of hydrocortisone to prevent virilization was probably a result of the lower placental transfer and adrenal suppression potency compared with dexamethasone (38).

Hydrocortisone has been used in attempts to enhance fetal lung maturation and, thus, prevent RDS (18,39–48). This therapy is relatively nontoxic to the fetus. However, hydrocortisone is no longer used for this purpose because very large doses are required to overcome placental metabolism and relatively short half-life of the corticosteroid in the fetus. Compared with a corticosteroid frequently used to prevent RDS (betamethasone 24 mg/treatment course), at least a 2000 mg/treatment course of hydrocortisone would have to be administered to achieve therapeutically equivalent results (48).

Both hydrocortisone and cortisone have been used to treat pregnancy-induced severe nausea and vomiting (i.e., hyperemesis gravidarum (21,49,50)). Although this therapy appears to be successful, its risks, especially in the 1st trimester (e.g., see reference 21), indicate that corticosteroids should not be used as primary therapy.

Hydrocortisone and other systemic and inhaled corticosteroids are frequently prescribed to control the symptoms of severe asthma during pregnancy (51–57). Most authorities believe that these agents are relatively safe in pregnancy and that their benefit to both the mother and her pregnancy clearly outweigh the potential risks to the fetus (51–56). One author, however, suggested caution in their use around the time of palate closure and in women with a family history of cleft lip (with or without cleft palate) (51). A recent study of 824 pregnant asthmatic patients matched with 678 controls (all singleton pregnancies in both groups) found no significant relationship between major congenital malformations and 1st trimester exposure to corticosteroids (oral, inhaled, or intranasal) (53). However, significant associations were found between corticosteroid use and preeclampsia (exposed 11.4% vs. controls 7.1%, p = 0.014), preterm birth (exposed 6.4% vs. controls 3.8%, p = 0.048), and low birth weight (exposed 6.0% vs. controls 3.3%, p = 0.032) (53). Other references have reported IUGR as a complication of systemic corticosteroids (54–56). The latter reference quantified the impaired fetal growth as about a 300- to 400-g decrease in birth weight (56).

BREASTFEEDING SUMMARY

Trace amounts of endogenous hydrocortisone (cortisol) are excreted into breast milk (57,58). The amount of the corticosteroid in milk varies from 0.2 to 32 ng/mL with the highest mean concentrations (25.5 ng/mL) measured in colostrum during late pregnancy (58). The concentration of hydrocortisone in colostrum averages 7.5% of the plasma level.

No reports describing the excretion of exogenous hydrocortisone or cortisone into human milk have been located. It is unlikely, however, that these agents pose a risk to a nursing infant. Prednisone, a corticosteroid more potent than hydrocortisone, is excreted in trace amounts into milk and is classified as compatible with breastfeeding (see Prednisone). Moreover, a 1997 review stated that corticosteroids have been used safely during lactation (54).

References

1. American Hospital Formulary Service. *Drug Information 1999*. Bethesda, MD: American Society of Health-System Pharmacists, 1999:2637.
2. Fraser FC, Fainstat TD. Production of congenital defects in the offspring of pregnant mice treated with cortisone. Progress report. Pediatrics 1951;8:527–33.
3. Fraser FC, Kalter H, Walker BE, Fainstat TD. The experimental production of cleft palate with cortisone and other hormones. J Cell Comp Physiol 1954;43(Suppl 1):235–59.
4. Fraser FC, Walker BE, Trasler DG. Experimental production of congenital cleft palate: genetic and environmental factors. Pediatrics 1957;19:782–7.
5. Kalter H, Fraser FC. Production of congenital defects in the offspring of pregnant mice treated with compound F. Nature 1952;169:665.
6. Kalter H. Factors influencing the frequency of cortisone-induced cleft palate in mice. J Exp Zool 1957;134:449–67.
7. Kalter H. Fetal growth restriction induced by cortisone 40 years ago. Am J Obstet Gynecol 1998;179:835.
8. Pinsky L, DiGeorge AM. Cleft palate in the mouse: a teratogenic index of glucocorticoid potency. Science 1965;147:402–3.
9. Rogoyski A, Trzcinska-Dabrowska Z. Corticosteroid-induced cataract and palatoschisis in the mouse fetus. Am J Ophthalmol 1969;68:128–33.
10. DeCosta EJ, Abelman MA. Cortisone and pregnancy. An experimental and clinical study of the effects of cortisone on gestation. Am J Obstet Gynecol 1952;64:746–67.
11. Fainstat T. Cortisone-induced congenital cleft palate in rabbits. Endocrinology 1954;55:502–8.
12. Kotas RV, Mims LC, Hart LK. Reversible inhibition of lung cell number after glucocorticoid injection into fetal rabbits to enhance surfactant appearance. Pediatrics 1974;53:358–61.
13. Van Geijn HP, Zuspan FP, Copeland SJ, Vorys AS, Zuspan MF, Scott GD. The effects of hydrocortisone on the development of the amine system in the fetal brain. Am J Obstet Gynecol 1979;135:743–50.
14. Crocker JFS, Ogborn MR. Glucocorticoid teratogenesis in the developing nephron. Teratology 1991;43:571–4.
15. Shepard TH. *Catalog of Teratogenic Agents*. 8th ed. Baltimore, MD: The Johns Hopkins University Press, 1995.
16. Beitins IZ, Bayard F, Ances IG, Kowarski A, Migeon CJ. The metabolic clearance rate, blood production, interconversion and transplacental passage of cortisol and cortisone in pregnancy near term. Pediatr Res 1973;7:509–19.
17. Pearson Murphy BE, Clark SJ, Donald IR, Pinsky M, Vedady D. Conversion of maternal cortisol to cortisone during placental transfer to the human fetus. Am J Obstet Gynecol 1974;118:538–41.
18. Levitz M, Jansen V, Dancis J. The transfer and metabolism of corticosteroids in the perfused human placenta. Am J Obstet Gynecol 1978;132:363–6.
19. Ballard PL, Liggins GC. Glucocorticoid activity in cord serum: comparison of hydrocortisone and betamethasone regimens. J Pediatr 1982;101:468–70.
20. Heinonen OP, Slone D, Shapiro S. *Birth Defects and Drugs in Pregnancy*. Littleton, MA: Publishing Sciences Group, 1977.
21. Guilbeau JA Jr. Effects of cortisone on fetus. Am J Obstet Gynecol 1953;64:227.
22. Reisman LE, Matheny A. Corticosteroids in pregnancy. Lancet 1968;1:592–3.
23. Khudr G, Olding L. Cyclopia. Am J Dis Child 1973;125:120–2.
24. Malpas P. Foetal malformation and cortisone therapy. Br Med J 1965;1:795.
25. Kraus AM. Congenital cataract and maternal steroid ingestion. J Pediat Ophthalmol 1975;12:107–8.
26. Fraser FC, Sajoo A. Teratogenic potential of corticosteroids in humans. Teratology 1995;51:45–6.
27. Harris JWS, Ross IP. Cortisone therapy in early pregnancy: relation to cleft palate. Lancet 1956;1:1045–7.
28. Doig RK, Coltman OM. Cleft palate following cortisone therapy in early pregnancy. Lancet 1956;2:730.
29. Popert AJ. Pregnancy and adrenocortical hormones. Some aspects of the interaction in rheumatic diseases. Br Med J 1962;1:967–72.
30. Bongiovanni AM, McPadden AJ. Steroids during pregnancy and possible fetal consequences. Fertil Steril 1960;11:181–6.
31. Robert E, Vollset SE, Botto L, Lancaster PAL, Merlob P, Mastroiacovo P, Cocchi G, Ashizawa M, Sakamoto S, Orioli I. Malformation surveillance and maternal drug exposure: the MADRE project. Int J Risk Safety Med 1994;6:75–118.
32. Pradat P, Robert-Gnansia E, Di Tanna GL, Rosano A, Lisi A, Mastroiacovo P, and all contributors to the MADRE database. First trimester exposure to corticosteroids and oral clefts. Birth Defects Res A Clin Mol Teratol 2003;67:968–70.
33. Rodriguez-Pinilla E, Martinez-Frias ML. Corticosteroids during pregnancy and oral clefts: a case-control study. Teratology 1998;58:2–5.
34. Czeizel AE, Rockenbauer M. Population-based case-control study of teratogenic potential of corticosteroids. Teratology 1997;56:335–40.
35. Carmichael SL, Shaw GM. Maternal corticosteroid use and risk of selected congenital anomalies. Am J Med Genet 1999;86:242–4.
36. Mygind H, Thulstrup AM, Pedersen L, Larsen H. Risk of intrauterine growth restriction, malformations and other birth outcomes in children after topical use of corticosteroids in pregnancy. Acta Obstet Gynecol Scand 2002;81:234–9.
37. Gur C, Diav-Citrin O, Shechtman S, Arnon J, Ornoy A. Pregnancy outcome after first trimester exposure to corticosteroids: a prospective controlled study. Reprod Toxicol 2004;18:93–101.
38. David M, Forest MG. Prenatal treatment of congenital adrenal hyperplasia resulting from 21-hydroxylase deficiency. J Pediatr 1984;105:799–803.
39. Taeusch HW Jr. Glucocorticoid prophylaxis for respiratory distress syndrome: a review of potential toxicity. J Pediatr 1975;87:617–23.
40. Dluholucky S, Babic J, Taufer I. Reduction of incidence and mortality of respiratory distress syndrome by administration of hydrocortisone to mother. Arch Dis Child 1976;51:420–3.
41. Zuspan FP, Cordero L, Semchyshyn S. Effects of hydrocortisone on lecithin-sphingomyelin ratio. Am J Obstet Gynecol 1977;128:571–4.
42. Morrison JC, Whybrew WD, Bucovaz ET, Schneider JM. Injection of corticosteroids into mother to prevent neonatal respiratory distress syndrome. Am J Obstet Gynecol 1978;131:358–66.
43. Beck JC, Johnson JWC. Maternal administration of glucocorticoids. Clin Obstet Gynecol 1980;23:93–113.
44. Semchyshyn S, Zuspan FP, Cordero L. Cardiovascular response and complications of glucocorticoid therapy in hypertensive pregnancies. Am J Obstet Gynecol 1983;145:530–3.
45. Schmidt PL, Sims ME, Strassner HT, Paul RH, Mueller E, McCart D. Effect of antepartum glucocorticoid administration upon neonatal respiratory distress syndrome and perinatal infection. Am J Obstet Gynecol 1984;148:178–86.
46. Iams JD, Barrows H. Management of preterm prematurely ruptured membranes: a retrospective comparison of observation versus use of steroids and timed delivery. Am J Obstet Gynecol 1984;150:977–81.
47. Iams JD, Talbert ML, Barrows H, Sachs L. Management of preterm prematurely ruptured membranes: a prospective randomized comparison of observation versus use of steroids and timed delivery. Am J Obstet Gynecol 1985;151:32–8.
48. Ward RM. Pharmacologic enhancement of fetal lung maturation. Clin Perinatol 1994;21:523–42.
49. Wells CN. Treatment of hyperemesis gravidarum with cortisone. I. Fetal results. Am J Obstet Gynecol 1953;66:598–601.
50. Taylor R. Successful management of hyperemesis gravidarum using steroid therapy. QJM 1996;89:103–7.
51. Greenberg F. The potential teratogenicity of allergy and asthma treatment in pregnancy. Immunol Aller Prac 1985;7:15–20.
52. D'Alonzo GE. The pregnant asthmatic patient. Sem Perinatol 1990;14:119–29.
53. Schatz M, Zeiger RS, Harden K, Hoffman CC, Chilingar L, Petitti D. The safety of asthma and allergy medications during pregnancy. J Allergy Clin Immunol 1997;100:301–6.
54. Venkataraman MT, Shanies HM. Pregnancy and asthma. J Asthma 1997;34:265–71.
55. Schatz M, Zeiger RS. Asthma and allergy in pregnancy. Clin Perinatol 1997;24:407–32.
56. Report of the Working Group on Asthma and Pregnancy. *Management of Asthma during Pregnancy*. National Institutes of Health. NIH Publication No. 93-3279, 1993:18–9.
57. Rosner W, Beers PC, Awan T, Khan MS. Identification of corticosteroid-binding globulin in human milk: measurement with a filter disk assay. J Clin Endocrinol Metab 1976;42:1064–73.
58. Kulski JK, Hartmann PE. Changes in the concentration of cortisol in milk during different stages of human lactation. Aust J Exp Biol Med Sci 1981;59:769–78.

HYDROFLUMETHIAZIDE

Diuretic

See Chlorothiazide.

HYDROMORPHONE

Narcotic Agonist Analgesic

PREGNANCY RECOMMENDATION: **Human Data Suggest Risk**
BREASTFEEDING RECOMMENDATION: **Limited Human Data—Potential Toxicity**

H

PREGNANCY SUMMARY

The National Birth Defects Prevention Study discussed below found evidence that opioid use during organogenesis is associated with a low absolute risk of congenital birth defects. In addition, withdrawal could occur in infants exposed in utero to prolonged maternal ingestion of hydromorphone. Use of the drug in pregnancy is primarily confined to labor. Respiratory depression in the neonate similar to that produced by meperidine or morphine should be expected (1) (see also Codeine).

FETAL RISK SUMMARY

Hydromorphone, an opioid analgesic, is a hydrogenated ketone of morphine. The drug is extensively metabolized in the liver to apparently inactive metabolites. It also is a metabolite of hydrocodone. Plasma protein binding of hydromorphone is low (about 8%–19%) and the elimination half-life is dose-dependent (about 2.6–2.8 hours) (2).

Results of a National Birth Defects Prevention Study (1997–2005) were published in 2011 (3). This population-based case–control study examined the association between maternal use of opioid analgesics and >30 types of major structural birth defects. In 17,449 case mothers, therapeutic opioid use was reported by 454 (2.6%) compared with 134 (2.0%) of 6701 control mothers. Indications for use of opioid analgesics were surgical procedures (41%), infections (34%), chronic diseases (20%), and injuries (18%). Dose, duration, and frequency were not evaluated. The exposure period evaluated was from 1 month before to 3 months after conception. Limiting the exposure period to the first 2 months after conception produced similar results. Infants with >1 defect were included in multiple birth defect categories. The following opioids were included (number of cases for each agent not specified): codeine, hydrocodone, hydromorphone, fentanyl, meperidine, methadone, morphine, oxycodone, pentazocine, propoxyphene, and tramadol. The birth defect, total number, number exposed, and the adjusted odds ratio (aOR) with 95% confidence interval (CI) were as follows:

Birth Defect	Total	Cases	aOR (95% CI)
Spina bifida	718	26	2.0 (1.3–3.2)
Any heart defect (20 types)	7724	211	1.4 (1.1–1.7)
Atrioventricular septal defect	175	9	2.4 (1.2–4.8)
Teratology of Fallot	672	21	1.7 (1.1–2.8)
Conotruncal defect	1481	41	1.5 (1.0–2.1)
Conoventricular septal defect	110	6	2.7 (1.1–6.3)
Left ventricular outflow tract obstruction defect	1195	36	1.5 (1.0–2.2)
Hypoplastic left heart syndrome	357	17	2.4 (1.4–4.1)
Right ventricular outflow tract obstruction defect	1175	40	1.6 (1.1–2.3)
Pulmonary valve stenosis	867	34	1.7 (1.2–2.6)
Atrial septal defect (ASD)	511	17	2.0 (1.2–3.6)
Ventricular septal defect + ASD	528	17	1.7 (1.0–2.9)
Hydrocephaly	301	11	2.0 (1.0–3.7)
Glaucoma/anterior chamber defects	103	5	2.6 (1.0–6.6)
Gastroschisis	726	26	1.8 (1.1–2.9)

The authors speculated that the activity of opioids and their receptors as growth regulators during development of the embryo might be a mechanism to explain the above findings. The exposure data were obtained by retrospective maternal self-report; the authors acknowledged that recall bias and misclassification might have affected their results. They concluded that the absolute risk was a modest absolute increase above the baseline risk for birth defects (3).

BREASTFEEDING SUMMARY

Hydromorphone is excreted into breast milk (4). Eight healthy lactating women were given a single dose of

2-mg hydromorphone by nasal spray and serial blood and milk samples were collected over 24 hours. Infants were not allowed to nurse during the study. Little of the drug was found in milk fat (skim milk:whole milk ratio 0.98). The milk:plasma ratio was about 2.6 and the estimated infant dose (based on 150 mL/kg/day) was 0.67% of the mother's weight-adjusted dose (3).

The effect of these amounts, if any, on a nursing infant are unknown but appear to be clinically insignificant. However, further study, especially with multiple dosing, is warranted (see also Hydrocodone).

References

1. Bonica J. *Principles and Practice of Obstetric Analgesia and Anesthesia*. Philadelphia, PA: FA Davis, 1967:251.
2. Product information. Dilaudid. Purdue Pharma, 2013.
3. Broussard CS, Rasmussen SA, Reefhuis J, Friedman JM, Jann MW, Riehle-Colarusso T, Honein MA, for the National Birth Defects Prevention Study. Maternal treatment with opioid analgesics and risk for birth defects. Am J Obstet Gynecol 2011;204:314–7.
4. Edwards JE, Rudy AC, Wermeling DP, Desai N, McNamara PJ. Hydromorphone transfer into breast milk after intranasal administration. Pharmacotherapy 2003;23:153–8.

HYDROQUINONE

Dermatologic Agent

PREGNANCY RECOMMENDATION: Limited Human Data—Probably Compatible
BREASTFEEDING RECOMMENDATION: No Human Data—Probably Compatible

PREGNANCY SUMMARY

In a 1998 study, approximately 45% of a dose from a 24-hour application of 2% topical hydroquinone cream was absorbed into the systemic circulation (1). In one of two animal species studied, an increased incidence of structural anomalies was noted but only at a maternal toxic dose. The difference between the oral doses used in animals and the topical human dose in terms of systemic exposure (i.e., AUC) is unknown. However, since the difference should be large, the animal data appear to suggest low risk. Moreover, the nearly complete absence of reported human pregnancy experience, combined with the expected frequent use in pregnancy, provides some reassurance that topical hydroquinone is not associated with embryo or fetal toxicity. Although more data are needed, the use of hydroquinone in pregnancy probably is low risk, but one review concluded that it was best to minimize exposure because of the amounts absorbed into the systemic circulation (2).

FETAL RISK SUMMARY

Hydroquinone, usually in combination with a sunscreen agent, is used topically to produce reversible depigmentation of the skin (3–5). Hydroquinone also occurs naturally in leaves, bark, and fruit of a number of plants and in some insects, and has several industrial uses (6). It is structurally related to monobenzone. Two commercial preparations (EpiQuin Micro and Claripel) are indicated for the gradual treatment of ultraviolet-induced dyschromia and discoloration resulting from the use of oral contraceptives, pregnancy, hormone replacement therapy, or skin trauma (3,4). A third product (Glyquin XM) is indicated for the gradual bleaching of hyperpigmented skin conditions such as chloasma, melasma, freckles, senile lentigines, and other unwanted areas of melanin hyperpigmentation (5). Hydroquinone is a strong base (pK_a 9.96) (3).

Animal reproductive tests have not been conducted with topical hydroquinone (3–5). However, oral doses of the drug have been tested in pregnant animals (6–8). In a rat study, gavage doses ≤300 mg/kg/day during organogenesis caused no adverse effects on reproductive indices (i.e., pregnancy rate, numbers of corpora lutea, implantation sites, preimplantation and postimplantation losses, early and late resorptions, viable fetuses, fetal sex ratio, and gravid uterine weights) (7). However, the highest dose did cause maternal toxicity (slightly reduced body weight) and an associated small decrease in mean fetal weight. Common vertebral variations also were observed in the fetuses at the highest dose. The no-observable-effect level (NOEL) for both maternal and developmental toxicity was 100 mg/kg/day (7). In a two-generation rat study, no evidence of impaired fertility or embryo–fetal harm was observed at oral doses up to 150 mg/kg/day given before and throughout gestation (6).

In a study with pregnant rabbits, gavage doses of 75 and 150 mg/kg/day during organogenesis were associated with maternal toxicity (reduced food consumption and/or body weight) (8). The NOEL for maternal toxicity was 25 mg/kg/day. At 150 mg/kg/day, in the presence of maternal toxicity, nonsignificant increases in the incidences of fetal ocular and minor skeletal malformations (microphthalmia, vertebral/rib defects, angulated hyoid arch) were observed. The NOEL for developmental toxicity was 75 mg/kg/day (8).

The relationship of the systemic hydroquinone exposures resulting from the oral doses used in these studies to the human systemic exposure resulting from topical application is not known. However, even though the amount absorbed systemically by the animals is unknown, the exposures most likely are significantly higher than those that humans experience from topical use.

It is not known if hydroquinone crosses the human placenta. The molecular weight (about 110) is low enough for passive diffusion. Because it is a strong base, most of the drug that reaches the systemic circulation should be in the ionized state.

In a 1996 study, a combination of glycolic acid and hydroquinone was used, but the outcomes of the pregnancy cases were not specified (9). The treatment of hyperpigmentation disorders, including melasma (also known as the "mask of pregnancy"), typically involves women of reproductive age (9–15). Hydroquinone is the most commonly used agent for melasma (16,17). Other topical agents in addition to glycolic acid, such as antioxidants, tretinoin, and fluocinolone (a corticosteroid), are sometimes combined with hydroquinone to increase the efficacy of melasma treatment (14,15). The use of topical tretinoin in pregnancy is controversial and best avoided (see Tretinoin [Topical]).

BREASTFEEDING SUMMARY

No reports describing the use of topical hydroquinone during lactation have been located. It is not known if hydroquinone is excreted into breast milk. The molecular weight (about 110) is low enough but, because it is a strong base, most of the compound, if it reaches the systemic circulation, would be in the ionized state and not available for excretion into milk. The potential effects on a nursing infant appear to be negligible.

References

1. Wester RC, Melendres J, Hui X, Cox R, Serranzana S, Zhai J, Quan D, Maibach HI. Human in vivo and in vitro hydroquinone topical bioavailability, metabolism, and disposition. J Toxicol Environ Health 1998;54:301–17.
2. Bozzo P, Chua-Gocheco A, Einarson A. Safety of skin care products during pregnancy. Can Fam Physician 2011;57:665–7.
3. Product information. Claripel Cream. Stiefel Laboratories, 2005.
4. Product information. EpiQuin Micro. SkinMedica, 2005.
5. Product information. Glyquin XM. Valeant Pharmaceuticals, 2005.
6. Blacker AM, Schroeder RE, English JC, Murphy SJ, Krasavage WJ, Simon GS. A two-generation reproduction study with hydroquinone in rats. Fundam Appl Toxicol 1993;21:420–4.
7. Krasavage WJ, Blacker AM, English JC, Murphy SJ. Hydroquinone: a developmental study in rats. Fundam Appl Toxicol 1992;18:370–5.
8. Murphy SJ, Schroeder RE, Blacker AM, Krasavage WJ, English JC. A study of developmental toxicity of hydroquinone in the rabbit. Fundam Appl Toxicol 1992;19:214–21.
9. Garcia A, Fulton JE Jr. The combination of glycolic acid and hydroquinone or kojic acid for the treatment of melasma and related conditions. Dermatol Surg 1996;22:443–7.
10. Engasser PG, Maibach HI. Cosmetics and dermatology: bleaching creams. J Am Acad Dermatol 1981;5:143–7.
11. Grimes PE. Melasma: etiologic and therapeutic considerations. Arch Dermatol 1995;131:1453–7.
12. Goh CL, Dlova CN, A retrospective study on the clinical presentation and treatment outcome of melasma in a tertiary dermatolofical referral centre in Singapore. Singapore Med J 1999;40:455–8.
13. Kauh YC, Zachian TF. Melasma. Adv Exp Med Biol 1999;455:491–9.
14. Guevara IL, Pandya AG. Safety and efficacy of 4% hydroquinone combined with 10% glycolic acid, antioxidants, and sunscreen in the treatment of melasma. Int J Dermatol 2003;42:966–72.
15. Stulberg DI, Clark N, Tovey D. Common hyperpigmentation disorders in adults. II. Melanoma, seborrheic keratoses, acanthosis nigricans, melasma, diabetic dermopathy, tinea versicolor, and postinflammatory hyperpigmentation. Am Fam Physician 2003;68:1963–8.
16. Bolanca I, Bolanca Z, Kuna K, Vukovic A, Tuckar N, Herman R, Grubisic G. Chloasma—the mask of pregnancy. Coll Antropol 2008;32(Suppl 2): 139–41.
17. Sehgal VN, Verma P, Srivastava G, Aggarwal AK, Verma S. Melasma: treatment strategy. J Cosmet Laser Ther 2011;13:265–79.

H

HYDROXYCHLOROQUINE

Antimalarial/Immunologic Agent (Antirheumatic)

PREGNANCY RECOMMENDATION: Limited Human Data—Probably Compatible
BREASTFEEDING RECOMMENDATION: Limited Human Data—Probably Compatible

PREGNANCY SUMMARY

Hydroxychloroquine does not appear to pose a significant risk to the fetus, especially with lower doses. No reports of retinal or ototoxicity after in utero exposure have been located. The CDC has stated that hydroxychloroquine may be used during pregnancy for antimalarial prophylaxis since, in prophylactic doses, the agent has not been shown to be harmful to the fetus (1,2). The adult antimalarial prophylactic dose is 400 mg/week (3). The use of higher doses for prolonged periods, such as those used for systemic lupus erythematosus (SLE), acute attacks of malaria, and rheumatoid arthritis, probably represents an increased fetal risk, but the magnitude of this increase is unknown. At least one source has recommended that the use of hydroxychloroquine for rheumatoid arthritis or SLE be avoided during pregnancy (4), but recent reports (5–7) do not support this conclusion. Moreover, stopping therapy when a pregnancy became known would not, as discussed below, stop exposure of the embryo–fetus to the drug, but could increase the risk because of a lupus flare. If hydroxychloroquine is used in pregnancy for the treatment of rheumatoid arthritis, health care professionals are encouraged to call the toll-free number (877-311-8972) for information about patient enrollment in the Organization of Teratology Information Specialists (OTIS) Rheumatoid Arthritis study.

FETAL RISK SUMMARY

Hydroxychloroquine is used for the treatment of malaria, SLE, and rheumatoid arthritis. A 1988 review described several references relating to animal studies with the closely related agent, chloroquine (4). In pregnant mice, rats, rabbits, and monkeys, chloroquine crosses the placenta to the fetus. In fetal mice and monkeys, the drug accumulates for long intervals, ≤5 months in mice, in the melanin structures of the eyes and inner ears (3,4). Teratogenicity studies with chloroquine using monkeys have not been published. However, in rats, only high doses were teratogenic, producing skeletal and ocular defects (4). In pregnant mice, chloroquine alone was not teratogenic, but in combination with radiation, a significant increase in cleft palates and tail anomalies was observed. No similar data are available for hydroxychloroquine.

Published data relating to the use of hydroxychloroquine during human pregnancy are scarce but do not indicate that the drug poses a significant risk to the fetus. The Collaborative Perinatal Project monitored 50,282 mother–child pairs, 2 of whom had 1st trimester exposure to hydroxychloroquine (8). Neither child had a congenital malformation. A 1974 reference reported no abnormalities in a fetus after a therapeutic abortion at 14 weeks' gestation (9). The fetus had been exposed to the antimalarial agent, 200 mg twice daily, since the time of conception. Examination of the temporal bones, the embryonal precartilage, the anlages of the auditory ossicles, and the membranous labyrinth demonstrated a normal 14-week stage of development, indicating an apparent lack of drug-induced ototoxicity in this fetus (9). A short 1983 communication described the use of 200 mg/day of hydroxychloroquine during the first 16 weeks of gestation for the treatment of maternal discoid lupus erythematosus (10). A male infant was eventually delivered who was alive and well at 2 years of age.

The use of hydroxychloroquine during 27 pregnancies in 23 women with mild to moderate SLE was described in a 1995 abstract (5). In 17 of the pregnancies, the drug was used at a dose of 200–400 mg daily throughout gestation. The outcomes of these cases included 2 miscarriages, 2 perinatal deaths, 1 infant with congenital heart block (in a Ro-positive mother), and 12 normal newborns. In six other pregnancies, hydroxychloroquine was started after conception, three during the 1st trimester. In the remaining three cases, therapy was stopped after diagnosis of pregnancy, resulting in a worsening of the disease and higher doses of prednisolone, and pregnancy termination in one because of severe renal lupus. No fetal or newborn adverse effects related to hydroxychloroquine were observed. A follow-up of 20 newborns for ≥3 years found that all were healthy. The authors concluded that hydroxychloroquine was safe in pregnancy, and because of the risk of lupus flare, discontinuing therapy during pregnancy represented a greater danger to the fetus (5).

Other investigators have reached similar conclusions as to the safety of hydroxychloroquine in the treatment of SLE during pregnancy (6,7). These authors described nine pregnancies (plus seven from an earlier paper) in which hydroxychloroquine (200 mg/day) was used throughout gestation without producing congenital malformations. In the present series of nine pregnancies, five newborns were delivered preterm and four at term. Long-term follow-up of the children exposed in utero has been normal. Because of the very long elimination half-life of the drug from maternal tissues (weeks to months), the authors concluded that discontinuing the drug when pregnancy was known would not eliminate fetal exposure but could jeopardize the pregnancy from a lupus flare (6,7).

The use of hydroxychloroquine as an antimalarial, instead of chloroquine, has been recommended because of the belief that hydroxychloroquine is less toxic (4). However, few data are available to substantiate this practice, either in terms of congenital malformations or in optic or otic toxicity. From published reports of fetal exposure to either chloroquine or hydroxychloroquine, one source cited an incidence of 7 infants with congenital anomalies from 188 live births—a rate of 4.5% (4). This value is within the expected 3%–6% incidence of congenital malformations in a nonexposed population.

BREASTFEEDING SUMMARY

Two reports have described the excretion of small amounts of hydroxychloroquine into breast milk. A 27-year-old woman was treated with hydroxychloroquine, 400 mg (310 mg base) each night, for an exacerbation of lupus erythematosus (11). She had been breastfeeding her infant for 9 months. No mention of the infant's condition or of the presence of toxic effects was made by the authors of this report. Milk samples were collected 2.0, 9.5, and 14.0 hours after one dose and 17.7 hours after a second dose. Milk concentrations of hydroxychloroquine base at the 4 times were 1.46, 1.09, 1.09, and 0.85 mcg/mL, respectively. A maternal blood sample was collected 15.5 hours after the first dose. Hydroxychloroquine base concentrations in whole blood and plasma were 1.76 and 0.20 mcg/mL, respectively. The authors estimated that the infant was consuming, based on 1000 mL of milk, a daily dose of 1.1 mg hydroxychloroquine base, or approximately 0.35% of the mother's daily dose (11).

Much lower milk concentrations of drug were obtained from a 28-year-old woman who was being treated with hydroxychloroquine, 200 mg twice daily, for rheumatoid arthritis (12). Treatment had been stopped for 6 months during pregnancy and then restarted 2 months later because of arthritis relapse. A total of 3.2 mcg of the drug was recovered from her milk over a 48-hour interval, representing 0.0005% of the mother's dose. The highest milk concentration of the agent, 10.6 ng/mL, was found in the 39–48-hour sample. It was not stated whether the infant was allowed to breastfeed.

Because of the slow elimination rate and the potential for accumulation of a toxic amount in the infant, breastfeeding during daily therapy with hydroxychloroquine should be undertaken cautiously (11–13). The administration of once-weekly doses, such as those used for malaria prophylaxis, would markedly reduce the amount of drug available to the nursing infant and, consequently, produce a much lower risk of accumulation and toxicity. Although breastfeeding during maternal malarial prophylaxis is not thought to be harmful, the amount of hydroxychloroquine in milk is insufficient to provide protection against malaria in the infant (10). The American Academy of Pediatrics classifies the drug as compatible with breastfeeding (14).

References

1. CDC. Adverse reactions and contraindications to antimalarials. MMWR 1988;37:282–3.
2. CDC. Recommendations for the prevention of malaria among travelers. MMWR 1990;39:1–10.
3. Product information. Plaquenil. Sanofi Winthrop Pharmaceuticals, 1997.
4. Roubenoff R, Hoyt J, Petri M, Hochberg MC, Hellmann DB. Effects of antiinflammatory and immunosuppressive drugs on pregnancy and fertility. Semin Arthr Rheum 1988;18:88–110.
5. Buchanan NMM, Toubi E, Khamashta MA, Lima F, Kerslake S, Hughes GRV. The safety of hydroxychloroquine in lupus pregnancy: experience in 27 pregnancies (abstract). Br J Rheumatol 1995;34(Suppl 1):14.
6. Parke AL, Rothfield NF. Antimalarial drugs in pregnancy—the North American experience. Lupus 1996;5(Suppl 1):567–9.
7. Parke A, West B. Hydroxychloroquine in pregnant patients with systemic lupus erythematosus. J Rheumatol 1996;23:1715–8.
8. Heinonen OP, Slone D, Shapiro S. *Birth Defects and Drugs in Pregnancy*. Littleton, MA: Publishing Sciences Group, 1977:299.
9. Ross JB, Garatsos S. Absence of choroquine-induced ototoxicity in a fetus. Arch Dermatol 1974;109:573.
10. Suhonen R. Hydroxychloroquine administration in pregnancy. Arch Dermatol 1983;119:185–6.

11. Nation RL, Hackett LP, Dusci LJ, Ilett KF. Excretion of hydroxychloroquine in human milk. Br J Clin Pharmacol 1984;17:368–9.
12. Ostensen M, Brown ND, Chiang PK, Aarbakke J. Hydroxychloroquine in human breast milk. Eur J Clin Pharmacol 1985;28:357.
13. Anderson PO. Drug use during breast-feeding. Clin Pharm 1991;10: 594–624.
14. Committee on Drugs, American Academy of Pediatrics. The transfer of drugs and other chemicals into human milk. Pediatrics 2001;108:776–89.

HYDROXYPROGESTERONE

Progestogenic Hormone

PREGNANCY RECOMMENDATION: Human Data Suggest Risk (0–16 Weeks), Compatible (After 16 Weeks)
BREASTFEEDING RECOMMENDATION: No Human Data—Probably Compatible

PREGNANCY SUMMARY

Hydroxyprogesterone (17α-hydroxyprogesterone [17α-HP]) is efficacious and safe for the prevention of preterm labor when it is used after 16 weeks' gestation. Use before this carries a small risk of female masculinization and hypospadias and/or ambiguous genitals in males. Development of the phallus occurs between the 7th and 16th week of gestation (1). Use of 17α-HP after this point cannot cause hypospadias because the urethral groove has fused. Because several issues still exist, including long-term safety and the ideal progesterone formulation (e.g., progesterone vs. 17α-HP; and dosage), the American College of Obstetricians and Gynecologists (ACOG) recommended in 2008 that the use of progesterone supplementation should be restricted to women with a singleton pregnancy and a prior spontaneous preterm birth due to spontaneous preterm labor or premature rupture of membranes (2).

FETAL RISK SUMMARY

17α-HP is not available commercially in the United States but is prepared by some compounding pharmacies. It is a naturally occurring metabolite of progesterone (3).

The Collaborative Perinatal Project monitored 866 mother–child pairs with 1st trimester exposure to progestational agents (including 162 with exposure to 17α-HP) (4, pp. 389, 391). An increase in the expected frequency of cardiovascular defects and hypospadias was observed for both estrogens and progestogens (4, p. 394; 5). Reevaluation of these data in terms of timing of exposure, vaginal bleeding in early pregnancy, and previous maternal obstetric history, however, failed to support an association between female sex hormones and cardiac malformations (6).

Dillon reported six infants with malformations exposed to 17α-HP during various stages of gestation (7,8). The congenital defects included spina bifida, anencephalus, hydrocephalus, tetralogy of Fallot, common truncus arteriosus, cataract, and ventricular septal defect. Complete absence of both thumbs and dislocated head of the right radius in a child has been associated with 17α-HP (8). However, the use of diazepam in early pregnancy and the lack of similar reports make an association doubtful.

In 2000, Schardein (9) reviewed the risk of progestogens for female masculinization and male feminization after 1st trimester use. He cited seven cases of female masculinization with 17α-HP. Although admitting that the relationship between progestogens and male feminization was still tenuous, among 78 cases there were 7 cases of hypospadias and/or ambiguous genitals associated with 17α-HP and 2 cases of hypospadias with progesterone (9).

A 1985 study described 2754 offspring born to mothers who had vaginal bleeding during the 1st trimester (10). Of the total group, 1608 of the newborns were delivered from mothers treated during the 1st trimester with either oral medroxyprogesterone (20–30 mg/day), 17-hydroxyprogesterone (500 mg/week by injection), or a combination of the two. Medroxyprogesterone was used exclusively in 1274 (79.2%) of the study group. The control group consisted of 1146 infants delivered from mothers who bled during the 1st trimester but who were not treated. There were no differences between the study and control groups in the overall rate of malformations (120 vs. 123.9/1000, respectively) or in the rate of major malformations (63.4 vs. 71.5/1000, respectively) (10). Another 1985 study compared 988 infants exposed in utero to various progesterones with a matched cohort of 1976 unexposed controls (11). No association between the use of progestins, primarily progesterone and 17α-HP, and fetal malformations was discovered.

Developmental changes in the psychosexual performance of boys have been attributed to in utero exposure to 17α-HP (12). The mothers received an estrogen–progestogen regimen for their diabetes. Hormone-exposed males demonstrated a trend to have less heterosexual experience and fewer masculine interests than controls (12).

A number of studies have reported the use of 17α-HP during pregnancy or its benefits to prevent premature labor (13–30). The hormone is not effective in twin pregnancies (3,22). A 2005 meta-analysis of randomized controlled trials of progestational agents, most of which (80%) involved 17α-HP, concluded that these agents reduced the incidence of preterm birth and low-birth-weight newborns (31). In another 2005 review, the clinical use of 17α-HP for the prevention of preterm delivery and its safety was summarized (3). No increase in the incidence of fetal adverse effects has been observed. The evidence supports the use of 17α-HP (250 mg IM every week) beginning as soon as possible after 16 weeks' gestation and continuing to 36 weeks' (3).

17α-HP also has been used in early gestation to prevent spontaneous abortion, but the results have been mixed (32,33).

BREASTFEEDING SUMMARY

No reports describing the use of 17α-HP during human lactation have been located. Because of its use for the prevention of preterm birth, it is doubtful if such reports will ever be available. However, progesterone is classified as compatible with breastfeeding (34).

References

1. Bingol N, Wasserman E. Hypospadias. In: Buyse ML, ed. *Birth Defects Encyclopedia*. Cambridge, MA: Blackwell Scientific Publications, 1990:931–2.
2. Committee on Obstetric Practice, American College of Obstetricians and Gynecologists. Use of progesterone to reduce preterm birth. *ACOG Committee Opinion*. No. 419, October 2008. Obstet Gynecol 2008;112:963–5.
3. Meis PJ. 17 Hydroxyprogesterone for the prevention of preterm delivery. Obstet Gynecol 2005;105:1128–35.
4. Heinonen OP, Slone D, Shapiro S. *Birth Defects and Drugs in Pregnancy*. Littleton, MA: Publishing Sciences Group, 1977.
5. Heinonen OP, Slone D, Monson RR, Hook EB, Shapiro S. Cardiovascular birth defects and antenatal exposure to female sex hormones. N Engl J Med 1977;296:67–70.
6. Wiseman RA, Dodds-Smith IC. Cardiovascular birth defects and antenatal exposure to female sex hormones: a reevaluation of some base data. Teratology 1984;30:359–70.
7. Dillon S. Congenital malformations and hormones in pregnancy. Br Med J 1976;2:1446.
8. Dillon S. Progestogen therapy in early pregnancy and associated congenital defects. Practitioner 1970;205:80–4.
9. Schardein JL. *Chemically Induced Birth Defects*. 3rd ed. New York, NY: Marcel Dekker, 2000:303–4.
10. Katz Z, Lancet M, Skornik J, Chemke J, Mogilner BM, Klinberg M. Teratogenicity of progestogens given during the first trimester of pregnancy. Obstet Gynecol 1985;65:775–80.
11. Resseguie LJ, Hick JF, Bruen JA, Noller KL, O'Fallon WM, Kurland LT. Congenital malformations among offspring exposed in utero to progestins, Olmsted County, Minnesota, 1936–1974. Fertil Steril 1985;43:514–9.
12. Yalom ID, Green R, Fisk N. Prenatal exposure to female hormones. Effect on psychosexual development in boys. Arch Gen Psychiatry 1973;28:554–61.
13. Johnson JWC, Austin KL, Jones GS, Davis GH, King TM. Efficacy of 17-hydroxyprogesterone caproate in the prevention of premature labor. N Engl J Med 1975;293:675–80.
14. Johnson JWC, Lee PA, Zachary AS, Calhoun S, Migeon CJ. High-risk prematurity-progestin treatment and steroid studies. Obstet Gynecol 1979;54:412–8.
15. Kauppila A, Hartikainen-Sorri AL, Janne O, Tuimala R, Jarvinen PA. Suppression of threatened premature labor by administration of cortisol and 17α-hydroxyprogesterone caproate: a comparison with ritodrine. Am J Obstet Gynecol 1980;138:404–8.
16. Varma TR, Morsman J. Evaluation of the use of proluton-depot (hydroxyprogesterone hexanoate) in early pregnancy. Int J Gynecol Obstet 1982;20:13–7.
17. Hauth JC, Gilstrap LC III, Brekken AL, Hauth JM. The effect of 17α-hydroxyprogesterone caproate on pregnancy outcome in an active-duty military population. Am J Obstet Gynecol 1983;146:187–90.
18. Yemini M, Borenstein R, Dreazen E, Apelman Z, Mogilner BM, Kessler I, Lancet M. Prevention of premature labor by 17α-hydroxyprogesterone caproate. Am J Obstet Gynecol 1985;151:574–7.
19. Keirse MJNC. Progesterone administration in pregnancy may prevent preterm delivery. Br J Obstet Gynecol 1990;97:149–54.
20. Meis PJ, Klebanoff M, Thom E, Dombrowski MP, Sibai B, Moawad AH, Spong CY, Hauth JC, Miodovnik M, Varner MW, Leveno KJ, Caritis SN, Iams JD, Wapner RJ, Conway D, O'Sullivan MJ, Carpenter M, Mercer B, Ramin SM, Thorp JM, Peaceman AM, for the National Institute of Child Health and Human Development Maternal-Fetal Medicine Units Network. Prevention of recurrent preterm delivery by 17 alpha-hydroxyprogesterone caproate. N Engl J Med 2003;348:2379–85.
21. Greene MF. Progesterone and preterm delivery—déjà vu all over again. N Engl J Med 2003;348:2453–5.
22. Hartikainen-Sorri AL, Kauppila A, Tuimala R. Inefficacy of 17-hydroxyprogesterone caproate in the prevention of prematurity in twin pregnancy. Obstet Gynecol 1980;56:692–5.
23. Petrini JR, Callaghan WM, Klebanoff M, Green NS, Lackritz EM, Howse JL, Schwarz RH, Damus K. Estimated effect of 17 alpha-hydroxyprogesterone caproate on preterm birth in the United States. Obstet Gynecol 2005;105:267–72.
24. Meis PJ, Klebanoff M, Dombrowski MP, Sibai BM, Leindecker S, Moawwad AH, Northen A, Iams JD, Varner MW, Caritis SN, O'Sullivan MJ, Miodovnik M, Leveno KJ, Conway D, Wapner RJ, Carpenter M, Mercer B, Ramin SM, Thorp JM, Peaceman AM, Gabbe S, for the National Institute of Child Health and Human Development Maternal-Fetal Medicine Units Network. Does progesterone treatment influence risk factors for recurrent preterm delivery? Obstet Gynecol 2005;106:557–61.
25. Spong CY, Meis PJ, Thom EA, Sibai B, Dombrowski MP, Moawad AH, Hauth JC, Iams JD, Varner MW, Caritis SN, O'Sullivan MJ, Miodovnik M, Leveno KJ, Conway D, Wapner RJ, Carpenter M, Mercer B, Ramin SM, Thorp JM, Peaceman AM, Gabbe S, for the National Institute of Child Health and Human Development Maternal-Fetal Medicine Units Network. Progesterone for prevention of recurrent preterm birth: impact of gestational age at previous delivery. Am J Obstet Gynecol 2005;193:1127–31.
26. Ness A, Dias T, Damus K, Burd I, Berghella V. Impact of the recent randomized trials on the use of progesterone to prevent preterm birth: a 2005 follow-up survey. Am J Obstet Gynecol 2006;195:1174–9.
27. Odibo AO, Stamilio DM, Macones GA, Polsky D. 17α-hydroxyprogesterone caproate for the prevention of preterm delivery. A cost-effectiveness analysis. Obstet Gynecol 2006;108:492–9.
28. Rebarber A, Ferrara LA, Hanley ML, Istwan NB, Rhea DJ, Stanziano GJ, Saltzman DH. Increased recurrence of preterm delivery with early cessation of 17-alpha-hydroxyprogesterone caproate. Am J Obstet Gynecol 2007;196:224.e1–4.
29. Bailit JL, Votruba ME. Medical cost savings associated with 17 alpha-hydroxyprogesterone caproate. Am J Obstet Gynecol 2007;196:219.e1–7.
30. Armstrong J. 17 progesterone for preterm birth prevention: a potential $2 billion opportunity. Am Obstet Gynecol 2007;196:194–5.
31. Sanchez-Ramos L, Kaunitz AM, Delke I. Progestational agents to prevent preterm births: a meta-analysis of randomized controlled trials. Obstet Gynecol 2005;105:273–9.
32. Reijnders FJ, Thomas CM, Doesburg WH, Rolland R, Eskes TK. Endocrine effects of 17 alpha-hydroxyprogesterone caproate during early pregnancy: a double-blind clinical trial. Br J Obstet Gynecol 1988;95:462–8.
33. Prietl G, Diedrich K, van der Ven HH, Luckhaus J, Krebs D. The effect of 17α-hydroxyprogesterone caproate/oestradiol valerate on the development and outcome of early pregnancies following in vitro fertilization and embryo transfer: a prospective and randomized controlled trial. Hum Reprod 1992;7:1–5.
34. Committee on Drugs, American Academy of Pediatrics. The transfer of drugs and other chemicals into human milk. Pediatrics 2001;108:776–89.

HYDROXYUREA

Antineoplastic

PREGNANCY RECOMMENDATION: Limited Human Data Suggest Low Risk
BREASTFEEDING RECOMMENDATION: Limited Human Data—Potential Toxicity

PREGNANCY SUMMARY

Although hydroxyurea is teratogenic in animals, almost all reported human pregnancy exposures have resulted in normal outcomes. In some of cases, however, hydroxyurea was discontinued very early in gestation or started after organogenesis. The available data prevent a better assessment of the embryo–fetal risk. In addition, although many children exposed in utero have had normal growth and development during their first few years, longer evaluation periods are warranted because the drug might be a human carcinogen. Nevertheless, if the drug is indicated, it should not be withheld because of pregnancy, but avoiding organogenesis would be best.

FETAL RISK SUMMARY

Hydroxyurea is an antineoplastic agent that causes cytotoxic and cytoreductive effects. It is indicated to reduce the frequency of painful crises and to reduce the need for blood transfusions in adult patients with sickle cell anemia with recurrent moderate to severe painful crises. It undergoes partial metabolism. Hydroxyurea is presumed to be a human carcinogen (1). The drug is also used for other indications as discussed below.

Hydroxyurea is teratogenic in several animal species including mice, hamsters, cats, miniature swine, dogs, and monkeys at doses within onefold of the human dose based on BSA (1). Shepard (2) reviewed nine studies describing the effects of this agent on the embryos and fetuses of various animal species. Anomalies observed included defects of the CNS, palate, and skeleton, depressed DNA synthesis, extensive cell death in limb buds and CNS, impaired postnatal learning, and decreased body and brain growth (rats); beak defects (chick embryos); and neural tube and cardiac defects (hamsters) (2). A 1999 report, evaluating the combined prenatal toxicity of hydroxyurea and 6-mercaptopurine riboside in mice, determined that the NOAEL (no-observed-adverse-effect level) of a single, intraperitoneal dose of hydroxyurea administered on day 11 of gestation was 250 mg/kg (3). An increase in gross structural abnormalities was observed at the 300- and 350-mg/kg dose levels.

A number of reports have described the use of hydroxyurea in human pregnancy (4–27). Two women, both with acute myelocytic leukemia, were treated with five-drug chemotherapy regimens at 17 and 27 weeks' gestation, respectively (4). In both cases, hydroxyurea (8 mg) was given as an initial, single IV dose. One woman underwent an elective abortion (EAB) of a grossly normal fetus 4 weeks after the start of chemotherapy. The second patient delivered a premature infant at 31 weeks with no evidence of birth defects, again 4 weeks after the start of therapy. Follow-up at 13.5 months revealed normal growth and development (4).

A 1991 report described the use of hydroxyurea, 0.5–1.0 g/day, throughout gestation in a woman with chronic myelocytic leukemia (CML) (5). A spontaneous vaginal delivery at 36 weeks' gestation resulted in the birth of a normal, healthy 2670-g male infant with normal blood counts. The infant's growth and development have been normal through 26 months of age (5). A subsequent brief report described a similar patient treated with 1–3 g/day orally before and throughout gestation (6). Hydroxyurea therapy was stopped (to prevent a potential cytopenia in the fetus) 1 week before a planned cesarean section at 38 weeks' gestation. A healthy 3100-g male infant was delivered, without evidence of hematologic abnormalities, whose growth and development remain normal at 32 months of age (6). A 1992 report listed a pregnant woman with CML who was treated in the 1st trimester with hydroxyurea and three other agents (7). She elected to terminate her pregnancy.

Several other studies have reported on the use of hydroxyurea for CML during pregnancy (8–14). A 1992 publication described two women who were treated before and throughout gestation with oral doses of 1.5 g/day (8). Eclampsia developed at 26 weeks' gestation in one woman resulting in the delivery of a stillborn male fetus without gross abnormalities who had a normal phenotype. The second patient had a vaginal delivery at 40 weeks of a healthy 3.2-kg male infant with normal phenotype. No follow-up evaluation of the infant was mentioned (8). The clinical course of a pregnant woman with CML was discussed in a 1993 report (9). She required 1.5–3 g/day during pregnancy for her disease. At 37 weeks' gestation, she delivered a healthy baby girl who had normal blood counts and no evidence of congenital defects (9). A second 1993 report described a woman with CML treated unsuccessfully with interferon alfa before pregnancy and then with hydroxyurea (10). At the patient's request, all therapies were stopped before conception. Hydroxyurea therapy (dose not specified) was reinstituted during the 2nd trimester and continued until 1 month before the delivery of a normal, term, 3.4-kg male infant. The infant was developing normally at approximately 11 months of age (10). In another case, a woman received hydroxyurea, 1.5–2.5 g/day, throughout gestation and delivered a term, 3.44-kg female infant who was normal at age 6 weeks (11). In a 2011 case report, the therapy of a 24-year-old patient with CML was changed at 10 weeks' from imatinib to hydroxyurea. She was maintained on the agent (2.0–2.5 g/day) for the remainder of her pregnancy (12). A healthy 2.5-kg female baby was born at 37 weeks. At 1-year follow-up, her growth and development were normal. In a 2006 report, a woman was treated for chronic-phase CML with imatinib before and during the first 6 weeks of gestation until her pregnancy was diagnosed (13). Therapy was stopped until the completion of the 1st trimester, at which time hydroxyurea was started. At 30 weeks', a fetal ultrasound revealed a meningocele and 4 weeks later the woman delivered a dead fetus. The defect was thought to have been caused by imatinib (13). A brief 2009 case report described the outcome of a 34-year-old woman with CML who was treated with imatinib (400 mg/day) during the first 4 months of an unplanned pregnancy (14). When pregnancy was diagnosed, imatinib was stopped and hydroxyurea was started. At 37 weeks', she delivered a healthy 3.12-kg infant with Apgar scores of 9 and 10. The child was doing well at 26 months of age (14).

A 1994 report described a woman with primary thrombocythemia who had lost two previous pregnancies from stillbirths (15). She was treated with hydroxyurea (1–2 g/day) before and during the first 6 weeks of her third pregnancy. She delivered a healthy male infant at 35 weeks' gestation. Two other publications have also reported the use of hydroxyurea in pregnant women with essential thrombocythemia (16,17). In one case, the dose and exposure time were not specified but the pregnancy was electively terminated due to maternal complications (15). In the other case, 0.5–1.0 g/day was used from 18 to 28 weeks' gestation and a healthy male infant was delivered at 37 weeks' gestation (17).

In another 1994 case report, a 28-year-old woman, known to have familial myeloproliferative syndrome, was treated successfully for essential thrombocythemia (ET) with hydroxyurea and aspirin with disappearance of her neurologic symptoms (18). After about 9–10 months of treatment, she was found to be pregnant and all therapy was stopped. About 2–3 months later, her symptoms reappeared and she was treated with interferon alpha and aspirin the remainder of pregnancy. At term, she gave birth to a growth-restricted baby with multiple malformations (ambiguous genitalia, hemivertebrae D6 to D10 with 11 pairs of ribs, and secondary scoliosis) (no other details on the baby were provided) (18).

A 1995 study described the outcomes of 34 pregnancies in 18 women with ET (19). Only one of the pregnancies was treated with hydroxyurea and that pregnancy was terminated by an EAB. In a 2001 study, 43 pregnancies occurred in 20 patients with ET but only were treated with hydroxyurea (20). The pregnancy outcome was "successful" (no further details given). A 2011 report described the pregnancy outcome of a 42-year-old woman with ET who had been treated with hydroxyurea and aspirin during the first 5 months of gestation (21). At term, she delivered a normal 2.7-kg male infant with Apgar scores of 8 and 9.

Four reports have described the use of hydroxyurea for the management of sickle cell disease in pregnant women (22–25). In a study published in 1995, three women conceived while receiving the drug (22). All stopped the therapy when pregnancy was diagnosed. One delivered a normal, full-term infant, and two had EABs. A 1999 report described one woman with sickle cell disease who had received hydroxyurea (1 g/day) and folic acid (5 mg/day) for 3 years before pregnancy (23). She discontinued hydroxyurea when pregnancy was confirmed at 9 weeks' gestation and delivered a normal male 3.24-kg baby at 39 weeks' with Apgar scores of 8 and 10 at 1 and 5 minutes, respectively. The infant was developing normally at 15 months. Another 1999 publication reported two pregnancies that were exposed to hydroxyurea very early in gestation (24). Both women were being treated for sickle cell disease with the drug (1 and 0.5 g/day), in addition to folic acid and other drugs, and both discontinued hydroxyurea when pregnancy was confirmed at approximately 5 and 4 weeks, respectively. One woman delivered a 2750-g male infant at 37 weeks' gestation with Apgar scores of 8 and 9 at 1 and 5 minutes, respectively. The infant was developing normally at age 17 months. The second woman delivered a premature, 1365-g, male baby at 32.5 weeks' gestation with Apgar scores of 8 and 9 at 1 and 5 minutes, respectively. Because of his prematurity, the infant required treatment for respiratory distress syndrome, hyperbilirubinemia, patent ductus arteriosus, and sepsis during the first 6 weeks, but was developing normally at age 21 months (24).

In a 2009 report from the Multicenter Study of Hydroxyurea in Sickle Cell Anemia, attempts were made to prevent pregnancies during the randomized double-blind placebo-controlled trial (25). Among the 299 study participants, 153 were females and, of these, 77 (50.3%) were in the hydroxyurea group. During the trial, there were six pregnancies in female participants taking the drug. When pregnancy was diagnosed, all were taken off of the drug. The outcomes of the six pregnancies were two live births, three EABs, and one spontaneous abortion (25).

A 2010 case report described the pregnancy outcome of a 25-year-old patient with sickle-β thalassemia who had been treated with hydroxyurea during the first 9 weeks of gestation (26). At that time, hydroxyurea was stopped and other therapy initiated. Although the remainder of her pregnancy was complicated, she eventually gave birth at 38 weeks' to a healthy 2.68-kg female infant who was growing normally at 1 year of age (26).

The outcomes of pregnancies exposed to chemotherapy for gestational trophoblastic disease before conception were evaluated in two reports (27,28). In 436 long-term survivors treated with chemotherapy between 1958 and 1978, 69 (16%) received hydroxyurea as part of their treatment regimens (27). Of the 69 women, 14 (20%) had at least one live birth (numbers in parentheses refer to mean/maximum hydroxyurea dose in grams) (3.6/8.0), 3 (4%) had no live births (6.3/16.0), 3 (4%) failed to conceive (3.0/6.0), and 49 (71%) did not try to conceive (9.4/47.0). Additional details, including congenital anomalies observed, are described in the monograph for methotrexate (see Methotrexate) (27). In the other report, 336 women, who had tried to conceive, had previously received various combinations of chemotherapeutic agents, some of which included hydroxyurea (28). In comparison with a group receiving single-agent therapy ($N = 392$; methotrexate), no differences in pregnancy outcome were observed in the number of live births, unsuccessful pregnancies, and an inability to become pregnant. Only 18 major or minor congenital abnormalities (affecting 1.7% of the births) were reported. However, the stillbirth rate in all women treated for gestational trophoblastic disease was significantly higher than that of the general population (odds ratio 2.87; 95% confidence interval 2.44–3.03; $p < 0.001$) (28).

A woman treated for acute lymphoid leukemia with a combination of nine antineoplastic agents, one of which was hydroxyurea, conceived two pregnancies, 2 and 4 years after chemotherapy was stopped (29). Apparently normal term infants, a 3850-g male and a 3550-g female, resulted and both were doing well at 7 and 4.5 years, respectively.

Hydroxyurea was used to treat polycythemia vera for 18 months before a 34-year-old woman became pregnant (30). Her pregnancy was diagnosed at 9 weeks' and hydroxyurea was stopped. Her erythrocytosis was controlled with phlebotomy. At 37 weeks' she gave birth to normal 2550-g male infant. The infant's development up to 12 months of age was normal (30).

Occupational exposure of the mother to antineoplastic agents during pregnancy may present a risk to the fetus. A position statement from the National Study Commission on Cytotoxic Exposure and a research article involving some antineoplastic agents are presented in the monograph for cyclophosphamide (see Cyclophosphamide).

BREASTFEEDING SUMMARY

Hydroxyurea is excreted into human milk. A 29-year-old breastfeeding woman with recently diagnosed chronic myelogenous leukemia was treated with hydroxyurea, 500 mg orally 3 times daily (31). Breastfeeding was halted before initiation of the chemotherapy. Milk samples were collected 2 hours after the last dose for 7 days. Because of technical difficulties with the analysis, milk concentrations of hydroxyurea could be determined only on days 1, 3, and 4. The mean level of hydroxyurea was 6.1 mg/L (range 3.8–8.4 mg/L). Based on a milk intake of 600 mL/day, the authors estimated that a nursing infant would have received 3–4 mg/day of the drug. Serum concentrations were not measured (31).

Because the mother's weight was not provided, a comparison to the maternal weight-adjusted dose could not calculated. Although the concentrations are low, the potential for adverse effects in the infant suggests that nursing should be considered contraindicated during hydroxyurea therapy.

References

1. Product information. Droxia. E.R. Squibb & Sons, 2012.
2. Shepard TH. *Catalog of Teratogenic Agents*. 7th ed. Baltimore, MD: The Johns Hopkins University Press, 1992:206–7.
3. Platzek T, Schwabe R. Combined prenatal toxicity of 6-mercaptopurine riboside and hydroxyurea in mice. Teratogenesis Carcinog Mutagen 1999;19:223–32.
4. Doney KC, Kraemer KG, Shepard TH. Combination chemotherapy for acute myelocytic leukemia during pregnancy: three case reports. Cancer Treat Rep 1979;63:369–71.
5. Patel M, Dukes IAF, Hull JC. Use of hydroxyurea in chronic myeloid leukemia during pregnancy: a case report. Am J Obstet Gynecol 1991;165:565–6.
6. Tertian G, Tchernia G, Papiernik E, Elefant E. Hydroxyurea and pregnancy. Am J Obstet Gynecol 1992;166:1868.
7. Zemlickis D, Lishner M, Degendorfer P, Panzarella T, Sutcliffe SB, Koren G. Fetal outcome after in utero exposure to cancer chemotherapy. Arch Intern Med 1992;152:573–6.
8. Delmer A, Rio B, Bauduer F, Ajchenbaum F, Marie J-P, Zittoun R. Pregnancy during myelosuppressive treatment for chronic myelogenous leukaemia. Br J Haematol 1992;82:783–4.
9. Jackson N, Shukri A, Ali K. Hydroxyurea treatment for chronic myeloid leukaemia during pregnancy. Br J Haematol 1993;85:203–4.
10. Fitzgerald JM, McCann SR. The combination of hydroxyurea and leucapheresis in the treatment of chronic myeloid leukaemia in pregnancy. Clin Lab Haematol 1993;15:63–5.
11. Szanto F, Kovacs L. Successful delivery following continuous cytostatic therapy of a leukemic pregnant woman. Ovr Hetil 1994;134:527–9 (article in Hungarian). As cited in Diav-Citrin O, Hunnisett L, Sher GD, Koren G. Hydroxyurea use during pregnancy: a case report in sickle cell disease and review of the literature. Am J Hematol 1999;60:148–50.
12. Martin J, Ramesh A, Devadasan L, Palaniappan N, Martin JJ. An uneventful pregnancy and delivery, in a case with chronic myeloid leukemia on imatinib. Indian J Med Paediatr Oncol 2011;32:109–11.
13. Choudhary DR, Mishra P, Kumar R, Mahapatra M, Choudhry VP. Pregnancy on imatinib: fatal outcome with meningocele. Ann Oncol 2006;17:178–9.
14. Dolai TK, Bhargava R, Mahapatra M, Mishra P, Seth T, Pati HP, Saxena R. Is imatinib safe during pregnancy? Leuk Res 2009;33:572–3.
15. Cinkotai KI, Wood P, Donnai P, Kendra J. Pregnancy after treatment with hydroxyurea in a patient with primary thrombocythaemia and a history of recurrent abortion. J Clin Pathol 1994;47:769–70.
16. Fernandez H. Essential thrombocythemia and pregnancy. J Gynecol Obstet Biol Reprod 1994;23:103–4 (article in French). As cited in Diav-Citrin O, Hunniset L, Sher GD, Koren G. Hydroxyurea use during pregnancy: a case report in sickle cell disease and review of the literature. Am J Hematol 1999;60:148–50.
17. Dell'Isola A, De Rosa G, Catalano D. Essential thrombocythemia in pregnancy. A case report and general considerations. Minerva Ginecol 1997;49:165–72 (article in Italian). As cited in Diav-Citrin O, Hunnisett L, Sher GD, Koren G. Hydroxyurea use during pregnancy: a case report in sickle cell disease and review of the literature. Am J Hematol 1999;60:148–50.
18. Perez-Encinas M, Bello JL, Perez-Crespo S, De Miguel R, Tome S. Familial myeloproliferative syndrome. Am J Hematol 1994;46:225–9.
19. Beressi AH, Tefferi A, Silverstein MN. Petitt RM, Hoagland HC. Outcome analysis of 34 pregnancies in women with essential thrombocythemia. Arch Intern Med 1995;155:1217–22.
20. Wright CA, Tefferi A. A single institutional experience with 43 pregnancies in essential thrombocythemia. Eur J Haematol 2001;66:152–9.
21. Oskuie AE, Valizadeh N. Successful outcome of pregnancy in a case of essential thrombocytosis treated with hydroxyurea. Indian J Cancer 2011;48:268–9.
22. Charache S, Terrin ML, Moore RD, Dover GJ, Barton FB, Eckert SV, McMahon RP, Bonds DR, and the Investigators of the Multicenter Study of Hydroxyurea in Sickle Cell Anemia. Effect of hydroxyurea on the frequency of painful crises in sickle cell anemia. N Engl J Med 1995;332:1317–22.
23. Diav-Citrin O, Hunnisett L, Sher GD, Koren G. Hydroxyurea use during pregnancy: a case report in sickle cell disease and review of the literature. Am J Hematol 1999;60:148–50.
24. Byrd DC, Pitts SR, Alexander CK. Hydroxyurea in two pregnant women with sickle cell anemia. Pharmacotherapy 1999;19:1459–62.
25. Ballas SK, McCarthy WF, Guo N, DeCastro L, Bellevue R, Barton BA, Waclawiw MA, and the investigators of the Multicenter Study of Hydroxyurea in Sickle Cell Anemia. Exposure to hydroxyurea and pregnancy outcomes in patients with sickle cell anemia. J Natl Med Assoc 2009;101:1046–51.
26. Italia KY, Jijina FF, Chandrakala S, Nadkami AH, Sawant P, Ghosh K, Colah RB. Exposure to hydroxyurea during pregnancy in sickle-ß thalassemia: a report of a case. J Clin Pharmacol 2010;30:231–4.
27. Rustin GJS, Booth M, Dent J, Salt S, Rustin F, Bagshawe KD. Pregnancy after cytotoxic chemotherapy for gestational trophoblastic tumours. Br Med J 1984;288:103–6.
28. Woolas RP, Bower M, Newlands ES, Seckl M, Short D, Holden L. Influence of chemotherapy for gestational trophoblastic disease on subsequent pregnancy outcome. Br J Obstet Gynaecol 1998;105:1032–5.
29. Pajor A, Zimonyi I, Koos R, Lehoczky D, Ambrus C. Pregnancies and offspring in survivors of acute lymphoid leukemia and lymphoma. Eur J Obstet Gynecol Reprod Biol 1991;40:1–5.
30. Pata O, Tok CE, Yazici G, Oata C, Oz AU, Aban M, Dilek S. Polycythemia vera and pregnancy: a case report with the use of hydroxyurea in the first trimester. Am J Perinatol 2004;21:135–7.
31. Sylvester RK, Lobell M, Teresi ME, Brundage D, Dubowy R. Excretion of hydroxyurea into milk. Cancer 1987;60:2177–8.

HYDROXYZINE

Antihistamine

PREGNANCY RECOMMENDATION: Human Data Suggest Low Risk
BREASTFEEDING RECOMMENDATION: No Human Data—Probably Compatible

PREGNANCY SUMMARY

In animal studies, high doses of hydroxyzine were associated with developmental toxicity (structural anomalies and death), but the human data suggest low risk. Although a surveillance study found an increased risk of oral clefts, this defect has not been observed in other studies. Withdrawal or seizures have been reported in two newborns exposed near term.

FETAL RISK SUMMARY

Hydroxyzine belongs to the same class of compounds as buclizine, cyclizine, and meclizine. The drug is teratogenic in mice and rats, but not in rabbits, at high doses (1–5). One report suggested that hydroxyzine teratogenicity was mediated by a metabolite (norchlorcyclizine) that was common to four antihistamines (hydroxyzine, buclizine, meclizine, and chlorcyclizine) (3). High-dose hydroxyzine (6–12 mg/kg/day) resulted in abortions in rhesus monkeys (6). The manufacturer considers hydroxyzine to be contraindicated in early pregnancy because of the lack of clinical data (1,2).

It is not known if hydroxyzine crosses the human placenta. The molecular weight of the free base (about 376) suggests that the drug will cross to the embryo and fetus.

In 100 patients treated in the 1st trimester with oral hydroxyzine (50 mg daily) for nausea and vomiting, no significant difference from nontreated controls was found in fetal wastage or anomalies (7). A woman treated with 60 mg/day of hydroxyzine during the 3rd trimester gave birth to a normal infant (8).

The Collaborative Perinatal Project monitored 50,282 mother–child pairs, 50 of whom had 1st trimester exposure to hydroxyzine (9, pp. 335–337, 341). For use anytime during pregnancy, 187 exposures were recorded (9, p. 438). Based on five malformed children, a possible relationship was found between 1st trimester use and congenital defects.

In a surveillance study of Michigan Medicaid recipients involving 229,101 completed pregnancies conducted between 1985 and 1992, 828 newborns had been exposed to hydroxyzine during the 1st trimester (F. Rosa, personal communication, FDA, 1993). A total of 48 (5.8%) major birth defects were observed (42 expected). Specific data were available for six defect categories, including (observed/expected) 9/8 cardiovascular defects, 1/0.4 spina bifida, 0/2 polydactyly, 2/1 limb reduction defects, 0/2 hypospadias, and 3/1 oral clefts. Only with the latter defect is there a suggestion of a possible association, but other factors, including the mother's disease, concurrent drug use, and chance, may be involved.

Withdrawal in a newborn exposed to hydroxyzine 600 mg/day throughout gestation has been reported (10). The mother, who was being treated for severe eczema and asthma, was also treated with phenobarbital, 240 mg/day for 4 days and then 60 mg/day, for mild preeclampsia during the 3-week period before delivery. Symptoms in the newborn, some beginning 15 minutes after birth, consisted of a shrill cry, jitteriness with clonic movements of the upper extremities, irritability, and poor feeding. The presumed drug-induced withdrawal persisted for approximately 4 weeks and finally resolved completely after 2 weeks of therapy with phenobarbital and methscopolamine. The infant was apparently doing well at 9 months of age. Although phenobarbital withdrawal could not be excluded, and neonatal withdrawal is a well-known complication of phenobarbital pregnancy use, the author concluded the symptoms in the infant were primarily caused by hydroxyzine (10).

A 1996 report described the use of hydroxyzine, droperidol, diphenhydramine, and metoclopramide in 80 women with hyperemesis gravidarum (11). The mean gestational age at the start of treatment was 10.9 weeks. All women received approximately 200 mg/day of hydroxyzine in divided dosage for up to a week after discharge from the hospital, and 12 (15%) required a second course of therapy for recurrence of their symptoms. Three of the mothers (all treated in the 2nd trimester) delivered offspring with congenital defects: Poland's syndrome, fetal alcohol syndrome, and hydrocephalus and hypoplasia of the right cerebral hemisphere. Only the latter anomaly is a potential drug effect, but the most likely cause was thought to be the result of an in utero fetal vascular accident or infection (11).

A 2001 study, using a treatment method similar to the above study, described the use of droperidol and diphenhydramine in 28 women hospitalized for hyperemesis gravidarum (12). Pregnancy outcomes in the study group were compared with a historical control of 54 women who had received conventional antiemetic therapy. Oral metoclopramide and hydroxyzine were used after discharge from the hospital. Therapy was started in the study and control groups at mean gestational ages of 9.9 and 11.1 weeks, respectively. The study group appeared to have more severe disease than controls as suggested by a greater mean loss from the prepregnancy weight, 2.07 kg vs. 0.81 kg (*ns*), and a slightly lower serum potassium level, 3.4 vs. 3.5 mmol/L (*ns*). Compared with controls, the droperidol group had a shorter duration of hospitalization (3.53 vs. 2.82 days, $p = 0.023$), fewer readmissions (38.9% vs. 14.3%, $p = 0.025$), and lower average daily nausea and vomiting scores (both $p < 0.001$). There were no statistical differences in outcomes (study vs. controls) in terms of spontaneous abortions ($N = 0$ vs. $N = 2$ [3.7%]), elective abortions ($N = 3$ [10.7%] vs. $N = 3$ [5.6%]), Apgar scores at 1, 5, and 10 minutes, age at birth (37.3 vs. 37.9 weeks), and birth weight (3114 vs. 3347 g) (12). In controls, there was one major malformation of unknown cause, an acardiac fetus in a set of triplets, and one newborn with a genetic defect (Turner syndrome). There was also one unexplained major birth defect in the droperidol group (bilateral hydronephrosis), and there were two genetic defects (translocation of chromosomes 3 and 7; tyrosinemia) (12).

A prospective controlled study published in 1997 evaluated the teratogenic risk of hydroxyzine and cetirizine (see also Cetirizine) in human pregnancy (13). A total of 120 pregnancies (two sets of twins) exposed to either hydroxyzine ($N = 81$) or cetirizine ($N = 39$) during pregnancy were identified and compared with 110 controls. The control group was matched for maternal age, smoking, and alcohol use. The drugs were taken during the 1st trimester in 53 (65%) of the hydroxyzine cases and in 37 (95%) of the cetirizine exposures for various indications (e.g., rhinitis, urticaria, pruritic urticarial papules and plaques of pregnancy, sedation, and other nonspecified reasons). Fourteen spontaneous abortions (hydroxyzine 3, cetirizine 6, controls 5) and 11 induced abortions (hydroxyzine 6, controls 5) occurred in the three groups. Among the live births, there were no statistical differences between the groups in birth weight, gestational age at delivery, rate of cesarean section, or neonatal distress. In the hydroxyzine group, two of the live births had major malformations: one with a ventricular septal defect and one with a complex congenital heart defect (also exposed to carbamazepine). A third infant, exposed after organogenesis, also had a ventricular septal defect. Minor abnormalities were observed in four hydroxyzine-exposed infants: one case each of hydrocele, inguinal hernia, hypothyroidism (mother also taking propylthiouracil), and strabismus. Two minor anomalies were observed in liveborn infants exposed to cetirizine during organogenesis: one with an ectopic kidney and one with undescended testes. No major abnormalities were seen in this group. In the control group, no major malformations were observed, but five infants had minor defects (dislocated hip, growth hormone deficiency, short lingual frenulum, and two unspecified defects). Statistically, there were no differences between the groups in outcome (13).

A 1997 article compared the published pregnancy outcomes, in terms of congenital malformations, of various first and second generation antihistamines (14). Based on 995 hydroxyzine-exposed liveborn infants, the relative risk for any congenital malformation ranged from 1.2 (95% confidence interval [CI] 0.4–0.9) to 3.4 (95% CI 1.6–17.9). Based on analysis of published reports, the authors concluded that in pregnancy, chlorpheniramine is the oral antihistamine of choice and that diphenhydramine should be used if a parenteral antihistamine is required (14).

A 2005 case report described seizures in a newborn exposed to hydroxyzine in late pregnancy (15). The 36-year-old mother began taking hydroxyzine 150 mg/day for anxiety at 35 weeks' gestation. Four weeks later, a scheduled cesarean section delivered a 4.120-kg male infant with Apgar scores of 9 and 10 at 1 and 5 minutes, respectively. Four hours after birth, the infant developed clonic movements of the upper extremities that spread to the entire body followed by a tonic-clonic seizure lasting 4 minutes. No further seizures were observed and an extensive workup revealed no cause for the seizures. A hydroxyzine plasma concentration in the mother, 6 hours after birth, was 7.3 ng/mL (therapeutic concentrations 50–90 ng/mL), whereas in the infant, levels at 6 and 24 hours of age were 7.4 and 2.3 ng/mL, respectively. At 6 months of age, the infant was well with normal neurodevelopmental testing (15).

During labor, hydroxyzine has been shown to be safe and effective for the relief of anxiety (16,17). No effect on the progress of labor or on neonatal Apgar scores was observed. In a study published in 1978, however, a 75-mg IM dose administered during labor caused a statistically significant decrease in fetal heart rate (FHR) variability in 10 of 16 cases (18). Maximal effects on the FHR were observed within 25 minutes after which they returned to normal values. Administration of hydroxyzine close to delivery reduces newborn platelet aggregation, but the clinical significance of this is unknown (19).

BREASTFEEDING SUMMARY

No reports describing the use of hydroxyzine during lactation have been located. The molecular weight (about 448) is low enough that excretion into breast milk should be expected. The effects, if any, on the nursing infant are unknown.

H

References

1. Product information. Vistaril. Pfizer, 1997.
2. Product information. Atarax. Pfizer, 1997.
3. King CTG, Howell J. Teratogenic effect of buclizine and hydroxyzine in the rat and chlorcyclizine in the mouse. Am J Obstet Gynecol 1966;95:109–11.
4. Posner HS, Darr A. Fetal edema from benzhydrylpiperazines as a possible cause of oral-facial malformations in rats. Toxicol Appl Pharmacol 1970;17:67–75.
5. Walker BE, Patterson A. Induction of cleft palate in mice by tranquilizers and barbiturates. Teratology 1974;10:159–64.
6. Steffek AJ, King CTG, Wilk AL. Abortive effects and comparative metabolism of chlorcyclizine in various mammalian species. Teratology 1968;1:399–406.
7. Erez S, Schifrin BS, Dirim O. Double-blind evaluation of hydroxyzine as an antiemetic in pregnancy. J Reprod Med 1971;7:57–9.
8. Romero R, Olsen TG, Chervenak FA, Hobbins JC. Pruritic urticarial papules and plaques of pregnancy. A case report. J Reprod Med 1983;28:615–9.
9. Heinonen OP, Slone D, Shapiro S. *Birth Defects and Drugs in Pregnancy*. Littleton, MA: Publishing Sciences Group, 1977.
10. Prenner BM. Neonatal withdrawal syndrome associated with hydroxyzine hydrochloride. Am J Dis Child 1977;131:529–30.
11. Nageotte MP, Briggs GG, Towers CV, Asrat T. Droperidol and diphenhydramine in the management of hyperemesis gravidarum. Am J Obstet Gynecol 1996;174:1801–6.
12. Turcotte V, Ferreira E, Duperron L. Utilité du dropéridol et de la diphenhydramine dans l'hyperemesis gravidarum. J Soc Obstet Gynaecol Can 2001;23:133–9.
13. Einarson A, Bailey B, Jung G, Spizzirri D, Baillie M, Koren G. Prospective controlled study of hydroxyzine and cetirizine in pregnancy. Ann Allergy Asthma Immunol 1997;78:183–6.
14. Schatz M, Petitti D. Antihistamines and pregnancy. Ann Allergy Asthma Immunol 1997;78:157–9.
15. Serreau R, Komiha M, Blanc F, Guillot F, Jacqz-Aigrain E. Neonatal seizures associated with maternal hydroxyzine in late pregnancy. Reprod Toxicol 2005;20:573–4.
16. Zsigmond EK, Patterson RL. Double-blind evaluation of hydroxyzine hydrochloride in obstetric anesthesia. Anesth Analg (Cleve) 1967;46:275–80.
17. Amato G, Corsini D, Pelliccia E. Personal experience with a combination of Althesin and Atarax in caesarean section. Minerva Anesteriol 1980;46:671–4.
18. Petrie RH, Yeh S-Y, Murata Y, Paul RH, Hon EH, Barron BA, Johnson RJ. The effects of drugs on fetal heart rate variability. Am J Obstet Gynecol 1978;130:294–9.
19. Whaun JM, Smith GR, Sochor VA. Effect of prenatal drug administration on maternal and neonatal platelet aggregation and PF_4 release. Haemostasis 1980;9:226–37.

l-HYOSCYAMINE

Parasympatholytic (Anticholinergic)

PREGNANCY RECOMMENDATION: Limited Human Data—No Relevant Animal Data
BREASTFEEDING RECOMMENDATION: No Human Data—Probably Compatible

PREGNANCY SUMMARY

l-Hyoscyamine is an anticholinergic agent. No published reports of its use in pregnancy have been located (see also Belladonna or Atropine).

FETAL RISK SUMMARY

In a surveillance study of Michigan Medicaid recipients involving 229,101 completed pregnancies conducted between 1985 and 1992, 281 newborns had been exposed to *l*-hyoscyamine during the 1st trimester (F. Rosa, personal communication, FDA, 1993). A total of 12 (4.3%) major birth defects were observed (11 expected). Specific data were available for six defect categories, including (observed/expected) 1/3 cardiovascular defects, 0/0.5 oral clefts, 0/0 spina bifida, 0/1 hypospadias, 2/1 polydactyly, and 2/0.5 limb reduction defects. Only with the latter two defects is there a suggestion of a possible association, but other factors, including the mother's disease, concurrent drug use, and chance, may be involved.

BREASTFEEDING SUMMARY

No reports describing the use of *l*-hyoscyamine during human lactation have been located (see also Atropine).

HYPERALIMENTATION, PARENTERAL

Nutrient

PREGNANCY RECOMMENDATION: Compatible
BREASTFEEDING RECOMMENDATION: No Human Data—Probably Compatible

PREGNANCY SUMMARY

The use of total parenteral hyperalimentation (TPN) does not pose a significant risk to the fetus or newborn provided that normal procedures, as with nonpregnant patients, are followed to prevent maternal complications.

FETAL RISK SUMMARY

TPN is the administration of an IV solution designed to provide complete nutritional support for a patient unable to maintain adequate nutritional intake. The solution is normally composed of dextrose (5%–35%), amino acids (3.5%–5%), vitamins, electrolytes, and trace elements. Lipids (IV fat emulsions) are often given with TPN to supply essential fatty acids and calories (see Lipids). A number of studies describing the use of TPN in pregnant women have been published (1–26). A report of four additional cases with a review of the literature appeared in 1986 (27), followed by another review in 1990 (28). This latter review also included an in-depth discussion of indications, fluid, caloric (including lipids), electrolyte, and vitamin requirements for gestation and lactation, and monitoring techniques (28).

Maternal indications for TPN have been varied, with duration of therapy ranging from a few days to the entire pregnancy. Eleven patients were treated during the 1st trimester (1–5). No fetal complications attributable to TPN, including newborn hypoglycemia, have been identified in any of the reports. Intrauterine growth restriction occurred in five infants, and one of them died, but the restricted growth and neonatal death were most likely caused by the underlying maternal disease (2–4,6–9,22). In a group of eight women treated with TPN for severe hyperemesis gravidarum who delivered live babies, the ratio of birth weight to standard mean weight for gestational age was >1.0 in each case (5).

Obstetric complications included the worsening of one mother's renal hypertension after TPN was initiated, but the relationship between the effect and the therapy is not known (8). In a second case, resistance to oxytocin-induced labor was observed, but again, the relationship to TPN is not clear (9).

Maternal and fetal death secondary to cardiac tamponade during central hyperalimentation has been reported (29). A 22-year-old woman in the 3rd trimester of pregnancy was treated with TPN for severe hyperemesis gravidarum. Seven days after commencing central TPN therapy, the patient experienced acute sharp retrosternal pain and dyspnea (29). Cardiac tamponade was subsequently diagnosed, but the mother and the fetus expired before the condition could be corrected. Percutaneous pericardiocentesis yielded 70 mL of fluid that was a mixture of the TPN and lipid solutions that the patient had been receiving.

A stillborn male fetus was delivered at 22 weeks' gestation from a 31-year-old woman with hyperemesis gravidarum following 8 weeks of parenteral hyperalimentation with lipid emulsion (fat composed 24% of total calories) (30). The tan-yellow placenta showed vacuolated syncytial cells and Hofbauer cells that stained for fat (30).

BREASTFEEDING SUMMARY

No problems should be expected in nursing infants whose mothers are receiving TPN.

References

1. Hew LR, Deitel M. Total parenteral nutrition in gynecology and obstetrics. Obstet Gynecol 1980;55:464–8.
2. Tresadern JC, Falconer GF, Turnberg LA, Irving MH. Successful completed pregnancy in a patient maintained on home parenteral nutrition. Br Med J 1983;286:602–3.
3. Tresadern JC, Falconer GF, Turnberg LA, Irving MH. Maintenance of pregnancy in a home parenteral nutrition patient. J Parenter Enteral Nutr 1984;8:199–202.
4. Breen KJ, McDonald IA, Panelli D, Ihle B. Planned pregnancy in a patient who was receiving home parenteral nutrition. Med J Aust 1987;146:215–7.
5. Levine MG, Esser D. Total parenteral nutrition for the treatment of severe hyperemesis gravidarum: maternal nutritional effects and fetal outcome. Obstet Gynecol 1988;72:102–7.
6. Gineston JL, Capron JP, Delcenserie R, Delamarre J, Blot M, Boulanger JC. Prolonged total parenteral nutrition in a pregnant woman with acute pancreatitis. J Clin Gastroenterol 1984;6:249–52.
7. Lakoff KM, Feldman JD. Anorexia nervosa associated with pregnancy. Obstet Gynecol 1972;39:699–701.
8. Lavin JP Jr, Gimmon Z, Miodovnik M, von Meyenfeldt M, Fischer JE. Total parenteral nutrition in a pregnant insulin-requiring diabetic. Obstet Gynecol 1982;59:660–4.
9. Weinberg RB, Sitrin MD, Adkins GM, Lin CC. Treatment of hyperlipidemic pancreatitis in pregnancy with total parenteral nutrition. Gastroenterology 1982;83:1300–5.
10. Di Costanzo J, Martin J, Cano N, Mas JC, Noirclerc M. Total parenteral nutrition with fat emulsions during pregnancy—nutritional requirements: a case report. JPEN 1982;6:534–8.
11. Young KR. Acute pancreatitis in pregnancy: two case reports. Obstet Gynecol 1982;60:653–7.
12. Rivera-Alsina ME, Saldana LR, Stringer CA. Fetal growth sustained by parenteral nutrition in pregnancy. Obstet Gynecol 1984;64:138–41.
13. Seifer DB, Silberman H, Catanzarite VA, Conteas CN, Wood R, Ueland K. Total parenteral nutrition in obstetrics. JAMA 1985;253:2073–5.
14. Benny PS, Legge M, Aickin DR. The biochemical effects of maternal hyperalimentation during pregnancy. NZ Med J 1978;88:283–5.
15. Cox KL, Byrne WJ, Ament ME. Home total parenteral nutrition during pregnancy: a case report. JPEN 1981;5:246–9.
16. Gamberdella FR. Pancreatic carcinoma in pregnancy: a case report. Am J Obstet Gynecol 1984;149:15–7.
17. Loludice TA, Chandrakaar C. Pregnancy and jejunoileal bypass: treatment complications with total parenteral nutrition. South Med J 1980;73: 256–8.
18. Main ANH, Shenkin A, Black WP, Russell RI. Intravenous feeding to sustain pregnancy in patient with Crohn's disease. Br Med J 1981;283:1221–2.
19. Webb GA. The use of hyperalimentation and chemotherapy in pregnancy: a case report. Am J Obstet Gynecol 1980;137:263–6.
20. Stowell JC, Bottsford JE Jr, Rubel HR. Pancreatitis with pseudocyst and cholelithiasis in third trimester of pregnancy: management with total parenteral nutrition. South Med J 1984;77:502–4.
21. Martin R, Trubow M, Bistrian BR, Benotti P, Blackburn GL. Hyperalimentation during pregnancy: a case report. JPEN 1985;9:212–5.
22. Herbert WNP, Seeds JW, Bowes WA, Sweeney CA. Fetal growth response to total parenteral nutrition in pregnancy: a case report. J Reprod Med 1986;31:263–6.
23. Hatjis CG, Meis PJ. Total parenteral nutrition in pregnancy. Obstet Gynecol 1985;66:585–9.
24. Adami GF, Friedman D, Cuneo S, Marinari G, Gandolfo P, Scopinaro N. Intravenous nutritional support in pregnancy. Experience following biliopancreatic diversion. Clin Nutr 1992;11:106–9.
25. Satin AJ, Twickler D, Gilstrap LC III. Esophageal achalasia in late pregnancy. Obstet Gynecol 1992;79:812–4.
26. Teuscher AU, Sutherland DER, Robertson RP. Successful pregnancy after pancreatic islet autotransplantation. Transplant Proc 1994;26:3520.
27. Lee RV, Rodgers BD, Young C, Eddy E, Cardinal J. Total parenteral nutrition during pregnancy. Obstet Gynecol 1986;68:563–71.
28. Wolk RA, Rayburn WF. Parenteral nutrition in obstetric patients. Nutr Clin Pract 1990;5:139–52.
29. Greenspoon JS, Masaki DI, Kurz CR. Cardiac tamponade in pregnancy during central hyperalimentation. Obstet Gynecol 1989;73:465–6.
30. Jasnosz KM, Pickeral JJ, Graner S. Fat deposits in the placenta following maternal total parenteral nutrition with intravenous lipid emulsion. Arch Pathol Lab Med 1995;119:555–7.

I

IBANDRONATE

Bisphosphonate

PREGNANCY RECOMMENDATION: No Human Data—Animal Data Suggest Moderate Risk
BREASTFEEDING RECOMMENDATION: No Human Data—Probably Compatible

PREGNANCY SUMMARY

No reports describing the use of ibandronate in human pregnancy have been located. In one animal species, the drug caused growth restriction at doses ≤10 times the human dose, but maternal deaths at these doses also were observed. The lack of human pregnancy experience with ibandronate and the very limited human data for the bisphosphonate class prevent further assessment of the risk. The amount of drug retained in bone and eventually released back into the systemic circulation is directly related to the dose and duration of treatment. Because ibandronate probably crosses the placenta, treatment of the mother before conception could result in continuous exposure of the embryo and fetus to an unknown amount of drug. Moreover, animal data suggest that fetal bone has a greater uptake of bisphosphonates than maternal bone. Therefore, the use of ibandronate is not recommended in women who may become pregnant or during pregnancy. There is a theoretical risk of fetal harm (e.g., skeletal and other abnormalities) (1), but the magnitude of this risk cannot be estimated. Infants exposed in utero to ibandronate should be monitored for hypocalcemia during the first few days after birth.

FETAL RISK SUMMARY

Ibandronate is a bisphosphonate in the same class as alendronate, etidronate, pamidronate, risedronate, tiludronate, and zoledronic acid. It is available as IV and oral formulations. Ibandronate is indicated for the treatment and prevention of osteoporosis in postmenopausal women. The drug is apparently not metabolized in humans. After IV or oral administration, ibandronate elimination is multiphasic, with plasma concentrations declining to 10% of the peak concentrations within 3 or 8 hours, respectively. The initial decrease in the plasma concentration results from renal clearance and distribution into bone. The apparent terminal half-life after a 150-mg oral dose is 37–157 hours (1).

Reproduction studies have been conducted in rats and rabbits. During organogenesis, giving pregnant rats an IV dose that was ≥47 times the human exposure at the recommended IV dose of 3 mg every 3 months based on AUC (HERD-IV) resulted in an increased incidence of renal pelvis ureter syndrome. Oral doses ≥30 times the human exposure at the recommended daily dose of 2.5 mg (HERD-DD) or ≥9 times the human exposure at the recommended once-monthly dose of 150 mg (HERD-MD), both based on AUC, also resulted in an increased incidence of renal pelvis ureter.

In other studies, an IV dose during gestation that was ≥5 times the HERD-IV was associated with decreased fetal weight and pup growth. Impaired pup neuromuscular development was noted when female rats were given, from 14 days before mating through lactation, oral doses that were 45 times the HERD-DD or 13 times the HERD-MD. However, maternal deaths were observed with doses that were ≥2 times the HERD-IV, ≥3 times the HERD-DD, or ≥1 times the HERD-MD (1).

In rabbits, an IV dose during organogenesis that was 19 times the recommended IV dose of 3 mg every 3 months based on BSA was associated with maternal deaths, reduced maternal body weight gain, increased resorption rates, and decreased fetal weights. Oral doses during gestation that were ≥8 times the recommended daily dose of 2.5 mg or ≥4 times the recommended once-monthly dose of 150 mg, both based on BSA, caused maternal death (1).

Ibandronate was not carcinogenic in long-term (104-week) studies in male and female rats, or in male and female mice studied up to 78 weeks. In a 90-week study, however, dose-related increases in adrenal subcapsular adenoma/carcinoma were observed in female mice. The drug was not mutagenic or clastogenic in a number of assays. Fertility was impaired in both male and female rats given high IV doses, ≥40 and 117 times the HERD-IV, respectively, for 2–4 weeks before mating. Fertility also was impaired in female rats given oral doses that were 45 times the HERD-DD or 13 times the HERD-MD (1).

It is not known if ibandronate crosses the human placenta. The molecular weight (about 318 for the free acid), prolonged elimination half-life, and lack of metabolism suggest that the active drug will cross to the embryo and fetus.

A 2008 review described 51 cases of exposure to bisphosphonates before or during pregnancy: alendronate (*N* = 32) pamidronate (*N* = 11), etidronate (*N* = 5), risedronate (*N* = 2), and zoledronic acid (*N* = 1) (2). The authors concluded that although these drugs may affect bone modeling and development in the fetus, no such toxicity has yet been reported.

BREASTFEEDING SUMMARY

No reports describing the use of ibandronate during lactation have been located. The molecular weight (about 318 for the free acid), prolonged elimination half-life (up to 157 hours), and lack of metabolism suggest that active drug will be excreted into breast milk. Although the oral bioavailability in infants differs from that of adults, the very low adult oral bioavailability (<1% if fasting, much less with food) and the binding of ibandronate by the calcium in milk suggest that the amount absorbed by the infant will be clinically insignificant. Thus, breastfeeding is probably compatible with ibandronate treatment.

References

1. Product information. Boniva. Roche Pharmaceuticals, 2007.
2. Djokanovic N, Klieger-Grossmann C, Koren G. Does treatment with bisphosphonates endanger the human pregnancy? J Obstet Gynaecol Can 2008;30:1146–8.

IBRITUMOMAB TIUXETAN

Antineoplastic

PREGNANCY RECOMMENDATION: No Human Data—No Relevant Animal Data
BREASTFEEDING RECOMMENDATION: Contraindicated

PREGNANCY SUMMARY

No reports describing the use of ibritumomab tiuxetan in human pregnancy have been located. Rituximab has limited human pregnancy experience and immunosuppression has been the only documented developmental toxicity. However, the ibritumomab tiuxetan therapeutic regimen includes radioactive components. Because of this, ibritumomab tiuxetan should not be used in pregnancy. If inadvertent pregnancy does occur, the woman should be informed of the potential for embryo–fetal harm.

FETAL RISK SUMMARY

Ibritumomab tiuxetan is an immunoconjugate consisting of ibritumomab and the linker-chelator tiuxetan. Ibritumomab, a murine immunoglobulin G_1 (IgG_1) κ monoclonal antibody, is directed against the CD20 antigen found on the surface of normal and malignant B lymphocytes. Tiuxetan provides a high-affinity chelation site for indium-111 and yttrium-90. The therapeutic regimen includes indium-111 ibritumomab tiuxetan and yttrium-90 ibritumomab tiuxetan, prepared immediately before administration, and preceding rituximab (see also Rituximab). Ibritumomab tiuxetan, as part of the therapeutic regimen, is indicated for the treatment of patients with relapsed or refractory low-grade, follicular, or transformed B-cell non-Hodgkin's lymphoma, including patients with rituximab refractory follicular non-Hodgkin's lymphoma. In patients receiving the therapeutic regimen, the mean effective half-life for yttrium-90 activity in blood was 39 hours (1).

The ibritumomab tiuxetan therapeutic regimen may cause severe, infusion-related toxicity, including hypotension and other adverse effects. Premedication with acetaminophen and an antihistamine (e.g., diphenhydramine) is recommended before each infusion of rituximab (1). Hypotension in a pregnant woman could have deleterious effects on placental perfusion resulting in embryo and fetal harm.

Animal reproduction studies have not been conducted with ibritumomab tiuxetan. Neither have studies been conducted for carcinogenicity, mutagenicity, or effects on fertility. However, radiation is a potential carcinogen and mutagen. Moreover, the ibritumomab tiuxetan therapeutic regimen results in a significant radiation dose to the testes. The radiation dose to the ovaries has not been determined. Although it has not been studied, the therapeutic regimen does have the potential to cause toxic effects on the male and female gonads (1).

It is not known if ibritumomab tiuxetan of the components of the therapeutic regimen cross the human placenta. The high molecular weight (about 148,000) of ibritumomab tiuxetan suggests that it will not cross. However, human IG does cross and, therefore, ibritumomab tiuxetan, with the tightly bound radioactive components, may also cross. Rituximab, a component of the therapeutic regimen, does cross the placenta, at least at term (see Rituximab).

BREASTFEEDING SUMMARY

No reports describing the use of ibritumomab tiuxetan or its therapeutic regimen during human lactation have been located. The high molecular weight (about 148,000) of ibritumomab tiuxetan suggests that it will not be excreted into breast milk. It also is not known if rituximab, a component of the therapeutic regimen, is excreted into milk (see Rituximab). However, human IG is excreted into milk and, therefore, both rituximab and ibritumomab tiuxetan, with the tightly bound radioactive components, may also be excreted. The effects of this potential exposure on a nursing infant are unknown, but immunosuppression and other severe adverse effects, including those from radiation, are potential complications.

Reference

1. Product information. Zevalin. Biogen Idec, 2006.

IBUPROFEN

Nonsteroidal Anti-inflammatory

PREGNANCY RECOMMENDATION: Human Data Suggest Risk in 1st and 3rd Trimesters
BREASTFEEDING RECOMMENDATION: Compatible

PREGNANCY SUMMARY

Constriction of the ductus arteriosus in utero is a pharmacologic consequence arising from the use of prostaglandin synthesis inhibitors during pregnancy (see also Indomethacin) (1). Persistent pulmonary hypertension of the newborn may occur if these agents are used in the 3rd trimester close to delivery (1–3). These drugs also have been shown to inhibit labor and prolong pregnancy, both in humans (4) and in animals (5). Women attempting to conceive should not use any prostaglandin synthesis inhibitor, including ibuprofen, because of the findings in a variety of animal models that indicate these agents block blastocyst implantation (6,7). Moreover, as noted below, nonsteroidal anti-inflammatory drugs (NSAIDs) also have been associated with spontaneous abortion (SAB) and with cardiac defects, oral clefts, and gastroschisis. The risk for these defects, however, appears to be small.

I

FETAL RISK SUMMARY

Ibuprofen is an NSAID that is indicated for the reduction of fever and mild-to-moderate pain. It is the same subclass (propionic acids) as five other NSAIDs (fenoprofen, flurbiprofen, ketoprofen, naproxen, and oxaprozin). No evidence of developmental abnormalities was observed in reproduction studies in rats and rabbits at doses slightly less than the maximum human clinical dose (8).

The manufacturer has received information by a voluntary reporting system on the use of ibuprofen in 50 pregnancies (9). Seven of these cases were reported retrospectively and 43 prospectively. The results of the retrospective cases included one fetal death (cause of death unknown, no abnormalities observed) after 3rd trimester exposure, and one SAB without abnormality. Five infants with defects were observed, including an anencephalic infant exposed during the 1st trimester to ibuprofen and Bendectin (doxylamine succinate and pyridoxine hydrochloride), petit mal seizures progressing to grand mal convulsions, cerebral palsy (the fetus had also been exposed to other drugs), a hearsay report of microphthalmia with nasal cleft and mildly rotated palate, and tooth staining (M. M. Westland, personal communication, The Upjohn Company, 1981) (9). A cause and effect relationship between the drug and these defects is doubtful.

Prospectively, 23 of the exposed pregnancies ended in normal outcomes, 1 infant was stillborn, and 1 ended in SAB, both without apparent abnormality (9). Seven of the pregnancies were electively terminated, 3 had unknown outcomes, and 8 of the pregnancies were progressing at the time of the report.

In a surveillance study of Michigan Medicaid recipients involving 229,101 completed pregnancies conducted between 1985 and 1992, 3178 newborns had been exposed to ibuprofen during the 1st trimester (F. Rosa, personal communication, FDA, 1993). A total of 143 (4.5%) major birth defects were observed (129 expected). Specific data were available for six defect categories, including (observed/expected) 33/30 cardiovascular defects, 7/5 oral clefts, 3/2 spina bifida, 11/9 polydactyly, 5/5 limb reduction defects, and 4/8 hypospadias.

A combined 2001 population-based observational cohort study and a case–control study estimated the risk of adverse pregnancy outcome from the use of NSAIDs (10). The studies were based on data from the Danish Birth Registry and the North Jutland County's hospital discharge registry collected between 1991 and 1998. Only those women who had received a prescription for a NSAID at doses equivalent to 400 or 600 mg of ibuprofen were classified as exposed (NSAID doses equivalent to 200 mg of ibuprofen are over-the-counter drugs in Denmark). The cohort involved 1462 pregnant women who had received an NSAID prescription in the interval from 30 days before conception to birth and a reference group of 17,259 pregnant women who had not been prescribed any drugs during pregnancy. In both groups, only pregnancies lasting >28 weeks were included. There were 1106 women (76%) who had received an NSAID prescription between 30 days before conception and the end of the 1st trimester. The prevalences of congenital malformations in infants of these women and the reference group were $N = 46$, 4.2%, 95% confidence interval [CI] 3.0–5.3% vs. $N = 564$, 3.3%, 95% CI 3.0–3.5%), respectively; adjusted odds ratio (aOR) 1.27 (95% CI 0.93–1.75). A total of 997 women received an NSAID prescription in the 2nd and/or 3rd trimesters. In this group, the OR for preterm delivery was 1.05 (95% CI 0.80–1.39) and that for low birth weight (excluding preterm infants) was 0.79 (95% CI 0.45–1.38). Adjusting the data for the use of indomethacin (the tocolytic of choice in Denmark) did not affect the results. There was no evidence of a specific grouping of defects or of a dose–response relationship for adverse birth outcome. Based on the analysis, the authors concluded that NSAIDs were not associated with adverse birth outcome (10).

In the case–control portion of the above study, cases were defined as first recorded SAB in women who had received a prescription for NSAIDs in the 12 weeks before the date of discharge from the hospital after the SAB (63 of 4268 women who had SAB) (10). The controls were 29,750 primiparous women who had live births, 318 of whom had received a prescription for NSAIDs in the 1st trimester. The data were analyzed for the time from receiving an NSAID prescription in the weeks before the SAB (or missed abortion), adjusted for maternal age. The aOR (95% CI) for 1 week, 2–3 weeks, 4–6 weeks, 7–9 weeks, and 10–12 weeks before the SAB were 6.99 (2.75–17.74), 3.00 (1.21–7.44), 4.38 (2.66–7.20), 2.69 (1.81–4.00), and 1.26 (0.85–1.87), respectively. The results indicated that NSAIDs were associated with SAB because the OR decreased as the interval from assumed NSAID exposure to SAB increased (10).

A 2003 population-based cohort study involving 1055 pregnant women investigated the prenatal use of aspirin, NSAIDs, and acetaminophen (11). Fifty-three women (5%) reported use of NSAIDs around the time of conception or during pregnancy, 13 of whom had an SAB. After adjustment, an 80% increased risk of SAB was found for NSAIDs (adjusted hazard ratio 1.8, 95% CI 1.0–3.2). Moreover, the association was stronger if the initial use of drugs was around conception of if they were used for >1 week. A similar association was found with aspirin, but it was weaker because there were only 22 exposures (5 SABs). No association was observed with acetaminophen (11).

A prospective study of drug use in the 1st trimester examined the relationship between NSAIDs (N = 2557 infants born to exposed women) and congenital malformations (12). After adjustment, the aOR for any birth defect was 1.04 (95% CI 0.84–1.29). However, the aOR for cardiac defects (N = 36) and orofacial clefts (N = 6) were 1.86 (95% CI 1.32–2.62) and 2.61 (95% CI 1.01–6.78), respectively. There was no drug specificity for cardiac malformations, but five of the six cases of orofacial clefts had been exposed to naproxen (12).

A 2003 case–control study was conducted to identify drug use in early pregnancy that was associated with cardiac defects (13). Cases (cardiovascular defects without known chromosome anomalies) were drawn from three Swedish health registers (N = 5015) and controls consisting of all infants born in Sweden (1995–2001) (N = 577,730). Among the NSAIDs, only naproxen had a positive association with the defects (see Naproxen). For ibuprofen, there were 4124 pregnant women exposed and 37 cases of cardiac defects (OR 1.08, 95% CI 0.78–1.50) (13).

A 1996 case–control study of gastroschisis found a significantly elevated risk for ibuprofen (N = 6; OR 4.0, 95% CI 1.0–16.0) and other medications and exposures (14). A significant association was also found for aspirin (N = 7; OR 4.67, 95% CI 1.21–18.05). The data supported a vascular hypothesis for the pathogenesis of gastroschisis (14).

A 2006 case–control study found a significant association between congenital anomalies, specifically cardiac septal defects, and the use of NSAIDs in the 1st trimester (15). A population-based pregnancy registry (N = 36,387) was developed by linking three databases in Quebec (see Naprosyn for other study details). Case infants were those with any congenital anomaly diagnosed in the first year of life and were compared with matched controls. There were 93 infants (8.8%) with congenital defects from 1056 mothers who had filled prescriptions for NSAIDs in the 1st trimester. In controls, there were 2478 infants (7%) with anomalies from 35,331 mothers who had not filled such a prescription. The aOR was 2.21 (95% CI 1.72–2.85). The aOR for cardiac septal closure was 3.34 (95% CI 1.87–5.98). There also was a significant association for anomalies of the respiratory system 9.55 (95% CI 3.08–29.63), but this association disappeared when cases coded as "unspecified anomaly of the respiratory system" were excluded. For the cases involving septal closure, 61% were atrial septal defects and 31% were ventricular septal defects (VSDs). There were no significant associations for oral clefts or defects involving other major organ systems. The five most common NSAIDs were naproxen (35%), ibuprofen (26%), rofecoxib (15%), diclofenac (9%), and celecoxib (9%). Among these agents, the only significant association was for ibuprofen prescriptions in the 1st trimester and congenital defects ($p < 0.01$) (15).

In contrast to the above study, a 2004 case–control study involved 168 infants with a nonsyndromic muscular VSD who were compared with 692 infants without birth defects (16). No significant associations were found between the occurrence of the VSD and maternal use of NSAIDs or acetaminophen after adjusting for maternal fever nor were they detected between maternal fever and the defect.

The use of ibuprofen as a tocolytic agent has been associated with reduced amniotic fluid volume (17–19). Fourteen (82.3%) of 17 women treated with an NSAID had decreased amniotic fluid volume (17). Of the 17 women, ibuprofen, 1200–2400 mg/day, was used alone in three pregnancies and was combined with ritodrine in one. The other 13 women were treated with indomethacin (see also Indomethacin). One woman who was treated with ibuprofen for 44 days returned to a normal amniotic fluid volume after the drug was stopped (time for reversal not specified) (17).

Ibuprofen, 600 mg every 6 hours, was used as a tocolytic in a woman with a triplet pregnancy at approximately 26 weeks' gestation (18). Terbutaline and magnesium sulfate were combined with ibuprofen at various times for tocolysis. Oligohydramnios in each sac (pockets <1 cm) was documented by ultrasonogram on the 20th day of therapy and ibuprofen therapy was stopped. Therapy was restarted 5 days later when normal fluid volume for the three fetuses was observed, but oligohydramnios was again evident after 4 days and ibuprofen was discontinued. Tocolysis was then maintained with terbutaline and normal fluid volumes were observed 5 days after the second course of ibuprofen. The triplets were eventually delivered by elective cesarean section at 35 weeks' gestation, but no details on the infants were given (18).

A brief 1992 abstract described the results of using ibuprofen, 1200–2400 mg/day, as a tocolytic agent in 52 pregnancies (61 fetuses) up to 32 weeks' gestation (19). Amniotic fluid volumes were evaluated every 1–2 weeks. No cases of true oligohydramnios were observed, although 3 cases of low-normal fluid occurred that resolved after discontinuation of ibuprofen. Periodic Doppler echocardiography during therapy revealed a non-dose-related mild constriction of the ductus arteriosus in 4 (6.6%) of the fetuses. Ductal constriction was observed in three of the fetuses within 1 week of starting ibuprofen. Normal echocardiograms were obtained in all four cases within 1 week of discontinuing therapy (19).

Ibuprofen is commonly used by pregnant women, according to a 2003 study that identified the medications taken by a rural population (20). Among 578 participants, 86 (15%) took ibuprofen during pregnancy, including 20 during the 3rd trimester. Ibuprofen was the fourth most commonly used over-the-counter medication (after acetaminophen, calcium carbonate, and cough drops) (20).

A 2012 report from the National Birth Defects Prevention Study found associations between exposures to NSAIDs (aspirin, ibuprofen, and naproxen) and several birth defects (21). The data for this case–control study came from approximately 20,470 women with expected due dates in 1997–2004. Among this group, 3173 women (15.5%) were exposed to NSAIDs in the 1st trimester. Although the results suggested that NSAIDs are not a major cause of birth defects, the study did find several small-to-moderate but statistically significant increases in nine defects. The drug, aOR, and 95% CI for each defect were as follows: anencephaly/craniorachischisis—aspirin (2.1; 1.1–4.3); spina bifida—ibuprofen (1.6; 1.2–2.1); encephalocele—naproxen (3.5; 1.2–10); anophthalmia/microphthalmia—aspirin (3.0; 1.3–7.3), ibuprofen (1.9; 1.1–3.3), and naproxen (2.8; 1.1–7.3); cleft lip ± cleft palate—ibuprofen (1.3; 1.1–1.6) and naproxen (1.7; 1.1–2.5); cleft palate—aspirin (1.8; 1.1–2.9); transverse limb deficiency—naproxen (2.0; 1.0–3.8); amniotic bands/limb body wall—aspirin (2.5; 1.1–5.6) and ibuprofen (2.2; 1.4–3.5); and a heart defect (isolated pulmonary valve stenosis)—naproxen (2.4; 1.3–4.5). The analysis of the latter defect was limited to term births only. The authors acknowledged that further studies were needed because most of these associations had not been reported from other databases (21).

A 2013 study evaluated the effect of prolonged use of ibuprofen and acetaminophen during pregnancy on the neurodevelopment of 3-year-old same-sex sibling pairs (22). The cases came from the prospective Norwegian Mother and Child Cohort Study (see Acetaminophen for study details and results with acetaminophen). Prenatal acetaminophen was associated with significantly poorer outcomes than nonexposed siblings. In contrast, ibuprofen prenatal exposure was not associated with adverse neurodevelopment outcomes (22).

BREASTFEEDING SUMMARY

Ibuprofen is excreted into human milk. Two studies were unable to detect the drug (23–25), but a third using a more sensitive assay (lower limit 2.5 ng/mL) was able to quantify ibuprofen in milk (26). In 12 patients taking 400 mg every 6 hours for 24 hours, an assay capable of detecting 1 mcg/mL failed to demonstrate ibuprofen in the milk (23,24). In a second report, a woman was treated with 400 mg twice daily for 3 weeks (25). Milk levels shortly before and up to 8 hours after drug administration were all <0.5 mcg/mL.

The third study involved a lactating woman who underwent maxillary surgery (26). After surgery, she took ibuprofen 400 mg six times over a 42.5-hour interval for postoperative pain. Ten breast milk samples were collected during this same period. Ibuprofen was detected (13 ng/mL) 30 minutes after the first dose. The maximum milk concentration, 181 ng/mL, was found 20.5 hours after the first dose (about 5 hours after the third dose). Although the infant was not nursing, the infant's weight-adjusted dose would have been an estimated 0.0008% of the mother's dose (26).

The American Academy of Pediatrics classifies ibuprofen as compatible with breastfeeding (27).

References

1. Levin DL. Effects of inhibition of prostaglandin synthesis on fetal development, oxygenation, and the fetal circulation. Semin Perinatol 1980;4:35–44.
2. Van Marter LJ, Leviton A, Allred EN, Pagano M, Sullivan KF, Cohen A, Epstein MF. Persistent pulmonary hypertension of the newborn and smoking and aspirin and nonsteroidal antiinflammatory drug consumption during pregnancy. Pediatrics 1996;97:658–63.
3. Alano MA, Ngougmna E, Ostrea EM Jr, Konduri GG. Analysis of nonsteroidal antiinflammatory drugs in meconium and its relation to persistent pulmonary hypertension of the newborn. Pediatrics 2001; 107:519–23.
4. Fuchs F. Prevention of prematurity. Am J Obstet Gynecol 1976;126:809–20.
5. Powell JG, Cochrane RL. The effects of a number of non-steroidal anti-inflammatory compounds on parturition in the rat. Prostaglandins 1982;23:469–88.
6. Matt DW, Borzelleca JF. Toxic effects on the female reproductive system during pregnancy, parturition, and lactation. In: Witorsch RJ, ed. *Reproductive Toxicology*. 2nd ed. New York, NY: Raven Press, 1995:175–93.
7. Dawood MY. Nonsteroidal antiinflammatory drugs and reproduction. Am J Obstet Gynecol 1993;169:1255–65.
8. Product information. Motrin. McNeil Consumer, 2000.
9. Barry WS, Meinzinger MM, Howse CR. Ibuprofen overdose and exposure in utero: results from a postmarketing voluntary reporting system. Am J Med 1984;77(1A):35–9.
10. Nielsen GL, Sorensen HT, Larsen H, Pedersen L. Risk of adverse birth outcome and miscarriage in pregnant users of non-steroidal anti-inflammatory drugs: population based observational study and case-control study. Br Med J 2001;322:266–70.
11. Li DK, Liu L, Odouli R. Exposure to non-steroidal anti-inflammatory drugs during pregnancy and risk of miscarriage: population based cohort study. Br Med J 2003;327:368–71.
12. Ericson A, Kallen BAJ. Nonsteroidal anti-inflammatory drugs in early pregnancy. Reprod Toxicol 2001;15:371–5.
13. Kallen BAJ, Olausson PO. Maternal drug use in early pregnancy and infant cardiovascular defect. Reprod Toxicol 2003;17:255–61.
14. Torfs CP, Katz EA, Bateson TF, Lam PK, Curry CJR. Maternal medications and environmental exposures as risk factors for gastroschisis. Teratology 1996;54:84–92.
15. Ofori B, Oraichi D, Blais L, Rey E, Bérard A. Risk of congenital anomalies in pregnant users of non-steroidal anti-inflammatory drugs: a nested case-control study. Birth Defects Res B Dev Reprod Toxicol 2006;77:268–79.
16. Cleves MA, Savell VH Jr, Raj S, Zhao W, Correa A, Werler MM, Hobbs CA, and the National Birth Defects Prevention Study. Maternal use of acetaminophen and nonsteroidal anti-inflammatory drugs (NSAIDs), and muscular ventricular septal defects. Birth Defects Res A Clin Mol Teratol 2004;70:107–13.
17. Hickok DE, Hollenbach KA, Reilley SF, Nyberg DA. The association between decreased amniotic fluid volume and treatment with nonsteroidal anti-inflammatory agents for preterm labor. Am J Obstet Gynecol 1989;160:1525–31.
18. Wiggins DA, Elliott JP. Oligohydramnios in each sac of a triplet gestation caused by Motrin—fulfilling Kock's postulates. Am J Obstet Gynecol 1990;162:460–1.
19. Hennessy MD, Livingston EC, Papagianos J, Killam AP. The incidence of ductal constriction and oligohydramnios during tocolytic therapy with ibuprofen (abstract). Am J Obstet Gynecol 1992;166:324.
20. Glover DD, Amonkar M, Rybeck BF, Tracy TS. Prescription, over-the-counter, and herbal medicine use in a rural, obstetric population. Am J Obstet Gynecol 2003;188:1039–45.
21. Hernandez RK, Werler MM, Romitti P, Sun L, Anderka M, National Birth Defects Prevention Study. Nonsteroidal antiinflammatory drug use among women and the risk of birth defects. Am J Obstet Gynecol 2012;206:228.e1–8.
22. Brandlistuen RE, Ystrom E, Nulman I, Koren G, Nordeng H. Prenatal paracetamol exposure and child neurodevelopment: a sibling-controlled cohort study. Int J Epidemiol 2013;42:1702–13.
23. Townsend RJ, Benedetti T, Erickson S, Gillespie WR, Albert KS. A study to evaluate the passage of ibuprofen into breast milk (abstract). Drug Intell Clin Pharm 1982;16:482–3.
24. Townsend RJ, Benedetti TJ, Erickson S, Cengiz C, Gillespie WR, Gschwend J, Albert KS. Excretion of ibuprofen into breast milk. Am J Obstet Gynecol 1984;149:184–6.
25. Weibert RT, Townsend RJ, Kaiser DG, Naylor AJ. Lack of ibuprofen secretion into human milk. Clin Pharm 1982;1:457–8.
26. Walter K, Dilger C. Ibuprofen in human milk. Br J Clin Pharmacol 1997; 44:209–13.
27. Committee on Drugs, American Academy of Pediatrics. The transfer of drugs and other chemicals into human milk. Pediatrics 2001;108:776–89.

IBUTILIDE

Antiarrhythmic

PREGNANCY RECOMMENDATION: Limited Human Data—Animal Data Suggest Moderate Risk
BREASTFEEDING RECOMMENDATION: No Human Data—Probably Compatible

PREGNANCY SUMMARY

Animal data in the one species tested suggest a moderate risk to the human embryo–fetus. Three women in the second half of pregnancy with atrial flutter or fibrillation were successfully converted to sinus rhythm and, although there was no information on the newborns, apparently gave birth to normal infants at term. The limited human pregnancy experience, however, prevents a complete assessment of the embryo–fetal risk, but the benefits of therapy appear to outweigh the unknown risk. This conclusion is based on two considerations. First, the indication for ibutilide (i.e., rapid conversion of atrial fibrillation or atrial flutter of recent onset to sinus rhythm) is indicative of severe maternal disease that would be, in itself, harmful to the fetus if not treated. Second, treatment with ibutilide would be short term and occur in a hospital with the fetus under surveillance.

I

FETAL RISK SUMMARY

Ibutilide is a cardiac antiarrhythmic agent with predominantly class III (cardiac action potential prolongation) properties (1). Other available class III antiarrhythmic agents are amiodarone, sotalol, and bretylium (2). Ibutilide is administered by IV injection only. It undergoes rapid and extensive hepatic metabolism to eight metabolites, only one of which is active. Ibutilide has an average elimination half-life of about 6 hours (range 2–12 hours) (1).

Dose-related teratogenic, embryocidal effects, and fetal toxicity were observed in rats given ibutilide orally on days 6–15 of gestation (1,3,4). The no-observed-adverse-effect level (NOAEL), corrected for the 3% oral bioavailability, was 5 mg/kg/day, approximately the same as the maximum recommended human dose based on BSA (MRHD). Scoliosis was observed at a dose double the MRHD, but the incidence was not significantly different from controls (4). At four and eight times the MRHD, a significant dose–response effect was observed for adactyly, interventricular septal defects, scoliosis, and pharynx and palate malformations. A significant increase in embryo resorptions and fetal toxicity occurred at eight times the MRHD (4).

It is not known if ibutilide crosses the human placenta. The molecular weight (about 443 for the fumarate salt) and long elimination half-life suggest that the drug, and possibly its active metabolite, will cross to the embryo–fetus.

Two 2007 reports have described the use of ibutilide during three pregnancies (5,6). In the first case, a 20-year-old woman at 24 weeks' gestation presented with atrial flutter (5). Propranolol, esmolol, and sotalol were ineffective and could not be continued due to hypotension. IV ibutilide 1 mg successfully converted the patient to a sinus rhythm. She was discharged home on flecainide 50 mg twice daily and metoprolol 25 mg/day. She carried her pregnancy to term without further complication (5). No information was provided on the status of the newborn.

In the second case, a 27-year-old woman at 30 weeks' gestation had atrial fibrillation attributable to Wolff–Parkinson–White syndrome that was converted to a sinus rhythm with two doses of IV doses of ibutilide (0.87 mg) given at 30-minute intervals (6). She was maintained on flecainide 100 mg twice daily and atenolol 50 mg/day and delivered a healthy baby at term. The third case involved a 34-year-old woman at 23 weeks' who presented with atrial fibrillation. IV ibutilide 0.25 mg converted her to a sinus rhythm. She was discharged home on atenolol 50 mg/day and delivered a healthy baby at term. Both women remained asymptomatic throughout the remainder of their pregnancies (6). No additional information was given for either of the newborns.

BREASTFEEDING SUMMARY

No reports describing the use of ibutilide during lactation have been located. Because of the indication for this drug, it is doubtful if such reports will occur. In addition, its low oral bioavailability suggests that a nursing infant would absorb minimal amounts.

References

1. Product information. Corvert, Pharmacia & Upjohn, 2000.
2. Granberry MC. Ibutilide: a new class III antiarrhythmic agent. Am J Health-Syst Pharm 1998;55:255–60.
3. Marks TA, Terry RD. Developmental toxicity of ibutilide fumarate in rats (abstract). Teratology 1995;49:406.
4. Marks TA, Terry RD. Developmental toxicity of ibutilide fumarate in rats after oral administration. Teratology 1996;54:157–64.
5. Burkart TA, Kron J, Miles WM, Conti JB, Gonzalez MD. Successful termination of atrial flutter by ibutilide during pregnancy. Pacing Clin Electrophysiol 2007;30:283–6.
6. Kockova R, Kocka V, Kiernan T, Fahy GJ. Ibutilide-induced cardioversion of atrial fibrillation during pregnancy. J Cardiovasc Electrophysiol 2007;18:545–7.

ICATIBANT

Hematologic (Bradykinin Inhibitor)

PREGNANCY RECOMMENDATION: No Human Data—Animal Data Suggest Risk
BREASTFEEDING RECOMMENDATION: No Human Data—Potential Toxicity

PREGNANCY SUMMARY

No reports describing the use of icatibant in human pregnancy have been located. Although the drug was not teratogenic in rats and rabbits, it did cause other forms of developmental toxicity. However, the absence of human pregnancy experience prevents a more complete assessment of embryo–fetal risk. Because of the lack of information, if a pregnant woman has an attack of hereditary angioedema, treatments other than icatibant should be considered. A 2013 review recommended plasma-derived C1-INH as the drug of choice for hereditary angioedema in pregnancy and, if not available, then fresh frozen plasma (1).

I

FETAL RISK SUMMARY

Icatibant, a bradykinin (a vasodilator) B_2 receptor inhibitor that is given SC, is a synthetic decapeptide with five proteinogenic amino acids. It is indicated for the treatment of acute attacks of hereditary angioedema in adults 18 years of age and older. Icatibant is extensively metabolized to inactive metabolites. The mean elimination half-life is 1.4 hours. The manufacturer did not mention if the drug binds to plasma proteins (2).

Reproduction studies have been conducted in rats and rabbits. In rats, delayed parturition and fetal death occurred at exposures that were 0.5 and 2 times, respectively, the maximum recommended human dose (MRHD) based on AUC (MRHD-AUC) and increased preimplantation loss occurred at 7 times the MRHD-AUC. Impairment of pup air-righting reflex and decreased pup hair growth also occurred at 7 times the MRHD-AUC. In rabbits, a dose <1/40th the MRHD based on BSA resulted in an increase in premature birth and abortion rates. Also, in rabbits, exposures that were 13 times the MRHD-AUC resulted in preimplantation loss and increased fetal deaths (2).

Long-term studies for carcinogenic effects have not been conducted. The drug was not mutagenic in three assays. Daily SC doses in rats and dogs caused ovarian, uterine, and testicular atrophy/degeneration, as well as adverse effects on the mammary and prostate glands. These toxicities were not observed in dogs with less frequent dosing. Daily dosing in male and female mice had no effects on fertility or reproductive performance (2).

It is not known if icatibant crosses the human placenta. The molecular weight (about 1305) should limit the amount crossing, but the mean elimination half-life and, possibly, the lack of plasma protein binding might allow exposure, especially in the 3rd trimester.

BREASTFEEDING SUMMARY

No reports describing the use of icatibant during human lactation have been located. The molecular weight (about 1305) should limit excretion into mature breast milk, but mean elimination half-life (1.4 hours) and, possibly, the lack of plasma protein binding might allow some excretion. The effect of this exposure on a nursing infant is unknown, but the drug is a peptide and might be digested in the infant's gut. Nevertheless, if a mother is taking this drug and breastfeeding, her nursing infant must be monitored for the most common (>1%) adverse reactions: pyrexia, transaminase increase, dizziness, and rash (2).

References

1. Geng B, Riedl MA. HAE update: special consideration in the female patient with hereditary angioedema. Allergy Asthma Proc 2013;34:13–8.
2. Product information. Firazyr. Shire Orphan Therapies, 2011.

IDARUBICIN

Antineoplastic

PREGNANCY RECOMMENDATION: Limited Human Data—Animal Data Suggest Risk
BREASTFEEDING RECOMMENDATION: Contraindicated

PREGNANCY SUMMARY

Limited pregnancy experience, all in the 2nd trimester, suggests that idarubicin may cause significant fetal toxicity. Exposure during organogenesis has not been reported.

FETAL RISK SUMMARY

Idarubicin, an anthracycline antineoplastic antibiotic agent, is a DNA-intercalating analog of daunorubicin. It is used in the treatment of acute myeloid leukemia. It is in the same antineoplastic subclass of anthracyclines as daunorubicin, doxorubicin, epirubicin, and valrubicin.

In pregnant rats, a dose 10% of the human dose (HD) produced embryotoxicity and teratogenicity without causing maternal toxicity. Embryotoxicity, but not teratogenicity, occurred in rabbits treated with doses up to about 20% of the HD. However, this dose caused maternal toxicity (1).

Shepard (2) reviewed three reproductive studies in which IV doses up to 0.2 mg/kg were given to rats. When treatment occurred early in pregnancy, fetal loss, intrauterine growth restriction (IUGR), decreased ossification, and skeletal defects such as fused ribs were observed at the highest dose. These effects were not seen when treatment occurred perinatally. Infertility may have occurred in the second generation.

A 26-year-old woman at 20 weeks' gestation who presented with acute myeloblastic leukemia, was treated with an induction course of cytarabine and daunorubicin that failed to halt the disease progression (3). At approximately 23 weeks' gestation, a second induction course was started with mitoxantrone and cytarabine. Complete remission was achieved 60 days from the start of therapy. Weekly ultrasound examinations documented normal fetal growth. Because of the long interval required for remission, treatment was changed to idarubicin (10 mg/m^2, days 1 and 2) and cytarabine. She tolerated this therapy and was discharged home, but returned 2 days later complaining of abdominal pain and the loss of fetal movements. A stillborn, 2200-g fetus (gestational age not specified) without evidence of congenital malformations was delivered after induction. Permission for an autopsy was denied. Although the authors did not specify a mechanism, they concluded that the cause of the fetal death was due to idarubicin.

A 1998 case report described a woman with acute myeloid leukemia who was treated with idarubicin and cytarabine during the 2nd trimester (4). Treatment was begun at 21 weeks' gestation with IV idarubicin 10 mg/m^2 on days 1, 3, and 5 and IV cytarabine 100 mg/m^2 on days 1–10. A 6-day consolidation course of IV cytarabine, 1000 mg/m^2 every 12 hours, was given 6 weeks later. Complete remission was documented after recovery from this course. IUGR and decreased fetal movements were diagnosed at 32 weeks' gestation and a week and half later, a 1408-g female infant was delivered by cesarean section. Apgar scores were 4, 7, and 10 at 1, 5, and 10 minutes, respectively. Except for hyperbilirubinemia, the infant was healthy and was doing well on discharge. An echocardiographic examination revealed no evidence of cardiac anomalies or signs of cardiomyopathy (4).

A 22-year-old woman at 22 weeks' gestation with acute lymphoblastic leukemia type T was treated with idarubicin (9 mg/m^2 on days 1, 2, 3, and 8), cyclophosphamide (750 mg/m^2 on days 1 and 8), vincristine (2 mg/day on days 1, 8, 15, and 22), and prednisone (60 mg/m^2 on days 1–7 and 15–21) (5). The patient tolerated the therapy except for agranulocytosis with fever, which was treated with antibiotics. A complete remission was documented by 27 weeks' gestation. Before consolidation chemotherapy, a 1024-g male infant was delivered by cesarean section 1 week later. Apgar scores were 6, 8, and 8 at 1, 5, and 10 minutes, respectively. Neonatal complications, related to prematurity, were respiratory distress syndrome, necrotizing enterocolitis, and grade II ventricular hemorrhage (5). In addition, acute heart failure occurred during the first 3 days after birth (5). Diffuse cardiomyopathy involving both ventricles and the interventricular septum without anomalies was revealed by echocardiography. The condition was thought to be related to the chemotherapy, especially, idarubicin. With supportive care, the cardiac function returned to normal within 3 days. Except for slight delay in the acquisition of language, the infant was progressing normally at 18 months of age (5).

In a 2009 case report, a woman with relapse of acute myeloid leukemia at 22 weeks' gestation was treated with idarubicin, fludarabine, cytarabine, mitoxantrone, and gemtuzumab ozogamicin (6). The fetus developed signs of idarubicin-induced cardiomyopathy, transient cerebral ventriculomegaly, anemia, and intrauterine growth restriction. The newborn, delivered at 33 weeks' by cesarean section, showed no congenital malformations.

Occupational exposure of the mother to antineoplastic agents during pregnancy may present a risk to the fetus. A position statement from the National Study Commission on Cytotoxic Exposure and a research article involving some antineoplastic agents are presented in the monograph for cyclophosphamide (see Cyclophosphamide).

BREASTFEEDING SUMMARY

No reports describing the use of idarubicin during lactation have been located. The molecular weight (about 498 for the free base) is low enough that excretion into breast milk should be expected. Because of the potential toxicity, a woman treated with this drug should not breastfeed until idarubicin and its cytoxic and presumed active metabolite, idarubicinol, have been eliminated from her system. Idarubicin has a mean terminal half-life of 20–22 hours (range 4–46 hours), but the estimated mean terminal half-life of idarubicinol exceeds 45 hours (1). Thus, elimination of the two agents may require 10 days or longer. The American Academy of Pediatrics classifies similar antineoplastic agents (e.g., doxorubicin) as contraindicated during breastfeeding because of the potential for immune suppression and an unknown effect on growth or association with carcinogenesis (7).

References

1. Product information. Idamycin. Pharmacia, 1996.
2. Shepard TH. *Catalog of Teratogenic Agents*. 8th ed. Baltimore, MD: The Johns Hopkins University Press, 1995:1290.
3. Reynoso EE, Huerta F. Acute leukemia and pregnancy—fatal fetal outcome after exposure to idarubicin during the second trimester. Acta Oncol 1994;33:703–16.
4. Claahsen HL, Semmekrot BA, van Dongen PWJ, Mattijssen V. Successful fetal outcome after exposure to idarubicin and cytosine-arabinoside during the second trimester of pregnancy—a case report. Am J Perinatol 1998;15:295–7.
5. Achtari C, Hohlfeld P. Cardiotoxic transplacental effect of idarubicin administered during the second trimester of pregnancy. Am J Obstet Gynecol 2000;183:511–2.
6. Baumgartner AK, Oberhoffer R, Jacobs VR, Ostermayer E, Menzel H, Voigt M, Schneider KT, Pildner von Steinburg S. Reversible foetal cerebral ventriculomegaly and cardiomyopathy under chemotherapy for maternal AML. Onkologie 2009;32:40–3.
7. Committee on Drugs, American Academy of Pediatrics. The transfer of drugs and other chemicals into human milk. Pediatrics 2001;108:776–89.

IDOXURIDINE

Antiviral

PREGNANCY RECOMMENDATION: No Human Data—Animal Data Suggest Risk
BREASTFEEDING RECOMMENDATION: No Human Data—Potential Toxicity

PREGNANCY SUMMARY

No reports describing the use of idoxuridine in human pregnancy have been located. The drug is teratogenic in some species of animals after injection and ophthalmic use (1–3).

FETAL RISK SUMMARY

Idoxuridine is a topical ophthalmic preparation that is indicated for the treatment of keratitis caused by the virus of herpes simplex (1). Systemic exposure after topical use was not reported by the manufacturer.

Reproduction studies have been conducted in rabbits, rats, and mice. In pregnant rabbits given the drug topically to the eyes in doses similar to those used in humans, idoxuridine crossed the placenta and caused fetal malformations. Fetal malformations also occurred in rats and mice given intraperitoneal, oral, or SC injections of the drug (1).

Adequate studies for carcinogenicity have not been conducted but is considered potentially carcinogenic. Idoxuridine has caused chromosome aberrations in mice and is mutagenic in mammalian cells in culture.

BREASTFEEDING SUMMARY

No reports describing the use idoxuridine during human lactation have been located. Systemic concentrations after topical use have apparently not been determined. The manufacturer states that the drug should not be used during breastfeeding because the drug and metabolites may be excreted into breast milk (1).

References

1. Product information. Dendrid. Alcon Laboratories (*downloaded from Daily Med in September 2013*).
2. Nishimura H, Tanimura T. *Clinical Aspects of the Teratogenicity of Drugs*. New York, NY: American Elsevier, 1976:148, 258–9.
3. Itoi M, Gefter JW, Kaneko N, Ishii Y, Ramer RM, Gasset AR. Teratogenicities of ophthalmic drugs. I. Antiviral ophthalmic drugs. Arch Ophthalmol 1975;93:46–51.

IFOSFAMIDE

Antineoplastic

PREGNANCY RECOMMENDATION: Contraindicated—1st Trimester
BREASTFEEDING RECOMMENDATION: Contraindicated

PREGNANCY SUMMARY

There is limited human pregnancy experience with ifosfamide. The drug is carcinogenic and mutagenic in experimental studies. In addition, it is teratogenic and embryotoxic in three animal species at doses far less than the recommended human dose. Because of the close relationship of ifosfamide to cyclophosphamide, a known human teratogen, ifosfamide should be considered an agent with a high potential for human teratogenicity and embryo–fetal toxicity.

FETAL RISK SUMMARY

Ifosfamide is chemically related to the nitrogen mustards and is a synthetic analog of cyclophosphamide (see also Cyclophosphamide). Ifosfamide is a prodrug that requires metabolic activation by microsomal liver enzymes to produce biologically active metabolites. It is indicated for the treatment of germ cell testicular cancer. Combination with a prophylactic agent such as mesna is recommended to prevent hemorrhagic cystitis (1).

Ifosfamide was carcinogenic in rats (including a significant incidence of leiomyosarcomas and mammary fibroadenomas in female rats) and mutagenic in several assays (1). Reproduction studies have been conducted in pregnant mice, rats, and rabbits. In mice, a single dose of 30 mg/m^2 (1/40 the daily recommended human dose of 1200 mg/m^2) administered on gestational day 11 caused an increase in the incidence of resorptions and anomalies (not specified). Evidence of embryolethality was observed in rats given 54-mg/m^2 doses on gestational days 6–15. Embryotoxic effects (not specified) were observed when a smaller dose (18 mg/m^2) was administered over the same period. Embryotoxicity and teratogenicity were observed in rabbits given 88 mg/m^2/day on gestational days 6–18 (1). Maternal toxicity was not mentioned in any of the above studies.

A 1973 study described the teratogenic and embryotoxic effects of various single intraperitoneal doses (5, 10, and 20 mg/kg) of ifosfamide given to mice on gestational day 11 (2). Only the 20-mg/kg dose was embryolethal (significantly increased resorption rates), but significant fetal toxicity (decreased body weight and/or crown–rump length) was observed with the 10- and 20-mg/kg doses. A number of anomalies were observed in the highest dose group: open eyes, internal and external hydrocephalus, microphakia, micromelia, adactyly, syndactyly, microcaudate, kinky tails, kidney ectopia, and hydronephrosis. Both 10- and 20-mg/kg doses increased the number of skeletal defects and the 5-mg/kg dose was associated with a significant increase in supernumerary ribs. Finally, a single SC dose of 45 mg/kg administered to 1-day-old mice resulted in reduced body weight and altered development (2).

In sexually mature male rabbits, single IV doses of ifosfamide (0, 60, 90, 120, or 240 mg/kg) caused transient and dose-dependent depression of spermatocytogenesis, spermiogenesis, and sperm maturation in comparison to controls (3). In the second part of this study, using the same methods, the investigators combined ifosfamide with mesna (an uroprotectant agent) (4). Three groups of male rabbits were given different doses of the combination (ifosfamide 30, 45, or 60 mg/kg plus mesna 6, 9, or 12 mg/kg, followed by a second equal dose of mesna 4 hours later). Each group received 10 weekly treatments. Controls were given either mesna alone (three groups) or saline (one group). Dose-related ifosfamide–mesna suppression of spermatogenesis and epididymal sperm maturation was observed. In addition, the investigators noted incomplete recovery of the germinal epithelium (4).

A 1997 review stated that ifosfamide is less toxic for stem cell spermatogonia (type A spermatogonia) than is cyclophosphamide (5). In 15 of 16 patients who received 15–30 g/m^2 of ifosfamide, the median follicle-stimulating hormone levels returned to normal. In addition, there was no evidence of an increased risk of malformations or malignancies in offspring fathered by patients with germ cell cancer after chemotherapy (5). However, a 2003 study confirmed that ifosfamide exposure is a potential cause of male infertility (6). A significant ($p = 0.005$) dose-dependent relationship was observed between increasing doses of ifosfamide and infertility in patients treated for osteosarcoma.

It is not known if ifosfamide or its active metabolites cross the placenta to the fetus. The low molecular weight of the parent prodrug (about 261) suggests that it reaches the fetal circulation.

A 20-year-old woman at 23 weeks' gestation was treated with ifosfamide (5 g/day on days 1 and 2), vincristine (2 mg/day on days 1 and 14), and dactinomycin (1 mg/day on days 1 and 2) for advanced rhabdomyosarcoma of the face (7). In addition to the antineoplastics, the patient also received mesna and urate oxidase (used for the treatment of hyperuricemia). A second course of therapy was given 4 weeks later. At initiation of the chemotherapy, the fetal weight was estimated to be at the 20th percentile with normal amniotic fluid volume and active movements. At the time of the second course of chemotherapy, ultrasound revealed a complete absence of amniotic fluid, an empty fetal bladder, cessation of fetal growth, and absence of fetal movements. An emergency cesarean section was performed 2 weeks later after evidence of continued anhydramnios, intrauterine growth arrest, and acute fetal hypoxia. A 720-g female was delivered with Apgar scores of 3, 7, and 7 at 1, 5, and 10 minutes, respectively. An ultrasound of the neonate revealed bilateral intraventricular hemorrhage and left occipital meningeal hematomas. Anuria persisted, and the girl died at age 7 days. Autopsy noted extensive cerebral lesions associated with prematurity but no renal lesions or chromosome abnormalities. The placenta had large areas of ischemic necrosis without evidence of chorioamnionitis. No cancer cells were found in the fetus or placenta. The authors speculated that the lack of renal lesions suggested that causes in addition to ifosfamide-induced toxicity should be considered to explain the anuria in the fetus and newborn (7).

In contrast to the above study, a 21-year-old woman was treated with three courses of ifosfamide/mesna (each 5 g/m^2 three times weekly) and doxorubicin (50 mg/m^2 three times weekly) for Ewing's sarcoma of the pelvis (8). The three courses were given in the 27th, 30th, and 33rd week of pregnancy. Mild intrauterine growth restriction was detected by ultrasound. A cesarean section at the beginning of the 36th gestational week delivered a 42-cm-long, 1300-g female infant. No adverse effects were noted in the infant, who was doing well at 2 years of age (8).

In a 2004 case report, a 17-year-old woman at 22 weeks' gestation was diagnosed with an extraskeletal Ewing's sarcoma (9). She was treated with doxorubicin 50 mg/m^2 by 48-hour continuous infusion and ifosfamide 2 g/m^2 as a single injection, both given at 25, 28 and 30 weeks'. Mild fetal growth restriction was noted from the 29th week of gestation. An elective cesarean section delivered a 1.245-kg male infant with Apgar scores of 7 and 9 at 1 and 5 minutes, respectively. Based on weight and length (38 cm), the infant was small for gestational age. The infant had no congenital anomalies and no respiratory distress syndrome, but did have mild hyperbilirubinemia. He was growing well at 8 months of age (9).

A 2006 case report described the pregnancy outcome of a 21-year-old woman with Burkitt's lymphoma who was treated with intensive chemotherapy (10). Beginning at 26 weeks, she was treated with two cycles of chemotherapy that included ifosfamide, cyclophosphamide, vincristine, doxorubicin, cytarabine, etoposide, cytarabine, and mesna. At 32 weeks, a cesarean section delivered a 1.731-kg male infant with Apgar scores of 8 and 9 at 1 and 5 minutes, respectively. His weight, length, and head circumference were within normal limits for gestational age. No anomalies were noted but respiratory distress was evident. At 9 months of age, his weight was 6.36 kg. He had mild delayed motor skills that were thought to result from his premature birth. Otherwise he was healthy (10).

BREASTFEEDING SUMMARY

No reports describing the use of ifosfamide during lactation have been located. Ifosfamide is excreted into breast milk (1). This is consistent with its low molecular weight (about 261). Although the amount of ifosfamide in milk was not stated, severe toxicity in a nursing infant is a potential concern (e.g., bone marrow depression, urinary system, and CNS toxicity). Therefore, women receiving ifosfamide should not breastfeed.

References

1. Product information. Ifex. Bristol-Myers Squibb, 2000.
2. Bus JS, Gibson JE. Teratogenicity and neonatal toxicity of Ifosfamide in mice. Proc Soc Exp Biol Med 1973;143:965–70.
3. Ypsilantis P, Papaioannou N, Psalla D, Politou M, Simopoulos C. Effects of single-dose administration of ifosfamide on testes and semen characteristics in the rabbit. Reprod Toxicol 2003;17:237–45.
4. Ypsilantis P, Papaioannou N, Psalla D, Politou M, Pitiakoudis M, Simopoulos C. Effects of subchronic ifosfamide-mesna treatment on testes and semen characteristics in the rabbit. Reprod Toxicol 2003;17:699–708.
5. Pont J, Albrecht W. Fertility after chemotherapy for testicular germ cell cancer. Fert Steril 1997;68:1–5.
6. Longhi A, Macchiagodena M, Vitali G, Bacci G. Fertility in male patients treated with neoadjuvant chemotherapy for osteosarcoma. J Pediatr Hematol Oncol 2003;25:292–6.
7. Fernandez H, Diallo A, Baume D, Papiernik E. Anhydramnios and cessation of fetal growth in a pregnant mother with polychemotherapy during the second trimester. Prenat Diag 1989;9:681–2.
8. Merimsky O, Chevalier TL, Missenard G, Lepechoux C, Cojean-Zelek I, Mesurolle B, Le Cesne A. Management of cancer in pregnancy: a case of Ewing's sarcoma of the pelvis in the third trimester. Ann Oncol 1999;10:345–50.
9. Nakajima W, Ishida A, Takahashi M, Hirayama M, Washino N, Ogawa M, Takahashi S, Okada K. Good outcome for infant of mother treated with chemotherapy for Ewing sarcoma at 25–30 weeks' gestation. J Pediatr Hematol Oncol 2004;26:308–11.
10. Lam MSH. Treatment of Burkitt's lymphoma during pregnancy. Ann Pharmacother 2006;40:2048–52.

ILOPERIDONE

Antipsychotic

PREGNANCY RECOMMENDATION: No Human Data—Animal Data Suggest Moderate Risk
BREASTFEEDING RECOMMENDATION: No Human Data—Potential Toxicity

PREGNANCY SUMMARY

No reports describing the use of iloperidone in human pregnancy have been located. Animal reproduction studies observed two types of developmental toxicity (death and decreased weight) in one animal species. There is no evidence with other agents in this subclass of embryo or fetal harm. However, because of the very limited human pregnancy experience with atypical antipsychotics, the American College of Obstetricians and Gynecologists does not recommend the routine use of these agents in pregnancy, but a risk–benefit assessment may indicate that such use is appropriate (1). Because iloperidone is indicated for severe debilitating mental disease, the benefits to the mother appear to outweigh the unknown risk. A 1996 review on the management of psychiatric illness concluded that patients with histories of chronic psychosis represent a high-risk group (for both the mother and the fetus) and should be maintained on pharmacologic therapy before and during pregnancy (2). Folic acid 4 mg/day has been recommended for women taking atypical antipsychotics because they may have a higher risk of neural tube defects due to inadequate folate intake and obesity (3).

FETAL RISK SUMMARY

The atypical antipsychotic iloperidone is a benzisoxazole derivative in the same subclass of antipsychotic agents as paliperidone, risperidone, and ziprasidone. Iloperidone is indicated for the acute treatment of schizophrenia in adults. It is extensively metabolized to two predominate metabolites, P88 and P95, one (P88) of which is active. The parent drug and the two metabolites are highly bound (about 95%) to serum proteins. The mean elimination half-lives of iloperidone and the two metabolites (P88 and P95) in extensive metabolizers were 18, 26, and 23 hours, respectively, whereas in poor metabolizers the half-lives were 33, 37, and 31 hours, respectively (4).

Reproduction studies have been conducted in rats and rabbits. During organogenesis, rats were given doses 1.6–26 times the maximum recommended human dose of 24 mg/day based on BSA (MRHD). The highest dose caused increased early intrauterine deaths, decreased fetal weight and length, decreased skeletal ossification, and an increased incidence of minor fetal skeletal anomalies and variations and also was maternal toxic (decreased food consumption and weight gain). In separate studies, rats were given doses 1.6–26 times the MRHD either before conception or from gestational day 17 through weaning. Adverse effects included prolonged pregnancy and parturition, increased stillbirth rates, increased incidence of fetal visceral variations, decreased fetal and pup weights, and decreased postpartum pup survival. Maternal toxicity occurred at the higher doses. An increase in stillbirths occurred at all doses. The no-effect dose for the other effects ranged from 1.6 to about 5 times the MRHD. No drug effects on neurobehavioral or reproductive development were noted in the surviving pups. In rabbits during organogenesis, the highest dose tested (20 times the MRHD) was not teratogenic but did cause increased early intrauterine deaths, decreased fetal viability at term, and maternal toxicity (4).

Because P95 is not present in significant amounts in rats, a separate study was conducted in this species with the metabolite. During organogenesis, doses resulting in plasma levels up to twice those in humans receiving the MRHD did not cause teratogenicity, but delayed skeletal ossification occurred at all doses. No significant maternal toxicity was noted (4).

Long-term studies for carcinogenicity have been conducted in mice and rats. An increased incidence of malignant mammary gland tumors occurred in female mice that were considered to be prolactin mediated. No drug-related carcinogenicity was observed in rats. Long-term exposure to the P95 metabolite in rats resulted in proliferative responses in several organs. Neither iloperidone nor P95 was mutagenic in various assays, but the parent drug did cause chromosomal aberrations in one in vitro assay that also resulted in cytotoxicity. Decreased fertility in male and females was observed at doses >≈5 times the MRHD. The no-effect dose for impaired fertility was 1.6 times the MRHD (4).

It is not known if iloperidone or the two metabolites cross the human placenta. The molecular weight of the parent drug (about 426) and the long elimination half-lives suggest that the parent drug and possibly the metabolites will cross to the embryo–fetus. The high serum protein binding of iloperidone might limit some of this exposure.

BREASTFEEDING SUMMARY

No reports describing the use of iloperidone during human lactation have been located. The molecular weight (about 426) and the long elimination half-lives (ranging from 18–36 hours) suggest that the drug will be excreted into breast milk. However, there are two major metabolites, one of which is active, and these may also be excreted into milk. The amount of iloperidone and metabolites in milk might be limited by their high (about 95%) serum protein binding. The effect of this exposure on a nursing infant is unknown.

The manufacturer recommends women receiving iloperidone should not breastfeed (4). Moreover, the American Academy of Pediatrics classifies other atypical antipsychotics (e.g., see Ziprasidone) as drugs whose effect on the nursing infant is unknown but may be of concern (5).

Because of the very limited human experience with atypical antipsychotics, the American College of Obstetricians and Gynecologists does not recommend the routine use of these agents during lactation, but a risk–benefit assessment may indicate that such use is appropriate (1).

References

1. American College of Obstetricians and Gynecologists. Use of psychiatric medications during pregnancy and lactation. *ACOG Practice Bulletin*. No. 92, April 2008. Obstet Gynecol 2008;111:1001–19.
2. Althuler LL, Cohen L, Szuba MP, Burt VK, Gitlin M, Mintz J. Pharmacologic management of psychiatric illness during pregnancy: dilemmas and guidelines. Am J Psychiatry 1996;153:592–606.
3. Koren G, Cohn T, Chitayat D, Kapur B, Remington G, Myles-Reid D, Zipursky RB. Use of atypical antipsychotics during pregnancy and the risk of neural tube defects in infants. Am J Psychiatry 2002;159:136–7.
4. Product information. Fanapt. Vanda Pharmaceuticals, 2009.
5. Committee on Drugs, American Academy of Pediatrics. The transfer of drugs and other chemicals into human milk. Pediatrics 2001;108:776–89.

I

ILOPROST

Vasodilator

PREGNANCY RECOMMENDATION: Limited Human Data—Animal Data Not Relevant
BREASTFEEDING RECOMMENDATION: No Human Data—Potential Toxicity

PREGNANCY SUMMARY

Pregnancy is not advised in women with pulmonary arterial hypertension (PAH) because of the high risk of morbidity and death. However, pregnancy exposures to iloprost have occurred apparently without embryo–fetal harm. The animal reproduction data are not relevant because the oral and IV doses were not compared with the human dose. Nevertheless, PAH is a high-risk condition and, if indicated, the drug should not be withheld because of pregnancy.

FETAL RISK SUMMARY

Iloprost is a synthetic analog of prostacyclin PGI_2 given by inhalation or IV (outside of the U.S.). Iloprost is indicated for the treatment of PAH. The agent dilates systemic and pulmonary arterial vascular beds. There are no other agents in its subclass of prostacyclin analogs. The absolute bioavailability of inhaled iloprost has not been determined, but it was generally not detectable in plasma 30–60 minutes after a dose. When given IV, the half-life is 20–30 minutes and the plasma protein binding was about 60%, mainly to albumin. The main metabolite was inactive in animals (1).

Reproduction studies have been conducted in rats, rabbits, and monkeys. In Han-Wistar rats, a continuous IV dose (serum levels not specified) caused shortened digits of the thoracic extremity in fetuses–pups. In comparable studies giving oral or IV iloprost to Sprague-Dawley rats, rabbits, and monkeys, these anomalies were not observed. However, a maternal toxic oral dose in Sprague-Dawley rats significantly increased the number of nonviable fetuses and an IV dose that was 10 times the teratogenic dose in Han-Wistar rats was embryolethal (1). None of the studies compared the exposures with the human exposure from inhalation or IV use.

Iloprost was not carcinogenic, mutagenic, or clastogenic in multiple studies and assays, and did not cause chromosomal aberrations. The fertility of male and female rats was not impaired with embryolethal IV doses (1).

It is not known if iloprost crosses the human placenta. The molecular weight (about 360) is low enough, but the very short plasma half-life suggests that exposure of the embryo–fetus will be limited.

A 2005 report described three women with PAH who were treated with inhaled iloprost (2). Treatment was initiated at 8, 19, and 17 weeks' with doses titrated to the patient's condition and administered 7 times daily. The first woman had been treated with bosentan and warfarin until the therapy was changed at 8 weeks'. This woman suffered a cardiorespiratory arrest at about 25 weeks but was successfully resuscitated after about 1 minute and was converted to IV iloprost for 5 days. At that time, a cesarean section delivered a 0.65-kg male infant with Apgar scores of 8 and 9. The child was progressing well at 16 months of age. Because of premature labor, the second woman underwent a cesarean section at 36 weeks' to deliver a 2.8-kg male infant with Apgar scores of 9 and 9. At 18 months, the mother and her son were doing well. Placenta previa was diagnosed in the third woman and a cesarean section at 35 weeks delivered a 2.16-kg female infant with Apgar scores of 9, 9, and 10. At 12 weeks, the mother and her daughter were doing well. No congenital anomalies were noted in the three infants (2).

A 21-year-old with idiopathic PAH was treated with inhaled iloprost from 24 to 34 weeks' gestation, at which time she underwent a cesarean section because of oligohydramnios (3). The mother and infant were clinically well and were discharged home 8 days after delivery. No other details about the infant were provided.

Bosentan (250/day), sildenafil (150 mg/day), hydroxychloroquine (200 mg/day), azathioprine (100 mg/day), and phenprocoumon were used up to 5 weeks' gestation in a 29-year-old woman with systemic lupus erythematosus-associated PAH (4). At that time, bosentan and phenprocoumon were discontinued and the other three agents were continued with low-molecular-weight heparin. At 35 weeks', inhaled iloprost was added. At 37 weeks, a planned cesarean section delivered a healthy 2.760-kg female infant with Apgar scores of 8, 9, and 10. Breastfeeding was declined. At the time of the report, the child was doing well (4).

A 2013 case report described a 30-year-old pregnant woman who was diagnosed with PAH at 24 weeks' (5). She was treated with inhaled iloprost, oral sildenafil, oxygen, and low-molecular-weight heparin. Five days before delivery, inhaled iloprost was replaced with IV iloprost. At about 32 weeks', a cesarean section gave birth to 1.7-kg male infant with Apgar scores of 8 and 9 at 1 and 5 minutes, respectively. Weight, length, and head circumference were within normal limits for gestational age. No congenital anomalies were noted, but the infant had sinusal tachycardia and mild respiratory distress syndrome. He was apparently doing well at 18 days of age (5).

BREASTFEEDING SUMMARY

No reports describing the use of iloprost during human lactation have been located. The molecular weight (about 360) is low enough, but the very short plasma half-life suggests that excretion of the drug into breast milk will be limited. The effect of exposure on a nursing infant is unknown.

References

1. Product information. Ventavis. Actelion Pharmaceuticals US, 2010.
2. Elliot CA, Stewart P, Webster VJ, Mills GH, Hutchinson SP, Howarth ES, Bu'lock FA, Lawson RA, Armstrong IJ, Kiely DG. The use of iloprost in early pregnancy in patients with pulmonary hypertension. Eur Respir J 2005;26:168–73.
3. Cotrim C, Simoes O, Loureiro MJ, Cordeiro P, Miranda R, Silva C, Avillez T, Carrageta M. Acute resynchronization with inhaled iloprost in a pregnant woman with idiopathic pulmonary artery hypertension. Rev Port Cardiol 2006;25:529–33.
4. Streit M, Speich R, Fischler M, Ulrich S. Successful pregnancy in pulmonary arterial hypertension associated with systemic lupus erythematosus: a case report. J Med Case Rep 2009;3:7255.
5. Terek D, Kayikcioglu M, Kultursay H, Ergenoglu M, Yalaz M, Musayev O, Mogulkoc N, Gunusen I, Akisu M, Kultursay N. Pulmonary arterial hypertension and pregnancy. J Res Med Sci 2013;18:73–6.

IMATINIB

Antineoplastic (Tyrosine Kinase Inhibitor)

PREGNANCY RECOMMENDATION: Human and Animal Data Suggest Risk
BREASTFEEDING RECOMMENDATION: Limited Human Data—Probably Compatible

PREGNANCY SUMMARY

After use of imatinib in pregnancy, both normal and abnormal outcomes have been reported.

Because agents in this subclass inhibit angiogenesis, a critical component of embryonic and fetal development, avoiding the drug in pregnancy, especially during organogenesis, is the safest course. However, leukemia is a serious disease that presents a risk to the mother and the eventual outcome of her pregnancy. Consequently, if indicated, treatment with imatinib should not be withheld because of pregnancy.

FETAL RISK SUMMARY

Imatinib (formerly ST1571) is an oral tyrosine kinase inhibitor that inhibits tumor growth, pathologic angiogenesis, and metastatic progression of cancer. There are several other agents in this subclass (see Appendix). Imatinib is indicated for the treatment of newly diagnosed adult patients with Philadelphia chromosome-positive chronic myeloid leukemia in chronic phase. Imatinib is extensively metabolized in the liver. One metabolite has activity that is equipotent to imatinib. The plasma AUC for the active metabolite is about 15% of the AUC for imatinib. The plasma elimination half-lives of imatinib and the active metabolite are about 18 and 40 hours, respectively. Elimination is primarily in the feces. Plasma protein binding is about 95%, mostly to albumin and α-1 glycoprotein (1).

Reproduction studies have been conducted in rats. During organogenesis, oral doses about equal to or greater than the maximum human clinical dose of 800 mg/day based on BSA (MHCD) caused teratogenic effects that included exencephaly or encephalocele, and absent/reduced frontal and absent parietal bones. Doses about half the MHCD during pregnancy were associated with significant postimplantation loss as evidenced by early fetal resorption or stillbirths, nonviable pups, and pup mortality within 4 days of birth. When a dose greater than the MHCD was given, total fetal loss occurred in all animals. Fetal death was not observed at doses one-third the MHCD (1).

Male and female rats were exposed in utero to daily maternal doses of imatinib that were about half the MHCD from day 6 of gestation and through milk during the lactation period. Body weights were reduced from birth. No drug exposure occurred over the next 2 months. Although fertility was not affected, fetal loss was observed when these animals were mated (1).

Imatinib was carcinogenic in 2-year studies in rats, causing renal adenomas/carcinomas, urinary bladder papillomas, and papillomas/carcinomas of the preputial and clitoral gland. Genotoxic and clastogenic effects were seen in some tests. Male rats given daily doses about three-fourths the MHCD for 70 days had decreased testicular and epididymal weights and percent motile sperm. These effects were not seen at one-fourth the MHCD. In female rats, no effects on mating or the number of pregnant females were observed at doses one-fourth the MHCD (1).

It is not known if imatinib or its active metabolite crosses the human placenta. The molecular weight (about 494 for the free base) for the parent compound and the long elimination half-lives for imatinib and its metabolite suggest that the drug will cross to the embryo and fetus.

A 2003 report from the manufacturer described the effects of imatinib on male fertility (2). Although spermatogenesis was impaired in rats, dogs, and monkeys, clinical experience had not confirmed this in humans. The authors cited 18 pregnancies in the partners of men under treatment with imatinib, 13 during clinical trials and 5 from voluntary reports. In the clinical trial group, eight were treated with 400 mg/day for chronic-phase chronic myelogenous (i.e., myeloid) leukemia (CML), four with 800 mg/day for accelerated-phase CML, and one with 800 mg/day for gastrointestinal stromal tumors (GISTs). The outcomes of the pregnancies that occurred during clinical trials were four normal infants, one SAB, two EAs (normal abortuses), one death in utero at 13 weeks' gestation, three with no information, and two with ongoing pregnancies. There was limited information on the five pregnancies in the voluntary reports, four of which were ongoing (2).

The manufacturer also had reports of 26 pregnancies exposed to imatinib, 15 in clinical trials and 11 from voluntary reports (2). In the first group, pregnancy was detected between 5 and 22 weeks' gestation and imatinib therapy was stopped. However, in one woman who was taking 600 mg/day for blast-crises CML and whose therapy was stopped at 22 weeks, imatinib was restarted when the leukemia relapsed. The woman ultimately delivered a normal infant at term. The remaining 14 women in the clinical trial were treated with 400 mg/day for chronic-phase CML. The pregnancy outcomes of these patients were one SAB, nine EAs (no information on abortuses), two pregnancies ongoing, one term normal infant, and one infant with hypospadias (timing of exposure not specified). In the voluntary reports group, pregnancy was detected at 5–23 weeks. Five of the women were being treated for chronic-phase CML (400 mg/day), three for accelerated-phase CML (600 mg/day), one for GIST (200 mg/day), and two unknown. The outcomes of these pregnancies were four SABs, two EAs (one because of hydrocephalus, congenital heart defect, and a two-vessel cord), two ongoing pregnancies, and three with no information (2).

In a 2004 case report, a woman with Philadelphia-positive chronic-phase CML was treated with imatinib 400 mg/day from before conception through the first 7 weeks of gestation (3). Imatinib was stopped immediately when the pregnancy was diagnosed and no further treatment was given until hydroxyurea was started at 29 weeks because of very high white blood cell count. A 2820-g female infant was delivered at 38 weeks' gestation. The infant was morphologically normal but developed pyloric stenosis at 8 weeks of age. She underwent successful surgical correction and is healthy and developing normally at 25 months of age (3).

In a 2005 case similar to the one above, the woman also had Philadelphia-positive chronic-phase CML (4). She had been treated with imatinib for 5 months when a pregnancy was detected at 8 weeks' gestation. Imatinib was stopped and the woman eventually delivered a healthy, 3200-g female in the 38th week. The infant was growing normally (4). Another 2005 report described two women, with the same diagnosis as above, who were treated with imatinib before and throughout three pregnancies (5). One patient taking 400 mg/day delivered a healthy but small (1870-g) infant that was doing well. This patient's second pregnancy ended in an SAB at about 2 months. The second woman took imatinib 200 mg/day and delivered not only a healthy but also small 2540-g infant (5).

A 2005 case report described two women with CML who were treated throughout pregnancy with imatinib 400 mg/day (6). Both women delivered healthy, term infants. The authors noted that long-term follow-up of the infants was required to look for late developing toxicity (6). In contrast, a fatal fetal outcome was reported in 2006 (7). The woman was treated for chronic-phase CML before and during the first 6 weeks of gestation until her pregnancy was diagnosed. Therapy was stopped until the completion of the 1st trimester, at which time hydroxyurea was started. At 30 weeks', a fetal ultrasound revealed a meningocele and 4 weeks later the woman delivered a dead fetus (7).

A 36-year-old woman with accelerated-phase CML was treated with imatinib 600 mg/day until pregnancy was diagnosed in the 12th week (8). Imatinib was discontinued and she was treated with interferon-α for the remainder of the pregnancy. A healthy baby girl weighing 3280-g was delivered at 38 weeks' gestation. The infant was growing and developing normally at 44 months (8).

A 2006 retrospective study reported 19 pregnancies involving 18 patients (10 females and 8 males) with CML who were treated with imatinib (9). In the female patients, receiving 300–800 mg/day, pregnancy was diagnosed between 4 and 9 weeks' gestation and imatinib therapy was discontinued. The pregnancy outcomes (other therapy during remainder of pregnancy) were two SABs (none), one EA (none), seven (1 set of twins) normal infants (hydroxyurea three, interferon one, leukapheresis one, none two), and one infant with hypospadias (hydroxyurea and anagrelide started at 5 weeks'). The male patients, receiving 400–1000 mg/day, fathered eight infants (one fathered two) and an SAB occurred in the 9th pregnancy. One of the infants, a female delivered at 40 weeks' with a birth weight of about 3.4 kg, had a mild rotation of the small intestine that was corrected surgically shortly after birth (9).

In a 2009 report, pregnancy was diagnosed at 21 weeks' in a patient with CML who had been on imatinib throughout (10). Her therapy was changed to interferon-α and she delivered a healthy, full-term male infant who was developing normally (10). A brief 2009 case report described the outcome of a 34-year-old woman with CML who was treated during the first 4 months of an unplanned pregnancy with imatinib (400 mg/day) (11). When pregnancy was diagnosed, imatinib was stopped and hydroxyurea was started. At 37 weeks', she delivered a healthy 3.12-kg infant with Apgar scores of 9 and 10. The child was doing well at 26 months of age. Nine months later, she became pregnant again while on 800 mg/day of imatinib. The therapy was continued throughout pregnancy. She gave birth to a healthy 2.98-kg baby at 37 weeks' with Apgar scores of 10 and 10. The infant was doing well at 9 months of age (11). In a 2011 case report, the therapy of a 24-year-old patient with CML was changed at 10 weeks' from imatinib to hydroxyurea and maintained on the agent for the remainder of her pregnancy (12). A healthy 2.5-kg female baby was born at 37 weeks. At 1-year follow-up, her growth and development were normal (12).

A 27-year-old pregnant woman was diagnosed with Philadelphia chromosome-positive chronic-phase CML (13). Imatinib 400 mg/day was given during 21–39 weeks' gestation, resulting in complete hematological and cytogenetic remission. Fetal growth was normal and a healthy male infant, without defects, was born at 39 weeks. Imatinib concentrations in cord blood and the infant's peripheral blood, 16 hours after the mother's last dose, were 338 ng/mL and 478 ng/mL, respectively (13).

BREASTFEEDING SUMMARY

Consistent with the molecular weight (about 494 for the free base) of the parent compound and the long elimination half-lives of imatinib (18 hours) and its active metabolite (40 hours), both are excreted into breast milk. In a brief 2007 report, a woman taking imatinib 400 mg/day was nursing her 1-month-old infant (14). Steady-state concentrations of the parent drug and metabolite were 1.1–1.4 mcg/mL and 0.8 mcg/mL, respectively. The milk:plasma ratios were 0.5 and 0.9, respectively. Based on the infant's weight, the estimated infant dose from milk was about 10% of the therapeutic dose. No adverse effects in the nursing infant were mentioned (14).

In a case described in the Fetal Risk Summary, a mother with Philadelphia chromosome-positive chronic-phase CML was receiving imatinib 400 mg/day (13). Breast milk concentrations were measured on postpartum days 7, 14, 15, and 16. The concentrations ng/mL (hours after a maternal dose) were 2385 (12 hours), 1430 (14 hours), 2623 (10 hours), 1921 (16 hours), and 2378 (12 hours). The baby had normal growth and development at 10 months of age (13).

A 34-year-old woman taking imatinib 400 mg/day for CML became pregnant and the drug was stopped (15). She delivered a healthy baby at term. Imatinib was immediately restarted and breastfeeding was not recommended. Plasma and milk concentrations of the parent drug and active metabolite were measured at 3, 27, 51, and 171 hours after the start of therapy. Plasma concentrations of imatinib and metabolite were 1301–2003 ng/mL and 177–301 ng/mL, respectively, whereas the milk concentrations were 751–1153 ng/mL and 409–1052 ng/mL, respectively (15).

References

1. Product information. Gleevec. Novartis Pharmaceuticals, 2007.
2. Hensley ML, Ford JM. Imatinib treatment: specific issues related to safety, fertility, and pregnancy. Semin Hematol 2003;40(2 Suppl 2):21–5.
3. Heartin E, Walkinshaw S, Clark RE. Successful outcome of pregnancy in chronic myeloid leukaemia treated with imatinib. Leuk Lymphoma 2004;45:1307–8.
4. Ali R, Ozkalemkas F, Ozcelik T, Ozkocaman V, Ozan U, Kimya Y, Koksal N, Gulten T, Yakut T, Tunali A. Pregnancy under treatment of imatinib and successful labor in a patient with chronic myelogenous leukemia (CML). Outcome of discontinuation of imatinib therapy after achieving a molecular remission. Leuk Res 2005;29:971–3.
5. AlKindi S, Dennison D, Pathare A. Imatinib in pregnancy. Eur J Haematol 2005;74:535–7.
6. Prabhash K, Sastry PSRK, Biswas G, Bakshi A, Prasad N, Menon H, Parikh PM. Pregnancy outcome of two patients treated with imatinib. Ann Oncol 2005;16:1983–4.
7. Choudhary DR, Mishra P, Kumar R, Mahapatra M, Choudhry VP. Pregnancy on imatinib: fatal outcome with meningocele. Ann Oncol 2006;17:178–9.
8. Koh LP, Kanagalingam D. Pregnancies in patients with chronic myeloid leukemia in the era of imatinib. Int J Hematol 2006;84:459–62.
9. Ault P, Kantarjian H, O'Brien S, Faderl S, Beran M, Rios MB, Koller C, Giles F, Keating M, Talpaz M, Cortes J. Pregnancy among patients with chronic myeloid leukemia treated with imatinib. J Clin Oncol 2006;24:1204–8.
10. Klamova J, Markova M, Moravcova J, Siskova M, Cetkovsky P, Polakova KM. Response to treatment in women with chronic myeloid leukemia during pregnancy and after delivery. Leuk Res 2009;33:1567–9.
11. Dolai TK, Bhargava R, Mahapatra M, Mishra P, Seth T, Pati HP, Saxena R. Is imatinib safe during pregnancy? Leuk Res 2009;33:572–3.
12. Martin J, Ramesh A, Devadasan L, Palaniappan N, Martin JJ. An uneventful pregnancy and delivery, in a case with chronic myeloid leukemia on imatinib. Indian J Med Paediatr Oncol 2011;32:109–11.
13. Ali R, Ozkalemkas F, Kimya Y, Koksal N, Ozkocaman V, Gulten T, Yorulmaz H, Tunali A. Imatinib use during pregnancy and breast feeding: a case report and review of the literature. Arch Gynecol Obstet 2009;280:169–75.
14. Gambacorti-Passerini CB, Tornaghi L, Marangon E, Franceschino A, Pogliani EM, D'Incalci M, Zucchhetti M. Imatinib concentrations in human milk. Blood 2007;109:1790.
15. Kronenberger R, Schleyer E, Bornhauser M, Ehninger G, Gattermann N, Blum S. Imatinib in breast milk. Ann Hematol 2009;88:1265–6.

IMIGLUCERASE

Endocrine/Metabolic Agent (Gaucher's Disease)

PREGNANCY RECOMMENDATION: Limited Human Data—Probably Compatible
BREASTFEEDING RECOMMENDATION: Limited Human Data—Probably Compatible

PREGNANCY SUMMARY

No imiglucerase-related adverse effects in embryos and fetuses have been reported in the limited data on pregnancies complicated by type I Gaucher's disease. Pregnancy may exacerbate existing disease or result in new disease manifestations, but the data suggest that treatment may reduce the risk of spontaneous abortion and bleeding complications. However, systematic human or animal studies have not been conducted. Nevertheless, a brief 2009 review cited a recommendation from the European Medicines Agency that in women receiving imiglucerase, treatment continuation throughout pregnancy should be considered (1).

FETAL RISK SUMMARY

Imiglucerase, an enzyme given by IV infusion, is used in the treatment of patients with type I Gaucher's disease. It is in the same pharmacologic subclass as alglucerase, taliglucerase alfa, and velaglucerase alfa. Imiglucerase replaces the endogenous enzyme β-glucocerebrosidase. Imiglucerase is produced by recombinant DNA technology and differs from the endogenous enzyme by one amino acid substitution. After infusion, the terminal elimination half-life is 3.6–10.4 minutes (2).

Reproduction studies with imiglucerase have apparently not been conducted. Moreover, the carcinogenic and mutagenic potential of imiglucerase has not been studied.

It is not known if imiglucerase crosses the human placenta. The relatively high molecular weight (about 55,600) and the short terminal half-life suggest that placental transfer will be limited.

A 2007 case report described the pregnancy outcome of a 23-year-old woman with Gaucher's disease who was treated throughout gestation with imiglucerase 30 U/kg every 2 weeks (3). She gave birth to a healthy female infant at term (additional details not provided).

Outcomes of exposed pregnancies treated with either imiglucerase or the similar enzyme, alglucerase, have been summarized from surveys gathered from international treatment centers, from reports in the literature, as well as from the manufacturer's pharmacovigilance database. The total number of exposed patients is unclear as there could be overlap between the various sources of reports. However, as reviewed in a 2010 publication, among 43 to 78 treated pregnancies compared with 71 to 388 untreated pregnancies with the same disease, the risk of spontaneous abortion, disease-related bleeding complications at delivery, and disease-related complications postpartum were reduced. No evidence of teratogenic risk was noted (4,5). An additional four case reports (which may or may not have been included in the larger review) described successful pregnancy outcome in patients treated with imiglucerase, including three healthy liveborn singletons and one set of healthy liveborn twins (6–8).

BREASTFEEDING SUMMARY

Although the relatively high molecular weight (about 55,600) and the short terminal elimination half-life (3.6–10.4 minutes) suggest that excretion of the enzyme in milk will be limited, one case report did detect imiglucerase. Samples were collected from maternal serum and breast milk before and up to 24 hours after an imiglucerase IV infusion (8). Slightly increased enzymatic activity was observed in the first breast milk sample after the infusion, but levels were undetectable thereafter.

In a 2007 case report discussed earlier, a 23-year-old woman took imiglucerase 30 U/kg every 2 weeks throughout pregnancy and during the first 3 months of breastfeeding (3). Because of Gaucher's disease progression, her dose was increased to 60 U/kg every 2 weeks. She continued this dose until breastfeeding was discontinued at 1 year. Apparently, no toxicity was noted in the infant, but the infant's condition was not mentioned (3).

The effect, if any, on a nursing infant is unknown. However, the enzyme is probably digested in the infant's gut and is unlikely to reach the systemic circulation (1).

References

1. Belmatoug N. Considerations for pregnant patients with Gaucher disease: challenges for the patient and physician. Clin Ther 2009;31(Suppl C):S192–3.
2. Product information. Cerezyme. Genzyme, 2011.
3. Mrsic M, Fumic K, Vrcic H, Potocki K, Stern-Padovan R, Prutki M, Durakoviae N. Successful pregnancy on enzyme replacement therapy with Cerezyme. Clin Ther 2007;29(Suppl C):S84.
4. Zimran A, Morris E, Mengel E, Kaplan P, Belmatoug N, Hughes DA, Malinova V, Heitner R, Sobreira E, Mrsic M, Granovsky-Frisaru S, Amato D, vom Dahl S. The female Gaucher patient: the impact of enzyme replacement therapy around key reproductive events (menstruation, pregnancy and menopause). Blood Cells Mol Dis 2009;43:264–88.
5. Granovsky-Grisaru S, Belmatoug N, vom Dahl S, Mengel E, Morris E, Zimran A. The management of pregnancy in Gaucher disease. Eur J Obstet Gynecol Reprod Biol 2011;156:3–8.
6. Sherer Y, Dulitzki M, Levy Y, Livneh A, Shoenfeld Y, Langevitz P. Successful pregnancy outcome in a patient with Gaucher's disease and antiphospholipid syndrome. Ann Hematol 2002;81:161–3.
7. Malinova V, Poupetova H, Dvorakova L, Zeman J. Enzyme replacement therapy for Gaucher disease in twin pregnancy. Int J Gynaecol Obstet 2009;106:64–6.
8. Sekijima Y, Ohashi T, Ohira S, Kosho T, Fukushima Y. Successful pregnancy and lactation outcome in a patient with Gaucher disease receiving enzyme replacement therapy, and the subsequent distribution and excretion of imiglucerase in human breast milk. Clin Ther 2010;32:2048–52.

IMIPENEM-CILASTATIN SODIUM

Antibiotic

PREGNANCY RECOMMENDATION: Limited Human Data—Animal Data Suggest LowRisk
BREASTFEEDING RECOMMENDATION: Limited Human Data—Probably Compatible

PREGNANCY SUMMARY

No reports describing the use of this antibiotic–enzyme inhibitor combination in the 1st trimester of nonterminated human pregnancies have been located. Four sources consider imipenem–cilastatin to be a safe and effective agent during the perinatal period (1–4).

FETAL RISK SUMMARY

Imipenem, a semisynthetic carbapenem related to the β-lactam antibiotics, is only available in the United States in a 1:1 combination with the enzyme inhibitor cilastatin sodium. The latter agent is a specific, reversible inhibitor of dehydropeptidase I, an enzyme that is present in the proximal renal tubular cells and inactivates imipenem. By inhibiting this enzyme, cilastatin results in higher urinary concentrations of imipenem (5).

Reproductive studies in pregnant rabbits and rats with imipenem at doses up to 2 and 30 times, respectively, and with cilastatin sodium at 10 and 33 times, respectively, the maximum recommended human dose showed no evidence of adverse fetal effects. Similar negative findings were found with imipenem–cilastatin sodium in pregnant mice and rats treated with doses up to 11 times the maximum human dose (5).

Adverse effects observed in pregnant monkeys given either 40 mg/kg/day (IV) or 160 mg/kg/day (SC) included loss of appetite, weight loss, emesis, diarrhea, abortion, and death in some animals. No significant toxicity was observed in nonpregnant monkeys given 180 mg/kg/day SC. An IV infusion of 100 mg/kg/day (approximately three times the maximum daily recommended human IM dose) in pregnant monkeys did not produce significant maternal toxicity or teratogenic effects, but it did result in an increase in embryonic loss (5).

Imipenem–cilastatin crosses the placenta to the fetus (1,6). Seven women at a mean gestational age of 8.6 weeks' gestation (immediately before pregnancy termination) and seven at a mean gestational age of 38.7 weeks were given a single 20-minute IV infusion of 500 mg of imipenem–cilastatin (6). A third, nonpregnant group was also studied. Maternal plasma and amniotic fluid samples were collected at frequent intervals for 8 hours. In comparison with nonpregnant women, imipenem concentrations in maternal plasma were significantly lower in both early and late pregnancy. The mean concentrations in the amniotic fluid in early and late pregnancy were 0.07 and 0.72 mcg/mL, respectively. At delivery, the mean cord venous and arterial blood concentrations were 1.72 and 1.64 mcg/mL, respectively, representing a fetal:maternal mean ratio of 0.33 (venous) and 0.31 (arterial). Transfer of both imipenem and cilastatin across the placenta at term was observed in two Japanese studies (1,2). Peak concentrations of both agents were about 30% of those measured in the maternal blood (2). Both drugs were also transferred to the amniotic fluid, with the highest concentrations occurring, after a single dose, at about 5–6 hours. Peak amniotic fluid:maternal blood ratios for imipenem and cilastatin were approximately 0.30 and 0.45, respectively (2).

In a 2005 study from Japan, the pregnancy outcomes of 100 women who had preterm premature rupture of membranes (PPROM) at 24–31 weeks' and who received imipenem/cilastatin sodium (plus betamethasone) were compared with a control group of 40 women with PPROM who were treated with other antibiotics, such as penicillins or cephalosporins, but not betamethasone (4). The mean time from PPROM to delivery in the study and control groups were 11 and 6 days, respectively. No infants died within 1 year of birth in the study group compared with five infants in controls (4).

BREASTFEEDING SUMMARY

Small amounts of imipenem–cilastatin are excreted into breast milk. These amounts are comparable to other β-lactam antibiotics (1). The effects, if any, on a nursing infant are unknown.

References

1. Matsuda S, Suzuki M, Oh K, Ishikawa M, Soma A, Takada H, Shimizu T, Makinoda S, Fujimoto S, Chimura T, Morisaki N, Matsuo M, Cho N, Fukunaga K, Kunii K, Tamaya T, Hayasaki M, Ito K, Izumi K, Takagi H, Ninomiya K, Tateno M, Okada H, Yamamoto T, Yasuda J, Kanao M, Hirabayashi K, Okada E. Pharmacokinetic and clinical studies on imipenem/cilastatin sodium in the perinatal period. Jpn J Antibiot 1988;11:1731–41.
2. Hirabayashi K, Okada E. Pharmacokinetic and clinical studies of imipenem/cilastatin sodium in the perinatal period. Jpn J Antibiot 1988;11: 1797–804.
3. Cho N, Fukunaga K, Kunii K, Kobayashi I, Tezuka K. Studies on imipenem/cilastatin sodium in the perinatal period. Jpn J Antibiot 1988;11:1758–73.
4. Ryo E, Ikeya M, Sugimoto M. Clinical study of the effectiveness of imipenem/cilastatin sodium as the antibiotics of first choice in the expectant management of patients with preterm premature rupture of membranes. J Infect Chemother 2005;11:32–6.
5. Product information. Primaxin. Merck & Co., 1994.
6. Heikkila A, Renkonen O-V, Erkkola R. Pharmacokinetics and transplacental passage of imipenem during pregnancy. Antimicrob Agents Chemother 1992;36:2652–5.

IMIPRAMINE

Antidepressant

PREGNANCY RECOMMENDATION: Human Data Suggest Low Risk
BREASTFEEDING RECOMMENDATION: Limited Human Data—Potential Toxicity

PREGNANCY SUMMARY

Although structural anomalies have been reported following 1st trimester exposure to imipramine, no pattern of defects is evident when all reports are examined. Neonatal withdrawal is a potential complication when the drug is used near birth.

FETAL RISK SUMMARY

Shepard reviewed six animal reproductive studies involving imipramine in 1989 (1). Some defects were observed in one investigation using rabbits, but other studies with mice, rats, rabbits, and monkeys revealed no evidence of drug-induced teratogenicity.

Bilateral amelia was reported in one child whose mother had ingested imipramine during pregnancy (2). An analysis of 546,505 births, 161 with 1st trimester exposure to imipramine, however, failed to find an association with limb reduction defects (3–15). Reported malformations other than limb reduction included: defective abdominal muscles (1 case); diaphragmatic hernia (2 cases); exencephaly, cleft palate, adrenal hypoplasia (1 case); cleft palate (2 cases); and renal cystic degeneration (1 case) (4–6). These reports indicate that imipramine is not a major cause of congenital limb deformities.

In a surveillance study of Michigan Medicaid recipients involving 229,101 completed pregnancies conducted between 1985 and 1992, 75 newborns had been exposed to imipramine during the 1st trimester (F. Rosa, personal communication, FDA, 1993). Six (8.0%) major birth defects were observed (three expected), including (observed/expected) 3/0.8 cardiovascular defects, 1/0.2 spina bifida, and 1/0.2 hypospadias. No anomalies were observed in three other defect categories (oral clefts, polydactyly, and limb reduction defects) for which specific data were available. Only with cardiovascular defects is there a suggestion of an association, but other factors, including the mother's disease, concurrent drug use, and chance, may be involved.

In a 1996 descriptive case series, the European Network of the Teratology Information Services (ENTIS) prospectively examined the outcomes of 689 pregnancies exposed to antidepressants (16). Multiple drug therapy occurred in about two-thirds of the mothers. Imipramine exposure occurred in 30 pregnancies (1 set of twins). The outcomes of these pregnancies were 1 elective abortion, 3 spontaneous abortions, 25 normal newborns, and 2 infants with congenital defects. The defects (all exposed in the 1st trimester or longer) were six fingers on right hand, and an omphalocele (16).

Neonatal withdrawal symptoms have been reported with the use of imipramine during pregnancy (17–19). Symptoms observed in the infants during the 1st month after birth were colic, cyanosis, rapid breathing, and irritability. Urinary retention in the neonate has been associated with maternal use of nortriptyline (chemically related to imipramine) (20).

A 2002 prospective study compared two groups of mother–child pairs exposed to antidepressants throughout gestation (46 exposed to tricyclics—12 to imipramine; 40 to fluoxetine) with 36 nonexposed, not depressed controls (21). Offspring between the ages 15 and 71 months were studied for effects of antidepressant exposure in terms of IQ, language, behavior, and temperament. Exposure to antidepressants did not adversely affect the measured parameters, but IQ was significantly and negatively associated with the duration of depression, and language was negatively associated with the number of depression episodes after delivery (21).

BREASTFEEDING SUMMARY

Imipramine and its metabolite, desipramine, enter breast milk in low concentrations (22–24). A milk:plasma ratio of 1 has been suggested (22). Assuming a therapeutic serum level of 200 ng/mL, an infant consuming 1000 mL of breast milk would ingest a daily dose of about 0.2 mg. Ten nursing infants of mothers taking antidepressants (four with imipramine 75–150 mg/day) were compared with 15 bottle-fed infants of mothers with depression who did not breastfeed (24). Concentrations of imipramine in fore- and hindmilk ranged from 34 to 408 ng/mL and from 48 to 622 ng/mL, respectively. The milk:maternal plasma ratios were 0.7–1.7 and 1.2–2.3, respectively. In two infants, plasma levels were 0.6 ng/mL (mother's dose 75 mg/day) and 3.3–7.4 ng/mL (mother's dose 75–100 mg/day). No toxic effects or delays in development were observed in the infants. The estimated daily dose consumed by the infants was about 1% of the mother's weight-adjusted dose (24).

The clinical significance of these amounts is unknown. The American Academy of Pediatrics classifies imipramine as an agent whose effect on the nursing infant is unknown but may be of concern (25).

References

1. Shepard TH. *Catalog of Teratogenic Agents*. 6th ed. Baltimore, MD: The Johns Hopkins University Press, 1989:345–6.
2. McBride WG. Limb deformities associated with iminodibenzyl hydrochloride. Med J Aust 1972;1:492.
3. Heinonen OP, Slone D, Shapiro S. *Birth Defects and Drugs in Pregnancy*. Littleton, MA: Publishing Sciences Group, 1977:336–7.
4. Kuenssberg EV, Knox JDE. Imipramine in pregnancy. Br Med J 1972;2:29.
5. Barson AJ. Malformed infant. Br Med J 1972;2:45.
6. Idanpaan-Heikkila J, Saxen L. Possible teratogenicity of imipramine/chloropyramine. Lancet 1973;2:282–3.
7. Crombie DL, Pinsent R, Fleming D. Imipramine in pregnancy. Br Med J 1972; 1:745.

8. Sim M. Imipramine and pregnancy. Br Med J 1972;2:45.
9. Scanlon FJ. Use of antidepressant drugs during the first trimester. Med J Aust 1969;2:1077.
10. Rachelefsky GS, Flynt JW, Eggin AJ, Wilson MG. Possible teratogenicity of tricyclic antidepressants. Lancet 1972;1:838.
11. Banister P, Dafoe C, Smith ESO, Miller J. Possible teratogenicity of tricyclic antidepressants. Lancet 1972;1:838–9.
12. Jacobs D. Imipramine (Tofranil). S Afr Med J 1972;46:1023.
13. Australian Drug Evaluation Committee. Tricyclic antidepressant and limb reduction deformities. Med J Aust 1973;1:766–9.
14. Morrow AW. Imipramine and congenital abnormalities. NZ Med J 1972;75:228–9.
15. Wilson JG. Present status of drugs as teratogens in man. Teratology 1973;7:3–15.
16. McElhatton PR, Garbis HM, Elefant E, Vial T, Bellemin B, Mastroiacovo P, Arnon J, Rodriguez-Pinilla E, Schaefer C, Pexieder T, Merlob P, Dal Verme S. The outcome of pregnancy in 689 women exposed to therapeutic doses of antidepressants. A collaborative study of the European Network of Teratology Information Services (ENTIS). Reprod Toxicol 1996;10:285–94.
17. Hill RM. Will this drug harm the unborn infant? South Med J 1977;67:1476–80.
18. Eggermont E. Withdrawal symptoms in neonate associated with maternal imipramine therapy. Lancet 1973;2:680.
19. Shrand H. Agoraphobia and imipramine withdrawal? Pediatrics 1982;70:825.
20. Shearer WT, Schreiner RL, Marshall RE. Urinary retention in a neonate secondary to maternal ingestion of nortriptyline. J Pediatr 1972;81:570–2.
21. Nulman I, Rovet J, Stewart DE, Wolpin J, Pace-Asciak P, Shuhaiber S, Koren G. Child development following exposure to tricyclic antidepressants or fluoxetine throughout fetal life: a prospective, controlled study. Am J Psychiatry 2002;159:1889–95.
22. Sovner R, Orsulak PJ. Excretion of imipramine and desipramine in human breast milk. Am J Psychiatry 1979;136:451–2.
23. Erickson SH, Smith GH, Heidrich F. Tricyclics and breast-feeding. Am J Psychiatry 1979;136:1483.
24. Yoshida K, Smith B, Craggs M, Kumar RC. Investigation of pharmacokinetics and of possible adverse effects in infants exposed to tricyclic antidepressants in breast-milk. J Affect Disord 1997;43:225–37.
25. Committee on Drugs, American Academy of Pediatrics. The transfer of drugs and other chemicals into human milk. Pediatrics 2001;108:776–89.

IMIQUIMOD

Immunomodulator

PREGNANCY RECOMMENDATION: Limited Human Data Suggest Low Risk
BREASTFEEDING RECOMMENDATION: No Human Data—Probably Compatible

PREGNANCY SUMMARY

The animal reproduction data suggest that the risk of embryo–fetal harm is low. Moreover, an in vitro study with cultured human placental trophoblasts found that the systemic imiquimod concentrations obtained clinically should not alter normal placental function. The human pregnancy experience, however, is limited. Although the combined data suggest that the potential for human developmental toxicity is low, the data are too limited for a more complete assessment. Until such data are available, the safest course is to avoid imiquimod in pregnancy, but if exposure does occur, the risk to the embryo and/or fetus appears to be low.

FETAL RISK SUMMARY

The topical immune response modifier imiquimod is indicated for the treatment of: clinically typical, nonhyperkeratotic, nonhypertrophic actinic keratoses on the face and scalp of immunocompetent adults; biopsy-confirmed primary superficial basal cell carcinoma in immunocompetent adults; and external genital and perianal warts/condyloma acuminata in individuals 12 years of age or older. Small amounts of imiquimod are absorbed systemically and are eliminated slowly with a half-life of about 20 hours. An average dose of 4.6 mg, applied to the affected skin of patients with genital/perianal warts, produced a mean peak serum drug concentration of 0.4 ng/mL. In patients with actinic keratoses treated for 16 weeks, peak serum drug concentrations were 0.1–3.5 ng/mL. The amount absorbed systemically appears to be more related to the surface area treated than to the dose (1).

In vitro studies conducted with imiquimod have shown that it stimulates the production of the cytokines interferon-α, interleukin-1α, interleukin-1β, interleukin-6, and interleukin-8 (2). Because placental trophoblasts also express many of these same cytokines, an in vitro study was conducted to determine if imiquimod exposure during pregnancy could alter normal placental function. In 1st trimester trophoblasts cultured with imiquimod concentrations up to 5.0 mcg/mL, no increase in any of the above interleukins was detected. The results suggested that imiquimod would not induce the expression of inflammatory cytokines in placenta trophoblasts (2).

Reproduction studies have been conducted with oral and IV doses in rats and rabbits. In rats during organogenesis, oral doses 577 times the maximum recommended human dose (MRHD) based on AUC (MRHD-AUC) caused maternal and fetal toxicity. The fetal effects included increased resorptions, decreased body weight, delays in skeletal ossification, and bent limb bones. Two fetuses, among 1567, had exencephaly, protruding tongues, and low-set ears. The no-observed-effect-level for embryo–fetal developmental toxicity was 98 times the MRHD-AUC. In rabbits during organogenesis, no embryo or fetal developmental toxicity was observed with IV doses up to 1.5 times the MRHD based on BSA or with a dose that was 407 times the MRHD-AUC (1).

When imiquimod was given to male and female rats before and during mating, no effects on fertility or mating were noted with oral doses up to 87 times the MRHD-AUC. When these doses were continued throughout pregnancy, parturition, and lactation, no effects were observed on growth or postnatal development. However, bent limb bones in the fetuses were noted, as they were with exposure during organogenesis, in the absence of maternal toxicity. No treatment-related effects were noted at 41 times the MRHD-AUC. Multiple tests with imiquimod revealed no evidence of mutagenic or clastogenic potential (1).

It is not known if imiquimod crosses the human placenta. The low molecular weight (about 240) and long elimination half-life after systemic absorption (about 20 hours) suggest that the drug will reach the embryo and/or fetus. However, because the systemic concentrations are very low, the actual exposure appears to be clinically insignificant.

A 2004 case report described the use of topical imiquimod for the treatment of condylomata acuminata in a woman at 16 weeks' gestation (3). The initial treatment was 3 nights a week for 4 weeks. Because there was very good clinical response, she was prescribed additional treatment, but the woman was lost to follow-up until she delivered vaginally at 41 weeks. The 3.74-kg normal female infant had Apgar scores of 6 and 10 at 1 and 10 minutes, respectively. Subsequent development was apparently normal (3).

A 2006 report described the outcomes of seven pregnancies exposed to topical imiquimod, all ending in live births with a mean birth weight of 3528 g (4). No major malformations or other adverse effects were noted in the infants. The drug had been used for genital warts in four cases and for warts of the hand, face, or foot in three. Doses of the 5% cream ranged from once daily to four times per week with durations ranging from 1 to 10 weeks (average 5 weeks). Two women used the drug in the 1st trimester, one in the 2nd trimester, two in the 2nd and 3rd trimesters, and two in the 3rd trimester only (4).

Two studies reported the use of imiquimod for the treatment of anogenital warts in a total of 21 pregnant women (5,6). No adverse pregnancy outcomes or fetal anomalies were observed.

BREASTFEEDING SUMMARY

No reports describing the use of imiquimod during lactation have been located. The relatively low molecular weight (about 240) and long elimination half-life (about 20 hours) suggest that the drug will be excreted into breast milk. However, the amount absorbed systemically and available for excretion into milk is very low and probably is clinically insignificant. Therefore, although the risk to a nursing infant is unknown, use of imiquimod by the mother appears to be compatible with breastfeeding.

References

1. Product information. Aldara. 3M Pharmaceuticals, 2006.
2. Manlove JM, Zaher FM, Tomai M, Gonik B, Svinarich DM. Effect of imiquimod on cytokine induction in first trimester trophoblasts. Infect Dis Obstet Gynecol 2000;8:105–11.
3. Maw RD. Treatment of external genital warts with 5% imiquimod cream during pregnancy: a case report. BJOG 2004;111:1475.
4. Einarson A, Costei A, Kalra S, Rouleau M, Koren G. The use of topical 5% imiquimod during pregnancy: a case series. Reprod Toxicol 2006;21:1–2.
5. Audisio T, Roca FC, Piatti C. Topical imiquimod therapy for external anogenital warts in pregnant women. Int J Gynaecol Obstet 2008;110:275–86.
6. Ciavattini A, Tsiroglou D, Vichi M, Di Giuseppe J, Cecchi S, Tranquilli AL. Topical imiquimod 5% cream therapy for external anogenital warts in pregnant women: report of four cases and review of the literature. J Matern Fetal Neonatal Med 2012;25:873–6.

IMMUNE GLOBULIN, HEPATITIS B

Serum

PREGNANCY RECOMMENDATION: Compatible
BREASTFEEDING RECOMMENDATION: No Human Data—Probably Compatible

PREGNANCY SUMMARY

The American College of Obstetricians and Gynecologists recommends use of hepatitis B immune globulin in pregnancy for postexposure prophylaxis (1).

FETAL RISK SUMMARY

Hepatitis B immune globulin is used to provide passive immunity following exposure to hepatitis B. When hepatitis B occurs during pregnancy, an increased rate of abortion and prematurity may be observed (1). No risk to the fetus from the immune globulin has been reported (1–3).

BREASTFEEDING SUMMARY

No reports describing the use of hepatitis B immune globulin during human lactation have been located.

References

1. American College of Obstetricians and Gynecologists. Viral hepatitis in pregnancy. *ACOG Practice Bulletin*. No. 86, October 2007. Obstet Gynecol 2007;110:941–55.
2. Amstey MS. Vaccination in pregnancy. Clin Obstet Gynaecol 1983;10:13–22.
3. CDC. Guidelines for vaccinating pregnant women. Available at www.cdc.gov/vaccines/pubs/preg-guide.htm. Accessed May 16, 2010.

IMMUNE GLOBULIN INTRAMUSCULAR

Serum

PREGNANCY RECOMMENDATION: Compatible
BREASTFEEDING RECOMMENDATION: No Human Data—Probably Compatible

PREGNANCY SUMMARY

The American College of Obstetricians and Gynecologists recommends the use of immune globulin intramuscular (IGIM) for postexposure prophylaxis of hepatitis A and measles (rubeola) (1). No risk to the fetus from this therapy has been reported (2).

FETAL RISK SUMMARY

A solution of immunoglobulin, primarily immunoglobulin G, IGIM is prepared from pooled plasma that takes 2–5 days to obtain adequate serum levels (3). It is indicated for postexposure prophylaxis of hepatitis A and measles (rubeola) and in the prevention of serious infections in patients with immunoglobulin deficiencies. In cases of rubella exposure of the pregnant woman, IGIM administered as soon as possible after exposure may prevent or modify maternal infection, but there is no evidence that it will prevent fetal infection (4). However, its use in such cases may be of benefit in women who will not consider therapeutic abortion.

BREASTFEEDING SUMMARY

No reports describing the use of IGIM during human lactation have been located.

References

1. American College of Obstetricians and Gynecologists. Immunization during pregnancy. *ACOG Committee Opinion*. No. 282, January 2003. Obstet Gynecol 2003;101:207–12.
2. CDC. Guidelines for vaccinating pregnant women. Available at www.cdc.gov/vaccines/pubs/preg-guide.htm. Accessed May 16, 2010.
3. Product information. Gammar. Armour Pharmaceutical Co., 1993.
4. American Academy of Pediatrics and the American College of Obstetricians and Gynecologists. *Guidelines for Perinatal Care*. 3rd ed. Elk Grove Village, IL: American Academy of Pediatrics, and Washington, DC: American College of Obstetricians and Gynecologists, 1992:129.

IMMUNE GLOBULIN INTRAVENOUS

Serum

PREGNANCY RECOMMENDATION: Compatible
BREASTFEEDING RECOMMENDATION: No Human Data—Probably Compatible

PREGNANCY SUMMARY

No embryo–fetal risk attributable to immune globulin IV has been identified.

FETAL RISK SUMMARY

Immune globulin IV (IGIV) is a solution of immunoglobulin, primarily immunoglobulin G (IgG), prepared from pooled plasma that, in contrast to the IM preparation, provides immediate serum concentrations of antibodies (1).

IgG administered IV was shown to cross the human placenta in significant amounts only if the gestational age was >32 weeks (2). Placental transfer was also a function of dose, as well as gestational age. Four subclasses of IgG and two different antibodies in the preparation also crossed to the fetus in a similar manner (2). Others have found that the placental transfer of exogenous IgG depends on the dose and duration of treatment and, possibly, on the method of IgG preparation (3).

A 1988 review of IGIV summarized the clinical indications for the product in pregnancy (4). The indications included hypogammaglobulinemia such as common variable immunodeficiency, autoimmune diseases such as chronic immune thrombocytopenic purpura, and alloimmune disorders such as severe Rh-immunization disease and alloimmune thrombocytopenia. Recent reports have described the use of IGIV for the prevention of intracranial hemorrhage in fetal alloimmune thrombocytopenia (5,6), recurrent abortions caused by antiphospholipid antibodies (7,8), neonatal congenital heart block caused by maternal antibodies to Ro (SS-A) and La (SS-B) autoantigens (9), and severe isoimmunization with either Rh or Kell antibodies (10). No adverse effects were observed in the fetus or newborns in any of the above reports, but caution has been advised in its use to prevent spontaneous abortion (11).

BREASTFEEDING SUMMARY

No reports describing the use of immune globulin IV during human lactation have been located.

References

1. Product information. Gamimune N. Miles, Inc., 1993.
2. Sidiropoulos D, Herrmann U Jr, Morell A, von Muralt G, Barandun S. Transplacental passage of intravenous immunoglobulin in the last trimester of pregnancy. J Pediatr 1986;109:505–8.
3. Smith CIE, Hammarström SL. Intravenous immunoglobulin in pregnancy. Obstet Gynecol 1985;66(Suppl):39S–40S.
4. Sacher RA, King JC. Intravenous gamma-globulin in pregnancy: a review. Obstet Gynecol Surv 1988;44:25–34.
5. Lynch L, Bussel JB, McFarland JG, Chitkara U, Berkowitz RL. Antenatal treatment of alloimmune thrombocytopenia. Obstet Gynecol 1992;80:67–71.
6. Wenstrom KD, Weiner CP, Williamson RA. Antenatal treatment of fetal alloimmune thrombocytopenia. Obstet Gynecol 1992;80:433–5.
7. Scott JR, Branch DW, Kochenour NK, Ward K. Intravenous immunoglobulin treatment of pregnant patients with recurrent pregnancy loss caused by antiphospholipid antibodies and Rh immunization. Am J Obstet Gynecol 1988;159:1055–6.
8. Orvieto R, Achiron A, Ben-Rafael Z, Achiron R. Intravenous immunoglobulin treatment for recurrent abortions caused by antiphospholipid antibodies. Fertil Steril 1991;56:1013–20.
9. Kaaja R, Julkunen H, Ämmälä P, Teppo A-M, Kurki P. Congenital heart block: successful prophylactic treatment with intravenous gamma globulin and corticosteroid therapy. Am J Obstet Gynecol 1991;165:1333–4.
10. Chitkara U, Bussel J, Alvarez M, Lynch L, Meisel RL, Berkowitz RL. High-dose intravenous gamma globulin: does it have a role in the treatment of severe erythroblastosis fetalis? Obstet Gynecol 1990;76:703–8.
11. Marzusch K, Tinneberg H, Mueller-Eckhardt G, Kaveri SV, Hinney B, Redman C. Is immunotherapy justified for recurrent spontaneous abortion? Lancet 1992;339:1543.

IMMUNE GLOBULIN, RABIES

Serum

PREGNANCY RECOMMENDATION: Compatible
BREASTFEEDING RECOMMENDATION: No Human Data—Probably Compatible

PREGNANCY SUMMARY

Rabies immune globulin is used to provide passive immunity following exposure to rabies combined with active immunization with rabies vaccine (1). Because rabies is nearly 100% fatal if contracted, both the immune globulin and the vaccine should be given for postexposure prophylaxis (1). No risk to the fetus from the immune globulin has been reported (see also Vaccine, Rabies [Human]) (1–3). The American College of Obstetricians and Gynecologists recommends use of rabies immune globulin in pregnancy for postexposure prophylaxis (1).

BREASTFEEDING SUMMARY

No reports describing the use of rabies immune globulin during human lactation have been located.

References

1. American College of Obstetricians and Gynecologists. Immunization during pregnancy. *Technical Bulletin*. No. 160, October 1991.
2. Amstey MS. Vaccination in pregnancy. Clin Obstet Gynaecol 1983;10:13–22.
3. CDC. Guidelines for vaccinating pregnant women. Available at www.cdc.gov/vaccines/pubs/preg-guide.htm. Accessed May 16, 2010.

IMMUNE GLOBULIN, TETANUS

Serum

PREGNANCY RECOMMENDATION: Compatible
BREASTFEEDING RECOMMENDATION: No Human Data—Probably Compatible

PREGNANCY SUMMARY

Tetanus immune globulin is used to provide passive immunity following exposure to tetanus combined with active immunization with tetanus toxoid (1). Tetanus produces severe morbidity and mortality in both the mother and the newborn. No risk to the fetus from the immune globulin has been reported (1–3). The American College of Obstetricians and Gynecologists recommends the use of tetanus immune globulin in pregnancy for postexposure prophylaxis (1).

BREASTFEEDING SUMMARY

No reports describing the use of tetanus immune globulin during human lactation have been located.

References

1. American College of Obstetricians and Gynecologists. Immunization during pregnancy. *Technical Bulletin*. No. 160, October 1991.
2. Amstey MS. Vaccination in pregnancy. Clin Obstet Gynaecol 1983;10:13–22.
3. CDC. Guidelines for vaccinating pregnant women. Available at www.cdc.gov/vaccines/pubs/preg-guide.htm. Accessed May 16, 2010.

IMMUNE GLOBULIN, VARICELLA-ZOSTER (HUMAN)

Serum

PREGNANCY RECOMMENDATION: Compatible
BREASTFEEDING RECOMMENDATION: No Human Data—Probably Compatible

PREGNANCY SUMMARY

The American College of Obstetricians and Gynecologists recommends that one IM dose of the immune globulin should be given to healthy pregnant women within 96 hours of exposure to varicella to protect against maternal, but not congenital, infection (1). There is no known fetal risk from exposure to immune globulin (2).

FETAL RISK SUMMARY

Varicella-zoster (human) immune globulin (VZIG) is obtained from the plasma of normal volunteer blood donors. In most of the United States, it is available from the American Red Cross Blood Services.

Varicella-zoster immune globulin is indicated for susceptible (seronegative) pregnant women exposed to chickenpox because of the increased severity of maternal chickenpox, including death, in adults compared with children (1,3–14). One reference cited the increased risk of complications in adults as 9- to 25-fold greater than in children (6). It is not known whether administration of VZIG to the mother will protect the fetus from infection or the low risk of defects associated with the congenital varicella syndrome (3,11,13,14). Moreover, VZIG may modify the mother's infection such that she has a subclinical, asymptomatic infection, but not prevent fetal infection or disease (3,11,12,14).

Congenital malformations following intrauterine varicella in pregnancy are relatively uncommon, but case reports have periodically appeared since 1947 (7–9,11,12,15–19). In addition to cicatricial skin lesions, defects associated with this syndrome involve the brain, eyes, skeleton, and gastrointestinal and genitourinary tracts, with the highest risk occurring if the mother has varicella between the 8th and 21st weeks of gestation (7,9,11,19), although one case occurred when the mother had varicella at 25.5 weeks' gestation (20). One review (11) found that the incidence of congenital malformations after 1st trimester chickenpox infection was 2.3% (3/131; 95% confidence intervals 0.5–6.5%), but a second review (9) found a lower rate of 1.3% (4/308) if all cases of intrauterine varicella infection were included.

There is no known fetal risk from passive immunization of pregnant women with varicella-zoster immune globulin (1–3). Administration of VZIG to newborns of mothers who develop varicella within a 5-day interval before or 48 hours after delivery is recommended (1,3,7,13,14).

BREASTFEEDING SUMMARY

No reports describing the use of varicella-zoster immune globulin during human lactation have been located.

References

1. American College of Obstetricians and Gynecologists. Immunization during pregnancy. *ACOG Committee Opinion*. No. 282, January 2003. Obstet Gynecol 2003;101:207–12.
2. CDC. Guidelines for vaccinating pregnant women. Available at www.cdc.gov/vaccines/pubs/preg-guide.htm. Accessed May 16, 2010.
3. Centers for Disease Control and Prevention. Immunization Practices Advisory Committee. Varicella-zoster immune globulin for the prevention of chickenpox. MMWR 1984;33:84–100.
4. Enders G. Management of varicella-zoster contact and infection in pregnancy using a standardized varicella-zoster ELISA test. Postgrad Med J 1985;61(Suppl 4):23–30.
5. McGregor JA, Mark S, Crawford GP, Levin MJ. Varicella zoster antibody testing in the care of pregnant women exposed to varicella. Am J Obstet Gynecol 1987;157:281–4.
6. Greenspoon JS, Masaki DI. Screening for varicella-zoster immunity and the use of varicella zoster immune globulin in pregnancy. Am J Obstet Gynecol 1989;160:1020–1.
7. Sterner G, Forsgren M, Enocksson E, Grandien M, Granstrom G. Varicella-zoster infections in late pregnancy. Scand J Infect Dis Suppl 1990;71:19–26.
8. Prober CG, Gershon AA, Grose C, McCracken GH Jr, Nelson JD. Consensus: varicella-zoster infections in pregnancy and the perinatal period. Pediatr Infect Dis J 1990;9:865–9.
9. Brunell PA. Varicella in pregnancy, the fetus, and the newborn: problems in management. J Infect Dis 1992;166(Suppl 1):S42–7.
10. Wallace MR, Hooper DG. Varicella in pregnancy, the fetus, and the newborn: problems in management. J Infect Dis 1993;167:254.
11. McIntosh D, Isaacs D. Varicella zoster virus infection in pregnancy. Arch Dis Child Fetal Neonatal 1993;68:1–2.
12. Faix RG. Maternal immunization to prevent fetal and neonatal infection. Clin Obstet Gynecol 1991;34:277–87.
13. Committee on Infectious Diseases, American Academy of Pediatrics. Varicella-zoster infections. In: *Report of the Committee on Infectious Diseases*. 22nd ed. Elk Grove Village, IL: American Academy of Pediatrics, 1991:521–2.
14. Brown ZA, Watts DH. Antiviral therapy in pregnancy. Clin Obstet Gynecol 1990;33:276–89.

15. Laforet EG, Lynch CL Jr. Multiple congenital defects following maternal varicella: report of a case. N Engl J Med 1947;236:534–7.
16. Brice JEH. Congenital varicella resulting from infection during second trimester of pregnancy. Arch Dis Child 1976;51:474–6.
17. Bai APV, John TJ. Congenital skin ulcers following varicella in late pregnancy. J Pediatr 1979;94:65–7.
18. Preblud SR, Cochi SL, Orenstein WA. Varicella-zoster infection in pregnancy. N Engl J Med 1986;315:1416–7.
19. Alkalay AL, Pomerance JJ, Rimoin DL. Fetal varicella syndrome. J Pediatr 1987;111:320–3.
20. Salzman MB, Sood SK. Congenital anomalies resulting from maternal varicella at 25½ weeks of gestation. Pediatr Infect Dis J 1992;11:504–5.

INDACATEROL

Respiratory Drug (Bronchodilator)

PREGNANCY RECOMMENDATION: No Human Data—Animal Data Suggest Low Risk
BREASTFEEDING RECOMMENDATION: No Human Data—Probably Compatible

PREGNANCY SUMMARY

No reports describing the use of indacaterol in human pregnancy have been located. The animal reproduction data suggest low risk, but the absence of human pregnancy experience prevents a more complete assessment of embryo–fetal risk. Nevertheless, only small amounts reach the systemic circulation, so if the drug is indicated, it should not be withheld because of pregnancy.

FETAL RISK SUMMARY

Indacaterol is a long-acting β_2-adrenergic agonist that is available as an inhalation powder. It is indicated for long-term, once-daily maintenance bronchodilator treatment of airflow obstruction in patients with chronic obstructive pulmonary disease (COPD), including chronic bronchitis and/or emphysema. The absolute bioavailability after an inhaled dose was, on average, 43–45%.

Indacaterol is extensively metabolized to apparently inactive metabolites. The human serum and plasma protein binding is about 95% and 96%, respectively. The average terminal half-life ranges from 45.5 to 126 hours (1).

Reproduction studies have been conducted with SC doses in rats and rabbits. In these species, indacaterol doses that were about 130 and 260 times, respectively, the human 75 mcg dose based on BSA were not teratogenic (1).

In carcinogenic studies, the drug showed no statistically significant increase in tumor formation in mice or rats. However, similar to other β_2-adrenergic agonists, lifetime treatment in female rats resulted in an increased incidence of benign ovarian leiomyomas. Multiple assays for mutagenic or clastogenic effects were negative. The drug did not impair fertility of rats in reproduction studies (1).

It is not known if indacaterol crosses the human placenta. The molecular weight (about 509) and long terminal half-life suggest that exposure of the embryo–fetus will occur. However, the high serum and plasma protein binding might limit the exposure. Moreover, a relatively small amount of the drug will reach the systemic circulation.

BREASTFEEDING SUMMARY

No reports describing the use of indacaterol during human lactation have been located. The molecular weight (about 509) and long terminal half-life (45.5–126 hours) suggest that the drug will be excreted into breast milk. However, the high serum and plasma protein binding (about 95% and 96%) might limit the exposure. Moreover, a relatively small amount of the drug will reach the systemic circulation. Taken in sum, the drug is probably compatible with breastfeeding.

Reference

1. Product information. Arcapta. Novartis Pharmaceuticals, 2011.

INDAPAMIDE

Diuretic

PREGNANCY RECOMMENDATION: Limited Human Data—Animal Data Suggest Low Risk
BREASTFEEDING RECOMMENDATION: No Human Data—Probably Compatible

PREGNANCY SUMMARY

Although not thought to be teratogenic, diuretics are not recommended for the treatment of gestational hypertension and preeclampsia because of the maternal hypovolemia characteristic of these conditions.

FETAL RISK SUMMARY

Indapamide is an oral active antihypertensive–diuretic of the indoline class that is closely related to the thiazide diuretics (see also Chlorothiazide for a discussion of this class of diuretics). No evidence of impaired fertility, fetal harm, or effect on postnatal development was observed in mice, rats, or rabbits given doses up to 6250 times the therapeutic human dose during pregnancy (1). However, fetal growth restriction has been reported in rats dosed at 1000 mg/kg/day (2).

In an FDA surveillance study of Michigan Medicaid recipients involving 229,101 completed pregnancies conducted between 1985 and 1992, 46 newborns had been exposed to indapamide during the 1st trimester (F. Rosa, personal communication, FDA, 1993). Three (6.5%) major birth defects were observed (two expected). Details on the malformations were not available, but no anomalies were observed in six defect categories (cardiovascular defects, oral clefts, spina bifida, polydactyly, limb reduction defects, and hypospadias) for which specific data were available.

BREASTFEEDING SUMMARY

No reports describing the use of indapamide during lactation have been located. The closely related thiazide diuretics have been used to suppress lactation (see Chlorothiazide).

References

1. Product information. Indapamide Tablets, USP. Mylan Pharmaceuticals, 2000.
2. Seki T, Fujitani M, Osumi S, Yamamoto T, Eguchi K, Inoue N, Sakka N, Suzuki MR. Reproductive studies of indapamide. Yakuri to Chiryo 1982;10:1325–35, 1337–53, 1355–1414. As cited in Shepard TH. *Catalog of Teratogenic Agents*. 6th ed. Baltimore, MD: The Johns Hopkins University Press, 1989:347.

I

INDIGO CARMINE

Dye (Diagnostic)

PREGNANCY RECOMMENDATION: Limited Human Data—No Relevant Animal Data
BREASTFEEDING RECOMMENDATION: No Human Data—Probably Compatible

PREGNANCY SUMMARY

Indigo carmine is used as a diagnostic dye. No reports linking its use with congenital defects have been located. Intra-amniotic injection has been conducted without apparent effect on the fetus (1–4). Because of its known toxicities after IV administration, however, the dye should not be considered totally safe (5).

FETAL RISK SUMMARY

A report of jejunal atresia, possibly secondary to the use of methylene blue (see Methylene Blue) during genetic amniocentesis in pregnancies with twins was published in 1992 (6). A portion of this report described 67 newborns treated for the defect, 20 of whom were one of a set of twins. Of these latter cases, 2nd trimester amniocentesis had been performed with indigo carmine in 1 case and with methylene blue in 18 cases. An accompanying commentary noted that indigo carmine, like methylene blue, is a vasoconstrictor and may also induce small bowel atresia (7).

A brief 1993 report described the use of indigo carmine in women with twins who underwent amniocentesis between 1977 and 1991 in the United States (8). A total of 195 women were included, 78 (40%) of whom were administered indigo carmine during the procedure. Of the 156 fetuses (total data included live births, stillbirths, intrauterine deaths, and fetuses that were electively terminated; specific data for indigo carmine were not given), 7 (4.5%) had a major birth defect. Included in this number were two infants from the same set of twins who had syndactyly, one clubfoot, one hydrocephaly, one urethral obstruction sequence, and two multiple congenital defects (8). None of the exposed infants had small intestinal atresia.

BREASTFEEDING SUMMARY

No reports describing the use of indigo carmine during human lactation have been located.

References

1. Elias S, Gerbie AB, Simpson JL, Nadler HL, Sabbagha RE, Shkolnik A. Genetic amniocentesis in twin gestations. Am J Obstet Gynecol 1980;138:169–74.
2. Horger EO III, Moody LO. Use of indigo carmine for twin amniocentesis and its effect on bilirubin analysis. Am J Obstet Gynecol 1984;150:858–60.
3. Pijpers L, Jahoda MGJ, Vosters RPL, Niermeijer MF, Sachs ES. Genetic amniocentesis in twin pregnancies. Br J Obstet Gynaecol 1988;95:323–6.
4. Quintero RA, Morales WJ, Allen M, Bornick PW, Arroyo J, LeParc G. Treatment of iatrogenic previable premature rupture of membranes with intra-amniotic injection of platelets and cryoprecipitate (amniopatch): preliminary experience. Am J Obstet Gynecol 1999;181:744–9.
5. Fribourg S. Safety of intraamniotic injection of indigo carmine. Am J Obstet Gynecol 1981;140:350–1.
6. Van Der Pol JG, Wolf H, Boer K, Treffers PE, Leschot NJ, Hey HA, Vos A. Jejunal atresia related to the use of methylene blue in genetic amniocentesis in twins. Br J Obstet Gynaecol 1992;99:141–3.
7. McFadyen I. The dangers of intra-amniotic methylene blue. Br J Obstet Gynaecol 1992;99:89–90.
8. Cragan JD, Martin ML, Khoury MJ, Fernhoff PM. Dye use during amniocentesis and birth defects. Lancet 1993;341:1352.

INDINAVIR

Antiviral

PREGNANCY RECOMMENDATION: Compatible—Maternal Benefit >> Embryo–Fetal Risk
BREASTFEEDING RECOMMENDATION: Contraindicated

PREGNANCY SUMMARY

The limited human data do not suggest a major embryo–fetal risk, but the animal data involving birth defects are a concern. The finding of anophthalmia in rat pups at a systemic exposure approximately equivalent to human exposure needs further investigation. The authors of that study also observed anophthalmia in a rat experiment with ritonavir (1 of 113 offspring, unpublished data), another protease inhibitor (1). An editorial, accompanying this study, reviewed how the changes in the treatment of HIV disease (e.g., multiple combinations of drugs and use of agents throughout gestation) were altering the risk:benefit ratio of antiretroviral therapy during pregnancy (2). However, if indicated, the drug should not be withheld because of pregnancy.

I

FETAL RISK SUMMARY

The antiretroviral agent, indinavir, is an inhibitor of the HIV protease, an enzyme that is required for the cleavage of viral polyprotein precursors into active functional proteins found in infectious HIV.

Indinavir was not teratogenic in rats and rabbits at doses comparable to or slightly higher than those used in humans (3). In rats, however, an increase in the incidence of supernumerary ribs (at exposures at or less than those in humans) and cervical ribs (at exposures at or slightly greater than those in humans) were observed. These changes were not observed in rabbits and no effects were noted on embryonic and/or fetal survival or on fetal weight in either rats or rabbits. A study in dogs (because fetal exposure was about 2% of maternal levels in rabbits) observed no indinavir-related effects on embryo or fetal survival, fetal weight, or teratogenicity. At the highest dose tested in dogs, 80 mg/kg/day, fetal drug levels were about 50% of the maternal levels (3).

A study of the developmental toxicity of indinavir in rats was reported in 2000 (1). Pregnant rats were given an oral dose of 500 mg/kg once daily during day 6 to 15 of gestation or twice daily from day 9 to 11 of gestation (a dose of 640 mg/kg/day produces systemic exposure in the rat that is comparable to or slightly greater than human exposure). In both groups, an increased incidence of supernumerary ribs and variations of the vertebral ossification centers occurred, but no effects on litter sizes, fetal weight, or viability were observed. Unilateral anophthalmia was observed in 7 pups (3%) from 2 of the 19 litters. On examination, the ocular bulbs were noted to be absent and the bulbar cavity was filled with an enlarged lacrimal gland. No such cases were noted in controls. Other postnatal abnormalities included delayed fur development, eye opening, and slightly earlier descent of the testis. In addition, some liver changes were noted in dams (hepatocellular inclusions of lipids and myelin figure-like structures) and in offspring (infiltration with granulocytes) (1).

It is not known if indinavir crosses the human placenta. The molecular weight (about 712 for the sulfate salt) is low enough that transfer to the fetus should be expected. The drug has been found in fetal plasma of rats, rabbits, dogs, and monkeys (3). In monkeys, fetal plasma drug levels were 1%–2% of maternal plasma levels about 1 hour after a dose given in the 3rd trimester (3).

The pharmacokinetics of indinavir during pregnancy has been reported in two women (800 mg every 8 hours) (4). A marked decrease in maternal drug concentrations occurred around 33–34 weeks' gestation, suggesting that women may be exposed to subtherapeutic levels late in pregnancy.

The Antiretroviral Pregnancy Registry reported, for the period January 1989 through July 2009, prospective data (reported before the outcomes were known) involving 4702 live births that had been exposed during the 1st trimester to one or more antiretroviral agents (5). Congenital defects were noted in 134, a prevalence of 2.8% (95% confidence interval [CI] 2.4–3.4). In the 6100 live births with earliest exposure in the 2nd/3rd trimester, there were 153 infants with defects (2.5%, 95% CI 2.1–2.9). The prevalence rates for the two periods did not differ significantly. There were 288 infants with birth defects among 10,803 live births with exposure anytime during pregnancy (2.7%, 95% CI 2.4–3.0). The prevalence rate did not differ significantly from the rate expected in a nonexposed population. There were 436 outcomes exposed to indinavir (276 in the 1st trimester and 160 in the 2nd/3rd trimester) in combination with other antiretroviral agents. There were nine birth defects (six in the 1st trimester and three in the 2nd/3rd trimester). In reviewing the birth defects of prospective and retrospective (pregnancies reported after the outcomes were known) registered cases, the Registry concluded that, except for isolated cases of neural tube defects with efavirenz exposure in retrospective reports, there was no other pattern of anomalies (isolated or syndromic) (5) (see Lamivudine for required statement).

In an unusual case, a woman was exposed to HIV through self-insemination with fresh semen obtained from a man with a high HIV ribonucleic acid viral load (>750,000 copies/mL plasma) (6). Ten days later, she was started on a prophylactic regimen of indinavir (2400 mg/day), zidovudine (600 mg/day), and lamivudine (300 mg/day). Pregnancy was confirmed 14 days after insemination. Four weeks after the start of therapy, the indinavir dose was reduced to 1800 mg/day because of the development of renal calculi. The antiretroviral therapy was stopped after 9 weeks because of negative tests for HIV. She gave birth at 40 weeks' gestation to a healthy 3490-g male infant, without evidence of HIV disease, who was developing normally at 2 years of age (6).

The experience of one perinatal center with the treatment of HIV-infected pregnant women was summarized in a 1999 abstract (7). Of 55 women receiving ≥3 antiviral drugs, 39 were treated with a protease inhibitor (5 with indinavir). The outcomes included 2 spontaneous abortions, 5 elective abortions, 27 newborns, and 5 ongoing pregnancies. One woman was taken off indinavir because of ureteral obstruction and another woman (drug therapy not specified) developed gestational diabetes. None of the newborns tested positive for HIV or had major congenital anomalies or complications (7).

A study published in 1999 evaluated the safety, efficacy, and perinatal transmission rates of HIV in 30 pregnant women receiving various combinations of antiretroviral agents (8). Many of the women were substance abusers. Protease inhibitors (indinavir $N = 6$, nelfinavir $N = 7$, and saquinavir $N = 1$ in combination with nelfinavir) were used in 13 of the women. Antiretroviral therapy was initiated at a median of 14 weeks' gestation (range preconception to 32 weeks). In spite of previous histories of extensive antiretroviral experience and of vertical transmission of HIV, combination therapy was effective in treating maternal disease and in preventing transmission to the current newborns. The outcomes of the pregnancies treated with protease inhibitors appeared to be similar to the 17 cases in which these were not used, except that the birth weights were lower (8).

Indinavir has frequently produced hyperbilirubinemia in adults, but it is not known whether treatment of the mother prior to delivery will exacerbate physiologic hyperbilirubinemia in the neonate (3). No such effects have been observed in monkey neonates exposed in utero to indinavir during the 3rd trimester.

A public health advisory was issued by the FDA on the association between protease inhibitors and diabetes mellitus (9). Because pregnancy is a risk factor for hyperglycemia, there was concern that these antiviral agents would exacerbate this risk. An abstract published in 2000 described the results of a study involving 34 pregnant women treated with protease inhibitors (4 with indinavir) compared with 41 controls that evaluated the association with diabetes (10). No relationship between protease inhibitors and an increased incidence of gestational diabetes was found.

A multicenter, retrospective survey of pregnancies exposed to protease inhibitors was published in 2000 (11). There were 92 liveborn infants delivered from 89 women (3 sets of twins) at six health care centers. One nonviable infant, born at 22 weeks' gestation, died. The surviving 91 infants were evaluated in terms of adverse effects, prematurity rate, and frequency of HIV-1 transmission. Most of the infants were exposed in utero to a single protease inhibitor, but a few were exposed to more than one because of sequential or double-combined therapy. The number of newborns exposed to each protease inhibitor was indinavir ($N = 23$), nelfinavir ($N = 39$), ritonavir ($N = 5$), and saquinavir ($N = 34$). Protease inhibitors were started before conception in 18, during the 1st, 2nd, or 3rd trimester in 12, 44, and 14, respectively, and not reported in one. Other antiretrovirals used with the protease inhibitors included four nucleoside reverse transcriptase inhibitors (NRTIs) (didanosine, lamivudine, stavudine, and zidovudine). The most common NRTI regimen was a combination of zidovudine and lamivudine (65% of women). In addition, seven women were enrolled in the AIDS Clinical Trials Group Protocol 316 and, at the start of labor, received either a single dose of the nonnucleoside reverse transcriptase inhibitor, nevirapine, or placebo. Maternal conditions, thought possibly or likely to be related to therapy, were mild anemia in eight, severe anemia in one (probably secondary to zidovudine), and thrombocytopenia in one. Gestational diabetes mellitus was observed in three women (3.3%), a rate similar to the expected prevalence of 2.6% in a nonexposed population. One mother developed postpartum cardiomyopathy and died 2 months after birth of twins, but the cause of death was not known. For the surviving newborns, there was no increase in adverse effects over that observed in previous clinical trials of HIV-positive women, including the prevalence of anemia (12%), hyperbilirubinemia (6%; none exposed to indinavir), and low birth weight (20.6%). Premature delivery occurred in 19.1% of the pregnancies (close to the expected rate). The percentage of infants infected with HIV was 0 (95% CI 0–3%) (11).

Two reviews, one in 1996 and the other in 1997, concluded that all women receiving antiretroviral therapy should continue to receive therapy during pregnancy and that treatment of the mother with monotherapy should be considered inadequate therapy (12,13). The same conclusion was reached in a 2003 review with the added admonishment that therapy must be continuous to prevent emergence of resistant viral strains (14). In 2009, the updated U.S. Department of Health and Human Services guidelines for the use of antiretroviral agents in HIV-1-infected patients continued the recommendation that therapy, with the exception of efavirenz, should be continued during pregnancy (15). If indicated, therefore, protease inhibitors, including indinavir, should not be withheld in pregnancy because the expected benefit to the HIV-positive mother outweighs the unknown risk to the fetus. Pregnant women taking protease inhibitors should be monitored for hyperglycemia. Updated guidelines for the use of antiretroviral drugs to reduce perinatal HIV-1 transmission also were released in 2010 (16). Women receiving antiretroviral therapy during pregnancy should continue the therapy but, regardless of the regimen, zidovudine administration is recommended during the intrapartum period to prevent vertical transmission of HIV to the newborn (16).

BREASTFEEDING SUMMARY

No reports describing the use of indinavir during lactation have been located. The molecular weight (about 712 for the sulfate salt) is low enough that excretion into breast milk should be expected.

Reports on the use of indinavir during lactation are unlikely because of the potential toxicity in the nursing infant, especially hyperbilirubinemia, and because the drug is indicated in the treatment of patients with HIV. HIV-1 is transmitted in milk, and in developed countries, breastfeeding is not recommended (12,13,15,17–19). In developing countries, breastfeeding is undertaken, despite the risk, because there are no affordable milk substitutes available. Until 1999, no studies have been published that examined the effect of any antiretroviral therapy on HIV-1 transmission in milk. In that year, a study involving zidovudine was published that measured a 38% reduction in vertical transmission of HIV-1 infection despite breastfeeding when compared with controls (see Zidovudine).

References

1. Riecke K, Schultz TG, Shakibaei M, Krause B, Chahoud I, Stahlmann R. Developmental toxicity of the HIV-protease inhibitor indinavir in rats. Teratology 2000;62:291–300.
2. Miller RK. Anti-HIV therapy during pregnancy: risk–benefit ratio. Teratology 2000;62:288–90.
3. Product information. Crixivan. Merck, 2001.
4. Hayashi S, Beckerman K, Homma M, Kosel BW, Aweeka FT. Pharmacokinetics of indinavir in HIV-positive pregnant women. AIDS 2000;14:1061–2.
5. Antiretroviral Pregnancy Registry Steering Committee. *Antiretroviral Pregnancy Registry International Interim Report for 1 January 1989 through 31 July 2009*. Wilmington, NC: Registry Coordinating Center; 2009. Available at www.apregistry.com. Accessed May 29, 2010.
6. Bloch M, Carr A, Vasak E, Cunningham P, Smith D. The use of human immunodeficiency virus postexposure prophylaxis after successful artificial insemination. Am J Obstet Gynecol 1999;181:760–1.
7. Stek A, Kramer F, Fassen M, Khoury M. The safety and efficacy of protease inhibitor therapy for HIV infection during pregnancy (abstract). Am J Obstet Gynecol 1999;180:S7.
8. McGowan JP, Crane M, Wiznia AA, Blum S. Combination antiretroviral therapy in human immunodeficiency virus-infected pregnant women. Obstet Gynecol 1999;94:641–6.
9. CDC. Public Health Service Task Force recommendations for the use of antiretroviral drugs in pregnant women infected with HIV-1 for maternal health and for reducing perinatal HIV-1 transmission in the United States. MMWR 1998;47:No. RR-2.
10. Fassett M, Kramer F, Stek A. Treatment with protease inhibitors in pregnancy is not associated with an increased incidence of gestational diabetes (abstract). Am J Obstet Gynecol 2000;182:S97.
11. Morris AB, Cu-Uvin S, Harwell JI, Garb J, Zorrilla C, Vajaranant M, Dobles AR, Jones TB, Carlan S, Allen DY. Multicenter review of protease inhibitors in 89 pregnancies. J Acquir Immune Defic Syndr 2000;25:306–11.
12. Carpenter CCJ, Fischi MA, Hammer SM, Hirsch MS, Jacobsen DM, Katzenstein DA, Montaner JSG, Richman DD, Saag MS, Schooley RT, Thompson MA, Vella S, Yeni PG, Volberding PA. Antiretroviral therapy for HIV infection in 1996. JAMA 1996;276:146–54.
13. Minkoff H, Augenbraun M. Antiretroviral therapy for pregnant women. Am J Obstet Gynecol 1997;176:478–89.
14. Minkoff H. Human immunodeficiency virus infection in pregnancy. Obstet Gynecol 2003;101:797–810.
15. Panel on Antiretroviral Guidelines for Adults and Adolescents. *Guidelines for the Use of Antiretroviral Agents in HIV-1-infected Adults and Adolescents*. Department of Health and Human Services. December 1, 2009:1–161. Available at http://www.aidsinfo.nih.gov/ContentFiles/AdultandAdolescentGL.pdf. Accessed September 17, 2010:60, 96–8.
16. Panel on Treatment of HIV-Infected Pregnant Women and Prevention of Perinatal Transmission. *Recommendations for Use of Antiretroviral Drugs in Pregnant HIV-1-Infected Women for Maternal Health and Interventions to Reduce Perinatal HIV Transmission in the United States.* May 24, 2010:1–117. Available at http://aidsinfo.nih.gov/ContentFiles/PerinatalGL.pdf. Accessed September 17, 2010:30 (Table 5).
17. Brown ZA, Watts DH. Antiviral therapy in pregnancy. Clin Obstet Gynecol 1990;33:276–89.
18. de Martino M, Tovo P-A, Pezzotti P, Galli L, Massironi E, Ruga E, Floreea F, Plebani A, Gabiano C, Zuccotti GV. HIV-1 transmission through breast-milk: appraisal of risk according to duration of feeding. AIDS 1992;6:991–7.
19. Van de Perre P. Postnatal transmission of human immunodeficiency virus type 1: the breast feeding dilemma. Am J Obstet Gynecol 1995;173:483–7.

INDOMETHACIN

Nonsteroidal Anti-inflammatory

PREGNANCY RECOMMENDATION: Human Data Suggest Risk in 1st and 3rd Trimesters
BREASTFEEDING RECOMMENDATION: Limited Human Data—Probably Compatible

PREGNANCY SUMMARY

Indomethacin use during the latter part of pregnancy may cause severe fetal toxicity. Short-term use, such as 24–48 hours, lessens the risk. Based on animal data, prostaglandin synthesis inhibitors, including indomethacin, might block blastocyst implantation. Nonsteroidal anti-inflammatory agents (NSAIDs) also have been associated with spontaneous abortions (SABs) and congenital malformations, but the absolute risk appears to be low.

FETAL RISK SUMMARY

Indomethacin is an NSAID. It is indicated for the relief of the signs and symptoms of moderate-to-severe rheumatoid arthritis, osteoarthritis, gouty arthritis, ankylosing spondylitis, and acute painful shoulder (bursitis and/or tendonitis). Indomethacin is in the same subclass (acetic acids) as three other NSAIDs (diclofenac, sulindac, and tolmetin).

Shepard (1) reviewed four reproduction studies on the use of indomethacin in mice and rats. Fused ribs, vertebral abnormalities, and other skeletal defects were seen in mouse fetuses, but no malformations were observed in rats except for premature closure of the ductus arteriosus in some fetuses. A 1990 report described an investigation on the effects of several nonsteroidal anti-inflammatory agents on mouse palatal fusion both in vivo and in vitro (2). All of the compounds were found to induce some degree of cleft palate, although indomethacin was associated with the lowest frequency of cleft palate of the five agents tested (diclofenac, indomethacin, mefenamic acid, naproxen, and sulindac).

Indomethacin crosses the placenta to the fetus with concentrations in the fetus equal to those in the mother (3). Twenty-six women, between 23 and 37 weeks' gestation, who were undergoing cordocentesis for varying indications, were given a single 50-mg oral dose approximately 6 hours before the procedure. Mean maternal and fetal indomethacin levels were 218 and 219 ng/mL, respectively, producing a mean ratio of 0.97. The mean amniotic fluid level, 21 ng/mL, collected during cordocentesis, was significantly lower than the maternal and fetal concentrations. Neither fetal nor amniotic fluid concentrations varied with gestational age.

In a surveillance study of Michigan Medicaid recipients involving 229,101 completed pregnancies conducted between 1985 and 1992, 114 newborns had been exposed to indomethacin during the 1st trimester (F. Rosa, personal communication, FDA, 1993). Seven (6.1%) major birth defects were observed (five expected), two of which were cardiovascular defects (one expected). No anomalies were observed in five other defect categories (oral clefts, spina bifida, polydactyly, limb reduction defects, and hypospadias) for which specific data were available.

A combined 2001 population-based, observational cohort study and a case–control study estimated the risk of adverse pregnancy outcome from the use of NSAIDs (4). The use of NSAIDs during pregnancy was not associated with congenital malformations, preterm delivery, or low birth weight, but a positive association was discovered with SABs. A similar study, also published in 2001, failed to find a relationship, in general, between NSAIDs and congenital malformations, but did find a significant association with cardiac defects and orofacial clefts (5), In addition, a 2003 study found a significant association between exposure to NSAIDs in early pregnancy and SABs (6) (see Ibuprofen for details on these three studies).

A brief 2003 editorial on the potential for NSAID-induced developmental toxicity concluded that NSAIDs, and specifically those with greater COX-2 affinity, had a lower risk of this toxicity in humans than aspirin (7).

Indomethacin is occasionally used in the treatment of premature labor (8–40). The drug acts as a prostaglandin synthesis inhibitor and is an effective tocolytic agent, including in those cases resistant to β-mimetics. Niebyl (33) reviewed this topic in 1981. Daily doses ranged from 100 to 200 mg usually by the oral route, but rectal administration was used as well. In most cases, indomethacin, either alone or in combination with other tocolytics, was successful in postponing delivery until fetal lung maturation had occurred. More recent reviews on the use of indomethacin as a tocolytic agent appeared in 1992 (37) and 1993 (38). The latter review concluded that the prostaglandin synthesis inhibitors, such as indomethacin, might be the only effective tocolytic drugs (38).

In a 1986 report, 46 infants exposed in utero to indomethacin for maternal tocolysis were compared with two control groups: (a) 43 infants exposed to other tocolytics and (b) 46 infants whose mothers were not treated with tocolytics (34). Indomethacin-treated women received one or two courses of 150 mg orally over 24 hours, all before 34 weeks' gestation. No significant differences were observed between the groups in Apgar scores, birth weight, or gestational age at birth. Similarly, no differences were found in the number of neonatal complications such as hypocalcemia, hypoglycemia, respiratory distress syndrome, need for continuous positive airway pressure, pneumothorax, patent ductus arteriosus, sepsis, exchange transfusion for hyperbilirubinemia, congenital anomalies, or mortality (34).

A 1989 study compared indomethacin, 100-mg rectal suppository followed by 25 mg orally every 4 hours for 48 hours, with IV ritodrine in 106 women in preterm labor with intact membranes who were at a gestational age of ≤32 weeks (39). Fifty-two women received indomethacin and 54 received ritodrine. Thirteen (24%) of the ritodrine group developed adverse drug reactions severe enough to require discontinuance of the drug and a change to magnesium sulfate: cardiac arrhythmia ($N = 1$), chest pain ($N = 2$), tachycardia ($N = 3$), and hypotension ($N = 7$). None of the indomethacin-treated women developed drug intolerance ($p < 0.01$). The outcomes of the pregnancies were similar, regardless of whether delivery occurred close to the time of therapy or not. Of those delivered within 48 hours of initiation of therapy, the mean glucose level in the ritodrine-exposed newborns ($N = 9$) was significantly higher than the level in those exposed to indomethacin ($N = 8$), 198 vs. 80 mg/dL ($p < 0.05$), respectively. No cases of premature closure of the ductus arteriosus or pulmonary hypertension were observed. A reduction in amniotic fluid volume was noted in 3 (5.6%) of the ritodrine group and in 6 (11.5%) of those treated with indomethacin. With regard to cost, tocolysis with indomethacin was 17 times less costly than tocolysis with ritodrine (39).

The tocolytic effects of indomethacin and magnesium sulfate ($MgSO_4$) were compared in a study of women in labor at less than 32 weeks' gestation (40). A total of 49 women were treated with indomethacin, 100 mg per rectum followed by 25 mg orally every 4 hours for 48 hours, whereas 52 women were administered IV $MgSO_4$. Women who had responded to the initial treatment were then changed to oral terbutaline. All women received betamethasone and vitamin K and some received IV phenobarbital as prophylaxis against hyaline membrane disease and neonatal intracranial hemorrhage. Both indomethacin and $MgSO_4$ were effective in delaying delivery more than 48 hours, 90% vs. 85%, respectively, and combined with terbutaline, in extending the gestation, 22.9 vs. 22.7 days, respectively (40). Renal function of the newborns delivering at ≤48 hours (indomethacin, $N = 5$; $MgSO_4$, $N = 8$) as measured by blood urea nitrogen, creatinine, and urine output during the first 2 days after birth were statistically similar between the groups. Other neonatal outcomes, including the incidence of respiratory distress syndrome, intraventricular hemorrhage (all grades), and intraventricular hemorrhage (grades 3 and 4), were also similar. Tocolytic therapy was discontinued in eight (15%) of the women treated with $MgSO_4$ because of maternal adverse reactions compared with none in the indomethacin group ($p < 0.05$) (40).

Complications associated with the use of indomethacin during pregnancy may include premature closure of the ductus arteriosus, which may result in primary pulmonary hypertension of the newborn and, in severe cases, neonatal death (8–12,37,38,41–48). Ductal constriction is dependent on the gestational age of the fetus, starting as early as 27 weeks (49,50), and increasing markedly at 27–32 weeks (50,51), and occur with similar frequencies in singleton and multiple gestations (51). Further, constriction is independent of fetal serum indomethacin levels (49,50). Primary pulmonary hypertension of the newborn is caused by the shunting of the right ventricular outflow into the pulmonary vessels when the fetal ductus arteriosus narrows. This results in pulmonary arterial hypertrophy (48). Persistent fetal circulation occurs after birth secondary to pulmonary hypertension shunting blood through the foramen ovale, bypassing the lungs and still patent ductus arteriosus, with resultant difficulty in adequate oxygenation of the neonate (48).

Using fetal echocardiography, researchers described the above effects in a study of 13 women (14 fetuses, 1 set of twins) between the gestational ages of 26.5 and 31.0 weeks (48). The patients were treated with 100–150 mg of indomethacin orally per day. Fetal ductal constriction occurred in 7 of 14 fetuses 9.5–25.5 hours after the first dose and was not correlated with either gestational age or maternal indomethacin serum levels. In two other cases not included in the present series, ductal constriction did not occur until several weeks after the start of therapy. Tricuspid regurgitation was observed in three of the fetuses with ductal constriction. This defect was caused by the constriction-induced elevated pressure in the right ventricular outflow tract producing mild endocardial ischemia with papillary muscle dysfunction (48). All cases of constriction, including two of the three with tricuspid regurgitation, resolved within 24 hours after indomethacin was discontinued. The third tricuspid case returned to normal 40 hours after resolution of the ductal constriction. No cases of persistent fetal circulation were observed in the 11 newborns studied. Some have questioned the methods used in the aforementioned study and whether the results actually reflected fetal ductal constriction (52). In response, the authors of the original paper defended their techniques based on both animal and human experimental findings (53).

A 1987 report described a patient with premature labor who was treated for 29 days between 27 and 32 weeks' gestation with a total indomethacin dose of 6.2 g (54). The woman delivered a female infant who had patent ductus arteriosus that persisted for 4 weeks. A macerated twin fetus, delivered at the same time as the surviving infant, was thought to have died before the initiation of treatment.

Administration of indomethacin to the mother results in reduced fetal urine output. Severe oligohydramnios, meconium staining, constriction of the ductus arteriosus, and death were reported in the offspring of three women treated for preterm labor at 32–33 weeks' gestation (55). Indomethacin doses were 100 mg (1 case) and 400 mg (2 cases) during the first 24 hours, followed by 100 mg/day for 2–5 days. Two of the fetuses were stillborn, and the third died within 3 hours of birth. A second report described a woman with preterm labor at 24 weeks' gestation, who was treated with IV ritodrine and indomethacin, 300 mg/day, for 8 weeks (56). A reduction in the amount of amniotic fluid was noted at 28 weeks' gestation (after 4 weeks of therapy), and severe oligohydramnios was present 4 weeks later. Filling of the fetal bladder could not be visualized at this time. The infant, who died 47 hours after birth, had the characteristic facies of Potter's syndrome (i.e., oligohydramnios sequence), but autopsy revealed a normal urinary tract with normal kidneys. Both cardiac ventricles were hypertrophic and the lungs showed no evidence of pulmonary hypertension (56).

In a 1987 study involving eight patients with polyhydramnios and premature uterine contractions, indomethacin, administered by oral tablets or vaginal suppositories in a dose of 2.2–3.0 mg/kg/day, resolved the condition in each case (57). Four of the patients had diabetes mellitus. The gestational age of the patients at the start of treatment ranged between 21.5 and 34 weeks. The duration of therapy, which was stopped between 34.5 and 38 weeks' gestation, ranged from 2 to 11 weeks. The average gestational age at birth was 38.6 weeks and none was premature. All infants were normal at birth and at follow-up for 2–6 months. In addition to the reduced urine output, indomethacin was thought to have minimized the amount of fluid produced by the amnion and chorion (57).

A case report described a 33-year-old woman with a low serum α-fetoprotein level at 16 weeks' gestation and symptomatic polyhydramnios and preterm labor at 26 weeks' gestation who was treated with indomethacin, 25 mg orally every 4 hours, after therapeutic decompression had removed 3000 mL of amniotic fluid (58). During the 9 weeks of therapy, periodic fetal echocardiography was conducted to ensure that the fetal ductus arteriosus remained patent. Fetal urine output declined significantly (<50%) as determined by ultrasound examinations during therapy. Therapy was stopped at 35 weeks' gestation, and a 2280-g female infant was delivered vaginally a week later. Chromosomal analysis of the amniotic fluid at 26 weeks and of the infant after birth revealed 46 chromosomes with an additional marker or ring chromosome. No structural defects were noted in the infant, who was developing normally at 3 months of age (58).

In two women treated for premature labor, indomethacin-induced oligohydramnios was observed at 1 and 3.5 weeks, respectively, after starting therapy (59). Treatment was continued for 3 weeks in one patient and for 8 weeks in the other, with therapy discontinued at 31 and 32 weeks' gestation, respectively. Within a week of stopping indomethacin, amniotic fluid volume had returned to normal in both patients. Ultrasonography revealed that both fetuses had regular filling of their bladders. The newborns, delivered 3–4 weeks after indomethacin treatment was halted, had normal urine output. Neither premature closure of the ductus arteriosus nor pulmonary hypertension was observed (59). Another case of reversible indomethacin-induced oligohydramnios was reported in 1989 (60). The woman was treated from 20 to 28 weeks' gestation with indomethacin, 100–200 mg/day, plus various other tocolytic agents for premature labor. Ten days after indomethacin therapy was stopped, the volume of amniotic fluid was normal. She was eventually delivered of a 2905-g female infant at 36 weeks' gestation. Development was normal at 1 year of age (60).

The effects of tocolytic therapy on amniotic fluid volume were the subject of a 1989 study (61). Of 27 women meeting the criteria for the study, 13 were treated either with indomethacin alone ($N = 9$) or indomethacin combined with ritodrine ($N = 2$), terbutaline ($N = 1$), or magnesium sulfate ($N = 1$). Indomethacin dosage varied from 100 to 200 mg/day with a mean duration of treatment of 15.3 days (range 5–44 days). Four other patients were treated with ibuprofen, another nonsteroidal anti-inflammatory agent. Fourteen of the seventeen patients (82.3%) either had a decrease in amniotic fluid volume to low-normal levels or had oligohydramnios compared with none of the 10 women treated only with terbutaline, ritodrine, or magnesium sulfate ($p < 0.001$). The mean time required to reaccumulate amniotic fluid in 7 women after stopping nonsteroidal anti-inflammatory therapy was 4.4 days. In one other woman who had an ultrasound examination after therapy was discontinued, amniotic fluid volume remained in the low-normal range (61).

A study published in 1988 described the treatment with indomethacin, 100–150 mg/day, for premature labor in eight women at 27–32 weeks' gestation (62). Fetal urine output fell from a mean pretreatment value of 11.2 to 2.2 mL/hour at 5 hours, then stabilized at 1.8 mL/hour at 12 and 24 hours. Mean output 24 hours after stopping indomethacin was 13.5 mL/hour. No correlation was found between maternal indomethacin serum levels and hourly fetal urine output. Three of the four fetuses treated with indomethacin every 4 hours had ductal constriction at 24 hours that apparently resolved after therapy was halted. All newborns had normal renal function in the neonatal period.

Fetal adverse effects described during treatment of premature labor with indomethacin in recent studies include primary pulmonary hypertension (four cases) (35,63), ductal constriction with or without tricuspid regurgitation (36,64–67), and, in infants less than 30 weeks' gestation, a significantly increased incidence compared with controls of intracranial hemorrhage, necrotizing enterocolitis, and patent ductus arteriosus requiring ligation (68,69). A possible interaction between cocaine abuse and indomethacin resulting in fetal anuria, generalized massive edema, and neonatal gastrointestinal hemorrhage has been reported (70).

A number of reports have described the use of indomethacin for the treatment of symptomatic polyhydramnios in singleton and multiple pregnancies (71–82), including a 1991 review of this indication (83). Indomethacin-induced constriction of the ductus arteriosus and tricuspid regurgitation were observed in some of the studies (70,72,74,80). In one report, indomethacin was used to treat polyhydramnios because of feto-fetal transfusion syndrome in two sets of twins (80). One twin survived from each pregnancy, but one was oliguric (urine output 0.5 mL/kg/hour) and the other was anuric requiring peritoneal dialysis. The authors speculated that the renal failure in both infants was secondary to indomethacin. A unilateral pleural effusion developed in one twin fetus after 28 days of indomethacin therapy for polyhydramnios, possibly because of ductus arteriosus constriction (82). The condition resolved completely within 48 hours of stopping the drug.

A probable drug interaction between indomethacin and β-blockers resulting in severe maternal hypertension was reported in two women in 1989 (84). One woman, with a history of labile hypertension of 6 years' duration, was admitted at 30 weeks' gestation for control of her blood pressure. She was treated with propranolol 80 mg/day with good response. Indomethacin was started because of premature uterine contractions occurring at 32 weeks' gestation. An initial 200-mg rectal dose was followed by 25 mg orally/day. On the 4th day of therapy, the patient suffered a marked change in blood pressure, which rose from 135/85 mmHg to 240/140 mmHg, with cardiotocographic signs of fetal distress. A cesarean section was performed, but the severely growth-restricted newborn died 72 hours later. The second patient developed signs and symptoms of preeclampsia at 31 weeks' gestation. She was treated with pindolol 15 mg/day with good blood pressure response. Two weeks later, indomethacin was started, as in the first case, for preterm labor. On the 5th day of therapy, blood pressure rose to 230/130 mmHg. Signs of fetal distress were evident and a cesarean section was performed. The low-weight infant survived (84). In a brief letter referring to the above study, one author proposed that the mechanism of nonsteroidal anti-inflammatory-induced hypertension may be related to the inhibition of prostaglandin synthesis in the renal vasculature (85). On the basis of this theory, the author recommended that all similar agents should be avoided in women with preeclampsia. Although the mechanism is unknown, one source has reviewed several cases of the interaction and observed that indomethacin may inhibit the effects of β-blockers, as well as antihypertensives in general (86).

Severe complications after in utero exposure to indomethacin were reported in three preterm infants (87). The three mothers had been treated with indomethacin, 200–300 mg/day, for 4 weeks, 3 days, and 2 days, respectively, immediately before delivery. Complications in the newborns included edema or hydrops, oliguric renal failure (<0.5 mL/kg/hour) lasting for 1–2 days, gastrointestinal bleeding occurring on the 4th and 6th days (2 infants), subcutaneous bruising, intraventricular hemorrhage (1 infant), absent platelet aggregation (2 infants; not determined in the third infant), and perforation of the terminal ileum. The authors attributed the problems to maternal indomethacin therapy because of (a) the absence of predisposing factors, and the lack of diagnostic evidence, for necrotizing enterocolitis, and (b) the close similarity and sequential pattern of the signs and symptoms in the three newborns (87).

A single case of phocomelia with agenesis of the penis has been described, but the relationship between indomethacin and this defect is unknown (88). Inhibition of platelet aggregation may have contributed to postpartum hemorrhage in 3 of 16 women given a 100-mg indomethacin suppository during term labor (19).

The use of indomethacin as a tocolytic agent during the latter half of pregnancy may cause constriction of the fetal ductus arteriosus, with or without tricuspid regurgitation. These effects are usually transient and reversible if therapy is stopped at an adequate time before delivery. Premature closure of the ductus arteriosus can result in primary pulmonary hypertension of the newborn that, in severe cases, may be fatal (89). Reduced fetal urine output should be expected when indomethacin is administered to the mother. This may be therapeutic in cases of symptomatic polyhydramnios, but the complications of this therapy may be severe. Oliguric renal failure, hemorrhage, and intestinal perforation have been reported in premature infants exposed immediately before delivery. Use of indomethacin with antihypertensive agents, particularly the β-blockers, has been associated with severe maternal hypertension and resulting fetal distress. Short courses of indomethacin, such as 24–48 hours with allowance of at least 24 hours or more between the last dose and delivery, should prevent complications of this therapy in the newborn. Use of the smallest effective dose is essential, although maternal serum levels of indomethacin that are effective for tocolysis have not yet been defined (48) and, at least one complication, ductal constriction, is independent of fetal drug serum levels (49,50). Restriction of indomethacin tocolysis to gestational ages between 24 and 32 completed weeks, when therapy for premature labor is most appropriate, will also lessen the incidence of complications (38), although a higher rate of newborn complications has been observed when delivery occurred before 30 weeks' gestation (68,69). Other uses of indomethacin, such as for analgesia or inflammation, have not been studied in pregnancy but should be approached with caution because of the effects described above. Moreover, women attempting to conceive should not use any prostaglandin synthesis inhibitor, including indomethacin, because of the findings in a variety of animal models that indicate these agents block blastocyst implantation (90,91).

BREASTFEEDING SUMMARY

Indomethacin is excreted in breast milk. Although an earlier reference speculated that milk levels were similar to maternal plasma levels (92), a study published in 1991 reported a median milk:plasma ratio of 0.37 in 7 of 16 women taking 75–300 mg/day (93). The other nine women did not have measurable drug levels in both milk and plasma. The investigators calculated that the total infant dose ingested (assuming 100% absorption) ranged from 0.07% to 0.98% (median 0.18%) of the weight-adjusted maternal dose (93).

A case report of possible indomethacin-induced seizures in a breastfed infant has been published (92), although the causal link between the two events has been questioned (94). The mother was taking 200 mg/day (3 mg/kg/day). The American Academy of Pediatrics noted the above possible adverse reaction but classified indomethacin as compatible with breastfeeding (95).

References

1. Shepard TH. *Catalog of Teratogenic Agents*. 6th ed. Baltimore, MD: The Johns Hopkins University Press, 1989:348–9.
2. Montenegro MA, Palomino H. Induction of cleft palate in mice by inhibitors of prostaglandin synthesis. J Craniofac Genet Dev Biol 1990;10:83–94.
3. Moise KJ Jr, Ou C-N, Kirshon B, Cano LE, Rognerud C, Carpenter RJ Jr. Placental transfer of indomethacin in the human pregnancy. Am J Obstet Gynecol 1990;162:549–54.
4. Nielsen GL, Sorensen HT, Larsen H, Pedersen L. Risk of adverse birth outcome and miscarriage in pregnant users of non-steroidal anti-inflammatory drugs: population based observational study and case-control study. Br Med J 2001;322:266–70.
5. Ericson A, Kallen BAJ. Nonsteroidal anti-inflammatory drugs in early pregnancy. Reprod Toxicol 2001;15:371–5.
6. Li DK, Liu L, Odouli R. Exposure to non-steroidal anti-inflammatory drugs during pregnancy and risk of miscarriage: population-based cohort study. Br Med J 2003;327:368–71.
7. Tassinari MS, Cook JC, Hurtt ME. NSAIDs and developmental toxicity. Birth Defects Res B Dev Reprod Toxicol 2003;68:3–4.
8. Atad J, David A, Moise J, Abramovici H. Classification of threatened premature labor related to treatment with a prostaglandin inhibitor: indomethacin. Biol Neonate 1980;37:291–6.
9. Gonzalez CHL, Jimenez PG, Pezzotti y R MA, Favela EL. Hipertension pulmonar persistente en el recien nacido por uso prenatal de inhibidores de las prostaglandinas (indometacina). Informe de un caso. Ginecol Obstet Mex 1980;48:103–10.
10. Sureau C, Piovani P. Clinical study of indomethacin for prevention of prematurity. Eur J Obstet Gynecol Reprod Biol 1983;46:400–2.
11. Van Kets H, Thiery M, Derom R, Van Egmond H, Baele G. Perinatal hazards of chronic antenatal tocolysis with indomethacin. Prostaglandins 1979;18:893–907.
12. Van Kets H, Thiery M, Derom R, Van Egmond H, Baele G. Prostaglandin synthase inhibitors in preterm labor. Lancet 1980;2:693.
13. Blake DA, Niebyl JR, White RD, Kumor KM, Dubin NH, Robinson JC, Egner PG. Treatment of premature labor with indomethacin. Adv Prostaglandin Thromboxane Res 1980;8:1465–7.
14. Grella P, Zanor P. Premature labor and indomethacin. Prostaglandins 1978;16:1007–17.
15. Karim SMM. On the use of blockers of prostaglandin synthesis in the control of labor. Adv Prostaglandin Thromboxane Res 1978;4:301–6.
16. Katz Z, Lancet M, Yemini M, Mogilner BM, Feigl A, Ben Hur H. Treatment of premature labor contractions with combined ritodrine and indomethacine. Int J Gynaecol Obstet 1983;21:337–42.
17. Niebyl JR, Blake DA, White RD, Kumor KM, Dubin NH, Robinson JC, Egner PG. The inhibition of premature labor with indomethacin. Am J Obstet Gynecol 1980;136:1014–9.
18. Peteja J. Indometacyna w zapobieganiu porodom przedwczesnym. Ginekol Pol 1980;51:347–53.
19. Reiss U, Atad J, Rubinstein I, Zuckerman H. The effect of indomethacin in labour at term. Int J Gynaecol Obstet 1976;14:369–74.
20. Souka AR, Osman N, Sibaie F, Einen MA. Therapeutic value of indomethacin in threatened abortion. Prostaglandins 1980;19:457–60.
21. Spearing G. Alcohol, indomethacin, and salbutamol. Obstet Gynecol 1979;53:171–4.
22. Chimura T. The treatment of threatened premature labor by drugs. Acta Obstet Gynaecol Jpn 1980;32:1620–4.
23. Suzanne F, Fresne JJ, Portal B, Baudon J. Essai therapeutique de l'indometacine dans les menaces d'accouchement premature: a propos de 30 observations. Therapie 1980;35:751–60.
24. Tinga DJ, Aranoudse JG. Post-partum pulmonary oedema associated with preventive therapy for premature labor. Lancet 1979;1:1026.
25. Dudley DKL, Hardie MJ. Fetal and neonatal effects of indomethacin used as a tocolytic agent. Am J Obstet Gynecol 1985;151:181–4.
26. Gamissans O, Canas E, Cararach V, Ribas J, Puerto B, Edo A. A study of indomethacin combined with ritodrine in threatened preterm labor. Eur J Obstet Gynecol Reprod Biol 1978;8:123–8.
27. Wiqvist N, Lundstrom V, Green K. Premature labor and indomethacin. Prostaglandins 1975;10:515–26.
28. Wiqvist N, Kjellmer I, Thiringer K, Ivarsson E, Karlsson K. Treatment of premature labor by prostaglandin synthetase inhibitors. Acta Biol Med Germ 1978;37:923–30.
29. Zuckerman H, Reiss U, Rubinstein I. Inhibition of human premature labor by indomethacin. Obstet Gynecol 1974;44:787–92.
30. Zuckerman H, Reiss U, Atad J, Lampert I, Ben Ezra S, Sklan D. The effect of indomethacin on plasma levels of prostaglandin $F_2\alpha$ in women in labour. Br J Obstet Gynaecol 1977;84:339–43.
31. Zuckerman H, Shalev E, Gilad G, Katzuni E. Further study of the inhibition of premature labor by indomethacin. Part I. J Perinat Med 1984;12:19–23.
32. Zuckerman H, Shalev E, Gilad G, Katzuni E. Further study of the inhibition of premature labor by indomethacin. Part II. Double-blind study. J Perinat Med 1984;12:25–9.
33. Niebyl JR. Prostaglandin synthetase inhibitors. Semin Perinatol 1981;5: 274–87.
34. Niebyl JR, Witter FR. Neonatal outcome after indomethacin treatment for preterm labor. Am J Obstet Gynecol 1986;155:747–9.
35. Besinger RE, Niebyl JR, Keyes WG, Johnson TRB. Randomized comparative trial of indomethacin and ritodrine for the long-term treatment of preterm labor. Am J Obstet Gynecol 1991;164:981–8.
36. Evans DJ, Kofinas AD, King K. Intraoperative amniocentesis and indomethacin treatment in the management of an immature pregnancy with completely dilated cervix. Obstet Gynecol 1992;79:881–2.
37. Leonardi MR, Hankins GDV. What's new in tocolytics. Clin Perinatol 1992;19:367–84.
38. Higby K, Xenakis EM-J, Pauerstein CJ. Do tocolytic agents stop preterm labor? A critical and comprehensive review of efficacy and safety. Am J Obstet Gynecol 1993;168:1247–59.
39. Morales WJ, Smith SG, Angel JL, O'Brien WF, Knuppel RA. Efficacy and safety of indomethacin versus ritodrine in the management of preterm labor: a randomized study. Obstet Gynecol 1989;74:567–72.
40. Morales WJ, Madhav H. Efficacy and safety of indomethacin compared with magnesium sulfate in the management of preterm labor: a randomized study. Am J Obstet Gynecol 1993;169:97–102.
41. Levin DL. Effects of inhibition of prostaglandin synthesis on fetal development, oxygenation, and the fetal circulation. Semin Perinatol 1980;4: 35–44.
42. Csaba IF, Sulyok E, Ertl T. Relationship of maternal treatment with indomethacin to persistence of fetal circulation syndrome. J Pediatr 1978;92:484.
43. Levin DL, Fixler DE, Morriss FC, Tyson J. Morphologic analysis of the pulmonary vascular bed in infants exposed in utero to prostaglandin synthetase inhibitors. J Pediatr 1978;92:478–83.
44. Rubaltelli FF, Chiozza ML, Zanardo V, Cantarutti F. Effect on neonate of maternal treatment with indomethacin. J Pediatr 1979;94:161.
45. Manchester D, Margolis HS, Sheldon RE. Possible association between maternal indomethacin therapy and primary pulmonary hypertension of the newborn. Am J Obstet Gynecol 1976;126:467–9.
46. Goudie BM, Dossetor JFB. Effect on the fetus of indomethacin given to suppress labour. Lancet 1979;2:1187–8.
47. Mogilner BM, Ashkenazy M, Borenstein R, Lancet M. Hydrops fetalis caused by maternal indomethacin treatment. Acta Obstet Gynecol Scand 1982;61:183–5.
48. Moise KJ Jr, Huhta JC, Sharif DS, Ou CN, Kirshon B, Wasserstrum N, Cano L. Indomethacin in the treatment of premature labor: effects on the fetal ductus arteriosus. N Engl J Med 1988;319:327–31.
49. Van Den Veyver I, Moise K Jr, Ou C-N, Carpenter R Jr. The effect of gestational age and fetal indomethacin levels on the incidence of constriction of the fetal ductus arteriosus (abstract). Am J Obstet Gynecol 1993; 168:373.
50. Van Den Veyver IB, Moise KJ Jr, Ou C-N, Carpenter RJ Jr. The effect of gestational age and fetal indomethacin levels on the incidence of constriction of the fetal ductus arteriosus. Obstet Gynecol 1993;82:500–3.
51. Moise KJ Jr. Effect of advancing gestational age on the frequency of fetal ductal constriction in association with maternal indomethacin use. Am J Obstet Gynecol 1993;168:1350–3.
52. Ovadia M. Effects of indomethacin on the fetus. N Engl J Med 1988;319:1484.
53. Moise KJ Jr, Huhta JC, Mari G. Effects of indomethacin on the fetus. N Engl J Med 1988;319:1485.
54. Atad J, Lissak A, Rofe A, Abramovici H. Patent ductus arteriosus after prolonged treatment with indomethacin during pregnancy: case report. Int J Gynaecol Obstet 1987;25:73–6.
55. Itskovitz J, Abramovici H, Brandes JM. Oligohydramnion, meconium and perinatal death concurrent with indomethacin treatment in human pregnancy. J Reprod Med 1980;24:137–40.

56. Veersema D, de Jong PA, van Wijck JAM. Indomethacin and the fetal renal nonfunction syndrome. Eur J Obstet Gynecol Reprod Biol 1983;16:113–21.
57. Cabrol D, Landesman R, Muller J, Uzan M, Sureau C, Saxena BB. Treatment of polyhydramnios with prostaglandin synthetase inhibitor (indomethacin). Am J Obstet Gynecol 1987;157:422–6.
58. Kirshon B, Cotton DB. Polyhydramnios associated with a ring chromosome and low maternal serum α-fetoprotein levels managed with indomethacin. Am J Obstet Gynecol 1988;158:1063–4.
59. De Wit W, Van Mourik I, Wiesenhaan PF. Prolonged maternal indomethacin therapy associated with oligohydramnios: case reports. Br J Obstet Gynecol 1988;95:303–5.
60. Goldenberg RL, Davis RO, Baker RC. Indomethacin-induced oligohydramnios. Am J Obstet Gynecol 1989;160:1196–7.
61. Hickok DE, Hollenbach KA, Reilley SF, Nyberg DA. The association between decreased amniotic fluid volume and treatment with nonsteroidal anti-inflammatory agents for preterm labor. Am J Obstet Gynecol 1989;160:1525–31.
62. Kirshon B, Moise KJ Jr, Wasserstrum N, Ou CN, Huhta JC. Influence of short-term indomethacin therapy on fetal urine output. Obstet Gynecol 1988;72:51–3.
63. Demandt E, Legius E, Devlieger H, Lemmens F, Proesmans W, Eggermont E. Prenatal indomethacin toxicity in one member of monozygous twins; a case report. Eur J Obstet Gynecol Reprod Biol 1990;35:267–9.
64. Eronen M, Pesonen E, Kurki T, Ylikorkala O, Hallman M. The effects of indomethacin and a β-sympathomimetic agent on the fetal ductus arteriosus during treatment of premature labor: a randomized double-blind study. Am J Obstet Gynecol 1991;164:141–6.
65. Hallak M, Reiter AA, Ayres NA, Moise KJ Jr. Indomethacin for preterm labor: fetal toxicity in a dizygotic twin gestation. Obstet Gynecol 1991;78:911–3.
66. Rosemond RL, Boehm FH, Moreau G, Karmo H. Tricuspid regurgitation: a method of monitoring patients treated with indomethacin (abstract). Am J Obstet Gynecol 1992;166:336.
67. Bivins HA Jr, Newman RB, Fyfe DA, Campbell BA, Stramm SL. Randomized comparative trial of indomethacin and terbutaline for the long term treatment of preterm labor (abstract). Am J Obstet Gynecol 1993;168:375.
68. Norton M, Merril J, Kuller J, Clyman R. Neonatal complications after antenatal indomethacin for preterm labor (abstract). Am J Obstet Gynecol 1993;168:303.
69. Norton ME, Merrill J, Cooper BAB, Kuller JA, Clyman RI. Neonatal complications after the administration of indomethacin for preterm labor. N Engl J Med 1993;329:1602–7.
70. Carlan SJ, Stromquist C, Angel JL, Harris M, O'Brien WF. Cocaine and indomethacin: fetal anuria, neonatal edema, and gastrointestinal bleeding. Obstet Gynecol 1991;78:501–3.
71. Kirshon B, Mari G, Moise KJ Jr. Indomethacin therapy in the treatment of symptomatic polyhydramnios. Obstet Gynecol 1990;75:202–5.
72. Mari G, Moise KJ Jr, Deter RL, Kirshon B, Carpenter RJ. Doppler assessment of the renal blood flow velocity waveform during indomethacin therapy for preterm labor and polyhydramnios. Obstet Gynecol 1990;75:199–201.
73. Mamopoulos M, Assimakopoulos E, Reece EA, Andreou A, Zheng X-Z, Mantalenakis S. Maternal indomethacin therapy in the treatment of polyhydramnios. Am J Obstet Gynecol 1990;162:1225–9.
74. Kirshon B, Mari G, Moise KJ Jr, Wasserstrum N. Effect of indomethacin on the fetal ductus arteriosus during treatment of symptomatic polyhydramnios. J Reprod Med 1990;35:529–32.
75. Smith LG Jr, Kirshon B, Cotton DB. Indomethacin treatment of polyhydramnios and subsequent infantile nephrogenic diabetes insipidus. Am J Obstet Gynecol 1990;163:98–9.
76. Ash K, Harman CR, Gritter H. TRAP sequence—successful outcome with indomethacin treatment. Obstet Gynecol 1990;76:960–2.
77. Malas HZ, Hamlett JD. Acute recurrent polyhydramnios—management with indomethacin. Br J Obstet Gynaecol 1991;98:583–7.
78. Nordstrom L, Westgren M. Indomethacin treatment for polyhydramnios. Effective but potentially dangerous? Acta Obstet Gynecol Scand 1992;71:239–41.
79. Dolkart LA, Eshwar KP, Reimers FT. Indomethacin therapy and chronic hemodialysis during pregnancy. A case report. J Reprod Med 1992;37:181–3.
80. Buderus S, Thomas B, Fahnenstich H, Kowalewski S. Renal failure in two preterm infants: toxic effect of prenatal maternal indomethacin treatment? Br J Obstet Gynaecol 1993;100:97–8.
81. Deeny M, Haxton MJ. Indomethacin use to control gross polyhydramnios complicating triplet pregnancy. Br J Obstet Gynaecol 1993;100:281–2.
82. Murray HG, Stone PR, Strand L, Flower J. Fetal pleural effusion following maternal indomethacin therapy. Br J Obstet Gynaecol 1993;100:277–82.
83. Moise KJ Jr. Indomethacin therapy in the treatment of symptomatic polyhydramnios. Clin Obstet Gynecol 1991;34:310–8.
84. Schoenfeld A, Freedman S, Hod M, Ovadia Y. Antagonism of antihypertensive drug therapy in pregnancy by indomethacin? Am J Obstet Gynecol 1989;161:1204–5.
85. Mousavy SM. Indomethacin induces hypertensive crisis in preeclampsia irrespective of prior antihypertensive drug therapy. Am J Obstet Gynecol 1991;165:1577.
86. Hansen PD. *Drug Interactions*. 5th ed. Philadelphia, PA: Lea & Febiger, 1985:36.
87. Vanhaesebrouck P, Thiery M, Leroy JG, Govaert P, de Praeter C, Coppens M, Cuvelier C, Dhont M. Oligohydramnios, renal insufficiency, and ileal perforation in preterm infants after intrauterine exposure to indomethacin. J Pediatr 1988;113:738–43.
88. Di Battista C, Landizi L, Tamborino G. Focomelia ed agenesia del pene in neonato. Minerva Pediatr 1975;27:675. As cited in Dukes MNG, ed. *Side Effects of Drugs Annual 1*. Amsterdam: Excerpta Medica, 1977:89.
89. Van Marter LJ, Leviton A, Allred EN, Pagano M, Sullivan KF, Cohen A, Epstein MF. Persistent pulmonary hypertension of the newborn and smoking and aspirin and nonsteroidal antiinflammatory drug consumption during pregnancy. Pediatrics 1996;97:658–63.
90. Matt DW, Borzelleca JF. Toxic effects on the female reproductive system during pregnancy, parturition, and lactation. In: Witorsch RJ, ed. *Reproductive Toxicology*. 2nd ed. New York, NY: Raven Press, 1995:175–93.
91. Dawood MY. Nonsteroidal antiinflammatory drugs and reproduction. Am J Obstet Gynecol 1993;169:1255–65.
92. Eeg-Olofsson O, Malmros I, Elwin CE, Steen B. Convulsions in a breast-fed infant after maternal indomethacin. Lancet 1978;2:215.
93. Lebedevs TH, Wojnar-Horton RE, Yapp P, Roberts MJ, Dusci LJ, Hackett LP, Ilett KF. Excretion of indomethacin in breast milk. Br J Clin Pharmacol 1991;32:751–4.
94. Fairhead FW. Convulsions in a breast-fed infant after maternal indomethacin. Lancet 1978;2:576.
95. Committee on Drugs, American Academy of Pediatrics. The transfer of drugs and other chemicals into human milk. Pediatrics 2001;108:776–89.

INFLIXIMAB

Antirheumatic Agent/Gastrointestinal Agent

PREGNANCY RECOMMENDATION: Human Data Suggest Low Risk (Contraindicated If Combined with Methotrexate)
BREASTFEEDING RECOMMENDATION: Compatible

PREGNANCY SUMMARY

The maternal benefits of therapy with infliximab appear to far outweigh embryo–fetal risks (1,2). In 2011, the World Congress of Gastroenterology stated "Infliximab in pregnancy is considered to be low risk and compatible with use during conception in men and women and during pregnancy in at least the first two trimesters" (3). Animal reproduction studies have not been conducted with infliximab because the mechanism of action is different from that in humans. However, the agent should be avoided if it is combined with methotrexate, a potential teratogen, for the treatment of rheumatoid arthritis. Because of the long elimination half-life, use before conception may result in inadvertent exposure of an unplanned pregnancy. An indirect risk during any stage of gestation may exist because of the potential for severe maternal toxicity in some patient populations. This includes increased incidence of mortality in patients with moderate-to-severe congestive heart failure and an increased risk of severe infections.

FETAL RISK SUMMARY

Infliximab, a chimeric (mouse/human) immune globulin G (IgG1) monoclonal antibody, is indicated for the treatment of rheumatoid arthritis (in combination with methotrexate) and for severe Crohn's disease, including fistulizing Crohn's disease. Infliximab binds specifically to human tumor necrosis factor alpha (TNFα) to inhibit its activity. TNFα is a proinflammatory cytokine with a central role in inflammatory processes. Infliximab is in the same subclass of immunomodulators (blockers of TNFα activity) as adalimumab, certolizumab pegol, and golimumab. The agent has an elimination half-life of 8.0–9.5 days (4).

Animal reproduction studies have not been conducted with infliximab because it does not cross-react with TNFα in species other than humans and chimpanzees (4). However, when a reproduction study was conducted in mice with an analogous antibody that binds specifically to mouse TNFα, no evidence of maternal toxicity, embryo toxicity, or teratogenicity was observed (4,5).

Although the molecular weight is very high (about 149,100), infliximab crosses the human placenta to the fetus in late gestation (6). As an IgG1 antibody, the drug would be transported actively across the placenta, especially in the 3rd trimester, but with minimal transfer in the 1st trimester. In 11 cases at a mean gestational age 40 weeks (range 38–41 weeks), the median and range of infliximab concentrations in cord blood as a percentage of maternal concentration were 160% (87%–400%). Moreover, infliximab was detected in the infants for 2–7 months. No birth defects nor neonatal intensive care unit stays occurred in any infant (6).

A 2001 case report described the pregnancy outcome of a 26-year-old woman with Crohn's disease who had received infliximab early in gestation (7). The woman had a 6-year history of Crohn's disease and was symptomatic with a rectovaginal fistula while receiving azathioprine, metronidazole, and mesalamine. She was given two infusions of infliximab (dose not specified); the first occurred at about 1–2 weeks' gestation and the second at about 2–3 weeks. A planned third infusion was canceled when her pregnancy was diagnosed. She eventually delivered a premature 681-g infant at 24 weeks of conception who died 3 days later (7).

The author of the above report also cited data received from the manufacturer on 27 women who had been treated with infliximab immediately before or during the 1st trimester (7). Of the 27 women, 3 aborted spontaneously (SAB), 1 had an elective abortion (EAB) (for personal reasons), and 6 delivered term infants. (No information was given on the condition of the infants.) Another woman had received infliximab during the 1st trimester and delivered an infant with tetralogy of Fallot. No data were provided on the remaining 16 pregnancies. The author noted the close relationship between infliximab's mechanism of action and that of thalidomide, a known human teratogen that decreases the production of TNFα (7). This relationship has been noted by others (8).

In an extension of the above report (some of the same data are reported), a 2001 abstract evaluated data from 59 women who had received infliximab before or during pregnancy for the treatment of Crohn's disease (N = 45), rheumatoid arthritis (N = 5; not specified if these cases also received methotrexate), or unknown disease (N = 9) (9). The cases were retrieved from the infliximab postmarketing safety database. Treating physicians were contacted to document pregnancy outcomes. The timing of exposures were 27 before pregnancy, 11 before pregnancy and during the 1st trimester, 5 during the 1st trimester, and 16 unknown. Pregnancy outcomes were known for 36 cases (time of exposure not specified): 26 live births, 5 SABs, and 5 EABs. Among the live births, two had complications: 681-g infant delivered at 23 weeks' and died at age 3 weeks; and an infant with tetralogy of Fallot (corrected surgically) that is otherwise currently healthy. The investigators concluded the outcomes were consistent with those expected in healthy women (9).

In a 2003 case report, a 29-year-old woman with chronic, severe Crohn's disease received three infusions of infliximab (600 mg/dose) over a 6-week period (10). Three months later, she received a fourth infusion of 500 mg. This dose was given approximately 3 days after conception. She eventually delivered a healthy infant at 36 weeks' gestation (birth weight and other details not specified). The child has normal growth and development at 20 months of age (10).

A survey of 600 members of the American College of Rheumatology, partially conducted to determine the outcomes of pregnancies exposed to disease-modifying antirheumatic drugs (DMARD) (etanercept, infliximab, leflunomide, and methotrexate), was published in 2003 (11). From the 175 responders, the outcomes of two pregnancies exposed to infliximab were one full-term, healthy infant and one unknown outcome (11).

The similarity between the mechanism of action of infliximab and thalidomide is of interest. However, decreased production of TNFα may not be a primary cause of the teratogenicity of thalidomide (see Thalidomide). Theoretically, TNFα antagonists could interfere with implantation and ovulation, but this has not been shown clinically (12).

The preliminary results of an ongoing prospective collaborative study of rheumatoid arthritis medicines in pregnancy conducted by the Organization of Teratology Information Specialists (OTIS) have been reported (13,14). The study covered the period 1999–2004. There were 33 women exposed in the 1st trimester to either etanercept (N = 29) or infliximab (N = 4). The outcomes of these pregnancies were compared with 77 prospectively ascertained disease-matched controls (did not use anti-TNF α agents) and 50 prospectively ascertained healthy controls. Three controls were lost to follow-up. There was no difference between the groups in the number of SABs and EABs. One malformation (1/33; 3.0%) was reported in the subject group (a chromosomal anomaly, trisomy 18; spontaneously aborted by a woman exposed to etanercept). Major malformations in the other groups were 4.0% (3/75) in disease-matched controls and 4.1% (2/49) in healthy controls. However, women exposed to etanercept or infliximab and disease-matched controls were significantly more likely to give birth to infants <37 weeks' gestation and to have lower-birth-weight full-term infants than healthy controls. These results suggested that the disease itself was the causal factor (13,14).

A 2004 study reported data from the manufacturer's database of pregnancies exposed to infliximab (15). Among 146 pregnancies, 131 were direct exposures (drug given to women) and 15 were indirect (drug given to male partners). Among the direct exposures, there were outcome data for 96 (73%); 82 involving mothers with Crohn's disease and 14 with rheumatoid arthritis. The timing of the direct exposures were 53 exposed within 3 months of conception with 28 of these also exposed during the 1st trimester; 30 exposed during the 1st trimester; 7 exposed more than 3 months before conception; and 6 exposed at an unknown time. The outcomes for the 96 direct exposures were 64 (67%) pregnancies with live births (68 infants—4 sets of twins), 14 (15%) SABs, and 18 (19%) EABs. For the 82 women with Crohn's disease, the outcomes were 55 (67%) pregnancies with live births (58 infants—3 sets of twins), 11 (13%) SABs, and 18 (22%) EABs. There were five fetal complications, including two structural anomalies, among the 96 live births: (a) birth at 24 weeks of a 681-g infant, died shortly thereafter of intracerebral and intrapulmonary hemorrhage; (b) neonate with respiratory distress, jaundice, and a seizure, reported to be doing well at 9 months of age; (c) twin with delayed development and hypothyroidism; (d) infant with tetralogy of Fallot, defect corrected surgically and infant doing well at 1 year of age, mother was treated with infliximab about 1 year before conception and during the 1st trimester; and (e) infant with intestinal malrotation, mother received infliximab and leflunomide before conception and in pregnancy. Taken in sum, the outcomes did not differ significantly from pregnancy outcomes in the U.S. population or from pregnant women with Crohn's disease not exposed to infliximab (15).

A 2006 communication from England described the pregnancy outcomes of 23 women directly exposed to TNFα agents at the time of conception (17 etanercept, 3 adalimumab, and 3 infliximab) (16). Additional therapy included methotrexate in nine women and leflunomide in two. There also were nine patients (4 etanercept, 5 infliximab) that discontinued therapy before conception. The outcomes for the 32 pregnancies were 7 SABs, 3 EABs, and 22 live births. No major anomalies were observed in the live births, including one infant exposed to adalimumab and methotrexate early in gestation (16).

A 32-year-old woman with Crohn's disease was treated throughout pregnancy with five infusions of infliximab 10 mg/kg (17). The last dose was given 2 weeks for the birth at term of a healthy 3.29-kg female infant. Apgar scores were 9 and 9. At 6 months of age, the infant's immune development was normal, including an appropriate immune response to routine childhood immunizations (17).

A 2008 case report described a 22-year-old woman with Crohn's disease who was treated with infliximab (10 mg/kg every 4 weeks) and daily mesalamine before and during pregnancy and during breastfeeding (18). She received six doses of infliximab in pregnancy with the last dose given about 2 weeks before birth of a term, healthy 3.35-kg male infant. At 27 months of age, no developmental abnormalities were noted in the child (18).

A report using data from the FDA database described 61 congenital anomalies in 41 children born to mothers taking a TNF antagonist (22 etanercept and 19 infliximab) (19). The authors concluded that 24 of the children had one or more of the congenital anomalies that are part of VACTERL association (vertebral anomalies, anal atresia, cardiac defects, tracheo-esophageal, renal, and limb abnormalities) and the rate was higher than historical controls (19). An accompanying editorial, however, concluded that the evidence for teratogenicity or with the VACTERL association was insufficient (20). Many of the anomalies reported occur commonly, such as ventricular septal defects. In addition, such databases have selection bias (only cases with adverse outcomes are reported and emphasis placed on exposures to new drugs) (20).

A 2009 study from France reported the outcomes of 15 women who took anti-TNF drugs during pregnancy (10 etanercept, 3 infliximab, and 2 adalimumab) (21). The drugs were given in the 1st, 2nd, and 3rd trimesters in 12, 3, and 2 cases, respectively. The outcomes were 2 SABs, 1 EAB, and 12 healthy babies without malformation or neonatal illness. They also reviewed the literature regarding the use of anti-TNF agents in pregnancy and found more than 300 cases. They concluded that, although only 29 were treated throughout gestation, the malformation rate was similar to the general population (21).

Three women with Crohn's disease were treated with infliximab 5 mg/kg before and during pregnancy (22). Two patients received infliximab every 8 weeks (4 doses) through gestational week 31 and 32, respectively, whereas the third patient received the drug at gestational weeks 19, 21, and 25. The first two patients gave birth at 38 and 39 weeks' gestation to healthy infants with birth weights of about 2.84 and 2.70 kg, respectively. The third patient gave birth at 36 weeks' to a healthy infant with birth weight of about 2.78 kg. All Apgar scores were in the normal range. At follow-up, all of the children were developing normally and had not developed atypical infections or more typical infections than expected for their age group. Moreover, all had seroconverted after childhood immunizations, suggesting normal immune responses (22).

BREASTFEEDING SUMMARY

In a case discussed above, a mother with Crohn's disease breastfed her infant while receiving infliximab (17). The mother's last dose during pregnancy was 2 weeks before birth of her female infant and her postpartum 10 mg/kg doses were at 2 and 10 weeks. Maternal serum infliximab concentrations at 6, 10, and 13 weeks were 40, 9.3, and 84 mcg/mL, respectively. In contrast, breast milk concentrations were not detectable. A serum sample obtained from the infant at 6 weeks had a concentration of 39.5 mcg/mL, identical to the mother's level. Although the drug was not detected in milk, breastfeeding was halted for 3 weeks and resumed when the mother received her second postpartum dose at 10 weeks. Infant serum infliximab levels continued to decline in spite of the mother's second dose, leading the investigators to conclude that breast milk was not the source (17).

In a second case, a mother with Crohn's disease was treated during pregnancy with infliximab (10 mg/kg every 4 weeks) (18). She decided to continue treatment while breastfeeding her infant. Breast milk samples were collected immediately before her first postpartum dose and daily postdose for 30 days. Infliximab was not detected in any of the samples (18).

Three mothers breastfed their infants while resuming treatment with infliximab on postpartum days 3, 10, and 14, respectively (22). Maternal serum samples were collected 6–43 days postdose and breast milk samples 7–43 days postdose. Infant serum samples were collected at 5 and 43 days postdose in two infants. Serum was not available in the third infant. The maternal serum concentrations ranged from about 60 to 74 mcg/mL, but all milk and infant serum concentrations were below the level of detection (0.10 mcg/mL) (22).

In the above reports, infliximab was not detected in any milk samples. It also was not detected in the serum of two nursing infants, but was in the serum of a third infant. The reason for this difference is unknown. Moreover, no adverse effects were observed on the immune function of four infants (17,22). Although the data are limited, these results suggest that the risk of toxicity for a nursing infant is low, if it exists at all. In 2011, the World Congress of Gastroenterology stated that infliximab was compatible with breastfeeding (3).

References

1. Gisbert JP. Safety of immunomodulators and biologics for the treatment of inflammatory bowel disease during pregnancy and breast-feeding. Inflamm Bowel Dis 2010;16:881–95.
2. El Mourabet M, El-Hachem S, Harrison JR, Binion DG. Anti-TNF antibody therapy for inflammatory bowel disease during pregnancy: a clinical review. Curr Drug Targets 2010;234–41.
3. Mahadevan U, Cucchiara S, Hyams JS, Steinwurz F, Nuti F, Travis SPL, Sandborn WJ, Colombel IH. The London position statement of the World Congress of Gastroenterology on biological therapy for IBD with the European Crohn's and Colitis Organization: pregnancy and pediatrics. Am J Gastroenterol 2011;106:214–23.
4. Product information. Remicade. Centocor, 2001.
5. Treacy G. Using an analogous monoclonal antibody to evaluate the reproductive and chronic toxicity potential for a humanized anti-TNFα monoclonal antibody. Hum Exp Toxicol 2000;19:226–8.
6. Mahadevan U, Wolf DC, Dubinsky M, Cortot A, Lee SD, Siegel CA, Ullman T, Glover S, Valentine JF, Rubin DT, Miller J, Abreu MT. Placental transfer of anti-tumor necrosis factor agents in pregnant patients with inflammatory bowel disease. Clin Gastroenterol Hepatol 2013;11:286–92.
7. Srinivasan R. Infliximab treatment and pregnancy outcome in active Crohn's disease. Am J Gastroenterol 2001;96:2274–5.
8. Stein RB, Hanauer SB. Comparative tolerability of treatments for inflammatory bowel disease. Drug Saf 2000;23:429–48.
9. Antoni CE, Furst D, Manger B, Lichtenstein GR, Keenan GF, Healy DE, Jacobs SJ, Katz Erlangen JA. Outcome of pregnancy in women receiving Remicade (infliximab) for the treatment of Crohn's disease or rheumatoid arthritis (abstract). Arthritis Rheum 2001;44(Suppl 9):S152.
10. Burt MJ, Frizelle FA, Barbezar GO. Pregnancy and exposure to infliximab (anti-tumor necrosis factor-alpha monoclonal antibody). J Gastroenterol Hepatol 2003;18:465–6.
11. Chakravarty EF, Sanchez-Yamamoto D, Bush TM. The use of disease-modifying antirheumatic drugs in women with rheumatoid arthritis of childbearing age: a survey of practice patterns and pregnancy outcomes. J Rheumatol 2003;30:241–6.
12. Khanna D, McMahon M, Furst DE. Safety of tumour necrosis factor-α antagonists. Drug Saf 2004;27:307–24.
13. Chambers CD, Johnson DL, Jones KL, The OTIS Collaborative Research Group. Pregnancy outcome in women exposed to anti-TNF-alpha medications: The OTIS Rheumatoid Arthritis in Pregnancy study (abstract). Arthritis Rheum 2004;50:S479.
14. Chambers CD, Johnson DL, Jones KL. Safety of anti-TNF-α medications in pregnancy (abstract). J Am Acad Dermatol 2005;52(Suppl 1):P196.
15. Katz JA, Antoni C, Keenan GF, Smith DE, Jacobs SJ, Lichtenstein GR. Outcome of pregnancy in women receiving infliximab for the treatment of Crohn's disease and rheumatoid arthritis. Am J Gastroenterol 2004;99:2385–92.
16. Hyrich KL, Symmons DPM, Watson KD, Silman AJ. Pregnancy outcome in women who were exposed to anti-tumor necrosis factor agents: results from a national population register. Arthritis Rheum 2006;54:2701–2.
17. Vasiliauskas EA, Church JA, Silverman N, Barry M, Targan SR, Dubinsky MC. Case report: evidence for transplacental transfer of maternally administered infliximab to the newborn. Clin Gastroenterol Hepatol 2006;4:1255–8.
18. Stengel JZ, Arnold HL. Is infliximab safe to use while breastfeeding? World J Gastroenterol 2008;14:3085–7.
19. Carter JD, Ladhani A, Ricca LR, Valeriano J, Vasey FB. A safety assessment of tumor necrosis factor antagonists during pregnancy: a review of the Food and Drug Administration database. J Rheumatol 2009;36:635–41.
20. Koren G, Inoue M. Do tumor necrosis factor inhibitors cause malformations in humans? J Rheumatol 2009;36:465–6.
21. Berthelot JM, De Bandt M, Goupille P, Solau-Gervais E, Liote F, Goeb V, Azais I, Martin A, Pallot-Prades B, Maugars Y, Mariette X, on behalf of CRI (Club Rhumatismes et Inflammation). Exposition to anti-TNF drugs during pregnancy: outcome of 15 cases and review of the literature. Joint Bone Spine 2009;76:28–34.
22. Kane S, Ford J, Cohen R, Wagner C. Absence of infliximab in infants and breast milk from nursing mothers receiving therapy for Crohn's disease before and after delivery. J Clin Gastroenterol 2009;43:613–6.

I

INGENOL MEBUTATE

Dermatological Agent

PREGNANCY RECOMMENDATION: No Human Data—Probably Compatible
BREASTFEEDING RECOMMENDATION: No Human Data—Probably Compatible

PREGNANCY SUMMARY

No reports describing the use of ingenol mebutate in human pregnancy have been located. Animal reproduction studies have been conducted with IV formulations and are not relevant. Moreover, systemic exposure to the drug and two metabolites was not detected in subjects with actinic keratosis. Consequently, the drug appears to be compatible for use in pregnancy.

FETAL RISK SUMMARY

Ingenol mebutate, an inducer of cell death, is a clear colorless gel (0.015% or 0.05%) for topical administration. It is indicated for the topical treatment of actinic keratosis. Blood levels of ingenol mebutate and two of its metabolites were below the lower limit of quantification (0.1 ng/mL) in 16 subjects with actinic keratosis when 1 g of the 0.05% gel was applied to an area of 100 cm^2 on the dorsal forearm once daily for 2 consecutive days (1).

Reproduction studies have been conducted in rats and rabbits given IV doses. During organogenesis in rats, no treatment-related effects on embryo–fetal toxicity or teratogenicity were observed. In rabbits during organogenesis, increases in embryo–fetal mortality were noted at the highest dose. When two lower doses were given, all 3 doses caused an increase in the incidence of fetal visceral and skeletal variations. However, the clinical relevance of these results is questionable since, as noted earlier, systemic exposure was not observed in human subjects (1).

Long-term animal studies for carcinogenic potential have not been conducted. Three assays for mutagenicity were negative but one assay was positive. Effects on fertility in animals have not been evaluated (1).

It is not known if ingenol mebutate or its metabolites cross the human placenta. The molecular weight (about 431) is low enough, but the absence of quantifiable levels suggest that clinically significant amounts of the drug and metabolites will not cross the embryo or fetus.

BREASTFEEDING SUMMARY

No reports describing the use of ingenol mebutate during human lactation have been located. The molecular weight (about 431) is low enough, but the absence of quantifiable levels of the parent drug and two metabolites suggest that clinically significant amounts will not be excreted into breast milk.

Reference

1. Product information. Picato. LEO Pharma, 2012.

I

INSULIN

Antidiabetic Agent

PREGNANCY RECOMMENDATION: Compatible
BREASTFEEDING RECOMMENDATION: Compatible

PREGNANCY SUMMARY

Insulin, a naturally occurring polypeptide hormone, is the drug of choice for the control of diabetes mellitus in pregnancy.

FETAL RISK SUMMARY

Because it is a very large molecule, it has been believed that insulin does not cross the human placenta. Research published in 1990, however, found that animal (bovine or porcine) insulin does cross the human placenta as an insulin–antibody complex, and that the amount of transfer directly correlated with the amount of anti-insulin antibody in the mother (1). Moreover, high concentrations of animal insulin in cord blood were significantly associated with the development of fetal macrosomia, suggesting that the transferred insulin had biologic activity and that the fetal condition was determined by factors other than the mother's glycemic control (1). This latter conclusion has been challenged (2,3) and defended (4) and it requires additional study. The results of the study do underscore the argument that immunogenic insulin should not be used in women who may become pregnant (1,2).

Human insulin does not cross the placenta in clinically significant amounts, probably because of its high molecular weight (5808) (5). However, there may be endogenous carrier proteins that allow passage of insulin to the embryo early in gestation. After that period, the fetus produces its own insulin as insulin-secreting cells in the fetal pancreas become differentiated near the end of the 1st trimester (6).

Infants of diabetic mothers are at risk for an increased incidence of congenital anomalies, 3 to 5 times that of normal controls (7–14). The rate of malformations appears to be related to maternal glycemic control in the 1st trimester of pregnancy, but the exact mechanisms causing structural defects are unknown. A 1996 review examined this issue and concluded that uncontrolled diabetes, occurring very early in gestation (i.e., <8 weeks of gestation), causes an abnormal metabolic fuel state and that this condition leads to a number of processes, operating via a common pathway, that results in cell injury (13).

Congenital malformations are now the most common cause of perinatal death in infants of diabetic mothers (7,8). Not only is the frequency of major defects increased, but so is the frequency of multiple malformations (affecting more than one organ system) (7). Malformations observed in infants of diabetic mothers include the following (11,12,14–16):

Caudal regression syndrome (includes anomalies of the lower neural tube resulting in sacral agenesis and defects of lumbar vertebrae; defects of lower extremities, and gastrointestinal and genitourinary tracts [17])
Femoral hypoplasia and unusual facies syndrome
Spina bifida, hydrocephalus, and other CNS defects
Anencephalus
Cardiovascular: transposition of great vessels; ventricular septal defect; atrial septal defect
Anal and rectal atresia

Renal: agenesis, multicystic dysplasia, ureter duplex
Gastrointestinal: situs inversus, tracheoesophageal fistula, bowel atresias, imperforate anus, small left colon

Infants of diabetic mothers may have significant perinatal morbidity, even when the mothers have been under close diabetic control (14). Perinatal morbidity in one series affected 65% (169/260) of the infants and included hypoglycemia, hyperbilirubinemia, hypocalcemia, and polycythemia (18).

In contrast to the data relating to the adverse fetal effects of poor maternal hyperglycemia control, animal studies have documented that short periods of hypoglycemia during early organogenesis are associated with malformations of the skeleton and heart (19–21), and reduced growth, including some major organs (22). Although hypoglycemia in humans has not been shown to be teratogenic (23,24), at least one author has concluded that this has not been adequately studied (25).

BREASTFEEDING SUMMARY

Insulin is a naturally occurring constituent of the blood and is excreted into breast milk. In a 2012 study, milk samples were obtained from breastfeeding mothers, five without diabetes, four with type 1 diabetes, and five with type 2 diabetes (26). Samples were analyzed for total and endogenous insulin and for c-peptide. The type 1 diabetics were treated with artificial insulin (aspart plus glargine), whereas the type 2 diabetics received a diabetic diet either with ($N = 3$) or without ($N = 2$) metformin. Insulin was present in all of the samples, but only artificial insulin was detected in the milk of type 1 diabetics. The results showed that insulin, both endogenous and exogenous, is actively transported from the blood into milk and is protected from degradation and, presumably, has a functional or developmental role in the infant. If so, the authors suggested, it might be beneficial for formula-fed infants if insulin was added to formula milk (26).

References

1. Menon RK, Cohen RM, Sperling MA, Cutfield WS, Mimouni F, Khoury JC. Transplacental passage of insulin in pregnant women with insulin-dependent diabetes mellitus. N Engl J Med 1990;323:309–15.
2. Kimmerle R, Chantelau EA. Transplacental passage of insulin. N Engl J Med 1991;324:198.
3. Ben-Shlomo I, Dor J, Zohar S, Mashiach S. Transplacental passage of insulin. N Engl J Med 1991;324:198.
4. Menon RK, Sperling MA, Cohen RM. Transplacental passage of insulin. N Engl J Med 1991;324:199.
5. Schardein JL. Insulin and oral hypoglycemic agents. In: *Chemically Induced Birth Defects*. 3rd ed. New York, NY: Marcel Dekker, 2000:458.
6. Buchanan TA, Kjos SL. Diabetes in women. Early detection, prevention, and management. Clin Updates Women's Health Care. 2002;1(4/Fall):47.
7. Dignan PSJ. Teratogenic risk and counseling in diabetes. Clin Obstet Gynecol 1981;24:149–59.
8. Friend JR. Diabetes. Clin Obstet Gynaecol 1981;8:353–82.
9. Miller E, Hare JW, Cloherty JP, Dunn PJ, Gleason RE, Soeldner JS, Kitzmiller JL. Elevated maternal hemoglobin A_{1c} in early pregnancy and major congenital anomalies in infants of diabetic mothers. N Engl J Med 1981;304:1331–4.
10. Soler NG, Walsh CH, Malins JM. Congenital malformations in infants of diabetic mothers. Q J Med 1976;45:303–13.
11. American College of Obstetricians and Gynecologists. Diabetes and pregnancy. *Technical Bulletin*. No. 200, December 1994.
12. Towner D, Kjos SL, Leung B, Montoro MM, Xiang A, Mestman JH, Buchanan TA. Congenital malformations in pregnancies complicated by NIDDM. Diabetes Care 1995;18:1446–51.
13. Reece EA, Homko CJ, Wu Y-K. Multifactorial basis of the syndrome of diabetic embryopathy. Teratology 1996;54:171–82.
14. Steel JM, Johnstone FD. Guidelines for the management of insulin-dependent diabetes mellitus in pregnancy. Drugs 1996;52:60–70.
15. Cousins L. Etiology and prevention of congenital anomalies among infants of overt diabetic women. Clin Obstet Gynecol 1991;34:481–93.
16. Hinson RM, Miller RC, Macri CJ. Femoral hypoplasia and maternal diabetes: consider femoral hypoplasia/unusual facies syndrome. Am J Perinatol 1996;13:433–6.
17. Escobar LF, Weaver DD. Caudal regression syndrome. In: Buyse ML, Editor-in-Chief. *Birth Defects Encyclopedia*. Vol. 1. Dover, MA: Center for Birth Defects Information Services, 1990:296–7.
18. Gabbe SG, Mestman JH, Freeman RK, Goebelsmann UT, Lowensohn RI, Nochimson D, Cetrulo C, Quilligan EJ. Management and outcome of pregnancy in diabetes mellitus, classes B to R. Am J Obstet Gynecol 1977;129:723–32.
19. Tanigawa K, Kawaguchi M, Tanaka O, Kato Y. Skeletal malformations in rat offspring. Long-term effect of maternal insulin-induced hypoglycemia during organogenesis. Diabetes 1991;40:1115–21.
20. Peet JH, Sadler TW. Mouse embryonic cardiac metabolism under euglycemic and hypoglycemic conditions. Teratology 1996;54:20–26.
21. Smoak IW. Brief hypoglycemia alters morphology, function, and metabolism of the embryonic mouse heart. Reprod Toxicol 1997;11:495–502.
22. Lueder FL, Buroker CA, Kim S-B, Flozak AS, Ogata ES. Differential effects of short and long durations of insulin-induced maternal hypoglycemia upon fetal rat tissue growth and glucose utilization. Pediatr Res 1992;32:436–40.
23. Kimmerle R, Heinemann L, Delecki A, Berger M. Severe hypoglycemia incidence and predisposing factors in 85 pregnancies of type I diabetic women. Diabetes Care 1992;15:1034–7.
24. Kalter H. Letter to the editor. Teratology 1996;54:266.
25. Sadler TW. Letter from the editor. Teratology 1996;54:266.
26. Whitmore TJ, Trengove NJ, Graham DF, Hartmann PE. Analysis of insulin in human breast milk in mothers with type 1 and type 2 diabetes mellitus. Int J Endocrinol 2012; 2012:296368, doi:10.1155/2012/296368.

INSULIN ASPART

Antidiabetic Agent

PREGNANCY RECOMMENDATION: Limited Human Data—Probably Compatible
BREASTFEEDING RECOMMENDATION: Compatible

PREGNANCY SUMMARY

There are no reasons to believe that insulin aspart would pose a risk to the embryo or fetus different from that of other insulins. Older forms of insulin, whether of human or of porcine origin, are considered compatible with pregnancy. Insulin aspart can be classified similarly. As with all insulins, the primary concern is severe maternal hypoglycemia.

FETAL RISK SUMMARY

Insulin aspart is a rapid-acting human insulin analog that differs from regular human insulin by a single substitution of the amino acid praline by aspartic acid at position B28. It is produced by recombinant DNA technology. Insulin aspart is indicated for the treatment of patients with diabetes mellitus, for the control of hyperglycemia. It may be given by SC injection, as an SC infusion by an external insulin pump, or IV. The mechanism of action of insulin aspart is similar to human insulin in that it binds to receptors in muscle and fat cells to facilitate the cellular uptake of glucose and, at the same time, inhibits glucose release from the liver. Because the substitution at position B28 reduces the tendency to form hexamers, as observed with regular human insulin, insulin aspart is absorbed more rapidly after SC injection and has a shorter duration of action. Similar to regular insulin, plasma protein binding of insulin aspart is low (0%–9%) (1).

The median times to maximum serum concentrations for insulin aspart and regular insulin after SC administration are 40–50 minutes and 80–120 minutes, respectively. The elimination half-life of insulin aspart also is shorter than regular insulin, 81 vs. 141 minutes, respectively (1).

Reproduction studies of SC insulin aspart have been conducted in rats and rabbits. In female rats, insulin aspart was given before and during mating, and throughout gestation. The embryo–fetal effects observed with insulin aspart did not differ from human insulin. These effects were pre- and postimplantation losses and visceral/skeletal malformations at a daily dose about 32 times the human dose based on BSA (HD). Similar results were obtained in rabbits given daily doses that were about three times the HD during organogenesis. The effects in both species probably were due to maternal hypoglycemia. No significant effects were observed in rats and rabbits at doses that were about eight times and equal to the HD, respectively (1).

In rats, insulin aspart given over a 52-week period resulted in an increased incidence of mammary gland tumors in females at the highest SC dose tested (about 32 times the HD). Similar effects have been observed with human regular insulin. Insulin aspart was not genotoxic in multiple tests, nor did it have any effect on fertility or reproductive performance in male and female rats, at SC doses up to 32 times the HD (1).

It is not known if insulin aspart crosses the human placenta. Human insulin does not cross the placenta in clinically significant amounts (2). Because of the very close similarity between insulin aspart and human insulin, and its high molecular weight (about 5826), insulin aspart probably does not cross either. However, there may be endogenous carrier proteins that allow passage of insulin, including insulin aspart, to the embryo early in gestation. After that period, the fetus produces its own insulin as insulin-secreting cells in the fetal pancreas become differentiated near the end of the 1st trimester (3).

A 2003 report compared the effects of single doses of insulin aspart and human regular insulin on alternate days in 15 women with gestational diabetes (4). Pregnancy outcomes were not discussed.

In 2007, the FDA approved a change in the risk factor for insulin aspart from C to B (Novo Nordisk, press release, January 30, 2007). Insulin aspart was compared with human regular insulin in a randomized controlled trial at 63 sites in 18 countries involving 322 pregnant women with type 1 diabetes. The rates of maternal hypoglycemia and changes in hemoglobin A_{1c} (HbA_{1c}) were comparable between the two groups. However, insulin aspart showed improved, though not statistically significant outcomes in terms of fewer preterm deliveries ($p < 0.053$), reduced risk of neonatal hypoglycemia requiring treatment, and consistently low rates of major hypoglycemia. The study was too small to evaluate the risk of congenital malformations (Novo Nordisk, data on file, January 30, 2007).

A 2008 study compared insulin aspart with human insulin, both combined with NPH insulin, in a randomized study involving 322 pregnant women (5). There was no difference between the groups with respect to fetal loss, perinatal mortality, congenital anomalies, and neonatal short-term complications,

One review concluded that rapid-acting insulin analogs (aspart and lispro) could be considered the insulin of choice in pregnancy (6).

BREASTFEEDING SUMMARY

Insulin is a naturally occurring constituent of the blood and is excreted into breast milk. In a 2012 study, milk samples were obtained from breastfeeding mothers, five without diabetes, four with type 1 diabetes, and five with type 2 diabetes (7). Samples were analyzed for total and endogenous insulin and for c-peptide. The type 1 diabetics were treated with artificial insulin (aspart plus lantis), whereas the type 2 diabetics received a diabetic diet either with ($N = 3$) or without ($N = 2$) metformin. Insulin was present in all of the samples at comparable concentration to serum, but only artificial insulin was detected in the milk of type 1 diabetics. The results showed that insulin, both endogenous and exogenous, is actively transported from the blood into milk and is protected from degradation and, presumably, has a functional or developmental role in the infant. If so, the authors suggested, it might be beneficial for formula-fed infants if insulin was added to formula milk (7).

References

1. Product information. Novolog. Novo Nordisk, 2007.
2. Schardein JL. Insulin and oral hypoglycemic agents. In: *Chemically Induced Birth Defects*. 3rd ed. New York, NY: Marcel Dekker, 2000:458.
3. Buchanan TA, Kjos SL. Diabetes in women. Early detection, prevention, and management. Clin Updates Women's Health Care. 2002;1(4/Fall):47.
4. Pettitt DJ, Ospina P, Kolaczynski JW, Jovanovic L. Comparison of an insulin analog, insulin aspart, and regular human insulin with no insulin in gestational diabetes mellitus. Diabetes Care 2003;26:183–6.
5. Hod M, Damm P, Kaaja R, Visser GHA, Dunne F, Demidova I, Hansen ASP, Mersebach H, for the Insulin Aspart Pregnancy Study group. Fetal and perinatal outcomes in type 1 diabetes pregnancy: a randomized study comparing insulin aspart with human insulin in 322 subjects. Am J Obstet Gynecol 2008;198:186.e1–7.
6. Gonzalez C, Santoro S, Salzberg S, Di Girolamo G, Alvarinas J. Insulin analogue therapy in pregnancies complicated by diabetes mellitus. Expert Opin Pharmacother 2005;6:735–42.
7. Whitmore TJ, Trengove NJ, Graham DF, Hartmann PE. Analysis of insulin in human breast milk in mothers with type 1 and type 2 diabetes mellitus. Int J Endocrinol 2012;2012:296368. doi:10.1155/2012/296368. Epub 2012 Mar 5.

INSULIN DETEMIR

Antidiabetic Agent

PREGNANCY RECOMMENDATION: Compatible
BREASTFEEDING RECOMMENDATION: Compatible

PREGNANCY SUMMARY

The human data presented by the manufacturer and other sources indicate that the effects of insulin detemir on the embryo and/or the fetus are similar to human insulin. The animal data suggest risk, but the embryotoxicity and teratogenicity was thought to be secondary to maternal hypoglycemia. Moreover, there was no difference in developmental toxicity between insulin detemir and human insulin (1). Older forms of insulin, whether of human or of porcine origin, are considered compatible with pregnancy. As with all insulins, the primary concern is severe maternal hypoglycemia.

FETAL RISK SUMMARY

Insulin detemir is a long-acting basal insulin analog that differs from regular human insulin by the omission of the amino acid threonine in position B30 and the attachment of a C14 fatty-acid chain to amino acid B29. It is produced by recombinant DNA technology. Insulin detemir is indicated for once- or twice-daily SC administration for the treatment of adult and pediatric patients with type 1 diabetes mellitus or adult patients with type 2 diabetes mellitus who require basal (long-acting) insulin for the control of hyperglycemia.

The mechanism of action of insulin detemir is similar to human insulin in that it binds to receptors in muscle and fat cells to facilitate the cellular uptake of glucose and, at the same time, inhibits glucose release from the liver. The duration of action ranges from 5.7 hours at the lowest dose to 23.2 hours at the highest dose. The long duration results from the slow systemic absorption of insulin detemir from the injection site caused by the strong self-association of the insulin molecules and the high binding to albumin in the blood. In contrast to human insulin, more than 98% of insulin detemir in the blood is bound to albumin (1).

Reproduction studies have been conducted in rats and rabbits. When female rats were given daily doses about 1.5 and 3 times the recommended human dose based on AUC (RHD) before and during mating and throughout pregnancy, an increased number of fetuses with visceral anomalies were observed at both doses. No effect on fertility was observed. In pregnant rabbits, a dose that was 135 times the RHD was associated with gall bladder abnormalities described as small, bilobed, bifurcated, and missing. When human insulin was used in control groups, the effects of insulin detemir and human insulin were similar in terms of embryotoxicity and teratogenicity. Carcinogenicity studies have not been conducted with insulin detemir, but no mutagenic or clastogenic effects were observed in tests (1).

It is not known if insulin detemir crosses the human placenta. Human insulin does not cross the placenta in clinically significant amounts (2). Because of the close similarity between insulin detemir and human insulin, and its high molecular weight (about 5917), insulin detemir probably does not cross either. However, there may be endogenous carrier proteins that allow passage of insulin, including insulin detemir, to the embryo early in gestation. After that period, the fetus produces its own insulin as insulin-secreting cells in the fetal pancreas become differentiated near the end of the 1st trimester (3).

The manufacturer reported an open-label, clinical study in 310 pregnant women with type 1 diabetes (1). The women, between 8 and 12 weeks' gestation, were divided into two groups, insulin detemir $N = 152$ and NPH $N = 158$. The pregnancy outcomes in the two groups were similar (1).

Several reports have described the use of insulin detemir in human pregnancy (4–8). These reports concluded that the insulin analog had maternal efficacy and safety similar to other insulins. No embryo–fetal adverse effects related to the drug were observed (4–8).

BREASTFEEDING SUMMARY

No reports describing the use of insulin detemir during human lactation have been located. Insulin is a natural component of the blood and is excreted into breast milk. Insulin detemir probably also is present in milk.

References

1. Product information. Levemir. Novo Nordisk, 2012.
2. Schardein JL. Insulin and oral hypoglycemic agents. In: *Chemically Induced Birth Defects*. 3rd ed. New York, NY: Marcel Dekker, 2000:458.
3. Buchanan TA, Kjos SL. Diabetes in women. Early detection, prevention, and management. Clin Updates Women's Health Care. 2002;1(4/Fall):47.
4. Todorova-Ananieva K, Genova M. Pregnancy outcomes in women with type 2 diabetes treated with long-acting insulin analogues. A case control study. Diabetologia 2008;51(Suppl 1):S456 (abstract 1120).
5. Lapolla A, Di Cianni G, Bruttomesso D, Dalfra MG, Fresa R, Mello G, Napoli A, Romanelli T, Sciacca L, Stefanelli G, Torlone E, Mannino G. Use of insulin detemir in pregnancy: a report on 10 type 1 diabetic women. Diabet Med 2009;26:1179–80.
6. Sciacca L, Marotta V, Insalaco F, Tumminia A, Squatrito S, Vigneri R, Ettore G. Use of insulin detemir during pregnancy. Nutr Metab Cardiovasc Dis 2010 May; 20(4):e15-6. doi:10.1016/j.numecd.2009.12.010.
7. Callesen NF, Damm J, Mathiesen JM, Ringholm L, Damm P, Mathiesen ER. Treatment with the long-acting insulin analogues detemir or glargine during pregnancy in women with type 1 diabetes: comparison of glycaemic control and pregnancy outcome. J Matern Fetal Neonatal Med 2013;26:588–92.
8. Lambert K, Holt RIG. The use of insulin analogues in pregnancy. Diabetes Obes Metab 2013;15:888–900.

INSULIN GLARGINE

Antidiabetic Agent

PREGNANCY RECOMMENDATION: Compatible
BREASTFEEDING RECOMMENDATION: Compatible

PREGNANCY SUMMARY

The human pregnancy experience with insulin glargine demonstrates that the risk of embryo or fetal harm is low, if it exists at all. The use of insulin glargine during organogenesis at a dose close to that used in humans was associated with developmental toxicity in one animal species but not in another. Although it was not stated, the observed toxicity in rabbits may have been related to maternal hypoglycemia. Older forms of insulin, whether of human or of porcine origin, are considered compatible with pregnancy and, most likely, insulin glargine can be classified similarly. As with all insulins, the primary concern is severe maternal hypoglycemia.

I

FETAL RISK SUMMARY

Insulin glargine is a long-acting basal insulin analog that differs from regular human insulin by the replacement of the amino acid asparagine at A21 with glycine and two arginines are added to the C-terminus of the B-chain. It is produced by recombinant DNA technology. Insulin glargine is indicated for once-daily SC administration for the treatment of adult and pediatric patients with type 1 diabetes mellitus or adult patients with type 2 diabetes mellitus who require basal (long-acting) insulin for the control of hyperglycemia. The mechanism of action of insulin glargine is similar to human insulin in that it binds to receptors in muscle and fat cells to facilitate the cellular uptake of glucose and, at the same time, inhibits glucose release from the liver. Insulin glargine is an acidic solution (pH of about 4) that is neutralized in SC tissues, leading to the formation of micro-precipitates. The precipitates are slowly and continuously released over a 24-hour period with no pronounced peak (1).

Reproduction studies have been conducted in rats and rabbits. Female rats were given daily doses about seven times the recommended human SC starting dose based on BSA (RHD) before and during mating, and throughout pregnancy. Pregnant rabbits were given daily doses during organogenesis that were about twice the RHD. In both species, the effects of insulin glargine did not generally differ from those resulting from human insulin. However, in rabbits, five fetuses from two litters had dilation of the cerebral ventricles. In female rats and rabbits, no effects on fertility were observed (1).

In mice and rats, 2-year carcinogenicity studies were conducted with doses up to 5 and 10 times the RHD, respectively. Excessive mortality in female mice prevented conclusive evaluation in that group. Histiocytomas were found at the injection sites in male rats (statistically significant) and male mice (not significant) receiving insulin glargine. The tumors were not found in groups receiving saline or comparative human insulin in a non-acid-containing vehicle. Insulin glargine was not mutagenic or clastogenic in tests (1).

It is not known if insulin glargine crosses the human placenta. Human insulin does not cross the placenta in clinically significant amounts (2). Because of the close similarity between insulin glargine and human insulin, and its high molecular weight (6063), insulin glargine probably does not cross either. However, there may be endogenous carrier proteins that allow passage of insulin, including insulin glargine, to the embryo early in gestation. After that period, the fetus produces its own insulin as insulin-secreting cells in the fetal pancreas become differentiated near the end of the 1st trimester (3).

Several reports have described the use of insulin glargine in human pregnancy (4–14). These reports concluded that the insulin analog had maternal efficacy and safety similar to other insulins. No embryo–fetal adverse effects related to the drug were observed (4–14).

BREASTFEEDING SUMMARY

Insulin is a naturally occurring constituent of the blood and is excreted into breast milk. In a 2012 study, milk samples were obtained from breastfeeding mothers, five without diabetes, four with type 1 diabetes, and five with type 2 diabetes (15). Samples were analyzed for total and endogenous insulin and for c-peptide. The type 1 diabetics were treated with artificial insulin (aspart plus glargine), whereas the type 2 diabetics received a diabetic diet either with ($N = 3$) or without ($N = 2$) metformin. Insulin was present in all of the samples at comparable concentration to serum, but only artificial insulin was detected in the milk of type 1 diabetics. The results showed that insulin, both endogenous and exogenous, is actively transported from the blood into milk and is protected from degradation and, presumably, has a functional or developmental role in the infant. If so, the authors suggested, it might be beneficial for formula-fed infants if insulin was added to formula milk (15).

References

1. Product information. Lantus. Sanofi-Aventis, 2007.
2. Schardein JL. Insulin and oral hypoglycemic agents. In: *Chemically Induced Birth Defects*. 3rd ed. New York, NY: Marcel Dekker, 2000:458.
3. Buchanan TA, Kjos SL. Diabetes in women. Early detection, prevention, and management. Clin Updates Women's Health Care. 2002;1(4/Fall):47.
4. Devlin JT, Hothersall L, Wilkis JL. Use of insulin glargine during pregnancy in a type 1 diabetic woman. Diabetes Care 2002;25:1095–6.
5. Holstein A, Plaschke A, Egberts EH. Use of insulin glargine during embryogenesis in a pregnant woman with type 1 diabetes. Diabet Med 2003;20:779–80.
6. Di Cianni G, Volpe L, Lencioni C, Chatzianagnostou K, Cuccuuru I, Ghio A, Benzi L, Del Prato S. Use of insulin glargine during the first weeks of pregnancy in five type 1 diabetic women. Diabetes Care 2005;28:982–3.
7. Dolci M, Mori M, Baccetti F. Use of glargine insulin before and during pregnancy in a woman with type 1 diabetes and Addison's disease. Diabetes Care 2005;28:2084–5.

8. Woolderink JM, Van Loon AJ, Storms F, De Heide L, Hoogenberg K. Use of insulin glargine during pregnancy in seven type 1 diabetic women. Diabetes Care 2005;28:2594–5.
9. Al-Shaikh AA. Pregnant women with type 1 diabetes mellitus treated by glargine insulin. Saudi Med J 2006;27:563–5.
10. Graves DE, White JC, Kirk JK. The use of insulin glargine with gestational diabetes mellitus. Diabetes Care 2006;29:471–2.
11. Pollex E, Moretti ME, Koren G, Feig DS. Safety of insulin glargine use in pregnancy: a systematic review and meta-analysis. An Pharmacother 2011;45:9–16.
12. Lepercq J, Lin J, Hall GC, Wang E, Dain MP, Riddle MC, Home PD. Meta-analysis of maternal and neonatal outcomes associated with the use of insulin glargine versus NPH insulin during pregnancy. Obstet Gynecol Int 2012;2012:649070. doi:10.1155/2012/649070.
13. Callesen NF, Damm J, Mathiesen JM, Ringholm L, Damm P, Mathiesen ER. Treatment with the long-acting insulin analogues detemir or glargine during pregnancy in women with type 1 diabetes: comparison of glycaemic control and pregnancy outcome. J Matern Fetal Neonatal Med 2013;26:588–92.
14. Lambert K, Holt RIG. The use of insulin analogues in pregnancy. Diabetes Obes Metab 2013;15:888–900.
15. Whitmore TJ, Trengove NJ, Graham DF, Hartmann PE. Analysis of insulin in human breast milk in mothers with type 1 and type 2 diabetes mellitus. Int J Endocrinol 2012;2012:296368. doi:10.1155/2012/296368. Epub 2012 Mar 5.

INSULIN GLULISINE

Antidiabetic Agent

PREGNANCY RECOMMENDATION: No Human Data—Probably Compatible
BREASTFEEDING RECOMMENDATION: Compatible

I

PREGNANCY SUMMARY

No reports describing the use of insulin glulisine in human pregnancy have been located. The animal data suggest that the risk to the embryo or fetus is low. Although there are no human data, there are no reasons to believe that insulin glulisine would pose a risk to the embryo or fetus different from that of other insulins. Older forms of insulin, whether of human or of porcine origin, are considered compatible with pregnancy. Insulin glulisine probably can be classified similarly. As with all insulins, the primary concern is severe maternal hypoglycemia.

FETAL RISK SUMMARY

Insulin glulisine is a rapid-acting human insulin analog that differs from regular human insulin by a single substitution of the amino acid asparagine by lysine at position B3. It is produced by recombinant DNA technology. Insulin glulisine is indicated for the treatment of adult patients with diabetes mellitus for the control of hyperglycemia. It may be given by SC injection or as an SC infusion by an external insulin pump. The mechanism of action of insulin glulisine is similar to human insulin, in that it binds to receptors in muscle and fat cells to facilitate the cellular uptake of glucose and, at the same time, inhibits glucose release from the liver. The apparent elimination half-life of insulin glulisine is 42 minutes, compared with 86 minutes for human regular insulin (1).

Reproduction studies have been conducted in rats and rabbits using regular human insulin as a comparator. In pregnant rats given daily SC doses up to twice the average human dose based on BSA (HD) throughout gestation, no embryo or fetal toxicity different from that observed with human insulin was noted. In pregnant rabbits, daily SC doses up to 0.5 times the HD were associated with developmental toxicity, but only at doses that induced maternal toxicity (hypoglycemia). At the highest dose, increased postimplantation losses and skeletal defects were observed, as was maternal mortality. The no-effect SC dose in rabbits was 0.1 times the HD. The embryo–fetal toxicity in rabbits did not differ from that observed with human insulin at the same dose (1).

In a 12-month carcinogenicity study, rats were given daily SC doses of 1–20 times the HD. A non-dose-dependent increased incidence of mammary gland tumors was observed in female rats compared with untreated controls. However, the incidence of mammary gland tumors was similar to that noted in female rats given human regular insulin. Insulin glulisine was not mutagenic or clastogenic in tests. In male and female rats given daily SC doses up to twice the HD, no clear evidence of impaired fertility or reproductive performance was observed (1).

It is not known if insulin glulisine crosses the human placenta. Human insulin does not cross the placenta in clinically significant amounts (2). Because of the close similarity between insulin glulisine and human insulin, and its high molecular weight (5823), insulin glulisine probably does not cross either. However, there may be endogenous carrier proteins that allow passage of insulin, including insulin glargine, to the embryo early in gestation. After that period, the fetus produces its own insulin as insulin-secreting cells in the fetal pancreas become differentiated near the end of the 1st trimester (3).

BREASTFEEDING SUMMARY

No reports describing the use of insulin glulisine during human lactation have been located. Insulin is a natural component of the blood and is excreted into breast milk (1). Insulin glulisine probably also is present in milk.

References

1. Product information. Apidra. Sanofi-Aventis, 2007.
2. Schardein JL. Insulin and oral hypoglycemic agents. In: *Chemically Induced Birth Defects*. 3rd ed. New York, NY: Marcel Dekker, 2000:458.
3. Buchanan TA, Kjos SL. Diabetes in women. Early detection, prevention, and management. Clin Updates Women's Health Care. 2002;1(4/Fall):47.

INSULIN LISPRO

Antidiabetic Agent

PREGNANCY RECOMMENDATION: Compatible
BREASTFEEDING RECOMMENDATION: Compatible

PREGNANCY SUMMARY

The animal and human data suggest that the use of insulin lispro during pregnancy can be considered low risk for the embryo–fetus. Insulin lispro is very closely related to human insulin, differing only in the reversal of two amino acids in the B chain. There is no reason to believe that insulin lispro would pose a risk to the embryo or fetus different from that of other insulins. Older forms of insulin, whether of human or of porcine origin, are considered compatible with pregnancy and insulin lispro can be classified similarly. As with all insulins, the primary concern is severe maternal hypoglycemia.

I

FETAL RISK SUMMARY

Insulin lispro is a rapid-acting human insulin analog that differs from regular human insulin by the reversal of the amino acids at positions B28 and B29. It is produced by recombinant DNA technology. Insulin lispro is indicated for the treatment of adult patients with diabetes mellitus for the control of hyperglycemia. It may be given by SC injection or as an SC infusion by an external insulin pump. The mechanism of action of insulin lispro is similar to human insulin, in that it binds to receptors in muscle and fat cells to facilitate the cellular uptake of glucose and, at the same time, inhibits glucose release from the liver. The elimination half-life of SC insulin lispro is 1 hour, compared with 1.5 hours for human regular insulin (1).

Reproduction studies have been conducted in pregnant rats and rabbits. In these species, SC doses up to 4 and 0.3 times the average human dose (40 U/day) based on BSA revealed no evidence of impaired fertility or fetal harm due to insulin lispro. Long-term studies of carcinogenicity have not been conducted. The drug was not mutagenic or clastogenic in tests (1).

A 2001 study briefly described the use of normal, term human placentas to determine if insulin lispro crossed to the fetal circulation (2). Two concentrations, 0.1 and 0.5 U/mL, were studied in the dual-perfused isolated cotyledon system. Time-dependent transfer of insulin lispro to the fetal side was observed, but the concentrations used were >50 times the normal human therapeutic doses (2).

A 2003 study used a similar system to determine the amount of insulin lispro crossing the placenta (3). Placental transfer was not observed during perfusions with 100 and 200 micro-U/mL, but did occur at concentrations ≥580 micro-U/mL. To determine clinically relevant levels, serum concentrations were measured in 11 women at 31–40 years of age (9 pregnant; 1 in 1st trimester, 8 in 2nd or 3rd trimester) receiving insulin lispro. Concentrations ranged from 2 to 576 micro-U/mL. There was an apparent linear relationship between dose and serum levels. Ten women had levels <200 micro-U/mL (single doses less than 50 U), whereas one woman, who received a 52-U dose, had a serum level of 576 micro-U/mL (3). Using a human-perfused placental cotyledon, a 2004 study found no detectable insulin lispro on the fetal side with the highest maternal steady-state concentration of 48 micro-U in the maternal artery (4). However, very high concentrations of insulin lispro (1836 micro-U *without specifying a denominator*) were found in placental tissue.

Based on the above studies, insulin lispro, depending on the dose, could cross to the embryo–fetus. Moreover, there may be endogenous carrier proteins that allow passage of insulin, including insulin lispro (molecular weight 5808; identical to human insulin), to the embryo early in gestation. After that period, the fetus produces its own insulin as insulin-secreting cells in the fetal pancreas become differentiated near the end of the 1st trimester (5).

A 1997 case report described the pregnancy outcomes of two women with type 1 diabetes who were treated with insulin lispro and NPH insulin during pregnancy (6). In the first case, insulin lispro was started before conception. The pregnancy was terminated at 20 weeks' gestation because of intrauterine growth restriction and severe fetal embryopathy but a normal karyotype. The female fetus had left-sided pulmonary and atrial isomerism, a right-sided aortic arch, a single atrium with one atrioventricular valve, a large ventricular septal defect, a double-outlet right ventricle, polysplenia, and abdominal situs inversus. In the second mother, insulin lispro was started in the third week of gestation. An elective cesarean section at 37 weeks delivered a 2.82-kg male infant with normal Apgar scores. No neonatal complications were noted, but the infant died suddenly at 3 weeks of age. At autopsy, a congenital diaphragmatic hernia with herniation of the stomach and intestine into the chest and bilateral undescended testes were found. The cause of the defects in the two cases was unknown, but the authors did not believe they were due to suboptimal glycemic control. They also mentioned four other cases involving insulin lispro during pregnancy. Three of the women were still in the 1st trimester. The fourth woman was started at 26 weeks and she gave birth to a normal infant at 38 weeks (6).

In reply to the above cases, representatives of the manufacturer noted that the risk of congenital defects was known to be increased in infants of women with diabetes, especially cardiac defects (7). During clinical trials with insulin lispro, pregnancy was an exclusion, but 19 women gave birth to live infants. Only one infant had a birth defect (a right dysplastic kidney). The representatives cautioned that although case reports were important to raise hypotheses, they could not be used to infer a causal relationship (7).

Eight studies that included fetal outcomes have described the use of insulin lispro during 836 pregnancies (8–16). Diabetic types included 735 pregestational (types 1 and 2) and 101 gestational (type 3). No embryo, fetal, or neonatal complications attributable to insulin lispro were reported in 303 of the pregnancies (8–15).

The remaining pregnancies came from a multinational, multicenter study (16). The medical charts of 533 pregnancies (496 women) complicated by pregestational diabetes were examined and anomalies were assessed by two independent dysmorphologists. There were 542 outcomes involving 500 live births, 31 spontaneous abortions, 7 elective abortions, and 4 stillbirths. The mothers had a mean age of 29.9 years, 85.6% were white, and 97.2% had type 1 diabetes. All of the women had used insulin lispro for at least 1 month before conception and during at least the 1st trimester. More than 96% continued insulin lispro during the 2nd and 3rd trimesters. Twenty-seven (5.4%) of the offspring, including two that were electively aborted, had major congenital defects and two (0.4%) had minor anomalies. The anomaly rate among pregnancies that resulted in a live or stillbirth was 5.2%. Comparing these rates with the current published rates of 2.1%–10.9% for major defects in infants of diabetic mothers treated with insulin, the investigators concluded that their results suggested no difference in the anomaly rates between insulin lispro and regular insulin (16).

The cases of congenital defects in infants of two women using insulin lispro cited above were most likely due to diabetes or unknown causes. Four reviews concluded that the use of insulin lispro in pregnancy was appropriate and often gave better glycemic control than regular human insulin (17–20). However, a fifth review, published in 2006, cautioned that more comparative data were needed before insulin lispro could be recommended in pregnancy or alternatively avoided (21).

A 2003 study compared the progression of retinopathy in pregnant women with type 1 diabetes who were treated with insulin lispro (N = 36) or human insulin (N = 33) (22). Patients treated with insulin lispro had improved glycemic control with no adverse impact on progression of diabetic retinopathy.

BREASTFEEDING SUMMARY

No reports describing the use of insulin lispro during human lactation have been located. Insulin is a natural component of the blood and is excreted into breast milk (1). Insulin lispro probably also is present in milk.

References

1. Product information. Humalog. Eli Lilly, 2007.
2. Rosenn B, Kosssenjans W, Eis A, Brockman D, Myatt L. Does lispro insulin cross the human placenta? Am J Obstet Gynecol 2001;184:S69.
3. Boskovic R, Knie B, Feig DS, Portnoi G, Derewlany L, Koren G. Transfer of insulin lispro across the human placenta. Diabetes Care 2003;26:1390–4.
4. Holcberg G, Tsadkin-Tamir M, Sapir O, Wiznizer A, Segal D, Polachek H. Transfer of insulin lispro across the human placenta. Eur J Obstet Gynecol Reprod Biol 2004;115:117–8.
5. Buchanan TA, Kjos SL. Diabetes in women. Early detection, prevention, and management. Clin Updates Women's Health Care. 2002;1(4/Fall):47.
6. Diamond T, Kormas N. Possible adverse fetal effect of insulin lispro. N Engl J Med 1997;337:1009.
7. Anderson JH Jr, Bastyr EJ, Wishner KL. Possible adverse fetal effects of insulin lispro. Reply. N Engl J Med 1997;337:1010.
8. Bhattacharyya A, Brown S, Hughes S, Vice PA. Insulin lispro and regular insulin in pregnancy. QJM 2001;94:255–60.
9. Scherbaum WA, Lankisch MR, Pawlowski B, Somville T. Insulin lispro in pregnancy—retrospective analysis of 33 cases and matched controls. Exp Clin Endocrinol Diabetes 2002;110:6–9.
10. Persson B, Swahn ML, Hjertberg R, Hanson U, Nord E, Nordlander E, Hansson LO. Insulin lispro therapy in pregnancies complicated by type 1 diabetes mellitus. Diabetes Res Clin Pract 2002;58:115–21.
11. Durand-Gonzalez KN, Guillausseau N, Anciaux ML, Hentschel V, Gayno JP. Allergy to insulin in a woman with gestational diabetes mellitus: transient efficiency of continuous subcutaneous insulin lispro infusion. Diabetes Metab 2003;29:432–4.
12. Cypryk K, Sobczak M, Pertynska-Marczewska M, Zawodniak-Szalapska M, Syzmczak W, Wilczynski J, Lewinski A. Pregnancy complications and perinatal outcomes in diabetic women treated with Humalog (insulin lispro) or regular human insulin during pregnancy. Med Sci Monit 2004;10:P129–32.
13. Mecacci F, Carignani L, Cioni R, Bartoli E, Parretti E, La Torre P, Scarselli G, Mello G. Maternal metabolic control and perinatal outcome in women with gestational diabetes treated with regular or lispro insulin: comparison with non-diabetic pregnant women. Eur J Obstet Gynecol Reprod Biol 2003;111:19–24.
14. Dolci M, Mori M, Baccetti F. Use of glargine insulin before and during pregnancy in a woman with type 1 diabetes and Addison's disease. Diabetes Care 2005;28:2084–5.
15. Masson EA, Patmore JE, Brash PD, Baxtert M, Caldwell G, Gallen IW, Price PA, Vice PA, Walker JD, Lindow SW. Pregnancy outcome in type 1 diabetes mellitus treated with insulin lispro (Humalog). Diabet Med 2003;20:46–50.
16. Wyatt JW, Frias JL, Hoymet HE, Jovanovic L, Kaaja R, Brown F, Garg S, Lee-Parritz A, Seely EW, Kerr L, Mattoo V, Tan M, and the IONS Study Group. Congenital anomaly rate in offspring of mothers with diabetes treated with insulin lispro during pregnancy. Diabet Med 2005;22:803–7.
17. Radermecker RP, Scheen AJ. Continuous subcutaneous insulin infusion with short-acting insulin analogues or human regular insulin: efficacy, safety, quality of life, and cost-effectiveness. Diabetes Metab Res Rev 2004;20:178–88.
18. Lapolla A, Dalfra MG, Fedele D. Insulin therapy in pregnancy complicated by diabetes: are insulin analogs a new tool? Diabetes Metab Res Rev 2005;21:241–52.
19. Gonzalez C, Santoro S, Salzberg S, Di Girolamo G, Alvarinas J. Insulin analogue therapy in pregnancies complicated by diabetes mellitus. Expert Opin Pharmacother 2005;6:735–42.
20. Homko CJ, Reech EA. Insulins and oral hypoglycemic agents in pregnancy. J Matern Fetal Neonatal Med 2006;19:679–86.
21. Carr KJE, Lindow SW, Masson EA. The potential for the use of insulin lispro in pregnancy complicated by diabetes. J Matern Fetal Neonatal Med 2006;19:323–9.
22. Loukovaara S, Immonen I, Teramo KA, Kaaja R. Progression of retinopathy during pregnancy in type 1 diabetic women treated with human lispro. Diabetes Care 2003;26:1193–8.

INTERFERON, ALFA

Antineoplastic/Immunologic Agent (Immunomodulator)

PREGNANCY RECOMMENDATION: Limited Human Data—Probably Compatible
BREASTFEEDING RECOMMENDATION: Limited Human Data—Probably Compatible

PREGNANCY SUMMARY

Based on a limited number of human cases, the maternal administration of interferon alfa does not appear to pose a significant risk to the developing embryo and fetus. There does not seem to be a difference in risk among the subtypes but, in many cases, the actual product used was not specified. Although very high doses are abortifacient in rhesus monkeys, doses used clinically apparently do not have this effect. No teratogenic or other reproductive toxicity, other than that noted above, has been observed in animals, and no toxicity of any type attributable to interferon alfa has been observed in humans. However, because of the antiproliferative activity of these agents, they should be used cautiously during gestation until more data are available to assess their risk.

FETAL RISK SUMMARY

Interferon alfa is a family of at least 23 structurally similar subtypes of human proteins and glycoproteins that have antiviral, antineoplastic, and immunomodulating properties (1). Five preparations are available in the United States: interferon alfa-n3, interferon alfa-N1 (orphan drug status), interferon alfa-2a, interferon alfa-2b, and peginterferon alfa-2B. Interferon alfa-2c has been used in pregnancy, but this product is not available in the United States. No reports describing the placental transfer of interferon alfa have been located.

Shepard reviewed four studies in which human interferon alfa (subtype not specified) was administered by various parenteral routes to rats and rabbits during pregnancy (2–5). No teratogenicity or adverse developmental changes were observed in the offspring.

Interferon alfa-2a produced a statistically significant increase in abortions in rhesus monkeys given 20–500 times the human dose (HD) (6). No teratogenic effects, however, were observed in this species when doses of 1–25 million IU/kg/day were administered during the early to mid-fetal period (days 22–70 of gestation) (6). Interferon alfa-2b also had abortifacient effects in rhesus monkeys treated with doses that were 90–360 times the human dose (7). Reproduction studies have not been conducted with interferon alfa-n3 (8).

Administration of interferon alfa to female sheep before conception resulted in an increased number of pregnant ewes and embryonic survival (9). This effect may have been the result of enhanced biochemical communication between the mother and conceptus (9). A study published in 1986 demonstrated that human fetal blood and organs, placenta, membranes, amniotic fluid, and decidua contain significant concentrations of interferon alfa (10). In contrast, maternal blood and blood and tissues from nonpregnant adults contained little or none of these proteins. The investigators concluded that one of the effects of interferon alfa may involve the preservation of the fetus as a homograft (10). Other effects and actions of endogenous interferons (alfa, beta, and gamma) in relation to animal and human pregnancies and the presence of these proteins in various maternal and fetal tissues have been summarized in two reviews (11,12).

A number of reports have described the use of interferon alfa in all phases of pregnancy for the treatment of leukemia (13–20). The first reported case involved a woman with chronic myelogenous leukemia (CML) who was treated before conception and throughout a normal pregnancy with 4 million U/m^2 (6.4 million U) of interferon alfa-2a every other day (13). She delivered a term, healthy, 3487-g female infant whose growth and development continued to be normal at 15 months of age. The newborn had an elevated white blood cell count (40,000/mm^3) that normalized at 48 hours of age with no signs or symptoms of infection. Since this report, 10 other pregnancies have been described in which interferon alfa was used for CML or hairy cell leukemia (14–20).

In one case, a woman was treated with interferon alfa-2c (not available in the United States) (16). In two of the pregnancies, the concentrations of interferon alfa in the newborns were <0.6 and <1 U/mL, respectively, while those in the mothers were 20.8 and 58 U/mL, respectively (18). Normal pregnancy outcomes were observed in all of the above cases and there were no fetal or newborn toxic effects attributable to interferon alfa (13–20). In addition, four infants have been followed for periods ranging from 6 to 44 months and all had normal growth and development (14).

A 1995 reference reported the use of interferon alfa-2a for the treatment of multiple myeloma before and during approximately the first 6 weeks of pregnancy (21). The woman delivered a normal male infant at 38 weeks' gestation.

As noted above, interferon alfa does not appear to cross the placenta to the fetus. A study published in 1995 specifically evaluated this in two HIV-seropositive women who were undergoing abortions at 19 and 24 weeks (22). Both women were given a single IM injection of 5 million U interferon alfa-2a. Peak blood concentrations of the drug were reached at 3 hours in both women, 100 U and 400 U, respectively. Fetal blood and amniotic fluid samples were drawn at 1 hour from one fetus and at 4 hours from the other. Concentrations in the four samples were all below the detection limit of the assay (<2 U).

A number of pregnant women have been treated with interferon alfa (usually interferon alfa-2a) for essential thrombocythemia (23–34), although not without controversy (35–37). In some of these cases, the women were receiving interferon therapy at the time of conception (23,24,26,28,29) and, in most, the treatment was continued throughout pregnancy (26,28,29). No adverse effects in the fetuses or in the newborns attributable to the drug therapy were reported.

An HIV-infected pregnant woman was treated with IM interferon alfa, 2 million units twice weekly, and oral and IV glycyrrhizin during the 3rd trimester (38). Two weeks after interferon alfa was started, an elective cesarean section was performed at 37 weeks' gestation. The healthy, 2320-g female was alive and well at 4 years of age without evidence of HIV infection.

Two reports have described the use of interferon alfa for the treatment of chronic hepatitis C (39,40). In both cases, treatment was started before conception and continued into the 2nd trimester. Interferon alfa treatment throughout the 1st trimester also occurred in a woman with advanced Hodgkin's disease (41). Normal newborns resulted in all three of these pregnancies.

BREASTFEEDING SUMMARY

Interferon alfa is excreted into breast milk. A study published in 1996 measured interferon alfa milk concentrations in two women who had been treated with the drug throughout the 2nd and 3rd trimesters for CML (18). Both women were receiving 8 million units SC 3 times a week at the time of delivery. Immediately postpartum, milk concentrations in the two patients were 1.4 and 6 U/mL (time of the last dose in relationship to milk sampling not specified), while the serum levels in the mothers were 20.8 and 58 U/mL, respectively. The authors did not specify if the infants were allowed to breastfeed.

Breastfeeding was allowed in a second reference (25). The woman was being treated with interferon alfa-2a, 3 million units SC 3 times weekly, for essential thrombocythemia. Nursing was halted 2 weeks postpartum because of the onset of bilateral mastitis. In a 2000 case report, a woman with malignant melanoma received 30 million IU IV over 30 minutes (42). Breast milk samples were collected before (to measure endogenous interferon alfa) and after the infusion. Only small amounts of interferon alfa were transferred into milk (peak level 1551 IU/mL vs. 1249 IU/mL before infusion). The infant did not breastfeed during the therapy.

The American Academy of Pediatrics classifies interferon alfa as compatible with breastfeeding (43).

References

1. American Hospital Formulary Service. *Drug Information 1997*. Bethesda, MD: American Society of Health-System Pharmacists, 1997:775–804.
2. Matsumoto T, Nakamura K, Imai M, Aoki H, Okugi M, Shimoi H, Hagita K. Reproduction studies of human interferon α (interferon alpha). (I) Teratological study in rabbits. Iyakuhin Kenkyu 1986;17:397–404. As cited by Shepard TH. *Catalog of Teratogenic Agents*. 7th ed. Baltimore, MD: The Johns Hopkins University Press, 1992:220–1.
3. Matsumoto T, Nakamura K, Imai M, Aoki H, Okugi M, Shimoi H, Hagita K. Reproduction studies of human interferon α (interferon alpha). (III) Teratological study in rats. Iyakuhin Kenkyu 1986;17:417–38. As cited by Shepard TH. *Catalog of Teratogenic Agents*. 7th ed. Baltimore, MD: The Johns Hopkins University Press, 1992:220–1.
4. Matsumoto T, Nakamura K, Imai M, Aoki H, Okugi M, Shimoi H, Hagita K. Perinatal studies of human interferon α (interferon alpha). (IV) Teratological study in rats. Iyakuhin Kenkyu 1986;17:439–57. As cited by Shepard TH. *Catalog of Teratogenic Agents*. 7th ed. Baltimore, MD: The Johns Hopkins University Press, 1992:220–1.
5. Shibutani Y, Hamada Y, Kurokawa M, Inoue K, Shichi S. Toxicity studies of human lymphoblastoid interferon α. Teratogenicity study in rats. Iyakuhin Kenkyu 1987;18:60–78. As cited by Shepard TH. *Catalog of Teratogenic Agents*. 7th ed. Baltimore, MD: The Johns Hopkins University Press, 1992:220–1.
6. Product information. Roferon-A. Roche Laboratories, 2001.
7. Product information. Intron A. Schering, 2001.
8. Product information. Alferon N. Interferon Sciences, 2001.
9. Nephew KP, McClure KE, Day ML, Xie S, Roberts RM, Pope WF. Effects of intramuscular administration of recombinant bovine interferon-alpha$_1$1 during the period of maternal recognition of pregnancy. J Anim Sci 1990;68:2766–70.
10. Chard T, Craig PH, Menabawey M, Lee C. Alpha interferon in human pregnancy. Br J Obstet Gynaecol 1986;93:1145–9.
11. Chard T. Interferon in pregnancy. J Develop Physiol 1989;11:271–6.
12. Roberts RM, Cross JC, Leaman DW. Interferons as hormones of pregnancy. Endocrine Rev 1992;13:432–52.
13. Baer MR. Normal full-term pregnancy in a patient with chronic myelogenous leukemia treated with α-interferon. Am J Hematol 1991;37:66.
14. Baer MR, Ozer H, Foon KA. Interferon-α therapy during pregnancy in chronic myelogenous leukaemia and hairy cell leukaemia. Br J Haematol 1992;81:167–9.
15. Crump M, Wang X-H, Sermer M, Keating A. Successful pregnancy and delivery during α-interferon therapy for chronic myeloid leukemia. Am J Hematol 1992;40:238–43.
16. Reichel RP, Linkesch W, Schetitska D. Therapy with recombinant interferon alpha-2c during unexpected pregnancy in a patient with chronic myeloid leukaemia. Br J Haematol 1992;82:472–3.
17. Delmer A, Rio B, Bauduer F, Ajchenbaum F, Marie J-P, Zittoun R. Pregnancy during myelosuppressive treatment for chronic myelogenous leukaemia. Br J Haematol 1992;82:783–4.
18. Haggstrom J, Adriansson M, Hybbinette T, Harnby E, Thorbert G. Two cases of CML treated with alpha-interferon during second and third trimester of pregnancy with analysis of the drug in the new-born immediately postpartum. Eur J Haematol 1996;57:101–2.
19. Lipton JH, Derzko CM, Curtis J. Alpha-interferon and pregnancy in a patient with CML. Hematol Oncol 1996;14:119–22.
20. Kuroiwa M, Gondo H, Ashida K, Kamimura T, Miyamoto T, Niho Y, Tsukimori K, Nakano H, Ohga S. Interferon-alpha therapy for chronic myelogenous leukemia during pregnancy. Am J Hematol 1998;59:101–2.
21. Sakata H, Karamitsos J, Kundaria B, DiSaia PJ. Case report of interferon alfa therapy for multiple myeloma during pregnancy. Am J Obstet Gynecol 1995;172:217–9.
22. Pons J-C, Lebon P, Frydman R, Delfraissy J-F. Pharmacokinetics of interferon-alpha in pregnant women and fetoplacental passage. Fetal Diagn Ther 1995;10:7–10.
23. Pardini S, Dore F, Murineddu M, Bontigli S, Longinotti M, Grigliotti B, Spano B. α2b-Interferon therapy and pregnancy—report of a case of essential thrombocythemia. Am J Hematol 1993;43:78–9.
24. Petit JJ, Callis M, Fernandez de Sevilla A. Normal pregnancy in a patient with essential thrombocythemia treated with interferon-α_{2b}. Am J Hematol 1992;40:80.
25. Thornley S, Manoharan A. Successful treatment of essential thrombocythemia with alpha interferon during pregnancy. Eur J Haematol 1994;52:63–4.
26. Williams JM, Schlesinger PE, Gray AG. Successful treatment of essential thrombocythaemia and recurrent abortion with alpha interferon. Br J Haematol 1994;88:647–8.
27. Vianelli N, Gugliotta L, Tura S, Bovicelli L, Rizzo N, Gabrielli A. Interferon-α2a treatment in a pregnant woman with essential thrombocythemia. Blood 1994;83:874–5.
28. Shpilberg O, Shimon I, Sofer O, Dolitski M, Ben-Bassat I. Transient normal platelet counts and decreased requirement for interferon during pregnancy in essential thrombocythaemia. Br J Haematol 1996;92:491–3.
29. Pulik M, Lionnet F, Genet P, Petitdidier C, Jary L. Platelet counts during pregnancy in essential thrombocythaemia treated with recombinant α-interferon. Br J Haematol 1996;93:495.
30. Delage R, Demers C, Cantin G, Roy J. Treatment of essential thrombocythemia during pregnancy with interferon-α. Obstet Gynecol 1996;87:814–7.
31. Schmidt HH, Neumeister P, Kainer F, Karpf EF, Linkesch W, Sill H. Treatment of essential thrombocythemia during pregnancy: antiabortive effect of interferon-α? Ann Hematol 1998;77:291–2.
32. Diez-Martin JL, Banas MH, Fernandez MN. Childbearing age patients with essential thrombocythemia: should they be placed on interferon? Am J Hematol 1996;52:331–2.
33. Cincotta R, Higgins JR, Tippett C, Gallery E, North R, McMahon LP, Brennecke SP. Management of essential thrombocythaemia during pregnancy. Aust NZ J Obstet Gynaecol 2000;40:33–7.
34. Vantroyen B, Vanstraelen D. Management of essential thrombocythemia during pregnancy with aspirin, interferon alpha-2a and no treatment. Acta Haematol 2002;107:158–69.
35. Randi ML, Barbone E, Girolami A. Normal pregnancy and delivery in essential thrombocythemia even without interferon therapy. Am J Hematol 1994;45:270–1.
36. Petit J. Normal pregnancy and delivery in essential thrombocythemia even without interferon therapy. In reply. Am J Hematol 1994;45:271.
37. Frezzato M, Rodeghiero F. Pregnancy in women with essential thrombocythaemia. Br J Haematol 1996;93:977.
38. Sagara Y. Management of pregnancy of HIV infected woman. Early Hum Dev 1992;29:231–2.
39. Ruggiero G, Andreana A, Zampino R. Normal pregnancy under inadvertent alpha-interferon therapy for chronic hepatitis C. J Hepatol 1996;24:646.
40. Trotter JF, Zygmunt AJ. Conception and pregnancy during interferon-alpha therapy for chronic hepatitis C. J Clin Gastroenterol 2001;32:76–8.
41. Ferrari VD, Jirillo A, Lonardi F, Pavanato G, Bonciarelli G. Pregnancy during alpha-interferon therapy in patients with advanced Hodgkin's disease. Eur J Cancer 1995;31A;2121–2.
42. Kimar AR, Hale TW, Mock RE. Transfer of interferon alfa into human breast milk. J Hum Lact 2000;16:226–8.
43. Committee on Drugs, American Academy of Pediatrics. The transfer of drugs and other chemicals into human milk. Pediatrics 2001;108:776–89.

INTERFERON BETA-1B

Immunologic Agent (Immunomodulator)

PREGNANCY RECOMMENDATION: Limited Human Data—Animal Data Suggest Moderate Risk
BREASTFEEDING RECOMMENDATION: No Human Data—Probably Compatible

PREGNANCY SUMMARY

Although no published reports of its use in human pregnancy have been located, the manufacturer states that spontaneous abortions occurred in four patients who were participating in the Betaseron Multiple Sclerosis clinical trial (1). The relationship between interferon beta-1b and the abortions cannot be determined, at least partially because of the lack of details involving this clinical trial, such as the timing of abortion to drug administration, the dose used, the clinical condition of the women, and the number of pregnant women in the trial. Also unknown is the effect of multiple sclerosis on early pregnancy, although it appears that the physiologic immunomodulation that occurs in pregnancy offers some protection from relapses of the disease during gestation (2,3).

I

FETAL RISK SUMMARY

Interferon beta-1b, prepared by recombinant DNA technology, is used for the symptomatic treatment of multiple sclerosis and investigationally in the therapy of AIDS, some neoplasms, and acute non-A/non-B hepatitis. No teratogenic effects were observed in rhesus monkeys given doses up to 40 times the recommended human dose based on BSA (RHD) on gestation days 20–70 (1). However, dose-related abortifacient activity occurred in these monkeys with doses that were 2.8–40 times the RHD.

BREASTFEEDING SUMMARY

No reports describing the use of interferon beta-1b during human lactation have been reported.

References

1. Product information. Betaseron. Berlex Laboratories, 1994.
2. Hutchinson M. Pregnancy in multiple sclerosis. J Neurol Neurosurg Psychiatry 1993;56:1043–5.
3. Roullet E, Verdier-Taillefer M-H, Armarenco P, Gharbi G, Alperovitch A, Marteau R. Pregnancy and multiple sclerosis: a longitudinal study of 125 remittent patients. J Neurol Neurosurg Psychiatry 1993;56:1062–5.

INTERFERON GAMMA-1B

Immunologic Agent (Immunomodulator)

PREGNANCY RECOMMENDATION: No Human Data—Animal Data Suggest Low Risk
BREASTFEEDING RECOMMENDATION: No Human Data—Probably Compatible

PREGNANCY SUMMARY

No reports describing the use of interferon gamma-1b in human pregnancy have been located. Interferon gamma-1b, produced by recombinant DNA technology, is used to reduce the frequency and severity of serious infections in patients who have chronic granulomatous disease (1). Because of this indication, the opportunities for its use in human pregnancy should be rare.

FETAL RISK SUMMARY

Interferon gamma-1b has abortifacient activity in nonhuman primates treated with a dose approximately 100 times the human dose (HD) (1). Similar activity was observed in mice treated with maternally toxic doses. Other effects noted in mice were an increased incidence of uterine bleeding and decreased neonatal viability (1). However, no evidence of teratogenicity was found in primates with doses of 2–100 times the HD (1).

Treatment of pregnant mice with 5000 U/day for 6 days produced maternal and fetal hematologic toxicity (2). In addition to an increase in aborted fetuses and decreased fetal weight, severe anomalies, consisting of inhibition or retardation of eye formation and brain hematomas, were observed in surviving fetuses (2).

Two reviews have summarized the effects and actions of endogenous interferons (alfa, beta, and gamma) in animal and human pregnancies and the presence of these proteins in various maternal and fetal tissues (3,4).

BREASTFEEDING SUMMARY

No reports describing the use of interferon gamma-1b during human lactation have been located.

References

1. Product information. Actimmune. Genentech, Inc., 1994.
2. Vassiliadis S, Athanassakis I. Type II interferon may be a potential hazardous therapeutic agent during pregnancy. Br J Haematol 1992;82:782–3.
3. Chard T. Interferon in pregnancy. J Dev Physiol 1989;11:271–6.
4. Roberts RM, Cross JC, Leaman DW. Interferons as hormones of pregnancy. Endocrine Rev 1992;13:432–52.

IOCETAMIC ACID

Diagnostic

PREGNANCY RECOMMENDATION: No Human Data—Probably Compatible
BREASTFEEDING RECOMMENDATION: No Human Data—Probably Compatible

PREGNANCY SUMMARY

Iocetamic acid contains a high concentration of organically bound iodine. See Diatrizoate for possible effects on the fetus and newborn.

BREASTFEEDING SUMMARY

See Diatrizoate.

IODAMID

[Withdrawn from the market. See 9th edition.]

IODINATED GLYCEROL

Respiratory Drug (Expectorant)

PREGNANCY RECOMMENDATION: Limited Human Data—Probably Compatible
BREASTFEEDING RECOMMENDATION: No Human Data—Probably Compatible

PREGNANCY SUMMARY

Iodinated glycerol is a stable complex containing 50% organically bound iodine (see Potassium Iodide).

FETAL RISK SUMMARY

In a surveillance study of Michigan Medicaid recipients involving 229,101 completed pregnancies conducted between 1985 and 1992, 1453 newborns had been exposed to iodinated glycerol during the 1st trimester (F. Rosa, personal communication, FDA, 1993). A total of 65 (4.5%) major birth defects were observed (61 expected). Specific data were available for six defect categories, including (observed/expected) 11/15 cardiovascular defects, 0/2 oral clefts, 1/1 spina bifida, 8/4 polydactyly, 1/2 limb reduction defects, and 1/3 hypospadias. An additional 1338 newborns were exposed to the general class of expectorants during the 1st trimester with 63 (4.7%) major birth defects observed (57 expected). Specific malformations were (observed/expected) 9/13 cardiovascular defects, 0/2 oral clefts, 1/1 spina bifida, 7/4 polydactyly, 1/2 limb reduction defects, and 3/3 hypospadias. These data do not support an association between 1st trimester use of either iodinated glycerol or the general class of expectorants and congenital defects.

BREASTFEEDING SUMMARY

See Potassium Iodide.

IODINE

Anti-infective

See Potassium Iodide.

IODIPAMIDE

Diagnostic

PREGNANCY RECOMMENDATION: No Human Data—Probably Compatible
BREASTFEEDING RECOMMENDATION: No Human Data—Probably Compatible

PREGNANCY SUMMARY

The various preparations of iodipamide contain a high concentration of organically bound iodine. See Diatrizoate for possible effects on the fetus and newborn.

BREASTFEEDING SUMMARY

See Diatrizoate.

IODOQUINOL

Amebicide

PREGNANCY RECOMMENDATION: Limited Human Data—No Relevant Animal Data
BREASTFEEDING RECOMMENDATION: Limited Human Data—Probably Compatible

PREGNANCY SUMMARY

Iodoquinol (di-iodohydroxyquinoline; diiodohydroxyquin) is used in the treatment of intestinal amebiasis. It has been used in pregnancy apparently without causing fetal harm.

FETAL RISK SUMMARY

Two case reports described the use of iodoquinol in pregnancy for the treatment of a rare skin disease. The first case involved a woman with chronic acrodermatitis enteropathica, who was treated with the amebicide in the 2nd and 3rd trimesters of her first pregnancy (1). She delivered a typical achondroplastic dwarf who died in 30 minutes. The second case also involved a woman with the same disorder who took iodoquinol throughout gestation (2). Dose during the 1st trimester, 1.3 g/day, was systematically increased during pregnancy in an attempt to control the cutaneous lesions, eventually reaching 6.5 g/day during the last 4 weeks. A normal male infant was delivered at term. Physical examinations of the infant, including ophthalmic examinations, were normal at birth and at 6 weeks follow-up.

The Collaborative Perinatal Project monitored 50,282 mother–child pairs, 169 of whom had 1st trimester exposure to iodoquinol (3, pp. 299, 302). Ten of the infants were born with a congenital malformation, corresponding to a hospital standardized relative risk (SRR) of 0.88. Based on three infants, an SRR of 6.6 for congenital dislocation of the hip was calculated, but this association is uninterpretable without confirming evidence (3, pp. 467, 473). For use anytime during pregnancy, 172 exposures were recorded (3, pp. 434, 435). With the same caution as noted earlier, an SRR of 1.68 (95% confidence interval 0.62–3.58) was estimated based on malformations in 6 infants. The SRR for congenital dislocation of the hip after use anytime during pregnancy was 6.5 (3, p. 486).

BREASTFEEDING SUMMARY

No reports describing the use of iodoquinol during lactation have been located. Although the oral bioavailability is low, the molecular weight (397) should allow transfer of some drug from the plasma into the milk. In addition, protein-bound serum iodine levels may be increased with the administration of iodoquinol and may persist for as long as 6 months after discontinuation of therapy (4). The effects on a nursing infant from this exposure are unknown, but because iodide is concentrated in breast milk, serum and urinary iodide levels in the infant may be elevated (see Potassium Iodide).

References

1. Vedder JS, Griem S. Acrodermatitis enteropathica (Danbolt–Closs) in five siblings: efficacy of diodoquin in its management. J Pediatr 1956;48:212–9.
2. Verburg DJ, Burd LI, Hoxtell EO, Merrill LK. Acrodermatitis enteropathica and pregnancy. Obstet Gynecol 1974;44:233–7.
3. Heinonen OP, Slone D, Shapiro S. *Birth Defects and Drugs in Pregnancy*. Littleton, MA: Publishing Sciences Group, 1977.
4. Product information. Yodoxin. Glenwood, 2000.

IODOTHYRIN

[Withdrawn from the market. See 8th edition.]

IODOXAMATE

Diagnostic

PREGNANCY RECOMMENDATION: No Human Data—Probably Compatible
BREASTFEEDING RECOMMENDATION: No Human Data—Probably Compatible

PREGNANCY SUMMARY

The various preparations of iodoxamate contain a high concentration of organically bound iodine. See Diatrizoate for possible effects on the fetus and newborn.

BREASTFEEDING SUMMARY

See Diatrizoate.

IOFLUPANE IODINE^{123}

Diagnostic

PREGNANCY RECOMMENDATION: Contraindicated
BREASTFEEDING RECOMMENDATION: Contraindicated

PREGNANCY SUMMARY

No reports describing the use ioflupane iodine^{123} in human pregnancy have been located. Reproduction studies in animals have not been performed. In 2012, the Society of Nuclear Medicine stated that the drug was contraindicated in pregnancy (1).

FETAL RISK SUMMARY

Ioflupane iodine^{123} is a radiopharmaceutical for IV injection. It is indicated for striatal dopamine transporter visualization using single photon emission computed tomography brain imaging to assist in the evaluation of adult patients with suspected parkinsonian syndromes. The recommended dose is 111–185 MBq (3–5 mCi). Only about 5% of the administered radioactivity remained in whole blood 5 minutes after injection. By 48 hours, about 60% of the radioactivity had been excreted in the urine and about 14% in the feces. The physical half-life of iodine^{123} is 13.2 hours (2).

Reproduction studies in animals have not been conducted. Studies for carcinogenic potential and reproductive toxicity of ioflupane have not been conducted, but there was no evidence of mutagenesis in multiple assays (2).

In humans, a dose of 185 MBq results in an absorbed radiation dose to the uterus of 0.3 rad, Radiation doses >15 rad have been associated with congenital anomalies but doses <5 rad generally have not. However, radioactive iodine products cross the placenta and, depending on the stage of fetal development, can permanently impair fetal thyroid function (2).

BREASTFEEDING SUMMARY

Although no specific reports describing the use of ioflupane iodine^{123} during lactation have been located, it is known that iodine^{123} is excreted into breast milk. The manufacturer recommends that breastfeeding should not be started before the radiopharmaceutical is administered, or if breastfeeding is already underway, it should be interrupted. Based on the physical half-life of iodine^{123} (13.2 hours), nursing women should pump and discard breast milk for 6 days to minimize risks to a nursing infant (2). The breasts should be emptied regularly and completely. Milk that has been pumped during this period should either be discarded or stored in a refrigerator. The stored milk can be given to infant after 10 physical half-lifes, or about 5.5 days have elapsed since pumping (3).

References

1. Djang DSW, Janssen MJR, Bohnen N, Booij J, Henderson TA, Herholz K, Minoshima S, Rowe CC, Sabri O, Seibyl J, Van Berckel BNM, Wanner M. SNM practice guideline for dopamine transporter imaging with ^{123}I-ioflupane SPECT 1.0. J Nucl Med 2012;53:154–63.
2. Product information. DaTscan. GE Healthcare, Medi-Physics, 2011.
3. Ioflupane I 123. National Library of Medicine LactMed Database. Available at http://toxnet.nlm.gov/cgi-bin/sis/htmlgen?LACT. Accessed May 29, 2013.

IOHEXOL

Diagnostic

PREGNANCY RECOMMENDATION: Compatible (Intravenous Use)
BREASTFEEDING RECOMMENDATION: Limited Human Data—Probably Compatible

PREGNANCY SUMMARY

The various preparations of iohexol contain a high concentration of organically bound iodine. In the two reports below, the authors concluded that IV iodinated contrast material did not harm the thyroid function of newborns.

FETAL RISK SUMMARY

Iohexol, a nonionic radiopaque agent, contains a high concentration of organically bound iodine (140–350 mg iodine/mL). Iohexol was not detected in the fetuses or amniotic fluid of mid-term rabbits (1).

A study published in 2010 described the thyroxine (T4) and/or thyroid stimulating hormone (TSH) concentrations in newborns whose mothers received IV iohexol during pregnancy (2). The data for the study came from 344 maternal and 343 newborn records. The mothers had undergone multidetector pulmonary computed tomographic angiography because of suspected pulmonary embolism between 2004 and 2008. The mean gestational age of the test was 27.8 weeks and the mean dose of total iodine administered was 45,000 mg/L. All newborns had a normal T4 concentration at birth. One newborn had a transiently abnormal TSH, which normalized at day 6 of life (2).

A 2012 study evaluated the thyroid function of 64 neonates who been exposed in utero when 61 mothers had received IV iodinated contrast material (not further identified) for computed tomographic scans (3). One neonate had a low T4 concentration but a normal TSH level. That infant was born at 25 weeks' and developed respiratory distress syndrome and sepsis (3).

BREASTFEEDING SUMMARY

Iohexol is excreted into breast milk (3). Four lactating women received the IV contrast media (1 mL/kg) (1 mL contained 350 mg iodine) in the postpartum period (1 week to 14 months) (4). Breastfeeding was stopped for 48 hours. The amount excreted over a 24-hour period was 0.5% of the maternal weight-adjusted dose. This amount did not appear to be clinically significant (4). The American Academy of Pediatrics classifies iohexol as compatible with breastfeeding (5).

References

1. Bourrinet P, Dencausse A, Havard P, Violas X, Bonnemain B. Transplacental passage and milk excretion of iobitridol. Invest Radiol 1995;30:156–8.
2. Bourjeily G, Chalhoub M, Phornphutkul C, Alleyne TC, Woodfield CA, Chen KK. Neonatal thyroid function: effect of a single exposure to iodinated contrast medium in utero. Radiology 2010;256:744–50.
3. Kochi MH, Kaloudis EV, Ahmed W, Moore WH. Effect of in utero exposure of iodinated intravenous contrast on neonatal thyroid function. J Comput Assist Tomogr 2012;36:165–9.
4. Nielsen ST, Matheson I, Rasmussen JN, Skinnemoen K, Andrew E, Hafsahl G. Excretion of iohexol and metrizoate in human breast milk. Acta Radiol 1987;28:523–6.
5. Committee on Drugs, American Academy of Pediatrics. The transfer of drugs and other chemicals into human milk. Pediatrics 2001;108:776–89.

IOPAMIDOL

Diagnostic Agent

PREGNANCY RECOMMENDATION: Limited Human Data—Probably Compatible
BREASTFEEDING RECOMMENDATION: No Human Data—Probably Compatible

PREGNANCY SUMMARY

There is limited information on the use of iopamidol during human pregnancy. The animal data suggest low risk but the results were based on body weight and may not be interpretable. The iodine in this agent is organically bound, but the formulations may contain some free iodine either from contamination or from deiodination. Even though iopamidol crosses the placenta, at least in the 3rd trimester, none of the four newborns exposed in utero had hypothyroidism or goiter. The guidelines of the Contrast Media Safety Committee of the European Society of Urogenital Radiology recommend that iodinated contrast media may be used in pregnancy if such use is essential (1). This is consistent with a 2008 reference that concluded that intravascular use of nonionic iodinated contrast media was probably safe in pregnancy (2). However, there was a potential for neonatal hypothyroidism if ionic iodinated contrast media was instilled into the amniotic cavity during amniofetography (2). Therefore, with any use of iodinated contrast media, the thyroid function of the newborn should be monitored in the 1st week (1).

I

FETAL RISK SUMMARY

Iopamidol is an aqueous, nonionic, radiopaque diagnostic agent that, depending on the formulation used, contains about 200–370 mg of organically bound iodine per mL. It is indicated for angiography throughout the cardiovascular system, including cerebral and peripheral arteriography, coronary arteriography and ventriculography, pediatric angiocardiography, selective visceral arteriography and aortography, peripheral venography (phlebography), and adult and pediatric intravenous excretory urography and intravenous adult and pediatric contrast enhancement of computed tomographic (CT) head and body imaging. There appears to be no significant deposition of iopamidol in tissues. The agent undergoes no significant metabolism or deiodination and the elimination serum or plasma half-life is about 2 hours (3).

Reproduction studies have been conducted in rats and rabbits. In these species, doses up to 2.7 and 1.4 times the maximum recommended human dose based on body weight, respectively, revealed no evidence of impaired fertility or harm to the fetus (3).

Long-term studies for carcinogenic effects have not been conducted. No evidence of genetic toxicity was obtained with in vitro assays (3).

Consistent with its molecular weight (about 777) and elimination half-life, iopamidol crosses the human placenta. A 2011 case report described the use of the agent in a woman in the 3rd trimester (specific date not given) for evaluation of chest pain (4). The woman received two doses of the 370-mg/mL formulation because the first dose was given through an infiltrated IV catheter. The second dose was given 24 hours later. The chest CT resulted in the diagnosis of pericardial effusion. Premature dizygotic twin males, 1490 g and 1150 g, were delivered at 29 weeks' gestation by cesarean section because of the mother's severe preeclampsia. Apgar scores of twin A were 7 and 8 at 1 and 5 minutes, respectively, whereas in twin B, the scores were 1, 3, and 7 at 1, 5, and 10 minutes, respectively. Both infants had abdominal radiopaque densities that made exclusion of necrotizing entercolitis difficult. Serial images showed the opacities progressing through multiple loops of intestine and made the bowel wall appear thickened. When twin A passed meconium, the presence of intraluminal radiopaque material was confirmed. Thyroid function tests in both infants during this period were normal (4).

In a 2008 retrospective report, two pregnant women received iopamidol (5). The first woman, at 33 weeks' gestation, received the formulation with 370 mg/mL of organically bound iodine for imaging of her chest and abdomen, whereas the second woman, at 23 weeks, received the formulation with 300 mg/mL for imaging of the chest. Both infants, born at 38 and 24 weeks', respectively, had normal TSH levels. Thirty-three months after birth, neither mother reported known thyroid illness in the children (5).

A 2009 retrospective study compared pulmonary CT angiography (CTA) using iopamidol (370 mg/mL) with lung scintigraphy using low-dose (90 MBq) technetium Tc-99m to diagnose pulmonary embolism in pregnancy (6). There were 25 pregnant patients in each group. The authors concluded that lung scintigraphy was more reliable than pulmonary CTA in pregnant patients. The mean gestational ages in the two groups were not statistically different (30.6 ± 6.4 weeks vs. 26.5 ± 8.9 weeks). No information was provided on newborn outcomes (6).

A 22-year-old woman at 33 2/7 weeks' gestation with a history of asthma and migraine headaches and documented allergies to penicillin and codeine was admitted for chest pain, shortness of breath, and tachycardia (7). She was evaluated for pulmonary embolism with a CT angiogram conducted with an infusion of iopamidol (300 mg/mL formulation). During the infusion, she developed facial flushing, throat tightness, and worsening dyspnea. The infusion was stopped and she was treated for an allergic reaction with complete resolution of her symptoms. The imaging was negative for pulmonary embolism and she was discharged home. Several hours later, she returned with bleeding from the IV site and numerous ecchymoses and petechiae. Her platelet count, which had been 172,000/microliter the night before, was now 4000. She was transferred to another hospital and treated with dexamethasone 40 mg IV for 4 days. Her platelet count rose to 33,000 24 hours after transfer and was 99,000 when discharged on day 5. Ten days later, her thrombocytopenia had resolved with count of 220,000. She had an uncomplicated repeat cesarean section at 39 weeks' (no information on the newborn was given) (7).

BREASTFEEDING SUMMARY

No reports describing the use of iopamidol during human lactation have been located. The molecular weight (about 777) and elimination half-life (about 2 hours) suggest that limited amounts of the agent will be excreted into breast milk. Although the iodine in the agent is organically bound and significant deiodination does not occur, ingestion of the agent by the infant might release iodine that would be absorbed systemically. However, it is doubtful if clinically significant amounts of either iopamidol or iodine would be absorbed by a nursing infant. A 2005 review concluded that breastfeeding may be continued normally when iodinated agents are given to the mother (1).

References

1. Webb JAW, Thomsen HS, Morcos SK. The use of iodinated and gadolinium contrast media during pregnancy and lactation. Eur Radiol 2005;15:1234–40.
2. Chen MM, Coakley FV, Kaimal A, Laros RK Jr. Guidelines for computed tomography and magnetic resonance imaging use during pregnancy and lactation. Obstet Gynecol 2008;112:333–40.
3. Product information. Isovue. Bracco Diagnostics, 2012.
4. Fitzpatrick J, Speakman J, Kapfer SA, Holston AM. Transplacental passage of the non-ionic contrast agent iopamidol in twins. Pediatr Radiol 2011;41:534–6.
5. Atwell TD, Lteif AN, Brown DL, McCann M, Townsend JE, LeRoy AJ. Neonatal thyroid function after administration of IV iodinated contrast agent to 21 pregnant patients. AJR Am J Roentgenol 2008;191:268–71.
6. Ridge CA, McDermott S, Freyne BJ, Brennan DJ, Collins CD, Skehan SJ. Pulmonary embolism in pregnancy: comparison of pulmonary CT angiography and lung scintigraphy. AJR Am J Roentgenol 2009;193:1223–7.
7. McCaulley JA, Deering SH, Pates JA. Severe thrombocytopenia after contrast infusion in pregnancy. Obstet Gynecol 2013;121:473–5.

I

IOPANOIC ACID

Diagnostic

PREGNANCY RECOMMENDATION: No Human Data—Probably Compatible
BREASTFEEDING RECOMMENDATION: Limited Human Data—Probably Compatible

PREGNANCY SUMMARY

Iopanoic acid contains a high concentration of organically bound iodine. See Diatrizoate.

BREASTFEEDING SUMMARY

Iopanoic acid is excreted into breast milk. Cholecystography was performed in 11 lactating patients with iopanoic acid (1). The mean amount of iodine administered to five patients was 2.77 g (range 1.98–3.96 g) and the mean amount excreted in breast milk during the next 19–29 hours was 20.8 mg (0.08%) (range 6.72–29.9 mg). The nursing infants showed no reaction to the contrast media. The American Academy of Pediatrics classifies iopanoic acid as compatible with breastfeeding (2). See Diatrizoate.

References

1. Holmdahl KH. Cholecystography during lactation. Acta Radiol 1956;45:305–7.
2. Committee on Drugs, American Academy of Pediatrics. The transfer of drugs and other chemicals into human milk. Pediatrics 2001;108:776–89.

IOTHALAMATE

Diagnostic

PREGNANCY RECOMMENDATION: Limited Human Data—Probably Compatible
BREASTFEEDING RECOMMENDATION: No Human Data—Probably Compatible

PREGNANCY SUMMARY

Iothalamate contains a high concentration organically bound iodine. See Diatrizoate for possible effects on the fetus and newborn.

FETAL RISK SUMMARY

Iothalamate has been used for diagnostic procedures during pregnancy. Amniography was performed in one patient to diagnose monoamniotic twinning shortly before an elective cesarean section (1). No effect on the two newborns was mentioned. In a second study, 17 women were given either iothalamate or metrizoate for ascending phlebography during various stages of pregnancy (2). Two patients, one exposed in the 1st trimester and the other in the 2nd trimester, were diagnosed as having deep vein thrombosis and were treated with heparin. The baby from the 2nd trimester patient was normal, but the other newborn had hyperbilirubinemia and undescended testis (2). The relationship between the diagnostic agents (or other drugs) and the defects is not known.

BREASTFEEDING SUMMARY

See Diatrizoate.

References

1. Dunnihoo DR, Harris RE. The diagnosis of monoamniotic twinning by amniography. Am J Obstet Gynecol 1966;96:894–5.
2. Kierkegaard A. Incidence and diagnosis of deep vein thrombosis associated with pregnancy. Acta Obstet Gynecol Scand 1983;62:239–43.

IPILIMUMAB

Antineoplastic

PREGNANCY RECOMMENDATION: Contraindicated
BREASTFEEDING RECOMMENDATION: Contraindicated

PREGNANCY SUMMARY

No reports describing the use of ipilimumab in human pregnancy have been located. Although the absence of human pregnancy experience prevents a better assessment of the risk, severe fetal toxicity was observed in pregnant monkeys. The drug should be considered contraindicated in pregnancy. However, melanoma is a potentially fatal disease. If a pregnant woman requires ipilimumab, she should be informed of the possible risk to her embryo and/or fetus.

FETAL RISK SUMMARY

Ipilimumab, an IgG1 kappa immunoglobulin, is a recombinant, human monoclonal antibody that binds to the cytotoxic T-lymphocyte–associated antigen 4 (CTLA-4). It is produced in mammalian (Chinese hamster ovary) cell culture. Ipilimumab is indicated for the treatment of unresectable or metastatic melanoma. Neither the metabolism nor plasma protein binding was reported by the manufacturer, but the terminal half-life was 14.7 days (1).

Cynomolgus monkeys were given IV ipilimumab every 21 days from the onset of organogenesis through parturition at doses that were 2.6 and 7.2 times the recommended human dose based on AUC. Severe toxicities including increased incidences of 3rd trimester abortion, stillbirth, premature delivery, low birth weight, and infant death were observed. In mice in which the gene for CTLA-4 had been deleted, offspring lacking CTLA-4 were born healthy, but died within 3–4 weeks due to multiorgan infiltration and damage by lymphocytes (1).

Studies evaluating carcinogenesis, mutagenesis, and impairment of fertility have not been conducted (1).

It is not known if ipilimumab crosses the human placenta. The molecular weight (about 148,000) suggests that it will not cross, at least early in pregnancy. However, human IgG1 is known to cross, and ipilimumab is an IgG1 (1). Moreover, the prolonged terminal half-life (14.5 days) will increase the opportunity for transfer. Thus, fetal exposure should be expected, especially in the latter part of pregnancy.

BREASTFEEDING SUMMARY

No reports describing the use of ipilimumab during human lactation have been located. The molecular weight (about 148,000) suggests that it will not be excreted into mature breast milk, However, human IgG1 is known to be excreted into colostrum, and ipilimumab is an IgG1 (1). Moreover, the prolonged terminal half-life (14.5 days) will increase the opportunity for excretion. The effect of this exposure on a nursing infant is unknown, but the best course is to not breastfeed if the mother requires ipilimumab.

Reference

1. Product information. Vervoy. Bristol-Myers Squibb, 2011.

IPODATE

Diagnostic

PREGNANCY RECOMMENDATION: No Human Data—Probably Compatible
BREASTFEEDING RECOMMENDATION: No Human Data—Probably Compatible

PREGNANCY SUMMARY

Ipodate contains a high concentration of organically bound iodine. See Diatrizoate for possible effects on the fetus and newborn.

BREASTFEEDING SUMMARY

See Diatrizoate.

IPRATROPIUM

Respiratory Drug (Bronchodilator)

PREGNANCY RECOMMENDATION: Human Data Suggest Low Risk
BREASTFEEDING RECOMMENDATION: No Human Data—Probably Compatible

I

PREGNANCY SUMMARY

A number of sources recommend the use of inhaled ipratropium for severe asthma, especially in patients not responding adequately to other therapy (1–4). The consensus appears to be that although human data are rare, there is no evidence that the drug is hazardous to the fetus. Moreover, it produces fewer systemic effects than atropine (1), and may have an additive bronchodilatory effect to β_2 agonists (2).

FETAL RISK SUMMARY

Ipratropium, an anticholinergic compound chemically related to atropine, is a quaternary ammonium bromide used as a bronchodilator for the treatment of bronchospasm. Its use during pregnancy is primarily confined to patients with severe asthma (1).

Ipratropium was not teratogenic in mice, rats, and rabbits when administered either orally or by inhalation (5). Oral doses used in the reproductive toxicity studies were 2000, 200,000, and 26,000 times the maximum recommended human daily dose (MRHDD), respectively. Doses used by inhalation in rats and rabbits were, respectively, 312 and 375 times the MRHDD. Schardein cited a German study that found no evidence of teratogenicity in mice, rats, and rabbits (6). A Japanese study involving rats and rabbits that found no adverse fetal effects except a slight weight reduction was described by Shepard (7).

Data from a surveillance study of Medicaid patients between 1982 and 1994 indicated that 37 women took this drug during the 1st trimester (F. Rosa, personal communication, FDA, 1996). One malformation, a renal obstruction, was observed. Preliminary analysis found no brain defects among 80 recipients following exposure anytime during pregnancy.

A brief 1991 report described the use of nebulized ipratropium, among other drugs, in the treatment of life-threatening status asthmaticus in a pregnant patient at 12.5 weeks' gestation (8). She eventually delivered a term 3440-g male infant (information on the condition of the newborn was not provided).

BREASTFEEDING SUMMARY

No reports describing the excretion of ipratropium into human milk have been located. A chemically related drug, atropine, is considered compatible with breastfeeding by the American Academy of Pediatrics (9), although definitive data on the appearance of atropine in milk have not been published. Ipratropium is lipid-insoluble and, similar to other quaternary ammonium bases, may appear in milk. The amounts, although unknown, are probably clinically insignificant, however, especially after inhalation.

References

1. Report of the Working Group on Asthma and Pregnancy. *Management of Asthma during Pregnancy*. Washington, DC: National Institutes of Health Publication No. 93-3279, Public Health Service, US Department of Health and Human Services, 1993:20.
2. D'Alonzo GE. The pregnant asthmatic patient. Semin Perinatol 1990;14:119–29.
3. Schatz M. Asthma during pregnancy:interrelationships and management. Ann Allergy 1992;68:123–33.
4. Moore-Gillon J. Asthma in pregnancy. Br J Obstet Gynaecol 1994;101: 658–60.
5. Product information. Atrovent. Boehringer Ingelheim Pharmaceuticals, 1996.
6. Schardein JL. *Chemically Induced Birth Defects*. 2nd ed. New York, NY: Marcel Dekker, 1993:343.
7. Shepard TH. *Catalog of Teratogenic Agents*. 8th ed. Baltimore, MD: The Johns Hopkins University Press, 1995:238.
8. Gilchrist DM, Friedman JM, Werker D. Life-threatening status asthmaticus at 12.5 weeks' gestation. Chest 1991;100:285–6.
9. Committee on Drugs, American Academy of Pediatrics. The transfer of drugs and other chemicals into human milk. Pediatrics 1994;93:137–50.

IPRONIAZID

[Withdrawn from the market. See 9th edition.]

IRBESARTAN

Antihypertensive

PREGNANCY RECOMMENDATION: **Human Data Suggest Risk in 2nd and 3rd Trimesters**
BREASTFEEDING RECOMMENDATION: **No Human Data—Probably Compatible**

PREGNANCY SUMMARY

The human pregnancy experience with irbesartan is limited. However, the antihypertensive mechanisms of action of irbesartan and angiotensin-converting enzyme (ACE) inhibitors are very close. That is, the former selectively blocks the binding of angiotensin II to AT_1 receptors, whereas the latter prevents the formation of angiotensin II itself. Therefore, use of this drug during the 2nd and 3rd trimesters may cause teratogenicity and severe fetal and neonatal toxicity that is identical to that seen with ACE inhibitors (e.g., see Captopril or Enalapril). Fetal toxic effects may include anuria, oligohydramnios, fetal hypocalvaria, intrauterine growth restriction, premature birth, and patent ductus arteriosus. Anuria-associated oligohydramnios may produce fetal limb contractures, craniofacial deformation, and pulmonary hypoplasia. Severe anuria and hypotension, that is resistant to both pressor agents and volume expansion, may occur in the newborn following in utero exposure to irbesartan. Newborn renal function and blood pressure should be closely monitored.

FETAL RISK SUMMARY

Irbesartan is a selective angiotensin II receptor blocker (ARB) that is used either alone, or in combination with other antihypertensive agents, for the treatment of hypertension. Irbesartan blocks the vasoconstrictor and aldosterone-secreting effects of angiotensin II by preventing angiotensin II from binding to AT_1 receptors.

Reproduction studies have been conducted in pregnant rats and rabbits (1). In the pregnant rat, doses approximately equal to or higher than the maximum recommended human dose of 300 mg/day based on BSA (MRHD) were associated with increased incidences of renal pelvic cavitation, hydroureter, and/or absence of renal papilla. At four times the MRHD, subcutaneous edema was observed in the fetuses. The anomalies appeared to be related to late, rather than early, gestational exposure (1). Doses approximately 1.5 times the MRHD in pregnant rabbits produced maternal mortality and abortion. Surviving rabbits had a slight increase in early resorptions (1). No adverse effects on fertility or reproductive performance were seen in male and female rats at an oral dose about 5 times the MRHD (1).

It is not known if irbesartan crosses the human placenta to the fetus. The molecular weight (about 429) is low enough that transfer to the fetus should be expected. The drug does cross the placentas of rats and rabbits in late gestation (1).

A 24-year-old woman with type 1 diabetes, hypothyroidism, and hypertension was being treated with irbesartan 300 mg/day, hydrochlorothiazide 12.5 mg/day, insulin (glargine and regular), levothyroxine 0.125 mg/day, and epoetin alfa (2). An unplanned pregnancy occurred that was diagnosed at 8 weeks and irbesartan and hydrochlorothiazide were replaced with methyldopa. The patient's HbA1c was 7%. Ultrasonography at 13 weeks' detected an exencephaly and the pregnancy was terminated. Autopsy revealed a partial exencephaly and unilateral renal agenesis. The cause of the defects could not be determined, but the authors suspected irbesartan (2). However, unilateral renal agenesis is possibly autosomal dominant inheritance with variable expressivity and penetrance (3).

A 35-year-old woman with hypertension was exposed to irbesartan, atorvastatin, and sibutramine from 6 weeks to 8 days before conception (4). She had a 1st trimester miscarriage. Examination of the embryo revealed delayed development of the upper extremities. The karyotype was 45,XO (Turner syndrome), a chromosomal abnormality.

A 2009 report described three cases of irbesartan exposure before and during pregnancy (5). In each case, the drug was used to treat hypertension and was stopped at 5, 9, and 18 weeks' gestation, respectively. The three pregnancy (gestational age at birth) outcomes were small-for-gestational-age (39 weeks), polydactyly (40 weeks), and complications of prematurity (29 weeks), respectively. In the latter case, oligohydramnios was observed at 18 weeks. Other than the polydactyly, no structural malformations were reported (5).

A 2012 review of the use of ACE inhibitors and ARBs in the 1st trimester concluded that there may be an elevated teratogenic risk, but the risk appeared to be related to other factors (6). The factors, which typically coexist with hypertension in pregnancy, included diabetes, advanced maternal age, and obesity.

BREASTFEEDING SUMMARY

No reports describing the use irbesartan during human lactation have been located. Because of the relatively low molecular weight (about 429), excretion into human breast milk should be expected. The effect of this exposure on a nursing infant is unknown. The American Academy of Pediatrics, however, classifies ACE inhibitors, a closely related group of antihypertensive agents, as compatible with breastfeeding (see Captopril or Enalapril).

References

1. Product information. Avapro. Bristol-Myers Squibb, 2000.
2. Boix E, Zapater P, Pico A, Moreno O. Teratogenicity with angiotensin II receptor antagonists in pregnancy. J Endocrinol Invest 2005;28:1029–31.
3. Moel DI. Renal agenesis, unilateral. In: Buyse ML, Editor-in-Chief. *Birth Defects Encyclopedia*. Dover, MA: Blackwell Scientific Publications, 1990:1461.
4. Velazquez-Armenta EY, Han JY, Choi JS, Yang KM, Nava-Ocampo AA. Angiotensin II receptor blockers in pregnancy: a case report and systematic review of the literature. Hypertens Pregnancy 2007;26:51–66.
5. Gersak K, Cvijic M, Cerar LK. Angiotensin II receptor blockers in pregnancy: a report of 5 cases. Reprod Toxicol 2009;28:109–12.
6. Polifka JE. Is there an embryopathy associated with first-trimester exposure to angiotensin-converting enzyme inhibitors and angiotensin receptor antagonists? A critical review of the evidence. Birth Defects Res (Part A) 2012;94:576–98.

IRINOTECAN

Antineoplastic

PREGNANCY RECOMMENDATION: Limited Human Data—Animal Data Suggest Risk
BREASTFEEDING RECOMMENDATION: Contraindicated

PREGNANCY SUMMARY

One report described the use of irinotecan, combined with 5-fluorouracil and folinic acid, in the 2nd and 3rd trimesters that ended with a healthy infant. The animal reproduction data suggest risk, but the near absence of human pregnancy experience prevents a more complete assessment of embryo–fetal risk. Because of the potential for embryo and fetal harm, women of childbearing potential should employ adequate contraceptive methods to prevent pregnancy. Moreover, the recommended regimen for irinotecan sometimes includes the antineoplastic fluorouracil; the combined therapy might increase the embryo–fetal risk, especially in the 1st trimester. However, the indications for irinotecan involve potentially fatal cancers, so if informed consent is obtained, treatment should not be withheld because of pregnancy. If an inadvertent pregnancy occurs during therapy, the woman should be advised of the unknown, but potentially severe risk for her embryo–fetus.

FETAL RISK SUMMARY

The DNA topoisomerase I-inhibitor, irinotecan, is a semisynthetic derivative of camptothecin, an alkaloid extract from plants such as *Camptotheca acuminata*. It is given as an IV infusion. Irinotecan is in the same antineoplastic subclass as topotecan. It is indicated, either as a single agent or in combination with 5-fluoruracil and leucovorin, for the treatment of metastatic carcinoma of the colon or rectum. The cytotoxicity of irinotecan and its active metabolite, SN-38, is thought to involve the inhibition of the enzyme responsible for the repair of normally occurring single-strand breaks in DNA. However, the plasma AUC values for the active metabolite are only 2%–8% of irinotecan, so the precise contribution of SN-38 to the cytotoxicity activity of irinotecan is unknown. Irinotecan is metabolized primarily in the liver. Binding of irinotecan and SN-38 to plasma proteins is about 50% and 95%, respectively. The mean terminal elimination half-lives are 6–12 hours and 10–20 hours, respectively (1).

Reproduction studies have been conducted in rats and rabbits. In pregnant rats, an IV dose during organogenesis that produced an AUC that was about 0.2 times the AUC obtained with a human dose of 125 mg/m^2 (HD) caused increased postimplantation loss and decreased numbers of live fetuses. Doses producing AUC values that were greater than about 0.025 times the HD caused structural defects, including a variety of external, visceral, and skeletal abnormalities. In pregnant rabbits, an IV dose during organogenesis that was about 0.5 times the weekly starting dose based on BSA (WSD) caused similar embryolethality and structural defects. In rats, when a dose producing an AUC that was about 0.2 times the HD was given after organogenesis through weaning, decreased learning ability and decreased female body weights in offspring were observed (1).

Standard tests for carcinogenicity have not been conducted with irinotecan. When rats were given an IV dose that produced an AUC that was about 1.3 times the HD or a lower dose that was 8% (based on body weight) of the higher dose once weekly for 13 weeks and then allowed to recover for 91 weeks, there was a significant linear trend with dose for the incidence of combined uterine horn endometrial stromal polyps and endometrial stromal sarcomas. Neither irinotecan nor SN-38 was mutagenic, but irinotecan was clastogenic. Irinotecan did not cause significant adverse effects on fertility or reproductive performance in rats and rabbits given IV doses up to 0.2 times the HD or 0.5 times the WSD, respectively. However, multiple daily doses in rodents and dogs that produced an AUC that was about 1 and 0.07 times the HD, respectively, were associated with atrophy of male reproductive organs (1).

It is not known if irinotecan crosses the human placenta. The molecular weight (about 587 for the nonhydrated free base), moderate plasma protein binding, and long elimination half-life suggest that the drug will cross to the embryo–fetus.

A 2009 case report described a 34-year-old woman who was diagnosed with an ovarian adenocarcinoma tumor metastatic from a colon cancer that had been previously treated with surgery (2). After left salpingooophorectomy, treatment was begun at 18 weeks' gestation with irinotecan, 5-fluorouracil, and folinic acid every 2 weeks until the 36th week of pregnancy (total 10 courses). At 37 5/7 weeks, 13 days after the final chemotherapy course, her membranes ruptured and she gave birth to 5 lb 14 oz (about 2667 g) female infant with Apgar scores of 9 and 9 at 1 and 5 minutes, respectively. The infant was developing normally at 4 months of age with no teratogenic effects (2).

BREASTFEEDING SUMMARY

No reports describing the use of irinotecan during human lactation have been located. The molecular weight (about 587 for the nonhydrated free base), moderate plasma protein binding, and long elimination half-life suggest that the drug will be excreted into breast milk. The potential effect of this exposure on a nursing infant is unknown, but may be severe. It is best that a woman receiving this agent does not breastfeed. However, if she chooses to do so, the infant should be closely monitored for the most common or serious adverse effects observed in adults treated with the drug, such as gastrointestinal tract effects (nausea, vomiting, diarrhea, anorexia), bone marrow suppression (leukopenia, neutropenia, anemia), headache, abdominal pain, alopecia, and hepatic toxicity.

References

1. Product information. Camptosar. Pharmacia & Upjohn, 2007.
2. Taylor J, Amanze A, Di Federico E, Verschraegen C. Irinotecan use during pregnancy. Obstet Gynecol 2009;114:451–2.

ISOCARBOXAZID

Antidepressant

PREGNANCY RECOMMENDATION: Limited Human Data—No Relevant Animal Data
BREASTFEEDING RECOMMENDATION: No Human Data—Potential Toxicity

PREGNANCY SUMMARY

Isocarboxazid is a monoamine oxidase inhibitor. Other agents in this subclass are iproniazid, nialamide, phenelzine, and tranylcypromine. The human pregnancy experience is limited. There are no animal reproduction data (see also Tranylcypromine).

FETAL RISK SUMMARY

The Collaborative Perinatal Project monitored 21 mother–child pairs exposed to these drugs during the 1st trimester, 1 of which was exposed to isocarboxazid (1). Three of the 21 infants had malformations (relative risk 2.26). Details of the single case with exposure to isocarboxazid were not given.

It is not known if isocarboxazid crosses the human placenta. The molecular weight (about 231) is low enough that exposure of the embryo–fetus should be expected.

BREASTFEEDING SUMMARY

No reports describing the use of isocarboxazid during human lactation have been located. The molecular weight (about 231) is low enough that excretion into breast milk should be expected.

Reference

1. Heinonen OP, Slone D, Shapiro S. *Birth Defects and Drugs in Pregnancy*. Littleton, MA: Publishing Sciences Group, 1977:336–7.

ISOETHARINE

[Withdrawn from the market. See 9th edition.]

ISOFLURANE

General Anesthetic

PREGNANCY RECOMMENDATION: Limited Human Data—Animal Data Suggest Low Risk
BREASTFEEDING RECOMMENDATION: No Human Data—Probably Compatible

PREGNANCY SUMMARY

Isoflurane was not teratogenic in three animal species at doses that did not cause maternal toxicity. No reports of its use early in human gestation have been located. The absence of human experience during organogenesis prevents a complete assessment of the risk for structural anomalies. In addition, general anesthesia usually involves the use of multiple pharmacological agents. Although no teratogenicity has been observed with two other halogenated general anesthetic agents (halothane and methoxyflurane), only halothane has 1st trimester human exposure data. Isoflurane has been used immediately prior to delivery for analgesia and anesthesia. This use does not appear to affect the newborn any differently from other general anesthetic agents. The uterine effects of isoflurane (relaxation and increased blood loss) also appear to be similar to other agents in this class. All anesthetic agents can cause depression in the newborn that may last for 24 hours or more. The potential reproductive toxicity (spontaneous abortion [SAB] and infertility) of occupational exposure to isoflurane has not been studied but is a concern based on the exposure concentration found in one study. Further, occupational exposure to nitrous oxide was also measured in that study, and indicated that the nurses were exposed to both nitrous oxide and volatile anesthetic agents at the same time.

FETAL RISK SUMMARY

The nonflammable general anesthetic isoflurane is in the same class of volatile liquid halogenated agents such as desflurane, enflurane, halothane, methoxyflurane, and sevoflurane. It is closely related to desflurane and enflurane. The only difference between isoflurane and desflurane is the presence of a chlorine atom in isoflurane instead of a fluorine atom. This small difference, however, produces marked pharmacokinetic and clinical effects. The potency of isoflurane is five times that of desflurane, the blood–gas partition coefficient is increased (i.e., increased solubility in blood) (1.46 vs. 0.42), tissue solubility is increased (brain–blood partition coefficient 1.6 vs. 1.3), and recovery from anesthesia is slower (1).

In an animal reproductive study, mean anesthetic concentrations (about 1.6%) of isoflurane were administered to male and female rats for 5-day intervals up to 15 days before pairing (2). No adverse effects on mating and fertility indices were observed. Studies for structural anomalies were conducted in pregnant rats and rabbits in the same way. Three groups of rats received mean anesthetic doses of 1.6%–1.7% for 5-day intervals between day 1 and day 15 of gestation, whereas three groups of rabbits received mean doses of 2.3% for 4- or 5-day intervals between day 6 and 18 of gestation. No congenital malformations related to the exposures were found in either animal species (2). In the third segment of this study, pregnant rats were exposed to isoflurane 1.74% for 1 hour/day on gestation days 15–20. Maternal weight gain was significantly less in the exposed group, and fetal survival was also decreased (2).

Three dose-levels of isoflurane were administered in a reproduction study with pregnant mice: trace (0.006%), subanesthetic (0.06%), and light anesthetic (0.6%) (3). No adverse maternal or fetal effects were observed when the two smaller concentrations were administered for 4 hours daily on days 6–15 of pregnancy. When given the same way, the light anesthetic dose, however, resulted in significantly lower maternal weight gain. Fetal toxicity included a significant decrease in fetal weight, decreased skeletal ossification, minor hydronephrosis, and increased pelvic cavitation (3). In addition, an increased incidence of cleft palate was observed (12.1% vs. 0.75% for controls). The incidence of cleft palate also was higher than that observed in previous experiments with halothane (1.2%) or enflurane (1.9%) (3).

In a second study by the authors of the above report, the effects of four general anesthetic agents were compared in pregnant rats (4). The doses and agents used were nitrous oxide (75%; 0.55 minimum alveolar anesthetic concentration [MAC]), enflurane (1.65%; 0.75 MAC), halothane (0.8%; 0.75 MAC), and isoflurane (1.05%; 0.75 MAC). (*Note: The MAC is the concentration that causes immobility in 50% of patients exposed to a noxious stimulus such as a surgical incision; it represents the* ED_{50} *[5]*). Each agent was administered for 6 hours on each of three consecutive days in one of three gestational periods: pregnancy days 8–10, 11–13, or 14–16. Compared with controls, significantly decreased maternal weight gain was observed in three of the groups (nitrous oxide, isoflurane, and enflurane) after exposure on days 14–16. Exposure on those days resulted in significantly decreased fetal weight in all four groups and, when exposure occurred on days 8–10, in three groups (all except nitrous oxide). Nitrous oxide exposure during days 14–16 resulted in significant increases (three-fold) in total fetal wastage and resorptions. However, no major or minor teratogenic effects were observed in any of the groups (4).

The teratogenic potential of isoflurane, enflurane, and sevoflurane was studied by evaluating the effect of each agent on the proliferation and differentiation of cells exiting from the G1-phase of the cell cycle (6). The theory behind the study was that normal development during embryogenesis, organogenesis, and histogenesis depended on the proliferation and differentiative processes of cell migration (6). For example, valproate, a known human teratogen, is a potent G1-phase inhibitor of the in vitro proliferation rate at concentrations <2 times the therapeutic plasma concentration. At anesthetic concentrations <2 times the MAC, the antiproliferative potency of the three agents was isoflurane =enflurane>>sevoflurane. However, in the growth-arrested cell population, there was no specific accumulation of any cell-cycle phase and no specific effect on the G1 phase. The investigators concluded that the three agents lacked the specific in vitro characteristics of valproate (6).

Three anesthetic agents, isoflurane, halothane, and methoxyflurane, were administered to pregnant (near term) and nonpregnant ewes in a study designed to determine the requirement for inhaled anesthetic agents (7). The MAC was decreased in the pregnant animals in each case, 40%, 25%, and 32% less, respectively. In a 1994 study, women at

8–12 weeks' gestation (all undergoing termination of pregnancy) were matched with women undergoing gynecologic surgery (8). The MAC was reduced by 28% in comparison with the nonpregnant controls (median end-tidal concentration 0.775% vs. 1.075%, respectively).

Two reviews concluded that, in general, inhalational anesthetics are freely transferred to fetal tissues (9,10) and, in most cases, the maternal and fetal concentrations are equivalent (10). The low molecular weight (about 185) and the presence of isoflurane in the maternal brain support this assertion. In agreement, research has demonstrated the rapid uptake of isoflurane by the fetus (11).

A 1991 case report described two liver transplant procedures, 3 days apart, in a pregnant woman at approximately 21 weeks' gestation (12). Isoflurane was the only inhaled anesthetic agent used, although a number of other drugs were administered during the combined 24.4 hours of anesthesia. The woman eventually delivered a healthy infant by cesarean section (12).

Subanesthetic doses of isoflurane have been used for labor analgesia (13–15). A study published in 1985 compared the self-administration of isoflurane (0.75% in oxygen) or 50% nitrous oxide in oxygen given in a random sequence in 32 women (13). Isoflurane use resulted in better analgesia but increased drowsiness. The condition of the newborns was not mentioned. A 1989 study used isoflurane (0.2%–0.7%) or 30%–60% nitrous oxide (30 in each group) for labor analgesia (14). Seven percent of the newborns in both groups were depressed (1-minute Apgar scores 5–7), but all had Apgar scores of 8–10 at 5 minutes. There was also no difference in neonatal neurobehavior as measured by the Neurologic and Adaptive Capacity Scores (NACS) at 15 minutes, 2 hours, and 24 hours of age. Although specific percentages were not given, it was stated that there was no significant difference between the groups in the percentage of infants who scored 35–40 on the NACS. Mothers in the isoflurane group had higher concentrations of fluoride in their urine at 12–24 hours postpartum than those who had received nitrous oxide (36.5 vs. 23.6 μmol/L), but the fluoride blood levels were similar (<5.6 μmol/L). The fluoride urine levels in the newborns (first void) also were similar (<5.6 μmol/L) (14). In a 1993 report, 17 laboring women received alternating doses of 0.2% isoflurane plus 50% nitrous oxide/oxygen or nitrous oxide/oxygen alone, each over 1-hour intervals, for a total of 3 hours (15). Analgesia was significantly better when the women were receiving isoflurane. Progressive drowsiness was noted over the 3-hour period, but it was not considered clinically significant. The newborns were delivered vaginally and all had 1- and 5-minute Apgar scores of 8 to 10. Neurobehavior assessment was not conducted (15).

Isoflurane has been used for anesthesia during cesarean section (11,16–19). As with vaginal delivery, some degree of neonatal depression may occur as indicated by Apgar scores <7 at 1 minute (11,16–18) or an NACS <35 at 2 and 24 hours of age (16). A small 1983 study compared the neonatal outcomes in four groups (10 patients each) of women receiving general anesthesia for cesarean section: 50% nitrous oxide and 50% oxygen either alone, or combined with 0.5% halothane, 1.0% enflurane, or 0.75% isoflurane (19). One newborn had an Apgar score <7 at 1 minute (enflurane group), but all newborns in all groups had scores of ≥7 at 5 minutes. There were no significant differences between the groups in neonatal neurobehavior assessment 2–4 hours after delivery or in maternal or umbilical blood gas analysis at delivery.

In a 1977 in vitro study, isoflurane was shown to have a statistically significant depressive effect on myometrial strips from nongravid and gravid uteri (20). Three anesthetic agents, isoflurane, enflurane, and halothane, were studied at three concentrations (0.5, 1.0, and 1.5 MAC). The amount of depression was dose-related for each agent and was similar with all agents (20). Another study also demonstrated a dose-related relaxing effect of isoflurane (0.5%, 1.0%, and 1.5%) on isolated gravid human uterine muscle (21). All doses caused a significant decrease in uterine activity, but oxytocin, in a dose similar to that used clinically, reversed the effects of the anesthetic (21). In another study, the subjective assessment of maternal blood loss and uterine relaxation was less for isoflurane than for halothane (16).

A study published in 1998 evaluated the exposure of nine nurses in a postanesthesia care unit (PACU) to exhaled isoflurane and desflurane and compared these exposures with the National Institute of Occupational Safety and Health (NIOSH)-recommended exposure limits (22). The NIOSH recommendation for volatile anesthetics (without concomitant nitrous oxide exposure) is a maximum of 2 parts per million, but has not been adopted by the Occupational Safety and Health Administration. Moreover, the recommended limit is controversial and is thought by some to be inappropriately low (22). However, a potential for reproductive risk (SAB and infertility) is thought to exist for some anesthetic agents. The study involved exposure in the PACU to exhaled anesthetic gases from 50 adult patients (isoflurane $N = 19$, desflurane $N = 31$) over an approximately 1-hour recovery time. About one-half of the patients were extubated in the PACU. Exposure was continuously measured from the shoulders (i.e., breathing-zone) of the nurses. Breathing-zone anesthetic concentrations of isoflurane and desflurane exceeded the NIOSH limits in 37% and 87% of the cases, respectively. These exposures were above the limit 12% of the time for isoflurane and 49% of the time for desflurane. The investigators listed several limitations to their study and concluded that the results might represent a "worst-case analysis" (22).

A 2004 study found a significant association between maternal occupational exposure to waste anesthetic gases during pregnancy and developmental deficits in their children, including gross and fine motor ability, inattention/hyperactivity, and IQ performance (see Nitrous Oxide).

BREASTFEEDING SUMMARY

Although isoflurane has been administered during labor and delivery, the effects of this exposure on the infant that begins nursing immediately after birth have not been described. Isoflurane is probably excreted into colostrum and milk as suggested by its presence in the maternal blood and its low molecular weight (about 185), but the toxic potential of this exposure for the infant is unknown. However, the risk to a nursing infant from exposure to isoflurane via milk is probably very low (24,25). Another halogenated inhalation anesthetic, halothane, is classified as compatible with breastfeeding by the American Academy of Pediatrics (see Halothane).

References

1. Eger EI II. Desflurane animal and human pharmacology: aspects of kinetics, safety, and MAC. Anesth Analg 1992;75:S3–9.
2. Kennedy GL Jr, Smith SH, Keplinger ML, Calandra JG. Reproductive and teratologic studies with isoflurane. Drug Chem Toxicol 1977–78;1:75–88.
3. Mazze RI, Wilson AI, Rice SA, Baden JM. Fetal development in mice exposed to isoflurane. Teratology 1985;32:339–45.
4. Mazze RI, Fujinaga M, Rice SA, Harris SB, Baden JM. Reproductive and teratogenic effects of nitrous oxide, halothane, isoflurane, and enflurane in Sprague-Dawley rats. Anesthesiology 1986;64:339–44.
5. Trevor AJ, Miller RD. General anesthetics. In: Katzung BG, ed. *Basic and Clinical Pharmacology*. 8th ed. New York, NY: McGraw-Hill, 2001:426.
6. O'Leary G, Bacon CL, Odumeru O, Fagan C, Fitzpatrick T, Gallagher HC, Moriarty DC, Regan CM. Antiproliferative actions of inhalational anesthetics: comparisons to the valproate teratogen. Int J Dev Neurosci 2000;18:39–45.
7. Palahniuk RJ, Shnider SM, Eger EI II. Pregnancy decreases the requirement for inhaled anesthetic agents. Anesthesiology 1974;41:82–3.
8. Gin T, Chan MTV. Decrease minimum alveolar concentration of isoflurane in pregnant humans. Anesthesiology 1994;81:829–32.
9. Friedman JM. Teratogen update: anesthetic agents. Teratology 1988;37:69–77.
10. Kanto J. Risk–benefit assessment of anaesthetic agents in the puerperium. Drug Saf 1991;6:285–301.
11. Dwyer R, Fee JPH, Moore J. Uptake of halothane and isoflurane by mother and baby during caesarean section. Br J Anaesthesia 1995;74:379–83.
12. Merritt WT, Dickstein R, Beattie C, Burdick J, Klein A. Liver transplantation during pregnancy: anesthesia for two procedures in the same patient with successful outcome of pregnancy. Transplant Proc 1991;23:1996–7.
13. McLeod DD, Ramayya GP, Tunstall ME. Self-administered isoflurane in labour. A comparative study with Entonox. Anaesthesia 1985;40:424–6.
14. Abboud TK, Gangolly J, Mosaad P, Crowell D. Isoflurane in obstetrics. Anesth Analg 1989;68:388–91.
15. Wee MYK, Hasan MA, Thomas TA. Isoflurane in labour. Anaesthesia 1993;48:369–72.
16. Ghaly RG, Flynn RJ, Moore J. Isoflurane as an alternative to halothane for caesarean section. Anaesthesia 1988;43:5–7.
17. Abboud TK, Zhu J, Richardson M, Peres Da Silva E, Donovan M. Intravenous propofol vs. thiamylal-isoflurane for caesarean section, comparative maternal and neonatal effects. Acta Anaesthesiol Scand 1995;39:205–9.
18. Stuart JC, Kan AF, Rowbottom SJ, Yau G, Gin T. Acid aspiration prophylaxis for emergency caesarean section. Anaesthesia 1996;51:415–21.
19. Warren TM, Datta S, Ostheimer GW, Naulty JS, Weiss JB, Morrison JA. Comparison of the maternal and neonatal effects of halothane, enflurane, and isoflurane for cesarean section. Anesth Analg 1983;62:516–20.
20. Munson ES, Embro WJ. Enflurane, isoflurane, and halothane and isolated human uterine muscle. Anesthesiology 1977;46:11–4.
21. Abadir AR, Humayun SG, Calvello D, Gintautas J. Effects of isoflurane and oxytocin on gravid human uterus in vitro (abstract). Anesth Analg 1987;66:S1.
22. Sessler DI, Badgwell JM. Exposure of postoperative nurses to exhaled anesthetic gases. Anesth Analg 1998;87:1083–8.
23. Lee JJ, Rubin AP. Breast feeding and anaesthesia. Anaesthesia 1993;48:616–25.
24. Spigset O. Anaesthetic agents and excretion in breast milk. Acta Anaesthesiol Scand 1994;38:94–103.

I

ISOFLUROPHATE

[Withdrawn from the market. See 9th edition.]

ISOMETHEPTENE

Sympathomimetic (Adrenergic)

PREGNANCY RECOMMENDATION: Limited Human Data—No Relevant Animal Data
BREASTFEEDING RECOMMENDATION: No Human Data—Probably Compatible

PREGNANCY SUMMARY

No reports of human developmental toxicity or animal reproductive studies have been located.

FETAL RISK SUMMARY

The sympathomimetic drug, isometheptene, is commercially available in combination with dichloralphenazone and acetaminophen (e.g., Isocom, Isopap, Midchlor, Midrin, and Migratine) for the treatment of tension and vascular (migraine) headaches (see also Dichloralphenazone and Acetaminophen).

The Collaborative Perinatal Project, conducted between 1958 and 1965, recorded eight 1st trimester exposures to isometheptene among 96 mothers who had consumed a miscellaneous group of sympathomimetics (1). From these 96 mothers, 7 children had congenital malformations giving a standardized relative risk (SRR) of 0.96. When only malformations showing uniform rates by hospital were analyzed, the number of children with defects decreased to 4 (SRR 0.81). The authors of this study concluded there was no association between these agents and congenital anomalies.

A 1984 source briefly reviewed isometheptene (2). Although citing no primary references, the authors concluded that the agent was not contraindicated in pregnancy because of the lack of reports of harmful effects on the fetus, the mother, and the pregnancy (2).

BREASTFEEDING SUMMARY

No reports describing the use of isometheptene during human lactation have been located.

References

1. Heinonen OP, Slone D, Shapiro S. *Birth Defects and Drugs in Pregnancy*. Littleton, MA: Publishing Sciences Group, 1977:346.
2. Onnis A, Grella P. *The Biochemical Effects of Drugs in Pregnancy*. Vol. 1. West Sussex, England: Ellis Horwood, 1984:179.

ISONIAZID

Antituberculosis Agent

PREGNANCY RECOMMENDATION: Compatible—Maternal Benefit >> Embryo–Fetal Risk
BREASTFEEDING RECOMMENDATION: Limited Human Data—Probably Compatible

PREGNANCY SUMMARY

Isoniazid does not appear to be a human teratogen. The American Thoracic Society recommends use of the drug for tuberculosis occurring during pregnancy because, "Untreated tuberculosis represents a far greater hazard to a pregnant woman and her fetus than does treatment of the disease" (1).

FETAL RISK SUMMARY

Isoniazid is used in the prevention and treatment of pulmonary tuberculosis. Reproduction studies in mice, rats, and rabbits have not revealed teratogenic effects, but embryocidal effects were observed in rats and rabbits (2).

An official statement of the American Thoracic Society published in 1986 recommends isoniazid as part of the treatment regimen for women who have tuberculosis during pregnancy (1). Other reviewers also consider isoniazid as part of the treatment of choice for tuberculosis occurring during pregnancy (3).

Isoniazid crosses the placenta to the fetus (4–6). In a 1955 study, 19 women in labor were given a single 100-mg dose of isoniazid 0.25–4.25 hours before delivery (4). The mean maternal serum concentration at birth was 0.32 mcg/mL compared with a cord blood level of 0.22 mcg/mL. The mean cord:maternal ratio was 0.73, but in seven of the patients, cord blood concentrations exceeded those in the maternal plasma. Another study examined the placental transfer of isoniazid in two women who had been treated with 300 mg/day during the 3rd trimester (5). One hour before delivery, the women were given a single 300-mg IM dose. Mean cord blood and maternal serum concentrations were 4 and 6.5 mcg/mL, respectively, a ratio of 0.62. These studies and the elimination kinetics of intrauterine-acquired isoniazid in the newborn were reviewed in 1987 (6).

Reports discussing fetal effects of isoniazid during pregnancy reflect multiple drug therapies. Early reports identified slow psychomotor activity, psychic retardation, convulsions, myoclonia, myelomeningocele with spina bifida and talipes, and hypospadias as possible effects related to isoniazid therapy during pregnancy (7,8). The Collaborative Perinatal Project monitored 85 patients who received isoniazid during the 1st trimester (9, pp. 299, 313). They observed 10 malformations, an incidence almost twice the expected rate, but they cautioned that their findings required independent confirmation. For use anytime during pregnancy, 146 mother–child pairs were exposed to isoniazid, with malformations that may have been produced after the 1st trimester observed in 4 infants (9, p. 435). This was close to the expected frequency. Adverse outcomes in the fetus and newborn after intrauterine exposure to isoniazid have not been confirmed by other studies (10–15). Retrospective analysis of >4900 pregnancies in which isoniazid was administered demonstrated rates of malformations similar to those in control populations (0.7%–2.3%). A 1980 review also found no association between isoniazid and fetal anomalies (16).

In a surveillance study of Michigan Medicaid recipients involving 229,101 completed pregnancies conducted between 1985 and 1992, 11 newborns had been exposed to isoniazid during the 1st trimester (F. Rosa, personal communication, FDA, 1993). One (9.1%) major birth defect was observed (0.5 expected), a case of polydactyly.

A case report of a malignant mesothelioma in a 9-year-old child who was exposed to isoniazid in utero was published in 1980 (17). The authors suggested a possible carcinogenic effect of isoniazid because of the rarity of malignant mesotheliomas during the first decade and supportive animal data. However, an earlier study examined 660 children up to 16 years of age and found no association with carcinogenic effects (18).

An association between isoniazid and hemorrhagic disease of the newborn has been suspected in two infants (19). The mothers were also treated with rifampin and ethambutol, and in a third case, only with these latter two drugs. Although other reports of this potentially serious reaction have not been found, prophylactic vitamin K_1 is recommended at birth (see Phytonadione).

BREASTFEEDING SUMMARY

No reports of isoniazid-induced effects in the nursing infant have been located, but the potential for interference with nucleic acid function and for hepatotoxicity may exist (20,21). Both isoniazid and its metabolite, acetylisoniazid, are excreted in breast milk (21–23). A woman was given a single oral dose of 300 mg after complete weaning of her infant (21). Both isoniazid and the metabolite were present in her milk within 1 hour, with peak levels of isoniazid (16.6 mcg/mL) occurring at 3 hours and those of the metabolite (3.76 mcg/mL) at 5 hours. At 5 and 12 hours after the dose, isoniazid levels in the milk were twice the levels in simultaneously obtained plasma. Levels of acetylisoniazid were similar in plasma and milk at 5 and 12 hours. The elimination half-life for milk isoniazid was calculated to be 5.9 hours, whereas that of the metabolite was 13.5 hours. Both were detectable in milk 24 hours after the dose. The 24-hour excretion of isoniazid was estimated to be 7 mg. Two other studies also reported substantial excretion of isoniazid into human milk (22,23). A milk:plasma ratio of 1.0 was reported in one of these studies (22). In another, milk levels 3 hours after a maternal dose of 5 mg/kg were 6 mcg/mL (23). Doubling the maternal dose doubled the milk concentration.

Based on the above information, at least one review concluded that women can safely breastfeed their infants while taking isoniazid if, among other precautions, the infant is periodically examined for signs and symptoms of peripheral neuritis or hepatitis (20). Moreover, the American Academy of Pediatrics classifies isoniazid as compatible with breastfeeding (24).

I

References

1. American Thoracic Society. Treatment of tuberculosis and tuberculosis infection in adults and children. Am Rev Respir Dis 1986;134:355–63.
2. Product information. Rifamate. Hoechst Marion Roussel, 2000.
3. Medchill MT, Gillum M. Diagnosis and management of tuberculosis during pregnancy. Obstet Gynecol Surv 1989;44:81–4.
4. Bromberg YM, Salzberger M, Bruderman I. Placental transmission of isonicotinic acid hydrazide. Gynaecologia 1955;140:141–4.
5. Miceli JN, Olson WA, Cohen SN. Elimination kinetics of isoniazid in the newborn infant. Dev Pharmacol Ther 1981;2:235–9.
6. Holdiness MR. Transplacental pharmacokinetics of the antituberculosis drugs. Clin Pharmacokinet 1987;13:125–9.
7. Weinstein L, Dalton AC. Host determinants of response to antimicrobial agents. N Engl J Med 1968;279:524–31.
8. Lowe CR. Congenital defects among children born to women under supervision or treatment for pulmonary tuberculosis. Br J Prev Soc Med 1964;18:14–6.
9. Heinonen OP, Slone D, Shapiro S. *Birth Defects and Drugs in Pregnancy*. Littleton, MA: Publishing Sciences Group, 1977.
10. Marynowski A, Sianozecka E. Comparison of the incidence of congenital malformations in neonates from healthy mothers and from patients treated because of tuberculosis. Ginekol Pol 1972;43:713.
11. Jentgens H. Antituberkulose Chimotherapie und Schwangerschaft sabbruch. Prax Klin Pneumol 1973;27:479.
12. Ludford J, Doster B, Woolpert SF. Effect of isoniazid on reproduction. Am Rev Respir Dis 1973;108:1170–4.
13. Scheinhorn DJ, Angelillo VA. Antituberculosis therapy in pregnancy; risks to the fetus. West J Med 1977;127:195–8.
14. Good JT, Iseman MD, Davidson PT, Lakshminarayan S, Sahn SA. Tuberculosis in association with pregnancy. Am J Obstet Gynecol 1981;140:492–8.
15. Kingdom JCP, Kennedy DH. Tuberculous meningitis in pregnancy. Br J Obstet Gynaecol 1989;96:233–5.
16. Snider DE Jr, Layde PM, Johnson MW, Lyle MA. Treatment of tuberculosis during pregnancy. Am Rev Respir Dis 1980;122:65–79.
17. Tuman KJ, Chilcote RR, Gerkow RI, Moohr JW. Mesothelioma in child with prenatal exposure to isoniazid. Lancet 1980;2:362.
18. Hammond DC, Silidoff IJ, Robitzek EH. Isoniazid therapy in relation to later occurrence of cancer in adults and in infants. Br Med J 1967;2:792–5.
19. Eggermont E, Logghe N, Van De Casseye W, Casteels-Van Daele M, Jaeken J, Cosemans J, Verstraete M, Renaer M. Haemorrhagic disease of the newborn in the offspring of rifampicin and isoniazid treated mothers. Acta Paediatr Belg 1976;29:87–90.
20. Snider DE Jr, Powell KE. Should women taking antituberculosis drugs breast-feed? Arch Intern Med 1984;144:589–90.
21. Berlin CM Jr, Lee C. Isoniazid and acetylisoniazid disposition in human milk, saliva and plasma. Fed Proc 1979;38:426.
22. Vorherr H. Drugs excretion in breast milk. Postgrad Med 1974;56:97–104.
23. Ricci G, Copaitich T. Modalta di eliminazione dili'isoniazide somministrata per via orale attraverso il latte di donna. Rass Clin Ter 1954–5;209:53–4.
24. Committee on Drugs, American Academy of Pediatrics. The transfer of drugs and other chemicals into human milk. Pediatrics 2001;108:776–89.

ISOPROPAMIDE

[Withdrawn from the market. See 9th edition.]

ISOPROTERENOL

Sympathomimetic/Bronchodilator

PREGNANCY RECOMMENDATION: Limited Human Data—Animal Data Suggest Moderate Risk
BREASTFEEDING RECOMMENDATION: No Human Data—Probably Compatible

PREGNANCY SUMMARY

No reports linking the human use of isoproterenol with congenital defects have been located. Isoproterenol was not teratogenic in rats and rabbits, but was in hamsters (1,2). Sympathomimetics are often administered in combination with other drugs to alleviate the symptoms of upper respiratory infections. Thus, the fetal effects of sympathomimetics, other drugs, and viruses cannot be totally separated.

FETAL RISK SUMMARY

The Collaborative Perinatal Project monitored 50,282 mother–child pairs, 31 of whom had 1st trimester exposure to isoproterenol (3, pp. 346–347). No evidence was found to suggest a relationship between large categories of major or minor malformations or to individual defects. However, an association in the 1st trimester was found between the sympathomimetic class of drugs as a whole and minor malformations (not life-threatening or major cosmetic defects), inguinal hernia, and clubfoot (3, pp. 345–356).

In a surveillance study of Michigan Medicaid recipients involving 229,101 completed pregnancies conducted between 1985 and 1992, 16 newborns had been exposed to isoproterenol during the 1st trimester (F. Rosa, personal communication, FDA, 1993). One (6.3%) major birth defect was observed (0.7 expected), an oral cleft.

Isoproterenol has been used during pregnancy to accelerate heart rhythm when high-grade atrioventricular block is present and to treat ventricular arrhythmias associated with prolonged QT intervals (4). Because of its β-adrenergic effect, the agent will inhibit contractions of the pregnant uterus (4). Of incidental interest, five-term, nonlaboring pregnant women were discovered to have an increased resistance to the chronotropic effect of isoproterenol in comparison to nonpregnant women (5). One fetus had an isolated 5-beats/minute late deceleration 2 minutes after the mother received 0.25 mcg of the drug (5).

BREASTFEEDING SUMMARY

No reports describing the use of isoproterenol during human lactation have been located.

References

1. Nishimura H, Tanimura T. *Clinical Aspects of the Teratogenicity of Drugs*. New York, NY: American Elsevier, 1976:231–2.
2. Shepard TH. *Catalog of Teratogenic Agents*. 3rd ed. Baltimore, MD: The Johns Hopkins University Press, 1980:191.
3. Heinonen OP, Slone D, Shapiro S. *Birth Defects and Drugs in Pregnancy*. Littleton, MA: Publishing Sciences Group, 1977.
4. Tamari I, Eldar M, Rabinowitz B, Neufeld HN. Medical treatment of cardiovascular disorders during pregnancy. Am Heart J 1982;104:1357–63.
5. DeSimone CA, Leighton BL, Norris MC, Chayen B, Menduke H. The chronotropic effect of isoproterenol is reduced in term pregnant women. Anesthesiology 1988;69:626–8.

ISOSORBIDE

Diuretic

PREGNANCY RECOMMENDATION: Limited Human Data—Probably Compatible
BREASTFEEDING RECOMMENDATION: No Human Data—Probably Compatible

PREGNANCY SUMMARY

Isosorbide is an osmotic diuretic used for the short-term reduction of intraocular pressure in acute glaucoma before and after intraocular surgery. No published reports describing the use of isosorbide in pregnancy have been located.

FETAL RISK SUMMARY

In an FDA surveillance study of Michigan Medicaid recipients involving 229,101 completed pregnancies conducted between 1985 and 1992, 13 newborns had been exposed to isosorbide during the 1st trimester (F. Rosa, personal communication, FDA, 1993). No major birth defects were observed (0.6 expected).

BREASTFEEDING SUMMARY

No reports describing the use of isosorbide during human lactation have been located.

ISOSORBIDE DINITRATE

Vasodilator

PREGNANCY RECOMMENDATION: Limited Human Data—Animal Data Suggest Moderate Risk
BREASTFEEDING RECOMMENDATION: No Human Data—Probably Compatible

PREGNANCY SUMMARY

Isosorbide is a nitric oxide donor, similar to nitroglycerin that is used in the management of angina pectoris and of heart failure. No reports have described pregnancy outcomes following therapeutic use of this agent.

FETAL RISK SUMMARY

Isosorbide is administered sublingually, as chewable tablets, and as oral tablets. An oral spray is also available outside of the United States. The molecular weight (about 236) is low enough that passage to the fetus should be expected.

The drug produces dose-related embryotoxicity in rabbits at doses 35 and 150 times the maximum recommended human dose (1) (see also Nitroglycerin and Amyl Nitrite).

Two full reports and one abstract have described the use of isosorbide dinitrate during human pregnancy (2–4). However, all of the pregnancies in these reports had prescheduled elective terminations for nonmedical reasons shortly after the drug exposure. In a 1996 study (first published as an abstract in 1995), 18 women in the 2nd trimester received a single 5-mg sublingual dose of isosorbide dinitrate (2,3). Statistically significant decreases in the maternal systolic and diastolic blood pressures were observed 6 minutes after the dose. The blood pressures gradually returned to control levels over the ensuing 30 minutes. The mean maternal heart rate significantly increased from about 85 beats/minute to 96 beats/minute at 6 minutes, but declined to near control levels at 8 minutes. The mean systolic–diastolic flow velocity ratios in the umbilical and uterine arteries declined significantly, reaching nadirs at 6 and 10 minutes, respectively, before gradually returning to predose levels. These findings suggested that isosorbide dinitrate may be beneficial in reversing the effects of endothelial cell dysfunction–induced generalized vasoconstriction and increased vascular resistance to flow in the uteroplacental circulation, such as that occurs in preeclampsia (2,3).

In a similar investigation by these same researchers, 11 women at a mean gestational age of 10.0 weeks (range 8.2–11.6 weeks) were given a single 5-mg sublingual dose of the drug (4). The results of this study were comparable to the researchers previous work and led them to a similar conclusion that isosorbide dinitrate may be effective in reversing the effects of the endothelial cell dysfunction that is observed in preeclampsia (4).

BREASTFEEDING SUMMARY

No reports describing the use of isosorbide dinitrate during lactation have been located. The molecular weight (about 236) is low enough that excretion into breast milk should be expected. The effect of this exposure on a nursing infant is unknown.

References

1. Product information. Isordil. Wyeth-Ayerst Laboratories, 1993.
2. Thaler I, Amit A, Itskovitz J. The effect of isosorbide dinitrate, a nitric oxide donor, on human uterine and placental vascular resistance in patients with preeclampsia (abstract). Am J Obstet Gynecol 1995;172:387.
3. Thaler I, Amit A, Jakobi P, Itskovitz-Eldor J. The effect of isosorbide dinitrate on uterine artery and umbilical artery flow velocity waveforms at mid-pregnancy. Obstet Gynecol 1996;88:838–43.
4. Amit A, Thaler I, Paz Y, Itskovity-Eldor J. The effect of a nitric oxide donor on Doppler flow velocity waveforms in the uterine artery during the first trimester of pregnancy. Ultrasound Obstet Gynecol 1998;11:94–8.

ISOSORBIDE MONONITRATE

Vasodilator

PREGNANCY RECOMMENDATION: Limited Human Data—Animal Data Suggest Moderate Risk
BREASTFEEDING RECOMMENDATION: No Human Data—Probably Compatible

PREGNANCY SUMMARY

The vasodilator isosorbide mononitrate is the major active metabolite of isosorbide dinitrate. The drug has been used for cervical ripening.

FETAL RISK SUMMARY

In rats and rabbits administered doses up to 250 mg/kg/day, no adverse effects on reproduction and development were observed, but doses of 500 mg/kg/day in rats caused significant increases in prolonged gestation, prolonged parturition, stillbirth, and neonatal death (1).

A number of reports have described the use of vaginal isosorbide mononitrate for cervical ripening at term (2–11). No adverse fetal effects were observed.

BREASTFEEDING SUMMARY

No reports describing the use of isosorbide mononitrate during human lactation have been located.

References

1. Product information. Ismo. Wyeth-Ayerst Laboratories, 1993.
2. Nicoll AE, MacKenzie F, Greer IA, Norman JE. Vaginal application of the nitric oxide donor isosorbide mononitrate for preinduction cervical ripening: a randomized controlled trial to determine effects on maternal and fetal hemodynamics. Am J Obstet Gynecol 2001;184:958–64.
3. Chanrachakul B, Herabutya Y, Punyavachira P. Randomized trial of isosorbide mononitrate versus misoprostol for cervical ripening at term. Int J Gynaecol Obstet 2002;78:139–45.
4. Ekerhovd E, Bullarbo M, Andersch B, Norstrom A. Vaginal administration of the nitric oxide donor isosorbide mononitrate for cervical ripening at term-a randomized controlled study. Am J Obstet Gynecol 2003;189:1692–7.
5. Wolfler MM, Facchinetti F, Venturini P, Huber A, Helmer H, Hussiein P, Tschugguel W. Induction of labor at term using isosorbide mononitrate simultaneously with dinoprostone compared to dinoprostone treatment alone: a randomized, controlled trial. Am J Obstet Gynecol 2006;195:1617–22.

6. Osman I, MacKenzie F, Norrie J, Murray HM, Greer IA, Norman JE. The "PRIM" study: a randomized comparison of prostaglandin E_2 gel with the nitric oxide donor isosorbide mononitrate for cervical ripening before the induction of labor at term. Am J Obstet Gynecol 2006;194:1012–21.
7. Bullarbo M, Orrskog ME, Andersch B, Granstrom L, Norstrom A, Ekerhovd E. Outpatient vaginal administration of the nitric oxide donor isosorbide mononitrate for cervical ripening and labor induction post-term: a randomized controlled study. Am J Obstet Gynecol 2007;196:50.e1–5.
8. Rameez MF, Goonewardene IM. Nitric oxide donor isosorbide mononitrate for pre-induction cervical ripening at 41 weeks' gestation: a randomized controlled trial. J Obstet Gynaecol Res 2007;33:452–6.
9. Habib SM, Emam SS, Saber AS. Outpatient cervical ripening with nitric oxide donor isosorbide mononitrate prior to induction of labor. Int J Gynaecol Obstet 2008;101:57–61.
10. Bollapragada SS, MacKenzie F, Norrie JD, Eddama O, Petrou S, Reid M, Norman JE. Randomized placebo-controlled trial of outpatient (at home) cervical ripening with isosorbide mononitrate (IMN) prior to induction of labour-clinical trial with analyses of efficacy and acceptability. The IMOP study. BJOG 2009;116;1185–95.
11. Eddama O, Petrou S, Schroeder L, Bollapragada SS, MacKenzie F, Norrie J, Reid M, Norman JE. The cost-effectiveness of outpatient (at home) cervical ripening with isosorbide mononitrate prior to induction of labour. BJOG 2009;116:1196–203.

ISOTRETINOIN

Vitamin

PREGNANCY RECOMMENDATION: Contraindicated
BREASTFEEDING RECOMMENDATION: No Human Data—Potential Toxicity

I

PREGNANCY SUMMARY

Isotretinoin is a potent human teratogen. Critically important is the fact that a high percentage of the recipients of this drug are women with childbearing potential. Estimates have indicated that 38% of isotretinoin users are women aged 13–19 years (1). Pregnancy must be excluded and prevented in these and other female patients before isotretinoin is prescribed.

FETAL RISK SUMMARY

Isotretinoin (Accutane) is a vitamin A isomer used for the treatment of severe, recalcitrant cystic acne. The animal teratogenicity of this drug was well documented before its approval for human use in 1982 (2,3). The mechanism of isotretinoin teratogenicity in animals may involve cytotoxic peroxyl free radical generation by metabolism with prostaglandin synthase (4). Newborn mice exposed in utero to isotretinoin at a critical point in gestation had characteristic craniofacial and limb malformations, but concurrent treatment with aspirin, a prostaglandin synthase inhibitor, resulted in a dose-dependent decrease in the overall incidence of abnormalities, the number of anomalies per fetus, and the incidence of specific craniofacial and limb defects (4).

Shortly after its approval, several publications appeared warning of the human teratogenic potential if isotretinoin was administered to women who were pregnant or who may become pregnant (5–10). In the 22 months following its introduction (September 1982 through July 5, 1984), the manufacturer, the FDA, and the CDC received reports on 154 isotretinoin-exposed pregnancies (11). Some of these cases had been described in earlier reports (1,12–20). Of the 154 pregnancies, 95 were electively aborted, 12 aborted spontaneously, 26 infants were born without major defects (some may not have been exposed during the critical gestational period), and 21 had major malformations (11). Three of the 21 infants were stillborn and 9 died after birth. A characteristic pattern of defects was observed in the 21 infants that closely resembled that seen in animal experiments (11). The syndrome of defects observed in these infants and in other reported cases (21–34) consists of all or part of the following:

Central nervous system
- Hydrocephalus
- Facial (VII nerve) palsy
- Posterior fossa structure defects
- Cortical and cerebellar defects
- Cortical blindness
- Optic nerve hypoplasia
- Retinal defects
- Microphthalmia

Craniofacial
- Microtia or anotia
- Low-set ears
- Agenesis or marked stenosis of external ear canals
- Micrognathia
- Small mouth
- Microcephaly
- Triangular skull
- Facial dysmorphism
- Depressed nasal bridge
- Cleft palate
- Hypertelorism

Cardiovascular
- Conotruncal malformations
- Transposition of great vessels
- Tetralogy of Fallot
- Double-outlet right ventricle
- Truncus arteriosus communis
- Ventricular septal defect
- Atrial septal defect
- Branchial-arch mesenchymal-tissue defects
- Interrupted or hypoplastic aortic arch
- Retroesophageal right subclavian artery

Thymic defects
- Ectopia, hypoplasia, or aplasia

Miscellaneous defects (sporadic occurrence)
- Spina bifida
- Nystagmus
- Hepatic abnormality

Hydroureter
Decreased muscle tone
Large scrotal sac
Simian crease
Limb reduction

Other defects have been reported with isotretinoin, but in these cases exposure had either been terminated before conception or was outside the critical period for the defect (33). These defects are thought to be nonteratogenic or have occurred by chance (33). Similarly, three reports of anomalies in children in which only the father was exposed (biliary atresia and ventricular septal defect; four-limb ectromelia and hydrocephalus; anencephaly) also probably occurred by chance (33).

A 1985 case report proposed that reduction deformities observed in all four limbs of a male infant were induced by isotretinoin (35,36). Other evidence suggested that these defects may have been secondary to amniotic bands (37). However, a 1991 reference described an infant and a fetus with limb reduction deformities after 1st trimester exposure to isotretinoin (38). A 17-year-old mother took 50 mg/day of isotretinoin for 10 days during the 2nd month of gestation. Abnormalities present in the infant were absence of the right clavicle and nearly absent right scapula, a short humerus, and a short, broad, completely synostotic right radius and ulna (38). Other defects present were asymmetrical ventriculomegaly, minor dysmorphic facial features, a short sternum with a sterno-umbilical raphe, and developmental delay (38). The second case involved an 18-year-old woman who took 60 mg/day of isotretinoin during the first 62 days of gestation (38). The pregnancy was terminated at 22 weeks' gestation because of fetal hydrocephalus and cystic kidney. Multiple defects were noted in the fetus, including an absent left thumb but with normal proximal bony structures, a single umbilical artery, anal and vaginal atresia, urethral agenesis with dysplastic, multicystic kidneys, and other malformations consistent with isotretinoin exposure (38).

Because isotretinoin causes CNS abnormalities, concern has been raised over the potential for adverse behavioral effects in infants who seemingly are normal at birth (39). Long-term studies are in progress to evaluate behavioral toxicities, such as mental retardation and learning disabilities, but have not been concluded because the exposed children are still too young for tests to produce meaningful results (40).

The teratogenic mechanism of isotretinoin and its main metabolite, 4-oxo-isotretinoin, is thought to result from an adverse effect on the initial differentiation and migration of cephalic neural crest cells (11,41). Daily doses in the range of 0.5–1.5 mg/kg were usually ingested in cases with adverse outcome (11), but doses as low as 0.2 mg/kg or lower may also have caused teratogenicity (34,42). The critical period of exposure is believed to be 2–5 weeks after conception, but clinically it is difficult to establish the exact dating in many cases (33). Because of the high proportion of spontaneous abortions in prospectively identified exposed women, the CDC commented that fetotoxicity may be a more common adverse outcome than liveborn infants with abnormalities (12).

The lack of reports of isotretinoin-induced abnormalities from areas other than the United States and Canada caused speculation that this was caused by the use of lower doses, more restricted use in women, or later marketing of the drug (43). Several groups of investigators have responded to this, and although under diagnosis and underreporting may contribute, the reasons are still unclear (44–47).

An autosomal or X-linked recessive syndrome with features of isotretinoin-induced defects has been described in three male siblings (48). Although the mother had no history of isotretinoin or vitamin A use, the authors did not rule out a defect in vitamin A metabolism.

In a follow-up to a previous report involving 36 pregnancies, investigators noted the outcome of an additional 21 pregnancies exposed in the 1st trimester to isotretinoin (49). The outcomes of the 57 pregnancies were 9 spontaneous abortions, 1 malformed stillborn, 10 malformed live births, and 37 normal live births. In this population, the absolute risk for a major defect in pregnancies extending to 20 weeks' gestation or longer was 23% (11 of 48) (49).

In a surveillance study of Michigan Medicaid recipients involving 229,101 completed pregnancies conducted between 1985 and 1992, 6 newborns had been exposed to isotretinoin during the 1st trimester (F. Rosa, personal communication, FDA, 1993). One (16.7%) major birth defect was observed (0.3 expected). Specific data were not available for the anomaly, but it was not one of six defect categories (cardiovascular defects, oral clefts, spina bifida, polydactyly, limb reduction defects, and hypospadias) for which specific data were available.

The outcome of pregnancies occurring after the discontinuation of isotretinoin was described in a 1989 article (50). Of 88 prospectively ascertained pregnancies, conception occurred in 77 within 60 days of the last dose of the drug. In 10 cases, the date of conception (defined as 14 days after the last menstrual period) occurred within 2–5 days after the last dose of isotretinoin. These 10 pregnancies ended in 2 spontaneous abortions and 8 normal infants. Three women who had taken their last dose within 2 days of the estimated date of conception delivered normal infants. The outcomes of all 88 pregnancies were as follows: 8 (9.1%) spontaneous abortions, 1 abnormal birth (details not provided), 75 (85.3%) normal infants, and 4 (4.5%) infants with congenital malformations. The defects observed were small anterior fontanelle (1 case), congenital cataract with premature hypertrophic vitreous membrane (1 case), congenital cataract (1 case), and hypospadias (1 case). The mothers had taken their last dose of isotretinoin 33, 22, 17, and 55 days before conception, respectively. These anomalies are not characteristic of those reported with in utero exposure to isotretinoin. In an additional 13 cases obtained retrospectively, 5 ended in spontaneous abortions, 4 normal infants were delivered, and 4 infants had congenital defects: syndactyly (1 case), Down's syndrome (1 case), hypoplasia of left side of heart (1 case), and unknown defects (1 case). In the cases of known defects, the mothers had stopped isotretinoin at least 9 months before conception. As with the prospective cases, the defects described in the three infants were not those typical of isotretinoin-induced anomalies. Moreover, retrospective reports are probably more likely to report abnormal outcomes and to underreport normal infants (50).

In one study the drug did not interfere with the action of oral contraceptive steroids (51). Initially, recommendations included stopping therapy at least 1 month before conception (1), but others indicated that shorter intervals between the last dose of isotretinoin and conception were apparently safe (50). Labeling by the manufacturer states that a negative serum pregnancy 2 weeks before beginning therapy is required (52,53). A recent statement by the Teratology Society supplemented the manufacturer's recommendations, for treatment of women of childbearing potential with isotretinoin, with additional recommendations and reviewed the animal and human teratogenicity of this agent (53).

BREASTFEEDING SUMMARY

It is not known whether isotretinoin or its metabolite, 4-oxo-isotretinoin, is excreted into human milk. The closely related retinoid, vitamin A, is excreted (see Vitamin A), and the presence of isotretinoin in breast milk should be expected.

References

1. Anonymous. Adverse effects with isotretinoin. FDA Drug Bull 1983;13:21–3.
2. Voorhees JJ, Orfanos CE. Oral retinoids. Arch Dermatol 1981;117:418–21.
3. Kamm JJ. Toxicology, carcinogenicity, and teratogenicity of some orally administered retinoids. J Am Acad Dermatol 1982;6:652–9.
4. Kubow S. Inhibition of isotretinoin teratogenicity by acetylsalicylic acid pretreatment in mice. Teratology 1992;45:55–63.
5. Perry MD, McEvoy GK. Isotretinoin: new therapy for severe acne. Clin Pharm 1983;2:12–9.
6. Henderson IWD, Rice WB. Accutane. Can Med Assoc J 1983;129:682.
7. Shalita AR, Cunningham WJ, Leyden JJ, Pochi PE, Strauss JS. Isotretinoin treatment of acne and related disorders: an update. J Am Acad Dermatol 1983;9:629–38.
8. Anonymous. Update on isotretinoin (Accutane) for acne. Med Lett Drugs Ther 1983;25:105–6.
9. Conner CS. Isotretinoin: a reappraisal. Drug Intell Clin Pharm 1984;18:308–9.
10. Ward A, Brogden RN, Heel RC, Speight TM, Avery GS. Isotretinoin. A review of its pharmacological properties and therapeutic efficacy in acne and other skin disorders. Drugs 1984;28:6–37.
11. Lammer EJ, Chen DT, Hoar RM, Agnish ND, Benke PJ, Braun JT, Curry CJ, Fernhoff PM, Grix AW Jr, Lott IT, Richard JM, Sun SC. Retinoic acid embryopathy. N Engl J Med 1985;313:837–41.
12. Anonymous. Isotretinoin—a newly recognized human teratogen. MMWR 1984;33:171–3.
13. Anonymous. Update on birth defects with isotretinoin. FDA Drug Bull 1984;14:15–6.
14. Rosa FW. Teratogenicity of isotretinoin. Lancet 1983;2:513.
15. Braun JT, Franciosi RA, Mastri AR, Drake RM, O'Neil BL. Isotretinoin dysmorphic syndrome. Lancet 1984;1:506–7.
16. Hill RM. Isotretinoin teratogenicity. Lancet 1984;1:1465.
17. Benke PJ. The isotretinoin teratogen syndrome. JAMA 1984;251:3267–9.
18. Fernhoff PM, Lammer EJ. Craniofacial features of isotretinoin embryopathy. J Pediatr 1984;105:595–7.
19. Lott IT, Bocian M, Pribram HW, Leitner M. Fetal hydrocephalus and ear anomalies associated with maternal use of isotretinoin. J Pediatr 1984;105:597–600.
20. De La Cruz E, Sun S, Vangvanichyakorn K, Desposito F. Multiple congenital malformations associated with maternal isotretinoin therapy. Pediatrics 1984;74:428–30.
21. Stern RS, Rosa F, Baum C. Isotretinoin and pregnancy. J Am Acad Dermatol 1984;10:851–4.
22. Marwick C. More cautionary labeling appears on isotretinoin. JAMA 1984;251:3208–9.
23. Zarowny DP. Accutane Roche: risk of teratogenic effects. Can Med Assoc J 1984;131:273.
24. Hall JG. Vitamin A: a newly recognized human teratogen. Harbinger of things to come? J Pediatr 1984;105:583–4.
25. Robertson R, MacLeod PM. Accutane-induced teratogenesis. Can Med Assoc J 1985;133:1147–8.
26. Willhite CC, Hill RM, Irving DW. Isotretinoin-induced craniofacial malformations in humans and hamsters. J Craniofac Genet Dev Biol 1986;2(Suppl):193–209.
27. Cohen M, Rubinstein A, Li JK, Nathenson G. Thymic hypoplasia associated with isotretinoin embryopathy. Am J Dis Child 1987;141:263–6.
28. Millan SB, Flowers FP, Sherertz EF. Isotretinoin. South Med J 1987;80: 494–9.
29. Jahn AF, Ganti K. Major auricular malformations due to Accutane (isotretinoin). Laryngoscope 1987;97:832–5.
30. Bigby M, Stern RS. Adverse reactions to isotretinoin: a report from the adverse drug reaction reporting system. J Am Acad Dermatol 1988;18:543–52.
31. Anonymous. Birth defects caused by isotretinoin—New Jersey. MMWR 1988;37:171–2,177.
32. Orfanos CE, Ehlert R, Gollnick H. The retinoids: a review of their clinical pharmacology and therapeutic use. Drugs 1987;34:459–503.
33. Rosa FW, Wilk AL, Kelsey FO. Teratogen update: vitamin A congeners. Teratology 1986;33:355–64.
34. Rosa FW. Retinoic acid embryopathy. N Engl J Med 1986;315:262.
35. McBride WG. Limb reduction deformities in child exposed to isotretinoin in utero on gestation days 26–40 only. Lancet 1985;1:1276.
36. McBride WG. Isotretinoin and reduction deformities. Lancet 1985;2:503.
37. Lammer EJ, Flannery DB, Barr M. Does isotretinoin cause limb reduction defects? Lancet 1985;2:328.
38. Rizzo R, Lammer EJ, Parano E, Pavone L, Argyle JC. Limb reduction defects in humans associated with prenatal isotretinoin exposure. Teratology 1991;44:599–604.
39. Vorhees CV. Retinoic acid embryopathy. N Engl J Med 1986;315:262–3.
40. Lammer EJ. Retinoic acid embryopathy (in reply). N Engl J Med 1986;315:263.
41. Webster WS, Johnston MC, Lammer EJ, Sulik KK. Isotretinoin embryopathy and the cranial neural crest: an in vivo and in vitro study. J Craniofac Genet Dev Biol 1986;6:211–22.
42. Ayme S, Julian C, Gambarelli D, Mariotti B, Maurin N. Isotretinoin dose and teratogenicity. Lancet 1988;1:655.
43. Rosa F. Isotretinoin dose and teratogenicity. Lancet 1987;2:1154.
44. Robert E. Isotretinoin dose and teratogenicity. Lancet 1988;1:236.
45. Lammer EJ, Schunior A, Hayes AM, Holmes LB. Isotretinoin dose and teratogenicity. Lancet 1988;2:503–4.
46. Hope G, Mathias B. Teratogenicity of isotretinoin and etretinate. Lancet 1988;2:1143.
47. Lancaster PAL. Teratogenicity of isotretinoin. Lancet 1988;2:1254.
48. Kawashima H, Ohno I, Ueno Y, Nakaya S, Kato E, Taniguchi N. Syndrome of microtia and aortic arch anomalies resembling isotretinoin embryopathy. J Pediatr 1987;111:738–40.
49. Lammer EJ, Hayes AM, Schunior A, Holmes LB. Risk for major malformation among human fetuses exposed to isotretinoin (13-cis-retinoic acid). Teratology 1987;35:68A.
50. Dai WS, Hsu M-A, Itri LM. Safety of pregnancy after discontinuation of isotretinoin. Arch Dermatol 1989;125:363–5.
51. Orme M, Back DJ, Shaw MA, Allen WL, Tjia J, Cunliffe WJ, Jones DH. Isotretinoin and contraception. Lancet 1984;2:752–3.
52. Product information. Accutane. Roche Dermatologics, 1993.
53. Public Affairs Committee, The Teratology Society. Recommendations for isotretinoin use in women of childbearing potential. Teratology 1991;44:1–6.

ISOXSUPRINE

Sympathomimetic (Vasodilator)

PREGNANCY RECOMMENDATION: Limited Human Data—No Relevant Animal Data
BREASTFEEDING RECOMMENDATION: No Human Data—Probably Compatible

PREGNANCY SUMMARY

No reports linking the use of isoxsuprine with congenital defects have been located.

FETAL RISK SUMMARY

Isoxsuprine, a β-sympathomimetic, is indicated for vasodilation, but it has been used to prevent premature labor (1–6). Uterine inhibitory effects usually require high IV doses, which increase the risk for serious adverse effects (7,8). Maternal heart rate increases and blood pressure decreases are usually mild at lower doses (2,4,6). A decrease in the incidence of neonatal respiratory distress syndrome has been observed (9). However, in one study, neonatal respiratory depression was increased if cord serum levels exceeded 10 ng/mL (10). The depression was always associated with hypotension, so the mechanism of the defect may have been related to pulmonary hypoperfusion.

Neonatal toxicity is generally rare if cord levels of isoxsuprine are <2 ng/mL (corresponding to a drug-free interval of >5 hours), but levels >10 ng/mL (drug-free interval of 2 hours of less) were associated with severe neonatal problems (10). These problems include hypocalcemia, hypoglycemia, ileus, hypotension, and death (10–12). Hypotension and neonatal death occurred primarily in infants of 26–31 weeks' gestation, especially if cord levels exceeded 10 ng/mL, and in infants whose mothers developed hypotension or tachycardia during isoxsuprine infusion (10,11). Neonatal ileus, up to 33% in some series, was not related to cord isoxsuprine concentrations, but hypotension and hypocalcemia were directly related, reaching 89% and 100%, respectively, when cord levels exceeded 10 ng/mL (10,12). Fetal tachycardia is a common side effect. As compared with controls, no increase in late or variable decelerations was seen (10). In contrast to the above, infusion of isoxsuprine 30 minutes before cesarean section under general anesthesia was not observed to produce adverse effects in the mother, fetus, or newborn (13). Cord concentrations were not measured.

Long-term evaluation of infants exposed to β-mimetics in utero has been reported but not specifically for isoxsuprine (14). No harmful effects in the infants resulting from this exposure were observed.

The Collaborative Perinatal Project monitored 50,282 mother–child pairs, 54 of whom were exposed to isoxsuprine during the 1st trimester (15, pp. 346–347). For use anytime during pregnancy, 858 exposures were recorded (15, p. 439). In neither case was evidence found for an association with malformations.

BREASTFEEDING SUMMARY

No reports describing the use of isoxsuprine during human lactation have been located.

References

1. Bishop EH, Woutersz TB. Isoxsuprine, a myometrial relaxant. A preliminary report. Obstet Gynecol 1961;17:442–6.
2. Hendricks CH, Cibils LA, Pose SV, Eskes TKAB. The pharmacological control of excessive uterine activity with isoxsuprine. Am J Obstet Gynecol 1961;82:1064–78.
3. Bishop EH, Woutersz TB. Arrest of premature labor. JAMA 1961;178: 812–4.
4. Stander RW, Barden TP, Thompson JF, Pugh WR, Werts CE. Fetal cardiac effects of maternal isoxsuprine infusion. Am J Obstet Gynecol 1964;89:792–800.
5. Hendricks CH. The use of isoxsuprine for the arrest of premature labor. Clin Obstet Gynecol 1964;7:687–94.
6. Allen HH, Short H, Fraleigh DM. The use of isoxsuprine in the management of premature labor. Appl Ther 1965;7:544–7.
7. Anonymous. Drugs acting on the uterus. Br Med J 1964;1:1234–6.
8. Briscoe CC. Failure of oral isoxsuprine to prevent prematurity. Am J Obstet Gynecol 1966;95:885–6.
9. Kero P, Hirvonen T, Valimaki I. Perinatal isoxsuprine and respiratory distress syndrome. Lancet 1973;2:198.
10. Brazy JE, Little V, Grimm J, Pupkin M. Risk:benefit considerations for the use of isoxsuprine in the treatment of premature labor. Obstet Gynecol 1981;58:297–303.
11. Brazy JE, Pupkin MJ. Effects of maternal isoxsuprine administration on preterm infants. J Pediatr 1979;94:444–8.
12. Brazy JE, Little V, Grimm J. Isoxsuprine in the perinatal period. II. Relationships between neonatal symptoms, drug exposure, and drug concentration at the time of birth. J Pediatr 1981;98:146–51.
13. Jouppila R, Kauppila A, Tuimala R, Pakarinen A, Moilanen K. Maternal, fetal and neonatal effects of beta-adrenergic stimulation in connection with cesarean section. Acta Obstet Gynecol Scand 1980;59:489–93.
14. Freysz H, Willard D, Lehr A, Messer J, Boog G. A long term evaluation of infants who received a beta-mimetic drug while in utero. J Perinat Med 1977;5:94–9.
15. Heinonen OP, Slone D, Shapiro S. *Birth Defects and Drugs in Pregnancy*. Littleton, MA: Publishing Sciences Group, 1977.

ISRADIPINE

Calcium Channel Blocker

PREGNANCY RECOMMENDATION: Limited Human Data—Animal Data Suggest Low Risk
BREASTFEEDING RECOMMENDATION: No Human Data—Probably Compatible

PREGNANCY SUMMARY

Several studies have described the use of isradipine in pregnant women (1–8). No adverse fetal effects attributable to the drug were observed. Isradipine crosses the placenta to the fetus at term (3).

FETAL RISK SUMMARY

Isradipine is a calcium channel-blocking agent used in the treatment of hypertension. The drug is not teratogenic in rats or rabbits at doses 150 and 25 times the maximum recommended human dose, respectively. Embryotoxicity was not observed in either species at doses that were not maternally toxic (9).

In a study to determine the effects of isradipine on maternal and fetal hemodynamics, 27 women with pregnancy-induced hypertension in the 3rd trimester were treated with the drug, 2.5 mg twice daily for 4 days and then 5 mg twice daily (1). Hemodynamic measurements, conducted before and after 1 week of therapy, demonstrated a significant reduction in mean arterial pressure without a significant change in uteroplacental or fetal blood flows. The lack of change in uteroplacental blood flow suggested that there was uterine vasodilation with decreased uterine vascular resistance. No fetal adverse effects were observed (1).

A 1992 study examined the effect of isradipine on three standardized physical stress tests in 14 women under treatment for hypertension (3 with essential hypertension, 11 with preeclampsia) (2). Treatment with isradipine, 5 mg once daily for 4 days and then 5 mg twice daily, was begun at a mean 33 weeks' gestation with delivery occurring at a mean of 38 weeks. The pregnancy outcomes were normal except for one newborn whose birth weight was below the 10th percentile and transient hyperbilirubinemia in two neonates (2).

A study reported in 1999 compared antihypertensive effect of isradipine ($N = 20$) with hydralazine and methyldopa ($N = 19$) in women with severe preeclampsia (8). There were no differences in the outcomes in terms of gestational age at birth, Apgar scores, and birth weight.

BREASTFEEDING SUMMARY

No reports describing the use of isradipine during human lactation have been located. The relatively low molecular weight (about 371), however, suggests that the drug is excreted into breast milk. The potential effects of this exposure on a nursing infant are unknown.

References

1. Lunell N-O, Garoff L, Grunewald C, Nisell H, Nylund L, Sarby B, Thornstrom S. Isradipine, a new calcium antagonist: effects on maternal and fetal hemodynamics. J Cardiovasc Pharmacol 1991;18(Suppl 3):S37–40.
2. Lunell NO, Grunewald C, Nisell H. Effect of isradipine on responses to standardized physical stress tests in hypertension of pregnancy. J Cardiovasc Pharmacol 1992;19(Suppl 3):S99–101.
3. Lunnell NO, Bondesson U, Grunewald C, Ingemarsson I, Nisell H, Wide-Swensson D. Transplacental passage of isradipine in the treatment of pregnancy-induced hypertension. Am J Hypertens 1993;6:110S–1S.
4. Wide-Swensson DH, Ingemarsson I, Lunell NO, Forman A, Skajaa K, Lindberg B, Lindeberg S, Marsal K, Andersson KE. Calcium channel blockade (isradipine) in treatment of hypertension in pregnancy: a randomized placebo-controlled study. Am J Obstet Gynecol 1995;173:872–8.
5. Maharaj B, Khedun SM, Moodley J, Madhanpall N, van der Byl K. Intravenous isradipine in the management of severe hypertension in pregnant and nonpregnant patients. A pilot study. Am J Hypertens 1994;7:61S–3S.
6. Kublickas M, Lunell NO, Grunewald C, Nisell H. Effect of isradipine on maternal renal artery pulsatility index in hypertensive pregnancy. Hypertens Pregnancy 1995;14:277–85.
7. Resch B, Mache CJ, Windhager T, Holzer H, Leitner G, Muller W. FK 506 and successful pregnancy in a patient after renal transplantation. Transplant Proc 1998;30:163–4.
8. Fletcher H, Roberts G, Mullings A, Forrester T. An open trial comparing isradipine with hydralazine and methyldopa in the treatment of patients with severe pre-eclampsia. J Obstet Gynaecol 2009;19:235–8.
9. Product information. DynaCirc. Sandoz Pharmaceuticals, 1993.

ITRACONAZOLE

Antifungal

PREGNANCY RECOMMENDATION: Human Data Suggest Low Risk
BREASTFEEDING RECOMMENDATION: Limited Human Data—Potential Toxicity

PREGNANCY SUMMARY

The human pregnancy experience suggests that the risk of itraconazole-induced structural anomalies is low. However, another triazole antifungal agent, fluconazole, has demonstrated a possible dose-related relationship with major malformations (see Fluconazole). For itraconazole, the animal data cannot be adequately interpreted because maternal toxicity was evident and comparisons with the human dose appeared to be based on body weight. Therefore, the safest course is to avoid itraconazole, if possible, during organogenesis. If inadvertent exposure does occur during the 1st trimester, or if itraconazole must be used during early pregnancy, the woman can be reassured that the risk to her embryo or fetus is low, if it exists at all.

FETAL RISK SUMMARY

Itraconazole is a triazole antifungal agent that is structurally related to a number of other antifungal agents, including the imidazole derivatives butoconazole, clotrimazole, and ketoconazole, and to the triazoles, fluconazole and terconazole (1). Other triazole antifungals are posaconazole and voriconazole.

A dose-related increase in toxicity and teratogenicity was found in both rats and mice (2). In pregnant rats treated with a dose 5–20 times the maximum recommended human dose

(MRHD), maternal and embryo toxicity was observed, as were major skeletal malformations. In mice given 10 times the MRHD, maternal toxicity, embryo toxicity, and malformations consisting of encephaloceles or macroglossia occurred.

It is not known if itraconazole crosses the human placenta. The molecular weight (about 706) is low enough that passage to the fetus should be expected.

Cohort data presented at a 1996 meeting on single-dose fluconazole or itraconazole exposures during organogenesis did not demonstrate adverse outcomes in approximately 70 exposed pregnancies (3). However, the FDA has received 14 case reports of malformations following use of itraconazole, 4 of which involved limb defects (includes 1 case of agenesis of the fingers and toes (3).

A 1998 noninterventional observational cohort study described the outcomes of pregnancies in women who had been prescribed one or more of 34 newly marketed drugs by general practitioners in England (4). Data were obtained by questionnaires sent to the prescribing physicians one month after the expected or possible date of delivery. In 831 (78%) of the pregnancies, a newly marketed drug was thought to have been taken during the 1st trimester, with birth defects noted in 14 (2.5%) singleton births of the 557 newborns (10 sets of twins). In addition, two birth defects were observed in aborted fetuses. However, few of the aborted fetuses were examined. Itraconazole was taken during the 1st trimester in 41 pregnancies. The outcomes of these pregnancies included 1 ectopic pregnancy, 2 spontaneous abortions (SABs), 6 elective abortions (EABs), 2 cases lost to follow-up, and 30 normal newborns (1 premature) (4). One of the normal, full-term newborns, however, had a minor congenital anomaly consisting of a thin, prominent, protruding left ear. Although no major congenital malformations were observed, the study lacked the sensitivity to identify minor anomalies because of the absence of standardized examinations. Late-appearing major defects may also have been missed due to the timing of the questionnaires.

A prospective cohort study published in 2000 evaluated the pregnancy outcomes of 198 women exposed to itraconazole in the 1st trimester (5). The pregnancy exposures had been reported to the manufacturer, before the outcomes were known, between April 1989 and June 1998. The median itraconazole dose was 200 mg (range 50–800 mg) with mean therapy duration of 8.5 days (range 1–90 days). A matched control group (N = 198) was formed from pregnant women who had contacted the Motherisk Program, a teratogen information service in Toronto, Canada. The control group had not been exposed to any known teratogens (acceptable exposures were acetaminophen, penicillins, prenatal vitamins, dental radiography, or no exposures). There were no statistical differences between the groups in gravidity, parity, alcohol use, or cigarette smoking, but the maternal age in the study group was significantly less than controls (30.1 vs. 31.0 years, $p = 0.02$). Among pregnancy outcomes, there were no statistical differences between the groups in delivery method, rates of term, preterm, and postterm deliveries, 1- and 5-minute Apgar scores, sex ratios, and rates of neonatal complications. Significantly more pregnancy losses occurred in the exposed group than in controls (relative risk 1.75, 95% confidence interval 1.47–2.09), including SABs (12.6% vs. 4.0%), EABs (7.5% vs 0.5%), and fetal deaths (1.5% vs. 1.0%). The authors attributed these differences to group differences, rather than to effects of itraconazole exposure (5). In addition, the birth weight of exposed newborns was significantly lower than controls (3.33 vs. 3.46 kg. $p = 0.048$), but this finding was probably not clinically significant (5). There was no statistical difference between the groups in major congenital malformations. Among the 156 live births in the study group, there were five infants (3.2%) with major anomalies (microphthalmia, dysplasia of the right hand, pyloric stenosis, hip joint dysplasia, and congenital heart disease [type not specified]). There were nine newborns (4.8%) with major defects among the 187 controls with live births (congenital heart disease [three cases—two with ventricular septal defect and one not specified], hypospadias requiring surgery [two cases], and one each of oversized tongue, congenital hip dislocation, cleft palate, and Down's syndrome with atrioventricular canal). The study had 80% power to detect a threefold increased risk of major defects (5), but no evaluation was conducted for minor defects.

The authors of the above study, in a letter correspondence that predated that study, demonstrated that retrospective reports to the manufacturer, at least for itraconazole, involved reporting bias (6). The rates for retrospective vs. prospective outcomes, all of which were significant, were live births (64% vs. 79%), EABs (15% vs. 8%), SABs (18% vs. 13%), major anomalies (13% vs. 3%), and major anomalies including EABs (15% vs. 3%). The authors concluded that women with poor outcomes were more likely to report the event than those with good outcomes (6).

A prospective cohort study involving itraconazole pregnancy exposure was published in 2009 (7). The data were collected by two teratology information services in Italy. During the period 2002–2006, 206 women called the services because of 1st trimester exposure to the drug and their pregnancy outcomes were compared with 207 controls. The rates of major congenital anomalies in the two groups were not significant (1.8% vs. 2.1%, respectively). The three anomalies in the exposed group and the maternal daily dose were cerebral calcification and hepatomegaly (200 mg), unilateral hydronephrosis (100 mg), and interatrial defect (100 mg). There were no significant differences in the rates of vaginal delivery, premature births, low birth weight, and high birth weight. However, significant differences were found for live births (79.1% vs. 91.8%), SABs (11.2% vs. 4.8%), and EABs (9.2% vs. 3.4%). The lower live birth rate was obviously due to the higher rates of abortion (7).

BREASTFEEDING SUMMARY

Itraconazole is excreted into breast milk. Two healthy lactating women each took two oral doses of 200 mg 12 hours apart (total dose 400 mg) (personal communication, EK Cazzaniga and A Chanlam, Janssen Pharmaceuticals, 1996). Neither infant was allowed to nurse during the study. At 4, 24, and 48 hours after the second dose, the average milk concentrations of itraconazole were 70, 28, and 16 ng/mL, respectively. At 72 hours, the milk level was 20 ng/mL in one woman and not detectable (<5 ng/mL) in the other. The average milk:plasma ratios at 4, 24, and 48 hours were 0.51, 1.61, and 1.77, respectively. Based on the 4-hour concentration (the approximate time of the peak plasma level), and assuming that the infants consumed 500 mL of milk/day, the maximum 24-hour average dose the infants would have received was 35 mcg.

Although the above amount seems small, peak plasma concentrations in healthy male volunteers taking itraconazole 200 mg twice daily were not reached until about 15 days (2). The mean peak concentration of the parent compound in these volunteers was 2282 ng/mL, or about 15 times the average peak concentration measured in the two women above. Moreover, the mean plasma concentration of one of the metabolites (hydroxyitraconazole) exceeded that of the parent compound. Continuous daily dosing, even with lower doses, should result in milk levels of the drug much higher than those found above and could result in widespread tissue accumulation in nursing infants. Because the potential effects of this exposure have not been studied, women taking itraconazole should probably not breastfeed.

References

1. American Hospital Formulary Service. *Drug Information 1997*. Bethesda, MD: American Society of Health-System Pharmacists, 1997:93–5.
2. Product information. Sporanox. Janssen Pharmaceutica, 2001.
3. Rosa F. *Azole Fungicide Pregnancy Risks*. Presented at the Ninth International Conference of the Organization of Teratology Information Services, May 2–4, 1996, Salt Lake City, Utah.
4. Wilton LV, Pearce GL, Martin RM, Mackay FJ, Mann RD. The outcomes of pregnancy in women exposed to newly marketed drugs in general practice in England. Br J Obstet Gynaecol 1998;105:882–9.
5. Bar-Oz B, Moretti ME, Bishai R, Mareels G, Van Tittelboom T, Verspeelt J, Koren G. Pregnancy outcome after in utero exposure to itraconnazole: a prospective cohort study. Am J Obstet Gynecol 2000;183:617–20.
6. Bar-Oz B, Moretti ME, Mareels G, Van Tittelboom T, Koren G. Reporting bias in retrospective ascertainment of drug-induced embryopathy. Lancet 1999;354:1700–1.
7. De Santis M, Gianantonio ED, Cesari E, Ambrosini G, Straface G, Clementi M. First-trimester itraconazole exposure and pregnancy outcome; a prospective cohort study of women contacting teratology information services in Italy. Drug Safety 2009;32:239–44.

IVACAFTOR

Endocrine/Metabolic Agent (Miscellaneous)

PREGNANCY RECOMMENDATION: No Human Data—Animal Data Suggest Low Risk
BREASTFEEDING RECOMMENDATION: No Human Data—Potential Toxicity

PREGNANCY SUMMARY

No reports describing the use of ivacaftor in human pregnancy have been located. The animal data suggest low risk, but the absence of human pregnancy experience prevents a more complete assessment of embryo–fetal risk. However, cystic fibrosis can be a debilitating chronic disease. If the drug is indicated it should not be withheld because of pregnancy, but the woman should be informed of the lack of human data.

FETAL RISK SUMMARY

Ivacaftor is an orally administered potentiator of the cystic fibrosis transmembrane conductance regulator (CFTR) protein. It is indicated for the treatment of cystic fibrosis in patients 6 years and older who have a G551D mutation in the CFTR gene. Ivacaftor is extensively metabolized to a partially active metabolite (1/6th the potency of the parent drug) and to inactive metabolites. Plasma protein binding (about 99%) is primarily to α-1-acid glycoprotein and albumin. The apparent terminal half-life is about 12 hours (1).

Reproduction studies have been conducted in rats and rabbits. In these species, ivacaftor was not teratogenic at exposures that were about 6 and 12 times, respectively, the maximum recommended human dose based on summed AUCs (MRHD) for ivacaftor and its metabolites. Placental transfer of ivacaftor was observed in rats and rabbits (1).

Two-year studies in mice and rats for carcinogenicity were negative, as were multiple assays for genotoxicity. Ivacaftor impaired fertility and reproductive performance indices in male and female rats at exposures that were about 5 and 6 times, respectively, the MRHD. In rats dosed before and during pregnancy, increases in prolonged dietrus and the number with all nonviable embryos were observed. Decreased corpora lutea, implantations, and viable embryos were also noted. The effects on the male and female indices were attributed to severe toxicity. No effects were observed on the indices at exposures that were about 3 times the MRHD (1).

It is not known if ivacaftor or its metabolites crosses the human placenta. The molecular weight of the parent drug (about 392) and the long terminal half-life suggest that the parent drug will cross to the embryo–fetus.

BREASTFEEDING SUMMARY

No reports describing the use of ivacaftor during human lactation have been located. The molecular weight of the parent drug (about 392) and the long terminal half-life (about 12 hours) suggest that the parent drug will be excreted into breast milk. The effect of this exposure on a nursing infant is not known. The most common ($\geq$8%) adverse effects in patients were headache, oropharyngeal pain, upper respiratory tract infection, nasal congestion, abdominal pain, nasopharyngitis, diarrhea, rash, nausea, and dizziness (1). If a woman taking this drug and breastfeeding, her infant should be monitored for these effects.

Reference

1. Product information. Kalydeco. Vertex Pharmaceuticals, 2012.

IVERMECTIN

Anthelmintic

PREGNANCY RECOMMENDATION: Human Data Suggest Low Risk
BREASTFEEDING RECOMMENDATION: Limited Human Data—Probably Compatible

PREGNANCY SUMMARY

Ivermectin was teratogenic in three animal species, but only at doses at or near those producing maternal toxicity. No teratogenicity or toxicity attributable to ivermectin has been observed in limited human pregnancy experience. A 1997 review, citing a World Health Organization reference, stated that because of the high risk of blindness from onchocerciasis, and the lack of reported adverse outcomes, the use of ivermectin after the 1st trimester was probably acceptable (1).

FETAL RISK SUMMARY

I

Ivermectin is a semisynthetic anthelmintic. It is a mixture of two components derived from the avermectins, a class of antiparasitic agents isolated from the fermentation of *Steptomyces avermitilis*. Ivermectin is indicated for the treatment of intestinal strongyloidiasis infections due to the nematode *Strongyloides stercoralis* and onchocerciasis due to the nematode *Onchocerca volvulus* (2).

In reproduction studies with mice, rats, and rabbits, ivermectin was teratogenic when given in repeated doses of 0.2, 8.1, and 4.5 times, respectively, the maximum recommended human dose based on BSA. The malformations observed, cleft palate (in all three species) and clubbed forepaws in rabbits, however, were only observed at or near doses producing maternal toxicity. The results were thought to indicate that ivermectin was not selectively toxic to the developing fetus (2).

It is not known if ivermectin crosses the human placenta. The molecular weights of the two components in the product, approximately 875 and 861, are low enough that some exposure of the embryo or fetus probably occurs.

A well-conducted study published in 1990 described the pregnancy outcomes of women who were inadvertently exposed to ivermectin during community-based ivermectin distribution programs (1987–1989) for onchocerciasis on a Liberian rubber plantation (14,000 people) (3). The average oral ivermectin dose was 150 mcg/kg as a single dose. Because the women did not recall the date of their last menstrual period before delivery, pregnancy exposure was defined as a delivery occurring within 40 weeks of treatment. During the distribution programs, 2884 women received treatment, including 200 (7%) that were inadvertently treated during pregnancy. Of those treated during pregnancy, 85% were treated in the first 12 weeks of pregnancy and 36% occurred within the first 4 weeks. The outcomes of all pregnancies were followed up by a field census team, systematic examination of all babies born at the hospital, and a year-round plantation-wide surveillance system of all births and deaths. All children under 12 months of age were examined by a physician and children aged 12–24 months were examined by a pediatrician. Among the 203 pregnancy outcomes from exposed pregnancies, there were 10 (4.9%) abnormal events—5 stillbirths and 5 congenital malformations (single-dose exposure in weeks before delivery shown in parentheses): anal atresia (34 weeks); cleft palate and lip (33 weeks); Pierre–Robin syndrome, micrognathia, glossoptosis, low-slung ears, and shortening of limbs in a stillborn infant (32 weeks); Turner's syndrome (24 weeks); and deafness plus probable ventricular septal defect (VSD) (33 weeks). Among the 1767 pregnancy outcomes not exposed to ivermectin, there were 76 (4.3%) abnormal events: 55 stillbirths or miscarriages and 21 congenital anomalies. The congenital anomalies were: polydactyly ($N = 6$), convergent strabismus ($N = 3$), talipes equinovarus ($N = 2$), unspecified ($N = 2$), and 1 each deafness, facial malformations, hypopigmented skin, hypospadias, microcephaly, Down's syndrome, syndactyly, and VSD. There were no significant differences between the treated and untreated groups in the rates of congenital malformations, stillbirths, or all abnormalities (congenital malformations, stillbirths, and miscarriages). Also, no statistical differences were found in terms of health status and malformations between infants (aged 2–7 months) and children (aged 12–24 months) whose mothers had been treated in comparison with untreated controls, matched for age, sex, and distance from the hospital (3).

A brief 1993 communication from Cameroon described the outcomes of pregnancies in 110 women who had inadvertently received ivermectin treatment during a mass treatment campaign for onchocerciasis (4). During the 2-year campaign, 401 of 2710 women were excluded from treatment because of pregnancy. Of the remaining 2309 women who were treated, 110 were discovered to be pregnant during regularly scheduled follow-up. Treatment was considered to have been given during pregnancy if delivery occurred within 40 weeks of ivermectin distribution. A comparison of the 110 women treated during gestation with the 401 pregnant women who did not receive treatment revealed no statistical differences in early abortion (<4 months) (3.6% vs. 2.2%), late abnormal events (abortion, miscarriage, stillbirth) (15.5% vs. 11%), children lost to follow-up (7.3% vs. 11.2%), infants with malformations (0 vs 0.5%), or normal infants (74.5% vs. 75.8%). The prevalence of all abnormal obstetric events of treated women was similar to that of those not treated ($p > 0.37$). Only two newborns with congenital malformations were observed, both in the untreated group. In a second analysis, pregnancy outcomes of 97 women treated in the 1st trimester were compared with the outcomes of 142 untreated women. As before, no statistical differences were observed. The authors concluded that ivermectin did not present a major risk to the fetus (4).

BREASTFEEDING SUMMARY

Ivermectin is excreted into breast milk, but its use during breastfeeding has not been reported. Four healthy women, who had lost their babies at birth, were given a single 150 mcg/kg oral ivermectin dose after an overnight fast (5). Ivermectin was detected in the plasma and breast milk within 1 hour. The mean peak concentration in plasma was 37.9 ng/mL and in milk was14.1 ng/mL. The mean milk:plasma ratio was 0.51 (range 0.39–0.57). The steady-state ivermectin concentration in milk over a 24-hour period was approximately 10 ng/mL. The investigators estimated that the dose a 1-month-old African infant would receive from breast milk was 2.75 mcg/kg. This dose is much lower than an estimated dose of 21.8 mcg/kg they calculated for a 1-month-old infant (5). (*Note: In the United States, because the safety and effectiveness have not been established, ivermectin is not recommended for children weighing <15 kg [1]*). In Nigeria, where the study was conducted, lactating women within the first week of breastfeeding were excluded from community-wide ivermectin distribution because of the concerns for infant safety (5). The investigators concluded, however, that the benefits of treatment for the lactating woman, combined with the impracticality of withholding nursing for a week, the low drug levels in milk, and the lack of reported adverse effects in nursing infants in their population, suggested that the drug should be given to the mother regardless of her lactation status (5). The American Academy of Pediatrics classifies ivermectin as compatible with breastfeeding (6).

References

1. de Silva N, Guyatt H, Bundy D. Anthelmintics. A comparative review of their clinical pharmacology. Drugs 1997;53:769–88.
2. Product information. Stromectol. Merck, 2002.
3. Pacque M, Munoz B, Poetschke G, Foose J, Greene BM, Taylor HR. Pregnancy outcome after inadvertent ivermectin treatment during community-based distribution. Lancet 1990;336:1486–9.
4. Chippaux JP, Gardon-Wendel N, Gardon J, Ernould JC. Absence of any adverse effect of inadvertent ivermectin treatment during pregnancy. Tran R Soc Trop Med Hyg 1993;87:318.
5. Ogbuokiri JE, Ozumba BC, Okonkwo PO. Ivermectin levels in human breast-milk. Eur J Clin Pharmacol 1993;45:389–90.
6. Committee on Drugs, American Academy of Pediatrics. The transfer of drugs and other chemicals into human milk. Pediatrics 2001;108:776–89.

IXABEPILONE

Antineoplastic

PREGNANCY RECOMMENDATION: **No Human Data—Animal Data Suggest Moderate Risk**
BREASTFEEDING RECOMMENDATION: **Contraindicated**

PREGNANCY SUMMARY

No reports describing the use of ixabepilone in human pregnancy have been located. Teratogenicity was not observed in two animal species. However, embryo death (in the absence of maternal toxicity) was noted in one species. Because of maternal toxicity, the highest doses that could be given were about 10% of the human exposure or dose. The absence of human pregnancy experience prevents a complete assessment of the embryo–fetal risk, but the drug should be avoided in pregnancy. If it must be administered for the mother's benefit, avoiding the 1st trimester should be considered.

FETAL RISK SUMMARY

Ixabepilone is a semisynthetic analog of epothilone B, a polypeptide macrolide isolated from the myxobacterium *Sorangium cellulosum*. There are no other agents in this antineoplastic subclass. Ixabepilone is a microtubule inhibitor that is given as an IV infusion every 3 weeks. It is indicated in combination with capecitabine (see Capecitabine) for the treatment of metastatic or locally advanced breast cancer resistant to an anthracycline and a taxane, or in patients whose cancer is taxane resistant and for whom further anthracycline therapy is contraindicated. It also is indicated as monotherapy for the treatment of metastatic or locally advanced breast cancer resistant to anthracyclines, taxanes, and capecitabine. The drug is extensively metabolized in the liver to inactive compounds. Binding to human serum proteins ranges between 67% and 77%, and the terminal elimination half-life is about 52 hours (1).

Reproductive studies have been conducted in rats and rabbits. No teratogenic effects were observed in rats with doses producing exposures up to about 0.1 times the human clinical exposure based on AUC (HCE). The highest dose was maternal toxic and resulted in fetal death and decreased fetal weight. In rabbits, no teratogenicity was observed at doses up to about 0.1 times the human clinical dose based on BSA, but maternal and fetal toxicity (death in both) was noted at the highest dose (1).

Carcinogenicity studies with ixabepilone have not been conducted. The drug was not mutagenic in one assay but was clastogenic in one of two tests. No effect on the fertility of male and female rats was observed with doses producing exposures that were about 0.07 times the HCE. However, when female rats were given an IV infusion at this dose during breeding and through the first 7 days of gestation, a significant increase in resorptions and pre- and postimplantation loss, and a decrease in the number of corpora lutea were observed. Testicular atrophy or degeneration was observed in male rats when IV doses that were 2.1 times the HCE were given every 21 days for 6 months. Similar toxicity was observed in male dogs when IV doses that were ≥0.2 times the HCE were given every 21 days for 9 months (1).

It is not known if ixabepilone crosses the human placenta. The molecular weight (about 507), the moderate serum protein binding, and the very long elimination half-life suggest that the drug will cross to the embryo–fetus.

BREASTFEEDING SUMMARY

No reports describing the use of ixabepilone during human lactation have been located. The molecular weight (about 507), the moderate serum protein binding (67%–77%), and the very long elimination half-life (about 52 hours) suggest that the drug will be excreted into breast milk. The effects of this exposure on a nursing infant are unknown, but there is potential for severe toxicity. The most common adverse reactions in adults were peripheral sensory neuropathy, fatigue/asthenia, myalgia/arthralgia, alopecia, nausea, vomiting, stomatitis/mucositis, diarrhea, and musculoskeletal pain (1). Because of the risk, women receiving ixabepilone should not breastfeed.

Reference

1. Product Information. Ixempra. Bristol-Myers Squibb, 2007.

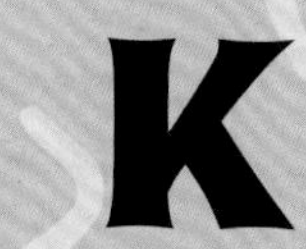

KANAMYCIN

Antibiotic (Aminoglycoside)

PREGNANCY RECOMMENDATION: Human Data Suggest Risk
BREASTFEEDING RECOMMENDATION: Limited Human Data—Probably Compatible

PREGNANCY SUMMARY

Except for ototoxicity, no reports of congenital defects due to kanamycin have been located. Embryos were examined from five patients who aborted during the 11th and 12th weeks of pregnancy and who had been treated with kanamycin during the 6th and 8th weeks (1). No abnormalities in the embryos were found.

FETAL RISK SUMMARY

Kanamycin is an aminoglycoside antibiotic. At term, the drug was detectable in cord serum 15 minutes after a 500-mg IM maternal dose (2). Mean cord serum levels at 3–6 hours were 6 mcg/mL. Amniotic fluid levels were undetectable during the first hour, and then rose during the next 6 hours to a mean value of 5.5 mcg/mL. No effects on the infants were mentioned.

Eighth cranial nerve damage has been reported following in utero exposure to kanamycin (1,3). In a retrospective survey of 391 mothers who received kanamycin, 50 mg/kg, for prolonged periods during pregnancy, 9 (2.3%) children were found to have hearing loss (1). Complete hearing loss in a mother and her infant was reported after the mother had been treated during pregnancy with IM kanamycin, 1 g/day for 4.5 days (3). Ethacrynic acid, an ototoxic diuretic, was also given to the mother during pregnancy.

BREASTFEEDING SUMMARY

Kanamycin is excreted into breast milk. Milk:plasma ratios of 0.05–0.40 have been reported (4). A 1-g IM dose produced peak milk levels of 18.4 mcg/mL (5). No effects were reported in the nursing infants. Because oral absorption of kanamycin is poor, ototoxicity would not be expected. However, three potential problems exist for the nursing infant: modification of bowel flora, direct effects on the infant, and interference with the interpretation of culture results if a fever workup is required. The American Academy of Pediatrics classifies kanamycin as compatible with breastfeeding (6).

References

1. Nishimura H, Tanimura T. *Clinical Aspects of the Teratogenicity of Drugs*. New York, NY: American Elsevier, 1976:131.
2. Good R, Johnson G. The placental transfer of kanamycin during late pregnancy. Obstet Gynecol 1971;38:60–2.
3. Jones HC. Intrauterine ototoxicity. A case report and review of literature. J Natl Med Assoc 1973;65:201–3.
4. Wilson JT. Milk/plasma ratios and contraindicated drugs. In: Wilson JT, ed. *Drugs in Breast Milk*. Balgowlah, Australia: ADIS Press, 1981:79.
5. O'Brien T. Excretion of drugs in human milk. Am J Hosp Pharm 1974; 31:844–54.
6. Committee on Drugs, American Academy of Pediatrics. The transfer of drugs and other chemicals into human milk. Pediatrics 2001;108: 776–89.

KAOLIN/PECTIN

Antidiarrheal

PREGNANCY RECOMMENDATION: No Human Data—Probably Compatible
BREASTFEEDING RECOMMENDATION: No Human Data—Probably Compatible

PREGNANCY SUMMARY

No reports have related the use of the kaolin/pectin mixture in pregnancy with adverse fetal outcome. There have been reports of iron-deficiency anemia and hypokalemia secondary to the eating of clays (i.e., geophagia) containing kaolin (1–3).

FETAL RISK SUMMARY

Kaolin is hydrated aluminum silicate clay used for its adsorbent properties in diarrhea, and pectin is a polysaccharide obtained from plant tissues that is used as a solidifying agent. Neither agent is absorbed into the systemic circulation.

The mechanism for iron deficiency anemia is thought to be either a reduction in the intake of foods containing absorbable iron or an interference with the absorption of iron. In humans, iron-deficiency anemia may significantly enhance the chance for a low-birth-weight infant and preterm delivery (4,5).

Rats fed a diet containing 20% kaolin became anemic and delivered pups with a significant decrease in birth weight (6). When an iron supplement was added to the kaolin-fortified diet, no anemia or reduced birth weight was observed.

BREASTFEEDING SUMMARY

Other than producing anemia in the mother after prolonged, chronic use, the kaolin/pectin mixture should have no effect on lactation or the nursing infant.

References

1. Mengel CE, Carter WA, Horton ES. Geophagia with iron deficiency and hypokalemia: *Cachexia africana*. Arch Intern Med 1964;114:470–4.
2. Talington KM, Gant NF Jr, Scott DE, Pritchard JA. Effect of ingestion of starch and some clays on iron absorption. Am J Obstet Gynecol 1970;108:262–7.
3. Roselle HA. Association of laundry starch and clay ingestion with anemia in New York City. Arch Intern Med 1970;125:57–61.
4. Scholl TO, Hediger ML, Fischer RL, Shearer JW. Anemia vs. iron deficiency: increased risk of preterm delivery in a prospective study. Am J Clin Nutr 1992;55:985–8.
5. Macgregor MW. Maternal anaemia as a factor in prematurity and perinatal mortality. Scott Med J 1963;8:134–40.
6. Patterson EC, Staszak DJ. Effects of geophagia (kaolin ingestion) on the maternal blood and embryonic development in the pregnant rat. J Nutr 1977;107:2020–5.

K

KETAMINE

General Anesthetic

PREGNANCY RECOMMENDATION: Limited Human Data—Animal Data Suggest Low Risk
BREASTFEEDING RECOMMENDATION: No Human Data—Probably Compatible

PREGNANCY SUMMARY

Although ketamine anesthesia close to delivery may induce dose-related, transient toxicity in the newborn, these effects are usually avoided with the use of lower maternal doses. No reports of malformations in humans (1) or in animals attributable to ketamine have been located, although experience with the anesthetic agent during human organogenesis apparently has not been published.

FETAL RISK SUMMARY

Ketamine is a rapid-acting IV general anesthetic agent related in structure and action to phencyclidine. No teratogenic or other adverse fetal effects have been observed in reproduction studies during organogenesis and near delivery with rats, mice, rabbits, and dogs (2–6). In one study with pregnant rats, a dose of 120 mg/kg/day for 5 days during organogenesis resulted in no malformations or effect on fetal weight (5).

Ketamine rapidly crosses the placenta to the fetus in animals and humans (7,8). Pregnant ewes were given 0.7 mg/kg IV, and 1 minute later the maternal and fetal concentrations of ketamine were 1230 ng/mL and 470 ng/mL (ratio 0.38), respectively (7). Maternal effects were slight, transitory increases in mean arterial pressure and cardiac output; respiratory acidosis; and an increase in uterine tone without changes in uterine blood flow. In humans, the placental transfer of ketamine was documented in a study in which a dose of 250 mg IM was administered when the fetal head reached the perineum (8). The ketamine concentration in cord venous plasma at the 0- to 10-minute dose-to-delivery interval was 0.61 mcg/mL, compared with 1.03 mcg/mL at the 10- to 30-minute interval, reflecting absorption following the IM route.

Pregnant monkeys were administered ketamine in IV doses of 2 mg/kg ($N = 3$) or 1 mg/kg ($N = 2$) in an investigation of the anesthetic's effects on the fetus and newborn (9). No fetal effects were observed from either dose. The newborns from the mothers given 2 mg/kg, but not those exposed to lower doses, had profound respiratory depression.

The use of ketamine (C-581) for obstetric anesthesia was first described in 1966 (10). Since then, a large number of references have documented its use for this purpose (11–39). Among the maternal and newborn complications reported with ketamine are oxytocic properties, an increase in maternal blood pressure, newborn depression, and an increased tone of newborn skeletal musculature. These adverse effects were usually related to higher IV doses (1.5–2.2 mg/kg) administered during early studies rather than to the lower IV doses (0.2–0.5 mg/kg) now commonly used.

Ketamine usually demonstrates a dose-related oxytocic effect with an increase in uterine tone, and in frequency and intensity of uterine contractions (10–13,23,38), but one investigator reported weakened uterine contractions following a 250-mg IM dose administered when the fetal head reached the perineum (8). Uterine tetany was observed in one case (13). Low IV doses (0.275–1.1 mg/kg) of ketamine increased only uterine contractions, whereas a higher IV dose (2.2 mg/kg) resulted in a marked increase in uterine tone (23). Maximum effects were observed within 2–4 minutes of the dose. In one study, however, the effect on uterine contractions from an IV dose of 1 mg/kg, followed by succinylcholine 1 mg/kg, was no different from thiopental (15). No effect on intrauterine pressure was measured in 12 term patients treated with IV ketamine 2 mg/kg, in contrast to a marked uterine pressure increase in patients in early pregnancy undergoing termination (40). Similarly, in 12 women given IV ketamine 2.2 mg/kg for termination of pregnancy at 8–19 weeks, uterine pressure and the intensity and frequency of contractions were increased (41).

Several investigators noted a marked increase in maternal blood pressure, up to 30%–40% in systolic and diastolic in some series, during ketamine induction (8,11,13,14,16,24,25). An increased maternal heart rate was usually observed. These effects are dose-related, with the greatest increases occurring when 2–2.2 mg/kg IV was administered, but smaller elevations of pressure and pulse were noted with lower IV doses.

Maternal ketamine anesthesia may cause depression of the newborn (8,13,16–19,22,24,27,33). As with the other complications, the use of higher IV doses (1.5–2.2 mg/kg) resulted in the highest incidence of low neonatal Apgar scores and requirements for newborn resuscitation. The induction-to-delivery (ID) interval is an important determinant for neonatal depression (8,22,33,35). In two studies, neonatal depression was markedly lower or absent if the ID interval was $<$10 minutes (8,33). In a third study, significant depression occurred with an ID interval of 9.2 minutes, but an IV dose of 2.1 mg/kg had been used (22).

The use of ketamine in low doses apparently has little effect on fetal cardiovascular status or acid–base balance as evidenced by neonatal blood gases (8,25,27,30,32–34). In one study, a ketamine dose of 25 mg IV administered with nitrous oxide and oxygen within 4 minutes of delivery did not adversely affect neonatal blood pressure (39).

Ketamine doses of 2 mg/kg IV have been associated with excessive neonatal muscle tone, sometimes with apnea (11,12,18). In some cases, the increased muscle tone made endotracheal intubation difficult. In contrast, lower doses (e.g., 0.25–1 mg/kg) have not been associated with this complication (25).

Neonatal neurobehavior, as measured by the Scanlon Group of Early Neonatal Neurobehavioral Tests during the first 2 days, is depressed following maternal ketamine (1 mg/kg IV) anesthesia but less than the effect measured after thiopental anesthesia (4 mg/kg IV) (42,43). In these studies, spinal anesthesia with 6–8 mg of tetracaine was associated with the best performance, general anesthesia with ketamine was intermediate, and that with thiopental was the poorest in performance.

BREASTFEEDING SUMMARY

Because ketamine is a general anesthetic agent, breastfeeding would not be possible during use of the drug, and no reports have been located that measured the amount of the agent in milk. The elimination half-life of ketamine has been reported to be 2.17 hours in unpremedicated patients (32). Thus, the drug should be undetectable in the mother's plasma approximately 11 hours after a dose. Nursing after this time should not expose the infant to pharmacologically significant amounts of ketamine.

References

1. Friedman JM. Teratogen update: anesthetic agents. Teratology 1988;37:69–77.
2. Nishimura H, Tanimura T. *Clinical Aspects of the Teratogenicity of Drugs*. New York, NY: American Elsevier, 1976:178.
3. Schardein JL. *Chemically Induced Birth Defects*. 2nd ed. New York, NY: Marcel Dekker, 1993:148.
4. Onnis A, Grella P. *The Biochemical Effects of Drugs in Pregnancy*. Vol. 1. West Sussex, England: Ellis Norwood, 1984:18–9.
5. El-Karum AHA, Benny R. Embryotoxic and teratogenic action of ketamine. Ain Shams Med J 1976;27:459–63.
6. Product information. Ketalar. Parke-Davis, 1993.
7. Craft JB Jr, Coaldrake LA, Yonekura ML, Dao SD, Co EG, Roizen MF, Mazel P, Gilman R, Shokes L, Trevor AJ. Ketamine, catecholamines, and uterine tone in pregnant ewes. Am J Obstet Gynecol 1983;146:429–34.
8. Nishijima M. Ketamine in obstetric anesthesia: special reference to placental transfer and its concentration in blood plasma. Acta Obstet Gynaecol Jpn 1972;19:80–93. As cited in Anonymous. Operative obstetrics and anesthesia. Obstet Gynecol Surv 1975;30:605–6.
9. Eng M, Bonica JJ, Akamatsu TJ, Berges PU, Ueland K. Respiratory depression in newborn monkeys at caesarean section following ketamine administration. Br J Anaesth 1975;47:917–21.
10. Chodoff P, Stella JG. Use of CI-581 a phencyclidine derivative for obstetric anesthesia. Anesth Analg 1966;45:527–30.
11. Bovill JG, Coppel DL, Dundee JW, Moore J. Current status of ketamine anaesthesia. Lancet 1971;1:1285–8.
12. Moore J, McNabb TG, Dundee JW. Preliminary report on ketamine in obstetrics. Br J Anaesth 1971;43:779–82.
13. Little B, Chang T, Chucot L, Dill WA, Enrile LL, Glazko AJ, Jassani M, Kretchmer H, Sweet AY. Study of ketamine as an obstetric anesthetic agent. Am J Obstet Gynecol 1972;113:247–60.
14. McDonald JS, Mateo CV, Reed EC. Modified nitrous oxide or ketamine hydrochloride for cesarean section. Anesth Analg 1972;51:975–83.
15. Peltz B, Sinclair DM. Induction agents for caesarean section. A comparison of thiopentone and ketamine. Anaesthesia 1973;28:37–42.
16. Meer FM, Downing JW, Coleman AJ. An intravenous method of anaesthesia for caesarean section. Part II: ketamine. Br J Anaesth 1973;45:191–6.
17. Galbert MW, Gardner AE. Ketamine for obstetrical anesthesia. Anesth Analg 1973;52:926–30.
18. Corssen G. Ketamine in obstetric anesthesia. Clin Obstet Gynecol 1974;17:249–58.
19. Janeczko GF, El-Etr AA, Younes S. Low-dose ketamine anesthesia for obstetrical delivery. Anesth Analg 1974;53:828–31.
20. Akamatsu TJ, Bonica JJ, Rehmet R, Eng M, Ueland K. Experiences with the use of ketamine for parturition. I. Primary anesthetic for vaginal delivery. Anesth Analg 1974;53:284–7.
21. Krantz ML. Ketamine in obstetrics: comparison with methoxyflurane. Anesth Analg 1974;53:890–3.
22. Downing JW, Mahomedy MC, Jeal DE, Allen PJ. Anaesthesia for caesarean section with ketamine. Anaesthesia 1976;31:883–92.
23. Galloon S. Ketamine for obstetric delivery. Anesthesiology 1976;44:522–4.
24. Ellingson A, Haram K, Sagen N. Ketamine and diazepam as anaesthesia for forceps delivery. A comparative study. Acta Anaesth Scand 1977;21:37–40.
25. Maduska AL, Hajghassemali M. Arterial blood gases in mothers and infants during ketamine anesthesia for vaginal delivery. Anesth Analg 1978;57:121–3.
26. Dich-Nielsen J, Holasek J. Ketamine as induction agent for caesarean section. Acta Anaesth Scand 1982;26:139–42.

K

27. White PF, Way WL, Trevor AJ. Ketamine—its pharmacology and therapeutic uses. Anesthesiology 1982;56:119–36.
28. Hill CR, Schultetus RR, Dharamraj CM, Banner TE, Berman LS. Wakefulness during cesarean section with thiopental, ketamine, or thiopental–ketamine combination (abstract). Anesthesiology 1993;59:A419.
29. Schultetus RR, Paulus DA, Spohr GL. Haemodynamic effects of ketamine and thiopentone during anaesthetic induction for caesarean section. Can Anaesth Soc J 1985;32:592–6.
30. Bernstein K, Gisselsson L, Jacobsson L, Ohrlander S. Influence of two different anaesthetic agents on the newborn and the correlation between foetal oxygenation and induction-delivery time in elective caesarean section. Acta Anaesthesiol Scand 1985;29:157–60.
31. Schultetus RR, Hill CR, Dharamraj CM, Banner TE, Berman LS. Wakefulness during cesarean section after anesthetic induction with ketamine, thiopental, or ketamine and thiopental combined. Anesth Analg 1986;65:723–8.
32. Reich DL, Silvay G. Ketamine: an update on the first twenty-five years of clinical experience. Can J Anaesth 1989;36:186–97.
33. Baraka A, Louis F, Dalleh R. Maternal awareness and neonatal outcome after ketamine induction of anaesthesia for caesarean section. Can J Anaesth 1990;37:641–4.
34. Rowbottom SJ, Gin T, Cheung LP. General anaesthesia for caesarean section in a patient with uncorrected complex cyanotic heart disease. Anaesth Intens Care 1994;22:74–8.
35. Krissel J, Dick WF, Leyser KH, Gervais H, Brockerhoff P, Schranz D. Thiopentone, thiopentone/ketamine, and ketamine for induction of anaesthesia in caesarean section. Eur J Anaesthesiol 1994;11:115–22.
36. Conway JB, Posner M. Anaesthesia for caesarean section in a patient with Watson's syndrome. Can J Anaesth 1994;41:1113–6.
37. Maleck W. Ketamine and thiopentone in caesarean section. Eur J Anaesthesiol 1995;12:533.
38. Marx GF, Hwang HS, Chandra P. Postpartum uterine pressures with different doses of ketamine. Anesthesiology 1979;50:163–6.
39. Marx GF, Cabe CM, Kim YI, Eidelman AI. Neonatal blood pressures. Anaesthesist 1976;25:318–22.
40. Oats JN, Vasey DP, Waldron BA. Effects of ketamine on the pregnant uterus. Br J Anaesth 1979;51:1163–6.
41. Galloon S. Ketamine and the pregnant uterus. Can Anaesth Soc J 1973;20:141–5.
42. Hodgkinson R, Marx GF, Kim SS, Miclat NM. Neonatal neurobehavioral tests following vaginal delivery under ketamine, thiopental, and extradural anesthesia. Anesth Analg 1977;56:548–53.
43. Hodgkinson R, Bhatt M, Kim SS, Grewal G, Marx GF. Neonatal neurobehavioral tests following cesarean section under general and spinal anesthesia. Am J Obstet Gynecol 1978;132:670–4.

KETOCONAZOLE

Antifungal

PREGNANCY RECOMMENDATION: Limited Human Data—Animal Data Suggest Risk (Oral)
No Human Data—Probably Compatible (Topical)
BREASTFEEDING RECOMMENDATION: No Human Data—Probably Compatible

PREGNANCY SUMMARY

Ketoconazole is a synthetic, broad-spectrum antifungal agent. It has been used, apparently without fetal harm, for the treatment of vaginal candidiasis occurring during pregnancy (1).

FETAL RISK SUMMARY

Ketoconazole is in the same antifungal class of imidazole derivatives as butoconazole, clotrimazole, econazole, miconazole, oxiconazole, sertaconazole, sulconazole, and tioconazole.

Ketoconazole is embryotoxic and teratogenic in rats, producing syndactyly and oligodactyly at a dose 10 times the maximum recommended human dose (weight basis) (2,3). However, the dose caused maternal toxicity.

In a surveillance study of Michigan Medicaid recipients involving 229,101 completed pregnancies conducted between 1985 and 1992, 20 newborns had been exposed to oral ketoconazole during the 1st trimester (F. Rosa, personal communication, FDA, 1993). No major birth defects were observed (one expected). Since this study, the FDA has received six reports of limb defects (F. Rosa, personal communication, FDA, 1996).

Limb malformations were reported in a 1985 abstract (4). A Turkish woman had used ketoconazole, 200 mg daily, during the first 7 weeks of gestation. Hydrops fetalis was diagnosed at 29 weeks' gestation and she delivered a female infant at 30.5 weeks'. The infant, with a normal karyotype (46,XX), had multiple anomalies of the limbs (further details not specified).

Women infected with HIV frequently have vaginal candidiasis. Maternal symptoms, such as pruritus, may require treatment; in these cases, therapeutic and prophylactic ketoconazole regimens are recommended, even though the fungal infection has little perinatal significance (5).

Ketoconazole inhibits steroidogenesis in fungal cells. In humans, high doses, such as those >400 mg/day, impair testosterone and cortisol synthesis (6–9). Because of this effect, ketoconazole has been used in the treatment of hypercortisolism (10). A review summarizing the treatment of 67 cases of Cushing's syndrome occurring during pregnancy did not find any cases treated with ketoconazole (10). A 1990 report, however, described a ketoconazole-treated 36-year-old pregnant woman with Cushing's syndrome (11). The pregnancy, in addition to Cushing's syndrome, was complicated by hypertension, diabetes mellitus diagnosed at 9 weeks' gestation, and intrauterine growth restriction. Ketoconazole, 200 mg every 8 hours, was started at 32 weeks' gestation and continued for 5 weeks because of maternal clinical deterioration resulting from the sustained hypercortisolism. Rapid clinical improvement was noted in the mother after therapy was begun. A growth-restricted, 2080-g, but otherwise normal, female infant was delivered by elective cesarean section at 37 weeks. The Apgar scores were 9 and 9 at 1 and 5 minutes, respectively. No clinical or biochemical evidence of adrenal insufficiency was found in the newborn. The infant's basal cortisol and adrenocorticotropic hormone levels, 306 nmol/L and 8.1 pmol/L, respectively, were normal. The child was growing normally at 18 months of age.

BREASTFEEDING SUMMARY

Ketoconazole is excreted into breast milk (12). A 41-year-old, 82-kg woman took 200 mg/day for 10 days while nursing her 1-month-old infant. Five manually expressed milk samples were collected over a 24-hour interval (1.75–24 hours postdose) on day 10. The maximum milk concentration (0.22 mcg/mL) was measured at 3.25 hours postdose. Ketoconazole was undetectable (detection limit 0.005 mcg/mL) at 24 hours postdose. The mean milk concentration, based on AUC for 0–24 hours, was 0.068 mcg/mL. The level corresponded to an estimated infant dose (based on 150 mL/kg/day) of 0.01 mg/kg/day (maximum estimated dose 0.033 mg/kg/day). The dose was about 0.4% of the mother's weight-adjusted dose. No adverse effects were observed in the infant (12).

The effects on the nursing infant from exposure to drug in the milk are unknown, but the exposure in the above case does not appear to be clinically significant. The American Academy of Pediatrics classifies ketoconazole as compatible with breastfeeding (13).

References

1. Luscher KP, Schneitter J, Vogt HP. Incidence of Candida infections during pregnancy and their treatment with ketoconazole ovula. Schweiz Rundsch Med Prax 1987;76:1285–7.
2. Product information. Nizoral. Janssen Pharmaceutics, 1997.
3. Nishikawa S, Hara T, Miyazaki H, Ohguro Y. Reproduction studies of KW-1414 in rats and rabbits. Clin Rep 1984;18:1433–88. As cited in Shepard TH. *Catalog of Teratogenic Agents*. 6th ed. Baltimore, MD: The Johns Hopkins University Press, 1989:1075.
4. Lind J. Limb malformations in a case of hydrops fetalis with ketoconazole use during pregnancy (abstract). Arch Gynecol 1985;237(Suppl):398.
5. Minkoff HL. Care of pregnant women infected with human immunodeficiency virus. JAMA 1987;258:2714–7.
6. Hobbs ER. Coccidioidomycosis. Dermatol Clin 1989;7:227–39.
7. Pont A, Williams PL, Loose DS, Feldman D, Reitz RE, Bochra C, Stevens DA. Ketoconazole blocks adrenal steroid synthesis. Ann Intern Med 1982;97:370–2.
8. Engelhardt D, Mann K, Hormann R, Braun S, Karl HJ. Ketoconazole inhibits cortisol secretion of an adrenal adenoma in vivo and in vitro. Klin Wochenschr 1983;61:373–5.
9. Divers MJ. Ketoconazole treatment of Cushing's syndrome in pregnancy. Am J Obstet Gynecol 1990;163:1101.
10. Aron DC, Schnall AM, Sheeler LR. Cushing's syndrome and pregnancy. Am J Obstet Gynecol 1990;162:244–52.
11. Amado JA, Pesquera C, Gonzalez EM, Otero M, Freijanes J, Alvarez A. Successful treatment with ketoconazole of Cushing's syndrome in pregnancy. Postgrad Med J 1990;66:221–3.
12. Moretti ME, Ito S, Koren G. Disposition of maternal ketoconazole in breast milk. Am J Obstet Gynecol 1995;173:1625–8.
13. Committee on Drugs, American Academy of Pediatrics. The transfer of drugs and other chemicals into human milk. Pediatrics 2001;108:776–89.

KETOPROFEN

Nonsteroidal Anti-inflammatory

PREGNANCY RECOMMENDATION: Human Data Suggest Risk in 1st and 3rd Trimesters
BREASTFEEDING RECOMMENDATION: No Human Data—Probably Compatible

PREGNANCY SUMMARY

Constriction of the ductus arteriosus in utero is a pharmacologic consequence arising from the use of prostaglandin synthesis inhibitors during pregnancy (see also Indomethacin) (1). Persistent pulmonary hypertension of the newborn may occur if these agents are used in the 3rd trimester close to delivery (1,2). These drugs also have been shown to inhibit labor and prolong pregnancy, in both humans (3) (see also Indomethacin) and animals (4). Women attempting to conceive should not use any prostaglandin synthesis inhibitor, including ketoprofen, because of the findings in a variety of animal models indicating that these agents block blastocyst implantation (5,6). As noted below, nonsteroidal anti-inflammatory drugs (NSAIDs) have been associated with spontaneous abortions (SABs) and congenital malformations (see also Ibuprofen), but the risk for these defects appears to be low.

FETAL RISK SUMMARY

Ketoprofen is an NSAID that is indicated for the management of the signs and symptoms of rheumatoid arthritis and osteoarthritis. It is in the same subclass (propionic acids) as five other NSAIDs (fenoprofen, flurbiprofen, ibuprofen, naproxen, and oxaprozin). The drug undergoes metabolism to an inactive metabolite but can be converted back to the parent compound. Plasma protein binding, mainly to albumin, is high (>99%) and the elimination half-life is about 2 hours (7).

Reproductive studies in mice and rats at about 0.2 times the maximum recommended human dose based on BSA revealed no teratogenic or embryotoxic effects (7). In rabbits, maternally toxic doses were embryotoxic but not teratogenic (7). Shepard (8) reviewed four animal studies that used mice, rats, and monkeys and found no adverse fetal effects or congenital malformations.

Consistent with the low molecular weight (about 254), ketoprofen crosses the human placenta. A 1998 study, using a human isolated perfused placenta, demonstrated transfer of the drug (9). The investigators had previously shown that the drug crosses to the fetus and is detectable in the newborn (10).

In a surveillance study of Michigan Medicaid recipients involving 229,101 completed pregnancies conducted between 1985 and 1992, 112 newborns had been exposed to ketoprofen during the 1st trimester (F. Rosa, personal communication, FDA, 1993). Three (2.7%) major birth defects were observed (five expected), including (expected/observed) 1/1 cardiovascular defect and 1/0.3 polydactyly. No anomalies were observed in four other categories of defects (oral clefts, spina bifida, limb reduction defects, and hypospadias) for which specific data were available.

A combined 2001 population-based, observational cohort study and a case–control study estimated the risk of adverse pregnancy outcome from the use of NSAIDs (11). The use of NSAIDs during pregnancy was not associated with congenital malformations, preterm delivery, or low birth weight, but a positive association was discovered with SABs. A similar study with NSAIDs found a significant association with cardiac defects and orofacial clefts (12). In addition, a 2003 study found a significant association between exposure to NSAIDs in early pregnancy and SABs (13). (See Ibuprofen for details on these three studies.)

A brief 2003 editorial on the potential for NSAID-induced developmental toxicity concluded that NSAIDs, and specifically those with greater cyclooxygenase 2 (COX-2) affinity, had a lower risk of this toxicity in humans than aspirin (14).

K

In a 2007 study, atosiban (an oxytocin inhibitor not available in the United States) was compared with ritodrine for the prevention of preterm labor (15). Ketoprofen was added to 51.1% of the atosiban group and 47.7% of the ritodrine group because the response to the single drug was unsatisfactory. The ketoprofen dose was 100 mg IV followed by 100–150 mg IV every 12 hours for a total duration up to 48 hours. Neonatal mortality and morbidity were unrelated to ketoprofen exposure (15).

BREASTFEEDING SUMMARY

No reports describing the use of ketoprofen during breastfeeding have been located. However, in a 2007 report, 18 non-breastfeeding women immediately after delivery were given IV ketoprofen (100 mg every 12 hours) and nalbuphine (0.2 mg/kg every 4 hours) for postpartum pain (16). The mean and maximum ketoprofen milk concentrations were 57 and 91 ng/mL, respectively. Assuming a milk volume of 150 mL/kg/day, the estimated mean and maximum infant doses were 8.5 and 13.6 mcg/kg/day, respectively. The relative infant dose as a percentage of the weight-adjusted maternal dose was 0.31% (16). (See Nalbuphine for additional data.)

The above data are consistent with the low molecular weight (about 254) of ketoprofen as well as the relatively short elimination half-life (about 2 hours) and the high plasma protein binding (>99%). Although the amounts measured in the above are low, an abstract from France reported that ketoprofen use during breastfeeding was associated with adverse renal and gastrointestinal effects (17). Based on this information, maternal use of other agents should be considered, such as ibuprofen, which is classified as compatible with breastfeeding by the American Academy of Pediatrics (see Ibuprofen).

References

1. Levin DL. Effects of inhibition of prostaglandin synthesis on fetal development, oxygenation, and the fetal circulation. Semin Perinatol 1980;4:35–44.
2. Van Marter LJ, Leviton A, Allred EN, Pagano M, Sullivan KF, Cohen A, Epstein MF. Persistent pulmonary hypertension of the newborn and smoking and aspirin and nonsteroidal antiinflammatory drug consumption during pregnancy. Pediatrics 1996;97:658–63.
3. Fuchs F. Prevention of prematurity. Am J Obstet Gynecol 1976;126:809–20.
4. Powell JG, Cochrane RL. The effects of a number of non-steroidal anti-inflammatory compounds on parturition in the rat. Prostaglandins 1982;23:469–88.
5. Matt DW, Borzelleca JF. Toxic effects on the female reproductive system during pregnancy, parturition, and lactation. In: Witorsch RJ, ed. *Reproductive Toxicology*. 2nd ed. New York, NY: Raven Press, 1995:175–93.
6. Dawood MY. Nonsteroidal antiinflammatory drugs and reproduction. Am J Obstet Gynecol 1993;169:1255–65.
7. Product information. Ketoprofen. Mylan Pharmaceuticals, 2011.
8. Shepard TH. *Catalog of Teratogenic Agents*. 6th ed. Baltimore, MD: The Johns Hopkins University Press, 1989:364.
9. Lagrange F, Pehourcq F, Bannwarth B, Leng JJ, Saux MC. Passage of S-(+)- and R-(−)-ketoprofen across the human isolated perfused placenta. Fundam Clin Pharmacol 1998;12:286–91.
10. Labat L, Llanas B, Demotes-Mainard F, Lagrange F, Demarquez JL, Bannwarth B. Accumulation of S-ketoprofen in neonates after maternal administration of the racemate. Fundam Clin Pharmacol 1995;9:62. As cited in Lagrange F, Pehourcq F, Bannwarth B, Leng JJ, Saux MC. Passage of S-(+)- and R-(−)-ketoprofen across the human isolated perfused placenta. Fundam Clin Pharmacol 1998;12:286–91.
11. Nielsen GL, Sorensen HT, Larsen H, Pedersen L. Risk of adverse birth outcome and miscarriage in pregnant users of non-steroidal anti-inflammatory drugs: population-based observational study and case-control study. Br Med J 2001;322:266–70.
12. Ericson A, Kallen BAJ. Nonsteroidal anti-inflammatory drugs in early pregnancy. Reprod Toxicol 2001;15:371–5.
13. Li DK, Liu L, Odouli R. Exposure to non-steroidal anti-inflammatory drugs during pregnancy and risk of miscarriage: population-based cohort study. Br Med J 2003;327:368–71.
14. Tassinari MS, Cook JC, Hurtt ME. NSAIDs and developmental toxicity. Birth Defects Res B Dev Reprod Toxicol 2003;68:3–4.
15. Grignaffini A, Soncini E, Ronzoni E, Lo Cane F, Anfuso S, Nardelli GB. Clinical practice evaluation of combination of atosiban, ritodrine and ketoprofen for inhibiting preterm labor. Minerva Ginecol 2007;59:481–9.
16. Jacqz-Aigrain E, Serreau R, Boissinot C, Popon M, Sobel A, Michel J, Sibony O. Excretion of ketoprofen and nalbuphine in human milk during treatment of maternal pain after delivery. Ther Drug Monit 2007;29:815–8.
17. Lacroix I, Soussan C, Portolan G, Montastruc JL. Drug-induced adverse reactions via breastfeeding: a study in the French Pharmacovigilance Database (abstract 26-01). Fundam Clin Pharmacol 2013;27(Suppl 1):42–3. doi:10.1111/fep.12025. As cited by National Library of Medicine LactMed Database. Ketoprofen, 2013.

KETOROLAC

Nonsteroidal Anti-inflammatory

PREGNANCY RECOMMENDATION: Human Data Suggest Risk in 1st and 3rd Trimesters
BREASTFEEDING RECOMMENDATION: Contraindicated

PREGNANCY SUMMARY

Because ketorolac is a prostaglandin synthesis inhibitor, constriction of the ductus arteriosus in utero and fetal renal impairment are potential complications when multiple doses of the drug are administered during the latter half of pregnancy (1) (see also Indomethacin). Premature closure of the ductus can result in primary pulmonary hypertension of the newborn that, in severe cases, may be fatal (1,2). Other complications that have been associated with nonsteroidal anti-inflammatory drugs (NSAIDs) are inhibition of labor and prolongation of pregnancy. Women attempting to conceive should not use any prostaglandin synthesis inhibitor, including ketorolac, because of the findings in a variety of animal models indicating that these agents block blastocyst implantation (3,4). Moreover, as noted above, NSAIDs have been associated with spontaneous abortions (SABs) and congenital malformations (see also Ibuprofen). The risk for these defects, however, appears to be low.

In a "black box" warning, the FDA stated that ketorolac was contraindicated in labor and delivery because its prostaglandin synthesis inhibitory effect may adversely affect fetal circulation and inhibit uterine contractions.

FETAL RISK SUMMARY

Ketorolac is an NSAID indicated for the short-term (≤5 days) treatment of pain. The drug is also available as a solution for ocular pain. Ketorolac is in an NSAID subclass (pyrrolizine carboxylic acid) with no other members.

Ketorolac was not teratogenic in rats (1.0 times the human AUC) and rabbits (0.37 times the human AUC) treated with daily oral doses of the drug during organogenesis. Oral dosing in rats at 0.14 times the human AUC after day 17 of gestation caused dystocia and decreased pup survivability (5).

In a study using chronically catheterized pregnant sheep, an infusion of ketorolac completely blocked the ritodrine-induced increase of prostaglandin $F_{2\alpha}$, a potent uterine stimulant, in the uterine venous plasma (6,7). The researchers speculated that ritodrine stimulation of prostaglandin synthesis in pregnant uterine tissue might contribute to the tachyphylaxis sometimes observed with the tocolytic agent.

It is not known if ketorolac crosses the human placenta. The molecular weight (about 376) is low enough that passage to the embryo and fetus should be expected.

A combined 2001 population-based, observational cohort study and a case–control study estimated the risk of adverse pregnancy outcome from the use of NSAIDs (8). The use of NSAIDs during pregnancy was not associated with congenital malformations, preterm delivery, or low birth weight, but a positive association was discovered with SABs. A similar study, also published in 2001, failed to find a relationship, in general, between NSAIDs and congenital malformations, but did find a significant association with cardiac defects and orofacial clefts (9), In addition, a 2003 study found a significant association between exposure to NSAIDs in early pregnancy and SABs (10). (See Ibuprofen for details on these three studies.)

A brief 2003 editorial on the potential for NSAID-induced developmental toxicity concluded that NSAIDs, and specifically those with greater cyclooxygenase 2 (COX-2) affinity, had a lower risk of this toxicity in humans than aspirin (11).

A randomized, double-blind study published in 1992 compared single IM doses of ketorolac 10 mg, meperidine 50 mg, and meperidine 100 mg in multiparous women in labor (12). All patients also received a single dose of prochlorperazine (for nausea and vomiting) and ranitidine for acid reflux. Ineffective pain relief was observed in all three treatment groups, but both doses of meperidine were superior to ketorolac. Duration of labor was similar among the three groups, as was the occurrence of adverse effects, including maternal blood loss. One-minute Apgar scores were significantly greater in the ketorolac group compared with the meperidine groups, most likely because of the lack of respiratory depressant effects of ketorolac, but this difference was not observed at 5 minutes (12).

A 1997 abstract and later full report described the use of ketorolac for acute tocolysis in preterm labor (13,14). Women, at ≤32 weeks' gestation, were randomized to receive either ketorolac (N = 45), 60 mg IM and then 30 mg IM every 4–6 hours, or magnesium sulfate (N = 43), 6 g IV and then 3–6 g/hour IV. Therapy was stopped if 48 hours lapsed, labor progressed (>4 cm), severe side effects occurred, or uterine quiescence was achieved. Ketorolac was significantly better than magnesium sulfate in the time required to stop uterine contractions (2.7 vs. 6.2 hours), but no difference was found between the two regimens for the other parameters (failed tocolysis, birth weight, gestational age at delivery, and neonatal morbidity). There was no difference in the incidence of maternal and neonatal adverse effects between the groups (13,14).

BREASTFEEDING SUMMARY

Ketorolac is excreted into breast milk (15). Ten women, 2–6 days postpartum, were given oral ketorolac, 10 mg four times daily for 2 days. Their infants were not allowed to breastfeed during the study. Four of the women had milk concentrations of the drug below the detection limit of the assay (<5 ng/mL) and were excluded from analysis. In the remaining six women, the mean milk:plasma ratios 2 hours after doses 1, 3, 5, and 7 ranged from 0.016 to 0.027, corresponding to mean milk concentrations ranging from 5.2 to 7.9 ng/mL. Based on a milk production of 400–1000 mL/day, the investigators estimated that the maximum amount of drug available to a nursing infant would range from 3.16 to 7.9 mcg/day (*Note: The cited reference indicated 3.16–7.9 mg/day, but this appears to be an error*), equivalent to 0.16%–0.40% of the mother's dose on a weight-adjusted basis. These amounts were considered clinically insignificant (15).

The FDA has placed a "Black Box" warning on ketorolac, stating that drug is contraindicated during breastfeeding because of the potential adverse effects of prostaglandin-inhibiting drugs on neonates.

K

References

1. Levin DL. Effects of inhibition of prostaglandin synthesis on fetal development, oxygenation, and the fetal circulation. Semin Perinatol 1980;4:35–44.
2. Van Marter LJ, Leviton A, Allred EN, Pagano M, Sullivan KF, Cohen A, Epstein MF. Persistent pulmonary hypertension of the newborn and smoking and aspirin and nonsteroidal antiinflammatory drug consumption during pregnancy. Pediatrics 1996;97:658–63.
3. Matt DW, Borzelleca JF. Toxic effects on the female reproductive system during pregnancy, parturition, and lactation. In: Witorsch RJ, ed. *Reproductive Toxicology*. 2nd ed. New York, NY: Raven Press, 1995:175–93.
4. Dawood MY. Nonsteroidal antiinflammatory drugs and reproduction. Am J Obstet Gynecol 1993;169:1255–65.
5. Product information. Toradol. Roche Laboratories, 2000.
6. Rauk PN, Laifer SA. Ketorolac blocks ritodrine-stimulated production of $PGF_{2\alpha}$ in pregnant sheep (abstract). Am J Obstet Gynecol 1992;166:274.
7. Rauk PN, Laifer SA. The prostaglandin synthesis inhibitor ketorolac blocks ritodrine-stimulated production of prostaglandin $F_{2\alpha}$ in pregnant sheep. Obstet Gynecol 1993;81:323–6.
8. Nielsen GL, Sorensen HT, Larsen H, Pedersen L. Risk of adverse birth outcome and miscarriage in pregnant users of non-steroidal anti-inflammatory drugs: population-based observational study and case-control study. Br Med J 2001;322:266–70.
9. Ericson A, Kallen BAJ. Nonsteroidal anti-inflammatory drugs in early pregnancy. Reprod Toxicol 2001;15:371–5.
10. Li DK, Liu L, Odouli R. Exposure to non-steroidal anti-inflammatory drugs during pregnancy and risk of miscarriage: population-based cohort study. Br Med J 2003;327:368–71.
11. Tassinari MS, Cook JC, Hurtt ME. NSAIDs and developmental toxicity. Birth Defects Res (Part B) 2003;68:3–4.
12. Walker JJ, Johnston J, Fairlie FM, Lloyd J, Bullingham R. A comparative study of intramuscular ketorolac and pethidine in labour pain. Eur J Obstet Gynecol Reprod Biol 1992;46:87–94.
13. Schorr SJ, Ascarelli MH, Rust OA, Ross EL, Calfee EF, Perry KG Jr, Morrison JC. Ketorolac is a safe and effective drug for acute tocolysis (abstract). Am J Obstet Gynecol 1997;176:S7.
14. Schorr SJ, Ascarelli MH, Rust OA, Ross EL, Calfee EL, Perry KG Jr, Morrison JC. A comparative study of ketorolac (Toradol) and magnesium sulfate for arrest of preterm labor. South Med J 1998;91:1028–32.
15. Wischnik A, Manth SM, Lloyd J, Bullingham R, Thompson JS. The excretion of ketorolac tromethamine into breast milk after multiple oral dosing. Eur J Clin Pharmacol 1989;36:521–4.

KUDZU

Herb

PREGNANCY RECOMMENDATION: No Human Data—Probably Compatible
BREASTFEEDING RECOMMENDATION: No Human Data—Probably Compatible

PREGNANCY SUMMARY

No studies describing the use of kudzu during animal or human pregnancy have been located. Because the herb has been used as a medicine for more than 2500 years, it is doubtful that it causes developmental toxicity. Moreover, many chemical constituents of kudzu can also be found in foods. Nevertheless, the safest course is to avoid high, frequent doses of the herb or its individual constituents during pregnancy.

FETAL RISK SUMMARY

Kudzu, a fast-growing vine native to Japan, China, and Fiji, was introduced to the United States in the late 1800s to control soil erosion. It is well established in moist southern regions and is now considered an invasive pest. In China, kudzu has been used as a medicine since the 6th century BC as therapy for alcoholism, muscular pain, and treatment of measles. Treatment of alcohol hangover, drunkenness, and alcoholism is its primary indications. It also has been used for numerous other indications, none of which have been adequately studied. Kudzu also has been investigated for its antiproliferative activity in some cancers (breast, ovarian, and cervical), its cardiovascular activity for arrhythmia, ischemia, and angina pectoris, and for hepatic protection, hyperlipidemia, and osteogenic activity. Some constituents of kudzu are phytoestrogens and antioxidants (1,2).

The chemical constituents identified from the root, flowers, and leaves include flavonoids, isoflavonoids, and isoflavones. Specific constituents that have been identified include kudzu saponins, robinin, tectoridin, kakkalide, formononetin, biochanin A, plant sterols, and the isoflavones daidzein, daidzin, genistein, genistin, and puerarin. Many of these agents are found in food, such as daidzein and genistein from soybeans (1,2).

A long-term study in mice evaluated the fertility and reproductive toxicity of kudzu (3). Toxicity with high daily doses (100 mg/kg) included prolonged estrous cycles, hyperplasia of the uterine endothelium, and a decrease in the number of growing ovarian follicles. This dose also resulted in a decrease in mating efficiency. The effects were attributed to decreases in the serum concentrations of luteinizing hormone (LH) and follicle-stimulating hormone (FSH). In contrast, a 10-mg/kg/day dose induced no changes in the hypothalamic–pituitary–ovarian–uterine axis (3).

BREASTFEEDING SUMMARY

No reports describing the use of kudzu during lactation have been located. Because the herb has been used as a medicine for more than 2500 years, it is doubtful that it causes harm during breastfeeding. Moreover, many chemical constituents of kudzu can also be found in foods. Nevertheless, nursing women should avoid high, frequent doses of the herb or its individual constituents.

References

1. Kudzu. In: *The Review of Natural Products*. St. Louis, MO: Wolters Kluwer Health, 2008.
2. Kudzu. In: *Natural Medicines Comprehensive Database*. 10th ed. Stockton, CA: Therapeutic Research Faculty, 2008:890–3.
3. Jaroenporn S, Malaivijitnond S, Wattanasirmkit K, Watanabe G, Taya K, Cherdshewasart W. Assessment of fertility and reproductive toxicity in adult female mice after long-term exposure to *Pueraria mirifica* herb. J Reprod Dev 2007;53:995–1005.

KUNECATECHINS

Dermatologic Agent

PREGNANCY RECOMMENDATION: No Human Data—Animal Data Suggest Low Risk
BREASTFEEDING RECOMMENDATION: No Human Data—Probably Compatible

PREGNANCY SUMMARY

No reports describing the use of kunecatechins ointment in human pregnancy have been located. The animal reproductive data suggest low risk, but the absence of human pregnancy experience prevents a complete assessment of the embryo–fetal risk. Kunecatechins is a water extract of green tea leaves. Moderate consumption of green tea during pregnancy is thought to be safe (1). If the recommended dose and directions are followed, the risk for an embryo or fetus appears to be low, if it exists at all.

FETAL RISK SUMMARY

Kunecatechins is a partially purified fraction of the water extract of green tea leaves [*Camellia sinensis (L.) O Kuntze*]. It is a mixture of eight catechins (85%–95% of the total weight) and other green tea components (about 2.5% of the total weight) including gallic acid, caffeine, and theobromine. It is available as a 15% ointment that is applied three times daily for a maximum of 16 weeks. The systemic absorption of repeated topical administration of kunecatechins has not been adequately studied but is thought to be less than that obtained after a single oral intake of 400 mL of green tea. Kunecatechins is indicated for the topical treatment of external genital and perianal warts (*Condylomata acuminata*) in immunocompetent patients 18 years and older. Treatment of urethral, intravaginal, cervical, rectal or intra-anal human papilloma viral disease has not been evaluated and the ointment should not be used for these conditions (2).

Reproductive studies have been conducted in rats and rabbits. Comparisons, based on body weight, were made based on the maximum recommended human dose of the ointment (250 mg three times daily; 750 mg of the ointment or 125.5 mg kunecatechins per day) (MRHD). During organogenesis, daily oral doses in rats and rabbits of ≤86 and ≤173 times, respectively, the MRHD revealed no effects on embryo or fetal development or teratogenicity. In rabbits during organogenesis, daily SC doses that were about 2.1 and 6.3 times the MRHD caused maternal toxicity (marked local irritation at the injection site and decreased body weight and food consumption) and fetal toxicity (reduced body weights and delayed skeletal ossification). The no-effect dose for fetal toxicity was 0.7 times the MRHD. In a combined fertility/embryo–fetal development test, female rats were given daily vaginal doses of the ointment that were ≤8 times the MRHD from day 4 before mating through day 17 of gestation. No adverse effects on mating performance or fertility or on the embryo–fetus were observed (2).

Carcinogenicity studies were conducted in mice with daily doses ≤22 times the MRHD for 26 weeks. There was an increased incidence of either neoplastic or non-neoplastic lesions in the organs and tissues examined. In mutagenicity tests, four assays were negative and one was positive (2).

It is not known if the major components (i.e., catechins) of kunecatechins cross the human placenta. The molecular weights of the eight catechins are varied but are <500 and would be expected to cross the placenta. However, systemic concentration of kunecatechins is thought to be low.

BREASTFEEDING SUMMARY

No reports describing the use of kunecatechins ointment during lactation have been located. It is not known if the major components (i.e., catechins) of kunecatechins are excreted into breast milk. The molecular weights of the eight catechins are varied but are <500 and would be expected to pass into milk. However, systemic concentrations of kunecatechins are thought to be low. Moreover, kunecatechins is a water extract of green tea leaves. Moderate consumption of green tea during breastfeeding is thought to be safe (1). If the recommended dose and directions are followed, the risk for a nursing infant appears to be low, if it exists at all.

References

1. Green tea. In: Jellin JM, ed. *Natural Medicines Comprehensive Database*. 10th ed. Stockton, CA: Therapeutic Research Faculty, 2008:733–43.
2. Product information. Veregen. Doak Dermatologics, 2006.

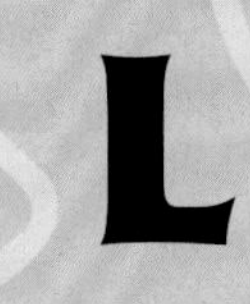

LABETALOL

Sympatholytic (Antihypertensive)

PREGNANCY RECOMMENDATION: Human Data Suggest Low Risk
BREASTFEEDING RECOMMENDATION: Limited Human Data—Probably Compatible

PREGNANCY SUMMARY

The use of labetalol for the treatment of maternal hypertension does not appear to pose a risk to the fetus, except possibly in the 1st trimester, and may offer advantages over the use of agents with only β-blocker activity. Most studies have found no effect on fetal growth, but one did find fetal growth restriction when used for the treatment of mild preeclampsia. Some β-blockers may cause intrauterine growth restriction (IUGR) and reduced placental weight, especially those lacking intrinsic sympathomimetic activity (ISA) (i.e., partial agonist). Labetalol does not possess ISA. IUGR and reduced placental weight may potential occur with all agents within this class and can be a consequence of maternal hypertension. Although IUGR is a serious concern, the benefits of maternal therapy with labetalol outweigh the risks to the fetus. If used near delivery, the newborn infant should be closely observed for 24–48 hours for signs and symptoms of β-blockade. Long-term effects of in utero exposure to labetalol have not been studied but warrant evaluation.

FETAL RISK SUMMARY

Labetalol, a combined α/β-adrenergic blocking agent, has been used for the treatment of hypertension occurring during pregnancy (1–29). No teratogenicity was observed in rats and rabbits at oral doses 6 and 4 times the maximum recommended human dose (MRHD), respectively (30). However, increased fetal resorptions occurred in both species at doses approximately equivalent to the MRHD. In rabbits, IV doses ≤1.7 times the MRHD revealed no drug-related fetal harm (30).

Labetalol crosses the human placenta to produce cord serum concentrations averaging 40%–80% of peak maternal levels (1–5). Maternal serum and amniotic fluid concentrations are approximately equivalent 1–3 hours after a single IV dose (4). After oral dosing (1–42 days) in eight women, amniotic fluid concentrations of labetalol were in the same range as, but lower than, the plasma concentrations in six of the women (6). The pharmacokinetics of labetalol in pregnant patients has been reported (7,8).

In a surveillance study of Michigan Medicaid recipients involving 229,101 completed pregnancies conducted between 1985 and 1992, 29 newborns had been exposed to labetalol during the 1st trimester (F. Rosa, personal communication, FDA, 1993). Four (13.8%) major birth defects were observed (one expected). Details on the malformations were not available, but no anomalies were observed in six defect categories (cardiovascular defects, oral clefts, spina bifida, polydactyly, limb reduction defects, and hypospadias) for which specific data were available. Although the number of exposures is small, the incidence of malformations is suggestive of an association, but other factors, including the mother's disease, concurrent drug use, and chance, may be involved.

No published reports of fetal malformations attributable to labetalol have been located, but experience during the 1st trimester, except for the surveillance study described above, is lacking. Most reports have found no adverse effects on birth weight, head circumference, Apgar scores, or blood glucose control after in utero exposure to labetalol (9–13). One case of neonatal hypoglycemia has been mentioned, but the mother was also taking a thiazide diuretic (2). Offspring of mothers treated with labetalol had a significantly higher birth weight than infants of atenolol-treated mothers, 3280 vs. 2750 g, respectively (14). However, in a study comparing labetalol plus hospitalization with hospitalization alone for the treatment of mild preeclampsia presenting at 26–35 weeks' gestation, labetalol treatment did not improve perinatal outcome, and a significantly higher number of labetalol-exposed infants were growth restricted, 19.1% (18 of 94) vs. 9.3% (9 of 97), respectively (15).

Fetal heart rate is apparently unaffected by labetalol treatment of hypertensive pregnant women. However, two studies have observed newborn bradycardia in five infants (16,17). In one of these infants, bradycardia was marked (<100 beats/minute) and persistent (17). All five infants survived. Hypotension was noted in another infant delivered by cesarean section at 28 weeks' gestation (1). In a study examining the effects of labetalol exposure on term (≥37 weeks) newborns, mild transient hypotension, which resolved within 24 hours, was observed in 11 infants compared with 11 matched controls (18). Maternal dosage varied from 100 to 300 mg 3 times daily with the last dose given within 12 hours of birth. The mean systolic blood pressures at 2 hours of age in exposed and nonexposed infants were 58.8 and 63.3 mmHg

($p < 0.05$), respectively. Other measures of β-blockade, such as heart and respiratory rates, palmar sweating, blood glucose control, and metabolic and vasomotor responses to cold stress, did not differ between the groups. The investigators concluded that labetalol did not cause clinically significant β-blockade in mature newborn infants (18).

Several investigations have shown a lack of effect of labetalol treatment on uterine contractions (1–3,16,19–21). One study did report a higher incidence of spontaneous labor in labetalol-treated mothers (6 of 10) than in a similar group treated with methyldopa (2 of 9) (22). In another report, 3 of 31 patients treated with labetalol experienced spontaneous labor, one of whom delivered prematurely (23). The authors attributed the uterine activity to the drug because no other causes were found. However, because most trials with labetalol in hypertensive women have not shown this effect, it is questionable whether the drug has any direct effect on uterine contractility.

Labetalol does not change uteroplacental blood flow despite a drop in blood pressure (2,4,5,24,25). The lack of effect on blood flow was probably caused by reduced peripheral resistance.

Labetalol apparently reduces the incidence of hyaline membrane disease in premature infants by increasing the production of pulmonary surfactant (1,2,4,16,26). The mechanism for this effect may be mediated through β_2-adrenoceptor agonist activity that the drug partially possesses (1,2,4,16,26).

Follow-up studies have been completed at 6 months of age on 10 infants exposed in utero to labetalol (27). All infants demonstrated normal growth and development. In addition, no ocular toxicity was observed in newborns, even though labetalol has an affinity for ocular melanin (1,2,26).

The experience with labetalol in pregnancy was briefly reviewed in a 1988 article (31). A 2000 meta-analysis concluded that IV labetalol for late-onset hypertension in pregnancy was safer than IV hydralazine or diazoxide in terms of drug-induced maternal hypotension and fewer cesarean sections (32).

BREASTFEEDING SUMMARY

Labetalol is excreted into breast milk (1,6). In 24 lactating women at 3 days postpartum, administration of 330–800 mg/day produced a mean milk level of 33 ng/mL. No adverse effects were observed in the nursing infants. One patient, consuming 1200 mg/day, had a mean milk concentration of 600 ng/mL, but this woman did not breastfeed. Three women at 6–9 days postpartum consumed daily doses of labetalol of 600, 600, and 1200 mg and produced peak milk concentrations of the drug of 129, 223, and 662 ng/mL, respectively (6). Peak concentrations of labetalol in the milk occurred between 2 and 3 hours after a dose. Measurable plasma concentrations of labetalol were found in only one infant: 18 ng/mL at 4 hours and 21 ng/mL at 8 hours. Although no adverse effects have been reported, nursing infants should be closely observed for bradycardia, hypotension, and other symptoms of α/β-blockade. Long-term effects of exposure to labetalol from milk have not been studied but warrant evaluation. The American Academy of Pediatrics classifies labetalol as compatible with breastfeeding (33).

References

1. Michael CA. Use of labetalol in the treatment of severe hypertension during pregnancy. Br J Clin Pharmacol 1979;8(Suppl 2):211S–5S.
2. Riley AJ. Clinical pharmacology of labetalol in pregnancy. J Cardiovasc Pharmacol 1981;3(Suppl 1):S53–9.
3. Andrejak M, Coevoet B, Fievet P, Gheerbrant JD, Comoy E, Leuillet P, Verhoest P, Boulanger JC, Vitse M, Fournier A. Effect of labetalol on hypertension and the renin–angiotensin–aldosterone and adrenergic systems in pregnancy. In: Riley A, Symonds EM, eds. *The Investigation of Labetalol in the Management of Hypertension in Pregnancy*. Amsterdam: Excerpta Medica, 1982:77–87.
4. Lunell NO, Hjemdahl P, Fredholm BB, Lewander R, Nisell H, Nylund L, Persson B, Sarby J, Wager J, Thornstrom S. Acute effects of labetalol on maternal metabolism and uteroplacental circulation in hypertension of pregnancy. In: Riley A, Symonds EM, eds. *The Investigation of Labetalol in the Management of Hypertension in Pregnancy*. Amsterdam, Netherlands: Excerpta Medica, 1982:34–45.
5. Nylund L, Lunell NO, Lewander R, Sarby B, Thornstrom S. Labetalol for the treatment of hypertension in pregnancy. Acta Obstet Gynecol Scand 1984;118(Suppl):71–3.
6. Lunell NO, Kulas J, Rane A. Transfer of labetalol into amniotic fluid and breast milk in lactating women. Eur J Clin Pharmacol 1985;28:597–9.
7. Rubin PC. Drugs in pregnancy. In: Riley A, Symonds EM, eds. *The Investigation of Labetalol in the Management of Hypertension in Pregnancy*. Amsterdam, Netherlands: Excerpta Medica, 1982:28–33.
8. Rubin PC, Butters L, Kelman AW, Fitzsimons C, Reid JL. Labetalol disposition and concentration–effect relationships during pregnancy. Br J Clin Pharmacol 1983;15:465–70.
9. Lamming GD, Broughton Pipkin F, Symonds EM. Comparison of the alpha and beta blocking drug, labetalol, and methyl dopa in the treatment of moderate and severe pregnancy-induced hypertension. Clin Exp Hypertens 1980;2:865–95.
10. Lotgering FK, Derkx FMH, Wallenburg HCS. Primary hyperaldosteronism in pregnancy. Am J Obstet Gynecol 1986;155:986–8.
11. Mabie WC, Gonzalez AR, Sibai BM, Amon E. A comparative trial of labetalol and hydralazine in the acute management of severe hypertension complicating pregnancy. Obstet Gynecol 1987;70:328–33.
12. Plouin P-F, Breart G, Maillard F, Papiernik E, Relier J-P. Comparison of antihypertensive efficacy and perinatal safety of labetalol and methyldopa in the treatment of hypertension in pregnancy: a randomized controlled trial. Br J Obstet Gynaecol 1988;95:868–76.
13. Pickles CJ, Symonds EM, Broughton Pipkin F. The fetal outcome in a randomized trial of labetalol versus placebo in pregnancy-induced hypertension. Br J Obstet Gynaecol 1989;96:38–43.
14. Lardoux H, Gerard J, Blazquez G, Chouty F, Flouvat B. Hypertension in pregnancy: evaluation of two beta blockers atenolol and labetalol. Eur Heart J 1983;4(Suppl G):35–40.
15. Sibai BM, Gonzalez AR, Mabie WC, Moretti M. A comparison of labetalol plus hospitalization versus hospitalization alone in the management of preeclampsia remote from term. Obstet Gynecol 1987;70:323–7.
16. Michael CA, Potter JM. A comparison of labetalol with other antihypertensive drugs in the treatment of hypertensive disease of pregnancy. In: Riley A, Symonds EM, eds. *The Investigation of Labetalol in the Management of Hypertension in Pregnancy*. Amsterdam, Netherlands: Excerpta Medica, 1982:111–22.
17. Davey DA, Dommisse J, Garden A. Intravenous labetalol and intravenous dihydralazine in severe hypertension in pregnancy. In: Riley A, Symonds EM, eds. *The Investigation of Labetalol in the Management of Hypertension in Pregnancy*. Amsterdam, Netherlands: Excerpta Medica, 1982:52–61.
18. MacPherson M, Broughton Pipkin F, Rutter N. The effect of maternal labetalol on the newborn infant. Br J Obstet Gynaecol 1986;93:539–42.
19. Redman CWG. A controlled trial of the treatment of hypertension in pregnancy: labetalol compared with methyldopa. In: Riley A, Symonds EM, eds. *The Investigation of Labetalol in the Management of Hypertension in Pregnancy*. Amsterdam, Netherlands: Excerpta Medica, 1982:101–10.
20. Walker JJ, Crooks A, Erwin L, Calder AA. Labetalol in pregnancy-induced hypertension: fetal and maternal effects. In: Riley A, Symonds EM, eds. *The Investigation of Labetalol in the Management of Hypertension of Pregnancy*. Amsterdam, Netherlands: Excerpta Medica, 1982:148–60.
21. Thulesius O, Lunell NO, Ibrahim M, Moberger B, Angilivilayil C. The effect of labetalol on contractility of human myometrial preparations. Acta Obstet Gynecol 1987;66:237–40.
22. Lamming GD, Symonds EM. Use of labetalol and methyldopa in pregnancy-induced hypertension. Br J Clin Pharmacol 1979;8(Suppl 2):217S–22S.

23. Jorge CS, Fernandes L, Cunha S. Labetalol in the hypertensive states of pregnancy. In: Riley A, Symonds EM, eds. *The Investigation of Labetalol in the Management of Hypertension of Pregnancy*. Amsterdam, Netherlands: Excerpta Medica, 1982:124–30.
24. Lunell NO, Nylund L, Lewander R, Sarby B. Acute effect of an antihypertensive drug, labetalol, on uteroplacental blood flow. Br J Obstet Gynaecol 1982;89:640–4.
25. Jouppila P, Kirkinen P, Koivula A, Ylikorkala O. Labetalol does not alter the placental and fetal blood flow or maternal prostanoids in pre-eclampsia. Br J Obstet Gynaecol 1986;93:543–7.
26. Michael CA. The evaluation of labetalol in the treatment of hypertension complicating pregnancy. Br J Clin Pharmacol 1982;13(Suppl):127S–31S.
27. Symonds EM, Lamming GD, Jadoul F, Broughton Pipkin F. Clinical and biochemical aspects of the use of labetalol in the treatment of hypertension in pregnancy: comparison with methyldopa. In: Riley A, Symonds EM, eds. *The Investigation of Labetalol in the Management of Hypertension in Pregnancy*. Amsterdam, Netherlands: Excerpta Medica, 1982:62–76.
28. Smith AM. Beta-blockers for pregnancy hypertension. Lancet 1983;1:708–9.
29. Walker JJ, Bonduelle M, Greer I, Calder AA. Antihypertensive therapy in pregnancy. Lancet 1983;1:932–3.
30. Product information. Normodyne. Schering, 2000.
31. Frishman WH, Chesner M. Beta-adrenergic blockers in pregnancy. Am Heart J 1988;115:147–52.
32. Magee LA, Elran E, Bull SB, Logan A, Koren G. Risks and benefits of β-receptor blockers for pregnancy hypertension: overview of the randomized trials. Eur J Obstet Gynecol Reprod Biol 2000;88:15–26.
33. Committee on Drugs, American Academy of Pediatrics. The transfer of drugs and other chemicals into human milk. Pediatrics 2001;108:776–89.

LACOSAMIDE

Anticonvulsant

PREGNANCY RECOMMENDATION: No Human Data—Animal Data Suggest Moderate Risk
BREASTFEEDING RECOMMENDATION: No Human Data—Potential Toxicity

PREGNANCY SUMMARY

No reports of human pregnancy experience have been located. Lacosamide was not teratogenic in two animal species but, in one, was associated with developmental neurobehavioral toxicity at plasma exposures close to those obtained in humans. Moreover, in vitro studies have shown that lacosamide interferes with the activity of collapsin response mediator protein-2 (CRMP-2), which is involved in neuronal differentiation and control of axonal outgrowth (1). Thus, lacosamide could cause adverse effects on CNS development if used in pregnancy. Until human data are available, the safest course is to avoid this drug in pregnancy.

FETAL RISK SUMMARY

Chemically, lacosamide is a functionalized amino acid that was approved by the FDA in 2008 as an anticonvulsant. It is available in both oral and IV formulations. The oral tablets are indicated as adjunctive therapy in the treatment of partial-onset seizures in patients with epilepsy aged ≥17 years. IV injection is indicated in the same population when oral administration is temporarily not feasible. It is partially metabolized before elimination into an inactive metabolite. Plasma protein binding is minimal (about 15%), but the elimination half-life (about 13 hours) is prolonged (1).

Reproduction studies have been conducted in rats and rabbits. In rats, oral doses given during organogenesis that resulted in plasma exposures that were about twice the human exposure (AUC) from the maximum recommended dose of 400 mg/day (MRHD) caused maternal toxicity and embryo–fetal death. No teratogenic effects were observed. This dose, when given throughout gestation, parturition, and lactation, increased perinatal mortality and decreased body weights in the offspring. The no-effect dose for prenatal and postnatal developmental toxicity produced plasma concentrations approximately equal to the MRHD. In rabbits, oral doses that produced plasma exposures about equal to the MRHD caused maternal toxicity but no teratogenicity (1).

Oral lacosamide also was given to rats during the neonatal and juvenile periods because the early postnatal period is thought to correspond to the 3rd trimester in humans in terms of brain development (1). This exposure resulted in decreased brain weights and long-term neurobehavioral changes (altered open field performance and deficits in learning and memory). The no-effect dose for developmental neurotoxicity was plasma concentrations about 0.5 times the MRHD (1).

Lacosamide was not carcinogenic in 2-year studies in mice and rats at doses producing plasma exposures up to about one and three times, respectively, the MRHD. Two of three mutagenicity studies were negative. In fertility studies, no adverse effects were observed on fertility or reproduction in male or female rats (1).

It is not known if lacosamide crosses the human placenta. The molecular weight (about 250), low plasma protein binding, and long elimination half-life suggest that it will cross to the embryo–fetus.

The manufacturer has established the UCB AED Pregnancy Registry in which either the healthcare provider or the patient can initiate enrollment by calling 1-888-537-7734. The manufacturer also recommends that patients enroll in the North American Antiepileptic Drug Pregnancy Registry by calling 1-888-233-2334. (This must be done by the patients themselves.) (1).

BREASTFEEDING SUMMARY

No reports describing the use of lacosamide during human lactation have been located. The molecular weight (about 250), low plasma protein binding (about 15%), and long elimination half-life (about 13 hours) suggest that the drug will be excreted into breast milk. The effects of this exposure on a nursing infant are unknown. However, consideration should be given to the neurobehavioral toxicity observed in neonatal rats at clinically relevant plasma exposures. Until human data are available, the safest course is for women taking this drug to not breastfeed.

Reference

1. Product information. Vimpat. UCB, 2008.

LACTULOSE

Laxative

PREGNANCY RECOMMENDATION: No Human Data—Probably Compatible
BREASTFEEDING RECOMMENDATION: No Human Data—Probably Compatible

PREGNANCY SUMMARY

Lactulose is a synthetic disaccharide that is biodegraded only by bacteria in the colon to the low-molecular-weight acids, lactic acid, formic acid, and acetic acid. Small amounts of lactulose, about 3% of a dose, are absorbed following oral administration (1).

FETAL RISK SUMMARY

No impairment of fertility or fetal harm has been observed in pregnant mice, rats, and rabbits at doses up to three or six times the usual human oral dose (2). No reports on the use of this product in human pregnancy or lactation have been located, but the risk to the fetus and the newborn appears to be negligible.

BREASTFEEDING SUMMARY

No reports describing the use of lactulose during human lactation have been located.

References

1. Product information. Cephulac. Marion Merrell Dow, 1992.
2. Product information. Duphalac. Solvay Pharmaceuticals, 2000.

L

LAETRILE

[See 9th edition.]

LAMIVUDINE

Antiviral

PREGNANCY RECOMMENDATION: Compatible—Maternal Benefit >> Embryo/Fetal Risk
BREASTFEEDING RECOMMENDATION: Contraindicated

PREGNANCY SUMMARY

The animal and human data suggest that lamivudine is a low risk to the developing fetus for structural malformations. Theoretically, exposure to agents in this class at the time of implantation could result in impaired fertility as a result of embryonic cytotoxicity, but this has not been studied in humans. The risk of mitochondrial dysfunction with nucleoside analog reverse transcriptase inhibitors (NRTIs) needs confirmation. However, even if an association is proven, the risk of mortality and morbidity from HIV infection outweighs the risk (1). If indicated, the drug should not be withheld because of pregnancy.

FETAL RISK SUMMARY

Lamivudine (2′,3′-dideoxy-3′-thiacytidine, 3TC), an antiviral agent structurally similar to zalcitabine, inhibits viral reverse transcription via viral DNA chain termination. It is classified as an NRTI that is used for the treatment of HIV infection. Lamivudine is believed to be converted by intracellular enzymes to the active metabolite, lamivudine-5′-triphosphate (3TC-TP) (2).

No teratogenic effects were observed in rats and rabbits administered lamivudine up to approximately 130 and 60 times, respectively, the usual human adult dose. Early embryo lethality was observed in rabbits at doses close to those used in humans and above. This effect was not observed in rats given ≥130 times the usual human dose. Lamivudine crossed the placenta to the fetus in both animal types (2).

Adverse effects on neurobehavior development in mice offspring resulting from a combination of lamivudine and zidovudine were described in a 2001 study (3). Pregnant mice received both drugs from day 10 of gestation to delivery. The effects on somatic and sensorimotor development were minor but more marked in exposed offspring than when either drug was given alone (2). Both developmental endpoints were delayed with respect to control animals. Further, alterations of social behavior were observed in both sexes of exposed offspring (3).

The low molecular weight (about 229) of lamivudine suggests that it will cross the placenta. A study published in 1997 described the human placental transfer of lamivudine using an *ex vivo* single cotyledon perfusion system (4). Lamivudine crossed the placenta to the fetal side by simple diffusion. Transfer did not appear to be affected by the presence of zidovudine. Confirming this, a 1998 study found that combination therapy with zidovudine did not affect the pharmacokinetics of lamivudine (5). Lamivudine freely crossed the placenta when given near term with nearly equivalent drug levels in the mother, cord blood, and newborn.

The Antiretroviral Pregnancy Registry reported, for the period January 1989 through July 2009, prospective data (reported before the outcomes were known) involving 4702 live births that had been exposed during the 1st trimester to one or more antiretroviral agents (6). Congenital defects were noted in 134, a prevalence of 2.8% (95% confidence interval [CI] 2.4–3.4). In the 6100 live births with earliest exposure in the 2nd/3rd trimesters, there were 153 infants with defects (2.5%, 95% CI 2.1–2.9). The prevalence rates for the two periods did not differ significantly. There were 288 infants with birth defects among 10,803 live births with exposure anytime during pregnancy (2.7%, 95% CI 2.4–3.0). The prevalence rate did not differ significantly from the rate expected in a nonexposed population. There were 8331 outcomes exposed to lamivudine (3314 in the 1st trimester and 5017 in the 2nd/3rd trimesters) in combination with other antiretroviral agents. There were 222 birth defects (96 in the 1st trimester and 126 in the 2nd/3rd trimesters). In reviewing the birth defects of prospective and retrospective (pregnancies reported after the outcomes were known) registered cases, the Registry concluded that, except for isolated cases of neural tube defects with efavirenz exposure in retrospective reports, there was no other pattern of anomalies (isolated or syndromic) (6). (See required statement below.)

A study published in 1999 evaluated the safety, efficacy, and perinatal transmission rates of HIV in 30 pregnant women receiving various combinations of antiretroviral agents (7). Many of the women were substance abusers. Lamivudine was taken by 29 women in various combinations that included zidovudine, nelfinavir, indinavir, stavudine, nevirapine, and saquinavir. Antiretroviral therapy was initiated at a median of 14 weeks' gestation (range preconception to 32 weeks). In spite of previous histories of extensive antiretroviral experience and of vertical transmission of HIV, combination therapy was effective in treating maternal disease and in preventing transmission to the current newborns. The outcomes of the pregnancies included one stillbirth, one case of microcephaly, and five infants with birth weights <2500 g, two of whom were premature (7).

In an unusual case, a woman was exposed to HIV through self-insemination with fresh semen obtained from a man with a high HIV ribonucleic acid viral load (>750,000 copies/mL plasma) (8). Ten days later, she was started on a prophylactic regimen of lamivudine (300 mg/day), zidovudine (600 mg/day), and indinavir (2400 mg/day). Pregnancy was confirmed 14 days after insemination. The indinavir dose was reduced to 1800 mg/day, 4 weeks after the start of therapy because of the development of renal calculi. All antiretroviral therapy was stopped after 9 weeks because of negative tests for HIV. She gave birth at 40 weeks' gestation to a healthy 3490-g male infant, without evidence of HIV disease, who was developing normally at 2 years of age (8).

Several reports have described the apparent safe use of lamivudine, usually in combination with other agents, during human pregnancy (9–12). Occasional mild adverse effects were observed in the newborns (e.g., anemia), but no birth defects attributable to drug therapy. In one report, lamivudine concentrations in the newborn were similar to those in the mother (11).

A 1999 report from France described the possible association of zidovudine and lamivudine (NRTIs) use in pregnancy with mitochondrial dysfunction in the offspring (13). Mitochondrial disease is relatively rare in France (estimated prevalence 1 in 5000–20,000 children). From an ongoing epidemiological survey of 1754 mother–child pairs exposed to zidovudine and other agents during pregnancy, however, 8 children with possible mitochondrial dysfunction were identified. None of the eight infants was infected with HIV, but all received prophylaxis for up to 6 weeks after birth with the same antiretroviral regimen as given during pregnancy. Four of the cases were exposed to zidovudine alone and four to a combination of zidovudine and lamivudine. Two from the combination group died at about 1 year of age. All eight cases had abnormally low respiratory-chain enzyme activities. The authors concluded that their results supported the hypothesis of a causative association between mitochondrial respiratory-chain dysfunction and NRTIs. Moreover, the toxicity may have been potentiated by combination of these agents (13).

In a paper following the above study, investigators noted that NRTIs inhibit DNA polymerase γ, the enzyme responsible for mitochondrial DNA replication (14). They then hypothesized that this inhibition would induce depletion of mitochondrial DNA and mitochondrial DNA-encoded mitochondrial enzymes, thus resulting in mitochondrial dysfunction. Moreover, they stated that support for their hypothesis was suggested by the closeness of the clinical manifestations of inherited mitochondrial diseases with the adverse effects attributed to NRTIs. These adverse effects included polyneuropathy, myopathy, cardiomyopathy, pancreatitis, bone marrow suppression, and lactic acidosis. They also postulated this mechanism was involved in the development of a lipodystrophy syndrome of peripheral fat wasting and central adiposity, a condition that has been thought to be related to protease inhibitors (14).

A commentary on the above two studies concluded that the evidence for NRTI-induced mitochondrial dysfunction was equivocal (1). First, the clinical presentations in the infants were varied and not suggestive of a single cause; indeed, three of infants were symptom-free and one had Leigh's syndrome, a classic mitochondrial disease. Second, the clinical features, in some cases, were not suggestive of mitochondrial dysfunction. Although three had neurological symptoms, none had raised levels of lactate in the cerebrospinal fluid. Moreover, histological or histochemical features of mitochondrial disease were found in only two cases. Finally, low mitochondrial DNA, which would have been direct evidence of NRTI toxicity, was not found in the three cases in which it was measured (1).

A case of combined transient mitochondrial and peroxisomal β-oxidation dysfunction after exposure to NRTIs (lamivudine and zidovudine) combined with protease inhibitors (ritonavir and saquinavir) throughout gestation was reported in 2000 (15). A male infant was delivered at 38 weeks' gestation. He received postnatal prophylaxis with lamivudine and zidovudine for 4 weeks until the agents were discontinued because of anemia. Other adverse effects that were observed in the infant (age at onset) were hypocalcemia (shortly after birth), Group B streptococcal sepsis, ventricular extrasystoles, prolonged metabolic acidosis, and lactic acidemia (8 weeks), a mild elevation of long chain fatty acids (9 weeks), and neutropenia (3 months). The metabolic acidosis required treatment until 7 months of age, whereas the elevated plasma lactate resolved over 4 weeks. Cerebrospinal fluid lactate was not determined nor was a muscle biopsy conducted. Both the neutropenia and the cardiac dysfunction had resolved by 1 year of age. The elevated plasma fatty acid level was confirmed in cultured fibroblasts, but other peroxisomal functions (plasmalogen biosynthesis and catalase staining) were normal. Although mitochondrial dysfunction has been linked to NRTIs, the authors were unable to identify the cause of the combined abnormalities in the infant. The child was reported to be healthy and developing normally at 26 months of age (15).

A case of life-threatening anemia following in utero exposure to antiretroviral agents was described in 1998 (16). A 30-year-old woman with HIV infection was treated with zidovudine, didanosine, and trimethoprim/sulfamethoxazole (three times weekly) during the 1st trimester. Vitamin supplementation was also given. Because of an inadequate response, didanosine was discontinued and lamivudine and zalcitabine were started in the 3rd trimester. Two weeks before delivery the HIV viral load was undetectable. At term, a pale, male infant was delivered who developed respiratory distress shortly after birth. Examination revealed a hyperactive precordium and hepatomegaly without evidence of hydrops. The hematocrit was 11% with a reticulocyte count of zero. An extensive work-up of the mother and infant failed to determine the cause of the anemia. Bacterial and viral infections, including HIV, parvovirus B19, cytomegalovirus, and others, were excluded. The infant received a transfusion and was apparently doing well at 10 weeks of age. Because no other cause of the anemia could be found, the authors attributed the condition to bone morrow suppression, most likely to zidovudine. A contribution of the other agents to the condition, however, could not be excluded (16).

Two reviews, one in 1996 and the other in 1997, concluded that all women currently receiving antiretroviral therapy should continue to receive therapy during pregnancy and that treatment of the mother with monotherapy should be considered inadequate therapy (17,18). The same conclusion was reached in a 2003 review with the added admonishment that therapy must be continuous to prevent emergence of resistant viral strains (19). In 2009, the updated United States Department of Health and Human Services guidelines for the use of antiretroviral agents in HIV type 1 (HIV-1) infected patients continued the recommendation that therapy, with the exception of efavirenz, should be continued during pregnancy (20). If indicated, lamivudine should not be withheld in pregnancy because the expected benefit to the HIV-positive mother outweighs the unknown risk to the fetus.

A review published in 2000 described seven clinical trials that have been effective in reducing perinatal transmission, five with zidovudine alone, one with zidovudine plus lamivudine, and one with nevirapine (22). Six of the trials were in less-developed countries. Prolonged use of zidovudine in the mother and infant was the most effective for preventing vertical transmission, but also was the most expensive. The combination of lamivudine and zidovudine, consisting of antepartum, intrapartum, and postpartum maternal therapy with continued therapy in the infant for 1 week, may have been as effective as prolonged zidovudine (22). The updated guidelines for the use of antiretroviral drugs to reduce perinatal HIV-1 transmission were released in 2010 (21). Women receiving antiretroviral therapy during pregnancy should continue the therapy but, regardless of the regimen, zidovudine administration is recommended during the intrapartum period to prevent vertical transmission of HIV to the newborn (21).

***Required Statement**: "The Registry's analytic approach is to evaluate specific classes of antiretroviral drugs (FIs [fusion inhibitor(s)], NRTIs [nucleoside analog reverse transcriptase inhibitor(s)], NNRTIs [nonnucleoside reverse transcriptase inhibitor(s)], NtRTIs [nucleotide reverse transcriptase inhibitors], and PIs [protease inhibitor(s)]). The following specific drugs have large enough groups of exposed women to warrant a separate analysis: abacavir, didanosine, efavirenz, lamivudine, lopinavir, nelfinavir, nevirapine, ritonavir, stavudine, tenofovir, and zidovudine.*

L

No increases in risk of overall birth defects or specific defects have been detected to date. For lamivudine and zidovudine sufficient numbers of 1st trimester exposures have been monitored to detect at least a 1.5-fold increase in risk of overall birth defects and a twofold increase in risk of birth defects in the more common classes, cardiovascular and genitourinary systems. No such increases have been detected to date. For abacavir, efavirenz, nelfinavir, nevirapine, ritonavir, and stavudine sufficient numbers of 1st trimester exposures have been monitored to detect at least a twofold increase in risk of overall birth defects. No such increases have been detected to date. Although no pattern of birth defects has been detected with didanosine, the Committee continues to monitor the apparent increased frequency of defects among infants exposed to didanosine in the 1st trimester of gestation.

To date, the Registry has not demonstrated an increased prevalence of birth defects overall, or in the specific classes studied, or among women exposed to abacavir, efavirenz, lamivudine, nelfinavir, nevirapine, ritonavir, stavudine, or zidovudine individually or in combination during the 1st trimester when compared with observed rates for "early diagnoses" in population-based birth defects surveillance systems. While the Registry to date has not detected a major teratogenic signal overall or within classes of drugs or the individual drugs analyzed separately, the population exposed and monitored to date is not sufficient to detect an increase in the risk of relatively rare defects. These findings should provide some assurance when counseling patients."

L

BREASTFEEDING SUMMARY

Lamivudine is excreted into breast milk. In 10 women on lamivudine monotherapy (300 mg/day), the mean drug concentrations in maternal serum and breast milk were 0.55 and 1.22 mcg/mL, respectively (5). The infants were not allowed to breastfeed.

Reports on the use of lamivudine during breastfeeding are unlikely because the antiviral agent is used in the treatment of HIV infection. HIV-1 is transmitted in milk, and in developed countries, breastfeeding is not recommended (17,18,20,23–25). In developing countries, breastfeeding is undertaken, despite the risk, because there are no affordable milk substitutes available. Until 1999, no studies had been published that examined the effect of any antiretroviral therapy on HIV-1 transmission in milk. In that year, a study involving zidovudine was published that measured a 38% reduction in vertical transmission of HIV-1 infection despite breastfeeding when compared with controls (see Zidovudine).

References

1. Morris AAM, Carr A. HIV nucleoside analogues: new adverse effects on mitochondria? Lancet 1999;354:1046–7.
2. Product information. Epivir. Glaxo Wellcome, 2001.
3. Venerosi A, Valanzano A, Alleva E, Calamandrei G. Prenatal exposure to anti-HIV drugs: neurobehavioral effects of zidovudine (AZT) + lamivudine (3TC) treatment in mice. Teratology 2001;63:26–37.
4. Bloom SL, Dias KM, Bawdon RE, Gilstrap LC III. The maternal-fetal transfer of lamivudine in the ex vivo human placenta. Am J Obstet Gynecol 1997;176:291–3.
5. Moodley J, Moodley D, Pillay K, Coovadia H, Saba J, van Leeuwen R, Goodwin C, Harrigan PR, Moore KHP, Stone C, Plumb R, Johnson MA. Pharmacokinetics and antiretroviral activity of lamivudine alone or when coadministered with zidovudine in human immunodeficiency virus type 1-infected pregnant women and their offspring. J Infect Dis 1998;178:1327–33.
6. Antiretroviral Pregnancy Registry Steering Committee. *Antiretroviral Pregnancy Registry International Interim Report for 1 January 1989 through 31 July 2009.* Wilmington, NC: Registry Coordinating Center, 2009. Available at www.apregistry.com. Accessed May 29, 2010.
7. McGowan JP, Crane M, Wiznia AA, Blum S. Combination antiretroviral therapy in human immunodeficiency virus-infected pregnant women. Obstet Gynecol 1999;94:641–6.
8. Bloch M, Carr A, Vasak E, Cunningham P, Smith D. The use of human immunodeficiency virus postexposure prophylaxis after successful artificial insemination. Am J Obstet Gynecol 1999;181:760–1.
9. Scott GB, Tuomala R. Combination antiretroviral therapy during pregnancy. AIDS 1998;12:2495–7.
10. Lorenzi P, Spicher VM, Laubereau B, Hirschel B, Kind C, Rudin C, Irion O, Kaiser L. Antiretroviral therapies in pregnancy: maternal, fetal and neonatal effects. Swiss HIV Cohort Study, the Swiss Collaborative HIV and Pregnancy Study, and the Swiss Neonatal HIV Study. AIDS 1998;12:F241–7.
11. Grubert TA, Wintergerst U, Lutz-Friedrich R, Belohradsky BH, Rolinski B. Long-term antiretroviral combination therapy including lamivudine in HIV-1 infected women during pregnancy. AIDS 1999;13:1430–1.
12. Ristola M, Salo E, Ammala P, Suni J. Combined stavudine and lamivudine during pregnancy. AIDS 1999;13:285.
13. Blanche S, Tardieu M, Rustin P, Slama A, Barret B, Firtion G, Ciraru-Vigneron N, Lacroix C, Rouzioux C, Mandelbrot L, Desguerre I, Rotig A, Mayaux MJ, Delfraissy JF. Persistent mitochondrial dysfunction and perinatal exposure to antiretroviral nucleoside analogues. Lancet 1999;354:1084–9.
14. Brinkman K, Smeitink JA, Romijn JA, Reiss P. Mitochondrial toxicity induced by nucleoside-analogue reverse-transcriptase inhibitors is a key factor in the pathogenesis of antiretroviral-therapy-related lipodystrophy. Lancet 1999;354:1112–5.
15. Stojanov S, Wintergerst U, Belohradsky BH. Mitochondrial and peroxisomal dysfunction following perinatal exposure to antiretroviral drugs. AIDS 2000;14:1669.
16. Watson WJ, Stevens TP, Weinberg GA. Profound anemia in a newborn infant of a mother receiving antiretroviral therapy. Pediatr Infect Dis J 1998;17:435–6.
17. Carpenter CCJ, Fischi MA, Hammer SM, Hirsch MS, Jacobsen DM, Katzenstein DA, Montaner JSG, Richman DD, Saag MS, Schooley RT, Thompson MA, Vella S, Yeni PG, Volberding PA. Antiretroviral therapy for HIV infection in 1996. JAMA 1996;276;146–54.
18. Minkoff H, Augenbraun M. Antiretroviral therapy for pregnant women. Am J Obstet Gynecol 1997;176:478–89.
19. Minkoff H. Human immunodeficiency virus infection in pregnancy. Obstet Gynecol 2003;101:797–810.
20. Panel on Antiretroviral Guidelines for Adults and Adolescents. *Guidelines for the Use of Antiretroviral Agents in HIV-1-infected Adults and Adolescents.* Department of Health and Human Services. December 1, 2009;1–161. Available at http://www.aidsinfo.nih.gov/ContentFiles/AdultandAdolescentGL.pdf. Accessed September 17, 2010:60, 96–8.
21. Panel on Treatment of HIV-Infected Pregnant Women and Prevention of Perinatal Transmission. *Recommendations for Use of Antiretroviral Drugs in Pregnant HIV-1-Infected Women for Maternal Health and Interventions to Reduce Perinatal HIV Transmission in the United States.* May 24, 2010:1–117. Available at http://aidsinfo.nih.gov/ContentFiles/PerinatalGL.pdf. Accessed September 17, 2010:30 (Table 5).
22. Mofenson LM, McIntrye JA. Advances and research directions in the prevention of mother-to-child HIV-1 transmission. Lancet 2000;355:2237–44.
23. Brown ZA, Watts DH. Antiviral therapy in pregnancy. Clin Obstet Gynecol 1990;33:276–89.
24. de Martino M, Tovo P-A, Tozzi AE, Pezzotti P, Galli L, Livadiotti S, Caselli D, Massironi E, Ruga E, Fioredda F, Plebani A, Gabiano C, Zuccotti GV. HIV-1 transmission through breast-milk: appraisal of risk according to duration of feeding. AIDS 1992;6:991–7.
25. Van de Perre P. Postnatal transmission of human immunodeficiency virus type 1: the breast feeding dilemma. Am J Obstet Gynecol 1995;173:483–7.

LAMOTRIGINE

Anticonvulsant

PREGNANCY RECOMMENDATION: Compatible—Maternal Benefit >> Embryo–Fetal Risk
BREASTFEEDING RECOMMENDATION: Limited Human Data—Potential Toxicity

PREGNANCY SUMMARY

Women with epilepsy may have a higher risk of delivering an infant with a malformation than those who do not have this condition. Reproduction studies with lamotrigine in two animal species showed evidence, in the presence of maternal toxicity, of developmental toxicity (growth restriction, behavioral deficits, and death) but not structural anomalies. Moreover, at least two reviews have concluded that this anticonvulsant may be associated with a lower risk of teratogenicity (1,2). However, a recent report has shown a significant risk for oral clefts following 1st trimester exposure (3). A 2012 review concluded that the absolute risk of lamotrigine-induced cleft lip and palate or cleft palate alone was between 0.1% and 0.4% (4). In addition, a significant increase in the risk for major defects has been reported when lamotrigine was combined with valproate (5).

FETAL RISK SUMMARY

Lamotrigine is an anticonvulsant, chemically unrelated to existing antiepileptic drugs, that is used as adjunctive therapy for the treatment of partial seizures in patients with epilepsy. It is also indicated for the maintenance treatment of bipolar disorder to delay the time to occurrence of mood episodes. Protein binding is moderate (about 55%) and the agent is metabolized to inactive metabolites (6).

Lamotrigine was not teratogenic in animal reproductive studies involving mice, rats, and rabbits using oral doses that were 1.2, 0.5, and 1.1 times, respectively, the highest usual human maintenance dose (500 mg/day) based on BSA (HUHMD). However, maternal toxicity and secondary fetal toxicity consisting of reduced fetal weight and/or delayed ossification were observed at these doses in mice and rats but not in rabbits. Behavioral deficits were observed in the offspring of rats dosed with 0.1 and 0.5 times the HUHMD during organogenesis. No structural defects were observed after IV bolus doses in rats and rabbits, but an increased incidence of intrauterine fetal death occurred in rats dosed at 0.6 times the HUHMD. Similarly, an increase in fetal deaths occurred in rats dosed orally at 0.1, 0.14, or 0.3 times the HUHMD during the latter part of gestation. These doses were maternally toxic (decreased food consumption and weight). Postnatal deaths also were observed with the two highest doses (6).

No evidence of carcinogenicity was observed in 2-year studies in mice and rats. In multiple other tests, there was no evidence of mutagenicity or clastogenicity, and no impairment of fertility in rats (6).

Lamotrigine reduces fetal folate levels in rats, an effect known to be associated with malformations in animals and humans (6). Human fetal folate levels have apparently not been investigated, but in studies with nonpregnant humans, the drug's inhibitory action of dihydrofolate reductase did not significantly reduce folate levels (7). Serum folate and red blood cell folate concentrations were within the 95% confidence interval (CI) of the baseline values.

Lamotrigine crosses the human placenta (8–10). A 24-year-old woman had been treated before and throughout gestation with the anticonvulsant (300 mg/day) in combination with valproic acid (8). The latter drug was discontinued during the 3rd week of pregnancy. Her lamotrigine serum levels decreased from 17.8 mcg/mL (2 weeks after her last dose of valproic acid) to 2.52 mcg/mL at week 34, but she remained seizure-free throughout pregnancy. She delivered a healthy, 3620-g male infant at 39 weeks' gestation. The umbilical cord blood lamotrigine concentration was 3.26 mcg/mL, indicating a probable cord:maternal serum ratio of 1 (maternal serum level at delivery not reported). On the second day after delivery and a few hours after commencing suckling, the serum concentrations in the infant and mother were 2.79 and 3.88 mcg/mL, respectively, a ratio of 0.7. A 1997 case report found that maternal lamotrigine plasma levels decreased during pregnancy (9). The woman in that case delivered a healthy infant (weight and sex not given) at term. At delivery, the umbilical cord:maternal plasma ratio was 1.2.

In a 2000 report, maternal and cord plasma concentrations of lamotrigine were determined at term delivery in nine women (10 pregnancies; 1 woman with 2 pregnancies also reported in reference 3) (10). Maternal and cord plasma levels were similar. At 72 hours postpartum, median lamotrigine plasma levels in the infants were 75% of the cord plasma levels (range 50%–100%). The placental transfer is consistent with the low molecular weight (about 256). Moreover, during the first 2 weeks after delivery, the median increase in maternal plasma concentration/dose ratio was 170%, a significant increase (10).

A 2004 report described 12 pregnancies in which women were treated with lamotrigine monotherapy for epilepsy (11). An increase in seizure frequency and/or severity occurred in nine pregnancies, attributed to a gradual decrease in the serum-to-dose ratio to 40% of baseline. Consequently, the doses were increased in seven pregnancies. Three to ten days after delivery, toxic symptoms (dizziness, diplopia, or ataxia) occurred in three of the women with dose increases. Lamotrigine serum levels were 12–14 mcg/mL, a high normal range. The symptoms resolved when the dose was decreased (11).

A 2005 abstract reported 62 pregnancy outcomes after exposure to gabapentin, lamotrigine, or topiramate (12).

The study included a blinded dysmorphology examination. Nineteen women used lamotrigine, one of whom had a major malformation: coarctation of the aorta with anomalous left coronary artery, frontal hair upsweep, and a long philtrum (monotherapy for seizures). Of the nine infants examined by a dysmorphologist, none had more than one feature consistent with anticonvulsant embryopathy (12).

The Lamotrigine Pregnancy Registry, an ongoing project conducted by the manufacturer, was closed to new enrollments in June 2009 and the final report was issued in July 2010 (5). The final report covers pregnancy exposures from September 1992 through March 2010. There were 3416 pregnancies registered prospectively (reported to the Registry before the pregnancy outcome was known), 2444 were closed with known outcomes, and 972 (28.5%) were lost to follow-up. In the 2444 known pregnancy outcomes, there were 43 sets of twins, 1 set of triplets and 1 set of quadruplets, for a total of 2492 fetal outcomes. Among the 1817 fetal outcomes involving lamotrigine monotherapy, there were 1636 live births (defects not reported but cannot be ruled out), 98 spontaneous abortions (SABs), 33 elective abortions (EABs), and 10 fetal deaths without defects. Major birth defects were observed in 36 live births, 3 EABs, and 1 fetal death. Excluding SABs, EABs, and fetal deaths without defects, the earliest exposure by trimester was 1554 (1st), 95 (2nd), 18 (3rd), and 5 not specified. Major birth defects were observed in 35 1st trimester exposures (31 live births, 1 fetal death, and 3 EABs), 4 live births in the 2nd trimester, and 1 live birth in the 3rd trimester. The rate of major birth defects in the 1st trimester exposures was 2.2% (35/1558 excluding fetal deaths and EABs without defects). The sample size of 1558 was sufficient to detect, with 80% power, at least a 1.39- to 1.48-fold increase over baseline in the overall rate of major birth defects (5).

Polytherapy (lamotrigine plus at least one other AED) with valproate involved 173 outcomes: 159 live births, 6 SABs, 6 EABs, and 2 fetal deaths. Among 161 1st trimester exposures, there were 14 live births and 2 EABs with birth defects, 6 SABs, and 139 outcomes without defects (134 live births, 4 EABs, and 1 fetal death). Excluding the 6 SABs, and the 4 EABs and 1 fetal death without defects, the rate of birth defects in the 1st trimester exposures was 10.7% (16/150). Polytherapy without valproate involved 502 outcomes: 457 live births, 22 SABs, 20 EABs, and 3 fetal deaths. Among 474 1st trimester exposures, there were 11 live births and 1 EAB with birth defects, 22 SABs, and 440 outcomes without defects (418 live births, 19 EABs, and 3 fetal deaths). Excluding the 22 SABs, and the 10 EABs and 3 fetal deaths without defects, the rate of birth defects in the 1st trimester exposures was 2.8% (12/430) (5).

The Registry listed the major birth defects observed in the monotherapy and polytherapy groups and concluded that there was no consistent pattern among the defects. Although the data were insufficient to reach a definite conclusion, the Registry found no evidence of a dose–response effect with daily doses of lamotrigine up to 1200 mg/day (5).

Retrospective cases (reported to the Registry after the pregnancy outcome was known) are often biased (only adverse outcomes are reported), but they are useful in identifying specific patterns of anomalies suggestive of a common cause. There were 164 pregnancies with birth defects reported retrospectively to the Registry, 142 involving earliest exposure to lamotrigine in the 1st trimester, 4 with earliest exposure in the 2nd trimester, and 18 with an unspecified trimester of exposure. Lamotrigine monotherapy was used in 94 pregnancies, while 70 involved polytherapy (5).

As of 1996, the FDA had received three disparate reports of birth defects, in which lamotrigine was used in combination with other anticonvulsants during the affected pregnancy (F. Rosa, personal communication, FDA, 1996).

A 1998 noninterventional, observational cohort study described the outcomes of pregnancies in women who had been prescribed ≥1 of 34 newly marketed drugs by general practitioners in England (13). Data were obtained by questionnaires sent to the prescribing physicians one month after the expected or possible date of delivery. In 831 of the pregnancies (78%), a newly marketed drug was thought to have taken during the 1st trimester with birth defects noted in 14 (2.5%) singleton births of the 557 newborns (10 sets of twins). In addition, two birth defects were observed in aborted fetuses. However, few of the aborted fetuses were examined. Lamotrigine was taken during the 1st trimester in 59 pregnancies. The outcomes of these pregnancies included 10 SABs, 1 missed abortion, 9 EABs, 35 normal newborns (4 premature), and 4 newborns with congenital malformations. The malformations observed were ventricular septal defect; congenital respiratory stridor; palatal cleft (soft palate only), hypospadias, and undescended testes (mother had convulsions early in gestation); and abdominal distension with possible congenital intestinal obstruction. In three of these cases, lamotrigine was given in various combinations with other anticonvulsants (e.g., carbamazepine, phenytoin, phenobarbital, and/or sodium valproate). In addition, the study lacked the sensitivity to identify minor anomalies because of the absence of standardized examinations. Late-appearing major defects may also have been missed due to the timing of the questionnaires (13).

A significant association between lamotrigine and isolated, nonsyndromic oral clefts has been reported (3). The findings were published in May 2006 and presented at the June 2006 annual meeting of the Teratology Society in Tucson, Arizona. The cases were collected between 1997 and 2006 by the North American Antiepileptic Drug Pregnancy Registry (North American AED Pregnancy Registry). Among 564 infants (including live births, stillbirths, and elective terminations for anomalies) exposed to lamotrigine monotherapy in the 1st trimester, 15 had major malformations. The prevalence was 2.7% (95% CI 1.5%–4.3%) compared with 1.62% in an unexposed comparison group (N = 221,746 births) (relative risk [RR] 1.7; 95% CI 1.0–2.7). Five infants in the lamotrigine-exposed group had oral clefts (8.9/1000 births): three isolated cleft palate and two isolated cleft lip. None had a recognized syndrome (3).

In the comparison group, the prevalence of the two defects was 1:6160 (0.16/1000) and 1:4820 (0.21/1000), respectively. The RRs attributed to lamotrigine for cleft palate and cleft lip were 32.8 (95% CI 10.6–101.3) and 17.1 (95% CI 4.3–68.2), respectively. The authors thought that the low rates of oral clefts in the comparison group reflected the limited identification of syndromes associated with cleft lip and/or palate. In five other registries that reported 1623 lamotrigine-exposed infants, four infants had oral clefts for a frequency of 2.5/1000 compared with 0.37/1000 in the comparison group. The combined findings showed a significant risk of oral clefts following 1st trimester exposure to lamotrigine monotherapy (3).

An update to the North American AED Pregnancy Registry was published in 2008 (14). Among 684 infants exposed in utero to lamotrigine monotherapy, 16 (2.3%) had major malformations identified at birth, well within the normal background rate. However, five infants (7.3/1000) had oral clefts: three with isolated cleft palate and one each with isolated cleft lip or cleft lip and palate. The rate was 10.4 times the rate among a comparison group of 206,224 unexposed infants (0.7/1000). A comparison also was made with 1623 infants exposed to lamotrigine monotherapy who had enrolled in five other registries. In that group there were four infants with oral clefts (2.5/1000) (RR 3.8, 95% CI 1.4–10.0) (14).

In a population-based case–control study, the EUROCAT Antiepileptic Drug Working Group evaluated data for 3.9 million births from 19 registries covering the period 1995–2005 (15). The data included congenital anomalies among live births, stillbirths, and terminations of pregnancy after prenatal diagnosis. Cases were 5511 nonsyndromic oral clefts, 4571 of whom were isolated oral clefts. In these, there were 1969 cases of cleft palate, 1532 of whom were isolated cleft palate. Controls were 80,052 nonchromosomal, nonepileptic, non-AED-use pregnancies. In the cases, there were 40 pregnancies exposed to lamotrigine monotherapy. Comparisons were made between the monotherapy and the control group for oral clefts relative to other malformations, for isolated oral clefts, cleft palate, and isolated cleft palate. None of the comparisons reached statistical significance. However, when the same comparisons were made between any AED use and no AED use, significant results were found for oral clefts relative to other malformations, cleft palate, and isolated cleft palate (15).

An editorial discussed the results from the above two studies, noting the small number of oral cleft cases in the two reports (five in the North American Registry and three in the EUROCAT) study (16). The editorial also listed the limitations in both. The conclusion was that although the overall risk for oral clefts from lamotrigine monotherapy was low, there was a specific signal that required clarification by additional studies.

A 2013 study reported dose-dependent associations with reduced cognitive abilities across a range of domains at 6 years of age after fetal valproate exposure (17). Analysis showed that IQ was significantly lower for valproate (mean 97, 95% CI 94–101) than for carbamazepine (mean 105, 95% CI 102–108; $p = 0.0015$), lamotrigine (mean 108, 95% CI 105–110; $p = 0.0003$), or phenytoin (mean 108, 95% CI 104–112; $p = 0.0006$). Mean IQs were higher in children whose mothers had taken folic acid (mean 108, 95% CI 106–111) compared with children whose mothers had not taken the vitamin (mean 101, 95% CI 98–104; $p = 0.0009$) (17).

In a 2009 case report, a 38-year-old woman took lamotrigine during the latter portion of one pregnancy and throughout another pregnancy (18). Both infants appeared to be normal, although a benign peripheral pulmonary stenosis was discovered at 16 days of age in the second infant. This infant also had an apneic episode and became cyanotic (see Breastfeeding Summary).

A 2006 review of prophylactic therapy of bipolar disorder briefly described the effects in pregnancy and breastfeeding of a number of drugs, including lamotrigine (19). Untreated pregnant and nursing women with the disorder are at an increased risk of poor obstetrical outcomes and relapse of affective symptoms. Although the limited data prevented conclusions on the relative safety of the drugs, the author did state that each case needed to be considered separately (19).

A study published in 2009 examined the effect of AEDs on the head circumference in newborns (20). Significant reductions in mean birth-weight-adjusted mean head circumference (bw-adj-HC) was noted for monotherapy with carbamazepine and valproic acid. No effect on bw-adj-HC was observed with gabapentin, phenytoin, clonazepam, and lamotrigine. A significant increase in the occurrence of microcephaly (bw-adj-HC smaller than 2 standard deviations below the mean) was noted after any AED polytherapy but not after any monotherapy, including carbamazepine and valproic acid. The potential effects of these findings on child development warrant study (20).

The pharmacokinetics of lamotrigine were described in 2002 (21). The clearance of the drug increases by >50% starting early in pregnancy and reverts to the nonpregnant state quickly after delivery. Lamotrigine blood levels should be checked before, during, and after pregnancy.

BREASTFEEDING SUMMARY

Lamotrigine is excreted into breast milk (6,8–10,18,22–25). A 24-year-old mother who had been treated throughout gestation with lamotrigine (see details above) began nursing her infant on the 2nd day after delivery (8). At this time, she was taking 300 mg/day, decreased to 200 mg/day approximately 6 weeks postpartum to lessen the drug exposure of the infant. From day 2 to day 145 after delivery, 11 maternal serum and 9 milk samples (about 2–3 hours after the morning dose) were drawn, with lamotrigine serum concentrations ranging from 3.59 to 9.61 mcg/mL and milk levels ranging from 1.26 to 6.51 mcg/mL. The mean milk:serum ratio was 0.56 with a high correlation ($r = 0.959$, $p < 0.01$) between the serum and milk. The infant's serum levels (about 1–2 hours after breastfeeding), determined at the same times as the mother's, ranged from <0.2 mcg/mL (during weaning) to 2.79 mcg/mL. No adverse effects were observed in the nursing infant either during breastfeeding or during weaning (8).

A 60-kg woman took lamotrigine 200 mg/day throughout gestation and during nursing (9). Two weeks after delivery, the milk:maternal plasma ratio was 0.6. The infant's plasma level, which had been similar to the mother's at birth, was now 25% of the maternal levels. No adverse effects were observed in the nursing infant (9).

In a 2000 report, nine women (10 pregnancies, one woman with two pregnancies also reported in reference 3) received lamotrigine throughout gestation (see Fetal Risk Summary above) and continued the drug during breastfeeding (10). The median milk:maternal plasma ratio 2–3 weeks after delivery was 0.61 (range 0.47–0.77). The lamotrigine plasma concentrations in the infants were approximately 30% (range 23%–50%) of the corresponding maternal plasma levels. The estimated infant lamotrigine dose was ≥0.2–1 mg/kg/day, assuming a milk intake of 150 mL/kg/day, about 9% of the weight-adjusted maternal daily dose. Because of the slow elimination in the infant (most likely due to reduced hepatic glucuronidation capacity), the marked increase in maternal plasma lamotrigine concentrations that occurred after birth (see Fetal Risk Summary above), and the fact that infant drug levels may not have reached steady-state concentrations, the infant exposure could eventually result in therapeutic plasma lamotrigine levels. No adverse effect in the nursing infants was observed (10).

A 38-year-old woman took lamotrigine throughout her third pregnancy for a seizure disorder caused by a pilocytic astrocytoma 6 years earlier (18). Although the brain tumor had been removed surgically, she had residual epilepsy that was treated with lamotrigine. In her second pregnancy, she started daily lamotrigine 550 mg toward the end of the pregnancy, and then gradually reduced the dose while breastfeeding to 425 mg. The highest serum concentration, measured at 45 days postpartum, was 8.96 mcg/mL. No adverse effects were observed in the fully breastfed infant. In her third pregnancy, the mother's daily dose was increased from 450 mg (pregestation) to 875 mg (term). The dose at term was 10.9 mg/kg/day. Serum concentrations during this interval were 5.12 mcg/mL (pregestation), 3.30 mcg/mL (3rd trimester), and 4.53 mcg/mL (day of birth). She had a focal epileptic seizure during the 5th gestational month and a generalized tonic–clonic seizure shortly after delivery. She took her last 875-mg dose 20.5 hours before giving birth to a full-term, 4200-g male infant with Apgar scores of 9 and 9. Because of the latest seizure, a dose reduction was not started until the 2nd week. The infant was exclusively breastfed. His lamotrigine concentration approximately 12.5 hours after birth was 7.71 mcg/mL (proposed pediatric therapeutic range 1–5 mcg/mL). At age 3 days, his serum concentration was 5.81 mcg/mL. At 16 days of age, his breathing became irregular and strenuous and he had a brief episode of apnea. Three hours after the first apneic episode, he became cyanotic while nursing. The mother, a physician, successfully resuscitated him and took him to the hospital. On admission, his lamotrigine serum concentration was 4.87 mcg/mL (4 hours after the mother's 850-mg dose and 3 hours after nursing). Except for periodic sinus tachycardia (170–180 beats/minute) and a benign peripheral pulmonary stenosis, his examination and laboratory tests were normal. Breastfeeding was discontinued on postpartum day 17. The mother's lamotrigine serum concentration at this time was 14.93 mcg/mL. Her dose was decreased to 600 mg on postpartum day 22, and then gradually reduced to 525 mg by day 64. Using a milk concentration of 7.68 mcg/mL obtained on day 22, the theoretical infant dose (1.15 mg/kg/day) as a percentage of the mother's weight-adjusted dose was 13%. The milk:plasma ratio determined 4 times during postpartum days 22–64 was 0.79–0.96. Based on blood samples obtained 22 and 25 days after birth, the estimated lamotrigine half-life in the infant was 56 hours, about twice that seen in adults. The infant had no further apneic or cyanotic episodes and was developing normally at 7 months of age. The authors could not determine why the infant developed apnea but concluded that lamotrigine was the probable cause (18).

A 2004 study reported lamotrigine serum concentrations in four nursing infants, all of whom had been exposed throughout pregnancy (22). All the women had full-term deliveries of healthy babies. The doses on day 10 postpartum, the sampling day, were 200–800 mg/day. The infant: maternal plasma concentration ratios were 0.2, 0.2, 0.43, and ≤0.17 (infant <1 mcg/mL and maternal 5.2 mcg/mL), respectively. For the first two cases, sampling was repeated at 2 months of age with nearly identical ratios of 0.22 and 0.23, respectively, but both nursing infants were being supplemented with formula 2–3 times per day. No adverse effects were observed in the infants, but the authors were concerned because of the drug concentrations reaching "therapeutic ranges" (22).

A 2005 case report described a woman treated for epilepsy with partial seizures with 300 mg/day lamotrigine throughout pregnancy and during breastfeeding (23). The healthy, 3.3-kg male infant was spontaneous delivered at term with Apgar scores of 8 and 9. Development of the infant was normal during the first 4 breastfed months and no toxicity was observed (23).

A 2006 report quantified the amount of lamotrigine in the breast milk of six mothers and in the plasma of their breastfed infants (mean age 4.1 months; range 0.4–5.1 months) (24). The mothers, who obtained the milk samples by hand expression, were taking a mean dose of 400 mg/day (range 75–800 mg) for epilepsy (N = 5) or bipolar disorder (N = 1). The duration of treatment before the study was not stated. The mean maternal dose based on body weight was 6.3 mg/kg/day, whereas the mean absolute infant dose was 0.45 mg/kg/day. The daily infant dose relative to the mother's weight-adjusted dose was 7.6%. The mean infant plasma concentration of lamotrigine was 0.60 mg/L, a level that was a mean of 18% of the maternal plasma concentration. The mothers and physicians observed no adverse effects in the infants (24).

A 2008 report described steady-state lamotrigine concentrations in 26 women who were breastfeeding while taking the drug (25). The mean age of the infants was 13.0 weeks and the mean maternal dose was 5.93 mg/kg/day. The mean breast milk concentration was 3.38 mcg/mL (based on sampling from one breast every 4 hours for 24 hours) and the milk:plasma ratio was 0.413. The mean theoretical infant dose was 0.51 mg/kg/day and the relative infant dose was 9.2%. No adverse events were noted among the mothers or their nursing infants, but seven infants had elevated platelet counts without adverse clinical consequences (25).

As with any drug, a mother who must take lamotrigine to control her disease and who chooses to nurse her infant should carefully monitor the infant for adverse effects. Some anticonvulsants have produced adverse effects in nursing infants (see Phenobarbital and Primidone); whereas others are considered compatible with breastfeeding. (See Carbamazepine, Phenytoin, and Valproic Acid.) No adverse effects have been seen in nursing infants of mothers taking lamotrigine. Monitoring infant lamotrigine concentrations should be considered, as well as close monitoring for sedation and rash (26).

In a 2010 study, 199 children who had been breastfed while their mothers were taking a single antiepileptic drug (carbamazepine, lamotrigine, phenytoin, or valproate) were evaluated at 3 years of age cognitive outcome (27). Mean adjusted IQ scores for exposed children were 99 (95% CI 96–103), whereas the mean adjusted IQ scores of nonbreastfed infants were 98 (95% CI 95–101).

Because of the potential for therapeutic serum concentrations in the infant, the American Academy of Pediatrics classifies lamotrigine as a drug for which the effect on a nursing infant is unknown but may be of concern (28).

References

1. Dichter MA, Brodie MJ. New antiepileptic drugs. N Engl J Med 1996;334:1583–90.
2. Morrell MJ. The new antiepileptic drugs and women: efficacy, reproductive health, pregnancy, and fetal outcome. Epilepsia 1996;37(Suppl 6):S34–S44.
3. Holmes LB, Wyszynski DF, Baldwin EJ, Habecker E, Glassman LH, Smith CR. Increased risk for non-syndromic cleft palate among infants exposed to lamotrigine during pregnancy (abstract). Birth Defects Res A Clin Mol Teratol 2006;76:318.
4. Holmes LB, Hernandez-Diaz S. Newer anticonvulsants: lamotrigine, topiramate, and gabapentin. Birth Defects Res A Clin Mol Teratol 2012;94:599–606.
5. The Lamotrigine Pregnancy Registry. Final Report. 1 September 1992 through 31 March 2010. GlaxoSmithKline, July 2010.
6. Product information. Lamictal. GlaxoSmithKline, 2004.
7. Betts T, Goodwin G, Withers RM, Yuen AWC. Human safety of lamotrigine. Epilepsia 1991;32(Suppl 2):S17–S21.
8. Rambeck B, Kurlemann G, Stodieck SRG, May TW, Jurgens U. Concentrations of lamotrigine in a mother on lamotrigine treatment and her newborn child. Eur J Clin Pharmacol 1997;51:481–4.
9. Tomson T, Ohman I, Vitols S. Lamotrigine in pregnancy and lactation: a case report. Epilepsia 1997;38:1039–41.
10. Ohman I, Vitols S, Tomson T. Lamotrigine in pregnancy: pharmacokinetics during delivery, in the neonate, and during lactation. Epilepsia 2000;41:709–13.
11. de Haan GJ, Edelbroek P, Segers J, Engelsman M, Lindhout D, Devile-Notschaele M, Augustijn P. Gestation-induced changes in lamotrigine pharmacokinetics: a monotherapy study. Neurology 2004;63:571–3.
12. Chambers CD, Kao KK, Felix RJ, Alvarado S, Chavez C, Ye N, Dick LM, Jones KL. Pregnancy outcome in infants prenatally exposed to newer anticonvulsants (abstract). Birth Defects Res A Clin Mol Teratol 2005;73:316.
13. Wilton LV, Pearce GL, Martin RM, Mackay FJ, Mann RD. The outcomes of pregnancy in women exposed to newly marketed drugs in general practice in England. Br J Obstet Gynaecol 1998;105:882–9.
14. Holmes LB, Baldwin EJ, Smith CR, Habecker E, Glassman L, Wong SL, Wyszynski DF. Increased frequency of isolated cleft palate in infants exposed to lamotrigine during pregnancy. Neurology 2008;70:2152–8.
15. Dolk H, Jentink J, Loane M, Morris J, de Jong-van den Berg LTW. Does lamotrigine use in pregnancy increase orofacial cleft risk relative to other malformations? Neurology 2008;71:714–22.
16. Meador KJ, Penovich P. What is the risk of orofacial clefts from lamotrigine exposure during pregnancy? Neurology 2008;71:706–7.
17. Meador KJ, Baker GA, Browning N, Cohen MJ, Bromley RL, Clayton-Smith J, Kalayjian LA, Kanner A, Liporace JD, Pennell PB, Privitera M, Loring DW., for the NEAD Study Group. Fetal antiepileptic drug exposure and cognitive outcomes at age 6 years (NEAD study): a prospective observational study. Lancet Neurol 2013;12:244–52.
18. Nordmo E, Aronsen L, Wasland K, Smabrekke L, Vorren S. Severe apnea in an infant exposed to lamotrigine in breast milk. Ann Pharmacother 2009;43:1983–7.
19. Gentile S. Prophylactic treatment of bipolar disorder in pregnancy and breastfeeding: focus on emerging mood stabilizers. Bipolar Disord 2006;8:207–20.
20. Almgren M, Kallen B, Lavebratt C. Population-based study of antiepileptic drug exposure in utero—influence on head circumference in newborns. Seizure 2009;18:672–5.
21. Tran TA, Leppik IE, Blesi K, Sathanandan ST, Remmel R. Lamotrigine clearance during pregnancy. Neurology 2002;59:251–5.
22. Liporace J, Kao A, D'Abreu A. Concerns regarding lamotrigine and breast-feeding. Epilepsy Behav 2004;5:102–5.
23. Gentile S. Lamotrigine in pregnancy and lactation. Arch Womens Ment Health 2005;8:57–8.
24. Page-Sharp M, Kristensen JH, Hackett IP, Beran RG, Rampono J, Hale TW, Kohan R, Ilett KF. Transfer of lamotrigine into breast milk. Ann Pharmacother 2006;40:1470–1.
25. Newport DJ, Pennell PB, Calamaras MR, Ritchie JC, Newman M, Knight B, Viguera AC, Liporace J, Stowe ZN. Lamotrigine in breast milk and nursing infants: determination of exposure. Pediatrics 2008;122:e223–31.
26. Bar-Oz B, Nulman I, Koren G, Ito S. Anticonvulsants and breast feeding—a critical review. Paediatr Drugs 2000;2:113–26.
27. Meador KJ, Baker GA, Browning N, Clayton-Smith J, Combs-Cantrell DT, Cohen M, Kalayjian LA, Kanner A, Liporace JD, Pennell PB, Privitera M, Loring DW, for the NEAD Study Group. Effects of breastfeeding in children of women taking antiepileptic drugs. Neurology 2010;75:1954–60.
28. Committee on Drugs, American Academy of Pediatrics. The transfer of drugs and other chemicals into human milk. Pediatrics 2001;108:776–89.

LANATOSIDE C

Cardiac Glycoside

See Digitalis.

LANSOPRAZOLE

Gastrointestinal Agent (Antisecretory)

PREGNANCY RECOMMENDATION: Human Data Suggest Low Risk
BREASTFEEDING RECOMMENDATION: No Human Data—Potential Toxicity

PREGNANCY SUMMARY

The human and animal data for proton pump inhibitors (PPIs) suggest that this class of drugs can be considered low risk in pregnancy, but the human pregnancy experience for lansoprazole alone is still limited. A study showing an association between in utero exposure to gastric acid-suppressing drugs and childhood allergy and asthma requires confirmation. Birth defects, including cardiac defects, have been reported in pregnancies exposed to a PPI (see also Omeprazole), but there is no evidence of a causal association. Most likely, the observed defects were the result of many factors, including possibly the severity of the disease and concurrent use of other drugs. The data do warrant continued investigation. In addition, the studies lacked the sensitivity to detect minor anomalies because of the absence of standardized examinations. Late-appearing major defects may also have been missed due to the timing of some data collection. If lansoprazole is required or if inadvertent exposure does occur early in gestation, the known risk to the embryo–fetus appears to be low. Long-term follow-up of offspring exposed during gestation is warranted.

FETAL RISK SUMMARY

Lansoprazole is a PPI that blocks gastric acid secretion by a direct inhibitory effect on the gastric parietal cell (1). It is used for the treatment of gastric and duodenal ulcer, erosive esophagitis, gastroesophageal reflux disease (GERD), and pathologic hypersecretory conditions, such as Zollinger-Ellison syndrome. It is also used in combination with amoxicillin and/or clarithromycin for *Helicobacter pylori* eradication to reduce the risk of duodenal ulcer recurrence. Lansoprazole is in the same class of PPIs as dexlansoprazole, esomeprazole, omeprazole, pantoprazole, and rabeprazole.

Reproductive studies have been conducted in pregnant rats and rabbits at oral doses ≤40 and 16 times, respectively, the recommended human dose based on BSA (1). No evidence was found that these doses impaired fertility or caused fetal harm. Similar to other PPIs, lansoprazole is carcinogenic in mice and rats, producing dose-related gastric, testicular, and liver tumors (1). In addition, positive results were seen with lansoprazole in the in vitro human lymphocyte chromosomal aberration assays, but the Ames mutation assay and other genotoxic animal tests were negative (1).

In a study published in 1990, lansoprazole at a dose of 50 or 300 mg/kg was not teratogenic in pregnant rats, but a decrease in fetal weight occurred (2). Schardein also cited a 1990 study, which appears to be similar to the one cited above, that found no evidence of teratogenicity in rats and rabbits (3).

It is not known if lansoprazole crosses the human placenta. The molecular weight (about 369) is low enough that passage to the fetus should be expected. Another PPI, omeprazole, has a molecular weight (about 345) and chemical structure that are very similar to lansoprazole, and it is known to cross the human placenta (see Omeprazole).

A 1998 noninterventional, observational cohort study described the outcomes of pregnancies in women who had been prescribed ≥1 of 34 newly marketed drugs by general practitioners in England (4). Data were obtained by questionnaires sent to the prescribing physicians one month after the expected or possible date of delivery. In 831 (78%) of the pregnancies, a newly marketed drug was thought to have been taken during the 1st trimester, with birth defects noted in 14 (2.5%) singleton births of the 557 live newborns (10 sets of twins). In addition, two birth defects were observed in aborted fetuses. However, few of the aborted fetuses were examined. Lansoprazole was taken during the 1st trimester in six pregnancies. Seven healthy newborns (one premature; one set of twins) were delivered (4).

Data from the Swedish Medical Birth Registry were presented in 1998 (5). A total of 553 infants (6 sets of twins) were delivered from 547 women who had used acid-suppressing drugs early in pregnancy. The odds ratio (OR) for malformations after PPI exposure was 0.91, 95% confidence interval (CI) 0.45–1.84. Of the 19 infants with birth defects, 10 had been exposed to PPIs alone and 1 was also exposed to ranitidine. Lansoprazole was the only acid-suppressing drug exposure in 13 infants. Two of these infants had birth defects: an atrial septum defect and an undescended testicle (see Omeprazole for additional details of this study (5).

In a study published in 1999, investigators linked data from a Danish prescription database to a birth registry to evaluate the risks of PPIs for congenital malformations, low birth weight, and preterm delivery (<37 weeks') (6). From a total of 51 women who had filled a prescription for these drugs sometime during pregnancy, 38 (omeprazole N = 35, lansoprazole N = 3) had done so during the interval of 30 days before conception to the end of the 1st trimester. A control group, consisting of 13,327 pregnancies in which the mother had not obtained a prescription for reimbursed medication from 30 days before conception to the end of her pregnancy, was used for comparison. The prevalence of major congenital anomalies in controls was 5.2%. Three major birth defects (7.9%), two of which were cardiovascular anomalies, were observed from the 38 pregnancies possibly exposed in the 1st trimester (specific drug exposure not given): ventricular septum defect; pyloric stenosis; and one case of patent ductus arteriosus, atrial septum defect, hydronephrosis, and agenesis of the iris. In comparison with controls, the adjusted (for maternal age, birth order, gestational age, and smoking, but not for alcohol abuse) relative risks for the three outcomes were congenital malformations 1.6 (95% CI 0.5–5.2), low birth weight 1.8 (95% CI 0.2–13.1), and preterm delivery (not adjusted for gestational age) 2.3 (95% CI 0.9–6.0). Although the study found no elevated risks for the three outcomes, the investigators cautioned that more data were needed to assess the possible association between PPIs and cardiac malformations or preterm delivery (6).

A 2002 study conducted a meta-analysis involving the use of PPIs in pregnancy (7). In the five cohort studies analyzed, there were 593 infants, mostly exposed to omeprazole, but also including lansoprazole and pantoprazole. The relative risk (RR) for major malformations was 1.18, 95% CI 0.72–1.94 (7).

A 2005 study by the European Network of Teratology Information Services reported the outcomes of pregnancies exposed to omeprazole (N = 295), lansoprazole (N = 62), or pantoprazole (N = 53) (8). In the pantoprazole group, the median duration of treatment was 14 days (range 7–23 days) and the dose used was 40 mg/day. The outcomes consisted of one spontaneous abortion (SAB), three elective abortions (EABs) (none for congenital anomalies), one stillbirth, and 48 live births. One infant exposed early in gestation (week 2 for 8 days) had congenital toxoplasmosis. Compared with a nonexposed control group, there was no difference in the rate of major malformations between the lansoprazole and control groups (RR 1.04, 95% CI 0.25–4.21). Similar results were observed for omeprazole and pantoprazole (8).

A 2007 case report described the use of lansoprazole in a woman with Zollinger-Ellison syndrome (9). In the 1st trimester, she underwent a left lobectomy of the liver to remove a gastrin-secreting neuroendocrine tumor. Lansoprazole (30 mg three times a day) was taken throughout gestation. Ultrasound scans revealed a single umbilical artery and bilateral choroid plexus cysts with no other malformations. In the 38th week, she gave birth to a 3.370-kg male infant with Apgar scores of 8 and 10. A routine physical examination of the infant was normal. At the time of the report, the woman was in her second pregnancy and receiving the same oral treatment (9).

A population-based observational cohort study formed by linking data from three Swedish national healthcare registers over a 10-year period (1995–2004) was reported in 2009 (10). The main outcome measures were a diagnosis of allergic disease or a prescription for asthma or allergy medications. The drug types included in the study were gastric acid suppressors, including H_2-receptor antagonists, prostaglandins, PPIs, combinations for eradication of *Helicobacter pylori*, and drugs for peptic ulcer and GERD. Of 585,716 children, 29,490 (5.0%) met the diagnosis and 5645 (1%) had been exposed to gastric acid suppression therapy in pregnancy. Of these children, 405 (0.07%) were treated for allergic disease. For developing allergy, the odds ratio (OR) was 1.43, 98% CI 1.29–1.59, irrespective of the drug, time of exposure during pregnancy, and maternal history of allergy. For developing childhood asthma, but not other allergic diseases, the OR was 1.51, 95% CI 1.35–1.69, irrespective of the type of acid-suppressive drug and the time of exposure in pregnancy. The authors proposed three possible mechanisms for their findings: (a) exposure to increased amounts of allergens could cause sensitization to digestion-labile antigens in the fetus; (b) maternal Th2 cytokine pattern could promote an allergy-prone phenotype in the fetus; and (c) maternal allergen-specific IgE could cross the placenta and sensitize fetal immune cells to food- and airborne allergens. Several limitations of the study that might have affected their findings were identified, including a general increase in childhood asthma but not necessarily an increase in allergic asthma (10). The study requires confirmation.

A second meta-analysis of PPIs in pregnancy was reported in 2009 (11). Based on 1530 exposed compared with 133,410 not exposed pregnancies, the OR for major malformations was 1.12, 95% CI 0.86–1.45. There also was no increased risk for SABs (OR 1.29, 95% CI 0.84–1.97) or preterm birth (OR 1.13, 95% CI 0.96–1.33) (11).

In a 2010 study from Denmark, covering the period 1996–2008, there were 840,968 live births among whom 5082 were exposed to PPIs between 4 weeks before conception to the end of the 1st trimester (12). In the exposed group, there were 174 (3.4%) major malformations compared with 21,811 (2.6%) not exposed to PPIs (adjusted prevalence odds ratio [aPOR] 1.23, 95 CI 1.05–1.44). When the analysis was limited to exposure in the 1st trimester, there were 118 (3.2%) major malformations among 3651 exposed infants (aPOR 1.10, 95% CI 0.91–1.34). For exposure to lansoprazole in the 1st trimester, there were 28 (3.5%) major birth defects among 794 live births (aPOR 1.13, 95% CI 0.77–1.67) (see Esomeprazole, Omeprazole, Pantoprazole, and Rabeprazole for their data). The data showed that exposure to PPIs in the 1st trimester was not associated with a significantly increased risk of major birth defects (12). An accompanying editorial discussed the strengths and weaknesses of the study (13).

In a 2012 publication, the National Birth Defects Prevention study, a multi-site population-based case–control study, examined whether nausea/vomiting of pregnancy (NVP) or its treatment were associated with the most common non-cardiac defects (nonsyndromic cleft lip with or without cleft palate [CL/P], cleft palate alone [CP], neural tube defects [NTDs], and hypospadias) (14). PPI exposure included esomeprazole, lansoprazole, and omeprazole. There were 4524 cases and 5859 controls. NVP was not associated with cleft palate or NTDs, but modest risk reductions were observed for CL/P and hypospadias. Increased risks were found for PPIs (N = 7) and hypospadias (adjusted OR [aOR] 4.36, 95% CI 1.21–15.81), steroids (N = 10) and hypospadias (aOR 2.87, 95% CI 1.03–7.97), and ondansetron (N = 11) and CP (aOR 2.37, 95% CI 1.18–4.76) (14).

Another 2012 reference, using the Danish nationwide registries, evaluated the risk of hypospadias after exposure to PPIs during the 1st trimester and throughout gestation (15). The study period, 1997 through 2009, included all liveborn boys that totaled 430,569, of whom 2926 were exposed to maternal PPI use. Hypospadias was diagnosed in 20 (0.7%) exposed boys, whereas 2683 (0.6%) of the nonexposed had hypospadias (adjusted prevalence ratio [aPR] 1.1, 95% CI 0.7–1.7). For the 5227 boys exposed throughout pregnancy, 32 (0.6%) had hypospadias (PR 1.0, 95% CI 0.7–1.4). When the analysis was restricted to mothers with 2 or more PPI prescriptions, the aPR of overall hypospadias was 1.7, 95% CI 0.9–3.3) and 1.6, 95% CI 0.7–3.9 for omeprazole. The authors concluded that PPIs were not associated with hypospadias (15).

A large retrospective cohort study from Israel covering 1998–2009 was published in 2012 (16). Among 114,960 live births, there were 110,783 singletons and 1239 EABs. Major malformations were observed in 6037 (5.5%) singletons and in 468 abortuses. Exposure to a PPI (lansoprazole, omeprazole, or pantoprazole) during the 1st trimester occurred in 1186 (1159 infants and 27 abortuses). In the exposed infants and abortuses, 80 (6.7%) had a major malformation compared with 6425 (5.9%) not exposed (adjusted OR [aOR] 1.06, 95% CI 0.84–1.33). In the 233 infants–abortuses exposed to lansoprazole, 13 (5.6%) had a major malformation compared with 6753 (6.1%) not exposed (aOR 0.83, 95% CI 0.48–1.46). The data showed that exposure to PPIs during the 1st trimester was not associated with an increased risk of major defects. Moreover, additional analysis revealed that exposure during the 3rd trimester was not associated with increased risk of perinatal mortality, premature delivery, low birth weight, or low Apgar scores (16).

Five reviews on the treatment of GERD have concluded that PPIs can be used in pregnancy with relative safety (17–21). Because there is either very limited or no human pregnancy data for the three newest agents in this class (dexlansoprazole, esomeprazole, and rabeprazole), other drugs in the class are preferred.

BREASTFEEDING SUMMARY

No reports describing the use of lansoprazole during human lactation have been located. The molecular weight (about 369) is low enough that excretion into breast milk should be expected. Because of the carcinogenicity observed in animals, and the potential for suppression of gastric acid secretion in the nursing infant, the use of lansoprazole during lactation is best avoided.

L

References

1. Product information. Prevacid. Tap Pharmaceuticals, 2001.
2. Schardein JL, Furuhashi T, Ooshima Y. Reproductive and developmental toxicity studies of lansoprazole (ag-1749) in rats and rabbits. Yakuri to Rinsho 1990;18:S2773–83. As cited in Shepard TH. *Catalog of Teratogenic Agents*. 8th ed. Baltimore, MD: Johns Hopkins University Press, 1995:245.
3. Schardein JL, Furuhashi T, Ooshima Y. Reproductive and developmental toxicity studies of lansoprazole (AG-1749) in rats and rabbits. Jpn Pharmacol Ther 1990;18(Suppl 10):119–29. As cited in Schardein JL. *Chemically Induced Birth Defects*. 2nd ed. New York, NY: Marcel Dekker, 1993:447.
4. Wilton LV, Pearce GL, Martin RM, Mackay FJ, Mann RD. The outcomes of pregnancy in women exposed to newly marketed drugs in general practice in England. Br J Obstet Gynaecol 1998;105:882–9.
5. Kallen B. Delivery outcome after the use of acid-suppressing drugs in early pregnancy with special reference to omeprazole. Br J Obstet Gynaecol 1998;105:877–81.
6. Nielsen GL, Sorensen HT, Thulstrup AM, Tage-Jensen U, Olesen C, Ekbom A. The safety of proton pump inhibitors in pregnancy. Aliment Pharmacol Ther 1999;13:1085–9.
7. Nikfar S, Abdollahi M, Moretti ME, Magee LA, Koren G. Use of proton pump inhibitors during pregnancy and rates of major malformations: a meta-analysis. Dig Dis Sci 2002;47:1526–9.
8. Diav-Citrin O, Arnon J, Shechtman S, Schaefer C, Van Tonningen MR, Clementi M, De Santis M, Robert-Gnansia E, Valti E, Malm H, Ornoy A. The safety of proton pump inhibitors in pregnancy: a multicentre prospective controlled trial. Aliment Pharmacol Ther 2005;21:269–75.
9. Mayer A, Sheiner E, Holcherg G. Zollinger Ellison syndrome, treated with lansoprazole, during pregnancy. Arch Gynecol Obstet 2007;276:171–3.
10. Dehlink E, Yen E, Leichtner AM, Hait EJ, Fiebiger E. First evidence of a possible association between gastric acid suppression during pregnancy and childhood asthma: a population-based register study. Clin Exp Allergy 2009;39:246–53.
11. Gill SK, O'Brien L, Einarson TR, Koren G. The safety of proton pump inhibitors (PPIs) in pregnancy: a meta-analysis. Am J Gastroenterol 2009;104:1541–5.
12. Pasternak B, Hviid A. Use of proton-pump inhibitors in early pregnancy and the risk of birth defects. N Engl J Med 2010;363:2114–23.
13. Mitchell AA. Proton-pump inhibitors and birth defects—some reassurance, but more needed. N Engl J Med 2010;363:2161–3.
14. Anderka M, Mitchell AA, Louik C, Werler MM, Hernandez-Diaz S, Rasmussen SA, and the National Birth Defects Prevention Study. Medications used to treat nausea and vomiting of pregnancy and the risk of selected birth defects. Birth Defects Res A Clin Mol Teratol 2012;94:22–30.
15. Erichsen R, Mikkelsen E, Pedersen L, Sorensen HT. Maternal use of proton pump inhibitors during early pregnancy and the prevalence of hypospadias in male offspring. Am J Ther 2012 (Feb 3) [Epub ahead of print].
16. Matok I, Levy A, Wiznitzer A, Uziel E, Koren G, Gorodischer R. The safety of fetal exposure to proton-pump inhibitors during pregnancy. Dig Dis Sci 2012;57:699–705.
17. Broussard CN, Richter JE. Treating gastro-oesophageal reflux disease during pregnancy and lactation. What are the safest therapy options? Drug Saf 1998;19:325–37.
18. Katz PO, Castell DO. Gastroesophageal reflux disease during pregnancy. Gastroenterol Clin N Am 1998;27:153–67.
19. Ramakrishnan A, Katz PO. Pharmacologic management of gastroesophageal reflux disease. Curr Treat Options Gastroenterol 2002;5:301–10.
20. Richter JE. Gastroesophageal reflux disease during pregnancy. Gastroenterol Clin N Am 2003;32:235–61.
21. Richter JE. Review article: the management of heartburn in pregnancy. Aliment Pharmacol Ther 2005;22:749–57.

LANTHANUM CARBONATE

Antidote (Phosphate Binder)

PREGNANCY RECOMMENDATION: No Human Data—Probably Compatible
BREASTFEEDING RECOMMENDATION: No Human Data—Probably Compatible

PREGNANCY SUMMARY

No reports describing the use of lanthanum carbonate in human pregnancy have been located. The indication for the drug suggests that human pregnancy experience will be very limited. The systemic bioavailability is minimal and should have no effect on the embryo or fetus.

FETAL RISK SUMMARY

Lanthanum carbonate, an oral phosphate binder, is indicated to reduce serum phosphate in patients with end-stage renal disease. In the acid environment of the upper gastrointestinal tract, lanthanum ions are released to bind dietary phosphate from food during digestion. The resulting lanthanum phosphate complexes are highly insoluble. The systemic bioavailability of lanthanum carbonate is very low (<0.002%) with a mean plasma concentration of 0.6 ng/mL. The drug is practically insoluble in water. Lanthanum carbonate is not metabolized. Plasma protein binding is >99% and the plasma elimination half-life is 53 hours. However, lanthanum is bound to bone and is slowly released with an estimated half-life of 2.0–3.6 years (1).

Reproduction studies have been conducted in rats and rabbits. In rats, oral doses up to 3.4 times the maximum recommended daily human dose (MRDHD) resulted in no evidence of fetal harm. When the highest dose was given from implantation through lactation, offspring had delayed eye opening, reduction in body weight gain, and delayed sexual development (preputial separation and vaginal opening). In rabbits, doses up to 5 times the MRDHD were maternal toxic (reduced body weight gain and food consumption) and were associated with increased postimplantation loss, reduced fetal weights, and delayed fetal ossification (1).

In long-term studies, lanthanum carbonate was not carcinogenic in rats but was associated with an increased incidence of glandular stomach adenomas in male mice. The drug did not cause mutagenicity or chromosomal aberrations in multiple tests. Fertility of male and female rats was not affected by doses up to 3.4 times the MRDHD (1).

It is not known if lanthanum carbonate crosses the human placenta. The molecular weight (about 458 for anhydrous form) is low enough, but the very low systemic bioavailability and high plasma protein binding suggest that exposure of the embryo–fetus will not be clinically significant.

BREASTFEEDING SUMMARY

No reports describing the use of lanthanum carbonate during human lactation have been located. The very low systemic bioavailability (<0.002%) and high plasma protein binding (>99%) suggest that insignificant amounts of the drug will be excreted into breast milk. Moreover, even the minimal amounts that might be excreted would bind with milk phosphate, resulting in a nonabsorbable complex. The effect of this binding on infant bone growth is unknown but is probably not clinically significant.

Reference

1. Product information. Fosrenol. Shire US Manufacturing, 2009.

LAPATINIB

Antineoplastic (Tyrosine Kinase Inhibitor)

PREGNANCY RECOMMENDATION: Contraindicated
BREASTFEEDING RECOMMENDATION: Contraindicated

PREGNANCY SUMMARY

The human pregnancy experience with lapatinib is very limited. The animal reproduction studies suggest moderate risk. The no-observed-effect-level (NOEL) in animals was ≤1 times the human clinical exposure based on AUC (HCE). Although the near absence of human pregnancy experience prevents a complete assessment of the embryo–fetal risk, the drug should be avoided in pregnancy. If it must be administered for the mother's benefit, avoiding the period of organogenesis should be considered.

FETAL RISK SUMMARY

Lapatinib is an intracellular tyrosine kinase inhibitor that is indicated, in combination with capecitabine (see Capecitabine), for the treatment of patients with advanced or metastatic breast cancer whose tumors overexpress human epidermal receptor type 2 (HER2) and who have received prior therapy, including an anthracycline, a taxane, and trastuzumab. There are no other agents in this subclass (see Appendix). Lapatinib is extensively metabolized to inactive metabolites. Plasma protein binding to albumin and α-1 acid glycoprotein is >99%. The terminal phase half-life following repeated dosing is 24 hours (1).

Reproduction studies have been conducted in rats and rabbits. Pregnant rats were given doses during organogenesis and through lactation that produced systemic exposures that were about 6.4 times the HCE. At this exposure, 91% of the pups died by the 4th day after birth, but this dose also caused maternal toxicity. When half of the dose was used (about 3.3 times the HCE), 34% of the pups died. The NOEL was about equal to the HCE. There were no teratogenic effects at the highest exposure, but minor anomalies observed were left-sided umbilical artery, cervical rib, and precocious ossification. In rabbits, maternal toxicity was observed at doses resulting in exposures that were about 0.07 and 0.2 times the HCE. Decreased fetal body weights and minor skeletal variations were noted at both doses, and abortions were observed at the higher dose (1).

Carcinogenicity studies have not been completed. Lapatinib was not clastogenic or mutagenic in a variety of assays. There were no effects on mating or fertility in female and male rats given doses producing exposures that were 6.4 and 2.6 times the HCE, respectively. However, in female rats, this exposure during breeding and through the first 6 days of gestation was associated with a significant decrease in the number of live fetuses. At about 3.3 times the HCE, there was a significant decrease in fetal body weights (1).

It is not known if lapatinib crosses the human placenta. Although the high plasma protein binding will inhibit transfer, the molecular weight (about 926 for the nonhydrated form) and the prolonged half-life suggest that embryo–fetus exposure will occur.

A 44-year-old woman with breast cancer conceived while being treated in a phase I clinical trial with lapatinib (2). During the previous 10 years, she had been treated with a number of antineoplastic agents, including cyclophosphamide, doxorubicin, fluorouracil, paclitaxel, trastuzumab, and vinorelbine. She also had undergone a left modified radical mastectomy, regional radiation, and 10 years of tamoxifen. When cancer was discovered in her right breast, she was enrolled in the clinical trial. She was initially treated with lapatinib 1500 mg/day, but the dose was reduced by 50% because of diarrhea and rash. Pregnancy was diagnosed at about 14 weeks' gestation; conception was thought to have occurred in the 3rd or 4th week of study drug. A modified radical mastectomy was conducted to avoid further antineoplastic treatment. Because of disease progression, labor was induced, and the woman gave birth to a healthy, 2.6-kg female infant with Apgar scores of 8 and 9 at 1 and 5 minutes, respectively. At 18 months of age, the infant was doing well, having reached all developmental milestones on schedule (2).

BREASTFEEDING SUMMARY

No reports describing the use of lapatinib during lactation have been located. Although the high plasma protein binding (>99%) should inhibit excretion, the molecular weight (about 926 for the nonhydrated form) and the prolonged half-life (24 hours) suggest that the drug will be excreted into breast milk. Women receiving lapatinib should not breastfeed because of the potential for toxicity in a nursing infant. The most common toxicities in adults were severe diarrhea, nausea and vomiting, and rash.

References

1. Product information. Tykerb. GlaxoSmithKline, 2007.
2. Kelly H, Graham M, Humes E, Dorflinger LJ, Boggess KA, O'Neil BH, Harris J, Spector NL, Dees EC. Delivery of a healthy baby after first-trimester maternal exposure to lapatinib. Clin Breast Cancer 2006;7:339–41.

LARONIDASE

Endocrine/Metabolic Agent (Enzyme)

PREGNANCY RECOMMENDATION: Limited Human Data—Animal Data Suggest Low Risk
BREASTFEEDING RECOMMENDATION: No Human Data—Potential Toxicity (≤7 Days after Birth)
Probably Compatible (>7 Days after Birth)

PREGNANCY SUMMARY

One report of laronidase in human pregnancy has been located, and that case involved exposure before the onset of organogenesis. The animal reproduction data, although based on body weight, suggest low risk. However, the absence of human pregnancy experience during organogenesis and later prevents a more complete assessment. Nevertheless, the benefits (improved pulmonary function and walking capacity) of treatment with laronidase to a pregnant woman with mucopolysaccharidosis I (MPS I) appear to outweigh the unknown risks to the embryo and/or fetus. Therefore, if a woman requires this therapy, it should not be withheld because of pregnancy.

L

FETAL RISK SUMMARY

Laronidase, a polymorphic variant of the human enzyme, α-L-iduronidase, is a glycoprotein prepared by recombinant DNA technology. It is indicated for patients with the Hurler and Hurler-Scheie forms of MPS I and for patients with the Scheie form who have moderate-to-severe symptoms. The predicted amino acid sequence of laronidase is identical to the polymorphic form of human α-L-iduronidase. Laronidase is given as a once-weekly 3–4 hour IV infusion. The mean elimination half-life ranges from 1.5 to 3.6 hours (1).

Hypersensitivity reactions, including anaphylaxis, may occur during laronidase IV infusions. Patients should receive antipyretics and/or antihistamines 60 minutes before the infusion. Hypotension was observed in 9% (2/22) of the patients receiving an infusion of laronidase in a placebo-controlled study (1). This adverse effect in a pregnant woman could have deleterious effects on placental perfusion, resulting in embryo and fetal harm.

Reproduction studies have been conducted in rats. No evidence of fetal harm was observed with a dose that was 6.2 times the human dose (assumed to be based on body weight). In addition, the same dose had no effect on male and female rat fertility (1).

It is not known if laronidase crosses the human placenta. The molecular weight is high (about 83,000), suggesting that the glycoprotein will not cross to the embryo or fetus.

A 2006 case report described a 21-year-old woman with MPS I, who became pregnant while receiving weekly infusions (100 U/kg) of laronidase (2). Exposure appears to have been no longer than 4 weeks. Further laronidase treatment was stopped. The woman went into spontaneous premature labor at 29 weeks' gestation and delivered a healthy, normal 1250-g female infant. Although the cause of the preterm labor was unknown, the authors speculated that it might have been secondary to the disease (2).

BREASTFEEDING SUMMARY

No reports describing the use of laronidase during human lactation have been located.

The high molecular weight (about 83,000) suggests that the glycoprotein will not be excreted into breast milk. However, many proteins (e.g., immunoglobulins) are excreted into milk and absorbed by the infant in the first few days after birth. Thus, laronidase could potentially be excreted and absorbed.

If laronidase is excreted into milk, one strategy to reduce the exposure of a nursing infant, especially during the first week after birth, involves using the pharmacokinetics and dosing schedule of the drug. Laronidase has a short elimination half-life (1.5–3.6 hours) and is infused once weekly over 3–4 hours. The woman could nurse immediately before the start of the infusion, and then pump and dump her milk for about 8–12 hours after the end of the infusion. During this period, the infant could be fed breast milk stored earlier. This strategy should markedly reduce laronidase exposure of the nursing infant. Nevertheless, if a woman receiving laronidase therapy chooses to nurse, especially during the first week after birth, her infant should be closely monitored for the adverse effects most commonly observed in adults (skin rash, upper respiratory tract infection, hyperreflexia, paresthesia, chest pain, edema, and hypotension).

References

1. Product information. Aldurazyme. Genentech, 2007.
2. Anbu AT, Mercer J, Wraith JE. Effect of discontinuing of laronidase in a patient with mucopolysaccharidosis type 1. J Inherit Metab Dis 2006;29:230–1.

LATANOPROST

Ophthalmic (Prostaglandin Agonist)

PREGNANCY RECOMMENDATION: Limited Human Data—Probably Compatible
BREASTFEEDING RECOMMENDATION: No Human Data—Probably Compatible

PREGNANCY SUMMARY

Neither the limited human pregnancy experience nor the animal reproduction data suggest that latanoprost is a clinically significant risk to the embryo–fetus. The amount of drug in the systemic circulation after ophthalmic use of the recommended dose is likely minimal. The limited data suggest that, if indicated, latanoprost should not be withheld because of pregnancy.

FETAL RISK SUMMARY

Latanoprost, a prostaglandin $F2_\alpha$ analog, is a topical ophthalmic solution indicated for the reduction of elevated intraocular pressure in patients with open-angle glaucoma or ocular hypertension. It is in the same class as bimatoprost, tafluprost, and travoprost. Latanoprost is a prostanoid selective FP receptor agonist, which is believed to reduce the intraocular pressure by increasing the outflow of aqueous humor. Latanoprost is a prodrug that is hydrolyzed by esterases in the cornea to the biologically active acid. Metabolites of the active acid are inactive. The elimination half-life of the active acid form is 17 minutes (1,2).

Reproduction studies have been performed in rats and rabbits. In rabbits, 4 of 16 dams had no viable fetuses at a dose that was about 80 times the maximum human dose (MHD) (*assumed to be based on body weight*). The no-effect dose for embryo death in rabbits was about 15 times the MHD (1,2). No information on studies conducted in pregnant rats was provided.

Latanoprost was not carcinogenic in mice and rats at doses up to 2800 times the MHD. Mutagenicity studies were also negative in multiple assays, but the drug did cause chromosome aberrations in an in vitro assay with human lymphocytes. The drug had no effect on male or female fertility in animal studies (1,2).

It is not known if latanoprost or its active acid crosses the human placenta. The molecular weight of the prodrug (about 433) is low enough, but plasma concentrations are probably very low and have a very short elimination half-life. These properties suggest that clinically significant exposure of the embryo–fetus is unlikely.

Prostaglandin $F2_\alpha$ has been used for pregnancy termination in humans via intrauterine extra-amniotic infusion to treat missed abortion or intrauterine death. However, there is no evidence that at doses given to reduce elevated ophthalmic pressure, an increased risk for uterine contractions would be seen (3,4).

Eleven 1st trimester latanoprost-exposed pregnancies were identified by a teratology information service in Italy (5). Exposure in the 1st trimester occurred for 4–70 days. Three women continued therapy throughout gestation and one discontinued the drug in the 3rd trimester. One pregnancy was lost to follow-up, one ended in a spontaneous abortion 2 weeks after therapy was discontinued (in a 46-year-old woman), and nine women gave birth at term to normal, healthy infants (5).

BREASTFEEDING SUMMARY

No reports describing the use of latanoprost during human lactation have been located. The molecular weight of the prodrug (about 433) is low enough, but plasma concentrations are probably very low and have a very short elimination half-life (17 minutes). These properties suggest that clinically significant amounts will not be excreted into breast milk.

References

1. Product information. Xalatan. Pharmacia & Upjohn, 2009.
2. Product information. Latanoprost. Apotex, 2011.
3. Lipitz S, Grisaru D, Libshiz A, Rotstein Z, Schiff E, Lidor A, Achiron R. Intra-amniotic prostaglandin F2 alpha for pregnancy termination in the second and early third trimesters of pregnancy. J Reprod Med 1997;42:235–8.
4. Salamalekis E, Kassanos D, Hassiakos D, Chrelias C, Ghristodoulakos G. Intra/extra-amniotic administration of prostaglandin F2α in fetal death, missed and therapeutic abortions. Clin Exp Obstet Gynecol 1990;17:17–21.
5. De Santis M, Lucchese A, Carducci B, Cavaliere AF, De Santis L, Merola A, Straface G, Caruso A. Latanoprost exposure in pregnancy. Am J Ophthalmol 2004;138:305–6.

LEFLUNOMIDE

Immunologic Agent (Antirheumatic)

PREGNANCY RECOMMENDATION: Contraindicated
BREASTFEEDING RECOMMENDATION: No Human Data—Potential Toxicity

PREGNANCY SUMMARY

Leflunomide is an animal teratogen and its use in pregnancy is contraindicated. The drug and its active metabolite are eliminated from the body very slowly and may take up to 2 years to reach nondetectable plasma metabolite levels. Nevertheless, the limited human pregnancy experience has not shown an increased risk of major or minor anomalies. Moreover, the risk of preterm delivery and lower birth weight of full-term infants appears to be related to the disease (rheumatoid arthritis) or concurrent drug therapy other than leflunomide. In women of childbearing age, pregnancy should be excluded and the woman should be on a reliable contraceptive before starting therapy. In the event of inadvertent conceptions, a drug elimination procedure using cholestyramine has been developed and is included in the product information. However, the procedure for preventing embryo exposure to therapeutic levels in unplanned pregnancies might be clinically ineffective. In inadvertent pregnancies, the procedure, to be at least partially effective, should be initiated no later than the time of the first missed menstrual period (1). Pregnancy loss and anomalies occurring early in organogenesis would still be a risk, but drug-induced microcephaly and mental retardation would be prevented (2). A pregnancy registry and cohort study has been established to monitor fetal outcomes of pregnant women exposed to leflunomide for the treatment of rheumatoid arthritis (RA) (3). Healthcare providers are encouraged to register their patients by calling the toll-free number (877-311-8972) (1).

FETAL RISK SUMMARY

Leflunomide, a pyrimidine synthesis inhibitor, is indicated for the treatment of active RA to reduce signs and symptoms and retard structural damage. The drug is metabolized to an active metabolite that has an elimination half-life of about 2 weeks (1).

Leflunomide is contraindicated in pregnancy because it has exhibited dose-related teratogenicity and embryo–fetal toxicity in animals at doses that resulted in systemic exposures at or below those obtained in humans. Therefore, in women of childbearing age, leflunomide should not be started until pregnancy has been excluded and the use of reliable contraception has been confirmed (1).

In reproduction studies with pregnant rats during organogenesis, an oral dose that produced systemic exposure approximately 10% of the human exposure level based on AUC (HE) was teratogenic (anophthalmia or microphthalmia and internal hydrocephalus). This dose also resulted in an increase in embryo death and a decrease in maternal and surviving fetuses' body weight. In rabbits, an oral dose equivalent to the maximum HE during organogenesis resulted in fused, dysplastic sternebrae. No teratogenic effects were noted at lower doses in either species. In rats treated with doses 1% of the HE for 14 days before mating and continued until the end of lactation, >90% of the offspring failed to survive the postnatal period (1).

Leflunomide was not carcinogenic in rats, but mice exhibited dose-related increases in lymphoma (males) and bronchoalveolar adenomas and carcinomas combined (females). The incidence of the lung tumors, however, was within the spontaneous range for the mouse strain. The drug was not mutagenic or clastogenic in various assays, although a minor metabolite (4-trifluoromethylaniline) was in some tests. Because of the very low amounts of this metabolite, the results were not thought to be clinically significant (1).

It is not known if leflunomide crosses the human placenta. The molecular weight (about 270) is low enough that passage to the fetus should be expected. It also is not known if the active metabolite can cross the placenta or if the fetus can metabolize the parent compound to the active metabolite.

Because it may take ≤2 years to reach nondetectable plasma levels (<0.02 mcg/mL) of the active metabolite, the manufacturer has developed a drug elimination procedure in the event that a woman taking leflunomide becomes pregnant: (a) administer cholestyramine 8 g 3 times daily for 11 days (not necessarily consecutive unless there is a need to lower the plasma level rapidly); (b) verify plasma levels <0.02 mcg/mL by two tests = 14 days apart. If plasma levels are >0.02 mcg/mL, additional cholestyramine treatment should be considered (1).

Information relating to the risks of leflunomide use in human pregnancy has been published. A 2000 review on the treatment of rheumatic diseases briefly mentioned the agent, stating that it was contraindicated in pregnancy (4). It also reviewed the drug elimination procedure in the manufacturer's product literature. A 2001 reference thoroughly reviewed the reproductive risks of leflunomide and provided detailed information on counseling of men and women who might have been exposed to the agent and were either contemplating fathering a child, were pregnant, or were planning a pregnancy (2). The drug blood level considered safe was 0.03 mcg/mL, which was 123 and 136 times lower than the no-effect blood levels in rats and rabbits, respectively. The safe concentration was about 0.1% of the average steady-state plasma level of the active metabolite. The author mentioned that approximately 30 women had become pregnant on leflunomide, 29 of whom were exposed to therapeutic levels of the drug during early organogenesis despite initiating the drug elimination protocol as soon as pregnancy was diagnosed. Only three pregnancies were continuing (no outcome data available), however, as 27 women had elected to undergo termination (2).

A survey of 600 members of the American College of Rheumatology, conducted partially to determine the outcomes of pregnancies exposed to disease-modifying antirheumatic drugs (DMARDs) (etanercept, infliximab, leflunomide, and methotrexate), was published in 2003 (5). From the 175 responders, the outcomes of 10 pregnancies exposed to leflunomide were two full-term healthy infants, one preterm delivery, one spontaneous abortion, two elective abortions, two unknown outcomes, and two women still pregnant. Cholestyramine was definitely used in two pregnancies and may have been used in all (5).

A 2004 study reported data from the manufacturer's database of pregnancies exposed to infliximab (see Infliximab for details of this study) (6). One woman had received infliximab and leflunomide before conception and in pregnancy and delivered an infant with intestinal malrotation (6).

An Italian teratogen information service described the outcomes of five pregnancies in women exposed to leflunomide and one case of paternal exposure (7). Exposures in three women who had elective abortions were until 1.5 months before conception, and until 5 weeks' and 9 weeks' gestation, respectively. A woman exposed until 6.5 months before conception gave birth to a normal 2600-g male infant at 39 weeks' and another woman exposed until the 9th week of gestation had a normal 2200-g male infant at 36 weeks'. The paternal exposure started 6 months before conception and continued throughout pregnancy without a condom being worn during intercourse. A normal 3350-g male infant was born at 38 weeks'. All three births were by cesarean section. None of six cases had a washout procedure (7).

In a 2007 case report from England, a 43-year-old woman with RA became pregnant about 8 months after starting leflunomide 20 mg/day (8). At 21 weeks', the drug was discontinued and cholestyramine treatment was started. A male infant was born 9 weeks prematurely and was found to be blind in the right eye, and to have cerebral palsy with left-sided spasticity. The mother's three previous pregnancies had involved a neonatal death within 24 hours of birth due to a congenital heart defect, a healthy daughter, and a son diagnosed with autism (8).

In a 2004 abstract, preliminary results of the on-going Organization of Teratology Information Specialists (OTIS) Rheumatoid Arthritis in Pregnancy study were reported (9). As of January, 2004, 168 infant outcomes were known: 43 exposed to leflunomide, 78 RA controls without leflunomide exposure, and 47 nondiseased controls. The proportion of major and minor malformations was similar between the groups. However, both RA groups were significantly more likely to deliver preterm infants than nondiseased controls: leflunomide group, adjusted odds ratio (OR) 12.0, 95% confidence interval (CI) 2.5–59.2; and RA group, OR 10.1, 95% CI 2.2–47.3. The mean birth weight of full-term infants also was significantly lower in both RA groups than in nondiseased controls: 3158, 3336, and 3487 g, respectively. The results suggested that RA itself, with a possible contribution from other medications, such as corticosteroids, was responsible for the increased rate of preterm delivery and lower birth weight of full-term infants (9).

In a continuation of the above prospective cohort study, 250 pregnancy outcomes were known: 64 exposed to leflunomide (61 [95.3%] of who received cholestyramine), 108 RA controls, and 78 healthy pregnant women (10). Women exposed to methotrexate or cyclophosphamide at any time during pregnancy were excluded. The number of live births in the three groups was 56, 95, and 72, respectively. Of these, 51 (91.1%), 90 (94.7%), and 65 (90.3%) were examined by a pediatric dysmorphologist blinded to the groups. There was no significant difference in the number of major defects in all pregnancies (live births plus losses): 4.8%, 6.6%, and 4.0%, respectively. The three major anomalies in the leflunomide-exposed infants were occult spinal dysraphism, unilateral uretero pelvic junction obstruction and multicystic kidney disease, and microcephaly. There also was no difference between the groups in terms of functional problems, but significantly more exposed infants had minor defects ($p = 0.05$) and a higher proportion of three or more minor defects (47.1% vs. 32.2% vs. 29.2%, $p = 0.10$). There was no specific pattern of major or minor anomalies. Infants in both RA groups were born smaller and earlier than infants from healthy mothers, but there were no significant differences between the RA groups. In addition, among 19 infants from leflunomide-treated mothers who were not eligible for the cohort study for various reasons, 2 had major anomalies: aplasia cutis congenita in a surviving twin; and multiple defects including the Pierre-Robin sequence, cleft of the soft palate, and chondrodysplasia punctata (mother treated for systemic lupus erythematosus). The data indicated that there was no substantial risk of adverse pregnancy outcome among leflunomide-treated women who undergo the cholestyramine elimination procedure early in pregnancy (10).

A 2010 report described a 22-year-old woman with Takayasu's arteritis who conceived while taking leflunomide 10 mg/day, adalimumab 40 mg SC every 4 weeks, prednisolone 5 mg/day, and dalteparin 500 IU/day (11). Leflunomide was discontinued by the patient at 8 weeks' gestation but the other agents were continued throughout pregnancy. At 37 weeks', a cesarean section was performed to deliver a healthy 2550-g male infant with Apgar scores of 9, 9, and 10 at 1, 5, and 10 minutes, respectively (11).

BREASTFEEDING SUMMARY

No reports describing the use of leflunomide during lactation have been located. The molecular weight (about 270) is low enough that excretion into breast milk should be expected. The effects of this exposure on a nursing infant are unknown. Because of the potential for serious adverse effects and without information on the amount of drug in milk, nursing mothers receiving this drug should probably not breastfeed (2).

References

1. Product information. Arava. Sanofi-Aventis, 2012.
2. Brent RL. Teratogen update: reproductive risks of leflunomide (Arava); a pyrimidine synthesis inhibitor: counseling women taking leflunomide before or during pregnancy and men taking leflunomide who are contemplating fathering a child. Teratology 2001;63:106–12.
3. Jones KL, Johnson DL, Chambers CD. Monitoring leflunomide (Arava) as a new potential teratogen. Teratology 2002;65:200–2.
4. Janssen NM, Genta MS. The effects of immunosuppressive and anti-inflammatory medications on fertility, pregnancy, and lactation. Arch Intern Med 2000;160:610–9.
5. Chakravarty EF, Sanchez-Yamamoto D, Bush TM. The use of disease-modifying antirheumatic drugs in women with rheumatoid arthritis of

childbearing age: a survey of practice patterns and pregnancy outcomes. J Rheumatol 2003;30:241–6.
6. Katz JA, Antoni C, Keenan GF, Smith DE, Jacobs SJ, Lichtenstein GR. Outcome of pregnancy in women receiving infliximab for the treatment of Crohn's disease and rheumatoid arthritis. Am J Gastroenterol 2004;99:2385–92.
7. De Santis M, Straface G, Cavaliere A, Carducci B, Caruso A. Paternal and maternal exposure to leflunomide: pregnancy and neonatal outcome. Ann Rheum Dis 2005;64:1096–7.
8. Neville CE, McNally J. Maternal exposure to leflunomide associated with blindness and cerebral palsy. Rheumatology 2007;46:1506.
9. Chambers CD, Johnson DL, Macaraeg GR, Jones KL. Pregnancy outcome following early gestational exposure to leflunomide: the OTIS Rheumatoid in Pregnancy study (abstract). Pharmacoepidemiol Drug Saf 2004;13: S126–7.
10. Chambers CD, Johnson DL, Robinson LK, Braddock SR, Xu R, Lopez-Jimenez J, Mirrasoul N, Salas E, Luo YJ, Jin S, Jones KL, and the Organizations of Teratology Information Specialists Collaborative Research Group. Birth outcomes in women who have taken leflunomide during pregnancy. Arthritis Rheum 2010;62:1494–503.
11. Kraemer B, Abele H, Hahn M, Rajab T, Kraemer E, Wallweiner D, Becker S. A successful pregnancy in a patient with Takayasu's arteritis. Hypertens Pregnancy 2008;27:247–52.

LENALIDOMIDE

Immunomodulator

PREGNANCY RECOMMENDATION: Contraindicated
BREASTFEEDING RECOMMENDATION: No Human Data—Potential Toxicity

PREGNANCY SUMMARY

No reports describing the use of lenalidomide in human pregnancy have been located. Thalidomide is a well-known potent human teratogen (see Thalidomide). As an analog of thalidomide, lenalidomide is contraindicated in human pregnancy and in women capable of becoming pregnant. It is available only under a restricted distribution program (RevAssist) (1).

L

FETAL RISK SUMMARY

Lenalidomide is an analog of thalidomide that is used for its immunomodulatory and antiangiogenic properties. It is indicated for the treatment of transfusion-dependent anemia due to low- or intermediate-1-risk myelodysplastic syndrome (MDS) associated with a deletion 5q cytogenetic abnormality with or without additional cytogenetic abnormalities. It also is indicated, in combination with dexamethasone, for the treatment of multiple myeloma patients who have received at least prior therapy. The only other immunomodulator with a similar indication is thalidomide. Lenalidomide is partly metabolized (about one-third), but the metabolites have not been characterized. Plasma protein binding also is low (about 30%) and the elimination half-life is about 3 hours. The pharmacokinetics in MDS patients has not been studied, but in multiple myeloma patients the exposure (AUC) was 57% higher than in healthy male volunteers (1).

Reproduction studies have been conducted in rats and rabbits. In pregnant rats, no evidence of teratogenicity was observed with daily doses up to about 600 times the human dose of 10 mg based on BSA (HD). Minimal maternal toxicity (slight, transient decrease in mean body weight gain and food intake) was observed at doses that were about 120–600 times the HD. Male offspring of pregnant rats given daily doses ≤600 times the HD exhibited slightly delayed sexual maturation. Female offspring had slightly lower body weight gains during gestation when bred with male offspring. In pregnant rabbits, a dose that was about 120 times the HD had an embryocidal effect (1).

Carcinogenicity studies have not been conducted with lenalidomide. The drug was not mutagenic in several assays. In studies in rats, doses up to about 600 times the HD had no effect on fertility (1).

It is not known if lenalidomide crosses the human placenta. The molecular weight (about 259), moderate metabolism and plasma protein binding, and the elimination half-life suggest that the drug will cross to the embryo and/or fetus.

Lenalidomide is contraindicated in pregnancy and in women who might become pregnant. However, when there is no other alternative, the drug can be used in women of reproductive age if specific conditions to avoid pregnancy are met. These conditions include abstention from heterosexual intercourse, or the use of two methods of reliable birth control. One of the birth control methods should be considered highly effective (e.g., intrauterine device, hormonal contraception, tubal ligation, or partner's vasectomy), whereas the second method should be considered effective (e.g., latex condom, diaphragm, or cervical cap). The birth control methods should be used continuously for 4 weeks before starting therapy, during therapy, during therapy delay, and for 4 weeks after the end of therapy. Pregnancy testing should be conducted within 10–14 days and a second test within 24 hours of starting therapy and then weekly during the 1st month. After the first month, pregnancy testing should be conducted monthly in women with regular menstrual cycles or every 2 weeks in women with irregular menstrual cycles.

BREASTFEEDING SUMMARY

No reports describing the use of lenalidomide during human lactation have been located.

The molecular weight (about 259), moderate metabolism (about one-third) and plasma protein binding (about 30%), and the elimination half-life (about 3 hours) suggest that the drug will be excreted into breast milk. The effects of this exposure on a nursing infant are unknown. However, serious toxicity has been observed in adult patients with del 5q MDS who were treated with lenalidomide. The most serious toxicities were neutropenia, thrombocytopenia, deep venous thrombosis, and pulmonary embolism, but other commonly observed (≥20%) adverse effects included pruritus, rash, diarrhea, constipation, nausea, nasopharyngitis, fatigue, pyrexia, peripheral edema, arthralgia, and back pain. Because of the uncertainty regarding the amount of drug in milk and the potential for severe toxicity, women being treated with lenalidomide should not breastfeed.

Reference

1. Product information. Revlimid. Celgene, 2007.

LEPIRUDIN

Hematologic Agent (Thrombin Inhibitor)

PREGNANCY RECOMMENDATION: Limited Human Data—Probably Compatible
BREASTFEEDING RECOMMENDATION: Limited Human Data—Probably Compatible

PREGNANCY SUMMARY

The animal data suggest low risk, but the near absence of human pregnancy experience prevents a more complete assessment of embryo/fetal risk. The passage of lepirudin across the rat placenta suggests that the agent might also cross the human placenta. The effects of this potential exposure on a human embryo or fetus, including hemorrhage, are unknown. However, if a pregnant woman requires lepirudin therapy for heparin-induced thrombocytopenia (HIT), the benefits to her appear to outweigh the theoretical risks to her embryo–fetus.

FETAL RISK SUMMARY

The polypeptide lepirudin (rDNA) is a recombinant hirudin derived from yeast cells that is indicated for anticoagulation in patients with HIT and associated thromboembolic disease. It is composed of 65 amino acids and is administered as a continuous IV infusion. Lepirudin binds to thrombin to directly block the thrombogenic activity of thrombin (1).

Reproduction studies with lepirudin have been conducted in rats and rabbits. In pregnant rats, IV doses up to 1.2 times the maximum recommended daily human dose based on BSA (MRHD) during organogenesis and the perinatal–postnatal period revealed no evidence of fetal harm. However, increased rat maternal mortality from undetermined causes was noted. Studies with pregnant rabbits at IV doses up to 2.4 times the MRHD also found no evidence of embryo or fetal harm (1).

Despite the high molecular weight of lepirudin (about 6970), the drug crosses the placenta of pregnant rats (1). Because of the similarities between rat and human placentas, exposure of the human embryo–fetus might occur.

Several case reports (2–6) and a review (7) have described the successful use of lepirudin for the treatment of HIT in pregnancy. In another case report, lepirudin was used in the 3rd trimester when heparin-induced thrombosis occurred (8). Developmental toxicity was not observed in any of these cases.

BREASTFEEDING SUMMARY

One report has described the use of lepirudin (recombinant hirudin) during lactation. A 34-year-old woman, breastfeeding a 7-week-old infant, developed a deep vein thrombosis in her calf and was treated with low-molecular-weight heparin (9). She developed HIT on day 20 of treatment. Therapy was changed to lepirudin 50 mg twice daily. Although therapeutic levels of hirudin were measured in her plasma (0.5–1.0 mg/L), it was not detected in her milk (detection level 0.1 mg/L). The woman continued breastfeeding for the next 6 months while being treated with lepirudin. No adverse effects were observed in the mother or infant (9).

The above report is consistent with the high molecular weight (about 6970) of lepirudin that suggests excretion into milk does not occur. Even if small amounts are excreted, the polypeptide probably would be digested in the stomach of the infant.

References

1. Product information. Refludan. Aventis Pharmaceuticals, 2002.
2. Huhle G, Geberth M, Hoffmann U, Heene DL, Harenberg J. Management of heparin-associated thrombocytopenia in pregnancy with subcutaneous r-hirudin. Gynecol Obstet Invest 2000;49:67–9.
3. Mehta R, Golichowski A. Treatment of heparin-induced thrombocytopenia and thrombosis during the first trimester of pregnancy. J Thromb Haemost 2004;2:1665–6.
4. Harenberg J, Jorg I, Bayer C, Fiehn C. Treatment of a woman with lupus pernio, thrombosis and cutaneous intolerance to heparins using lepirudin during pregnancy. Lupus 2005;14:411–2.
5. Furlan A, Vianello F, Clementi M, Prandoni P. Heparin-induced thrombocytopenia occurring in the first trimester of pregnancy: successful treatment with lepirudin. A case report. Haematologica 2006;91(8 Suppl):ECR40.
6. Plesinac S, Babovic I, Plesinac Karapandzic V. Successful pregnancy after pulmonary embolism and heparin-induced thrombocytopenia—case report. Clin Exp Obstet Gynecol 2013;40:307–8.
7. Lindhoff-Last E, Bauersachs R. Heparin-induced thrombocytopenia—alternative anticoagulation in pregnancy and lactation. Semin Thromb Hemost 2002;28:439–46.
8. Chapman ML, Martinez-Borges AR, Mertz HL. Lepirudin for treatment of acute thrombosis during pregnancy. Obstet Gynecol 2008;112:432–3.
9. Lindhoff-Last E, Willeke A, Thalhammer C, Nowak G, Bauersachs R. Hirudin treatment in a breastfeeding woman. Lancet 2000;355:467–8.

LETROZOLE

Antineoplastic

PREGNANCY RECOMMENDATION: Contraindicated
BREASTFEEDING RECOMMENDATION: Contraindicated

PREGNANCY SUMMARY

No published reports describing the use of letrozole in human pregnancy have been located.

The animal data suggest risk. However, several reports and reviews have described the use of letrozole for ovulation stimulation, an off-label indication. In a 2005 letter from Novartis to healthcare professionals, the manufacturer warned that the drug should not be used for pregnancy induction because it was teratogenic (Novartis issues breast cancer drug warning. December 1, 2005). Novartis was aware of 13 women exposed to the drug during pregnancy resulting in two spontaneous abortions and two infants with birth defects (no additional details are available). Because the drug inhibits estrogen synthesis in all tissues, it is contraindicated during pregnancy.

FETAL RISK SUMMARY

Letrozole is an aromatase inhibitor indicated for postmenopausal women as (a) adjuvant treatment with hormone receptor positive breast cancer; (b) extended adjuvant treatment of early breast cancer in those who have received prior standard adjuvant tamoxifen therapy; and (c) first- and second-line treatment of those with hormone receptor positive or unknown advanced breast cancer. It also has been used off-label to induced ovulation in infertile women. Letrozole inhibits the aromatase enzyme, resulting in a reduction of estrogen synthesis in all tissues. It is metabolized to inactive metabolites, weakly bound to plasma proteins, and the terminal elimination half-life is about 2 days (1).

Reproduction studies have been conducted in rats and rabbits. In rats, doses during organogenesis that were ≥0.01 times the daily maximum recommended human dose based on BSA (MRHD) caused increased resorptions and postimplantation loss, decreased numbers of live fetuses, and fetal anomalies including absence and shortening of renal papilla, dilation of ureter, edema, and incomplete ossification of frontal skull and metatarsals. Doses that were 0.1 times MRHD caused fetal domed head and cervical/centrum vertebral fusion. In rabbits, doses that were 0.0001–0.00001 times the MRHD caused embryo–fetal toxicity and anomalies that included incomplete ossification of the skull, sternebrae, and fore- and hindlegs (1).

In 2-year studies, letrozole was carcinogenic in mice and rats. The drug was not mutagenic but was a potential clastogen in an in vitro test but not in an in vivo test. In mice, rats, and dogs, letrozole caused sexual inactivity in females and atrophy of the reproductive tract in male and female animals (1).

It is not known if letrozole crosses the human placenta. The molecular weight (about 285), low plasma protein binding, and long terminal elimination half-life suggest that exposure of the embryo and/or fetus will occur.

A number of studies (2–14) and reviews (15–20) have reported the use of letrozole, alone or with gonadotropins, follicle-stimulating hormone, or metformin for ovarian stimulation. The effectiveness of letrozole for this use was comparable to other agents. No increase in the incidence of congenital malformations was observed and pregnancy outcomes were comparable or better than when clomiphene citrate was used.

BREASTFEEDING SUMMARY

No reports describing the use of letrozole during human lactation have been located. Such reports are unlikely because of its indication for breast cancer. Moreover, the molecular weight (about 285), low plasma protein binding, and long terminal elimination half-life (about 2 days) suggest that it will be excreted into breast milk. Women requiring this agent should not breastfeed.

References

1. Product information. Femara. Novartis Pharmaceuticals, 2010.
2. Mitwally MF, Biljan MM, Casper RF. Pregnancy outcome after the use of an aromatase inhibitor for ovarian stimulation. Am J Obstet Gynecol 2005;192:381–6.
3. Thatcher SS, Jackson EM. Pregnancy outcome in infertile patients with polycystic ovary syndrome who were treated with metformin. Fertil Steril 2006;85:1002–9.
4. Tulandi T, Martin J, Al-Fadhli R, Kabli N, Forman R, Hitkari J, Librach C, Greenblatt E, Casper RF. Congenital malformations among 911 newborns conceived after infertility treatment with letrozole or clomiphene citrate. Fertil Steril 2006;85:1761–5.
5. Dickerson RD, Pinto AB, Putman JM, Lee-Messinger JR. Use of letrozole in polycystic ovary syndrome patients resistant to clomiphene (abstract). Obstet Gynecol 2006;107(Suppl);41S.
6. Forman R, Gill S, Moretti M, Tulandi T, Koren G, Casper R. Fetal safety of letrozole and clomiphene citrate for ovulation induction. J Obstet Gynaecol Can 2007;29:668–71.
7. Badawy A, Shokeir T, Allam FA, Abdelhady H. Pregnancy outcome after ovulation induction with aromatase inhibitors or clomiphene citrate in unexplained infertility. Acta Obstet Gynecol Scand 2009;88:187–91.
8. Hashim HA, Shokeir T, Badawy A. Letrozole versus combined metformin and clomiphene citrate for ovulation induction in clomiphene-resistant women with polycystic ovary syndrome: a randomized controlled trial. Fertil Steril 2010;94:1405–9.
9. Kamath MS, Aleyamma TK, Chandy A, George K. Aromatase inhibitors in women with clomiphene citrate resistance: a randomized, double-blind, placebo-controlled trial. Fertil Steril 2010;94:2857–9.
10. Badawy A, Elnashar A, Totongy M. Clomiphene citrate or aromatase inhibitors combined with gonadotropins for superovulation in women undergoing intrauterine inseminations: a prospective randomised trial. J Obstet Gynaecol 2010;30:617–21.
11. Zeinalzadeh M, Basirat Z, Esmailpour M. Efficacy of letrozole in ovulation induction compared to that of clomiphene citrate in patients with polycystic ovarian syndrome. J Reprod Med 2010;55:36–40.

L

12. Akar ME, Johnston-MacAnanny EB, Carrillo AJ, Miller J, Yalcinkaya TM. The pregnancy outcome of retrieved excess eggs collected during selective follicular reduction from patients with three or more preovulatory follicles undergoing controlled ovarian stimulation and IUI. Hum Reprod 2010;25:2931.
13. Wagman I, Levin I, Kapustiansky R, Shrim A, Amit A, Almog B, Azem F. Clomiphene citrate vs. letrozole for cryopreserved-thawed embryo transfer; a randomized, controlled trial. J Reprod Med 2010;55:134–8.
14. Abdellah MS. Reproductive outcome after letrozole versus laparoscopic ovarian drilling for clomiphene-resistant polycystic ovary syndrome. Int J Gynecol Obstet 2011;113:218–21.
15. Requena A, Herrero J, Landeras J, Navarro E, Neyro JL, Salvador C, Tur R, Callejo J, Checa MA, Farre M, Espinos JJ, Fabregues F, Grana-Barcia M, Reproductive Endocrinology Interest Group of the Spanish Society of Fertility. Use of letrozole in assisted reproduction: a systematic review and meta-analysis. Human Reprod Update 2008;14:571–82.
16. Elizur SE, Tulandi T. Drugs in infertility and fetal safety. Fertil Steril 2008;89:1595–602.
17. Gill SK, Moretti M, Koren G. Is the use of letrozole to induce ovulation teratogenic? Can Fam Physician 2008;54:353–4.
18. Eckmann KR, Kockler DR. Aromatase inhibitors for ovulation and pregnancy in polycystic ovary syndrome. Ann Pharmacother 2009;43:1338–46.
19. Polyzos NP, Tzioras S, Badawy AM, Valachis A, Dritsas C, Mauri D. Aromatase inhibitors for female infertility: a systematic review of the literature. Reprod Biomed Online 2009;19:456–71.
20. Pritts EA. Letrozole for ovulation induction and controlled ovarian hyperstimulation. Curr Opin Obstet Gynecol 2010;22:289–94.

LEUCOVORIN

Vitamin

PREGNANCY RECOMMENDATION: Compatible
BREASTFEEDING RECOMMENDATION: Compatible

PREGNANCY SUMMARY

Leucovorin (folinic acid) is an active metabolite of folic acid (1). It has been used for the treatment of megaloblastic anemia during pregnancy (2). See Folic Acid.

BREASTFEEDING SUMMARY

Leucovorin (folinic acid) is an active metabolite of folic acid (1). See Folic Acid.

References

1. American Hospital Formulary Service. *Drug Information 1997*. Bethesda, MD: American Society of Health-System Pharmacists, 1997:2890–93.
2. Scott JM. Folinic acid in megaloblastic anaemia of pregnancy. Br Med J 1957:2:270–2.

LEUPROLIDE

Antineoplastic/Hormone

PREGNANCY RECOMMENDATION: Contraindicated
BREASTFEEDING RECOMMENDATION: Contraindicated

PREGNANCY SUMMARY

Although the human data are limited, daily injections of leuprolide early in gestation do not appear to be associated with an increased risk of spontaneous abortions (SABs), intrauterine growth restriction (IUGR), or major congenital malformations.

FETAL RISK SUMMARY

Leuprolide is a synthetic nonapeptide analog of naturally occurring gonadotropin-releasing hormone that inhibits the secretion of gonadotropin when given continuously and in therapeutic doses.

Leuprolide causes a dose-related increase in the incidence of major malformations in pregnant rabbits, but not in rats (1). The most frequently observed malformations in rabbits were vertebral anomalies and hydrocephalus (J.D. Miller, personal communication, Tap Pharmaceuticals, Inc., 1992). The doses tested were 1/300th to 1/3rd of the typical human dose. Increased fetal mortality and decreased fetal weights were observed in both animal species with the higher test doses.

In humans, SABs or IUGR are theoretically possible because leuprolide suppresses endometrial proliferation. The risk of these adverse outcomes is considered greater than the risk of congenital malformations because the affected organs in animal studies do not depend on the presence of gonadal steroids for normal development (J.D. Miller, personal communication, Tap Pharmaceuticals, Inc., 1992).

A 1991 case report described a woman who was treated with leuprolide from days 21 to 38 after her last menstrual period (2). She had received the drug in preparation for in vivo fertilization. At 38 weeks' gestation, she delivered a healthy, 3300-g male infant who was doing well at 6 months of age (2).

The manufacturer is maintaining a registry of inadvertent human exposures during pregnancy to leuprolide and currently has more than 100 such cases (J.D. Miller, personal communication, Tap Pharmaceuticals, Inc., 1992). No cases of congenital defects attributable to the drug have been reported, although the numbers are too small to draw conclusions as to the risk for perinatal mortality, low birth weight, or teratogenicity.

The outcomes of 18 pregnancies in 17 women who had been exposed to leuprolide early in gestation were described in a 1993 report (3). The outcomes included five 1st trimester SABs, one of which was a fetus with trisomy 18, and the loss of a normal fetus at 20 weeks' because of cervical incompetence. The other 12 cases involved delivery of normal infants; 11 at term and 1 at 36 weeks'. The results suggested no increased risk for birth defects or pregnancy wastage (3).

BREASTFEEDING SUMMARY

No reports describing the use of leuprolide during human lactation have been located.

References

1. Product information. Lupron. Tap Pharmaceuticals, Inc., 1990.
2. Ghazi DM, Kemmann E, Hammond JM. Normal pregnancy outcome after early maternal exposure to gonadotropin releasing hormone agonist. A case report. J Reprod Med 1991;36:173–4.
3. Wilshire GB, Emmi AM, Gagliardi CC, Weiss G. Gonadotropin-releasing hormone agonist administration in early human pregnancy is associated with normal outcomes. Fert Steril 1993;60:980–3.

LEVALLORPHAN

[Withdrawn from the market. See 8th edition.]

L

LEVALBUTEROL

Respiratory Drug (Bronchodilator)

PREGNANCY RECOMMENDATION: No Human Data—Probably Compatible
BREASTFEEDING RECOMMENDATION: No Human Data—Probably Compatible

PREGNANCY SUMMARY

No reports describing the use of levalbuterol (levosalbutamol), an (R)-enantiomer of racemic albuterol, in human pregnancy have been located. However, racemic albuterol is considered compatible in pregnancy, and there is no apparent reason not to classify levalbuterol the same. If levalbuterol is used in pregnancy for the treatment of asthma, healthcare professionals are encouraged to call the toll-free number (877-311-8972) for information about patient enrollment in an Organization of Teratology Specialists (OTIS) study.

FETAL RISK SUMMARY

Levalbuterol (levosalbutamol) is a β_2-adrenergic receptor agonist that acts as a bronchodilator. It is an (R)-enantiomer of the racemic albuterol. Levalbuterol inhalation is indicated for the treatment or prevention of bronchospasm in adults, adolescents, and children ≥6 years of age with reversible obstructive airway disease. It is in the same subclass of β_2-adrenergic bronchodilators as albuterol, arformoterol, formoterol, metaproterenol, pirbuterol, salmeterol, and terbutaline. The drug is partially metabolized to an inactive metabolite before elimination. The plasma elimination half-life in adults after four doses was 4.0 hours (1).

Reproduction studies have been conducted in rabbits. Oral doses up to 110 times the maximum recommended daily inhalation dose were not teratogenic. However, racemic albuterol was teratogenic in mice and rabbits (see also Albuterol).

Studies for carcinogenicity and fertility have not been conducted with levalbuterol (see Albuterol). Levalbuterol was not mutagenic in two assays (1).

It is not known if levalbuterol crosses the human placenta. The molecular weight (about 240 for the free base) and elimination half-life suggest that the drug will cross to the embryo–fetus. However, the plasma concentrations after inhalation are very low.

BREASTFEEDING SUMMARY

No reports describing the use of levalbuterol during human lactation have been located. The molecular weight (about 240 for the free base) and elimination half-life (4 hours) suggest that the drug will be excreted into breast milk. However, the plasma concentrations (ng/mL) after inhalation are very low. The effect of this exposure on a nursing infant is unknown, but the drug is probably compatible with breastfeeding.

Reference

1. Product information. Xopenex. Sepracor, 2005.

LEVETIRACETAM

Anticonvulsant

PREGNANCY RECOMMENDATION: Limited Human Data—Animal Data Suggest Risk
BREASTFEEDING RECOMMENDATION: No Human Data—Probably Compatible

PREGNANCY SUMMARY

The animal data suggest risk, but the limited human pregnancy experience with levetiracetam has not shown an increased risk of major congenital malformations. Although confirmation is needed, severe growth restriction has been observed. Additional data are required before a more complete assessment of embryo–fetal risk can be derived. It is not known if levetiracetam causes folic acid deficiency, but it will usually be combined with other anticonvulsants, some of which may cause folic acid deficiency. Therefore, daily supplementation with 4–5 mg of folic acid, combined with multivitamins that include adequate amounts of other B vitamins, is recommended. If a pregnant patient is receiving levetiracetam, clinicians are encouraged to register her, before pregnancy outcome is known, in the Antiepileptic Drug Pregnancy Registry by calling the toll-free number (888-233-2334) (1).

FETAL RISK SUMMARY

Levetiracetam is an anticonvulsant used as adjunctive therapy in the treatment of partial-onset seizures in epilepsy. It is chemically unrelated to other anticonvulsant agents. Levetiracetam is minimally protein bound (<10%) and is not metabolized by the liver (1,2). Major metabolism occurs by enzymatic hydrolysis of the acetamide group to produce the carboxylic acid metabolite (1). Levetiracetam does not inhibit and is not a high affinity substrate for epoxide hydrolase (1). Reports describing the effects (if any) of levetiracetam on folic acid have not been located.

In reproduction studies with pregnant rats, maternal doses approximately equivalent to the maximum recommended human dose (3000 mg) based on BSA (MRHD) administered throughout pregnancy and lactation were associated with an increased incidence of minor fetal skeletal abnormalities and restricted growth prenatally and postnatally (1). When doses six times the MRHD were used, increased pup mortality and behavioral alterations were observed. The developmental no-effect dose administered throughout pregnancy and lactation was 0.2 times the MRHD. Dosing at 12 times the MRHD given only during organogenesis resulted in reduced fetal weights and an increased incidence of fetal skeletal variations. The developmental no-effect dose during organogenesis was four times the MRHD. No evidence of fetal or neonatal harm was observed with doses up to six times the MRHD during the last third of pregnancy and throughout lactation. None of the studied doses produced maternal toxicity (1).

In pregnant rabbits, increased embryo/fetal mortality and an increased incidence of minor skeletal abnormalities were observed at maternal doses four times the MRHD administered during organogenesis. When a dose 12 times the MRHD was used, decreased fetal weight and increased incidences of fetal malformations were noted, but maternal toxicity was also evident at this dose. The developmental no-effect dose was 1.3 times the MRHD (1).

It is not known if levetiracetam crosses the human placenta. The low molecular weight (about 170) and the lack of protein binding suggest that exposure of the embryo and fetus should be expected.

An estimated 20%–30% of epileptic patients have seizures not well controlled by monotherapy and require anticonvulsant polytherapy (2). Clinical studies of levetiracetam have demonstrated efficacy in partial-onset seizures with a good tolerability profile. In addition, its lack of hepatic metabolism and low protein binding result in a low risk of interaction with other drugs, including other anticonvulsants and oral contraceptives. Although comparison studies with other adjunctive anticonvulsants (e.g., felbamate, gabapentin, lamotrigine, tiagabine, topiramate, and vigabitrin) have not been conducted, it should be added to the list of agents to consider in cases of treatment-refractory partial-onset seizures (2).

A 2005 report described the outcomes of 11 pregnancies exposed to levetiracetam that were enrolled in the European Registry of Antiepileptic Drugs and Pregnancy (3). Levetiracetam was used alone in two pregnancies and combined with other antiepileptic agents in nine. The outcomes were one spontaneous abortion, one elective abortion, and nine infants without birth defects. However, three of the infants, one of whom was premature, had very low birth weight (≤5th percentile) (3).

The Lamotrigine Pregnancy Registry, an ongoing project conducted by the manufacturer, was first published in January 1997 (4). The final report was published in July 2010. The Registry is now closed. Among 57 prospectively enrolled pregnancies exposed to levetiracetam and lamotrigine, with or without other anticonvulsants, 54 were exposed in the 1st trimester resulting in 48 live births without birth defects, 3 SABs, 1 fetal death, and 2 birth defects. There were three exposures in the 2nd/3rd trimesters resulting in live births without defects (4).

BREASTFEEDING SUMMARY

No reports describing the use of levetiracetam during lactation have been located. The molecular weight (about 170) and low protein binding (<10%) suggest that levetiracetam will be excreted into breast milk. The effects of this exposure on a nursing infant are unknown. Of note, however, other anticonvulsants (see Carbamazepine, Phenytoin, and Valproic

Acid) are classified as compatible with breastfeeding by the American Academy of Pediatrics.

References

1. Product information. Keppra. UCB Pharma, 2002.
2. Dooley M, Plosker GL. Levetiracetam. A review of its adjunctive use in the management of partial-onset seizures. Drugs 2000;60:871–93.
3. Ten Berg K, Samren EB, van Oppen AC, Engelsman M, Lindhout D. Levetiracetam use and pregnancy outcome. Reprod Toxicol 2005;20:175–8.
4. The Lamotrigine Pregnancy Registry. Final Report. 1 September 1992 through 31 March 2010. GlaxoSmithKline, July 2010.

LEVOCETIRIZINE

Antihistamine

PREGNANCY RECOMMENDATION: No Human Data—Animal Data Suggest Low Risk
BREASTFEEDING RECOMMENDATION: No Human Data—Probably Compatible

PREGNANCY SUMMARY

No reports describing the use of levocetirizine in human pregnancy have been located. The animal reproduction data suggest low risk, but the absence of human pregnancy experience prevents a more complete assessment of the embryo–fetal risk. There are no data suggesting that antihistamines, in general, are associated with human developmental toxicity, and the embryo–fetal risk from exposure levocetirizine appears to be low, if it exists at all. Nevertheless, if an antihistamine is required during pregnancy, agents with human pregnancy experience, such as chlorpheniramine or diphenhydramine, appear to be a better choice.

L

FETAL RISK SUMMARY

The antihistamine levocetirizine is a H_1-receptor antagonist. It is the (R)-enantiomer and principal pharmacologically active component of the racemic compound cetirizine. (See also Cetirizine.) Levocetirizine is indicated for the relief of symptoms associated with allergic rhinitis (seasonal and perennial) and, for the treatment of uncomplicated skin manifestations of chronic idiopathic urticaria, both indications in adults and children 6 years of age or older. The drug is only partially metabolized (<14%) but plasma protein binding is high (91%–92%). The plasma half-life is about 8–9 hours (1,2).

Reproduction studies have been conducted in pregnant rats and rabbits. In these species, oral doses up to 320 and 390 times, respectively, the maximum recommended daily dose in adults based on BSA (MRDD), were not teratogenic (1,2).

Although carcinogenicity studies have not been conducted with levocetirizine, they have been with cetirizine. This drug was not carcinogenic in 2-year studies in rats. In a similar study in mice, cetirizine caused an increased incidence of benign hepatic tumors in males. Levocetirizine was not mutagenic or clastogenic in multiple assays. The antihistamine had no effect on fertility and general reproductive performance in mice at a dose that was about 25 times the MRDD (1,2).

It is not known if levocetirizine crosses the human placenta. The molecular weight (about 390 for the free base), minimum metabolism, and long plasma half-life suggest that the drug will reach the embryo–fetus, but the high plasma protein binding might lessen the amount crossing the placenta.

BREASTFEEDING SUMMARY

No reports describing the use of levocetirizine during human lactation have been located. The molecular weight (about 390 for the free base), minimum metabolism, and long plasma half-life suggest that the drug will be excreted into breast milk, but the high plasma protein binding might lessen the amount excreted. The effects of this exposure on a nursing infant are unknown, but sedation or irritability is a potential minor adverse effect.

Antihistamines are a large pharmacologic class of drugs, only one of which, when used alone, has been associated with major toxicity in a nursing infant. (See Clemastine.) Milk concentrations have been determined for only four antihistamines (see Fexofenadine, Loratadine, Terfenadine, and Triprolidine), and these four agents are considered compatible with breastfeeding by the American Academy of Pediatrics. The theoretical infant dose, as a percentage of the mother's weight-adjusted dose, was calculated for three of drugs and was ≤0.45%. Because there is no reason to believe that levocetirizine should be any different, the drug probably is compatible with breastfeeding.

References

1. Product information. Xyzal. UCB, 2008.
2. Product information. Xyzal. Sanofi-Aventis, 2008.

LEVODOPA

Antiparkinson Agent

PREGNANCY RECOMMENDATION: Human Data Suggest Low Risk
BREASTFEEDING RECOMMENDATION: Limited Human Data—Probably Compatible

PREGNANCY SUMMARY

Levodopa-induced teratogenicity and dose-related toxicity have been observed in animals, but no adverse outcomes associated with this drug have been observed in a limited number of human pregnancies. Although conditions requiring the use of levodopa during the childbearing years are relatively uncommon, exposure to this agent during gestation does not appear to present a major risk to the fetus. (See also Carbidopa.) However, evaluation of the effect of chronic in utero exposure to dopamine, the active metabolite of levodopa, on neurodevelopment is warranted.

FETAL RISK SUMMARY

Levodopa, a metabolic precursor to dopamine, is primarily used for the treatment and prevention of symptoms related to Parkinson's disease. The active agent for this purpose is thought to be dopamine, which is formed in the brain after metabolism of levodopa. Levodopa crosses the blood–brain barrier, but dopamine does not. Combination with carbidopa (see also Carbidopa), an agent that inhibits the decarboxylation of extracerebral levodopa, allows for lower doses of levodopa, fewer adverse drug effects related to peripheral dopamine, and higher amounts of levodopa available for passage to the brain and eventual conversion to dopamine.

Levodopa, either alone or in combination with carbidopa, has caused visceral and skeletal malformations in rabbits (1). Doses of 125 or 250 mg/kg/day in pregnant rabbits produced malformations of the fetal circulatory system (2). This teratogenicity was not observed at 75 mg/kg/day, but all three doses produced fetal toxicity manifested by decreased litter weight and an increased incidence of stunted and resorbed fetuses. In mice, no teratogenicity was observed with doses of 125, 250, and 500 mg/kg/day, but at the highest dose, fetuses were significantly smaller than controls (2). A similar, significant decrease in the weights of newborn mice was observed in a study in which pregnant mice were fed levodopa 40 mg/g of food, but not at lower doses (3). The number of pregnancies and the number of newborns were also significantly decreased in those treated at 40 mg/g of food compared with those treated with 0, 10, or 20 mg/g of food.

Levodopa, in oral doses of 1–1000 mg/kg/day administered to pregnant rats during the 1st week of gestation, produced a dose-related occurrence in brown fat (interscapular brown adipose tissue) hemorrhage and vasodilation in the newborns (4). A similar response was observed with dopamine. The addition of carbidopa (MK-486) to levodopa resulted in a significant decrease in this toxicity, implying that the causative agent was dopamine.

A study published in 1978 examined the effect of carbidopa (20 mg/kg SC every 12 hours × 7 days) and levodopa plus carbidopa (200/20 mg/kg SC every 12 hours × 7 days) on the length of gestation in pregnant rats (5). Only the combination had a statistically significant effect on pregnancy duration, causing a delay in parturition of 12 hours. The results were thought to be consistent with dopamine inhibition of oxytocin release.

Because Parkinson's disease is relatively uncommon in women of childbearing age, only a few reports, some involving uses other than for parkinsonism, have been located that describe the use of levodopa, with or without carbidopa, in human pregnancy.

Placental transfer of levodopa at term was documented in a 1989 report (6). A 34-year-old multiparous woman, with a 6-year history of Parkinson's disease, was treated with a proprietary combination of levodopa and benserazide (Madopar, not available in the United States), three 250-mg tablets/day. When pregnancy was diagnosed (15th day postconception), the combination therapy was discontinued and treatment with levodopa (≤500 mg/day) alone was started. After 5 months, because of worsening parkinsonism, she was again treated with levodopa/benserazide (six 250-mg tablets/day). She eventually gave birth to a normal, 3070-g female infant who had no signs or symptoms of toxicity from the drug therapy during the first 8 days of life. Her 1-minute Apgar score was 2; then improved to 7 and 10 at 3 and 5 minutes, respectively. The cord plasma level of levodopa was 0.38 mcg/mL compared with 2.7 mcg/mL in the mother's plasma, a ratio of 0.14.

A 1995 reference described the placental transfer of levodopa and the possible fetal metabolism of the drug to dopamine, its active metabolite (7). A 34-year-old woman with juvenile Parkinson's disease was treated with carbidopa/levodopa (200/800 mg/day) during two pregnancies (see also Carbidopa). Both pregnancies were electively terminated, one at 8 weeks' gestation and the other at 10 weeks' gestation. Mean concentrations of levodopa (expressed as ng/mg protein) in the maternal serum, placental tissue (including umbilical cord), fetal peripheral organs (heart, kidney, muscle), and fetal neural tissue (brain and spinal cord) were 8.5, 33.6, 7.4, and 7.7, respectively. Corresponding mean concentrations of dopamine at these sites were 0.10, <0.03, 0.29, and 1.01, respectively. The levels in the placentas and fetuses for both levodopa and dopamine were much higher than those measured in control tissue. Moreover, the relatively high concentrations of dopamine in fetal peripheral organs and neural tissue implied that the fetuses had metabolized levodopa. The investigators cautioned that, because neurotransmitters were known to alter early neural development in animals and in cultured cells, the increased amounts of dopamine found in their study suggested that chronic use of levodopa during gestation could induce long-term damage (7).

The pregnancy outcomes of two women who were treated with levodopa or carbidopa/levodopa during three pregnancies were described in a 1985 paper (8). The first woman, with at least a 7-year history of parkinsonism, conceived while being treated with carbidopa/levodopa (five 25/250-mg tablets/day) and amantadine (100 mg twice daily). She had delivered a normal male infant approximately 6 years earlier, but no medical treatment had been given during that pregnancy. Amantadine was immediately discontinued when the current pregnancy was diagnosed. Other than slight vaginal bleeding in the 1st trimester, there were no maternal or fetal complications. She gave birth to a normal-term infant (sex and weight not specified) who was doing well at 1.5 years of age. The second patient, a 32-year-old woman with parkinsonism first diagnosed at age 23, was being treated with levodopa (4 g/day) when a pregnancy of about 6 months' duration was diagnosed. Attempts to lower her levodopa dose were unsuccessful. She delivered a term, male, 7-lb 2-oz (about 3235-g) infant. Two years later, while still undergoing treatment with levodopa, she delivered a term, female, 2951-g infant. Both children were alive and well at 7 and 5 years, respectively.

A 1987 retrospective report described the use of carbidopa/levodopa, starting before conception, in five women during seven pregnancies, one of which was electively terminated during the 1st trimester (9). A sixth woman, taking levodopa plus amantadine, had a miscarriage at 4 months. All of the other pregnancies went to term (newborn weights and sexes not specified). Maternal complications in three pregnancies included slight 1st trimester vaginal bleeding, nausea, and vomiting during the 8th and 9th months (the only patient who reported nausea and vomiting after the 1st trimester) and depression that resolved postpartum, and preeclampsia. One infant, whose mother took amantadine and carbidopa/levodopa and whose pregnancy was complicated by preeclampsia, had an inguinal hernia. No adverse effects or congenital anomalies were noted in the other five newborns and all remained healthy at follow-up (approximately 1–5 years of age).

A 27-year-old woman, with a history of chemotherapy and radiotherapy for non-Hodgkin's lymphoma occurring approximately 4 years earlier had developed a progressive parkinsonism syndrome that was treated with a proprietary preparation of carbidopa/levodopa (co-careldopa, Sinemet Plus; 375 mg/day) (10). She conceived 5 months after treatment began and eventually delivered a healthy, 3540-g male infant at term. Apgar scores were both 9 at 1 and 10 minutes. Co-careldopa had been continued throughout her pregnancy.

A brief case report, published in 1997, described a normal outcome in the 3rd pregnancy of a woman with levodopa-responsive dystonia (Segawa's type) who was treated throughout gestation with 500 mg/day of levodopa alone (11). The male infant weighed 2350 g at birth and was developing normally at the time of the report. Two previous pregnancies had occurred while the woman was being treated with daily doses of levodopa 100 mg and carbidopa 10 mg. Spontaneous abortions had occurred in both pregnancies; one at 6 weeks and the other at 12 weeks. An investigation failed to find any cause for the miscarriages (11).

A successful pregnancy in a 27-year-old woman with Segawa disease was reported in 2009 (12). The woman was treated throughout gestation with levodopa 1250 mg/day and, at 36 weeks', gave birth to a healthy, 2298-g male infant with an Apgar score of 9 at 5 minutes. The infant was doing well at 6 months of age. The authors cited eight other cases of the disease in five pregnant women. Five of the pregnancies were treated with levodopa monotherapy and ended in healthy newborns. In one of those patients, her first two pregnancies were treated with carbidopa/levodopa and both ended in abortions (see reference 11 above). The ninth pregnancy was not treated with any agent and the severely asphyxiated newborn died after birth (12).

Two 1998 case reports described the use of levodopa, in combination with selegiline and benserazide, during human pregnancy (see Selegiline for details) (13,14). In another 1998 case report, a woman took levodopa/carbidopa (Sinemet CR 50/200) four times daily throughout gestation (15). Healthy male infants were delivered in all three pregnancies.

A brief 1996 communication included data obtained from a manufacturer (the Roche Drug Safety database) on the effects of levodopa on the fetus during human pregnancy (16). This database, current up to March 31, 1995, had six reports involving the use of levodopa/benserazide during gestation. The outcomes of these pregnancies included two elective terminations, one spontaneous abortion, two normal outcomes, and one lost to follow-up. No information was available on the condition of the fetuses in the three abortions. Another normal pregnancy outcome, without further details, from a mother who used levodopa/benserazide during gestation, was also cited (17). To the knowledge of these authors, two of whom were representatives of the manufacturer, no reports of human birth defects resulting from use of levodopa had been discovered.

A woman with a 12-year history of Parkinson's disease was treated throughout gestation with levodopa, carbidopa, entacapone, and bromocriptine (18). She gave birth at term to a 3175-g female infant, without deformities, with Apgar scores of 9, 10, and 10. Generalized seizures occurred in the infant 1 hour after birth, followed by repeated episodes of shivering throughout the first day that responded to diazepam. Slowly improving hypotonia also was observed during the first week. Pneumonia was diagnosed, but an extensive workup for the cause of seizures was negative. The child was developing normally at 1 year of age and has not had any other seizures (18).

A 2002 case report described the use of levodopa/pergolide in a 35-year-old woman throughout gestation (19). The woman was started on levodopa (200 mg/day) and pergolide (3 mg/day) about 3 years before conception. She continued these doses until delivery of a normal-term infant (sex and weight not specified), with Apgar scores of 9 (assumed to mean 9 and 9 at 1 and 5 minutes, respectively). The healthy child was developing normally at 13 months of age (19).

In a 2005 report, a woman with Parkinson's disease took levodopa/carbidopa 330 mg/day and cabergoline 1 mg/day throughout an uncomplicated pregnancy and gave birth at term to a healthy baby girl (20). A few years later, now at age 34 and receiving levodopa/carbidopa 625 mg/day and cabergoline 4 mg/day, she became pregnant again. At 32 weeks', she underwent a cesarean section because of placenta abruption. The baby girl was doing well (20).

A study designed to investigate the inhibitory effect of levodopa on prolactin levels in late pregnancy was reported in 1973 (21). Four women in the 3rd trimester of pregnancy were given a single oral dose of levodopa, 1000 mg.

A statistically significant decrease in serum prolactin occurred, with the lowest levels measured 4 hours after the dose, but 2 hours later the levels had returned to pretreatment values, similar to nontreated controls. No further decreases in prolactin were measured during the next 3 days. All of the treated women eventually delivered normal infants at or near term.

Levodopa has been used in the treatment of coma resulting from fulminant hepatic failure occurring during pregnancy (22,23). A 22-year-old woman, in her 6th month of pregnancy, had severe viral hepatitis with a grade IV coma (22). She was successfully treated with levodopa, 1 g orally every 6 hours, neomycin, vitamins, and parenteral hydrocortisone (1000 mg/day). Recovery from the coma occurred 24–48 hours after the start of levodopa. Approximately 3 months later, she delivered a full-term infant (details of the infant and its condition were not included). In the second case, a 30-year-old woman in her 5th month of gestation was treated for 1 week with levodopa, 1 g orally every 6 hours (23). This patient, who also had viral hepatitis, began to recover consciousness 1 hour after the first dose of levodopa and was fully awake within 24–48 hours. She delivered a term, healthy infant (sex and weight not specified).

Angiotensin pressor responsiveness (vascular sensitivity) was decreased by the administration of levodopa in pregnancy (mean 29–30 weeks, range 24–36 weeks' gestation) (24). Five patients were treated with a single 500-mg oral dose and 16 received 1000 mg. Only the higher dose produced a significant decrease in angiotensin sensitivity. The authors hypothesized that chronic treatment with levodopa might not only decrease angiotensin sensitivity but also decrease pregnancy-induced hypertension. No data were provided on the outcome of these pregnancies following the study. The effect of levodopa on plasma prolactin secretion and inhibition of the renin–aldosterone axis was reported in a subsequent paper by this same group of investigators (25). Using methods and a patient population nearly identical with those of their previous study, the investigators found that a 1000-mg oral dose of levodopa produced a significant decrease in serum prolactin, plasma renin activity, and plasma aldosterone.

BREASTFEEDING SUMMARY

Levodopa is excreted into breast milk. A 1998 case report described a woman who took levodopa/carbidopa (Sinemet CR 50/200) four times daily throughout gestation (15). She continued the therapy after delivery and during breastfeeding. At about 5 months postpartum, the peak concentration of levodopa in milk (based on 5-mL milk samples) was 1.6 nmol/mL, 3 hours after a dose. The milk:plasma ratio, based on AUC (6 hours for plasma and milk) was 0.28. When the dose was changed to two tablets of Sinemet 25/100 four times daily, the peak milk concentration (3 hours after a dose) was 3.47 nmol/mL and the milk:plasma ratio was 0.32. With both tablet strengths, the milk concentrations returned to baseline in 6 hours. The authors estimated that the nursing infant was ingesting 0.127–0.181 mg/day (0.016–0.023 mg/kg/day) of levodopa. No adverse effects were observed in the infant and he was developing normally at 2 years of age (15).

Levodopa inhibits prolactin release in both animals (26) and humans (21,25). In lactating rats, levodopa injected intraperitoneally in doses of 1.25, 2.5, 5, and 10 mg/100 g body weight produced a dose-related inhibition of milk ejection (26). Doses of 5 and 10 mg/100 g body weight, but not lower doses, prevented the release of prolactin induced by suckling. Small doses of oxytocin given immediately before suckling produced a normal milk-ejection response, indicating that the mechanism of inhibition by levodopa was not caused by mammary gland response but to an increase in catecholamines at the hypothalamic–hypophysial axis (26).

In one study, four women in the 3rd trimester of pregnancy received a single 1000-mg oral dose of levodopa (21). A significant decrease in serum prolactin occurred with the lowest concentration at 4 hours. Two hours later, the level had returned to pretreatment values. After delivery at or near term, all of the women had completely normal lactation. A second study also found that a single 1000-mg oral dose of levodopa produced a significant decrease in serum prolactin (25).

Clinical evidence of lactation inhibition was provided in a 1974 study (27). Ten female patients with a history of inappropriate galactorrhea were treated orally with levodopa, 500–3500 mg/day. Partial-to-complete suppression of lactation was observed in the women, but when treatment was stopped, lactation returned to normal levels.

References

1. Product information. Sinemet. DuPont Pharmaceuticals, 1997.
2. Staples RE, Mattis PA. Teratology of L-dopa (abstract). Teratology 1973;8:238.
3. Cotzia GC, Miller ST, Tang LC, Papavila PS. Levodopa, fertility, and longevity. Science 1977;196:549–50.
4. Kitchin KT, DiStefano V. L-Dopa and brown fat hemorrhage in the rat pup. Toxicol Appl Pharmacol 1976;38:251–63.
5. Seybold VS, Miller JW, Lewis PR. Investigation of a dopaminergic mechanism for regulating oxytocin release. J Pharmacol Exp Ther 1978;207:605–10.
6. Allain H, Bentue-Ferrer D, Milon D, Moran P, Jacquemard F, Defawe G. Pregnancy and parkinsonism. A case report without problem. Clin Neuropharmacol 1989;12:217–9.
7. Merchant CA, Cohen G, Mytilineou C, DiRocco A, Moros D, Molinari S, Yahr MD. Human transplacental transfer of carbidopa/levodopa. J Neural Transm Park Dis Dement Sect 1995;9:239–42.
8. Cook DG, Klawans HL. Levodopa during pregnancy. Clin Neuropharmacol 1985;8:93–5.
9. Golbe LI. Parkinson's disease and pregnancy. Neurology 1987;37:1245–9.
10. Ball MC, Sagar HJ. Levodopa in pregnancy. Mov Disord 1995;10:115.
11. Nomoto M, Kaseda S, Iwata S, Osame M, Fukuda T. Levodopa in pregnancy. Mov Disord 1997;12:261.
12. Watanabe T, Matsubara S, Baba Y, Tanaka H, Suzuki T, Suzuki M. Successful management of pregnancy in a patient with Segawa disease: case report and literature review. J Obstet Gynaecol Res 2009; 35:562–4.
13. Hagell P, Odin P, Vinge E. Pregnancy in Parkinson's disease: a review of the literature and a case report. Mov Disord 1998;13:34–8.
14. Kupsch A, Oertel WH. Selegiline, pregnancy, and Parkinson's disease. Mov Disord 1998;13:175–94.
15. Thulin PC, Woodward WR, Carter JH, Nutt JG. Levodopa in human breast milk: clinical implications. Neurology 1998;50:1920–1.
16. von Graeventiz KS, Shulman LM, Revell SP. Levodopa in pregnancy. Mov Disord 1996;11:115–6.
17. Bauherz G. Pregnancy and Parkinson's disease. A case report. N Trends Clin Neuropharmacol 1994;8:142. As cited by von Graeventiz KS, Shulman LM, Revell SP. Levodopa in pregnancy. Mov Disord 1996;11:115–6.
18. Lindh J. Short episode of seizures in a newborn of mother treated with levodopa/carbidopa/entacapone and bromocriptine. Mov Disord 2007;22:1515.
19. De Mari M, Zenzola A, Lamberti P. Antiparkinsonian treatment in pregnancy. Mov Disord 2002;17:428–9.
20. Scott M, Chowdhury M. Pregnancy in Parkinson's disease: unique case report and review of the literature. Mov Disord 2005;20:1078–9.
21. Pujol-Amat P, Gamissans O, Calaf J, Benito E, Perez-Lopez FR, L'Hermite M, Robyn C. Influence of L-dopa on serum prolactin, human chorionic

L

somatomammotrophin (HCS) and human chorionic gonadotrophin (HCG) during the last trimester of pregnancy. In: *Human Prolactin. Proceedings of the International Symposium on Human Prolactin*, Brussels, June 12–14, 1973. New York, NY: American Elsevier, 1973:316–20.
22. Datta DV, Maheshwari YK, Aggarwal ML. Levodopa in fulminant hepatic failure: preliminary report. Am J Med Sci 1976;272:95–9.
23. Chajek T, Friedman G, Berry EM, Abramsky O. Treatment of acute hepatic encephalopathy with L-dopa. Postgrad Med J 1977;53:262–5.
24. Kaulhausen H, Oney T, Feldmann R, Leyendecker G. Decrease of vascular angiotensin sensitivity by L-dopa during human pregnancy. Am J Obstet Gynecol 1981;140:671–5.
25. Kaulhausen H, Oney T, Leyendecker G. Inhibition of the renin-aldosterone axis and of prolactin secretion during pregnancy by L-dopa. Br J Obstet Gynaecol 1982;89:483–8.
26. Prilusky J, Deis RP. Effect of L-dopa on milk ejection and prolactin release in lactating rats. J Endocrinol 1975;67:397–401.
27. Ayalon D, Peyser MR, Toaff R, Cordova T, Harell A, Franchimont P, Lindner HR. Effect of L-dopa on galactopoiesis and gonadotropin levels in the inappropriate lactation syndrome. Obstet Gynecol 1974;44:159–70.

LEVOFLOXACIN

Anti-infective (Quinolone)

PREGNANCY RECOMMENDATION: Human Data Suggest Low Risk
BREASTFEEDING RECOMMENDATION: Limited Human Data—Probably Compatible

PREGNANCY SUMMARY

Although only a few reports describing the use of levofloxacin during human gestation have been located, the available evidence for other members of this class suggests that the risk of major malformations is low. However, a causal relationship with birth defects cannot be excluded (see Ofloxacin), although the lack of a pattern among the anomalies is reassuring (see Ciprofloxacin). Because of these concerns and the available animal data, levofloxacin should be used cautiously during pregnancy, especially during the 1st trimester. A 1993 review on the safety of fluoroquinolones concluded that these antibacterials should be avoided during pregnancy because of the difficulty in extrapolating animal mutagenicity results to humans and because interpretation of this toxicity is still controversial (1). The authors of this review were not convinced that fluoroquinolone-induced fetal cartilage damage and subsequent arthropathies were a major concern, even though this effect had been demonstrated in several animal species after administration to both pregnant and immature animals and in occasional human case reports involving children (1). Others have also concluded that fluoroquinolones should be considered contraindicated in pregnancy, because safer alternatives are usually available (2). A 2013 review stated that fluoroquinolones are usually avoided in pregnancy because of concerns for fetal cartilage damage, but there were no human studies to validate this concern (3).

FETAL RISK SUMMARY

Levofloxacin is a synthetic, broad-spectrum antibacterial agent that is the optical isomer of ofloxacin. As a fluoroquinolone, it is in the same class as ciprofloxacin, enoxacin, lomefloxacin, norfloxacin, ofloxacin, and sparfloxacin. Nalidixic acid is also a quinolone drug. Levofloxacin undergoes limited metabolism and plasma protein binding only is 24%–38%. The mean terminal plasma elimination half-life is about 6–8 hours (4).

Reproduction studies have been conducted in rats and rabbits. In rats given oral and IV doses that were ≤4.2 and ≤1.2 times the maximum recommended human dose based on BSA (MRHD), respectively, no evidence of impaired fertility or reproductive performance was noted. No teratogenicity was observed in pregnant rats with oral and IV doses that were ≤9.4 and ≤1.9 times the MRHD, respectively. However, an oral dose 9.4 times the MRHD caused decreased fetal weight and increased fetal mortality. In pregnant rabbits, no teratogenicity was observed with oral and IV doses that were ≤1.1 and ≤0.5 times the MRHD, respectively (4).

A 2005 study measured the amount of three fluoroquinolones (ciprofloxacin, ofloxacin, levofloxacin) that crossed the perfused human placenta (5). All three agents crossed the placenta from the maternal to the fetal compartment, but the amounts crossing were small: 3.2%, 3.7%, and 3.9%, respectively. The transfer of levofloxacin across the placenta is consistent with the molecular weight (about 370). Moreover, in vivo transfer should be expected because of the low metabolism and plasma protein binding, and the moderately long plasma elimination half-life.

In a 2010 study, 12 women scheduled for a cesarean section were given IV levofloxacin 500 mg over 60 minutes (6). The transplacental passage rate calculated as a percentage of fetal venous concentration to maternal blood concentration was about 67%, whereas the transfetal passage rate calculated as a percentage of fetal arterial drug concentration to fetal venous concentration was about 84% (6).

A second study by the same group as above, measured levofloxacin amniotic fluid concentrations in 10 women given a 500-mg oral dose about 2 hours before amniocentesis (7). The study was conducted between the 16th and 20th gestational weeks. The mean concentrations of levofloxacin in maternal blood and amniotic fluid were 3.95 mcg/mL and 0.60 mcg/mL, an amniotic fluid passage rate of about 16% (7).

In a prospective follow-up study conducted by the European Network of Teratology Information Services (ENTIS), data on 549 pregnancies exposed to fluoroquinolones (none to levofloxacin; 93 to ofloxacin) (see also Ofloxacin) were described in a 1996 reference (2). Data on another 116 prospective and 25 retrospective pregnancy exposures to the antibacterials were also included. Of the 666 cases with known outcome, 32 (4.8%) of the embryos, fetuses, or newborns had congenital malformations. From previous epidemiologic data, the authors concluded that the 4.8% frequency of malformations did not exceed the background rate. Finally, 25 retrospective reports of infants with anomalies, who had been exposed in utero to fluoroquinolones, were described, but no specific patterns of major congenital malformations were detected (2).

The authors of the above study concluded that pregnancy exposure to quinolones was not an indication for termination, but that this class of antibacterials should still be considered contraindicated in pregnant women. Moreover, this study did not address the issue of cartilage damage from quinolone exposure and the authors recognized the need for follow-up studies of this potential toxicity in children exposed in utero. Because of their own and previously published findings, they further recommended that the focus of future studies should be on malformations involving the abdominal wall and urogenital system and on limb reduction defects (2).

BREASTFEEDING SUMMARY

When first marketed, the use of levofloxacin during lactation was not recommended because of the potential for arthropathy and other serious toxicity in the nursing infant (4). Phototoxicity has been observed with quinolones when exposure to excessive sunlight (i.e., ultraviolet [UV] light) has occurred. Well-differentiated squamous cell carcinomas of the skin has been produced in mice who were exposed chronically to some fluoroquinolones and periodic UV light (e.g., see Lomefloxacin), but studies to evaluate the carcinogenicity of ofloxacin in this manner have not been conducted (4).

Levofloxacin is excreted into breast milk (8). A lactating woman received levofloxacin 500 mg/day during the first 23 days postpartum. Milk samples were collected at various times at steady state. The peak concentration in milk, 8.2 mcg/mL, occurred 5 hours after a dose. The pharmacokinetics in milk was similar to those in the plasma. Minimal levels of the drug were detectable 65 hours after the last dose. The infant was not allowed to breastfeed (8). The effect of this exposure on a nursing infant is unknown, but other fluoroquinolones are classified as compatible with breastfeeding by the American Academy of Pediatrics (see Ofloxacin and Ciprofloxacin).

References

1. Norrby SR, Lietman PS. Safety and tolerability of fluoroquinolones. Drugs 1993;45(Suppl 3):59–64.
2. Schaefer C, Amoura-Elefant E, Vial T, Ornoy A, Garbis H, Robert E, Rodriguez-Pinilla E, Pexieder T, Prapas N, Merlob P. Pregnancy outcome after prenatal quinolone exposure. Evaluation of a case registry of the European Network of Teratology Information Services (ENTIS). Eur J Obstet Gynecol Reprod Biol 1996;69:83–9.
3. Meaney-Delman D, Rasmussen SA, Beigi RH, Zotti ME, Hutchings Y, Bower WA, Treadwell TA, Jamieson DJ. Prophylaxis and treatment of anthrax in pregnant women. Obstet Gynecol 2013;122:885–900.
4. Product information. Levaquin. Ortho-McNeil Pharmaceutical, 2007.
5. Polachek H, Holcberg G, Sapir G, Tsadkin-Tamir M, Polacheck J, Katz M, Ben-Zvi Z. Transfer of ciprofloxacin, ofloxacin and levofloxacin across the perfused human placenta in vitro. Eur J Obstet Gynecol Reprod Biol 2005;122:61–5.
6. Ozyuncu O, Nemutlu E, Katlan D, Kir S, Beksac MS. Maternal and fetal blood levels of moxifloxacin, levofloxacin, cefepime and cefoperazone. Int J Antimicrob Agents 2010;36:175–8.
7. Ozyuncu O, Beksac MS, Nemutlu E, Katlan D, Kir S. Maternal blood and amniotic fluid levels of moxifloxacin, levofloxacin and cefixime. J Obstet Gynecol 2010;36:484–7.
8. Cahill JB Jr, Bailey EM, Chien S, Johnson GM. Levofloxacin secretion in breast milk: a case report. Pharmacotherapy 2005;25:116–8.

LEVORPHANOL

Narcotic Agonist Analgesic

PREGNANCY RECOMMENDATION: Human Data Suggest Risk in 3rd Trimester
BREASTFEEDING RECOMMENDATION: No Human Data—Probably Compatible

PREGNANCY SUMMARY

The use of levorphanol during labor should be expected to produce neonatal depression to the same degree as other narcotic analgesics (1). If levorphanol is used in pregnancy, healthcare professionals are encouraged to call the toll-free number (800-670-6126) for information about patient enrollment in the Motherisk study.

FETAL RISK SUMMARY

No reports linking the use of levorphanol with human congenital defects have been located. A single oral dose of 25 mg/kg was teratogenic in mice (2). At this dose, nearly 50% of the mouse embryos died.

BREASTFEEDING SUMMARY

No reports describing the use of levorphanol during lactation have been located. The molecular weight (about 444) is low enough that passage into breast milk should be expected. Moreover, the drug is structurally similar to morphine, which is excreted into milk (see Morphine). The potential for long-term effects on neurobehavior and development in a nursing infant from exposure to levorphanol in milk are unknown but warrant study.

References

1. Bonica JJ. *Principles and Practice of Obstetric Analgesia and Anesthesia.* Philadelphia, PA: FA Davis, 1967:251.
2. Product information. Levo-Dromoran. ICN Pharmaceuticals, 2000.

LEVOTHYROXINE

Thyroid

PREGNANCY RECOMMENDATION: Compatible
BREASTFEEDING RECOMMENDATION: Compatible

PREGNANCY SUMMARY

Levothyroxine (T4) is compatible with all stages of pregnancy. Untreated or undertreated maternal hypothyroidism is associated with low birth weight secondary to medically indicated preterm delivery, preeclampsia or placental abruption (1), and with lower neuropsychological development of their offspring (2).

FETAL RISK SUMMARY

T4 is a naturally occurring thyroid hormone produced by the mother and the fetus. It is used during pregnancy for the treatment of hypothyroidism (see also Liothyronine [T3] and Thyroid). Earlier investigations concluded that there was negligible transplacental passage of T4 at physiologic serum concentrations (3–8), but a 1989 study found that sufficient amounts of T4 cross the placenta to protect the congenital hypothyroid fetus and newborn (see below) (9). A 1994 review summarized the evidence that T4 crosses to the embryo and fetus throughout gestation (10).

In a surveillance study of Michigan Medicaid recipients involving 229,101 completed pregnancies conducted between 1985 and 1992, 554 newborns had been exposed to levothyroxine during the 1st trimester (F. Rosa, personal communication, FDA, 1993). A total of 25 (4.5%) major birth defects were observed (24 expected). Specific data were available for six defect categories, including (observed/expected) 5/6 cardiovascular defects, 0/1 oral clefts, 0/0.3 spina bifida, 1/2 polydactyly, 1/1 limb reduction defects, and 1/1 hypospadias. These data do not support an association between the drug and congenital defects.

In a study of 25 neonates born with an autosomal recessive disorder that completely prevents iodination of thyroid proteins and thus the synthesis of T4, the thyroid hormone was measured in their cord serum in concentrations ranging from 35 to 70 nmol/L (9). Because the newborns were unable to synthesize the hormone, the T4 must have come from the mothers. The investigators then studied 15 newborns with thyroid agenesis and measured similar cord levels of T4. The mean serum half-life of T4 in the neonates was only 3.6 days, indicating that T4 would be below the level of detection between 8 and 19 days after birth. Although the amounts measured were below normal values of T4 (80–170 nmol/L), the amounts were sufficient to protect the infants initially from impaired mental development. A possible mechanism for this protection may involve increased conversion of T4 to T3 in the cerebral cortex in hypothyroid fetuses, and when combined with a decreased rate of T3 degradation, the net effect is to normalize intracellular levels of the active thyroid hormone in the brain (9).

Several reports have described the direct administration of T4 to the fetus and amniotic fluid (2,7,9,11–15). In almost identical cases, two fetuses were treated in the 3rd trimester with IM injections of T4, 120 mcg, every 2 weeks for four doses in an attempt to prevent congenital hypothyroidism (2,7). Their mothers had been treated with radioactive iodine (I^{131}) at 13 and 13.5 weeks' gestation. Both newborns were hypothyroid at birth and developed respiratory stridor, but neither had physical signs of cretinism. At the time of the reports, one child had mild developmental retardation at 3 years of age (7). The second infant was stable with a tracheostomy tube in place at 6 months of age (11). In a third mother who inadvertently received I^{131} at 10–11 weeks' gestation, intra-amniotic T4, 500 mcg, was given weekly during the last 7 weeks of pregnancy (12). Evidence was found that the T4 was absorbed by the fetus. A male infant who developed normally was delivered. In a study to determine the metabolic fate of T4 in utero, 700 mcg of T4 were injected intra-amniotically 24 hours before delivery in five full-term healthy patients (13). Serum T4 levels were increased in all infants. Intra-amniotic T4, 200 mcg, was given to eight women in whom premature delivery was inevitable or was indicated to enhance fetal lung maturity (14). The patients ranged in gestational age between 29 and 32 weeks. No respiratory distress syndrome was found in the eight newborn infants. Delivery occurred 1–49 days after the injection. The dimensions of a large fetal goiter, secondary to propylthiouracil, were decreased but not eliminated within 5 days of an intra-amniotic 200-mcg dose of T4 administered at 34.5 weeks' gestation (15). Serial lecithin:sphingomyelin (L:S) ratios before and after the injection demonstrated no effect of T4 on fetal lung maturity.

In a large prospective study, 537 mother–child pairs were exposed to levothyroxine and thyroid (desiccated) during the 1st trimester (16, pp. 388–400). For use anytime during pregnancy, 780 exposures were reported (16, p. 443). After 1st trimester exposure, possible associations were found with cardiovascular anomalies (nine cases), Down's syndrome (three cases), and polydactyly in blacks (three cases). Because of the small numbers involved, the statistical significance of these findings is unknown and independent confirmation is required. Maternal hypothyroidism itself has been reported to be responsible for poor pregnancy outcome (17–19). Others have not found this association, claiming that fetal development is not directly affected by maternal thyroid function (20). However, untreated maternal hypothyroidism during pregnancy has been shown to result in lower scores relating to intelligence, attention, language, reading ability, school performance, and visual–motor performance in children 7–9 years of age (21).

Combination therapy with thyroid–antithyroid drugs was advocated at one time for the treatment of hyperthyroidism but is now considered inappropriate (see Propylthiouracil).

BREASTFEEDING SUMMARY

Levothyroxine (T4) is excreted into breast milk in low concentrations. The effect of this hormone on the nursing infant is controversial (see also Liothyronine and Thyrotropin). Two reports have claimed that sufficient quantities are present to partially treat neonatal hypothyroidism (22,23). A third study measured high T4 levels in breastfed infants but was unsure of its significance (24). In contrast, four competing studies have found that breastfeeding does not alter either T4 levels or thyroid function in the infant (25–28). Although all of the investigators on both sides of the issue used sophisticated available methods to arrive at their conclusions, the balance of evidence weighs in on the side of those claiming lack of effect because they have relied on increasingly refined means to measure the hormone (29–31). The reports are briefly summarized below.

In 19 healthy euthyroid mothers not taking thyroid replacement therapy, mean milk T4 concentrations in the 1st postpartum week were 3.8 ng/mL (22). Between 8 and 48 days, the levels rose to 42.7 ng/mL and then decreased to 11.1 ng/mL after 50 days postpartum. The daily excretion of T4 at the higher levels is about the recommended daily dose for hypothyroid infants (22). An infant was diagnosed as athyrotic shortly after breastfeeding was stopped at age 10 months (23). Growth was at the 97th percentile during breastfeeding, but the bone age remained that of a newborn. In this study, mean levels of T4 in breast milk during the last trimester (12 patients) and within 48 hours of delivery (22 patients) were 14 and 7 ng/mL, respectively (23). A 1983 report measured significantly greater serum levels of T4 in 22 breastfed infants than those in 25 formula-fed babies, 131.1 vs. 118.4 ng/mL, respectively (24). The overlap between the two groups, however, casts doubt on the physiologic significance of the differences.

In 77 euthyroid mothers, measurable amounts of T4 were found in only 5 of 88 milk specimens collected over 43 months of lactation, with 4 of the positive samples occurring within 4 days of delivery. Concentrations ranged from 8 to 13 ng/mL (25). A 1980 report described four exclusively breastfed infants with congenital hypothyroidism who were diagnosed between the ages of 2 and 79 days. Breastfeeding did not hinder making the diagnosis (26). Another report, evaluating clinical and biochemical thyroid parameters in hypothyroid infants, found no differences between breastfed (N = 12) and bottle-fed (N = 33) babies. These results lead to the conclusion that breast milk does not offer protection against the effects of congenital hypothyroidism (27). In a 1985 study, serum concentrations of T4 were similar in breastfed and bottle-fed infants at 5, 10, and 15 days postpartum (28).

The discrepancies described above can be partially explained by the various techniques used to measure milk T4 concentrations. Japanese researchers failed to detect milk T4 using four different methods of radioimmunoassay (RIA) (29). Using three competitive protein-binding assays, highly variable T4 levels were recovered from milk and a standard solution. Although the RIA methods were not completely reliable because recovery from a standardized solution exceeded 100% with one method, the researchers concluded that milk T4 concentrations must be very low and had no influence on the pituitary–thyroid axis of normal babies. No difficulty was encountered with measuring serum T4 levels, which were not significantly different between breastfed and bottle-fed infants (29). Swedish investigators using RIA methods also failed to find T4 in milk (30). A second group of Swedish researchers used a gas chromatography–mass spectrometry technique to determine that the concentration of T4 in milk was <4 ng/mL (31).

Levothyroxine breast milk levels, as determined by modern laboratory techniques, are too low to protect a hypothyroid infant completely from the effects of the disease. The levels are also too low to interfere with neonatal thyroid screening programs (28). The American Academy of Pediatrics classifies levothyroxine as compatible with breastfeeding (32).

References

1. American College of Obstetricians and Gynecologists. Thyroid disease in pregnancy. *ACOG Practice Bulletin*. No. 37, August 2002. Obstet Gynecol 2002;100:387–96.
2. Jafek BW, Small R, Lillian DL. Congenital radioactive iodine–induced stridor and hypothyroidism. Arch Otolaryngol 1974;99:369–71.
3. Grumbach MM, Werner SC. Transfer of thyroid hormone across the human placenta at term. J Clin Endocrinol Metab 1956;16:1392–5.
4. Kearns JE, Hutson W. Tagged isomers and analogues of thyroxine (their transmission across the human placenta and other studies). J Nucl Med 1963;4:453–61.
5. Fisher DA, Lehman H, Lackey C. Placental transport of thyroxine. J Clin Endocrinol Metab 1964;24:393–400.
6. Fisher DA, Klein AH. Thyroid development and disorders of thyroid function in the newborn. N Engl J Med 1981;304:702–12.
7. Van Herle AJ, Young RT, Fisher DA, Uller RP, Brinkman CR III. Intrauterine treatment of a hypothyroid fetus. J Clin Endocrinol Metab 1975;40: 474–7.
8. Bachrach LK, Burrow GN. Maternal–fetal transfer of thyroxine. N Engl J Med 1989;321:1549.
9. Vulsma T, Gons MH, de Vijlder JJM. Maternal–fetal transfer of thyroxine in congenital hypothyroidism due to a total organification defect or thyroid agenesis. N Engl J Med 1989;321:13–6.
10. Burrow GN, Fisher DA, Larsen PR. Maternal and fetal thyroid function. N Engl J Med 1994;331:1072–8.
11. Larsen PR. Maternal thyroxine and congenital hypothyroidism. N Engl J Med 1989;321:44–6.
12. Lightner ES, Fisher DA, Giles H, Woolfenden J. Intra-amniotic injection of thyroxine (T4) to a human fetus. Am J Obstet Gynecol 1977;127:487–90.
13. Klein AH, Hobel CJ, Sack J, Fisher DA. Effect of intraamniotic fluid thyroxine injection on fetal serum and amniotic fluid iodothyronine concentrations. J Clin Endocrinol Metab 1978;47:1034–7.
14. Mashiach S, Barkai G, Sach J, Stern E, Goldman B, Brish M, Serr DM. Enhancement of fetal lung maturity by intra-amniotic administration of thyroid hormone. Am J Obstet Gynecol 1978;130:289–93.
15. Weiner S, Scharf JI, Bolognese RJ, Librizzi RJ. Antenatal diagnosis and treatment of fetal goiter. J Reprod Med 1980;24:39–42.
16. Heinonen OP, Slone D, Shapiro S. *Birth Defects and Drugs in Pregnancy*. Littleton, MA: Publishing Sciences Group, 1977.
17. Potter JD. Hypothyroidism and reproductive failure. Surg Gynecol Obstet 1980;150:251–5.
18. Pekonen F, Teramo K, Ikonen E, Osterlund K, Makinen T, Lamberg BA. Women on thyroid hormone therapy: pregnancy course, fetal outcome, and amniotic fluid thyroid hormone level. Obstet Gynecol 1984;63:635–8.
19. Man EB, Shaver BA Jr, Cooke RE. Studies of children born to women with thyroid disease. Am J Obstet Gynecol 1958;75:728–41.
20. Montoro M, Collea JV, Frasier SD, Mestman JH. Successful outcome of pregnancy in women with hypothyroidism. Ann Intern Med 1981;94:31–4.
21. Haddow JE, Palomaki GE, Allan WC, Williams JR, Knight GJ, Gagnon J, O'Heir CE, Mitchell ML, Hermos RJ, Waisbren SE, Faix JD, Klein RZ. Maternal thyroid deficiency during pregnancy and subsequent neuropsychological development of the child. N Engl J Med 1999;341:549–55.
22. Sack J, Amado O, Lunenfeld B. Thyroxine concentration in human milk. J Clin Endocrinol Metab 1977;45:171–3.
23. Bode HH, Vanjonack WJ, Crawford JD. Mitigation of cretinism by breastfeeding. Pediatrics 1978;62:13–6.

L

24. Hahn HB Jr, Spiekerman AM, Otto WR, Hossalla DE. Thyroid function tests in neonates fed human milk. Am J Dis Child 1983;137:220–2.
25. Varma SK, Collins M, Row A, Haller WS, Varma K. Thyroxine, triiodothyronine, and reverse triiodothyronine concentrations in human milk. J Pediatr 1978;93:803–6.
26. Abbassi V, Steinour TA. Successful diagnosis of congenital hypothyroidism in four breast-fed neonates. J Pediatr 1980;97:259–61.
27. Letarte J, Guyda H, Dussault JH, Glorieux J. Lack of protective effect of breast-feeding in congenital hypothyroidism: report of 12 cases. Pediatrics 1980;65:703–5.
28. Franklin R, O'Grady C, Carpenter L. Neonatal thyroid function: comparison between breast-fed and bottle-fed infants. J Pediatr 1985;106:124–6.
29. Mizuta H, Amino N, Ichihara K, Harada T, Nose O, Tanizawa O, Miyai K. Thyroid hormones in human milk and their influence on thyroid function of breast-fed babies. Pediatr Res 1983;17:468–71.
30. Jansson L, Ivarsson S, Larsson I, Ekman R. Tri-iodothyronine and thyroxine in human milk. Acta Paediatr Scand 1983;72:703–5.
31. Moller B, Bjorkhem I, Falk O, Lantto O, Larsson A. Identification of thyroxine in human breast milk by gas chromatography–mass spectrometry. J Clin Endocrinol Metab 1983;56:30–4.
32. Committe on Drugs, American Academy of Pediatrics. The transfer of drugs and other chemicals into human milk. Pediatrics 2001;108:776–89.

LIDOCAINE

Local Anesthetic/Cardiac Drug

PREGNANCY RECOMMENDATION: Compatible
BREASTFEEDING RECOMMENDATION: Limited Human Data—Probably Compatible

PREGNANCY SUMMARY

Lidocaine is a local anesthetic that also is used for the treatment of cardiac ventricular arrhythmias. The majority of the information on the drug in pregnancy derives from its use as a local anesthetic during labor and delivery. Reproduction studies have revealed no evidence of fetal harm in pregnant rats at doses up to 6.6 times the human dose (1).

L

FETAL RISK SUMMARY

Lidocaine rapidly crosses the placenta to the fetus, appearing in the fetal circulation within a few minutes after administration to the mother. Cord:maternal serum ratios range between 0.50 and 0.70 after IV and epidural anesthesia (2–12). In 25 women just before delivery, a dose of 2–3 mg/kg was given by IV infusion at a rate of 100 mg/minute (2). The mean cord:maternal serum ratio in 9 patients who received 3 mg/kg was 0.55. A mean ratio of 1.32 was observed in nonacidotic newborns following local infiltration of the perineum for episiotomy (13). A similarly elevated ratio was measured in an acidotic newborn (14). The infant had umbilical venous/arterial pH values of 7.23/7.08 and a lidocaine cord:maternal serum ratio of 1.32 following epidural anesthesia. Because lidocaine is a weak base, the high ratio may have been caused by ion trapping (14).

Both the fetus and the newborn are capable of metabolizing lidocaine (8,9). The elimination half-life of lidocaine in the newborn following maternal epidural anesthesia averaged 3 hours (8). After local perineal infiltration for episiotomy, lidocaine was found in neonatal urine for at least 48 hours after delivery (13).

A number of studies have examined the effect of lidocaine on the newborn. In one report, offspring of mothers receiving continuous lumbar epidural blocks had significantly lower scores on tests of muscle strength and tone than did controls (15). Results of other tests of neurobehavior did not differ from those of controls. In contrast, four other studies failed to find adverse effects on neonatal neurobehavior following lidocaine epidural administration (10–12,16). Continuous infusion epidural analgesia with lidocaine has been used without effect on the fetus or newborn (17).

Lidocaine may produce central nervous system depression in the newborn with high serum levels. Of eight infants with lidocaine levels greater than 2.5 mcg/mL, four had Apgar scores of 6 or less (3). Three infants with levels above 3.0 mcg/mL were mildly depressed at birth (3). A 1973 study observed fetal tachycardia (3 cases) and bradycardia (3 cases) after paracervical block with lidocaine in 12 laboring women (18). The authors were unable to determine whether these effects were a direct effect of the drug. Accidental direct injection into the fetal scalp during local infiltration for episiotomy led to apnea; hypotonia; and fixed, dilated pupils 15 minutes after birth in one infant (19). Lidocaine-induced seizures occurred at 1 hour. The lidocaine concentration in the infant's serum at 2 hours was 14 mcg/mL. The heart rate was 180 beats/minute. Following successful treatment, physical and neurologic examinations at 3 days and again at 7 months were normal.

Lidocaine is the treatment of choice for ventricular arrhythmias (20,21). A 1984 report described the use of therapeutic lidocaine doses (100 mg IV injection followed by 4 mg/minute infusion) in a woman who was successfully resuscitated after a cardiac arrest at 18 weeks' gestation (22). A normal infant was delivered at 38 weeks' gestation. Neurologic development was normal at 17 months of age, but growth was below the 10th percentile.

The Collaborative Perinatal Project monitored 50,282 mother–child pairs, 293 of whom had exposure to lidocaine during the 1st trimester (23, pp. 358–363). No evidence of an association with large classes of malformations was found. Greater than expected risks were found for anomalies of the respiratory tract (three cases), tumors (two cases), and inguinal hernias (eight cases), but the statistical significance is unknown and independent confirmation is required (23, pp. 358–363, 477). For use anytime during pregnancy, 947 exposures were recorded (23, pp. 440, 493). From these data, no evidence of an association with large categories of major or minor malformations or to individual defects was found.

BREASTFEEDING SUMMARY

Small amounts of lidocaine are excreted into breast milk (24). A 37-year-old, lactating woman was treated with intravenous lidocaine for acute-onset ventricular arrhythmia secondary to chronic mitral valve prolapse. The woman had been nursing her 10-month-old infant up to the time of treatment. She was treated with lidocaine, 75 mg over 1 minute, followed by a continuous infusion of 2 mg/minute (23 mcg/kg/minute). A second 50-mg dose was given 5 minutes after the first bolus dose. The woman's serum lidocaine level 5 hours after initiation of therapy was 2 mcg/mL. The drug concentration in a milk sample, obtained 2 hours later when therapy was stopped, was 0.8 mcg/mL (40% of maternal serum). Although the infant was not allowed to nurse during and immediately following the mother's therapy, the potential for harm of the infant from exposure to lidocaine in breast milk is probably very low. The American Academy of Pediatrics classifies lidocaine as compatible with breastfeeding (25).

References

1. Product information. Xylocaine. Astrazeneca, 2000.
2. Shnider SM, Way EL. The kinetics of transfer of lidocaine (Xylocaine) across the human placenta. Anesthesiology 1968;29:944–50.
3. Shnider SM, Way EL. Plasma levels of lidocaine (Xylocaine) in mother and newborn following obstetrical conduction anesthesia: clinical applications. Anesthesiology 1968;29:951–8.
4. Lurie AO, Weiss JB. Blood concentrations of mepivacaine and lidocaine in mother and baby after epidural anesthesia. Am J Obstet Gynecol 1970;106:850–6.
5. Petrie RH, Paul WL, Miller FC, Arce JJ, Paul RH, Nakamura RM, Hon EH. Placental transfer of lidocaine following paracervical block. Am J Obstet Gynecol 1974;120:791–801.
6. Zador G, Lindmark G, Nilsson BA. Pudendal block in normal vaginal deliveries. Clinical efficacy, lidocaine concentrations in maternal and foetal blood, foetal and maternal acid-base values and influence on uterine activity. Acta Obstet Gynecol Scand Suppl 1974;34:51–64.
7. Blankenbaker WL, DiFazio CA, Berry FA Jr. Lidocaine and its metabolites in the newborn. Anesthesiology 1975;42:325–30.
8. Brown WU Jr, Bell GC, Lurie AO, Weiss JB, Scanlon JW, Alper MH. Newborn blood levels of lidocaine and mepivacaine in the first postnatal day following maternal epidural anesthesia. Anesthesiology 1975;42:698–707.
9. Kuhnert BR, Knapp DR, Kuhnert PM, Prochaska AL. Maternal, fetal, and neonatal metabolism of lidocaine. Clin Pharmacol Ther 1979;26:213–20.
10. Abboud TK, Sarkis F, Blikian A, Varakian L. Lack of adverse neurobehavioral effects of lidocaine. Anesthesiology 1982;57(Suppl):A404.
11. Kileff M, James FM III, Dewan D, Floyd H, DiFazio C. Neonatal neurobehavioral responses after epidural anesthesia for cesarean section with lidocaine and bupivacaine. Anesthesiology 1982;57(Suppl):A403.
12. Abboud TK, David S, Costandi J, Nagappala S, Haroutunian S, Yeh SY. Comparative maternal, fetal and neonatal effects of lidocaine versus lidocaine with epinephrine in the parturient. Anesthesiology 1984;61(Suppl):A405.
13. Philipson EH, Kuhnert BR, Syracuse CD. Maternal, fetal, and neonatal lidocaine levels following local perineal infiltration. Am J Obstet Gynecol 1984;149:403–7.
14. Brown WU Jr, Bell GC, Alper MH. Acidosis, local anesthetics, and the newborn. Obstet Gynecol 1976;48:27–30.
15. Scanlon JW, Brown WU Jr, Weiss JB, Alper MH. Neurobehavioral responses of newborn infants after maternal epidural anesthesia. Anesthesiology 1974;40:121–8.
16. Abboud TK, Williams V, Miller F, Henriksen EH, Doan T, Van Dorsen JP, Earl S. Comparative fetal, maternal, and neonatal responses following epidural analgesia with bupivacaine, chloroprocaine, and lidocaine. Anesthesiology 1981;55(Suppl):A315.
17. Chestnut DH, Bates JN, Choi WW. Continuous infusion epidural analgesia with lidocaine: efficacy and influence during the second stage of labor. Obstet Gynecol 1987;69:323–7.
18. Liston WA, Adjepon-Yamoah KK, Scott DB. Foetal and maternal lignocaine levels after paracervical block. Br J Anaesth 1973;45:750–4.
19. Kim WY, Pomerance JJ, Miller AA. Lidocaine intoxication in a newborn following local anesthesia for episiotomy. Pediatrics 1979;64:643–5.
20. Tamari I, Eldar M, Rabinowitz B, Neufeld HN. Medical treatment of cardiovascular disorders during pregnancy. Am Heart J 1982;104:1357–63.
21. Rotmensch HH, Elkayam U, Frishman W. Antiarrhythmic drug therapy during pregnancy. Ann Intern Med 1983;98:487–97.
22. Stokes IM, Evans J, Stone M. Myocardial infarction and cardiac arrest in the second trimester followed by assisted vaginal delivery under epidural analgesia at 38 weeks gestation. Case report. Br J Obstet Gynaecol 1984;91:197–8.
23. Heinonen OP, Slone D, Shapiro S. *Birth Defects and Drugs in Pregnancy*. Littleton, MA: Publishing Sciences Group, 1977.
24. Zeisler JA, Gaarder TD, De Mesquita SA. Lidocaine excretion in breast milk. Drug Intell Clin Pharm 1986;20:691–3.
25. Committee on Drugs, American Academy of Pediatrics. The transfer of drugs and other chemicals into human milk. Pediatrics 2001;108:776–89.

LINACLOTIDE

Gastrointestinal Agent (Laxative)

PREGNANCY RECOMMENDATION: No Human Data—Probably Compatible
BREASTFEEDING RECOMMENDATION: No Human Data—Probably Compatible

PREGNANCY SUMMARY

No reports describing the use of linaclotide during human pregnancy have been located. Although the animal reproduction data are reassuring, the comparisons to human doses were based on body weight and may not be interpretable. Nevertheless, the absence of quantifiable plasma concentrations of linaclotide and its active metabolite suggest that clinically significant amounts of these agents will not cross to the embryo or fetus.

FETAL RISK SUMMARY

Linaclotide, guanylate cyclase-C agonist, and its active metabolite act locally on the luminal surface of the intestinal epithelium. The parent drug is a 14-amino-acid peptide. Linaclotide is indicated in adults for treatment of irritable bowel syndrome with constipation and for chronic idiopathic constipation. Both linaclotide and its active metabolite are minimally absorbed with plasma concentrations below the limit of quantitation (1).

Reproduction studies have been conducted in rats, rabbits, and mice. In rats and rabbits, oral doses up to 20,000 and 8000 times, respectively, the maximum recommended human dose of about 5 mcg/kg/day based on a 60-kg body weight (MRHD) produced no maternal toxicity and no effects on embryo–fetal development. In mice, oral doses at least 8000 times the MRHD caused severe maternal toxicity including death, reduction of gravid uterine and fetal weights, and effects on fetal morphology. A dose 1000 times the MRHD in mice was not maternal toxic and caused no adverse effects on embryo–fetal development (1).

In 2-year studies, linaclotide was not carcinogenic in rats and mice. Assays for mutagenicity also were negative and the drug had no effect on fertility or reproductive function in male and female rats (1).

It is not known if linaclotide or its active metabolite cross the human placenta. The molecular weight of the parent drug (about 1527) and the absence of quantifiable concentrations of either agent suggest that exposure of the embryo or fetus will be nil. However, both agents are proteolytically degraded within the intestinal lumen to smaller peptides and naturally occurring amino acids and these may be absorbed and cross the placenta.

BREASTFEEDING SUMMARY

No reports describing the use of linaclotide during human lactation have been located. The molecular weight of the parent drug (about 1527) and the absence of quantifiable plasma concentrations of linaclotide or its active metabolite suggest that excretion into breast milk of clinically significant amounts of either agent is unlikely. However, both agents are proteolytically degraded within the intestinal lumen to smaller peptides and naturally occurring amino acids and these may be absorbed and excreted into milk. Nevertheless, the use of linaclotide during breastfeeding appears to be compatible.

Reference

1. Product information. Linzess. Forest Pharmaceuticals, 2012.

L

LINAGLIPTIN

Antidiabetic Agent

PREGNANCY RECOMMENDATION: No Human Data—Animal Data Suggest Low Risk
BREASTFEEDING RECOMMENDATION: No Human Data—Probably Compatible

PREGNANCY SUMMARY

No reports describing the use of linagliptin in human pregnancy have been located. The animal reproduction data suggest low risk, but the absence of human pregnancy experience prevents a complete assessment of the embryo–fetal risk. Although the use of linagliptin may help decrease the incidence of fetal and newborn morbidity and mortality in developing countries where the proper use of insulin is problematic, insulin still is the treatment of choice for this disease during pregnancy. Moreover, insulin does not cross the placenta, which eliminates the additional concern that the drug therapy will adversely affect the fetus. Carefully prescribed insulin therapy will provide better control of the mother's blood glucose, thereby preventing the fetal and neonatal complications that occur with this disease. High maternal glucose levels, as might occur in diabetes mellitus, are associated with a number of maternal and fetal adverse effects, including fetal structural anomalies if the hyperglycemia occurs early in gestation. To prevent this toxicity, the American College of Obstetricians and Gynecologists recommends that insulin be used for types 1 and 2 diabetes occurring during pregnancy and, if diet therapy alone is not successful, for gestational diabetes (1,2). If a woman becomes pregnant while taking linagliptin, changing the therapy to insulin should be considered.

FETAL RISK SUMMARY

Linagliptin is an oral antidiabetic agent. It is in same class of dipeptidyl peptidase-4 (DPP-4) inhibitors as saxagliptin and sitagliptin. Linagliptin is indicated as an adjunct to diet and exercise to improve glycemic control in adults with type 2 diabetes mellitus. Linagliptin undergoes minimal metabolism to inactive metabolites. Plasma protein binding at steady state is 70%–80%. Although the terminal half-life is >100 hours, relating to saturable binding to DPP-4, the effective half-life is about 12 hours (3).

Reproduction studies have been conducted in rats and rabbits. No teratogenic effects were observed when the drug was given to these species during organogenesis in doses up to about 49 and 1943 times, respectively, the human clinical dose based on AUC exposure (HCD). In rats, a dose that was 1000 times HCD caused maternal toxicity and developmental delays in skeletal ossification and slightly increased embryo–fetal loss. When the maternal toxic dose was administered to rats from gestation day 6 to lactation day 21, decreased body weight and delays in physical and behavioral development in male and female offspring were observed. No functional, behavioral, or reproductive toxicity was observed in the offspring of rats exposed to 49 times the HCD. In rabbits, a dose 1943 times the HCD caused increased fetal resorptions and visceral and skeletal variations. The drug crossed the placenta in pregnant rats and rabbits (3).

In 2-year carcinogenesis studies, linagliptin did not increase the incidence of tumors in male and female rats and mice, but a higher dose in female mice did increase the incidence of lymphoma. Mutagenic clastogenic effects were not observed in various assays. In fertility studies with rats, no adverse effects on early embryonic development, mating, fertility, or bearing live young were observed with doses up to about 943 times the HCD (3).

It is not known if linagliptin crosses the human placenta. The molecular weight (about 473), minimal metabolism, moderate plasma protein binding, and long elimination half-life all suggest that the drug will cross to the embryo–fetus.

BREASTFEEDING SUMMARY

No reports describing the use of linagliptin during human lactation have been located. The molecular weight of the parent compound (about 473), minimal metabolism, moderate plasma protein binding (70%–80%), and effective half-life (about 12 hours) suggest that linagliptin will be excreted into breast milk. The effect of this exposure on a nursing infant is unknown. Single doses of linagliptin up to 600 mg (120 times the maximum recommended human dose in healthy adults) caused no dose-related adverse reactions (3). Thus, hypoglycemia in a nursing infant might be unlikely but should be monitored. The most common (≥5%) adverse reaction in adults receiving monotherapy was nasopharyngitis (3).

References

1. American College of Obstetricians and Gynecologists. Pregestational diabetes mellitus. *ACOG Practice Bulletin* No. 60, March 2005. Obstet Gynecol 2005;105:675–85.
2. American College of Obstetricians and Gynecologists. Gestational diabetes. *ACOG Practice Bulletin*. No. 30. September 2001. Obstet Gynecol 2001;98:525–38.
3. Product information. Tradjenta. Boehringer Ingelheim Pharmaceuticals and Eli Lilly, 2012.

LINCOMYCIN

Antibiotic

PREGNANCY RECOMMENDATION: Compatible
BREASTFEEDING RECOMMENDATION: Compatible

PREGNANCY SUMMARY

No reports linking the use of lincomycin with congenital defects have been located.

FETAL RISK SUMMARY

Lincomycin crosses the placenta, achieving cord serum levels about 25% of the maternal serum level (1,2). Multiple IM injections of 600 mg did not result in accumulation in the amniotic fluid (2). No effects on the newborn were observed.

The progeny of 302 patients treated at various stages of pregnancy with oral lincomycin, 2 g/day for 7 days, were evaluated at various intervals up to 7 years after birth (3). As compared with a control group, no increases in malformations or in delayed developmental defects were observed.

BREASTFEEDING SUMMARY

Lincomycin is excreted into breast milk. Six hours following oral dosing of 500 mg every 6 hours for 3 days, serum and milk levels in nine patients averaged 1.37 and 1.28 mcg/mL, respectively, a milk:plasma ratio of 0.9 (1). Much lower milk:plasma ratios of 0.13–0.17 have also been reported (4). Although no adverse effects have been reported, three potential problems exist for the nursing infant: modification of bowel flora, direct effects on the infant, and interference with the interpretation of culture results if a fever workup is required.

References

1. Medina A, Fiske N, Hjelt-Harvey I, Brown CD, Prigot A. Absorption, diffusion, and excretion of a new antibiotic, lincomycin. Antimicrob Agents Chemother 1963:189–96.
2. Duignan NM, Andrews J, Williams JD. Pharmacological studies with lincomycin in late pregnancy. Br Med J 1973;3:75–8.
3. Mickal A, Panzer JD. The safety of lincomycin in pregnancy. Am J Obstet Gynecol 1975;121:1071–4.
4. Wilson JT. Milk/plasma ratios and contraindicated drugs. In: Wilson JT, ed. *Drugs in Breast Milk*. Balgowlah, Australia: ADIS Press, 1981: 78–9.

LINDANE

Scabicide/Pediculicide

PREGNANCY RECOMMENDATION: Limited Human Data—Animal Data Suggest Low Risk
BREASTFEEDING RECOMMENDATION: Limited Human Data—Probably Compatible

PREGNANCY SUMMARY

If maternal treatment is required, the manufacturers recommend using lindane no more than twice during a pregnancy (1,2). However, because of lindane's potentially serious toxicity, the CDC recommends, in pregnant women, permethrin or pyrethrins with piperonyl butoxide for the treatment of lice infestations and permethrin for the treatment of scabies (see Permethrin and Pyrethrins with Piperonyl Butoxide) (3).

FETAL RISK SUMMARY

Lindane (γ-benzene hexachloride) is used topically for the treatment of lice and scabies. Small amounts are absorbed through the intact skin and mucous membranes (4).

No published reports linking the use of this drug with toxic or congenital defects have been located, but one reference suggested that it should be used with caution because of its potential to produce neurotoxicity, convulsions, and aplastic anemia (5). Animal studies have not shown a teratogenic effect (6,7) and in one, lindane seemed to have a protective effect when given with known teratogens (8). Multigeneration reproduction studies in mice, rats, rabbits, pigs, and dogs at oral doses up to 10 times the human dose have revealed no evidence of impaired fertility or fetal harm (1).

In a surveillance study of Michigan Medicaid recipients involving 229,101 completed pregnancies conducted between 1985 and 1992, 1417 newborns had been exposed to topical lindane during the 1st trimester (F. Rosa, personal communication, FDA, 1993). A total of 64 (4.5%) major birth defects were observed (60 expected). Specific data were available for six defect categories, including (observed/expected) 17/14 cardiovascular defects, 4/2 oral clefts, 0/0.7 spina bifida, 1/4 polydactyly, 2/2 limb reduction defects, and 7/3 hypospadias. Only with the latter defect is there a suggestion of a possible association, but other factors, including concurrent drug use and chance, may be involved.

BREASTFEEDING SUMMARY

Lindane is excreted into breast milk after ingestion of the agent from treated foods (1). Concentrations in milk ranged from 0 to 113 parts per billion.

No reports describing the use of lindane in lactating women have been located. Based on theoretical considerations, a manufacturer estimated the upper limit of lindane levels in breast milk to be approximately 30 ng/mL after maternal application (E.D. Rickard, personal communication, Reed & Carnrick Pharmaceuticals, 1983). A nursing infant consuming 1000 mL of milk/day would thus ingest about 30 mcg/day of lindane. This is in the same general range that the infant would absorb after direct topical application (E.D. Rickard, personal communication, 1983). These amounts are probably clinically insignificant. Waiting 4 days after discontinuing lindane lotion, however, should prevent exposure of a nursing infant to any drug in the milk (1).

References

1. Product information. Lindane Lotion USP 1%. Alpharma, 2001.
2. Product information. Kwell. Reed & Carnrick Pharmaceuticals, 1990.
3. CDC. 1998 guidelines for treatment of sexually transmitted diseases. MMWR 1998;47(RR-1):106–8.
4. American Hospital Formulary Service. *Drug Information 1997*. Bethesda, MD: American Society of Health-System Pharmacists, 1997:2711–3.
5. Sanmiguel GS, Ferrer AP, Alberich MT, Genaoui BM. Consideraciones sobre el tratamiento de la infancia y en el embarazo. Actas Dermosifilogr 1980;71:105–8.
6. Palmer AK, Cozens DD, Spicer EJF, Worden AN. Effects of lindane upon reproduction function in a 3-generation study of rats. Toxicology 1978;10:45–54.
7. Palmer AK, Bottomley AM, Worden AN, Frohberg H, Bauer A. Effect of lindane on pregnancy in the rabbit and rat. Toxicology 1978;10:239–47.
8. Shtenberg AI, Torchinski I. Adaptation to the action of several teratogens as a consequence of preliminary administration of pesticides to females. Biull Eksp Biol Med 1977;83:227–8.

LINEZOLID

Anti-infective

PREGNANCY RECOMMENDATION: Compatible—Maternal Benefit >> Embryo/Fetal Risk
BREASTFEEDING RECOMMENDATION: No Human Data—Potential Toxicity

PREGNANCY SUMMARY

No reports describing the use of linezolid during human pregnancy have been located. Because of the lack of human pregnancy data, other antibiotics with this experience should be used if possible. If no other alternatives are available and linezolid must be used, the maternal benefit appears to outweigh the unknown fetal risk.

FETAL RISK SUMMARY

Linezolid is a synthetic, oxalodinone class, antibacterial agent that is indicated for the treatment of gram-positive bacteria, including vancomycin-resistant enterococcus (VRE). It is available in both oral and IV formulations.

Reproduction studies have been conducted in pregnant mice and rats (1). No evidence of teratogenicity was seen in mice and rats at doses that were 4 and 1 times the expected human exposure based on AUC (EHE), respectively. However, in mice, embryo and fetal toxicity (embryo death, including total litter loss, decreased fetal weight, and an increased incidence of costal cartilage fusion) and maternal toxicity (clinical signs and reduced weight gain) were seen at this dose. In pregnant rats, doses 0.13 and 0.64 times the EHE resulted in slight fetal toxicity (reduced fetal weight and ossification of sternebrae). The higher dose (0.64 times the EHE) caused slight maternal toxicity consisting of reduced body weight gain. When this dose was given during pregnancy and lactation, pup survival was decreased on postnatal days 1 to 4. In addition, when surviving pups reached maturity and were mated, they had decreased fertility as evidenced by an increase in preimplantation loss (1).

It is not known if linezolid crosses the human placenta. The molecular weight (about 337) is low enough that transfer to the fetus should be expected.

BREASTFEEDING SUMMARY

No reports describing the use of linezolid during human lactation have been located. The molecular weight (about 337) is low enough that excretion into breast milk should be expected. The effects of this exposure on a nursing infant are unknown, but myelosuppression and reversible thrombocytopenia are potential complications. Women taking linezolid should probably not breastfeed.

Reference

1. Product information. Zyvox. Pharmacia & Upjohn, 2001.

L

LIOTHYRONINE

Thyroid

PREGNANCY RECOMMENDATION: Compatible
BREASTFEEDING RECOMMENDATION: Compatible

PREGNANCY SUMMARY

Liothyronine (T3) is compatible with all stages of pregnancy. Untreated or undertreated maternal hypothyroidism is associated with low birth weight secondary to medically indicated preterm delivery, preeclampsia, or placental abruption (1) and with lower neuropsychological development of their offspring (2).

FETAL RISK SUMMARY

T3 is a naturally occurring thyroid hormone produced by the mother and the fetus. It is used during pregnancy for the treatment of hypothyroidism (see also Levothyroxine and Thyroid). Although early studies found little or no transplacental passage of T3 at physiologic serum concentrations (3–5), as well as limited passage following very high doses (6,7), a 1994 review cited evidence that small amounts of T3 do cross the human placenta (8).

In a large prospective study, 34 mother–child pairs were exposed to T3 during the 1st trimester. No association between the drug and fetal defects was found (9). Maternal hypothyroidism itself has been reported to be responsible for poor pregnancy outcome (10). Others have not found this association, claiming that fetal development is not directly affected by maternal thyroid function (11). However, untreated maternal hypothyroidism during pregnancy has been shown to result in lower scores relating to intelligence, attention, language, reading ability, school performance, and visual–motor performance in children 7–9 years of age (2).

Combination therapy with thyroid–antithyroid drugs was advocated at one time for the treatment of hyperthyroidism but is now considered inappropriate (see Propylthiouracil).

BREASTFEEDING SUMMARY

T3 is excreted into breast milk in low concentrations. The effect on the nursing infant is not thought to be physiologically significant, although at least one report concluded otherwise (12). An infant was diagnosed as athyrotic shortly after breastfeeding was stopped at age 10 months. Growth was at the 97th percentile during breastfeeding, but the bone age remained that of a newborn. Mean levels of T3 in breast milk during the last trimester (12 patients) and within 48 hours of delivery (22 patients) were 1.36 and 2.86 ng/mL, respectively (12).

A 1978 study reported milk concentrations varying between 0.4 and 2.38 ng/mL (range 0.1–5 ng/mL) from the day of delivery to 148 days postpartum (13). No T3 was detected in a number of samples. Levels in three instances, collected 16, 20, and 43 months postpartum, ranged from 0.68 to 4.5 ng/mL with the highest concentration measured at 20 months. From the first week through 148 days postdelivery, the calculated maximum amount of T3 that a nursing infant would have ingested was 2.1–2.6 mcg/day, far less than the dose required to treat congenital hypothyroidism. However, it was concluded that this was enough to mask the symptoms of the disease without halting its progression (13).

In a study comparing serum T3 levels between 22 breastfed and 29 formula-fed infants, significantly higher levels were found in the breastfeeding group. The levels, 2.24 and 1.79 ng/mL, were comparable with previous reports and probably were of doubtful clinical significance (14).

A 1980 report described four exclusively breastfed infants with congenital hypothyroidism who were diagnosed between the ages of 2 and 79 days. Breastfeeding did not hinder making the diagnosis (15). Another report, evaluating clinical and biochemical thyroid parameters in hypothyroid infants, found no differences between breastfed (N = 12) and bottle-fed (N = 33) babies. These results lead to the conclusion that breast milk does not offer protection against the effects of congenital hypothyroidism (16). As reported in a 1985 paper, serum concentrations of T3 were similar in breastfed and bottle-fed infants at 5, 10, and 15 days postpartum. The levels were too low to interfere with neonatal thyroid screening programs (17).

Japanese researchers found a T3 milk:plasma ratio of 0.36 (18). No correlation was discovered between serum T3 and milk T3 or total daily T3 excretion, nor was there a correlation between milk T3 levels and milk protein concentration or daily volume of milk. They concluded that breastfeeding has no influence on the pituitary–thyroid axis of normal babies (18). A Swedish investigation measured higher levels of T3 in milk 1–3 months after delivery as compared with T3 levels in early colostrum (19). The concentrations were comparable with those in the studies cited above.

T3 breast milk concentrations are too low to protect a hypothyroid infant completely from the effects of the disease.

References

1. American College of Obstetricians and Gynecologists. Thyroid disease in pregnancy. *ACOG Practice Bulletin*. No. 37, August 2002.
2. Haddow JE, Palomaki GE, Allan WC, Williams JR, Knight GJ, Gagnon J, O'Heir CE, Mitchell ML, Hermos RJ, Waisbren SE, Faix JD, Klein RZ. Maternal thyroid deficiency during pregnancy and subsequent neuropsychological development of the child. N Engl J Med 1999;341:549–55.
3. Grumbach MM, Werner SC. Transfer of thyroid hormone across the human placenta at term. J Clin Endocrinol Metab 1956;16:1392–5.
4. Kearns JE, Hutson W. Tagged isomers and analogues of thyroxine (their transmission across the human placenta and other studies). J Nucl Med 1963;4:453–61.
5. Fisher DA, Lehman H, Lackey C. Placental transport of thyroxine. J Clin Endocrinol Metab 1964;24:393–400.
6. Raiti S, Holzman GB, Scott RI, Blizzard RM. Evidence for the placental transfer of tri-iodothyronine in human beings. N Engl J Med 1967;277: 456–9.
7. Dussault J, Row VV, Lickrish G, Volpe R. Studies of serum triiodothyronine concentration in maternal and cord blood: transfer of triiodothyronine across the human placenta. J Clin Endocrinol Metab 1969;29:595–606.
8. Burrow GN, Fisher DA, Larsen PR. Maternal and fetal thyroid function. N Engl J Med 1994;331:1072–8.
9. Heinonen OP, Slone D, Shapiro S. *Birth Defects and Drugs in Pregnancy*. Littleton, MA: Publishing Sciences Group, 1977:388–400.
10. Potter JD. Hypothyroidism and reproductive failure. Surg Gynecol Obstet 1980;150:251–5.
11. Montoro M, Collea JV, Frasier SD, Mestman JH. Successful outcome of pregnancy in women with hypothyroidism. Ann Intern Med 1981;94:31–4.
12. Bode HH, Vanjonack WJ, Crawford JD. Mitigation of cretinism by breast-feeding. Pediatrics 1978;62:13–6.
13. Varma SK, Collins M, Row A, Haller WS, Varma K. Thyroxine, triiodothyronine, and reverse triiodothyronine concentrations in human milk. J Pediatr 1978;93:803–6.
14. Hahn HB Jr, Spiekerman AM, Otto WR, Hossalla DE. Thyroid function tests in neonates fed human milk. Am J Dis Child 1983;137:220–2.
15. Abbassi V, Steinour TA. Successful diagnosis of congenital hypothyroidism in four breast-fed neonates. J Pediatr 1980;97:259–61.
16. Letarte J, Guyda H, Dussault JH, Glorieux J. Lack of protective effect of breast-feeding in congenital hypothyroidism: report of 12 cases. Pediatrics 1980;65:703–5.
17. Franklin R, O'Grady C, Carpenter L. Neonatal thyroid function: comparison between breast-fed and bottle-fed infants. J Pediatr 1985;106:124–6.
18. Mizuta H, Amino N, Ichihara K, Harade T, Nose O, Tanizawa O, Miyai K. Thyroid hormones in human milk and influence on thyroid function of breast-fed babies. Pediatr Res 1983;17:468–71.
19. Jansson L, Ivarsson S, Larsson I, Ekman R. Tri-iodothyronine and thyroxine in human milk. Acta Paediatr Scand 1983;72:703–5.

LIOTRIX

Thyroid

Liotrix is a synthetic combination of levothyroxine and liothyronine (see Levothyroxine and Liothyronine).

LIPIDS

Nutrient

PREGNANCY RECOMMENDATION: Compatible
BREASTFEEDING RECOMMENDATION: No Human Data—Probably Compatible

PREGNANCY SUMMARY

Based on limited clinical experience, IV lipids apparently do not pose a significant risk to the mother or fetus, although two cases of fetal death indicate that the therapy is not without danger. Standard precautions, as taken with nonpregnant patients, should be followed when administering these solutions during pregnancy.

FETAL RISK SUMMARY

Lipids (IV fat emulsions) are a mixture of neutral triglycerides, primarily unsaturated fatty acids, prepared from either soybean or safflower oil. Egg yolk phospholipids are used as an emulsifier. Most fatty acids readily cross the placenta to the fetus (1,2).

A number of reports have described the use of lipids during pregnancy in conjunction with dextrose/amino acid solutions (see Hyperalimentation, Parenteral) (3–14). However, one investigator concluded in 1977 that lipid infusions were contraindicated during pregnancy for several reasons: (a) an excessive increase in serum triglycerides, often with ketonemia, would result because of the physiologic hyperlipemia present during pregnancy; (b) premature labor would occur; and (c) placental infarctions would occur from fat deposits and cause placental insufficiency (15). A brief 1986 correspondence also stated that lipids were contraindicated because of the danger of inducing premature uterine contractions with the potential for abortion or premature delivery (16). This conclusion was based on the observation that lipids contain arachidonic acid, a precursor to prostaglandins E_2 and $F_{2\alpha}$ (16). However, another investigator concluded that concentrations of arachidonic acid must arise from decidual membranes or amniotic fluid (i.e., must be very close to the myometrium) to produce this effect (17).

A 1986 report described four women in whom parenteral hyperalimentation was used during pregnancy, two of whom also received lipids, and, in addition, reviewed the literature for both total parenteral nutrition and lipid use during gestation (18). These authors concluded that there was no evidence that lipid emulsions had an adverse effect on pregnancy (18).

The effect of oral administration of a triglyceride emulsion on the fetal breathing index was described in a 1982 publication (19). Six women, at 32 weeks' gestation, ingested 100 mL of the emulsion containing 67 g of triglycerides and were compared with six women, also at 32 weeks' gestation, who drank mineral water. No correlation was noted between the fetal breathing index and plasma free fatty acids, glucose, insulin, glucagon, total cortisol, free cortisol, or triglyceride levels (19).

Cardiac tamponade, resulting in maternal and fetal death, was reported in a woman receiving central hyperalimentation with lipids for severe hyperemesis gravidarum (20) (see Hyperalimentation, Parenteral, for details of this case).

A stillborn male fetus was delivered at 22 weeks' gestation from a 31-year-old woman with hyperemesis gravidarum who had been treated with total IV hyperalimentation and lipid emulsion for 8 weeks (21). The tan-yellow placenta showed vacuolated syncytial cells and Hofbauer cells that stained for fat. The placental fat deposits, the first to be described with parenteral lipids, were thought to be the cause of the fetal demise.

BREASTFEEDING SUMMARY

Although there are no reports describing the use of IV lipids during lactation, there does not appear to be any risk to the nursing infant.

References

1. Elphick MC, Filshie GM, Hull D. The passage of fat emulsion across the human placenta. Br J Obstet Gynaecol 1978;85:610–8.
2. Hendrickse W, Stammers JP, Hull D. The transfer of free fatty acids across the human placenta. Br J Obstet Gynaecol 1985;92:945–52.
3. Hew LR, Deitel M. Total parenteral nutrition in gynecology and obstetrics. Obstet Gynecol 1980;55:464–8.
4. Tresadern JC, Falconer GF, Turnberg LA, Irving MH. Successful completed pregnancy in a patient maintained on home parenteral nutrition. Br Med J 1983;286:602–3.
5. Tresadern JC, Falconer GF, Turnberg LA, Irving MH. Maintenance of pregnancy in a home parenteral nutrition patient. JPEN 1984;8:199–202.
6. Seifer DB, Silberman H, Catanzarite VA, Conteas CN, Wood R, Ueland K. Total parenteral nutrition in obstetrics. JAMA 1985;253;2073–5.
7. Lavin JP Jr, Gimmon Z, Miodovnik M, von Meyenfeldt M, Fischer JE. Total parenteral nutrition in a pregnant insulin-requiring diabetic. Obstet Gynecol 1982;59:660–4.
8. Rivera-Alsina ME, Saldana LR, Stringer CA. Fetal growth sustained by parenteral nutrition in pregnancy. Obstet Gynecol 1984;64:138–41.
9. Di Costanzo J, Martin J, Cano N, Mas JC, Noirclerc M. Total parenteral nutrition with fat emulsions during pregnancy—nutritional requirements: a case report. JPEN 1982;6:534–8.
10. Young KR. Acute pancreatitis in pregnancy: two case reports. Obstet Gynecol 1982;60:653–7.
11. Breen KJ, McDonald IA, Panelli D, Ihle B. Planned pregnancy in a patient who was receiving home parenteral nutrition. Med J Aust 1987;146:215–7.
12. Levine MG, Esser D. Total parenteral nutrition for the treatment of severe hyperemesis gravidarum: maternal nutritional effects and fetal outcome. Obstet Gynecol 1988;72:102–7.
13. Herbert WNP, Seeds JW, Bowes WA, Sweeney CA. Fetal growth response to total parenteral nutrition in pregnancy: a case report. J Reprod Med 1986;31:263–6.
14. Hatjis CG, Meis PJ. Total parenteral nutrition in pregnancy. Obstet Gynecol 1985;66:585–9.
15. Heller L. Parenteral nutrition in obstetrics and gynecology. In: Greep JM, Soeters PB, Wesdorp RIC, Grant JP, eds. *Current Concepts in Parenteral Nutrition*. The Hague: Martinus Nijhoff Medical Division, 1977:179–86.
16. Neri A. Fetal growth sustained by parenteral nutrition in pregnancy. Obstet Gynecol 1986;67:753.
17. Saldana LR. Fetal growth sustained by parenteral nutrition in pregnancy (in reply). Obstet Gynecol 1986;67:753.
18. Lee RV, Rodgers BD, Young C, Eddy E, Cardinal J. Total parenteral nutrition during pregnancy. Obstet Gynecol 1986;68:563–71.
19. Neldam S, Hornnes PJ, Kuhl C. Effect of maternal triglyceride ingestion on fetal respiratory movements. Obstet Gynecol 1982;59:640–2.
20. Greenspoon JS, Masaki DI, Kurz CR. Cardiac tamponade in pregnancy during central hyperalimentation. Obstet Gynecol 1989;73:465–6.
21. Jasnosz KM, Pickeral JJ, Graner S. Fat deposits in the placenta following maternal total parenteral nutrition with intravenous lipid emulsion. Arch Pathol Lab Med 1995;119:555–7.

LIRAGLUTIDE

Antidiabetic Agent

PREGNANCY RECOMMENDATION: No Human Data—Animal Data Suggest Risk
BREASTFEEDING RECOMMENDATION: No Human Data—Probably Compatible (NEW)

PREGNANCY SUMMARY

No reports describing the use of liraglutide in human pregnancy have been located. The drug caused developmental toxicity (decreased body weight and structural anomalies) in two animal species at systemic exposures less than the human exposure. The absence of human pregnancy experience prevents a complete assessment of the embryo–fetal risk. Until such data are available, the best course is to avoid liraglutide in pregnancy.

FETAL RISK SUMMARY

Liraglutide is a glucagon-like peptide-1 receptor agonist that enhances glucose-dependent insulin secretion, suppresses inappropriately elevated glucagon secretion and slows gastric emptying. It is in the same subclass of antidiabetic agents as exenatide. Liraglutide is indicated as an adjunct to diet and exercise to improve glycemic control in adults with type 2 diabetes mellitus. It is given as an SC injection once daily. The low metabolism is similar to large proteins without a specific organ as a major route of elimination. The drug is extensively bound to plasma protein (>98%) and the elimination half-life is about 13 hours (1).

Reproduction studies have been conducted in rats and rabbits. Rats were given daily SC doses beginning 2 weeks before mating to gestation day 17 that resulted in estimated systemic exposures that were 0.8–11 times the human exposure resulting from the maximum recommended human dose based on plasma AUC (MRHD). The highest dose caused maternal toxicity (reduced body weight gain and food consumption). All doses were associated with fetal abnormalities and variations in kidneys and blood vessels, irregular ossification of the skull, and a more complete state of ossification. The incidences of misshapen oropharynx and/or narrowed opening into the larynx, and umbilical hernia were increased at the lowest dose. At the highest dose, the number of early embryonic deaths increased slightly, and mottled liver and minimally kinked ribs were observed. Daily SC doses given from gestation day 6 through weaning or termination of nursing on lactation day 24 were associated with a slight delay in parturition and a decrease in group mean body weight of neonatal rats. Bloody scabs and agitated behavior occurred in male rats descended from dams treated with the highest dose. A nonsignificant trend toward lower group mean body weight from birth to postpartum day 14 was seen in F_2 generation rats (1).

Pregnant rabbits were given three different daily SC doses from gestation days 6 through 18 that resulted in estimated systemic exposures that were all less than the MRHD. Decreased fetal weight and a dose-dependent increase in fetal abnormalities were observed at all doses. The malformations involved the kidneys, scapula, eyes, forelimb, brain, tail, sacral vertebrae, major blood vessels, heart, umbilicus, sternum, and parietal bones. Irregular ossification and/or skeletal abnormalities occurred in the skull and jaw, vertebrae and ribs, sternum, pelvis, tail, and scapula. Dose-dependent minor skeletal variations also were observed. Visceral abnormalities occurred in blood vessels, lung, liver, and esophagus, and bilobed or bifurcated gallbladder (1).

Studies for carcinogenicity potential have been conducted in mice and rats. In both of these species, a dose-related increase in benign thyroid C-cell adenomas and malignant C-cell carcinomas were observed. Thyroid C-cell tumors are rare findings during carcinogenicity testing in mice and rats. Liraglutide was negative with and without metabolic activation in multiple tests for mutagenicity and clastogenicity. In rats, the drug had no effect on male fertility. In female rats, a maternal toxic dose that was 11 times the MRHD caused an increase in early embryonic deaths.

It is not known if liraglutide crosses the human placenta. The high molecular weight (about 3751) and plasma protein binding suggest that the agent will not cross in clinically significant amounts, but the low metabolism and long elimination half-life are favorable factors for exposure of the embryo–fetus.

BREASTFEEDING SUMMARY

No reports describing the use of liraglutide during human lactation have been located. The high molecular weight (about 3751) and plasma protein binding (>98%) suggest that clinically significant amounts of the agent will not be excreted into breast milk. However, the low metabolism and long elimination half-life (about 13 hours) might increase these amounts. What little is excreted will probably be digested in the stomach of the nursing infant. Therefore, although the effect of the exposure on a nursing infant is unknown, the risk appears to be negligible. Nevertheless, blood glucose monitoring of the infant should be considered.

Reference

1. Product information. Victoza. Novo Nordisk, 2010.

LISDEXAMFETAMINE

Central Stimulant

PREGNANCY RECOMMENDATION: Human and Animal Data Suggest Risk
BREASTFEEDING RECOMMENDATION: Limited Human Data—Potential Toxicity

PREGNANCY SUMMARY

No reports describing the use of lisdexamfetamine in human pregnancy have been located. However, the prodrug is rapidly metabolized upon absorption to dextroamphetamine (see Amphetamine for human data).

FETAL RISK SUMMARY

Lisdexamfetamine is a prodrug that is rapidly metabolized upon absorption to dextroamphetamine (see Amphetamine) and *l*-lysine. It is indicated for the treatment of attention deficit hyperactivity disorder. The average plasma elimination half of lisdexamfetamine is <1 hour (1).

Animal reproduction studies have not been conducted with lisdexamfetamine. Studies have been conducted with amphetamine (D- to L-enantiomer ratio of 3:1) in rats, rabbits, and mice, but comparisons to the recommended human dose based on BSA or AUC was not given. No adverse effects on embryo–fetal morphological development or survival were observed in rats and rabbits given the drug throughout organogenesis. In mice, fetal malformations and death resulted from parenteral doses that caused severe maternal toxicity (1).

Several studies in animals, using doses similar to those used clinically, have shown that prenatal or early postnatal exposure can result in long-term neurochemical and behavioral alterations (learning and memory deficits, altered locomotor activity, and changes in sexual function) (1).

Carcinogenicity studies have not been conducted with lisdexamfetamine, but no evidence of carcinogenicity was found in mice and rats with dl-amphetamine. Several studies for mutagenic or clastogenic effects with lisdexamfetamine were negative. Amphetamine (d- to l-enantiomer ratio of 3:1) did not adversely affect fertility or early embryonic development in rats (1).

It is not known if lisdexamfetamine crosses the human placenta. The molecular weight of the dimesylate formulation (about 456) is low enough, but the prodrug is rapidly metabolized to dexamphetamine (molecular weight about 135) and this agent probably crosses to the embryo–fetus.

There are numerous reports of amphetamine use in human pregnancy (see Amphetamine).

BREASTFEEDING SUMMARY

No reports describing the use of the prodrug lisdexamfetamine during human lactation have been located. However, the prodrug is rapidly metabolized upon absorption to dextroamphetamine and this agent is concentrated in breast milk (see Amphetamine for human data).

Reference

1. Product information. Vyvanse. Shire, 2009.

LISINOPRIL

Antihypertensive

PREGNANCY RECOMMENDATION: Human Data Suggest Risk in the 2nd and 3rd Trimesters
BREASTFEEDING RECOMMENDATION: No Human Data—Probably Compatible

PREGNANCY SUMMARY

The fetal toxicity of lisinopril in the 2nd and 3rd trimesters is similar to other angiotensin-converting enzyme (ACE) inhibitors. The use of this drug during the 2nd and 3rd trimesters may cause teratogenicity and severe fetal and neonatal toxicity. Fetal toxic effects may include anuria, oligohydramnios, fetal hypocalvaria, intrauterine growth restriction (IUGR), prematurity, and patent ductus arteriosus. Stillbirth or neonatal death may occur. Anuria-associated oligohydramnios may produce fetal limb contractures, craniofacial deformation, and pulmonary hypoplasia. Severe anuria and hypotension, which is resistant to both pressor agents and volume expansion, may occur in the newborn following in utero exposure. Newborn renal function and blood pressure should be closely monitored.

FETAL RISK SUMMARY

Lisinopril is a long-acting ACE inhibitor used for the treatment of hypertension. The drug is not teratogenic in mice, rats, and rabbits treated with doses ≤55, 33, and 0.15 times, respectively, the maximum recommended human daily dose based on BSA (1).

Use of lisinopril limited to the 1st trimester does not appear to present a significant risk to the fetus, but fetal exposure after this time has been associated with teratogenicity and severe toxicity in the fetus and newborn, including death. The pattern of fetal toxicity, including teratogenicity, appears to be similar to that experienced with captopril and enalapril.

In a surveillance study of Michigan Medicaid recipients involving 229,101 completed pregnancies conducted between 1985 and 1992, 15 newborns had been exposed to lisinopril during the 1st trimester (F. Rosa, personal communication, FDA, 1993). Two (13.3%) major birth defects were observed (0.6 expected), one of which was polydactyly (none expected). No anomalies were observed in five other categories of defects (cardiovascular defects, oral clefts, spina bifida, limb reduction defects, and hypospadias) for which specific data were available.

Two cases of lisinopril-induced perinatal renal failure in newborns were published in a 1991 abstract (2). Additional details were not provided other than that both infants had been exposed in utero to the agent. The authors noted, however, that the effects of ACE inhibitors in the newborn are prolonged unless removed by dialysis, because 95% of the active metabolites are eliminated by renal excretion (2).

In a 2000 report, a woman with normal amniotic fluid volume and fetal measurements by ultrasound consistent with 18 weeks' gestation presented with severe chronic hypertension (3). She had been treated before conception and during the first 16 weeks with lisinopril but had self-stopped therapy 2 weeks before presentation. Because a combination of methyldopa, nifedipine, and labetalol failed to control her blood pressure, lisinopril was re-added to her regimen. At 22 weeks' gestation, the amniotic fluid index was 8 but declined to 0 at 24 weeks'. A cesarean section was performed at about 27 weeks' because of deteriorating maternal and fetal condition. The growth restricted, 680-g (3rd percentile) female infant had minimal respiratory distress syndrome. Severe renal impairment (maximum urine output 0.3 mL/kg/hr) was present during the first 6 days before improving after corrective surgery for bowel perforations secondary to necrotizing enterocolitis. She was discharged home on day 102 (3).

An 18-year-old woman received lisinopril, 10 mg/day, throughout gestation for the treatment of essential hypertension (4). No mention of amniotic fluid levels during pregnancy was made in this brief report. She delivered a premature, 1.48-kg, anuric infant at 33 weeks' gestation. Fetal calvarial hypoplasia was present. The normal-sized kidneys showed no evidence of perfusion on renal ultrasonography. An open biopsy at 11 weeks of age showed extensive atrophy and loss of tubules with interstitial fibrosis. The findings were compatible with exposure to a nephrotoxic agent. Peritoneal dialysis was instituted on day 8. Measurements of the drug in the dialysate indicated that removal of lisinopril was occurring. At 12 months of age, the infant continued to require dialysis (4).

Three cases of in utero exposure to ACE inhibitors, one of which was lisinopril, were reported in a 1992 abstract (5). The infant, delivered at 32 weeks' gestation because of severe oligohydramnios and fetal distress, suffered from IUGR, hypocalvaria, renal tubular dysplasia, and persistent renal insufficiency. The profound neonatal hypotension and anuria observed at birth improved only after dialysis. At the time of the report, the 15-month-old infant was maintained on dialysis.

Six pregnancies treated with lisinopril were reported in a 1997 study of 19 pregnancies exposed to ACE inhibitors (6). Lisinopril therapy was stopped in the 1st trimester in four pregnancies and at 20 and 25 weeks', respectively, in the others. No congenital anomalies or renal dysfunction were noted in the six neonates (6).

A case of lisinopril-induced fetopathy and hypocalvaria was included in a study examining the causes of fetal skull hypoplasia (7). Among 14 known cases of hypocalvaria or acalvaria, 5 were caused by ACE inhibitors. The authors speculated that the underlying pathogenetic mechanism in these cases is fetal hypotension (7).

A 1991 article examining the teratogenesis of ACE inhibitors cited evidence linking fetal calvarial hypoplasia with the use of these agents after the 1st trimester (8). The proposed mechanism was drug-induced oligohydramnios that allowed the uterine musculature to exert direct pressure on the fetal skull. This mechanical insult, combined with drug-induced fetal hypotension, could inhibit peripheral perfusion and ossification of the calvaria (8).

A retrospective study using pharmacy-based data from the Tennessee Medicaid program identified 209 infants, born between 1985 and 2000, that had 1st trimester exposure to ACE inhibitors (9). Infants of mothers with evidence of diabetes, either before or during pregnancy, were excluded, as were those exposed to angiotensin-receptor antagonists (ARBs), ACE inhibitors, or other antihypertensives beyond the 1st trimester, and those exposed to known teratogens. Two comparison groups, other antihypertensives (N = 202) and no antihypertensives (N = 29,096), were formed. The number of major birth defects in each of the three groups was 18 (8.6%), 4 (2%), and 834 (2.9%), respectively. Compared with the no-antihypertensives group, exposure to ACE inhibitors was associated with a significantly increased risk of major defects (relative risk [RR] 2.71, 95% confidence interval [CI] 1.72–4.27). When the analysis was conducted by the type of defect, the highest rates were with cardiovascular defects, 9, 2, and 294 respectively, RR 3.72, 95% CI 1.89–7.30, and with CNS defects, 3, 0, and 80, respectively, RR 4.39, 95% CI 1.37–14.02. The major defects observed in the subject group were as follows: atrial septal defect (N = 6) (includes three with pulmonic stenosis and/or three with patent ductus arteriosus (PDA), renal dysplasia (N = 2), PDA alone (N = 2), and one each of ventricular septal defect, spina bifida, microcephaly with eye anomaly, coloboma, hypospadias, intestinal and choanal atresia, Hirschsprung disease, and diaphragmatic hernia (9). In an accompanying editorial, it was noted that neither previous reports of 1st trimester exposure to ACE inhibitors nor the animal studies had observed an increased risk of birth defects (10). It also was noted that no mechanism for ACE inhibitor-induced teratogenicity was known. A subsequent communication raising concerns about the validity of the study in terms of adequate exclusion of diabetes, charting and coding errors in busy medical practices, and the effects of maternal obesity (11), was addressed by the investigators (12).

Lisinopril and other ACE inhibitors are human teratogens when used in the 2nd and 3rd trimesters, producing fetal hypocalvaria and renal defects. The cause of the defects and other toxicity is probably related to fetal hypotension and decreased renal blood flow. The compromise of the fetal renal system may result in severe, and at times fatal, anuria, both in the fetus and in the newborn. Anuria-associated oligohydramnios may produce pulmonary hypoplasia, limb contractures, persistent PDA, craniofacial deformation, and neonatal death (13,14). IUGR, prematurity, and severe neonatal hypotension may also be observed. Two reviews of fetal and newborn renal function indicated that both renal perfusion and glomerular plasma flow are low during gestation and that high levels of angiotensin II are physiologically necessary to maintain glomerular filtration at low perfusion pressures (15,16). Lisinopril prevents the conversion of angiotensin I to angiotensin II and, thus, may lead to in utero renal failure. Since the primary means of removal of the drug is renal, the impairment of this system in the newborn prevents elimination of the drug resulting in prolonged hypotension. Newborn renal function and blood pressure should be closely monitored. If oligohydramnios occurs, stopping lisinopril may resolve the problem but may not improve infant outcome because of irreversible fetal damage (13). In those cases in which lisinopril must be used to treat the mother's disease, the lowest possible dose should be used combined with close monitoring of amniotic fluid levels and fetal well-being. Guidelines for counseling exposed pregnant patients have been published and should be of benefit to health professionals faced with this task (8,13).

The observation in Tennessee Medicaid data of an increased risk of major congenital defects after 1st trimester exposure to ACE inhibitors raises concerns about teratogenicity that have not been seen in other studies (10). Medicaid data are a valuable tool for identifying early signals of teratogenicity, but are subject to a number of shortcomings and their findings must be considered hypotheses until confirmed by independent studies.

A 2012 review of the use of ACE inhibitors and ARBs in the 1st trimester concluded that there may be an elevated teratogenic risk, but the risk appeared to be related to other factors (17). The factors, that typically coexist with hypertension in pregnancy, included diabetes, advanced maternal age, and obesity.

BREASTFEEDING SUMMARY

No reports describing the use of lisinopril during human lactation have been located. The molecular weight (about 442) is low enough that excretion into breast milk should be expected. Two similar agents (captopril and enalapril) are present in milk in low concentrations and are classified by the American Academy of Pediatrics as compatible with breastfeeding (see Captopril and Enalapril).

References

1. Product information. Prinivil. Merck, 2001.
2. Rosa F, Bosco L. Infant renal failure with maternal ACE inhibition (abstract). Am J Obstet Gynecol 1991;164:273.
3. Tomlinson AJ, Campbell J, Walker JJ, Morgan C. Malignant primary hypertension in pregnancy treated with lisinopril. Ann Pharmacother 2000;34:180–2.
4. Bhatt-Mehta V, Deluga KS. *Chronic Renal Failure (CRF) in a Neonate Due to in-utero Exposure to Lisinopril.* Presented at the 12th Annual Meeting of the American College of Clinical Pharmacy, August 20, 1991, Minneapolis, MN. Abstract No. 43.
5. Pryde PG, Nugent CE, Sedman AB, Barr M Jr. ACE inhibitor fetopathy (abstract). Am J Obstet Gynecol 1992;166:348.
6. Lip GYH, Churchill D, Beevers M, Auckett A, Beevers DG. Angiotensin-converting-enzyme inhibitors in early pregnancy. Lancet 1997;350: 1446–7.
7. Barr M Jr, Cohen MM Jr. ACE inhibitor fetopathy and hypocalvaria: the kidney–skull connection. Teratology 1991;44:485–95.
8. Brent RL, Beckman DA. Angiotensin-converting enzyme inhibitors, an embryopathic class of drugs with unique properties: information for clinical teratology counselors. Teratology 1991;43:543–6.
9. Cooper WO, Hernandez-Diaz S, Arbogast PG, Dudley JA, Dyer S, Gideon PS, Hall K, Ray WA. Major congenital malformations after first-trimester exposure to ACE inhibitors. N Engl J Med 2006;354:2443–51.
10. Friedman JM. ACE inhibitors and congenital anomalies. N Engl J Med 2006;354:2498–2500.
11. Scialli AR, Lione A. ACE inhibitors and major congenital malformations. N Engl J Med 2006;355:1280.
12. Cooper WO, Ray WA. ACE inhibitors and major congenital malformations. Reply. N Engl J Med 2006;355:1281.
13. Barr M Jr. Teratogen update: angiotensin-converting enzyme inhibitors. Teratology 1994;50:399–409.
14. Shotan A, Widerhorn J, Hurst A, Elkayam U. Risks of angiotensin-converting enzyme inhibition during pregnancy: experimental and clinical evidence, potential mechanisms, and recommendations for use. Am J Med 1994;96:451–6.
15. Robillard JE, Nakamura KT, Matherne GP, Jose PA. Renal hemodynamics and functional adjustments to postnatal life. Semin Perinatol 1988;12: 143–50.
16. Guignard J-P, Gouyon J-B. Adverse effects of drugs on the immature kidney. Biol Neonate 1988;53:243–52.
17. Polifka JE. Is there an embryopathy associated with first-trimester exposure to angiotensin-converting enzyme inhibitors and angiotensin receptor antagonists? A critical review of the evidence. Birth Defects Res (Part A) 2012;94:576–98.

LITHIUM

Antipsychotic

PREGNANCY RECOMMENDATION: Human Data Suggest Risk
BREASTFEEDING RECOMMENDATION: Limited Human Data—Potential Toxicity

L

PREGNANCY SUMMARY

If possible, lithium should be avoided during pregnancy, especially during the period of organogenesis. In those cases in which 1st trimester use is unavoidable, adequate screening tests, including level II ultrasound and fetal echocardiography (e.g., at 18–20 weeks' gestation [1]), should be performed (1–3). Serum levels should also be monitored. Daily folic acid (5 mg/day) is also recommended. Use of the drug near term may produce severe toxicity in the newborn, which is usually reversible. The long-term effects of in utero lithium exposure on postnatal development are unknown but warrant investigation.

FETAL RISK SUMMARY

Lithium is used for the treatment of manic episodes of manic-depressive illness. The drug is available as either lithium carbonate or lithium citrate.

The use of lithium during the 1st trimester may be related to an increased incidence of congenital defects, particularly of the cardiovascular system. A 1987 review of psychotherapeutic drugs in pregnancy evaluated several reproduction studies of lithium in animals, including mice, rats, rabbits, and monkeys, and observed no teratogenicity except in rats (4).

Lithium freely crosses the placenta, equilibrating between maternal and cord serum (4–9). Amniotic fluid concentrations exceed cord serum levels (6).

A 1992 report described the outcomes of 11 women taking lithium during pregnancy, five of whom had two pregnancies (10). All gave birth to healthy babies.

Frequent reports have described the fetal effects of lithium, the majority from data accumulated by the Lithium Baby Register (4,5,11–19). The Register, founded in Denmark in 1968 and later expanded internationally, collects data on known cases of 1st trimester exposure to lithium (17). By 1977, the Register included 183 infants, 20 (11%) with major congenital anomalies. Of the 20 malformed infants, 15 involved cardiovascular defects, including 5 with the rare Ebstein's anomaly. Others have also noted the increased incidence of Ebstein's anomaly in lithium-exposed babies (20). Two new case reports bring the total number of infants with cardiovascular defects to 17, or 77% (17 of 22) of the known malformed children (21,22). Ebstein's anomaly has been diagnosed in the fetus during the 2nd trimester by echocardiography (23). Details on 16 of the malformed infants are given below.

Author	Case No.	Defect
Weinstein and Goldfield (16)	1	Coarctation of aorta
	2	High intraventricular septal defect
	3	Stenosis of aqueduct with hydrocephalus, spina bifida with sacral meningo-myelocele, bilateral talipes equinovarus with paralysis; atonic bladder, patulous rectal sphincter and rectal prolapse (see also reference 7)
	4	Unilateral microtia
	5	Mitral atresia, rudimentary left ventricle without inlet or outlet, aorta and pulmonary artery arising from right ventricle, patent ductus arteriosus, left superior vena cava
	6	Mitral atresia
	7	Ebstein's anomaly
	8	Single umbilical artery, bilateral hypoplasia of maxilla
	9	Ebstein's anomaly
	10	Atresia of tricuspid valve
	11	Ebstein's anomaly
	12	Patent ductus arteriosus, ventricular septal defect
	13	Ebstein's anomaly
Rane et al. (21)	14	Dextrocardia and situs solitus, patent ductus arteriosus, juxtaductal aortic coarctation
Weinstein (17)	15	Ebstein's anomaly
Arnon et al. (22)	16	Massive tricuspid regurgitation, atrial flutter, congestive heart failure

In 60 of the children born without malformations, follow-up comparisons with nonexposed siblings did not show an increased frequency of physical or mental anomalies (24).

The fetal toxicity of lithium, particularly in regard to cardiac abnormalities and the Ebstein's anomaly, was discussed in two 1988 references (25,26). As an indication of the rarity of Ebstein's anomaly, only approximately 300 cases of the defect have been recorded in the literature since Ebstein first described it approximately 100 years ago (25). One author concluded that the majority of tricuspid valve malformations, such as Ebstein's anomaly, are not related to drug therapy and, thus, the association between lithium and Ebstein's anomaly is weak (26).

A 1996 case report described multiple anomalies in an aborted male fetus of a woman treated with lithium carbonate monotherapy for a schizodepressive disorder (27). Maternal plasma levels before pregnancy varied between 0.58 and 0.73 mmol/L, but were not determined during gestation. Following diagnosis of multiple defects, the pregnancy was terminated at 22 weeks. The findings in the fetus were deep-seated ears, clubfeet, bilateral agenesis of the kidneys (Potter's syndrome), and a septal defect with transposition of the great vessels (26). In addition, the placenta had portions that were poorly vascularized and villi of different sizes. A causal association in this case between lithium and the defects cannot be determined. Moreover, Potter's syndrome is thought to be a genetic defect (28).

A prospective study published in 1992 gathered data from four teratogen information centers in Canada and the United States on lithium exposure in pregnancy (2). A total of 148 pregnant women using lithium (mean daily dose 927 mg) during the 1st trimester were matched by age with 148 controls. Ten women using lithium were lost to postnatal follow-up, but information was available on the fetal echocardiograms performed. The number of live births in the two groups was 76% (105/138) and 83% (123/148), respectively. One stillbirth, in the exposed group, was observed. Other outcomes (figures based on 148 women in each group) included spontaneous abortion (9% vs. 8%), therapeutic abortion (10% vs. 6%), and ectopic pregnancy (1 case vs. 0 case). None of these differences were statistically significant. However, the birth weight of lithium-exposed infants was significantly higher than that of controls, 3475 vs. 3383 g, $p = 0.02$), even though significantly many of their mothers smoked cigarettes than did controls (31.8% vs. 15.5%, $p = 0.002$). Three exposed infants and three controls had congenital malformations. The defects observed after lithium exposure were two infants with neural tube defects (hydrocephalus and meningomyelocele—also exposed to carbamazepine during the 1st trimester—spina bifida and tethered cord) and one with meromelia who was delivered at 23 weeks' gestation and died shortly after birth. Defects in the offspring of control mothers were a ventricular septal defect (one), congenital hip dislocation (one), and cerebral palsy and torticollis (one). In addition to the above cases, one of the therapeutic abortions in the lithium group was a pregnancy terminated at 16 weeks' gestation for a severe form of Ebstein's anomaly. The mother had also taken fluoxetine, trazodone, and L-thyroxine in the 1st trimester. Ebstein's anomaly has an incidence of 1 in 20,000 in the general population; thus, the appearance of this case is consistent with an increased risk for the heart defect among infants of women using lithium. However, a larger sample size is still needed to define the actual magnitude of the risk. The investigators concluded that lithium is not an important human teratogen and that, because it is beneficial in the therapy of major affective disorders, women may continue the drug during pregnancy. They cautioned, however, that adequate screening tests, including level II ultrasound and fetal echocardiography, were required when lithium is used during gestation (2).

A 1994 reference evaluated the teratogenic risk of 1st trimester exposure to lithium and summarized the treatment recommendations for lithium use in women with bipolar disorder (3). Included in their assessment were four case-controlled studies in which no cases of Ebstein's anomaly occurred among 207 lithium-exposed pregnancies as compared with 2 cases of the defects among 398 nonexposed controls. These data led them to the conclusion that the risk of teratogenicity after 1st trimester exposure to lithium was lower than previously reported (3). Reaching a similar conclusion, another review, published in 1995, concluded that the risk of teratogenicity with lithium was low in women with carefully controlled therapy, but that therapy should probably be avoided during the period of cardiac organogenesis (2nd–4th month of pregnancy) (29).

Concerning nonteratogenic effects, lithium toxicity in the fetus and newborn has been reported frequently:

Cyanosis (6,21,30–35)
Hypotonia (6,15,30–38)
Bradycardia (21,31,34,35,37,39)
Thyroid depression with goiter (6,15,38)
Atrial flutter (40)
Hepatomegaly (34,35)
Hyperbilirubinemia (42)
Electrocardiogram abnormalities
 (T-wave inversion) (31,39)
Cardiomegaly (32,34,35,40,42)
Gastrointestinal bleeding (39)
Diabetes insipidus (6,34,35,41,42)
Hypoglycemia (42)
Polyhydramnios (35,41)
Polyuria (42)
Poor respiratory effort (42)
Seizures (35)
Shock (34)

Most of these toxic effects are self-limiting, returning to normal in 1–2 weeks. This corresponds with the renal elimination of lithium from the infant. The serum half-life of lithium in newborns is prolonged, averaging 68–96 hours, as compared with the adult value of 10–20 hours (7,21). Two of the reported cases of nephrogenic diabetes insipidus persisted for 2 months or longer (6,34).

Premature labor, loss of fetal cardiac variability and acceleration, an unusual fetal heart rate pattern (double phase baseline), and depression at birth (Apgar scores of 4 and 7 at 1 and 5 minutes, respectively) were observed in a comatose mother and her infant after an acute overdose of an unknown amount of lithium and haloperidol at 31 weeks' gestation (43). Because of progressive premature labor, the female, 1526-g infant was delivered about 3 days after the overdose. The lithium concentrations of the maternal plasma, amniotic fluid, and cord vein plasma were all greater than 4 mmol/L (severe toxic effect >2.5 mmol/L), while the maternal level of haloperidol at delivery was about 1.6 ng/mL. The effects observed in the fetus and newborn were attributed to cardiac and cerebral manifestations of lithium intoxication. No follow-up on the infant was reported (43).

In a surveillance study of Michigan Medicaid recipients involving 229,101 completed pregnancies conducted between 1985 and 1992, 62 newborns had been exposed to lithium during the 1st trimester (F. Rosa, personal communication, FDA, 1993). Two (3.2%) major birth defects were observed (three expected), one of which was a polydactyly (0.2 expected). No anomalies were observed in five other categories of defects (cardiovascular defects, oral clefts, spina bifida, limb reduction defects, and hypospadias) for which specific data were available.

A 2014 case study described the use of phenelzine (105 mg/day), lithium (900 mg/day), and quetiapine (600 mg/day) in a 31-year-old woman with bipolar affective disorder (44). She was also taking metformin (1 g/day) for polycystic ovarian syndrome with oligomenorrhea. Her pregnancy was confirmed at 17 weeks' gestation. A glucose tolerance test was negative at 26 weeks'. Lithium was suspended 24–48 hours before induction of labor at 39 weeks'. Because of obstructed labor, a cesarean section was performed to give birth to a 4.2-kg male infant with Apgar scores of 5 and 9 at 1 and 5 minutes, respectively. The baby required initial resuscitation during the first 10 minutes. He was discharged home with the mother on day 5 and, at 10 weeks of age, his growth and development were normal (44).

Fetal red blood cell choline levels are elevated during maternal therapy with lithium (45). The clinical significance of this effect on choline, the metabolic precursor to acetylcholine, is unknown but may be related to the teratogenicity of lithium because of its effect on cellular lithium transport (45). In an in vitro study, lithium had no effect on human sperm motility (46).

A review published in 1995 used a unique system to assess the reproductive toxicity of lithium in animals and humans (47). Following an extensive evaluation of the available literature, for both experimental animals and humans, up through the early 1990s, a committee concluded that lithium, at concentrations within the human therapeutic range, could induce major malformations (particularly cardiac) and may be associated with neonatal toxicity. The evaluation included an assessment of human reproductive toxicity from lithium exposure in food, mineral supplements, swimming pools and spas, and drinking water, as well as from other environmental or occupational exposures. Because a linear relationship between lithium and toxicity was assumed, these exposures, which produce concentrations of lithium well below therapeutic levels, were not thought to produce human toxicity (47).

In the mother, renal lithium clearance rises during pregnancy, returning to prepregnancy levels shortly after delivery (48). In four patients, the mean clearance before delivery was 29 mL/minute, declining to 15 mL/minute 6–7 weeks after delivery, a statistically significant difference ($p < 0.01$). These data emphasize the need to monitor lithium levels closely before and after pregnancy (48).

BREASTFEEDING SUMMARY

Lithium is excreted into breast milk (9,31,49–52). Milk levels are approximately 40%–50% of the maternal serum concentration (31,50,51). Infant serum and milk levels are approximately equal. In a 2003 study, milk lithium levels were determined in 11 lactating women (daily dose 600–1500 mg) that were taking the drug for the management of bipolar disorder (52). No adverse effects were observed in the infants. The estimated infant dose from milk ranged from 0% to 30% of the mother's weight adjusted dose. These data suggested that monitoring lithium levels in milk and/or the infant's blood, combined with close observation of the nursing infant for adverse effects, was a rational approach (52).

Although no toxic effects in the nursing infant have been reported, long-term effects from this exposure have not been studied. Because of the near therapeutic blood concentrations in infants, the American Academy of Pediatrics classifies lithium as a drug that should be given to nursing mothers with caution (53).

References

1. Committee on Drugs. American Academy of Pediatrics. Use of psychoactive medication during pregnancy and possible effects on the fetus and newborn. Pediatrics 2000;105:880–7.
2. Jacobson SJ, Jones K, Johnson K, Ceolin L, Kaur P, Sahn D, Donnenfeld AE, Rieder M, Santelli R, Smythe J, Pastuszak A, Einarson T, Koren G. Prospective multicentre study of pregnancy outcome after lithium exposure during first trimester. Lancet 1992;339:530–3.
3. Cohen LS, Friedman JM, Jefferson JW, Johnson EM, Weiner ML. A reevaluation of risk of in utero exposure to lithium. JAMA 1994;271:146–50.
4. Elia J, Katz IR, Simpson GM. Teratogenicity of psychotherapeutic medications. Psychopharmacol Bull 1987;23:531–86.
5. Weinstein MR, Goldfield M. Lithium carbonate treatment during pregnancy: report of a case. Dis Nerv Syst 1969;30:828–32.
6. Mizrahi EM, Hobbs JF, Goldsmith DI. Nephrogenic diabetes insipidus in transplacental lithium intoxication. J Pediatr 1979;94:493–5.
7. Mackay AVP, Loose R, Glen AIM. Labour on lithium. Br Med J 1976;1:878.
8. Schou M, Amdisen A. Lithium and placenta. Am J Obstet Gynecol 1975;122:541.
9. Sykes PA, Quarrie J, Alexander FW. Lithium carbonate and breast-feeding. Br Med J 1976;2:1299.
10. van Gent EM, Verhoeven WMA. Bipolar illness, lithium prophylaxis, and pregnancy. Pharmacopsychiatry 1992;25:187–91.
11. Schou M, Amdisen A. Lithium in pregnancy. Lancet 1970;1:1391.
12. Aoki FY, Ruedy J. Severe lithium intoxication: management without dialysis and report of a possible teratogenic effect of lithium. Can Med Assoc J 1971;105:847–8.
13. Goldfield M, Weinstein MR. Lithium in pregnancy: a review with recommendations. Am J Psychiatry 1971;127:888–93.
14. Goldfield MD, Weinstein MR. Lithium carbonate in obstetrics: guidelines for clinical use. Am J Obstet Gynecol 1973;116:15–22.
15. Schou M, Goldfield MD, Weinstein MR, Villeneuve A. Lithium and pregnancy. I. Report from the register of lithium babies. Br Med J 1973;2:135–6.
16. Weinstein MR, Goldfield MD. Cardiovascular malformations with lithium use during pregnancy. Am J Psychiatry 1975;132:529–31.
17. Weinstein MR. Recent advances in clinical psychopharmacology. I. Lithium carbonate. Hosp Form 1977;12:759–62.
18. Linden S, Rich CL. The use of lithium during pregnancy and lactation. J Clin Psychiatry 1983;44:358–61.
19. Pitts FN. Lithium and pregnancy (editorial). J Clin Psychiatry 1983;44:357.
20. Nora JJ, Nora AH, Toews WH. Lithium, Ebstein's anomaly, and other congenital heart defects. Lancet 1974;2:594–5.
21. Rane A, Tomson G, Bjarke B. Effects of maternal lithium therapy in a newborn infant. J Pediatr 1978;93:296–7.
22. Arnon RG, Marin-Garcia J, Peeden JN. Tricuspid valve regurgitation and lithium carbonate toxicity in a newborn infant. Am J Dis Child 1981;135:941–3.
23. Allan LD, Desai G, Tynan MJ. Prenatal echocardiographic screening for Ebstein's anomaly for mothers on lithium therapy. Lancet 1982;2:875–6.
24. Schou M. What happened later to the lithium babies? A follow-up study of children born without malformations. Acta Psychiatr Scand 1976;54:193–7.
25. Warkany J. Teratogen update: lithium. Teratology 1988;38:593–6.
26. Källén B. Comments on teratogen update: lithium. Teratology 1988;38:597.
27. Eikmeier G. Fetal malformations under lithium treatment. Eur Psychiatry 1996;11:376–7.
28. Moel DI. Renal agenesis, bilateral. In: Buyse ML, ed. *Birth Defects Encyclopedia*. Volume II. Dover, MA: Center for Birth Defects Information Service, 1990:1460–1.
29. Leonard A, Hantson Ph, Gerber GB. Mutagenicity, carcinogenicity and teratogenicity of lithium compounds. Mutat Res 1995;339:131–7.
30. Woody JN, London WL, Wilbanks GD Jr. Lithium toxicity in a newborn. Pediatrics 1971;47:94–6.
31. Tunnessen WW Jr, Hertz CG. Toxic effects of lithium in newborn infants: a commentary. J Pediatr 1972;81:804–7.
32. Piton M, Barthe ML, Laloum D, Davy J, Poilpre E, Venezia R. Acute lithium intoxication. Report of two cases: mother and her newborn. Therapie 1973;28:1123–44.
33. Wilbanks GD, Bressler B, Peete CH Jr, Cherny WB, London WL. Toxic effects of lithium carbonate in a mother and newborn infant. JAMA 1970;213:865–7.
34. Morrell P, Sutherland GR, Buamah PK, Oo M, Bain HH. Lithium toxicity in a neonate. Arch Dis Child 1983;58:539–41.
35. Krause S, Ebbesen F, Lange AP. Polyhydramnios with maternal lithium treatment. Obstet Gynecol 1990;75:504–6.

36. Silverman JA, Winters RW, Strande C. Lithium carbonate therapy during pregnancy: apparent lack of effect upon the fetus. Am J Obstet Gynecol 1971;109:934–6.
37. Strothers JK, Wilson DW, Royston N. Lithium toxicity in the newborn. Br Med J 1973;3:233–4.
38. Karlsson K, Lindstedt G, Lundberg PA, Selstam U. Transplacental lithium poisoning: reversible inhibition of fetal thyroid. Lancet 1975;1:1295.
39. Stevens D, Burman D, Midwinter A. Transplacental lithium poisoning. Lancet 1974;2:595.
40. Wilson N, Forfar JC, Godman MJ. Atrial flutter in the newborn resulting from maternal lithium ingestion. Arch Dis Child 1983;58:538–9.
41. Ang MS, Thorp JA, Parisi VM. Maternal lithium therapy and polyhydramnios. Obstet Gynecol 1990;76:517–9.
42. Pinelli JM, Symington AJ, Cunningham KA, Paes BA. Case report and review of the perinatal implications of maternal lithium use. Am J Obstet Gynecol 2002;187:245–9.
43. Nishiwaki T, Tanaka K, Sekiya S. Acute lithium intoxication in pregnancy. Int J Gynecol Obstet 1996;52:191–2.
44. Frayne J, Nguyen T, Kohan R, De Felice N, Rampono J. The comprehensive management of pregnant women with major mood disorders: a case study involving phenelzine, lithium, and quetiapine. Arch Womens Ment Health 2014;17:73–5.
45. Mallinger AG, Hanin I, Stumpf RL, Mallinger J, Kopp U, Erstling C. Lithium treatment during pregnancy: a case study of erythrocyte choline content and lithium transport. J Clin Psychiatry 1983;44:381–4.
46. Levin RM, Amsterdam JD, Winokur A, Wein AJ. Effects of psychotropic drugs on human sperm motility. Fertil Steril 1981;36:503–6.
47. Moore JA, and an IEHR Expert Scientific Committee. An assessment of lithium using the IEHR evaluative process for assessing human developmental and reproductive toxicity of agents. Reprod Toxicol 1995;9:175–210.
48. Schou M, Amdisen A, Steenstrup OR. Lithium and pregnancy. II. Hazards to women given lithium during pregnancy and delivery. Br Med J 1973;2:137–8.
49. Fries H. Lithium in pregnancy. Lancet 1970;1:1233.
50. Schou M, Amdisen A. Lithium and pregnancy. III. Lithium ingestion by children breast-fed by women on lithium treatment. Br Med J 1973;2:138.
51. Kirksey A, Groziak SM. Maternal drug use: evaluation of risks to breast-fed infants. World Rev Nutr Diet 1984;43:60–79.
52. Moretti ME, Koren G, Verjee Z, Ito S. Monitoring lithium in breast milk: an individualized approach for breast-feeding mothers. Ther Drug Monit 2003;25:364–6.
53. Committee on Drugs, American Academy of Pediatrics. The transfer of drugs and other chemicals into human milk. Pediatrics 2001;108:776–89.

LODOXAMIDE

Ophthalmic (Mast Cell Stabilizer)

PREGNANCY RECOMMENDATION: No Human Data—Probably Compatible
BREASTFEEDING RECOMMENDATION: No Human Data—Probably Compatible

PREGNANCY SUMMARY

No reports describing the use of lodoxamide in human pregnancy have been located. The animal data suggest low risk. Moreover, the drug is available as an ophthalmic solution and such use has not resulted in detectable levels in the plasma. The drug appears to be compatible in pregnancy.

FETAL RISK SUMMARY

Lodoxamide is a mast cell stabilizer that is available as an ophthalmic 0.1% solution. It is indicated in the treatment of ocular disorders referred to by the terms vernal keratoconjunctivitis, vernal conjunctivitis, and vernal keratitis. In healthy adult volunteers, administration of one drop in each eye four times daily for 10 days did not result in measurable lodoxamide plasma concentrations (detection limit 2.5 ng/mL) (1).

Reproduction studies have been conducted in rats and rabbits. Oral doses in these species that were more than 5000 times the proposed human clinical dose produced no evidence of developmental toxicity (1)

No evidence of carcinogenicity was observed in long-term studies with oral doses in rats. There also was no evidence of mutagenicity or genetic damage in multiple assays or evidence of impaired reproductive function in laboratory animal studies (1).

It is not known if lodoxamide crosses the human placenta. The molecular weight (about 554) is low enough, but the absence of detectable plasma levels suggests that embryo–fetal exposure will be very low or nil.

BREASTFEEDING SUMMARY

No reports describing the use of lodoxamide during lactation have been located. The molecular weight (about 554) is low enough for excretion into breast milk, but the absence of detectable plasma levels suggests that the effects on a nursing infant are probably nil.

Reference

1. Product information. Alomide. Alcon Laboratories, 2003.

LOMEFLOXACIN

Anti-infective (Quinolone)

PREGNANCY RECOMMENDATION: Human Data Suggest Low Risk
BREASTFEEDING RECOMMENDATION: No Human Data—Probably Compatible

PREGNANCY SUMMARY

Although no reports describing the use of lomefloxacin during human gestation have been located, the available evidence for other members of this class suggests that the risk of major malformations is low. However, a causal relationship with birth defects cannot be excluded (see Ciprofloxacin or Ofloxacin), although the lack of a pattern among the anomalies is reassuring. Because of these concerns and the available animal data, the use of lomefloxacin should be limited in pregnancy, especially during the 1st trimester. A 1993 review on the safety of fluoroquinolones concluded that these antibacterials should be avoided during pregnancy because of the difficulty in extrapolating animal mutagenicity results to humans and because interpretation of this toxicity is still controversial (1). The authors of this review were not convinced that fluoroquinolone-induced fetal cartilage damage and subsequent arthropathies were a major concern, even though this effect had been demonstrated in several animal species after administration to both pregnant and immature animals and in occasional human case reports involving children. Others have also concluded that fluoroquinolones should be considered contraindicated in pregnancy, because safer alternatives are usually available (2).

FETAL RISK SUMMARY

Lomefloxacin is an oral, synthetic, broad-spectrum antibacterial agent. As a fluoroquinolone, it is in the same class of agents as ciprofloxacin, enoxacin, levofloxacin, norfloxacin, ofloxacin, and sparfloxacin. Nalidixic acid is also a quinolone drug.

Reproductive studies have been conducted in rats, rabbits, and monkeys. No evidence of impaired fertility, in male or female rats, or fetal harm in pregnant rats was observed at doses up to 8 times the recommended human dose (RHD) based on BSA (RHD-BSA) (34 times the RHD based on body weight [RHD-BW]). In rabbits, maternal and fetal toxicity was evident at a dose twice the RHD-BSA, consisting of reduced placental weight and variations of the coccygeal vertebrae. Pregnant monkeys dosed at 3–6 times the RHD-BSA (6–12 times the RHD-BW) had an increased incidence of fetal loss, but no teratogenic effects were observed. As with other quinolones, multiple doses of lomefloxacin produced permanent lesions and erosion of cartilage in weight-bearing joints, leading to lameness in immature rats and dogs (3).

It is not known whether lomefloxacin crosses the placenta to the human fetus, but the molecular weight (about 388) is low enough that transfer to the fetus should be expected. No reports describing the use of the antibacterial in human gestation have been located.

In a prospective follow-up study conducted by the European Network of Teratology Information Services (ENTIS), data on 549 pregnancies exposed to fluoroquinolones (none to lomefloxacin) were described in a 1996 reference (2). Data on another 116 prospective and 25 retrospective pregnancy exposures to the antibacterials were also included. Of the 666 cases with known outcome, 32 (4.8%) of the embryos, fetuses, or newborns had congenital malformations. From previous epidemiologic data, the authors concluded that the 4.8% frequency of malformations did not exceed the background rate (2). Finally, 25 retrospective reports of infants with anomalies, who had been exposed in utero to fluoroquinolones, were analyzed, but no specific patterns of major congenital malformations were detected.

The authors of the above study concluded that pregnancy exposure to quinolones was not an indication for termination, but that this class of antibacterial agents should still be considered contraindicated in pregnant women. Moreover, this study did not address the issue of cartilage damage from quinolone exposure and the authors recognized the need for follow-up studies of this potential toxicity in children exposed in utero. Because of their own and previously published findings, they further recommended that the focus of future studies should be on malformations involving the abdominal wall and urogenital system and on limb reduction defects (2).

BREASTFEEDING SUMMARY

When first marketed, the administration of lomefloxacin during breastfeeding was not recommended because of the potential for arthropathy and other serious toxicity in the nursing infant, such as phototoxicity and the eventual development of squamous cell carcinoma of the skin that had been observed in mice (3).

No reports describing the use of lomefloxacin in human lactation have been located. Other quinolones are excreted into milk and, because of its relatively low molecular weight (about 388), the passage of lomefloxacin into milk should be expected. The American Academy of Pediatrics classifies ciprofloxacin and ofloxacin as compatible with breastfeeding (see Ciprofloxacin and Ofloxacin).

References

1. Norrby SR, Lietman PS. Safety and tolerability of fluoroquinolones. Drugs 1993;45(Suppl 3):59–64.
2. Schaefer C, Amoura-Elefant E, Vial T, Ornoy A, Garbis H, Robert E, Rodriguez-Pinilla E, Pexieder T, Prapas N, Merlob P. Pregnancy outcome after prenatal quinolone exposure. Evaluation of a case registry of the European Network of Teratology Information Services (ENTIS). Eur J Obstet Gynecol Reprod Biol 1996;69:83–9.
3. Product information. Maxaquin. G.D. Searle, 1997.

LOMITAPIDE

Antilipemic Agent (Miscellaneous)

PREGNANCY RECOMMENDATION: No Human Data—Animal Data Suggest High Risk
BREASTFEEDING RECOMMENDATION: No Human Data—Potential Toxicity

PREGNANCY SUMMARY

No reports describing the use of lomitapide in human pregnancy have been located. The animal data suggest risk, but the absence of human pregnancy experience prevents a more complete assessment of the embryo–fetal risk. The manufacturer classifies the drug as contraindicated because of the toxicity observed in three animal species.

FETAL RISK SUMMARY

Lomitapide is an oral synthetic lipid-lowering agent that directly binds and inhibits microsomal triglyceride transfer protein. It is indicated as an adjunct to a low-fat diet and other lipid-lowering treatments, including low-density lipoprotein (LDL) apheresis where available, to reduce LDL cholesterol, total cholesterol, apolipoprotein B, and non-high-density lipoprotein cholesterol in patients with homozygous familial hypercholesterolemia. It is extensively metabolized by the liver to inactive metabolites. The drug is highly (99.8%) bound to plasma protein and the mean terminal half-life is about 40 hours (1).

Reproduction studies have been conducted in rats, rabbits, and ferrets. In rats, oral doses that were ≥2 times the human exposure at the maximum recommended human dose of 60 mg based on AUC (MRHD-AUC) given from gestation day 6 through organogenesis caused fetal malformations. The defects included umbilical hernia, gastroschisis, imperforate anus, alterations in heart shape and size, limb malrotations, skeletal malformations of the tail, and delayed ossification of cranial, vertebral and pelvic bones. When given from gestation day 7 through termination of nursing on lactation day 20, systemic exposures that were equivalent to the human exposure at the MRND-AUC were associated with malformations. Increased pup mortality occurred at 4 times the MRHD-AUC. In rabbits, exposures up to 3 times the MRHD based on BSA (MRHD-BSA) from gestational day 6 through organogenesis were not associated with adverse effects. However, exposures that were ≥6 times the MRHD-BSA resulted in embryo–fetal death. In ferrets given the drug from gestation day 12 through organogenesis, exposures that were <1–5 times the human exposure at the MRHD-AUC were associated with maternal toxicity and fetal malformations. Defects included umbilical hernia, medially rotated or short limbs, absent or fused digits on paws, cleft palate, open eye lids, low-set ears, and kinked tail (1).

In a 2-year dietary carcinogenicity study in mice, lomitapide caused significant increases of liver adenomas and small intestine carcinomas in males and combined adenomas and carcinomas in females. In 2-year studies in rats, there were no statistically significant drug-related increases in tumor incidences. Various assays for mutagenicity were negative. The drug had no effects on fertility in male and female rats at exposures up to 4–5 times the MRHD-AUC (1).

It is not known if lomitapide crosses the human placenta. The molecular weight (about 790) and high plasma protein binding suggest that exposure of the embryo–fetus will be limited, but the long terminal half-life might allow the drug to cross.

BREASTFEEDING SUMMARY

No reports describing the use of lomitapide during human lactation have been located. The molecular weight (about 790) and high (99.8%) plasma protein binding suggest that excretion of the drug into breast milk will be limited, but the long terminal half-life (about 40 hours) might allow excretion of the drug into milk. The effect of the exposure on a nursing infant is unknown. The potential for tumorigenicity in a mouse study suggests that the drug should not be used during breastfeeding. However, if a mother receiving the drug chooses to breastfeed, the infant should be monitored for the most common (incidence ≥28%) adverse effect seen in adults. These effects include diarrhea, nausea, vomiting, dyspepsia, and abdominal pain (1).

Reference

1. Product information. Juxtapid. Aegerion Pharmaceuticals, 2012.

LOPERAMIDE

Antidiarrheal

PREGNANCY RECOMMENDATION: Limited Human Data—Animal Data Suggest Low Risk
BREASTFEEDING RECOMMENDATION: Limited Human Data—Probably Compatible

PREGNANCY SUMMARY

The animal data suggest low risk, but the human pregnancy experience is too limited to allow a more complete assessment of embryo/fetal risk. Nevertheless, an abstract suggests that the human risk also is low.

FETAL RISK SUMMARY

Loperamide is a synthetic opioid analog that is used for the treatment of diarrhea. It is available without a prescription. No published reports linking the use of loperamide with congenital defects have been located.

Reproduction studies with rats and rabbits at doses up to 30 times the human dose have revealed no evidence of impaired fertility, teratogenicity, or other fetal harm (1).

In a surveillance study of Michigan Medicaid recipients involving 229,101 completed pregnancies conducted between 1985 and 1992, 108 newborns had been exposed to loperamide during the 1st trimester (F. Rosa, personal communication, FDA, 1993). Six (5.6%) major birth defects were observed (five expected), three of which were cardiovascular defects (one expected). No anomalies were observed in five other defect categories (oral clefts, spina bifida, polydactyly, limb reduction defects, and hypospadias) for which specific data were available. The number of cardiovascular defects suggests a possible association, but other factors, including the mother's disease, concurrent drug use, and chance, may be involved.

In a 1999 abstract, the pregnancy outcomes of 89 women exposed to loperamide in the 1st trimester were compared with matched controls (2). There were no significant differences between the groups in terms of major and minor malformations, spontaneous abortions, elective abortions, preterm delivery, and birth weights. However, in 21 mothers who took loperamide throughout gestation, birth weights tended to be lower (200 g) (*ns*) (2).

BREASTFEEDING SUMMARY

No reports describing the use of loperamide during lactation have been located. However, one study investigated loperamide oxide, a pharmacologically inactive prodrug that is reduced to loperamide as it progresses through the intestinal tract, during lactation (3). Six women in the immediate postpartum period, who were not nursing, were given two 4-mg oral doses of loperamide oxide 12 hours apart. Simultaneous plasma and milk samples were collected 12 hours after the first dose, and 6 and 24 hours after the second dose. Small amounts of loperamide oxide were measured in some of the plasma samples, but the mean loperamide oxide milk concentrations were <0.10 ng/mL (detection limit) at each sampling time. Mean loperamide milk concentrations for the three samples were 0.18, 0.27, and 0.19 ng/mL, respectively, corresponding to milk:plasma ratios of 0.50, 0.37, and 0.35, respectively (3). The American Academy of Pediatrics classifies loperamide as compatible with breastfeeding (4).

References

1. Product information. Imodium. McNeil Consumer, 2000.
2. Einarson A, Mastroiacovo P, Arnon J, Ornoy A, Addis A, Ritvanen A, Koren G. A prospective controlled multicentre study of loperamide in pregnancy (abstract). Teratology 1999;59:377.
3. Nikodem VC, Hofmeyr GJ. Secretion of the antidiarrhoeal agent loperamide oxide in breast milk. Eur J Clin Pharmacol 1992;42:695–6.
4. Committee on Drugs, American Academy of Pediatrics. The transfer of drugs and other chemicals into human milk. Pediatrics 2001;108:776–89.

LOPINAVIR

Antiviral

PREGNANCY RECOMMENDATION: Compatible—Maternal Benefit >> Embryo/Fetal Risk
BREASTFEEDING RECOMMENDATION: Contraindicated

PREGNANCY SUMMARY

The human pregnancy experience with lopinavir, always in combination with ritonavir and other antiretroviral agents, suggests that the embryo–fetal risk is low. The animal data are suggestive of moderate risk because the exposure for lopinavir was less than the human therapeutic exposure. If indicated, the drug should not be withheld because of pregnancy.

FETAL RISK SUMMARY

Lopinavir, an inhibitor of HIV protease, prevents cleavage of the Gag-Pol polyproteins, resulting in the production of immature, noninfectious viral particles. The agent is only available in a fixed combination (200 mg lopinavir/50 mg ritonavir per capsule; 80 mg lopinavir/20 mg ritonavir per mL oral solution). Ritonavir is a potent inhibitor of CYP3A isozyme from the hepatic cytochrome P450 system that is responsible for the metabolism of lopinavir, thereby increasing the plasma levels of lopinavir. The plasma levels of ritonavir are very low; therefore, the antiviral activity of the combination is due to lopinavir. Plasma protein binding of lopinavir is high (98%–99%), primarily by α_1-acid glycoprotein, but some is bound to albumin. The average half-life of lopinavir over a 12-hour dosing interval is 5–6 hours (1).

Reproduction studies have been conducted in rats and rabbits. In rats, doses producing systemic exposures that were approximately 0.7 (lopinavir)/1.8 (ritonavir) times the human exposure obtained with the recommended dose of 400/100 mg twice daily based on AUC (HE) resulted in embryonic and fetal toxicity (early resorption, decreased fetal viability and body weight, increased incidences of skeletal variations and skeletal ossification delays). This dose was maternal toxic. Developmental toxicity (decreased pup survival) also was observed in a perinatal and postnatal rat study at doses producing exposures equal to or greater than about 0.3 (lopinavir)/0.7 (ritonavir) times the HE. In rabbits, maternal toxic doses (0.6 [lopinavir]/1.0 [ritonavir]) did not result in embryonic or fetal development toxicity (1).

Consistent with the molecular weight (about 629) and lipid solubility, lopinavir crosses the human placenta. A 2006 study using the ex vivo human cotyledon perfusion model found that placental transfer of lopinavir (combined with ritonavir) was compatible with passive diffusion, even in the presence of physiologic concentrations of human albumin (2). The amount entering the fetal compartment was well above the 50% inhibitory concentration (2). In an earlier study, the cord:maternal blood ratio 12.25 hours after lopinavir (533 mg twice daily in combination with lamivudine and abacavir) in a woman delivering at term (38 weeks) was <0.1 (<250 ng/mL/3105 ng/mL) (3,4).

The Antiretroviral Pregnancy Registry reported, for January 1989 through July 2009, prospective data (reported before the outcomes were known) involving 4702 live births that had been exposed during the 1st trimester to one or more antiretroviral agents (5). Congenital defects were noted in 134, a prevalence of 2.8% (95% confidence interval [CI] 2.4–3.4). In the 6100 live births with earliest exposure in the 2nd/3rd trimesters, there were 153 infants with defects (2.5%, 95% CI 2.1–2.9). The prevalence rates for the two periods did not differ significantly. There were 288 infants with birth defects among 10,803 live births with exposure anytime during pregnancy (2.7%, 95% CI 2.4–3.0). The prevalence rate did not differ significantly from the rate expected in a nonexposed population. There were 1794 outcomes exposed to lopinavir (526 in the 1st trimester and 1268 in the 2nd/3rd trimesters) in combination with other antiretroviral agents. There were 39 birth defects (9 in the 1st trimester and 30 in the 2nd/3rd trimesters). In reviewing the birth defects of prospective and retrospective (pregnancies reported after the outcomes were known) registered cases, the Registry concluded that, except for isolated cases of neural tube defects with efavirenz exposure in retrospective reports, there was no other pattern of anomalies (isolated or syndromic) (5). (See Lamivudine for required statement.)

In 1998, a public health advisory was issued by the FDA on the association between protease inhibitors and diabetes mellitus (6). Because pregnancy is a risk factor for hyperglycemia, there was concern that these antiretroviral agents would exacerbate this risk. The manufacturer's product information also notes the potential risk for new-onset diabetes, exacerbation of preexisting diabetes, and hyperglycemia in HIV-infected patients receiving protease inhibitor therapy (1). An abstract published in 2000 described the results of a study involving 34 pregnant women treated with protease inhibitors compared with 41 controls that evaluated the association with diabetes (7). No association between protease inhibitors and an increased incidence of gestational diabetes was found.

Two reviews, one in 1996 and the other in 1997, concluded that all women currently receiving antiretroviral therapy should continue to receive therapy during pregnancy and that treatment of the mother with monotherapy should be considered inadequate therapy (8,9). The same conclusion was reached in a 2003 review with the added admonishment that therapy must be continuous to prevent emergence of resistant viral strains (10). In 2009, the updated U.S. Department of Health and Human Services guidelines for the use of antiretroviral agents in HIV type 1 (HIV-1)-infected patients continued the recommendation that therapy, with the exception of efavirenz, should be continued during pregnancy (11). If indicated, therefore, protease inhibitors, including lopinavir, should not be withheld in pregnancy because the expected benefit to the HIV-positive mother outweighs the unknown risk to the fetus. Pregnant women taking protease inhibitors should be monitored for hyperglycemia. Updated guidelines for the use of antiretroviral drugs to reduce perinatal HIV-1 transmission also were released in 2010 (12). Women receiving antiretroviral therapy during pregnancy should continue the therapy but, regardless of the regimen, zidovudine administration is recommended during the intrapartum period to prevent vertical transmission of HIV to the newborn (12).

BREASTFEEDING SUMMARY

No reports have been located that describe the use of the combination product, lopinavir/ritonavir, during human lactation. The molecular weights of lopinavir (about 629) and ritonavir (about 721), combined with their lipid solubility, suggest that the drugs will be excreted into human breast milk, although the extensive plasma protein binding (98%–99%) should limit this excretion. The effects of this exposure on a nursing infant are unknown.

However, reports on the use of lopinavir/ritonavir during lactation are unlikely because the combination is indicated in the treatment of patients with HIV. HIV-1 is transmitted in milk, and in developed countries, breastfeeding is not recommended (8,9,11,13–16). In developing countries, breastfeeding is undertaken, despite the risk, because there are no affordable milk substitutes available.

References

1. Product information. Kaletra. Abbott Laboratories, 2004.
2. Gavard L, Gil S, Peytavin G, Ceccaldi PF, Ferreira C, Farinotti R, Mandelbrot L. Placental transfer of lopinavir/ritonavir in the ex vivo human cotyledon perfusion model. Am J Obstet Gynecol 2006;195:296–301.
3. Marzolini C, Rudin C, Decosterd LA, Telenti A, Schreyer A, Biollaz J, Buclin T, and the Swiss Mother + Child HIV Cohort Study. Transplacental passage of protease inhibitors at delivery. AIDS 2002;16:889–93.
4. Marzolini C, Beguin A, Telenti A, Schreyer A, Buclin T, Biollaz J, Decosterd LA. Determination of lopinavir and nevirapine by high-performance liquid chromatography after solid-phase extraction: application for the assessment of their transplacental passage at delivery. J Chromatogr B Analyt Technol Biomed Life Sci 2002;774:127–40.
5. Antiretroviral Pregnancy Registry Steering Committee. *Antiretroviral Pregnancy Registry International Interim Report for 1 January 1989 through 31 July 2009*. Wilmington, NC: Registry Coordinating Center; 2009. Available at www.apregistry.com. Accessed May 29, 2010.

6. CDC. Public Health Service Task Force recommendations for the use of antiretroviral drugs in pregnant women infected with HIV-1 for maternal health and for reducing perinatal HIV-1 transmission in the United States. MMWR 1998;47:No. RR-2.
7. Fassett M, Kramer F, Stek A. Treatment with protease inhibitors in pregnancy is not associated with an increased incidence of gestational diabetes (abstract). Am J Obstet Gynecol 2000;182:S97.
8. Carpenter CCJ, Fischi MA, Hammer SM, Hirsch MS, Jacobsen DM, Katzenstein DA, Montaner JSG, Richman DD, Saag MS, Schooley RT, Thompson MA, Vella S, Yeni PG, Volberding PA. Antiretroviral therapy for HIV infection in 1996. JAMA 1996;276:146–54.
9. Minkoff H, Augenbraun M. Antiretroviral therapy for pregnant women. Am J Obstet Gynecol 1997;176:478–89.
10. Minkoff H. Human immunodeficiency virus infection in pregnancy. Obstet Gynecol 2003;101:797–810.
11. Panel on Antiretroviral Guidelines for Adults and Adolescents. *Guidelines for the Use of Antiretroviral Agents in HIV-1-infected Adults and Adolescents.* Department of Health and Human Services. December 1, 2009:1–161. Available at http://www.aidsinfo.nih.gov/ContentFiles/AdultandAdolescentGL.pdf. Accessed September 17, 2010:60, 96–8.
12. Panel on Treatment of HIV-Infected Pregnant Women and Prevention of Perinatal Transmission. *Recommendations for Use of Antiretroviral Drugs in Pregnant HIV-1-Infected Women for Maternal Health and Interventions to Reduce Perinatal HIV Transmission in the United States.* May 24, 2010:1–117. Available at http://aidsinfo.nih.gov/ContentFiles/PerinatalGL.pdf. Accessed September 17, 2010:30 (Table 5).
13. Brown ZA, Watts DH. Antiviral therapy in pregnancy. Clin Obstet Gynecol 1990;33:276–89.
14. De Martino M, Tovo P-A, Pezzotti P, Galli L, Massironi E, Ruga E, Floreea F, Plebani A, Gabiano C, Zuccotti GV. HIV-1 transmission through breast-milk: appraisal of risk according to duration of feeding. AIDS 1992;6:991–7.
15. Van de Perre P. Postnatal transmission of human immunodeficiency virus type 1: the breast-feeding dilemma. Am J Obstet Gynecol 1995;173: 483–7.
16. American College of Obstetricians and Gynecologists. Breastfeeding: Maternal and infant aspects. *Educational Bulletin.* No. 258, July 2000.

LORACARBEF

[Withdrawn from the market. See 9th edition.]

LORATADINE

Antihistamine

PREGNANCY RECOMMENDATION: Limited Human Data—Animal Data Suggest Low Risk
BREASTFEEDING RECOMMENDATION: Limited Human Data—Probably Compatible

PREGNANCY SUMMARY

No evidence of increased teratogenicity has been found in animals or humans. The human pregnancy experience is adequate to show that the drug is not a major human teratogen. Moreover, a significant increase in loratadine-induced congenital malformations would be unusual, as no other antihistamine has been shown to be a major human teratogen. If an oral antihistamine agent is required during pregnancy, first-generation agents such as chlorpheniramine or tripelennamine should be considered. Previous reviews published before the availability of the studies discussed below concluded that loratadine and cetirizine were acceptable alternatives, except during the 1st trimester, if a first-generation drug was not tolerated (1–3).

FETAL RISK SUMMARY

Loratadine, a second-generation histamine H_1-receptor antagonist, is used for the treatment of symptoms related to seasonal allergic rhinitis. Studies with rats and rabbits with oral doses up to 75 and 150 times, respectively, the maximum recommended human daily oral dose based on BSA found no evidence of teratogenicity (4). Treatment of pregnant rats from gestational day 7 through postpartum day 4 with doses up to 26 times the human clinical exposure revealed no evidence of antiandrogenic activity, as demonstrated by a lack of effect on androgen-dependent development in male offspring (5).

It is not known if loratadine crosses the human placenta. The molecular weight (about 383) is low enough that passage to the fetus should be expected.

The FDA has received six reports of adverse outcomes following exposure during pregnancy, including two cases of cleft palate, and one case each of microtia and microphthalmia, deafness, tricuspid dysplasia, and diaphragmatic hernia (F. Rosa, personal communication, FDA, 1996). A relationship, if any, between loratadine and the outcomes cannot be determined from these data.

A 1998 noninterventional, observational cohort study described the outcomes of pregnancies in women who had been prescribed one or more of 34 newly marketed drugs by general practitioners in England (6). Data were obtained by questionnaires sent to the prescribing physicians one month after the expected or possible date of delivery. In 831 (78%) of the pregnancies, a newly marketed drug was thought to have been taken during the 1st trimester with birth defects noted in 14 (2.5%) singleton births of the 557 newborns (10 sets of twins). In addition, two birth defects were observed in aborted fetuses. However, few of the aborted fetuses were examined. Loratadine was taken during the 1st trimester in

18 pregnancies. The outcomes of these pregnancies included 2 elective abortions and 16 normal, term infants (6).

A 2002 study found no increased risk of teratogenicity or other pregnancy or newborn complications for antihistamines when used in early pregnancy for the treatment of nausea and vomiting (*N* = 12,394) and allergy (*N* = 5041) (7). In the study, 1769 women used loratadine.

A collaborative 2003 report gathered data from four teratology information services (Canada, Israel, Italy, and Brazil) pertaining to 1st trimester loratadine exposures in 161 pregnancies (8). The outcomes of these pregnancies were compared with 161 nonexposed controls. The average daily dose of loratadine was 11.3 mg. The live birth rate, gestational age at delivery, and birth weight in the two groups were similar. There were five congenital malformations (kidney defect, aortic valve stenosis, unspecified chromosomal abnormalities, bilateral inguinal hernia, and congenital hip dislocation) in the loratadine group and six in the controls. The sample size had an 80% power to detect a 3.5-fold increase in the overall rate of defects (8).

In 2004, the CDC summarized their analysis of data from The National Birth Defects Prevention Study that examined the association between loratadine and hypospadias (9). The study population consisted of 563 male infants with hypospadias and 1444 male infants with no major birth defects. Cases and controls were born between October 1997 and June 2001. In the cases, 46 (8.2%) had multiple congenital malformations that were not recognized as phenotypes, and in 517 (91.8%) hypospadias was an isolated defect. Exposure to loratadine occurred in 11 cases and 22 controls (adjusted odds ratio [OR] 0.96, 95% confidence interval [CI] 0.41–2.22). For nonsedating (including loratadine) and sedating antihistamines, the OR (and 95% CI) were 0.95 (0.48–1.89) and 1.02 (0.68–1.53), respectively. Thus, neither type of antihistamine was associated with hypospadias (9).

BREASTFEEDING SUMMARY

Loratadine and its metabolite, descarboethoxyloratadine, are excreted into human milk (4,10). Six lactating women were given a single 40-mg dose (10). The peak milk concentration, 29.2 ng/mL, occurred within 2 hours of the dose, whereas the peak plasma level, 30.5 ng/mL, was measured 1 hour after the dose. The mean milk:plasma area under the concentration curve (AUC) ratios for the parent compound and the active metabolite, measured during 48 hours, were 1.17 and 0.85, respectively (4,10). During 48 hours, the mean amounts of loratadine and metabolite recovered from the milk were 4.2 mcg (0.010% of the dose) and 6.0 mcg (equivalent to 7.5 mcg of loratadine; 0.019% of the dose), respectively. A 4-kg infant ingesting this milk would have received a dose equivalent to 0.46% of the mother's dose on an mg/kg basis (10). Based on this estimate, and the fact that the dose used in the study was four times the current recommended dose, there is probably little clinical risk to a nursing infant whose mother was taking 10 mg of loratadine per day. The American Academy of Pediatrics classifies loratadine as compatible with breastfeeding (11).

References

1. Mazzotta P, Loebstein R, Koren G. Treating allergic rhinitis in pregnancy. Safety considerations. Drug Saf 1999;20:361–75.
2. Horak F, Stubner UP. Comparative tolerability of second generation antihistamines. Drug Saf 1999;20:385–401.
3. Joint committee of the American College of Obstetricians and Gynecologists (ACOG) and the American College of Allergy, Asthma and Immunology (ACAAI). Position statement. The use of newer asthma and allergy medications during pregnancy. Ann Allergy Asthma Immunol 2000;84:475–80.
4. Product information. Claritin. Schering, 2001.
5. McIntyre BS, Vancutsem PM, Treinen KA, Morrissey RE. Effects of perinatal loratadine exposure on male rat reproductive organ development. Reprod Toxicol 2003;17:691–7.
6. Wilton LV, Pearce GL, Martin RM, Mackay FJ, Mann RD. The outcomes of pregnancy in women exposed to newly marketed drugs in general practice in England. Br J Obstet Gynaecol 1998;105:882–9.
7. Kallen B. Use of antihistamine drugs in early pregnancy and delivery outcome. J Matern Fetal Neonatal Med 2002;11:146–52.
8. Moretti ME, Caprara D, Coutinho CJ, Bar-Oz B, Berkovitch M, Addis A, Jovanovski E, Schuler-Faccini L, Koren G. Fetal safety of loratadine use in the first trimester of pregnancy: a multicenter study. J Allergy Clin Immunol 2003;111:479–83.
9. Werler M, McCloskey C, Edmonds LD, Olney R, Honein MA, Reefhuis J. Evaluation of an association between loratadine and hypospadias—United States, 1997–2001. MMWR 2004;53:219–21.
10. Hilbert J, Radwanski E, Affrime MB, Perentesis G, Symchowicz S, Zampaglione N. Excretion of loratadine in human breast milk. J Clin Pharmacol 1988;28:234–9.
11. Committee on Drugs, American Academy of Pediatrics. The transfer of drugs and other chemicals into human milk. Pediatrics 2001;108: 776–89.

LORAZEPAM

Sedative

PREGNANCY RECOMMENDATION: Human Data Suggest Risk in the 1st and 3rd Trimesters
BREASTFEEDING RECOMMENDATION: Limited Human Data—Probably Compatible*
*Potential toxicity if combined with other CNS depressants

PREGNANCY SUMMARY

Lorazepam is a benzodiazepine indicated for the treatment of status epilepticus and as a preanesthetic sedative. One report found a significant association with anal atresia. When used close to delivery, "floppy infant" syndrome has been reported. The long-term effects of in utero exposure on neurobehavior, especially when the exposure occurs in the latter half of pregnancy, have not been studied but are of concern.

FETAL RISK SUMMARY

Reproduction studies with lorazepam have been conducted in mice, rats, and two strains of rabbits. Occasional, non-dose-related malformations (reduction of tarsals, tibia, metatarsals, malrotated limbs, gastroschisis, malformed skull, and microphthalmia) were observed in rabbits, but these defects have also randomly occurred in controls. Fetal resorptions and increased fetal loss occurred in rabbits at oral (40 mg/kg) and IV (4 mg/kg) doses and higher (1).

Lorazepam crosses the placenta, achieving cord levels similar to maternal serum concentrations (2–5). Placental transfer is slower than that of diazepam, but high IV doses may produce the "floppy infant" syndrome (3). (See Diazepam for a description of this syndrome.)

A case reported in 1996 described an otherwise healthy male infant, exposed throughout gestation to lorazepam (7.5–12.5 mg/day) and clozapine (200–300 mg/day), who developed transient, mild floppy infant syndrome after delivery at 37 weeks' gestation (6). The mother had taken the combination therapy for the treatment of schizophrenia. The hypotonia, attributed to lorazepam because of the absence of such reports in pregnancies exposed to clozapine alone, resolved 5 days after birth.

An abstract published in 1999 found an association between lorazepam and anal atresia (7). Using data from a French pregnancy registry, the investigators reported that among infants exposed to benzodiazepines 5 of 6 cases of anal atresia were exposed to lorazepam ($p = 0.01$).

Lorazepam has been used in labor to potentiate the effects of narcotic analgesics (8). Although not statistically significant, a higher incidence of respiratory depression occurred in the exposed newborn infants.

BREASTFEEDING SUMMARY

Lorazepam is excreted into breast milk in low concentrations (9,10). In one study, no effects on the nursing infant were reported (9), but the slight delay in establishing feeding was a cause for concern (11). Milk:plasma ratios in four women who had received 3.5 mg orally of lorazepam 4 hours earlier ranged from 0.15 to 0.26 (9). The mean milk concentration was 8.5 ng/mL. In another study, 5 mg of oral lorazepam was given 1 hour before labor induction and the effects on feeding behavior were measured in the newborn infants (12). During the first 48 hours, no significant effect was observed on volume of milk consumed or duration of feeding.

The effects of exposure to benzodiazepines during breastfeeding were reported in a 2012 study (13). In a 15-month period spanning 2010–2011, 296 women called the Motherisk Program in Toronto, Ontario, seeking advice on the use of these drugs during lactation and 124 consented to the study. The most commonly used benzodiazepines were lorazepam (52%), clonazepam (18%), and midazolam (15%). Neonatal sedation was reported in only two infants. Lorazepam was not used by either mother. There was no significant difference between the characteristics of these 2 and the 122 that reported no sedation in terms of maternal age, gestational age at birth, daily amount of time nursing, amount of time infant slept each day, and the benzodiazepine dose (mg/kg/day). The only difference was in the number of CNS depressants that the mothers were taking: 3.5 vs. 1.7 ($p = 0.0056$). The investigators concluded that their results supported the recommendation that the use benzodiazepines was not a reason to avoid breastfeeding (13).

The American Academy of Pediatrics classifies the effects of lorazepam on the nursing infant as unknown but may be of concern if exposure is prolonged (14).

References

1. Product information. Ativan. Wyeth-Ayerst Pharmaceuticals, 2000.
2. De Groot G, Maes RAA, Defoort P, Thiery M. Placental transfer of lorazepam. IRCS Med Sci 1975;3:290.
3. McBride RJ, Dundee JW, Moore J, Toner W, Howard PJ. A study of the plasma concentrations of lorazepam in mother and neonate. Br J Anaesth 1979;51:971–8.
4. Kanto J, Aaltonen L, Liukko P, Maenpaa K. Transfer of lorazepam and its conjugate across the human placenta. Acta Pharmacol Toxicol (Copenh) 1980;47:130–4.
5. Kanto JH. Use of benzodiazepines during pregnancy, labour and lactation, with particular reference to pharmacokinetic considerations. Drugs 1982;23:354–80.
6. Di Michele V, Ramenghi LA, Sabatino G. Clozapine and lorazepam administration in pregnancy. Eur Psychiatry 1996;11:214.
7. Bonnot O, Vollset SE, Godet PF, Robert E. Maternal exposure to lorazepam and anal atresia in newborns? Results from a hypothesis generating study of benzodiazepines and malformations (abstract). Teratology 1999;59:439–40.
8. McAuley DM, O'Neill MP, Moore J, Dundee JW. Lorazepam premedication for labour. Br J Obstet Gynaecol 1982;89:149–54.
9. Whitelaw AGL, Cummings AJ, McFadyen IR. Effect of maternal lorazepam on the neonate. Br Med J 1981;282:1106–8.
10. Summerfield RJ, Nielsen MS. Excretion of lorazepam into breast milk. Br J Anaesth 1985;57:1042–3.
11. Johnstone M. Effect of maternal lorazepam on the neonate. Br Med J 1981;282:1973.
12. Johnstone MJ. The effect of lorazepam on neonatal feeding behaviour at term. Pharmatherapeutica 1982;3:259–62.
13. Kelly LE, Poon S, Madadi P, Koren G. Neonatal benzodiazepines exposure during breastfeeding. J Pediatr 2012;161:448–51.
14. Committee on Drugs, American Academy of Pediatrics. The transfer of drugs and other chemicals into human milk. Pediatrics 2001;108:776–89.

LORCASERIN

Anorexiant

PREGNANCY RECOMMENDATION: Contraindicated
BREASTFEEDING RECOMMENDATION: No Human Data—Potential Toxicity

PREGNANCY SUMMARY

No reports describing the use of lorcaserin in human pregnancy have been located. The animal reproduction data suggest moderate risk, but the absence of human pregnancy experience prevents a more complete assessment of embryo–fetal risk. However, the manufacturer classifies the drug as contraindicated in pregnancy because weight loss offers no potential benefit to a pregnant woman and may result in fetal harm (1).

FETAL RISK SUMMARY

Lorcaserin is an oral selective agonist of serotonin 2C receptors that are located in the hypothalamus. It is indicated as an adjunct to a reduced-calorie diet and increased physical activity for chronic weight management in adult patients with an initial body mass index (BMI) of 30 kg/m^2 or greater (obese) or 27 kg/m^2 or greater (overweight) in the presence of at least one weight-related comorbid condition (e.g., hypertension, dyslipidemia, and type 2 diabetes). Lorcaserin is extensively metabolized to inactive metabolites. The drug is moderately (about 70%) bound to plasma proteins and has a plasma half-life of about 11 hours (1).

Reproduction studies have been conducted in rats and rabbits. In these species, plasma exposures during organogenesis that were 44 and 19 times, respectively, the human exposure (HE) revealed no evidence of teratogenicity or embryolethality. In a separate study, rats were given the drug from gestation through postnatal day 21 with doses resulting in exposures up to about 44 times the HE. The highest dose resulted in stillborns and lower pup viability, but all doses lowered pup body weight at birth, which persisted to adulthood. However, no developmental abnormalities or effects on reproductive performance in the offspring were observed at any dose (1).

Two-year carcinogenicity studies in mice were negative. In a similar study in rats, mammary adenocarcinoma and mammary fibroadenoma occurred in females. These findings may have been associated with drug-induced changes in prolactin homeostasis and their relevance to humans is unknown. In male rats, treatment-related neoplastic changes were noted in the subcutis (fibroadenoma, Schwannoma), the skin (squamous cell carcinoma), mammary gland, and the brain (astrocytoma). Lorcaserin was not mutagenic or genotoxic in multiple assays. No effects on fertility in male and female rats were observed (1).

It is not known if lorcaserin crosses the human placenta. The molecular weight (about 197 for the free base), moderate plasma protein binding, and the long plasma half-life suggest that the drug will cross to the embryo–fetus.

BREASTFEEDING SUMMARY

No reports describing the use of lorcaserin during human lactation have been located. The molecular weight (about 197 for the free base), moderate (about 70%) plasma protein binding, and the long (about 11 hours) plasma half-life suggest that the drug will be excreted into breast milk. The effect of the exposure on a nursing infant is unknown. The most common (>5%) adverse effects in nondiabetic patients were headache, dizziness, fatigue, nausea, dry mouth, and constipation (1). If a woman is receiving lorcaserin and chooses to nurse, her infant should be monitored for these adverse effects.

Reference

1. Product information. Belviq. Arena Pharmaceuticals GmbH, 2012.

L

LOSARTAN

Antihypertensive

PREGNANCY RECOMMENDATION: Human Data Suggest Risk in the 2nd and 3rd Trimesters
BREASTFEEDING RECOMMENDATION: No Human Data—Probably Compatible

PREGNANCY SUMMARY

The antihypertensive mechanisms of action of losartan and angiotensin-converting enzyme (ACE) inhibitors are very close. That is, the former selectively blocks the binding of angiotensin II to AT$_1$ receptors, whereas the latter prevents the formation of angiotensin II itself. Therefore, use of this drug during the 2nd and 3rd trimesters may cause teratogenicity and severe fetal and neonatal toxicity that is identical to that seen with ACE inhibitors (e.g., see Captopril or Enalapril). Fetal toxic effects may include anuria, oligohydramnios, fetal hypocalvaria, intrauterine growth restriction (IUGR), prematurity, and patent ductus arteriosus. Anuria-associated oligohydramnios may produce fetal limb contractures, craniofacial deformation, and pulmonary hypoplasia. Severe anuria and hypotension, which is resistant to both pressor agents and volume expansion, may occur in the newborn following in utero exposure to losartan. Newborn renal function and blood pressure should be closely monitored.

FETAL RISK SUMMARY

Losartan is a selective angiotensin II receptor blocker (ARB) that is used, either alone or in combination, with other antihypertensive agents, for the treatment of hypertension. Losartan, and its active metabolite, block the vasoconstrictor and aldosterone-secreting effects of angiotensin II by preventing angiotensin II from binding to AT_1 receptors.

Reproduction studies have been conducted in pregnant rats (1–3). At oral doses greater than three times the maximum recommended human dose of 100 mg based on BSA (MRHD), reduced body weight, delayed physical and behavioral development, mortality, and renal toxicity were observed in rat fetuses and neonates (1–3). These adverse effects were attributed to exposure during late pregnancy (gestational days 15–20) and/or during lactation (1,2). The irreversible renal abnormalities in the newborn pups included dilatation of the renal pelvis, edema of the renal papilla, medial hypertrophy of intracortical arterioles, chronic renal inflammation, and irregular scarring of the renal parenchyma (2).

In fertility and reproductive performance studies, a significant decrease in fetal implants in rats was noted at a maternally toxic oral dose, approximately 24 times the MRHD. No effects on implants/pregnant female, percent postimplantation loss, or live pups/litter at parturition were observed at an oral dose approximately 12 times the MRHD (1–3).

It is not known if losartan or its active metabolite crosses the human placenta to the fetus. Because the molecular weight of losartan (about 461) is low enough, passage to the human fetus should be expected.

A postmarketing safety surveillance study of losartan, published in 1999, described the outcomes of four human pregnancies (4). Three of the pregnancies were exposed to the drug in the 1st trimester and the fourth pregnancy was diagnosed about 2 months after stopping the drug. In the first case, the woman became pregnant while taking losartan and the drug was discontinued at approximately 8 weeks' gestation. Because of worsening renal failure, dialysis was required during pregnancy. She delivered a growth-restricted infant at 29 weeks who died at 9 days of age. In the second case, losartan was stopped 6 weeks after the last menstrual period. The woman delivered prematurely at 30 weeks because of preeclampsia. The infant was reported to be doing well. The third pregnancy ended with a spontaneous abortion (no specific embryo data) at 6–8 weeks' gestation while the woman was receiving losartan. Finally, a spontaneous abortion (no specific embryo data) occurred at 6 weeks' gestation in a woman who had stopped losartan about 2 months before the pregnancy was diagnosed. Because of the timing of the exposures, none of the outcomes appear to be related to the use of losartan. They are probably a consequence of the women's severe hypertension (4).

In a 2001 case report, anhydramnios was diagnosed at 31 weeks' gestation in a 31-year-old woman with periarteritis nodosa (5). Hypertension had developed at 17 weeks' gestation and losartan, 50 mg/day, had been started. Therapy was changed to methyldopa (750 mg/day), but 2 days later the woman noticed no fetal movements. Ultrasound confirmed intrauterine fetal death and she delivered a stillborn 1592-g male infant the next day. The infant had facial and limb deformities characteristic of oligohydramnios. At autopsy, pulmonary hypoplasia and hypoplastic skull bones with wide sutures were observed, but no other apparent abnormalities, including the kidneys and urinary tract, were noted. The anhydramnios and resulting fatal fetal abnormalities were attributed to losartan (5).

A 42-year-old woman was treated with losartan (dose not specified), hydrochlorothiazide, felodipine, and metoprolol throughout gestation (6). Oligohydramnios was diagnosed at 33 weeks' gestation. A 2180-g female infant was born at 36 weeks' with limb deformities (varus of left foot, right clubfoot, and fixed external rotation of the right knee). Potter's facies, pulmonary hypertension, and anuria were present and the infant died of respiratory distress on day 4. Autopsy revealed a patent ductus arteriosus and abnormal kidneys (6).

In another case, a 35-year-old woman with hypertension was treated with losartan (50 mg/day) throughout gestation (7). An examination at 22 weeks' was normal, but oligohydramnios was noted at 34 weeks'. Losartan was stopped and an amnioinfusion was given, but the woman developed signs of infection and a hypotonic male infant (weight not given) was delivered. Apgar scores were 1, 4, and 4 at 1, 5, and 10 minutes, respectively. The infant had persistent hypotension, anuria, and multivisceral failure and died on day 4 (7).

In an unusual case, a 45-year-old woman with type 2 diabetes and chronic hypertension developed anhydramnios (amniotic fluid index [AFI] 0) at about 28 weeks' gestation while receiving losartan (8). Losartan was discontinued and 4 days later, a transabdominal amnioinfusion produced an AFI of 6. Normal amniotic fluid levels were maintained for the remainder of the pregnancy. At 32 weeks', ultrasound revealed a thrombus in the fetal vena cava at the level of the right renal vein. Labor was induced at 38 weeks' to deliver 2960-g male infant with Apgar scores of 8 and 9 at 1 and 5 minutes, respectively. Further ultrasound studies revealed an inclusive inferior vena cava thrombus with up to three collateral vessels providing flow around the clot. At 10 days of age, additional examination of the asymptomatic infant revealed a single dominant collateral vessel (8).

A 41-year-old woman with hypertension was treated throughout gestation with losartan (9). At 29 weeks' gestation, anhydramnios was detected. A cesarean section delivered a 1223-g (50th–60th percentile) female infant was delivered with Apgar scores of 2, 5, and 7 at 1, 5, and 10 minutes, respectively. The flaccid newborn had apnea, bradycardia, and was cyanotic. The neonatal course was complicated by marked renal impairment, hypotension, respiratory depression, joint contractures, and a large anterior fontanelle with widely separated sutures. Follow-up at 7 months of age revealed a growth-restricted infant (≤5th percentile) and renal disease, including apparent renal tubular acidosis (9).

A brief teratogen update in 2005 summarized the adverse outcomes of pregnancies exposed to losartan and three other similar agents (10). Exposure in the second half of pregnancy resulted in fetal toxicity that was very similar to that observed with ACE inhibitors. Although the number of reported 1st trimester exposures was limited, there was no suggestion of an increased risk of major congenital defects (10).

A 2009 report described two cases of losartan exposure before and during pregnancy (11). The drug was used to treat hypertension and was stopped at 8 and 23 weeks' gestation, respectively. The pregnancy outcome in the first patient was a healthy, 3.730-kg female infant born at 39 weeks. In the second woman, pregnancy woman was diagnosed at 25 weeks' and losartan was stopped, but oligohydramnios was noted on ultrasound. A repeat ultrasound 1 week later showed worsening oligohydramnios (AFI 1.5). At 27 weeks', she spontaneously gave birth to a 1.040-kg female infant with Apgar scores of 9 and 9. In addition to the complications of prematurity, impaired renal function was noted but spontaneously resolved by day 6 of age. A renal ultrasound on day 9 was normal. The infant was discharged home on day 52, at which time a small umbilical hernia was discovered. A neurological examination revealed slightly increased muscle tone and mild tremor (11).

A 2012 review of the use of ACE inhibitors and ARBs in the 1st trimester concluded that there may be an elevated teratogenic risk, but the risk appeared to be related to other factors (12). The factors, which typically coexist with hypertension in pregnancy, included diabetes, advanced maternal age, and obesity.

BREASTFEEDING SUMMARY

No reports describing the use of losartan during human lactation have been located. Because the molecular weight (about 461) of losartan is low enough, excretion into human breast milk should be expected. The effects of this exposure on a nursing infant are unknown. The American Academy of Pediatrics, however, classifies ACE inhibitors, a closely related group of antihypertensive agents, as compatible with breastfeeding (see Captopril or Enalapril).

References

1. Product information. Cozaar. Merck, 2001.
2. Spence SG, Allen HL, Cukierski MA, Manson JM, Robertson RT, Eydelloth RS. Defining the susceptible period of developmental toxicity for the AT_1-selective angiotensin II receptor antagonist losartan in rats. Teratology 1995;51:367–82.
3. Spence SG, Cukierski MA, Manson JM, Robertson RT, Eydelloth RS. Evaluation of the reproductive and developmental toxicity of the AT_1-selective angiotensin II receptor antagonist losartan in rats. Teratology 1995;51:383–97.
4. Mann RD, Mackay F, Pearce G, Freemantle S, Wilton LV. Losartan: a study of pharmacovigilance data on 14 522 patients. J Hum Hyperten 1999;13: 551–7.
5. Saji H, Yamanaka M, Hagiwara A, Ijiri R. Losartan and fetal toxic effects. Lancet 2001;357:363.
6. Lambot MA, Vermeylen D, Noel JC. Angiotensin-II-receptor inhibitors in pregnancy. Lancet 2001;357:1619–20.
7. Martinovic J, Benachi A, Laurent N, Daikha-Dahmane F, Gubler MC. Fetal toxic effects and angiotensin-II-receptor antagonists. Lancet 2001;358: 241–2.
8. Bakkum JN, Brost BC, Johansen KL, Johnston BW, Watson WJ. In utero losartan withdrawal and subsequent development of fetal inferior vena cava thrombosis. Obstet Gynecol 2006;108:739–40.
9. Bass JK, Faix RG. Gestational therapy with an angiotensin II receptor antagonist and transient renal failure in a premature infant. Am J Perinatol 2006;23:313–8.
10. Alwan S, Polifka JE, Friedman JM. Addendum: sartan treatment during pregnancy. Birth Defects Res A Clin Mol Teratol 2005;73:904–5.
11. Gersak K, Cvijic M, Cerar LK. Angiotensin II receptor blockers in pregnancy: a report of 5 cases. Reprod Toxicol 2009;28:109–12.
12. Polifka JE. Is there an embryopathy associated with first-trimester exposure to angiotensin-converting enzyme inhibitors and angiotensin receptor antagonists? A critical review of the evidence. Birth Defects Res (Part A) 2012;94:576–98.

LOVASTATIN

Antilipemic Agent

PREGNANCY RECOMMENDATION: Contraindicated
BREASTFEEDING RECOMMENDATION: Contraindicated

PREGNANCY SUMMARY

Infants with malformations following in utero exposure to lovastatin have been described in published and unpublished reports. A causal relationship between the drug and some of the defects is possible, but some might have occurred by chance. Additional data are needed. Because there is apparently no maternal benefit for the use of lovastatin during gestation and because of the human cases and the teratogenicity observed in one animal species, the drug should be avoided during pregnancy.

FETAL RISK SUMMARY

Lovastatin, a 3-hydroxy-3-methylglutaryl-coenzyme A (HMG-CoA) reductase inhibitor ("statins") that is lipophilic, is used to lower elevated levels of cholesterol. It has the same mechanism of action as other available drugs in this class, atorvastatin, fluvastatin, pitavastatin, pravastatin, rosuvastatin, and simvastatin (cerivastatin was withdrawn from the market in 2001).

The drug is teratogenic in mice and rats, producing decreased fetal weight and skeletal malformations in exposed fetuses, at doses of 800 mg/kg/day (40 and 80 times the maximum recommended human dose based on BSA [MRHD], respectively) (1,2). However, the skeletal malformations were thought to be due to maternal toxicity that involved gastric lesions and not due to the drug (3). No teratogenic effects were observed in rabbits administered doses ≤15 mg/kg/day (3 times the MRHD), the maximum tolerated dose (1,2).

A surveillance study of lovastatin and simvastatin exposures during pregnancy, conducted by the manufacturer, was reported in 1996 (2) and updated in 2005 (4). Of the 477 reports, all involving 1st trimester exposure, 386 were prospective (67 lovastatin, 319 simvastatin) and 91 were retrospective (38 lovastatin, 53 simvastatin). The pregnancy outcomes were known for 225 (58%) of the prospective reports. There were congenital defects in five liveborn and one stillborn, all involving simvastatin. (See Simvastatin.) Other outcomes were 18 spontaneous abortions (SABs), 49 elective abortions (EABs), 4 fetal deaths, and 148 live births without defects. All of the outcomes, with the exception of fetal deaths, were similar to the population background rate. Although the number of fetal deaths was increased, there was no specific pattern to suggest a common cause. One death involved a nuchal cord and another was a trisomy 18. No congenital defects were reported in the SABs or EABs (4).

There were 13 cases of congenital defects in retrospective reports; 7 involving lovastatin and 6 with simvastatin (4). The details of the congenital defects after exposure to lovastatin (daily dose and exposure in weeks from last menstrual period) were as follows:

(a) atrial and ventricular septal defect, aortic hypoplasia, infant died on day 32 (40 mg, 0–5 weeks)
(b) features of VATER association with other abnormalities, mother also took dextroamphetamine at the same time (10 mg, 6–11 weeks)
(c) spina bifida, EAB (20 mg, 1st trimester)
(d) rudimentary right thumb, skull defects (40 mg, 0–4 weeks)
(e) "severe deformity" (dose and exposure not reported)
(f) open neural tube defect, duplication of spinal cord, cleft palate, EAB (20 mg, 0–18 weeks)
(g) deformed right ear, no auditory canal (microtia) (dose not reported, 0–8 weeks)

The case involving the VATER association is also described below. There was no specific patterns observed in the above reports (4).

In a surveillance study of Michigan Medicaid recipients involving 229,101 completed pregnancies conducted between 1985 and 1992, 3 newborns had been exposed to lovastatin during the 1st trimester (F. Rosa, personal communication, FDA, 1993). One (33.3%) major birth defect was observed (none expected), a cardiovascular defect. Eight other exposures to lovastatin occurred after the 1st trimester without apparent fetal harm (5).

Three retrospective spontaneous reports of birth defects suspected of being associated with 1st trimester use of lovastatin have been received by the FDA (5). The anomalies described were aortic hypoplasia, ventricular septal defect with cerebral dysfunction, death (one case); anal atresia and renal dysplasia (one case); and short forearm, absent thumb, and thoracic scoliosis (one case).

A 1992 case report described the use of lovastatin in a human pregnancy (6). A woman was treated for 5 weeks with lovastatin and dextroamphetamine, starting approximately 6 weeks from her last menstrual period, for progressive weight gain and hypercholesterolemia. Therapy was discontinued when her pregnancy was diagnosed at 11 weeks' gestation. A female infant was delivered by cesarean section at 39 weeks' gestation. Gestational age was confirmed by an ultrasound examination at 21 weeks' gestation and the Dubowitz score at birth. The infant had a constellation of malformations termed the VATER association (vertebral anomalies, anal atresia, tracheoesophageal fistula with esophageal atresia, renal and radial dysplasias). Specific anomalies included an asymmetric chest, thoracic scoliosis, absent left thumb, foreshortened left forearm, left elbow contracture, fusion of the ribs on the left, butterfly vertebrae in the thoracic and lumbar spine, left radial aplasia, and a lower esophageal stricture. Chromosomal analysis was normal, and the family history was noncontributory (6). This case is also described above (see reference 2).

The cause of the defects in the above infant is unknown, but drug-induced teratogenicity cannot be excluded as in utero exposure to both drugs occurred during organogenesis. Experiments with mice and rabbits indicated that amphetamines are teratogenic, but the anomalies primarily involve the heart and CNS (7). Moreover, the use of amphetamines during human pregnancy for medical indications has not been found to present a significant risk to the fetus in terms of fetotoxicity or teratogenicity (see Amphetamines).

A 1995 abstract reported an extensive NTD in a fetus exposed during the 1st trimester to lovastatin (8). A causal relationship could not be established.

A 2004 report evaluated 20 cases of adverse pregnancy outcomes reported to the FDA after exposures to statins (9). The cases were among 178 cases of 1st trimester pregnancy exposure to cholesterol-lowering statin drugs reported to the FDA. There were 52 cases suitable for evaluation after exclusion for spontaneous abortions, elective abortions, pregnancy loss due to maternal diseases, fetal genetic disorders, transient neonatal disorders, or loss to follow-up. In the 52 cases, there were 20 reports of malformation as follows (drug, dose, and exposure time in weeks after last menstrual period shown in parentheses):

CNS

(a) Holoprosencephaly (cerivastatin, 0.25 mg/day, 0–8 weeks)
(b) Holoprosencephaly (see reference 10) (defective septum separating lateral cerebral ventricles), atrial septal defect, aortic hypoplasia, death at 1 month of age (lovastatin, 40 mg/day, 0–7 weeks)
(c) Aqueductal stenosis with hydrocephalus, limb deficiency (right banded, atretic thumb) (lovastatin, 40 mg/day, 0–4.5 weeks)
(d) NTD, myelocele, duplication of spinal cord, cerebellar herniation with hydrocephalus, apparent agenesis of palate (lovastatin, 20 mg/day, 1st trimester)
(e) spina bifida, right arm abnormality (mother also type 1 diabetic) (atorvastatin, unknown dose, until pregnancy recognized)

Limb deficiency

(a) same as c above
(b) right leg fibula and tibia 9% shorter than left side, agenesis of one tarsal bone, right foot 16% shorter than left (reported at 4 years of age) (simvastatin, 20 mg/day, 0–6 weeks)

(c) left leg femur 16% shorter than right, foot with aplasia of metatarsals and phalanges 3, 4, and 5, additional VACTERL defects—left renal dysplasia, reversed laterality of aorta, disorganized lumbosacral vertebrae, single umbilical artery, additional findings—clitoral hypertrophy, vaginal and uterine agenesis (mother also took drug similar to progesterone 10 days/month, 0–13 weeks) (simvastatin, 10 mg/day, 0–13 weeks)

(d) left arm aplasia of radius and thumb, shortened ulna, additional VACTERL defects—left arthrogryposis, thoracic scoliosis, fusion of ribs on left, butterfly vertebrae in thoracic and lumbar region, esophageal stricture, anal atresia, renal dysplasia, additional findings—hemihypertrophy of entire left side, craniofacial anomalies (including asymmetric ears, ptosis of eyelids, high arched palate), torticollis (mother also took dextroamphetamine, 6–11 weeks) (lovastatin, 10 mg/day, 6–11 weeks)

(e) limb reduction deficiency, transverse deficiency of otherwise normal radius and ulna superior to wrist structures, with aplasia of all distal structures (atorvastatin, 10 mg/day, 0–9 weeks) (9)

The other 11 cases of malformations were simvastatin: cleft lip with intrauterine growth restriction; cleft lip; polydactyly; duodenal atresia; hypospadias; clubfoot; and unspecified major abnormalities; atorvastatin: cleft palate; esophageal atresia; lovastatin: microtia with absent auditory canal and severe unspecified deformity (9). All of the 20 defects involved a lipophilic statin (i.e., atorvastatin, cerivastatin, lovastatin, and simvastatin). There were no malformations in the 14 cases of exposure to pravastatin, a hydrophilic agent with low tissue penetration that is not related to reproductive toxicity in animals (see Pravastatin). Because of the voluntary nature of the reports to the FDA, the authors thought that the reports were likely to be biased toward severe outcomes. However, the nature of some of the CNS and limb deficiency malformations (i.e., primarily the cases of holoprosencephaly and VACTERL association) might be consistent with the inhibition of cholesterol biosynthesis (9,10).

In 2005, the authors of the above study reexamined the clinical report of the case listed as holoprosencephaly (CNS, case b) and discovered a coding error (11). The infant had a "ventricular septal defect," not a "defective septum separating lateral cerebral ventricles," thus reducing the number of lovastatin fetuses with midline CNS anomalies from three to two (11).

BREASTFEEDING SUMMARY

No human studies describing the use of lovastatin during lactation have been located. Because there is potential for adverse effects in the infant, the drug should not be used by women who are nursing.

References

1. Product information. Mevacor. Merck, 2000.
2. Manson JM, Freyssinges C, Ducrocq MB, Stephenson WP. Postmarketing surveillance of lovastatin and simvastatin exposure during pregnancy. Reprod Toxicol 1996;10:439–46.
3. Wise LD, Cukierski MA, Lankas GR, Skiles GL. The predominant role of maternal toxicity in lovastatin-induced developmental toxicity (abstract). Teratology 2000;61:444.
4. Pollack PS, Shields KE, Burnett DM, Osborne MJ, Cunningham ML, Stepanavage ME. Pregnancy outcomes after maternal exposure to simvastatin and lovastatin. Birth Defects Res A Clin Mol Teratol 2005;73:888–96.
5. Rosa F. *Anti-cholesterol Agent Pregnancy Exposure Outcomes*. Presented at the 7th International Organization for Teratology Information Services, Woods Hole, MA, April 1994.
6. Ghidini A, Sicherer S, Willner J. Congenital abnormalities (VATER) in baby born to mother using lovastatin. Lancet 1992;339:1416–7.
7. Shepard TH. *Catalog of Teratogenic Agents*. 6th ed. Baltimore, MD: Johns Hopkins University Press, 1989:197–8.
8. Hayes A, Gilbert A, Lopez G, Miller WA. Mevacor—a new teratogen? Am J Hum Genet 1995;57(4 Suppl):A92.
9. Edison RJ, Muenke M. Central nervous system and limb anomalies in case reports of first-trimester statin exposure. N Engl J Med 2004;350:1579–82.
10. Edison RJ, Muenke M. Mechanistic and epidemiologic considerations in the evaluation of adverse birth outcomes following gestational exposure to statins. Am J Med Genetics 2004;131A:287–98.
11. Edison RJ, Muenke M. Gestational exposure to lovastatin followed by cardiac malformation misclassified as holoprosencephaly. N Engl J Med 2005;352:2759.

LOXAPINE

Antipsychotic

PREGNANCY RECOMMENDATION: Limited Human Data—Animal Data Suggest Moderate Risk
BREASTFEEDING RECOMMENDATION: No Human Data—Potential Toxicity

PREGNANCY SUMMARY

There is limited human pregnancy experience with loxapine. Animal reproductive data suggest risk. Because of the very limited human pregnancy experience with atypical antipsychotics, the American College of Obstetricians and Gynecologists does not recommend the routine use of these agents in pregnancy, but a risk–benefit assessment may indicate that such use is appropriate (1). Because loxapine is indicated for severe debilitating mental disease, the benefits to the mother appear to outweigh the unknown risk. A 1996 review on the management of psychiatric illness concluded that patients with histories of chronic psychosis represent a high-risk group (for both the mother and the fetus) and should be maintained on pharmacologic therapy before and during pregnancy (2). Folic acid 4 mg/day has been recommended for women taking atypical antipsychotics because they may have a higher risk of NTDs due to inadequate folate intake and obesity (3). Moreover, neonates exposed to antipsychotic drugs in the 3rd trimester are at risk of extrapyramidal and/or withdrawal symptoms (4).

FETAL RISK SUMMARY

Loxapine is an atypical antipsychotic that is indicated for the treatment of schizophrenia (4). The drug is extensively metabolized to apparently inactive metabolites. The manufacturer did not state the amount of plasma protein binding or the elimination half-life, but did state that loxapine was rapidly removed from the plasma and distributed in tissues (4). Loxapine belongs to the antipsychotic subclass of dibenzapine derivatives that includes asenapine, clozapine, olanzapine, and quetiapine.

In reproductive studies with rats, rabbits, and dogs, no embryotoxicity or teratogenicity was observed. However, with the exception of one rabbit study, the dose used was ≤ 2 times the maximum recommended human dose (*presumably based on* weight) (4,5). Renal papillary abnormalities were found in offspring of rats treated from mid-gestation with doses approximately equivalent to the usual human dose (4).

It is not known if loxapine crosses the human placenta. The molecular weight (about 328 for the free base) suggests that it will cross to the embryo–fetus.

A 2009 review cited information received from the manufacturer regarding the outcomes of three pregnancies exposed to loxapine (6). The retrospective outcomes were one baby with achondroplasia; one with multiple unspecified anomalies; and one infant, exposed throughout pregnancy, with tremors at 15 weeks of age (6). However, achondroplasia is a known autosomal dominant inheritance defect and is not related to drug exposure.

BREASTFEEDING SUMMARY

No reports describing the use of loxapine during human lactation have been located. The relatively low molecular weight of loxapine (about 328 for the free base) suggests that the drug will be excreted into breast milk. The effect of this exposure on a nursing infant is unknown. The American Academy of Pediatrics classifies other antipsychotics (e.g., see Clozapine) as drugs whose effect on the nursing infant is unknown but may be of concern (7). Because of the very limited human experience with atypical antipsychotics, the American College of Obstetricians and Gynecologists does not recommend the routine use of these agents during lactation, but a risk–benefit assessment may indicate that such use is appropriate (1).

References

1. American College of Obstetricians and Gynecologists. Use of psychiatric medications during pregnancy and lactation. *ACOG Practice Bulletin*. No. 92, April 2008. Obstet Gynecol 2008;111:1001–19.
2. Althuler LL, Cohen L, Szuba MP, Burt VK, Gitlin M, Mintz J. Pharmacologic management of psychiatric illness during pregnancy: dilemmas and guidelines. Am J Psychiatry 1996;153:592–606.
3. Koren G, Cohn T, Chitayat D, Kapur B, Remington G, Myles-Reid D, Zipursky RB. Use of atypical antipsychotics during pregnancy and the risk of neural tube defects in infants. Am J Psychiatry 2002;159:136–7.
4. Product information. Loxitane. Watson Laboratories, 2010.
5. Mineshita T, Hasewaga Y, Inoue Y, Kozen T, Yamamoto A. Teratological studies on fetuses and suckling young mice and rats of S-805. Oyo Yakuri 1970;4:305–16. As cited in Shepard TH. *Catalog of Teratogenic Agents*. 6th ed. Baltimore, MD: Johns Hopkins University Press, 1989:378.
6. Einarson A, Boskovic R. Use and safety of antipsychotic drugs during pregnancy. J Psychiatr Pract 2009;15:183–92.
7. Committee on Drugs, American Academy of Pediatrics. The transfer of drugs and other chemicals into human milk. Pediatrics 2001;108:776–89.

LUBIPROSTONE

Gastrointestinal Agent (Laxative)

PREGNANCY RECOMMENDATION: Limited Human Data—Probably Compatible
BREASTFEEDING RECOMMENDATION: No Human Data—Probably Compatible

PREGNANCY SUMMARY

The human pregnancy experience with lubiprostone is limited. In animal reproduction studies, no teratogenicity was observed in two species. In a third species, the drug caused fetal loss, but the cause of the loss is unknown because systemic absorption of lubiprostone, at least in humans, is minimal, although one metabolite is absorbed systemically. The limited human data prevent a complete assessment of the embryo–fetal risk.

FETAL RISK SUMMARY

Lubiprostone, a locally acting chloride channel activator, increases intestinal fluid secretion that results in increased motility of the intestine, thereby increasing the passage of stool and alleviating symptoms associated with constipation (1). It is a prostaglandin E_1 derivative (2). Lubiprostone is indicated for the treatment of chronic idiopathic constipation in adults. It has low systemic bioavailability with plasma concentrations below the level of quantitation (10 pg/mL). Rapid and extensive metabolism occurs in the stomach and jejunum. One of the metabolites, M3, is absorbed into the plasma, but at very low levels (peak plasma concentration about 42 pg/mL). The plasma elimination half-life of M3 ranges from 0.9 to 1.4 hours. In vitro studies indicate that lubiprostone is about 94% bound to human plasma proteins (1).

Reproduction studies have been conducted in rats, rabbits, and guinea pigs. In pregnant rats and rabbits, oral doses up to about 332 and 32 times, respectively, the recommended human dose based on BSA (RHD) revealed no evidence of teratogenicity. In pregnant guinea pigs, repeated doses that were two and six times, respectively, the RHD caused fetal loss (1).

Long-term (2-year) carcinogenicity studies were conducted in mice and rats. Doses up to about 42 times the RHD in mice were not associated with a significant increase in any tumor incidences. In rats at the highest dose tested (about 68 times the RHD), there was a significant increase in the incidence of interstitial cell adenoma of the testes in male rats. Hepatocellular adenomas were observed at the highest dose in female rats. Lubiprostone was not genotoxic in several tests, and had no effect on male and female fertility or on reproductive function at daily doses that were about 166 times the RHD (1).

It is not known if lubiprostone or the metabolite M3 crosses the human placenta. The molecular weight of the parent compound (about 391) is low enough, but plasma levels are below the level of quantitation. M3 has been detected in the plasma at low levels and may cross to the embryo–fetus. However, the very short elimination half-life and presumably high plasma protein binding should limit the amount crossing the placenta.

In clinical trials, four women became pregnant while taking the recommended human dose of 24 mg twice daily. Therapy was stopped when the pregnancies were detected. Three of the women gave birth to healthy infants, but the fourth woman, with an apparent normal pregnancy, was lost to follow-up (1).

The manufacturer recommends that before treatment, women of reproductive age should have a negative pregnancy test and should use effective contraception during treatment (1,3). However, based on the pharmacokinetics of lubiprostone, the embryo–fetal risk from inadvertent exposure during pregnancy appears to be low.

BREASTFEEDING SUMMARY

No reports describing the use of lubiprostone during human lactation have been located.

It is not known if lubiprostone or the metabolite M3 is excreted into human breast milk. The molecular weight of the parent compound (about 391) is low enough, but plasma levels are below the level of quantitation. M3 has been detected in the plasma at low levels and may be excreted into milk. However, the very short elimination half-life (0.9–1.4 hours) and presumably high plasma protein binding (parent drug 94%) should limit the amount excreted. Although the risk to a nursing infant probably is very low, if it exists at all, nursing women taking lubiprostone should monitor their infants for adverse effects commonly observed in adults (e.g., headache, nausea, and diarrhea).

References

1. Product information. Amitiza. Takeda Pharmaceuticals America, 2007.
2. Ginzburg R, Ambizas EM. Clinical pharmacology of lubiprostone, a chloride channel activator in defecation disorders. Expert Opin Drug Metab Toxicol 2008;4:1091–7.
3. Anonymous. Lubiprostone (Amitiza) for chronic constipation. Med Lett Drugs Ther 2006;48:428. As cited in Obstet Gynecol 2006;108:1026–7.

LURASIDONE

Antipsychotic

PREGNANCY RECOMMENDATION: No Human Data—Potential Risk in the 3rd Trimester
BREASTFEEDING RECOMMENDATION: No Human Data—Potential Toxicity

PREGNANCY SUMMARY

No reports describing the use of lurasidone in human pregnancy have been located. The animal data suggest low risk in early pregnancy, but the absence of human pregnancy experience prevents further assessment of the embryo–fetal risk. The use of other atypical antipsychotics during the 3rd trimester has been associated with a risk of abnormal muscle movements (extrapyramidal symptoms) and withdrawal symptoms in newborns. Symptoms may be self-limiting and include agitation, feeding disorder, hypertonia, hypotonia, respiratory distress, somnolence, and tremor (1,2).

FETAL RISK SUMMARY

Lurasidone is an atypical antipsychotic indicated for the treatment of schizophrenia. The drug is in the benzoisothiazol subclass of antipsychotics. There are no other approved drugs in this class. The activity of the agent is primarily due to the parent drug, but it is metabolized to two active metabolites. Lurasidone is highly bound (about 99%) to plasma proteins. The mean elimination half-life is 18 hours (1).

Reproduction studies have been conducted in rats and rabbits. When these species were given lurasidone during organogenesis, no evidence of teratogenicity was observed at doses up to 3 and 12 times, respectively, the maximum recommended human dose of 80 mg/day based on BSA (MRHD). There was no evidence of adverse developmental effects in rats given doses up to approximately equal to the MRHD during organogenesis and continued through weaning (1).

In carcinogenicity studies, significant increases in the incidences of malignant mammary gland tumors and pituitary gland adenomas were observed in female mice. Similar increases in mammary gland carcinomas were seen in female rats. No increases in these tumors were observed in male mice or rats. These neoplastic changes are considered to be prolactin mediated with chronic administration of atypical antipsychotics. It is not known whether this increased risk of the tumors is relevant to human risk. Lurasidone was not genotoxic in multiple assays. Estrous cycle irregularities were seen in female rats and fertility was reduced but reversible. Fertility was not affected in male rats (1).

It is not known if lurasidone or its active metabolites cross the human placenta. The molecular weight of the parent drug (about 493 for the free base) and the elimination half-life suggest that the drug will cross to the embryo–fetus. However, the very high plasma protein binding may limit the exposure.

BREASTFEEDING SUMMARY

No reports describing the use of lurasidone during human lactation have been located. The molecular weight of the parent drug (about 493 for the free base) and the elimination half-life (18 hours) suggest that the drug will be excreted into human milk, although the very high plasma protein binding (about 99%) might limit excretion. However, lurasidone is a weak base, and when used during lactation, accumulation in the milk may occur with concentrations significantly greater than corresponding plasma levels. The American Academy of Pediatrics classifies other antipsychotics as agents whose effect on the nursing infant is unknown but may be of concern (3). Lurasidone should be classified the same way.

References

1. Product information. Latuda. Sunovion, 2011.
2. Koren G, Cohn T, Chitayat D, Kapur B, Remington G, Myles-Reid D, Zipursky RB. Use of atypical antipsychotics during pregnancy and the risk of neural tube defects in infants. Am J Psychiatry 2002;159:136–7.
3. Committee on Drugs, American Academy of Pediatrics. The transfer of drugs and other chemicals into human milk. Pediatrics 2001;108:776–89.

L

LYNESTRENOL

[Withdrawn from the market. See 9th edition.]

LYPRESSIN

[Withdrawn from the market. See 9th edition.]

LYSERGIC ACID DIETHYLAMIDE

Hallucinogen

PREGNANCY RECOMMENDATION: Contraindicated
BREASTFEEDING RECOMMENDATION: Contraindicated

PREGNANCY SUMMARY

The available data suggest that pure lysergic acid diethylamide (LSD) does not cause chromosomal abnormalities, spontaneous abortions, or congenital malformations. There have been no cases published of fetal anomalies when only pure LSD was administered under medical supervision. Early descriptions of congenital abnormalities involved patients who had used or were using illicit LSD and are believed to be examples of reporting bias, the effects of multiple drugs, or other nondrug factors. However, long-term follow-up of exposed infants has never been reported. This is an area that warrants additional research.

FETAL RISK SUMMARY

LSD (lysergide) is a chemical used for its hallucinogenic properties. The drug does not have a legal indication in the United States. Illicitly obtained LSD is commonly adulterated with a variety of other chemicals (e.g., amphetamines) (1,2). In some cases, doses sold illicitly as LSD may contain little or none of the chemical; as a result, the actual amount of LSD ingested cannot be determined (1). In addition, persons consuming the hallucinogen often consume multiple abuse drugs simultaneously, such as marijuana, opiates, alcohol, amphetamines, STP (2,5-dimethoxy-4-methylamphetamine, or DOM, a synthetic hallucinogen), barbiturates, cocaine, and other prescription and nonprescription substances. Further complicating the situation are the lifestyles that some of these persons live, which are often not conducive to good fetal health. As a consequence, the effects of pure LSD on the human fetus can only be evaluated by examining those cases in which the chemical was administered under strict medical supervision. These cases, however, are few in number. Most data are composed of sample populations who ingested the chemical in an unsupervised environment. Correct interpretation of this latter material is extremely difficult and, although cited in this monograph, must be viewed cautiously.

The passage of LSD across the human placenta has not been studied. The molecular weight of the chemical (about 323) is low enough that passage to the fetus should be expected. LSD has been shown to cross the placenta in mice with early 1st trimester fetal levels averaging five times the levels measured in late gestation (3).

Concerns with fetal exposure to LSD have primarily focused on chromosomal damage (both chromatid-type and chromosome-type abnormalities), an increased risk of spontaneous abortions, and congenital malformations. These topics are discussed in the sections below.

A 1967 report was the first to claim that the use of LSD could cause chromosomal abnormalities in human leukocytes (4). Because these abnormalities could potentially result in carcinogenic, mutagenic, and teratogenic effects in current or future generations, at least 25 studies were published in the next 7 years. These studies were the subject of three reviews published in the 1970s with all three arriving at similar conclusions (2,5,6). First, in the majority of studies, the addition of LSD to cells in vitro caused chromosomal breakage, but a dose–response relationship was not always apparent. The clinical relevance of the in vitro studies was questionable because pure LSD was used, usually with much higher levels than could be achieved in humans, and the in vitro systems lacked the normal protective mechanisms of metabolism and excretion that are present in the body. Second, only a slight transitory increase in chromosomal breaks was seen in a small percentage (14%) of the subjects administered pure LSD. A much higher percentage of persons (49%) consuming illicit LSD was observed to have chromosomal damage. The abnormalities in this latter group were probably related to the effects of multiple drug abuse and not to LSD alone. Four prospective studies found no definitive evidence that LSD damages lymphocyte chromosomes in vitro (2). Third, there was no evidence that the chromosomal defects observed in illicit LSD users were expressed as an increased incidence of leukemias or other neoplasia. Fourth, mutagenic changes were only observed in experimental organisms (e.g., Drosophila) when massive doses (2000–10,000 mcg/mL) were used. Because of this, LSD was believed to be a weak mutagen, but mutagenicity was thought to be unlikely after exposure to any concentration used by humans (5). Finally, the reviewers found no compelling evidence for a teratogenic effect of LSD, either in animals or in humans.

A 1974 investigation involving 50 psychiatric patients, who had been treated for varying intervals under controlled conditions with pure LSD, provided further confirmation that the chemical does not cause chromosomal damage (7). Chromosomal analyses of these patients were compared with those of 50 nonexposed controls matched for age, sex, and marital status. The analysis was blinded so that the investigators did not know the origin of the samples. No significant difference between the groups in chromosomal abnormalities was observed. In another 1974 reference (not included in the previously cited reviews), involving only two subjects, no evidence of chromosomal damage was found in their normal offspring (8). The two women had been treated medically with pure LSD before pregnancy. Thus, the predominance of evidence indicates that LSD does not induce chromosomal aberrations, and even if it did, it has no clinical significance to the fetus.

The question of whether fetal wastage could be induced by LSD exposure was investigated in a study published in 1970 (9). This investigation involved 148 pregnancies (81 patients) in which either the father (*N* = 60) or the mother (*N* = 21) had ingested LSD. In 12 pregnancies, exposure occurred both before and during pregnancy. In the 136 pregnancies in which the exposure occurred only before conception, 118 involved the administration of pure LSD (the medical group) and 18 involved both medical and illicit LSD exposure (the combined group). The spontaneous abortion rates for these two populations were 14% (17 of 118) and 28% (5 of 18), respectively. In 83 of the pregnancies, only the father had been exposed to LSD. Excluding these, the incidences of fetal loss for the medical and combined groups are 26% (11 of 43) and 40% (4 of 10), respectively. In the 12 pregnancies in which LSD was consumed both before and during gestation, 3 were in the medical group and 9 were in the combined group. The frequency of spontaneous abortions in these cases was 33% (1 of 3) and 56% (5 of 9). In the combined sample, however, one woman accounted for five abortions and one liveborn infant. If she is excluded, the incidence of fetal wastage in the combined group is zero.

In the medical group, the number of women (12 of 46; 26%) with fetal wastage was high. However, 25 of these pregnancies occurred in women undergoing psychotherapy, and 21 occurred in an experimental setting (9). The number of spontaneous abortions in the psychotherapy group (*N* = 9, 36%) was more than twice the incidence in the experimental sample (*N* = 3, 14%). The authors speculated that the greater frequency of fetal wastage in the women undergoing psychotherapy may have been caused by the greater emotional stress that often accompanies such therapy. The increased

L

rate in the combined sample (9 of 19; 47%) was probably caused by the use of multiple abuse drugs, other nondrug factors, and the inclusion of one woman with five abortions and one live birth. Exclusion of this latter patient decreases the combined sample incidence to 31% (4 of 13). Thus, although other studies examining the incidence of spontaneous abortions in LSD-exposed women have not been located, it appears unlikely that pure LSD administered in a controlled condition is an abortifacient. The increased rate of fetal wastage that was observed in the 1970 study was probably caused by a combination of factors, rather than only to the ingestion of LSD.

A number of case reports have described LSD use in pregnancies ending with poor outcomes since the first report in 1967 of an exposed infant with major malformations (10–25). All of these reports, however, are biased in the respect that malformed infants exposed in utero to LSD are much more likely to be reported than exposed normal infants and are also more frequently reported than nonexposed malformed infants (2). Most of the reports either involved multiple drug exposures, including abuse drugs, or other drug exposures could probably be deduced because of the illicit nature of LSD. With these cautions, the reports are briefly described below.

The first mention of an anomaly observed in an infant exposed in utero to LSD appeared in a 1967 editorial (10). The editorial, citing a report in a lay publication, briefly described a case of LSD exposure in a pregnancy that ended in a malformed infant with megacolon. Apparently, details of this case have never been published in the medical literature.

The first case report in the medical literature also appeared in 1967 and involved a female infant with unilateral fibular aplastic syndrome (11,12). The mother had taken LSD four times between the 25th and 98th days of gestation with one dose occurring during the time of most active lower limb differentiation (11). Defects in the infant, which were characteristic of the syndrome, included absence of the fibula and lateral rays of the foot, anterior bowing of the shortened tibia, shortening of the femur, and dislocated hip. A second case involving limb defects and LSD exposure was published in 1968 (13). The infant, with a right terminal transverse acheiria defect (absence of the hand), was the offspring of a woman who had taken LSD both before and during early gestation. She had also smoked marijuana throughout the pregnancy and had taken a combination product containing dicyclomine, doxylamine, and pyridoxine for 1st trimester nausea. Another infant with a terminal transverse deficit, also exposed to LSD and marijuana, was described in 1969 (14). The defect involved portions of the fingers on the left hand, syndactyly of the right hand with shortened fingers, and talipes equinovarus of the left foot. Two of these same authors described another exposed infant with amputation deformities of the third finger of the right hand and the third toe of the left foot (15). A critique of these latter three case histories concluded that the defects in the infants could have been caused by amniotic band syndrome (26). Limb defects and intrauterine growth restriction were observed in an offspring of a malnourished mother who had used LSD, marijuana, methadone, and cigarettes during gestation (16). The anomalies consisted of partial adactyly of the hands and feet, syndactyly of the remaining fingers, and defective formation of the legs and forearms.

In a study of 140 women using LSD and marijuana followed up through 148 pregnancies, 8 of 83 liveborn infants had major defects as did 4 of 14 embryos examined after induced abortion (17). The incidence of defects in this sample was 8.1% (12/148) and may have been higher if the other abortuses had been examined. Only one of the liveborn infants had a limb defect (absence of both feet) combined with spina bifida occulta and hemangiomas. Defects in the other seven infants were as follows: myelomeningocele with hydrocephalus in three (one with clubfoot); tetralogy of Fallot; hydrocephalus; right kidney neuroblastoma; and hydrocephalus and congestive heart failure. A limb defect was one of several anomalies found in a male infant whose mother ingested LSD both before and during gestation (18). The abnormalities included absent left arm, syndactyly, anencephaly with ectopic placenta, cleft lip and palate, coloboma of the iris, cataract, and corneal opacity with vascularization. At least one author thought that the limb and cranial defects in this latter case may have been caused by amniotic band syndrome (27). This opinion was contested by the original authors, who stated that the limb defects were true aplasia and not an amputation deformity (28). Similarly, they claimed that the cranial anomaly was not a form of encephalocele, which an amniotic band could have caused, but a true anencephaly (28). Congenital anomalies were observed in 11 of 120 liveborn infants in a previously cited study that examined the effects of LSD on spontaneous abortions and other pregnancy outcomes (9). Nine of the 11 infants had limb defects that were, in most cases, easily correctable with either special shoes or casts. None of the 11 cases appear to be related to LSD exposure. The defects were (the number of cases and possible causes are shown in parentheses): turned-in feet (6 cases, 4 familial, 2 unknown); "crimped" ureter (1 case, familial); tibial rotation (2 cases, 2 familial); pyloric stenosis (1 case, possibly genetic); bone deformity of legs and deafness (1 case, postrubella syndrome) (9).

Other infants with ocular defects, in addition to the case mentioned immediately above, have been described. A mother who ingested LSD, marijuana, meprobamate, amphetamines, and hydrochlorothiazide throughout pregnancy delivered an infant with generalized hypotonia, a high-pitched cry, brachycephaly with widely separated sutures, bilateral cephalohematomas, a right eye smaller than the left and with a cataract, and overlapping second and third toes (19). Two other cases of ocular defects were published in 1978 and 1980 (20,21). In one case, a premature female infant was delivered from a 16-year-old mother who had consumed LSD, cocaine, and heroin during the 1st trimester (20). The infant, who died 1 hour after birth, had microphthalmos, intraocular cartilage, cataract, persistent hyperplastic primary vitreous, and retinal dysplasia. A hypoplastic left lung and a defect in the diaphragm were also noted. The second case involved another premature female infant born to a mother enrolled in a methadone program who also used LSD (21). The infant had left anophthalmia but no other defects.

Various other malformations have been reported after in utero LSD exposure (22–25). Complete exstrophy of the bladder, epispadias, widely separated pubic rami, and bilateral inguinal hernias were observed in a newborn exposed to LSD, marijuana, and mephentermine (22). The mother had consumed LSD 12–15 times during an interval extending from 2 months before conception to 2.5 months into pregnancy. A mother, who ingested LSD at the time of conception, produced a female infant with multiple defects, including a short neck, left hemithorax smaller than the right, protuberant abdomen because of a severe thoracolumbar lordosis, a thoracolumbar rachischisis, craniolacunia, long fingers, clubfeet, and defects of the urinary tract and brain (23). The infant died at 41 days of age. Other drug exposures consisted of cigarettes, an estrogen preparation (type not specified) that was used unsuccessfully to induce menstruation, and medroxyprogesterone for 1st trimester bleeding. Because the case resembled a previously described cluster of unusual defects (i.e., spondylothoracic dysplasia and Jarcho–Levin syndrome), which is caused by an autosomal recessive mode of inheritance, the authors could not exclude this mechanism. In a case of a female infant with multiple anomalies compatible with trisomy 13 with D/D translocation, the mother had last used LSD 9 months before conception (24). She had also used marijuana, barbiturates, and amphetamines throughout gestation and, presumably, before conception. The authors theorized that the defect may have been caused by LSD-induced damage to maternal germ cells before fertilization. A 1971 study evaluated 47 infants born to parents who had used LSD (25). Maternal use of the drug could be documented in only 30 of the cases and multiple other abuse drugs were consumed. Abnormalities observed in 8 (17%) of the infants were transient hearing loss and ventricular septal defect, cortical blindness, tracheoesophageal fistula, congenital heart disease (type not specified), congenital neuroblastoma, spastic diplegia, and seizure disorders in 2 infants.

Two other case reports involving the combined use of LSD and marijuana with resulting adverse fetal outcomes do not appear to have any relationship to either drug (29,30). One of these involved a report of six infants with persistent ductus arteriosus, one of whom was exposed to LSD and marijuana during early gestation (29). The history of maternal drug use was coincidental. The second case described an infant who died at 2.5 months of age of a bilateral in utero cerebral vascular accident and resulting porencephaly (30). The mother had used LSD, marijuana, alcohol, and other abuse drugs, including cocaine. This latter drug was thought to be the causative agent.

In contrast to the above reports, a large body of research has been published describing the maternal (and paternal) ingestion of LSD without apparent fetal consequences (1,7–9,31–36). A number of reviews have also examined the teratogenic potential of the chemical and have concluded that a causal relationship between congenital malformations and LSD does not exist (2,5,6,37–45). (See reference 6 for an excellent critique of the early investigations in laboratory animals.)

BREASTFEEDING SUMMARY

No reports have been located concerning the passage of lysergic acid diethylamide into breast milk. Because the drug has a relatively low molecular weight (about 323), which should allow its transfer into milk, and because its psychotomimetic effects are produced at extremely low concentrations, the use of LSD during lactation is contraindicated.

References

1. Warren RJ, Rimoin DL, Sly WS. LSD exposure in utero. Pediatrics 1970;45:466–9.
2. Matsuyama SS, Jarvik LF. Cytogenetic effects of psychoactive drugs. Mod Probl Pharmacopsychiatry 1975;10:99–132.
3. Idanpaan-Heikkila JE, Schoolar JC. LSD: autoradiographic study on the placental transfer and tissue distribution in mice. Science 1969;164:1295–7.
4. Cohen MM, Marinello MJ, Back N. Chromosomal damage in human leukocytes induced by lysergic acid diethylamide. Science 1967;155:1417–9.
5. Dishotsky NI, Loughman WD, Mogar RE, Lipscomb WR. LSD and genetic damage: is LSD chromosome damaging, carcinogenic, mutagenic, or teratogenic? Science 1971;172:431–40.
6. Long SY. Does LSD induce chromosomal damage and malformations? A review of the literature. Teratology 1972;6:75–90.
7. Robinson JT, Chitham RG, Greenwood RM, Taylor JW. Chromosome aberrations and LSD: a controlled study in 50 psychiatric patients. Br J Psychiatry 1974;125:238–44.
8. Fernandez J, Brennan T, Masterson J, Power M. Cytogenetic studies in the offspring of LSD users. Br J Psychiatry 1974;124:296–8.
9. McGlothlin WH, Sparkes RS, Arnold DO. Effect of LSD on human pregnancy. JAMA 1970;212:1483–7.
10. Anonymous. Hallucinogen and teratogen? Lancet 1967;2:504–5.
11. Zellweger H, McDonald JS, Abbo G. Is lysergic-acid diethylamide a teratogen? Lancet 1967;2:1066–8.
12. Zellweger H, McDonald JS, Abbo G. Is lysergide a teratogen? Lancet 1967;2:1306.
13. Hecht F, Beals RK, Lees MH, Jolly H, Roberts P. Lysergic-acid-diethylamide and cannabis as possible teratogens in man. Lancet 1968;2:1087.
14. Carakushansky G, Neu RL, Gardner LI. Lysergide and cannabis as possible teratogens in man. Lancet 1969;1:150–1.
15. Assemany SR, Neu RL, Gardner LI. Deformities in a child whose mother took L.S.D. Lancet 1970;1:1290.
16. Jeanbart P, Berard MJ. A propos d'un cas personnel de malformations congenitales possiblement dues au LSD-25: revue de la litterature. Union Med Can 1971;100:919–29.
17. Jacobson CB, Berlin CM. Possible reproductive detriment in LSD users. JAMA 1972;222:1367–73.
18. Apple DJ, Bennett TO. Multiple systemic and ocular malformations associated with maternal LSD usage. Arch Ophthalmol 1974;92:301–3.
19. Bogdanoff B, Rorke LB, Yanoff M, Warren WS. Brain and eye abnormalities: possible sequelae to prenatal use of multiple drugs including LSD. Am J Dis Child 1972;123:145–8.
20. Chan CC, Fishman M, Egbert PR. Multiple ocular anomalies associated with maternal LSD ingestion. Arch Ophthalmol 1978;96:282–4.
21. Margolis S, Martin L. Anophthalmia in an infant of parents using LSD. Ann Ophthalmol 1980;12:1378–81.

L

22. Gelehrter TD. Lysergic acid diethylamide (LSD) and exstrophy of the bladder. J Pediatr 1970;77:1065–6.
23. Eller JL, Morton JM. Bizarre deformities in offspring of user of lysergic acid diethylamide. N Engl J Med 1970;283:395–7.
24. Hsu LY, Strauss L, Hirschhorn K. Chromosome abnormality in offspring of LSD user: D trisomy with D/D translocation. JAMA 1970;211:987–90.
25. Dumars KW Jr. Parental drug usage: effect upon chromosomes of progeny. Pediatrics 1971;47:1037–41.
26. Blanc WA, Mattison DR, Kane R, Chauhan P. L.S.D., intrauterine amputations, and amniotic-band syndrome. Lancet 1971;2:158–9.
27. Holmes LB. Ocular malformations associated with maternal LSD usage. Arch Ophthalmol 1975;93:1061.
28. Apple DJ. Ocular malformations associated with maternal LSD usage. Reply. Arch Ophthalmol 1975;93:1061.
29. Brown R, Pickering D. Persistent transitional circulation. Arch Dis Child 1974;49:883–5.
30. Tenorio GM, Nazvi M, Bickers GH, Hubbird RH. Intrauterine stroke and maternal polydrug abuse. Clin Pediatr 1988;27:565–7.
31. Cohen MM, Hirschhorn K, Frosch WA. In vivo and in vitro chromosomal damage induced by LSD-25. N Engl J Med 1967;277:1043–9.
32. Sato H, Pergament E. Is lysergide a teratogen? Lancet 1968;1:639–40.
33. Egozcue J, Irwin S, Maruffo CA. Chromosomal damage in LSD users. JAMA 1968;204:214–8.
34. Cohen MM, Hirschhorn K, Verbo S, Frosch WA, Groeschel MM. The effect of LSD-25 on the chromosomes of children exposed in utero. Pediatr Res 1968;2:486–92.
35. Hulten M, Lindsten J, Lidberg L, Ekelund H. Studies on mitotic and meiotic chromosomes in subjects exposed to LSD. Ann Genet (Paris) 1968;11:201–10.
36. Aase JM, Laestadius N, Smith DW. Children of mothers who took L.S.D. in pregnancy. Lancet 1970;2:100–1.
37. Hoffer A. Effect of LSD on chromosomes. Can Med Assoc J 1968;98:466.
38. Smart RG, Bateman K. The chromosomal and teratogenic effects of lysergic acid diethylamide: a review of the current literature. Can Med Assoc J 1968;99:805–10.
39. Rennert OM. Drug-induced somatic alterations. Clin Obstet Gynecol 1975;18:185–98.
40. Glass L, Evans HE. Perinatal drug abuse. Pediatr Ann 1979;8:84–92.
41. VanBlerk GA, Majerus TC, Myers RAM. Teratogenic potential of some psychopharmacologic drugs: a brief review. Int J Gynaecol Obstet 1980;17:399–402.
42. Chernoff GF, Jones KL. Fetal preventive medicine: teratogens and the unborn baby. Pediatr Ann 1981;10:210–7.
43. Stern L. In vivo assessment of the teratogenic potential of drugs in humans. Obstet Gynecol 1981;58:3S–8S.
44. Lee CC, Chiang CN. Maternal–fetal transfer of abused substances: pharmacokinetic and pharmacodynamic data. Natl Inst Drug Abuse Res Monogr Ser 1985;60:110–47.
45. McLane NJ, Carroll DM. Ocular manifestations of drug abuse. Surv Ophthalmol 1986;30:298–313.

L

L-LYSINE

Nutrient (Amino Acid)

PREGNANCY RECOMMENDATION: No Human Data—Probably Compatible
BREASTFEEDING RECOMMENDATION: No Human Data—Probably Compatible

PREGNANCY SUMMARY

L-Lysine is an essential amino acid that has been occasionally used for the treatment and prophylaxis of herpes simplex infections (the effectiveness of this indication is questionable). No reports on the use of the commercial formulation in human pregnancy have been located.

FETAL RISK SUMMARY

L-Lysine is actively transported across the human placenta to the fetus with a steady-state fetal:maternal ratio of approximately 1.6:1 (1,2). Fetal tissues retain most of the essential amino acids, including *l*-lysine, in preference to the nonessential amino acids (3).

One published case has been located that described a woman with familial hyperlysinemia because of deficiency of the enzymes lysine ketoglutarate reductase and saccharopine dehydrogenase (4). The woman gave birth to a normal child. No details of the pregnancy or the child were provided other than that the child was normal. Serum lysine levels, which were regularly >10 mg/dL and may have been as high as 20 mg/dL or more when the disorder was detected, were not measured during the pregnancy or in the baby.

BREASTFEEDING SUMMARY

No reports describing the use of *l*-lysine during human lactation have been located.

References

1. Schneider H, Mohlen KH, Dancis J. Transfer of amino acids across the in vitro perfused human placenta. Pediatr Res 1979;13:236–40.
2. Schneider H, Mohlen KH, Challier JC, Dancis J. Transfer of glutamic acid across the human placenta perfused in vitro. Br J Obstet Gynaecol 1979;86:299–306.
3. Velazquez A, Rosado A, Bernal A, Noriega L, Arevalo N. Amino acid pools in the feto-maternal system. Biol Neonate 1976;29:28–40.
4. Dancis J, Hutzler J, Ampola MG, Shih VE, van Gelderen HH, Kirby LT, Woody NC. The prognosis of hyperlysinemia: an interim report. Am J Hum Genet 1983;35:438–42.

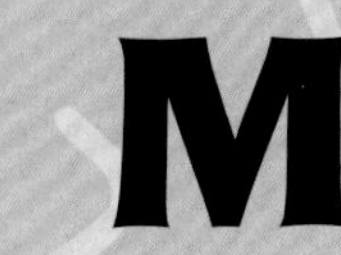

M

MAFENIDE

Anti-infective

PREGNANCY RECOMMENDATION: No Human Data—Probably Compatible
BREASTFEEDING RECOMMENDATION: No Human Data—Potential Toxicity

PREGNANCY SUMMARY

No reports describing the use of mafenide during human pregnancy have been located. The cream formulation is absorbed into the systemic circulation and exposure of the embryo–fetus probably occurs. The anti-infective did not cause fetal toxicity in the only animal species tested. Although the mechanism of action is different from the sulfonamides, it is closely related to that class of agents (see also Sulfonamides). Because of its indication for severe burns, it should not be withheld because of pregnancy.

FETAL RISK SUMMARY

Mafenide is an anti-infective available as a topical 11.2% cream or 5% solution. The cream is indicated for adjunctive therapy of patients with second- and third-degree burns. The solution is indicated for use as an adjunctive topical antimicrobial agent to control bacterial infection when used under moist dressings over meshed autografts on excised burn wounds. The mechanism of action of mafenide is not known but is different from the sulfonamides. In addition, it is not known if there is cross-sensitivity to other sulfonamides. (See also Sulfonamides.) The cream formulation is absorbed into the systemic circulation where the agent is converted to an inactive metabolite. Peak blood concentrations ranged from 26 to 197 mcg/mL 2 hours after application (1,2).

A reproduction study has been conducted in rats. In pregnant rats given oral doses of mafenide up to 600 mg/kg/day, no evidence of fetal harm was observed. No animal studies evaluating the potential for carcinogenicity or for effects on fertility have been conducted. However, the drug was not mutagenic in one assay (1).

It is not known if mafenide crosses the human placenta. The molecular weight of the free base (about 186) is low enough that passage to the embryo–fetus should be expected.

BREASTFEEDING SUMMARY

No reports describing the use of mafenide during human lactation have been located. The molecular weight of the free base (about 186) is low enough that excretion into breast milk should be expected. Although the mechanism of action is different from the sulfonamides, it is closely related to that class of agents (see also Sulfonamides). Mafenide and its metabolite inhibit carbonic anhydrase, which has caused metabolic acidosis in patients treated with the drug. Hemolytic anemia, presumably related to glucose-6-phosphate dehydrogenase deficiency, has also been reported during treatment. Because the indications for this agent suggest long-term exposure from milk that could increase the possibility of toxicity, nursing is best avoided if the mother requires treatment.

References

1. Product information. Sulfamylon. Mylan Pharmaceuticals, 2008.
2. Product information. Sulfamylon Cream. Mylan Pharmaceuticals, 2007.

MAGNESIUM SULFATE

Anticonvulsant/Laxative

PREGNANCY RECOMMENDATION: Compatible
BREASTFEEDING RECOMMENDATION: Compatible

PREGNANCY SUMMARY

The administration of magnesium sulfate to the mother for anticonvulsant or tocolytic effects does not usually pose a risk to the fetus or newborn. Long-term infusions of magnesium may be associated with sustained hypocalcemia in the fetus resulting in congenital rickets. Neonatal neurologic depression may occur with respiratory depression, muscle weakness, and loss of reflexes. The toxicity is not usually correlated with cord serum magnesium levels. Offspring of mothers treated with this drug close to delivery should be closely observed for signs of toxicity during the first 24–48 hours after birth. Caution is also advocated with the use of aminoglycoside antibiotics during this period.

FETAL RISK SUMMARY

Magnesium sulfate ($MgSO_4$) is commonly used as an anticonvulsant for toxemia and as a tocolytic agent for premature labor during the last half of pregnancy. Concentrations of magnesium, a natural constituent of human serum, are readily increased in both the mother and fetus following maternal therapy with cord serum levels ranging from 70% to 100% of maternal concentrations (1–6). Elevated levels in the newborn may persist for up to 7 days with an elimination half-life of 43.2 hours (2). The elimination rate is the same in premature and full-term infants (2). IV magnesium sulfate did not cause lower Apgar scores in a study of women treated for pregnancy-induced hypertension, although the magnesium levels in the newborns reflected hypermagnesemia (6). The mean cord magnesium level, 5.3 mEq/dL, was equal to the mean maternal serum level.

No reports linking the use of magnesium sulfate with congenital defects have been located. The Collaborative Perinatal Project monitored 50,282 mother–child pairs, 141 of which had exposure to magnesium sulfate during pregnancy (7). No evidence was found to suggest a relationship to congenital malformations.

In a 1987 report, 17 women, who had been successfully treated with IV magnesium sulfate for preterm labor, were given 1 g of magnesium gluconate every 4 hours after the IV magnesium had been discontinued (8). A mean serum magnesium level before any therapy was 1.44 mg/dL. Two hours after an oral dose (12–24 hours after discontinuation of IV magnesium) the mean magnesium serum level was 2.16 mg/dL, a significant increase ($p < 0.05$). A group of 568 women was randomly assigned to receive either 15 mmol of magnesium-aspartate hydrochloride ($N = 278$) or 13.5 mmol of aspartic acid ($N = 290$) per day (9). Therapy was started as early as possible in the pregnancies, but not later than 16 weeks' gestation. Women receiving the magnesium tablets had fewer hospitalizations ($p < 0.05$), fewer preterm deliveries, and less frequent referral of the newborn to the neonatal intensive care unit ($p < 0.01$) (9). In a double-blind randomized, controlled clinical study, 374 young women (mean age approximately 18 years) were treated with either 365 mg of elemental magnesium/day (provided by six tablets of magnesium-aspartate hydrochloride each containing 60.8 mg of elemental magnesium) ($N = 185$) or placebo tablets containing aspartic acid only ($N = 189$) (10). Treatment began at approximately a mean gestational age of 18 weeks (range 13–24 weeks). In addition, both groups received prenatal vitamins containing 100 mg of elemental magnesium. In contrast to the reference cited above, the magnesium therapy did not improve the outcome of the pregnancies as judged by the nonsignificant differences between the groups in incidences of preeclampsia, fetal growth restriction, preterm labor, birth weight, gestational age at delivery, or number of infants admitted to the special care unit (10).

Most studies have been unable to find a correlation between cord serum magnesium levels and newborn condition (2,5,11–15). In a study of 7000 offspring of mothers treated with $MgSO_4$ for toxemia, no adverse effects from the therapy were noted in fetuses or newborns (5). Other studies have also observed a lack of toxicity (16,17). A 1983 investigation of women at term with pregnancy-induced hypertension compared newborns of magnesium-treated mothers with newborns of untreated mothers (15). No differences in neurologic behavior were observed between the two groups except that exposed infants had decreased active tone of the neck extensors on the first day after birth.

Newborn depression and hypotonia have been reported as effects of maternal magnesium therapy in some series, but intrauterine hypoxia could not always be eliminated as a potential cause or contributing factor (2,11,12,18–20). In a study reporting on the effects of IV magnesium on Apgar scores, the most common negative score was assigned for color, rather than for muscle tone (6).

A 1971 report described two infants with magnesium levels >8 mg/dL who were severely depressed at birth (13). Spontaneous remission of toxic symptoms occurred after 12 hours in one infant, but the second had residual effects of anoxic encephalopathy. In a 1982 study, activities requiring sustained muscle contraction, such as head lag, ventral suspension, suck reflex, and cry response, were impaired up to 48 hours after birth in infants exposed in utero to magnesium (14). A hypertensive woman, treated with 11 g of magnesium sulfate within 3.5 hours of delivery, gave birth to a depressed infant without spontaneous respirations, movement, or reflexes (21). An exchange transfusion at 24 hours reversed the condition. In another study, decreased gastrointestinal motility, ileus, hypotonia, and patent ductus arteriosus occurring in the offspring of mothers with severe hypertension were thought to be caused by maternal drug therapy, including magnesium sulfate (22). However, the authors could not relate their findings to any particular drug or drugs and could not completely eliminate the possibility that the effects were caused by the severe maternal disease.

A mild decrease in cord calcium concentrations has been reported in mothers treated with magnesium (3,13,15). In contrast, a 1980 study reported elevated calcium levels in cord blood following magnesium therapy (4). No newborn symptoms were associated with either change in serum calcium concentrations. However, long-term maternal tocolysis with IV magnesium sulfate may cause injury to the newborn as described below.

In an investigation of five newborn infants whose mothers had been treated with IV magnesium sulfate for periods ranging from 5 to 14 weeks, radiographic bony abnormalities were noted in two of the infants (18). One of the mothers, a class C diabetic who had been insulin-dependent for 12 years, was treated with IV magnesium, beginning at 21 weeks' gestation, for 14 weeks. A 2030-g female infant was delivered vaginally at 35 weeks' gestation following spontaneous rupture of the mother's membranes. The maternal histories of this and another mother treated for 6 weeks were described in 1986 (19). The infant had frank rachitic changes of the long bones and the calvaria. Serum calcium at 6 hours of age was normal. The infant was treated with IV calcium gluconate for 3 days, then given bottle feedings without additional calcium or vitamin D. Scout films for an IV pyelogram taken at 4 months of age because of a urinary tract infection showed no bony abnormalities. Growth over the first 3 years has been consistently at the 3rd percentile for height, weight, and head circumference. Dental enamel hypoplasia, especially of the central upper incisors, was the only physical abnormality noted at 3 years of age. The second infant's mother had been treated with IV magnesium for 9 weeks beginning at 25 weeks' gestation. The 2190-g female infant was delivered vaginally at 34 weeks because of spontaneous rupture of membranes. Hypocalcemia (5.8 mg/dL, normal 6.0–10.0 mg/dL) was measured at 6 hours of age. A chest radiograph taken on the 1st day revealed lucent bands at the distal ends of the metaphyses (18). She was treated with IV calcium for 5 days and then given bottle feedings without additional calcium or vitamin D. A scout film for an IV pyelogram at 5 months of age showed no bony abnormalities. In the remaining three cases, the mothers had been treated with IV magnesium for 4–6 weeks, and their infants were normal on examination. The authors hypothesized that the fetal hypermagnesemia produced by the long-term maternal administration of magnesium caused a depression of parathyroid hormone release that resulted in fetal hypocalcemia (18).

In another study of long-term IV magnesium tocolysis, 22 women were treated for an average of 26.3 days (maximum duration in any patient was 75 days) (20). Two infants delivered from this group were noted to have wide-spaced fontanelles and parietal bone thinning. These effects returned to normal with time. A third newborn, delivered from a mother belonging to an intermediate group treated with IV magnesium for an average of 6.3 days, suffered a parietal bone fracture during an instrumental delivery and developed spastic quadriplegia (20).

More recent studies have also described the adverse effects of prolonged magnesium therapy on fetal bone mineralization (23–27). The mechanism of this reaction appears to be increased and persistent urinary calcium losses in the mother and her fetus (26,27). In one investigation, increases in 1,25-dihydroxyvitamin D and parathyroid hormone in both the mother and the fetus may have prevented more severe hypocalcemia (27).

Clinically significant drug interactions have been reported, one in a newborn and three in mothers, after maternal administration of $MgSO_4$. In one case, an interaction between in utero acquired magnesium and gentamicin was reported in a newborn 24 hours after birth (28,29). The mother had received 24 g of $MgSO_4$ during the 32 hours preceding birth of a neurologically depressed female infant. Gentamicin, 2.5 mg/kg IM every 12 hours, was begun at 12 hours of age for presumed sepsis. The infant developed respiratory arrest following the second dose of gentamicin, which resolved after the antibiotic was stopped. Animal experiments confirmed the interaction. The maternal cases involved an interaction between magnesium and nifedipine (30,31). One report described two women who were hospitalized at 30 and 32 weeks' gestation, respectively, for hypertension (30). In both cases, oral methyldopa, 2 g, and IV $MgSO_4$, 20 g, daily were ineffective in lowering the mother's blood pressure. Oral nifedipine, 10 mg, was given and a marked hypotensive response occurred 45 minutes later. The blood pressures before nifedipine in the women were 150/110 and 140/105 mmHg, respectively, and decreased to 80/50 and 90/60 mmHg, respectively, after administration of the calcium channel blocker. Blood pressure returned to previous levels 25–30 minutes later. Both infants were delivered following the hypotensive episodes, but only one survived. In the third maternal case, a woman in premature labor at 32 weeks' gestation was treated with oral nifedipine, 60 mg over 3 hours, then 20 mg every 8 hours (31). Because uterine contractions returned, intravenous $MgSO_4$ was begun 12 hours later followed by the onset of pronounced muscle weakness after 500 mg had been administered. Her symptoms included jerky movements of the extremities, difficulty in swallowing, paradoxical respirations, and an inability to lift her head from the pillow. The magnesium was stopped and the symptoms resolved in the next 25 minutes. The reaction was attributed to nifedipine potentiation of the neuromuscular blocking action of magnesium.

Maternal hypothermia with maternal and fetal bradycardia apparently caused by IV magnesium sulfate has been reported (32). The 30-year-old woman, at about 31 weeks' gestation, was being treated for premature labor. She had received a single, 12-mg IM dose of betamethasone at the same time that magnesium therapy was started. Her oral temperature fell from 99.8°F to 97°F 2 hours after the infusion had been increased from 2 to 3 g/hr. Twelve hours after admission to the hospital, her heart rate fell to 64 beats/minute (baseline 80 beats/minute), whereas the fetal heart rate decreased to 110 beats/minute (baseline 140–150 beats/minute). A rectal temperature at this time was 95.8°F and the patient complained of lethargy and diplopia. Her serum magnesium level was 6.6 mg/dL. Magnesium therapy was discontinued and all signs and symptoms returned to baseline values within 6 hours. Neither the mother nor the fetus suffered adversely from the effects attributed to magnesium.

BREASTFEEDING SUMMARY

Magnesium salts may be encountered by nursing mothers using over-the-counter laxatives. A study in which 50 mothers received an emulsion of magnesium and liquid petrolatum or mineral oil found no evidence of changes or frequency of stools in nursing infants (33). In 10 preeclamptic patients receiving magnesium sulfate 1 g/hr IV during the first 24 hours after delivery, magnesium levels in breast milk were 64 mcg/mL as compared with 48 mcg/mL in nontreated controls (34). Twenty-four hours after stopping the drug, magnesium levels in breast milk in treated and nontreated patients were 38 and 32 mcg/mL, respectively. By 48 hours, the levels were identical in the two groups. Milk:plasma ratios were 1.9

and 2.1 in treated and nontreated patients, respectively. The American Academy of Pediatrics classifies magnesium sulfate as compatible with breastfeeding (35).

References

1. Chesley LC, Tepper I. Plasma levels of magnesium attained in magnesium sulfate therapy for preeclampsia and eclampsia. Surg Clin North Am 1957;37:353–67.
2. Dangman BC, Rosen TS. Magnesium levels in infants of mothers treated with $MgSO_4$ (abstract #262). Pediatr Res 1977;11:415.
3. Cruikshank DP, Pitkin RM, Reynolds WA, Williams GA, Hargis GK. Effects of magnesium sulfate treatment on perinatal calcium metabolism. I. Maternal and fetal responses. Am J Obstet Gynecol 1979;134:243–9.
4. Donovan EF, Tsang RC, Steichen JJ, Strub RJ, Chen IW, Chen M. Neonatal hypermagnesemia: effect on parathyroid hormone and calcium homeostasis. J Pediatr 1980;96:305–10.
5. Stone SR, Pritchard JA. Effect of maternally administered magnesium sulfate on the neonate. Obstet Gynecol 1970;35:574–7.
6. Pruett KM, Kirshon B, Cotton DB, Adam K, Doody KJ. The effects of magnesium sulfate therapy on Apgar scores. Am J Obstet Gynecol 1988;159:1047–8.
7. Heinonen OP, Slone D, Shapiro S. *Birth Defects and Drugs in Pregnancy*. Littleton, MA: Publishing Sciences Group, 1977:440.
8. Martin RW, Gaddy DK, Martin JN Jr, Lucas JA, Wiser WL, Morrison JC. Tocolysis with oral magnesium. Am J Obstet Gynecol 1987;156: 433–4.
9. Spatling L, Spatling G. Magnesium supplementation in pregnancy: a double-blind study. Br J Obstet Gynaecol 1988;95:120–5.
10. Sibai BM, Villar L. MA, Bray E. Magnesium supplementation during pregnancy: a double-blind randomized controlled clinical trial. Am J Obstet Gynecol 1989;161:115–9.
11. Lipsitz PJ, English IC. Hypermagnesemia in the newborn infant. Pediatrics 1967;40:856–62.
12. Lipsitz PJ. The clinical and biochemical effects of excess magnesium in the newborn. Pediatrics 1971;47:501–9.
13. Savory J, Monif GRG. Serum calcium levels in cord sera of the progeny of mothers treated with magnesium sulfate for toxemia of pregnancy. Am J Obstet Gynecol 1971;110:556–9.
14. Rasch DK, Huber PA, Richardson CJ, L'Hommedieu CS, Nelson TE, Reddi R. Neurobehavioral effects of neonatal hypermagnesemia. J Pediatr 1982;100:272–6.
15. Green KW, Key TC, Coen R, Resnik R. The effects of maternally administered magnesium sulfate on the neonate. Am J Obstet Gynecol 1983;146:29–33.
16. Sibai BM, Lipshitz J, Anderson GD, Dilts PV Jr. Reassessment of intravenous $MgSO_4$ therapy in preeclampsia-eclampsia. Obstet Gynecol 1981;57: 199–202.
17. Hutchinson HT, Nichols MM, Kuhn CR, Vasicka A. Effects of magnesium sulfate on uterine contractility, intrauterine fetus, and infant. Am J Obstet Gynecol 1964;88:747–58.
18. Lamm CI, Norton KI, Murphy RJC, Wilkins IA, Rabinowitz JG. Congenital rickets associated with magnesium sulfate infusion for tocolysis. J Pediatr 1988;113:1078–82.
19. Wilkins IA, Goldberg JD, Phillips RN, Bacall CJ, Chervenak FA, Berkowitz RL. Long-term use of magnesium sulfate as a tocolytic agent. Obstet Gynecol 1986;67:38S–40S.
20. Dudley D, Gagnon D, Varner M. Long-term tocolysis with intravenous magnesium sulfate. Obstet Gynecol 1989;73:373–8.
21. Brady JP, Williams HC. Magnesium intoxication in a premature infant. Pediatrics 1967;40:100–3.
22. Brazy JE, Grimm JK, Little VA. Neonatal manifestations of severe maternal hypertension occurring before the thirty-sixth week of pregnancy. J Pediatr 1982;100:265–71.
23. Holcomb WL Jr, Shackelford GD, Petrie RH. Prolonged magnesium therapy affects fetal bone (abstract). Am J Obstet Gynecol 1991;164:386.
24. Smith LG Jr, Schanler RJ, Burns P, Moise KJ Jr. Effect of magnesium sulfate therapy ($MgSO_4$) on the bone mineral content of women and their newborns (abstract). Am J Obstet Gynecol 1991;164:427.
25. Holcomb WL Jr, Shackelford GD, Petrie RH. Magnesium tocolysis and neonatal bone abnormalities: a controlled study. Obstet Gynecol 1991;78:611–4.
26. Smith LG Jr, Burns PA, Schanler RJ. Calcium homeostasis in pregnant women receiving long-term magnesium sulfate therapy for preterm labor. Am J Obstet Gynecol 1992;167:45–51.
27. Cruikshank DP, Chan GM, Doerrfeld D. Alterations in vitamin D and calcium metabolism with magnesium sulfate treatment of preeclampsia. Am J Obstet Gynecol 1993;168:1170–7.
28. L'Hommedieu CS, Nicholas D, Armes DA, Jones P, Nelson T, Pickering LK. Potentiation of magnesium sulfate-induced neuromuscular weakness by gentamicin, tobramycin, and amikacin. J Pediatr 1983;102:629–31.
29. L'Hommedieu CS, Huber PA, Rasch DK. Potentiation of magnesium-induced neuromuscular weakness by gentamicin. Crit Care Med 1983;11:55–6.
30. Waisman GD, Mayorga LM, Camera MI, Vignolo CA, Martinotti A. Magnesium plus nifedipine: potentiation of hypotensive effect in preeclampsia? Am J Obstet Gynecol 1988;159:308–9.
31. Snyder SW, Cardwell MS. Neuromuscular blockade with magnesium sulfate and nifedipine. Am J Obstet Gynecol 1989;161:35–6.
32. Rodis JF, Vintzileos AM, Campbell WA, Deaton JL, Nochimson DJ. Maternal hypothermia: an unusual complication of magnesium sulfate therapy. Am J Obstet Gynecol 1987;156:435–6.
33. Baldwin WF. Clinical study of senna administration to nursing mothers: assessment of effects on infant bowel habits. CMAJ 1963;89:566–8.
34. Cruikshank DP, Varner MW, Pitkin RM. Breast milk magnesium and calcium concentrations following magnesium sulfate treatment. Am J Obstet Gynecol 1982;143:685–8.
35. Committee on Drugs, American Academy of Pediatrics. The transfer of drugs and other chemicals into human milk. Pediatrics 2001;108:776–89.

MANDELIC ACID

[Withdrawn from the market. See 9th edition.]

MANNITOL

Diuretic

PREGNANCY RECOMMENDATION: No Human Data—Probably Compatible
BREASTFEEDING RECOMMENDATION: No Human Data—Probably Compatible

PREGNANCY SUMMARY

Mannitol is an osmotic diuretic. No reports of its use in pregnancy following IV administration have been located. Mannitol, given by intra-amniotic injection, has been used to induce abortion (1).

BREASTFEEDING SUMMARY

No reports describing the use of mannitol during human lactation have been located.

Reference

1. Craft IL, Mus BD. Hypertonic solutions to induce abortions. Br Med J 1971;2:49.

MAPROTILINE

Antidepressant

PREGNANCY RECOMMENDATION: Limited Human Data—Animal Data Suggest Low Risk
BREASTFEEDING RECOMMENDATION: Limited Human Data—Potential Toxicity

PREGNANCY SUMMARY

No published reports linking the use of maprotiline with congenital defects have been located.

FETAL RISK SUMMARY

Maprotiline is a tetracyclic antidepressant. Animal studies have failed to demonstrate teratogenicity, carcinogenicity, mutagenicity, or impairment of fertility (1,2).

In a surveillance study of Michigan Medicaid recipients involving 229,101 completed pregnancies conducted between 1985 and 1992, 13 newborns had been exposed to maprotiline during the 1st trimester (F. Rosa, personal communication, FDA, 1993). Two (15.4%) major birth defects were observed (0.6 expected), one of which was an oral cleft (none expected). No anomalies were observed in five other defect categories (cardiovascular defects, spina bifida, polydactyly, limb reduction defects, and hypospadias) for which specific data were available. The number of exposures is too small for an assessment of the embryo–fetal risk.

In a 1996 descriptive case series, the European Network of the Teratology Information Services (ENTIS) prospectively examined the outcomes of 689 pregnancies exposed to antidepressants (3). Multiple drug therapy occurred in about two-thirds of the mothers. Maprotiline was used in 107 pregnancies. The outcomes of these pregnancies were 17 elective abortions, 11 spontaneous abortions, 2 stillbirths, 72 normal newborns (includes 7 premature infants), 3 normal infants with neonatal disorder (hypotonia in 2; diabetes associated disorder in 1), and 2 infants with congenital defects. The defects (all exposed in the 1st trimester or longer; both exposed to multiple other agents) were facial dysmorphology, nasal hypoplasia, bone immaturity; and bilateral talipes.

A 2002 prospective study compared two groups of mother–child pairs exposed to antidepressants throughout gestation (46 exposed to tricyclics or tetracyclics—1 to maprotiline; 40 to fluoxetine) with 36 nonexposed, not depressed controls (4). Offspring were studied between the ages 15 and 71 months for effects of antidepressant exposure in terms of IQ, language, behavior, and temperament. Exposure to antidepressants did not adversely affect the measured parameters, but IQ was significantly and negatively associated with the duration of depression, and language was negatively associated with the number of depression episodes after delivery (4).

BREASTFEEDING SUMMARY

Maprotiline is excreted into breast milk (5). Milk:plasma ratios of 1.5 and 1.3 have been reported following a 100-mg single dose and 150 mg in divided doses for 120 hours. Multiple dosing resulted in milk concentrations of unchanged maprotiline of 0.2 mcg/mL. Although this amount is low, the significance to the nursing infant is not known.

References

1. Product information. Ludiomil. CIBA, 1993.
2. Esaki K, Tanioka Y, Tsukada M, Izumiyama K. Teratogenicity of maprotiline tested by oral administration to mice and rats. (Japanese) CIEA Preclinical Report 1976;2:69–77. As cited in Shepard TH. *Catalog of Teratogenic Agents*. 6th ed. Baltimore, MD: Johns Hopkins University Press, 1989:384.
3. McElhatton PR, Garbis HM, Elefant E, Vial T, Bellemin B, Mastroiacovo P, Arnon J, Rodriguez-Pinilla E, Schaefer C, Pexieder T, Merlob P, Dal Verme S. The outcome of pregnancy in 689 women exposed to therapeutic doses of antidepressants. A collaborative study of the European Network of Teratology Information Services (ENTIS). Reprod Toxicol 1996;10:285–94.
4. Nulman I, Rovet J, Stewart DE, Wolpin J, Pace-Asciak P, Shuhaiber S, Koren G. Child development following exposure to tricyclic antidepressants or fluoxetine throughout fetal life: a prospective, controlled study. Am J Psychiatry 2002;159:1889–95.
5. Reiss W. The relevance of blood level determinations during the evaluation of maprotiline in man. In Murphy JE, ed. *Research and Clinical Investigation in Depression*. Northampton, England: Cambridge Medical Publications, 1980;19–38.

MARAVIROC

Antiviral

PREGNANCY RECOMMENDATION: Compatible—Maternal Benefit >> Embryo–Fetal Risk
BREASTFEEDING RECOMMENDATION: Contraindicated

PREGNANCY SUMMARY

Although the animal data suggest low risk, the absence of detailed human pregnancy experience prevents an assessment of the embryo–fetal risk. If indicated, the drug should not be withheld because of pregnancy.

FETAL RISK SUMMARY

Maraviroc, a cellular chemokine receptor (CCR5) antagonist, is in the same antiviral subclass of entry inhibitors as enfuvirtide. It is indicated for combination antiretroviral treatment of adults infected with only CCR5-tropic detectable HIV-1, who have evidence of viral replication and HIV-1 strains resistant to multiple antiretroviral agents. The drug is metabolized to inactive compounds by the cytochrome P450 system and is moderately (76%) bound to plasma proteins, including both albumin and α_1-acid glycoprotein. The terminal half-life at steady state is 14–18 hours (1).

Reproduction studies have been conducted in rats and rabbits. No increase in the incidence of fetal variations and malformations was observed in these species at exposures (AUC) that were 20 and 5 times, respectively, the human exposure from the recommended daily dose (HE). No effects of the exposure were observed in the offspring during prenatal and postnatal development studies, including fertility and reproductive performance (1).

Carcinogenicity studies have been conducted in mice and rats and no drug-related increases in tumor incidence were observed. Maraviroc was not genotoxic in multiple assays and did not impair mating or fertility of male and female rats at exposures that were about 20 times the HE (1).

M

Consistent with the molecular weight (514), moderate protein binding, and long elimination half-life, maraviroc crosses the human placenta. A woman with HIV became pregnant and was treated with multiple antiviral agents (2). Maraviroc (150 mg twice daily) was started at 29 weeks' gestation. At 38 weeks', a cesarean section gave birth to a baby with no abnormalities. At birth, maraviroc concentrations in the maternal plasma and cord blood, 13 hours after a dose, were 186 and 69 ng/mL, respectively, a ratio of 0.37 (2). Another study using an ex vivo human cotyledon perfusion model also found that the drug crosses the human placenta (3).

The Antiretroviral Pregnancy Registry has reported one 2nd/3rd trimester exposure to maraviroc. An apparently normal outcome was observed (4).

Two reviews, one in 1996 and the other in 1997, concluded that all women receiving antiretroviral therapy should continue to receive the therapy during pregnancy and that treatment of the mother with monotherapy should be considered inadequate (5,6). The same conclusion was reached in a 2003 review with the added admonishment that therapy must be continuous to prevent emergence of resistant viral strains (7). In 2009, the updated U.S. Department of Health and Human Services guidelines for the use of antiretroviral agents in HIV-1 infected patients continued the recommendation that therapy, with the exception of efavirenz, should be continued during pregnancy (8). If indicated, maraviroc should not be withheld in pregnancy because the expected benefit to the HIV-positive mother outweighs the unknown risk to the fetus. Updated guidelines for the use of antiretroviral drugs to reduce perinatal HIV transmission also were released in 2010 (9). Women receiving antiretroviral therapy during pregnancy should continue the therapy but, regardless of the regimen, zidovudine administration is recommended during the intrapartum period to prevent vertical transmission of HIV to the newborn (9). Physicians are encouraged to register exposed patients in the Antiretroviral Pregnancy Registry by calling 1-800-258-4263 (1).

BREASTFEEDING SUMMARY

No reports have been located that describe the use of maraviroc during human lactation. The molecular weight (about 514) and long elimination half-life (14–18 hours) suggest that the drug will be excreted into breast milk. The effect on a nursing infant is unknown.

Reports on the use of maraviroc during human lactation are unlikely because the drug is used in the treatment of HIV infections. HIV is transmitted in milk, and in developed countries, breastfeeding is not recommended (5,6,8–12). In developing countries, breastfeeding is undertaken, despite the risk, because milk substitutes are not affordable. Until 1999, no studies had been published that examined the effect of any antiretroviral therapy on HIV transmission in milk. In that year, a study involving zidovudine was published that measured a 38% reduction in vertical transmission of HIV-1 infection despite breastfeeding when compared with controls. (See Zidovudine.)

References

1. Product information. Selzentry. Pfizer. 2007.
2. Calcagno A, Trentini L, Marinaro L, Montrucchio C, D'Avolio A, Ghisetti V, Di Perri G, Bonora S. Transplacental passage of etravirine and maraviroc in a multidrug-experienced HIV-infected woman failing on darunavir-based HAART in late pregnancy. J Antimicrob Chemother 2013;68: 1938–9.
3. Vinot C, Gavard L, Treluyer JM, Manceau S, Courbon E, Scherrmann JM, Decleves X, Duro D, Peytavin G, Mandelbrot L, Giraud C. Placental transfer of maraviroc in an *ex vivo* human cotyledon perfusion model and influence of ABC transporter expression. Antimicrob Agents Chemother 2013;57:1415–20.
4. Antiretroviral Pregnancy Registry Steering Committee. Antiretroviral Pregnancy Registry International Interim Report for 1 January 1989 through 31 July 2009. Wilmington, NC: Registry Coordinating Center; 2009. Available at www.apregistry.com. Accessed May 29, 2010.
5. Carpenter CCJ, Fischi MA, Hammer SM, Hirsch MS, Jacobsen DM, Katzenstein DA, Montaner JSG, Richman DD, Saag MS, Schooley RT, Thompson MA, Vella S, Yeni PG, Volberding PA. Antiretroviral therapy for HIV infection in 1996. JAMA 1996;276:146–54.
6. Minkoff H, Augenbraun M. Antiretroviral therapy for pregnant women. Am J Obstet Gynecol 1997;176:478–89.
7. Minkoff H. Human immunodeficiency virus infection in pregnancy. Obstet Gynecol 2003;101:797–810.
8. Panel on Antiretroviral Guidelines for Adults and Adolescents. Guidelines for the use of antiretroviral agents in HIV-1-infected adults and adolescents. Department of Health and Human Services. December 1, 2009;1–161. Available at http://www.aidsinfo.nih.gov/ContentFiles/AdultandAdolescentGL.pdf. Accessed September 17, 2010:60, 96–8.
9. Panel on Treatment of HIV-Infected Pregnant Women and Prevention of Perinatal Transmission. Recommendations for Use of Antiretroviral Drugs in Pregnant HIV-1-Infected Women for Maternal Health and Interventions

to Reduce Perinatal HIV Transmission in the United States. May 24, 2010:1–117. Available at http://aidsinfo.nih.gov/ContentFiles/PerinatalGL.pdf. Accessed September 17, 2010:30, Table 5.

10. Brown ZA, Watts DH. Antiviral therapy in pregnancy. Clin Obstet Gynecol 1990;33:276–89.

11. De Martino M, Tovo P-A, Pezzotti P, Galli L, Massironi E, Ruga E, Floreea F, Plebani A, Gabiano C, Zuccotti GV. HIV-1 transmission through breast-milk: appraisal of risk according to duration of feeding. AIDS 1992;6:991–7.

12. Van de Perre P. Postnatal transmission of human immunodeficiency virus type 1: the breast-feeding dilemma. Am J Obstet Gynecol 1995;173:483–7.

MARIJUANA

Hallucinogen

PREGNANCY RECOMMENDATION: Contraindicated
BREASTFEEDING RECOMMENDATION: Contraindicated

PREGNANCY SUMMARY

The use of marijuana in pregnancy has produced conflicting reports on the length of gestation, the quality and duration of labor, fetal growth, congenital defects, and neurobehavior in the newborn. These effects have been the subject of a number of reviews. A meta-analysis and a longitudinal study could not find associations between marijuana and low birth weight or growth in adolescents, but an association with lower birth weight and length was found when biomarkers were used to document maternal exposure. The possible association of in utero marijuana exposure with leukemia in children should be a major concern of any woman who chooses to use this drug during pregnancy. No pattern of malformations has been observed that could be considered characteristic of in utero marijuana exposure. However, there is evidence that marijuana might potentiate the fetal effects of alcohol and may be associated with an increased risk of ventricular septal defects. Two research centers have concluded that prenatal marijuana use adversely effects neurobehavior in infants and adolescents. In the neonatal period, exposed infants may have symptoms similar to mild narcotic withdrawal. In older children, the negative effects included decreased problem-solving ability, inattention, increased hyperactivity, impulsivity and delinquency, and externalization of problems. Some of these results were found even after controlling for the home environment. In most studies, the use of marijuana is closely associated with the use of nicotine and alcohol; and the abuse of other drugs, both prescription and illicit, occurs frequently. Moreover, maternal self-reporting of the amounts and timing of the exposures to marijuana and other abuse substances is common. Separating the effects of these confounding exposures from the effects of marijuana is a daunting task. In addition, failure to account for the varying concentrations of delta-9-tetrahydrocannabinol (Δ-9-THC, THC) contained in the natural product, the presence of contaminants, and the underreporting of maternal marijuana use could very well have changed the findings of many studies. Therefore, the associations with structural and neurobehavior defects require continued study.

FETAL RISK SUMMARY

Marijuana (cannabis; hashish) is a natural substance that is smoked for its hallucinogenic properties. (One marijuana cigarette is commonly referred to as a "joint.") Hashish is a potent concentrated form of marijuana. The main psychoactive ingredient, THC is also available in a commercial oral formulation (dronabinol) for use as an antiemetic agent. Natural preparations of marijuana may vary widely in their potency and, except for the commercial preparation, no standardization exists either for the THC content or for the presence of contaminants. Only the commercially available oral formulation can be legally used in the United States.

The use of marijuana by pregnant women is common. Most investigators have reported incidences of 3%–16% (1–17). Other researchers have proposed that even these figures represent underreporting, especially in the 1st month when pregnancy may not be suspected (18–20). Because of the illicit nature of marijuana, many women will simply not admit to its use (4,8). Data from the Ottawa Prenatal Prospective Study in Canada indicated that 20% of their patients used marijuana during the year before pregnancy with the incidence declining to about 10% after the women knew they were pregnant (13). In addition, heavy marijuana usage (>5 joints/week or the use of hashish), when compared with alcohol or nicotine usage, was the least reduced of the three agents during pregnancy (21).

Although the use of marijuana by pregnant women is common, the effects of this use on the pregnancies and the fetuses are unclear. Part of this problem is attributable to the close association between marijuana, alcohol, cigarette smoking, other abuse drugs, and lifestyles that may increase perinatal risk (1–3,6,7). Moreover, studies have relied on maternal self-reporting of the amount and timing of exposures to marijuana and the other substances. Controlling for these confounders becomes a daunting task of almost all studies. However, sufficient data appear to be available to allow classification of the major concerns surrounding exposure to marijuana during pregnancy. These concerns are

- Placental passage of Δ-9-THC
- Pregnancy complications
  - Length of gestation
  - Quality and duration of labor
  - Effect on maternal hormone levels
- Fetal or newborn complications
  - Intrauterine growth
  - Structural defects

M

Neurobehavioral defects
Leukemia
Miscellaneous effects

Placental Passage

Δ-9-THC and a metabolite, 9-carboxy-THC, cross the placenta to the fetus at term (4,22). Data for other periods of gestation and for other metabolites are not available. A 1982 study found measurable amounts of 9-carboxy-THC, but not THC, in two cord blood samples but did not quantify the concentrations (4). In a study of 10 women who daily smoked up to five marijuana cigarettes, maternal serum samples were drawn 10–20 minutes before corresponding cord blood samples (22). The time interval between last exposure and sampling ranged from 5 to 26 hours. This is well beyond the time of peak THC levels that occur 3–8 minutes after beginning to smoke (23). Maternal levels of THC were below the limit of sensitivity (0.2 ng/mL) in five samples and ranged from 0.4 to 6 ng/mL in the others. Measurable cord blood concentrations of THC were found in three samples and varied between 0.3 and 1.0 ng/mL. The maternal plasma:cord blood ratios for these three samples were 2.7, 4, and 6. The metabolite, 9-carboxy-THC, which was measured in all maternal and cord blood samples, ranged between 2.3 and 125 ng/mL and 0.4 and 18 ng/mL, respectively. Plasma:cord blood ratios for the metabolite varied from 1.7 to 7.8.

Pregnancy Complications

LENGTH OF GESTATION Marijuana-induced complications of pregnancy are controversial, with different studies producing conflicting results. One of these areas of controversy involves the effect of marijuana on length of gestation. A 1980 prospective study of 291 women found no relationship between maternal use of marijuana and gestational length (3). Similar results were reported from two studies, one in 1982 involving 1690 women (24) and one in 1989 with 1226 women (25). Of interest, marijuana use by the women in the later study was confirmed with urine assays (25). A significantly shorter gestational period was found in 1246 users in a retrospective study of 12,424 pregnancies, but this difference disappeared when the data were controlled for nicotine exposure, demographic characteristics, and medical and obstetric histories (9).

In contrast to the above reports, three groups of investigators associated regular marijuana use with shorter gestations (1,10,14) and one group with longer gestations (26). In 36 women using marijuana ≥2 times/week, 9 (25%) delivered prematurely, a rate much higher than the 5.1% for users of marijuana ≤1/week and the 5.6% for nonusers (1). Investigation of 583 women who delivered single live births, a continuation of the 1980 study mentioned above, now revealed that heavy use of marijuana (more than five marijuana cigarettes/week) was significantly associated with a reduction of 0.8 week's gestational length after adjustment for the mother's prepregnancy weight (10). A total of 84 women (14.4%) used marijuana in this population, 18 of whom were classified as heavy users. A large prospective study of 3857 pregnancies ending in singleton live births found that regular marijuana use (2–3 times/month or more) was associated with an increased risk of preterm (<37 weeks) delivery for white women but not for nonwhite women (14). For the 122 regular white users, 8.2% delivered prematurely compared with 3.8% of 105 occasional users (one marijuana cigarette or less/month) and 4.0% of 2778 nonusers. In the nonwhite groups, the incidences of shortened gestation for the 86 regular, 53 occasional, and 706 nonusers were 10.5%, 11.3%, and 8.8%, respectively. In a population of lower socioeconomic-status women, the total amount of marijuana used during pregnancy was positively correlated with an average 2 days' prolongation of gestation (26). However, the authors of this study noted that their evidence for a longer gestational period was weak in terms of magnitude.

QUALITY AND DURATION OF LABOR A second pregnancy complication examined frequently is the effect of marijuana on the quality and duration of labor. No association between marijuana and duration of labor, including precipitate labor and the type of presentation at birth, was found in the Ottawa Prenatal Prospective Study (3,5,8) or in another study (26). In contrast, other investigators found a significant difference in precipitate labor (<3 hours total) between users (29%) and nonusers (3%) (4,27). Although not significant, 31% of users (11 of 35) had prolonged, protracted, or arrested labor as compared with 19% (7 of 36) nonusers (4,27). Because of the dysfunctional labor, 57% of the newborn infants in the user group had meconium staining vs. 25% among nonusers, a situation that probably resulted in the observation that 41% of newborn infants of users required resuscitation compared with 21% of infants of nonusers. Adjustment of the data for race, income, smoking, alcohol use, and first physician visit did not change the findings. A second study by these latter investigators using a different group of patients produced similar results in the incidence of dysfunctional labor, precipitate labor, and meconium staining, but the differences between users and nonusers were not significant (7).

MATERNAL HORMONE LEVELS In nonhuman primates, marijuana disrupts the menstrual cycle by inhibiting ovulation through its effects on the pituitary trophic hormones (luteinizing hormone and follicle-stimulating hormone), prolactin, and resulting decreases in estrogen and progesterone levels (16). Tolerance to these effects has been reported (16). Similar effects have been observed in human clinical studies (16).

Thirteen pregnant women, who were regular users of marijuana (once/month to 4 times/day), were matched with controls (28). No effect of this exposure was measured on the levels of human chorionic gonadotropin (hCG), pregnancy-specific β-1-glycoprotein, placental lactogen, progesterone, 17-hydroxyprogesterone, estradiol, and estriol.

Fetal or Newborn Complications

Concerns with the fetal complications arising from maternal marijuana use center around the effects on intrauterine growth restriction, structural anomalies, and neurobehavioral complications in the newborn infant. A recent report indicates that induction of leukemia in childhood must also be considered. As with pregnancy complications, conflicting reports are common.

INTRAUTERINE GROWTH Data of the Ottawa Prenatal Prospective Study indicated no significant reduction in birth weight or head circumference (after adjustment for other factors) in babies of marijuana users (3,5,8,10,13). Compared with infants of nonusers, birth weight actually increased by an average of 67 g in irregular users (one marijuana cigarette/week or less) and 117 g in moderate users (two to five/week), whereas heavy use (more than five/week) was associated with a nonsignificant reduction of 52 g (10). Other studies observed no effect on growth after adjustment of their data (1,7,9,26,29–33). However, in one study, a reduction of 0.55 cm in infant length, but not head circumference, was correlated with maternal use of three marijuana cigarettes/day in the 1st trimester (26). Use during the remainder of pregnancy or the total amount smoked during pregnancy did not significantly affect the infants' length or head circumference. One study, however, did find a significantly smaller head size in offspring of mothers who were heavy marijuana users (32). In addition, one group of investigators found no association between marijuana and preterm delivery or abruptio placentae (30).

A number of researchers have reported positive correlations with reduced intrauterine growth (after adjustment). In one study, use of <3 joints/week was associated with a significant decrease in birth weight of 95 g compared with that of controls, and use of ≥3 cigarettes/week was associated with a significant reduction of 139 g (24,34). A related 1989 study found that marijuana use during pregnancy, when confirmed by positive urine assays, was independently associated with impaired fetal growth, and that the effects of cocaine abuse were additive but not synergistic (25). However, they could not demonstrate a cause-and-effect relationship with marijuana because of other factors, such as the markedly elevated blood levels of carbon monoxide that occur with marijuana use (blood carboxyhemoglobin levels after smoking marijuana are about 5 times those observed after smoking tobacco) (25). Of 1226 mothers who were studied, 331 (27%) used marijuana during gestation as determined by history and positive urine assay. Only 278 (84%) of these would have been detected by history alone. After controlling for potential confounding variables, infants of marijuana users with positive urine assays (*N* = 202), compared with infants of nonusers (*N* = 895), were found to have significantly lower birth weight (79 g) and length (0.52 cm) but not head circumference. The birth weight and length measurements did not differ statistically if only self-reported marijuana use was considered, demonstrating the importance of a biologic marker in studies involving this drug (25).

A study, conducted from 1975 to 1983 in two phases, found decreased birth weight only in the second phase (17). The two phases, involving 1434 and 1381 patients, respectively, differed primarily in their assessment of marijuana use early in pregnancy. In the first phase, 9.3% used marijuana, with consumption of two to four joints/month associated with a significant increase in birth weight. No trend was observed with more or less frequent use. The second phase, with 10.3% users, found weight reductions in all classifications of marijuana exposure: 127 g for two to three joints/week, 143 g for four to six joints/week, and 230 g for daily use (17). The authors speculated that the difference between the groups may have been related to the use of other abuse drugs (e.g., cocaine) or changes in the composition or contaminants of marijuana. In a 1986 study, regular marijuana use (2 to 3 times/month or more) was correlated with an increased risk of low-birth-weight (<2500 g) and small-for-gestational-age (SGA) infants in whites only (14). The rates of low-birth-weight and SGA infants in users (*N* = 122) and nonusers (*N* = 3490) were 8.2% vs. 2.7%, and 12.5% vs. 4.9%, respectively. In 845 nonwhites, no differences between users and nonusers were observed. In a 1984 report, examination of 462 infants, 16% of whom were exposed to marijuana and alcohol during early gestation, revealed a significant correlation between maternal marijuana use and decreased body length at 8 months of age (11). Body weight and head circumference were not significantly affected.

In three case reports on the same five infants, low birth weight (all <2500 g) with reduced head circumference and length were observed (35–37). Two of the infants were premature (<37 weeks). The mothers of these infants smoked 2–14 marijuana cigarettes/day during pregnancy with one also using alcohol, cocaine, and nicotine, and two mothers also using nicotine. In a 1999 study, positive pregnancy test urine samples were screened for several drugs, including marijuana (38). Those testing positive for marijuana had babies with significantly lower birth weight, an increased risk of prematurity, and a lower gestational age at delivery.

A 1997 meta-analysis on the effect of marijuana on birth weight identified 10 studies in which the results were adjusted for cigarette smoking and 5 of these met their criteria for analysis (39). The pooled odds ratio (OR) for any use of marijuana and low birth weight was 1.09 (95% confidence interval [CI] 0.94–1.27). They concluded that, in the amounts typically used by pregnant women, there was insufficient evidence that marijuana caused low birth weight (39). In a 2001 study, exposure to marijuana during pregnancy was not associated with any growth measurement or timing of pubertal milestones in a group of 152 adolescents (13- to 16-year-olds) that had been followed longitudinally since birth (40).

STRUCTURAL DEFECTS

Animal research in the 1960s and 1970s yielded inconclusive evidence on the teratogenicity of marijuana and its active ingredients unless high doses were used in certain species (41–44). In humans, most investigators and reviewers have concluded either that marijuana does not produce structural defects or that insufficient data exist to reach any conclusion (1,13,25,26,29,45–56). However, one reviewer cautioned that marijuana-induced birth defects could be rare and easily missed (55), and another observed that marijuana could potentiate known teratogens by lowering the threshold for their effects (49). A previously mentioned study that used urine assays to document marijuana exposure found that the drug was not associated with minor (either singly or as a constellation of three) or major congenital anomalies (25).

Because marijuana use is so common in women during pregnancy, and because of its frequent association with alcohol and other abuse drugs, it is not surprising that a number of studies and case reports have described congenital malformations in infants whose mothers were smoking marijuana. With some exceptions, most of these investigators did not attribute the observed defects to marijuana, but they are chronicled here mainly for a complete record.

Several reports have described the combined maternal use of marijuana and lysergic acid diethylamide (LSD) in cases ending with poor fetal outcome (57–65). A 1968 report described an infant with right terminal transverse acheiria (absence of hand) (57). The mother had taken LSD early in gestation before she knew she was pregnant. She had also smoked marijuana throughout the pregnancy and had taken a combination product containing dicyclomine, doxylamine, and pyridoxine for 1st trimester nausea. A second infant with a terminal transverse deficit, who was also exposed to the two hallucinogens, was described in 1969 (58). The defect involved portions of fingers of the left hand. Syndactyly of the right hand with shortened fingers and talipes equinovarus of the left foot were also present. A critique of these case reports and others concluded that the defects in the two infants might have been caused by amniotic band syndrome (59). Complete exstrophy of the bladder, epispadias, widely separated pubic rami, and bilateral inguinal hernias were observed in a newborn exposed to LSD, marijuana, and mephentermine (60). Marijuana was allegedly used only twice by the mother. In another case, a female infant with multiple anomalies compatible with trisomy 13 with D/D translocation was delivered from a 22-year-old mother who had last used LSD 9 months before conception (61). The mother used marijuana, barbiturates, and amphetamines throughout gestation and, presumably, before conception. The authors speculated that the defect may have been caused by LSD-induced damage of maternal germ cells before fertilization. A 1972 case report described an infant with multiple eye and central nervous system defects consisting of brachycephaly with widely separated sutures, bilateral cephalohematomas, a right eye smaller than the left, a possible cataract, and multiple brain anomalies (62). The mother had taken marijuana, LSD, and other drugs throughout pregnancy. In a study of 140 women using LSD and marijuana followed through 148 pregnancies, 8 of 83 liveborn infants had major defects as did 4 of 14 embryos examined after induced abortion (63). The incidence of defects in this sample is high (8.1%), but many of the women were using multiple other abuse drugs and had lifestyles that probably were not conducive to good fetal health. Two other reports involving the combined use of marijuana and LSD with resulting adverse fetal outcomes do not appear to have any relationship to either drug (64,65). One of these involved a report of six cases of persistent ductus arteriosus, one of which involved exposure to marijuana in utero (64). The history of maternal marijuana use was coincidental. The second case described an infant who died at 2.5 months of age of a bilateral in utero cerebral vascular accident and resulting porencephaly (65). The mother had used marijuana, LSD, alcohol, and other abuse drugs, including cocaine. This latter drug was thought to be the causative agent.

In one of two fatal cases of congenital hypothalamic hamartoblastoma tumor, an infant exposed to marijuana also had congenital heart disease and skeletal anomalies suggestive of the Ellis-von Creveld syndrome (i.e., chondroectodermal dysplasia syndrome) (66). In addition to marijuana, the mother had used cocaine and methaqualone during early pregnancy, but the authors did not attribute the defects to a particular agent. In a report of an infant with a random pattern of amputations and constrictions consistent with the amniotic band sequence, the mother's occasional use of marijuana was coincidental (67).

In contrast to the above case reports, in which marijuana use was apparently not related to structural defects, studies have reported possible associations with the drug (9,24,35–37,68,69). In a large study involving 12,424 women of whom 1246 (10%) used marijuana during pregnancy, a crude association between one or more major malformations and marijuana was discovered; no association was found with minor malformations (9). Logistic regression was used to control confounding variables, and although the OR (1.36) was suggestive, the association between marijuana and the defects was not significant. In 1690 mother–child pairs, women who smoked marijuana, but who only drank small amounts of alcohol, were 5 times more likely than nonusers to deliver an infant with features compatible with the fetal alcohol syndrome (see Ethanol) (24). The relative risk for this defect in marijuana users was 12.7 compared with 2.0 in nonusers. In a series of case reports, five infants were described with congenital defects suggestive of the fetal alcohol syndrome (35–37). In addition to daily marijuana use by the mothers, one used alcohol, cocaine, and nicotine; two used nicotine only; and two denied the use of other drugs (35). One study compared 25 marijuana users with 25 closely matched nonusing controls in a search for minor anomalies (68). Infants were examined at a mean age of 28.8 months. No relationship between the drug and minor malformations was found, but the authors could not exclude the existence of a possible relationship at birth because some minor anomalies disappear with age. Of interest, three infants had severe epicanthal folds, three had true ocular hypertelorism, and all were the offspring of heavy users (more than five joints/week) (68).

A 2004 report from the Atlanta Birth Defects Case–Control Study identified an association between maternal marijuana use and ventricular septal defects (VSD) in the offspring (69). The cases, 122 infants with isolated simple VSD, were compared with 3029 control infants. Maternal marijuana use was determined by self-report combined with paternal proxy-reports of the mother's exposure. The OR for maternal use of marijuana and VSD, after adjustment, was 1.90, 95% CI 1.29–2.81. The risk of VSD increased with regular (≥3 days/week) marijuana use. A similar analysis for heavy (≥10 drinks/week) maternal alcohol consumption produced an OR of 2.10, 95% CI 0.75–5.87 (69).

Strabismus was diagnosed in 24% (7 of 29) of the infants delivered from mothers maintained on methadone throughout pregnancy in a 1987 report (70). This percentage was approximately 4–8 times the expected incidence of the eye defect in the general population. Two (29%) of the seven infants were also exposed in utero to marijuana vs. three (14%) of the nonaffected infants. Although use of other abuse drugs was common, the authors attributed the eye condition to low birth weight and, possibly, an unknown contribution from methadone (70). However, in the Ottawa Prenatal Prospective Study, 35% of the marijuana-exposed infants compared with 6% of the controls had significantly more than one of the following eye problems: myopia, strabismus, abnormal oculomotor functioning, or unusual discs (13). The examiner was blinded to the prenatal histories of the infants.

NEUROBEHAVIOR DEFICITS Significant alterations in neurobehavior in offspring of regular marijuana users were noted in the Ottawa Prenatal Prospective Study (3,5,13,15,71–80). After adjustment for nicotine and alcohol use, in utero exposure to marijuana was associated with increased tremors and exaggerated startles, both spontaneous and in response to minimal stimuli (13,15). Decreased visual responses, including poorer visual habituation to light, were also observed in these infants. In addition, a slight increase in irritability was noted. In early data from the Ottawa group, a distinctive shrill, high-pitched, cat-like cry, reminiscent of the cry considered to be symptomatic of drug withdrawal, was heard from a large number of the offspring of regular users (3). No differences were noted between exposed and nonexposed infants in terms of lateralization, muscle tone, hand-to-mouth behavior, general activity, alertness, or lability of states (3). On follow-up examinations, the abnormalities in neonatal neurobehavior apparently did not result in poorer performance on cognitive and motor tests at 18 and 24 months (13). The investigators cautioned that they were unable to determine whether the follow-up results were truly indicative of a return to normal or were related to insensitivity of the available tests (13).

In a longitudinal analysis of exposed offspring, a series of additional reports from the Ottawa Prenatal Prospective Study appeared covering the period 1989–2001 (71–80). Offspring exposed prenatally to marijuana were evaluated at 9 and 30 days of age (71). Exposure was associated with symptoms similar to those of mild narcotic withdrawal (tremors associated with Moro reflex, increased fine tremor, and startles). Children exposed in utero were evaluated by a series of tests at 12 and 24 months of age (72). A positive association was found between maternal use of marijuana and the cognitive composite score at 12 months but not at 24 months. At 36- and 48-month follow-up, significantly lower scores in verbal and memory were associated with maternal use of the drug during pregnancy (73). However, no association was found with lower verbal or cognitive scores at 60- and 72-month evaluation (74), although in the latter evaluation, a dose–response association was found with a possible deficit in sustained attention and a higher rating by the mothers on the impulsive/hyperactive scale (75). In children 6–9 years of age, parental ratings of behavior problems, visuoperceptual tasks, language comprehension, and distractibility, after adjustment for the home environment condition, were not associated with marijuana exposure (76). No association was found between marijuana and reading or language outcomes in children 9–12 years of age (77). Although subsequent analysis found no association between exposure and global or verbal intelligence, it did find a negative association with executive function tasks that require impulse control and visual analysis/hypothesis testing (78). Prenatal marijuana exposure did not adversely affect basic visuoperceptual tasks in 9–12-year-olds, but a negative association was found with performance in visual problem solving situations (79). This latter finding could be explained by marijuana's negative impact on problem-solving situations requiring integration, analysis, and synthesis (i.e., executive functions) (79). In 13–16-year-olds, prenatal marijuana exposure was associated with the stability of attention over time (increased errors of omissions) (80). This finding was similar to what was found in 6-year-olds (75). Several reviews by the above investigators have summarized their findings (81–86).

A 1984 report examining maternal drinking and neonatal withdrawal found that marijuana use had no effect on the signs of withdrawal in their patients (87). In another study, no increase in startles, tremors, or other neurobehavioral measures at birth was noted in exposed infants (26). Marijuana exposure also had no effect on muscle tone. Evaluation at 1 year of age found no significant differences in growth or in mental and motor development between infants exposed in utero to either none or varying amounts of the drug (26).

A 1994 study of children exposed to marijuana during the 1st and 2nd trimesters found significant negative effects on the performance of 3-year-old children on the Stanford-Binet Intelligence Scale (88). Although the effects were small, they indicated that, on average, exposed children had a lower IQ compared with nonexposed children. In another study, infants were assessed at 9 and 19 months of age (88). At 9 months, 3rd trimester marijuana use (>1 joint/day) was associated with delayed mental development, but not on infants at 19 months of age (89). In a third study from this group, children exposed prenatally were evaluated at 10 years of age (90). A significant relationship between prenatal exposure to marijuana and increased hyperactivity, impulsivity, inattention, increased delinquency, and externalizing problems was found.

Leukemia

The development of leukemia in children exposed to marijuana during gestation was suggested in a 1989 report (91). In a multicenter study conducted between 1980 and 1984 by the Childrens Cancer Study Group, in utero marijuana exposure was significantly related to the development of acute nonlymphoblastic leukemia (ANLL). Of the 204 cases that were analyzed, marijuana use was found in 10 mothers, only 1 of whom used other (LSD) mind-altering drugs. An 11th case mother used methadone. Only 1 of the 203 closely matched healthy controls was exposed to abuse drugs. The 10-fold risk induced by marijuana exposure was statistically significant. The mean age of ANLL diagnosis was significantly younger in the exposed children than in nonexposed children: 37.7 vs. 96.1 months, respectively. Based on the French–American–British system of classification, the morphology of the leukemias also differed significantly, with 70% of the exposed cases presenting with monocytic (M5) or myelomonocytic (M4) morphology compared with 31% of the nonexposed cases. Additionally, only 10% of the exposed children had M1 or M2 (myelocytic) morphology vs. 58% of the nonexposed children. The authors were able to exclude reporting bias but could not exclude the possibility that the association was related to other factors, such as the presence of herbicides or pesticides on the marijuana (91).

Miscellaneous Effects

Early concerns (92,93) that marijuana-induced chromosomal damage could eventually lead to congenital defects have been largely laid to rest (46,55,56). The clinical significance of any drug-induced chromosomal abnormality is doubtful (55). Finally, heavy marijuana use in males has been associated with decreased sperm production (16,93). However, the clinical significance of this finding has been questioned because no evidence indicates that the reduction in sperm counts is related to infertility (16,93).

Review Articles

A number of reviews have examined the conflicting reports on the association between marijuana and developmental toxicity (16,42,43,45–49,52–56,81–86,94–96).

BREASTFEEDING SUMMARY

THC, the main active ingredient of marijuana (cannabis, hashish), is excreted into breast milk (26,49,97,98). Analyses of THC and its two metabolites, 11-hydroxy-THC and 9-carboxy-THC, were conducted on the milk of two women who had been nursing for 7 and 8 months and who smoked marijuana frequently (97). A THC concentration of 105 ng/mL, but no metabolites, was found in the milk of the woman smoking one pipe of marijuana daily. In the second woman, who smoked seven pipes/day, concentrations of THC, 11-hydroxy-THC, and 9-carboxy-THC were 340 ng/mL,

M

4 ng/mL, and none, respectively. The analysis was repeated in the second mother, approximately 1 hour after the last use of marijuana, using simultaneously obtained samples of milk and plasma. Concentrations (in ng/mL) of the active ingredient and metabolites in milk and plasma (ratios shown in parenthesis) were 60.3 and 7.2 (8.4), 1.1 and 2.5 (0.4), and 1.6 and 19 (0.08), respectively. The marked differences in THC found between the milk samples was thought to be related to the amount of marijuana smoked and the interval between smoking and sample collection. A total fecal sample from the infant yielded levels of 347 ng of THC, 67 ng of 11-hydroxy-THC, and 611 ng of 9-carboxy-THC. Because of the large concentration of metabolites, the authors interpreted this as evidence that the nursing infant was absorbing and metabolizing the THC from the milk. Despite the evidence that the fat-soluble THC was concentrated in breast milk, both nursing infants were developing normally (97).

In animals, THC decreases the amount of milk produced by suppressing the production of prolactin and, possibly, by a direct action on the mammary glands (49). Human data on this effect are not available.

Two studies have examined the long-term effects of marijuana exposure on nursing infants (26,98).

A 1985 study evaluated 27 infants at 1 year of age who were exposed to marijuana via the milk (26). Compared with 35 nonexposed infants, no significant differences were found in terms of age at weaning, growth, and mental or motor development. In contrast, a 1990 study that evaluated the development at 1 year of age of 68 breastfed infants exposed to marijuana in the mother's milk in the first month postpartum compared with 68 infants not exposed, found that the exposure appeared to be associated with a decrease in infant motor development (98). Based on these reports, additional research on the long-term effects of marijuana exposure from breast milk is warranted. The American Academy of Pediatrics classifies marijuana as a drug that should not be used by nursing mothers (99).

M

References

1. Gibson GT, Baghurst PA, Colley DP. Maternal alcohol, tobacco and cannabis consumption and the outcome of pregnancy. Aust NZ J Obstet Gynaecol 1983;23:15–9.
2. Fried PA, Watkinson B, Grant A, Knights RM. Changing patterns of soft drug use prior to and during pregnancy: a prospective study. Drug Alcohol Depend 1980;6:323–43.
3. Fried PA. Marihuana use by pregnant women: neurobehavioral effects in neonates. Drug Alcohol Depend 1980;6:415–24.
4. Greenland S, Staisch KJ, Brown N, Gross SJ. The effects of marijuana use during pregnancy. I. A preliminary epidemiologic study. Am J Obstet Gynecol 1982;143:408–13.
5. Fried PA. Marihuana use by pregnant women and effects on offspring: an update. Neurobehav Toxicol Teratol 1982;4:451–4.
6. Rayburn W, Wible-Kant J, Bledsoe P. Changing trends in drug use during pregnancy. J Reprod Med 1982;27:569–75.
7. Greenland S, Richwald GA, Honda GD. The effects of marijuana use during pregnancy. II. A study in a low-risk home-delivery population. Drug Alcohol Depend 1983;11:359–66.
8. Fried PA, Buckingham M, Von Kulmiz P. Marijuana use during pregnancy and perinatal risk factors. Am J Obstet Gynecol 1983;146:992–4.
9. Linn S, Schoenbaum SC, Monson RR, Rosner R, Stubblefield PC, Ryan KJ. The association of marijuana use with outcome of pregnancy. Am J Public Health 1983;73:1161–4.
10. Fried PA, Watkinson B, Willan A. Marijuana use during pregnancy and decreased length of gestation. Am J Obstet Gynecol 1984;150:23–7.
11. Barr HM, Streissguth AP, Martin DC, Herman CS. Infant size at 8 months of age: relationship to maternal use of alcohol, nicotine, and caffeine during pregnancy. Pediatrics 1984;74:336–41.
12. Zuckerman BS, Hingson RW, Morelock S, Amaro H, Frank D, Sorenson JR, Kayne HL, Timperi R. A pilot study assessing maternal marijuana use by urine assay during pregnancy. Natl Inst Drug Abuse Res Monogr Ser 1985;57:84–93.
13. Fried PA. Postnatal consequences of maternal marijuana use. Natl Inst Drug Abuse Res Monogr Ser 1985;59:61–72.
14. Hatch EE, Bracken MB. Effect of marijuana use in pregnancy on fetal growth. Am J Epidemiol 1986;124:986–93.
15. Fried PA, Makin JE. Neonatal behavioural correlates of prenatal exposure to marihuana, cigarettes and alcohol in a low risk population. Neurotoxicol Teratol 1987;9:1–7.
16. Smith CG, Asch RH. Drug abuse and reproduction. Fertil Steril 1987;48:355–73.
17. Kline J, Stein Z, Hutzler M. Cigarettes, alcohol and marijuana: varying associations with birthweight. Int J Epidemiol 1987;16:44–51.
18. Day NL, Wagener DK, Taylor PM. Measurement of substance use during pregnancy: methodologic issues. Natl Inst Drug Abuse Res Monogr Ser 1985;59:36–47.
19. Hingson R, Zuckerman B, Amaro H, Frank DA, Kayne H, Sorenson JR, Mitchell J, Parker S, Morelock S, Timperi R. Maternal marijuana use and neonatal outcome: uncertainty posed by self-reports. Am J Public Health 1986;76:667–9.
20. Little RE, Uhl CN, Labbe RF, Abkowitz JL, Phillips ELR. Agreement between laboratory tests and self-reports of alcohol, tobacco, caffeine, marijuana and other drug use in post-partum women. Soc Sci Med 1986;22:91–8.
21. Fried PA, Barnes MV, Drake ER. Soft drug use after pregnancy compared to use before and during pregnancy. Am J Obstet Gynecol 1985;151:787–92.
22. Blackard C, Tennes K. Human placental transfer of cannabinoids. N Engl J Med 1984;311:797.
23. Busto U, Bendayan R, Sellers EM. Clinical pharmacokinetics of non-opiate abused drugs. Clin Pharmacokinet 1989;16:1–26.
24. Hingson R, Alpert JJ, Day N, Dooling E, Kayne H, Morelock S, Oppenheimer E, Zuckerman B. Effects of maternal drinking and marijuana use on fetal growth and development. Pediatrics 1982;70:539–46.
25. Zuckerman B, Frank DA, Hingson R, Amaro H, Levenson SM, Kayne H, Parker S, Vinci R, Aboagye K, Fried LE, Cabral H, Timperi R, Bauchner H. Effects of maternal marijuana and cocaine use on fetal growth. N Engl J Med 1989;320:762–8.
26. Tennes K, Avitable N, Blackard C, Boyles C, Hassoun B, Holmes L, Kreye M. Marijuana: prenatal and postnatal exposure in the human. Natl Inst Drug Abuse Res Monogr Ser 1985;59:48–60.
27. Greenland S, Staisch KJ, Brown N, Gross SJ. Effects of marijuana on human pregnancy, labor, and delivery. Neurobehav Toxicol Teratol 1982;4:447–50.
28. Braunstein GD, Buster JE, Soares JR, Gross SJ. Pregnancy hormone concentrations in marijuana users. Life Sci 1983;33:195–9.
29. Rosett HL, Weiner L, Lee A, Zuckerman B, Dooling E, Oppenheimer E. Patterns of alcohol consumption and fetal development. Obstet Gynecol 1983;61:539–46.
30. Shiono PM, Klebanoff MA, Nugent RP, Cotch MF, Wilkins DG, Rollins DE, Carey JC, Behrman RE. The impact of cocaine and marijuana use on low birth weight and preterm birth. A multicenter study. Am J Obstet Gynecol 1995;172:19–27.
31. Cornelius MD, Taylor PM, Geva D, Day NL. Prenatal tobacco and marijuana use among adolescents: effect on offspring gestational age, growth, and morphology. Pediatrics 1995;95:738–43.
32. Fried PA, Watkinson B, Gray R. Growth from birth to early adolescence in offspring prenatally exposed to cigarettes and marijuana. Neurotoxicol Teratol 1999;21:513–25.
33. Fergusson DM, Horwood LJ, Northstone K, ALSPAC Team. Maternal use of cannabis and pregnancy outcome. BJOG 2002;109:21–7.
34. Zuckerman B, Alpert JJ, Dooling E, Oppenheimer E, Hingson R, Day N, Rosett H. Substance abuse during pregnancy and newborn size. Pediatr Res 1980;15:524.
35. Qazi QH, Mariano E, Milman DH, Beller E, Crombleholme W. Abnormalities in offspring associated with prenatal marihuana exposure. Dev Pharmacol Ther 1985;8:141–8.
36. Qazi QH, Mariano E, Beller E, Milman DH, Crombleholme W. Abnormalities in offspring associated with prenatal marihuana exposure. Pediatr Res 1983;17:153A.
37. Qazi QH, Milman DH. Nontherapeutic use of psychoactive drugs. N Engl J Med 1983;309:797–8.
38. Sherwood RA, Keating J, Kavvadia V, Greenough A, Peters TJ. Substance misuse in early pregnancy and relationship to fetal outcome. Eur J Pediatr 1999;158:488–92.

39. English DR, Hulse GK, Milne E, Holman CDJ, Bower CI. Maternal cannabis use and birth weight: a meta-analysis. Addiction 1997;92:1553–60.
40. Fried PA, James DS, Watkinson B. Growth and pubertal milestones during adolescence in offspring prenatally exposed to cigarettes and marihuana. Neurotoxicol Teratol 2001;23:431–6.
41. Abel EL. Prenatal exposure to cannabis: a critical review of effects on growth, development, and behavior. Behav Neural Biol 1980;29:137–56.
42. VanBlerk GA, Majerus TC, Myers RAM. Teratogenic potential of some psychopharmacologic drugs: a brief review. Int J Gynaecol Obstet 1980;17:399–402.
43. Lee CC, Chiang CN. Maternal-fetal transfer of abused substances: pharmacokinetic and pharmacodynamic data. Natl Inst Drug Abuse Res Monogr Ser 1985;60:110–47.
44. Shepard TH. *Catalog of Teratogenic Agents*. 5th ed. Baltimore, MD: Johns Hopkins University Press, 1986:353–6.
45. Rennert OM. Drug-induced somatic alterations. Clin Obstet Gynecol 1975;18:185–98.
46. Matsuyama S, Jarvik L. Effects of marihuana on the genetic and immune systems. Natl Inst Drug Abuse Res Monogr Ser 1977;14:179–93.
47. Nahas GG. Current status of marijuana research: symposium on marijuana held July 1978 in Reims, France. JAMA 1979;242:2775–8.
48. Glass L, Evans HE. Perinatal drug abuse. Pediatr Ann 1979;8:84–92.
49. Harclerode J. The effect of marijuana on reproduction and development. Natl Inst Drug Abuse Res Monogr Ser 1980;31:137–66.
50. Chernoff GF, Jones KL. Fetal preventive medicine: teratogens and the unborn baby. Pediatr Ann 1981;10:210–7.
51. Stern L. In vivo assessment of the teratogenic potential of drugs in humans. Obstet Gynecol 1981;58:3S–8S.
52. Shy KK, Brown ZA. Maternal and fetal well-being. West J Med 1984;141:807–15.
53. Tennes K. Effects of marijuana on pregnancy and fetal development in the human. Natl Inst Drug Abuse Res Monogr Ser 1984;44:115–23.
54. Mullins CL, Gazaway PM III. Alcohol and drug use in pregnancy: a case for management. Md Med J 1985;34:991–6.
55. Hollister LE. Health aspects of cannabis. Pharmacol Rev 1986;38:1–20.
56. O'Connor MC. Drugs of abuse in pregnancy—an overview. Med J Aust 1987;147:180–3.
57. Hecht F, Beals RK, Lees MH, Jolly H, Roberts P. Lysergic-acid-diethylamide and cannabis as possible teratogens in man. Lancet 1968;2:1087.
58. Carakushansky G, Neu RL, Gardner LI. Lysergide and cannabis as possible teratogens in man. Lancet 1969;1:150–1.
59. Blanc WA, Mattison DR, Kane R, Chauhan P. L.S.D., intrauterine amputations, and amniotic-band syndrome. Lancet 1971;2:158–9.
60. Gelehrter TD. Lysergic acid diethylamide (LSD) and exstrophy of the bladder. J Pediatr 1970;77:1065–6.
61. Hsu LY, Strauss L, Hirschorn K. Chromosome abnormality in offspring of LSD user. JAMA 1970;211:987–90.
62. Bogdanoff B, Rorke LB, Yanoff M, Warren WS. Brain and eye abnormalities. Am J Dis Child 1972;123:145–8.
63. Jacobson CB, Berlin CM. Possible reproductive detriment in LSD users. JAMA 1972;222:1367–73.
64. Brown R, Pickering D. Persistent transitional circulation. Arch Dis Child 1974;49:883–5.
65. Tenorio GM, Nazvi M, Bickers GH, Hubbird RH. Intrauterine stroke and maternal polydrug abuse. Clin Pediatr 1988;27:565–7.
66. Huff DS, Fernandes M. Two cases of congenital hypothalamic hamartoblastoma, polydactyly, and other congenital anomalies (Pallister-Hall syndrome). N Engl J Med 1982;306:430–1.
67. Lage JM, VanMarter LJ, Bieber FR. Questionable role of amniocentesis in the etiology of amniotic band formation. A case report. J Reprod Med 1988;33:71–3.
68. O'Connell CM, Fried PA. An investigation of prenatal cannabis exposure and minor physical anomalies in a low risk population. Neurobehav Toxicol Teratol 1984;6:345–50.
69. Williams LJ, Correa A, Rasmussen S. Maternal lifestyle factors and risk for ventricular septal defects. Birth Defects Res A Clin Mol Teratol 2004;70: 59–64.
70. Nelson LB, Ehrlich S, Calhoun JH, Matteucci T, Finnegan LP. Occurrence of strabismus in infants born to drug-dependent women. Am J Dis Child 1987;141:175–8.
71. Fried PA, Watkinson B, Dillon RF, Dulberg CS. Neonatal neurological status in a low-risk population after prenatal exposure to cigarettes, marijuana, and alcohol. J Dev Behav Pediatr 1987;8:318–26.
72. Fried PA, Watkinson B. 12- and 24-month neurobehavioural follow-up of children prenatally exposed to marihuana, cigarettes and alcohol. Neurotoxicol Teratol 1988;10:305–13.
73. Fried PA, Watkinson B. 36- and 48-month neurobehavioral follow-up of children prenatally exposed to marijuana, cigarettes, and alcohol. J Dev Behav Pediatr 1990;11:49–58.
74. Fried PA, O'Connell CM, Watkinson B. 60- and 72-month follow-up of children prenatally exposed to marijuana, cigarettes, and alcohol: cognitive and language assessment. J Dev Behav Pediatr 1992;13:383–91.
75. Fried PA, Watkinson B, Gray R. A follow-up study of attentional behavior in 6-year-old children exposed prenatally to marihuana, cigarettes, and alcohol. Neurotoxicol Teratol 1992;14:299–311.
76. O'Connell CM, Fried PA. Prenatal exposure to cannabis: a preliminary report of postnatal consequences in school-age children. Neurotoxicol Teratol 1991;13:631–9.
77. Fried PA, Watkinson B, Siegel LS. Reading and language in 9- to 12-year olds prenatally exposed to cigarettes and marijuana. Neurotoxicol Teratol 1997;19:171–83.
78. Fried PA, Watkinson B, Gray R. Differential effects on cognitive functioning in 9- to 12-year-olds prenatally exposed to cigarettes and marihuana. Neurotoxicol Teratol 1998;20:293–306.
79. Fried PA, Watkinson B. Visuoperceptual functioning differs in 9- to 12-year-olds prenatally exposed to cigarettes and marihuana. Neurotoxicol Teratol 2000;22:11–20.
80. Fried PA, Watkinson B. Differential effects on facets of attention in adolescents prenatally exposed to cigarettes and marihuana. Neurotoxicol Teratol 2001;23:421–30.
81. Fried PA. Cigarettes and marijuana: are there measurable long-term neurobehavioral teratogenic effects? Neurotoxicol 1989;10:577–83.
82. Fried PA. Postnatal consequences of maternal marijuana use in humans. Ann NY Acad Sci 1989;562:123–32.
83. Fried PA. Marijuana use during pregnancy: consequences for the offspring. Seminars Perinatol 1991;15:280–7.
84. Fried PA. Behavioral outcomes in preschool and school-age children exposed prenatally to marijuana: a review and speculative interpretation. NIDA Res Monogr 1996;164:242–60.
85. Fried PA, Smith AM. A literature review of the consequences of prenatal marihuana exposure. An emerging theme of a deficiency in aspects of executive function. Neurotoxicol Teratol 2001;23:1–11.
86. Fried PA. Conceptual issues in behavioral teratology and their application in determining long-term sequelae of prenatal marihuana exposure. J Child Psychol Psychiatry 2002;43:81–102.
87. Coles CD, Smith IE, Fernhoff PM, Falek A. Neonatal ethanol withdrawal: characteristics in clinically normal, nondysmorphic neonates. J Pediatr 1984;105:445–51.
88. Day NL, Richardson GA, Goldschmidt L, Robles N, Taylor PM, Stoffer DS, Cornelius MD, Geva D. Effect of prenatal marijuana exposure on the cognitive development of offspring at age three. Neurotoxicol Teratol 1994;16:169–75.
89. Richardson GA, Day NL, Goldschmidt L. Prenatal alcohol, marijuana, and tobacco use: infant mental and motor development. Neurotoxicol Teratol 1995;17:479–87.
90. Goldschmidt L, Day NL, Richardson GA. Effects of prenatal marijuana exposure on child behavior problems at age 10. Neurotoxicol Teratol 2000;22:325–36.
91. Robison LL, Buckley JD, Daigle AE, Wells R, Benjamin D, Arthur DC, Hammond GD. Maternal drug use and risk of childhood nonlymphoblastic leukemia among offspring: an epidemiologic investigation implicating marijuana (a report from the Childrens Cancer Study Group). Cancer 1989;63:1904–11.
92. Stenchever MA, Kunysz TJ, Allen MA. Chromosome breakage in users of marihuana. Am J Obstet Gynecol 1974;118:106–13.
93. Matsuyama SS, Jarvik LF. Cytogenetic effects of psychoactive drugs. Mod Probl Pharmacopsychiatry 1975;10:99–132.
94. Abel EL. Marihuana and sex: a critical survey. Drug Alcohol Depend 1981;8:1–22.
95. Nahas GG. Cannabis: toxicological properties and epidemiological aspects. Med J Aust 1986;145:82–7.
96. Walker A, Rosenberg M, Balaban-Gil K. Neurodevelopmental and neurobehavioral sequelae of selected substances of abuse and psychiatric medications in utero. Child Adolesc Psychiatr Clin N Am 1999;8:845–67.
97. Perez-Reyes M, Wall ME. Presence of delta-9-tetrahydrocannabinol in human milk. N Engl J Med 1982;307:819–20.
98. Astley SJ, Little RE. Maternal marijuana use during lactation and infant development at one year. Neurotoxicol Teratol 1990;12:161–8.
99. Committee on Drugs, American Academy of Pediatrics. The transfer of drugs and other chemicals into human milk. Pediatrics 2001;108: 776–89.

MAZINDOL

[Withdrawn from the market. See 9th edition.]

MEBENDAZOLE

Anthelmintic

PREGNANCY RECOMMENDATION: Human Data Suggest Low Risk
BREASTFEEDING RECOMMENDATION: Limited Human Data—Probably Compatible

PREGNANCY SUMMARY

A 1985 review of intestinal parasites and pregnancy concluded that treatment of the pregnant patient should only be considered if the "parasite is causing clinical disease or may cause public health problems" (1). When indicated, mebendazole was recommended for the treatment of *Trichuris trichiura* (whipworm) occurring during pregnancy. A 1986 review recommended mebendazole therapy, when indicated, for the treatment of *Ascaris lumbricoides* (roundworm) and *Enterobius vermicularis* (threadworm, seatworm, or pinworm) (2), although another review recommended piperazine for this purpose, despite the known poor absorption of mebendazole (3).

FETAL RISK SUMMARY

Mebendazole is a synthetic anthelminthic agent. Although embryotoxic and teratogenic in rats at single oral doses approximately equal to the human dose based on BSA (4), this effect has not been observed in multiple other animal species (5).

One manufacturer has reports of 1st trimester mebendazole exposure in 170 pregnancies going to term without an identifiable teratogenic risk (4). There was also no increased risk of spontaneous abortion following 1st trimester exposure. Earlier, another manufacturer knew of only one malformation, a digital reduction of one hand, in 112 infants exposed in utero to the drug (6).

In a surveillance study of Michigan Medicaid recipients involving 229,101 completed pregnancies conducted between 1985 and 1992, 64 newborns had been exposed to mebendazole during the 1st trimester (F. Rosa, personal communication, FDA, 1993). Four (6.3%) major birth defects were observed (three expected), one of which was a limb reduction defect (none expected). No anomalies were observed in five other defect categories (cardiovascular defects, oral clefts, spina bifida, polydactyly, and hypospadias) for which specific data were available.

During a 1984 outbreak of trichinosis (*Trichinella spiralis*) in Lebanon, four pregnant patients were treated with mebendazole and corticosteroids (7). Two women, both in the 1st trimester, had miscarriages. The authors did not mention if this was caused by the disease or the drug. Neither fetus was examined. The remaining two patients, both in the 3rd trimester, delivered healthy infants. In a separate case, a pregnant patient, also with trichinosis, was treated with mebendazole and delivered a normal infant (8). The period of pregnancy when the infection and treatment occurred was not specified.

In Sri Lanka, *Necator americanus*, one of the two known causes of hookworm, is endemic and it is an important contributor to iron-deficiency anemia in pregnancy (9). Consequently, the routine use of mebendazole is recommended in the 2nd trimester of pregnancy. A study published in 1999 compared the pregnancy outcomes of women treated with mebendazole (N = 5275) to a control group (N = 1737) that was not treated. There was no significant difference in the rate of major congenital malformations for exposures anytime during pregnancy, 1.8% (97 of 5275) vs. 1.5% (26 of 1737), odds ratio (OR) 1.24, 95% confidence interval (CI) 0.8–1.91. For 1st trimester exposure, the incidence was 2.5% (10 of 407), OR 1.66, 95% CI0.81–3.56, $p = 0.23$. In other comparisons between the two groups, significant decreases occurred in the exposed group in the incidence of stillbirths and perinatal deaths (1.9% vs. 3.3%, $p = 0.0004$), and low (≤1500 g) birth weights (1.1% vs. 2.3%, $p = 0.0003$). The researchers concluded that although there was no significant increase in the number of major defects associated with mebendazole, the agent should not be used during the 1st trimester, and a small increased risk of defects could not be excluded (9).

A 2003 prospective controlled cohort study reported the outcomes of 192 pregnancies exposed to mebendazole, most of which (71.5%) involved 1st trimester exposure (10). The rate of major birth defects, spontaneous abortions, and median birth weight did not differ significantly between the exposed and matched control groups, 3.3% vs. 1.7%, 11.5% vs. 9.4%, and 3222 g vs. 3258 g, respectively. However, more pregnancies were electively terminated in the study group than in controls, 11.5% vs. 1.6%. There was no pattern in the defects to suggest a single cause. Moreover, the timing of the exposures made a causative association with the malformations implausible (10).

BREASTFEEDING SUMMARY

A nursing woman, in her 10th week of lactation, was treated with mebendazole (100 mg twice daily for 3 days) for a roundworm infection (11). Immediately before this, she had been treated for 7 days with metronidazole for genital *Trichomonas vaginalis*. Milk production decreased markedly on the 2nd day of mebendazole therapy and stopped completely within 1 week. Although no mechanism was suggested, the author concluded that the halt in lactation was mebendazole induced.

In contrast to the above report, a 1994 reference described no effect on lactation or breastfeeding in four postpartum women treated with mebendazole, 100 mg twice daily for 3 days, for various intestinal parasites (12). In one of the patients, the maternal plasma concentration of mebendazole at the end of therapy was <20 ng/mL, and milk levels were undetectable. The decreased milk production in the above case was attributed to maternal anxiety from having passed a roundworm per rectum (12).

Based on the more recent data, breastfeeding should not be withheld during mebendazole therapy. Only about 2%–10% of an oral dose is absorbed (13) and, as expected, the amounts of the drug excreted into milk are below the level of detection and appear to be clinically insignificant.

References

1. D'Alauro F, Lee RV, Pao-In K, Khairallah M. Intestinal parasites and pregnancy. Obstet Gynecol 1985;66:639–43.
2. Ellis CJ. Antiparasitic agents in pregnancy. Clin Obstet Gynecol 1986;13:269–75.
3. Leach FN. Management of threadworm infestation during pregnancy. Arch Dis Child 1990;65:399–400.
4. Product information. Vermox. McNeil Consumer, 2000.
5. Beard TC, Rickard MD, Goodman HT. Medical treatment for hydatids. Med J Aust 1978;1:633–5.
6. Shepard TH. *Catalog of Teratogenic Agents*, 8th ed. Baltimore, MD: Johns Hopkins University Press, 1995:261.
7. Blondheim DS, Klein R, Ben-Dror G, Schick G. Trichinosis in southern Lebanon. Isr J Med Sci 1984;20:141–4.
8. Draghici O, Vasadi T, Draghici G, Codrea A, Mihuta A, Dragan S, Biro S, Mocuja D, Mihuja S. Comments with reference to a trichinellosis focus. Rev Ig (Bacteriol) 1976;21:99–104.
9. de Silva NR, Sirisena JLGJ, Gunasekera DPS, Ismail MM, de Silva HJ. Effect of mebendazole therapy during pregnancy on birth outcome. Lancet 1999;353:1145–9.
10. Diav-Citrin O, Shechtman S, Arnon J, Lubart I, Ornoy A. Pregnancy outcome after gestational exposure to mebendazole: a prospective controlled cohort study. Am J Obstet Gynecol 2003;188:282–5.
11. Rao TS. Does mebendazole inhibit lactation? NZ Med J 1983;96:589–90.
12. Kurzel RB, Toot PJ, Lambert LV, Mihelcic AS. Mebendazole and postpartum lactation. NZ Med J 1994;107:439.
13. American Hospital Formulary Service. *Drug Information 1997*. Bethesda, MD: American Society of Health System Pharmacists, 1997:44–6.

MECAMYLAMINE

[Withdrawn from the market. See 9th edition.]

MECHLORETHAMINE

Antineoplastic

PREGNANCY RECOMMENDATION: Contraindicated—1st Trimester
BREASTFEEDING RECOMMENDATION: Contraindicated

PREGNANCY SUMMARY

Mechlorethamine is an alkylating antineoplastic agent. Other agents in this class (e.g., see also Busulfan, Chlorambucil, and Cyclophosphamide) are known to be human teratogens and, combined with the animal data, strongly suggest that mechlorethamine should not be given in the 1st trimester.

FETAL RISK SUMMARY

Mechlorethamine produced congenital malformations in rats and ferrets when given as a single SC injection of 1 mg/kg (2–3 times the maximum recommended human dose) (1).

Mechlorethamine has been used in pregnancy, usually in combination with other antineoplastic drugs. Most reports have not shown an adverse effect in the fetus even when mechlorethamine was given during the 1st trimester (2–6). However, structural anomalies and toxicity were observed in two infants exposed to mechlorethamine during the 1st trimester: oligodactyly of both feet with webbing of the third and fourth toes, four metatarsals on the left, three on the right, bowing of the right tibia, and cerebral hemorrhage (7); and malformed kidneys that were markedly reduced in size and malpositioned (8). The relationship between these outcomes and the drug is uncertain.

Data from one review indicated that 40% of the infants exposed to anticancer drugs were of low birth weight (4). Long-term studies of growth and mental development in offspring exposed to mechlorethamine during the 2nd trimester, the period of neuroblast multiplication, have not been conducted (9).

Ovarian function has been evaluated in 27 women previously treated with mechlorethamine and other antineoplastic drugs (10). Excluding 3 patients who received pelvic radiation, 13 (54%) maintained regular cyclic menses and, overall, 13 normal children were born after therapy. Other successful pregnancies have been reported following combination chemotherapy with mechlorethamine (11–17). Ovarian failure is apparently often gradual in onset and is age related (10). Mechlorethamine therapy in males has been observed to produce testicular germinal cell depletion and azoospermia (15,16,18,19).

Occupational exposure of the mother to antineoplastic agents during pregnancy may present a risk to the fetus. A position statement from the National Study Commission on Cytotoxic Exposure and a research article involving some antineoplastic agents are presented in the monograph for cyclophosphamide (see Cyclophosphamide).

BREASTFEEDING SUMMARY

No reports describing the use of mechlorethamine during lactation have been located. The low molecular weight (about 157 for the free base) suggests that the drug passes into milk. Although it undergoes rapid chemical transformation in water and body fluids, it is not known if exposure to this biologic alkylating agent in breast milk poses a significant risk to a nursing infant. Because of the potential for serious adverse reactions, however, breastfeeding should be discontinued while the mother is receiving therapy.

References

1. Product information. Mustargen. Merck, 2000.
2. Hennessy JP, Rottino A. Hodgkin's disease in pregnancy with a report of twelve cases. Am J Obstet Gynecol 1952;63:756–64.
3. Riva HL, Andreson PS, O'Grady JW. Pregnancy and Hodgkin's disease: a report of eight cases. Am J Obstet Gynecol 1953;66:866–70.
4. Nicholson HO. Cytotoxic drugs in pregnancy: review of reported cases. J Obstet Gynaecol Br Commonw 1968;75:307–12.
5. Jones RT, Weinerman ER. MOPP (nitrogen mustard, vincristine, procarbazine, and prednisone) given during pregnancy. Obstet Gynecol 1979;54:477–8.
6. Johnson IR, Filshie GM. Hodgkin's disease diagnosed in pregnancy: case report. Br J Obstet Gynaecol 1977;84:791–2.
7. Garrett MJ. Teratogenic effects of combination chemotherapy. Ann Intern Med 1974;80:667.
8. Mennuti MT, Shepard TH, Mellman WJ. Fetal renal malformation following treatment of Hodgkin's disease during pregnancy. Obstet Gynecol 1975;46:194–6.
9. Dobbing J. Pregnancy and leukaemia. Lancet 1977;1:1155.
10. Schilsky RL, Sherins RJ, Hubbard SM, Wesley MN, Young RC, DeVita VT Jr. Long-term follow-up of ovarian function in women treated with MOPP chemotherapy for Hodgkin's disease. Am J Med 1981;71:552–6.
11. Ross GT. Congenital anomalies among children born of mothers receiving chemotherapy for gestational trophoblastic neoplasms. Cancer 1976;37:1043–7.
12. Johnson SA, Goldman JM, Hawkins DF. Pregnancy after chemotherapy for Hodgkin's disease. Lancet 1979;2:93.
13. Whitehead E, Shalet SM, Blackledge G, Todd I, Crowther D, Beardwell CG. The effect of combination chemotherapy on ovarian function in women treated for Hodgkin's disease. Cancer 1983;52:988–93.
14. Andrieu JM, Ochoa-Molina ME. Menstrual cycle, pregnancies and offspring before and after MOPP therapy for Hodgkin's disease. Cancer 1983;52:435–8.
15. Dein RA, Mennuti MT, Kovach P, Gabbe SG. The reproductive potential of young men and women with Hodgkin's disease. Obstet Gynecol Surv 1984;39:474–82.
16. Schilsky RL, Lewis BJ, Sherins RJ, Young RC. Gonadal dysfunction in patients receiving chemotherapy for cancer. Ann Intern Med 1980;93:109–14.
17. Shalet SM, Vaughan Williams CA, Whitehead E. Pregnancy after chemotherapy induced ovarian failure. Br Med J 1985;290:898.
18. Sherins RJ, Olweny CLM, Ziegler JL. Gynecomastia and gonadal dysfunction in adolescent boys treated with combination chemotherapy for Hodgkin's disease. N Engl J Med 1978;299:12–6.
19. Sherins RJ, DeVita VT Jr. Effect of drug treatment for lymphoma on male reproductive capacity: studies of men in remission after therapy. Ann Intern Med 1973;79:216–20.

MECLIZINE

Antihistamine/Antiemetic

PREGNANCY RECOMMENDATION: Compatible
BREASTFEEDING RECOMMENDATION: No Human Data—Probably Compatible

PREGNANCY SUMMARY

Meclizine is a piperazine antihistamine that is frequently used as an antiemetic (see also Buclizine and Cyclizine). In general, antihistamines are considered low risk in pregnancy. However, exposure near birth of premature infants has been associated with an increased risk of retrolental fibroplasia.

FETAL RISK SUMMARY

Meclizine is teratogenic in animals, causing cleft palates in rats at 25–50 times the human dose, but apparently not in humans (1). Since late 1962, the question of meclizine's effect on the fetus has been argued in numerous communications, the bulk of which are case reports and letters (2–28). Three studies involving large numbers of patients have concluded that meclizine is not a human teratogen (29–31).

The Collaborative Perinatal Project (CPP) monitored 50,282 mother–child pairs, 1014 of whom had exposure to meclizine in the 1st trimester (29, p. 328). For use anytime during pregnancy, 1463 exposures were recorded (29, p. 437). In neither group was evidence found to suggest a relationship to large categories of major or minor malformations. Several possible associations with individual malformations were found (see below), but their statistical significance is unknown (29, pp. 328, 437, 475). Independent confirmation is required to determine the actual risk.

Respiratory defects (7 cases)
Eye and ear defects (7 cases)
Inguinal hernia (18 cases)
Hypoplasia cordis (3 cases)
Hypoplastic left heart syndrome (3 cases)

The CPP study indicated a possible relationship to ocular malformations, but the authors warned that the results must be interpreted with extreme caution (32). The FDA's

Over-The-Counter Laxative Panel, acting on the data from the CPP study, concluded that meclizine was not teratogenic (33). A second large prospective study covering 613 1st trimester exposures supported these negative findings (30). No harmful effects were found in the exposed offspring as compared with the total sample. Finally, in a 1971 report, significantly fewer infants with malformations were exposed to antiemetics in the 1st trimester as compared with controls (31). Meclizine was the third most commonly used antiemetic.

An association between exposure during the last 2 weeks of pregnancy to antihistamines in general and retrolental fibroplasia in premature infants has been reported. See Brompheniramine for details.

BREASTFEEDING SUMMARY

No reports describing the use of meclizine during lactation have been located. The molecular weight (about 464) is low enough that passage into milk should be anticipated. The potential effects of this exposure on a nursing infant are unknown. Some agents in this class (e.g., see Brompheniramine and Diphenhydramine) have been classified by their manufacturers as contraindicated during nursing because of the increased sensitivity of newborn or premature infants to antihistamines.

References

1. Product information. Antivert. Pfizer, 2000.
2. Watson GI. Meclozine ("Ancoloxin") and foetal abnormalities. Br Med J 1962;2:1446.
3. Smithells RW. "Ancoloxin" and foetal abnormalities. Br Med J 1962;2:1539.
4. Diggorg PLC, Tomkinson JS. Meclozine and foetal abnormalities. Lancet 1962;2:1222.
5. Carter MP, Wilson FW. "Ancoloxin" and foetal abnormalities. Br Med J 1962;2:1609.
6. Macleod M. "Ancoloxin" and foetal abnormalities. Br Med J 1962;2:1609.
7. Lask S. "Ancoloxin" and foetal abnormalities. Br Med J 1962;2:1609.
8. Leck IM. "Ancoloxin" and foetal abnormalities. Br Med J 1962;2:1610.
9. McBride WG. Drugs and foetal abnormalities. Br Med J 1962;2:1681.
10. Fagg CG. "Ancoloxin" and foetal abnormalities. Br Med J 1962;2:1681.
11. Barwell TE. "Ancoloxin" and foetal abnormalities. Br Med J 1962;2:1681–2.
12. Woodall J. "Ancoloxin" and foetal abnormalities. Br Med J 1962;2:1682.
13. McBride WG. Drugs and congenital abnormalities. Lancet 1962;2:1332.
14. Lenz W. Drugs and congenital abnormalities. Lancet 1962;2:1332–3.
15. David A, Goodspeed AH. "Ancoloxin" and foetal abnormalities. Br Med J 1963;1:121.
16. Gallagher C. "Ancoloxin" and foetal abnormalities. Br Med J 1963;1:121–2.
17. Watson GI. "Ancoloxin" and foetal abnormalities. Br Med J 1963;1:122.
18. Mellin GW, Katzenstein M. Meclozine and foetal abnormalities. Lancet 1963;1:222–3.
19. Salzmann KD. "Ancoloxin" and foetal abnormalities. Br Med J 1963;1:471.
20. Burry AF. Meclozine and foetal abnormalities. Br Med J 1963;1:1476.
21. Smithells RW, Chinn ER. Meclozine and foetal abnormalities. Br Med J 1963;1:1678.
22. O'Leary JL, O'Leary JA. Nonthalidomide ectromelia. Report of a case. Obstet Gynecol 1964;23:17–20.
23. Smithells RW, Chinn ER. Meclozine and foetal malformations: a prospective study. Br Med J 1964;1:217–8.
24. Pettersson F. Meclozine and congenital malformations. Lancet 1964;1:675.
25. Yerushalmy J, Milkovich L. Evaluation of the teratogenic effect of meclizine in man. Am J Obstet Gynecol 1965;93:553–62.
26. Sadusk JF Jr, Palmisano PA. Teratogenic effect of meclizine, cyclizine, and chlorcyclizine. JAMA 1965;194:987–9.
27. Lenz W. Malformations caused by drugs in pregnancy. Am J Dis Child 1966;112:99–106.
28. Lenz W. How can the teratogenic action of a factor be established in man? South Med J 1971;64(Suppl 1):41–7.
29. Heinonen OP, Slone D, Shapiro S. *Birth Defects and Drugs in Pregnancy*. Littleton, MA: Publishing Sciences Group, 1977.
30. Milkovich L, Van den Berg BJ. An evaluation of the teratogenicity of certain antinauseant drugs. Am J Obstet Gynecol 1976;125:244–8.
31. Nelson MM, Forfar JO. Associations between drugs administered during pregnancy and congenital abnormalities of the fetus. Br Med J 1971;1:523–7.
32. Shapiro S, Kaufman DW, Rosenberg L, Slone D, Monson RR, Siskind V, Heinonen OP. Meclizine in pregnancy in relation to congenital malformations. Br Med J 1978;1:483.
33. Anonymous. Pink Sheets. Meclizine, cyclizine not teratogenic. FDC Rep 1974;2.

MECLOFENAMATE

Nonsteroidal Anti-inflammatory

PREGNANCY RECOMMENDATION: Human Data Suggest Risk in 1st and 3rd Trimesters
BREASTFEEDING RECOMMENDATION: No Human Data—Probably Compatible

PREGNANCY SUMMARY

Constriction of the ductus arteriosus in utero is a pharmacologic consequence arising from the use of prostaglandin synthesis inhibitors during pregnancy, as is inhibition of labor, prolongation of pregnancy, and suppression of fetal renal function (see also Indomethacin) (1). Persistent pulmonary hypertension of the newborn may occur if these agents are used in the 3rd trimester close to delivery (1,2). Women attempting to conceive should not use any prostaglandin synthesis inhibitor, including meclofenamate, because of the findings in a variety of animal models that indicate these agents block blastocyst implantation (3,4). Moreover, nonsteroid anti-inflammatory drugs (NSAIDs) have been associated with spontaneous abortions (SABs) and congenital malformations. The risk for these defects, however, appears to be small.

FETAL RISK SUMMARY

The NSAID, meclofenamate sodium, is used in the treatment of acute and chronic pain, arthritis, and primary dysmenorrhea. It is in the same NSAID subclass (fenamates) as mefenamic acid.

Reproduction studies in mice, rats, and rabbits during organogenesis found no teratogenic effects (5–7), but postimplantation losses were observed in rats (7). Although apparently not reported, animal reproductive toxicities, such as prolonged gestation, dystocia, intrauterine growth restriction, and decreased fetal and neonatal survival, which were observed with other agents in the class, should also be expected with meclofenamate.

It is not known if meclofenamate crosses the human placenta. The molecular weight of the free acid (about 313) is low enough that passage to the embryo and fetus should be expected.

In a surveillance study of Michigan Medicaid recipients involving 229,101 completed pregnancies conducted between 1985 and 1992, 166 newborns had been exposed to meclofenamate during the 1st trimester (F. Rosa, personal communication, FDA, 1993). Six (3.6%) major birth defects were observed (seven expected), including one cardiovascular defect (two expected) and one oral cleft (three expected). No anomalies were observed in four other categories of defects (spina bifida, polydactyly, limb reduction defects, and hypospadias) for which specific data were available. These data do not support an association between the drug and congenital defects.

A combined 2001 population-based observational cohort study and a case–control study estimated the risk of adverse pregnancy outcome from the use of NSAIDs (8). The use of NSAIDs during pregnancy was not associated with congenital malformations, preterm delivery, or low birth weight, but a positive association was discovered with SABs. A similar study, also published in 2001, failed to find a relationship, in general, between NSAIDs and congenital malformations, but did find a significant association with cardiac defects and orofacial clefts (9). In addition, a 2003 study found a significant association between exposure to NSAIDs in early pregnancy and SABs (10). (See Ibuprofen for details on these three studies.)

A brief 2003 editorial on the potential for NSAID-induced developmental toxicity concluded that NSAIDs, and specifically those with greater COX-2 affinity, had a lower risk of this toxicity in humans than aspirin (11).

Two reviews, both on antirheumatic drug therapy in pregnancy, recommended that if a NSAID was needed, agents with short elimination adult half-lives should be used at the maximum tolerated dosage interval, using the lowest effective dose, and that therapy should be stopped within 8 weeks of the expected delivery date (12,13). Meclofenamate has a short plasma elimination half-life (2 hours), but other factors, such as its toxicity profile, need to be considered.

BREASTFEEDING SUMMARY

No reports describing the use of meclofenamate sodium during lactation have been located. The molecular weight of the free acid (about 313) suggests that the drug will be excreted into breast milk. The effects of this exposure on a nursing infant are unknown, but other NSAIDs are classified as compatible with breastfeeding by the American Academy of Pediatrics (see Ibuprofen and Indomethacin).

References

1. Levin DL. Effects of inhibition of prostaglandin synthesis on fetal development, oxygenation, and the fetal circulation. Semin Perinatol 1980;4:35–44.
2. Van Marter LJ, Leviton A, Allred EN, Pagano M, Sullivan KF, Cohen A, Epstein MF. Persistent pulmonary hypertension of the newborn and smoking and aspirin and nonsteroidal antiinflammatory drug consumption during pregnancy. Pediatrics 1996;97:658–63.
3. Matt DW, Borzelleca JF. Toxic effects on the female reproductive system during pregnancy, parturition, and lactation. In Witorsch RJ, ed. *Reproductive Toxicology*. 2nd ed. New York, NY: Raven Press, 1995:175–93.
4. Dawood MY. Nonsteroidal antiinflammatory drugs and reproduction. Am J Obstet Gynecol 1993;169:1255–65.
5. Product information. Meclomen. Parke-Davis, 1993.
6. Schardein JL, Blatz AT, Woosley ET, Kaump DH. Reproduction studies on sodium meclofenamate in comparison to aspirin and phenylbutazone. Toxicol Appl Pharmacol 1969;15:46–55. As cited in Schardein JL. *Chemically Induced Birth Defects*. 2nd ed. New York, NY: Marcel Dekker, Inc., 1993:131.
7. Petrere JA, Humphrey RR, Anderson JA, Fitzgerald JE, De La Iglesia FA. Studies on reproduction in rats with meclofenamate sodium, a nonsteroidal antiinflammatory agent. Fund Appl Toxicol 1985;5:665–71. As cited in Shepard TH. *Catalog of Teratogenic Agents*. 7th ed. Baltimore, MD: Johns Hopkins University Press, 1992:244–5.
8. Nielsen GL, Sorensen HT, Larsen H, Pedersen L. Risk of adverse birth outcome and miscarriage in pregnant users of non-steroidal anti-inflammatory drugs: population based observational study and case-control study. Br Med J 2001;322:266–70.
9. Ericson A, Kallen BAJ. Nonsteroidal anti-inflammatory drugs in early pregnancy. Reprod Toxicol 2001;15:371–5.
10. Li DK, Liu L, Odouli R. Exposure to non-steroidal anti-inflammatory drugs during pregnancy and risk of miscarriage: population based cohort study. Br Med J 2003;327:368–71.
11. Tassinari MS, Cook JC, Hurtt ME. NSAIDs and developmental toxicity. Birth Defects Res B Dev Reprod Toxicol 2003;68:3–4.
12. Needs CJ, Brooks PM. Antirheumatic medication in pregnancy. Br J Rheumatol 1985;24:282–90.
13. Ostensen M. Optimisation of antirheumatic drug treatment in pregnancy. Clin Pharmacokinet 1994;27:486–503.

MEDROXYPROGESTERONE

Progestogenic Hormone

PREGNANCY RECOMMENDATION: Contraindicated
BREASTFEEDING RECOMMENDATION: Compatible

PREGNANCY SUMMARY

Medroxyprogesterone acetate (MPA) demonstrates dose-related teratogenicity and toxicity in animals. Although the hormone is contraindicated in human pregnancy, inadvertent exposure to therapeutic doses does not appear to represent a significant risk of structural defects. Fetal growth restriction might be a low-risk complication if MPA is administered within 4 weeks of conception. However, confirmation of this finding is needed.

FETAL RISK SUMMARY

MPA is a derivative of progesterone that is available in both parenteral and oral formulations. The indications for this hormone include contraception (either alone or in combination with an estrogen), secondary amenorrhea and abnormal uterine bleeding due to hormonal imbalance in the absence of organic pathology, and in combination with estrogens for the treatment of vasomotor symptoms associated with menopause, vulvar and vaginal atrophy, and the prevention of osteoporosis. There are no pregnancy-related indications for this hormone.

A 1977 report described reproduction tests conducted with MPA in mice, rats, and rabbits (1). In each species, once daily SC doses of 0.1–3000 mg/kg/day were given during organogenesis for 3, 6, or 9 consecutive days. Untreated controls were used for each species. No congenital defects attributable to the hormone were observed in mice and rats. In two breeds of rabbits, however, a dose-related increase in cleft palate was observed at doses of 3, 10, and 30 mg/kg/day. The absence of a significant dose–response relationship at doses >30 mg/kg/day was thought to be due to the mortality caused by the higher doses (1).

In an attempt to explain the teratogenic effects observed in rabbits, the same investigative group examined the binding of MPA to glucocorticoid receptors in appropriate rat and rabbit target tissues (2). Their results indicated that, in rabbits but not in rats, MPA was as effective as natural glucocorticoids in competing for selected binding sites. They theorized that the MPA-induced cleft palates in their original experiment might have been caused by the hormone binding to specific glucocorticoid receptors and by its progestational activity (2).

An experiment to determine a possible mechanism for progestogen-induced hypospadias was reported in 1982 (3). Pregnant rats were given MPA at doses of 1, 10, and 100 times, respectively, the human contraceptive dose equivalent based on body weight (HCDE) on days 13–20 of gestation. Norethisterone, alone or in combination with ethnylestradiol, was also given to other pregnant rats at similar doses. Compared with untreated controls, no effect was observed from these agents on dehydroepiandrosterone metabolism by fetal Wolffian ducts. Inhibition of this testosterone precursor had been shown previously to cause severe hypospadias in male rats and was thought to be a possible mechanism for similar defects in human males (3).

Mice given SC MPA (5–900 mg/kg) before implantation (day 2 of pregnancy) had sporadic increases in dead and resorbed fetuses, decreased fetal weight, and an increase in the incidence of cleft palate and malformed fetuses (4). These effects were not dose-related. Treatment with 30 mg/kg on gestational day 9 was associated with increased rates of respiratory and urinary tract defects. In addition, increased incidences of cleft palate were observed with this dose on several days between gestational days 1 and 12 (4). The methods used in this animal study have been criticized and its findings considered to have questionable relevancy (5) and defended (6).

The fetal effects of IM MPA were studied in pregnant baboons given doses during organogenesis that were 1, 10, and 40 times the HCDE (7). Only the two highest doses were teratogenic, causing anomalies only in the target organs: male external genitalia (short penis, hypospadias, underdeveloped glans and prepuce, bilateral cryptorchidism), female external genitalia (clitoral hypertrophy, labial fusion, female pseudohermaphroditism), and adrenal gland hypoplasia (only at 40 times the HCDE) (7).

Pregnant mice were treated during organogenesis with subdermal pellets that delivered MPA at daily doses 25, 250, and 2500 times the human dose equivalent (HDE) (8). No increase in nongenital malformations was noted at any dose, but the two highest doses caused embryotoxicity (resorptions and decreased weight). In addition, no evidence was found for limb reduction defects even when endochondral bone growth was inhibited (8).

An in vivo model in pregnant mice of intrauterine inflammation was developed using lipopolysaccharide (LPS) from *Escherichia coli* (9). At a gestational length corresponding to about 28–29 weeks in human, the animals were pretreated with either MPA or progesterone before LPS was infused into the uterus. The preterm delivery rates were 91% (LPS alone), 63% (LPS + progesterone), and 0% (LPS + MPA). All of the undelivered fetuses in the first two groups died within 48 hours, whereas most fetuses survived in the LPS + MPA group. The investigators concluded that the progestational and anti-inflammatory properties of MPA prevented inflammation-induced preterm parturition and preserved fetal viability (9).

Although the FDA mandated deletion of pregnancy-related indications from all progestins years ago because of concerns for congenital anomalies, MPA was once used to prevent early abortions. A 1964 report described the use of the hormone for that purpose in 239 women (10). Of the 203 women who went to term, 172 were treated with MPA (oral or IM) before the 12th week of gestation. The average daily dose was 5–50 mg orally with a total dose ranging from <50 to >7000 mg. In six cases, MPA (IM) was the only agent used. Among the 174 infants (2 sets of twins), there were 92 males and 82 females. The outcomes included one stillborn, one newborn with congenital heart disease (no details provided), and one case of mild, transient clitoral enlargement. The infant's mother had received oral MPA 25 mg/day for 7 days during the 6th week of gestation. At 6 months of age, the clitoral hypertrophy had resolved (10).

An unusual cluster of multiple anomalies was observed in a newborn female exposed in utero during the 1st trimester to MPA (for 1st trimester bleeding), lysergic acid diethylamide (LSD), and cigarette smoking (11). The authors of the report could not exclude an autosomal recessive mode of inheritance as a cause of the defects (see Lysergic Acid Diethylamide).

A total of 259 1st trimester exposures to MPA were reported in a 1975 letter (12). Pregnancies exposed to estrogens or progesterones were identified prospectively over a 3-year period (1966–1968). Women were interviewed during pregnancy about early drug use and their outcomes were compared with women who were not exposed to sex hormones. Of those exposed to MPA, 30 infants had congenital malformations, some of which were minor anomalies. Among major defects, there were eight cases involving male genitalia (undescended testis [*N* = 4], hypospadias [*N* = 2], and hydrocele [*N* = 2]), four infants with talipes, two heart defects, and three infants with defects of blood-vessel development (hemangioma, telangiectasia [*N* = 2]). No causal association could be determined because of the nature of indications for the hormones (e.g., threatened or previous abortions) (12).

As of 1981, 14 cases of ambiguous genitalia of the fetus had been reported to the FDA, although the literature is more supportive of the 19-nortestosterone derivatives (see Norethindrone, Norethynodrel) (13). Moreover, a 1979 review proposed that the use of progestins during the 1st trimester was a possible cause of hypospadias (14).

A brief 1982 correspondence described the use of oral MPA (40 mg/day) to support an in vitro fertilization procedure (15). The drug was given for 10 days after fertilization was confirmed and restarted about 3 weeks later for threatened abortion (vaginal bleeding and a fall in basal temperature). The second course was continued until 16 weeks' gestation by menstrual dates. A 2340-g male infant was delivered at term that, except for growth restriction, was otherwise healthy (15). The potential adverse consequences of the drug therapy on female (virilization) and male (hypospadias) fetuses were the subject of later correspondence on this report (16).

The Collaborative Perinatal Project monitored 866 mother–child pairs with 1st trimester exposure to progestational agents, including 130 with exposure to MPA (17, p. 389). An increase in the expected frequency of cardiovascular defects (also see FDA data below) and hypospadias was observed for the progestational agents as a group (17, p. 394). The cardiovascular defects included a ventricular septal defect and tricuspid atresia (18). Reevaluation of these data in terms of timing of exposure, vaginal bleeding in early pregnancy, and previous maternal obstetric history, however, failed to support an association between female sex hormones and cardiac malformations (19). Other studies have also failed to find any relationship with nongenital malformations (20,21).

M

In a surveillance study of Michigan Medicaid recipients involving 229,101 completed pregnancies conducted between 1985 and 1992, 407 newborns had been exposed to MPA during the 1st trimester (F. Rosa, personal communication, FDA, 1993). A total of 15 (3.7%) major birth defects were observed (13 expected), including (observed/expected) 7/4 cardiovascular defects and 1/1 oral clefts. No malformations were observed in four other defect categories (spina bifida, polydactyly, limb reduction defects, and hypospadias) for which specific data were available. Only the number of cardiovascular defects is suggestive of an association, but other factors, including the mother's disease, concurrent drug use, and chance, may be involved.

One infant of a set of triplets was found to have an additional lumbar rib and hemi vertebrae at two levels of the spinal column (22). In addition, the infant had a small, deformed right ear. The pregnancy had resulted from in vitro fertilization following ovulation induction with clomiphene citrate. Because of threatened abortion, the mother had been treated with oral MPA (80 mg/day) from the 4th week after embryo transfer throughout the 30 weeks' gestation. The authors thought the combination of ear, spinal, and rib malformations was probably consistent with the Goldenhar syndrome (oculoauriculovertebral anomaly) (22).

A 1985 study described 2754 infants born to mothers who had vaginal bleeding during the 1st trimester (23). Of the total group, 1608 of the newborns were delivered from mothers treated during the 1st trimester with either oral MPA (20–30 mg/day), 17-hydroxyprogesterone (500 mg/week by injection), or a combination of the two. MPA was used exclusively in 1274 (79.2%) of the study group. The control group consisted of 1146 infants delivered from mothers who bled during the 1st trimester but who were not treated. There were no differences between the study and control groups in the overall rate of malformations (120 vs. 123.9/1000, respectively) or in the rate of major malformations (63.4 vs. 71.5/1000, respectively) (23). Another 1985 study compared 988 infants exposed in utero to various progesterones with a matched cohort of 1976 unexposed controls (24). Only 60 infants were exposed to MPA. No association between progestins, primarily progesterone and 17-hydroxyprogesterone, and fetal malformations was discovered.

A 1988 report from Thailand described the outcomes of pregnancies of 1229 women who had used MPA before the index pregnancy compared with 4023 women who had used no contraception (controls) and 3038 who had used oral contraceptives (pill) (25). No differences were observed between the groups in terms of stillbirths, multiple pregnancies, or birth weight. Women who had used MPA had a similar incidence of major and minor malformations and deformations as controls, but both groups had significantly increased incidences of these outcomes compared with pill users. There was a significantly increased association of polysyndactyly in the MPA group compared with the other two groups (rate per 1000: 8.1 vs. 1.7 and 1.2). However, only 3 of the 10 cases had exposure to MPA during gestation and in 5 cases, the last injection of the hormone had occurred more than 9 months before conception. Thus, a causal association between MPA and syndactyly was thought to be unlikely. Another unexpected finding was an increase in the number of chromosomal anomalies ($N = 5$) found in the MPA group relative to the controls ($N = 3$) and pill users ($N = 2$). Adjustment by maternal age did not affect these results. Because of the unrelated nature of the defects, the lack of confirming studies, and the distant timing of the exposure in some cases, the authors concluded that the association had occurred by chance (25).

Using the same population base as above, the same investigators studied the effects of in utero exposure to steroid contraceptives on birth weight (26). A total of 1573 pregnancies were exposed to injectable MPA (830 accidental pregnancies and 743 infants conceived before the use of the steroid), 601 to oral contraceptives, and 2578 planned pregnancies (controls). Both the injectable and oral contraceptive groups had increased risks for low-birth-weight infants (<2500 g), but this result was thought to be partial due to confounders. However, the risk of low-birth-weight infants was significantly increased in accidental pregnancies when MPA was given within 4 weeks of conception (odds ratio [OR] 1.9, 95% confidence interval [CI] 1.4–3.2) (26). The researchers then investigated the effect of steroid contraceptives on neonatal and infant survival (27). As above, three groups were formed consisting of 1431 children of women who had received injectable MPA during pregnancy, 565 children exposed in utero to oral contraceptives, and 2307 control infants with no exposure to hormonal contraceptives. After adjustment (including adjustment for birth weight), the neonatal and infant death rates in those exposed to MPA were nonsignificant. However, there was a relation between shorter injection-to-conception intervals and an increased risk of death: OR 2.5 (95% CI 1.1–5.7), interval ≤4 weeks; OR 2.1 (95% CI 1.0–4.6), interval 5–8 weeks, and OR 0.9 (95% CI 0.4–2.4), interval ≥9 weeks

(27). The investigators concluded that infants of pregnancies that occur 1–2 months after an injection of MPA might be at increased risk of low birth weight and death (26,27).

A commentary on the methodology used in the above two studies raised concerns about the validity of the results (28). In particular, criticism involved the comparison groups, establishing the timing of conception, and the biologic plausibility of the effects on birth weight. The authors, however, defended the methods used in the studies and their findings (29).

In the fourth study from the research group in Thailand, no increased risk of impaired growth in height, after adjustment for socioeconomic factors, was found in children (up to the age of 17 years) exposed to MPA during pregnancy (*N* = 1207) and/or during breastfeeding (*N* = 1215) (30). However, there was a delay in the onset of reported pubic hair growth among girls exposed to MPA during pregnancy. No other effects on attainment of puberty (i.e., menarche and breast development) were observed (30).

Another 1988 report focused on the potential teratogenicity of MPA (31). Three groups of women were formed: subfertile women with a history of recurrent spontaneous abortion (*N* = 180) or threatened abortion (*N* = 269), and matched subfertile controls (*N* = 464). The women in the first groups were treated with oral MPA (80–120 mg/day) from the 5th or 7th week of pregnancy until the 18th week. The number of pregnancies in each group was 199, 309, and 508, respectively, and the total number of infants was 161, 205, and 428, respectively. Early pregnancy wastage was high in all groups. Congenital malformations were noted in 15/366 (4.1%) in the treated groups and 15/428 (3.5%) in the controls (difference not significant). Of note, there were two cases of hypospadias, one in the treated group and one in controls. The investigators concluded that MPA was not teratogenic (31).

A possible association between MPA and epispadias, with or without bladder exstrophy, was reported in 1991 (32). Among 20,650 infants delivered at one hospital over a 5-year period, 4 male infants had epispadias and 2 of the 4 also had bladder exstrophy. In each case, MPA had been given to the mother to prevent 1st trimester threatened abortion. The infants were delivered at term with a mean birth weight of 2980 g. The cluster of these rare defects suggested to the authors that a relationship to the drug was possible (32).

BREASTFEEDING SUMMARY

Medroxyprogesterone (MPA) has not been shown to affect lactation adversely (33,34). A 1981 review concluded that use of the drug by the mother would not have a significant effect on the nursing infant (35). Milk production and duration of lactation may be increased if the drug is given in the puerperium. This effect might be secondary to the increase in basal serum prolactin levels that has been shown to occur with depot-MPA (36). If breastfeeding is desired, MPA may be used safely (37,38). A 1996 study found no effect on the urine hormonal profiles of male infants nursing from mothers receiving a depot injection of MPA (38). The American Academy of Pediatrics classifies MPA as compatible with breastfeeding (39).

References

1. Andrew FD, Staples RE. Prenatal toxicity of medroxyprogesterone acetate in rabbits, rats, and mice. Teratology 1977;15:25–32.
2. Kimmel GL, Hartwell BS, Andrew FD. A potential mechanism in medroxyprogesterone acetate teratogenesis. Teratology 1979;19:171–6.
3. Briggs MH. Hypospadias, androgen biosynthesis, and synthetic progestogens during pregnancy. Int J Fertil 1982;27:70–2.
4. Eibs HG, Spielmann H, Hagele M. Teratogenic effects of cyproterone acetate and medroxyprogesterone treatment during the pre- and postimplantation period of mouse embryos. I. Teratology 1982;25:27–36.
5. Marks TA. Comments on two recent papers dealing with the teratogenicity of medroxyprogesterone acetate. Teratology 1984;31:313–5.
6. Spielmann H. Reply to comments on two articles dealing with the teratogenicity of cyproterone acetate (CA) and medroxyprogesterone acetate (MPA). Teratology 1985;32:319–20.
7. Prahalada S, Carroad E, Hendrickx AG. Embryotoxicity and maternal serum concentrations of medroxyprogesterone acetate (MPA) in baboons (*Papio cynocephalus*). Contraception 1985;32:497–515.
8. Carbone JP, Figurska K, Buck S, Brent RL. Effect of gestational sex steroid exposure on limb development and endochondral ossification in the pregnant C57B1/6J mouse: I. Medroxyprogesterone acetate. Teratology 1990;42:121–30.
9. Elovitz M, Wang Z. Medroxyprogesterone acetate, but not progesterone, protects against inflammation-induced parturition and intrauterine fetal demise. Am J Obstet Gynecol 2004;190:693–701.
10. Burstein R, Wasserman HC. The effect of Provera on the fetus. Obstet Gynecol 1964;23:931–4.
11. Eller JL, Morton JM. Bizarre deformities in offspring of user of lysergic acid diethylamide. N Engl J Med 1970;283:395–7.
12. Harlap S, Prywes R, Davies AM. Birth defects and oestrogens and progesterones in pregnancy. Lancet 1975;1:682–3.
13. Dayan E, Rosa FW. Fetal ambiguous genitalia associated with sex hormones use early in pregnancy. Food and Drug Administration, Division of Drug Experience. ADR Highlights 1981:1–14.
14. Aarskog D, Maternal progestins as a possible cause of hypospadias. N Engl J Med 1979;300:75–8.
15. Yovich J, Puzey A, De'Atta R, Roberts R, Reid S, Grauaug A. In-vitro fertilisation pregnancy with early progestogen support. Lancet 1982;2:378–9.
16. Barlow SM. Medroxyprogesterone in in-vitro fertilisation. Lancet 1982;2:1408.
17. Heinonen OP, Slone D, Shapiro S. *Birth Defects and Drugs in Pregnancy*. Littleton, MA: Publishing Sciences Group, 1977.
18. Heinonen OP, Slone D, Monson RR, Hook EB, Shapiro S. Cardiovascular birth defects and antenatal exposure to female sex hormones. N Engl J Med 1977;296:67–70.
19. Wiseman RA, Dodds-Smith IC. Cardiovascular birth defects and antenatal exposure to female sex hormones: a reevaluation of some base data. Teratology 1984;30:359–70.
20. Wilson JG, Brent RL. Are female sex hormones teratogenic? Am J Obstet Gynecol 1981;141:567–80.
21. Dahlberg K. Some effects of depo-medroxyprogesterone acetate (DMPA): observations in the nursing infant and in the long-term user. Int J Gynaecol Obstet 1982;20:43–8.
22. Yovich JL, Stanger JD, Grauaug AA, Lunay GG, Hollingsworth P, Mulcahy MT. Fetal abnormality (Goldenhar syndrome) occurring in one of triplet infants derived from in vitro fertilization with possible monozygotic twinning. J In Vitro Fert Embryo Transf 1985;2:27–32.
23. Katz Z, Lancet M, Skornik J, Chemke J, Mogilner BM, Klinberg M. Teratogenicity of progestogens given during the first trimester of pregnancy. Obstet Gynecol 1985;65:775–80.
24. Resseguie LJ, Hick JF, Bruen JA, Noller KL, O'Fallon WM, Kurland LT. Congenital malformations among offspring exposed in utero to progestins, Olmsted County, Minnesota, 1936–74. Fertil Steril 1985;43:514–9.
25. Pardthaisong T, Gray RH, McDaniel EB, Chandacham A. Steroid contraceptive use and pregnancy outcome. Teratology 1988;38:51–8.
26. Pardthaisong T, Gray RH. In utero exposure to steroid contraceptives and outcome of pregnancy. Am J Epidemiol 1991;134:795–803.
27. Gray RH, Pardthaisong T. In utero exposure to steroid contraceptives and survival during infancy. Am J Epidemiol 1991;134:804–11.
28. Hogue CJR. Invited commentary: the contraceptive technology tightrope. Am J Epidemiol 1991;134:812–5.

29. Gray RH, Pardthaisong T. The author's response to Hogue. Am J Epidemiol 1991;134:816–7.
30. Pardthaisong T, Yenchit C, Gray R. The long-term growth and development of children exposed to Depo-Provera during pregnancy and lactation. Contraception 1992;45:313–24.
31. Yovich JL, Turner SR, Draper R. Medroxyprogesterone acetate therapy in early pregnancy has no apparent fetal effects. Teratology 1988;38:135–44.
32. Blickstein I, Katz Z. Possible relationship of bladder exstrophy and epispadias with progestins taken during early pregnancy. Br J Urol 1991;68:105–6.
33. Guiloff E, Ibarra-Polo A, Zanartu J, Toscanini C, Mischler TW, Gomez-Rogers C. Effect of contraception on lactation. Am J Obstet Gynecol 1974;118:42–5.
34. Karim M, Ammar R, El Mahgoub S, El Ganzoury B, Fikri F, Abdou Z. Injected progesterone and lactation. Br Med J 1971;1:200–3.
35. Schwallie PC. The effect of depot-medroxyprogesterone acetate on the fetus and nursing infant: a review. Contraception 1981;23:375–86.
36. Ratchanon S, Taneepanichskul S. Depot medroxyprogesterone acetate and basal serum prolactin levels in lactating women. Obstet Gynecol 2000;96:926–8.
37. Sapire KE, Dommisse J. Injectable contraception and lactation. S Afr Med J 1995;85:1302–3.
38. Virutamasen P, Leepipatpaiboon S, Kriengsinyot R, Vichaidith P, Ndavi Muia P, Sekadde-Kigondu CB, Mati JKG, Forest MG, Dikkeschei LD, Wolthers BG, d'Arcangues C. Pharmacodynamic effects of depot-medroxyprogesterone acetate (DMPA) administered to lactating women on their male infants. Contraception 1996;54:153–7.
39. Committee on Drugs, American Academy of Pediatrics. The transfer of drugs and other chemicals into human milk. Pediatrics 2001;108:776–89.

MEFENAMIC ACID

Nonsteroidal Anti-inflammatory

PREGNANCY RECOMMENDATION: Human Data Suggest Risk in 1st and 3rd Trimesters
BREASTFEEDING RECOMMENDATION: Limited Human Data—Probably Compatible

PREGNANCY SUMMARY

Constriction of the ductus arteriosus in utero is a pharmacologic consequence arising from the use of prostaglandin synthesis inhibitors during pregnancy, as is inhibition of labor, prolongation of pregnancy, and suppression of fetal renal function (see also Indomethacin) (1). Persistent pulmonary hypertension of the newborn may occur if these agents are used in the 3rd trimester close to delivery (1,2). Women attempting to conceive should not use any prostaglandin synthesis inhibitor, including mefenamic acid, because of the findings in a variety of animal models that indicate these agents block blastocyst implantation (3,4). Moreover, nonsteroidal anti-inflammatory drugs (NSAIDs) have been associated with spontaneous abortions (SABs) and congenital malformations. The risk for these defects, however, appears to be small.

M

FETAL RISK SUMMARY

Mefenamic acid, a NSAID, is used for the short-term treatment of pain and for primary dysmenorrhea. It is in the same NSAID subclass (fenamates) as meclofenamate.

Although mefenamic acid causes toxic effects in pregnant animals similar to those produced by other agents in this class (decreased fertility, delayed parturition, increase in the number of resorptions, and decreased pup survival), no congenital malformations were observed in studies involving rats, rabbits, and dogs at doses up to 10 times those used in humans (5). In one study of pregnant rats, inhibition of parturition by mefenamic acid appeared to be dose-related (6).

Consistent with its low molecular weight (about 241), mefenamic acid crosses the human placenta to the fetus. Fetal concentrations of the drug, 40–180 minutes after a 500-mg dose administered to 13 women at 15–22 weeks' gestation, were 32%–54% of the maternal plasma concentrations (7).

A combined 2001 population-based observational cohort study and a case–control study estimated the risk of adverse pregnancy outcome from the use of NSAIDs (8). The use of NSAIDs during pregnancy was not associated with congenital malformations, preterm delivery, or low birth weight, but a positive association was discovered with SABs. A similar study, also published in 2001, failed to find a relationship, in general, between NSAIDs and congenital malformations, but did find a significant association with cardiac defects and orofacial clefts (9). In addition, a 2003 study found a significant association between exposure to NSAIDs in early pregnancy and SABs (10). (See Ibuprofen for details on these three studies.)

A brief 2003 editorial on the potential for NSAID-induced developmental toxicity concluded that NSAIDs, and specifically those with greater COX-2 affinity, had a lower risk of this toxicity in humans than aspirin (11).

Mefenamic acid, 500 mg 3 times a day, was used as a tocolytic in a double-blind, randomized human study (12). Compared with controls, preterm delivery occurred less in the mefenamic acid group (15% vs. 40%, $p < 0.005$), and birth weights were higher. No adverse effects were observed in the newborns exposed in utero to mefenamic acid.

An infant, delivered by urgent cesarean section at 34 weeks' gestation, had marked cyanosis after in utero exposure to mefenamic acid used to prevent premature delivery (13). Echocardiography of the infant demonstrated a small (1- to 2-mm) patent ductus arteriosus. The authors concluded that the maternal drug therapy was responsible for the premature closure of the ductus.

BREASTFEEDING SUMMARY

Small amounts of mefenamic acid are excreted into breast milk and absorbed by the nursing infant (14). Ten nursing mothers in the immediate postpartum period were given a 500-mg oral loading dose followed by 250 mg 3 times daily for 3 days. Blood and milk samples were obtained 2 hours after the first daily dose on postpartum days 2–4. Blood and urine samples were obtained from the infants 1 hour after nursing on postpartum day 4. The averages of the mean daily concentrations of mefenamic acid in maternal plasma and milk were 0.94 and 0.17 mcg/mL, respectively, corresponding to a milk:plasma ratio of 0.18. In three of the mothers, breast milk concentrations of mefenamic acid plus metabolites ranged from 0.62 to 1.99 mcg/mL. The mean infant blood concentration of mefenamic acid was 0.08 mcg/mL, whereas the mean urine concentration of mefenamic acid plus metabolites was 9.8 mcg/mL (14).

One reviewer concluded that because of the potential toxicity of mefenamic acid, other agents (diclofenac, fenoprofen, flurbiprofen, ibuprofen, ketoprofen, ketorolac, and tolmetin) were safer alternatives if a NSAID was required during nursing (15). However, the American Academy of Pediatrics classifies mefenamic acid as usually compatible with breastfeeding (16).

References

1. Levin DL. Effects of inhibition of prostaglandin synthesis on fetal development, oxygenation, and the fetal circulation. Semin Perinatol 1980;4:35–44.
2. Van Marter LJ, Leviton A, Allred EN, Pagano M, Sullivan KF, Cohen A, Epstein MF. Persistent pulmonary hypertension of the newborn and smoking and aspirin and nonsteroidal antiinflammatory drug consumption during pregnancy. Pediatrics 1996;97:658–63.
3. Matt DW, Borzelleca JF. Toxic effects on the female reproductive system during pregnancy, parturition, and lactation. In Witorsch RJ, ed. *Reproductive Toxicology*. 2nd ed. New York, NY: Raven Press, 1995:175–93.
4. Dawood MY. Nonsteroidal antiinflammatory drugs and reproduction. Am J Obstet Gynecol 1993;169:1255–65.
5. Product information. Ponstel. Parke-Davis, 1995.
6. Powell JG Jr, Cochrane RL. The effects of a number of non-steroidal anti-inflammatory compounds on parturition in the rat. Prostaglandins 1982;23:469–88.
7. MacKenzie IZ, Graf AK, Mitchell MD. Prostaglandins in the fetal circulation following maternal ingestion of a prostaglandin synthetase inhibitor during mid-pregnancy. Int J Gynaecol Obstet 1985;23:455–8.
8. Nielsen GL, Sorensen HT, Larsen H, Pedersen L. Risk of adverse birth outcome and miscarriage in pregnant users of non-steroidal anti-inflammatory drugs: population based observational study and case-control study. Br Med J 2001;322:266–70.
9. Ericson A, Kallen BAJ. Nonsteroidal anti-inflammatory drugs in early pregnancy. Reprod Toxicol 2001;15:371–5.
10. Li DK, Liu L, Odouli R. Exposure to non-steroidal anti-inflammatory drugs during pregnancy and risk of miscarriage: population based cohort study. Br Med J 2003;327:368–71.
11. Tassinari MS, Cook JC, Hurtt ME. NSAIDs and developmental toxicity. Birth Defects Res B Dev Reprod Toxicol 2003;68:3–4.
12. Mital P, Garg S, Khuteta RP, Khuteta S, Mital P. Mefenamic acid in prevention of premature labor. J R Soc Health 1992;112:214–6.
13. Menahem S. Administration of prostaglandin inhibitors to the mother; the potential risk to the fetus and neonate with duct-dependent circulation. Reprod Fertil Dev 1991;3:489–94.
14. Buchanan RA, Eaton CJ, Koeff ST, Kinkel AW. The breast milk excretion of mefenamic acid. Curr Ther Res Clin Exp 1968;10:592–6.
15. Anderson PO. Medication use while breast feeding a neonate. Neonatal Pharmacol Q 1993;2:3–14.
16. Committee on Drugs, American Academy of Pediatrics. The transfer of drugs and other chemicals into human milk. Pediatrics 2001;108:776–89.

MEFLOQUINE

Antimalarial

PREGNANCY RECOMMENDATION: Compatible
BREASTFEEDING RECOMMENDATION: Limited Human Data—Probably Compatible

PREGNANCY SUMMARY

Mefloquine is a quinoline-methanol antimalarial agent used in the prevention and treatment of malaria caused by *Plasmodium falciparum*, including chloroquine-resistant strains, or by *Plasmodium vivax*. If indicated, mefloquine should not be withheld in pregnancy because the maternal and embryo–fetal risk from malaria far outweighs the unknown potential of developmental toxicity.

FETAL RISK SUMMARY

At high doses (80–160 mg/kg/day), mefloquine is teratogenic in mice, rats, and rabbits, and, at one dose (160 mg/kg/day), it is embryotoxic in rabbits (1). Smaller doses (20–50 mg/kg/day) impaired fertility in rats, but no adverse effect was observed on spermatozoa in humans taking 250 mg/week for 22 weeks (1).

A study published in 1990 examined the pharmacokinetics of mefloquine during the 3rd trimester of pregnancy (2). Twenty women were treated with either 250 mg of mefloquine base (N = 10) or 125 mg of base (N = 10) weekly until delivery at term. Peak and trough concentrations of mefloquine were lower than those measured in nonpregnant adults, and the terminal elimination half-life was 11.6 days. The half-life reported in nonpregnant adults is 15–33 days (1). No obstetric complications were observed at either dosage level, including during labor, and no toxicity was observed in the exposed infants. Normal infant development was observed during a 2-year follow-up.

The risks of complications from malarial infection occurring during pregnancy are increased, especially in women not living in endemic areas (i.e., nonimmune women) (3–6). Infection is associated with a number of severe maternal and fetal outcomes: maternal death, anemia, abortion, stillbirth, prematurity, low birth weight, fetal distress, and congenital malaria (3–7). However, one of these outcomes, low birth weight with the resulting increased risk of infant mortality, may have other causes inasmuch as it has not been established that antimalarial chemoprophylaxis can prevent this complication (4). Increased maternal morbidity and mortality includes adult respiratory distress syndrome, pulmonary edema, massive hemolysis, disseminated intravascular coagulation, acute renal failure, and hypoglycemia (5–7). Severe *P. falciparum* malaria in pregnant nonimmune women has a poor prognosis and may be associated with asymptomatic uterine contractions, intrauterine growth restriction, fetal tachycardia, fetal distress, placental insufficiency because of intense parasitization, and hypoglycemia (4,7). The exacerbation of this latter adverse effect has not been reported with mefloquine (7), but it occurs frequently with quinine (7–9). Because of the severity of this disease in pregnancy, chemoprophylaxis is recommended for women of childbearing age traveling in areas where malaria is present (3–5). However, some authors state that mefloquine should not be used for prophylaxis during pregnancy, especially during the 1st trimester, because of the potential for fetotoxicity (3–5,7,10–14), except in areas where chloroquine-resistant *P. falciparum* is present (11). An editorial comment to one reference stated that recent data indicated the use of mefloquine during early pregnancy could result in congenital defects, but no other information was provided (15).

Two reports have described the therapeutic use of mefloquine during pregnancy without causing adverse fetal effects (4,16). A 24-year-old woman presented at 33 weeks' gestation with fever, scleral icterus, and tender splenomegaly secondary to *P. falciparum* infection involving 3% of her erythrocytes (16). After two attempts to administer doses of mefloquine (750 and 500 mg), both of which were vomited, predosing with IV metoclopramide allowed the woman to tolerate three 250-mg doses spaced 4 hours apart and two 250-mg doses the following day (total dose 1250 mg). Maternal fever resolved the day after therapy and, at 5 days, no parasites were observed in the mother's blood. Two months later, a 3405-g infant (sex not specified) was delivered by cesarean section for pelvic disproportion and poor beat-to-beat fetal heart rate variability. Apgar scores at 1 and 5 minutes were 6 and 9, respectively. The child was developing normally at 2 months.

An unpublished double-blind, randomized controlled study from Thailand conducted between 1983 and 1989 was briefly described in a World Health Organization (WHO) publication (4) and a 1993 review (13). A total of 178 pregnant women were randomized to two groups; one group received mefloquine 500 mg every 8 hours for two doses (*N* = 87), and the other group received quinine 600 mg every 8 hours for 7 days (*N* = 91). Although the exact stages of pregnancy at the time of treatment were not specified, a small number of the women in the mefloquine group were in the 1st trimester (4,13). All of the women were followed to term. The incidence of uterine contractions, premature labor, and fetal distress in the mefloquine and quinine groups were 18% vs. 25%, 1% vs. 5%, and 2% vs. 4%, respectively (4). None of the differences was statistically significant. No stillbirths occurred, but one spontaneous abortion was observed in each group, 21 days after mefloquine and 37 days after quinine; neither was thought to be related to drug treatment (4). The 21-day cure rate was 97% among those treated with mefloquine compared with 86% of those treated with quinine. Three newborns had congenital malformations, but these were believed to be unrelated to the drug therapy (13). The study investigators concluded that the therapeutic use of mefloquine during pregnancy was safe and effective. The WHO Scientific Group concluded, however, that because of the small number of patients, treatment with mefloquine should be undertaken cautiously during the first 12–14 weeks of gestation (4).

Two trials of mefloquine prophylaxis in pregnancy were reviewed in a 1993 reference (13). An unpublished study compared weekly prophylaxis with either mefloquine (*N* = 468) or chloroquine (*N* = 1312) in asymptomatic pregnant women (13). Mefloquine was more effective than chloroquine in preventing fetal growth restriction and was also effective in reducing placental *P. falciparum* infections. In another double-blind, placebo-controlled trial, prophylaxis during the second half of pregnancy with 250 mg/week for 1 month followed by 125 mg/week until delivery in 360 Karen women (living on the Thailand–Burma border) was 95% effective in preventing malaria (13). The incidence of stillbirths was similar between mefloquine (*N* = 4) and placebo (*N* = 5).

A presentation made at a 1991 conference described the follow-up of 98 prospectively recorded pregnancy exposures to mefloquine (17). Five diverse congenital malformations were observed, an incidence that does not support mefloquine-induced teratogenicity.

BREASTFEEDING SUMMARY

Mefloquine is excreted into human milk (1,18). Two women, who were not breastfeeding, were given a single 250-mg dose, 2–3 days after delivery (18). Milk samples were collected from both women during the first 4 days after dosing, and from one woman at various intervals up to 56 days. The milk:plasma ratios in the two women during the first 4 days were 0.13 and 0.16, respectively. In one woman, the ratio was 0.27 calculated over 56 days. The investigators estimated that a 4-kg infant consuming 1000 mL of milk daily would ingest 0.08 mg/day of the mother's dose (18), or approximately 4% of the dose would be recovered from the milk (1,18). Although these amounts are not thought to be harmful to the nursing infant, they are insufficient to provide adequate protection against malaria (3).

Long-term effects of mefloquine exposure via breast milk have not been studied. Because the antimalarial agent has a long plasma half-life, averaging nearly 12 days during pregnancy (2) and 14.4–18.0 days during and after lactation (18), weekly prophylactic doses of mefloquine will result in continuous exposure of a nursing infant. Moreover, higher milk concentrations of mefloquine than those reported should be expected after therapeutic or weekly prophylactic doses (18).

References

1. Product information. Lariam. Roche Laboratories, 1993.
2. Nosten F, Karbwang J, White NJ, Honeymoon, Na Bangchang K, Bunnag D, Harinasuta T. Mefloquine antimalarial prophylaxis in pregnancy: dose finding and pharmacokinetic study. Br J Clin Pharmacol 1990;30:79–85.
3. Centers for Disease Control. Recommendations for the prevention of malaria among travelers. MMWR 1990;39:1–10.
4. World Health Organization. Practical chemotherapy of malaria. WHO Tech Rep Ser 1990;805:1–141.
5. Subramanian D, Moise KJ Jr, White AC Jr. Imported malaria in pregnancy: report of four cases and review of management. Clin Infect Dis 1992;15:408–13.
6. World Health Organization. Severe and complicated malaria. Trans R Soc Trop Med Hyg 1990;84(Suppl 2):1–65.
7. Nathwani D, Currie PF, Douglas JG, Green ST, Smith NC. *Plasmodium falciparum* malaria in pregnancy: a review. Br J Obstet Gynaecol 1992;99: 118–21.

8. Phillips RE, Looareesuwan S, White NJ, Silamut K, Kietinun S, Warrell DA. Quinine pharmacokinetics and toxicity in pregnant and lactating women with falciparum malaria. Br J Clin Pharmacol 1986;21:677–83.
9. White NJ, Warrell DA, Chanthavanich P, Looareesuwan S, Warrell MJ, Krishna S, Williamson DH, Turner RC. Severe hypoglycemia and hyperinsulinemia in falciparum malaria. N Engl J Med 1983;309:61–6.
10. Bradley D. Prophylaxis against malaria for travelers from the United Kingdom. Br Med J 1993;306:1247–52.
11. Barry M, Bia F. Pregnancy and travel. JAMA 1989;261:728–31.
12. Lackritz EM, Lobel HO, Howell BJ, Bloland P, Campbell CC. Imported *Plasmodium falciparum* malaria in American travelers to Africa. JAMA 1991;265:383–5.
13. Palmer KJ, Holliday SM, Brogden RN. Mefloquine. A review of its antimalarial activity, pharmacokinetic properties and therapeutic efficacy. Drugs 1993;45:430–75.
14. Baker L, Van Schoor JD, Bartlett GA, Lombard JH. Malaria prophylaxis—the South African viewpoint. S Afr Med J 1993;83:126–9.
15. Raccurt CP, Le Bras M, Ripert C, Cuisinier-Raynal JC, Carteron B, Buestel ML. Paludisme d'importation à Bordeaux: évaluation du risque d'infectation par Plasmodium falciparum en fonction de la destination. Bull WHO 1991;69:85–91.
16. Collignon P, Hehir J, Mitchell D. Successful treatment of falciparum malaria in pregnancy with mefloquine. Lancet 1989;1:967.
17. Elefant E, Boyer M, Roux C. Presentation at the 4th International Conference of Teratogen Information Services, Chicago, IL, April 18–20, 1991 (F. Rosa, personal communication, 1993).
18. Edstein MD, Veenendaal JR, Hyslop R. Excretion of mefloquine in human breast milk. Chemotherapy (Basel) 1988;34:165–9.

MELATONIN

Hormone (Pineal Gland)/Nutritional Supplement

PREGNANCY RECOMMENDATION: No Human Data—Animal Data Suggest Moderate Risk
BREASTFEEDING RECOMMENDATION: Limited Human Data—Probably Compatible (Low Doses)
No Human Data—Potential Toxicity (High Doses)

PREGNANCY SUMMARY

No reports of human pregnancy exposure to exogenous melatonin have been located. Moreover, there have been no long-term studies of the safety of melatonin in nonpregnant humans. This neurohormone is available as an OTC nutritional supplement, as well as a drug. Thus, the use in human pregnancy has most likely occurred but apparently has not been reported. The lack of noticeable toxicity and structural defects in rat fetuses and newborn pups exposed in utero to maternal doses higher than those used in humans is reassuring, but the dose comparison is based on body weight, not BSA or AUC. Moreover, melatonin doses very near the human dose (again based on body weight) did adversely affect the development of the neuroendocrine reproductive axis in female rat fetuses, a toxicity that would not be immediately apparent. There is probably no relationship of this toxicity in pregnant humans consuming occasional low (≤10 mg) doses, but high doses or frequent use during gestation should be avoided. One source recommends avoiding the agent in pregnancy (1). High daily doses have been shown to inhibit ovulation. In addition, maternal consumption of melatonin may affect the fetal suprachiasmatic nucleus with resulting adverse effects for the prenatal and postnatal expression and entrainment of circadian rhythms (2). If melatonin is used, synthetic preparations should be chosen. Animal-derived products should be avoided because of the risk of contamination and/or the transmission of infectious agents.

FETAL RISK SUMMARY

Melatonin is a neurohormone produced by the pineal gland (pineal body) under the control of the suprachiasmatic nucleus located in the anterior hypothalamus (3,4). Secretion of melatonin from the pineal body occurs in a diurnal pattern (during periods of darkness) and affects sleep pattern (3–5). The endogenous hormone is thought to have a wide range of effects. These include increased concentrations of serotonin and aminobutyric acid in the brain; enhanced activity of an enzyme (pyridoxal-kinase) that is involved in the synthesis of serotonin, aminobutyric acid, and dopamine; inhibition of gonadal development; and a role in the control of estrus (5).

Melatonin is commercially available as a nutritional supplement, either as a synthetic or animal-derived product (6). Two sources recommend avoiding the product produced from animal pineal tissue (beef cattle) because of the theoretical risk of contamination or viral transmission (1,6).

A 1981 study evaluated the effect on female offspring of maternal administration of melatonin to rats (7). Pregnant rats were given daily SC doses of 250 mcg/100 g (2.5 mg/kg); about 2–10 times the usual recommended human dose of 10–100 mg in a 70-kg person (RHD) throughout gestation and compared with two control groups (nonmedicated and pinealectomized pregnant rats). Female offspring of melatonin-treated rats showed significantly later vaginal opening compared with the control groups. In addition, they also had significantly lower luteinizing hormones blood levels. The concentrations of melatonin in the three offspring groups did not differ. The investigators concluded that the exogenous melatonin crossed the placenta and demonstrated an inhibitory influence on the development of the neuroendocrine reproductive axis in the fetus (7).

In another animal study, pregnant rats were administered up to 200 mg/kg/day (about 143–1430 times the RHD) from gestational day 6 to day 19 (8,9). No maternal or fetal toxicity was observed. The developmental toxicity NOAEL (no-observed-adverse-effect level) was ≥200 mg/kg/day (8,9).

A 2000 study suggested that melatonin might be useful in protecting the fetal brain from neurodegenerative conditions, such as fetal hypoxia and preeclampsia (10). These conditions may involve free radical production, and melatonin is known to be scavenger of oxygen free radicals. The investigators gave melatonin intraperitoneal injections to rats on gestational day 20 and then measured the concentrations of the substance in fetal brains over the next 3 hours. Melatonin rapidly crossed the rat placenta, with peak levels in maternal serum and fetal brain occurring 1 hour after the dose. Moreover, over the 3-hour period, the fetal brain had significant increases in the activities of two free radical scavenging enzymes, superoxide dismutase and glutathione peroxidase. The investigators concluded that the changes in melatonin concentrations and enzyme activity might protect the fetal brain from oxidation of cerebral lipids and DNA, thereby preventing central nervous system injury (10).

Because of its enhancement of circadian rhythm, melatonin has been used for treating jet lag and other sleep disorders (1,4–6). In the United States, melatonin has orphan drug status for circadian rhythm sleep disorders in blind persons without light perception (6,11). Other possible indications that have been studied, without establishing efficacy, are an anticancer action, chemotherapy-induced thrombocytopenia, cluster headaches, tinnitus, and as an antiaging hormone with antioxidant and immune system–boosting properties to extend life (6,12).

High doses of melatonin also have been studied as a human contraceptive. A 1992 study compared the contraceptive effect of melatonin (75 or 300 mg/day) either alone or in combination with the synthetic progestin, norethisterone (0.3 or 0.75 mg/day) (13). Both melatonin groups, compared with controls, inhibited ovarian function with significant decreases in blood levels of luteinizing hormone, estradiol, and progesterone.

Two publications, one in 1997 (2) and the other in 2000 (3), reviewed the role of melatonin in animal and human development. The human embryo and fetus have multiple binding melatonin sites in the pituitary and hypothalamus, actually more than in adults (2,3). As early as the 18th week of gestation, melatonin receptors can be found in the fetal suprachiasmatic nucleus. However, the effects of the neurohormone during this period are thought primarily to involve melatonin of maternal origin (2). Melatonin is a lipophilic hormone that easily crosses the placenta and is present in human fetal blood and amniotic fluid (2,3). The two main functions of melatonin during human prenatal development are thought to be: (a) establishment of periodicity by communicating information about photoperiod; and (b) entrainment of the developing circadian pacemaker (2). However, circadian rhythms (such as sleep and the secretion of cortisol and melatonin) are not expressed until several months after birth (2,4).

One author critically reviewed the literature on the consequences of abnormal melatonin rhythmicity development in infancy as a result of either prenatal or postnatal events (3). These consequences included sudden infant death syndrome, fetal onset of adult disease (e.g., cardiovascular disease), and scoliosis. In none of these conditions, however, has a causative association with abnormal melatonin rhythmicity been established (3).

M

BREASTFEEDING SUMMARY

Although no reports describing the use of exogenous melatonin during lactation have been located, endogenous melatonin is excreted into human breast milk (14). In 10 mothers, 3–4 days after delivery, blood and milk samples were collected between 1400 and 1700 (day samples) and between 0200 and 0400 (night samples). No melatonin was detected in the day samples (<43 pmol/L for blood and milk), but the mean levels in the blood and milk of the night samples were 280 and 99 pmol/L, respectively. Milk samples were collected after each feeding from another group of six women within 3 months after delivery. A marked daily rhythm of melatonin excretion was detected; undetectable levels during the day and high levels at night. The investigators speculated that the circadian rhythm of melatonin in milk might be involved in postnatal development by communicating the time of day to the nursing infant (14). The effects of potentially higher milk concentrations when the mother is taking melatonin are unknown, but the best course is to avoid the hormone during lactation. One source recommends avoiding the agent because of the lack of information (1).

References

1. Melatonin. *Natural Medicines Comprehensive Database*. Stockton, CA: Therapeutic Research Faculty, 2003:910–15.
2. Davis FC. Melatonin: role in development. J Biol Rhythms 1997;12: 498–508.
3. Kennaway DJ. Melatonin and development: physiology and pharmacology. Semin Perinatal 2000;24:258–66.
4. Cavallo A. The pineal gland in human beings: relevance to pediatrics. J Pediatr 1993;123:843–51.
5. Melatonin. Reynolds JEF, ed. *Martindale: The Extra Pharmacopoeia*. 34th ed. London: Royal Pharmaceutical Society of Great Britain, 2005: 1710–1.
6. Melatonin. *The Review of Natural Products*. St. Louis, MO: Facts and Comparisons, July 2004.
7. Colmenero MD, Diaz B, Miguel JL, Gonzalez MLI, Esquifino A, Marin B. Melatonin administration during pregnancy retards sexual maturation of female offspring in the rat. J Pineal Res 1991;11:23–7.
8. Price CJ, Marr MC, Myers CB, Jahnke GD. Developmental toxicity evaluation of melatonin in rats (abstract). Teratology 1998;57:245.
9. Jahnke G, Marr M, Myers C, Wilson R, Travlos G, Price C. Maternal and developmental toxicity evaluation of melatonin administered orally to pregnant Sprague-Dawley rats. Toxicol Sci 1999;50:271–9.
10. Okatani Y, Wakatsuki A, Kaneda C. Melatonin increases activities of glutathione peroxidase and superoxide dismutase in fetal rat brain. J Pineal Res 2000;28:89–96.
11. Orphan drugs. Melatonin. *Drug Facts and Comparisons*. St. Louis: Facts and Comparisons, December, 2006:KU-14g.
12. Pepping J, Alternative therapies: melatonin. Am J Health-System Pharm 1999;56:2520, 2523–4, 2527.
13. Voordouw BCG, Euser R, Verdonk RER, Alberda BTH, De Jong FH, Drogendijk AC, Fauser BCJM, Cohen M. Melatonin and melatonin-progestin combinations alter pituitary-ovarian function in women and can inhibit ovulation. J Clin Endocrinol Metab 1992;74:108–17.
14. Illnerova H, Buresova M, Presi J. Melatonin rhythm in human milk. J Clin Endocrinol Metab 1993;77:838–41.

MELOXICAM

Nonsteroidal Anti-inflammatory

PREGNANCY RECOMMENDATION: Human Data Suggest Risk in 1st and 3rd Trimesters
BREASTFEEDING RECOMMENDATION: No Human Data—Probably Compatible

PREGNANCY SUMMARY

Constriction of the ductus arteriosus in utero is a pharmacologic consequence arising from the use of prostaglandin synthesis inhibitors during pregnancy (see also Indomethacin) (1). Persistent pulmonary hypertension of the newborn may occur if these agents are used in the 3rd trimester close to delivery (1,2). These drugs have also been shown to inhibit labor and prolong gestation, both in humans (3) (see also Indomethacin) and in animals (4,5). Women attempting to conceive should not use any prostaglandin synthesis inhibitor, including meloxicam, because of the findings in a variety of animal models that indicate these agents block blastocyst implantation (6,7). Moreover, as noted, nonsteroidal anti-inflammatory drugs (NSAIDs) have been associated with spontaneous abortions (SABs) and congenital malformations. The risk for these defects, however, appears to be small.

FETAL RISK SUMMARY

The NSAID meloxicam shares the same mechanism of action and uses as other agents in this class. It is an oxicam derivative in the same subclass as piroxicam. No published reports linking meloxicam to human congenital malformations have been located.

Reproduction studies have been conducted in the rat and rabbit. In rabbits, oral doses 64.5 times the human dose at 15 mg/day for a 50-kg adult based on BSA (HD) given throughout organogenesis resulted in an increased incidence of cardiac septal defects. Embryo lethality was observed at ≥5.4 times the HD. In pregnant rats, no teratogenicity was noted at doses up to 2.2 times the HD. An increase in stillbirths, however, occurred at oral doses about ≥0.5 times the HD and a decrease in pup survival at 2.1 times the HD, when these doses were administered throughout organogenesis. At ≥0.5 times the HD in late gestation, meloxicam was associated with stillbirths, an increased length of delivery time, and delayed parturition. At doses ≥0.07 times the HD during late gestation and lactation, reductions in birth index, live births, and neonatal survival were seen in rats (4).

It is not known if meloxicam crosses the human placenta. The molecular weight (about 351) is low enough that transfer to the fetus should be expected. Meloxicam does cross the rat placenta (1).

A combined 2001 population-based observational cohort study and a case–control study estimated the risk of adverse pregnancy outcome from the use of NSAIDs (8). The use of NSAIDs during pregnancy was not associated with congenital malformations, preterm delivery, or low birth weight, but a positive association was discovered with SABs. A similar study, also published in 2001, failed to find a relationship, in general, between NSAIDs and congenital malformations, but did find a significant association with cardiac defects and orofacial clefts (9). In addition, a 2003 study found a significant association between exposure to NSAIDs in early pregnancy and SABs (10). (See Ibuprofen for details on these three studies.)

A brief 2003 editorial on the potential for NSAID-induced developmental toxicity concluded that NSAIDs, and specifically those with greater COX-2 affinity, had a lower risk of this toxicity in humans than aspirin (11).

BREASTFEEDING SUMMARY

No reports describing the use of meloxicam during lactation have been located. The molecular weight (about 351) is low enough that excretion into breast milk should be expected. The effects of this exposure on a nursing infant are unknown, but a similar agent, piroxicam, is classified as compatible with breastfeeding by the American Academy of Pediatrics (see Piroxicam).

References

1. Levin DL. Effects of inhibition of prostaglandin synthesis on fetal development, oxygenation, and the fetal circulation. Semin Perinatol 1980;4:35–44.
2. Van Marter LJ, Leviton A, Allred EN, Pagano M, Sullivan KF, Cohen A, Epstein MF. Persistent pulmonary hypertension of the newborn and smoking and aspirin and nonsteroidal antiinflammatory drug consumption during pregnancy. Pediatrics 1996;97:658–63.
3. Fuchs F. Prevention of prematurity. Am J Obstet Gynecol 1976;126:809–20.
4. Product information. Mobic. Boehringer Ingelheim Pharmaceuticals, 2001.
5. Powell JG, Cochrane RL. The effects of a number of non-steroidal anti-inflammatory compounds on parturition in the rat. Prostaglandins 1982;23:469–88.
6. Matt DW, Borzelleca JF. Toxic effects on the female reproductive system during pregnancy, parturition, and lactation. In Wilorsch RJ, ed. *Reproductive Toxicology*. 2nd ed. New York, NY: Raven Press, 1995:175–93.
7. Dawood MY. Nonsteroidal antiinflammatory drugs and reproduction. Am J Obstet Gynecol 1993;169:1255–65.
8. Nielsen GL, Sorensen HT, Larsen H, Pedersen L. Risk of adverse birth outcome and miscarriage in pregnant users of non-steroidal anti-inflammatory drugs: population based observational study and case-control study. Br Med J 2001;322:266–70.
9. Ericson A, Kallen BAJ. Nonsteroidal anti-inflammatory drugs in early pregnancy. Reprod Toxicol 2001;15:371–5.
10. Li DK, Liu L, Odouli R. Exposure to non-steroidal anti-inflammatory drugs during pregnancy and risk of miscarriage: population based cohort study. Br Med J 2003;327:368–71.
11. Tassinari MS, Cook JC, Hurtt ME. NSAIDs and developmental toxicity. Birth Defects Res B Dev Reprod Toxicol 2003;68:3–4.

MELPHALAN

Antineoplastic

PREGNANCY RECOMMENDATION: Contraindicated—1st Trimester
BREASTFEEDING RECOMMENDATION: Contraindicated

PREGNANCY SUMMARY

Melphalan, a phenylalanine derivative of nitrogen mustard, is a bifunctional alkylating antineoplastic agent. Other agents in this class (e.g., see also Busulfan, Chlorambucil, and Cyclophosphamide) are known to be human teratogens and, combined with the animal data, strongly suggest that melphalan should not be given in the 1st trimester.

FETAL RISK SUMMARY

No reports linking the use of melphalan with congenital defects have been located. The drug is mutagenic as well as carcinogenic (1–8). These effects have not been described in infants following in utero exposure.

Reproduction studies in rats with oral doses of 6–18 mg/m^2/day for 10 days, or with a single intraperitoneal dose of 18 mg/m^2 revealed embryolethal and teratogenic effects (9). Congenital anomalies included those of the brain (underdevelopment, deformation, meningocele, and encephalocele), eye (anophthalmia and microphthalmos), reduction of the mandible and tail, and hepatocele.

Studies examining the placental transfer of melphalan have not been found. The molecular weight (about 305) is low enough that exposure of the embryo and/or fetus should be expected.

Data from one review indicated that 40% of the infants exposed to anticancer drugs were of low birth weight (10). Long-term studies of growth and mental development in offspring exposed to melphalan and other antineoplastic drugs during the 2nd trimester, the period of neuroblast multiplication, have not been conducted (11).

Melphalan has caused suppression of ovarian function resulting in amenorrhea (11–14). These effects should be considered before administering the drug to patients in their reproductive years. However, of 436 long-term survivors treated with chemotherapy between 1958 and 1978 for gestational trophoblastic tumors, 15 received melphalan as part of their treatment regimens (15). Three of these women had at least one live birth (mean melphalan dose 18 mg; maximum dose 24 mg), and the remaining 12 did not attempt to conceive. Complete details of this study are discussed in the monograph for methotrexate (see Methotrexate).

Occupational exposure of the mother to antineoplastic agents during pregnancy may present a risk to the fetus. A position statement from the National Study Commission on Cytotoxic Exposure and a research article on some antineoplastic agents are presented in the monograph for cyclophosphamide (see Cyclophosphamide).

BREASTFEEDING SUMMARY

No reports describing the use of melphalan during lactation have been located. The molecular weight (about 305) is low enough that excretion into breast milk should be expected. Because of the potential for severe toxicity in the nursing infant, women receiving this antineoplastic agent should not nurse.

References

1. Sharpe HB. Observations on the effect of therapy with nitrogen mustard or a derivative on chromosomes of human peripheral blood lymphocytes. Cell Tissue Kinet 1971;4:501–4.
2. Kyle RA, Pierre RV, Bayrd ED. Multiple myeloma and acute myelomonocytic leukemia. N Engl J Med 1970;283:1121–5.
3. Kyle RA. Primary amyloidosis in acute leukemia associated with melphalan. Blood 1974;44:333–7.
4. Burton IE, Abbott CR, Roberts BE, Antonis AH. Acute leukemia after four years of melphalan treatment for melanoma. Br Med J 1976;1:20.
5. Peterson HS. Erythroleukemia in a melphalan treated patient with primary macroglobulinaemia. Scand J Haematol 1973;10:5–11.
6. Stavem P, Harboe M. Acute erythroleukaemia in a patient treated with melphalan for the cold agglutinin syndrome. Scand J Haematol 1971;8:375–9.
7. Einhorn N. Acute leukemia after chemotherapy (melphalan). Cancer 1978;41:444–7.
8. Reimer RR, Hover R, Fraumen JF, Young RC. Acute leukemia after alkylating agent therapy of ovarian cancer. N Engl J Med 1977;297:177–81.
9. Product information. Alkeran. Glaxo Wellcome, 2000.
10. Nicholson HO. Cytotoxic drugs in pregnancy: review of reported cases. J Obstet Gynaecol Br Commonw 1968;75:307–12.
11. Dobbing J. Pregnancy and leukaemia. Lancet 1977;1:11–15.
12. Rose DP, David PE. Ovarian function in patients receiving adjuvant chemotherapy for breast cancer. Lancet 1977;1:1174–6.
13. Ahmann DL. Repeated adjuvant chemotherapy with phenylalanine mustard or 5-fluorouracil, cyclophosphamide and prednisone with or without radiation. Lancet 1978;1:893–6.
14. Schilsky RL, Lewis BJ, Sherins RJ, Young RC. Gonadal dysfunction in patients receiving chemotherapy for cancer. Ann Intern Med 1980;93:109–14.
15. Rustin GJS, Booth M, Dent J, Salt S, Rustin F, Bagshawe KD. Pregnancy after cytotoxic chemotherapy for gestational trophoblastic tumours. Br Med J 1984;288:103–6.

MENADIONE

[Withdrawn from the market. See 9th edition.]

MEPENZOLATE

Parasympatholytic (Anticholinergic)

PREGNANCY RECOMMENDATION: Limited Human Data—No Relevant Animal Data
BREASTFEEDING RECOMMENDATION: No Human Data—Probably Compatible

PREGNANCY SUMMARY

The very limited pregnancy experience showing a possible association with minor malformations requires confirmation. In general, however, anticholinergics appear to be low risk in pregnancy (see Atropine).

FETAL RISK SUMMARY

Mepenzolate is an anticholinergic quaternary ammonium bromide. In a large prospective study, 2323 patients were exposed to this class of drugs during the 1st trimester, 1 of whom took mepenzolate (1). A possible association was found between the total group and minor malformations.

BREASTFEEDING SUMMARY

No reports describing the use of mepenzolate during human lactation have been located (see Atropine).

Reference

1. Heinonen OP, Slone D, Shapiro S. *Birth Defects and Drugs in Pregnancy*. Littleton, MA: Publishing Sciences Group, 1977:346–53.

MEPERIDINE

Narcotic Agonist Analgesic

PREGNANCY RECOMMENDATION: Human Data Suggest Risk
BREASTFEEDING RECOMMENDATION: Compatible

PREGNANCY SUMMARY

The National Birth Defects Prevention Study discussed below found evidence that opioid use during organogenesis is associated with a low absolute risk of congenital birth defects. As with all opioids, maternal and neonatal addiction is possible from inappropriate use. Neonatal depression, at times fatal, has historically been the primary concern following obstetric meperidine analgesia. Controversy has arisen over the potential long-term adverse effects resulting from this use.

FETAL RISK SUMMARY

The placental transfer of meperidine is very rapid, appearing in cord blood within 2 minutes following IV administration (1). It is detectable in amniotic fluid 30 minutes after IM injection (2). Cord blood concentrations average 70%–77% (range 45%–106%) of maternal plasma levels (3,4). The drug has been detected in the saliva of newborns for 48 hours following maternal administration during labor (5). Concentrations in pharyngeal aspirates were higher than in either arterial or venous cord blood.

In a surveillance study of Michigan Medicaid recipients involving 229,101 completed pregnancies conducted between 1985 and 1992, 62 newborns had been exposed to meperidine during the 1st trimester (F. Rosa, personal communication, FDA, 1993). Three (4.8%) major birth defects were observed (three expected), including (observed/expected) 1/0 polydactyly and 1/0 hypospadias. No malformations were observed in four other defect categories (cardiovascular defects, oral clefts, spina bifida, and limb reduction defects) for which specific data were available.

Respiratory depression in the newborn following use of the drug in labor is time- and dose-dependent. The incidence of depression increases markedly if delivery occurs 60 minutes or longer after injection, reaching a peak around 2–3 hours after injection (6,7). Whether this depression is caused by metabolites of meperidine (e.g., normeperidine) or the drug itself is not known (2,8–10). However, recent work suggests that these effects are related to unmetabolized meperidine and not to normeperidine (7).

Impaired behavioral response and electroencephalographic changes persisting for several days have been observed (11,12). These persistent effects may be partially explained by the slow elimination of meperidine and normeperidine from the neonate over several days (13,14). One group of investigators related depressed attention and social responsiveness during the first 6 weeks of life to high cord blood levels of meperidine (15). An earlier study reported long-term follow-up of 70 healthy neonates born to mothers who had received meperidine within 2 hours of birth (16,17). Psychologic and physical parameters at 5 years of age were similar in both exposed and control groups. Academic progress and behavior during the 3rd and 4th years in school were also similar.

The Collaborative Perinatal Project monitored 50,282 mother–child pairs, 268 of whom had 1st trimester exposure to meperidine (18, pp. 287–295). For use anytime during pregnancy, 1100 exposures were recorded (18, p. 434). No evidence was found to suggest a relationship to large categories of major or minor malformations. A possible association between the use of meperidine in the 1st trimester and inguinal hernia was found based on six cases (18, p. 471). The statistical significance of this association is unknown and independent confirmation is required.

Results of a National Birth Defects Prevention Study (1997–2005) were published in 2011 (19). This population-based case–control study examined the association between maternal use of opioid analgesics and >30 types of major structural birth defects. In 17,449 case mothers, therapeutic opioid use was reported by 454 (2.6%) compared with 134 (2.0%) of 6701 control mothers. Indications for use of opioid analgesics were surgical procedures (41%), infections (34%), chronic diseases (20%), and injuries (18%). Dose, duration, or frequency were not evaluated. The exposure period evaluated was from 1 month before to 3 months after conception. Limiting the exposure period to the first 2 months after conception produced similar results. Infants with >1 defect were included in multiple birth defect categories. The following opioids were included (number of cases for each agent not specified): codeine, hydrocodone, hydromorphone, fentanyl, meperidine, methadone, morphine, oxycodone, pentazocine, propoxyphene, and tramadol. The birth defect, total number, number exposed, and the adjusted odds ratio (aOR) with 95% confidence interval (CI) were as follows:

Birth Defect	Total	Cases	aOR (95% CI)
Spina bifida	718	26	2.0 (1.3–3.2)
Any heart defect (20 types)	7724	211	1.4 (1.1–1.7)
Atrioventricular septal defect	175	9	2.4 (1.2–4.8)
Teratology of Fallot	672	21	1.7 (1.1–2.8)
Conotruncal defect	1481	41	1.5 (1.0–2.1)
Conoventricular septal defect	110	6	2.7 (1.1–6.3)
Left ventricular outflow tract obstruction defect	1195	36	1.5 (1.0–2.2)
Hypoplastic left heart syndrome	357	17	2.4 (1.4–4.1)
Right ventricular outflow tract obstruction defect	1175	40	1.6 (1.1–2.3)
Pulmonary valve stenosis	867	34	1.7 (1.2–2.6)
Atrial septal defect (ASD)	511	17	2.0 (1.2–3.6)
Ventricular septal defect + ASD	528	17	1.7 (1.0–2.9)
Hydrocephaly	301	11	2.0 (1.0–3.7)
Glaucoma/anterior chamber defects	103	5	2.6 (1.0–6.6)
Gastroschisis	726	26	1.8 (1.1–2.9)

The authors speculated that the activity of opioids and their receptors as growth regulators during development of the embryo might be a mechanism to explain the above findings. The exposure data were obtained by retrospective maternal self-report; the authors acknowledged that recall bias and misclassification might have affected their results. They concluded that the absolute risk was a modest absolute increase above the baseline risk for birth defects (19).

BREASTFEEDING SUMMARY

Meperidine is excreted into breast milk (20,21). In a group of mothers who had received meperidine during labor, the breastfed infants had higher saliva levels of the drug for up to 48 hours after birth than a similar group that was bottle-fed (5). In nine nursing mothers, a single 50-mg IM dose produced peak levels of 0.13 mcg/mL at 2 hours (21). After 24 hours, the concentrations decreased to 0.02 mcg/mL. Average milk:plasma ratios for the nine patients were greater than 1.0. No adverse effects in nursing infants were reported in any of the above studies.

The American Academy of Pediatrics classifies meperidine as compatible with breastfeeding (22).

References

1. Crawford JS, Rudofsky S. The placental transmission of pethidine. Br J Anaesth 1965;37:929–33.
2. Szanto HH, Zervoudakis IA, Cederquist LL, Inturrise CE. Amniotic fluid transfer of meperidine from maternal plasma in early pregnancy. Obstet Gynecol 1978;52:59–62.
3. Apgar V, Burns JJ, Brodie BB, Papper EM. The transmission of meperidine across the human placenta. Am J Obstet Gynecol 1952;64:1368–70.
4. Snider SM, Way EL, Lord MJ. Rate of appearance and disappearance of meperidine in fetal blood after administration of narcotic to the mother. Anesthesiology 1966;27:227–8.
5. Freeborn SF, Calvert RT, Black P, MacFarlane T, D'Souza SW. Saliva and blood pethidine concentrations in the mother and the newborn baby. Br J Obstet Gynaecol 1980;87:966–9.
6. Morrison JC, Wiser WL, Rosser SI, Gayden JO, Bucovaz ET, Whybrew WD, Fish SA. Metabolites of meperidine related to fetal depression. Am J Obstet Gynecol 1973;115:1132–7.
7. Belfries P, Boreus LO, Hartvig P, Irestedt L, Raabe N. Neonatal depression after obstetrical analgesia with pethidine. The role of the injection-delivery time interval and the plasma concentrations of pethidine and norpethidine. Acta Obstet Gynecol Scand 1981;60:43–9.
8. Morrison JC, Whybrew WD, Rosser SI, Bucovaz ET, Wiser WL, Fish SA. Metabolites of meperidine in the fetal and maternal serum. Am J Obstet Gynecol 1976;126:997–1002.
9. Clark RB, Lattin DL. Metabolites of meperidine in serum. Am J Obstet Gynecol 1978;130:113–5.
10. Morrison JC. Reply to Drs. Clark and Lattin. Am J Obstet Gynecol 1978;130:115–7.
11. Borgstede AD, Rosen MG. Medication during labor correlated with behavior and EEG of the newborn. Am J Dis Child 1968;115:21–4.
12. Hodgkinson R, Bhatt M, Wang CN. Double-blind comparison of the neurobehaviour of neonates following the administration of different doses of meperidine to the mother. Can Anaesth Soc J 1978;25:405–11.
13. Cooper LV, Stephen GW, Aggett PJA. Elimination of pethidine and bupivacaine in the newborn. Arch Dis Child 1977;52:638–41.
14. Kushner BR, Kuhnert PM, Prochaska AL, Sokol RJ. Meperidine disposition in mother, neonate and nonpregnant females. Clin Pharmacol Ther 1980;27:486–91.
15. Betsey EM, Rosenblatt DB, Lieberman BA, Redshaw M, Caldwell J, Notarianni L, Smith RL, Beard RW. The influence of maternal analgesia on neonatal behaviour. I. Pethidine. Br J Obstet Gynaecol 1981;88:398–406.
16. Buck C, Gregg R, Stavraky K, Subrahmaniam K, Brown J. The effect of single prenatal and natal complications upon the development of children of mature birthweight. Pediatrics 1969;43:942–55.
17. Buck C. Drugs in pregnancy. Can Med Assoc J 1975;112:1285.
18. Heinonen O, Slone D, Shapiro S. *Birth Defects and Drugs in Pregnancy*. Littleton, MA: Publishing Sciences Group, 1977.
19. Broussard CS, Rasmussen SA, Reefhuis J, Friedman JM, Jann MW, Riehle-Colarusso T, Honein MA; National Birth Defects Prevention Study. Maternal treatment with opioid analgesics and risk for birth defects. Am J Obstet Gynecol 2011;204:314–7.

20. Vorherr H. Drug excretion in breast milk. Postgrad Med 1974;56:97–104.
21. Peiker G, Muller B, Ihn W, Noschel H. Excretion of pethidine in mother's milk. Zentralbl Gynaekol 1980;102:537–41.
22. Committee on Drugs, American Academy of Pediatrics. The transfer of drugs and other chemicals into human breast milk. Pediatrics 2001;108:776–89.

MEPHENTERMINE

[Withdrawn from the market. See 9th edition.]

MEPHENYTOIN

[Withdrawn from the market. See 9th edition.]

MEPHOBARBITAL

[Withdrawn from the market. See 9th edition.]

MEPINDOLOL

[Withdrawn from the market. See 9th edition.]

MEPROBAMATE

Sedative

PREGNANCY RECOMMENDATION: Human Data Suggest Low Risk
BREASTFEEDING RECOMMENDATION: Limited Human Data—Potential Toxicity

PREGNANCY SUMMARY

Few indications exist for meprobamate in the pregnant woman. If therapy is required, avoiding the 1st trimester is the safest course, but inadvertent exposure does not appear to represent a major risk. Two large surveillance studies did not support the associations with defects reported in earlier studies. In those studies, the defects may have occurred by chance or have been caused by unidentified factors. Moreover, meprobamate is the active metabolite of the central acting muscle relaxant, carisoprodol. That agent has been used in pregnancy without causing birth defects (see Carisoprodol). Nevertheless, until additional data are available, avoiding meprobamate in the 1st trimester is best.

FETAL RISK SUMMARY

Meprobamate is used in the treatment of anxiety disorders or for the short-term treatment of the symptoms of anxiety. It has hypnotic, sedative, and sedative-related muscle-relaxant properties (1). It is partially metabolized to inactive metabolites before excretion in the urine. Meprobamate also is the active metabolite of carisoprodol (see Carisoprodol). The elimination half-life is in the range of 6–17 hours, but may be prolonged after chronic administration (1).

Schardein (2) reviewed seven reproduction studies in mice, rats, and rabbits. Meprobamate caused digital defects in mice and neurobehavior toxicity in rats. However, because most of the studies involved parenteral administration, the findings cannot be used to assess the degree of human risk (2).

Meprobamate crosses the placenta to the fetus and has been measured in umbilical cord blood at or near maternal plasma levels (3). The low molecular weight (about 218) and long elimination half-life are in agreement with that finding.

Four reports have associated the use of meprobamate in pregnancy with an increased risk of congenital anomalies (4–7). In a study of 395 patients (402 live births) who took meprobamate during pregnancy, 115 infants had been exposed during the 1st trimester (4). Ten of the 115 infants had birth defects, but only 5 of the defects, all involving different defects of the heart, could be potentially related to drugs or other unidentified factors. The other non-meprobamate-related defects were Down's syndrome, partial deafness (a toxicity not known to be associated with meprobamate), deformed elbows and joints (a probable deformation), and two unspecified defects. A second report described multiple anomalies, including congenital heart defects, in a newborn exposed to meprobamate (5). The mother of this patient was treated very early in the 1st trimester with meprobamate and propoxyphene. Malformations observed were omphalocele, defective anterior abdominal wall, defect in diaphragm, congenital heart disease with partial ectopic cordis secondary to sternal cleft, and dysplastic hips. Multiple defects of the eye and central nervous system were observed in a newborn exposed to multiple drugs, including meprobamate and lysergic acid diethylamide (LSD) (6). A brief 1975 report summarized the findings of a combined England–France study on the fetal effects of tranquilizers (7). Of the 84 women that took meprobamate during the 1st trimester, 4 delivered infants with congenital malformations. None of the defects were cardiac malformations. In addition, three of the four mothers had experienced a previous pregnancy with a poor outcome (abortion, stillbirth, or malformation) (7).

The Collaborative Perinatal Project monitored 50,282 mother–child pairs, 356 of whom were exposed in the 1st trimester to meprobamate (8). No association of meprobamate with large classes of malformations or to individual defects was found. In a follow-up to this study, there was no evidence that exposure to meprobamate in the 1st trimester was related to congenital malformations (20 of 356 infants; expected 17.4; *ns*), deaths (stillbirth to the fourth birthday), adverse effects on mental and motor scores at the age of 8 months, or intelligence quotient scores at 4 years of age (9). Others also have failed to find a relationship between the use of meprobamate and congenital malformations (10).

In a surveillance study of Michigan Medicaid recipients involving 229,101 completed pregnancies conducted between 1985 and 1992, 75 newborns had been exposed to meprobamate during the 1st trimester (F. Rosa, personal communication, FDA, 1993). Three (4.0%) major birth defects were observed (three expected), including (observed/expected) 1/0 oral cleft and 2/0 polydactyly. No anomalies were observed in four other defect categories (cardiovascular defects, spina bifida, limb reduction defects, and hypospadias) for which specific data were available. Only with the cases of polydactyly is there a suggestion of a possible association, but other factors, such as the mother's disease, concurrent drug use, and chance, may be involved.

A 1997 report described the pregnancy outcomes of 12 women who had taken large doses of various medications during the first postconception month and who had delivered live infants (11). Four of the cases involved the ingestion of meprobamate either alone or with other drugs. No birth defects were observed in three cases (dose and other drugs in parentheses): meprobamate (1400 mg), meprobamate (5000 mg), and meprobamate (2000 mg, plus chlordiazepoxide 25 mg). A nondrug-induced defect (bilateral undescended testis) was observed in one case in which the mother took meprobamate 1000 mg, promethazine 250 mg, diazepam 120 mg, and metoprolol 1000 mg (11).

BREASTFEEDING SUMMARY

Meprobamate is excreted into breast milk with concentrations 2–4 times that of maternal plasma (1,12). Two case reports described mothers who took carisoprodol throughout gestation and during breastfeeding. Both carisoprodol and meprobamate, the active metabolites, were found in milk. Meprobamate had the highest concentration (see Carisoprodol). The lack of detectable adverse effects in both infants suggested that the risk of toxicity is low, at least in infants that also were exposed during pregnancy. Starting meprobamate during breastfeeding may have different results in a nursing infant. Women taking meprobamate and who elect to nurse should closely monitor their infants for sedation and other changes in behavior or functions.

References

1. Sweetman SC, Editor. *Martindale. The Complete Drug Reference*. 34th ed. London: Pharmaceutical Press, 2005:706.
2. Schardein JL. *Chemically Induced Birth Defects*. 3rd ed. New York, NY: Marcel Dekker, 2000:243.
3. Product information. Miltown. Wallace Laboratories, 2000.
4. Milkovich L, van den Berg BJ. Effects of prenatal meprobamate and chlordiazepoxide hydrochloride on human embryonic and fetal development. N Engl J Med 1974;291:1268–71.
5. Ringrose CAD. The hazard of neurotropic drugs in the fertile years. CMAJ 1972;106:1058.
6. Bogdanoff B, Rorke LB, Yanoff M, Warren WS. Brain and eye abnormalities: possible sequelae to prenatal use of multiple drugs including LSD. Am J Dis Child 1972;123:145–8.
7. Crombie DL, Pinsent RJ, Fleming DM, Rumeau-Rouguette C, Goujard J, Huel G. Fetal effects of tranquilizers in pregnancy. N Engl J Med 1975;293:198–9.
8. Heinonen OP, Slone D, Shapiro S. *Birth Defects and Drugs in Pregnancy*. Littleton, MA: Publishing Sciences Group, 1977:336–7.
9. Hartz SC, Heinonen OP, Shapiro S, Siskind V, Slone D. Antenatal exposure to meprobamate and chlordiazepoxide in relation to malformations, mental development, and childhood mortality. N Engl J Med 1975;292:726–8.
10. Belafsky HA, Breslow S, Hirsch LM, Shangold JE, Stahl MB. Meprobamate during pregnancy. Obstet Gynecol 1969;34:378–86.
11. Czeizel AE, Mosonyi A. Monitoring of early human fetal development in women exposed to large doses of chemicals. Environ Mol Mutagen 1997;30:240–4.
12. Wilson JT, Brown RD, Cherek DR, Dailey JW, Hilman B, Jobe PC, Manno BR, Manno JE, Redetzki HM, Stewart JJ. Drug excretion in human breast milk: principles, pharmacokinetics and projected consequences. Clin Pharmacokinet 1980;5:1–66.

MERCAPTOPURINE

Antineoplastic

PREGNANCY RECOMMENDATION: Human Data Suggest Risk in 3rd Trimester
BREASTFEEDING RECOMMENDATION: No Human Data—Potential Toxicity

PREGNANCY SUMMARY

Mercaptopurine (6-MP) is an antimetabolite antineoplastic agent. It is the active metabolite of azathioprine (see also Azathioprine). 6-MP is in the same subclass of purine analogs and related agents as cladribine, clofarabine, fludarabine, pentostatin, and thioguanine. Although the data are limited, 6-MP does not appear to be a major human teratogen, but the agent has been associated with newborn toxicity when used near delivery.

FETAL RISK SUMMARY

References citing the use of mercaptopurine in 79 human pregnancies have been located, including 34 cases in which the drug was used in the 1st trimester (1–21). Excluding those pregnancies that ended in abortion or stillbirths, congenital abnormalities were observed in only one infant (10). Defects noted in the infant were cleft palate, microphthalmia, hypoplasia of the ovaries and thyroid gland, corneal opacity, cytomegaly, and intrauterine growth restriction. The anomalies were attributed to busulfan.

Neonatal toxicity as a result of combination chemotherapy has been observed in three infants: pancytopenia (6), microangiopathic hemolytic anemia (9), and transient severe bone marrow hypoplasia (12). In the latter case, administration of mercaptopurine was stopped 3.5 weeks before delivery because of severe maternal myelosuppression. No chemotherapy was given during this period and the patient's peripheral blood counts were normal during the final 2 weeks of her pregnancy (12).

In another case, a 34-year-old woman with acute lymphoblastic leukemia was treated with multiple antineoplastic agents from 22 weeks' gestation until delivery of a healthy female infant 18 weeks later (14). Mercaptopurine was administered throughout the 3rd trimester. Chromosomal analysis of the newborn revealed a normal karyotype (46,XX) but with gaps and a ring chromosome. The clinical significance of these findings is unknown, but because these abnormalities may persist for several years, the potential existed for an increased risk of both cancer and genetic damage in the next generation (14).

Data from one review indicated that 40% of the infants exposed to anticancer drugs were of low birth weight (2). This finding was not related to the timing of exposure. In addition, except in a few cases, long-term studies of growth and mental development in infants exposed to mercaptopurine during the 2nd trimester, the period of neuroblast multiplication, have not been conducted (22). However, growth and development were normal in 13 infants (one set of twins) examined for 6 months to 10 years (12,15,16,18–21).

Severe oligospermia has been described in a 22-year-old male receiving sequential chemotherapy of cyclophosphamide, methotrexate, and mercaptopurine for leukemia (23). After treatment was stopped, the sperm count returned to normal and the patient fathered a healthy female child. Others have also observed reversible testicular dysfunction (24).

Ovarian function in women exposed to mercaptopurine does not seem to be affected adversely (25–29). An investigator noted in 1980 that long-term analysis of human reproduction following mercaptopurine therapy had not been reported (30). However, a brief 1979 correspondence described the reproductive performance of 314 women after treatment of gestational trophoblastic tumors, 159 of whom had conceived with a total of 218 pregnancies (28). Excluding the 17 women still pregnant at the time of the report, 38 (79%) of 48 women, exposed to mercaptopurine as part of their therapy, delivered live, term infants. A more detailed report of these and additional patients was published in 1984 (31). This latter study and another published in 1988 (32), both involving women treated for gestational trophoblastic neoplasms, are discussed below.

In 436 long-term survivors treated with chemotherapy between 1958 and 1978, 95 (22%) received mercaptopurine as part of their treatment regimens (31). Of the 95 women, 33 (35%) had at least one live birth (numbers given in parentheses refer to mean/maximum mercaptopurine dose in grams) (5.9/30.0), 3 (3%) conceived but had no live births (5.3/14.0), 3 (3%) failed to conceive (1.3/2.0), and 56 (59%) did not try to conceive (5.4/30.0). Additional details, including congenital anomalies observed, are described in the monograph for methotrexate (see Methotrexate).

A 1988 report described the reproductive results of 265 women who had been treated from 1959 to 1980 for gestational trophoblastic disease (32). Single-agent chemotherapy was administered to 91 women, including 26 cases in which mercaptopurine was the only agent used, whereas sequential (single agent) and combination therapy was administered to 67 and 107 women, respectively. Of the total group, 241 were exposed to pregnancy and 205 (85%) of these women conceived, with a total of 355 pregnancies. The time interval between recovery and pregnancy was 1 year or less (8.5%), 1–2 years (32.1%), 2–4 years (32.4%), 4–6 years (15.5%), 6–8 years (7.3%), 8–10 years (1.4%), and >10 years (2.8%). A total of 303 (4 sets of twins) liveborn infants resulted from the 355 pregnancies, 3 of whom had congenital malformations: anencephaly, hydrocephalus, and congenital heart disease (1 in each case). No gross developmental abnormalities were observed in the dead fetuses. Cytogenetic studies were conducted on the peripheral lymphocytes of 94 children and no significant chromosomal abnormalities were noted. Moreover, follow-up of the children, with >80% of the group >5 years of age (the oldest was 25 years), revealed normal development. The reproductive histories and pregnancy outcomes of the treated women were comparable to those of the normal population (32).

A 2012 case described a 27-year-old woman with ulcerative colitis who was treated throughout pregnancy with allopurinol 100 mg/day, mercaptopurine 25 mg/day, and mesalazine 4 g/day (33). Pregnancy was complicated by diarrhea and blood loss in the 2nd trimester. An elective cesarean section was performed at 39 weeks to give birth to a healthy 3550-g infant (sex not specified) with Apgar score of 9, 10, and 10 at 1, 5, and 10 minutes, respectively. No anomalies were observed in the infant (33).

Occupational exposure of the mother to antineoplastic agents during pregnancy may present a risk to the fetus. A position statement from the National Study Commission on Cytotoxic Exposure and a research article involving some antineoplastic agents are presented in the monograph for cyclophosphamide (see Cyclophosphamide).

BREASTFEEDING SUMMARY

No reports describing the use of mercaptopurine during lactation have been located. The molecular weight (about 170) suggests that the drug will be excreted into milk. Because of the potential for severe toxicity in the nursing infant, women receiving this antineoplastic agent should not nurse. However, if the mother chooses to breastfeed, the infant's complete blood count and liver function tests should be monitored.

References

1. Moloney WC. Management of leukemia in pregnancy. Ann NY Acad Sci 1964;114:857–67.
2. Nicholson HO. Cytotoxic drugs in pregnancy: review of reported cases. J Obstet Gynaecol Br Commonw 1968;75:307–12.
3. Gililland J, Weinstein L. The effects of cancer chemotherapeutic agents on the developing fetus. Obstet Gynecol Surv 1983;38:6–13.
4. Wegelius R. Successful pregnancy in acute leukaemia, Lancet 1975;2:1301.
5. Nicholson HO. Leukaemia and pregnancy: a report of five cases and discussion of management. J Obstet Gynaecol Br Commonw 1968;75:517–20.
6. Pizzuto J, Aviles A, Noriega L, Niz J, Morales M, Romero F. Treatment of acute leukemia during pregnancy: presentation of nine cases. Cancer Treat Rep 1980;64:679–83.
7. Burnier AM. Discussion. In Plows CW. Acute myelomonocytic leukemia in pregnancy: report of a case. Am J Obstet Gynecol 1982;143:41–3.
8. Dara P, Slater LM, Armentrout SA. Successful pregnancy during chemotherapy for acute leukemia. Cancer 1981;47:845–6.
9. McConnell JF, Bhoola R. A neonatal complication of maternal leukemia treated with 6-mercaptopurine. Postgrad Med J 1973;49:211–3.
10. Diamond J, Anderson MM, McCreadie SR. Transplacental transmission of busulfan (Myleran) in a mother with leukemia: production of fetal malformation and cytomegaly. Pediatrics 1960;25:85–90.
11. Khurshid M, Saleem M. Acute leukaemia in pregnancy. Lancet 1978;2:534–5.
12. Okun DB, Groncy PK, Sieger L, Tanaka KR. Acute leukemia in pregnancy: transient neonatal myelosuppression after combination chemotherapy in the mother. Med Pediatr Oncol 1979;7:315–9.
13. Doney KC, Kraemer KG, Shepard TH. Combination chemotherapy for acute myelocytic leukemia during pregnancy: three case reports. Cancer Treat Rep 1979;63:369–71.
14. Schleuning M, Clemm C. Chromosomal aberrations in a newborn whose mother received cytotoxic treatment during pregnancy. N Engl J Med 1987;317:1666–7.
15. Turchi JJ, Villasis C. Anthracyclines in the treatment of malignancy in pregnancy. Cancer 1988;61:435–40.
16. Feliu J, Juarez S, Ordonez A, Garcia-Paredes ML, Gonzalez-Baron M, Montero JM. Acute leukemia and pregnancy. Cancer 1988;61:580–4.
17. Haerr RW, Pratt AT. Multiagent chemotherapy for sarcoma diagnosed during pregnancy. Cancer 1985;56:1028–33.
18. Frenkel EP, Meyers MC. Acute leukemia and pregnancy. Ann Intern Med 1960;53:656–71.
19. Loyd HO. Acute leukemia complicated by pregnancy. JAMA 1961;178:1140–3.
20. Lee RA, Johnson CE, Hanlon DG. Leukemia during pregnancy. Am J Obstet Gynecol 1962;84:455–8.
21. Coopland AT, Friesen WJ, Galbraith PA. Acute leukemia in pregnancy. Am J Obstet Gynecol 1969;105:1288–9.
22. Dobbing J. Pregnancy and leukaemia. Lancet 1977;1:1155.
23. Hinkes E, Plotkin D. Reversible drug-induced sterility in a patient with acute leukemia. JAMA 1973;223:1490–1.
24. Lendon M, Palmer MK, Hann IM, Shalet SM, Jones PHM. Testicular histology after combination chemotherapy in childhood for acute lymphoblastic leukaemia. Lancet 1978;2:439–41.
25. Schilsky RL, Lewis BJ, Sherins RJ, Young RC. Gonadal dysfunction in patients receiving chemotherapy for cancer. Ann Intern Med 1980;93:109–14.
26. Gasser C. Long-term survival (cures) in childhood acute leukemia. Paediatrician 1980;9:344–57.
27. Bacon C, Kernahan J. Successful pregnancy in acute leukaemia. Lancet 1975;2:515.
28. Walden PAM, Bagshawe KD. Pregnancies after chemotherapy for gestational trophoblastic tumours. Lancet 1979;2:1241.
29. Sanz MH, Rafecas FJ. Successful pregnancy during chemotherapy for acute promyelocytic leukemia. N Engl J Med 1982;306:939.
30. Steckman ML. Treatment of Crohn's disease with 6-mercaptopurine: what effects on fertility? N Engl J Med 1980;303:817.
31. Rustin GJS, Booth M, Dent J, Salt S, Rustin F, Bagshawe KD. Pregnancy after cytotoxic chemotherapy for gestational trophoblastic tumours. Br Med J 1984;288:103–6.
32. Song H, Wu P, Wang Y, Yang X, Dong S. Pregnancy outcomes after successful chemotherapy for choriocarcinoma and invasive mole: long-term follow-up. Am J Obstet Gynecol 1988;158:538–45.
33. Seinen ML, de Boer NKH, van Hoorn ME, van Bodegraven AA, Bouma G. Safe use of allopurinol and low-dose mercaptopurine therapy during pregnancy in an ulcerative colitis patient. Inflamm Bowel Dis 2012;Mar 8;doi:10,1002/ibd. 22945 [Epub ahead of print].

MEROPENEM

Antibiotic

PREGNANCY RECOMMENDATION: Limited Human Data—Animal Data Suggest Low Risk
BREASTFEEDING RECOMMENDATION: Limited Human Data—Probably Compatible

PREGNANCY SUMMARY

Two reports have described the use of meropenem in human pregnancy. Although the limited human pregnancy experience does not allow a full assessment of the embryo–fetal risk, another carbapenem antibiotic is considered safe to use during the perinatal period (i.e., 28 weeks' gestation or later), and, most likely, meropenem can be classified similarly. The fetal risk of use before this period is unknown.

FETAL RISK SUMMARY

Meropenem is a broad-spectrum, carbapenem antibiotic given IV. The drug belongs to the same class of antibiotics as imipenem. Meropenem is indicated as single-agent therapy for the treatment of complicated skin and skin structure infections (adult patients and pediatric patients ≥3 months only), complicated intra-abdominal infections (adult patients and pediatric patients ≥3 months only), and bacterial meningitis (pediatric patients ≥3 months only). The drug is metabolized to an inactive metabolite. Plasma protein binding is minimal (about 2%) and the elimination half-life is about 1 hour (1).

Reproduction studies in rats and cynomolgus monkeys at doses up to 1.8 and 3.7 times, respectively, the usual human dose (1 g every 8 hours), found no evidence of impaired fertility or fetal harm, except for slight changes in fetal weight in rats at doses of 0.4 times the usual human dose or greater (1).

Placental passage in humans has apparently not been studied, but the molecular weight (about 384) suggests that the drug will cross to the embryo–fetus. Moreover, the drug is distributed into many human tissues, including the endometrium, fallopian tubes, and ovaries (1).

Vancomycin-resistant *Enterococcus faecium* pyelonephritis occurred in a woman at 27 weeks' gestation (2). She also had positive cultures for *Ralstonia pickettii*, methicillin-resistant *Staphylococcus epidermidis*, and *Enterobacter gergoviae* from blood drawn through a peripherally inserted central catheter (PICC) line. The woman was successfully treated with a 14-day course of IV daptomycin (4 mg/kg/day) and meropenem 1 g every 8 hours. The woman went into premature labor 1 month after completion of the therapy and delivered a baby without evidence of infection or abnormalities (no other details were provided) (2).

In a 2013 case report, a 24-year-old woman at 22 weeks' gestation was treated with 6 weeks of meropenem (3 g/day) and cefotaxime (2 g/day) for a brain abscess (3). Glycerin (20 g/day) was given to reduce intracranial pressure. She responded well to the therapy and was then given amoxicillin (750 mg/day) for 4 weeks. At term, she gave birth to a normal 2890-g female infant (3).

BREASTFEEDING SUMMARY

Consistent with the molecular weight (about 384), meropenem is excreted into breast milk. A 2012 case report described the use of meropenem (3 g/day) for 7 days starting on postpartum day 6 by a mother exclusively breastfeeding her infant (4). Five hindmilk samples were collected over a 48-hour period. The average and maximum meropenem concentrations were 0.48 and 0.644 mcg/mL, respectively. The theoretical maximum infant dose was 97 mcg/kg/day which was 0.18% of the maternal weight-adjusted dose. No dermatologic or gastrointestinal adverse effects were noted in the infant (4).

In another case, a mother breastfed her infant until the 4th postpartum month (5). At 2 months, the mother was treated with a 2-week course of meropenem and tobramycin (doses not specified) for a cystic fibrosis exacerbation. There was no change in the infant's stool pattern and it had normal renal function at 6 months of age (5).

In the above cases, the absence of toxic effects in the nursing infants, even with prolonged therapy, suggests that use of meropenem during breastfeeding is probably compatible. However, additional data are warranted and, until such data are available, infants should be monitored for the most common (≥2%) adverse effects observed in adult patients (headache, nausea, constipation, diarrhea, anemia, vomiting, and rash (1)).

References

1. Product information. Meropenem. APP Pharmaceuticals, 2013.
2. Shea K, Hilburger E, Baroco A, Oldfield E. Successful treatment of vancomycin-resistant *Enterococcus faecium* pyelonephritis with daptomycin during pregnancy. Ann Pharmacother 2008;42:722–5.
3. Yoshida M, Matsuda H, Furuya K. Successful prognosis of brain abscess during pregnancy. J Reprod Infertil 2013;14:152–5.
4. Sauberan JB, Bradley JS, Blumer J, Stellwagen LM. Transmission of meropenem in breast milk. Pediatr Infect Dis J 2012;31:832–4.
5. Festini F, Ciuti R, Repetto T, et al. Safety of breast-feeding during an IV tobramycin course for infants of CF women (abstract). Pediatr Pulmonol Suppl 2004;27:288–9. As cited in Meropenem—National Library of Medicine LactMed database, November 6, 2013.

M

MESALAMINE

Anti-inflammatory Bowel Disease Agent

PREGNANCY RECOMMENDATION: Compatible
BREASTFEEDING RECOMMENDATION: Limited Human Data—Potential Toxicity

PREGNANCY SUMMARY

The maternal benefits of therapy with mesalamine appear to outweigh the potential risks to the fetus. No teratogenic effects due to mesalamine have been described and, although toxicity in the fetus has been reported in one case, a causal relationship between the drug and the outcome is controversial.

FETAL RISK SUMMARY

Mesalamine (5-aminosalicylic acid, 5-ASA) is administered by either rectal suspension or suppository for the treatment of distal ulcerative colitis, proctosigmoiditis, and proctitis. It also results from metabolism in the large intestine of the oral preparation sulfasalazine, which is split to mesalamine and sulfapyridine, and from balsalazide and olsalazine, oral formulations that are metabolized in the colon to mesalamine. The history, pharmacology, and pharmacokinetics of mesalamine and olsalazine were extensively reviewed in a 1992 reference (1).

Reproduction studies in rats and rabbits at oral doses of 480 mg/kg/day observed no fetal toxicity or teratogenicity (2).

Sulfasalazine and one of the metabolites, sulfapyridine, readily cross the placenta and could displace bilirubin from albumin if the concentrations were great enough. Mesalamine is bound to different sites on albumin than bilirubin and, thus, has no bilirubin-displacing ability (3). Moreover, only small amounts of mesalamine are absorbed from the cecum and colon into the systemic circulation, and most of this is rapidly excreted in the urine (4).

A 1987 reference reported the concentrations of mesalamine and its metabolite, acetyl-5-aminosalicylic acid, in amniotic fluid at 16 weeks' gestation and in maternal and cord plasma at term in women treated prophylactically with sulfasalazine 3 g/day (5). The drug and metabolite levels (all in mcg/mL) and the number of patients were as follows: amniotic fluid (N = 4), 0.02–0.08 and 0.07–0.77, respectively; maternal plasma (N = 5), 0.08–0.29 and 0.31–1.27, respectively; and cord plasma (N = 5), <0.02–0.10 and 0.29–1.80, respectively. No effects on the fetus or newborn from the maternal drug therapy were mentioned. At delivery in a woman taking 1 g of mesalamine 3 times daily, the concentrations of the drug and its metabolite, 3.3 hours after the last dose, in the mother's serum were 1.2 and 2.8 mcg/mL, respectively, and in the umbilical cord serum 0.4 and 5.7 mcg/mL, respectively (6). The cord:maternal serum ratios were 0.33 and 2.0, respectively.

A review of drug therapy for ulcerative colitis recommended that women taking mesalamine to maintain remission of the disease should continue the drug when trying to conceive or when pregnant (7). A study published in 1993 described the course of 19 pregnancies in 17 women (ulcerative colitis N = 10; Crohn's disease N = 7) who received mesalamine (mean dose 1.7 g/day; range 0.8–2.4 g/day) throughout gestation (8). Full-term deliveries occurred in 18, and 1 patient, with a history of 4 previous miscarriages, suffered a spontaneous abortion. No congenital malformations were observed.

Only one report has described possible in utero mesalamine-induced toxicity that may have occurred during 2nd trimester exposure to the drug (9). The 24-year-old mother was treated, between the 13th and 24th week of gestation, for Crohn's disease with 4 g/day of mesalamine for 5 weeks, then tapered to 2 g/day for 6 weeks, then stopped. A fetal ultrasound at 17 weeks' gestation was normal, but a second examination at 21 weeks' showed bilateral renal hyperechogenicity (9). The term male infant had a serum creatinine at birth of 115 μmol/L (normal 18–35 μmol/L). Renal hyperechogenicity was confirmed at various times up to 6 months of age. At this age, the serum creatinine was 62 μmol/L with a creatinine clearance of 52 mL/min (normal 80–90 mL/min). A renal biopsy at 6 months of age showed focal tubulointerstitial lesions with interstitial fibrosis and tubular atrophy in the absence of cell infiltration (9). Because no other cause of the renal lesions could be found and there was some resemblance to lesions induced by the prostaglandin synthesis inhibitor, indomethacin, the authors attributed the defect to mesalamine (9). A letter published in response to this study, however, questioned the association between the drug and observed renal defect because of the lack of toxicity in an unpublished series of 60 exposed pregnancies and the lack of evidence that mesalamine causes renal prostaglandin synthesis inhibition in utero (10).

A 1997 report described the successful outcomes of 19 pregnancies followed prospectively in 16 women with proven distal colitis (11). The women received either 4-g mesalamine enemas 3 times weekly or a 500-mg mesalamine suppository every night throughout gestation. No fetal abnormalities were observed during pregnancy and all of the full-term offspring were normal at birth and at a median follow-up of 2 years (range 2 months to 5 years) (11).

A 1998 prospective study reported the pregnancy outcomes of 165 women exposed to mesalamine (146 during the 1st trimester) who had contacted a teratogen information service (TIS) (12). The study patients were compared with 165 matched controls who had called the TIS concerning nonteratogenic exposures. There were no significant differences between the two groups in spontaneous abortions (6.7% vs. 8.5%), ectopic pregnancies (0.6% vs. 0%), or elective abortions (none were associated with malformed fetuses) (4.2% vs. 1.8%). There was one major defect (an extra right thumb) in the study group compared with five major anomalies in controls (*ns*). Eight subjects had minor malformations compared with five controls (*ns*). However, compared with controls, significantly more preterm deliveries occurred in subjects (13.0% vs. 4.7%), the mean birth weight was lower (3253 vs. 3461 g), and the mean maternal weight gain was lower (13.1 vs. 15.6 kg) (12).

A 2004 report described the pregnancy outcomes of 113 women who were being treated for inflammatory bowel disease (39 ulcerative colitis; 73 Crohn's disease; and 1 indeterminate colitis) (13). In the group, there were 207 pregnancies, 100 during treatment with a 5-ASA agent (mesalamine, sulfasalazine, balsalazide, or olsalazine) at sometime during pregnancy. Other agents used included 49 cases with prednisone, 101 with azathioprine or mercaptopurine, 27 with metronidazole, 18 with ciprofloxacin, and 2 with cyclosporine. The pregnancy outcomes of the first eligible pregnancy in the 113 women were 2 ectopic pregnancies, 2 elective abortions, 16 spontaneous abortions, 6 premature infants, 85 full-term infants (1 set of twins), and 3 major defects (2.7%). However, one of the "defects" was a case of immature lungs, which is not considered a congenital defect. The other two defects were imperforate anus and an unspecified heart defect. In addition, the two elective abortions were for unspecified fetal defects. The study concluded that there was no evidence that any of the drugs used either alone or in combination was associated with poor pregnancy outcomes (13).

A 2012 case described a 27-year-old woman with ulcerative colitis who was treated throughout pregnancy with allopurinol 100 mg/day, mercaptopurine 25 mg/day, and mesalazine 4 g/day (14). Pregnancy was complicated by diarrhea and blood loss in the 2nd trimester. An elective cesarean section was performed at 39 weeks to give birth to a healthy 3550-g infant (sex not specified) with Apgar score of 9, 10, and 10 at 1, 5, and 10 minutes, respectively. No anomalies were observed in the infant (14).

In contrast to sulfasalazine, mesalamine apparently has no adverse effect on spermatogenesis. Treatment of males with sulfasalazine may adversely affect spermatogenesis (15–19), but either stopping therapy or changing to mesalamine allows recovery of sperm production, usually within 3 months (16–19).

BREASTFEEDING SUMMARY

Small amounts of mesalamine are excreted into human milk. A 1990 report described the excretion of mesalamine and its metabolite, acetyl-5-aminosalicylic acid, into breast milk (20). The woman was receiving 500 mg 3 times daily for ulcerative colitis. In a single plasma and milk sample obtained 5.25 hours after a dose, milk and plasma levels of mesalamine were 0.11 and 0.41 mcg/mL, respectively, a milk:plasma ratio of 0.27. Milk and plasma levels of acetyl-5-aminosalicylic acid were 12.4 and 2.44 mcg/mL, respectively, a ratio of 5.1. In another study, women treated prophylactically with 3 g/day of sulfasalazine had milk levels of mesalamine and acetyl-5-aminosalicylic acid of 0.02 and 1.13–3.44 mcg/mL, respectively (5). No adverse effects on the nursing infants were mentioned.

Low concentrations of mesalamine and its metabolite were also found in a woman taking 1 g 3 times daily (6). Maternal serum levels of the drug and metabolite, determined at 7 and 11 days postpartum, were 0.6 and 1.1 mcg/mL (day 7) and 1.1 and 1.8 mcg/mL (day 11), respectively. Milk concentrations of the drug and metabolite at these times were 0.1 and 18.1 mcg/mL (day 7) and 0.1 and 12.3 mcg/mL (day 11), respectively, representing milk:plasma ratios for mesalamine of 0.17 and 0.09 (day 7 and 11), respectively, and for the metabolite of 16.5 and 6.8 (day 7 and 11), respectively. The estimated daily intake by the infant of mesalamine and metabolite was 0.065 mg (0.015 mg/kg) and 10 mg (2.3 mg/kg), respectively, considered to be negligible amounts (6).

A study published in 1993 described the excretion of olsalazine, a prodrug that is partially (2.4%) absorbed into the systemic circulation before conversion of the remainder by colonic bacteria into two molecules of mesalamine (see Olsalazine), in the breast milk of a woman 4 months postpartum (21). Following a 500-mg oral dose, olsalazine, olsalazine sulfate, and mesalamine were undetectable in breast milk up to 48 hours (detection limits 0.5, 0.2, and 1.0 μmol/L, respectively). Acetyl-5-aminosalicylic concentrations at 10, 14, and 24 hours, were 0.8, 0.86, and 1.24 μmol/L, respectively, but undetectable (detection limit 1.0 μmol/L) during the first 6 hours and after 24 hours. The quantities detected were considered clinically insignificant (21).

Diarrhea in a nursing infant, apparently because of the rectal administration of mesalamine to the mother, has been reported (22). The mother had relapsing ulcerative proctitis. Six weeks after childbirth, treatment was begun with 500-mg mesalamine suppositories twice daily. Her exclusively breastfed infant developed watery diarrhea 12 hours after the mother's first dose. After 2 days of therapy, the mother stopped the suppositories and the infant's diarrhea stopped 10 hours later. Therapy was reinstituted on four occasions with diarrhea developing each time in the infant 8–12 hours after the mother's first dose and stopping 8–12 hours after therapy was halted. Because of the severity of the mother's disease, breastfeeding was discontinued and no further episodes of diarrhea were observed in the infant (22).

Because of the adverse effect described above, a possible allergic reaction, nursing infants of women being treated with mesalamine or olsalazine should be closely observed for changes in stool consistency. The American Academy of Pediatrics classifies 5-aminosalicylic acid (i.e., mesalamine) as a drug that has produced adverse effects in a nursing infant and should be used with caution during breastfeeding (23).

References

1. Segars LW, Gales BJ. Mesalamine and olsalazine: 5-aminosalicylic acid agents for the treatment of inflammatory bowel disease. Clin Pharm 1992;11:514–28.
2. Product information. Asacol. Procter & Gamble Pharmaceuticals, 2000.
3. Jarnerot G, Andersen S, Esbjorner E, Sandstrom B, Brodersen R. Albumin reserve for binding of bilirubin in maternal and cord serum under treatment with sulphasalazine. Scand J Gastroenterol 1981;16:1049–55.
4. Berlin CM Jr, Yaffe SJ. Disposition of salicylazosulfapyridine (Azulfidine) and metabolites in human breast milk. Dev Pharmacol Ther 1980;1:31–9.
5. Christensen LA, Rasmussen SN, Hansen SH, Bondesen S, Hvidberg EF. Salazosulfapyridine and metabolites in fetal and maternal body fluids with special reference to 5-aminosalicylic acid. Acta Obstet Gynecol Scand 1987;66:433–435.
6. Klotz U, Harings-Kaim A. Negligible excretion of 5-aminosalicylic acid in breast milk. Lancet 1993;342:618–9.
7. Kamm MA, Senapati A. Drug management of ulcerative colitis. Br Med J 1992;305:35–8.
8. Habal FM, Hui G, Greenberg GR. Oral 5-aminosalicylic acid for inflammatory bowel disease in pregnancy: safety and clinical course. Gastroenterology 1993;105:1057–60.
9. Colombel J-F, Brabant G, Gubler M-C, Locquet A, Comes M-C, Dehennault M, Delcroix M. Renal insufficiency in infant: side-effect of prenatal exposure to mesalazine? Lancet 1994;344:620–1.
10. Marteau P, Devaux CB. Mesalazine during pregnancy. Lancet 1994;344:1708–9.
11. Bell CM, Habal FM. Safety of topical 5-aminosalicylic acid in pregnancy. Am J Gastroenterol 1997;92:2201–2.
12. Diav-Citrin O, Park Y-H, Veerasuntharam G, Polachek H, Bologa M, Pastuszak A, Koren G. The safety of mesalamine in human pregnancy: a prospective controlled cohort study. Gastroenterology 1998;114:23–8.
13. Moskovitz DN, Bodian C, Chapman ML, Marion JF, Rubin PH, Scherl E, Present DH. The effect on the fetus of medications used to treat pregnant inflammatory bowel-disease patients. Am J Gastroenterol 2004;99:656–61.
14. Seinen ML, de Boer NKH, van Hoorn ME, van Bodegraven AA, Bouma G. Safe use of allopurinol and low-dose mercaptopurine therapy during pregnancy in an ulcerative colitis patient. Inflamm Bowel Dis 2013;19:E37.
15. Freeman JG, Reece VAC, Venables CW. Sulphasalazine and spermatogenesis. Digestion 1982;23:68–71.
16. Toovey S, Hudson E, Hendry WF, Levi AJ. Sulphasalazine and male infertility: reversibility and possible mechanism. Gut 1981;22:445–51.
17. O'Morain C, Smethurst P, Dore CJ, Levi AJ. Reversible male infertility due to sulphasalazine: studies in man and rat. Gut 1984;25:1078–84.
18. Chatzinoff M, Guarino JM, Corson SL, Batzer FR, Friedman LS. Sulfasalazine-induced abnormal sperm penetration assay reversed on changing to 5-aminosalicylic acid enemas. Dig Dis Sci 1988;33:108–10.
19. Delaere KP, Strijbos WE, Meuleman EJ. Sulphasalazine-induced reversible male infertility. Acta Urol Belg 1989;57:29–33.
20. Jenss H, Weber P, Hartmann F. 5-Aminosalicylic acid and its metabolite in breast milk during lactation. Am J Gastroenterol 1990;85:331.
21. Miller LG, Hopkinson JM, Motil KJ, Corboy JE, Andersson S. Disposition of olsalazine and metabolites in breast milk. J Clin Pharmacol 1993;33:703–6.
22. Nelis GF. Diarrhoea due to 5-aminosalicylic acid in breast milk. Lancet 1989;1:383.
23. Committee on Drugs, American Academy of Pediatrics. The transfer of drugs and other chemicals into human milk. Pediatrics 2001;108:776–89.

MESCALINE

Hallucinogenic

See Peyote.

MESNA

Cytoprotective Agent (Antineoplastic)

PREGNANCY RECOMMENDATION: Compatible—Maternal Benefit >> Embryo–Fetal Risk
BREASTFEEDING RECOMMENDATION: Contraindicated

PREGNANCY SUMMARY

The limited animal and human data and the pharmacokinetic properties of mesna suggest that the drug poses little, if any, risk to a human fetus. There is no experience, however, in the 1st trimester. Moreover, mesna is probably not protective against ifosfamide- or cyclophosphamide-induced birth defects if these chemotherapy agents are used in the 1st trimester. However, the maternal benefits from use of the agent with ifosfamide or cyclophosphamide to lessen or prevent hemorrhagic cystitis appear to outweigh the unknown fetal risks.

FETAL RISK SUMMARY

Mesna (sodium 2-mercaptoethane sulfonate) is a cytoprotective agent that is used to prevent hemorrhagic cystitis caused by ifosfamide (approved indication) and cyclophosphamide (off label indication). Upon administration, the agent is rapidly oxidized to its only metabolite, mesna disulfide (dimesna). Dimesna remains in the intravascular compartment and is rapidly eliminated by the kidneys where it is changed back to mesna. The elimination half-lives of mesna and dimesna in the blood are 0.36 and 1.17 hours, respectively (1).

Reproduction studies have been conducted in rats and rabbits. Both species were given doses up to 1000 mg/kg during pregnancy without evidence of fetal harm (1). Two studies investigated the reproductive effects of mesna in pregnant rats and rabbits (2,3). In rats, IV doses up to 800 mg/kg on days 7–17 were associated with lumbar ribs at 400 mg/kg and decreased fetal weight at 800 mg/kg (2). Increased open field activity was observed in rat pups exposed in utero to doses of 400 mg/kg or higher. In pregnant rabbits treated similarly, decreased fetal weights and lumbar ribs were observed with doses of 600 mg/kg or higher (3).

In a 1986 study with rats, two doses of mesna were evaluated to determine if they were protective against cyclophosphamide-induced teratogenicity (4). The low dose (5 mg/kg) offered no protection, but the high dose (30 mg/kg) significantly decreased the number of fetuses with external and skeletal malformations. However, the protection was not extensive enough to be considered effective in protecting pregnant women exposed to cyclophosphamide (4).

In a 2003 study, mesna was combined with ifosfamide to determine if the cytoprotective agent could decrease the toxic effects of ifosfamide on the testes and semen characteristics of rabbits (5). Three groups of male rabbits were given different doses of the combination (ifosfamide 30, 45, or 60 mg/kg plus mesna 6, 9, or 12 mg/kg, followed by a second equal dose of mesna 4 hours later, respectively). Each group received 10 weekly treatments. Controls were given either mesna alone (three groups) or saline (one group). Dose-related ifosfamide-mesna suppression of spermatogenesis and epididymal sperm maturation was observed. In addition, the investigators noted incomplete recovery of the germinal epithelium (5).

It is not known if mesna crosses the human placenta. The molecular weight (about 164) is low enough to cross the placenta, but the short elimination half-life of the parent compound and its rapid metabolism to a metabolite that is restricted to the intravascular compartment suggest that little, if any, exposure of embryo or fetus occurs.

Two reports have described the use of mesna in human pregnancy. In both cases, mesna was combined with ifosfamide in the 2nd and/or 3rd trimesters (see Ifosfamide).

BREASTFEEDING SUMMARY

No reports describing the use of mesna during lactation have been located. The molecular weight (about 164) is low enough for excretion into breast milk, but the short elimination half-life of the parent compound (0.36 hours) and its rapid metabolism to a metabolite that is restricted to the intravascular compartment suggest that little, if any, of the drug will appear in milk. However, mesna is always combined with ifosfamide or cyclophosphamide and women receiving these antineoplastic agents should not breastfeed.

References

1. Product information. Mesna. Gensia Sicor Pharmaceuticals, 2000.
2. Komai Y, Itoh I, Iriyam K, Ishimura K, Fuchigami K, Kobayashi F. Reproduction study of mesna—teratogenicity study in rats by intravenous administration. Kiso to Rinsho 1990;24:6553–94. As cited by Shepard TH.

Catalog of Teratogenic Agents. 10th ed. Baltimore, MD: The Johns Hopkins University Press, 2001:323.
3. Komai Y, Itoh I, Ishimura K, Fuchigami K, Kobayashi F. Reproduction study of mesna—teratogenicity study in rabbits by intravenous administration. Kiso to Rinsho 1990;24:6596–602. As cited in Shepard TH. *Catalog of Teratogenic Agents.* 10th ed. Baltimore, MD: The Johns Hopkins University Press, 2001:323.
4. Slott VL, Hales BF. Sodium 2-mercaptoethane sulfonate protection against cyclophosphamide-induced teratogenicity in rats. Toxicol Appl Pharmacol 1986;82:80–6.
5. Ypsilantis P, Papaioannou N, Psalla D, Politou M, Pitiakoudis M, Simopoulos C. Effects of subchronic ifosfamide-mesna treatment on testes and semen characteristics in the rabbit. Reprod Toxicol 2003;17:699–708.

MESORIDAZINE

[Withdrawn from the market. See 9th edition.]

MESTRANOL

Estrogenic Hormone

PREGNANCY RECOMMENDATION: Contraindicated
BREASTFEEDING RECOMMENDATION: Limited Human Data—Probably Compatible

PREGNANCY SUMMARY

Mestranol is the 3-methyl ester of ethinyl estradiol. Mestranol is used frequently in combination with progestins for oral contraception (see Oral Contraceptives). Congenital malformations attributed to the use of mestranol alone have not been reported.

FETAL RISK SUMMARY

The Collaborative Perinatal Project monitored 614 mother–child pairs with 1st trimester exposure to estrogenic agents (including 179 with exposure to mestranol) (1, pp. 389, 391). An increase in the expected frequency of cardiovascular defects, eye and ear anomalies, and Down's syndrome was found for estrogens as a group but not for mestranol (1, pp. 389, 391, 395). Reevaluation of these data in terms of timing of exposure, vaginal bleeding in early pregnancy, and previous maternal obstetric history, however, failed to support an association between estrogens and cardiac malformations (2). An earlier study also failed to find any relationship with nongenital malformations (3). The use of estrogenic hormones during pregnancy is contraindicated.

In a surveillance study of Michigan Medicaid recipients involving 229,101 completed pregnancies conducted between 1985 and 1992, 190 newborns had been exposed to mestranol during the 1st trimester (F. Rosa, personal communication, FDA, 1993). A total of 13 (6.8%) major birth defects were observed (8 expected). Specific data were available for six defect categories, including (observed/expected) 1/2 cardiovascular defects, 1/0.5 oral clefts, 0/0 spina bifida, 0/0.5 polydactyly, 1/0.5 limb reduction defects, and 0/0.5 hypospadias.

BREASTFEEDING SUMMARY

Estrogens are frequently used for suppression of postpartum lactation (4). Doses of 100–150 mcg of ethinyl estradiol (equivalent to 160–240 mcg of mestranol) for 5–7 days are used (4). Mestranol, when used in oral contraceptives with doses of 30–80 mcg, has been associated with decreased milk production, lower infant weight gain, and decreased composition of nitrogen and protein content of human milk (5–7). The magnitude of these changes is low. However, the changes in milk production and composition may be of nutritional importance in malnourished mothers. If breastfeeding is desired, the lowest dose of oral contraceptives should be chosen. Monitoring of infant weight gain and the possible need for nutritional supplementation should be considered (see Oral Contraceptives).

References

1. Heinonen OP, Slone D, Shapiro S. *Birth Defects and Drugs in Pregnancy*. Littleton, MA: Publishing Sciences Group, 1977.
2. Wiseman RA, Dodds-Smith IC. Cardiovascular birth defects and antenatal exposure to female sex hormones: a reevaluation of some base data. Teratology 1984;30:359–70.
3. Wilson JG, Brent RL. Are female sex hormones teratogenic? Am J Obstet Gynecol 1981;141:567–80.
4. Gilman AG, Goodman LS, Gilman A. *The Pharmacological Basis of Therapeutics*. New York, NY: MacMillan, 1980:1431.
5. Kora SJ. Effect of oral contraceptives on lactation. Fertil Steril 1969;20:419–23.
6. Miller GH, Hughs LR. Lactation and genital involution effects of a new low-dose oral contraceptive on breast-feeding mothers and their infants. Obstet Gynecol 1970;35:44–50.
7. Lonnerdal B, Forsum E, Hambraeus L. Effect of oral contraceptives on composition and volume of breast milk. Am J Clin Nutr 1980;33:816–24.

METAPROTERENOL

Respiratory Drug (Bronchodilator)

PREGNANCY RECOMMENDATION: Compatible
BREASTFEEDING RECOMMENDATION: No Human Data—Probably Compatible

PREGNANCY SUMMARY

No published reports linking the use of metaproterenol with congenital defects have been located. Selective β_2-agonists, including metaproterenol, are commonly used during gestation for the treatment of asthma (1). Fetal tachycardia may occur, but because there is no evidence of fetal injury, there is no contraindication to their use in pregnancy (1). If metaproterenol is used in pregnancy for the treatment of asthma, health care professionals are encouraged to call the toll-free number (877-311-8972) for information about patient enrollment in an Organization of Teratology Information Specialists (OTIS) study.

FETAL RISK SUMMARY

Metaproterenol, a selective β_2-adrenergic agonist, is used as a bronchodilator for bronchial asthma and for reversible bronchospasm occurring in bronchitis and emphysema.

Reproduction studies in mice, rats, and rabbits have been conducted. No embryotoxic or fetotoxic effects, or teratogenicity was observed in rats at a dose that was about 25 times the maximum recommended human oral dose (MRHOD), but embryo toxicity was observed in mice at 31 times the MRHOD. In rabbits, oral doses 620 times the human inhalation dose and 62 times the MRHOD caused both embryotoxic and teratogenic (skeletal anomalies, hydrocephalus, and skull bone separation) effects (2).

In a surveillance study of Michigan Medicaid recipients involving 229,101 completed pregnancies conducted between 1985 and 1992, 361 newborns had been exposed to metaproterenol during the 1st trimester (F. Rosa, personal communication, FDA, 1993). A total of 17 (4.7%) major birth defects were observed (15 expected). Specific data were available for six defect categories, including (observed/expected) 3/4 cardiovascular defects, 1/1 oral clefts, 0/0 spina bifida, 1/1 limb reduction defects, 0/1 hypospadias, and 3/1 polydactyly. Only with the latter defect is there a suggestion of a possible association, but other factors, including the mother's disease, concurrent drug use, and chance, may be involved.

Metaproterenol has been used to prevent premature labor (3–5). Its use for this purpose has been largely assumed by ritodrine, albuterol, or terbutaline. As with all β-mimetics, metaproterenol causes maternal and, to a lesser degree, fetal tachycardia. Maternal hypotension and hyperglycemia and neonatal hypoglycemia should be expected (see also Ritodrine, Albuterol, and Terbutaline). Long-term evaluation of infants exposed in utero to β-mimetics has been reported, but not specifically for metaproterenol (6). No harmful effects in the infants were observed.

BREASTFEEDING SUMMARY

No reports describing the use of metaproterenol during lactation have been located. However, agents in this class, including metaproterenol, are commonly used in the treatment of asthma and there is no contraindication to their use during breastfeeding (1). Neonatal tachycardia, hypoglycemia, or tremor are potential adverse effects (1).

References

1. Report of the Working Group on Asthma and Pregnancy. Management of Asthma During Pregnancy. U.S. Department of Health and Human Services, NIH Publication No. 93-3279, September 1993:19.
2. Product information. Alupent. Boehringer Ingelheim, 2000.
3. Baillie P, Meehan FP, Tyack AJ. Treatment of premature labour with orciprenaline. Br Med J 1970;4:154–5.
4. Tyack AJ, Baillie P, Meehan FP. In-vivo response of the human uterus to orciprenaline in early labour. Br Med J 1971;2:741–3.
5. Zilianti M, Aller J. Action of orciprenaline on uterine contractility during labor, maternal cardiovascular system, fetal heart rate, and acid-base balance. Am J Obstet Gynecol 1971;109:1073–9.
6. Freysz H, Willard D, Lehr A, Messer J, Boog G. A long term evaluation of infants who received a β-mimetic drug while in utero. J Perinat Med 1977;5:94–9.

METARAMINOL

[Withdrawn from the market. See 9th edition.]

METAXALONE

Skeletal Muscle Relaxant

PREGNANCY RECOMMENDATION: No Human Data—No Relevant Animal Data
BREASTFEEDING RECOMMENDATION: No Human Data—Potential Toxicity

PREGNANCY SUMMARY

No reports describing the use of metaxalone in human pregnancy have been located. The manufacturer states that post-marketing experience has not revealed evidence of fetal harm (1), but additional details are not provided. The very limited, incomplete animal data and absence of reported human pregnancy experience prevents an assessment of human embryo–fetal risk. Therefore, avoid in the 1st trimester, if possible, if metaxalone is required in pregnancy.

FETAL RISK SUMMARY

Metaxalone is a skeletal muscle relaxant that is indicated as an adjunct to rest and physical therapy and other measures for the relief of discomforts associated with acute, painful musculoskeletal conditions. The agent has no direct effect on muscles. It is thought to act centrally as a sedative. Metaxalone is metabolized by the liver and the unidentified metabolites are excreted in the urine. The mean terminal elimination half-life is approximately 2.4 hours (1).

Reproduction studies in rats revealed no evidence of impaired fertility or fetal harm (1). Further details of these studies have apparently not been published.

It is not known if metaxalone crosses the human placenta. The molecular weight (about 221) suggests that transfer to the fetal compartment should be expected.

BREASTFEEDING SUMMARY

No reports describing the use of metaxalone during lactation have been located. The molecular weight (about 221) suggests the drug will be excreted into breast milk. The effects of this exposure on a nursing infant are unknown. Because the drug is to be a centrally acting sedative, nursing infants should be closely observed for sedation.

Reference

1. Product information. Skelaxin. Monarch Pharmaceuticals, 2004.

M

METFORMIN

Antidiabetic Agent

PREGNANCY RECOMMENDATION: Human Data Suggest Low Risk
BREASTFEEDING RECOMMENDATION: Compatible

PREGNANCY SUMMARY

Both the animal and human data suggest that metformin is low risk in pregnancy. There also appears to be benefit for the use of metformin in women with polycystic ovary syndrome (PCOS). However, for the treatment of diabetes, although metformin may be beneficial for decreasing the incidence of fetal and/or newborn morbidity and mortality in developing countries where the proper use of insulin is problematic, insulin is still the treatment of choice. Moreover, insulin, unlike metformin, does not cross the placenta and, thus, eliminates the additional concern that the drug therapy itself is adversely affecting the fetus. Carefully prescribed insulin therapy will provide better control of the mother's blood glucose, thereby preventing the fetal and neonatal complications that occur with this disease. High maternal glucose levels, as may occur in diabetes mellitus, are associated with a number of maternal and fetal adverse effects, including fetal structural anomalies if the hyperglycemia occurs early in gestation. To prevent this toxicity, the American College of Obstetricians and Gynecologists recommends that insulin be used for types 1 and 2 diabetes occurring during pregnancy and, if diet therapy alone is not successful, for gestational diabetes (1,2).

FETAL RISK SUMMARY

Metformin is an oral, biguanide, antihyperglycemic agent that is chemically and pharmacologically unrelated to the sulfonylureas. Its mechanism of action is thought to include decreased hepatic glucose production, decreased intestinal absorption of glucose, and increased peripheral uptake and utilization of glucose. The latter two mechanisms result in improved insulin sensitivity (i.e., decreased insulin requirements) (3,4).

Reproduction studies found no evidence of impaired fertility in male and female rats and no evidence of teratogenicity in rats and rabbits at doses up to 600 mg/kg/day, approximately 2 times the maximum recommended human dose based on BSA. A partial placental barrier to metformin was observed, however, based on fetal concentrations (3).

Shepard (5) and Schardein (6) cited a study in rats that observed teratogenesis (neural tube closure defects and edema) in rat fetuses exposed to metformin. The drug did not appear to be a major teratogen because less than 0.5% of the rat fetuses in mothers fed 500–1000 mg/kg developed anophthalmia and anencephaly (5). Higher doses in this study were embryotoxic (7).

A 1994 abstract described the teratogenic effects of high metformin concentrations on early somite mouse embryos exposed in vitro (8). At levels much higher than those obtained clinically, metformin produced neural tube defects and malformations of the heart and eye. In contrast, a study that also appeared in 1994 observed no major malformations in mouse embryos exposed in culture to similar concentrations of metformin (9). About 10% of the embryos, however, demonstrated a transient delay in closure of cranial neuropores.

M

Several studies have documented that metformin crosses the placenta to the embryo and fetus. In an experiment using the human single-cotyledon model with placentas obtained from diabetic patients and normal controls, researchers measured the effect of metformin on the uptake and transport of glucose in both the maternal-to-fetal and fetal-to-maternal directions (10). A second publication described only the results of the experiments studying the effect of metformin on the maternal-to-fetal direction of glucose (11). Compared with controls, metformin had no effect on the movement of glucose in either direction (10,11). In a third study, a dually perfused human placental lobule was used (12). Metformin was rapidly transferred to the fetal side and was the same in placentas obtained from uncomplicated pregnancies and pregnancies with gestational diabetes. A fourth study measured metformin in women and cord blood at delivery (13). All 15 women had PCOS and were taking 850 mg twice daily. The median maternal, umbilical vein, and umbilical artery serum concentrations were 1.50, 2.81, and 3.16 μmol/L, respectively. Metformin had no effect on the pH of umbilical artery blood. No teratogenic effects were observed in the offspring (13).

Among 26 women undergoing treatment for PCOS with metformin, 1.5 g/day for 8 weeks, 3 became pregnant during treatment (14). The women were involved in a study to determine whether metformin was effective in normalizing the condition that is characterized by insulin resistance and hyperandrogenism. One of the pregnancies aborted after 2 months, but the outcomes of the other two were not mentioned. In three reports from the same center, women who had successfully conceived while taking metformin for PCOS were continued on the agent during pregnancy (15–17). Metformin reduced the incidences of 1st trimester spontaneous abortion and gestational diabetes without causing birth defects or neonatal or maternal complications. The therapy had no adverse effect on birth weight or height, or growth and development at 3 and 6 months of age (16).

A number of references have described the use of metformin during all stages of gestation for the control of maternal diabetes (18–26). A 1979 reference described the therapy of gestational diabetes that included the use of metformin alone (*N* = 15), glyburide alone (*N* = 9), or metformin plus glyburide (*N* = 6) in women who were not controlled on diet alone and did not require insulin (20). None of the newborns developed symptomatic hypoglycemia, and only one infant had a congenital defect (ventricular septal defect). Although the treatment group was not specified, ventricular septal defects are commonly associated with poorly controlled diabetes occurring early in gestation (26).

A 1979 reference described the pregnancy outcomes of 60 obese women who received metformin in the 2nd and the 3rd trimester for diabetes (preexisting [*N* = 39] or gestational [*N* = 21]) that was not controlled by diet alone (21). The drug was not effective in 21 (54%) and 6 (29%) of the patients, respectively. The pregnancy outcomes, in terms of hyperbilirubinemia, polycythemia, necrotizing enterocolitis, and major congenital abnormalities, were not better than those observed in another group of insulin-dependent and non-insulin-dependent diabetic women treated by the investigators, except for perinatal mortality. None of the newborns had symptoms of hypoglycemia. The three infants with congenital malformations had defects (two heart defects and one sacral agenesis) that were most likely caused by poorly controlled diabetes occurring early in gestation (21).

Metformin in combination with diet (*N* = 22) and glyburide (*N* = 45) was used during pregnancy for the treatment of preexisting diabetes (22). No cases of lactic acidosis or neonatal hypoglycemia were observed with metformin and diet alone, but the latter complication did occur when glyburide was added. Although neonatal hypoglycemia is a well-known complication of sulfonylurea agents ingested close to delivery (e.g., see Chlorpropamide), this effect is unusual with glyburide (see Glyburide). In an earlier reference, 56 patients received metformin up to 24 hours of delivery without adverse effects in the newborns (19).

Metformin was used during the 1st trimester in 21 pregnancies in a 1984 report (23). A minor abnormality (polydactyly) was observed in a newborn whose mother had taken metformin and glyburide (23). Based on this and previous experience, a treatment regimen was proposed for the management of women with non-insulin-dependent diabetes mellitus (NIDDM) (i.e., type 2 diabetes mellitus) who become pregnant consisting of diet and treatment with metformin and glyburide as necessary (24). If this regimen did not provide control of the blood glucose, a change to insulin therapy was recommended. It was concluded that the drug therapy was not teratogenic, did not cause ketosis, and that neonatal hypoglycemia was preventable if the therapy was changed to insulin before delivery (24).

A 1990 reference addressed the problem of treating diabetes in tropical countries where the availability of medical support and facilities is poor (25). It was recommended that gestational diabetes, not responding to diet alone, could be treated with sulfonylurea agents or metformin or both because of the difficulty in initiating insulin therapy in developing countries (25).

The fetal effects of oral hypoglycemic agents on the fetuses of women attending a diabetes and pregnancy clinic were reported in 1991 (26). All of the women ($N = 21$) had NIDDM and were treated during organogenesis with oral agents (1 with metformin, 2 with phenformin, 17 with sulfonylureas, and 1 with an unknown agent), with a duration of exposure of 3–28 weeks. A control group ($N = 40$) of similar women with NIDDM who were also attending the clinic, matched for age, race, parity, and glycemic control, was used for comparison. Both groups of patients were changed to insulin therapy at the first prenatal visit. From the study group, 11 infants (52%) had congenital malformations, compared with 6 (15%) from the controls ($p < 0.002$). Moreover, six of the newborns from the study group (none in the control group) had ear defects, a malformation that is observed, albeit uncommonly, in diabetic embryopathy. No defects were seen in the one infant exposed to metformin. Sixteen live births occurred in the exposed group, compared with 36 in controls. The groups did not differ in the incidence of hypoglycemia at birth (53% vs. 53%), but three of the exposed newborns had severe hypoglycemia lasting 2, 4, and 7 days, respectively, even though the mothers had not used the oral agents close to delivery. In one of these cases, the mother had been taking metformin 1500 mg daily for 28 weeks. Hyperbilirubinemia was noted in 10 (67%) of 15 exposed liveborn infants, compared with 13 (36%) of the controls, and polycythemia and hyperviscosity requiring partial exchange transfusions were observed in 4 (27%) of 15 exposed vs. 1 (3.0%) control (one exposed infant was not included in these data because the child presented after completion of the study) (26).

A 2004 report described the outcomes of 90 women with PCOS who conceived on metformin (27). Metformin was not associated with preeclampsia. Of the 100 live births, there were no major birth defects (27).

In a second 2004 study, the growth and motor-social development during the first 18 months of 126 live births to 109 women (122 pregnancies) with PCOS was assessed (28). All of the women had conceived while on metformin (1.5–2.55 g/day) and 104 (85%) continued the drug throughout pregnancy. There were two (1.6%) birth defects: a sacrococcygeal teratoma and a tethered spinal cord. Gestational diabetes was significantly lower in the PCOS group than in controls, 7/6% vs. 15.9%. In the 52 male neonates, the birth weight and length did not differ from controls, whereas the 74 female neonates weighed less (3.09 vs. 3.29 kg) and were shorter (48.9 vs. 50.6 cm) than controls. However, there were no systematic differences in growth between the PCOS group and controls over 18 months. At 3, 6, 9, 12, and 18 months, motor-social development scores were >94% and no metformin-exposed infant had motor-social development delays (28).

BREASTFEEDING SUMMARY

Consistent with its molecular weight (about 166), metformin is excreted into breast milk. In seven women taking metformin (500 mg 3 times daily), the mean milk:plasma ratio was 0.35 and the average metformin concentration over the dosing interval was 0.27 mcg/mL (29). The average infant dose received from the milk was about 0.28% of the mother's weight-adjusted dose. A second study involving eight women (three at steady state and five after a single 500-mg dose) estimated that nursing infants would ingest about 0.11%–0.21% of the mother's weight-adjusted dose (30). For the women at steady state, the milk:plasma ratios (based on AUC) were 0.37–0.71. The concentration–time profile of the drug was relatively flat in all subjects (30).

A 2005 study measured metformin in the milk of five women and the effects of this exposure in three of their infants (31). The women were started on metformin (500 mg twice daily) on the first day after cesarean delivery. Peak and trough serum and milk samples were drawn at steady state. The mean serum peak and trough levels in four women (one woman was excluded because her trough level was below the level of detection) were 1.06 and 0.42 mcg/mL, respectively, whereas similar samples from milk yielded mean concentrations of 0.42 and 0.39 mcg/mL, respectively. The mean milk:serum ratio was 0.63. The mean estimated dose as a percentage of the mother's weight-adjusted dose was 0.65% (range 0.43%–1.08%). In three infants, the blood glucose concentrations 4 hours after a feeding were normal (47–77 mg/dL) (31).

References

1. American College of Obstetricians and Gynecologists. Pregestational diabetes mellitus. *ACOG Practice Bulletin*. No. 60. March 2005. Obstet Gynecol 2005;105:675–85.
2. American College of Obstetricians and Gynecologists. Gestational diabetes. *ACOG Practice Bulletin*. No. 30. September 2001. Obstet Gynecol 2001;98:525–38.
3. Product information. Glucophage. Bristol-Myers Squibb, 1997.
4. Klepser TB, Kelly MW. Metformin hydrochloride: an antihyperglycemic agent. Am J Health-Syst Pharm 1997;54:893–903.
5. Shepard TH. *Catalog of Teratogenic Agents*. 8th ed. Baltimore, MD: Johns Hopkins University Press, 1995:270.
6. Schardein JL. *Chemically Induced Birth Defects*. 2nd ed. New York, NY: Marcel Dekker, 1993:417–8.
7. Onnis A, Grella P. *The Biochemical Effects of Drugs in Pregnancy*. Volume 2. West Sussex, England: Ellis Horwood, 1984:179.
8. Miao J, Smoak IW. In vitro effects of the biguanide, metformin, on early-somite mouse embryos (abstract). Teratology 1994;49:389.
9. Denno KM, Sadler TW. Effects of the biguanide class of oral hypoglycemic agents on mouse embryogenesis. Teratology 1994;49:260–6.
10. Elliott B, Schuessling F, Langer O. The oral antihyperglycemic agent metformin does not affect glucose uptake and transport in the human diabetic placenta (abstract). Am J Obstet Gynecol 1997;176:S182.
11. Elliott B, Langer O, Schuessling F. Human placental glucose uptake and transport are not altered by the oral antihyperglycemic agent metformin. Am J Obstet Gynecol 1997;176:527–30.
12. Nanovskaya TN, Nekhayeva IA, Patrikeeva SL, Hankins GDV, Ahmed MS. Transfer of metformin across the dually perfused human placenta lobule. Am J Obstet Gynecol 2006;195:1081–5.
13. Vanky E, Zahlsen K, Spigset O, Carlsen SM. Placental passage of metformin in women with polycystic ovary syndrome. Fert Steril 2005;83:1575–8.
14. Velazquez EM, Mendoza S, Hamer T, Sosa F, Glueck CJ. Metformin therapy in polycystic ovary syndrome reduces hyperinsulinemia, insulin resistance, hyperandrogenemia, and systolic blood pressure, while facilitating normal menses and pregnancy. Metabolism 1994;43:647–54.
15. Glueck CJ, Phillips H, Cameron D, Sieve-Smith L, Wang P. Continuing metformin throughout pregnancy in women with polycystic ovary syndrome appears to safely reduce first-trimester spontaneous abortion: a pilot study. Fertil Steril 2001;75:46–52.
16. Glueck CJ, Wang P, Goldenberg, Sieve-Smith L. Pregnancy outcomes among women with polycystic ovary syndrome treated with metformin. Hum Reprod 2002;17:2858–64.
17. Glueck CJ, Wang P, Kobayashi S, Phillips H, Sieve-Smith L. Metformin therapy throughout pregnancy reduces the development of gestational diabetes in women with polycystic ovary syndrome. Fertil Steril 2002;77:520–5.
18. Brearley BF. The management of pregnancy in diabetes mellitus. Practitioner 1975;215:644–52.

M

19. Jackson WPU, Coetzee EJ. Side-effects of metformin. S Afr Med J 1979;56:1113–4.
20. Coetzee EJ, Jackson WPU. Diabetes newly diagnosed during pregnancy. A 4-year study at Groote Schuur Hospital. S Afr Med J 1979;56:467–75.
21. Coetzee RJ, Jackson WPU. Metformin in management of pregnant insulin-independent diabetics. Diabetologia 1979;16:241–45.
22. Coetzee EJ, Jackson WPU. Pregnancy in established non-insulin-dependent diabetics. A five-and-a-half year study at Groote Schuur Hospital. S Afr Med J 1980;58:795–802.
23. Coetzee EJ, Jackson WPU. Oral hypoglycaemics in the first trimester and fetal outcome. S Afr Med J 1984;65:635–7.
24. Coetzee EJ, Jackson WPU. The management of non-insulin-dependent diabetes during pregnancy. Diabetes Res Clin Pract 1986;5:281–7.
25. Gill G. Practical management of diabetes in the tropics. Trop Doct 1990;20:4–10.
26. Piacquadio K, Hollingsworth DR, Murphy H. Effects of in-utero exposure to oral hypoglycaemic drugs. Lancet 1991;338:866–9.
27. Glueck CJ, Bornovak S, Pranikoff J, Goldenberg N, Dharashivkar S, Wang P. Metformin, pre-eclampsia, and pregnancy outcomes in women with polycystic ovary syndrome. Diabet Med 2004;21:829–36.
28. Glueck CJ, Goldenberg N, Pranikoff J, Loftspring M, Sieve I, Wang P. Height, weight, and motor-social development during the first 18 months of life in 126 infants born to 109 mothers with polycystic ovary syndrome who conceived on and continued metformin through pregnancy. Hum Reprod 2004;19:1323–30.
29. Hale TW, Kristensen JH, Hackett LP, Kohan R, Ilett KF. Transfer of metformin into human milk. Diabetologia 2002;45:1509–14.
30. Gardiner SJ, Kirkpatrick CMJ, Begg EJ, Zhang M, Moore MP, Saville DJ. Transfer of metformin into human milk. Clin Pharmacol Ther 2003;73:71–7.
31. Briggs GG, Ambrose PJ, Nageotte MP, Padilla G, Wan S. Excretion of metformin into breast milk and the effect on nursing infants. Obstet Gynecol 2005;105:1437–41.

METHACYCLINE

[Withdrawn from the market. See 9th edition.]

METHADONE

Narcotic Agonist Analgesic

PREGNANCY RECOMMENDATION: Human Data Suggest Risk
BREASTFEEDING RECOMMENDATION: Limited Human Data—Probably Compatible

M

PREGNANCY SUMMARY

The reported use in pregnancy of methadone is almost exclusively related to the treatment of heroin addiction, but the drug also is used in patients addicted to other opioid agonists. The National Birth Defects Prevention Study discussed below found evidence that opioid use during organogenesis is associated with a low absolute risk of congenital birth defects. A second study also found a similar association. Because patients taking methadone usually consume a wide variety of drugs, it is not always possible to separate completely the effects of methadone from the effects of other agents. Neonatal narcotic withdrawal and low birth weight appear to be major problems.

FETAL RISK SUMMARY

Withdrawal symptoms occur in approximately 60%–90% of the infants exposed in utero to methadone (1–6). One study concluded that the intensity of withdrawal was increased if the daily maternal dosage exceeded 20 mg (5). When withdrawal symptoms do occur, they normally start within 48 hours after delivery, but a small percentage may be delayed up to 7–14 days (1). One report observed initial withdrawal symptoms appearing up to 28 days after birth, but the authors do not mention if mothers of these infants were breastfeeding (6). Methadone concentrations in breast milk are reported to be sufficient to prevent withdrawal in addicted infants (see Breastfeeding Summary below). Some authors believe methadone withdrawal is more intense than that occurring with heroin (1). Less than one-third of symptomatic infants, require therapy (1–5). A lower incidence of hyaline membrane disease is seen in infants exposed in utero to chronic methadone and may be due to elevated blood levels of prolactin (7).

Infants of drug-addicted mothers are often small for gestational age (SGA). In some series, one-third or more of the infants weigh less than 2500 g (1,2,4). The newborns of methadone addicts may have a higher birth weight than comparable offspring of heroin addicts for reasons that remain unclear (4).

Other problems occurring in the offspring of methadone addicts are increased mortality, sudden infant death syndrome (SIDS), jaundice, and thrombocytosis. A correlation between drug addiction and SIDS has been suggested with 20 cases (2.8%) in a group of 702 infants, but the data could not attribute the increase to a single drug (8,9). Another study of 313 infants of methadone-addicted mothers reported 2 cases (0.6%) of SIDS, an incidence similar to the overall experience of that location (4). In one study, a positive correlation was found between severity of neonatal withdrawal and the incidence of SIDS (9). Maternal withdrawal during pregnancy has been observed to produce a marked response of the fetal adrenal glands and sympathetic nervous system (10). An increased stillborn and neonatal mortality rate has also been reported (11). Both reports recommend against detoxification of the mother during gestation. Jaundice is comparatively infrequent in both heroin- and methadone-exposed newborns. However, a higher rate of severe hyperbilirubinemia in methadone-exposed infants than in a comparable group of heroin-exposed infants has been observed (1). Thrombocytosis developing in the 2nd week of life, with some platelet counts exceeding 1,000,000/mm^3 and persisting for more than 16 weeks has been reported (12). The condition was not related to withdrawal symptoms or neonatal treatment. Some of these infants also had increased circulating platelet aggregates.

Respiratory depression is not a significant problem, and Apgar scores are comparable to those of a nonaddicted population (1–5). Long-term effects on the behavior and gross motor development skills are not known.

Results of a National Birth Defects Prevention Study (1997–2005) were published in 2011 (13). This population-based case–control study examined the association between maternal use of opioid analgesics and >30 types of major structural birth defects. In 17,449 case mothers, therapeutic opioid use was reported by 454 (2.6%) compared with 134 (2.0%) of 6701 control mothers. Indications for use of opioid analgesics were surgical procedures (41%), infections (34%), chronic diseases (20%), and injuries (18%). Dose, duration, or frequency were not evaluated. The exposure period evaluated was from 1 month before to 3 months after conception. Limiting the exposure period to the first 2 months after conception produced similar results. Infants with >1 defect were included in multiple birth defect categories. The following opioids were included (number of cases for each agent not specified): codeine, hydrocodone, hydromorphone, fentanyl, meperidine, methadone, morphine, oxycodone, pentazocine, propoxyphene, and tramadol. The birth defect, total number, number exposed, and the adjusted odds ratio (aOR) with 95% confidence interval (CI) were as follows:

Birth Defect	Total	Cases	aOR (95% CI)
Spina bifida	718	26	2.0 (1.3–3.2)
Any heart defect (20 types)	7724	211	1.4 (1.1–1.7)
Atrioventricular septal defect	175	9	2.4 (1.2–4.8)
Teratology of Fallot	672	21	1.7 (1.1–2.8)
Conotruncal defect	1481	41	1.5 (1.0–2.1)
Conoventricular septal defect	110	6	2.7 (1.1–6.3)
Left ventricular outflow tract obstruction defect	1195	36	1.5 (1.0–2.2)
Hypoplastic left heart syndrome	357	17	2.4 (1.4–4.1)
Right ventricular outflow tract obstruction defect	1175	40	1.6 (1.1–2.3)
Pulmonary valve stenosis	867	34	1.7 (1.2–2.6)
Atrial septal defect (ASD)	511	17	2.0 (1.2–3.6)
Ventricular septal defect + ASD	528	17	1.7 (1.0–2.9)
Hydrocephaly	301	11	2.0 (1.0–3.7)
Glaucoma/anterior chamber defects	103	5	2.6 (1.0–6.6)
Gastroschisis	726	26	1.8 (1.1–2.9)

The authors speculated that the activity of opioids and their receptors as growth regulators during development of the embryo might be a mechanism to explain the above findings. The exposure data were obtained by retrospective maternal self-report; the authors acknowledged that recall bias and misclassification might have affected their results. They concluded that the absolute risk was a modest absolute increase above the baseline risk for birth defects (13).

In a 2011 retrospective cohort study from Ireland, there were 61,030 singleton births from one hospital in 2000–2007 (14). Among these births, there were 618 (1%) on methadone at delivery who were more likely to be younger and smokers. Exposure to methadone was associated with increased risk of preterm birth <32 weeks' gestation (aOR 2.47, 95% CI 1.40–4.34), SGA (<10th percentile) (aOR 3.27, 95% CI 2.49–4.28), admission to the neonatal unit (aOR 9.14, 95% CI 7.21–11.57), and a major birth anomaly (aOR 1.94, 95% CI 1.10–3.43). There was a dose–response relationship between methadone and neonatal abstinence syndrome (14).

A 1980 case report described a female infant born at 34 weeks' to a mother enrolled in a methadone program for heroin addiction and who also used LSD (15). Both drugs were used throughout gestation. The infant had left anophthalmia but no other defects. The authors thought that LSD was the most likely cause of the defect (15).

Two reports described the occurrence of strabismus in infants exposed in utero to methadone (primarily) and other opioids (16,17). The incidence of the eye defect was 8–10 times the occurrence in a nonexposed population.

M

BREASTFEEDING SUMMARY

Methadone is excreted into breast milk and claims have been made that it could prevent withdrawal in addicted infants. One study reported an average milk concentration in 10 patients of 0.27 mcg/mL, representing an average milk:plasma ratio of 0.83 (18). The same investigators earlier reported levels ranging from 0.17 to 5.6 mcg/mL in the milk of mothers on methadone maintenance (2). At least one infant death has been attributed to methadone obtained through breast milk (19). However, a recent report claimed that methadone enters breast milk in very low quantities that are clinically insignificant (20).

A 1997 report described two cases where the mothers were taking high maintenance doses of methadone (73 and 60 mg/day) (21). Both mothers breastfed their infants. The average milk:plasma ratios were 0.66 and 1.22, respectively. The amounts of methadone in milk were considered to be negligible (21). A 2000 study evaluated eight lactating women who were taking methadone (25–180 mg/day) (22). The mean amount of methadone in milk was 95 ng/mL (range 27–260 ng/mL). Based on an estimated newborn milk intake of 475 mL/day, the estimated mean daily methadone dose was 0.05 mg/day. No adverse effects of the exposure were observed during the duration of breastfeeding (2.5–21 months) or during weaning (22).

In another 1997 study, 12 breastfeeding women were taking methadone in single daily doses of 20–80 mg (23). The mean milk:plasma ratio was 0.44 (95% CI 0.24–0.64). The mean infant dose as a percentage of the mother's dose was 2.79% (2.07%–3.51%). In blood samples obtained from eight infants, seven had methadone concentrations below the limit of detection. The plasma concentration in the eighth infant was 6.5 mcg/L. Milk methadone was insufficient to prevent the development of neonatal abstinence syndrome in seven infants. No drug-induced adverse effects were observed in the 12 infants (23).

The American Academy of Pediatrics classifies methadone as compatible with breastfeeding (24).

References

1. Zelson C, Lee SJ, Casalino M. Neonatal narcotic addiction. N Engl J Med 1973;289:1216–20.
2. Blinick G, Jerez E, Wallach RC. Methadone maintenance, pregnancy and progeny. JAMA 1973;225:477–9.
3. Strauss ME, Andresko M, Stryker JC, Wardell JN, Dunkel LD. Methadone maintenance during pregnancy: pregnancy, birth and neonate characteristics. Am J Obstet Gynecol 1974;120:895–900.
4. Newman RG, Bashkow S, Calko D. Results of 313 consecutive live births of infants delivered to patients in the New York City methadone maintenance program. Am J Obstet Gynecol 1975;121:233–7.
5. Ostrea EM, Chavez CJ, Strauss ME. A study of factors that influence the severity of neonatal narcotic withdrawal. J Pediatr 1976;88:642–5.
6. Kandall SR, Gartner LM. Delayed presentation of neonatal methadone withdrawal. Pediatr Res 1973;7:320.
7. Parekh A, Mukherjee TK, Jhaveri R, Rosenfeld W, Glass L. Intrauterine exposure to narcotics and cord blood prolactin concentrations. Obstet Gynecol 1981;57:447–9.
8. Pierson PS, Howard P, Kleber HD. Sudden deaths in infants born to methadone-maintained addicts. JAMA 1972;220:1733–4.
9. Chavez CJ, Ostrea EM, Stryker JC, Smialek Z. Sudden infant death syndrome among infants of drug-dependent mothers. J Pediatr 1979;95:407–9.
10. Zuspan FP, Gumpel JA, Mejia-Zelaya A, Madden J, David R. Fetal stress from methadone withdrawal. Am J Obstet Gynecol 1975;122:43–6.
11. Rementeria JL, Nunag NN. Narcotic withdrawal in pregnancy: stillbirth incidence with a case report. Am J Obstet Gynecol 1973;116:1152–6.
12. Burstein Y, Giardina PJV, Rausen AR, Kandall SR, Siljestrom K, Peterson CM. Thrombocytosis and increased circulating platelet aggregates in newborn infants of polydrug users. J Pediatr 1979;94:895–9.
13. Broussard CS, Rasmussen SA, Reefhuis J, Friedman JM, Jann MW, Riehle-Colarusso T, Honein MA; National Birth Defects Prevention Study. Maternal treatment with opioid analgesics and risk for birth defects. Am J Obstet Gynecol 2011;204:314–7.
14. Cleary BJ, Donnelly JM, Strawbridge JD, Gallagher PJ, Fahey T, White MJ, Murphy DJ. Methadone and perinatal outcomes: a retrospective cohort study. Am J Obstet Gynecol 2011;204:139–41.
15. Margolis S, Martin L. Anophthalmia in an infant of parents using LSD. Ann Ophthalmol 1980;12:1378–81.
16. Nelson LB, Ehrlich S, Calhoun JH, Matteucci T, Finnegan LP. Occurrence of strabismus in infants born to drug-dependent women. AJDC 1987;141:175–8.
17. Gill AC, Oei J, Lewis NL, Younan N, Kennedy I, Lui K. Strabismus in infants of opiate-dependent mothers. Acta Paediatr 2003;92:379–85.
18. Blinick G, Inturrisi CE, Jerez E, Wallach RC. Methadone assays in pregnant women and progeny. Am J Obstet Gynecol 1975;121:617–21.
19. Smialek JE, Monforte JR, Aronow R, Spitz WU. Methadone deaths in children—a continuing problem. JAMA 1977;238:2516–7.
20. Anonymous. Methadone in breast milk. Med Lett Drugs Ther 1979;21:52.
21. Geraghty B, Graham EA, Logan B, Weiss EL. Methadone levels in breast milk. J Hum Lact 1997;13:227–30.
22. McCarthy JJ, Posey BL. Methadone levels in human milk. J Hum Lact 2000;16:115–20.
23. Wojnar-Horton RE, Kristensen JH, Yapp P, Ilett KF, Dusci LJ, Hackett LP. Methadone distribution and excretion into breast milk of clients in a methadone maintenance programme. Br J Clin Pharmacol 1997;44:543–7.
24. Committee on Drugs, American Academy of Pediatrics. The transfer of drugs and other chemicals into human milk. Pediatrics 2001;108:776–89.

METHAMPHETAMINE

Central Stimulant

See Amphetamine.

METHANTHELINE

[Withdrawn from the market. See 9th edition.]

METHAQUALONE

[Withdrawn from the market. See 9th edition.]

METHARBITAL

[Withdrawn from the market. See 8th edition.]

METHAZOLAMIDE

Diuretic (Carbonic Anhydrase Inhibitor)

PREGNANCY RECOMMENDATION: No Human Data—Probably Compatible
BREASTFEEDING RECOMMENDATION: No Human Data—Probably Compatible

PREGNANCY SUMMARY

Methazolamide is a carbonic anhydrase inhibitor used in glaucoma to lower intraocular pressure. No reports describing the use of methazolamide in human pregnancy have been located. The drug is teratogenic in some animal species (1). (See also Acetazolamide.)

BREASTFEEDING SUMMARY

No reports describing the use of methazolamide during human lactation have been located.

Reference

1. Product information. Neptazane. Lederle Laboratories, 1988.

METHDILAZINE

[Withdrawn from the market. See 9th edition.]

METHENAMINE

Urinary Germicide

PREGNANCY RECOMMENDATION: Compatible
BREASTFEEDING RECOMMENDATION: Limited Human Data—Probably Compatible

PREGNANCY SUMMARY

Methenamine, in either the mandelate or the hippurate salt forms, is used for chronic suppressive treatment of bacteriuria. The limited human data do not suggest risk.

FETAL RISK SUMMARY

In two studies, the mandelate form was given to 120 patients and the hippurate to 70 patients (1,2). No increases in congenital defects or other problems as compared with controls were observed.

The Collaborative Perinatal Project reported 49 1st trimester exposures to methenamine (3, pp. 299, 302). For use anytime in pregnancy, 299 exposures were recorded (3, p. 435). Only in the latter group was a possible association with malformations found. Independent confirmation is required.

In a surveillance study of Michigan Medicaid recipients involving 229,101 completed pregnancies conducted between 1985 and 1992, 209 newborns had been exposed to methenamine during the 1st trimester (F. Rosa, personal communication, FDA, 1993). Eight (3.8%) major birth defects were observed (nine expected). Specific data were available for six defect categories, including (observed/expected) 1/2 cardiovascular defects, 1/0.5 oral clefts, 0/0 spina bifida, 1/1 polydactyly, 1/0.5 limb reduction defects, and 0/0.5 hypospadias. These data do not support an association between the drug and congenital defects.

Methenamine interferes with the determination of urinary estrogen (4). Urinary estrogen was formerly used to assess the condition of the fetoplacental unit, depressed levels being associated with fetal distress. This assessment is now made by measuring unconjugated estriol, which is not affected by methenamine.

BREASTFEEDING SUMMARY

Methenamine is excreted into breast milk. Peak levels occur at 1 hour (5). No adverse effects on the nursing infant have been reported.

References

1. Gordon SF. Asymptomatic bacteriuria of pregnancy. Clin Med 1972;79: 22–4.
2. Furness ET, McDonald PJ, Beasley NV. Urinary antiseptics in asymptomatic bacteriuria of pregnancy. NZ Med J 1975;81:417–9.
3. Heinonen OP, Slone D, Shapiro S. *Birth Defects and Drugs in Pregnancy*. Littleton, MA: Publishing Sciences Group, 1977.
4. Kivinen S, Tuimala R. Decreased urinary oestriol concentrations in pregnant women during hexamine hippurate treatment. Br Med J 1977;2:682.
5. Sapeika N. The excretion of drugs in human milk—a review. J Obstet Gynaecol Br Emp 1947;54:426–31.

METHICILLIN

[Withdrawn from the market. See 9th edition.]

METHIMAZOLE

Antithyroid

PREGNANCY RECOMMENDATION: Human Data Suggest Risk
BREASTFEEDING RECOMMENDATION: Compatible

PREGNANCY SUMMARY

Structural anomalies that have been observed after exposure during organogenesis have suggested a phenotype for methimazole embryopathy (1,2), but the complete spectrum of anomalies may need further definition (3). Carbimazole is converted in vivo to methimazole. Some of the anomalies have also been seen in untreated hyperthyroidism. If methimazole or carbimazole is used, the lowest possible dose to control the maternal disease should be given. One review recommended that the dosage should be adjusted to maintain the maternal free thyroxine levels in a mildly thyrotoxic range (4).

M

FETAL RISK SUMMARY

Methimazole, a thiourea antithyroid agent, is used for the treatment of hyperthyroidism. It readily crosses the placenta to the fetus. Two patients undergoing 2nd trimester therapeutic abortions were given a single 10-mg ^{35}S-labeled oral dose 2 hours before pregnancy termination (5). Fetal:maternal serum ratios were 0.72 and 0.81, representing 0.22% and 0.24% of the administered dose. In the same study, three patients at 14, 14, and 20 weeks' gestation were given an equimolar dose of carbimazole (16.6 mg). Fetal:maternal serum ratios were 0.80–1.09 with 0.17%–0.87% of the total radioactivity in the fetus. The highest serum and tissue levels were found in the 20-week-old fetus (5).

A comparison of the placental transfer of methimazole and propylthiouracil (PTU) in the perfused human term placental lobule was reported in 1997 (6). Because there were no significant differences between the drugs, the investigators concluded that the drugs have similar placental transfer kinetics.

Early references reported 11 cases of scalp defects (aplasia cutis congenita) in newborns exposed in utero to methimazole or carbimazole (converted in vivo to methimazole) (7–11). In 2 of the 11 infants, umbilical defects (patent urachus in one; patent vitelline duct in another) were also observed, suggesting to one investigator, because of the rarity of these defects, that the combination of anomalies represented a possible malformation syndrome (9). In one of the above cases, á-fetoprotein was elevated in both the maternal serum (3–18 standard deviations [SD] above normal) and the amniotic fluid (2.4–4 SD above normal) (11). The 6-cm scalp defect was the only defect found in the newborn who had been exposed during the 1st trimester to methimazole (10 mg/day).

In contrast, a 1987 study examined the records of 49,091 live births for cases of congenital skin defects (12). Of such cases 25 (0.05%) were identified, 13 (0.03%) of which were confined to the scalp. In the sample of 48,057 women, 24 were treated with methimazole or carbimazole during the 1st trimester, but none of these mothers produced children with the skin defects. The authors concluded that they could not exclude an association between the therapy and scalp defects, but if it existed, it was a weak association (12).

Defects observed in two infants exposed to the antithyroid agents in two other reports were imperforate anus (8) and transposition of the great arteries (died at 3 days of age) (13). In a large prospective study, 25 patients were exposed to one or more noniodide thyroid suppressants during the 1st trimester, 9 of whom took methimazole (14). From the total group, 4 children with nonspecified malformations were found, suggesting that the drugs may be teratogenic. However, since 16 of the group took other antithyroid drugs, the relationship between methimazole and the anomalies cannot be determined. In a study of 25 infants exposed to carbimazole, 2 were found to have defects: bilateral congenital cataracts and partial adactyly of the right foot (15). Because no pattern of malformations has emerged from these reports, it appears that these malformations were not associated with the drug therapy. In addition, other reports have described the use of methimazole and carbimazole during pregnancy without fetal anomalies (16–30).

In a surveillance study of Michigan Medicaid recipients involving 229,101 completed pregnancies conducted between 1985 and 1992, 5 newborns had been exposed to methimazole during the 1st trimester (F. Rosa, personal communication, FDA, 1993). One (20.0%) major birth defect was observed (none expected), a hypospadias.

A 1984 report described the relationship between maternal Graves' disease and major structural malformations of external organs, including the oral cavity, in 643 newborns (31). Of 167 newborns delivered from mothers who were hyperthyroid during gestation, 117 were exposed in utero to methimazole. In 50 newborns, the mothers received no treatment, other than subtotal thyroidectomy before or during pregnancy. The incidences of anomalies in these two groups were 1.7% (2 of 117) and 6.0% (3 of 50), respectively. For 476 neonates the mothers were euthyroid during gestation, with 126 receiving treatment with methimazole and 350 receiving no treatment (other than surgery). No malformations were observed in the methimazole-exposed infants and only 1 (0.3%) occurred in the patients not receiving drug therapy. The difference in malformation rates between the nonexposed neonates in the hyperthyroid and euthyroid groups was significant (6% vs. 0.3%, $p < 0.01$). Similarly, the difference between the two groups in total malformations, 3% (5 of 167) vs. 0.2% (1 of 476) was also significant ($p < 0.01$). The defects observed were malformation of the earlobe (methimazole-exposed, hyperthyroid), omphalocele (methimazole-exposed, hyperthyroid), imperforate anus (hyperthyroid), anencephaly (hyperthyroid), harelip (hyperthyroid), and polydactyly (euthyroid). The authors concluded that the disease itself causes congenital malformations and that the use of methimazole lessened the risk for adverse outcome (31).

A 1987 case report described a female infant (46,XX) who had been exposed throughout gestation to methimazole and propranolol given for maternal hyperthyroidism (32). Choanal atresia was noted at birth and treated surgically. At 6 months of age, she was noted to be developmentally delayed, especially in gross motor development, and had mild neurosensory hearing loss bilaterally and recurrent dacryocystitis. By 3.5 years, her development continued to be markedly delayed. Her height and weight were below the 3rd percentile and a small area of alopecia was noted in the parietal region close to the midline on the otherwise normal scalp. Although the chest was symmetrical, both nipples were absent (athelia). Other abnormalities noted at this time were upper slanting palpebral fissures and epicanthal folds, a broad nasal bridge with slightly anteverted nostrils, and a tented upper lip with a short philtrum (32).

Two cases of esophageal atresia and tracheoesophageal fistula in newborn infants exposed throughout gestation to methimazole (30 mg/day) were reported in 1992 (33). The mothers were euthyroid during pregnancy. Both newborns were small for gestational age and had palpable goiters with laboratory evidence of hypothyroidism. Surgical correction of the defects was attempted but the infants died from postoperative sepsis and renal failure. At autopsy, in addition to the defects noted above, one infant had a ventricular septal defect and a Meckel's diverticulum, and both had diffuse goiters. Because of the relatively low frequency of esophageal atresia and tracheoesophageal fistula (1:3000–1:4500), the authors attributed the defects to methimazole (33).

A 1992 study reported no difference in the intellectual capacity of offspring of 31 mothers with Graves' disease who were treated during gestation with either methimazole (N = 15) or PTU (N = 16) when compared with nonexposed controls (34). The ages of the subjects ranged from 4 to 23 years. None was hypothyroid or had goiter at birth. There were no differences between the antithyroid drugs, and there was no correlation between dosage used and intelligence (34).

Two reports, one in 1994 and the other in 1995, described aplasia cutis in two newborns exposed during pregnancy to methimazole (35,36). In reviewing their case and previously published cases, the authors of the 1994 publication were uncertain of a causal association between the drug and the scalp defect (35). The other group of authors concluded that the evidence indicated a strong association between the drug and aplasia cutis (36). Both groups concluded, because no such cases had been reported with PTU, that this drug was preferred for the treatment of hyperthyroidism during pregnancy (35,36).

A female infant exposed in utero to methimazole during the first 2 months of pregnancy and then to PTU until term was described in a 1997 abstract (37). Birth weight and length were normal as was the chromosomal analysis (46,XX). Malformations observed in the infant were choanal atresia, right iris/retinal coloboma, right renal pelvis ectasia, and minor facial anomalies (37).

A brief 1996 report described multiple malformations in a newborn of a woman who was treated with methimazole (38). Metoprolol (150 mg/day) and methimazole (30 mg/day) were taken throughout most of the 1st trimester. Levothyroxine was also administered during most of the pregnancy. Metoprolol was discontinued at about 9 weeks' gestation and the methimazole dose was gradually tapered until a subtotal thyroidectomy was performed at 18 weeks'. Premature labor could not be arrested and a 750-g male infant was delivered at 27 weeks' with Apgar scores of 1, 0, and 3 at 1, 5, and 10 minutes, respectively. Major malformations evident were choanal atresia, esophageal atresia with tracheoesophageal fistula, omphaloenteric connection, and multiple ventricular septal defects. The infant died at 6 weeks of age secondary to complications arising from corrective surgery (38).

A 1998 case report described a 3-year-old boy with choanal atresia (surgically corrected shortly after birth), hypoplastic nipples (hypothelia; see also reference 32 for a case of athelia), and developmental delay (1). He had been exposed throughout a 34 weeks' gestation to carbimazole, but was euthyroid at birth. He was hypotonic at birth and remained so at 3 years of age. He had mild global but predominantly motor developmental delay. His height and weight were at the 10th percentile or less. Other features noted were short upslanting palpebral fissures (length <3rd percentile), small nose and mouth, and a short philtrum. The nipples were hypoplastic and inverted. The mother had a normal, healthy child before and after the subject case. The authors suggested that the combination of malformations represented a rare but distinct syndrome of methimazole teratogenicity (1).

A case of multiple defects in a newborn infant exposed in utero to methimazole (20 mg/day) was reported in 1999 (2). The mother, who was euthyroid on therapy, had taken methimazole for 9 years prior to conception and was continued on the drug during the first 7 gestational weeks (i.e., 9 weeks after the first day of the last menstrual period). At

M

that time, she was changed to PTU for the remainder of her pregnancy. A 1475-g (25th–50th percentile) male preterm infant was delivered at 31 gestational weeks because of premature rupture of the membranes. The Apgar scores, length, and head circumference were not recorded, but severe respiratory distress required assisted ventilation. Anomalies observed in the infant were bilateral choanal atresia, esophageal atresia and tracheoesophageal fistula, patent ductus arteriosus (closed spontaneously at 2 months), and periventricular leukomalacia with bilateral parieto-occipital cavitations. The latter defect was confirmed by magnetic resonance imaging (MRI) at age 2 years and was thought to be of possible hypoxic-ischemic origin and related to prematurity. At 7 months of age, abdominal sonography, chromosomal analysis, and brain-stem auditory evoked responses were normal. An eye examination revealed bilateral convergent strabismus, mildly pale papillae, and diffuse depigmentation of the fundi. Severe psychomotor retardation with mixed tetraparesis was evident. At 4.25 years, the weight and height were both below the 3rd percentile for age, he was unable to walk or sit without support, and language was absent. Physical examination noted dolichocephaly, bilateral ptosis of the eyelid with inner epicanthal fold, convergent squint, mild malar hypoplasia, small nose with moderately anteverted nostrils, long and flat philtrum, a highly arched palate, bilateral bridged palmar creases, axial hypotonia and limb hypertonia, poor head control, Moro-like reflexes, and bilateral talipes varus. A localized (6 × 6 cm) patchy defect consisting of short, sparse, kinky, and hypopigmented hair in the occipital region was also noted. Based on previously reported cases, the defects suggested to the authors that they represented a specific teratogenic malformation syndrome (2).

A 2000 report described various congenital abnormalities observed in a term, female infant of a woman who was kept euthyroid throughout pregnancy with methimazole 30 mg/day (3). Aplasia cutis congenita was noted at birth. Seizures were noted at 18 months of age. At 3 years of age, the child's height, weight, and head circumference were normal (75th–80th percentile) as was her psychomotor development. Minor facial abnormalities consisted of hypertrichosis of the eyelashes and synophrys. There were areas of hyperpigmented skin on the back; two supernumerary nipples' bilateral syndactylies between the third and fourth fingers and between the second and third toes; dystrophic, small and shortened fingernails; and longitudinal ridges on a finger of each hand. Brain MRI, electroencephalogram, and karyotyping findings were normal. The authors considered this case to represent a new combination of signs, including abnormalities of various tissues of ectodermal origin (fingernails and skin anomalies) and epilepsy that were associated with in utero exposure to methimazole (3).

Several reports have studied pregnancies complicated by hyperthyroidism and the effects of methimazole and carbimazole on maternal and fetal thyroid indexes (4,27,39–41). In separate pregnancies in a mother with Graves' disease, fetal thyrotoxicosis was treated with 20–40 mg/day of carbimazole with successful resolution of fetal tachycardia in both cases and disappearance of fetal goiter in the first infant (27). A woman with hyperthyroidism was treated with a partial thyroidectomy before pregnancy (40). She subsequently had four pregnancies, all of which were complicated by fetal hyperthyroidism. No antithyroid therapy was administered during her first two pregnancies. The first ended in a late stillbirth, and the second resulted in a child with skull deformities. Both adverse outcomes were compatible with fetal hyperthyroidism. Carbimazole was administered in the next two pregnancies and both resulted in normal infants (40).

A 1992 abstract and a later full report described a retrospective evaluation of hyperthyroid pregnancy outcomes treated with either methimazole (*N* = 36) or PTU (*N* = 99) (42,43). One newborn (2.8%) in the methimazole group had a birth defect (inguinal hernia) whereas 3 (3.0%) defects were observed in those exposed to PTU (ventricular septal defect, pulmonary stenosis, patent ductus arteriosus in a term infant). No scalp defects were observed.

A 2001 report described the pregnancy outcomes of 241 women counseled by Teratology Information Services (TIS) associated with the European Network of Teratology Information Services because of exposure to carbimazole (20–40 mg/day) or methimazole (8–50 mg/day) during the 1st trimester (44). The control group consisted of 1089 pregnant women who had contacted the TIS concerning exposures to nonteratogenic agents. There was no increase in the rate of major birth defects in the exposed pregnancies compared with controls. However, two newborns had defects (choanal atresia; esophageal atresia) that were consistent with the anomalies postulated for methimazole embryopathy (44).

A 2003 case report described the outcomes of two pregnancies with hyperthyroidism (45). Diagnosis of the disease was made in the 2nd trimester and methimazole was started at 14 and 16 weeks' gestation, respectively. In the first case, discordant female twins (2000 and 1200 g) were delivered at 33.5 weeks'. Twin A was normal but twin B had esophageal atresia and tracheoesophageal fistula. After corrective surgery, she was growing adequately at 9 months of age. In the second case, intrauterine growth restriction occurred and a 1400-g female infant was delivered at 33 weeks'. Apgar scores were 6 and 10 at 1 and 5 minutes, respectively. The infant developed jaundice and examination revealed a complete absence of the biliary ducts and tree. The infant is now 18 months old and is waiting for a liver transplantation. Both affected infants were euthyroid at birth. Because the observed defects were associated with 1st trimester methimazole exposure, the authors raised the question of whether the actual teratogen was untreated hyperthyroidism (45).

Two cases of major congenital defects were described in another 2003 report (46). Both pregnancies (one with twins) were treated with methimazole in the 1st trimester. In one case, methimazole (10 mg/day) was replaced with propylthiouracil at 8 weeks'. A 2550-g, euthyroid female infant was delivered at 36 weeks' with Apgar scores of 5, 7, and 7 at 1, 5, and 10 minutes, respectively. Defects recognized in the infant included choanal atresia, aplasia cutis, umbilical hernia, sacral pilonidal sinus, limb hypertonia, and downslanting palpebral fissures. Additional follow-up could not be obtained. In the second case (twins), the mother received methimazole 40 mg/day until the 18th week when the dose was decreased to 20 mg/day. The male twins were euthyroid with birth weights of 1850 and 1900 g with Apgar scores of 9 and 9 at 1 and 5 minutes, respectively. No malformations were detected in the larger twin. However, the smaller twin had a full-thickness defect of the parietal scalp and a small omphalocele. At 12 months of age, the small twin had mild global (mostly motor) developmental delay, whereas development in the larger twin was normal (46).

Treatment of maternal hyperthyroidism may result in mild fetal hypothyroidism because of increased levels of fetal pituitary thyrotropin (21,24,41,47). This usually resolves within a few days without treatment (20). An exception to this occurred in one newborn exposed to 30 mg of carbimazole daily to term who appeared normal at birth but who developed hypothyroidism evident at 2 months of age with subsequent mental retardation (16).

A brief 1992 report from Spain examined the relationship between the illicit and uncontrolled use of methimazole in cattle feed as a weight enhancer and the appearance of congenital scalp aplasia cutis in humans (48). Seven cases of the rare malformation were observed in 1990–1991 in regions thought to have used methimazole in cattle food. The investigators speculated that pregnant women eating the meat of methimazole-exposed cattle would expose their fetuses to the drug (48).

Small, usually nonobstructing goiters in the newborn have been reported frequently with PTU (see Propylthiouracil). Only two goiters have been reported in carbimazole-exposed newborns and none with methimazole (13). Long-term follow-up of 25 children exposed in utero to carbimazole showed normal growth and development (15).

Combination therapy with thyroid–antithyroid drugs was advocated at one time but is now considered inappropriate (see also Propylthiouracil) (22,25,47,49,50). Two reasons contributed to this change: (a) use of thyroid hormones may require higher doses of the antithyroid drug to be used, and (b) placental transfer of levothyroxine and liothyronine is minimal and not sufficient to reverse fetal hypothyroidism (see also Levothyroxine and Liothyronine) (24).

A 2002 review of the fetal effects of antithyroid drugs concluded that the evidence for a specific methimazole syndrome is inadequate (51). However, the cluster of case reports of aplasia cutis congenita cases suggests a weak association but additional studies are required.

A 2007 case report described a male child whose mother had taken methimazole throughout most of pregnancy; 50 mg/day from conception to 5.5 weeks', no medication until 9 weeks', then 30 mg/day until delivery (52). At 40 weeks', a 2.270-kg (3rd percentile) male was delivered with Apgar scores of 9 and 10 at 1 and 5 minutes, respectively. Examination at 19 months of age revealed the following: height 75 cm (3rd percentile), weight 8.9 kg (<3rd percentile), and head circumference 44 cm (<3rd percentile). Relevant features included upward slanted palpebral fissures, arched flared eyebrows, small nose with broad nasal bridge, restriction of supination–rotation in both arms, and bilateral radioulnar synostosis. No choanal stenosis was found. Developmental delay was documented at 4 years 5 months of age (52).

Because of the possible association with aplasia cutis and other malformations, and the passage of methimazole into breast milk, many investigators, including two in 1984 (53), consider PTU to be the drug of choice for the medical treatment of hyperthyroidism during pregnancy. However, this opinion is not universal (50).

BREASTFEEDING SUMMARY

Methimazole is excreted into breast milk (54–57). In a patient given 10 mg of radiolabeled carbimazole (converted in vivo to methimazole), the milk:plasma ratio was a fairly constant 1.05 over 24 hours (54). This represented about 0.47% of the given radioactive dose. In a second study, a patient was administered 2.5 mg of methimazole every 12 hours (55). The mean milk:plasma ratio was 1.16, representing 16–39 mcg of methimazole in the daily milk supply. Extrapolation of these results to a daily dose of 20 mg indicated that approximately 3 mg/day would be excreted into the milk (55). Five lactating women were given 40 mg of carbimazole, producing a mean milk:plasma ratio at 1 hour of 0.72 (56). For the 8-hour period after dosing, the milk:plasma ratio was 0.98. A new radioimmunoassay was used to measure methimazole milk levels after a single 40-mg oral dose in four lactating women. The mean milk:plasma ratio during the first 8 hours was 0.97, with 70 mcg excreted in the milk (56).

A 1987 publication described the results of carbimazole therapy in a woman breastfeeding twins (57). Two months after delivery, the mother was started on carbimazole, 30 mg/day. The dose was decreased as she became euthyroid. Three paired milk:plasma levels revealed ratios of 0.30–0.70. The mean free methimazole concentration in milk, determined between 2 and 16 weeks of therapy, was 43 ng/mL (range 0–92 ng/mL). Peak milk levels occurred 2–4 hours after a dose. Mean plasma levels in the twins were 45 ng/mL (range 0–105 ng/mL) and 52 ng/mL (range 0–156 ng/mL), with the highest concentrations occurring while the mother was taking 30 mg/day. No evidence of thyroid suppression was found clinically or after thyroid function tests in the nursing twins (57).

Two other studies also found no effect on clinical status or thyroid function in nursing infants of mothers taking carbimazole or methimazole (58,59). In one report, no adverse effects were observed during a 3-week study of 11 infants whose mothers were taking carbimazole 5–15 mg/day (58). In the other study, normal thyroid function in 35 nursing infants, whose mothers were taking methimazole, was documented over periods ranging from 1 to 6 months (59). Most mothers were taking 5–10 mg/day, but six received 20 mg/day for 1 month and then tapered to 5 mg/day.

Because the amounts found in some studies may cause thyroid dysfunction in the nursing infant, methimazole and carbimazole have, in the past, been considered contraindicated during lactation. If antithyroid drug therapy was required, PTU was considered the treatment of choice, partially because PTU is ionized at physiologic pH and because 80% of the drug is protein bound (60). Methimazole is neither ionized nor protein bound, but small doses of methimazole (e.g., 10–20 mg/day or less) do not appear to pose a major risk to the nursing infant if thyroid function is monitored at frequent (e.g., weekly or biweekly) intervals (58–60).

In 2000, a long-term study confirmed the lack of toxicity in infants of mothers being treated with methimazole (61). A total of 139 thyrotoxic lactating mothers and their nursing infants were studied, 51 of the mothers were treated with methimazole during pregnancy and continued their treatment during lactation. The other 88 women started methimazole

M

therapy during lactation with 10–20 mg/day for 1 month, 10 mg/day during the second month, then 5–10 mg/day thereafter. Methimazole serum levels in six infants whose mothers were taking 20 mg/day were <0.03 mcg/mL, 2 hours after breastfeeding. No effects on infant thyroid function were detected at various times up to 12 months. In a blinded assessment, the total IQ scores, including verbal and performance IQ, of 14 children (age 48–74 months) exposed to methimazole in milk did not differ from 17 nonexposed controls (61).

The American Academy of Pediatrics classifies methimazole and carbimazole as compatible with breastfeeding (62).

References

1. Wilson LC, Kerr BA, Wilkinson R, Fossard C, Donnai D. Choanal atresia and hypothelia following methimazole exposure in utero: a second report. Am J Med Genet 1998;75:220–2.
2. Clementi M, Di Gianantonio E, Pelo E, Mammi I, Basile RT, Tenconi R. Methimazole embryopathy: delineation of the phenotype. Am J Med Genet 1999;83:43–6.
3. Martin-Danavit T, Edery P, Plauchu H, Attia-Sobol J, Raudrant D, Aurand JM, Thomas L. Ectodermal abnormalities associated with methimazole intrauterine exposure. Am J Med Genet 2000;94:338–40.
4. Momotani N, Noh J, Oyanagi H, Ishikawa N, Ito K. Antithyroid drug therapy for Graves' disease during pregnancy: optimal regimen for fetal thyroid status. N Engl J Med 1986;315:24–8.
5. Marchant B, Brownlie EW, Hart DM, Horton PW, Alexander WD. The placental transfer of propylthiouracil, methimazole and carbimazole. J Clin Endocrinol Metab 1977;45:1187–93.
6. Mortimer RH, Cannell GR, Addison RS, Johnson LP, Roberts MS, Bernus I. Methimazole and propylthiouracil equally cross the perfused human term placental lobule. J Clin Endocrinol Metab 1997;82:3099–102.
7. Milham S Jr, Elledge W. Maternal methimazole and congenital defects in children. Teratology 1972;5:125.
8. Mujtaba Q, Burrow GN. Treatment of hyperthyroidism in pregnancy with propylthiouracil and methimazole. Obstet Gynecol 1975;46:282–6.
9. Milham S Jr. Scalp defects in infants of mothers treated for hyperthyroidism with methimazole or carbimazole during pregnancy. Teratology 1985;32:321.
10. Kalb RE, Grossman ME. The association of aplasia cutis congenita with therapy of maternal thyroid disease. Pediatr Dermatol 1986;3:327–30.
11. Farine D, Maidman J, Rubin S, Chao S. Elevated alpha-fetoprotein in pregnancy complicated by aplasia cutis after exposure to methimazole. Obstet Gynecol 1988;71:996–7.
12. Van Dijke CP, Heydendael RJ, De Kleine MJ. Methimazole, carbimazole, and congenital skin defects. Ann Intern Med 1987;106:60–1.
13. Sugrue D, Drury MI. Hyperthyroidism complicating pregnancy: results of treatment by antithyroid drugs in 77 pregnancies. Br J Obstet Gynaecol 1980;87:970–5.
14. Heinonen OP, Slone D, Shapiro S. *Birth Defects and Drugs in Pregnancy*. Littleton, MA: Publishing Sciences Group, 1977:388–400.
15. McCarroll AM, Hutchinson M, McAuley R, Montgomery DAD. Long-term assessment of children exposed in utero to carbimazole. Arch Dis Child 1976;51:532–6.
16. Hawe P, Francis HH. Pregnancy and thyrotoxicosis. Br Med J 1962;2:817–22.
17. Herbst AL. Selenkow HA. Combined antithyroid-thyroid therapy of hyperthyroidism in pregnancy. Obstet Gynecol 1963;21:543–50.
18. Reveno WS, Rosenbaum H. Observation on the use of antithyroid drugs. Ann Intern Med 1964;60:982–9.
19. Herbst AL, Selenkow HA. Hyperthyroidism during pregnancy. N Engl J Med 1965;273:627–33.
20. Talbert LM, Thomas CG Jr, Holt WA, Rankin P. Hyperthyroidism during pregnancy. Obstet Gynecol 1970;36:779–85.
21. Refetoff S, Ochi Y, Selenkow HA, Rosenfield RL. Neonatal hypothyroidism and goiter in one infant of each of two sets of twins due to maternal therapy with antithyroid drugs. J Pediatr 1974;85:240–4.
22. Mestman JH, Manning PR, Hodgman J. Hyperthyroidism and pregnancy. Ann Intern Med 1974;134:434–9.
23. Ramsay I. Attempted prevention of neonatal thyrotoxicosis. Br Med J 1976;2:1110.
24. Low L, Ratcliffe W, Alexander W. Intrauterine hypothyroidism due to antithyroid-drug therapy for thyrotoxicosis during pregnancy. Lancet 1978;2:370–1.
25. Robinson PL, O'Mullane NH, Alderman B. Prenatal treatment of fetal thyrotoxicosis. Br Med J 1979;1:383–4.
26. Kock HCLV, Merkus JMWM. Graves' disease during pregnancy. Eur J Obstet Gynecol Reprod Biol 1983;14:323–30.
27. Pekonen F, Teramo K, Makinen T, Ikonen E, Osterlund K, Lamberg BA. Prenatal diagnosis and treatment of fetal thyrotoxicosis. Am J Obstet Gynecol 1984;150:893–4.
28. Jeffcoate WJ, Bain C. Recurrent pregnancy-induced thyrotoxicosis presenting as hyperemesis gravidarum. Case report. Br J Obstet Gynaecol 1985;92:413–5.
29. Johnson IR, Filshie GM. Hodgkin's disease diagnosed in pregnancy: case report. Br J Obstet Gynaecol 1977;84:791–2.
30. Ramsay I, Kaur S, Krassas G. Thyrotoxicosis in pregnancy: results of treatment by antithyroid drugs combined with T4. Clin Endocrinol (Oxf) 1983;18:73–85.
31. Momotani N, Ito K, Hamada N, Ban Y, Nishikawa Y, Mimura T. Maternal hyperthyroidism and congenital malformation in the offspring. Clin Endocrinol (Oxf) 1984;20:695–700.
32. Greenberg, F. Choanal atresia and athelia: methimazole teratogenicity or a new syndrome? Am J Med Genet 1987;28:931–4.
33. Ramirez A, Espinosa de los Monteros A, Parra A, De Leon B. Esophageal atresia and tracheoesophageal fistula in two infants born to hyperthyroid women receiving methimazole (Tapazol) during pregnancy. Am J Med Genet 1992;44:200–2.
34. Eisenstein Z, Weiss M, Katz Y, Bank H. Intellectual capacity of subjects exposed to methimazole or propylthiouracil in utero. Eur J Pediatr 1992;151:558–9.
35. Mandel SJ, Brent GA, Larsen PR. Review of antithyroid drug use during pregnancy and report of a case of aplasia cutis. Thyroid 1994;4:129–33.
36. Vogt T, Stolz W, Landthaler M. Aplasia cutis congenita after exposure to methimazole: a causal relationship? Br J Dermatol 1995;133:994–6.
37. Hall BD. Methimazole as a teratogenic etiology of choanal atresia/multiple congenital anomaly syndrome (abstract). Am J Hum Genet 1997;61(Suppl):A100. As cited in Clementi M, Di Gianantonio E, Pelo E, Mammi I, Basile RT, Tenconi R. Methimazole embryopathy: delineation of the phenotype. Am J Med Genet 1999;83:43–6.
38. Johnsson E, Larsson G, Ljunggren M. Severe malformations in infant born to hyperthyroid woman on methimazole. Lancet 1997;350:1520.
39. Hardisty CA, Munro DS. Serum long acting thyroid stimulator protector in pregnancy complicated by Graves' disease. Br Med J 1983;286:934–5.
40. Cove DH, Johnston P. Fetal hyperthyroidism: experience of treatment in four siblings. Lancet 1985;1:430–2.
41. Burrow GN. The management of thyrotoxicosis in pregnancy. N Engl J Med 1985;313:562–5.
42. Wing D, Millar L, Koonings P, Montoro M, Mestman J. A comparison of PTU versus Tapazole in the treatment of hyperthyroidism (abstract). Am J Obstet Gynecol 1992;166:308.
43. Wing DA, Millar LK, Koonings PP, Montoro MN, Mestman JH. A comparison of propylthiouracil versus methimazole in the treatment of hyperthyroidism in pregnancy. Am J Obstet Gynecol 1994;170:90–5.
44. Di Gianantonio E, Schaefer C, Mastroiacovo PP, Cournot MP, Benedicenti F, Reuvers M, Occupati B, Robert E, Bellemin B, Addis A, Arnon J, Clementi M. Adverse effects of prenatal methimazole exposure. Teratology 2001;64:262–6.
45. Seoud M, Nassar A, Usta I, Mansour M, Salti I, Younes K. Gastrointestinal malformations in two infants born to women with hyperthyroidism untreated in the first trimester. Am J Perinatol 2003;20:59–62.
46. Ferraris S, Valenzise M, Lerone M, Divizia MT, Rosaia L, Blaid D, Nemelka O, Ferrero GB, Silengo M. Malformations following methimazole exposure in utero: an open issue. Birth Defects Res A Clin Mol Teratol 2003;67:989–92.
47. Burr WA. Thyroid disease. Clin Obstet Gynecol 1981;8:341–51.
48. Martinez-Frias ML, Cereijo A, Rodriguez-Pinilla E, Urioste M. Methimazole in animal feed and congenital aplasia cutis. Lancet 1992;339:742–3.
49. Anonymous. Transplacental passage of thyroid hormones. N Engl J Med 1967;277:486–7.
50. Mestman JH. Hyperthyroidism in pregnancy. Clin Obstet Gynecol 1997;40:45–64.
51. Diav-Citrin O, Ornoy A. Teratogen update: antithyroid drugs—methimazole, carbimazole, and propylthiouracil. Teratology 2002;65:38–44.
52. Valdez RM, Barbero PM, Liascovich RC, De Rosa LF, Aguirre MA, Alba LG. Methimazole embryopathy: a contribution to defining the phenotype. Reprod Toxicol 2007;23:253–5.

M

53. Bachrach LK, Burrow GN. Aplasia cutis congenita and methimazole. CMAJ 1984;130:1264.
54. Low LCK, Lang J, Alexander WD. Excretion of carbimazole and propylthiouracil in breast milk. Lancet 1979;2:1011.
55. Tegler L, Lindstrom B. Antithyroid drugs in milk. Lancet 1980;2:591.
56. Johansen K, Andersen AN, Kampmann JP, Hansen JM, Mortensen HB. Excretion of methimazole in human milk. Eur J Clin Pharmacol 1982;23:339–41.
57. Rylance GW, Woods CG, Donnelly MC, Oliver JS, Alexander WD. Carbimazole and breastfeeding. Lancet 1987;1:928.
58. Lamberg BA, Ikonen E, Osterlund K, Teramo K, Pekonen F, Peltola J, Valimaki M. Antithyroid treatment of maternal hyperthyroidism during lactation. Clin Endocrinol 1984;21:81–7.
59. Azizi F. Effect of methimazole treatment of maternal thyrotoxicosis on thyroid function in breast-feeding infants. J Pediatr 1996;128:855–8.
60. Cooper DS. Antithyroid drugs: to breast-feed or not to breast-feed. Am J Obstet Gynecol 1987;157:234–5.
61. Azizi F, Khoshniat M, Bahrainian M, Hedayati M. Thyroid function and intellectual development of infants nursed by mothers taking methimazole. J Clin Endocrinol Metab 2000;85:3233–8.
62. Committee on Drugs, American Academy of Pediatrics. The transfer of drugs and other chemicals into human milk. Pediatrics 2001;108:776–89.

METHIXENE

[Withdrawn from the market. See 9th edition.]

METHOCARBAMOL

Muscle Relaxant

PREGNANCY RECOMMENDATION: Human Data Suggest Low Risk
BREASTFEEDING RECOMMENDATION: No Human Data—Probably Compatible

PREGNANCY SUMMARY

No evidence of human developmental toxicity attributable to methocarbamol has been located.

FETAL RISK SUMMARY

The centrally acting muscle relaxant, methocarbamol, is not teratogenic in animals (A.H. Robins Company, personal communication, 1987). It is not known if the drug crosses the human placenta. The agent crosses the placenta of dogs (1).

One manufacturer has an unpublished case on file relating to a mother who consumed methocarbamol, 1 g 4 times/day, throughout gestation (A.H. Robins Company, personal communication, 1987). The mother also used marijuana, and possibly other illicit substances, during her pregnancy. No physical or developmental abnormalities were noted at birth, but the infant did exhibit withdrawal symptoms consisting of prolonged crying, restlessness, easy irritability, and seizures. The infant was hospitalized for 2 months following birth to treat these symptoms. No further withdrawal symptoms or seizures were observed following discharge from the hospital. Follow-up neurologic examination indicated that developmental patterns were normal.

The above manufacturer also has informal data on file obtained from the Boston Collaborative Drug Surveillance Program (A.H. Robins Company, personal communication, 1987). These data, compiled between 1977 and 1981, relate to the use of methocarbamol by pregnant patients of the Puget Sound Group Health Cooperative in Seattle, Washington. During the data collection interval, 27 1st trimester exposures to the muscle relaxant were documented. None of the exposed infants had a congenital malformation.

The Collaborative Perinatal Project monitored 50,282 mother–child pairs, 22 of whom were exposed to methocarbamol during the 1st trimester (2, pp. 358, 360). One of these infants had an inguinal hernia. For use anytime during pregnancy, 119 exposures were recorded (2, p. 493). In this latter group, six infants had an inguinal hernia. An association between the drug and the defect cannot be determined from these data.

In a surveillance study of Michigan Medicaid recipients involving 229,101 completed pregnancies conducted between 1985 and 1992, 340 newborns had been exposed to methocarbamol during the 1st trimester (F. Rosa, personal communication, FDA, 1993). A total of 13 (3.8%) major birth defects were observed (14 expected), including (observed/expected) 1/1 polydactyly and 1/1 limb reduction defect. No anomalies were observed in four other defect categories (cardiovascular defects, oral clefts, spina bifida, and hypospadias) for which specific data were available. These data do not support an association between the drug and congenital defects.

The authors of a 1982 study of 350 patients with congenital contractures of the joints (arthrogryposis) concluded that only 15 had been exposed to a possible teratogen (3). One of the 15 cases involved a 24-year-old woman who at 2 months of gestation had consumed methocarbamol and propoxyphene, 750 and 65 mg, respectively, 2–3 times/day for 3 days to treat severe back pain. The term female infant was noted at birth to have multiple joint contractures involving the thumbs, wrists, elbows, knees, and feet. The latter was described as a bilateral equinovarus deformity. There were practically no foot creases. Other abnormalities present were frontal bosselation, a midline hemangioma, and weak abdominal musculature. Development was normal at 3 years of age except for the joint contractures, which had improved with time and a grade I/VI systolic murmur.

The authors of the above study attributed the multiple joint contractures in the infant to methocarbamol because of its muscle relaxant properties. However, their review of the literature and of the records of the Centers for Disease Control and Prevention failed to find any other cases of arthrogryposis with maternal methocarbamol ingestion. Moreover, no reports have appeared since then relating the defect to maternal use of the drug. A case of arthrogryposis, however, had been previously described with propoxyphene ingestion (see Propoxyphene for details) (4). Thus, based on the present information, it is unlikely that a relationship exists between maternal use of methocarbamol and congenital contractures in the newborn.

BREASTFEEDING SUMMARY

No reports describing the use of methocarbamol during human lactation have been located. Because newborns have been directly treated for tetanus with methocarbamol, any amount excreted in milk is probably clinically insignificant.

References

1. Campbell AD, Coles FK, Eubank LL, Huf EG. Distribution and metabolism of methocarbamol. J Pharmacol Exp Ther 1961;131:18–25.
2. Heinonen OP, Slone D, Shapiro S. *Birth Defects and Drugs in Pregnancy*. Littleton, MA: Publishing Sciences Group, 1977.
3. Hall JG, Reed SD. Teratogens associated with congenital contractures in humans and in animals. Teratology 1982;25:173–91.
4. Barrow MV, Souder DE. Propoxyphene and congenital malformations. JAMA 1971;217:1551–2.

METHOHEXITAL SODIUM

General Anesthetic

PREGNANCY RECOMMENDATION: Compatible
BREASTFEEDING RECOMMENDATION: Limited Human Data—Probably Compatible

PREGNANCY SUMMARY

Methohexital sodium is commonly used for induction of general anesthesia for cesarean sections and for electroconvulsive therapy (ECT). The drug can cause dose-related fetal heart rate slowing and respiratory depression and sedation in the newborn. Moreover, reported experience in the 1st trimester is lacking. The animal reproduction studies found no fetal harm.

FETAL RISK SUMMARY

Methohexital sodium is a rapid, ultra short-acting barbiturate anesthetic. It is indicated for IV induction of anesthesia before the use of other general anesthetic agents. In pediatric patients older than 1 month it is given either rectally or as an IM injection (1).

Reproduction studies have been conducted in pregnant rats and rabbits. Doses that were 4 and 7 times the human dose revealed no fetal harm. Studies for carcinogenic or mutagenic potential have not been conducted. There was no evidence of impaired fertility in animals (1).

Consistent with the molecular weight (about 284), methohexital sodium crosses the human placenta (2,3). Women undergoing a cesarean section were given a 1 mg/kg IV dose (2). The mean umbilical vein serum concentration in newborns 5 minutes after injection was 0.02 mcg/mL. No adverse effects in the newborns were observed (2). In a 2000 report, perfused human term placentas were used to study the bidirectional (mother to fetus and fetus to mother) transfer of methohexital sodium (3). Although protein binding significantly affected the degree of transfer, the drug readily crossed the placenta in both directions.

A study reported in 1974 evaluated two doses of methohexital sodium, 1.0 and 1.4 mg/kg, in 26 women undergoing an elective cesarean section (4). In the group that received the lower dose, fewer infants required assisted ventilation, took less time to establish regular respiration, and had higher Apgar scores. A letter to the editor commented on this study and thought that the data suggested a greater degree of acidemia in the infants exposed to the higher maternal dose (5).

A 2009 review of ECT in pregnancy noted that the most frequently used anesthetic agent for ECT was methohexital sodium (6). Although not teratogenic, the agent does cause dose-related fetal heart rate slowing and newborn sedation. These effects can be minimized, however, by using low doses (0.5–1.0 mg/kg).

BREASTFEEDING SUMMARY

Methohexital sodium is excreted into breast milk. Nine women undergoing tubal sterilization 32–341 days after giving birth received 120 or 150 mg IV methohexital sodium for induction of general anesthesia (7). Milk and maternal blood samples were drawn 1–2 hours after induction in five women and 2–4 hours in four. Subsequent samples were drawn at 8–10 hours and 24–28 hours. The highest milk concentration (407 ng/mL) was drawn 63 minutes after induction. The mean milk:blood ratio was 1.1 at 1–2 hours. The drug was undetectable in milk in four women at 8–10 hours and undetectable in milk or blood at 24 hours. The maximum dose to a nursing infant in a 100-mL feeding 1 hour after induction was estimated to be 0.04 mg. This amount did not warrant interruption of breastfeeding (7).

References

1. Product information. Brevital. JHP Pharmaceuticals, 2009.
2. Varga VJ, Machay T, Paulin F, Balazs M, Fedak L. Changes in serum level of methohexital (Brietal) in mothers and newborns during cesarean section. Zbl Gynakol 1983;105:297–9.
3. Herman NL, Li A-T, Johnson RF, Bjoraker RW, Downing JW, Jones D. Transfer of methohexital across the perfused human placenta. J Clin Anesth 2000;12:25–30.
4. Holdcroft A, Robinson MJ, Gordon H, Whitwam JG. Comparison of effect of two induction doses of methohexitone on infants delivered by elective caesarean section. Br Med J 1974;2:472–5.
5. Downing JW. Effect of methohexitone on infants delivered by caesarean section. Br Med J 1974;3:411.
6. Anderson EL, Reti IM. ECT in pregnancy: a review of the literature from 1941 to 2007. Psychosom Med 2009;71:235–42.
7. Borgatta L, Jenny RW, Gruss L, Ong C, Barad D. Clinical significance of methohexital, meperidine, and diazepam in breast milk. J Clin Pharmacol 1997;37:186–92.

METHOTREXATE

Antineoplastic/Immunologic Agent (Antirheumatic)

PREGNANCY RECOMMENDATION: Contraindicated
BREASTFEEDING RECOMMENDATION: Contraindicated

PREGNANCY SUMMARY

The use of methotrexate during organogenesis is associated with a spectrum of congenital defects collectively called methotrexate embryopathy or the fetal aminopterin-methotrexate syndrome. The critical period of exposure is 6–8 weeks postconception (8–10 weeks after the first day of the last menstrual period) and the critical dose is thought to be ≥10 mg/week. Typical characteristics of the syndrome are intrauterine growth restriction (IUGR); a marked decrease in ossification of the calvarium; hypoplastic supraorbital ridges; small, low-set ears; micrognathia; limb abnormalities; and occasional mental retardation (1). Exposure in the 2nd and 3rd trimesters may be associated with fetal toxicity and mortality. Although methotrexate may persist in tissues for long periods, pregnancies occurring after treatment with methotrexate do not appear to be at a risk any different from that of an unexposed population. If methotrexate is used in pregnancy for the treatment of rheumatoid arthritis, health care professionals are encouraged to call the toll-free number 877-311-8972 for information about patient enrollment in the Organization of Teratology Information Specialists (OTIS) Rheumatoid Arthritis study.

FETAL RISK SUMMARY

Methotrexate is a folic acid antagonist. It is in the same antineoplastic subclass as aminopterin, pemetrexed, and pralatrexate.

A number of references describing the use of this antineoplastic agent in pregnancy have been located (1–28). Methotrexate-induced congenital defects (also known as the aminopterin-methotrexate syndrome) are similar to those produced by another folic acid antagonist, aminopterin (see also Aminopterin) (7). Anomalies in two infants were absence of lambdoid and coronal sutures, oxycephaly, absence of frontal bone, low-set ears, hypertelorism, dextroposition of heart, absence of digits on feet, growth restriction, very wide posterior fontanelle, hypoplastic mandible, multiple anomalous ribs (3); and oxycephaly caused by absent coronal sutures, large anterior fontanelle, depressed and wide nasal bridge, low-set ears, long webbed fingers, wide-set eyes (4).

A 1990 report described the pregnancy outcomes of eight women who were treated with low-dose oral methotrexate for rheumatic disease during 10 pregnancies (18). The outcomes included two elective abortions (EABs) (no details given for these cases), three spontaneous abortions (SABs), and five normal full-term live births. In the eight pregnancies (six women) with details, the methotrexate weekly dose (usually given as a single dose) was 7.5 mg in seven and 10 mg in one. In the live birth group, the mean methotrexate exposure was 6.8 weeks postconception (range 2–15 weeks), whereas in the SAB group the mean exposure was 7 weeks (range 4–9 weeks). The mean cumulative methotrexate dose prior to conception was 1384 mg (range 165–3545 mg) (live births) and 333 mg (range 45–775 mg) (SAB). Other drugs taken by the women included aspirin, nonsteroidal anti-inflammatory agents, prednisone (<10 mg/day), and hydroxychloroquine. Folate supplements had been taken in three of the five pregnancies ending in live births and in all three of the SAB cases. No obvious differences were apparent between the live birth and SAB groups in terms of smoking, use of alcohol, or the use of other drugs. Information on the long-term development of the five live births was obtained by telephone interview at a mean age of 11.5 years (range 3.7–16.7 years). All of the children were healthy and had experienced normal physical and mental development (one child had a minor speech impediment that had resolved with speech therapy) (18).

A 1993 case report and review described the pregnancy outcome of a 39-year-old woman with severe rheumatoid arthritis who was exposed to methotrexate and other drugs shortly after conception (19). For about 6 months before conception she had been taking methotrexate (7.5 mg once weekly), ibuprofen (6.4 g/day), misoprostol (0.4 mg/day), and cimetidine (600 mg) or sucralfate (3 g) per day. All medications were stopped within 10 days of the last menstrual period (as determined by ultrasound at 5–6 weeks' gestation). A healthy full-term, 3962-g male infant was delivered by cesarean section (breech presentation) with Apgar scores of 8 and 9 at 1 and 5 minutes, respectively. Examination by a dysmorphologist at 12 weeks of age revealed a healthy, normal infant with no evidence of embryopathy (19).

A 25-year-old woman at 30 weeks' gestation was diagnosed with metastatic choriocarcinoma of the vagina and lungs (20). The woman was treated with IV methotrexate 20 mg/day for 5 days. Five days later, she delivered a preterm male infant with an Apgar of 10 (no other details given). The mother and infant were alive and well at 12 months' follow-up (20).

In a 1994 reference, data relating to methotrexate use before or during pregnancy were gathered from programs participating in the Organization of Teratology Information Services (OTIS) and the European Network of Teratology Information Services (ENTIS) (21). The survey resulted in data for 21 prospectively ascertained cases. Seven exposures occurred more than 1 year before conception and they were excluded from the analysis. In the remaining 14 cases, 9 were exposed within 1 year of conception and 5 were exposed during pregnancy. Four of the five pregnancy exposures occurred within the first 6 weeks of gestation with a duration of exposure of 1–3 weeks and one single dose exposure occurred at 37–38 weeks' gestation. Doses ranged from 7.5 mg/week (one woman had been taking this dose for 3 years) to a single 42 mg IV dose. All of these outcomes resulted in healthy infants without birth defects (one delivered at 36 weeks'). In the women exposed within 1 year of pregnancy, the duration of exposures ranged from a few weeks to 6 years. The doses were known in four cases (7.5 mg/week in three, 12.5 mg/week in one). The outcomes of these nine cases were four SABs, four healthy infants, and one infant born at term with a cavernous hemangioma. The authors concluded that the limited data confirmed that the critical time for methotrexate-induced defects was 6–8 weeks postconception and the critical dose was ≥10 mg/week (21).

A 1997 case report described an adverse pregnancy outcome in a 20-year-old woman with polyarticular rheumatoid arthritis who had been treated with oral doses of methotrexate (10–12.5 mg/week) for about 5–6 years (22). Folic acid (1 mg/day) was also prescribed but her compliance was unclear. The woman discontinued treatment at about 8 weeks' gestation (estimated dose during gestation about 100 mg). At 35 weeks' she gave birth to a 1.79-kg female (normal 46,XX karyotype) infant with IUGR and multiple congenital anomalies. The defects included brachycephaly, 0.5-cm anterior fontanelle, coronal ridging, shallow orbits with hypertelorism, retrognathia, malformed ears, palate with a posterior groove and a bifid uvula, umbilical hernia, spinal defects (dorsal kyphosis with L5 and S1 hemivertebrae), deformed thumb, bilateral simian creases, hypoplastic nails, reduction of radial ray on right side, syndactyly of fourth and fifth toes, absent fifth metatarsal bone, and cardiovascular defects (double-outlet right ventricle, doubly committed ventricular septal defect, transposed great vessels, restrictive atrial septal defect, pulmonary stenosis, and an aberrant right subclavian artery). The infant died at 6 months of age. The authors concluded that the anomalies were consistent with methotrexate-induced embryopathy (22).

A 26-year-old man with fetal methotrexate syndrome and two children with mild manifestations of the syndrome were described in 1998 (23). In the adult's case, his mother (who gave him up for adoption) had attempted to terminate the pregnancy at 6–8 weeks' gestation with an unknown amount of methotrexate. His malformations included hypertelorism, ptosis of the eyelids, short palpebral fissures, sparse eyebrows, prominent nose, low-set ears, a widow's peak at the frontal hairline, flexion contractures of the metacarpophalangeal joints of both thumbs and syndactyly of all fingers (all repaired surgically), four metacarpals, and a single fused hypoplastic nub of tissue at the forefoot (corrected surgically with reconstruction of all toes). His physical growth was restricted, but his psychomotor development was normal, as is his intelligence. The first child, a 9-year-old male, was exposed to 80 mg/week of methotrexate for 6 doses at 7.5–28.5 weeks' gestation. His mother, with an undetected pregnancy, had been treated for breast cancer with methotrexate, fluorouracil (1200 mg/week × 10 doses), and radiation (total dose estimated to be 14 rads). He was born at 29 weeks with a birth weight of 820 g (small for gestational age) and he remains growth restricted. Malformations included hypertelorism, a frontal hair whorl, upsweep of the frontal hairline, microcephaly, low-set ears, micrognathia, right palmar simian crease, and borderline mental retardation (composite IQ of 70). The second child is a 3.5-year-old male infant who was born at 29 weeks' gestation with a normal weight (1160 g; 50th percentile). His mother had undergone a failed EAB (dilatation, suction, and curettage; 11 weeks after the last menstrual period [LMP]) and then, because of large uterine myomas, had chosen to have a medical abortion with methotrexate. She received 100 mg bi-weekly from about 13 to 19 weeks' and 200 mg bi-weekly from 19 to 25 weeks', but this abortion attempt also failed. Birth defects noted were a bulging forehead, bitemporal narrowing, upward slanting palpebral fissures, sparse hair on the temporal areas, low-set ears, broad nasal tip, and a high arched palate. He has had chronic diarrhea since 9 months of age. An intestinal biopsy revealed villous atrophy. His psychomotor development has been normal. At 34 months, his weight and length were restricted, but his head circumference was normal (75th percentile) (23).

A 1999 report described the outcomes of pregnancies in 20 women with breast cancer who were treated with antineoplastic agents (24). (See also Fluorouracil.) Methotrexate (25 mg/m^2), in combination with epirubicin and vincristine, was administered to one woman at 6 weeks' gestation. The pregnancy ended in an SAB (24).

Another 1999 reference reported the outcome of a male infant (normal karyotype 46,XY) whose mother had been treated for chronic severe psoriasis with 12.5 mg methotrexate 3 times weekly during the first 8 weeks postconception (1). He was delivered at 40 weeks' gestation with Apgar scores of 2, 5, and 6 at 1, 5, and 10 minutes, respectively. Birth weight, length, and head circumference were severely restricted (<3rd percentile). Malformations included widely separated sutures and large fontanels; bilateral epicanthal folds and sparse eyebrows laterally with hypoplastic supraorbital ridges; broad nasal bridge; anteverted nares; smooth long philtrum; hypoplastic nipples; small umbilical hernia; diastasis recti; a shawl scrotum; decreased extension of the elbows; short bilateral proximal phalanges of the third, fourth, and fifth fingers; and mildly hypoplastic fingernails. The only neurologic abnormality noted was mild hypotonia. At 20 months, he was still growth restricted. He had a triangular face (trigonocephaly) with a prominent metopic suture and the open anterior fontanel finally closed at age 30 months. Generalized tonic-clonic seizures associated with fever were noted at 1 and 2 years (both of his older sisters had a similar episode during the first 2 years of life). Developmental testing revealed mental retardation with significant early motor and cognitive delays (1).

A 23-year-old woman underwent an attempted EAB at 8 weeks' gestation with IM methotrexate 100 mg followed by misoprostol 800 mcg 4 days later (25). Four weeks later she still had a viable pregnancy but could not afford hospitalization for surgical termination. She eventually delivered a 2050-g female infant at term with Apgar scores of 4 and 8 at 1 and 5 minutes, respectively. The infant was hypotonic. All growth parameters (weight, height, and head circumference) were severely growth restricted. Multiple malformations were noted including a disproportionately long head (dolichocephaly), a prominent broad nose, hypertelorism, short palpebral fissure, small mouth, micrognathia, fifth-finger clinodactyly, extra flexion creases on the thumbs, mild syndactyly of the second and third toes with fourth and fifth toe clinodactyly, and hypoplastic toenails. Severe growth restriction was evident at the 12- and 18-month examinations. The mother declined developmental testing of the child, but stated that the usual developmental milestones were normal (25).

A 2002 case report described the pregnancy outcome of a woman who was treated for psoriasis with two doses of methotrexate 7.5 mg/day at 3.5 weeks postconception (26). She also was taking sertraline and smoked cigarettes. An ultrasound examination at 18 weeks' gestation revealed multiple anomalies and the pregnancy was terminated 2 weeks later. The male fetus (normal 46,XY karyotype) had a wide anterior fontanelle, sloping forehead, under mineralization of the skull, low-set and poorly formed ears, absent auditory canals, flat nose, micrognathia, multiple skeletal abnormalities (absent and slender ribs, a hemivertebrae, and fusion of the third through fifth lumbar vertebral bodies), limb defects (absent left radius, hypoplastic right radius, bilaterally short forearms, hypoplastic left thumb, and clinodactyly of the fifth digit bilaterally), tracheal atresia, markedly hypoplastic lungs, cardiovascular defects (left ventricle mildly hypoplastic, ventricular septal defect, persistent right subclavian artery with an arterial ring, and absent left and right pulmonary arteries), malrotated intestines, duodenal atresia, a Meckel's diverticulum, multiple accessory spleens, enlarged left liver lobe, and a two-vessel umbilical cord (26).

A 2003 case reported a failed pregnancy termination attempt at 6 weeks' gestation with IM methotrexate 75 mg and oral misoprostol 400 mcg (27). The pregnancy was terminated at 27 weeks' secondary to ultrasound diagnosis of methotrexate embryopathy. Autopsy revealed a 918-g female (normal karyotype) fetus with upper extremities that were asymmetric in length, bilateral shortening of the radii and ulnae, asymmetric in length lower extremities with bilateral absent fibulae, polydactyly of the right foot, small head, prominent eyes, low-set ears, micrognathia, and a two-vessel umbilical cord (27).

A survey of 600 members of the American College of Rheumatology, partially conducted to determine the outcomes of pregnancies exposed to disease-modifying antirheumatic drugs (etanercept, infliximab, leflunomide, and methotrexate), was published in 2003 (28). From the 175 responders, the outcomes of 39 pregnancies exposed to methotrexate were 21 full-term healthy infants, 7 spontaneous abortions (1 with a congenital malformation), 8 elective abortions, 1 woman still pregnant, and 2 liveborn infants with birth defects. No information was available on the three cases with malformations or if they were thought to have resulted from methotrexate exposure (28).

Possible retention of methotrexate in maternal tissues before conception was suggested as the cause of a rare pulmonary disorder in a newborn, desquamating fibrosing alveolitis (29). The infant's mother had conceived within 6 months of completing treatment with the antineoplastic. (*Note: A later publication from these investigators, which included this case, noted that the newborn was conceived within 2 months of treatment termination [41]*). In addition, a sister of the infant born 3 years later developed the same disorder, although a third child born from the mother 1 year later developed normally.) Previous studies have shown that methotrexate may persist for prolonged periods in human tissues (30). However, conception occurred 3 months after discontinuance of therapy in one case (31), after 6 months in a second (14), and after 7 months in a third (32). Four (one set of twins) normal infants resulted from these latter pregnancies. Thus, the association between methotrexate and the pulmonary disorder is unknown.

Two cases of severe newborn myelosuppression have been reported after methotrexate use in pregnancy. In one case, pancytopenia was discovered in a 1000-g male newborn after exposure to six different antineoplastic agents, including methotrexate, in the 3rd trimester (5). The second infant, delivered at 31 weeks' gestation, was exposed to methotrexate only during the 12th week of pregnancy (10). The severe bone marrow hypoplasia was most likely caused by the use of mercaptopurine near delivery.

Data from one review indicated that 40% of the infants exposed to cytotoxic drugs were of low birth weight (2). This finding was not related to the timing of the exposure. Long-term studies of growth and mental development in offspring exposed to antineoplastic agents during the 2nd trimester, the period of neuroblast multiplication, have not been conducted (32–34). Several studies, however, have followed individual infants for periods ranging from 2 to 84 months and have not discovered any problems (10–14,16,17).

Methotrexate crosses the placenta to the fetus (15). A 34-year-old mother was treated with multiple antineoplastic agents for acute lymphoblastic leukemia beginning in her 22nd week of pregnancy. Weekly intrathecal methotrexate (10 mg/m^2) was administered from approximately 26–29 weeks' gestation; the dose was then increased to 20 mg/m^2 weekly until delivery at 40 weeks' gestation. Methotrexate levels in cord serum and red cells were 1.86×10^{-9} mol/L, and 2.6×10^{-9} mol/g of hemoglobin, respectively, with 29% as the polyglutamate metabolite (15).

In the case described above, chromosomal analysis of the newborn revealed a normal karyotype (46,XX), but with gaps and a ring chromosome (15). The clinical significance of these findings is unknown, but because these abnormalities may persist for several years, the potential existed for an increased risk of cancer as well as for a risk of genetic damage in the next generation (15).

Successful pregnancies have followed the use of methotrexate before conception (14,29,31,32,35–41). Apparently,

M

ovarian and testicular dysfunction are reversible (34,42–45). Two studies, one in 1984 and one in 1988, both involving women treated for gestational trophoblastic neoplasms, have analyzed reproductive function after methotrexate therapy and are described below (41,46).

In 438 long-term survivors treated with chemotherapy between 1958 and 1978, 436 received methotrexate either alone or in combination with other antineoplastic agents (41). This report was a continuation of a brief 1979 correspondence that discussed some of the same patients (29). The mean duration of chemotherapy was 4 months with a mean interval from completion of therapy to the first pregnancy of 2.7 years. Conception occurred within 1 year of therapy completion in 45 women, resulting in 31 live births, 1 anencephalic stillbirth, 7 SABs, and 6 EABs. Of the 436 women, 187 (43%) had at least one live birth (numbers given in parentheses refer to mean/maximum methotrexate dose in grams when used alone; mean/maximum dose in grams when used in combination) (1.26/6.0; 1.22/6.8), 23 (5%) had no live births (1.56/2.6; 1.33/6.5), 7 (2%) failed to conceive (1.30/1.6; 1.95/4.5), and 219 (50%) did not try to conceive (1.10/2.0; 2.20/34.5). The average ages at the end of treatment in the four groups were 24.9, 24.4, 24.4, and 31.5 years, respectively. Congenital abnormalities noted were anencephaly (2), spina bifida (1), tetralogy of Fallot (1), talipes equinovarus (1), collapsed lung (1), umbilical hernia (1), desquamative fibrosing alveolitis (1; same case as described above), asymptomatic heart murmur (1), and mental retardation (1). An 11th child had tachycardia but developed normally after treatment. One case of sudden infant death syndrome occurred in a female infant at 4 weeks of age. None of these outcomes differed statistically from that expected in a normal population (41).

The 1988 report described the reproductive results of 265 women who had been treated from 1959 to 1980 for gestational trophoblastic disease (46). Single-agent chemotherapy was administered to 91 women, only 2 of whom received methotrexate. Sequential (single agent) and combination therapy were administered to 67 and 107 women, respectively, but the individual agents used were not specified. Further details of this study are provided in the monograph for mercaptopurine (see Mercaptopurine).

The long-term effects of combination chemotherapy on menstrual and reproductive function have also been described in women treated for malignant ovarian germ cell tumors (47). Only 2 of the 40 women treated received methotrexate. The results of this study are discussed in the monograph for cyclophosphamide (see Cyclophosphamide).

A 34-year-old man, being treated with oral methotrexate for Reiter's syndrome, fathered a normal full-term female infant (48). The man had been receiving treatment with the drug intermittently for approximately 5 years and continuously for 5 months before conception.

Occupational exposure of the mother to antineoplastic agents during pregnancy may present a risk to the fetus. A position statement from the National Study Commission on Cytotoxic Exposure and a research article involving some antineoplastic agents are presented in the monograph for cyclophosphamide (see Cyclophosphamide).

BREASTFEEDING SUMMARY

Methotrexate is excreted into breast milk in low concentrations (49). After a dose of 22.5 mg/day, milk concentrations of 0.26 mcg/dL have been measured with a milk:plasma ratio of 0.08. The significance of this small amount is not known. However, because the drug may accumulate in neonatal tissues, breastfeeding is contraindicated. The American Academy of Pediatrics classifies methotrexate as a cytotoxic drug that may interfere with cellular metabolism of the nursing infant (50).

References

1. Del Campo M, Kosaki K, Bennett FC, Jones KL. Developmental delay in fetal aminopterin/methotrexate syndrome. Teratology 1999;60:10–2.
2. Nicholson HO. Cytotoxic drugs in pregnancy: review of reported cases. J Obstet Gynaecol Br Commonw 1968;75:307–12.
3. Milunsky A, Graef JW, Gaynor MF. Methotrexate-induced congenital malformations. J Pediatr 1968;72:790–5.
4. Powell HR, Ekert H. Methotrexate-induced congenital malformations. Med J Aust 1971;2:1076–7.
5. Pizzuto J, Aviles A, Noriega L, Niz J, Morales M, Romero F. Treatment of acute leukemia during pregnancy: presentation of nine cases. Cancer Treat Rep 1980;64:679–83.
6. Dara P, Slater LM, Armentrout SA. Successful pregnancy during chemotherapy for acute leukemia. Cancer 1981;47:845–6.
7. Warkany J. Teratogenicity of folic acid antagonists. Cancer Bull 1981;33:76–7.
8. Burnier AM. Discussion. In Plows CW. Acute myelomonocytic leukemia in pregnancy: report of a case. Am J Obstet Gynecol 1982;143:41–3.
9. Khurshid M, Saleem M. Acute leukaemia in pregnancy. Lancet 1978;2: 534–5.
10. Okun DB, Groncy PK, Sieger L, Tanaka KR. Acute leukemia in pregnancy: transient neonatal myelosuppression after combination chemotherapy in the mother. Med Pediatr Oncol 1979;7:315–9.
11. Doney KC, Kraemer KG, Shepard TH. Combination chemotherapy for acute myelocytic leukemia during pregnancy: three case reports. Cancer Treat Rep 1979;63:369–71.
12. Karp GI, von Oeyen P, Valone F, Khetarpal VK, Israel M, Mayer RJ, Frigoletto FD, Garnick MB. Doxorubicin in pregnancy: possible transplacental passage. Cancer Treat Rep 1983;67:773–7.
13. Feliu J, Juarez S, Ordonez A, Garcia-Paredes ML, Gonzalez-Baron M, Montero JM. Acute leukemia and pregnancy. Cancer 1988;61:580–4.
14. Turchi JJ, Villasis C. Anthracyclines in the treatment of malignancy in pregnancy. Cancer 1988;61:435–40.
15. Schleuning M, Clemm C. Chromosomal aberrations in a newborn whose mother received cytotoxic treatment during pregnancy. N Engl J Med 1987;317:1666–7.
16. Frenkel EP, Meyers MC. Acute leukemia and pregnancy. Ann Intern Med 1960;53:656–71.
17. Coopland AT, Friesen WJ, Galbraith PA. Acute leukemia in pregnancy. Am J Obstet Gynecol 1969;105:1288–9.
18. Kozlowski RD, Steinbrunner JV, MacKenzie AH, Clough JD, Wilke WS, Segal AM. Outcome of first-trimester exposure to low-dose methotrexate in eight patients with rheumatic disease. Am J Med 1990;88:589–92.
19. Feldkamp M, Carey JC. Clinical teratology counseling and consultation case report: low dose methotrexate exposure in the early weeks of pregnancy. Teratology 1993;47:533–9.
20. Gangadharan VP, Chitrathara K, Satishkumar K, Rajan B, Nair MK. Successful management of choriocarcinoma with pregnancy. Acta Oncol 1994;33:76–7.
21. Donnenfeld AE, Pastuszak A, Noah JS, Schick B, Rose NC, Koren G. Methotrexate exposure prior to and during pregnancy. Teratology 1994;49:79–81.
22. Buckley LM, Bullaboy CA, Leichtman L, Marquez M. Multiple congenital anomalies associated with weekly low-dose methotrexate treatment of the mother. Arthritis Rheum 1997;40:971–3.
23. Bawle EV, Conard JV, Weiss L. Adult and two children with fetal methotrexate syndrome. Teratology 1998;57:51–5.
24. Giacalone PL, Laffargue F, Benos P. Chemotherapy for breast carcinoma during pregnancy. Cancer 1999;86:2266–72.

25. Wheeler M, O'Meara P, Stanford M. Fetal methotrexate and misoprostol exposure: the past revisited. Teratology 2002;66:73–6.
26. Nguyen C, Duhl AJ, Escallon CS, Blakemore KJ. Multiple anomalies in a fetus exposed to low-dose methotrexate in the first trimester. Obstet Gynecol 2002;99:599–602.
27. Chapa JB, Hibbard JU, Weber EM, Abramowicz JS, Verp MS. Prenatal diagnosis of methotrexate embryopathy. Obstet Gynecol 2003;101:1104–7.
28. Chakravarty EF, Sanchez-Yamamoto D, Bush TM. The use of disease modifying antirheumatic drugs in women with rheumatoid arthritis of childbearing age: a survey of practice patterns and pregnancy outcomes. J Rheumatol 2003;30:241–6.
29. Walden PAM, Bagshawe KD. Pregnancies after chemotherapy for gestational trophoblastic tumours. Lancet 1979;2:1241.
30. Charache S, Condit PT, Humphreys SR. Studies on the folic acid vitamins. IV. The persistence of amethopterin in mammalian tissues. Cancer 1960;13:236–40.
31. Barnes AB, Link DA. Childhood dermatomyositis and pregnancy. Am J Obstet Gynecol 1983;146:335–6.
32. Sivanesaratnam V, Sen DK. Normal pregnancy after successful treatment of choriocarcinoma with cerebral metastases: a case report. J Reprod Med 1988;33:402–3.
33. Dobbing J.Pregnancy and leukaemia. Lancet 1977;1:1155.
34. Schilsky RL, Lewis BJ, Sherins RJ, Young RC. Gonadal dysfunction in patients receiving chemotherapy for cancer. Ann Intern Med 1980;93:109–14.
35. Bacon C, Kernahan J. Successful pregnancy in acute leukaemia. Lancet 1975;2:515.
36. Wegelius R. Successful pregnancy in acute leukaemia. Lancet 1975;2:1301.
37. Ross GT. Congenital anomalies among children born of mothers receiving chemotherapy for gestational trophoblastic neoplasms. Cancer 1976;37:1043–7.
38. Gasser C. Long-term survival (cures) in childhood acute leukemia. Paediatrician 1980;9:344–57.
39. Sanz MA, Rafecas FJ. Successful pregnancy during chemotherapy for acute promyelocytic leukemia. N Engl J Med 1982;306:939.
40. Deeg HJ, Kennedy MS, Sanders JE, Thomas ED, Storb R. Successful pregnancy after marrow transplantation for severe aplastic anemia and immunosuppression with cyclosporine. JAMA 1983;250:647.
41. Rustin GJS, Booth M, Dent J, Salt S, Rustin F, Bagshawe KD. Pregnancy after cytotoxic chemotherapy for gestational trophoblastic tumours. Br Med J 1984;288:103–6.
42. Hinkes E, Plotkin D. Reversible drug-induced sterility in a patient with acute leukemia. JAMA 1973;223:1490–1.
43. Sherins RJ, DeVita VT Jr. Effect of drug treatment for lymphoma on male reproductive capacity. Ann Intern Med 1973;79:216–20.
44. Lendon M, Palmer MK, Hann IM, Shalet SM, Jones PHM. Testicular histology after combination chemotherapy in childhood for acute lymphoblastic leukaemia. Lancet 1978;2:439–41.
45. Evenson DP, Arlin Z, Welt S, Claps ML, Melamed MR. Male reproductive capacity may recover following drug treatment with the L-10 protocol for acute lymphocytic leukemia. Cancer 1984;53:30–6.
46. Song H, Wu P, Wang Y, Yang X, Dong S. Pregnancy outcomes after successful chemotherapy for choriocarcinoma and invasive mole: long-term follow-up. Am J Obstet Gynecol 1988;158:538–45.
47. Gershenson DM. Menstrual and reproductive function after treatment with combination chemotherapy for malignant ovarian germ cell tumors. J Clin Oncol 1988;6:270–5.
48. Perry WH. Methotrexate and teratogenesis. Arch Dermatol 1983;119:874.
49. Johns DG, Rutherford LD, Keighton PC, Vogel CL. Secretion of methotrexate into human milk. Am J Obstet Gynecol 1972;112:978–80.
50. Committee on Drugs, American Academy of Pediatrics. The transfer of drugs and other chemicals into human milk. Pediatrics 2001;108:776–89.

METHOTRIMEPRAZINE

[Withdrawn from the market. See 9th edition.]

METHOXAMINE

[Withdrawn from the market. See 9th edition.]

METHOXSALEN

Dermatologic Agent

PREGNANCY RECOMMENDATION: Compatible (Oral and Topical Lotion)
Contraindicated (Extracorporeal Solution)
BREASTFEEDING RECOMMENDATION: Hold Breastfeeding

PREGNANCY SUMMARY

Although methoxsalen combined with ultraviolet A (UV-A) is mutagenic, clastogenic, carcinogenic, and cataractogenic in humans, it does not appear to be a significant human teratogen. However, the long-term effects of in utero exposure to methoxsalen, such as cancer, have not been studied but warrant investigation.

FETAL RISK SUMMARY

Methoxsalen (8-methoxypsoralen; 8-MOP), available in oral capsules and as a topical lotion, is used as a photosensitizer in conjunction with long-wave UV-A radiation (PUVA) for the symptomatic control of severe psoriasis (1). The drug also is available as a sterile solution that is indicated for extracorporeal photopheresis in the palliative treatment of the skin manifestations of cutaneous T-cell lymphoma that is unresponsive to other forms of treatment (2).

Reproductive toxicity testing of the oral agent in animals has not been conducted (1). However, the extracorporeal product was studied in pregnant rats (2). Doses given during organogenesis that were ≥4000 times the single human dose based on BSA were maternal (weight loss, anorexia, and increased relative liver weight) and fetal toxic. Fetal toxicity included increased fetal death and resorptions, late fetal death, fewer fetuses per litter, and decreased fetal weight. An increase in skeletal malformations and variations also was observed (2).

Shepard (3) reviewed a closely related compound, 5-methoxypsoralen (5-MOP), that was not teratogenic in mice given up to 500 mg/kg/day, but was teratogenic in rabbits (type of malformations not specified) fed 70 or 560 mg/kg/day. A 2003 reference cited evidence suggesting that the developmental toxicity of 8-MOP and 5-MOP given in the diet of female rats was due to enhanced metabolism of estrogens (4).

Because PUVA treatments are mutagenic, a 1991 report described the pregnancy outcomes among 1380 patients (892 men and 488 women) who had received the therapy (5). Of the men, 99 (11.1%) reported 167 pregnancies in their partners, whereas 94 (19.3%) of the women reported 159 pregnancies. Among the men, 34% (55 of 163; data missing for 4 pregnancies) received PUVA therapy near the time of conception. In the women, 20% (31 of 158; data missing for 1 pregnancy) received treatment at the time of conception or during pregnancy. The difference in the incidence of spontaneous abortions among those exposed (men 3.6% vs. women 12.9%) was thought to be related to reporting bias, but the total rate of abortions is no different from that expected in a nonexposed population. No congenital malformations were reported in the offspring of the exposed patients (5).

A 1993 publication described the outcome of 689 infants born before maternal PUVA treatment, 502 infants conceived and born after treatment, and 14 infants whose mothers had received the therapy during pregnancy (6). No difference among the three groups was noted in sex ratio, twinning, and mortality rate after birth. A significant increase in low-birth-weight infants was observed in those conceived and born after maternal treatment, an effect, the authors concluded, that may have resulted from the mother's disease. No congenital abnormalities were observed in the 14 infants exposed in utero to PUVA therapy. In the other two groups, 3.6% (25 of 689) and 3.2% (16 of 502) of the infants had congenital defects (6).

Treatment with PUVA occurred around the time of conception or during the 1st trimester of pregnancy (none treated after the 1st trimester) in 41 women identified by the European Network of Teratology Information Services (7). Of these cases, 32 were treated before conception and during the 1st trimester, 8 were treated only during the 1st trimester, and 1 stopped treatment 2 weeks before conception. The number of treatments was described as normal (two to three per week) in 27 cases, less than normal in 6 cases, greater than normal in 2 cases, and unknown in 6 women. The maximum daily dose of methoxsalen was 40 mg. Four (10%) of the pregnancies terminated with a spontaneous abortion (a normal incidence), 6 were voluntarily terminated, 1 woman was lost to follow-up, and 31 infants (1 set of twins) were liveborn. Two of the infants had low birth weights (2120 and 2460 g), but neither was attributable to the mother's therapy or to psoriasis. No malformations were observed at birth or in the neonatal period. The sample size in this study allowed the authors to exclude a sixfold increase in the risk for all malformations (7).

M

BREASTFEEDING SUMMARY

No reports describing the use of methoxsalen during breastfeeding have been located, nor is it known whether the drug is excreted into breast milk. Because the drug acts as a photosensitizer, breastfeeding should be stopped and the milk discarded, probably for at least 24 hours (approximately 95% of a dose is excreted in the urine as metabolites within 24 hours (1,2)), if the drug is administered.

References

1. Product information. Oxsoralen. ICN Pharmaceuticals, 1995.
2. Product information. Uvadex. Therakos, 2009.
3. Shepard TH. *Catalog of Teratogenic Agents*. 7th ed. Baltimore, MD: Johns Hopkins University Press, 1992:257.
4. Diawara MM, Kulkosky PJ. Reproductive toxicity of the psoralens. Pediatr Pathol Mol Med 2003;22:247–58.
5. Stern RS, Lange R, Members of The Photochemotherapy Follow-up Study. Outcomes of pregnancies among women and partners of men with a history of exposure to methoxsalen photochemotherapy (PUVA) for the treatment of psoriasis. Arch Dermatol 1991;127:347–50.
6. Gunnarskog JG, Källén AJB, Lindelöf BG, Sigurgeirsson B. Psoralen photochemotherapy (PUVA) and pregnancy. Arch Dermatol 1993;129:320–3.
7. Garbis H, Eléfant E, Bertolotti E, Robert E, Serafini MA, Prapas N. Pregnancy outcome after periconceptional and first-trimester exposure to methoxsalen photochemotherapy. Arch Dermatol 1995;131:492–3.

METHSCOPOLAMINE

Parasympatholytic (Anticholinergic)

PREGNANCY RECOMMENDATION: Limited Human Data—No Relevant Animal Data
BREASTFEEDING RECOMMENDATION: No Human Data—Probably Compatible

PREGNANCY SUMMARY

The very limited pregnancy experience showing a possible association with minor malformations requires confirmation. In general, however, anticholinergics appear to be low risk in pregnancy (see Atropine).

FETAL RISK SUMMARY

Methscopolamine is an anticholinergic quaternary ammonium bromide derivative of scopolamine (see also Scopolamine). In a large prospective study, 2323 patients were exposed to this class of drugs during the 1st trimester, 2 of whom took methscopolamine (1). A possible association was found in the total group between this class of drugs and minor malformations.

BREASTFEEDING SUMMARY

No reports describing the use of methscopolamine during human lactation have been located (see also Atropine).

Reference

1. Heinonen OP, Slone D, Shapiro S. *Birth Defects and Drugs in Pregnancy.* Littleton, MA: Publishing Sciences Group, 1977:346–53.

METHSUXIMIDE

Anticonvulsant

PREGNANCY RECOMMENDATION: Limited Human Data—No Relevant Animal Data
BREASTFEEDING RECOMMENDATION: No Human Data—Probably Compatible

PREGNANCY SUMMARY

Methsuximide is a succinimide anticonvulsant used in the treatment of petit mal epilepsy. The use of methsuximide during the 1st trimester has been reported in only five pregnancies (1,2). No evidence of adverse fetal effects was found. Methsuximide has a much lower teratogenic potential than the oxazolidinedione class of anticonvulsants (see Trimethadione) (3,4). The succinimide anticonvulsants have been considered the anticonvulsants of choice for the treatment of petit mal epilepsy during the 1st trimester (see Ethosuximide).

M

BREASTFEEDING SUMMARY

No reports describing the use of methsuximide during human lactation have been located. Other agents in this class have been classified as compatible with breastfeeding (see Ethosuximide).

References

1. Annegers JF, Elveback LR, Hauser WA, Kurland LT. Do anticonvulsants have a teratogenic effect? Arch Neurol 1974;31:364–73.
2. Heinonen OP, Slone D, Shapiro S. *Birth Defects and Drugs in Pregnancy.* Littleton, MA: Publishing Sciences Group, 1977:358–9.
3. Fabro S, Brown NA. Teratogenic potential of anticonvulsants. N Engl J Med 1979;300:1280–1.
4. The National Institutes of Health. Anticonvulsants found to have teratogenic potential. JAMA 1981;241:36.

METHYCLOTHIAZIDE

Diuretic

PREGNANCY RECOMMENDATION: Limited Human Data—Probably Compatible
BREASTFEEDING RECOMMENDATION: Limited Human Data—Probably Compatible

PREGNANCY SUMMARY

There is no evidence that thiazide diuretics are teratogenic. However, diuretics are not recommended for the treatment of gestational hypertension–preeclampsia because of the maternal hypovolemia characteristic of this disease.

FETAL RISK SUMMARY

Methyclothiazide is a member of the thiazide class of diuretics (see Chlorothiazide). Reproduction studies in rats and rabbits at doses up to about 20 times the maximum recommended human dose did not observe any evidence of impaired fertility or fetal harm (1).

BREASTFEEDING SUMMARY

See Chlorothiazide.

Reference

1. Product information. Enduron. Abbott Laboratories, 2000.

METHYLDOPA

Antihypertensive

PREGNANCY RECOMMENDATION: Compatible
BREASTFEEDING RECOMMENDATION: Limited Human Data—Probably Compatible

PREGNANCY SUMMARY

Methyldopa is a centrally acting, antiadrenergic agent used in the treatment of hypertension. It has been used frequently in pregnancy for this indication. There is no confirmed evidence that use of this agent presents a risk to the embryo or fetus.

FETAL RISK SUMMARY

Reproduction studies in mice, rats, and rabbits at doses 1.4, 0.2, and 1.1 times, respectively, the maximum recommended human dose based on BSA (MRHD), revealed no fetal harm (1). No impairment of fertility was noted in male or female rats at 0.2 times the MRHD. At higher doses (0.5 and 1 times the MRHD) in male rats, however, methyldopa decreased sperm count, sperm motility, the number of late spermatids, and the male fertility index (1).

Methyldopa crosses the placenta and achieves fetal concentrations similar to the maternal serum concentration (2–4). The Collaborative Perinatal Project monitored only one mother–child pair in which 1st trimester exposure to methyldopa was recorded (5). No abnormalities were found.

In a surveillance study of Michigan Medicaid recipients involving 229,101 completed pregnancies conducted between 1985 and 1992, 242 newborns had been exposed to methyldopa during the 1st trimester (F. Rosa, personal communication, FDA, 1993). A total of 11 (4.5%) major birth defects were observed (10 expected). Specific data were available for six defect categories, including (observed/expected) 1/2 cardiovascular defects, 1/0 oral clefts, 0/0 spina bifida, 1/1 polydactyly, 0/0 limb reduction defects, and 0/1 hypospadias. These data do not support an association between the drug and congenital defects.

A decrease in intracranial volume has been reported after 1st trimester exposure to methyldopa (6,7). Children evaluated at 4 years of age showed no association between small head size and slow mental development (8). Review of 1157 hypertensive pregnancies demonstrated no adverse effects from methyldopa administration (9–21). A reduced systolic blood pressure of 4–5 mmHg in 24 infants for the first 2 days after delivery has been reported (22). This mild reduction in blood pressure was not considered significant. An infant born with esophageal atresia with fistula, congenital heart disease, absent left kidney, and hypospadias was exposed to methyldopa throughout gestation (23). The mother also took clomiphene early in the 1st trimester.

BREASTFEEDING SUMMARY

Methyldopa is excreted into breast milk in small amounts. In four lactating women taking 750–2000 mg/day, milk levels of free and conjugated methyldopa ranged from 0.1 to 0.9 mcg/mL (2). A milk:plasma ratio could not be determined because simultaneous plasma levels were not obtained. The American Academy of Pediatrics classifies methyldopa as compatible with breastfeeding (24).

References

1. Product information. Aldomet. Merck, 2000.
2. Jones HMR, Cummings AJ. A study of the transfer of á-methyldopa to the human foetus and newborn infant. Br J Clin Pharmacol 1978;6:432–4.
3. Jones HMR, Cummings AJ, Setchell KDR, Lawson AM. Pharmacokinetics of methyldopa in neonates. Br J Clin Pharmacol 1979;8:433–40.
4. Cummings AJ, Whitelaw AGL. A study of conjugation and drug elimination in the human neonate. Br J Clin Pharmacol 1981;12:511–5.
5. Heinonen OP, Slone D, Shapiro S. *Birth Defects and Drugs in Pregnancy*. Littleton, MA: Publishing Sciences Group, 1977:372.
6. Myerscough PR. Infant growth and development after treatment of maternal hypertension. Lancet 1980;1:883.
7. Moar VA, Jefferies MA, Mutch LMM, Dunsted MK, Redman CWG. Neonatal head circumference and the treatment of maternal hypertension. Br J Obstet Gynaecol 1978;85:933–7.
8. Dunsted M, Moar VA, Redman CWG. Infant growth and development following treatment of maternal hypertension. Lancet 1980;1:705.
9. Redman CWG, Beilin LJ, Bonnar J, Ounsted MK. Fetal outcome in trial of antihypertensive treatment in pregnancy. Lancet 1976;2:753–6.
10. Hamilton M, Kopelman H. Treatment of severe hypertension with methyldopa. Br Med J 1963;1:151–5.
11. Abramowsky CR, Vegas ME, Swinehart G, Gyves MT. Decidual vasculopathy of the placenta in lupus erythematosus. N Engl J Med 1980;303:668–72.
12. Gallery EDM, Sounders DM, Hunyor SN, Gyory AZ. Randomised comparison of methyldopa and oxprenolol for treatment of hypertension in pregnancy. Br Med J 1979;1:1591–4.
13. Gyory AZ, Gallery ED, Hunyor SN. Effect of treatment of maternal hypertension with oxprenolol and α-methyldopa on plasma volume, placental and birth weights (abstract 1098). Presented at Eighth World Congress of Cardiology, Tokyo, 1978.
14. Arias F, Zamora J. Antihypertensive treatment and pregnancy outcome in patients with mild chronic hypertension. Obstet Gynecol 1979;53:489–94.
15. Redman CWG, Beilin LJ, Bonnar J. A trial of hypotensive treatment in pregnancy. Clin Sci Mol Med 1975;49:3–4.

16. Tcherdakoff P, Milliez P. Traitement de l'hypertension arterielle par alpha-methyldopa au cours de la grossesse. In Proceedings Premier Symposium National, Hypertension Arterielle, Cannes, 1970:207–9.
17. Lselve A, Berger R, Vial JY, Gaillard MF. Alpha-methyldopa/Aldomet and reserpine/Serpasil: treatment of pregnancy hypertensions. J Med Lyon 1968;1369–75.
18. Leather HM, Humphreys DM, Baker P, Chadd MA. A controlled trial of hypotensive agents in hypertension in pregnancy. Lancet 1968;2:488–90.
19. Hamilton H. Some aspects of the long-term treatment of severe hypertension with methyldopa. Postgrad Med J 1968;44:66–9.
20. Skacel K, Sklendvsky A, Gazarek F, Matlocha Z, Mohapl M. Therapeutic use of alpha-methyldopa in cases of late toxemia of pregnancy. Cesk Gynekol 1967;32:78–80.
21. Kincaid-Smith P, Bullen M. Prolonged use of methyldopa in severe hypertension in pregnancy. Br Med J 1966;1:274–6.
22. Whitelaw A. Maternal methyldopa treatment and neonatal blood pressure. Br Med J 1981;283:471.
23. Ylikorkala O. Congenital anomalies and clomiphene. Lancet 1975;2:1262–3.
24. Committee on Drugs, American Academy of Pediatrics. The transfer of drugs and other chemicals into human milk. Pediatrics 2001;108:776–89.

METHYLENE BLUE

Urinary Germicide/Diagnostic Dye

PREGNANCY RECOMMENDATION: Human Data Suggest Risk in 2nd and 3rd Trimesters
BREASTFEEDING RECOMMENDATION: No Human Data—Probably Compatible

PREGNANCY SUMMARY

The intraamniotic injection of methylene blue to detect ruptured membranes should be discouraged. If indicated, other dyes, such as indigo carmine or Evans blue appear to be safer alternatives, although both have limited pregnancy data (see Indigo Carmine and Evans Blue) (1).

FETAL RISK SUMMARY

Methylene blue has been administered orally for its weak urinary germicide properties or injected into the amniotic fluid to diagnose premature rupture of the membranes. For oral dosing, nine exposures in the 1st trimester have been reported (2, p. 299). No congenital abnormalities were observed. For use anytime during pregnancy, 46 exposures were reported (2, pp. 434–435). Based on three malformed infants, a possible association with malformations (type not specified) was found.

Diagnostic intraamniotic injection of methylene blue has resulted in hemolytic anemia, hyperbilirubinemia, and methemoglobinemia in the newborn (3–12). Doses of the dye in most reports ranged from 10 to 70 mg, but in one case, 200 mg was injected into the amniotic cavity (9). Deep blue staining of the newborn may occur after injection of the agent into the amniotic fluid (8–10,12). One author suggested that smaller doses, such as 1.6 mg, would be adequate to confirm the presence of ruptured membranes without causing hemolysis (3).

In a 1989 report, 1 mL of a 1% solution (10 mg) was used to diagnose suspected membrane rupture in a woman with premature labor at 26 weeks of gestation (13). A 920-g girl was born 18 hours later who was stained a deep blue. The clinical assessment of hypoxia was impaired by the skin color as was pulse oximetry. A transcutaneous oxygen monitor was eventually used to measure arterial blood gas so that ventilator therapy could be regulated. No evidence of hemolysis was observed. The bluish tinge persisted for more than 2 weeks despite frequent baths (13).

Inadvertent intrauterine injection in the 1st trimester has been reported (14). No adverse effects were reported in the full-term neonate.

Multiple ileal occlusions were found in seven newborns born to mothers with twin pregnancies, at three different medical centers, who had received diagnostic intraamniotic methylene blue into one of the amniotic sacs at 15–17 weeks' gestation (15). The doses in these cases ranged from 10 to 30 mg. Four of the infants required surgery for intestinal obstruction, but no information was given on the other three. The authors speculated that the mechanism of the adverse effect was related either to hemolysis or to acute intestinal hypoxia secondary to methylene blue–induced release of norepinephrine and subsequent vasoconstriction (15).

In an abstract published in 1992, data on jejunal and ileal atresia in twins were reported from Australia (16). Higher risks of atresia were found in twins, compared with singletons, and in twins delivered from older mothers. When undiluted 1% methylene blue was used in one group, 1 of 9 twins of 40 (22.5%) twin pregnancies had atresia, compared with 3 cases among 53 (5.7%) in those exposed to a 0.25% solution (16).

A third report of the above complication appeared in 1992 (17). Intraamniotic methylene blue, 10–20 mg, was used in 86 of 89 consecutive twin pregnancies for prenatal diagnosis. No dye was used in three pregnancies for technical reasons. Jejunal atresia occurred in 17 (19%) of the pregnancies; in 15 of the affected cases, it was possible to determine that the affected fetus had been the one exposed to the dye. All of the infants required surgery to relieve the intestinal obstruction. A portion of this report also described 67 newborns that were treated for jejunal atresia, 20 of whom were one of a set of twins. Of the 20 newborns from twins, 18 had been exposed to methylene blue during 2nd trimester amniocentesis. Because the incidence of jejunal atresia was much higher than expected and because the dye appears to cause the defect, the authors of the study (17) and an accompanying commentary (18) recommended avoidance of methylene blue for this purpose. The commentary also alluded to the vasoconstrictor properties of methylene blue as a possible mechanism (18).

A brief 1993 report described the use of methylene blue dye in women with twins who underwent amniocentesis in

M

the Atlanta, Georgia, area between 1977 and 1991 (19). A total of 195 women were included, 4 (2%) of whom were administered methylene blue during the procedure. Of the eight fetuses, one had anencephaly (no association with the dye), but no cases of small intestinal atresia were observed.

A 1993 article reviewed the teratogenicity and newborn adverse effects resulting from intraamniotic injection of methylene blue (1). The most frequent adverse effects in newborns were hyperbilirubinemia, hemolytic anemia with or without Heinz body formation, blue staining of the skin, and occasionally methemoglobinemia and fetal death. Respiratory distress was also frequently observed but may have been related to other causes. The structural defects observed were jejunal-ileal atresias, but the mechanism of the bowel injury is unknown. Based on the pharmacologic properties of the dye, the most likely mechanism was thought to be vascular disruption caused by methylene blue–induced arterial constriction. However, methemoglobinemia- and hemolytic anemia–induced hypoxia causing a shunting of blood away from the intestine with resulting ischemia and atresia, or a direct toxic effect from the dye when swallowed with amniotic fluid were other possible mechanisms (1).

BREASTFEEDING SUMMARY

No reports describing the use of methylene blue during human lactation have been located. However, the dye does not appear to present a risk to a nursing infant.

References

1. Cragan JD. Teratogen update: methylene blue. Teratology 1999;60:42–48.
2. Heinonen OP, Slone D, Shapiro S. *Birth Defects and Drugs in Pregnancy*. Littleton, MA: Publishing Sciences Group, 1977.
3. Plunkett GD. Neonatal complications. Obstet Gynecol 1973;41:476–7.
4. Cowett RM, Hakanson DO, Kocon RW, Oh W. Untoward neonatal effect of intraamniotic administration of methylene blue. Obstet Gynecol 1976;48:74S–5S.
5. Kirsch IR, Cohen HJ. Heinz body hemolytic anemia from the use of methylene blue in neonates. J Pediatr 1980;96:276–8.
6. Crooks J. Haemolytic jaundice in a neonate after intra-amniotic injection of methylene blue. Arch Dis Child 1982;57:872–3.
7. McEnerney JK. McEnerney LN. Unfavorable neonatal outcome after intraamniotic injection of methylene blue. Obstet Gynecol 1983;61: 35S–6S.
8. Serota FT, Bernbaum JC, Schwartz E. The methylene-blue baby. Lancet 1979;2:1142–3.
9. Vincer MJ, Allen AC, Evans JR, Nwaesei C, Stinson DA. Methylene-blue-induced hemolytic anemia in a neonate. CMAJ 1987;136:503–4.
10. Spahr RC, Salsburey DJ, Krissberg A, Prin W. Intraamniotic injection of methylene blue leading to methemoglobinemia in one of twins. Int J Gynaecol Obstet 1980;17:477–8.
11. Poinsot J, Guillois B, Margis D, Carlhant D, Boog G, Alix D. Neonatal hemolytic anemia after intra-amniotic injection of methylene blue. Arch Fr Pediatr 1988;45:657–60.
12. Fish WH, Chazen EM. Toxic effects of methylene blue on the fetus. Am J Dis Child 1992;146:1412–3.
13. Troche BI. The methylene-blue baby. N Engl J Med 1989;320:1756–7.
14. Katz Z, Lancet M. Inadvertent intrauterine injection of methylene blue in early pregnancy. N Engl J Med 1981;304:1427.
15. Nicolini U, Monni G. Intestinal obstruction in babies exposed in utero to methylene blue. Lancet 1990;336:1258–9.
16. Lancaster PAL, Pedisich EL, Fisher CC, Robertson RD. Intra-amniotic methylene blue and intestinal atresia in twins (abstract). J Perinat Med 1992;20 (Suppl 1):262.
17. Van Der Pol JG, Wolf H, Boer K, Treffers PE, Leschot NJ, Hey HA, Vos A. Jejunal atresia related to the use of methylene blue in genetic amniocentesis in twins. Br J Obstet Gynaecol 1992;99:141–3.
18. McFadyen I. The dangers of intra-amniotic methylene blue. Br J Obstet Gynaecol 1992;99:89–90.
19. Cragan JD, Martin ML, Khoury MJ, Fernhoff PM. Dye use during amniocentesis and birth defects. Lancet 1993;341:1352.

METHYLERGONOVINE MALEATE

Oxytocic

PREGNANCY RECOMMENDATION: Contraindicated
BREASTFEEDING RECOMMENDATION: Compatible

PREGNANCY SUMMARY

Methylergonovine does not appear to be a major teratogen in either animals or humans, but the data are too limited for any conclusion. The drug is contraindicated during pregnancy because of its propensity to cause sustained, tetanic uterine contractions that result in fetal hypoxia. Because of this, it is used as an alternate drug to oxytocin for management of the third stage of labor (i.e., from delivery of the infant to delivery of the placenta) and for the treatment of postpartum or postabortion hemorrhage. Care must be taken before administering this agent to confirm that the intended recipient has delivered her fetus.

FETAL RISK SUMMARY

Methylergonovine maleate (methylergometrine maleate; methylergobasine maleate) is an ergot alkaloid derivative used in the treatment of postpartum and postabortion hemorrhage. It is contraindicated during pregnancy because it may cause sustained, tetanic uterine contractions and resulting fetal compromise.

Only one animal reproductive study has been located that investigated the effect of methylergonovine on the fetus (1). Thirteen albino rats were administered 0.5 mg/kg intraperitoneally twice daily from the 12th day through the 21st day (second half of gestation) after sperm were found in the vaginal smears of the animals (1). Three other groups received different ergot alkaloids and another group acted as controls. Three (23%) of the methylergonovine group failed to conceive or resorbed their conception compared with an average of 17% (10 of 58) in the other three treated groups and 17% (2 of 12) in the controls. The surviving pups were not examined for congenital malformations (drug-induced anomalies not expected) but their birth weights were similar to those of pups in the control group.

The Collaborative Perinatal Project monitored 50,282 mother–child pairs, 32 of whom were exposed to ergot derivatives other than ergotamine during the 1st trimester (2). Five of this group were exposed to methylergonovine maleate, 18 to ergonovine, 5 to ergot, 3 to dihydroergotamine, and 1 to methysergide. Three children with any malformation were observed in the total group, but only 1 had a malformation considered easily recognizable among the 12 medical centers participating in the study. The authors concluded that, although the numbers were small, there was no evidence that these agents were teratogenic (2).

A 1979 report described the effects of methylergonovine on a woman in the first stage of labor (i.e., from onset of labor to full dilation of the cervix) at 43 weeks' gestation (3). The woman was accidentally given 0.2 mg methylergonovine IM that had been ordered for a postpartum patient. Within 20 minutes, uterine hypertonus was evident, and the fetal heart rate (FHR) decreased to 80–90 beats/minute (bpm) with increased variability. IV epinephrine (0.5 mL of 1:1000) was administered with a rapid decline in excessive uterine activity but the FHR fell to 40–50 bpm (most likely because of epinephrine-induced vasoconstriction) before slowly returning to baseline. When uterine tetany returned, a second dose of epinephrine (1/6 mL) was required, producing similar effects on uterine activity and the FHR, but of shorter duration. An approximate 2731-g male infant was delivered 6 hours later with Apgar scores of 5 and 7 at 1 and 5 minutes, respectively. Examinations of the infant over the next 9 months were normal.

A similar case of accidental (i.e., a dose intended for another patient) methylergonovine administration resulting in uterine hypertonus was reported in 1988 (4). The 18-year-old woman at 37 weeks' gestation in the first stage of labor with uterine contractions every 2–3 minutes and a partially dilated and effaced cervix received 0.2 mg methylergonovine IM. Six minutes later, the FHR fell from 150 to 70 bpm and uterine hypertonus was detected on palpation. Terbutaline, 0.25 mg IV reversed the fetal bradycardia but did not relax the uterus. Magnesium sulfate, 4-g IV loading dose followed by 2 g/hr, also failed to reverse the hypertonus. Adverse changes in the fetus, including loss of FHR beat-to-beat variability, late decelerations, development of tachycardia (170 bpm), and acidosis (scalp pH 7.12), impelled the authors to perform a cesarean section, under general anesthesia, to deliver the approximate 3604-g male infant. Apgar scores were 8 and 9 at 1 and 5 minutes, respectively. At delivery, the umbilical artery blood had a pH of 7.13, confirming the diagnosis of metabolic acidosis (4). The infant did well after delivery and was discharged home at 4 days of age.

BREASTFEEDING SUMMARY

Methylergonovine is excreted into breast milk in very small quantities. No accumulation of the drug in breast milk has been measured. This ergot derivative appears to inhibit release of prolactin, including that induced by suckling, resulting in a decreased milk production, but not to the same degree as the structurally related drug bromocriptine. The clinical significance of the lactation suppression and the exposure of the nursing infant to the drug, however, is most likely nil. This may be a result of its usual short-term use after delivery and its lower potency (on a milligram-to-milligram basis) as a prolactin-release inhibitor. No adverse effects attributable to methylergonovine in a nursing infant have been reported. Moreover, methylergonovine is one of the most commonly prescribed drugs during the first postpartum week.

Small amounts of methylergonovine are excreted into breast milk. During the first 4 days postpartum, eight lactating women (not stated whether the women were nursing) were treated with the drug, 0.125 mg orally 3 times daily, because of incomplete uterine involution (5). On the 5th postpartum day, a 0.25-mg oral dose was administered, and milk and plasma samples were collected 1 and 8 hours later. Methylergonovine concentrations in the milk were determined by radioimmunoassay. Measurable (test sensitivity 0.5 ng/mL) amounts were found in four of the eight milk samples at 1 hour (average 0.8 ng/mL; range 0.6–1.3 ng/mL) and in one sample at 8 hours (1.2 ng/mL). Seven other milk samples had detectable amounts of the drug, but the concentrations were <0.5 ng/mL. In contrast, all eight of the plasma samples had measurable drug (average 2.5 ng/mL; range 0.6–4.4 ng/mL). At 8 hours after the dose, two plasma samples had measurable drug (0.5 and 0.6 ng/mL), and one had detectable drug (<0.5 ng/mL). In the four cases at 1 hour that had measurable drug in both the plasma and milk, the milk:plasma ratio was about 0.3. Based on the lack of accumulation of methylergonovine in the plasma or milk, the authors concluded that the use of the drug during breastfeeding would not affect the infant (5).

M

Higher plasma and, presumably, milk drug levels may have occurred at 3 hours after a dose based on other research conducted by these investigators (6). In this study, conducted in the same manner as the study described above but with drug levels determined on the 3rd and 6th postpartum days, maternal plasma levels of methylergonovine at 1 and 3 hours after a 0.25-mg oral dose were about 1.7 and 2 ng/mL, respectively (5,6). The authors, however, did not believe that measurement of the higher drug levels would have changed their conclusion (5).

The effect of methylergonovine, which is structurally related to bromocriptine, a known inhibitor of prolactin secretion and human lactation, on suckling-induced release of prolactin and subsequent milk production is controversial. In a study published in 1975, 14 women received a 0.2-mg IM dose of the drug after delivery of the placenta and 15 other women acted as controls (7). Serum prolactin levels before drug administration in the two groups were 90.1 and 93.6 ng/mL, respectively. At 80–90 minutes after delivery, the mean serum prolactin concentration in the treated group was 141 ng/mL (difference not significant from baseline). In contrast, the level in the controls was 266 ng/mL, significantly higher than baseline and the methylergonovine group.

Similar effects of methylergonovine on prolactin release were published in a 1975 reference (8). A 0.2-mg IM dose administered on the 3rd postpartum day produced a statistically significant decrease in serum prolactin between 45 and 60 minutes after injection. At 180 minutes after the dose, the prolactin levels began to rise, but they still had not returned to baseline by 240 minutes.

In another 1975 report, 10 breastfeeding mothers in the immediate postpartum period were treated with methylergonovine, 0.2 mg orally 3 times daily for 7 days (9). A similar group of 10 breastfeeding women received no medication. Plasma prolactin concentrations in both groups were measured each morning. No significant difference between the groups in prolactin concentrations was measured with plasma levels of prolactin decreasing from a mean of 144 ng/mL (both groups) to 41 ng/mL (methylergonovine) and 37 ng/mL (controls) at 7 days. Milk let-down occurred between the 2nd and 4th postpartum day in both groups. Moreover, the mean milk volume production (estimated by infant weight gain and residual milk obtained by electric breast pump) on the 7th postpartum day was 386 mL in the treated group and 367 mL in the controls.

Contrary to the above study, two reports, one in 1976 (10) and one in 1979 (11), described the inhibitory effects of ergot derivatives on prolactin secretion and lactation. In the 1976 paper, ergonovine, an agent closely related to methylergonovine, was given to 10 women in a dose of 0.2 mg orally 3 times daily from the 1st through the 7th postpartum day (10). None of the women nursed their infants. Six other women who were not breastfeeding acted as controls. Blood samples for serum prolactin measurement were drawn each morning in both groups. Before-treatment mean serum prolactin concentrations in the ergonovine and control groups were 537 and 562 ng/mL, respectively, and on postpartum day 7 they were 89.7 and 218.0 ng/mL, respectively. Moreover, the serum prolactin concentrations were significantly lower each day than the levels in the ergonovine group. Three of the ergonovine-treated women showed progressive lactation inhibition, whereas the other seven women had painful breast engorgement and spontaneous milk let-down.

Two other women in the above study received ergonovine 0.2 mg IV before nursing on the 5th postpartum day (10). One of these women also received ergonovine, 0.2 mg orally 3 times daily, before and after the IV dose. In the woman who received both IV and oral doses, the normal rise in serum prolactin induced by suckling was abolished.

The 1979 report described the effects of methylergonovine, 0.2 mg orally 3 times daily, in 30 breastfeeding women compared with 30 nonmedicated, breastfeeding control women (11). Plasma prolactin concentrations were determined in both groups on postpartum days 1, 3, and 7. Milk yields, estimated by weighing the nursing baby before and after suckling, were determined on postpartum days 3 and 7. In the control group, mean plasma prolactin levels on days 1, 3, and 7 were 374.1, 226.2, and 166.3 ng/mL, respectively. Mean plasma prolactin levels in the treated group on these days were 352.9, 219.6, and 88.7 ng/mL, respectively. Only the levels on day 7 were statistically different (11). Milk production (in g/day) was significantly less in the treated group compared with the controls on days 3 and 7 (specific weights of milk not stated).

References

1. Sommer AF, Buchanan AR. Effects of ergot alkaloids on pregnancy and lactation in the albino rat. Am J Physiol 1955;180:296–300.
2. Heinonen OP, Slone D, Shapiro S. *Birth Defects and Drugs in Pregnancy*. Littleton, MA: Publishing Sciences Group, 1977:357–65.
3. Wong R, Paul RH. Methergine-induced uterine tetany treated with epinephrine: case report. Am J Obstet Gynecol 1979;134:602–3.
4. Moise KJ Jr, Carpenter RJ Jr. Methylergonovine-induced hypertonus in term pregnancy. A case report. J Reprod Med 1988;33:771–3.
5. Erkkola R, Kanto J, Allonen H, Kleimola T, Mantyla R. Excretion of methylergometrine (methylergonovine) into the human breast milk. Int J Clin Pharmacol Biopharm 1978;16:579–80.
6. Allonen H, Juvakoski R, Kanto J, Laitinen S, Mantyla R, Kleimola T. Methylergometrine: comparison of plasma concentrations and clinical response of two brands. Int J Clin Pharmacol Biopharm 1978;16:340–2.
7. Weiss G, Klein S, Shenkman L, Kataoka K, Hollander CS. Effect of methylergonovine on puerperal prolactin secretion. Obstet Gynecol 1975;46:209–10.
8. Perez-Lopez FR, Delvoye P, Denayer P, L'Hermite M, Roncero MC, Robyn C. Effect of methylergobasine maleate on serum gonadotrophin and prolactin in humans. Acta Endocrinol 1975;79:644–57.
9. Del Pozo E, Brun Del Re R, Hinselmann M. Lack of effect of methyl-ergonovine on postpartum lactation. Am J Obstet Gynecol 1975;123:845–6.
10. Canales ES, Garrido JT, Zarate A, Mason M, Soria J. Effect of ergonovine on prolactin secretion and milk let-down. Obstet Gynecol 1976;48:228–9.
11. Peters F, Lummerich M, Breckwoldt M. Inhibition of prolactin and lactation by methylergometrine hydrogenmaleate. Acta Endocrinol 1979;91:213–6.

METHYLNALTREXONE

Narcotic Antagonist

PREGNANCY RECOMMENDATION: No Human Data—Animal Data Suggest Low Risk
BREASTFEEDING RECOMMENDATION: No Human Data—Probably Compatible

PREGNANCY SUMMARY

Published human pregnancy experience with methylnaltrexone has not been located. The animal reproduction data suggest low risk, but the absence of human data prevents a complete assessment of the embryo–fetal risk. Orthostatic hypotension, an effect that could decrease placental perfusion, is a potential risk if the drug is inadvertently given IV. Close attention to the dose and SC administration technique is warranted.

FETAL RISK SUMMARY

Methylnaltrexone, a selective antagonist of opioid binding at the mu-opioid receptor, is given by SC injection. It is a quaternary amine that because of its restricted ability to cross the blood–brain barrier acts peripherally without affecting opioid-mediated analgesic effects in the central nervous system. Methylnaltrexone is indicated for the treatment of opioid-induced constipation in patients with advanced illness who are receiving palliative care, when response to laxative therapy has not been sufficient. The drug undergoes partial metabolism before elimination. Plasma protein binding is about 15% or less and the elimination half-life is about 8 hours (1).

Reproduction studies have been conducted in pregnant rats and rabbits. In these species, IV doses up to about 14 and 17 times, respectively, the maximum recommended human SC dose of 0.3 mg/kg based on BSA (MRHD) revealed no evidence of impaired fertility or fetal harm. There were no effects on the mother, labor, delivery, offspring survival, or growth in rats (1).

Carcinogenicity studies have not been conducted, but the drug was not mutagenic in multiple assays. SC doses up to 81 times the MRHD had no adverse effect on fertility or reproductive performance in male or female rats (1).

It is not known if methylnaltrexone crosses the human placenta. The molecular weight (about 436), minimal plasma protein binding, and long elimination half-life suggest that the drug will cross. However, quaternary amines cross biological membranes poorly; this should limit the exposure of the embryo or fetus.

Orthostatic hypotension, an effect that could decrease placental perfusion if it occurred in pregnancy, has been noted in healthy volunteers given an IV bolus of 0.64 mg/kg. However, this dose is twice the recommended maximum SC dose. Moreover, a 0.5 mg SC dose was well tolerated by healthy volunteers (1).

BREASTFEEDING SUMMARY

No reports describing the use of methylnaltrexone, a quaternary amine, during human lactation have been located. The molecular weight (about 436), minimal plasma protein binding (<15%), and long elimination half-life (about 8 hours) suggest that the drug will be excreted into breast milk. The effects of this exposure on a nursing infant are unknown, but are probably clinically insignificant.

Reference

1. Product information. Relistor. Progenics Pharmaceuticals, 2009.

METHYLPHENIDATE

Central Stimulant

PREGNANCY RECOMMENDATION: Limited Human Data—Animal Data Suggest Moderate Risk
BREASTFEEDING RECOMMENDATION: Limited Human Data—Potential Toxicity

PREGNANCY SUMMARY

Although the animal data suggest moderate risk, the limited human data prevent a more complete assessment of embryo–fetal risk. Neither the isolated cases of structural defects nor the outcomes observed with methylphenidate abuse are suggestive of methylphenidate-induced developmental toxicity.

FETAL RISK SUMMARY

Methylphenidate is a mild central nervous system stimulant used in the treatment of attention-deficit disorders and in narcolepsy.

Reproductive testing with methylphenidate in mice found no teratogenicity (1). In rabbits, doses about 40 times the maximum recommended human dose based on BSA (MRHD) were teratogenic (increased incidence of spina bifida) (2). The no-effect dose for embryo–fetal development was about 11 times the MRHD. No teratogenic effects were observed in rats, but a dose 7 times the MRHD caused maternal toxicity and fetal skeletal variations. The no-effect dose in rats was 2 times the MRHD. Dosing in rats throughout gestation and lactation at 4 times the MRHD resulted in decreased body weight gain in the offspring. In this case, the no-effect dose was equal to the MRHD (2).

The Collaborative Perinatal Project monitored 3082 mother–child pairs with exposure to sympathomimetic drugs, 11 of which were exposed to methylphenidate (3). No evidence for an increased malformation rate was found.

In a surveillance study of Michigan Medicaid recipients involving 229,101 completed pregnancies conducted between 1985 and 1992, 13 newborns had been exposed to methylphenidate during the 1st trimester (F. Rosa, personal communication, FDA, 1993). One (7.7%) major birth defect was observed (one expected), a cardiovascular defect (none expected).

A report of an infant with microtia following in utero exposure to methylphenidate from the 3rd to the 6th week of pregnancy appeared in a 1962 publication (4). No other details of the case were provided, other than the fact that the mother did not take antiemetic medication and had no virus infection during gestation.

A 1975 report described a male infant, delivered at 30 weeks' gestation, with multiple congenital limb malformations. The infant had been exposed during the first 7 weeks of pregnancy to haloperidol (15 mg/day), methylphenidate (30 mg/day), and phenytoin (300 mg/day) (5). The mother had also taken tetracycline and a decongestant for a cold during the 1st trimester. The infant died at 2 hours of age of a subdural hemorrhage. Limb malformations included a thumb and two fingers on each hand, syndactyly of the two fingers on the right hand, deformed radius and missing ulna in the left forearm, four toes on the right foot, shortened right tibia, and incomplete development of the right midfoot ossification centers. A defect of the aortic valve (bicuspid with a notch in one of the valve leaflets) was also found. The chromosomal analysis was normal and the mother had no family history of limb malformations (5).

A study published in 1993 examined the effects on the fetus and newborn of IV pentazocine and methylphenidate abuse during pregnancy (6). During a 2-year (1987–1988) period, 39 infants (38 pregnancies, 1 set of twins) were identified in the study population as being subjected to the drug abuse during gestation, a minimum incidence of 5 cases per 1000 live births. Many of the mothers had used cigarettes (34%), alcohol (71%), or abused other drugs (26%). The median duration of IV pentazocine and methylphenidate abuse was 3 years (range 1–9 years), with a median frequency of 14 injections/week (range 1–70 injections/week). Among the infants, 8 were delivered prematurely, 12 were growth restricted, and 11 had withdrawal symptoms after birth. Four of the infants had birth defects including twins with fetal alcohol syndrome, one with a ventricular septal defect, and one case of polydactyly. Of the 21 infants that had formal developmental testing, 17 had normal development and 4 had low–normal developmental quotients (6).

BREASTFEEDING SUMMARY

Methylphenidate is excreted into breast milk (7). A 26-year-old mother was taking methylphenidate 80 mg/day (40 mg 4 hours apart in the morning) for 5 days each week for attention-deficit disorder. At the time of the study, she had been taking the drug for 5.5 weeks and for 7 consecutive days. The mother's male infant was 6.4 months old and was obtaining his primary sustenance from breast milk. His weight was at the 50th percentile and he had been feeding and sleeping well. Using an electric pump, breast milk samples were collected immediately before the first morning dose and at each of the 7 times the infant breastfed over the next 24 hours. Over the 24-hour interval, the average milk and maternal plasma concentrations were 15.4 and 5.8 mcg/L, respectively, a milk:plasma ratio of 2.7. The absolute infant dose of 2.3 mcg/kg/day was 0.2% of the weight-adjusted maternal dose. Methylphenidate was not detected in the infant's plasma 5.3 hours after the first morning dose. The mother had not observed any adverse effects in her infant (7).

The excretion of methylphenidate into milk is consistent with its molecular weight (about 270). The absolute infant dose was very low in comparison to the maternal dose and no adverse effects were observed in the infant. However, toxicity from exposure to drugs in breast milk is infrequent in nursing infants who are >6 months of age, accounting only for 4% of 100 reported cases involving adverse effects (8). If a mother chooses to breastfeed while taking methylphenidate, the greatest risk of toxicity probably will occur in the first month after birth. However, regardless of the infant's age, the mother should be counseled to observe her nursling for signs and symptoms of central nervous system stimulation, such as decreased appetite, insomnia, and irritability.

References

1. Takano K, Tanimura T, Nishimura H. Effects of some psychoactive drugs administered to pregnant mice upon the development of their offspring. Congenital Anom 1963;3:2. As cited in Schardein JL. *Chemically Induced Birth Defects*. 2nd ed. New York, NY: Marcel Dekker, 1993:223.
2. Product information. Ritalin LA. Novartis Pharmaceuticals, 2004.
3. Heinonen OP, Slone D, Shapiro S. *Birth Defects and Drugs in Pregnancy*. Littleton, MA: Publishing Sciences Group, 1977:346–7.
4. Smithells RW. Thalidomide and malformations in Liverpool. Lancet 1962;1:1270–3.
5. Kopelman AE, McCullar FW, Heggeness L. Limb malformations following maternal use of haloperidol. JAMA 1975;231:62–4.
6. Debooy VD, Seshia MMK, Tenenbein M, Casiro OG. Intravenous pentazocine and methylphenidate abuse during pregnancy. Maternal lifestyle and infant outcome. Am J Dis Child 1993;147:1062–5.
7. Hackett LP, Kristensen JH, Hale TW, Paterson R, Ilet KF. Methylphenidate and breast-feeding. Ann Pharmacother 2006;40:1890–1.
8. Anderson PO, Pochop SL, Manoguerra AS. Adverse drug reactions in breastfed infants: less than imagined. Clin Pediatr 2003;42:325–40.

METHYLTESTOSTERONE

Androgenic Hormone

See Testosterone.

METOCLOPRAMIDE

Antiemetic/Gastrointestinal Stimulant

PREGNANCY RECOMMENDATION: Compatible
BREASTFEEDING RECOMMENDATION: Limited Human Data—Potential Toxicity

PREGNANCY SUMMARY

Metoclopramide has been used during all stages of pregnancy. No evidence of embryo, fetal, or newborn harm has been found in human and animal studies.

FETAL RISK SUMMARY

Metoclopramide has been used during pregnancy as an antiemetic and to decrease gastric emptying time (1–24). Reproductive studies in mice, rats, and rabbits at doses up to 250 times the human dose have revealed no evidence of impaired fertility or fetal harm as a result of the drug (25). Metoclopramide (10 mg) given IV to pregnant sheep increased maternal heart rate, but had no effect on maternal blood pressure, uterine blood flow, or fetal hemodynamic variables (26).

No congenital malformations or other fetal or newborn adverse effects attributable to the drug have been observed. Except for the one study noted below (7), long-term evaluation of infants exposed in utero to metoclopramide has not been reported.

Metoclopramide crosses the placenta at term (1–3). Cord:maternal plasma ratios were 0.57–0.84 after IV doses just before cesarean section. Placental transfer during other stages of pregnancy has not been studied.

Nine reports described the use of metoclopramide for the treatment of nausea and vomiting occurring in early pregnancy (4–7, 20–24). Administration of the drug was begun at 7–8 weeks' gestation in two of these studies (4,5) and at 6 weeks in another (6). The exact timing of pregnancy was not specified in one report (7). Daily doses ranged between 10 and 60 mg. Metoclopramide was as effective as other antiemetics for this indication and superior to placebo (8,9). Normal infant development for up to 4 years was mentioned in one study, but no details were provided (7).

In another case of metoclopramide use for nausea and vomiting, the drug was started at 10 weeks' gestation (20). Dose was not specified. At 18 weeks, after 8 weeks of therapy, the patient developed a neuropsychiatric syndrome with acute asymmetrical axonal motor-sensory polyneuropathy and marked anxiety, depression, irritability, and memory and concentration difficulties (20). Acute porphyria was diagnosed based on the presence of increased porphyrin precursors in the patient's urine. Metoclopramide was discontinued and the patient was treated with a high-carbohydrate diet. Eventually, a normal, 3500-g infant was delivered at term. The woman recovered except for slight residual weakness in the lower extremities. The investigators speculated that the pregnancy itself, the starvation, the drug, or a combination of these may have precipitated the acute attack (20).

A 1996 report described the use of metoclopramide, droperidol, diphenhydramine, and hydroxyzine in 80 women with hyperemesis gravidarum (21). The mean gestational age at the start of treatment was 10.9. All of the women received metoclopramide 40 mg/day orally for approximately 7 days, and 12 (15%) required a second course because of the recurrence of their symptoms of nausea and vomiting. Three of the mothers (all treated in the 2nd trimester) delivered offspring with congenital defects: Poland's syndrome, fetal alcohol syndrome, and hydrocephalus and hypoplasia of the right cerebral hemisphere. Only the latter anomaly is a potential drug effect, but the most likely cause was thought to be the result of an in utero fetal vascular accident or infection (21).

A 2001 study, using a treatment method similar to the above study, described the use of droperidol and diphenhydramine in 28 women hospitalized for hyperemesis gravidarum (22). Pregnancy outcomes in the study group were compared with a historical control of 54 women who had received conventional antiemetic therapy. Oral metoclopramide and hydroxyzine were used after discharge from the hospital. Therapy was started in the study and control groups at mean gestational ages of 9.9 and 11.1 weeks, respectively. The study group appeared to have more severe disease than controls as suggested by a greater mean loss from the prepregnancy weight, 2.07 vs. 0.81 kg (*ns*), and a slightly lower serum potassium level, 3.4 vs. 3.5 mmol/L (*ns*). Compared with controls, the droperidol group had a shorter duration of hospitalization (3.53 vs. 2.82 days, $p = 0.023$), fewer readmissions (38.9% vs. 14.3%, $p = 0.025$), and lower average daily nausea and vomiting scores (both $p < 0.001$). There were no statistical differences ($p > 0.05$) in outcomes (study vs. controls) in terms of spontaneous abortions ($N = 0$ vs. $N = 2$ [4.3%]), elective abortions ($N = 3$ [12.0%] vs. $N = 3$ [6.5%]), Apgar scores at 1, 5, and 10 minutes, age at birth (37.3 vs. 37.9 weeks'), and birth weight (3114 vs. 3347 g) (22). In controls, there was one (2.4%) major malformation of unknown cause, an acardiac fetus in a set of triplets, and one newborn with a genetic defect (Turner syndrome). There was also one unexplained major birth defect (4.4%) in the droperidol group (bilateral hydronephrosis), and two genetic defects (translocation of chromosomes 3 and 7; tyrosinemia) (22).

The Pharmaco-Epidemiological Prescription Database of North Jutland County (Denmark) identified 309 women with singleton pregnancies who filled prescriptions for metoclopramide during a 6-year period (1991–1996) (23). The pregnancy outcomes of this group were compared with 13,327 women who did not receive prescriptions of any kind during pregnancy. The mean birth weights of the metoclopramide and control groups were nearly identical, 3480 vs. 3470 g, respectively. No significant differences were found between the groups in terms of congenital malformations (odds ratio [OR] 1.11, 95% confidence interval [CI] 0.6–2.1), low birth weight (OR 1.79, 95% CI 0.8–3.9), or preterm delivery (OR 1.02, 95% CI 0.6–1.7) (23).

A brief 2000 communication examined the outcome of 126 women who had received metoclopramide for nausea and vomiting of pregnancy during the 1st trimester (24). The pregnancy outcomes of these women, who had called one of five teratogen information centers (one each in Italy and Brazil and three in Israel), were compared with a control group of 126 women who had contacted the centers for information on nonteratogenic and nonembryotoxic drug exposures, matched for age, smoking status, and alcohol use. The pregnancy outcomes were similar between the groups in terms of live births, spontaneous abortions, gestational age at delivery, rate of prematurity, birth weight, fetal distress, and major malformations. Both groups had five infants with major birth defects. In the metoclopramide group, two infants had patent ductus arteriosus, two had ventricular septal defects (VSD), and one had hypospadias. The birth defects in the infants born to the control group were two cases of VSD and one each of bilateral syndactyly of the foot, hypospadias, and an inguinal hernia. The gross motor development (as measured by the Denver Development Scale) of the infants in the two groups at ages 4–15 months was also similar (24).

In a surveillance study of Michigan Medicaid recipients involving 229,101 completed pregnancies conducted between 1985 and 1992, 192 newborns had been exposed to metoclopramide during the 1st trimester (F. Rosa, personal communication, FDA, 1993). Ten (5.2%) major birth defects were observed (8 expected), including (observed/expected) 1/2 cardiovascular defects and 1/1 polydactyly. No anomalies were observed in four other defect categories (oral clefts, spina bifida, limb reduction defects, and hypospadias) for which specific data were available. These data do not support an association between the drug and congenital defects.

A 1997 case report described the signs and symptoms of acute intermittent porphyria in a 29-year-old woman at 13 weeks' gestation (27). The patient presented with abdominal pain, constipation, and vomiting and was treated with IV metoclopramide. Her symptoms worsened with treatment and included weakness of the lower extremities and a severe neuropsychiatric syndrome consisting of both autonomic and neurologic functions. Metoclopramide was stopped and she was treated with high-dose IV glucose and a high-carbohydrate diet. Evaluation of urine and stool porphyrin precursors confirmed the diagnosis. She eventually delivered a normal 2760-g infant at term. The authors concluded that the severe maternal symptoms were brought on by metoclopramide, a porphyrinogenic agent, and starvation resulting from hyperemesis (27).

Several studies have examined the effect of metoclopramide on gastric emptying time during labor for the prevention of Mendelson's syndrome (i.e., pulmonary aspiration of acid gastric contents and resulting chemical pneumonitis and pulmonary edema) (1,3,10–16,28,29). Gastroesophageal reflux was decreased as was the gastric emptying time. The drug was effective in preventing vomiting during anesthesia. No effects were noted on the course of labor or the fetus. Apgar scores and results of neurobehavioral tests did not differ from those of controls (1,3,10,16) nor did newborn heart rates or blood pressures (1).

The effect of metoclopramide on maternal and fetal prolactin secretion during pregnancy and labor has been studied (2,17,18). The drug is a potent stimulator of prolactin release from the anterior pituitary by antagonism of hypothalamic dopaminergic receptors. However, transplacentally acquired metoclopramide did not cause an increased prolactin release from the fetal pituitary nor did maternal prolactin cross the placenta to the fetus (2,17). In two other studies, 10 mg of intravenous metoclopramide administered during labor did not affect the levels of maternal or fetal thyroid-stimulating hormone or thyroid hormones (19), or maternal growth hormone concentrations (30).

M

BREASTFEEDING SUMMARY

Metoclopramide is excreted into breast milk. Because of ion trapping of the drug in the more acidic (as compared with plasma) milk, accumulation occurs with milk:plasma ratios of 1.8–1.9 after steady state conditions are reached (31–33).

Several studies have examined the effect of metoclopramide as a lactation stimulant in women with inadequate or decreased milk production (31–43). One study involved 23 women who had delivered prematurely (mean gestational length, 30.4 weeks) (41). The drug, by stimulating the release of prolactin from the anterior pituitary, was effective in increasing milk production with doses of 20–45 mg/day (9,32–42). Doses of 15 mg/day were not effective (37). In one study, metoclopramide caused a shift in the amino acid composition of milk, suggesting an enhanced rate of transition from colostrum to mature milk (38). No effect on the serum levels of prolactin, thyroid-stimulating hormone, or free thyroxin was observed in nursing infants in a 1985 study of 11 women with lactational insufficiency (39). A 1994 investigation found a positive response in 78% (25 of 32) of treated women, but the increase in daily milk production was inversely correlated with maternal age (43).

The total daily dose that would be consumed by a nursing infant during the maternal use of 30 mg/day has been estimated to be 1–45 mcg/kg (31–33). This is much less than the maximum daily dose of 500 mcg/kg recommended in infants (9) or the 100 mcg/kg/day dosage that has been given to premature infants (44). Metoclopramide was detected in the plasma of one of five infants whose mothers were taking 10 mg 3 times daily (32,33). Adverse effects have been observed in only two infants—both with mild intestinal discomfort (36,37). In one case, the mother was consuming 30 mg/day (36) and in the other, 45 mg/day (37).

Metoclopramide apparently represents a small risk to the nursing infant with maternal doses of 45 mg/day or less. Mild adverse effects only have been reported in two nursing infants. One review stated that the drug should not be used during breastfeeding because of the potential risks to the neonate (45), but there are no published studies to substantiate this caution. The American Academy of Pediatrics classifies metoclopramide as a drug for which the effect on a nursing infant is unknown but may be of concern because it is a dopaminergic blocking agent (46).

References

1. Bylsma-Howell M, Riggs KW, McMorland GH, Rurak DW, Ongley R, McErlane B, Price JDE, Axelson JE. Placental transport of metoclopramide: assessment of maternal and neonatal effects. Can Anaesth Soc J 1983;30:487–92.
2. Arvela P, Jouppila R, Kauppila A, Pakarinen A, Pelkonen O, Tuimala R. Placental transfer and hormonal effects of metoclopramide. Eur J Clin Pharmacol 1983;24:345–8.
3. Cohen SE, Jasson J, Talafre M-L, Chauvelot-Moachon L, Barrier G. Does metoclopramide decrease the volume of gastric contents in patients undergoing cesarean section? Anesthesiology 1984;61:604–7.
4. Lyonnet R, Lucchini G. Metoclopramide in obstetrics. J Med Chir Prat 1967;138:352–5.
5. Sidhu MS, Lean TH. The use of metoclopramide (Maxolon) in hyperemesis gravidarum. Proc Obset Gynaecol Soc Singapore 1970;1:1–4.
6. Guikontes E, Spantideas A, Diakakis J. Ondansetron and hyperemesis gravidarum. Lancet 1992;340:1223.
7. Martynshin MYA, Arkhengel'skii AE. Experience in treating early toxicoses of pregnancy with metoclopramide. Akush Ginekol 1981;57:44–5.
8. Pinder RM, Brogden RN, Sawyer PR, Speight TM, Avery GS. Metoclopramide: a review of its pharmacological properties and clinical use. Drugs 1976;12:81–131.
9. Harrington RA, Hamilton CW, Brogden RN, Linkewich JA, Romankiewicz JA, Heel RC. Metoclopramide: an update review of its pharmacological properties and clinical use. Drugs 1983;25:451–94.
10. McGarry JM. A double-blind comparison of the anti-emetic effect during labour of metoclopramide and perphenazine. Br J Anaesth 1971;43:613–5.
11. Howard FA, Sharp DS. Effect of metoclopramide on gastric emptying during labour. Br Med J 1973;1:446–8.
12. Brock-Utne JG, Dow TGB, Welman S, Dimopoulos GE, Moshal MG. The effect of metoclopramide on the lower oesophageal sphincter in late pregnancy. Anaesth Intensive Care 1978;6:26–9.
13. Hey VMF, Ostick DG. Metoclopramide and the gastro-oesophageal sphincter. Anaesthesia 1978;33:462–5.
14. Feeney JG. Heartburn in pregnancy. Br Med J 1982;284:1138–9.
15. Murphy DF, Nally B, Gardiner J, Unwin A. Effect of metoclopramide on gastric emptying before elective and emergency caesarean section. Br J Anaesth 1984;56:1113–6.

16. Vella L, Francis D, Houlton P, Reynolds F. Comparison of the antiemetics metoclopramide and promethazine in labour. Br Med J 1985;290:1173–5.
17. Messinis IE, Lolis DE, Dalkalitsis N, Kanaris C, Souvatzoglou A. Effect of metoclopramide on maternal and fetal prolactin secretion during labor. Obstet Gynecol 1982;60:686–8.
18. Bohnet HG, Kato K. Prolactin secretion during pregnancy and puerperium: response to metoclopramide and interactions with placental hormones. Obstet Gynecol 1985;65:789–92.
19. Roti E, Robuschi G, Emanuele R, d'Amato L, Gnudi A, Fatone M, Benassi L, Foscolo MS, Gualerzi C, Braverman LE. Failure of metoclopramide to affect thyrotropin concentration in the term human fetus. J Clin Endocrinol Metab 1983;56:1071–5.
20. Milo R, Neuman M, Klein C, Caspi E, Arlazoroff A. Acute intermittent porphyria in pregnancy. Obstet Gynecol 1989;73:450–2.
21. Nageotte MP, Briggs GG, Towers CV, Asrat T. Droperidol and diphenhydramine in the management of hyperemesis gravidarum. Am J Obstet Gynecol 1996;174:1801–6.
22. Turcotte V, Ferreira E, Duperron L. Utilité du dropéridol et de la diphenhydramine dans l'hyperemesis gravidarum. J Soc Obstet Gynaecol Can 2001;23:133–9.
23. Sorensen HT, Nielsen GL, Christensen K, Tage-Jensen U, Ekborn A, Baron J, and the Euromap study group. Birth outcome following maternal use of metoclopramide. Br J Clin Pharmacol 2000;49:264–8.
24. Berkovitch M, Elbirt D, Addis A, Schuler-Faccini L, Ornoy A. Fetal effects of metoclopramide therapy for nausea and vomiting of pregnancy. N Engl J Med 2000;343:445–6.
25. Product information. Reglan. A.H. Robins, 1997.
26. Eisenach JC, Dewan DM. Metoclopramide exaggerates stress-induced tachycardia in pregnant sheep. Anesth Analg 1996;82:607–11.
27. Shenhav S, Gemer O, Sassoon E, Segal S. Acute intermittent porphyria precipitated by hyperemesis and metoclopramide treatment in pregnancy. Acta Obstet Gynecol Scand 1997;76:484–5.
28. Orr DA, Bill KM, Gillon KRW, Wilson CM, Fogarty DJ, Moore J. Effects of omeprazole, with and without metoclopramide, in elective obstetric anaesthesia. Anaesthesia 1993;48:114–9.
29. Stuart JC, Kan AF, Rowbottom SJ, Yau G, Gin T. Acid aspiration prophylaxis for emergency caesarean section. Anaesthesia 1996;51:415–21.
30. Robuschi G, Emanuele R, d'Amato L, Salvi M, Montermini M, Gnudi A, Roti E. Failure of metoclopramide to release GH in pregnant women. Horm Metab Res 1983;15:460–1.
31. Lewis PJ, Devenish C, Kahn C. Controlled trial of metoclopramide in the initiation of breast feeding. Br J Clin Pharmacol 1980;9:217, 219.
32. Pelkonen O, Arvela P, Kauppila A, Koivisto M, Kivinen S, Ylikorkala O. Metoclopramide in breast milk and newborn (abstract). Acta Physiol Scand 1982;(Suppl 502):62.
33. Kauppila A, Arvela P, Koivisto M, Kivinen S, Ylikorkala O, Pelkonen O. Metoclopramide and breast feeding: transfer into milk and the newborn. Eur J Clin Pharmacol 1983;25:819–23.
34. Sousa PLR. Metoclopramide and breast-feeding. Br Med J 1975;1:512.
35. Guzman V, Toscano G, Canales ES, Zarate A. Improvement of defective lactation by using oral metoclopramide. Acta Obstet Gynecol Scand 1979;58:53–5.
36. Kauppila A, Kivinen S, Ylikorkala O. Metoclopramide increases prolactin release and milk secretion in puerperium without stimulating the secretion of thyrotropin and thyroid hormones. J Clin Endocrinol Metab 1981;52:436–9.
37. Kauppila A, Kivinen S, Ylikorkala O. A dose response relation between improved lactation and metoclopramide. Lancet 1981;1:1175–7.
38. de Gezelle H, Ooghe W, Thiery M, Dhont M. Metoclopramide and breast milk. Eur J Obstet Gynecol Reprod Biol 1983;15:31–6.
39. Kauppila A, Anunti P, Kivinen S, Koivisto M, Ruokonen A. Metoclopramide and breast feeding: efficacy and anterior pituitary responses of the mother and the child. Eur J Obstet Gynecol Reprod Biol 1985;19:19–22.
40. Gupta AP, Gupta PK. Metoclopramide as a lactogogue. Clin Pediatr 1985;24:269–72.
41. Ehrenkranz RA, Ackerman BA. Metoclopramide effect on faltering milk production by mothers of premature infants. Pediatrics 1986;78:614–20.
42. Budd SC, Erdman SH, Long DM, Trombley SK, Udall JN Jr. Improved lactation with metoclopramide. Clin Pediatr 1993;32:53–7.
43. Toppare MF, Laleli Y, Senses DA, Kitaper F, Kaya IS, Dilmen U. Metoclopramide for breast milk production. Nutrition Research 1994;14:1019–29.
44. Sankaran K, Yeboah E, Bingham WT, Ninan A. Use of metoclopramide in preterm infants. Dev Pharmacol Ther 1982;5:114–9.
45. Lewis JH, Weingold AB, The Committee on FDA-Related Matters, American College of Gastroenterology. The use of gastrointestinal drugs during pregnancy and lactation. Am J Gastroenterol 1985;80:912–23.
46. Committee on Drugs, American Academy of Pediatrics. The transfer of drugs and other chemicals into human milk. Pediatrics 2001;108:776–89.

METOLAZONE

Diuretic

PREGNANCY RECOMMENDATION: No Human Data—Probably Compatible
BREASTFEEDING RECOMMENDATION: Limited Human Data—Probably Compatible

PREGNANCY SUMMARY

Metolazone is structurally related to the thiazide diuretics. (See also Chlorothiazide.) There is no evidence that thiazide diuretics are teratogenic. However, diuretics are not recommended for the treatment of gestational hypertension–preeclampsia because of the maternal hypovolemia characteristic of this disease.

FETAL RISK SUMMARY

Reproduction studies in mice, rats, and rabbits at doses up to 50 mg/kg/day revealed no evidence of fetal harm (1).

BREASTFEEDING SUMMARY

See Chlorothiazide.

Reference

1. Product information. Mykrox. Medeva Pharmaceuticals, 2000.

METOPROLOL

Sympatholytic (Antihypertensive)

PREGNANCY RECOMMENDATION: Human Data Suggest Risk in 2nd and 3rd Trimesters
BREASTFEEDING RECOMMENDATION: Limited Human Data—Potential Toxicity

PREGNANCY SUMMARY

Although the use of metoprolol for maternal disease does not seem to pose a major risk to the fetus, the long-term effects of in utero exposure to β-blockers have not been studied. Persistent β-blockade has been observed in newborns exposed near delivery to other members of this class (see Acebutolol, Atenolol, and Nadolol). Therefore, newborns exposed in utero to metoprolol should be closely observed during the first 24–48 hours after birth for bradycardia and other symptoms. Some β-blockers may cause intrauterine growth restriction (IUGR) (as may have occurred in some of the cases) and reduced placental weight, especially those lacking intrinsic sympathomimetic activity (ISA) (i.e., partial agonist). Metoprolol does not possess ISA. Treatment beginning early in the 2nd trimester results in the greatest weight reductions, whereas treatment restricted to the 3rd trimester primarily affects only placental weight. Although growth restriction is a serious concern, the benefits of maternal therapy, in some cases, might outweigh the risks to the fetus and must be judged on a case-by-case basis.

FETAL RISK SUMMARY

Metoprolol, a cardioselective β_1-adrenergic blocking agent, has been used during pregnancy for the treatment of maternal hypertension and tachycardia (1–10). Reproductive studies in mice and rats have found no evidence of impaired fertility or teratogenicity (11). In rats, however, increases in fetal loss and decreases in neonatal survival were observed at doses up to 55.5 times the maximum daily human dose (11).

M

The drug readily crosses the placenta, producing approximately equal concentrations of metoprolol in maternal and fetal serum at delivery (1–3). The serum half-lives of metoprolol determined in five women during the 3rd trimester and repeated 3–5 months after delivery were similar (1.3 vs. 1.7 hours, respectively), but peak levels during pregnancy were only 20%–40% of those measured later (4). Neonatal serum levels of metoprolol increase up to fourfold in the first 2–5 hours after birth, then decline rapidly during the next 15 hours (2,3).

No fetal malformations attributable to metoprolol have been reported, but experience during the 1st trimester is limited. Twins, exposed throughout gestation to metoprolol 200 mg/day plus other antihypertensive agents for severe maternal hypertension, were reported to be doing well at 10 months of age (7).

In a surveillance study of Michigan Medicaid recipients involving 229,101 completed pregnancies conducted between 1985 and 1992, 52 newborns had been exposed to metoprolol during the 1st trimester (F. Rosa, personal communication, FDA, 1993). Three (5.8%) major birth defects were observed (two expected). No anomalies were observed in six defect categories (cardiovascular defects, oral clefts, spina bifida, polydactyly, limb reduction defects, and hypospadias) for which specific data were available.

A 1978 study described 101 hypertensive pregnant patients treated with metoprolol alone (57 patients) or combined with hydralazine (44 patients) compared with 97 patients treated with hydralazine alone (1). The duration of pregnancy at the start of antihypertensive treatment was 34.1 weeks (range 13–41 weeks) for the metoprolol group and 32.5 weeks (range 12–40 weeks) for the hydralazine group. The metoprolol group experienced a lower rate of perinatal mortality (2% vs. 8%) and a lower incidence of IUGR (11.7% vs. 16.3%). No signs or symptoms of β-blockade were noted in the fetuses or newborns in this or other studies (1,2,5).

The use of metoprolol in a pregnant patient with pheochromocytoma has been reported (5). High blood pressure had been controlled with prazosin, an α-adrenergic blocking agent, but the onset of maternal tachycardia required the addition of metoprolol during the last few weeks of pregnancy. No adverse effects were observed in the newborn.

The acute effects of metoprolol on maternal hemodynamics have been studied (12). Nine women at a mean gestational age of 36.7 weeks with a diagnosis of gestational hypertension were given a single oral dose of 100 mg of metoprolol. Statistically significant ($p < 0.01$) decreases were observed in maternal heart rate, systolic and diastolic blood pressure, and cardiac output. No significant change was noted in mean blood volume or intervillous blood flow. An improvement was observed in four women for the latter parameter, but a reduction occurred in another four. The intervillous blood flow did not change in the ninth patient.

Cardiac palpitations, accompanied by lightheadedness and dyspnea but without syncope, developed in a previously healthy 33-year-old woman at 10 weeks' gestation (13). A diagnosis of ventricular tachycardia and mitral valve prolapse with mild mitral regurgitation was diagnosed at 22 weeks, and treatment with metoprolol, 50 mg twice daily, was begun. Four weeks later, quinidine was added to the regimen because of recurrent palpitations. Growth restriction was noted during her obstetric care and she eventually gave birth at term to a healthy newborn weighing about 2242 g. Follow-up of the infant was not mentioned (13).

New-onset ventricular tachycardia was diagnosed in seven pregnant women among whom four were treated with metoprolol (250–450 mg/day) throughout the remainder of their pregnancy (14). Metoprolol therapy in a fifth patient did not resolve the arrhythmia and it was discontinued. Treatment was started in the 1st trimester in one, during the 2nd trimester in one, and in the 3rd trimester in two. All four were delivered at term of healthy newborns with birth weights (in grams) (daily metoprolol dose shown in parentheses) of 3380 (250 mg), 3462 (350 mg), 3560 (250 mg), and 2535 (450 mg), respectively (14).

A retrospective study published in 1992 reported the follow-up of 35 very low birth weight (≤1500 g) infants who had been exposed in utero to maternal antihypertensive therapy (15). Nineteen of the infants (mean birth weight 1113 g) had been exposed to β-blockers (metoprolol *N* = 15, propranolol *N* = 4; combination with hydralazine or clonidine in 17 cases) whereas in 16 cases (mean birth weight 1102 g), other antihypertensives (hydralazine alone *N* = 11, hydralazine plus clonidine *N* = 3, hydralazine plus methyldopa *N* = 1, and diuretics *N* = 1) had been used. The metoprolol dose ranged from 100 to 200 mg/day while that of hydralazine varied from 30 to 150 mg/day. The mean duration of therapy was similar in both groups (12 vs. 11 days). Among the 19 infants exposed to β-blockers, 7 died, 4 within 15 days of birth, compared with no deaths in the other group ($p = 0.006$). The authors speculated that the β-blockade might have impaired the infant's adaptation to the postnatal environment by inhibition of the sympathoadrenal system (15).

BREASTFEEDING SUMMARY

Metoprolol is concentrated in breast milk (1,3,16–18). Milk concentrations are approximately 3 times (range 2.0–3.7) those found simultaneously in the maternal serum. No adverse effects have been observed in nursing infants exposed to metoprolol in milk. Based on calculations from a 1984 study, a mother ingesting 200 mg/day of metoprolol would provide only about 225 mcg in 1000 mL of her milk (3). To minimize this exposure even further, one reference suggested waiting 3–4 hours after a dose to breastfeed (18). Although these levels are probably clinically insignificant, nursing infants should be closely observed for signs or symptoms of β-blockade. The long-term effects of exposure to β-blockers from milk have not been studied but warrant evaluation. The American Academy of Pediatrics classifies metoprolol as compatible with breastfeeding (19).

References

1. Sandstrom B. Antihypertensive treatment with the adrenergic beta-receptor blocker metoprolol during pregnancy. Gynecol Invest 1978;9:195–204.
2. Lundborg P, Agren G, Ervik M, Lindeberg S, Sandstrom B. Disposition of metoprolol in the newborn. Br J Clin Pharmacol 1981;12:598–600.
3. Lindeberg S, Sandstrom B, Lundborg P, Regardh CG. Disposition of the adrenergic blocker metoprolol in the late-pregnant woman, the amniotic fluid, the cord blood and the neonate. Acta Obstet Gynecol Scand 1984;118(Suppl):61–4.
4. Hogstedt S, Lindberg B, Rane A. Increased oral clearance of metoprolol in pregnancy. Eur J Clin Pharmacol 1983;24:217–20.
5. Venuto R, Burstein P, Schneider R. Pheochromocytoma: antepartum diagnosis and management with tumor resection in the puerperium. Am J Obstet Gynecol 1984;150:431–2.
6. Robson DJ, Jeeva Ray MV, Storey GAC, Holt DW. Use of amiodarone during pregnancy. Postgrad Med J 1985;61:75–7.
7. Coen G, Cugini P, Gerlini G, Finistauri D, Cinotti GA. Successful treatment of long-lasting severe hypertension with captopril during a twin pregnancy. Nephron 1985;40:498–500.
8. Gallery EDM. Hypertension in pregnant women. Med J Aust 1985;143:23–7.
9. Hogstedt S, Lindeberg S, Axelsson O, Lindmark G, Rane A, Sandstrom B, Lindberg BS. A prospective controlled trial of metoprolol-hydralazine treatment in hypertension during pregnancy. Acta Obstet Gynecol Scand 1985;64:505–10.
10. Frishman WH, Chesner M. Beta-adrenergic blockers in pregnancy. Am Heart J 1988;115:147–52.
11. Product information. Lopressor. CibaGeneva Pharmaceuticals, 1997.
12. Suonio S, Saarikoski S, Tahvanainen K, Paakkonen A, Olkkonen H. Acute effects of dihydralazine mesylate, furosemide, and metoprolol on maternal hemodynamics in pregnancy-induced hypertension. Am J Obstet Gynecol 1985;155:122–5.
13. Braverman AC, Bromley BS, Rutherford JD. New onset ventricular tachycardia during pregnancy. Int J Cardiol 1991;33:409–12.
14. Brodsky M, Doria R, Allen B, Sato D, Thomas G, Sada M. New-onset ventricular tachycardia during pregnancy. Am Heart J 1992;123:933–41.
15. Kaaja R, Hiilesmaa V, Holma K, Jarvenpaa A-L. Maternal antihypertensive therapy with beta-blockers associated with poor outcome in very-low birth-weight infants. Int J Gynecol Obstet 1992;38:195–9.
16. Sandstrom B, Regardh CG. Metoprolol excretion into breast milk. Br J Clin Pharmacol 1980;9:518–9.
17. Liedholm H, Melander A, Bitzen PO, Helm G, Lonnerholm G, Mattiasson I, Nilsson B. Accumulation of atenolol and metoprolol in human breast milk. Eur J Clin Pharmacol 1981;20:229–31.
18. Kulas J, Lunell NO, Rosing U, Steen B, Rane A. Atenolol and metoprolol. A comparison of their excretion into human breast milk. Acta Obstet Scand 1984;118(Suppl):65–9.
19. Committee on Drugs, American Academy of Pediatrics. The transfer of drugs and other chemicals into human milk. Pediatrics 2001;108:776–89.

METRIZAMIDE

[Withdrawn from the market. See 9th edition.]

METRIZOATE

[Withdrawn from the market. See 9th edition.]

METRONIDAZOLE

Anti-infective/Amebicide/Trichomonacide

PREGNANCY RECOMMENDATION: Human Data Suggest Low Risk
BREASTFEEDING RECOMMENDATION: Hold Breastfeeding (Single Dose)
Limited Human Data—Potential Toxicity (Divided Dose)

PREGNANCY SUMMARY

Although some of the available reports have arrived at conflicting conclusions as to the safety of metronidazole in pregnancy, most of the published evidence suggests that the anti-infective does not represent a significant risk of structural defects to the fetus. At present, it is not possible to assess the risk to the fetus from the carcinogenic potential of metronidazole. The answer to the question of transplacental carcinogenic potential of metronidazole has major public health implications, but may never be answered because of the rarity of childhood cancers and the inability to identify potentially confounding environmental factors in older children and adults. The manufacturer considers metronidazole to be contraindicated during the 1st trimester in patients with trichomoniasis or bacterial vaginosis (1). The use of metronidazole for trichomoniasis or vaginosis during the 2nd and 3rd trimesters is acceptable. For other indications, metronidazole can be used during pregnancy if there are no other alternatives with established safety profiles.

FETAL RISK SUMMARY

Metronidazole possesses trichomonacidal and amebicidal activity as well as effectiveness against certain bacteria. The drug crosses the placenta to the fetus throughout gestation with a cord:maternal plasma ratio at term of approximately 1.0 (2–4). The pharmacokinetics of metronidazole in pregnant women has been reported (5,6).

Reproduction studies conducted in mice (at oral doses about 0.1 times the human dose) and in rats (at doses up to 5 times the human dose) revealed no fetal harm. After intraperitoneal administration in mice, however, some fetal deaths were noted (1).

The use of metronidazole in pregnancy is controversial. The drug is mutagenic in bacteria and carcinogenic in rodents, and although these properties have never been shown in humans, concern for these toxicities have led some to advise against the use of metronidazole in pregnancy (7,8). However, no association with human cancer has been proven (8,9).

A 1995 case report described a 32-year-old woman who was treated with metronidazole during the 12th and 13th weeks of pregnancy with 500 mg/day orally plus 500 mg/day intravaginally for 10 days (10). She eventually delivered an apparently normal, 3640-g male infant at term. Fifteen days later, the infant was diagnosed with adrenal neuroblastoma with hepatic metastasis (eventual outcome not mentioned). The authors acknowledged that neuroblastoma was the second most common malignant solid tumor in childhood and that a causal relationship between the tumor and metronidazole in this case could not be established (10).

A retrospective cohort study of childhood cancer and in utero exposure to metronidazole was reported in 1998 (11). The cohort included 328,846 children under 5 years of age who had been born to women (ages 15–44 years) enrolled from 1975 through 1992 in Tennessee Medicaid at any time between the last menstrual period and the date of delivery. Exposure to metronidazole was based on Medicaid pharmacy prescription records. A statewide childhood cancer database was developed to identify study cases. In the cohort, 8.1% were exposed in utero to metronidazole and 91.9% were not exposed. From 952 children younger than 5 years of age in the cancer database, 175 met the criteria for the study (first primary cancer before age 5 years, a Tennessee resident, and seen at a Tennessee hospital at the time of diagnosis). The study was limited to children under the age of 5 years to minimize the loss to out-of-state migration (expected to be no more than 6% (12)). None of the study cases had a history of therapeutic radiation or exposure to chemotherapy before their cancer diagnosis. The cancer type, number of cases, adjusted relative risk (RR), and 95% confidence interval (CI) were, for all cancers: $N = 175$, RR 0.81, 95% CI 0.41–1.59; for leukemia: $N = 42$, no exposed cases; for central nervous system tumors: $N = 30$, RR 1.23, 95% CI 0.29–5.21; for neuroblastoma: $N = 28$, RR 2.60, 95% CI 0.89–7.59; and other cancers: $N = 75$, RR 0.57, 95% CI 0.18–1.82. Although none of the observed relative risks were statistically significant, the authors stated that the increased risk for neuroblastoma needed further evaluation (11).

In a brief comment, other investigators agreed with the conclusions of the above study but expressed concern that the frequent use of medications during pregnancy combined with the rarity of childhood cancer made it difficult to establish a carcinogenic effect (12). In addition, limiting the study to children less than 5 years of age prevented the identification of potential effects on later developing cancers such as Hodgkin's disease, Ewing's sarcomas, and osteosarcoma.

Several studies, individual case reports, and reviews have described the safe use of metronidazole during pregnancy (13–27). Included among these is a 1972 review summarizing 20 years of experience with the drug and involving 1469 pregnant women, 206 of whom were treated during the 1st trimester (27). No association with congenital malformations, abortions, or stillbirths was found. Some investigations, however, found an increased risk when the agent was used early in pregnancy (9,28–30).

In a 1979 report, metronidazole was used in 57 pregnancies including 23 during the 1st trimester (9). Three of the 1st trimester exposures ended in spontaneous abortion (a normal incidence), and in the remaining 20 births, there were 5 congenital anomalies: hydrocele (two), congenital dislocated hip (female twin), metatarsus varus, and mental retardation (both parents mentally slow). Analysis of the data is not possible because of the small numbers and possible involvement of genetic factors (9).

The Collaborative Perinatal Project monitored 50,282 mother–child pairs, 31 of whom had 1st trimester exposure to metronidazole (28). A possible association with malformations was found (RR 2.02) based on defects in four children, but independent confirmation is required.

Two mothers, treated with metronidazole during the 5th–7th weeks of gestation for amebiasis, gave birth to infants with midline facial defects (29). Diiodohydroxyquinoline was also used in one of the pregnancies. One of the infants had holotelencephaly and one had unilateral cleft lip and palate.

A mother treated for trichomoniasis between the 6th and 7th weeks of gestation gave birth to a male infant with a

M

cleft of the hard and soft palate, optic atrophy, a hypoplastic, short philtrum, and a Sydney crease on the left hand (30). The mother was also taking an antiemetic medication (Bendectin) on an "as needed" basis. Chromosomal analysis of the infant was normal. The relationship between metronidazole and the defects is unknown.

As of May 1987, the FDA had received reports of 26 adverse outcomes with metronidazole: spontaneous abortions (*N* = 3), brain defects (*N* = 6), limb defects (*N* = 5), genital defects (*N* = 3), unspecified defects (*N* = 3), and 1 each of craniostenosis, peripheral neuropathy, ventricular septal defect, retinoblastoma, obstructive uropathy, and a chromosomal defect (31). In this same report, the authors, from data obtained from the Michigan Medicaid program between 1980 and 1983, cited 1020 other cases in which metronidazole use in the 1st trimester for treatment of vaginitis was not linked with birth defects. In an additional 63 cases, use of the agent for this indication was linked to a birth defect diagnosis. Based on these data, the estimated RR of a birth defect was 0.92 (95% CI 0.7–1.2). Of the 122 infants with oral clefts, none was exposed to metronidazole. An estimated RR for spontaneous abortion of 1.67 (95% CI 1.4–2.0) was determined from 135 exposures among 4264 spontaneous abortions compared to 1020 exposures among 55,736 deliveries (31).

In a continuation of the study cited immediately above, 229,101 completed pregnancies of Michigan Medicaid recipients were evaluated between 1985 and 1992 (F. Rosa, personal communication, FDA, 1993). Of this group, 2445 newborns had been exposed to metronidazole during the 1st trimester. A total of 100 (4.1%) major birth defects were observed (97 expected). Specific data were available for six defect categories, including (observed/expected) 23/24 cardiovascular defects, 1/1 spina bifida, 4/7 polydactyly, 2/4 limb reduction defects, 7/6 hypospadias, and 8/4 oral clefts. Only with oral clefts is there a suggestion of a possible association, but in view of the outcomes observed between 1980 and 1983, other factors, such as the mother's disease, concurrent drug use, and chance, are probably involved.

Using data from the Tennessee Medicaid program, pregnancy outcomes of women (*N* = 1307) who had filled a prescription for metronidazole between 30 days before and 120 days after the onset of their last normal menstrual period were compared with those of women who had not filled such a prescription (32). The groups were matched for age, race, year of delivery, and hospital. Data were available for 1322 exposed (1318 live births; 4 stillbirths) and 1328 nonexposed (1320 live births; 8 stillbirths) infants. The occurrence of birth defects was similar in the two groups; 96 in the exposed group and 80 in the nonexposed group (adjusted odds ratio [OR] 1.2; 95% CI 0.9–1.6). Similar results were obtained when congenital malformations were analyzed by specific types, including those of the central nervous system, heart, gastrointestinal tract, musculoskeletal system, urogenital system, respiratory tract, chromosomal, and by multiple organ systems. The investigators concluded that the use of metronidazole was not associated with an increased risk for birth defects (32).

A study published in 1995 conducted a meta-analysis of seven studies (from a total of 32 references identified in their search) that met their criteria for assessing the safety of metronidazole use in human pregnancy (33). The criteria required exposure during the 1st trimester and comparison of these outcomes with the outcomes of pregnancies that were not exposed or only exposed during the 3rd trimester. Six of the studies were prospective and one was retrospective. The OR (exposure vs. no exposure during the 1st trimester) for the seven studies was 0.93 (95% CI 0.73–1.18) and for the six prospective studies was 1.02 (95% CI 0.48–2.18). Based on these findings, the investigators concluded that the use of metronidazole during the 1st trimester was not associated with an increased risk of congenital defects (33).

A second meta-analysis, similar in design to the study above, evaluated the risk for birth defects after the use of metronidazole early in pregnancy (34). A total of five studies, one unpublished case–control study and four published cohort studies, met the inclusion criteria. As in the study immediately above, the OR 1.08 (95% CI 0.90–1.29) indicated that exposure to metronidazole during the 1st trimester was not associated with birth defects (34).

A large ethnically homogeneous population-based dataset (Hungarian Case–Control Surveillance of Congenital Abnormalities, 1980–1991) was used in a study published in 1998 to evaluate whether the use of metronidazole in the 1st trimester was associated with congenital anomalies (35). The background rate of congenital malformations in the dataset was 4.0%–4.7% (liveborn, stillborn, and selectively terminated fetuses). Minor abnormalities and congenital abnormality syndromes of known origin were excluded. Among 17,300 cases with birth defects, 665 (3.8%) were treated with metronidazole (oral and IV) in the 2nd to 3rd months of gestation (dating from last menstrual period). In comparison, among 30,663 matched controls, 1041 (3.4%) were treated with metronidazole (oral and IV) during this period of gestation. Using the McNemar analysis of case–control pairs, the only defect with a positive association was cleft lip ± palate (nine cases) (adjusted OR 8.54, 95% CI 1.06–68.86). The investigators concluded that the most likely reasons for the association were recall bias or chance alone, but that a true association could not be ruled out. However, based on the prevalence of isolated cleft lip (with or without cleft palate) in their population and the prevalence of exposure to metronidazole during the 2nd and 3rd months of pregnancy, their analysis suggested that even a true association would only increase the prevalence of the defect from 100 cases/100,000 births to 103 cases/100,000 births. Moreover, the finding was not confirmed when the comparison was made with the total control group (35).

In a second study from the above group, the teratogenic potential of vaginal metronidazole plus miconazole treatment during the 2nd and 3rd months of pregnancy was evaluated using the 1980–1996 dataset of the Hungarian Case–Control Surveillance of Congenital Abnormalities (36). Their analysis included 21 groups of congenital anomalies. They compared 22,843 women who had newborn infants or fetuses with congenital anomalies (cases) with 38,151 pregnant women who had newborns without defects (controls). Vaginal treatment with the drug combination occurred in 2.5% (576) cases and 2.2% (846) controls. The analysis of cases and their matched controls found an association between the drug combination and polysyndactyly (21 cases) with an adjusted prevalence OR 6.0, 95% CI 2.4–15.2. The authors thought that recall bias was unlikely and considered their findings to be a signal of the defect, although they had no plausible biological mechanism (36).

A population-based cohort study on the use of metronidazole during pregnancy from 1991 to 1996 was conducted in Denmark and reported in 1999 (37). An estimated 35,000 pregnancies were used in the risk analysis for the specific outcomes of congenital abnormalities, low birth weight (<2500 g), and preterm birth (<37 weeks). Data on the use of metronidazole were determined from a prescription database and classified as either exposure from 30 days before conception to the end of the 1st trimester (group 1) or during the 2nd and 3rd trimesters (group 2). A total of 138 prescriptions to the agent were obtained by 124 women during the study period. A control group of 13,327 pregnancies was used for comparison. Outcome data were determined independently from exposure information. Based on prevalence rates of congenital anomalies in the exposed (group 1) and control groups of 2.4% and 5.2%, respectively, no increased risk for malformations was found (OR 0.44, 95% CI 0.11–1.81). The two birth defects in group 1 were transposition vasorum with ventricular septum defect and hypertelorism. Preterm birth occurred in 6 of the 124 exposed women (4.8%) and in 793 of 13,327 controls (6.0%) (adjusted OR 0.80, 95% CI 0.35–1.83). After adjustment for maternal age, birth order, gestational age, and smoking, there was no difference in mean birth weight between those exposed and the controls. The investigators acknowledged the major limitations of their study: low statistical power due to the small number of exposed subjects; the inability to control for potentially confounding factors; and the lack of information on spontaneous abortions and fetuses aborted for prenatal diagnosis of malformations. They concluded, however, that their results showed no evidence of major teratogenicity and no indication for the termination of pregnancies because of exposure to metronidazole (37).

Metronidazole has been shown to markedly potentiate the fetotoxicity and teratogenicity of alcohol in mice (38). Human studies of this possibly clinically significant interaction have not been reported.

A 2001 prospective, controlled cohort study evaluated the pregnancy outcomes of 217 women exposed to metronidazole (86.2% exposed in 1st trimester) (39). The women had consulted a Teratogen Information Service concerning their exposure to the drug. A matched control group consisted of 612 women who had called about nonteratogenic exposures. There were no statistical differences between the groups in terms of spontaneous abortions (7.8% vs. 7.2%), stillbirths (0.0% vs. 0.2%), preterm delivery (6.8% vs. 5.7%), or rate of major birth defects (2.6% vs. 2.1%). However, exposed cases had a lower birth weight than controls (3253 vs. 3375 g, $p = 0.004$) (39).

A number of reports have described the use of metronidazole in pregnant women with bacterial vaginosis in attempts to reduce the incidence of preterm births (40–50). A 1994 randomized, double-blind, placebo-controlled study found that two courses of oral metronidazole (400 mg twice daily for 2 days) administered at 24 and 29 weeks' gestation, respectively, were effective in suppressing *Gardnerella vaginalis* for 2–3 months in the majority of women with bacterial vaginosis (40).

A prospective, randomized, double-blind, placebo-controlled study first published in abstract form in 1993 (41) and then in full in 1994 (42) compared a 7-day course of oral metronidazole (750 mg/day) to a 7-day course of placebo in women with bacterial vaginosis and a history of preterm birth (<37 weeks' gestation) in the preceding pregnancy from either idiopathic preterm labor or premature rupture of membranes. The women were enrolled between 13 and 20 weeks' gestation. Compared to the placebo group ($N = 36$), the pregnancy outcomes of the active drug group ($N = 44$) included significantly fewer admissions for preterm labor (27% vs. 78%, $p <0.05$), fewer preterm births (18% vs. 39%, $p <0.05$), fewer newborns with birth weight <2500 g (14% vs. 33%, $p <0.05$), and fewer cases of premature rupture of membranes (5% vs. 33%, $p <0.05$) (42).

Another prospective randomized, double-blind, placebo-controlled study first published in abstract form in 1993 (43) and then in full in 1995 (44) described the effect of a 7-day course of oral metronidazole (750 mg/day) combined with a 14-day course of oral erythromycin base (999 mg/day) in pregnant women at increased risk for preterm delivery (based on a history of spontaneous preterm delivery or prepregnancy body weight less than 50 kg). At enrollment (at a mean 23 weeks' gestation for both groups), 41% of the 433 women in the active drug group had bacterial vaginosis compared with 46% of the 191 women receiving placebo. If a second examination (at a mean 27.6 weeks' gestation for both groups) revealed bacterial vaginosis, a second course of active drugs or placebo was administered. Eight women were lost to follow-up. A total of 110 women (26%) in the active group delivered preterm (<37 weeks) compared with 68 women (36%) in the placebo group ($p = 0.01$). However, the rates of preterm delivery in those without bacterial vaginosis were nearly identical (22% in the active drug group vs. 25% in the placebo group, $p = 0.55$). In contrast, in those with bacterial vaginosis, the rates of preterm delivery were 31% for the active drug group compared with 49% in those receiving placebo, $p = 0.006$. The positive association with anti-infective treatment existed both for women with a history of preterm birth (39% vs. 57%, $p = 0.02$) and prepregnancy body weight less than 50 kg (14% vs. 33%, $p = 0.04$) (44).

A 1997 randomized, placebo-controlled study also found that the beneficial effect of a 2-day course of oral metronidazole (400 mg twice daily) on prolonging pregnancy was restricted to those women with bacterial vaginosis and a previous history of spontaneous preterm birth (45). Metronidazole therapy was started at 24 weeks' gestation and repeated at 29 weeks' if *G. vaginalis* was still present.

Another 1997 randomized, double blind, placebo-controlled study administered a combination of metronidazole and ampicillin to 59 women and placebo to 51 women (46). The subjects in both groups had threatened idiopathic preterm labor and intact membranes. The anti-infective regimen was an 8-day course of metronidazole (500 mg IV every 8 hours for 24 hours, then 400 mg orally every 8 hours for 7 days) and ampicillin (2 g IV every 6 hours for 24 hours, then pivampicillin 500 mg orally every 8 hours for 7 days). The women were enrolled in the study at 26–34 weeks' gestation from six clinics in the Copenhagen area. Treatment with the anti-infectives was associated with prolongation of gestation (47.5 vs. 27 days, $p <0.05$), higher gestational age at birth (37 vs. 34 weeks, $p <0.05$), reduced preterm birth rate (40% vs. 63%, $p <0.05$), and a lower rate of admission to neonatal intensive care unit (40% vs. 63%, $p <0.05$). The incidences of maternal (5% vs. 0%, $p = 0.30$) and neonatal (10% vs. 22%, $p = 0.18$) infectious morbidity, however, were statistically similar between the groups (46). In four other reports, all from the same source, gestational metronidazole treatment of women with asymptomatic bacterial vaginosis, but without a history of previous preterm birth, either did not reduce the risk of preterm birth (47–49) or increased the risk for that outcome (50).

Metronidazole was not effective in preventing preterm delivery among pregnant women with asymptomatic *Trichomonas vaginalis* infection in a 2001 report (51). Women were screened for the infection at 16–23 weeks' gestation and then randomized to either metronidazole (N = 320) or placebo (N = 297). The metronidazole group received two 2-g doses 48 hours apart at randomization and then again at 24–29 weeks'. Preterm delivery (<37 weeks') occurred in 19% of the treated group and about 11% of the controls (51).

BREASTFEEDING SUMMARY

Metronidazole is excreted into breast milk. Following a single 2-g oral dose in three patients, peak milk concentrations in the 50–60 mcg/mL range were measured at 2–4 hours (52). With normal breastfeeding, infants would have received about 25 mg of metronidazole during the next 48 hours. By interrupting feedings for 12 hours, infant exposure to the drug would have been reduced to 9.8 mg, or 3.5 mg if feeding had been stopped for 24 hours (52).

In women treated with divided oral doses of either 600 or 1200 mg/day, the mean milk levels were 5.7 and 14.4 mcg/mL, respectively (53). The milk:plasma ratios in both groups were approximately 1.0. The mean plasma concentrations in the exposed infants were about 20% of the maternal plasma drug level. Eight women treated with metronidazole rectal suppositories, 1 g every 8 hours, produced a mean milk drug level of 10 mcg/mL with maximum concentrations of 25 mcg/mL (54).

One report described diarrhea and secondary lactose intolerance in a breastfed infant whose mother was receiving metronidazole (55). The relationship between the drug and the events is unknown. Except for this one case, no reports of adverse effects in metronidazole-exposed nursing infants have been located. However, because the drug is mutagenic and carcinogenic in some test species (see Fetal Risk Summary), unnecessary exposure to metronidazole should be avoided. However, topical or vaginal use of metronidazole during breastfeeding does not appear to represent a risk to a nursing infant.

A 1988 report analyzed the milk and plasma concentrations of metronidazole and its metabolite (hydroxymetronidazole) in 12 breastfeeding women who had been taking 400 mg 3 times daily for 4 days (56). The mean milk:plasma ratios for the parent drug and metabolite were 0.9 and 0.76, respectively. In seven of the nursing infants, the plasma concentrations for the parent drug and metabolite ranged from 1.27 to 2.41 mcg/mL and 1.1 to 2.4 mcg/mL, respectively. The investigators also monitored 35 other women under treatment with metronidazole while nursing. There were no significant increases in adverse effects in their infants that could be attributed to the drug therapy (56).

If a single, 2-g oral dose of metronidazole is used for trichomoniasis, the American Academy of Pediatrics recommends discontinuing breastfeeding for 12–24 hours to allow excretion of the drug (57).

References

1. Product information. Flagyl. G.D. Searle, 2000.
2. Amon K, Amon I, Huller H. Maternal-fetal passage of metronidazole. In *Advances in Antimicrobial and Antineoplastic Chemotherapy*. Proceedings of the VII International Congress of Chemotherapy, Prague, 1971:113–5.
3. Heisterberg L. Placental transfer of metronidazole in the first trimester of pregnancy. J Perinat Med 1984;12:43–5.
4. Karhunen M. Placental transfer of metronidazole and tinidazole in early human pregnancy after a single infusion. Br J Clin Pharmacol 1984;18: 254–7.
5. Amon I, Amon K, Franke G, Mohr C. Pharmacokinetics of metronidazole in pregnant women. Chemotherapy 1981;27:73–9.
6. Visser AA, Hundt HKL. The pharmacokinetics of a single intravenous dose of metronidazole in pregnant patients. J Antimicrob Chemother 1984;13:279–83.
7. Anonymous. Is Flagyl dangerous? Med Lett Drugs Ther 1975;17:53–4.
8. Finegold SM. Metronidazole. Ann Intern Med 1980;93:585–7.
9. Beard CM, Noller KL, O'Fallon WM, Kurland LT, Dockerty MB. Lack of evidence for cancer due to use of metronidazole. N Engl J Med 1979;301:519–22.
10. Carvajal A, Sanchez A, Hurtarte G. Metronidazole during pregnancy. Int J Gynecol Obstet 1995;48:323–4.
11. Thapa PB, Whitlock JA, Brockman Worrell KG, Gideon P, Mitchel EF Jr, Roberson P, Pais R, Ray WA. Prenatal exposure to metronidazole and risk of childhood cancer. A retrospective cohort study of children younger than 5 years. Cancer 1998;83:1461–8.
12. Berbel-Tornero O, Lopez-Andreu JA, Ferris-Tortajada J. Prenatal exposure to metronidazole and risk of childhood cancer. A retrospective cohort study of children younger than 5 years. Cancer 1999;85:2494–5.
13. Gray MS. Trichomonas vaginalis in pregnancy: the results of metronidazole therapy on the mother and child. J Obstet Gynaecol Br Commonw 1961;68:723–9.
14. Robinson SC, Johnston DW. Observations on vaginal trichomoniasis. II. Treatment with metronidazole. Can Med Assoc J 1961;85:1094–6.
15. Luthra R, Boyd JR. The treatment of trichomoniasis with metronidazole. Am J Obstet Gynecol 1962;83:1288–93.
16. Schram M, Kleinman H. Use of metronidazole in the treatment of trichomoniasis. Am J Obstet Gynecol 1962;83:1284–7.
17. Andrews MC, Andrews WC. Systemic treatment of trichomonas vaginitis. South Med J 1963;56:1214–8.
18. Zacharias LF, Salzer RB, Gunn JC, Dierksheide EB. Trichomoniasis and metronidazole. Am J Obstet Gynecol 1963;86:748–52.
19. Kotcher E, Frick CA, Giesel LO, Jr. The effect of metronidazole on vaginal microbiology and maternal and neonatal hematology. Am J Obstet Gynecol 1964;88:184–9.
20. Scott-Gray M. Metronidazole in obstetric practice. J Obstet Gynaecol Br Commonw 1964;71:82–5.
21. Perl G. Metronidazole treatment of trichomoniasis in pregnancy. Obstet Gynecol 1965;25:273–6.
22. Peterson WF, Stauch JE, Ryder CD. Metronidazole in pregnancy. Am J Obstet Gynecol 1966;94:343–9.
23. Robinson SC, Mirchandani G. Trichomonas vaginalis. V. Further observations on metronidazole (Flagyl) (including infant follow-up). Am J Obstet Gynecol 1965;93:502–5.
24. Mitchell RW, Teare AJ. Amoebic liver abscess in pregnancy. Case reports. Br J Obstet Gynaecol 1984;91:393–5.
25. Morgan I. Metronidazole treatment in pregnancy. Int J Gynaecol Obstet 1978;15:501–2.
26. Sands RX. Pregnancy, trichomoniasis, and metronidazole. Am J Obstet Gynecol 1966;94:350–3.
27. Berget A, Weber T. Metronidazole and pregnancy. Ugeskr Laeger 1972;134:2085–9. As cited in Shepard TH. *Catalog of Teratogenic Agents*. 6th ed. Baltimore, MD: Johns Hopkins University Press, 1989:426.
28. Heinonen OP, Slone D, Shapiro S. *Birth Defects and Drugs in Pregnancy*. Littleton, MA: Publishing Sciences Group, 1977:298, 299, 302.
29. Cantu JM, Garcia-Cruz D. Midline facial defect as a teratogenic effect of metronidazole. Birth Defects 1982;18:85–8.
30. Greenberg F. Possible metronidazole teratogenicity and clefting. Am J Med Genet 1985;22:825.

M

31. Rosa FW, Baum C, Shaw M. Pregnancy outcomes after first-trimester vaginitis drug therapy. Obstet Gynecol 1987;69:751–5.
32. Piper JM, Mitchel EF, Ray WA. Prenatal use of metronidazole and birth defects: no association. Obstet Gynecol 1993;82:348–52.
33. Burtin P, Taddio A, Ariburnu O, Einarson TR, Koren G. Safety of metronidazole in pregnancy: a meta-analysis. Am J Obstet Gynecol 1995;172:525–9.
34. Caro-Paton T, Carvajal A, Martin de Diego I, Martin-Arias LH, Alvarez Requejo A, Rodriguez Pinilla E. Is metronidazole teratogenic? A meta-analysis. Br J Clin Pharmacol 1997;44:179–82.
35. Czeizel AE, Rockenbauer M. A population based case-control teratologic study of oral metronidazole treatment during pregnancy. Br J Obstet Gynaecol 1998;105:322–7.
36. Kazy Z, Puho E, Czeizel AE. The possible association between the combination of vaginal metronidazole and miconazole treatment and poly-syndactyly population-based case-control teratologic study. Reprod Toxicol 2005;20:89–94.
37. Sorensen HT, Larsen H, Jensen ES, Thulstrup AM, Schonheyder HC, Nielsen GL, Czeizel A, and the EUROMAP Study Group. Safety of metronidazole during pregnancy: a cohort study of risk of congenital abnormalities, preterm delivery and low birth weight in 124 women. J Antimicrob Chemother 1999;44:854–5.
38. Damjanov I. Metronidazole and alcohol in pregnancy. JAMA 1986;256:472.
39. Diav-Citrin O, Shechtman S, Gotteiner T, Arnon J, Ornoy A. Pregnancy outcome after gestational exposure to metronidazole: a prospective controlled cohort study. Teratology 2001;63:186–92.
40. McDonald HM, O'Loughlin JA, Vigneswaran R, Jolley PT, McDonald PJ. Bacterial vaginosis in pregnancy and efficacy of short-course oral metronidazole treatment: a randomized controlled trial. Obstet Gynecol 1994;84:343–8.
41. Morales WJ, Schorr S, Albritton J. Effect of metronidazole in patients with history of preterm birth and bacterial vaginosis: a placebo control double blind study (abstract). Am J Obstet Gynecol 1993;168:377.
42. Morales WJ, Schorr S, Albritton J. Effect of metronidazole in patients with preterm birth in preceding pregnancy and bacterial vaginosis: a placebo-controlled, double-blind study. Am J Obstet Gynecol 1994;171:345–9.
43. Hauth J, Goldenberg R, Andrews W, Copper R, Schmid T. Efficacy of metronidazole plus erythromycin to decrease bacterial vaginosis and other markers of altered vaginal flora (abstract). Am J Obstet Gynecol 1993;168:421.
44. Hauth JC, Goldenberg RL, Andrews WW, DuBard MB, Copper RL. Reduced incidence of preterm delivery with metronidazole and erythromycin in women with bacterial vaginosis. N Engl J Med 1995;333:1732–6.
45. McDonald HM, O'Loughlin JA, Vigneswaran R, Jolley PT, Harvey JA, Bof A, McDonald PJ. Impact of metronidazole therapy on preterm birth in women with bacterial vaginosis flora (Gardnerella vaginalis): a randomized, placebo controlled trial. Br J Obstet Gynaecol 1997;104:1391–7.
46. Svare J, Langhoff-Roos J, Andersen LF, Kryger-Baggesen N, Borch-Christensen H, Heisterberg L, Kristensen J. Ampicillin-metronidazole treatment in idiopathic preterm labour: a randomized controlled multicentre trial. Br J Obstet Gynaecol 1997;104:892–7.
47. Klebanoff M, Carey JC, for the NICHD MFMU Network, Bethesda, MD. Metronidazole did not prevent preterm birth in asymptomatic women with bacterial vaginosis (abstract). Am J Obstet Gynecol 1999;180:S2.
48. Hauth JC, for the NICHD MFMU Network, Bethesda, MD. Response of the three components of a vaginal gram stain score to metronidazole treatment and in relation to preterm birth (abstract). Am J Obstet Gynecol 2000;182:S56.
49. Carey J, Klebanoff MA, Hauth JC, Hillier SL, Thom EA, Ernest JM, Heine RP, Nugent RP, Fischer ML, Leveno KJ, Wapner R, Varner M, and the National Institute of Child Health and Human Development Network of Maternal-Fetal Medicine Units. Metronidazole to prevent preterm delivery in pregnant women with asymptomatic bacterial vaginosis. N Engl J Med 2000;342:534–40.
50. Carey JC, Klebanoff M, for the NICHD MFMU Network, Bethesda MD. Metronidazole treatment increased the risk of preterm birth in asymptomatic women with trichomonas (abstract). Am J Obstet Gynecol 2000;182:Ss13.
51. Klebanoff MA, Carey JC, Hauth JC, Hillier SL, Nugent RP, Thom EA, Ernest JM, Heine RP, Wapner RJ, Trout W, Moawad A, Leveno KJ, and the National Institute of Child Health and Human Development Network of Maternal-Fetal Medicine Units. Failure of metronidazole to prevent preterm delivery among pregnant women with asymptomatic *Trichomonas vaginalis* infection. N Engl J Med 2001;345:487–93.
52. Erickson SH, Oppenheim GL, Smith GH. Metronidazole in breast milk. Obstet Gynecol 1981;57:48–50.
53. Heisterberg L, Branebjerg PE. Blood and milk concentrations of metronidazole in mothers and infants. J Perinat Med 1983;11:114–20.
54. Moore B, Collier J. Drugs and breast-feeding. Br Med J 1979;2:211.
55. Clements CJ. Metronidazole and breast feeding. NZ Med J 1980;92:329.
56. Passmore CM, McElnay JC, Rainey EA, D'Arcy PF. Metronidazole excretion in human milk and its effect on the suckling neonate. Br J Clin Pharmacol 1988;26:45–51.
57. Committee on Drugs, American Academy of Pediatrics. The transfer of drugs and other chemicals into human milk. Pediatrics 2001;108:776–89.

M

METYROSINE

Antihypertensive

PREGNANCY RECOMMENDATION: Limited Human Data—No Relevant Animal Data
BREASTFEEDING RECOMMENDATION: No Human Data—Potential Toxicity

PREGNANCY SUMMARY

Metyrosine, an enzyme inhibitor, is used for preoperative preparation in patients with pheochromocytoma management when surgery is contraindicated, or as chronic treatment of malignant pheochromocytoma. Because these indications are relatively rare in pregnancy, the human pregnancy experience is very limited and there are no animal reproduction data. However, if required, the drug should not be withheld because of pregnancy.

FETAL RISK SUMMARY

Metyrosine inhibits tyrosine hydroxylase, the enzyme that catalyzes the conversion of tyrosine to dihydroxyphenylalanine, the first transformation in catecholamine biosynthesis (1).

No reproduction studies in animals have been located. The molecular weight of the compound (195) is low enough that transfer to the fetus should be expected.

A case report published in 1986 described the pregnancy of a 24-year-old woman at 30 weeks' gestation who was treated for recurrent pheochromocytoma with a combination of metyrosine, prazosin (α_1-adrenergic blocker), and timolol (β-adrenergic blocker) (2). Hypertension had been noted at her first prenatal visit at 12 weeks' gestation. Because of declines in fetal breathing, body movements, and amniotic fluid volume that began 2 weeks after the start of therapy, a cesarean section was conducted at 33 weeks'. The 1450-g female infant had Apgar scores of 3 and 5 at 1 and 5 minutes, respectively. Mild metabolic acidosis was found on analysis of umbilical cord blood gases. Multiple infarcts were noted in the placenta but no evidence of metastatic tumor. The growth-restricted infant did well and was discharged home on day 53 of life (2).

BREASTFEEDING SUMMARY

No reports describing the use of metyrosine during human lactation have been located. The molecular weight (195) is low enough that excretion into breast milk probably occurs. The effects of this exposure on a nursing infant are unknown.

References

1. Product information. Demser. Merck, 2001.
2. Devoe LD, O'Dell BE, Castillo RA, Hadi HA, Searle N. Metastatic pheochromocytoma in pregnancy and fetal biophysical assessment after maternal administration of alpha-adrenergic, beta-adrenergic, and dopamine antagonists. Obstet Gynecol 1986;68:15S–8S.

MEXILETINE

Antiarrhythmic

PREGNANCY RECOMMENDATION: Limited Human Data—Animal Data Suggest Low Risk
BREASTFEEDING RECOMMENDATION: Limited Human Data—Probably Compatible

PREGNANCY SUMMARY

Based on the very limited published information in humans, mexiletine does not appear to present a significant risk to the fetus. However, three reviews on the use of cardiovascular drugs during pregnancy caution that too few data are available to assess the safety of this agent during pregnancy (1–3).

FETAL RISK SUMMARY

Mexiletine is a local anesthetic, orally active, antiarrhythmic agent structurally similar to lidocaine. It is indicated for the treatment of documented ventricular arrhythmias, such as sustained ventricular tachycardia. The drug is metabolized to inactive metabolites. Depending on hepatic or renal function, the elimination half-life is in the range of about 13–25 hours (6).

The drug is not teratogenic in pregnant mice, rats, and rabbits given doses up to and including maternal toxicity (4–6). Human pregnancy experience with mexiletine is limited to three women, one treated throughout gestation, one starting during the 14th week, and one at 32 weeks (7–9). No adverse effects attributable to mexiletine were mentioned in these reports.

A healthy 2600-g male infant was delivered at 39 weeks' gestation (Apgar scores 9 and 10 at 1 and 5 minutes, respectively) to a 26-year-old primigravida woman who had been treated throughout her pregnancy with mexiletine (200 mg 3 times daily) and atenolol (50 mg/day) for ventricular tachycardia with multifocal ectopic beats (7). A serum mexiletine level obtained from the infant 9 hours after birth was 0.4 mcg/mL (normal therapeutic range 0.75–2.0 mcg/mL). Heart rates during a normal newborn course were 120–160 beats/minute (bpm). Postpartum, the mother continued both mexiletine and atenolol. The infant was fed breast milk only, and by 17 days of age, his weight had decreased to 2155 g. The weight loss was attributed to failure to feed and was corrected with maternal education and formula supplementation. Breastfeeding was halted at 3 months of age. Gastroesophageal reflux, presenting with seizure-like episodes but with a normal neurologic examination and electroencephalogram, was diagnosed at 8 months of age. The condition responded to corrective measures, and growth and development were appropriate at 10 months of age (7).

A 1981 report described the treatment of a 30-year-old woman with cardiac palpitations with mexiletine (600 mg/day) and propranolol (60 mg/day) starting at approximately 14 weeks' gestation (8). A healthy infant (birth weight and sex not specified) was delivered 5 months later.

A 34-year-old woman was treated at 32 weeks' gestation with a combination of mexiletine 200 mg 3 times daily and propranolol 40 mg 3 times daily for paroxysmal ventricular tachycardia (9). A normal male infant (birth weight not given) was delivered by spontaneous vaginal birth at 39 weeks' gestation. Bradycardia, most likely as a result of propranolol, was noted in the infant during the first 6 hours after birth. The heart rate was 90 bpm, before increasing to a normal rate of 120 bpm. An electrocardiogram was normal. The cord blood and maternal serum mexiletine concentrations at birth were both 0.3 mcg/mL.

A 27-year-old woman was treated with mexiletine during pregnancy (10). Her initial dose was 100 mg 3 times daily but her symptoms required higher doses as her pregnancy progressed, eventually requiring 200 mg every 4 hours. At about 38 weeks', a repeat cesarean section was performed to deliver a 3750-g male infant with Apgar scores of 4 and 9 at 1 and 5 minutes, respectively. After 5 minutes, the infant's extremities were still blue. The low 1-minute Apgar was explained by the 9-minute general anesthesia induction to delivery time. The infant was large for gestational age and had hypoglycemia. The mother had no history of diabetes and there was no glucosuria noted during pregnancy. At delivery, maternal and fetal cord blood mexiletine concentrations were 0.6 and 0.4 mcg/mL (therapeutic concentrations are 0.7–2.0 mcg/mL), respectively. At 2 years of life, the child was developing normally (10).

A 1990 case report described the postoperative use of mexiletine (200 mg 3 times a day) in a 27-year-old woman who had undergone an aortic valve replacement under general anesthesia at 29 weeks' gestation (11). A normal 2510-g female infant was born by cesarean section at 28 weeks' with Apgar scores of 8 and 9 at 1 and 5 minutes, respectively. The postoperative course after delivery was uneventful (11).

BREASTFEEDING SUMMARY

Mexiletine is excreted into breast milk in concentrations exceeding those in the maternal serum (8,9). Three cases have been reported in which a nursing infant was exposed to the drug via the milk with drug levels determined in two of these cases. All three infants had been exposed to mexiletine in utero, and no adverse effects attributable to the drug were noted.

Milk and serum mexiletine concentrations in a woman described above, who was taking 600 mg/day in divided doses, were 0.6 and 0.3 mcg/mL, respectively, 2 days postpartum, and 0.8 and 0.7 mcg/mL, respectively, 6 weeks after delivery (9). These levels represented milk:plasma ratios of 2.0 and 1.1, respectively. Mexiletine was not detected in serum samples from the breastfed infant at either sampling time, nor were adverse effects observed in the infant. A second report, appearing 1 year later, described the excretion of the antiarrhythmic agent into breast milk of a woman also taking 600 mg/day in divided doses (8). Again, no adverse effects were noted in the breastfed infant. Twelve paired milk and serum levels, collected from the mother between the 2nd and 5th postpartum days, yielded peak concentrations of 0.959 mcg/mL in the milk compared with 0.724 mcg/mL in the serum, a ratio of 1.32 (mean ratio 1.45, range 0.78–1.89) (8).

Failure to feed was observed in a wholly breastfed infant whose mother was taking mexiletine (600 mg/day) and atenolol (50 mg/day) (7). The infant's weight dropped from 2600 g at birth to 2155 g at 17 days of age. An acceptable growth curve was obtained with maternal education and formula supplementation for the next 2.5 months, after which breastfeeding was stopped (7).

The American Academy of Pediatrics classifies mexiletine as compatible with breastfeeding (12).

References

1. Tamari I, Eldar M, Rabinowitz B, Neufeld HN. Medical treatment of cardiovascular disorders during pregnancy. Am Heart J 1982;104:1357–63.
2. Rotmensch HH, Rotmensch S, Elkayam U. Management of cardiac arrhythmias during pregnancy. Current concepts. Drugs 1987;33:623–33.
3. Brodsky M, Doria R, Allen B, Sato D, Thomas G, Sada M. New-onset ventricular tachycardia during pregnancy. Am Heart J 1992;123:933–41.
4. Matsuo A, Kast A, Tsunenari Y. Reproduction studies of mexiletine hydrochloride by oral administration. Iyakuhin Kenkyu 1983;14:527–49. As cited in Shepard TH. *Catalog of Teratogenic Agents*. 6th ed. Baltimore, MD: Johns Hopkins University Press, 1989:427.
5. Nishimura M, Kast A, Tsunenari Y. Reproduction studies of mexiletine hydrochloride by intravenous administration. Iyakuhin Kenkyu 1983;14:550–70. As cited in Shepard TH. *Catalog of Teratogenic Agents*. 6th ed. Baltimore, MD: Johns Hopkins University Press, 1989:427.
6. Product information. Mexiletine. Watson Laboratories, 2006.
7. Lownes HE, Ives TJ. Mexiletine use in pregnancy and lactation. Am J Obstet Gynecol 1987;157:446–7.
8. Lewis AM, Patel L, Johnston A, Turner P. Mexiletine in human blood and breast milk. Postgrad Med J 1981;57:546–7.
9. Timmis AD, Jackson G, Holt DW. Mexiletine for control of ventricular dysrhythmias in pregnancy. Lancet 1980;2:647–8.
10. Gregg AR, Tomich PG. Mexilitene use in pregnancy. J Perinatol 1988 Winter;8:33–5.
11. Ben-Ami M, Battino S, Rosenfeld T, Marin G, Shalev E. Aortic valve replacement during pregnancy—a case report and review of the literature. Acta Obstet Gynecol Scand 1990;69:651–3.
12. Committee on Drugs, American Academy of Pediatrics. The transfer of drugs and other chemicals into human milk. Pediatrics 2001;108:776–89.

MICAFUNGIN

Antifungal

PREGNANCY RECOMMENDATION: No Human Data—Animal Data Suggest Moderate Risk
BREASTFEEDING RECOMMENDATION: No Human Data—Probably Compatible

PREGNANCY SUMMARY

No reports describing the use of micafungin in human pregnancy have been located. The single animal species studied for developmental toxicity suggests moderate risk. However, the absence of pregnancy experience prevents an assessment of the risk in human embryos and fetuses. Although animal data do not always predict human risk, the safest course is to avoid micafungin in the 1st trimester.

FETAL RISK SUMMARY

Micafungin is a semisynthetic lipopeptide (echinocandin) hydrophilic antifungal agent derived from *Coleophoma empetri* F-11899 that is administered by IV infusion. It is in the same antifungal class as caspofungin. Micafungin is indicated for the treatment of patients with esophageal candidiasis and for the prophylaxis of *Candida* infections in patients undergoing hematopoietic stem cell transplantation. The mean elimination half-life ranges from 14 to 17 hours. Micafungin is highly bound to plasma proteins (>99%), mainly to albumin. At therapeutic concentrations, it does not competitively displace bilirubin binding from albumin. The antifungal agent undergoes partial metabolism before excretion in the feces (primary route) and urine (1).

Reproduction studies have been conducted in rabbits. During organogenesis, an IV dose equivalent to about 4 times the recommended human dose based on BSA (RHD) resulted in visceral abnormalities and abortions. The visceral abnormalities observed included abnormal lobation of the lung, levocardia, retrocaval ureter, anomalous right subclavian artery, and dilatation of the ureter (1).

Micafungin was not mutagenic or clastogenic in a number of assays. In male rats, IV dosing at 0.6 times the RHD over 9 weeks resulted in vacuolation of the epididymal ductal epithelial cells. Doses about twice the RHD resulted in higher epididymis weights and reduced numbers of sperm cells. In a 39-week study in dogs, doses about 2 and 7 times the RHD resulted in seminiferous tubular atrophy and decreased sperm in the epididymis, respectively. However, fertility was not impaired in these species (1).

It is not known if micafungin crosses the human placenta. The high molecular weight (about 1292 for the sodium salt), low lipid solubility, and very high protein binding should limit transfer to the embryo–fetus.

BREASTFEEDING SUMMARY

No reports describing the use of micafungin during human lactation have been located. The high molecular weight (about 1292 for the sodium salt), low lipid solubility, and very high protein binding suggest that excretion into breast milk will be limited. The antifungal agent is given as an IV infusion and this may imply that the oral bioavailability is low. Although the effect of exposure to micafungin in breast milk on a nursing infant is unknown, the risk appears to be low, if it exists at all.

Reference

1. Product information. Mycamine. Astellas Pharma US, 2006.

MICONAZOLE

Antifungal

PREGNANCY RECOMMENDATION: Compatible (Topical)
BREASTFEEDING RECOMMENDATION: No Human Data—Probably Compatible

PREGNANCY SUMMARY

Miconazole is normally used as a topical antifungal agent. Small amounts are absorbed from the vagina (1). Use in pregnant patients with vulvovaginal candidiasis (moniliasis) has not been associated with an increase in congenital malformations (1–7). Effects following IV use are unknown. However, one study did find a significant increase in the risk of spontaneous abortions (SABs) with 1st trimester vaginitis treatment (8). A later study speculated that this effect might have been due to inhibition of the critical enzyme aromatase (9). Until there are data on this potential association, the best course is to avoid the use of miconazole for vaginitis treatment in the 1st trimester or the application of the antifungal to large areas of skin at any time in pregnancy.

M

FETAL RISK SUMMARY

Miconazole is in the same antifungal class of imidazole derivatives as butoconazole, clotrimazole, econazole, ketoconazole, oxiconazole, sertaconazole, sulconazole, and tioconazole.

In data obtained from the Michigan Medicaid program between 1980 and 1983, a total of 2092 women were exposed to miconazole during the 1st trimester from a total sample of 97,775 deliveries not linked to a birth defect diagnosis (8). Of 6564 deliveries linked to such a diagnosis, miconazole was used in 144 cases. The estimated relative risk for birth defects from these data was 1.02 (95% confidence interval [CI] 0.9–1.2). An estimated relative risk for SABs of 1.38 (95% CI 1.2–1.5) was calculated based on 250 miconazole exposures among 4264 abortions compared with 2236 1st trimester exposures among 55,736 deliveries. No association was found between miconazole use and oral clefts, spina bifida, or cardiovascular defects. Although the relative risks for total birth defects or the three specific defects were not increased, the authors could not exclude the possibility of an association with other specific defects (8).

In an extension of the above investigation, data were obtained for 229,101 completed pregnancies between 1985 and 1992, in which 7266 newborns had been exposed to miconazole administered vaginally during the 1st trimester (F. Rosa, personal communication, FDA, 1993). A total of 304 (4.2%) major birth defects were observed (273 expected). Specific data were available for six defect categories, including (observed/expected) 77/73 cardiovascular defects, 14/12 oral clefts, 3/4 spina bifida, 22/21 polydactyly, 12/12 limb reduction defects, and 20/17 hypospadias. These data do not support an association between the drug and congenital defects.

A 2002 study evaluated azole antifungals commonly used in pregnancy for their potential to inhibit placental aromatase, an enzyme that is critical for the production of estrogen and for the maintenance of pregnancy (9). The authors speculated that the embryotoxicity observed in animals and humans (see also Clotrimazole and Sulconazole) might be explained by inhibition of placental aromatase. They found that the most potent inhibitors of aromatase were (shown in order of decreasing potency) econazole, bifonazole (not available in the United States), sulconazole, clotrimazole, and miconazole. However, an earlier study reported a pregnancy that was maintained even when there was severe fetal and placental aromatase deficiency (<0.3% of that of controls) caused by a rare genetic defect (10). In this case, both the fetus and mother were virilized because of diminished conversion of androgens to estrogen. Because the pregnancy was maintained and because of the virilization, the case suggested that the main function of placental aromatase was to protect the mother and fetus from exposure to adrenal androgens (10).

A 2005 report evaluated the teratogenic potential of vaginal metronidazole + miconazole treatment during the 2nd and 3rd months of pregnancy using the population-based dataset of the Hungarian Case–Control Surveillance of Congenital Abnormalities, 1980–1996 (11). Their analysis included 21 groups of congenital anomalies. They compared 22,843 women who had newborn infants or fetuses with congenital anomalies (cases) with 38,151 pregnant women who had newborns without defects (controls). Vaginal treatment with the drug combination occurred in 2.5% (576) cases and 2.2% (846) controls. The analysis of cases and their matched controls found an association between the drug combination and poly/syndactyly (21 cases) with an adjusted prevalence odds ratio of 6.0, 95% CI 2.4–15.2. The authors thought that recall bias was unlikely and considered their findings to be a signal, although they had no plausible biological mechanism (11).

BREASTFEEDING SUMMARY

No reports describing the use of miconazole during human lactation have been located. No risk for a nursing infant is expected if the mother is applying the agent topically.

References

1. Product information. Monistat. Ortho Pharmaceutical, 1990.
2. Culbertson C. Monistat: a new fungicide for treatment of vulvovaginal candidiasis. Am J Obstet Gynecol 1974;120:973–6.
3. Wade A, ed. *Martindate. The Extra Pharmacopoeia*. 27th ed. London: Pharmaceutical Press, 1977:648.
4. Davis JE, Frudenfeld JH, Goddard JL. Comparative evaluation of Monistat and Mycostatin in the treatment of vulvovaginal candidiasis. Obstet Gynecol 1974;44:403–6.
5. Wallenburg HCS, Wladimiroff JW. Recurrence of vulvovaginal candidosis during pregnancy. Comparison of miconazole vs nystatin treatment. Obstet Gynecol 1976;48:491–4.
6. McNellis D, McLeod M, Lawson J, Pasquale SA. Treatment of vulvovaginal candidiasis in pregnancy: a comparative study. Obstet Gynecol 1977;50:674–8.
7. Weisberg M. Treatment of vaginal candidiasis in pregnant women. Clin Ther 1986;8:563–7.
8. Rosa FW, Baum C, Shaw M. Pregnancy outcomes after first-trimester vaginitis drug therapy. Obstet Gynecol 1987;69:751–5.
9. Kragie L, Turner SD, Patten CJ, Crespi CL, Stresser DM. Assessing pregnancy risks of azole antifungals using a high throughput aromatase inhibition assay. Endocr Res 2002;28:129–40.
10. Harada N. Genetic analysis of human placental aromatase deficiency. J Steroid Biochem Mol Biol 1993;44:331–40.
11. Kazy Z, Puho E, Czeizel AE. The possible association between the combination of vaginal metronidazole and miconazole treatment and poly-syndactyly population-based case-control teratologic study. Reprod Toxicol 2005;20:89–94.

MIDAZOLAM

Sedative

PREGNANCY RECOMMENDATION: Limited Human Data—Animal Data Suggest Low Risk
BREASTFEEDING RECOMMENDATION: Compatible*
*Potential Toxicity If Combined with Other CNS Depressants

M

PREGNANCY SUMMARY

Midazolam is a short-acting benzodiazepine used for anesthetic induction. No reports have been located that describe the use of midazolam in humans during the 1st or 2nd trimesters. Use immediately near birth has resulted in adverse neonatal neurobehavior.

FETAL RISK SUMMARY

Reproduction studies in rats and rabbits at 10 and 5 times the human dose, respectively, found no evidence of teratogenicity in either species or impairment of fertility in rats (1).

Midazolam crosses the human placenta, but this transfer, at least after oral and IM use, appears to be slower than that experienced with other benzodiazepines, such as diazepam, oxazepam, or lorazepam (2). In 13 patients given 15 mg of midazolam orally a mean of 11.4 hours (range 10.5–12.4 hours) before cesarean section, only 1 had measurable levels of the drug at the time of surgery. Maternal venous level was 12 ng/mL and cord venous level was 7 ng/mL. No patient had detectable levels of the drug in the amniotic fluid. A second group of patients (N = 11) was administered 15 mg of midazolam orally a mean of 34.3 minutes (15–60 minutes) before cesarean section. The mean serum concentrations in maternal venous, umbilical venous, and umbilical arterial blood were 12.7, 8.4, and 5.7 ng/mL, respectively. The cord venous:maternal venous and cord arterial:maternal venous ratios were 0.74 and 0.45, respectively. Six patients in a third group were administered midazolam, 0.05 mg/kg IM, 18–45 minutes (mean 30.5 minutes) before cesarean section. Drug levels from the same sampling sites and ratios obtained in the second group were measured in this group, with results of 40.0, 21.7, and 12.8 ng/mL, respectively, and 0.56 and 0.32, respectively. None of the 1- and 5-minute Apgar scores of the 30 infants was less than 7, and no adverse effects attributable to midazolam were observed in the newborns (2).

The placental transfer of midazolam and its metabolite, α-hydroxymidazolam, was described in a 1989 reference (3). (See reference 7 for the clinical and physiologic condition of the newborns.) Twenty women were given 0.03 mg/kg of midazolam IV for anesthesia induction before cesarean section. The mean concentrations of midazolam in the mothers' serum and cord blood were 339 and 318 ng/mL (ratio 0.66), respectively. Similar measurements of the metabolite produced values of 22 and 5 (ratio 0.28), respectively. The elimination half-life of midazolam in the newborn infants was 6.3 hours (3).

Plasma levels of midazolam were measured at frequent intervals up to 2 hours after a 5-mg IV dose administered to two groups of pregnant patients in a study published in 1985 (4). Levels were significantly higher in 12 patients in early labor than in 8 women undergoing elective cesarean section. No reason was given for the significant difference. Data on the exposed newborns were not given.

Midazolam, 0.2 mg/kg (*N* = 26), or thiopental, 3.5 mg/kg (*N* = 26), was combined with succinylcholine for rapid-sequence IV induction before cesarean section in a study examining the effects of these agents on the newborn (5). Five of the newborns exposed to midazolam required tracheal intubation compared with one in the thiopental group, a significant difference ($p < 0.05$). The authors concluded that thiopental was superior to midazolam for this procedure.

A 1989 study compared the effects of midazolam 0.3 mg/kg (*N* = 20) with thiopental 4 mg/kg (*N* = 20) in mothers undergoing induction of anesthesia before cesarean section (6). The only difference found between the groups was a significantly higher (mean 7.9 mmHg) diastolic blood pressure in the midazolam group during, but not after, induction. Characteristics of the newborns from the midazolam and thiopental groups (both *N* = 19) were compared in the second part of this study (7). Oxygen via face mask was required in five midazolam-exposed newborns compared with three in the thiopental group. Respiratory depression on day 1 and hypoglycemia and jaundice on day 3 were also observed in the midazolam group. Moreover, three statistically significant ($p < 0.05$) neurobehavioral adverse effects, from the 19 tested, consisting of body temperature, general body tone, and arm recoil, were noted after midazolam exposure during the first 2 hours after birth. Other parameters that were inferior in the midazolam group, but that did not reach statistical significance, were palmar grasp, resistance against pull, and startle reaction (7). Although these differences do not meet all of the criteria for "floppy infant syndrome" (see Diazepam), they do indicate that the use of midazolam before cesarean section has a depressant effect on the newborn that is greater than that observed with thiopental.

BREASTFEEDING SUMMARY

Midazolam is excreted into breast milk. In a study published in 1990, 12 women in the immediate postpartum period took 15 mg midazolam orally at night for 5 nights (8). No measurable concentrations of midazolam or the metabolite, hydroxy-midazolam, were detected (<10 nmol/L) in milk samples collected a mean 7 hours (range 6–8 hours) after drug intake during the 5-day period. One mother, however, who was accidentally given a second dose (total dose 30 mg) did have a milk concentration of 30 nmol/L (milk:plasma ratio 0.20) at 7 hours. The authors estimated that the exposure of the infant would be nil in early breast milk if nursing was held for 4 hours after a 15-mg dose. Two women also were studied at 2–3 months postpartum. In six paired milk and serum samples collected up to 6 hours after a 15-mg dose, the mean milk:plasma ratio was 0.15. Based on an average milk concentration of 10 nmol/L, a nursing infant would ingest an estimated 0.33 mcg of midazolam and 0.34 mcg of metabolite per 100 mL of milk if nursed within 4–6 hours of the maternal dose (8).

The effects of exposure to benzodiazepines during breastfeeding were reported in a 2012 study (9). In a 15-month period, spanning 2010–2011, 296 women called the Motherisk Program in Toronto, Ontario, seeking advice on the use of these drugs during lactation and 124 consented to the study. The most commonly used benzodiazepines were lorazepam (52%), clonazepam (18%), and midazolam (15%). Neonatal sedation was reported in only two infants. Midazolam was not used by either mother. There was no significant difference between the characteristics of these 2 and the 122 that reported no sedation in terms of maternal age, gestational age at birth, daily amount of time nursing, amount of time infant slept each day, and the benzodiazepine dose (mg/kg/day). The only difference was in the number of CNS depressants that the mothers were taking: 3.5 vs. 1.7 ($p = 0.0056$). The investigators concluded that their results supported the recommendation that the use of benzodiazepines was not a reason to avoid breastfeeding (9).

The American Academy of Pediatrics classifies midazolam as a drug for which the effect on a nursing infant is unknown but may be of concern if exposure is prolonged (10).

M

References

1. Product information. Versed. Roche Laboratories, 1997.
2. Kanto J, Sjovall S, Erkkola R, Himberg J-J, Kangas L. Placental transfer and maternal midazolam kinetics. Clin Pharmacol Ther 1983;33:786–91.
3. Bach V, Carl P, Ravlo O, Crawford ME, Jensen AG, Mikkelsen BO, Crevoisier C, Heizmann P, Fattinger K. A randomized comparison between midazolam and thiopental for elective cesarean section anesthesia. III. Placental transfer and elimination in neonates. Anesth Analg 1989;68:238–42.
4. Wilson CM, Dundee JW, Moore J, Collier PS, Mathews HLM, Thompson EM. A comparison of plasma midazolam levels in non-pregnant and pregnant women at parturition. Br J Clin Pharmacol 1985;20:256P–7P.
5. Bland BAR, Lawes EG, Duncan PW, Warnell I, Downing JW. Comparison of midazolam and thiopental for rapid sequence anesthetic induction for elective cesarean section. Anesth Analg 1987;66:1165–8.
6. Crawford ME, Carl P, Bach V, Ravlo O, Mikkelsen BO, Werner M. A randomized comparison between midazolam and thiopental for elective cesarean section anesthesia. I. Mothers. Anesth Analg 1989;68:229–33.
7. Ravlo O, Carl P, Crawford ME, Bach V, Mikkelsen BO, Nielsen HK. A randomized comparison between midazolam and thiopental for elective cesarean section anesthesia: II. Neonates. Anesth Analg 1989;68:234–7.
8. Matheson I, Lunde PKM, Bredesen JE. Midazolam and nitrazepam in the maternity ward: milk concentrations and clinical effects. Br J Clin Pharmac 1990;30:787–93.
9. Kelly LE, Poon S, Madadi P, Koren G. Neonatal benzodiazepines exposure during breastfeeding. J Pediatr 2012;161:448–51.
10. Committee on Drugs, American Academy of Pediatrics. The transfer of drugs and other chemicals into human milk. Pediatrics 2001;108:776–89.

MIDODRINE

Sympathomimetic (Adrenergic)

PREGNANCY RECOMMENDATION: Limited Human Data—Animal Data Suggest Moderate Risk
BREASTFEEDING RECOMMENDATION: No Human Data—Potential Toxicity

PREGNANCY SUMMARY

One report has described the use of midodrine during human pregnancy. The active metabolite, desglymidrodrine, is an α_1-adrenergic receptor agonist that increases the vascular tone to raise blood pressure. It is indicated for the treatment of symptomatic orthostatic hypotension. Marked increases in systolic blood pressure greater than 200 mmHg may occur, which in itself could jeopardize the fetus. *(Withdrawn from the market in September 2010).*

FETAL RISK SUMMARY

Reproduction studies have been conducted in pregnant rats and rabbits (1). At doses 13 and 7 times, respectively, the maximum human dose based on BSA, embryo toxicity (resorptions) and reduced fetal weights occurred in both species, and decreased fetal survival was noted in rabbits. No teratogenicity was observed in either species.

It is not known if midodrine or its metabolite cross the human placenta. The molecular weight (about 255 for the free base) is low enough that transfer to the fetus should be expected.

A 26-year-old woman with postural orthostatic tachycardia syndrome (POTS) became pregnant while taking midodrine 10 mg 5 times daily (2). Because her disease was partially controlled, she continued the midodrine throughout pregnancy. She had hyperemesis gravidarum that was treated with ondansetron. A scheduled cesarean section at 37 weeks' gave birth to a healthy, about 3.5-kg, male infant (2).

BREASTFEEDING SUMMARY

No reports describing the use of midodrine in human lactation have been located. The molecular weight (about 255 for the free base) suggests that the drug will be excreted into breast milk. The effect of this exposure on a nursing infant is unknown. Because severe systolic hypertension is a potential effect in an infant, women who are taking midodrine should probably not breastfeed.

Reference

1. Product information. ProAmatine. Shire US, 2001.
2. Glatter KA, Tuteja D, Chiamvimonvat N, Hamdan M, Park JK. Pregnancy in postural orthostatic tachycardia syndrome. Pacing Clin Electrophysiol 2005;28:591–3.

M

MIFEPRISTONE

Antiprogestogen

PREGNANCY RECOMMENDATION: Contraindicated
BREASTFEEDING RECOMMENDATION: Contraindicated

PREGNANCY SUMMARY

Mifepristone (RU 486) is a potent antiprogestogen compound that is mainly used for the termination of pregnancy, usually in combination with a prostaglandin agent. It has also been used for cervical ripening before abortion and is currently being studied as an aid in the induction of labor at term. It is teratogenic in one animal species, but not in two others, one of which is a primate species. Data are too limited to determine whether the drug is a human teratogen. Because the incidence of successful abortion after mifepristone is high, but not total, women should be informed of the risk for embryotoxicity if their pregnancy continues after use of this drug.

FETAL RISK SUMMARY

Mifepristone (RU 38486; RU 486) is an orally active, synthetic antiprogestogen that has been used primarily to terminate pregnancy. At higher doses, the drug also has antiglucocorticoid effects. The mechanism of action of mifepristone, which exerts its antiprogestogen effect at the level of the receptor, and the physiologic effects it produces in both animals and humans have been studied and reviewed in a number of references (1–16). A 1993 review summarized the drug's antiprogestin and other pharmacologic effects in humans (17).

Mifepristone rapidly crosses the placenta to the fetus in both monkeys (18) and humans (19,20). The fetal:maternal ratio decreased from 0.31 to 0.18 in monkeys between the 2nd and 3rd trimesters (18). In 13 women undergoing 2nd trimester abortions, a single 100-mg oral dose produced fetal cord blood concentrations of mifepristone ranging from 20 ng/mL (30 minutes) to 400 ng/mL (18 hours) (19). The peak maternal concentration (1500 ng/mL) was attained in 1–2 hours, and the average fetal:maternal ratio was approximately 0.33. In contrast to a simple diffusion process observed in monkeys (18), an active transport mechanism was suggested because the fetal concentration increased exponentially (19). In the second human study, a lower mean fetal:maternal ratio (0.11) was measured at 17.2 hours in six women treated with 600 mg of mifepristone for 2nd trimester abortion (20). Maternal plasma concentrations of aldosterone, progesterone, estradiol, or cortisol did not change significantly 4 hours after mifepristone, but a significant increase in fetal aldosterone occurred at this time, rising from 999 to 1699 pmol/L. Mean changes in the fetal levels of the other three steroids were not significant.

A large number of studies have investigated the use of mifepristone as an abortive agent, either when given alone (21–36), or when combined with a prostaglandin analog (24,30,37–51). The drug has also been studied for labor induction after 2nd trimester intrauterine death (52,53), and as a cervical ripening agent in the 1st trimester (54–59), in the 2nd trimester (60), and at term (61–63). Although mifepristone, especially when combined with a prostaglandin analog, is an effective abortive agent, it has not been effective when used for the termination of ectopic pregnancies (64,65). The use of mifepristone as a postcoital contraceptive or for routine administration during the mid- to late luteal phase to prevent a potential early pregnancy by induction of menses (i.e., contragestation) has also been frequently investigated (22,66–79).

Mifepristone is teratogenic in rabbits and the effect is both dose and duration dependent (80). Abnormalities observed included growth restriction, nonfused eyelids and large fontanelle, opened cranial vault with exposure of the meninges and hemorrhagic or necrotic nervous tissue, necrotic destruction of the upper part of the head and brain, and absence of closure of the vertebral canal (80). At doses approximating those used in clinical practice, no evidence of teratogenicity was observed in postimplantation rat embryos exposed to mifepristone in culture (81). Similarly, no teratogenicity was observed after in vitro exposure of monkey embryos to mifepristone (82,83).

In humans, only six cases have been reported of exposure to mifepristone that was not followed by subsequent abortion. Although specific details were not provided, in the United Kingdom Multicenter Trial (gestational age <36–69 days from last menstrual period), one woman changed her mind after taking mifepristone and her pregnancy continued until a normal infant was delivered at term (41). In 1989, brief mention was made of fetal malformations discovered after pregnancy termination at 18 weeks' gestation (84). Additional information on this and one other case was published in 1991 (85–87). A 25-year-old primigravida was treated with 600 mg of mifepristone at 5 weeks' gestation, but then decided not to proceed with termination (85,86). Severe malformations were observed by ultrasound examination at 17 weeks' gestation, consisting of an absence of amniotic sac, stomach, gallbladder, and urinary tract, and the pregnancy was stopped with prostaglandin at 18 weeks' (85). The 190-g fetus had typical features of the sirenomelia sequence (sympodia; caudal regression syndrome): fused lower limbs with a single flexed foot containing seven toes; no external genitalia or anal or urethral openings; and absence of internal reproductive organs, lower urinary tract, and kidneys. Other anomalies were hypoplastic lungs, a cleft palate, and a cleft lip. Sirenomelia is thought to date back to the primitive streak stage during the 3rd week of gestation, and, thus, in this case, before exposure to mifepristone (85). However, induction of cleft palate and cleft lip occurs at approximately 36 days of gestation (85) and may have been a consequence of drug exposure.

A normal outcome was achieved in the second case in which a 30-year-old woman was treated with 400 mg of mifepristone 6 weeks after her last menstrual period, but then decided to continue her pregnancy (85). She eventually delivered a healthy, 3030-g male baby at 41 weeks' gestation. Three other normal infants have been described after in utero exposure to mifepristone (59,88). All three were participants in clinical trials who decided to continue their pregnancies after treatment with mifepristone at 8, 8, and 9 weeks' gestation (88). The latter patient vomited 1.5 hours after taking the drug and reported seeing at least one partially digested tablet in the vomit. Delivery occurred at 40 weeks (4150-g male), 39 weeks (3930-g male), and 41 weeks (3585 g, female), respectively. Follow-ups of the infants at 15, 9, and 6 months, respectively, were completely normal.

BREASTFEEDING SUMMARY

No data have been located on the excretion of mifepristone in breast milk. Because the drug is well absorbed after oral administration, it should not be used during breastfeeding because of its potent antihormonal effects. However, as a result of the limited indications for this agent, the opportunities for its use during lactation should be infrequent.

References

1. Garfield RE, Gasc JM, Baulieu EE. Effects of the antiprogesterone RU 486 on preterm birth in the rat. Am J Obstet Gynecol 1987;157:1281–5.
2. Roblero LS, Fernandez O, Croxatto HB. The effects of RU486 on transport, development and implantation of mouse embryos. Contraception 1987;36:549–55.
3. Burgess KM, Jenkin G, Ralph MM, Thorburn GD. Effect of the antiprogestin RU486 on uterine sensitivity to oxytocin in ewes in late pregnancy. J Endocrinol 1992;134:353–60.
4. Haluska GJ, Stanczyk FZ, Cook MJ, Novy MJ. Temporal changes in uterine activity and prostaglandin response to RU486 in rhesus macaques in late gestation. Am J Obstet Gynecol 1987;157:1487–95.
5. Cullingford TE, Pollard JW. RU 486 completely inhibits the action of progesterone on cell proliferation in the mouse uterus. J Reprod Fertil 1988;83:909–14.
6. Haluska GJ, West NB, Novy MJ, Brenner RM. Uterine estrogen receptors are increased by RU486 in late pregnant rhesus macaques but not after spontaneous labor. J Clin Endocrinol Metab 1990;70:181–6.
7. Haluska GJ, Mitchell MD, Novy MJ. Amniotic fluid lipoxygenase metabolites during spontaneous labor and after RU486 treatment during late pregnancy in rhesus macaques. Prostaglandins 1990;40:99–105.
8. Juneja SC, Dodson MG. In vitro effect of RU 486 on sperm-egg interaction in mice. Am J Obstet Gynecol 1990;163:216–21.
9. Cabrol D, Carbonne B, Bienkiewicz A, Dallot E, Alj AE, Cedard L. Induction of labor and cervical maturation using mifepristone (RU 486) in the late pregnant rat. Influence of a cyclooxygenase inhibitor (diclofenac). Prostaglandins 1991;42:71–9.
10. Smith SK, Kelly RW. The effect of the antiprogestins RU 486 and ZK 98734 on the synthesis and metabolism of prostaglandins $F_{2\alpha}$ and E_2 in separated cells from early human decidua. J Clin Endocrinol Metab 1987;65:527–34.
11. Das C, Catt KJ. Antifertility actions of the progesterone antagonist RU 486 include direct inhibition of placental hormone secretion. Lancet 1987;2:599–601.
12. Anonymous. Mifepristone—contragestive agent or medical abortifacient. Lancet 1987;2:1308–10.
13. Hill NCW, Selinger M, Ferguson J, Lopez Bernal A, Mackenzie IZ. The physiological and clinical effects of progesterone inhibition with mifepristone (RU 486) in the second trimester. Br J Obstet Gynaecol 1990;97:487–92.

14. Baulieu EE. RU-486 as an antiprogesterone steroid. From receptor to contragestion and beyond. JAMA 1989;262:1808–14.
15. Guillebaud J. Medical termination of pregnancy. Combined with prostaglandin RU 486 is effective. Br Med J 1990;301:352–4.
16. Brogden RN, Goa KL, Faulds D. Mifepristone. A review of its pharmacodynamic and pharmacokinetic properties, and therapeutic potential. Drugs 1993;45:384–409.
17. Spitz IM, Bardin CW. Mifepristone (RU 486)—a modulator of progestin and glucocorticoid action. N Engl J Med 1993;329:404–12.
18. Wolf JP, Chillik CF, Itskovitz J, Weyman D, Anderson TL, Ulmann A, Baulieu EE, Hodgen GD. Transplacental passage of a progesterone antagonist in monkeys. Am J Obstet Gynecol 1988;159:238–42.
19. Frydman R, Taylor S, Ulmann A. Transplacental passage of mifepristone. Lancet 1985;2:1252.
20. Hill NCW, Selinger M, Ferguson J, MacKenzie IZ. The placental transfer of mifepristone (RU 486) during the second trimester and its influence upon maternal and fetal steroid concentrations. Br J Obstet Gynaecol 1990;97:406–11.
21. Kovacs L, Sas M, Resch BA, Ugocsai G, Swahn ML, Bygdeman M, Rowe PJ. Termination of very early pregnancy by RU 486—an antiprogestational compound. Contraception 1984;29:399–410.
22. Haspels AA. Interruption of early pregnancy by an anti-progestational compound, RU 486. Eur J Obstet Gynecol Reprod Biol 1985;20:169–75.
23. Vervest HAM, Haspels AA. Preliminary results with the antiprogestational compound RU-486 (mifepristone) for interruption of early pregnancy. Fertil Steril 1985;44:627–32.
24. Bygdeman M, Swahn ML. Progesterone receptor blockage. Effect on uterine contractility and early pregnancy. Contraception 1985;32:45–51.
25. Couzinet B, Strat NL, Ulmann A, Baulieu EE, Schaison G. Termination of early pregnancy by the progesterone antagonist RU 486 (mifepristone). N Engl J Med 1986;315:1565–70.
26. Shoupe D, Mishell DR Jr, Brenner PF, Spitz IM. Pregnancy termination with a high and medium dosage regimen of RU 486. Contraception 1986;33: 455–61.
27. Mishell DR Jr, Shouupe D, Brenner PF, Lacarra M, Horenstein J, Lahteenmaki P, Spitz IM. Termination of early gestation with the anti-progestin steroid RU 486: medium versus low dose. Contraception 1987;35:307–21.
28. Urquhart DR, Templeton AA. Mifepristone (RU 486) and second-trimester termination. Lancet 1987;2:1405.
29. Birgerson L, Odlind V. Early pregnancy termination with antiprogestins: a comparative clinical study of RU 486 given in two dose regimens and epostane. Fertil Steril 1987;48:565–70.
30. Cameron IT, Michie AF, Baird DT. Therapeutic abortion in early pregnancy with antiprogestogen RU486 alone or in combination with prostaglandin analogue (Gemeprost). Contraception 1986;34:459–68.
31. Grimes DA, Mishell DR Jr, Shoupe D, Lacarra M. Early abortion with a single dose of the antiprogestin RU-486. Am J Obstet Gynecol 1988;158: 1307–12.
32. Cameron IT, Baird DT. Early pregnancy termination: a comparison between vacuum aspiration and medical abortion using prostaglandin (16,16 dimethyl-trans-$Ä_2$-PGE$_1$ methyl ester) or the antiprogestogen RU 486. Br J Obstet Gynaecol 1988;95:271–6.
33. Maria B, Stampf F, Goepp A, Ulmann A. Termination of early pregnancy by a single dose of mifepristone (RU 486), a progesterone antagonist. Eur J Obstet Gynecol Reprod Biol 1988;28:249–55.
34. Frydman R, Fernandez H, Pons JC, Ulmann A. Mifepristone (RU486) and therapeutic late pregnancy termination: a double-blind study of two different doses. Hum Reprod 1988;3:803–6.
35. Ylikorkala O, Alfthan H, Kaariainen M, Rapeli T, Lahteenmaki P. Outpatient therapeutic abortion with mifepristone. Obstet Gynecol 1989;74:653–7.
36. Gottlieb C, Bygdeman M. The use of antiprogestin (RU 486) for termination of second trimester pregnancy. Acta Obstet Gynecol Scand 1991;70:199–203.
37. Rodger MW, Baird DT. Induction of therapeutic abortion in early pregnancy with mifepristone in combination with prostaglandin pessary. Lancet 1987;2:1415–8.
38. Swahn ML, Bygdeman M. The effect of the antiprogestin RU 486 on uterine contractility and sensitivity to prostaglandin and oxytocin. Br J Obstet Gynaecol 1988;95:126–34.
39. Hill NCW, Ferguson J, MacKenzie IZ. The efficacy of oral mifepristone (RU 38,486) with a prostaglandin E_1 analog vaginal pessary for the termination of early pregnancy: complications and patient acceptability. Am J Obstet Gynecol 1990;162:414–7.
40. Silvestre L, Dubois C, Renault M, Rezvani Y, Baulieu EE, Ulmann A. Voluntary interruption of pregnancy with mifepristone (RU 486) and a prostaglandin analogue. N Engl J Med 1990;322:645–8.
41. UK Multicentre Trial. The efficacy and tolerance of mifepristone and prostaglandin in first trimester termination of pregnancy. Br J Obstet Gynaecol 1990;97:480–6.
42. Norman JE, Thong KJ, Baird DT. Uterine contractility and induction of abortion in early pregnancy by misoprostol and mifepristone. Lancet 1991;338:1233–6.
43. Anonymous. Misoprostol and legal medical abortion. Lancet 1991;338:1241–2.
44. World Health Organization. Pregnancy termination with mifepristone and gemeprost: a multicenter comparison between repeated doses and a single dose of mifepristone. Fertil Steril 1991;56:32–40.
45. Norman JE, Thong KJ, Rodger MW, Baird DT. Medical abortion in women of ≤56 days amenorrhoea: a comparison between gemeprost (a PGE$_1$ analogue) alone and mifepristone and gemeprost. Br J Obstet Gynaecol 1992;99:601–6.
46. Ulmann A, Silvestre L, Chemama L, Rezvani Y, Renault M, Aguillaume CJ, Baulieu EE. Medical termination of early pregnancy with mifepristone (RU 486) followed by a prostaglandin analogue: study in 16,369 women. Acta Obstet Gynecol Scand 1992;71:278–283.
47. Baird DT, Norman JE, Thong KJ, Glasier AF. Misoprostol, mifepristone, and abortion. Lancet 1992;339:313.
48. Thong KJ, Baird DT. A study of gemeprost alone, dilapan or mifepristone in combination with gemeprost for the termination of second trimester pregnancy. Contraception 1992;46:11–7.
49. Thong KJ, Baird DT. Induction of abortion with mifepristone and misoprostol in early pregnancy. Br J Obstet Gynaecol 1992;99:1004–7.
50. Heard M, Guillebaud J. Medical abortion. Safe, effective, and legal in Britain. Br Med J 1992;304:195–6.
51. Peyron R, Aubeny E, Targosz V, Silvestre L, Renault M, Elkik F, Leclerc P, Ulmann A, Baulieu E-E. Early termination of pregnancy with mifepristone (RU 486) and the orally active prostaglandin misoprostol. N Engl J Med 1993;328:1509–13.
52. Cabrol D, Bouvier D'Yvoire M, Mermet E, Cedard L, Sureau C, Baulieu EE. Induction of labour with mifepristone after intrauterine fetal death. Lancet 1985;2:1019.
53. Cabrol D, Dubois C, Cronje H, Gonnet JM, Guillot M, Maria B, Moodley J, Oury JF, Thoulon JM, Treisser A, Ulmann D, Correl S, Ulmann A. Induction of labor with mifepristone (RU 486) in intrauterine fetal death. Am J Obstet Gynecol 1990;163:540–2.
54. Radestad A, Christensen NJ, Stromberg L. Induced cervical ripening with mifepristone in first trimester abortion: a double-blind randomized biomechanical study. Contraception 1988;38:301–12.
55. Durlot F, Dubois C, Brunerie J, Frydman R. Efficacy of progesterone antagonist RU486 (mifepristone) for pre-operative cervical dilatation during first trimester abortion. Hum Reprod 1988;3:583–4.
56. Lefebvre Y, Proulx L, Elie R, Poulin O, Lanza E. The effects of RU-38486 on cervical ripening. Clinical studies. Am J Obstet Gynecol 1990;162:61–5.
57. Johnson N, Bryce FC. Could antiprogesterones be used as alternative cervical ripening agents? Am J Obstet Gynecol 1990;162:688–90.
58. World Health Organization. The use of mifepristone (RU 486) for cervical preparation in first trimester pregnancy termination by vacuum aspiration. Br J Obstet Gynaecol 1990;97:260–6.
59. Cohn M, Stewart P. Pretreatment of the primigravid uterine cervix with mifepristone 30 h prior to termination of pregnancy: a double blind study. Br J Obstet Gynaecol 1991;98:778–82.
60. Frydman R, Taylor S, Pons JC, Forman RG, Ulmann A. Obstetrical indications for mifepristone. Adv Contracept 1986;2:269–70.
61. Li Y, Perezgrovas R, Gazal OS, Schwabe C, Anderson LL. Antiprogesterone, RU 486, facilitates parturition in cattle. Endocrinology 1991;129: 765–70.
62. Wolf JP, Sinosich M, Anderson TL, Ulmann A, Baulieu EE, Hodgen GD. Progesterone antagonist (RU 486) for cervical dilation, labor induction, and delivery in monkeys; effectiveness in combination with oxytocin. Am J Obstet Gynecol 1989;160:45–7.
63. Frydman R, Lelaidier C, Baton-Saint-Mleux C, Fernandez H, Vial M, Bourget P. Labor induction in women at term with mifepristone (RU 486): a double-blind randomized, placebo-controlled study. Obstet Gynecol 1992;80:972–5.
64. Levin JH, Lacarra M, d'Ablain G, Grimes DA, Vermesh M. Mifepristone (RU 486) failure in an ovarian heterotopic pregnancy. Am J Obstet Gynecol 1990;163:543–4.
65. Pansky M, Golan A, Bukovsky I, Caspi E. Nonsurgical management of tubal pregnancy. Necessity in view of the changing clinical appearance. Am J Obstet Gynecol 1991;164:888–95.
66. Ulmann A. Uses of RU 486 for contragestion: an update. Contraception 1987;36(Suppl):27–31.

67. Nieman LK, Choate TM, Chrousos GP, Healy DL, Morin M, Renquist D, Merriam GR, Spitz IM, Bardin CW, Baulieu EE, Loriaux DL. The progesterone antagonist RU 486: a potential new contraceptive agent. N Engl J Med 1987;316:187–91.
68. Psychoyos A, Prapas I. Inhibition of egg development and implantation in rats after post-coital administration of the progesterone antagonist RU 486. J Reprod Fertil 1987;80:487–91.
69. Baulieu EE, Ulmann A, Philibert D. Contragestion by antiprogestin RU 486: a review. Arch Gynecol Obstet 1987;241:73–85.
70. Lahteenmaki P, Rapeli T, Kaariainen M, Alfthan H, Ylikorkala O. Late postcoital treatment against pregnancy with antiprogesterone RU 486. Fertil Steril 1988;50:36–8.
71. Dubois C, Ulmann A, Baulieu EE. Contragestion with late luteal administration of RU 486 (mifepristone). Fertil Steril 1988;50:593–6.
72. Couzinet B, Le Strat N, Silvestre L, Schaison G. Late luteal administration of the antiprogesterone RU486 in normal women: effects on the menstrual cycle events and fertility control in a long-term study. Fertil Steril 1990;54:1039–44.
73. Swahn ML, Gemzell K, Bygdeman M. Contraception with mifepristone. Lancet 1991;338:942–3.
74. Glasier A, Thong KJ, Dewar M, Mackie M, Baird DT. Postcoital contraception with mifepristone. Lancet 1991;337:1414–5.
75. Batista MC, Bristow TL, Mathews J, Stokes WS, Loriaux DL, Nieman LK. Daily administration of the progesterone antagonist RU 486 prevents implantation in the cycling guinea pig. Am J Obstet Gynecol 1991;165:82–6.
76. Glasier A, Thong KJ, Dewar M, Mackie M, Baird DT. Mifepristone (RU 486) compared with high-dose estrogen and progestogen for emergency postcoital contraception. N Engl J Med 1992;327:1041–4.
77. Grimes DA, Cook RJ. Mifepristone (RU 486)—an abortifacient to prevent abortion? N Engl J Med 1992;327:1088–9.
78. Hamel RP, Lysaught MT. Mifepristone (RU 486)—an abortifacient to prevent abortion? N Engl J Med 1993;328:354.
79. Grimes DA, Cook RJ. Mifepristone (RU 486)—an abortifacient to prevent abortion? Reply. N Engl J Med 1993;328:355.
80. Jost A. New data on the hormonal requirement of the pregnant rabbit: partial pregnancies and fetal anomalies resulting from treatment with a hormonal antagonist, given at a sub-abortive dosage. C R Acad Sci (Paris) 1986;303:281–4.
81. Hardy RP, New DAT. Effects of the anti-progestin RU 38486 on rat embryos growing in culture. Food Chem Toxicol 1991;29:361–2.
82. Avrech OM, Golan A, Weinraub Z, Bukovsky I, Caspi E. New tools for the trade. Reply. Fertil Steril 1992;57:1139–40.
83. Wolf JP, Chillik CF, Dubois C, Ulmann A, Baulieu EE, Hodgen GD. Tolerance of perinidatory primate embryos to RU486 exposure in vitro and in vivo. Contraception 1990;41:85–92.
84. Henrion R. RU 486 abortions. Nature 1989;338:110.
85. Pons JC, Imbert MC, Elefant E, Roux C, Herschkorn P, Papiernik E. Development after exposure to mifepristone in early pregnancy. Lancet 1991;338:763.
86. Ulmann A, Rubin I, Barnard J. Development after in-utero exposure to mifepristone. Lancet 1991;338:1270.
87. Pons JC, Papiernik E. Mifepristone teratogenicity. Lancet 1991;338:1332–3.
88. Lim BH, Lees DAR, Bjornsson S, Lunan CB, Cohn MR, Stewart P, Davey A. Normal development after exposure to mifepristone in early pregnancy. Lancet 1990;336:257–8.

MIGLITOL

Antidiabetic Agent

PREGNANCY RECOMMENDATION: No Human Data—Probably Compatible
BREASTFEEDING RECOMMENDATION: Limited Human Data—Probably Compatible

PREGNANCY SUMMARY

No reports describing the use of miglitol during human pregnancy have been located. Miglitol is normally used either alone or in combination with oral hypoglycemic agents, and these hypoglycemic drugs are not indicated for the pregnant diabetic as they may not provide good control in patients who cannot be controlled by diet alone. Carefully prescribed insulin therapy provides better control of the mother's glucose, thereby preventing the fetal and neonatal complications that occur with this disease. Moreover, insulin, unlike most oral agents, does not cross the placenta to the fetus, thus eliminating the additional concern that the drug therapy itself will adversely affect the fetus. High maternal glucose levels, as may occur in diabetes mellitus, are closely associated with a number of maternal and fetal adverse effects, including fetal structural anomalies if the hyperglycemia occurs early in gestation. To prevent this toxicity, the American College of Obstetricians and Gynecologists recommends that insulin be used for types 1 and 2 diabetes in pregnancy and, if diet therapy alone is not successful, for gestational diabetes (1,2).

FETAL RISK SUMMARY

Miglitol is an oral α-glucosidase inhibitor, in the same class as acarbose (see Acarbose), that delays the digestion of ingested carbohydrates within the gastrointestinal tract, thereby reducing the rise in blood glucose following meals. It is used either alone or in combination with a sulfonylurea as an adjunct to diet in the management of type 2 diabetes (non-insulin-dependent diabetes mellitus). In contrast to acarbose, miglitol is readily absorbed into the systemic circulation, but the absorption is saturable at high doses. In addition, miglitol is not metabolized and is excreted unchanged in the urine with an elimination half-life of approximately 2 hours (3).

Reproduction studies have been conducted in animals with miglitol. In rats and rabbits at doses up to 12 and 10 times, respectively, the maximum recommended human exposure based on BSA (MRHE), no evidence of teratogenicity was observed. In addition, no evidence of impaired fertility or fetal harm was noted at doses up to 4 and 3 times the MRHE, respectively, in these species. At 12 and 10 times the MRHE in rats and rabbits, respectively, maternal and/or fetal toxicity were noted. In rats, fetotoxicity was characterized by a slight but significant reduction in fetal weight. In rabbits, a slight reduction in fetal weight, an increased number of nonviable fetuses, and delayed ossification of the fetal skeleton were evident. In the rat peri-postnatal study, an increase in stillborns occurred at 4 times the MRHE (3).

It is not known if miglitol crosses the human placenta. The molecular weight (about 207) is low enough that exposure of the embryo and/or fetus should be expected.

BREASTFEEDING SUMMARY

Miglitol is excreted into breast milk. This is consistent with its relatively low molecular weight (about 207). The total amount excreted, however, is very small, accounting only for 0.02% of a 100-mg dose (only 50%–70% of a 100-mg dose is bioavailable). The estimated exposure of a nursing infant was about 0.4% of the mother's dose (3).

The effects of this exposure on a nursing infant are unknown, but the manufacturer recommends that miglitol should not be used during lactation (3). A 2000 review also stated that miglitol should not be used during breastfeeding (4). Nevertheless, based on the single study above, the exposure of a nursing infant appears to be clinically insignificant.

References

1. American College of Obstetricians and Gynecologists. Pregestational diabetes mellitus. *ACOG Practice Bulletin*. No. 60. March 2005. Obstet Gynecol 2005;105:675–85.
2. American College of Obstetricians and Gynecologists. Gestational diabetes. *ACOG Practice Bulletin*. No. 30. September 2001. Obstet Gynecol 2001;98:525–38.
3. Product information. Glyset. Pharmacia & Upjohn, 2000.
4. Campbell LK, Baker DE, Campbell RK. Miglitol: assessment of its role in the treatment of patients with diabetes mellitus. Ann Pharmacother 2000;34:1291–301.

MIGLUSTAT

Endocrine/Metabolic Agent (Gaucher Disease)

PREGNANCY RECOMMENDATION: No Human Data—Contraindicated
BREASTFEEDING RECOMMENDATION: No Human Data—Potential Toxicity

PREGNANCY SUMMARY

No reports describing the use of miglustat in human pregnancy have been located. The animal data suggest risk for embryotoxicity and decreased fetal weight at exposure levels comparable to human systemic exposure.

M

FETAL RISK SUMMARY

Miglustat is an oral medication that inhibits the enzyme glucosylceramide synthase and is used for the treatment of type I Gaucher disease in individuals for whom enzyme replacement therapy is not an option. Miglustat does not bind to plasma proteins. The effective elimination half-life is 6–7 hours (1).

Reproduction studies have been conducted in rats and rabbits. In rats, miglustat was given by oral gavage at doses up to ≥2 times the human therapeutic systemic exposure based on BSA (HTSE) beginning 14 days before mating and continuing through day 17 (organogenesis). At the mid-to-high doses that were ≥2 times the HTSE, decreased fetal survival, including complete litter loss, and decreased fetal weights were observed. Delayed parturition and dystocia were observed in another rat study that used the same mid-to-high doses and route of administration from gestation day 6 through lactation. In addition, decreased survival and reduced fetal weights were seen at doses comparable to or below the HTSE. In rabbits, doses that were less than the HTSE during gestation days 6–18 resulted in maternal toxicity and death (1).

In 2-year carcinogenicity studies conducted in mice, mucinous adenocarcinomas of the large intestine were observed in male and female mice given oral doses that were 3 and 6 times the recommended human dose (RHD), respectively. In rats, an increased incidence of interstitial cell adenomas of the testis was observed in males at doses equivalent to the RHD. Miglustat was not mutagenic or clastogenic in multiple in vitro and in vivo assays. Fertility studies in rats demonstrated decreased spermatogenesis in males who were treated 14 days prior to mating and at doses below the HTSE. In females, decreased corpora lutea were noted, as well as increased postimplantation loss at the lowest dose (1). However, in a study conducted in seven normal human males who were administered 100 mg of miglustat twice a day for 6 weeks, no effects on sperm concentration, motility, and morphology were seen (2).

It is not known if miglustat crosses the human placenta. The molecular weight (about 200), lack of plasma protein binding, and prolonged elimination half-life suggest that the drug will cross the placenta throughout gestation.

No reports of human pregnancy exposure to miglustat have been located. Because the drug is contraindicated in pregnancy, pregnancy exposures should be rare. One pharmacovigilance study in Europe followed 122 type I Gaucher disease patients for 5 years and identified 1 woman who discontinued the drug for a planned pregnancy (3).

BREASTFEEDING SUMMARY

No reports describing the use miglustat during human lactation have been located. The molecular weight (about 200), lack of plasma protein binding, and relatively long elimination half-life (6–7 hours) suggest that the drug will be excreted into breast milk.

References

1. Product information. Zavesca. Actelion Pharmaceuticals, 2010.
2. Amory JK, Muller CH, Page ST, Leifke E, Pagel ER, Bhandari A, Subramanyam B, Bone W, Radlmaier A, Bremner WJ. Miglustat has no apparent effect on spermatogenesis in normal men. Hum Reprod 2007;22:702–7.
3. Hollak CE, Hughes D, van Schaik IN, Schwierin B, Bembi B. Miglustat (Zavesca) in type I Gaucher disease: 5-year results of a post-authorisation safety surveillance programme. Pharmacoepidemiol Drug Saf 2009;18:770–7.

MILNACIPRAN

Antidepressant

PREGNANCY RECOMMENDATION: Human Data Suggest Risk in 3rd Trimester
BREASTFEEDING RECOMMENDATION: No Human Data—Potential Toxicity

PREGNANCY SUMMARY

No reports describing the use of milnacipran in human pregnancy have been located. Neither the animal reproduction data nor the human data from other selective norepinephrine and serotonin reuptake inhibitors (SNRIs) suggest that this class of drugs is a risk for structural anomalies. However, other SNRIs (e.g., see Venlafaxine) as well as selective serotonin reuptake inhibitors (SSRIs) have been associated with developmental toxicity, including spontaneous abortions, low birth weight, prematurity, neonatal serotonin syndrome, neonatal behavioral syndrome (withdrawal including seizures), possibly sustained abnormal neurobehavior beyond the neonatal period, and respiratory distress. Persistent pulmonary hypertension of the newborn (PPHN) is an additional potential risk, but confirmation is needed.

FETAL RISK SUMMARY

Milnacipran is an SNRI that is indicated for the management of fibromyalgia. Although not indicated for depression, it is in the same class of SNRI antidepressants as desvenlafaxine, duloxetine, and venlafaxine. The drug partially undergoes metabolism before urinary excretion. Plasma protein binding is low (13%). Milnacipran is racemic mixture with an elimination half-life of about 6–8 hours. However, the half-life of the active enantiomer, *d*-milnacipran, is 8–10 hours, whereas it is 4–6 hours for the *l*-enantiomer (1).

Reproduction studies have been conducted in rats, mice, and rabbits. In rats, doses that were 0.25 times the maximum recommended human dose based on BSA (MRHD) increased the incidence of dead fetuses in utero. In mice and rabbits during organogenesis, doses up to 3 and 6 times, respectively, the MRHD did not cause embryotoxicity or teratogenicity. However, a dose one-fourth of the above dose in rabbits increased the incidence of an extra single rib, a skeletal variation (1).

In a 2-year carcinogenicity study in rats, a dose twice the MRHD caused a statistically significant increase in the incidence of thyroid C-cell adenomas and combined adenomas and carcinomas in males. A 6-month study in mice did not induce tumors at any dose tested. Milnacipran was not mutagenic or clastogenic in various assays. No significant effects on mating or fertility were observed in males and females given doses up to 4 times the MRHD. However, there was an apparent dose-related decrease in the fertility index at clinically relevant doses based on BSA (1).

It is not known if milnacipran crosses the human placenta. The molecular weight (about 247 for the free base), the terminal elimination half-life of 6–8 hours (both enantiomers), and the very low plasma protein binding suggest that the drug will cross to the embryo–fetus.

BREASTFEEDING SUMMARY

No reports describing the use milnacipran during human lactation have been located. The molecular weight (about 247 for the free base), the terminal elimination half-life of 6–8 hours (both enantiomers), and the very low plasma protein binding suggest that the drug will be excreted into breast milk. The effects of this exposure on a nursing infant are unknown. However, the long-term effects on neurobehavior and cognitive development from exposure to SNRIs during a period of rapid central nervous system development have not been adequately studied. The American Academy of Pediatrics classifies other antidepressants as drugs for which the effect on nursing infants is unknown but may be of concern (2).

References

1. Product information. Savella. Forest Pharmaceuticals, 2009.
2. Committee on Drugs, American Academy of Pediatrics. The transfer of drugs and other chemicals into human milk. Pediatrics 2001;108:776–89.

MILRINONE

Cardiac Agent

PREGNANCY RECOMMENDATION: No Human Data—Animal Data Suggest Risk
BREASTFEEDING RECOMMENDATION: No Human Data—Probably Compatible

PREGNANCY SUMMARY

Milrinone is used IV in the treatment of congestive heart disease. No reports describing the use of this drug in human pregnancy have been located.

FETAL RISK SUMMARY

Reproductive studies in rats (doses up to 40 mg/kg/day) and rabbits (doses up to 12 mg/kg/day) have revealed an increased resorption rate, but no teratogenic effects (1).

In an experiment with four pregnant baboons at 155–165 days' gestation (term 175 days), milrinone was given as an IV bolus of 75 mcg/kg followed by a continuous infusion of 1 mcg/kg/minute for 180 minutes (loading and maintenance doses considered maximal in humans) (2). Placental transfer was demonstrated as early as 5 minutes after beginning. At steady state (60 minutes), the maternal:fetal concentration ratio was 4:1. Although a significant increase in maternal heart rate was measured during the experiment, no significant changes were observed in the maternal mean arterial pressure or in the fetal heart rate and arterial blood gasses or pH values. All four fetuses appeared normal at birth.

BREASTFEEDING SUMMARY

No reports describing the use of milrinone during human lactation have been located.

References

1. Product information. Primacor. Sanofi Pharmaceuticals, 2000.
2. Atkinson BD, Fishburne JI Jr, Hales KA, Levy GH, Rayburn WF. Placental transfer of milrinone in the nonhuman primate (baboon). Am J Obstet Gynecol 1996;174:895–6.

MINERAL OIL

Laxative

PREGNANCY RECOMMENDATION: Compatible
BREASTFEEDING RECOMMENDATION: Compatible

PREGNANCY SUMMARY

Mineral oil is an emollient laxative. The drug is generally considered nonabsorbable. Chronic use may lead to decreased absorption of fat-soluble vitamins.

M

BREASTFEEDING SUMMARY

No reports describing the use of mineral oil during lactation have been located. The product probably is harmless, but chronic use may cause deficiencies of fat-soluble vitamins in the mother.

MINOCYCLINE

Antibiotic (Tetracycline)

See Tetracycline.

MINOXIDIL

Antihypertensive

PREGNANCY RECOMMENDATION: Limited Human Data—Animal Data Suggest Moderate Risk
BREASTFEEDING RECOMMENDATION: Limited Human Data—Probably Compatible

PREGNANCY SUMMARY

Minoxidil is not teratogenic in rats and rabbits, but some fetotoxicity was observed in rabbits. The human pregnancy experience is too limited, after both oral dosing and topical application, to determine the risk of teratogenicity. A possible exception involves the two infants exposed in utero to oral minoxidil who had hypertrichosis. This is a known adverse effect in adults and, indeed, one of the mothers had hypertrichosis. However, the causes of the multiple congenital malformations observed in one of these infants and the heart defects in the other are unknown. Similarly, the causes of the multiple anomalies observed in two fetuses after minoxidil topical application also are unknown. Although the doses applied in these two cases were not specified, only small amounts of topically applied minoxidil are absorbed into the systemic circulation. Of interest, both mothers had a flu-like illness in the 1st trimester. Even if these malformations are not related to drug exposure, the potential toxicity of oral minoxidil is severe enough to preclude its use in pregnancy. One of these toxicities includes large orthostatic decreases in blood pressure that could severely jeopardize placental perfusion. Although the possibility of a causal relationship to malformations after topical application appears to be remote, the safest course is to avoid applying the agent during the 1st trimester.

FETAL RISK SUMMARY

Minoxidil is a potent antihypertensive peripheral vasodilator. It is indicated for the treatment of hypertension that is symptomatic or associated with target organ damage. Minoxidil is considered a second-line antihypertensive therapy because of the potential for severe adverse effects. After oral dosing, minoxidil is nearly completely (90%) metabolized to metabolites that have much less antihypertensive effects. The average plasma elimination half-life of the parent compound is 4.2 hours (1).

Minoxidil is also used topically for the treatment of androgenetic alopecia (male baldness) and alopecia areata. After topical application, it is poorly absorbed from normal intact skin, with an average of 1.4% (range 0.3%–4.5%) entering the systemic circulation. Steady state concentrations in the plasma are reached at the end of the third dosing interval (36 hours) (2).

Reproduction studies have been conducted in rats and rabbits (1–3). In rats, no evidence of teratogenicity or fetotoxicity was observed after an oral dose that was 5 times the human dose (1,2). Similarly, no teratogenicity was observed with an SC dose (80 mg/kg/day) that produced maternal toxicity (1). The oral dose, however, reduced the conception rate (2). There also was no teratogenicity in the offspring of pregnant rabbits given an oral dose that was 5 times the human dose, but an increased incidence of fetal resorptions was noted (1,2).

Pregnant rats were administered minoxidil at doses of 3 and 10 mg/kg/day on gestational days 6–15 (3). No evidence of teratogenicity or acute toxicity was observed. However, in the 10 mg/kg/day group, there was a higher than expected incidence of retinal folds in the eyes of offspring. Additional studies did not confirm this finding. In pregnant rabbits, similar doses administered on gestational days 6–18 resulted in fewer live pups per litter. At the highest dose, there was a higher incidence of resorptions (3).

It is not known if minoxidil crosses the human placenta. The molecular weight (about 209) is low enough that fetal exposure should be expected. Moreover, the moderately long elimination half-life (4.2 hours) should increase the opportunity for the drug to cross to the fetal compartment. In addition, the two cases of hypertrichosis described below suggest that minoxidil crosses the placenta.

Information on the use of oral minoxidil in human pregnancy is very limited, and only four cases of fetal exposure have been located (4–6). In one report, minoxidil was used throughout gestation with no effect seen in the healthy newborn (4). A second report involved a mother with a history of renal artery stenosis and malignant hypertension who was treated throughout gestation with minoxidil, captopril, and propranolol (5). Three of her four previous pregnancies had ended in midgestation stillbirths. The most recent stillbirth, her fourth pregnancy, involved a 500-g male infant with low-set ears but no gross anomalies. The mother had been treated with the above regimen plus furosemide. In her second pregnancy, she was treated only with hydrochlorothiazide, and delivered a normal term infant. No information was available on the first and third pregnancies, both of which ended in stillbirths.

In her current pregnancy, daily doses of the three drugs were 10, 50, and 160 mg, respectively. The infant, delivered by cesarean section at 38 weeks' gestation, had multiple abnormalities, including an omphalocele (repaired on the 2nd day), pronounced hypertrichosis of the back and extremities, depressed nasal bridge, low-set ears, micrognathia, bilateral fifth finger clinodactyly, undescended testes, a circumferential midphallic constriction, a large ventriculoseptal defect, and a brain defect consisting of slightly prominent sulci, especially the basal cisterns and interhemispheric fissure. Growth restriction was not evident, but the weight (3170 g, 60th percentile), length (46 cm, 15th percentile), and head circumference (32.5 cm, 25th percentile) were disproportionate. Neurologic, skeletal, and kidney examinations were normal. Marked hypotension (30–50 mmHg systolic) was present, which resolved after 24 hours. Heart rate, blood glucose, and renal function were normal.

The infant's hospital course was marked by failure to thrive, congestive heart failure, prolonged physiologic jaundice, and eight episodes of hyperthermia (>38.5°C without apparent cause) at 2–6 weeks of age. The hypertrichosis, which was much less prominent at 2 months of age, is a known side effect of minoxidil therapy in both children and adults, and the condition in this infant was thought to be caused by that drug. The cause of the other defects could not be determined, but a chromosomal abnormality was excluded based on a normal male karyotype (46,XY) determined after a midgestation amniocentesis (5).

It is interesting that captopril (see Captopril) is known to cause structural defects (hypocalvaria or acalvaria) and severe renal toxicity (anuria), but none of the anomalies observed in the above infant have been reported with captopril. The relatively low dose of 50 mg/day (recommended dose 50–150 mg/day) may have protected the fetus from the characteristic renal toxicity observed with angiotensin 1-converting enzyme inhibitors.

Two additional cases of in utero exposure to oral minoxidil were reported to the FDA and published in 1987 (6). The first infant was the product of a 32 weeks' gestation in a 22-year-old woman with severe uncontrolled renal hypertension who was treated during pregnancy with minoxidil, methyldopa, hydralazine, furosemide, and phenobarbital. The 1770-g infant died of congenital heart disease the day after delivery. Defects noted at autopsy were transposition of the great vessels and pulmonic bicuspid valvular stenosis. Hypertrichosis was not observed. No conclusions can be drawn on the cause of the cardiac defects. The second infant, delivered near term and weighing 3220 g, was exposed throughout gestation to minoxidil (5 mg/day) plus metoprolol (100 mg/day) and prazosin (20 mg/day). The mother had severe hypertension secondary to chronic nephritis. Hypertrichosis was evident in both the mother and the newborn, but no other abnormalities were noted in the infant. The excessive hair growth, which was longest in the sacral area, gradually disappeared during the following 2–3 months. Normal development was noted at 2 years of age (6).

Two reports have described the outcomes of pregnancies exposed to topical minoxidil (7,8). A 14 weeks' gestation was diagnosed in a nondiabetic 28-year-old, primigravid, woman who had used minoxidil 2% topical solution to treat hair loss during the 1st trimester (7). Her pregnancy was terminated at 17 weeks' gestation because an ultrasound examination had revealed oligohydramnios, a single umbilical artery, and multiple, severe anomalies. The woman also had experienced a flu-like upper respiratory disease during the 7th to 9th weeks of gestation which had been treated with trimethoprim-sulfamethoxazole (2 tablets twice daily for 2 weeks) and erythromycin (500 mg 4 times daily for 1 week). At termination, no evidence of infection was found, with a negative TORCH (toxoplasmosis, other infections, rubella, cytomegalovirus, and herpes simplex) test. Malformations in the male fetus included a transverse reduction deformity of the lower limbs and pelvis, agenesis of the cloacal membrane, imperforate anus, absence of external genitalia and bladder, renal agenesis, esophageal atresia, tracheoesophageal fistula, hypoplastic left thumb and thenar eminence, 11 ribs and absence of L5, sacrum and pelvis (7). There was no evidence of an amniotic band, and the cause of the malformations remained unknown. Trimethoprim is a folate antagonist and is believed to cause congenital anomalies but not of the type observed in this infant. (See Trimethoprim.) The constellation of defects was thought to represent a severe form of caudal regression syndrome, although the most severe form of this syndrome, the sirenomelia complex, could not be completely excluded (7).

A 28-year-old woman applied a 2% solution of minoxidil on her whole scalp to treat a diffuse bristly hair condition for at least 1 year and throughout her current pregnancy (8). She experienced a brief flu-like syndrome at the 9th week of gestation (maximum temperature 38.5°C). The woman elected to terminate her pregnancy at about 22 weeks' gestation after an ultrasound examination had revealed a fetus with multiple anomalies. The 450-g female fetus had extradural occipital hematomas, funnel-like posterior cranial base, hypoplastic middle cranial base, underdeveloped cerebellar lobes, fourth ventricle dilation, and diffuse intracerebral hemorrhages. Other defects included a globose heart, partial subaortic stenosis, mesentery commune, and a significantly increased length of the sigmoid colon. Histologic examination of the brain revealed multiple areas of necrosis, diffuse areas of white matter demyelinization with reactive gliosis, with capillary agglomerates. There also was dilation and congestion of cerebral small vessels and capillaries. The woman stopped the minoxidil and gave birth to a normal infant 2 years later. The cause of the malformations could not be determined, but the authors thought they were secondary to minoxidil (8).

BREASTFEEDING SUMMARY

Minoxidil is excreted into breast milk (4). Levels in the milk ranged from 41.7 ng/mL (1 hour) to 0.3 ng/mL (12 hours), with milk:plasma ratios during this interval varying from 0.67 to 1.0. No adverse effects were observed in the infant. The American Academy of Pediatrics classifies minoxidil as compatible with breastfeeding (9).

References

1. Product information. Loniten. Pharmacia & Upjohn, 2002.
2. Product information. Rogaine. RxMed: Pharmaceutical Information, 2004.
3. Carlson RG, Feenstra ES. Toxicologic studies with the hypotensive agent minoxidil. Toxicol Appl Pharmacol 1977;39:1–11.
4. Valdivieso A, Valdes G, Spiro TE, Westerman RL. Minoxidil in breast milk. Ann Intern Med 1985;102:135.
5. Kaler SG, Patrinos ME, Lambert GH, Myers TF, Karlman R, Anderson CL. Hypertrichosis and congenital anomalies associated with maternal use of minoxidil. Pediatrics 1987;79:434–6.
6. Rosa FW, Idanpaan-Heikkila J, Asanti R. Fetal minoxidil exposure. Pediatrics 1987;80:120.
7. Rojansky N, Fasouliotis SJ, Ariel H, Nadjari M. Extreme caudal agenesis. Possible drug-related etiology? J Reprod Med 2002;47:241–5.
8. Smorlesi C, Caldarella A, Caramelli L, Di Lollo S, Moroni F. Topically applied minoxidil may cause fetal malformation: a case report. Birth Defects Res A Clin Mol Teratol 2003;67:997–1001.
9. Committee on Drugs, American Academy of Pediatrics. The transfer of drugs and other chemicals into human milk. Pediatrics 2001;108:776–89.

MIRABEGRON

Urinary Tract Agent (Antispasmodic)

PREGNANCY RECOMMENDATION: No Human Data—Animal Data Suggest Low Risk
BREASTFEEDING RECOMMENDATION: No Human Data—Potential Toxicity

PREGNANCY SUMMARY

No reports describing the use of mirabegron in human pregnancy have been located. The animal data suggest low risk, but the absence of human pregnancy experience prevents a more complete assessment of the embryo–fetal risk.

FETAL RISK SUMMARY

Mirabegron is an oral agonist of the human β_3-adrenergic receptor but, at higher doses, also stimulates the β_1-adrenergic receptor. The primary action increases bladder capacity. It is indicated for the treatment of overactive bladder with symptoms of urge urinary incontinence.

The drug is metabolized to inactive metabolites. Plasma protein binding to albumin and α-1 acid glycoprotein is about 71% and the terminal elimination half-life is about 50 hours (1).

Reproduction studies have been conducted in rats and rabbits. No embryo or fetal toxicity was observed in rats given daily oral doses from implantation to closure of the fetal hard palate (gestational days 7–17) that resulted in maternal exposures that were 1–6 times the systemic exposure in women treated with the maximum recommended human dose of 50 mg based on AUC (MRHD). At systemic exposures 22 times the MRHD, an increased incidence of delayed ossification and wavy ribs were observed. These findings were reversible. When the drug was given daily from day 7 of gestation until 20 days after birth, maternal exposures up to 6 times the MRHD had no discernable adverse effects on the offspring. At exposures 22 times the MRHD, a slight but statistically significant decrease in pup survival, as well as a decrease in pup body weight gain were noted. In utero or lactational exposure at exposures 22 times the MRHD had no effect on behavior or fertility of offspring (1).

No embryo or fetal toxicity was noted in rabbits given daily oral doses from implantation to closure of the fetal hard palate (gestational days 6–20) that resulted in maternal exposures similar to those in women at the MRHD. Reduced fetal body weight was observed at exposures that were 14 times exposures at the MRHD. At exposures that were 36 times the systemic exposures at the MRHD, maternal toxicity (reduced maternal body weight gain and food consumption, and 1 of 17 pregnant rabbits died), an increased incidence of fetal death, and fetal findings of dilated aorta and cardiomegaly were reported (1).

In long-term studies in mice and rats, mirabegron showed no carcinogenic potential. Assays for mutagenic and clastogenic effects also were negative. No impairment of fertility was observed in male and female rats given high but nonlethal doses (1).

It is not known if mirabegron crosses the human placenta. The molecular weight (about 397), long terminal elimination half-life, and moderate plasma protein binding suggest that the drug will cross to the embryo–fetus.

BREASTFEEDING SUMMARY

No reports describing the use of mirabegron during human lactation have been located. The molecular weight (about 397), long terminal elimination half-life (50 hours), and moderate plasma protein binding (about 71%) suggest that the drug will be excreted into breast milk. Moreover, the drug is concentrated in the milk of rats (twice the maternal plasma level) (1) and may be in humans. The effect of this exposure on a nursing infant is unknown. The most common (>2%) adverse reactions in adults were hypertension, nasopharyngitis, urinary tract infections, and headache. If the mother receiving this drug is nursing, her infant should be monitored for these effects.

M

Reference

1. Product information. Myrbetriq. Astellas Pharma US, 2012.

MIRTAZAPINE

Antidepressant

PREGNANCY RECOMMENDATION: Limited Human Data—Animal Data Suggest Moderate Risk
BREASTFEEDING RECOMMENDATION: Limited Human Data—Potential Toxicity

PREGNANCY SUMMARY

Although the limited human pregnancy experience suggests that the embryo–fetal risk is low, at least for the more common major defects, additional data are needed to make a better assessment of the overall risk of developmental toxicity.

FETAL RISK SUMMARY

Mirtazapine is a tetracyclic antidepressant in the same subclass as maprotiline. It is chemically unrelated to selective serotonin reuptake inhibitors, tricyclic antidepressants, and monoamine oxidase inhibitors. Mirtazapine is also a potent inhibitor of histamine (H_1) receptors, a property that probably explains the marked sedation often seen with this agent (1).

Mirtazapine has an active metabolite, desmethylmirtazapine. Plasma protein binding is 85% and the mean plasma elimination half-life is 20–40 hours (2).

No teratogenic effects were observed in rats and rabbits given doses up to 20 and 17 times, respectively, the maximum recommended human dose based on BSA (MRHD). However, toxicity was observed in rats at the maximum dose that included an increase in postimplantation losses, increased pup deaths during the first 3 days of lactation, and lower pup birth weights. This developmental toxicity was not observed with a dose that was 15% of the maximum dose (about 3 times the MRHD) (1).

It is not known whether mirtazapine crosses the placenta to the fetus. Because of its low molecular weight (about 265) and prolonged elimination half-life, transfer to the embryo and/or fetus should be anticipated.

A brief 2002 report described the use of mirtazapine in two women very early in gestation (3). The first patient took mirtazapine 60 mg/day and trifluoperazine 8 mg/day in gestational weeks 1–5. The second woman took mirtazapine 30 mg/day for three consecutive days and trifluoperazine 4 mg/day for two consecutive days in the 4th gestational week. In both cases, healthy infants were delivered at term (one female and one male). The infants were followed for 6 months and were developing normally (3).

A 2003 study reported the use mirtazapine in the 1st trimester of 41 pregnancies (4). The pregnancy outcomes were 8 spontaneous abortions (SABs), 8 elective abortions (EABs), 1 unknown outcome, and 24 live births. Four of the live births were premature, one of whom had patent ductus arteriosus. No birth defects were observed (4).

A woman at 15 weeks' gestation with treatment-resistant hyperemesis gravidarum requested termination of her pregnancy because of the severe symptoms (5). Treatment with IV mirtazapine 6 mg/day stopped the nausea/vomiting and she no longer desired termination. After 3 days of IV therapy, she was changed to oral 30 mg/day. The oral dose was weaned over 4 weeks and then stopped. A second course was required at 27 weeks' gestation. Healthy male twins were delivered at 36 weeks' with normal Apgar scores. At 6 months of age, the twins were normal (5). A second report involving three women with intractable hyperemesis treated with mirtazapine resulted in similar outcomes (6).

M

A 2004 report described the pregnancy outcomes of nine women who had taken mirtazapine (doses 30 mg/day in eight, 60 mg/day in one) during the 1st trimester (7). None of the exposures went beyond 12 weeks' gestation. In five cases, mirtazapine was combined with other psychotropic agents and one patient took illicit drugs. The outcomes included one EAB, two SABs, and seven healthy infants that were normal at 12 months of age (7).

An international prospective study compared pregnancy outcomes in mirtazapine-exposed women with two control groups (disease-matched pregnant women with depression taking other antidepressants and nonteratogen exposed) (8). There were 104 pregnancy outcomes in each of the three groups. Mirtazapine was taken in the 1st trimester by 95% of the women with 25% taking it throughout gestation. The outcomes in subjects were 20 SABs, 6 EABs, 1 stillbirth, and 77 live births. Two major malformations were observed (no details provided), but the prevalence was similar to the two control groups. There were significantly fewer live births in subjects compared with nonteratogen-exposed controls and the number of SABs were higher, but not significantly so, in both antidepressant groups. Compared with nonteratogen-exposed controls, the mirtazapine group had significantly more preterm births. There were no significant differences between the groups in terms of EABs, stillbirths, gestational age at birth, or birth weight (8).

A prospective cohort study evaluated a large group of pregnancies exposed to antidepressants in the 1st trimester to determine if there was an association with major malformations (9). The patient population came from the Motherisk database and involved 928 cases that met their criteria. The 928 matched (for age, smoking, and alcohol use) controls were pregnancies not exposed to antidepressants or known teratogens. In addition to the 68 mirtazapine cases, the other cases were 113 bupropion, 184 citalopram, 21 escitalopram, 61 fluoxetine, 52 fluvoxamine, 39 nefazodone, 148 paroxetine, 61 sertraline, 17 trazodone, and 154 venlafaxine. In the antidepressant group, there were 24 (2.5%) major defects compared with 25 (2.6%) in controls (odds ratio 0.9, 95% CI 0.5–1.61). There were two major anomalies in the mirtazapine group: tracheomalacia and vesicoureteral reflux. There were no major defects in the pregnancies exposed to bupropion, escitalopram, or trazodone (9).

BREASTFEEDING SUMMARY

Mirtazapine is excreted into breast milk (9,10). A 27-year-old woman, 3 weeks postpartum, suffered a severe depressive episode with suicidal thoughts and was admitted to a psychiatric hospital (10). She was treated with mirtazapine 30 mg/day while breastfeeding her infant 6 times a day. Maternal blood and milk samples were drawn at steady state 22 and 15 hours postdose. At 22 hours, the maternal plasma level was 7 ng/mL (therapeutic range 5–100 ng/mL) and fore- and hind-milk levels were 7 and 18 ng/mL, respectively. At 15 hours, the three levels were 25, 28, and 34 ng/mL, respectively, and the infant's plasma level was 0.2 ng/mL. No adverse effects in the nursing infant were observed over a 6-week interval while the woman was hospitalized (10).

A 2007 study investigated the excretion of mirtazapine into milk of eight breastfeeding women (11). The median dose was 38 mg/day. The mean milk:plasma ratio based on AUC was 1.1 for mirtazapine and 0.6 for the active metabolite, desmethylmirtazapine. The mean relative infant dose for mirtazapine and the active metabolite were 1.5% and 0.4%, respectively, of the maternal weight-adjusted dose. Only one of the four infants tested had a detectable mirtazapine plasma level (1.5 mcg/L). No toxicity was observed in the nursing infants (11).

Although no adverse effects have been reported, the long-term effects on neurobehavior and development from exposure to this class of agents during a period of rapid central nervous system development have not been studied. The American Academy of Pediatrics classifies other antidepressants as drugs for which the effect on nursing infants is unknown but may be of concern (12).

References

1. Product information. Remeron. Organon, 1997.
2. Mirtazapine. In Sweetman SC, ed. *Martindale. The Complete Drug Reference*. 34th ed. London: Pharmaceutical Press, 2005:307–8.
3. Kesim M, Yaris F. Mirtazapine use in two pregnant women: is it safe? Teratology 2002;66:204.
4. Biswas PN, Wilton LV, Shakir SAW. The pharmacovigilance of mirtazapine: results of a prescription event monitoring study on 13,554 patients in England. J Psychopharmacol 2003;17:121–6.
5. Rohde A, Dembinski J, Dorn C. Mirtazapine (Remergil) for treatment resistant hyperemesis gravidarum: rescue of a twin pregnancy. Arch Gynecol Obstet 2003;268:219–21.
6. Guclu S, Gol M, Dogan E, Saygili U. Mirtazapine use in resistant hyperemesis gravidarum: report of three cases and review of the literature. Arch Gynecol Obstet 2005;272:298–300.
7. Yaris F, Kadioglu M, Kesim M, Ulku C, Yaris E, Kalyoncu NI, Unsal M. Newer antidepressants in pregnancy: prospective outcome of a case series. Reprod Toxicol 2004;19:235–8.
8. Djulus J, Koren G, Einarson TR, Wilton L, Shakir S, Diav-Citrin O, Kennedy D, Lavigne SV, De Santis M, Einarson A. Exposure to mirtazapine during

pregnancy: a prospective, comparative study of birth outcomes. J Clin Psychiatry 2006;67:1280–4.

9. Einarson A, Choi J, Einarson TR, Koren G. Incidence of major malformations in infants following antidepressant exposure in pregnancy: results of a large prospective cohort study. Can J Psychiatry 2009;54:242–6.
10. Aichhorn W, Whitworth AB, Weiss U, Stuppaeck C. Mirtazapine and breastfeeding. Am J Psychiatry 2004;161:2325.
11. Kristensen JH, Ilett KF, Rampono J, Kohan R, Hackett LP. Transfer of the antidepressant mirtazapine into breast milk. Br J Clin Pharmacol 2007;63:322–7.
12. Committee of Drugs, American Academy of Pediatrics. The transfer of drugs and other chemicals into human milk. Pediatrics 2001;108:776–89.

MISOPROSTOL

Gastrointestinal Agent (Antisecretory)

PREGNANCY RECOMMENDATION: Contraindicated (Oral)
Human Data Suggest Low Risk (Term Cervical Ripening)
BREASTFEEDING RECOMMENDATION: No Human Data—Potential Toxicity

PREGNANCY SUMMARY

Misoprostol is a potent uterine stimulant that induces abortion after either oral or vaginal administration early in pregnancy. The drug has been used as an illicit abortifacient and most cases of birth defects have been associated with abortion attempts. However, congenital malformations have also been associated with the therapeutic use of the drug. The teratogenic mechanism appears to be related to the induction of uterine contractions that deform the embryo, resulting in vascular disruption, hemorrhage, and cell death. Investigational and clinical use during the 2nd and 3rd trimesters has demonstrated the utility of misoprostol for labor induction and cervical ripening. Misoprostol appears to be superior, in terms of maternal morbidity and cost, to prostaglandin E_2 (PGE_2) when used for 2nd trimester pregnancy terminations and for cervical ripening.

FETAL RISK SUMMARY

Misoprostol, a synthetic prostaglandin E_1 analog, is used to prevent gastric ulcers induced by nonsteroidal anti-inflammatory agents. It is contraindicated in pregnancy because of the risk of uterine bleeding and contractions that may result in abortion. Although not indicated for such, misoprostol is routinely used for cervical ripening in term pregnancies and for 2nd trimester pregnancy termination.

In reproduction studies reported by the manufacturer, misoprostol was not teratogenic in rats and rabbits at doses 625 and 63 times the maximum recommended human dose (MRHD), respectively (1). At 6.25–625 times the MRHD, dose-related pre- and postimplantation losses and a significant decrease in the number of live pups were seen in rats (1). In another study, teratogenicity observed in pregnant rabbits given doses of 300–1500 mcg/kg on days 7–19 included spinal bifida, caudal vertebral defects, umbilical hernia, and gastroschisis (2).

In a surveillance study of Michigan Medicaid recipients involving 229,101 completed pregnancies conducted between 1985 and 1992, 5 newborns had been exposed to misoprostol during the 1st trimester (F. Rosa, personal communication, FDA, 1993). One (20.0%) major birth defect was observed (none expected)—a cardiovascular defect.

During the initial clinical trials, menstrual complaints were higher among nonpregnant women treated with misoprostol (3.7%) than with placebo (1.7%) (3). In a clinical study designed to assess the effect of misoprostol on the pregnant uterus, 111 women, who had consented to an elective 1st trimester abortion, were treated with either placebo or one or two 400-mcg doses of the prostaglandin. All six of the women who aborted spontaneously the day following treatment had received misoprostol. Uterine bleeding occurred in 45% (25 of 56) of the women treated with misoprostol compared with 4% (2 of 55) of the placebo-treated women (3).

Misoprostol has been combined with the antiprogestogen mifepristone (RU 486) to induce legal abortion (see also Mifepristone) (4–7). Some of the advantages of this prostaglandin analog over similar agents are that it is effective, active by the oral route, inexpensive, and stable at room temperature (4,5). In one study, 40 women were treated with 400 mcg of the drug 7 days before surgical termination of pregnancy (6). Only two of the women from this group had a complete abortion. In a second part of the study, 21 women were given 200–1000 mcg of misoprostol 48 hours after a 200-mg dose of mifepristone, resulting in a complete abortion in 18 women (6). Similar effectiveness was found in a large study published in 1993 involving 895 women who received misoprostol either 4 or 48 hours after a dose of mifepristone (7).

A 1991 reference cited the use of misoprostol as an illegal abortifacient in Brazil (8). The drug is freely available as an over-the-counter product in the country, where abortions are illegal. At one university hospital maternity unit, 20 women sought emergency treatment for uterine bleeding in 1988 after an unsuccessful attempt to induce abortion with misoprostol. In 1990, the number rose to 525. The usual dose consumed was 800 mcg (two 200-mcg tablets orally plus two tablets vaginally), but some women may have taken as much as 9200 mcg (46 tablets) (8).

Five infants with congenital malformations who had been exposed during the 1st trimester to misoprostol in unsuccessful attempts at abortion were described in a 1991 case report (9). The total dose was 1200 mcg in two of the mothers and 400–600 mcg in the other three cases. The five infants had an unusual defect of the frontotemporal region of the skull consisting of an asymmetric, well-circumscribed anomaly of the cranium and overlying scalp, exposing the dura mater and underlying cerebrum. Surgical correction of the defect was attempted within 4 days of birth in each of the cases, but one infant died of severe infection. Although the authors conceded that a later-acting agent was suggested by the nature of the defect, three of the mothers denied any further attempts to terminate their pregnancies after the use of misoprostol (9). In a later publication, two of the authors described more fully the defects of the scalp and cranium in three of the newborns (10).

Two additional reports describing the use of misoprostol as an abortifacient by Brazilian women appeared in 1993 (11,12). In Rio de Janeiro during a 9-month period of 1991, of 803 women admitted to hospitals with abortion complications, 458 (57%) had self-administered misoprostol to induce abortion (11). Most (80%) of these women had used the drug alone. The median dose used was 800 mcg (range 200–16,800 mcg) with 65% taking it orally, 29% orally and vaginally, and 6% vaginally only. The most frequently cited reasons by the women for seeking medical care were vaginal bleeding (80%) and uterine cramps (78%). Only 8% of the women reported vomiting and diarrhea. Morbidity among the 458 women included heavy bleeding (19%) (1% required blood transfusion), infection (17%), curettage required (85%), uterine perforation after curettage (1%), and systemic collapse (1%). In Fortaleza, Brazil, misoprostol use accounted for 444 (75%) of 593 incomplete abortions treated in a hospital by uterine evacuation during 1991 (12). Complications observed in the 444 women included 144 (32%) with infection, 1 with septic shock, 3 with hypovolemic shock, and 1 with uterine perforation.

A 1992 report from Brazil questioned the teratogenicity of misoprostol (13). Since 1990, 29 women had contacted a teratogen information counseling service after unsuccessful attempts at inducing abortion with misoprostol during the 1st trimester. The mean dose used by these women was 4000 mcg (20 tablets), with a range of 200 mcg (one tablet) to 11,200 mcg (56 tablets). The women were monitored with ultrasonography during the remainder of their pregnancies. The results of the pregnancies were: spontaneous abortions (2nd trimester)—3; still pregnant—3; lost to follow-up—6; normal infants—17 (one with preauricular tag). Of the 17 normal infants, 8 were examined by the authors, 4 were examined by pediatricians not associated with the authors, and in 5 cases verbal information was received from the mothers (13). The absence of data for the 9 (31%) cases, however, lessens the ability to interpret this report.

Seven cases of limb defects involving the hands and feet following 1st trimester use of misoprostol (dose range 600–1800 mcg) as an unsuccessful abortifacient were described in a 1993 report (14). Four of the infants demonstrated bilateral palsy of cranial nerves, leading to a diagnosis of Möbius sequence (6th and 7th nerve palsies). An additional five cases (one with limb deficiency, one with limb deficiency and Möbius sequence, and three with Möbius sequence) following failed abortion attempts with misoprostol were appended to the report, but specific details were not given. In the seven pregnancies with sufficient detail, misoprostol exposure was thought to have occurred between 30 and 60 days following conception. The investigators attributed the anomalies to misoprostol-induced vascular disruption (14). In a 1993 invited editorial on the strengths and weaknesses of case reports, the publication of the above research was thought to be valid because the association with birth defects was biologically plausible and there were other reports supporting a causal association (15).

A brief report (16) and abstract (17) suggested that a possible mechanism for Möbius syndrome was flexion of the embryo in the area of cranial nuclei 6 and 7 that resulted in vascular disruption of the region bent. The cranial nuclei 6 and 7 are located in a region of the embryo that would be bent if there was pressure in a cephalocaudal direction. The hypothesis proposed that flexing of the region would result in decreased blood flow and hemorrhage and/or cell death of the cranial nuclei. It was hypothesized that misoprostol-induced uterine contractions early in gestation, before there was sufficient amniotic fluid to cushion the embryo, would cause the flexing if the embryo was correctly positioned. Experiments in rat embryos confirmed that hemorrhage would occur in this region after mechanical flexion in the proposed direction. Although limb reduction defects are often associated with Möbius syndrome and may also be due to mechanical factors, the author's hypothesis could not reasonably explain these defects (16,17).

A 1998 study (18) and earlier abstract (19) compared the frequency of 1st trimester misoprostol use in 96 infants with Möbius syndrome with 96 infants with neural tube defects (NTD). In the 96 infants with Möbius syndrome, there were no differences in the clinical appearance between those exposed to misoprostol ($N = 47$; 46 for attempted abortion) and those not exposed ($N = 49$): bilateral facial-nerve (cranial nerve VII) paralysis, 34 vs. 36; unilateral facial-nerve paralysis, 13 vs. 13; abducens-nerve (cranial nerve VI) paralysis, 39 vs. 37; other cranial nerve palsy, 10 vs. 8; all limb defects, 31 vs. 28; club feet only, 25 vs. 18; limb reduction, 6 vs. 10; orofacial anomalies, 18 vs. 11; mental retardation, 26 vs. 26; other defects, 15 vs. 14 (all *ns*). Misoprostol was used in 47 cases of Möbius syndrome and 3 cases of NTD (odds ratio 29.7, 95% confidence interval [CI] 11.6–76.0). Among the 47 cases of misoprostol use, 20 took the drug orally, 20 took it both orally and vaginally, 3 took it vaginally only, and 4 could not recall how they took the drug. The authors concluded that attempted abortion with misoprostol was associated with an increased risk of Möbius syndrome (18,19).

A 1994 abstract reported a case of a woman who took misoprostol 600 mcg/day for 2 days at 7 weeks' gestation in an unsuccessful attempt to induce abortion (20). An elective abortion at 17 weeks' gestation revealed a male fetus with an omphalocele, left leg below-the-knee amputation, absence of the middle and distal phalanges of four fingers of the right hand with distal fusion by amniotic band, and evidence of early amniotic rupture. Although the mother had had chicken pox at 12 weeks, there was no evidence in the placenta or fetus of viral infection.

The Latin-America Collaborative Study of Congenital Malformations found 12 misoprostol-exposed newborns among 5708 malformed and 5708 nonmalformed matched controls (21). Each of the exposures involved unsuccessful attempts by the women to induce abortion. Four of the infants were in the control group, but the maternal dose (1000 mcg) was known in only one case. Of the eight exposed infants, two had Down's syndrome (doses 1400 and 4000 mcg) and two had minor anomalies (café-au-lait spot on right leg, dose 600 mcg; extranumerary nipple on left, dose 400 mcg). These cases do not appear to be related to misoprostol. In the remaining four infants, the authors characterized the defects as suggestive of misoprostol-induced in utero vascular disruption (maternal dose shown in parentheses) (21):

Missing metacarpals and phalanges; hypoplasia of thumbs and two fingers; partial syndactyly of two fingers; peculiar face with prominent nasal bridge and ocular hypertelorism; weak cry (400 mcg)

Complete bilateral cleft lip and palate; ocular hypertelorism; short limbs; absence of thumbs and 5th fingers; skin tags on one finger; stiff knees; bilateral talipes equinovarus (dose unknown)

Skin scar over T2–T3; no evidence of spina bifida by x-ray (dose unknown) Gastroschisis (1400 mcg)

In a second report from the above group, they found 57 newborn infants exposed to misoprostol among 9653 newborns: 34 in 4673 malformed infants and 23 in 4980 control infants (*ns*) (22). In comparing exposed vs. nonexposed malformed infants, significant differences were measured for four vascular disruption malformations that had been reported by others: arthrogryposis (5.88% vs. 0.73%), hydrocephalus (11.76% vs. 3.04%), terminal transverse limb reduction (8.82% vs. 0.67%), and limb constriction ring or skin scars (8.82% vs. 0.24%). No cases of cranial nerve palsies (e.g., Möbius sequence) were in the registry because these types of defects would not be obvious at birth. Significant associations with two other malformations that had not been reported previously were holoprosencephaly (5.88% vs. 0.34%) and bladder exstrophy (2.94% vs. 0.06%). However, the authors recommended caution in interpreting these latter defects as causal associations. They concluded that there was a causal association between the four vascular disruption defects and the use of misoprostol as an abortifacient (22).

Of note, a 1996 report provided detailed descriptions of three cases of arthrogryposis (i.e., arthrogryposis multiplex congenita; the use of the shorter term, arthrogryposis, implies multiple, nonprogressive congenital joint contractures) after failed mechanical attempts at pregnancy termination (23). The cause of the defect was thought to be vascular disruption resulting in nerve damage that led to fetal akinesia and subsequent contractures (23).

A relative risk of >7.0 for congenital malformations, particularly Möbius sequence, was found among 732 children born after 1990 who were attending 5 outpatient genetic clinics in Brazil (24). About 10% of the children had been exposed in utero to misoprostol. There were 25 cases of Möbius syndrome, 24 cases of reduction of phalanges, and 227 cases with isolated malformations. Associations with misoprostol occurred in 17 (68%), 7 (29%), and 15 (6.6%), respectively, of the cases (24).

A below-the-knee amputation was observed in a female newborn delivered at 29 weeks' gestation because of fetal distress (25). An abortion had been attempted at about 13 weeks' under medical supervision. A single misoprostol tablet (strength not specified) had been inserted vaginally for 4 days, but only some vaginal bleeding had occurred on day 4. Spontaneous rupture of the membranes was documented at about 26 weeks' gestation (25).

A 1998 study proposed that the abnormalities observed in children exposed in utero during the 1st trimester to misoprostol were induced by uterine contractions that caused vascular disruption in the fetuses, including ischemia of the brain-stem (26). Of the 42 infants with congenital malformations, 17 had equinovarus with cranial nerve defects (usually of nerves V, VI, and VII), 10 had equinovarus as part of a more extensive arthrogryposis, and 9 had terminal transverse limb defects. Five children had a distinctive arthrogryposis, without cranial nerve injury, that was confined to the legs. Severe amyoplasia of the legs was confirmed in five children by electromyography, and two of the cases had deficient anterior horn cell activity. Eight had hydrocephalus associated with increased pressure that required shunt placement to relieve. One child had an omphalocele, but no evidence of cranial nerve defects of arthrogryposis (26).

A 1997 abstract and 1999 full report described a prospective, observational cohort study of 86 misoprostol-exposed pregnancies compared with 86 pair-matched controls (27,28). All of the women had called a teratogen information service regarding pregnancy exposure to either misoprostol or nonteratogenic agents. There were no statistical differences between the groups in the rates of major (2/67 vs. 2/81) or minor (7/67 vs. 3/81) malformations, gestational age at birth, prematurity, birth weight, low birth weight, sex ratio, or rates of cesarean section. However, there were more abortions in the exposed group, 17.1% vs. 5.8%, relative risk 2.97, 95% CI 1.12–7.88. The sample size had limited power as it was only able to detect an eightfold increase in the risk of major malformations (28).

A study published in 2000 reported the clinical evaluations of 15 children (8 males, 7 females; average age 2 years) from Salvador and Brazil with misoprostol-induced arthrogryposis (29). Their mothers had taken 400–4800 mcg of misoprostol, orally or vaginally, from 8 to 12 weeks' gestation for attempted abortions. Common pathologic features in the children were growth restriction, underdeveloped bones, short feet with equinovarus, rigidity of joints with skin dimples and webs, neurologic impaired leg movement, bilateral symmetrical hypoplasia or atrophy of limb muscles, and absent tendon reflexes. Twelve had normal intelligence (information not available for the other three). Other abnormalities included neurogenic bladder/bowel (N = 9), hip dislocation (N = 6), upper and lower limb deformity (N = 5), cryptorchidism (N = 2), inguinal hernia (N = 2), and single cases of medullar stenosis/syringomyelia, spina bifida, abdominal muscle hypoplasia, and nail hypoplasia. Neurogenic patterns suggestive of anterior horn cell defects were observed on electromyogram in five children (29).

In another 2000 report, a multicenter, case–control study compared the frequency of misoprostol exposure in 93 children with vascular disruption anomalies (subjects) and 279 children with other types of defects (controls) (30). All of the children were born after 1992. Congenital malformations classified as vascular disruptions in the subject cases were Möbius syndrome (N = 29), transverse limb reduction (N = 27), hemifacial microsomia (N = 16), arthrogryposis

(*N* = 9), microtia (*N* = 9), porencephalic cyst (*N* = 2), and hypoglossia hypodactyly (*N* = 1). Misoprostol exposure (all for attempted abortion) occurred in 32 subject cases (34.4%) compared with 12 controls (4.3%), $p < 0.0000001$. In 16 subjects, misoprostol was used between the 5th and 8th week after the last menstrual period, and in two the exposure occurred after the 1st trimester. There was no difference between the two groups in the misoprostol dose taken. Based on their data, the investigators concluded that misoprostol was associated with vascular disruption defects (30).

A case of maternal misoprostol overdosage resulting in fetal death was reported in 1994 (31). In a suicide attempt, a 19-year-old woman at 31 weeks' gestation ingested 6000 mcg (thirty 200-mcg tablets) and 8 mg of trifluoperazine. She was seen 2 hours later at a hospital complaining of feeling hot, chills, shortness of breath, restlessness, and discomfort. A tetanic uterus was observed, and physical examination revealed her cervix to be dilated to 5 cm with 80% effacement. Fetal movements and heart motion (by sonogram) were absent 1 hour after admission (3 hours after ingestion), and 1 hour later she delivered a stillborn 1800-g fetus that was diffusely ecchymotic. Postmortem examination was remarkable only for diffuse head and upper body bruising (31).

A 2006 meta-analysis reviewed the risk of specific birth defects when misoprostol was used in the 1st trimester (32). The data source consisted of case–control studies through June 2005. The analysis of 4899 cases of congenital malformations and 5742 controls revealed the following odds ratios (OR): any congenital defect OR 3.56, 95% CI 0.98–12.98; Möbius sequence OR 25.31, 95% CI 11.11–57.66; and terminal transverse limb defects OR 11.86, 95% CI 4.86–28.90 (32).

M

Misoprostol has been used for the induction of labor in cases involving intrauterine fetal death (IUFD) or when medical or genetic reasons existed for pregnancy termination (33–35). In 20 cases of IUFD, pregnancy termination was conducted a mean 9.2 hours after the start of oral misoprostol, 400 mcg every 4 hours (mean total dose 1000 mcg) (33). Maternal adverse effects were common. A second study, involving 72 women with IUFD at 18–40 weeks' gestation, used a lower dose (100 mcg) introduced into the vaginal posterior fornix every 12 hours (up to 48 hours) until effective contractions and cervical dilatation were obtained (34). Only 6 women (8%) required treatment between 24 and 48 hours and all had delivered within 48 hours (mean 12.6 hours; range 2–48 hours). None of the women required surgical intervention. Other than one case of abruptio placentae, no complications were observed. A dose of 200 mcg, also administered vaginally, was used in a third study with a comparison group receiving a 20-mg PGE_2 vaginal suppository every 3 hours (35). Successful abortions were obtained within 24 hours in 89% (25 of 28) of women treated with misoprostol and in 81% (22 of 27) of women administered PGE_2 (*ns*). The remaining three misoprostol-treated women had successful abortions within 38 hours (similar data for PGE_2 were not given). Complete abortions (passage of the fetus and the placenta simultaneously) occurred in 43% and 32% of the misoprostol- and PGE_2-treated groups, respectively. Significantly more women experienced adverse effects (pyrexia, uterine pain, vomiting, and diarrhea) with PGE_2 than with misoprostol, and the difference in average cost between the treatments was large ($315.30 for PGE_2 vs. $0.97 for misoprostol). Two other studies have described the use of intravaginal misoprostol (200–800 mcg) to successfully induce legal abortion at gestational ages ranging from 11 to 23 weeks (36,37).

Several reports and communications have described the use of misoprostol for cervical ripening and labor induction in the 3rd trimester (38–44). The doses used were 50–100 mcg administered either as a single dose or at 4-hour intervals, but one group of investigators was studying a 25-mcg dose (43). Tachysystole was observed in some cases, but the uterine hyperstimulation was not associated with an increased incidence of fetal distress or a higher rate of operative deliveries. The American College of Obstetricians and Gynecologists considers low-dose (e.g., 25 mcg) intravaginal misoprostol to be effective for inducing labor in pregnant women who have unfavorable cervices (45,46).

Some authors consider the potential teratogenicity of misoprostol following an unsuccessful abortion attempt a reason to proceed cautiously with the use of the drug for this purpose, particularly in countries with limited medical services (47).

BREASTFEEDING SUMMARY

No studies describing the use of misoprostol during human lactation have been located. The manufacturer considers the drug to be contraindicated during nursing because of the potential for severe, drug-induced diarrhea in the nursing infant (1). Naturally occurring PGE_1, however, is excreted into milk in concentrations similar to that in maternal plasma and may have an important function (e.g., cytoprotection) in the gastrointestinal tract of the nursing infant (48).

References

1. Product information. Cytotec. G.D. Searle, 2001.
2. Clemens GR, Hilbish KG, Hartnagel RE Jr, Schluter G, Reynolds JA. Developmental toxicity including teratogenicity of E_1 prostaglandins in rabbits. The Toxicologist 1997;36:260. As cited in Gonzalez CH, Marques-Dias MJ, Kim CA, Sugayama SMM, Da Paz JA, Huson SM, Holmes LB. Congenital abnormalities in Brazilian children associated with misoprostol misuse in first trimester of pregnancy. Lancet 1998;351:1624–7.
3. Lewis JH. Summary of the 29th meeting of the Gastrointestinal Drugs Advisory committee, Food and Drug Administration—June 10, 1985. Am J Gastroenterol 1985;80:743–5.
4. Anonymous. Misoprostol and legal medical abortion. Lancet 1991;338:1241–2.
5. Baird DT, Norman JE, Thong KJ, Glasier AF. Misoprostol, mifepristone, and abortion. Lancet 1992;339:313.
6. Norman JE, Thong KJ, Baird DT. Uterine contractility and induction of abortion in early pregnancy by misoprostol and mifepristone. Lancet 1991;338:1233–6.
7. Peyron R, Aubeny E, Targosz V, Silvestre L, Renault M, Elkik F, Leclerc P, Ulmann A, Baulieu E-E. Early termination of pregnancy with mifepristone (RU 486) and the orally active prostaglandin misoprostol. N Engl J Med 1993;328:1509–13.
8. Schonhofer PS. Brazil: misuse of misoprostol as an abortifacient may induce malformations. Lancet 1991;337:1534–5.
9. Fonseca W, Alencar AJC, Mota FSB, Coelho HLL. Misoprostol and congenital malformations. Lancet 1991;338:56.
10. Fonseca W, Alencar AJC, Pereira RMM, Misago C. Congenital malformation of the scalp and cranium after failed first trimester abortion attempt with misoprostol. Clin Dysmorphol 1993;2:76–80.
11. Costa SH, Vessey MP. Misoprostol and illegal abortion in Rio de Janeiro, Brazil. Lancet 1993;341:1258–61.
12. Coêlho HLL, Teixeira AC, Santos AP, Forte EB, Morais SM, Vecchia CL, Tognoni G, Herxheimer A. Misoprostol and illegal abortion in Fortaleza, Brazil. Lancet 1993;341:1261–3.
13. Schuler L, Ashton PW, Sanseverino MT. Teratogenicity of misoprostol. Lancet 1992;339:437.

14. Gonzalez CH, Vargas FR, Perez ABA, Kim CA, Brunoni D, Marques-Dias MJ, Leone CR, Neto JC, Llerena JC Jr, Cabral de Almeida JC. Limb deficiency with or without Möbius sequence in seven Brazilian children associated with misoprostol use in the first trimester of pregnancy. Am J Med Genet 1993;47:59–64.
15. Brent RL. Congenital malformation case reports: the editor's and reviewer's dilemma. Am J Med Genet 1993;47:872–4.
16. Shepard TH. Möbius syndrome after misoprostol: a possible teratogenic mechanism. Lancet 1995;346:780.
17. Shepard TH, Lemire RJ. Möbius syndrome: a possible teratogenic mechanism (abstract). Teratology 1996;53:86.
18. Pastuszak AL, Schuler L, Speck-Martins CE, Coelho KEFA, Cordello SM, Vargas F, Brunoni D, Schwarz IVD, Larrandaburu M, Safattle H, Meloni VFA, Koren G. Use of misoprostol during pregnancy and Möbius' syndrome in infants. N Engl J Med 1998;338:1881–5.
19. Pastuszak AL, Schuler L, Coelho KA, Vargas F, Brunoni D, Speck-Martin C, Larrandaburu M. Misoprostol use during pregnancy is associated with an increased risk for Möbius sequence (abstract). Teratology 1997;55:36.
20. Genest DR, Richardson A, Rosenblatt M, Holmes L. Limb defects and omphalocele in a 17 week fetus following first trimester misoprostol exposure (abstract). Teratology 1994;49:418.
21. Castilla EE, Orioli IM. Teratogenicity of misoprostol: data from the Latin-American Collaborative Study of Congenital Malformations (ECLAMC). Am J Med Genet 1994;51:161–2.
22. Orioli IM, Castilla EE. Epidemiological assessment of misoprostol teratogenicity. Br J Obstet Gynaecol 2000;107:519–23.
23. Hall JG. Arthrogryposis associated with unsuccessful attempts at termination of pregnancy. Am J Med Genet 1996;63:293–300.
24. Vargas FR, Brunoni D, Gonzalez C, Kim C, Meloni V, Conte A, Bortolotto E, Almeida JCC, Llerena JC, Duarte A, Albano L, Oliveira S, Cavalcanti D, Castilla EE. Investigation of the teratogenic potential of misoprostol (abstract). Teratology 1997;55:104.
25. Hofmeyr GJ, Milos D, Nikodem VC, de Jager M. Limb reduction anomaly after failed misoprostol abortion. S Afr Med J 1998;88:566–7.
26. Gonzalez CH, Marques-Dias MJ, Kim CA, Sugayama SMM, Da Paz JA, Huson SM, Holmes LB. Congenital abnormalities in Brazilian children associated with misoprostol misuse in first trimester of pregnancy. Lancet 1998;351:1624–7.
27. Schuler L, Pastuszak A, Sanseverino MT, Orioli IM, Brunoni D, Koren G. Pregnancy outcome after abortion attempt with misoprostol (abstract). Teratology 1997;55:36.
28. Schuler L, Pastuszak A, Sanseverino MTV, Orioli IM, Brunoni D, Ashton-Prolla P, Da Costa FS, Giugliani R, Couto AM, Brandao SB, Koren G. Pregnancy outcome after exposure to misoprostol in Brazil: a prospective, controlled study. Reprod Toxicol 1999;13:147–51.
29. Coelho KEFA, Sarmento MVF, Veiga CM, Speck-Martins CE, Safatle HPN, Castro CV, Niikawa N. Misoprostol embryotoxicity: clinical evaluation of fifteen patients with arthrogryposis. Am J Med Genet 2000;95: 297–301.
30. Vargas FR, Schuler-Faccini L, Brunoni D, Kim C, Meloni VFA, Sugayama SMM, Albano L, Llerena JC Jr, Almeida JCC, Duarte A, Cavalcanti DP, Goloni-Bertollo E, Conte A, Koren G, Addis A. Prenatal exposure to misoprostol and vascular disruption defects: a case-control study. Am J Med Genet 2000;95:302–6.
31. Bond GR, Zee AV. Overdosage of misoprostol in pregnancy. Am J Obstet Gynecol 1994;171:561–2.
32. de Silva Dal Pizzol T, Knop FP, Mengu SS. Prenatal exposure to misoprostol and congenital anomalies: systematic review and meta-analysis. Reprod Toxicol 2006;22:666–71.
33. Mariani-Neto C, Leao EJ, Barreto EMCP, Kenj G, Aquino MMA, Tuffi VHB. Use of misoprostol for labor induction in stillbirth. Rev Paul Med 1987;105:325–8.
34. Bugalho A, Bique C, Machungo F, Faúndes A. Induction of labor with intravaginal misoprostol in intrauterine fetal death. Am J Obstet Gynecol 1994;171:538–41.
35. Jain JK, Mishell DR Jr. A comparison of intravaginal misoprostol with prostaglandin E_2 for termination of second-trimester pregnancy. N Engl J Med 1994;331:290–3.
36. Bugalho A, Bique C, Almeida L, Bergström S. Pregnancy interruption by vaginal misoprostol. Gynecol Obstet Invest 1993;36:226–9.
37. Bugalho A, Bique C, Almeida L, Faúndes A. The effectiveness of intravaginal misoprostol (Cytotec) in inducting abortion after eleven weeks of pregnancy. Stud Fam Plann 1993;24:319–23.
38. Margulies M, Perez GC, Voto LS. Misoprostol to induce labour. Lancet 1992;339:64.
39. Sanchez-Ramos L, Kaunitz AM, Del Valle GO, Delke I, Schroeder A, Briones DK. Labor induction with the prostaglandin E_1 methyl analogue misoprostol versus oxytocin: a randomized trial. Obstet Gynecol 1993;81:332–6.
40. Fletcher HM, Mitchell S, Frederick J, Brown D. Intravaginal misoprostol as a cervical ripening agent. Br J Obstet Gynaecol 1993;100:641–44.
41. Sanchez-Ramos L, Chen A, Briones D, Del Valle GO, Gaudier FL, Delke I. Premature rupture of membranes at term: induction of labor with intravaginal misoprostol tablets (PGE_1) or intravenous oxytocin (abstract). Am J Obstet Gynecol 1994;170:380.
42. Fletcher H, Mitchell S, Frederick J, Simeon D, Brown D. Intravaginal misoprostol versus dinoprostone as cervical ripening and labor-inducing agents. Obstet Gynecol 1994;83:244–7.
43. Sanchez-Ramos L, Kaunitz A. Intravaginal misoprostol versus dinoprostone as cervical ripening and labor-inducing agents. Obstet Gynecol 1994;83:799–800.
44. Fletcher H. Intravaginal misoprostol versus dinoprostone as cervical ripening and labor-inducing agents (reply). Obstet Gynecol 1994;83:800–1.
45. Committee on Obstetric Practice, American College of Obstetricians and Gynecologists. Induction of labor with misoprostol. *Committee Opinion*. No. 228, November 1999.
46. Committee on Obstetric Practice, American College of Obstetricians and Gynecologists. Response to Searle's drug warning on misoprostol. *Committee Opinion*. No. 248, December 2000.
47. Fonseca W, Misago C, Kanji N. Misoprostol plus mifepristone. Lancet 1991;338:1594.
48. Shimizu T, Yamashiro Y, Yabuta K. Prostaglandins E_1, E_2, and $F_{2á}$ in human milk and plasma. Biol Neonate 1992;61:222–5.

M

MITOMYCIN

Antineoplastic

PREGNANCY RECOMMENDATION: No Human Data—Animal Data Suggest High Risk
BREASTFEEDING RECOMMENDATION: Hold Breastfeeding

PREGNANCY SUMMARY

No reports describing the use of mitomycin in human pregnancy have been located. Although the doses were not compared with the human dose in terms of BSA or AUC, the drug was teratogenic or embryolethal in three animal species. If the drug is indicated in a pregnant woman, avoidance of the 1st trimester should be considered.

FETAL RISK SUMMARY

Mitomycin (mitomycin-C) is an antibiotic with antitumor activity isolated from *Streptomyces caespitosus*. It is in the same antineoplastic subclass of antibiotics as bleomycin and dactinomycin. Mitomycin is indicated in the therapy of disseminated adenocarcinoma of the stomach and pancreas in proven combinations with other approved chemotherapeutic agents and as palliative treatment when other modalities have failed. It is given as a single IV dose at 6–8-week intervals. The drug is primarily metabolized in the liver, but metabolism occurs in other tissues as well. However, metabolic pathways are saturated at relatively low doses. After a 30-mg IV bolus injection, the serum half-life was 17 minutes (1).

A number of reproduction studies in mice, rats, and dogs have been cited by Shepard and Lemire (2) and Schardein (3). Mitomycin caused either congenital malformations or embryolethality in these species when given during pregnancy (2,3). The studies specified doses based on weight, but apparently did compare them with the human dose based on BSA or AUC.

Mitomycin was carcinogenic in male rats and female mice. At doses approximating the recommended human clinical dose (*assumed to be based on body weight*), the tumor incidence in these species was increased by >100% and >50%, respectively. Assays for mutagenicity and tests for impaired fertility have not been conducted (1).

It is not known if mitomycin crosses the human placenta. The molecular weight (about 334) and the high lipid solubility suggest that it will, but the short serum half-life will limit the embryo–fetal exposure.

A 28-year-old nulliparous woman with squamous cell carcinoma of the uterine cervix was treated with four courses of low-dose mitomycin, cisplatin, bleomycin, and vincristine (4). The therapy produced a complete response. Two years later, she became pregnant and gave birth to a healthy infant.

BREASTFEEDING SUMMARY

No reports describing the use of mitomycin during human lactation have been located. The molecular weight (about 334) and the high lipid solubility suggest that it will be excreted into breast milk, but the short serum half-life (17 minutes) will limit the amount in milk. Because the drug is given as a single IV dose at 6–8-week intervals, pumping and dumping for a few hours after a dose should prevent exposure of a nursing infant.

References

1. Product information. Mitomycin For Injection, USP. Bedford Laboratories, 2000.
2. Shepard TH, Lemire RJ. *Catalog of Teratogenic Agents*. 12th ed. Baltimore: The Johns Hopkins University Press, 2007:297.
3. Schardein JL. *Chemically Induced Birth Defects*. 3rd ed. New York, NY: Marcel Dekker, 2000:567, 574.
4. Kobayashi Y, Aklyama F, Hasumi K. A case of successful pregnancy after treatment of invasive cervical cancer with systemic chemotherapy and conization. Gynecol Oncol 2006;100:213–5.

MITOXANTRONE

Antineoplastic

PREGNANCY RECOMMENDATION: Contraindicated—1st Trimester
BREASTFEEDING RECOMMENDATION: Contraindicated

PREGNANCY SUMMARY

This synthetic anthracenedione, structurally related to doxorubicin, is an antineoplastic antibiotic used in the treatment of acute nonlymphocytic leukemia, refractory lymphomas, and cancers of the breast, ovary, and liver. Reports describing the use of this agent in five pregnancies, all in the 2nd trimester, have been located. Mitoxantrone is toxic to DNA and has a cytocidal effect on both proliferating and nonproliferating human cells (1).

FETAL RISK SUMMARY

The mean half-life of mitoxantrone is 5.8 days (range 2.3–13.0 days) and may be longer in tissue. Moreover, the drug accumulates after multiple dosing in plasma and tissue (1).

Mitoxantrone administration to pregnant rats at a dose 0.05 times the recommended human dose based on BSA (RHD) caused decreased fetal weight and retarded development of the fetal kidney (1). Although not teratogenic in rabbits, a dose 0.01 times the RHD was associated with an increased incidence of premature delivery (1).

Two case reports, both during the 2nd trimester, have described the use of mitoxantrone in human pregnancy (2,3). A 26-year-old woman at 20 weeks' gestation presented with acute myeloblastic leukemia and was treated with an induction course of cytarabine and daunorubicin that failed to halt the disease progression (2). At approximately 23 weeks' gestation, a second induction course was started with mitoxantrone (12 mg/m^2, days 1–3) and cytarabine (days 1–4). Complete remission was achieved 60 days from the start of therapy. Weekly ultrasound examinations documented normal fetal growth. Because of the long interval required for remission, treatment was changed to idarubicin and cytarabine for the consolidation phase. Shortly after the start of this therapy, the woman delivered a 2200-g stillborn infant (gestational age not specified). No apparent congenital malformations were observed but permission for an autopsy was refused. The authors speculated that the fetal death was secondary to the use of idarubicin (2).

In the second case, a 28-year-old woman at 24 week's gestation with acute promyelocytic leukemia was treated with an induction course of behenoyl-cytosine arabinoside (enocitabine; converted in vivo to cytarabine), daunorubicin, and 6-mercaptopurine (3). Following a rapid, complete remission and her first consolidation therapy with cytarabine and mitoxantrone (dose not specified), a cesarean section was performed at 34 weeks' gestation to deliver a healthy 2960-g female infant who was alive and well at 16 months of age (3).

A 1999 report from France described the outcomes of pregnancies in 20 women with breast cancer who were treated with antineoplastic agents (4). The first cycle of chemotherapy occurred at a mean gestational age of 26 weeks with delivery occurring at a mean 34.7 weeks. A total of 38 cycles were administered during pregnancy with a median of two cycles per woman. None of the women received radiation therapy during pregnancy. The pregnancy outcomes included two spontaneous abortions (both exposed in the 1st trimester), one intrauterine death (exposed in the 2nd trimester), and 17 live births, one of whom died at 8 days of age without apparent cause. The 16 surviving children were developing normally at a mean follow-up of 42.3 months (4). Mitoxantrone, in combination with cyclophosphamide and fluorouracil, was administered to two of the women at a mean dose of 12 mg/m^2. The outcomes were two surviving liveborn infants, both exposed in the 2nd trimester. One of the infants was growth restricted (1460 g, born at 33 weeks' gestation after two cycles of chemotherapy) (4).

In a 2009 case report, a woman with relapse of acute myeloid leukemia at 22 weeks' gestation was treated with mitoxantrone, fludarabine, cytarabine, idarubicin, and gemtuzumab ozogamicin (5). The fetus developed signs of idarubicin-induced cardiomyopathy, transient cerebral ventriculomegaly, anemia, and intrauterine growth restriction. The newborn, delivered at 33 weeks' by cesarean section, showed no congenital malformations (5).

Occupational exposure of the mother to antineoplastic agents during pregnancy may present a risk to the fetus. A position statement from the National Study Commission on Cytotoxic Exposure and a research article involving some antineoplastic agents are presented in the monograph for cyclophosphamide (see Cyclophosphamide).

BREASTFEEDING SUMMARY

Mitoxantrone is excreted in breast milk (3). After delivery at 34 weeks' gestation, a 28-year-old woman with acute promyelocytic leukemia in remission (case described above) was treated with a second consolidation therapy course of cytarabine and mitoxantrone. She maintained milk secretion by pumping her breasts during this and a third consolidation course consisting of mitoxantrone (6 mg/m^2, days 1–3), etoposide, and behenoyl-cytosine arabinoside (enocitabine; converted in vivo to cytarabine). The milk concentration of mitoxantrone on the 3rd day of this last course of therapy was 120 ng/mL and was still high (18 ng/mL) 28 days later. Although data on the drug concentration in milk were not yet available, and against the authors' advisement, the patient voluntarily began to breastfeed her infant 21 days after drug administration. Her infant, exposed to mitoxantrone in utero and during nursing was doing well at 16 months of age (3).

Although no adverse effects were observed in the above infant, the long-term consequences of such exposure are unknown. Mitoxantrone accumulates in the plasma and tissue after multiple doses and is slowly eliminated from the body (1). Because of its long elimination time and the uncertainty over the potential toxicity, women who have been treated with this agent should not breastfeed. The American Academy of Pediatrics classifies doxorubicin, an antineoplastic agent structurally related to mitoxantrone, as contraindicated during breastfeeding (see Doxorubicin).

References

1. Product information. Novantrone. Immunex, 2000.
2. Reynoso EE, Huerta F. Acute leukemia and pregnancy—fatal fetal outcome after exposure to idarubicin during the second trimester. Acta Oncologica 1994;33:703–16.
3. Azuno Y, Kaku K, Fujita N, Okubo M, Kaneko T, Matsumoto N. Mitoxantrone and etoposide in breast milk. Am J Hematol 1995;48:131–2.
4. Giacalone PL, Laffargue F, Benos P. Chemotherapy for breast carcinoma during pregnancy. Cancer 1999;86:2266–72.
5. Baumgartner AK, Oberhoffer R, Jacobs VR, Ostermayer E, Menzel H, Voigt M, Schneider KT, Pildner von Steinburg S. Reversible foetal cerebral ventriculomegaly and cardiomyopathy under chemotherapy for maternal AML. Onkologie 2009;32:40–3.

MODAFINIL

Central Stimulant

PREGNANCY RECOMMENDATION: Limited Human Data—Animal Data Suggest Moderate Risk
BREASTFEEDING RECOMMENDATION: No Human Data—Potential Toxicity

PREGNANCY SUMMARY

Only one report, in addition to the nine cases mentioned by the manufacturer, describing the use of modafinil in human pregnancy has been located. The animal data suggest moderate risk, but the limited human pregnancy experience prevents a full assessment of the embryo–fetal risk. Avoiding modafinil during pregnancy is the best course, but inadvertent exposure does not appear to represent a major risk of embryo–fetal harm.

FETAL RISK SUMMARY

Modafinil is a mixture of R- and S-enantiomers and the R-enantiomer, armodafinil, also is available (see Armodafinil). Modafinil is indicated to improve wakefulness in patients with excessive daytime sleepiness associated with narcolepsy. Its pharmacologic profile is not identical to that of sympathomimetic agents. Plasma protein binding, primarily to albumin, is moderate (about 60%). Modafinil is extensively (>90%) metabolized by the liver. After chronic dosing, the elimination half-life is about 15 hours (1).

Reproduction studies have been conducted in rats and rabbits. In rats, doses 10 times the maximum recommended human daily dose of 200 mg based on BSA (MRHDD) given throughout organogenesis were associated with increased resorptions, hydronephrosis, and skeletal variations. No maternal toxicity was observed at this dose. The no-effect dose for these effects was 5 times the MRHDD. Doses up to 4.8 times the MRHDD given to male and female rats before and during gestation had no effect on fertility. In rabbits, no embryotoxicity was observed at doses up to 10 times the MRHDD during organogenesis. However, the sample sizes and doses were inadequate to assess the toxic effects on fertility or reproduction (1). (See Armodafinil for additional animal data.)

It is not known if modafinil crosses the human placenta. The molecular weight (about 273), moderate plasma protein binding, and long elimination half-life suggest that the drug will cross to the embryo–fetus.

The manufacturer cited the outcomes of nine pregnancies that were exposed to modafinil, but few details were given. There were seven normal births, one healthy male infant delivered 3 weeks before the expected range of delivery dates (based on ultrasound), and one spontaneous abortion (woman had history of previous spontaneous abortions) (1).

A 16-year-old primigravid woman with narcolepsy, cataplexy, and glutaric aciduria type II, an autosomal recessive disorder, was treated throughout pregnancy with modafinil 200 mg/day, fluoxetine 20 mg/day, L-carnitine, and riboflavin (2). Because the episodes of narcolepsy and cataplexy increased in frequency, a cesarean section was conducted at 38 weeks' to deliver 2.360-kg infant (sex not specified) with Apgar scores of 7, 8, and 9. No signs of withdrawal or abnormalities in vital signs or behaviour were noted in the infant. The infant was discharged home with the mother after 3 days (2).

BREASTFEEDING SUMMARY

No reports describing the use of modafinil during human lactation have been located. The relatively low molecular weight (about 273), moderate plasma protein binding (about 60%), and long elimination half-life (about 15 hours) suggest that the drug will be excreted in breast milk. The effects of this exposure on a nursing infant are unknown. However, if a lactating woman uses modafinil, her infant should be closely observed for adverse effects that are commonly seen in adults (i.e., headache, nausea, nervousness, anxiety, and insomnia).

References

1. Product information. Provigil. Cephalon, 2004.
2. Williams SF, Alvarez JR, Pedro HF, Apuzzio JJ. Glutaric aciduria type II and narcolepsy in pregnancy. Obstet Gynecol 2008;111:522–4.

M

MOEXIPRIL

Antihypertensive

PREGNANCY RECOMMENDATION: Human Data Suggest Risk in 2nd and 3rd Trimesters
BREASTFEEDING RECOMMENDATION: No Human Data—Probably Compatible

PREGNANCY SUMMARY

The fetal toxicity of moexipril in the 2nd and 3rd trimesters is similar to other angiotensin-converting enzyme (ACE) inhibitors. The use of this drug during the 2nd and 3rd trimesters may cause teratogenicity and severe fetal and neonatal toxicity. Fetal toxic effects may include anuria, oligohydramnios, fetal hypocalvaria, intrauterine growth restriction (IUGR), prematurity, and patent ductus arteriosus. Stillbirth or neonatal death may occur. Anuria-associated oligohydramnios may produce fetal limb contractures, craniofacial deformation, and pulmonary hypoplasia. Severe anuria and hypotension, which is resistant to both pressor agents and volume expansion, may occur in the newborn following in utero exposure. Newborn renal function and blood pressure should be closely monitored.

FETAL RISK SUMMARY

The prodrug, moexipril, is rapidly metabolized to the active drug, moexiprilat. It is indicated in the management of hypertension either alone, or in combination with thiazide diuretics. The active metabolite, moexiprilat, is an ACE inhibitor, thus preventing the conversion of angiotensin I to angiotensin II.

Reproduction studies have been conducted in pregnant rats and rabbits (1). Doses up to 90.9 and 0.7 times, respectively, the maximum recommended human dose based on BSA revealed no embryotoxic, fetotoxic, or teratogenic effects.

It is not known if moexipril or moexiprilat crosses the human placenta. The molecular weight (about 535 for the hydrochloride salt forms) is low enough that transfer to the fetus should be expected.

A retrospective study using pharmacy-based data from the Tennessee Medicaid program identified 209 infants, born between 1985 and 2000, that had 1st trimester exposure to ACE inhibitors (2). Infants of mothers with evidence of diabetes, either before or during pregnancy, were excluded, as were those exposed to angiotensin-receptor antagonists (ARBs), ACE inhibitors or other antihypertensives beyond the 1st trimester, and exposure to known teratogens. Two comparison groups, other antihypertensives (*N* = 202) and no antihypertensives (*N* = 29,096), were formed. The number of major birth defects in each of the three groups was 18 (8.6%), 4 (2%), and 834 (2.9%), respectively. Compared with the no-antihypertensives group, exposure to ACE inhibitors was associated with a significantly increased risk of major defects (relative risk [RR] 2.71, 95% confidence interval [CI] 1.72–4.27). When the analysis was conducted by the type of defect, the highest rates were with cardiovascular defects, 9, 2, and 294, respectively, RR 3.72, 95% CI 1.89–7.30, and with CNS defects, 3, 0, and 80, respectively, RR 4.39, 95% CI 1.37–14.02. The major defects observed in the subject group were atrial septal defect (*N* = 6) (includes three with pulmonic stenosis and/or three with patent ductus arteriosus [PDA]), renal dysplasia (*N* = 2), PDA alone (*N* = 2), and one each of ventricular septal defect, spina bifida, microcephaly with eye anomaly, coloboma, hypospadias, intestinal and choanal atresia, Hirschsprung disease, and diaphragmatic hernia (2).

In an accompanying editorial, it was noted that neither previous reports of 1st trimester exposure to ACE inhibitors nor the animal studies had observed an increased risk of birth defects (3). It also was noted that no mechanism for ACE inhibitor-induced teratogenicity was known. A subsequent communication raising concerns about the validity of the study in terms of adequate exclusion of diabetes, charting and coding errors in busy medical practices, and the effects of maternal obesity (4) was addressed by the investigators (5).

Moexipril and other ACE inhibitors are human teratogens when used in the 2nd and 3rd trimesters, producing fetal hypocalvaria and renal defects. The cause of the defects and other toxicity is probably related to fetal hypotension and decreased renal blood flow. The compromise of the fetal renal system may result in severe, and at times fatal, anuria, both in the fetus and in the newborn. Anuria-associated oligohydramnios may produce pulmonary hypoplasia, limb contractures, persistent patent ductus arteriosus, craniofacial deformation, and neonatal death (6,7). IUGR, prematurity, and severe neonatal hypotension may also be observed. Two reviews of fetal and newborn renal function indicated that both renal perfusion and glomerular plasma flow are low during gestation and that high levels of angiotensin II may be physiologically necessary to maintain glomerular filtration at low perfusion pressures (8,9). Moexipril prevents the conversion of angiotensin I to angiotensin II and, thus, may lead to in utero renal failure. Because the primary means of removal of the drug is renal, impairment of this system in the newborn prevents elimination of the drug resulting in prolonged hypotension. Newborn renal function and blood pressure should be closely monitored. If oligohydramnios occurs, stopping moexipril may resolve the problem but may not improve infant outcome because of irreversible fetal damage (6). In those cases in which moexipril must be used to treat the mother's disease, the lowest possible dose should be used combined with close monitoring of amniotic fluid levels and fetal well-being. Guidelines for counseling exposed pregnant patients have been published and should be of benefit to health professionals faced with this task (6,10).

The observation in Tennessee Medicaid data of an increased risk of major congenital defects after 1st trimester exposure to ACE inhibitors raises concerns about teratogenicity that have not been seen in other studies (3). Medicaid data are a valuable tool for identifying early signals of teratogenicity, but are subject to a number of shortcomings and their findings must be considered hypotheses until confirmed by independent studies.

A 2012 review of the use of ACE inhibitors and ARBs in the 1st trimester concluded that there may be an elevated teratogenic risk, but the risk appeared to be related to other factors (11). The factors, that typically coexist with hypertension in pregnancy, included diabetes, advanced maternal age, and obesity.

BREASTFEEDING SUMMARY

No reports describing the use of moexipril in human lactation have been located. The molecular weight (about 535 for the salt forms of the parent drug and metabolite) suggests that excretion into breast milk should be expected. The effects of this exposure on a nursing infant are unknown. However, other ACE inhibitors are excreted into breast milk and are considered compatible with breastfeeding by the American Academy of Pediatrics (see Captopril and Enalapril).

M

References

1. Product information. Univasc. Schwarz Pharma, 2001.
2. Cooper WO, Hernandez-Diaz S, Arbogast PG, Dudley JA, Dyer S, Gideon PS, Hall K, Ray WA. Major congenital malformations after first-trimester exposure to ACE inhibitors. N Engl J Med 2006;354:2443–51.
3. Friedman JM. ACE inhibitors and congenital anomalies. N Engl J Med 2006;354:2498–2500.
4. Scialli AR, Lione A. ACE inhibitors and major congenital malformations. N Engl J Med 2006;355:1280.
5. Cooper WO, Ray WA. Reply—ACE inhibitors and major congenital malformations. N Engl J Med 2006;355:1281.
6. Barr M Jr. Teratogen update: angiotensin-converting enzyme inhibitors. Teratology 1994;50:399–409.
7. Shotan A, Widerhorn J, Hurst A, Elkayam U. Risks of angiotensin-converting enzyme inhibition during pregnancy: experimental and clinical evidence, potential mechanisms, and recommendations for use. Am J Med 1994;96:451–6.
8. Robillard JE, Nakamura KT, Matherne GP, Jose PA. Renal hemodynamics and functional adjustments to postnatal life. Semin Perinatol 1988;12:143–50.
9. Guignard J-P, Gouyon J-B. Adverse effects of drugs on the immature kidney. Biol Neonate 1988;53:243–52.
10. Brent RL, Beckman DA. Angiotensin-converting enzyme inhibitors, an embryopathic class of drugs with unique properties: information for clinical teratology counselors. Teratology 1991;43:543–6.
11. Polifka JE. Is there an embryopathy associated with first-trimester exposure to angiotensin-converting enzyme inhibitors and angiotensin receptor antagonists? A critical review of the evidence. Birth Defects Res (Part A) 2012;94:576–98.

MOLINDONE

[Withdrawn from the market. See 9th edition.]

MOMETASONE

Corticosteroid

PREGNANCY RECOMMENDATION: No Human Data—Probably Compatible
BREASTFEEDING RECOMMENDATION: No Human Data—Probably Compatible

PREGNANCY SUMMARY

No reports describing the use of mometasone in human pregnancy have been located. The animal data suggest risk, but the observed developmental toxicity is similar to that observed after systemic exposure to other corticosteroids (e.g., see Hydrocortisone). In addition, the animal reproduction studies were not conducted with the inhaled or nasal spray formulation of mometasone. These products are known to have very low systemic bioavailability. Moreover, several large studies involving asthma patients have found no association between inhaled corticosteroids and adverse pregnancy outcomes, such as congenital anomalies (1), intrauterine growth restriction (2), or preterm delivery, low birth weight, small size for gestational age, and major malformations (3). Although mometasone was not included in any of these studies, and allergic rhinitis was not a condition studied, there is no reason to believe that the use of this corticosteroid or the additional diagnosis would have resulted in different outcomes. Because asthma is known to cause maternal and fetal harm, the use of mometasone should not be withheld because of pregnancy. However, beclomethasone or budesonide have been considered the inhaled corticosteroids of choice for use during pregnancy (4).

FETAL RISK SUMMARY

Mometasone is a corticosteroid in inhaled and nasal spray formulations. The inhaled product is indicated for the maintenance treatment of asthma as prophylactic therapy. It also is used to reduce or eliminate the need for oral corticosteroids (5). The nasal spray is indicated for the treatment of the nasal symptoms of seasonal allergic and perennial allergic rhinitis and for prophylaxis in patients with a known seasonal allergen that precipitates nasal symptoms of seasonal allergic rhinitis (6).

The mean absolute systemic bioavailability of a single inhaled 400-mcg dose, compared with a similar IV dose, is less than 1% (5). Plasma concentrations in most subjects were near or below the lower limit of quantitation (50 pg/mL). After administration of the recommended highest inhaled dose (400 mcg twice daily) for 28 days, the mean peak plasma concentrations were 94–114 pg/mL (5). Systemic bioavailability after use of the nasal spray also is low, with concentrations virtually undetectable at the quantitation limit (6). Moreover, any of the drug that is swallowed and absorbed undergoes extensive metabolism in the liver.

Reproduction studies have been conducted in mice, rats, and rabbits but not with the inhaled or nasal spray formulations (5,6). In mice, SC doses less than the maximum recommended daily inhaled dose in humans based on BSA (MRDID-BSA) caused cleft palate. Fetal survival was reduced at doses about equal to the MRDID-BSA. The no-toxicity dose was one-third the dose causing cleft palate. In rats, a topical dermal dose about 6 times more than the MRDID-BSA or higher resulted in umbilical hernia. A dose about 3 times the MRDID-BSA produced delays in ossification, but no malformations. An SC dose about 6 times the maximum recommended daily inhalation dose based on AUC (MRDID-AUC) or less than the MRDID-BSA, given throughout pregnancy or during the later stages of pregnancy, caused prolonged and difficult labor. In addition, this dose reduced the number of live births, birth weight, and early pup survival. These effects were not observed when the dose was halved. In rabbits, topical dermal doses about 3 times the MRDID-BSA caused multiple anomalies including flexed front paws, gallbladder agenesis, umbilical hernia, and hydrocephaly. When given orally in a dose less than the MRDID-AUC, mometasone increased resorptions and caused cleft palate and/or head defects (hydrocephaly and domed head). When the dose was increased to about twice the MRDID-AUC, most litters were aborted or resorbed. The no-toxicity dose was 20% of the dose causing cleft palate and/or head defects (5,6).

It is not known if mometasone crosses the animal or human placenta. The molecular weight (about 513) is low enough for passage, but the very low systemic bioavailability suggests that little, if any, drug will reach the embryo or fetus.

BREASTFEEDING SUMMARY

No reports describing the use of mometasone during human lactation have been located. Other corticosteroids are excreted into breast milk in low concentrations. (See Prednisone.) The molecular weight (about 513) suggests that the drug, if it reached the plasma, would be excreted into breast milk. However, the very low systemic concentrations obtained after use of the inhaled or nasal spray formulations suggest that any excretion into milk will be clinically insignificant.

References

1. Schatz M, Zeiger RS, Harden K, Hoffman CC, Chilingar L, Petitti D. The safety of asthma and allergy medications during pregnancy. J Allergy Clin Immunol 1997;100:301–6.
2. Namazy J, Schatz M, Long L, Lipkowitz M, Lillie MA, Voss M, Deitz RJ, Petitti D. Use of inhaled steroids by pregnant women does not reduce intrauterine growth. J Allergy Clin Immunol 2004;113:427–32.
3. Schatz M, Dombrowski MP, Wise R, Momirova V, Landon M, Mabie W, Newman RB, Hauth JC, Lindheimer M, Caritis SN, Leveno KJ, Meis P, Miodovnik M, Wapner RJ, Paul RH, Varner MW, O'Sullivan MJ, Thurnau GR, Conway DL, for The National Institute of Child Health and Development Maternal-Fetal Medicine Units Network and the National Heart, Lung, and Blood Institute. The relationship of asthma medication use to perinatal outcomes. J Allergy Clin Immunol 2004;113:1040–5.
4. Joint Committee of the American College of Obstetricians and Gynecologists (ACOG) and the American College of Allergy, Asthma, and Immunology

(ACAAI). Position statement. The use of newer asthma and allergy medications during pregnancy. Ann Allergy Asthma Immunol 2000;84:475–80.

5. Product information. Asmanex Twisthaler. Schering Corporation, 2005.
6. Product information. Nasonex. Schering Corporation, 2005.

MONTELUKAST

Respiratory (Leukotriene Receptor Antagonist)

PREGNANCY RECOMMENDATION: Limited Human Data—Probably Compatible
BREASTFEEDING RECOMMENDATION: No Human Data—Probably Compatible

PREGNANCY SUMMARY

Montelukast is not teratogenic in animals, and the few adverse outcomes in humans do not demonstrate a pattern that suggests a common etiology. One source states that montelukast may be safe to use during pregnancy, but this conclusion was based solely on animal studies (1). A 2000 position statement of the American College of Obstetricians and Gynecologists and the American College of Allergy, Asthma and Immunology recommended that montelukast could be considered in patients with recalcitrant asthma who had shown a uniquely favorable response to the drug prior to becoming pregnant (2). The available data support this assessment. The manufacturer maintains a pregnancy registry for women exposed to montelukast. Health care professionals are encouraged to report pregnancy exposures to the registry by calling the toll-free number 800-986-8999.

FETAL RISK SUMMARY

Montelukast, an oral inhibitor of the cysteinyl leukotriene $CysLT_1$ receptor, is indicated for the prophylaxis and chronic treatment of asthma. It is extensively metabolized and plasma protein binding is >99%. Excretion of montelukast and its metabolites is almost exclusively via the bile with a mean plasma elimination half-life of 2.7–5.5 hours (3).

Reproduction studies in rats and rabbits at doses up to about 100 and 110 times the maximum recommended human daily oral dose based on AUC (MRHD), respectively, found no evidence of teratogenicity (1). The drug impaired the fertility and fecundity of female rats at about 70 times, but not at about 20 times, the MRHD. Fertility in male rats was not affected by oral doses up to 160 times the MRHD. No evidence of carcinogenicity was found in long-term animal studies, and assays for mutagenic and clastogenic effects were negative (3).

It is not known if montelukast crosses the human placenta. The drug crosses the placenta in rats and rabbits (3). The molecular weight (about 608) and elimination half-life suggest that transfer to the embryo and fetus should be expected. However, the extensive metabolism and high plasma protein binding should limit the exposure.

The manufacturer maintains a pregnancy registry for montelukast (4). As of July 2009, there were 391 prospective (reported before outcome of pregnancy known) reports of exposure during gestation. The outcomes of these pregnancies were: 3 pending, 140 lost to follow-up, 3 spontaneous abortions (SABs), 2 elective abortions (EABs), and 245 live births (2 sets of twins). Of the live births, 193 were known to have been exposed in the 1st trimester. Congenital anomalies were observed in eight cases, seven in live births, exposed in the 1st trimester: absent left hand (amniotic band deformity); two cases of hypospadias; slight valgus foot deviation; mild chordee; polydactyly (a tiny pedicle [skin] on the small finger of the left hand); multicystic dysplasia of right kidney with compensatory left kidney hypertrophy and hydronephrosis, small congenital hydroceles, and a cleft tongue; and triploidy 69XXY (EAB). There were 11 congenital defects in retrospective reports (reported after the outcome of pregnancy known), 5 of which involved 1st trimester exposures: bilateral sensorineural hearing loss; partial right hand (thumb, three-fourths of the palm and finger nubbins); large hole in heart (exposed in 2nd trimester; no other details); 2 cases of polydactyly; cleft palate; 2 cases of hypospadias (1 required corrective surgery); 3 chromosomal abnormalities (trisomy 18 [SAB], Down's syndrome and fetal alcohol syndrome, and unspecified chromosomal abnormalities [SAB]). When national and international studies were combined, there were six reports of potential limb reduction defects after 1st trimester exposure, two of which are described above. The other four (all from retrospective reports) were: no left hand, left radius and cubitus were incomplete; hypoplasia of distal phalanx of the thumb; missing or hypoplastic fingers, camptodactyly, and syndactyly; and reduction defect of left arm. No additional reports of limb reduction defects were received by the registry from August 2006 through July 2009. A health insurance claims database study with medical record review identified 1535 women dispensed montelukast during pregnancy; none of their infants had a limb reduction defect. The report noted that there was no plausible mechanism by which montelukast could have caused limb reduction defects (4).

A 2007 report described the pregnancy outcomes of 96 women exposed to leukotriene receptor antagonists (montelukast and zafirlukast) (5). The women were enrolled in the Organization of Teratology Information Specialists (OTIS) Asthma Medications in Pregnancy study. Two comparison groups were formed consisting of 122 pregnant women who exclusively took short-acting β_2-sympathomimetics or 346 pregnant women without asthma (control group). Among the 96 subjects, 72 took montelukast, 22 took zafirlukast, and 2 took both drugs. Most subjects (89.6%) were exposed in the 1st trimester and 50% were exposed throughout gestation. There were no differences between the three groups in terms of preterm delivery, Apgar scores at 1 and 5 minutes, birth weight and height ≤10th percentile, or ponderal index <2.2. The adjusted mean birth weight in subject infants was significantly lower than that in infants from controls without asthma, 3384 vs. 3529 g (p <0.05). There were also no significant differences in pregnancy loss (SABs, ectopic pregnancies, and stillbirths), gestational diabetes, preeclampsia, and maternal weight gain. There was significantly (p <0.05) more birth defects in subjects (5.95%) compared with the control group (0.3%), but the prevalence in the control group was abnormally low. There was no significant difference in the prevalence of defects between subjects and those treated with β_2-agonists (3.9%). No birth defects were reported in stillbirths, SABs, or EABs. Birth defects in liveborn infants of subjects (specific exposure not given) were: Sturge-Weber sequence, congenital hip dislocation, bilateral club foot, neurofibromatosis type 1 (an autosomal-dominant inheritance pattern), and imperforate anus. The causes of the other four defects are either unknown or multifactorial, but no specific pattern of defects is evident (5).

A 2009 study enrolled 180 asthmatic pregnant women using montelukast (usually in combination with other drugs such as short- and long-acting β-agonists and inhaled corticosteroids) from six teratogen information services in Canada, Israel, Italy, and the United States (6). The outcomes of these pregnancies were compared with the outcomes from two controls: 180 disease-matched using inhalers and 180 healthy not exposed to any known teratogens. In the montelukast group, 166 (92%) used the drug in the 1st trimester and 56 (31%) continued to use it throughout pregnancy. There were 160 live births (3 sets of twins), 20 (11%) SABs, and 3 (1.7%) EABs (1 for a trisomy 21). The only major birth defect among live births exposed in utero to montelukast was a twin with patent ductus arteriosus, atrial septal defect, and congestive heart failure. There were no statistical differences between the three groups in the number of live births, SABs, and major birth defects, but the number of birth defects in the montelukast and healthy control groups (1 vs. 0) were unusually low. Compared with healthy controls, the montelukast group had lower mean gestational age (37.8 vs. 39.3 weeks) and birth weight (3214 vs. 3425 g) among singleton outcomes. There were also significantly more cases of fetal distress at birth compared with both control groups (25.6% vs. 13.6% vs. 8.7%). However, in a sub-analysis of women who continued to use montelukast until the end of pregnancy, only birth weight remained significantly lower than the healthy controls and that was thought to be due to disease severity (6).

BREASTFEEDING SUMMARY

No reports describing the use of montelukast during human lactation have been located. The molecular weight (about 608) and elimination half-life (2.7–5.5 hours) suggest that the drug will be excreted into breast milk. However, the extensive metabolism and high plasma protein binding (>99%) should limit the exposure. The effect on this potential exposure on a nursing infant is unknown.

References

1. Anonymous. Drugs for asthma. Med Lett Drugs Ther 2000;42:19–24.
2. Joint Committee of the American College of Obstetricians and Gynecologists (ACOG) and the American College of Allergy, Asthma and Immunology (ACAAI). The use of newer asthma and allergy medications during pregnancy. Ann Allergy Asthma Immunol 2000;84:475–80.
3. Product information. Singulair. Merck, 2000.
4. Eleventh annual report from the Merck Pregnancy Registry for Singulair (montelukast sodium) covering the period from U.S. approval (February 20, 1998) through July 31, 2009.
5. Bakhireva LN, Jones KL, Schatz M, Klonoff-Cohen HS, Johnson D, Slymen DJ, Chambers CD, and the Organization of Teratology Information Specialists Collaborative Research Group. Safety of leukotriene receptor antagonists in pregnancy. J Allergy Clin Immunol 2007;119:618–25.
6. Sarkar M, Koren G, Kalra S, Ying A, Smorlesi C, De Santis M, Diav-Citrin, Avgil M, Voyer Lavigne S, Berkovich M, Einarson A. Montelukast use during pregnancy: a multicentre, prospective, comparative study of infant outcomes. Eur J Clin Pharmacol 2009;65:1259–64.

MORICIZINE

Antiarrhythmic

PREGNANCY RECOMMENDATION: No Human Data—Animal Data Suggest Low Risk
BREASTFEEDING RECOMMENDATION: Limited Human Data—Probably Compatible

PREGNANCY SUMMARY

No reports of the use of moricizine in human pregnancy have been located. It is an orally active agent used in the treatment of ventricular tachycardia. The drug is neither teratogenic nor fetotoxic in rats and rabbits at doses up to 6.7 and 4.7 times the maximum recommended human dose, respectively (1).

BREASTFEEDING SUMMARY

The excretion of moricizine in human milk has been documented in one patient (data on file, Roberts Pharmaceutical Corporation, 1993), but no details on the amount in milk or its relationship to maternal levels are available. The clinical significance to the nursing infant is unknown.

Reference

1. Product information. Ethmozine. Roberts Pharmaceutical, 2000.

MORPHINE

Narcotic Agonist Analgesic

PREGNANCY RECOMMENDATION: Human Data Suggest Risk
BREASTFEEDING RECOMMENDATION: Limited Human Data—Potential Toxicity

PREGNANCY SUMMARY

The National Birth Defects Prevention Study discussed below found evidence that opioid use during organogenesis is associated with a low absolute risk of congenital birth defects. Similar to other opioid analgesics, the use of morphine late in pregnancy has the potential to cause respiratory depression and withdrawal in the newborn.

FETAL RISK SUMMARY

Morphine is not teratogenic in rats at a dose 35 times the usual human dose (1).

Bilateral horizontal nystagmus persisting for 1 year was reported in one addicted newborn (2). Like all narcotics, placental transfer of morphine is very rapid (3,4). Maternal addiction with subsequent neonatal withdrawal is well known following illicit use (see also Heroin) (2,5,6). Morphine was widely used in labor until the 1940s, when it was largely displaced by meperidine. Clinical impressions that meperidine caused less respiratory depression in the newborn were apparently confirmed (7,8). Other clinicians reported no difference between narcotics in the degree of neonatal depression when equianalgesic IV doses were used (4). Epidural use of morphine has been reported in women in labor but with unsatisfactory analgesic effects (9). The intrathecal route, however, has provided safe and effective analgesia without fetal or newborn toxicity (10–12).

The Collaborative Perinatal Project monitored 50,282 mother–child pairs, 70 of whom had 1st trimester exposure to morphine (13, pp. 287–295). For use anytime during pregnancy, 448 exposures were recorded (13, p. 434). No evidence was found to suggest a relationship to large categories of major or minor malformations. A possible association with inguinal hernia (10 cases) after anytime use was observed (13, p. 484). The statistical significance of this association is unknown and independent confirmation is required.

Results of a National Birth Defects Prevention Study (1997–2005) were published in 2011 (14). This population-based case–control study examined the association between maternal use of opioid analgesics and >30 types of major structural birth defects. In 17,449 case mothers, therapeutic opioid use was reported by 454 (2.6%) compared with 134 (2.0%) of 6701 control mothers. Indications for use of opioid analgesics were surgical procedures (41%), infections (34%), chronic diseases (20%), and injuries (18%). Dose, duration, or frequency were not evaluated. The exposure period evaluated was from 1 month before to 3 months after conception. Limiting the exposure period to the first 2 months after conception produced similar results. Infants with >1 defect were included in multiple birth defect categories. The following opioids were included (number of cases for each agent not specified): codeine, hydrocodone, hydromorphone, fentanyl, meperidine, methadone, morphine, oxycodone, pentazocine, propoxyphene, and tramadol. The birth defect, total number, number exposed, and the adjusted odds ratio (aOR) with 95% confidence interval (CI) were as follows:

Birth Defect	Total	Cases	aOR (95% CI)
Spina bifida	718	26	2.0 (1.3–3.2)
Any heart defect (20 types)	7724	211	1.4 (1.1–1.7)
Atrioventricular septal defect	175	9	2.4 (1.2–4.8)
Teratology of Fallot	672	21	1.7 (1.1–2.8)
Conotruncal defect	1481	41	1.5 (1.0–2.1)
Conoventricular septal defect	110	6	2.7 (1.1–6.3)
Left ventricular outflow tract obstruction defect	1195	36	1.5 (1.0–2.2)
Hypoplastic left heart syndrome	357	17	2.4 (1.4–4.1)
Right ventricular outflow tract obstruction defect	1175	40	1.6 (1.1–2.3)
Pulmonary valve stenosis	867	34	1.7 (1.2–2.6)
Atrial septal defect (ASD)	511	17	2.0 (1.2–3.6)
Ventricular septal defect + ASD	528	17	1.7 (1.0–2.9)
Hydrocephaly	301	11	2.0 (1.0–3.7)
Glaucoma/anterior chamber defects	103	5	2.6 (1.0–6.6)
Gastroschisis	726	26	1.8 (1.1–2.9)

The authors speculated that the activity of opioids and their receptors as growth regulators during development of the embryo might be a mechanism to explain the above findings. The exposure data were obtained by retrospective maternal self-report; the authors acknowledged that recall bias and misclassification might have affected their results. They concluded that the absolute risk was a modest absolute increase above the baseline risk for birth defects (14).

BREASTFEEDING SUMMARY

Although earlier reports had indicated that only trace amounts of morphine enter breast milk and that the clinical significance of this was unknown (15–17), in a 1990 report, much higher concentrations of morphine were measured in the breast milk of one woman and in her infant's serum (18). A 30-year-old, 75-kg woman with systemic lupus erythematosus and severe arthritic back pain was treated with morphine, 50 mg every 6 hours, during the 3rd trimester and then with tapering doses during breastfeeding. At the time of the study, the normal, healthy 3.5-kg infant was 21 days of age. One day before the study, the dose was 10 mg every 6 hours and then was tapered to 5 mg every 6 hours on the study day. Milk sampling times and morphine concentrations were: 4.5 hours after a dose (before feeding), 100 ng/mL; 4.75 hours after a dose (at end of feeding), 10 ng/mL; and 0.5 hours after a dose, 12 ng/mL (reported as 12 ng/L). A blood sample drawn from the infant 1 hour after a feeding (4 hours after a dose) had a morphine concentration of 4 ng/mL, a close approximation to the estimated therapeutic level. It was presumed that the infant had been exposed to much higher morphine concentrations from the milk before dose tapering and, thus, had higher therapeutic serum concentrations. Using pharmacokinetic calculations, the authors estimated that the infant was receiving between 0.8% and 12% of the maternal dose. No adverse effects of the exposure were observed in the infant (18).

The American Academy of Pediatrics classifies morphine as compatible with breastfeeding (19). However, the long-term effects on neurobehavior and development are unknown but warrant study.

References

1. Product information. Duramorph. Elkins-Sinn, 2000.
2. Perlstein MA. Congenital morphinism. A rare cause of convulsions in the newborn. JAMA 1947;135:633.
3. Fisher DE, Paton JB. The effect of maternal anesthetic and analgesic drugs on the fetus and newborn. Clin Obstet Gynaecol 1974;17:275–87.
4. Bonica JJ. *Principles and Practice of Obstetric Analgesia and Anesthesia*. Philadelphia, PA: FA Davis, 1967:247.
5. McMullin GP, Mobarak AN. Congenital narcotic addiction. Arch Dis Child 1970;45:140–1.
6. Cobrinik RW, Hodd RT Jr, Chusid E. The effect of maternal narcotic addiction on the newborn infant. Pediatrics 1959;24:288–304.
7. Gilbert G, Dixon AB. Observations on Demerol as an obstetric analgesic. Am J Obstet Gynecol 1943;45:320–6.
8. Way WL, Costley EC, Way EL. Respiratory sensitivity of the newborn infant to meperidine and morphine. Clin Pharmacol Ther 1965;6:454–61.
9. Nybell-Lindahl G, Carlsson C, Ingemarsson I, Westgren M, Paalzow L. Maternal and fetal concentrations of morphine after epidural administration during labor. Am J Obstet Gynecol 1981;139:20–1.
10. Baraka A, Noueihid R, Hajj S. Intrathecal injection of morphine for obstetric analgesia. Anesthesiology 1981;54:136–40.
11. Bonnardot JP, Maillet M, Colau JC, Millot F, Deligne P. Maternal and fetal concentration of morphine after intrathecal administration during labour. Br J Anaesth 1982;54:487–9.
12. Brizgys RV, Shnider SM. Hyperbaric intrathecal morphine analgesia during labor in a patient with Wolff-Parkinson-White syndrome. Obstet Gynecol 1984;64:44S–6S.
13. Heinonen OP, Slone D, Shapiro S. *Birth Defects and Drugs in Pregnancy*. Littleton, MA: Publishing Sciences Group, 1977.
14. Broussard CS, Rasmussen SA, Reefhuis J, Friedman JM, Jann MW, Riehle-Colarusso T, Honein MA; National Birth Defects Prevention Study. Maternal treatment with opioid analgesics and risk for birth defects. Am J Obstet Gynecol 2011;204:314–7.
15. Terwilliger WG, Hatcher RA. The elimination of morphine and quinine in human milk. Surg Gynecol Obstet 1934;58:823–6.
16. Kwit NT, Hatcher RA. Excretion of drugs in milk. Am J Dis Child 1935;49:900–4.
17. Anonymous. Drugs in breast milk. Med Lett Drugs Ther 1979;21:21–4.
18. Robieux I, Koren G, Vandenbergh H, Schneiderman J. Morphine excretion in breast milk and resultant exposure of a nursing infant. J Toxicol Clin Toxicol 1990;28:365–70.
19. Committee on Drugs, American Academy of Pediatrics. The transfer of drugs and other chemicals into human milk. Pediatrics 2001;108: 776–89.

MOXALACTAM

[Withdrawn from the market. See 9th edition.]

MOXIFLOXACIN

Anti-infective (Quinolone)

PREGNANCY RECOMMENDATION: Human Data Suggest Low Risk
BREASTFEEDING RECOMMENDATION: No Human Data—Probably Compatible

PREGNANCY SUMMARY

There is limited human pregnancy experience with moxifloxacin. Only two reports have been located and both involved single doses, one report in the 2nd trimester and the other just before delivery, to measure amniotic concentrations and placental passage, respectively. There is no evidence that fluoroquinolones are a major risk of developmental toxicity. Some reviewers, however, have concluded that all fluoroquinolones should be considered contraindicated in pregnancy (e.g., see Ciprofloxacin and Norfloxacin), because safer alternatives are usually available. A 2013 review stated that fluoroquinolones are usually avoided in pregnancy because of concerns for fetal cartilage damage, but there were no human studies to validate this concern (1).

FETAL RISK SUMMARY

Moxifloxacin is a synthetic, broad-spectrum, fluoroquinolone anti-infective agent that is available in oral and IV formulations. It is in the same anti-infective class as ciprofloxacin, enoxacin, gatifloxacin, lomefloxacin, levofloxacin, norfloxacin, ofloxacin, sparfloxacin, and trovafloxacin. About 52% of a dose is metabolized and the plasma protein binding is moderate (30%–50%). Depending on the number of doses and route, the elimination half-life varies between about 8 and 15 hours (2).

In reproduction studies with pregnant rats, oral doses up to 0.24 times the maximum recommended human dose (MRHD) based on AUC (MRHD-AUC) were not teratogenic. At this dose, fetal toxicity was observed, as indicated by decreased fetal body weight and slightly delayed fetal skeletal development. Moreover, in a pre- and postnatal development study, the highest dose (0.24 times the MRHD-AUC) was associated with increases in pregnancy duration and prenatal loss, reduced pup birth weight, decreased neonatal survival, and treatment-related maternal death during gestation. In rats, IV doses that were about 2 times the MRHD based on BSA resulted in maternal toxicity and a marginal effect on fetal and placental weights but no evidence of teratogenicity. In pregnant rabbits given an IV dose during organogenesis that was about equal to the MRHD-AUC (a maternal toxic dose), decreased fetal body weights and delayed fetal skeletal ossification were observed. In addition, there was an increased fetal and litter incidence of rib and vertebral malformations when these effects were combined. No evidence of teratogenicity was seen when cynomolgus monkeys were given oral doses up to 2.5 times the MRHD-AUC, but fetal growth restriction was observed (2).

Consistent with the molecular weight (about 401 for the free base), moxifloxacin crosses the human placenta. In a 2010 study, 10 women scheduled for a cesarean section were given IV moxifloxacin 400 mg over 60 minutes (3). The transplacental passage rate calculated as a percentage of fetal venous concentration to maternal blood concentration was about 75%, whereas the transfetal passage rate calculated as a percentage of fetal arterial drug concentration to fetal venous concentration was about 91% (3).

A second study, by the same group as above, measured moxifloxacin amniotic fluid concentrations in 10 women given a 400 mg oral dose about 2 hours before amniocentesis (4). The study was conducted between the 16th and 20th gestational weeks. The mean concentrations of moxifloxacin in maternal blood and amniotic fluid were 3.53 mcg/mL and 0.27 mcg/mL, respectively; a amniotic fluid passage rate of about 8% (4).

BREASTFEEDING SUMMARY

No reports describing the use of moxifloxacin in human lactation have been located. The molecular weight (about 401 for the free base), moderate metabolism (52%) and plasma protein binding (30%–50%), and long elimination half-life (about 8–15 hours) suggest that the agent will be excreted into breast milk. The effect of this exposure on a nursing infant is unknown. However, two other fluoroquinolones are classified as compatible with breastfeeding by the American Academy of Pediatrics (see Ciprofloxacin and Ofloxacin).

References

1. Meaney-Delman D, Rasmussen SA, Beigi RH, Zotti ME, Hutchings Y, Bower WA, Treadwell TA, Jamieson DJ. Prophylaxis and treatment of anthrax in pregnant women. Obstet Gynecol 2013;122:885–900.
2. Product information. Avelox. Schering Plough, 2013.
3. Ozyuncu O, Nemutlu E, Katlan D, Kir S, Beksac MS. Maternal and fetal blood levels of moxifloxacin, levofloxacin, cefepime and cefoperazone. Int J Antimicrob Agents 2010;36:175–8.
4. Ozyuncu O, Beksac MS, Nemutlu E, Katlan D, Kir S. Maternal blood and amniotic fluid levels of moxifloxacin, levofloxacin and cefixime. J Obstet Gynecol 2010;36:484–7.

MUPIROCIN

Antibiotic

PREGNANCY RECOMMENDATION: No Human Data—Probably Compatible
BREASTFEEDING RECOMMENDATION: No Human Data—Probably Compatible

PREGNANCY SUMMARY

No reports describing the use of any of the three mupirocin formulations in human pregnancy have been located. The animal data and the minimal systemic concentrations in humans suggest that the embryo–fetal risk, if it exists at all, is probably nil.

FETAL RISK SUMMARY

Mupirocin is an antibacterial agent produced by fermentation from *Pseudomonas fluorescens*. It is active against many gram-positive bacteria, including methicillin-resistant *Staphylococcus aureus* (MRSA), and some gram-negative bacteria. Mupirocin is bactericidal at concentrations achieved by topical application. Mupirocin cream is indicated for the treatment of secondarily infected traumatic skin lesions (up to 10 cm in length or 100 cm^2 in area) due to susceptible strains of *S. aureus* and *Streptococcus pyogenes*. The ointment formulation is indicated for the topical treatment of impetigo due to *S. aureus* and *S. pyogenes*, whereas the nasal spray is indicated for the eradication of nasal colonization with MRSA in adult patients and health care workers (1).

Minimal amounts of mupirocin are absorbed into the systemic circulation after use of cream, but not after use of the ointment. For the nasal spray, the extrapolated systemic exposure, based on the concentration of the inactive metabolite monic acid in urine, was 3.3% of the dose. Any antibiotic reaching the circulation is rapidly metabolized to monic acid that is excreted in the urine. The elimination half-lives of mupirocin and monic acid after IV administration in healthy adults were 20–40 and 30–80 minutes, respectively (1).

Reproduction studies have been conducted in rats and rabbits. During pregnancy in these species, SC doses up to 78 and 154 times, respectively, the daily human topical dose of the cream based on BSA revealed no evidence of fetal harm. For the ointment, the dose comparisons were 22 and 43 times, respectively, the daily human topical dose based on BSA and, for the nasal spray, 65 and 130 times, respectively, the daily human intranasal dose based on BSA (1).

Studies for carcinogenicity have not been conducted with mupirocin. Multiple assays for mutagenicity were negative. SC doses in male and female rats revealed no evidence of impaired fertility or reproductive performance (1).

It is not known if mupirocin crosses the human placenta. The molecular weight of the free acid (about 501) is low enough for passage, but the minimal plasma concentrations and rapid metabolism and elimination suggest that clinically significant amounts of the antibiotic will not reach the embryo or the fetus.

BREASTFEEDING SUMMARY

No reports describing the use of mupirocin during human lactation have been located. The molecular weight of the free acid (about 501) is low enough for excretion into breast milk, but the minimal plasma concentrations and rapid metabolism and elimination suggest that clinically significant amounts of the antibiotic will not reach the milk.

Reference

1. Product information. Bactroban. GlaxoSmithKline, 2004.

MUROMONAB-CD3

Immunologic Agent (Immunosuppressant)

PREGNANCY RECOMMENDATION: Compatible—Maternal Benefit >> Embryo–Fetal Risk
BREASTFEEDING RECOMMENDATION: Contraindicated

M

PREGNANCY SUMMARY

No reports describing the use of muromonab-CD3 in pregnancy have been located. The absence of animal and human data prevents an assessment of the risk to the embryo or fetus. If the antibody crosses the placenta, the effects of cytokine release and immunosuppression in the embryo or fetus are unknown. Preterm delivery is a potential complication because there are increased amniotic fluid levels of cytokines in women with intra-amniotic infections and subsequent preterm labor (1). The manufacturer lists known or suspected pregnancy as a contraindication to the use of this agent (2). Nonetheless, if a pregnant woman's condition requires muromonab-CD3, and there are no alternatives, the maternal benefit appears to outweigh the unknown embryo or fetal effects.

FETAL RISK SUMMARY

The immunosuppressant muromonab-CD3 is a murine monoclonal antibody to the CD3 antigen of human T cells. It is an IgG_{2a} immunoglobulin that is given IV. Muromonab-CD3 is indicated for the treatment of acute allograft rejection in renal transplant patients. It is also indicated for the treatment of steroid-resistant acute allograft rejection in cardiac and hepatic transplant patients.

Neither the effects on reproduction nor the carcinogenic potential has been studied in animals (2) .

The placental passage of muromonab-CD3 has not been studied. However, because it is an IgG antibody, it may cross the placenta (2).

BREASTFEEDING SUMMARY

No reports describing the use of muromonab-CD3 during lactation have been located. As an IgG antibody, it probably is excreted into breast milk. The effects of this exposure on a nursing infant are unknown, but it might be broken down to its constituent amino acids or fragments thereof in the infant's digestive tract. However, the adverse effects observed in adults during clinical trials involved most body systems and may be severe (2). In addition, the manufacturer lists breastfeeding as a contraindication to the use of muromonab-CD3 (2). Because of the potential for severe toxicity in a nursing infant, women who require this agent should not breastfeed.

References

1. Norwitz ER, Robinson JN, Challis JRG. The control of labor. N Engl J Med 1999;341:660–6.
2. Product information. Orthoclone OKT 3. Ortho Biotech Products, 2005.

MYCOPHENOLATE

Immunologic Agent (Immunosuppressive)

PREGNANCY RECOMMENDATION: Human and Animal Data Suggest Risk
BREASTFEEDING RECOMMENDATION: Contraindicated

PREGNANCY SUMMARY

The use of mycophenolate mofetil (MMF) during early pregnancy is associated with spontaneous abortions (SABs) and major birth defects that may represent a characteristic phenotype. Specific malformations involved the external ear, facial anomalies, cleft lip/palate, and defects of the distal limbs, heart, esophagus, and kidney. The animal data for both MMF and mycophenolate sodium also suggest risk of embryo–fetal death and structural defects. Although all of the reported adverse pregnancy outcomes involved MMF, the lack of reports with mycophenolate sodium is probably due to its later availability. MMF was approved by the FDA in 1995, whereas mycophenolate sodium was approved in 2004. The embryo–fetal toxicity of the two agents probably is similar. Indeed, the manufacturer of mycophenolate sodium states that there are no relevant qualitative or quantitative differences in the teratogenic potential of the two products (1). More data are needed to confirm the full spectrum of defects and especially its magnitude, but women of childbearing potential should be informed of the risks, and both agents should be avoided during pregnancy (1–3). The manufacturers recommend that women of reproductive potential should use effective contraception before and during therapy and for 6 weeks after therapy is stopped (1,2). However, the apparent half-lives suggest that a shorter waiting period might be appropriate. If mycophenolate is used in pregnancy, health care professionals are encouraged to call the toll-free number 877-311-8972 for information about patient enrollment in an Organization of Teratology Information Specialists (OTIS) study.

FETAL RISK SUMMARY

Mycophenolate is a purine synthesis inhibitor that is used as an immunosuppressant agent in the prophylaxis of organ rejection in patients receiving allogeneic renal and liver transplants (1,2,4). It is available as MMF (the 2-morpholinoethyl ester of mycophenolic acid) and mycophenolate sodium. Following oral administration, mycophenolate mofetil undergoes rapid and complete metabolism to mycophenolic acid (MPA), the active moiety. MPA is further metabolized to an inactive metabolite, the phenolic glucuronide of MPA (MPAG). Both MPA and MPAG are bound to plasma albumin, 97% and 82%, respectively. The mean apparent half-life of MPA when mycophenolate mofetil is used is 17.9 hours (2), whereas it ranges between 8 and 16 hours when mycophenolate sodium is taken (1).

Reproductive studies have been conducted in rats and rabbits. In both species, in the absence of maternal toxicity, fetal resorptions and malformations were observed at MMF doses that were 0.03–0.92 times the recommended clinical dose in renal transplant recipients based on BSA (RCD-R) and 0.02–0.61 times the recommended clinical dose in cardiac transplant recipients based on BSA (RCD-C). In rats, a dose 0.02 times the RCD-R or 0.1 times the RCD-C produced malformations, principally of the head and eyes (2). Similar results have been observed with mycophenolate sodium (1).

In 2-year studies, mycophenolate was not carcinogenic in mice and rats but was genotoxic in two of five assays. The drug had no adverse effects on fertility or reproductive performance in male and female rats (2).

It is not known if MPA crosses the human placenta to the embryo–fetus. The molecular weight of MPA (about 319) and the moderately long elimination half-life suggest that exposure of the embryo–fetus will occur. The animal and human data support this assessment.

A 2001 case report described the use of MMF during pregnancy (5). The 33-year-old woman, with an unknown pregnancy at the time of surgery, had received a renal transplant at about 6–7 weeks' gestation. Postoperatively, she had been treated with MMF, tacrolimus, corticosteroids, cefepime, and vancomycin. After discharge from the hospital, she was maintained on acyclovir, nifedipine, trimethoprim/sulfamethoxazole, tacrolimus (14 mg/day), MMF (2 g/day), and prednisone (25 mg/day). The pregnancy was diagnosed on posttransplant day 100, at which time the two anti-infectives were discontinued and the MMF dose reduced to 1 g/day. The woman delivered a 2250-g female infant at about 34 weeks' with Apgar scores of 5 and 8 at 1 and 5 minutes, respectively. The birth weight, length, and head circumference were at the 75th, 75th–90th, and 10th–25th percentile, respectively. The infant had hypoplastic fingernails and toenails and shortened fifth fingers bilaterally. An aberrant blood vessel between the trachea and esophagus was found later. The infant was hospitalized 3 times during her first year with pneumonia (thought to have been due in part to aspiration of stomach contents). Since then, the child has been healthy and growing and developing normally at 3 years of age (5).

Severe congenital malformations were detailed in a 2004 case report (6). A 27-year-old woman had received a renal transplant 2 years before her pregnancy and had been maintained on MMF (500 mg/day), tacrolimus (9 mg/day), and prednisone (15 mg/day). Her pregnancy was diagnosed at 13 weeks' gestation. At this time, azathioprine (50 mg/day) was substituted for MMF. Multiple malformations were detected at 22 weeks, and the pregnancy was terminated. Defects included complete agenesis of the corpus callosum, cleft lip/palate, micrognathia, ocular hypertelorism, microtia and external auditory duct atresia, and a left pelvic ectopic kidney. The fetus had a normal male karyotype. One year later, the woman had another pregnancy and delivered a normal 2640-g male infant who was growing and developing normally at follow-up. During this pregnancy, she had been maintained on azathioprine, tacrolimus, and prednisone (6).

A renal transplant unit in Spain reported the outcomes of 43 pregnancies in 35 recipients of a renal transplant that had occurred during 1976–2004 (7). Four of the pregnancies were exposed to MMF and sirolimus. In 1996, immunotherapy with these agents was stopped before conception and replaced with other immunosuppressants, such as cyclosporine, azathioprine, tacrolimus, and corticosteroids. There were 9 SABs, 10 elective abortions (EABs), and 24 successful pregnancies with healthy newborns (7).

A report from the National Transplantation Pregnancy Registry (NTPR) was published in 2005 (8). MMF was used in 26 pregnancies in 18 women who had received a kidney transplant. However, only 10 pregnancies were exposed to MMF throughout gestation, whereas in 16, the dose was decreased, discontinued, or changed to azathioprine. MMF also was used in three pregnancies in three women after a liver transplant, and three pregnancies in two women after a heart transplant. In the kidney transplant group, one or more immunosuppressants were combined with MMF. These agents were cyclosporine (N = 5), tacrolimus (N = 13), sirolimus (N = 1), and prednisone (N = 15). The pregnancy outcomes in this group were 11 SABs (61%) and 15 live births. Congenital malformations were observed in four newborns delivered from four women (exposures in addition to MMF shown in parentheses): hypoplastic nails with shortened fifth fingers (tacrolimus and prednisone) (*might be the same case described in reference 4*); cleft lip and palate, microtia (tacrolimus, sirolimus, and prednisone); multiple malformations, infant died on day 1 (tacrolimus and prednisone); and microtia (tacrolimus and prednisone). In the liver transplant group, there was one SAB (also exposed to tacrolimus), and two live births without defects (also exposed to tacrolimus and prednisone in one and tacrolimus in one). MMF was discontinued in two pregnancies, one with a live birth and the other with an SAB (8).

In the heart transplant group, the pregnancy of one woman ended in an SAB, as did the first pregnancy of a second woman. In her second pregnancy, the latter woman had a live birth without defects. All three pregnancies also were exposed to tacrolimus. The combined outcomes of the 32 pregnancies were 14 SABs (44%), 14 live births (44%) without defects, and 4 newborns (4 of 18; 22%) with birth defects. The average gestational age for the live births was 35.6 weeks (range 31–39), and the average birth weight was 2397 g (range 822–3487 g) (8).

A second report from the NTPR, published in 2006, described the same pregnancy outcomes of the 26 pregnancies after kidney transplant but with additional details on the dose and timing of the exposures (9). MMF was continued in 11 pregnancies, not 10 as stated above, and the dose was decreased in 1, discontinued in 9, changed to azathioprine in 4, or changed to sirolimus in 1. Additional details were available on two of the four newborns with birth defects. The infant with cleft lip/palate and microtia had surgical repair of the clefts and, except for the need for bone conduction hearing aids, was doing well at 4 years of age. The multiple defects in the infant who died at 1 day of age were cleft lip/palate, congenital diaphragmatic hernia, and congenital heart defects. The defects might have been associated with Fryn's syndrome, an autosomal recessive anomaly (8). In addition to the six liver or heart transplants mentioned in the 2005 report, an SAB at 6 weeks occurred in a seventh woman that had been treated with MMF, tacrolimus, and prednisone after a kidney–pancreas transplant. There were 15 SABs (45%) in the combined 33 pregnancies and 4 (22%) of the 18 liveborn infants had birth defects. The authors noted the higher incidence of birth defects in those exposed to MMF compared with the overall incidence observed in kidney transplant recipient offspring (9).

A brief 2006 report from the Sindh Institute of Urology and Transplantation in Pakistan described 47 pregnancy outcomes from 31 women after kidney transplant (10). All of the women received cyclosporine and prednisone, 82% also received azathioprine, and four had MMF added. There were 7 SABs (15%), 2 EABs, 6 preterm infants, and 32 full-term newborns. The specific therapy in the pregnancies of these outcomes was not mentioned, but none of the 38 live births had a birth defect (10).

A 36-year-old woman, 4 years after a kidney transplant, was treated with MMF and prednisolone throughout gestation (11). The woman had a history of psychoses that were treated with diazepam and haloperidol from the 4th month of pregnancy. In the last months of her pregnancy (exact dates not specified), she received darbepoetin alfa for anemia and methyldopa for hypertension. Because of fetal distress, a cesarean section was performed at 35 weeks' gestation to deliver a 2330-g male infant with Apgar scores of 5, 8, and 8 at 1, 5, and 10 minutes, respectively. Abnormalities found in the infant were severe anemia, nonimmune hydrops fetalis, and a malformed right ear. An infectious disease workup was negative. The infant had a normal 46,XY karyotype. Myoclonic movements of both arms and legs were attributed to withdrawal from diazepam and haloperidol. A magnetic resonance imaging scan of the cerebrum revealed a complete absence of the right auditory pathway, without other defects. Unable to find any other causes, the authors attributed the anemia and resulting hydrops fetalis and the ear malformation to MMF (11).

A 21-year-old woman with lupus nephritis had been treated with two 6-month courses of cyclophosphamide separated by 2 years (12). She had been on MMF (2000 mg/day) maintenance therapy for 10 months when pregnancy was diagnosed at 25 weeks' gestation. She also was receiving prednisone, hydroxychloroquine, and perindopril. The pregnancy was terminated because of multiple malformations. The fetus had a normal karyotype. Malformations affected the head (bilateral anotia, external auditory duct atresia), lower limb (polydactylia and nail hypoplasia), heart (anterior positioning of the aorta, interventricular communication), and kidneys (asymmetric) (12).

A 2008 case report described the pregnancy outcome of a woman, with systemic lupus erythematosus involving the kidney, who had been treated with cyclophosphamide and MMF before conception, and then with MMF (1500 mg/day) until pregnancy was diagnosed at 8 2/7 weeks' gestation (13). MMF was then discontinued and azathioprine 100 mg/day was started. The pregnancy was electively terminated at 17 weeks because of major congenital anomalies. The chromosomally normal female fetus (46,XX) had a large square skull with extension of facial clefts that resulted in an almost complete defect of the midface in the presence of severe mandibulofacial dysostosis and ophthalmic anomalies. Preaxial limb defects with digitalization of the thumbs also were observed, as was hypoplasia of the thymus and lungs, a subaortic ventricular septal defect with overriding common truncus arteriosus of the heart, an aberrant right subclavian artery, a single umbilical artery, esophageal atresia with tracheoesophageal fistula, left renal agenesis with ipsilateral streak gonad, agenesis of the corpus callosum, and mild hydrocephaly (13).

A woman with lupus nephritis took MMF (1000 mg/day) and adalimumab (40 mg every other week) during the first 8 weeks of pregnancy (14). She underwent a cesarean section for transverse position at 32 weeks' gestation to give birth to a 4422-g female infant with normal karyotype (46,XX). The infant had multiple birth defects including arched eyebrows, hypertelorism, epicanthic folds, micrognathia, thick everted lower lip, cleft palate, bilateral microtia with aural atresia, congenital tracheomalacia, and brachydactyly. Shortly after birth, a tracheostomy was done for respiratory distress and a G-tube was placed because of feeding difficulties. The cleft palate was repaired surgically. At 20 months of age, the infant had normal growth and slightly delayed motor development. The tracheostomy was still required as were G-tube feedings. She seemed to have some hearing, but had significant expressive speech delay. The defects were attributed to MMF (14).

The 10-year experience of a renal transplant center in Iran was reported in 2008 (15). A total of 61 pregnancies were reported in 53 patients. In 38 patients (72%), immunosuppressive therapy consisted of MMF, cyclosporine, and prednisolone, whereas in 15 patients (28%), therapy was azathioprine, cyclosporine, and prednisone. Adverse outcomes included 11 small-for-gestational-age newborns, 1 infant with a club foot, and 1 infant with a large facial hemangioma. Early neonatal death occurred in four infants, one from extreme prematurity. There were no significant differences in outcomes between the MMF- and azathioprine-treated groups (15).

Additional evidence that MMF exposure during the 1st trimester is associated with a recognizable phenotype was presented in a 2008 report (16). A 25-year-old Spanish woman became pregnant for the first time 2 years after receiving her second renal transplant. Immunosuppressive therapy consisted of MMF 500 mg/day and tacrolimus 12 mg/day until pregnancy was diagnosed at 10 weeks. MMF was discontinued while tacrolimus was continued until delivery by cesarean section at 41 weeks. The infant, with a normal 46,XX female karyotype, weighed 3050 g with a length of 52 cm and a head circumference of 33.5 cm. Structural anomalies evident at birth were a bilateral upper cleft lip with complete cleft palate, bilateral microtia, hypertelorism, micrognathia, and mild left ptosis. Later examinations revealed a large chorioretinal coloboma in both eyes, bilateral absence of external ear canals, and small tympanic cavities with abnormal auditory ossicles. Bilateral conductive hearing loss was diagnosed. At 9 months of age, the infant wore hearing aids, but her physical and neurodevelopment were normal for her age. The authors considered the abnormalities to be a characteristic phenotype caused by exposure to MMF (16).

In October 2007, the manufacturer of MMF and the FDA reported that postmarketing data from the NTPR and the Roche worldwide adverse-event reporting system had revealed that 1st trimester use of MMF was associated with pregnancy loss and an increased risk of congenital malformations (17). The FDA risk category was changed from C to D. The specific malformations involved the external ear, facial anomalies, including cleft lip/palate, and anomalies of the distal limbs, heart, esophagus, and kidney (17).

BREASTFEEDING SUMMARY

No reports describing the use of MMF or mycophenolate sodium during human lactation have been located. The relatively low molecular weight of MPA (about 319), the active metabolite of MMF, and its moderately long elimination half-lives (17.9 hours when MMF is taken and 8–16 hours when mycophenolate sodium is used) suggest that excretion of MPA into breast milk should be expected. There is a potential for serious adverse effects in a nursing infant, including an increased frequency of infections and the possible development of lymphoma that has been observed in adults. Until human data are available, MMF and mycophenolate sodium should be classified as contraindicated during breastfeeding.

References

1. Product information. Myfortic. Novartis Pharmaceuticals, 2004.
2. Product information. CellCept. Roche Pharmaceuticals, 2007.
3. Pisoni CN, D'Cruz DP. The safety of mycophenolate mofetil in pregnancy. Expert Opin Drug Saf 2008;7:219–22.
4. Casele HL, Laifer SA. Pregnancy after liver transplantation. Semin Perinatol 1998;22:149–55.
5. Pergola PE, Kancharla A, Riley DJ. Kidney transplantation during the first trimester of pregnancy: immunosuppression with mycophenolate mofetil, tacrolimus, and prednisone. Transplantation 2001;71:994–7.
6. Le Ray C, Coulomb A, Elefant E, Frydman R, Audibert F. Mycophenolate mofetil in pregnancy after renal transplantation: a case of major fetal malformations. Obstet Gynecol 2004;103:1091–4.
7. Gutierrez MJ, Acebedo-Ribo M, Garcia-Donaire JA, Manzanera MJ, Molina A, Gonzalez E, Nungaray N, Andres A, Morales JM. Pregnancy in renal transplant recipients. Transplant Proc 2005;37:3721–2.
8. Armenti VT, Radomski JS, Moritz MJ, Gaughan WJ, Gulati R, McGrory CH, Coscia LA. Report from the National Transplantation Pregnancy Registry (NTPR): outcomes of pregnancy after transplantation. Clin Transpl 2005: 69–83.
9. Sifontis NM, Coscia LA, Constantinescu S, Lavelanet AF, Moritz MJ, Armenti VT. Pregnancy outcomes in solid organ transplant recipients with exposure to mycophenolate mofetil or sirolimus. Transplantation 2006;82:1698–702.
10. Naqvi R, Nor H, Ambaries S, Khan H, Halder A, Jeri N, Alam A, Asia R, Manor K, Asia T, Ahmed E, Akhter F, Naqvi A, Rive A. Outcome of pregnancy in renal allograft recipients: SIUT experience. Transplant Proc 2006;38:2001–2.
11. Tjeertes IFA, Bastiaans DET, van Ganzewinkel CJLM, Zegers SHJ. Neonatal anemia and hydrops fetalis after maternal mycophenolate mofetil use. J Perinatal 2007;27:62–4.
12. El Sebaaly Z, Charpentier B, Snanoudj R. Fetal malformations associated with mycophenolate mofetil for lupus nephritis. Nephrol Dial Transplant 2007;22:2722.
13. Schoner K, Steinhard J, Figiel J, Rehder H. Severe facial clefts in acrofacial dysostosis. Obstet Gynecol 2008;111:483–6.
14. Velinov M, Zellers N. The fetal mycophenolate mofetil syndrome. Clin Dysmorphol 2008;17:77–8.
15. Ghafari A, Sanadgol H. Pregnancy after renal transplantation: ten-year single-center experience. Transplant Proc 2008;40:251–2.
16. Perez-Aytes A, Ledo A, Boso V, Saenz P, Roma E, Poveda JL, Vento M. In utero exposure to mycophenolate mofetil: a characteristic phenotype? Am J Med Genet A 2008;146A:1–7.
17. MedWatch—2007 Safety Information Alerts. CellCept (mycophenolate mofetil). http://www.fda.gov/medwatch/safety/2007/safety07.htm. Accessed July 19, 2008.

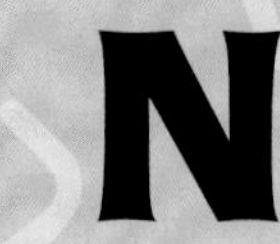

NABILONE

Gastrointestinal Agent (Antiemetic)

PREGNANCY RECOMMENDATION: No Human Data—Animal Data Suggest Risk
BREASTFEEDING RECOMMENDATION: No Human Data—Potential Toxicity

PREGNANCY SUMMARY

No reports describing the use of nabilone in human pregnancy have been located. Dose-related developmental toxicity consisting of growth restriction and death was observed in two animal species. In addition, unspecified postnatal toxicity was observed in one species. Nabilone is structurally related to delta-9-tetrahydrocannabinol (delta-9-THC), the active ingredient in marijuana. Although additional studies are needed, there is evidence that marijuana use in pregnancy is associated with developmental toxicity, such as growth restriction, long-term neurobehavioral deficits, and potentiation of the fetal effects of alcohol. (See Marijuana.) Because of the potential for adverse effects in the embryo and fetus, as well as the absence of human pregnancy experience, the best course is to avoid nabilone during gestation. Nevertheless, the use of this drug may be acceptable if other therapies, including hospitalization and treatment with IV antiemetics, have failed.

FETAL RISK SUMMARY

Nabilone is a synthetic cannabinoid that is indicated for the treatment of nausea and vomiting associated with cancer chemotherapy in patients who have failed to respond to other antiemetic regimens. The chemical structure is similar to delta-9-THC, the active ingredient in marijuana. The drug may produce disturbing psychotomimetic reactions and psychological dependence, and has the potential to be abused. Nabilone is extensively metabolized, but the activity of the metabolites has not been characterized. The plasma half-lives of nabilone and its metabolites are 2 and 35 hours, respectively. Terminal elimination, mainly in the feces (67%) with smaller amounts in the urine (22%), occurs within 7 days. Although no accumulation of nabilone after repeated doses has been observed, accumulation of the metabolites may occur (1).

Reproduction studies have been conducted in rats and rabbits. There was no evidence of structural defects in pregnant rats and rabbits receiving oral doses up to about 16 and 9 times, respectively, the human dose based on BSA (HD). However, dose-related developmental toxicity, consisting of embryo death, fetal resorptions, decreased fetal weight, and pregnancy disruptions, was observed. Unspecified postnatal developmental toxicity also was observed in rats (1,2).

Studies for carcinogenicity have not been conducted with nabilone, but assays for genotoxicity were negative (2). Doses up to six times the HD had no effect on fertility or reproductive performance of male and female rats (1,2).

It is not known if nabilone crosses the human placenta. The molecular weight (about 373) and lipid solubility suggest that the drug will cross to the embryo and fetus, but the very short plasma half-life of the parent compound should limit the exposure.

BREASTFEEDING SUMMARY

No reports describing the use of nabilone during human lactation have been located. Nabilone is structurally similar to delta-9-THC, the active ingredient of marijuana (2). Delta-9-THC is known to be excreted into breast milk. (See Marijuana.) The molecular weight (about 373) and lipid solubility of nabilone suggest that it also will be excreted into breast milk, but the very short plasma half-life (2 hours) should limit the amount. The metabolites, whose activity has not been characterized, have a longer plasma half-life (35 hours) and, therefore, a greater potential for clinically significant concentrations in milk. However, the metabolites of delta-9-THC have not been detected in milk; this also could be the case for the metabolites of nabilone. The effects on the nursing infant from exposure to nabilone or its metabolites in the milk are unknown, but are of concern. Although no adverse effects of marijuana exposure from breast milk have been reported, follow-up of exposed infants is inadequate. Because of the potential for long-term toxicity in nursing infants, women taking nabilone should not breastfeed.

References

1. Markham JK, Hanasono GK, Adams ER, Owen NV. Reproduction studies on nabilone, a synthetic 9-keto-cannabinoid (abstract). Toxicol Appl Pharmacol 1979;48:A119.
2. Product information. Cesamet. Valeant Pharmaceuticals, 2007.

NABUMETONE

Nonsteroidal Anti-inflammatory

PREGNANCY RECOMMENDATION: Human Data Suggest Risk in 1st and 3rd Trimesters
BREASTFEEDING RECOMMENDATION: No Human Data—Potential Toxicity

PREGNANCY SUMMARY

Constriction of the ductus arteriosus in utero is a pharmacologic consequence arising from the use of prostaglandin synthesis inhibitors during pregnancy, as is inhibition of labor, prolongation of pregnancy, and suppression of fetal renal function (see also Indomethacin) (1). Persistent pulmonary hypertension of the newborn may occur if these agents are used in the 3rd trimester close to delivery (1,2). Women attempting to conceive should not use any prostaglandin synthesis inhibitor, including nabumetone, because of the findings in several animal models that indicate these agents block blastocyst implantation (3,4). Moreover, as noted in the discussion below, nonsteroidal anti-inflammatory drugs (NSAIDs) have been associated with spontaneous abortions (SABs) and congenital malformations. The risk for these defects, however, appears to be small.

FETAL RISK SUMMARY

The NSAID nabumetone is used in the acute and chronic treatment of arthritis. Nabumetone is a prodrug that partially undergoes hepatic conversion to an active metabolite. It is in an NSAID subclass (naphthylalkanones) that contains no other agents.

The drug was not teratogenic in rats and rabbits but did produce toxicity similar to other agents in this class, including delayed parturition, dystocia, decreased fetal growth, and decreased fetal survival (5,6). Increased postimplantation loss in rats was observed at a dose equal to the average human exposure at the maximum recommended dose (1).

It is not known if nabumetone crosses the human placenta. The molecular weight (about 228) is low enough that passage to the embryo and fetus should be expected.

A combined 2001 population-based, observational cohort study and a case–control study estimated the risk of adverse pregnancy outcome from the use of NSAIDs (7). The use of NSAIDs during pregnancy was not associated with congenital malformations, preterm delivery, or low birth weight, but a positive association was discovered with SABs. A similar study, also published in 2001, failed to find a relationship, in general, between NSAIDs and congenital malformations, but did find a significant association with cardiac defects and orofacial clefts (8). In addition, a 2003 study found a significant association between exposure to NSAIDs in early pregnancy and SABs (9). (See Ibuprofen for details on these three studies.)

A brief 2003 editorial on the potential for NSAID-induced developmental toxicity concluded that NSAIDs, and specifically those with greater cyclooxygenase 2 (COX-2) affinity, had a lower risk of this toxicity in humans than aspirin (10).

BREASTFEEDING SUMMARY

No reports describing the use of nabumetone during human lactation have been located. The molecular weight (about 228) is low enough that excretion into breast milk should be expected.

One reviewer listed several NSAIDs (diclofenac, fenoprofen, flurbiprofen, ibuprofen, ketoprofen, ketorolac, and tolmetin) that were considered safer alternatives to other agents (nabumetone not mentioned) if these drugs were required during nursing (11). Because of the long serum elimination half-life (≥22.5 hours) of the active metabolite in adults and the unknown amounts of the drug that are excreted into milk, any of these choices probably is preferable.

N

References

1. Levin DL. Effects of inhibition of prostaglandin synthesis on fetal development, oxygenation, and the fetal circulation. Semin Perinatol 1980;4:35–44.
2. Van Marter LJ, Leviton A, Allred EN, Pagano M, Sullivan KF, Cohen A, Epstein MF. Persistent pulmonary hypertension of the newborn and smoking and aspirin and nonsteroidal antiinflammatory drug consumption during pregnancy. Pediatrics 1996;97:658–63.
3. Matt DW, Borzelleca JF. Toxic effects on the female reproductive system during pregnancy, parturition, and lactation. In: Witorsch RJ, ed. *Reproductive Toxicology*. 2nd ed. New York, NY: Raven Press, 1995:175–93.
4. Dawood MY. Nonsteroidal antiinflammatory drugs and reproduction. Am J Obstet Gynecol 1993;169:1255–65.
5. Product information. Relafen. SmithKline Beecham Pharmaceuticals, 2001.
6. Toshiyaki F, Kadoh Y, Fujimoto Y, Tenshio A, Fuchigami K, Ohtsuka T. Toxicity study of nabumetone (iii)—teratological studies. Kiso to Rinsho 1988;22:2975–85. As cited in Shepard TH. *Catalog of Teratogenic Agents*. 7th ed. Baltimore, MD: The Johns Hopkins University Press, 1992:275–6.
7. Nielsen GL, Sorensen HT, Larsen H, Pedersen L. Risk of adverse birth outcome and miscarriage in pregnant users of non-steroidal anti-inflammatory drugs: population-based observational study and case–control study. Br Med J 2001;322:266–70.
8. Ericson A, Kallen BAJ. Nonsteroidal anti-inflammatory drugs in early pregnancy. Reprod Toxicol 2001;15:371–5.
9. Li DK, Liu L, Odouli R. Exposure to non-steroidal anti-inflammatory drugs during pregnancy and risk of miscarriage: population based cohort study. Br Med J 2003;327:368–71.
10. Tassinari MS, Cook JC, Hurtt ME. NSAIDs and developmental toxicity. Birth Defects Res B Dev Reprod Toxicol 2003;68:3–4.
11. Anderson PO. Medication use while breast feeding a neonate. Neonatal Pharmacol Q 1993;2:3–14.

NADOLOL

Sympatholytic (Antihypertensive)

PREGNANCY RECOMMENDATION: Human Data Suggest Risk in 2nd and 3rd Trimesters
BREASTFEEDING RECOMMENDATION: Limited Human Data—Potential Toxicity

PREGNANCY SUMMARY

Some β-blockers may cause intrauterine growth restriction (IUGR) and reduced placental weight, especially those lacking intrinsic sympathomimetic activity (ISA) (i.e., partial agonist). Treatment beginning early in the 2nd trimester results in the greatest weight reductions, whereas treatment restricted to the 3rd trimester primarily affects only placental weight. Nadolol does not possess ISA. However, IUGR and reduced placental weight may potentially occur with all agents within this class. Although growth restriction is a serious concern, the benefits of maternal therapy with β-blockers, in some cases, might outweigh the risks to the fetus and must be judged on a case-by-case basis.

FETAL RISK SUMMARY

Nadolol is a nonselective β_1,β_2-adrenergic blocking agent used for hypertension and angina pectoris. The drug is not teratogenic in rats, hamsters, and rabbits, but embryotoxicity and fetotoxicity were observed in the latter species (1,2).

In a surveillance study of Michigan Medicaid recipients involving 229,101 completed pregnancies conducted between 1985 and 1992, 71 newborns had been exposed to nadolol during the 1st trimester (F. Rosa, personal communication, FDA, 1993). One (1.4%) major birth defect was observed (three expected), a cardiovascular defect (one expected).

Only one published case of the use of nadolol in pregnancy has been located (3). A mother with immunoglobulin A nephropathy and hypertension was treated throughout pregnancy with nadolol, 20 mg/day, plus a diuretic (triamterene/hydrochlorothiazide) and thyroid. The infant, delivered by emergency cesarean section at 35 weeks' gestation, was growth restricted and exhibited tachypnea (68 breaths/minute) and mild hypoglycemia (20 mg/dL). Depressed respirations (23 breaths/minute), slowed heart rate (112 beats/minute), and hypothermia (96.5°F) occurred at 4.5 hours of age. The lowered body temperature responded to warming, but the cardiorespiratory depression, with brief episodes of bradycardia, persisted for 72 hours. Nadolol serum concentrations in cord blood and in the infant at 12 and 38 hours after delivery were 43, 145, and 80 ng/mL, respectively. The cause of some or all of the effects observed in this infant may have been β-blockade (3). However, maternal disease could not be excluded as the sole or contributing factor behind the IUGR and hypoglycemia (3). In addition, hydrochlorothiazide may have contributed to the low blood glucose (see Chlorothiazide).

The authors identified several characteristics of nadolol in the adult that could potentially increase its toxicity in the fetus and newborn, including a long serum half-life (17–24 hours), lack of metabolism (excreted unchanged by the kidneys), and low protein binding (30%) (3). Because of these factors, other β-blockers may be safer for use during pregnancy, although persistent β-blockade has also been observed with acebutolol and atenolol. As with other agents in this class, long-term effects of in utero β-blockade have not been studied but warrant evaluation.

BREASTFEEDING SUMMARY

Nadolol is excreted into breast milk (3,4). A mother taking 20 mg of nadolol/day had a concentration in her milk of 146 ng/mL 38 hours after delivery (3). In 12 lactating women ingesting 80 mg once daily for 5 days, mean steady-state levels of nadolol, approximately 357 ng/mL, were attained at 3 days. This level was approximately 4.6 times higher than simultaneously measured maternal serum levels (4). By calculation, a 5-kg infant would have received 2%–7% of the adult therapeutic dose, but the infants were not allowed to breastfeed (4).

Because experience is lacking, nursing infants of mothers consuming nadolol should be closely observed for symptoms of β-blockade. Long-term effects of exposure to β-blockers from milk have not been studied but warrant evaluation. The American Academy of Pediatrics classifies nadolol as compatible with breastfeeding (5).

References

1. Product information. Corgard. Bristol Laboratories, 1993.
2. Saegusa T, Suzuki T, Narama I. Reproduction studies of nadolol a new β-adrenergic blocking agent. Yakuri to Chiryo 1983;11:5119–38. As cited in Shepard TH, Lemire RJ. *Catalog of Teratogenic Agents*. 12th ed. Baltimore, MD: The Johns Hopkins University Press, 2007:304.
3. Fox RE, Marx C, Stark AR. Neonatal effects of maternal nadolol therapy. Am J Obstet Gynecol 1985;152:1045–6.
4. Devlin RG, Duchin KL, Fleiss PM. Nadolol in human serum and breast milk. Br J Clin Pharmacol 1981;12:393–6.
5. Committee on Drugs, American Academy of Pediatrics. The transfer of drugs and other chemicals into human milk. Pediatrics 2001;108:776–89.

NADROPARIN

[Withdrawn from the market. See 9th edition.]

NAFCILLIN

Antibiotic (Penicillin)

PREGNANCY RECOMMENDATION: Compatible
BREASTFEEDING RECOMMENDATION: Compatible

PREGNANCY SUMMARY

Although the reported pregnancy experience with nafcillin is limited, all penicillins are considered low risk in pregnancy.

FETAL RISK SUMMARY

Nafcillin is a penicillin antibiotic (see also Penicillin G). No reports linking its use with congenital defects have been located. The Collaborative Perinatal Project monitored 50,282 mother–child pairs, 3546 of whom had 1st trimester exposure to penicillin derivatives (1, pp. 297–313). For use anytime during pregnancy, 7171 exposures were recorded (1, p. 435). In neither group was evidence found to suggest a relationship to large categories of major or minor malformations or to individual defects.

BREASTFEEDING SUMMARY

No reports describing the use of nafcillin during human lactation have been located. (See also Penicillin G.)

Reference

1. Heinonen OP, Slone D, Shapiro S. *Birth Defects and Drugs in Pregnancy*. Littleton, MA: Publishing Sciences Group, 1977.

N

NAFTIFINE

Antifungal

PREGNANCY RECOMMENDATION: No Human Data—Animal Data Suggest Low Risk
BREASTFEEDING RECOMMENDATION: No Human Data—Probably Compatible

PREGNANCY SUMMARY

No reports describing the use of naftifine in human pregnancy have been located. The animal data, although based on body weight, suggest low risk, but the absence of human pregnancy experience prevents a more complete assessment of the pregnancy risk. However, the low systemic bioavailability suggests that the amounts reaching the embryo and/or fetus are clinically insignificant. The topical use of this agent during pregnancy probably is low risk.

FETAL RISK SUMMARY

Naftifine is a broad-spectrum, antifungal agent that is available as a 1% topical cream. It has both fungicidal and fungistatic activity. Chemically, naftifine is a synthetic allylamine derivative in the same class as terbinafine. Approximately 6% of an applied dose is absorbed systemically from healthy skin. The plasma elimination half-lives of naftifine and its metabolites are about 2–3 days (1).

Reproduction studies have been conducted with oral doses in rats and rabbits. In these species, oral doses 150 or more times the human topical dose revealed no evidence of impaired fertility or fetal harm. Studies for carcinogenicity have not been performed, but in vitro and animal studies did not demonstrate mutagenicity (1).

It is not known if naftifine and/or its metabolites cross the human placenta. The molecular weight of the parent drug (about 324) and the prolonged elimination half-life suggest that the drug will cross to the embryo and/or fetus. The low systemic bioavailability should prevent clinically significant exposure of the embryo/fetus.

BREASTFEEDING SUMMARY

No reports describing the use of naftifine during human lactation have been located. The low molecular weight (about 324) and the prolonged elimination half-life from the systemic circulation suggest that it will be excreted into breast milk. The systemic bioavailability after topical application of the 1% cream is low (about 6%), so the amount in milk, if any, probably is clinically insignificant. The cream should not be applied to the nipples or breasts if breastfeeding.

Reference

1. Product information. Naftin. Merz Pharmaceuticals, 2004.

NALBUPHINE

Narcotic Agonist–Antagonist Analgesic

PREGNANCY RECOMMENDATION: Human Data Suggest Risk in 3rd Trimester
BREASTFEEDING RECOMMENDATION: Limited Human Data—Probably Compatible

PREGNANCY SUMMARY

No congenital defects have been reported in humans or in experimental animals following the use of nalbuphine in pregnancy (1). Nalbuphine has both narcotic agonist and antagonist effects. Prolonged use during pregnancy could theoretically result in fetal addiction with subsequent withdrawal in the newborn (see also Pentazocine). The use of the drug in labor may produce fetal distress and neonatal respiratory depression comparable with that produced by meperidine (1–6).

FETAL RISK SUMMARY

Nalbuphine is indicated for the relief of moderate-to-severe pain. It also is used as a supplement to balanced anesthesia, for preoperative and postoperative analgesia, and for obstetrical analgesia during labor and delivery. The plasma half-life is 5 hours (2).

Reproduction studies in rats and rabbits at doses up to 6 and 4 times, respectively, the maximum recommended human dose (MRHD) revealed no evidence of impaired fertility or fetal harm (2). Administration to rats at doses 4 times the MRHD during at least the last third of gestation and during lactation reduced both neonatal body weight and survival (2).

Nalbuphine crosses the placenta to the fetus (6–8). The cord:maternal serum ratio in five women in active labor given 20 mg as an IV bolus ranged from 0.37 to 6.03 (7). A sixth patient given 15 mg had a ratio of 1.24. Umbilical cord concentrations of nalbuphine obtained 3–10 hours after a dose varied from "not detectable" to 46 ng/mL. The terminal half-life of the drug in the mothers was 2.4 hours. In another study, the fetal:maternal ratio was 0.74 at delivery and the estimated neonatal plasma half-life was 4.1 hours (8).

A sinusoidal fetal heart rate pattern was observed after a 10-mg IV dose administered to a woman in labor at 42 weeks' gestation (9). The sinusoidal pattern persisted for at least 2.25 hours, and periodic late decelerations became evident. A cesarean section was performed to deliver a healthy female infant with Apgar scores of 8 and 9 at 1 and 5 minutes, respectively, who did well following delivery. The authors attributed the persistent sinusoidal pattern to the prolonged plasma half-life in adults (9).

A 1987 reference compared the use of nalbuphine administered during labor via either a patient-controlled analgesia (PCA) IV pump or by direct IV-push doses (10). No differences were observed between the groups in terms of fetal distress, as evidenced by late decelerations or abnormal scalp blood pH, or in Apgar scores, but specific details on the newborns were not given. However, the fetuses of women receiving nalbuphine by the PCA system had a higher incidence of variable heart rate decelerations (10).

In a 1991 study, IV nalbuphine ($N = 70$; 10 mg) and meperidine ($N = 67$; 50 mg) were compared for analgesia during the active phase of labor at term (11). Neither regimen had an advantage over the other, but, in the nalbuphine group, there were significantly more newborns with a 1-minute Apgar score <7 (10.6% vs. 1.7%, $p < 0.05$). Of note, the time interval between the dose of the two drugs and delivery was not provided although it was >1 hour (11).

BREASTFEEDING SUMMARY

No reports describing the use of nalbuphine during breastfeeding have been located. The manufacturer states that small amounts (<1% of the mother's dose) are excreted into breast milk and these amounts are clinically insignificant (2).

In a 2007 report, 18 non-breastfeeding women immediately after delivery were given IV nalbuphine (0.2 mg/kg every 4 hours) and ketoprofen (100 mg every 12 hours) for postpartum pain (12). The mean and maximum nalbuphine milk concentrations were 42 and 61 ng/mL, respectively. Assuming a milk volume of 150 mL/kg/day, the estimated mean and maximum infant doses were 7.0 and 9.0 mcg/kg/day, respectively. The relative infant dose as a percentage of the weight-adjusted maternal dose was 0.59% (12). (See Ketoprofen for additional data.)

Because nalbuphine has poor oral absorption, it is unlikely to adversely affect a nursing infant.

References

1. Miller RR. Evaluation of nalbuphine hydrochloride. Am J Hosp Pharm 1980;37:942–9.
2. Product information. Nalbuphine hydrochloride. Hospira, 2007.
3. Guillonneau M, Jacqz-Aigrain E, De Grepy A, Zeggout H. Perinatal adverse effects of nalbuphine given during parturition. Lancet 1990;335:1588.

4. Sgro C, Escousse A, Tennenbaum D, Gouyon JB. Perinatal adverse effects of nalbuphine given during labour. Lancet 1990;336:1070.
5. Wilson CM, McClean E, Moore J, Dundee JW. A double-blind comparison of intramuscular pethidine and nalbuphine in labour. Anaesthesia 1986;41:1207–13.
6. Frank M, McAteer EJ, Cattermole R, Loughnan B, Stafford LB, Hitchcock AM. Nalbuphine for obstetric analgesia. Anaesthesia 1987;42:697–703.
7. Wilson SJ, Errick JK, Balkon J. Pharmacokinetics of nalbuphine during parturition. Am J Obstet Gynecol 1986;155:340–4.
8. Nicolle E, Devillier P, Delanoy B, Durand C, Bessard G. Therapeutic monitoring of nalbuphine: transplacental transfer and estimated pharmacokinetics in the neonate. Eur J Clin Pharmacol 1996;49:485–9.
9. Feinstein SJ, Lodeiro JG, Vintzileos AM, Campbell WA, Montgomery JT, Nochimson DJ. Sinusoidal fetal heart rate pattern after administration of nalbuphine hydrochloride: a case report. Am J Obstet Gynecol 1986;154:159–60.
10. Podlas J, Breland BD. Patient-controlled analgesia with nalbuphine during labor. Obstet Gynecol 1987;70:202–4.
11. Dan U, Rabinovici Y, Barkai G, Modan M, Etchin A, Mashiach S. Intravenous pethidine and nalbuphine during labor: a prospective double-blind comparative study. Gynecol Obstet Invest 1991;32:39–43.
12. Jacqz-Aigrain E, Serreau R, Boissinot C, Popon M, Sobel A, Michel J, Sibony O. Excretion of ketoprofen and nalbuphine in human milk during treatment of maternal pain after delivery. Ther Drug Monit 2007;29:815–8.

NALIDIXIC ACID

Urinary Germicide

PREGNANCY RECOMMENDATION: Limited Human Data—Animal Data Suggest Moderate Risk
BREASTFEEDING RECOMMENDATION: Compatible

PREGNANCY SUMMARY

The animal data suggest moderate risk, but the human data are limited. In a large case–control study, a possible association, based on seven cases, was found with pyloric stenosis. However, the association might have occurred by chance. Because nalidixic acid has been available for many years, the lack of other reports of developmental toxicity is reassuring.

FETAL RISK SUMMARY

No reports linking the use of nalidixic acid, a quinolone antibacterial agent, with congenital defects have been located. At oral doses six times the human dose, nalidixic acid was embryocidal and teratogenic in rats (1). Prolongation of pregnancy was also noted, especially at four times the human dose. Similar to other agents in this class, nalidixic acid causes arthropathy in immature animals (1).

Chromosomal damage was not observed in human leukocytes cultured with various concentrations of the drug (2). One author cautioned that the drug should be avoided in late pregnancy because it may produce hydrocephalus (3). However, a subsequent report examined the newborns of 63 patients treated with nalidixic acid at various stages of gestation (4). No defects attributable to the drug or intracranial hypertension were observed.

A study using the population-based dataset of the Hungarian Case-Control Surveillance of Congenital Abnormalities 1980–1996 was published in 2001 (5). There were 22,865 cases with congenital malformations and 38,151 controls without birth defects in the dataset. The control group was 1.8% of the total number of births (2,146,574) in Hungary during the study period. Exposure to nalidixic acid during gestation occurred in 242 (1.1%) cases compared with 377 (1.0%) controls (crude odds ratio [OR] 1.1, 95% confidence interval [CI] 0.9–1.3). Seventeen congenital abnormality groups were analyzed and OR and 95% CI were calculated for exposure in the 2nd and 3rd months and the entire pregnancy. No increased risk was found with use of nalidixic acid in the 1st trimester. However, there was an increased prevalence of pyloric stenosis when the mother took the drug in the last few months of gestation (7 cases; OR 8.0, 95% CI 1.0–66.4). Although the results suggested an association, a chance relationship could not be excluded (5).

BREASTFEEDING SUMMARY

Nalidixic acid is excreted into breast milk in low concentrations (6–8). Hemolytic anemia was reported in one infant with glucose-6-phosphate dehydrogenase deficiency whose mother was taking 1 g 4 times a day (6). Milk levels were not measured in this case, but the author noted data from the manufacturer in which milk levels from four women taking a similar dose were found to be 4 mcg/mL. The milk:plasma ratio has been reported as 0.08–0.13 (7).

A 1980 report described the excretion of unmetabolized nalidixic acid into the breast milk of 13 women, 3–8 days postpartum, following a 2-g oral dose (8). Nursing was suspended on the day of the test. Milk was collected from each woman for a 24-hour period and serum samples were taken 7 hours after the dose. The highest milk concentration of the drug occurred in the sample collected from 0 to 4 hours, 0.64 mcg/mL, but the total unchanged drug excreted over 24 hours was only 0.003% of the mother's dose. The milk:serum ratio at 7 hours was 0.061, and the minimal inhibitory concentration of about 3 mcg/mL was never reached (8).

The quantities measured above are normally considered insignificant (9). Although noting the single case of hemolytic anemia described above, the American Academy of Pediatrics classifies nalidixic acid as compatible with breastfeeding (10).

References

1. Product information. NegGram. Sanofi Winthrop Pharmaceuticals, 1997.
2. Stenchever MA, Powell W, Jarvis JA. Effect of nalidixic acid on human chromosome integrity. Am J Obstet Gynecol 1970;107:329–30.
3. Asscher AW. Diseases of the urinary system. Urinary tract infections. Br Med J 1977;1:1332.
4. Murray EDS. Nalidixic acid in pregnancy. Br Med J 1981;282:224.
5. Czeizel AE, Sorensen HT, Rockenbauer M, Olsen J. A population-based case–control teratologic study of nalidixic acid. Int J Gynaecol Obstet 2001;73:221–8.

N

6. Belton EM, Jones RV. Hemolytic anemia due to nalidixic acid. Lancet 1965;2:691.
7. Wilson JT. Milk/plasma ratios and contraindicated drugs. In: Wilson JT, ed. *Drugs in Breast Milk*. Balgowlah, Australia: ADIS Press, 1981:78–9.
8. Traeger A, Peiker G. Excretion of nalidixic acid via mother's milk. Arch Toxicol 1980;4(Suppl):388–90.
9. Takyi BE. Excretion of drugs in human milk. J Hosp Pharm 1970;28: 317–25.
10. Committee on Drugs, American Academy of Pediatrics. The transfer of drugs and other chemicals into human milk. Pediatrics 2001;108: 776–89.

NALORPHINE

[Withdrawn from the market. See 9th edition.]

NALOXONE

Narcotic Antagonist

PREGNANCY RECOMMENDATION: Compatible
BREASTFEEDING RECOMMENDATION: No Human Data—Probably Compatible

PREGNANCY SUMMARY

Naloxone is a narcotic antagonist that is used to reverse the effects of narcotic overdose. The drug has no intrinsic respiratory depressive actions or other narcotic effects of its own (1).

FETAL RISK SUMMARY

Reproduction studies in mice and rats at doses up to 50 times the usual human dose revealed no evidence of impaired fertility or fetal harm (2).

Naloxone crosses the human placenta, appearing in fetal blood 2 minutes after a maternal dose and gradually increasing over 10–30 minutes (3).

In three reports, naloxone was given to mothers in labor after the administration of meperidine (4–6). One study found that 18–40 mcg/kg (maternal weight) given IV provided the best results in comparison with controls who did not receive meperidine or naloxone (5). In measurements of newborn neurobehavior, groups treated in labor with either meperidine or meperidine plus naloxone (0.4 mg) were compared with a nontreated control group (6). The control group scored better in the first 24 hours than either of the treated groups and, after 2 hours, no difference was found between meperidine and meperidine plus naloxone-treated patients. Women in active labor received 1.0 mg of morphine intrathecal followed in 1 hour by a 0.4-mg IV bolus of naloxone plus 0.6 mg/hr or placebo as constant infusion for 23 hours (7). A reduction in some morphine-induced maternal side effects was seen with naloxone, but no significant differences with placebo were found for fetal heart rate or variability, Apgar scores, umbilical venous and arterial gases, neonatal respirations, or neurobehavioral examination scores. The cord blood:maternal serum ratio for naloxone was 0.50. Naloxone has also been safely given to newborns within a few minutes of delivery (8–13).

Naloxone has been used at term to treat fetal heart rate baselines with low beat-to-beat variability not caused by maternally administered narcotics (14). This use was based on the assumption that the heart rate patterns were caused by elevated fetal endorphins. In one case, however, naloxone may have enhanced fetal asphyxia, leading to fatal respiratory failure in the newborn (14). Based on the above data, naloxone should not be given to the mother just before delivery to reverse the effects of narcotics in the fetus or newborn unless narcotic toxicity is evident. Information on its fetal effects during pregnancy, other than labor, is not available.

In a study of the effects of naloxone on fetal behavior, 54 pregnant women with gestational ages between 37 and 39 weeks were evenly divided into two groups (15). One group received 0.4 mg of naloxone and the other received an equal volume of saline placebo. In the group receiving naloxone, significant increases were observed in the number, duration, and amplitude of fetal heart rate accelerations. Significant increases were also observed in the number of fetal body movements and the percentage of time spent breathing. Moreover, significantly more fetuses exposed to naloxone were actively awake than those not exposed. The investigators attributed their findings to reversal of the effects of fetal endorphins.

BREASTFEEDING SUMMARY

No reports describing the use of naloxone during human lactation have been located.

References

1. Jaffe JH, Martin WR. Opioid analgesics and antagonists. In: Gilman AG, Goodman LS, Gilman A, eds. *The Pharmacological Basis of Therapeutics*. 6th ed. New York, NY: MacMillan, 1980:522–5.
2. Product information. Narcan. Endo Pharmaceuticals, 2000.
3. Finster M, Gibbs C, Dawes GS, et al. *Placental Transfer of Meperidine (Demerol) and Naloxone (Narcan)*. Presented at the Annual Meeting of the American Society of Anesthesiologists, October 4, 1972, Boston, MA. Cited in Clark RB, Beard AG, Greifenstein FE, Barclay DL. Naloxone in the parturient and her infant. South Med J 1976;69:570–5.

4. Clark RB. Transplacental reversal of meperidine depression in the fetus by naloxone. J Arkansas Med Soc 1971;68:128–30.
5. Clark RB, Beard AG, Greifenstein FE, Barclay DL. Naloxone in the parturient and her infant. South Med J 1976;69:570–5.
6. Hodgkinson R, Bhatt M, Grewal G, Marx GF. Neonatal neurobehavior in the first 48 hours of life: effect of the administration of meperidine with and without naloxone in the mother. Pediatrics 1978;62:294–8.
7. Brookshire GL, Shnider SM, Abboud TK, Kotelko DM, Nouiehed R, Thigpen JW, Khoo SS, Raya JA, Foutz SE, Brizgys RV. Effects of naloxone on the mother and neonate after intrathecal morphine for labor analgesia. Anesthesiology 1983;59:A417.
8. Evans JM, Hogg MIJ, Rosen M. Reversal of narcotic depression in the neonate by naloxone. Br Med J 1976;2:1098–100.
9. Wiener PC, Hogg MIJ, Rosen M. Effects of naloxone on pethidine-induced neonatal depression. II. Intramuscular naloxone. Br Med J 1977;2:229–31.
10. Wiener PC, Hogg MIJ, Rosen M. Effects of naloxone on pethidine-induced neonatal depression. I. Intravenous naloxone. Br Med J 1977;2:228–9.
11. Gerhardt T, Bancalari E, Cohen H, Rocha LF. Use of naloxone to reverse narcotic respiratory depression in the newborn infant. J Pediatr 1977;90:1009–12.
12. Bonta BW, Gagliardi JV, Williams V, Warshaw JB. Naloxone reversal of mild neurobehavioral depression in normal newborn infants after routine obstetric analgesia. J Pediatr 1979;94:102–5.
13. Welles B, Belfrage P, de Chateau P. Effects of naloxone on newborn infant behavior after maternal analgesia with pethidine during labor. Acta Obstet Gynecol Scand 1984;63:617–9.
14. Goodlin RC. Naloxone and its possible relationship to fetal endorphin levels and fetal distress. Am J Obstet Gynecol 1981;139:16–9.
15. Arduini D, Rizzo G, Dell'Acqua S, Mancuso S, Romanini C. Effect of naloxone on fetal behavior near term. Am J Obstet Gynecol 1987;156:474–8.

NALTREXONE

Narcotic Antagonist

PREGNANCY RECOMMENDATION: Limited Human Data—Animal Data Suggest Moderate Risk
BREASTFEEDING RECOMMENDATION: Limited Human Data—Probably Compatible

PREGNANCY SUMMARY

Except for the following reports in which the naltrexone was discontinued very early in gestation, no other references describing the use of the agent during human pregnancy have been located. Although naltrexone did not produce gross structural abnormalities in any of the animal studies, it did alter some opioid receptors in the brain that appeared to have long-lasting consequences. This potential for behavioral alteration in humans cannot be assessed because of the lack of data, but concern is warranted.

FETAL RISK SUMMARY

Naltrexone is an opioid antagonist that is indicated in the treatment of alcohol dependence and for the blockade of the effects of exogenously administered opioids. The agent is a synthetic congener of oxymorphone and is also related to another opioid antagonist, naloxone. The major metabolite is 6-β-naltrexol. Plasma protein binding is low (21%) and the mean elimination half-lives for naltrexone and its major metabolite are 4 and 13 hours, respectively (1).

In fertility studies, a significant increase in pseudopregnancy and a decrease in the pregnancy rate after mating were observed in rats given a dose that was 16 times the recommended human therapeutic dose based on BSA (RHTD). No adverse effects on male rat fertility were seen at this dose. A significant increase in early fetal loss was observed in rats and rabbits at 5 and 18 times the RHTD, respectively. No evidence of teratogenicity was found in either species at doses up to 32 and 65 times the RHTD, respectively, administered during organogenesis. Because rats do not form appreciable amounts of the major metabolite found in humans (6-β-naltrexol), the potential reproductive toxicity of the metabolite is unknown (1).

An animal study published in 1984 evaluated the reproductive effects of naltrexone in rats and rabbits (2). In rats, prolonged administration of naltrexone at doses that did not affect body weight produced excitatory signs in both sexes, increased production of seminal plugs in males, and decreased estrus cycling and fertility in females. No adverse effect on mating activity was observed, but there was an increase in pseudopregnancy in those receiving 100 mg/kg/day. Fertility was also reduced (i.e., fewer females became pregnant) when both sexes received this dose. No evidence of teratogenicity or embryo toxicity was noted in either pregnant rats or rabbits (2).

When administered to rats near term (20 days' gestation), naltrexone crossed the placenta and was measured in all fetal tissues (3).

In an experiment with stressed (noise and light at unpredictable frequency) pregnant rats, a continuous infusion of naltrexone (10 mg/kg/day) was administered by implanted minipumps from day 17 of gestation (4). Compared with controls receiving an infusion of vehicle only, naltrexone prevented the reduction in anogenital distance in male pups and restored the growth rate in both sexes. Other adverse fetal effects of prenatal stress were also prevented by naltrexone, leading the authors to conclude that some of the morphologic and behavioral changes induced by prenatal stress may result from excess opioid activity (4).

The effects of daily injections of naltrexone (50 mg/kg) administered to rats throughout gestation on fetal growth were described in a 1997 publication (5). Compared with controls given daily injections of saline, naltrexone-exposed pups had greater body weights, crown–rump lengths, and organ and skeletal muscle weights. Naltrexone had no effect on the length of gestation, course of pregnancy, litter size, or viability of the mother or offspring (5). The effects on growth were attributed to the blocking of endogenous opioids.

Decreased sensitivity to morphine has been observed in rat offspring exposed in utero to naltrexone (6,7). The appreciation of pain was not affected. However, insensitivity was not observed to butorphanol (7). These results raise the possibility that, later in life, morphine would provide less-effective analgesia in human offspring who were exposed during gestation to naltrexone.

Other rat studies have also demonstrated that naltrexone can modify behavior of both the mother and the offspring (8–10). Naltrexone was administered at parturition to ewes lambing for the first time (8). Compared with controls, naltrexone significantly delayed the onset of maternal behavior (licking and bleating) toward the newborn. The drug facilitated sexual behavior in adult male rats who had been exposed in utero (9). Another study found that naltrexone exposure throughout gestation modified postnatal behavioral development of rat offspring (10). The investigators concluded that blocking the endogenous opioid systems during embryogenesis altered the somatic, physical, and behavioral development after birth. Of interest, a 1998 study found that naltrexone was present in the brains and hearts of newborn rats after maternal administration during gestation, but it was not present on postnatal days 2 and 10 (11). The investigators concluded that the somatic and neurobiological acceleration observed in previous studies was not due to opioid receptor blockade during the postnatal period (11).

It is not known if naltrexone or its metabolite crosses the human placenta. The molecular weight of naltrexone (about 342 for the free base), low plasma protein binding, and long elimination half-lives of naltrexone and the major metabolite suggest that one or both agents will cross to the embryo–fetus.

Two 1993 reports, from the same research group, described the use of naltrexone (25–150 mg/day for 4–100 weeks) in 138 women with various grades of hypothalamic or hyperandrogenic ovarian failure (12,13). A total of 24 pregnancies in 22 women were achieved. Naltrexone was discontinued as soon as pregnancy had been diagnosed. Four pregnancies ended in an early spontaneous abortion (SAB), six women had given birth (no data provided on newborn condition), eight pregnancies were ongoing, and no information was given for six cases. A 1995 study of women with functional hypothalamic amenorrhea, however, found that even after priming with exogenous estradiol and progesterone or pulsatile gonadotropin-releasing hormone, the continued use of naltrexone alone did not maintain gonadotropin secretion and eventual ovulation (14).

Continuous naltrexone (50 mg/day), either alone or with intermittent clomiphene, has been used successfully in women with clomiphene-resistant normogonadotrophic anovulation (15). In this study, 19 of 22 women achieved ovulation and 12 singleton pregnancies were documented. Naltrexone was discontinued when pregnancy was diagnosed. The outcomes of the pregnancies included two SABs and eight ongoing pregnancies (15).

BREASTFEEDING SUMMARY

Consistent with the molecular weight of naltrexone (about 342), low plasma protein binding (21%), and long elimination half-lives of naltrexone (4 hours) and 6-β-naltrexone (major metabolite) (13 hours), both agents are excreted into breast milk.

In a 2004 case report, a 30-year-old woman was taking naltrexone (50 mg/day) for opiate addiction while breastfeeding her 1.5-month-old male infant (16). The mother had started the drug during the latter part of pregnancy and had been taking it for 135 days before the study. The mean milk concentrations of the parent drug and metabolite were 1.6 and 46 mcg/L, respectively. The measured relative infant doses as a percentage of the maternal dose were 0.03% (naltrexone) and 0.83% (metabolite). The healthy infant was achieving expected milestones and had no adverse effects (16). Although this report is reassuring, additional data are warranted and use during lactation should be evaluated on a case-by-case basis.

References

1. Product information. Revia. Duramed Pharmaceuticals, 2009.
2. Christian MS. Reproductive toxicity and teratology evaluations of naltrexone. J Clin Psychiatry 1984;45:7–10.
3. Zagon IS, Hurst WJ, McLaughlin PJ. Transplacental transfer of naltrexone in rats. Life Sci 1997;61:1261–7.
4. Keshet GI, Weinstock M. Maternal naltrexone prevents morphological and behavioral alterations induced in rats by prenatal stress. Pharmacol Biochem Behav 1995;50:413–9.
5. McLaughlin PJ, Tobias SW, Lang CM, Zagon IS. Chronic exposure to the opioid antagonist naltrexone during pregnancy: maternal and offspring effects. Physiol Behav 1997;62:501–8.
6. Harry GJ, Rosecrans JA. Behavioral effects of perinatal naltrexone exposure: a preliminary investigation. Pharmacol Biochem Behav 1979;11(Suppl):19–22.
7. Zagon IS, Tobias SW, Hytrek SD, McLaughlin PJ. Opioid receptor blockade throughout prenatal life confers long-term insensitivity to morphine and alters μ opioid receptors. Pharmacol Biochem Behav 1998;59:201–7.
8. Caba M, Poindron P, Krehbiel D, Levy F, Romeyer A, Venier G. Naltrexone delays the onset of maternal behavior in primiparous parturient ewes. Pharmacol Biochem Behav 1995;52:743–8.
9. Cohen E, Keshet G, Shavit Y, Weinstock M. Prenatal naltrexone facilitates male sexual behavior in the rat. Pharmacol Biochem Behav 1996;54:183–8.
10. McLaughlin PJ, Tobias SW, Lang CM, Zagon IS. Opioid receptor blockade during prenatal life modifies postnatal behavioral development. Pharmacol Biochem Behav 1997;58:1075–82.
11. Zagon IS, Hurst WJ, McLaughlin PJ. Naltrexone is not detected in preweaning rats following transplacental exposure: implications for growth modulation. Life Sci 1998;62:221–8.
12. Wildt L, Leyendecker G, Sir-Petermann T, Waibel-Treber S. Treatment with naltrexone in hypothalamic ovarian failure: induction of ovulation and pregnancy. Hum Reprod 1993;8;350–8.
13. Wildt L, Sir-Petermann T, Leyendecker G, Waibel-Treber S, Rabenbauer B. Opiate antagonist treatment of ovarian failure. Hum Reprod 1993;8(Suppl 2):168–74.
14. Couzinet B, Young J, Brailly S, Chanson P, Schaison G. Even after priming with ovarian steroids or pulsatile gonadotropin-releasing hormone administration, naltrexone is unable to induce ovulation in women with functional hypothalamic amenorrhea. J Clin Endocrinol Metab 1995;80:2102–7.
15. Roozenburg BJ, van Dessel HJHM, Evers JLH, Bots RSGM. Successful induction of ovulation in normogonadotrophic clomiphene-resistant anovulatory women by combined naltrexone and clomiphene citrate treatment. Hum Reprod 1997;12:1720–2.
16. Chan CF, Page-Sharp M, Kristensen JH, O'Neil G, Ilett KF. Transfer of naltrexone and its metabolite 6,ß-naltrexol into human milk. J Hum Lact 2004;20:322–6.

N

NAPHAZOLINE

Ophthalmic (Sympathomimetic)

PREGNANCY RECOMMENDATION: Limited Human Data—No Relevant Animal Data
BREASTFEEDING RECOMMENDATION: No Human Data—Probably Compatible

PREGNANCY SUMMARY

The human pregnancy experience with naphazoline is very limited and animal reproduction studies have not been conducted. In addition, reports describing the amount of drug in the systemic circulation after nasal or ophthalmic use have not been located. However, it is doubtful if appropriate short-term use results in clinically significant systemic concentrations. Thus, the occasional use of naphazoline does not appear to represent a risk to the embryo and/or fetus.

FETAL RISK SUMMARY

Naphazoline is an α-adrenergic agonist that is used as a topical vasoconstrictor to relieve eye redness and as an intranasal spray to treat symptoms of nasal congestion. The drug is available over the counter (1,2).

Reproduction studies in animals have not been conducted (1,2). In addition, no studies evaluating the carcinogenicity or mutagenicity of naphazoline, or its effects on fertility have been located.

It is not known if clinically significant amounts of naphazoline cross the human placenta. The molecular weight (about 210 for the free base) is low enough, but the systemic concentrations after ocular or nasal use should be low.

The Collaborative Perinatal Project monitored 50,282 mother–child pairs, 20 of whom had 1st trimester exposure to naphazoline (3, pp. 346–347). No evidence was found to suggest a relationship between large categories of major or minor malformations or to individual defects. However, an association in the 1st trimester was found between the sympathomimetic class of drugs as a whole and minor malformations (not life-threatening or major cosmetic defects), inguinal hernia, and clubfoot (3, pp. 345–356).

A 1995 report described a case in which naphazoline nasal spray was used repeatedly throughout pregnancy (4). The newborn had cyanosis, hypertension, and ischemia of the foot. The cause of the outcome could not be determined (4).

BREASTFEEDING SUMMARY

No reports describing the use of naphazoline during human lactation have been located. The molecular weight (about 210 for the free base) is low enough for excretion into breast milk, but the expected low systemic concentrations after ocular or nasal use should limit the exposure of the infant. Thus, occasional use of naphazoline during breastfeeding appears to be compatible.

N

References

1. Product information. Albalon. Allergan, 2003.
2. Product information. Vasocon. CIBA Vision, 2006.
3. Heinonen OP, Slone D, Shapiro S. *Birth Defects and Drugs in Pregnancy*. Littleton, MA: Publishing Sciences Group, 1977.
4. Dageville C, Joly E, Spreux A, Berard E. Toxicite neonatale de la naphazoline administree durant la grossesse. Therapie 1995;50:463–84.

NAPROXEN

Nonsteroidal Anti-inflammatory

PREGNANCY RECOMMENDATION: Human Data Suggest Risk in 1st and 3rd Trimesters
BREASTFEEDING RECOMMENDATION: Limited Human Data—Probably Compatible

PREGNANCY SUMMARY

Exposure to nonsteroidal anti-inflammatory drugs (NSAIDs), including naproxen, during the 1st trimester appears to be a risk for structural anomalies and spontaneous abortions (SABs). The structural defects usually involve the heart, especially septal defects, but associations with oral clefts also have been reported. The absolute risk for these defects, however, appears to be low. When used in the 3rd trimester, NSAIDs have the potential to cause premature closure of the ductus arteriosus, which, in some cases, may result in primary pulmonary hypertension of the newborn (PPHN). In addition, the use of NSAIDs as tocolytics has been associated with an increased risk of neonatal complications, such as necrotizing enterocolitis, patent ductus arteriosus, and intraventricular hemorrhage (1), but further studies are required to confirm the magnitude of these toxicities. Because of the potential newborn toxicity, naproxen should not be used late in the 3rd trimester (1–3). Moreover, women attempting to conceive should not use any prostaglandin synthesis inhibitor, including naproxen, because of the findings in various animal models, indicating that these agents block blastocyst implantation (4,5).

Women who are pregnant or are at risk of pregnancy should be counseled on these risks. Such counseling is especially important because the use of NSAIDs during pregnancy, either prescribed or over the counter (OTC), is very common. One report stated that the use of ibuprofen in pregnancy occurred in 14.9% of the patients studied, 52% (45 of 86) of whom were exposed in the first trimester (6). NSAIDs available as OTC products in the United States include ibuprofen and naproxen, either as single-ingredient products or in decongestant/analgesic combinations. Thus, women might be exposed to NSAIDs at any time in gestation without realizing they are taking a drug with the potential for developmental toxicity.

FETAL RISK SUMMARY

Naproxen is an NSAID used in the management of the signs and symptoms of rheumatoid arthritis, osteoarthritis, ankylosing spondylitis, and juvenile arthritis. It is in the same subclass (propionic acids) as five other NSAIDs (fenoprofen, flurbiprofen, ibuprofen, ketoprofen, and oxaprozin). Drugs in this class have been shown to inhibit labor and to prolong the length of pregnancy (1,7).

Animal reproduction studies have been conducted in mice, rats, and rabbits. At 0.23–0.28 times, the human systemic exposure at the recommended dose, no evidence of impaired fertility or fetal harm was seen in these species (1). It was not stated if maternal toxicity prevented higher doses. A 1990 report described an investigation on the effects of several NSAIDs on mouse palatal fusion both in vivo and in vitro (8). The compounds, including naproxen, were found to induce cleft palate.

Consistent with the relatively low molecular weight (about 230), naproxen readily crosses the placenta to the fetal circulation. Twenty-eight women received two 500-mg naproxen doses, the first within 10.5–15 hours and the second within 4 hours of an elective 1st trimester pregnancy termination (9). Mean naproxen levels in maternal serum, fetal tissue, coelomic fluid, and amniotic fluid were 69.5, 6.4, 1.85, and 0.14 mcg/mL, respectively. The mean fetal:maternal drug ratio was 0.092 (9). In a woman at 30 weeks' gestation treated with 250 mg of naproxen every 8 hours for four doses, plasma levels in twins 5 hours after the last dose were 59.5 and 68 mcg/mL (10).

In a surveillance study of Michigan Medicaid recipients involving 229,101 completed pregnancies conducted between 1985 and 1992, 1448 newborns had been exposed to naproxen during the 1st trimester (F. Rosa, personal communication, FDA, 1993). A total of 70 (4.8%) major birth defects were observed (62 expected). Specific data were available for six defect categories, including (observed/expected) 14/14 cardiovascular defects, 2/2 oral clefts, 0/1 spina bifida, 3/4 polydactyly, 2/2 limb reduction defects, and 3/3 hypospadias. These data do not support an association between the drug and congenital defects.

A combined 2001 population-based, observational cohort study and a case–control study estimated the risk of adverse pregnancy outcome from the use of NSAIDs (2). The use of NSAIDs during pregnancy was not associated with congenital malformations, preterm delivery, or low birth weight, but a positive association was discovered with SABs. A similar study, also published in 2001, failed to find a relationship, in general, between NSAIDs and congenital malformations but did find a significant association with cardiac defects and orofacial clefts (11). In addition, a 2003 study found a significant association between exposure to NSAIDs in early pregnancy and SABs (12). (See Ibuprofen for details on these three studies.)

A brief 2003 editorial on the potential for NSAID-induced developmental toxicity concluded that NSAIDs, and specifically those with greater cyclooxygenase 2 (COX-2) affinity, had a lower risk of this toxicity in humans than aspirin (13).

A 2003 study using data from three Swedish health registers (1995–2001) that included maternal drug history collected prospectively identified 1142 infants with orofacial clefts (isolated or with other malformations, excluding chromosome anomalies) (14). Compared with the expected number (2.9) of orofacial clefts, there were eight naproxen-exposed cases, a relative risk of 2.72 (95% confidence interval [CI] 1.17–5.36).

A 2003 case–control study, using data from the same Swedish registers as the above study, was conducted to identify drug use in early pregnancy that was associated with cardiac defects (15). Cases (cardiovascular defects without known chromosome anomalies) (N = 5015) were compared with controls consisting of all infants born in Sweden from 1995 to 2001 (N = 577,730). Associations were identified for several drugs, some of which were probably due to confounding from the underlying disease or complaint or multiple testing, but some were thought to be true drug effects. For NSAIDs, the total exposed, number of cases, and odds ratios (ORs) with 95% CI were NSAIDs (all) (7698; 80 cases; 1.24, 0.99–1.55), naproxen (1679; 24 cases; 1.70, 1.14–2.54), diclofenac (1362; 15 cases; 1.30, 0.78–2.16), ibuprofen (4124; 37 cases; 1.08, 0.78–1.50), and aspirin (5920; 52 cases; 1.01, 0.76–1.33). Five of the defects observed with naproxen were two infants with transposition of the great vessels and three with endocardial cushion defects (one infant had both defects). The authors noted that further studies were needed to verify or reject the hypothesis (15).

A 2004 case report described a 24-year-old woman who took naproxen (550 mg about twice a week), bisoprolol (5 mg/day), and sumatriptan (100 mg about once a week) for migraine headaches during the first 5 weeks of pregnancy (16). An elective cesarean section was performed at 37 weeks' for breech presentation to deliver a 3125-g male infant. The infant had a wide bilateral cleft lip/palate, marked hypertelorism, a broad nose, and bilateral but asymmetric toe abnormalities (missing and hypoplastic phalanges) (16).

A 2006 case–control study found a significant association between congenital anomalies, specifically cardiac septal defects, and the use of NSAIDs in the 1st trimester (17). A population-based pregnancy registry (N = 36,387) was developed by linking three databases in Quebec. The combined database covered all of the pregnancies that occurred in Quebec from January 1997 through June 2003. Inclusion criteria were mothers of singleton infants, 15–45 years of age, who were prescribed an NSAID or other medications during pregnancy. The use of OTC NSAIDs was a potential confounder but the investigators provided reasonable arguments that such exposure was unlikely. The data were adjusted for chronic comorbidities, including rheumatoid arthritis and disease-modifying anti-rheumatic drugs, hypothyroidism and thyroid drugs, and chronic or gestational hypertension. Adjustment also was made for 1st trimester use of known human teratogens (17).

Case infants were those with any congenital anomaly diagnosed in the first year of life (17). Up to 10 controls (infants without a congenital anomaly) were selected for each case and matched with cases for maternal age, urban or rural residence, gestational age, and diabetes status. There were 93 infants (8.8%) with congenital defects from 1056 mothers who had filled prescriptions for NSAIDs in the 1st trimester. In controls, there were 2478 infants (7%) with anomalies from 35,331 mothers who had not filled such a prescription. The adjusted OR (aOR) was 2.21 (95% CI 1.72–2.85). The aOR for cardiac septal closure was 3.34 (95% CI 1.87–5.98). There also was a significant association for anomalies of the respiratory system 9.55 (95% CI 3.08–29.63), but this association disappeared when cases coded as "unspecified anomaly of the respiratory system" were excluded. For the cases involving septal closure, 61% were atrial septal defects and 31% were ventricular septal defects. There were no significant associations for oral clefts or defects involving other major organ systems. The five most common NSAIDs were naproxen (35%), ibuprofen (26%), rofecoxib (15%), diclofenac (9%), and celecoxib (9%). Among these agents, the only significant association was for ibuprofen prescriptions in the 1st trimester and congenital defects ($p < 0.01$) (17).

Prostaglandin synthesis inhibitors may cause constriction of the ductus arteriosus in utero, which may result in PPHN (18–22). The dose, duration, and period of gestation are important determinants of these effects. Most studies of NSAIDs used as tocolytics have indicated that the fetus is relatively resistant to premature closure of the ductus before the 34th or 35th week of gestation (see Indomethacin). However, three fetuses (one set of twins) exposed to naproxen at 30 weeks for 2–6 days in an unsuccessful attempt to halt premature labor had markedly decreased plasma concentrations of prostaglandin E. PPHN with severe hypoxemia, increased blood clotting times, hyperbilirubinemia, and impaired renal function were observed in the newborns. One infant died 4 days after birth, probably because of subarachnoid hemorrhage. Autopsy revealed a short and constricted ductus arteriosus. Use in other patients for premature labor at 34 weeks or earlier has not resulted in neonatal problems (23,24).

In a case report published in 2000, a mother took an OTC preparation of naproxen 220 mg twice a day over the 4 days immediately preceding birth of a term 3790-g male infant (25). Within 2 hours of birth, the infant developed typical signs and symptoms of PPHN with a closed ductus arteriosus. Conservative management was initiated and the infant was improving by the sixth postnatal day. At 6 weeks of age, the infant was doing well clinically without cyanosis (25).

A 2012 report from the National Birth Defects Prevention Study found associations between exposures to NSAIDs (aspirin, ibuprofen, and naproxen) and several birth defects (26). The data for this case–control study came from approximately 20,470 women with expected due dates in 1997–2004. Among this group, 3173 women (15.5%) were exposed to NSAIDs in the 1st trimester. Although the results suggested that NSAIDs are not a major cause of birth defects, the study did find several small-to-moderate but statistically significant increases in nine defects. The drug, aOR, and 95% CI for each defect were anencephaly/craniorachischisis—aspirin (2.1; 1.1–4.3); spina bifida—ibuprofen (1.6; 1.2–2.1); encephalocele—naproxen (3.5; 1.2–10); anophthalmia/microphthalmia—aspirin (3.0; 1.3–7.3), ibuprofen (1.9; 1.1–3.3), and naproxen (2.8; 1.1–7.3); cleft lip ± cleft palate—ibuprofen (1.3; 1.1–1.6) and naproxen (1.7; 1.1–2.5); cleft palate—aspirin (1.8; 1.1–2.9); transverse limb deficiency—naproxen (2.0; 1.0–3.8); amniotic bands/limb body wall—aspirin (2.5; 1.1–5.6) and ibuprofen (2.2; 1.4–3.5); and a heart defect (isolated pulmonary valve stenosis)—naproxen (2.4; 1.3–4.5). The analysis of the latter defect was limited to term births only. The authors acknowledged that further studies were needed because most of these associations had not been reported from other databases (26).

BREASTFEEDING SUMMARY

Naproxen passes into breast milk in very small quantities. The milk:plasma ratio is approximately 0.01 (1). Following 250 or 375 mg twice daily, maximum milk levels were found 4 hours after a dose and ranged from 0.7 to 1.25 mcg/mL and 1.76 to 2.37 mcg/mL, respectively (27,28). The total amount of naproxen excreted in the infant's urine was 0.26% of the mother's dose. The effect on the infant from these amounts is unknown.

The American Academy of Pediatrics classifies naproxen as compatible with breastfeeding (29).

References

1. Product information. Naprosyn. Roche Laboratories, 2000.
2. Nielsen GL, Sorensen HT, Larsen H, Pedersen L. Risk of adverse birth outcome and miscarriage in pregnant users of non-steroidal anti-inflammatory drugs: population-based observational study and case-control study. Br Med J 2001;322:266–70.
3. Anonymous. PG-synthetase inhibitors in obstetrics and after. Lancet 1980;2:185–6.
4. Matt DW, Borzelleca JF. Toxic effects on the female reproductive system during pregnancy, parturition, and lactation. In: Witorsch RJ, ed. *Reproductive Toxicology*. 2nd ed. New York, NY: Raven Press, 1995: 175–93.
5. Dawood MY. Nonsteroidal antiinflammatory drugs and reproduction. Am J Obstet Gynecol 1993;169:1255–65.
6. Glover DD, Amonkar M, Rybeck BF, Tracy TS. Prescription, over-the-counter, and herbal medicine use in a rural, obstetric population. Am J Obstet Gynecol 2003;188:1039–45.
7. Fuchs F. Prevention of prematurity. Am J Obstet Gynecol 1976;126: 809–20.
8. Montenegro MA, Palomino H. Induction of cleft palate in mice by inhibitors of prostaglandin synthesis. J Craniofac Genet Del Biol 1990;10:83–94.
9. Siu SSN, Yeung JHK, Lau TK. An in-vivo study on placental transfer of naproxen in early human pregnancy. Hum Reprod 2002;17:1056–9.
10. Wilkinson AR. Naproxen levels in preterm infants after maternal treatment. Lancet 1980;2:591–2.
11. Ericson A, Kallen BAJ. Nonsteroidal anti-inflammatory drugs in early pregnancy. Reprod Toxicol 2001;15:371–5.
12. Li DK, Liu L, Odouli R. Exposure to non-steroidal anti-inflammatory drugs during pregnancy and risk of miscarriage: population based cohort study. Br Med J 2003;327:368–71.
13. Tassinari MS, Cook JC, Hurtt ME. NSAIDs and developmental toxicity. Birth Defects Res B Dev Reprod Toxicol 2003;68:3–4.
14. Kallen B. Maternal drug use and infant cleft lip/palate with special reference to corticoids. Cleft Palate Craniofac J 2003;40:624–8.
15. Kallen BAJ, Olausson PO. Maternal drug use in early pregnancy and infant cardiovascular defect. Reprod Toxicol 2003;17:255–61.

16. Kajantie E, Somer M. Bilateral cleft lip and palate, hypertelorism and hypoplastic toes. Clin Dysmorphol 2004;13:195–6.
17. Ofori B, Oraichi D, Blais L, Rey E, Bérard A. Risk of congenital anomalies in pregnant users of non-steroidal anti-inflammatory drugs: a nested case-control study. Birth Defects Res B Dev Reprod Toxicol 2006;77:268–79.
18. Levin DL. Effects of inhibition of prostaglandin synthesis on fetal development, oxygenation, and the fetal circulation. Semin Perinatol 1980;4:35–44.
19. Rudolph AM. The effects of nonsteroidal antiinflammatory compounds on fetal circulation and pulmonary function. Obstet Gynecol 1981;58(Suppl):63s–7s.
20. Van Marter LJ, Leviton A, Allred EN, Pagano M, Sullivan KF, Cohen A, Epstein MF. Persistent pulmonary hypertension of the newborn and smoking and aspirin and nonsteroidal antiinflammatory drug consumption during pregnancy. Pediatrics 1996;97:658–63.
21. Wilkinson AR, Aynsley-Green A, Mitchell MD. Persistent pulmonary hypertension and abnormal prostaglandin E levels in preterm infants after maternal treatment with naproxen. Arch Dis Child 1979;54:942–5.
22. Alano MA, Ngougmna E, Ostrea EM Jr, Konduri GG. Analysis of nonsteroidal antiinflammatory drugs in meconium and its relation to persistent pulmonary hypertension of the newborn. Pediatrics 2001;107:519–23.
23. Gerris J, Jonckheer M, Sacre-Smits L. Acute hyperthyroidism during pregnancy: a case report and critical analysis. Eur J Obstet Gynecol Reprod Biol 1981;12:271–80.
24. Wiqvist N, Kjellmer I, Thiringer K, Ivarsson E, Karlsson K. Treatment of premature labor by prostaglandin synthetase inhibitors. Acta Biol Med Germ 1978;37:923–30.
25. Talati AJ, Salim MA, Korones SB. Persistent pulmonary hypertension after maternal naproxen ingestion in a term newborn: a case report. Am J Perinatol 2000;17:69–71.
26. Hernandez RK, Werler MM, Romitti P, Sun L, Anderka M, National Birth Defects Prevention Study. Nonsteroidal antiinflammatory drug use among women and the risk of birth defects. Am J Obstet Gynecol 2012;206: 228.e1–8.
27. Jamali F, Tam YK, Stevens RD. Naproxen excretion in breast milk and its uptake by suckling infant (abstract). Drug Intell Clin Pharm 1982;16:475.
28. Jamali F, Stevens DRS. Naproxen excretion in milk and its uptake by the infant. Drug Intell Clin Pharm 1983;17:910–11.
29. Committee on Drugs, American Academy of Pediatrics. The transfer of drugs and other chemicals into human milk. Pediatrics 2001;108: 776–89.

NARATRIPTAN

Antimigraine

PREGNANCY RECOMMENDATION: Limited Human Data—Animal Data Suggest Moderate Risk
BREASTFEEDING RECOMMENDATION: No Human Data—Probably Compatible

PREGNANCY SUMMARY

Naratriptan is not an animal teratogen but does produce dose-related embryo and fetal developmental toxicity. Human pregnancy experience, however, is too limited to assess the embryo–fetal risk. Although a 2008 review of triptans in pregnancy found no evidence for teratogenicity, the data did suggest a possible increase in the rate of preterm birth (1).

N

FETAL RISK SUMMARY

Naratriptan is an oral selective serotonin (5-hydroxytryptamine; 5-HT) receptor subtype agonist used for the acute treatment of migraine headaches. The safety and effectiveness of naratriptan have not been established for cluster headaches. Plasma protein binding is low (28%–31%) and the elimination half-life is 6 hours (2).

Developmental toxicity was observed in pregnant rats and rabbits at oral doses producing maternal plasma drug levels as low as 11 and 2.5 times, respectively, the plasma levels in humans receiving the maximum recommended daily dose of 5 mg (MRDD). Toxicity consisted of embryo lethality, minor fetal structural variations, pup mortality, and offspring growth restriction. In pregnant rats during the period of organogenesis, daily oral doses of 10, 60, and 340 mg/kg/day that resulted in maternal plasma levels 11, 70, and 470 times the human plasma levels obtained with the MRDD, respectively, were associated with dose-related increases in embryonic death and in the incidence of fetal structural variations: incomplete, irregular ossification of skull bones, sternebrae, and ribs. A no-effect dose for these toxicities was not established. The highest dose was associated with maternal toxicity as evidenced by decreased body weight gain. When naratriptan was administered before and throughout the mating period at ≥60 mg/kg/day, there was an increase in preimplantation loss. Impairment of fertility in both male (testicular effects) and female (anestrus) rats occurred at higher doses. Exposure to the two highest doses—60 and 340 mg/kg/day—late in gestation and during lactation resulted in offspring behavioral impairment (tremors) and decreased viability and growth (2).

Pregnant rabbits received daily oral doses during organogenesis, which produced maternal plasma levels ranging from 2.5 to 140 times the human levels produced by the MRDD. Developmental toxicity, observed at all doses, consisted of embryonic death and fetal variations (major blood vessel variations, supernumerary ribs, and incomplete skeletal ossification). Fetal skeletal malformation (fused sternebrae) was observed in one rabbit subspecies at the highest dose. A no-effect dose for these toxicities was not established (2).

It is not known if naratriptan crosses the human placenta. The molecular weight (about 336 for the free base), low plasma protein binding, and long elimination half-life suggest that the drug will cross.

The Sumatriptan/Naratriptan/Treximet Pregnancy Registry, covering the period January 1, 1996, through April 30, 2009, has outcome data for 57 prospectively enrolled (reported before pregnancy outcome was known) pregnancies exposed to naratriptan. There were 52 with earliest exposure in the 1st trimester and 5 in the 2nd trimester. Among those with earliest exposure in the 1st trimester, the outcomes included 45 live births without defects, 1 induced abortion without defect, 5 spontaneous abortions (SABs), and 1 infant (also exposed to sumatriptan in the 1st trimester) with a small ventricular septal defect that was expected to close spontaneously. There were no birth defects in the five cases with earliest exposure in the 2nd trimester. Excluding the fetal death and SABs, the observed proportion of birth defects in the 1st trimester group was 2.2% (95% confidence interval 0.1%–13.0%). The prevalence of birth defects in women with migraine has been estimated at 3.4% (3,4).

Retrospective reports (reported after the outcome was known) are often biased (only adverse outcomes are reported). There were three retrospective reports of birth defects exposed in the 1st trimester. Review of all birth defects from prospective and retrospective reports revealed no signal or consistent pattern to suggest a common cause (4). (See Sumatriptan for required statement.)

Data from the Norwegian Mother and Child Cohort Study were published in 2010 (5). Of the 1535 pregnant women exposed to triptans, 36 were exposed to naratriptan. The exposed group was compared with 68,021 women who did not use triptans. There were no significant associations between 1st trimester exposure to triptans and major congenital anomalies (adjusted odds ratio [OR] 1.0, 95% confidence interval [CI] 0.7–1.2) or other adverse pregnancy outcomes. However, exposure in the 2nd and 3rd trimesters was significantly associated with atonic uterus (OR 1.4, 95% CI 1.1–1.8) and >500 mL blood loss during labor (OR1.3, 95% CI 1.1–1.5) (5).

BREASTFEEDING SUMMARY

No reports describing the use of naratriptan during human lactation have been located. The molecular weight (about 336 for the free base), low plasma protein binding (28%–31%), and the long elimination half-life (6 hours) suggest that the drug will be excreted into breast milk. The effect of this exposure, if any, on a nursing infant is unknown. However, a brief 2010 review concluded that the minimal amounts of other triptans excreted into breast milk are insufficient to cause adverse effects in breastfeeding infants (6).

References

1. Soldin OP, Dahlin J, O'Mara DM. Triptans in pregnancy. Ther Drug Monit 2008;30:5–9.
2. Product information. Amerge. GlaxoSmithKline, 2007.
3. Cunnington M, Ephross S, Churchill P. The safety of sumatriptan and naratriptan in pregnancy: what have we learned. Headache 2009;49:1414–22.
4. Sumatriptan/Naratriptan/Treximet Pregnancy Registry. Interim Report. 1 January 1996 through 30 April 2009. GlaxoSmithKline, August 2009.
5. Nezvalova-Henriksen K, Spigset O, Nordeng H. Triptan exposure during pregnancy and the risk of major congenital malformations and adverse pregnancy outcomes: results from the Norwegian Mother and Child Cohort Study. Headache 2010;50:563–75.
6. Duong S, Bozzo P, Nordeng H, Einarson A. Safety of triptans for migraine headaches during pregnancy and breastfeeding. Can Fam Physician 2010;56:537–9.

NATALIZUMAB

Immunologic Agent (Immunomodulator)

PREGNANCY RECOMMENDATION: Compatible
BREASTFEEDING RECOMMENDATION: No Human Data—Probably Compatible

PREGNANCY SUMMARY

The extensive human pregnancy experience has not shown an increase in structural anomalies, spontaneous abortions (SABs), or fetal death. However, a study described below did find that exposure in the second half of pregnancy impaired the immune system of two newborns, a finding similar to the effect observed in adults treated with the drug. The clinical significance of this impairment requires supportive data. In 2011, the World Congress of Gastroenterology stated, "The safety of natalizumab during pregnancy is unknown. Although human data show no increased risk of birth defects, the agent is too new for adequate supportive data and there are no drugs of similar mechanism with which to compare." (1). Nevertheless, if the maternal condition indicates that the drug is required, it should not be withheld because of pregnancy. If natalizumab is used in pregnancy, physicians are encouraged to enroll patients in the Tysabri pregnancy exposure registry by calling 800-456-2255.

FETAL RISK SUMMARY

Natalizumab is a recombinant humanized immunoglobu lin G4-kappa ($IgG4_K$) monoclonal antibody produced in murine myeloma cells. It is an α-4 integrin inhibitor that is indicated as monotherapy for the treatment of relapsing forms of multiple sclerosis (MS) to delay the accumulation of physical disability and reduce the frequency of clinical exacerbations. It also is indicated for inducing and maintaining clinical response and remission in adult patients with moderately to severely active Crohn's disease and evidence of inflammation, and who have had an inadequate response to, or are unable to tolerate, conventional therapies. The recommended dose is 300 mg IV every 4 weeks. The elimination half-life is approximately 10–11 days (2).

Reproduction studies have been conducted in pregnant guinea pigs and cynomolgus monkeys. In these species, there was no evidence of teratogenicity at doses up to seven times the human clinical dose based on body weight (HCD). In guinea pigs given a dose seven times the HCD during the second half of pregnancy, a small reduction in pup survival was noted at postnatal day 14. At doses seven times the HCD, a doubling of abortions (33% vs. 17%) was observed in one of five studies with monkeys, but no association with abortion was seen in guinea pigs. At this dose in both species, serum levels in fetal animals at delivery were approximately 35% of maternal levels. A dose that was 2.3 times the HCD in monkeys produced drug-related changes in the fetuses: mild anemia, reduced platelet count, increased spleen weights, and reduced liver and thymus weights associated with increased splenic extramedullary hematopoiesis, thymic atrophy, and decreased hepatic hematopoiesis. Reduced platelet counts also were observed in offspring of mothers given seven times the HCD, but this effect was reversed upon clearance of the drug. Offspring exposed in utero had no drug-related changes in the lymphoid organs and had normal immune response (2).

No carcinogenic, clastogenic, or mutagenic effects were observed in various assays and tests conducted with natalizumab. The drug had no effect on male guinea pig fertility, but, at a dose seven times the HCD, a 47% decrease in pregnancy rate relative to controls was observed in females. No such effect was observed at a dose that was 2.3 times the HCD (2).

A series of four research reports, conducted by the manufacturer, on the effects of natalizumab in guinea pigs and cynomolgus monkeys was published in 2009 (3–6). One concern was that the drug would interfere with pregnancy because α-4 integrins and their ligands appear to be critically involved in mammalian fertilization, implantation, and placental and cardiac development (3–6). The results and conclusions of the four studies were similar to those described above. However, the increase in monkey abortions in one cohort was 39.3% vs. 7.1% in controls but, in a second cohort, no increase was observed (33.3% vs. 37.5%). In cynomolgus monkeys treated with doses up to seven times the HCD, no adverse effects on the general health, survival, development, or immunologic structure and function of exposed offspring were observed (6).

Natalizumab crosses the placentas of guinea pigs and monkeys producing fetal drug concentrations approximately 35% of maternal concentrations at birth (2). Because of the similarity to the human placenta and the very long elimination half-life, passage to the fetus should be expected, regardless of the very high molecular weight (about 149,000). Moreover, immune globulin crosses the human placenta in significant amounts near term (see Immune Globulin Intravenous).

Several reports have described the use of natalizumab during pregnancy (1,7–12).

A 2011 review mentioned 164 pregnancies treated with natalizumab during the 1st trimester for either Crohn's disease ($N = 35$) or MS ($N = 129$) (1). There was no increase in the rate of birth defects compared with the expected background occurrence.

In another 2011 report, 35 women with MS became accidentally pregnant while receiving natalizumab (7). Six of the women received the last dose before the last menstrual period (21.3 ± 13.7 days) and 29 after the last menses (22.6 ± 20 days). All of the women stopped the drug when they became aware of the pregnancy. The mean number of doses before pregnancy was 11.7 (range 2–35). The pregnancy outcomes were 28 healthy children, 1 case of hexadactyly, 5 SABs, and 1 elective abortion. There were no significant differences between the outcomes of those exposed and a control group of 23 women with MS who were not exposed to disease-modifying treatments (7).

In a 2011 case report, a 17-year-old patient, who had been treated with natalizumab for MS since she was 16, received seven doses of the drug during an unknown pregnancy (8). Pregnancy was diagnosed in the 31st gestational week. She gave birth to a healthy 2830-g female infant at term with Apgar scores of 10. The infant was doing well at 10 months of age (8).

The outcomes of two planned pregnancies were reported in 2011 (9). In the first case, a 28-year-old woman with MS became pregnant while receiving natalizumab; her last dose was on day 9 of the menstrual cycle. At 37 3/7 weeks, she gave birth to a healthy 3160-g baby girl with Apgar scores of 10 and 10. No abnormalities in the infant were found. The second case involved a 24-year-old woman with MS who did not notify her physician of her pregnancy until 20 weeks' gestation. Natalizumab, 300 mg every 4 weeks, was continued throughout pregnancy. A cesarean section at 41 weeks' delivered a 2940-g female infant with Apgar scores of 5 and 8 at 1 and 5 minutes, respectively. The infant was doing well at 6 weeks of age (9).

A preliminary report from the Tysabri (Natalizumab) Pregnancy Register was described in two references (10,11). As of May 2011, 341 pregnant patients had been prospectively enrolled with 277 known outcomes. There did not appear to be a pattern of drug-related malformations and the rate of SAB (11%) were consistent with the background rate (15%) in the US general population (10,11). Several other pregnancy outcomes following use of natalizumab were also described in one of the references (11).

A 2013 report described the effect of natalizumab on the immune system of two neonates, both born at 38 weeks, whose mothers received the drug until 34 weeks' for MS (12). In the first case, the mother received four doses starting at 21 weeks' gestation. The 2640-g infant had Apgar scores of 9, 10, and 10. No structural anomalies were evident, but a minor intracerebral hemorrhage was detected by ultrasound that later resolved. The infant was anemic and had moderate thrombocytopenia. At age of 6 weeks, the infant was admitted to the hospital with respiratory syncitial virus bronchiolitis that resolved within a few days with symptomatic treatment. The infant was still anemic but the platelet count had normalized. At 12 weeks of age, the infant had mild anemia but otherwise was doing well. The mother in the second case was treated with methylprednisolone up to 13 weeks but, because of relapsing MS, was given four doses of natalizumab starting at 21 weeks' similar to the first case. The 2755-g newborn had Apgar scores of 9, 10, and 10. Because adults treated with natalizumab have a significant decrease in T-lymphocyte chemotaxis, both infants were examined for this decrease. The impaired effects on the immune system were found in both infants at 2 weeks of age but, in both cases, the impairment had resolved by 12 weeks of age. The authors concluded that the clinical relevance of the impaired chemotaxis in the context of host defense, especially against viral pathogens, was unclear because chemotaxis was just one of several features of altered immune cell functions under treatment with natalizumab (12).

BREASTFEEDING SUMMARY

No reports describing the use of natalizumab during human lactation have been located. The molecular weight is very high (about 149,000), but immunoglobulins are excreted into breast milk. Although given once every 4 weeks, the long elimination half-life (10–11 days) will assure that the drug is available for excretion throughout the dosing period. The effects of this potential exposure on a nursing infant are unknown.

References

1. Mahadevan U, Cucchiara S, Hyams JS, Steinwurz F, Nuti F, Travis SPL, Sandborn WJ, Colombel IH. The London position statement of the World Congress of Gastroenterology on biological therapy for IBD with the European Crohn's and Colitis Organization: pregnancy and pediatrics. Am J Gastroenterol 2011;106:214–23.
2. Product information. Tysabri. Biogen Idec, 2008.
3. Wehner NG, Shopp G, Rocca MS, Clarke J. Effects of natalizumab, an α4 integrin inhibitor, on the development of Hartley guinea pigs. Birth Defects Res B Dev Reprod Toxicol 2009;86:98–107.
4. Wehner NG, Skov M, Shopp G, Rocca MS, Clarke J. Effects of natalizumab, an α4 integrin inhibitor, on fertility in male and female guinea pigs. Birth Defects Res B Dev Reprod Toxicol 2009;86:108–16.
5. Wehner NG, Shopp G, Oneda S, Clarke J. Embryo/fetal development in cynomolgus monkeys exposed to natalizumab, an α4 integrin inhibitor. Birth Defects Res B Dev Reprod Toxicol 2009;86:117–30.
6. Wehner NG, Shopp G, Osterburg I, Fuchs A, Buse E, Clarke J. Postnatal development in cynomolgus monkeys following prenatal exposure to natalizumab, an α4 integrin inhibitor. Birth Defects Res B Dev Reprod Toxicol 2009;86:144–56.
7. Hellwig K, Haghikia A, Gold R. Pregnancy and natalizumab: results of an observational study in 35 accidental pregnancies during natalizumab treatment. Mult Scler 2011;17:958–63.
8. Bayas A, Penzien J, Hellwig K. Accidental natalizumab administration to the third trimester of pregnancy in an adolescent patient with multiple sclerosis. Acta Neurol Scand 2011;124:290–2.
9. Hoevenaren IA, de Vries LC, Rijnders RJP, Lotgering FK. Delivery of healthy babies after natalizumab use for multiple sclerosis: a report of two cases. Acta Neurol Scand 2011;123:430–3.
10. Bayas A, Penzien J, Hellwig K. Accidental natalizumab administration in pregnancy in multiple sclerosis. Acta Neurol Scand 2012;126:e5–6. doi:10.1111/j.1600-0404.2011.01636.x.
11. Houtchens MK, Kolb CM. Multiple sclerosis and pregnancy: therapeutic considerations. J Neurol 2013;260:1202–14.
12. Schneider H, Weber CE, Hellwig K, Schroten H, Tenenbaum T. Natalizumab treatment during pregnancy—effects on the neonatal immune system. Acta Neurol Scand 2013;127:e1–4. doi:10.1111/ane.12004.

NATEGLINIDE

Antidiabetic Agent

PREGNANCY RECOMMENDATION: Limited Human Data—Animal Data Suggest Low Risk
BREASTFEEDING RECOMMENDATION: No Human Data—Potential Toxicity

PREGNANCY SUMMARY

The animal data suggest a low risk for developmental toxicity, but only one report of human pregnancy experience has been located. Insulin is the treatment of choice for pregnant diabetics if diet and exercise cannot control the maternal hyperglycemia. Insulin does not cross the placenta to the fetus and, thus, eliminates the additional concern that the drug therapy itself may adversely affect the fetus. Although a potential role in gestational diabetes may exist for some oral hypoglycemics (e.g., see Glyburide), carefully prescribed insulin therapy will provide better control of the mother's blood glucose, thereby preventing the fetal and neonatal complications that occur with this disease. In general, if oral hypoglycemics are used during pregnancy, consideration should be given to changing the therapy to insulin to lessen the possibility of prolonged hypoglycemia in the newborn. The rapid elimination and extensive protein binding of nateglinide, however, may lessen the potential for this adverse effect.

FETAL RISK SUMMARY

Nateglinide is an amino acid derivative that is used as an oral insulin secretagogue. It is structurally unrelated to the oral sulfonylurea agents. Nateglinide is indicated for the management of type 2 diabetes mellitus (non-insulin-dependent) as monotherapy to lower blood glucose when hyperglycemia cannot be adequately controlled by diet and exercise. The drug is rapidly cleared from the plasma with an elimination half-life of approximately 1.5 hours. It is protein bound (98%) primarily by serum albumin and to a lesser degree by α_1-acid glycoprotein. Although the major metabolites are less-potent antidiabetic agents, a minor metabolite has antidiabetic potency similar to that of the parent compound (1).

Reproduction studies with nateglinide have been conducted in rats and rabbits. In rats, no evidence of teratogenicity was observed at doses up to approximately 60 times the human therapeutic exposure from the recommended dose of 120 mg 3 times daily before meals (HTE). Decreased body weights in offspring were observed when these doses were administered in the perinatal and postnatal periods. In rabbits, a dose approximately 40 times the HTE adversely affected embryonic development and increased the incidence of gallbladder agenesis or small gallbladder (1).

It is not known if nateglinide crosses the human placenta. The molecular weight (about 317) suggests that exposure of the embryo and fetus is possible, but the short plasma elimination half-life and extensive protein binding should limit the amount of drug available to cross to the fetal compartment.

In a 2004 case report, a 39-year-old woman took pravastatin (80 mg/day), metformin (2 g/day), and nateglinide (360 mg/day) during the first 24 weeks of gestation (2). All therapy was discontinued and insulin was started for her diabetes. At term, the woman delivered a healthy 2.4-kg male infant (head circumference 34 cm, length 46 cm) with Apgar scores of 8 and 9 at 1 and 5 minutes, respectively. The infant's growth and development were normal at follow-up examinations during the first 6 months of life (2).

N

BREASTFEEDING SUMMARY

No reports describing the use of nateglinide during human lactation have been located. The molecular weight (about 317) suggests that excretion into breast milk may occur, but the short elimination half-life (1.5 hours) and extensive protein binding (98%) should limit the amount of drug and active metabolites available in milk. The effect on a nursing infant is unknown, but hypoglycemia is a potential complication. Thus, if a woman plans to breastfeed, changing her therapy to other agents, such as insulin or a second-generation sulfonylurea (see Glipizide and Glyburide) might be appropriate. In any case, monitoring the infant's blood glucose should be conducted.

References

1. Product information. Starlix. Novartis Pharmaceuticals, 2007.
2. Teelucksingh S, Youssef JE, Sohan K, Ramsewak S. Prolonged inadvertent pravastatin use in pregnancy. Reprod Toxicol 2004;18:299–300.

NEBIVOLOL

Sympatholytic (Antihypertensive)

PREGNANCY RECOMMENDATION: Human Data Suggest Risk in 2nd and 3rd Trimesters
BREASTFEEDING RECOMMENDATION: No Human Data—Potential Toxicity

PREGNANCY SUMMARY

No reports describing the use of nebivolol in human pregnancy have been located.

Based on studies with other agents in the class, the use of nebivolol for maternal disease probably does not pose a major risk of structural defects, but the long-term effects of in utero exposure to β-blockers have not been studied. Persistent β-blockade has been observed in newborns exposed near delivery to other members of this class (see Acebutolol, Atenolol, and Nadolol). Newborns exposed in utero to nebivolol should be closely observed during the first 24–48 hours after birth for bradycardia and other symptoms. Some β-blockers may cause intrauterine growth restriction (IUGR) and reduced placental weight, especially those lacking intrinsic sympathomimetic activity (ISA) (i.e., partial agonist), and nebivolol does not possess ISA. Treatment beginning early in the 2nd trimester results in the greatest weight reductions, whereas treatment restricted to the 3rd trimester primarily affects only placental weight. Although growth restriction is a serious concern, the benefits of maternal therapy, in some cases, might outweigh the risks to the fetus and must be judged on a case-by-case basis.

N

FETAL RISK SUMMARY

Nebivolol, a β-adrenergic receptor blocking agent, is a racemic mixture of d- and l-nebivolol. The active isomer (d-nebivolol) has an effective half-life of about 12 hours in CYP2D6-extensive metabolizers and 19 hours in poor metabolizers. In extensive metabolizers (most of the population) and at doses ≤10 mg, the drug is preferentially β_1 selective, but at higher doses and in poor metabolizers, it is a β_1/β_2 blocker. Nebivolol is indicated for the treatment of hypertension, either alone or in combination with other antihypertensives. The drug has no ISA but does have active metabolites. Plasma protein binding, primarily to albumin, is about 98% and is independent of plasma concentrations (1).

Reproduction studies have been conducted in rats and rabbits. Pregnant rats given nebivolol during organogenesis at maternally toxic doses that were 5 and 10 times the maximum recommended human dose of 40 mg/day based on BSA (MRHD) resulted in reduced fetal body weights. Additionally, at 10 times the MRHD, small reversible delays in sternal and thoracic ossification and a small increase in resorptions were observed. Doses given during late gestation, parturition, and lactation that were ≥1.2 times the MRHD caused decreased birth and pup weights, prolonged gestation, dystocia, and reduced maternal care with corresponding increases in late fetal deaths and stillbirths and decreased pup survival. Insufficient numbers of pups survived at 1.2 times the MRHD to evaluate the offspring for reproductive performance. In contrast, no adverse effects on embryo–fetal viability, sex, weight, or morphology were observed in pregnant rabbits given doses up to 10 times the MRHD (1).

Two-year studies for carcinogenicity were conducted in mice and rats. In mice given a dose that was 5 times the MRHD, a significant increase in testicular Leydig cell hyperplasia and adenomas was observed. The findings were not observed with doses up to 1.2 times the MRHD. The Leydig cell hyperplasia was consistent with an indirect luteinizing hormone–mediated effect of the drug and was not thought to be clinically relevant in humans. No evidence of carcinogenicity was observed in rats with doses up to 10 times the MRHD. No evidence of mutagenicity was noted in several assays (1).

It is not known if nebivolol crosses the human placenta. The molecular weight (about 406 for the free base) and moderately long effective half-life suggest that the drug will cross to the embryo–fetus. Moreover, other β-blockers readily cross the placenta (e.g., see Atenolol, Metoprolol, and Propranolol).

BREASTFEEDING SUMMARY

No reports describing the use of nebivolol during human lactation have been located. The molecular weight (about 406 for the free base) and moderately long effective half-life

(12 or 19 hours) suggest that the drug will be excreted into breast milk. Moreover, other β-blockers are excreted into milk (e.g., see Atenolol, Metoprolol, and Propranolol). Although the amount in milk might not be clinically significant, nursing infants should be closely observed for signs or symptoms of β-blockade. The long-term effects of exposure to β-blockers from milk have not been studied but warrant evaluation. The American Academy of Pediatrics classifies other similar agents as compatible with breastfeeding (e.g., see Metoprolol and Propranolol).

Reference

1. Product information. Bystolic. Forest Pharmaceuticals, 2007.

NEDOCROMIL SODIUM

Respiratory Anti-inflammatory (Inhaled)

PREGNANCY RECOMMENDATION: Limited Human Data—Animal Data Suggest Low Risk
BREASTFEEDING RECOMMENDATION: No Human Data—Probably Compatible

PREGNANCY SUMMARY

The absence of animal embryo–fetal toxicity, the limited human systemic bioavailability, and the outcomes of the exposed human pregnancies appear to suggest that nedocromil sodium is not a major teratogenic risk. Although this assessment is based on limited pregnancy experience, the benefits in preventing maternal asthma probably outweigh any potential fetal harm. Because of the greater pregnancy experience, cromolyn sodium may be the preferred choice (see Cromolyn Sodium).

FETAL RISK SUMMARY

Nedocromil sodium is an inhaled anti-inflammatory agent used in the prevention of asthma. Because of its mast cell–stabilizing properties, it is also available as a 2% ophthalmic solution for the treatment of itching associated with allergic conjunctivitis. Its respiratory action appears to be similar to that of cromolyn sodium. Each activation of the meter delivers 1.75 mg nedocromil from the mouthpiece. In asthmatic patients, the absolute bioavailability after chronic dosing (two activations 4 times a day for 1 month) was approximately 5% of the administered dose (1). No accumulation was observed after chronic use. With chronic administration in the eye, <4% of the total dose is absorbed systemically (2).

No effects on fertility in male and female mice and rats were observed with an SC dose of nedocromil sodium that was about 30 and 60 times, respectively, the maximum recommended human daily inhalation dose based on BSA (MRHID), respectively (1). In reproduction studies, no evidence of teratogenicity or fetal harm was revealed when an SC dose was given to pregnant mice, rats, and rabbits that was about 30, 60, and 116 times the MRHID, respectively (1). The SC dose was >1600 times the maximum recommended human daily ocular dose on a body weight basis (2).

It is not known if nedocromil sodium crosses the human placenta. The molecular weight of the drug (about 415) is low enough that transfer to the fetus should be expected. The low systemic bioavailability (e.g., mean peak plasma concentrations in the 1.6- to 2.8-ng/mL range [1]) suggests that the amounts reaching the embryo or fetus are clinically insignificant.

A report published in 1988 described three women who became pregnant while enrolled in a trial of nedocromil (3). All three were withdrawn from the study because of their pregnancy. One woman stopped the therapy 5 weeks after her last menstrual period. She and another woman (gestational age when therapy stopped not specified) had normal pregnancies. The third woman stopped nedocromil therapy at 8 weeks' gestation and had a spontaneous abortion 5 days later. The abortion was thought to be unrelated to treatment (3).

A 1998 noninterventional observational cohort study described the outcomes of pregnancies in women who had been prescribed one or more of 34 newly marketed drugs by general practitioners in England (4). Data were obtained by questionnaires sent to the prescribing physicians 1 month after the expected or possible date of delivery. In 831 (78%) of the pregnancies, a newly marketed drug was thought to have been taken during the 1st trimester with birth defects noted in 14 (2.5%) singleton births of the 557 newborns (10 sets of twins). In addition, two birth defects were observed in aborted fetuses. However, few of the aborted fetuses were examined. Nedocromil was taken during the 1st trimester in 35 pregnancies. The outcomes of these pregnancies included 1 spontaneous abortion, 8 elective abortions, 3 cases lost to follow-up, 22 normal-term infants, and 1 newborn with a birth defect (4). The birth defect, in an infant born to a 22-year-old woman, was categorized as congenital heart disease (no details given). Other maternal drug exposures in this case included aminophylline, corticosteroids, and salbutamol. Although the cause of the one major congenital malformation observed is unknown, the study lacks the sensitivity to identify minor anomalies because of the absence of standardized examinations. Late-appearing major defects may also have been missed because of the timing of the questionnaires.

BREASTFEEDING SUMMARY

No reports describing the use of nedocromil sodium during human lactation have been located. Although the molecular weight of the drug (about 415) is low enough to allow excretion into breast milk, the very small amounts in the systemic circulation (see above) suggests that the potential for harm in a nursing infant is nil.

References

1. Product information. Tilade. Rhone-Poulenc Rorer Pharmaceuticals, 2000.
2. Product information. Alocril. Allergan, 2001.
3. Carrasco E, Sepulveda R. The acceptability, safety and efficacy of nedocromil sodium in long-term clinical use in patients with perennial asthma. J Int Med Res 1988;16:394–401.
4. Wilton LV, Pearce GL, Martin RM, Mackay FJ, Mann RD. The outcomes of pregnancy in women exposed to newly marketed drugs in general practice in England. Br J Obstet Gynaecol 1998;105:882–9.

NEFAZODONE

Antidepressant

PREGNANCY RECOMMENDATION: Limited Human Data—Animal Data Suggest Moderate Risk
BREASTFEEDING RECOMMENDATION: Limited Human Data—Potential Toxicity

PREGNANCY SUMMARY

Nefazodone, a phenylpiperazine antidepressant, is structurally related to trazodone. Although its exact mechanism of action is unknown, it inhibits neuronal reuptake of serotonin and norepinephrine. Although the animal data suggest moderate risk, the limited human pregnancy experience suggests that the risk of developmental toxicity is low. However, long-term studies on functional and/or neurobehavioral deficits have not been conducted.

FETAL RISK SUMMARY

No teratogenic effects were observed with the use of nefazodone in reproductive toxicity studies involving rats and rabbits dosed, respectively, at 5 and 6 times the maximum human daily dose based on BSA (MHDD) (1). Increased early pup mortality was observed, however, when dosing at 5 times the MHDD in rats began during gestation and continued until weaning. Moreover, decreased pup weights were seen at this and lower doses. The no-effect dose for pup mortality was 1.3 times the MHDD (1).

A 2003 prospective controlled study described the outcomes of 147 pregnancies exposed in the 1st trimester (52 exposed throughout gestation) to either nefazodone or trazodone (2). The outcomes were compared with two control groups (one exposed to other antidepressants and the other exposed to nonteratogens). There were no significant differences among the three groups in terms of spontaneous abortions, elective abortions, stillbirths, major malformations, gestational age at birth, or birth weights. In the study group, there were two (1.4%) major malformations: neural tube defect and Hirschsprung's disease (2).

A 2005 meta-analysis of seven prospective comparative cohort studies involving 1774 patients was conducted to quantify the relationship between seven newer antidepressants and major malformations (3). The antidepressants were bupropion, fluoxetine, fluvoxamine, nefazodone, paroxetine, sertraline, and trazodone. There was no statistical increase in the risk of major birth defects above the baseline of 1%–3% in the general population for the individual or combined studies (3).

A prospective cohort study evaluated a large group of pregnancies exposed to antidepressants in the 1st trimester to determine if there was an association with major malformations (4). The patient population came from the Motherisk database and involved 928 cases that met their criteria. The 928 matched (for age, smoking, and alcohol use) controls were pregnancies not exposed to antidepressants or known teratogens. In addition to the 39 nefazodone cases, the other cases were 113 bupropion, 184 citalopram, 21 escitalopram, 61 fluoxetine, 52 fluvoxamine, 68 mirtazapine, 148 paroxetine, 61 sertraline, 17 trazodone, and 154 venlafaxine. In the antidepressant group, there were 24 (2.5%) major defects compared with 25 (2.6%) in controls (odds ratio 0.9, 95% confidence interval 0.5–1.61). There was one major anomaly, Hirschsprung disease, in the nefazodone group. There were no major defects in the pregnancies exposed to bupropion, escitalopram, or trazodone (4).

BREASTFEEDING SUMMARY

Nefazodone is excreted into breast milk. A 1999 report described an analytical method for determining the concentrations of nefazodone and its metabolites in human plasma and milk (5). In addition, in one woman taking 200 mg twice daily, the paired concentrations of nefazodone in milk and plasma (trough) were 57 and 617 ng/mL, respectively; the milk:plasma ratio was 0.09. In two other subjects, one taking 50 mg twice daily and the other 50 mg in the morning and 100 mg in the evening, the trough plasma levels were <50 ng/mL, whereas the paired milk concentrations were 687 and 213 ng/mL, respectively (5).

Two mothers breastfeeding their infants 21 and 4 weeks postpartum, respectively, were being treated with nefazodone for depression (6). One patient was taking 150 mg/day (50 mg in the morning and 100 mg in the evening) and the other 400 mg/day (200 mg in the morning and evening). Milk and plasma samples were obtained from both patients. Two of the metabolites were not detected in any sample, and hydroxynefazodone was not detected in the plasma of the first patient or in the milk of the second patient (concentrations in both <50 ng/mL). Based on 150 mL/kg/day of milk consumption, the infant doses as a percentage of the mothers' weight-adjusted doses were 2.2% and 0.4%. No adverse effects were observed in the two nursing infants (6).

A 35-year-old woman gave birth to a premature female infant at 27 weeks' gestation (7). The infant was fed the mother's breast milk from a bottle while in the hospital. The mother was started on nefazodone, 200 mg in the morning and 100 mg at night, because of depression 7 weeks after delivery. One week later, the mother began breastfeeding. At 9 weeks of age, the 2.1-kg infant was readmitted to the hospital because of drowsiness, lethargy, failure to maintain body temperature, and poor feeding. Breastfeeding was stopped 1 week later and the infant's symptoms resolved gradually over 72 hours. Maternal blood and breast milk were collected immediately before the 200-mg morning dose and at intervals ≤6 hours (for milk) or 12 hours (for blood). The milk:plasma ratio (based on AUC over 12 hours) for nefazodone was 0.27, and 0.02–0.19 for three metabolites that were identified. The maximum concentrations in milk and plasma were 358 ng/mL (at 3 hours) and 1270 ng/mL (at 1 hour), respectively. The estimated infant dose, relative to the weight-adjusted total daily maternal dose, was 0.3% for nefazodone and 0.45% for the parent drug plus metabolites. The investigators speculated that the sedative effects might have resulted from reduced clearance of the drug secondary to the infant's prematurity (7).

The long-term effects on neurobehavior and development from exposure to antidepressants during a period of rapid CNS development have not been studied. The American Academy of Pediatrics classifies the effects of other antidepressants on nursing infants as unknown but may be of concern (8).

References

1. Product information. Serzone. Bristol-Myers Squibb, 1996.
2. Einarson A, Bonari L, Voyer-Lavigne S, Addis A, Matsui D, Johnson Y, Koren G. A multicentre prospective controlled study to determine the safety of trazodone and nefazodone use during pregnancy. Can J Psychiatry 2003;48:106–9.
3. Einarson TR, Einarson A. Newer antidepressants in pregnancy and rates of major malformations: a meta-analysis of prospective comparative studies. Pharmacoepidemiol Drug Saf 2005;14:823–7.
4. Einarson A, Choi J, Einarson TR, Koren G. Incidence of major malformations in infants following antidepressant exposure in pregnancy: results of a large prospective cohort study. Can J Psychiatry 2009;54:242–6.
5. Dodd S, Buist A, Burrows GD, Maguire KP, Norman TR. Determination of nefazodone and its pharmacologically active metabolites in human blood plasma and breast milk by high-performance liquid chromatography. J Chromatogr B Biomed Sci Appl 1999;730:249–55.
6. Dodd S, Maguire KP, Burrows GD, Norman TR. Nefazodone in the breast milk of nursing mothers: a report of two patients. J Clin Psychopharmacol 2000;20:717–8.
7. Yapp P, Ilett KF, Kristensen JH, Hackett LP, Paech MJ, Rampono J. Drowsiness and poor feeding in a breast-fed infant: association with nefazodone and its metabolites. Ann Pharmacother 2000;34:1269–72.
8. Committee on Drugs, American Academy of Pediatrics. The transfer of drugs and other chemicals into human milk. Pediatrics 2001;108:776–89.

NELARABINE

Antineoplastic

PREGNANCY RECOMMENDATION: No Human Data—Animal Data Suggest Risk
BREASTFEEDING RECOMMENDATION: Contraindicated

N

PREGNANCY SUMMARY

No reports describing the use of nelarabine in human pregnancy have been located. The animal reproduction data and the properties of the drug suggest that there are significant embryo–fetal risks. Nelarabine should be avoided in pregnancy, especially in the 1st trimester. If a pregnant woman requires this agent or if an inadvertent pregnancy occurs, the woman should be advised of the potential risk for severe adverse effects in the embryo and fetus.

FETAL RISK SUMMARY

Nelarabine is a prodrug of a cytotoxic deoxyguanosine analog, 9-β-D-arabinofuranosylguanine (ara-G) that is given as an IV infusion. As a DNA demethylation agent, it is in the same antineoplastic subclass as azacitidine and decitabine. Nelarabine is indicated for the treatment of T-cell acute lymphoblastic leukemia and T-cell lymphoblastic lymphoma that have not responded to or have relapsed following treatment with at least two chemotherapy regimens. Nelarabine is rapidly converted in vivo to ara-G, and then to the active compound, 5′-triphosphate, ara-GTP. The ara-GTP accumulates in leukemic blasts where the drug produces cell death. The plasma half-lives of nelarabine and ara-G are about 30 minutes and 3 hours, respectively, but the terminal elimination half-life could not be accurately estimated because of the prolonged intracellular levels of ara-GTP. Plasma protein binding is less than 25% (1).

Reproduction studies have been conducted in rabbits. Pregnant rabbits given IV infusions of doses ranging from 0.25 to 2 times the human dose based on BSA (HD) had increased incidences of fetal malformations and variations: absent gall bladder, absent accessory lung lobes, fused or extra sternebrae, and delayed ossification (all doses); cleft palates (about 2 times the HD); and absent digits (about 0.75 times the HD). Maternal body weight gain and fetal body weight were reduced at about 3 times the HD, but this toxicity could not account for the increased incidence of malformations (1).

It is not known if nelarabine or ara-G can cross the human placenta. The molecular weight (about 297) of nelarabine and the lack of protein binding suggest that these agents will reach the embryo and fetus. The short plasma half-lives should decrease the exposure.

BREASTFEEDING SUMMARY

No reports describing the use of nelarabine during lactation have been located. The molecular weight (about 297) and lack of protein binding suggest that nelarabine and ara-G will be excreted into breast milk. The short plasma half-lives,

30 minutes and 3 hours, respectively, should decrease the exposure, but the terminal elimination half-life of the intracellular active metabolite ara-GTP has not been determined. Severe neurologic toxicity has been observed in adults receiving this drug, including severe somnolence, convulsions, peripheral neuropathy, and ascending peripheral neuropathies similar in appearance to Guillain-Barré syndrome (1). Therefore, the best course is to not breastfeed while receiving nelarabine.

Reference

1. Product information. Arranon. GlaxoSmithKline, 2006.

NELFINAVIR

Antiviral

PREGNANCY RECOMMENDATION: Compatible—Maternal Benefit >> Embryo/Fetal Risk
BREASTFEEDING RECOMMENDATION: Contraindicated

PREGNANCY SUMMARY

The lack of animal toxicity and the human pregnancy data suggest that nelfinavir is not a major teratogen. If indicated, the drug should not be withheld because of pregnancy.

FETAL RISK SUMMARY

Nelfinavir is an inhibitor of HIV protease. In in vitro tests, the agent was found to be active against both HIV types 1 and 2 (HIV-1 and HIV-2) (1). Other drugs in this class are amprenavir, indinavir, ritonavir, and saquinavir. Protease is an enzyme that is required for the cleavage of viral polyprotein precursors into active functional proteins found in infectious HIV. Nelfinavir, usually in combination with other antiretroviral agents, is indicated for the treatment of HIV infections.

Reproduction studies with nelfinavir have been conducted in rats and rabbits (1). No effects on fertility, mating, embryo survival, or fetal development were observed in rats given doses that produced plasma concentrations comparable with those measured in humans with therapeutic doses. Exposure of pregnant rats from mid-gestation through lactation had no effect on survival, growth, development to weaning, or subsequent fertility of the offspring (1). In rabbits, doses up to a maternal toxic dose (decreased maternal body weight) had no effect on fetal development. However, even at the highest dose, the systemic exposure in rabbits was significantly less than that observed in humans (1).

It is not known if nelfinavir crosses the human placenta to the fetus. The molecular weight of the free base (about 568) is low enough that transfer to the embryo and fetus should be expected.

A 2004 study, using data (through July 2002) from the Antiretroviral Pregnancy Registry (see below), reported 301 1st trimester exposures to nelfinavir (2). The prevalence rate of birth defects, based on nine cases, was 3.0% (95% confidence interval [CI] 1.4–5.6). This rate was similar to the expected rate of 3.1% in the CDC population-based surveillance system (2).

The Antiretroviral Pregnancy Registry reported, for the period January 1989 through July 2009, prospective data (reported before the outcomes were known) involving 4702 live births that had been exposed during the 1st trimester to one or more antiretroviral agents (3). Congenital defects were noted in 134, a prevalence of 2.8% (95% CI 2.4–3.4). In the 6100 live births with earliest exposure in the 2nd/3rd trimesters, there were 153 infants with defects (2.5%, 95% CI 2.1–2.9). The prevalence rates for the two periods did not differ significantly. There were 288 infants with birth defects among 10,803 live births with exposure anytime during pregnancy (2.7%, 95% CI 2.4–3.0). The prevalence rate did not differ significantly from the rate expected in a nonexposed population. There were 3272 outcomes exposed to nelfinavir (1075 in the 1st trimester and 2197 in the 2nd/3rd trimesters) in combination with other antiretroviral agents. There were 98 birth defects (37 in the 1st trimester and 61 in the 2nd/3rd trimesters). In reviewing the birth defects of prospective and retrospective (pregnancies reported after the outcomes were known) registered cases, the Registry concluded that, except for isolated cases of neural tube defects with efavirenz exposure in retrospective reports, there was no other pattern of anomalies (isolated or syndromic) (3). (See Lamivudine for required statement.)

A study published in 1999 evaluated the safety, efficacy, and perinatal transmission rates of HIV in 30 pregnant women receiving various combinations of antiretroviral agents (4). Many of the women were substance abusers. Protease inhibitors (nelfinavir [$N = 7$], indinavir [$N = 6$], and saquinavir [$N = 1$] in combination with nelfinavir) were used in 13 of the women. Antiretroviral therapy was initiated at a median of 14 weeks' gestation (range preconception to 32 weeks). In spite of previous histories of extensive antiretroviral experience and of vertical transmission of HIV, combination therapy was effective in treating maternal disease and in preventing transmission to the current newborns. The outcomes of the pregnancies treated with protease inhibitors appeared to be similar to the 17 cases that did not receive these agents, except that the birth weights were lower (4).

The FDA issued a public health advisory in 1998 on the association between protease inhibitors and diabetes mellitus (5). Because pregnancy is a risk factor for hyperglycemia, there was concern that these antiviral agents would exacerbate this risk. The manufacturer's product information also notes the potential risk for new-onset diabetes, exacerbation of preexisting diabetes, and hyperglycemia in HIV-infected patients receiving protease inhibitor therapy (1). An abstract published in 2000 described the results of a study involving 34 pregnant women treated with protease inhibitors (30 with nelfinavir) compared with 41 controls that evaluated the association with diabetes (6). No association between protease inhibitors and an increased incidence of gestational diabetes was found.

A 1999 abstract reported the effect of protease inhibitors (nelfinavir, indinavir, ritonavir, or saquinavir) in combination with two or more other antiretroviral agents in 39 pregnant women (7). Nelfinavir was the most commonly used protease inhibitor. The mean gestational age at the start of protease inhibitor therapy was 31 weeks (range 8–39 weeks). All of the newborns tested HIV-negative. Based on these outcomes, and the lack of congenital anomalies and serious neonatal complications, and the mother's response to therapy, the authors concluded that protease inhibitor therapy during pregnancy was effective for maternal HIV disease and contributed to the very low rate of perinatal HIV transmission (7).

A multicenter, retrospective survey of pregnancies exposed to protease inhibitors was published in 2000 (8). There were 92 liveborn infants delivered from 89 women (3 sets of twins) at six healthcare centers. One nonviable infant, born at 22 weeks' gestation, died. The surviving 91 infants were evaluated in terms of adverse effects, prematurity rate, and frequency of HIV-1 transmission. Most of the infants were exposed in utero to a single protease inhibitor, but a few were exposed to more than one because of sequential or double combined therapy. The number of newborns exposed to each protease inhibitor was indinavir ($N = 23$), nelfinavir ($N = 39$), ritonavir ($N = 5$), and saquinavir ($N = 34$). Protease inhibitors were started before conception in 18, and during the 1st, 2nd, or 3rd trimester in 12, 44, and 14, respectively, and not reported in 1. Other antiretrovirals used with the protease inhibitors included four nucleoside reverse transcriptase inhibitors (NRTIs) (didanosine, lamivudine, stavudine, and zidovudine). The most common NRTI regimen was a combination of zidovudine and lamivudine (65% of women). In addition, seven women were enrolled in the AIDS Clinical Trials Group Protocol 316 and, at the start of labor, received either a single dose of the non-NTRI nevirapine, or placebo. Maternal conditions thought possibly or likely to be related to therapy were mild anemia in eight, severe anemia in one (probably secondary to zidovudine), and thrombocytopenia in one. Gestational diabetes mellitus was observed in three women (3.3%), a rate similar to the expected prevalence of 2.6% in a nonexposed population. One mother developed postpartum cardiomyopathy and died 2 months after birth of twins, but the cause of death was not known. For the surviving newborns, there was no increase in adverse effects over that observed in previous clinical trials of HIV-positive women, including the prevalence of anemia (12%), hyperbilirubinemia (6%; none exposed to indinavir), and low birth weight (20.6%). Premature delivery occurred in 19.1% of the pregnancies (close to the expected rate). The percentage of infants infected with HIV was 0 (95% CI 0%–3%) (8).

Two reviews, one in 1996 and the other in 1997, concluded that all women currently receiving antiretroviral therapy should continue to receive therapy during pregnancy and that treatment of the mother with monotherapy should be considered inadequate therapy (9,10). The same conclusion was reached in a 2003 review with the added admonishment that therapy must be continuous to prevent emergence of resistant viral strains (11). In 2009, the updated U.S. Department of Health and Human Services guidelines for the use of antiretroviral agents in HIV-1-infected patients continued the recommendation that therapy, with the exception of efavirenz, should be continued during pregnancy (12). If indicated, therefore, protease inhibitors, including nelfinavir, should not be withheld in pregnancy because the expected benefit to the HIV-positive mother outweighs the unknown risk to the fetus. Pregnant women taking protease inhibitors should be monitored for hyperglycemia. Updated guidelines for the use of antiretroviral drugs to reduce perinatal HIV-1 transmission also were released in 2010 (13). Women receiving antiretroviral therapy during pregnancy should continue the therapy, but, regardless of the regimen, zidovudine administration is recommended during the intrapartum period to prevent vertical transmission of HIV to the newborn (13).

BREASTFEEDING SUMMARY

No reports describing the use of nelfinavir during human lactation have been located. The molecular weight of the free base (about 568) is low enough that excretion into breast milk should be expected.

Reports on the use of nelfinavir during human lactation are unlikely because the antiviral agent is used in the treatment of HIV infections. HIV-1 is transmitted in milk, and in developed countries, breastfeeding is not recommended (9,10,12,14–16). In developing countries, breastfeeding is undertaken, despite the risk, because there are no affordable milk substitutes available. Until 1999, no studies had been published that examined the effect of any antiretroviral therapy on HIV-1 transmission in milk. In that year, a study of zidovudine measured a 38% reduction in vertical transmission of HIV-1 infection in spite of breastfeeding when compared with controls (see Zidovudine).

N

References

1. Product information. Viracept. Pfizer, 2006.
2. Covington DL, Conner SD, Doi PA, Sinson J, Daniels EM. Risk of birth defects associated with nelfinavir exposure during pregnancy. Obstet Gynecol 2004;103:1181–9.
3. Antiretroviral Pregnancy Registry Steering Committee. *Antiretroviral Pregnancy Registry International Interim Report for 1 January 1989 through 31 July 2009*. Wilmington, NC: Registry Coordinating Center; 2009. Available at www.apregistry.com. Accessed May 29, 2010.
4. McGowan JP, Crane M, Wiznia AA, Blum S. Combination antiretroviral therapy in human immunodeficiency virus-infected pregnant women. Obstet Gynecol 1999;94:641–6.
5. CDC. Public Health Service Task Force recommendations for the use of antiretroviral drugs in pregnant women infected with HIV-1 for maternal health and for reducing perinatal HIV-1 transmission in the United States. MMWR 1998;47:No. RR-2.
6. Fassett M, Kramer F, Stek A. Treatment with protease inhibitors in pregnancy is not associated with an increased incidence of gestational diabetes (abstract). Am J Obstet Gynecol 2000;182:S97.
7. Stek A, Kramer F, Fassett M, Khoury M. The safety and efficacy of protease inhibitor therapy for HIV infection during pregnancy (abstract). Am J Obstet Gynecol 1999;180:S7.
8. Morris AB, Cu-Uvin S, Harwell JI, Garb J, Zorrilla C, Vajaranant M, Dobles AR, Jones TB, Carlan S, Allen DY. Multicenter review of protease inhibitors in 89 pregnancies. J Acquir Immune Defic Syndr 2000;25:306–11.

9. Carpenter CCJ, Fischi MA, Hammer SM, Hirsch MS, Jacobsen DM, Katzenstein DA, Montaner JSG, Richman DD, Saag MS, Schooley RT, Thompson MA, Vella S, Yeni PG, Volberding PA. Antiretroviral therapy for HIV infection in 1996. JAMA 1996;276;146–54.
10. Minkoff H, Augenbraun M. Antiretroviral therapy for pregnant women. Am J Obstet Gynecol 1997;176:478–89.
11. Minkoff H. Human immunodeficiency virus infection in pregnancy. Obstet Gynecol 2003;101:797–810.
12. Panel on Antiretroviral Guidelines for Adults and Adolescents. *Guidelines for the Use of Antiretroviral Agents in HIV-1-Infected Adults and Adolescents*. Department of Health and Human Services. December 1, 2009:1–161. Available at http://www.aidsinfo.nih.gov/ContentFiles/AdultandAdolescentGL.pdf. Accessed September 17, 2010:60, 96–8.
13. Panel on Treatment of HIV-Infected Pregnant Women and Prevention of Perinatal Transmission. *Recommendations for Use of Antiretroviral Drugs in Pregnant HIV-1-Infected Women for Maternal Health and Interventions to Reduce Perinatal HIV Transmission in the United States*. May 24, 2010:1–117. Available at http://aidsinfo.nih.gov/ContentFiles/PerinatalGL.pdf. Accessed September 17, 2010:30 (Table 5).
14. Brown ZA, Watts DH. Antiviral therapy in pregnancy. Clin Obstet Gynecol 1990;33:276–89.
15. De Martino M, Tovo P-A, Pezzotti P, Galli L, Massironi E, Ruga E, Floreea F, Plebani A, Gabiano C, Zuccotti GV. HIV-1 transmission through breast-milk: appraisal of risk according to duration of feeding. AIDS 1992;6:991–7.
16. Van de Perre P. Postnatal transmission of human immunodeficiency virus type 1: the breast-feeding dilemma. Am J Obstet Gynecol 1995;173:483–7.

NEOMYCIN

Antibiotic (Aminoglycoside)

PREGNANCY RECOMMENDATION: Human Data Suggest Low Risk
BREASTFEEDING RECOMMENDATION: No Human Data—Probably Compatible

PREGNANCY SUMMARY

Neomycin is an aminoglycoside antibiotic. Ototoxicity, which is known to occur in patients after oral, topical, and parenteral neomycin therapy, has not been reported as an effect of in utero exposure. However, eighth cranial nerve toxicity in the fetus is well known following exposure to kanamycin and streptomycin and may potentially occur with neomycin.

FETAL RISK SUMMARY

Small amounts of neomycin (about 3%) are absorbed from the normal gastrointestinal (GI) tract after oral and rectal administration (1). Larger systemic amounts may be obtained if GI motility is impaired. A single 4-g oral dose has produced peak plasma concentrations of 2.5–6.1 mcg/mL 1–4 hours after the dose (1).

No reports describing the passage of neomycin across the placenta to the embryo and fetus have been located, but this should be expected (see other aminoglycosides: Amikacin, Gentamicin, Kanamycin, Streptomycin, and Tobramycin).

Oral neomycin therapy, 2 g daily, depresses urinary estrogen excretion, apparently by inhibiting steroid conjugate hydrolysis in the gut (2). The fall in estrogen excretion resembles the effect produced by ampicillin but occurs about 2 days later. Urinary estriol was formerly used to assess the condition of the fetoplacental unit with depressed levels being associated with fetal distress.

The Collaborative Perinatal Project monitored 50,282 mother–child pairs, 30 of whom had 1st trimester exposure to neomycin (3). No evidence was found to suggest a relationship to large categories of major or minor malformations or to individual defects.

The population-based dataset of the Hungarian Case-Control Surveillance of Congenital Abnormalities, covering 1980–1996, was used to evaluate the teratogenicity of aminoglycoside antibiotics (parenteral gentamicin, streptomycin, tobramycin, and oral neomycin) in a study published in 2000 (4). A case group of 22,865 women who had fetuses or newborns with congenital malformations were compared with 38,151 women who had newborns with no structural defects. A total of 38 cases and 42 controls were treated with aminoglycosides. There were 12 cases (0.05%) and 14 controls (0.04%) treated with oral neomycin (odds ratio 1.4, 95% confidence interval 0.7–3.1). A case–control pair analysis for the 2nd and 3rd months of gestation also failed to show a risk for teratogenicity. The investigators concluded that there was no detectable teratogenic risk for structural defects for any of the aminoglycoside antibiotics (4). They also concluded, although it was not investigated in this study, that the risk of deafness after in utero aminoglycoside exposure was small.

BREASTFEEDING SUMMARY

No reports describing the use of neomycin during human lactation have been located. Small amounts of other aminoglycosides (e.g., see Gentamicin) are excreted into breast milk and absorbed by the nursing infant. The very limited systemic bioavailability of oral neomycin (about 3% for a normal GI tract) suggests that the amounts of neomycin in breast milk are clinically insignificant.

References

1. American Hospital Formulary Service. *Drug Information 2000*. Bethesda, MD: American Society of Health-System Pharmacists, 2000:73–4.
2. Pulkkinen M, Willman K. Reduction of maternal estrogen excretion by neomycin. Am J Obstet Gynecol 1973;115:1153.
3. Heinonen OP, Slone D, Shapiro S. *Birth Defects and Drugs in Pregnancy*. Littleton, MA: Publishing Sciences Group, 1977:297–301.
4. Czeizel AE, Rockenbauer M, Olsen J, Sorensen HT. A teratological study of aminoglycoside antibiotic treatment during pregnancy. Scand J Infect Dis 2000;32:309–13.

NEOSTIGMINE

Parasympathomimetic (Cholinergic)

PREGNANCY RECOMMENDATION: Limited Human Data—No Relevant Animal Data
BREASTFEEDING RECOMMENDATION: Limited Human Data—Probably Compatible

PREGNANCY SUMMARY

Neostigmine is a quaternary ammonium compound with anticholinesterase activity used in the diagnosis and treatment of myasthenia gravis and to reverse muscle relaxation from competitive (nondepolarizing) muscle relaxants. Multiple studies have reported its use for this indication without observing embryo–fetal harm.

FETAL RISK SUMMARY

Although neostigmine is ionized at physiologic pH, the molecular weight (about 223) is low enough that transfer of the nonionized fraction to the embryo and fetus should be expected. Circumstantial evidence for neostigmine placental transfer was presented in a 1996 case report (1). A woman at 31 weeks' gestation, undergoing surgery for a fractured elbow, was given IV neostigmine (5 mg) and glycopyrrolate (1 mg) to reverse muscle paralysis at the end of the procedure. The fetal heart rate immediately decreased from 115–130 beats/minute to 90–110 beats/minute and then gradually returned to 130 bpm within 1 hour. Four days later, surgical repair of the elbow was again required. At the end of this surgery, neostigmine (5 mg) and atropine (0.4 mg) were given IV and no change in the fetal heart rate was observed. The authors attributed the different effects on the fetal heart rate to the greater placental transfer of atropine in comparison with glycopyrrolate (see also Glycopyrrolate), which resulted in blocking the transplacental muscarinic effects of neostigmine (1).

The safe use of neostigmine in the treatment of maternal myasthenia gravis or other conditions has been reported (2–12). One study described 22 exposures to neostigmine in the 1st trimester (2). No relationship to congenital defects was found. A 1973 study reported the use of IM neostigmine (0.5 mg/day) for 3 days as a pregnancy test in 27 women with "uncertain pregnancies" at 5–14 weeks' gestation (3). Although vaginal bleeding occurred in 7 (26%) patients, only 1 aborted and the remaining 26 went to term without complications. In a 1983 report, two women with myasthenia gravis were treated throughout gestation with neostigmine, 105 mg/day (combined with pyridostigmine and ambenonium) and 300 mg/day (combined with pyridostigmine), respectively, without apparent fetal harm (12).

One investigator considers neostigmine to be one of the drugs of choice for pregnant patients with myasthenia gravis (4). This author also cautioned that IV anticholinesterases should not be used in pregnancy because of the potential for inducing premature labor and suggested that IM neostigmine be used in place of IV edrophonium for diagnostic purposes (4). This recommendation, however, should be approached with caution in view of the high rate of vaginal bleeding following IM neostigmine described above.

Transient muscular weakness has been observed in about 20% of newborns of mothers with myasthenia gravis (10). The neonatal myasthenia is caused by transplacental passage of anti-acetylcholine receptor immunoglobulin G antibodies (10).

BREASTFEEDING SUMMARY

No reports describing the use of neostigmine during lactation have been located. Two publications have stated that the drug is not excreted into breast milk (11,13). However, pyridostigmine, another quaternary ammonium compound, is found in breast milk (see Pyridostigmine). Thus, although neostigmine is ionized at physiologic pH, the molecular weight (about 223) is low enough that the nonionized fraction should be excreted into milk. The effects, if any, on a nursing infant from exposure to neostigmine in milk are unknown.

N

References

1. Clark RB, Brown MA, Lattin DL. Neostigmine, atropine, and glycopyrrolate: does neostigmine cross the placenta? Anesthesiology 1996;84:450–2.
2. Heinonen OP, Slone D, Shapiro S. *Birth Defects and Drugs in Pregnancy*. Littleton, MA: Publishing Sciences Group, 1977:345–56.
3. Brunclik V, Hauser GA. Short-term therapy in secondary amenorrhea. Ther Umsch 1973;30:496–502.
4. McNall PG, Jafarnia MR. Management of myasthenia gravis in the obstetrical patient. Am J Obstet Gynecol 1965;92:518–25.
5. Foldes FF, McNall PG. Myasthenia gravis: a guide for anesthesiologists. Anesthesiology 1962;23:837–72.
6. Chambers DC, Hall JE, Boyce J. Myasthenia gravis and pregnancy. Obstet Gynecol 1967;29:597–603.
7. Hay DM. Myasthenia gravis and pregnancy. J Obstet Gynaecol Br Commonw 1969;76:323–9.
8. Blackhall MI, Buckley GA, Roberts DV, Roberts JB, Thomas BH, Wilson A. Drug-induced neonatal myasthenia. J Obstet Gynaecol Br Commonw 1969;76:157–62.
9. Eden RD, Gall SA. Myasthenia gravis and pregnancy: a reappraisal of thymectomy. Obstet Gynecol 1983;62:328–33.
10. Plauche WC. Myasthenia gravis in pregnancy: an update. Am J Obstet Gynecol 1979;135:691–7.
11. Fraser D, Turner JWA. Myasthenia gravis and pregnancy. Proc R Soc Med 1963;56:379–81.
12. Lefvert AK, Osterman PO. Newborn infants to myasthenic mothers: a clinical study and an investigation of acetylcholine receptor antibodies in 17 children. Neurology 1983;33:133–8.
13. Wilson JT. Pharmacokinetics of drug excretion. In: Wilson JT, ed. *Drugs in Breast Milk*. Balgowlah, Australia: ADIS Press, 1981:17.

NEPAFENAC

Ophthalmic Nonsteroidal Anti-inflammatory

PREGNANCY RECOMMENDATION: No Human Data—Animal Data Suggest Low Risk
BREASTFEEDING RECOMMENDATION: No Human Data—Probably Compatible

PREGNANCY SUMMARY

No reports describing the use of the nonsteroidal anti-inflammatory drug (NSAID) nepafenac in human pregnancy have been located. The animal reproduction data suggest low risk, but the absence of human pregnancy experience prevents a more complete assessment of the embryo–fetal risk. The manufacturer recommends avoiding use of the drug in late pregnancy because of the known toxicity on the fetal cardiovascular system (premature closure of the ductus arteriosus) (1).

FETAL RISK SUMMARY

Nepafenac is an NSAID available as an ophthalmic suspension. It is indicated for the treatment of pain and inflammation associated with cataract surgery. The drug penetrates the cornea and is converted by ocular tissue enzymes to the NSAID drug amfenac, the active agent. After bilateral 3-times-daily dosing, low concentrations of nepafenac and amfenac were detected in the plasma with peak concentrations of 0.3 and 0.4 ng/mL, respectively, 2–3 hours postdose. No information on plasma protein binding or elimination half-life was provided (1).

Reproduction studies with nepafenac and amfenac have been conducted in rats and rabbits. When rats were given oral doses of nepafenac and amfenac that produced plasma exposures up to about 260 and 2400 times, respectively, the human plasma exposures at the recommended human ophthalmic dose (RHOD), no evidence of teratogenicity was observed. However, maternal toxicity, observed at the highest dose or higher, was associated with dystocia, increased postimplantation loss, reduced fetal weights and growth, and reduced fetal survival. No evidence of teratogenicity was observed in rabbits with oral doses producing exposures up to about 80 and 680 times, respectively, the human plasma exposures at the RHOD. Maternal toxicity also was observed at the highest dose (1).

Nepafenac has not been evaluated in long-term carcinogenicity studies. The drug increased chromosomal aberrations in hamster ovary cells but was not mutagenic in multiple assays. No effects on fertility in male and female rats were observed with nepafenac or amfenac (1).

It is not known if nepafenac or amfenac crosses the human placenta. The molecular weight of nepafenac (about 254) is low enough to cross the placenta. Although the molecular weight of amfenac was not provided, it is probably similar to the prodrug and also should cross. However, the systemic concentrations of both drugs are very low.

BREASTFEEDING SUMMARY

No reports describing the use nepafenac during human lactation have been located. The molecular weight of nepafenac (about 254) is low enough for excretion into breast milk. Although the molecular weight of the active agent, amfenac, was not provided, it is probably similar to the prodrug and also should be excreted into milk. However, the systemic concentrations of both drugs are very low. Consequently, the risk to a nursing infant from exposure is probably low or nonexistent.

Reference

1. Product information. Nevanac. Alcon Laboratories, 2008.

NESIRITIDE

Vasodilator

PREGNANCY RECOMMENDATION: No Human Data—Animal Data Suggest Low Risk
BREASTFEEDING RECOMMENDATION: No Human Data—Probably Compatible

PREGNANCY SUMMARY

No reports describing the use of nesiritide in human pregnancy have been located. The animal data suggest low risk, but the absence of human pregnancy experience prevents an accurate assessment of the embryo–fetal risk. However, nesiritide is a recombinant formulation of human B-type natriuretic peptide, a naturally occurring peptide produced in the ventricular myocardium. Although the indication suggests that use in pregnancy will be uncommon; if indicated, it should not be withheld because of pregnancy.

FETAL RISK SUMMARY

Nesiritide is indicated for the IV treatment of patients with acutely decompensated congestive heart failure who have dyspnea at rest or with minimal activity. Nesiritide is metabolized to inactive metabolites and the terminal elimination half-life is about 18 minutes (1).

Reproduction studies have been conducted in rabbits. In this species, no adverse effects on live births or fetal development were observed at a dose given by continuous infusion for 13 days, producing exposures that were about 70 times higher than the human exposure at the recommended dose (1).

Studies of carcinogenicity or effects on fertility have not been conducted. The drug was not mutagenic in an in vitro assay (1).

It is not known if nesiritide crosses the human placenta. The relatively high molecular weight (3464) and very short terminal elimination half-life suggest that exposure of the embryo and/or fetus will be minimal.

BREASTFEEDING SUMMARY

No reports describing the use of nesiritide during human lactation have been located. The relatively high molecular weight (3464) and very short terminal elimination half-life (about 18 minutes) suggest that the peptide will not be excreted into breast milk in clinically significant amounts. Moreover, as a peptide, any amounts in milk probably will be digested in the infant's gut.

Reference

1. Product information. Natrecor. Scios, 2009.

NEVIRAPINE

Antiviral

PREGNANCY RECOMMENDATION: Compatible—Maternal Benefit >> Embryo/Fetal Risk
BREASTFEEDING RECOMMENDATION: Contraindicated

PREGNANCY SUMMARY

The human data for nevirapine suggest that the risk for embryo–fetal harm is low. At least at term, the drug readily crosses the human placenta. If indicated, the drug should not be withheld because of pregnancy.

N

FETAL RISK SUMMARY

Nevirapine is used in combination with other antiviral agents in the treatment of HIV infections. It is a non-nucleoside reverse transcriptase inhibitor (nnRTI). Other agents in this class include delavirdine and efavirenz (1).

No teratogenic effects were observed in reproductive studies with rats and rabbits. In rats, however, a significant decrease in fetal weight occurred at doses producing systemic levels approximately 50% higher (based on AUC) than those seen with the recommended human dose. Moreover, impaired fertility was noted in female rats at doses producing levels approximately equal to those seen with the recommended human dose (1).

Nevirapine readily crosses the human placenta to the fetus. In a study reported by the manufacturer, nevirapine crossed the placentas of 10 HIV type 1 (HIV-1)-infected women given a single oral dose of 100 or 200 mg a mean 5.8 hours before delivery (1). The placental transfer is consistent with the low molecular weight of about 266.

A study published in 1998 described the pharmacokinetics of nevirapine in 18 HIV-1-infected women who received the drug in active labor (2). In the first cohort, 10 women were treated with 100 or 200 mg of nevirapine, but no drug was given to their infants. Based on the pharmacokinetic data in the first cohort, eight additional women were given a 200-mg dose of nevirapine during active labor and their infants received a 2-mg/kg dose 48–72 hours after birth. In this latter cohort, delivery was a median 5.4 hours after dosing. The median cord blood nevirapine concentration was 1106 ng/mL, resulting in a median ratio of cord blood:maternal plasma of 82.9% (range 71.9%–120.2%). The median calculated nevirapine concentration 7 days after birth was 215 ng/mL (range 112–275 ng/mL). Maintaining the concentration above 100 ng/mL (10 times the in vitro 50% inhibitory concentration [IC_{50}] against HIV) during labor and in the neonate during the 7 days of life was a specific goal of the study. No adverse effects due to nevirapine or HIV-infected infants were observed (2).

A 1999 study also described the pharmacokinetics of a single 200-mg dose of nevirapine given to 20 HIV-infected women during labor and to 13 of the neonates at 72 hours (3). The median cord:maternal blood ratio was 0.75. The target drug level (>100 ng/mL; 10 times the IC_{50}) in the neonates was maintained in all infants at 7 days of age, whether or not they received nevirapine at 72 hours. No serious adverse effects attributable to nevirapine were observed (3).

The Antiretroviral Pregnancy Registry reported, for January 1989 through July 2009, prospective data (reported before the outcomes were known) involving 4702 live births that had been exposed during the 1st trimester to one or more antiretroviral agents (4). Congenital defects were noted in 134, a prevalence of 2.8% (95% confidence interval [CI] 2.4–3.4). In the 6100 live births with earliest exposure in the 2nd/3rd trimesters, there were 153 infants with defects (2.5%, 95% CI 2.1–2.9). The prevalence rates for the two periods did not differ significantly. There were 288 infants with birth defects among 10,803 live births with exposure anytime during pregnancy (2.7%, 95% CI 2.4–3.0). The prevalence rate did not differ significantly from the rate expected in a nonexposed population. There were 2007 outcomes exposed to nevirapine (842 in the 1st trimester and 1165 in the 2nd/3rd trimesters) in combination with other antiretroviral agents. There were 45 birth defects (18 in the 1st trimester and 27 in the 2nd/3rd trimesters). In reviewing the birth defects of prospective and retrospective (pregnancies reported after the outcomes were known) registered cases, the Registry concluded that, except for isolated cases of neural tube defects with efavirenz exposure in retrospective reports, there was no other pattern of anomalies (isolated or syndromic) (4). (See Lamivudine for required statement.)

A 2000 case report described the pregnancy outcomes of two pregnant women with HIV infection who were treated with the anti-infective combination, trimethoprim/sulfamethoxazole, for prophylaxis against *Pneumocystis carinii*, concurrently with antiretroviral agents (5). One of the cases involved a 31-year-old woman, who presented at 15 weeks' gestation. She was receiving trimethoprim/sulfamethoxazole, didanosine, stavudine, nevirapine, and vitamin B supplements (specific vitamins and dosage not given) that had been started before conception. A fetal ultrasound at 19 weeks' gestation revealed spina bifida and ventriculomegaly. The patient elected to terminate her pregnancy. The fetus did not have HIV infection. Defects observed at autopsy included ventriculomegaly, an Arnold-Chiari malformation, sacral spina bifida, and a lumbosacral meningomyelocele. The authors attributed the neural tube defects to the antifolate activity of trimethoprim (5).

A study published in 1999 evaluated the safety, efficacy, and perinatal transmission rates of HIV in 30 pregnant women receiving various combinations of antiretroviral agents (6). Many of the women were substance abusers. Nevirapine was used in combination with zidovudine, didanosine, and/or lamivudine in two of the women. Antiretroviral therapy was initiated at a median of 14 weeks' gestation (range preconception to 32 weeks). Despite previous histories of extensive antiretroviral experience and of vertical transmission of HIV, combination therapy was effective in treating maternal disease and in preventing transmission to the current newborns. No adverse outcomes were noted in the two nevirapine-exposed cases (6).

A 1999 study compared the safety and efficacy of a short course of nevirapine to zidovudine for the prevention of mother-to-child transmission of HIV-1 (7). At the onset of labor, women were randomly assigned to receive either a single dose of nevirapine (200 mg) plus a single dose (2 mg/kg) to their infants 24–72 hours after birth ($N = 310$) or zidovudine (600 mg then 300 mg every 3 hours until delivery) plus 4 mg/kg twice daily for 7 days to their infants ($N = 308$). Nearly all (98.8%) of the women breastfed their infants immediately after birth. Up to age 14–16 weeks, significantly fewer infants in the nevirapine group were HIV-1 infected, lowering the risk of infection or death, compared with zidovudine, by 48% (95% CI, 24–65) (7). The prevalence of maternal and infant adverse effects was similar in the two groups. In an accompanying study, the nevirapine regimen was shown to be cost-effective in various seroprevalence settings (8).

If nevirapine is used in the 2nd/3rd trimesters, in utero exposure may induce hepatic cytochrome P450 CYP3A metabolism, thereby increasing the drug's clearance in the newborn (9). Therefore, offspring of pregnant women chronically treated with nevirapine may not receive protection from HIV infection for the full 7 days observed in those not exposed to chronic dosing (9).

A review published in 2000 reviewed seven clinical trials that have been effective in reducing perinatal transmission, five with zidovudine alone, one with zidovudine plus lamivudine, and one with nevirapine (10). Six of the trials were in developing countries. Prolonged use of zidovudine in the mother and infant was not only the most effective for preventing vertical transmission, but also the most expensive. Single-dose nevirapine (in the mother and infant) was the least expensive and the simplest regimen to administer (10).

Two reviews, one in 1996 and the other in 1997, concluded that all women currently receiving antiretroviral therapy should continue to receive therapy during pregnancy and that treatment of the mother with monotherapy should be considered inadequate therapy (11,12). The same conclusion was reached in a 2003 review with the added admonishment that therapy must be continuous to prevent emergence of resistant viral strains (13). In 2009, the updated U.S. Department of Health and Human Services guidelines for the use of antiretroviral agents in HIV-1-infected patients continued the recommendation that therapy, with the exception of efavirenz, should be continued during pregnancy (14). If indicated, nevirapine should not be withheld in pregnancy because the expected benefit to the HIV-positive mother outweighs the unknown risk to the fetus. Updated guidelines for the use of antiretroviral drugs to reduce perinatal HIV-1 transmission also were released in 2010 (15). Women receiving antiretroviral therapy during pregnancy should continue the therapy, but, regardless of the regimen, zidovudine administration is recommended during the intrapartum period to prevent vertical transmission of HIV to the newborn (15).

BREASTFEEDING SUMMARY

Nevirapine is excreted into breast milk. In a study reported by the manufacturer, nevirapine was found in the breast milk of 10 women with HIV-1 infection given a single oral dose of 100 or 200 mg a mean 5.8 hours before delivery (1). In 21 HIV-infected women who had received a single 200-mg dose of nevirapine during labor, the median milk:maternal plasma ratio was 60.5% (range 25.3%–122.2%) (3). At 48 hours after birth, the median breast milk concentration was 454 ng/mL (range 219–972 ng/mL), declining to 103 ng/mL (range 50–309 ng/mL) 7 days after birth (3).

HIV-1 is transmitted in milk, and in developed countries, breastfeeding is not recommended (11,12,14,16–18). In developing countries, breastfeeding is undertaken, despite the risk, because there are no affordable milk substitutes available. Zidovudine, zidovudine plus lamivudine, and nevirapine have all been shown to reduce, but not eliminate, the risk of HIV-1 transmission during breastfeeding (see also Lamivudine and Zidovudine) (10).

References

1. Product information. Viramune. Roxane Laboratories, 2001.
2. Mirochnick M, Fenton T, Gagnier P, Pav J, Gwynne M, Siminski S, Sperling RS, Beckerman K, Jimenez E, Yogev R, Spector SA, Sullivan JL, for the Pediatric AIDS Clinical Trials Group Protocol 250 Team. Pharmacokinetics

of nevirapine in human immunodeficiency virus type 1-infected pregnant women and their neonates. J Infect Dis 1998;178:368–74.
3. Musoke P, Guay LA, Bagenda D, Mirochnick M, Nakabiito C, Fleming T, Elliott T, Horton S, Dransfield K, Pav JW, Murarka A, Allen M, Fowler MG, Mofenson L, Hom D, Mmiro F, Jackson JB. A phase I/II study of the safety and pharmacokinetics of nevirapine in HIV-1-infected pregnant Ugandan women and their neonates (HIVNET 006). AIDS 1999;13:479–86.
4. Antiretroviral Pregnancy Registry Steering Committee. *Antiretroviral Pregnancy Registry International Interim Report for 1 January 1989 through 31 July 2009*. Wilmington, NC: Registry Coordinating Center; 2009. Available at www.apregistry.com. Accessed May 29, 2010.
5. Richardson MP, Osrin D, Donaghy S, Brown NA, Hay P, Sharland M. Spinal malformations in the fetuses of HIV infected women receiving combination antiretroviral therapy and co-trimoxazole. Eur J Obstet Gynecol Reprod Biol 2000;93:215–7.
6. McGowan JP, Crane M, Wiznia AA, Blum S. Combination antiretroviral therapy in human immunodeficiency virus-infected pregnant women. Obstet Gynecol 1999;94:641–6.
7. Guay LA, Musoke P, Fleming T, Bagenda D, Allen M, Nakabiito C, Sherman J, Bakaki P, Ducar C, Deseyve M, Emel L, Mirochnick M, Fowler MG, Mofenson L, Miotti P, Dransfield K, Bray D, Mmiro F, Jackson JB. Intrapartum and neonatal single-dose nevirapine compared with zidovudine for prevention of mother-to-child transmission of HIV-1 in Kampala, Uganda: HIVNET 012 randomised trial. Lancet 1999;354:795–802.
8. Marseille E, Kahn JG, Mmiro F, Guay L, Musoke P, Fowler MG, Jackson JB. Cost effectiveness of single-dose nevirapine regimen for mothers and babies to decrease vertical HIV-1 transmission in sub-Saharan Africa. Lancet 1999;354:803–9.
9. Taylor GP, Lyall EGH, Back D, Ward C, Tudor-Williams G. Pharmacological implications of lengthened in-utero exposure to nevirapine. Lancet 2000;355:2134–5.
10. Mofenson LM, McIntyre JA. Advances and research directions in the prevention of mother-to-child HIV-1 transmission. Lancet 2000;355: 2237–44.
11. Carpenter CCJ, Fischi MA, Hammer SM, Hirsch MS, Jacobsen DM, Katzenstein DA, Montaner JSG, Richman DD, Saag MS, Schooley RT, Thompson MA, Vella S, Yeni PG, Volberding PA. Antiretroviral therapy for HIV infection in 1996. JAMA 1996;276:146–54.
12. Minkoff H, Augenbraun M. Antiretroviral therapy for pregnant women. Am J Obstet Gynecol 1997;176:478–89.
13. Minkoff H. Human immunodeficiency virus infection in pregnancy. Obstet Gynecol 2003;101:797–810.
14. Panel on Antiretroviral Guidelines for Adults and Adolescents. *Guidelines for the Use of Antiretroviral Agents in HIV-1-Infected Adults and Adolescents*. Department of Health and Human Services. December 1, 2009:1–161. Available at http://www.aidsinfo.nih.gov/ContentFiles/AdultandAdolescentGL.pdf. Accessed September 17, 2010:60, 96–8.
15. Panel on Treatment of HIV-Infected Pregnant Women and Prevention of Perinatal Transmission. *Recommendations for Use of Antiretroviral Drugs in Pregnant HIV-1-Infected Women for Maternal Health and Interventions to Reduce Perinatal HIV Transmission in the United States*. May 24, 2010:1–117. Available at http://aidsinfo.nih.gov/ContentFiles/PerinatalGL.pdf. Accessed September 17, 2010:30 (Table 5).
16. Brown ZA, Watts DH. Antiviral therapy in pregnancy. Clin Obstet Gynecol 1990;33:276–89.
17. De Martino M, Tovo P-A, Pezzotti P, Galli L, Massironi E, Ruga E, Floreea F, Plebani A, Gabiano C, Zuccotti GV. HIV-1 transmission through breast-milk: appraisal of risk according to duration of feeding. AIDS 1992;6:991–7.
18. Van de Perre P. Postnatal transmission of human immunodeficiency virus type 1: the breast feeding dilemma. Am J Obstet Gynecol 1995;173: 483–7.

NIACIN

Vitamin/Antilipemic Agent

PREGNANCY RECOMMENDATION: Compatible
BREASTFEEDING RECOMMENDATION: Compatible

PREGNANCY SUMMARY

Niacin, a B complex vitamin, is converted in humans to niacinamide, the active form of vitamin B_3. See Niacinamide.

BREASTFEEDING SUMMARY

See Niacinamide.

NIACINAMIDE

Vitamin

PREGNANCY RECOMMENDATION: Compatible
BREASTFEEDING RECOMMENDATION: Compatible

PREGNANCY SUMMARY

Niacinamide, a water-soluble B complex vitamin, is an essential nutrient required for lipid metabolism, tissue respiration, and glycogenolysis (1). Both niacin, which is converted to niacinamide in vivo, and niacinamide are available commercially and are collectively known as vitamin B_3. The National Academy of Sciences' recommended dietary allowance (RDA) for niacin in pregnancy is 17 mg (1).

N

FETAL RISK SUMMARY

Only two reports have been located that link niacinamide with maternal or fetal complications. A 1948 study observed an association between niacinamide deficiency and pregnancy-induced hypertension (PIH) (2). Other B complex vitamins have also been associated with this disease, but any relationship between vitamins and PIH is controversial (see other B complex vitamins). One patient with hyperemesis gravidarum presented with neuritis, reddened tongue, and psychosis (3). She was treated with 100 mg of niacin plus other B complex vitamins, resulting in the rapid disappearance of her symptoms. The authors attributed her response to the niacin.

Niacinamide is actively transported to the fetus (4,5). Higher concentrations are found in the fetus and newborn, rather than in the mother (5–8). Deficiency of niacinamide in pregnancy is uncommon except in women with poor nutrition (6,7). At term, the mean niacinamide value in 174 mothers was 3.9 mcg/mL (range 2.0–7.2 mcg/mL) and in their newborns was 5.8 mcg/mL (range 3.0–10.5 mcg/mL) (6). Conversion of the amino acid, tryptophan, to niacin and then to niacinamide is enhanced in pregnancy (9).

BREASTFEEDING SUMMARY

Niacin, the precursor to niacinamide, is actively excreted into breast milk (10). Reports on the excretion of niacinamide in milk have not been located, but it is probable that it also is actively transferred. In a study of lactating women with low nutritional status, supplementation with niacin in doses of 2.0–60.0 mg/day resulted in mean milk concentrations of 1.17–2.75 mcg/mL (10). Milk concentrations were directly proportional to dietary intake. A 1983 English study measured niacin levels in pooled human milk obtained from mothers of preterm (26 mothers, 29–34 weeks) and term (35 mothers, ≥39 weeks) infants (11). Niacin in milk from preterm mothers rose from 0.65 (colostrum) to 2.05 mcg/mL (16–196 days), whereas that in milk from term mothers increased during the same period from 0.50 to 1.82 mcg/mL.

The National Academy of Sciences' RDA for niacin during lactation is 20 mg (1). If the diet of the lactating woman adequately supplies this amount, supplementation with niacinamide is not needed. Maternal supplementation with the RDA for niacinamide is recommended for those patients with inadequate nutritional intake.

References

1. American Hospital Formulary Service. *Drug Information 1997*. Bethesda, MD: American Society of Health-System Pharmacists, 1997:2811–13.
2. Hobson W. A dietary and clinical survey of pregnant women with particular reference to toxaemia of pregnancy. J Hyg 1948;46:198–216.
3. Hart BF, McConnell WT. Vitamin B factors in toxic psychosis of pregnancy and the puerperium. Am J Obstet Gynecol 1943;46:283.
4. Hill EP, Longo LD. Dynamics of maternal-fetal nutrient transfer. Fed Proc 1980;39:239–44.
5. Kaminetzky HA, Baker H, Frank O, Langer A. The effects of intravenously administered water-soluble vitamins during labor in normovitaminemic and hypovitaminemic gravidas on maternal and neonatal blood vitamin levels at delivery. Am J Obstet Gynecol 1974;120:697–703.
6. Baker H, Frank O, Thomson AD, Langer A, Munves ED, De Angelis B, Kaminetzky HA. Vitamin profile of 174 mothers and newborns at parturition. Am J Clin Nutr 1975;28:59–65.
7. Baker H, Frank O, Deangelis B, Feingold S, Kaminetzky HA. Role of placenta in maternal-fetal vitamin transfer in humans. Am J Obstet Gynecol 1981;141:792–6.
8. Baker H, Thind IS, Frank O, DeAngelis B, Caterini H, Lquria DB. Vitamin levels in low-birth-weight newborn infants and their mothers. Am J Obstet Gynecol 1977;129:521–4.
9. Wertz AW, Lojkin ME, Bouchard BS, Derby MB. Tryptophan–niacin relationships in pregnancy. Am J Nutr 1958;64:339–53.
10. Deodhar AD, Rajalakshmi R, Ramakrishnan CV. Studies on human lactation. Part III. Effect of dietary vitamin supplementation on vitamin contents of breast milk. Acta Paediatr Scand 1964;53:42–8.
11. Ford JE, Zechalko A, Murphy J, Brooke OG. Comparison of the B vitamin composition of milk from mothers of preterm and term babies. Arch Dis Child 1983;58:367–72.

NIALAMIDE

[Withdrawn from the market. See 8th edition.]

NICARDIPINE

Calcium Channel Blocker

PREGNANCY RECOMMENDATION: Limited Human Data—Animal Data Suggest Risk
BREASTFEEDING RECOMMENDATION: No Human Data—Probably Compatible

PREGNANCY SUMMARY

Nicardipine has caused dose-related embryo toxicity, but not teratogenicity, in animals. Human data early in gestation are insufficient to assess the risk to the embryo or fetus. Only a few of the 10 calcium channel blockers have any human data on exposure during early gestation. Based on this very limited information, these agents do not appear to be major human teratogens. However, more information is required before any conclusion can be reached as to the potential teratogenic risk of these agents. In addition, maternal hypotension caused by nicardipine is a theoretical complication that could jeopardize the fetus.

FETAL RISK SUMMARY

Nicardipine is a calcium channel-blocking agent used in the treatment of angina and hypertension. The drug has also been used as a tocolytic in premature labor.

Dose-related embryotoxicity, but not teratogenicity, was observed in reproduction studies using IV nicardipine in rats and rabbits (1). Embryotoxic doses were about 2.5 and 0.5 times, respectively, the maximum recommended human dose (MRHD). At 50 times the MRHD in rats, dystocia, reduced birth weights, reduced neonatal survival, and reduced neonatal weight gain were noted (1). In one type of rabbit, but not in another, high doses (about 75 times the MRHD) were embryocidal (1). Two studies with rats reported that in utero exposure had no effect on postnatal function or subsequent fertility (2,3).

Nicardipine 20 mcg/kg/minute was infused for 2 minutes in 15 near-term ewes given angiotensin II 5 mcg/minute (4). Transient bradycardia was observed in the fetuses, followed by hypercapnia and acidemia. These changes were associated with a decrease in fetal placental blood flow and an increase in fetal vascular resistance, and five fetuses died 65 minutes after nicardipine was given. In the second part of this study in the pregnant ewe, nicardipine was found to reverse maternal angiotensin II-induced systemic vasoconstriction, including that of the renal and endomyometrial vascular beds, but it caused a significant increase in placental vascular resistance (5).

The use of nicardipine as a tocolytic agent was first investigated in an experiment using excised rabbit uterus and in laboring (either spontaneous or induced) rats (6). In both species, the calcium channel blocker was effective in abolishing uterine contractions. A 1983 study investigated the effect of nicardipine and nifedipine on isolated human pregnant-term and nonpregnant myometrium (7). Nicardipine was a more potent tocolytic than nifedipine in pregnant myometrium, but its onset of action was slower.

Because the cardiovascular and myometrial responses of pregnant rabbits are similar to those observed in human pregnancies (8), a series of studies was conducted in the rabbit with nicardipine to determine its effectiveness as a tocolytic agent and its safety for the mother and the fetus (8–10). A statistically significant inhibition of uterine contractions was recorded in each study, but this effect was accompanied by maternal tachycardia, an increase in cardiac output, a drop in both diastolic and systolic blood pressure and mean arterial pressure, and a decrease in uteroplacental blood flow. The authors of these studies cautioned that further trials were necessary because the decrease in uteroplacental blood flow would seriously jeopardize the fetus (9,10).

In a study to determine the tocolytic effects of nicardipine in a primate species, pregnant rhesus monkeys with spontaneous uterine contractions were treated with an IV bolus of 500 mcg, followed by a continuous infusion of 6 mcg/kg/minute for 1 hour (11). Placental transfer of nicardipine was demonstrated with peak fetal concentrations ranging from 7 to 35 ng/mL compared with maternal peak levels of 175 to 865 ng/mL. Although a marked tocolytic effect was observed, significant acidemia and hypoxemia developed in the fetuses.

It is not known if nicardipine crosses the human placenta. The molecular weight (about 480 for the free base) suggests that exposure of the embryo–fetus should be expected.

The tocolytic effects of nicardipine have been reported (12–14). The agent compared favorably with albuterol (12) and magnesium sulfate (13,14). No adverse effects in the newborns attributable to nicardipine were observed.

The direct effects of nicardipine on the fetus were investigated in a study using fetal sheep (15). Infusions of nicardipine, either 50 or 100 mcg, had minimal, nonsignificant effects on mean arterial and diastolic blood pressure and no effect on fetal heart rate, fetal arterial blood gas values, and maternal cardiovascular variables. The authors concluded that the fetal hypoxia observed in other animal studies, when nicardipine was administered to the mother, was not due to changes in umbilical or ductal blood flow but to a decrease in maternal uterine blood flow (15).

A single 10-mg dose of nicardipine was given to eight women with acute hypertension (diastolic blood pressure >105 mmHg) in the 3rd trimester of pregnancy (16). A significant decrease in maternal diastolic, but not in systolic, pressure was observed during the next 60 minutes with an onset at 15 minutes.

Nicardipine has been used in human pregnancy for the treatment of hypertension (17,18). Forty women with mild or moderate hypertension (25 with gestational hypertension, 3 with preeclampsia, and 12 with chronic hypertension) were treated with oral nicardipine 20 mg 3 times a day, beginning at 28 weeks' gestation through the 7th postpartum day, a mean duration of 9 weeks (17). An additional 20 women were treated with IV nicardipine for severe preeclampsia, 5 of whom also had chronic hypertension, beginning at a mean 33 weeks' gestation (range 27–40 weeks). The IV dose used was based on body weight: 2 mg/hr (N = 9; <80 kg), 4 mg/hr (N = 8; 80–90 kg), and 6 mg/hr (N = 3; >90 kg). The mean duration of IV therapy was 5.3 days (range 2–15 days). Low placental passage of nicardipine was demonstrated in 10 women, 7 on oral therapy, and 3 receiving IV therapy, but no accumulation of the drug was observed in the fetus. No perinatal deaths, fetal adverse effects, or adverse neonatal outcomes attributable to nicardipine were observed during treatment. Both umbilical and cerebral Doppler velocimetry remained stable throughout the study (17).

A study published in 1994 compared nicardipine and metoprolol in the treatment of hypertension (gestational, preeclampsia, and chronic) during pregnancy (18). Fifty patients were treated in each group starting at a gestational age of about 29 weeks. Nicardipine decreased maternal systolic and diastolic blood pressure and umbilical artery resistance significantly more than metoprolol and significantly fewer patients required a cesarean section for fetal distress (6% vs. 28%). The difference in birth weights in the two groups was 201 g (2952 vs. 2751 g) (*ns*) (18).

A prospective, multicenter, cohort study of 78 women (81 outcomes; 3 sets of twins) who had 1st trimester exposure to calcium channel blockers (none of whom took nicardipine) was reported in 1996 (19). Compared with controls, no increased risk of congenital malformations was found.

BREASTFEEDING SUMMARY

No reports describing the use of nicardipine during human lactation have been located. The molecular weight (about 480 for the free base) suggests that the drug will be excreted into breast milk. The effect of this exposure on a nursing infant is unknown.

N

References

1. Product information. Cardene. Wyeth-Ayerst Pharmaceuticals, 2000.
2. Sejima Y, Sado T. Teratological study of 2-(*N*-benzyl-*N*-methylamino) ethyl methyl 2,6-dimethyl-4-m-nitrophenyl)-1,4-dihydropyridine-3,5-dicarboxylate hydrochloride (YC-93) in rats. Kiso to Rinsho 1979;13:1149–59. As cited in Shepard TH. *Catalog of Teratogenic Agents*. 6th ed. Baltimore, MD: The Johns Hopkins University Press, 1989:447.
3. Sato T, Nagaoka T, Fuchigami K, Ohsuga F, Hatano M. Reproductive studies of 2-(*N*-benzyl-*N*-methylamino) ethyl methyl 2,6-dimethyl-4-m-nitrophenyl)-1,4-dihydropyridine-3,5-dicarboxylate hydrochloride (YC-93) in rats and rabbits. Kiso to Rinsho 1979;13:1160–76. As cited in Shepard TH. *Catalog of Teratogenic Agents*. 6th ed. Baltimore, MD: The Johns Hopkins University Press, 1989:447.
4. Parisi VM, Salinas J, Stockmar EJ. Fetal vascular responses to maternal nicardipine administration in the hypertensive ewe. Am J Obstet Gynecol 1989;161:1035–9.
5. Parisi VM, Salinas J, Stockmar EJ. Placental vascular responses to nicardipine in the hypertensive ewe. Am J Obstet Gynecol 1989;161:1039–43.
6. Csapo AI, Puri CP, Tarro S, Henzel MR. Deactivation of the uterus during normal and premature labor by the calcium antagonist nicardipine. Am J Obstet Gynecol 1982;142:483–91.
7. Maigaard S, Forman A, Andersson KE, Ulmsten U. Comparison of the effects of nicardipine and nifedipine on isolated human myometrium. Gynecol Obstet Invest 1983;16:354–66.
8. Lirette M, Holbrook RH, Katz M. Effect of nicardipine HCl on prematurely induced uterine activity in the pregnant rabbit. Obstet Gynecol 1985;65:31–6.
9. Litette M, Holbrook RH, Katz M. Cardiovascular and uterine blood flow changes during nicardipine HCl tocolysis in the rabbit. Obstet Gynecol 1987;69:79–82.
10. Holbrook RH Jr, Lirette M, Katz M. Cardiovascular and tocolytic effects of nicardipine HCl in the pregnant rabbit: comparison with ritodrine HCl. Obstet Gynecol 1987;69:83–7.
11. Ducsay CA, Thompson JS, Wu AT, Novy MJ. Effects of calcium entry blocker (nicardipine) tocolysis in rhesus macaques: fetal plasma concentrations and cardiorespiratory changes. Am J Obstet Gynecol 1987;157:1482–6.
12. Jannet D, Abankwa A, Guyard B, Carbonne B, Marpeau L, Milliez J. Nicardipine versus salbutamol in the treatment of premature labor. A prospective randomized study. Eur J Obstet Gynaecol Reprod Med 1997;73:11–6.
13. Ross EL, Ross BS, Dickerson GA, Fischer RG, Morrison JC. Oral nicardipine versus intravenous magnesium sulfate for the treatment of preterm labor (abstract). Am J Obstet Gynecol 1998;178:S181.
14. Larmon JE, Ross BS, May WL, Dickerson GA, Fischer RG, Morrison JC. Oral nicardipine versus intravenous magnesium sulfate for the treatment of preterm labor. Am J Obstet Gynecol 1999;181:1432–7.
15. Holbrook RH, Voss EM, Gibson RN. Ovine fetal cardiorespiratory response to nicardipine. Am J Obstet Gynecol 1989;161:718–21.
16. Walker JJ, Mathers A, Bjornsson S, Cameron AD, Fairlie FM. The effect of acute and chronic antihypertensive therapy on maternal and fetoplacental Doppler velocimetry. Eur J Obstet Gynecol Reprod Biol 1992;43:193–9.
17. Carbonne B, Jannet D, Touboul C, Khelifati Y, Milliez J. Nicardipine treatment of hypertension during pregnancy. Obstet Gynecol 1993;81:908–14.
18. Jannet D, Carbonne B, Sebban E, Milliez J. Nicardipine versus metoprolol in the treatment of hypertension during pregnancy: a randomized comparative trial. Obstet Gynecol 1994;84:354–9.
19. Magee LA, Schick B, Donnenfeld AE, Sage SR, Conover B, Cook L, McElhatton PR, Schmidt MA, Koren G. The safety of calcium channel blockers in human pregnancy: a prospective, multicenter cohort study. Am J Obstet Gynecol 1996;174:823–8.

NICOTINE REPLACEMENT THERAPY

Central Nervous System Agent (Smoking Deterrent)

N

PREGNANCY RECOMMENDATION: Compatible—Maternal Benefit >> Embryo/Fetal Risk
Contraindicated (with any use of tobacco)
BREASTFEEDING RECOMMENDATION: No Human Data—Potential Toxicity

PREGNANCY SUMMARY

Nicotine is a toxic, highly addictive compound. Although additional studies are needed to determine the magnitude of the embryo/fetal risk from using nicotine replacement therapy (NRT), the risk from cigarette smoking is well known. Cigarette smoke contains more than 3000 different compounds, including nicotine, carbon monoxide, ammonia, polycyclic aromatic hydrocarbons, hydrogen cyanide, and vinyl chloride (see Cigarette Smoking).

Nonpharmacologic approaches to smoking cessation are the safest for the mother and her embryo/fetus, but if these methods have failed, the use of nicotine replacement therapy (NRT) during pregnancy might be reasonable. Women must be counseled that if they continue to smoke while using NRT, such as the dermal patch, the risk to their embryo and/or fetus might be greater than when either is used alone. Reducing smoking before or early in gestation and before starting the dermal patch should be attempted. Other strategies that might lessen the fetal risk include starting the patches after organogenesis, wearing the patches for 16 hours a day, and adherence to the tapering schedule so that the patches can be discontinued after 8–10 weeks. These strategies apply to all NRTs. Nevertheless, a pregnant woman should be informed that exposure to any nicotine, whatever the source, carries a risk of embryo and/or fetal harm.

FETAL RISK SUMMARY

Nicotine is a stimulant that is a major component of tobacco smoke. NRT is used to reduce withdrawal symptoms, including nicotine craving, associated with quitting smoking. The products include skin patches (nicotine transdermal patches), chewing gum (nicotine polacrilex [nicotine resin complex]), nicotine inhaler, and nicotine nasal sprays. Only the inhaler and nasal sprays require a prescription in the United States.

Shepard (1) briefly reviewed a number of animal studies that found widespread nicotine-induced toxicity during pregnancy. The animal species included mice, rats, and rabbits, and accidentally exposed swine. Toxicity included stillbirths, reduced fetal body weight, skeletal defects, cleft palate, limb deformities, hydrocephalus, changes in the brain, toxicity to germ cells and oocytes, and retarded placental development. Schardein also discusses the teratogenicity of tobacco in livestock and experimental animals (2).

The pharmacokinetics of nicotine, its effects on uterine blood flow, and its presence in the fetal compartment are described in the review of cigarette smoking (see Cigarette Smoking). NRT avoids the high nicotine levels associated with cigarette smoking (1). However, it may actually deliver more nicotine to the embryo and fetus (see reference 12 below).

In 2006, a study using data from the Danish National Birth Cohort (1997–2003) evaluated the outcomes of 20,603 women who smoked during the first 12 weeks of pregnancy compared with 56,165 nonexposed controls (3). In the smoking group, there were 1034 (5.0%) liveborn infants with congenital malformations compared with 2733 (4.9%) liveborn infants in the control group (not significant). Malformations of cleft lip, the digestive tract, and the cardiovascular system had significantly high odds ratios. There were 19 (7.6%) liveborn infants with congenital malformations among 250 women who used NRT during the first 12 weeks of pregnancy. Six of the defects were major musculoskeletal congenital malformations. After exclusion of seven cases of dislocation of the hip and one minor defect, the relative prevalence rate ratio (RPR) for major malformations was 1.13 (95% confidence interval [CI] 0.62–2.07) and for musculoskeletal defects was 2.05 (95% CI 0.91–4.63). For smokers, the RPR ranged from 1.01 to 1.09 with no indication of a dose–response association. However, early spontaneous abortions in smokers may have altered the findings. The authors concluded that the data suggested an increased risk of congenital defects in nonsmokers using NRT (3).

Four groups of authors criticized the above study for various reasons, but all were most concerned over the study's conclusion that smoking may be safer for the fetus than NRT (4–7). Other concerns included the small size of the NRT group, the absence of maternal history, when the NRT was started, the levels of nicotine obtained with smoking compared with NRT, lack of a statistical power estimation, lack of statistical significance, differences between subjects and controls, and the potential for misclassification. In a reply, the authors responded to the concerns and stated that while they did not claim the association to be causal, causality could not be excluded (8).

Women who are attempting to conceive and those who are pregnant should be encouraged to stop smoking (9–13). In addition to the obvious health benefits for the woman, smoking cessation can significantly decrease the known risks to the embryo, fetus, newborn, infant, and adolescent. For example, women who quit smoking in the first 3 or 4 months of pregnancy can lower the risk of a low-birth-weight infant to that of nonsmoking women (9). Smoking cessation also reduces the risk of prematurity and perinatal deaths, and results in fewer infant/adolescent complications (9). Many different strategies have been developed to promote smoking cessation (9–13). A nonpharmacologic approach is preferred, but many women may be heavily addicted to smoking and require NRT and other agents. However, NRT has not been adequately studied in pregnancy. One concern is the potential for nicotine-induced decreased uterine blood flow and increased uterine vascular resistance that could result in impaired fetal growth and other complications.

Transdermal systems appear to be more effective than chewing gum because of improper use and taste of the latter (10). On the other hand, transdermal patches may actually deliver more nicotine to the embryo/fetus because continuous blood levels of nicotine, in contrast to periodic levels from episodic smoking, are available to cross the placenta (12). One strategy to reduce the amount of embryo–fetal nicotine exposure is to apply the patches for only 16 hours a day (4).

Based on four published studies of NRT in pregnancy, two involving patches, gum in one, and any type of NRT in one, a 2010 review concluded that the therapy decreased the risk for low birth weight and preterm delivery compared with continued smoking (14).

BREASTFEEDING SUMMARY

No reports describing the use of NRT during lactation have been located. Nicotine is excreted into breast milk (see Cigarette Smoking). Although there are significant risks from cigarette smoking for the mother and her nursing infant, the risks of exposure to NRT have not been defined. The American Academy of Pediatrics encourages smoking cessation during lactation, but makes no recommendation for or against NRT because of insufficient data (15).

References

1. Shepard TH. *Catalog of Teratogenic Agents*. 10th ed. Baltimore, MD: The Johns Hopkins University Press, 2001:361–2.
2. Schardein JL. *Chemically Induced Birth Defects*. 3rd ed. New York, NY: Marcel Dekker, 2000:981–2.
3. Morales-Suarez-Varela MM, Bille C, Christensen K, Olsen J. Smoking habits, nicotine use, and congenital malformations. Obstet Gynecol 2006;107: 51–7.
4. Le Houezec J, Benowitz NL. Smoking habits, nicotine use, and congenital malformations. Obstet Gynecol 2006;107:1166.
5. Davidson P. Smoking habits, nicotine use, and congenital malformations. Obstet Gynecol 2006;107:1166–7.
6. Einarson A, Sarkar M, Djulus J, Koren G. Smoking habits, nicotine use, and congenital malformations. Obstet Gynecol 2006;107:1167.
7. Dempsey DA, Stewart SI. Smoking habits, nicotine use, and congenital malformations. Obstet Gynecol 2006;107:1167–8.
8. Morales-Suarez-Varela MM, Olsen J, Bille C, Christensen K. Smoking habits, nicotine use, and congenital malformations. Obstet Gynecol 2006;107:1168.
9. Adams J. Statement of the Public Affairs Committee of the Teratology Society on the importance of smoking cessation during pregnancy. Birth Defects Res A Clin Mol Teratol 2003;67:895–9.
10. Kendrick JS, Merritt RK. Women and smoking: an update for the 1990s. Am J Obstet Gynecol 1996;175:528–35.
11. Floyd RL, Rimer BK, Giovino GA, Mullen PD, Sullivan SE. A review of smoking in pregnancy: effects on pregnancy outcomes and cessation efforts. Annu Rev Publ Health 1993;14:379–411.
12. Slotkin TA. Fetal nicotine or cocaine exposure: which one is worse? J Pharmacol Exp Ther 1998;285:931–45.
13. American College of Obstetricians and Gynecologists. Smoking cessation during pregnancy. *Committee Opinion*. No. 471, November 2010. Obstet Gynecol 2010;116:1241–4.
14. Forinash AB, Pitlick JM, Clark K, Alsat V. Nicotine replacement therapy's effect on pregnancy outcome. Ann Pharmacother 2010;44: published online, 26 Oct 2010, theannals.com. doi:10.1345/aph.1P279.
15. Committee on Drugs, American Academy of Pediatrics. The transfer of drugs and other chemicals into human milk. Pediatrics 2001;108:776–89.

N

NICOTINYL ALCOHOL

[Withdrawn from the market. See 9th edition.]

NICOUMALONE

Anticoagulant

See Coumarin Derivatives.

NIFEDIPINE

Calcium Channel Blocker

PREGNANCY RECOMMENDATION: Human Data Suggest Low Risk
BREASTFEEDING RECOMMENDATION: Limited Human Data—Probably Compatible

PREGNANCY SUMMARY

The experience with nifedipine in human pregnancy is limited, although the agent has been used for tocolysis and as an antihypertensive agent in pregnant women. The agent does not appear to be a major human teratogen based on the results of two studies. Severe adverse reactions, however, have occurred when the drug was combined with IV magnesium sulfate.

FETAL RISK SUMMARY

N

The use of nifedipine, a calcium channel-blocking agent, during pregnancy is controversial. Studies in pregnant sheep with IV infusions of the drug indicate that a progressive decrease in mean maternal arterial blood pressure occurs without a significant alteration of uterine vascular resistance (1). The hypotensive effect of nifedipine resulted in a decrease in uterine blood flow and fetal arterial oxygen content. Other investigators have reported similar results in animals with other calcium channel blockers (2). Although these studies indicated the potential problems with nifedipine, the investigators cautioned that their findings were preliminary and needed to be confirmed in humans (1,3).

Reproduction studies with nifedipine have been conducted in mice, rats, and rabbits (4). The drug was teratogenic (digital anomalies similar to those reported with phenytoin) in rats and rabbits, an effect that might have resulted from compromised uterine blood flow. Other toxicities were noted in the embryos and fetuses of mice, rats, and rabbits at doses 3.5 to 42 times the maximum recommended human dose (MRHD) on a weight basis, or doses higher or lower than the MRHD based on BSA (4). These toxicities included stunted fetuses (mice, rats, rabbits), rib deformities (mice), cleft palate (mice), embryo and fetal deaths (mice, rats, rabbits), and prolonged pregnancy and decreased neonatal survival (rats; not evaluated in other species) (4). Small placentas and underdeveloped chorionic villi were observed in monkeys at doses equivalent to or less than the MRHD based on BSA (4). IV nifedipine in pregnant rhesus monkeys has been associated with fetal hypoxemia and acidosis (5).

In a surveillance study of Michigan Medicaid recipients involving 229,101 completed pregnancies conducted between 1985 and 1992, 37 newborns had been exposed to nifedipine during the 1st trimester (F. Rosa, personal communication, FDA, 1993). Two (5.4%) major birth defects were observed (two expected), one of which was a cardiovascular defect (0.5 expected). No anomalies were observed in five other categories of defects (oral clefts, spina bifida, polydactyly, limb reduction defects, and hypospadias) for which specific data were available.

A human study was reported in 1988 in which nine hypertensive pregnant women in the 3rd trimester were treated with 5 mg of nifedipine sublingually and compared with nine hypertensive women treated with placebo (6). The women were randomly assigned to the two groups, but treatment was not blinded. Both maternal arterial blood pressure and uterine artery perfusion pressure were significantly lowered by nifedipine, but no apparent reduction in uteroplacental blood flow was detected. The investigators interpreted their findings as suggestive of a relative uterine vasodilation and a relative decrease in uterine vascular resistance that was proportional to the decrease in blood pressure (6).

Nifedipine has been used during the 2nd and 3rd trimesters for the treatment of severe hypertension (7). No fetal heart rate changes were observed after reduction of maternal blood pressure, nor were other adverse effects noted in the fetus or newborn. In a 1987 study, 23 women with severe hypertension of various causes (4 gestational, 17 essential, 1 renal, and 1 systemic lupus erythematosus) who either failed to respond to first-line therapy (atenolol, methyldopa, or hydralazine) and had slow-release nifedipine, 40–120 mg/day, added to their regimens

(N = 22), or nifedipine, 40 mg/day, was used as initial therapy (N = 1) (8). Good blood pressure control was obtained in 20 women. The mean duration of therapy was 8.75 weeks (range 1–24 weeks). There were three perinatal deaths (rate 130/1000), but none could be attributed to drug therapy. The mean gestational age at delivery was 35 weeks (range 29–39 weeks), and 15 (71%) of the 21 liveborn infants were delivered by cesarean section. A high percentage of the 22 infants with accessible data were growth restricted, 9 (41%) had birth weights at or below the 3rd percentile, and 20 (91%) were at or below the 10th percentile for body weight. The investigators could not determine whether this outcome was caused by the severe maternal disease, drug therapy, or a combination of both (8).

Nifedipine has been used as a tocolytic agent. An in vitro study using pregnant human myometrium found that nifedipine caused a dose-related decrease in contraction strength and lengthened the period of contraction in a non-dose-related manner (9). In three studies totaling 31 women, nifedipine was used for this purpose (10–12). In one patient, nifedipine, 20 mg 3 times daily combined with terbutaline, was given for a total of 55 days (11). A study involving 60 women in presumed early labor was reported in 1986 (12). Women were included in this open trial if they had a singleton pregnancy and intact membranes, were between 20 and 35 weeks' gestation, and were contracting at least once every 10 minutes, and if their cervix was <4 cm dilated. Included among the various exclusions was a history of mid-trimester abortion or previous preterm delivery. The women were equally divided into three groups: nifedipine, ritodrine, and no treatment. Nifedipine dosage was 30 mg orally followed by 20 mg every 8 hours for 3 days. Ritodrine was initially administered as a standard IV infusion, followed by 48 hours of oral therapy. The days from presentation to delivery in the nifedipine, ritodrine, and no treatment groups were 36.3, 25.1, and 19.3 days (p <0.001 nifedipine compared with the other two groups), respectively (12). No complications of the therapy were found in any of the infants from the three studies. Two of the studies conducted follow-up examinations of the infants at 5–12 months of age and all were alive and well (10,11).

Two apparently clinically significant drug interactions when nifedipine and magnesium were used concurrently have been reported (13,14). A woman, at 32 weeks' gestation in premature labor, was treated with 60 mg of nifedipine orally for 3 hours, followed by 20 mg every 8 hours. Uterine contractions returned 12 hours later and IV magnesium sulfate was started, followed by the onset of pronounced muscle weakness after 500 mg had been administered. Her symptoms consisted of jerky movements of the extremities, difficulty in swallowing, paradoxical respirations, and an inability to raise her head from the pillow (13). The muscle weakness resolved 25 minutes after the magnesium was stopped. The effects were attributed to nifedipine potentiation of the neuromuscular-blocking action of magnesium. In a second report, two women were hospitalized for hypertension at 30 and 32 weeks' gestation (14). In both cases, oral methyldopa (2 g) and IV magnesium sulfate (20 g) daily were ineffective in lowering the mother's blood pressure. Oral nifedipine 10 mg was given and a marked hypotensive response occurred 45 minutes later. The blood pressures before nifedipine were 150/110 and 140/105 mmHg, respectively, and then decreased to 80/50 and 90/60 mmHg, respectively, after administration of the calcium channel blocker. The blood pressures returned to the previous levels 25–30 minutes later. Both infants were delivered following the hypotensive episodes, but only one survived.

The pharmacokinetics of nifedipine in pregnant women have been studied (15).

A prospective, multicenter, cohort study of 78 women (81 outcomes; 3 sets of twins) who had 1st trimester exposure to calcium channel blockers, including 44% to nifedipine, was reported in 1996 (16). Compared with controls, no increase in the risk of major congenital malformations was found.

BREASTFEEDING SUMMARY

Nifedipine is excreted into breast milk (17). A woman with persistent hypertension after premature delivery at 26 weeks' gestation was treated with nifedipine 30 mg every 8 hours for 48 hours, then 20 mg every 8 hours for 48 hours, then 10 mg every 8 hours for 36 hours. Concentrations of the drug in milk were related to dosage and the time interval between the dose and milk collection. Peak concentrations and time of occurrence were 53.35 ng/mL 30 minutes after 30 mg, 16.35 ng/mL 1 hour after 20 mg, and 12.89 ng/mL 30 minutes after 10 mg. The estimated milk half-lives after the three doses were 2.4 hours (30 mg), 3.1 hours (20 mg), and 1.4 hours (10 mg). In comparison with controls, nifedipine had no effect on milk composition. The authors concluded that these amounts, representing <5% of a therapeutic dose, posed little risk to a nursing infant. If desired, delaying breastfeeding by 3–4 hours after a dose would significantly decrease the amount of drug ingested by the infant (17). The American Academy of Pediatrics classifies nifedipine as compatible with breastfeeding (18).

N

References

1. Harake B, Gilbert RD, Ashwal S, Power GG. Nifedipine: effects on fetal and maternal hemodynamics in pregnant sheep. Am J Obstet Gynecol 1987;157:1003–8.
2. Holbrook RH Jr. Effects of calcium antagonists during pregnancy. Am J Obstet Gynecol 1989;160:1018.
3. Gilbert RD. Effects of calcium antagonists during pregnancy. Reply. Am J Obstet Gynecol 1989;160:1018–9.
4. Product information. Procardia. Pfizer, 2000.
5. Ducsay CA, Cook MJ, Veille JC, Novy MJ. *Nifedipine Tocolysis in Pregnant Rhesus Monkeys: Maternal and Fetal Cardiorespiratory Effects*. Society of Perinatal Obstetricians Annual Meeting, Las Vegas, NV, February 1985, Abstract No. 79.
6. Lindow SW, Davies N, Davey DA, Smith JA. The effect of sublingual nifedipine on uteroplacental blood flow in hypertensive pregnancy. Br J Obstet Gynaecol 1988;95:1276–81.
7. Walters BNJ, Redman CWG. Treatment of severe pregnancy-associated hypertension with the calcium antagonist nifedipine. Br J Obstet Gynaecol 1984;91:330–6.
8. Constantine G, Beevers DG, Reynolds AL, Luesley DM. Nifedipine as a second line antihypertensive drug in pregnancy. Br J Obstet Gynaecol 1987;94;1136–42.
9. Bird LM, Anderson NC Jr, Chandler ML, Young RC. The effects of aminophylline and nifedipine on contractility of isolated pregnant human myometrium. Am J Obstet Gynecol 1987;157:171–7.
10. Ulmsten U, Andersson K-E, Wingerup L. Treatment of premature labor with the calcium antagonist nifedipine. Arch Gynecol 1980;229:1–5.
11. Kaul AF, Osathanondh R, Safon LE, Frigoletto FD Jr, Friedman PA. The management of preterm labor with the calcium channel-blocking agent nifedipine combined with the â-mimetic terbutaline. Drug Intell Clin Pharm 1985;19:369–71.
12. Read MD, Wellby DE. The use of a calcium antagonist (nifedipine) to suppress preterm labour. Br J Obstet Gynaecol 1986;93:933–7.
13. Snyder SW, Cardwell MS. Neuromuscular blockade with magnesium sulfate and nifedipine. Am J Obstet Gynecol 1989;161:35–6.

14. Waisman GD, Mayorga LM, Camera MI, Vignolo CA, Martinotti A. Magnesium plus nifedipine: potentiation of hypotensive effect in preeclampsia? Am J Obstet Gynecol 1988;159:308–9.
15. O'Neill S, Osathanondh R, Kaul AF, Scavone JM, Bromley BS, Malin MA. The pharmacokinetics of nifedipine in pregnant women (abstract). Drug Intell Clin Pharm 1986;20:460–1.
16. Magee LA, Schick B, Donnenfeld AE, Sage SR, Conover B, Cook L, McElhatton PR, Schmidt MA, Koren G. The safety of calcium channel blockers in human pregnancy: a prospective, multicenter cohort study. Am J Obstet Gynecol 1996;174:823–8.
17. Ehrenkranz RA, Ackerman BA, Hulse JD. Nifedipine transfer into human milk. J Pediatr 1989;114:478–80.
18. Committee on Drugs, American Academy of Pediatrics. The transfer of drugs and other chemicals into human milk. Pediatrics 2001;108:776–89.

NILOTINIB

Antineoplastic (Tyrosine Kinase Inhibitor)

PREGNANCY RECOMMENDATION: Contraindicated
BREASTFEEDING RECOMMENDATION: Contraindicated

PREGNANCY SUMMARY

No reports describing the use of nilotinib in human pregnancy have been located.

In animal studies, developmental toxicity (embryo–fetal death) without maternal toxicity was observed in one species. The absence of human pregnancy experience prevents a complete assessment of the embryo–fetal risk. However, the drug should be avoided in pregnancy. If it must be given for the mother's benefit, avoiding the 1st trimester should be considered.

FETAL RISK SUMMARY

Nilotinib is an oral tyrosine kinase inhibitor. It is in the same subclass as several other agents (see Appendix). Nilotinib is indicated for the treatment of chronic-phase and accelerated-phase Philadelphia chromosome-positive chronic myelogenous leukemia in adults resistant to or intolerant to prior therapy that include imatinib. It is metabolized to inactive metabolites. Serum protein binding is about 98%, and the apparent elimination half-life is about 17 hours (1).

Reproduction studies have been conducted in rats and rabbits. In pregnant rats, doses producing systemic exposures that were about ≥1.7 times the exposure (AUC) from the recommended human dose (RHD) resulted in increased resorptions and postimplantation losses. Maternal toxicity (decreased body weight, uterine weight, weight gain, and food consumption) was evident at exposures that were about 5.7 times the RHD. At this exposure, there was a decrease in viable fetuses. In pregnant rabbits, a dose about half of the RHD was maternal toxic (death and decreased weight and food consumption) and was associated with embryo death (resorptions) and minor skeletal anomalies. Nilotinib did not cause structural anomalies in these two species (1).

Carcinogenicity studies have not been conducted with nilotinib. The drug was not mutagenic or clastogenic in multiple assays. Nilotinib had no effect on mating or fertility in male and female rats at doses up to about 4–7 times the RHD or in female rabbits at doses that were about half the RHD. When male and female rats were given doses that were about 1–6.6 times the RHD during pre-mating and mating and then continued in pregnant rats through gestation day 6, there was an increase in postimplantation loss and early resorption, and a decrease in the number of viable fetuses and litter size at all doses tested (1).

It is not known if nilotinib crosses the human placenta. Although the serum protein binding is high, the molecular weight (about 512 for the nonhydrated free base) and long elimination half-life suggest that the drug will cross to the embryo–fetus.

BREASTFEEDING SUMMARY

No reports describing the use of nilotinib during human lactation have been located. Although the serum protein binding (98%) is high, the molecular weight (about 512 for the nonhydrated free base) and long elimination half-life (about 17 hours) suggest that the drug will be excreted into breast milk. The effects of this exposure on a nursing infant are unknown, but there is potential for severe toxicity based on the adult data. The most common adverse reactions in adults were rash, pruritus, nausea, vomiting, fatigue, headache, and constipation and/or diarrhea. Thrombocytopenia and neutropenia also have been observed (1). Because of the risk, women receiving nilotinib should not breastfeed.

Reference

1. Product information. Tasigna. Novartis Pharmaceuticals, 2007.

NIMODIPINE

Calcium Channel Blocker

PREGNANCY RECOMMENDATION: Limited Human Data—Animal Data Suggest Risk
BREASTFEEDING RECOMMENDATION: Limited Human Data—Probably Compatible

N

PREGNANCY SUMMARY

Nimodipine is teratogenic and toxic in experimental animals. However, human data early in gestation are insufficient to assess the risk to the embryo or fetus. Only a few of the 10 calcium channel blockers have any human data on exposure during early gestation. Based on this very limited information, these agents do not appear to be major human teratogens. However, more information is required before any conclusion can be reached as to the potential teratogenic risk of these agents.

FETAL RISK SUMMARY

Nimodipine is a dihydropyridine calcium channel blocker used to reduce the incidence and severity of ischemic deficits in patients with subarachnoid hemorrhage after rupture of congenital aneurysms. Nimodipine shares similar hemodynamic effects with other calcium channel blockers, but does not usually produce a marked lowering of blood pressure. In clinical studies involving nonpregnant patients, only about 5% of the subjects experienced a marked lowering of blood pressure (1).

In studies with male and female rats, nimodipine had no effect on fertility or reproductive performance at doses up to about four times the equivalent human dose of 60 mg every 4 hours in a 50-kg patient (EHD) (1). Reproduction studies have been conducted in rats and rabbits. Nimodipine was teratogenic in rabbits, producing an increase in the incidence of malformations and stunted fetuses at oral doses of 1–10 mg/kg/day (1). In rats, nimodipine dosing during organogenesis was embryotoxic, causing resorptions and stunted fetal growth, but except for skeletal variations, caused no malformations (1). The dose used in rats was about 12 times the EHD. Oral doses about 4 times the EHD administered late in organogenesis and continued to nearly the end of gestation or for 21 days after delivery were associated with an increase in skeletal variations, stunted fetuses, and stillbirths but no malformations (1).

The placental transfer of nimodipine early in human gestation has apparently not been studied. Consistent with its molecular weight (about 418), nimodipine crosses the human placenta at term.

An abstract and later full report described the use of nimodipine for the management of preeclampsia (2,3). Ten women at about 38 weeks' gestation with preeclampsia were treated with nimodipine, 30 mg orally every 4 hours. Delivery occurred within 24 hours of starting nimodipine and continued for 24 hours after delivery. Both systolic and diastolic blood pressures were significantly reduced after nimodipine administration without evidence of fetal distress. At delivery, the median nimodipine concentrations in the maternal and umbilical cord serum were 7.32 and 2.6 ng/mL, respectively (fetal:maternal ratio 0.36). In four patients who were delivered by cesarean section within 2 hours of the first dose, the maternal and cord serum levels were 9.68 and 3.46 ng/mL, respectively (fetal:maternal ratio 0.36). The median Apgar scores were 8 (range 6–10) and 9 (range 8–10) at 1 and 5 minutes, respectively. No adverse effects of the drug treatment were observed in the newborns and all were doing well at 6-week follow-up (3). One newborn was excluded from the above data because the mother suffered a ruptured uterus. Although severely depressed at birth (Apgar scores 1 and 5 at 1 and 5 minutes, respectively), the infant was successfully resuscitated and was developing normally at 6 weeks of age (3).

A prospective, multicenter, cohort study of 78 women (81 outcomes; 3 sets of twins) who had 1st trimester exposure to calcium channel blockers, including 11% to nimodipine, was reported in 1996 (4). Compared with controls, the women experienced no increase in major congenital malformations.

Nimodipine also has been used for its cerebral vasodilator characteristics in the treatment of eclampsia complicated by cerebral vasospasm and edema (5–7). In the first two cases, delivery of the fetus had occurred before initiation of therapy (5,6). The use of nimodipine in combination with magnesium sulfate was not recommended because of the risk for maternal heart block (6). In the third report, seizures in four pregnant patients were halted with IV clonazepam (average dose 3 mg, range 1–5 mg), followed by IV nimodipine (1 mg/hr for 20 minutes, then 2 mg/hr) to control blood pressure (mean dose 1.83 mg) (7). The four liveborn infants were delivered by cesarean section once maternal blood pressure was controlled. The mean birth weight was 1822 g (range 1460–2800 g). Individual Apgar scores were not provided, but two infants had 5-minute Apgar scores <7. One mother died of severe postpartum complications, and another developed multiorgan disease secondary to severe preeclampsia/eclampsia (7).

A 1998 abstract described an ongoing international, multicenter, randomized, controlled trial comparing the effects of nimodipine and magnesium sulfate in the prevention of eclampsia (8). Another study involving 21 women with severe preeclampsia compared oral nimodipine with IV magnesium sulfate for the prevention of seizures (9). Neither report provided data on newborns.

Maternal hypotension caused by nimodipine is a potential, but yet unreported, complication that could jeopardize the fetus. An in vitro study has examined the potential use of nimodipine as a tocolytic agent (10). Thus, additional data on the potential for nimodipine-induced maternal hypotension may be forthcoming.

BREASTFEEDING SUMMARY

Nimodipine is excreted into breast milk. In a 1996 case report, a 36-year-old woman at 3 weeks postpartum experienced a transient clinical syndrome of paresthesias (arm and face) associated with motor dysphasia (11). The symptoms resolved, but perioral dysesthesia and motor dysphasia recurred after cerebral angiography. Because the symptoms were thought possibly to be vascular spasm secondary to angiographic examination, the woman was treated with IV nimodipine (formulation not available in the United States). Over a 24-hour interval, she received a total dose of 46 mg (1 mg/hr for 2 hours, then 2 mg/hr). Milk samples were collected (50–60 mL/collection) by the patient every 3–4 hours during nimodipine therapy and blood samples were drawn about every 6 hours. The infant was not allowed to nurse during this

N

period. Nimodipine milk concentrations ranged from 0.42 ng/mL (0.5 hours) to 4.70 ng/mL (26 hours; 2 hours after the infusion ended), whereas the maternal serum concentrations ranged from 3.54 to 10.83 ng/mL. The milk:serum ratios at 0.5, 7.5, and 13.5 hours were 0.12, 0.06, and 0.15, respectively. Assuming a milk intake of 150 mL/kg/day, the authors estimated that the infant would have received 0.008% to 0.092% of the mother's weight-adjusted dose. This exposure was thought to be clinically insignificant (11).

References

1. Product information. Nimotop. Bayer, 2002.
2. Belfort M, Saade G, Cruz A, Adam K, Kirshon B, Kramer W, Moise K Jr. Nimodipine as an alternative to magnesium sulfate in the management of severe preeclampsia: maternal and fetal effects (abstract). Am J Obstet Gynecol 1994;170:412.
3. Belfort MA, Saade GR, Moise KJ Jr, Cruz A, Adam K, Kramer W, Kirshon B. Nimodipine in the management of preeclampsia: maternal and fetal effects. Am J Obstet Gynecol 1994;171:417–24.
4. Magee LA, Schick B, Donnenfeld AE, Sage SR, Conover B, Cook L, McElhatton PR, Schmidt MA, Koren G. The safety of calcium channel blockers in human pregnancy: a prospective, multicenter cohort study. Am J Obstet Gynecol 1996;174:823–8.
5. Horn EH, Filshie M, Kerslake RW, Jaspan T, Worthington BS, Rubin PC. Widespread cerebral ischaemia treated with nimodipine in a patient with eclampsia. Br Med J 1990;301:794.
6. Belfort MA, Carpenter RJ Jr, Kirshon B, Saade GR, Moise KJ Jr. The use of nimodipine in a patient with eclampsia: color flow Doppler demonstration of retinal artery relaxation. Am J Obstet Gynecol 1993;169:204–6.
7. Anthony J, Mantel G, Johanson R, Dommisse J. The haemodynamic and respiratory effects of intravenous nimodipine used in the treatment of eclampsia. Br J Obstet Gynaecol 1996;103:518–22.
8. Belfort M, Anthony J, Saade G and the Nimodipine Study Group. Interim report of the nimodipine vs. magnesium sulfate for seizure prophylaxis in severe preeclampsia study: an international, randomized, controlled trial (abstract). Am J Obstet Gynecol 1998;178:S7.
9. Belfort MA, Saade GR, Yared M, Grunewald C, Herd JA, Varner MA, Nisell H. Change in estimated cerebral perfusion pressure after treatment with nimodipine or magnesium sulfate in patients with preeclampsia. Am J Obstet Gynecol 1999;181:402–7.
10. Kaya T, Cetin A, Cetin M, Sarioglu Y. Effects of endothelin-1 and calcium channel blockers on contractions in human myometrium. A study on myometrial strips from normal and diabetic pregnant women. J Reprod Med 1999;44:115–21.
11. Carcas AJ, Abad-Santos F, de Rosendo JM, Frias J. Nimodipine transfer into human breast milk and cerebrospinal fluid. Ann Pharmacother 1996;30:148–50.

NISOLDIPINE

Calcium Channel Blocker

PREGNANCY RECOMMENDATION: No Human Data—Animal Data Suggest Risk
BREASTFEEDING RECOMMENDATION: No Human Data—Probably Compatible

N

PREGNANCY SUMMARY

Although the lack of human pregnancy experience prevents a complete assessment of the embryo–fetal risk, the absence of teratogenicity and the observance of fetotoxicity only at maternal toxic doses in animals are reassuring. Other calcium channel blockers have been extensively used in human pregnancy as antihypertensives and tocolytics without evidence of major congenital defects or fetal toxicity (see Nicardipine, Nifedipine, and Verapamil).

FETAL RISK SUMMARY

Nisoldipine is a calcium channel blocker indicated for the treatment of hypertension, either alone or in combination with other antihypertensive agents. The elimination half-life (about 7–12 hours) of this agent allows for once-daily dosing.

Animal reproduction studies have been conducted in three species (1). No teratogenicity was observed in rats and rabbits, but fetotoxicity, most likely due to maternal toxicity, did occur in both species. Decreased fetal weight was observed in pregnant rats given doses about 5 and 16 times the maximum recommended human dose based on BSA (MRHD). At the higher dose, increased postimplantation loss (resorption) was also noted. In pregnant rabbits, decreased fetal and placental weights occurred at doses approximately 10 times the MRHD. At a dose 30 times the MRHD in pregnant monkeys, the only surviving fetus had forelimb and vertebral abnormalities not previously seen in control monkeys of the same strain (1). In this particular study, control monkeys also had increased rates of abortion and mortality (1).

It is not known if nisoldipine crosses the human placenta. The molecular weight (about 388) is low enough that placental transfer should be expected.

No reports describing the use of nisoldipine during human pregnancy have been located. A 1992 abstract did report the successful use of the agent in 12 women for the treatment of severe postpartum pregnancy-induced hypertension (2). Other calcium channel blockers (e.g., see Nicardipine, Nifedipine, and Verapamil) have been used for maternal hypertension and as tocolytic agents.

BREASTFEEDING SUMMARY

No reports describing the use of nisoldipine in human lactation have been reported. The molecular weight (about 388) is low enough that excretion into breast milk should be expected. The effect of this exposure on a nursing infant is unknown. Other calcium channel blockers are excreted in milk and are classified as compatible with breastfeeding by the American Academy of Pediatrics (see Diltiazem, Nifedipine, and Verapamil).

References

1. Product information. Sular. AstraZeneca Pharmaceuticals, 2001.
2. Belfort M. Nisoldipine: preliminary results using a new orally administered calcium antagonist in the treatment of severe postpartum pregnancy induced hypertension (PIH) (abstract). Am J Obstet Gynecol 1992;166:440.

NITAZOXANIDE

Anti-Infective (Antiprotozoal)

PREGNANCY RECOMMENDATION: No Human Data—Animal Data Suggest Low Risk
BREASTFEEDING RECOMMENDATION: No Human Data—Probably Compatible

PREGNANCY SUMMARY

No reports describing the use of nitazoxanide in human pregnancy have been located. Although the animal data are suggestive of low risk, the absence of human pregnancy experience prevents an assessment of risk that the drug represents to an embryo or fetus. If indicated, nitazoxanide should not be withheld during pregnancy. However, until human pregnancy data are available, exposure to the agent should be avoided in the 1st trimester, if possible.

FETAL RISK SUMMARY

Nitazoxanide is an oral synthetic antiprotozoal agent approved for the treatment of diarrhea caused by *Cryptosporidium parvum* and *Giardia lamblia* in pediatric patients between the ages of 1 and 11 years (1). However, the drug has been used in children and adults for a wide variety of gastrointestinal and hepatic infections, including those associated with AIDS (2–10). Nitazoxanide is a prodrug that is rapidly hydrolyzed during absorption to the active metabolites, tizoxanide and tizoxanide glucuronide (1). The parent compound, nitazoxanide, is not detected in plasma. Tizoxanide is extensively bound to plasma proteins (>99.9%) (1). The terminal elimination half-life of tizoxanide is 7.3 hours (11).

Reproduction studies have been conducted in rats and rabbits. In rats, doses up to 48 times the human clinical dose based on BSA (HCD) revealed no evidence of fetal harm. Higher doses (up to 66 times the HCD) had no effect on fertility in male and female rats. In rabbits, doses up to three times the HCD revealed no evidence of impaired fertility or fetal harm (1).

It is not known if the active metabolites of nitazoxanide cross the human placenta (nitazoxanide itself is not detected in the plasma). The molecular weight of one of the active metabolites, tizoxanide (about 265), is low enough for placental passage, but the extensive plasma protein binding will limit the amount of drug transferred to the embryo or fetus.

BREASTFEEDING SUMMARY

No reports describing the use of nitazoxanide during human lactation have been located. It is not known if the active metabolites of nitazoxanide are excreted into breast milk (nitazoxanide itself is not detected in the plasma). The molecular weight of one of the active metabolites, tizoxanide (about 265), is low enough to be excreted into breast milk, but the extensive plasma protein binding (>99.9%) will limit the amount. The effect of this exposure on a nursing infant is unknown, but probably is not clinically significant. However, the nursing infant should be monitored for gastrointestinal symptoms.

References

1. Product information. Alinia. Romark Pharmaceuticals, 2004.
2. Rossignol JF, Maisonneuve H. Nitazoxanide in the treatment of *Taenia saginata* and *Hymenolepis nana* infections. Am J Trop Med Hyg 1984;33:511–2.
3. Murphy JR, Friedman JC. Pre-clinical toxicology of nitazoxanide—a new antiparasitic compound. J Appl Toxicol 1985;5:49–52.
4. Dubreuil L, Houcke I, Mouton Y, Rossignol JF. In vitro evaluation of activities of nitazoxanide and tizoxanide against anaerobes and aerobic organisms. Antimicrob Agents Chemother 1996;40:2266–70.
5. Romero Cabello R, Guerrero LR, Munoz Garcia MDR, Geyne Cruz A. Nitazoxanide for the treatment of intestinal protozoan and helminthic infections in Mexico. Trans R Soc Trop Med Hyg 1997;91:701–3.
6. Doumbo O, Rossignol JF, Pichard E, Traore HA, Dembele M, Diakite M, Traore F, Diallo DA. Nitazoxanide in the treatment of cryptosporidial diarrhea and other intestinal parasitic infections associated with acquired immunodeficiency syndrome in tropical Africa. Am J Trop Med Hyg 1997;56:637–9.
7. Megraud F, Occhialini A, Rossignol JF. Nitazoxanide, a potential drug for eradication of *Helicobacter pylori* with no cross-resistance to metronidazole. Antimicrob Agents Chemother 1998;42:2836–40.
8. Rossignol JF, Abaza H, Friedman H. Successful treatment of human fascioliasis with nitazoxanide. Trans R Soc Trop Med Hyg 1998;92:103–4.
9. Yamamoto Y, Hakki A, Friedman H, Okubo S, Shimamura T, Hoffman PS, Rossignol JF. Nitazoxanide, a nitrothiazolide antiparasitic agent with anti-vacuolating toxin activity. Chemotherapy 1999;45:303–12.
10. Bicart-See A, Massip P, Linas MD, Datry A. Successful treatment with nitazoxanide of *Enterocytozoon bieneusi* microsporidiosis in a patient with AIDS. Antimicrob Agents Chemother 2000;44:167–8.
11. Stockis A, Deroubaix X, Lins R, Jeanbaptiste B, Calderon P, Rossignol JF. Pharmacokinetics of nitazoxanide after single oral dose administration in 6 healthy volunteers. Int J Clin Pharmacol Ther 1996;34:349–51.

NITROFURANTOIN

Urinary Germicide

PREGNANCY RECOMMENDATION: Human Data Suggest Risk in 3rd Trimester
BREASTFEEDING RECOMMENDATION: Limited Human Data—Probably Compatible

PREGNANCY SUMMARY

Nitrofurantoin is not an animal teratogen with doses close to those used in humans and, although two retrospective studies reported associations with congenital anomalies, there are no confirmed data suggesting that it is a human teratogen. The two studies require confirmation. However, there appears to be risk of hemolytic anemia in newborns, including those who are not glucose-6-phosphate dehydrogenase (G6PD) deficient, who are exposed in utero to nitrofurantoin close to delivery. Although the incidence is unknown, the rare reports of this toxicity combined with the popularity of the drug for urinary tract infections in pregnant women suggest that the risk is rare. The safest course, however, is to avoid nitrofurantoin close to delivery.

FETAL RISK SUMMARY

The anti-infective agent nitrofurantoin is commonly used in pregnancy for the treatment and prophylaxis of urinary tract infections.

Neither impaired fertility, teratogenicity, nor other fetal adverse effects were observed in rats and rabbits treated with nitrofurantoin before and during gestation (1,2). Doses used were up to six times the human dose based on body weight (HD) (1). In mice, a dose 68 times the HD was associated with fetal growth restriction and a low incidence of minor and common malformations (1). When a dose 25 times the HD was administered, fetal malformations were not observed (1). A dose 19 times the HD induced lung papillary adenomas in mice offspring, but the relationship of this to potential human carcinogenesis is unknown (1).

In a surveillance study of Michigan Medicaid recipients involving 229,101 completed pregnancies conducted between 1985 and 1992, 1292 newborns had been exposed to nitrofurantoin during the 1st trimester (F. Rosa, personal communication, FDA, 1993). A total of 52 (4.0%) major birth defects were observed (55 expected). Specific data were available for six defect categories, including (observed/expected) 15/12 cardiovascular defects, 1/2 oral clefts, 0/2 spina bifida, 4/4 polydactyly, 3/2 limb reduction defects, and 5/3 hypospadias. These data do not support an association between the drug and congenital defects.

One manufacturer (Norwich-Eaton Laboratories) has collected more than 1700 case histories describing the use of this drug during various stages of pregnancy (95 references) (personal communication, 1981). None of the reports observed deleterious effects on the fetus. In a published study, a retrospective analysis of 91 pregnancies in which nitrofurantoin was used yielded no evidence of fetal toxicity (3). Other studies have also supported the safety of this drug in pregnancy (4).

In a 1995 report, 22 studies of nitrofurantoin use in pregnancy were evaluated for a meta-analysis (5). Only four of the studies met the inclusion criteria of the investigators. The pooled odds ratio (OR) for malformations after use of the drug in the 1st trimester was 1.29 (95% confidence interval [CI] 0.25–6.57). These results demonstrated no significant correlation between nitrofurantoin use in early gestation and congenital malformations (5).

In contrast to the above reports, a 2003 case–control study, using data from three Swedish health registers, was conducted to identify drug use in early pregnancy that was associated with cardiac defects (6). Cases (cardiovascular defects without known chromosome anomalies) ($N = 5015$) were compared with controls consisting of all infants born in Sweden from 1995 to 2001 ($N = 577,730$). Associations were identified for several drugs, some of which were probably due to confounding from the underlying disease or complaint or multiple testing, but some were thought to be true drug effects. For nitrofurantoin, there were 30 cases in 2060 exposures (OR 1.68, 95% CI 1.17–2.40) (6).

A 2009 report from the National Birth Defects Prevention Study estimated the association between antibacterial agents and more than 30 selected birth defects (7). The authors conducted a population-based, multiple site, case–control study of women who gave birth to an infant with one of >30 selected defects. The outcomes were identified in a 10-state birth defect surveillance program and involved 13,155 cases and 4941 controls selected from the same geographical regions. Exposure to an antibacterial was determined by a detailed telephone interview conducted within 24 months after the estimated date of delivery. Women were considered exposed if they had used an antibacterial drug during the month before the estimated date of conception through the end of the 1st trimester (defined as the end of the 3rd month of pregnancy). Significant associations with multiple selected birth defects were found (total number of exposed cases/controls) with sulfonamides (145/42) (probably combined with trimethoprim) and nitrofurantoin (150/42). The adjusted ORs and 95% CIs (in parentheses) for nitrofurantoin were anophthalmia or microphthalmos 3.7 (1.1–12.2), hypoplastic left heart syndrome 4.2 (1.9–9.1), atrial septal defects 1.9 (1.1–3.4), and cleft lip with cleft palate 2.1 (1.2–3.9). Significant associations (total number of exposed cases–controls; number of associations) also were found for penicillins (716–293; 1), erythromycins (202–78; 2), cephalosporins (128–47; 1), quinolones (42–14; 1) and tetracyclines (36–6; 1). The results for quinolones and tetracyclines, however, were based on small numbers of exposed cases and controls (7).

As with all retrospective case–control studies, the data can determine associations, but not causative associations (7).

Moreover, several limitations were identified by the authors, including spurious associations caused by the large number of analyses, interviews were conducted 6 weeks to 2 years after the pregnancy making recall difficult for cases and controls, recall bias, and inability to distinguish between drug-induced defects and defects resulting from the infection (7).

Nitrofurantoin may induce hemolytic anemia in G6PD-deficient patients and in patients whose red blood cells are deficient in reduced glutathione (8). One manufacturer considers nitrofurantoin to be contraindicated in pregnant women at term (38–42 weeks' gestation), when the onset of labor is imminent, or during labor and delivery, because of the risk of hemolytic anemia in the newborn secondary to immature erythrocyte enzyme systems (glutathione instability) (1). A 1990 reference, citing data from a manufacturer's database, mentioned nine cases of hemolytic anemia in newborns whose mothers had taken the drug late in pregnancy (9). None of the mothers or infants were tested for G-6-PD deficiency and there was no information available as to whether the mothers were also affected. A 2000 case report published in France described hemolytic anemia in a full-term newborn whose mother had taken nitrofurantoin during the last month of pregnancy (10). The authors attributed the toxicity to the drug.

Nitrofurantoin has been reported to cause discoloration of the primary teeth when given to an infant; by implication, this could occur from in utero exposure (11). However, the fact that the baby was also given a 14-day course of tetracycline, an antibiotic known to cause this adverse effect, and the lack of other confirming reports make the likelihood of a causal relationship remote (12).

The effect of postcoital prophylaxis with a single oral dose of either cephalexin (250 mg) or nitrofurantoin macrocrystals (50 mg) starting before or during pregnancy in 33 women (39 pregnancies) with a history of recurrent urinary tract infections was described in a 1992 reference (13). A significant decrease in the number of infections was documented without fetal toxicity.

Long-term, low-dose (50 mg at bedtime) nitrofurantoin for prophylaxis after acute pyelonephritis was shown to be effective in pregnant women (14). Nitrofurantoin was started after treatment of the infection and continued until 1 month after delivery. There were no additional cases of pyelonephritis (14). No mention was made on the fetal outcomes.

When given orally in high doses of 10 mg/kg/day to young males, nitrofurantoin may produce slight-to-moderate transient spermatogenic arrest (15). The lower doses used clinically do not seem to have this effect.

BREASTFEEDING SUMMARY

Nitrofurantoin is excreted into breast milk. In one study, the drug could not be detected in 20 samples from mothers receiving 100 mg 4 times daily (16). In a second study, nine mothers were given 100 mg every 6 hours for 1 day, then either 100 mg or 200 mg the next morning (17). Only two of the four patients receiving the 200-mg dose excreted measurable amounts of nitrofurantoin, 0.3–0.5 mcg/mL. Although these amounts are negligible, infants with G6PD deficiency may develop hemolytic anemia from this exposure (17).

A 2001 study concluded that nitrofurantoin is actively transported into milk, by an unknown mechanism, resulting in a milk:plasma ratio of 6.21 (18). The observed milk:plasma ratio was about 22-fold greater than the predicted ratio (0.28) that was determined in the study. Four lactating women, who did not breastfeed during the study, were given a single 100-mg capsule of nitrofurantoin macrocrystals with a standardized high-fat breakfast. Nine serum and milk samples were drawn after the dose over a 12-hour interval. The mean milk drug concentration in each patient during the 12-hour interval was approximately 1.3 mcg/mL. Based on this, the investigators estimated that if a 60-kg woman was taking 100 mg twice daily, the infant dose would be 0.2 mg/kg, or about 6% of the mother's weight-adjusted dose. Although this exposure was thought to be low, nursing infants younger than 1 month of age and those with a high frequency of G6PD deficiency or sensitivity to nitrofurantoin may be at risk for toxicity (18).

In a 1993 cohort study, diarrhea was reported in 32 (19.3%) nursing infants of 166 breastfeeding mothers who were taking antibiotics (19). For the six women taking nitrofurantoin, decreased milk volume was observed in one woman and diarrhea was observed in two (33%) infants. Both effects were considered minor because they did not require medical attention (19).

The above studies suggest that there is a potential for nitrofurantoin-induced toxicity from exposure to the drug in breast milk. Determining the magnitude of the risk will require more data, but the risk appears to be rare. The American Academy of Pediatrics classifies nitrofurantoin as compatible with breastfeeding (20).

References

1. Product information. Macrodantin. Procter & Gamble Pharmaceuticals, 2001.
2. Prytherch JP, Sutton ML, Denine EP. General reproduction, perinatal–postnatal and teratology studies of nitrofurantoin macrocrystals in rats and rabbits. J Toxicol Environ Health 1984;13:811–23. As cited in Shepard TH. *Catalog of Teratogenic Agents.* 6th ed. Baltimore, MD: The Johns Hopkins University Press, 1989:454.
3. Hailey FJ, Fort H, Williams JC, Hammers B. Foetal safety of nitrofurantoin macrocrystals therapy during pregnancy: a retrospective analysis. J Int Med Res 1983;11:364–9.
4. Lenke RR, VanDorsten JP, Schifrin BS. Pyelonephritis in pregnancy: a prospective randomized trial to prevent recurrent disease evaluating suppressive therapy with nitrofurantoin and close surveillance. Am J Obstet Gynecol 1983;146:953–7.
5. Ben David S, Einarson T, Ben David Y, Nulman I, Pastuszak A, Koren G. The safety of nitrofurantoin during the first trimester of pregnancy: meta-analysis. Fundam Clin Pharmacol 1995;9:503–7.
6. Kallen BAJ, Olausson PO. Maternal drug use in early pregnancy and infant cardiovascular defect. Reprod Toxicol 2003;17:255–61.
7. Crider KS, Cleves MA, Reefhuis J, Berry RJ, Hobbs CA, Hu DJ. Antibacterial medication use during pregnancy and risk of birth defects. Arch Pediatr Adolesc Med 2009;163:978–85.
8. Powell RD, DeGowin RL, Alving AS. Nitrofurantoin-induced hemolysis. J Lab Clin Med 1963;62:1002–3.
9. Gait JE. Hemolytic reactions to nitrofurantoin in patients with glucose-6-phosphate dehydrogenase deficiency: theory and practice. DICP Ann Pharmacother 1990;24:1210–3.
10. Bruel H, Guillemant V, Saladin-Thiron C, Chabrolle JP, Lahary A, Poinsot J. Hemolytic anemia in a newborn after maternal treatment with nitrofurantoin at the end of pregnancy. Arch Pediatr 2000;7:745–7.
11. Ball JS, Ferguson AN. Permanent discoloration of primary dentition by nitrofurantoin. Br Med J 1962;2:1103.
12. Duckworth R, Swallow JN. Nitrofurantoin and teeth. Br Med J 1962;2:1617.
13. Pfau A, Sacks TG. Effective prophylaxis for recurrent urinary tract infections during pregnancy. Clin Infect Dis 1992;14:810–4.
14. Sandberg T, Brorson JE. Efficacy of long-term antimicrobial prophylaxis after acute pyelonephritis in pregnancy. Scan J Infect Dis 1991;23:221–3.

N

15. Nelson WO, Bunge RG. The effect of therapeutic dosages of nitrofurantoin (Furadantin) upon spermatogenesis in man. J Urol 1957;77:275–81.
16. Hosbach RE, Foster RB. Absence of nitrofurantoin from human milk. JAMA 1967;202:1057.
17. Varsano I, Fischl J, Shochet SB. The excretion of orally ingested nitrofurantoin in human milk. J Pediatr 1973;82:886–7.
18. Gerk PM, Kuhn RJ, Desai NS, McNamara PJ. Active transport of nitrofurantoin into human milk. Pharmacotherapy 2001;21:669–75.
19. Ito S, Blajchman A, Stephenson M, Eliopoulos C, Koren G. Prospective follow-up of adverse reactions in breast-fed infants exposed to maternal medication. Am J Obstet Gynecol 1993;168:1393–9.
20. Committee on Drugs, American Academy of Pediatrics. The transfer of drugs and other chemicals into human milk. Pediatrics 2001;108:776–89.

NITROFURAZONE

Anti-infective

PREGNANCY RECOMMENDATION: Limited Human Data—Probably Compatible
BREASTFEEDING RECOMMENDATION: No Human Data—Probably Compatible

PREGNANCY SUMMARY

The reported human pregnancy experience is limited to one large surveillance study that found 1 (0.4%) major defect among 234 1st trimester exposures. The animal studies in one species used systemic exposures that probably were much higher than those obtained in humans from topical application and, most likely, have little clinical significance. Based on these data, if the drug is indicated, it should not be withheld because of pregnancy.

FETAL RISK SUMMARY

Nitrofurazone is a bactericidal nitrofuran anti-infective that is used topically (1) and as bladder irrigation (2). It is available as 0.2% topical solution, ointment, and cream. Nitrofurazone is indicated as adjunctive therapy for patients undergoing treatment for severe burns when bacterial resistance to other agents is a real or potential problem. It also is indicated for patients undergoing skin grafting when contamination with resistant bacteria might cause graft rejection (1,2).

In mice, reproduction studies with systemic nitrofurazone induced a low frequency of limb reduction defects in one study (3,4), but not in another (3). In rabbits, doses up to 30 times the usual human dose (*assumed to be based on weight*) were embryocidal (5).

It is not known if nitrofurazone is absorbed into the systemic circulation or if it crosses the human placenta. However, some absorption should be expected when it is used topically for burns or as bladder irrigation. The molecular weight (about 198) and lipid solubility suggest that the drug will cross the placenta if it is absorbed, but the clinical significance of this is unknown.

The Collaborative Perinatal Project monitored 50,282 mother–child pairs, 234 of whom had exposure to nitrofurazone in lunar months 1–4 (6). Structural anomalies were observed in seven cases, one major and six minor defects. These outcomes were not statistically significant.

BREASTFEEDING SUMMARY

No reports describing the use of nitrofurazone during human lactation have been located. It is not known if nitrofurazone is absorbed into the systemic circulation or if it is excreted into breast milk. However, some absorption should be expected when it is used topically for burns or as bladder irrigation. The molecular weight (about 198) and lipid solubility suggest that the drug will be excreted into milk, but the clinical significance of this is unknown.

References

1. Nitrofurazone. *Drug Facts and Comparisons*. St. Louis, MO: Wolters Kluwer Health, 2009:1630–1.
2. Nitrofurazone. In: Sweetman SC, ed. *Martindale. The Complete Drug Reference*. 34th ed. London, UK: Pharmaceutical Press, 2005:238.
3. Schardein JL. *Chemically Induced Birth Defects*. 3rd ed. New York, NY: Marcel Dekker, 2000:403, 406.
4. Shepard TH, Lemire RJ. Nitrofurazone. *Catalog of Teratogenic Agents*. 12th ed. Baltimore, MD: The Johns Hopkins University Press, 2007:313.
5. Product information. Furacin. Roberts, 1997.
6. Heinonen OP, Slone D, Shapiro S. *Birth Defects and Drugs in Pregnancy*. Littleton, MA: Publishing Sciences Group, 1977:300–11.

NITROGLYCERIN

Vasodilator

PREGNANCY RECOMMENDATION: Human Data Suggest Low Risk
BREASTFEEDING RECOMMENDATION: No Human Data—Probably Compatible

PREGNANCY SUMMARY

The use of nitroglycerin during pregnancy does not seem to present a risk to the fetus. However, the number of women treated during pregnancy is limited, especially during the 1st trimester. With the smaller doses reported, transient decreases in the mother's blood pressure may occur, but these do not appear to be sufficient to jeopardize placental perfusion. Nitroglycerin appears to be a safe, effective, rapid-onset, short-acting tocolytic agent. The use of transdermal nitroglycerin patches may also prove to be effective when longer periods of tocolysis are required. With any route of administration, however, additional studies are required to determine the safest effective dose.

FETAL RISK SUMMARY

Nitroglycerin (glyceryl trinitrate) is primarily indicated for the treatment or prevention of angina pectoris. Because of the nature of this use, experience in pregnancy is limited. The drug, a rapid-onset, short-acting vasodilator, has been used to control severe hypertension during cesarean section (1,2). The use of nitroglycerin sublingually for angina during pregnancy without fetal harm has also been reported (3). Recent investigations, discussed below, have explored the use of nitroglycerin as both an emergency and a routine tocolytic agent.

Reproductive studies in rats and rabbits have been conducted with nitroglycerin (4–6). No adverse fetal effects or postnatal changes were observed in these experiments.

The Collaborative Perinatal Project recorded seven 1st trimester exposures to nitroglycerin and amyl nitrite plus eight other patients exposed to other vasodilators (7). From this small group of 15 patients, 4 malformed children were produced, a statistically significant incidence. The data did not indicate whether nitroglycerin was taken by any of the mothers of the affected infants. Because of the lack of specific information and the small number of patients, no conclusions as to the relative safety of nitroglycerin in the 1st trimester can be made from this study. Moreover, the authors of this study emphasized that statistical significance could not be used to infer causal relationships and that independent confirmation from other studies was required.

The use of nitroglycerin in gestational hypertension has been described (8–11). In three patients, IV infusions of nitroglycerin were effective in rapidly correcting the hemodynamic disturbances of gestational hypertension complicated by hydrostatic pulmonary edema, but a rapid improvement in arterial oxygenation did not occur (8). In another study by the same investigators, the effectiveness of IV nitroglycerin to decrease blood pressure in six women with gestational hypertension was dependent on the patient's volume status (9). When volume expansion was combined with nitroglycerin therapy, a marked resistance to the hypotensive effect of the drug was observed. In two of the women treated with IV nitroglycerin alone, significant reductions in blood pressure occurred, resulting in fetal heart rate changes that included late decelerations and bradycardia. Recovery occurred after nitroglycerin therapy was terminated and then restarted at a lower dose. In three other fetuses, a loss of beat-to-beat variability (average variability <5 beats/minute) was noted. Therapy was continued and no abnormalities were observed in the umbilical blood gases or Apgar scores.

An abstract published in 1996 described the use of transdermal nitroglycerin patches (releasing 10 mg in 24 hours) in the treatment of gestational hypertension (10). The 24-hour mean systemic and diastolic blood pressures were significantly decreased (5% and 7%, respectively). In a 1995 study, 12 women with severe preeclampsia received an infusion of nitroglycerin starting at 0.25 mcg/kg/minute with stepwise dosage increases until a diastolic blood pressure of 100 mmHg was achieved (11). The mean systolic blood pressure decreased from 161 to 138 mmHg, whereas diastolic pressure decreased from a mean of 116 to 103 mmHg. The umbilical artery pulsatility index changed significantly but not the uterine pulsatility index, implying vasodilation in the umbilical circulation and avoidance of adverse impairment of fetoplacental perfusion (11).

Lowering of maternal blood pressure and a lessening of the hemodynamic responses to endotracheal intubation were beneficial effects obtained from IV nitroglycerin in six women with severe preeclampsia (12). A progressive flattening of fetal heart rate beat-to-beat variability was observed in all six patients. Prevention of an increase in mean arterial pressure of >20% was achieved in only two of the women, and all had nausea, retching, and vomiting that was apparently not dose-related.

Myocardial infarction, secondary to development of a thrombus on an artificial aortic valve, occurred in a 25-year-old woman at 26 weeks' gestation (13). A portion of her initial treatment consisted of both oral and IV nitroglycerin, with the latter being continued for an unspecified interval. Maternal diastolic blood pressure was maintained above 50 mmHg while on nitroglycerin and, apparently, no fetal distress was observed. A viable 2608-g male infant was eventually delivered at 35 weeks' gestation, but specific details were not provided on his condition.

A 1993 reference described two women, one with triplets, who suffered myocardial infarctions during pregnancy, at 16 and 28 weeks' gestation, and who were treated with IV nitroglycerin and other agents (14). In addition, mild chest pain occurring during labor was successfully treated with sublingual nitroglycerin in one of the women. Both patients survived and eventually delivered infants apparently unaffected by the treatment. Another report described a woman at 26 weeks' gestation who was treated with IV nitroglycerin and other agents for a myocardial infarction (15). She eventually delivered a healthy female infant by cesarean section at 39 weeks.

In gravid ewes, IV nitroglycerin was effective in counteracting norepinephrine-induced uterine vasoconstriction (16). The antihypertensive effect resulted in a significantly decreased mean aortic pressure but did not significantly change uterine blood flow or uterine vascular conductance. A 1994 abstract reported no adverse effects on fetal cardiorespiratory function in sheep from a 2-hour IV infusion of nitroglycerin at 3 times the minimum effective tocolytic dose (17).

The use of nitroglycerin during cesarean section to allow delivery of babies entrapped by a contracted uterus has been described in two case reports (18,19). In the first case, the head of a baby presenting as a double footling breech was trapped in the hypertonic upper segment (18). Uterine relaxation was achieved with a 1000-mcg IV bolus of nitroglycerin. The mother's blood pressure fell to 70/30 mmHg but responded to ephedrine. The Apgar scores of the 3090-g, term infant were 5 and 9 at 1 and 5 minutes, respectively. In the second case, a woman received a 100-mcg bolus of nitroglycerin to quickly relax a contracted uterus and to allow the successful delivery of her twins (19). Other than a systolic blood pressure decrease (preoperative pressure 120 mmHg; after nitroglycerin 85 mmHg) that responded rapidly to ephedrine, no other adverse effects from nitroglycerin were encountered in the mother or her newborns.

Two references have discussed the use of IV nitroglycerin as a short-acting tocolytic agent during intrapartum external cephalic version (20,21) and one involving internal podalic version (22). A woman in premature labor (uterine contractions every 2 minutes with the cervix dilated to 9 cm) at 30 weeks 5 days was given a 50-mcg IV bolus of nitroglycerin (20). The uterus relaxed palpably within 20 seconds and the fetus was repositioned to allow for vaginal delivery. A decrease in the maternal blood pressure was noted (145/100 to 130/75 mmHg, then stabilizing at 130/85 mmHg within 2 minutes), but the heart rate and oxygen saturation remained unchanged. The premature infant was delivered vaginally shortly after rupture of the membranes and start of an oxytocin infusion. A second mother at 39 weeks 4 days of gestation received a 100-mcg IV bolus dose before external cephalic version (blood pressure decreased from 120/60 to 112/60 mmHg within 1 minute) and subsequently underwent a vaginal delivery of a healthy infant.

N

In the second report, a woman delivered one twin vaginally and then received a 50-mcg IV nitroglycerin bolus to allow external version of the second transverse-lie twin (21). No significant maternal adverse effects (e.g., headache or dizziness) or changes in blood pressure or heart rate were observed. The healthy twin was delivered vaginally 45 minutes after the version.

Internal podalic version and total breech extraction of the second twin was accomplished in a third case with sublingual nitroglycerin by aerosol after the uterus had contracted down on the operator's forearm (22). Two 400-mcg boluses were given, resulting in uterine relaxation within 30 seconds. No adverse effects on the newborn were observed.

Three cases of total breech extraction, with internal podalic version in two, of the second twin were aided by the use of nitroglycerin spray (0.4 mg) administered sublingually after either contraction of the uterine corpus and lower segment or uterine or cervical contractions with failure of the fetal head to engage (23). Minimal changes were observed in the maternal blood pressures and pulses. All three newborns were doing well.

A 1996 report described nine cases of internal podalic version of a second nonvertex twin with the assistance of an IV bolus of nitroglycerin (1 mg in eight and 1.5 mg in one) (24). One of the women had a panic attack that required general anesthesia for sedation, although the version was successful. In another case, nitroglycerin failed to induce uterine relaxation and an emergency cesarean section was required for fetal distress. Postpartum hemorrhage (2000 mL) occurred in a third woman. A significant fall in maternal blood pressure was observed in all cases, but no adverse effects from the decrease occurred in the mothers or newborns (24).

Transdermal patches of nitroglycerin have been tested as tocolytics in 13 women in preterm labor (23–33 weeks' gestation) (25). Most of the women received a single patch that delivered 10 mg of nitroglycerin for 24 hours, but some patients were given a second patch if uterine contractions had not subsided within 1 hour. Patches were changed every 24 hours. The mean prolongation of pregnancy, as of the date of a subsequent report (one woman was still pregnant), was 59 days (26). The babies who had been delivered were all doing well.

Small IV bolus doses of nitroglycerin (60 or 90 mcg for one or two doses) were used in 24 laboring women for severe fetal distress, related to uterine hyperactivity that was unresponsive to standard measures (27). Six of the patients developed hypotension with a mean nadir of 93.2 mmHg (minimum 85 mmHg) that was reversed with a single dose of ephedrine (4.5–6 mg). Four newborns had low 1-minute Apgar scores (3, 4, 5, and 6, respectively), but all newborns had Apgar scores of 9 or 10 and were vigorous at 5 minutes.

Nitroglycerin has also been used to relax the uterus in postpartum cases with retained placenta (28–31), two of which occurred in patients with an inverted uterus (30,31). The IV bolus dose was 500 mcg in 15 women (28), 50 mcg (some patients required two doses) in 23 cases (29,30), and 100 mcg in 1 woman (31). No significant changes in blood pressure or heart rate were recorded, and no adverse effects, such as headache, palpitations, or prolonged uterine relaxation, were observed.

BREASTFEEDING SUMMARY

No reports describing the use of nitroglycerin during human lactation have been located. The molecular weight (about 227) suggests that the drug will be excreted into breast milk.

References

1. Snyder SW, Wheeler AS, James FM III. The use of nitroglycerin to control severe hypertension of pregnancy during cesarean section. Anesthesiology 1979;51:563–4.
2. Hood DD, Dewan DM, James FM III, Bogard TD, Floyd HM. The use of nitroglycerin in preventing the hypertensive response to tracheal intubation in severe preeclamptics. Anesthesiology 1983;59:A423.
3. Diro M, Beydown SN, Jaramillo B, O'Sullivan MJ, Kieval J. Successful pregnancy in a woman with a left ventricular cardiac aneurysm: a case report. J Reprod Med 1983;28:559–63.
4. Oketani Y, Mitsuzono T, Ichikawa K, Itono Y, Gojo T, Gofuku M, Konoha N. Toxicological studies on nitroglycerin (NK-843). 6. Teratological studies in rabbits. Oyo Yakuri 1981;22:633–38. As cited in Schardein JL. *Chemically Induced Birth Defects*. 2nd ed. New York, NY: Marcel Dekker, 1993:91.
5. Oketani Y, Mitsuzono T, Ichikawa K, Itono Y, Gojo T, Gofuku M, Konoha N. Toxicological studies on nitroglycerin (NK-843). 8. Teratological study in rats. Oyo Yakuri 1981;22:737–51. As cited in Schardein JL. *Chemically Induced Birth Defects*. 2nd ed. New York, NY: Marcel Dekker, 1993:91.
6. Sato K, Taniguchi H, Ohtsuka T, Himeno Y, Uchiyama K, Koide M, Hoshino K. Reproductive studies of nitroglycerin applied dermally to pregnant rats and rabbits. Clin Report 1984;18:3511–86. As cited in Shepard TH. *Catalog of Teratogenic Agents*. 7th ed. Baltimore, MD: The Johns Hopkins University Press, 1992:285.
7. Heinonen OP, Slone D, Shapiro S. *Birth Defects and Drugs in Pregnancy*. Littleton, MA: Publishing Sciences Group, 1977:371–3.
8. Cotton DB, Jones MM, Longmire S, Dorman KF, Tessem J, Joyce TH III. Role of intravenous nitroglycerin in the treatment of severe pregnancy-induced hypertension complicated by pulmonary edema. Am J Obstet Gynecol 1986;154:91–3.

9. Cotton DB, Longmire S, Jones MM, Dorman KF, Tessem J, Joyce TH III. Cardiovascular alterations in severe pregnancy-induced hypertension: effects of intravenous nitroglycerin coupled with blood volume expansion. Am J Obstet Gynecol 1986;154:1053–9.
10. Facchinetti F, Neri I, Volpe A. Glyceryl trinitrate lowers blood pressure in patients with gestational hypertension (abstract). Am J Obstet Gynecol 1996;174:455.
11. Grunewald C, Kublickas M, Carlstrom K, Lunell N-O, Nisell H. Effects of nitroglycerin on the uterine and umbilical circulation in severe preeclampsia. Obstet Gynecol 1995;86:600–4.
12. Longmire S, Leduc L, Jones MM, Hawkins JL, Joyce TH III, Cotton DB. The hemodynamic effects of intubation during nitroglycerin infusion in severe preeclampsia. Am J Obstet Gynecol 1991;164:551–6.
13. Ottman EH, Gall SA. Myocardial infarction in the third trimester of pregnancy secondary to an aortic valve thrombus. Obstet Gynecol 1993;81:804–5.
14. Sheikh AU, Harper MA. Myocardial infarction during pregnancy: management and outcome of two pregnancies. Am J Obstet Gynecol 1993;169:279–84.
15. Sanchez-Ramos L, Chami YG, Bass TA, DelValle GO, Adair CD. Myocardial infarction during pregnancy: management with transluminal coronary angioplasty and metallic intracoronary stents. Am J Obstet Gynecol 1994;171:1392–3.
16. Wheeler AS, James FM III, Meis PJ, Rose JC, Fishburne JI, Dewan DM, Urban RB, Greiss FC Jr. Effects of nitroglycerin and nitroprusside on the uterine vasculature of gravid ewes. Anesthesiology 1980;52:390–4.
17. Bootstaylor B, Roman C, Heymann MA, Parer JT. Fetal cardiorespiratory effects of nitroglycerin in the near-term pregnant sheep (abstract). Am J Obstet Gynecol 1994;170:281.
18. Roblin SH, Hew EM, Bernstein A. Uterine relaxation can be life saving. Can J Anaesth 1991;38:939–40.
19. Mayer DC, Weeks SK. Antepartum uterine relaxation with nitroglycerin at caesarean delivery. Can J Anaesth 1992;39:166–9.
20. Belfort MA. Intravenous nitroglycerin as a tocolytic agent for intrapartum external cephalic version. S Afr Med J 1993;83:656.
21. Abouleish AE, Corn SB. Intravenous nitroglycerin for intrapartum external version of the second twin. Anesth Analg 1994;78:808–9.
22. Greenspoon JS, Kovacic A. Breech extraction facilitated by glyceryl trinitrate sublingual spray. Lancet 1991;338:124–5.
23. Rosen DJD, Velez J, Greenspoon JS. Total breech extraction of the second twin with uterine relaxation induced by nitroglycerin sublingual spray. Israel J Obstet Gynecol 1994;5:18–21.
24. Dufour PH, Vinatier D, Vanderstichele S, Subtil D, Ducloy JC, Puech F, Codaccionni X, Monnier JC. Intravenous nitroglycerin for intrapartum internal podalic version of the second non-vertex twin. Eur J Obstet Gynecol Reprod Biol 1996;70:29–32.
25. Lees C, Campbell S, Jauniaux E, Brown R, Ramsay B, Gibb D, Moncada S, Martin JF. Arrest of preterm labour and prolongation of gestation with glyceryl trinitrate, a nitric oxide donor. Lancet 1994;343:1325–6.
26. Lees C, Campbell S, Martin J, Moncada S, Brown R, Jauniaux E, Ramsay B, Gibb D. Glyceryl trinitrate in management of preterm labour. Authors' reply. Lancet 1994;344:553–4.
27. Mercier FJ, Dounas M, Bouaziz H, Lhuissier C, Benhamou D. Intravenous nitroglycerin to relieve intrapartum fetal distress related to uterine hyperactivity: a prospective observational study. Anesth Analg 1997;84:1117–20.
28. Peng ATC, Gorman RS, Shulman SM, DeMarchis E, Nyunt K, Blancato LS. Intravenous nitroglycerin for uterine relaxation in the postpartum patient with retained placenta. Anesthesiology 1989;71:172–3.
29. DeSimone CA, Norris MC, Leighton BL. Intravenous nitroglycerin aids manual extraction of a retained placenta. Anesthesiology 1990;73:787.
30. Altabef KM, Spencer JT, Zinberg S. Intravenous nitroglycerin for uterine relaxation of an inverted uterus. Am J Obstet Gynecol 1992;166:1237–8.
31. Dayan SS, Schwalbe SS. The use of small-dose intravenous nitroglycerin in a case of uterine inversion. Anesth Anal 1996;82:1091–3.

NITROPRUSSIDE

Antihypertensive

PREGNANCY RECOMMENDATION: Human and Animal Data Suggest Risk
BREASTFEEDING RECOMMENDATION: No Human Data—Potential Toxicity

PREGNANCY SUMMARY

No reports linking the use of sodium nitroprusside with congenital defects have been located. Nitroprusside has been used in pregnancy to produce deliberate hypotension during aneurysm surgery or to treat severe hypertension (1–8). Transient fetal bradycardia was the only adverse effect noted (1). One advantage of nitroprusside is the very rapid onset of action and the return to pretreatment blood pressure levels when the drug is stopped (8). Balanced against this is the potential accumulation of cyanide in the fetus.

FETAL RISK SUMMARY

Nitroprusside crosses the placenta and produces fetal cyanide concentrations higher than maternal levels in animals (9). This effect has not been studied in humans.

A 1984 article reviewed the potential fetal toxicity of nitroprusside (6). Avoidance of prolonged use and the monitoring of serum pH, plasma cyanide, red blood cell cyanide, and methemoglobin levels in the mother were recommended. Standard doses of nitroprusside apparently do not pose a major risk of excessive accumulation of cyanide in the fetal liver (6).

BREASTFEEDING SUMMARY

No reports describing the use of nitroprusside during human lactation have been located.

References

1. Donchin Y, Amirav B, Sahar A, Yarkoni S. Sodium nitroprusside for aneurysm surgery in pregnancy. Br J Anaesth 1978;50:849–51.
2. Paull J. Clinical report of the use of sodium nitroprusside in severe preeclampsia. Anesth Intensive Care 1975;3:72.
3. Rigg D, McDonogh A. Use of sodium nitroprusside for deliberate hypotension during pregnancy. Br J Anaesth 1981;53:985–7.
4. Willoughby JS. Case reports: sodium nitroprusside, pregnancy and multiple intracranial aneurysms. Anaesth Intensive Care 1984;12:358–60.
5. Stempel JE, O'Grady JP, Morton MJ, Johnson KA. Use of sodium nitroprusside in complications of gestational hypertension. Obstet Gynecol 1982;60:533–8.
6. Shoemaker CT, Meyers M. Sodium nitroprusside for control of severe hypertensive disease of pregnancy: a case report and discussion of potential toxicity. Am J Obstet Gynecol 1984;149:171–3.
7. Willoughby JS. Review article: sodium nitroprusside, pregnancy and multiple intracranial aneurysms. Anaesth Intensive Care 1984;12:351–7.
8. de Swiet M. Antihypertensive drugs in pregnancy. Br Med J 1985;291:365–6.
9. Lewis PE, Cefalo RC, Naulty JS, Rodkey RL. Placental transfer and fetal toxicity of sodium nitroprusside. Gynecol Invest 1977;8:46.

NITROUS OXIDE

General Anesthetic

PREGNANCY RECOMMENDATION: Human and Animal Data Suggest Risk
BREASTFEEDING RECOMMENDATION: Compatible

PREGNANCY SUMMARY

The animal reproduction data suggest risk, but the exposures to the gas were usually much higher and longer than the exposures that occur in humans. In animals, nitrous oxide is an embryo and fetal toxin that may have long-lasting consequences. The evidence for human reproductive and developmental toxicity is not as clear. Much of the data relating to spontaneous abortions (SABs), infertility, and decreased birth weight are based on voluntary responses to surveys that involved self-reported outcomes. These retrospective reports are subject to self-selection and/or recall bias. Moreover, many studies have evaluated exposure to nitrous oxide in operating rooms or dental offices, rather than in individuals and have not quantified the amount and type of anesthetic gas exposure (1,2). In addition, the studies have not always accounted for confounding variables, such as the introduction of scavenging equipment and ventilation, maternal age, smoking, and other drug exposures, and have characterized nitrous oxide exposure based only on job title (3). Nevertheless, there does appear to be an increase in the incidence of SAB and infertility related to chronic exposure to nitrous oxide, but the dose and magnitude of these effects need further study. Moreover, general anesthesia in the 1st and 2nd trimesters has been associated with reduced birth weight, but the causative agents have not been identified.

The information for nitrous oxide and congenital malformations is less confusing, but many of the limitations identified earlier also apply to this population. However, the available data do not appear to suggest that acute or chronic exposure to nitrous oxide at any time in pregnancy represents a major risk for structural anomalies. Although nitrous oxide is the most commonly used general anesthetic agent, it is never administered alone, being combined with several other agents. Therefore, the safest course is to postpone elective surgical procedures until after pregnancy or, at the minimum, until after the period of organogenesis. Moreover, because even operating rooms that are scavenged and ventilated are not entirely free of waste anesthetic gases, women who might become pregnant and are working in these areas should be counseled as to the potential risks and offered positions in areas free of nitrous oxide contamination. Recent data have shown that offspring of mothers with occupational exposure could have long-term neurodevelopmental deficits. Finally, long-term neurotoxicity studies of infants exposed in utero to nitrous oxide during the 3rd trimester or during the first few years after birth are warranted.

FETAL RISK SUMMARY

Nitrous oxide (N_2O; laughing gas) is a nonflammable, nonexplosive gas that is widely used as an analgesic and general anesthetic. It is always administered with at least 20% oxygen to prevent hypoxia. The blood–gas coefficient is relatively low (0.47) as is tissue solubility (brain–gas coefficient 0.50) (4).

Animal Studies

In a 1967 study, pregnant rats were exposed to 45%–50% nitrous oxide for 2, 4, or 6 days starting on gestational day 8 (5). Compared with nonexposed controls, there was a dose-related increase in embryonic death and resorptions, growth restriction, and skeletal malformations (vertebrae and ribs), and the male–female sex ratio of surviving fetuses was lower (5). Resorptions and fetal deaths were significantly increased in rats exposed to nitrous oxide (0.1% or 1.5%) mixed with oxygen for 8 or 24 hours per day for several days during mid-gestation (6). A lower concentration (0.01%) had no effect on the incidence of resorptions but did increase the number of fetal deaths.

A 1978 study did not observe teratogenic effects, changes in surviving fetal sex ratio, or increased fetal loss in pregnant rats exposed 8 hours/day throughout gestation to nitrous oxide (1%, 10%, or 50%) or nitrous oxide (10%) plus halothane (0.16%) (7). However, fetal growth restriction was observed in all four groups exposed to nitrous oxide. Exposure of pregnant rats to 50% nitrous oxide for 25 minutes/day for three consecutive days in mid-gestation resulted in an increase in fetal death rate, but no effects on fetal growth were observed (8). In another study, pregnant rats were exposed to nitrous oxide either alone (0.005% or 0.05%) or a mixture of nitrous oxide (0.05%) and halothane (0.001%) for 7 hours/day during the first 15 days of gestation (9,10). No adverse embryo or fetal effects were observed.

Continuous exposure of gravid rats to nitrous oxide (0.5%) from gestational day 1 to day 19 resulted in a significant increase in the incidence of resorptions, growth restriction, and skeletal anomalies, and a lower male–female sex ratio of surviving fetuses (11). In a follow-up to this study, the threshold dose required to produce some of these effects was determined using exposures of 0%, 0.1%, 0.05% and 0.025% (12). Only the group exposed to 0.1% had an increased incidence of resorptions and growth restriction. The same group of investigators reported a third study in which gravid rats were intermittently exposed (6 hours per day, 5 days per week) to nitrous oxide 0%, 0.025%, 0.05%, 0.1%, and 0.5% throughout gestation (13). A significant reduction in litter size was noted only in the highest exposure group, but no signs of fetal resorption or skeletal malformations were found in any group.

Pregnant hamsters were exposed to nitrous oxide (70%–95%) mixed with oxygen for 24 hours during organogenesis (14). An increased incidence of fetal death was observed only at concentrations of 90%–95%, but hypoxia-induced mortality could not be excluded. A small but significant number of fetuses had malformations (cleft palate, limb defects, gut herniation, and fetal edema), but a dose–effect relationship was not observed (14). The effects on pregnant hamsters from exposure to a combination of nitrous oxide (60%) and halothane (0.6%) for 3 hours per day on gestational days 9, 10, or 11 was reported in 1974 (15). No effects were noted on the sex ratio of surviving fetuses. Compared with controls, resorptions were increased on day 11, and decreased fetal weight was noted in the groups exposed on days 10 and 11 (15).

In a 1980 study, pregnant rats were exposed to nitrous oxide (70%–75%) or xenon (70%–75%) for 24 hours on gestational day 9 (16). Compared with controls and the xenon-exposed group, the nitrous oxide group had a significant increase in the incidence of resorptions and congenital malformations (delayed maturation of the skeletal system, fused ribs, encephalocele, hydrocephalus, anophthalmia, microphthalmia, gastroschisis, and gonadal agenesis) (16). The above experiment was repeated by another group with four different concentrations of nitrous oxide: 0.75%, 7.5%, 25%, and 75% (17). The threshold for toxicity was determined to be >25% because only those animals exposed to the 75% concentration had increased incidences of resorptions and both major and minor congenital malformations. However, all exposures caused a significant increase in minor variants involving the ribs and sternum (17).

In another study by the above investigators, the effect of nitrous oxide in pregnant rats was compared with three other general anesthetic agents (see also Enflurane, Halothane, and Isoflurane) (18). The nitrous oxide dose was 75% (0.55 minimum alveolar anesthetic concentration [MAC]). (*Note: MAC is the concentration that causes immobility in 50% of patients exposed to a noxious stimulus such as a surgical incision; it represents the ED_{50} [19].*) Each agent was administered for 6 hours on each of three consecutive days in one of three periods: gestational days 8–10, 11–13, or 14–16. Compared with controls, significantly decreased maternal weight gain was observed in three of the groups (nitrous oxide, isoflurane, and enflurane) after exposure on days 14–16. Exposure on those days resulted in significantly decreased fetal weight in all four groups; when exposure occurred on days 8–10, the effect was noted in three groups (all except nitrous oxide). Nitrous oxide exposure during days 14–16 resulted in significant increases in total fetal wastage and resorptions (threefold increase). However, no major or minor congenital defects were observed in any of the groups (18).

No evidence of reproductive toxicity was observed in mice exposed to nitrous oxide (0.5%, 5%, or 50%) for 4 hours per day on days 6–15 of gestation (20). In the same experiment, the fertility of male mice exposed in the same way for 9 weeks was not affected. Based on their previous work, they concluded that the order of reproductive toxicity was halothane > enflurane > methoxyflurane > nitrous oxide (20). Of interest, a 1990 study found that brief exposure of two-cell mouse preimplantation embryos to nitrous oxide/oxygen (60%/40%) caused disruption to subsequent embryo cleavage and blastocyst development (21).

A 1989 study determined the susceptible period for nitrous oxide teratogenicity in rats (22). Pregnant rats were exposed to 60% nitrous oxide for 24 hours on each of gestational days 6–12. There were no differences among the seven groups in the number of live fetuses, fetal weight, and sex ratio. However, compared with controls, there was a significant increase in the mean percentage of resorptions/litter and number of litters with resorptions on days 8 and 11. Major skeletal anomalies (ribs and vertebrae) were increased only on day 9, but minor skeletal defects were increased on days 8 and 9. Right-sided aortic arch and left-sided umbilical artery, defects indicative of altered laterality, were increased on day 8 and hydrocephalus was increased on gestational day 9 (22).

A 1986 mouse study tested the hypothesis that prenatal nitrous oxide exposure (75% with 25% oxygen for 6 hours on gestational day 14) or postnatal exposure (same mixture for 4 hours on postnatal day 2) would cause permanent damage to the developing brain and behavioral effects (23). Compared with controls, offspring (postnatal day 6 to 6 months of age) exposed prenatally or postnatally were noted to have several abnormal behavioral effects that included preweaning motor development and general activity. When they reached adulthood, their brains were also noted to have significant morphologic changes (23). A 1986 rat study also found that in utero exposure caused permanent alterations in the spontaneous motor output of the brain that affected females more than males (24). Using a slightly different exposure protocol during rat pregnancy, these same investigators did observe subtle differences from controls in growth rates at 14 and 21 days and reduced reflex suspension, indicating that normal development had been interrupted (25). In a fourth study, mouse offspring exposed in utero to nitrous oxide during organogenesis had hyporeactivity of the startle reflex at 60 and 95 days of age (26).

The effects of nitrous oxide on growing neural tips (growth cones) in the forebrains of neonatal rat pups were described in a 1993 report (27). The pups were exposed to three concentrations of nitrous oxide (25%, 50%, and 75%) over a 6-hour period on postnatal day 1. A dose–response on the activity of a growth cone enzyme (protein kinase C, PKC) was found, with the lowest concentration having no effect on the enzyme. The 75% concentration, however, reduced the activity to about 63%. The 50% dose also reduced the PKC activity but to a lesser degree. The authors thought that the reduced enzyme activity could be related to long-term morphologic or behavioral neuroabnormalities in the pups (27).

The effect of nitrous oxide on rat fertility was described in a 1990 study (28). Adult virgin female rats were exposed to the gas during their 4-day ovulatory cycles. Nitrous oxide disrupted luteinizing hormone-releasing hormone (LH-RH) (*now known as gonadotropin-releasing hormone*) cells in the hypothalamus. This disruption resulted in the inhibition of LH-RH release and, thus, ovulation (28).

Human Studies

PLACENTAL PASSAGE Nitrous oxide rapidly crosses the human placenta to the fetus obtaining amounts in the fetal circulation nearly equivalent to those in the mother (29–34). In a 1970 study, umbilical vein and artery nitrous oxide concentrations ranged up to 91% of maternal levels and increased progressively with increasing duration of anesthesia (30).

SPONTANEOUS ABORTION A number of reports have described the association between SAB and exposure to anesthetic gasses in the operating room, the dental office, or during surgery (1,35–48). In addition, several reviews have examined this topic (49–57).

The principal concern for chronic exposure to anesthetic gasses relates to unscavenged environments in which high concentrations of gases, such as nitrous oxide, have been measured. A 1972 reference cited studies that measured levels of nitrous oxide in the operating room averaging 130 ppm (0.013%) but with peak concentrations as high as 428 ppm (0.048%) (35). Even higher levels (e.g., 9700 ppm or 0.97%) were measured in the anesthesiologist's inhalational zone. A 1970 report described the results of a survey from a group of nurses (67 operating room/92 general duty) and physicians (50 anesthetists/81 specialists other than anesthesia) that were routinely exposed to anesthetics in the operating room (36). In the first group, 29.7% of the pregnancies of operating room nurses ended in SAB, compared with 8.8% in the controls. In the second group, the SAB incidence was 37.8% and 10.3%, respectively. In both exposed groups, the SAB occurred earlier than that in the controls (8th vs. 10th week). However, the study could not identify a specific anesthetic agent, nor could it establish a cause-and-effect relationship (36).

The results of a national survey of operating room personnel was reported in 1974 (37). The survey included the memberships of four organizations, essentially covering all personnel in the United States who were continuously exposed to low levels of anesthetic gases: the American Society of Anesthesiologists (ASA), the American Association of Nurse Anesthetists (AANA), the Association of Operating Room Nurses (AORN), and the Association of Operating Room Technicians (AORT). Two control groups were surveyed: the American Academy of Pediatrics (AAP) and the American Nurses Association (ANA). At the time of the survey, about 21% of the operating rooms were ventilated and anesthetic-scavenged. The rates of SAB among the respondents (organization and total number of pregnancies shown in parentheses) were 17.1% (ASA; 468), 17.0% (AANA; 1826), and 19.5% (AORN/AORT; 2781). The results were statistically significant when compared with women working outside of the operating room. However, no difference was found with the controls for the time (in gestational weeks) of the abortions or for a decrease in the sex ratio of exposed pregnancies (37).

A survey of women physicians in England and Wales to determine the outcome of pregnancies was reported in 1977 (38). The analysis involved 9044 pregnancies that were classified into three groups: working anesthetists (N = 670), other medical specialties (includes medical students but excludes radiologists) (N = 6377), and physicians not currently working (N = 1997). The adjusted SAB rates were 13.8%, 13.8%, and 12.0%, respectively. For stillbirths, the rates were 17.3%, 8.3%, and 10.3% (*ns*), respectively (38). Another survey in England of anesthetists exposed to anesthetics, male and female, appeared in 1979 (39). The SAB rates (percentages of known conceptions) for exposed fathers, mothers, both parents, and nonexposed controls were 15.7%, 34.4%*, 23.1%*, and 9.8%, respectively (*significant compared with controls).

Because dentists and their assistants may be exposed to even higher concentrations of anesthetic gases than personnel in hospital operating rooms, a survey of this population was undertaken and reported in 1980 (40). The responding sample size involved >22,000 dentists (98.5% male) and >21,000 chairside assistants (99.1% female). Only about 19% of the individuals were exposed to halogenated anesthetic gases in addition to nitrous oxide. The two groups were further classified by the amount of exposure in the year before conception (nonusers, light [1–2999 hours in the past decade], and heavy [>3000 hours in the past decade]). After adjustment for smoking, age, and pregnancy history, a significant association was found between use of anesthetics and the rate of SAB in chairside assistants (8.1% nonusers, 14.2% light, and 19.1% heavy). The association also was significant for wives of dentists but the rates of SAB were about half of those for the assistants (40). In a brief 1986 report, six SAB were observed in four female personnel over a 17-month interval (41). These persons worked in an oral surgery department that used 35% nitrous oxide in oxygen as a sedative during procedures. In the operating rooms, the range of nitrous oxide concentrations were 0.01%–0.04% but were as high as 0.07% when the patient talked (41). A 1995 study found a significant increase in SAB among female dental assistants who worked for 3 or more hours per week in offices not using scavenging equipment (42). After adjustment for age, smoking, and number of amalgams prepared, the relative risk (RR) was 2.6 (95% confidence interval [CI] 1.3–5.0).

In contrast to the above reports, two studies found no association between chronic exposure to nitrous oxide and SAB, and a third found only a partial association (43–45). In comparison with unexposed controls, the adjusted odds ratios (ORs) for SAB in dental assistants working in unscavenged clinics or dental school services in Denmark were 0.9 (95% CI 0.4–2.1) and 0.3 (95% CI 0.0–1.8), respectively (43). In a Swedish study of 1711 midwives, the use of nitrous oxide (>50% of deliveries) was not associated with an increased risk of SAB (OR 0.95, 95% CI 0.62–1.47) (44). The study could not determine if scavenging equipment for waste gas was used. The investigators concluded that night work and high workload increased the risk of SAB (44). In an earlier study, the rates of SAB were compared for 563 married female anesthetists, working and not working, to 828 female physician controls (45). The rates were 18.3%, 13.7%, and 14.7%, respectively.

A 1980 report described the outcomes of 187 women who had been exposed to inhalational anesthetics (mostly nitrous oxide) during work or by their husbands, and who had surgery during pregnancy (46). This was an extension of the study involving occupational exposure to inhalational anesthetics and SAB in wives of dentists and dental assistants (N = 12,929) (see reference 37). The rates of 1st trimester SAB in four groups classified as controls (N = 8654; no exposure or surgery), exposure/no surgery (N = 4088), no exposure/surgery (N = 122), and exposure/surgery (N = 65) were 5.1%, 8.6%, 8.0%, and 14.8%, respectively. The rates for 2nd trimester SAB were 1.4%, 2.6%, 6.9%, and 0, respectively (46). A Canadian study compared pregnant women undergoing incidental surgery with pregnant women not undergoing surgery (47). Surgery (usually gynecologic) under general anesthesia in the 1st or 2nd trimester was associated with an increased risk of SAB (estimated risk ratio [ERR] 2.0, 95% CI 1.10–3.64). The risk was also increased following procedures under general anesthesia that were remote from the conceptus (ERR 1.54, 95% CI 1.03–2.30) (47). A 1986 study of general anesthesia with nitrous oxide in 433 women (9 sets of twins) given in the 1st and 2nd trimesters was unable to find an association between the anesthetic and SAB (48).

Finally, a 1985 study combined the data from six studies to determine the risk of SAB in operating room personnel (1). The low RR was 1.3 (95% CI 1.2–1.4) for pregnant physicians and nurses.

INFERTILITY—FEMALE An increased rate of infertility in anesthetists was noted in a 1972 study (45). In this survey of women anesthetists in the United Kingdom, 65 (12%) of the 563 married anesthetists reported infertility of unknown cause compared with 6% of controls. However, 36 (44%) eventually conceived even though 92% of them continued to work (45). A 1979 survey reported that 30% of anesthetists (includes both sexes) had difficulty in conceiving, but unexpected infertility occurred in only 3% (40).

A 1992 study examined the effect of environmental nitrous oxide on the fertility of dental assistants (58). A group of 7000 female dental assistants was surveyed and 459 were determined to be eligible for the study because they had met all inclusion criteria, including conception within the previous 4 years. Of those eligible, 418 (91%) completed the telephone interview. Data were collected over 13 menstrual cycles (about 1 year). The primary statistical analysis involved a comparison of the adjusted fecundability ratio (an estimate of the conception rate for exposed women relative to that for unexposed women in each menstrual cycle of unprotected intercourse). No difference in the ratio was observed in the 121 assistants who worked <5 hours/week (N = 85; ratio 1.05) or ≥5 hours/week (N = 36; ratio 1.15) in scavenged offices. In contrast, among the 60 assistants who worked in unscavenged offices, the 41 working <5 hours/week had a significantly higher adjusted ratio (1.01) than the 19 working ≥5 hours/week (0.41). Thus, the latter group was only 41% as likely as unexposed women to conceive during each menstrual cycle. In addition, the study examined the occurrence of SAB. Among the 325 pregnancies (93 excluded because they were pregnant at the time of data collection), 10 were in the "high exposure" unscavenged group. Their SAB rate was 50% (5/10), whereas 25 (8%) of the remaining 315 pregnancies aborted (58). An accompanying editorial and later correspondence discussed the implications of the study (59–63).

A 1996 study involving Swedish midwives obtained results similar to those above (64). As in the above study, data were collected over 13 menstrual cycles. In the 84% of responders (N = 3985) to a mailed questionnaire, the adjusted fecundability ratios of three groups, compared with those working in the day time, were two-shift rotations 0.78, three-shift rotations 0.77, night-shift only 0.82, respectively. The effect of nitrous oxide was noted only for midwives exposed to >30 deliveries/month where the gas was used (ratio 0.64) (64).

The effects of general anesthesia on pregnancy rates in patients undergoing embryo transfer after in vitro fertilization were described in a 1995 study (65). Analgesia for ovum retrieval and embryo transfer was sedation (opiates, diazepam, promethazine)/local anesthesia (120 cycles; 88 patients), epidural block (139 cycles; 111 patients), and general anesthesia (nitrous oxide, halothane, opiates, and barbiturates) (173 cycles; 112 patients). The groups did not differ in embryo yield or number or quality of embryos transferred. However, the clinical pregnancy rates for the general anesthesia group were significantly lower than the other two groups: 25.8%, 23.7%, and 14.5%, respectively. The delivery rate also was significantly lower for the general anesthesia group: 19.2%, 20.1%, and 8.7%, respectively. The authors concluded that the adverse effect of general anesthesia occurred after embryo transfer and was probably related to nitrous oxide exposure (65). However, a 1999 study with data from seven fertility programs involving gamete intrafallopian transfer found no significant difference in the clinical pregnancy or delivery rates between women who had received nitrous oxide (or other anesthetic agents) and those who did not (66).

INFERTILITY—MALE A survey of 5507 male anesthetists in the United Kingdom found no association between paternal work in operating rooms and SAB, infertility, or the frequency of congenital anomalies (67). However, if the mother is also exposed, the risk of SAB may be increased by 158%–271%. A 1987 review suggested that male fertility could be affected by direct nitrous oxide-inactivation of vitamin B_{12} (cyanocobalamine) (68). The inactivation of this vitamin could result in a reduction of methionine synthetase that is essential for normal cell division (68). A later review discussed the effect of nitrous oxide on cyanocobalamine-dependent methionine synthetase and other factors that eventually impair DNA synthesis and could cause infertility (69).

CONGENITAL MALFORMATIONS Several studies have examined the relationship between 1st trimester exposure to nitrous oxide and congenital malformations (1,37–39,45–48,70–76). Two early studies did not find such a relationship, but the number of exposed cases was small (70,71). A larger study also found no relationship between surgical anesthesia and congenital malformations (47). In another previously cited study, the overall rate of birth defects in live births was no different in 583 anesthetists (5.2%) and 828 controls (4.9%) (45). However, when analyzed separately, working anesthetists had a significantly higher rate of offspring with defects (6.5%) than those who were not working (2.5%), but not significantly higher than controls.

A 1974 survey of 621 female nurse-anesthetists, with a response rate of 84.5%, found an incidence of birth defects (major and minor) in offspring of working mothers of 16.4%, compared with 5.7% when the mother was not working (72). Nearly one-half of the defects in the exposed group were cutaneous anomalies. In another 1974 national survey cited above, the congenital abnormality rates (all skin anomalies were excluded) in the groups (unexposed vs. exposed) were ASA (3.4% vs. 5.9%), AANA (5.9% vs. 9.6%), and AORN/AORT (7.0% vs 7.7%) (37). The first two comparisons were statistically significant. The survey also provided the congenital malformation rates (excluding skin anomalies) for wives of the male survey respondents in the three groups: 5.4%, 8.2%, and 6.4%, respectively (37). A 1977 survey found a significant rate of heart/great vessels defects in working anesthetists (13.8%) in comparison with a combined group of other physicians (3.6%), or an earlier population-based study (6.6%) (38). However, no differences were found for other congenital anomalies (neural tube defects [NTDs], oral clefts, talipes, congenital hip dislocation, hydrocele, hypospadias, and epispadias, and genitourinary). The rates of development or congenital abnormalities (percentage of live births) in a 1979 survey of anesthetists exposed to anesthetics were 9.3%

N

($N = 22$) for exposed fathers, 4.8% ($N = 1$) for exposed mothers, and 15.0% ($N = 3$) when both parents were exposed (39). These rates did not differ significantly from nonexposed controls.

No significant increase in the incidence of birth defects was found in a 1980 study of surgery during early pregnancy (46). Anesthetics for surgery were used in 187 women during the 1st trimester and in 100 women during the 2nd trimester. The rates of defects in the offspring of mothers who had surgery in the 1st and 2nd trimesters, but no occupational exposure to inhalational anesthetics, were 3.1% and 5.8%, respectively. For surgery plus occupational exposure, the rates were 7.2% and 2.3%, respectively. The differences were not significant (46). A 1986 study analyzed the outcomes of 375 cases (8 sets of twins) of cervical cerclage and 58 other surgeries (1 set of twins) conducted under general anesthesia with nitrous oxide (48). Cases were further stratified by the gestational week when surgery was conducted (>16 weeks or ≤16 weeks). None of the observed birth defects could be attributed to anesthetic exposure (48). A 1985 study combined the results from six studies to derive an RR for congenital abnormalities of 1.2 (95% CI 1.0–1.4) for pregnant physicians and nurses working in operating rooms (1).

Using data from three Swedish health care registries for 1973–1981, a 1989 study analyzed 5405 cases of nonobstetric surgical operations that occurred during pregnancy (73). The types of anesthesia were general (about 54%; 99% using combinations with nitrous oxide), regional (about 14%), and unknown (32%). The rates of congenital malformations, stillbirths, infant death within 7 days of birth, and decreased birth weights were determined by the trimester of operation. For congenital malformations, the RR and 95% CI (in parentheses) for the 1st, 2nd, and 3rd trimesters and the total group were 1.0 (0.8–1.4), 0.9 (0.6–1.2), 1.5 (1.1–2.2) and 1.1 (0.9–1.3), respectively. The rate for all defects was about 5%; and 1.9% for major anomalies. Both rates were similar to those in the total Swedish population. The risk for stillbirths also was not significantly different from the general population (RR 1.4, 95% CI 1.0–1.8), but the risk of infant death within 7 days of birth was increased (RR 2.1, 95% CI 1.6–2.7). Most of the infant deaths (70%) occurred in infants of very low birth weight. The rates of low-birth-weight (<2500 g) and very-low-birth-weight (<1500 g) infants were increased in all trimesters and for the total the RRs (95% CI) were 2.0 (1.8–2.2) and 2.2 (1.8–2.8). The reduced weights were due to prematurity and intrauterine growth restriction. For all mothers operated on, the prematurity rate was 7.47% vs. 5.13% in controls ($p < 0.001$) (73).

Using the same data as in the above study, a possible association between surgery in the 1st trimester and NTDs was published in 1990 (74). The investigators studied 2252 infants whose mothers had surgery during the 1st trimester. Six of the infants had NTD (expected 2.5), one of whom was thought to have Meckel's syndrome. An additional infant had a diagnosis of hydranencephaly, but the autopsy report indicated the diagnosis was uncertain and it may have been a very large encephalocele. In the total group, 572 infants had operations during the period of neural tube closure (gestational weeks 4 and 5). Mothers of five of the six infants with NTD (expected 0.6) had surgery during this period, but only three had been exposed to nitrous oxide. The mother of the hydranencephaly case had surgery in gestational week 8 and was not exposed to nitrous oxide. The authors could not determine whether the findings represented a causal association with surgery or just a random occurrence (74).

In a 1994 population-based, case–control study, 12 (1.7%) of 694 mothers of infants with CNS defects had surgery under general anesthesia in the 1st trimester, compared with 34 (1.1%) of 2984 controls (75). Analysis of total CNS defects and 1st trimester exposure to general anesthesia revealed the following: NTD (345 cases; 3 exposed), OR 0.7, 95% CI 0.2–2.4; microcephaly (91 cases; 1 exposed), OR 1.7, 95% CI 0.2–13.5; and hydrocephalus (198 cases; 7 exposed), OR 3.8, 95% CI 1.6–9.1. When isolated CNS defects were analyzed, the OR and 95% CI for the three defects were 1.1 (0.3–4.9), 3.8 (0.4–33.0), and 0.0 (0.00–4.1) (all *ns*). However, when the analysis included multiple CNS defects, there were 70 cases (7 exposed) of hydrocephalus (OR 9.6, 95% CI 3.8–24.6), 8 cases (3 exposed) of hydrocephalus and eye defects (OR 39.6, 95% CI 7.5, 209.2), and 2 cases (2 exposed) of hydrocephalus and cataracts (OR infinity, 95% CI 1329, infinity). Although the investigators identified several limitations of their study, including the inability to identify the specific medications used for general anesthesia, the findings do warrant additional study (75).

The Collaborative Perinatal Project monitored 50,282 mother–child pairs, 76 of whom were exposed to nitrous oxide during the 1st trimester (76). Four malformed infants were observed, a hospital standardized RR of 0.75. There was no evidence of an association between the gas and the defects (76).

NEUROTOXICITY The mechanism of the action of nitrous oxide, at anesthetic concentrations, is thought to involve blockade of *N*-methyl-D-aspartate (NMDA) glutamate receptors (77–81). This action also produces neurotoxic effects, which can be prevented by drugs (e.g., benzodiazepines, barbiturates, halothane, isoflurane, propofol, scopolamine, and atropine) that enhance GABAergic (γ-amino-*n*-butyric acid) inhibition (77,79). However, the addition of ketamine, another NMDA antagonist, to nitrous oxide without concomitant use of a GABA agonist has been shown in animals to potentiate the neurotoxicity of nitrous oxide (82). Recent evidence has shown that the neurotoxicity of ethanol, an NMDA antagonist and a potentiator of GABA transmission, is different in immature brains from what it is in adult brains (83). Therefore, the potential exists that the common use of nitrous oxide and GABAergic agents together during general anesthesia in obstetrics and pediatrics could cause neuroteratogenicity during human brain growth spurts (synaptogenesis; 3rd trimester to several years after birth) (83–85). Animal studies in 7-day-old rats have demonstrated this teratogenicity as evidenced by widespread apoptotic neurodegeneration, deficits in hippocampal synaptic function, and persistent impairment of memory and learning (86).

A 2004 study examined the association between exposure of mothers to waste anesthetic gases during pregnancy and development of their offspring (87). Although the specific gases were not identified, the timing of the exposures (1983–1996) and practice patterns suggested that nitrous oxide, halothane, and isoflurane were the most likely agents.

Forty children (age 5–13 years) born to female anesthesiologists and operating room nurses who were exposed to waste anesthetic gases were compared with 40 female physicians and nurses (matched for children's age, gender, and maternal occupation) who worked in hospitals during their pregnancies but did not work in operating rooms (unexposed controls). All children underwent standardized developmental tests to evaluate their medical and neurodevelopmental state and the mothers were interviewed. The developmental milestones in the two groups were similar, but the exposed children had a significantly lower gross motor ability and more evidence of inattention/hyperactivity. Moreover, the level of exposure was significantly and negatively correlated with fine motor ability and IQ performance. The investigators concluded that the results supported the hypothesis that occupational exposure to waste anesthetic gases during pregnancy might be a risk factor for minor neurological deficits in the offspring (87).

MISCELLANEOUS EFFECTS Subanesthetic doses of nitrous oxide have been used for analgesia in laboring patients (88–95). The effects on the fetus do not appear to be any different from other general anesthetics (94). When used as an analgesic, nitrous oxide has no direct effect on uterine activity (89,96). In contrast, prolonged general anesthesia with nitrous oxide may cause neonatal acidosis and an increased incidence of low Apgar scores (97). A 1988 study concluded that the use of high intermittent doses of nitrous oxide used for obstetric analgesia was associated with a risk of developing amphetamine addiction in later life (98). The mechanism was thought to be an effect of imprinting. However, this study has been criticized for several design flaws and conclusions (90).

A 2-minute inhalation dose of 30% nitrous oxide with oxygen for analgesia at term resulted in a decrease in both maternal and fetal central vascular resistance (99). Although this dose is usually safe for the mother or fetus, the cerebral hyperemia induced by nitrous oxide might increase the risk of intracranial hemorrhage in preterm infants (99).

Decreased birth weight, but not preterm birth, was associated with occupational exposure to nitrous oxide in a 1999 study based on a survey of the Swedish Midwives Association (100). Chronic nitrous oxide exposure during the 2nd trimester was associated with a 77-g decrease in birth weight (95% CI −129, −24) and an increase in the odds of infants being small for gestational age (OR 1.8, 95% CI 1.1–2.8) (98). In a 1977 survey, the offspring of working anesthetists had significantly lower birth weights and a higher proportion of infants weighing ≤2500 g than two other physician groups (38). Lower birth weights also were observed in offspring of female anesthetists in a 1979 survey (39). Female infants were particularly underweight. Moreover, there was a lower male:female sex ratio in the offspring of female anesthetists (36). The author, however, has had to defend his research (101).

A 1991 population-based case–control study conducted in Sweden found an association between childhood leukemia and nitrous oxide anesthesia during delivery (102). Mothers of the 411 cases were more likely than controls to have received the anesthetic (OR 1.3, 95% CI 1.0–1.6).

BREASTFEEDING SUMMARY

No reports describing the use of nitrous oxide during lactation have been located. The solubility in blood and tissue is low. Moreover, the plasma half-life is very short (<3 minutes) and, thus, it is unlikely that a nursing infant would be exposed to the agent in milk or that it would be orally bioavailable to the infant (103).

References

1. Buring JE, Hennekens CH, Mayrent SL, Rosner B, Greenberg ER, Colton T. Health experience of operating room personnel. Anesthesiology 1985;62:325–30.
2. Dale O, Husum B. Nitrous oxide: at threat to personnel and global environment? Acta Anaesthesiol Scand 1994;38:777–9.
3. Jones HE, Balster RL. Inhalant abuse in pregnancy. Obstet Gynecol Clin North Am 1998;25:153–67.
4. Steward A, Allott PR, Cowles AL, Mapleson WW. Solubility coefficients for inhaled anaesthetics for water, oil and biological media. Br J Anaesth 1973;45:282–93.
5. Fink BR, Shepard TH, Blandau RJ. Teratogenic activity of nitrous oxide. Nature 1967;214:146–8.
6. Corbett TH, Cornell RG, Endres JL, Millard RI. Effect of low concentrations of nitrous oxide on rat pregnancy. Anesthesiology 1973;39:299–301.
7. Pope WDB, Halsey MJ, Phil D, Lansdown ABG, Simmonds A, Bateman PE. Fetotoxicity in rats following chronic exposure to halothane, nitrous oxide, or methoxyflurane. Anesthesiology 1978;48:11–6.
8. Ramazzotto LJ, Carlin RD, Warchalowski GA. Effects of nitrous oxide during organogenesis in the rat. J Dent Res 1979;58:1940–3.
9. Coate WB, Kapp RW Jr, Lewis TR. Chronic exposure to low concentrations of halothane-nitrous oxide. Anesthesiology 1979;50:310–8.
10. Coate WB, Kapp RW Jr, Ulland BM, Lewis TR. Toxicity of low concentration long-term exposure to an airborne mixture of nitrous oxide and halothane. J Environ Pathol Toxicol 1979;2:209–31.
11. Vieira E. Effect of the chronic administration of nitrous oxide 0.5% to gravid rats. Br J Anaesth 1979;51:283–7.
12. Vieira E, Cleaton-Jones P, Austin JC, Moyes DG, Shaw R. Effects of low concentrations of nitrous oxide on rat fetuses. Anesth Analg 1980;59:175–7.
13. Vieira E, Cleaton-Jones P, Moyes D. Effects of low intermittent concentrations of nitrous oxide on the developing rat fetus. Br J Anaesth 1983;55:67–9.
14. Shah RM, Burdett DN, Donaldson D. The effects of nitrous oxide on the developing hamster embryos. Can J Physiol Pharmacol 1979;57:1229–32.
15. Bussard DA, Stoelting RK, Peterson C, Ishaq M. Fetal changes in hamsters anesthetized with nitrous oxide and halothane. Anesthesiology 1974;41:275–8.
16. Lane GA, Nahrwold ML, Tait AR, Taylor-Busch M, Cohen PJ, Beaudoin AR. Anesthetics as teratogens: nitrous oxide is fetotoxic, xenon is not. Science 1980;210:899–901.
17. Mazze RI, Wilson AI, Rice SA, Baden JM. Reproduction and fetal development in rats exposed to nitrous oxide. Teratology 1984;30:259–65.
18. Mazze RI, Fujinaga M, Rice SA, Harris SB, Baden JM. Reproductive and teratogenic effects of nitrous oxide, halothane, isoflurane, and enflurane in Sprague-Dawley rats. Anesthesiology 1986;64:339–44.
19. Trevor AJ, Miller RD. General anesthetics. In: Katzung BG, ed. *Basic and Clinical Pharmacology*. 8th ed. New York, NY: McGraw-Hill, 2001:426.
20. Mazze RI, Wilson AI, Rice SA, Baden JM. Reproduction and fetal development in mice chronically exposed to nitrous oxide. Teratology 1982;26:11–6.
21. Warren JR, Shaw B, Steinkampf MP. Effects of nitrous oxide on preimplantation mouse embryo cleavage and development. Biol Reprod 1990;43:158–61.
22. Fujinaga M, Baden JM, Mazze RI. Susceptible period of nitrous oxide teratogenicity in Sprague-Dawley rats. Teratology 1989;40:439–44.
23. Rodier PM. Inhalant anesthetics as neuroteratogens. Ann NY Acad Sci 1986;477:42–8.

24. Mullenix PJ, Moore PA, Tassinari MS. Behavioral toxicity of nitrous oxide in rats following prenatal exposure. Toxicol Ind Health 1986;2:273–87.
25. Tassinari MS, Mullenix PJ, Moore PA. The effects of nitrous oxide after exposure during middle and late gestation. Toxicol Ind Health 1986;2: 261–71.
26. Rice SA. Effect of prenatal N_2O exposure on startle reflex reactivity. Teratology 1990;42:373–81.
27. Saito S, Fujita T, Igarashi M. Effects of inhalational anesthetics on biochemical events in growing neuronal tips. Anesthesiology 1993;79: 1338–47.
28. Kugel G, Letelier C, Zive MA, King JC. Nitrous oxide and infertility. Anesth Prog 1990;37:176–80.
29. Cohen EN, Paulson WJ, Wall J, Elert B. Thiopental, curare, and nitrous oxide anesthesia for cesarean section with studies on placental transmission. Surg Gynecol Obstet 1953;97:456–62.
30. Marx GF, Joshi CW, Orkin LR. Placental transmission of nitrous oxide. Anesthesiology 1970;32:429–32.
31. Morgan CA, Paull J. Drugs in obstetric anaesthesia. Anaesth Intens Care 1980;8:278–88.
32. Nandi PR, Morrison PF, Morgan BM. Effects of general anaesthesia on the fetus during caesarean section. Anaesth Rev 1991;8:103–22.
33. Friedman JM. Teratogen update: anesthetic agents. Teratology 1988;37:69–77.
34. Kanto J. Risk–benefit assessment of anaesthetic agents in the puerperium. Drug Saf 1991;6:285–301.
35. Corbett TH. Anesthetics as a cause of abortion. Fertil Steril 1972;23: 866–9.
36. Cohen EN, Bellville JW, Brown BW Jr. Anesthesia, pregnancy, and miscarriage: a study of operating room nurses and anesthetists. Anesthesiology 1971;35:343–7.
37. Ad Hoc Committee on the Effect of Trace Anesthetics on the Health of Operating Room Personnel, American Society of Anesthesiologists. Occupational disease among operating room personnel: a national study. Anesthesiology 1974;41:321–40.
38. Pharoah POD, Alberman E, Doyle P. Outcome of pregnancy among women in anaesthetic practice. Lancet 1977;1:34–6.
39. Tomlin PJ. Health problems of anaesthetists and their families in the West Midlands. Br Med J 1979;1:779–84.
40. Cohen EN, Brown BW, Wu ML, Whitcher CE, Brodsky JB, Gift HC, Greenfield W, Jones TW, Driscoll EJ. Occupational disease in dentistry and chronic exposure to trace anesthetic gases. J Am Dent Assoc 1980;101:21–31.
41. Schuyt HC, Brakel K, Oostendorp SGLM, Schiphorst BJM. Abortion among dental personnel exposed to nitrous oxide. Anaesthesia 1986;41:82–3.
42. Rowland AS, Baird DD, Shore DL, Weinberg CR, Savitz DA, Wilcox AJ. Nitrous oxide and spontaneous abortion in female dental assistants. Am J Epidemiol 1995;141:531–8.
43. Heidam LZ. Spontaneous abortions among dental assistants, factory workers, painters, and gardening workers: a follow up study. J Epidemiol Comm Health 1984;38:149–55.
44. Axelsson G, Ahlborg G Jr, Bodin L. Shift work, nitrous oxide exposure, and spontaneous abortion among Swedish midwives. Occup Environ Med 1996;53:374–8.
45. Knill-Jones RP, Rodrigues LV, Moir DD, Spence AA. Anaesthetic practice and pregnancy—controlled survey of women anaesthetists in the United Kingdom. Lancet 1972;1:1326–8.
46. Brodsky JB, Cohen EN, Brown BW Jr, Wu ML, Whitcher C. Surgery during pregnancy and fetal outcome. Am J Obstet Gynecol 1980;138:1165–7.
47. Duncan PG, Pope WDB, Cohen MM, Greer N. Fetal risk of anesthesia and surgery during pregnancy. Anesthesiology 1986;64:790–4.
48. Crawford JS, Lewis M. Nitrous oxide in early human pregnancy. Anaesthesia 1986;41:900–5.
49. Spence AA, Knill-Jones RP. Is there a health hazard in anaesthetic practice? Br J Anaesth 1978;50:713–9.
50. Brodsky JB. Anesthesia and surgery during early pregnancy and fetal outcome. Clin Obstet Gynecol 1983;26:449–57.
51. Alridge LM, Tunstall ME. Nitrous oxide and the fetus. Br J Anaesth 1986;58:1348–56.
52. Eger EI II. Fetal injury and abortion associated with occupational exposure to inhaled anesthetics. AANA J 1991;59:309–12.
53. Shortridge-McCauley LA. Reproductive hazards: an overview of exposures to health care workers. AAOHN J 1995;43:614–21.
54. Donaldson D, Meechan JG. The hazards of chronic exposure to nitrous oxide: an update. Br Dent J 1995;178:95–100.
55. Sessler DI. Risks of occupational exposure to waste-anesthetic gases. Acta Anaesthesiol Scand 1997;41(Suppl 111):237–9.
56. Wasylko L, Matsui D, Dykxhoorn SM, Rieder MJ, Weinberg S. A review of common dental treatments during pregnancy: implications for patients and dental personnel. J Can Dent Assoc 1998;64:434–9.
57. Smith DA. Hazards of nitrous oxide exposure in healthcare personnel. AANA J 1998;66:390–3.
58. Rowland AS, Baird DD, Weinberg CR, Shore DL, Shy CM, Wilcox AJ. Reduced fertility among women employed as dental assistants exposed to high levels of nitrous oxide. N Engl J Med 1992;327:993–7.
59. Baird PA. Occupational exposure to nitrous oxide—not a laughing matter. N Engl J Med 1992;327:1026–7.
60. Gray RH. Nitrous oxide and fertility. N Engl J Med 1993;328:284.
61. Rowland AS, Baird DD, Weinberg CR. Nitrous oxide and fertility. Reply. N Engl J Med 1993;328:284.
62. Brodsky JB. Nitrous oxide and fertility. N Engl J Med 1993;328:284–5.
63. Baird PA. Nitrous oxide and fertility (reply). N Engl J Med 1993;328:285.
64. Ahlborg G Jr, Axelsson G, Bodin L. Shift work, nitrous oxide exposure and subfertility among Swedish midwives. Int J Epidemiol 1996;25:783–90.
65. Gonen O, Shulman A, Ghetler Y, Shapiro A, Judeiken R, Beyth Y, Ben-Nun I. The impact of different types of anesthesia on in vitro fertilization-embryo transfer treatment outcome. J Assist Reprod Genet 1995;12: 678–82.
66. Beilin Y, Bodian CA, Mukherjee T, Andres LA, Vincent RD Jr, Hock DL, Sparks AET, Munson AK, Minnich ME, Steinkampf MP, Christman GM, McKay RSF, Eisenkraft JB. The use of propofol, nitrous oxide, or isoflurane does not affect the reproductive success rate following gamete intrafallopian transfer (GIFT). Anesthesiology 1999;90:36–41.
67. Knill-Jones RP, Newman BJ, Spence AA. Anaesthetic practice and pregnancy. Lancet 1975;2:807–9.
68. Buckley DN, Brodsky JB. Nitrous oxide and male fertility. Reprod Toxicol 1987;1:93–7.
69. Louis-Ferdinand RT. Myelotoxic, neurotoxic and reproductive adverse effects of nitrous oxide. Adverse Drug React Toxicol Rev 1994;13: 193–206.
70. Shnider SM, Webster GM. Maternal and fetal hazards of surgery during pregnancy. Am J Obstet Gynecol 1965;92:891–900.
71. Mellin GW. Comparative teratology. Anesthesiology 1968;29:1–4.
72. Corbett TH, Cornell RG, Endres JL, Lieding K. Birth defects among children of nurse-anesthetists. Anesthesiology 1974;41:341–4.
73. Mazze RI, Kallen B. Reproductive outcome after anesthesia and operation during pregnancy: a registry study of 5405 cases. Am J Obstet Gynecol 1989;161:1178–85.
74. Kallen B, Mazze RI. Neural tube defects and first trimester operations. Teratology 1990;41:717–20.
75. Sylvester GC, Khoury MJ, Lu X, Erickson JD. First-trimester anesthesia exposure and the risk of central nervous system defects: a population-based case-control study. Am J Public Health 1994;84:1757–60.
76. Heinonen OP, Sloan D, Shapiro S. *Birth Defects and Drugs in Pregnancy*. Littleton, MA: Publishing Sciences Group, 1977:358–60.
77. Jevtovic-Todorovic V, Todorovic SM, Mennerick S, Powell S, Dikranian K, Benshoff N, Zorumski CF, Olney JW. Nitrous oxide (laughing gas) is an NMDA antagonist, neuroprotectant and neurotoxin. Nat Med 1998;4:460–3.
78. Mennerick S, Jevtovic-Todorovic V, Todorovic SM, Shen W, Olney JW, Zorumski CF. Effect of nitrous oxide on excitatory and inhibitory synaptic transmission in hippocampal cultures. J Neurosci 1998;18:9716–26.
79. Jevtovic-Todorovic V, Beals J, Benshoff N, Olney JW. Prolonged exposure to inhalational anesthetic nitrous oxide kills neurons in adult rat brain. Neuroscience 2003;122:609–16.
80. Jevtovic-Todorovic V, Wozniak DF, Benshoff ND, Olney JW. A comparative evaluation of the neurotoxic properties of ketamine and nitrous oxide. Brain Res 2001;895:264–7.
81. Olney JW, Wozniak DF, Farber NB, Jevtovic-Todorovic V, Bittigau P, Ikonomidou C. The enigma of fetal alcohol neurotoxicity. Ann Med 2002;34:109–19.
82. Jevtovic-Todorovic V, Benshoff N, Olney JW. Ketamine potentiates cerebrocortical damage induced by the common anaesthetic agent nitrous oxide in adult rats. Br J Pharmacol 2000;130:1692–8.
83. Olney JW, Farber NB, Wozniak DF, Jevtovic-Todorovic V, Ikonomidou C. Environmental agents that have the potential to trigger massive apoptotic neurodegeneration in the developing brain. Environ Health Perspect 2000;108(Suppl 3):383–8.

84. Olney JW, Wozniak DF, Jevtovic-Todorovic V, Farber NB, Bittigau P, Ikonomidou C. Drug-induced apoptotic neurodegeneration in the developing brain. Brain Pathol 2002;12:488–98.
85. Ikonomidou C, Bittigau P, Koch C, Genz K, Hoerster F, Felderhoff-Mueser U, Tenkova T, Dikranian K, Olney JW. Neurotransmitters and apoptosis in the developing brain. Biochem Pharmacol 2001;62:401–5.
86. Jevtovic-Todorovic V, Hartman RE, Izumi Y, Benshoff ND, Dikranian K, Zorumski CF, Olney JW, Wozniak DF. Early exposure to common anesthetic agents causes widespread neurodegeneration in the developing rat brain and persistent learning deficits. J Neurosci 2003;23:876–82.
87. Ratzon NZ, Ornoy A, Pardo A, Rachel M, Hatch M. Development evaluation of children born to mothers occupationally exposed to waste anesthetic gases. Birth Defects Res A Clin Mol Teratol 2004;70:476–82.
88. Harrison RF, Shore M, Woods T, Mathews G, Gardiner J, Unwin A. A comparison study of transcutaneous electrical nerve stimulation (TENS), Entonox, pethidine + promazine and lumbar epidural for pain relief in labor. Acta Obstet Gynecol Scand 1987;66:914.
89. Marx GF, Katsnelson T. The introduction of nitrous oxide analgesia into obstetrics. Obstet Gynecol 1992;80:715–8.
90. Irestedt L. Current status of nitrous oxide for obstetric pain relief. Acta Anaesthesiol Scand 1994;38:771–2.
91. Ross JAS, Tunstall ME, Campbell DM, Lemon JS. The use of 0.25% isoflurane premixed in 50% nitrous oxide and oxygen for pain relief in labour. Anaesthesia 1999;54:1166–72.
92. King R, Hepp M. Isoflurane Entonox mixtures for pain relief during labour. Anaesthesia 2000;55:711.
93. Ross JAS. Isoflurane Entonox mixtures for pain relief during labour. Reply. Anaesthesia 2000;55:711–2.
94. Stefani SJ, Hughes SC, Shnider SM, Levinson G, Abboud TK, Henriksen EH, Williams V, Johnson J. Neonatal neurobehavioral effects of inhalation analgesia for vaginal delivery. Anesthesiology 1982;56:351–5.
95. Abboud TK, Swart F, Zhu J, Donovan MM, Peres Da Silva E, Yakal K. Desflurane analgesia for vaginal delivery. Acta Anaesthesiol Scand 1995;39:259–61.
96. Baxi LV, Petrie RH. Pharmacologic effects on labor: effects of drugs on dystocia, labor, and uterine activity. Clin Obstet Gynecol 1987;30:19–32.
97. Datta S, Ostheimer GW, Weiss JB, Brown WU Jr, Alper MH. Neonatal effect of prolonged anesthetic induction for cesarean section. Obstet Gynecol 1981;58:331–5.
98. Jacobson B, Nyberg K, Eklund G, Bygdeman M, Rydberg U. Obstetric pain medication and eventual adult amphetamine addiction in offspring. Acta Obstet Gynecol Scand 1988;67:677–82.
99. Polvi HJ, Pirhonen JP, Erkkola RU. Nitrous oxide inhalation: effects on maternal and fetal circulations at term. Obstet Gynecol 1996;87:1045–8.
100. Bodin L, Axelsson G, Ahlborg G Jr. The association of shift work and nitrous oxide exposure in pregnancy with birth weight and gestational age. Epidemiology 1999;10:429–36.
101. Tomlin PJ. Health problems of anaesthetists and their families. Br Med J 1979;1:1280–1.
102. Zack M, Adam HO, Ericson A. Maternal and perinatal risk factors for childhood leukemia. Cancer Res 1991;51:3696–701.
103. Hale TW. Anesthetic medications in breastfeeding mothers. J Hum Lact 1999;15:185–94.

NIZATIDINE

Gastrointestinal Agent (Antisecretory)

PREGNANCY RECOMMENDATION: Limited Human Data—Animal Data Suggest Low Risk
BREASTFEEDING RECOMMENDATION: Limited Human Data—Probably Compatible

N

PREGNANCY SUMMARY

Nizatidine is an H_2-receptor antagonist (H2 blocker) that inhibits gastric acid secretion. Although the animal reproduction data suggest low risk, the limited human pregnancy experience prevents a complete assessment of the embryo–fetal risk. A study showing an association between in utero exposure to gastric acid-suppressing drugs and childhood allergy and asthma requires confirmation.

FETAL RISK SUMMARY

Nizatidine is a competitive, reversible H2 blocker, particularly those in the gastric parietal cells. It is indicated for the treatment of active duodenal and gastric ulcer, esophagitis, including erosive and ulcerative esophagitis, and associated heartburn due to gastroesophageal reflux disease (GERD). Nizatidine undergoes minimal metabolism (<7%) to an active metabolite. Plasma protein binding, primarily to α_1-acid glycoprotein, is low (about 35%) and the elimination half-life is 1–2 hours (1).

In reproduction studies reported by the manufacturer, no evidence of impaired fertility or fetal harm was observed in rats given oral doses up to 40.5 times the recommended human dose based on BSA (RHD) or rabbits at doses up to 14.6 times the RHD (1). In a 1987 animal study, pregnant rats and rabbits were given oral doses ≤506 mg/kg/day (2). No adverse effects were observed on fertility, and no teratogenic effects occurred with doses ≤1500 mg/kg/day, although some abortions occurred in rabbits, but not in rats, at the highest dose (*highest dose in rabbits is about 80 times the RHD*) .

A single cotyledon perfusion model was used to determine the placental transfer of nizatidine in both term human and preterm baboon placentas (3). In both systems, nizatidine was transferred at about 40% of the freely diffusible reference compound. Nizatidine transfer across the placentas was the same in both directions (i.e., mother to fetus and fetus to mother). The transfer across the placenta is consistent with the low molecular weight (about 331) and plasma protein binding.

Based on studies in male humans (4) and animals (5,6), nizatidine does not appear to have antiandrogenic effects like those observed with cimetidine (see Cimetidine). Reversible impotence, however, has been described in men treated with nizatidine for therapeutic indications (7).

A genetic counselor was consulted about a woman who had taken nizatidine during the 14th through the 16th postconception weeks (T.M. Gardner, personal communication, Jefferson Medical College, 1996). The woman delivered a healthy, about 3547-g, male infant at 37 weeks' gestation who was doing well at 1 month of age.

A 1996 prospective cohort study compared the pregnancy outcomes of 178 women who were exposed during pregnancy to H2 blockers with 178 controls matched for maternal age, smoking, and heavy alcohol consumption (8). All of the women had contacted a teratology information service concerning gestational exposure to H2 blockers (subjects) or nonteratogenic or nonfetotoxic agents (controls). Among subjects (mean daily dose in parentheses), 71% took ranitidine (258 mg), 16% cimetidine (487 mg), 8% famotidine (32 mg), and 5% nizatidine (283 mg). There were no significant differences between the outcomes of subjects and controls in terms of live births, spontaneous abortions (SABs) and elective abortions (EABs), gestational age at birth, delivery method, birth weight, infants small for gestational age, or major malformations. Among subjects, there were 3 birth defects (2.1%) among the 142 exposed to H2 blockers in the 1st trimester: one each of atrial septal defect, ventricular septal defect, and tetralogy of Fallot. There were 5 birth defects (3.0%) among the 165 exposed anytime during pregnancy. For controls, the rates of defects were 3.5% (1st trimester) and 3.1% (anytime). There were also no differences between the groups in neonatal health problems and developmental milestones, but two children (one subject and one control) were diagnosed as developmentally delayed. The investigators concluded that 1st trimester exposure to H2 blockers did not represent a major teratogenic risk (8).

Data from the Swedish Medical Birth Registry were presented in 1998 (9). A total of 553 infants (6 sets of twins) were delivered from 547 women who had used acid-suppressing drugs early in pregnancy. Nizatidine was the only acid-suppressing drug exposure in three infants, none of whom had birth defects (see Omeprazole for additional details of this study) (9).

N

A population-based, observational cohort study formed by linking data from three Swedish national healthcare registers over a 10-year period (1995–2004) was reported in 2009 (10). The main outcome measures were a diagnosis of allergic disease or a prescription for asthma or allergy medications. The drug types included in the study were gastric acid suppressors, including H2 blockers, prostaglandins, proton pump inhibitors, combinations for eradication of *Helicobacter pylori*, and drugs for peptic ulcer and gastroesophageal reflux disease. Of 585,716 children, 29,490 (5.0%) met the diagnosis and 5645 (1%) had been exposed to gastric acid suppression therapy in pregnancy. Of these children, 405 (0.07%) were treated for allergic disease. For developing allergy, the odds ratio (OR) was 1.43, 98% confidence interval (CI) 1.29–1.59, irrespective of the drug, time of exposure during pregnancy, and maternal history of allergy. For developing childhood asthma, but not other allergic diseases, the OR was 1.51, 95% CI 1.35–1.69, irrespective of the type of acid-suppressive drug and the time of exposure in pregnancy. The authors proposed three possible mechanisms for their findings: (a) exposure to increased amounts of allergens could cause sensitization to digestion labile antigens in the fetus; (b) the maternal Th2 cytokine pattern could promote an allergy-prone phenotype in the fetus; and (c) maternal allergen-specific immunoglobulin E could cross the placenta and sensitize fetal immune cells to food- and airborne allergens. Several limitations of the study that might have affected their findings were identified, including a general increase in childhood asthma but not necessarily an increase in allergic asthma (10). The study requires confirmation.

A 2005 study evaluated the outcomes of 553 pregnancies after exposure to H2 blockers, 501 (91%) in the 1st trimester (11). The data were collected by the European Network of Teratology Information Services (ENTIS). The agents and number of cases were nizatidine 15, cimetidine 113, famotidine 75, ranitidine 335, and roxatidine 15. No increase in the number of major malformations were noted (11).

A 2009 meta-analysis of published studies was conducted to assess the safety of H2 blockers that were used in 2398 pregnancies (12). Compared with 119,892 nonexposed pregnancies, the OR for congenital malformations was 1.14 (95% CI 0.89–1.45), whereas the ORs and 95% CIs for SABs, preterm birth, and small for gestational age were 0.62 (0.36–1.05), 1.17 (0.94–1.147), and 0.28 (0.06–1.22), respectively. The authors concluded that H2 blockers could be used safely in pregnancy (12).

Five reviews on the treatment of GERD have concluded that H2 blockers, with the possible exception of nizatidine, could be used in pregnancy with relative safety (13–17). Nizatidine was not recommended because of the adverse animal reproduction data (16). However, no consideration of the high doses used in animals was mentioned. Nevertheless, the very limited human pregnancy data suggest that other agents in this class are preferred.

A 2010 study from Israel identified 1148 infants exposed in the 1st trimester to H2 blockers (18). No association with congenital malformations was found (OR 1.03, 95% CI 0.80–1.32). Moreover, no association was found with EABs, perinatal mortality, premature delivery, low birth weight, or low Apgar scores (18).

BREASTFEEDING SUMMARY

Small amounts of nizatidine are excreted into breast milk (19). Three women, who had been breastfeeding for 3–8 months, were administered nizatidine (150 mg) as a single dose and as multiple doses given every 12 hours for five doses. Serum and milk samples from both breasts were collected at intervals ≤12 hours after a dose. The mean total amount of drug measured in the milk from both breasts during a 12-hour interval was 96.1 mcg. This amount represented 0.064% of the maternal dose. Peak concentrations of the drug in milk occurred between 1 and 2 hours after a dose (19).

Although the infants were not allowed to breastfeed during the above study, the small amounts excreted into the milk are probably not clinically significant. Other drugs in this class are excreted into milk (see Cimetidine and Ranitidine). The American Academy of Pediatrics classifies one of these agents as compatible with breastfeeding (see Cimetidine).

References

1. Product information. Nizatidine. Genpharm, 2002.
2. Morton DM. Pharmacology and toxicology of nizatidine. Scand J Gastroenterol 1987;22(Suppl 136):1–8.
3. Dicke JM, Johnson RF, Henderson GI, Kuehl TJ, Schenker S. A comparative evaluation of the transport of H_2-receptor antagonists by the human and baboon placenta. Am J Med Sci 1988;295:198–206.
4. Van Thiel DH, Gavaler JS, Heyl A, Susen B. An evaluation of the anti-androgen effects associated with H_2 antagonist therapy. Scand J Gastroenterol 1987;22(Suppl 136):24–8.

5. Neubauer BL, Goode RL, Best KL, Hirsch KS, Lin T-M, Pioch RP, Probst KS, Tinsley FC, Shaar CJ. Endocrine effects of new histamine H_2-receptor antagonist, nizatidine (LY139037), in the male rat. Toxicol Appl Pharmacol 1990;102:219–32.
6. Probst KS, Higdon GL, Fisher LF, McGrath JP, Adams ER, Emmerson JL. Preclinical toxicology studies with nizatidine, a new H_2-receptor antagonist: acute, subchronic, and chronic toxicity evaluations. Fundam Appl Toxicol 1989;13:778–92.
7. Kassianos GC. Impotence and nizatidine. Lancet 1989;1:963.
8. Magee LA, Inocencion G, Kamboj L, Rosetti F, Koren G. Safety of first trimester exposure to histamine H_2 blockers. A prospective cohort study. Dig Dis Sci 1996;41:1145–9.
9. Kallen B. Delivery outcome after the use of acid-suppressing drugs in early pregnancy with special reference to omeprazole. Br J Obstet Gynaecol 1998;105:877–81.
10. Dehlink E, Yen E, Leichtner AM, Hait EJ, Fiebiger E. First evidence of a possible association between gastric acid suppression during pregnancy and childhood asthma: a population-based register study. Clin Exp Allergy 2009;39:246–53.
11. Garbis H, Elefant E, Diav-Citrin O, Mastroiacovo P, Schaefer C, Vial T, Clementi M, Valti E, McElhatton P, Smorlesij C, Rodriguez EP, Robert-Gnansia E, Merlob P, Peiker G, Pexieder T, Schueler L, Ritvanen A, Mathieu-Nolf M. Pregnancy outcome after exposure to ranitidine and other H2-blockers—a collaborative study of the European Network of Teratology Information Services. Reprod Toxicol 2005;453–8.
12. Gill SK, O'Brien L, Koren G. The safety of histamine 2 (H2) blockers in pregnancy: a meta-analysis. Dig Dis Sci 2009;54:1835–8.
13. Broussard CN, Richter JE. Treating gastro-oesophageal reflux disease during pregnancy and lactation. What are the safest therapy options? Drug Saf 1998;19:325–37.
14. Katz PO, Castell DO. Gastroesophageal reflux disease during pregnancy. Gastroenterol Clin N Am 1998;27:153–67.
15. Ramakrishnan A, Katz PO. Pharmacologic management of gastroesophageal reflux disease. Curr Treat Options Gastroenterol 2002;5:301–10.
16. Richter JE. Gastroesophageal reflux disease during pregnancy. Gastroenterol Clin N Am 2003;32:235–61.
17. Richter JE. Review article: the management of heartburn in pregnancy. Aliment Pharmacol Ther 2005;22:749–57.
18. Matok I, Gorodischer R, Koren G, Sheiner E, Wiznitzer A, Uziel E, Levy A. The safety of H_2-blockers use during pregnancy. J Clin Pharmacol 2010;50:81–7.
19. Obermeyer BD, Bergstrom RF, Callaghan JT, Knadler MP, Golichowski A, Rubin A. Secretion of nizatidine into human breast milk after single and multiple doses. Clin Pharmacol Ther 1990;47:724–30.

NONOXYNOL-9/OCTOXYNOL-9

Vaginal Spermicides

PREGNANCY RECOMMENDATION: Contraindicated
BREASTFEEDING RECOMMENDATION: No Human Data—Possible Toxicity

PREGNANCY SUMMARY

The available evidence indicates that the use of vaginal spermicides, either before or during early pregnancy, does not pose a risk of congenital malformations to the fetus. Three authors of the original 1981 paper reporting a relationship between spermicides and congenital defects (1) have commented that available data now argue against a causal association (2). In addition, the FDA has issued a statement that spermicides do not cause birth defects (3). There is also controversy on whether the 1981 study should have been published (4,5). The data for spontaneous abortions (SABs), low birth weight, stillbirths, sex ratios at birth, frequency of multiple births, and premature delivery also indicate that it is unlikely that these factors are influenced by spermicide use.

FETAL RISK SUMMARY

Nonoxynol-9 and octoxynol-9 are vaginal spermicides used to prevent conception. These agents, applied intravaginally, act by inactivating sperm after direct contact. Although human data are lacking, nonoxynol-9 rapidly crossed the vaginal wall into the systemic circulation in animals (6). Octoxynol should also be expected to act in a similar manner. The use of vaginal spermicides just before conception or inadvertently during the early stages of pregnancy has led to investigations of their effects on the fetus. The effects studied include congenital malformations, SABs, low birth weight, stillbirth, sex ratio at birth, frequency of multiple births, and premature delivery.

A causal relationship between vaginal spermicides and congenital abnormalities was first tentatively proposed in a 1981 study comparing 763 spermicide users and 3902 nonuser controls (1). The total number of infants with malformations was low: 17 (2.2%) in the exposed group and 39 (1.0%) in the nonexposed group. Malformations thought to be associated with spermicide use were limb reduction deformities (3 cases), neoplasms (2 cases), chromosomal abnormalities (Down's syndrome) (3 cases), and hypospadias (2 cases). An earlier investigation, published in 1977, had concluded there was no causal relationship between spermicides and congenital defects, although there was an increased incidence of limb reduction defects in infants of users (11 of 93) as compared with nonusers (8 of 186) (7). Three reports appeared in 1982 that suggested a possible relationship between spermicide use and congenital malformations (8–10). In a case–control study conducted by one of the co-authors of the 1981 investigation, a positive association with Down's syndrome was proposed when in a group of 16 affected infants, 4 were from users of spermicides (8). In another case–control study, increased risk ratios after spermicide use, although not statistically significant, were reported for limb reduction defects (relative risk 2.00; six infants) and hypospadias (relative risk 4.00; eight infants) (9). Finally, an English study observed, among other defects, 2 cases each of hypospadias, limb reduction deformity, and Down's syndrome among infants of 1103 spermicide users (10). The authors stated that their data were not conclusive, but the occurrence rates of these particular defects were higher than those observed in a comparative nonuser group.

Several criticisms have been directed at the original 1981 study (11–14). First, an infant was presumed exposed if the mother had a prescription filled at a designated pharmacy within 600 days of delivery. No attempt was made to ascertain actual use of the product or whether the mothers, either users or nonusers, had purchased a spermicide without a prescription (11–13). In a subsequent correspondence, all of the study's exposed cases of limb reduction deformity (three cases), Down's syndrome (three cases), and neoplasm (two cases) were reexamined in terms of the exact timing of spermicide use (14). The data suggested that spermicides were not used near the time of conception in these cases. However, this does not eliminate the possibility that spermicides may act directly on the ovum before conception (15). Second, the four types of malformations lack a common cause and time of occurrence (13). Even a single type of defect, such as limb reduction deformity, has a varied origin (13). Third, the total number of infants with malformations was low (2.2% vs. 1.0%). Because these values are comparable with the 2%–5% reported incidence of major malformations in hospital-based studies, the apparent association may have been caused by a lower than expected rate of defects in the nonexposed group rather than an increase in the exposed infants (11,13). Fourth, no confounding variables other than maternal age were adjusted (13).

A number of investigators have been unable to reproduce the results published in 1981 (12,16–23). In a study examining 188 infants with chromosomal abnormalities or limb reduction defects, no relationship between periconceptual use of spermicides and these defects was observed (12). No association between spermicide use at conception and any congenital malformation was observed in a study comparing 1427 cases with 3001 controls (16). In a prospective study of 34,660 women controlled for age, time in pregnancy, concentration of spermicide used, and other confounding variables, the malformation rate of spermicide users was no greater than in users of other contraceptive methods (17–19). A cohort study, the Collaborative Perinatal Project involving 50,282 mother–child pairs, found no greater risk for limb reduction deformities, neoplasm, Down's syndrome, or hypospadias in children exposed in utero to spermicides (20). One group of investigators interviewed 12,440 women during delivery and found no relationship between the last contraceptive method used and congenital malformations (21). Spermicides were the last contraceptive method used by 3891 (31%) of the women. A 1987 case–control study of infants with Down's syndrome (N = 265), hypospadias (N = 396), limb reduction defects (N = 146), neoplasms (N = 116), or neural tube defects (N = 215) compared with 3442 control infants with a wide variety of other defects was unable to establish any causal relationship to maternal spermicide use (22). The authors investigated spermicide usage at three different time intervals—preconceptional (1 month before to 1 month after the last menstrual period), first trimester (first 4 lunar months), and any use during lifetime—without producing a positive association. A similar study, involving 13,729 women who had produced 154 fetuses with trisomy, 98 with trisomy 21 (i.e., Down's syndrome), also failed to find any association with spermicides (23). In addition, a letter correspondence from one researcher argued that an association between vaginal spermicides, or any environmental risk factor for that matter, and trisomies was implausible based on an understanding of the origin of these defects (24).

An association between vaginal spermicides and SABs was found in five studies (25–29). A strong association was found among subjects who had obtained a spermicide within 12 weeks of conception (25). Another study demonstrated approximately twice the rate of SABs in women who continued to use spermicides after conception compared with users before or close to the time of conception (26). However, a 1985 critique concluded that both sets of investigators had seriously biased their results by failing to adjust for potentially confounding variables (13). In a study involving women aborting spontaneously before the 28th week of gestation and controls delivering after the 28th week, women who used spermicides at the time of conception demonstrated a five-fold increase in chromosomal anomalies on karyotype examinations in 929 cases (27). Although no association between spermicide use and chromosomally normal abortion was found in a study involving 6339 women, spermicide use of more than 1 year was more common in cases aborting trisomic conception than in controls (28). In an earlier report, the same authors observed an odds ratio of 4.8 for the association between abortuses with anomalies and unexposed controls (29). Two of these latter studies (27,29) did not adjust for confounding variables.

Three studies have found no association with SABs (10,18,30). No significant risk for SAB was observed in a large cohort study involving 17,032 subjects (10) or in another study examining periconceptional spermicide use (18). In a well-designed, large prospective study involving 32,123 subjects, spermicide use before conception was associated with a significant reduction in SAB during the 2nd trimester (30).

Three studies found no association between spermicide use and birth weight (10,18,26), but one study did find such an association (9). In this latter investigation, spermicide use after the last menstrual period was significantly associated with a lower mean birth weight among female infants of both smoking and nonsmoking mothers. For male births, an association with lower birth weight was found only when the mothers smoked. The authors were unable to determine whether these relationships were causal. Spermicide use before the last menstrual period had no effect on birth weight (9).

Under miscellaneous effects, a case–control study of 73 nontraumatic stillbirths found no relationship with the use of vaginal spermicides (31). No association between sex ratio at birth or frequency of multiple births and spermicides was found in one study (10). However, in a 1976 national survey, female births were approximately 25% higher among women using spermicides near the time of conception compared with nonusers, a statistically significant difference (26). Finally, a 1985 study found no evidence of a relationship between spermicide use and preterm delivery (18).

A 1990 reference reported the meta-analysis of previous studies to determine whether maternal spermicide use is detrimental to the developing fetus (32). Negative associations were found between the periconceptual or postconceptual maternal use of spermicides and teratogenicity, SAB, stillbirth, reduced fetal weight, prematurity, or an increased incidence of female births.

BREASTFEEDING SUMMARY

No reports describing the use of nonoxynol-9 during human lactation have been located. If excretion into milk occurs, the effect on the nursing infant is unknown.

References

1. Jick H, Walker AM, Rothman KJ, Hunter JR, Holmes LB, Watkins RN, D'Ewart DC, Danford A, Madsen S. Vaginal spermicides and congenital disorders. JAMA 1981;245:1329–32.
2. Jick H, Walker AM, Rothman KJ. The relation between vaginal spermicides and congenital disorders. Reply. JAMA 1987;258:2066.
3. Anonymous. Data do not support association between spermicides, birth defects. FDA Drug Bull 1986;16:21.
4. Mills JL. Reporting provocative results; can we publish "hot" papers without getting burned? JAMA 1987;258:3428–9.
5. Holmes LB. Vaginal spermicides and congenital disorders: the validity of a study—in reply. JAMA 1986;256:3096.
6. Chvapil M, Eskelson CD, Stiffel V, Owen JA, Droegemueller W. Studies on nonoxynol-9. II. Intravaginal absorption, distribution, metabolism and excretion in rats and rabbits. Contraception 1980;22:325–39.
7. Smith ESO, Dafoe CS, Miller JR, Banister P. An epidemiological study of congenital reduction deformities of the limbs. Br J Prev Soc Med 1977;31:39–41.
8. Rothman KJ. Spermicide use and Down's syndrome. Am J Public Health 1982;72:399–401.
9. Polednak AP, Janerich DT, Glebatis DM. Birth weight and birth defects in relation to maternal spermicide use. Teratology 1982;26:27–38.
10. Huggins G, Vessey M, Flavel R, Yeates D, McPherson K. Vaginal spermicides and outcome of pregnancy: findings in a large cohort study. Contraception 1982;25:219–30.
11. Oakley GP Jr. Spermicides and birth defects. JAMA 1982;247:2405.
12. Cordero JF, Layde PM. Vaginal spermicides, chromosomal abnormalities and limb reduction defects. Fam Plann Perspect 1983;15:16–8.
13. Bracken MB. Spermicidal contraceptives and poor reproductive outcomes: the epidemiologic evidence against an association. Am J Obstet Gynecol 1985;151:552–6.
14. Watkins RN. Vaginal spermicides and congenital disorders: the validity of a study. JAMA 1986;256:3095.
15. Jick H, Walker A, Rothman KJ. Vaginal spermicides and congenital disorders: the validity of a study. Reply. JAMA 1986;256:3095–6.
16. Bracken MB, Vita K. Frequency of non-hormonal contraception around conception and association with congenital malformations in offspring. Am J Epidemiol 1983;117:281–91.
17. Mills JL, Harley EE, Reed GF, Berendes HW. Are spermicides teratogenic? JAMA 1982;248:2148–51.
18. Mills JL, Reed GF, Nugent RP, Harley EE, Berendes HW. Are there adverse effects of periconceptional spermicide use? Fertil Steril 1985;43:442–6.
19. Harlap S, Shiono PH, Ramcharan S. Congenital abnormalities in the offspring of women who used oral and other contraceptives around the time of conception. Int J Fertil 1985;30:39–47.
20. Shapiro S, Slone D, Heinonen OP, Kaufman DW, Rosenberg L, Mitchell AA, Helmrich SP. Birth defects and vaginal spermicides. JAMA 1982;247:2381–4.
21. Linn S, Schoenbaum SC, Monson RR, Rosner B, Stubblefield PG, Ryan KJ. Lack of association between contraceptive usage and congenital malformations in offspring. Am J Obstet Gynecol 1983;147:923–8.
22. Louik C, Mitchell AA, Werler MM, Hanson JW, Shapiro S. Maternal exposure to spermicides in relation to certain birth defects. N Engl J Med 1987;317:474–8.
23. Warburton D, Neugut RH, Lustenberger A, Nicholas AG, Kline J. Lack of association between spermicide use and trisomy. N Engl J Med 1987;317:478–82.
24. Bracken MB. Vaginal spermicides and congenital disorders: study reassessed, not retracted. JAMA 1987;257:2919.
25. Jick H, Shiota K, Shepard TH, Hunter JR, Stergachis A, Madsen S, Porter JB. Vaginal spermicides and miscarriage seen primarily in the emergency room. Teratogenesis Carcinog Mutagen 1982;2:205–10.
26. Scholl TO, Sobel E, Tanfer K, Soefer EF, Saidman B. Effects of vaginal spermicides on pregnancy outcome. Fam Plann Perspect 1983;15:244, 249–50.
27. Warburton D, Stein Z, Kline J, Strobino B. Environmental influences on rates of chromosome anomalies in spontaneous abortions (abstract). Am J Hum Genet 1980;32:92A.
28. Strobino B, Kline J, Lai A, Stein Z, Susser M, Warburton D. Vaginal spermicides and spontaneous abortion of known karyotype. Am J Epidemiol 1986;123:431–43.
29. Strobino B, Kline J, Stein Z, Susser M, Warburton D. Exposure to contraceptive creams, jellies and douches and their effect on the zygote (abstract). Am J Epidemiol 1980:112:434.
30. Harlap S, Shiono PH, Ramcharan S. Spontaneous foetal losses in women using different contraceptives around the time of conception. Int J Epidemiol 1980;9:49–56.
31. Porter JB, Hunter-Mitchell J, Jick H, Walker AM. Drugs and stillbirth. Am J Public Health 1986;76:1428–31.
32. Einarson TR, Koren G, Mattice D, Schechter-Tsafriri O. Maternal spermicide use and adverse reproductive outcome: a meta-analysis. Am J Obstet Gynecol 1990;162:655–60.

N

NOREPINEPHRINE

Sympathomimetic (Adrenergic)

PREGNANCY RECOMMENDATION: Human and Animal Data Suggest Risk
BREASTFEEDING RECOMMENDATION: No Human Data—Potential Toxicity

PREGNANCY SUMMARY

Uterine vessels are normally maximally dilated, and they have only α-adrenergic receptors (1). Use of the α- and β-adrenergic stimulant, norepinephrine, could cause constriction of these vessels and reduce uterine blood flow, thereby producing fetal hypoxia (bradycardia). Norepinephrine may also interact with oxytocics or ergot derivatives to produce severe persistent maternal hypertension (1). Rupture of a cerebral vessel is possible. If a pressor agent is indicated, other drugs, such as ephedrine, should be considered.

FETAL RISK SUMMARY

Norepinephrine (noradrenaline; levarterenol) is a direct-acting adrenergic agent that is used for acute hypotension and as an adjunct in the treatment of cardiac arrest. It is a mixture of the racemic stereoisomer and is given by IV infusion. Norepinephrine readily crosses the placenta (2), consistent with its relatively low molecular weight (about 169).

In animal reproduction studies, norepinephrine has caused situs inversus (rat embryos) (*l*-isomer only; no effect from *d*-form) (3); cataract (rat embryos) (4); hemorrhages of cephalic, skin, and extremity structures (chick embryo) (5); and microscopic liver abnormalities and delayed skeletal ossification (hamsters) (6).

In a 1995 study in pregnant ewes (123–137 days gestation), a high maternal dose (40 mcg/minute) of norepinephrine given by IV infusion caused a significant decrease in maternal placental blood flow (7). Although fetal arterial pressure did not change, transient (≤2.5 hours) but statistically significant decreases in fetal oxygenation, fetal urine flow, and lung liquid flow were observed. Because the average human maintenance dose is much less (about 2–4 mcg/minute), the clinical significance of these changes to a human fetus is unknown.

BREASTFEEDING SUMMARY

No reports describing the use of norepinephrine in lactation have been located. Use of the agent during breastfeeding would not be expected because of the indications for use.

References

1. Smith NT, Corbascio AN. The use and misuse of pressor agents. Anesthesiology 1970;33:58–101.
2. Morgan CD, Sandler M, Panigel M. Placental transfer of catecholamines in vitro and in vivo. Am J Obstet Gynecol 1972;112:1068–75.
3. Fujinaga M, Maze M, Hoffman BB, Baden JM. Activation of α-1 adrenergic receptors modulates the control of left/right sidedness in rat embryos. Dev Biol 1992;150:419–21. As cited in Shepard TH. *Catalog of Teratogenic Agents*. 9th ed. Baltimore, MD: The Johns Hopkins University Press, 1998:340.
4. Pitel M, Lerman S. Studies on the fetal rat lens. Effects of intrauterine adrenalin and noradrenalin. Invest Ophthalmol 1962;1:406–12. As cited in Shepard TH. *Catalog of Teratogenic Agents*. 9th ed. Baltimore, MD: The Johns Hopkins University Press, 1998:340.
5. Gatling RR. The effect of sympathomimetic agents on the chick embryo. Am J Pathol 1962;40:113–27.
6. Hirsch KS, Fritz HI. A comparison of mescaline with epinephrine and norepinephrine in the hamster. Teratology 1974;9:A19–20. As cited in Schardein TH. *Chemically Induced Birth Defects*. 3rd ed. New York, NY: Marcel Dekker, 2000:360, 364.
7. Stevens AD, Lumbers ER. Effects of intravenous infusions of noradrenaline into the pregnant ewe on uterine blood flow, fetal renal function, and lung liquid flow. Can J Physiol Pharmacol 1995;73:202–8.

NORETHINDRONE

Progestogenic Hormone

PREGNANCY RECOMMENDATION: Contraindicated
BREASTFEEDING RECOMMENDATION: Limited Human Data—Probably Compatible

PREGNANCY SUMMARY

Norethindrone is a progestogen derived from 19-nortestosterone. It is used in oral contraceptives and hormonal pregnancy tests (no longer available in the United States). Masculinization of the female fetus has been associated with norethindrone (1–3). One researcher observed an 18% incidence of masculinization of female infants born to mothers given norethindrone (2). A more conservative estimate for the incidence of masculinization caused by synthetic progestogens has been reported as 0.3% (4).

FETAL RISK SUMMARY

The Collaborative Perinatal Project monitored 866 mother–child pairs with 1st trimester exposure to progestational agents (including 132 with exposure to norethindrone) (5, pp. 389, 391). Evidence of an increased risk of malformation was found for norethindrone. An increase in the expected frequency of cardiovascular defects and hypospadias was also observed for progestational agents as a group (5, p. 394; 6). Reevaluation of these data in terms of timing of exposure, vaginal bleeding in early pregnancy, and previous maternal obstetric history, however, failed to support an association between female sex hormones and cardiac malformations (7). An earlier study also failed to find any relationship with nongenital malformations (3). One investigator observed two infants with malformations who were exposed to norethindrone (8). The congenital defects included spina bifida and hydrocephalus. The relationship between norethindrone and the anomalies is unknown.

In a surveillance study of Michigan Medicaid recipients involving 229,101 completed pregnancies conducted between 1985 and 1992, 238 newborns had been exposed to norethindrone (see also Oral Contraceptives) shortly before or after conception (F. Rosa, personal communication, FDA, 1993). A total of 20 (8.4%) major birth defects were observed (10 expected). Specific data were available for six defect categories, including (observed/expected) 2/2 cardiovascular defects, 1/0.5 oral clefts, 0/0 spina bifida, 0/1 polydactyly, 0/0.5 limb reduction defects, and 1/1 hypospadias. The total number of congenital malformations suggests a moderate association between the drug and the incidence of congenital defects, but the study could not determine the percentage of women who presumably stopped the hormone before conception or the number of anomalies as a result of prematurity (F. Rosa, personal communication, FDA, 1993).

BREASTFEEDING SUMMARY

Norethindrone exhibits a dose-dependent suppression of lactation (9). Lower infant weight gain, decreased milk production, and decreased composition of nitrogen and protein content of human milk have been associated with norethindrone and estrogenic agents (10–13). The magnitude of these changes is low. However, the changes in milk production and composition may be of nutritional importance in malnourished mothers. If breastfeeding is desired, the lowest dose of oral contraceptives should be chosen. Monitoring of infant weight gain and the possible need for nutritional supplementation should be considered. The American Academy of Pediatrics classifies norethindrone as compatible with breastfeeding (14).

References

1. Hagler S, Schultz A, Hankin H, Kunstadter RN. Fetal effects of steroid therapy during pregnancy. Am J Dis Child 1963;106:586–90.
2. Jacobson BD. Hazards of norethindrone therapy during pregnancy. Am J Obstet Gynecol 1962;84:962–8.
3. Wilson JG, Brent RL. Are female sex hormones teratogenic? Am J Obstet Gynecol 1981;141:567–80.
4. Bongiovanni AM, McFadden AJ. Steroids during pregnancy and possible fetal consequences. Fertil Steril 1960;11:181–4.
5. Heinonen OP, Slone D, Shapiro S. *Birth Defects and Drugs in Pregnancy*. Littleton, MA: Publishing Sciences Group, 1977.
6. Heinonen OP, Slone D, Monson RR, Hook EB, Shapiro S. Cardiovascular birth defects and antenatal exposure to female sex hormones. N Engl J Med 1977;296:67–70.
7. Wiseman RA, Dodds-Smith IC. Cardiovascular birth defects and antenatal exposure to female sex hormones: a reevaluation of some base data. Teratology 1984;30:359–70.
8. Dillon S. Congenital malformations and hormones in pregnancy. Br Med J 1976;2:1446.
9. Guiloff E, Ibarra-Polo A, Zanartu J, Toscanini C, Mischler TW, Gomez-Rogers C. Effect of contraception on lactation. Am J Obstet Gynecol 1974;118:42–5.
10. Karim M, Ammarr R, El-Mahgoubh S, El-Ganzoury B, Fikri F, Abdou I. Injected progestogen and lactation. Br Med J 1971;1:200–3.
11. Kora SJ. Effect of oral contraceptives on lactation. Fertil Steril 1969;20:419–23.
12. Miller GH, Hughes LR. Lactation and genital involution effects of a new low-dose oral contraceptive on breast-feeding mothers and their infants. Obstet Gynecol 1970;35:44–50.
13. Lonnerdal B, Forsum E, Hambraeus L. Effect of oral contraceptives on composition and volume of breast milk. Am J Clin Nutr 1980;33:816–24.
14. Committee on Drugs, American Academy of Pediatrics. Transfer of drugs and other chemicals into human milk. Pediatrics 2001;108:776–89.

NORETHYNODREL

[Withdrawn from the market. See 9th edition.]

NORFLOXACIN

Anti-infective (Quinolone)

PREGNANCY RECOMMENDATION: Human Data Suggest Low Risk
BREASTFEEDING RECOMMENDATION: No Human Data—Probably Compatible

PREGNANCY SUMMARY

The use of norfloxacin during human gestation does not appear to be associated with an increased risk of major congenital malformations. Although various birth defects have occurred in the offspring of women who had taken this drug during pregnancy, the lack of a pattern among the anomalies is reassuring. However, a causal relationship with some of the birth defects cannot be excluded. Because of this and the available animal data, the use of norfloxacin during pregnancy, especially during the 1st trimester, should be approached with caution. A 1993 review on the safety of fluoroquinolones concluded that these antibacterials should be avoided during pregnancy because of the difficulty in extrapolating animal mutagenicity results to humans and because interpretation of this toxicity is still controversial (1). The authors of this review were not convinced that fluoroquinolone-induced fetal cartilage damage and subsequent arthropathies were a major concern, even though this effect had been demonstrated in several animal species after administration to both pregnant and immature animals and in occasional human case reports involving children (1). Others have also concluded that fluoroquinolones should be considered contraindicated in pregnancy, because safer alternatives are usually available (2).

FETAL RISK SUMMARY

Norfloxacin is an oral, synthetic, broad-spectrum antibacterial agent. As a fluoroquinolone, it is in the same class as ciprofloxacin, enoxacin, levofloxacin, lomefloxacin, ofloxacin, and sparfloxacin. Nalidixic acid is also a quinolone drug.

In rats, high doses of norfloxacin administered before and at various intervals during gestation, including during organogenesis, did not produce an increase in congenital abnormalities, adverse effects on fertility, fetotoxicity, or changes in postnatal function in the offspring (3,4). Embryo lethality, but not teratogenicity, was observed in rabbits given 100 mg/kg (1), and in cynomolgus monkeys given 200 or 300 mg/day (≥200 mg/kg/day) (5). In the monkeys, plasma concentrations (about three times human therapeutic levels) were high enough to produce maternal toxicity (5). In the second part of this study, the cause of the embryotoxicity was found to be directly related to a decrease in placental-derived progesterone production (6).

In reproductive studies reported by the manufacturer, no evidence of teratogenicity was found in mice, rats, rabbits, or monkeys at 6–50 times the maximum daily human dose on a weight basis (MDHD). Embryonic loss was observed in monkeys with doses 10 times the MDHD (peak plasma levels about twice those obtained in humans) (7).

A 1991 reference evaluated the toxic effects of norfloxacin on rat liver and kidney DNA in mothers and their fetuses (8). Single oral doses of the antibiotic, ranging from 1 to 8 mmol/kg (319–2552 mg/kg), about 30 times the human dose, were administered to pregnant rats on the 17th day of gestation. No DNA damage was observed in the female rats at any dose, but at 4 and 8 mmol/kg, a statistically significant decrease in the percentage of double-stranded DNA (i.e., an increase in DNA damage) was observed in fetal tissues. Because a dose–response relationship with the DNA fragmentation was lacking, and because of the very high doses administered, the investigators concluded that the results did not indicate genotoxicity, but most likely a nonspecific consequence of fetal toxicity. Thus, the potential for mutagenic and carcinogenic risk in humans was probably nil (8).

The effects of norfloxacin on spermatogenesis and sperm abnormalities were studied using a mouse sperm morphology test following either single or five consecutive daily doses of 2 and 4 mmol/kg (9). Norfloxacin stimulated spermatogenesis, presumably through a hormonal action, and may have had a mutagenic effect that resulted in an increase in abnormal sperm morphology. However, because a significant dose–response relationship for adverse morphology was not observed, the investigators could not conclude with certainty that the antibiotic induced abnormal sperm (9).

In humans, norfloxacin crosses the placenta, appearing in cord blood and in amniotic fluid (T.P. Dowling, personal communication, Merck & Co, Inc., 1987). Following a single oral 200-mg dose given to nine patients, cord blood and amniotic fluid levels varied from undetectable to 0.18 mcg/mL and undetectable to 0.19 mcg/mL, respectively. Cord blood levels were about one-half of maternal serum levels. In another 14 women administered a single 200-mg dose, the peak maternal serum, cord blood, and amniotic fluid levels were 1.1, 0.38, and 0.92 mcg/mL, respectively.

N

No congenital malformations were observed in the infants of 38 women who received either norfloxacin ($N = 28$) or ciprofloxacin ($N = 10$) during pregnancy (35 in the 1st trimester) (10). Most ($N = 35$) received the drugs for the treatment of urinary tract infections. Matched to a control group, the fluoroquinolone-exposed pregnancies had a significantly higher rate of cesarean section for fetal distress and their infants were significantly heavier. No differences were found between the groups in infant development or in the musculoskeletal system.

A surveillance study on the use of fluoroquinolones during pregnancy was conducted by the Toronto Motherisk Program among members of the Organization of Teratology Information Specialists (OTIS) and briefly reported in 1995 (11). Pregnancy outcome data were available for 134 cases, of which 61 were exposed to norfloxacin, 68 to ciprofloxacin, and 5 to both drugs. Most (90%) were exposed during the first 13 weeks postconception. Fluoroquinolone-exposed pregnancies were compared with matched controls and there were no differences in live births (87% vs. 86%), terminations (3% vs. 5%), miscarriages (10% vs. 9%), abnormal outcomes (7% vs. 4%), cesarean section rate (12% vs. 22%), fetal distress (15% vs. 15%), and pregnancy weight gain (15 kg vs. 16 kg). The birth weights of exposed infants were a mean 162 g higher than those in the control group and their gestations were a mean 1 week longer (11).

In a prospective follow-up study conducted by the European Network of Teratology Information Services (ENTIS), data on 549 pregnancies exposed to fluoroquinolones (318 to norfloxacin) were described in a 1996 reference (2). Data on another 116 prospective and 25 retrospective pregnancy exposures to the antibacterials were also included. From the 549 follow-up cases, 509 were treated during the 1st trimester, 22 after the 1st trimester, and in 18 cases the exposure occurred at an unknown gestational time. The liveborn infants were delivered at a mean gestational age of 39.4 weeks and had a mean birth weight of 3302 g, length of 50.3 cm, and head circumference of 34.9 cm. Of the 549 pregnancies, there were 415 liveborn infants (390 exposed during the 1st trimester), 356 of which were normal-term deliveries (including 1 set of twins), 15 were premature, 6 were small for gestational age (intrauterine growth restriction [IUGR], <10th percentile), 20 had congenital anomalies (19 from mothers exposed during the 1st trimester; 4.9%), and 18 had postnatal disorders unrelated to either prematurity, low birth weight, or malformations. Of the remaining 135 pregnancies, there were 56 spontaneous abortions or fetal deaths (none late) (1 malformed fetus), and 79 elective abortions (4 malformed fetuses) (2). A total of 116 (all involving ciprofloxacin) prospective cases were obtained from a manufacturer's registry (10). Among these, there were 91 liveborn infants, 6 of whom had malformations. Of the remaining 25 pregnancies, 15 were terminated (no malformations reported), and 10 aborted spontaneously (1 embryo with acardia, no data available on a possible twin). Thus, of the 666 cases with known outcome, 32 (4.8%) of the embryos, fetuses, or newborns had congenital malformations. From previous epidemiologic data, the authors concluded that the 4.8% frequency of malformations did not exceed the background rate. Finally, 25 retrospective reports of infants with anomalies, who had been exposed in utero to fluoroquinolones, were analyzed, but no specific patterns of major congenital malformations were detected (2).

The defects observed in 12 infants followed up prospectively and in 16 infants reported retrospectively who were exposed to norfloxacin were as follows (2):

Source: Prospective ENTIS
- Trisomy 18, heart defect
- Diastasis recti, mild hypospadias
- Patient ductus arteriosus (term)
- CNS calcification, cataract
- Urogenital malformation (no uterus and gonad)
- Fossa posterior hypoplasia
- Bilateral uretero-vesical reflux, hydronephrosis
- Herniation of abdominal viscera, rudimentary umbilical cord, severe kyphoscoliosis, absent diaphragma and pericardium, ectopia cordis, imperforated anus, ambiguous genitalia, urinary bladder not identifiable (pregnancy terminated)
- Anencephaly (pregnancy terminated)
- Trisomy 21
- Unilateral cryptorchidism
- Macroglossia (2nd trimester exposure) (pregnancy terminated)

Source: Retrospective Reports

1st trimester exposure:
- Abdominal and thoracic wall defects, lungs outside of thoracic cavity, pericardium visible (pregnancy terminated)
- Achondroplastic dwarfism (pregnancy terminated)
- Renal and ureteral agenesis, pulmonary hypoplasia
- Supraumbilical hernia

Intestinal cystic duplication
Ventricular septal defect
Penoscrotal hypospadias
2nd trimester exposure:
Dysplastic hips
Hypertelorism, cryptorchism, small penis, short thorax, heart valves dysplasia
Urachal abnormality
3rd trimester exposure:
Microretrognathia
Two nevi, 4 × 2 and 2 × 2 cm
Talipes valgus
Hands and feet syndactyly
Trisomy 21
Short limbs (possibly familial)

The authors of the above study concluded that pregnancy exposure to quinolones was not an indication for termination, but that this class of antibacterials should still be considered contraindicated in pregnant women (2). Moreover, this study did not address the issue of cartilage damage from quinolone exposure, and the authors recognized the need for follow-up studies of this potential toxicity in children exposed in utero. Because of their own and previously published findings, they further recommended that the focus of future studies should be on malformations involving the abdominal wall and urogenital system, and on limb reduction defects (2).

In a surveillance study of Michigan Medicaid recipients involving 229,101 completed pregnancies conducted between 1985 and 1992, 139 newborns had been exposed to norfloxacin, 79 during the 1st trimester (F. Rosa, personal communication, FDA, 1994). Among those exposed in the 1st trimester, four (5.1%) had a major birth defect (three expected). In addition, a brain defect was noted in an infant whose mother consumed the drug after the 1st trimester. Details of the remaining cases were not available, but none of the abnormalities was included in seven other categories of defects (cardiovascular defects, oral clefts, spina bifida, polydactyly, limb reduction defects, hypospadias, and eye defects) for which specific data were available.

A 1998 prospective, multicenter study reported the pregnancy outcomes of 200 women exposed to fluoroquinolones compared with 200 matched controls (12). Subjects were pregnant women who had called one of four teratogen information services concerning their exposure to fluoroquinolones. The agents and number of subjects, and daily doses (in parentheses) were ciprofloxacin (N = 105; 500–1000 mg), norfloxacin (N = 93; 400–800 mg), and ofloxacin (N = 2; 200–400 mg). The most common infections involved the urinary tract (69.4%) or the respiratory tract (24%). The fewer live births in the fluoroquinolone group (173 vs. 188, $p = 0.02$) were attributable to the greater number of spontaneous abortions (18 vs. 10, $p = 0.17$) and induced abortions (9 vs. 2, $p = 0.06$). There were no differences between the groups in terms of premature birth, fetal distress, method of delivery, low birth weight (<2500 g), or birth weight. Among the liveborn infants exposed during organogenesis, major malformations were observed in 3 infants of 133 subjects and 5 of 188 controls ($p = 0.54$). The defects in subject infants were two cases of ventricular septal defect and one case of patent ductus arteriosus, whereas those in controls were two cases of ventricular septal defect, one case of atrial septal defect with pulmonic valve stenosis, one case of hypospadias, and one case of displaced hip. There were also no differences between the children of the groups in gross motor development milestone achievements (musculoskeletal functions: lifting, sitting, crawling, standing, or walking) as measured by the Denver Developmental Scale (12).

BREASTFEEDING SUMMARY

The administration of norfloxacin during breastfeeding is not recommended because of the potential for arthropathy and other serious toxicity in the nursing infant (7). Phototoxicity has been observed with some members of the quinolone class of drugs when exposure to excessive sunlight (i.e., ultraviolet [UV] light) has occurred. Well-differentiated squamous cell carcinomas of the skin have been produced in mice who were exposed chronically to some quinolones and periodic UV light (e.g., see Lomefloxacin), but studies to evaluate the carcinogenicity of norfloxacin in this manner have not been conducted (7).

The manufacturer reports that the drug was not detected in milk following a single 200-mg oral dose administered to nursing mothers (7). However, this dose is one-fourth of the normal recommended daily dose and, thus, may not be indicative of excretion after normal use. Similarly, a 1991 review cited a study that the antibacterial was undetectable in milk, but no details on dosage were given (13).

Although it is not known whether norfloxacin is excreted into human milk, the relatively low molecular weight (about 319), and the excretion of other quinolones suggest that the drug will probably be present in milk. Both ciprofloxacin and ofloxacin are classified by the American Academy of Pediatrics as compatible with breastfeeding (see individual agents).

N

References

1. Norrby SR, Lietman PS. Safety and tolerability of fluoroquinolones. Drugs 1993;45(Suppl 3):59–64.
2. Schaefer C, Amoura-Elefant E, Vial T, Ornoy A, Garbis H, Robert E, Rodriguez-Pinilla E, Pexieder T, Prapas N, Merlob P. Pregnancy outcome after prenatal quinolone exposure. Evaluation of a case registry of the European Network of Teratology Information Services (ENTIS). Eur J Obstet Gynecol Reprod Biol 1996;69:83–9.
3. Irikura T, Imada O, Suzuki H, Abe Y. Teratological study of 1-ethyl-6-fluoro-1, 4-dihydro-4-oxo-7-(1-piperazinyl)-3-quinolinecarboxilic acid (AM-715). Kiso to Rinsho 1981;15:5251–63. As cited in Shepard TH. *Catalog of Teratogenic Agents*. 7th ed. Baltimore, MD: The Johns Hopkins University Press, 1992:290.
4. Irikura T, Suzuki H, Sugimoto T. Reproductive studies of AM-715. Chemotherapy 1981:29:886–931. As cited in Shepard TH. *Catalog of Teratogenic Agents*. 7th ed. Baltimore, MD: The Johns Hopkins University Press, 1992:290.
5. Cukierski MA, Prahalada S, Zacchei AG, Peter CP, Rodgers JD, Hess DL, Cukierski MJ, Tarantal AF, Nyland T, Robertson RT, Hendrickx AG. Embryotoxicity studies of norfloxacin in cynomolgus monkeys. I. Teratology studies and norfloxacin plasma concentrations in pregnant and nonpregnant monkeys. Teratology 1989;39:39–52. As cited in Shepard TH. *Catalog of Teratogenic Agents*. 7th ed. Baltimore, MD: The Johns Hopkins University Press, 1992:290.
6. Cukierski MA, Hendrickx AG, Prahalada S, Tarantal AF, Hess DL, Lasley BL, Peter CP, Tarara R, Robertson RT. Embryotoxicity studies of norfloxacin in cynomolgus monkeys. II. Role of progesterone. Teratology 1992;46:429–38.
7. Product information. Noroxin. Merck & Company, 1997.
8. Pino A, Maura A, Villa F, Masciangelo L. Evaluation of DNA damage induced by norfloxacin in liver and kidney of adult rats and in fetal tissues after transplacental exposure. Mutat Res Lett 1991;264:81–5.
9. Maura A, Pino A. Induction of sperm abnormalities in mice by norfloxacin. Mutat Res Lett 1991;264:197–200.

10. Berkovitch M, Pastuszak A, Gazarian M, Lewis M, Koren G. Safety of the new quinolones in pregnancy. Obstet Gynecol 1994;84:535–8.
11. Pastuszak A, Andreou R, Schick B, Sage S, Cook L, Donnenfeld A, Koren G. New postmarketing surveillance data supports a lack of association between quinolone use in pregnancy and fetal and neonatal complications. Reprod Toxicol 1995;9:584.
12. Loebstein R, Addis A, Ho E, Andreou R, Sage S, Donnenfeld AE, Schick B, Bonati M, Mortetti M, Lalkin A, Pastuszak A, Koren G. Pregnancy outcome following gestational exposure to fluoroquinolones: a multicenter prospective controlled study. Antimicrob Agents Chemother 1998;42:1336–9.
13. Takase Z, Shirafuji H, Uchida M. Basic and clinical studies of AM-715 in the field of obstetrics and gynecology. Chemotherapy (Tokyo) 1981;29(Suppl 4):697–704. As cited by Anderson PO. Drug use during breast-feeding. Clin Pharmacol 1991;10:594–624.

NORGESTREL

Progestogenic Hormone

Norgestrel is commonly used as an oral contraceptive either alone or in combination with estrogens (see Oral Contraceptives).

NORTRIPTYLINE

Antidepressant

PREGNANCY RECOMMENDATION: Human Data Suggest Low Risk
BREASTFEEDING RECOMMENDATION: Limited Human Data—Potential Toxicity

PREGNANCY SUMMARY

Nortriptyline is a tricyclic antidepressant. The limited human pregnancy experience does not support a major association with congenital defects.

N

FETAL RISK SUMMARY

Limb reduction anomalies have been reported with nortriptyline (1,2). However, one of these children was not exposed until after the critical period for limb development (3). The second infant was also exposed to sulfamethizole and heavy cigarette smoking (1). Evaluation of data from 86 patients with 1st trimester exposure to amitriptyline, the active precursor of nortriptyline, does not support the drug as a major cause of congenital limb deformities (see Amitriptyline). Urinary retention in the neonate has been associated with maternal use of nortriptyline (4).

In a surveillance study of Michigan Medicaid recipients involving 229,101 completed pregnancies conducted between 1985 and 1992, 61 newborns had been exposed to nortriptyline during the 1st trimester (F. Rosa, personal communication, FDA, 1993). Two (3.3%) major birth defects were observed (two expected), both cardiovascular anomalies (0.5 expected).

In a 1996 descriptive case series, the European Network of the Teratology Information Services (ENTIS) prospectively examined the outcomes of 689 pregnancies exposed to antidepressants (5). Multiple drug therapy occurred in about two-thirds of the mothers. There were four exposures to nortriptyline. The outcomes of these pregnancies were four normal newborns (one premature) without birth defects (5).

A 2002 prospective study compared two groups exposed to antidepressants throughout gestation, either to tricyclics ($N = 46$ including 3 to nortriptyline) or to fluoxetine ($N = 40$), with 36 nonexposed, not depressed controls (6). Offspring were studied between the ages 15 and 71 months for effects of antidepressant exposure in terms of IQ, language, behavior, and temperament. Exposure to antidepressants did not adversely affect the measured parameters, but IQ was significantly and negatively associated with the duration of depression, and language was negatively associated with the number of depression episodes after delivery (6).

BREASTFEEDING SUMMARY

Nortriptyline is excreted into breast milk in low concentrations (7–11). A milk level in one patient was 59 ng/mL, representing a milk:serum ratio of 0.7 (8). A second patient was treated with nortriptyline 100 mg daily during the 2nd and 3rd trimesters, and then stopped 2 weeks before an elective cesarean section (10). Treatment was restarted at 125 mg every night on the first postpartum day, then decreased to 75 mg nightly over the next 7 weeks. The mother was also receiving flupenthixol. Milk concentrations of nortriptyline, measured 11–13.5 hours after a dose on postpartum days 6 (four samples), 20 (two samples), and 48 (two samples), ranged from 90 to 404 ng/mL, mean 230 ng/mL. The milk:serum ratios for these samples ranged from 0.87 to 3.71 (mean 1.62). No effects of the drug exposure were observed in the nursing infant, who had normal motor development for the first 4 months. Infant serum concentrations were not determined (10).

Nortriptyline was not detected in the serum of other breastfed infants when their mothers were taking the drug (8,9,11); however, low levels (5–11 ng/mL) of the metabolite,

10-hydroxynortriptyline, were measured in the serum of two infants in one study (11). In this latter study, no evidence of accumulation in nursing infants after long-term (e.g., >50 days) maternal use of the antidepressant was observed (11). A 1996 review of antidepressant treatment during breast-feeding found no information that nortriptyline exposure during nursing resulted in quantifiable amounts of the parent compound in an infant or that the exposure caused adverse effects (12).

The significance of chronic exposure of the nursing infant to the antidepressant is unknown, but concern has been expressed about the effects of long-term exposure on the infant's neurobehavioral mechanisms (10). The American Academy of Pediatrics classifies nortriptyline as a drug for which the effect on nursing infants is unknown but may be of concern (13).

References

1. Bourke GM. Antidepressant teratogenicity? Lancet 1974;1:98.
2. McBride WG. Limb deformities associated with iminobenzyl hydrochloride. Med J Aust 1972;1:492.
3. Australian Drug Evaluation Committee. Tricyclic antidepressants and limb reduction deformities. Med J Aust 1973;1:768–9.
4. Shearer WT, Schreiner RL, Marshall RE. Urinary retention in a neonate secondary to maternal ingestion of nortriptyline. J Pediatr 1972;81:570–2.
5. McElhatton PR, Garbis HM, Elefant E, Vial T, Bellemin B, Mastroiacovo P, Arnon J, Rodriguez-Pinilla E, Schaefer C, Pexieder T, Merlob P, Dal Verme S. The outcome of pregnancy in 689 women exposed to therapeutic doses of antidepressants. A collaborative study of the European Network of Teratology Information Services (ENTIS). Reprod Toxicol 1996;10:285–94.
6. Nulman I, Rovet J, Stewart DE, Wolpin J, Pace-Asciak P, Shuhaiber S, Koren G. Child development following exposure to tricyclic antidepressants or fluoxetine throughout fetal life: a prospective, controlled study. Am J Psychiatry 2002;159:1889–95.
7. Bader TF, Newman K. Amitriptyline in human breast milk and the nursing infant's serum. Am J Psychiatry 1980;137:855–6.
8. Erickson SH, Smith GH, Heidrich F. Tricyclics and breast feeding. Am J Psychiatry 1979;136:1483.
9. Brixen-Rasmussen L, Halgrener J, Jorgensen A. Amitriptyline and nortriptyline excretion in human breast milk. Psychopharmacology (Berlin) 1982;76:94–5.
10. Matheson I, Skjaeraasen J. Milk concentrations of flupenthixol, nortriptyline and zuclopenthixol and between-breast differences in two patients. Eur J Clin Pharmacol 1988;35:217–20.
11. Wisner KL, Perel JM. Serum nortriptyline levels in nursing mothers and their infants. Am J Psychiatry 1991;148:1234–6.
12. Wisner KL, Perel JM, Findling RL. Antidepressant treatment during breast-feeding. Am J Psychiatry 1996;153:1132–7.
13. Committee on Drugs, American Academy of Pediatrics. The transfer of drugs and other chemicals into human milk. Pediatrics 2001;108:776–89.

NOVOBIOCIN

[Withdrawn from the market. See 9th edition.]

NUTMEG

Herb

PREGNANCY RECOMMENDATION: Compatible
BREASTFEEDING RECOMMENDATION: No Human Data—Probably Compatible

PREGNANCY SUMMARY

Nutmeg, the dried aromatic seeds of the tree *Myristica fragrans*, is used as a common spice. The seeds contain a toxic chemical, myristicin, that has anticholinergic properties.

FETAL RISK SUMMARY

A 1987 case report described an accidental overdose of grated nutmeg in a pregnant woman at 30 weeks' gestation (1). The woman used 1 tablespoon of the spice (equivalent to approximately 7 g, or one whole grated nutmeg) instead of the suggested amount of 1/8 teaspoon in a recipe for cookies (1). After ingesting some of the cookies, she developed a sinus tachycardia (170 beats/minute), hypertension (170/80 mmHg), and a sensation of impending doom, but no mydriasis. The fetal heart rate was 160–170 beats/minute with loss of long-term variability. It returned to its normal baseline of 120–140 beats/minute within 12 hours. A diagnosis of atropine-like poisoning was made based on the history and physical findings (1). Following nonspecific treatment for poisoning, the mother made an uneventful recovery and was discharged home after 24 hours. Approximately 10 weeks later, she delivered a healthy infant.

BREASTFEEDING SUMMARY

No reports describing the use of nutmeg during human lactation have been located. Because the herb is commonly used as a spice, the risk to a nursing infant is probably nil.

Reference

1. Lavy G. Nutmeg intoxication in pregnancy; a case report. J Reprod Med 1987;32:63–4.

NYLIDRIN

[Withdrawn from the market. See 9th edition.]

NYSTATIN

Antifungal

PREGNANCY RECOMMENDATION: Compatible
BREASTFEEDING RECOMMENDATION: Compatible

PREGNANCY SUMMARY

Nystatin is poorly absorbed after oral administration and from intact skin and mucous membranes. Animal studies have not been conducted with this antifungal agent.

FETAL RISK SUMMARY

The Collaborative Perinatal Project found a possible association with congenital malformations after 142 1st trimester exposures to nystatin, but this was probably related to its use as an adjunct to tetracycline therapy (1, p. 313). No association was found following 230 exposures anytime in pregnancy (1, p. 435). Other investigators have reported its safe use in pregnancy (2–5).

In a surveillance study of Michigan Medicaid recipients involving 229,101 completed pregnancies conducted between 1985 and 1992, 489 newborns had been exposed to nystatin during the 1st trimester (F. Rosa, personal communication, FDA, 1993). A total of 20 (4.1%) major birth defects were observed (21 expected). Specific data were available for six defect categories, including (observed/expected) 3/5 cardiovascular defects, 1/1 oral clefts, 0/0 spina bifida, 1/1 polydactyly, 1/1 limb reduction defects, and 2/1 hypospadias. These data do not support an association between the drug and congenital defects.

BREASTFEEDING SUMMARY

Because nystatin is poorly absorbed, if at all, serum and milk levels would not occur.

References

1. Heinonen OP, Slone D, Shapiro S. *Birth Defects and Drugs in Pregnancy*. Littleton, MA: Publishing Sciences Group, 1977.
2. Culbertson C. Monistat: a new fungicide for treatment of vulvovaginal candidiasis. Am J Obstet Gynecol 1974;120:973–6.
3. David JE, Frudenfeld JH, Goddard JL. Comparative evaluation of Monistat and Mycostatin in the treatment of vulvovaginal candidiasis. Obstet Gynecol 1974;44:403–6.
4. Wallenburg HCS, Wladimiroff JW. Recurrence of vulvovaginal candidosis during pregnancy. Comparison of miconazole vs. nystatin treatment. Obstet Gynecol 1976;48:491–4.
5. Rosa FW, Baum C, Shaw M. Pregnancy outcomes after first-trimester vaginitis drug therapy. Obstet Gynecol 1987;69:751–5.

N

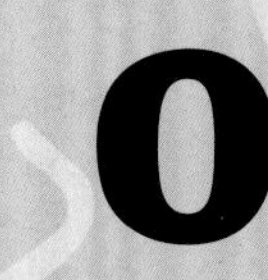

OCRIPLASMIN

Ophthalmic

PREGNANCY RECOMMENDATION: No Human Data—Probably Compatible
BREASTFEEDING RECOMMENDATION: No Human Data—Probably Compatible

PREGNANCY SUMMARY

No reports describing the use of ocriplasmin in human pregnancy have been located. Animal reproduction studies have not been conducted. However, detectable concentrations of the drug in the systemic circulation drug are not expected. Use of the drug during pregnancy appears to be compatible.

FETAL RISK SUMMARY

Ocriplasmin, given as a single intravitreal injection, is a recombinant truncated form of human plasmin produced by recombinant DNA technology. It is indicated for the treatment of symptomatic vitreomacular adhesion. Ocriplasmin has proteolytic activity against components of the vitreous body and the vitreoretinal interface, thereby dissolving the protein matrix responsible for the vitreomacular adhesion. Because of the small dose (0.125 mg) and its rapid inactivation, detectable concentrations in the systemic circulation are not expected (1).

Animal reproduction studies have not been conducted. No carcinogenicity, mutagenicity, or impairment of fertility studies have been conducted (1).

It is not known if ocriplasmin crosses the human placenta. The molecular weight (about 27,000) and the predicted absence of detectable concentrations in the systemic circulation indicate that exposure of the embryo–fetus to clinically significant amounts will not occur.

BREASTFEEDING SUMMARY

No reports describing the use of ocriplasmin during human lactation have been located. The molecular weight (about 27,000) and the predicted absence of detectable concentrations in the systemic circulation indicate that the drug will not be excreted into breast milk.

Reference

1. Product information. Jetrea. ThromboGenics, 2012.

OCTREOTIDE

Endocrine/Metabolic (Somatostatin Analog)

PREGNANCY RECOMMENDATION: Limited Human Data—Animal Data Suggest Low Risk
BREASTFEEDING RECOMMENDATION: No Human Data—Probably Compatible

PREGNANCY SUMMARY

Octreotide is not teratogenic or toxic in two animal species, but published reports have described only five women who were treated during portions of their pregnancies. Although all of the outcomes were normal, the data are too limited to assess the human embryo–fetal risk. The drug crosses the placenta to the fetus and has been measured in the newborn.

FETAL RISK SUMMARY

This cyclic octapeptide (Octreotide; SMS-201-995), an analog of the natural hormone somatostatin, is used to reduce blood levels of growth hormone and somatomedin C in patients with acromegaly and for the symptomatic treatment of patients with profuse watery diarrhea as a result of metastatic carcinoid tumors or vasoactive intestinal peptide-secreting tumors. It has also been used to reduce insulin requirements for patients with diabetes mellitus; to reduce output from gastrointestinal, enteric, and pancreatic fistulas; to treat variceal bleeding; and for various other indications.

No evidence of impaired fertility, teratogenicity, or fetal harm was observed in pregnant rats and rabbits given up to 16 times the highest human dose based on BSA (1).

Octreotide crosses the human placenta to the fetus (2,3). A 31-year-old infertile woman was treated with octreotide 300 mcg/day for hyperthyroidism induced by a thyroid-stimulating hormone (TSH)–secreting macroadenoma (2,3). The patient became euthyroid, with return of normal menstruation, after 3 months of therapy. She was found to be pregnant 1 month later and octreotide treatment was stopped. Because her symptoms recurred, therapy was reinstated at 6 months' gestation and continued until an elective cesarean section at 8 months' gestation delivered a normal infant (weight 3300 g, length 51 cm, sex not specified). The concentration of octreotide in umbilical cord serum at delivery was 359 pg/mL compared with the mean maternal level (measured on two different occasions 1 month earlier) of 890 pg/mL (range 764–1191 pg/mL) (2). Although the amount of drug in the newborn was only about 40% that in the mother, the authors concluded that octreotide crossed the placenta by passive diffusion for two reasons (3). First, only the unbound fraction of octreotide is available for placental transfer and, second, the drug is 60%–65% bound to maternal lipoprotein. Thus, assuming that the mother's concentration had not changed significantly, the unbound maternal fraction and the infant's serum level were close to unity. Subsequently, the concentration of octreotide in the infant's serum decreased to 251 pg/mL at 3 hours of age and was undetectable (<20 pg/mL) when next measured (at 40 days).

The cord serum concentrations of TSH, thyroid hormones, prolactin, and growth hormone were normal at birth, at 3 hours, and at 40 and 104 days of age (3). Because the infant's pituitary–thyroid function was not affected by exposure to octreotide at these concentrations, the authors speculated that the somatostatin receptors on thyrotroph cells, as suggested by studies in animals, are not completely functional at birth (3).

The pregnancy of a previously infertile 37-year-old woman who was treated with octreotide for acromegaly during the first 8 weeks of gestation was described in a 1989 reference (4). Treatment (100 mcg) SC 3 times daily, was started within approximately 4 days of conception and discontinued when pregnancy was diagnosed at 8 weeks. A healthy male infant (weight 2530 g, length 46.0 cm) was delivered by cesarean section 2 weeks before term because of the mother's age and imminent fetal asphyxia. No malformations were apparent and his subsequent development at the time of report (age not specified but estimated to be about 9 months) was normal.

A 37-year-old woman with primary amenorrhea was discovered to have acromegaly as a result of pituitary macroadenoma (5). She was treated with octreotide and bromocriptine with reappearance of her menses occurring 7 months later. Treatment with octreotide (300 mcg) 3 times daily and bromocriptine (20 mg/day) was continued for an additional 7 months until a 1-month pregnancy was diagnosed. She eventually delivered, by emergency cesarean section for fetal distress, a term 3540 g, 50 cm male infant with no evidence of congenital defects. Except for requiring mechanical ventilation for 3 days because of neonatal asphyxia, his subsequent development was satisfactory.

A 1999 case report described the pregnancy of a 36-year-old woman who was treated with octreotide (240 mcg/day) for a pituitary adenoma (6). The woman had clinical and laboratory signs of acromegaly. Treatment was started at 13 weeks' gestation and continued until delivery at 40 weeks' of a 3288-g normal female infant with Apgar scores of 8 and 9 at 1 and 5 minutes, respectively, who was developing normally. Cord concentrations of growth hormone, thyrotropin, and prolactin were within normal limits.

In another 1999 case report, a 27-year-old woman with acromegaly was treated throughout the 1st trimester of an unknown pregnancy with SC octreotide (7). At 4 months of pregnancy, she received a continuous infusion of octreotide immediately before surgical resection of the tumor. Postoperative treatment consisted of hydrocortisone, thyroxine, and bromocriptine. Pregnancy was diagnosed at 6 months and at 39 weeks, she delivered a 3780-g healthy female infant who was doing well (7).

BREASTFEEDING SUMMARY

It is not known whether octreotide is transferred to breast milk, but this should be expected because of the documented placental passage. No reports have been located that described the use of this agent during lactation. However, because of probable digestion following oral therapy, the risk to the nursing infant appears to be nonexistent.

References

1. Product information. Sandostatin. Novartis Pharmaceuticals, 2000.
2. Caron P, Gerbeau C, Pradayrol L. Maternal-fetal transfer of octreotide. N Engl J Med 1995;333:601–2.
3. Caron P, Gerbeau C, Pradayrol L, Cimonetta C, Bayard F. Successful pregnancy in an infertile woman with a thyrotropin-secreting macroadenoma treated with somatostatin analog (octreotide). J Clin Endocrinol Metab 1996;81:1164–8.
4. Landolt AM, Schmid J, Karlsson ERC, Boerlin V. Successful pregnancy in a previously infertile woman treated with SMS-201-995 for acromegaly. N Engl J Med 1989;320:621–2.
5. Montini M, Pagani G, Gianola D, Pagani MD, Piolini R, Camboni MG. Acromegaly and primary amenorrhea: ovulation and pregnancy induced by SMS 201-995 and bromocriptine. J Endocrinol Invest 1990;13:193.
6. Takeuchi K, Funakoshi T, Oomori S, Maruo T. Successful pregnancy in an acromegalic woman treated with octreotide. Obstet Gynecol 1999; 93:848.
7. Mozas J, Ocon E, Lopez de la Torre M, Suarez AM, Miranda JA, Herruzo AJ. Successful pregnancy in a woman with acromegaly treated with somatostatin analog (octreotide) prior to surgical resection. Int J Gynecol Obstet 1999;65:71–3.

OFATUMUMAB

Antineoplastic

PREGNANCY RECOMMENDATION: No Human Data—Animal Data Suggest Risk
BREASTFEEDING RECOMMENDATION: No Human Data—Probably Compatible

PREGNANCY SUMMARY

No reports describing the use of ofatumumab in human pregnancy have been located. In monkeys, the antibody caused fetal B-cell depletions, and decreased placental, spleen, and thymus weights at doses similar to those used in humans. The potential long-term effects of these toxic effects have not been studied in animals. However, refractory chronic lymphocytic leukemia is a serious disease and the maternal benefit appears to outweigh the risks to the fetus. If the antibody must be used in pregnancy, the woman should be informed of the absence of human pregnancy data and the potential fetal risks.

FETAL RISK SUMMARY

Ofatumumab is an IgG1k human monoclonal antibody. It is indicated for the treatment of chronic lymphocytic leukemia refractory to fludarabine and alemtuzumab. The mean half-life, between the 4th and 12th IV infusion doses was about 14 days (range 2.3–61.5 days). The antibody does not bind normal human tissues other than B lymphocytes (1). Data on metabolism have not been found.

Reproduction studies have been conducted in monkeys. Doses that were 0.7 and 3.5 times the recommended human dose (*assumed to be based on body weight*) were given weekly during organogenesis (gestation days 20–50). No maternal toxicity or teratogenicity was observed. However, both doses depleted circulating B cells in the dams. Ofatumumab crossed the placenta and fetuses, delivered at gestational day 100, had decreased mean peripheral B-cell counts (about 10% of control values), splenic B-cell counts (about 15%–20% of control values), spleen weights (15% for the low dose and 30% for the high dose, compared with control values), and thymus weight (15% compared with controls). In addition, there also was a 10% decrease in placental weights. The potential long-term effects of B-cell depletions or decreases in spleen and thymus weights have not been studied in animals (1).

Studies for carcinogenic or mutagenic potential or effects on fertility have not been conducted (1).

It is not known if ofatumumab crosses the human placenta. The molecular weight (about 149,000) is high, but immunoglobulin G crosses the placenta late in pregnancy (see Immune Globulin Intravenous). Placental transfer of IgG was a function of dose, as well as gestational age. Moreover, ofatumumab crossed to the fetus in monkeys and, because the placentas in monkeys are similar to those in humans, the antibody should be expected to cross to the human fetus.

BREASTFEEDING SUMMARY

No reports describing the use of ofatumumab during human lactation have been located. It is not known if the antibody is excreted into breast milk. The molecular weight (about 149,000) is high, but the terminal half-life is very long (about 14 days). Because immunoglobulins are excreted into milk, exposure of a nursing infant might occur. The effect of this exposure is unknown, but published data suggest that neonatal and infant consumption of breast milk does not result in substantial absorption of maternal antibodies into the circulation (1). Nevertheless, cytopenia, progressive multifocal leukoencephalopathy, and small intestine obstruction have been observed in human adults treated with ofatumumab and, if a woman chooses to nurse while receiving this agent, her infant should be monitored for these toxicities.

Reference

1. Product information. Arzerra. GlaxoSmithKline, 2009.

OFLOXACIN

Anti-infective (Quinolone)

PREGNANCY RECOMMENDATION: Human Data Suggest Low Risk
BREASTFEEDING RECOMMENDATION: Limited Human Data—Probably Compatible

PREGNANCY SUMMARY

The use of ofloxacin during human gestation does not appear to be associated with an increased risk of major congenital malformations. Although a number of birth defects have occurred in the offspring of women who had taken this drug during pregnancy, the lack of a pattern among the anomalies is reassuring. However, a causal relationship with some of the birth defects cannot be excluded. Because of this and the available animal data, the use of ofloxacin during pregnancy, especially during the 1st trimester, should be approached with caution. A 1993 review on the safety of fluoroquinolones concluded that these antibacterials should be avoided during pregnancy because of the difficulty in extrapolating animal mutagenicity results to humans and because interpretation of this toxicity is controversial (1). The authors of this review were not convinced that fluoroquinolone-induced fetal cartilage damage and subsequent arthropathies were a major concern, even though this effect had been demonstrated in several animal species after administration to both pregnant and immature animals and in occasional human case reports involving children (1). Others have also concluded that fluoroquinolones should be considered contraindicated in pregnancy, because safer alternatives are usually available (2).

FETAL RISK SUMMARY

Ofloxacin is a synthetic, broad-spectrum antibacterial agent available in oral and parenteral formulations. As a fluoroquinolone, it is in the same class as ciprofloxacin, enoxacin, lomefloxacin, norfloxacin, and sparfloxacin.

A study published in 1986 observed no ofloxacin-induced malformations with high doses in pregnant rats and rabbits (3). Similarly, no evidence of teratogenicity was observed in pregnant rats and rabbits at doses 11 times the recommended maximum human dose based on BSA (RMHD) or 4 times the RMHD, respectively (4). These doses were fetotoxic, however, causing reduced birth weight, increased mortality, and, in rats only, minor skeletal variations. In rats dosed at 5 times the RMHD, no adverse effects were seen on late fetal development, labor, delivery, lactation, neonatal viability, or subsequent growth of the newborn (4).

In a study investigating the pharmacokinetics of ofloxacin, 20 pregnant women, between 19 and 25 weeks' gestation (mean 22.2 weeks), were scheduled for pregnancy termination because the fetuses were affected with β-thalassemia major (5). Two doses of ofloxacin, 400 mg IV every 12 hours, were given before abortion. Serum and amniotic fluid concentrations were determined concomitantly at 6, 10, and 12 hours after dosing. Mean maternal serum concentrations at these times were 0.68, 0.21, and 0.07 mcg/mL, respectively, compared with mean amniotic fluid levels of 0.25, 0.15, and 0.13 mcg/mL, respectively. The amniotic fluid:maternal serum ratios were 0.37, 0.71, and 1.86, respectively (5).

A 2005 study measured the amount of three fluoroquinolones (ciprofloxacin, ofloxacin, levofloxacin) that crossed the perfused human placenta (6). All three agents crossed the placenta from the maternal to the fetal compartment, but the amounts crossing were small: 3.2%, 3.7%, and 3.9%, respectively.

In a prospective follow-up study conducted by the European Network of Teratology Information Services (ENTIS), data on 549 pregnancies exposed to fluoroquinolones (93 to ofloxacin) were described in a 1996 reference (2). Data on another 116 prospective and 25 retrospective pregnancy exposures to the antibacterials were also included. From the 549 follow-up cases, 509 were treated during the 1st trimester, 22 after the 1st trimester, and in 18 cases, the exposure occurred at an unknown gestational time. The liveborn infants were delivered at a mean gestational age of 39.4 weeks' and had a mean birth weight of 3302 g, length of 50.3 cm, and head circumference of 34.9 cm. Of the 549 pregnancies, there were 415 liveborn infants (390 exposed during the 1st trimester), 356 of which were normal term deliveries (including 1 set of twins), 15 were premature, 6 were small for gestational age (intrauterine growth restriction [IUGR], <10th percentile), 20 had congenital anomalies (19 from mothers exposed during the 1st trimester; 4.9%), and 18 had postnatal disorders unrelated to either prematurity, low birth weight, or malformations. Of the remaining 135 pregnancies, there were 56 spontaneous abortions or fetal deaths (none late) (1 malformed fetus), and 79 elective abortions (4 malformed fetuses). A total of 116 (all involving ciprofloxacin) prospective cases were obtained from the manufacturer's registry. Among these, there were 91 liveborn infants, 6 of whom had malformations. Of the remaining 25 pregnancies, 15 were terminated (no malformations reported), and 10 aborted spontaneously (1 embryo with acardia, no data available on a possible twin). Thus, of the 666 cases with known outcome, 32 (4.8%) of the embryos, fetuses, or newborns had congenital malformations. From previous epidemiologic data, the authors concluded that the 4.8% frequency of malformations did not exceed the background rate. Finally, 25 retrospective reports of infants with anomalies, who had been exposed in utero to fluoroquinolones, were analyzed but no specific patterns of major congenital malformations were detected (2).

The defects observed in seven infants followed up prospectively (no ofloxacin-exposed cases among the retrospective reports), all exposed to ofloxacin during the 1st trimester, were as follows (2):

Myelomeningocele, hydrocephaly
Ureterostenosis
Maldescensus testis
Hypospadias
Hernia inguinalis left side
Bilateral hip dysplasia
Small atrial septal defect

The authors of the above study concluded that pregnancy exposure to quinolones was not an indication for pregnancy termination, but that this class of antibacterials should still be considered contraindicated in pregnant women. Moreover, this study did not address the issue of cartilage damage from quinolone exposure and the authors recognized the need for follow-up studies of this potential toxicity in children exposed in utero. Because of their own and previously published findings, they further recommended that the focus of future studies should be on malformations involving the abdominal wall and urogenital system, and on limb reduction defects (2).

A 1998 prospective multicenter study reported the pregnancy outcomes of 200 women exposed to fluoroquinolones compared with 200 matched controls (7). Subjects were pregnant women who had called one of four teratogen information services concerning their exposure to fluoroquinolones. The agents, number of subjects, and daily doses were ciprofloxacin, (N = 105; 500–1000 mg), norfloxacin (N = 93; 400–800 mg), and ofloxacin (N = 2; 200–400 mg). The most common infections involved the urinary tract (69.4%) or the respiratory tract (24%). The fewer live births in the fluoroquinolone group (173 vs. 188, $p = 0.02$) were attributable to the greater number of spontaneous abortions (18 vs. 10, *ns*) and induced abortions (9 vs. 2, *ns*). There were no differences between the groups in terms of premature birth, fetal distress, method of delivery, low birth weight (<2500 g), or birth weight. Among the liveborn infants exposed during organogenesis, major malformations were observed in 3 infants of 133 subjects and 5 of 188 controls (*ns*). The defects in subject infants were two cases of ventricular septal defect and one case of patent ductus arteriosus, whereas those in controls were two cases of ventricular septal defect, one case of atrial septal defect with pulmonic valve stenosis, one case of hypospadias, and one case of displaced hip. There were also no differences between the children of the groups in gross motor development milestone achievements (musculoskeletal functions: lifting, sitting, crawling, standing, or walking) as measured by the Denver Developmental Scale (7).

BREASTFEEDING SUMMARY

When first marketed, ofloxacin use during lactation was not recommended because of the potential for arthropathy and other serious toxicity in the nursing infant (4). Phototoxicity has been observed with quinolones when exposure to excessive sunlight (i.e., ultraviolet [UV] light) has occurred (4). Well-differentiated squamous cell carcinomas of the skin have been produced in mice exposed chronically to some fluoroquinolones and periodic UV light (e.g., see Lomefloxacin), but studies to evaluate the carcinogenicity of ofloxacin in this manner have not been conducted.

Ofloxacin is excreted into breast milk in concentrations approximately equal to those in maternal serum (4,5). The manufacturer reports that following a single 200-mg dose, milk and serum concentrations of ofloxacin were similar (4). Ten lactating women were given three oral doses of ofloxacin, 400 mg each (5). Six simultaneous serum and milk samples were drawn between 2 and 24 hours after the third dose of the antibiotic. The mean peak serum level occurred at 2 hours (2.45 mcg/mL), then steadily fell to 0.03 mcg/mL at 24 hours. Milk concentrations exhibited a similar pattern, with a mean peak level measured at 2 hours (2.41 mcg/mL), and the lowest amount at 24 hours (0.05 mcg/mL). The mean milk:serum ratio varied from 0.98 to 1.66, with the highest ratio occurring 24 hours after the last dose (5).

The American Academy of Pediatrics classifies ofloxacin as compatible with breastfeeding (8).

References

1. Norrby SR, Lietman PS. Safety and tolerability of fluoroquinolones. Drugs 1993;45(Suppl 3):59–64.
2. Schaefer C, Amoura-Elefant E, Vial T, Ornoy A, Garbis H, Robert E, Rodriguez-Pinilla E, Pexieder T, Prapas N, Merlob P. Pregnancy outcome after prenatal quinolone exposure. Evaluation of a case registry of the European Network of Teratology Information Services (ENTIS). Eur J Obstet Gynecol Reprod Biol 1996;69:83–9.
3. Takayama S, Watanabe T, Akiyama Y, Ohura K, Harada S, Matsuhashi K, Mochida K, Yamashita N. Reproductive toxicity of ofloxacin. Arzneim Forsch 1986;36:1244–8. As cited in Shepard TH. *Catalog of Teratogenic Agents*. 7th ed. Baltimore, MD: The Johns Hopkins University Press, 1992:296.
4. Product information. Floxin. Ortho-McNeil Pharmaceutical, 2000.
5. Giamarellou H, Kolokythas E, Petrikkos G, Gazis J, Aravantinos D, Sfikakis P. Pharmacokinetics of three newer quinolones in pregnant and lactating women. Am J Med 1989;87(Suppl 5A):49S–51S.
6. Polachek H, Holcberg G, Sapir G, Tsadkin-Tamir M, Polacheck J, Katz M, Ben-Zvi Z. Transfer of ciprofloxacin, ofloxacin and levofloxacin across the perfused human placenta in vitro. Eur J Obstet Gynecol Reprod Biol 2005;122:61–5.
7. Loebstein R, Addis A, Ho E, Andreou R, Sage S, Donnenfeld AE, Schick B, Bonati M, Mortetti M, Lalkin A, Pastuszak A, Koren G. Pregnancy outcome following gestational exposure to fluoroquinolones: a multicenter prospective controlled study. Antimicrob Ag Chemother 1998;42:1336–9.
8. Committee on Drugs, American Academy of Pediatrics. The transfer of drugs and other chemicals into human milk. Pediatrics 2001;108:776–89.

OLANZAPINE

Antipsychotic

PREGNANCY RECOMMENDATION: Compatible—Maternal Benefit >> Embryo–Fetal Risk
BREASTFEEDING RECOMMENDATION: Limited Human Data—Potential Toxicity

PREGNANCY SUMMARY

Although no structural malformations attributable to olanzapine or other agents in this subclass have been reported, the number of exposures is too low to fully assess the embryo–fetal risk. In addition, there is a risk of extrapyramidal and/or withdrawal symptoms in the newborn if the drug is used in the 3rd trimester. Nevertheless, olanzapine is indicated for severe debilitating mental disease and the benefits to the mother appear to outweigh the potential embryo–fetal risks. One inadvertent pregnancy was attributed to olanzapine-induced normalization of prolactin levels, but the opposite effect (i.e., hyperprolactinemia) is reported by the manufacturer. More study of this potential concern is warranted. Olanzapine has been associated with hyperglycemia and new-onset diabetes, and blood glucose levels should be monitored because poorly controlled diabetes mellitus is a well-known cause of developmental toxicity. A 1996 review on the management of psychiatric illness concluded that patients with histories of chronic psychosis or severe bipolar illness represent a high-risk group (for both the mother and the fetus) and should be maintained on pharmacologic therapy before and during pregnancy (1). However, a 2000 review stated that the human pregnancy data were too limited to recommend olanzapine (2). Folic acid 4 mg/day has been recommended for women taking atypical antipsychotics because they may have a higher risk of neural tube defects due to inadequate folate intake and obesity (3).

FETAL RISK SUMMARY

Olanzapine, a thienobenzodiazepine-class psychotropic agent, is indicated for the management of schizophrenia and bipolar mania. The drug has a relatively long elimination half-life (mean 30 hours, range 21–54 hours) (4). The long half-life is partially a result of extensive protein binding to albumin (90%) and to α_1-acid glycoprotein (77%) (5).

In reproduction studies in rats and rabbits, no evidence of teratogenicity was observed at doses up to 9 and 30 times the maximum recommended human dose based on BSA (MRHD), respectively. In rats, early resorption and increased numbers of nonviable fetuses were observed at 9 times the MRHD. In addition, prolonged gestations were noted at 5 times the MRHD. In rabbits administered a maternal toxic dose (30 times the MRHD), increased resorptions and decreased fetal weight were indications of fetotoxicity (4).

Consistent with the molecular weight (about 312), an in vitro experiment demonstrated that olanzapine crosses the human placenta (5). In a 1999 study that used a near-term human placenta-perfused single-cotyledon system, up to 14% of [^{14}C]-olanzapine crossed from the maternal to the fetal compartment over 4 hours. The initial concentration (10 ng/mL) was equal to the peak human plasma concentration observed after a 10-mg dose. Although no placental oxidative metabolites were found, the glucuronide metabolite did cross the placenta, but at a slightly slower rate than the parent drug (5). In another study, 14 women taking a staple dose (mean 8.9 mg/day) of olanzapine for a mean 18.4 weeks before delivery had maternal and cord concentrations of the drug determined at birth (6). The cord blood concentration was 72.1% of the maternal concentration. The pregnancy outcomes include three premature infants (<37 weeks) and four growth-restricted infants (<2500 g). The mean Apgar scores were 7.6 and 8.8 at 1 and 5 minutes, respectively. There were eight neonatal complications (three cardiovascular, four respiratory, one hypotonia; complications were not further described), and four infants were admitted to the neonatal intensive care unit (reasons not provided) (6).

In its product information, the manufacturer reported seven pregnancies exposed to olanzapine during clinical trials (4). The outcomes of these pregnancies were one spontaneous abortion (SAB), three elective abortions (EAs), one neonatal death due to a cardiovascular defect (no specific data given), and two normal births.

A 2000 report expanded the above database, describing the outcomes of 37 prospectively identified pregnancies that had been exposed to olanzapine during clinical trials (7). The mean daily maternal dose, in 30 of these pregnancies, was 12.9 mg (range 5–25 mg/day). There were 3 SABs, 13 EAs, and 1 ectopic pregnancy that was aborted. There was one stillbirth at 37 weeks' gestation after premature rupture of the membranes. This pregnancy, exposed to an unknown dose in the 2nd and 3rd trimesters, had been complicated by gestational diabetes, thrombocytopenia, hepatitis, and polydrug abuse. In 19 pregnancies, there were 16 normal newborns without complications (exposure times: 8 in 1st trimester, 1 in 1st and 2nd trimesters, 6 throughout, and 1 unknown). Among the remaining three outcomes, one infant exposed in utero to 20 mg/day was delivered by cesarean section at 30 weeks. The birth weight and length were 2.13 kg and 40 cm, respectively. The pregnancy had been complicated by gestational diabetes, hypothyroidism, preeclampsia, and abnormal liver enzymes. The infant recovered from respiratory distress and hypoglycemia after 2 weeks of therapy. A second infant, whose mother had taken 10 mg/day throughout gestation, was delivered 10 days after term because of fetal distress (birth weight 3.66 kg). The neonatal examination was normal. Finally, one infant, exposed only during the 1st trimester to an unknown dose, had meconium aspiration after a cesarean section for postmaturity. The eventually neonatal outcome of this case was not given. No congenital malformations were observed in the 19 newborns (7).

In addition to the prospective cases, the above report also described the outcomes of 11 retrospectively identified olanzapine-exposed pregnancies (7). Although retrospective reports are considered to be biased, they are useful as early indicators of fetal risks if a cluster of defects or abnormalities is observed. The results of these pregnancies were as follows: SABs (two cases; 1st trimester, dose unknown); fetal death (olanzapine and risperidone overdose, timing and doses unknown); unilateral dysplastic kidney (1st trimester, dose unknown); and Down's syndrome (timing and dose unknown). The case of unilateral dysplastic kidney does not appear to be related to the drug exposure. Most likely, a chemical insult during development would have produced bilateral kidney damage. Three infant complications also are worth noting, but their relationship to olanzapine is unknown: (a) cardiomegaly, jaundice, somnolence, heart murmur (1st and 3rd trimesters, 5 mg/day); (b) convulsion at 12 days of age (1st and 3rd trimesters, 20 mg/day; electroencephalogram and laboratory tests were normal); and (c) heart murmur, sudden infant death at 2 months of age (throughout gestation, 10 mg/day) (7).

In a 2002 reference, the authors briefly reported the outcomes of 96 olanzapine-exposed pregnancies in a further expansion of the above prospective case registry (8). The new material was based on a 2001 written communication with the manufacturer. The outcomes included 69 normal births, 12 SABs, 3 stillbirths, 2 premature births, 7 had perinatal complications, and 1 major malformation. Neither the perinatal complications nor the malformation were provided (8).

Another report of olanzapine use in human pregnancy appeared in 2000 (9). A 40-year-old obese woman with a 24-year complicated history of schizophrenia and chronic hypertension was treated throughout pregnancy with olanzapine. During the first month she received 20 mg/day and then, because of sedation, 15 mg/day for the remainder of gestation. Her mental disease was stable throughout, but pregnancy was complicated by excessive weight gain (79 lb; 35.9 kg), gestational diabetes, and severe preeclampsia (hypertension, proteinuria, and elevated liver function tests). Because of worsening preeclampsia, a cesarean section was performed at 30 weeks' gestation to deliver a female 2128-g infant. Apgar scores were 7 and 9 at 1 and 5 minutes, respectively. No other information on the infant was provided (9).

A 31-year-old woman with paranoid schizophrenia was treated with olanzapine (10 mg/day) from the 2nd trimester until delivery and then continued during breastfeeding (10). The patient was hospitalized for treatment of a psychotic episode in the 18th gestational week and olanzapine was started at this time. Hospitalization was continued for over 3 months. A normal 3190-g female infant was born at term with Apgar scores of 9, 10, and 10 at 1, 5, and 10 minutes, respectively. Olanzapine plasma levels in the mother and infant on the first day after delivery were 33.4 and 11.3 ng/mL. The infant was breastfed (see Breastfeeding Summary). At 7 months of age, the infant was not able to roll from the back to the ventral position, possibly suggesting impaired motor development. No impairment, however, was noted at 11 months. At this age, head circumference was approximately at the 50th percentile, whereas height and weight were around the 97th percentile (10).

A 2001 case report described the pregnancy of a 38-year-old woman who was treated with olanzapine (7.5 mg/day) for maintenance treatment of schizoaffective disorder (11). She took the drug throughout a 38-week pregnancy, eventually delivering a 3883-g female infant by cesarean section. Apgar scores were 9 and 9 at 1 and 5 minutes, respectively. The infant's length and head circumference were 21.75 and 14.75 inches, respectively. No abnormalities were noted. The mother, who was advised not to breastfeed, required a dose increase to 12.5 mg/day after delivery. The infant's growth was described as normal with weights at 6, 18, and 24 months of age of 6.8 kg (25th percentile), 10.4 kg (50th percentile), and 12.2 kg (75th percentile), respectively. No other measurements were available. She was doing well at age 26 months (11).

A postmarketing surveillance study of olanzapine that was conducted in England identified 18 pregnancies, 11 of the women took the drug in the 1st trimester and 3 during the 2nd/3rd trimesters (12). The outcomes were 11 live births, 2 SABs, 3 EAs, and 1 unknown outcome. In another case, exposure to the drug was uncertain. One of the EAs was for a fetus with a lumbar myelomeningocele (12).

A 37-year-old woman with paranoid schizophrenia was started on olanzapine in the 8th week of gestation (13). She had not received antipsychotics for 3 months prior to this time. Her daily dose was titrated to 25 mg over the next 3 months. She discontinued therapy against medical advice at 32 weeks' gestation because she felt well. She remained well and eventually delivered a healthy 3-kg male infant at 39 weeks' gestation. The Apgar scores were 9 and 10 at 1 and 5 minutes, respectively (13).

Concern that switching a patient from typical neuroleptics (e.g., fluphenazine) to an atypical agent, such as olanzapine, may result in pregnancy was expressed in a brief 1998 communication (14). An unmarried 41-year-old woman with a 22-year history of schizophrenia, paranoid type, and bipolar disorder had been unsuccessfully treated with multiple agents. Her regimen, immediately prior to olanzapine, was depot fluphenazine decanoate (75 mg IM every 2 weeks) and carbamazepine (400 mg/day). Because she remained chronically delusional and thought disordered, her regimen was changed to olanzapine, eventually reaching a maintenance dose of 12.5 mg/day. An 8-week pregnancy was diagnosed 14 weeks after the start of olanzapine. An EA was performed at the patient's request. The authors attributed the pregnancy to a normalization of prolactin levels, such as that observed with clozapine, another atypical neuroleptic (14). However, the manufacturer states that hyperprolactinemia does occur with olanzapine and that a modest elevation of prolactin levels persists during chronic therapy (4).

A 27-year-old woman at 24 weeks' gestation was started on olanzapine when she developed a recurrence of her psychosis (15). The initial dose of 2.5 mg/day had to be gradually increased to 20 mg/day to control her symptoms. After 1 month at 20 mg/day, her dose was tapered over a period of 8 weeks and then discontinued 10 days before delivery. At term, she delivered 2.9-kg male infant with Apgar scores of 8 and 9 at 1 and 5 minutes, respectively. The infant was growing and developing normally at 3 months of age (15).

A 2005 study, involving women from Canada, Israeli, and England, described 151 pregnancy outcomes in women using atypical antipsychotic drugs (16). The exposed group was matched with a comparison group ($N = 151$) who had not been exposed to these agents. The drugs and number of pregnancies were olanzapine ($N = 60$), risperidone ($N = 49$), quetiapine ($N = 36$), and clozapine ($N = 6$). In those exposed, there were 110 live births (72.8%), 22 SABs (14.6%), 15 EAs (9.9%), and 4 stillbirths (2.6%). Among the live births, one infant exposed in utero to olanzapine had multiple anomalies including midline defects (cleft lip, encephalocele, and aqueductal stenosis). The mean birth weight was 3341 g. There were no statistically significant differences, including rates of neonatal complications, between the cases and controls, with the exceptions of low birth weight (10% vs. 2%, $p = 0.05$) and EAs (9.9% vs. 1.3%, $p = 0.003$). The low birth weight may have been caused by the increased rate of cigarette smoking (38% vs. 13%, $p \leq 0.001$) and heavy/binge alcohol use (5 vs. 1) in the exposed group (16).

A 2006 review of prophylactic therapy of bipolar disorder briefly described the effects in pregnancy and breastfeeding of a number of drugs, including olanzapine (17). Untreated pregnant and nursing women with the disorder are at an increased risk of poor obstetrical outcomes and relapse of affective symptoms. Although the limited data prevented conclusions on the relative safety of the drugs, the author did state that each case needed to be considered separately (17).

BREASTFEEDING SUMMARY

Consistent with the molecular weight (about 312) and the prolonged elimination half-life (mean 30 hours, range 21–54 hours), olanzapine is excreted into breast milk (18–20). Several reports have described the use of olanzapine in lactating women.

One mother took 5 mg/day in the 1st and 3rd trimesters and continued the drug during breastfeeding (7). The infant had cardiomegaly, jaundice, somnolence, and a heart murmur. At 7 days of age, the infant was changed to bottle-feeding, but sedation and jaundice continued. No other details were provided, but the authors stated that the continued sedation and jaundice suggested that they were not drug-induced. However, the elimination half-life of olanzapine in adults is prolonged and, although the neonatal half-life is unknown, it may be longer because of immature hepatic and renal function. If comparable, it would take about 4–11 days for the infant to eliminate from its system approximately 97% of the drug that was obtained during pregnancy and/or nursing. Thus, a causal relationship cannot be excluded without knowing additional information. In a second case, the mother started olanzapine 10 mg/day for paranoid schizophrenia 2 months after delivery (7). She was also taking paroxetine, trifluoperazine, and procyclidine. No adverse effects were reported in the infant.

The third case involved a woman who took olanzapine 10 mg/day throughout the second half of pregnancy and during 2 months of lactation (10). Plasma levels in the mother and infant 1 day after delivery were 33.4 and 11.3 ng/mL, respectively. The infant's level is attributable to drug acquired while in utero. During nursing, the mother's and infant's plasma levels were determined at 2 and 6 weeks postpartum. Maternal levels were 39.5 and 32.8 ng/mL, respectively, whereas those in the infant were <2 and <2 ng/mL, respectively. No adverse effects of this exposure were noted in the infant (see Fetal Risk Summary for development and growth measures at 11 months of age) (10).

In a 2002 study, five lactating women were started on olanzapine for postpartum psychosis (18). After 5 days of therapy, one to three paired samples per patient (nine samples) of maternal plasma and milk were drawn 11–23 hours after a dose. The mean milk:plasma ratio was 0.46 (range 0.2–0.84). The median infant dose was 1.6% (range 0%–2.5%) of the weight-adjusted maternal dose. The highest milk concentrations (21 mg/L at 11 hours postdose and 16 mg/mL at 23 hours postdose) occurred in the woman taking the highest dose (10 mg/day). The other women were taking 2.5 mg/day and their milk levels ranged from <1 to 8 mg/L. The olanzapine plasma level in one infant 15 hours after the mother's 2.5-mg dose was <1 mcg/L. No adverse effects in the infants were observed (18).

A 2003 study reported the milk concentrations of olanzapine in seven women, two of whom started treatment during pregnancy (19). The women had been taking olanzapine for a mean of 114 days (range 19–395 days) and the mean age of the infants was 2.4 months (range 0.1–4.3 months). Multiple maternal plasma and milk samples were collected over 12- or 24-hour intervals. In six women, the median maternal dose was 7.5 mg/day (range 5–20 mg/day) or 131.5 mcg/kg (range 75–286 mcg/kg) and the median peak plasma concentration and time postdose were 29 mcg/L (range 15–73 mcg/L) and 2.5 hours (1.5–4.5 hours), respectively. The median peak drug concentration in milk occurred 5.2 hours (range 0.7–13.2 hours) after the dose and the median concentration was 8.8 mcg/L (range 1.2–22.7 mcg/L). The median milk:plasma AUC ratio was 0.38. Olanzapine plasma levels in the infants were below the detection limit (1–5 mcg/L). No adverse effects were observed or measured in the nursing infants. For the seventh woman, the milk:plasma ratio was 0.75 at 6 hours postdose based on a single sample collection. Sedation had been noted in her infant 3 weeks before the study and her dose had been halved to 5 mg/day. Sedation was not observed in infant at the time of the study (19).

Olanzapine 20 mg/day was given to a 32-year-old woman hospitalized 9 days after delivery for a postpartum psychotic disorder (20). Although she had been breastfeeding her infant, she decided to stop nursing on admission. Serial milk samples were drawn for 10 days with olanzapine concentrations ranging from 7.6 (day 2) to 27.5 ng/mL. The milk:plasma ratio ranged from 0.35 to 0.42. If nursing had been continued, the infant would have consumed a dose that was approximately 4% of the maternal weight-adjusted dose, or about 0.011 mg/kg/day (18). Therefore, the infant exposure would have been very low (20).

Sedation is a frequent adverse effect in adults treated with olanzapine and has occurred in nursing infants whose mothers were taking the drug. Reducing the maternal dose may eliminate this problem, but the potential effect on control of the mother's disease must be considered. The prolonged adult elimination half-life and the potential for long-term neurodevelopment toxicity in a nursing infant should be considered before olanzapine is prescribed during lactation. The American Academy of Pediatrics classifies other antipsychotics (e.g., see Clozapine) as drugs whose effect on the nursing infant is unknown but may be of concern (21).

References

1. Altshuler LL, Cohen L, Szuba MP, Burt VK, Gitlin M, Mintz J. Pharmacologic management of psychiatric illness during pregnancy: dilemmas and guidelines. Am J Psychiatry 1996;153:592–606.
2. Committee on Drugs, American Academy of Pediatrics. Use of psychoactive medication during pregnancy and possible effects on the fetus and newborn. Pediatrics 2000;105:880–7.
3. Koren G, Cohn T, Chitayat D, Kapur B, Remington G, Myles-Reid D, Zipursky RB. Use of atypical antipsychotics during pregnancy and the risk of neural tube defects in infants. Am J Psychiatry 2002;159:136–7.
4. Product information. Zyprexa. Eli Lilly, 2001.
5. Schenker S, Yang Y, Mattiuz E, Tatum D, Lee M. Olanzapine transfer by human placenta. Clin Exp Pharmacol Physiol 1999;26:691–7.
6. Newport DJ, Calamaras MR, DeVane CL, Donovan J, Beach AJ, Winn S, Knight BT, Gibson BB, Viguera AC, Owens MJ, Nemeroff CB, Stowe ZN. Atypical antipsychotic administration during late pregnancy: placental passage and obstetrical outcomes. Am J Psychiatry 2007;164:1214–20.
7. Goldstein DJ, Corbin LA, Fung MC. Olanzapine-exposed pregnancies and lactation: early experience. J Clin Psychopharmacol 2000;20:399–403.
8. Ernst CL, Goldberg JF. The reproductive safety profile of mood stabilizers, atypical antipsychotics, and broad-spectrum psychotropics. J Clin Psychiatry 2002;63(Suppl 4):42–55.
9. Littrell KH, Johnson CG, Peabody CD, Hilligoss N. Antipsychotics during pregnancy. Am J Psychiatry 2000;157:1342.
10. Kirchheiner J, Berghofer A, Bolk-Weischedel D. Healthy outcome under olanzapine treatment in a pregnant woman. Pharmacopsychiatry 2000;33:78–80.
11. Malek-Ahmadi P. Olanzapine in pregnancy. Ann Pharmacother 2001;35:1294–5.
12. Biwsas PN, Wilton LV, Pearce GL, Freemantle S, Shakir SAW. The pharmacovigilance of olanzapine: results of a post-marketing surveillance study on 8858 patients in England. J Psychopharmacol 2001;15:265–71.
13. Lim LM. Olanzapine and pregnancy. Aust N Z J Psychiatry 2001;35:856–7.
14. Dickson RA, Dawson DT. Olanzapine and pregnancy. Can J Psychiatry 1998;43:196–7.
15. Mendhekar DN, War L, Sharma JB, Jiloha RC. Olanzapine and pregnancy. Pharmacopsychiatry 2002;35:122–3.
16. McKenna K, Koren G, Tetelbaum M, Wilton L, Shakir S, Diav-Citrin O, Levinson A, Zipursky RB, Einarson A. Pregnancy outcome of women using atypical antipsychotic drugs: a prospective comparative study. J Clin Psychiatry 2005;66:444–9.
17. Gentile S. Prophylactic treatment of bipolar disorder in pregnancy and breastfeeding: focus on emerging mood stabilizers. Bipolar Disord 2006;8:207–20.
18. Croke S, Buist A, Hackett LP, Ilett KF, Norman TR, Burrows GD. Olanzapine excretion in human breast milk: estimation of infant exposure. Int J Neuropsychopharmacol 2002;5:243–7.
19. Gardiner SJ, Kristensen JH, Begg EJ, Hackett LP, Wilson DA, Ilett KF, Kohan R, Rampono J. Transfer of olanzapine into breast milk, calculation of infant drug dose, and effect on breast-fed infants. Am J Psychiatry 2003;160:1428–31.
20. Ambresin G, Berney P, Schulz P, Bryois C. Olanzapine excretion into breast milk: a case report. J Clin Psychopharmacol 2004;24:93–5.
21. Committee on Drugs, American Academy of Pediatrics. The transfer of drugs and other chemicals into human milk. Pediatrics 2001;108:776–89.

OLEANDOMYCIN

[Withdrawn from the market. See 9th edition.]

OLMESARTAN

Antihypertensive

PREGNANCY RECOMMENDATION: Human Data Suggest Risk in 2nd and 3rd Trimesters
BREASTFEEDING RECOMMENDATION: No Human Data—Probably Compatible

PREGNANCY SUMMARY

The antihypertensive mechanisms of action of olmesartan and angiotensin-converting enzyme (ACE) inhibitors are very close. That is, the former selectively blocks the binding of angiotensin II to AT_1 receptors, whereas the latter prevents the formation of angiotensin II itself. Therefore, use of this drug during the 2nd and 3rd trimesters may cause teratogenicity and severe fetal and neonatal toxicity identical to that seen with ACE inhibitors (see Captopril or Enalapril). Fetal toxic effects may include anuria, oligohydramnios, fetal hypocalvaria, intrauterine growth restriction, prematurity, and patent ductus arteriosus. Anuria-associated oligohydramnios may produce fetal limb contractures, craniofacial deformation, and pulmonary hypoplasia. Severe anuria and hypotension, resistant to both pressor agents and volume expansion, may occur in the newborn following in utero exposure to olmesartan. Newborn renal function and blood pressure should be closely monitored.

FETAL RISK SUMMARY

The prodrug olmesartan medoxomil is hydrolyzed to olmesartan during absorption from the gastrointestinal tract. No additional metabolism occurs. Olmesartan is a selective angiotensin II receptor blocker (ARB) that is indicated, either alone or in combination with other antihypertensive agents, for the treatment of hypertension. Olmesartan blocks the vasoconstrictor and aldosterone-secreting effects of angiotensin II by preventing angiotensin II from binding to the AT_1 receptors. Other drugs in this class include candesartan, eprosartan, irbesartan, telmisartan, and valsartan. The terminal elimination half-life is about 13 hours (1).

Reproduction studies with olmesartan have been conducted in rats and rabbits. No evidence of teratogenicity was observed in either species at doses up 240 and 0.5 times, respectively, the maximum recommended human dose based on BSA (MRHD). Higher doses in rabbits could not be administered because they caused maternal death. In rats, doses equal to or greater than about 0.4 times the MRHD caused fetal toxicity (decreases in pup birth weight and weight gain). Higher doses (equal to or greater than about twice the MRHD) resulted in delays in developmental milestones and dose-related increases in the incidence of dilation of the renal pelvis. The no-observed effect dose for developmental toxicity was about 0.1 times the MRHD (1).

The case report below strongly suggests that olmesartan crosses the human placenta. This would be consistent with the molecular weight (about 559) and relatively long terminal elimination half-life.

A woman took olmesartan (dose not specified) for hypertension in the last month of pregnancy (2). Severe oligohydramnios developed and she delivered a 3.045-kg female infant by cesarean section at 36 weeks' gestation. Apgar scores were 7 and 7. The infant received dialysis for renal failure but died on day 45. Autopsy revealed severe tubular dysgenesis and the renal arteries and arteriole walls were thickened (2).

A 2012 review of the use of ACE inhibitors and ARBs in the 1st trimester concluded that there may be an elevated teratogenic risk, but the risk appeared to be related to other factors (3). The factors, that typically coexist with hypertension in pregnancy, included diabetes, advanced maternal age, and obesity.

BREASTFEEDING SUMMARY

No reports describing the use of olmesartan during human lactation have been located. The molecular weight (about 559) is low enough that excretion into breast milk should be expected. The effect of this exposure on a nursing infant is unknown. The American Academy of Pediatrics, however, classifies ACE inhibitors, a closely related group of antihypertensive agents, as compatible with breastfeeding (see Captopril or Enalapril).

References

1. Product information. Benicar. Sankyo Pharma, 2004.
2. Sinelli MT, Cattarelli D, Cortinovis S, Maroccolo D, Chirico G. Severe neonatal renal failure after maternal use of angiotensin II type 1 receptor antagonists. Ped Med Chir 2008;30:306–8.
3. Polifka JE. Is there an embryopathy associated with first-trimester exposure to angiotensin-converting enzyme inhibitors and angiotensin receptor antagonists? A critical review of the evidence. Birth Defects Res (Part A) 2012;94:576–98.

OLOPATADINE

Antihistamine

PREGNANCY RECOMMENDATION: No Human Data—Probably Compatible
BREASTFEEDING RECOMMENDATION: No Human Data—Probably Compatible

PREGNANCY SUMMARY

No reports describing the use of olopatadine in human pregnancy have been located. The animal reproduction data and the very low plasma concentrations suggest that the risk in humans is negligible. Moreover, antihistamines, in general, are not thought to cause human developmental toxicity at recommended doses.

FETAL RISK SUMMARY

The antihistamine olopatadine is administered topically to the eye for treatment of the signs and symptoms of allergic conjunctivitis. Low concentrations, ranging from 0.5 to 1.3 ng/mL, have been detected in the plasma of nonpregnant volunteers within 2 hours of a dose. The plasma elimination half-life was about 3 hours (1).

Reproduction studies have been conducted in rats and rabbits. No evidence of teratogenicity was observed in either species at oral doses up to 93,750 and 62,500 times, respectively, the maximum recommended ocular human dose (MROHD). However, at the maximum dose during organogenesis, there was a decrease in live fetuses. In male and female rats, an oral dose 62,500 times the MROHD resulted in a slight decrease in the fertility index and implantation rate. The no-effect dose on animal reproductive function was 7800 times the MROHD (1).

It is not known if olopatadine crosses the human placenta. The molecular weight (about 374) is low enough, but the very small amounts in the systemic circulation suggest that clinically significant amounts of the antihistamine will not reach the embryo and/or fetus.

BREASTFEEDING SUMMARY

No reports describing the use olopatadine during human lactation have been located. Because ocular use in humans results in very low plasma concentrations, the risk to a nursing infant is probably negligible.

Reference

1. Product information. Patanol. Alcon Laboratories, 2005.

O

OLSALAZINE

Anti-inflammatory Bowel Disease Agent

PREGNANCY RECOMMENDATION: Compatible
BREASTFEEDING RECOMMENDATION: Limited Human Data—Potential Toxicity

PREGNANCY SUMMARY

No reports describing adverse fetal effects following the use of olsalazine in human pregnancy have been located. The use of 5-aminosalicylic acid, the active metabolite of olsalazine, in human pregnancy is discussed under Mesalamine.

FETAL RISK SUMMARY

Olsalazine is used to maintain remission of ulcerative colitis in patients who cannot tolerate sulfasalazine. It is poorly absorbed, approximately 2.4% after oral administration, with the remainder reaching the colon intact where it is converted into two molecules of 5-aminosalicylic acid (mesalamine) by colonic bacteria (1). The history, pharmacology, and pharmacokinetics of mesalamine and olsalazine were extensively reviewed in a 1992 reference (2).

Reproductive studies with olsalazine in rats have revealed reduced fetal weights, retarded ossifications, and immaturity of the fetal visceral organs with doses 5–20 times the recommended human dose on a weight basis (1).

BREASTFEEDING SUMMARY

The active metabolite of olsalazine, 5-aminosalicylic acid (mesalamine), is excreted into human milk (see Mesalamine). In one study, however, only a metabolite of mesalamine, acetyl-5-aminosalicylic acid, was detected in breast milk after the ingestion of olsalazine (see Mesalamine) (3). Because diarrhea has occurred in a nursing infant of a mother receiving mesalamine (see Mesalamine), nursing infants of women being treated with olsalazine should be closely observed for changes in stool consistency.

References

1. Product information. Dipentum. Pharmacia & Upjohn, 2000.

2. Segars LW, Gales BJ. Mesalamine and olsalazine: 5-aminosalicylic acid agents for the treatment of inflammatory bowel disease. Clin Pharm 1992;11:514–28.

3. Miller LG, Hopkinson JM, Motil KJ, Corboy JE, Andersson S. Disposition of olsalazine and metabolites in breast milk. J Clin Pharmacol 1993;33:703–6.

OMACETAXINE

Antineoplastic (Protein Synthesis Inhibitor)

PREGNANCY RECOMMENDATION: Contraindicated
BREASTFEEDING RECOMMENDATION: Contraindicated

PREGNANCY SUMMARY

No reports describing the use omacetaxine in human pregnancy have been located. Reproduction studies conducted in one species suggest risk, but the absence of human pregnancy experience prevents a more complete assessment of embryo–fetal risk. Moreover, based on the mechanism of action, the drug may cause fetal harm.

FETAL RISK SUMMARY

Omacetaxine is a protein synthesis inhibitor that is given by SC injection. It is indicated for the treatment of adult patients with chronic or accelerated phase chronic myeloid leukemia with resistance and/or intolerance to two or more tyrosine kinase inhibitors. The drug is metabolized by plasma esterases to apparently inactive metabolites. Plasma protein binding is ≤50% and the mean half-life is about 6 hours (1).

Reproduction studies have been conducted in mice. In this species during organogenesis, doses that were about 50% of the recommended daily human dose based on BSA (RDHD) caused fetal toxicity, including embryo death, an increase in unossified bones/reduced bone ossification, and decreased fetal weights (1).

Carcinogenicity studies have not been conducted with omacetaxine. The drug was genotoxic in one assay but negative in two other assays. Studies in mice demonstrated adverse effects on male reproductive organs. SC doses that were about 2–3 times the clinical dose based on BSA caused bilateral degeneration of the seminiferous tubular epithelium in testes and hypospermia/aspermia in the epididymides.

It is not known if omacetaxine crosses the human placenta. The molecular weight (about 546), moderate plasma protein binding, and the mean half-life suggest that the drug will cross to the embryo–fetus.

BREASTFEEDING SUMMARY

No reports describing the use of omacetaxine during human lactation have been located.

The molecular weight (about 546), moderate plasma protein binding (≤50%), and the mean half-life (about 6 hours) suggest that the drug will be excreted into breast milk. The effect of this exposure on a nursing infant is unknown, but the infant should be monitored for the most common (frequency ≥20%) adverse effects seen in adults. These effects include thrombocytopenia, anemia, neutropenia, diarrhea, nausea, fatigue, asthenia, pyrexia, infection, and lymphopenia (1).

O

Reference

1. Product information. Synribo. Teva Pharmaceuticals USA, 2012.

OMALIZUMAB

Respiratory Drug (Monoclonal Antibody)

PREGNANCY RECOMMENDATION: Limited Human Data—Animal Data Suggest Low Risk
BREASTFEEDING RECOMMENDATION: No Human Data—Potential Toxicity

PREGNANCY SUMMARY

The limited animal data suggest that the risk of human embryo–fetal harm is low. The rate of spontaneous abortions (SABs) (14%) in women who conceived while under treatment with omalizumab is within the normal background rate for clinically recognized pregnancies. However, the minimal information regarding the other outcomes of the early pregnancy exposures prevents a better assessment of the risk. Other immunoglobulins have been used in pregnancy without causing embryo–fetal harm (see Immune Globulin Intramuscular and Intravenous). Therefore, if indicated, omalizumab should not be withheld because of pregnancy. If a woman has received omalizumab within 8 weeks prior to conception or during pregnancy, health care professionals or patients are encouraged to call 1-866-496-5247 for information about enrollment in the Xolair Pregnancy Registry (EXPECT).

FETAL RISK SUMMARY

Omalizumab is a recombinant DNA-derived humanized immunoglobulin ($IgG1_k$) monoclonal antibody that is administered SC for patients with moderate to severe persistent asthma. Omalizumab selectively binds to human IgE. Patients should have had a positive skin test or in vitro reactivity to a perennial aeroallergen and symptoms inadequately controlled by inhaled corticosteroids. Because of its slow absorption, it takes an average of 7–8 days to reach peak serum concentrations. The serum elimination half-life averaged 26 days (1).

Reproduction studies have been conducted in cynomolgus monkeys. At SC doses up to 12 times the maximum human dose based on body weight (MHD) throughout organogenesis, no evidence of maternal toxicity, embryotoxicity, or teratogenicity was observed. The same dose administered throughout late gestation, delivery, and nursing did not cause adverse effects on fetal or neonatal growth. In fertility studies with monkeys, no effect was observed on male or female reproductive capability, including implantation in females, with weekly SC doses 2–5 times the human exposure based on AUC over the range of adult clinical doses (1).

The transplacental passage of omalizumab in humans has not been studied. Although the molecular weight (about 149,000) is high, immune globulin G is known to cross the human placenta and, combined with the long elimination half-life, exposure of the human embryo or fetus should be expected.

No published reports describing the use of omalizumab in human pregnancy have been located. In its safety data, the manufacturer reported 29 pregnancies exposed to omalizumab during clinical trials, but in each case, the drug was discontinued when pregnancy was diagnosed (2). In the completed studies, the outcomes of 17 pregnancies were 3 SABs, 3 elective abortions, and 11 normal deliveries. Of the12 pregnancies in ongoing studies, 1 ended in a SAB. The outcomes of the remaining 11 were normal deliveries or awaiting delivery (number of each not specified). The 4 SABs occurred within 3 months of the last menstrual period. In one case, the woman had a prior history of a SAB. No information (e.g., sex, weight, anomalies, or abnormalities) on the newborn infants was provided (2).

BREASTFEEDING SUMMARY

No reports describing the use of omalizumab during human lactation have been located. If the drug is excreted into milk, the effect of this exposure on a nursing infant is unknown.

References

1. Product information. Xolair. Genentech, 2005.
2. BLA STN 103976/0. Review of Clinical Safety Data. Omalizumab for allergic asthma. Food and Drug Administration—Center for Drug Evaluation and Research website. Available at http://www.fda.gov/cder/biologics/review/omalgen062003r1.pdf. Accessed January 2005.

O

OMEGA-3 FATTY ACID SUPPLEMENTS

Dietary Supplement

PREGNANCY RECOMMENDATION: Compatible
BREASTFEEDING RECOMMENDATION: Compatible

PREGNANCY SUMMARY

Omega-3 fatty acids, including alpha-linoleic acid (ALA), docosahexaenoic acid (DHA), and eicosapentaenoic acid (EPA), are present in foods, particularly fish. Omega-3 fatty acids are thought to play a role in normal development of the central nervous system, retina, inflammatory and immune responses (1). Although there is no recommended daily allowance (RDA) for omega-3 fatty acids, the "adequate intake" level for pregnant women, as established by the U.S. Institute of Medicine and the Food and Nutrition Board, is 1.4 g/day (2). It is thought that many pregnant women do not achieve this level of intake from the diet due in part to the recommendation to limit fish consumption during pregnancy to no more than two servings per week (3). Additional sources of omega-3 fatty acids include fish oil supplements and some prenatal vitamin supplements that contain DHA. Evolving evidence suggests that use of supplements in addition to dietary sources of omega-3 fatty acids to achieve the recommended adequate intake level has positive benefits for pregnancy outcome (4).

FETAL RISK SUMMARY

Omega-3 fatty acids are polyunsaturated fatty acids (PUFAs) consisting of three types. The parent compound, ALA, is found in plant foods such as nuts, seeds, and vegetable oils and is an essential fatty acid because it cannot be synthesized by humans and prevents symptoms of deficiency (1). DHA and EPA are long-chain PUFAs (LC-PUFAs) that can be synthesized from ALA; however, the process of conversion is not very efficient in humans, and therefore fish in the diet is the major source of LC-PUFAs (5). Recent population trends in reduced dietary fat intake have led to the likelihood of suboptimal levels of omega-3 fatty acids in pregnancy, in particular DHA and EPA (6). In addition, dietary intake of LC-PUFAs is limited in pregnant women because they are advised to restrict intake of fish to no more than two servings per week due to concerns for mercury contamination (3).

Although no official RDA for omega-3 fatty acids has been established to date, the U.S. Institute of Medicine and the Food and Nutrition Board have suggested an adequate intake of 1.4 g/day during pregnancy, and the International Society for the Study of Fatty Acids and Lipids (ISSFAL) has established a recommended minimum dose of 500 mg EPA+DHA for adults and 200–300 mg DHA daily for pregnant and lactating women (2,7).

Although research is still evolving regarding the effects of LC-PUFA during pregnancy, the majority of human studies show that increased intake of EPA and DHA has potential benefits on maternal and fetal health outcomes including reduced incidence of preterm birth (8), increased birth length, weight, and head circumference (9), improved infant and child cognitive development (6,9), improved visual development (10), and reduced risk of allergies in infants (11). Although it is generally agreed that more studies are needed, there is broad consensus that improving LC-PUFA status during pregnancy is desirable (7,12).

Similar to dietary fish, omega-3 fatty acid supplements made from fish oil may be contaminated by mercury and other toxins; however, evidence suggests that with high-quality manufacturing processes, the level of contamination and the amount of mercury consumed with the recommended supplement dose is far less than that in fish and unlikely to be of any concern (13). No studies have been located that report substantial adverse effects of LC-PUFA supplementation when given in the recommended doses during pregnancy (12).

BREASTFEEDING SUMMARY

DHA and EPA are present in breast milk. The infant need for DHA during breastfeeding is about 70–80 mg daily (14). Levels of maternal DHA decline during pregnancy and decrease even further during the lactation period. Recent studies have established that the diet of Western pregnant and lactating women contains only 20%–60% of the recommended DHA+EPA daily intake of 200–300 mg/day and these low levels are reflected in breast milk composition. Supplementation with omega-3 fatty acids results in increased levels in breast milk (15).

Although no official RDA for omega-3 fatty acids during lactation has been established to date, the U.S. Institute of Medicine and the Food and Nutrition Board have suggested an adequate intake of 1.3 g/day during lactation which may be achieved through a combination of diet and supplements (2).

References

1. Benatti P, Peluso G, Nicolai R, Calvani M. Polyunsaturated fatty acids: biochemical, nutritional and epigenetic properties. J Am Coll Nutr 2004;23:281–302.
2. Otten JJ, Hellway JP, Meyers LD, eds. *Dietary Reference Intakes IOM and Food and Nutrition Board*. New York, NY: National Academies Press, 2006:122–39.
3. Greenberg JA, Bell SJ, Ausdal WV. Omega-3 Fatty Acid supplementation during pregnancy. Rev Obstet Gynecol 2008;1:162–9.
4. Coletta JM, Bell SJ, Roman AS. Omega-3 fatty acids and pregnancy. Rev Obstet Gynecol 2010;3:163–71.
5. Koletzko B, Lien E, Agostoni C, Bohles H, Campoy C, Cetin I, Decsi T, Dudenhausen JW, Dupont C, Forsyth S, Hoesli I, Holzgreve W, Lapillonne A, Putet G, Secher NJ, Symonds M, Szajewska H, Willatts P, Uauy R; World Association of Perinatal Medicine Dietary Guidelines Working Group. The roles of long-chain polyunsaturated fatty acids in pregnancy, lactation and infancy: review of current knowledge and consensus recommendations. J Perinat Med 2008;36:5–14.
6. Koletzko B, Larque E, Demmelmair H. Placental transfer of long-chain polyunsaturated fatty acids (LC-PUFA). J Perinat Med 2007;35(Suppl 1):S5–11.
7. Koletzko B, Cetin I, Brenna JT. Dietary fat intakes for pregnant and lactating women. Br J Nutr 2007;98:873–7.
8. Horvath A, Koletzko B, Szajewska H. Effect of supplementation of women in high-risk pregnancies with long-chain polyunsaturated fatty acids on pregnancy outcomes and growth measures at birth: a meta-analysis of randomized controlled trials. Br J Nutr 2007;98:253–9.
9. Morse NL. Benefits of docosahexaenoic acid, folic acid, vitamin D and iodine on foetal and infant brain development and function following maternal supplementation during pregnancy and lactation. Nutrients 2012;4:799–840.
10. Innis SM. Perinatal biochemistry and physiology of long-chain polyunsaturated fatty acids. J Pediatr 2003;143(4 Suppl):S1–8.
11. Dunstan JA, Prescott SL. Does fish oil supplementation in pregnancy reduce the risk of allergic disease in infants? Curr Opin Allergy Clin Immunol 2005;5:215–21.
12. Brenna JT, Lapillonne A. Background paper on fat and fatty acid requirements during pregnancy and lactation. Ann Nutr Metab 2009;55:97–122.
13. Foran SE, Flood JG, Lewandrowski KB. Measurement of mercury levels in concentrated over-the-counter fish oil preparations: is fish oil healthier than fish? Arch Pathol Lab Med 2003;127:1603–5.
14. Makrides M, Gibson RA. Long-chain polyunsaturated fatty acid requirements during pregnancy and lactation. Am J Clin Nutr 2000;71(1 Suppl):307S–11S.
15. Koletzko B, Rodriguez-Palmero M, Demmelmair H, Fidler N, Jensen R, Sauerwald T. Physiological aspects of human milk lipids. Early Hum Dev 2001;65(Suppl):S3–18.

OMEPRAZOLE

Gastrointestinal Agent (Antisecretory)

PREGNANCY RECOMMENDATION: Human Data Suggest Low Risk
BREASTFEEDING RECOMMENDATION: Limited Human Data—Potential Toxicity

PREGNANCY SUMMARY

The lack of teratogenicity in animals and the bulk of the human 1st trimester exposure data suggest that omeprazole can be classified as low risk in pregnancy. A study showing an association between in utero exposure to gastric acid–suppressing drugs and childhood allergy and asthma requires confirmation. None of the other studies measured a significant increase in the rates of major birth defects with proton pump inhibitors (PPIs), but they lacked the power to detect small increases in birth defects or rare malformations. The small cluster of cardiac defects observed in one study after omeprazole exposure appears to be an errant signal because it has not been confirmed in other studies. Most likely, cardiac and other defects observed in all studies were the result of many factors, including possibly the severity of the disease and concurrent use of other drugs. The data, however, do warrant continued investigation. In addition, the studies lacked the sensitivity to detect minor anomalies because of the absence of standardized examinations. Late appearing major defects may also have been missed due to the timing of some of the data collection. If omeprazole is required or if inadvertent exposure does occur early in gestation, the known risk to the embryo–fetus appears to be low. Long-term follow-up of offspring exposed during gestation is warranted.

FETAL RISK SUMMARY

The antisecretory agent, omeprazole, a PPI, suppresses gastric acid secretion by a direct inhibitory effect on the gastric parietal cell (1). It is used for the treatment of duodenal and gastric ulcers, erosive esophagitis, and pathologic hypersecretory conditions, such as Zollinger-Ellison syndrome. Omeprazole is in the same class of PPIs as dexlansoprazole, esomeprazole, lansoprazole, pantoprazole, and rabeprazole. The drug has a short plasma half-life (0.5–1.0 hour) and is extensively metabolized to metabolites that have little or no antisecretory activity (1).

In reproductive studies in pregnant rats and rabbits, doses up to approximately 345 and 172 times, respectively, the normal human dose produced no evidence of teratogenicity, but dose-related embryo and fetal mortality was observed (1). A dose-dependent increase in gastric cell carcinoid tumors has been observed in rats (1). The in vitro Ames mutagen assay was negative. Other tests for genotoxicity in mice and rats were either borderline or negative (1).

O

Omeprazole crosses the placenta to the fetus in sheep (2) and in humans (3). In sheep, the fetal:maternal ratio of total omeprazole, after both low and high dose, was 0.2, but the ratio of unbound drug was 0.5 (2). Urinary clearance of the drug was low in both the mother and the fetus.

Placental passage of omeprazole in humans was demonstrated in a study published in 1989 (3). Twenty women were administered a single 80-mg oral dose of omeprazole the night before scheduled cesarean sections with a mean dosing-to-general anesthesia induction time interval of 853 minutes (range 765–977 minutes) (3). At the time of surgery, maternal omeprazole levels ranged from 0 to 271 nmol/L. The drug concentration in 13 of the 20 infants (both arterial and venous umbilical samples were drawn in most cases) was either 0 or below the minimum detection limit (20 nmol/L). In the remaining seven infants, omeprazole cord blood concentrations ranged from 21 to 109 nmol/L. No adverse effects attributable to the drug were observed either at birth or at follow-up in 7 days (3).

The FDA has received reports of 11 birth defects following pregnancy exposure to omeprazole, 4 of which were anencephaly and 1 of which was a hydranencephaly that developed de novo after starting omeprazole in the 13th gestational week (F. Rosa, personal communication, FDA, 1996).

A paper published in 1995 described the use of omeprazole, 20 mg daily for esophageal reflux, by a woman in two consecutive pregnancies that were terminated because of severe congenital anomalies—anencephaly in one and severe talipes in the other (4). The first pregnancy was the result of a gamete intrafallopian transfer (GIFT) procedure, and the second occurred after a natural conception. Both aborted fetuses had normal chromosomal patterns.

A woman with Zollinger-Ellison syndrome was treated in two of her three pregnancies with omeprazole (5). In her first pregnancy, she had been treated with ranitidine (300 mg/day) and with other therapy during the 2nd and 3rd trimesters and delivered a healthy, 2560-g boy at 37 weeks' gestation. She then presented at 11 weeks' gestation in her second pregnancy, complaining of abdominal pain and vomiting. Her symptoms were controlled with omeprazole (120 mg/day) which was continued until delivery of a healthy, 2610-g girl. During the third pregnancy, she was treated throughout gestation with omeprazole (180 mg/day) and cimetidine (450 mg/day) and delivered a healthy term 2550-g male infant (5).

Data from the Swedish Medical Birth Registry were presented in 1998 (6). A total of 553 infants (6 sets of twins) were delivered from 547 women who had used acid-suppressing drugs early in pregnancy. A number of other pharmaceutical agents, identified only by drug category, were also used by these women. Nineteen infants with birth defects were identified (3.1%, 95% confidence interval [CI] 1.8–4.9) compared with the crude malformation rate of 3.9% in the Registry. The odds ratio (OR) for a congenital malformation, stratified for birth year, maternal age, parity, and smoking was 0.72 (95% CI 0.41–1.24) (6). The OR for malformations after PPI exposure was 0.91 (95% CI 0.45–1.84) compared with 0.46 (95% CI 0.17–1.20) for H_2-receptor antagonists (OR 0.86, 95% CI 0.33–2.23; $p = 0.13$). Of the 19 infants with birth defects, 10 had been exposed to PPIs, 8 to H_2 antagonists, and 1 to both classes of drug. Six of the defects in the PPI group were cardiovascular defects (see also Lansoprazole), whereas only one such defect occurred in those exposed to H_2 antagonists. Omeprazole was the only acid-suppressing drug exposure in 262 infants. Twenty other offspring were exposed in utero to omeprazole combined either with cimetidine (2 infants) or ranitidine (18 infants). Eight birth defects (3.1%) were observed in the group where omeprazole was the only acid-suppressing agent used (defects described below) (6).

A 2001 study expanded the above data to 955 infants who had been exposed to omeprazole during pregnancy (7).

Of these, 863 infants were exposed during the 1st trimester and 39 of these, plus an additional 92 infants, were exposed after the 1st trimester. Twenty-eight infants (3.2%) had congenital malformations, 16 of which were exposed to other medications. Eight infants had cardiac defects, seven of which were considered mild or unspecified: ventricular septal defects (*N* = 5), unspecified (*N* = 2). The infant with the severe cardiac defect had tetralogy of Fallot plus an eye defect (coloboma plus posterior segment malformation). The other, noncardiac defects were (one each) hypospadias, urethral stenosis, bladder exstrophy, plagiocephaly, facial anomaly, Down's syndrome, valgus foot deformity, jejunal atresia, and nevus. Defects that appeared two or more times were persistent ductus arteriosus at term (*N* = 2), hydronephrosis (*N* = 2), undescended testicle (*N* = 2), unstable hip (*N* = 3), and pylorostenosis (*N* = 2). The adjusted OR for any malformation was 0.82, 95% CI 0.50–1.34. In addition to the defects, five infants were stillborn. The author thought that the slight increase in cardiac malformations and the stillbirths may have been random effects (7).

A prospective cohort study published in 1998 described the pregnancy outcomes of 113 women exposed to omeprazole (101 during organogenesis) matched with 113 disease-paired controls (exposed to H_2-receptor antagonists) and 113 controls who were exposed to nonteratogenic agents (8). All of the subjects and controls had contacted a teratogen information service to inquire about drug exposures during their pregnancy. Omeprazole-exposed women were from Canada (*N* = 59), Italy (*N* = 41), and France (*N* = 13), whereas all of the 226 controls were from Canada (Motherisk Program in Toronto). There were no significant differences between the groups in alcohol use and smoking. However, omeprazole-exposed women used significantly more antipeptic and prokinetic agents (histamine blockers, antacids, sucralfate, bismuth subsalicylate, calcium carbonate, and cisapride) than women in the two control groups. Pregnancy outcomes were determined from information supplied by the women shortly after delivery. No significant differences between the three groups in terms of live births, spontaneous abortions (SABs), elective abortions (EABs), gestational age at birth, preterm delivery, Cesarean section, and birth weight were observed (8). The incidence of major anomalies in live births exposed during the 1st trimester in the three groups were 4 of 78 (5.1%), 3 of 98 (3.1%), and 2 of 66 (3.0%), respectively. The four malformations in omeprazole-exposed infants were ventricular septal defect, polycystic kidneys, ureteropelvic junction stenosis, and patent ductus arteriosus. In disease-paired controls, the three defects were atrial septal defect and two cases of ventricular septal defect, whereas in nonteratogenic controls the two malformations were atrial septal defect with pulmonary stenosis and developmental delay. Although the study lacked the statistical power to detect a small increase in major malformations, the authors concluded that it was unlikely that omeprazole was a major teratogen (8).

A 1998 noninterventional observational cohort study described the outcomes of pregnancies in women who had been prescribed ≥1 of 34 newly marketed drugs by general practitioners in England (9). Data were obtained by questionnaires sent to the prescribing physicians 1 month after the expected or possible date of delivery. In 831 (78%) of the pregnancies, a newly marketed drug was thought to had been taken during the 1st trimester with birth defects noted in 14 (2.5%) singleton births of the 557 newborns (10 sets of twins). In addition, two birth defects were observed in aborted fetuses. However, few of the aborted fetuses were examined. Omeprazole was taken during the 1st trimester in five pregnancies. The outcomes of these pregnancies included one EAB and four normal, full-term infants (9).

The pregnancy outcomes of nine women who had taken omeprazole (20–60 mg/day) during gestation were described in a 1998 publication (10). Four of the women took omeprazole during the 1st trimester and five started treatment in the 2nd or 3rd trimesters. No complications or congenital malformations were observed in the offspring or during subsequent follow-up periods ranging from 2 to 12 years (10).

In a study published in 1999, investigators linked data from a Danish prescription database to a birth registry to evaluate the risks of PPIs for congenital malformations, low birth weight, and preterm delivery (<37 weeks') (11). From a total of 51 women who had filled a prescription for these drugs sometime during pregnancy, 38 (omeprazole *N* = 35, lansoprazole *N* = 3) had done so during the interval of 30 days before conception to the end of the 1st trimester. A control group, consisting of 13,327 pregnancies in which the mother had not obtained a prescription for reimbursed medication from 30 days before conception to the end of her pregnancy, was used for comparison. The prevalence of major congenital anomalies in the controls was 5.2%. Three major birth defects (7.9%), two of which were cardiovascular anomalies, were observed from the 38 pregnancies possibly exposed in the 1st trimester (specific drug exposure not given): ventricular septum defect; pyloric stenosis; and one case of patent ductus arteriosus, atrial septum defect, hydronephrosis, and agenesis of the iris. Compared with controls, the adjusted (for maternal age, birth order, gestational age, and smoking, but not for alcohol abuse) relative risks for the three outcomes were congenital malformations 1.6 (95% CI 0.5–5.2), low birth weight 1.8 (95% CI 0.2–13.1), and preterm delivery (not adjusted for gestational age) 2.3 (95% CI 0.9–6.0). Although the study found no elevated risks for the three outcomes, the investigators cautioned that more data were needed to assess the possible association between PPIs and cardiac malformations or preterm delivery (11).

Two databases, one from England and the other from Italy, were combined in a study published in 1999 that was designed to assess the incidence of congenital malformations in women who had received a prescription for an acid-suppressing drug (omeprazole, cimetidine, or ranitidine) during the 1st trimester (12). Nonexposed women were selected from the same databases to form a control group. SABs and EABs (except two cases of prenatally diagnosed congenital anomalies that were grouped with stillbirths) were excluded from the analysis. Stillbirths were defined as any pregnancy loss occurring at 28 weeks' gestation or later. Omeprazole was taken in 134 pregnancies, resulting in 139 live births (11 [7.9%] premature), 5 (3.7%) of whom had a congenital malformation. There were no stillbirths or neonatal deaths. The malformations were (shown by system): head/face (tongue tie), heart (septal defects *N* = 2), muscle/skeletal (dysplastic hip/dislocation/clicking hip), and genital/urinary (congenital hydrocele/inguinal hernia). In addition, three newborns had a small head circumference for gestational age. In comparison, the outcomes of 1547 nonexposed pregnancies included 1560 live births (115 [7.4%] premature),

15 stillbirths (includes 2 EABs for anomalies), and 10 neonatal deaths. Sixty-four (4.1%) of the newborns had malformations that involved the central nervous system (*N* = 2), head/face (*N* = 13), eye (*N* = 2), heart (*N* = 7), muscle/skeletal (*N* = 13), genital/urinary (*N* = 18), and gastrointestinal (*N* = 2), or were polyformation (*N* = 3) or known genetic anomalies (*N* = 4). Twenty-one newborns were small for gestational age and 78 had a small head circumference for gestational age. The relative risk of malformation (adjusted for mother's age and prematurity) associated with omeprazole was 0.9 (95% CI 0.4–2.4), with cimetidine 1.3 (95% CI 0.7–2.6), and with ranitidine 1.5 (95% CI 0.9–2.6) (12).

A 1998 case report described a 41-year-old woman with refractory gastroesophageal reflux disease (GERD) who was treated with omeprazole (20 mg/day) starting at 29 weeks' gestation (13). Previous treatment with ranitidine (late 1st trimester), cisapride (2nd trimester), or a combination of the two had been unsuccessful. A slightly premature male child (birth weight not given) with fetal bradycardia was delivered in the 36th week with Apgar scores of 6 and 9 at 1 and 5 minutes, respectively. He was doing well at 1 year of age (13).

A 2002 study conducted a meta-analysis involving the use of PPIs in pregnancy (14). In the five cohort studies analyzed, there were 593 infants, mostly exposed to omeprazole, but also including lansoprazole and pantoprazole. The relative risk (RR) for major malformations was 1.18, 95% CI 0.72–1.94 (14).

A 2005 study by the European Network of Teratology Information Services reported the outcomes of pregnancies exposed to omeprazole (*N* = 295), lansoprazole (*N* = 62), or pantoprazole (*N* = 53) (15). In the pantoprazole group, the median duration of treatment was 14 days (range 7–23 days) and the dose used was 40 mg/day. The outcomes consisted of 1 SAB, 3 EABs (none for congenital anomalies), 1 stillbirth, and 48 live births. One infant exposed early in gestation (week 2 for 8 days) had congenital toxoplasmosis. Compared with a nonexposed control group, there was no difference in the rate of major malformations between the pantoprazole and control groups (RR 0.95, 95% CI 0.46–1.98). Similar results were observed for lansoprazole and pantoprazole (15).

A population-based observational cohort study formed by linking data from three Swedish national health care registers over a 10-year period (1995–2004) was reported in 2009 (16). The main outcome measure was a diagnosis of allergic disease or a prescription for asthma or allergy medications. The drug types included in the study were gastric acid suppressors, including H_2-receptor antagonists, prostaglandins, PPIs, combinations for eradication of *Helicobacter pylori*, and drugs for peptic ulcer and gastro-esophageal reflux disease. Of 585,716 children, 29,490 (5.0%) met the diagnosis and 5645 (1%) had been exposed to gastric acid–suppression therapy in pregnancy. Of these children, 405 (0.07%) were treated for allergic disease. For developing allergy, the odds ratio (OR) was 1.43, 98% confidence interval (CI) 1.29–1.59, irrespective of the drug, time of exposure during pregnancy, and maternal history of allergy. For developing childhood asthma, but not other allergic diseases, the OR was 1.51 95% CI 1.35–1.69, irrespective of the type of acid-suppressive drug and the time of exposure in pregnancy. The authors proposed three possible mechanisms for their findings: (a) exposure to increased amounts of allergens could cause sensitization to digestion labile antigens in the fetus; (b) maternal Th2 cytokine pattern could promote an allergy-prone phenotype in the fetus; and (c) maternal allergen-specific IgE could cross the placenta and sensitize fetal immune cells to food and airborne allergens. Several limitations of the study that might have affected their findings were identified, including a general increase in childhood asthma but not necessarily an increase in allergic asthma (16). The study requires confirmation.

Several investigations have studied the effect of omeprazole for prophylaxis against aspiration pneumonitis in emergency cesarean section (17–22). No adverse effects were noted in the newborns.

A second meta-analysis of PPIs in pregnancy was reported in 2009 (23). Based on 1530 exposed compared with 133,410 not exposed pregnancies, the OR for major malformations was 1.12, 95% CI 0.86–1.45. There also was no increased risk for SABs (OR 1.29, 95% CI 0.84–1.97) or preterm birth (OR 1.13, 95% CI 0.96–1.33). When the analysis was conducted for exposure to omeprazole alone, the OR for major malformations was 1.17, 95% CI 0.90–1.53 (23).

In a 2010 study from Denmark, covering the period 1996–2008, there were 840,968 live births among whom 5082 were exposed to PPIs between 4 weeks before conception to the end of the 1st trimester (24). In the exposed group there were 174 (3.4%) major malformations compared with 21,811 (2.6%) not exposed to PPIs (adjusted prevalence odds ratio [aPOR] 1.23, 95 CI 1.05–1.44). When the analysis was limited to exposure in the 1st trimester, there were 118 (3.2%) major malformations among 3651 exposed infants (aPOR 1.10, 95% CI 0.91–1.34). For exposure to omeprazole in the 1st trimester, there were 52 (2.9%) major birth defects among 1800 live births (aPOR 1.05, 95% CI 0.79–1.40) (see Esomeprazole, Lansoprazole, Pantoprazole, and Rabeprazole for their data). The data showed that exposure to PPIs in the 1st trimester was not associated with a significantly increased risk of major birth defects (24). An accompanying editorial discussed the strengths and weaknesses of the study (25).

In a 2012 publication, the National Birth Defects Prevention study, a multisite population-based case–control study, examined whether nausea/vomiting of pregnancy (NVP) or its treatment were associated with the most common noncardiac defects (nonsyndromic cleft lip with or without cleft palate [CL/P], cleft palate alone [CP], neural tube defects [NTDs], and hypospadias) (26). PPI exposure included esomeprazole, lansoprazole, and omeprazole. There were 4524 cases and 5859 controls. NVP was not associated with cleft palate or NTDs, but modest risk reductions were observed for CL/P and hypospadias. Increased risks were found for PPIs (*N* = 7) and hypospadias (adjusted OR [aOR] 4.36, 95% CI 1.21–15.81), steroids (*N* = 10) and hypospadias (aOR 2.87, 95% CI 1.03–7.97), and ondansetron (*N* = 11) and CP (aOR 2.37, 95% CI 1.18–4.76) (26).

Another 2012 study, using the Danish nationwide registries, evaluated the risk of hypospadias after exposure to PPIs during the 1st trimester and throughout gestation (27). The study period, 1997 through 2009, included all liveborn boys that totaled 430,569 of whom 2926 were exposed to maternal PPI use. Hypospadias was diagnosed in 20 (0.7%) exposed boys, whereas 2683 (0.6%) of the nonexposed had hypospadias (adjusted prevalence ratio [aPR] 1.1, 95% CI 0.7–1.7). For the 5227 boys exposed throughout pregnancy, 32 (0.6%) had hypospadias (PR 1.0, 95% CI 0.7–1.4). When the analysis was restricted to mothers with two or more PPI prescriptions, the aPR of overall hypospadias was 1.7 (95% CI 0.9–3.3) and 1.6

(95% CI 0.7–3.9) for omeprazole. The authors concluded that PPIs were not associated with hypospadias (27).

A large retrospective cohort study from Israel covering the period 1998–2009 was published in 2012 (28). Among 114,960 live births, there were 110,783 singletons and 1239 elective abortions. Major malformations were observed in 6037 (5.5%) singletons and in 468 abortuses. Exposure to a PPI (lansoprazole, omeprazole, or pantoprazole) during the 1st trimester occurred in 1186 (1159 infants and 27 abortuses). In the exposed infants and abortuses, 80 (6.7%) had a major malformation compared with 6425 (5.9%) not exposed (aOR 1.06, 95% CI 0.84–1.33). In the 955 infants–abortuses exposed to omeprazole, 67 (7.0%) had a major malformation compared with 6438 (5.9%) not exposed (aOR 1.11, 95% CI 0.87–1.43). The data showed that exposure to PPIs during the 1st trimester was not associated with an increased risk of major defects. Moreover, additional analysis revealed that exposure during the 3rd trimester was not associated with increased risk of perinatal mortality, premature delivery, low birth weight, or low Apgar scores (28).

Five reviews on the treatment of GERD have concluded that PPIs can be used in pregnancy with relative safety (29–33). Because there are either very limited or no human pregnancy data for the three newest agents in this class (dexlansoprazole, esomeprazole, and rabeprazole), other drugs in the class are preferred.

BREASTFEEDING SUMMARY

Only one report describing the use of omeprazole during human lactation has been located. A woman with refractory GERD was treated with omeprazole (20 mg/day) for 7–8 weeks before delivering a premature male infant (birth weight not given) at 36 weeks' gestation (see above) (13). Treatment was continued during breastfeeding. During this time, she fed her infant son just before taking her dose at 8 AM, refrained from nursing for 4 hours, then expressed and discarded her milk at 12 noon. At 3 weeks postpartum, blood and milk samples were obtained at 8 AM and then every 30 minutes for 4 hours (i.e., until 12 noon). The milk was obtained by expressing but the volume of the samples was not specified. Maternal serum concentrations began to rise 90 minutes after the dose, reached 950 nM at 12 noon, and appeared to be still rising. Breast milk levels also began to rise at 90 minutes and peaked at 180 minutes at 58 nM. The infant was doing well at 1 year of age (13).

The above case report estimated a maximum daily omeprazole exposure of 4 mcg, but the calculation was based on a consumption of only 200 mL of milk/day for a 5-kg infant (40 mL/kg/day). A more acceptable value is 150 mL/kg/day (34). Moreover, the milk samples were obtained by expression and the volumes expressed were not given. This is clinically relevant because hindmilk obtained at the end of a feeding is 4–5 times higher in fat than foremilk (35). For lipid-soluble drugs, such as omeprazole, hindmilk would be expected to contain most of the drug in milk.

In concurrence with the above case report, the molecular weight of omeprazole (about 345) suggests that it will be excreted into human milk. One source stated that the safety of a drug during breastfeeding can be arbitrarily defined as no more than 10% of the adult dose standardized by weight if a therapeutic dose for infants is not known (34). Until additional studies show that omeprazole meets this criterion, the use of omeprazole during breastfeeding should probably be avoided. Other concerns, such as the carcinogenicity observed in animals and the potential for suppression of gastric acid secretion in the nursing infant, also warrant further study.

References

1. Product information. Prilosec. AstraZeneca, 2002.
2. Ching MS, Morgan DJ, Mihaly GW, Hardy KF, Smallwood RA. Placental transfer of omeprazole in maternal and fetal sheep. Dev Pharmacol Ther 1986;9:323–31.
3. Moore J, Flynn RJ, Sampaio M, Wilson CM, Gillon KRW. Effect of single-dose omeprazole on intragastric acidity and volume during obstetric anaesthesia. Anaesthesia 1989;44:559–62.
4. Tsirigotis M, Yazdani N, Craft I. Potential effects of omeprazole in pregnancy. Hum Reprod 1995;10:2177–8.
5. Harper MA, McVeigh JE, Thompson W, Ardill JES, Buchanan KD. Successful pregnancy in association with Zollinger-Ellison syndrome. Am J Obstet Gynecol 1995;173:863–4.
6. Kallen B. Delivery outcome after the use of acid-suppressing drugs in early pregnancy with special reference to omeprazole. Br J Obstet Gynaecol 1998;105:877–81.
7. Kallen BAJ. Use of omeprazole during pregnancy—no hazard demonstrated in 955 infants exposed during pregnancy. Eur J Obstet Gynecol Reprod Biol 2001;98:63–8.
8. Lalkin A, Loebstein R, Addis A, Ramezani-Namin F, Mastroiacovo P, Mazzone T, Vial T, Bonati M, Koren G. The safety of omeprazole during pregnancy: a multicenter prospective controlled study. Am J Obstet Gynecol 1998;179:727–30.
9. Wilton LV, Pearce GL, Martin RM, Mackay FJ, Mann RD. The outcomes of pregnancy in women exposed to newly marketed drugs in general practice in England. Br J Obstet Gynaecol 1998;105:882–9.
10. Brunner G, Meyer H, Athmann C. Omeprazole for peptic ulcer disease in pregnancy. Digestion 1998;59:651–4.
11. Nielsen GL, Sorensen HT, Thulstrup AM, Tage-Jensen U, Olesen C, Ekbom A. The safety of proton pump inhibitors in pregnancy. Aliment Pharmacol Ther 1999;13:1085–9.
12. Ruigomez A, Rodriguez LAG, Cattaruzzi C, Troncon MG, Agostinis L, Wallander MA, Johansson S. Use of cimetidine, omeprazole, and ranitidine in pregnant women and pregnancy outcomes. Am J Epidemiol 1999;150:476–81.
13. Marshall JK, Thomson ABR, Armstrong D. Omeprazole for refractory gastroesophageal reflux disease during pregnancy and lactation. Can J Gastroenterol 1998;12:225–7.
14. Nikfar S, Abdollahi M, Moretti ME, Magee LA, Koren G. Use of proton pump inhibitors during pregnancy and rates of major malformations: a meta-analysis. Dig Dis Sci 2002;47:1526–9.
15. Diav-Citrin O, Arnon J, Shechtman S, Schaefer C, Van Tonningen MR, Clementi M, De Santis M, Robert-Gnansia E, Valti E, Malm H, Ornoy A. The safety of proton pump inhibitors in pregnancy: a multicentre prospective controlled trial. Aliment Pharmacol Ther 2005;21:269–75.
16. Dehlink E, Yen E, Leichtner AM, Hait EJ, Fiebiger E. First evidence of a possible association between gastric acid suppression during pregnancy and childhood asthma: a population-based register study. Clin Exp Allergy 2009;39:246–53.
17. Yau G, Kan AF, Gin T, Oh TE. A comparison of omeprazole and ranitidine for prophylaxis against aspiration pneumonitis in emergency caesarean section. Anaesthesia 1992;47:101–4.
18. Orr DA, Bill KM, Gillon KRW, Wilson CM, Fogarty DJ, Moore J. Effects of omeprazole, with and without metoclopramide, in elective obstetric anaesthesia. Anaesthesia 1993;48:114–9.
19. Rocke DA, Rout CC, Gouws E. Intravenous administration of the proton pump inhibitor omeprazole reduces the risk of acid aspiration at emergency cesarean section. Anesth Analg 1994;78:1093–8.
20. Gin T. Intravenous omeprazole before emergency cesarean section. Anesth Analg 1995;80:848.
21. Rocke DA, Rout CC. Intravenous omeprazole before emergency cesarean section. Anesth Analg 1995;80:848–9.
22. Stuart JC, Kan AF, Rowbottom SJ, Gin T. Acid aspiration prophylaxis for emergency caesarean section. Anaesthesia 1996;51:415–21.
23. Gill SK, O'Brien L, Einarson TR, Koren G. The safety of proton pump inhibitors (PPIs) in pregnancy: a meta-analysis. Am J Gastroenterol 2009;104:1541–5.

O

24. Pasternak B, Hviid A. Use of proton-pump inhibitors in early pregnancy and the risk of birth defects. N Engl J Med 2010;363:2114–23.
25. Mitchell AA. Proton-pump inhibitors and birth defects—some reassurance, but more needed. N Engl J Med 2010;363:2161–3.
26. Anderka M, Mitchell AA, Louik C, Werler MM, Hernandez-Diaz S, Rasmussen SA, and the National Birth Defects Prevention Study. Medications used to treat nausea and vomiting of pregnancy and the risk of selected birth defects. Birth Defects Res A Clin Mol Teratol 2012;94:22–30.
27. Erichsen R, Mikkelsen E, Pedersen L, Sorensen HT. Maternal use of proton pump inhibitors during early pregnancy and the prevalence of hypospadias in male offspring. Am J Ther 2012 (Feb 3). [Epub ahead of print].
28. Matok I, Levy A, Wiznitzer A, Uziel E, Koren G, Gorodischer R. The safety of fetal exposure to proton-pump inhibitors during pregnancy. Dig Dis Sci 2012;57:699–705.
29. Broussard CN, Richter JE. Treating gastro-oesophageal reflux disease during pregnancy and lactation. What are the safest therapy options? Drug Saf 1998;19:325–37.
30. Katz PO, Castell DO. Gastroesophageal reflux disease during pregnancy. Gastroenterol Clin N Am 1998;27:153–67.
31. Ramakrishnan A, Katz PO. Pharmacologic management of gastroesophageal reflux disease. Curr Treat Options Gastroenterol 2002;5:301–10.
32. Richter JE. Gastroesophageal reflux disease during pregnancy. Gastroenterol Clin N Am 2003;32:235–61.
33. Richter JE. Review article: the management of heartburn in pregnancy. Aliment Pharmacol Ther 2005;22:749–57.
34. Ito S. Drug therapy for breast-feeding women. N Engl J Med 2000;343:118–26.
35. Lawrence RA, Lawrence RM. *Breastfeeding. A Guide for The Medical Profession*. 5th ed. St. Louis, MO: Mosby, 1999:360.

ONDANSETRON

Antiemetic

PREGNANCY RECOMMENDATION: Human Data Suggest Low Risk
BREASTFEEDING RECOMMENDATION: No Human Data—Probably Compatible

PREGNANCY SUMMARY

Consistent with the animal data, most human pregnancy data for ondansetron suggest that the risk of birth defects is low. However, in many studies ondansetron was started after organogenesis. Moreover, a large Danish study reported a 2-fold increased risk of cardiac anomalies. Thus, additional data are required to determine the risk. Consequently, if indicated, starting ondansetron therapy after 10 weeks of gestation should be considered.

FETAL RISK SUMMARY

Ondansetron is a selective 5-HT_3 receptor antagonist. It is an antiemetic that is indicated for the prevention and treatment of nausea and vomiting induced by chemotherapy, radiotherapy, and postoperative. The drug is extensively metabolized to metabolites that are unlikely to contribute to the parent drug's biological activity. The mean elimination half-life of a single 8-mg dose in women of reproductive age (18–40 years) is 3.5 hours (1).

No adverse effects on fertility or on the fetus were observed in reproduction studies in rats and rabbits with oral doses up to 15 and 30 mg/kg/day, respectively (1).

It is not known if ondansetron crosses the human placenta. The molecular weight (about 293) and the moderate elimination half-life suggest that the drug will cross to the embryo–fetus, but the extensive metabolism may limit the amount of parent drug crossing the placenta.

Ondansetron has been used in the treatment of hyperemesis gravidarum (2–6). A 21-year-old primigravida with severe nausea and vomiting was treated unsuccessfully for approximately 4 weeks, beginning at 6 weeks' gestation, with IV metoclopramide, 10 mg 3 times daily, rectal dimenhydrinate, 100 mg twice daily, and IV fluids (2). Because her condition was considered life-threatening for both her and her fetus, ondansetron 8 mg IV 3 times daily was instituted at 11 weeks' gestation and continued for 14 days. Significant improvement was noted in the patient's condition from the second day of therapy. The woman eventually gave birth at term to a healthy 3.2-kg girl.

A second report on the use of ondansetron for severe NVP involved a 22-year-old woman with renal impairment and nephrotic syndrome (3). Treatment with the antiemetic was begun at 30 weeks' gestation with 8 mg IV 3 times daily for 1 day, then orally (dose not specified) until 33 weeks' gestation. A healthy 2052-g female infant was delivered at 36 weeks by elective cesarean section. The infant remained in good health at an unspecified follow-up period.

A randomized, double-blind study, first published as an abstract (4) and then as a full report (5), compared IV ondansetron (10 mg) (N = 15) with IV promethazine (50 mg) (N = 15) for the treatment of hyperemesis gravidarum. Both drugs were given as an initial dose followed by as-needed doses every 8 hours. The mean gestational ages of the two groups at the start of therapy were 11.0 and 10.2 weeks, respectively. No differences were observed between the two groups in terms of duration of hospitalization, nausea score, number of doses received, treatment failures, and daily weight gain. The only adverse effect observed was sedation in 8 women who received promethazine compared with none in the ondansetron group. No mention was made of the pregnancy outcomes in either group.

Ondansetron, 8 mg IV twice daily, was administered to a woman at 14 weeks' gestation after 6 weeks of unsuccessful therapy with intermittent use of promethazine, prochlorperazine, metoclopramide, and IV hydration (6). IV ondansetron was able to control her vomiting, but not her nausea, and 2 days later she was converted to oral therapy (4 mg) that was taken intermittently (1–2 times daily) until 33 weeks' gestation. Nausea occurred throughout her pregnancy, with occasional episodes of vomiting. She eventually delivered a healthy, 2.7-kg male infant at 39 weeks' who was doing well at early follow-up.

A prospective comparative observational study, published in 2004, compared three groups of pregnant women ($N = 176$ in each group) for the treatment of NVP: ondansetron, other antiemetics, and nonteratogen exposures (7). There were no significant differences between the three groups in terms of life births, spontaneous abortions (SABs), elective abortions, stillbirths, birth weight, and gestational age at birth. In the ondansetron group, there were six (3.5%) major anomalies compared with three (1.8%) in each of the other two groups ($p = 0.52$). There were three cases of hypospadias in the ondansetron group compared with one in the other groups ($p = 0.25$) (7).

A 2012 study, using data from the National Birth Defects Prevention Study (NBDPS), examined whether NVP or its treatment was associated with the most common noncardiac birth defects in the NBDPS: nonsyndromic cleft lip with or without cleft palate, cleft palate alone, neural tube defects, and hypospadias (8). For NVP, there were modest risk reductions for cleft lip/palate (adjusted odds ratio [aOR] 0.87, 95% confidence interval [CI] 0.77–0.98) and hypospadias (aOR 0.84, 95% CI 0.72–0.98). For NVP treatments in the 1st trimester, there were increased risks for proton pump inhibitors and hypospadias (aOR 4.36, 95% CI 1.21–15.81), corticosteroids and hypospadias (aOR 2.87, 95% CI 1.03–7.97), and ondansetron and cleft palate (aOR 2.37, 95% CI 1.18–4.76), whereas antacids had a reduced risk for cleft lip/palate (aOR 0.58, 95% CI 0.38–0.89). The authors commented that the three associations could be chance findings but warranted further study (8).

In a 2013 study from Denmark, pregnant women exposed to ondansetron were compared in a 1:4 ratio with women not exposed (9). There was no increased risk for SAB that occurred in 1.1% of exposed compared with 3.7% of unexposed women during weeks 7–12 (hazard ratio [HR] 0.49, 95% CI 0.27–0.91) or for weeks 13–22 (1.0% vs. 2.1%, respectively, HR 0.60, 95% CI 0.29–1.21). There also was no increased risk for stillbirth (0.3% vs. 0.40%, respectively, HR 0.42, 95% CI 0.10–1.73), any major birth defect (2.9% vs. 2.9%, prevalence OR [pOR] 1.12, 95% CI 0.69–1.82), preterm birth (6.2% vs. 5.2%, pOR 0.90, 95% CI 0.66–1.25), low-birth-weight infant (4.1% vs. 3.7%, pOR 0.76, 95% CI 0.51–1.13), or small-for-gestational-age infant (10.4% vs. 9.2%, pOR 1.13, 95% CI 0.89–1.44)(9).

Although this study found no association with an increased risk of some adverse fetal outcomes, the question whether ondansetron causes birth defects remains unanswered. This is true because the median gestational age when the first ondansetron prescription was filled was 10 weeks. Thus, half of the exposed women were beyond the period (i.e., organogenesis) when a drug could cause structural anomalies.

A 2014 letter noted that the above study and a second study from Denmark were presented at the 2013 International Society of Pharmacoepidemiology meeting in Montreal (10). The second Danish study (11), using the same national registries but covering more years (1997–2010 vs. 2004–2011) and more pregnant women (897,108 vs. 608,835), reported a 2-fold increased risk of cardiac anomalies (OR 2.0, 95% CI 1.3–3.1). Other issues raised in the letter were concerns for maternal harm caused from QT prolongation, torsade de pointes, and serotonin syndrome (10).

BREASTFEEDING SUMMARY

No reports describing the use of ondansetron during human lactation have been located. The molecular weight (about 293) and the moderate elimination half-life (3.5 hours) suggest that the drug will be excreted into breast milk, but the extensive metabolism may limit the amount in milk. The effect of this exposure on a nursing infant is unknown.

References

1. Product information. Zofran. GlaxoSmithKline, 2012.
2. Guikontes E, Spantideas A, Diakakis J. Ondansetron and hyperemesis gravidarum. Lancet 1992;340:1223.
3. World MJ. Ondansetron and hyperemesis gravidarum. Lancet 1993;341:185.
4. Sullivan CA, Johnson CA, Roach H, Martin RW, Stewart DK, Morrison JC. A prospective, randomized, double-blind comparison of the serotonin antagonist ondansetron to a standardized regimen of promethazine for hyperemesis gravidarum. A preliminary investigation (abstract). Am J Obstet Gynecol 1995;172:299.
5. Sullivan CA, Johnson CA, Roach H, Martin RW, Stewart DK, Morrison JC. A pilot study of intravenous ondansetron for hyperemesis gravidarum. Am J Obstet Gynecol 1996;174:1565–8.
6. Tincello DG, Johnstone MJ. Treatment of hyperemesis gravidarum with the 5-HT_3 antagonist ondansetron (Zofran). Postgrad Med J 1996;72:688–9.
7. Einarson A, Maltepe C, Navioz Y, Kennedy D, Tan MP, Koren G. The safety of ondansetron for nausea and vomiting of pregnancy: a prospective comparative study. Br J Obstet Gynaecol 2004;111:940–3.
8. Anderka M, Mitchell AA, Louik C, Werler MM, Hernandez-Diaz S, Rasmussen SA, and the National Birth Defects Prevention Study. Medications use to treat nausea and vomiting of pregnancy and the risk of selected birth defects. Birth Defects Res (Part A) 2012;94:22–30.
9. Pasternak B, Svanstrom H, Hviid A. Ondansetron in pregnancy and risk of adverse fetal outcomes. NEJM 2013;368:814–23.
10. Koren G. Scary science: ondansetron safety in pregnancy – two opposing results from the same Danish registry. Ther Drug Monit 2014;36:1–2.
11. Andersen JT, Jimenez-Solem E, Andersen NL, et al. Ondansetron use in early pregnancy and the risk of congenital malformations—a registry based nationwide control study. International Society of Pharmaco-epidemiology. Montreal, Canada; 2013. Abstract 25, Pregnancy Session 1. As cited by Koren G. Scary science: ondansetron safety in pregnancy—two opposing results from the same Danish registry. Ther Drug Monit 2014;36:1–2.

O

OPIPRAMOL

[Withdrawn from the market. See 9th edition.]

OPIUM

Narcotic Antidiarrheal

PREGNANCY RECOMMENDATION: Human Data Suggest Risk in 3rd Trimester
BREASTFEEDING RECOMMENDATION: No Human Data—Probably Compatible

PREGNANCY SUMMARY

The effects of opium are caused by morphine (see Morphine). Neonatal withdrawal is a potential complication if used for prolonged periods or in high doses close to term.

FETAL RISK SUMMARY

The Collaborative Perinatal Project monitored 50,282 mother–child pairs, 36 of whom had 1st trimester exposure to opium (1, pp. 287–95). For use anytime during pregnancy, 181 exposures were recorded (1, p. 434). Four of the 1st trimester exposed infants had congenital defects, but these numbers are too small to draw any conclusion about a relationship between the drug and major or minor malformations. A possible association with inguinal hernia based on seven cases after anytime exposure was suggested (1, p. 485) (see also Morphine for similar findings). The statistical significance of these associations is unknown and independent confirmation is required.

Narcotic withdrawal was observed in a newborn whose mother was treated for regional ileitis with deodorized tincture of opium during the 2nd and 3rd trimesters (2). Symptoms of withdrawal in the infant began at 48 hours of age.

BREASTFEEDING SUMMARY

No reports describing the use of opium during human lactation. (See Morphine.)

References

1. Heinonen OP, Slone D, Shapiro S. *Birth Defects and Drugs in Pregnancy*. Littleton, MA: Publishing Sciences Group, 1977.
2. Fisch GR, Henley WL. Symptoms of narcotic withdrawal in a newborn infant secondary to medical therapy of the mother. Pediatrics 1961;28: 852–3.

OPRELVEKIN

Hematopoietic

PREGNANCY RECOMMENDATION: No Human Data—Animal Data Suggest Risk
BREASTFEEDING RECOMMENDATION: No Human Data—Probably Compatible

PREGNANCY SUMMARY

No reports describing the use of oprelvekin in human pregnancy have been located. The animal data suggest a risk of toxicity but not teratogenicity. However, the absence of human pregnancy experience prevents an assessment of the risk the drug represents to the embryo and fetus.

FETAL RISK SUMMARY

Oprelvekin is a protein, produced by recombinant DNA technology from *Escherichia coli* that differs from natural interleukin-11 (IL-11) by one terminal amino acid. This difference does not affect its bioactivity as a thrombopoietic growth factor that indirectly stimulates increased platelet production. It is indicated to prevent severe thrombocytopenia and to reduce the need for platelet transfusions following myelosuppressive chemotherapy. The terminal half-life is about 6.9 hours (1).

Reproduction studies have been conducted in rats and rabbits. Oprelvekin was embryocidal in rats at doses 2–20 times the human dose based on body weight (HD). Maternal toxicity (transient hypoactivity and dyspnea) and prolonged estrus cycle were evident at these doses. Embryo–fetal effects included increased early embryonic deaths and decreased numbers of live fetuses. At 20 times the HD, retarded fetal development occurred as evidenced by low fetal weight, and reduced number of ossified sacral and caudal vertebrae. Doses $\geq$2 times the HD used throughout gestation and lactation resulted in increased newborn mortality, decreased viability index on day 4 of lactation, and decreased pup body weights. In pregnant rabbits, doses 0.02–2 times the HD were maternal toxic (decreased fecal/urine eliminations, decreased food consumption and body weight loss). These doses caused abortion, increased embryonic and fetal deaths, and decreased numbers of live fetuses. No teratogenicity was observed in rabbits at doses $\leq$0.6 times HD (1).

It is not known if oprelvekin crosses the human placenta. Oprelvekin is a 177-amino acid protein with a molecular weight of about 19,000, but proteins can cross to the embryo and fetus.

BREASTFEEDING SUMMARY

No reports describing the use of oprelvekin during lactation have been located. Oprelvekin is a 177-amino acid protein with a molecular weight of about 19,000. Although it may be excreted into breast milk, it would most likely be digested in the infant's gastrointestinal tract. Therefore, the risk to a nursing infant from exposure to the drug in milk appears to be very low or nonexistent.

Reference

1. Product information. Neumega. Wyeth Pharmaceuticals, 2004.

ORAL CONTRACEPTIVES

Estrogenic/Progestogenic Hormones

PREGNANCY RECOMMENDATION: Contraindicated
BREASTFEEDING RECOMMENDATION: Compatible

PREGNANCY SUMMARY

The use of oral contraceptives is contraindicated in pregnancy primarily because there are no benefits for such use. The absolute risk of embryo–fetal harm after inadvertent exposure early in gestation appears to be low. Use later in pregnancy of products containing synthetic progestogens may be associated with masculinization of female fetuses.

FETAL RISK SUMMARY

Oral contraceptives contain a 19-nortestosterone progestin and a synthetic estrogen (see Mestranol, Norethindrone, Norethynodrel, Ethinyl Estradiol, Hydroxyprogesterone, Ethisterone). Because oral contraceptives are primarily combination products, it is difficult to separate entirely the fetal effects of progestogens and estrogens. Two groups of investigators have reviewed the effects of these hormones on the fetus (133 references) (1,2). Several potential problems were discussed: congenital heart defects, central nervous system defects, limb reduction malformations, general malformations, and modified development of sexual organs. Except for the latter category, no firm evidence has appeared that establishes a causal relationship between oral contraceptives and various congenital anomalies.

The acronym VACTERL (**v**ertebral, **a**nal, **c**ardiac, **t**racheal, **e**sophageal, **r**enal or **r**adial, and **l**imb) has been used to describe the fetal malformations produced by oral contraceptives or the related hormonal pregnancy test preparations (no longer available in the United States) (2,3). The use of this acronym should probably be abandoned in favor of more conventional terminology because a large variety of malformations has been reported with estrogen–progestogen-containing products (1–11). The Population Council estimates that even if the study findings for VACTERL malformations are accurate, such abnormalities would occur in only 0.07% of the pregnancies exposed to oral contraceptives (12). Some reviewers have concluded that the risk to the fetus for nongenital malformations after in utero exposure to these agents is small, if indeed it exists at all (2).

In contrast to the above, the effect of estrogens and some synthetic progestogens on the development of the sexual organs is well established (2). Masculinization of the female infant has been associated with norethindrone, norethynodrel, hydroxyprogesterone, medroxyprogesterone, and diethylstilbestrol (2,13,14). The incidence of masculinization of female infants exposed to synthetic progestogens is reported to be approximately 0.3% (15). Pseudohermaphroditism in the male infant is not a problem, because of the low doses of estrogen employed in oral contraceptives (14).

Increased serum bilirubin in neonates of mothers taking oral contraceptives or progestogens before and after conception has been observed (16). Icterus occasionally reached clinically significant levels in infants whose mothers were exposed to the progestogens.

Concern that oral contraceptives may be a risk factor for preeclampsia has been suggested based on the known effects of oral contraceptives on blood pressure (17). However, a retrospective controlled review of 341 patients found no association between this effect and the drugs (17).

Possible interactions between oral contraceptives and tetracycline, rifampin, ampicillin, or chloramphenicol resulting in pregnancy have been reported (18–25). The mechanism for this interaction may involve the interruption of the enterohepatic circulation of contraceptive steroids by inhibiting gut hydrolysis of steroid conjugates, resulting in lower concentrations of circulating steroids.

BREASTFEEDING SUMMARY

Use of oral contraceptives during lactation has been associated with shortened duration of lactation, decreased infant weight gain, decreased milk production, and decreased composition of nitrogen and protein content of milk (26–29). The American Academy of Pediatrics has reviewed this subject (30) (37 references). Although the magnitude of these changes is low, the changes in milk production and composition may be of nutritional importance in malnourished mothers.

In general, progestin-only contraceptives demonstrate no consistent alteration of breast milk composition, volume, or duration of lactation (30). The composition and volume of breast milk varies considerably even in the absence of steroidal contraceptives (29). Both estrogens and progestins

O

cross into milk. An infant consuming 600 mL of breast milk daily from a mother using contraceptives containing 50 mcg of ethinyl estradiol will probably receive a daily dose in the range of 10 ng (30). This is in the same range as the amount of natural estradiol received by infants of mothers not using oral contraceptives. Progestins also pass into breast milk, although naturally occurring progestins have not been identified. One study estimated 0.03, 0.15, and 0.3 mcg of *d*-norgestrel/600 mL in milk from mothers receiving 30, 150, and 250 mcg of the drug, respectively (31). A milk:plasma ratio of 0.15 for norgestrel was calculated by the authors (31). A ratio of 0.16 was calculated for lynestrenol (31,32).

Reports of adverse effects are lacking except for one child with mild breast tenderness and hypertrophy who was exposed to large doses of estrogen (30). If breastfeeding is desired, the lowest effective dose of oral contraceptives should be chosen. Infant weight gain should be monitored, and the possible need for nutritional supplements should be considered. The American Academy of Pediatrics classifies combination oral contraceptives as compatible with breastfeeding (33).

References

1. Ambani LM, Joshi NJ, Vaidya RA, Devi PK. Are hormonal contraceptives teratogenic? Fertil Steril 1977;28:791–7.
2. Wilson JG, Brent RL. Are female sex hormones teratogenic? Am J Obstet Gynecol 1981;141:567–80.
3. Corcoran R, Entwistle GC. VACTERL congenital malformations and the male fetus. Lancet 1975;2:981–2.
4. Nora JJ, Nora AH. Can the pill cause birth defects? N Engl J Med 1974;294:731–2.
5. Kasan PN, Andrews J. Oral contraceptives and congenital abnormalities. Br J Obstet Gynaecol 1980;87:545–51.
6. Kullander S, Kallen B. A prospective study of drugs and pregnancy. Acta Obstet Gynecol Scand 1976;55:221–4.
7. Oakley GP, Flynt JW. Hormonal pregnancy test and congenital malformations. Lancet 1973;2:256–7.
8. Savolainen E, Saksela E, Saxen L. Teratogenic hazards of oral contraceptives analyzed in a national malformation register. Am J Obstet Gynecol 1981;140:521–4.
9. Frost O. Tracheo-oesophageal fistula associated with hormonal contraception during pregnancy. Br Med J 1976;3:978.
10. Redline RW, Abramowsky CR. Transposition of the great vessels in an infant exposed to massive doses of oral contraceptives. Am J Obstet Gynecol 1981;141:468–9.
11. Farb HF, Thomason J, Carandang FS, Sampson MB, Spellacy WH. Anencephaly twins and HLA-B27. J Reprod Med 1980;25:166–9.
12. Department of Medical and Public Affairs. *Population Reports*. Washington, DC: George Washington University Medical Center, 1975;2:A29–51.
13. Bongiovanni AM, DiGeorge AM, Grumbach MM. Masculinization of the female infant associated with estrogenic therapy alone during gestation: four cases. J Clin Endocrinol Metab 1959;19:1004–11.
14. Hagler S, Schultz A, Hankin H, Kunstadter RH. Fetal effects of steroid therapy during pregnancy. Am J Dis Child 1963;106:586–90.
15. Bongiovanni AM, McFadden AJ. Steroids during pregnancy and possible fetal consequences. Fertil Steril 1960;11:181–4.
16. McConnell JB, Glasgow JF, McNair R. Effect on neonatal jaundice of oestrogens and progestogens taken before and after conception. Br Med J 1973;3:605–7.
17. Bracken MB, Srisuphan W. Oral contraception as a risk factor for preeclampsia. Am J Obstet Gynecol 1982;142:191–6.
18. Bacon JF, Shenfield GM. Pregnancy attributable to interaction between tetracycline and oral contraceptives. Br Med J 1980;1:283.
19. Stockley I. Interactions with oral contraceptives. Pharm J 1976;216:140.
20. Reiners D, Nockefinck L, Breurer H. Rifampin and the "pill" do not go well together. JAMA 1974;227:608.
21. Dosseter EJ. Drug interactions with oral contraceptives. Br Med J 1975;1:1967.
22. Pullskinnen MO, Williams K. Reduced maternal plasma and urinary estriol during ampicillin treatment. Am J Obstet Gynecol 1971;109:895–6.
23. Friedman GI, Huneke AL, Kim MH, Powell J. The effect of ampicillin on oral contraceptive effectiveness. Obstet Gynecol 1980;55:33–7.
24. Back DJ, Breckenridge AM. Drug interactions with oral contraceptives. IPFF Med Bull 1978;12:1–2.
25. Orme ML, Back DJ. Therapy with oral contraceptive steroids and antibiotics J Antimicrob Chemother 1979;5:124–6.
26. Miller GH, Hughes LR. Lactation and genital involution effects of a new low-dose oral contraceptive on breast-feeding mothers and their infants. Obstet Gynecol 1970;35:44–50.
27. Kora SJ. Effect of oral contraceptives on lactation. Fertil Steril 1969;20: 419–23.
28. Guiloff E, Ibarra-Polo A, Zanartu J, Tuscanini C, Mischler TW, Gomez-Rodgers C. Effect of contraception on lactation. Am J Obstet Gynecol 1974;118:42–5.
29. Lonnerdal B, Forsum E, Hambraeus L. Effect of oral contraceptives on consumption and volume of breast milk. Am J Clin Nutr 1980;33:816–24.
30. Committee on Drugs, American Academy of Pediatrics. Breast-feeding and contraception. Pediatrics 1981;68:138–40.
31. Nilsson S, Nygren KC, Johansson EDB. D-Norgestrel concentrations in maternal plasma, milk, and child plasma during administration of oral contraceptives to nursing women. Am J Obstet Gynecol 1977;129:178–83.
32. van der Molen HJ, Hart PG, Wijmenga HG. Studies with 4-$_{14}$C-lynestrol in normal and lactating women. Acta Endocrinol 1969;61:255–74.
33. Committee on Drugs, American Academy of Pediatrics. The transfer of drugs and other chemicals into human milk. Pediatrics 2001;108: 776–89.

ORLISTAT

Gastrointestinal Agent (Lipase Inhibitor)

PREGNANCY RECOMMENDATION: Limited Human Data—Animal Data Suggest Low Risk
BREASTFEEDING RECOMMENDATION: No Human Data—Probably Compatible

PREGNANCY SUMMARY

One report describing the use of orlistat during human pregnancy has been located. Because of its minimal systemic bioavailability, orlistat appears to present a very low risk, if any, to the embryo or fetus. Orlistat may cause a deficiency of fat-soluble vitamins (vitamins A [both retinol and β-carotene], D, and E) if a daily multiple vitamin supplement is not taken. The vitamin should be taken 2 hours either before or after an orlistat dose (1). Maternal deficiency of these vitamins may result in fetal adverse effects (see also Vitamin A, Vitamin D, and Vitamin E). If orlistat is used in pregnancy, health care professionals are encouraged to call the toll-free number 800-670-6126 for information about patient enrollment in the Motherisk study.

FETAL RISK SUMMARY

Orlistat is a lipase inhibitor used in the management of obesity. The agent inhibits the absorption of dietary fats. The mechanism of action of orlistat involves bonding to gastric and pancreatic lipases, thereby inactivating these enzymes. The inactive enzymes are unable to hydrolyze dietary fat to absorbable free fatty acids and monoglycerides (1). The systemic bioavailability of orlistat is minimal (1).

Reproduction studies in rats and rabbits at doses up to 23 and 47 times the recommended human daily dose based on BSA (RHD) revealed no evidence of embryotoxicity or teratogenicity (1). In two rat studies, but not in two others, doses of 6 and 23 times the RHD were associated with an increased incidence of dilated cerebral ventricles. At 12 times the RHD in rats, no evidence of impaired fertility was observed (1).

It is not known if orlistat crosses the placenta. Although the molecular weight (about 496) is low enough for passage to the fetus, the minimal systemic bioavailability of the agent following oral administration suggests that little, if any, of the agent would be available for transfer from the maternal circulation.

A 2005 case report described the pregnancy outcome of a 33-year-old woman treated with orlistat in the first 8 weeks of an unplanned pregnancy (2). Diseases in the patient included morbid obesity, type 2 diabetes mellitus, hypertension, and hypercholesterolemia. Other drugs used by the woman were glimepiride, ramipril, thiocolchicoside (a muscle relaxant), simvastatin, metformin, ciprofloxacin, and aspirin. When pregnancy was diagnosed at 8 weeks all medications were stopped, and she was started on methyldopa and insulin. She gave birth at 38 weeks to a 3.470-kg female infant with Apgar scores of 5 and 7 at 1 and 5 minutes, respectively. No minor or major malformations were observed in the infant (2).

BREASTFEEDING SUMMARY

No reports describing the use of orlistat during human lactation have been located. The minimal systemic bioavailability suggests that the drug would not be found in breast milk, but maternal hypovitaminosis A, D, and E may occur (see above).

References

1. Product information. Xenical. Roche Laboratories, 2000.
2. Kalyoncu NI, Yaris F, Kadioglu M, Kesim M, Ulku C, Yaris E, Unsal M, Dikici M. Pregnancy outcome following exposure to orlistat, ramipril, glimepiride in a woman with metabolic syndrome. Saudi Med J 2005;26:497–9.

ORPHENADRINE

Skeletal Muscle Relaxant

PREGNANCY RECOMMENDATION: Limited Human Data—No Relevant Animal Data
BREASTFEEDING RECOMMENDATION: No Human Data—Probably Compatible

PREGNANCY SUMMARY

Orphenadrine is an anticholinergic agent used in the treatment of painful skeletal muscle conditions. No published reports of its use in human pregnancy have been located (see also Atropine).

FETAL RISK SUMMARY

An animal study in pregnant rats using large oral doses (15 and 30 mg) produced enlarged bladders containing blood but no other anomalies in 8 of 159 fetuses (1).

In a surveillance study of Michigan Medicaid recipients involving 229,101 completed pregnancies conducted between 1985 and 1992, 411 newborns had been exposed to orphenadrine during the 1st trimester (F. Rosa, personal communication, FDA, 1993). A total of 11 (2.7%) major birth defects were observed (16 expected), including (observed/expected) 2/4 cardiovascular defects and 1/1 polydactyly. No anomalies were observed in four other defect categories (oral clefts, spina bifida, limb reduction defects, and hypospadias) for which specific data were available. These data do not support an association between the drug and congenital defects.

BREASTFEEDING SUMMARY

No reports describing the use of orphenadrine during human lactation have been located (see also Atropine).

Reference

1. Beall JR. A teratogenic study of chlorpromazine, orphenadrine, perphenazine, and LSD-25 in rats. Toxicol Appl Pharmacol 1972;21:230–6. As cited in Shepard TH. *Catalog of Teratogenic Agents*. 6th ed. Baltimore, MD: The Johns Hopkins University Press, 1989:476–7.

OSELTAMIVIR

Antiviral

PREGNANCY RECOMMENDATION: Compatible—Maternal Benefit >> Embryo–Fetal Risk
BREASTFEEDING RECOMMENDATION: Compatible

PREGNANCY SUMMARY

Limited reports describing the use of oseltamivir during human pregnancy do not suggest a significant risk of developmental toxicity. The drug is used for the treatment and prophylaxis of influenza, including novel influenza A (H1N1). Because influenza infection in pregnancy is a high-risk condition, the maternal benefit far outweighs the unknown risk, if any, to the embryo or fetus. Moreover, hyperthermia, a common condition of influenza infections, occurring during the 1st trimester doubles the risk of neural tube defects (1). In addition, maternal hyperthermia during labor is a risk factor for neonatal seizures, encephalopathy, cerebral palsy, and neonatal death. Thus, in either case, hyperthermia should be promptly treated with acetaminophen and, in the 1st trimester, combined with multivitamins containing folic acid (1).

FETAL RISK SUMMARY

Oseltamivir is an ethyl ester prodrug that is rapidly metabolized by hepatic esterases to oseltamivir carboxylate, the active antiviral agent. Systemic exposure to oseltamivir is <5% of the total exposure. It is a neuraminidase inhibitor in the same antiviral subclass as zanamivir. Plasma protein binding of oseltamivir carboxylate is low (3%), but the elimination half-life is prolonged (6–10 hours). Oseltamivir is indicated for the treatment of uncomplicated acute illness due to influenza infection in patients 1 year of age and older who have been symptomatic for no more than 2 days. It also is indicated for the prophylaxis of influenza in patients aged 1 year and older (2). In April 2009, the FDA issued an Emergency Use Authorization to allow the drug to be used to treat and prevent influenza in children under 1 year of age, and to provide alternate dosing recommendations for children older than 1 year (3). Oseltamivir is active against novel influenza A (H1N1) (*formerly known as swine flu*), either as treatment of acute illness or as chemoprophylaxis in patients at high risk of complications, such as pregnant women (4).

In reproduction studies, doses up to 100 times the human systemic exposure based on AUC of oseltamivir carboxylate (HSE) had no effects on fertility or mating performance in male and female rats, or on embryo–fetal development. The highest dose was associated with minimal maternal toxicity. In rabbits, doses up to 50 times the HSE also had no effect on embryo–fetal development. Maternal toxicity was observed in rabbits with doses 15 times the HSE or higher. In both species, fetal exposure to the antiviral agent was documented. Although a dose-dependent increase in the incidence rates of skeletal abnormalities and variants was observed in both species, the individual incidence rate of each defect remained within the expected background rate of occurrence (2).

Oseltamivir and its active metabolite were not carcinogenic in 2-year studies in mice and rats. Oseltamivir was not mutagenic in several assays, but was positive in one. The active metabolite was negative in all assays (2).

Although the relatively low molecular weight (about 312 and 284 for the parent drug free base and metabolite, respectively), minimal plasma protein binding, and prolonged elimination half-life suggest that both the parent drug and the metabolite will cross to the embryo–fetus, a 2008 study (5) found otherwise. In the ex vivo human placenta model, extensive metabolism of oseltamivir to the active metabolite was observed, but neither the parent drug nor its metabolite could be detected on the fetal side when concentrations 5–6-fold above the therapeutic concentration were used. Concentrations 20–830-fold above the therapeutic range were required for detectable levels on the fetal side. The mean clearance index for these high levels was 0.13 and fetal accumulation was minimal (5).

The Centers for Disease Control and Prevention has published information on two cases of H1N1 virus infection in pregnancy that were treated with oseltamivir (4). A 29-year-old woman at 23 weeks' gestation presented at a family practice clinic. She had a 1-day history of cough, sore throat, chills, fever, and weakness. Rapid influenza diagnostic testing was positive, and H1N1 virus was later confirmed. The mother was prescribed oseltamivir and her symptoms were resolving without complication. Her pregnancy was proceeding normally. The clinic physician who evaluated the mother was also pregnant (13 weeks' gestation). She began prophylactic oseltamivir and had remained asymptomatic (4).

A 2005 report from the manufacturer briefly mentioned the use of oseltamivir in 61 pregnant women without specifying the timing of the exposures (6). Among these, there were four spontaneous abortions (SABs) and six elective abortions (EABs). In addition, there were single cases of trisomy 21 (Down's syndrome) and anencephaly, neither of which was thought to be related to the drug therapy. The remaining cases resulted in the birth of normal infants (6).

A 2009 report summarized the safety of neuraminidase inhibitors in pregnant and breastfeeding women (7). The data, from two Japanese teratogen information services, involved 90 pregnancies exposed during the 1st trimester to therapeutic doses of oseltamivir (75 mg twice a day for up to 5 days). The outcomes of the pregnancies were three SABs, one EAB, four preterm births, seven infants with low birth weight, and one major malformation (ventricular septal defect). The malformation incidence (1.2%; 1 in 86 live births) is well within the background incidence of major malformations (7).

A retrospective cohort study, covering the period 2003–2008, described 239 pregnancies that were treated with antiviral agents during pregnancy (8). Of these, 104 women received M2 ion channel inhibitors (rimantadine, amantadine, or both) and 135 received oseltamivir. The pregnancy outcomes of these patients were compared with 82,097 controls from the site's overall obstetric patient population. The exposure timing for the combined treated groups was 13% 1st trimester, 32% 2nd trimester, and 55% 3rd trimester. There were no significant differences between the treated groups and controls in terms of maternal and delivery characteristics except that M2 inhibitors had more multiple gestations. For M2 inhibitors, oseltamivir vs. controls, there also was no differences in stillbirths (0%, 0% vs. 1%), major defects (1% [trisomy 21], 0% vs. 2%), and minor defects (19%, 15% vs. 22%). The only significant finding in the characteristics of liveborn, singleton neonates, after exclusion of twins and major anomalies, was a higher risk of necrotizing enterocolitis in both treatment groups compared with controls—1.0%, 0.8% vs. 0.02% (8).

BREASTFEEDING SUMMARY

Oseltamivir and its active metabolite are excreted into breast milk. A woman who was breastfeeding her 9-month-old child twice daily accidentally stuck herself with a novel influenza A (H1N1)-contaminated needle (9). She was treated with oseltamivir 75 mg twice daily for 5 days. Breastfeeding was stopped during this period because of possible adverse effects in the infant. Milk samples (*N* = 11) were collected twice daily over the 5-day period by completely emptying both breasts. The timings of the samples were distributed at various times, with eight of the samples collected 30 minutes before or after a dose. The steady state concentration of the metabolite (37–39 ng/mL) was reached after 3 days. The authors estimated that the maximum relative infant dose (oseltamivir plus the metabolite) was 0.012 mg/kg/day or about 0.5% of the mother's weight-adjusted dose (based on an assumed maternal weight of 60 kg) (9).

Based on the above study, in which the infant did not nurse, the concentration of the drug in breast milk appears to be clinically insignificant. In addition, the potential dose for a nursing infant is much less than the pediatric dose. Moreover, breastfeeding is recommended for women infected with novel influenza A (H1N1), regardless of whether they are being treated, because of the advantages of breast milk for the infant's immune system (10).

References

1. Rasmussen SA, Jamieson DJ, MacFarlane K, Cragan JD, Williams J, Henderson Z, for the Pandemic Influenza Pregnancy Working Group. Pandemic influenza and pregnant women: summary of a meeting of experts. Am J Public Health 2009;99(Suppl 2):S248–54.
2. Product information. Tamiflu. Roche Laboratories, 2008.
3. FDA News Release. FDA authorizes emergency use of influenza medicines, diagnostic test in response to swine flu outbreak in humans. Available at http://www.fda.gov/NewsEvents/Newsroom/PressAnnouncements/ucm149571.htm. Accessed June 8, 2009.
4. Centers for Disease Control and Prevention (CDC). Novel influenza A (H1N1) virus infections in three pregnant women—United States, April–May 2009. MMWR Morb Mortal Wkly Rep 2009 May 15;58(18):497–500.
5. Worley KC, Roberts SW, Bawdon RE. The metabolism and transplacental transfer of oseltamivir in the ex vivo human model. Inf Dis Obstet Gynecol 2008;2008(Article ID 927574):1–5.
6. Ward P, Small I, Smith J, Suter P, Dutkowski R. Oseltamivir (Tamiflu) and its potential for use in the event of an influenza pandemic. J Antimicrob Chemother 2005;55(Suppl S1):i5–i21.
7. Tanaka T, Nakajima K, Murashima A, Garcia-Bournissen F, Koren G, Ito S. Safety of neuraminidase inhibitors against novel influenza A (H1N1) in pregnant and breastfeeding women. CMAJ 2009;181:55–8.
8. Greer LG, Sheffield JS, Rogers VL, Roberts SW, McIntire DD, Wendel GD Jr. Maternal and neonatal outcomes after antepartum treatment of influenza with antiviral medications. Obstet Gynecol 2010;115:711–6.
9. Wentges-van Holthe N, van Eijkeren M, van der Laan JW. Oseltamivir and breastfeeding. Int J Infect Dis 2008;12:451.
10. CDC. What pregnant women should know about H1N1 (formerly called swine flu) virus. Available at: http://www.cdc.gov/h1n1flu/guidance/pregnant.htm. Accessed June 8, 2009.

OUABAIN

[Withdrawn from the market. See 9th edition.]

OXACILLIN

Antibiotic (Penicillin)

PREGNANCY RECOMMENDATION: Compatible
BREASTFEEDING RECOMMENDATION: Compatible

PREGNANCY SUMMARY

Although the reported pregnancy experience with oxacillin is limited, all penicillins are considered low risk in pregnancy.

FETAL RISK SUMMARY

Oxacillin is a penicillin antibiotic (see also Penicillin G). The drug crosses the placenta in low concentrations. Cord serum and amniotic fluid levels were <0.3 mcg/mL in 15 of 18 patients given 500 mg orally 0.5–4 hours before cesarean section (1). No effects were seen in the infants.

The Collaborative Perinatal Project monitored 50,282 mother–child pairs, 3546 of whom had 1st trimester exposure to penicillin derivatives (2, pp. 297–313). For use anytime during pregnancy, 7171 exposures were recorded (2, p. 435). In neither group was evidence found to suggest a relationship to large categories of major or minor malformations or to individual defects.

A 1999 study used the population-based database of the Hungarian Case–Control Surveillance of Congenital Abnormalities (1980–1996) to evaluate the teratogenicity of oxacillin (3). The database contained 22,865 fetuses or newborns with congenital malformations and 38,151 matched control newborns without birth defects. The mothers of 14 cases (4 in the 1st trimester) and 19 controls (8 in the 1st trimester) were treated with oxacillin during pregnancy. No associations were discovered based on a comparison with the expected rates in 24 congenital anomaly groups (3).

An interaction between oxacillin and oral contraceptives resulting in pregnancy has been reported (4). Other penicillins (e.g., see Ampicillin) have been suspected of this interaction, but not all investigators believe that it occurs. Although controversial, an alternate means of contraception may be a practical solution if both drugs are consumed at the same time.

BREASTFEEDING SUMMARY

Oxacillin is excreted in breast milk in low concentrations (1). Although no adverse effects have been reported, three potential problems exist for the nursing infant: modification of bowel flora, direct effects on the infant (e.g., allergic response), and interference with the interpretation of culture results if a fever workup is required.

References

1. Prigot A, Froix C, Rubin E. Absorption, diffusion, and excretion of new penicillin, oxacillin. Antimicrob Agents Chemother 1962:402–10.
2. Heinonen OP, Slone D, Shapiro S. *Birth Defects and Drugs in Pregnancy*. Littleton, MA: Publishing Sciences Group, 1977.
3. Czeizel AE, Rockenbauer M, Sorensen HT, Olsen J. Teratogenic evaluation of oxacillin. Scan J Infect Dis 1999;31:311–2.
4. Silber TJ. Apparent oral contraceptive failure associated with antibiotic administration. J Adolesc Health Care 1983;4:287–9.

OXALIPLATIN

Antineoplastic

PREGNANCY RECOMMENDATION: Contraindicated (1st Trimester)
BREASTFEEDING RECOMMENDATION: Contraindicated

PREGNANCY SUMMARY

The human pregnancy experience is limited and the animal data in one species suggest risk. Although two infants exposed in utero had no complications attributable to oxaliplatin, both were exposed only in the 2nd and 3rd trimesters. Exposure during organogenesis and/or in any portion of the 1st trimester has the potential for causing embryo–fetal harm and should be avoided.

FETAL RISK SUMMARY

Oxaliplatin is indicated, in combination with infusional fluorouracil/leucovorin (5-FU/LV), for the treatment of patients with metastatic carcinoma of the colon or rectum whose disease has recurred or progressed during or within 6 months of completion of first-line therapy with the combination of 5-FU/LV and irinotecan. The drug undergoes rapid and extensive nonenzymatic biotransformation to several reactive oxaliplatin derivatives. Preceded by two relatively short distribution phases (0.43 and 16.8 hours), the terminal elimination half-life is 391 hours (about 16 days). Following a 2-hour infusion, only about 15% of the dose is in the systemic circulation, with the remaining 85% in tissues or eliminated in the urine. Plasma protein binding (>90%) primarily to albumin and γ-globulins is irreversible (1).

Reproduction studies have been conducted in rats. In this species, a dose <0.1 times the recommended human dose based on BSA (RHD) given before implantation and before and during organogenesis was associated with early resorptions, decreased body weight, and delayed ossification (1).

Long-term carcinogenicity studies have not been conducted. The drug was mutagenic and clastogenic in animal and human assays. A dose <1/7th the RHD in male and female rats did not affect pregnancy rates, but did cause increased early resorptions, decreased live fetuses, decreased live births, and decreased fetal weight. In dogs, a dose about 1/6th the RHD given for 5 days every 28 days for three cycles caused testicular damage (characterized by degeneration, hypoplasia, and atrophy) (1).

It is not known if oxaliplatin or any of its reactive derivatives cross the human placenta. The molecular weight of oxaliplatin (about 397 and about 309 without the oxalate ligand) and the long terminal half-life suggest that the parent drug and/or its derivatives will cross to the embryo–fetus. However, the relatively small amount of the dose in the systemic circulation and the irreversible binding to albumin and γ-globulins should limit the amount transferred.

A 2009 case report described the use of oxaliplatin at 20 weeks' gestation in a 25-year-old woman with metastatic rectal cancer (2). Therapy involved a modified FOLFOX-6 regimen consisting of oxaliplatin 85 mg/m^2 and leucovorin 400 mg/m^2, and 5-fluorouracil 400 mg/m^2 bolus followed by a 5-fluorouracil 2400 mg/m^2 46-hour infusion given biweekly. After six biweekly courses, the woman gave birth vaginally at 33.6 weeks' gestation to a normal, about 2440-g (5 pounds, 6 ounces), female infant with Apgar scores of 8 and 8 at 1 and 5 minutes, respectively. At 3.5 years of age, the child was growing normally with her height and weight at the 60th and 45th percentile, respectively (2).

A 40-year-old woman (gravida 4, para 3) was diagnosed at 23 weeks' gestation with advanced metastatic colorectal cancer (3). At 27 weeks', treatment was begun with the same FOLFOX-6 regimen described above at 2-week intervals except that the oxaliplatin dose was 100 mg/m^2. The woman received four treatments before a planned cesarean section was performed at 31.5 weeks' to give birth to a small-for-gestational-age 1175-g female infant. In addition to the typical complications associated with prematurity, the infant also was hypothyroid. At 11.75 months of age, the infant's height, weight, and head circumference were at the 50th, 80th, and 90th percentiles (corrected for prematurity), respectively. The infant had a flaky red spot on the top of her head but no other abnormalities. Except for gastroesophageal reflux (treated with lansoprazole) and hypothyroidism (treated with levothyroxine), the infant was developing normally (3).

BREASTFEEDING SUMMARY

No reports describing the use of oxaliplatin during human lactation have been located. The molecular weight of oxaliplatin (about 397 and about 309 without the oxalate ligand) and the long terminal half-life (391 hours) suggest that the parent drug and/or its derivatives will be excreted into breast milk. However, the relatively small amount of a dose in the systemic circulation and the irreversible binding to albumin and γ-globulins should limit the amount excreted. The effect of the potential exposure on a nursing infant is not known. However, the safest course for the infant is to not breastfeed if the mother is receiving this antineoplastic.

References

1. Product information. Eloxatin. Sanofi-Synthelabo, 2002.
2. Gensheimer M, Jones CA, Graves CR, Merchant NB, Lockhart AC. Administration of oxaliplatin to a pregnant woman with rectal cancer. Cancer Chemother Pharmacol 2009;63:371.
3. Kanate AS, Auber ML, Higa GM. Priorities and uncertainties of administering chemotherapy in a pregnant woman with newly diagnosed colorectal cancer. J Oncol Pharm Pract 2009;15:5–8.

OXAPROZIN

Nonsteroidal Anti-inflammatory

PREGNANCY RECOMMENDATION: Human Data Suggest Risk in 1st and 3rd Trimesters
BREASTFEEDING RECOMMENDATION: No Human Data—Potential Toxicity

PREGNANCY SUMMARY

Constriction of the ductus arteriosus in utero is a pharmacologic consequence arising from the use of prostaglandin synthesis inhibitors during pregnancy, as is inhibition of labor, prolongation of pregnancy, and suppression of fetal renal function (see also Indomethacin) (1). Persistent pulmonary hypertension of the newborn may occur if these agents are used in the 3rd trimester close to delivery (1,2). Women attempting to conceive should not use any prostaglandin synthesis inhibitor, including oxaprozin, because of the findings in a variety of animal models that indicate these agents block blastocyst implantation (3,4). Moreover, as noted below, nonsteroidal anti-inflammatory drugs (NSAIDs) have been associated with spontaneous abortions (SABs) and congenital malformations. The absolute risk for these defects, however, appears to be low.

FETAL RISK SUMMARY

Oxaprozin is an NSAID used in the treatment of acute and chronic arthritis. It is in the same subclass (propionic acids) as five other NSAIDs (fenoprofen, flurbiprofen, ibuprofen, ketoprofen, and naproxen).

The drug produced infrequent congenital malformations in rabbits treated with doses in the usual human range, but not in mice and rats (5). No teratogenic effects were observed in two other studies of pregnant rats and rabbits (6–9). A dose-dependent constriction of the ductus arteriosus, similar to that produced by other nonsteroidal anti-inflammatory agents, was observed in fetal rats (9).

It is not known if oxaprozin crosses the human placenta. The molecular weight (about 293) is low enough that passage to the fetus should be expected.

A combined 2001 population-based observational cohort study and a case–control study estimated the risk of adverse pregnancy outcome from the use of NSAIDs (10). The use of NSAIDs during pregnancy was not associated with congenital malformations, preterm delivery, or low birth weight, but a positive association was discovered with SABs. A similar study, also published in 2001, failed to find a relationship, in general, between NSAIDs and congenital malformations, but did find a significant association with cardiac defects and orofacial clefts (11). In addition, a 2003 study found a significant association between exposure to NSAIDs in early pregnancy and SABs (12). (See Ibuprofen for details on these three studies.)

A brief 2003 editorial on the potential for NSAID-induced developmental toxicity concluded that NSAIDs, and specifically those with greater COX-2 affinity, had a lower risk of this toxicity in humans than aspirin (13).

BREASTFEEDING SUMMARY

No reports describing the use of oxaprozin during human lactation have been located. The molecular weight (about 293) is low enough that excretion into breast milk should be expected. One reviewer listed several NSAIDs (diclofenac, fenoprofen, flurbiprofen, ibuprofen, ketoprofen, ketorolac, and tolmetin) that were considered safer alternatives to other agents (oxaprozin not mentioned) if a NSAID was required while nursing (14). Because of the long terminal elimination half-life (approximately 42 hours or longer) in adults and the unknown amount of oxaprozin that is excreted into milk, any of these choices is probably preferable.

References

1. Levin DL. Effects of inhibition of prostaglandin synthesis on fetal development, oxygenation, and the fetal circulation. Semin Perinatol 1980;4:35–44.

2. Van Marter LJ, Leviton A, Allred EN, Pagano M, Sullivan KF, Cohen A, Epstein MF. Persistent pulmonary hypertension of the newborn and smoking and aspirin and nonsteroidal antiinflammatory drug consumption during pregnancy. Pediatrics 1996;97:658–63.
3. Matt DW, Borzelleca JF. Toxic effects on the female reproductive system during pregnancy, parturition, and lactation. In: Witorsch RJ, ed. *Reproductive Toxicology*. 2nd ed. New York, NY: Raven Press, 1995:175–93.
4. Dawood MY. Nonsteroidal antiinflammatory drugs and reproduction. Am J Obstet Gynecol 1993;169:1255–65.
5. Product information. Daypro. G.D. Searle, 2001.
6. Yamada T, Nishiyama T, Sasajima M, Nakane S. Reproduction studies of oxaprozin in the rat and rabbit. Iyakuhin Kenkyu 1984;15:207–92. As cited in Shepard TH. *Catalog of Teratogenic Agents*. 7th ed. Baltimore, MD: The Johns Hopkins University Press, 1992:299–300.
7. Yamada T, Norariya T, Sasajima M, Nakane S. Reproduction studies of oxaprozin. II. Teratology study in rats. Iyakuhin Kenkyu 1984;15:225–49. As cited in Schardein JL. *Chemically Induced Birth Defects*. 2nd ed. New York, NY: Marcel Dekker, 1993:132–3.
8. Yamada T, Uchida H, Sasajima M, Nakane S. Reproduction studies of oxaprozin. III. Teratogenicity study in rabbits. Iyakuhin Kenkyu 1984;15: 250–64. As cited in Schardein JL. *Chemically Induced Birth Defects*. 2nd ed. New York, NY: Marcel Dekker, 1993:132–3.
9. Yamada T, Inoue T, Hara M, Ohba Y, Nakame S, Uchida H. Reproductive studies of oxaprozin and studies on the fetal ductus arteriosus. Clin Report 1984;18:514–25, 528–36. As cited in Shepard TH. *Catalog of Teratogenic Agents*. 7th ed. Baltimore, MD: The Johns Hopkins University Press, 1992:299–300.
10. Nielsen GL, Sorensen HT, Larsen H, Pedersen L. Risk of adverse birth outcome and miscarriage in pregnant users of non-steroidal anti-inflammatory drugs: population based observational study and case-control study. Br Med J 2001;322:266–70.
11. Ericson A, Kallen BAJ. Nonsteroidal anti-inflammatory drugs in early pregnancy. Reprod Toxicol 2001;15:371–5.
12. Li DK, Liu L, Odouli R. Exposure to non-steroidal anti-inflammatory drugs during pregnancy and risk of miscarriage: population based cohort study. Br Med J 2003;327:368–71.
13. Tassinari MS, Cook JC, Hurtt ME. NSAIDs and developmental toxicity. Birth Defects Res (Part B) 2003;68:3–4.
14. Anderson PO. Medication use while breast feeding a neonate. Neonatal Pharmacol Q 1993;2:3–14.

OXAZEPAM

Sedative

PREGNANCY RECOMMENDATION: Human Data Suggest Risk in 1st and 3rd Trimesters
BREASTFEEDING RECOMMENDATION: No Human Data—Potential Toxicity

PREGNANCY SUMMARY

The effects of benzodiazepines, including oxazepam, on the human embryo and fetus are controversial. Although a number of studies have reported an association with various types of congenital defects including the study below, other studies with this class of drugs have not found such associations. Maternal denial of exposure and the concurrent exposure to other toxic drugs and substances (e.g., alcohol and smoking) may be confounding factors. Continuous use during gestation or close to delivery might result in neonatal withdrawal or a dose-related syndrome similar to that observed with diazepam. The safest course is to avoid oxazepam during gestation. (See Diazepam.)

FETAL RISK SUMMARY

Oxazepam is an active metabolite of diazepam (see also Diazepam). It is a member of the benzodiazepine group. The drug, both free and conjugated forms, crosses the placenta achieving average cord:maternal serum ratios of 0.6 during the 2nd trimester and 1.1 at term (1). Large variations between patients for placental transfer have been observed (1–3). Passage of oxazepam is slower than that of diazepam, but the clinical significance of this is unknown (4). Two reports have suggested that the use of oxazepam in preeclampsia would be safer for the newborn infant than diazepam (5,6). However, it is doubtful whether either drug is indicated for this condition.

A 1989 report described characteristic dysmorphic features, growth restriction, and central nervous system defects in eight infants exposed either to oxazepam (≥75 mg/day) or diazepam (≥30 mg/day) (7) (see Diazepam for a detailed description of the infants). The authors concluded that the clinical characteristics observed in the infants probably represented a teratogenic syndrome related to benzodiazepines (7).

BREASTFEEDING SUMMARY

Specific data relating to oxazepam use in lactating women have not been located. Oxazepam, an active metabolite of diazepam, was detected in the urine of an infant exposed to high doses of diazepam during lactation (8). The infant was lethargic and demonstrated an electroencephalographic pattern compatible with sedative medication (see Diazepam).

References

1. Kangas L, Erkkola R, Kanto J, Eronen M. Transfer of free and conjugated oxazepam across the human placenta. Eur J Clin Pharmacol 1980;17: 301–4.
2. Kanto J, Erkkola R, Sellman R. Perinatal metabolism of diazepam. Br Med J 1974;1:641–2.
3. Mandelli M, Morselli PL, Nordio S, Pardi G, Principi N, Seveni F, Tognoni G. Placental transfer of diazepam and its disposition in the newborn. Clin Pharmacol Ther 1975;17:564–72.
4. Kanto JH. Use of benzodiazepines during pregnancy, labour and lactation, with particular reference to pharmacokinetic considerations. Drugs 1982;23:354–80.
5. Gillberg C. "Floppy infant syndrome" and maternal diazepam. Lancet 1977;2:612–3.
6. Drury KAD, Spalding E, Donaldson D, Rutherford D. Floppy-infant syndrome: Is oxazepam the answer? Lancet 1977;2:1126–7.
7. Laegreid L, Olegard R, Walstrom J, Conradi N. Teratogenic effects of benzodiazepine use during pregnancy. J Pediatr 1989;114:126–31.
8. Patrick MJ, Tilstone WJ, Reavey P. Diazepam and breast-feeding. Br Med J 1972;1:542–3.

OXCARBAZEPINE

Anticonvulsant

PREGNANCY RECOMMENDATION: Limited Human Data—Animal Data Suggest Risk
BREASTFEEDING RECOMMENDATION: Limited Human Data—Probably Compatible

PREGNANCY SUMMARY

Oxcarbazepine is embryo and fetal toxic and teratogenic in some animal species. Mild facial defects have been observed with oxcarbazepine and, a closely related agent carbamazepine has been associated with neural tube defects and minor craniofacial malformations (see Carbamazepine). The human data are too limited to assess the risk to the embryo–fetus. The effect of oxcarbazepine on folic acid levels or metabolism is unknown (1). Until this information is available, the safest course is to give folic acid supplementation with oxcarbazepine, as is done with other antiepileptic agents. In addition, metabolism of oxcarbazepine does not result in epoxide metabolites (1–3). Because these intermediate arene oxide metabolites have been associated with teratogenicity (see Carbamazepine, Phenytoin, and Valproic Acid), this may indicate a lower risk of teratogenicity with oxcarbazepine compared with the other agents.

FETAL RISK SUMMARY

Oxcarbazepine is an orally active anticonvulsant agent used as either monotherapy or adjunctive therapy in the treatment of partial seizures. The chemical structure of oxcarbazepine is closely related to that of another anticonvulsant, carbamazepine. Oxcarbazepine is rapidly metabolized to an active 10-monohydroxy metabolite (10-hydroxy-10,11-dihydrocarbamazepine; MHD) that is primarily responsible for the anticonvulsant activity (4).

In fertility studies with the active metabolite MHD, an oral dose, 2 times the maximum recommended human dose based on BSA (MRHD) administered to rats before and during mating and during early gestation caused disruption of the estrous cyclicity and a reduction in the numbers of corpora lutea, implantations, and live embryos. In pregnant rats, the administration of oral oxcarbazepine during organogenesis, at doses approximately 1.2 and 4 times the MRHD, caused increased incidences of fetal malformations (craniofacial, cardiovascular, and skeletal) and variations. Developmental toxicity (embryo–fetal death and growth restriction) was observed with oxcarbazepine at 4 times the MRHD. Oxcarbazepine (0.6 times the MRHD) or its active metabolite (equal to the MRHD) given during the latter part of gestation and throughout lactation were associated with persistent reductions in offspring body weights and, in the case of oxcarbazepine, altered behavior (decreased activity). Embryo and fetal death but no birth defects were observed in rabbits given oral doses of the active metabolite (1.5 times the MRHD) during organogenesis (4).

In a strain of mice susceptible to the teratogenic effects of carbamazepine, the highest tolerable oral dose of oxcarbazepine (1100 mg/kg/day) produced a lower incidence of teratogenicity (8% vs. 5% in controls; *ns*) than the epoxide metabolite of carbamazepine (14%–27% vs. 6% in controls; $p < 0.05$). Concurrent treatment with phenobarbital did not increase the incidence of congenital malformations over that observed with oxcarbazepine alone (5).

In agreement with the molecular weight (about 252) of the parent drug, oxcarbazepine and its metabolite have been found in the fetus (2,6). In a woman who was taking oxcarbazepine monotherapy (300 mg 3 times daily) throughout gestation, maternal and term newborn plasma concentrations of the drug and its metabolite MHD were approximately equal (6). The healthy 3700-g female infant had mild facial dysmorphism with a discrete epicanthus and a broad nasal bridge. Her development at 13 months of age was normal without signs of mental retardation or neurologic deficit.

In three women taking oxcarbazepine (600–1800 mg/day; time of last dose not specified), maternal and cord blood were obtained at delivery and analyzed for the parent drug, active metabolite MHD, and the inactive metabolite of MHD (2). The three agents were detected in all samples. In another part of the study, oxcarbazepine was metabolized to MHD in a dual recirculating human placental perfusion system, suggesting that the same metabolic process occurs in vivo. MHD, however, was not metabolized to the inactive metabolite by the placenta. No placental metabolism of carbamazepine was observed in the perfusion system (2).

The author of a 1994 report very briefly reviewed the pregnancy outcomes of 27 women treated with oxcarbazepine (7). The outcomes included 1 infant born with "some dysmorphic features" (which disappeared later in life), 3 spontaneous abortions (SABs), 1 infant with spina bifida (whose mother also received valproate), 1 newborn with "amniotic bands," and 22 normal infants (including 1 set of twins).

A 1996 review discussed the effects of oxcarbazepine and other anticonvulsants (1). Compared with carbamazepine, oxcarbazepine causes less induction of the cytochrome P450 enzyme system. However, oxcarbazepine may compromise the efficacy of hormonal contraception. The outcomes of 12 pregnancies treated with oxcarbazepine (3 SABs and 9 normal newborns) were listed without further details (1).

The Lamotrigine Pregnancy Registry, an ongoing project conducted by the manufacturer, was first published in January 1997 (8). The final report was published in July 2010. The Registry is now closed. Among 34 prospectively enrolled pregnancies exposed to oxcarbazepine and lamotrigine, with or without other anticonvulsants, 31 were exposed in the 1st trimester resulting in 27 live births without defects, 2 SABs, and 2 birth defects. There were three exposures in the 2nd/3rd trimesters resulting in live births without defects (8).

A 2006 review of prophylactic therapy of bipolar disorder briefly described the effects in pregnancy and breastfeeding of a number of drugs, including oxcarbazepine (9). Untreated pregnant and nursing women with the disorder are at an increased risk of poor obstetrical outcomes and relapse of affective symptoms. Although the limited data prevented conclusions on the relative safety of the drugs, the author did state that each case needed to be considered separately (9).

BREASTFEEDING SUMMARY

Only one published report describing the use of oxcarbazepine during human lactation has been located. In a woman who took oxcarbazepine (900 mg/day) throughout gestation and during lactation (see case discussion above), the milk:plasma ratios of the drug and its active metabolite MHD were 0.5 (6). No adverse effects in the nursing infant from the exposure were mentioned. The manufacturer also states that the milk:plasma ratio for both agents is 0.5 (4). Nursing infants should be monitored for poor suckling, vomiting, and sedation (10). However, because the American Academy of Pediatrics classifies carbamazepine as compatible with breastfeeding (see Carbamazepine), oxcarbazepine can probably be similarly classified.

References

1. Morrell MJ. The new antiepileptic drugs and women: efficacy, reproductive health, pregnancy, and fetal outcome. Epilepsia 1996;37(Suppl 6): S34–44.
2. Pienimaki P, Lampela E, Hakkola J, Arvela P, Raunio H, Vahakangas K. Pharmacokinetics of oxcarbazepine and carbamazepine in human placenta. Epilepsia 1997;38:309–16.
3. Grant SM, Faulds D. Oxcarbazepine. A review of its pharmacology and therapeutic potential in epilepsy, trigeminal neuralgia and affective disorders. Drugs 1992;43:873–88.
4. Product information. Trileptal. Novartis Pharmaceuticals, 2001.
5. Bennett GD, Amore BM, Finnell RH, Wlodarczyk B, Kalhorn TF, Skiles GL, Nelson SD, Slattery JT. Teratogenicity of carbamazepine-10,11-epoxide and oxcarbazepine in the SWV mouse. J Pharmacol Exp Ther 1996;279: 1237–42.
6. Bulau P, Paar WD, von Unruh GE. Pharmacokinetics of oxcarbazepine and 10-hydroxy-carbazepine in the newborn child of an oxcarbazepine-treated mother. Eur J Clin Pharmacol 1988;34:311–3.
7. Andermann E. Pregnancy and oxcarbazepine. Epilepsia 1994;35 (Suppl 3):S26.
8. The Lamotrigine Pregnancy Registry. Final Report. 1 September 1992 through 31 March 2010. GlaxoSmithKline, July 2010.
9. Gentile S. Prophylactic treatment of bipolar disorder in pregnancy and breastfeeding: focus on emerging mood stabilizers. Bipolar Disord 2006;8:207–20.
10. Bar-Oz, B, Nulman I, Koren G, Ito S. Anticonvulsants and breast feeding—a critical review. Paediatr Drugs 2000;2:113–26.

OXICONAZOLE

Antifungal

PREGNANCY RECOMMENDATION: No Human Data—Probably Compatible
BREASTFEEDING RECOMMENDATION: No Human Data—Probably Compatible

O

PREGNANCY SUMMARY

No reports describing the use of oxiconazole in human pregnancy have been located. The drug is used topically and the systemic bioavailability is minimal. The animal reproduction data suggest that the risk to the embryo or fetus is low. Moreover, there is no evidence suggesting that similar topical imidazole derivative antifungal agents cause embryo–fetal harm, and there is no reason to believe that oxiconazole would be different.

FETAL RISK SUMMARY

Oxiconazole is available for topical use as a cream or lotion. It is in the same antifungal class of imidazole derivatives as butoconazole, clotrimazole, econazole, ketoconazole, miconazole, sertaconazole, sulconazole, and tioconazole. Oxiconazole is indicated for the treatment of tinea pedis, tinea cruris, and tinea corporis due to *Trichophyton rubrum*, *T. mentagrophytes*, or *Epidermophyton floccosum*. The cream also is indicated for the treatment of tinea (pityriasis) versicolor due to *Malassezia furfur*. Neither the cream nor the lotion should be applied intravaginally. Systemic absorption from the skin is low, with <0.3% of the applied dose recovered in the urine of healthy adults (1). Information regarding the metabolism, plasma protein binding, and elimination half-life has not been located.

Reproduction studies with orally administered oxiconazole have been conducted in pregnant mice, rats, and rabbits. No evidence of fetal harm was observed in these species at doses that were 27, 40, and 57 times, respectively, the human dose based on BSA (1).

Studies evaluating the carcinogenic potential of oxiconazole have not been conducted by the manufacturer. No evidence of mutagenicity was found in multiple assays. In female and male rats, oral doses that were 1 and 4 times, respectively, the human dose based on BSA did not impair fertility. At higher doses, there was a decrease in fertility parameters in both females and males, decreased number of sperm in vaginal smears, extended estrous cycle, and a decrease in mating frequency (1).

It is not known if oxiconazole crosses the human placenta. The molecular weight (about 492) is low enough for passage, but the minimal systemic bioavailability suggests that exposure of the embryo or fetus is clinically insignificant.

BREASTFEEDING SUMMARY

No reports describing the use of oxiconazole during human lactation have been located. The molecular weight (about 492) is low enough for excretion into breast milk, but the minimal systemic bioavailability suggests that exposure of the nursing infant would be clinically insignificant.

Reference

1. Product information. Oxistat. PharmaDerm, 2008.

OXPRENOLOL

[Withdrawn from the market. See 9th edition.]

OXTRIPHYLLINE

[Withdrawn from the market. See 9th edition.]

OXYBUTYNIN

Urinary Tract Agent (Antispasmodic)

PREGNANCY RECOMMENDATION: Limited Human Data—Animal Data Suggest Low Risk
BREASTFEEDING RECOMMENDATION: No Human Data—Probably Compatible

PREGNANCY SUMMARY

One report described the use of oxybutynin throughout pregnancy. The drug is a tertiary amine that is a direct inhibitor of smooth muscle spasm of the urinary tract. It also possesses antimuscarinic activity (about one-fifth of the anticholinergic activity of atropine). Oxybutynin is used for the relief of symptoms associated with bladder instability and nocturnal enuresis. It is in the same subclass as darifenacin, flavoxate, solifenacin, tolterodine, and trospium.

FETAL RISK SUMMARY

Reproduction studies in the hamster, mouse, rat, and rabbit have not demonstrated definite evidence of impaired fertility or fetal harm (1–3). No fetal harm was noted in female rats dosed orally with oxybutynin, 20–160 mg/kg/day (maximum recommended human dose is 20 mg/day or less than 0.5 mg/kg/day for an average adult) (4).

It is not known if the drug crosses the placenta to the fetus. The molecular weight (about 358 for the free base) is low enough that exposure of the embryo–fetus should be expected.

A 2001 case report described a paraplegic woman who had used baclofen 80 mg/day (*the maximum recommended daily oral dose*), oxybutynin 9 mg/day, and trimethoprim 100 mg/day throughout an uneventful pregnancy (5). The fetus developed tachycardia at an unspecified gestational age and an apparently healthy female infant was delivered (birth weight not given). Apgar scores were 10 at 1 and 5 minutes. At 7 days of age, the infant was admitted to the hospital for generalized seizures, but the mother had noted abnormal movements 2 days after birth. All diagnostic test results were negative and the seizures did not respond to phenytoin, phenobarbital, clonazepam, lidocaine, or pyridoxine. Because seizures had been reported in adults after abrupt withdrawal of baclofen, a dose of 1 mg/kg divided into four daily doses was started and the seizures stopped 30 minutes after the first dose. Baclofen was slowly tapered and then discontinued after 2 weeks. Magnetic resonance imaging of the infant's brain on day 17 suggested a short hypoxic ischemic insult that was thought to have been secondary to the seizures (5).

BREASTFEEDING SUMMARY

No reports describing the use of oxybutynin during human lactation have been located. The molecular weight (about 358 for the free base) is low enough that excretion into milk should be expected. The effect of this exposure on a nursing infant is unknown. However, other anticholinergics are classified by the American Academy of Pediatrics as compatible with breastfeeding (see Atropine and Scopolamine).

References

1. Product information. Ditropan. ALZA Pharmaceuticals, 2000.
2. Schardein JL. *Chemically Induced Birth Defects*. 2nd ed. New York, NY: Marcel Dekker, 1993:645.
3. Edwards JA, Reid YJ, Cozens DD. Reproductive toxicity studies with oxybutynin hydrochloride. Toxicology 1986;40:31–44.
4. Department of Research and Development, Marion Laboratories. *A Compendium. Ditropan. A New Urinary Tract Antispasmodic*. Kansas City, MO: Marian Laboratories, 1975:16.
5. Ratnayaka BDM, Dhaliwal H, Watkin S. Neonatal convulsions after withdrawal of baclofen. BMJ 2001;323:85.

OXYCODONE

Narcotic Agonist Analgesic

PREGNANCY RECOMMENDATION: Human Data Suggest Risk
BREASTFEEDING RECOMMENDATION: Limited Human Data—Potential Toxicity

PREGNANCY SUMMARY

The National Birth Defects Prevention Study discussed below found evidence that opioid use during organogenesis is associated with a low absolute risk of congenital birth defects. Use for prolonged periods or in high doses at term has the potential to cause withdrawal or respiratory depression in the newborn.

FETAL RISK SUMMARY

Oxycodone is a narcotic analgesic available as a single agent or in combination with nonnarcotic analgesics, such as acetaminophen or aspirin. The drug is rapidly metabolized in the liver to noroxycodone (weakly active), oxymorphone (active), and their glucuronides. Plasma protein binding is about 45%. The elimination half-lives of the extended-release and immediate-release formulations are 4.5 and 3.2 hours, respectively (1).

Reproduction studies in rats and rabbits at doses up to 3 and 46 times the human dose of 160 mg/day based on BSA, respectively, found no evidence of fetal harm (1).

The Collaborative Perinatal Project monitored 50,282 mother–child pairs, 8 of whom had 1st trimester exposure to oxycodone (2). No evidence was found to suggest a relationship to large categories of major or minor malformations or to individual defects.

In a surveillance study of Michigan Medicaid recipients involving 229,101 completed pregnancies conducted between 1985 and 1992, 281 newborns had been exposed to oxycodone during the 1st trimester (F. Rosa, personal communication, FDA, 1993). A total of 13 (4.6%) major birth defects were observed (12 expected), including (observed/expected) 3/3 cardiovascular defects and 1/1 hypospadias. No anomalies were observed in four other defect categories (oral clefts, spina bifida, polydactyly, and limb reduction defects) for which specific data were available. These data do not support an association between the drug and congenital defects.

At a 1996 meeting, data were presented on 118 women using oxycodone ($N = 78$) or hydrocodone ($N = 40$) during the 1st trimester for postoperative pain, general pain, or upper respiratory infection who were matched with a similar group using codeine for these purposes (3). Six (5.1%) of the infants exposed to oxycodone or hydrocodone had malformations, an odds ratio of 2.61 (95% confidence interval 0.6–11.5, $p = 0.13$). There was no pattern evident among the six malformations (3).

A 26-year-old woman with chronic pain and depression took oxycodone 60 mg/day, quetiapine 400 mg/day, and fluoxetine 40 mg/day throughout pregnancy (4). She gave birth at 37 weeks' gestation to an apparently normal 3.4-kg (50th percentile) male infant, and then continued these drugs during breastfeeding. The infant's weight at 3 months of age was 5.6 kg (25th percentile), but the Denver development assessment was consistent with his chronological age (4).

Neonatal withdrawal associated with maternal use of oxycodone has been reported (5,6). A 37-year-old woman underwent a cesarean section to give birth to a normal 3685-g female infant with Apgar scores of 8 and 9 (5). The infant was excessively irritable during the first 48 hours but did not require any therapeutic intervention. When the mother suffered an acute abstinence syndrome after delivery, it was discovered that she had taken Percodan (oxycodone + aspirin) daily throughout pregnancy (5). The second case involved a 24-year-old woman who had used IV oxycodone (120–500 mg/day) and oral methadone during pregnancy (6). At 39 weeks', she gave birth to a 2864-g (>25th percentile) male infant, Apgar scores 7 and 10, without structural anomalies. The infant's length (47 cm, <5th percentile) and head circumference (33 cm, <5th percentile) were restricted. The infant had a shrill cry at birth and developed severe neonatal abstinence syndrome. The infant's urine was positive for oxymorphone (a metabolite of oxycodone) but not for methadone. The infant was discharged to foster care on day 16 of life (6).

Results of a National Birth Defects Prevention Study (1997–2005) were published in 2011 (7). This population-based case–control study examined the association between maternal use of opioid analgesics and >30 types of major structural birth defects. In 17,449 case mothers, therapeutic opioid use was reported by 454 (2.6%) compared with 134 (2.0%) of 6701 control mothers. Indications for use of opioid analgesics were surgical procedures (41%), infections (34%), chronic diseases (20%), and injuries (18%). Dose, duration, and frequency were not evaluated. The exposure period evaluated was from 1 month before to 3 months after conception. Limiting the exposure period to the first 2 months after conception produced similar results. Infants with >1 defect were included in multiple birth defect categories. The following opioids were included (number of cases for each agent not specified): codeine, hydrocodone, hydromorphone, fentanyl, meperidine, methadone, morphine, oxycodone, pentazocine, propoxyphene, and tramadol. The birth defect, total number, number exposed, and the adjusted odds ratio (aOR) with 95% confidence interval (CI) were as follows:

Birth Defect	Total	Cases	aOR (95% CI)
Spina bifida	718	26	2.0 (1.3–3.2)
Any heart defect (20 types)	7724	211	1.4 (1.1–1.7)
Atrioventricular septal defect	175	9	2.4 (1.2–4.8)
Teratology of Fallot	672	21	1.7 (1.1–2.8)
Conotruncal defect	1481	41	1.5 (1.0–2.1)
Conoventricular septal defect	110	6	2.7 (1.1–6.3)
Left ventricular outflow tract obstruction defect	1195	36	1.5 (1.0–2.2)
Hypoplastic left heart syndrome	357	17	2.4 (1.4–4.1)
Right ventricular outflow tract obstruction defect	1175	40	1.6 (1.1–2.3)
Pulmonary valve stenosis	867	34	1.7 (1.2–2.6)
Atrial septal defect (ASD)	511	17	2.0 (1.2–3.6)
Ventricular septal defect + ASD	528	17	1.7 (1.0–2.9)
Hydrocephaly	301	11	2.0 (1.0–3.7)
Glaucoma/anterior chamber defects	103	5	2.6 (1.0–6.6)
Gastroschisis	726	26	1.8 (1.1–2.9)

The authors speculated that the activity of opioids and their receptors as growth regulators during development of the embryo might be a mechanism to explain the above findings. The exposure data were obtained by retrospective maternal self-report; the authors acknowledged that recall bias and misclassification might have affected their results. They concluded that the absolute risk was a modest absolute increase above the baseline risk for birth defects (7).

BREASTFEEDING SUMMARY

Oxycodone is excreted into breast milk. Six healthy postpartum women received a combination product of oxycodone and acetaminophen, one or two capsules every 4–7 hours, while breastfeeding their newborn infants (8). Maternal plasma levels were in the expected range of 14–35 ng/mL and milk concentrations ranged from <5 to 226 ng/mL. Peak milk concentrations occurred 1.5–2.0 hours after the first dose, and then at variable times after multiple doses. Although a large degree of variability was present, the mean milk:plasma ratio was 3.4:1. No mention was made of any effects observed in the nursing infants (8).

In a 2012 report, neonatal central nervous system (CNS) depression was assessed in three cohorts of breastfeeding mother–infant pairs exposed to oxycodone (N = 139), codeine (N = 210), or acetaminophen only (N = 184) (9). More infants had CNS depression with oxycodone (20.1%) compared with 0.5% in the acetaminophen cohort (20.1%; OR 46.16, 95% CI 6.2–344.2; $p < 0.0001$) and 16.7% in the codeine cohort (16.7%; OR 0.79, 95% CI 0.46-1.38; $p > 0.05$). In the oxycodone and codeine cohorts, mothers of infants with symptoms took significantly higher doses compared with mother of infants with no symptoms in the same cohorts: oxycodone—median 0.4 mg/kg/day (range 0.03–4.06 mg/kg/day) vs. median 0.15 mg/kg/day (range 0.02–2.25 mg/kg/day); $p = 0.005$; codeine—median 1.4 mg/kg/day (range 0.7–10.5 mg/kg/day) vs. median 0.9 mg/kg/day (range 0.18–5.8 mg/kg/day); $p \leq 0.001$. In addition, significantly more mothers in the oxycodone cohort had sedation compared with the codeine cohort. Based on these results, the authors concluded that oxycodone was not a safer alternative to codeine in breastfed infants (9).

If a mother is receiving oxycodone, her nursing infant should be monitored for sedation and other adverse effects, such as gastrointestinal effects and changes in feeding patterns.

References

1. Product information. Oxycontin. Endo Pharmaceuticals, 2004.
2. Heinonen OP, Slone D, Shapiro S. *Birth Defects and Drugs in Pregnancy*. Littleton, MA: Publishing Sciences Group, 1977:287.
3. Schick B, Hom M, Tolosa J, Librizzi R, Donnfeld A. *Preliminary Analysis of First Trimester Exposure to Oxycodone and Hydrocodone* (abstract). Presented at the Ninth International Conference of the Organization of Teratology Information Services, Salt Lake City, Utah, May 2–4, 1996. Reprod Toxicol 1996;10:162.
4. Rampono J, Kristensen JH, Ilett KF, Hackett LP, Kohan R. Quetiapine and breast feeding. Ann Pharmacother 2007;41:711–4.
5. Weintraub SJ, Naulty JS. Acute abstinence syndrome after epidural injection of butorphanol. Anesth Analg 1985;64:452–3.
6. Rao R, Desai NS. OxyContin and neonatal abstinence syndrome. J Perinatol 2002;22:324–5.
7. Broussard CS, Rasmussen SA, Reefhuis J, Friedman JM, Jann MW, Riehle-Colarusso T, Honein MA, for the National Birth Defects Prevention Study. Maternal treatment with opioid analgesics and risk for birth defects. Am J Obstet Gynecol 2011;204:314–7.
8. Marx CM, Pucino F, Carlson JD, Driscoll JW, Ruddock V. Oxycodone excretion in human milk in the puerperium (abstract). Drug Intell Clin Pharm 1986;20:474.
9. Lam J, Kelly L, Ciszkowski C, Landsmeer MLA, Nauta M, Carleton BC, Hayden MR, Madadi P, Koren G. Central nervous system depression of neonates breastfed by mothers receiving oxycodone for postpartum analgesia. J Pediatr 2012;160:33–7.

OXYMETAZOLINE

Sympathomimetic (Adrenergic)

PREGNANCY RECOMMENDATION: Limited Human Data—No Relevant Animal Data
BREASTFEEDING RECOMMENDATION: No Human Data—Probably Compatible

PREGNANCY SUMMARY

Oxymetazoline, an α-adrenergic agent, is a long-acting vasoconstrictor used topically in nasal decongestant sprays. No reports associating oxymetazoline with congenital abnormalities have been located.

FETAL RISK SUMMARY

The Collaborative Perinatal Project recorded only 2 cases of exposure from 50,282 mother–child pairs (1). Although there was no indication of risk for malformations, the number of women exposed is too small for any conclusion.

Uterine vessels are normally maximally dilated and have only α-adrenergic receptors (2). Use of the α-adrenergic agent, oxymetazoline, could cause constriction of these vessels and reduce uterine blood flow, thus producing fetal hypoxia and bradycardia. A 1985 case report illustrated this toxicity when a nonreactive nonstress test and a positive contraction stress test were discovered in a 20-year-old woman at 41 weeks' gestation (3). Persistent late fetal heart rate decelerations were observed, and blood obtained from the fetal scalp revealed a pH of 7.23. The mother had self-administered a nasal spray containing 0.05% oxymetazoline, two sprays in each nostril, 6 times in a 15.5-hour interval before the nonstress test with the last dose administered 0.5 hour before testing. The recommended dosage interval for the preparation was every 12 hours. Approximately 6 hours after the last dose, the late decelerations disappeared and the normal beat-to-beat variability returned about 0.5 hour later. A normal male infant with Apgar scores of 9 and 9 at 1 and 5 minutes, respectively, was spontaneously delivered 14 hours after the last dose.

In contrast to the above case, a 1990 report described the results of a single dose (two full squirts) of 0.05% oxymetazoline (4). The drug was self-administered by 12 women with allergic rhinitis, sinusitis, or an upper respiratory tract infection. The otherwise healthy women were between 27 and 39 weeks' gestation. The effects of this dose on the maternal and fetal circulations were measured at 15-minute intervals for 2 hours after the dose. No significant changes were observed for maternal blood pressures or pulse rates, fetal aortic blood flow velocity, and fetal heart rate, or for the systolic to diastolic ratios in the uterine arcuate artery and umbilical artery. The investigators concluded that oxymetazoline, when administered at the recommended frequency, did not pose a risk for the healthy patient. Women with borderline placental reserve, however, should use the agent cautiously (4).

BREASTFEEDING SUMMARY

No reports describing the use of oxymetazoline during human lactation have been located.

References

1. Heinonen OP, Slone D, Shapiro S. *Birth Defects and Drugs in Pregnancy*. Littleton, MA: Publishing Sciences Group, 1977:346.
2. Smith NT, Corbascio AN. The use and misuse of pressor agents. Anesthesiology 1970;33:58–101.
3. Baxi LV, Gindoff PR, Pregenzer GJ, Parras MK. Fetal heart rate changes following maternal administration of a nasal decongestant. Am J Obstet Gynecol 1985;153:799–800.
4. Rayburn WF, Anderson JC, Smith CV, Appel LL, Davis SA. Uterine and fetal Doppler flow changes from a single dose of a long-acting intranasal decongestant. Obstet Gynecol 1990;76:180–2.

O

OXYMORPHONE

Narcotic Agonist Analgesic

PREGNANCY RECOMMENDATION: Human Data Suggest Risk
BREASTFEEDING RECOMMENDATION: No Human Data—Potential Toxicity

PREGNANCY SUMMARY

Although oxymorphone was not included in a National Birth Defects Prevention Study, the use of other opioid agonists during organogenesis was associated with a low absolute risk of congenital birth defects (see Morphine). In addition, the use of any opioid agonist during labor or close to delivery may cause neonatal respiratory depression.

FETAL RISK SUMMARY

Oxymorphone is an opioid agonist that is available in both oral and injectable formulations. It is highly metabolized in the liver to active and inactive metabolites (1).

Reproduction studies have been conducted in rats, rabbits, and hamsters. Oxymorphone did not cause malformations in rats and rabbits at daily oral doses that were about 2 and 8 times, respectively, the total human daily oral dose of 120 mg based on BSA (THDD). Fetal weights were decreased in both species at doses that were about 0.8 and 4 times the THDD. In rats given the drug daily during gestation and postnatally at a dose that was about 2 times the THDD, there was an increase in stillborn pups and neonatal deaths, as well as low pup birth weight and a decrease in postnatal weight gain. In hamsters, a single SC dose that was about 10 times the THDD produced malformations in offspring but also produced 83% maternal death (1).

Although no studies have been found indicating that oxymorphone crosses the human placenta, the molecular weight (about 338) and experience with other opioid analgesics (e.g., see Morphine) indicates that the drug will rapidly cross to the embryo–fetus.

Use of oxymorphone during labor produces neonatal respiratory depression to the same degree as other narcotic analgesics (2–5).

BREASTFEEDING SUMMARY

No reports describing the use of oxymorphone during human lactation have been located. However, the molecular weight (about 338) and experience with other opioid analgesics (e.g., see Morphine) indicates that the drug will be excreted into breast milk. Although occasional maternal doses would probably not produce adverse effects in the nursing infant, higher doses and prolonged use could cause toxicity. Moreover, long-term effects on neurobehavior and development are unknown but warrant study.

References

1. Product information. Opana. Endo Pharmaceuticals, 2013.
2. Simeckova M, Shaw W, Pool E, Nichols EE. Numorphan in labor. A preliminary report. Obstet Gynecol 1960;16:119–23.
3. Sentnor MH, Solomons E, Kohl SG. An evaluation of oxymorphone in labor. Am J Obstet Gynecol 1962;84:956–61.
4. Eames GM, Pool KRS. Clinical trial of oxymorphone in labor. Br Med J 1964; 2:353–5.
5. Ransom S. Oxymorphone as an obstetric analgesic. A clinical trial. Anesthesia 1966;21:464–71.

OXYPHENBUTAZONE

Nonsteroidal Anti-inflammatory

See Phenylbutazone.

OXYPHENCYCLIMINE

[Withdrawn from the market. See 9th edition.]

OXYPHENONIUM

[Withdrawn from the market. See 9th edition.]

OXYTETRACYCLINE

Antibiotic (Tetracycline)

See Tetracycline.

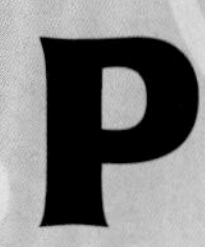

P

PACLITAXEL

Antineoplastic

PREGNANCY RECOMMENDATION: Limited Human Data—Animal Data Suggest Risk
BREASTFEEDING RECOMMENDATION: Contraindicated

PREGNANCY SUMMARY

Paclitaxel produces embryo–fetal toxicity, including teratogenicity, in animals. In addition, the drug was clastogenic with in vitro and in vivo tests. In animals, compared with the free drug, liposome encapsulation of paclitaxel appears to markedly increase the dose at which toxicity and teratogenicity are observed. Whether this also would occur in human pregnancy is not known. The human pregnancy experience is limited to use in the 2nd and 3rd trimesters. No fetal or newborn toxicity have been reported following this use. Based on the animal data, the use of paclitaxel during organogenesis should be avoided if possible. Use after this period appears to be relatively low risk, but the fetus should be monitored appropriately. (*See Carboplatin for additional data*.)

FETAL RISK SUMMARY

Paclitaxel, an antineoplastic agent, is indicated for the treatment of advanced ovarian cancer but also is used in other malignancies. The drug is a natural product obtained by extraction from *Taxus brevifolia* (Pacific yew tree) (1,2). Paclitaxel is an antimicrotubule agent, an action that results in the inhibition of the normal reorganization of the microtubule network that is essential for vital interphase and mitotic cellular functions. It is in the same subclass of taxoids as docetaxel and cabazitaxel. The pharmacokinetics of paclitaxel are markedly affected by the dose and infusion rate with elimination half-lives varying from approximately 13 to 53 hours. Approximately 89%–98% of the agent is protein bound (1). The free commercial form of paclitaxel contains the vehicle polyoxyethylated castor oil (also known as polyoxyl 35 castor oil) (1,2).

Reproduction studies in pregnant rabbits at doses about 0.2 times the maximum recommended human daily dose based on BSA (MRHDD) caused embryo and fetal toxicity (increased resorptions and intrauterine deaths). However, maternal toxicity was observed at this dose. No teratogenic effects were noted at a dose about 0.07 times the MRHDD, but the teratogenic potential of higher doses could not be assessed because of extensive fetal mortality (1).

The carcinogenic potential of paclitaxel has not been studied. The drug was not mutagenic in one test but was clastogenic in vitro (human lymphocytes) and in vivo (micronucleus test in mice). Fertility in male and female rats was impaired at doses about 0.04 times the MRHDD, and at this dose, increased embryo and fetal toxicity was observed (1).

Interestingly, a 1995 research report concluded that some, paclitaxel-induced, embryotoxicity in animals might be due to the polyoxyethylated castor oil vehicle (2). In an experiment with chick embryos, the researchers compared free paclitaxel containing the vehicle with liposome-encapsulated paclitaxel. At a dose of 1.5 mcg per egg, 60% of the embryos either died or were malformed. A 20-fold higher dose was required to produce the same degree of toxicity with the liposome-encapsulated product (2).

In a follow-up to the above study, the same group of researchers compared the developmental toxicity in rats of free and encapsulated paclitaxel (3). Free paclitaxel, at a dose of 10 mg/kg (approximately 0.4 times the MRHDD) given IV once on gestation day 8 (determined to be the most sensitive day for the production of paclitaxel-induced malformations), produced maternal toxicity and resorption of all embryos in surviving dams. At 2 mg/kg (about 0.08 times the MRHDD) of free paclitaxel, embryo–fetal toxicity (increased resorptions and reduced fetal weight) and anomalies (exencephaly, anencephaly, ventral wall defects, facial clefts, anophthalmia, diaphragmatic hernia, and malformations of the kidney, cardiovascular system, and tail) were observed (3). In contrast, no toxicity or anomalies were observed with a 2 mg/kg IV dose of encapsulated paclitaxel. At 10 mg/kg, toxicity and malformations were noted that were similar to those observed with the free drug at 2 mg/kg. Thus, encapsulation appeared to increase the dose needed to produce toxicity and malformations (3). However, encapsulation of paclitaxel could markedly increase or decrease the amount of drug crossing the placenta to the fetus. The authors of the study cited examples in perfused in vitro human placentas in which liposome encapsulation reduced placental transfer. In contrast, they also cited studies in intact rats and rabbits that have shown that encapsulation enhanced placental transfer, possibly by a process involving placental intracellular sequestration and degradation of liposomes (3).

Although the molecular weight (about 854) suggests that paclitaxel will cross the placenta, the extensive protein binding might limit the exposure of the embryo or fetus. Of interest, in an in vitro model, paclitaxel slowly crossed the human placenta to the fetal side (4).

In a novel case report, a 21-year-old woman was diagnosed with metastatic ovarian cancer that was initially treated with surgery that left her uterus, right fallopian tube, and ovary in situ (5). She was then enrolled into a phase I transplant protocol and received three cycles of paclitaxel (225 mg/m^2) and carboplatin (dose specified as AUC 6). Subsequent high-dose chemotherapy was then given (paclitaxel, carboplatin, and/or cyclophosphamide). After her chemotherapy, the woman received a successful transplant of autologous peripheral blood stem cells. Approximately 16 months after the transplant, she conceived but had a 1st trimester miscarriage. She conceived again several months later and eventually delivered a healthy full-term 3000-g female infant. The child was developing normally at 17 months of age (5).

A 33-year-old woman was diagnosed with ovarian carcinoma at 27 weeks' gestation (6). Six days after debulking surgery that preserved the pregnancy, she received the first cycle of paclitaxel (135 mg/m^2) over 24 hours and cisplatin (75 mg/m^2) over 4 hours. She received two more cycles of chemotherapy at 3-week intervals. Appropriate fetal growth was documented by ultrasound. Fetal lung maturity was demonstrated at 37 weeks' gestation and a cesarean section was performed to deliver a 2800-g female with Apgar scores of 9 and 10 at 1 and 5 minutes, respectively, and normal blood counts. The infant has had normal growth and development to 30 months of age (6).

A 2003 report described the pregnancy outcome of a 30-year-old woman treated with carboplatin and paclitaxel during the 2nd and 3rd trimesters (7). She was diagnosed with an advanced stage of serous papillary adenocarcinoma of the ovary in the 1st trimester. The woman underwent an exploratory laparotomy at 7.5 weeks' gestation and consented to chemotherapy beginning at 16–17 weeks. She received six cycles of carboplatin (dose specified as AUC 5) and paclitaxel (175 mg/m^2) and was delivered by cesarean hysterectomy 3 weeks after the last cycle, at 35.5 weeks. The newborn (sex not specified) had Apgar scores of 9, 9, and 9 at 1, 5, and 10 minutes, respectively. Birth weight was 2500 g (44th percentile), and the physical examination and laboratory tests were normal. In addition, the placenta appeared grossly normal. The infant was doing well at 15 months of age with no evidence of neurologic, renal, growth, or hematologic effects from the exposure (7).

In another 2003 report, a 36-year-old woman with breast cancer was treated with paclitaxel (175 mg/m^2 every 3 weeks for three cycles) and epirubicin (120 mg/m^2 every 3 weeks for four cycles) from the 14th to the 32nd week of pregnancy (8). At 36 weeks', she delivered by cesarean section a normal 2.280-kg female infant with a 5-minute Apgar score of 9. The child had normal development and growth at 36 months of age (8).

A 30-year-old woman became pregnant approximately 2 years after treatment of stage IIB fallopian tube carcinoma with paclitaxel and cisplatin (9). She was diagnosed with an asymptomatic intra-abdominal recurrence at 16 weeks' gestation but refused additional therapy. A 2888-g male infant was delivered by cesarean section at 37 weeks. No additional information about the infant was given (9).

A 38-year-old woman with breast cancer had been treated with a radical mastectomy followed by four cycles of doxorubicin and cyclophosphamide before pregnancy (10). Starting at about 21 weeks' gestation, she received 12 weekly cycles of paclitaxel (80 mg/m^2). At 37 weeks', she delivered by cesarean section a normal 2.45-kg male infant with Apgar scores of 9 at 1, 5, and 10 minutes. The infant's birth weight was at the 5th–10th percentile for gestational age. The infant had normal development and growth at 12 months of age (10).

A 2009 report described the use of paclitaxel (90 mg/m^2 on days 1, 8, and 15 of a 28-day cycle) for six cycles starting at 29 weeks' gestation for recurrent breast cancer (11). An elective cesarean section at 38 weeks' delivered a healthy infant (no other details were provided).

A 2007 report described the pregnancy outcome of 30-year-old woman with cervical cancer who was treated with paclitaxel (175 mg/m^2) and cisplatin (75 mg/m^2) at 19 weeks' gestation (12). Paclitaxel was discontinued after the first course because of a severe allergic reaction, but cisplatin was continued every 3 weeks until a cesarean section at 35 weeks'. The normal 2.400-kg female infant had Apgar scores of 7 and 9 at 1 and 5 minutes, respectively. The infant was doing well at 10 months of age (12).

Ovarian cancer was diagnosed in a 42-year-old woman at 18 weeks' gestation (13). Following surgery that preserved the pregnancy, she was treated with four courses of paclitaxel plus carboplatin (AUC 5) from 22 to 35 weeks'. A cesarean section delivered 2.600-kg male infant with Apgar scores of 9 at 1 and 5 minutes. The healthy infant was doing well at 6 months of age (13).

Another case involving the treatment of ovarian cancer with paclitaxel in pregnancy was reported in 2007 (14). Following diagnosis of the tumor at 25 weeks' gestation, the patient was treated with paclitaxel (175 mg/m^2) and carboplatin (AUC 5) every 3 weeks for 3 cycles with the last cycle during the 32nd gestational week. At 35 weeks', a cesarean section delivered a healthy 2.450-kg male infant with Apgar scores of 9, 10, and 10. At 20 months, the child continued to show no abnormalities (14).

A third case of ovarian cancer in pregnancy was treated with paclitaxel (120 mg/m^2) and carboplatin (AUC 3) in (bi-weekly cycles (15). Five cycles were given starting at) 24 weeks' gestation. An elective cesarean section at 36 weeks' delivered a 2.062-kg female infant with Apgar scores of 8 and 9 at 1 and 5 minutes, respectively. The child remained healthy at 40 months of age (15).

A 39-year-old woman in the 17th week of pregnancy was diagnosed with non–small-cell lung cancer (16). In the 21st week, paclitaxel (175 mg/m^2) and cisplatin (75 mg/m^2) every 21 days were started. Three cycles had been given when she presented in the 30th week with tonic-clonic seizures caused by brain metastases. An emergency cesarean section was performed to deliver a 1.720-kg male infant with Apgar scores of 3 and 4 at 1 and 5 minutes, respectively. Although the infant developed acute respiratory distress shortly after birth, no other abnormalities were found and he was doing well with normal development and growth after 15 months (16).

A second case of non–small-cell lung cancer occurring in pregnancy was reported in 2009 (17). Starting in the

19th week of pregnancy, the 33-year-old woman was treated with paclitaxel (60 mg/m^2) weekly and carboplatin (AUC 5) every 3 weeks. The patient had received 5 weeks of treatment when brain metastases were discovered. Following corticosteroids for fetal lung maturity, she underwent a cesarean section to deliver a healthy male baby (no other details provided). At 5 months of age, the infant's development was normal (17).

BREASTFEEDING SUMMARY

Consistent with its molecular weight (about 854), paclitaxel is excreted into breast milk. In a 2012 case report, a 40-year-old woman at about 4 months postpartum was exclusively breastfeeding when she began treatment with 6 weekly doses of IV paclitaxel and carboplatin for recurrent papillary thyroid cancer (18). Her infant was fed donor milk during treatment. After the 6th dose, milk samples were collected at 0, 4, 28, 172, and 316 hours. For paclitaxel, the level at 172 hours was 0.97 mg/L but was undetectable at 316 hours. Carboplatin levels remained detectable (0.16 mg/L) at 316 hours. The relative infant dose for paclitaxel was 16.7%, whereas the relative infant dose for carboplatin was 2.0%. The authors concluded that although these levels were probably too low to cause toxicity, potential toxicity could include myelosuppression (especially neutropenia and thrombocytopenia), severe hypersensitivity reactions, nephrotoxicity, and neurotoxicity (18). Because of the potential toxicity, women receiving these agents should not nurse (19).

References

1. Product information. Paclitaxel Injection. Faulding Pharmaceutical, 2003.
2. Scialli AR, DeSesso JM, Rahman A, Husain SR, Goeringer GC. Embryotoxicity of free and liposome-encapsulated Taxol in the chick. Pharmacology 1995;51:145–51.
3. Scialli AR, Waterhouse TB, DeSesso JM, Rahman A, Goeringer GC. Protective effect of liposome encapsulation on paclitaxel developmental toxicity in the rat. Teratology 1997;56:305–10.
4. Nekhayeva IA, Nanovskaya TN, Hankins GDV, Ahmed MS. Role of human placental efflux transporter P-glycoprotein in the transfer of buprenorphine, levo-α-acetylmethadol, and paclitaxel. Am J Perinatol 2006;23:423–30.
5. Seiden MV, Spitzer TR, McAfee S, Fuller AF. Successful pregnancy after high-dose cyclophosphamide, carboplatinum, and Taxol with peripheral blood stem cell transplant in a young woman with ovarian cancer. Gynecol Oncol 2001;83:412–4.
6. Sood AK, Shahin MS, Sorosky JI. Paclitaxel and platinum chemotherapy for ovarian carcinoma during pregnancy. Gynecol Oncol 2001;83: 599–600.
7. Méndez LE, Mueller A, Salom E, González-Quintero VH. Paclitaxel and carboplatin chemotherapy administered during pregnancy for advanced epithelial ovarian cancer. Obstet Gynecol 2003;102:1200–2.
8. Gadducci A, Cosio S, Fanucchi A, Nardini V, Roncella M, Conte PF, Genazzani AR. Chemotherapy with epirubicin and paclitaxel for breast cancer during pregnancy: case report and review of the literature. Anticancer Res 2003;23:5225–9.
9. Adolph A, Le T, Khan K, Biem S. Recurrent metastatic fallopian tube carcinoma in pregnancy. Gynecol Oncol 2001;81:110–2.
10. Gonzalez-Angulo AM, Walters RS, Carpenter RJ Jr, Ross MI, Perkins GH, Gwyn K, Theriault RL. Paclitaxel chemotherapy in a pregnant patient with bilateral breast cancer. Clin Breast Cancer 2004;5:317–9.
11. Morris PG, King F, Kennedy MJ. Cytotoxic chemotherapy for pregnancy-associated breast cancer: a single institution case series. J Oncol Pharm Practice 2009;15:241–7.
12. Palaia I, Pernice M, Graziano M, Bellati F, Panici PB. Neoadjuvant chemotherapy plus radical surgery in locally advance cervical cancer during pregnancy: a case report. Am J Obstet Gynecol 2007;197:e5–6.
13. Modares Giliani M, Karimi Zarchi M, Behtash N, Ghaemmaghami F, Mousavi AS, Behnamfar F. Preservation of pregnancy in a patient with advanced ovarian cancer at 20 weeks of gestation: case report and literature review. Int J Gynecol Cancer 2007;17:1140–3.
14. Hubalek M, Smekal-Schindelwig C, Zeimet AG, Brezinka CSC, Mueller-Holzner E, Marth C. Chemotherapeutic treatment of a pregnant patient with ovarian dysgerminoma. Arch Gynecol Obstet 2007;276: 179–83.
15. Doi D, Boh Y, Konishi H, Asakura H, Takeshita T. Combined chemotherapy with paclitaxel and carboplatin for mucinous cystadenocarcinoma of the ovary during pregnancy. Arch Gynecol Obstet 2009;280:633–6.
16. Garcia-Gonzalez J, Cueva J, Lamus MJ, Curiel T, Grana B, Lopez-Lopez R. Paclitaxel and cisplatin in the treatment of metastatic non-small-cell lung cancer during pregnancy. Clin Transl Oncol 2008;10:375–6.
17. Azim HA Jr, Scarfone G, Peccatori FA. Carboplatin and weekly paclitaxel for the treatment of non-small cell lung cancer (NSCLC) during pregnancy. J Thorac Oncol 2009;4:559–60.
18. Griffin SJ, Milla M, Baker TE, Liu T, Wang H, Hale TW. Transfer of carboplatin and paclitaxel into breast milk. J Hum Lact 2012;28:457–9.
19. Leslie KK. Chemotherapy and pregnancy. Clin Obstet Gynecol 2002;45: 153–64.

P

PALIFERMIN

Keratinocyte Growth Factor

PREGNANCY RECOMMENDATION: No Human Data—Animal Data Suggest Risk
BREASTFEEDING RECOMMENDATION: Contraindicated

PREGNANCY SUMMARY

No reports describing the use of palifermin in human pregnancy have been located. The animal reproduction data suggest risk of developmental toxicity, but the embryo–fetal effects (growth restriction and death) might have been secondary to maternal toxicity. Importantly, the no-effect doses in two animal species were close to the human dose (based on body weight). A more informative dose comparison (BSA or AUC) was not provided by the manufacturer. The use of this agent by a pregnant patient implies that she also will receive or has received chemotherapy that is toxic to the bone marrow and oral mucosa, and possibly to her embryo or fetus as well. The addition of palifermin to decrease maternal oral mucosal toxicity and to allow a more rapid return to a normal intake of food and fluids appears to be an overall embryo–fetal benefit. In this context, although the absence of human pregnancy experience prevents an assessment of the potential for embryo–fetal harm, the maternal benefit appears to outweigh this unknown risk.

FETAL RISK SUMMARY

Palifermin, a water-soluble, 140 amino acid protein produced by recombinant DNA technology, is a human keratinocyte growth factor (KGF). It is indicated to decrease the incidence and duration of severe oral mucositis in patients with hematologic malignancies receiving myelotoxic therapy requiring hematopoietic stem cell support (1). KGF is an endogenous protein in the fibroblast growth factor family. It binds to the KGF receptor that is present on epithelial cells in many tissues (e.g., throughout the gastrointestinal tract), resulting in proliferation, differentiation, and migration of epithelial cells. Palifermin is given as a daily IV bolus dose for 3 days before and after myelotoxic therapy (total of six doses). The elimination half-life is about 4.5 hours (range 3.3–5.7 hours) (1).

Reproduction studies have been conducted in rats and rabbits. In pregnant rats, IV doses 8 or more times the recommended human dose based on body weight (RHD) were associated with increased postimplantation loss, decreased fetal body weight, and/or increased skeletal variations. These doses also were maternal toxic (clinical signs and decreased body weight gain/food consumption). The no-effect dose for developmental toxicity was 4.8 times the RHD. Systemic toxicity in male and female rats was observed at a dose 5 times the RHD, and the fertility index was decreased at a dose about 16 times the RHD. In pregnant rabbits, increased postimplantation losses and decreased fetal body weights were observed at IV doses 2.5 times the RHD. This dose produced maternal toxicity similar to that observed in rats. The no-effect dose for developmental toxicity in the rabbit was equal to the RHD (1).

The carcinogenic potential of palifermin has not been studied in animals. Palifermin has been shown to enhance the growth of human epithelial tumor cell lines in vitro and to increase the rate of tumor cell line growth in a human xenograft model (1). No clastogenic or mutagenic effects were observed in assays (1).

It is not known if palifermin crosses the human placenta. The molecular weight of the protein (about 16,300) should preclude passive diffusion, but active transfer, such as occurs with immunoglobulins, is possible. Moreover, as an endogenous protein, KGF is present in the embryo and fetus.

BREASTFEEDING SUMMARY

No reports describing the use of palifermin during human lactation have been located. Although this protein has a high molecular weight (16,300), it might be excreted into breast milk, as are other proteins (e.g., antibodies). The effects of this exposure on a nursing infant are unknown, but palifermin would most likely be broken down to its constituent amino acids or fragments thereof in the infant's digestive tract. However, because it stimulates the proliferation, differentiation, and migration of epithelial cells, including epithelial tumor cell lines, the best course is to stop breastfeeding when the mother is being treated. Moreover, the use of palifermin implies that the mother also has received or is receiving myelotoxic chemotherapy, and exposure of a nursing infant to these agents should be avoided.

Reference

1. Product information. Kepivance. Amgen, 2004.

PALIPERIDONE

Antipsychotic

PREGNANCY RECOMMENDATION: No Human Data—Animal Data Suggest Low Risk
BREASTFEEDING RECOMMENDATION: Limited Human Data—Potential Toxicity

PREGNANCY SUMMARY

No reports describing the use of paliperidone, the active metabolite of risperidone, in human pregnancy have been located. Developmental toxicity, in the absence of maternal toxicity, was not observed in two animal species. Risperidone was carcinogenic in rodents, but the relationship of this effect to humans has not been studied. Although there are no human pregnancy data with paliperidone, there are limited data for risperidone. (See Risperidone.) However, the absence of specific information for paliperidone prevents a complete assessment of the embryo–fetal risk. Nevertheless, if the mother's disease requires the use of paliperidone, the benefits to her probably outweigh any fetal risk. Folic acid 4 mg/day has been recommended for women taking atypical antipsychotics because they may have a higher risk of neural tube defects due to inadequate folate intake and obesity (1). If paliperidone is used in pregnancy, health care professionals are encouraged to call the toll-free number 800-670-6126 for information about patient enrollment in the Motherisk study.

FETAL RISK SUMMARY

Paliperidone (9-hydroxyrisperidone), an atypical antipsychotic, is the major active metabolite of risperidone. (See also Risperidone.) It is a benzisoxazole derivative in the same antipsychotic subclass as iloperidone, risperidone, and ziprasidone. Paliperidone is indicated for the acute and maintenance treatment of schizophrenia. The plasma protein binding is 74%, and the metabolites are inactive. The terminal elimination half-life is about 23 hours (2).

Reproduction studies have been conducted in rats and rabbits. No increases in fetal abnormalities were observed in these species at oral doses that were 8 times the maximum recommended human dose based on BSA (MRHD) (2).

Carcinogenicity studies have not been performed with paliperidone. However, in mice and rats, the parent compound risperidone produced pituitary gland adenomas, endocrine pancreas adenomas, and mammary gland adenocarcinomas. This effect in rodents from risperidone and other antipsychotics is thought to be mediated by prolonged dopamine D_2 antagonism and hyperprolactinemia. The no-observed-effect-level (NOEL) for these tumors was equal to or less than the maximum recommended human dose of risperidone based on BSA (2).

Paliperidone was not mutagenic in three assays. Fertility of male and female rats was not affected by oral doses up to about 2 times the MRHD. However, preimplantation and postimplantation losses were increased at the maximum dose that also caused slight maternal toxicity. No decrease in live embryos was observed at a dose that was about 0.5 times the MRHD (2).

It is not known if paliperidone crosses the human placenta. The molecular weight (about 426), moderate plasma protein binding, and long elimination half-life suggest that the drug will cross to the embryo–fetus.

Antipsychotics, especially those classified as high potency, can cause extrapyramidal reactions (e.g., acute dystonia, akathisia, parkinsonism, and tardive dyskinesia) in those taking the drug and, if large doses are taken by the mother, also in the newborn. The American Academy of Pediatrics (AAP) classifies risperidone as high potency; its active metabolite should be classified similarly. However, the AAP did note that high-potency antipsychotics were preferred to minimize maternal anticholinergic, hypotensive, and antihistamine adverse effects (3).

BREASTFEEDING SUMMARY

No reports describing the use of paliperidone during human lactation have been located.

However, risperidone and its active metabolite, 9-hydroxyrisperidone (paliperidone), are excreted into breast milk (4–6). (See also Risperidone.)

P

A 21-year-old mother with a 2-year history of bipolar disorder stopped all medication when her pregnancy was diagnosed (4). She did well during pregnancy and delivered a healthy infant at 38 weeks' gestation. When her disease relapsed, she was admitted to the hospital 2.5 months after birth of her infant, stopped breastfeeding, and started on risperidone, eventually reaching a steady-state dose of 6 mg/day. Concentrations of risperidone and paliperidone were determined in the plasma and milk. The milk:plasma ratios, based on AUC_{0-24}, were 0.42 and 0.24, respectively. Based on a daily milk intake of 150 mL/kg, a nursing infant would have received 0.84% of the mother's risperidone dose (mg/kg/day) and an additional 3.46% from the paliperidone (as risperidone equivalents), or about 4.3% of the weight-adjusted maternal dose. Although the combined amounts of risperidone and paliperidone measured in breast milk appear to be too low to cause extrapyramidal effects, concern was expressed for other effects, such as neuroleptic malignant syndrome, and effects on cognitive development (4).

A 2004 study measured the steady-state plasma and milk concentrations of risperidone and 9-hydroxyrisperidone in two breastfeeding women and one woman with risperidone-induced galactorrhea (5). A 29-year-old woman with galactorrhea was taking risperidone 3 mg at night (37.5 mcg/kg/day) for schizophrenia. The galactorrhea was attributed to elevated prolactin concentrations due to the D_2 antagonist effects of risperidone. Milk and plasma samples were collected 20 hours postdose, and then milk only on days 2 and 3, each at 21 hours postdose. The plasma concentrations of risperidone and the metabolite were <1 and 14 mcg/L, respectively. All milk risperidone concentrations were <1 mcg/L, whereas the mean concentration of the metabolite was 5.1 mcg/L (range 4.4–5.6 mcg/L). Although the woman was not nursing, the absolute and relative infant doses were 0.88 mcg/kg/day or 2.3% (as risperidone equivalents) (5).

The two women who were breastfeeding were treated for psychosis with risperidone doses of 42.1 (2 mg every 12 hours) and 23.1 mcg/kg/day (0.5 mg in the morning and 1 mg at night), respectively (5). The nursing infants were a 3.3-month-old female and a 6-week-old male, respectively. In the first woman, milk concentrations of the parent drug and metabolite were 49 and 142 mcg•hr/L (AUC), respectively, whereas the average concentrations were 2.1 and 6 mcg/L, respectively. The absolute infant doses were 0.32 and 0.9 mcg/kg/day, respectively. In the second woman, milk concentrations were 3.1 and 56.5 mcg•hr/L (AUC), respectively, whereas the average concentrations over 24 hours were 0.39 and 7.06 mcg/L, respectively. The absolute infant doses were 0.06 and 1.06 mcg/kg/day, respectively. The milk:plasma ratios were 0.1 and 0.5, respectively. Neither risperidone nor the metabolite was detected in the plasma of the infants and both were developing normally at 9 and 12 months, respectively (5).

A 23-year-old woman, nursing a 4.2-kg male infant 6 times daily, was diagnosed with paranoid schizophrenia 1 week after birth (6). She was hospitalized and started on risperidone 1 mg twice daily. The dose was changed to 2 mg every evening on day 7 and then to 3 mg every evening on day 10. Milk (fore and hind) and maternal plasma concentrations of risperidone and paliperidone were determined on days 6, 10, and 20. No drug accumulation was observed and the concentrations of paliperidone always exceeded those of risperidone. The ranges of risperidone and paliperidone milk concentrations were 0–3 and 1.2–11 ng/mL, respectively, whereas the plasma concentrations were 0.4–10 and 4–43 ng/mL, respectively. Moreover, the concentrations in fore- and hind-milk were comparable. On day 10, 15 hours after a 2 mg dose, the concentrations of risperidone and paliperidone in infant plasma were 0 and 0.1 ng/mL, respectively. The mother was discharged home on risperidone after 5 weeks. The psychomotor development of the infant during the mother's hospitalization was normal and no adverse effects or sedation in the infant were observed. The mother and infant were doing well 2 months after discharge (6).

The AAP classifies other antipsychotic drugs as agents for which the effect on nursing infants is unknown but may be of concern, especially when given for long periods (7). Neither risperidone nor paliperidone was mentioned, but the AAP noted that antipsychotics are excreted into breast milk and could conceivably alter both short-term and long-term CNS function (7). Although no adverse effects from exposure to risperidone and paliperidone have been observed, studies have not been conducted to determine if there are long-term effects.

References

1. Koren G, Cohn T, Chitayat D, Kapur B, Remington G, Myles-Reid D, Zipursky RB. Use of atypical antipsychotics during pregnancy and the risk of neural tube defects in infants. Am J Psychiatry 2002;159:136–7.
2. Product information. Invega. Janssen, 2008.
3. Committee on Drugs, American Academy of Pediatrics. Use of psychoactive medication during pregnancy and possible effects on the fetus and newborn. Pediatrics 2000;105:880–7.
4. Hill RC, McIvor RJ, Wojnar-Horton RE, Hackett LP, Ilett KF. Risperidone distribution and excretion into human milk: case report and estimated infant exposure during breast-feeding. J Clin Psychopharmacol 2000;20:285–6.
5. Ilett KF, Hackett LP, Kristensen JH, Vaddadi KS, Gardiner SJ, Begg EJ. Transfer of risperidone and 9-hydroxyrisperidone into human milk. Ann Pharmacother 2004;38:273–6.
6. Aichhorn W, Stuppaeck C, Whitworth AB. Risperidone and breast-feeding. J Psychopharmacol 2005;19:211–3.
7. Committee on Drugs, American Academy of Pediatrics. The transfer of drugs and other chemicals into human milk. Pediatrics 2001;108:776–89.

PALIVIZUMAB

Respiratory Drug (Monoclonal Antibody)

PREGNANCY RECOMMENDATION: No Human Data—No Relevant Animal Data
BREASTFEEDING RECOMMENDATION: No Human Data—Probably Compatible

PREGNANCY SUMMARY

No reports describing the use of palivizumab in human pregnancy have been located. However, such reports are unlikely because the drug is indicated only for pediatric patients.

FETAL RISK SUMMARY

Palivizumab is a recombinant humanized monoclonal antibody antiviral that acts against respiratory syncytial virus (RSV). After IM injection, it acts by binding the RSV envelope fusion protein on the surface of the virus and blocking a critical step in the membrane fusion process. It also prevents cell-to-cell fusion of RSV-infected cells. Palivizumab is indicated for the prevention of serious lower respiratory tract disease caused by RSV in children at high risk for RSV disease. In children <24 months of age, the mean half-life was 20 days (1).

Animal reproduction studies and studies for carcinogenicity, mutagenicity, and fertility have not been conducted (1).

It is not known if palivizumab crosses the human placenta. The molecular weight (about 148,000) suggests that it will not cross, at least in the 1st and 2nd trimesters.

BREASTFEEDING SUMMARY

No reports describing the use of palivizumab during human lactation have been located. Such reports are unlikely because the drug is indicated only for pediatric patients. Moreover, after the colostral phase, even if a lactating woman inadvertently received the drug, the high molecular weight (about 148,000) should prevent excretion of the monoclonal antibody into breast milk.

Reference

1. Product information. Synagis. MedImmune, 2012.

P

PALONOSETRON

Antiemetic

PREGNANCY RECOMMENDATION: No Human Data—Animal Data Suggest Low Risk
BREASTFEEDING RECOMMENDATION: No Human Data—Probably Compatible

PREGNANCY SUMMARY

No reports describing the use of palonosetron in human pregnancy have been located. The animal data suggest that the risk to the human embryo–fetus is low, but the lack of human pregnancy experience prevents a more complete assessment of the risk. Regarding other agents in this class, there is no human pregnancy experience with dolasetron and granisetron, but limited experience with ondansetron has not demonstrated embryo or fetal toxicity. Based on this experience and the lack of developmental toxicity in two animal species, palonosetron appears to represent a minimal risk to the human embryo or fetus.

FETAL RISK SUMMARY

Palonosetron is a selective serotonin (5-HT_3) receptor antagonist that is in the same pharmacologic class as dolasetron, granisetron, and ondansetron. IV doses of this agent are indicated for the prevention of acute nausea and vomiting associated with initial and repeat courses of moderately and highly emetogenic cancer chemotherapy, and for the prevention of delayed nausea and vomiting associated with initial and repeat courses of moderately emetogenic cancer chemotherapy. Only moderate amounts (about 62%) of palonosetron are bound to plasma proteins and about 50% is metabolized to two inactive compounds. The mean terminal elimination half-life is about 40 hours (1).

Reproduction studies have been conducted in pregnant rats and rabbits. In these species, oral doses up to 1894 and 3789 times, respectively, the recommended human IV dose based on BSA revealed no evidence of impaired fertility or harm to the fetus. In male and female rats, the highest dose had no effect on fertility or reproductive performance (1).

In a 2-year study with mice, palonosetron was not tumorigenic at oral doses up to those producing systemic exposures about 150–289 times the human exposure based on AUC resulting from the recommended IV dose (HE). In a 2-year study with male and female rats, oral doses up to those producing systemic exposures 308 times the HE were carcinogenic. In other tests, palonosetron was not genotoxic but did have clastogenic effects (1).

It is not known if palonosetron crosses the human placenta. The molecular weight of the free base (about 297), the moderate protein binding and metabolism, and the extended plasma half-life suggest that substantial amounts of active drug will be at the maternal–fetal interface for prolonged periods.

BREASTFEEDING SUMMARY

No reports describing the use of palonosetron during human lactation have been located. The molecular weight of the free base (about 297), the moderate protein binding and metabolism, and the extended plasma half-life suggest that the drug will be excreted into breast milk. The effects of this exposure on a nursing infant are unknown. Because the use of palonosetron is normally for short periods, the risk of any toxicity in a nursing infant appears remote.

Reference

1. Product information. Aloxi. MGI Pharma, 2006.

PAMIDRONATE

Bisphosphonate

PREGNANCY RECOMMENDATION: Limited Human Data—Animal Data Suggest Risk
BREASTFEEDING RECOMMENDATION: Limited Human Data—Probably Compatible

PREGNANCY SUMMARY

Although the dose comparisons in animal species were based on body weight, and maternal toxicity was evident, pamidronate, at doses close to those used in humans, did cause nonteratogenic toxicity in the embryo–fetus. The human data are limited to eight cases. In two of the cases, pamidronate was given during the 2nd trimester. Hypocalcemia was noted in one of the newborns but not the other. The amount of drug retained in bone and eventually released back into the systemic circulation is directly related to the dose and duration of treatment. Because pamidronate probably crosses the placenta, continuous exposure most likely occurred throughout gestation in six cases. However, these embryos were exposed during organogenesis to the low plasma concentrations resulting from the slow release of pamidronate from bone, not to the much higher concentrations obtained in the first few days after an IV dose. The use of pamidronate is not recommended in women who may become pregnant or during pregnancy. However, based solely on the limited human pregnancy experience, inadvertent exposure does not appear to represent a major risk to the embryo or fetus, but infants should be monitored for hypocalcemia during the first few days after birth.

FETAL RISK SUMMARY

Pamidronate, a hydrophilic bisphosphonate, is a synthetic analog of pyrophosphate that binds to the hydroxyapatite found in bone to inhibit bone resorption. Pamidronate has three indications: (a) for the treatment of moderate or severe hypercalcemia associated with malignancy, with or without bone metastases; (b) for the treatment of moderate to severe Paget's disease of bone; and (c) in conjunction with standard antineoplastic therapy, for the treatment of osteolytic bone metastases of breast cancer and osteolytic lesions of multiple myeloma. Other agents in this pharmacologic class are alendronate, etidronate, ibandronate, risedronate, tiludronate, and zoledronic acid. Pamidronate is not metabolized. After IV infusion, about 46% of the dose is excreted as unchanged drug in the urine over 120 hours with a mean elimination half-life of 28 hours. The remainder of the dose is retained in the body. The amount bound to plasma proteins apparently has not been determined (1). Based on preclinical studies, the oral bioavailability is $<2\%$ (2).

Reproduction studies have been conducted in pregnant rats and rabbits. In these species, IV bolus doses 0.6–8.3 times the highest recommended human dose (based on body weight) produced toxicity in the mother (decreased body-weight gain and survival during parturition), embryo (death and general underdevelopment), and fetus (marked skeletal restriction) (1,2).

In 2-year carcinogenic studies with oral doses, male rats, but not females, had a significant increase in benign adrenal pheochromocytoma. After adjustment for the limited oral bioavailability, the lowest dose causing this effect was similar to the human IV dose. Pamidronate was not carcinogenic in mice. Tests for mutagenic effects have been negative (1).

It is not known if pamidronate crosses the human placenta. The molecular weight of the free acid (about 233), lack of metabolism, and prolonged elimination half-life suggest that the drug will cross the placenta to the embryo–fetus. The low lipid solubility may limit the exposure.

A 1990 report described a woman who received a 30-mg infusion of pamidronate at 34 weeks' for malignant hypercalcemia due to metastatic breast cancer (3). Two weeks later, she gave birth to healthy 3.06-kg male infant who developed transient hypocalcemia that resolved by 5 days of age. The infant's subsequent growth and development were normal.

A 42-year-old woman presented with newly diagnosed metastatic breast cancer at 24 weeks' gestation (4). Over the next 4 weeks, she was treated with oral dexamethasone (16 mg/day) and SC heroin (100 mg/day). At 28 weeks', she developed severe hypercalcemia that was treated with a single IV dose of pamidronate (90 mg over 8 hours). One week later, a 1412-g male infant was delivered by cesarean section. The Apgar score was 8 at 1 minute. The infant was treated for respiratory distress syndrome, narcotic withdrawal, and hypocalcemia. He was discharged home at 13 weeks of age weighing 3228 g. At 1 year, he was developing normally and his weight, length, and head circumference were at 50th percentile (4).

A 2004 report described two women with osteogenesis imperfecta who were treated with IV pamidronate before conception (5). The timing of the last IV dose in relation to conception was not provided in either case. The first case involved a 17-year-old woman who had received a cumulative IV dose of 49.5 mg/kg (9 mg/kg/year) over a 5-year period. Treatment was stopped when she became pregnant. Her only complication during pregnancy was hyperemesis gravidarum in the 1st trimester. She received daily doses of elemental calcium (1000 mg) and vitamin D (400 IU) throughout gestation. A 3600-g male infant was delivered vaginally at term. Apgar scores were 8 and 9 at 1 and 5 minutes, respectively. Blue sclera, but no dysmorphic features, fractures, or long bone deformities, were noted. The infant inherited osteogenesis imperfecta. Asymptomatic hypocalcemia (ionized calcium below the age-related reference range) was found at 24 hours of age but had resolved at 11 days of age without specific treatment. At that age, a skeletal survey found no evidence of fracture, abnormal bone development, modeling defect, or wormian bones (*small irregular bones along the sutures of the cranium, particularly related to the parietal bone*) in the skull. At 16 months, the baby's growth (weight and length) was normal, and he remained free of fracture (5).

In the second case, pregnancy occurred in a 17.8-year-old woman who had received a cumulative IV dose of 48 mg/kg (9 mg/kg/year) over 5.3 years (5). Treatment was stopped when she became pregnant. Similar to the above case, the woman received the same dose of calcium and vitamin D throughout gestation. Her pregnancy was uneventful, and she delivered a 2860-g female infant by cesarean section at 38 weeks' gestation. The infant inherited osteogenesis imperfecta and had bilateral talipes equinovarus but no fractures. Otherwise, the limbs were straight. Her plasma calcium was not measured in the first few days after birth. Blue sclera was noted at age 13 days, as were wormian bones on the skull radiograph. Otherwise, her physical examination was normal. At 14 months of age, her growth (weight and length) was normal and she remained free of fracture. The authors cited an incidence for talipes equinovarus of 0.93–6.8 per 1000 live births in the general population. Although the prevalence of the deformity in osteogenesis imperfecta is unknown, they had observed a second case among 400 children with the disorder. They concluded that an association between pamidronate and talipes equinovarus could not be excluded but that the possibility of such an association was unlikely (5). Another source thought the defect had a genetic component (6).

A 40-year-old woman with breast cancer was treated with doxorubicin and paclitaxel over a 3-week interval starting at 24 weeks' gestation (7). At 28 weeks', deteriorating renal function, uterine contractions, and hypercalcemia (17.6 mg/dL) were noted. When other therapies for the hypercalcemia failed, she was treated with IV pamidronate, 90 mg over 6 hours. At 48 hours posttreatment, her calcium concentration had decreased to 12.8 mg/dL and the uterine contractions had stopped. No effects were noted on the fetal heart rate. Her calcium level decreased to 9.9 mg/dL on day 3. At this time, preeclampsia developed and a cesarean section was conducted to give birth to a 1.147-kg female infant with a normal calcium concentration. The infant did well and was discharged from the neonatal intensive care unit at a gestational age of 36 weeks. The mother died 13 days after birth of her infant (7).

A 2006 report described the use of pamidronate before four uneventful pregnancies from three women (8). Treatment durations—interval between the last dose and conception (both in months) were: 46–3; 26–3 (first pregnancy) and 26–48 (second pregnancy); and 19–21. The four infants were healthy at birth and were developing normally. No evidence of biochemical or skeletal abnormality was found in the infants (8).

A woman with hereditary hyperphosphatasia was treated with pamidronate 1 mg/kg on 3 consecutive days every 4 months for 42 months (9). One month after the last cycle she conceived. The patient was given 1000 mg/day of elemental calcium but no vitamin D throughout pregnancy. The pregnancy was uneventful except for premature rupture of the membrane at 36 weeks' gestation, resulting in the birth of a 3130-g female infant with Apgar scores of 8 and 9. No structural anomalies, fractures or long bone deformities were noted in the infant. All laboratory tests were normal in the mother and infant shortly after birth and after 14 days of breastfeeding (9).

A 2008 review described 51 cases of exposure to bisphosphonates before or during pregnancy: alendronate ($N = 32$), pamidronate ($N = 11$), etidronate ($N = 5$), risedronate ($N = 2$), and zoledronic acid ($N = 1$) (10). The authors concluded that although these drugs may affect bone modeling and development in the fetus, no such toxicity has yet been reported.

BREASTFEEDING SUMMARY

Although the low molecular weight of the free acid (about 233), lack of metabolism, and prolonged elimination half-life suggest that pamidronate will be excreted into breast milk, a 2000 study was unable to detect the drug in milk. A 39-year-old woman with reflex sympathetic dystrophy delivered a healthy male infant at 40 weeks' gestation (11). She began breastfeeding, and several weeks later (exact time not stated), she began monthly treatments of IV pamidronate 30 mg/infusion. After the infusion, she pumped and discarded her breast milk for 48 hours and then resumed nursing her infant. After the first dose, her breast milk was collected and separated into two pooled samples (0–24 and 25–48 hours). Pamidronate was not detected in either sample (detection limit 0.4 μmol/L) (11).

Breastfeeding during pamidronate treatment does not appear to place the nursing infant at risk.

Failure to detect the drug in milk in the above case might have been due to its low lipid solubility and acidic nature. Although the oral bioavailability of pamidronate in infants is not known, in adults it is very low, about 2% in the fasting state (2). Moreover, the drug is highly bound by calcium and should not be absorbable from milk. Based on these data, breastfeeding appears to be compatible with pamidronate therapy, but withholding nursing for 12–24 hours should ensure that the infant is exposed to little or no drug.

References

1. Product information. Aredia. Novartis Pharmaceuticals, 2006.
2. Graepel P, Bentley P, Fritz H, Miyamoto M, Slater SR. Reproduction toxicity studies with pamidronate. Arzneimittelforschung 1992;42:654–67.
3. Dunlop DJ, Soukop M, McEwan HP. Antenatal administration of aminopropylidene diphosphate. Ann Rheum Dis 1990;49:955.
4. Illidge TM, Hussey M, Godden CW. Malignant hypercalcaemia in pregnancy and antenatal administration of intravenous pamidronate. Clin Oncol (R Coll Radiol) 1996;8:257–8.
5. Munns CFJ, Rauch F, Ward L, Glorieux FH. Maternal and fetal outcome after long-term pamidronate treatment before conception: a report of two cases. J Bone Miner Res 2004;19:1742–5.
6. Fleischnick EA, Kasser JR. Foot, talipes equinovarus (TEV). In Buyse ML, ed. *Birth Defects Encyclopedia*. Volume 1. Dover, ME: Blackwell Scientific Publications. Center for Birth Defects Information Services, 1990:744–6.
7. Culbert EC, Schfirin BS. Malignant hypercalcemia in pregnancy. Effect of pamidronate on uterine contractions. Obstet Gynecol 2006;108: 789–91.
8. Chan B, Zacharin M. Maternal and infant outcome after pamidronate treatment of polyostotic fibrous dysplasia and osteogenesis imperfecta before conception: a report of four cases. J Clin Endocrinol Metab 2006;91: 2017–20.
9. Cabar ER, Nomura RMY, Zugaib M. Maternal and fetal outcome of pamidronate treatment before conception: a case report. Clin Exp Rheumatol 2007;25:344–5.
10. Djokanovic N, Klieger-Grossmann C, Koren G. Does treatment with bisphosphonates endanger the human pregnancy? J Obstet Gynaecol Can 2008;30:1146–8.
11. Siminoski K, Fitzgerald AA, Flesch G, Gross MS. Intravenous pamidronate for treatment of reflex sympathetic dystrophy during breast feeding. J Bone Miner Res 2000;15:2052–5.

PANCURONIUM

Skeletal Muscle Relaxant

PREGNANCY RECOMMENDATION: Limited Human Data—Animal Data Suggest Low Risk
BREASTFEEDING RECOMMENDATION: No Human Data—Probably Compatible

P

PREGNANCY SUMMARY

Pancuronium has been administered directly to the fetus during the last half of pregnancy and to the mother at cesarean section without causing fetal harm. Although no teratogenicity was observed in two animal species, the use of pancuronium in early human pregnancy has not been reported. The drug is known to cross the human placenta to the fetus, at least near term. Placental transfer early in pregnancy has not been reported. Large or repetitive doses and/or prolonged dose-to-delivery intervals may potentially result in newborn depression, but the clinical significance of this appears to be low. Moreover, other anesthetic agents may contribute to the condition. In addition, transient fetal heart rate (FHR) changes, such as decreased accelerations and beat-to-beat variability, and an occasional sinusoidal-like pattern, have been observed after direct fetal administration, but apparently this does not indicate fetal compromise.

FETAL RISK SUMMARY

Pancuronium (pancuronium bromide) is a competitive (nondepolarizing) neuromuscular blocking agent. Structurally, it is a bisquaternary ammonium compound (i.e., contains two quaternary ammonium groups) and is commercially available as the dibromide. Pancuronium is used to induce skeletal muscle relaxation during anesthesia and other procedures and has been used to produce fetal muscle paralysis during intrauterine procedures.

Unpublished reproduction studies in rats and rabbits with pancuronium did not reveal any effect on the number of resorptions, litter size, birth weight and vitality, or the frequency of malformations (gross, skeletal, and internal organs) (1). Pregnant rats (average gestational length 21–22 days (2)) received intraperitoneal doses of 0.16 mg/kg/day either from 7th to 14th day or from 1st to 20th day of gestation, whereas pregnant rabbits (average gestational length 31–34 days (2)) were given IV doses of 0.02 mg/kg/day from day 8 to day 16 of gestation.

Theoretically, the combination of relatively high molecular weight (about 733 for the dibromide) and the presence of two quaternary ammonium groups that are ionized at physiologic pH should limit the placental transfer of pancuronium. An animal study published in 1973 appeared to confirm the lack of significant transfer when cumulative IV doses up to 16.3 mg/kg administered to pregnant ferrets (neuromuscular blockade in the mother is complete at 0.015 mg/kg) did not cause neuromuscular blockade in the fetus during a 1-hour observation period (3). The fetus was responsive to pancuronium-induced blockade by direct administration. Further, the lack of adverse effects in newborns after mean doses of 0.0875 mg/kg at cesarean section led some authors to conclude that the drug did not cross the placenta (4). However, several human studies have demonstrated placental transfer, at least near term, when pancuronium was used during cesarean section (5–11).

Maternal IV bolus doses between 0.04 and 0.12 mg/kg (approximately 2.8–8.6 times the maternal ED_{50}, the dose producing a 50% depression of evoked twitch tension (12)) resulted in mean umbilical vein:maternal vein ratios ranging from 0.19 to 0.26. These ratios were higher than those measured with atracurium, fazadinium, pipecuronium, rocuronium, *d*-tubocurarine, and vecuronium (13). No clinical evidence of neuromuscular blockade was observed in five studies in which the neonatal condition was noted (5–9), but in one of the studies (9), the Neurological and Adaptive Capacity Scores (NACS) system indicated that neonatal depression was present. The NACS evaluates adaptive capacity, passive and active muscular tone, primary reflexes, and general assessment (13). The maximum score possible is 40 with a score of 35–40 denoting a normal, vigorous baby.

The NACS was measured at 15 minutes, 2 hours, and 24 hours in seven newborns whose mothers had been given IV doses of *d*-tubocurarine (3 mg), thiopental (4 mg/kg), succinylcholine (1.5 mg/kg), and pancuronium (0.04 mg/kg) immediately prior to cesarean section (9). Five newborns (71%) had an NACS value <35 at 15 minutes, three were <35 at 2 hours, and none were <35 at 24 hours (9). Although the NACS indicated depression, no neonatal adverse effects were actually observed (9). A 1998 review, commenting on this and other studies of neuromuscular relaxants in pregnancy, thought the low NACS values might have been caused by a contribution from the other anesthetic agents (13).

The direct administration of pancuronium has been reported in animals and humans (14–38). A 1989 report compared the effects of pancuronium (0.5 mg/kg IV over 5 minutes) and *d*-tubocurarine (3.0 mg/kg IV over 5 minutes) on the heart rate and mean arterial pressure of fetal lambs (14). Whereas pancuronium significantly increased both rate and pressure, both measures were significantly decreased by *d*-tubocurarine. Only pancuronium affected fetal pH and Pco_2, increasing the former and decreasing the latter. The human studies, discussed below, all involve pancuronium administration during the second half of gestation.

In a study published in 1988, the baseline FHR, number of accelerations, and beat-to-beat variability were assessed before and after an IV bolus dose of pancuronium (0.05–0.10 mg/kg) was given to 17 fetuses before transfusion (15). Twenty minutes after transfusion, no changes were noted in the baseline FHR, although some heart rate patterns appeared "sinusoidal-like," but significant decreases in accelerations ($p = 0.003$) and variability ($p = 0.0003$) were observed (15). The transient FHR changes were not indicative of fetal compromise and returned to normal when the fetus "awakened" (15). A 1991 abstract reported significantly less bradycardia with the use of pancuronium (0.3 mg/kg) compared with no muscle relaxant after cordocentesis (3.6% [8/224] vs. 8.2% [27/329], $p = 0.04$) and a near significant difference after intravascular transfusion (7.9% [9/114] vs. 40% [2/5], $p = 0.06$) (16).

Pancuronium (0.1 mg/kg IV) was administered to 20 fetuses immediately before blood transfusion at 28–34 weeks' gestation (17). A control group of 20 fetuses matched for gestational age and hematocrit who did not receive pancuronium was used for comparison. After transfusion, compared with controls, fetuses receiving pancuronium had significantly fewer FHR accelerations (mean 0 vs. 3.0, $p < 0.0005$), less change in the baseline FHR (increase 1.5 beats/minute vs. decrease 4 beats/minute, $p < 0.0005$), lower mean minute range in FHR variation (17.3 vs. 34.7, $p < 0.0001$), and less short-term variation (3.4 vs. 7.35, $p = 0.0001$). Another study compared FHR changes after the use of pancuronium or vecuronium for intravascular transfusion, fetal thoracentesis, or paracentesis (18). Specific details were not provided for the pancuronium group, but the authors concluded that the pancuronium-induced increase in FHR and decrease in variability made it less desirable than vecuronium, which caused no FHR changes.

Fetal death at 25.5 weeks' gestation, that was apparently the result of a cord hematoma, occurred 2 hours after an intravascular intrauterine transfusion (19). The authors thought that the accident was related to the injection of pancuronium before confirmation of needle placement by aspiration of fetal blood. The results of an autopsy confirmed that the cause of death was compression of the umbilical vein by the hematoma with subsequent umbilical venous thrombosis.

Fetal administration of pancuronium immediately preceding magnetic resonance imaging has been described in a number of publications (20–28). Most used doses varying from 0.08 to 0.3 mg/kg (IV into the umbilical vein or IM) (20–25), two used 0.5 mg IM (26,27), and one reported 100 mg (sic) into the intrahepatic vein of each twin (28).

Direct fetal administration of pancuronium for intrauterine procedures, such as cordocentesis and intravascular transfusion, has been reported (29–38). The fetal dose ranged from 0.1 to 0.3 mg/kg IV or IM, but in one report, a single 0.5-mg IM dose was administered (29). In another study, pancuronium (0.15 mg/kg of the estimated total fetal body weights of twins) was administered in two cases to the smaller of a set of twins (38). The procedure was undertaken in an attempt to diagnose twin–twin transfusion syndrome. In the first case, the FHR patterns of both twins showed lack of accelerations and decreased variability and, in addition, the larger twin had a "sinusoidal-like" pattern. In the second case, absent accelerations and decreased variability occurred only in the smaller twin (38).

A continuous infusion of morphine, midazolam, and pancuronium was administered for 10 hours to allow mechanical ventilation in a seriously ill, pregnant (about 35 weeks) woman with pneumonia due to *Legionella pneumophila* (39). No evidence of fetal harm was observed during the infusion, but the fetus was noted to have a consistent pattern of "sleeping." Approximately 3–4 weeks later, at 40 weeks' gestation, the mother gave birth to a healthy female infant.

BREASTFEEDING SUMMARY

No reports describing the use of pancuronium in a lactating woman have been located. Because of the nature of the drug and its indications, such reports are unlikely to occur. Moreover, because pancuronium is a bisquaternary ammonium compound, it is ionized at physiologic pH. Only the nonionized form would be available for excretion into milk, and this would probably be only trace amounts (40). In addition, compounds of this type are poorly absorbed from the gastrointestinal tract (40).

References

1. Speight TM, Avery GS. Pancuronium bromide: a review of its pharmacological properties and clinical application. Drugs 1972;4:163–226.
2. Shepard TH. *Catalog of Teratogenic Agents*. 9th ed. Baltimore, MD: The Johns Hopkins University Press, 1998.
3. Evans CA, Waud DR. Do maternally administered neuromuscular blocking agents interfere with fetal neuromuscular transmission? Anesth Analg 1973;52:548–52.
4. Neeld JB Jr, Seabrook PD Jr, Chastain GM, Frederickson EL. A clinical comparison of pancuronium and tubocurarine for cesarean section anesthesia. Anest Analg 1974;53:7–11.
5. Speirs I, Sim AW. The placental transfer of pancuronium bromide. Br J Anaesth 1972;44:370–3.
6. Booth PN, Watson MJ, McLeod K. Pancuronium and the placental barrier. Anaesthesia 1977;32:320–3.
7. Duvaldestin P, Demetriou M, Henzel D, Desmonts JM. The placental transfer of pancuronium and its pharmacokinetics during caesarian section. Acta Anaesthiol Scand 1978;22:327–33.
8. Abouleish E, Wingard LB Jr, De La Vega S, Uy N. Pancuronium in caesarean section and its placental transfer. Br J Anaesth 1980;52:531–6.
9. Dailey PA, Fisher DM, Shnider SM, Baysinger CL, Shinohara Y, Miller RD, Abboud TK, Kim KC. Pharmacokinetics, placental transfer, and neonatal effects of vecuronium and pancuronium administered during cesarean section. Anesthesiology 1984;60:569–74.
10. Heaney GAH. Pancuronium in maternal and foetal serum. Br J Anaesth 1974;46:282–7.
11. Wingard LB Jr, Abouleish E, West DC, Goehl TJ. Modified fluorometric quantitation of pancuronium bromide and metabolites in human maternal and umbilical serums. J Pharm Sci 1979;68:914–5.
12. Agoston S, Crul JF, Kersten UW, Scaf AHJ. Relationship of the serum concentration of pancuronium to its neuromuscular activity in man. Anesthesiology 1977;47:509–12.
13. Guay J, Grenier Y, Varin F. Clinical pharmacokinetics of neuromuscular relaxants in pregnancy. Clin Pharmacokinet 1998;34:483–96.
14. Chestnut DH, Weiner CP, Thompson CS, McLaughlin GL. Intravenous administration of *d*-tubocurarine and pancuronium in fetal lambs. Am J Obstet Gynecol 1989;160:510–3.
15. Pielet BW, Socol ML, MacGregor SN, Dooley SL, Minogue J. Fetal heart rate changes after fetal intravascular treatment with pancuronium bromide. Am J Obstet Gynecol 1988;159:640–3.
16. Weiner C. Pancuronium protects against fetal bradycardia following umbilical cord puncture (abstract). Am J Obstet Gynecol 1991;164:335.
17. Spencer JAD, Ronderos-Dumit D, Rodeck CH. The effect of neuromuscular blockade on human fetal heart rate and its variation. Br J Obstet Gynaecol 1994;101:121–4.
18. Watson WJ, Atchison SR, Harlass FE. Comparison of pancuronium and vecuronium for fetal neuromuscular blockade during invasive procedures. J Matern Fetal Med 1996;5:151–4.
19. Seeds JW, Chescheir NC, Bowes WA Jr, Owl-Smith FA. Fetal death as a complication of intrauterine intravascular transfusion. Obstet Gynecol 1989;74:461–3.
20. Williamson RA, Weiner CP, Yuh WTC, Abu-Yousef MM. Magnetic resonance imaging of anomalous fetuses. Obstet Gynecol 1989;73: 952–6.
21. Lituania M, Passamonti U, Cordone MS, Magnano GM, Toma P. Schizencephaly: prenatal diagnosis by computed sonography and magnetic resonance imaging. Prenat Diagn 1989;9:649–55.
22. Toma P, Lucigrai G, Dodero P, Lituania M. Prenatal detection of an abdominal mass by MR imaging performed while the fetus is immobilized with pancuronium bromide. Am J Roentgenol 1990;154:1049–50.
23. Toma P, Costa A, Magnano GM, Cariati M, Lituania M. Holoprosencephaly: prenatal diagnosis by sonography and magnetic resonance imaging. Prenat Diagn 1990;10:429–36.
24. Wenstrom KD, Williamson RA, Weiner CP, Sipes SL, Yuh WTC. Magnetic resonance imaging of fetuses with intracranial defects. Obstet Gynecol 1991;77:529–32.
25. Okamura K, Murotsuki J, Sakai T, Matsumoto K, Shirane R, Yajima A. Prenatal diagnosis of lissencephaly by magnetic resonance image. Fetal Diagn Ther 1993;8:56–9.
26. Lenke RR, Persutte WH, Nemes JM. Use of pancuronium bromide to inhibit fetal movement during magnetic resonance imaging. A case report. J Reprod Med 1989;34:315–7.
27. Horvath L, Seeds JW. Temporary arrest of fetal movement with pancuronium bromide to enable antenatal magnetic resonance imaging of holoprosencephaly. Am J Perinatol 1989;6:418–20.
28. Zoppini C, Vanzulli A, Kustermann A, Rizzuti T, Selicorni A, Nicolini U. Prenatal diagnosis of anatomical connections in conjoined twins by use of contrast magnetic resonance imaging. Prenat Diag 1993;13: 995–9.
29. Seeds JW, Corke BC, Spielman FJ. Prevention of fetal movement during invasive procedures with pancuronium bromide. Am J Obstet Gynecol 1986;155:818–9.
30. Moise KJ Jr, Carpenter RJ Jr, Deter RL, Kirshon B, Diaz SF. The use of neuromuscular blockade during intrauterine procedures. Am J Obstet Gynecol 1987;157:874–9.
31. Copel JA, Grannum PA, Harrison D, Hobbins JC. The use of intravenous pancuronium bromide to produce fetal paralysis during intravascular transfusion. Am J Obstet Gynecol 1988;158:170–1.
32. Moise KJ Jr, Deter RL, Kirshon B, Adam K, Patton DE, Carpenter RJ Jr. intravenous pancuronium bromide for fetal neuromuscular blockade during intrauterine transfusion for red-cell alloimmunization. Obstet Gynecol 1989;74:905–8.
33. Fan SZ, Huang, FY, Lin SY, Wang YP, Hsieh FJ. Intrauterine neuromuscular blockade in fetus. Anaesth Sinica 1990;28:31–4.
34. Weiner CP, Wenstrom KD, Sipes SL, Williamson RA. Risk factors for cordocentesis and fetal intravascular transfusion. Am J Obstet Gynecol 1991;165:1020–5.
35. Fan SZ, Susetio L, Tsai MC. Neuromuscular blockade of the fetus with pancuronium or pipecuronium for intra-uterine procedures. Anaesthesia 1994;49:284–6.
36. Mouw RJC, Hermans J, Brandenburg HCR, Kanhai HHH. Effects of pancuronium or atracurium on the anemic fetus during and directly after intrauterine transfusion (IUT): a double blind randomized study (abstract). Am J Obstet Gynecol 1997;176:S18.
37. Mouw RJC, Klumper F, Hermans J, Brandenburg HCR, Kanhai HHH. Effect of atracurium or pancuronium on the anemic fetus during and directly after intravascular intrauterine transfusion. A double blind randomized study. Acta Obstet Gynecol Scand 1999;78:763–7.
38. Tanaka M, Natori M, Ishimoto H, Kohno H, Kobayashi T, Nozawa S. Intravascular pancuronium bromide infusion for prenatal diagnosis of twin-twin transfusion syndrome. Fetal Diagn Ther 1992;7:36–40.
39. Eisenberg VH, Eidelman LA, Arbel R, Ezra Y. Legionnaire's disease during pregnancy: a case presentation and review of the literature. Eur J Obstet Gynecol Reprod Biol 1997;72:15–8.
40. Spigset O. Anaesthetic agents and excretion in breast milk. Acta Anaesthesiol Scand 1994;38:94–103.

PANITUMUMAB

Antineoplastic

PREGNANCY RECOMMENDATION: No Human Data—Animal Data Suggest Risk
BREASTFEEDING RECOMMENDATION: Contraindicated

P

PREGNANCY SUMMARY

No reports describing the use of panitumumab in human pregnancy have been located. The animal reproduction data suggest risk, but the absence of human pregnancy experience prevents a more complete assessment of embryo and fetal risk. Until such data are available, the best course is to avoid the use of this antineoplastic in pregnancy. Women of reproductive age should use effective contraception. However, colorectal cancer can be fatal, so if a woman requires therapy with panitumumab and informed consent is obtained, treatment should not be withheld because of pregnancy. If an inadvertent pregnancy occurs, the woman should be advised of the potential risk for severe adverse effects in the embryo and fetus.

FETAL RISK SUMMARY

Panitumumab is a recombinant, human immunoglobulin G2 (IgG2) kappa monoclonal antibody. Panitumumab specifically binds to the human epidermal growth factor receptor (EGFR). It is indicated for the treatment of EGFR-expressing, metastatic colorectal carcinoma with disease progression on or following fluoropyrimidine-, oxaliplatin-, and irinotecan-containing chemotherapy regimens.

Panitumumab may cause severe, infusion-related toxicity, including hypotension and other adverse effects. The use of premedication before infusion was not standardized in clinical trials, so the efficacy of premedication to prevent infusion reactions is unknown (1). However, since premedication is recommended with other monoclonal antibodies, it is reasonable to use acetaminophen and an antihistamine (e.g., diphenhydramine) before each infusion of panitumumab. Moreover, hypotension in a pregnant woman could have deleterious effects on placental perfusion resulting in embryo and fetal harm.

Reproduction studies have been conducted in cynomolgus monkeys. When panitumumab was given to monkeys during organogenesis (gestational days 20–50) in weekly doses that were 1.25–5 times the recommended human dose based on body weight (RHD), significant increases in embryolethal or abortifacient effects were observed. No structural anomalies in the offspring were observed (1).

The carcinogenic or mutagenic effects of panitumumab have not been studied. Panitumumab may adversely affect fertility. In female cynomolgus monkeys given weekly doses that were 1.25–5 times the RHD, prolonged menstrual cycles and/or amenorrhea were observed. The menstrual cycle irregularities were accompanied by both a decrease and delay in peak progesterone and 17β-estradiol levels. Normal menstrual cycles returned in most monkeys when panitumumab was stopped. A no-effect dose for menstrual cycle irregularities was not determined. No adverse effects were observed microscopically in reproductive organs of male cynomolgus monkeys given doses up to about 5 times the RHD for 26 weeks. However, the effects of this exposure on male fertility were not studied (1).

It is not known if panitumumab crosses the human placenta. The high molecular weight (about 147,000) suggests that it will not cross. As IgG does cross and, therefore, panitumumab may also cross. However, panitumumab was not detected in the serum of neonates from panitumumab-treated cynomolgus monkeys, but anti-panitumumab antibody titers were present in 14 of 27 offspring (1).

BREASTFEEDING SUMMARY

No reports describing the use of panitumumab during lactation have been located. The very high molecular weight (about 147,000) suggests that it will not be excreted into breast milk. However, human IgG is excreted into milk and, therefore, panitumumab may also be excreted (1). The effects of this potential exposure on a nursing infant are unknown, but immunosuppression and other severe adverse effects are potential complications.

P

Reference

1. Product information. Vectibix. Amgen, 2006.

PANTOPRAZOLE

Gastrointestinal Agent (Antisecretory)

PREGNANCY RECOMMENDATION: Human Data Suggest Low Risk
BREASTFEEDING RECOMMENDATION: Limited Human Data—Probably Compatible

PREGNANCY SUMMARY

The animal and limited human data suggest that pantoprazole represents a low risk in pregnancy. A study showing an association between in utero exposure to gastric acid–suppressing drugs and childhood allergy and asthma requires confirmation. Moreover, the human pregnancy experience with other proton pump inhibitors (PPIs) has not shown a causal relationship with congenital malformations. However, malformations may have been missed, because of the design and size of the studies. If pantoprazole is required or if inadvertent exposure does occur early in gestation, the known risk to the embryo–fetus appears to be low. Long-term follow-up of offspring exposed during gestation is warranted.

FETAL RISK SUMMARY

Pantoprazole is a PPI that blocks gastric acid secretion by a direct inhibitory effect on the gastric parietal cell. It is used for the short-term treatment of erosive esophagitis associated with gastroesophageal reflux disease (GERD). Pantoprazole is in the same class of PPIs as dexlansoprazole, esomeprazole, lansoprazole, omeprazole, and rabeprazole. It is extensively metabolized to inactive metabolites. The terminal elimination half-life is about 1 hour but is 3.5–10 hours in patients with altered metabolism (slow metabolizers). Serum protein binding, primarily to albumin, is about 98% (1).

Reproductive studies have been conducted in pregnant rats and rabbits at doses up to 88 and 16 times, respectively, the recommended human dose based on BSA. No evidence was found at these doses of impaired fertility or fetal harm (1).

Similar to other PPIs, pantoprazole is carcinogenic in mice and rats (gastrointestinal, liver, and thyroid) (1). The dose-related nature of the tumors and the presumably limited in utero exposure to the drug during human gestation probably suggest a negligible risk. In addition, positive results were seen with pantoprazole in the in vitro human lymphocyte chromosomal aberration assays and in some mutagenic tests with mice, rats, and hamsters. In contrast, negative results were obtained in the in vitro Ames mutation assay, the mammalian cell-forward gene mutation assay, and in several other tests of mutagenicity (1).

It is not known if pantoprazole crosses the human placenta. The molecular weight (about 432 for the hydrated form) is low enough, but the short elimination half-life and high protein binding will limit the amount of drug available to cross at the maternal–fetal interface. Embryo–fetal exposure, however, may be higher in slow metabolizers because of the longer elimination half-life. Of interest, another PPI, omeprazole, has a similar molecular weight (about 345), elimination half-life (1 hour), and protein binding (about 95%), and is known to cross the human placenta. (See Omeprazole.)

A 2002 study conducted a meta-analysis involving the use of PPIs in pregnancy (2). In the 5 cohort studies analyzed, there were 593 infants, mostly exposed to omeprazole, but also including lansoprazole and pantoprazole. The relative risk (RR) for major malformations was 1.18, 95% confidence interval (CI) 0.72–1.94 (2).

A 2005 study by the European Network of Teratology Information Services reported the outcomes of pregnancies exposed to omeprazole ($N = 295$), lansoprazole ($N = 62$), or pantoprazole ($N = 53$) (3). In the pantoprazole group, the median duration of treatment was 14 days (range 7–23 days), and the dose used was 40 mg/day. The outcomes consisted of 1 spontaneous abortion (SAB), 3 elective abortions (EABs) (none for congenital anomalies), 1 stillbirth, and 48 live births. One infant exposed early in gestation (week 2 for 8 days) had congenital toxoplasmosis. Compared with a nonexposed control group, there was no difference in the rate of major malformations between the pantoprazole and control groups (RR 0.55, 95% CI 0.08–3.95). Similar results were observed for omeprazole and lansoprazole (3).

A population-based observational cohort study formed by linking data from three Swedish national health care registers over a 10-year period (1995–2004) was reported in 2009 (4). The main outcome measures were a diagnosis of allergic disease or a prescription for asthma or allergy medications. The drug types included in the study were gastric acid suppressors, including H_2-receptor antagonists, prostaglandins, PPIs, combinations for eradication of *Helicobacter pylori*, and drugs for peptic ulcer disease and GERD. Of 585,716 children, 29,490 (5.0%) met the diagnosis and 5645 (1%) had been exposed to gastric acid–suppression therapy in pregnancy. Of these children, 405 (0.07%) were treated for allergic disease. For developing allergy, the odds ratio (OR) was 1.43, 98% CI 1.29–1.59, irrespective of the drug, time of exposure during pregnancy, and maternal history of allergy. For developing childhood asthma, but not other allergic diseases, the OR was 1.51, 95% CI 1.35–1.69, irrespective of the type of acid-suppressive drug and the time of exposure in pregnancy. The authors proposed three possible mechanisms for their findings: (a) exposure to increased amounts of allergens could cause sensitization to digestion labile antigens in the fetus, (b) maternal Th2 cytokine pattern could promote an allergy-prone phenotype in the fetus, and (c) maternal allergen-specific immunoglobulin E could cross the placenta and sensitize fetal immune cells to food and airborne allergens. Several limitations of the study that might have affected their findings were identified, including a general increase in childhood asthma but not necessarily an increase in allergic asthma (4). The study requires confirmation.

A second meta-analysis of PPIs in pregnancy was reported in 2009 (5). Based on 1530 exposed compared with 133,410 not-exposed pregnancies, the OR for major malformations was 1.12, 95% CI 0.86–1.45. There also was no increased risk for SABs (OR 1.29, 95% CI 0.84–1.97) or preterm birth (OR 1.13, 95% CI 0.96–1.33) (5).

In a 2010 study from Denmark, covering the period 1996–2008, there were 840,968 live births among whom 5082 were exposed to PPIs between 4 weeks before conception to the end of the 1st trimester (6). In the exposed group there were 174 (3.4%) major malformations compared with 21,811 (2.6%) not exposed to PPIs (adjusted prevalence odds ratio [aPOR] 1.23, 95 CI 1.05–1.44). When the analysis was limited to exposure in the 1st trimester, there were 118 (3.2%) major malformations among 3651 exposed infants (aPOR 1.10, 95% CI 0.91–1.34). For exposure to pantoprazole in the 1st trimester, there were 21 (3.8%) major birth defects among 549 live births (aPOR 1.33, 95% CI 0.85–2.08) (see Esomeprazole, Lansoprazole, Omeprazole, and Rabeprazole for their data). The data showed that exposure to PPIs in the 1st trimester was not associated with a significantly increased risk of major birth defects (6). An accompanying editorial discussed the strengths and weaknesses of the study (7).

In a 2012 publication, the National Birth Defects Prevention study, a multisite population-based case–control study, examined whether nausea/vomiting of pregnancy (NVP) or its treatment were associated with the most common noncardiac defects (nonsyndromic cleft lip with or without cleft palate [CL/P], cleft palate alone [CP], neural tube defects [NTDs], and hypospadias) (8). PPI exposure included esomeprazole, lansoprazole, and omeprazole. There were 4524 cases and 5859 controls. NVP was not associated with cleft palate or NTDs, but modest risk reductions were observed for CL/P and hypospadias. Increased risks were found for PPIs ($N = 7$) and hypospadias (adjusted OR [aOR] 4.36, 95% CI 1.21–15.81), steroids ($N = 10$) and hypospadias (aOR 2.87,

95% CI 1.03–7.97), and ondansetron ($N = 11$) and CP (aOR 2.37, 95% CI 1.18–4.76) (8).

Another 2012 study, using the Danish nationwide registries, evaluated the risk of hypospadias after exposure to PPIs during the 1st trimester and throughout gestation (9). The study period, 1997 through 2009, included all liveborn boys that totaled 430,569 of whom 2926 were exposed to maternal PPI use. Hypospadias was diagnosed in 20 (0.7%) exposed boys, whereas 2683 (0.6%) of the nonexposed had hypospadias (adjusted prevalence ratio [aPR] 1.1, 95% CI 0.7–1.7). For the 5227 boys exposed throughout pregnancy, 32 (0.6%) had hypospadias (PR 1.0, 95% CI 0.7–1.4). When the analysis was restricted to mothers with 2 or more PPI prescriptions, the aPR of overall hypospadias was 1.7 (95% CI 0.9–3.3), and 1.6 (95% CI 0.7–3.9) for omeprazole. The authors concluded that PPIs were not associated with hypospadias (9).

A large retrospective cohort study from Israel covering the period 1998–2009 was published in 2012 (10). Among 114,960 live births, there were 110,783 singletons and 1239 EABs. Major malformations were observed in 6037 (5.5%) singletons and in 468 abortuses. Exposure to a PPI (lansoprazole, omeprazole, or pantoprazole) during the 1st trimester occurred in 1186 (1159 infants and 27 abortuses). In the exposed infants and abortuses, 80 (6.7%) had a major malformation compared with 6425 (5.9%) not exposed (aOR 1.06, 95% CI 0.84–1.33). A separate analysis with pantoprazole was not possible because of the limited number of exposures. However, the overall data showed that exposure to PPIs during the 1st trimester was not associated with an increased risk of major defects. Moreover, additional analysis revealed that exposure during the 3rd trimester was not associated with increased risk of perinatal mortality, premature delivery, low birth weight, or low Apgar scores (10).

Five reviews on the treatment of GERD have concluded that PPIs can be used in pregnancy with relative safety (11–15). Because there is either very limited or no human pregnancy data for the three newest agents in this class (dexlansoprazole, esomeprazole, and rabeprazole), other drugs in the class are preferred.

BREASTFEEDING SUMMARY

Small amounts of pantoprazole are excreted into breast milk. A 43-year-old mother, partially nursing a healthy 10-month-old, 8.2-kg, female infant was given a single 40-mg enteric-coated pantoprazole tablet (16). Breastfeeding was held while nine samples of maternal serum and six of breast milk were obtained over a 24-hour interval. The milk samples, about 10 mL each, were obtained at 0, 2, 4, 6, 8, and 24 hours postdose. Pantoprazole was detected only in the 2-hour (0.036 mg/L) and 4-hour (0.024 mg/L) samples, resulting in an estimated AUC of 0.103 mg·hr/L. The milk AUC was about 2.8% of the AUC for plasma. The peak maternal plasma concentration, 1.65 mg/L, occurred at 2 hours, but the levels were <0.025 mg/L at 8 and 24 hours postdose. If the infant had been nursing, the authors estimated that the infant dose would have been ≤0.14% of the weight-adjusted maternal dose (16).

The results of the above case are consistent with the relatively low molecular weight (about 432 for the hydrated form) that suggests pantoprazole will be excreted into breast milk. In addition, pantoprazole is unstable at acidic pH so the amount actually absorbed by the infant may have been less than estimated (16).

References

1. Product information. Protonix. Wyeth-Ayerst Pharmaceuticals, 2001.
2. Nikfar S, Abdollahi M, Moretti ME, Magee LA, Koren G. Use of proton pump inhibitors during pregnancy and rates of major malformations: a meta analysis. Dig Dis Sci 2002;47:1526–9.
3. Diav-Citrin O, Arnon J, Shechtman S, Schaefer C, Van Tonningen MR, Clementi M, De Santis M, Robert-Gnansia E, Valti E, Malm H, Ornoy A. The safety of proton pump inhibitors in pregnancy: a multicentre prospective controlled trial. Aliment Pharmacol Ther 2005;21:269–75.
4. Dehlink E, Yen E, Leichtner AM, Hait EJ, Fiebiger E. First evidence of a possible association between gastric acid suppression during pregnancy and childhood asthma: a population-based register study. Clin Exp Allergy 2009;39:246–53.
5. Gill SK, O'Brien L, Einarson TR, Koren G. The safety of proton pump inhibitors (PPIs) in pregnancy: a meta-analysis. Am J Gastroenterol 2009;104:1541–5.
6. Pasternak B, Hviid A. Use of proton-pump inhibitors in early pregnancy and the risk of birth defects. N Engl J Med 2010;363:2114–23.
7. Mitchell AA. Proton-pump inhibitors and birth defects—some reassurance, but more needed. N Engl J Med 2010;363:2161–3.
8. Anderka M, Mitchell AA, Louik C, Werler MM, Hernandez-Diaz S, Rasmussen SA, and the National Birth Defects Prevention Study. Medications used to treat nausea and vomiting of pregnancy and the risk of selected birth defects. Birth Defects Res A Clin Mol Teratol 2012;94:22–30.
9. Erichsen R, Mikkelsen E, Pedersen L, Sorensen HT. Maternal use of proton pump inhibitors during early pregnancy and the prevalence of hypospadias in male offspring. Am J Ther 2012 Feb 3; [Epub ahead of print].
10. Matok I, Levy A, Wiznitzer A, Uziel E. Koren G, Gorodischer R. The safety of fetal exposure to proton-pump inhibitors during pregnancy. Dig Dis Sci 2012;57:699–705.
11. Broussard CN, Richter JE. Treating gasto-oesophageal reflux disease during pregnancy and lactation. What are the safest therapy options? Drug Saf 1998;19:325–37.
12. Katz PO, Castell DO. Gastroesophageal reflux disease during pregnancy. Gastroenterol Clin North Am 1998;27:153–67.
13. Ramakrishnan A, Katz PO. Pharmacologic management of gastroesophageal reflux disease. Curr Treat Options Gastroenterol 2002;5:301–10.
14. Richter JE. Gastroesophageal reflux disease during pregnancy. Gastroenterol Clin N Am 2003;32:235–61.
15. Richter JE. Review article: the management of heartburn in pregnancy. Aliment Pharmacol Ther 2005;22:749–57.
16. Plante L, Ferron GM, Unruh M, Mayer PR. Excretion of pantoprazole in human breast milk. J Reprod Med 2004;49:825–7.

P

PANTOTHENIC ACID

Vitamin

PREGNANCY RECOMMENDATION: Compatible
BREASTFEEDING RECOMMENDATION: Compatible

PREGNANCY SUMMARY

No reports of maternal or fetal complications associated with pantothenic acid have been located.

FETAL RISK SUMMARY

Pantothenic acid, a water-soluble B-complex vitamin, acts as a coenzyme in the metabolism or synthesis of a number of carbohydrates, proteins, lipids, and steroid hormones (1). The U.S. recommended daily allowance (RDA) for pantothenic acid or its derivatives (dexpanthenol and calcium pantothenate) in pregnancy is 10.0 mg (2).

Deficiency of this vitamin was not found in two studies evaluating maternal vitamin levels during pregnancy (3,4). Like other B-complex vitamins, newborn pantothenic acid levels are significantly greater than maternal levels (3–6). At term, mean pantothenate levels in 174 mothers were 430 ng/mL (range 250–710 ng/mL) and in their newborns 780 ng/mL (range 400–1480 ng/mL) (3). Placental transfer of pantothenate to the fetus is by active transport, but it is slower than transfer of other B-complex vitamins (7,8). In one report, low-birth-weight infants had significantly lower levels of pantothenic acid than did normal-weight infants (6).

BREASTFEEDING SUMMARY

Pantothenic acid is excreted in breast milk with concentrations directly proportional to intake (9,10). With a dietary intake of 8–15 mg/day, mean milk concentrations average 1.93–2.35 mcg/mL (9). In a group of mothers who had delivered premature babies (28–34 weeks' gestational age), pantothenic acid milk levels were significantly greater than a comparable group with term babies (39–41 weeks) (10). Milk levels in the preterm group averaged 3.91 mcg/mL up to 40 weeks' gestational age and then fell to 3.16 mcg/mL. For the term group, levels at 2 and 12 weeks postpartum were 2.57 and 2.55 mcg/mL, respectively. A 1983 English study measured pantothenic acid levels in pooled human milk obtained from preterm (26 mothers: 29–34 weeks) and term (35 mothers: ≥39 weeks) patients (11). Milk from mothers of preterm infants rose from 1.29 mcg/mL (colostrum) to 2.27 mcg/mL (16–196 days), whereas milk from mothers of term infants increased during the same period from 1.26 to 2.61 mcg/mL.

An RDA for pantothenic acid during lactation has not been established. However, because this vitamin is required for good health, amounts at least equal to the RDA recommendation for pregnancy are recommended. If the diet of the lactating woman adequately supplies this amount, maternal supplementation with pantothenic acid is probably not required. Supplementation with the pregnancy RDA recommendation for pantothenic acid is recommended for those women with inadequate nutritional intake.

References

1. American Hospital Formulary Service. *Drug Information 1997*. Bethesda, MD: American Society of Health-System Pharmacists, 1997:2813–5.
2. *Recommended Dietary Allowances*. 9th ed. Washington, DC: National Academy of Sciences, 1980:122–4.
3. Baker H, Frank O, Thomson AD, Langer A, Munves ED, De Angelis B, Kaminetzky HA. Vitamin profile of 174 mothers and newborns at parturition. Am J Clin Nutr 1975;28:59–65.
4. Baker H, Frank O, Deangelis B, Feingold S, Kaminetzky HA. Role of placenta in maternal–fetal vitamin transfer in humans. Am J Obstet Gynecol 1981;141:792–6.
5. Cohenour SH, Calloway DH. Blood, urine, and dietary pantothenic acid levels of pregnant teenagers. Am J Clin Nutr 1972;25:512–7.
6. Baker H, Thind IS, Frank O, DeAngelis B, Caterini H, Louria DB. Vitamin levels in low-birth-weight newborn infants and their mothers. Am J Obstet Gynecol 1977;129:521–4.
7. Hill EP, Longo LD. Dynamics of maternal–fetal nutrient transfer. Fed Proc 1980;39:239–44.
8. Kaminetsky HA, Baker H, Frank O, Langer A. The effects of intravenously administered water-soluble vitamins during labor in normovitaminemic and hypovitaminemic gravidas on maternal and neonatal blood vitamin levels at delivery. Am J Obstet Gynecol 1974;120:697–703.
9. Deodhar AD, Rajalakshmi R, Ramakrishnan CV. Studies on human lactation. Part III. Effect of dietary vitamin supplementation on vitamin contents of breast milk. Acta Paediatr Scand 1964;53:42–8.
10. Song WO, Chan GM, Wyse BW, Hansen RG. Effect of pantothenic acid status on the content of the vitamin in human milk. Am J Clin Nutr 1984;40: 317–24.
11. Ford JE, Zechalko A, Murphy J, Brooke OG. Comparison of the B vitamin composition of milk from mothers of preterm and term babies. Arch Dis Child 1983;58:367–72.

PARAMETHADIONE

[Withdrawn from the market. See 8th edition.]

PAREGORIC

Antidiarrheal

PREGNANCY RECOMMENDATION: Human Data Suggest Risk
BREASTFEEDING RECOMMENDATION: Limited Human Data—Probably Compatible

P

PREGNANCY SUMMARY

Paregoric is a mixture of opium powder, anise oil, benzoic acid, camphor, glycerin, and ethanol. Its action is mainly caused by morphine (see also Morphine). High or chronic use near term could result in neonatal depression and/or withdrawal. There also is concern that exposure to opioids during organogenesis, including morphine, results in a low absolute risk of congenital anomalies.

FETAL RISK SUMMARY

Paregoric is indicated for the treatment of diarrhea. Animal reproduction studies have not been conducted with paregoric or morphine. Although long-term animal studies have not been conducted, paregoric has no known carcinogenic or mutagenic potential (1).

The Collaborative Perinatal Project monitored 50,282 mother–child pairs, 90 of whom had 1st trimester exposure to paregoric (2, pp. 287–295). For use anytime during pregnancy, 562 exposures were recorded (2, p. 434). No evidence was found to suggest a relationship to large categories of major or minor malformations or to individual defects.

BREASTFEEDING SUMMARY

The active component of paregoric, morphine, is thought to be compatible with breastfeeding (see Morphine). However, high doses or chronic use might have long-term effects on a nursing infant.

References

1. Product information. Paregoric. Hi-Tech Pharmacal, 2012.
2. Heinonen OP, Slone D, Shapiro S. *Birth Defects and Drugs in Pregnancy*. Littleton, MA: Publishing Sciences Group, 1977.

PARGYLINE

[Withdrawn from the market. See 9th edition.]

PARICALCITOL

Vitamin

PREGNANCY RECOMMENDATION: **No Human Data—Probably Compatible**
BREASTFEEDING RECOMMENDATION: **No Human Data—Probably Compatible**

PREGNANCY SUMMARY

No reports describing the use of paricalcitol in human pregnancy have been located. The drug did not cause structural anomalies in animals, but high doses did cause toxicity that was thought to be secondary to hypercalcemia. Human pregnancy experience with vitamin D and calcitriol indicates that recommended doses are safe in pregnancy. There is no evidence that the effects of recommended doses of paricalcitol would be any different. However, if the mother is taking paricalcitol, she should not take pharmacologic doses of vitamin D and its derivatives (1).

FETAL RISK SUMMARY

Paricalcitol is a synthetic analog of calcitriol, the physiologically active form of vitamin D. (See also Calcitriol and Vitamin D.) Paricalcitol, oral or IV, is indicated for the prevention and treatment of secondary hyperparathyroidism associated with chronic kidney disease. The vitamin is well absorbed (72%) and is extensively bound to plasma proteins (≥99.8%). Paricalcitol also is extensively metabolized. The plasma half-life in healthy individuals is 4–6 hours, but it is 17–20 hours in patients with chronic kidney disease (1).

Reproduction studies have been conducted in pregnant rabbits and rats. In these species, daily doses 0.5 and 2 times, respectively, the recommended human dose based on BSA (RHD) were associated with minimal decreases (5%) in fetal viability. In rats, a dose 13 times the RHD given 3 times weekly caused a significant increase in the mortality of newborn pups, but this dose also was maternally toxic. Long-term studies for carcinogenicity revealed an increased incidence of uterine leiomyoma and leiomyosarcoma in mice and uterine leiomyoma and benign adrenal pheochromocytoma in rats. Assays for mutagenic or clastogenic effects were negative, as was impairment of fertility in male and female rats (1).

Paricalcitol crosses the rat placenta (1), but studies in humans have not been located. The molecular weight (about 417) and the elimination half-life suggest that paricalcitol will cross to the embryo and fetus. Moreover, both vitamin

D and calcitriol cross the human placenta (see Vitamin D) but do so slowly. Therefore, paricalcitol probably crosses placenta, but the extensive metabolism and plasma protein binding should limit the amount reaching the embryo and/or fetus.

BREASTFEEDING SUMMARY

No reports describing the use of paricalcitol during human lactation have been located. The molecular weight (about 417) and the long elimination half-life in patients with chronic kidney disease (17–20 hours) suggest that the vitamin will be excreted into breast milk. However, the extensive metabolism and plasma protein binding should limit the amount in milk. Women who are nursing and taking paricalcitol should consider not taking vitamin supplements containing vitamin D. Whether such a woman does or does not, serum calcium levels in the nursing infant should be monitored.

Reference

1. Product information. Zemplar. Abbott Laboratories, 2006.

PARNAPARIN

[Withdrawn from the market. See 9th edition.]

PAROMOMYCIN

Antibiotic (Aminoglycoside)/Amebicide

PREGNANCY RECOMMENDATION: Limited Human Data—Probably Compatible
BREASTFEEDING RECOMMENDATION: No Human Data—Probably Compatible

PREGNANCY SUMMARY

Paromomycin is an aminoglycoside antibiotic used for intestinal amebiasis. No reports linking this agent with congenital malformations have been located. Because it is poorly absorbed, with almost 100% of an oral dose excreted unchanged in the feces, little if any of the drug will reach the fetus.

FETAL RISK SUMMARY

Two women, one at 13 weeks' and the other at 23 weeks' gestation, were treated for a symptomatic intestinal infection caused by *Giardia lamblia* (1). Both delivered normal female infants at term. A 1985 review of intestinal parasites and pregnancy concluded that treatment of the pregnant patient should only be considered if the "parasite is causing clinical disease or may cause public health problems" (2). When indicated, paromomycin has been recommended for the treatment of protozoan infections caused by *G. lamblia* and *Entamoeba histolytica* and for tapeworm infestations occurring during pregnancy (2).

BREASTFEEDING SUMMARY

Paromomycin excretion in human milk is not expected as the drug is not absorbed into the systemic circulation after oral dosing.

References

1. Kreutner AK, Del Bene VE, Amstey MS. Giardiasis in pregnancy. Am J Obstet Gynecol 1981;140:895–901.
2. D'Alauro F, Lee RV, Pao-In K, Khairallah M. Intestinal parasites and pregnancy. Obstet Gynecol 1985;66:639–43.

PAROXETINE

Antidepressant

PREGNANCY RECOMMENDATION: Human Data Suggest Risk
BREASTFEEDING RECOMMENDATION: Limited Human Data—Potential Toxicity

PREGNANCY SUMMARY

A public health advisory was issued by the FDA regarding paroxetine on December 8, 2005 (1). The advisory cited evidence from two epidemiologic studies (2,3) that paroxetine use in the 1st trimester was associated with a 1.8-fold increased risk for congenital malformations overall and a 1.5- to 2.0-fold increased risk for cardiac defects (most were atrial or ventricular septal defects). The advisory noted that the pregnancy category for paroxetine had been changed from C to D and that paroxetine should be avoided, if possible, in the 1st trimester of pregnancy (1). The results of two 2007 case–control studies suggested that the absolute risk of any birth defect with paroxetine and other selective serotonin reuptake inhibitors (SSRIs) is low (4,5). One study found an increased risk from SSRIs (the highest risk was with paroxetine alone) for a group of three defects (anencephaly, craniosynostosis, and omphalocele) (5), but the other did not (3), and neither found a relationship with ventricular septal defects. In addition, one study found an association between paroxetine and four specific defects: anencephaly, gastroschisis, omphalocele, and right ventricular outflow tract obstruction lesions (4). The second study did not find an increased risk with the first three defects but did so for the cardiac defect (5). That study also reported that paroxetine was associated with neural tube defects and clubfoot. Although developmental toxicity is well known to be dose related, only one study has considered dosage, finding that doses >25 mg/day were related to major malformations and cardiac defects (6). An accompanying editorial highlighted the findings and limitations of these studies, concluding that the absolute risk of major malformations was likely to be low (7). For right ventricular outflow tract obstruction defects and all congenital heart defects, it was thought to be unlikely that the absolute risks would exceed 1% and 2%, respectively (7). There also is evidence, but not conclusive, that SSRI antidepressants, including paroxetine, are associated with higher risks of other developmental toxicities, including spontaneous abortions (SABs), low birth weight, prematurity, neonatal serotonin syndrome, neonatal behavioral syndrome (withdrawal), possibly sustained abnormal neurobehavior beyond the neonatal period, respiratory distress, and persistent pulmonary hypertension of the newborn (PPHN).

Although more data have accumulated since publication of the above references, the issue whether or not paroxetine and other SSRIs cause structural anomalies is still being debated. One reason cited in a joint statement from the American Psychiatric Association and the American College of Obstetricians and Gynecologists (see reference 60) is the adequacy of the research that has not completely controlled for other factors that could influence birth outcomes, such as maternal illness or problematic health behaviors that could adversely affect pregnancy. Although avoiding the use of paroxetine in pregnancy, especially high doses, may be an option, the apparently low risk of embryo–fetal harm must be balanced against the risk of untreated or undertreated depression. The decision to use or not use paroxetine, or any other antidepressant, must be made on a case-by-case basis. If paroxetine is used in pregnancy, or if inadvertent exposure occurs, the woman should be counseled as to the potential, albeit low, risks for birth defects and the higher risks for complications in the newborn.

FETAL RISK SUMMARY

Paroxetine is an SSRI antidepressant. Its chemical structure is unrelated to other antidepressants, including those classified as SSRI agents. Paroxetine is metabolized to inactive metabolites. About 95% is bound to plasma protein and the mean plasma elimination half-life is about 21 hours (2).

All of the antidepressant agents in the SSRI class (citalopram, escitalopram, fluoxetine, fluvoxamine, paroxetine, and sertraline) share a similar mechanism of action but have different chemical structures. These differences could be construed as evidence against any conclusion that they share similar effects on the embryo, fetus, or newborn. In the mouse embryo, however, craniofacial morphogenesis appears to be regulated, at least in part, by serotonin. Interference with serotonin regulation by chemically different inhibitors produces similar craniofacial defects (8). Regardless of the structural differences, therefore, some of the potential adverse effects on pregnancy outcome may also be similar.

In reproduction studies with rats and rabbits, paroxetine was not teratogenic at doses that were equivalent to 9.7 and 2.2 times, respectively, the maximum recommended human dose based on BSA (MRHD) for depression and social anxiety disorder (DSAD), and 8.1 and 1.9 times, respectively, the MRHD for obsessive-compulsive disorder (OCD). In rats dosed at 0.19 times the MRHD for DSAD and 0.16 times the MRHD for OCD, there was an increase in pup deaths when paroxetine was used during the last trimester and continued during lactation. The cause of the deaths was not known (2). In another study, no embryotoxic or teratogenic effects were observed in either of these species at doses similar to those used above (9).

The effects of paroxetine on behavioral changes in developing mice have been studied (10,11). The drug was administered for 2 weeks before conception and throughout gestation. A similar group of mice were administered placebo for comparison. The daily dose was known to achieve levels in the mouse serum equivalent to the upper human therapeutic level and to obtain levels in the fetal mouse brain equivalent to those in the adult mouse (11). No drug-induced facial abnormalities were seen nor were there any differences between the exposed and control groups in terms of pregnancy duration, litter size, and sex ratio. Body weights, however, were significantly lower for the exposed pups (both male and female) at least through postnatal day 5. Most of the behavioral tests showed no differences between the groups, but subtle differences in anxiety testing and adult male aggressiveness were noted. These effects may have resulted from the effect of paroxetine on the development of the postsynaptic serotonin (1A) receptors (11).

Consistent with the molecular weight (about 329 for the free base), paroxetine crosses the human placenta. A 2003 study of the placental transfer of SSRI antidepressants found cord blood:maternal serum ratios of 0.05–0.91 (12). The dose-to-delivery interval was 6–40 hours with the highest ratio occurring at 21 hours.

Congenital Malformations

By 1995, the FDA had received 10 reports of birth defects involving paroxetine, including 4 involving clubfoot and 2 cases of cutaneous hemangioma (F. Rosa, personal communication, FDA, 1995).

The results of a postmarketing survey of paroxetine, conducted in England between March 1991 and March 1992, were published in 1993 (13). A total of 137 pregnancies were identified, including 66 in which the drug was stopped before the last menstrual period. In this group, there were 12 deliveries, 9 SABs, 5 elective abortions (EABs), and 40 unknown outcomes. Among the remaining 71 pregnancies, 63 were known to be exposed during the 1st trimester, but the dates of exposure were uncertain in 8. The outcomes in the combined exposed group were 44 newborns (3 sets of twins; 1 twin stillborn [cause not specified]), 9 SABs, 12 EABs, and 9 unknown outcomes. There were no congenital anomalies in the liveborn infants (data not provided for the abortions or stillborn) (13).

A 1998 noninterventional observational cohort study described the outcomes of pregnancies in women who had been prescribed ≥1 of 34 newly marketed drugs by general practitioners in England (14). Data were obtained by questionnaires sent to the prescribing physicians 1 month after the expected or possible date of delivery. In 831 (78%) of the pregnancies, a newly marketed drug was thought to had been taken during the 1st trimester with birth defects noted in 14 (2.5%) singleton births of the 557 newborns (10 sets of twins). In addition, two birth defects were observed in aborted fetuses. However, few of the aborted fetuses were examined. Paroxetine was taken during the 1st trimester in 63 pregnancies. The outcomes of these pregnancies included 8 SABs, 11 EABs, 1 intrauterine death, 2 stillborns (twins), 3 cases lost to follow-up, 41 normal infants (3 premature plus 2 sets of full-term twins). No birth defects were noted in any of the outcomes (14).

In a 1996 descriptive case series, the European Network of the Teratology Information Services (ENTIS) prospectively examined the outcomes of 689 pregnancies exposed to antidepressants (15). Multiple drug therapy occurred in about two-thirds of the mothers. Paroxetine was used in three pregnancies, all with normal outcomes.

A prospective, multicenter, controlled cohort study published in 1998 evaluated the pregnancy outcomes of 267 women exposed to ≥1 of 3 SSRI antidepressants during the 1st trimester: fluvoxamine (N = 26); paroxetine (N = 97); and sertraline (N = 147) (16). The women were combined into a study group without differentiation as to the drug they had consumed. A randomly selected control group (N = 267) was formed from women who had exposures to nonteratogenic agents. In most cases, the pregnancy outcomes were determined 6–9 months after delivery. No significant differences were measured in the number of live births, SABs, EABs, stillbirths, major malformations, birth weight, or gestational age at birth. Nine major malformations were observed in each group. The relative risk (RR) for major anomalies was 1.06 (95% confidence interval [CI] 0.43–2.62). No clustering of defects was apparent. The outcomes of women who took an antidepressant throughout gestation were similar to those who took an antidepressant only during the 1st trimester (16). All of the women in the study group had taken an antidepressant during embryogenesis (17).

A 2005 meta-analysis of 7 prospective comparative cohort studies involving 1774 patients was conducted to quantify the relationship between 7 newer antidepressants and major malformations (18). The antidepressants were bupropion, fluoxetine, fluvoxamine, nefazodone, paroxetine, sertraline, and trazodone. There was no statistical increase in the risk of major birth defects above the baseline of 1%–3% in the general population for the individual or combined studies (18).

A brief 2005 report described significant associations between the use of SSRIs in the 1st trimester and congenital defects (19). The data were collected by the CDC-sponsored National Birth Defects Prevention Study in an ongoing case–control study of birth defect risk factors. Case infants (N = 5357) with major birth defects were compared with 3366 normal controls. A positive association was found with omphalocele (161 cases; odds ratio [OR] 3.0, 95% CI 1.4–6.1). Paroxetine, which accounted for 36% of all SSRI exposures, had the strongest association with the defect (OR 6.3, 95% CI 2.0–19.6). The study also found a significant association between the use of any SSRI and craniosynostosis (372 cases; OR 1.8, 95% CI 1.0–3.2) (19).

In an expansion of the above CDC-sponsored study, 9622 case infants with major birth defects were compared with 4092 control infants selected randomly from the same geographic areas (4). The reported use of SSRIs in the period 1 month before to 3 months after conception was 2.4% (230 case mothers) and 2.1% (86 control mothers). Although the study found no significant associations between early gestational exposure to SSRIs overall and congenital heart defects (includes four types and eight subtypes), spina bifida, oral clefts, or nine other defects, significant associations were found with anencephaly (OR 2.4, 95% CI 1.1–5.1, p 0.02), craniosynostosis (OR 2.5, 95% CI 1.5–4.0, p <0.001), and omphalocele (OR 2.8, 95% CI 1.3–5.7, p 0.005). The use of paroxetine (OR 4.2, 95% CI 2.1–8.5) or citalopram (OR 4.0, 95% CI 1.3–11.9) significantly increased the risk for the combined three defects. For the three most commonly used SSRIs and individual defects, increased risks were found with fluoxetine (craniosynostosis N = 10, OR 2.8, 95% CI 1.3–6.1), sertraline (anencephaly N = 4, OR 3.2, 95% CI 1.1–9.3), and paroxetine (anencephaly N = 5, OR 5.1, 95% CI 1.7–15.3; right ventricular outflow tract obstruction N = 7, OR 2.5, 95% CI 1.0–6.0; omphalocele N = 6, OR 8.1, 95% CI 3.1–20.8; and gastroschisis N = 5, OR 2.9, 95% CI 1.0–8.4). However, the absolute risks for these defects are small and require confirmation (4).

In a multicenter, prospective controlled study, the pregnancy outcomes of three groups of women were evaluated: (a) paroxetine 330 (286 in the 1st trimester); (b) fluoxetine 230 (206 in the 1st trimester); and (c) 1141 exposures not known to cause birth defects (20). Compared with controls, there was a higher rate of congenital defects among those exposed to 1st trimester paroxetine, 5.1% vs. 2.6%, RR 1.92, 95% CI 1.01–3.65. There also was a higher rate for cardiovascular anomalies, 1.9% vs. 0.6%, RR 3.46, 95% CI 1.06–11.42. In addition, perinatal complications were more prevalent in both SSRI groups than in controls (20).

A meta-analysis of clinical trials (1990–2005) with SSRIs was reported in 2006 (21). The SSRI agents included were citalopram, fluoxetine, fluvoxamine, paroxetine, and sertraline. The specific outcomes analyzed were major, minor, cardiac malformations, and SABs. The OR with 95% CI for the four outcomes were 1.394 (0.906–2.145), 0.97 (0.13–6.93), 1.193 (0.531–2.677), and 1.70 (1.28–2.25), respectively. Only the risk of SABs was significantly increased (21).

In 1999, the Swedish Medical Birth Registry compared the use of antidepressants in early pregnancy and delivery outcomes for the years 1995–1997 (22). There were no significant differences for birth defects, infant survival, or risk of low birth weight (<2500 g) among singletons between those exposed to any antidepressant, SSRIs only, or non-SSRIs only, but a shorter gestational duration (<37 weeks) was observed for any antidepressant exposure (OR 1.43, 95% CI 1.14–1.80) (22). A second Registry report, published in 2006 covering the years 1995–2003, analyzed the relationship between antidepressants and major malformations or cardiac defects (3). There was no significant increase in the risk of major malformations with any antidepressant. The strongest effect among cardiac defects was with ventricular or atrial septum defects (VSDs-ASDs). Significant increases were found with paroxetine (OR 2.22, 95% CI 1.39–3.55) and clomipramine (OR 1.87, 95% CI 1.16–2.99 (3). In 2007, the analysis was expanded to include the years 1995–2004 (23). There were 6481 women (6555 infants) who had reported the use of SSRIs in early pregnancy. The number of women using a single SSRI during the 1st trimester was 2579 citalopram, 1807 sertraline, 908 paroxetine, 860 fluoxetine, 66 escitalopram, and 36 fluvoxamine. After adjustment, only paroxetine was significantly associated with an increased risk of cardiac defects (N = 13, RR 2.62, 95% CI 1.40–4.50) or VSDs-ASDs (N = 8, RR 3.07, 95% CI 1.32–6.04). Analysis of the combined SSRI group, excluding paroxetine, revealed no associations with these defects. The study found no association with omphalocele or craniostenosis (23).

In 2006, the manufacturer reported the findings of a retrospective cohort study using United States United Healthcare data (2). There were 5956 infants of mothers dispensed paroxetine or other antidepressants during the 1st trimester, including 815 for paroxetine. Compared with other antidepressants, there was a trend for increased risk of cardiovascular defects with paroxetine (12 cases, OR 1.5, 95% CI 0.8–2.9). Nine of the paroxetine cases had VSDs. There also was an increased risk of overall major anomalies with paroxetine compared with other antidepressants (OR 1.8, 95% CI 1.2–2.8). The prevalence of all congenital defects was 4% for paroxetine vs. 2% for other antidepressants (2).

A cohort study from Denmark compared the number of infants with congenital malformations from mothers who either took or did not take an SSRI during the first 3 months of pregnancy (24). The 1051 women who filled a prescription for an SSRI from 30 days before conception to the end of the 1st trimester gave birth to 51 (4.9%) infants with a defect compared with 5112 (3.4%) infants from 150,780 control mothers (RR 1.34, 95% CI 1.00–1.79). For 453 women who filled such a prescription in the 2nd and 3rd months of pregnancy, 31 (6.8%) of whom had an infant with a defect, the RR was 1.84, 95% CI 1.25–2.71 (24).

A 2007 study evaluated the association between 1st trimester exposure to paroxetine and cardiac defects by quantifying the dose–response relationship (6). A population-based pregnancy registry was used by linking three administrative databases so that it included all pregnancies in Quebec between 1997 and 2003. There were 101 infants with major congenital defects, 24 involving the heart, among the 1403 women using only one type of antidepressant during the 1st trimester. The use of paroxetine or other SSRIs did not significantly increase the risk of major defects or cardiac defects compared with non-SSRI antidepressants. However, a paroxetine dose >25 mg/day during the 1st trimester was significantly associated with an increased risk of major defects (OR 2.23, 95% CI 1.19–4.17) and of cardiac defects (OR 3.07, 95% CI 1.00–9.42) (6).

A study published in 2007 was conducted to determine if paroxetine exposure in the 1st trimester was associated with congenital malformations (25). Exposure to the antidepressants was based on drug dispensing and timing was based on estimated dates of conception for singleton and multi-gestations. Using data collected in 1995–2004, the study cohorts included 1020 infants exposed to paroxetine monotherapy or polytherapy in the 1st trimester, and a subset of 815 infants exposed only to paroxetine monotherapy in the 1st trimester. The comparison cohorts, exposed to other antidepressants, were 4936 exposed to monotherapy or polytherapy, and a subset of 4198 infants exposed only to monotherapy in the 1st trimester. The adjusted odds ratios (AORs) for all paroxetine-associated congenital malformations were 1.89 (95% CI 1.20–2.98) for monotherapy, and 1.76 (95% CI 1.18–2.64) for monotherapy or polytherapy. For cardiovascular malformations, the AORs for the two groups were 1.46 (95% CI 0.74–2.88) and 1.68 (95% CI 0.95–2.97), respectively. A number of study limitations were discussed, such as missing data from charts that could not be assessed and the inability to document actual consumption of the antidepressants. The investigators concluded that the findings suggested a possible modest increased occurrence of congenital defects compared with other antidepressants (25).

A 2007 review conducted a literature search to determine the risk of major congenital malformations after 1st trimester exposure to SSRIs and SNRIs (26). Fifteen controlled studies were analyzed. The data were adequate to suggest that citalopram, fluoxetine, sertraline, and venlafaxine were not associated with an increased risk of congenital defects. In contrast, the analysis did suggest an increased risk with paroxetine. The data were inadequate to determine the risk for the other SSRIs and SNRIs (26).

Data collected in the period 1993–2004 by the Slone Epidemiology Center Birth Defects Study and reported in 2007 evaluated associations between 1st trimester use of SSRIs (defined as exposure 28 days before to 112 days after the last menstrual period) and the risk of major birth defects (5). There were 9849 case infants with major malformations and 5860 control infants without malformations. Two analyses were conducted: one on defects previously associated with SSRIs (craniosynostosis, omphalocele, and cardiac defects) and the other on some defects not previously reported to be associated with SSRI exposure. For outcomes previously reported, only the cardiac anomaly, right ventricular outflow tract obstruction defect, was associated with the use of any SSRI (OR 2.0, 95% CI 1.1–3.6). Paroxetine also was associated with that defect (OR 3.3, 95% CI 1.3–8.8). Sertraline was associated with an increased risk of omphalocele

(OR 5.7, 95% CI 1.6–20.7) and septal defects (OR 2.0, 95% 1.2–4.0). For defects not previously associated with SSRIs, increased risks were found with sertraline (anal atresia, OR 4.4, 95% CI 1.2–16.4; and limb reduction defects, OR 3.9, 95% CI 1.1–13.5) and paroxetine (neural tube defects, OR 3.3, 95% CI 1.1–10.4; and clubfoot, OR 5.8, 95% CI 2.6–12.8). The use of any SSRI also was associated with clubfoot (OR 2.2, 95% CI 1.4–3.6). Additional studies are required but, even if confirmed, the absolute risks are small because the estimated prevalence of the defects also is small (e.g., the prevalence of anal atresia and right ventricular outflow tract obstruction defect are both thought to be 5.5 cases per 10,000 live births). Thus, an increased risk of four would mean an absolute risk of 0.2% (5).

A 2003 prospective study evaluated the pregnancy outcomes of 138 women treated with SSRIs antidepressants during gestation (27). The number of women using each agent was 73 fluoxetine, 36 sertraline, 19 paroxetine, 7 citalopram, and 3 fluvoxamine. Most (62%) took an SSRI throughout pregnancy and 95% were taking an SSRI at delivery. Birth complications were observed in 28 infants, including preterm birth (9 cases), meconium aspiration, nuchal cord, floppy at birth, and low birth weight. Four infants (2.9%) had low birth weight, all exposed to fluoxetine (40–80 mg/day) throughout pregnancy, including two of the three infants of mothers taking 80 mg/day. One infant had Hirschsprung disease, a major defect, and another had cavum septi pellucidi (neither the size of the cavum nor the SSRI agents were specified) (27). The clinical significance of cavum septi pellucidi is doubtful as it is nearly always present at birth but resolves in the first several months (28).

A 2008 retrospective case–control study from the province of Quebec involved 2329 women who had used antidepressants, 189 (8.1%) of whom had a baby with a major defect (29). The antidepressants were SSRIs, tricyclics, and newer classes of antidepressants. No association was found between the duration of antidepressant use during the 1st trimester and major congenital defects (29).

In 2008, Teratogen Information Services (TISs) in Jerusalem, Italy, and Germany reported a prospective, case-controlled, multicenter, observational study for major congenital anomalies (30). Women taking paroxetine (N = 348) or fluoxetine (N = 253) in the 1st trimester were compared with women exposed to nonteratogens (N = 1467). Significant increases in major anomalies were found for paroxetine (5.5%) and fluoxetine (5.9%) compared with controls (2.9%). After logistic regression analysis, cigarette smoking of ≥10 cigarettes/day (OR 5.4, 95% CI 1.76–16.54) and fluoxetine (OR 4.47, 95% CI 1.31–15.27) were significant variables for cardiovascular anomalies but not paroxetine (2.66, 95% CI 0.80–8.90) (30).

In a 2008 report, investigators gathered unpublished data from eight TISs on 1174 infants exposed in utero to paroxetine during the 1st trimester (31). In addition, information was obtained from five published database studies regarding 2061 cases of 1st trimester exposure to paroxetine. The control group consisted of pregnancy outcomes of women who had called a TIS inquiring about exposures to drugs thought to be safe in pregnancy. The rate of cardiovascular anomalies in the exposed TISs group was 0.7% compared with 0.7% in controls. In the database, the rate was 1.5%. When the TISs and database groups were combined, the mean rate of cardiovascular defects was 1.2% (95% CI 1.1–2.1). Although the investigators did not categorize the data by dose because there was insufficient variability to conduct a dose–response analysis, most of the women were taking ≤20 mg/day (31).

A 2009 study from Israel investigated the prevalence of nonsyndromic congenital heart defects in infants exposed in utero to SSRIs (32). The prospective case–control study involved 235 women who took the agents during the 1st trimester and who gave birth in the years 2000–2007 at one center. Controls (N = 67,636) were infants not exposed in utero to SSRIs. All infants with a persistent cardiac murmur were evaluated by echocardiography. In the cases, nonsyndromic heart defects (6 VSDs, 1 bicuspid aortic valve, and 1 right superior vena cava to coronary sinus) were found in 8 (3.40%) compared with 1083 (1.60%) controls. The difference was significant (RR 2.17, 95% CI 1.07–4.39). The prevalence rates for paroxetine and fluoxetine were 4.3% and 3.0%, respectively. Although there was a twofold higher risk for cardiac defects, all of the defects in the exposed group were considered mild (32).

A 2010 case report described abnormalities in naturally conceived, monozygotic twin females born at 33 weeks' gestation from a pregnancy complicated by gestational diabetes, polyhydramnios, and preterm premature rupture of the membranes (33). The birth weights were 1420 g (10–25th percentile) and 1250 g (<3rd percentile). Their mother had used paroxetine 5 mg/day during the first 2 months of pregnancy and 20 mg/day in the last 3 weeks. Ultrasound at 20 weeks' had shown right aortic arch in the first twin and a single umbilical artery in the second twin. At birth, facial dysmorphism, consisting of hypertelorism, proptosis, hypoplastic nasal pyramid, and wide nostrils were noted. Neurobehavioral and motor signs were noted on the 2nd day of life (hyperactivity, irritability, jitteriness, hyperextension of the trunk and limbs with worsening dyspnea during handling). At 6 months of life, the twins had adequate psychomotor development with no neurobehavioral or respiratory symptoms (33).

In a population-based case–control study from the Netherlands, 678 cases (fetuses and children with isolated heart defects) were compared with 615 controls (fetuses and children with a genetic disorder with no heart defect) (34). Exposure to paroxetine only in the 1st trimester was not associated with a significantly increased risk for heart defects overall (10 cases) (adjusted OR 1.5, 95% CI 0.5–4.0) but, based on three cases, was for atrium septum defects (adjusted OR 5.7, 95% CI 1.4–23.7) (34).

A 2010 meta-analysis of epidemiological studies evaluated 1st trimester exposures to paroxetine and congenital defects, particularly cardiac defects (35). The investigators analyzed published data from 1992 to 2008 and, in some instances, involved additional information that was requested and received from the original authors. The meta-analysis found little evidence of publication bias or overall statistical heterogeneity. The prevalence OR for 1st trimester paroxetine use and combined cardiac defects was 1.46, 95% CI 1.17–1.82, whereas for aggregated congenital defects it was 1.24, 95% CI 1.08–1.43. However, the increased prevalence of aggregated defects may have resulted, in part, from the increased prevalence of cardiac defects (35). Immediately following this meta-analysis were two sophisticated commentaries, one supporting an association between paroxetine and cardiac defects (36) and one opposing such an association (37).

A prospective cohort study evaluated a large group of pregnancies exposed to antidepressants in the 1st trimester to determine if there was an association with major malformations (38). The patient population came from the Motherisk database and involved 928 cases that met their criteria. The 928 matched (for age, smoking, and alcohol use) controls were pregnancies not exposed to antidepressants or known teratogens. In addition to the 149 paroxetine cases, the other cases were 113 bupropion, 184 citalopram, 21 escitalopram, 61 fluoxetine, 52 fluvoxamine, 68 mirtazapine, 39 nefazodone, 61 sertraline, 17 trazodone, and 154 venlafaxine. In the antidepressant group, there were 24 (2.5%) major defects compared with 25 (2.6%) in controls (odds ratio 0.9, 95% CI 0.5–1.61). There were five major anomalies in the paroxetine group: bilateral pulmonary hypoplasia, ventricular septal defect, clinodactyly, cleft lip and palate, and an omphalocele. There were no major defects in the pregnancies exposed to bupropion, escitalopram, or trazodone (38).

Complications in Neonates

(Includes references 22 and 27 above.)

A 2001 case report described complications consistent with neonatal withdrawal in four neonates exposed to paroxetine during pregnancy (39). The infants were delivered at 37–38 weeks' gestation and one mother breastfed her infant. The maternal doses were 10–120 mg/day. The symptoms in the four infants included jitteriness, irritability, lethargy, myoclonus, vomiting, and hypothermia. In one infant, serum levels of paroxetine and desipramine on days 5 and 15 of age were 48 and 70 ng/mL, respectively, and <10 and <10 ng/ mL, respectively. In a second infant, the serum paroxetine concentration on day 2 was 66 ng/mL, whereas trazodone was undetectable. Two infants were hypoglycemic (one shortly after birth and one at 40 hours of age), but both mothers had gestational diabetes mellitus. Necrotizing enterocolitis was also observed in two infants. The withdrawal symptoms in one infant resolved over a few days, but some symptoms in the other three were still apparent at discharge on days 5, 22, and 24 of age, respectively (39).

Another 2001 report described withdrawal symptoms in newborn infants exposed in utero to SSRIs (40). Male infants exposed to paroxetine ($N = 3$; 10–40 mg/day), citalopram ($N = 1$; 30 mg/day), or fluoxetine ($N = 1$; 20 mg/day) during gestation exhibited withdrawal symptoms at or within a few days of birth and lasting up to 1 month. Symptoms included irritability, constant crying, shivering, increased tonus, eating and sleeping problems, and convulsions (40).

Paroxetine withdrawal was suspected in a third 2001 case report (41). The mother had taken paroxetine (40 mg/day) throughout pregnancy and delivered a 2690-g female infant at 35 weeks' gestation. Apgar scores were 9, 10, and 10 at 1, 5, and 10 minutes, respectively. The premature infant was bottle-fed and did well during the first few days, but then became irritable, lethargic, hypertonic, apathetic, and jittery. Tube feeding was required. The infant improved without therapy and was discharged home at 18 days of age. After delivery, the mother's serum paroxetine concentration was 126 mcg/L (therapeutic levels 10–150 mcg/L) (41).

The pregnancy outcomes of 55 women taking paroxetine (median dose 20 mg/day) in the 3rd trimester were reported in 2002 (42). Twelve neonates had complications requiring short-term intensive treatment and prolonged hospitalization. The complications, all resolving within 1–2 weeks, included respiratory distress ($N = 9$; 3 preterm infants), hypoglycemia ($N = 2$), and jaundice ($N = 1$). Compared with controls, significantly more infants were premature. In contrast, only three complications were observed in 54 matched controls. Twenty-seven women in the comparison group had used paroxetine (median dose 20 mg/day) in the 1st and 2nd trimesters, but not in the 3rd trimester. Only 3rd trimester exposure was associated with respiratory distress (OR 9.53, 95% CI 1.14–79.30) (42).

The effect of SSRIs on birth outcomes and postnatal neurodevelopment of children exposed prenatally was reported in 2003 (43). Thirty-one children (mean age 12.9 months) exposed during pregnancy to SSRIs (15 sertraline, 8 paroxetine, 7 fluoxetine, and 1 fluvoxamine) were compared with 13 children (mean age 17.7 months) of mothers with depression who elected not to take medications during pregnancy. All of the mothers had healthy lifestyles. The timing of the exposures was 71% in the 1st trimester, 74% in the 3rd trimester, and 45% throughout. The average duration of breastfeeding in the subjects and controls was 6.4 and 8.5 months. Twenty-eight (90%) subjects nursed their infants, 17 of who took SSRIs (10 sertraline, 4 paroxetine, and 3 fluoxetine) compared with 11 (85%) controls, 3 of whom took sertraline. There were no significant differences between the groups in terms of gestational age at birth, premature births, birth weight and length or, at follow-up, in sex distribution or gain in weight and length (expressed at percentage). Seven (23%) of the exposed infants were admitted to a neonatal intensive care unit (NICU) (six respiratory distress, four meconium aspiration, and one cardiac murmur) compared with none of the controls (*ns*). Follow-up examinations were conducted by a pediatric neurologist, psychologist, and a dysmorphologist who were blinded as to the mother's mediations status. The mean Apgar scores at 1 and 5 minutes were lower in the exposed group than in controls, 7.0 vs. 8.2, and 8.4 vs. 9.0, respectively. There was one major defect in each group: small asymptomatic ventricular septal defect (exposed); bilateral lacrimal duct stenosis that required surgery (control). The test outcomes for mental development were similar in the groups, but significant differences in the subjects included a slight delay in psychomotor development and lower behavior motor quality (tremulousness and fine motor movements) (43).

A 2004 case report described a term 3750-g male newborn who had a normal examination at birth except that he did not cry in the delivery room or afterward (44). The mother had taken paroxetine 20 mg/day throughout the pregnancy. The infant was bottle-fed and had a normal appetite. He was discharged home at 48 hours of age, but was readmitted 2 days later because of lethargy and the absence of cry. The only abnormality detected on examination was the lack of reaction to pain stimulation. On the day 6 of life, an electroencephalogram (EEG) was abnormal ("...depressed background activity with trace alternance and independent spike and wave activity; somatosensory-evoked potentials on the posterior tibial were impossible to elicit"). The infant began crying and responded to pain stimulation on day 13 of life and an EEG on day 14 showed marked improvement. Physical examination at 6 weeks of age was normal (44).

A 2004 prospective study examined the effect of four SSRIs (citalopram, fluoxetine, paroxetine, and sertraline) on newborn neurobehavior, including behavioral state, sleep organization, motor activity, heart rate variability, tremulousness, and startles (45). Seventeen SSRI-exposed, healthy, full-birth-weight newborns and 17 nonexposed, matched controls were studied. A wide range of disrupted neurobehavioral outcomes were shown in the subject infants. After adjustment for gestational age, the exposed infants were found to differ significantly from controls in terms of tremulousness, behavioral states, and sleep organization. The effects observed on motor activity, startles, and heart rate variability were not significant after adjustment (45).

A 37-year-old woman with depression was treated with paroxetine 30 mg/day and chlorpromazine 100 mg/day throughout gestation (46). The woman delivered a 4.46-kg female infant at 39 weeks' gestation with Apgar scores of 6 and 9 at 1 and 5 minutes, respectively. Both the birth weight and head circumference (38 cm) were >97th percentile. The infant was not breastfed. At 12 hours of age, the infant developed a mild fever and respiratory distress (tachypnea, respiratory rate 80/minute, and intercostal recession). At 60 hours of age, rhythmical jerking of the left arm and leg was observed. Investigations for infectious and metabolic causes were negative. On day 6, a blood sample for paroxetine was negative (detection level 5 mcg/L). The infant continued to display jitteriness, tremor, focal jerking movements of all four limbs with hypertonia, opisthotonus posturing, hyper-reflexia, and a hyperactive Moro reflex. Abnormal posture with neck retraction and generalized hypertonia persisted until day 8, but by day 11, the infant was feeding well and all symptoms had resolved (46).

A 2004 case report described severe symptoms in a newborn consisting of tremor, rigidity, and diarrhea during the first 4 days after birth (47). The mother had taken chlorpromazine 20 mg/day up to 32 weeks' gestation, at which time she began paroxetine 30 mg/day. The 4080-g female was delivered by cesarean section at 42 weeks' with Apgar scores of 7, 8, and 9 presumably at 1, 5, and 10 minutes, respectively. The symptoms began 1.5 hours after birth. Paroxetine levels in the infant and mother 17 hours after birth were 30 and 94 nmol/L (trough), respectively. Genetic analysis of the infant revealed that she had two defective CYP2D6 alleles, the enzyme responsible for metabolizing paroxetine, thus classifying her as a poor metabolizer. Nevertheless, the mother breastfed the infant while taking paroxetine 30 mg/day and at 4 months of age, the infant's growth and development were normal (47).

The database of the World Health Organization (WHO) was used in a 2005 report on neonatal SSRI withdrawal syndrome (48). Ninety-three suspected cases with either neonatal convulsions or withdrawal syndrome were identified in the WHO database. Mothers had taken paroxetine in 64 of the cases. The analysis suggested that paroxetine might have an increased risk of convulsions or withdrawal compared with other SSRIs (48).

Evidence for a neonatal behavioral syndrome associated with in utero exposure to SSRIs and serotonin and norepinephrine reuptake inhibitors (SNRIs) (collectively called serotonin reuptake inhibitors [SRIs]) in late pregnancy was reviewed in 2005 (49). The report followed a recent agreement by the FDA and manufacturers for a class labeling change about the neonatal syndrome. Analysis of case reports, case series, and cohort studies revealed that late exposure to SRIs carried an overall risk ratio of 3.0 (95% CI 2.0–4.4) for the syndrome compared with early exposure. The case reports (*N* = 18) and case series (*N* = 131) involved 97 cases of paroxetine, 18 fluoxetine, 16 sertraline, 12 citalopram, 4 venlafaxine, and 2 fluvoxamine. There were nine cohort studies analyzed. The typical neonatal syndrome consisted of central nervous system (CNS), motor, respiratory, and gastrointestinal signs that were mild and usually resolved within 2 weeks. Only 1 of 313 quantifiable cases involved a severe syndrome consisting of seizures, dehydration, excessive weight loss, hyperpyrexia, and intubation. There were no neonatal deaths attributable to the syndrome (49).

Possible sustained neurobehavioral outcomes beyond the neonatal period were reported in 2005 (50). Based on previous findings that prenatally exposed newborns had reduced pain responses, biobehavioral responses to acute pain (heel lance) were prospectively studied in 2-month-old infants. The responses included facial action (Neonatal Facial Coding System) and cardiac autonomic reactivity (derived from respiratory activity and heart rate variability). Three groups of infants were formed: 11 infants with prenatal SSRI exposure alone (2 fluoxetine and 9 paroxetine); 30 infants with prenatal and postnatal (from breast milk) SSRI exposure (6 fluoxetine, 20 paroxetine, and 4 sertraline); and 22 nonexposed controls (mothers not depressed). The exposure during breastfeeding was considered to be very low. Heel lance–induced facial action increased in all three groups but was significantly lowered (blunted) in the first group. Heart rate was significantly lower in the exposed infants during recovery. Moreover, exposed infants had a greater return of parasympathetic cardiac modulation, whereas controls had a sustained sympathetic response. The findings were consistent with the patterns of pain reactivity observed in exposed newborns and suggested sustained neurobehavioral outcomes (50).

A 2006 case report described serotonin toxicity in a newborn that was correlated with serum levels of paroxetine (51). The 29-year-old mother had taken paroxetine, 15 mg/day, from 28 weeks' gestation to delivery at 40 weeks'. The 3-kg male infant had Apgar scores of 9 and 9 at 1 and 5 minutes, respectively. At birth, the infant was pale and flaccid, with an irregular heartbeat (premature atrial contractions), and had signs of respiratory distress. Subsequent examinations revealed a pneumomediastinum and pneumothorax. The hypotonicity was replaced by hypertonicity at about 5 hours of age. Most of the symptoms had resolved within about 24 hours and the infant began breastfeeding at 52 hours of age. A cord blood paroxetine level, about 23 hours after the last dose, was 368 nmol/L (therapeutic range for adults at the author's institution 12–155 nmol/L). Serial drug levels in the infant during the first 24 hours decreased from about 400 nmol/L at birth to 125 nmol/L at 24 hours. The decrease paralleled the decrease in hypertonicity (51).

A significant increase in the risk of low birth weight (<10th percentile) and respiratory distress after prenatal exposure to SSRIs was reported in 2006 (52). The population-based study, representing all live births (*N* = 119,547) during a 39-month period in British Columbia, Canada, compared pregnancy outcomes of depressed mothers treated with SSRIs with outcomes in depressed mothers not treated with medication and in nonexposed controls. The severity of depression in the depressed groups was accounted for by propensity score matching (52).

A 30% incidence of SSRI-induced neonatal abstinence syndrome was found in a 2006 cohort study (53). Sixty neonates with prolonged in utero exposure to SSRIs were compared with nonexposed controls. The agents used were paroxetine (62%), fluoxetine (20%), citalopram (13%), venlafaxine (3%), and sertraline (2%). Assessment was conducted by the Finnegan score. Ten of the infants had mild and eight had severe symptoms of the syndrome. The maximum mean score in infants with severe symptoms occurred within 2 days of birth, but some occurred as long as 4 days after birth. Because of the small numbers, a dose–response analysis could only be conducted with paroxetine. Infants exposed to mean maternal doses that were <19 mg/day had no symptoms, <23 mg/day had mild symptoms, and 27 mg/day had severe symptoms (53).

A 2007 case report described seizures in a newborn infant whose mother had taken paroxetine 30 mg/day throughout pregnancy (54). At birth, the infant was floppy with respiratory distress. Tonic seizures were noted 5 minutes after vaginal birth and continued intermittently, in spite of treatment, until about 48 hours. Other symptoms included hypertonia, fluctuating temperature, and hypoglycemia. He was weaned off of phenobarbital by 2 months of age. His growth and neurodevelopment at 15 months were appropriate (54).

A 2007 retrospective cohort study examined the effects of exposure to SSRIs or venlafaxine in the 3rd trimester on 21 premature and 55 term newborns (55). The randomly selected unexposed control group consisted of 90 neonates of mothers not taking antidepressants, psychotropic agents, or benzodiazepines at the time of delivery. There were significantly more premature infants among the subjects (27.6%) than in controls (8.9%), but the groups were not matched. The antidepressants, number of subjects, and daily doses in the exposed group were paroxetine (46; 5–40 mg), fluoxetine (10; 10–40 mg), venlafaxine (9; 74–150 mg), citalopram (6; 10–30 mg), sertraline (3; 125–150 mg), and fluvoxamine (2; 50–150 mg). The behavioral signs that were significantly increased in exposed compared with nonexposed infants were: CNS—abnormal movements, shaking, spasms, agitation, hypotonia, hypertonia, irritability, and insomnia; respiratory system—indrawing, apnea/bradycardia, and tachypnea; and other—vomiting, tachycardia, and jaundice. In exposed infants, CNS (63.2%) and respiratory system (40.8%) signs were most common, appearing during the first day of life and lasting for a median duration of 3 days. All of the exposed premature infants exhibited behavioral signs compared with 69.1% of exposed term infants. The duration of hospitalization was significantly longer in exposed premature compared with nonexposed premature infants, 14.5 vs. 3.7 days, respectively. In 75% of the term and premature infants, the signs resolved within 3 and 5 days, respectively. There were six infants in each group with congenital malformations, but the drugs involved were not specified (55).

A case–control study, published in 2006, was conducted to test the hypothesis that exposure to SSRIs in late pregnancy was associated with persistent pulmonary hypertension of the newborn (56). A total of 1213 women were enrolled in the study, 377 cases whose infants had PPHN and 836 matched controls and their infants. Mothers were interviewed by nurses that were blinded to the hypothesis. Fourteen case infants had been exposed to an SSRI after the 20th week of gestation compared with six control infants (adjusted OR 6.1, 95% CI 2.2–16.8). The numbers were too small to analyze the effects of dosage, SSRI used, or reduction of the length of exposure before delivery. No increased risk of PPHN was found with the use of SSRIs before the 20th week or with the use of non-SSRI antidepressants at any time in pregnancy. If the relationship was causal, the absolute risk was estimated to be about 1% (56).

A 2008 reference found that, after controlling for maternal illness, longer prenatal exposure to SSRIs significantly increased the risks of lower birth weight, respiratory distress, and reduced gestational age (57).

In a 2009 retrospective study, the medical records of 25,214 births that occurred at the Mayo Clinic from 1993 to 2205 were reviewed for use of SSRIs during pregnancy (58). A total of 808 mothers took an SSRI (122 citalopram, 8 escitalopram, 184 fluoxetine, 134 paroxetine, 296 sertraline, 53 venlafaxine, and 1 to more than 1 SSRI) and 24,406 did not. The prevalence of congenital heart disease in the two groups was 3 (0.4%) and 205 (0.8%). There were 16 infants with PPHN, none of whom had been exposed to SSRIs (58).

A prospective cohort study from Denmark evaluated the effects of SSRIs on pregnancy outcomes (59). Three groups of women that gave birth at a single hospital in 1989–2006 were identified: 329 exposed to SSRIs during pregnancy, 4902 with a history of psychiatric illness but not treated with SSRIs, and 51,770 reported no history of psychiatric illness. Compared with the other groups, SSRI exposure was significantly associated with an increased risk of preterm birth, a low 5-minute Apgar score, and admission to an NICU. The NICU admissions were not explained by the lower Apgar score or gestational age (59).

Representatives of the American Psychiatric Association and the American College of Obstetricians and Gynecologists issued a joint statement on the management of depression during pregnancy in 2009 (60). The objective of the statement was to analyze the maternal and neonatal risks of depression and antidepressant exposure and to develop algorithms for periconceptional and antenatal management. Three algorithms were developed: (i) patients considering pregnancy who were currently being treated; (ii) pregnant patients having a recurrent major depressive disorder (MDD) who were not taking an antidepressant; and (iii) pregnant patients with MDD who were taking an antidepressant. The conclusion of the joint statement was that research had not adequately controlled for other factors that could influence birth outcomes such as maternal illness or problematic health behaviors that could adversely affect pregnancy (60).

A large 2009 review of SSRIs and SNRIs in pregnancy concluded that use of these agents was associated with adverse effects and such use required careful follow-up of infants exposed in utero (61).

Spontaneous Abortions

A nested case–control study in Quebec found that the use of antidepressants during pregnancy were significantly associated with SABs (62). Significant increases were observed for SSRIs alone, SNRIs alone, combined use of different classes of antidepressants, paroxetine, and venlafaxine. The ranges for the OR were 1.68–3.51, with the highest in the combined use group. Because of the smaller number of exposures among other SSRIs and in other antidepressant classes, the authors thought that their data suggested a class effect of SSRIs, rather than a specific drug effect (62). An accompanying commentary discussed the difficulties of measuring the effects of antidepressants in pregnancy and concluded that if a risk of SAB existed, it was small (63).

A 2010 review evaluated 15 prospective studies involving antidepressants that had been published in 1975–2009 to determine if there was an association between specific agents and SAB (64). The majority of the studies involved tricyclic antidepressants or SSRIs. After adjustment, only paroxetine (OR 1.7, 95% CI 1.3–2.3) and venlafaxine (OR 2.1, 95% CI 1.3–3.3) were significantly associated with the risk of SABs (64).

BREASTFEEDING SUMMARY

Paroxetine is excreted into breast milk. A brief 1996 correspondence described a 39-year-old, 60-kg woman with a recurrent depressive and obsessive disorder who was started on paroxetine 20 mg/day (333 mcg/kg/day) 3 days after delivery (65). One week later, analysis of a milk sample for paroxetine revealed a concentration of 7.6 ng/mL. Assuming that the infant ingested 0.15 L/kg of milk per day, the estimated daily weight-adjusted dose was 0.34% of the mother's dose. The minimum milk:plasma ratio (obtained 4 hours after a dose) was estimated to be 0.09. No data were available on the effects of this exposure on the nursing infant (65).

Breast milk concentrations of paroxetine in seven lactating women were reported in a 1999 publication (66). In six women receiving a paroxetine dose of 10–40 mg/day, milk and maternal serum samples were obtained 4–7 and 24 hours after a dose. The samples corresponded to either close to peak milk concentrations or trough levels. Based on AUC calculations, the mean estimated daily infant dose was 1.4% (range 0.7%–2.9%) of the weight-adjusted maternal dose. The mean milk:serum ratio was 0.69 (range 0.39–1.11). In a seventh woman, frequent sampling during two 24-hour periods (one at 20 mg/day and one at 40 mg/day, 7 weeks apart) resulted in estimated daily infant doses of 1.0% and 2.0%, respectively, of the weight-adjusted maternal dose. The milk:serum ratios were 0.69 and 0.72, respectively. The study also measured paroxetine concentrations in fore-milk and hind-milk at two steady-state doses (20 and 40 mg/day) in one subject. Drug levels in hind-milk were a mean 78% (range 16%–169%) higher than those in fore-milk. The increase paralleled the increase in milk triglycerides and was thought to be consistent with the lipophilic properties of the drug. No adverse effects of the exposure were observed in the seven nursing infants (66).

In a two-phase study published in 1999, the dose of paroxetine received by 10 nursing infants from breast milk was estimated (67). In six subjects sampled over 24 hours, the mean daily estimated infant dose was 1.13% (range 0.5%–1.7%) of the weight-adjusted maternal dose (based on AUC). The mean milk:plasma ratio was 0.39 (range 0.32–0.51). In the second phase, milk and serum samples were obtained from four subjects around a normal infant feeding time. In this case, the mean infant dose was 1.25% (range 0.38%–2.24%) of the maternal dose and the mean milk:plasma ratio was 0.96 (range 0.31–3.33). The milk:plasma ratio was similar for fore- and hind-milk. Paroxetine was detected (limit 2 ng/mL) in the plasma of one of the eight infants tested, but the concentration was below the level of quantification for the assay (4 ng/mL). No adverse effects were noted in any of the infants (67).

A 2000 study described the excretion of paroxetine into breast milk (68). Sixteen women on a stable paroxetine dose (mean 23.1 mg/day; range 10–50 mg/day) were studied during the postpartum period (4–55.2 weeks). Seven of the women had continued their prenatal paroxetine, four had started the antidepressant postpartum, and data were not available for five subjects. Milk samples were collected after a dose at 4- to 6-hour intervals over a 24-hour period. The mean milk concentration was 41.6 ng/mL (range 2–101 ng/mL). Paroxetine concentrations were higher in hind-milk than in fore-milk. No detectable levels of paroxetine (all <2 ng/mL) were found in the infants serum, including the 10 infants who were exclusively breastfed. No adverse effects in the nursing infants were reported by the mothers upon direct interview (68).

In another 2000 report, maternal serum, breast milk, and infant serum samples were obtained from 24 mother–infant pairs (mean infant age 4.5 months) 6 hours after a paroxetine dose (69). In 13 of the pairs, the infants were exclusively breastfed. All of the mothers were on a stable dose of paroxetine (10–40 mg/day for at least 30 days). One mother–infant pair was tested twice; once at 10 mg/day and again at 40 mg/day. The mean maternal serum, breast milk, and infant serum concentrations (ng/mL) were 45.2, 19.2, and not detectable (<0.1 ng/mL), respectively. The mean milk:plasma ratio, infant dose, and percent of maternal dose were 0.53, 2.88 mcg/kg/day, and 1.1%, respectively. No adverse effects of the drug exposure were noted in the nursing infants (69).

In a 2002 report, the pregnancy outcomes of 55 women who had taken paroxetine during the 3rd trimester were reported (see Fetal Risk Summary) (42). Thirty-six of the women breastfed their infants. Eight of the women reported adverse symptoms in their infants: alertness ($N = 6$), constipation ($N = 3$), sleepiness ($N = 1$), and irritability ($N = 1$). No adverse events were reported in 44 breastfed infants in the comparison group (42).

A 2004 study was conducted in 25 women (nursing 26 infants) to quantify the concentration of the SSRI or SNRI in their breast milk (70). The antidepressants taken by the women were citalopram (nine), paroxetine (six), sertraline (six), fluoxetine (one), and venlafaxine (three). The maternal mean dose of paroxetine was 20 mg/day (10–30 mg/day). The mean milk concentration was 88 nmol/L (18–152 nmol/L), resulting in a theoretical maximum infant dose that was 1.4% of the mother's weight-adjusted dose. Paroxetine was not detected in the infant's serum, even though one mother–infant pair was identified as CYP2D6 poor metabolizers. There was no evidence of adverse effects in the breastfeeding infants (70).

A 1999 review of SSRI agents concluded that if there were compelling reasons to treat a mother for postpartum depression, a condition in which a rapid antidepressant effect is important, the benefits of therapy with SSRIs would most likely outweigh the risks (71). However, because the long-term effects of exposure to SSRI antidepressants in breast milk on the infant's neurobehavioral development are unknown,

P

stopping or reducing the frequency of breastfeeding should be considered if therapy with these agents is required. Avoiding nursing around the time of peak maternal concentration (about 4 hours after a dose) may limit infant exposure. However, the long elimination half-lives of all SSRIs and their weakly basic properties, which are conducive to ion trapping in the relatively acidic milk, probably will lessen the effectiveness of this strategy. The American Academy of Pediatrics classifies paroxetine as a drug for which the effect on nursing infants is unknown but may be of concern (72).

A 2010 study, using human and animal models, found that drugs that disturb serotonin balance such as SSRIs and SNRIs can impair lactation (73). The authors concluded that mothers taking these drugs may need additional support to achieve breastfeeding goals.

References

1. FDA Public Health Advisory. Paroxetine. December 8, 2005. Available at http://www.fda.gov/cder/drug/advisory/paroxetine200512.htm. Accessed May 19, 2007.
2. Product information. Paxil. GlaxoSmithKline, 2006.
3. Kallen B, Olausson PO. Antidepressant drugs during pregnancy and infant congenital heart defect. Reprod Toxicol 2006;21:221–2.
4. Alwan S, Reefhuis J, Rasmussen SA, Olney RS, Friedman JM, for the National Birth Defects Prevention Study. Use of selective serotonin-reuptake inhibitors in pregnancy and the risk of birth defects. N Engl J Med 2007;356:2684–92.
5. Louik C, Lin AE, Werler MM, Hernandez-Diaz S, Mitchell AA. First-trimester use of selective serotonin-reuptake inhibitors and the risk of birth defects. N Engl J Med 2007;356:2675–83.
6. Berard A, Ramos E, Rey E, Blais L, St.-Andre M, Oraichi D. First trimester exposure to paroxetine and risk of cardiac malformations in infants: the importance of dosage. Birth Defects Res B Dev Reprod Toxicol 2007;80:18–27.
7. Greene MF. Teratogenicity of SSRIs—Serious concern or much ado about little? N Engl J Med 2007;356:2732–3.
8. Shuey DL, Sadler TW, Lauder JM. Serotonin as a regulator of craniofacial morphogenesis: site-specific malformations following exposure to serotonin uptake inhibitors. Teratology 1992;46:367–78.
9. Baldwin JA, Davidson EJ, Pritchard AL, Ridings JE. The reproductive toxicology of paroxetine. Acta Psychiatrica Scand Suppl 1989;350:37–9.
10. Coleman F, Christensen D, Gonzalez C, Rayburn W. Behavioral changes in developing mice after prenatal exposure to paroxetine (Paxil) (abstract). Am J Obstet Gynecol 1999;180:S61.
11. Coleman FH, Christensen HD, Gonzalez CL. Rayburn WF. Behavioral changes in developing mice after prenatal exposure to paroxetine (Paxil). Am J Obstet Gynecol 1999;181:1166–71.
12. Hendrick V, Stowe ZN, Altshuler LL, Hwang S, Lee E, Haynes D. Placental passage of antidepressant medications. Am J Psychiatry 2003;160:993–6.
13. Inman W, Kubota K, Pearce G, Wilton L. PEM report number 6. Paroxetine. Pharmacoepidemiol Drug Saf 1993;2:393–422.
14. Wilton LV, Pearce GL, Martin RM, Mackay FJ, Mann RD. The outcomes of pregnancy in women exposed to newly marketed drugs in general practice in England. Br J Obstet Gynaecol 1998;105:882–9.
15. McElhatton PR, Garbis HM, Elefant E, Vial T, Bellemin B, Mastroiacovo P, Arnon J, Rodriguez-Pinilla E, Schaefer C, Pexieder T, Merlob P, Dal Verme S. The outcome of pregnancy in 689 women exposed to therapeutic doses of antidepressants. A collaborative study of the European Network of Teratology Information Services (ENTIS). Reprod Toxicol 1996;10:285–94.
16. Kulin NA, Pastuszak A, Sage SR, Schick-Boschetto B, Spivey G, Feldkamp M, Ormond K, Matsui D, Stein-Schechman AK, Cook L, Brochu J, Rieder M, Koren G. Pregnancy outcome following maternal use of the new selective serotonin reuptake inhibitors. A prospective controlled multicenter study. JAMA 1998;279:609–10.
17. Koren G. In reply. Risk of fetal anomalies with exposure to selective serotonin reuptake inhibitors. JAMA 1998;279:1873–4.
18. Einarson TR, Einarson A. Newer antidepressants in pregnancy and rates of major malformations: a meta-analysis of prospective comparative studies. Pharmacoepidemiol Drug Saf 2005;14:823–7.
19. Alwan S, Reefhuis J, Rasmussen S, Olney R, Friedman JM. Maternal use of selective serotonin reuptake inhibitors and risk for birth defects (abstract). Birth Defects Res A Clin Mol Teratol 2005;73:291.
20. Diav-Citrin O, Shechtman S, Weinbaum D, Arnon J, Gianantonio ED, Clementi M, Ornoy A. Paroxetine and fluoxetine in pregnancy: a multicenter, prospective, controlled study (abstract). Reprod Toxicol 2005;20:459.
21. Rahimi R, Nikfar S, Abdollahi M. Pregnancy outcomes following exposure to serotonin reuptake inhibitors: a meta-analysis of clinical trials. Reprod Toxicol 2006;22:571–5.
22. Ericson A, Kallen B, Wiholm BE. Delivery outcome after the use of antidepressants in early pregnancy. Eur J Clin Pharmacol 1999;55:503–8.
23. Kallen BAJ, Olausson PO. Maternal use of selective serotonin re-uptake inhibitors in early pregnancy and infant congenital malformations. Birth Defects Res A Clin Mol Teratol 2007;79:301–8.
24. Wogelius P, Norgaard M, Gislum M, Pedersen L, Munk E, Mortensen PB, Lipworth L, Sorensen HT. Maternal use of selective serotonin reuptake inhibitors and risk of congenital malformations. Epidemiology 2006;17:701–4.
25. Cole JA, Ephross SA, Cosmatos IS, Walker AM. Paroxetine in the first trimester and the prevalence of congenital malformations. Pharmacoepidemiol Drug Saf 2007;16:1075–85.
26. Bellantuono C, Migliarese G, Gentile S. Serotonin reuptake inhibitors in pregnancy and the risk of major malformations: a systematic review. Hum Psychopharmacol Clin Exp 2007;22:121–8.
27. Hendrick V, Smith LM, Suri R, Hwang S, Haynes D, Altshuler L. Birth outcomes after prenatal exposure to antidepressant medication. Am J Obstet Gynecol 2003;188:812–5.
28. DeMyer W. Brain, midline caves. In Buyse ML, ed. *Birth Defects Encyclopedia*. Cambridge, MA: Blackwell Scientific Publications, 1990:238.
29. Ramos E, St-Andre M, Rey E, Oraichi D, Berard A. Duration of antidepressant use during pregnancy and risk of major congenital malformations. Br J Psychiatry 2008;192:344–50.
30. Diav-Citrin O, Shechtman S, Weinbaum D, Wajnberg R, Avgil M, Di Gianantonio E, Clementi M, Weber-Schoendorfer C, Schaefer C, Ornoy A. Paroxetine and fluoxetine in pregnancy: a prospective, multicentre, controlled, observational study. Br J Clin Pharmacol 2008;66:695–705.
31. Einarson A, Pistelli A, DeSantis M, Malm H, Paulus WD, Panchaud A, Kennedy D, Einarson TR, Koren G. Evaluation of the risk of congenital cardiovascular defects associated with use of paroxetine during pregnancy. Am J Psychiatry 2008;165:749–52.
32. Merlob P, Birk E, Sirota, Linder N, Berant M, Stahl B, Klinger G. Are selective serotonin reuptake inhibitors cardiac teratogens? Echocardiographic screening of newborns with persistent heart murmur. Birth Defects Res A Clin Mol Teratol 2009;85:837–41.
33. Marsella M, Ubaldini E, Solinas A, Guerrini P. Prenatal exposure to serotonin reuptake inhibitors: a case report. Ital J Pediatr 2010;36:27.
34. Bakker MK, Kerstjens-Frederikse WS, Buys CHCM, de Walle HEK, de Jong-van den Berg LTW. First-trimester use of paroxetine and congenital heart defects: a population-base case-control study. Birth Defects Res A Clin Mol Teratol 2010;88:94–100.
35. Wurst KE, Poole C, Ephross SA, Olshan AF. First trimester paroxetine use and the prevalence of congenital, specifically cardiac, defects: a meta-analysis of epidemiological studies. Birth Defects Res A Clin Mol Teratol 2010;88:159–70.
36. Berard A. Paroxetine exposure during pregnancy and the risk of cardiac malformations: what is the evidence? Birth Defects Res A Clin Mol Teratol 2010; 88:171–4.
37. Scialli AR. Paroxetine exposure during pregnancy and cardiac malformations. Birth Defects Res (Part A) 2010; 88:175–7.
38. Einarson A, Choi J, Einarson TR, Koren G. Incidence of major malformations in infants following antidepressant exposure in pregnancy: results of a large prospective cohort study. Can J Psychiatry 2009;54:242–6.
39. Stiskal JA, Kulin N, Koren G, Ho T, Ito S. Neonatal paroxetine withdrawal syndrome. Arch Dis Child Fetal Neonatal Ed 2001;84:F134–5.
40. Nordeng H, Lindemann R, Perminov KV, Reikvam A. Neonatal withdrawal syndrome after in utero exposure to selective serotonin reuptake inhibitors. Acta Paediatr 2001;90:288–91.
41. Nijhuis IJM, Kok-Van Rooij GWM, Bosschaart AN. Withdrawal reactions of a premature neonate after maternal use of paroxetine. Arch Dis Child Neonatal Ed 2001;84:F77.
42. Costei AM, Kozer E, Ho T, Ito S, Koren G. Perinatal outcome following third trimester exposure to paroxetine. Arch Pediatr Adolesc Med 2002;156:1129–32.
43. Casper RC, Fleisher BE, Lee-Ancajas JC, Gilles A, Gaylor E, DeBattista A, Hoyme HE. Follow-up of children of depressed mothers exposed or not exposed to antidepressant drugs during pregnancy. J Pediatr 2003;142: 402–8.
44. Morag I, Batash D, Keidar R, Bulkowstein M, Heyman E. Paroxetine use throughout pregnancy: does it pose any risk to the neonate? J Toxicol Clin Toxicol 2004;42:97–100.

45. Zeskind PS, Stephens LE. Maternal selective serotonin reuptake inhibitor use during pregnancy and newborn neurobehavior. Pediatrics 2004;113: 368–75.
46. Haddad PM, Pal BR, Clarke P, Wieck A, Sridhiran S. Neonatal symptoms following maternal paroxetine treatment: serotonin toxicity or paroxetine discontinuation syndrome? J Psychopharmacol 2005;19:554–7.
47. Laine K, Kytola J, Bertilsson L. Severe adverse effects in a newborn with two defective CYP2D6 alleles after exposure to paroxetine during late pregnancy. Ther Drug Monit 2004;26:685–7.
48. Sanz EJ, De-las-Cuevas C, Kiuru A, Edwards R. Selective serotonin reuptake inhibitors in pregnant women and neonatal withdrawal syndrome: a database analysis. Lancet 2005;365:482–7.
49. Moses-Kolko EL, Bogen D, Perel J, Bregar A, Uhl K, Levin B, Wisner KL. Neonatal signs after late in utero exposure to serotonin reuptake inhibitors. JAMA 2005;293:2372–83.
50. Oberlander TF, Grunau RE, Fitzgerald C, Papsdorf M, Rurak D, Riggs W. Pain reactivity in 2-month-old infants after prenatal and postnatal selective serotonin reuptake inhibitor medication exposure. Pediatrics 2005;115: 411–25.
51. Knoppert DC, Nimkar R, Principi T, Yuen D. Paroxetine toxicity in a newborn after in utero exposure: clinical symptoms correlate with serum levels. Ther Drug Monit 2006;28:5–7.
52. Oberlander TF, Warburton W, Misri S, Aghajanian J, Hertzman C. Neonatal outcomes after prenatal exposure to selective serotonin reuptake inhibitor antidepressants and maternal depression using population-based linked health data. Arch Gen Psychiatry 2006;63:898–906.
53. Levinson-Castiel R, Merlob P, Linder N, Sirota L, Klinger G. Neonatal abstinence syndrome after in utero exposure to selective serotonin reuptake inhibitors in term infants. Arch Pediatr Adoles Med 2006;160:173–6.
54. Ahmed M, Parameshwaran A, Swamy P. Neonatal convulsions secondary to paroxetine withdrawal. J Pak Med Assoc 2007;57:162.
55. Ferreira E, Carceller AM, Agogue C, Martin BZ, St-Andre M, Francoeur D, Berard A. Effects of selective serotonin reuptake inhibitors and venlafaxine during pregnancy in term and preterm neonates. Pediatrics 2007;119:52–9.
56. Chambers CD, Hernandez-Diaz S, Van Marter LJ, Werler MM, Louik C, Jones KL, Mitchell AA. Selective serotonin-reuptake inhibitors and risk of persistent pulmonary hypertension of the newborn. N Engl J Med 2006;354:579–87.
57. Oberlander TF, Warburton W, Misri S, Aghajanian J, Hertzman C. Effects of timing and duration of gestational exposure to serotonin reuptake inhibitor antidepressants: population-based study. Br J Psychiatry 2008;192: 338–43.
58. Wichman CL, Moore KM, Lang TR, St. Sauver JL, Heise RH Jr, Watson WJ. Congenital heart disease associated with selective serotonin reuptake inhibitor use during pregnancy. Mayo Clin Proc 2009;84:23–7.
59. Lund N, Pederson LH, Henriksen TB. Selective serotonin reuptake inhibitor exposure in utero and pregnancy outcomes. Arch Pediatr Adolesc Med 2009;163:949–54.
60. Yonkers KA, Wisner KL, Stewart DE, Oberlander TF, Dell DL, Stotland N, Ramin S, Chaudron L, Lockwood C. The management of depression during pregnancy: a report from the American Psychiatric Association and the American College of Obstetricians and Gynecologists. Obstet Gynecol 2009;114:703–13.
61. Tuccori M, Testi A, Antonioli L, Fornai M, Montagnani S, Ghisu N, Colucci R, Corona T, Blandizzi C, Del Tacca M. Safety concerns associated with the use of serotonin reuptake inhibitors and other serotonergic/noradrenergic antidepressants during pregnancy: a review. Clin Therapeutics 2009;31:1426–53.
62. Nakhai-Pour HR, Broy P, Berard A. Use of antidepressants during pregnancy and the risk of spontaneous abortion. CMAJ 2010;182:1031–7.
63. Einarson A. Antidepressants and pregnancy: complexities of producing evidence-based information. CMAJ 2010;182:1079.
64. Broy P, Berard A. Gestational exposure to antidepressants and the risk of spontaneous abortion: a review. Curr Drug Deliv 2010;7:76–92.
65. Spigset O, Carleborg L, Norstrom A, Sandlund M. Paroxetine level in breast milk. J Clin Psychiatry 1996;57:39.
66. Ohman R, Hagg S, Carleborg L, Spigset O. Excretion of paroxetine into breast milk. J Clin Psychiatry 1999;60:519–23.
67. Begg EJ, Duffull SB, Saunders DA, Buttimore RC, Ilett KF, Hackett LP, Yapp P, Wilson DA. Paroxetine in human milk. Br J Clin Pharmacol 1999;48: 142–7.
68. Stowe ZN, Cohen LS, Hostetter A, Ritchie JC, Owens MJ, Nemeroff CB. Paroxetine in human breast milk and nursing infants. Am J Psychiatry 2000;157:185–9.
69. Misri S, Kim J, Riggs KW, Kostaras X. Paroxetine levels in postpartum depressed women, breast milk, and infant serum. J Clin Psychiatry 2000;61:828–32.
70. Berle JO, Steen VM, Aamo TO, Breilid H, Zahlsen K, Spigset O. Breastfeeding during maternal antidepressant treatment with serotonin reuptake inhibitors: infant exposure, clinical symptoms, and cytochrome P450 genotypes. J Clin Psychiatry 2004;65:1228–34.
71. Edwards JG, Anerson I. Systematic review and guide to selection of selective serotonin reuptake inhibitors. Drugs 1999;57:507–33.
72. Committee on Drugs, American Academy of Pediatrics. The transfer of drugs and other chemicals into human milk. Pediatrics 2001;108: 776–89.
73. Marshall AM, Nommsen-Rivers LA, Hernandez LI, Dewey KG, Chantry CJ, Gregerson KA, Horseman ND. Serotonin transport and metabolism in the mammary gland modulates secretory activation and involution. J Clin Endocrin Metab 2010;95:837–46.

PASIREOTIDE

Endocrine/Metabolic (Somatostatin Analog)

PREGNANCY RECOMMENDATION: No Human Data—Animal Data Suggest Risk
BREASTFEEDING RECOMMENDATION: No Human Data—Potential Toxicity

PREGNANCY SUMMARY

No reports describing the use of pasireotide in human pregnancy have been located. The animal data suggest risk, but the absence of human pregnancy experience prevents a full assessment of the embryo–fetal risk. If a woman becomes pregnant while receiving the drug, she should be informed of the potential risk, including abortion, to her embryo and/or fetus.

FETAL RISK SUMMARY

Pasireotide is a cyclohexapeptide somatostatin analog that is given as an SC injection. It is in the same subclass as octreotide. Pasireotide is indicated for the treatment of adult patients with Cushing's disease for whom pituitary surgery is not an option or has not been curative. The drug is not metabolized. Plasma protein binding is moderate (88%) and the calculated effective half-life is about 12 hours (1).

Reproduction studies have been conducted in rats and rabbits. In rats throughout organogenesis, doses resulting in exposures that were 4 times or higher than the maximum therapeutic dose based on AUC (MHD) caused maternal toxicity. Exposures less than the human clinical exposure based on BSA caused a significant increase in implantation loss and decreased viable fetuses, corpora lutea, and implantation sites. In addition, restricted growth was noted in rat pups exposed during prenatal and postnatal studies but was reversible after weaning. In rabbits through organogenesis, an exposure that was 7 times the MHD caused maternal toxicity. At exposures less than the MHD, an increased incidence of skeletal malformations was observed in offspring (1).

Long-term studies for carcinogenesis were negative in rats and mice. Pasireotide was not mutagenic or genotoxic in several assays. As noted above, fertility studies in rats caused harm. In addition, abnormal cycles or acyclicity were observed (1).

It is not known if pasireotide crosses the human placenta. The molecular weight (about 1313) suggests that passage would be limited, but the moderate plasma protein binding and long effective half-life could increase the possibility for crossing to the embryo–fetus.

BREASTFEEDING SUMMARY

No reports describing the use of pasireotide during human breastfeeding have been located. The molecular weight (about 1313) suggests that excretion into breast milk will be limited, but the moderate plasma protein binding (88%) and long effective half-life (12 hours) could increase the possibility for excretion. The effect of this exposure on a nursing infant is unknown. The most common (≥20%) adverse reactions in adults were diarrhea, nausea, hyperglycemia, cholelithiasis, headache, abdominal pain, fatigue, and diabetes mellitus (1). Because of these potential risks, the best course is to not breastfeed.

Reference

1. Product information. Signifor. Novartis Pharmaceuticals, 2012.

PASSION FLOWER

Herb

PREGNANCY RECOMMENDATION: No Human Data—No Relevant Animal Data
BREASTFEEDING RECOMMENDATION: No Human Data—Potential Toxicity

PREGNANCY SUMMARY

No reports describing the use of passion flower during human pregnancy have been located. As with most herbal products, a large number of chemicals have been identified in this herb and none has undergone reproductive testing. Since passion flower has been used for hundreds of years or longer, it is doubtful that a major teratogenic effect or other significant reproductive toxicity would have escaped notice. More subtle or low-incidence effects, however, including structural and behavioral teratogenicity, the induction of abortions due to its uterine stimulant properties, and infertility, may have escaped detection, and further study is required before human reproductive risk or safety can be assessed. In addition to the above concerns, standardization of any herbal product is often questionable (1). As such, the presence of therapeutic or subtherapeutic amounts of active ingredients, or their complete absence, in a given preparation cannot be predicted. Commercial herbal products may also be adulterated with unlabeled ingredients (1). Because of these uncertainties, the consumption of passion flower during gestation should be avoided.

FETAL RISK SUMMARY

The herbal product used for medicinal purposes usually refers to the plant, *Passiflora incarnata*, but the common name, passion flower, may refer to many of the approximately 400 species of the genus *Passiflora*. Some species are grown for their flowers. In addition, some species produce edible fruit, such as *P. incarnata*, *P. edulis*, and *P. quadrangularis*. The plant is a perennial vine that may reach 10 meters in length. It is indigenous to the southeastern United States to South America. The medicinal parts include the whole or cut dried herb and the fresh aerial parts (2,3). In this review, the term passion flower will only refer to *P. incarnata*, the product used in herbal medicine.

Commercial products of passion flower are available for both oral and topical administration. A number of indications have been claimed for passion flower, including nervousness (e.g., hysteria, nervous exhaustion, pediatric nervousness, and excitability), neuralgia, insomnia, pain, asthma and other bronchial disorders, generalized seizures, compresses for burns, hemorrhoids (externally), and for menopausal complaints (2–5).

As with most herbs, a relatively large number of chemical compounds are contained in the commercial product: flavonoids (content 2.5%; includes flavone di-C-glycosides shaftoside, isoshaftoside, isovitexin, iso-orientin, vicenin, lucenin, saponarin, and passiflorine), maltol (0.05%), cyanogenic glycosides (gynocardine [<0.1%]), and indole alkaloids (harman, harmine, harmaline, harmalol, and harmin) are the primary constituents (2–5). The alkaloids, however, are reportedly present in subtherapeutic amounts (6). Other constituents include free flavonoids (apigenin, luteolin, quercetin, and campherol), several acid compounds (phenolic, linoleic, linolenic, palmitic, oleic, myristic, formic, and butyric acids), coumarins, phytosterols, and essential oil (2).

The pharmacologic activity of passion flower apparently derives from the flavonoids and alkaloids (2,4). A few studies have apparently documented the sedative action of passion flower in animals and humans. The FDA prohibited the use of passion flower in over-the-counter (OTC) products in 1978 because it had not been proven to be safe and effective (6), but the product is apparently available as a herbal remedy.

No reports have been located describing the use of passion flower in human pregnancy. However, two sources have cited reports that the herb is contraindicated during pregnancy because of the uterine stimulant action of the harman (harmala) alkaloids (harman, harmaline) shown in animals and because of the presence of cyanogenic glycoside gynocardine (2,4). In contrast, the German Commission E monographs state that there are no contraindications (5).

BREASTFEEDING SUMMARY

No reports describing the use of passion flower during lactation have been located. Because of the large number of chemical compounds in the herb, the lack of standardization of commercial products, and the complete lack of information on the effects of exposure to these substances in a nursing infant, the use of passion flower during breastfeeding should be avoided.

References

1. Miller LG, Hume A, Harris IM, Jackson EA, Kanmaz TJ, Cauffield JS, Chin TWF, Knell M. White paper on herbal products. American College of Clinical Pharmacy. Pharmacotherapy 2000;20:877–91.
2. Passion flower. In *The Review of Natural Products*. St. Louis, MO: Facts and Comparisons, March 1999.
3. Passiflora incarnata. In *PDR for Herbal Medicines*. Montvale, NJ: Medical Economics, 1998:1015–6.
4. Passion flower. In *Natural Medicines Comprehensive Database*. Stockton, CA: Therapeutic Research Faculty, 1999:645–6.
5. Passionflower herb. In Blumenthal M, ed. *The Complete German Commission E Monographs. Therapeutic Guide to Herbal Medicines*. Austin, TX: American Botanical Council, 1998:179–80.
6. Robbers JE, Tyler VE. *Tyler's Herbs of Choice. The Therapeutic Use of Phytomedicinals*. Binghamton, NY: Haworth Press, 2000:159–60.

PAZOPANIB

Antineoplastic (Tyrosine Kinase Inhibitor)

PREGNANCY RECOMMENDATION: Contraindicated
BREASTFEEDING RECOMMENDATION: Contraindicated

P

PREGNANCY SUMMARY

No reports describing the use of pazopanib in human pregnancy have been located. The animal reproduction data suggest risk because developmental toxicity (growth restriction, structural anomalies, and death) was observed in two species at systemic exposures that were much lower than those in humans. The absence of human pregnancy experience prevents a full assessment of the embryo–fetal risk. The manufacturer advises women to avoid becoming pregnant while taking pazopanib (1). However, renal cell carcinoma may be fatal without appropriate treatment. If a woman becomes pregnant while receiving everolimus she should be advised of the potential for embryo–fetal harm. If possible, avoiding the 1st trimester should be considered.

FETAL RISK SUMMARY

Pazopanib is a tyrosine kinase inhibitor antineoplastic that is available as oral tablets. It is indicated for the treatment of advanced renal cell carcinoma. Pazopanib is in the same subclass as several other agents (see Appendix). The drug is metabolized, but the activity of the metabolites (*assumed to be inactive*) was not stated. Plasma protein binding is >99% and the mean elimination half-life is about 31 hours (1).

Reproduction studies have been conducted in rats and rabbits. In rats, doses given during organogenesis that resulted in exposures that were about 0.1 times the human clinical exposure based on AUC (HCE) caused cardiovascular malformations (retroesophageal subclavian artery, missing innominate artery, changes in the aortic arch) and incomplete or absent ossification. Other toxicities were reduced fetal body weight, and pre- and postimplantation embryolethality. In rabbits, doses resulting in exposures that were about 0.007 times the HCE caused maternal toxicity (reduced food consumption, increased postimplantation loss, and abortion). At 0.02 times the HCE, severe maternal body weight loss and 100% litter loss were observed. Fetal body weight was reduced at a dose 1% (AUC not calculated) of the dose causing 100% litter loss (1).

Carcinogenicity studies have not been conducted, but in a 13-week mouse study, proliferative lesions in the liver including eosinophilic foci in two females and a single case of adenoma in another female were noted. The drug was not mutagenic or clastogenic in various assays. In female fats, various doses all resulting in exposures less than the HCE, caused decreased fertility, increased pre- and postimplantation losses, and decreased fetal body weight. Decreased corpora lutea and increased cysts were noted in mice given a dose that was about 1.3 times the HCE for 13 weeks, and in a 26-week study, ovarian atrophy was seen in rats at a dose that was about 0.85 times the HCE. Decreased corpora lutea were also noted in monkeys given a dose that was about 0.4 times the HCE for up to 34 weeks. The drug did not affect mating or fertility in male rats, but did cause decreases in sperm production and concentrations, as well as decreased testicular and epididymal weights. In a 6-month toxicity study with male rats, atrophy and degeneration of the testes with aspermia, hypospermia, and cribiform change in the epididymis were observed (1).

It is not known if pazopanib crosses the human placenta. The molecular weight (about 438 for the free base) and long elimination half-life suggest that the drug will cross, but the high plasma protein binding might limit the amount crossing.

BREASTFEEDING SUMMARY

No reports describing the use of pazopanib during human lactation have been located. The molecular weight (about 438 for the free base) and long elimination half-life (about 31 hours) suggest that the drug will be excreted into breast milk, but the high plasma protein binding (>99%) might limit the amount. The effect of this exposure on a nursing infant is unknown. In adults, adverse reactions occurring in ≥10% of patients were diarrhea, hypertension, hair color changes, nausea and vomiting, anorexia, fatigue, asthenia, abdominal pain, and headache. Other serious toxicities, such as hepatotoxicity, were also observed (1). Because the potential for severe toxicity in a nursing infant is a concern, women receiving pazopanib should not breastfeed.

Reference

1. Product information. Votrient. GlaxoSmithKline, 2009.

PEGAPTANIB

Ophthalmic

PREGNANCY RECOMMENDATION: No Human Data—Probably Compatible
BREASTFEEDING RECOMMENDATION: No Human Data—Probably Compatible

PREGNANCY SUMMARY

No reports describing the use of pegaptanib in human pregnancy have been located. The animal data suggest low risk, but the absence of human pregnancy experience prevents a more complete assessment. However, the very low plasma levels probably prevent clinically significant amounts of the drug from reaching the embryo or fetus. Thus, if a woman requires pegaptanib, it should not be withheld because of pregnancy.

FETAL RISK SUMMARY

Pegaptanib is an aptamer—a pegylated modified oligonucleotide that is a selective vascular endothelial growth factor (VEGF) antagonist. It is in the same class as ranibizumab. Pegaptanib is indicated for the treatment of neovascular (wet) age-related macular degeneration. It is administered as a 0.3-mg intravitreous injection every 6 weeks. When a 3-mg dose (10 times the recommended dose) was given, the mean maximum plasma concentration, about 80 ng/mL, occurred within 1–4 days. The mean AUC was about 25 mcg·hr/mL and the plasma elimination half-life was about 10 days. Pegaptanib is metabolized but the amount of metabolism apparently has not been determined (1).

Reproduction studies have been conducted in mice. In pregnant mice, no evidence of maternal toxicity, teratogenicity, or fetal mortality was observed with daily IV doses up to about 7000 times the recommended human monocular ophthalmic dose of 0.3 mg based on body weight (1).

Studies for carcinogenicity and fertility have not been conducted with pegaptanib. Mutagenicity and clastogenicity assays with pegaptanib and its monomer component nucleotides have been negative (1).

It is not known if pegaptanib crosses the human placenta. The molecular weight (about 50,000) suggests that exposure of the embryo and/or fetus is unlikely. The drug does cross the mouse placenta after IV administration (1). Moreover, the plasma elimination half-life is very long. Nevertheless, if the drug does cross the human placenta, the very low plasma levels will limit the amount reaching the embryo and/or fetus.

BREASTFEEDING SUMMARY

No reports describing the use of pegaptanib during human lactation have been located. Although the long plasma elimination half-life (about 10 days) favors excretion, the molecular weight (about 50,000) and very low plasma concentrations suggest that the drug will not be excreted into breast milk. The effects of any exposure on a nursing infant are unknown, but probably are clinically insignificant. Thus, if a lactating woman requires pegaptanib, it should not be withheld because she is breastfeeding.

Reference

1. Product information. Macugen. Eyetech Pharmaceuticals, 2006.

PEGFILGRASTIM

Hematopoietic

PREGNANCY RECOMMENDATION: No Human Data—Animal Data Suggest Low Risk
BREASTFEEDING RECOMMENDATION: No Human Data—Probably Compatible

PREGNANCY SUMMARY

No reports describing the use of pegfilgrastim in human pregnancy have been located. Although the animal data do not suggest fetal risk, the absence of human pregnancy experience prevents an assessment of the embryo–fetal risk. Filgrastim has been used in the pregnancy without apparent fetal harm. (See Filgrastim.) Therefore, until human data are available, filgrastim would be preferred over pegfilgrastim in pregnancy.

FETAL RISK SUMMARY

Pegfilgrastim is a covalent conjugate of monomethoxypolyethylene glycol and filgrastim that results in reduced renal elimination and prolonged persistence in the serum. (See also Filgrastim.) Pegfilgrastim is indicated to decrease the incidence of infection, as manifested by febrile neutropenia, in patients with nonmyeloid malignancies receiving myelosuppressive chemotherapy associated with a clinically significant incidence of febrile neutropenia. The serum half-life depends on the dose and the number of neutrophils, ranging from 15 to 80 hours after SC injection (1).

Reproduction studies have been conducted in rats and rabbits. In rats, pegfilgrastim given SC in doses up to 1000 mcg/kg/dose every other day during organogenesis caused no embryotoxic or fetotoxic outcome. However, an increased incidence of wavy ribs was observed at the maximum dose. When doses up to 1000 mcg/kg/dose were given once weekly from gestation day 6 through lactation day 18, no maternal toxicity or adverse effects on the growth or development of offspring were observed. The highest dose was about 23 times the recommended human dose (RHD). In addition, the once-weekly dose in male and nonpregnant female rats had no effect on reproductive performance, fertility, or sperm parameters. In rabbits, SC doses as low as 4 times the RHD given every other day were maternally toxic (decreased food consumption and maternal weight gain) and fetotoxic (decreased body weights). At about 16 times the RHD or higher, there was an increased incidence of resorptions and abortions with a corresponding decrease in the number of live fetuses (1).

It is not known if pegfilgrastim crosses the human placenta, but filgrastim apparently reaches the fetus late in gestation in amounts sufficient to produce a biologic effect. (See Filgrastim.) The molecular weight of pegfilgrastim (about 39,000) is twice that of filgrastim (about 19,000) because of the polyethylene glycol. The addition of this nonamino acid moiety may prevent the transfer of pegfilgrastim in amounts sufficient to produce a biologic effect in the fetus.

BREASTFEEDING SUMMARY

No reports describing the use of pegfilgrastim during human lactation have been located. Pegfilgrastim is composed of monomethoxypolyethylene glycol and filgrastim that are chemically bound together. This produces a compound with a very long half-life (15–80 hours) and a very high molecular weight (about 39,000). Excretion into breast milk is doubtful, but even if the drug were excreted, it probably would be digested in a nursing infant's stomach. The risk to a nursing infant is unknown but appears to be low to nonexistent. Therefore, treatment with pegfilgrastim should not be withheld because of breastfeeding.

Reference

1. Product information. Neulasta. Amgen, 2004.

PEGINESATIDE

Hematologic Agent (Hematopoietic)

PREGNANCY RECOMMENDATION: No Human Data—Animal Data Suggest Risk
BREASTFEEDING RECOMMENDATION: No Human Data—Probably Compatible

PREGNANCY SUMMARY

No reports describing the use of peginesatide in human pregnancy have been located. Animal reproduction tests suggest risk, but the absence of human pregnancy experience prevents a more complete assessment of embryo–fetal risk.

FETAL RISK SUMMARY

Peginesatide is given as an IV or SC injection. It is a dimeric peptide that is covalently linked to a PEG chain. Peginesatide is indicated for the treatment of anemia due to chronic kidney disease in adult patients on dialysis. The agent binds to and activates the human erythropoietin receptor and stimulates erythropoiesis in human red blood cell precursors. Peginesatide is not metabolized. The mean half-life in dialysis patients is 47.9 ± 17.7 hours (1).

Reproduction studies have been conducted in rats and rabbits. In rats given an IV every 3 days for a total of five doses, and every 5th day in rabbits for a total of three doses, adverse embryo–fetal effects included reduced fetal weights, increased resorption, embryo–fetal death, cleft palate (rats only), sternoschisis (rats only), variations in blood vessels (rats only), sternum anomalies, fused sternebrae (rabbits only), unossification of sternebrae and metatarsals, and reduced ossification of some bones. In rats, embryo–fetal toxicity was evident at doses of ≥1 mg/kg resulting in exposures (AUC) comparable to or higher than those in humans after IV administration at a dose of 0.35 mg/kg in patients on dialysis. In rabbits, adverse effects were observed at doses lower (5%–50%) than the dose of 0.35 mg/kg in patients (1).

Long-term carcinogenicity studies in rats were negative as were assays for mutagenic or clastogenic effects. In males and females given IV doses, peginesatide produced adverse effects in males including reduced weight of seminal vesicles and prostate. In females, decreased viable fetuses appeared to be due to preimplantation and postimplantation losses. There were no apparent drug-related effects on estrous cycles or the number of corpora lutea (1).

It is not known if peginesatide crosses the human placenta. The molecular weight (about 4900 for the dimeric peptide alone) suggests that the drug will not cross the placenta in spite of a relative long mean half-life. However, exposure during the 3rd trimester might still occur.

BREASTFEEDING SUMMARY

No reports describing the use of peginesatide during human lactation have been located. The molecular weight (about 4900 for the dimeric peptide alone) suggests that clinically significant amounts of the drug will not be excreted into breast milk in spite of a relative long (about 48 hours) mean half-life. Moreover, even if small amounts were excreted, they probably would be digested in the infant's gut. Nonetheless, if the drug is used during lactation, the nursing infant should be monitored for the most common (≥10%) adverse effects in patients. These effects were dyspnea, diarrhea, nausea, and cough (1).

Reference

1. Product information. Omontys. Affymax, 2012.

PEGLOTICASE

Antigout (Uricosuric)

PREGNANCY RECOMMENDATION: No Human Data—Animal Data Suggest Low Risk
BREASTFEEDING RECOMMENDATION: No Human Data—Probably Compatible

P

PREGNANCY SUMMARY

No reports describing the use of pegloticase in human pregnancy have been located. Although animal data suggest low risk, the absence of human pregnancy experience prevents a more complete assessment of the embryo–fetal risk. If the drug is used in a pregnancy, the woman should be informed of the lack of data.

FETAL RISK SUMMARY

Pegloticase is a PEGylated, recombinant, mammalian urate oxidase enzyme given as an IV infusion every 2 weeks. It is indicated for the treatment of chronic gout in adult patients who are refractory to conventional therapy. No information was provided by the manufacturer on plasma protein binding, metabolism, or elimination half-life (1). However, in two studies, the mean elimination half-life was 12.5 (range 3.5–21.5 days) and 14 days (range 7–44 days) (2,3).

Reproduction studies have been conducted in rats. In this species, doses given on gestation days 6–16 that were 6–50 times higher than the maximum recommended human dose based on BSA were not teratogenic (1).

Pegloticase has not been evaluated for carcinogenesis, mutagenesis, or impairment of fertility.

It is not known if pegloticase crosses the human placenta. The high molecular weight (about 540,000) suggests that exposure of the embryo–fetus is unlikely to occur.

BREASTFEEDING SUMMARY

No reports describing the use of pegloticase during human lactation have been located.

The high molecular weight (about 540,000) suggests that the enzyme will not be excreted into breast milk. If excretion does occur, the enzyme most likely would be digested in the infant's gut. Consequently, although the risk to a nursing infant is unknown, it appears to be negligible.

References

1. Product information. Krystexxa. Savient Pharmaceuticals, 2010.

2. Sundy JS, Ganson NJ, Kelly SJ, Scarlett EL, Rehrig CD, Huang W, Hershfield MS. Pharmacokinetics and pharmacodynamics of intravenous PEGylated recombinant mammalian urate oxidase in patients with refractory gout. Arthritis Rheum 2007;56:1021–8.
3. Yue CS, Huang W, Alton M, Maroli AN, Wright D, Marco MD. Population pharmacokinetic and pharmacodynamic analysis of pegloticase in subjects with hyperuricemia and treatment-failure gout. J Clin Pharmacol. 2008;48:708–18.

PEGVISOMANT

Metabolic Agent (Growth Hormone Receptor Antagonist)

PREGNANCY RECOMMENDATION: Limited Human Data—Animal Data Suggest Low Risk
BREASTFEEDING RECOMMENDATION: Limited Human Data—Probably Compatible

PREGNANCY SUMMARY

The limited human data, as well as the animal data, suggest that use of pegvisomant during human pregnancy represents a low risk of embryo–fetal harm.

FETAL RISK SUMMARY

Pegvisomant, an analog of human growth hormone (GH) that has been structurally altered to act as a GH antagonist, is given as a daily SC injection. The protein is covalently bound to various amounts of polyethylene glycol (PEG) polymers to reduce its clearance rate. Pegvisomant is indicated for the treatment of acromegaly in patients who have had an inadequate response to surgery and/or radiation therapy and/or other medical therapies, or for whom these therapies are not appropriate. The goal of treatment is to normalize serum insulin-like growth factor-1 (IGF-1). The mean serum elimination half-life is about 6 days (1).

Reproduction studies have been conducted in rabbits. No evidence of teratogenic effects was observed with SC doses up to 10 times the maximum human therapeutic dose based on BSA (MHTD) during organogenesis. However, at the highest dose, a slight increase in postimplantation loss was observed (1).

In long-term studies for carcinogenic potential in rats, an increase in malignant fibrous histiocytoma at injection sites in male rats but not in female rats was observed. The tumors were thought to have been caused by irritation and the high sensitivity of the rat to repeated SC injections. Multiple assays for mutagenicity were negative. There was no effect on fertility or reproductive performance of female rabbits at SC doses up to 10 times the MHTD (1).

It is not known if pegvisomant crosses the human placenta. Although the elimination half-life is prolonged, the protein is bound to various amounts of PEG polymers yielding predominant molecular weights of 42,000–52,000. This suggests that little if any of the drug will cross to the embryo–fetus. In a case discussed below, analysis of a cord blood sample at term revealed a minimal concentration of the protein.

A 2006 case report described the use of pegvisomant (20 mg SC daily) in a 29-year-old woman with active acromegaly who underwent in vitro fertilization (2). A positive pregnancy test was documented 2 weeks later and pegvisomant was discontinued. She eventually gave birth to a healthy, 3.5-kg male infant who was physically and developmentally normal at 1 year of age (2).

Another case report described the use of pegvisomant throughout the pregnancy of a 26-year-old woman with acromegaly (3). The woman conceived during the 13th month of pegvisomant therapy while receiving 15 mg/day. The dose was increased to 20 mg/day at 1 month and to 25 mg/day at 3 months for the remainder of the pregnancy. At 40 weeks' gestation, she underwent a cesarean section to give birth to 3.8 kg female infant with Apgar scores of 9 and 9. The infant's weight, length, and head circumference were at the 75th percentile. GH and IGF-1 concentrations in cord blood were within the normal range and a pegvisomant concentration was minimal (112 ng/mL). These findings suggested that pegvisomant had no effect on fetal GH or IGF-1 interactions. At 6 months of age, the infant was healthy and achieving normal developmental milestones (3).

A 2005 review of acromegaly pharmacotherapy stated that pegvisomant should not be used in pregnancy (4). However, no studies of the drug in pregnancy were cited. In contrast, a 2012 review of acromegaly concluded that treatment of the disease in pregnancy does not cause teratogenicity or significant complications (5).

BREASTFEEDING SUMMARY

No reports describing the use of pegvisomant during human breastfeeding have been located. However, in a case report discussed earlier, a mother receiving 25 mg/day of the protein had undetectable concentrations (<50 ng/mL) in her milk (4). The timing of the sample relative to the last dose or the time after birth was not reported. The concentration of GH in her breast milk was 0.6 ng/mL, whereas the GH concentration in three milk samples from normal healthy mothers was consistently <0.1 ng/mL (4).

In the above study, the undetectable pegvisomant concentration in milk is consistent with the high molecular weights (42,000–52,000) of PEG-bound pegvisomant. Moreover, even if some of the protein is excreted into milk, it would most likely be digested in the infant's gut and not absorbed.

References

1. Product information. Somavert. Pharmacia & Upjohn, 2010.

2. Qureshi A, Kalu E, Ramanathan G, Bano G, Croucher C, Panahloo A. IVF/ICSI in a woman with active acromegaly: successful outcome following treatment with pegvisomant. J Assist Reprod Genet 2006;23:439–42.
3. Brian SR, Bidlingmaier M, Wajnrajch MP, Weinzimer SA, Inzucchi SE. Treatment of acromegaly with pegvisomant during pregnancy: maternal and fetal effects. J Clin Endocrinol Metab 2007;92:3374–7.
4. Biermasz NR, Romijn JA, Pereira AM, Roelfsema F. Current pharmacotherapy for acromegaly: a review. Expert Opin Pharmacother 2005;6:2393–405.
5. Cheng S, Grasso L, Martinez-Orozco JA, Al-Agha R, Pivonello R, Colao A, Ezzat S. Pregnancy in acromegaly: experience from two referral centers and systematic review of the literature. Clin Endocrinol (Oxf) 2012;76:264–71.

PEMETREXED

Antineoplastic (Antimetabolite)

PREGNANCY RECOMMENDATION: Contraindicated—1st Trimester
Contraindicated (If Combined with Cisplatin)
BREASTFEEDING RECOMMENDATION: Hold Breastfeeding
Contraindicated (If Combined with Cisplatin)

PREGNANCY SUMMARY

No reports describing the use of pemetrexed in human pregnancy have been located. The animal data suggest risk based on the only animal species tested. The drug is often combined with cisplatin, another antineoplastic. The drug should be avoided in pregnancy, especially during the 1st trimester. Use after that period may be appropriate if the mother's condition requires use of the drug, but severe fetal toxicity (e.g., bone marrow suppression observed in adults) is a potential risk.

FETAL RISK SUMMARY

Pemetrexed is a folate analog metabolic inhibitor that is given as a 10-minute IV infusion on day 1 of each 21-day cycle. It is in the same antineoplastic subclass of folic acid antagonists (antimetabolites) as aminopterin, methotrexate, and pralatrexate. Pemetrexed is indicated for nonsquamous non–small-cell lung cancer and mesothelioma either alone or in combination with cisplatin. (See also Cisplatin.) Pemetrexed is not metabolized to an appreciable extent and is primarily eliminated unchanged in the urine. Plasma protein binding is about 81%. In patients with normal renal function, the elimination half-life is 3.5 hours (1).

Reproduction studies have been conducted in mice. Repeated intraperitoneal doses given to mice during organogenesis caused dose-related fetal malformations: incomplete ossification of talus and skull bone at about 1/833rd the recommended IV human dose based on BSA (RHD) and cleft palate at about 1/33rd the RHD. Embryo–fetal deaths and reduced litter sizes also were observed (1).

Carcinogenicity studies have not been conducted with pemetrexed. The drug was clastogenic in an in vivo mouse assay, but was not mutagenic in multiple in vivo tests. IV doses administered to male mice that were about ≥1/1666th the RHD resulted in reduced fertility, hypospermia, and testicular atrophy (1).

It is not known if pemetrexed crosses the human placenta. The molecular weight (about 471 for the nonhydrated form), moderate plasma protein binding, and the elimination half-life suggest that the drug will cross to the embryo–fetus.

BREASTFEEDING SUMMARY

No reports describing the use of pemetrexed during human lactation have been located. The molecular weight (about 471 for the nonhydrated form), moderate (81%) plasma protein binding, and the elimination half-life (3.5 hours) suggest that the drug will be excreted into breast milk. The effect of this exposure on a nursing infant is unknown, but severe toxicity such as that observed in patients receiving the drug (e.g., bone marrow suppression, hepatic and renal toxicities, and gastrointestinal disturbances) is a potential complication. Holding breastfeeding for 18–24 hours while "pumping and dumping," would allow the drug to be nearly eliminated from the mother's circulation and lessen the risk to a nursing infant. However, breastfeeding is not recommended if the therapy includes cisplatin (see Cisplatin).

Reference

1. Product information. Alimta. Eli Lilly, 2009.

PEMOLINE

[Withdrawn from the market. See 9th edition.]

P

PENBUTOLOL

Sympatholytic (Antihypertensive)

PREGNANCY RECOMMENDATION: Human Data Suggest Risk in 2nd and 3rd Trimesters
BREASTFEEDING RECOMMENDATION: No Human Data—Potential Toxicity

PREGNANCY SUMMARY

No reports describing the use of penbutolol in human pregnancy have been located. If used near delivery, the newborn infant should be closely observed for 24–48 hours for signs and symptoms of β-blockade. Long-term effects of in utero exposure to β-blockers have not been studied but warrant evaluation.

Some β-blockers may cause intrauterine growth restriction (IUGR) and reduced placental weight, especially those lacking intrinsic sympathomimetic activity (ISA) (i.e., partial agonist). Treatment beginning early in the 2nd trimester results in the greatest weight reductions, whereas treatment restricted to the 3rd trimester primarily affects only placental weight. Penbutolol does possess ISA. However, IUGR and reduced placental weight may potentially occur with all agents within this class. Although growth restriction is a serious concern, the benefits of maternal therapy with β-blockers, in some cases, might outweigh the risks to the fetus and must be judged on a case-by-case basis.

FETAL RISK SUMMARY

Penbutolol is a nonselective β_1, β_2-adrenergic blocking agent used in the treatment of hypertension. No teratogenic effects were noted in mice, rats, and rabbits treated with doses up to 250 times the maximum recommended human dose (MRHD) (1,2). A slight increase in fetal and newborn mortality was observed in rabbits given 156 times the MRHD (2). In rats dosed at 200 times the MRHD, decreased pup body weight and survival were observed (2). In mice, the drug produced no behavioral changes in the exposed offspring (1).

BREASTFEEDING SUMMARY

No reports describing the use of penbutolol during human lactation have been located. If penbutolol is used during nursing, the infant should be closely monitored for hypotension, bradycardia, and other signs or symptoms of β-blockade. Long-term effects of exposure to β-blockers from milk have not been studied but warrant evaluation.

References

1. Sugisaki T, Takagi S, Seshimo M, Hayashi S, Miyamoto M. Reproductive studies of penbutolol sulfate given orally to mice. Oyo Yakuri 1981;22:289–305. As cited in Shepard TH. *Catalog of Teratogenic Agents*. 6th ed. Baltimore, MD: The Johns Hopkins University Press, 1989:487.
2. Product information. Levatol. Schwarz Pharma, 1997.

P

PENCICLOVIR

Antiviral

PREGNANCY RECOMMENDATION: Limited Human Data—Probably Compatible
BREASTFEEDING RECOMMENDATION: No Human Data—Probably Compatible

PREGNANCY SUMMARY

One study reported the use of penciclovir in human pregnancy and found no statistically significant association with major birth defects (1). Penciclovir is the active metabolite of the prodrug famciclovir (see also Famciclovir). Animal reproductive data suggest low risk. In addition, the drug has not been detected in the plasma or urine after single or repeated topical doses in healthy males. Thus, the risk to an embryo or fetus from maternal use of the agent appears to be nil.

FETAL RISK SUMMARY

Penciclovir is an antiviral agent indicated for the treatment of recurrent herpes labialis (cold sores) in adults and children 12 years of age and older. Penciclovir is available for topical administration as a 1% cream that is active against herpes simplex types 1 and 2. The agent was not detected in the plasma (detection level 0.1 mcg/mL) or urine (detection level 10 mcg/mL) of healthy male adults following single or repeat applications of the cream (2).

Reproduction studies with penciclovir have been conducted in rats and rabbits. In these species, IV doses that were 260 and 355 times, respectively, the maximum recommended human topical dose caused no adverse effects on the course and outcome of pregnancy or on fetal development (2).

Two-year carcinogenicity studies have been conducted with famciclovir (the prodrug) in rats and mice. At a dose about 395 times the maximum theoretical human exposure from topical penciclovir based on AUC (MTHE), an increase in the incidence of mammary adenocarcinoma was observed in female rats. This tumor is common in female rats of the strain used. No increases in tumor incidence were observed in male rats or in male and female mice at doses producing exposures that were about 190 and 100 times, respectively, the MTHE. High doses of penciclovir produced mixed results in mutagenic assays. In fertility studies with rats and dogs, high IV doses that were about 1155 and 3255 times, respectively, the MTHE caused testicular toxicity that included atrophy of the seminiferous tubules and decreased sperm counts. These effects were not observed with lower doses, nor have they been observed in clinical trials in immunocompetent men treated with famciclovir for recurrent genital herpes (2).

It is not known if penciclovir crosses the human placenta. The molecular weight (about 253) is low enough, but the systemic concentration is below the limit of detection. Consequently, clinically significant exposure of the embryo or fetus is not expected.

A 2010 study compared the pregnancy outcomes of 118 women exposed to penciclovir topical cream in the 1st trimester with 837,677 unexposed cases (1). The number of infants with birth defects in the two groups were 5 (4.2%) and 19,965 (2.4%), respectively. There was no significant association between exposure to penciclovir and the risk of major birth defects (prevalence odds ratio 1.88, 95% confidence interval 0.76–4.62) (1).

BREASTFEEDING SUMMARY

No reports describing the use of penciclovir during lactation have been located. The molecular weight (about 253) is low enough for excretion into breast milk, but the systemic concentration is below the limit of detection. Consequently, the effects on a nursing infant are probably nil.

References

1. Pasternak B, Hviid A. Use of acyclovir, valacyclovir, and famciclovir in the first trimester of pregnancy and the risk of birth defects. JAMA 2010;304:859–66.
2. Product information. Denavir. New American Therapeutics, 2010.

PENICILLAMINE

Chelating Agent

PREGNANCY RECOMMENDATION: Human Data Suggest Risk
BREASTFEEDING RECOMMENDATION: No Human Data—Potential Toxicity

PREGNANCY SUMMARY

Although the evidence is incomplete, maintaining the daily dose at ≤500 mg may reduce the incidence of penicillamine-induced toxicity in the newborn (1,2). The manufacturer recommends that the dose should be limited to 1 g/day and, if a cesarean section is planned, to 250 mg/day for 6 weeks before delivery and postoperatively until wound healing is complete (3).

FETAL RISK SUMMARY

Penicillamine is a chelating agent used in the treatment of Wilson's disease, cystinuria, and severe rheumatoid arthritis. Reproductive studies in rats at doses 6 times higher than the maximum recommended human dose revealed fetal anomalies consisting of skeletal defects, cleft palates, and fetal resorptions (3).

The use of penicillamine during pregnancy has been observed in >100 pregnancies (1,2,4–20). The mothers were treated for rheumatoid arthritis, cystinuria, or Wilson's disease. Most of the pregnancies resulted in healthy newborns who developed normally, but anomalies were observed in 10 infants:

- Cutis laxa, hypotonia, hyperflexion of hips and shoulders, pyloric stenosis, vein fragility, varicosities, impaired wound healing, death (5)
- Cutis laxa, growth restriction, inguinal hernia, simian crease, perforated bowel, death (8)
- Cutis laxa (6)
- Cutis laxa, mild micrognathia, low-set ears, inguinal hernia (12)
- Cutis laxa, inguinal hernia (13)
- Marked flexion deformities of extremities, dislocated hips, hydrocephalus, intraventricular hemorrhage, death (14)
- Cerebral palsy, blindness, bilateral talipes, sudden infant death at 3 months (14)
- Hydrocephalus (14)
- Ventricular septal defect (small) (9)
- Bilateral cleft lip with totally cleft palate (19)

The relationship of the last five cases listed above to penicillamine is controversial because they did not include connective tissue anomalies. The drug may be partially responsible, but other factors, such as maternal infections and surgery, may have a stronger association with the defects (14).

A 2000 review cited data from the literature involving 111 women with Wilson's disease who had 153 pregnancies

(20). The outcomes included 144 normal neonates (1 premature), 4 elective abortions, 1 spontaneous abortion, and 4 cases of birth defects (mannosidosis; cleft lip and palate; 2 transient cutis laxa).

Penicillamine crosses the placenta to the fetus. A mother was treated for cystinuria throughout gestation with penicillamine hydrochloride 1050 mg/day (843 mg of penicillamine base) (4). The drug was found in the urine of her newborn infant. The baby's physical and mental development was normal at 3 months.

A 1993 report described the effects of untreated Wilson's disease on a fetus (21). A 23-year-old woman, diagnosed with Wilson's disease at 12 years of age, had been treated with penicillamine but she had stopped the therapy when she was 15 years old. Liver cirrhosis, thrombocytopenia, and low serum proteins developed during the 2nd trimester and, when the diagnosis of Wilson's disease was remade (the patient had withheld information about her past history), an elective cesarean section was performed at 36 weeks' gestation. The 2380-g male infant had hepatomegaly, elevated liver enzymes, slightly low serum ceruloplasmin, and high excretion of urinary copper. His development during the first year was normal, as was his current serum ceruloplasmin concentration, but his liver enzymes remained elevated, possibly because of copper accumulation in the fetal liver (21).

Several conflicting recommendations have appeared in the literature concerning the use of penicillamine during pregnancy. The authors of one review believe the drug should be avoided during pregnancy (22). Another suggests that therapy with penicillamine should be continued during pregnancy in women with Wilson's disease, but stopped in those with rheumatoid arthritis (23). Still others recommend continuing therapy during the treatment of Wilson's disease, except during the 1st trimester (24).

BREASTFEEDING SUMMARY

No reports describing the use of penicillamine during lactation have been located. Authors of one review recommend avoiding penicillamine during lactation (21). However, a 2000 review stated that no adverse effects in nursing infants have been reported by mothers taking penicillamine, even though one study did find lower amounts of zinc and copper in milk (20).

References

1. Marecek Z, Graf M. Pregnancy in penicillamine-treated patients with Wilson's disease. N Engl J Med 1976;295:841–2.
2. Endres W. D-penicillamine in pregnancy—to ban or not to ban? Klin Wochenschr 1981;59:535–7.
3. Product information. Cuprimine. Merck & Co, 1997.
4. Crawhall JC, Scowen EF, Thompson CJ, Watts RWE. Dissolution of cystine stones during d-penicillamine treatment of a pregnant patient with cystinuria. Br Med J 1967;2:216–8.
5. Mjolnerod OK, Rasmussen K, Dommerud SA, Gjeruldsen ST. Congenital connective-tissue defect probably due to d-penicillamine treatment in pregnancy. Lancet 1971;1:673–5.
6. Laver M, Fairley KF. D-penicillamine treatment in pregnancy. Lancet 1971;1:1019–20.
7. Scheinberg IH, Sternlieb I. Pregnancy in penicillamine-treated patients with Wilson's disease. N Engl J Med 1975;293:1300–3.
8. Solomon L, Abrams G, Dinner M, Berman L. Neonatal abnormalities associated with d-penicillamine treatment during pregnancy. N Engl J Med 1977;296:54–5.
9. Walshe JM. Pregnancy in Wilson's disease. Q J Med 1977;46:73–83.
10. Lyle WH. Penicillamine in pregnancy. Lancet 1978;1:606–7.
11. Linares A, Zarranz JJ, Rodriguez-Alarcon J, Diaz-Perez JL. Reversible cutis laxa due to maternal d-penicillamine treatment. Lancet 1979;2:43.
12. Harpey JP, Jaudon MC, Clavel JP, Galli A, Darbois Y. Cutis laxa and low serum zinc after antenatal exposure to penicillamine. Lancet 1983; 2:858.
13. Beck RB, Rosenbaum KN, Byers PH, Holbrook KA, Perry LW. Ultrastructural findings in the fetal penicillamine syndrome (abstract). Presented at the 13th Annual Birth Defects Conference, June 1980, March of Dimes and University of California, San Diego.
14. Gal P, Ravenel SD. Contractures and hydrocephalus with penicillamine and maternal hypotension. J Clin Dysmorphol 1984;2:9–12.
15. Gregory MC, Mansell MA. Pregnancy and cystinuria. Lancet 1983;2: 1158–60.
16. Dupont P, Irion O, Béguin F. Pregnancy in a patient with treated Wilson's disease: a case report. Am J Obstet Gynecol 1990;163:1527–8.
17. Hartard C, Kunze K. Pregnancy in a patient with Wilson's disease treated with D-penicillamine and zinc sulfate. Eur Neurol 1994;34:337–40.
18. Berghella V, Steele D, Spector T, Cambi F, Johnson A. Successful pregnancy in a neurologically impaired woman with Wilson's disease. Am J Obstet Gynecol 1997;176:712–4.
19. Martinez-Frias ML, Rodriguez-Pinilla E, Bermejo E, Blanco M. Prenatal exposure to penicillamine and oral clefts: case report. Am J Med Genet 1998;76:274–5.
20. Sternlieb I. Wilson's disease and pregnancy. Hepatology 2000;31:531–2.
21. Oga M, Matsui N, Anai T, Yoshimatsu J, Inoue I, Miyakawa I. Copper disposition of the fetus and placenta in a patient with untreated Wilson's disease. Am J Obstet Gynecol 1993;169:196–8.
22. Ostensen M, Husby G. Antirheumatic drug treatment during pregnancy and lactation. Scand J Rheumatol 1985;14:1–7.
23. Miehle W. Current aspects of D-penicillamine and pregnancy. Z Rheumatol 1988;47(Suppl 1):20–3.
24. Woods SE, Colón VF. Wilson's disease. Am Fam Physician 1989;40:171–8.

PENICILLIN G

Antibiotic (Penicillin)

PREGNANCY RECOMMENDATION: Compatible
BREASTFEEDING RECOMMENDATION: Compatible

PREGNANCY SUMMARY

Penicillin G is used routinely for maternal infections during pregnancy. Reproduction studies in mice, rats, and rabbits revealed no evidence of impaired fertility or fetal harm (1). The antibiotic is considered low risk in pregnancy.

FETAL RISK SUMMARY

Several investigators have documented the rapid passage of penicillin G into the fetal circulation and amniotic fluid (2–6). Therapeutic levels are reached in both sites except for the amniotic fluid during the 1st trimester (6). At term, maternal serum and amniotic fluid concentrations are equal 60–90 minutes after IV administration (3). Continuous IV infusions (10,000 U/hr) produce equal concentrations of penicillin G at 20 hours in maternal serum, cord serum, and amniotic fluid (3).

The early use of penicillin G was linked to increased uterine activity and abortion (7–11). It is not known whether this was related to impurities in the drug or to penicillin itself. No reports of this effect have appeared since a report published in 1950 (11). An anaphylactic reaction in a pregnant patient reportedly led to the death of her fetus in utero (12).

Only one reference has linked the use of penicillin G with congenital abnormalities (13). An examination of hospital records indicated that in three of four cases the administration of penicillin G had been followed by the birth of a malformed baby. A retrospective review of additional patients exposed to antibiotics in the 1st trimester indicated an increase in congenital defects. Unfortunately, the authors did not analyze their data for each antibiotic, so no causal relationship to penicillin G could be shown (13,14).

In another case, a patient was treated in early pregnancy with high doses of penicillin G procaine IV,* cortisone, and sodium salicylate (15). A cyclopic male was delivered at term but died 5 minutes later. The defect was attributed to salicylates, cortisone, or maternal viremia. In a controlled study, 110 patients received one to three antibiotics during the 1st trimester for a total of 589 weeks (16). Penicillin G was given for a total of 107 weeks. The incidence of birth defects was no different from that in a nontreated control group. *(*Penicillin G procaine should not be given IV. Presumably, the drug was either given IM or the procaine form was not used. Attempts to clarify this with the authors have been unsuccessful.)*

The Collaborative Perinatal Project monitored 50,282 mother–child pairs, 3546 of whom had 1st trimester exposure to penicillin derivatives (17, pp. 297–313). For use anytime during pregnancy, 7171 exposures were recorded (17, p. 435). In neither group was evidence found to suggest a relationship to large categories of major or minor malformations or to individual defects. From these data, it is unlikely that penicillin G is teratogenic.

BREASTFEEDING SUMMARY

Penicillin G is excreted into breast milk in low concentrations. Milk:plasma ratios following IM doses of 100,000 U in 11 patients varied between 0.02 and 0.13 (18). The maximum concentration measured in milk was 0.6 U/mL after this dose. Although no adverse effects were reported, three potential problems exist for the nursing infant: modification of bowel flora, direct effects on the infant (e.g., allergic response), and interference with the interpretation of culture results if a fever workup is required.

References

1. Product information. Pfizerpen. Pfizer, 2000.
2. Herrel W, Nichols D, Heilman D. Penicillin. Its usefulness, limitations, diffusion and detection, with analysis of 150 cases in which it was employed. JAMA 1944;125:1003–11.
3. Woltz J, Zintel H. The transmission of penicillin to amniotic fluid and fetal blood in the human. Am J Obstet Gynecol 1945;50:338–40.
4. Hutter A, Parks J. The transmission of penicillin through the placenta. A preliminary report. Am J Obstet Gynecol 1945;49:663–5.
5. Woltz J, Wiley M. The transmission of penicillin to the previable fetus. JAMA 1946;131:969–70.
6. Wasz-Hockert O, Nummi S, Vuopala S, Jarvinen P. Transplacental passage of azidocillin, ampicillin and penicillin G during early and late pregnancy. Acta Paediatr Scand (Suppl) 1970;206:109–10.
7. Lentz J, Ingraham N Jr, Beerman H, Stokes J. Penicillin in the prevention and treatment of congenital syphilis. JAMA 1944;126:408–13.
8. Leavitt H. Clinical action of penicillin on the uterus. J Vener Dis Inf 1945;26:150–3.
9. McLachlan A, Brown D. The effects of penicillin administration on menstrual and other sexual functions. Br J Vener Dis 1947;23:1–10.
10. Mazingarbe A. Le pencilline possede-t-elle une action abortive? Gynecol Obstet 1946;45:487.
11. Perin L, Sissmann R, Detre F, Chertier A. La pencilline a-t-elle une action abortive? Bull Soc Fr Dermatol 1950;57:534–8.
12. Kosim H. Intrauterine fetal death as a result of anaphylactic reaction to penicillin in a pregnant woman. Dapim Refuiim 1959;18:136–7.
13. Carter M, Wilson F. Antibiotics and congenital malformations. Lancet 1963;1:1267–8.
14. Carter M, Wilson F. Antibiotics in early pregnancy and congenital malformations. Dev Med Child Neurol 1965;7:353–9.
15. Khudr G, Olding L. Cyclopia. Am J Dis Child 1973;125:120–2.
16. Ravid R, Toaff R. On the possible teratogenicity of antibiotic drugs administered during pregnancy-a prospective study. In Klingberg M, Abramovici A, Chemki J, eds. *Drugs and Fetal Development*. New York, NY: Plenum Press, 1972:505–10.
17. Heinonen OP, Slone D, Shapiro S. *Birth Defects and Drugs in Pregnancy*. Littleton, MA: Publishing Sciences Group, 1977.
18. Greene H, Burkhart B, Hobby G. Excretion of penicillin in human milk following parturition. Am J Obstet Gynecol 1946;51:732–3.

P

PENICILLIN G, BENZATHINE

Antibiotic (Penicillin)

PREGNANCY RECOMMENDATION: Compatible
BREASTFEEDING RECOMMENDATION: Compatible

PREGNANCY SUMMARY

Benzathine penicillin G is a combination of an ammonium base and penicillin G suspended in water (see also Penicillin G). Reproduction studies in mice, rats, and rabbits have revealed no evidence of impaired fertility or fetal harm (1). The antibiotic is considered low risk in pregnancy.

FETAL RISK SUMMARY

The pharmacokinetics of benzathine penicillin G in healthy women at 38–39 weeks' gestation, 1–7 days before delivery, have been described (2). Penicillin concentrations were measured in maternal serum, maternal cerebrospinal fluid, cord serum, and amniotic fluid. Because of the wide range of concentrations measured, the authors concluded that the altered pharmacokinetics occurring at this time may adversely affect the efficacy of the drug to prevent congenital syphilis.

BREASTFEEDING SUMMARY

See Penicillin G.

References

1. Product information. Bicillin L-A. Wyeth-Ayerst Pharmaceuticals, 2000.
2. Nathan L, Bawdon RE, Sidawi JE, Stettler RW, McIntire DM, Wendel GD Jr. Penicillin levels following the administration of benzathine penicillin G in pregnancy. Obstet Gynecol 1993;82:338–42.

PENICILLIN G, PROCAINE

Antibiotic (Penicillin)

PREGNANCY RECOMMENDATION: Compatible
BREASTFEEDING RECOMMENDATION: Compatible

PREGNANCY SUMMARY

Procaine penicillin G is an equimolar combination of procaine and penicillin G suspended in water (1). The combination is broken down in vivo into the two components. Reproduction studies in mice, rats, and rabbits have revealed no evidence of impaired fertility or fetal harm (2) (see also Penicillin G). The antibiotic is considered low risk in pregnancy.

P

FETAL RISK SUMMARY

A case report described the use of high doses of penicillin G procaine IV,* cortisone, and sodium salicylate in early pregnancy followed by the delivery at term of a cyclopic male infant (3). The lethal defect was attributed to salicylates, cortisone, or maternal viremia. *(*Penicillin G procaine should not be given IV. Presumably, the drug was either given IM or the procaine form was not used. Attempts to clarify this with the authors have been unsuccessful.)"*

BREASTFEEDING SUMMARY

See Penicillin G.

References

1. Mandel G, Sande M. Antimicrobial agents (continued). Penicillins and cephalosporins. In Gilman AG, Goodman LS, Gilman A, eds. *The Pharmacological Basis of Therapeutics*. 6th ed. New York, NY: MacMillan, 1980:1137.
2. Product information. Bicillin C-R. Wyeth-Ayerst Pharmaceuticals, 2000.
3. Khudr G, Olding L. Cyclopia. Am J Dis Child 1973;125:120–2.

PENICILLIN V

Antibiotic (Penicillin)

PREGNANCY RECOMMENDATION: Compatible
BREASTFEEDING RECOMMENDATION: Compatible

PREGNANCY SUMMARY

No reports linking the use of penicillin V with congenital defects have been located. The antibiotic is considered low risk in pregnancy.

FETAL RISK SUMMARY

The Collaborative Perinatal Project monitored 50,282 mother–child pairs, 3546 of whom had 1st trimester exposure to penicillin derivatives (1, pp. 297–313). For use anytime during pregnancy, 7171 exposures were recorded (1, p. 435). In neither group was evidence found to suggest a relationship to large categories of major or minor malformations or to individual defects.

In a surveillance study of Michigan Medicaid recipients involving 229,101 completed pregnancies conducted between 1985 and 1992, 4597 newborns had been exposed to penicillin V during the 1st trimester (F. Rosa, personal communication, FDA, 1993). A total of 202 (4.4%) major birth defects were observed (195 expected). Specific data were available for six defect categories, including (observed/expected) 46/56 cardiovascular defects, 5/7 oral clefts, 3/2 spina bifida, 17/13 polydactyly, 7/8 limb reduction defects, and 8/11 hypospadias. These data do not support an association between the drug and congenital defects.

Penicillin V depresses both plasma-bound and urinary excreted estriol (2). Urinary estriol was formerly used to assess the condition of the fetoplacental unit, with depressed levels being associated with fetal distress. This assessment is now made by measuring plasma-unconjugated estriol, which is not usually affected by penicillin V.

The pharmacokinetics of penicillin V during the 2nd and 3rd trimesters have been reported (3). Elimination of the drug is enhanced at these stages of pregnancy.

BREASTFEEDING SUMMARY

No reports describing the use of penicillin V during human lactation have been located. (See also Penicillin G.)

References

1. Heinonen OP, Slone D, Shapiro S. *Birth Defects and Drugs in Pregnancy*. Littleton, MA: Publishing Sciences Group, 1977.
2. Pulkkinen M, Willman K. Maternal oestrogen levels during penicillin treatment. Br Med J 1971;4:48.
3. Heikkilä AM, Erkkola RU. The need for adjustment of dosage regimen of penicillin V during pregnancy. Obstet Gynecol 1993;81:919–21.

PENTAERYTHRITOL TETRANITRATE

[Withdrawn from the market. See 9th edition.]

PENTAMIDINE

Antiprotozoal

PREGNANCY RECOMMENDATION: Compatible—Maternal Benefit >> Embryo–Fetal Risk
BREASTFEEDING RECOMMENDATION: Contraindicated

PREGNANCY SUMMARY

Pentamidine is an antiprotozoal agent indicated for the treatment of pneumonia caused by *Pneumocystis carinii,* a common opportunistic infection in patients suffering from HIV disease. Although no developmental toxicity has been observed with this agent, some sources consider it contraindicated in pregnancy. Nevertheless, the maternal benefit appears to outweigh the unknown embryo–fetal risk.

FETAL RISK SUMMARY

The mechanism of action of pentamidine is not fully known. In vitro tests have indicated that pentamidine inhibits the synthesis of DNA, RNA, phospholipids, and proteins, and may be a folic acid antagonist by inhibiting dihydrofolate reductase (1,2).

Pentamidine was not teratogenic in pregnant rats treated with doses similar to those used in humans (3). However, these doses were embryocidal when administered during embryogenesis (3). Significant placental transfer was observed in rats administered pentamidine in late pregnancy (4). By the 12th hour, fetal brain tissue concentrations of pentamidine were statistically similar to the maternal serum levels achieved 2 hours after the dose.

In an experiment using in vitro–perfused human placentas, the placental transfer of pentamidine in humans was undetectable with therapeutic maternal concentrations of approximately 2 mcg/mL (5). The level of sensitivity of the high-performance liquid chromatography method was 0.05 mcg/mL. When peak concentrations of pentamidine on the maternal side were increased to approximately 14 mcg/mL, fetal levels were consistently 0.2 mcg/mL at 30 minutes. Pentamidine did concentrate in placental tissue at all drug levels studied, but the clinical significance of this to placental function is unknown (5).

In contrast to the above, a study published in 1995 used a more sensitive test to document the placental transfer of pentamidine at about 33 weeks' gestation (6). A 21-year-old HIV-infected woman received pentamidine, 200 mg (3.4 mg/kg) IV daily, for 7 days before a cesarean section. A maternal serum sample, drawn 8 hours after her seventh dose, was 0.0813 mcg/mL (free base). The pentamidine concentration in the cord blood sample, obtained 16.5 hours after the dose, was 0.0132 mcg/mL.

The CDC recommends aerosolized pentamidine as one of two treatment regimens for prophylaxis against *P. carinii* in persons infected with HIV (7,8). However, because the safety of this treatment has not been established in human pregnancies, the CDC advises against this use in pregnant women (7,8). Others have cited information from the manufacturer that the use of aerosolized pentamidine is contraindicated in pregnancy (9).

A 1988 reference cited a concern that pregnant health care workers involved in the care of patients treated with aerosolized pentamidine might be at risk for fetal harm (10). An estimation of this risk, based on a pharmacokinetic model, was published in 1994 (11). The maximum exposure of health care workers, at two different hospitals, to aerosolized pentamidine was estimated to be 1.7 and 9.8 mcg/kg/day (IV equivalent). The authors then calculated the embryolethal and teratogenic IV-equivalent reference doses, based on pregnant rat data, to be 0.08 and 4 mcg/kg/day, respectively. Comparison of the estimated actual exposures to the predicted toxic levels led to the conclusion that improvement was needed in the methods used to reduce pentamidine exposure of health care workers (11).

An argument favoring the use of pentamidine in the pregnant patient with active *P. carinii* pneumonia, when other treatment regimens had failed, was put forth in a 1987 article (12). Moreover, this same source, in a 1990 reference, argued that the availability of aerosolized pentamidine for prophylaxis should be disclosed to the pregnant HIV-seropositive patient "as part of the informed consent process" (13). This latter position is strengthened by the in vitro data cited above relating to the placental transfer of the agent. Because aerosolized pentamidine results in very low systemic concentrations, fetal exposure to the drug by this route is probably minimal and below the level of detection.

The use of aerosolized and IV pentamidine during gestation in women with HIV infection has been described (14–17). A 1992 abstract described the use of aerosolized pentamidine, 300 mg/month, in 15 women during the 2nd and 3rd trimesters (14). No significant effects on the course of pregnancy or on the fetus or newborn were observed. The second reference reported five pregnancies (six fetuses, one set of twins) that were treated with aerosolized pentamidine, zidovudine, and other drugs (15). One woman was treated throughout her 39-week gestation, one from 10 to 39 weeks' gestation, and three during the 2nd and 3rd trimesters. The outcomes of the exposed pregnancies included one growth-restricted infant, one with albinism, one with congenital cytomegalovirus infection, and three normal infants. The latter two references described IV pentamidine in five women (16) and aerosolized drug in nine (16,17). No adverse fetal effects of the drug were reported.

BREASTFEEDING SUMMARY

Because systemic concentrations achieved with aerosolized pentamidine are very low, breast milk levels of the drug after administration via this route are probably nil. No reports of lactating women administered pentamidine by any route (IM, IV, or by inhalation) have been located.

References

1. Product information. Pentam. Lyphomed, Inc., 1991.
2. Drake S, Lampasona V, Nicks HL, Schwarzmann SW. Pentamidine isethionate in the treatment of *Pneumocystis carinii* pneumonia. Clin Pharm 1985;4:507–16.
3. Harstad TW, Little BB, Bawdon RE, Knoll K, Roe D, Gilstrap LC III. Embryofetal effects of pentamidine isethionate administered to pregnant Sprague-Dawley rats. Am J Obstet Gynecol 1990;163:912–6.
4. Little BB, Harstad TH, Bawdon RE, Sobhi S, Roe DA, Knoll KA, Ghali FE. Pharmacokinetics of pentamidine in Sprague-Dawley rats in late pregnancy. Am J Obstet Gynecol 1991;164:927–30.
5. Fortunato SJ, Bawdon RE. Determination of pentamidine transfer in the in vitro perfused human cotyledon with high-performance liquid chromatography. Am J Obstet Gynecol 1989;160:759–61.
6. Schwebke K, Fletcher CV, Acosta EP, Henry K. Pentamidine concentrations in a mother with AIDS and in her neonate. Clin Infect Dis 1995;20:1569–70.
7. CDC. Guidelines for prophylaxis against *Pneumocystis carinii* pneumonia for persons infected with human immunodeficiency virus. MMWR 1989;38 (Suppl 5):1–9.
8. CDC. Guidelines for prophylaxis against *Pneumocystis carinii* pneumonia for persons infected with human immunodeficiency virus. JAMA 1989;262:335–9.
9. Sarti GM. Aerosolized pentamidine in HIV; promising new treatment for *Pneumocystis carinii* pneumonia. Postgrad Med 1989;86:54–69.
10. Conover B, Goldsmith JC, Buehler BA, Maloley BA, Windle ML. Aerosolized pentamidine and pregnancy. Ann Intern Med 1988;109:927.
11. Ito S, Koren G. Estimation of fetal risk from aerosolized pentamidine in pregnant healthcare workers. Chest 1994;106:1460–2.
12. Minkoff HL. Care of pregnant women infected with human immunodeficiency virus. JAMA 1987;258:2714–7.
13. Minkoff HL, Moreno JD. Drug prophylaxis for human immunodeficiency virus-infected pregnant women; ethical considerations. Am J Obstet Gynecol 1990;163:1111–4.
14. Nana D, Tannenbaum I, Landesman S, Mendez H, Moroso G, Minkoff H. Pentamidine prophylaxis in pregnancy (abstract). Am J Obstet Gynecol 1992;166:387.
15. Sperling RS, Stratton P, O'Sullivan MJ, Boyer P, Watts DH, Lambert JS, Hammill H, Livingston EG, Gloeb DJ, Minkoff H, Fox HE. A survey of zidovudine use in pregnant women with human immunodeficiency virus infection. N Engl J Med 1992;326:857–61.
16. Stratton P, Mofenson LM, Willoughby AD. Human immunodeficiency virus infection in pregnant women under care at AIDS clinical trials centers in the United States. Obstet Gynecol 1992;79:364–8.
17. Gates HS Jr, Barker CD. Pneumocystis carinii pneumonia in pregnancy. A case report. J Reprod Med 1993;38:483–6.

P

PENTAZOCINE

Narcotic Agonist–Antagonist Analgesic

PREGNANCY RECOMMENDATION: Human Data Suggest Risk
BREASTFEEDING RECOMMENDATION: No Human Data—Probably Compatible

PREGNANCY SUMMARY

The National Birth Defects Prevention Study discussed below found evidence that opioid use during organogenesis is associated with a low absolute risk of congenital birth defects. In addition, pentazocine is associated with behavioral teratogenicity, either from the drug itself, the mother's lifestyle, other drug abuse, or a combination of these factors. Moreover, its abuse during pregnancy is associated with intrauterine growth restriction and withdrawal in the newborn.

FETAL RISK SUMMARY

Oral pentazocine is only available in the United States in combination with naloxone or acetaminophen. However, an injectable form of the drug is available. Reproductive studies in animals did not find embryotoxic or teratogenic effects (1). In a 1975 reference, however, increasing single SC doses of pentazocine (98–570 mg/kg) administered to hamsters during the critical period of CNS organogenesis resulted in a significant increase in the number of offspring with malformations (exencephaly, cranioschisis, and various other CNS lesions). Maternal death was observed in 10% of the mothers at the highest dose, but not with the lower doses (2).

The drug rapidly crosses the placenta, resulting in cord blood levels of 40%–70% of maternal serum (3). Withdrawal has been reported in infants exposed in utero to chronic maternal ingestion of pentazocine (4–8). Symptoms, presenting within 24–48 hours of birth, consist of trembling and jitteriness, marked hyperirritability, hyperactivity with hypertonia, high-pitched cry, diaphoresis, diarrhea, vomiting, and opisthotonic posturing.

During labor, increased overall uterine activity has been observed after pentazocine, but without changes in fetal heart rate (9). In equianalgesic doses, most studies report no significant differences between meperidine and pentazocine in pain relief, length of labor, or Apgar scores (10–15). However, meperidine in one study was observed to produce significantly lower Apgar scores than pentazocine, especially in repeated doses (16). Severe neonatal respiratory depression may also occur with pentazocine (10,16).

A 1982 report from New Orleans described 24 infants born of mothers using the IV combination of pentazocine/tripelennamine (T's and blue's) (17). Doses were unknown but probably ranged from 200 to 600 mg of pentazocine and 100 to 250 mg of tripelennamine. Six of the newborns were exposed early in pregnancy. Birth weights for 11 of the infants were <2500 g; 9 of these were premature (<37 weeks) and 2 were small for gestational age. Daily or weekly exposure throughout pregnancy produced withdrawal symptoms, occurring ≤7 days of birth, in 15 of 16 infants. Withdrawal was thought to be related to pentazocine, but antihistamine withdrawal has been reported (see Diphenhydramine). Thirteen of 15 infants became asymptomatic 3–11 days following onset of withdrawal, but symptoms persisted for up to 6 months in 2 (17).

Three cases of maternal bacterial endocarditis were observed following IV drug abuse, one of which involved the injection of pentazocine/tripelennamine intermittently throughout pregnancy (18). Following satisfactory antibiotic treatment for the infection, the mother gave birth at term to a healthy, male infant.

In a study published in 1983, three groups of pregnant women were evaluated in a perinatal addiction program in the Chicago area (19). One group (N = 13) was composed of women addicted to pentazocine/tripelennamine. A second group consisted of women who conceived while self-administering heroin, and who were then converted to low-dose (5–40 mg/day) methadone (N = 46). The third group consisted of drug-free controls (N = 27). The three groups were statistically similar as to mean maternal age, educational level, gravidity, cigarette smoking, and mean weight gain during pregnancy. Heavy alcohol users were excluded. All infants were delivered at term. Apgar scores were similar among the three groups of newborns, and no significant perinatal complications were observed. Mean birth weight, length, and head circumference were similar between the two drug groups. Compared with the drug-free controls, the pentazocine/tripelennamine-exposed infants had significantly lower weights (2799 vs. 3479 g), lengths (48.1 vs. 51.1 cm), and head circumferences (32.9 vs. 34.7 cm). Neonatal withdrawal was observed in both drug-exposed infant groups. Withdrawal characteristics observed in the pentazocine/tripelennamine infants were similar to those seen in the methadone group, consisting of irritability, voracious sucking, and feeding difficulties (19). However, none of these infants required therapy for their symptoms. Neonatal behavior was evaluated using the Brazelton Neonatal Behavioral Assessment Scale. Results of these tests indicated that the infants exposed to the drug combination had interactive deficits and withdrawal similar to the methadone-addicted babies (19).

In 1986, nearly the same data as above were published but with the addition of a group exposed to mixed sedative/stimulant (N = 22) and a group exposed to phencyclidine (N = 9) (20). The outcomes of the pentazocine/tripelennamine group were the same as above.

Another study described the effects of pentazocine/tripelennamine abuse in 50 pregnancies identified retrospectively from 23,779 deliveries occurring between 1981 and 1983 (21). Compared with matched controls, users of the

P

combination were significantly more likely to have no prenatal care; to be anemic; and to have syphilis, gonorrhea, or hepatitis. Moreover, their infants were significantly more likely to be small for gestational age, to have lower birth weights (3260 vs. 2592 g), to have a 1-minute Apgar score <7, and to have neonatal withdrawal. No congenital abnormalities were observed in the infants exposed to the drug combination.

A study published in 1993 examined the effects on the fetus and newborn of IV pentazocine and methylphenidate abuse during pregnancy (22). During a 2-year (1987–1988) period, 39 infants (38 pregnancies, 1 set of twins) were identified in the study population as being subjected to the drug abuse during gestation, a minimum incidence of 5 cases per 1000 live births. Many of the mothers had used cigarettes (34%) or alcohol (71%) or abused other drugs (26%). The median duration of IV pentazocine and methylphenidate abuse was 3 years (range 1–9 years) with a median frequency of 14 injections/week (range 1–70 injections/week). Among the infants, 8 were delivered prematurely, 12 were growth restricted, and 11 had withdrawal symptoms. Four of the infants had birth defects, including twins with fetal alcohol syndrome, one with a ventricular septal defect, and one case of polydactyly. Of the 21 infants who had formal developmental testing, 17 had normal development and 4 had low–normal developmental quotients (22).

Results of a National Birth Defects Prevention Study (1997–2005) were published in 2011 (23). This population-based case–control study examined the association between maternal use of opioid analgesics and >30 types of major structural birth defects. In 17,449 case mothers, therapeutic opioid use was reported by 454 (2.6%) compared with 134 (2.0%) of 6701 control mothers. Indications for use of opioid analgesics were surgical procedures (41%), infections (34%), chronic diseases (20%), and injuries (18%). Dose, duration, or frequency were not evaluated. The exposure period evaluated was from 1 month before to 3 months after conception. Limiting the exposure period to the first 2 months after conception produced similar results. Infants with >1 defect were included in multiple birth defect categories. The following opioids were included (number of cases for each agent not specified): codeine, hydrocodone, hydromorphone, fentanyl, meperidine, methadone, morphine, oxycodone, pentazocine, propoxyphene, and tramadol. The birth defect, total number, number exposed, and the adjusted odds ratio (aOR) with 95% confidence interval (CI) were as follows:

Birth Defect	Total	Cases	aOR (95% CI)
Spina bifida	718	26	2.0 (1.3–3.2)
Any heart defect (20 types)	7724	211	1.4 (1.1–1.7)
Atrioventricular septal defect	175	9	2.4 (1.2–4.8)
Teratology of Fallot	672	21	1.7 (1.1–2.8)
Conotruncal defect	1481	41	1.5 (1.0–2.1)
Conoventricular septal defect	110	6	2.7 (1.1–6.3)
Left ventricular outflow tract obstruction defect	1195	36	1.5 (1.0–2.2)
Hypoplastic left heart syndrome	357	17	2.4 (1.4–4.1)
Right ventricular outflow tract obstruction defect	1175	40	1.6 (1.1–2.3)
Pulmonary valve stenosis	867	34	1.7 (1.2–2.6)
Atrial septal defect (ASD)	511	17	2.0 (1.2–3.6)
Ventricular septal defect + ASD	528	17	1.7 (1.0–2.9)
Hydrocephaly	301	11	2.0 (1.0–3.7)
Glaucoma/anterior chamber defects	103	5	2.6 (1.0–6.6)
Gastroschisis	726	26	1.8 (1.1–2.9)

The authors speculated that the activity of opioids and their receptors as growth regulators during development of the embryo might be a mechanism to explain the above findings. The exposure data were obtained by retrospective maternal self-report; the authors acknowledged that recall bias and misclassification might have affected their results. They concluded that the absolute risk was a modest absolute increase above the baseline risk for birth defects (23).

BREASTFEEDING SUMMARY

No reports describing the use of pentazocine during lactation have been located. The molecular weight (about 285) suggests that the drug will be excreted into breast milk. The effects of this exposure on a nursing infant are unknown, but small, infrequent doses most likely present a minimal risk.

References

1. Product information. Talwin. Hospira, 2010.
2. Geber WF, Schramm LC. Congenital malformations of the central nervous system produced by narcotic analgesics in the hamster. Am J Obstet Gynecol 1975;123:705–13.
3. Beckett AH, Taylor JF. Blood concentrations of pethidine and pentazocine in mother and infant at time of birth. J Pharm Pharmacol 1967;19(Suppl):50s–2s.
4. Goetz RL, Bain RV. Neonatal withdrawal symptoms associated with maternal use of pentazocine. J Pediatr 1974;84:887–8.
5. Scanlon JW. Pentazocine and neonatal withdrawal symptoms. J Pediatr 1974;85:735–6.
6. Kopelman AE. Fetal addiction to pentazocine. Pediatrics 1975;55:888–9.
7. Reeds TO. Withdrawal symptoms in a neonate associated with maternal pentazocine abuse. J Pediatr 1975;87:324.
8. Preis O, Choi SJ, Rudolph N. Pentazocine withdrawal syndrome in the newborn infant. Am J Obstet Gynecol 1977;127:205–6.
9. Filler WW, Filler NW. Effect of a potent non-narcotic analgesic agent (pentazocine) on uterine contractility and fetal heart rate. Obstet Gynecol 1966;28:224–32.
10. Freedman H, Tafeen CH, Harris H. Parenteral Win 20,228 as analgesic in labor. NY State J Med 1967;67:2849–51.
11. Duncan SLB, Ginsburg J, Morris NF. Comparison of pentazocine and pethidine in normal labor. Am J Obstet Gynecol 1969;105:197–202.
12. Moore J, Carson RM, Hunter RJ. A comparison of the effects of pentazocine and pethidine administered during labor. J Obstet Gynaecol Br Commonw 1970;77:830–6.
13. Mowat J, Garrey MM. Comparison of pentazocine and pethidine in labour. Br Med J 1970;2:757–9.
14. Levy DL. Obstetric analgesia. Pentazocine and meperidine in normal primiparous labor. Obstet Gynecol 1971;38:907–11.
15. Moore J, Ball HG. A sequential study of intravenous analgesic treatment during labour. Br J Anaesth 1974;46:365–72.
16. Refstad SO, Lindbaek E. Ventilatory depression of the newborn of women receiving pethidine or pentazocine. Br J Anaesth 1980;52:265–70.

17. Dunn DW, Reynolds J. Neonatal withdrawal symptoms associated with "T's and Blue's" (pentazocine and tripelennamine). Am J Dis Child 1982;136:644–5.
18. Pastorek JG, Plauche WC, Faro S. Acute bacterial endocarditis in pregnancy: a report of three cases. J Reprod Med 1983;28:611–4.
19. Chasnoff IJ, Hatcher R, Burns WJ, Schnoll SH. Pentazocine and tripelennamine ("T's and blue's"): effects on the fetus and neonate. Dev Pharmacol Ther 1983;6:162–9.
20. Chasnoff IJ, Burns KA, Burns WJ, Schnoll SH. Prenatal drug exposure: effects on neonatal and infant growth and development. Neurobehavior Toxicol Teratol 1986;8:357–62.
21. Von Almen WF II, Miller JM Jr. "Ts and blues" in pregnancy. J Reprod Med 1986;31:236–9.
22. Debooy VD, Seshia MMK, Tenenbein M, Casiiro OG. Intravenous pentazocine and methylphenidate abuse during pregnancy. Maternal lifestyle and infant outcome. Am J Dis Child 1993;147:1062–5.
23. Broussard CS, Rasmussen SA, Reefhuis J, Friedman JM, Jann MW, Riehle- Colarusso T, Honein MA; National Birth Defects Prevention Study. Maternal treatment with opioid analgesics and risk for birth defects. Am J Obstet Gynecol 2011;204:314–7.

PENTOBARBITAL

Sedative/Hypnotic

PREGNANCY RECOMMENDATION: Limited Human Data—Probably Compatible
BREASTFEEDING RECOMMENDATION: Limited Human Data—Potential Toxicity

PREGNANCY SUMMARY

No reports linking the use of pentobarbital with congenital defects have been located. However, the data are limited and there are no relevant animal reproduction studies.

FETAL RISK SUMMARY

The Collaborative Perinatal Project monitored 50,282 mother–child pairs, 250 of whom had 1st trimester exposure to pentobarbital (1). No evidence was found to suggest a relationship to large categories of major or minor malformations or to individual defects. Hemorrhagic disease and barbiturate withdrawal in the newborn are theoretical possibilities (see also Phenobarbital).

BREASTFEEDING SUMMARY

Pentobarbital is excreted into breast milk (2). Breast milk levels of 0.17 mcg/mL have been detected 19 hours after a dose of 100 mg daily for 32 days. The effect on the nursing infant is not known.

References

1. Heinonen OP, Slone D, Shapiro S. *Birth Defects and Drugs in Pregnancy*. Littleton, MA: Publishing Sciences Group, 1977:336–7.
2. Wilson JT, Brown RD, Cherek DR, Dailey JW, Hilman B, Jobe PC, Manno BR, Manno JE, Redetzki HM, Stewart JJ. Drug excretion in human breast milk: principles, pharmacokinetics and projected consequences. Clin Pharmacokinet 1980;5:1–66.

P

PENTOSAN

Urinary Tract Agent (Analgesic)

PREGNANCY RECOMMENDATION: Limited Human Data—Animal Data Suggest Low Risk
BREASTFEEDING RECOMMENDATION: No Human Data—Probably Compatible

PREGNANCY SUMMARY

Except for the one case (discussed below), no reports describing the use of pentosan in human pregnancy have been located. The animal data suggest low risk but the absence of human pregnancy experience prevents a more complete assessment. The drug does not appear to cross the placenta, at least in amounts that could affect fetal coagulation. The prevalence of interstitial cystitis in pregnancy is unknown. Studies have found that nearly one in four women in the general population has the disease (1). Thus, the prevalence in pregnancy may be higher than suggested by the lack of reported exposures. Based only on the animal data and the pharmacokinetics of the drug, inadvertent or planned exposure during gestation appears to represent a low risk to the embryo–fetus.

FETAL RISK SUMMARY

Pentosan polysulfate is an oral semi-synthetic heparin-like macromolecular carbohydrate derivative that chemically and structurally resembles glycosaminoglycans. It is a low-molecular-weight heparinoid compound with anticoagulant and fibrinolytic effects. Pentosan is indicated for the relief of bladder pain or discomfort associated with interstitial cystitis. The oral absorption is low, about 3%, and drug reaching the systemic circulation is partly metabolized in the liver, spleen, and kidney. The elimination half-life from urine following oral administration is 4.8 hours (2).

Reproduction studies have been conducted in mice, rats, and rabbits. In mice and rats, daily IV doses 0.42 times the daily oral human dose based on BSA (DOHD) revealed no evidence of impaired fertility or fetal harm. A similar negative result was observed in rabbits given daily IV doses 0.14 times the DOHD. Bathing of in vitro–cultured mouse embryos with a concentration of 1 mg/mL caused reversible limb bud abnormalities (2). However, this finding has no clinical significance because the concentration was far in excess of the potential human embryo exposure.

Animal studies for carcinogenicity have not been conducted. However, assays for mutagenic and clastogenic effects were negative (2).

The high molecular weight (4000–6000) and low oral absorption suggest that pentosan does not reach the embryo or the fetus. A 1986 study found no evidence of placental transfer in eight women undergoing elective abortions between the 18th and 23rd week of gestation for chromosomal abnormalities (3). All women were given a single 50-mg IV dose of pentosan polysulfate. Blood samples drawn 30 minutes later showed a marked change in the mean activated partial thromboplastin time (APTT), which increased from 35 to 88 seconds, and factor V level, decreasing from 87% to 33%. Fetal samples, drawn from the umbilical cord before abortion in controls and at the same time as the maternal samples in exposed fetuses, showed no differences in these parameters (93 vs. 91 seconds and 42% vs. 48%, respectively) (3).

BREASTFEEDING SUMMARY

No reports describing the use of pentosan polysulfate during human lactation have been located. The high molecular weight (4000–6000) and low oral bioavailability suggest that the drug will not be detected in breast milk. Moreover, at least in adults, the oral absorption is only about 3%. Thus, the risk to a nursing infant from the drug probably is nil.

References

1. Rosenberg MT, Moldwin RM, Stanford EJ. Early diagnosis and management of interstitial cystitis. Women's Health Primary Care 2004;7:456–63.
2. Product information. Elmiron. Ortho Women's Health & Urology, Ortho-McNeil Pharmaceutical, 2006.
3. Forestier F, Fischer AM, Daffos F, Beguin S, Diner H. Absence of transplacental passage of pentosan polysulfate during mid-trimester of pregnancy. Thromb Haemost 1986;56:247–9.

PENTOSTATIN

Antineoplastic

PREGNANCY RECOMMENDATION: No Human Data—Animal Data Suggest Risk
BREASTFEEDING RECOMMENDATION: No Human Data—Potential Toxicity

PREGNANCY SUMMARY

No reports describing the use of pentostatin in human pregnancy have been located. The animal reproduction data suggest risk, but the absence of human pregnancy experiences prevents a complete assessment of the embryo–fetal risk. However, pentostatin inhibits the synthesis of DNA and RNA, and increases DNA damage. Because hairy cell leukemia usually has an indolent course, deferring treatment until after delivery may be appropriate (1).

FETAL RISK SUMMARY

Pentostatin is a hydrophilic, cytotoxic agent that is classified as an antimetabolite. It is in the same antineoplastic subclass of purine analogs and related agents as cladribine, clofarabine, fludarabine, mercaptopurine, and thioguanine. Pentostatin is indicated as single-agent treatment for both untreated and alpha-interferon-refractory hairy cell leukemia patients with active disease as defined by clinically significant anemia, neutropenia, thrombocytopenia, or disease-related symptoms. It inhibits DNA and RNA synthesis and causes increased DNA damage. The agent is partially metabolized before urinary excretion, but the activity of the metabolites (*assumed to be inactive*) has not been stated. Plasma protein binding is very low (about 4%) and the terminal elimination half-life is 5.7 hours (2).

Reproduction studies have been conducted in rats, mice, and rabbits. In rats, daily IV doses (days 6–15) that were about (based on total dose) 1.5 and 11 times the recommended human dose given every 2 weeks based on BSA (RHD) caused maternal toxicity and the highest dose was associated with various fetal skeletal malformations. Other defects observed in rats were omphalocele at about 0.75 times the RHD, gastroschisis at about 11 and 15 times the RHD, and flexure defect of the hindlimbs at about 11 times the RHD. The drug was teratogenic (defects not specified) in mice given a single intraperitoneal dose that was about 1.5 times the RHD. No teratogenicity was observed in rabbits with daily IV doses (days 6–18) that were about (based on total dose) 0.05–0.2 times the RHD. However, maternal toxicity, abortions, early deliveries, and deaths occurred in all dose groups (2).

Carcinogenic studies have not been conducted. Pentostatin was mutagenic in some assays but not others, and was clastogenic in one test. Fertility studies have not been conducted, but in a 5-day IV toxicity study in dogs, mild seminiferous tubular degeneration was observed (2).

It is not known if pentostatin crosses the human placenta. The molecular weight (about 268), low plasma protein binding, and moderate elimination half-life suggest that exposure of the embryo–fetus will occur.

BREASTFEEDING SUMMARY

No reports describing the use of pentostatin during human lactation have been located. The molecular weight (about 268), low plasma protein binding (about 4%), and moderate elimination half-life (5.7 hours) suggest that the drug will be excreted into breast milk. However, the hydrophilic properties of the drug may limit excretion. The effect of this exposure on a nursing infant is unknown, but the drug has caused severe toxicity in treated patients, such as gastrointestinal upset, rash, fever, and fatigue. If a woman elects to breastfeed in spite of this potential risk, pumping and dumping for about 30 hours after a dose should significantly reduce the exposure.

References

1. Robak T. Current treatment options in hairy cell leukemia and hairy cell leukemia variant. Cancer Treat Rev 2006;32:365–76.
2. Product information. Pentostatin for injection. Bedford Laboratories, 2006.

PENTOXIFYLLINE

Hemorrheologic Agent

PREGNANCY RECOMMENDATION: Limited Human Data—Animal Data Suggest Moderate Risk
BREASTFEEDING RECOMMENDATION: Limited Human Data—Probably Compatible

PREGNANCY SUMMARY

Pentoxifylline is a synthetic xanthine derivative used to lower blood viscosity in peripheral vascular and cerebrovascular diseases. No published reports of its use in human pregnancy have been located. The drug caused embryo death in rats at a dose near the human therapeutic dose.

FETAL RISK SUMMARY

Reproduction studies in rats and rabbits at oral doses up to 4.2 and 3.5 times the maximum recommended human dose based on BSA revealed no evidence of teratogenicity. In rats, however, an increased incidence of resorptions was seen at the maximum dose (1).

In a surveillance study of Michigan Medicaid recipients involving 229,101 completed pregnancies conducted between 1985 and 1992, 34 newborns had been exposed to pentoxifylline during the 1st trimester (F. Rosa, personal communication, FDA, 1993). Five (14.7%) major birth defects were observed (one expected), including (observed/expected) 2/0 cardiovascular defects and 1/0 spina bifida. No anomalies were observed in four other defect categories (oral clefts, polydactyly, limb reduction defects, and hypospadias) for which specific data were available. Although the number of exposures is small, the total number of defects and both specific defects are suggestive of possible associations, but other factors, including the mother's disease, concurrent drug use, and chance, may be involved.

Pentoxifylline causes a significant increase in sperm motility, but not concentration, and may be useful in patients with normogonadotrophic asthenozoospermia (2).

BREASTFEEDING SUMMARY

Pentoxifylline is excreted into human milk. Five healthy women who had been breastfeeding for at least 6 weeks were given a single 400-mg sustained-release tablet of pentoxifylline after a 4-hour fast (3). The mean milk:plasma ratio of unmetabolized pentoxifylline at 4 hours was 0.87. Mean milk:plasma ratios for the three major metabolites at 4 hours were 0.76, 0.54, and 1.13. Mean milk concentration of pentoxifylline at 2 hours (73.9 ng/mL) was approximately twice as much as that occurring at 4 hours (35.7 ng/mL) (3). Pentoxifylline and its metabolites are stable in breast milk for 3 weeks when stored at −15°C (4).

References

1. Product information. Trental. Hoechst Roussel, 2000.
2. Shen M-R, Chiang P-H, Yang R-C, Hong C-Y, Chen S-S. Pentoxifylline stimulates human sperm motility both in vitro and after oral therapy. Br J Clin Pharmacol 1991;31:711–4.
3. Witter FR, Smith RV. The excretion of pentoxifylline and its metabolites into human breast milk. Am J Obstet Gynecol 1985;151:1094–7.
4. Bauza MT, Smith RV, Knutson DE, Witter FR. Gas chromatographic determination of pentoxifylline and its major metabolites in human breast milk. J Chromatogr 1984;310:61–9.

PEPPERMINT

Herb

PREGNANCY RECOMMENDATION: Limited Human Data—Probably Compatible
BREASTFEEDING RECOMMENDATION: No Human Data—Probably Compatible

PREGNANCY SUMMARY

Peppermint and its oil have been used for hundreds of years. These products are available as teas, liquid extract, capsules, lozenges, throat sprays, flavorings, liniments, and inhalants. Several sources state that ingestion of large doses of peppermint/peppermint oil is unsafe in pregnancy because of possible emmenagogue and abortifacient effects. Although scientific documentation of increased uterine bleeding and abortion associated with peppermint/peppermint oil has not been located, high oral doses of menthol (e.g., 2–9 g) are considered lethal (1). However, this should not be concern for topical preparations and ingesting recommended doses of oral products. The absence in the medical literature of adverse reports involving a commonly used substance suggests that there is little risk from the typical use of this herb in pregnancy.

FETAL RISK SUMMARY

A variety of peppermint plants are cultivated in Europe and North America. Peppermint (*Mentha x piperita*) and its essential oil, first described in England in 1696, have been used in the treatment of cancers, colds, cramps, indigestion, nausea, sore throat, and toothaches (2). The plants contain 0.1%–1.5% essential oil (2,3). More than 100 compounds have been isolated from peppermint oil, but the primary pharmacologically active agents are menthol (29%–48%), menthone (20%–31%), and menthyl acetate (3%–10%), and lesser amounts of caffeic acid, flavonoids, and tannins (2). Menthol is a common ingredient in over-the-counter mouth and throat products and liniments.

The ingestion of large doses of peppermint or peppermint oil in pregnancy is considered by some reviewers to be unsafe because of a possible emmenagogue and abortifacient properties (1,2,4–6), but another source does not mention these effects (7). No original reports describing this toxicity have been located.

A 2000 review conducted an extensive search of the literature regarding the use of herbal products for nausea/vomiting of pregnancy (8). Finding little information in scientific and medical databases, the author continued the search in Web sites and the lay literature. From this source, the most commonly recommended herbs, all in the form of teas, were red raspberry leaf, ginger, peppermint, and chamomile (Roman and/or German). There were 33 sources recommending peppermint and 6 stating that it was unsafe in pregnancy. However, none of the sources provided scientific or clinical evidence to support their recommendations or warnings (8).

In a 2004 nonrandomized study conducted in Canada, 20 of 27 women (74%) experienced pregnancy-induced nausea/vomiting 10 of whom were being treated with herbal remedies (9). The herbal remedies were ginger ($N = 3$), ginger plus peppermint ($N = 3$), peppermint ($N = 3$), and cannabis ($N = 1$). Although the peak incidence of nausea/vomiting of pregnancy is usually in the 1st trimester, no information was given on the timing or quantity of the exposures or the outcomes of the pregnancies (9).

BREASTFEEDING SUMMARY

No reports describing the use of peppermint, peppermint oil, or menthol during lactation have been located. Peppermint and its oil have been used for hundreds of years. These products are available as teas, liquid extract, capsules, lozenges, throat sprays, flavorings, liniments, and inhalants. The absence in the medical literature of adverse reports involving a commonly used substance suggests that there is little risk to a nursing infant from the mother's use of this herb during breastfeeding. Because infants may be sensitive to menthol (1,2), rubs and liniments containing menthol should not be applied to the mother's breast or nipples.

References

1. Peppermint leaf. Peppermint oil. In *Natural Medicines Comprehensive Database*. 5th ed. Stockton, CA: Therapeutic Research Faculty, 2003:1028–9; 1029–31.
2. Peppermint. In *The Review of Natural Products*. Facts and Comparisons. St. Louis, MO: Wolters Kluwer Health, November 2006.
3. Charrois TL, Hrudey J, Garniner P, Vohra S. Peppermint oil. Pediatr Rev 2006;27:e49–51.
4. Ernst E. Herbal medicinal products during pregnancy: are they safe? Br J Obstet Gynaecol 2002;109:227–35.
5. Peppermint oil (*Mentha x piperita* L) Natural Standard Monograph 2007. Available at http://www.naturalstand.com. Accessed April 30, 2007.
6. Gallo M, Koren G, Smith MJ, Boon H. The use of herbal medicine in pregnancy and lactation. Koren G, ed. In *Maternal–Fetal Toxicology. A Clinician's Guide*. 3rd ed. New York, NY: Marcel Dekker, 2001:583.
7. Peppermint leaf. Peppermint oil. Blumenthal M, ed. In *The Complete German Commission E Monographs*. Austin, TX: American Botanical Council, 1998:180–2.
8. Wilkinson JM. What do we know about herbal morning sickness treatments? A literature survey. Midwifery 2000;16:224–8.
9. Westfall RE. Use of anti-emetic herbs in pregnancy: women's choices, and the question of safety and efficacy. Complement Ther Nurs Midwifery 2004;10:30–6.

PERAMPANEL

Anticonvulsant

PREGNANCY RECOMMENDATION: No Human Data—Animal Data Suggest Risk
BREASTFEEDING RECOMMENDATION: No Human Data—Potential Toxicity

PREGNANCY SUMMARY

No reports describing the use of perampanel in human pregnancy have been located. The animal data suggest risk, but the absence of human pregnancy experience prevents a more complete assessment of the embryo–fetal risk. If the drug is used in pregnancy, physicians are encouraged to recommend that their patient enroll in the North American Antiepileptic Drug Pregnancy Registry by calling the toll free number 1-888-233-2334. Information on the Registry can also be found at the website: http://www.aedpregnancyregistry.com.

FETAL RISK SUMMARY

Perampanel is a noncompetitive antagonist of a glutamate receptor on postsynaptic neurons. It is indicated as adjunctive therapy for the treatment of partial-onset seizures with or without secondarily generalized seizures in patients with epilepsy 12 years or older. It is extensively metabolized to apparently inactive metabolites. Plasma protein binding, mainly to albumin and α1-acid glycoprotein, is about 95%–96% and the half-life is about 105 hours (1).

Reproduction studies have been conducted in rats and rabbits. In pregnant rats during organogenesis, all doses (1, 3, or 10 mg/kg/day) tested resulted in visceral abnormalities (diverticulum of the intestine). The lowest dose was similar to the human dose of 8 mg/day based on BSA (HD). Embryo lethality and reduced fetal body weight were observed at the mid and high doses. When all doses tested were given throughout gestation and lactation, fetal and pup deaths were observed at the mid and high doses and delayed sexual maturation in males and females at the highest dose. No effects were observed on measures of neurobehavioral or reproductive function in the offspring. The no-effect dose for prenatal and postnatal developmental toxicity was similar to the HD. In pregnant rabbits given the drug throughout organogenesis at the same three doses as above, embryo lethality was observed at the mid to high doses; the no-effect dose was about 2 times the HD (1).

Long-term studies for carcinogenicity in mice and rats were negative as were the assays for mutagenicity. No clear effects on fertility were observed in male and female rats given perampanel (1, 10, or 30 mg/kg/day) before and throughout mating and continuing in females to gestation day 6. Prolonged and/or irregular estrus cycles were observed at all doses tested, but especially at the highest dose (1).

It is not known if perampanel crosses the human placenta. The molecular weight (about 349 for the nonhydrated form) and the long half-life suggest that the drug will cross to the embryo and fetus in spite of the high plasma protein binding.

BREASTFEEDING SUMMARY

No reports describing the use of perampanel during human lactation have been located.

The molecular weight (about 349 for the nonhydrated form) and the long half-life (105 hours) suggest that the drug will be excreted into breast milk in spite of the high (95%–96%) plasma protein binding. The effect of this exposure on a nursing infant is unknown. If the drug is used during breastfeeding, the infant should be monitored for some of the most common adverse reactions observed in adults, such as dizziness, somnolence, fatigue, irritability, and nausea.

Reference

1. Product information. Fycompa. Eisai, 2012.

P

PERGOLIDE

[Withdrawn from the market. See 9th edition.]

PERINDOPRIL

Antihypertensive

PREGNANCY RECOMMENDATION: Human Data Suggest Risk in 2nd and 3rd Trimesters
BREASTFEEDING RECOMMENDATION: No Human Data—Probably Compatible

PREGNANCY SUMMARY

The fetal toxicity of perindopril in the 2nd and 3rd trimesters is similar to other angiotensin-converting enzyme (ACE) inhibitors. The use of this drug during the 2nd and 3rd trimesters may cause teratogenicity and severe fetal and neonatal toxicity. Fetal toxic effects may include anuria, oligohydramnios, fetal hypocalvaria, intrauterine growth restriction (IUGR), prematurity, and patent ductus arteriosus. Stillbirth or neonatal death may occur. Anuria-associated oligohydramnios may produce fetal limb contractures, craniofacial deformation, and pulmonary hypoplasia. Severe anuria and hypotension, which is resistant to both pressor agents and volume expansion, may occur in the newborn following in utero exposure. Newborn renal function and blood pressure should be closely monitored.

FETAL RISK SUMMARY

Perindopril, an ACE inhibitor, is a prodrug that is hydrolyzed in vivo to the active agent, perindoprilat. The agent is used in the management of essential hypertension.

Reproduction studies have been conducted with perindopril in mice, rats, rabbits, and cynomolgus monkeys (1). No evidence of teratogenicity was observed in these species at doses 6, 670, 50, and 17 times, respectively, the maximum recommended human dose based on BSA for a 50-kg adult (MRHD). At 6 times the MRHD in rats, no adverse effects on reproductive performance or fertility were observed in male and female rats (1).

It is not known if either perindopril or its metabolite, perindoprilat, crosses the human placenta to the fetus. The molecular weights of perindopril (about 368 for the free acid or 442 for the salt form) and perindoprilat (less than the prodrug) suggest that transfer to the embryo and fetus will occur.

A retrospective study using pharmacy-based data from the Tennessee Medicaid program identified 209 infants, born between 1985 and 2000, who had 1st trimester exposure to ACE inhibitors (2). Infants of mothers with evidence of diabetes, either before or during pregnancy, were excluded, as were those exposed to angiotensin-receptor antagonists (ARBs), ACE inhibitors, or other antihypertensives beyond the 1st trimester, and exposure to known teratogens. Two comparison groups, other antihypertensives (N = 202) and no antihypertensives (N = 29,096), were formed. The number of major birth defects in each of the three groups was 18 (8.6%), 4 (2%), and 834 (2.9%), respectively. Compared with the no antihypertensives group, exposure to ACE inhibitors was associated with a significantly increased risk of major defects (relative risk [RR] 2.71, 95% confidence interval [CI] 1.72–4.27). When the analysis was conducted by the type of defect, the highest rates were with cardiovascular defects, 9, 2, and 294, respectively, RR 3.72, 95% CI 1.89–7.30, and with CNS defects, 3, 0, and 80, respectively, RR 4.39, 95% CI 1.37–14.02. The major defects observed in the subject group were atrial septal defect (N = 6, includes three with pulmonic stenosis and/or three with ductus arteriosus [PDA]), renal dysplasia (N = 2), PDA alone (N = 2), and one each of ventricular septal defect, spina bifida, microcephaly with eye anomaly, coloboma, hypospadias, intestinal and choanal atresia, Hirschsprung disease, and diaphragmatic hernia (2). In an accompanying editorial, it was noted that neither previous reports of 1st trimester exposure to ACE inhibitors nor the animal studies had observed an increased risk of birth defects (3). It also was noted that no mechanism for ACE inhibitor–induced teratogenicity was known. A subsequent communication raising concerns about the validity of the study in terms of adequate exclusion of diabetes, charting and coding errors in busy medical practices, and the effects of maternal obesity (4) was addressed by the investigators (5).

Perindopril and other ACE inhibitors are human teratogens when used in the 2nd and 3rd trimesters, producing fetal hypocalvaria and renal defects. The cause of the defects and other toxicity is probably related to fetal hypotension and decreased renal blood flow. The compromise of the fetal renal system may result in severe, and at times fatal, anuria, both in the fetus and in the newborn. Anuria-associated oligohydramnios may produce pulmonary hypoplasia, limb contractures, persistent PDA, craniofacial deformation, and neonatal death (6,7). IUGR, prematurity, and severe neonatal hypotension may also be observed. Two reviews of fetal and newborn renal function indicated that both renal perfusion and glomerular plasma flow are low during gestation and that high levels of angiotensin II may be physiologically necessary to maintain glomerular filtration at low perfusion pressures (8,9). Perindopril prevents the conversion of angiotensin I to angiotensin II and, thus, may lead to in utero renal failure. Since the primary means of removal of the drug is renal, the impairment of this system in the newborn prevents elimination of the drug resulting in prolonged hypotension. Newborn renal function and blood pressure should be closely monitored. If oligohydramnios occurs, stopping perindopril may resolve the problem but may not improve infant outcome because of irreversible fetal damage (6). In those cases in which perindopril must be used to treat the mother's disease, the lowest possible dose should be used combined with close monitoring of amniotic fluid levels and fetal well-being. Guidelines for counseling exposed pregnant patients have been published and should be of benefit to health professionals faced with this task (6,10).

The observation in Tennessee Medicaid data of an increased risk of major congenital defects after 1st trimester exposure to ACE inhibitors raises concerns about teratogenicity that have not been seen in other studies (3). Medicaid data are a valuable tool for identifying early signals of teratogenicity, but are subject to a number of shortcomings and their findings must be considered hypotheses until confirmed by independent studies.

A 2012 review of the use of ACE inhibitors and ARBs in the 1st trimester concluded that there may be an elevated teratogenic risk, but the risk appeared to be related to other factors (11). The factors, that typically coexist with hypertension in pregnancy, included diabetes, advanced maternal age, and obesity.

BREASTFEEDING SUMMARY

No reports describing the use of the prodrug perindopril during human lactation have been located. The molecular weights of perindopril (about 368 for the free acid and 442 for the salt form) and its active metabolite, perindoprilat (molecular weight less than perindopril), suggest that both will be excreted into breast milk. The effects on a nursing infant from exposure to perindopril or perindoprilat in milk are unknown. However, other agents in this class are excreted into milk and, because the amounts are low and no adverse effects have been observed in nursing infants, are classified as compatible with breastfeeding by the American Academy of Pediatrics (see also Captopril and Enalapril).

References

1. Product information. Aceon. Solvay Pharmaceuticals, 2000.
2. Cooper WO, Hernandez-Diaz S, Arbogast PG, Dudley JA, Dyer S, Gideon PS, Hall K, Ray WA. Major congenital malformations after first-trimester exposure to ACE inhibitors. N Engl J Med 2006;354:2443–51.
3. Friedman JM. ACE inhibitors and congenital anomalies. N Engl J Med 2006;354:2498–500.
4. Scialli AR, Lione A. ACE inhibitors and major congenital malformations. N Engl J Med 2006;355:1280.
5. Cooper WO, Ray WA. Reply—ACE inhibitors and major congenital malformations. N Engl J Med 2006;355:1281.
6. Barr M Jr. Teratogen update: angiotensin-converting enzyme inhibitors. Teratology 1994;50:399–409.
7. Shotan A, Widerhorn J, Hurst A, Elkayam U. Risks of angiotensin-converting enzyme inhibition during pregnancy: experimental and clinical evidence, potential mechanisms, and recommendations for use. Am J Med 1994;96:451–6.
8. Robillard JE, Nakamura KT, Matherne GP, Jose PA. Renal hemodynamics and functional adjustments to postnatal life. Semin Perinatol 1988;12: 143–50.
9. Guignard J-P, Gouyon J-B. Adverse effects of drugs on the immature kidney. Biol Neonate 1988;53:243–52.
10. Brent RL, Beckman DA. Angiotensin-converting enzyme inhibitors, an embryopathic class of drugs with unique properties: information for clinical teratology counselors. Teratology 1991;43:543–6.
11. Polifka JE. Is there an embryopathy associated with first-trimester exposure to angiotensin-converting enzyme inhibitors and angiotensin receptor antagonists? A critical review of the evidence. Birth Defects Res (Part A) 2012;94:576–98.

PERMETHRIN

Scabicide

PREGNANCY RECOMMENDATION: Compatible
BREASTFEEDING RECOMMENDATION: Compatible

PREGNANCY SUMMARY

Neither the animal data nor the limited human pregnancy data suggest risk for the embryo or fetus. The CDC considers permethrin or pyrethrins with piperonyl butoxide to be the treatments of choice for pubic lice in pregnant women (1). Although not specifically mentioned, permethrin or pyrethrins with piperonyl butoxide should also be used if other body areas of a pregnant woman, such as the head, are infested with lice. For pregnant women with scabies, permethrin is considered the treatment of choice in the United States and the United Kingdom (1,2).

FETAL RISK SUMMARY

Permethrin, a pyrethroid, is indicated for the topical treatment of *Sarcoptes scabiei* (scabies) infestations. The drug is also active against lice, ticks, fleas, mites, and other arthropods. In patients with moderate to severe scabies, systemic absorption was estimated to be ≤2% of the dose (3,4).

Oral reproduction studies with permethrin have been conducted in mice, rats, and rabbits at doses of 200–400 mg/kg/day (3,4). No adverse effects on fertility or evidence of fetal harm were observed in these studies. Species-specific carcinogenesis was observed in mouse studies but negative results were seen in rats. Genetic toxic studies revealed no evidence of mutagenicity (3,4). Only the highest oral concentrations (2500–4000 ppm) of permethrin administered after implantation were found to lower significantly the protein and glycogen contents of rat placentas, but this had no statistical effect on the number of live fetuses (5).

Although no studies of permethrin placental transfer have been located, the molecular weight (about 391) is low enough that transfer should occur. However, because only small amounts are absorbed systemically and these are rapidly metabolized by ester hydrolysis to inactive metabolites, the opportunity for fetal exposure to permethrin appears to be minimal, if it occurs at all.

A 1995 case report described the use of multiple courses of permethrin and other agents in a pregnant woman who had developed crusted scabies (6). She was initially treated at 2 months' gestation with monosulfiram (a pesticide not available in the United States). Relapse occurred at 5 months' gestation and she was treated with two total-body (24-hour) applications of malathion 0.5% liquid and one total-body (24-hour) application of monosulfiram 25% solution. Three weeks later another relapse occurred and she was treated with permethrin 5% cream to the whole body for 12 hours. Because live mites were found the next day, a sulfur/tar/coconut oil soak to the scalp was used 3 times daily followed by two total-body benzyl benzoate 25% treatments within 24 hours. Then permethrin cream was used weekly for 3 weeks. A healthy male infant was delivered at term (6).

A 2005 observational study compared 113 pregnancies exposed to permethrin sometime in gestation with 113 matched controls (7). There were no differences between the groups in pregnancy outcomes in terms of live births, spontaneous abortions, therapeutic abortions, major malformations, birth weight, and gestational age at delivery.

BREASTFEEDING SUMMARY

No reports describing the use of topical permethrin during lactation have been located. Although the molecular weight (about 391) is low enough for excretion into breast milk, the minimal systemic absorption and rapid metabolism suggests that little, if any, of the drug will be found in milk. The CDC considers permethrin or pyrethrins with piperonyl butoxide to be the treatment of choice for pubic lice during lactation (1). For lactating women with scabies, permethrin is considered the treatment of choice in the United States and the United Kingdom (1,2).

References

1. CDC. 1998 Guidelines for treatment of sexually transmitted diseases. MMWR 1998;47:1–116.
2. Clinical Effectiveness Group (Association of Genitourinary Medicine and the Medical Society for the Study of Venereal Diseases). National guideline for the management of scabies. Sex Transm Inf 1999;75(Suppl):S76–7.
3. Product information. Elimite. Allergan, 2001.
4. Product information. Acticin. Bertek Pharmaceuticals, 2001.
5. Spencer F, Berhane Z. Uterine and fetal characteristics in rats following a post-implantational exposure to permethrin. Bull Environm Contam Toxicol 1982;29:84–8.
6. Judge MR, Kobza-Black A. Crusted scabies in pregnancy. Br J Dermatol 1995;132:116–9.
7. Kennedy D, Hurst V, Konradsdottir E, Einarson A. Pregnancy outcome following exposure to permethrin and use of teratogen information. Am J Perinatol 2005;22:87–90.

PERPHENAZINE

Antipsychotic

PREGNANCY RECOMMENDATION: Limited Human Data—No Relevant Animal Data
BREASTFEEDING RECOMMENDATION: Limited Human Data—Potential Toxicity

PREGNANCY SUMMARY

Although occasional published reports have attempted to link various phenothiazine compounds with congenital defects, the bulk of the evidence suggests that the therapeutic use of these drugs are safe for the mother and fetus (see also Chlorpromazine). A possible association between perphenazine, amitriptyline, or both and congenital defects is suggested by a single case, but without confirming evidence no conclusions can be reached.

FETAL RISK SUMMARY

Perphenazine is a piperazine phenothiazine in the same group as prochlorperazine (see Prochlorperazine). The phenothiazines readily cross the placenta to the fetus (1).

The Collaborative Perinatal Project monitored 50,282 mother–child pairs, 63 of whom had 1st trimester exposure to perphenazine (2). For use anytime during pregnancy, 166 exposures were recorded. No evidence was found in either group to suggest either a relationship to malformations, or an effect on perinatal mortality rates, birth weight, or IQ scores at 4 years of age.

In a surveillance study of Michigan Medicaid recipients involving 229,101 completed pregnancies conducted between 1985 and 1992, 140 newborns had been exposed to perphenazine during the 1st trimester (F. Rosa, personal communication, FDA, 1993). Five (3.6%) major birth defects were observed (six expected), four of which were cardiovascular defects (one expected). No anomalies were observed in five other defect categories (oral clefts, spina bifida, polydactyly, limb reduction defects, and hypospadias) for which specific data were available. The number of cardiovascular defects is suggestive of a possible association, but other factors, including the mother's disease, concurrent drug use, and chance, may be involved.

A case of maternal suicide attempt with a combination of amitriptyline (725 mg) and perphenazine (58 mg) at 8 days' gestation was described in a 1980 abstract (3). An infant was eventually delivered with multiple congenital defects. The abnormalities included microcephaly, "cotton-like" hair with pronounced shedding, cleft palate, micrognathia, ambiguous genitalia, foot deformities, and undetectable dermal ridges (3).

Perphenazine has been used as an antiemetic during normal labor without producing any observable effect on the newborn (4).

BREASTFEEDING SUMMARY

Perphenazine is excreted into human milk (5). A 50-kg, lactating 22-year-old woman was taking perphenazine 12 mg twice daily (480 mcg/kg) for postpartum psychosis. She had a 1-month-old child. During a 24-hour interval, she produced 510 mL of milk that contained 3.2 ng/mL (7.8 nmol/L) of perphenazine. Because of toxicity, her dose was decreased to 8 mg twice daily, with a proportionate decrease in the concentration in milk to 2.1 ng/mL. The mean milk:plasma ratio from samples drawn at various times during the day was approximately 1. Calculated on the infant's weight of 3.5 kg, the authors estimated that the infant would consume about 0.1% of the weight-adjusted maternal dose. Because they did not consider this exposure to be clinically significant, breastfeeding was started. For the next 3.5 months while the mother was on perphenazine, the infant's growth and development were normal. Although no adverse effects were observed in this single case, the American Academy of Pediatrics classifies perphenazine as a drug for which the effect on nursing infants is unknown but may be of concern (6).

References

1. Moya F, Thorndike V. Passage of drugs across the placenta. Am J Obstet Gynecol 1962;84:1778–98.
2. Slone D, Siskind V, Heinonen OP, Monson RR, Kaufman DW, Shapiro S. Antenatal exposure to the phenothiazines in relation to congenital malformations, perinatal mortality rate, birth weight, and intelligence quotient score. Am J Obstet Gynecol 1977;128:486–8.
3. Wertelecki W, Purvis-Smith SG, Blackburn WR. Amitriptyline/perphenazine maternal overdose and birth defects (abstract). Teratology 1980;21:74A.
4. McGarry JM. A double-blind comparison of the anti-emetic effect during labour of metoclopramide and perphenazine. Br J Anaesth 1971;43:613–5.
5. Olesen OV, Bartels U, Poulsen JH. Perphenazine in breast milk and serum. Am J Psychiatry 1990;147:1378–9.
6. Committee on Drugs, American Academy of Pediatrics. The transfer of drugs and other chemicals into human milk. Pediatrics 2001;108:776–89.

P

PERTUZUMAB

Antineoplastic (Monoclonal Antibody)

PREGNANCY RECOMMENDATION: Contraindicated
BREASTFEEDING RECOMMENDATION: Contraindicated

PREGNANCY SUMMARY

No reports describing the use of pertuzumab in human pregnancy have been located. The animal data suggest risk, but the absence of human pregnancy experience prevents a more complete assessment of embryo–fetal risk. However, the drug is given in combination with two other antineoplastics, so the embryo–fetus could potentially be exposed to three agents. The manufacturer recommends that women of reproductive potential should use effective contraception while receiving therapy and for 6 months after the last dose. If the drug is given during pregnancy or a woman becomes pregnant during therapy, the manufacturer encourages enrollment in the MotHER Pregnancy Registry by calling 1-800-690-6720 (1).

FETAL RISK SUMMARY

Pertuzumab is a recombinant humanized monoclonal antibody. It is indicated for use in combination with trastuzumab and docetaxel (see also Trastuzumab and Docetaxel) for the treatment of patients with HER2-positive metastatic breast cancer who have not received prior anti-HER2 therapy or chemotherapy for metastatic disease. Pertuzumab is given as an IV infusion every 3 weeks. The median half-life is 18 days. Metabolism and plasma protein binding were not specified in the product information (1).

Reproduction studies have been conducted in cynomolgus monkeys. In this species, IV bi-weekly doses that were 2.5–20 times the recommended human dose based on C_{max} (RHD) during organogenesis (gestational days 19–50) were embryotoxic with dose-dependent increases (33%–85%) in embryo–fetal death occurring in gestational days 25–70. At cesarean section on gestational day 100, oligohydramnios, decreased relative lung and kidney weights, and microscopic evidence of renal hypoplasia consistent with delayed renal development were seen in all dose groups (1).

Studies for carcinogenic and mutagenic potential have not been conducted. Although specific fertility studies have not been performed, no adverse effects on male and female reproductive organs were observed in repeat-dose toxicity studies up to 6 months duration in cynomolgus monkeys (1).

It is not known if pertuzumab crosses the human placenta. Even though the half-life is long, the high molecular weight (about 148,000) probably precludes passage to the embryo–fetus, at least during early pregnancy. However, the monkey and human placentas are similar (both are hemomonochorial) and the drug did cause embryo–fetal toxicity in monkeys.

BREASTFEEDING SUMMARY

No reports describing the use of pertuzumab during human lactation have been located. The molecular weight (about 148,000) suggests that the drug will not be excreted into mature breast milk. However, immunoglobulins, such as IgG, readily pass into milk during the colostral phase (first 48 hours) and, because pertuzumab has a long half-life (18 days), doses received late in pregnancy will be excreted into colostrum and possibly into early milk. Moreover, the drug is given in combination with trastuzumab and docetaxel, so a nursing infant might be exposed to three antineoplastics. Consequently, the safest course for the infant is to not breastfeed if the mother is receiving this therapy.

P

Reference

1. Product information. Perjeta. Genentech, 2012.

PEYOTE

Hallucinogen

PREGNANCY RECOMMENDATION: Limited Human Data—Probably Compatible (Low Dose)
Contraindicated (Recreational Use)
BREASTFEEDING RECOMMENDATION: No Human Data—Potential Toxicity (Low Dose)
Contraindicated (Recreational Use)

PREGNANCY SUMMARY

Peyote is a hallucinogenic agent that is used legally in certain religious ceremonies. An active alkaloid in peyote is mescaline, an agent that causes developmental toxicity in animals. The use of peyote for religious rituals by certain Indian populations involves low doses and does not appear, based on limited data, to cause developmental toxicity. If true, this would be consistent with the principle that developmental toxicity is dose related. However, the apparent low risk of developmental toxicity in Native American populations using carefully monitored amounts of peyote probably is not transferable to the recreational use of peyote, and certainly not to the use of mescaline. Although the recreational use of peyote or mescaline in pregnancy has not been studied, the presumed higher doses might represent a risk to the embryo or fetus. In addition, the lifestyle of recreational users and the probable use of other hallucinogenic or abuse drugs might not be conducive to a healthy pregnancy. Therefore, such use should be discouraged in pregnancy and is classified as contraindicated.

FETAL RISK SUMMARY

The aboveground parts of peyote (*Lophophora williamsii*) are used primarily for their hallucinogenic properties. Other uses include orally for the treatment of fever, rheumatism, and paralysis, and topically for treating fractures, wounds, and snakebite (1). Scientific documentation of these uses has not been located. The active ingredient in peyote is mescaline, a chemical structurally related to amphetamines. It causes CNS and sympathetic stimulation. The effect on the CNS is similar to that of lysergic acid diethylamide (LSD) (1). (See also Lysergic Acid Diethylamide.)

A 1967 study used a single SC dose of mescaline (0.45, 1.33, or 3.25 mg/kg) in pregnant hamsters on day 8 (organogenesis) (2). Congenital malformations of the brain, spinal cord, liver, and other viscera were increased. The incidence of defects, however, was not dose-related as the lowest dose caused the greatest number of defects (28%), whereas the highest dose caused the fewest (9%). Resorptions (7%–25%), dead fetuses (5%–10%), and runts (5%–12%) were dose related (2).

A 1981 reproduction study with mescaline was conducted in hamsters (3). Oral doses of 16 and 32 mg/kg on the 7th through the 10th day of gestation resulted in dose-dependent increases in resorptions and corresponding decreases in litter size. The number of resorptions in controls and the two doses were 6.4%, 12.0%, and 48.8%, respectively. There also was a dose-related increased delay in the ossification of the skull, sternum, and metatarsals. No gross abnormalities were observed at necropsy (3).

Using an IV combination of carbon-14 labeled and unlabeled mescaline, investigators found that the drug crossed the placenta to the fetus in monkeys (4). Although the passage was limited by the high ionization at physiologic pH (99.3%) (pK_a 9.56) and the low lipid solubility of nonionized mescaline, the drug crossed the placenta and concentrated, at various postinjection times, in the fetal organs. Low concentrations were found in fetal blood, brain, and cerebrospinal fluid (4). A similar study in mice, using only labeled mescaline given intraperitoneally, found that the drug crossed the placenta and concentrated in fetal organs with the lowest concentrations in fetal brain (5). Although one author stated that mescaline is known to cross the human placenta (6), such studies have not been located. The molecular weight (about 211) is low enough that exposure of the embryo and fetus should be expected. Passage across the human placenta should be limited by the ionization at physiologic pH and the low solubility of unionized mescaline found in the above monkey study.

A 1979 case report described a pregnancy in which the mother and father regularly used LSD, peyote, and marijuana during the first 4 months of gestation (7). The woman delivered a healthy 2951-g male infant without any abnormalities at about 38 weeks' gestation. The infant was doing well at 8 months of age.

A brief 1970 review summarized the history, dosage, effects, and adverse effects of mescaline (8). Mescaline was only one of the then-known eight alkaloids present in peyote. Peyote has been used by some Mexican and American Indian tribes for hundreds of years and still is being used legally for religious rituals by the Native American Church. The author thought that mescaline, based on dosage, was the least potent of the commonly used hallucinogens (other hallucinogens not specified). The author also thought that mescaline might be teratogenic based on animal studies (8).

A 2001 review provided more information on the legal use of peyote and its pharmacology (6). Although *L. williamsii* is the cactus legally available and cultivated by the Native American Church, other members of the cactaceae family including *Trichocercus pachanoi* (San Pedro cactus) and *Opuntia cylindrical* also contain mescaline and other alkaloids. In addition to mescaline, about 50 alkaloids have been identified in these cacti. When peyote is used according to recommendations of the Native American Church, the risk for developmental toxicity was not thought to be increased. No increase in malformations was observed in Huichol Indians, a tribe that has used peyote as part of its religious rituals for centuries. However, based on the 1967 animal study cited above, the author concluded that risk of human developmental toxicity was associated with the recreational use of peyote and/or mescaline in which much higher doses than those in religious rituals are used. In addition, mescaline obtained on the street is often mislabeled and may not contain any mescaline at all. For example, phencyclidine (PCP), a much more potent and longer-lasting hallucinogen, is often labeled as mescaline (6). (See also Phencyclidine.)

BREASTFEEDING SUMMARY

No reports describing the use of peyote or its active alkaloid mescaline during human lactation have been located. The molecular weight of mescaline (about 211) is low enough that excretion into breast milk should be expected. The effect of this exposure on a nursing infant is unknown. However, the use of low doses of peyote by adults in religious rituals often is associated with adverse effects, such as nausea, vomiting, and sympathomimetic effects (mydriasis, mild tachycardia, mild hypertension, diaphoresis, ataxia, and hyperreflexia) (6). Higher maternal doses that may be associated with recreational use of peyote, and certainly with mescaline, could cause these effects in a nursing infant. Thus, the recreational use of peyote or mescaline should be considered contraindicated.

References

1. Peyote. *Natural Medicines Comprehensive Database*. 5th ed. Stockton, CA: Therapeutic Research Faculty, 2003:1034–5.
2. Geber WF. Congenital malformations induced by mescaline, lysergic acid diethylamide, and bromolysergic acid in the hamster. Science 1967;158:265–7.

P

3. Hirsch KS, Fritz HI. Teratogenic effects of mescaline, epinephrine, and norepinephrine in the hamster. Teratology 1961;23:287–91.
4. Taska RJ, Schoolar JC. Placental transfer and fetal distribution of mescaline-^{14}C in monkeys. J Pharmacol Exp Ther 1972;183:427–32.
5. Shah NS, Neely AE, Shah KR, Lawrence RS. Placental transfer and tissue distribution of mescaline-^{14}C in the mouse. J Pharmacol Exp Ther 1973;184:489–93.
6. Gilmore HT. Peyote use during pregnancy. S D J Med 2001;54:27–9.
7. Warren RJ, Rimoin DL, Sly WS. LSD exposure in utero. Pediatrics 1970;45:466–9.
8. Olney RK. Mescaline. Tex Med 1972;68:80–2.

PHENACETIN

[Withdrawn from the market. See 9th edition.]

PHENAZOPYRIDINE

Urinary Tract Agent (Analgesic)

PREGNANCY RECOMMENDATION: Compatible
BREASTFEEDING RECOMMENDATION: Contraindicated

PREGNANCY SUMMARY

No reports linking the use of phenazopyridine with congenital defects have been located. There are no relevant animal reproduction data. However, the human pregnancy experience suggest low risk for the embryo–fetus.

FETAL RISK SUMMARY

The Collaborative Perinatal Project monitored 50,282 mother–child pairs, 219 of whom had 1st trimester exposure to phenazopyridine (1, pp. 299–308). For use anytime during pregnancy, 1109 exposures were recorded (1, p. 435). In neither group was evidence found to suggest a relationship to large categories of major or minor malformations or to individual defects. A brief 2008 review of urinary tract infections in pregnancy also cited the above data (2).

In a surveillance study of Michigan Medicaid recipients involving 229,101 completed pregnancies conducted between 1985 and 1992, 496 newborns had been exposed to phenazopyridine during the 1st trimester (F. Rosa, personal communication, FDA, 1993). A total of 27 (5.4%) major birth defects were observed (21 expected), including (observed/expected) 7/5 cardiovascular defects and 1/1 oral cleft. No anomalies were observed in four other defect categories (spina bifida, polydactyly, limb reduction defects, and hypospadias) for which specific data were available. These data do not support an association between the drug and congenital defects.

It is not known if phenazopyridine crosses the human placenta. The molecular weight (about 214 for the free base) suggests that the drug will cross to the embryo–fetus.

In a large 1985 study involving 6509 women with live births, 217 were exposed to phenazopyridine in the 1st trimester (3). One infant had a congenital disorder. Although the defect was not described, the incidence (0.5%) was very low.

BREASTFEEDING SUMMARY

No reports describing the use of phenazopyridine during human lactation have been located. The molecular weight (about 214 for the free base) suggests that the drug will be excreted into breast milk. Because phenazopyridine can cause methemoglobinemia, sulfhemoglobinemia, and hemolytic anemia, it should not be used during breastfeeding, especially with an infant under 1 month of age or with G-6-PD deficiency (4).

References

1. Heinonen OP, Slone D, Shapiro S. *Birth Defects and Drugs in Pregnancy*. Littleton, MA: Publishing Sciences Group, 1977.
2. Lee M, Bozzo P, Einarson A, Koren G. Urinary tract infections in pregnancy. Can Fam Physician 2008;54:853–4.
3. Aselton P, Jick H, Milunsky A, Hunter JR, Stergachis A. First-trimester drug use and congenital disorders. Obstet Gynecol 1985;65:451–5.
4. Phenazopyridine. September 7, 2013. Available at NIH LactMed database at http://toxnet.nih.nih.gov/cgi-bin/sis/search/f?./temp/~jTTJol:1. Accessed March 19, 2014.

PHENCYCLIDINE

Hallucinogen

PREGNANCY RECOMMENDATION: Contraindicated
BREASTFEEDING RECOMMENDATION: Contraindicated

PREGNANCY SUMMARY

Phencyclidine (PCP) is an illicit drug used for its hallucinogenic effects. Although the drug does not appear to cause structural anomalies, its use in pregnancy has been associated with functional/neurobehavioral defects.

FETAL RISK SUMMARY

Exposure of the fetus to PCP has been demonstrated in humans with placental metabolism of the drug (1–7). Qualitative analysis of the urine from two newborns revealed phencyclidine levels of 75 ng/mL or greater up to 3 days after birth (2). In 24 (12%) of 200 women evaluated at a Los Angeles hospital, cord blood PCP levels ranged from 0.10 to 5.80 ng/mL (3). Cord blood concentrations were twice as high as maternal serum—1215 vs. 514 pg/mL in one woman who allegedly consumed her last dose approximately 53 days before delivery (4). PCP in the newborn's urine was found to be 5841 pg/mL (4).

Relatively few studies have appeared on the use of PCP during pregnancy, but fetal exposure may be more common than this lack of reporting indicates. During a 9-month period in 1980–1981 at a Cleveland hospital, 30 of 519 (5.8%) consecutively screened pregnant patients were discovered to have PCP exposure (8). In a subsequent report from this same hospital, 2327 pregnant patients were screened for PCP exposure between 1981 and 1982 (6). Only 19 patients (0.8%) had positive urine samples, but up to 256 (11%) or more may have tested positive with more frequent checking (6). In the Los Angeles study cited above, 12% were exposed (3). However, the specificity of the chemical screening methods used in this latter report has been questioned (7).

Most pregnancies in which the mother used PCP apparently end with healthy newborns (3,4,9). However, case reports involving four newborns indicate that the use of this agent may result in long-term damage (2,9,10):

- Depressed at birth, jittery, hypertonic, poor feeding (2) (two infants)
- Irritable, poor feeding and sucking reflex (9) (one infant)
- Triangular-shaped face with pointed chin, narrow mandibular angle, antimongoloid slanted eyes, poor head control, nystagmus, inability to track visually, respiratory distress, hypertonic, jitteriness (10) (one infant)

Irritability, jitteriness, hypertonicity, and poor feeding were common features in the affected infants. In three of the neonates, most of the symptoms had persisted at the time of the report. In the case with the malformed child, no causal relationship with PCP could be established. Marijuana was also taken, which is a known teratogen in some animal species (11). However, marijuana is not considered to be a human teratogen (see Marijuana).

A study published in 1992 described the effects of PCP on human fetal cerebral cortical neurons in culture (12). High levels of the drug caused progressive degeneration and death of the neurons, whereas sublethal concentrations inhibited axonal outgrowth. Because the fetal CNS can concentrate and retain PCP, these results suggested that PCP exposure during pregnancy could produce profound functional impairments (12).

Abnormal neurobehavior in the newborn period was observed in nine infants delivered from mothers who had used PCP during pregnancy (13). The abnormality was significantly more than that observed in control infants and those exposed in utero to opiates, sedative/stimulants, or the combination of pentazocine and tripelennamine (i.e., T's and blue's). However, by 2 years of age, the mental and psychomotor development of all drug-exposed infants, including those exposed to PCP, were similar to controls.

BREASTFEEDING SUMMARY

PCP is excreted into breast milk (14). One lactating mother, who took her last dose 40 days previously, excreted 3.90 ng/mL in her milk. Women consuming PCP should not breastfeed. The American Academy of Pediatrics considers the drug to be contraindicated during breastfeeding (15).

References

1. Nicholas JM, Lipshitz J, Schreiber EC. Phencyclidine: its transfer across the placenta as well as into breast milk. Am J Obstet Gynecol 1982;143:143–6.
2. Strauss AA, Modanlou HD, Bosu SK. Neonatal manifestations of maternal phencyclidine (PCP) abuse. Pediatrics 1981;68:550–2.
3. Kaufman KR, Petrucha RA, Pitts FN Jr, Kaufman ER. Phencyclidine in umbilical cord blood: preliminary data. Am J Psychiatry 1983;140:450–2.
4. Petrucha RA, Kaufman KR, Pitts FN. Phencyclidine in pregnancy: a case report. J Reprod Med 1982;27:301–3.
5. Rayburn WF, Holsztynska EF, Domino EF. Phencyclidine: biotransformation by the human placenta. Am J Obstet Gynecol 1984;148:111–2.
6. Golden NL, Kuhnert BR, Sokol RJ, Martier S, Bagby BS. Phencyclidine use during pregnancy. Am J Obstet Gynecol 1984;148:254–9.
7. Lipton MA. Phencyclidine in umbilical cord blood: some cautions. Am J Psychiatry 1983;140:449.
8. Golden NL, Sokol RJ, Martier S, Miller SI. A practical method for identifying angel dust abuse during pregnancy. Am J Obstet Gynecol 1982;142: 359–61.
9. Lerner SE, Burns RS. Phencyclidine use among youth: history, epidemiology, and acute and chronic intoxication. In Petersen R, Stillman R, eds. *Phencyclidine (PCP) Abuse: An Appraisal*. Washington, DC: National Institute on Drug Abuse Research Monograph No. 21, US Government Printing Office, 1978.
10. Golden NL, Sokol RJ, Rubin IL. Angel dust: possible effects on the fetus. Pediatrics 1980;65:18–20.
11. Persaud TVN, Ellington AC. Teratogenic activity of cannabis resin. Lancet 1968;2:406–7.
12. Mattson MP, Rychlik B, Cheng B. Degenerative and axon outgrowth-altering effects of phencyclidine in human fetal cerebral cortical cells. Neuropharmacology 1992;31:279–91.
13. Chasnoff IJ, Burns KA, Burns WJ, Schnoll SH. Prenatal drug exposure: effects on neonatal and infant growth and development. Neurobehavior Toxicol Teratol 1986;8:357–62.
14. Kaufman KR, Petrucha RA, Pitts FN Jr, Weekes ME. PCP in amniotic fluid and breast milk: case report. J Clin Psychiatry 1983;44:269–70.
15. Committee on Drugs, American Academy of Pediatrics. The transfer of drugs and other chemicals into human milk. Pediatrics 2001;108:776–89.

PHENDIMETRAZINE

Central Stimulant/Anorexiant

PREGNANCY RECOMMENDATION: Contraindicated
BREASTFEEDING RECOMMENDATION: Contraindicated

PREGNANCY SUMMARY

It is doubtful if any real benefit is derived from the use of phendimetrazine for weight control during pregnancy, and its use during gestation, especially during the 1st trimester, should be considered contraindicated. (See also Phentermine or Amphetamine.)

FETAL RISK SUMMARY

Phendimetrazine is a sympathomimetic amine that has pharmacologic activity similar to the amphetamines. No animal or human reproductive data are available. It is indicated for the management of exogenous obesity as a short-term adjunct (a few weeks) in a regimen of weight reduction based on caloric restriction. Its activity is similar to amphetamines. Animal reproduction studies have not been conducted (1).

It is not known if phendimetrazine crosses the human placenta. The molecular weight (about 191 for the free base) is low enough, but its hydrophilic nature should limit the exposure of the embryo–fetus.

BREASTFEEDING SUMMARY

No reports describing the use phendimetrazine during lactation have been located. The molecular weight (191 for the free base) is low enough for excretion into breast milk. Milk is slightly acidic compared with plasma and ion trapping could result in milk:plasma ratios >1. Because CNS stimulation and other adverse reactions may occur in a nursing infant exposed to this drug in milk, breastfeeding should be considered a contraindication if the mother is taking phendimetrazine.

Reference

1. Product information. Phendimetrazine tartrate. Milkart, 1996.

PHENELZINE

Antidepressant

PREGNANCY RECOMMENDATION: Limited Human Data—Animal Data Suggest Moderate Risk
BREASTFEEDING RECOMMENDATION: No Human Data—Potential Toxicity

PREGNANCY SUMMARY

Phenelzine is a monoamine oxidase (MAO) inhibitor used in the treatment of depression. Other agents in this subclass are iproniazid, isocarboxazid, nialamide, and tranylcypromine. The human pregnancy experience is too limited to assess the embryo–fetal risk. (See also Tranylcypromine.)

FETAL RISK SUMMARY

Phenelzine has been found to be effective in depressed patients clinically characterized as atypical, nonendogenous, or neurotic. It is extensively metabolized to apparently inactive metabolites. Plasma protein binding was not reported by the manufacturer, but the mean elimination half-life after a single 30-mg dose was 11.6 hours (1).

In reproduction studies with mice at doses above the maximum recommended human dose, a significant decrease in the number of viable offspring per mouse was observed (1).

It is not known if phenelzine crosses the human placenta. The molecular weight of the sulfate form (about 234) and elimination half-life suggest that exposure of the embryo–fetus should be expected.

The Collaborative Perinatal Project monitored 21 mother–child pairs exposed to MAO inhibitors during the 1st trimester, 3 of which were exposed to phenelzine (2). Three of the 21 infants had malformations (relative risk 2.26). Details of the three cases with phenelzine exposure were not specified (2).

A 1995 report described a 25-year-old woman who had been treated for depression with phenelzine (45 mg/day) for 6 years before becoming pregnant (3). The drug was continued throughout gestation. Because labor failed to progress, a cesarean section was performed to give birth to a healthy male infant with Apgar scores of 9 at 1 and 5 minutes (3).

A 31-year-old white female with severe recurrent major depression took phenelzine 45 mg/day before and throughout her pregnancy (4). Attempts to taper her dose were unsuccessful and the patient declined to change to other depression therapy. An ultrasound at 10 weeks' gestation revealed nonidentical twins. A repeat examination at 16 weeks' showed resorption of one fetus, an event that was considered spontaneous and not related to the patient's drug therapy. Because of worsening depression in the 2nd trimester, her daily dose was increased to 52.5 mg. At 37 weeks', she gave birth to a normal healthy 2.651-kg male infant with Apgar scores of 6, 8, and 9 at 1, 5, and 10 minutes, respectively. The infant was discharged home on day 3 and growth and development were normally at 16 months of age (4).

A 2014 case study described the use of phenelzine (105 mg/day), lithium (900 mg/day), and quetiapine (600mg/ day) in a 31-year-old woman with bipolar affective disorder (5). She was also taking metformin (1 g/day) for polycystic ovarian syndrome with oligomenorrhea. Despite her oligomenorrhea, a pregnancy was confirmed at 17 weeks' gestation. A glucose tolerance test was negative at 26 weeks'. Lithium was suspended 24–48 hours before induction of labor at 39 weeks' Because of obstructed labor, a cesarean section was performed to give birth to a 4.2-kg male infant with Apgar scores of 5 and 9 at 1 and 5 minutes, respectively. The baby required initial resuscitation during the first 10 minutes. The baby was discharged home with the mother at 5 days. At 10 weeks of age, the baby's growth and development were normal (5).

BREASTFEEDING SUMMARY

No reports describing the use of phenelzine during breastfeeding have been located. The molecular weight (about 234) and moderately long elimination half-life (11.6 hours) suggest that the drug will be excreted into breast milk. If the drug is used during breastfeeding, the infant should be monitored for the most common adverse reactions observed in adults (dizziness, headache, drowsiness, sleep disturbances, fatigue, weakness, tremors, twitching, myoclonic movements, hyperreflexia, constipation, dry mouth, and edema).

References

1. Product information. Nardil. Parke-Davis, 2000.
2. Heinonen OP, Slone D, Shapiro S. *Birth Defects and Drugs in Pregnancy*. Littleton, MA: Publishing Sciences Group, 1977:336–7.
3. Pavy TJG, Kliffer AP, Douglas MJ. Anaesthetic management of labour and delivery in a woman taking long-term MAOI. Can J Anaesth 1995;42:618–20.
4. Gracious BL, Wisner KL. Phenelzine use throughout pregnancy and the puerperium: case report, review of the literature, and management recommendations. Depress Anxiety 1997;6:124–8.
5. Frayne J, Nguyen T, Kohan R, De Felice N, Rampono J. The comprehensive management of pregnant women with major mood disorders: a case study involving phenelzine, lithium, and quetiapine. Arch Womens Ment Health 2014;17:73–5.

PHENINDIONE

Anticoagulant

See Coumarin Derivatives.

PHENIRAMINE

Antihistamine

PREGNANCY RECOMMENDATION: Limited Human Data—Probably Compatible
BREASTFEEDING RECOMMENDATION: No Human Data—Probably Compatible

PREGNANCY SUMMARY

In general, antihistamines are considered low risk in pregnancy. However, exposure near birth of premature infants has been associated with an increased risk of retrolental fibroplasia.

FETAL RISK SUMMARY

The Collaborative Perinatal Project monitored 50,282 mother–child pairs, 831 of whom were exposed to pheniramine during the 1st trimester (1, pp. 322–334). A possible relationship between this use and respiratory malformations and eye/ear defects was found, but independent confirmation is required. For use anytime during pregnancy, 2442 exposures were recorded (1, pp. 436–437). No evidence was found in this group to suggest a relationship to congenital anomalies.

It is not known if pheniramine crosses the human placenta. The molecular weight (about 240) is low enough that exposure of the embryo–fetus should be expected.

An association between exposure during the last 2 weeks of pregnancy to antihistamines in general and retrolental fibroplasia in premature infants has been reported. See Brompheniramine for details.

BREASTFEEDING SUMMARY

No reports describing the use of pheniramine during human lactation have been located. The molecular weight (about 240) is low enough for excretion into breast milk.

Reference

1. Heinonen OP, Slone D, Shapiro S. *Birth Defects and Drugs in Pregnancy*. Littleton, MA: Publishing Sciences Group, 1977.

PHENOBARBITAL

Sedative/Anticonvulsant

PREGNANCY RECOMMENDATION: Human Data Suggest Risk
BREASTFEEDING RECOMMENDATION: Limited Human Data—Potential Toxicity

PREGNANCY SUMMARY

Phenobarbital therapy in the epileptic pregnant woman presents a risk to the fetus in terms of major and minor congenital defects, hemorrhage at birth, and addiction. Adverse effects on neurobehavioral development have also been reported. The risk to the mother, however, is greater if the drug is withheld and seizure control is lost. The risk:benefit ratio, in this case, favors continued use of the drug during pregnancy at the lowest possible level to control seizures. Use of the drug in nonepileptic patients does not seem to pose a significant risk for structural defects, but neurodevelopment, hemorrhage, and addiction in the newborn are still concerns.

FETAL RISK SUMMARY

Phenobarbital has been used widely in clinical practice as a sedative and anticonvulsant since 1912 (1). The drug crosses the placenta to the fetus at birth (2). Factors significantly influencing placental transfer were duration of maternal treatment, gestational age, and arterial cord pH (2).

The potential teratogenic effects of phenobarbital were recognized in 1964 along with phenytoin (3). Since this report, there have been numerous reviews and studies on the teratogenic effects of phenobarbital either alone or in combination with phenytoin and other anticonvulsants. Based on this literature, the epileptic pregnant woman taking phenobarbital in combination with other antiepileptics has a two- to threefold greater risk for delivering a child with congenital defects over the general population (4–11).

It has not always been known if the increased risk of congenital anomalies was caused by antiepileptic drugs, the disease itself, genetic factors, or a combination of these factors. A 1991 study of epileptic mothers who had been treated with either phenobarbital or carbamazepine, or the two agents in combination during pregnancy concluded that major and minor anomalies appeared to be more related to the mother's disease than to the drugs (11). An exception to this was the smaller head circumference observed in infants exposed in utero to either phenobarbital alone or in combination with carbamazepine. However, an earlier publication thought there was evidence that drugs were the causative factor (12).

A prospective study published in 1999 described the outcomes of 517 pregnancies of epileptic mothers identified at one Italian center from 1977 (13). Excluding genetic and chromosomal defects, malformations were classified as severe structural defects, mild structural defects, and deformations. Minor anomalies were not considered. Spontaneous ($N = 38$) and early ($N = 20$) voluntary abortions were excluded from the analysis, as were seven pregnancies that delivered at other hospitals. Of the remaining 452 outcomes, 427 were exposed to anticonvulsants of which 313 involved monotherapy: phenobarbital ($N = 83$), carbamazepine ($N = 113$), valproate ($N = 44$), primidone ($N = 35$), phenytoin ($N = 31$), clonazepam ($N = 6$), and other ($N = 1$). There were no defects in the 25 pregnancies not exposed to anticonvulsants. Of the 42 (9.3%) outcomes with malformations, 24 (5.3%) were severe, 10 (2.2%) were mild, and 8 (1.8%) were deformities. There were four malformations with phenobarbital monotherapy: two (2.4%) severe (Fallot's tetralogy, hydronephrosis), one (1.2%) mild (umbilical and inguinal hernia), and one (1.2%) deformation (hip dislocation). The investigators concluded that the anticonvulsants were the primary risk factor for an increased incidence of congenital malformations (see also Carbamazepine, Clonazepam, Phenytoin, Primidone, and Valproic Acid) (13).

A 2001 prospective study provides further evidence that the congenital defects observed in the offspring of epileptic mothers treated with anticonvulsants are caused by drugs (14). The prospective cohort study, conducted from 1986 to 1993 at five maternity hospitals, was designed to determine if anticonvulsant agents or other factors (e.g., genetic) were responsible for the constellation of abnormalities seen in infants of mothers treated with anticonvulsants during pregnancy. A total of 128,049 pregnant women were screened at delivery for exposure to anticonvulsant drugs. Three groups of singleton infants were identified: (a) exposed to anticonvulsant drugs, (b) not exposed to anticonvulsant drugs but with a maternal history of seizures, and (c) not exposed to anticonvulsant drugs and with no maternal history of seizures (control group). For a variety of reasons, including exposure to other teratogens, many identified infants were excluded, leaving 316, 98, and 508 infants, respectively, in the three groups for analysis. Anticonvulsant monotherapy occurred in 223 women: phenytoin ($N = 87$), phenobarbital ($N = 64$), carbamazepine ($N = 58$), and too few cases for analysis with valproic acid, clonazepam, diazepam, and lorazepam. Ninety-three infants were exposed to two or more anticonvulsant drugs. All infants were examined systematically (blinded as to group in 93% of the cases) for embryopathy associated with anticonvulsant exposure (major malformations, hypoplasia of the midface and fingers, microcephaly, and intrauterine growth restriction). Compared with controls, statistically significant associations between anticonvulsants and anticonvulsant embryopathy were phenobarbital monotherapy, 26.6% (17/64); phenytoin monotherapy, 20.7% (18/87); all infants exposed to anticonvulsant monotherapy, 20.6% (46/223); those exposed to two or more anticonvulsants, 28.0% (26/93); and all infants exposed to anticonvulsants (monotherapy and polytherapy), 22.8% (72/316). Nonsignificant associations were found for carbamazepine monotherapy, 13.8% (8/58); nonexposed infants with a maternal history of seizures, 6.1% (6/98); and controls, 8.5% (43/508).

The investigators concluded that the distinctive pattern of physical abnormalities observed in infants exposed to anticonvulsants during gestation was due to the drugs rather than to epilepsy itself (14).

A phenotype, as described for phenytoin in the fetal hydantoin syndrome (FHS), apparently does not occur with phenobarbital. (See Phenytoin for details of FHS.) However, as summarized by Janz (15), some of the minor malformations composing the FHS have been occasionally observed in infants of epileptic mothers treated only with phenobarbital.

The effects of prenatal exposure to phenobarbital on CNS development of offspring have been studied in both animals (16–18) and humans (11,19–22). The neural development in 90-day-old offspring of female rats given phenobarbital in doses of 0, 20, 40, or 60 mg/kg/day before and throughout gestation were described in a 1992 study (16). The drug produced dose- and sex-dependent changes in the electroencephalograms of the offspring. Lower doses resulted in adverse changes in learning and attentional focus, whereas higher doses also adversely affected neural function related to slow-wave sleep and receptor homeostasis. An earlier study measured the long-term effects on the offspring of rats from exposure to 40 mg/kg/day of phenobarbital from day 12 to day 19 of gestation (17). The effects included delays in the onset of puberty; disorders in the estrous cycle; infertility; and altered concentrations of sex steroids, gonadotropic hormones, and estrogen receptors. The changes represented permanent alterations in sexual maturation. A similar study measured decreases in the concentration of testosterone in the plasma and brain of exposed fetal rats (18). These changes persisted into adult life, indicating that phenobarbital may lead to sexual dysfunction in mature animals.

In a 1991 human study, the cognitive development (as measured by school career, reading, spelling, and arithmetic skills) of children who had been exposed in utero to either phenobarbital alone or in combination with carbamazepine was significantly impaired in comparison with children of nonepileptic mothers (11). A similar finding, but not significant, was suggested when the phenobarbital-exposed children were compared with children exposed only to carbamazepine.

In a 1988 study designed to evaluate the effect of in utero exposure to anticonvulsants on intelligence, 148 Finnish children of epileptic mothers were compared with 105 controls (19). Previous studies had either shown intellectual impairment from this exposure or no effect. Of the 148 children of epileptic mothers, 129 were exposed to anticonvulsant therapy during the first 20 weeks of pregnancy, 2 were only exposed after 20 weeks, and 17 were not exposed. In those mothers treated during pregnancy, 22 received phenobarbital in combination with other anticonvulsants, all during the first 20 weeks. The children were evaluated at 5.5 years of age for both verbal and nonverbal measures of intelligence. A child was considered mentally deficient if the results of both tests were <71. Two of the 148 children of epileptic mothers were diagnosed as mentally deficient and 2 others had borderline intelligence (the mother of one of these latter children had not been treated with anticonvulsant medication). None of the controls was considered mentally deficient. Both verbal (110.2 vs. 114.5) and nonverbal (108.7 vs. 113.2) intelligence scores were significantly lower in the study group children than in controls. In both groups, intelligence scores were significantly lower when seven or more minor anomalies were present. However, the presence of hypertelorism and digital hypoplasia, two minor anomalies considered typical of exposure to phenytoin, was not predictive of low intelligence (19).

A 1996 study also described the effects of in utero phenobarbital exposure on cognitive performance (20). Intelligence scores of Danish adult men, born between 1959 and 1961, who had been exposed to prenatal phenobarbital were measured. Their mothers had no history of CNS disorder and there was no exposure to other psychopharmacological drugs. Two double-blind studies using different measures of general intelligence were conducted on subjects (total = 114) and controls (total = 153). The test scores of matched controls were used to predict scores for each exposed subject. The exposure effects were then estimated by comparing the predicted to the observed scores. Phenobarbital exposure was associated with significantly lower verbal intelligence scores (about 0.5 standard deviations). Exposure in the 3rd trimester was the most detrimental. The magnitude of the intelligence deficit was increased by lower socioeconomic status and being the offspring of an unwanted pregnancy (20).

A two-part 2000 study evaluated the effects of prenatal phenobarbital and phenytoin exposure on brain development and cognitive functioning in adults (21). Subjects and matched controls, delivered at a mean 40 weeks' gestation, were retrospectively identified from birth records covering the years between 1957 and 1972. Maternal diseases of the subjects included epilepsy (treated with anticonvulsants) and other conditions in which anticonvulsants were used as sedatives (nausea, vomiting, or emotional problems), whereas the control group had no maternal pathologies. Only those exposed prenatally to phenobarbital alone or phenobarbital plus phenytoin had sufficient subjects to analyze. The mean occipitofrontal circumference for phenobarbital-exposed neonates was not different from controls (34.49 vs. 34.50 cm), but it was significantly smaller (33.82 cm) for phenobarbital plus phenytoin subjects compared with phenobarbital alone or controls. In the follow-up part of the study, no differences in adult cognitive functioning (intelligence, attention, and memory) were found between the exposed and control groups. More subjects than controls, however, were mentally slow (4 vs. 2; causes of retardation not known except for 1 case of autism in controls) and more had persistent learning problems (12% vs. 1%). The investigators concluded that phenobarbital plus phenytoin reduced occipitofrontal circumference but may affect cognitive capacity only in susceptible offspring (21).

The relationship between maternal anticonvulsant therapy, neonatal behavior, and neurologic function in children was reported in a 1996 study (22). Among newborns exposed to maternal monotherapy, 18 were exposed to phenobarbital (including primidone), 13 to phenytoin, and 8 to valproic acid. Compared with controls, neonates exposed to phenobarbital had significantly higher mean apathy and optimality scores. Phenytoin-exposed neonates also had a significantly higher mean apathy score. However, the neonatal optimality and apathy scores did not correlate with neurologic outcome of the children at 6 years of age. In contrast, those exposed to valproic acid had optimality and apathy scores statistically similar to controls but a significantly higher hyperexcitability score. Moreover, the hyperexcitability score correlated with later minor and major neurologic dysfunction at age 6 years (22).

The Collaborative Perinatal Project monitored 50,282 mother–child pairs, 1415 of whom had 1st trimester exposure to phenobarbital (23, pp. 336–339). For use anytime during pregnancy, 8037 exposures were recorded (23, p. 438). In neither group was evidence found to suggest a relationship to large categories of major or minor malformations, although a possible association with Down's syndrome was shown statistically. However, a relationship between phenobarbital and Down's syndrome is unlikely.

In a surveillance study of Michigan Medicaid recipients involving 229,101 completed pregnancies conducted between 1985 and 1992, 334 newborns had been exposed to phenobarbital during the 1st trimester (F. Rosa, personal communication, FDA, 1993). A total of 20 (6.0%) major birth defects were observed (14 expected). Specific data were available for six defect categories, including (observed/expected) 8/3 cardiovascular defects, 1/1 oral clefts, 1/0 spina bifida, 1/1 polydactyly, 0/1 limb reduction defects, and 1/1 hypospadias. Only the data for cardiovascular defects are suggestive of a possible association.

The effects of exposure (at any time during the 2nd or 3rd month after the last menstrual period) to folic acid antagonists on embryo–fetal development were evaluated in a large, multicenter, case–control surveillance study published in 2000 (24). The report was based on data collected between 1976 and 1998 from 80 maternity or tertiary care hospitals. Mothers were interviewed within 6 months of delivery about their use of drugs during pregnancy. Folic acid antagonists were categorized into two groups: group I—dihydrofolate reductase inhibitors (aminopterin, methotrexate, sulfasalazine, pyrimethamine, triamterene, and trimethoprim); and group II—agents that affect other enzymes in folate metabolism, impair the absorption of folate, or increase the metabolic breakdown of folate (carbamazepine, phenytoin, primidone, and phenobarbital). The case subjects were 3870 infants with cardiovascular defects, 1962 with oral clefts, and 1100 with urinary tract malformations. Infants with defects associated with a syndrome were excluded as were infants with coexisting neural tube defects (NTDs; known to be reduced by maternal folic acid supplementation). Too few infants with limb reduction defects were identified to be analyzed. Controls (N = 8387) were infants with malformations other than oral clefts and cardiovascular, urinary tract, limb reduction, and NTDs but included infants with chromosomal and genetic defects. The risk of malformations in control infants would not have been reduced by vitamin supplementation, and none of the controls used folic acid antagonists. For group I cases, the relative risks (RRs) of cardiovascular defects and oral clefts were 3.4 (95% confidence interval [CI] 1.8–6.4) and 2.6 (95% CI 1.1–6.1), respectively. For group II cases, the RRs of cardiovascular and urinary tract defects, and oral clefts were 2.2 (95% CI 1.4–3.5), 2.5 (95% CI 1.2–5.0), and 2.5 (95% CI 1.5–4.2), respectively. Maternal use of multivitamin supplements with folic acid (typically 0.4 mg) reduced the risks in group I cases, but not in group II cases (24).

Thanatophoric dwarfism was found in a stillborn infant exposed throughout gestation to phenobarbital (300 mg/day), phenytoin (200 mg/day), and amitriptyline (>150 mg/day) (25). The cause of the malformation could not be determined, but both drug and genetic causes were considered.

A 2000 study, using data from the MADRE (an acronym for malformation and drug exposure) surveillance project, assessed the human teratogenicity of anticonvulsants (26). Among 8005 malformed infants, cases were defined as infants with a specific malformation, whereas controls were infants with other anomalies. Of the total group, 299 were exposed in the 1st trimester to anticonvulsants. Among these, exposure to monotherapy occurred in the following: phenobarbital (N = 65), mephobarbital (N = 10), carbamazepine (N = 46), valproic acid (N = 80), phenytoin (N = 24), and other agents (N = 16). Statistically significant associations were found with phenobarbital monotherapy and cardiac defects (N = 12), and cleft lip/palate (N = 11). When all 1st trimester exposures (monotherapy and polytherapy) were evaluated, significant associations were found between phenobarbital and cardiac defects (N = 20), cleft lip/palate (N = 19), and persistent left superior vena cava/other anomalies of the circulatory system (N = 3). Although the study confirmed some previously known associations, several new associations with anticonvulsants were discovered and require independent confirmation (see also Carbamazepine, Mephobarbital, Phenytoin, and Valproic Acid) (26).

The Lamotrigine Pregnancy Registry, an ongoing project conducted by the manufacturer, was first published in January 1997 (27). The final report was published in July 2010. The Registry is now closed. Among 24 prospectively enrolled pregnancies exposed to phenobarbital and lamotrigine, with or without other anticonvulsants, 22 were exposed in the 1st trimester resulting in 16 live births without defects, 4 elective abortions, and 2 birth defects. There were two exposures in the 2nd/3rd trimesters resulting in live births without defects (27).

Phenobarbital and other anticonvulsants (e.g., phenytoin) may cause early hemorrhagic disease of the newborn (28–37). Hemorrhage occurs during the first 24 hours after birth and may be severe or even fatal. The exact mechanism of the defect is unknown but may involve phenobarbital induction of fetal liver microsomal enzymes that deplete the already low reserves of fetal vitamin K (37). This results in suppression of the vitamin K-dependent coagulation factors II, VII, IX, and X. A 1985 review summarized the various prophylactic treatment regimens that have been proposed (see Phenytoin for details) (37).

Barbiturate withdrawal has been observed in newborns exposed to phenobarbital in utero (38). The average onset of symptoms in 15 addicted infants was 6 days (range 3–14 days). These infants had been exposed during gestation to doses varying from 64 to 300 mg/day with unknown amounts in four patients.

Phenobarbital may induce folic acid deficiency in the pregnant woman (39–41). A discussion of this effect and the possible consequences for the fetus are presented under Phenytoin (see also reference 24 above).

High-dose phenobarbital, contained in an antiasthmatic preparation, was reported in a mother giving birth to a stillborn full-term female infant with complete triploidy (42). The authors speculated on the potential for phenobarbital-induced chromosomal damage. However, an earlier in vitro study found no effect of phenobarbital on the incidence of chromosome gaps, breaks, or abnormal forms (43). Any relationship between the drug and the infant's condition is probably coincidental.

P

Phenobarbital and cholestyramine have been used to treat cholestasis of pregnancy (44,45). Although no drug-induced fetal complications were noted, the therapy was ineffective for this condition. An earlier study, however, reported the successful treatment of intrahepatic cholestasis of pregnancy with phenobarbital, resulting in the normalization of serum bilirubin concentrations (46). The drug has also been used in the last few weeks of pregnancy to reduce the incidence and severity of neonatal hyperbilirubinemia (47).

Antenatal phenobarbital, either alone or in combination with vitamin K, has been used to reduce the incidence and severity of intraventricular hemorrhage in very-low-birth-weight infants (48–55). The therapy seemed to consistently reduce the frequency of grade 3 and grade 4 hemorrhage, and infant mortality from this condition. A 1991 review of this therapy summarized several proposed mechanisms by which phenobarbital might produce this beneficial effect (56). However, three studies (51,53,55), one involving 668 infants (treated and controls) (55), have concluded that the risk of intraventricular hemorrhage or early death in preterm infants is not decreased by antenatal phenobarbital.

In a study using the same subjects and controls as in reference (54) above, antenatal phenobarbital (10 mg/kg IV, then 100 mg orally every 24 hours until delivery or until completion of 34 weeks' gestation) had no effect, compared with nonexposed controls, on neurodevelopment as measured serially up to age 3 years (57). In contrast, another study using the same subjects and controls as a previous study (reference 53) found that antenatal phenobarbital (720–780 mg IV, then 60 mg IV every 6 hours until delivery or 34 weeks' gestation) significantly impaired developmental outcome as measured at age 2 years (58,59).

BREASTFEEDING SUMMARY

P

Phenobarbital is excreted into breast milk (60–65). In two reports, the milk:plasma ratio varied between 0.4 and 0.6 (61,62). The amount of phenobarbital ingested by the nursing infant has been estimated to reach 2–4 mg/day (63). The pharmacokinetics of phenobarbital during lactation have been reviewed (62). Because of slower elimination in the nursing infant, accumulation may occur to the point that blood levels in the infant may actually exceed those of the mother (62). Phenobarbital-induced sedation has been observed in three nursing infants probably caused by this accumulation (60).

A case of withdrawal in a 7-month-old nursing infant after abrupt weaning from a mother taking phenobarbital, primidone, and carbamazepine has been reported (65). The mother had taken the anticonvulsant agents throughout gestation and during lactation. The baby's serum phenobarbital level at approximately 8 weeks of age was 14.8 μmol/L, near the lower level of the therapeutic range. At 7 months of age, the mother abruptly stopped nursing her infant; shortly thereafter withdrawal symptoms were observed in the infant consisting of episodes of "startle" responses and infantile spasms confirmed by electroencephalography. The infant was treated with phenobarbital, with prompt resolution of her symptoms and she was gradually weaned from the drug during a 6-month interval. Her neurologic and mental development were normal during the subsequent 5-year follow-up period (65).

Women consuming phenobarbital during breastfeeding, especially those on high doses, should be instructed to observe their infants for sedation. Phenobarbital levels in the infant should also be monitored to avoid toxic concentrations (62,66). The American Academy of Pediatrics classifies phenobarbital as a drug that has caused major adverse effects in some nursing infants, and it should be given to nursing women with caution (66).

References

1. Hauptmann A. Luminal bei epilepsie. Munchen Med Wochenschr 1912;59:1907–8.
2. De Carolis MP, Romagnoli C, Frezza S, D'Urzo E, Muzil U, Mezza A, Ferrazzani S, De Carolis S. Placental transfer of phenobarbital: what is new? Dev Pharmacol Ther 1992;19:19–26.
3. Janz D, Fuchs V. Are anti-epileptic drugs harmful when given during pregnancy? German Med Monogr 1964;9:20–3.
4. Hill RB. Teratogenesis and anti-epileptic drugs. N Engl J Med 1973;289: 1089–90.
5. Bodendorfer TW. Fetal effects of anticonvulsant drugs and seizure disorders. Drug Intell Clin Pharm 1978;12:14–21.
6. Committee on Drugs, American Academy of Pediatrics. Anticonvulsants and pregnancy. Pediatrics 1977;63:331–3.
7. Nakane Y, Okoma T, Takahashi R, Sato Y, Wada T, Sato T, Fukushima Y, Kumashiro H, Ono T, Takahashi T, Aoki Y, Kazamatsuri H, Inami M, Komai S, Seino M, Miyakoshi M, Tanimura T, Hazama H, Kawahara R, Otuski S, Hosokawa K, Inanaga K, Nakazawa Y, Yamamoto K. Multi-institutional study of the teratogenicity and fetal toxicity of anti-epileptic drugs: a report of a collaborative study group in Japan. Epilepsia 1980;21:633–80.
8. Andermann E, Dansky L, Andermann F, Loughnan PM, Gibbons J. Minor congenital malformations and dermatoglyphic alterations in the offspring of epileptic women: a clinical investigation of the teratogenic effects of anticonvulsant medication. In *Epilepsy, Pregnancy and the Child.* Proceedings of a Workshop in Berlin, September 1980. New York, NY: Raven Press, 1981.
9. Dansky L, Andermann E, Andermann F. Major congenital malformations in the offspring of epileptic patients. In *Epilepsy, Pregnancy and the Child.* Proceedings of a Workshop in Berlin, September 1980. New York, NY: Raven Press, 1981.
10. Janz D. The teratogenic risks of antiepileptic drugs. Epilepsia 1975;16: 159–69.
11. Van der Pol MC, Hadders-Algra M, Huisjes HJ, Touwen BCL. Antiepileptic medication in pregnancy: late effects on the children's central nervous system development. Am J Obstet Gynecol 1991;164:121–8.
12. Hanson JW, Buehler BA. Fetal hydantoin syndrome: current status. J Pediatr 1982;101:816–8.
13. Canger R, Battino D, Canevini MP, Fumarola C, Guidolin L, Vignoli A, Mamoli D, Palmieri C, Molteni F, Granata T, Hassibi P, Zamperini P, Pardi G, Avanzini G. Malformations in offspring of women with epilepsy: a prospective study. Epilepsia 1999;40:1231–6.
14. Holmes LB, Harvey EA, Coull BA, Huntington KB, Khoshbin S, Hayes AM, Ryan LM. The teratogenicity of anticonvulsant drugs. N Engl J Med 2001;344:1132–8.
15. Janz D. Antiepileptic drugs and pregnancy: altered utilization patterns and teratogenesis. Epilepsia 1982;23(Suppl 1):S53–63.
16. Livezey GT, Rayburn WF, Smith CV. Prenatal exposure to phenobarbital and quantifiable alterations in the electroencephalogram of adult rat offspring. Am J Obstet Gynecol 1992;167:1611–5.
17. Gupta C, Sonawane BR, Yaffe SJ, Shapiro BH. Phenobarbital exposure in utero: alterations in female reproductive function in rats. Science 1980;208:508–10.
18. Gupta C, Yaffe SJ, Shapiro BH. Prenatal exposure to phenobarbital permanently decreases testosterone and causes reproductive dysfunction. Science 1982;216:640–2.
19. Gaily E, Kantola-Sorsa E, Granstrom ML. Intelligence of children of epileptic mothers. J Pediatr 1988;113:677–84.
20. Reinisch JM, Sanders SA, Mortensen EL, Rubin DB. In utero exposure to phenobarbital and intelligence deficits in adult men. JAMA 1995;274:1518–25.
21. Dessens AB, Cohen-Kettenis PT, Mellenbergh GJ, Koppe JG, van de Poll NE, Boer K. Association of prenatal phenobarbital and phenytoin exposure with small head size at birth and with learning problems. Acta Paediatr 2000;89:533–41.

22. Koch S, Jager-Roman E, Losche G, Nau H, Rating D, Helge H. Antiepileptic drug treatment in pregnancy: drug side effects in the neonate and neurological outcome. Acta Paediatr 1996;84:739–46.
23. Heinonen OP, Slone D, Shapiro S. *Birth Defects and Drugs in Pregnancy*. Littleton, MA: Publishing Sciences Group, 1977.
24. Hernandez-Diaz S, Werler MM, Walker AM, Mitchell AA. Folic acid antagonists during pregnancy and the risk of birth defects. N Engl J Med 2000;343:1608–14.
25. Rafla NM, Meehan FP. Thanatophoric dwarfism; drugs and antenatal diagnosis; a case report. Eur J Obstet Gynecol Reprod Biol 1990;38:161–5.
26. Arpino C, Brescianini S, Robert E, Castilla EE, Cocchi G, Cornel MC, de Vigan C, Lancaster PAL, Merlob P, Sumiyoshi Y, Zampino G, Renzi C, Rosano A, Mastroiacovo P. Teratogenic effects of antiepileptic drugs: use of an international database on malformations and drug exposure (MADRE). Epilepsia 2000;41:1436–43.
27. The Lamotrigine Pregnancy Registry. Final Report. September 1, 1992 through March 31, 2010. GlaxcoSmithKline, July 2010.
28. Spiedel BD, Meadow SR. Maternal epilepsy and abnormalities of the fetus and the newborn. Lancet 1972;2:839–43.
29. Bleyer WA, Skinner AL. Fatal neonatal hemorrhage after maternal anticonvulsant therapy. JAMA 1976;235:826–7.
30. Lawrence A. Anti-epileptic drugs and the foetus. Br Med J 1963;2:1267.
31. Kohler HG. Haemorrhage in the newborn of epileptic mothers. Lancet 1966;1:267.
32. Mountain KR, Hirsh J, Gallus AS. Neonatal coagulation defect due to anticonvulsant drug treatment in pregnancy. Lancet 1970;1:265–8.
33. Evans AR, Forrester RM, Discombe C. Neonatal haemorrhage during anticonvulsant therapy. Lancet 1970;1:517–8.
34. Margolin FG, Kantor NM. Hemorrhagic disease of the newborn. An unusual case related to maternal ingestion of an anti-epileptic drug. Clin Pediatr (Phila) 1972;11:59–60.
35. Srinivasan G, Seeler RA, Tiruvury A, Pildes RS. Maternal anticonvulsant therapy and hemorrhagic disease of the newborn. Obstet Gynecol 1982;59:250–2.
36. Payne NR, Hasegawa DK. Vitamin K deficiency in newborns: a case report in α-1-antitrypsin deficiency and a review of factors predisposing to hemorrhage. Pediatrics 1984;73:712–6.
37. Lane PA, Hathaway WE. Vitamin K in infancy. J Pediatr 1985;106:351–9.
38. Desmond MM, Schwanecke RP, Wilson GS, Yasunaga S, Burgdorff I. Maternal barbiturate utilization and neonatal withdrawal symptomatology. J Pediatr 1972;80:190–7.
39. Pritchard JA, Scott DE, Whalley PJ. Maternal folate deficiency and pregnancy wastage. IV. Effects of folic acid supplements, anticonvulsants, and oral contraceptives. Am J Obstet Gynecol 1971;109:341–6.
40. Hiilesmaa VK, Teramo K, Granstrom ML, Bardy AH. Serum folate concentrations during pregnancy in women with epilepsy: relation to antiepileptic drug concentrations, number of seizures, and fetal outcome. Br Med J 1983;287:577–9.
41. Biale Y, Lewenthal H. Effect of folic acid supplementation on congenital malformations due to anticonvulsive drugs. Eur J Obstet Reprod Biol 1984;18:211–6.
42. Halbrecht I, Komlos L, Shabtay F, Solomon M, Book JA. Triploidy 69, XXX in a stillborn girl. Clin Genet 1973;4:210–2.
43. Stenchever MA, Jarvis JA. Effect of barbiturates on the chromosomes of human cells in vitro—a negative report. J Reprod Med 1970;5:69–71.
44. Heikkinen J, Maentausta O, Ylostalo P, Janne O. Serum bile acid levels in intrahepatic cholestasis of pregnancy during treatment with phenobarbital or cholestyramine. Eur J Obstet Reprod Biol 1982;14:153–62.
45. Shaw D, Frohlich J, Wittmann BAK, Willms M. A prospective study of 18 patients with cholestasis of pregnancy. Am J Obstet Gynecol 1982;142:621–5.
46. Espinoza J, Barnafi L, Schnaidt E. The effect of phenobarbital on intrahepatic cholestasis of pregnancy. Am J Obstet Gynecol 1974;119:234–8.
47. Valaes T, Kipouros K, Petmezaki S, Solman M, Doxiadis SA. Effectiveness and safety of prenatal phenobarbital for the prevention of neonatal jaundice. Pediatr Res 1980;14:947–52.
48. Morales WJ, Koerten J. Prevention of intraventricular hemorrhage in very low birth weight infants by maternally administered phenobarbital. Obstet Gynecol 1986;68:295–9.
49. Shankaran S, Cepeda EE, Ilagan N, Mariona F, Hassan M, Bhatia R, Ostrea E, Bedard MP, Poland RL. Antenatal phenobarbital for the prevention of neonatal intracerebral hemorrhage. Am J Obstet Gynecol 1986; 154:53–7.
50. De Carolis S, De Carolis MP, Caruso A, Oliva GC, Romagnoli C, Ferrazzani S, Umberto M, Luciano R, Mancuso S. Antenatal phenobarbital in preventing intraventricular hemorrhage in premature newborns. Fetal Ther 1988;3:224–9.
51. Kaempf JW, Porreco R, Molina R, Hale K, Pantoja AF, Rosenberg AA. Antenatal phenobarbital for the prevention of periventricular and intraventricular hemorrhage: a double-blind, randomized, placebo-controlled, multihospital trial. J Pediatr 1990;117:933–8.
52. Thorp JA, Parriott J, Ferrette-Smith D, Holst V, Meyer BA, Cohen GR, Yeast JD, Johnson J, Anderson J. Antepartum vitamin K (VK) and phenobarbital (PB) for preventing intraventricular hemorrhage (IVH) in the premature newborn: a randomized double blind placebo controlled trial (abstract). Am J Obstet Gynecol 1993;168:367.
53. Thorp JA, Parriott J, Ferrette-Smith D, Meyer BA, Cohen GR, Johnson J. Antepartum vitamin K and phenobarbital for preventing intraventricular hemorrhage in the premature newborn: a randomized, double-blind, placebo-controlled trial. Obstet Gynecol 1994;83:70–6.
54. Shankaran S, Cepeda E, Muran G, Mariona F, Johnson S, Kazzi SN, Poland R, Bedard MP. Antenatal phenobarbital therapy and neonatal outcome I: effect on intracranial hemorrhage. Pediatrics 1996;97:644–8.
55. Shankaran S, Papile LA, Wright LL, Ehrenkranz RA, Mele L, Lemons JA, Korones SB, Stevenson DK, Donovan EF, Stoll BJ, Fanaroff AA, Oh W. The effect of antenatal phenobarbital therapy on neonatal intracranial hemorrhage in preterm infants. N Engl J Med 1997;337:466–71.
56. Morales WJ. Antenatal therapy to minimize neonatal intraventricular hemorrhage. Clin Obstet Gynecol 1991;34:328–35.
57. Shankaran S, Woldt E, Nelson J, Bedard M, Delaney-Black V. Antenatal phenobarbital therapy and neonatal outcome II: neurodevelopmental outcome at 36 months. Pediatrics 1996;97:649–52.
58. Thorpe JA, Yeast JD, Cohen GR, Poskin M, Peng V, Hoffman E. Does in-utero phenobarbital lower IQ: follow up of the intracranial hemorrhage prevention trial (abstract). Am J Obstet Gynecol 1997;176:S117.
59. Thorp JA, O'Connor M, Jones AMH, Hoffman EL, Belden B. Does perinatal phenobarbital exposure affect developmental outcome at age 2? Am J Perinatol 1999;16:51–60.
60. Tyson RM, Shrader EA, Perlman HN. Drugs transmitted through breast-milk. II. Barbiturates. J Pediatr 1938;13:86–90.
61. Kaneko S, Sata T, Suzuki K. The levels of anticonvulsants in breast milk. Br J Clin Pharmacol 1979;7:624–7.
62. Nau H, Kuhnz W, Egger HJ, Rating D, Helge H. Anticonvulsants during pregnancy and lactation: transplacental, maternal and neonatal pharmacokinetics. Clin Pharmacokinet 1982;7:508–43.
63. Horning MG, Stillwell WG, Nowlin J, Lertratanangkoon K, Stillwell RN, Hill RM. Identification and quantification of drugs and drug metabolites in human breast milk using GC-MS-COM methods. Mod Probl Paediatr 1975;15:73–9.
64. Reith H, Schafer H. Antiepileptic drugs during pregnancy and the lactation period. Pharmacokinetic data. Dtsch Med Wochenschr 1979;104:818–23.
65. Knott C, Reynolds F, Clayden G. Infantile spasms on weaning from breast milk containing anticonvulsants. Lancet 1987;2:272–3.
66. Committee on Drugs, American Academy of Pediatrics. The transfer of drugs and other chemicals into human breast milk. Pediatrics 2001;108:776–89.

PHENOLPHTHALEIN

[Withdrawn from the market. See 9th edition.]

PHENOXYBENZAMINE

Antihypertensive

PREGNANCY RECOMMENDATION: Compatible—Maternal Benefit >> Embryo–Fetal Risk
BREASTFEEDING RECOMMENDATION: No Human Data—Potential Toxicity

PREGNANCY SUMMARY

The use of phenoxybenzamine during pregnancy to treat hypertension secondary to pheochromocytoma is indicated for the reduction of maternal and fetal mortality, especially after 24 weeks' gestation when surgical intervention is associated with high rates of these outcomes (1). Maternal α-blockade may also reduce or eliminate the adverse effect of hypertension on placental perfusion and subsequent poor fetal growth. No adverse fetal effects related to this drug treatment have been observed, but drug-induced hypotension in a newborn might have occurred.

FETAL RISK SUMMARY

Phenoxybenzamine, a long-acting α-adrenergic blocking agent, is used for the treatment of hypertension caused by pheochromocytoma. Because of the lack of well-controlled studies, the effect of phenoxybenzamine on pregnant animals is not known (B.A. Wallin, personal communication, Smith Kline & French Laboratories, 1987). Animal and in vitro experiments conducted by the manufacturer, however, have indicated that the drug has carcinogenic and mutagenic activity. Neither of these adverse outcomes, nor other fetal harm, has been reported in the relatively few human studies that have been published.

In a study using pregnant rats, phenoxybenzamine, with or without the β-blocker propranolol, had no effect on implantation of the fertilized ovum, nor was there any interference with the antifertility effect of an intrauterine contraceptive device placed in the uterus of rats (2).

One study has evaluated the human transplacental passage of phenoxybenzamine (3). A 22-year-old woman with pheochromocytoma was treated with phenoxybenzamine, 10 mg 3 times daily, and labetalol, 100 mg 3 times daily, for 26 days beginning at 33 weeks' gestation. She received her last dose of phenoxybenzamine 2 hours before delivery. The mean concentrations of the drug in the cord and maternal plasma and in the amniotic fluid were 103.3, 66, and 79.3 ng/mL, respectively, representing a cord:maternal plasma ratio of 1.6. Serum samples for phenoxybenzamine obtained from the infant at 32 and 80 hours of age contained mean concentrations of 22.3 ng/mL and none detected (limit of detection 10 ng/mL), respectively. The 2475-g male infant had depressed respiratory effort and hypotonia at birth and was hypotensive during the first 2 days of life. The cause of the hypotension could not be determined, but may have been caused by both drugs. He subsequently did well and was discharged home 14 days after birth (3).

No reports describing the use of phenoxybenzamine early in the 1st trimester of pregnancy have been located. Early in vitro studies of phenoxybenzamine indicated the drug abolished the *l*-norepinephrine-stimulated contractile activity of animal and human myometrium (4,5). However, a phenoxybenzamine infusion for 3 hours had no significant effect on the uterine activity in two pregnant women (5). One study included the use of phenoxybenzamine for the treatment of essential hypertension, toxemia, and cardiovascular renal disease occurring during pregnancy (4). No adverse fetal effects were observed.

Because of the relative rarity of pheochromocytoma, only a small number of cases have been found in which phenoxybenzamine was used during pregnancy. In 24 pregnancies, phenoxybenzamine administration was begun in the 2nd or 3rd trimesters and continued for periods ranging from 1 day to 35 weeks (1,6–22). Therapy was started at 10 weeks' gestation in a 24th case and continued for approximately 25 weeks when a healthy 2665-g male infant was delivered by cesarean section (23). Eighteen other pregnancies ended with either a cesarean section (N = 14) or vaginal delivery (N = 4) of a healthy infant before resection of the pheochromocytoma. In some of the cases the infant was growth restricted, probably secondary to uncontrolled maternal hypertension before treatment, but all survived. One fetus apparently survived the initial surgery to remove the mother's tumor, but the outcome of the pregnancy was not discussed (18). In another case, phenoxybenzamine was begun at 17 weeks' gestation and continued for 7 days before surgery (1). Following successful tumor resection, the patient's pregnancy went to term and terminated with the vaginal birth of a normal healthy female infant.

Fetal death has been reported in four cases, but only two occurred during pharmacologic therapy of the mother's disease (6,9,16). In one case, fetal death occurred when the mother, in her 5th to 6th month of pregnancy, died 2 days after extensive surgery to remove a metastatic pheochromocytoma (6). Another involved a therapeutic abortion performed at approximately 12 weeks' gestation during the surgical removal of the mother's tumor (16). The third fetal loss involved a woman whose pheochromocytoma was diagnosed at 7 months' gestation. Therapy with phenoxybenzamine was begun, but the fetus died in utero (details of therapy were not given) (16). In the fourth case, a 15-year-old patient at 25.5 weeks' gestation was treated for 3 days with oral phenoxybenzamine in preparation for surgery. On the 3rd day of therapy, her membranes spontaneously ruptured followed by a hypertensive crisis requiring a phentolamine infusion. A spontaneous abortion occurred shortly thereafter of a severely growth-restricted fetus (9).

The low incidences of maternal (4%; 1 of 24) and fetal (9%; 2 of 22) mortality when α-blockade with phenoxybenzamine is used is much better than the mortality observed in undiagnosed pheochromocytoma complicating pregnancy. A 1971 review of 89 cases of unsuspected tumor found that maternal and fetal mortality rates were 48% and 54.4%, respectively (24). A more recent review cited incidences of maternal and fetal mortality without α-blockade of 9% and 50%, respectively (20). When all cases of α-blockade (i.e., those receiving phenoxybenzamine, phentolamine, or both) administered during pregnancy were considered, maternal mortality was 3% (1 of 29) and fetal loss was 19% (5 of 27) (2 cases were excluded because fetal death in utero had occurred at the time of diagnosis) (20).

Long-term follow-up of infants exposed in utero to phenoxybenzamine has only been reported in three cases (8,11,14). The follow-up periods ranged from 2 to 8 years, and all three were normal healthy children.

BREASTFEEDING SUMMARY

No reports describing the use of phenoxybenzamine during human lactation have been located. The molecular weight of the drug (about 340) is low enough that excretion into breast milk should be expected. The potential effects of this exposure on a nursing infant, including but not limited to, hypotension are unknown.

References

1. Combs CA, Easterling TR, Schmucker BC, Benedetti TJ. Hemodynamic observations during paroxysmal hypertension in a pregnancy with pheochromocytoma. Obstet Gynecol 1989;74:439–41.
2. Sethi A, Chaudhury RR. Effect of adrenergic receptor-blocking drugs in pregnancy in rats. J Reprod Fertil 1970;21:551–4.
3. Santeiro ML, Stromquist C, Wyble L. Phenoxybenzamine placental transfer during the third trimester. Ann Pharmacother 1996;30:1249–51.
4. Maughan GB, Shabanah EH, Toth A. Experiments with pharmacologic sympatholysis in the gravid. Am J Obstet Gynecol 1967;97:764–76.
5. Wansbrough H, Nakanishi H, Wood C. The effect of adrenergic receptor blocking drugs on the human uterus. J Obstet Gynaecol Br Commonw 1968;75:189–98.
6. Brown RB, Borowsky M. Further observations on intestinal lesions associated with pheochromocytomas. A case of malignant pheochromocytoma in pregnancy. Ann Surg 1960;151:683–92.
7. Lawee D. Pheochromocytoma associated with pregnancy. Can Med Assoc J 1970;103:1185–7.
8. Simanis J, Amerson JR, Hendee AE, Anton AH. Unresectable pheochromocytoma in pregnancy. Pharmacology and biochemistry. Am J Med 1972;53:381–5.
9. Brenner WE, Yen SSC, Dingfelder JR, Anton AH. Pheochromocytoma: serial studies during pregnancy. Am J Obstet Gynecol 1972;113:779–88.
10. Smith AM. Phaeochromocytoma and pregnancy. J Obstet Gynaecol Br Commonw 1973;80:848–51.
11. Griffith MI, Felts JH, James FM, Meyers RT, Shealy GM, Woodruff LF Jr. Successful control of pheochromocytoma in pregnancy. JAMA 1974;229:437–9.
12. Awitti-Sunga SA, Ursell W. Phaeochromocytoma in pregnancy. Case report. Br J Obstet Gynaecol 1975;82:426–8.
13. Coombes GB. Phaeochromocytoma presenting in pregnancy. Proc R Soc Med 1976;69:224–5.
14. Leak D, Carroll JJ, Robinson DC, Ashworth EJ. Management of pheochromocytoma during pregnancy. Can Med Assoc J 1977;116:371–5.
15. Burgess GE III. Alpha blockade and surgical intervention of pheochromocytoma in pregnancy. Obstet Gynecol 1979;53:266–70.
16. Modlin IM, Farndon JR, Shepherd A, Johnston IDA, Kennedy TL, Montgomery DAD, Welbourn RB. Phaeochromocytomas in 72 patients: clinical and diagnostic features, treatment and long term results. Br J Surg 1979;66:456–65.
17. Fudge TL, McKinnon WMP, Geary WL. Current surgical management of pheochromocytoma during pregnancy. Arch Surg 1980;115:1224–5.
18. Coetzee A, Hartwig N, Erasmus FR. Feochromositoom tydens swangerskap. Die narkosehantering van 'n pasient. S Afr Med J 1981;59:861–2.
19. Stonham J, Wakefield C. Phaeochromocytoma in pregnancy: caesarean section under epidural analgesia. Anaesthesia 1983;38:654–8.
20. Stenstrom G, Swolin K. Pheochromocytoma in pregnancy. Experience of treatment with phenoxybenzamine in three patients. Acta Obstet Gynecol Scand 1985;64:357–61.
21. Bakri YN, Ingemansson SE, Ali A, Parikh S. Pheochromocytoma and pregnancy: report of three cases. Acta Obstet Gynecol Scand 1992;71:301–4.
22. Miller C, Bernet V, Elkas JC, Dainty L, Gherman RB. Conservative management of extra-adrenal pheochromocytoma during pregnancy. Obstet Gynecol 2005;105:1185–8.
23. Lyons CW, Colmorgen GHC. Medical management of pheochromocytoma in pregnancy. Obstet Gynecol 1988;72:450–1.
24. Schenker JG, Chowers I. Pheochromocytoma and pregnancy. Review of 89 cases. Obstet Gynecol Surv 1971;26:739–47.

PHENPROCOUMON

Anticoagulant

See Coumarin Derivatives.

PHENSUXIMIDE

[Withdrawn from the market. See 9th edition.]

PHENTERMINE

Anorexiant

PREGNANCY RECOMMENDATION: Contraindicated
BREASTFEEDING RECOMMENDATION: Contraindicated

PREGNANCY SUMMARY

It is doubtful if any real benefit is derived from the use of phentermine for weight control during pregnancy, and its use during gestation, especially during the 1st trimester, should be considered contraindicated. Moreover, although the causes of the stillbirths cited in one human study were not fully elucidated and may not have been caused by maternal phentermine treatment, the high incidence is disturbing and is another reason to withhold use of the drug during pregnancy.

FETAL RISK SUMMARY

Phentermine (phenyl-tertiary-butylamine) is a sympathomimetic amine that has activity as a CNS stimulant. Similar to other drugs in this class, such as the amphetamines, it is used as an appetite suppressant in the treatment of obesity. In addition to other adverse effects, hypertension has occurred in adults treated with this agent.

Reproduction studies in animals with phentermine have not been conducted. A closely related compound, chlorphentermine (30 mg/kg/day SC), was administered to pregnant rats during the last 5 days of gestation (1). Phospholipidosis was evident in the lungs of the mothers and the newborn rats, and 83% of the latter died within 24 hours of birth. Another group treated with phentermine (30 mg/kg/day SC) in a similar manner did not develop the complication and did not die. A subsequent reference suggested that the chlorphentermine-induced pup mortality was consistent with retardation of fetal pulmonary maturity (2).

No studies have been located that described the placental transfer of phentermine in animals or humans. The molecular weight (about 186) is low enough that exposure of the embryo–fetus should be expected.

A study published in 1962 described the use of phentermine in 118 women who were treated for obesity during the 3rd trimester of pregnancy up to delivery (3). Women weighing <200 pounds were given 30 mg each morning, whereas those >200 pounds were given 30 mg twice daily. The weights of the patients before treatment ranged from 180 to 315 pounds. Adverse outcomes occurred in five women with stillborn infants, one of whom was caused by abruptio placentae. The cause of the other stillborns, whose weights ranged from 9 to 10 pounds, was not mentioned, other than the statement that one mother had mild preeclampsia.

As of 1997, the FDA had received two reports involving the use of the combination, fenfluramine and phentermine, in early pregnancy (F. Rosa, personal communication, FDA, 1997). A spontaneous abortion occurred in one of the pregnancies. In the other, an infant with bilateral valvular abnormalities, both aortic and pulmonary, with moderate stenosis and displacement was born. Because valvular toxicity has been reported in adults taking the combination, a causal relationship in the pregnancy case is potentially possible. No other details of these cases were available.

A 2002 controlled prospective cohort study compared 98 women who had taken phentermine/fenfluramine for weight loss (product withdrawn in 1997) during portions or all of the 1st trimester with 233 nonteratogen-exposed controls (4). About 88% of the subjects had begun the drug combination before conception and the remainder started after conception. The phentermine and fenfluramine daily doses ranged 15–45 mg and 20–60 mg, respectively. Most (96%) stopped the drug combination before the 12th week of gestation. In the two groups, 71% and 65% of the liveborn infants were examined by a dysmorphologist for the presence of major or minor malformations who was blinded to the exposures. There were no statistical differences between the groups in terms of major malformations or ≥3 or more minor malformations, spontaneous abortions, elective abortions, ectopic pregnancies, or preterm delivery. No pattern of malformations was identified. The increased rate of gestational diabetes (11% vs. 4%, $p = 0.05$) probably reflects the significantly greater prepregnancy body weight and pregnancy weight gain of exposed subjects. The significantly higher mean birth weight and head circumference in full-term infants of subjects were most likely due to the significantly greater mean prepregnancy body weight and weight gain during pregnancy of their mothers as well as to the increased rate of gestational diabetes (4).

BREASTFEEDING SUMMARY

No reports describing the use of phentermine during lactation have been located. The molecular weight (about 186) is low enough that excretion of phentermine into breast milk should be expected. Because CNS stimulation and other adverse reactions may occur in a nursing infant exposed to this drug in milk, breastfeeding should be considered a contraindication if the mother is taking phentermine.

References

1. Thoma-Laurie D, Walker ER, Reasor MJ. Neonatal toxicity in rats following in utero exposure to chlorphentermine or phentermine. Toxicology 1982;24:85–94.
2. Kacew S, Reasor MJ. Newborn response to cationic amphiphilic drugs. Fed Proc 1985;44:2323–7.
3. Sands RX. Obesity and pregnancy. Weight control with a resinate. Am J Obstet Gynecol 1962;83:1617–21.
4. Jones KL, Johnson KA, Dick LM, Felix RJ, Kao KK, Chambers CD. Pregnancy outcomes after first trimester exposure to phentermine/fenfluramine. Teratology 2002;65:125–30.

PHENTOLAMINE

Antihypertensive

PREGNANCY RECOMMENDATION: Compatible—Maternal Benefit >> Embryo–Fetal Risk
BREASTFEEDING RECOMMENDATION: No Human Data—Potential Toxicity

PREGNANCY SUMMARY

Phentolamine has been used for the short-term management of severe hypertension caused by pheochromocytoma, including those cases occurring during surgery to deliver a fetus or to resect the tumor (1–4). No adverse effects on the fetus or newborn attributable to phentolamine from this use have been reported, but fetal hypoxia is a potential complication.

FETAL RISK SUMMARY

Phentolamine, a short-acting α-adrenergic blocker, is used for the treatment of severe hypertension secondary to maternal pheochromocytoma. Animal studies with phentolamine have observed neither teratogenicity nor embryotoxicity (5). No reports of adverse fetal outcome in humans have been located, but 1st trimester experience with this agent has not been documented, nor have studies describing the placental transfer of phentolamine in humans been found. However, although apparently not teratogenic, phentolamine must be used with caution because of the marked decrease in maternal blood pressure that can occur with resulting fetal anoxia.

Early in vitro and in vivo investigations of phentolamine indicated the drug inhibited the *l*-norepinephrine-stimulated contractile activity of human myometrium (6–8). A 1971 investigation examined the effect of combined α-adrenergic blockade (phentolamine) and β-adrenergic stimulation (isoxsuprine) on oxytocin-stimulated uterine activity in six women just before undergoing therapeutic abortion at 16–20 weeks' gestation (9). The results indicated that phentolamine had no effect on uterine activity, while isoxsuprine inhibited uterine contractions. Moreover, the uterine inhibitory effect of β-stimulation was independent of α-blockade.

In one study, phentolamine was used for approximately 10 weeks for the treatment of toxemia (6). No adverse effects in the fetus were observed and the infant was alive and well at 18 months. The authors commented that they had stopped using phentolamine for this purpose because prolonged use in a few cases had resulted in "jitters" in the newborns, especially in premature infants (6).

The most common use of phentolamine in pregnancy is for the diagnosis of pheochromocytoma. Administration of phentolamine to patients with this disease causes a marked drop in blood pressure. Because of the drug's very short half-life (19 minutes), the return to the pretest blood pressures usually occurs in <30 minutes (5). A 1971 review article of pheochromocytoma in pregnancy cited 22 cases of the disease identified in 1955–1966 in which the diagnosis was made during pregnancy with phentolamine (10). Three additional cases were published in 1969 (11) and 1973 (12). Reflecting the high maternal and fetal mortality that can occur with this disease, 21% (3 of 14) of the mothers and 43% (6 of 14) of the fetuses died.

BREASTFEEDING SUMMARY

No reports describing the use of phentolamine during human lactation have been located. Because of its indication, it is unlikely that such reports will appear. Moreover, the drug has a very short half-life (19 minutes), so if it is used in a lactating woman, waiting a few hours and then pumping and discarding the milk should prevent exposure of a nursing infant.

References

1. Anton AH, Brenner WE, Yen SS, Dingfelder JR. Pheochromocytoma: studies during pregnancy, premature delivery and surgery. Presented at the 5th International Congress on Pharmacology, July 23–28, 1972, San Francisco, CA, Abstract No. 43, 8.
2. Simanis J, Amerson JR, Hendee AE, Anton AH. Unresectable pheochromocytoma in pregnancy. Pharmacology and biochemistry. Am J Med 1972;53:381–5.
3. Brenner WE, Yen SSC, Dingfelder JR, Anton AH. Pheochromocytoma: serial studies during pregnancy. Am J Obstet Gynecol 1972;113: 779–88.
4. Burgess GE III. Alpha blockade and surgical intervention of pheochromocytoma in pregnancy. Obstet Gynecol 1979;53:266–70.
5. Product information. Regitine. Ciba-Geigy Corporation, 1991.
6. Maughan GB, Shabanah EH, Toth A. Experiments with pharmacologic sympatholysis in the gravid. Am J Obstet Gynecol 1967;97:764–76.
7. Wansbrough H, Nakanishi H, Wood C. The effect of adrenergic receptor blocking drugs on the human uterus. J Obstet Gynaecol Br Commonw 1968;75:189–98.
8. Althabe O Jr, Schwarcz RL Jr, Sala NL, Fisch L. Effect of phentolamine methanesulfonate upon uterine contractility induced by l-norepinephrine in pregnancy. Am J Obstet Gynecol 1968;101:1083–8.
9. Jenssen H. Inhibition of oxytocin-induced uterine activity in midpregnancy by combined adrenergic α-blockade and β-stimulation. Acta Obstet Gynecol Scand 1971;50:135–9.
10. Schenker JG, Chowers I. Pheochromocytoma and pregnancy. Review of 89 cases. Obstet Gynecol Surv 1971;26:739–47.
11. Hendee AE, Martin RD, Waters WC III. Hypertension in pregnancy: toxemia or pheochromocytoma? Am J Obstet Gynecol 1969;105:64–72.
12. Smith AM. Phaeochromocytoma and pregnancy. J Obstet Gynaecol Br Commonw 1973;80:848–51.

PHENYLBUTAZONE

[Withdrawn from the market. See 9th edition.]

PHENYLEPHRINE

Sympathomimetic (Adrenergic)

PREGNANCY RECOMMENDATION: Human Data Suggest Risk
BREASTFEEDING RECOMMENDATION: No Human Data—Probably Compatible

PREGNANCY SUMMARY

Phenylephrine is a sympathomimetic used in emergency situations to treat hypotension and to alleviate allergic symptoms of the eye and ear. Uterine vessels are normally maximally dilated and they have only α-adrenergic receptors (1). Use of the predominantly α-adrenergic stimulant, phenylephrine, could cause constriction of these vessels and reduce uterine blood flow, thereby producing fetal hypoxia (bradycardia). Phenylephrine may also interact with oxytocics or ergot derivatives to produce severe persistent maternal hypertension (1). Rupture of a cerebral vessel is possible. If a pressor agent is indicated, other drugs such as ephedrine should be considered. Sympathomimetic amines are teratogenic in some animal species, but human teratogenicity has not been suspected (2,3).

FETAL RISK SUMMARY

No studies describing the placental passage of phenylephrine have been located. The molecular weight (about 167) of the drug is low enough that exposure of the embryo–fetus should be expected.

The Collaborative Perinatal Project monitored 50,282 mother–child pairs, 1249 of whom had 1st trimester exposure to phenylephrine (4, pp. 345–356). For use anytime during pregnancy, 4194 exposures were recorded (4, p. 439). An association was found between 1st trimester use of phenylephrine and malformations; association with minor defects was greater than with major defects (4, pp. 345–356). For individual malformations, several possible associations were found (4, pp. 345–356, 476, 491):

- 1st trimester
  - Eye and ear (8 cases)
  - Syndactyly (6 cases)
  - Preauricular skin tag (4 cases)
  - Clubfoot (3 cases)
- Anytime use
  - Congenital dislocation of hip (15 cases)
  - Other musculoskeletal defects (4 cases)
  - Umbilical hernia (6 cases)

Independent confirmation of these findings is required. For the sympathomimetic class of drugs as a whole, an association was found between 1st trimester use and minor malformations (not life-threatening or major cosmetic defects), inguinal hernia, and clubfoot (4, pp. 345–356).

Sympathomimetics are often administered in combination with other drugs to alleviate the symptoms of upper respiratory infections. Thus, the fetal effects of sympathomimetics, other drugs, and viruses cannot be totally separated. However, indiscriminate use of this class of drugs, especially in the 1st trimester, is not without risk.

Phenylephrine has been used as a stress test to determine fetal status in high-risk pregnancies (5). In the United States, however, this test is normally conducted with oxytocin.

BREASTFEEDING SUMMARY

No reports describing the use of phenylephrine during human lactation have been located. The molecular weight (about 167) of the drug is low enough that passage into breast milk should be expected. The effect of this exposure on a nursing infant is unknown.

References

1. Smith NT, Corbascio AN. The use and misuse of pressor agents. Anesthesiology 1970;33:58–101.
2. Nashimura H, Tanimura T. *Clinical Aspects of the Teratogenicity of Drugs*. Amsterdam, Netherlands: Excerpta Medica, 1976:231.
3. Shepard TH. *Catalog of Teratogenic Agents*. 3rd ed. Baltimore, MD: The Johns Hopkins University Press, 1980:134–5.
4. Heinonen OP, Slone D, Shapiro S. *Birth Defects and Drugs in Pregnancy*. Littleton, MA: Publishing Sciences Group, 1977.
5. Eguchi K, Yonezawa M, Hagegawa T, Lin TT, Ejiri K, Kudo T, Sekiba K, Takeda Y. Fetal activity determination and Neo-Synephrine test for evaluation of fetal well-being in high risk pregnancies. Nippon Sank Fujinka Gakkai Zasshi 1980;32:663–8.

PHENYLPROPANOLAMINE

[Withdrawn from the market. See 9th edition.]

PHENYLTOLOXAMINE

Antihistamine

PREGNANCY RECOMMENDATION: No Human Data—No Relevant Animal Data
BREASTFEEDING RECOMMENDATION: No Human Data—Probably Compatible

PREGNANCY SUMMARY

No reports describing the use of phenyltoloxamine in human pregnancy have been located. In general, antihistamines are considered low risk in pregnancy. However, exposure near birth of premature infants has been associated with an increased risk of retrolental fibroplasia.

FETAL RISK SUMMARY

It is not known if phenyltoloxamine crosses the human placenta. The molecular weight (about 448 for phenyltoloxamine citrate) is low enough that exposure of the embryo–fetus should be expected.

An association between exposure during the last 2 weeks of pregnancy to antihistamines in general and retrolental fibroplasia in premature infants has been reported. See Brompheniramine for details.

BREASTFEEDING SUMMARY

No reports describing the use of phenyltoloxamine during human lactation have been located. The molecular weight (about 448 for phenyltoloxamine citrate) is low enough for excretion into breast milk.

PHENYTOIN

Anticonvulsant

PREGNANCY RECOMMENDATION: Compatible—Maternal Benefit >> Embryo–Fetal Risk
BREASTFEEDING RECOMMENDATION: Compatible

PREGNANCY SUMMARY

The use of phenytoin during pregnancy involves significant risk to the fetus in terms of major and minor congenital abnormalities and hemorrhage at birth. Adverse effects on neurodevelopment have also been reported. The risk to the mother, however, is also great if the drug is not used to control her seizures. The risk:benefit ratio, in this case, favors continued use of the drug during pregnancy. Frequent determinations of phenytoin levels are recommended to maintain the lowest level required to prevent seizures and possibly to lessen the likelihood of fetal anomalies. Based on recent research, consideration should also be given to monitoring folic acid levels simultaneously with phenytoin determinations and administering folic acid very early in pregnancy or before conception to those women shown to have low folate concentrations. Alternatively, adding folic acid, such as 4–5 mg/day (the dose recommended for women with a history of a fetus or infant with a neural tube defect [NTD]), should be considered.

FETAL RISK SUMMARY

Phenytoin is a hydantoin anticonvulsant introduced in 1938. The teratogenic effects of phenytoin were recognized in 1964 (1). Since this report there have been numerous reviews and studies on the teratogenic effects of phenytoin and other anticonvulsants. Based on this literature, the epileptic pregnant woman taking phenytoin, either alone or in combination with other anticonvulsants, has a 2–3 times greater risk for delivering a child with congenital defects over the general population (2–9).

It was not always known whether this increased risk was caused by antiepileptic drugs, the disease itself, genetic factors, or a combination of these, although past evidence indicated that drugs were the causative factor. Fifteen epidemiologic studies cited by reviewers in 1982 found an incidence of defects in treated epileptics varying from 2.2% to 26.1% (9). In each case, the rate for treated patients was higher than for untreated epileptics or normal controls. Animal studies have also implicated drugs and have suggested that a dose-related response may occur (9). Two studies cited below provide further evidence that the congenital defects observed in the offspring of epileptic mothers treated with anticonvulsants are caused by drugs.

A prospective study published in 1999 described the outcomes of 517 pregnancies of epileptic mothers identified at one Italian center from 1977 (10). Excluding genetic and chromosomal defects, malformations were classified as severe structural defects, mild structural defects, and deformations. Minor anomalies were not considered. Spontaneous (N = 38) and early (N = 20) voluntary abortions were excluded from the analysis, as were seven pregnancies that delivered at other hospitals. Of the remaining 452 outcomes, 427 were exposed to anticonvulsants of which 313 involved monotherapy: phenytoin (N = 31), carbamazepine (N = 113), phenobarbital (N = 83), valproate (N = 44), primidone (N = 35), clonazepam (N = 6), and other (N = 1). There were no defects in the 25 pregnancies not exposed to anticonvulsants. Of the 42 (9.3%) outcomes with malformations, 24 (5.3%) were severe, 10 (2.2%) were mild, and 8 (1.8%) were deformities. There were three malformations with phenytoin monotherapy: none were severe, one (3.2%) was mild (umbilical hernia), and two (6.4%) deformations (clubfoot and hip dislocation). The investigators concluded that the anticonvulsants were the primary risk factor for an increased incidence of congenital malformations (see also Carbamazepine, Clonazepam, Phenobarbital, Primidone, and Valproic Acid) (10).

A prospective cohort study, conducted from 1986 to 1993 at five maternity hospitals, was designed to determine if anticonvulsant agents or other factors (e.g., genetic) were responsible for the constellation of abnormalities seen in infants of mothers treated with anticonvulsants during pregnancy (11). A total of 128,049 pregnant women were screened at delivery for exposure to anticonvulsant drugs. Three groups of singleton infants were identified: (a) exposed to anticonvulsant drugs, (b) not exposed to anticonvulsant drugs but with a maternal history of seizures, and (c) not exposed to anticonvulsant drugs and with no maternal history of seizures (control group). After applying exclusion criteria, including exposure to other teratogens, 316, 98, and 508 infants, respectively, were analyzed. Anticonvulsant monotherapy occurred in 223 women: phenytoin (N = 87), phenobarbital (N = 64), carbamazepine (N = 58), and too few cases for analysis with valproic acid, clonazepam, diazepam, and lorazepam. Ninety-three infants were exposed to two or more anticonvulsant drugs. All infants were examined systematically (blinded as to group in 93% of the cases) for embryopathy associated with anticonvulsant exposure (major malformations, hypoplasia of the midface and fingers, microcephaly, and intrauterine growth restriction). Compared with controls, significant associations between anticonvulsants and anticonvulsant embryopathy were as follows: phenytoin monotherapy 20.7% (18/87), phenobarbital monotherapy 26.6% (17/64), any monotherapy 20.6% (46/223), exposed to ≥2 anticonvulsants 28.0% (26/93), and all infants exposed to anticonvulsants (monotherapy and polytherapy) 22.8% (72/316). Nonsignificant associations were found for carbamazepine monotherapy 13.8% (8/58), nonexposed infants with a maternal history of seizures 6.1% (6/98), and controls 8.5% (43/508). The investigators concluded that the distinctive pattern of physical abnormalities observed in infants exposed to anticonvulsants during gestation was due to the drugs, rather than to epilepsy itself (11).

A study published in 1990 provided evidence that, at least in some cases, the teratogenic effects of phenytoin are secondary to elevated levels of oxidative metabolites (epoxides) (12). Epoxides are normally eliminated by the enzyme epoxide hydrolase, but in some individuals, low activity of this enzyme is present. By measuring the enzyme's activity in a number of subjects, the investigators proposed a trimodal distribution that is regulated by a single gene with two allelic forms. The three phenotypes proposed were: low activity (homozygous for the recessive allele), intermediate activity (heterozygous), and high activity (homozygous for the dominant allele). In the prospective portion of the study, 19 pregnant women with epilepsy, who were being treated with phenytoin monotherapy, had an amniocentesis performed and the microsomal epoxide hydrolase activity in amniocytes was determined. Four of the 19 had low activity (<30% of standard), whereas 15 had normal activity (>30% of standard). As predicted, only the four fetuses with low activity had clinical evidence of the fetal hydantoin syndrome (FHS) (12).

In contrast to the above study, a 1999 study with mice involving fluconazole and phenytoin was unable to provide support for the theory that toxic intermediates, such as epoxides, were the cause of phenytoin-induced congenital defects (13). Because fluconazole inhibits the cytochrome P450 pathway responsible for phenytoin metabolism, the authors of this study reasoned that the drug combination could provide a test of the hypothesis. Pretreatment of mice with a nonembryotoxic fluconazole dose, however, significantly doubled (from 6.2% to 13.3%) the incidence of phenytoin-induced cleft palate. Administering both drugs closely together significantly increased the incidence of resorptions but not malformations. This lack of effect on malformations may have been related to the increased embryolethality of the combination. The mechanism for the teratologic interaction between the drugs was unknown (13).

In a surveillance study of Michigan Medicaid recipients involving 229,101 completed pregnancies conducted between 1985 and 1992, 332 newborns had been exposed to phenytoin during the 1st trimester (F. Rosa, personal communication, FDA, 1993). A total of 15 (4.5%) major birth defects were observed (13 expected), including (observed/expected) 5/3 cardiovascular defects, 1/0 spina bifida, and 1/1 hypospadias. No anomalies were observed in three other defect categories (oral clefts, polydactyly, and limb reduction defects) for which specific data were available.

A recognizable pattern of malformations, now known as the FHS, was partially described in 1968 when Meadow (14) observed distinct facial abnormalities in infants exposed to phenytoin and other anticonvulsants. In 1973, two groups of investigators, in independent reports, described unusual anomalies of the fingers and toes in exposed infants (15,16). The basic syndrome consists of variable degrees of hypoplasia and ossification of the distal phalanges and craniofacial abnormalities. Clinical features of the FHS, not all of which are apparent in every infant, are as follows (14–16):

- Craniofacial
  - Broad nasal bridge
  - Wide fontanelle
  - Low-set hairline
  - Broad alveolar ridge
  - Metopic ridging
  - Short neck
  - Ocular hypertelorism
  - Microcephaly
  - Cleft lip and/or palate
  - Abnormal or low-set ears

Epicanthal folds
Ptosis of eyelids
Coloboma
Coarse scalp hair

Limbs
Small or absent nails
Hypoplasia of distal phalanges
Altered palmar crease
Digital thumb
Dislocated hip

Impaired growth (physical and mental) and congenital heart defects are often observed in conjunction with FHS.

Numerous other defects have been reported to occur after phenytoin exposure in pregnancy. Janz, in a 1982 review (17), stated that nearly all possible types of malformations may be observed in the offspring of epileptic mothers. This statement is supported by the large volume of literature describing various anomalies that have been attributed to phenytoin with or without other anticonvulsants (1–9,14–58).

In one of the above cases the mother took phenytoin (300 mg/day) during the first 7 months of gestation and phenobarbital (90 mg/day) during the last 2 months (54). The full-term female infant had features of FHS (hypoplastic nails and flat nasal bridge), hydrocephalus, a left porencephalic cyst, and an encephalocele. She died at 2.5 months of age of bronchopneumonia. An autopsy of the brain revealed both gross and microscopic abnormalities. The defects were consistent with changes produced early in fetal development and with tissue destruction resulting in the second half of gestation (54).

A possible association between phenytoin and the rare defect, holoprosencephaly, was reported in 1993 (56). Because of psychomotor and petit mal seizures, the mother was treated with phenytoin (350 mg/day) and primidone (500 mg/day) during gestation. Except for microcephaly, fetal sonography detected no pathology. The female infant was born after 36 weeks of gestation with both weight and length above the 50th percentile. The Apgar scores were 3, 9, and 10 at 1, 5, and 10 minutes, respectively. The occipitofrontal head circumference (31 cm) was below the 25th percentile. Malformations evident on examination were microcephaly, narrow forehead, hypertelorism, hypoplastic midface with anteverted nostrils, smooth philtrum, and thin vermillion border lip. Distal phalanges and nails on all fingers and toes were noted to be hypoplastic. A sacral dimple was also noted. Ultrasound examination revealed a right-sided renal duplication, hepatomegaly, a mild ventricular septal defect, and bilateral hip dysplasia. An electroencephalogram revealed significantly delayed visual-evoked potentials. A partial lobar holoprosencephaly with ventral fusion of the cerebral hemispheres was noted on magnetic resonance imaging of the brain. Coarse gyri and horizontal cleavage, but no sagittal cleavage, was noted in the frontal lobe. The corpus callosum was absent. Although both parents suffered from epilepsy, there was no consanguinity and the infant's karyotype was normal (46,XX), thus a genetic cause of the holoprosencephaly was thought to be unlikely (56).

Authors of correspondence relating to the above report noted that they had also identified a case of holoprosencephaly in a stillborn infant exposed in utero to anticonvulsants (59). Unfortunately, the clinical examination did not record the presence or absence of minor physical features characteristic of the FHS. Based on their experience, however, establishing an association between phenytoin and the defect would be very difficult because of the infrequent in utero exposure to anticonvulsants (1:250 births), the even lower frequency of exposure to phenytoin monotherapy (1:844 births), and the rarity of holoprosencephaly (1:10,000) (59).

Thanatophoric dwarfism was found in a stillborn infant exposed throughout gestation to phenytoin (200 mg/day), phenobarbital (300 mg/day), and amitriptyline (>150 mg/day) (60). The cause of the malformation could not be determined, but drug and genetic causes were considered.

A 2000 study, using data from the MADRE (an acronym for malformation and drug exposure) surveillance project, assessed the human teratogenicity of anticonvulsants (61). Among 8005 malformed infants, cases were defined as infants with a specific malformation, whereas controls were infants with other anomalies. Of the total group, 299 were exposed in the 1st trimester to anticonvulsants. Among these, exposure to monotherapy occurred in the following: phenytoin (N = 24), phenobarbital (N = 65), mephobarbital (N = 10), carbamazepine (N = 46), valproic acid (N = 80), and other agents (N = 16). No statistically significant associations were found with phenytoin monotherapy or polytherapy. Although the study confirmed some previously known associations, several new associations with anticonvulsants were discovered that require independent confirmation (see also Carbamazepine, Mephobarbital, Phenobarbital, and Valproic Acid) (61).

The Lamotrigine Pregnancy Registry, an ongoing project conducted by the manufacturer, was first published in January 1997. The final report was published in July 2010 (62). The Registry is now closed. Among 68 prospectively enrolled pregnancies exposed to phenytoin and lamotrigine, with or without other anticonvulsants, 62 were exposed in the 1st trimester resulting in 56 live births, 1 birth defect, 1 spontaneous abortion, and 4 elective abortions. There were six exposures in the 2nd/3rd trimesters resulting in six live births without birth defects (62).

Twelve case reports have been located that, taken in sum, suggest phenytoin is a human transplacental carcinogen (18–28,63). Tumors reported to occur in infants after in utero exposure to phenytoin include the following:

Neuroblastoma (6 cases) (18–22,63)
Ganglioneuroblastoma (1 case) (23)
Melanotic neuroectodermal tumor (1 case) (24)
Extrarenal Wilms' tumor (1 case) (25)
Mesenchymoma (1 case) (26)
Lymphangioma (1 case) (27)
Ependymoblastoma (1 case) (28)

Children exposed in utero to phenytoin should be closely observed for several years because tumor development may take that long to express itself. A 1989 study, however, found no in utero exposures to phenytoin among 188 cases of childhood neuroblastoma diagnosed between 1969 and 1988 at their center (64). But the investigators did conclude that an increased risk of the neoplasm in children with FHS was still a possibility.

Phenytoin and other anticonvulsants (e.g., phenobarbital) may cause early hemorrhagic disease of the newborn (18,65–79). Hemorrhage occurs during the first 24 hours after birth and may be severe or even fatal. The exact mechanism of the defect is unknown but may involve phenytoin induction of fetal liver microsomal enzymes that deplete the already low reserves of fetal vitamin K (79). This results in suppression of the vitamin K-dependent coagulation factors II, VII, IX, and X. Phenytoin-induced thrombocytopenia has also been reported as a mechanism for hemorrhage in the newborn (76). A 1985 review summarized the various prophylactic treatment regimens that have been proposed (79):

Administering 10 mg of oral vitamin K daily during the last 2 months of pregnancy
Administering 20 mg of oral vitamin K daily during the last 2 weeks of pregnancy
Avoiding salicylates and administering vitamin K during labor
Cesarean section if a difficult or traumatic delivery is anticipated
Administering IV vitamin K to the newborn in the delivery room plus cord blood clotting studies

Although all of the above suggestions are logical, none has been tested in controlled trials. The reviewers recommended immediate IM vitamin K and close observation of the infant (see also Phytonadione) (79).

Of interest, a 1995 study suggested that anticonvulsant-induced vitamin K deficiency may be the mechanism that causes the maxillonasal hypoplasia seen in the FHS (80). They proposed early vitamin K supplementation of at-risk pregnancies to prevent this disfiguring malformation.

Liver damage was observed in an infant exposed during gestation to phenytoin and valproic acid (81). Although they were unable to demonstrate which anticonvulsant caused the injury, the authors concluded that valproic acid was the more likely offending agent.

Phenytoin may induce folic acid deficiency in the epileptic patient by impairing gastrointestinal absorption or by increasing hepatic metabolism of the vitamin (82–84). Whether phenytoin also induces folic acid deficiency in the fetus is less certain because the fetus seems to be efficient in drawing on available maternal stores of folic acid (see Folic Acid). Low maternal folate levels, however, have been proposed as one possible mechanism for the increased incidence of defects observed in infants exposed in utero to phenytoin. In a 1984 report, two investigators studied the relationship between folic acid, anticonvulsants, and fetal defects (82). In the retrospective part of this study, a group of 24 women treated with phenytoin and other anticonvulsants produced 66 infants, 10 (15%) with major anomalies. Two of the mothers with affected infants had markedly low red blood cell folate concentrations. A second group of 22 epileptic women was then supplemented with daily folic acid, 2.5–5.0 mg, starting before conception in 26 pregnancies and within the first 40 days in 6. This group produced 33 newborns (32 pregnancies—1 set of twins) with no defects, a significant difference from the nonsupplemented group. Loss of seizure control caused by folic acid lowering of phenytoin serum levels, which is known to occur, was not a problem in this small series (82).

Negative associations between phenytoin and folate deficiency have been reported (83,84). In one study, mothers were given supplements with an average folic acid dose of 0.5 mg/day from the 6th to 16th week of gestation until delivery (84). Defects were observed in 20 infants (15%) from the 133 women taking anticonvulsants, which is similar to the reported frequency in pregnant patients not given supplements. Folate levels were usually within the normal range for pregnancy.

The effects of exposure (at any time during the 2nd or 3rd month after the last menstrual period) to folic acid antagonists on embryo–fetal development were evaluated in a large, multicenter, case–control surveillance study published in 2000 (85). The report was based on data collected between 1976 and 1998 from 80 maternity or tertiary care hospitals. Mothers were interviewed within 6 months of delivery about their use of drugs during pregnancy. Folic acid antagonists were categorized into two groups: group I—dihydrofolate reductase inhibitors (aminopterin, methotrexate, sulfasalazine, pyrimethamine, triamterene, and trimethoprim); group II—agents that affect other enzymes in folate metabolism, impair the absorption of folate, or increase the metabolic breakdown of folate (carbamazepine, phenytoin, primidone, and phenobarbital). The case subjects were 3870 infants with cardiovascular defects, 1962 with oral clefts, and 1100 with urinary tract malformations. Infants with defects associated with a syndrome were excluded as were infants with coexisting NTDs (known to be reduced by maternal folic acid supplementation). Too few infants with limb reduction defects were identified to be analyzed. Controls (N = 8387) were infants with malformations other than oral clefts and cardiovascular, urinary tract, and limb reduction defects and NTDs, but included infants with chromosomal and genetic defects. The risk of malformations in control infants would not have been reduced by vitamin supplementation, and none of the controls used folic acid antagonists. For group I cases, the relative risks (RRs) of cardiovascular defects and oral clefts were 3.4 (95% confidence interval [CI] 1.8–6.4) and 2.6 (95% CI 1.1–6.1), respectively. For group II cases, the RRs of cardiovascular and urinary tract defects, and oral clefts were 2.2 (95% CI 1.4–3.5), 2.5 (95% CI 1.2–5.0), and 2.5 (95% CI 1.5–4.2), respectively. Maternal use of multivitamin supplements with folic acid (typically 0.4 mg) reduced the risks in group I cases, but not in group II cases (85).

The pharmacokinetics and placental transport of phenytoin have been extensively studied and reviewed (86–88). Plasma concentrations of phenytoin may fall during pregnancy. Animal studies and recent human reports suggest a dose-related teratogenic effect of phenytoin (89,90). Although these results are based on a small series of patients, it is reasonable to avoid excessively high plasma concentrations of phenytoin. Close monitoring of plasma phenytoin concentrations is recommended to maintain adequate seizure control and prevent potential fetal hypoxia.

Placental function in women taking phenytoin has been evaluated (91). No effect was detected from phenytoin as measured by serum human placental lactogen, 24-hour urinary total estriol excretion, placental weight, and birth weight.

In a study evaluating thyroid function, no differences were found between treated epileptic pregnant women and normal pregnant controls (92). Thyroxine levels in the cord blood of anticonvulsant-exposed infants were significantly lower than in controls, but this was shown to be caused by altered protein binding and not altered thyroid function. Other parameters studied—thyrotropin, free thyroxine, and triiodothyronine—were similar in both groups.

The effect of phenytoin on maternal and fetal vitamin D metabolism was examined in a 1984 study (93). In comparison to normal controls, several significant differences were found in the level of various vitamin D compounds and in serum calcium, but the values were still within normal limits. No alterations were found in alkaline phosphatase and phosphate concentrations. The authors doubted whether the observed differences were of major clinical significance.

Phenytoin may be used for the management of digitalis-induced arrhythmias that are unresponsive to other agents and for refractory ventricular tachyarrhythmias (94–96). This short-term use has not been reported to cause problems in the exposed fetuses. The drug has also been used for anticonvulsant prophylaxis in severe preeclampsia (97).

A study published in 2009 examined the effect of antiepileptic drugs (AEDs) on the head circumference in newborns (98). Significant reductions in mean birth-weight-adjusted mean head circumference (bw-adj-HC) was noted for monotherapy with carbamazepine and valproic acid. No effect on bw-adj-HC was observed with gabapentin, phenytoin, clonazepam, and lamotrigine. A significant increase in the occurrence of microcephaly (bw-adj-HC smaller than 2 standard deviations below the mean) was noted after any AED polytherapy but not after any monotherapy, including carbamazepine and valproic acid. The potential effects of these findings on child development warrant study (98).

In a 1988 study designed to evaluate the effect of in utero exposure to anticonvulsants on intelligence, 148 Finnish children of epileptic mothers were compared with 105 controls (99). Previous studies had either shown intellectual impairment from this exposure or no effect. Of the 148 children of epileptic mothers, 129 were exposed to anticonvulsant therapy during the first 20 weeks of pregnancy, 2 were only exposed after 20 weeks, and 17 were not exposed. In those mothers treated during pregnancy, 103 received phenytoin (monotherapy in 54 cases), all during the first 20 weeks. The children were evaluated at 5.5 years of age for both verbal and nonverbal measures of intelligence. A child was considered mentally deficient if the results of both tests were <71. Two of the 148 children of epileptic mothers were diagnosed as mentally deficient and 2 others had borderline intelligence (the mother of 1 of these latter children had not been treated with anticonvulsant medication). None of the controls was considered mentally deficient. Both verbal (110.2 vs. 114.5) and nonverbal (108.7 vs. 113.2) intelligence scores were significantly lower in the study group children than in controls. In both groups, intelligence scores were significantly lower when seven or more minor anomalies were present. However, the presence of hypertelorism and digital hypoplasia, two minor anomalies considered typical of exposure to phenytoin, was not predictive of low intelligence (99).

A prospective, controlled, blinded observational 1994 study compared the global IQ and language development of children exposed in utero to either phenytoin ($N = 36$) or carbamazepine ($N = 34$) monotherapy to their respective matched controls (100). The cognitive tests were administered to the children between the ages of 18 and 36 months. The maternal IQ scores and socioeconomic status in the phenytoin subjects and their controls were similar (90 vs. 93.9 and 40.8 vs. 40.9, respectively) as they were in the carbamazepine subjects and controls (96.5 vs. 96.0 and 44.7 vs. 46.1, respectively). Compared with controls, phenytoin-exposed children had a significantly lower mean global IQ than their matched controls (113.4 vs. 103.1). The verbal comprehension and expressive language scores were also significantly lower (0.2 vs. 1.1 and −0.47 vs. 0.2, respectively). In contrast, no significant differences were measured either in IQ or language development scores between carbamazepine-exposed children and their matched controls. No correlation between the daily dose (mg/kg) of either anticonvulsant and global IQ was found. Major malformations were observed in two phenytoin-exposed children (cleft palate and hypospadias; meningomyelocele and hydrocephalus), none of the phenytoin controls, two carbamazepine-exposed children (missing last joint of right index finger and nail hypoplasia; hypospadias), and one carbamazepine control (pulmonary atresia). The study results suggested that phenytoin had a clinically important negative effect on neurobehavioral development that was independent of maternal or environmental factors (100). In subsequent correspondence relating to the above study (101,102), various perceived problems were cited and were addressed in a reply (103).

A 2013 study reported dose-dependent associations with reduced cognitive abilities across a range of domains at 6 years of age after fetal valproate exposure (104). Analysis showed that IQ was significantly lower for valproate (mean 97, 95% CI 94–101) than for carbamazepine (mean 105, 95% CI 102–108; $p = 0.0015$), lamotrigine (mean 108, 95% CI 105–110; $p = 0.0003$), or phenytoin (mean 108, 95% CI 104–112; $p = 0.0006$). Mean IQs were higher in children whose mothers had taken folic acid (mean 108, 95% CI 106–111) compared with children whose mothers had not taken the vitamin (mean 101, 95% CI 98–104; $p = 0.0009$) (104).

The relationship between maternal anticonvulsant therapy, neonatal behavior, and neurologic function in children was reported in a 1996 study (105). Among newborns exposed to maternal monotherapy, 18 were exposed to phenobarbital (including primidone), 13 to phenytoin, and 8 to valproic acid. Compared with controls, neonates exposed to phenobarbital had significantly higher mean apathy and optimality scores. Phenytoin-exposed neonates also had a significantly higher mean apathy score. However, the neonatal optimality and apathy scores did not correlate with neurologic outcome of the children at 6 years of age. In contrast, those exposed to valproic acid had optimality and apathy scores statistically similar to controls but a significantly higher hyperexcitability score. Moreover, the hyperexcitability score correlated with later minor and major neurologic dysfunction at age 6 years (105).

A two-part 2000 study evaluated the effects of prenatal phenobarbital and phenytoin exposure on brain development and cognitive functioning in adults (106). Subjects and controls, delivered at a mean 40 weeks' gestation, were retrospectively identified from birth records covering the years between 1957 and 1972. Maternal diseases of the subjects included epilepsy (treated with anticonvulsants) and other conditions in which anticonvulsants were used as sedatives (nausea, vomiting, or emotional problems), whereas the matched control group had no maternal pathologies. Only those exposed prenatally to phenobarbital alone or phenobarbital plus phenytoin had sufficient subjects to analyze. The mean occipitofrontal circumference for phenobarbital-exposed neonates was not different from controls (34.49 vs. 34.50 cm), but it was

P

significantly smaller for phenobarbital plus phenytoin subjects compared with phenobarbital alone or controls (33.82 cm). In the follow-up part of the study, no differences in adult cognitive functioning (intelligence, attention, and memory) were found between the exposed and control groups. More subjects than controls, however, were mentally slow (4 vs. 2; 1 control had autism) and more had persistent learning problems (12% vs. 1%). The investigators concluded that phenobarbital plus phenytoin reduced occipitofrontal circumference but may only affect cognitive capacity in susceptible offspring (106).

BREASTFEEDING SUMMARY

Phenytoin is excreted into breast milk. Milk:plasma ratios range from 0.18 to 0.54 (86,106–110). The pharmacokinetics of phenytoin during lactation have been reviewed (86). The reviewers concluded that little risk to the nursing infant was present if maternal levels were kept in the therapeutic range. However, methemoglobinemia, drowsiness, and decreased sucking activity were reported in one infant (111). Except for this one case, no other reports of adverse effects with the use of phenytoin during lactation have been located.

In a 2010 study, 199 children, who had been breastfed while their mothers were taking a single antiepileptic drug (carbamazepine, lamotrigine, phenytoin, or valproate), were evaluated at 3 years of age cognitive outcome (112). Mean adjusted IQ scores for exposed children were 99 (95% CI 96–103), whereas the mean adjusted IQ scores of nonbreastfed infants were 98 (95% CI 95–101).

The American Academy of Pediatrics classifies phenytoin as compatible with breastfeeding (113).

References

1. Janz D, Fuchs V. Are anti-epileptic drugs harmful when given during pregnancy? German Med Monogr 1964;9:20–3.
2. Hill RB. Teratogenesis and antiepileptic drugs. N Engl J Med 1973;289: 1089–90.
3. Janz D. The teratogenic risk of antiepileptic drugs. Epilepsia 1975;16:159–69.
4. Bodendorfer TW. Fetal effects of anticonvulsant drugs and seizure disorders. Drug Intell Clin Pharm 1978;12:14–21.
5. Committee on Drugs, American Academy of Pediatrics. Anticonvulsants and pregnancy. Pediatrics 1977;63:331–3.
6. Nakane Y, Okuma T, Takahashi R, Sato Y, Wada T, Sato T, Fukushima Y, Kumashiro H, Ono T, Takahashi T, Aoki Y, Kazamatsuri H, Inami M, Komai S, Seino M, Miyakoshi M, Tanimura T, Hazama H, Kawahara R, Otuski S, Hosokawa K, Inanaga K, Nakazawa Y, Yamamoto K. Multi-institutional study of the teratogenicity and fetal toxicity of antiepileptic drugs: a report of a collaborative study group in Japan. Epilepsia 1980;21:663–80.
7. Andermann E, Dansky L, Andermann F, Loughnan PM, Gibbons J. Minor congenital malformations and dermatoglyphic alterations in the offspring of epileptic women: a clinical investigation of the teratogenic effects of anticonvulsant medication. In *Epilepsy, Pregnancy and the Child*. Proceedings of a Workshop in Berlin, September 1980. New York, NY: Raven Press, 1981.
8. Dansky L, Andermann E, Andermann F. Major congenital malformations in the offspring of epileptic patients. In *Epilepsy, Pregnancy and the Child*. Proceedings of a Workshop in Berlin, September 1980. New York, NY: Raven Press, 1981.
9. Hanson JW, Buehler BA. Fetal hydantoin syndrome: current status. J Pediatr 1982;101:816–8.
10. Canger R, Battino D, Canevini MP, Fumarola C, Guidolin L, Vignoli A, Mamoli D, Palmieri C, Molteni F, Granata T, Hassibi P, Zamperini P, Pardi G, Avanzini G. Malformations in offspring of women with epilepsy: a prospective study. Epilepsia 1999;40:1231–6.
11. Holmes LB, Harvey EA, Coull BA, Huntington KB, Khoshbin S, Hayes AM, Ryan LM. The teratogenicity of anticonvulsant drugs. N Engl J Med 2001;344:1132–8.
12. Buehler BA, Delimont D, Van Waes M, Finnell RH. Prenatal prediction of risk of the fetal hydantoin syndrome. N Engl J Med 1990;322:1567–72.
13. Tiboni GM, Iammarrone E, Giampietro F, Lamonaca D, Bellati U, Di Ilio C. Teratological interaction between the bis-triazole antifungal agent fluconazole and the anticonvulsant drug phenytoin. Teratology 1999;59:81–7.
14. Meadow SR. Anticonvulsant drugs and congenital abnormalities. Lancet 1968;2:1296.
15. Loughnan PM, Gold H, Vance JC. Phenytoin teratogenicity in man. Lancet 1973;1:70–2.
16. Hill RM, Horning MG, Horning EC. Antiepileptic drugs and fetal well-being. In Boreus L, ed. *Fetal Pharmacology*. New York, NY: Raven Press, 1973:375–9.
17. Janz D. Antiepileptic drugs and pregnancy: altered utilization patterns and teratogenesis. Epilepsia 1982;23(Suppl 1):S53–63.
18. Allen RW Jr, Ogden B, Bentley FL, Jung AL. Fetal hydantoin syndrome, neuroblastoma, and hemorrhagic disease in a neonate. JAMA 1980;244: 1464–5.
19. Ramilo J, Harris VJ. Neuroblastoma in a child with the hydantoin and fetal alcohol syndrome. The radiographic features. Br J Radiol 1979;52:993–5.
20. Pendergrass TW, Hanson JW. Fetal hydantoin syndrome and neuroblastoma. Lancet 1976;2:150.
21. Sherman S, Roizen N. Fetal hydantoin syndrome and neuroblastoma. Lancet 1976;2:517.
22. Ehrenbard LT, Chaganti RSK. Cancer in the fetal hydantoin syndrome. Lancet 1981;2:97.
23. Seeler RA, Israel JN, Royal JE, Kaye CI, Rao S, Abulaban M. Ganglioneuroblastoma and fetal hydantoin-alcohol syndromes. Pediatrics 1979;63:524–7.
24. Jimenez JF, Seibert RW, Char F, Brown RE, Seibert JJ. Melanotic neuroectodermal tumor of infancy and fetal hydantoin syndrome. Am J Pediatr Hematol Oncol 1981;3:9–15.
25. Taylor WF, Myers M, Taylor WR. Extrarenal Wilms' tumour in an infant exposed to intrauterine phenytoin. Lancet 1980;2:481–2.
26. Blattner WA, Hanson DE, Young EC, Fraumeni JF. Malignant mesenchymoma and birth defects. JAMA 1977;238:334–5.
27. Kousseff BG. Subcutaneous vascular abnormalities in fetal hydantoin syndrome. Birth Defects 1982;18:51–4.
28. Lipson A. Bale P. Ependymoblastoma associated with prenatal exposure to diphenylhydantoin and methylphenobarbitone. Cancer 1985;55:1859–62.
29. Corcoran R, Rizk MW. VACTERL congenital malformation and phenytoin therapy? Lancet 1976;2:960.
30. Pinto W Jr, Gardner LI, Rosenbaum P. Abnormal genitalia as a presenting sign in two male infants with hydantoin embryopathy syndrome. Am J Dis Child 1977;131:452–5.
31. Hoyt CS, Billson FA. Maternal anticonvulsants and optic nerve hypoplasia. Br J Ophthalmol 1978;62:3–6.
32. Wilson RS, Smead W, Char F. Diphenylhydantoin teratogenicity: ocular manifestations and related deformities. J Pediatr Ophthalmol Strabismus 1970;15:137–40.
33. Dabee V, Hart AG, Hurley RM. Teratogenic effects of diphenylhydantoin. Can Med Assoc J 1975;112:75–7.
34. Anderson RC. Cardiac defects in children of mothers receiving anticonvulsant therapy during pregnancy. J Pediatr 1976;89:318–9.
35. Hill RM, Verniaud WM, Horning MG, McCulley LB, Morgan NF. Infants exposed in utero to antiepileptic drugs. A prospective study. Am J Dis Child 1974;127:645–53.
36. Stankler L, Campbell AGM. Neonatal acne vulgaris: a possible feature of the fetal hydantoin syndrome. Br J Dermatol 1980;103:453–5.
37. Ringrose CAD. The hazard of neurotropic drugs in the fertile years. Can Med Assoc J 1972;106:1058.
38. Pettifor JM, Benson R. Congenital malformations associated with the administration of oral anticoagulants during pregnancy. J Pediatr 1975;86: 459–61.
39. Biale Y, Lewenthal H, Aderet NB. Congenital malformations due to anticonvulsant drugs and congenital abnormalities. Obstet Gynecol 1975; 45:439–42.
40. Aase JM. Anticonvulsant drugs and congenital abnormalities. Am J Dis Child 1974;127:758.
41. Lewin PK. Phenytoin associated congenital defects with Y-chromosome variant. Lancet 1973;I:559.
42. Yang TS, Chi CC, Tsai CJ, Chang MJ. Diphenylhydantoin teratogenicity in man. Obstet Gynecol 1978;52:682–4.
43. Mallow DW, Herrick MK, Gathman G. Fetal exposure to anticonvulsant drugs. Arch Pathol Lab Med 1980;104:215–8.
44. Hirschberger M, Kleinberg F. Maternal phenytoin ingestion and congenital abnormalities: report of a case. Am J Dis Child 1975;129:984.

45. Hanson JW, Myrianthopoulos NC, Sedgwick Harvey MA, Smith DW. Risks to the offspring of women treated with hydantoin anticonvulsants, with emphasis on the fetal hydantoin syndrome. J Pediatr 1976;89:662–8.
46. Shakir RA, Johnson RH, Lambie DG, Melville ID, Nanda RN. Comparison of sodium valproate and phenytoin as single drug treatment in epilepsy. Epilepsia 1981;22:27–33.
47. Michalodimitrakis M, Parchas S, Coutselinis A. Fetal hydantoin syndrome: congenital malformation of the urinary tract—a case report. Clin Toxicol 1981;18:1095–7.
48. Phelan MC, Pellock JM, Nance WE. Discordant expression of fetal hydantoin syndrome in heteropaternal dizygotic twins. N Engl J Med 1982;307:99–101.
49. Kousseff BG, Root ER. Expanding phenotype of fetal hydantoin syndrome. Pediatrics 1982;70:328–9.
50. Wilker R, Nathenson G. Combined fetal alcohol and hydantoin syndromes. Clin Pediatr 1982;21:331–4.
51. Kogutt MS. Fetal hydantoin syndrome. South Med J 1984;77:657–8.
52. Krauss CM, Holmes LB, VanLang QN, Keith DA. Four siblings with similar malformations after exposure to phenytoin and primidone. J Pediatr 1984;105:750–5.
53. Pearl KN, Dickens S, Latham P. Functional palatal incompetence in the fetal anticonvulsant syndrome. Arch Dis Child 1984;59:989–90.
54. Trice JE, Ambler M. Multiple cerebral defects in an infant exposed in utero to anticonvulsants. Arch Pathol Lab Med 1985;109:521–3.
55. D'Souza SW, Robertson IG, Donnai D, Mawer G. Fetal phenytoin exposure, hypoplastic nails, and jitteriness. Arch Dis Child 1990;65:320–4.
56. Kotzot D, Weigl J, Huk W, Rott HD. Hydantoin syndrome with holoprosencephaly: a possible rate teratogenic effect. Teratology 1993;48:15–19.
57. Shaw GM, Wasserman CR, O'Malley CD, Lammer EJ, Finnell RH. Orofacial clefts and maternal anticonvulsant use. Reprod Toxicol 1995;9:97–8.
58. Sabry MA, Farag TI. Hand anomalies in fetal-hydantoin syndrome: from nail/phalangeal hypoplasia to unilateral acheiria. Am J Med Genet 1996;62:410–2.
59. Holmes LB, Harvey EA. Holoprosencephaly and the teratogenicity of anticonvulsants. Teratology 1994;49:82.
60. Rafla NM, Meehan FP. Thanatophoric dwarfism: drugs and antenatal diagnosis: a case report. Eur J Obstet Gynecol Reprod Biol 1990;38:161–5.
61. Arpino C, Brescianini S, Robert E, Castilla EE, Cocchi G, Cornel MC, de Vigan C, Lancaster PAL, Merlob P, Sumiyoshi Y, Zampino G, Renzi C, Rosano A, Mastroiacovo P. Teratogenic effects of antiepileptic drugs: use of an international database on malformations and drug exposure (MADRE). Epilepsia 2000;41:1436–43.
62. The Lamotrigine Pregnancy Registry. Final Report. September 1, 1992 through March 31, 2010. GlaxoSmithKline, July 2010.
63. Al-Shammri S, Guberman A, Hsu E. Neuroblastoma and fetal exposure to phenytoin in a child without dysmorphic features. Can J Neurol Sci 1992;19:243–5.
64. Koren G, Demitrakoudis D, Weksberg R, Reider M, Shear NH, Sonely M, Shandling B, Spielberg SP. Neuroblastoma after prenatal exposure to phenytoin: cause and effect? Teratology 1989;40:157–62.
65. Lawrence A. Antiepileptic drugs and the foetus. Br Med J 1963;2:1267.
66. Kohler HG. Haemorrhage in newborn of epileptic mothers. Lancet 1966;1:267.
67. Douglas H. Haemorrhage in the newborn. Lancet 1966;1:816–7.
68. Monnet P, Rosenberg D, Bovier-Lapierre M. Terapeutique anticomitale administree pendant la grosses et maladie hemorragique du nouveau-ne. As cited in Bleyer WA, Skinner AL. Fetal neonatal hemorrhage after maternal anticonvulsant therapy. JAMA 1976;235:626–7.
69. Davis PP. Coagulation defect due to anticonvulsant drug treatment in pregnancy. Lancet 1970;1:413.
70. Evans AR, Forrester RM, Discombe C. Neonatal haemorrhage following maternal anticonvulsant therapy. Lancet 1970;1:517–8.
71. Stevensom MM, Bilbert EF. Anticonvulsants and hemorrhagic diseases of the newborn infant. J Pediatr 1970;77:516.
72. Speidel BD, Meadow SR. Maternal epilepsy and abnormalities of the foetus and newborn. Lancet 1972;2:839–40.
73. Truog WE, Feusner JH, Baker DL. Association of hemorrhagic disease and the syndrome of persistent fetal circulation with the fetal hydantoin syndrome. J Pediatr 1980;96:112–4.
74. Solomon GE, Hilgartner MW, Kutt H. Coagulation defects caused by diphenylhydantoin. Neurology 1972;22:1165–71.
75. Griffiths AD. Neonatal haemorrhage associated with maternal anticonvulsant therapy. Lancet 1981;2:1296–7.
76. Page TE, Hoyme HE, Markarian M, Jones KL. Neonatal hemorrhage secondary to thrombocytopenia: an occasional effect of prenatal hydantoin exposure. Birth Defects 1982;18:47–50.
77. Srinivasan G, Seeler RA, Tiruvury A, Pildes RS. Maternal anticonvulsant therapy and hemorrhagic disease of the newborn. Obstet Gynecol 1982;59:250–2.
78. Payne NR, Hasegawa DK. Vitamin K deficiency in newborns: a case report in α-1-antitrypsin deficiency and a review of factors predisposing to hemorrhage. Pediatrics 1984;73:712–6.
79. Lane PA, Hathaway WE. Vitamin K in infancy. J Pediatr 1985;106:351–9.
80. Howe AM, Lipson AH, Sheffield LJ, Haan EA, Halliday JL, Jenson F, David DJ, Webster WS. Prenatal exposure to phenytoin, facial development, and a possible role for vitamin K. Am J Med Genet 1995;58: 238–44.
81. Felding I, Rane A. Congenital liver damage after treatment of mother with valproic acid and phenytoin? Acta Paediatr Scand 1984;73:565–8.
82. Biale Y, Lewenthal H. Effect of folic acid supplementation on congenital malformations due to anticonvulsive drugs. Eur J Obstet Reprod Biol 1984;18:211–6.
83. Pritchard JA, Scott DE, Whalley PJ. Maternal folate deficiency and pregnancy wastage. IV. Effects of folic acid supplements, anticonvulsants, and oral contraceptives. Am J Obstet Gynecol 1971;109:341–6.
84. Hiilesmaa VK, Teramo K, Granstrom ML, Bardy AH. Serum folate concentrations during pregnancy in women with epilepsy: relation to antiepileptic drug concentrations, number of seizures, and fetal outcome. Br Med J 1983;287:577–9.
85. Hernandez-Diaz S, Werler MM, Walker AM, Mitchell AA. Folic acid antagonists during pregnancy and the risk of birth defects. N Engl J Med 2000;343:1608–14.
86. Nau H, Kuhnz W, Egger HJ, Rating D, Helge H. Anticonvulsants during pregnancy and lactation: transplacental, maternal and neonatal pharmacokinetics. Clin Pharmacokinet 1982;7:508–43.
87. Chen SS, Perucca E, Lee JN, Richens A. Serum protein binding and free concentrations of phenytoin and phenobarbitone in pregnancy. Br J Clin Pharmacol 1982;13:547–52.
88. Van der Kligh E, Schobben F, Bree TB. Clinical pharmacokinetics of antiepileptic drugs. Drug Intell Clin Pharm 1980;14:674–85.
89. Dansky L, Andermann E, Sherwin AL, Andermann F. Plasma levels of phenytoin during pregnancy and the puerperium. In *Epilepsy, Pregnancy and the Child*. Proceedings of a Workshop held in Berlin, September 1980. New York, NY: Raven Press, 1981.
90. Dansky L, Andermann E, Andermann F, Sherwin AL, Kinch RA. Maternal epilepsy and congenital malformation: correlation with maternal plasma anticonvulsant levels during pregnancy. In *Epilepsy, Pregnancy and the Child*. Proceedings of a Workshop held in Berlin, September 1980. New York, NY: Raven Press, 1981.
91. Hiilesmaa VK. Evaluation of placental function in women on antiepileptic drugs. J Perinat Med 1983;11:187–92.
92. Carriero R, Andermann E, Chen MF, Eeg-Oloffson O, Kinch RAH, Klein G, Pearson Murphy BE. Thyroid function in epileptic mothers and their infants at birth. Am J Obstet Gynecol 1985;151:641–4.
93. Markestad T, Ulstein M, Strandjord RE, Aksnes L, Aarskog D. Anticonvulsant drug therapy in human pregnancy: effects on serum concentrations of vitamin D metabolites in maternal and cord blood. Am J Obstet Gynecol 1984;150:254–8.
94. Tamari I, Eldar M, Rabinowitz B, Neufeld HN. Medical treatment of cardiovascular disorders during pregnancy. Am Heart J 1982;104:1357–63.
95. Rotmensch HH, Elkayam U, Frishman W. Antiarrhythmic drug therapy during pregnancy. Ann Intern Med 1983;98:487–97.
96. Rotmensch HH, Rotmensch S, Elkayam U. Management of cardiac arrhythmias during pregnancy: current concepts. Drugs 1987;33:623–33.
97. Ryan G, Lange IR, Naugler MA. Clinical experience with phenytoin prophylaxis in severe preeclampsia. Am J Obstet Gynecol 1989;161: 1297–304.
98. Almgren M, Kallen B, Lavebratt C. Population-based study of antiepileptic drug exposure *in utero*—influence on head circumference in newborns. Seizure 2009;18:672–5.
99. Gaily E, Kantola-Sorsa E, Granstrom M-L. Intelligence of children of epileptic mothers. J Pediatr 1988;113:677–84.
100. Scolnik D, Nulman I, Rovet J, Gladstone D, Czuchta D, Gardner HA, Gladstone R, Ashby P, Weksberg R, Einarson T, Koren G. Neurodevelopment of children exposed in utero to phenytoin and carbamazepine monotherapy. JAMA 1994;271:767–70.
101. Jeret JS. Neurodevelopment after in utero exposure to phenytoin and carbamazepine. JAMA 1994;272:850.
102. Loring DW, Meador KJ, Thompson WO. Neurodevelopment of children exposed in utero to phenytoin and carbamazepine. JAMA 1994;272: 850–1.

103. Koren G. Neurodevelopment of children exposed in utero to phenytoin and carbamazepine. JAMA 1994;272:851.
104. Meador KJ, Baker GA, Browning N, Cohen MJ, Bromley RL, Clayton-Smith J, Kalayjian LA, Kanner A, Liporace JD, Pennell PB, Privitera M, Loring DW, for the NEAD Study Group. Fetal antiepileptic drug exposure and cognitive outcomes at age 6 years (NEAD study): a prospective observational study. Lancet Neurol 2013;12:244–52.
105. Koch S, Jager-Roman E, Losche G, Nau H, Rating D, Helge H. Antiepileptic drug treatment in pregnancy: drug side effects in the neonate and neurological outcome. Acta Paediatr 1996;84:739–46.
106. Dessens AB, Cohen-Kettenis PT, Mellenbergh GJ, Koppe JG, van de Poll NE, Boer K. Association of prenatal phenobarbital and phenytoin exposure with small head size at birth and with learning problems. Acta Paediatr 2000;89:533–41.
107. Horning MG, Stillwell WG, N owling J, Lertratanangkoon K, Stillwell RN, Hill RM. Identification and quantification of drugs and drug metabolites in human breast milk using GC-MS-COM methods. Mod Probl Pediatr 1975;15:73–9.
108. Svensmark O, Schiller PJ. 5-5-Diphenylhydantoin (Dilantin) blood level after oral or intravenous dosage in man. Acta Pharmacol Toxicol 1960;16:331–46.
109. Kok THHG, Taitz LS, Bennett MJ, Holt DW. Drowsiness due to clemastine transmitted in breast milk. Lancet 1982;1:914–5.
110. Steen B, Rane A, Lonnerholm G, Falk O, Elwin CE, Sjoqvist F. Phenytoin excretion in human breast milk and plasma levels in nursed infants. Ther Drug Monit 1982;4:331–4.
111. Finch E, Lorber J. Methaemoglobinaemia in the newborn: probably due to phenytoin excreted in human milk. J Obstet Gynaecol Br Emp 1954;61:833.
112. Meador KJ, Baker GA, Browning N, Clayton-Smith J, Combs-Cantrell DT, Cohen M, Kalayjian LA, Kanner A, Liporace JD, Pennell PB, Privitera M, Loring DW, for the NEAD Study Group. Effects of breastfeeding in children of women taking antiepileptic drugs. Neurology 2010;75:1954–60.
113. Committee on Drugs, American Academy of Pediatrics. The transfer of drugs and other chemicals into human milk. Pediatrics 2001;108:776–89.

PHYSOSTIGMINE

Parasympathomimetic (Cholinergic)

PREGNANCY RECOMMENDATION: Limited Human Data—No Relevant Animal Data
BREASTFEEDING RECOMMENDATION: No Human Data—Probably Compatible

PREGNANCY SUMMARY

Physostigmine is rarely used in pregnancy. No reports linking its use with congenital defects have appeared.

FETAL RISK SUMMARY

Physostigmine is an anticholinesterase agent, but it does not contain a quaternary ammonium element. It crosses the blood–brain barrier and should be expected to cross the placenta (1). Crossing to the embryo–fetus would be consistent with its relatively low molecular weight (about 275).

One report described the use of the drug in 15 women at term to reverse scopolamine-induced twilight sleep (2). Apgar scores of 14 of the newborns ranged from 7 to 9 at 1 minute and 8 to 10 at 5 minutes. One infant was depressed at birth and required resuscitation, but the mother had also received meperidine and diazepam. No other effects in the infants were mentioned.

Transient muscular weakness has been observed in about 20% of newborns of mothers with myasthenia gravis (3–5). The neonatal myasthenia is caused by transplacental passage of anti-acetylcholine receptor immunoglobulin G antibodies (5).

BREASTFEEDING SUMMARY

No reports describing the use of physostigmine during human lactation have been located. The relatively low molecular weight (about 275) suggests that it will be excreted into breast milk. The effect of this exposure on a nursing infant is unknown.

References

1. Taylor P. Anticholinesterase agents. In Gilman AG, Goodman LS, Gilman A, eds. *The Pharmacological Basis of Therapeutics*. 6th ed. New York, NY: Macmillan, 1980:100–19.
2. Smiller BG, Bartholomew EG, Sivak BJ, Alexander GD, Brown EM. Physostigmine reversal of scopolamine delirium in obstetric patients. Am J Obstet Gynecol 1973;116:326–9.
3. McNall PG, Jafarnia MR. Management of myasthenia gravis in the obstetrical patient. Am J Obstet Gynecol 1965;92:518–25.
4. Blackhall MI, Buckley GA, Roberts DV, Roberts JB, Thomas BH, Wilson A. Drug-induced neonatal myasthenia. J Obstet Gynaecol Br Commonw 1969;76:157–62.
5. Plauche WC. Myasthenia gravis in pregnancy: an update. Am J Obstet Gynecol 1979;135:691–7.

PHYTONADIONE

Vitamin

PREGNANCY RECOMMENDATION: Compatible
BREASTFEEDING RECOMMENDATION: Compatible

PREGNANCY SUMMARY

Phytonadione (vitamin K_1) is the treatment of choice for maternal hypoprothrombinemia and for the prevention of hemorrhagic disease of the newborn (HDN). Maternal supplements are not needed except for those patients deemed at risk for vitamin K deficiency. A recommended dietary intake of 45 mcg (100 nmol) of vitamin K_1 from food during pregnancy has been proposed (1).

FETAL RISK SUMMARY

Phytonadione is a synthetic, fat-soluble substance identical to vitamin K_1, the natural vitamin found in a variety of foods. It is used for the prevention and treatment of hypoprothrombinemia caused by vitamin K deficiency (2). Animal reproduction studies have not been conducted with phytonadione.

In a surveillance study of Michigan Medicaid recipients involving 229,101 completed pregnancies conducted between 1985 and 1992, 5 newborns had been exposed to phytonadione during the 1st trimester (F. Rosa, personal communication, FDA, 1993). Four (80.0%) major birth defects were observed (none expected), including 2/0 cardiovascular defects and 1/0 spina bifida. No anomalies were observed in four other defect categories (oral clefts, polydactyly, limb reduction defects, and hypospadias) for which specific data were available.

The use of phytonadione (vitamin K_1) during pregnancy and in the newborn has been the subject of several large reviews (3–6). Administration of vitamin K during pregnancy is usually not required because of the abundance of natural sources in food and the synthesis of the vitamin by the normal intestinal flora. Vitamin K_1 is indicated for maternal hypoprothrombinemia and for the prevention of HDN induced by maternal drugs, such as anticonvulsants, warfarin, rifampin, and isoniazid (3–6).

Only low amounts of vitamin K_1 cross the placenta (7,8). A 1982 study found no detectable vitamin K (<0.10 ng/mL) in the cord blood of nine term infants, although adequate levels (mean 0.20 ng/mL) were present in eight of the nine mothers (7). Vitamin K_1, 1 mg IV, was then given to six additional mothers shortly before delivery (11–47 minutes) resulting in plasma vitamin K_1 values of 45–93 ng/mL. Vitamin K_1 was detected in only four of the six cord blood samples (ranging from 0.10 to 0.14 ng/mL), and its appearance did not seem to be time dependent. In a 1990 study, women were administered one or two doses of vitamin K_1 10 mg IM at 4-day intervals, and if not delivered, followed by daily oral 20-mg doses until the end of the 34th week or delivery (8). Treated subjects had significantly higher vitamin K_1 maternal and cord plasma levels than controls (11.592 vs. 0.102 ng/mL and 0.024 vs. 0.010 ng/mL, respectively). Although the median plasma vitamin K_1 levels in the mothers treated only with IM doses were similar to those treated with IM and oral doses, cord plasma levels in the latter group were significantly higher (0.42 vs. 0.017 ng/ mL). No correlation was found between cord plasma levels of vitamin K_1 and gestational age or duration of therapy (8).

Vitamin K_1 is nontoxic in doses <20 mg (4). In a double-blind trial, 933 women at term were given 20 mg of either K_1 or K_2, the naturally occurring vitamins (9). No toxicity from either vitamin was found, including any association with low birth weight, asphyxia, neonatal jaundice, or perinatal mortality.

Oral vitamin K_1 has been suggested during the last 2 weeks of pregnancy for women taking anticonvulsants to prevent hypoprothrombinemia and hemorrhage in their newborns, but the effectiveness of this therapy has not been proven (3,4). In a group of mothers receiving phenindione, an oral anticoagulant, 10–30 mg of vitamin K_1 was given either IV or intra-amniotically 2–4 days before delivery (10). In a separate group, 2.5–3.0 mg of vitamin K_1 was injected IM into the fetuses at the same interval before delivery. Only in this latter group were coagulation factors significantly improved.

BREASTFEEDING SUMMARY

The natural vitamin K content of breast milk is too low to protect the newborn from vitamin K deficiency and resulting hemorrhagic disease. The administration of vitamin K to the mother to increase milk concentrations may be possible but needs further study. All newborns should receive parenteral prophylactic therapy at birth consisting of 0.5–1.0 mg of phytonadione. Larger or repeat doses may be required for infants whose mothers are consuming anticonvulsants or oral anticoagulants (3,11). The American Academy of Pediatrics classifies vitamin K_1 as compatible with breastfeeding (12).

Levels of phytonadione (vitamin K_1) in breast milk are naturally low with most samples having <20 ng/mL and many having <5 ng/mL (3,4). In 20 lactating women, colostrum and mature milk concentrations were 2.3 and 2.1 ng/mL, less than half that found in cow's milk (13). Administration of a single 20-mg oral dose of phytonadione to one mother produced a concentration of 140 ng/mL at 12 hours with levels at 48 hours still about double normal values (13). In another study, 40-mg oral doses of vitamin K_1 or K_3 (menadione) were given to mothers within 2 hours after delivery (14). Effects from either vitamin on the prothrombin time of the breastfed newborns were nil to slight during the first 3 days.

Natural levels of vitamin K_1 or K_2 in milk will not provide adequate supplies of the vitamin for the breastfed infant (3,4). The vitamin K_1-dependent coagulation factors II, VII, IX, and X are dependent on gestational age (3). In the newborn, these factors are approximately 30%–60% of normal and do not reach adult levels until about 6 weeks (3). Although not all newborns are vitamin K_1 deficient, many are because of poor placental transfer of the vitamin. Exclusive breastfeeding will not prevent further decline of these already low stores and the possible development of deficiency in 48–72 hours (3,4). In addition, the intestinal flora of breastfed infants may produce less vitamin K than the flora of formula-fed infants (3). The potential consequence of this deficiency is HDN.

The American Academy of Pediatrics has suggested that HDN be defined as "a hemorrhagic disorder of the first days of life caused by a deficiency of vitamin K and characterized by deficiency of prothrombin and proconvertin (stable factor, factor VII), and probably of other factors" (11). The hemorrhage is frequently life-threatening with intracranial bleeds common. A 1985 review (3) identified three types of HDN:

Early HDN (onset 0–24 hours)
Classic HDN (onset 2–5 days)
Late HDN (onset 1–12 months)

The maternal ingestion of certain drugs, such as anticonvulsants, warfarin, or antituberculous agents, is one of the known causes of early and classic HDN, whereas breastfeeding has been shown to be a cause of classic and late HDN (3). The administration of phytonadione to the newborn prevents HDN by preventing further decline of factors II, VII, IX, and X (3).

The use of prophylactic vitamin K_1 in all newborns is common in the United States but is controversial in other countries (3). The American Academy of Pediatrics Committee on Nutrition recommended in 1961 and again in 1980 that all newborns receive 0.5–1.0 mg of parenteral vitamin K_1 (11,15). The Committee recommended that administration to the mother prenatally should not be substituted for newborn prophylaxis (11). The bleeding risk in breastfed infants who did not receive prophylactic vitamin K_1 is 15–20 times greater than in infants fed cow's milk, given vitamin K_1, or both (3). Despite this evidence, new cases of HDN are still reported (4,16). In a recent report, 10 breastfed infants with intracranial hemorrhage as a result of vitamin K deficiency were described (16). Onset of the bleeding was between 27 and 47 days of age with three infants dying and three having permanent brain injury. Milk levels of total vitamin K (K_1 + K_2) varied between 1.36 and 9.17 ng/mL. None of the infants had been given prophylactic therapy at birth.

References

1. Olson JA. Recommended dietary intakes (RDI) of vitamin K in humans. Am J Clin Nutr 1987;45:687–92.
2. American Hospital Formulary Service. *Drug Information 1997*. Bethesda, MD: American Society of Health-System Pharmacists, 1997:2834–36.
3. Lane PA, Hathaway WE. Vitamin K in infancy. J Pediatr 1985;106:351–9.
4. Payne NR, Hasegawa DK. Vitamin K deficiency in newborns: a case report in α-1-antitrypsin deficiency and a review of factors predisposing to hemorrhage. Pediatrics 1984;73:712–6.
5. Wynn RM. The obstetric significance of factors affecting the metabolism of bilirubin, with particular reference to the role of vitamin K. Obstet Gynecol Surv 1963;18:333–54.
6. Finkel MJ. Vitamin K_1 and the vitamin K analogues. J Clin Pharmacol Ther 1961;2:795–814.
7. Shearer MJ, Rahim S, Barkhan P, Stimmler L. Plasma vitamin K_1 in mothers and their newborn babies. Lancet 1982;2:460–3.
8. Kazzi NJ, Ilagan NB, Liang K-C, Kazzi GM, Grietsell LA, Brans YW. Placental transfer of vitamin K_1 in preterm pregnancy. Obstet Gynecol 1990;75:334–7.
9. Blood Study Group of Gynecologists. Effect of vitamins K_2 and K_1 on the bleeding volume during parturition and the blood coagulation disturbance of newborns by a double blind controlled study. Igaku no Ayumi 1971;76:818. As cited in Nishimura H, Tanimura T. *Clinical Aspects of the Teratogenicity of Drugs*. New York, NY: American Elsevier, 1976:253.
10. Larsen JF, Jacobsen B, Holm HH, Pedersen JF, Mantoni M. Intrauterine injection of vitamin K before delivery during anticoagulant therapy of the mother. Acta Obstet Gynecol Scand 1978;57:227–30.
11. Committee on Nutrition, American Academy of Pediatrics. Vitamin K compounds and the water-soluble analogues. Pediatrics 1961;28:501–7.
12. Committee on Drugs, American Academy of Pediatrics. The transfer of drugs and other chemicals into human milk. Pediatrics 2001;108:776–89.
13. Haroon Y, Shearer MJ, Rahim S, Gunn WG, McEnery G, Barkhan P. The content of phylloquinone (vitamin K_1) in human milk, cows' milk and infant formula foods determined by high-performance liquid chromatography. J Nutr 1982;112:1105–17.
14. Dyggve HV, Dam H, Sondergaard E. Influence on the prothrombin time of breast-fed newborn babies of one single dose of vitamin K_1 or Synkavit given to the mother within 2 hours after birth. Acta Obstet Gynecol Scand 1956;35:440–4.
15. Committee on Nutrition, American Academy of Pediatrics. Vitamin and mineral supplement needs in normal children in the United States. Pediatrics 1980;66:1015–21.
16. Motohara K, Matsukura M, Matsuda I, Iribe K, Ikeda T, Kondo Y, Yonekubo A, Yamamoto Y, Tsuchiya F. Severe vitamin K deficiency in breast-fed infants. J Pediatr 1984;105:943–5.

P

PILOCARPINE

Parasympathomimetic (Cholinergic)

PREGNANCY RECOMMENDATION: Limited Human Data—Probably Compatible
BREASTFEEDING RECOMMENDATION: No Human Data—Probably Compatible

PREGNANCY SUMMARY

Pilocarpine is used topically in the eye for glaucoma or as oral tablets in the treatment of dry mouth. No reports of developmental toxicity attributable to the drug have been located. However, animal reproduction studies have observed toxicity with oral doses ≤10 times the human dose.

FETAL RISK SUMMARY

In reproduction studies in rats at a dose about 26 times the maximum human oral dose of pilocarpine based on BSA (MRHD), adverse effects consisting of a decrease in fetal weight and an increase in the incidence of skeletal variations were observed. These effects may have been secondary to maternal toxicity (1). In another study with rats, doses approximately 10 times the MRHD during gestation and lactation were associated with an increased incidence of stillbirths, whereas doses ≥5 times the MRHD were associated with decreased neonatal survival and reduced pup body weights (1).

A single report of the topical use during pregnancy has been located. A woman with glaucoma was treated throughout gestation with topical pilocarpine (two drops twice daily), timolol (two drops each eye), and oral acetazolamide (2). Within 48 hours of delivery at 36 weeks' gestation, the infant presented with hyperbilirubinemia, hypocalcemia, hypomagnesemia, and metabolic acidosis. The toxic effects, attributed to the carbonic anhydrase inhibitor acetazolamide (see

Acetazolamide), resolved quickly on treatment. Mild hypertonicity requiring physiotherapy was observed at examinations at 1, 3, and 8 months of age.

BREASTFEEDING SUMMARY

No reports describing the use of pilocarpine during lactation have been located. Because of the molecular weight (about 209 for the free base), excretion into breast milk should be expected, at least after oral doses.

References

1. Product information. Salagen. MGI Pharma, 2000.
2. Merlob P, Litwin A, Mor N. Possible association between acetazolamide administration during pregnancy and metabolic disorders in the newborn. Eur J Obstet Gynecol Reprod Biol 1990;35:85–8.

PIMECROLIMUS

Immunologic Agent (Immunomodulator)

PREGNANCY RECOMMENDATION: No Human Data—Animal Data Suggest Low Risk
BREASTFEEDING RECOMMENDATION: No Human Data—Probably Compatible

PREGNANCY SUMMARY

No reports describing the use of pimecrolimus in human pregnancy have been located. The systemic absorption after topical application of the cream is minimal. Moreover, the animal reproduction data suggest low risk. Based on this information, the topical use of the drug during pregnancy appears to represent a low, if any, risk to the embryo or fetus.

FETAL RISK SUMMARY

Pimecrolimus, a selective inhibitor of inflammatory cytokine release, is an immunosuppressant that is available as a 1% cream for topical application. It is the same subclass of topical calcineurin inhibitor immunomodulators as tacrolimus. Pimecrolimus is indicated as second-line therapy for the short-term and noncontinuous chronic treatment of mild to moderate atopic dermatitis in nonimmunocompromised adults and children ≥2 years of age. Systemic absorption was minimal with blood concentrations <0.5 ng/mL in 91% of adult subjects (1244/1362) tested. The maximum blood concentration observed in these subjects was 1.4 ng/mL. Based on in vitro tests, plasma protein binding of drug reaching the systemic circulation was 99.5%. Following a single oral dose given to volunteers, pimecrolimus was extensively metabolized to inactive metabolites and primarily excreted in the feces (1). Based on oral studies in adult patients with psoriasis, the terminal elimination half-life after 28 days of therapy was 50–100 hours (2).

Reproduction studies have been conducted in rats and rabbits. No maternal or fetal toxicity was observed in these species exposed during organogenesis to dermal doses that were 0.14 times the maximum recommended human dose of the cream (MRHD) based on BSA and 0.65 times the MRHD based on AUC, respectively. A second dermal study in pregnant rats at doses up to 0.66 times the MRHD based on AUC revealed no maternal, reproductive, or embryo–fetal toxicity, including teratogenicity, attributable to the drug. When pimecrolimus was given orally to pregnant rats and rabbits, no evidence of developmental toxicity was observed at doses up to 38 and 3.9 times the MRHD based on AUC, respectively. In rabbits, an oral dose that was 12 times the MRHD based on AUC caused maternal, embryo, and fetal toxicity. No toxicity was observed at 5 times the MRHD based on AUC. Pimecrolimus crossed the placentas of rats and rabbits given oral doses (1).

In a 2-year dermal carcinogenicity study conducted in rats, a significant increase in the incidence of follicular cell adenoma of the thyroid was observed. In mice, lymphoproliferative changes, including lymphoma, were observed. A 39-week oral study in monkeys also observed dose-related and duration-related changes that could progress to lymphoma. A dose-dependent increase in opportunistic infections also was noted. No evidence of mutagenicity or clastogenicity was observed in several tests. No effect on fertility in female and male rats was observed with oral doses that were 12 and 23 times the MRHD based on AUC, respectively. In a second oral fertility study, the no effect doses were 5 and 0.7 times the MRHD based on AUC, respectively (1).

It is not known if pimecrolimus crosses the human placenta. The molecular weight (about 810) and the long elimination half-life suggest that if the drug reaches the maternal circulation, exposure of the embryo–fetus will occur. However, the minimal blood concentrations, high plasma protein binding, and extensive metabolism suggest that such exposure will be limited, if it occurs at all.

BREASTFEEDING SUMMARY

No reports describing the use of pimecrolimus during human lactation have been located. The molecular weight (about 810) and the long elimination half-life (50–100 hours after 28 days of therapy) suggest that if the drug reaches the maternal circulation, excretion into breast milk will occur. However, the minimal blood concentrations, high plasma protein binding (99.5%), and extensive metabolism to inactive metabolites suggest that such excretion will be limited, if it occurs at all. The risk to a nursing infant is unknown but does not appear to be clinically significant.

References

1. Product information. Elidel. Novartis Pharmaceuticals, 2009.
2. Scott G, Osborne SA, Greig G, Hartmann S, Ebelin ME, Burtin P, Rappersberger K, Komar M, Wolff K. Pharmacokinetics of pimecrolimus, a novel nonsteroid anti-inflammatory drug, after single and multiple oral administration. Clin Pharmacokinet 2003;42:1305–14.

P

PIMOZIDE

Antipsychotic

PREGNANCY RECOMMENDATION: Limited Human Data—Animal Data Suggest Low Risk
BREASTFEEDING RECOMMENDATION: No Human Data—Potential Toxicity

PREGNANCY SUMMARY

The human pregnancy experience with pimozide is limited, but no embryo–fetal harm has been reported. The animal data do not suggest a risk of teratogenicity, but the lack of a meaningful comparison with the human dose limits the data's usefulness. The use of antipsychotics, including pimozide, close to delivery may cause extrapyramidal effects (Parkinson-like symptoms; akinesia) in the newborn (1). Until adequate human pregnancy experience has been reported, the safest course is to avoid pimozide in pregnancy, especially in the 1st trimester and close to delivery. However, it should not be withheld because of pregnancy if it is the best drug for the patient.

FETAL RISK SUMMARY

Pimozide is an orally active antipsychotic agent that blocks dopaminergic receptors on neurons in the CNS. It is indicated for the suppression of motor and phonic tics in patients with Tourette's syndrome who have failed to respond satisfactorily to standard treatment. Pimozide is extensively metabolized, primarily in the liver, but the antipsychotic activity of the metabolites has not been determined. In schizophrenic patients, the mean serum elimination half-life was about 55 hours (2).

Reproduction studies have been conducted in rats and rabbits. In rats, oral doses up to 8 times the maximum human dose (HD) were not teratogenic, but decreased rates of pregnancies and increased rates of retarded fetal development were observed. The decreased pregnancy rates were thought to be due to an inhibition or delay in implantation, an effect in rodents that has been observed with other antipsychotic drugs. Although rat fertility studies were not adequate to assess all aspects of fertility, pimozide caused prolonged estrus cycles similar to those observed with other antipsychotics. In the rabbit, dose-related (doses not specified) maternal toxicity, mortality, decreased weight gain, and embryo toxicity, including increased resorptions, were noted (2).

Dose-related increases in pituitary and mammary gland tumors in female mice were observed in long-term studies. The latter tumors may have been related to drug-induced elevated prolactin levels. Doses up to 50 times the HD were not tumorigenic in rats, but the limited number of animals surviving this study makes the findings unclear (2).

It is not known if pimozide crosses the human placenta. The molecular weight (about 462) and prolonged elimination half-life suggest that the drug will cross to the embryo–fetus.

A 2006 case report described the use of pimozide throughout pregnancy (3). The 26-year-old woman had been diagnosed with Tourette's syndrome at the age of 12–13 years and was treated with pimozide 1–3 mg/day. At age 19 years, in addition to the occurrence of tics from Tourette's syndrome, she began to experience symptoms of obsessive-compulsive disorder (OCD). Fluoxetine 20 mg daily partially controlled the new disorder. Pimozide 1 mg/day (the usual maintenance dose is 2–6 mg/day) and fluoxetine were continued until the 27th week of pregnancy at which time she discontinued fluoxetine. Ultrasound examinations of the fetus conducted 7 times from weeks 8 through 27 were normal. A cesarean section was planned for week 38 and, to prevent potential toxicity in the newborn, pimozide was discontinued at 36 weeks' gestation. However, 1 week after stopping pimozide the patient developed continuous, severe tics with drastic movements and grimaces always followed by coughing tics. In addition, she experienced intense symptoms of OCD and pulled out her hair. During this period, the woman took several doses of oxazepam. Because of the severity of the combined symptoms, an emergency cesarean section was performed to deliver a healthy, 2448-g male infant with Apgar scores of 7, 8, and 10 at 1, 5, and 10 minutes, respectively. Results of physical and neurologic examinations of the infant at delivery and on day 3 of life were normal. On day 3, an electroencephalogram was obtained, and although the infant was asleep during most of the examination, no abnormalities were observed. The mother restarted pimozide after delivery and decided not to breastfeed (3).

In a brief 2009 report, a 29-year-old woman with Tourette's syndrome was treated with pimozide 4 mg/day throughout gestation (4). She gave birth to a healthy female infant (no other data available).

BREASTFEEDING SUMMARY

No reports describing the use of pimozide during human lactation have been located. The molecular weight (about 462) and prolong elimination half-life (about 55 hours) suggest that the drug will be excreted into breast milk. The effects, including effects on neurodevelopment, of this exposure on a nursing infant are unknown. If a woman taking this drug decides to breastfeed, her infant should be closely monitored for adverse effects seen in adults, such as extrapyramidal reactions (Parkinson-like symptoms; akinesia), sedation, and constipation.

References

1. Committee on Drugs. American Academy of Pediatrics. Use of psychoactive medication during pregnancy and possible effects on the fetus and newborn. Pediatrics 2000;105:880–7.
2. Product information. Orap. Gate Pharmaceuticals, 2004.
3. Bjarnason NH, Rode L, Dalhoff K. Fetal exposure to pimozide: a case report. J Reprod Med 2006;51:443–4.
4. Prowler ML, Kim DR. Perinatal akathisia: implications for pharmacokinetic changes during pregnancy. Am J Psychiatry 2009;166:1296–7.

P

PINDOLOL

Sympatholytic (Antihypertensive)

PREGNANCY RECOMMENDATION: Human Data Suggest Risk in 2nd and 3rd Trimesters
BREASTFEEDING RECOMMENDATION: No Human Data—Potential Toxicity

PREGNANCY SUMMARY

β-Blockade in the newborn has not been reported in the offspring of pindolol-treated mothers. However, because this complication has been observed in infants exposed to other β-blockers (see Acebutolol, Atenolol, and Nadolol), close observation of the newborn is recommended during the first 24–48 hours after birth. Long-term effects of in utero exposure to β-blockers have not been studied but warrant evaluation.

Some β-blockers may cause intrauterine growth restriction (IUGR) and reduced placental weight, especially those lacking intrinsic sympathomimetic activity (ISA) (i.e., partial agonist). Treatment beginning early in the 2nd trimester results in the greatest weight reductions, whereas treatment restricted to the 3rd trimester primarily affects only placental weight. Pindolol does possess ISA. However, IUGR and reduced placental weight may potentially occur with all agents within this class. Although IUGR is a serious concern, the benefits of maternal therapy with β-blockers, in some cases, might outweigh the risks to the fetus and must be judged on a case-by-case basis.

FETAL RISK SUMMARY

Pindolol, a nonselective β-adrenergic blocking agent, has been used for the treatment of hypertension occurring during pregnancy (1–7). Reproductive studies in rats and rabbits at doses >100 times the maximum recommended human dose (MRHD) found no evidence of embryotoxicity or teratogenicity (8). Impaired mating behavior and increased mortality of offspring were observed in female rats given doses 35 times the MRHD before and through 21 days of lactation (8). At 118 times the MRHD, increased fetal resorptions were noted (8).

A 1988 review compared the effects of β-blockers, including pindolol, in pregnancy and concluded that these agents are relatively safe (9) (see comment below).

Pindolol crosses the placenta to the fetus with maternal serum levels higher than cord concentrations (10). Cord:maternal serum ratios at 2 and 6 hours after the last dose were 0.37 and 0.67, respectively. Elimination half-lives in fetal and maternal serum were 1.6 and 2.2 hours, respectively.

The effect of pindolol on uteroplacental blood flow was studied in 10 women with gestational hypertension given a 10-mg oral dose (11). A significant fall in the mean maternal blood pressure and mean arterial blood pressure occurred, but no significant changes were observed in maternal or fetal heart rates, uteroplacental blood flow index, or uteroplacental vascular resistance. In contrast, a 1992 study, comparing the effects of pindolol and propranolol in women with preeclampsia, found a significant reduction in uterine artery vascular resistance, prompting the authors to conclude that pindolol acted, at least in part, through a peripheral vascular mechanism (12).

No fetal malformations attributable to pindolol have been reported, but experience in the 1st trimester is lacking. In a study comparing three β-blockers for the treatment of hypertension during pregnancy, the mean birth weight of pindolol-exposed babies was slightly higher than that of the acebutolol group and much higher than that of the offspring of atenolol-treated mothers (3375 vs. 3160 vs. 2745 g) (2). It is not known whether these differences were caused by the degree of maternal hypertension, the potency of the drugs used, or a combination of these and other factors.

The preliminary results of another study found that more than a third of the infants delivered from hypertensive women treated with pindolol were of low birth weight, but the authors thought this did not differ significantly from the expected rate for this population (3). In mothers treated with pindolol or atenolol, a decrease in the basal fetal heart rate was noted only in the atenolol-exposed fetuses (4). Additionally, in a prospective randomized study comparing 27 pindolol-treated women with 24 atenolol-treated women, no differences between the groups were found in gestational length, birth weight, Apgar scores, rates of cesarean section, or umbilical cord blood glucose levels (5). Treatment in both groups started at about 33 weeks' gestation.

A 1986 reference described the comparison of pindolol plus hydralazine with hydralazine alone for the treatment of maternal hypertension (6). Treatment in both groups was started at about 25 weeks' gestation. The newborn outcomes of the two groups, including birth weights, were similar.

A 1992 report described the outcomes of 29 women with gestational hypertension in the 3rd trimester (7). The women were randomized to receive either the cardioselective β-blocker, atenolol ($N = 13$), or the nonselective β-blocker, pindolol ($N = 16$). The mean maternal arterial blood pressure decrease in the two groups was 9 and 7.8 mmHg, respectively (*ns*). In comparing before and after therapy, several significant changes were measured in fetal hemodynamics with atenolol but, except for fetal heart rate, no significant changes were measured with pindolol. The atenolol-induced changes included a decrease in fetal heart rate, increases in the pulsatility indexes (and thus, the peripheral vascular resistance) of the fetal thoracic descending aorta, the abdominal aorta, and the umbilical artery and a decrease in the umbilical venous blood flow. Although no difference was observed in the birth weights in the two groups, the placental weight in atenolol-treated pregnancies was significantly less (529 vs. 653 g, respectively).

An apparently significant drug interaction occurred when a woman, who was being treated with pindolol for preeclampsia, had indomethacin added for tocolysis to her therapy (13). Two weeks after starting pindolol, 15 mg/day, indomethacin was started with a 200-mg rectal loading dose followed by 25 mg daily for 5 days. A sudden rise in blood pressure (230/130 mmHg) occurred on the fifth day with cardiotocographic changes in fetal vitality (13). A low-birth-weight newborn infant was delivered by cesarean section and the mother's blood pressure returned to normal (125/85 mmHg) in the postpartum period. A similar interaction occurred in another patient who was being treated with propranolol (13).

BREASTFEEDING SUMMARY

No reports describing the use of pindolol during human lactation have been located. The manufacturer, however, states that pindolol is excreted in human milk (8). Because β-blockade has been observed in nursing infants exposed to other β-blockers (see Acebutolol and Atenolol), infants should be closely observed for bradycardia and other symptoms of β-blockade. Long-term effects of exposure to β-blockers from milk have not been studied but warrant evaluation.

References

1. Dubois D, Petitcolas J, Temperville B, Klepper A. Beta blockers and high-risk pregnancies. Int J Biol Res Pregnancy 1980;1:141–5.
2. Dubois D, Petitcolas J, Temperville B, Klepper A, Catherine PH. Treatment of hypertension in pregnancy with β-adrenoceptor antagonists. Br J Clin Pharmacol 1982;13(Suppl):375S–8S.
3. Sukerman-Voldman E. Pindolol therapy in pregnant hypertensive patients. Br J Clin Pharmacol 1982;13(Suppl):379S.
4. Ingemarsson I, Liedholm H, Montan S, Westgren M, Melander A. Fetal heart rate during treatment of maternal hypertension with beta-adrenergic antagonists. Acta Obstet Gynecol Scand 1984;118(Suppl):95–7.
5. Tuimala R, Hartikainen-Sorri A-L. Randomized comparison of atenolol and pindolol for treatment of hypertension in pregnancy. Curr Ther Res 1988;44:579–84.
6. Rosenfeld J, Bott-Kanner G, Boner G, Nissenkorn A, Friedman S, Ovadia J, Merlob P, Reisner S, Paran E, Zmora E, Biale Y, Insler V. Treatment of hypertension during pregnancy with hydralazine monotherapy or with combined therapy with hydralazine and pindolol. Eur J Obstet Gynecol Reprod Biol 1986;22:197–204.
7. Montan S, Ingemarsson I, Marsal K, Sjoberg N-O. Randomized controlled trial of atenolol and pindolol in human pregnancy: effects on fetal haemodyndamics. Br Med J 1992;304:946–9.
8. Product information. Visken. Sandoz Pharmaceuticals, 1997.
9. Frishman WH, Chesner M. Beta-adrenergic blockers in pregnancy. Am Heart J 1988;115:147–52.
10. Grunstein S, Ellenbogen A, Anderman S, Davidson A, Jaschevatsky O. Transfer of pindolol across the placenta in hypertensive pregnant women. Curr Ther Res 1985;37:587–91.
11. Lunell NO, Nylund L, Lewander R, Sarby B, Wager J. Uteroplacental blood flow in pregnancy hypertension after the administration of a beta-adrenoceptor blocker, pindolol. Gynecol Obstet Invest 1984;18:269–74.
12. Meizner I, Paran E, Katz M, Holcberg G, Insler V. Flow velocity analysis of umbilical and uterine artery flow in pre-eclampsia treated with propranolol or pindolol. J Clin Ultrasound 1992;20:115–9.
13. Schoenfeld A, Freedman S, Hod M, Ovadia Y. Antagonism of antihypertensive drug therapy in pregnancy by indomethacin? Am J Obstet Gynecol 1989;161:1204–5.

PIOGLITAZONE

Antidiabetic Agent

PREGNANCY RECOMMENDATION: No Human Data—Animal Data Suggest Moderate Risk
BREASTFEEDING RECOMMENDATION: No Human Data—Probably Compatible

P

PREGNANCY SUMMARY

No reports describing the use of pioglitazone during human pregnancy have been located. Insulin is the treatment of choice for pregnant diabetic patients because, in general, other hypoglycemic agents do not provide adequate glycemic control. Moreover, insulin, unlike most oral agents, does not cross the placenta to the fetus, thus eliminating the additional concern that the drug therapy itself will adversely affect the fetus. Carefully prescribed insulin therapy provides better control of the mother's glucose, thereby preventing the fetal and neonatal complications that occur with this disease. High maternal glucose levels, as may occur in diabetes mellitus, are closely associated with a number of maternal and fetal adverse effects, including fetal structural anomalies if the hyperglycemia occurs early in gestation. To prevent this toxicity, the American College of Obstetricians and Gynecologists recommends that insulin be used for types 1 and 2 diabetes occurring during pregnancy and, if diet therapy alone is not successful, for gestational diabetes (1,2).

FETAL RISK SUMMARY

Pioglitazone, a thiazolidinedione antidiabetic agent, is used as an adjunct to diet and exercise to improve glycemic control in patients with type 2 diabetes mellitus. It is used either alone or in combination with other antidiabetic agents (insulin, metformin, or sulfonylureas). Pioglitazone is not an insulin secretagogue, but acts to decrease insulin resistance in the periphery and in the liver (i.e., decreases insulin requirements). It requires the presence of insulin for its action. Pioglitazone undergoes extensive metabolism by hydroxylation and oxidation, and at least three of the metabolites are pharmacologically active (3).

Reproduction studies with pioglitazone have been conducted in rats and rabbits at doses up to 17 and 40 times, respectively, the maximum recommended human dose based on BSA (MRHD) (1). In pregnant rats, at ≥10 times the MRHD, pioglitazone was embryotoxic as evidenced by increased postimplantation losses, delayed development, and reduced fetal weights. At ≥2 times the MRHD during late gestation and in the lactation period, delayed development was observed that was attributed to decreased body weights. Embryotoxicity was observed in rabbits dosed at 40 times the MRHD (3).

It is not known if pioglitazone or its active metabolites cross the placenta to the fetus. The molecular weight of the parent compound (about 357 for the free base) is low enough that transfer to the fetus should be expected.

BREASTFEEDING SUMMARY

No reports describing the use of pioglitazone during human lactation have been located. The molecular weight of pioglitazone (about 357 for the free base) is low enough that secretion into breast milk should be expected. At least three active metabolites have been identified and these also may be transferred into milk. The effect on a nursing infant from these exposures is unknown. However, weak bases are known to accumulate in milk with concentrations higher than those in maternal plasma.

References

1. American College of Obstetricians and Gynecologists. Pregestational diabetes mellitus. *ACOG Practice Bulletin*. No. 60. March 2005. Obstet Gynecol 2005;105:675–85.
2. American College of Obstetricians and Gynecologists. Gestational diabetes. *ACOG Practice Bulletin*. No. 30. September 2001. Obstet Gynecol 2001;98:525–38.
3. Product information. Actos. Takeda Pharmaceuticals America, 2000.

PIPERACETAZINE

[Withdrawn from the market. See 8th edition.]

PIPERACILLIN

Antibiotic (Penicillin)

PREGNANCY RECOMMENDATION: Compatible
BREASTFEEDING RECOMMENDATION: Compatible

PREGNANCY SUMMARY

Although the reported pregnancy experience with piperacillin is limited, all penicillins are considered low risk in pregnancy.

FETAL RISK SUMMARY

Piperacillin, a piperazine derivative of ampicillin, is a broad-spectrum penicillin (see also Ampicillin). Animal reproduction studies in mice and rats at doses up to 4 times the human dose have shown no evidence of impaired fertility or fetal harm (1).

No reports linking the use of piperacillin with congenital defects in humans have been located. Piperacillin has been used between 24 and 35 weeks' gestation in women with premature rupture of the membranes to delay delivery (2). No adverse maternal or fetal effects were observed.

Piperacillin rapidly crosses the placenta to the fetus (3). Three women, between 22 and 33 weeks' gestation, were administered a single 4-g IV dose of the antibiotic immediately before intrauterine exchange transfusion for Rh isoimmunization. The mean concentrations of piperacillin in fetal serum, maternal serum, and amniotic fluid were 20, 121, and 0.9 mcg/mL, respectively. The fetal:maternal ratio was 0.17.

The pharmacokinetics of piperacillin during pregnancy have been reported (4). Women were administered a 4-g IV dose just before cesarean section. The mean venous cord concentration was 9.7 mcg/mL, representing a mean fetal:maternal ratio of 0.27. As with other penicillins, an increased clearance of the antibiotic was observed during pregnancy.

BREASTFEEDING SUMMARY

Piperacillin is excreted in small amounts into breast milk (1). Although concentrations are low, three potential problems exist for the nursing infant: modification of bowel flora, direct effects on the infant, and interference with the interpretation of culture results if a fever workup is required.

References

1. Product information. Pipracil. Lederle Laboratories, 2000.
2. Lockwood CJ, Costigan K, Ghidini A, Wein R, Cetrulo C, Alvarez M, Berkowitz RL. Double-blind, placebo-controlled trial of piperacillin sodium in preterm membrane rupture (abstract). Am J Obstet Gynecol 1993;168:378.
3. Brown CEL, Christmas JT, Bawdon RE. Placental transfer of cefazolin and piperacillin in pregnancies remote from term complicated by Rh isoimmunization. Am J Obstet Gynecol 1990;163:938–43.
4. Heikkilä A, Erkkola R. Pharmacokinetics of piperacillin during pregnancy. J Antimicrob Chemother 1991;28:419–23.

PIPERAZINE

Anthelmintic

PREGNANCY RECOMMENDATION: Limited Human Data—No Relevant Animal Data
BREASTFEEDING RECOMMENDATION: Hold Breastfeeding

PREGNANCY SUMMARY

No reports associating the use of piperazine with congenital defects have been located, but the data are very limited. There are no relevant animal data.

FETAL RISK SUMMARY

A review of the treatment of threadworm infestation during pregnancy cited a personal communication involving two infants with congenital malformations who were exposed to piperazine (1). One of the infants had bilateral hare lip, cleft palate, and anophthalmia, but exposure to piperazine had occurred at 12 and 14 weeks' gestation, after the period when an exposure could have caused the defects. The mother in the second case had taken the anthelmintic at 6 and 8 weeks' gestation and her infant had a defect of the right foot (1). Based on the timing and scarcity of reports, the possibility of a causal relationship in the both cases is doubtful.

The Collaborative Perinatal Project monitored 50,282 mother–child pairs, 3 of whom had 1st trimester exposure to piperazine. No evidence was found to suggest a relationship to malformations (2).

BREASTFEEDING SUMMARY

Piperazine is excreted in breast milk (1), but specific data have not been located. According to one reviewer, the mother should take her dose immediately following feeding her infant, and then express and discard her milk during the next 8 hours (1).

References

1. Leach FN. Management of threadworm infestation during pregnancy. Arch Dis Child 1990;65:399–400.
2. Heinonen OP, Slone D, Shapiro S. *Birth Defects and Drugs in Pregnancy*. Littleton, MA: Publishing Sciences Group, 1977:299.

PIPERIDOLATE

P

[Withdrawn from the market. See 9th edition.]

PIRBUTEROL

Respiratory Drug (Bronchodilator)

PREGNANCY RECOMMENDATION: No Human Data—Probably Compatible
BREASTFEEDING RECOMMENDATION: No Human Data—Probably Compatible

PREGNANCY SUMMARY

No reports describing the use of pirbuterol in human pregnancy have been located. The animal reproduction data suggest low risk. Other agents in this class (see below) are considered low risk or compatible. Because of its β-2 adrenergic activity, the drug probably inhibits uterine contractions. However, this effect is not seen clinically because the drug has not been detected in blood after inhalation. Nevertheless, pirbuterol inhalers should only be used during labor if clearly indicated. If pirbuterol is used in pregnancy for the treatment of asthma, health care professionals are encouraged to call the toll-free number 877-311-8972 for information about patient enrollment in an Organization of Teratology Information Specialists (OTIS) study.

FETAL RISK SUMMARY

Pirbuterol is an inhaled sympathomimetic amine that has a preferential effect on β-2 adrenergic receptors (1). Other agents in this class are albuterol, metaproterenol, salmeterol, and terbutaline. Pirbuterol is indicated for the prevention and reversal of bronchospasm in patients ≥12 years of age with reversible bronchospasm including asthma. It may be used with or without concurrent theophylline and/or corticosteroid therapy. Each activation delivers a total dose of 453 mcg of pirbuterol acetate. Systemic blood concentrations of pirbuterol following inhalation of doses up to 800 mcg were below the level of detection (2–5 ng/mL). When the drug was given orally, the plasma elimination half-life was about 2 hours (1).

Reproduction studies have been conducted in rats and rabbits. In rats, no teratogenicity was observed with oral doses up to 1000 times the maximum recommended daily inhalation dose in adults based on BSA (MRDID). Pirbuterol was not teratogenic in rabbits given oral doses up to 680 times the MRDID. At 2000 times the MRDID, abortions and fetal death were observed in rabbits (1).

In long-term studies with rats and mice, no evidence of carcinogenicity was seen with dietary doses up to 35 and 15 times the MRDID, respectively. Assays for mutagenicity and cytogenicity were negative. There also was no evidence of impaired fertility in rats given oral doses up to 35 times the MRDID (1).

It is not known if pirbuterol crosses the human placenta. Although the molecular weight (about 300) is low enough, the drug has not been detected in blood when administered by inhalation.

BREASTFEEDING SUMMARY

No reports describing the use of pirbuterol inhalers during human lactation have been located. Although the molecular weight (about 300) is low enough, the drug has not been detected in blood when administered by inhalation. Consequently, there should be no drug in breast milk.

Reference

1. Product information. Maxair. Graceway Pharmaceuticals, 2009.

PIROXICAM

Nonsteroidal Anti-inflammatory

PREGNANCY RECOMMENDATION: **Human Data Suggest Risk in 1st and 3rd Trimesters**
BREASTFEEDING RECOMMENDATION: **Compatible**

PREGNANCY SUMMARY

Constriction of the ductus arteriosus in utero is a pharmacologic consequence arising from the use of prostaglandin synthesis inhibitors during pregnancy (see also Indomethacin) (1). Persistent pulmonary hypertension of the newborn may occur if these agents are used in the 3rd trimester close to delivery (1,2). These drugs also have been shown to inhibit labor and prolong pregnancy, both in humans (3) (see also Indomethacin) and in animals (4). Women attempting to conceive should not use any prostaglandin synthesis inhibitor, including piroxicam, because of the findings in a variety of animal models that indicate these agents block blastocyst implantation (5,6). Moreover, as noted below, nonsteroidal anti-inflammatory drugs (NSAIDs) have been associated with spontaneous abortions (SABs) and congenital malformations. The absolute risk for these defects, however, appears to be low.

FETAL RISK SUMMARY

Piroxicam is an NSAID used for relief of the signs and symptoms of rheumatoid arthritis and osteoarthritis. It is in the same NSAID subclass (oxicams) as meloxicam.

Animal reproduction studies in rabbits and rats have not shown drug-related embryotoxicity or teratogenicity (7–9). However, decreased fetal growth was observed in some species (8).

In a surveillance study of Michigan Medicaid recipients involving 229,101 completed pregnancies conducted between 1985 and 1992, 161 newborns had been exposed to piroxicam during the 1st trimester (F. Rosa, personal communication, FDA, 1993). Six (3.7%) major birth defects were observed (seven expected). Specific data were available for six defect categories, including (observed/expected) 1/2 cardiovascular defects, 1/0 oral clefts, 1/0 spina bifida, 1/0.5 polydactyly, 0/0 limb reduction defects, and 0/0 hypospadias. These data do not support an association between the drug and congenital defects.

A combined 2001 population-based observational cohort study and a case–control study estimated the risk of adverse pregnancy outcome from the use of NSAIDs (10). The use of NSAIDs during pregnancy was not associated with congenital malformations, preterm delivery, or low birth weight, but a positive association was discovered with SABs. A similar study, also published in 2001, failed to find a relationship, in general, between NSAIDs and congenital malformations, but did find a significant association with cardiac defects and orofacial clefts (11). In addition, a 2003 study found a significant association between exposure to NSAIDs in early pregnancy and SABs (12). (See Ibuprofen for details on these three studies.)

A brief 2003 editorial on the potential for NSAID-induced developmental toxicity concluded that NSAIDs, and specifically those with greater cyclooxygenase 2 (COX-2) affinity, had a lower risk of this toxicity in humans than aspirin (13).

BREASTFEEDING SUMMARY

Piroxicam is excreted into breast milk. A nursing woman, 9 months postpartum, was treated with piroxicam 20 mg/day for 4 months (14). Maternal serum concentrations of the drug 2.5 and 15.0 hours after a dose were 5.85 and 4.79 mcg/mL, respectively. Milk levels varied between 0.05 and 0.17 mcg/mL. Based on an ingested volume of 600 mL/day, the investigators estimated the infant would have received a daily dose of about 0.05 mg. However, no drug was detectable in the infant's serum. A second woman stopped nursing her 8-month-old infant when she was treated with piroxicam 40 mg/day (14). Milk concentrations of the drug ranged from 0.11 to 0.22 mcg/mL, with the highest level measured 2.5 hours after the second dose. In both cases, the concentration of the drug in milk was approximately 1% of the mother's serum levels. These amounts probably do not present a risk to the nursing infant (15). The American Academy of Pediatrics classifies piroxicam as compatible with breastfeeding (16).

References

1. Levin DL. Effects of inhibition of prostaglandin synthesis on fetal development, oxygenation, and the fetal circulation. Semin Perinatol 1980;4:35–44.
2. Van Marter LJ, Leviton A, Allred EN, Pagano M, Sullivan KF, Cohen A, Epstein MF. Persistent pulmonary hypertension of the newborn and smoking and aspirin and nonsteroidal antiinflammatory drug consumption during pregnancy. Pediatrics 1996;97:658–63.
3. Fuchs F. Prevention of prematurity. Am J Obstet Gynecol 1976;126:809–20.
4. Powell JG, Cochrane RL. The effects of a number of non-steroidal anti-inflammatory compounds on parturition in the rat. Prostaglandins 1982;23:469–88.
5. Matt DW, Borzelleca JF. Toxic effects on the female reproductive system during pregnancy, parturition, and lactation. In Witorsch RJ, ed. *Reproductive Toxicology*. 2nd ed. New York, NY: Raven Press, 1995:175–93.
6. Dawood MY. Nonsteroidal antiinflammatory drugs and reproduction. Am J Obstet Gynecol 1993;169:1255–65.
7. Product information. Feldene. Pfizer, 2001.
8. Sakai T, Ofsuki I, Noguchi F. Reproduction studies on piroxicam. Yakuri to Chiryo 1980;8:4655–71. As cited in Shepard TH. *Catalog of Teratogenic Agents*. 6th ed. Baltimore, MD: The Johns Hopkins University Press, 1989:513.
9. Perraud J, Stadler J, Kessedjian MJ, Monro AM. Reproductive studies with the anti-inflammatory agent, piroxicam: modification of classical protocols. Toxicology 1984;30:59–63.
10. Nielsen GL, Sorensen HT, Larsen H, Pedersen L. Risk of adverse birth outcome and miscarriage in pregnant users of non-steroidal anti-inflammatory drugs: population based observational study and case-control study. Br Med J 2001;322:266–70.
11. Ericson A, Kallen BAJ. Nonsteroidal anti-inflammatory drugs in early pregnancy. Reprod Toxicol 2001;15:371–5.
12. Li DK, Liu L, Odouli R. Exposure to non-steroidal anti-inflammatory drugs during pregnancy and risk of miscarriage: population based cohort study. Br Med J 2003;327:368–71.
13. Tassinari MS, Cook JC, Hurtt ME. NSAIDs and developmental toxicity. Birth Defects Res B Dev Reprod Toxicol 2003;68:3–49.
14. Ostensen M. Piroxicam in human breast milk. Eur J Clin Pharmacol 1983;25:829–30.
15. Ostensen M, Husby G. Antirheumatic drug treatment during pregnancy and lactation. Scand J Rheumatol 1985;14:1–7.
16. Committee on Drugs, American Academy of Pediatrics. The transfer of drugs and other chemicals into human milk. Pediatrics 2001;108:776–89.

PITAVASTATIN

Antilipemic Agent

PREGNANCY RECOMMENDATION: Contraindicated
BREASTFEEDING RECOMMENDATION: Contraindicated

P

PREGNANCY SUMMARY

No reports describing the use of pitavastatin in human pregnancy have been located. The absence of human pregnancy experience prevents an assessment of the embryo and/or fetal risk. Because the interruption of cholesterol-lowering therapy during pregnancy should have no apparent effect on the long-term treatment of hyperlipidemia, pitavastatin should not be used during pregnancy. Moreover, cholesterol and other products of cholesterol biosynthesis are essential components for fetal development (1). Women taking this agent before conception should stop the therapy before becoming pregnant and certainly on recognition of pregnancy. Accidental use of the drug during gestation, though, apparently has no proven consequences for the fetus.

FETAL RISK SUMMARY

Pitavastatin, a synthetic 3-hydroxy-3-methyl-coenzyme A (HMG-CoA) reductase inhibitor (a statin) that is lipophilic, is indicated as an adjunctive therapy to diet to reduce elevated total cholesterol, low-density lipoprotein cholesterol, apolipoprotein B, and triglycerides and to increase high-density lipoprotein cholesterol. It has the same mechanism of action as other agents available in this class, atorvastatin, fluvastatin, lovastatin, pravastatin, rosuvastatin, and simvastatin (cerivastatin was withdrawn from the market in 2001). Pitavastatin is metabolized to inactive metabolites. Plasma protein binding is high (>99%), mainly to albumin and α-1-acid glycoprotein, and the mean plasma elimination half-life is about 12 hours (1).

Reproduction studies have been conducted in rats and rabbits. In rats during organogenesis, doses resulting in systemic exposures up to 22 times the human systemic exposure at 4 mg/day based on AUC (HSE), the lowest dose tested, caused no adverse effects. When the drug was given from organogenesis through weaning, maternal toxicity (mortality at about ≥3 times the HSE and impaired lactation at about ≥1 times the HSE) contributed to the decreased survival of neonates. In rabbits, maternal toxicity (reduced body weight and abortions) were observed at 4 times the HSE (1).

Carcinogenicity studies in mice were negative, but high doses (295 times the HSE) caused thyroid follicular cell tumors in rats. Pitavastatin was not mutagenic in several assays but high doses that also caused cytotoxicity were clastogenic. High doses caused no adverse effects on male and female rat fertility (1).

It is not known if pitavastatin crosses the human placenta. The molecular weight (about 813 for the free acid) and elimination half-life suggest that it will cross, but the high plasma protein binding might limit the exposure. The drug does cross the rat placenta (1).

BREASTFEEDING SUMMARY

No reports describing the use of pitavastatin during human lactation have been located. The molecular weight (about 813 for the free acid) and elimination half-life (about 12 hours) suggest that it will be excreted into breast milk, but the high plasma protein binding might limit the amount. At least two similar agents (fluvastatin and pravastatin) appear in human milk. Because of the potential for adverse effects in the nursing infant, the drug should not be used during lactation.

Reference

1. Product information. Livalo. Kowa Pharmaceuticals America, 2009.

PLERIXAFOR

Hematologic (Hematopoietic)

PREGNANCY RECOMMENDATION: No Human Data—Animal Data Suggest Moderate Risk
BREASTFEEDING RECOMMENDATION: No Human Data—Potential Toxicity

PREGNANCY SUMMARY

No reports describing the use of plerixafor during human pregnancy have been located. The animal reproduction data suggest risk but only one species was studied. If a pregnant woman's disease requires the use of this agent, she should be informed of the potential risk to her embryo or fetus.

FETAL RISK SUMMARY

Plerixafor, a hematopoietic stem cell mobilizer, is an inhibitor of the CXCR4 chemokine receptor and blocks binding of its cognate ligand, stromal cell-derived factor-1α. It is indicated in combination with granulocyte-colony stimulating factor to mobilize hematopoietic stem cells to the peripheral blood for collection and subsequent autologous transplantation in patients with non-Hodgkin's lymphoma and multiple myeloma. Plerixafor is not metabolized. Plasma protein binding is up to 58% and the terminal half-life is 3–5 hours in patients with normal renal function (1).

Reproduction studies have been conducted in rats. In this species, embryo–fetal toxicity was observed mainly at a dose that was about 10 times the recommended human dose of 0.24 mg/kg based on BSA or 10 times the AUC in subjects with normal renal function who received a single of 0.24 mg/kg. The embryo–fetal toxicities included fetal death, increased resorptions and postimplantation loss, decreased fetal weights, anophthalmia, shortened digits, cardiac interventricular septal defect, ringed aorta, globular heart, hydrocephaly, dilation of olfactory ventricles, and retarded skeletal development (1).

Carcinogenicity studies have not been conducted with plerixafor. The drug was not genotoxic in various assays. Studies in animals on male or female fertility have not been conducted. However, no adverse effects were observed on spermatogenesis in rats in a 28-day repeated dose toxicity study, nor was there any evidence of toxicity in male or female reproductive organs (1).

It is not known if plerixafor crosses the human placenta. However, the molecular weight (about 503), lack of metabolism, moderate plasma protein binding, and moderately long terminal half-life suggest that the drug will cross to the embryo or fetus.

BREASTFEEDING SUMMARY

No reports describing the use of plerixafor during human lactation have been located. The molecular weight (about 503), lack of metabolism, moderate plasma protein binding (up to 58%), and moderately long terminal half-life (3–5 hours) suggest that the drug will be excreted into breast milk. The effect of this exposure on a nursing infant is unknown. The safest course for the infant would be to hold nursing for about 24 hours after a dose. If the mother is given this drug and continues nursing, her infant should be closely monitored for the most common adverse reactions seen in adults: diarrhea, nausea, fatigue, headache, arthralgia, dizziness, and vomiting.

Reference

1. Product information. Mozobil. Genzyme, 2010.

P

PLICAMYCIN

[Withdrawn from the market. See 9th edition.]

PODOFILOX

Keratolytic Agent

PREGNANCY RECOMMENDATION: Contraindicated
BREASTFEEDING RECOMMENDATION: No Human Data—Potential Toxicity

PREGNANCY SUMMARY

Podofilox (podophyllotoxin) is the active compound in podophyllum resin. (See Podophyllum.)

FETAL RISK SUMMARY

No teratogenicity was observed in pregnant rabbits after once daily topical use for 13 days at doses up to 5 times the maximum human dose (1).

BREASTFEEDING SUMMARY

No reports describing the use of podofilox during human lactation have been located.

Reference

1. Product information. Condylox. Oclassen Pharmaceuticals, 2000.

PODOPHYLLUM

Keratolytic Agent

PREGNANCY RECOMMENDATION: Contraindicated
BREASTFEEDING RECOMMENDATION: No Human Data—Potential Toxicity

PREGNANCY SUMMARY

Although it is uncertain whether podophyllum is a human teratogen, products containing this drug should not be used during pregnancy for the treatment of genital warts (human papillomavirus infections) because of the potential severe myelotoxicity and neurotoxicity in the mother. Although one author believes the topical application of podophyllum resin is safe during pregnancy (1), most other sources consider it a dangerous agent to use during this period, especially because of the availability of alternative, safer treatments. The American College of Obstetricians and Gynecologists (2) and other reviews (3) and reference sources (4) all state that the drug is contraindicated during pregnancy. The contraindications to the use of podophyllum agents include the use of podophyllotoxin (podofilox) during pregnancy and in the vagina or cervix at any time (2).

FETAL RISK SUMMARY

Podophyllum is the dried rhizomes and roots of *Podophyllum peltatum* (American mandrake, May apple) (4). Podophyllum resin is the dried mixture of resins extracted from podophyllum (4). Podophyllotoxin (podofilox), the major active compound in podophyllum resin, and podophyllum are keratolytic agents whose caustic action is thought to be caused by the arrest of mitosis in metaphase. In addition to its antimitotic effect, podophyllum also has cathartic action, but should not be used for this purpose because of the potential for severe drug-induced toxicity (5).

Three reproductive studies in rats and mice with podophyllum or podophyllotoxin found no teratogenic effects, but resorptions occurred when the agents were used early in gestation (6–8). A 1952 study observed no teratogenic changes in mice, rats, and rabbits with podophyllotoxin (9). Two other studies involving podophyllum reported embryotoxicity, but not teratogenicity, in mice (10) and only minor skeletal changes in rats (11). Another agent derived from *P. peltatum* that is present in podophyllum resin, peltatin (α and β forms), was not teratogenic in mice (12).

The first report of human teratogenicity related to podophyllum appeared in 1962 (13). A 24-year-old woman took herbal "slimming tablets," containing podophyllum and other extracts, from the 5th to 9th weeks of gestation, a total of 3.5 weeks. The estimated daily dose of podophyllum was 180 mg. The term, female infant had multiple anomalies, including an absent right thumb and radius, a supernumerary left thumb, a probable septal defect of the heart, a defect of the right external ear, and skin tags. The malformations were attributed to the antimitotic action of podophyllum (13).

In contrast to the above outcome, a woman at 26 weeks' gestation was treated with multiple applications of 20% podophyllum resin in compound benzoin tincture for condylomata acuminata (genital human papillomavirus infection) that covered the entire vulva, the minor and major labia, and a portion of the vagina (14). In addition, the woman was accidentally given 5 mL of the preparation orally, a potentially fatal dose. Toxic symptoms in the mother included persistent, severe coughing, nausea and vomiting, and hypotension, all of which had resolved within 72 hours. Three months later, the mother delivered a normal 3560-g male infant who was doing well.

A 1972 report described severe peripheral neuropathy and intrauterine fetal death in a woman at either 32 or 34 weeks' (both dates were used) gestation following the administration of 7.5 mL (1.88 g of podophyllum) of 25% podophyllum resin to florid vulval warts that were friable and bled easily (15). General anesthesia (nitrous oxide and oxygen) was used during application of podophyllum. Fetal heart sounds were lost 2 days after the application of podophyllum, and 10 days later a stillborn female infant was delivered. The woman's symptoms and death of her fetus were attributed to podophyllum poisoning, apparently from systemic absorption of the drug. She eventually recovered and within a year or two she had an uneventful pregnancy and normal infant (15).

Minor congenital malformations consisting of a simian crease on the left hand and a preauricular skin tag were observed in a newborn whose mother had been treated with five applications of 25% podophyllum resin between the 23rd and 29th weeks of pregnancy for condyloma acuminata (16). Although the authors attributed the skin tag to the drug, podophyllum was not related to either anomaly because of the late timing of exposure (17).

The Collaborative Perinatal Project recorded 14 1st trimester exposures to podophyllum (presumably oral) among 50 mothers who had used a group of miscellaneous gastrointestinal drugs (18). From this group, one (2%) infant with an unspecified congenital malformation was observed (standardized relative risk 0.27). It was not stated whether podophyllum was taken by the mother of the affected infant.

BREASTFEEDING SUMMARY

No reports describing the use of podophyllum during human lactation have been located.

References

1. Bargman H. Is podophyllin a safe drug to use and can it be used during pregnancy? Arch Dermatol 1988;124:1718–20.
2. American College of Obstetricians and Gynecologists. Genital human papillomavirus infections. *Technical Bulletin*, No. 193, June 1994.
3. Patsner B, Baker DA, Orr JW Jr. Human papillomavirus genital tract infections during pregnancy. Clin Obstet Gynecol 1990;33:258–67.
4. American Hospital Formulary Service. *Drug Information 1997*. Bethesda, MD: American Society of Health-System Pharmacists, 1997:2754–5.
5. Rosenstein G, Rosenstein H, Freeman M, Weston N. Podophyllum—a dangerous laxative. Pediatrics 1976;57:419–21.
6. Wiesner BP, Yudkin J. Control of fertility by antimitotic agents. Nature (London) 1955;176:249–50. As cited in Shepard TH. *Catalog of Teratogenic Agents*. 7th ed. Baltimore, MD: The Johns Hopkins University Press, 1992:322.
7. Thiersch JB. Effects of podophyllin (P) and podophyllotoxin (PT) on the rat litter in utero. Proc Soc Exp Biol Med 1963;113:124–7. As cited in Shepard TH. *Catalog of Teratogenic Agents*. 7th ed. Baltimore, MD: The Johns Hopkins University Press, 1992:322.
8. Chaube S, Murphy ML. The teratogenic effects of the recent drugs active in cancer chemotherapy. In Woollam DHM, ed. *Advances in Teratology*. New York, NY: Logos and Academic Press, 1968;3:181–237. As cited in Shepard TH. *Catalog of Teratogenic Agents*. 7th ed. Baltimore, MD: The Johns Hopkins University Press, 1992:322.
9. Didcock KA, Picard CW, Robson JM. The action of podophyllotoxin on pregnancy. J Physiol (London) 1952;117:65P–6P. As cited in Schardein JL. *Chemically Induced Birth Defects*. 2nd ed. New York, NY: Marcel Dekker, 1993:491.
10. Joneja MG, LeLiever WC. Effects of vinblastine and podophyllin on DBA mouse fetuses. Toxicol Appl Pharmacol 1974;27:408–14. As cited in Schardein JL. *Chemically Induced Birth Defects*. 2nd ed. New York, NY: Marcel Dekker, 1993:446.
11. Dwornik JJ, Moore KL. Congenital anomalies produced in the rat by podophyllin. Anat Rec 1967;157:237. As cited in Schardein JL. *Chemically Induced Birth Defects*. 2nd ed. New York, NY: Marcel Dekker, 1993:446.
12. Wiesner BP, Wolfe M, Yudkin J. The effects of some antimitotic compounds on pregnancy in the mouse. Stud Fertil 1958;9:129–36. As cited in Schardein JL. *Chemically Induced Birth Defects*. 2nd ed. New York, NY: Marcel Dekker, 1993:805.
13. Cullis JE. Congenital deformities and herbal "slimming tablets." Lancet 1962;2:511–2.
14. Balucani M, Zellers DD. Podophyllum resin poisoning with complete recovery. JAMA 1964;189:639–40.
15. Chamberlain MJ, Reynolds AL, Yeoman WB. Toxic effect of podophyllum application in pregnancy. Br Med J 1972;3:391–2.
16. Karol MD, Conner CS, Watanabe AS, Murphrey KJ. Podophyllum: suspected teratogenicity from topical application. Clin Toxicol 1980;16:283–6.
17. Fraser FC. Letter to the editor. Mod Med Canada 1981;36:1508.
18. Heinonen OP, Slone D, Shapiro S. *Birth Defects and Drugs in Pregnancy*. Littleton, MA: Publishing Sciences Group, 1977:385.

P

POLIDOCANOL

Sclerosing Agent

PREGNANCY RECOMMENDATION: Limited Human Data—Probably Compatible
BREASTFEEDING RECOMMENDATION: No Human Data—Probably Compatible

PREGNANCY SUMMARY

The human pregnancy experience with polidocanol is limited. In animals, polidocanol was associated with both maternal and fetal toxicity in one species, but there was no evidence of an increase in structural abnormalities. The absence of human pregnancy experience prevents a better assessment of the risk to the embryo–fetus.

FETAL RISK SUMMARY

Polidocanol is given IV. It is a sclerosing agent indicated to treat uncomplicated spider veins (varicose veins ≤1 mm in diameter) and uncomplicated reticular veins (varicose veins 1–3 mm in diameter) in the lower extremities. Polidocanol causes local endothelial damage and occlusion of the varicose vein. In four patients, the mean half-life was 1.5 hours (1).

Reproduction studies have been conducted in rats and rabbits. No teratogenic or fetal toxic effects were noted in rats given IV doses up to the maximum human dose based on BSA (MHD) during gestation days 6–17. Polidocanol did not affect the ability of rats to deliver and rear pups when IV doses up to the MHD were given from gestation day 17 to postpartum day 21. In rabbits, IV doses up to the MHD during gestation days 6–20 caused maternal and fetal toxicity, including lower fetal weights and reduced fetal survival, but not skeletal or visceral abnormalities. No adverse maternal or fetal effects in rabbits were observed with a dose one-fifth the MHD (1).

Carcinogenicity studies have not been conducted with polidocanol. The drug was not genotoxic in multiple assays, but it induced numerical chromosomal aberrations in cultured newborn Chinese hamster lung fibroblasts. No effect on reproductive performance was observed in rats given intermittent IV doses equivalent to the MHD (1).

It is not known if polidocanol crosses the human placenta. The molecular weight (about 600) suggests that the drug will cross, but the short elimination half-life may limit the embryo–fetal exposure. Low systemic blood levels have been noted in some patients treated for spider or reticular veins (1). This might result in very-low-level exposure of the embryo–fetus.

A 1991 case report described a woman who was treated for a variceal hemorrhage with endoscopic intravasal injection of polidocanol in mid-pregnancy (2). No adverse effects were observed in her infant. A 2008 case report involved 3rd trimester in utero treatment of two fetuses with polidocanol for congenital cystic adenomatoid malformation of the lung (3). No apparent treatment-related adverse effects were noted in the infants.

BREASTFEEDING SUMMARY

No reports describing the use of polidocanol during lactation have been located. The low-level systemic blood levels and the molecular weight (about 600) suggest that the drug may be excreted into human milk. The effects of this exposure on a nursing infant are unknown but most likely lack clinical significance.

References

1. Product information. Asclera. Merz Aesthetics, 2011.
2. Potzi R, Ferenci P, Gangl A. Endoscopic sclerotherapy of esophageal varices during pregnancy—a case report. Z Gastroenterol 1991;29:246–7.
3. Bermudez C, Perez-Wulff J, Arcadipane M, Bufalino G, Gomez L, Flores L, Sosa C, Bornick PW, Kontopoulus E, Quintero RA. Percutaneous fetal sclerotherapy for congenital cystic adenomatoid malformation of the lung. Fetal Diagn Ther 2008;24:237–40.

P

POLYETHYLENE GLYCOL (3350 & 4000)

Laxative

PREGNANCY RECOMMENDATION: Compatible
BREASTFEEDING RECOMMENDATION: No Human Data—Probably Compatible

PREGNANCY SUMMARY

Although the published human pregnancy experience is limited, the substances are compatible in pregnancy because only minimal amounts are absorbed without significant change in fluid or electrolyte balance. Several sources have concluded that polyethylene glycol (PEG), either PEG-3350 or PEG-4000 (numbers refer to the average molecular weight) are safe and effective and should be considered as first-line therapy for constipation in pregnancy (1–3).

FETAL RISK SUMMARY

PEG-3350 with electrolytes is a white powder that is dissolved in water. It is indicated for bowel cleansing prior to colonoscopy. The osmotic activity of PEG-3350 and the electrolytes result in virtually no net absorption or excretion of ions so that large volumes can be given without significant change in fluid or electrolyte balance (4,5). Similar properties should be expected for PEG-4000.

Reproduction studies in animals have not been conducted. Studies for carcinogenic effects and impairment of fertility in animals have not been performed (4,5).

It is not known if PEG-3350 or PEG-4000 cross the human placenta. Although the average molecular weights are high (3350 and 4000), only minimal amounts are absorbed and clinically significant exposure of the embryo–fetus should not occur.

In a survey on the choice of colonoscopy preparations for pregnant patients, gastroenterologists favored the use of the PEG solution and avoided oral sodium phosphate, whereas obstetricians tended to prefer oral sodium phosphate over the PEG product (6). However, the majority in both groups avoided the sodium phosphate laxative.

In a 2004 observational open label study, 40 pregnant women with constipation were enrolled at 6–37 weeks' gestation (mean 21.0 weeks) and given a solution of PEG-4000 for 15 days at a dose of 250 mL once or twice daily (7). Pregnancy outcomes included one spontaneous abortion at 11 weeks' and two preterm deliveries at 26 weeks'; one for failure of a cervical cerclage and the other for severe gestational hypertension. Of the remaining 37 women, the mean gestational age at delivery was 39.2 weeks. No neonatal complications were observed (7).

A brief 1989 case report described the use of PEG (molecular weight not specified) electrolyte solution in a 18-year-old woman at 38 weeks' gestation who had ingested 55 tablets of a prenatal iron supplement (8). An x-ray demonstrated many iron tablets in her stomach. A whole bowel irrigation with PEG through a nasogastric tube at 2.0 L/hr was started and continued until the bowels were clear. Deferoxamine also was given for chelation. The patient was subsequently discharged in good health and, 5 weeks later, gave birth to a normal 3550-g female infant with no perinatal complications (8).

BREASTFEEDING SUMMARY

No reports describing the use of PEG-3350 or PEG-4000 during human lactation have been located. However, the substances probably are compatible with breastfeeding because only minimal amounts are absorbed. Large volumes can be given without significant change in fluid or electrolyte balance (4,5).

References

1. Tytgat GN, Heading RC, Muller-Lissner S, Kamm MA, Scholmerich J, Berstad A, Fried M, Chaussade S, Jewell D, Briggs A. Contemporary understanding and management of reflux and constipation in the general population and pregnancy: a consensus meeting. Aliment Pharmacol Ther 3003;18:291–301.
2. Mahadevan U, Kane S. American Gastroenterological Association Institute medical position statement on the use of gastrointestinal medications in pregnancy. Gastroenterology 2006;131:278–82.
3. Mahadevan U, Kane S. American Gastroenterological Association Institute technical review on the use of gastrointestinal medications in pregnancy. Gastroenterology 2006;131:283–311.
4. Product information. Nulytely. Braintree Laboratories, 2008.
5. Product information. Trilyte. Alaven Pharmaceutical, 2008.
6. Vinod J, Bonheur J, Korelitz BI, Panagopoulos G. Choice of laxatives and colonoscopic preparation in pregnant patients from the viewpoint of obstetricians and gastroenterologists. World J Gastroenterol 2007;13:6549–52.
7. Neri I, Blasi I, Castro P, Grandinetti G, Ricchi A, Facchinetti F. Polyethylene glycol electrolyte solution (Isocolan) for constipation during pregnancy: an observational open-label study. J Midwifery Women's Health 2004;49:355–8.
8. Van Ameyde KJ, Tenenbein M. Whole bowel irrigation during pregnancy. Am J Obstet Gynecol 1989;160:646–7.

POLYMYXIN B

Antibiotic

PREGNANCY RECOMMENDATION: Compatible (Topical)
BREASTFEEDING RECOMMENDATION: Compatible (Topical)

PREGNANCY SUMMARY

No reports linking the use of polymyxin B with congenital defects have been located. Although available for injection, polymyxin B is used almost exclusively by topical administration.

FETAL RISK SUMMARY

In one study, seven polymyxin B exposures were recorded in the 1st trimester (1). No association with congenital defects was observed. In a brief 2005 report from the Hungarian Case–Control Surveillance of Congenital Abnormalities (1980–1996) database, 6 infants, among 22,843 cases (fetus or newborn) with birth defects, were exposed in utero to parenteral polymyxin B (2). Two of the cases, exposed in the 1st trimester (one in the 1st and the other in the 3rd month of gestation), had cardiovascular malformations. The other four cases, neural tube defect, microcephaly, limb reduction defect, and talipes equinovarus, were exposed after the 1st trimester. There were 13 exposed infants in the matched controls. The crude odds ratio for 1st trimester exposure was 0.8, 95% confidence interval 0.3–2.0 (2).

BREASTFEEDING SUMMARY

No reports describing the use of polymyxin B during human lactation have been reported.

References

1. Heinonen OP, Slone D, Shapiro S. *Birth Defects and Drugs in Pregnancy*. Littleton, MA: Publishing Sciences Group, 1977:297.
2. Kazy Z, Puho E, Czeizel AE. Parenteral polymyxin B treatment during pregnancy. Reprod Toxicol 2005;20:181–2.

P

POLYTHIAZIDE

[Withdrawn from the market. See 9th edition.]

PONATINIB

Antineoplastic (Tyrosine Kinase Inhibitor)

PREGNANCY RECOMMENDATION: Contraindicated
BREASTFEEDING RECOMMENDATION: Contraindicated

PREGNANCY SUMMARY

No reports describing the use of ponatinib in human pregnancy have been located. Embryo–fetal toxicity was observed in the only species studied at a dose about one-fourth the human dose. The lack of human pregnancy experience prevents a more complete assessment of the embryo–fetal risk. If a woman who is or may be pregnant is given this drug, she must be informed of the potential embryo–fetal risk.

FETAL RISK SUMMARY

Ponatinib is an oral tyrosine kinase inhibitor. There are several other agents in this same subclass (see Appendix). It is indicated for the treatment of adult patients with chronic phase, accelerated phase, or blast phase chronic myeloid leukemia that is resistant or intolerant to prior tyrosine kinase inhibitor or Philadelphia chromosome positive acute lymphoblastic leukemia that is resistant or intolerant to prior tyrosine kinase inhibitor therapy. The drug undergoes partial metabolism to apparently inactive metabolites. Plasma protein binding is high (>99%) and the mean elimination half-life is about 24 hours (range 12–66 hours) (1).

Reproduction studies have been conducted in rats. In this species during organogenesis, a dose that was about 24% of the AUC in patients receiving the recommended dose (AUC-RD) caused embryo–fetal toxicities that involved multiple fetal soft-tissue and skeletal alterations, including reduced ossification. A dose equivalent to the AUC-RD was maternal toxic and caused embryo–fetal toxicity as shown by increased resorptions, reduced body weight, external alterations, multiple soft-tissue and skeletal alterations, and reduced ossification (1).

Carcinogenicity studies have not been conducted with ponatinib. The drug was not mutagenic or clastogenic in multiple assays. Although fertility studies in animals have not been conducted, the drug has caused degeneration of epithelium of the testes in rats and monkeys and follicular atresia in monkey ovary with associated endometrial atrophy. The effects seen in rats were at a dose that was about equivalent to the AUC-RD, whereas those in monkeys were seen at about 4 times the AUC-RD (1).

It is not known if ponatinib crosses the human placenta. The molecular weight (about 569) and long elimination half-life suggest that the drug will cross to the embryo–fetus. However, the high plasma protein binding might limit the exposure.

BREASTFEEDING SUMMARY

No reports describing the use of ponatinib during human lactation have been located. The molecular weight (about 569) and long elimination half-life (mean 24 hours, range 12–66 hours) suggest that the drug will be excreted into breast milk. However, the high (>99%) plasma protein binding might limit the exposure. The effect of exposure to the drug on a nursing infant is unknown. However, in adults, the drug has caused multiple hematologic and nonhematologic adverse effects. A nursing infant of a woman who is taking this drug should be closely monitored.

Reference

1. Product information. Iclusig. ARIAD Pharmaceuticals, 2013.

PORFIMER

Antineoplastic

PREGNANCY RECOMMENDATION: No Human Data—Animal Data Suggest Moderate Risk
BREASTFEEDING RECOMMENDATION: No Human Data—Potential Toxicity

P

PREGNANCY SUMMARY

No reports describing the use of porfimer in human pregnancy have been located. Although the dose comparisons used in the animal reproduction studies were based on body weight, there was no association with structural anomalies in two species at doses less than the human dose. Other aspects of developmental toxicity could not be assessed because the tested doses caused maternal toxicity. When the dose was decreased by 50% in one species and continued throughout lactation, there was a reduction in the body weights of the offspring. The absence of human pregnancy experience prevents a more complete assessment of the embryo–fetal risk. Nevertheless, if porfimer is required by a woman, the drug should not be withheld because of pregnancy. If inadvertent pregnancy does occur, the woman should be informed of the potential for embryo and fetal harm.

FETAL RISK SUMMARY

Porfimer is a mixture of oligomers formed by ether and ester linkages of up to eight porphyrin units. It is given IV as a photosensitizing agent used in photodynamic therapy. Photodynamic therapy with porfimer is indicated for cases of esophageal cancer, endobronchial non–small-cell lung cancer, and high-grade Barrett's esophagus. In patients with cancer, the plasma elimination half-life was 250 ± 285 hours (about 10 ± 12 days), but in healthy volunteers, the half-life was 415 ± 104 hours (about 17 ± 4.3 days). Porfimer is about 90% protein bound in human serum.

Reproduction studies with porfimer have been conducted in rats and rabbits. In pregnant rats, an IV dose 0.64 times the human clinical dose based on BSA (HCD) given daily during organogenesis did not cause congenital malformations but did result in maternal and fetal toxicity (resorptions, decreased litter size, delayed ossification, and reduced fetal weight). An IV dose that was 0.32 times the HCD given daily to pregnant rats during late pregnancy through lactation caused a reversible decrease in growth of offspring. An IV dose 0.65 times the HCD, given daily to pregnant rabbits during organogenesis did not cause fetal anomalies, but did cause maternal toxicity resulting in resorptions, decreased litter size, and reduced fetal weight (1).

Long-term studies for carcinogenicity have not been conducted. Porfimer was not mutagenic or clastogenic in several tests. In studies with male and female rats, an IV dose 0.32 times the HCD caused no impairment of fertility. Long-term dosing resulted in discoloration of the testes and ovaries, hypertrophy of the testes, and decreased body weights (1).

It is not known if porfimer crosses the human placenta. Because it is a mixture of oligomers, the exact molecular weight, which is high, cannot be determined. The long elimination half-life, however, does increase the possibility that some may cross to the embryo or fetus.

BREASTFEEDING SUMMARY

No reports describing the use of porfimer during human lactation have been located.

Because it is a mixture of oligomers, the exact molecular weight, which is high, cannot be determined,. The long elimination half-life, however, does increase the possibility that some drug may be excreted into breast milk. The effect of this potential exposure on a nursing infant is unknown, but this agent is a photosensitizer.

Reference

1. Product information. Photofrin. Axcan Scandipharm, 2007.

P

POSACONAZOLE

Antifungal

PREGNANCY RECOMMENDATION: No Human Data—Animal Data Suggest Risk
BREASTFEEDING RECOMMENDATION: No Human Data—Potential Toxicity

PREGNANCY SUMMARY

No reports describing the use of posaconazole in human pregnancy have been located. The animal reproduction data suggest risk, but the absence of human pregnancy experience prevents a more complete assessment of embryo–fetal risk. However, the drug will most likely cross the placenta to the embryo and/or fetus. High-dose fluconazole (400 mg/day) is suspected of causing birth defects (see Fluconazole), but doses <400 mg/day appear to be low risk. Developmental toxicity has not been associated with itraconazole. Thus, the best course is to avoid posaconazole during pregnancy, especially in the 1st trimester. However, if the woman's condition requires posaconazole, the benefit probably outweighs the unknown risk. The lowest possible dose should be used.

FETAL RISK SUMMARY

Posaconazole is a triazole antifungal agent in the same class as fluconazole, itraconazole, terconazole, and voriconazole. Oral posaconazole is indicated for prophylaxis of invasive *Aspergillus* and *Candida* infections in patients who are at high risk of developing these infections due to being severely immunocompromised, such as hematopoietic stem cell transplant recipients with graft-versus-host disease or those with hematologic malignancies with prolonged neutropenia from chemotherapy. It is also indicated for the treatment of oropharyngeal candidiasis, including oropharyngeal candidiasis refractory to itraconazole and/or fluconazole. Posaconazole is only partially metabolized (about 17%) but is highly protein bound (>98%) in the plasma, primarily to albumin. The mean elimination half-life of posaconazole is 35 hours (range 20–66 hours) (1).

Reproduction studies have been conducted in rats and rabbits. In pregnant rats, doses ≥1.4 times the human dose of 400 mg twice daily based on steady-state plasma concentrations in healthy volunteers (HD) resulted in skeletal malformations (cranial malformations and missing ribs). The no-effect dose was 0.7 times the HD. In pregnant rabbits, a dose 2.9 times the HD or higher caused an increase in resorptions. At 5.2 times the HD, maternal toxicity (reduction in body weight gain) and a reduction in litter size were seen. The no-effect dose in rabbits was about 1.4 times the HD (1).

No carcinogenicity was observed in 2-year studies in male and female rats and mice. In addition, the drug was not mutagenic or clastogenic in several tests. Posaconazole had no effect on fertility in male and female rats given doses that were 1.7 and 2.2 times the HD, respectively (1).

It is not known if posaconazole crosses the human placenta. The molecular weight (about 701), low metabolism, and long elimination half-life suggest that the drug will cross to the embryo and/or fetus. The high plasma protein binding, however, should limit the exposure.

BREASTFEEDING SUMMARY

No reports describing the use of posaconazole during human lactation have been located.

The molecular weight (about 701), low metabolism (about 17%), and long elimination half-life (35 hours; range 20–66 hours) suggest that the drug will be excreted into breast milk. The high plasma protein binding (>98%) should limit the amount in milk. The effects, if any, of this potential exposure on a nursing infant are unknown, but severe treatment-related toxicity has been reported in adults, particularly hepatic toxicity, and nausea and vomiting.

Reference

1. Product information. Noxafil. Schering, 2007.

POTASSIUM CHLORIDE

Electrolyte

PREGNANCY RECOMMENDATION: Compatible
BREASTFEEDING RECOMMENDATION: Compatible

P

PREGNANCY SUMMARY

Potassium chloride is a natural constituent of human tissues and fluids. Exogenous potassium chloride may be indicated as replacement therapy for pregnant women with low serum potassium levels, such as those receiving diuretics. Because high or low levels are detrimental to maternal and fetal cardiac function, serum levels should be closely monitored.

FETAL RISK SUMMARY

In a surveillance study of Michigan Medicaid recipients involving 229,101 completed pregnancies conducted between 1985 and 1992, 35 newborns had been exposed to oral potassium salts during the 1st trimester (F. Rosa, personal communication, FDA, 1993). One (2.9%) infant with major birth defects was observed (one expected), a case of limb reduction and hypospadias.

BREASTFEEDING SUMMARY

Breast milk is naturally high in potassium with levels that are 3–4 times those in plasma (1). The concentration of potassium in mature milk is about 55–57 mg/dL (*about 14–15 mEq/L*) (1). Because potassium freely passes into and out of milk, the use of potassium chloride by a lactating woman with normal plasma potassium levels would have no adverse effect on a nursing infant.

Reference

1. Lawrence RA, Lawrence RM. Biochemistry of human milk. In *Breastfeeding. A Guide for the Medical Profession*. 5th ed. St. Louis, MO: Mosby, 1999:127–9.

POTASSIUM CITRATE

Electrolyte/Urinary Alkalinizer

PREGNANCY RECOMMENDATION: Limited Human Data—Probably Compatible
BREASTFEEDING RECOMMENDATION: No Human Data—Probably Compatible

PREGNANCY SUMMARY

Except for the case discussed below, no other reports describing the use of potassium citrate in human pregnancy have been located. In four animal species, no teratogenicity was observed with very high doses of citric acid. Citric acid is widely distributed in nature and is a key ingredient in intermediary metabolism. In addition, potassium is a natural constituent of human tissues and fluids. The primary risk appears to be from hyperkalemia, as this product could produce this in patients who have a condition predisposing them to high blood potassium levels. Because high levels are detrimental to maternal and embryo–fetal cardiac function, maternal serum potassium levels should be closely monitored.

FETAL RISK SUMMARY

Potassium citrate, the potassium salt of citric acid, is given orally to raise the urinary pH. Citric acid is the acid of citrus fruits and is widely distributed in nature. After absorption, metabolism of citrate increases the alkaline load. Potassium citrate is indicated for the management of renal tubular acidosis with calcium stones, hypocitraturic calcium oxalate nephrolithiasis of any etiology, and uric acid lithiasis with or without calcium stones (1).

Reproduction studies have been conducted with citric acid in mice, rats, rabbits, and hamsters. The highest doses studied were 241, 295, 425, and 272 mg/kg, respectively. No teratogenicity was observed in these species (2).

A 1964 report mentioned the use of potassium citrate in one pregnant patient (3). The liveborn infant had an unspecified malformation, but no other details, such as the timing of the exposure, dose, other drugs used, and the medical and obstetric history, were provided.

BREASTFEEDING SUMMARY

No reports describing the use of potassium citrate during lactation have been located. Breast milk is naturally high in potassium with levels that are 3–4 times those in plasma (4). The concentration of potassium in mature milk is about 55–57 mg/dL (*about 14–15 mEq/L*) (4). Because potassium freely passes into and out of milk, the use of potassium citrate by a lactating woman with normal plasma potassium levels would have no adverse effect on a nursing infant. However, if the woman has hyperkalemia, this could result in higher milk potassium concentrations. In this case, nursing infants should be observed for gastrointestinal complaints commonly observed in adults with oral potassium and plasma potassium concentrations should be monitored.

References

1. Product information. Potassium Citrate. Upsher-Smith Laboratories, 2006.
2. Anonymous. Food and Drug Research Labs, Inc.: Teratologic evaluation of FDA 71–54 (citric acid). NTIS Report PB-223 814, 1973. As cited in Shepard TH. *Catalog of Teratogenic Agents*. 10th ed. Baltimore, MD: The Johns Hopkins University Press, 2001:115.
3. Mellin GW. Drugs in the first trimester of pregnancy and the fetal life of Homo sapiens. Am J Obstet Gynecol 1964;90:1169–80.
4. Lawrence RA, Lawrence RM. Biochemistry of human milk. In *Breastfeeding. A Guide for the Medical Profession*. 5th ed. St. Louis, MO: Mosby, 1999:127.

P

POTASSIUM GLUCONATE

Electrolyte

See Potassium Chloride.

POTASSIUM IODIDE

Respiratory Drug (Expectorant)

PREGNANCY RECOMMENDATION: Human Data Suggest Risk in 2nd and 3rd Trimesters
BREASTFEEDING RECOMMENDATION: Limited Human Data—Probably Compatible

PREGNANCY SUMMARY

Because a large number of prescription and over-the-counter medications contain iodide or iodine, pregnant patients should consult with their physician before using these products. The American Academy of Pediatrics considers the use of iodides as expectorants during pregnancy to be contraindicated (1).

FETAL RISK SUMMARY

The primary concern with the use of potassium iodide and the anti-infective, iodine, during pregnancy relates to the effect of iodide on the fetal thyroid gland. Because aqueous solutions of iodine are in equilibrium with the ionized form, all iodide or iodine products are considered as one group.

Iodide readily crosses the placenta to the fetus (2). When used for prolonged periods or close to term, iodide may cause hypothyroidism and goiter in the fetus and newborn. Short-term use, such as a 10-day preparation course for maternal thyroid surgery, does not carry this risk and is apparently safe (3,4). A 1983 review tabulated 49 cases of congenital iodide goiter dating back to 1940 (66 references) (5). In 14 cases, the goiter was large enough to cause tracheal compression resulting in death. Cardiomegaly was present in three surviving newborns and in one of the fatalities. In a majority of the cases, exposure to the iodide was a result of maternal asthma treatment.

Four studies have shown the potential hazard resulting from the use of povidone-iodine during pregnancy (6–9). In each case, significant absorption of iodine occurred in the mother and fetus following topical, vaginal, or perineal use before delivery. Transient hypothyroidism was demonstrated in some newborns (6,9).

BREASTFEEDING SUMMARY

Iodide is concentrated in breast milk (5,10,11). In one report, a breastfeeding mother used povidone-iodine vaginal gel daily for 6 days without douching (10). Two days after stopping the gel, the mother noted an odor of iodine on the 7.5-month-old baby. The free iodide serum:milk ratio 1 day later was approximately 23:1. By day 7, the ratio had fallen to about 4:1 but then rose again on day 8 to 10:1. Serum and urine iodide levels in the infant were grossly elevated. No problems or alterations in thyroid tests were noted in the baby.

In a 2000 case report, a woman delivered a female infant at 29 weeks' gestation by cesarean section (11). An abscess of the abdominal wall 1 week after delivery was treated with IV antibiotics and iodine tampons (each tampon contained about 10.5 mg of iodine). Full breastfeeding of the infant was begun approximately 20 days after birth. At 29 days, neonatal hypothyroidism was diagnosed: the thyroid-stimulating hormone (TSH) level was 287.9 μU/mL (normal range 0.45–10.0 microU/mL). Iodine levels in the mother's milk and infant urine were 4410 mcg/L (normal range 29–490 mcg/L) and 3932 mcg/L (normal <185 mcg/L), respectively. At 32 days, iodine tampons and breastfeeding were stopped and the infant was given levothyroxine (25 mcg/day). Six days later, thyroid function had normalized and breastfeeding was restarted. The infant's thyroid function remained normal over a 4-month follow-up period (11).

The use of povidone-iodine immediately before delivery as a topical anesthetic for epidural anesthesia or cesarean section produced iodine overload in newborn infants who were breastfed as evidenced by increased neonatal TSH concentrations (12). Breastfed infants had a 25- to 30-fold increase in the recall rate at screening for congenital hypothyroidism (TSH >50 mU/L) compared with bottle-fed infants.

The normal iodine content of human milk has been recently assessed (13). Mean iodide levels in 37 lactating women were 178 mcg/L. This is approximately 4 times the recommended daily allowance (RDA) for infants. The RDA for iodine was based on the amount of iodine found in breast milk in earlier studies (13). The higher levels now are probably caused by dietary supplements of iodine (e.g., salt, bread, cow's milk). The significance to the nursing infant from the chronic ingestion of higher levels of iodine is not known. The American Academy of Pediatrics, although recognizing that the maternal use of iodides during lactation may affect the infant's thyroid activity by producing elevated iodine levels in breast milk, classifies the agents as compatible with breastfeeding (14).

References

1. Committee on Drugs. American Academy of Pediatrics. Adverse reactions to iodide therapy of asthma and other pulmonary diseases. Pediatrics 1976;57:272–4.
2. Wolff J. Iodide goiter and the pharmacologic effects of excess iodide. Am J Med 1969;47:101–24.
3. Herbst AL, Selenkow HA. Hyperthyroidism during pregnancy. N Engl J Med 1965;273:627–33.
4. Selenkow HA, Herbst AL. Hyperthyroidism during pregnancy. N Engl J Med 1966;274:165–6.
5. Mehta PS, Mehta SJ, Vorherr H. Congenital iodide goiter and hypothyroidism: a review. Obstet Gynecol Surv 1983;38:237–47.
6. l'Allemand D, Gruters A, Heidemann P, Schurnbrand P. Iodine-induced alterations of thyroid function in newborn infants after prenatal and perinatal exposure to povidone iodine. J Pediatr 1983;102:935–8.
7. Bachrach LK, Burrow GN, Gare DJ. Maternal–fetal absorption of povidone-iodine. J Pediatr 1984;104:158–9.
8. Jacobson JM, Hankins GV, Young RL, Hauth JC. Changes in thyroid function and serum iodine levels after prepartum use of a povidone-iodine vaginal lubricant. J Reprod Med 1984;29:98–100.
9. Danziger Y, Pertzelan A, Mimouni M. Transient congenital hypothyroidism after topical iodine in pregnancy and lactation. Arch Dis Child 1987;62:295–6.
10. Postellon DC, Aronow R. Iodine in mother's milk. JAMA 1982;247:463.
11. Casteels K, Punt S, Bramswig J. Transient neonatal hypothyroidism during breastfeeding after post-natal maternal topical iodine treatment. Eur J Pediatr 2000;159:716–7.
12. Chanoine JP, Boulvain M, Bourdoux P, Pardou A, Van Thi HV, Ermans AM, Delange F. Increased recall rate at screening for congenital hypothyroidism in breast fed infants born to iodine overloaded mothers. Arch Dis Child 1988;63:1207–10.
13. Gushurst CA, Mueller JA, Green JA, Sedor F. Breast milk iodide: reassessment in the 1980s. Pediatrics 1984;73:354–7.
14. Committee on Drugs. American Academy of Pediatrics. The transfer of drugs and other chemicals into human milk. Pediatrics 2001;108:776–89.

POVIDONE-IODINE

Anti-infective

See Potassium Iodide.

PRALATREXATE

Antineoplastic (Antimetabolite)

PREGNANCY RECOMMENDATION: Contraindicated
BREASTFEEDING RECOMMENDATION: Contraindicated

PREGNANCY SUMMARY

No reports describing the use of pralatrexate in human pregnancy have been located. The animal data suggest risk based on the two animal species studied. Although the drug did not cause structural anomalies, it did cause embryo and fetal death. Moreover, pralatrexate is a folic acid antagonist in the same subclass of antimetabolites as aminopterin and methotrexate, agents known to cause embryo–fetal harm. Another agent in this subclass is pemetrexed. Pralatrexate should be avoided in pregnancy. If indicated during pregnancy for maternal benefit, the mother should be informed of the potential risk to her embryo and/or fetus.

FETAL RISK SUMMARY

Pralatrexate is a folate analog metabolic inhibitor that is given as weekly IV push doses. It is in the same antineoplastic subclass of folic acid antagonists (antimetabolites) as methotrexate and pemetrexed. Pralatrexate is indicated for the treatment of patients with relapsed or refractory peripheral T-cell lymphoma. The drug is partially metabolized (about a third of a dose excreted unchanged in urine), but the amount of plasma protein binding was not specified. The terminal elimination half-life is 12–18 hours (1).

Reproduction studies have been conducted in rats and rabbits. In rats, daily doses given on gestation days 7–20 that were about 1.2% of the clinical dose based on BSA (CD) were embryotoxic and fetotoxic. A dose-dependent decrease in fetal viability manifested as an increase in early, late, and total resorptions was observed. There was also a dose-dependent increase in postimplantation loss. In rabbits, similar daily doses given on gestation days 8–21 caused abortion and fetal lethality. The toxicity was manifested as early and total resorptions, postimplantation loss, and a decrease in the total number of live fetuses (1).

Neither carcinogenicity nor fertility studies have been conducted with pralatrexate. The drug was not mutagenic in multiple tests (1).

It is not known if pralatrexate crosses the human placenta. The molecular weight (about 477) and the long terminal elimination half-life suggest that the drug will cross to the embryo–fetus.

BREASTFEEDING SUMMARY

No reports describing the use of pralatrexate during human lactation have been located. The molecular weight (about 477) and the long terminal elimination half-life (12–18 hours) suggest that the drug will be excreted into breast milk. Moreover, the long half-life makes a "pump and dump" method impractical (i.e., the mother would have to wait about 60–90 hours to eliminate most of the drug from her circulation). The effect of this exposure on a nursing infant is unknown, but serious toxicities observed in adults (e.g., pyrexia, bone marrow depression, mucositis, nausea, and vomiting) are potential complications. Based on the potential risk, the best course is not to breastfeed.

Reference

1. Product information. Folotyn. Allos Therapeutics, 2009.

PRALIDOXIME

Antidote

PREGNANCY RECOMMENDATION: Compatible—Maternal Benefit >> Embryo–Fetal Risk
BREASTFEEDING RECOMMENDATION: Hold Breastfeeding

PREGNANCY SUMMARY

Reproduction studies with pralidoxime have not been conducted and the human pregnancy experience is limited to two cases. No other reports describing the use of this drug in human pregnancy have been located. Although the risk this agent represents in pregnancy cannot be assessed, the maternal benefit clearly outweighs any concern regarding embryo or fetal toxicity. Therefore, pralidoxime should not be withheld because of pregnancy.

FETAL RISK SUMMARY

Pralidoxime (2-PAM) reactivates cholinesterase (mainly outside of the CNS) that has been inactivated by phosphorylation due to an organophosphate pesticide or related compound. Its most critical effect is relieving the paralysis of the muscles of respiration. Pralidoxime is short-acting (apparent half-life 74–77 minutes) and is not bound to plasma proteins. Pralidoxime is available in an auto-injector that can be used rapidly in cases of exposure to nerve agents possessing anticholinesterase activity (organophosphate poisoning) (1).

Animal reproduction studies have not been conducted with pralidoxime.

It is not known if pralidoxime crosses the human placenta to the embryo or fetus. Pralidoxime chloride is a quaternary ammonium compound, but the molecular weight of the free base (about 137) is low enough for passage across the placenta. The rapid elimination of the drug should mitigate this transfer.

A 1988 report described the pregnancy outcomes of two women who were treated with pralidoxime for self-induced organophosphorus insecticide poisoning (2). In the first case, a 22-year-old primigravida at 36 weeks' gestation was admitted to the hospital 3 hours after ingesting methamidophos. She was treated with pralidoxime and atropine and eventually recovered. Forty-four days after poisoning, she delivered a healthy 2.85-kg male infant with an Apgar score of 8 at 1 minute. The second case involved a 25-year-old woman at 16 weeks' gestation who ingested fenthion. She also was treated with pralidoxime and atropine and made a full recovery. She delivered a healthy 3.83-kg infant (Apgar 10 at 1 minute) 24 weeks after intoxication (2).

BREASTFEEDING SUMMARY

No reports describing the use of pralidoxime during lactation have been located. Pralidoxime chloride is a quaternary ammonium compound, but the molecular weight of the free base (about 137) is low enough for excretion into breast milk. The rapid elimination of the drug should mitigate this transfer into milk. Moreover, the emergency nature of its use suggests that nursing is unlikely when it has been used. In any event, the maternal benefit is clear and breastfeeding should be held for at least 6–7 hours (about five half-lives) after a dose is given.

References

1. Product information. Pralidoxime Chloride Injection (Auto-Injector). Meridian Medical Technologies, 2002.
2. Karalliedde L, Senanayake N, Ariaratnam A. Acute organophosphorus insecticide poisoning during pregnancy. Hum Toxicol 1988;7:363–4.

P

PRAMIPEXOLE

Antiparkinson Agent

PREGNANCY RECOMMENDATION: Limited Human Data—Animal Data Suggest Low Risk
BREASTFEEDING RECOMMENDATION: No Human Data—Potential Toxicity

PREGNANCY SUMMARY

One report described the use of pramipexole throughout pregnancy with the birth of a normal infant. The limited animal data do not suggest a significant risk for teratogenicity or toxicity. The toxicity observed in rats apparently was caused by mechanisms not present in human pregnancy. However, the near absence of human pregnancy experience prevents an assessment of the embryo–fetal risk. Since Parkinson disease is relatively uncommon during the childbearing years, the use of pramipexole during pregnancy also will be uncommon. Until data on such use are available, the safest course is to avoid, if possible, the use of pramipexole during the 1st trimester.

FETAL RISK SUMMARY

Pramipexole is a nonergoline dopamine agonist indicated for the treatment of the signs and symptoms of idiopathic Parkinson disease. The drug has high specificity for the D_2 and D_3 receptor subtypes. Pramipexole undergoes little if any metabolism, and no metabolites in plasma or urine have been identified. The plasma protein binding of the agent is low (about 15%) and the elimination half-life, in young healthy adults, is about 8 hours. Pramipexole is commonly used in combination with levodopa (1).

Reproduction studies have been conducted in rats and rabbits. In pregnant rats given pramipexole throughout gestation, a dose 5.4 times the highest recommended human clinical dose (1.5 mg 3 times daily) based on BSA (HRHCD) inhibited implantation. A lower dose (3.2 times the HRHCD), administered during organogenesis, caused a high incidence of total resorptions. At this dose, the AUC was 4.3 times the AUC of adults taking 1.5 mg 3 times daily. These adverse effects were thought to be secondary to the prolactin-lowering effect of the drug and prevented an adequate evaluation of the teratogenic potential of pramipexole. Prolactin is required for implantation and pregnancy maintenance in rats but not in rabbits or humans. Offspring postnatal growth was inhibited when pramipexole, at doses approximately equal to the HRHCD or higher, was given to rats during the latter half of pregnancy and throughout lactation. In pregnant rabbits treated during organogenesis with doses 71 times the AUC of adults taking 1.5 mg 3 times daily, no evidence of adverse effects on embryo or fetal development was observed (1).

In a 2-year carcinogenicity study in mice, dietary administration of pramipexole, at doses up to 11 times the HRHCD, was not associated with a significant increase in tumors. A similar study in rats, at doses up to 12.5 times the AUC of adults taking 1.5 mg 3 times daily, also was negative for tumors (1).

It is not known if pramipexole crosses the human placenta. The low molecular weight (about 211 for the free base), low protein binding, and prolonged elimination half-life suggest that the drug will cross to the embryo–fetus.

A 2004 case report described the use of pramipexole throughout pregnancy in a 41-year-old woman with movement disorder caused by Parkinson disease (2). She gave birth by cesarean section to a normal female infant at term with an Apgar score of 9. At 6 months of age, the infant was doing well with normal development (2).

BREASTFEEDING SUMMARY

No reports describing the use of pramipexole during human lactation have been located. The molecular weight (about 211 for the free base) and low protein binding (about 15%) suggest that it will be excreted into breast milk. Because it is a base, accumulation in milk should be expected. The effect of this exposure on a nursing infant is unknown. Infants should be monitored for adverse events commonly observed in adults, such as extrapyramidal disorders (e.g., dyskinesia), hallucinations, somnolence, nausea, and constipation. Pramipexole inhibits prolactin secretion and may inhibit lactation. Until data on its safe use are available, pramipexole should not be used during lactation.

References

1. Product information. Mirapex. Pharmacia & Upjohn, 2003.
2. Mucchiut M, Belgrado E, Cutuli D, Antonini A, Bergonzi P. Pramipexole-treated Parkinson's disease during pregnancy. Mov Disord 2004;19:1114–5.

PRAMLINTIDE

Antidiabetic Agent

PREGNANCY RECOMMENDATION: No Human Data—Animal Data Suggest Moderate Risk
BREASTFEEDING RECOMMENDATION: No Human Data—Probably Compatible

PREGNANCY SUMMARY

No reports describing the use of pramlintide in human pregnancy have been located. The developmental toxicity (structural anomalies) that was observed in one animal species suggests moderate risk. Although pramlintide is an analog of a naturally occurring hormone and the human risk is probably low, the absence of any human pregnancy experience prevents a better assessment of the embryo–fetal risk.

FETAL RISK SUMMARY

Pramlintide, a synthetic analog of human amylin, acts as an amylinomimetic agent that slows the rate of gastric emptying, prevents the postprandial rise in plasma glucagon, and promotes satiety leading to decreased caloric intake and potential weight loss (1). Amylin is a naturally occurring neuroendocrine hormone that is synthesized by pancreatic beta cells. It is located with insulin in beta cells and is excreted with insulin in response to food intake. Pramlintide is 37-amino acid peptide that slightly differs in the amino acid sequence found in human amylin. The agent, given by SC injection, is indicated for type 1 and type 2 diabetes as an adjunct treatment in patients who use mealtime insulin therapy and have not achieved desired glucose control despite optimal insulin therapy. For type 2 diabetes, pramlintide can be given with or without a concurrent sulfonylurea agent and/or metformin. Pramlintide is metabolized primarily by the kidneys, and about 60% is bound to blood cells and albumin. The elimination half-life is about 48 minutes (1).

Reproduction studies with pramlintide have been conducted in rats and rabbits. In rats during organogenesis, increases in structural anomalies (neural tube defects, cleft palate, and exencephaly) were observed at doses producing systemic exposures 10 or more times the exposure from the maximum recommended human dose based on AUC (MRHD). In pregnant rabbits, no evidence of fetal harm was observed with doses producing exposures 9 times the MRHD (1).

No evidence of carcinogenicity was observed in mice and rats given doses over a 2-year period that produced exposures up to 159 and 25 times the MRHD, respectively. Neither mutagenic nor clastogenic effects have been observed in tests with pramlintide. Fertility in male and female rats was not impaired at doses up to 82 times the maximum recommended human dose based on BSA. However, the highest dose resulted in dystocia in 67% of female rats secondary to significant decreases in serum calcium levels (1).

A 2003 ex vivo study using single human cotyledons from term placentas investigated if pramlintide crossed the placenta (2). Consistent with the drug's high molecular weight (about 3949) and the very short elimination half-life, the fetal:maternal ratio was ≤0.006. Although these results might not be reproducible throughout gestation, it is likely that embryo and/or fetal exposure to pramlintide is negligible.

BREASTFEEDING SUMMARY

No reports describing the use of pramlintide during lactation have been located. The high molecular weight (about 3949) and the very short elimination half-life (48 minutes) suggest that little, if any, of the polypeptide will be excreted into breast milk. Even if the polypeptide were excreted into milk, it should be digested in the stomach of the nursing infant. Therefore, although the effect of exposure on a nursing infant is unknown, the risk appears to be negligible.

References

1. Product information. Symlin. Amylin Pharmaceuticals, 2005.
2. Hiles RA, Bawdon RE, Petrella EM. *Ex vivo* human placental transfer of the peptides pramlintide and exenatide (synthetic exendin-4). Hum Exp Toxicol 2003;22:623–8.

PRAMOXINE

Local Anesthetic

PREGNANCY RECOMMENDATION: Compatible
BREASTFEEDING RECOMMENDATION: No Human Data—Probably Compatible

PREGNANCY SUMMARY

Even though no studies describing the use of pramoxine during animal or human pregnancy have been located (1,2), since symptomatic hemorrhoids occur frequently in pregnancy, products containing pramoxine probably have been used during gestation. Because there is insignificant systemic absorption, there does not appear to be a risk to the embryo or fetus from pramoxine.

FETAL RISK SUMMARY

Pramoxine is a local anesthetic used for topical anesthesia. It is administered either alone or combined with hydrocortisone or other ingredients for the temporary relief of pain and itching secondary to minor skin irritations resulting from burns, sunburn, cuts, abrasions, insect bites, and hemorrhoids and other anorectal disorders. Pramoxine is typically formulated in a 1% concentration. Animal reproduction studies with pramoxine have not been conducted.

The molecular weight of pramoxine (about 294 for the free base) is low enough to cross the placenta, but the amount, if any, that is absorbed after topical administration into the systemic circulation is unknown. A 1985 review stated that pramoxine and similar anorectal products were not absorbed (1). However, even if some were absorbed systemically, the maternal plasma concentration would be very low, thus the amount available for transfer to the embryo or fetus should be negligible.

BREASTFEEDING SUMMARY

No studies describing the use of pramoxine during lactation have been located. The molecular weight of the free base (about 294) is low enough for excretion into breast milk, but the drug is not thought to be absorbed (1). Even if some absorption does occur, the amount in the maternal plasma should be very low so that little, if any, drug would appear in milk. The risk to a nursing infant is probably nil.

References

1. Lewis JH, Weingold AB, The Committee on FDA-Related Matters, American College of Gastroenterology. The use of gastrointestinal drugs during pregnancy and lactation. Am J Gastroenterol 1985;80:912–23.
2. Friedman JM. Teratogen update: anesthetic agents. Teratology 1988;37:69–77.

PRASUGREL

Hematologic Agent (Antiplatelet)

PREGNANCY RECOMMENDATION: No Human Data—Animal Data Suggest Low Risk
BREASTFEEDING RECOMMENDATION: No Human Data—Probably Compatible

PREGNANCY SUMMARY

No reports describing the use of prasugrel in human pregnancy have been located. The drug did not cause developmental toxicity (in the absence of maternal toxicity) in two animal species, but the recommended combination of prasugrel and aspirin was not used in animal studies. (See also Aspirin.) The lack of human pregnancy experience prevents a complete assessment of the embryo–fetal risk. Prasugrel is a prodrug that has not been detected in the system circulation, but the active and inactive metabolites have been detected and exposure of the embryo–fetus to these compounds may occur. However, if a woman's condition requires prasugrel combined with aspirin, the benefits appear to outweigh the unknown fetal risks and the drug should not be withheld because of pregnancy.

FETAL RISK SUMMARY

Prasugrel is an irreversible inhibitor of platelet activation and aggregation that is in the same subclass of aggregation inhibitors as cilostazol, clopidogrel, ticlopidine, and treprostinil. It is indicated to reduce the rate of thrombotic cardiovascular events (including stent thrombosis) in patients with acute coronary syndrome who are to be managed with percutaneous coronary intervention. Combination with aspirin (75–325 mg/day) is recommended. Prasugrel is a prodrug that is hydrolyzed in the intestine and converted to the active metabolite before reaching the plasma. The active metabolite has an elimination half-life of about 7 hours (range 2–15 hours) and is highly bound (98%) to serum albumin. The two major inactive metabolites also are highly bound plasma proteins (1,2).

Reproduction studies have been conducted in rats and rabbits. In these species, oral doses up to 30 times the recommended therapeutic human exposure based on plasma exposures to the major circulating human metabolite (RTHE) revealed no evidence of fetal harm. When the doses were increased to a maternal toxic dose, 40 times the RTHE, a slight decrease in pup body weight was observed. At doses >150 times the RTHE, no effect on the behavioral or reproductive development of the offspring was noted (1,2).

In 2-year carcinogenicity studies with high doses, there was an increase in hepatocellular adenomas in mice but no tumors in rats. The drug was not genotoxic or clastogenic in several assays. It had no effect on the fertility of male and female rats at daily doses that were 80 times the human major metabolite exposure at a daily dose of 10 mg (1,2).

The prodrug prasugrel is not detected in plasma. It is not known if the active metabolite crosses the human placenta. The molecular weight of the active metabolite was not stated, but it should be close to the molecular weight of prasugrel (about 374 for the free base). Combined with the long elimination half-life, this suggests that the active metabolite will cross, although the high binding to albumin should limit the exposure.

BREASTFEEDING SUMMARY

No reports describing the use of prasugrel, a prodrug, during human lactation have been located. The prodrug is not detected in plasma, but the active and inactive metabolites have been detected. The molecular weight of the active metabolite was not stated, but it should be close to the molecular weight of prasugrel (about 374 for the free base). Combined with the long elimination half-life (7 hours; range 2–15 hours), this suggests that the active metabolite will be excreted into breast milk, although the high binding to albumin (98%) should limit the amount excreted. Moreover, daily aspirin is recommended for patients taking prasugrel. The effects of these possible exposures on a nursing infant are unknown. However, the American Academy of Pediatrics recommends that aspirin should be used cautiously by the mother during lactation because of potential adverse effects in the nursing infant (see Aspirin).

P

References

1. Product information. Effient. Eli Lilly, 2009.
2. Product information. Effient. Daiichi Sankyo, 2009.

PRAVASTATIN

Antilipemic Agent

PREGNANCY RECOMMENDATION: Contraindicated
BREASTFEEDING RECOMMENDATION: Contraindicated

PREGNANCY SUMMARY

Because the interruption of cholesterol-lowering therapy during pregnancy should have no effect on the long-term treatment of hyperlipidemia, and because of the human data reported with lovastatin, the use of pravastatin is contraindicated during pregnancy. However, evidence suggesting that pravastatin has a lower risk of developmental toxicity because of its hydrophilic properties has been published (see Lovastatin).

FETAL RISK SUMMARY

Pravastatin is used to lower elevated levels of cholesterol. It is a hepatic 3-hydroxy-3-methylglutaryl-coenzyme A (HMG-CoA) reductase inhibitor (a statin). It has the same mechanism of action as other available drugs in this class, atorvastatin, fluvastatin, lovastatin, pitavastatin, rosuvastatin, and simvastatin (cerivastatin was withdrawn from the market in 2001). Pravastatin is structurally related to lovastatin and simvastatin but, in contrast to the lipophilic properties of these agents, it is hydrophilic.

Pravastatin was not teratogenic in rats and rabbits administered doses up to 240 times and 20 times, respectively, the human exposure based on BSA (HE) (1). Similarly, no adverse effects on fertility or reproductive performance were observed in rats with doses up to 120 times the HE (1).

The FDA has received a single report of a fetal loss in a mother taking pravastatin, but further details are not available (F. Rosa, personal communication, FDA, 1995).

In a 2004 case report, a 39-year-old woman took pravastatin (80 mg/day), metformin (2 g/day), and nateglinide (360 mg/day) during the first 24 weeks of gestation (2). All therapy was discontinued and insulin was started for her diabetes. At term, the woman delivered a healthy 2.4-kg male infant (head circumference 34 cm, length 46 cm) with Apgar scores of 8 and 9 at 1 and 5 minutes, respectively. The infant's growth and development were normal at follow-up examinations during the first 6 months of life (2).

A 2004 report described the outcomes of pregnancy that had been exposed to statins and reported to the FDA (see Lovastatin).

Among 19 cases followed by a teratology information service in England, 4 involved 1st trimester exposure to pravastatin (3). The pregnancy outcomes included four healthy newborns (3).

BREASTFEEDING SUMMARY

No reports describing the use of pravastatin during lactation have been located. The manufacturer reports that pravastatin is excreted into breast milk in small amounts (1). Because of the potential for adverse effects in the nursing infant, the drug should not be used during lactation.

References

1. Product information. Pravachol. Bristol-Myers Squibb, 2000.
2. Teelucksingh S, Youssef JE, Sohan K, Ramsewak S. Prolonged inadvertent pravastatin use in pregnancy. Reprod Toxicol 2004;18:299–300.
3. McElhatton P. Preliminary data on exposure to statins during pregnancy (abstract). Reprod Toxicol 2005;20:471–2.

PRAZIQUANTEL

Anthelmintic

PREGNANCY RECOMMENDATION: Limited Human Data—Animal Data Suggest Moderate Risk
BREASTFEEDING RECOMMENDATION: No Human Data—Potential Toxicity

P

PREGNANCY SUMMARY

Praziquantel is not an animal teratogen, but human data are limited to one case. The lack of published human data prevents any assessment of a human risk. Recent data have indicated that the agent may be mutagenic and carcinogenic in humans, especially in developing countries where infections of trematodes and cestodes are frequent and multiple treatment courses may be prescribed. Moreover, the presence of other environmental mutagens combined with praziquantel may increase the risk for mutagenicity (1). Because of this potential toxicity, the use of praziquantel during pregnancy should be reserved for those cases in which the parasite is causing clinical illness or public health problems.

FETAL RISK SUMMARY

Praziquantel is a systemic anthelmintic used in the treatment of parasitic infections involving cestodes (tapeworms), including neurocysticercosis, and trematode (flukes) infestations of the liver and other tissues. The drug is rapidly and nearly completely (80%) absorbed following oral administration. The various metabolites are excreted primarily by the kidneys (2).

Praziquantel was not carcinogenic in rats and hamsters but mutagenic effects in Salmonella tests were observed in one laboratory. The mutagenicity was not confirmed in the same tested strain by other laboratories (2). Similarly, a study published in 1982 found no mutagenic effects in five strains of Salmonella exposed to praziquantel (3). A 1984 review also described negative mutagenic results in a variety of tests, including those with mice, rats, and humans, and negative carcinogenic results in tests with rats and hamsters (4). A 1997 review, however, cited studies that observed a co-mutagenic effect between praziquantel and several mutagens and carcinogens (5). Praziquantel has also been shown in in vitro studies to induce micronuclei in hamster embryonic cells and lymphocytes. Moreover, in some pigs and humans, praziquantel was found to induce hyperploid lymphocytes and structural chromosomal aberrations (5).

Reproduction studies in mice, rats, and rabbits at doses up to 40 times the human dose (60–75 mg/kg over 1 day) showed no evidence of impaired fertility or teratogenicity (2,4). An increase in the abortion rate in rats, however, was observed at doses 3 times the single human therapeutic dose (2). No teratogenicity was observed in other studies in rats and rabbits with doses up to 300 mg/kg (5,6) or in rats with doses up to 450 mg/kg (3). Compared with controls, the administration of praziquantel and ivermectin (another anthelmintic agent) to possums at 8- to 10-week intervals throughout the breeding season to the time of emergence of young from the pouch had no significant effect on the number of births or survival of the young to emergence (7).

A study published in 1985 concluded that treatment of parasitic disease with potentially teratogenic or toxic drugs might not always be indicated in otherwise healthy pregnant women (8). For example, in their study, the authors found that treatment of some gastrointestinal parasites, including some tapeworms and liver flukes, could be postponed until after delivery unless the parasite was causing clinical disease or public health problems (8). Similarly, reviews in 1996 and 1997 recommended avoiding praziquantel during pregnancy (9,10).

There were two cases of neurocysticercosis treated with praziquantel during gestation, but no outcome information is available in either case. A 1996 case report, however, described the use of praziquantel for the treatment of neurocysticercosis in a 17-year-old pregnant woman (11).

She received praziquantel, 1050 mg 3 times daily, for 21 days starting at about 8 weeks' gestation. Seizures, which occurred at the time of presentation and again 4 days after the start of anticysticercus therapy, were successfully controlled with phenytoin and carbamazepine. She eventually delivered a 2.5-kg female at term. Other than documented anemia, no other abnormalities or malformations were found. The placenta appeared normal on gross examination.

BREASTFEEDING SUMMARY

Because praziquantel is excreted into breast milk at a concentration of about one-fourth that of the maternal serum, the manufacturer advises holding nursing on the day of treatment and during the subsequent 72 hours (2). The drug is excreted primarily in the urine with 80% of the dose being eliminated within 4 days (12). About 90% of this elimination, however, occurs in the first 24 hours (12).

No reports describing the use of praziquantel during nursing have been located, but a 1996 review recommended avoiding praziquantel during lactation (9). The effects, if any, on a healthy, noninfected nursing infant from exposure to the drug via breast milk are unknown. Because adverse reactions induced by the death of an infecting parasite have been observed in treated adults (7), nursing infants with parasitic infections sensitive to praziquantel may be at risk for similar adverse effects. Moreover, the potential for mutagenic and carcinogenic effects of the drug should be considered (see Fetal Risk Summary).

References

1. Montero R, Ostrosky P. Genotoxic activity of praziquantel. Mutat Res 1997;387:123–39.
2. Product information. Biltricide. Bayer Corporation, 1999.
3. Ni YC, Shao BR, Zhan CQ, Xu YQ, Ha SH, Jiao PY. Mutagenic and teratogenic effects of anti-schistosomal praziquantel. Chin Med J 1982;95:494–8.
4. Frohberg H. Results of toxicological studies on praziquantel. Arzneimittelforschung 1984;34:1137–44.
5. Muermann P, Von Eberstein M, Frohberg H. Notes on the tolerance of Droncit. Summary of trial results. Ved Med Rev 1976;2:142–65. As cited by Schardein JL. *Chemical Induced Birth Defects*. 2nd ed. New York, NY: Marcel Dekker, 1993:402–15.
6. Muermann P, Von Eberstein M, Frohberg H. Notes on the tolerance of Droncit. Summary of trial results. Vet Med Rev 1976;2:142–65. As cited by Shepard TH. *Catalog of Teratogenic Agents*. 8th ed. Baltimore, MD: The Johns Hopkins University Press, 1995:350.
7. Viggers KL, Lindenmayer DB, Cunningham RB, Donnelly CF. The effects of parasites on a wild population of the Mountain Brushtail possum (*Trichosurus caninus*) in south-eastern Australia. Int J Parasitol 1998;28:747–55.
8. D'Alauro F, Lee RV, Pao-In K, Khairallah M. Intestinal parasites and pregnancy. Obstet Gynecol 1985;66:639–43.
9. Volkheimer G. Intestinal helminthiasis—general practice problem of the gastroenterologist. Z Gastroenterol 1996;34:534–41.
10. De Silva N, Guyatt H, Bundy D. Anthelmintics. A comparative review of their clinical pharmacology. Drugs 1997;53:769–88.
11. Paparone PW, Menghetti RA. Case report: neurocysticercosis in pregnancy. N J Med 1996;93:91–4.
12. Reynolds JEF, ed. *Martindale. The Extra Pharmacopoeia*. 31st ed. London, UK: Royal Pharmaceutical Society, 1996:123–5.

P

PRAZOSIN

Sympatholytic (Antihypertensive)

PREGNANCY RECOMMENDATION: **Limited Human Data—Animal Data Suggest Low Risk**
BREASTFEEDING RECOMMENDATION: **Limited Human Data—Potential Toxicity**

PREGNANCY SUMMARY

Prazosin is an α_1-adrenergic blocking agent used for hypertension. The limited human pregnancy experience and the animal reproduction data suggest low embryo–fetal risk.

FETAL RISK SUMMARY

No evidence of teratogenicity was observed in reproduction studies with rats, rabbits, and monkeys at doses more than 225, 225, and 12 times, respectively, the usual maximum recommended human dose (1). A decreased litter size at birth in rats, however, was observed at the maximum dose.

The molecular weight of prazosin (about 384 for the free base) is low enough that transfer across the placenta to the embryo–fetus is likely. Consistent with this, a 1995 study using a 5-mg delayed-release formulation in three women measured umbilical cord blood concentrations at delivery that were 9%–23% of the maternal plasma levels 8–15 hours after the last dose (2).

In two studies, prazosin was combined with oxprenolol or atenolol, β-adrenergic blockers, in the treatment of pregnant women with severe essential hypertension or gestational hypertension (3,4). The combinations were effective in the first group but less so in the patients with gestational hypertension. No adverse effects attributable to the drugs were noted. Prazosin, 20 mg/day, was combined with minoxidil and metoprolol throughout gestation to treat severe maternal hypertension secondary to chronic nephritis (5). The child, normal except for hypertrichosis as a result of minoxidil, was doing well at 2 years of age.

Prazosin has been used during the 3rd trimester in patients with pheochromocytoma (6,7). In one case, blood pressure was well controlled, but maternal tachycardia required the addition of a β-blocker. A healthy male infant was delivered by cesarean section (6).

A case report published in 1986 described the pregnancy of a 24-year-old woman at 30 weeks' gestation who was managed for recurrent pheochromocytoma with a combination of prazosin, metyrosine (a tyrosine hydroxylase inhibitor), and timolol (a β-adrenergic blocker) (7). Hypertension had been noted at her first prenatal visit at 12 weeks' gestation. Because of declines in fetal breathing, body movements, and amniotic fluid volume that began 2 weeks after the start of therapy, a cesarean section was conducted at 33 weeks'. The 1450-g female infant had Apgar scores of 3 and 5 at 1 and 5 minutes, respectively. Mild metabolic acidosis was found on analysis of umbilical cord blood gases. Multiple infarcts were noted in the placenta but there was no evidence of metastatic tumor. The growth-restricted infant did well and was discharged home on day 53 of life (7).

BREASTFEEDING SUMMARY

No reports describing the use of prazosin during lactation have been located. The manufacturer reports that small amounts are excreted into human milk (1). This is consistent with the molecular weight (about 384 for the free base) of prazosin. The effects on a nursing infant from exposure to the drug from breast milk are unknown.

References

1. Product information. Minipress. Pfizer, 2000.
2. Bourget P, Fernandez H, Edouard D, Lesne-Hulin A, Ribou F, Baton-Saint-Mleux C, Lelaidier C. Disposition of a new rate-controlled formulation of prazosin in the treatment of hypertension during pregnancy: transplacental passage of prazosin. Eur J Drug Metab Pharmacokinet 1995;20:233–41.
3. Lubbe WF, Hodge JV. Combined alpha- and beta-adrenoceptor antagonism with prazosin and oxprenolol in control of severe hypertension in pregnancy. NZ Med J 1981;94:169–72.
4. Lubbe WF. More on beta-blockers in pregnancy. N Engl J Med 1982;307:753.
5. Rosa FW, Idanpaan-Heikkila J, Asanti R. Fetal minoxidil exposure. Pediatrics 1987;80:120.
6. Venuto R, Burstein P, Schneider R. Pheochromocytoma: antepartum diagnosis and management with tumor resection in the puerperium. Am J Obstet Gynecol 1984;150:431–2.
7. Devoe LD, O'Dell BE, Castillo RA, Hadi HA, Searle N. Metastatic pheochromocytoma in pregnancy and fetal biophysical assessment after maternal administration of alpha-adrenergic, beta-adrenergic, and dopamine antagonists. Obstet Gynecol 1986;68:15S–8S.

PREDNISOLONE

Corticosteroid

PREGNANCY RECOMMENDATION: Human Data Suggest Risk
BREASTFEEDING RECOMMENDATION: Compatible

P

PREGNANCY SUMMARY

Prednisolone is the biologically active form of prednisone (see Prednisone). The placenta can oxidize prednisolone to inactive prednisone or less active cortisone (see Cortisone).

BREASTFEEDING SUMMARY

See Prednisone.

PREDNISONE

Corticosteroid

PREGNANCY RECOMMENDATION: Human Data Suggest Risk
BREASTFEEDING RECOMMENDATION: Compatible

PREGNANCY SUMMARY

Prednisone and prednisolone apparently pose a small risk to the developing fetus. One of these risks appears to be orofacial clefts. Although the available evidence supports their use to control various maternal diseases, the mother should be informed of this risk so that she can actively participate in the decision on whether to use these agents during her pregnancy. If prednisone (or prednisolone) is used in pregnancy for the treatment of rheumatoid arthritis, health care professionals are encouraged to call the toll-free number (877-311-8972) for information about patient enrollment in the Organization of Teratology Information Specialists (OTIS) Rheumatoid Arthritis study.

FETAL RISK SUMMARY

Prednisone is metabolized to prednisolone. There are a number of studies in which pregnant patients received either prednisone or prednisolone (see also various antineoplastic agents for additional references) (1–14).

Although most reports describing the use of prednisone or prednisolone during gestation have not observed abnormal outcomes, four large epidemiologic studies have associated the use of corticosteroids in the 1st trimester with nonsyndromic orofacial clefts. Specific agents were not identified in three of these studies (see Hydrocortisone for details), but in one 1999 study, discussed below, the corticosteroids were listed.

In a case–control study, the California Birth Defects Monitoring Program evaluated the association between selected congenital anomalies and the use of corticosteroids 1 month before to 3 months after conception (periconceptional period) (15). Case infants or fetal deaths diagnosed with orofacial clefts, conotruncal defects, neural tubal defects (NTDs), and limb anomalies were identified from a total of 552,601 births that occurred from 1987 through the end of 1989. Controls, without birth defects, were selected from the same database. Following exclusion of known genetic syndromes, mothers of case and control infants were interviewed by telephone, an average of 3.7 years (cases) or 3.8 years (controls) after delivery, to determine various exposures during the periconceptional period. The number of interviews completed were orofacial cleft case mothers (*N* = 662, 85% of eligible), conotruncal case mothers (*N* = 207, 87%), NTD case mothers (*N* = 265, 84%), limb anomaly case mothers (*N* = 165, 82%), and control mothers (*N* = 734, 78%) (15). Orofacial clefts were classified into four phenotypic groups: isolated cleft lip with or without cleft palate (ICLP, *N* = 348), isolated cleft palate (ICP, *N* = 141), multiple cleft lip with or without cleft palate (MCLP, *N* = 99), and multiple cleft palate (MCP, *N* = 74). A total of 13 mothers reported using corticosteroids during the periconceptional period for a wide variety of indications. Six case mothers of infants with ICLP and three of infants with ICP used corticosteroids (unspecified corticosteroid *N* = 1, prednisone *N* = 2, cortisone *N* = 3, triamcinolone acetonide *N* = 1, dexamethasone *N* = 1, and cortisone plus prednisone *N* = 1). One case mother of an infant with NTD used cortisone and an injectable unspecified corticosteroid, and three controls used corticosteroids (hydrocortisone *N* = 1 and prednisone *N* = 2). The odds ratio (OR) for corticosteroid use and ICLP was 4.3 (95% confidence interval [CI] 1.1–17.2), whereas the OR for ICP and corticosteroid use was 5.3 (95% CI 1.1–26.5). No increased risks were observed for the other anomaly groups. Commenting on their results, the investigators thought that recall bias was unlikely because they did not observe increased risks for other malformations, and it was also unlikely that the mothers would have known of the suspected association between corticosteroids and orofacial clefts (15).

A prospective cohort study and meta-analysis of corticosteroid use in pregnancy was reported in 2000 (16). In the prospective study, 187 outcomes (184 pregnancies, 3 sets of twins) exposed to prednisone were compared with the outcomes in 188 controls. Prednisone-exposed infants were delivered at a lower gestational age (38 vs. 39.5 weeks), had an increased rate of premature delivery (17% vs. 5%), and had a lower birth weight (3112 vs. 3429 g) (all statistically significant). There was no significant difference in the rate of major birth defects (3.6% vs. 2%) and there was no cluster of malformations suggesting a common cause. The defects in the prednisone-exposed cases were: Hirschsprung disease; double outlet right ventricle, valvar and subvalvar pulmonary stenosis, hypothyroidism, hypospadias; undescended testicle; and cleft palate, hypospadias. Two cases were excluded from the analysis because the cause of the defects was known (genetic history and maternal infection) (16). In their meta-analysis, they found a small increase in major malformations (OR 3.03, 95% CI 1.08–8.54) for 1st trimester corticosteroid exposure (16). In addition, case–control studies showed a significant association with oral clefts (OR 3.35, 95% CI 1.97–5.69) (16).

In a surveillance study of Michigan Medicaid recipients involving 229,101 completed pregnancies conducted between 1985 and 1992, 143, 236, and 222 newborns had been exposed to prednisolone, prednisone, and methylprednisolone, respectively, during the 1st trimester (F. Rosa, personal communication, FDA, 1993). The number of birth defects, the number expected, and the percent for each drug were 11/6 (7.7%), 11/10 (4.7%), and 14/9 (6.3%), respectively. Specific details were available for six defect categories (observed/expected): cardiovascular defects (2/1, 2/2, 3/2), oral clefts (0/0, 0/0, 0/0), spina bifida (0/0, 0/0, 0/0), polydactyly (0/0, 0/1, 0/1), limb reduction defects (0/0, 0/0, 1/0), and hypospadias (1/0, 0/1, 1/1), respectively. These data do not support an association between the drugs and congenital defects, except for a possible association between prednisolone and the total number of defects. In the latter case, other factors, such as the mother's disease, concurrent drug use, and chance may be involved.

Immunosuppression was observed in a newborn exposed to high doses of prednisone with azathioprine throughout gestation (17). The newborn had lymphopenia, decreased survival of lymphocytes in culture, absence of immunoglobulin M and reduced levels of immunoglobulin G. Recovery occurred at 15 weeks of age. However, these effects were not observed in a larger group of similarly exposed newborns

(18). A 1968 study reported an increase in the incidence of stillbirths following prednisone therapy during pregnancy (7). Increased fetal mortality has not been confirmed by other investigators.

An infant exposed to prednisone throughout pregnancy was born with congenital cataracts (1). The eye defect was consistent with reports of subcapsular cataracts observed in adults receiving corticosteroids. The relationship in this case between the cataracts and prednisone is unknown, but other reports have also described cataracts after corticosteroid use during gestation (see Hydrocortisone).

In a 1970 case report, a female infant with multiple deformities was described (19). Her father had been treated several years before conception with prednisone, azathioprine, and radiation for a kidney transplant. The authors speculated that the child's defects might have been related to the father's immunosuppressive therapy. A relationship to prednisone seems remote because previous studies have shown that the drug has no effect on chromosome number or morphology (20). High, prolonged doses of prednisolone (30 mg/day for at least 4 weeks) may damage spermatogenesis (21). Recovery may require 6 months after the drug is stopped.

Prednisone has been used successfully to prevent neonatal respiratory distress syndrome when premature delivery occurs between 28 and 36 weeks of gestation (22). Therapy between 16 and 25 weeks of gestation had no effect on lecithin:sphingomyelin ratios (23).

BREASTFEEDING SUMMARY

Trace amounts of prednisone and prednisolone have been measured in breast milk (24–27). Following a 10-mg oral dose of prednisone, milk concentrations of prednisone and prednisolone at 2 hours were 26.7 and 1.6 ng/mL, respectively (24). The authors estimated the infant would ingest approximately 28.3 mcg in 1000 mL of milk. In a second study using radioactive-labeled prednisolone in seven patients, a mean of 0.14% of a 5-mg oral dose was recovered per liter of milk during 48–61 hours (25).

In six lactating women, prednisolone doses of 10–80 mg/day resulted in milk concentrations ranging from 5% to 25% of maternal serum levels (26). The milk:plasma ratio increased with increasing serum concentrations. For maternal doses of 20 mg 1–2 times daily, the authors concluded that the nursing infant would be exposed to minimal amounts of steroid. At higher doses, they recommended waiting at least 4 hours after a dose before nursing was performed. However, even at 80 mg/day, the nursing infant would ingest <0.1% of the dose, which corresponds to <10% of the infant's endogenous cortisol production (26).

A 1993 report described the pharmacokinetics of prednisolone in milk (27). Following a 50-mg IV dose, an average of 0.025% (range 0.010%–0.049%) was recovered from the milk. The data suggested a rapid, bidirectional transfer of unbound prednisolone between the milk and serum (27). The investigators concluded that the measured milk concentrations of the steroid did not pose a clinically significant risk to a nursing infant.

Although nursing infants were not involved in the above studies, it is doubtful whether the amounts measured are clinically significant. The American Academy of Pediatrics classifies prednisolone and prednisone as compatible with breastfeeding (28).

References

1. Kraus AM. Congenital cataract and maternal steroid injection. J Pediatr Ophthalmol 1975;12:107–8.
2. Durie BGM, Giles HR. Successful treatment of acute leukemia during pregnancy: Combination therapy in the third trimester. Arch Intern Med 1977;137:90–1.
3. Nolan GH, Sweet RL, Laros RK, Roure CA. Renal cadaver transplantation followed by successful pregnancies. Obstet Gynecol 1974;43:732–9.
4. Grossman JH III, Littner MR. Severe sarcoidosis in pregnancy. Obstet Gynecol 1977;50(Suppl):81s–4s.
5. Cutting HO, Collier TM. Acute lymphocytic leukemia during pregnancy: report of a case. Obstet Gynecol 1964;24:941–5.
6. Hanson GC, Ghosh S. Systemic lupus erythematosus and pregnancy. Br Med J 1965;2:1227–8.
7. Warrell DW, Taylor R. Outcome for the foetus of mothers receiving prednisolone during pregnancy. Lancet 1968;1:117–8.
8. Walsh SD, Clark FR. Pregnancy in patients on long-term corticosteroid therapy. Scott Med J 1967;12:302–6.
9. Zulman JI, Talal N, Hoffman GS, Epstein WV. Problems associated with the management of pregnancies in patients with systemic lupus erythematosus. J Rheumatol 1980;7:37–49.
10. Hartikainen-Sorri AL, Kaila J. Systemic lupus erythematosus and habitual abortion: case report. Br J Obstet Gynaecol 1980;87:729–31.
11. Minchinton RM, Dodd NJ, O'Brien H, Amess JAL, Waters AH. Autoimmune thrombocytopenia in pregnancy. Br J Haematol 1980;44:451–9.
12. Tozman ECS, Urowitz MB, Gladman DD. Systemic lupus erythematosus and pregnancy. J Rheumatol 1980;7:624–32.
13. Karpatkin M, Porges RF, Karpatkin S. Platelet counts in infants of women with autoimmune thrombocytopenia: effect of steroid administration to the mother. N Engl J Med 1981;305:936–9.
14. Pratt WR. Allergic diseases in pregnancy and breast feeding. Ann Allergy 1981;47:355–60.
15. Carmichael SL, Shaw GM. Maternal corticosteroid use and risk of selected congenital anomalies. Am J Med Genet 1999;86:242–4.
16. Park-Wyllie L, Mazzotta P, Pastuszak A, Moretti ME, Beique L, Hunnisett L, Friesen MH, Jacobson S, Kasapinovic S, Chang D, Diav-Citrin O, Chitayat D, Nulman I, Einarson TR, Koren G. Birth defects after maternal exposure to corticosteroids: prospective cohort study and meta-analysis of epidemiological studies. Teratology 2000;62:385–82.
17. Cote CJ, Meuwissen HJ, Pickering RJ. Effects on the neonate of prednisone and azathioprine administered to the mother during pregnancy. J Pediatr 1974;85:324–8.
18. Cederqvist LL, Merkatz IR, Litwin SD. Fetal immunoglobulin synthesis following maternal immunosuppression. Am J Obstet Gynecol 1977;129:687–90.
19. Tallent MB, Simmons RL, Najarian JS. Birth defects in child of male recipient of kidney transplant. JAMA 1970;211:1854–5.
20. Jensen MK. Chromosome studies in patients treated with azathioprine and amethopterin. Acta Med Scand 1967;182:445–55.
21. Mancini RE, Larieri JC, Muller F, Andrada JA, Saraceni DJ. Effect of prednisolone upon normal and pathologic human spermatogenesis. Fertil Steril 1966;17:500–13.
22. Szabo I, Csaba I, Novak P, Drozgyik I. Single-dose glucocorticoid for prevention of respiratory-distress syndrome. Lancet 1977;2:243.
23. Szabo I, Csaba I, Bodis J, Novak P, Drozgyik J, Schwartz J. Effect of glucocorticoid on fetal lecithin and sphingomyelin concentrations. Lancet 1980;1:320.
24. Katz FH, Duncan BR. Entry of prednisone into human milk. N Engl J Med 1975;293:1154.
25. McKenzie SA, Selley JA, Agnew JE. Secretion of prednisone into breast milk. Arch Dis Child 1975;50:894–6.
26. Ost L, Wettrell G, Bjorkhem I, Rane A. Prednisolone excretion in human milk. J Pediatr 1985;106:1008–11.
27. Greenberger PA, Odeh YK, Frederiksen MC, Atkinson AJ Jr. Pharmacokinetics of prednisolone transfer to breast milk. Clin Pharmacol Ther 1993;53:324–8.
28. Committee on Drugs, American Academy of Pediatrics. The transfer of drugs and other chemicals into human milk. Pediatrics 2001;108:776–89.

PREGABALIN

Anticonvulsant

PREGNANCY RECOMMENDATION: No Human Data—Animal Data Suggest Moderate Risk
BREASTFEEDING RECOMMENDATION: No Human Data—Potential Toxicity

PREGNANCY SUMMARY

No reports describing the use of pregabalin in human pregnancy have been located. The animal reproduction data suggest moderate risk, but the absence of human pregnancy experience prevents an assessment of the embryo–fetal risk. Until human pregnancy experience is available, the best course is to avoid pregabalin during gestation.

FETAL RISK SUMMARY

Pregabalin is a structural derivative of the inhibitory neurotransmitter gamma-aminobutyric acid (GABA). However, it does not directly bind to GABA or benzodiazepine receptors, augment GABA responses, alter rat brain GABA concentrations, or have acute effects on GABA uptake or degradation. Pregabalin is indicated as oral adjunctive therapy for adult patients with partial-onset seizures. It is also indicated for the management of neuropathic pain associated with diabetic peripheral neuropathy and postherpetic neuralgia. Pregabalin is freely soluble in water and in both acidic and basic aqueous solutions. It undergoes minimal metabolism and the elimination half-life is about 6 hours. The drug is not bound to plasma proteins (1).

Reproduction studies have been conducted in rats and rabbits. Skull alterations secondary to abnormally advanced ossification were observed in the embryos of rats given an oral dose of pregabalin during organogenesis that produced plasma exposures (AUC) about 42 times the human exposure at the maximum recommended dose of 600 mg/day (HE-MRD). Doses producing exposures about 17–85 times the HE-MRD resulted in increased incidences of skeletal variations and retarded ossification. Decreased fetal body weights were observed at about 85 times the HE-MRD. A no-effect dose for rat embryo–fetal developmental toxicity was not established (1).

When rats were dosed throughout gestation and lactation, offspring growth and survival were decreased at exposures about ≥4 and ≥10 times the HE-MRD, respectively. Mortality was 100% at exposures about 85 times the HE-MRD. Neurobehavioral deficits (decreased auditory startle response) and reproductive impairment (decreased fertility and litter size) were observed in the adult offspring of rats given doses producing exposures about ≥10 and 42 times the HE-MRD, respectively. The no-effect dose for prenatal and postnatal developmental toxicity in rats produced a plasma exposure about 2 times the HE-MRD (1).

In pregnant rabbits given doses during organogenesis that produced plasma exposures about 40 times the HE-MRD, decreased fetal body weight and increased incidences of skeletal malformations, visceral variations, and retarded ossification were observed. The no-effect dose for developmental toxicity was about 16 times the HE-MRD (1).

Pregabalin produced dose-related carcinogenicity (hemangiosarcomas) in two strains of mice. The lowest dose resulting in the malignant vascular tumors was about equal to the HE-MRD; a no-effect dose in mice was not established. No carcinogenic effects were observed in rats. Mutagenic and clastogenic effects were not observed in various assays (1).

Pregabalin caused reproductive toxicity in male rats: decreased sperm counts and motility, increased sperm abnormalities, and reduced fertility. When the males were mated with untreated females, increased preimplantation embryo loss, decreased litter size, decreased fetal body weights, and an increased incidence of fetal abnormalities were observed. The no-effect dose for male reproductive toxicity was about 3 times the HE-MRD. Adverse effects were also noted on male reproductive organs (testes, epididymides) histopathology. The no-effect dose for male fertility toxicity produced plasma exposures about 8 times the HE-MRD. Pregabalin also impaired the fertility of female rats (disrupted estrous cyclicity) and increased the number of days to mating at exposures as low as 9 times the HE-MRD. A no-effect dose for female fertility toxicity was not established (1).

It is not known if pregabalin crosses the human placenta. The low molecular weight (about 159), minimal metabolism, lack of plasma protein binding, and the moderately long elimination half-life suggest that the drug will reach the embryo and fetus.

BREASTFEEDING SUMMARY

No reports describing the use of pregabalin during lactation have been located. The molecular weight (about 159), minimal metabolism, lack of plasma protein binding, and the moderately long elimination half-life (6 hours) suggest that the drug will be excreted into breast milk. Because it is freely soluble in water, the highest concentrations of the drug should be found in fore-milk. In adults, increased incidences of several adverse effects have been observed, including dizziness and somnolence, blurred vision, peripheral edema, myopathy, and decreased platelet count. The lack of data on the excretion of pregabalin into breast milk, combined with the potential for serious toxicity in a nursing infant, suggest that the drug should not be used by women who are breastfeeding.

Reference

1. Product information. Lyrica. Parke-Davis, 2006.

PRIMAQUINE

Antimalarial

PREGNANCY RECOMMENDATION: Contraindicated
BREASTFEEDING RECOMMENDATION: No Human Data—Potential Toxicity

PREGNANCY SUMMARY

No reports describing the use of primaquine in human pregnancy have been located. Primaquine may cause hemolytic anemia in patients with glucose-6-phosphate dehydrogenase (G6PD) deficiency. Two 1978 references stated that pregnant patients at risk for this disorder should be tested accordingly (1), but if the G6PD status was unknown the drug should be withheld until after delivery (2). However, because the fetus is relatively G6PD-deficient (see below), the drug should not be used in pregnancy regardless of the mother's status.

FETAL RISK SUMMARY

Primaquine phosphate is indicated for the radical cure (prevention of relapse) of vivax malaria. Animal reproduction studies were not provided by the manufacturer (3).

It is not known if primaquine phosphate crosses the human placenta. The molecular weight (about 455 for primaquine) is low enough that exposure of the embryo–fetus should be expected.

A 1982 article stated that if prophylaxis or treatment is required with primaquine, it should not be withheld (4). However, more recent reviews have concluded that the drug should not be used in pregnancy because primaquine causes acute hemolysis in those who are G6PD-deficient and because the fetus is relatively G6PD-deficient (5–7).

BREASTFEEDING SUMMARY

No reports describing the use of primaquine during human lactation have been located. The molecular weight (about 259 primaquine) is low enough for excretion into breast milk. The effect of this exposure on a nursing infant is unknown. However, the mother and the infant should be tested for G6PD deficiency before the drug is used during breastfeeding.

References

1. Trenholme GM, Parson PE. Therapy and prophylaxis of malaria. JAMA 1978;240:2293–5.
2. Anonymous. Chemoprophylaxis of malaria. MMWR 1978;27:81–90.
3. Product information. Primaquine Phosphate. Sanofi-Aventis U.S, 2013.
4. Diro M, Beydoun SN. Malaria in pregnancy. South Med J 1982;75:959–62.
5. Phillips-Howard PA, Wood D. The safety of antimalarial drugs in pregnancy. Drug Saf 1996;14:131–45.
6. Nosten F, McGready R, d'Alessandro U, Bonell A, Verhoeff F, Menendez C, Mutabingwa T, Brabin B. Antimalarial drugs in pregnancy: a review. Curr Drug Saf 2006;1:1–15.
7. Irvine MH, Einarson A, Bozzo P. Prophylactic use of antimalarials during pregnancy. Can Fam Physician 2011;57:1279–81.

PRIMIDONE

Anticonvulsant

PREGNANCY RECOMMENDATION: Human Data Suggest Risk
BREASTFEEDING RECOMMENDATION: Limited Human Data—Potential Toxicity

PREGNANCY SUMMARY

Primidone, a structural analog of phenobarbital (see also Phenobarbital), is effective against generalized convulsive seizures and psychomotor attacks. The epileptic patient on anticonvulsant medication is at a higher risk for having a child with developmental toxicity compared with the general population (1–7).

FETAL RISK SUMMARY

A total of 323 infants who were exposed to primidone during the 1st trimester have been noted in various publications (4,8–17). Of the 41 malformed infants described in these reports, only 3 infants were exposed to primidone alone during gestation (8,15,16). The anomalies observed in these three infants were similar to those observed in the fetal hydantoin syndrome (see Phenytoin).

Acardia, a rare congenital defect, was described in a 1996 case report (18). The 28-year-old mother with two healthy children and a long history of epilepsy had taken primidone (500 mg/day) until the 3rd month of pregnancy. She stopped the drug at this time because of concern for malformations. Her pregnancy history included three epileptic seizures in months 4, 5, and 8. She had no prenatal care during the pregnancy until she presented at term. An ultrasound revealed a twin pregnancy. A cesarean section was performed to deliver a normal 2300-g female infant and a female acardiac acephalic monster. Both were in a single amniotic cavity. The normal female infant did well with no problems in the neonatal period. Genetic studies on the anomalous twin could not be conducted because of delay in receiving permission to study it. At autopsy, the head and upper extremities were totally absent and the major internal organs (heart, lungs, liver, spleen, pancreas, and the upper gastrointestinal tract) could not be identified. Structures that were identified included the small intestine with a blind proximal ending, colon with an anal opening, two adrenal glands, two hypoplastic kidneys and ureters, bladder, uterus and tubes, two ovaries, and a single umbilical artery and vein. The cause of the rare defect could not be determined.

In a surveillance study of Michigan Medicaid recipients involving 229,101 completed pregnancies conducted between 1985 and 1992, 36 newborns had been exposed to primidone during the 1st trimester (F. Rosa, personal communication, FDA, 1993). One (2.8%) major birth defect was observed (two expected). Details were not available on the single case, but no anomalies were observed in six defect categories (cardiovascular defects, oral clefts, spina bifida, polydactyly, limb reduction defects, and hypospadias) for which specific data were available.

The effects of exposure (at any time during the 2nd or 3rd month after the last menstrual period) to folic acid antagonists on embryo–fetal development were evaluated in a large, multicenter, case–control surveillance study published in 2000 (19). The report was based on data collected between 1976 and 1998 from 80 maternity or tertiary care hospitals. Mothers were interviewed within 6 months of delivery about their use of drugs during pregnancy. Folic acid antagonists were categorized into two groups: group I—dihydrofolate reductase inhibitors (aminopterin, methotrexate, sulfasalazine, pyrimethamine, triamterene, and trimethoprim); group II—agents that affect other enzymes in folate metabolism, impair the absorption of folate, or increase the metabolic breakdown of folate (carbamazepine, phenytoin, primidone, and phenobarbital) (18). The case subjects were 3870 infants with cardiovascular defects, 1962 with oral clefts, and 1100 with urinary tract malformations. Infants with defects associated with a syndrome were excluded, as were infants with coexisting neural tube defects (NTDs; known to be reduced by maternal folic acid supplementation). Too few infants with limb reduction defects were identified to be analyzed. Controls (N = 8387) were infants with malformations other than oral clefts and cardiovascular, urinary tract, and limb reduction defects and NTDs, but included infants with chromosomal and genetic defects. The risk of malformations in control infants would not have been reduced by vitamin supplementation, and none of the controls used folic acid antagonists. For group I cases, the relative risks (RRs) of cardiovascular defects and oral clefts were 3.4 (95% confidence interval [CI] 1.8–6.4) and 2.6 (95% CI 1.1–6.1), respectively. For group II cases, the RRs of cardiovascular and urinary tract defects, and oral clefts were 2.2 (95% CI 1.4–3.5), 2.5 (95% CI 1.2–5.0), and 2.5 (95% CI 1.5–4.2), respectively. Maternal use of multivitamin supplements with folic acid (typically 0.4 mg) reduced the risks in group I cases, but not in group II cases (19).

A prospective study published in 1999 described the outcomes of 517 pregnancies of epileptic mothers identified at one Italian center from 1977 (20). Excluding genetic and chromosomal defects, malformations were classified as severe structural defects, mild structural defects, and deformations. Minor anomalies were not considered. Spontaneous (N = 38) and early (N = 20) voluntary abortions were excluded from the analysis, as were 7 pregnancies that delivered at other hospitals. Of the remaining 452 outcomes, 427 were exposed to anticonvulsants of which 313 involved monotherapy: primidone (N = 35), carbamazepine (N = 113), phenobarbital (N = 83), valproate (N = 44), phenytoin (N = 31), clonazepam (N = 6), and other (N = 1). There were no defects in the 25 pregnancies not exposed to anticonvulsants. Of the 42 (9.3%) outcomes with malformations, 24 (5.3%) were severe, 10 (2.2%) were mild, and 8 (1.8%) were deformities. There were three malformations with primidone monotherapy: two (5.7%) were severe (intraventricular defect and hypospadias), and one (2.8%) was mild (undescended testis and inguinal hernia). The investigators concluded that the anticonvulsants were the primary risk factor for an increased incidence of congenital malformations (see also Carbamazepine, Clonazepam, Phenobarbital, Phenytoin, and Valproic Acid) (20).

The Lamotrigine Pregnancy Registry, an ongoing project conducted by the manufacturer, was first published in January 1997 (21). The final report was published in July 2010. The Registry is now closed. In nine prospectively enrolled pregnancies exposed in the 1st trimester to primidone and lamotrigine, with or without other anticonvulsants, the outcomes were seven live births without birth defects, one elective abortion, and one birth defect (21).

There are other potential complications associated with the use of primidone during pregnancy. Neurologic manifestations in the newborn, such as overactivity and tumors, have been associated with use of primidone in pregnancy (16,22). Neonatal hemorrhagic disease with primidone alone or in combination with other anticonvulsants has been reported (14,23–27). Suppression of vitamin K_1-dependent clotting factors is the proposed mechanism of the hemorrhagic effect (14,23). Administration of prophylactic vitamin K_1 to the infant immediately after birth is recommended (see Phytonadione, Phenytoin, and Phenobarbital).

BREASTFEEDING SUMMARY

Primidone is excreted into breast milk. Because primidone undergoes limited conversion to phenobarbital, breast milk concentrations of phenobarbital should be anticipated (see Phenobarbital). A milk:plasma ratio of 0.8 for primidone has been reported (28). The amount of primidone available to the nursing infant is small, with milk concentrations of 2.3 mcg/mL. No reports linking adverse effects to the nursing infant have been located, however, patients who breastfeed should be instructed to watch for potential sedative effects in the infant. The American Academy of Pediatrics classifies primidone as an agent that has been associated with significant effects in some nursing infants and should be used with caution in the lactating woman (29).

References

1. Hill RB. Teratogenesis and antiepileptic drugs. N Engl J Med 1973;289: 1089–90.
2. Bodendorfer TW. Fetal effect of anticonvulsant drugs and seizure disorders. Drug Intell Clin Pharm 1978;12:14–21.
3. Committee on Drugs, American Academy of Pediatrics. Anticonvulsants and pregnancy. Pediatrics 1977;63:331–3.
4. Nakane Y, Okuma T, Takahashi R, Sato Y, Wada T, Sato T, Fukushima Y, Kumashiro H, Ono T, Takahashi T, Aoki Y, Kazamatsuri H, Inami M, Komai S, Seino M, Miyakoshi M, Tanimura T, Hazama H, Kawahara R, Otuski S, Hosokawa K, Inanaga K, Nakazawa Y, Yamamoto K. Multi-institutional study on the teratogenicity and fetal toxicity of antiepileptic drugs: a report of a collaborative study group in Japan. Epilepsia 1980;21:663–80.
5. Andermann E, Dansky L, Andermann F, Loughnan PM, Gibbons J. Minor congenital malformations and dermatoglyphic alterations in the offspring of epileptic women: a clinical investigation of the teratogenic effects of anticonvulsant medication. In *Epilepsy, Pregnancy and the Child*. Proceedings of a Workshop held in Berlin, September 1980. New York, NY: Raven Press, 1981.
6. Danksy L, Andermann F. Major congenital malformations in the offspring of epileptic patients. In *Epilepsy, Pregnancy and the Child*. Proceedings of a Workshop held in Berlin, September 1980. New York, NY: Raven Press, 1981.
7. Janz D. The teratogenic risks of antiepileptic drugs. Epilepsia 1975;16: 159–69.
8. Lowe CR. Congenital malformations among infants born to epileptic women. Lancet 1973;1:9–10.
9. Lander CM, Edwards BE, Eadie MJ, Tyrer JH. Plasma anticonvulsants concentrations during pregnancy. Neurology 1977;27:128–31.
10. Speidel BD, Meadow SR. Maternal epilepsy and abnormalities of the fetus and newborn. Lancet 1972;2:839–43.
11. McMullin GP. Teratogenic effects of anticonvulsants. Br Med J 1971;4:430.
12. Fedrick J. Epilepsy and pregnancy: a report from the Oxford Record Linkage Study. Br Med J 1973;2:442–8.
13. Biale Y, Lewenthal H, Aderet NB. Congenital malformations due to anticonvulsant drugs. Obstet Gynecol 1975;45:439–42.
14. Thomas P, Buchanan N. Teratogenic effect of anticonvulsants. J Pediatr 1981;99:163.
15. Myhree SA, Williams R. Teratogenic effects associated with maternal primidone therapy. J Pediatr 1981;99:160–2.
16. Rudd NL, Freedom RM. A possible primidone embryopathy. J Pediatr 1979;94:835–7.
17. Heinonen OP, Slone D, Shapiro S. *Birth Defects and Drugs in Pregnancy*. Littleton, MA: Publishing Sciences Group, 1977:358.
18. Kutlay B, Bayramoglu S, Kutlar AI, Yesildaglar N. An acardiac acephalic monster following in-utero anti-epileptic drug exposure. Eur J Obstet Gynecology Reprod Med 1996;65:245–8.
19. Hernandez-Diaz S, Werler MM, Walker AM, Mitchell AA. Folic acid antagonists during pregnancy and the risk of birth defects. N Engl J Med 2000;343:1608–14.
20. Canger R, Battino D, Canevini MP, Fumarola C, Guidolin L, Vignoli A, Mamoli D, Palmieri C, Molteni F, Granata T, Hassibi P, Zamperini P, Pardi G, Avanzini G. Malformations in offspring of women with epilepsy: a prospective study. Epilepsia 1999;40:1231–6.
21. The Lamotrigine Pregnancy Registry. Final Report. September 1, 1992 through March 31, 2010. GlaxoSmithKline, July 2010.
22. Martinez G, Snyder RD. Transplacental passage of primidone. Neurology 1973;23:381–3.
23. Kohler HG. Haemorrhage in the newborn of epileptic mothers. Lancet 1966;1:267.
24. Bleyer WA, Skinner AL. Fatal neonatal hemorrhage after maternal anticonvulsant therapy. JAMA 1976;235:826–7.
25. Mountain KR, Hirsh J, Gallus AS. Neonatal coagulation defect due to anticonvulsant drug treatment in pregnancy. Lancet 1970;1:265–8.
26. Evans AR, Forrester RM, Discombe C. Neonatal hemorrhage following maternal anticonvulsant therapy. Lancet 1970;1:517–8.
27. Margolin DO, Kantor NM. Hemorrhagic disease of the newborn: an unusual case related to maternal ingestion of antiepileptic drug. Clin Pediatr (Phila) 1972;11:59–60.
28. Kaneko S, Sato T, Suzuki K. The levels of anticonvulsants in breast milk. Br J Clin Pharmacol 1979;7:624–7.
29. Committee on Drugs, American Academy of Pediatrics. The transfer of drugs and other chemicals into human milk. Pediatrics 2001;108:776–89.

PROBENECID

Antigout (Uricosuric)

P

PREGNANCY RECOMMENDATION: Limited Human Data—Probably Compatible
BREASTFEEDING RECOMMENDATION: Limited Human Data—Probably Compatible

PREGNANCY SUMMARY

No reports linking the use of probenecid with congenital defects have been located. Probenecid has been used during pregnancy without producing adverse effects in the fetus or in the infant (1–7).

FETAL RISK SUMMARY

Probenecid is a uricosuric and renal tubular blocking agent. It is indicated for the treatment of the hyperuricemia associated with gout and gouty arthritis. It also is indicated as an adjuvant to therapy with penicillin or with ampicillin, methicillin, ocacillin, cloxacillin, or nafcillin, for elevation and prolongation of plasma levels by whatever route the antibiotic is given (8).

Animal reproduction studies have apparently not been conducted.

The manufacturer reports that the drug crosses the placenta and appears in cord blood (8). This is consistent with its relatively low molecular weight (about 285).

In a surveillance study of Michigan Medicaid recipients involving 229,101 completed pregnancies conducted between 1985 and 1992, 339 newborns had been exposed to probenecid during the 1st trimester (F. Rosa, personal communication, FDA, 1993). A total of 17 (5.0%) major birth defects were observed (14 expected). Specific data were available for six defect categories, including (observed/expected) 5/3 cardiovascular defects, 1/1 oral clefts, 0/0 spina bifida, 1/1 polydactyly, 0/1 limb reduction defects, and 1/1 hypospadias. These data do not support an association between the drug and congenital defects.

BREASTFEEDING SUMMARY

Consistent with its molecular weight (about 285), probenecid is excreted into breast milk. A 30-year-old, penicillin-allergic, breastfeeding woman developed erysipelas/cellulitis in her breasts 9 days after a cesarean section (9). She was treated with IV cephalothin, 1 g every 6 hours for 3 days, then oral cephalexin and probenecid (both 500 mg 4 times daily). Severe diarrhea, discomfort, and crying was observed in the nursing infant during IV therapy and continued with oral therapy, but at a decreased level. The symptoms had nearly resolved after partial replacement of breast milk with goat's milk for 7 days. Sixteen days after initiation of oral therapy, the woman collected 12 milk samples (6 pairs of fore- and hind-milk) by manual expression over a 16-hour interval. The average concentrations of probenecid and cephalexin were 964 and 745 mcg/L, respectively. The concentrations of the two substances in fore- and hind-milk were not significantly different. The infant doses, based on the milk AUC and an estimated intake of 150 mL/kg/day, of probenecid and cephalexin were 0.7% and 0.5%, respectively, of the mother's weight-adjusted dose. Although these doses were thought to be low enough to exclude systemic effects, it was concluded that cephalexin was the most likely cause of the diarrhea (9).

References

1. Beidleman B. Treatment of chronic hypoparathyroidism with probenecid. Metabolism 1958;7:690–8.
2. Lee FI, Loeffler FE. Gout and pregnancy. J Obstet Gynaecol Br Commonw 1962;69:299.
3. Batt RE, Cirksena WJ, Lebhertz TB. Gout and salt-wasting renal disease during pregnancy. Diagnosis, management and follow-up. JAMA 1963;186:835–8.
4. Hayashi TT. The effect of Benemid on uric acid excretion in normal pregnancy and in pre-eclampsia. Am J Obstet Gynecol 1957;73:17–22.
5. Czaczkes WJ, Ullmann TD, Sadowsky E. Plasma uric acid levels, uric acid excretion, and response to probenecid in toxemia of pregnancy. J Lab Clin Med 1958;51:224–9.
6. Harris RE, Gilstrap LC III, Pretty A. Single-dose antimicrobial therapy for asymptomatic bacteriuria during pregnancy. Obstet Gynecol 1982;59: 546–9.
7. Cavenee MR, Farris JR, Spalding TR, Barnes DL, Castaneda YS, Wendel GD Jr. Treatment of gonorrhea in pregnancy. Obstet Gynecol 1993;81: 33–8.
8. Product information. Probenecid. Mylan Pharmaceuticals, 2006.
9. Ilett KF, Hackett LP, Ingle B, Bretz PJ. Transfer of probenecid and cephalexin into breast milk. Ann Pharmacother 2006;40:986–9.

PROBUCOL

[Withdrawn from the market. See 9th edition.]

PROCAINAMIDE

Antiarrhythmic

PREGNANCY RECOMMENDATION: Limited Human Data—No Relevant Animal Data
BREASTFEEDING RECOMMENDATION: Limited Human Data—Probably Compatible

PREGNANCY SUMMARY

Procainamide is a cardiac drug used for the termination and prophylaxis of atrial and ventricular tachyarrhythmias (1). The limited human pregnancy data suggest low risk for the embryo–fetus, but there is no 1st trimester or animal reproduction data.

FETAL RISK SUMMARY

Animal reproduction studies with procainamide have not been conducted. The use of procainamide during human pregnancy has not been associated with congenital anomalies or other adverse fetal effects (1–9).

Successful cardioversion with procainamide of a fetal supraventricular tachycardia presenting at 30 weeks' gestation has been reported (4). Therapy with digoxin alone and digoxin combined with propranolol failed to halt the arrhythmia. Procainamide was then combined with digoxin, resulting in cardioversion to a sinus rhythm and resolution of fetal ascites and pericardial effusion. During the following 3 weeks, the mother was maintained on oral procainamide, 1 g every 6 hours, and digoxin. Maternal serum levels of procainamide varied from 2.4 to 4.1 mcg/mL. The abnormal rhythm returned at 33 weeks' gestation, and control became increasingly difficult. Additional therapy with procainamide increased the maternal serum concentration to 6.8 mcg/mL. During the last 24 hours, four IV bolus doses of procainamide (700 mg 3 times, 650 mg once) were administered plus a maintenance dose of 3 mg/minute. Three hours after the last bolus dose, a 2650-g female infant was delivered by cesarean section. Serum procainamide concentrations in the newborn and mother were 4.3 and 15.6 mcg/mL, respectively, a ratio of 0.28. During the subsequent neonatal course, the infant was successfully treated for congestive heart failure and persistent supraventricular tachycardia. The electrocardiogram was normal at 6 months of age.

In a case similar to the one described above, therapy with digoxin, verapamil, and procainamide failed to control fetal supraventricular tachycardia presenting at 24 weeks' gestation (5). At cordocentesis, procainamide concentrations in the fetus and mother were 11.7 and 12.8 mcg/mL (ratio 0.91), respectively. Levels of the active metabolite, *N*-acetylprocainamide, were 3.0 and 3.5 mcg/mL (ratio 0.86), respectively. Cardioversion was eventually accomplished with direct fetal digitalization by periodic IM injection.

Procainamide was prescribed for a woman in her 24th week of gestation for ventricular tachycardia (7). She was treated with doses up to 2000 mg every 6 hours, combined with metoprolol 100 mg every 12 hours, until delivery of a healthy 3155-g female at 38 weeks' gestation. Maternal and mixed cord blood concentrations of procainamide were 6.0 and 6.4 mcg/mL (fetal:maternal ratio 1.1), respectively. Similar analysis for *N*-acetylprocainamide yielded levels of 9.4 and 8.7 mcg/mL (ratio 0.9), respectively. No fetal or newborn adverse effects were observed.

BREASTFEEDING SUMMARY

Procainamide and its active metabolite, *N*-acetylprocainamide, are accumulated in breast milk (10). A woman was treated with procainamide, 375 mg 4 times daily, for premature ventricular contractions during the 3rd trimester (10). The dose was increased to 500 mg 4 times daily 1 week before delivery at 39 weeks' gestation. Simultaneous serum and milk samples were obtained in the postpartum period (exact time not specified) every 3 hours for a total of 15 hours. Procainamide (500 mg) was administered orally at hours 0, 6, and 12 immediately after samples were obtained. Mean serum concentrations of procainamide and *N*-acetylprocainamide were 1.1 and 1.6 mcg/mL, respectively, while the concentrations in the milk were 5.4 and 3.5 mcg/mL, respectively. The mean milk:serum ratios for the parent drug and the metabolite were 4.3 (range 1.0–7.3) and 3.8 (range 1.0–6.2), respectively. The amount of drug available to the nursing infant based on a hypothetical serum level of 8 mcg/mL was estimated to be 64.8 mcg/mL (procainamide plus metabolite). Assuming the infant could ingest 1000 mL of milk/day (thought to be unlikely), this would only provide about 65 mg of total active drug. This amount was not expected to yield clinically significant serum concentrations (10).

The American Academy of Pediatrics classifies procainamide as compatible with breastfeeding (11). However, the long-term effects of exposure in the nursing infant to procainamide and its metabolites are unknown, particularly in regard to potential drug toxicity (e.g., development of antinuclear antibodies and lupus-like syndrome).

References

1. Rotmensch HH, Elkayam U, Frishman W. Antiarrhythmic drug therapy during pregnancy. Ann Intern Med 1983;98:487–97.
2. Mendelson CL. Disorders of the heartbeat during pregnancy. Am J Obstet Gynecol 1956;72:1268–301.
3. Tamari I, Eldar M, Rabinowitz B, Neufeld HN. Medical treatment of cardiovascular disorders during pregnancy. Am Heart J 1982;104:1357–63.
4. Dumesic DA, Silverman NH, Tobias S, Golbus MS. Transplacental cardioversion of fetal supraventricular tachycardia with procainamide. N Engl J Med 1982;307:1128–31.
5. Weiner CP, Thompson MIB. Direct treatment of fetal supraventricular tachycardia after failed transplacental therapy. Am J Obstet Gynecol 1988;158:570–3.
6. Little BB, Gilstrap LC III. Cardiovascular drugs during pregnancy. Clin Obstet Gynecol 1989;32:13–20.
7. Allen NM, Page RL. Procainamide administration during pregnancy. Clin Pharm 1993;12:58–60.
8. Kanzaki T, Murakami M, Kobayashi H, Takahashi S, Chiba Y. Hemodynamic changes during cardioversion in utero: a case report of supraventricular tachycardia and atrial flutter. Fetal Diagn Ther 1993;8:37–44.
9. Hallak M, Neerhof MG, Perry R, Nazir M, Huhta JC. Fetal supraventricular tachycardia and hydrops fetalis: combined intensive, direct, and transplacental therapy. Obstet Gynecol 1991;78:523–5.
10. Pittard WB III, Glazier H. Procainamide excretion in human milk. J Pediatr 1983;102:631–3.
11. Committee on Drugs, American Academy of Pediatrics. The transfer of drugs and other chemicals into human milk. Pediatrics 2001;108:776–89.

P

PROCARBAZINE

Antineoplastic

PREGNANCY RECOMMENDATION: Contraindicated—1st Trimester
BREASTFEEDING RECOMMENDATION: Contraindicated

PREGNANCY SUMMARY

Although combined with other antineoplastics, structural anomalies have been observed when procarbazine was used in the 1st trimester. The drug is best avoided during organogenesis.

FETAL RISK SUMMARY

The use of procarbazine, in combination with other antineoplastic agents, during pregnancy has been described in nine patients, five during the 1st trimester (1–8). One of the 1st trimester exposures was electively terminated, but no details on the fetus were given (5). Congenital malformations were observed in the remaining four 1st trimester exposures (1–4):

Multiple hemangiomas (1)
Oligodactyly of both feet with webbing of third and fourth toes, four metatarsals on left, three on right, bowing of right tibia, cerebral hemorrhage, spontaneously aborted at 24 weeks' gestation (2)
Malformed kidneys—markedly reduced size and malposition (3)
Small secundum atrial septal defect, intrauterine growth restriction (4)

A patient in her 12th week of pregnancy received procarbazine, 50 mg daily, in error for 30 days when she was given the drug instead of an iron/vitamin supplement (6). A normal 3575-g male infant was delivered at term.

Long-term studies of growth and mental development in offspring exposed to procarbazine during the 2nd trimester, the period of neuroblast multiplication, have not been conducted (9). Data from one review indicated that 40% of the infants exposed to anticancer drugs were of low birth weight (10). This finding was not related to the timing of exposure.

Procarbazine is mutagenic and carcinogenic in animals (11). In combination with other antineoplastic drugs, procarbazine may produce gonadal dysfunction in males and females (12–17). Ovarian and testicular function may return to normal, with successful pregnancies possible, depending on the patient's age at the time of therapy and the total dose of chemotherapy received (16–20).

It is not known if procarbazine crosses the human placenta. The molecular weight (about 222 for the free base) is low enough that exposure of the embryo–fetus should be expected.

Occupational exposure of the mother to antineoplastic agents during pregnancy may present a risk to the fetus. A position statement from the National Study Commission on Cytotoxic Exposure and a research article involving some antineoplastic agents are presented in the monograph for cyclophosphamide (see Cyclophosphamide).

BREASTFEEDING SUMMARY

No reports describing the use of procarbazine during lactation have been located. The molecular weight (about 222 for the free base) is low enough that excretion into breast milk should be expected. Because of the potential for tumorigenicity, women receiving this drug should not nurse (21).

References

1. Wells JH, Marshall JR, Carbone PP. Procarbazine therapy for Hodgkin's disease in early pregnancy. JAMA 1968;205:935–7.
2. Garrett MJ. Teratogenic effects of combination chemotherapy. Ann Intern Med 1974;80:667.
3. Mennuti MT, Shepard TH, Mellman WJ. Fetal renal malformation following treatment of Hodgkin's disease during pregnancy. Obstet Gynecol 1975;46:194–6.
4. Thomas PRM, Peckham MJ. The investigation and management of Hodgkin's disease in the pregnant patient. Cancer 1976;38:1443–51.
5. Daly H, McCann SR, Hanratty TD, Temperley IJ. Successful pregnancy during combination chemotherapy for Hodgkin's disease. Acta Haematol (Basel) 1980;64:154–6.
6. Daw EG. Procarbazine in pregnancy. Lancet 1970;2:984.
7. Johnson IR, Filshie GM. Hodgkin's disease diagnosed in pregnancy: case report. Br J Obstet Gynaecol 1977;84:791–2.
8. Jones RT, Weinerman ER. MOPP (nitrogen mustard, vincristine, procarbazine, and prednisone) given during pregnancy. Obstet Gynecol 1979;54:477–8.
9. Dobbing J. Pregnancy and leukaemia. Lancet 1977;1:1155.
10. Nicholson HO. Cytotoxic drugs in pregnancy: review of reported cases. J Obstet Gynecol Br Commonw 1968;75:307–12.
11. Lee IP, Dixon RL. Mutagenicity, carcinogenicity and teratogenicity of procarbazine. Mutat Res 1978;55:1–14.
12. Sherins RJ, DeVita VT Jr. Effect of drug treatment for lymphoma on male reproductive capacity: studies of men in remission after therapy. Ann Intern Med 1973;79:216–20.
13. Sherins RJ, Olweny CLM, Ziegler JL. Gynecomastia and gonadal dysfunction in adolescent boys treated with combination chemotherapy for Hodgkin's disease. N Engl J Med 1978;299:12–6.
14. Johnson SA, Goldman JM, Hawkins DF. Pregnancy after chemotherapy for Hodgkin's disease. Lancet 1979;2:93.
15. Card RT, Holmes IH, Sugarman RG, Storb R, Thomas ED. Successful pregnancy after high dose chemotherapy and marrow transplantation for treatment of aplastic anemia. Exp Hematol 1980;8:57–60.
16. Schilsky RL, Sherins RJ, Hubbard SM, Wesley MN, Young RC, DeVita VT Jr. Long-term follow-up of ovarian function in women treated with MOPP chemotherapy for Hodgkin's disease. Am J Med 1981;71:552–6.
17. Shalet SM, Vaughan Williams CA, Whitehead E. Pregnancy after chemotherapy induced ovarian failure. Br Med J 1985;290:898.
18. Whitehead E, Shalet SM, Blackledge G, Todd I, Crowther D, Beardwell CG. The effect of combination chemotherapy on ovarian function in women treated for Hodgkin's disease. Cancer 1983;52:988–93.
19. Andrieu JM, Ochoa-Molina ME. Menstrual cycle, pregnancies and offspring before and after MOPP therapy for Hodgkin's disease. Cancer 1983;52:435–8.
20. Schapira DV, Chudley AE. Successful pregnancy following continuous treatment with combination chemotherapy before conception and throughout pregnancy. Cancer 1984;54:800–3.
21. Product information. Matulane. Sigma-Tau Pharmaceuticals, 2000.

PROCHLORPERAZINE

Antipsychotic/Antiemetic

PREGNANCY RECOMMENDATION: Compatible
BREASTFEEDING RECOMMENDATION: No Human Data—Potential Toxicity

PREGNANCY SUMMARY

Although there are isolated reports of congenital defects in children exposed to prochlorperazine in utero, the majority of the evidence indicates that this drug and the general class of phenothiazines are low risk for both mother and fetus if used occasionally in low doses. Other reviewers have also concluded that the phenothiazines are not teratogenic (1,2).

FETAL RISK SUMMARY

Prochlorperazine is a piperazine phenothiazine. In one rat study, prochlorperazine produced significant postnatal weight decrease, increased fetal mortality, and minor behavioral changes, but no structural defects (3). In a second rat study, an increased incidence of cleft palate, a few anencephalic fetuses, and one double monster was observed (4).

The drug readily crosses the placenta (5). Prochlorperazine has been used to treat nausea and vomiting of pregnancy. Most studies have found the drug to be safe for this indication (see also Chlorpromazine) (6–8).

The Collaborative Perinatal Project (CPP) monitored 50,282 mother–child pairs, 877 of whom had 1st trimester exposure to prochlorperazine (8). For use anytime during pregnancy, 2023 exposures were recorded. No evidence was found in either group to suggest a relationship to malformations or an effect on perinatal mortality rate, birth weight, or IQ scores at 4 years of age (8).

In a separate study using data from the CPP, offspring of psychotic or neurotic mothers who had consumed prochlorperazine for 1–2 months during gestation ($N = 30$) were significantly taller than nonexposed controls ($N = 71$) at 4 months and at 1 year of age (9). Those who had been exposed for longer than 2 months ($N = 8$) were also taller than controls at both ages, but not significantly so. Offspring ($N = 21$) of normal women, who had taken the drug for more than 2 months during pregnancy, were significantly taller than nonexposed controls ($N = 68$) at 1 year of age but no difference was measured at 7 years of age. Moreover, the mean weight of exposed children of normal mothers was significantly greater than controls at 1 year of age, but not at 7 years of age. The mechanisms behind these effects were not clear, but may have been related to the dopamine receptor-blocking action of the drug (9).

Five infants exposed to prochlorperazine, and, in some cases, to multiple other drugs, during the 1st trimester are described below:

Cleft palate, micrognathia, congenital heart defects, skeletal defects (10)
Thanatophoric dwarfism (short limb anomaly) (11)
Hypoplasia of radium and ulnar bones with a vestigial wrist and hand (12)
Below-the-elbow amputation in one arm and small atrophic hand attached to the stump (13)
Below-the-knee amputation in one limb, with rudimentary foot attached to stump (one twin) (13)

The relationship between prochlorperazine and the above defects is unknown. The case of dwarfism was probably caused by genetic factors. No evidence of amniotic bands was observed in the two cases involving amputations, both of whom were exposed during the mothers' treatment for hyperemesis gravidarum (13).

A 1963 report described phocomelia of the upper limbs in a male infant exposed to two phenothiazines during gestation (14). The mother had not taken prochlorperazine until approximately the 13th week of gestation, so no association between the drug and the defect is possible. However, the other agent, trifluoperazine, was taken early in pregnancy (see also Trifluoperazine). In another study, no increase in defects or pattern of malformations were observed in 76 infants (2 sets of twins) exposed in utero to the antiemetic (15).

In a surveillance study of Michigan Medicaid recipients involving 229,101 completed pregnancies conducted between 1985 and 1992, 704 newborns had been exposed to prochlorperazine during the 1st trimester (F. Rosa, personal communication, FDA, 1993). A total of 24 (3.4%) major birth defects were observed (29 expected). Specific data were available for six defect categories, including (observed/expected) 6/7 cardiovascular defects, 1/1 oral clefts, 0/0 spina bifida, 1/2 polydactyly, 1/1 limb reduction defects, and 0/2 hypospadias. These data do not support an association between the drug and congenital defects.

BREASTFEEDING SUMMARY

No reports describing the excretion of prochlorperazine into breast milk have been located. Because other phenothiazines appear in human milk (e.g., chlorpromazine), excretion of prochlorperazine should be expected. Sedation is a possible effect in the nursing infant.

References

1. Ayd FJ Jr. Children born of mothers treated with chlorpromazine during pregnancy. Clin Med 1964;71:1758–63.
2. Ananth J. Congenital malformations with psychopharmacologic agents. Compr Psychiatry 1975;16:437–45.
3. Vorhees CV, Brunner RL, Butcher RE. Psychotropic drugs as behavioral teratogens. Science 1979;205:1220–5. As cited in Shepard TH. *Catalog of Teratogenic Agents*. 6th ed. Baltimore, MD: The Johns Hopkins University Press, 1989:525–6.
4. Roux C. Action teratogene de la prochlorpemazine. Arch Fr Pediatr 1959;16:968–71. As cited in Shepard TH. *Catalog of Teratogenic Agents*. 6th ed. Baltimore, MD: The Johns Hopkins University Press, 1989:525–6.
5. Moya F, Thorndike V. Passage of drugs across the placenta. Am J Obstet Gynecol 1962;84:1778–98.
6. Reider RO, Rosenthal D. Wender P, Blumenthal H. The offspring of schizophrenics. Fetal and neonatal deaths. Arch Gen Psychiatry 1975;32:200–11.
7. Milkovich L, Van den Berg BJ. An evaluation of the teratogenicity of certain antinauseant drugs. Am J Obstet Gynecol 1976;125:244–8.
8. Slone D, Siskind V, Heinonen OP, Monson RR, Kaufman DW, Shapiro S. Antenatal exposure to the phenothiazines in relation to congenital malformations, perinatal mortality rate, birth weight, and intelligence quotient score. Am J Obstet Gynecol 1977;128:486–8.
9. Platt JE, Friedhoff AJ, Broman SH, Bond RN, Laska E, Lin SP. Effects of prenatal exposure to neuroleptic drugs on children's growth. Neuropsychopharmacology 1988;1:205–12.
10. Ho CK, Kaufman RL, McAlister WH. Congenital malformations. Cleft palate, congenital heart disease, absent tibiae, and polydactyly. Am J Dis Child 1975;129:714–6.
11. Farag RA, Ananth J. Thanatophoric dwarfism associated with prochlorperazine administration. N Y State J Med 1978;78:279–82.
12. Freeman R. Limb deformities: possible association with drugs. Med J Aust 1972;1:606–7.
13. Rafla N. Limb deformities associated with prochlorperazine. Am J Obstet Gynecol 1987;156:1557.
14. Hall G. A case of phocomelia of the upper limbs. Med J Aust 1983;1: 449–50.
15. Mellin GW. Report of prochlorperazine during pregnancy from the fetal life study bank (abstract). Teratology 1975;11:28A.

P

PROCYCLIDINE

[Withdrawn from the market. See 9th edition.]

PROGUANIL

Antimalarial

PREGNANCY RECOMMENDATION: Compatible—Maternal Benefit >> Embryo–Fetal Risk
BREASTFEEDING RECOMMENDATION: Limited Human Data—Probably Compatible

PREGNANCY SUMMARY

No adverse fetal or newborn effects attributable to the use of proguanil during gestation have been reported. It is considered by some to be the least toxic prophylactic agent available (1).

FETAL RISK SUMMARY

Proguanil is not available in the United States as a single agent, but is available in combination with atovaquone (see also Atovaquone). Proguanil, a biguanide compound that inhibits plasmodial dihydrofolate reductase, has been frequently used in other parts of the world for causal prophylaxis (defined as absolute prevention) of falciparum malaria since 1948. It is now known, however, that no chemoprophylaxis regimen ensures complete protection against infection with malaria (2). Proguanil is also indicated for the suppression of other forms of malaria and reduced transmission of infection, but because of its slow action it is not used for the acute treatment of malaria. Combination with other antimalarial agents such as chloroquine is common because of the rapid development of drug resistance. Proguanil is converted in vivo to cycloguanil, the active metabolite. Because it is a folate antagonist, pregnant women taking proguanil should also take folic acid supplements (3–7). One reviewer recommended either 5 mg/day of folic acid or 5 mg/week of folinic acid (leucovorin) at least during the 1st trimester (7). Moreover, because iron-deficiency anemia is often present in some regions, a combination of proguanil, iron, and folic acid has been recommended (8).

A reproductive study in pregnant rats given proguanil and the active metabolite, cycloguanil, was summarized by Shepard (9) and also cited by Schardein (10). Proguanil, 30 mg/kg every 4 hours, was given by gavage on days 1, 9, and 13 of gestation. No effects on the embryos or fetuses were observed. In contrast, the same dose of cycloguanil on day 1 of gestation caused death in 90% of the embryos. As with proguanil, no effects were observed from exposure to cycloguanil on days 9 and 13.

Antimalarial agents, including proguanil, are used routinely during pregnancy because the risks from the disease far outweigh the risks to the fetus from drug therapy (4,5). The risks of complications from maternal malarial infection are increased during pregnancy, especially in primigravidas and in women not living in endemic areas (i.e., nonimmune women) (11–14). Infection is associated with a number of severe maternal and fetal outcomes: maternal death, anemia, abortion, stillbirth, prematurity, low birth weight, intrauterine growth restriction, fetal tachycardia, fetal distress, and congenital malaria (11–16). One of these outcomes, low birth weight with the resulting increased risk of infant mortality, may have other causes, however, inasmuch as it has not been established that antimalarial chemoprophylaxis can completely prevent this complication (12). Increased maternal morbidity and mortality includes adult respiratory distress syndrome, pulmonary edema, massive hemolysis, disseminated intravascular coagulation, acute renal failure, and hypoglycemia (13–15). Severe *Plasmodium falciparum* malaria in pregnant nonimmune women has a poor prognosis and may be associated, in addition to the toxicities noted above, with asymptomatic uterine contractions, placental insufficiency because of intense parasitization, and hypoglycemia (12,15). Because of the severity of this disease in pregnancy, chemoprophylaxis is recommended for women of childbearing age traveling in areas where malaria is present (6,11–13).

Of 200 Nigerian women enrolled in a randomized double-blind trial, 160 were given an initial curative chloroquine course (600 mg base once), followed by prophylaxis regimens consisting of proguanil, 100 mg/day, with or without daily iron supplements, or 1 mg/day of folic acid (17,18). A control group of 40 women received no treatment. All patients were primigravidas seen before 24 weeks' gestation. In the treated groups, the prevalence of falciparum parasitemia was decreased from 32%–35% to about 2% at gestational weeks 28 and 36. Benefits of the regimens that included iron and/or folic acid were reductions in (a) severe anemia during pregnancy (from 18% to 3%), (b) megaloblastic erythropoiesis at or before delivery (from 56% to 25%), and (c) anemia at 6 weeks postpartum (from 61% to 29%). However, the mean birth weight was increased by only 132 g in treated compared with untreated pregnancies (difference not significant). Other than a single case of talipes and two infants with umbilical hernias, no other birth defects were observed. The authors stated that no association with the maternal treatment groups was evident, but the groups the infants were in was not specified (17).

In the first of a series of four reports, a study published in 1993 described the use of proguanil, either alone (*N* = 124) (200 mg once daily) or in combination with chloroquine (*N* = 90) (300 mg base once weekly), or of chloroquine alone (*N* = 113) (300 mg base once weekly) as malarial chemoprophylaxis during pregnancy in Tanzania (19). Chemoprophylaxis was begun after a single curative dose of pyrimethamine/sulfadoxine (Fansidar) was administered to clear preexisting parasitemia. Both proguanil chemoprophylaxis regimens were superior to chloroquine alone. The proguanil regimens were well tolerated by the mothers, with no cases of mouth ulcers and palmar or plantar skin scaling, although a few of the women complained of nausea. Based on urinary levels of proguanil and cycloguanil, they concluded that better protection from infection would have been achieved if a 12-hour dosing regimen with proguanil had been used (19).

In the second report, the effects of drug therapy on maternal hemoglobin, placental malaria, and birth weight were examined (20). As above, either proguanil alone or proguanil in combination with chloroquine was superior to chloroquine alone, producing higher levels of maternal hemoglobin, higher birth weights, and less placental malaria. The difference in outcomes between the two proguanil groups was not significant, however, leading the investigators to the conclusion that chemoprophylaxis with proguanil alone was suitable for this particular region (20).

The third and fourth reports in the series related to the effects of the therapy on the maternal malaria immunity and the transfer of maternal antibodies to the fetus and subsequent immunity of the offspring during early infancy (21,22). The data demonstrated that the chemoprophylaxis regimens did not significantly interfere with the maternal–fetal transfer of antisporozoite antibodies but that antibody levels at birth did not alter the first occurrence of malaria parasitemia in the infant (22).

The pharmacokinetics of proguanil in pregnant and postpartum women was described in a 1993 report (23). Ten healthy women in the 3rd trimester were given a single 200-mg oral dose and four of the women were restudied 2 months after delivery. The pharmacokinetics of proguanil during pregnancy and postpartum were similar, but the blood concentrations of the active metabolite, cycloguanil, were markedly decreased during late gestation. The mean maximum concentration (ng/mL) of cycloguanil in plasma and whole blood during pregnancy was 12.5 and 11.9, respectively, compared with postpartum levels of 28.4 and 22.4, respectively. Moreover, the proguanil:cycloguanil ratio based on the area under the plasma concentration curve (AUC) was 16.7 during pregnancy and 7.8 following pregnancy. The decreased conversion to the active antimalarial metabolite may have been caused by estrogen inhibition of the enzyme that metabolizes proguanil. Although the antimalarial prophylaxis concentration of cycloguanil is not known with certainty, these data indicate that the currently recommended dose of 200 mg/day may need to be doubled during late pregnancy to achieve the same blood levels as those obtained 2 months postpartum (23).

Most investigators have concluded that proguanil is safe to use during pregnancy (1–7,11,19,24,25).

BREASTFEEDING SUMMARY

No reports quantifying the amount of proguanil excreted in breast milk have been located. At least two reports have stated that agents used for malaria prophylaxis, such as proguanil, are excreted in small amounts in milk (3,11). These amounts, however, are too low for adequate malaria chemoprophylaxis of a nursing infant (3,11). Because proguanil is recommended for malaria protection in infants of any age (3,11,25), the use of the agent by a nursing woman is probably safe. Studies are needed, however, to measure the amount of proguanil and the active metabolite, cycloguanil, in milk and to determine the safety of this exposure in the nursing infant.

References

1. Olsen VV. Why not proguanil in malaria prophylaxis? Lancet 1983;1:649.
2. Barry M, Bia F. Pregnancy and travel. JAMA 1989;261:728–31.
3. Luzzi GA, Peto TEA. Adverse effects of antimalarials. An update. Drug Saf 1993;8:295–311.
4. Cook GC. Prevention and treatment of malaria. Lancet 1988;1:32–7.
5. Bradley DJ, Phillips-Howard PA. Prophylaxis against malaria for travelers from the United Kingdom. Br Med J 1989;299:1087–9.
6. Ellis CJ. Antiparasitic agents in pregnancy. Clin Obstet Gynaecol 1986;13:269–75.
7. Spracklen FHN. Malaria 1984. Part I. Malaria prophylaxis. S Afr Med J 1984;65:1037–41.
8. Fleming AF. The aetiology of severe anaemia in pregnancy in Ndola, Zambia. Ann Trop Med Parasitol 1989;83:37–49.
9. Shepard TH. *Catalog of Teratogenic Agents*. 8th ed. Baltimore, MD: The Johns Hopkins University Press, 1995:118.
10. Schardein JL. *Chemically Induced Birth Defects*. 2nd ed. New York, NY: Marcel Dekker, 1993:403.
11. CDC. Recommendations for the prevention of malaria among travelers. MMWR 1990;39(RR-3):1–10.
12. World Health Organization. Practical chemotherapy of malaria. WHO Tech Rep Ser 1990;805:1–141.
13. Subramanian D, Moise KJ Jr, White AC Jr. Imported malaria in pregnancy: report of four cases and review of management. Clin Infect Dis 1992;15:408–13.
14. World Health Organization. Severe and complicated malaria. Trans R Soc Trop Med Hyg 1990;84(Suppl 2):1–65.
15. Nathwani D, Currie PF, Douglas JG, Green ST, Smith NC. *Plasmodium falciparum* malaria in pregnancy: a review. Br J Obstet Gynaecol 1992;99:118–21.
16. Steketee RW, Wirima JJ, Slutsker L, Heymann DL, Breman JG. The problem of malaria and malaria control in pregnancy in sub-Saharan Africa. Am J Trop Med Hyg 1996;55(Suppl):2–7.
17. Fleming AF, Ghatoura GBS, Harrison KA, Briggs ND, Dunn DT. The prevention of anaemia in pregnancy in primigravidae in the Guinea Savanna of Nigeria. Ann Trop Med Parasitol 1986;80:211–33.
18. Fleming AF. Antimalarial prophylaxis in pregnant Nigerian women. Lancet 1990;335:45.
19. Mutabingwa TK, Malle LN, de Geus A, Oosting J. Malaria chemosuppression in pregnancy. I. The effect of chemosuppressive drugs on maternal parasitaemia. Trop Geogr Med 1993;45:6–14.
20. Mutabingwa TK, Malle LN, de Geus A, Oosting J. Malaria chemosuppression in pregnancy. II. Its effect on maternal haemoglobin levels, placental malaria and birth weight. Trop Geogr Med 1993;45:49–55.
21. Mutabingwa TK, Malle LN, Eling WMC, Verhave JP, Meuwissen JHETh, de Geus A. Malaria chemosuppression in pregnancy. III. Its effects on the maternal malaria immunity. Trop Geogr Med 1993;45:103–9.
22. Mutabingwa TK, Malle LN, Verhave JP, Eling WMC, Meuwissen JHETh, de Geus A. Malaria chemosuppression during pregnancy. IV. Its effects on the newborn's passive malaria immunity. Trop Geogr Med 1993;45:150–6.
23. Wangboonskul J, White NJ, Nosten F, ter Kuile F, Moody RR, Taylor RB. Single dose pharmacokinetics of proguanil and its metabolites in pregnancy. Eur J Clin Pharmacol 1993;44:247–51.
24. Anonymous. Malaria in pregnancy. Lancet 1983;2:84–5.
25. Anonymous. Prevention of malaria in pregnancy and early childhood. Br Med J 1984;289:1296–7.

PROMAZINE

[Withdrawn from the market. See 9th edition.]

PROMETHAZINE

Antihistamine/Antiemetic

PREGNANCY RECOMMENDATION: Compatible
BREASTFEEDING RECOMMENDATION: No Human Data—Probably Compatible

PREGNANCY SUMMARY

Promethazine is a phenothiazine antihistamine that is sometimes used as an antiemetic in pregnancy and as an adjunct to narcotic analgesics during labor. There are reports of embryo–fetal harm but confirming studies are required. In general, use of the drug in pregnancy appears to be low risk for the embryo–fetus.

FETAL RISK SUMMARY

The Collaborative Perinatal Project monitored 50,282 mother–child pairs, 114 of whom had promethazine exposure in the 1st trimester (1, pp. 323–324). For use anytime during pregnancy, 746 exposures were recorded (1, p. 437). In neither group was evidence found to suggest a relationship to large categories of major or minor malformations or to individual defects. A 1964 report also failed to show an association between 165 cases of promethazine exposure in the 1st trimester and malformations (2). In a 1971 reference, infants of mothers who had ingested antiemetics during the 1st trimester actually had significantly fewer abnormalities when compared with controls (3). Promethazine was the most commonly used antiemetic in this latter study.

In a surveillance study of Michigan Medicaid recipients involving 229,101 completed pregnancies conducted between 1985 and 1992, 1197 newborns had been exposed to promethazine during the 1st trimester (F. Rosa, personal communication, FDA, 1993). A total of 61 (5.1%) major birth defects were observed (51 expected). Specific data were available for six defect categories, including (observed/expected) 1/2 oral clefts, 0/1 spina bifida, 4/3 polydactyly, 1/2 limb reduction defects, 1/3 hypospadias, and 17/12 cardiovascular defects. Only with the latter defect is there a suggestion of a possible association, but other factors, including the mother's disease, concurrent drug use, and chance, may be involved.

At term, the drug rapidly crosses the placenta, appearing in cord blood within 1.5 minutes of an IV dose (4). Fetal and maternal blood concentrations are at equilibrium in 15 minutes, with infant levels persisting for at least 4 hours.

Several investigators have studied the effect of promethazine on labor and the newborn (5–13). Significant neonatal respiratory depression was seen in a small group of patients (5). However, in three large series, no clinical evidence of promethazine-induced respiratory depression was found (6–8). In a series of 33 mothers at term, 28 received either promethazine alone (1 patient) or a combination of meperidine with promethazine or phenobarbital (27 patients). Transient behavioral and electroencephalographic changes, persisting for <3 days, were seen in all newborns (10). These and other effects prompted one author to recommend that promethazine should not be used during labor (14).

Maternal tachycardia as a result of promethazine (mean increase 30 beats/minute) or promethazine-meperidine (mean increase 42 beats/minute) was observed in one series (9). The maximum effect occurred about 10 minutes after injection. The fetal heart rate did not change significantly.

The antiemetic effects of promethazine 25 mg and metoclopramide 10 mg following the use of meperidine in labor were described in a study involving 477 women (13). Both drugs were superior to placebo as antiemetics, but significantly more of the promethazine-treated mothers had persistent sedation that extended into the immediate postpartum period. Moreover, an antianalgesic effect, as evidenced by pain score, duration of analgesia, and an increased need for meperidine, was observed when promethazine was used.

Fatal shock was reported in a pregnant woman with an undiagnosed pheochromocytoma given promethazine (15). A precipitous drop in blood pressure resulted from administration of the drug, probably secondary to unmasking of hypovolemia (15).

Effects on the uterus have been mixed, with both increases and decreases in uterine activity reported (8,9,11).

Promethazine used during labor has been shown to markedly impair platelet aggregation in the newborn but less so in the mother (12,16). Although the clinical significance of this is unknown, the degree of impairment in the newborn is comparable to those disorders associated with a definite bleeding state.

Promethazine has been used to treat hydrops fetalis in cases of anti-erythrocytic isoimmunization (17). Six patients were treated with 150 mg/day orally between the 26th and 34th weeks of gestation while undergoing intraperitoneal transfusions. No details on the infants' conditions were given except that all were born alive. Other authors have reported similarly successful results in Rh-sensitized pregnancies (18,19).

As described by some authors, doses up to 6.5 mg/kg/day may be required (18). However, a 1991 review concluded that the benefits of promethazine in the treatment of Rh immunization were marginal and may be hazardous to the fetus (20).

Two female anencephalic infants were born to mothers after ovulatory stimulation with clomiphene (21). One of the mothers had taken promethazine for morning sickness. No association between promethazine and this defect has been suggested.

BREASTFEEDING SUMMARY

Available laboratory methods for the accurate detection of promethazine in breast milk are not clinically useful because of the rapid metabolism of phenothiazines (M. Lipshutz, personal communication, Wyeth Laboratories, 1981). Because of the low molecular weight (about 284), excretion into breast milk should be expected. The potential effects of this exposure on a nursing infant are unknown.

References

1. Heinonen OP, Slone D, Shapiro S. *Birth Defects and Drugs in Pregnancy*. Littleton, MA: Publishing Sciences Group, 1977.
2. Wheatley D. Drugs and the embryo. Br Med J 1964;1:630.
3. Nelson MM, Forfar JO. Association between drugs administered during pregnancy and congenital abnormalities of the fetus. Br Med J 1971;1:523–7.
4. Moya F, Thorndike V. The effects of drugs used in labor on the fetus and newborn. Clin Pharmacol Ther 1963;4:628–53.
5. Crawford JS, as quoted by Moya F, Thorndike V. The effects of drugs used in labor on the fetus and newborn. Clin Pharmacol Ther 1963;4:628–53.
6. Powe CE, Kiem IM, Fromhagen C, Cavanagh D. Propiomazine hydrochloride in obstetrical analgesia. JAMA 1962;181:290–4.
7. Potts CR, Ullery JC. Maternal and fetal effects of obstetric analgesia. Am J Obstet Gynecol 1961;81:1253–9.
8. Carroll JJ, Moir RS. Use of promethazine (Phenergan) hydrochloride in obstetrics. JAMA 1958;168:2218–24.
9. Riffel HD, Nochimson DJ, Paul RH, Hon EH. Effects of meperidine and promethazine during labor. Obstet Gynecol 1973;42:738–45.
10. Borgstedt AD, Rosen MG. Medication during labor correlated with behavior and EEG of the newborn. Am J Dis Child 1968;115:21–4.
11. Zakut H, Mannor SM, Serr DM. Effect of promethazine on uterine contractions. Harefuah 1970;78:61–2. As cited in Anonymous. References and reviews. JAMA 1970;211:1572.
12. Corby DG, Shulman I. The effects of antenatal drug administration on aggregation of platelets of newborn infants. J Pediatr 1971;79:307–13.
13. Vella L, Francis D, Houlton P, Reynolds F. Comparison of the antiemetics metoclopramide and promethazine in labour. Br Med J 1985;290:1173–5.
14. Hall PF. Use of promethazine (Phenergan) in labour. Can Med Assoc J 1987;136:690–1.
15. Montminy M, Teres D. Shock after phenothiazine administration in a pregnant patient with a pheochromocytoma: a case report and literature review. J Reprod Med 1983;28:159–62.
16. Whaun JM, Smith GR, Sochor VA. Effect of prenatal drug administration on maternal and neonatal platelet aggregation and PF_4 release. Haemostasis 1980;9:226–37.
17. Bierme S, Bierme R. Antihistamines in hydrops foetalis. Lancet 1967;1:574.
18. Gusdon JP Jr. The treatment of erythroblastosis with promethazine hydrochloride. J Reprod Med 1981;26:454–8.
19. Charles AG, Blumenthal LS. Promethazine hydrochloride therapy in severely Rh-sensitized pregnancies. Obstet Gynecol 1982;60:627–30.
20. Bowman JM. Antenatal suppression of Rh alloimmunization. Clin Obstet Gynecol 1991;34:296–303.
21. Dyson JL, Kohler HC. Anencephaly and ovulation stimulation. Lancet 1973;1:1256–7.

PROPAFENONE

Antiarrhythmic

PREGNANCY RECOMMENDATION: Limited Human Data—Animal Data Suggest Moderate Risk
BREASTFEEDING RECOMMENDATION: Limited Human Data—Probably Compatible

P

PREGNANCY SUMMARY

Four reports and a review have described the use of propafenone in late pregnancy (1–5). There is no reported experience in the 1st trimester. No adverse effects were observed in the fetus or the newborn.

FETAL RISK SUMMARY

Propafenone is an orally active antiarrhythmic used in the treatment of ventricular tachycardia. The agent has an active metabolite, 5-OH-propafenone. No teratogenic effects have been observed in studies with rabbits and rats, but propafenone was embryotoxic in both species when given in doses of 10 and 40 times the maximum recommended human dose, respectively (6).

Propafenone crosses the human placenta at term (1). A woman, delivering at 36 weeks' gestation, was taking 300 mg 3 times daily in the 3rd trimester. Trough concentrations of propafenone and its active metabolite in the mother were 145 and 69 ng/mL, respectively, and in the newborn were 30 and 29 ng/mL, respectively.

BREASTFEEDING SUMMARY

Propafenone is excreted into breast milk. A woman took propafenone 300 mg 3 times a day during the latter part of pregnancy and during breastfeeding (1). Three days postpartum, trough concentrations of propafenone and its active metabolite were 32 and 47 ng/mL, respectively, whereas the maternal plasma levels were 219 and 86 ng/mL, respectively.

In a 2005 study, a single oral dose of propafenone 150 mg was given to a nursing mother (7). The infant was not allowed to breastfeed during the study. Six paired samples of milk and maternal plasma were drawn over 12 hours. The milk:plasma ratio, based on AUC, was 0.25, and the relative infant dose was 0.1% of the mother's weight-adjusted dose (7).

References

1. Libardoni M, Piovan D, Busato E, Padrini R. Transfer of propafenone and 5-OH-propafenone to foetal plasma and maternal milk. Br J Clin Pharmacol 1991;32:527–8.
2. Brunozzi LT, Meniconi L, Chiocchi P, Liberati R, Zuanetti G, Latini R. Propafenone in the treatment of chronic ventricular arrhythmias in a pregnant patient. Br J Clin Pharmacol 1988;26:489–90.
3. Santinelli V, De Paola M, Turco P, Smimmo D, Chiariello M, Condorelli M. Wolff-Parkinson-White at risk and propafenone. J Am Coll Cardiol 1988;11:1138.
4. Gembruch U, Manz M, Bald R, Rüddel H, Redel DA, Schlebusch H, Nitsch J, Hansmann M. Repeated intravascular treatment with amiodarone in a fetus with refractory supraventricular tachycardia and hydrops fetalis. Am Heart J 1989;118:1335–8.
5. Capucci A. Boriani G. Propafenone in the treatment of cardiac arrhythmias. A risk-benefit appraisal. Drug Saf 1995;12:55–72.
6. Product information. Rythmol. Knoll Pharmaceuticals, 2000.
7. Wakaumi M, Tsuruoka S, Sakamoto K, Shigal T, Fujimura A. Pilsicainide in breast milk from a mother: comparison with disopyramide and propafenone. Br J Clin Pharmacol 2005;59:120–2.

PROPANTHELINE

Parasympatholytic (Anticholinergic)

PREGNANCY RECOMMENDATION: Limited Human Data—No Relevant Animal Data
BREASTFEEDING RECOMMENDATION: No Human Data—Probably Compatible

PREGNANCY SUMMARY

Propantheline is an anticholinergic quaternary ammonium bromide. There are no reports associating the use of this drug with developmental toxicity, but the data are limited. There also are no relevant animal data. (See also Atropine.)

FETAL RISK SUMMARY

The Collaborative Perinatal Project monitored 50,282 mother–child pairs, 33 of whom used propantheline in the 1st trimester (1). No evidence was found for an association with congenital malformations. When the group of parasympatholytics were taken as a whole (2323 exposures), a possible association with minor malformations was found (1).

BREASTFEEDING SUMMARY

No reports describing the use of propantheline during human lactation have been located. (See also Atropine.)

Reference

1. Heinonen OP, Slone D, Shapiro S. *Birth Defects and Drugs in Pregnancy*. Littleton, MA: Publishing Sciences Group, 1977:346–53.

P

PROPOFOL

Hypnotic

PREGNANCY RECOMMENDATION: Limited Human Data—Animal Data Suggest Low Risk
BREASTFEEDING RECOMMENDATION: Limited Human Data—Probably Compatible

PREGNANCY SUMMARY

A number of studies have described the use of propofol during cesarean section. The drug has caused transient newborn depression. No reports describing the use of the drug during the 1st and 2nd trimesters have been located.

FETAL RISK SUMMARY

Propofol is a hypnotic agent used for the IV induction and maintenance of anesthesia (1–20). Reproduction studies in rats and rabbits at doses 6 times the recommended human induction dose have revealed no evidence of impaired fertility or fetal harm (21).

The pharmacokinetics of propofol in women undergoing cesarean section was reported in 1990 (1). Propofol rapidly crosses the placenta and distributes in the fetus (2–12). The fetal:maternal (umbilical vein:maternal vein) ratio is approximately 0.7. Doses were administered either by IV bolus, by continuous infusion, or by both methods.

Several studies have examined the effect of maternal propofol anesthesia on infant Apgar scores, time to sustained spontaneous respiration, and Neurological and Adaptive Capacity Score (NACS) or the Early Neonatal Neurobehavioural Scale (ENNS) (1,2,4,5,7,8,11–18). Most investigators reported no difference in the Apgar scores of infants exposed to propofol either alone or when compared with other general anesthesia techniques, such as thiopental with enflurane or isoflurane (2,5,7,8,14–18). Moreover, no correlation was found between the Apgar scores and umbilical arterial or venous concentration of propofol (2,5,8,11,15).

In one study, infants (N = 20) exposed to a maternal propofol dose of 2.8 mg/kg had significantly lower Apgar scores at 1 and 5 minutes compared with infants (N = 20) whose mothers were treated with thiopental 5 mg/kg (13). The Apgar scores in both groups were significantly lower when compared with infants born by spontaneous vaginal delivery. The induction-to-delivery and uterine incision-to-delivery intervals in the two treatment groups were nearly identical. Five propofol-exposed infants had profound muscular hypotonus at birth and at 5 minutes, and one newborn was somnolent (13). Propofol-exposed infants were evaluated using the ENNS and were found to have a depression in alert state, pinprick and placing reflexes, and mean decremental count in Moro and light reflexes 1 hour after birth but not at 4 hours (13). Five (25%) of the infants exhibited generalized irritability and continuous crying at 1 hour, but not at 4 hours.

In contrast, most studies found no difference in the NACS or time to sustained spontaneous respiration between various groups with propofol IV bolus doses of 2.5 mg/kg or when continuous infusion doses were no higher than 6 mg/kg/hr (2,5,8,14–16). Higher doses, such as 9 mg/kg/hr, were correlated with a depressed NACS (8,12,14–16,18).

BREASTFEEDING SUMMARY

Small amounts of propofol are excreted into breast milk and colostrum following use of the agent for the induction and maintenance of maternal anesthesia during cesarean section (3). Two groups of women were studied. The first group consisted of four women who had received a mean IV propofol dose of 2.55 mg/kg at a mean of 25.9 minutes before delivery. The mean total dose received by patients in this group was 155.5 mg. The second group consisted of three women who had received a mean IV dose of 2.51 mg/kg plus a mean infusion of 5.08 mg/kg/hr. The mean total dose in this group was 247.4 mg, and the mean time to delivery was 20.2 minutes. Breast milk or colostrum samples were collected at various intervals from 4 to 24 hours after delivery. Propofol concentrations in the seven patients varied between 0.048 and 0.74 mcg/mL, with the highest levels predictably occurring at 4–5 hours in group 2. In one patient from group 2, the milk/colostrum concentration was 0.74 mcg/mL at 5 hours and fell to 0.048 mcg/mL (6% of the initial sample) at 24 hours. These amounts were considered negligible when compared with the amounts the infants received before birth from placental transfer of the drug (3).

References

1. Gin T, Gregory MA, Chan K, Buckley T, Oh TE. Pharmacokinetics of propofol in women undergoing elective caesarean section. Br J Anaesth 1990;64:148–53.
2. Dailland P, Lirzin JD, Cockshott ID, Jorrot JC, Conseiller C. Placental transfer and neonatal effects of propofol administered during cesarean section (abstract). Anesthesiology 1987;67:A454.
3. Dailland P, Cockshott ID, Lirzin JD, Jacquinot P, Jorrot JC, Devery J, Harmey JL, Conseiller C. Intravenous propofol during cesarean section: placental transfer, concentrations in breast milk, and neonatal effects. A preliminary study. Anesthesiology 1989;71:827–34.
4. Moore J, Bill KM, Flynn RJ, McKeating KT, Howard PJ. A comparison between propofol and thiopentone as induction agents in obstetric anaesthesia. Anaesthesia 1989;44:753–7.
5. Dailland P, Jacquinot P, Lirzin JD, Jorrot JC. Neonatal effects of propofol administered to the mother in anesthesia in cesarean section. Can Anesthesiol 1989;37:429–33.
6. Dailland P, Jacquinot P, Lirzin JD, Jorrot JC, Conseiller C. Comparative study of propofol with thiopental for general anesthesia in cesarean section. Ann Fr Anesth Reanim 1989;8 (Suppl):R65.
7. Valtonen M, Kanto J, Rosenberg P. Comparison of propofol and thiopentone for induction of anaesthesia for elective caesarean section. Anaesthesia 1989;44:758–62.
8. Gin T, Gregory MA. Propofol for caesarean section. Anaesthesia 1990;45:165.
9. Pagnoni B, Casalino S, Monzani R, Lazzarini A, Tiengo M. Placental transfer of propofol in elective cesarean section. Minerva Anestesiol 1990;56:877–9.
10. Maglione F, Guarini MC, Montanari A, Cirillo F, Postiglione M, Pica M, Amorena M, De Liguoro M. Determination of propofol blood levels in mothers and newborns in anesthesia for cesarean section. Minerva Anestesiol 1990;56:881–3.
11. Gin T, Gregory MA, Chan K, Oh TE. Maternal and fetal levels of propofol at caesarean section. Anaesth Intensive Care 1990;18:180–4.
12. Gin T, Yau G, Chan K, Gregory MA, Oh TE. Disposition of propofol infusions for caesarean section. Can J Anaesth 1991;38:31–6.
13. Celleno D, Capogna G, Tomassetti M, Costantino P, Di Feo G, Nisini R. Neurobehavioural effects of propofol on the neonate following elective caesarean section. Br J Anaesth 1989;62:649–54.
14. Gin T, Yau G, Gregory MA. Propofol during cesarean section. Anesthesiology 1990;73:789.
15. Gin T, Yau G, Chan K, Gregory MA, Kotur CF. Recovery from propofol infusion anaesthesia for caesarean section. Neurosci Lett (Suppl) 1990;37:S44.
16. Gregory MA, Gin T, Yau G, Leung RKW, Chan K, Oh TE. Propofol infusion anaesthesia for caesarean section. Can J Anaesth 1990;37:514–20.
17. Gin T, Gregory MA, Oh TE. The haemodynamic effects of propofol and thiopentone for induction of caesarean section. Anaesth Intensive Care 1990;18:175–9.
18. Yau G, Gin T, Ewart MC, Kotur CF, Leung RKW, Oh TE. Propofol for induction and maintenance of anaesthesia at caesarean section. Anaesthesia 1991;46:20–3.
19. Costantino P, Emanuelli M, Muratori F, Sebastiani M. Propofol versus thiopentone as induction agents in cesarean section. Minerva Anestesiol 1990;56:865–70.
20. Alberico FP. Propofol in anesthesia induction for cesarean section. Minerva Anestesiol 1990;56:871.
21. Product information. Diprivan. AstraZeneca, 2000.

PROPOXYPHENE

[Withdrawn from the market. See 9th edition.]

PROPRANOLOL

Sympatholytic (Antihypertensive)

PREGNANCY RECOMMENDATION: Human Data Suggest Risk in 2nd and 3rd Trimesters
BREASTFEEDING RECOMMENDATION: Limited Human Data—Potential Toxicity

PREGNANCY SUMMARY

Propranolol has been used during pregnancy for maternal and fetal indications. The drug is apparently not a teratogen, but fetal and neonatal toxicity may occur. Some β-blockers, including propranolol, may cause intrauterine growth restriction (IUGR) and reduced placental weight, especially those lacking intrinsic sympathomimetic activity (ISA) (partial agonist). Treatment beginning early in the 2nd trimester results in the greatest weight reductions, whereas treatment restricted to the 3rd trimester primarily affects only placental weight. Propranolol does not possess ISA. However, IUGR and reduced placental weight may potentially occur with all agents within this class. Although growth restriction is a serious concern, the benefits of maternal therapy with β-blockers, in some cases, might outweigh the risks to the fetus and must be judged on a case-by-case basis. Newborn infants of women consuming the drug near delivery should be closely observed during the first 24–48 hours after birth for bradycardia, hypoglycemia, and other symptoms of β-blockade. Long-term effects of in utero exposure to β-blockers have not been studied but warrant evaluation.

FETAL RISK SUMMARY

Propranolol, a nonselective β-adrenergic blocking agent, has been used for various indications in pregnancy:

- Maternal hyperthyroidism (1–7)
- Pheochromocytoma (8)
- Maternal cardiac disease (6,7,9–20)
- Fetal tachycardia or arrhythmia (21,22)
- Maternal hypertension (7,20,23–30)
- Dysfunctional labor (31)
- Termination of pregnancy (32)

Reproduction studies, all apparently based on body weight, have been conducted in rats and rabbits. In rats, embryotoxicity (increased resorption sites and reduced litter sizes) and reduced neonatal survival were observed at doses ≤10 times the maximum recommended human dose (MRHD) (33). No embryotoxicity was observed in rabbits at doses ≤20 times the MRHD. No teratogenicity was noted in either species.

The drug readily crosses the placenta (2,6,12,16,22,29,34,35). Cord serum levels varying between 19% and 127% of maternal serum have been reported (2,16,22,29). Oxytocic effects have been demonstrated following IV, extra-amniotic injections, and high oral dosing (17, 31,32,36,37). IV propranolol has been shown to block or decrease the marked increase in maternal plasma progesterone induced by vasopressin or theophylline (38). The pharmacokinetics of propranolol in pregnancy have been described (39). Plasma levels and elimination were not significantly altered by pregnancy.

A number of fetal and neonatal adverse effects have been reported following the use of propranolol in pregnancy. Whether these effects were caused by propranolol, maternal disease, other drugs consumed concurrently, or a combination of these factors is not always clear. Daily doses of ≥160 mg seem to produce the more serious complications, but lower doses have also resulted in toxicity. Analysis of 23 reports involving 167 liveborn infants exposed to chronic propranolol in utero is shown in below table (1–4,6,7,9,11–14,20,22–24,26–29,40–43):

	Number of Cases	Percent (%)
Intrauterine growth restriction (IUGR)	23	14
Hypoglycemia	16	10
Bradycardia	12	7
Respiratory depression at birth	6	4
Hyperbilirubinemia	6	4
Small placenta (size not always noted)	4	2
Polycythemia	2	1
Thrombocytopenia (40,000/mm^3)	1	0.6
Hyperirritability	1	0.6
Hypocalcemia with convulsions	1	0.6
Blood coagulation defect	1	0.6

Two infants were reported to have anomalies (pyloric stenosis; crepitus of hip), but the authors did not relate these to propranolol (27,40). In another case, a malformed fetus was spontaneously aborted from a 30-year-old woman with chronic renovascular hypertension (44). The patient had been treated with propranolol, amiloride, and captopril for her severe hypertension. Malformations included absence of the left leg below the midthigh and no obvious skull formation above the brain tissue. The authors attributed the defect either to captopril alone or to a combination effect of the three drugs (44), but recent reports have associated fetal calvarial hypoplasia with captopril (see Captopril).

In a surveillance study of Michigan Medicaid recipients involving 229,101 completed pregnancies conducted between 1985 and 1992, 274 newborns had been exposed to propranolol during the 1st trimester (F. Rosa, personal communication, FDA, 1993). A total of 11 (4.0%) major birth defects were observed (12 expected), including (observed/expected) 3/3 cardiovascular defects and 2/1 hypospadias. No anomalies were observed in four other defect categories (oral

P

clefts, spina bifida, polydactyly, and limb reduction defects) for which specific data were available.

Respiratory depression was noted in four of five infants whose mothers were given 1 mg of propranolol IV just before cesarean section (45). None of the five controls in the double-blind study was depressed at birth. The author suggested the mechanism may have been β-adrenergic blockade of the cervical sympathetic discharge that occurs at cord clamping.

Fetal bradycardia was observed in 2 of 10 patients treated with propranolol, 1 mg/minute for 4 minutes, for dysfunctional labor (31). No lasting effects were seen in the babies. In a retrospective study, 8 markedly hypertensive patients (9 pregnancies) treated with propranolol were compared with 15 hypertensive controls not treated with propranolol (25). Other antihypertensives were used in both groups. A significant difference was found between the perinatal mortality rates, with seven deaths in the propranolol group (78%) and five deaths in the controls (33%). A possible explanation for the difference may have been the more severe hypertension and renal disease in the propranolol group than in the controls (46).

IUGR may be related to propranolol. Several possible mechanisms for this effect have been reviewed (47). Premature labor has been suggested as a possible complication of propranolol therapy in patients with gestational hypertension (42). In nine women treated with propranolol for gestational hypertension, three delivered prematurely. The author speculated that these patients were relatively hypovolemic and when a compensatory increase in cardiac output failed to occur, premature delivery resulted. However, another report on chronic propranolol use in 14 women did not observe premature labor (43).

In a randomized, double-blind trial, 36 patients at term were given either 80 mg of propranolol or placebo (48). Fetal heart rate reaction to a controlled sound stimulus was then measured at 1, 2, and 3 hours. The heart rate reaction in the propranolol group was significantly depressed, compared with placebo, at all three time intervals.

The reactivity of nonstress tests (NSTs) was affected by propranolol in two hypertensive women in the 2nd and 3rd trimesters (49). One woman was taking 20 mg every 6 hours and the other 10 mg 3 times daily. Repeated NSTs were nonreactive in both women, but immediate follow-up contraction stress tests were negative. The NSTs became reactive 2 and 10 days, respectively, after propranolol was discontinued.

A 1988 review on the use of β-blockers including propranolol, during pregnancy, concluded that these agents are relatively safe (50).

BREASTFEEDING SUMMARY

Propranolol is excreted into breast milk. Peak concentrations occur 2–3 hours after a dose (12,20,43,51). Milk levels have ranged from 4 to 64 ng/mL, with milk:plasma ratios of 0.2–1.5 (12,20,29,50). Although such adverse effects as respiratory depression, bradycardia, and hypoglycemia have not been reported, nursing infants exposed to propranolol in breast milk should be closely observed for these symptoms of β-blockade. Long-term effects of exposure to β-blockers from milk have not been studied but warrant evaluation. The American Academy of Pediatrics classifies propranolol as compatible with breastfeeding (52).

References

1. Jackson GL. Treatment of hyperthyroidism in pregnancy. Pa Med 1973;76:56–7.
2. Langer A, Hung CT, McA'Nulty JA, Harrigan JT, Washington E. Adrenergic blockade: a new approach to hyperthyroidism during pregnancy. Obstet Gynecol 1974;44:181–6.
3. Bullock JL, Harris RE, Young R. Treatment of thyrotoxicosis during pregnancy with propranolol. Am J Obstet Gynecol 1975;121:242–5.
4. Lightner ES, Allen HD, Loughlin G. Neonatal hyperthyroidism and heart failure: a different approach. Am J Dis Child 1977;131:68–70.
5. Levy CA, Waite JH, Dickey R. Thyrotoxicosis and pregnancy. Use of preoperative propranolol for thyroidectomy. Am J Surg 1977;133:319–21.
6. Habib A, McCarthy JS. Effects on the neonate of propranolol administered during pregnancy. J Pediatr 1977;91:808–11.
7. Pruyn SC, Phelan JP, Buchanan GC. Long-term propranolol therapy in pregnancy: maternal and fetal outcome. Am J Obstet Gynecol 1979;135: 485–9.
8. Leak D, Carroll JJ, Robinson DC, Ashworth EJ. Management of pheochromocytoma during pregnancy. Can Med Assoc J 1977;116:371–5.
9. Turner GM, Oakley CM, Dixon HG. Management of pregnancy complicated by hypertrophic obstructive cardiomyopathy. Br Med J 1968;4:281–4.
10. Barnes AB. Chronic propranolol administration during pregnancy: a case report. J Reprod Med 1970;5:79–80.
11. Schroeder JS, Harrison DC. Repeated cardioversion during pregnancy. Am J Cardiol 1971;27:445–6.
12. Levitan AA, Manion JC. Propranolol therapy during pregnancy and lactation. Am J Cardiol 1973;32:247.
13. Reed RL, Cheney CB, Fearon RE, Hook R, Hehre FW. Propranolol therapy throughout pregnancy: a case report. Anesth Analg (Cleve) 1974;53: 214–8.
14. Fiddler GI. Propranolol and pregnancy. Lancet 1974;2:722–3.
15. Kolibash AE, Ruiz DE, Lewis RP. Idiopathic hypertrophic subaortic stenosis in pregnancy. Ann Intern Med 1975;82:791–4.
16. Cottrill CM, McAllister RG Jr, Gettes L, Noonan JA. Propranolol therapy during pregnancy, labor, and delivery: evidence for transplacental drug transfer and impaired neonatal drug disposition. J Pediatr 1977;91:812–4.
17. Datta S, Kitzmiller JL, Ostheimer GW, Schoenbaum SC. Propranolol and parturition. Obstet Gynecol 1978;51:577–81.
18. Diaz JH, McDonald JS. Propranolol and induced labor: anesthetic implications. Anesth Rev 1979;6:29–32.
19. Oakley GDG, McGarry K, Limb DG, Oakley CM. Management of pregnancy in patients with hypertrophic cardiomyopathy. Br Med J 1979;1: 1749–50.
20. Bauer JH, Pape B, Zajicek J, Groshong T. Propranolol in human plasma and breast milk. Am J Cardiol 1979;43:860–2.
21. Eibschitz I, Abinader EG, Klein A, Sharf M. Intrauterine diagnosis and control of fetal ventricular arrhythmia during labor. Am J Obstet Gynecol 1975;122:597–600.
22. Teuscher A, Boss E, Imhof P, Erb E, Stocker FP, Weber JW. Effect of propranolol on fetal tachycardia in diabetic pregnancy. Am J Cardiol 1978;42: 304–7.
23. Gladstone GR, Hordof A, Gersony WM. Propranolol administration during pregnancy: effects on the fetus. J Pediatr 1975;86:962–4.
24. Tcherdakoff PH, Colliard M, Berrard E, Kreft C, Dupry A, Bernaille JM. Propranolol in hypertension during pregnancy. Br Med J 1978;2:670.
25. Lieberman BA, Stirrat GM, Cohen SL, Beard RW, Pinker GD, Belsey E. The possible adverse effect of propranolol on the fetus in pregnancies complicated by severe hypertension. Br J Obstet Gynaecol 1978;85:678–83.
26. Eliahou HE, Silverberg DS, Reisin E, Romen I, Mashiach S, Serr DM. Propranolol for the treatment of hypertension in pregnancy. Br J Obstet Gynaecol 1978;85:431–6.
27. Bott-Kanner G, Schweitzer A, Schoenfeld A, Joel-Cohen J, Rosenfeld JB. Treatment with propranolol and hydralazine throughout pregnancy in a hypertensive patient: a case report. Isr J Med Sci 1978;14:466–8.

28. Bott-Kanner G, Reisner SH, Rosenfeld JB. Propranolol and hydralazine in the management of essential hypertension in pregnancy. Br Obstet Gynaecol 1980;87:110–4.
29. Taylor EA, Turner P. Anti-hypertensive therapy with propranolol during pregnancy and lactation. Postgrad Med J 1981;57:427–30.
30. Serup J. Propranolol for the treatment of hypertension in pregnancy. Acta Med Scand 1979;206:333.
31. Mitrani A, Oettinger M, Abinader EG, Sharf M, Klein A. Use of propranolol in dysfunctional labour. Br J Obstet Gynaecol 1975;82:651–5.
32. Amy JJ, Karim SMM. Intrauterine administration of 1-noradrenaline and propranolol during the second trimester of pregnancy. J Obstet Gynaecol Br Commonw 1974;81:75–83.
33. Product information. Inderal. Wyeth-Ayerst Laboratories, 1997.
34. Smith MT, Livingstone I, Eadie MJ, Hooper WD, Triggs EJ. Metabolism of propranolol in the human maternal–placental–foetal unit. Eur J Clin Pharmacol 1983;24:727–32.
35. Erkkola R, Lammintausta R, Liukko P, Anttila M. Transfer of propranolol and sotalol across the human placenta. Acta Obstet Gynecol Scand 1982;61:31–4.
36. Barden TP, Stander RW. Myometrial and cardiovascular effects of an adrenergic blocking drug in human pregnancy. Am J Obstet Gynecol 1968;101:91–9.
37. Wansbrough H, Nakanishi H, Wood C. The effect of adrenergic receptor blocking drugs on the human fetus. J Obstet Gynaecol Br Commonw 1968;75:189–98.
38. Fylling P. Dexamethasone or propranolol blockade of induced increase in plasma progesterone in early human pregnancy. Acta Endocrinol (Copenh) 1973;72:569–72.
39. Smith MT, Livingstone I, Eadie MJ, Hooper WD, Triggs EJ. Chronic propranolol administration during pregnancy: maternal pharmacokinetics. Eur J Clin Pharmacol 1983;25:481–90.
40. O'Connor PC, Jick H, Hunter JR, Stergachis A, Madsen S. Propranolol and pregnancy outcome. Lancet 1981;2:1168.
41. Caldroney RD. Beta-blockers in pregnancy. N Engl J Med 1982;306:810.
42. Goodlin RC. Beta blocker in pregnancy-induced hypertension. Am J Obstet Gynecol 1982;143:237.
43. Livingstone I, Craswell PW, Bevan EB, Smith MT, Eadie MJ. Propranolol in pregnancy: three year prospective study. Clin Exp Hypertens (B) 1983;2:341–50.
44. Duminy PC, Burger PD. Fetal abnormality associated with the use of captopril during pregnancy. S Afr Med J 1981;60:805.
45. Tunstall ME. The effect of propranolol on the onset of breathing at birth. Br J Anaesth 1969;41:792.
46. Rubin PC. Beta-blockers in pregnancy. N Engl J Med 1981;305:1323–6.
47. Redmond GP. Propranolol and fetal growth restriction. Semin Perinatol 1982;6:142–7.
48. Jensen OH. Fetal heart rate response to a controlled sound stimulus after propranolol administration to the mother. Acta Obstet Gynecol Scand 1984;63:199–202.
49. Margulis E, Binder D, Cohen AW. The effect of propranolol on the nonstress test. Am J Obstet Gynecol 1984;148:340–1.
50. Frishman WH, Chesner M. Beta-adrenergic blockers in pregnancy. Am Heart J 1988;115:147–52.
51. Karlberg B, Lundberg O, Aberg H. Excretion of propranolol in human breast milk. Acta Pharmacol Toxicol (Copenh) 1974;34:222–4.
52. Committee on Drugs, American Academy of Pediatrics. The transfer of drugs and other chemicals into human milk. Pediatrics 2001;108: 776–89.

PROPYLTHIOURACIL

Antithyroid

PREGNANCY RECOMMENDATION: Compatible—Maternal Benefit >> Embryo–Fetal Risk
BREASTFEEDING RECOMMENDATION: Compatible

PREGNANCY SUMMARY

Propylthiouracil (PTU) is routinely used in pregnancy for the treatment of hyperthyroidism. The maternal benefit outweighs the potential embryo–fetal risk.

FETAL RISK SUMMARY

PTU has been used for the treatment of hyperthyroidism during pregnancy since its introduction in the 1940s (1–39). The drug prevents synthesis of thyroid hormones and inhibits peripheral deiodination of levothyroxine (T4) to liothyronine (T3) (40).

PTU crosses the placenta. Four patients undergoing therapeutic abortion were given a single 15-mg ^{35}S-labeled oral dose 2 hours before pregnancy termination (41). Serum could not be obtained from two 8-week-old fetuses, but 0.0016%–0.0042% of the given dose was found in the fetal tissues. In two other fetuses at 12 and 16 weeks of age, the fetal:maternal serum ratios were 0.27 and 0.35, respectively, with 0.020% and 0.025% of the dose in the fetuses. A 1986 report described the pharmacokinetics of PTU in six pregnant, hyperthyroid women (42). Serum concentrations of PTU consistently decreased during the 3rd trimester. At delivery in five patients, 1–9 hours after the last dose of 100–150 mg, the mean maternal serum concentration of PTU was 0.19 mcg/mL (range <0.02–0.52 mcg/mL) compared with a mean cord blood level of 0.36 mcg/mL (range 0.03–0.67 mcg/mL). The cord:maternal serum ratio was 1.9 (42).

The primary effect on the fetus from transplacental passage of PTU is the production of a mild hypothyroidism when the drug is used close to term. This usually resolves within a few days without treatment (34). Clinically, the hypothyroid state may be observed as a goiter in the newborn and is the result of increased levels of fetal pituitary thyrotropin (24). The incidence of fetal goiter after PTU treatment in reported cases is approximately 12% (29 goiters/241 patients) (1–37,43). Some of these cases may have been caused by co-administration of iodides (9,11,18,22). The use of PTU early in pregnancy does not produce fetal goiter, as the fetal thyroid does not begin hormone production until approximately the 11th or 12th week of gestation (44). Goiters from PTU exposure are usually small and do not obstruct the airway as do iodide-induced goiters (see also Potassium Iodide) (43–45). However, two reports have been located that described PTU-induced goiters in newborns that were sufficiently massive to produce tracheal compression resulting in death in one infant and moderate respiratory distress in the second (7,10). In two other PTU-exposed fetuses, clinical hypothyroidism was evident at birth with subsequent slow mental and physical development (10–12). One of these infants was also exposed to high doses of iodide during gestation (12). PTU-induced goiters are not predictable or dose dependent, but the smallest possible dose of PTU should be used, especially during the 3rd trimester (19,33,44–46). No effect on intellectual or physical development from PTU-induced hypothyroxinemia was observed in comparison studies between exposed and nonexposed siblings (19,47).

Congenital anomalies have been reported in seven newborns exposed to PTU in utero (14,17,21,27,34). This incidence is well within the expected rate of malformations. Maternal hyperthyroidism itself has been shown to be a cause of malformations (48). No association between PTU and defects has been suggested. The reported defects were as follows: congenital dislocation of hip (14), cryptorchidism (17), muscular hypotonicity (17), syndactyly of hand and foot (I^{131} also used) (21), hypospadias (27), aortic atresia (27), and choanal atresia (34).

In a large prospective study, 25 patients were exposed to ≥1 noniodide thyroid suppressants during the 1st trimester, 16 of whom took PTU (49). From the total group, four children with nonspecified malformations were found, suggesting that this group of drugs may be teratogenic. However, because of the maternal disease and the use of other drugs (i.e., methimazole in nine women and other thiouracil derivatives in two), the relationship between PTU and the anomalies cannot be determined. This study also noted that independent confirmation of the data was required (49).

In a surveillance study of Michigan Medicaid recipients involving 229,101 completed pregnancies conducted between 1985 and 1992, 35 newborns had been exposed to PTU during the 1st trimester (F. Rosa, personal communication, FDA, 1993). One (2.9%) major birth defect was observed (one expected), a case of hypospadias (none expected).

A 1992 abstract and a later full report described a retrospective evaluation of hyperthyroid pregnancy outcomes treated with either PTU ($N = 99$) or methimazole ($N = 36$) (50,51). Three (3.0%) defects were observed in those exposed to PTU (ventricular septal defect; pulmonary stenosis; patent ductus arteriosus in a term infant), whereas one newborn (2.8%) had a defect (inguinal hernia) in the methimazole group. No scalp defects were observed.

A 2002 review of the fetal effects of antithyroid drugs concluded that the risk of congenital defects with PTU is not increased over that of nontreated controls (52). However, PTU was more likely than methimazole to cause suppression of fetal thyroid function that could result in fetal thyroid hyperplasia and goiter. Suppression of the fetal thyroid function occurred in 1%–5% of newborns of PTU-treated mothers, and many exhibited goiter. In addition, little is known of the long-term consequences of suppression of the fetal thyroid gland on postnatal brain development (52).

In comparison with other antithyroid drugs, PTU is considered the drug of choice for the medical treatment of hyperthyroidism during pregnancy (see also Carbimazole, Methimazole, Potassium Iodide) (34,36,44–46). Combination therapy with thyroid–antithyroid drugs was advocated at one time but is now considered inappropriate (25,26,34,36,44–46,53). Two reasons contributed to this change: (a) use of thyroid hormones may require higher doses of PTU to be used, and (b) placental transfer of T4 and T3 is minimal and not sufficient to reverse fetal hypothyroidism (see also Levothyroxine and Liothyronine).

BREASTFEEDING SUMMARY

PTU is excreted into breast milk in low amounts. In a patient given 100 mg of radiolabeled PTU, the milk:plasma ratio was a constant 0.55 for a 24-hour period, representing about 0.077% of the given radioactive dose (54). In a second study, nine patients were given an oral dose of 400 mg (55). Mean serum and milk levels at 90 minutes were 7.7 and 0.7 mcg/mL, respectively. The average amount excreted in milk during 4 hours was 99 mcg, about 0.025% of the total dose. One mother took 200–300 mg daily while breastfeeding. No changes in any of the infant's thyroid parameters were observed (55).

Based on these two reports, PTU does not seem to pose a significant risk to the breastfed infant, but periodic evaluation of the infant's thyroid function would be prudent. A 1987 review of antithyroid medication during lactation considered PTU the drug of choice because it is ionized at phyiologic pH and protein bound (80%), both limiting its transfer into milk (56).

An interesting study published in 2000 found that the physician's advice was the only significant predictor of a woman's choice to breastfeed during PTU therapy (57). In the postpartum period, a group of 36 hyperthyroid women who required PTU were compared with 30 women who no longer required PTU therapy and 36 healthy women (controls). The breastfeeding initiation rates in the three groups were 44%, 83%, and 83%, respectively. In 15 of the women receiving PTU who breastfed, advice on breastfeeding was given by 22 physicians (20 in favor, 1 against, and 1 equivocal). In those women taking PTU who formula-fed, 11 received advice from 17 physicians (4 in favor, 12 against, and 1 equivocal) (57).

The American Academy of Pediatrics classifies PTU as compatible with breastfeeding (58).

References

1. Astwood EB, VanderLaan WP. Treatment of hyperthyroidism with propylthiouracil. Ann Intern Med 1946;25:813–21.
2. Bain L. Propylthiouracil in pregnancy: report of a case. South Med J 1947;40:1020–1.
3. Lahey FH, Bartels EC. The use of thiouracil, thiobarbital and propylthiouracil in patients with hyperthyroidism. Ann Surg 1947;125:572–81.
4. Reveno WS. Propylthiouracil in the treatment of toxic goiter. J Clin Endocrinol Metab 1948;8:866–74.
5. Eisenberg L. Thyrotoxicosis complicating pregnancy. NY State J Med 1950;50:1618–9.
6. Astwood EB. The use of antithyroid drugs during pregnancy. J Clin Endocrinol Metab 1951;11:1045–56.
7. Aaron HH, Schneierson SJ, Siegel E. Goiter in newborn infant due to mother's ingestion of propylthiouracil. JAMA 1955;159:848–50.
8. Waldinger C, Wermer OS, Sobel EH. Thyroid function in infant with congenital goiter resulting from exposure to propylthiouracil. J Am Med Wom Assoc 1955;10:196–7.
9. Bongiovanni AM, Eberlein WR, Thomas PZ, Anderson WB. Sporadic goiter of the newborn. J Clin Endocrinol Met 1956;16:146–52.
10. Krementz ET, Hooper RG, Kempson RL. The effect on the rabbit fetus of the maternal administration of propylthiouracil. Surgery 1957:41:619–31.
11. Branch LK, Tuthill SW. Goiters in twins resulting from propylthiouracil given during pregnancy. Ann Intern Med 1957;46:145–8.

12. Man EB, Shaver BA Jr, Cooke RE. Studies of children born to women with thyroid disease. Am J Obstet Gynecol 1958;75:728–41.
13. Becker WF, Sudduth PG. Hyperthyroidism and pregnancy. Ann Surg 1959;149:867–74.
14. Greenman GW, Gabrielson MO, Howard-Flanders J, Wessel MA. Thyroid dysfunction in pregnancy. N Engl J Med 1962;267:426–31.
15. Herbst AL, Selenkow HA. Combined antithyroid-thyroid therapy of hyperthyroidism in pregnancy. Obstet Gynecol 1963;21:543–50.
16. Reveno WS, Rosenbaum H. Observations on the use of antithyroid drugs. Ann Intern Med 1964;60:982–9.
17. Herbst AL, Selenkow HA. Hyperthyroidism during pregnancy. N Engl J Med 1965;273:627–33.
18. Burrow GN. Neonatal goiter after maternal propylthiouracil therapy. J Clin Endocrinol Metab 1965;25:403–8.
19. Burrow GN, Bartsocas C, Klatskin EH, Grunt JA. Children exposed in utero to propylthiouracil. Am J Dis Child 1968;116:161–5.
20. Talbert LM, Thomas CG Jr, Holt WA, Rankin P. Hyperthyroidism during pregnancy. Obstet Gynecol 1970;36:779–85.
21. Hollingsworth DR, Austin E. Thyroxine derivatives in amniotic fluid. J Pediatr 1971;79:923–9.
22. Ayromlooi J. Congenital goiter due to maternal ingestion of iodides. Obstet Gynecol 1972;39:818–22.
23. Worley RJ, Crosby WM. Hyperthyroidism during pregnancy. Am J Obstet Gynecol 1974;119:150–5.
24. Refetoff S, Ochi Y, Selenkow HA, Rosenfield RL. Neonatal hypothyroidism and goiter in one infant of each of two sets of twins due to maternal therapy with antithyroid drugs. J Pediatr 1974;85:240–4.
25. Mestman JH, Manning PR, Hodgman J. Hyperthyroidism and pregnancy. Arch Intern Med 1974;134:434–9.
26. Goluboff LG, Sisson JC, Hamburger JI. Hyperthyroidism associated with pregnancy. Obstet Gynecol 1974;44:107–16.
27. Mujtaba Q, Burrow GN. Treatment of hyperthyroidism in pregnancy with propylthiouracil and methimazole. Obstet Gynecol 1975;46:282–6.
28. Serup J, Petersen S. Hyperthyroidism during pregnancy treated with propylthiouracil. Acta Obstet Gynecol Scand 1977;56:463–6.
29. Petersen S, Serup J. Case report: neonatal thyrotoxicosis. Acta Paediatr Scand 1977;66:639–42.
30. Serup J. Maternal propylthiouracil to manage fetal hyperthyroidism. Lancet 1978;2:896.
31. Wallace EZ, Gandhi VS. Triiodothyronine thyrotoxicosis in pregnancy. Am J Obstet Gynecol 1978;130:106–7.
32. Weiner S, Scharf JI, Bolognese RJ, Librizzi RJ. Antenatal diagnosis and treatment of a fetal goiter. J Reprod Med 1980;24:39–42.
33. Sugrue D, Drury MI. Hyperthyroidism complicating pregnancy: results of treatment by antithyroid drugs in 77 pregnancies. Br J Obstet Gynaecol 1980;87:970–5.
34. Cheron RG, Kaplan MM, Larsen PR, Selenkow HA, Crigler JF Jr. Neonatal thyroid function after propylthiouracil therapy for maternal Graves' disease. N Engl J Med 1981;304:525–8.
35. Check JH, Rezvani I, Goodner D, Hopper B. Prenatal treatment of thyrotoxicosis to prevent intrauterine growth retardation. Obstet Gynecol 1982;60:122–4.
36. Kock HCLV, Merkus JMWM. Graves' disease during pregnancy. Eur J Obstet Gynecol Reprod Biol 1983;14:323–30.
37. Hollingsworth DR, Austin E. Observations following I^{131} for Graves disease during first trimester of pregnancy. South Med J 1969;62:1555–6.
38. Burrow GN. The management of thyrotoxicosis in pregnancy. N Engl J Med 1985;313:562–5.
39. Momotani N, Noh J, Oyanagi H, Ishikawa N, Ito K. Antithyroid drug therapy for Graves' disease during pregnancy. Optimal regiment for fetal thyroid status. N Engl J Med 1986;315:24–8.
40. American Hospital Formulary Service. *Drug Information 1997*. Bethesda, MD: American Society of Health-System Pharmacists, 1997:2487–8.
41. Marchant B, Brownlie EW, Hart DM, Horton PW, Alexander WD. The placental transfer of propylthiouracil, methimazole and carbimazole. J Clin Endocrinol Metab 1977;45:1187–93.
42. Gardner DF, Cruikshank DP, Hays PM, Cooper DS. Pharmacology of propylthiouracil (PTU) in pregnant hyperthyroid women: correlation of maternal PTU concentrations with cord serum thyroid function tests. J Clin Endocrinol Metab 1986;62:217–20.
43. Ramsay I, Kaur S, Krassas G. Thyrotoxicosis in pregnancy: results of treatment by antithyroid drugs combined with T4. Clin Endocrinol (Oxf) 1983;18:73–85.
44. Burr WA. Thyroid disease. Clin Obstet Gynecol 1981;8:341–51.
45. Burrow GN. Hyperthyroidism during pregnancy. N Engl J Med 1978; 298:150–3.
46. Burrow GN. Maternal–fetal considerations in hyperthyroidism. Clin Endocrinol Metab 1978;7:115–25.
47. Burrow GN, Klatskin EH, Genel M. Intellectual development in children whose mothers received propylthiouracil during pregnancy. Yale J Biol Med 1978;51:151–6.
48. Momotani N, Ito K, Hamada N, Ban Y, Nishikawa Y, Mimura T. Maternal hyperthyroidism and congenital malformations in the offspring. Clin Endocrinol (Oxf) 1984;20:695–700.
49. Heinonen OP, Slone D, Shapiro S. *Birth Defects and Drugs in Pregnancy*. Littleton, MA: Publishing Sciences Group, 1977:388–400.
50. Wing D, Millar L, Koonings P, Montoro M, Mestman J. A comparison of PTU versus Tapazole in the treatment of hyperthyroidism (abstract). Am J Obstet Gynecol 1992;166:308.
51. Wing DA, Millar LK, Koonings PP, Montoro MN, Mestman JH. A comparison of propylthiouracil versus methimazole in the treatment of hyperthyroidism in pregnancy. Am J Obstet Gynecol 1994;170:90–5.
52. Diav-Citrin O, Ornoy A. Teratogen update: antithyroid drugs—methimazole, carbimazole, and propylthiouracil. Teratology 2002;65:38–44.
53. Anonymous. Transplacental passage of thyroid hormones. N Engl J Med 1967;277:486–7.
54. Low LCK, Lang J, Alexander WD. Excretion of carbimazole and propylthiouracil in breast milk. Lancet 1979;2:1011.
55. Kampmann JP, Johansen K, Hansen JM, Helweg J. Propylthiouracil in human milk. Lancet 1980;1:736–8.
56. Cooper DS. Antithyroid drugs: to breast-feed or not to breast-feed. Am J Obstet Gynecol 1987;157:234–5.
57. Lee A, Moretti ME, Collantes A, Chong D, Mazzotta P, Koren G, Merchant SS, Ito S. Choice of breastfeeding and physicians' advice: a cohort study of women receiving propylthiouracil. Pediatrics 2000;106: 27–30.
58. Committee on Drugs, American Academy of Pediatrics. The transfer of drugs and other chemicals into human milk. Pediatrics 2001;108: 776–89.

P

PROTAMINE

Antiheparin

PREGNANCY RECOMMENDATION: Compatible—Maternal Benefit >> Embryo–Fetal Risk
BREASTFEEDING RECOMMENDATION: No Human Data—Probably Compatible

PREGNANCY SUMMARY

Protamine is used to neutralize the anticoagulant effect of heparin. No reports of its use in pregnancy have been located. Reproduction studies in animals have not been conducted (1).

BREASTFEEDING SUMMARY

No reports describing the use of protamine during human lactation have been located. Such reports are unlikely due to its indication.

Reference

1. Product information. Protamine sulfate. Eli Lilly, 1993.

PROTIRELIN

[Withdrawn from the market. See 9th edition.]

PROTRIPTYLINE

Antidepressant

PREGNANCY RECOMMENDATION: No Human Data—Animal Data Suggest Low Risk
BREASTFEEDING RECOMMENDATION: No Human Data—Potential Toxicity

PREGNANCY SUMMARY

No reports on the use of protriptyline during human pregnancy have been located. (See also Amitriptyline and Nortriptyline.)

FETAL RISK SUMMARY

Protriptyline, a dibenzocycloheptene derivative, is a tricyclic antidepressant. Other antidepressants in this class are amitriptyline and its metabolite, nortriptyline.

Reproduction studies in mice, rats, and rabbits at doses about 10 times greater than the recommended human dose had no apparent adverse effects on reproduction (1).

It is not known if protriptyline crosses the human placenta. The molecular weight (about 264 for the free base) is low enough that exposure of the embryo–fetus should be expected.

BREASTFEEDING SUMMARY

No reports describing the use of protriptyline during lactation have been located. The molecular weight (about 264 for the free base) is low enough that excretion into breast milk should be expected. The effect on a nursing infant from exposure to the drug in breast milk is unknown. The American Academy of Pediatrics classifies amitriptyline, a similar antidepressant, as a drug whose effect on the nursing infant is unknown but may be of concern (see Amitriptyline).

Reference

1. Product information. Vivactil. Merck, 2000.

PSEUDOEPHEDRINE

Sympathomimetic (Adrenergic)

PREGNANCY RECOMMENDATION: Human Data Suggest Risk
BREASTFEEDING RECOMMENDATION: Limited Human Data—Probably Compatible

PREGNANCY SUMMARY

Although the limited human data suggest there may be a risk of gastroschisis and small intestinal atresia (SIA) from 1st trimester exposure to pseudoephedrine, the risk is low and may only be identifiable in case–control studies. Moreover, the risk may only be present when pseudoephedrine is combined with other agents, not when it used alone. Confirmation of these findings is required. Until such data are available, the best course is to avoid pseudoephedrine during the 1st trimester.

FETAL RISK SUMMARY

Pseudoephedrine is a sympathomimetic used to alleviate the symptoms of allergic disorders or upper respiratory infections. It is a common component of proprietary mixtures containing antihistamines and other ingredients. Thus, it is difficult to separate the effects of pseudoephedrine on the fetus from those of other drugs, disease states, and viruses.

Sympathomimetic amines are teratogenic in some animal species, but human teratogenicity has not been suspected (1). The Collaborative Perinatal Project monitored 50,282 mother–child pairs, 3082 of whom had 1st trimester exposure to sympathomimetic drugs (2, pp. 345–356). For use anytime during pregnancy, 9719 exposures were recorded (2, p. 439). An association in the 1st trimester was found between the sympathomimetic class of drugs as a whole and minor malformations (not life-threatening or major cosmetic defects), inguinal hernia, and clubfoot (2, pp. 345–356). However, independent confirmation of these results is required (2, pp. 345–356).

In a surveillance study of Michigan Medicaid recipients involving 229,101 completed pregnancies conducted between 1985 and 1992, 940 newborns had been exposed to pseudoephedrine during the 1st trimester (F. Rosa, personal communication, FDA, 1993). A total of 37 (3.9%) major birth defects were observed (40 expected). Specific data were available for six defect categories, including (observed/expected) 3/9 cardiovascular defects, 2/2 oral clefts, 0/0 spina bifida, 3/3 polydactyly, 0/2 limb reduction defects, and 0/2 hypospadias. These data do not support an association between the drug and congenital defects.

A case–control surveillance study published in 1992 reported a significantly elevated relative risk of 3.2 (95% confidence interval [CI] 1.3–7.7) for the use of pseudoephedrine during the 1st trimester and 76 exposed cases with gastroschisis (3). A total of 2142 infants with other malformations formed a control group. Relative risks for other drugs were salicylates, 1.6; acetaminophen, 1.7; ibuprofen, 1.3; and phenylpropanolamine, 1.5. Because some of these drugs are vasoactive substances, and because the cause of gastroschisis is thought to involve vascular disruption of the omphalomesenteric artery (3), the investigators compared the use of 1st trimester pseudoephedrine and other drugs in relation to a heterogeneous group of malformations, other than gastroschisis, suspected of also having a vascular origin. In this case, however, the relative risk for the drugs approximated unity. These data suggested that the association between pseudoephedrine and the other drugs and gastroschisis may have been caused by an underlying maternal illness (3).

In a 2002 retrospective case–control study, conducted in 1995–1999, mothers of 206 gastroschisis cases, 126 SIA cases, and 798 controls were interviewed about medication use and illnesses (4). The interval of between birth and interview was <6 months for all cases. The risk of gastroschisis was increased for aspirin (odds ratio [OR] 2.7, 95% CI 1.1–5.9), all pseudoephedrine (OR 1.8, 95% CI 1.0–3.2), all acetaminophen (OR 1.5, 95% CI 1.1–2.2), and pseudoephedrine plus acetaminophen (OR 4.2, 95% CI 1.9–9.2). The risk for SIA was increased for all pseudoephedrine (OR 2.0, 95% CI 1.0–4.0), and pseudoephedrine plus acetaminophen (OR 3.0, 95% CI 1.1–9.0). However, when pseudoephedrine was used as a single agent, the ORs and 95% CIs for gastroschisis and SIA were 0.7 (0.2–2.1) and 1.1 (0.5–2.9), respectively. Fever (as reported by the patient), upper respiratory infection, and allergy were not associated with increased risks of gastroschisis or SIA. There were also no significant associations with phenylpropanolamine, ibuprofen, antihistamines, guaifenesin, or dextromethorphan. The results confirmed the association of an increased risk of gastroschisis with aspirin shown in previous studies. However, the data for pseudoephedrine raised questions concerning interactions between drugs and possible confounding by underlying illness (4).

A 2005 abstract reviewed the fetal effects of pseudoephedrine after 1st trimester exposure (5). Two analyses of pharmacy data from health maintenance organizations revealed 9 malformed infants among 902 exposures, suggesting no association with congenital malformations overall. However, case–control studies have shown that 1st trimester exposure to decongestants is associated with small to moderate increases in the risk of gastroschisis, SIA, and hemifacial microsomia. Moreover, these risks are increased if the mother also smokes cigarettes (5).

Data from the Swedish Medical Birth Registry regarding pregnancy exposure to oral decongestants were reported in 2006 (6). The 1st trimester pregnancy exposures reported by 2474 women were 2304 phenylpropanolamine alone, 136 phenylpropanolamine plus cinnarizine, 23 pseudoephedrine alone, and 11 used 2 of these preparations. Compared with 1771 women who were prescribed an oral decongestant later in pregnancy, the risk ratio for any congenital malformation among the 2474 subjects was 0.96, 95% CI 0.80–1.16 (6).

A 1981 report described a woman who consumed, throughout pregnancy, 480–840 mL/day of a cough syrup (7). The potential maximum daily doses based on 840 mL of syrup were 5.0 g of pseudoephedrine, 16.8 g of guaifenesin, 1.68 g of dextromethorphan, and 79.8 mL of ethanol. The infant had features of the fetal alcohol syndrome (see Ethanol) and displayed irritability, tremors, and hypertonicity (7). It is not known whether the ingredients, other than the ethanol, were associated with the adverse effects observed in the infant.

BREASTFEEDING SUMMARY

Pseudoephedrine is excreted into breast milk (8,9). Three mothers, who were nursing healthy infants, were given an antihistamine-decongestant preparation containing 60 mg of pseudoephedrine and 2.5 mg of triprolidine (8). Two of the mothers had been nursing for 14 weeks, and one had been nursing for 18 months. Milk concentrations of pseudoephedrine were higher than plasma levels in all three patients, with peak milk concentrations occurring at 1.0–1.5 hours. The milk:plasma ratios at 1, 3, and 12 hours in one subject were 3.3, 3.9, and 2.6, respectively. The investigators calculated that 1000 mL of milk produced during 24 hours would contain 0.25–0.33 mg of pseudoephedrine base, approximately 0.5%–0.7% of the maternal dose (8).

A single-blind, cross-over study of pseudoephedrine 60 mg vs. placebo was conducted in eight lactating women (9). The mean milk volume was significantly reduced by pseudoephedrine, falling from 784 mL/day (placebo period) to 623 mL/day (pseudoephedrine period). The effect on milk volume was not due to breast blood flow, but the slightly reduced (*ns*) serum prolactin concentrations in the women may have contributed. The mean average milk concentration was 829 mcg/L. Assuming a pseudoephedrine 60 mg 4 times daily dose (maximum recommended dose), the estimated infant dose, based on AUC and 150 mL/kg/day, was 4.3% of the mother's weight-adjusted dose (9).

The American Academy of Pediatrics classifies pseudoephedrine as compatible with breastfeeding (10).

References

1. Nishimura H, Tanimura T. *Clinical Aspects of the Teratogenicity of Drugs*. Amsterdam, The Netherlands: Excerpta Medica, 1976:231.
2. Heinonen OP, Slone D, Shapiro S. *Birth Defects and Drugs in Pregnancy*. Littleton, MA: Publishing Sciences Group, 1977.
3. Werler MM, Mitchell AA, Shapiro S. First trimester maternal medication use in relation to gastroschisis. Teratology 1992;45:361–7.
4. Werler MM, Sheehan JE, Mitchell AA. Maternal medication use and risks of gastroschisis and small intestinal atresia. Am J Epidemiol 2002;155:26–31.
5. Werler MM. Teratogen update: pseudoephedrine. Birth Defects Res A Clin Mol Teratol 2005;73:328.
6. Kallen BAJ, Olausson PO. Use of oral decongestants during pregnancy and delivery outcome. Am J Obstet Gynecol 2006;194:480–5.
7. Chasnoff IJ, Diggs G. Fetal alcohol effects and maternal cough syrup abuse. Am J Dis Child 1981;135:968.
8. Findlay JWA, Butz RF, Sailstad JM, Warren JT, Welch RM. Pseudoephedrine and triprolidine in plasma and breast milk of nursing mothers. Br J Clin Pharmacol 1984;18:901–6.
9. Aljazaf K, Hale TW, Hett KF, Hartmann PE, Mitoulas LR, Kritensen JH, Hackett LP. Pseudoephedrine: effects on milk production in women and estimation of infant exposure via breastmilk. Br J Clin Pharmacol 2003;56:18–24.
10. Committee on Drugs, American Academy of Pediatrics. The transfer of drugs and other chemicals into human milk. Pediatrics 2001;108:776–89.

PUMPKIN SEED

Herb

PREGNANCY RECOMMENDATION: No Human Data—Probably Compatible
BREASTFEEDING RECOMMENDATION: No Human Data—Probably Compatible

PREGNANCY SUMMARY

No reports describing the use of pumpkin seed in human pregnancy have been located. Animal reproduction data also are lacking. However, this product has been used worldwide as a food and in traditional medicine for centuries (1). When used as a food, pumpkin seed probably is harmless for the embryo–fetus. High doses, such as those that might be used in traditional medicine or in eating disorders should be avoided.

FETAL RISK SUMMARY

Several subspecies of pumpkin are widely consumed as food and used in traditional medicine. The subspecies belong to the family Cucurbitaceae and include *Cucurbita pepo* (also known as *C. galeotti, C. mammeata,* and *Cucumis pepo*), *C. maxima* Duchesne (autumn squash), and *C. moschata* Poir (crookneck squash). Pumpkin seeds are used as a food, an anthelmintic and, in combination with other herbal products, in the treatment of dysuria caused by benign prostatic hyperplasia. The anthelmintic agent in pumpkin seeds is cucurbitin, a carboxypyrrolidine. The concentration of cucurbitin in pumpkin seeds depends on the subspecies, varying from 0.18% to 1.94%, with the highest concentrations in *C. maxima*. Other chemicals in pumpkin seeds are fatty acids (primarily palmitic, stearic, oleic, and linoleic), carotenoids (primarily β-carotene), amino acids and protein, and carbohydrates. In addition to β-carotene, the seeds are high in vitamin E (primarily γ-tocopherol) (1,2).

Animal reproduction studies involving pumpkin seed have not been located.

Vitamin A (i.e., from conversion of β-carotene), vitamin E, and fatty acids are known to cross the placenta and the other components of pumpkin probably also cross.

BREASTFEEDING SUMMARY

No reports describing the use of pumpkin seed during human lactation have been located. When used as a food, pumpkin seed probably is harmless for the nursing infant. High doses, such as those that might be used in traditional medicine or in eating disorders should be avoided.

References

1. Pumpkin. In DerMarderosian A, Beutler JA, eds. The Review of Natural Products. St. Louis, MO: Wolters Kluwer Health, July 2004.
2. Pumpkin. In Jellin JM, ed. *Natural Medicines Comprehensive Database*. 10th ed. Stockton, CA: Therapeutic Research Faculty, 2008:1219–20.

PYRANTEL PAMOATE

Anthelmintic

PREGNANCY RECOMMENDATION: No Human Data—Animal Data Suggest Low Risk
BREASTFEEDING RECOMMENDATION: No Human Data—Probably Compatible

PREGNANCY SUMMARY

No reports on the use of this drug in human pregnancy have been located. Shepard cited two studies in which no congenital defects or postnatal effects were observed in pregnant rats fed doses up to 3000 mg/kg or in pregnant rabbits given 1000 mg/kg (1,2).

FETAL RISK SUMMARY

It is not known if pyrantel pamoate crosses the human placenta. The molecular weight (about 595) is low enough that exposure of the embryo–fetus should be expected.

BREASTFEEDING SUMMARY

No reports describing the use of pyrantel pamoate during human lactation have been located. The molecular weight (about 595) is low enough for excretion into breast milk. The effect of this exposure on a nursing infant is unknown.

References

1. Owaki Y, Sakai T, Momiyama H. Teratological studies on pyrantel pamoate in rats. Oyo Yakuri 1971;5:41–50. As cited in Shepard TH. *Catalog of Teratogenic Agents*. 6th ed. Baltimore, MD: The Johns Hopkins University Press, 1989:536.
2. Owaki Y, Sakai T, Momiyama H. Teratological studies on pyrantel pamoate in rabbits. Oyo Yakuri 1971;5:33–39. As cited in Shepard TH. *Catalog of Teratogenic Agents*. 6th ed. Baltimore, MD: The Johns Hopkins University Press, 1989:536.

PYRAZINAMIDE

Antituberculosis Agent

PREGNANCY RECOMMENDATION: Compatible—Maternal Benefit >> Embryo–Fetal Risk
BREASTFEEDING RECOMMENDATION: Limited Human Data—Probably Compatible

PREGNANCY SUMMARY

Pyrazinamide is a synthetic antituberculosis agent derived from niacinamide. There is no relevant animal data, but a small number of human pregnancy exposures without fetal harm have been reported (1). Therefore, because active tuberculosis is a far greater risk to the embryo–fetus than the drug, pyrazinamide, if indicated should not be withheld in pregnancy (2).

FETAL RISK SUMMARY

Pyrazinamide is indicated for the initial treatment of active tuberculosis in adults and children when combined with other antituberculosis agents. Plasma protein binding (about 10%) is low and the elimination half-life in patients with normal renal and hepatic function is 9–10 hours. The drug is metabolized in the liver to an active metabolite (3).

Animal reproduction studies have not been conducted with pyrazinamide. The drug was not carcinogenic in rats and male mice (data lacking for female mice) or mutagenic in one test. However, pyrazinamide did induce chromosomal aberrations in human lymphocyte cell cultures (3).

It is not known if pyrazinamide crosses the human placenta. The molecular weight (about 123), low plasma protein binding, and prolonged elimination half-life suggest that exposure of the embryo–fetus will occur.

A 1994 report described the use of pyrazinamide in a pregnant woman (4). She had been treated for cavitary pulmonary tuberculosis with three other agents for 5 months before the addition of pyrazinamide at 26 weeks' gestation for persistent positive sputum cultures. No drug-related fetal toxicity was mentioned (4). Although past investigators have cautioned that pyrazinamide should not be routinely used because of the lack of information pertaining to its fetal effects (4–7), a more recent recommendation states that the drug can be used in pregnancy (2).

In a 1999 study involving 33 pregnant women with extrapulmonary tuberculosis, 6 (21%) were treated with isoniazid, rifampin, and pyrazinamide (8). Pyrazinamide was stopped after 2 months and all therapy was stopped after 9 months. No cases of congenital tuberculosis or fetal malformations were observed (8).

A 2003 report described the use of pyrazinamide in a pregnant woman with multidrug-resistant tuberculosis (9). The 22-year-old woman was diagnosed with the infection at 23 weeks' and daily treatment was initiated with rifampin (600 mg), isoniazid (300 mg), and ethambutol (700 mg). Because of lack of response, her therapy was changed after 3 weeks to capreomycin (IV 1000 mg 5 days/week), cycloserine (750 mg/day), levofloxacin (1000 mg/day), *para*-aminosalicylic acid (12 g/day), and pyrazinamide (1500 mg/day). After spontaneous rupture of the membranes, she gave birth at 35 weeks' to a healthy 2003-g infant. The results of a tuberculin skin test and three nasogastric aspiration cultures were negative, as were a neurologic examination and electrophysiology hearing studies. The infant was kept separated from the mother (9).

Pyrazinamide, in combination with isoniazid, rifampin, and ethambutol, was used in five pregnancies in a 2008 report (10). No adverse effects on the fetuses or newborns were observed.

BREASTFEEDING SUMMARY

Pyrazinamide is excreted into human milk. A patient who was not breastfeeding (days postpartum not stated) was given an oral 1-g dose of pyrazinamide (11). The peak milk concentration, 1.5 mcg/mL, occurred at 3 hours. The peak maternal plasma concentration, 42.0 mcg/mL, occurred at 2 hours (10).

In the above case, the milk:plasma ratio was approximately 0.04. The weight of the woman was not specified, but if her weight was 70 kg and a nursing infant consumed 150 mL/kg/day of breast milk, then the theoretically maximum infant dose as a percentage of the mother's weight-adjusted dose would be 1.6%. This suggests that if similar results are eventually reported in other studies, the risk of toxicity to a nursing infant is probably nil. Based on the one case, maternal treatment with pyrazinamide appears to be compatible with breastfeeding. However, nursing infants should be monitored for the rare toxicity observed in patients taking the drug, such as jaundice, fever, loss of appetite, nausea and vomiting, thrombocytopenia, rash, and arthralgia.

References

1. Ormerod P. Tuberculosis in pregnancy and the puerperium. Thorax 2001;56:494–9.
2. API Consensus Expert Committee. API TB consensus guidelines 2006: management of pulmonary tuberculosis, extra-pulmonary tuberculosis and tuberculosis in special situations. J Assoc Physicians India 2006;54:219–34.
3. Product information. Pyrazinamide. Mikart, 1994.
4. Bothamley G, Elston W. Pregnancy does not mean that patients with tuberculosis must stop treatment. BMJ 1991;318:1286,
5. Margono F, Mroueh J, Garely A, White D, Duerr A, Minkoff HL. Resurgence of active tuberculosis among pregnant women. Obstet Gynecol 1994;83:911–4.
6. American Thoracic Society. Treatment of tuberculosis and tuberculosis infection in adults and children. Am Rev Respir Dis 1986;134:355–63.
7. Hamadeh MA, Glassroth J. Tuberculosis and pregnancy. Chest 1992;101:1114–20.
8. Jana N, Vasishta K, Saha SC, Ghosh K. Obstetrical outcomes among women with extrapulmonary tuberculosis. N Engl J Med 1999;341:645–9.
9. Klaus-Dieter KLL, Qarah S. Multidrug-resistant tuberculosis in pregnancy—case report and review of the literature. Chest 2003;123:953–6.
10. Keskin N, Yilmaz S. Pregnancy and tuberculosis: to assess tuberculosis cases in pregnancy in a developing region retrospectively and two case reports. Arch Gynecol Obstet 2008;278:451–5
11. Holdiness MR. Antituberculosis drugs and breast-feeding. Arch Intern Med 1984;144:1888.

PYRETHRINS WITH PIPERONYL BUTOXIDE

Pediculicide

PREGNANCY RECOMMENDATION: No Human Data—Probably Compatible
BREASTFEEDING RECOMMENDATION: No Human Data—Probably Compatible

PREGNANCY SUMMARY

Pyrethrins with piperonyl butoxide is a synergistic combination product used topically for the treatment of lice infestations. It is considered the drug of choice for lice (1). Although no reports of its use in pregnancy have been located, topical absorption is poor, so potential toxicity should be less than that of lindane (see also Lindane) (2). For this reason, use of the combination is probably preferred over lindane in the pregnant patient.

BREASTFEEDING SUMMARY

No reports describing the use of pyrethrins with piperonyl butoxide during human lactation have been located. Because the drug is absorbed poorly after topical application, exposure of a nursing infant from breast milk is probably nil.

References

1. Anonymous. Drugs for parasitic infections. In *Handbook for Antimicrobial Therapy*. New Rochelle, NY: The Medical Letter, Inc., 1984:100.
2. Robinson DH, Shepherd DA. Control of head lice in schoolchildren. Curr Ther Res 1980;27:1–6.

PYRIDOSTIGMINE

Parasympathomimetic (Cholinergic)

PREGNANCY RECOMMENDATION: Limited Human Data—Animal Data Suggest Low Risk
BREASTFEEDING RECOMMENDATION: Limited Human Data—Probably Compatible

PREGNANCY SUMMARY

Pyridostigmine is a quaternary ammonium compound with anticholinesterase activity used in the treatment of myasthenia gravis. Most reports have described no fetal harm and the animal data suggest low risk.

FETAL RISK SUMMARY

Pyridostigmine was not teratogenic in rats at doses up to 30 mg/kg/day, but maternal and fetal toxicity (reduced weight) were observed at the highest dose (1).

Although it is ionized at physiologic pH, the low molecular weight of pyridostigmine (about 261) allows the nonionized fraction to cross to the fetus. Pyridostigmine concentrations have been determined at birth in maternal plasma, cord blood, and amniotic fluid (2). Two women with long-term myasthenia gravis were treated throughout gestation with pyridostigmine, 360 and 420 mg per day, respectively. The latter woman was also treated with neostigmine (105 mg/day) and ambenonium (60 mg/day). In the first case, the maternal plasma, cord blood, and amniotic drug concentrations were 77, 65, and 290 ng/mL, respectively, and in the second, 53, 39, and 300 ng/mL, respectively. Thus, the cord blood:maternal plasma ratios were 0.84 and 0.74, respectively, whereas the amniotic fluid:maternal plasma ratios were 3.8 and 5.7 respectively (2).

Caution has been advised against the use in pregnancy of IV anticholinesterases because they may cause premature labor (3,4). This effect on the pregnant uterus increases near term.

A number of reports have described the apparent safe use of pyridostigmine during human gestation (2–16). However, a case report published in 2000 described microcephaly and CNS injury in a newborn that was attributed to high-dose pyridostigmine (17). The infant's mother was a 24-year-old primigravida with a 14-year history of myasthenia gravis. She required high-dose pyridostigmine (1500–3000 mg/day) throughout gestation to control her diplopia and ptosis. In comparison, the average recommended daily dose is 600 mg, with daily doses ≤1500 mg required in severe cases (18). The mother denied smoking and the use of other drugs during pregnancy. At 36 weeks' gestation, an emergency cesarean section for fetal bradycardia was conducted, delivering a severely growth-restricted (1880 g, <2nd percentile), hypotonic male infant with Apgar scores of 3 and 8 at 1 and 5 minutes, respectively. Shortly after birth, neonatal myasthenia gravis was diagnosed, two exchange transfusions were used to lower his acetylcholine receptor antibody titer, and IV immunoglobulin was administered. The infant required immediate intubation because of poor respiratory effort and was continued on the respirator until age 3.5 months. Mild finger and wrist contractures and bilateral cryptorchidism were noted at birth, but he had no abnormal ocular findings (17). The head circumference was 33.5 cm at birth and 37 cm (<5th percentile) at 3 months of age. By about 5 months of age, a number of dysmorphic features were noted, including a broad nasal bridge with a prominent nose, slight downslanting palpebral fissures, high arched palate, short neck, broad chest, campylodactyly, and hammer toes (17). He continued to do poorly, requiring additional hospitalizations and mechanical ventilation. At 4.5 months, he was discharged home but readmitted 1 week later because of prolonged apnea and cyanosis. His weight (5.1 kg, 10th percentile) and head circumference (38 cm, <2nd percentile) were still restricted and he remained hypotonic. A cranial ultrasound, karyotyping, and TORCH titers (i.e., toxoplasmosis, other infections, rubella, cytomegalovirus, and herpes simplex) were normal or negative and there was no evidence of craniosynostosis. A brain magnetic resonance imaging scan at 5 months revealed apparent brachycephaly and mild ventriculomegaly. At 9 months of age, he still required nasal oxygen, tone was normal, and the joint contractures had resolved, but his reflexes were brisk and ankle clonus was evident. Because no other cause could be identified, the authors attributed the microcephaly and CNS injury to pyridostigmine (17).

Both antenatal and neonatal myasthenia gravis have been reported and either may result in perinatal death. Both forms of the disorder are caused by transplacental passage of anti-acetylcholine receptor immunoglobulin G antibodies (11,19). The inhibited fetal skeletal muscle movement and development may result in pulmonary hypoplasia, arthrogryposis multiplex, and polyhydramnios (19).

Transient muscular weakness has been observed in about 20% of newborns of mothers with myasthenia gravis (11,19).

BREASTFEEDING SUMMARY

Pyridostigmine is excreted into breast milk. Levels in two women receiving 120–300 mg/day were 2–25 ng/mL, representing milk:plasma ratios of 0.36–1.13 (15). Although pyridostigmine is an ionized quaternary ammonium compound, these values indicate that the nonionized fraction crosses easily into breast milk. The drug was not detected in the infants nor were any adverse effects noted. The authors estimated that the two infants were ingesting 0.1% or less of the maternal doses (15). The American Academy of Pediatrics classifies pyridostigmine as compatible with breastfeeding (20).

P

References

1. Levine BS, Parker RM. Reproductive and developmental toxicity studies of pyridostigmine bromide in rats. Toxicology 1991;69:291–300.
2. Lefvert AK, Osterman PO. Newborn infants to myasthenic mothers: a clinical study and an investigation of acetylcholine receptor antibodies in 17 children. Neurology 1983;33:133–8.
3. Foldes FF, McNall PG. Myasthenia gravis: a guide for anesthesiologists. Anesthesiology 1962;23:837–72.
4. McNall PG, Jafarnia MR. Management of myasthenia gravis in the obstetric patient. Am J Obstet Gynecol 1965;92:518–25.
5. Plauche WC. Myasthenia gravis in pregnancy. Am J Obstet Gynecol 1964;88:404–9.
6. Chambers DC, Hall JE, Boyce J. Myasthenia gravis and pregnancy. Obstet Gynecol 1967;29:597–603.
7. Hay DM. Myasthenia gravis and pregnancy. J Obstet Gynaecol Br Commonw 1969;76:323–9.
8. Heinonen OP, Slone D, Shapiro S. *Birth Defects and Drugs in Pregnancy*. Littleton, MA: Publishing Sciences Group, 1977:345–56.
9. Blackhall MI, Buckley GA, Roberts DV, Roberts JB, Thomas BH, Wilson A. Drug-induced neonatal myasthenia. J Obstet Gynaecol Br Commonw 1969;76:157–62.

10. Rolbin SH, Levinson G, Shnider SM, Wright RG. Anesthetic considerations for myasthenia gravis and pregnancy. Anesth Analg (Cleve) 1978;57:441–7.
11. Plauche WC. Myasthenia gravis in pregnancy: an update. Am J Obstet Gynecol 1979;135:691–7.
12. Eden RD, Gall SA. Myasthenia gravis and pregnancy: a reappraisal of thymectomy. Obstet Gynecol 1983;62:328–33.
13. Cohen BA, London RS, Goldstein PJ. Myasthenia gravis and preeclampsia. Obstet Gynecol 1976;48(Suppl):35S–7S.
14. Catanzarite VA, McHargue AM, Sandberg EC, Dyson DC. Respiratory arrest during therapy for premature labor in a patient with myasthenia gravis. Obstet Gynecol 1984;64:819–22.
15. Hardell LI, Lindstrom B, Lonnerholm G, Osterman PO. Pyridostigmine in human breast milk. Br J Clin Pharmacol 1982;14:565–7.
16. Carr SR, Gilchrist JM, Abuelo DN, Clark D. Treatment of antenatal myasthenia gravis. Obstet Gynecol 1991;78:485–9.
17. Niesen CE, Shah NS. Pyridostigmine-induced microcephaly. Neurology 2000;54:1873–4.
18. Product information. Mestinon. ICN Pharmaceuticals, 2000.
19. Gilchrist JM. Muscle disease in the pregnant woman. Adv Neurol 1994;64:193–208.
20. Committee on Drugs, American Academy of Pediatrics. The transfer of drugs and other chemicals into human milk. Pediatrics 2001;108:776–89.

PYRIDOXINE

Vitamin

PREGNANCY RECOMMENDATION: Compatible
BREASTFEEDING RECOMMENDATION: Compatible

PREGNANCY SUMMARY

Pyridoxine (vitamin B_6) deficiency during pregnancy is a common problem in unsupplemented women. Supplementation with oral pyridoxine reduces but does not eliminate the frequency of deficiency. No definitive evidence has appeared that indicates mild to moderate deficiency of this vitamin is a cause of maternal or fetal complications. Most of the studies with this vitamin have been open and uncontrolled. If a relationship does exist with poor pregnancy outcome, it is probable that a number of factors, of which pyridoxine may be one, contribute to the problem. A significant reduction in nausea and vomiting of pregnancy, however, appears to occur with pyridoxine. The available data are sufficient to conclude that the combination of pyridoxine and doxylamine is safe and effective for nausea and vomiting of pregnancy. Severe deficiency or abnormal metabolism is related to fetal and infantile convulsions and possibly to other conditions. However, the association of pyridoxine deficiency, with or without folate deficiency, and oral clefts requires confirmation. High doses apparently pose little risk to the fetus. Because pyridoxine is required for good maternal and fetal health, and an increased demand for the vitamin occurs during pregnancy, supplementation of the pregnant woman with the recommended dietary allowance (RDA) for pyridoxine is recommended.

P

FETAL RISK SUMMARY

Pyridoxine, a water-soluble B-complex vitamin, acts as an essential coenzyme involved in the metabolism of amino acids, carbohydrates, and lipids (1). The National Academy of Sciences' RDA for pyridoxine in pregnancy is 2.2 mg (1).

Pyridoxine is actively transported to the fetus (2–4). Like other B-complex vitamins, concentrations of pyridoxine in the fetus and newborn are higher than in the mother and are directly proportional to maternal intake (5–16). Actual pyridoxine levels vary from report to report because of the nutritional status of the populations studied and the microbiologic assays used, but usually indicate an approximate newborn:maternal ratio of 2:1 with levels ranging from 22 to 87 ng/mL for newborns and 13–51 ng/mL for mothers (4,14–16).

Pyridoxine deficiency without clinical symptoms is common during pregnancy (10,16–34). Clinical symptoms consisting of oral lesions have been reported, however, in severe B_6 deficiency (35). Supplementation with multivitamin products reduces, but does not always eliminate, the incidence of pyridoxine hypovitaminemia (16).

Severe vitamin B_6 deficiency is teratogenic in experimental animals (36,37). No reports of human malformations linked to B_6 deficiency have been located. A brief report in 1976 described an anencephalic fetus resulting from a woman treated with high doses of pyridoxine and other vitamins and nutrients for psychiatric reasons, but the relationship between the defect and the vitamins is unknown (38).

The effects on the mother and fetus resulting from pyridoxine deficiency or excess are controversial. These effects can be summarized as follows:

- Gestational hypertension (GH)
- Gestational diabetes mellitus
- Infantile convulsions
- Nausea and vomiting of pregnancy
- Congenital malformations
- Miscellaneous effects

Gestational Hypertension

Several researchers have claimed that pyridoxine deficiency is associated with the development of GH (12,39–41). Others have not found this relationship (10,19,42,43). One group of investigators demonstrated that women with GH excreted larger amounts of xanthurenic acid in their urine after a loading dose of *dl*-tryptophan than did normal pregnant women (39). Although the test only was partially specific for GH, they theorized that it could be of value for early detection of the disease and was indicative of abnormal pyridoxine–niacin–protein metabolism. In another study, 410 women treated with 10 mg of pyridoxine daily were compared with 410 controls (40).

GH occurred in 18 (4.4%) of the untreated controls and in 7 (1.7%) of the pyridoxine-supplemented patients, a significant difference. In an earlier report, no significant differences were found between women with GH and normal controls in urinary excretion of 4-pyridoxic acid, a pyridoxine metabolite, after a loading dose of the vitamin (19). Some investigators have measured lower levels of pyridoxine in mothers with GH than in mothers without GH (12). The difference in levels between the newborns of GH and normal mothers was more than twofold and highly significant. In a 1961 Swedish report, pyridoxine levels in 10 women with GH were compared with those in 26 women with uncomplicated pregnancies (42). The difference between the mean levels of the two groups, 25 and 33 ng/mL, respectively, was not significant. Similarly, others have been unable to find a correlation between pyridoxine levels and GH (10,43).

Gestational Diabetes Mellitus

Pyridoxine levels were studied in 14 pregnant women with an abnormal glucose tolerance test (GTT), and 13 of these patients were shown to be pyridoxine deficient (44). All were placed on a diet and given 100 mg of pyridoxine per day for 14 days, after which only two were diagnosed as having gestational diabetes mellitus. The effect of the diet on the GTT was said to be negligible, although a control group was not used. Other investigators duplicated these results in 13 women using the same dose of pyridoxine but without mentioning any dietary manipulation and without controls (45). However, a third study was unable to demonstrate a beneficial effect in four patients with an abnormal GTT using 100 mg of vitamin B_6 for 21 days (46). Moreover, all of the mothers had large-for-gestational-age infants, an expected complication of diabetic pregnancies. In 13 gestational diabetic women treated with the doses of pyridoxine described above, an improvement was observed in the GTT in 2 patients, a worsening was seen in 6, and no significant change occurred in the remaining 5 (47).

Infantile Convulsions

An association between pyridoxine and infantile convulsions was first described in the mid-1950s (48–52). Some infants fed a diet deficient in this vitamin developed intractable seizures that responded only to pyridoxine. A 1967 publication reviewed this complication in infants and differentiated between the states of pyridoxine deficiency and dependency (53). Whether or not these states can be induced in utero is open to question. As noted earlier, pyridoxine deficiency is common during pregnancy, even in well-nourished women, but the fetus accumulates the vitamin, although at lower levels, even in the face of maternal hypovitaminemia. Reports of seizures in newborn infants delivered from mothers with pyridoxine deficiency have not been located. On the other hand, high doses of pyridoxine early in gestation in one patient were suspected of altering the normal metabolism of pyridoxine, leading to intractable convulsions in the newborn (54). The woman, in whom two pregnancies were complicated by hyperemesis gravidarum, was treated with frequent injections of pyridoxine and thiamine, 50 mg each (54). The first newborn began convulsing 4 hours after birth and died within 30 hours. The second infant began mild twitching at 3 hours of age and progressed to severe generalized convulsions on the 5th day. Successful treatment was eventually accomplished with pyridoxine but not before marked mental retardation had occurred. The authors of this report postulated that the fetus, exposed to high doses of pyridoxine, developed an adaptive enzyme system that was capable of rapidly metabolizing the vitamin; following delivery, this adaptation was manifested by pyridoxine dependency and convulsions (54). Since this case, more than 50 additional cases of pyridoxine dependency have been reported, and the disease is now thought to be an inherited autosomal recessive disorder (55).

A 1967 report described in utero dependency-induced convulsions in three successive pregnancies in one woman (56). The first two newborns died—one during the 7th week and one on day 2—as a result of intractable convulsions. During the third pregnancy, in utero convulsions stopped after the mother was treated with 110 mg/day of pyridoxine 4 days before delivery. Following birth, the newborn was treated with pyridoxine. Convulsions occurred on three separate occasions when vitamin therapy was withheld and then abated when therapy was restarted. Late-onset seizures in a female infant were reported in 1999 (57). The mother had taken pyridoxine 80 mg/day throughout pregnancy and intermittently when the nursing infant was between 1 and 10 weeks of age. Four days after birth, the infant had two generalized colonic seizures. Then, at 3.5 months of age, the infant became irritable and fussy and had a cluster of 12 generalized seizures, each lasting 2–5 minutes, over 4 days. Laboratory tests and an electroencephalogram, taken when the infant was not seizing, were normal. A single dose of pyridoxine 100 mg IV was given and she was seizure-free for 3 weeks. Then three more seizures occurred over 4 days. She was given 100 mg oral pyridoxine and then 12.5 mg/day thereafter. At 7 months old, the infant was seizure free with normal temperament and development since starting oral pyridoxine (57).

Nausea and Vomiting of Pregnancy

The first use of pyridoxine for severe nausea and vomiting of pregnancy (hyperemesis gravidarum) was reported in 1942 (58). Individual injections ranged from 10 to 100 mg, with total doses up to 1500 mg being given. Satisfactory relief was obtained in most cases. In one study, patients were successfully treated with IM doses of 50–100 mg 3 times weekly (59). Another report described a single patient with hyperemesis who responded to an IV mixture of high-dose B-complex vitamins, including 50 mg of pyridoxine, each day for 3 days (60). Much smaller doses were used in a study of 17 patients (61). IM doses of 5 mg every 2–4 days were administered to these patients, with an immediate response observed in 12 women and all responding by the second dose. Oral doses of 60–80 mg/day up to a total dose of 2500 mg gave partial or complete relief from nausea and vomiting in 68 patients; an additional 10 patients required oral plus injectable pyridoxine (62). A success rate of 95% was claimed in a study of 62 women treated with a combination of pyridoxine and suprarenal cortex (adrenal cortex extract) (63). None of the preceding six studies was double-blind or controlled. The effect of pyridoxine on blood urea concentrations in hyperemesis has been investigated (64). Blood urea was decreased below normal adult levels in pregnant women and even lower in patients with hyperemesis. Pyridoxine, 40 mg/day orally for 3 days, significantly increased blood urea only in women with hyperemesis. In another measure of the effect of pyridoxine on hyperemesis, elevated serum glutamic acid levels observed with this condition were returned to normal pregnant values after pyridoxine therapy (65). However, another investigator could not demonstrate any value from pyridoxine therapy in 16 patients (66). Placebos were used but the study was not blinded. In addition, only 1 of 16 patients had hyperemesis gravidarum with the remaining 15 presenting with lesser degrees of nausea and vomiting. Based on the above studies, it is impossible to judge the effectiveness of the vitamin in allaying true hyperemesis gravidarum. More than likely, the effect of hydration, possibly improved prenatal care, the attention of health care personnel, the transitory nature of hyperemesis, the lack of strict diagnostic criteria in classifying patients with the disease, and other factors were involved in the reversal of the symptoms of the women involved in these studies. The vitamin, however, does appear to reduce nausea and vomiting of pregnancy as demonstrated in the two investigations described below.

Two studies have demonstrated that oral doses of pyridoxine are effective in alleviating nausea and vomiting of pregnancy (67–69). A randomized, double-blind, placebo-controlled study, found that pyridoxine, 25 mg orally every 8 hours for 72 hours, administered to 31 women at a mean gestational age of 9.3 weeks, significantly reduced severe nausea and vomiting of pregnancy (67,68). A second study, using pyridoxine 10 mg orally every 8 hours for 5 days in 167 women at a mean gestational age of 10.9 weeks, produced a significant reduction in nausea and nearly a significant decrease in the number of vomiting episodes (69).

Congenital Malformations

A case report suggested a link between high doses of pyridoxine and phocomelia (70). The mother, who weighed only 47 kg, took 50 mg of pyridoxine daily plus unknown doses of lecithin and vitamin B_{12} through the first 7 months of pregnancy. The full-term female infant was born with a near-total amelia of her left leg at the knee. A relationship between any of the drugs and the defect is doubtful.

The combination of doxylamine and pyridoxine (Bendectin, others) has been the focus of considerable debate in the past. The debate centered on whether the preparation was teratogenic. The combination had been used by millions of women for pregnancy-induced nausea and vomiting but was removed from the market by the manufacturer because of a number of large legal awards against the company. Jury decisions notwithstanding, the available scientific evidence indicates the combination is not teratogenic (see Doxylamine).

Pyridoxine has been shown to protect fetal rats from β-aminoproprionitrile-induced palatal clefting when given before and during administration of the chemical (71). The same protection may occur in humans. In a case–control study from two sites in the Philippines, women with offspring with an oral cleft (cleft lip, with or without cleft palate) had worst pyridoxine deficiency than controls (72). The association was strongest if the mother also had lower folate levels. However, folate–oral cleft associations were inconsistent and were thought to be due to differing pyridoxine status in the two populations studied. In contrast, poor maternal pyridoxine status was consistently associated with an increased risk of oral clefts (72).

Miscellaneous Effects

Among miscellaneous effects, two studies were unable to associate low maternal concentrations of pyridoxine with premature labor (29,43). Similarly, no correlation was found between low levels and stillbirths (10,40). However, 1-minute Apgar scores were significantly related to low maternal and newborn pyridoxine concentrations (14,73). The effects of pyridoxine supplementation in black pregnant women have been studied (74). Lower maternal serum lipid, fetal weight, and placental weight and the frequency of placental vascular sclerosis were observed. Others have not found a correlation between pyridoxine levels and birth weight (15,43,73). In an unusual report, pregnant women given daily 20-mg supplements of pyridoxine by either lozenges or capsules had less dental disease than untreated controls (75). The best cariostatic effect was seen in patients in the lozenge group.

BREASTFEEDING SUMMARY

Pyridoxine is excreted into breast milk (14,76–82). Concentrations in milk are directly proportional to intake (76–82). In well-nourished women, pyridoxine levels varied, depending on intake, from 123 to 314 ng/mL (76–78). Peak pyridoxine milk levels occurred 3–8 hours after ingestion of a vitamin supplement (76,78,79). A 1983 study measured pyridoxine levels in pooled human milk obtained from preterm (26 mothers: 29–34 weeks) and term (35 mothers: 39 weeks or longer) patients (80). Levels in milk obtained from preterm mothers rose from 11.1 ng/mL (colostrum) to 62.2 ng/mL (16–196 days), whereas levels in milk from term mothers increased during the same period from 17.0 to 107.1 ng/mL. In a 1985 study, daily supplements of 0–20 mg resulted in milk concentrations of 93–413 ng/mL, corresponding to an infant intake of 0.06–0.28 mg/day (79). A significant correlation was found between maternal intake and infant intake. Most infants, however, did not receive the RDA for infants (0.3 mg) even when the mother was consuming 8 times the RDA for lactating women (2.5 mg) (79). In lactating women with low nutritional status, supplementation with pyridoxine, 0.4–40 mg/day, resulted in mean milk concentrations of 80–158 ng/mL (81).

Convulsions have been reported in infants fed a pyridoxine-deficient diet (see discussion in the Fetal Risk Summary) (49–54). Seizures were described in two breastfed infants, one of whom was receiving only 67 mcg/day in the milk (83). Intake in the second infant was not determined. A similar report involved three infants whose mothers had levels <20 ng/mL (at 7 days postpartum) or <60 ng/mL (at 4 weeks) of pyridoxine in their milk (84). The convulsions responded promptly to pyridoxine therapy in all five of these infants.

Very large doses of pyridoxine have been reported to have a lactation-inhibiting effect (85). Using oral doses of 600 mg/day, lactation was successfully inhibited in 95% of patients within 1 week as compared with only 17% of placebo-treated controls. Very high IV doses of pyridoxine, 600 mg infused for 1 hour in healthy, nonlactating young adults, successfully suppressed the rise in prolactin induced by exercise (86). However, because use of this dose and method of administration in lactating women would be unusual, the relevance of these data to breastfeeding is limited. With dosage much closer to physiologic levels, such as 20 mg/day, no effect on lactation has been observed (79). In addition, two separate trials, using 450 mg and 600 mg/day in divided oral doses, failed to reproduce the lactation-inhibiting effect observed earlier or to show any suppression of serum prolactin levels (87,88). One writer, however, has suggested that pyridoxine be removed from multivitamin supplements intended for lactating women (89). This proposal has invoked sharp opposition from other correspondents who claimed the available evidence does not support a milk-inhibiting property for pyridoxine (90,91). Moreover, a study published in 1985 examined the effects of pyridoxine supplements, 0.5 or 4.0 mg/day started 24 hours after delivery, on lactation (92). Women receiving the higher dose of pyridoxine had significantly higher concentrations of plasma pyridoxal phosphate ($p < 0.01$) and milk total vitamin B_6 ($p < 0.05$) at 1, 3, 6, and 9 months. Plasma prolactin concentrations were similar between the two groups throughout the study.

The American Academy of Pediatrics classifies pyridoxine as compatible with breastfeeding (93). The National Academy of Sciences' RDA for pyridoxine during lactation is 2.1 mg (1). If the diet of the lactating woman adequately supplies this amount, maternal supplementation with pyridoxine is not required (82). Supplementation with the RDA for pyridoxine is recommended for those women with inadequate nutritional intake.

References

1. American Hospital Formulary Service. *Drug Information 1997*. Bethesda, MD: American Society of Health-System Pharmacists, 1997:2815–7.
2. Frank O, Walbroehl G, Thomson A, Kaminetzky H, Kubes Z, Baker H. Placental transfer: fetal retention of some vitamins. Am J Clin Nutr 1970;23:662–3.
3. Hill EP, Longo LD. Dynamics of maternal–fetal nutrient transfer. Fed Proc 1980;39:239–44.
4. Baker H, Frank O, Deangelis B, Feingold S, Kaminetzky HA. Role of placenta in maternal–fetal vitamin transfer in humans. Am J Obstet Gynecol 1981;141:792–6.
5. Wachstein M, Moore C, Graffeo LW. Pyridoxal phosphate (B_6-al-PO_4) levels of circulating leukocytes in maternal and cord blood. Proc Soc Exp Biol Med 1957;96:326–8.
6. Wachstein M, Kellner JD, Ortiz JM. Pyridoxal phosphate in plasma and leukocytes of normal and pregnant subjects following B_6 load tests. Proc Soc Exp Biol Med 1960;103:350–3.
7. Brin M. Thiamine and pyridoxine studies of mother and cord blood. Fed Proc 1966;25:245.
8. Contractor SF, Shane B. Blood and urine levels of vitamin B_6 in the mother and fetus before and after loading of the mother with vitamin B_6. Am J Obstet Gynecol 1970;107:635–40.
9. Brin M. Abnormal tryptophan metabolism in pregnancy and with the oral contraceptive pill. II. Relative levels of vitamin B_6-vitamers in cord and maternal blood. Am J Clin Nutr 1971;24:704–8.
10. Heller S, Salkeld RM, Korner WF. Vitamin B_6 status in pregnancy. Am J Clin Nutr 1973;26:1339–48.
11. Kaminetzky HA, Baker H, Frank O, Langer A. The effects of intravenously administered water-soluble vitamins during labor in normovitaminemic and hypovitaminemic gravidas on maternal and neonatal blood vitamin levels at delivery. Am J Obstet Gynecol 1974;120:697–703.
12. Brophy MH, Siiteri PK. Pyridoxal phosphate and hypertensive disorders of pregnancy. Am J Obstet Gynecol 1975;121:1075–9.
13. Bamji MS. Enzymic evaluation of thiamin, riboflavin and pyridoxine status of parturient women and their newborn infants. Br J Nutr 1976;35:259–65.
14. Roepke JLB, Kirksey A. Vitamin B_6 nutriture during pregnancy and lactation. I. Vitamin B_6 intake, levels of the vitamin in biological fluids, and condition of the infant at birth. Am J Clin Nutr 1979;32:2249–56.
15. Baker H, Thind IS, Frank O, DeAngelis B, Caterini H, Louria DB. Vitamin levels in low-birth-weight newborn infants and their mothers. Am J Obstet Gynecol 1977;129:521–4.
16. Baker H, Frank O, Thomason AD, Langer A, Munves ED, De Angelis B, Kaminetzky HA. Vitamin profile of 174 mothers and newborns at parturition. Am J Clin Nutr 1975;28:59–65.
17. Wachstein M, Gudaitis A. Disturbance of vitamin B_6 metabolism in pregnancy. J Lab Clin Med 1952;40:550–7.
18. Wachstein M, Gudaitis A. Disturbance of vitamin B_6 metabolism in pregnancy. II. The influence of various amounts of pyridoxine hydrochloride upon the abnormal tryptophane load test in pregnant women. J Lab Clin Med 1953;42:98–107.
19. Wachstein M, Gudaitis A. Disturbance of vitamin B_6 metabolism in pregnancy. III. Abnormal vitamin B_6 load test. Am J Obstet Gynecol 1953;66:1207–13.
20. Wachstein M, Lobel S. Abnormal tryptophan metabolites in human pregnancy and their relation to deranged vitamin B_6 metabolism. Proc Soc Exp Biol Med 1954;86:624–7.
21. Zartman ER, Barnes AC, Hicks DJ. Observations on pyridoxine metabolism in pregnancy. Am J Obstet Gynecol 1955;70:645–9.
22. Turner ER, Reynolds MS. Intake and elimination of vitamin B_6 and metabolites by women. J Am Diet Assoc 1955;31:1119–20.
23. Page EW. The vitamin B_6 requirement for normal pregnancy. West J Surg Obstet Gynecol 1956;64:96–103.
24. Coursin DB, Brown VC. Changes in vitamin B_6 during pregnancy. Am J Obstet Gynecol 1961;82:1307–11.
25. Brown RR, Thornton MJ, Price JM. The effect of vitamin supplementation on the urinary excretion of tryptophan metabolites by pregnant women. J Clin Invest 1961;40:617–23.
26. Hamfelt A, Hahn L. Pyridoxal phosphate concentration in plasma and tryptophan load test during pregnancy. Clin Chim Acta 1969;25:91–6.
27. Rose DP, Braidman IP. Excretion of tryptophan metabolites as affected by pregnancy, contraceptive steroids, and steroid hormones. Am J Clin Nutr 1971;24:673–83.
28. Kaminetzky HA, Langer A, Baker H, Frank O, Thomson AD, Munves ED, Opper A, Behrle FC, Glista B. The effect of nutrition in teen-age gravidas on pregnancy and the status of the neonate. I. A nutritional profile. Am J Obstet Gynecol 1973;115:639–46.
29. Shane B, Contractor SF. Assessment of vitamin B_6 status. Studies on pregnant women and oral contraceptive users. Am J Clin Nutr 1975;28:739–47.
30. Cleary RE, Lumeng L, Li TK. Maternal and fetal plasma levels of pyridoxal phosphate at term: adequacy of vitamin B_6 supplementation during pregnancy. Am J Obstet Gynecol 1975;121:25–8.
31. Lumeng L, Cleary RE, Wagner R, Yu PL, Li TK. Adequacy of vitamin B_6 supplementation during pregnancy: a prospective study. Am J Clin Nutr 1976;29:1376–83.
32. Anonymous. Requirement of vitamin B_6 during pregnancy. Nutr Rev 1976;34:15–6.
33. Dostalova L. Correlation of the vitamin status between mother and newborn during delivery. Dev Pharmacol Ther 1982;4(Suppl I):45–57.
34. Hunt IF, Murphy NJ, Martner-Hewes PM, Faraji B, Swendseid ME, Reynolds RD, Sanchez A, Mejia A. Zinc, vitamin B-6, and other nutrients in pregnant women attending prenatal clinics in Mexico. Am J Clin Nutr 1987;46:563–9.
35. Bapurao S, Raman L, Tulpule PG. Biochemical assessment of vitamin B_6 nutritional status in pregnant women with orolingual manifestations. Am J Clin Nutr 1982;36:581–6.
36. Davis SD. Immunodeficiency and runting syndrome in rats from congenital pyridoxine deficiency. Nature 1974;251:548–50. As cited in Shepard TH. *Catalog of Teratogenic Agents*. 6th ed. Baltimore, MD: The Johns Hopkins University Press, 1989:537–8.
37. Davis SD, Nelson T, Shepard TH. Teratogenicity of vitamin B_6 deficiency: omphalocele, skeletal and neural defects, and splenic hypoplasia. Science 1970;169:1329–30. As cited in Shepard TH. *Catalog of Teratogenic Agents*. 6th ed. Baltimore, MD: The Johns Hopkins University Press, 1989:537–8.
38. Averback P. Anencephaly associated with megavitamin therapy. Can Med Assoc J 1976;114:995.
39. Sprince H, Lowy RS, Folsome CE, Behrman J. Studies on the urinary excretion of "xanthurenic acid" during normal and abnormal pregnancy: a survey of the excretion of "xanthurenic acid" in normal nonpregnant, normal pregnant, pre-eclamptic, and eclamptic women. Am J Obstet Gynecol 1951;62:84–92.
40. Wachstein M, Graffeo LW. Influence of vitamin B_6 on the incidence of preeclampsia. Obstet Gynecol 1956;8:177–80.
41. Kaminetzky HA, Baker H. Micronutrients in pregnancy. Clin Obstet Gynecol 1977;20:363–80.
42. Diding NA, Melander SEJ. Serum vitamin B_6 level in normal and toxaemic pregnancy. Acta Obstet Gynecol Scand 1961;40:252–61.
43. Hillman RW, Cabaud PG, Nilsson DE, Arpin PD, Tufano RJ. Pyridoxine supplementation during pregnancy. Clinical and laboratory observations. Am J Clin Nutr 1963;12:427–30.

44. Coelingh Bennink HJT, Schreurs WHP. Improvement of oral glucose tolerance in gestational diabetes by pyridoxine. Br Med J 1975;3:13–5.
45. Spellacy WN, Buhi WC, Birk SA. Vitamin B_6 treatment of gestational diabetes mellitus. Studies of blood glucose and plasma insulin. Am J Obstet Gynecol 1977;127:599–602.
46. Perkins RP. Failure of pyridoxine to improve glucose tolerance in gestational diabetes mellitus. Obstet Gynecol 1977;50:370–2.
47. Gillmer MDG, Mazibuko D. Pyridoxine treatment of chemical diabetes in pregnancy. Am J Obstet Gynecol 1979;133:499–502.
48. Snyderman SE, Holt LE, Carretero R, Jacobs K. Pyridoxine deficiency in the human infant. J Clin Nutr 1953;1:200–7.
49. Molony CJ, Parmalee AH. Convulsions in young infants as a result of pyridoxine (vitamin B_6) deficiency. JAMA 1954;154:405–6.
50. Coursin DB. Vitamin B_6 deficiency in infants. Am J Dis Child 1955;90:344–8.
51. Coursin DB. Effects of vitamin B_6 on the central nervous activity in childhood. Am J Clin Nutr 1956;4:354–63.
52. Molony CJ, Parmelee AH. Convulsions in young infants as a result of pyridoxine (vitamin B_6) deficiency. JAMA 1954;154:405–6.
53. Scriver CR. Vitamin B_6 deficiency and dependency in man. Am J Dis Child 1967;113:109–14.
54. Hunt AD Jr, Stokes J Jr, McCrory WW, Stroud HH. Pyridoxine dependency: report of a case of intractable convulsions in an infant controlled by pyridoxine. Pediatrics 1954;13:140–5.
55. Bankier A, Turner M, Hopkins IJ. Pyridoxine dependent seizures—a wider clinical spectrum. Arch Dis Child 1983;58:415–8.
56. Bejsovec MIR, Kulenda Z, Ponca E. Familial intrauterine convulsions in pyridoxine dependency. Arch Dis Child 1967;42:201–7.
57. South M. Neonatal seizures after use of pyridoxine in pregnancy. Lancet 1999;353:1940.
58. Willis RS, Winn WW, Morris AT, Newsom AA, Massey WE. Clinical observations in treatment of nausea and vomiting in pregnancy with vitamins B_1 and B_6. A preliminary report. Am J Obstet Gynecol 1942;44:265–71.
59. Weinstein BB, Mitchell GJ, Sustendal GF. Clinical experiences with pyridoxine hydrochloride in treatment of nausea and vomiting of pregnancy. Am J Obstet Gynecol 1943;46:283–5.
60. Hart BF, McConnell WT. Vitamin B factors in toxic psychosis of pregnancy and the puerperium. Am J Obstet Gynecol 1943;46:283.
61. Varas O. Treatment of nausea and vomiting of pregnancy with vitamin B_6. Bol Soc Chilena Obstet Ginecol 1943;8:404. As abstracted in Am J Obstet Gynecol 1945;50:347–8.
62. Weinstein BB, Wohl Z, Mitchell GJ, Sustendal GF. Oral administration of pyridoxine hydrochloride in the treatment of nausea and vomiting of pregnancy. Am J Obstet Gynecol 1944;47:389–94.
63. Dorsey CW. The use of pyridoxine and suprarenal cortex combined in the treatment of the nausea and vomiting of pregnancy. Am J Obstet Gynecol 1949;58:1073–8.
64. McGanity WJ, McHenry EW, Van Wyck HB, Watt GL. An effect of pyridoxine on blood urea in human subjects. J Biol Chem 1949;178:511–6.
65. Beaton JR, McHenry EW. Observations on plasma glutamic acid. Fed Proc 1951;10:161.
66. Hesseltine HC. Pyridoxine failure in nausea and vomiting of pregnancy. Am J Obstet Gynecol 1946;51:82–6.
67. Sahakian V, Rouse DJ, Rose NB, Niebyl JR. Vitamin B6 for nausea and vomiting of pregnancy (abstract). Am J Obstet Gynecol 1991;164:322.
68. Sahakian V, Rouse D, Sipes S, Rose NB, Niebyl J. Vitamin B6 is effective therapy for nausea and vomiting of pregnancy: a randomized double-blind placebo-controlled study. Obstet Gynecol 1991;78:33–6.
69. Vutyavanich T, Wongtra-ngan S, Ruangsri R-a. Pyridoxine for nausea and vomiting of pregnancy: a randomized, double-blind, placebo-controlled trial. Am J Obstet Gynecol 1995;173:881–4.
70. Gardner LI, Welsh-Sloan J, Cady RB. Phocomelia in infant whose mother took large doses of pyridoxine during pregnancy. Lancet 1985;1:636.
71. Jacobsson C, Granstrom G. Effects of vitamin B_6 on beta-aminoproprionitrile-induced palatal cleft formation in the rat. Cleft Palate-Craniofacial J 1997;34:95–100.
72. Munger RG, Sauberlich HE, Corcoran C, Nepomuceno B, Daack-Hirsch S, Solon FS. Maternal vitamin B-6 and folate status and risk of oral cleft birth defects in the Philippines. Birth Defects Res A Clin Mol Teratol 2004;70:464–71.
73. Schuster K, Bailey LB, Mahan CS. Vitamin B_6 status of low-income adolescent and adult pregnant women and the condition of their infants at birth. Am J Clin Nutr 1981;34:1731–5.
74. Swartwout JR, Unglaub WG, Smith RC. Vitamin B_6, serum lipids and placental arteriolar lesions in human pregnancy. A preliminary report. Am J Clin Nutr 1960;8:434–44.
75. Hillman RW, Cabaud PG, Schenone RA. The effects of pyridoxine supplements on the dental caries experience of pregnant women. Am J Clin Nutr 1962;10:512–5.
76. West KD, Kirksey A. Influence of vitamin B_6 intake on the content of the vitamin in human milk. Am J Clin Nutr 1976;29:961–9.
77. Thomas MR, Kawamoto J, Sneed SM, Eakin R. The effects of vitamin C, vitamin B_6, and vitamin B_{12} supplementation on the breast milk and maternal status of well-nourished women. Am J Clin Nutr 1979;32: 1679–85.
78. Sneed SM, Zane C, Thomas MR. The effects of ascorbic acid, vitamin B_6, vitamin B_{12}, and folic acid supplementation on the breast milk and maternal nutritional status of low socioeconomic lactating women. Am J Clin Nutr 1981;34:1338–46.
79. Styslinger L, Kirksey A. Effects of different levels of vitamin B-6 supplementation on vitamin B-6 concentrations in human milk and vitamin B-6 intakes of breastfed infants. Am J Clin Nutr 1985;41:21–31.
80. Ford JE, Zechalko A, Murphy J, Brooke OG. Comparison of the B vitamin composition of milk from mothers of preterm and term babies. Arch Dis Child 1983;58:367–72.
81. Deodhar AD, Rajalakshmi R, Ramakrishnan CV. Studies on human lactation. Part III. Effect of dietary vitamin supplementation vitamin contents of breast milk. Acta Pediatr 1964;53:42–8.
82. Thomas MR, Sneed SM, Wei C, Nail PA, Wilson M, Sprinkle EE III. The effects of vitamin C, vitamin B_6, vitamin B_{12}, folic acid, riboflavin, and thiamine on the breast milk and maternal status of well-nourished women at 6 months postpartum. Am J Clin Nutr 1980;33:2151–6.
83. Bessey OA, Adam DJD, Hansen AE. Intake of vitamin B_6 and infantile convulsions: a first approximation of requirements of pyridoxine in infants. Pediatrics 1957;20:33–44.
84. Kirksey A, Roepke JLB. Vitamin B-6 nutriture of mothers of three breast-fed neonates with central nervous system disorders. Fed Proc 1981; 40:864.
85. Foukas MD. An antilactogenic effect of pyridoxine. J Obstet Gynaecol Br Commonw 1973;80:718–20.
86. Moretti C, Fabbri A, Gnessi L, Bonifacio V, Fraioli F, Isidori A. Pyridoxine (B6) suppresses the rise in prolactin and increases the rise in growth hormone induced by exercise. N Engl J Med 1982;307:444–5.
87. MacDonald HN, Collins YD, Tobin MJW, Wijayaratne, DN. The failure of pyridoxine in suppression of puerperal lactation. Br J Obstet Gynaecol 1976;83:54–5.
88. Canales ES, Soria J, Zarate A, Mason M, Molina M. The influence of pyridoxine on prolactin secretion and milk production in women. Br J Obstet Gynaecol 1976;83:387–8.
89. Greentree LB. Dangers of vitamin B_6 in nursing mothers. N Engl J Med 1979;300:141–2.
90. Lande NI. More on dangers of vitamin B_6 in nursing mothers. N Engl J Med 1979;300:926–7.
91. Rivlin RS. More on dangers of vitamin B_6 in nursing mothers. N Engl J Med 1979;300:927.
92. Andon MB, Howard MP, Moser PB, Reynolds RD. Nutritionally relevant supplementation of vitamin B6 in lactating women: effect on plasma prolactin. Pediatrics 1985;76:769–73.
93. Committee on Drugs, American Academy of Pediatrics. The transfer of drugs and other chemicals into human milk. Pediatrics 2001;108: 776–89.

P

PYRILAMINE

Antihistamine

PREGNANCY RECOMMENDATION: Limited Human Data—Probably Compatible
BREASTFEEDING RECOMMENDATION: No Human Data—Probably Compatible

PREGNANCY SUMMARY

Pyrilamine is used infrequently during pregnancy. One source found an increased risk of structural anomalies, but confirmation has not been reported. In general, antihistamines are considered low risk in pregnancy. However, exposure near birth of premature infants has been associated with an increased risk of retrolental fibroplasia.

FETAL RISK SUMMARY

The Collaborative Perinatal Project monitored 50,282 mother–child pairs, 121 of whom had pyrilamine exposure in the 1st trimester (1, pp. 323–324). No evidence was found to suggest a relationship to large categories of major or minor malformations. For use anytime during pregnancy, 392 exposures were recorded (1, pp. 436–437). A possible association with malformations was found on the basis of 12 defects, 6 of which involved benign tumors (1, p. 489).

It is not known if pyrilamine crosses the human placenta. The molecular weight (about 402) is low enough that exposure of the embryo–fetus should be expected.

An association between exposure during the last 2 weeks of pregnancy to antihistamines in general and retrolental fibroplasia in premature infants has been reported. See Brompheniramine for details.

BREASTFEEDING SUMMARY

No reports describing the use of pyrilamine during human lactation have been reported. The molecular weight (about 402) is low enough for excretion into breast milk. The effect of this exposure on a nursing infant is unknown.

Reference

1. Heinonen OP, Slone D, Shapiro S. *Birth Defects and Drugs in Pregnancy*. Littleton, MA: Publishing Sciences Group, 1977.

PYRIMETHAMINE

Antimalarial

PREGNANCY RECOMMENDATION: Compatible—Maternal Benefit >> Embryo–Fetal Risk
BREASTFEEDING RECOMMENDATION: Limited Human Data—Probably Compatible

PREGNANCY SUMMARY

Two reviews of toxoplasmosis (*Toxoplasma gondii*) in pregnancy were published in 1994 (1,2). Pyrimethamine, in combination with sulfadiazine, was recommended in both as the most effective treatment after the infection had reached the fetus. No fetal adverse effects of this therapy have been observed. Despite one animal study that described increased embryotoxicity after oral folic acid, if pyrimethamine is used during pregnancy, folic acid (5 mg/day) or folinic acid (leucovorin; 5 mg/day) supplementation is recommended, especially during the 1st trimester, to prevent folate deficiency (1,3–9).

FETAL RISK SUMMARY

Pyrimethamine is a folic acid antagonist (inhibitor of dihydrofolate reductase) used in combination with other agents primarily for the treatment and prophylaxis of malaria, but also for toxoplasmosis. Shepard (10) reviewed 15 studies that evaluated the reproductive effects of pyrimethamine in rats, mice, and hamsters. Malformations in fetal rats included cleft palate, mandibular hypoplasia, limb defects, and neural tube defects. In some cases, the teratogenic dose was similar to the human dose. At slightly higher doses in rats, pyrimethamine caused chromosomal aberrations such as trisomy or chromosomal mosaicism (10).

A 1993 study found in pregnant rats and mice that oral folic acid potentiated the embryotoxicity of pyrimethamine but that decreased embryotoxicity was observed when folic acid was given intraperitoneally (11). The mechanism of the increased toxicity appeared to be reduced plasma levels of 5-methyltetrahydrofolic acid in the dams. 5-Methyltetrahydrofolic acid is the principal active folate in plasma and it undergoes a large amount of enterohepatic circulating (11). Folic acid inhibited the absorption of the active folate from the intestine.

Reproduction studies, reported by the manufacturer, revealed teratogenicity in rats, hamsters, and miniature pigs (12). In rats, oral doses 7 times the human dose for chemoprophylaxis of malaria (HDCM) or 2.5 times the human dose for toxoplasmosis (HDT), caused cleft palate, brachygnathia, oligodactyly, and microphthalmia. Meningocele was seen in hamsters, given doses 170 times the HDCM or HDT, and cleft palate occurred in miniature pigs at 5 times the HDCM or HDT (12).

In an in vitro study using human perfused placentas, the transfer rate of pyrimethamine was about 30% (13). The results suggested that the placental transfer was independent of maternal concentration and the transfer occurred by passive diffusion.

Antimalarial agents, including pyrimethamine, are used routinely during pregnancy because the risks from the disease far outweigh the risks to the fetus from drug therapy (see Proguanil for a discussion on the maternal and fetal risks of malaria during pregnancy).

Although some folic acid antagonists are human teratogens (e.g., see Methotrexate), this does not seem to occur with pyrimethamine (3–7,14,15). One case report, however, did describe a severe defect of the abdominal and thoracic wall (exteriorization of the heart, lungs, and most of the abdominal viscera; possible variant of ectopia cordis) and a missing left arm in an infant exposed to the drug (16). The woman had been treated with chloroquine, 100 mg/day, plus a combination of dapsone (100 mg) and pyrimethamine (12.5 mg) (Maloprim) on postconception days 10, 20, and 30. However, an association between the drug and the defect has been questioned (8,17). Moreover, most studies describing the use of pyrimethamine in pregnant women for the treatment or prophylaxis of malaria have found the drug to be relatively safe and effective (8,9,18–31), although some recommend avoiding the drug during the 1st trimester (9).

BREASTFEEDING SUMMARY

Pyrimethamine is excreted into breast milk (32,33). Mothers treated with 25–75 mg orally produced peak concentrations of 3.1–3.3 mcg/mL at 6 hours (32). The drug was detectable up to 48 hours after a dose. Malaria parasites were completely eliminated in infants up to 6 months of age who were entirely breastfed. In a 1986 study, three women were treated with a combination tablet containing 100 mg of dapsone and 12.5 mg of pyrimethamine at 2–5 days postpartum (33). Blood and milk samples were collected up to 227 hours after the dose. The milk:plasma AUC ratios ranged from 0.46 to 0.66. Based on an estimated ingestion of 1000 mL of milk per day, the infants would have consumed between 16.8% and 45.6% of the maternal doses during a 9-day period.

The American Academy of Pediatrics classifies pyrimethamine as compatible with breastfeeding (34).

References

1. Wong S-Y, Remington JS. Toxoplasmosis in pregnancy. Clin Infect Dis 1994;18:853–62.
2. Matsui D. Prevention, diagnosis, and treatment of fetal toxoplasmosis. Clin Perinatol 1994;21:675–88.
3. Anonymous. Prevention of malaria in pregnancy and early childhood. Br Med J 1984;1296–7.
4. Spracklen FHN. Malaria 1984. Part I. Malaria prophylaxis. S Afr Med J 1984;65:1037–41.
5. Spracklen FHN, Monteagudo FSE. Therapeutic protocol no. 3. Malaria prophylaxis. S Afr Med J 1986;70:316.
6. Brown GV. Chemoprophylaxis of malaria. Med J Aust 1986;144:696–702.
7. Cook GC. Prevention and treatment of malaria. Lancet 1988;1:32–7.
8. Main EK, Main DM, Krogstad DJ. Treatment of chloroquine-resistant malaria during pregnancy. JAMA 1983;249:3207–9.
9. Luzzi GA, Peto TEA. Adverse effects of antimalarials. An update. Drug Saf 1993;8:295–311.
10. Shepard TH. *Catalog of Teratogenic Agents*. 8th ed. Baltimore, MD: The Johns Hopkins University Press, 1995:362–3.
11. Kudo G, Tsunematsu K, Shimoda M, Kokue E. Effects of folic acid on pyrimethamine teratogenesis in rats. Adv Exp Med Biol 1993;338:469–72.
12. Product information. Daraprim. Glaxo Wellcome, 2000.
13. Peytavin G, Leng JJ, Forestier F, Saux MC, Hohlfeld P, Farinotti R. Placental transfer of pyrimethamine studied in an ex vivo placental perfusion model. Biol Neonate 2000;78:83–5.
14. Barry M, Bia F. Pregnancy and travel. JAMA 1989;261:728–31.
15. Stekette RW, Wirima JJ, Slutsker L, Heymann DL, Breman JG. The problem of malaria and malaria control in pregnancy in sub-Saharan Africa. Am J Trop Med Hyg 1996;55:2–7.
16. Harpey J-P, Darbois Y, Lefebvre G. Teratogenicity of pyrimethamine. Lancet 1983;2:399.
17. Smithells RW, Sheppard S. Teratogenicity of Debendox and pyrimethamine. Lancet 1983;2:623–4.
18. Anonymous. Pyrimethamine combinations in pregnancy. Lancet 1983;2:1005–7.
19. Morley D, Woodland M, Cuthbertson WFJ. Controlled trial of pyrimethamine in pregnant women in an African village. Br Med J 1964;1:667–8.
20. Gilles HM, Lawson JB, Sibelas M, Voller A, Allan N. Malaria, anaemia and pregnancy. Ann Trop Med Parasitol 1969;63:245–63.
21. Heinonen OP, Slone D, Shapiro. *Birth Defects and Drugs in Pregnancy*. Littleton, MA: Publishing Sciences Group, 1977;299, 302.
22. Bruce-Chwatt LJ. Malaria and pregnancy. Br Med J 1983;286:1457–8.
23. Anonymous. Malaria in pregnancy. Lancet 1983;2:84–5.
24. Strang A, Lachman E, Pitsoe SB, Marszalek A, Philpott RH. Malaria in pregnancy with fatal complications. Case report. Br J Obstet Gynaecol 1984;91:399–403.
25. Nahlen BL, Akintunde A, Alakija T, Nguyen-Dinh P, Ogunbode O, Edungbola LD, Adetoro O, Breman JG. Lack of efficacy of pyrimethamine prophylaxis in pregnant Nigerian women. Lancet 1989;2:830–4.
26. Keuter M, van Eijk A, Hoogstrate M, Raasveld M, van de Ree M, Ngwawe WA, Watkins WM, Were JBO, Brandling-Bennett AD. Comparison of chloroquine, pyrimethamine and sulfadoxine, and chlorproguanil and dapsone as treatment for falciparum malaria in pregnant and non-pregnant women, Kakamega district, Kenya. Br Med J 1990;301:466–70.
27. Greenwood AM, Armstrong JRM, Byass P, Snow RW, Greenwood BM. Malaria chemoprophylaxis, birth weight and child survival. Trans Roy Soc Trop Med Hyg 1992;86:483–5.
28. Greenwood AM, Menendez C, Todd J, Greenwood BM. The distribution of birth weights in Gambian women who received malaria chemoprophylaxis during their first pregnancy and in control women. Trans Roy Soc Trop Med Hyg 1994;88:311–2.
29. Schultz LJ, Steketee RW, Macheso A, Kazembe P, Chitsulo L, Wirima JJ. The efficacy of antimalarial regimens containing sulfadoxine-pyrimethamine and/or chloroquine in preventing peripheral and placental *Plasmodium falciparum* infection among pregnant women in Malawi. Am J Trop Med Hyg 1994;51:515–22.
30. Menendez C, Todd J, Alonso PL, Lulat S, Francis N, Greenwood BM. Malaria chemoprophylaxis, infection of the placenta and birth weight in Gambian primigravidae. J Trop Med Hyg 1994;97:244–8.
31. Sowunmi A, Akindele JA, Omitowoju GO, Omigbodun AO, Oduola AMJ, Salako LA. Intramuscular sulfadoxine-pyrimethamine in uncomplicated chloroquine-resistant falciparum malaria during pregnancy. Trans Roy Soc Trop Med Hyg 1993;87:472.
32. Clyde DF, Shute GT, Press J. Transfer of pyrimethamine in human milk. J Trop Med Hyg 1956;59:277–84.
33. Edstein MD. Veerendaal JR, Newman K, Hyslop R. Excretion of chloroquine, dapsone and pyrimethamine in human milk. Br J Clin Pharmacol 1986;22:733–5.
34. Committee on Drugs, American Academy of Pediatrics. The transfer of drugs and other chemicals into human milk. Pediatrics 2001;108:776–89.

PYRVINIUM PAMOATE

[Withdrawn from the market. See 9th edition.]

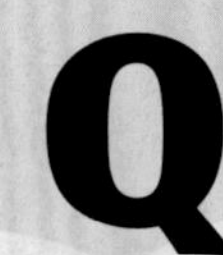

QUAZEPAM

Hypnotic

PREGNANCY RECOMMENDATION: Human Data Suggest Risk in 1st and 3rd Trimesters
BREASTFEEDING RECOMMENDATION: Limited Human Data—Potential Toxicity

PREGNANCY SUMMARY

No reports of human use of quazepam during human pregnancy have been located, but the effects of this agent on the fetus following prolonged use should be similar to those observed with other benzodiazepines (see also Diazepam). Maternal use near delivery may potentially cause neonatal motor depression and withdrawal.

FETAL RISK SUMMARY

Quazepam is a benzodiazepine that is used as a hypnotic for the short-term management of insomnia. No major abnormalities were observed in mice and rabbits at doses up to 400 and 134 times the human dose, respectively. Minor defects observed in mice were delayed ossification of the sternum, vertebrae, distal phalanges, and supraoccipital bones. The manufacturer considers the drug to be contraindicated during pregnancy (1).

BREASTFEEDING SUMMARY

Quazepam is excreted into breast milk (2). Four healthy, lactating volunteers, who agreed not to breastfeed their infants, were given a single 15-mg dose of the hypnotic. After the dose, blood and milk samples were collected at scheduled times during a 48-hour interval. Mean cumulative amounts of quazepam and its two major active metabolites excreted into milk during the 48-hour period were 11.6 mcg (range 2.4–32.8 mcg) quazepam, 4.0 mcg (range 1.3–10.0 mcg) 2-oxoquazepam, and 1.0 mcg (range 0.4–1.6 mcg) *N*-desalky-2-oxoquazepam. These amounts represented 0.08%, 0.02%, and 0.09% of the dose, respectively. Milk concentrations of quazepam and 2-oxoquazepam were always higher than those in the plasma, with milk:plasma ratios of 4.18 and 2.02, respectively. Because of the lipophilic properties of quazepam, these ratios are much higher than those observed with diazepam (see Diazepam). The investigators estimated that following a multiple-dose regimen, only 28.7 mcg/day of the three compounds combined would be excreted into milk, representing 0.19% of the daily dose. Moreover, they concluded that the pharmacokinetics of quazepam indicated that accumulation would not occur except for *N*-desalky-2-oxoquazepam, the metabolite excreted in milk in the smallest amounts (2).

Although the amounts measured in the above study are small, the effects, if any, on a nursing infant's central nervous system function are unknown. The American Academy of Pediatrics classifies quazepam, especially when taken by nursing mothers for long periods, as a drug for which the effect on nursing infants is unknown but may be of concern (3).

References

1. Product information. Doral. Wallace Laboratories, 1994.
2. Hilbert JM, Gural RP, Symchowicz S, Zampaglione N. Excretion of quazepam into human breast milk. J Clin Pharmacol 1984;24:457–62.
3. Committee on Drugs, American Academy of Pediatrics. The transfer of drugs and other chemicals into human milk. Pediatrics 2001;108: 776–89.

QUETIAPINE

Antipsychotic

PREGNANCY RECOMMENDATION: Compatible—Maternal Benefit >> Embryo–Fetal Risk
BREASTFEEDING RECOMMENDATION: Limited Human Data—Potential Toxicity

PREGNANCY SUMMARY

Although no structural malformations attributable to quetiapine or other agents in this subclass have been reported, the number of exposures is too low to fully assess the embryo–fetal risk. In addition, there is a risk of extrapyramidal and/or withdrawal symptoms in the newborn if the drug is used in the 3rd trimester. Nevertheless, quetiapine is indicated for severe debilitating mental disease and the benefits to the mother appear to outweigh the potential embryo–fetal risks. Because of the limited human pregnancy experience with atypical antipsychotics, the American College of Obstetricians and Gynecologists does not recommend the routine use of these agents in pregnancy, but a risk–benefit assessment may indicate that such use is appropriate (1). However, the benefits to the mother appear to outweigh the unknown risk to the embryo-fetus (2). A 1996 review on the management of psychiatric illness concluded that patients with histories of chronic psychosis or severe bipolar illness represent a high-risk group (for both the mother and the fetus) and should be maintained on pharmacologic therapy before and during pregnancy (3). Folic acid 4 mg/day has been recommended for women taking atypical antipsychotics because they may have a higher risk of neural tube defects due to inadequate folate intake and obesity (4). A 2010 review of antipsychotic use in pregnancy concluded that most studies reported no adverse effects, including congenital anomalies in the offspring of mothers who had taken quetiapine during pregnancy (5).

FETAL RISK SUMMARY

Quetiapine is an atypical antipsychotic agent that is indicated for the treatment of schizophrenia. The drug is an antagonist of histamine H_1 and adrenergic α_1-receptors and may cause somnolence and orthostatic hypotension, respectively. Other antipsychotic agents in the same subclass of dibenzapine derivatives are asenapine, clozapine, loxapine, and olanzapine. The drug is extensively metabolized to primarily inactive metabolites and one active metabolite. Plasma protein binding to albumin is 83% and the mean terminal half-life is about 6 hours (6).

Reproduction studies have been conducted in rats and rabbits. No evidence of teratogenicity was observed in pregnant rats or rabbits at oral doses up to 2.4 times the maximum human dose based on BSA (MHD) during organogenesis. However, minor soft-tissue malformations (carpal/tarsal flexure) were noted in rabbit fetuses at 2.4 times the MHD. Embryo–fetal toxicity was observed in both species but the doses used (in rats only with the highest dose and in rabbits with all doses) also caused maternal toxicity (decreased weight gain and/or death). Delays in skeletal ossification were observed in rats at doses equivalent to 0.6 and 2.4 times the MHD. Similar fetal effects were observed in rabbits at doses 1.2 and 2.4 times the MHD. Reduced fetal body weights were noted at the highest doses in both species. No drug-related effects were noted in rat offspring in a perinatal/postnatal study using oral doses that were 0.1–0.24 times the MHD (6).

Quetiapine decreased mating and fertility in male rats given oral doses up to 1.8 times the MHD. Adverse effects (increased interval to mate and number of matings required for successful impregnation) continued to be observed in the high-dose group 2 weeks after treatment had been stopped. In male rats, the no-effect dose for impaired mating and fertility was 0.3 times the MHD. Quetiapine also adversely effected mating and fertility in female rats. At an oral dose 0.6 times the MHD, drug effects included decreases in mating and in matings resulting in pregnancy, and increases in the interval to mate and in irregular estrus cycles (also noted at 0.1 times the MHD). The no-effect dose in female rats was 0.01 times the MHD (6).

In an in vitro study using dually perfused human placentas, small amounts (about 4%) of quetiapine crossed from the maternal side to the fetal venous outflow (7). This is consistent with the molecular weight (about 767 for the free base), moderate protein binding, and the moderately long elimination half-life. In another study, 21 women taking a staple dose (mean 336.9 mg/day) of quetiapine for a mean 28.9 weeks before delivery had maternal and cord concentrations of the drug determined at birth (8). The cord blood concentration was 24.1% of the maternal concentration. The pregnancy outcomes include one premature infant (<37 weeks) and one growth-restricted infant (<2500 g). The mean Apgar scores were 7.6 and 8.9 at 1 and 5 minutes, respectively. There were nine neonatal complications, two cardiovascular and 7 respiratory (complications were not further described), and two infants were admitted to the neonatal intensive care unit (reasons not provided) (8).

A 38-year-old woman with paranoid-type schizophrenia was started on quetiapine (300 mg/day) after an unsuccessful trial with zuclopenthixol (9). After a marked improvement in her symptoms, she conceived with her pregnancy being diagnosed at 17 weeks' gestation when she reported amenorrhea. At 20 weeks' her dose was lowered to 200 mg/day, and then 2 weeks later to 150 mg/day. She eventually gave birth to a healthy 3120-g male infant with Apgar scores of 9 and 10 at 1 and 5 minutes, respectively. Birth length was 48 cm. The infant was developing normally at 6 months of age (9).

A 33-year-old woman with psychosis was treated with quetiapine (300 mg/day) beginning 2 weeks before conception and continuing during gestation (10). The dose was decreased to 200 mg/day at week 21. The dose was further reduced by 50 mg/day each week starting 4 weeks before her estimated due date to enable breastfeeding. At 39 weeks' gestation, she gave birth to a healthy, 3.61-kg female infant with Apgar scores of 8 and 9 at 1 and 5 minutes, respectively. The infant was doing well in the first month after birth (10).

A woman took quetiapine (200 mg/day) throughout pregnancy and gave birth to a term, male infant (11). No information was provided on the pregnancy outcome, but the mother planned to continue the drug while breastfeeding her infant (see below).

A 2005 study, involving women from Canada, Israeli, and England, described 151 pregnancy outcomes in women using atypical antipsychotic drugs (12). The exposed group was matched with a comparison group (N = 151) who had not been exposed to these agents. The drugs and number of pregnancies were olanzapine ($N = 60$), risperidone ($N = 49$), quetiapine ($N = 36$), and clozapine ($N = 6$). In those exposed, there were 110 live births (72.8%), 22 spontaneous abortions (14.6%), 15 elective abortions (9.9%), and 4 stillbirths (2.6%). Among the live births, one infant exposed in utero to olanzapine had multiple anomalies including midline defects (cleft lip, encephalocele, and aqueductal stenosis). The mean birth weight was 3341 g. There were no statistically significant differences, including rates of neonatal complications, between the cases and controls, with the exceptions of low birth weight (10% vs. 2%, $p = 0.05$) and elective abortions (9.9% vs. 1.3%, $p = 0.003$). The low birth weight may have been caused by the increased rate of cigarette smoking (38% vs. 13%, $p \leq 0.001$) and heavy/binge alcohol use (5 vs. 1) in the exposed group (12).

A 2006 report mentioned three women treated with quetiapine and other agents during gestation (13). The drug therapy was continued during breastfeeding (see below).

In a second 2006 report, a 33-year-old woman with severe psychotic depression was treated with quetiapine (400 mg/day) and fluvoxamine (200 mg/day) (14). After appropriate counseling, she continued this therapy and conceived; after a normal pregnancy, she delivered a healthy, 2600-g, length 49 cm, female infant with Apgar scores of 9 and 10 at 1 and 5 minutes, respectively. The infant was developing normally a 3 months (14).

A 26-year-old woman was treated with quetiapine for resistant depression with comorbid chronic pain (15). She took 300 mg/day during the 1st trimester. The dose was increased to 400 mg/day in the 4th month and continued for the remainder of her pregnancy. Other drugs taken throughout pregnancy included oxycodone (20 mg 3 times daily) and fluoxetine (40 mg daily). She delivered a 3.4-kg (50th percentile) male infant at 37 weeks' gestation, but other details were not provided. She continued the three drugs during breastfeeding (see below) (15).

A 2006 review of prophylactic therapy of bipolar disorder briefly described the effects in pregnancy and breastfeeding of a number of drugs, including (16). Untreated pregnant and nursing women with the disorder are at an increased risk of poor obstetrical outcomes and relapse of affective symptoms. Although the limited data prevented conclusions on the relative safety of the drugs, the author did state that each case needed to be considered separately (16).

A 17-year-old pregnant adolescent with bipolar disorder was treated throughout gestation with quetiapine 300 mg/day, venlafaxine 75 mg/day, and trazodone 150 mg/day (17). In the 1st, 2nd, and 3rd trimesters, plasma concentrations of quetiapine were –27%, –42%, and –18%, respectively, of the concentrations at 6 months postpartum. She gave birth to a healthy 3-kg male infant with Apgar scores of 9, 10, and 10. The infant had jitteriness during the first 4 days of life that did not require intervention. He was seen monthly and met developmental milestones during the first year (17).

A woman with schizophrenia was treated with quetiapine 250 mg/day throughout two consecutive pregnancies (18). In the first pregnancy, she gave birth at term to a healthy 2.5-kg female infant. She conceived again about 1 year later and again delivered a healthy 2.4-kg female infant. Both infants were breastfed while the mother continued quetiapine. Both girls were healthy, the first one at about 2 years of age and the other at about 9 months (18).

A 2014 case study described the use of phenelzine (105 mg/day), lithium (900 mg/day), and quetiapine (600 mg/day) in a 31-year-old woman with bipolar affective disorder (19). She was also taking metformin (1 g/day) for polycystic ovarian syndrome with oligomenorrhea. Despite her oligomenorrhea, a pregnancy was confirmed at 17 weeks' gestation. A glucose tolerance test was negative at 26 weeks'. Lithium was suspended 24–48 hours before induction of labor at 39 weeks'. Because of obstructed labor, a cesarean section was performed to give birth to a 4.2-kg male infant with Apgar scores of 5 and 9 at 1 and 5 minutes, respectively. The baby required initial resuscitation during the first 10 minutes. The baby was discharged home with the mother at 5 days. At 10 weeks of age, the baby's growth and development were normal (19).

BREASTFEEDING SUMMARY

Consistent with its molecular weight (about 767 for the free base), protein binding (83%), and mean terminal half-life (about 6 hours), quetiapine is excreted into breast milk. A 36-year-old woman took quetiapine (200 mg/day) throughout gestation and planned to continue the drug while breastfeeding her term, male infant (11). However, the infant was initially given formula because it was not known how much of the drug was excreted in milk. At 3 weeks postpartum, manually expressed milk samples were obtained before a dose and again at 1, 2, 4, and 6 hours after a dose. The average milk AUC over 6 hours was 13 mcg/L, with a maximum concentration of 62 mcg/L measured at 1 hour. At 2 hours, the milk concentrations were almost predose levels. Based on a milk intake of 150 mL/kg/day, it was estimated that an exclusively breastfed infant would ingest 0.09% of the weight-adjusted maternal dose. Even at the maximum concentration, the estimated infant dose was only 0.43% of the maternal dose. When the mother was told of these findings, she began exclusive breastfeeding at 8 weeks. No adverse effects of quetiapine were reported and the infant was developing normally at 4.5 months (11).

A 2006 report described six women treated with quetiapine and other agents during lactation (13). In three cases, therapy was started before or during pregnancy (gestational age shown in parentheses): quetiapine (50 mg) and paroxetine (40 mg) (18 weeks); quetiapine (75 mg), trazodone (75 mg), and venlafaxine (75 mg) (before conception); and quetiapine (100 mg) and venlafaxine (225 mg) (35.5 weeks). In the other three cases, quetiapine was added after delivery (postpartum weeks shown in parentheses): quetiapine (25 mg), paroxetine (60 mg), and clonazepam (0.5 mg) (16.5 weeks); quetiapine (25 mg) and paroxetine (12.5 mg) (3 weeks); and quetiapine (400 mg) and paroxetine (50 mg) (10.5 weeks). Breast milk samples, drawn at variable times after the dose, were obtained between 6.5 and 18.5 weeks postpartum. Quetiapine was not detected (<30 nmol/L) in the breast milk of four women (doses 25–75 mg). The estimated infant exposures in these four cases were <0.01 mg/kg/day. In the two women taking 100 or 400 mg doses, the quetiapine milk levels were 32 and 264 nmol/L, respectively, and the estimated infant exposures were <0.01 and <0.10 mg/kg/day, respectively. Milk levels for the other agents were clonazepam (not detected), paroxetine (not detected in three; 776 nmol/L in one;

Q

estimated infant exposure <0.26 mg/kg/day), trazodone (108 nmol/L; estimated infant exposure <0.01 mg/kg/day), and venlafaxine (371 and 1179 nmol/L; estimated infant exposure <0.01 mg/kg/day for both) (13).

At 9–18 months of age, infant behavior was evaluated using the Bayley Scales of Infant Development, Second Edition (13). Four scored within normal limits, whereas two showed mild developmental delay (evaluated at 9 and 12.72 months, respectively). Both infants were exposed to quetiapine and paroxetine; one from 18 weeks' gestation and the other starting at 3 weeks postpartum. Neither agent was detected in the breast milk of the mothers. Based on the limited sample, the authors concluded that there appeared to be no association between developmental outcomes and exposure to the drugs in breast milk (13).

In a case described in the Fetal Risk Summary section, a woman took quetiapine 400 mg/day and fluvoxamine 200 mg/day throughout a normal pregnancy (14). She continued this therapy while attempting to breastfeed her healthy female infant. Because of insufficient milk production, formula supplementation was required. The infant was developing normally and meeting all milestones at 3 months of age (14).

Another case, also described in the Fetal Risk Summary section, involved a 26-year-old mother taking quetiapine 400 mg/day, oxycodone 60 mg/day, and fluoxetine 40 mg/day during pregnancy and while breastfeeding her 3-month-old male infant (15). The infant's weight, 3.4 kg (50th percentile) at birth, was now 5.6 kg (25th percentile). Blood and milk samples were collected before the night quetiapine dose was administered and at various times over a 24-hour period. Sixteen milk samples were collected by manual expression at regular feeding times. The average milk concentration of quetiapine was 41 mcg/L and the milk:plasma ratio was 0.29. Using 150 mL/kg/ day as an estimated milk intake, the infant's dose was 0.09% of the maternal weight-adjusted dose. The infant's plasma level, 1.4 mcg/L, was about 6% of the corresponding maternal plasma concentration. No adverse effects were noted in the infant. The results of a Denver developmental assessment were consistent with the chronologic age (15).

The long-term effects of these exposures on nursing infants are unknown. The manufacturer recommends women receiving quetiapine should not breastfeed (6). Moreover, the American Academy of Pediatrics classifies other antipsychotics (e.g., see Clozapine) as drugs whose effect on the nursing infant is unknown but may be of concern (20).

References

1. American College of Obstetricians and Gynecologists. Use of psychiatric medications during pregnancy and lactation. *ACOG Practice Bulletin*. No. 92, April 2008. Obstet Gynecol 2008;111:1001–19.
2. Cutler AJ, Goldstein JM, Tumas JA. Dosing and switching strategies for quetiapine fumarate. Clin Ther 2002;24:209–22.
3. Althuler LL, Cohen L, Szuba MP, Burt VK, Gitlin M, Mintz J. Pharmacologic management of psychiatric illness during pregnancy: dilemmas and guidelines. Am J Psychiatry 1996;153:592–606.
4. Koren G, Cohn T, Chitayat D, Kapur B, Remington G, Myles-Reid D, Zipursky RB. Use of atypical antipsychotics during pregnancy and the risk of neural tube defects in infants. Am J Psychiatry 2002;159:136–7.
5. McCauley-Elsom K, Gurvich C, Elsom SJ, Kulkarni J. Antipsychotics in pregnancy. J Psychiatr Ment Health Nurs 2010;17:97–104.
6. Product information. Seroquel. AstraZeneca Pharmaceuticals, 2013.
7. Rahi M, Heikkinen T, Hartter S, Hakkola J, Hakala K, Wallerman O, Wadelius M, Wadelius C, Laine K. Placental transfer of quetiapine in relation to P-glycoprotein activity. J Psychopharmacol 2007;21:751–6.
8. Newport DJ, Calamaras MR, DeVane CL, Donovan J, Beach AJ, Winn S, Knight BT, Gibson BB, Viguera AC, Owens MJ, Nemeroff CB, Stowe ZN. Atypical antipsychotic administration during late pregnancy: placental passage and obstetrical outcomes. Am J Psychiatry 2007;164:1214–20.
9. Tenyi T, Trixler M, Keresztes Z. Quetiapine and pregnancy. Am J Psychiatry 2002;159:674.
10. Taylor TM, O'Toole MS, Ohlsen RI, Walters J, Pilowsky LS. Safety of quetiapine during pregnancy. Am J Psychiatry 2003;160:588–9.
11. Lee A, Giesbrecht E, Dunn E, Ito S. Excretion of quetiapine in breast milk. Am J Psychiatry 2004;161:1715–6.
12. McKenna K, Koren G, Tetelbaum M, Wilton L, Shakir S, Diav-Citrin O, Levinson A, Zipursky RB, Einarson A. Pregnancy outcome of women using atypical antipsychotic drugs: a prospective comparative study. J Clin Psychiatry 2005;66:444–9.
13. Misri S, Corral M, Wardrop AA, Kendrick K. Quetiapine augmentation in lactation. A series of case reports. J Clin Psychopharmacol 2006;26:508–11.
14. Gentile S. Quetiapine-fluvoxamine combination during pregnancy and while breastfeeding. Arch Womens Ment Health 2006;9:158–9.
15. Rampono J, Kristensen JH, Ilett KF, Hackett LP, Kohan R. Quetiapine and breast feeding. Ann Pharmacother 2007;41:711–4.
16. Gentile S. Prophylactic treatment of bipolar disorder in pregnancy and breastfeeding: focus on emerging mood stabilizers. Bipolar Disord 2006;8:207–20.
17. Klier CM, Mossaheb N, Saria A, Schloegelhofer M, Zernig G. Pharmacokinetics and elimination of quetiapine, venlafaxine, and trazodone during pregnancy and postpartum. J Clin Psychopharmacol 2007;27:720–2.
18. Grover S, Madam R. Successful use of quetiapine in two successive pregnancies. J Neuropsychiatry Clin Neurosci 2012(Winter);24:E38.
19. Frayne J, Nguyen T, Kohan R, De Felice N, Rampono J. The comprehensive management of pregnant women with major mood disorders: a case study involving phenelzine, lithium, and quetiapine. Arch Womens Ment Health 2014;17:73–5.
20. Committee on Drugs, American Academy of Pediatrics. The transfer of drugs and other chemicals into human milk. Pediatrics 2001;108:776–89.

QUINACRINE

[Withdrawn from the market. See 9th edition.]

QUINAPRIL

Antihypertensive

PREGNANCY RECOMMENDATION: Human Data Suggest Risk in 2nd and 3rd Trimesters
BREASTFEEDING RECOMMENDATION: Limited Human Data—Probably Compatible

PREGNANCY SUMMARY

The fetal toxicity of quinapril in the 2nd and 3rd trimesters is similar to other angiotensin-converting enzyme (ACE) inhibitors. The use of this drug during the 2nd and 3rd trimesters may cause teratogenicity and severe fetal and neonatal toxicity. Fetal toxic effects may include anuria, oligohydramnios, fetal hypocalvaria, intrauterine growth restriction (IUGR), prematurity, and patent ductus arteriosus. Stillbirth or neonatal death may occur. Anuria-associated oligohydramnios may produce fetal limb contractures, craniofacial deformation, and pulmonary hypoplasia. Severe anuria and hypotension, which is resistant to both pressor agents and volume expansion, may occur in the newborn following in utero exposure. Newborn renal function and blood pressure should be closely monitored.

FETAL RISK SUMMARY

Quinapril is an ACE inhibitor. No teratogenic effects were observed in reproduction studies in rats and rabbits with doses 180 and 1 times the maximum recommended human dose, respectively (1).

A retrospective study using pharmacy-based data from the Tennessee Medicaid program identified 209 infants, born between 1985 and 2000, who had 1st trimester exposure to ACE inhibitors (2). Infants of mothers with evidence of diabetes, either before or during pregnancy, were excluded, as were those exposed to angiotensin-receptor antagonists (ARBs), ACE inhibitors or other antihypertensives beyond the 1st trimester, and exposure to known teratogens. Two comparison groups, other antihypertensives (N = 202) and no antihypertensives (N = 29,096), were formed. The number of major birth defects in each of the three groups was 18 (8.6%), 4 (2%), and 834 (2.9%), respectively. Compared with the no-antihypertensives group, exposure to ACE inhibitors was associated with a significantly increased risk of major defects (relative risk [RR] 2.71, 95% confidence interval [CI] 1.72–4.27). When the analysis was conducted by the type of defect, the highest rates were with cardiovascular defects, 9, 2, and 294, respectively, RR 3.72, 95% CI 1.89–7.30, and with CNS defects, 3, 0, and 80, respectively, RR 4.39, 95% CI 1.37–14.02. The major defects observed in the subject group were: atrial septal defect (N = 6) (includes three with pulmonic stenosis and/or three with patent ductus arteriosus [PDA]), renal dysplasia (N = 2), PDA alone (N = 2), and one each of ventricular septal defect, spina bifida, microcephaly with eye anomaly, coloboma, hypospadias, intestinal and choanal atresia, Hirschsprung disease, and diaphragmatic hernia (2). In an accompanying editorial, it was noted that neither previous reports of 1st trimester exposure to ACE inhibitors nor the animal studies had observed an increased risk of birth defects (3). It also was noted that no mechanism for ACE inhibitor–induced teratogenicity was known. A subsequent communication raising concerns about the validity of the study in terms of adequate exclusion of diabetes, charting and coding errors in busy medical practices, and the effects of maternal obesity (4) was addressed by the investigators (5).

Quinapril and other ACE inhibitors are human teratogens when used in the 2nd and 3rd trimesters, producing fetal hypocalvaria and renal defects. The cause of the defects and other toxicity is probably related to fetal hypotension and decreased renal blood flow. The compromise of the fetal renal system may result in severe, and at times fatal, anuria, both in the fetus and in the newborn. Anuria-associated oligohydramnios may produce pulmonary hypoplasia, limb contractures, persistent PDA, craniofacial deformation, and neonatal death (6,7). IUGR, prematurity, and severe neonatal hypotension may also be observed. Two reviews of fetal and newborn renal function indicated that both renal perfusion and glomerular plasma flow are low during gestation and that high levels of angiotensin II may be physiologically necessary to maintain glomerular filtration at low perfusion pressures (8,9). Quinapril prevents the conversion of angiotensin I to angiotensin II and, thus, may lead to in utero renal failure. Because the primary means of removal of the drug is renal, the impairment of this system in the newborn prevents elimination of the drug resulting in prolonged hypotension. Newborn renal function and blood pressure should be closely monitored. If oligohydramnios occurs, stopping quinapril may resolve the problem but may not improve infant outcome because of irreversible fetal damage (6). In those cases in which quinapril must be used to treat the mother's disease, the lowest possible dose should be used combined with close monitoring of amniotic fluid levels and fetal well-being. Guidelines for counseling exposed pregnant patients have been published and should be of benefit to health professionals faced with this task (6,10).

The observation in Tennessee Medicaid data of an increased risk of major congenital defects after 1st trimester exposure to ACE inhibitors raises concerns about teratogenicity that have not been seen in other studies (3). Medicaid data are a valuable tool for identifying early signals of teratogenicity, but are subject to a number of shortcomings, and their findings must be considered hypotheses until confirmed by independent studies.

A 2012 review of the use of ACE inhibitors and ARBs in the 1st trimester concluded that there may be an elevated teratogenic risk, but the risk appeared to be related to other factors (11). The factors, that typically coexist with hypertension in pregnancy, included diabetes, advanced maternal age, and obesity.

BREASTFEEDING SUMMARY

Quinapril is excreted into breast milk. Six healthy mothers who had been breastfeeding for at least 2 weeks were given a single 20 mg oral dose of quinapril (12). Serial blood and milk samples were collected over 24 hours. The mean milk:plasma ratio was 0.12 based on AUC, but no drug was detected in milk after 4 hours. The metabolite (quinaprilat) was not detected in any of the milk samples. The estimated infant dose was 1.6% of the mother's weight-adjusted dose (12).

The amount of quinapril measured in the above study is clinically insignificant. Although data from women receiving daily doses of the drug are needed, quinapril is probably compatible with nursing. The American Academy of Pediatrics classifies captopril and enalapril as compatible with breastfeeding (see Captopril and Enalapril).

References

1. Product information. Accupril. Parke-Davis, 2000.
2. Cooper WO, Hernandez-Diaz S, Arbogast PG, Dudley JA, Dyer S, Gideon PS, Hall K, Ray WA. Major congenital malformations after first-trimester exposure to ACE inhibitors. N Engl J Med 2006;354:2443–51.
3. Friedman JM. ACE inhibitors and congenital anomalies. N Engl J Med 2006;354:2498–500.
4. Scialli AR, Lione A. ACE inhibitors and major congenital malformations. N Engl J Med 2006;355:1280.
5. Cooper WO, Ray WA. Reply—ACE inhibitors and major congenital malformations. N Engl J Med 2006;355:1281.
6. Barr M Jr. Teratogen update: angiotensin-converting enzyme inhibitors. Teratology 1994;50:399–409.
7. Shotan A, Widerhorn J, Hurst A, Elkayam U. Risks of angiotensin-converting enzyme inhibition during pregnancy: experimental and clinical evidence, potential mechanisms, and recommendations for use. Am J Med 1994;96:451–6.
8. Robillard JE, Nakamura KT, Matherne GP, Jose PA. Renal hemodynamics and functional adjustments to postnatal life. Semin Perinatol 1988;12:143–50.
9. Guignard J-P, Gouyon J-B. Adverse effects of drugs on the immature kidney. Biol Neonate 1988;53:243–52.
10. Brent RL, Beckman DA. Angiotensin-converting enzyme inhibitors, an embryopathic class of drugs with unique properties: information for clinical teratology counselors. Teratology 1991;43:543–6.
11. Polifka JE. Is there an embryopathy associated with first-trimester exposure to angiotensin-converting enzyme inhibitors and angiotensin receptor antagonists? A critical review of the evidence. Birth Defects Res (Part A) 2012;94:576–98.
12. Begg EJ, Robson RA, Gardiner SJ, Hudson LF, Reece PA, Olson SC, Posvar EL, Sedman AJ. Quinapril and its metabolite quinaprilat in human milk. Br J Clin Pharmacol 2001;51:478–81.

QUINETHAZONE

[Withdrawn from the market. See 9th edition.]

QUINIDINE

Antiarrhythmic/Antimalarial

PREGNANCY RECOMMENDATION: Compatible
BREASTFEEDING RECOMMENDATION: Limited Human Data—Probably Compatible

PREGNANCY SUMMARY

The use of quinidine during pregnancy has been classified in reviews of cardiovascular drugs as relatively low risk for the fetus (1–4). In therapeutic doses, the oxytocic properties of quinidine have been rarely observed, but high doses can produce this effect and may result in abortion (3,5).

FETAL RISK SUMMARY

No reports linking the use of quinidine with congenital defects have been located. Animal reproduction studies apparently have not been conducted with quinidine.

Quinidine has been in use as an antiarrhythmic drug for more than 100 years (6) and in pregnancy, at least back to the 1920s (7–13). Eighth cranial nerve damage has been associated with high doses of the optical isomer, quinine, but not with quinidine (9). Neonatal thrombocytopenia has been reported after maternal use of quinidine (10).

Quinidine crosses the placenta and achieves fetal serum levels similar to maternal levels (6,11–13). In a 1979 case, a woman taking 600 mg every 8 hours plus an additional dose of 300 mg (2100 mg/day) had serum and amniotic fluid levels of 5.8 and 10.6 mcg/mL, respectively, 10 days before term (11). Three days later, 10 hours after the last dose, a healthy male infant was delivered by elective cesarean section. Quinidine concentrations in the serum, cord blood, and amniotic fluid were 3.4, 2.8, and 9.3 mcg/mL, respectively. The cord blood:serum ratio was 0.82 (11). The cord blood level was greater than those measured in three other reports (6,12,13).

In a 1984 study, three women maintained on quinidine (300 mg every 6 hours) and digoxin had serum levels of quinidine at delivery ranging from 0.7 to 2.1 mcg/mL (12). A quinidine level in one amniotic fluid sample was 0.9 mcg/mL, whereas cord blood levels ranged from <0.5 to 1.6 mcg/mL. In two of the three cases, cord blood:serum ratios were 0.2 and 0.9 (12).

In a 1985 report, a woman taking quinidine (400 mg every 6 hours) plus digoxin and propranolol had an elective cesarean section 18 hours after the last dose (13). The quinidine concentration in the cord blood was 0.8 mcg/mL.

One case involved a woman in whom quinidine doses were escalated during a 6-day interval from 300 mg every 6 hours to 1500 mg every 6 hours (6). On day 8, the dosage was reduced to 1500 mg every 8 hours, then to 1200 mg every 8 hours on day 9, and then stopped on day 10. Amniotic fluid levels of quinidine and the metabolite, 3-hydroxyquinidine, on day 10 were 2.2 and 9.7 mcg/mL, respectively. At delivery 2 days later, cord blood contained 0.5 mcg/mL of quinidine and 0.7 mcg/mL of the metabolite (6).

In a surveillance study of Michigan Medicaid recipients involving 229,101 completed pregnancies conducted between 1985 and 1992, 17 newborns had been exposed to quinidine during the 1st trimester (F. Rosa, personal communication, FDA, 1993). One (5.9%) major birth defect was observed (one expected). No anomalies were observed in six defect categories (cardiovascular defects, oral clefts, spina bifida, polydactyly, limb reduction defects, and hypospadias) for which specific data were available.

The drug has been used in combination with digoxin to treat fetal supraventricular and reciprocating atrioventricular tachycardia (12,13). The authors of one of these reports consider quinidine to be the drug of choice after digoxin for the treatment of persistent fetal tachyarrhythmias (13). A 1990 report described an unsuccessful attempt of maternal transplacental cardioversion with quinidine for a rare case of fetal ventricular tachycardia associated with nonimmune hydrops fetalis at 30 weeks' gestation (14). A dose of 200 mg quinidine 4 times daily was given for 3 days before worsening preeclampsia with breech presentation required delivery by cesarean section. The newborn died 5 hours after birth.

A 33-year-old woman with new-onset, sustained ventricular tachycardia was treated with metoprolol (50 mg twice daily) at 22 weeks' gestation (15). Because of recurrent palpitations, quinidine (dose not specified) was added to the regimen at 26 weeks' gestation, and with the attainment of a therapeutic quinidine level, the combination was successful in controlling the ectopic beats. Combination therapy was continued until term when a healthy, growth-restricted, approximately 2240-g infant was delivered. Intrauterine growth restriction apparently developed after maternal combination therapy was initiated, but a discussion of the cause was not included in the reference, nor was maternal blood pressures given (15).

A mother treated with quinidine for a fetal supraventricular tachycardia developed symptoms of quinidine toxicity consisting of severe nausea and vomiting, diarrhea, lightheadedness, and tinnitus (6). Electrocardiographic changes were consistent with quinidine toxicity. Her dosage had been increased during an interval of 6 days in a manner described above, producing serum quinidine levels of 1.4–3.3 mcg/mL (therapeutic range in the author's laboratory was 1.5–5.0 mcg/mL). At the highest dose, her serum level was 2.3 mcg/mL. Levels of the metabolite, 3-hydroxyquinidine, rose from 1.1 to 6.8 mcg/mL during the 6-day interval, eventually reaching 9.7 mcg/mL 1 day after quinidine was discontinued. The 3-hydroxyquinidine:quinidine ratio varied from 0.8 (on day 2) to 3.7 (on day 10). These ratios were much higher than those observed in previously reported patients (1). Because the fetal heart rate continued to be elevated, with only occasional reductions to 120–130 beats/minute, and fetal lung maturity had been demonstrated; labor was induced, resulting in the delivery of a 3540-g infant with hydrops fetalis. The infant required pharmacologic therapy to control the supraventricular tachycardia. The maternal toxicity was attributed to the elevated levels of 3-hydroxyquinidine, because concentrations of quinidine were in the low- to mid-therapeutic range (6).

In an in vitro study using plasma from 16 normal pregnant women, quinidine concentrations between 0.5 and 5.0 mcg/mL were shown to inhibit plasma pseudocholinesterase activity (16). Inhibition varied from 29% (0.5 mcg/mL) to 71% (5.0 mcg/mL). Pseudocholinesterase is responsible for the metabolism of succinylcholine and ester-type local anesthetics (e.g., procaine, tetracaine, cocaine, and chloroprocaine) (16). The quinidine-induced inhibition of this enzyme, which is already significantly decreased by pregnancy itself, could potentially result in toxicity if these agents were used in a mother maintained on quinidine.

A 21-year-old woman in premature labor at 31 weeks' gestation was treated with IV quinidine and exchange transfusion for severe, apparently chloroquine-resistant, malaria (17). Parasitemia with *Plasmodium falciparum* >12% was shown on blood smears before treatment and then fell to 1% after treatment. Initial therapy with 1 g oral chloroquine was unsuccessful and approximately 12 hours later, she was given an IV loading dose of quinidine,10 mg base/kg during 2 hours, followed by a continuous infusion of 0.02 mg/kg/minute and exchange transfusion. No potentiation of labor was observed during quinidine therapy, although the mother was receiving IV magnesium sulfate for tocolysis. Because of fetal distress, thought to be caused by uteroplacental insufficiency as a result of maternal parasitemia or fever, a cesarean section was performed to deliver a 1570-g male infant with Apgar scores of 5 and 7 at 1 and 5 minutes, respectively. Except for respiratory difficulty during the first 6 hours, the infant had an uneventful hospital course, including a negative blood smear for malaria (17).

BREASTFEEDING SUMMARY

Quinidine is excreted into breast milk (11). A woman taking 600 mg every 8 hours had milk and serum concentrations determined on the 5th postpartum day, 3 hours after a dose. Levels in the two samples were 6.4 and 9.0 mcg/mL, respectively, a milk:serum ratio of 0.71. A quinidine level of 8.2 mcg/mL was noted in a milk sample on the preceding day (time relationship to the dose not specified) but a simultaneous serum concentration was not determined. The infant in this case did not breastfeed (11). The American Academy of Pediatrics classifies quinidine as compatible with breastfeeding (18).

References

1. Rotmensch HH, Elkayam U, Frishman W. Antiarrhythmic drug therapy during pregnancy. Ann Intern Med 1983;98:487–97.
2. Tamari I, Eldar M, Rabinowitz B, Neufeld HN. Medical treatment of cardiovascular disorders during pregnancy. Am Heart J 1982;104:1357–63.
3. Rotmensch HH, Rotmensch S, Elkayam U. Management of cardiac arrhythmias during pregnancy: current concepts. Drugs 1987;33:623–33.
4. Ward RM. Maternal drug therapy for fetal disorders. Semin Perinatol 1992;16:12–20.
5. Bigger JT, Hoffman BF. Antiarrhythmic drugs. In: Gilman AG, Goodman LS, Gilman A, eds. *The Pharmacological Basis of Therapeutics*. 6th ed. New York, NY: MacMillan, 1980:768.
6. Killeen AA, Bowers LD. Fetal supraventricular tachycardia treated with high-dose quinidine: toxicity associated with marked elevation of the metabolite, 3(S)-3-hydroxyquinidine. Obstet Gynecol 1987;70:445–9.
7. Meyer J, Lackner JE, Schochet SS. Paroxysmal tachycardia in pregnancy. JAMA 1930;94:1901–4.
8. McMillan TM, Bellet S. Ventricular paroxysmal tachycardia: report of a case in a pregnant girl of sixteen years with an apparently normal heart. Am Heart J 1931;7:70–8.
9. Mendelson CL. Disorders of the heartbeat during pregnancy. Am J Obstet Gynecol 1956;72:1268–301.
10. Domula VM, Weissach G, Lenk H. Uber die auswirkung medikamentoser Behandlung in der Schwangerschaft auf das Gerennungspotential des Neugeborenen. Zentralbl Gynaekol 1977;99:473.
11. Hill LM, Malkasian GD Jr. The use of quinidine sulfate throughout pregnancy. Obstet Gynecol 1979;54:366–8.
12. Spinnato JA, Shaver DC, Flinn GS, Sibai BM, Watson DL, Marin-Garcia J. Fetal supraventricular tachycardia: in utero therapy with digoxin and quinidine. Obstet Gynecol 1984;64:730–5.
13. Guntheroth WG, Cyr DR, Mack LA, Benedetti T, Lenke RR, Petty CN. Hydrops from reciprocating atrioventricular tachycardia in a 27-week fetus requiring quinidine for conversion. Obstet Gynecol 1985;66(Suppl):29S–33S.

14. Sherer DM, Sadovksy E, Menashe M, Mordel N, Rein AJJT. Fetal ventricular tachycardia associated with nonimmunologic hydrops fetalis: a case report. J Reprod Med 1990;35:292–4.
15. Braverman AC, Bromely BS, Rutherford JD. New onset ventricular tachycardia during pregnancy. Int J Cardiol 1991;33:409–12.
16. Kambam JR, Franks JJ, Smith BE. Inhibitory effect of quinidine on plasma pseudocholinesterase activity in pregnant women. Am J Obstet Gynecol 1987;157:897–9.
17. Wong RD, Murthy ARK, Mathisen GE, Glover N, Thornton PJ. Treatment of severe Falciparum malaria during pregnancy with quinidine and exchange transfusion. Am J Med 1992;92:561–2.
18. Committee on Drugs, American Academy of Pediatrics. The transfer of drugs and other chemicals into human milk. Pediatrics 2001; 108:776–89.

QUININE

Antimalarial

PREGNANCY RECOMMENDATION: Human Data Suggest Risk
BREASTFEEDING RECOMMENDATION: Limited Human Data—Probably Compatible

PREGNANCY SUMMARY

Quinine has effectively been replaced by newer agents for the treatment of malaria. Although no increased teratogenic risk can be documented for therapeutic doses, its use during pregnancy should be avoided. One manufacturer considers the drug to be contraindicated in pregnancy (1). However, some investigators believe quinine should be used for the treatment of chloroquine-resistant *Plasmodium falciparum* malaria (2).

FETAL RISK SUMMARY

Nishimura and Tanimura (3) summarized the human case reports of teratogenic effects linked with quinine in 21 infants who were exposed during the 1st trimester after unsuccessful abortion attempts (some infants had multiple defects and are listed more than once):

Central nervous system (CNS) anomalies (6 with hydrocephalus) (10 cases)
Limb defects (3 dysmelias) (8 cases)
Facial defects (7 cases)
Heart defects (6 cases)
Digestive organ anomalies (5 cases)
Urogenital anomalies (3 cases)
Hernias (3 cases)
Vertebral anomaly (1 case)

The malformations noted are varied, although CNS anomalies and limb defects were the most frequent. Auditory defects and optic nerve damage have also been reported (3–7). These reports usually concern the use of quinine in toxic doses as an abortifacient. Quinine has also been used to induce labor in women with intrauterine fetal death (8). Epidemiologic observations do not support an increased teratogenic risk or increased risk of congenital deafness over nonquinine-exposed patients (3,9). Neonatal and maternal thrombocytopenia purpura and hemolysis in glucose-6-phosphate dehydrogenase–deficient newborns has been reported (10,11).

In a surveillance study of Michigan Medicaid recipients involving 229,101 completed pregnancies conducted between 1985 and 1992, 35 newborns had been exposed to quinine during the 1st trimester (F. Rosa, personal communication, FDA, 1993). Two (5.7%) major birth defects were observed (one expected). No anomalies were observed in six defect categories (cardiovascular defects, oral clefts, spina bifida, polydactyly, limb reduction defects, and hypospadias) for which specific data were available.

BREASTFEEDING SUMMARY

Quinine is excreted into breast milk. Following 300- and 640-mg oral doses in six patients, the drug was detectable in milk up to 23 hours after a dose with concentrations ranging from trace to 2.2 mcg/mL (12). No adverse effects were reported in the nursing infants. Patients at risk for glucose-6-phosphate dehydrogenase deficiency should not be breastfed until this disease can be ruled out. The American Academy of Pediatrics classifies quinine as compatible with breastfeeding (13).

References

1. Product information. Quinamm. Merrell Dow, 1990.
2. Strang A, Lachman E, Pitsoe SB, Marszalek A, Philpott RH. Malaria in pregnancy with fatal complications: case report. Br J Obstet Gynaecol 1984;91:399–403.
3. Nishimura H, Tanimura T. *Clinical Aspects of the Teratogenicity of Drugs*. New York, NY: American Elsevier, 1976:140–3.
4. Robinson GC, Brummitt JR, Miller JR. Hearing loss in infants and preschool children. II. Etiological considerations. Pediatrics 1963;32:115–24.
5. West RA. Effect of quinine upon auditory nerve. Am J Obstet Gynecol 1938;36:241–8.
6. McKinna AJ. Quinine induced hypoplasia of the optic nerve. Can J Ophthalmol 1966;1:261.
7. Morgon A, Charachon D, Brinquier N. Disorders of the auditory apparatus caused by embryopathy or foetopathy. Prophylaxis and treatment. Acta Otolaryngol (Stockh) 1971;291(Suppl):5.
8. Mukherjee S, Bhose LN. Induction of labor and abortion with quinine infusion in intrauterine fetal deaths. Am J Obstet Gynecol 1968;101:853–4.
9. Heinonen OP, Slone D, Shapiro S. *Birth Defects and Drugs in Pregnancy*. Littleton, MA: Publishing Sciences Group, 1977:299, 302, 333.
10. Mauer MA, DeVaux W, Lahey ME. Neonatal and maternal thrombocytopenic purpura due to quinine. Pediatrics 1957;19:84–7.
11. Glass L, Rajegowda BK, Bowne E, Evans HE. Exposure to quinine and jaundice in a glucose-6-phosphate dehydrogenase-deficient newborn infant. Pediatrics 1973;82:734–5.
12. Terwilliger WG, Hatcher RA. The elimination of morphine and quinine in human milk. Surg Gynecol Obstet 1934;58:823–6.
13. Committee on Drugs, American Academy of Pediatrics. The transfer of drugs and other chemicals into human milk. Pediatrics 2001; 108:776–89.

QUINUPRISTIN/DALFOPRISTIN

Antibiotic

PREGNANCY RECOMMENDATION: Compatible—Maternal Benefit >> Embryo–Fetal Risk
BREASTFEEDING RECOMMENDATION: No Human Data—Potential Toxicity

PREGNANCY SUMMARY

No reports describing the use of quinupristin/dalfopristin in human pregnancy have been located. The drug does not cause teratogenicity or embryo–fetal toxicity in experimental animals. However, in pregnant rats the antibiotic combination may not reach the embryo or fetus in significant amounts. Placental passage in humans has not been studied. Because the indication for the combination involves potentially life-threatening infections, the maternal benefit of therapy appears to far outweigh the unknown embryo or fetal risk.

FETAL RISK SUMMARY

The semisynthetic pristinamycin derivatives quinupristin/dalfopristin are streptogramin antibacterial agents that are combined in a ratio of 30:70 (weight/weight). The antibacterial combination is indicated for the treatment of vancomycin-resistant *Enterococcus faecium*. It also is active against *Staphylococcus aureus* and *Streptococcus pyogenes*. Depending on the bacterium, the combination exhibits both bacteriostatic and bactericidal action. Although quinupristin and dalfopristin are the main active components circulating in the plasma, both agents are converted to several active metabolites (1).

In reproduction studies with rats, no adverse effects on fertility, or perinatal/postnatal development were observed with the combination at doses up to approximately 0.4 times the human dose based on BSA (HD). In addition, no evidence of impaired fertility or fetal harm was observed in pregnant mice, rats, and rabbits at approximately 0.5, 2.5, and 0.5 times the HD, respectively (1). In four genetic toxicity assays, the results with the combination and the individual antibacterial agents were negative. In a fifth test (Chinese hamster ovary cell chromosome aberration assay), dalfopristin was associated with structural chromosome aberrations but the combination and quinupristin were not (1).

It is not known whether quinupristin or dalfopristin crosses the human placenta to the fetus. Quinupristin is a combination of three peptide macrolactones in which the main component (>88%) has a molecular weight of about 1022. Dalfopristin has a molecular weight of about 691 (1). It is possible, therefore, that both agents and/or their metabolites could cross to the embryo and fetus. In a study with rats, the combination did not cross the placenta in significant amounts (2). Other than the fact that the antibiotic was given on gestation day 17, specific data, such as the dosage and amount crossing the placenta, were lacking.

BREASTFEEDING SUMMARY

The use of quinupristin/dalfopristin during human lactation has not been reported. The relatively high molecular weights for the two components (about 1022 and 691, respectively), suggest that only small amounts, if any, will pass into human milk. A 2000 review concluded that quinupristin/dalfopristin was unlikely to pass into breast milk because of its molecular size and weakly acidic nature (3). However, if the antibiotic were present in milk it could alter the bowel flora of a nursing infant. Because of the special indication for the antibiotic (vancomycin-resistant *E. faecium*) and the potential for the development of strains resistant to quinupristin/dalfopristin, breastfeeding is not recommended.

References

1. Product information. Synercid. Aventis Pharmaceuticals, 2002.
2. Bergeron M, Montay G. The pharmacokinetics of quinupristin/dalfopristin in laboratory animals and in humans. J Antimicrob Chemother 1997;39(Suppl A):129–38.
3. Chin KG, Mactal-Haaf C, McPherson CE III. Use of anti-infective agents during lactation: Part I: Beta-lactam antibiotics, vancomycin, quinupristin-dalfopristin, and linezolid. J Hum Lact 2000;16:351–8.

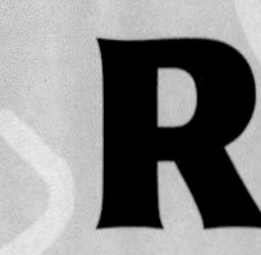

RABEPRAZOLE

Gastrointestinal Agent (Antisecretory)

PREGNANCY RECOMMENDATION: Limited Human Data—Animal Data Suggest Low Risk
BREASTFEEDING RECOMMENDATION: No Human Data—Potential Toxicity

PREGNANCY SUMMARY

No reports describing the use of rabeprazole during human pregnancy have been located. A study showing an association between in utero exposure to gastric acid–suppressing drugs and childhood allergy and asthma requires confirmation. Human pregnancy experience with three other proton pump inhibitors (PPIs) (see Lansoprazole, Omeprazole, and Pantoprazole) has not shown a causal relationship with congenital malformations. In some cases, malformations may have been missed because of the design and size of the studies. The carcinogenic and mutagenic data are a potential concern, but the absence of follow-up studies prevents a risk assessment for exposed offspring. As with all drug therapy, avoidance of rabeprazole during pregnancy, especially during the 1st trimester, is the safest course. If rabeprazole is required or if inadvertent exposure does occur early in gestation, the known risk to the embryo–fetus for congenital defects, based on animal data for rabeprazole and the published experience with other PPIs, appears to be low. Long-term follow-up of offspring exposed during gestation is warranted.

FETAL RISK SUMMARY

Rabeprazole is a PPI that blocks gastric acid secretion by a direct inhibitory effect on the gastric parietal cell (1). It is used for the treatment of duodenal ulcer, erosive or ulcerative gastroesophageal reflux disease (GERD), and the long-term treatment of pathologic hypersecretory conditions, such as Zollinger-Ellison syndrome. Rabeprazole is in the same class of PPIs as dexlansoprazole, esomeprazole, lansoprazole, omeprazole, and pantoprazole.

Reproductive studies have been conducted in rats and rabbits with IV doses up to 13 and 8 times, respectively, the recommended human dose based on AUC (1). No evidence was found at these doses of impaired fertility or fetal harm. In male and female rats, rabeprazole caused gastric cell hyperplasia and, in female rats, gastric cell tumors, at all doses tested (1). In addition, positive results with the drug and its inactive metabolite were demonstrated in hamsters and mice with the in vitro Ames mutation assay and in some other mutagenicity tests (1).

It is not known if rabeprazole crosses the human placenta. The molecular weight (about 381 for the sodium salt) is low enough that passage to the fetus should be expected. Another PPI, omeprazole, has a similar molecular weight and chemical structure and it is known to cross the human placenta (see Omeprazole).

A population-based observational cohort study formed by linking data from three Swedish national health care registers over a 10-year period (1995–2004) was reported in 2009 (2). The main outcome measures were a diagnosis of allergic disease or a prescription for asthma or allergy medications. The drug types included in the study were gastric acid suppressors, including H_2-receptor antagonists, prostaglandins, PPIs, combinations for eradication of *Helicobacter pylori*, and drugs for peptic ulcer and GERD. Of 585,716 children, 29,490 (5.0%) met the diagnosis and 5645 (1%) had been exposed to gastric acid–suppression therapy in pregnancy. Of these children, 405 (0.07%) were treated for allergic disease. For developing allergy, the odds ratio (OR) was 1.43, 98% confidence interval (CI) 1.29–1.59, irrespective of the drug, time of exposure during pregnancy, and maternal history of allergy. For developing childhood asthma, but not other allergic diseases, the OR was 1.51, 95% CI 1.35–1.69, irrespective of the type of acid-suppressive drug and the time of exposure in pregnancy. The authors proposed three possible mechanisms for their findings: (a) exposure to increased amounts of allergens could cause sensitization to digestion labile antigens in the fetus; (b) maternal Th2 cytokine pattern could promote an allergy-prone phenotype in the fetus; and (c) maternal allergen-specific immunoglobulin E could cross the placenta and sensitize fetal immune cells to food and airborne allergens. Several limitations of the study that might have affected their findings were identified, including a general increase in childhood asthma but not necessarily an increase in allergic asthma (2). The study requires confirmation.

A meta-analysis of PPIs in pregnancy was reported in 2009 (3). Based on 1530 exposed compared with 133,410 not-exposed pregnancies, the OR for major malformations was 1.12, 95% CI 0.86–1.45. There also was no increased risk for spontaneous abortions (OR 1.29, 95% CI 0.84–1.97) or preterm birth (OR 1.13, 95% CI 0.96–1.33) (3).

In a 2010 study from Denmark, covering the period 1996–2008, there were 840,968 live births among whom

5082 were exposed to PPIs between 4 weeks before conception and the end of the 1st trimester (4). In the exposed group there were 174 (3.4%) major malformations compared with 21,811 (2.6%) not exposed to PPIs (adjusted prevalence odds ratio [aPOR] 1.23, 95 CI 1.05–1.44). When the analysis was limited to exposure in the 1st trimester, there were 118 (3.2%) major malformations among 3651 exposed infants (aPOR 1.10, 95% CI 0.91–1.34). For exposure to rabeprazole in the 1st trimester, there were 3 (7.1%) major birth defects among 42 live births (aPOR 2.14, 95% CI 0.60–7.68; see Esomeprazole, Lansoprazole, Omeprazole, and Pantoprazole for their data). The data showed that exposure to PPIs in the 1st trimester was not associated with a significantly increased risk of major birth defects (4). An accompanying editorial discussed the strengths and weaknesses of the study (5).

In a 2012 publication, the National Birth Defects Prevention study, a multisite population-based case–control study, examined whether nausea/vomiting of pregnancy (NVP) or its treatment were associated with the most common noncardiac defects (nonsyndromic cleft lip with or without cleft palate [CL/P], cleft palate alone [CP], neural tube defects [NTDs], and hypospadias) (6). PPI exposure included esomeprazole, lansoprazole, and omeprazole. There were 4524 cases and 5859 controls. NVP was not associated with cleft palate or NTDs, but modest risk reductions were observed for CL/P and hypospadias. Increased risks were found for PPIs ($N = 7$) and hypospadias (adjusted OR [aOR] 4.36, 95% CI 1.21–15.81), steroids ($N = 10$) and hypospadias (aOR 2.87, 95% CI 1.03–7.97), and ondansetron ($N = 11$) and CP (aOR 2.37, 95% CI 1.18–4.76) (6).

Another 2012 study, using the Danish nationwide registries, evaluated the risk of hypospadias after exposure to PPIs during the 1st trimester and throughout gestation (7). The study period, 1997 through 2009, included all liveborn boys that totaled 430,569 of whom 2926 were exposed to maternal PPI use. Hypospadias was diagnosed in 20 (0.7%) exposed boys, whereas 2683 (0.6%) of the nonexposed had hypospadias (adjusted prevalence ratio [aPR] 1.1, 95% CI 0.7–1.7). For the 5227 boys exposed throughout pregnancy, 32 (0.6%) had hypospadias (PR 1.0, 95% CI 0.7–1.4). When the analysis was restricted to mothers with 2 or more PPI prescriptions, the aPR of overall hypospadias was 1.7, 95% CI 0.9–3.3 and 1.6, 95% CI 0.7–3.9 for omeprazole. The authors concluded that PPIs were not associated with hypospadias (7).

Several reports and reviews describing the use of PPIs during human pregnancy have observed no increased risk of developmental toxicity (see Lansoprazole, Omeprazole, and Pantoprazole).

BREASTFEEDING SUMMARY

No reports describing the use of rabeprazole during human lactation have been located. The molecular weight (about 381 for the sodium salt) suggests that the drug will be excreted into breast milk. Because of the positive carcinogenic tests and the potential for suppression of gastric acid secretion in the nursing infant, the use of rabeprazole during lactation should probably be avoided until clinical data are available.

References

1. Product information. Rapeprazole. Eisai, 2001.
2. Dehlink E, Yen E, Leichtner AM, Hait EJ, Fiebiger E. First evidence of a possible association between gastric acid suppression during pregnancy and childhood asthma: a population-based register study. Clin Exp Allergy 2009;39:246–53.
3. Gill SK, O'Brien L, Einarson TR, Koren G. The safety of proton pump inhibitors (PPIs) in pregnancy: a meta-analysis. Am J Gastroenterol 2009; 104:1541–5.
4. Pasternak B, Hviid A. Use of proton-pump inhibitors in early pregnancy and the risk of birth defects. N Engl J Med 2010;363:2114–23.
5. Mitchell AA. Proton-pump inhibitors and birth defects—some reassurance, but more needed. N Engl J Med 2010;363:2161–3.
6. Anderka M, Mitchell AA, Louik C, Werler MM, Hernandez-Diaz S, Rasmussen SA, and the National Birth Defects Prevention Study. Medications used to treat nausea and vomiting of pregnancy and the risk of selected birth defects. Birth Defects Res A Clin Mol Teratol 2012;94:22-30.
7. Erichsen R, Mikkelsen E, Pedersen L, Sorensen HT. Maternal use of proton pump inhibitors during early pregnancy and the prevalence of hypospadias in male offspring. Am J Ther 2012 Feb 3; [Epub ahead of print].

RALOXIFENE

Selective Estrogen Receptor Modulator

PREGNANCY RECOMMENDATION: Contraindicated
BREASTFEEDING RECOMMENDATION: Contraindicated

R

PREGNANCY SUMMARY

No reports describing the use of raloxifene in human pregnancy have been located, but the animal reproduction studies suggest risk. The indications for this drug suggest that human pregnancy experience is unlikely. Moreover, raloxifene is an estrogen antagonist in uterine tissue and estrogen is required to maintain pregnancy. Therefore, the drug is contraindicated in pregnancy. If a woman inadvertently becomes pregnant while taking raloxifene, she should be informed of the risk to her embryo and/or fetus.

FETAL RISK SUMMARY

Raloxifene is an estrogen agonist/antagonist that is in the benzothiophene class of selective estrogen receptor modulators. It is indicated for the treatment and prevention of osteoporosis in postmenopausal women, reduction in risk of invasive breast cancer in postmenopausal women with osteoporosis, and reduction in risk of invasive breast cancer in postmenopausal women at high risk for invasive breast cancer. Raloxifene produces estrogen-like effects on bone and lipid metabolism, while antagonizing the effects of estrogen on uterine and mammary tissue. The drug undergoes hepatic metabolism to apparently inactive metabolites. Plasma protein binding is 95% to albumin and α_1-acid glycoprotein, and the elimination half-life after multiple doses is 32.5 hours (1).

Reproduction studies have been performed in rats and rabbits. In rats, doses that were ≥0.2 times the human dose based on BSA (HD) caused retarded fetal development and developmental abnormalities (wavy ribs and kidney cavitation). Doses 0.02–1.6 times the HD during gestation and lactation resulted in delayed and disrupted parturition, decreased neonatal survival, and altered physical development; sex- and age-specific reductions in growth and changes in pituitary hormone content; and decreased lymphoid compartment size in offspring. The highest dose disrupted parturition resulting in maternal and offspring death and morbidity. In rabbits, doses that were ≥0.04 times the HD caused abortions and a low rate of ventricular septal defects. At ≥4 times the HD, hydrocephaly was observed in fetuses (1).

In a study with female rats before mating, minor delays in development of offspring without affecting viability or growth were observed (2). Raloxifene produced estrous cycle disruption in this study. When female rats were given the drug for 5 days after mating, delayed or inhibited implantation, an effect consistent with anti-estrogen administration in rodents was noted (3,4). Although pups were born up to a week late, they were morphologically and developmentally normal. Raloxifene given to pregnant rats from postimplantation until a few days before term caused impaired fetal growth. A higher dose decreased fetal viability without an increase in malformations (5,6). None of these studies compared the doses with the human dose.

In a 21-month carcinogenicity study in female mice with doses that produced systemic exposures that were 0.3–34 times the exposure in postmenopausal women taking 60 mg/day, an increased incidence of ovarian tumors, benign and malignant, were observed. In male mice, doses that were 4.7–24 times the AUC in humans were associated with an increase in testicular and prostatic tumors. Raloxifene was not genotoxic in multiple assays (1).

In fertility studies, no pregnancies resulted when daily doses ≥0.8 times the HD were given to male and female rats. Daily doses up to 16 times the HD had no effect on sperm production or quality, or reproductive performance in male rats. However, in female rats, daily doses that were 0.02–1.6 times the HD disrupted estrous cycles and inhibited ovulation. Doses that were ≥0.02 times the HD given during the preimplantation period caused delayed and disrupted embryo implantation, resulting in prolonged gestation and reduced litter size. These reproductive and developmental effects are consistent with the estrogen receptor activity of the drug (1).

It is not known whether raloxifene crosses the human placenta. The molecular weight (about 474 for the free base) and the long elimination half-life suggest that the drug will cross to the embryo–fetus. However, the high plasma protein binding might limit the exposure.

BREASTFEEDING SUMMARY

No reports describing the use of raloxifene during human lactation have been located. However, such reports are unlikely because of the drug's indications. The molecular weight (about 474 for the free base) and the long elimination half-life (32.5 hours) suggest that the drug will be excreted into breast milk, but the high plasma protein binding (95%) might limit the exposure. However, as with other weak bases, accumulation in the relatively acidic milk may occur. Raloxifene is an estrogen antagonist in breast tissue. We agree with the manufacturer that it is contraindicated during breastfeeding.

References

1. Product information. Evista. Eli Lilly, 2011.
2. Hoyt JA, Fisher LF, Buelke-Sam JL, Hoffman WP, Francis PC. The selective estrogen receptor modulator, raloxifene: reproductive assessments following premating exposure in female rats. Teratology 1996;53:103.
3. Clarke DO, Griffey KI, Buelke-Sam JL, Francis PC. The selective estrogen receptor modulator, raloxifene: reproductive assessments following preimplantation exposure in mated female rats. Teratology 1996;53:103–4.
4. Clarke DO, Griffey KI, Buelke-Sam J, Francis PC. The selective estrogen receptor modulator, raloxifene: reproductive assessments following preimplantation exposure in mated female rats. Reprod Toxicol 1998;12:247–59.
5. Buelke-Sam J, Bryant HU, Francis PC. The selective estrogen receptor modulator, raloxifene: an overview of nonclinical pharmacology and reproductive and developmental testing. Reprod Toxicol 1998;12:217–21.
6. Byrd RA, Francis PC. The selective estrogen receptor modulator raloxifene: segment II studies in rats and rabbits. Teratology 1996;53:104.

RALTEGRAVIR

Antiviral

PREGNANCY RECOMMENDATION: Compatible—Maternal Benefit >> Embryo–Fetal Risk
BREASTFEEDING RECOMMENDATION: Contraindicated

PREGNANCY SUMMARY

No reports describing the use of raltegravir in human pregnancy have been located. Although the animal data suggest low risk, the absence of human pregnancy experience prevents an assessment of the embryo–fetal risk. If indicated, the drug should not be withheld because of pregnancy.

FETAL RISK SUMMARY

Raltegravir is an HIV type 1 (HIV-1) integrase strand transfer inhibitor. There are no other antiviral agents in this class. Raltegravir, in combination with other antiretroviral agents, is indicated for the treatment of HIV-1 infection in treatment-experienced adult patients who have evidence of viral replication and HIV-1 strains resistant to multiple antiretroviral agents. The drug is partially metabolized by glucuronidation. Plasma protein binding is about 83% and the apparent terminal half-life is about 9 hours (1).

Reproduction studies have been conducted in rats and rabbits. In these species, at doses producing systemic exposures up to 3–4 times the human exposure at the recommended human dose (HERHD), no treatment-related effects on embryo–fetal survival or fetal weights were observed. In pregnant rats, an exposure 3 times the HERHD caused an increased incidence of supernumerary ribs. In pregnant rabbits receiving exposures that were 3–4 times the HERHD, no treatment-related external, visceral, or skeletal changes were observed (1).

Raltegravir crosses the placenta in rats and rabbits. In rats, doses producing systemic exposures that were 3–4 times the HERHD resulted in fetal plasma concentrations that were about 1.5–2.5 times the maternal plasma at 1 and 24 hours postdose, respectively. In rabbits, a similar maternal exposure produced mean drug concentrations in fetal plasma that were 2% of the mean maternal concentration at both 1 and 24 hours postdose (1).

It is not known if raltegravir crosses the human placenta. Although the molecular weight (about 483), moderate plasma protein binding, and terminal half-life suggest that exposure of the embryo–fetus will occur, the low lipid solubility might mitigate the amount of exposure.

The Antiretroviral Pregnancy Registry reported, for the period January 1989 through July 2009, prospective data (reported before the outcomes were known) involving 4702 live births that had been exposed during the 1st trimester to one or more antiretroviral agents (2). Congenital defects were noted in 134, a prevalence of 2.8% (95% confidence interval [CI] 2.4–3.4). In the 6100 live births with earliest exposure in the 2nd/3rd trimesters, there were 153 infants with defects (2.5%, 95% CI 2.1–2.9). The prevalence rates for the two periods did not differ significantly. There were 288 infants with birth defects among 10,803 live births with exposure anytime during pregnancy (2.7%, 95% CI 2.4–3.0). The prevalence rate did not differ significantly from the rate expected in a nonexposed population. There were 18 outcomes exposed to raltegravir (8 in the 1st trimester and 10 in the 2nd/3rd trimesters) in combination with other antiretroviral agents. There were no birth defects. In reviewing the birth defects of prospective and retrospective (pregnancies reported after the outcomes were known) registered cases, the Registry concluded that except for isolated cases of neural tube defects with efavirenz exposure in retrospective reports, there was no other pattern of anomalies (isolated or syndromic) (2). Health care professionals are encouraged to register patients exposed to raltegravir during pregnancy in the Antiviral Pregnancy Registry by calling the toll-free number 800-258-4263. (See Lamivudine for required statement.)

Two reviews, one in 1996 and the other in 1997, concluded that all women currently receiving antiretroviral therapy should continue to receive therapy during pregnancy and that treatment of the mother with monotherapy should be considered inadequate (3,4). The same conclusion was reached in a 2003 review with the added admonishment that therapy must be continuous to prevent emergence of resistant viral strains (5). In 2009, the updated U.S. Department of Health and Human Services guidelines for the use of antiretroviral agents in HIV-1 infected patients continued the recommendation that therapy, with the exception of efavirenz, should be continued during pregnancy (6). If indicated, raltegravir should not be withheld in pregnancy since the expected benefit to the HIV-positive mother outweighs the unknown risk to the fetus. Updated guidelines for the use of antiretroviral drugs to reduce perinatal HIV-1 transmission also were released in 2010 (7). Women receiving antiretroviral therapy during pregnancy should continue the therapy but, regardless of the regimen, zidovudine administration is recommended during the intrapartum period to prevent vertical transmission of HIV to the newborn (7).

BREASTFEEDING SUMMARY

No reports describing the use of raltegravir during lactation have been located. The molecular weight (about 483), moderate plasma protein binding (about 83%), and long terminal half-life (about 9 hours) suggest that the drug will be excreted into breast milk, but the low lipid solubility might mitigate the amount of exposure. The effect on a nursing infant is unknown.

Reports on the use of raltegravir during human lactation are unlikely, however, because the antiviral agent is used in the treatment of HIV infection. HIV-1 is transmitted in milk, and in developed countries, breastfeeding is not recommended (3,4,6,8–10). In developing countries, breastfeeding is undertaken, despite the risk, because there are no affordable milk substitutes available. Until 1999, no studies had been published that examined the effect of any antiretroviral therapy on HIV-1 transmission in milk. In that year, a study involving zidovudine was published that measured a 38% reduction in vertical transmission of HIV-1 infection despite breastfeeding when compared with controls (see Zidovudine).

R

References

1. Product information. Isentress. Merck & Company, 2008.
2. Antiretroviral Pregnancy Registry Steering Committee. *Antiretroviral Pregnancy Registry International Interim Report for 1 January 1989 through 31 July 2009*. Wilmington, NC: Registry Coordinating Center; 2009. Available at www.apregistry.com. Accessed May 29, 2010.
3. Carpenter CCJ, Fischi MA, Hammer SM, Hirsch MS, Jacobsen DM, Katzenstein DA, Montaner JSG, Richman DD, Saag MS, Schooley RT, Thompson MA, Vella S, Yeni PG, Volberding PA. Antiretroviral therapy for HIV infection in 1996. JAMA 1996;276:146–54.
4. Minkoff H, Augenbraun M. Antiretroviral therapy for pregnant women. Am J Obstet Gynecol 1997;176:478–89.
5. Minkoff H. Human immunodeficiency virus infection in pregnancy. Obstet Gynecol 2003;101:797–810.
6. Panel on Antiretroviral Guidelines for Adults and Adolescents. *Guidelines for the Use of Antiretroviral Agents in HIV-1-infected Adults and Adolescents*. Department of Health and Human Services. December 1,

2009:1–161. Available at http://www.aidsinfo.nih.gov/ContentFiles/AdultandAdolescentGL.pdf. Accessed September 17, 2010:60, 96–8.

7. Panel on Treatment of HIV-Infected Pregnant Women and Prevention of Perinatal Transmission. *Recommendations for Use of Antiretroviral Drugs in Pregnant HIV-1-Infected Women for Maternal Health and Interventions to Reduce Perinatal HIV Transmission in the United States*. May 24, 2010:1–117. Available at http://aidsinfo.nih.gov/ContentFiles/PerinatalGL.pdf. Accessed September 17, 2010:30 (Table 5).
8. Brown ZA, Watts DH. Antiviral therapy in pregnancy. Clin Obstet Gynecol 1990;33:276–89.
9. De Martino M, Tovo P-A, Pezzotti P, Galli L, Massironi E, Ruga E, Floreea F, Plebani A, Gabiano C, Zuccotti GV. HIV-1 transmission through breast-milk: appraisal of risk according to duration of feeding. AIDS 1992;6:991–7.
10. Van de Perre P. Postnatal transmission of human immunodeficiency virus type 1: the breast feeding dilemma. Am J Obstet Gynecol 1995;173:483–7.

RAMELTEON

Hypnotic

PREGNANCY RECOMMENDATION: No Human Data—Animal Data Suggest Low Risk
BREASTFEEDING RECOMMENDATION: No Human Data—Potential Toxicity

PREGNANCY SUMMARY

No reports describing the use of ramelteon in human pregnancy have been located. The drug has caused developmental toxicity in one animal species, but only at maternally toxic doses and exposures that were much higher than those used or obtained in humans. Although the animal data are reassuring, the complete lack of human pregnancy experience prevents a more-complete assessment of the embryo–fetal risk. However, long-term exposure in rodents has been associated with carcinogenic effects and this should be considered if ramelteon is used frequently in pregnancy. Infrequent or inadvertent exposure during gestation does not appear to represent a significant risk to the embryo or fetus.

FETAL RISK SUMMARY

Ramelteon is a melatonin receptor agonist with high affinity for melatonin MT_1 and MT_2 receptors. It is indicated for the treatment of insomnia characterized by difficulty with sleep onset. Other than melatonin itself (available as an orphan drug and as a nutritional supplement), there are no other hypnotic agents commercially available with this mechanism of action. Ramelteon undergoes extensive first-pass hepatic metabolism and one of the metabolites is active. About 82% of ramelteon is bound to serum proteins, primarily albumin. The elimination half-life of ramelteon is 1–2.6 hours, whereas the elimination half-life of the active metabolite is 2–5 hours (1).

R

Reproduction studies have been conducted in rats and rabbits. During organogenesis in rats, a dose 197 times higher than the maximum recommended human dose (MRHD) based on BSA (MRHD-BSA) was teratogenic, but this dose also caused maternal toxicity (decreased weight). Structural defects noted in the fetuses were diaphragmatic hernia and minor anatomical variations of the skeleton (irregularly shaped scapula). At 786 times the MRHD-BSA, reductions in fetal body weight and cysts on the external genitalia were additionally observed. The no-effect levels for teratogenicity for the parent compound and its active metabolite were 1892 and 45 times, respectively, the MRHD based on AUC (MRHD-AUC). The no-effect level for pre- and postnatal development (dosing from day 6 of gestation through weaning on postpartum day 21) in the rat was 39 times the MRHD-BSA (1).

During organogenesis in rabbits, doses producing exposures of the parent compound and metabolite that were 11,862 and 99 times, respectively, the MRHD-AUC caused maternal toxicity but no fetal effects. Therefore, these exposure comparisons were the no-effect levels for teratogenicity in rabbits (1).

In 2-year studies, ramelteon demonstrated dose-related carcinogenicity in mice and rats. The drug was not mutagenic in various tests, but a chromosomal aberration assay was positive. No effects were observed in mating behavior or fertility in male rats at doses up to 786 times the MRHD-BSA. In female rats, doses 79 times the MRHD-BSA were associated with irregular estrus cycles, reductions in the number of implants, and reductions in the number of live embryos. The no-effect dose for fertility endpoints in female rats was 26 times the MRHD-BSA (1).

It is not known if ramelteon or its active metabolite crosses the human placenta. The molecular weight of ramelteon (about 259) and the elimination half-lives of ramelteon and its active metabolite suggest that exposure of the embryo–fetus to both will probably occur.

BREASTFEEDING SUMMARY

No reports describing the use of ramelteon during human lactation have been located. The molecular weight (about 259) and the elimination half-lives of ramelteon (1–2.6 hours) and its active metabolite (2–5 hours) suggest that both will be excreted into breast milk. The effect of this exposure on a nursing infant is unknown, but sedation is a potential complication.

Reference

1. Product information. Rozerem. Takeda Pharmaceuticals North America, 2005.

RAMIPRIL

Antihypertensive

PREGNANCY RECOMMENDATION: Human Data Suggest Risk in 2nd and 3rd Trimesters
BREASTFEEDING RECOMMENDATION: No Human Data—Probably Compatible

PREGNANCY SUMMARY

The fetal toxicity of ramipril in the 2nd and 3rd trimesters is similar to other angiotensin-converting enzyme (ACE) inhibitors. The use of this drug during the 2nd and 3rd trimesters may cause teratogenicity and severe fetal and neonatal toxicity. Fetal toxic effects may include anuria, oligohydramnios, fetal hypocalvaria, intrauterine growth restriction (IUGR), prematurity, and patent ductus arteriosus. Stillbirth or neonatal death may occur. Anuria-associated oligohydramnios may produce fetal limb contractures, craniofacial deformation, and pulmonary hypoplasia. Severe anuria and hypotension, which is resistant to both pressor agents and volume expansion, may occur in the newborn following in utero exposure. Newborn renal function and blood pressure should be closely monitored.

FETAL RISK SUMMARY

Ramipril is an ACE inhibitor. Reproduction studies in rats, rabbits, and monkeys at doses 400, 2, and 400 times, respectively, the recommended human dose based on BSA revealed no teratogenic effects (1).

It is not known if ramipril crosses the human placenta. The molecular weight (about 417) is low enough that exposure of the embryo–fetus should be expected.

A 2005 case report described the pregnancy outcome of a 33-year-old woman treated with ramipril in the first 8 weeks of an unplanned pregnancy (2). Diseases in the patient included hypertension, morbid obesity, type 2 diabetes mellitus, and hypercholesterolemia. Other drugs used by the woman were glimepiride, orlistat, thiocolchicoside (a muscle relaxant), simvastatin, metformin, ciprofloxacin, and aspirin. When pregnancy was diagnosed at 8 weeks, all medications were stopped and she was started on methyldopa and insulin. She gave birth at 38 weeks to a 3470-g female infant with Apgar scores of 5 and 7 at 1 and 5 minutes, respectively. No minor or major malformations were observed in the infant (2).

A retrospective study using pharmacy-based data from the Tennessee Medicaid program identified 209 infants, born between 1985 and 2000, who had 1st trimester exposure to ACE inhibitors (3). Infants of mothers with evidence of diabetes, either before or during pregnancy, were excluded, as were those exposed to angiotensin-receptor antagonists (ARBs), ACE inhibitors or other antihypertensives beyond the 1st trimester, and exposure to known teratogens. Two comparison groups, other antihypertensives (N = 202) and no antihypertensives (N = 29,096), were formed. The number of major birth defects in each of the three groups was 18 (8.6%), 4 (2%), and 834 (2.9%), respectively. Compared with the no-antihypertensives group, exposure to ACE inhibitors was associated with a significantly increased risk of major defects (relative risk [RR] 2.71, 95% confidence interval [CI] 1.72–4.27). When the analysis was conducted by the type of defect, the highest rates were with cardiovascular defects, 9, 2, and 294, respectively, RR 3.72, 95% CI 1.89–7.30, and with CNS defects, 3, 0, and 80, respectively, RR 4.39, 95% CI 1.37–14.02. The major defects observed in the subject group were: atrial septal defect (N = 6) (includes three with pulmonic stenosis and/or three with patent ductus arteriosus [PDA]), renal dysplasia (N = 2), PDA alone (N = 2), and one each of ventricular septal defect, spina bifida, microcephaly with eye anomaly, coloboma, hypospadias, intestinal and choanal atresia, Hirschsprung disease, and diaphragmatic hernia (3). In an accompanying editorial, it was noted that neither previous reports of 1st trimester exposure to ACE inhibitors nor the animal studies had observed an increased risk of birth defects (4). It also was noted that no mechanism for ACE inhibitor–induced teratogenicity was known. A subsequent communication raising concerns about the validity of the study in terms of adequate exclusion of diabetes, charting and coding errors in busy medical practices, and the effects of maternal obesity (5) was addressed by the investigators (6).

A 2005 case report described a 28-year-old woman with chronic renal disease and hypertension (7). She presented at 25.5 weeks' gestation and had been taking before and throughout pregnancy ramipril 50 mg/day, nifedipine 60 mg/day, atenolol 50 mg/day, and hydroxychloroquine 200 mg/day. Severe oligohydramnios was noted and estimated fetal weight was at the 15th percentile. Ramipril was stopped and the dose of atenolol was increased. Three weeks later, the amniotic fluid volume had returned to normal (amniotic fluid index 15.3). At 30 weeks, worsening hypertension and renal function was noted and the woman gave birth by cesarean section to an 880-g female infant with Apgar scores of 8 and 9. The infant had respiratory distress, but there was no evidence of cerebral hemorrhage and her renal impairment was resolving (7).

In a 2009 case report, a 42-year-old woman with type 2 diabetes and hypertension was treated during the first 17 weeks' gestation with gliclazide 30 mg/day and ramipril 10 mg/day (8). This therapy was discontinued and replaced with insulin and methyldopa. At 36 weeks', she gave birth by cesarean section to a healthy 3200-g female infant with Apgar scores of 8 and 10. No malformations were noted and the infant was doing well at 1.5 years of age (8).

Ramipril and other ACE inhibitors are human teratogens when used in the 2nd and 3rd trimesters, producing fetal

R

hypocalvaria and renal defects. The cause of the defects and other toxicity is probably related to fetal hypotension and decreased renal blood flow. The compromise of the fetal renal system may result in severe, and at times fatal, anuria, both in the fetus and in the newborn. Anuria-associated oligohydramnios may produce pulmonary hypoplasia, limb contractures, persistent PDA, craniofacial deformation, and neonatal death (9,10). IUGR, prematurity, and severe neonatal hypotension may also be observed. Two reviews of fetal and newborn renal function indicated that both renal perfusion and glomerular plasma flow are low during gestation and that high levels of angiotensin II may be physiologically necessary to maintain glomerular filtration at low perfusion pressures (11,12). Ramipril prevents the conversion of angiotensin I to angiotensin II and, thus, may lead to in utero renal failure. Since the primary means of removal of the drug is renal, the impairment of this system in the newborn prevents elimination of the drug resulting in prolonged hypotension. Newborn renal function and blood pressure should be closely monitored. If oligohydramnios occurs, stopping ramipril may resolve the problem but may not improve infant outcome because of irreversible fetal damage (9). In those cases in which ramipril must be used to treat the mother's disease, the lowest possible dose should be used combined with close monitoring of amniotic fluid levels and fetal well-being. Guidelines for counseling exposed pregnant patients have been published and should be of benefit to health professionals faced with this task (9,13).

The observation in Tennessee Medicaid data of an increased risk of major congenital defects after 1st trimester exposure to ACE inhibitors raises concerns about teratogenicity that have not been seen in other studies (4). Medicaid data are a valuable tool for identifying early signals of teratogenicity, but are subject to a number of shortcomings and their findings must be considered hypotheses until confirmed by independent studies.

A 2012 review of the use of ACE inhibitors and ARBs in the 1st trimester concluded that there may be an elevated teratogenic risk, but the risk appeared to be related to other factors (14). The factors, that typically coexist with hypertension in pregnancy, included diabetes, advanced maternal age, and obesity.

BREASTFEEDING SUMMARY

No reports describing the use of ramipril during lactation have been located. The molecular weight (about 417) is low enough that excretion into breast milk should be expected. Other ACE inhibitors are excreted into breast milk and the American Academy of Pediatrics classifies them as compatible with breastfeeding (see Captopril and Enalapril).

References

1. Product information. Altace. Monarch Pharmaceuticals, 2000.
2. Kalyoncu NI, Yaris F, Kadioglu M, Kesim M, Ulku C, Yaris E, Unsal M, Dikici M. Pregnancy outcome following exposure to orlistat, ramipril, glimepiride in a woman with metabolic syndrome. Saudi Med J 2005;26:497–9.
3. Cooper WO, Hernandez-Diaz S, Arbogast PG, Dudley JA, Dyer S, Gideon PS, Hall K, Ray WA. Major congenital malformations after first-trimester exposure to ACE inhibitors. N Engl J Med 2006;354:2443–51.
4. Friedman JM. ACE inhibitors and congenital anomalies. N Engl J Med 2006;354:2498–500.
5. Scialli AR, Lione A. ACE inhibitors and major congenital malformations. N Engl J Med 2006;355:1280.
6. Cooper WO, Ray WA. Reply—ACE inhibitors and major congenital malformations. N Engl J Med 2006;355:1281.
7. Shrim A, Berger H, Kingdom J, Hamoudi A, Shah PS, Koren G. Prolonged exposure to angiotensin-converting enzyme inhibitors during pregnancy. Can Fam Physician 2005;51:1335–7.
8. Kolagasi O, Sari F, Akar M, Sari R. Normal pregnancy and healthy child after continued exposure to gliclazide and ramipril during pregnancy. Ann Pharmacother 2009;43:147–9.
9. Barr M Jr. Teratogen update: angiotensin-converting enzyme inhibitors. Teratology 1994;50:399–409.
10. Shotan A, Widerhorn J, Hurst A, Elkayam U. Risks of angiotensin-converting enzyme inhibition during pregnancy: experimental and clinical evidence, potential mechanisms, and recommendations for use. Am J Med 1994;96:451–6.
11. Robillard JE, Nakamura KT, Matherne GP, Jose PA. Renal hemodynamics and functional adjustments to postnatal life. Semin Perinatol 1988;12:143–50.
12. Guignard J-P, Gouyon J-B. Adverse effects of drugs on the immature kidney. Biol Neonate 1988;53:243–52.
13. Brent RL, Beckman DA. Angiotensin-converting enzyme inhibitors, an embryopathic class of drugs with unique properties: information for clinical teratology counselors. Teratology 1991;43:543–6.
14. Polifka JE. Is there an embryopathy associated with first-trimester exposure to angiotensin-converting enzyme inhibitors and angiotensin receptor antagonists? A critical review of the evidence. Birth Defects Res (Part A) 2012;94:576–98.

RANIBIZUMAB

Ophthalmic

PREGNANCY RECOMMENDATION: No Human Data—Probably Compatible
BREASTFEEDING RECOMMENDATION: No Human Data—Probably Compatible

PREGNANCY SUMMARY

No reports describing the use of ranibizumab in human pregnancy have been located. There also is no animal reproduction data. The predicted amount of antibody in the systemic circulation, however, is about 90,000-fold lower than the amounts in the vitreous and is below the estimated therapeutic concentration (1). Based on this estimation, the exposure and effect on an embryo or fetus probably is nil. Thus, if a woman requires ranibizumab, it should not be withheld because of pregnancy.

FETAL RISK SUMMARY

Ranibizumab binds to and inhibits vascular endothelial growth factor A (VEGF-A). It is a recombinant humanized immunoglobulin G1 (IgG1) kappa isotype monoclonal antibody fragment that is indicated for the treatment of neovascular (wet) age-related macular degeneration. It is in the same class as pegaptanib. Ranibizumab is administered as a once-monthly, 0.5-mg intravitreal injection. After monthly injections, the maximum ranibizumab serum concentrations are low (0.3–2.36 ng/mL) occurring about 1 day after a dose. These concentrations are less than the therapeutic levels (11–27 ng/mL) thought to be necessary to inhibit the biological activity of VEGF-A. The estimated average vitreous elimination half-life is about 9 days (1).

Reproduction, carcinogenicity, mutagenicity, and fertility studies in animals or humans have not been conducted (1).

It is not known if ranibizumab crosses the human placenta. The high molecular weight (48,000) and very low concentrations in the systemic circulation suggest that the antibody will not cross to the embryo or fetus. However, IgG crosses the placenta and so might ranibizumab.

BREASTFEEDING SUMMARY

No reports describing the use of ranibizumab during lactation have been located. Although the long plasma elimination half-life (about 9 days) favors excretion, the molecular weight (48,000) and very low plasma concentrations suggest that the antibody will not be detected in milk. However, IgG is excreted into milk. Nevertheless, even if excretion does occur it should be in clinically insignificant amounts. If a lactating woman requires ranibizumab, it should not be withheld because she is breastfeeding.

Reference

1. Product information. Lucentis. Genentech, 2007.

RANITIDINE

Gastrointestinal Agent (Antisecretory)

PREGNANCY RECOMMENDATION: Compatible
BREASTFEEDING RECOMMENDATION: Limited Human Data—Probably Compatible

PREGNANCY SUMMARY

The absence of teratogenicity or toxicity in animals and the available human pregnancy data suggest that ranitidine is not a major teratogen. Because it has no antiandrogenic activity in animals or nonpregnant humans, ranitidine may be a safer choice than cimetidine for chronic use during pregnancy. The antiandrogenic activity of cimetidine, however, has not been observed or studied following in utero exposure (see Cimetidine). Ranitidine-induced anaphylactoid shock has been reported in four laboring women. A study showing an association between in utero exposure to gastric acid–suppressing drugs and childhood allergy and asthma requires confirmation.

FETAL RISK SUMMARY

Ranitidine is a competitive, reversible inhibitor of histamine H_2-receptors (H_2 blockers) used in treatment and maintenance of patients with duodenal or gastric ulcers, pathologic hypersecretory conditions such as Zollinger-Ellison syndrome, and gastroesophageal reflux disease (GERD). The drug is partially metabolized to apparently inactive metabolites. Serum protein binding is minimal (average 15%) and the elimination half-life is 2.5–3.0 hours (1).

Reproduction studies with ranitidine in rats and rabbits at doses up to 160 times the human dose have revealed no evidence of impaired fertility or fetal harm (1–3). In contrast to the controversy surrounding cimetidine, ranitidine apparently has no antiandrogenic activity in humans (4) or in animals (5,6) (see also Cimetidine).

Consistent with the molecular weight (about 351), limited metabolism, and elimination half-life, ranitidine crosses the human placenta. At term, mean fetal:maternal ratios after 50 mg IV and 150 mg orally were 0.9 and 0.38, respectively (7–9). An in vitro study also documented transfer in term human placentas (10).

In a surveillance study of Michigan Medicaid recipients involving 229,101 completed pregnancies conducted between 1985 and 1992, 516 newborns had been exposed to ranitidine during the 1st trimester (F. Rosa, personal communication, FDA, 1993). A total of 23 (4.5%) major birth defects were observed (22 expected). Specific data were available for six defect categories, including (observed/expected) 6/5 cardiovascular defects, 1/1 oral clefts, 1/0.5 spina bifida, 1/1 polydactyly, 0/1 limb reduction defects, and 1/1 hypospadias. These data do not support an association between the drug and congenital defects.

Ranitidine has been used alone and in combination with antacids to prevent gastric acid aspiration (Mendelson's syndrome) before vaginal delivery or cesarean section (7–9, 11–14). No effect was observed in the frequency and strength of uterine contractions, in fetal heart rate pattern, or in Apgar scores (7). Neonatal gastric acidity was not affected at 24 hours. No problems in the newborn attributable to ranitidine were reported in these studies.

Ranitidine has been studied for its effectiveness in alleviating the symptoms of heartburn during pregnancy (15–17).

A twice-daily dosage regimen of ranitidine was effective for this indication (15–17), including in those cases resistant to antacids alone (17). Ranitidine was also effective in controlling gastric acid secretion in pregnant women with Zollinger-Ellison syndrome (18).

In a 1991 report, 23 women were exposed in the 1st trimester to ranitidine (*N* = 13), cimetidine (*N* = 9), or both (*N* = 1) (19). The pregnancy outcomes were 2 spontaneous abortions (SABs), 2 elective abortions (EABs), 18 normal births, and 1 infant with a large hemangioma of the upper eye lid (removed without incidence). The outcomes suggested that the agents were not teratogenic (19).

A 1996 prospective cohort study compared the pregnancy outcomes of 178 women who were exposed during pregnancy to H_2 blockers with 178 controls matched for maternal age, smoking, and heavy alcohol consumption (20). All of the women had contacted a teratology information service concerning gestational exposure to H_2 blockers (subjects) or nonteratogenic or nonfetotoxic agents (controls). Among subjects (mean daily dose in parentheses), 71% took ranitidine (258 mg), 16% cimetidine (487 mg), 8% famotidine (32 mg), and 5% nizatidine (283 mg). There were no significant differences between the outcomes of subjects and controls in terms of live births, SABs, EABs, gestational age at birth, delivery method, birth weight, infants small for gestational age, or major malformations. Among subjects, there were 3 birth defects (2.1%) among the 142 exposed to H_2 blockers in the 1st trimester: one each of atrial septal defect, ventricular septal defect, and tetralogy of Fallot. There were 5 birth defects (3.0%) among the 165 exposed anytime during pregnancy. For controls, the rates of defects were 3.5% (1st trimester) and 3.1% (anytime). There were also no differences between the groups in neonatal health problems and developmental milestones, but two children (one subject and one control) were diagnosed as developmentally delayed. The investigators concluded that 1st trimester exposure to H_2 blockers did not represent a major teratogenic risk (20).

Data from the Swedish Medical Birth Registry were presented in 1998 (21). A total of 553 infants (6 sets of twins) were delivered from 547 women who had used acid-suppressing drugs early in pregnancy. The odds ratio (OR) for malformations after H_2 blockers was 0.86, 95% confidence interval (CI) 0.33–2.23. Of the 19 infants with birth defects, 9 had been exposed to H_2 blockers, 1 of whom was also exposed to omeprazole. Ranitidine was the only acid-suppressing drug exposure in 156 infants. Twenty other offspring were exposed in utero to ranitidine combined either with famotidine (2 infants) or with omeprazole (18 infants). Seven infants with birth defects were exposed to ranitidine: six where ranitidine was the only acid-suppressing agent used and one exposed to ranitidine combined with omeprazole. The defects were cerebral arteriovenous malformation, unspecified cardiac defect, hydronephrosis, undescended testicle, hypospadias, and unstable hip. Hypospadias was also observed in a newborn exposed to a combination of ranitidine and omeprazole (see Omeprazole for additional details of this study) (21).

Two databases, one from England and the other from Italy, were combined for a study published in 1999 that was designed to assess the incidence of congenital malformations in women who had received a prescription during the 1st trimester for an acid-suppressing drug (ranitidine, cimetidine, and omeprazole) (22). Nonexposed women were selected from the same databases to form a control group. SABs and EABs (except two cases for anomalies that were grouped with stillbirths) were excluded from the analysis. Stillbirths were defined as any pregnancy loss occurring at 28 weeks' gestation or later. Ranitidine was taken in 322 pregnancies, resulting in 330 live births (29 premature), 2 stillbirths, and 1 neonatal death. Twenty (6.1%) of the newborns had a congenital malformation (shown by system): CNS (spina bifida/hydrocephaly), craniofacial (cleft palate only; asymmetric skull/plagiocephaly; tongue tie), eye (Duane's eye syndrome), cardiac (septal defect; anomaly of cardiac valve), musculoskeletal (dysplastic hip/dislocation/clicking hip, *N* = 3; syndactyly; sacral sinus), genital and urinary (undescended testes, *N* = 2; congenital hydrocele/inguinal hernia, *N* = 2; ovarian cyst), multiple (pyloric stenosis and talipes equinovarus), and two genetic anomalies (Hallerman-Streiff and Down's syndromes). In addition, two newborns were small for gestational age and nine had a small head circumference for gestational age. In comparison, the outcomes of 1547 nonexposed pregnancies included 1560 live births (115 premature), 15 stillbirths (includes 2 EABs for anomalies), and 10 neonatal deaths. Sixty-four (4.1%) of the newborns had malformations involving the following: CNS (*N* = 2), head/face (*N* = 13), eye (*N* = 2), heart (*N* = 7), muscle/skeletal (*N* = 13), genital/urinary (*N* = 18), gastrointestinal (*N* = 2), and those of polyformation (*N* = 3), or known genetic defects (*N* = 4). There were 21 newborns that were small for gestational age and 78 had a small head circumference for gestational age. The relative risk of malformation (adjusted for mother's age and prematurity) associated with ranitidine was 1.5 (95% CI 0.9–2.6), with cimetidine 1.3 (95% CI 0.7–2.6), and with omeprazole 0.9 (95% CI 0.4–2.4) (22).

A population-based observational cohort study formed by linking data from three Swedish national health care registers over a 10-year period (1995–2004) was reported in 2009 (23). The main outcome measures were a diagnosis of allergic disease or a prescription for asthma or allergy medications. The drug types included in the study were gastric acid suppressors, including H_2 blockers, prostaglandins, proton pump inhibitors, combinations for eradication of *Helicobacter pylori*, and drugs for peptic ulcer and GERD. Of 585,716 children, 29,490 (5.0%) met the diagnosis and 5645 (1%) had been exposed to gastric acid–suppression therapy in pregnancy. Of these children, 405 (0.07%) were treated for allergic disease. For developing allergy, the OR was 1.43, 98% CI 1.29–1.59, irrespective of the drug, time of exposure during pregnancy, and maternal history of allergy. For developing childhood asthma, but not other allergic diseases, the OR was 1.51, 95% CI 1.35–1.69, irrespective of the type of acid-suppressive drug and the time of exposure in pregnancy. The authors proposed three possible mechanisms for their findings: (a) exposure to increased amounts of allergens could cause sensitization to digestion labile antigens in the fetus; (b) the maternal Th2 cytokine pattern could promote an allergy-prone phenotype in the fetus; and (c) maternal allergen-specific immunoglobulin could cross the placenta and sensitize fetal immune cells to food and airborne allergens. Several limitations of the study that might have affected their findings were identified, including a general increase in

R

childhood asthma but not necessarily an increase in allergic asthma (23). The study requires confirmation.

Severe anaphylactoid reactions were observed in four women who had received IV or oral ranitidine during labor (24–27). Fetal bradycardia was observed in two cases, but the heart rates normalized before birth. The two cases as well as a third newborn had normal Apgar scores and did well (24–26). An emergency cesarean section was required in the fourth case when the mother developed severe systolic hypotension and the fetal heart rate decreased to 70 beats/minute (27). Apgar scores in the newborn were 1 and 4 at 1 and 5 minutes, respectively. The female infant had seizure-like movement in the NICU and was discharged home on day 19 on phenobarbital. At 8 months of age, the baby was still receiving phenobarbital but no seizures or physical or developmental abnormalities were noted (27).

A 2005 study evaluated the outcomes of 553 pregnancies after exposure to H_2 blockers, 501 (91%) in the 1st trimester (28). The data were collected by the European Network of Teratology Information Services (ENTIS). The agents and number of cases were ranitidine 335, cimetidine 113, famotidine 75, nizatidine 15, and roxatidine 15. No increase in the number of major malformations were noted (28).

Four reviews on the treatment of GERD have concluded that H_2 blockers, with the possible exception of nizatidine, could be used in pregnancy with relative safety (29–32).

A 2009 meta-analysis of published studies was conducted to assess the safety of H_2 blockers that were used in 2398 pregnancies (33). Compared with 119,892 nonexposed pregnancies, the OR for congenital malformations was 1.14 (95% CI 0.89–1.45), whereas the ORs and 95% CIs for SABs, preterm birth, and small for gestational age were 0.62 (0.36–1.05), 1.17 (0.94–1.147), and 0.28 (0.06–1.22), respectively. The authors concluded that H_2 blockers could be used safely in pregnancy (33).

A 2010 study from Israel identified 1148 infants exposed in the 1st trimester to H_2 blockers (34). No association with congenital malformations was found (OR 1.03, 95% CI 0.80–1.32). Moreover, no association was found with EABs, perinatal mortality, premature delivery, low birth weight, or low Apgar scores (34).

BREASTFEEDING SUMMARY

Following a single oral dose of 150 mg in six subjects, ranitidine milk concentrations increased with time, producing mean milk:plasma ratios at 2, 4, and 6 hours of 1.9, 2.8, and 6.7, respectively (35).

Markedly different results were observed in 1985 study (36). Ranitidine milk and blood concentrations were determined in a woman breastfeeding her healthy 54-day-old infant. The woman had taken four 150-mg (2.44 mg/kg) doses at 12-hour intervals immediately before sampling. Pooled milk/maternal blood concentrations (ng/mL) (milk:serum ratio) were: predose 993/53 (18.73), 1.5 hours postdose 722/106 (6.81), 5.5 hours postdose 2610/309 (8.44), and 1569/66 (23.77). The data suggested that steady-state conditions had not yet been achieved. No adverse effects in the nursing infant were noted (36).

The effects from long-term exposure to the above concentrations on the nursing infant are not known. Ranitidine decreases gastric acidity, but this effect has not been studied in nursing infants. However, cimetidine, an agent with similar activity, is classified as compatible during breastfeeding by the American Academy of Pediatrics (see Cimetidine).

References

1. Product information. Zantac. Glaxo Wellcome, 2011.
2. Higashida N, Kamada S, Sakanove M, Takeuchi M, Simpo K, Tanabe T. Teratogenicity studies in rats and rabbits. J Toxicol Sci 1983;8:101–50. As cited in Shepard TH. *Catalog of Teratogenic Agents*. 6th ed. Baltimore, MD: The Johns Hopkins University Press, 1989:550.
3. Higashida N, Kamada S, Sakanove M, Takeuchi M, Simpo K, Tanabe T. Teratogenicity studies in rats and rabbits. J Toxicol Sci 1984;9:53–72. As cited in Shepard TH. *Catalog of Teratogenic Agents*. 6th ed. Baltimore, MD: The Johns Hopkins University Press, 1989:550.
4. Wang C, Wong KL, Lam KC, Lai CL. Ranitidine does not affect gonadal function in man. Br J Clin Pharmacol 1983;16:430–2.
5. Parker S, Udani M, Gavaler JS, Van Thiel DH. Pre- and neonatal exposure to cimetidine but not ranitidine adversely affects adult sexual functioning of male rats. Neurobehav Toxicol Teratol 1984;6:313–8.
6. Parker S, Schade RR, Pohl CR, Gavaler JS, Van Thiel DH. Prenatal and neonatal exposure of male rat pups to cimetidine but not ranitidine adversely affects subsequent adult sexual functioning. Gastroenterology 1984;86:675–80.
7. McAuley DM, Moore J, Dundee JW, McCaughey W. Preliminary report on the use of ranitidine as an antacid in obstetrics. Ir J Med Sci 1982;151:91–2.
8. McAuley DM, Moore J, McCaughey W, Donnelly BD, Dundee JW. Ranitidine as an antacid before elective caesarean section. Anaesthesia 1983;38:108–14.
9. McAuley DM, Moore J, Dundee JW, McCaughey W. Oral ranitidine in labour. Anaesthesia 1984;39:433–8.
10. Dicke JM, Johnson RF, Henderson GI, Kuehl TJ, Schenker S. A comparative evaluation of the transport of H_2-receptor antagonists by the human and baboon placenta. Am J Med Sci 1988;295:198–206.
11. Gillett GB, Watson JD, Langford RM. Prophylaxis against acid aspiration syndrome in obstetric practice. Anesthesiology 1984;60:525.
12. Mathews HML, Wilson CM, Thompson EM, Moore J. Combination treatment with ranitidine and sodium bicarbonate prior to obstetric anaesthesia. Anaesthesia 1986;41:1202–6.
13. Ikenoue T, Iito J, Matsuda Y, Hokanishi H. Effects of ranitidine on maternal gastric juice and neonates when administered prior to caesarean section. Aliment Pharmacol Ther 1991;5:315–8.
14. Rout CC, Rocke DA, Gouws E. Intravenous ranitidine reduces the risk of acid aspiration of gastric contents at emergency cesarean section. Anest Analg 1993;76:156–61.
15. Larson J, Patatanian E, Miner P, Rayburn W, Robinson M. Double-blind, placebo controlled study of ranitidine (Zantac) for gastroesophageal reflux symptoms during pregnancy (abstract). Am J Obstet Gynecol 1997;176:S23.
16. Larson JD, Patatanian E, Miner PB Jr, Rayburn WF, Robinson MG. Double-blind, placebo-controlled study of ranitidine for gastroesophageal reflux symptoms during pregnancy. Obstet Gynecol 1997;90:83–7.
17. Rayburn W, Liles E, Christensen H, Robinson M. Antacids vs. antacids plus non-prescription ranitidine for heartburn during pregnancy. Int J Gynaecol Obstet 1999;66:35–7.
18. Stewart CA, Termanini B, Sutliff VE, Corleto VD, Weber HC, Gibril F, Jensen RT. Management of the Zollinger-Ellison syndrome in pregnancy. Am J Obstet Gynecol 1997;176:224–33.
19. Koren G, Zemlickis DM. Outcome of pregnancy after first trimester exposure to H2 receptor antagonists. Am J Perinatol 1991;8:37–8.
20. Magee LA, Inocencion G, Kamboj L, Rosetti F, Koren G. Safety of first trimester exposure to histamine H_2 blockers. A prospective cohort study. Dig Dis Sci 1996;41:1145–9.
21. Kallen B. Delivery outcome after the use of acid-suppressing drugs in early pregnancy with special reference to omeprazole. Br J Obstet Gynaecol 1998;105:877–81.
22. Ruigomez A, Rodriguez LAG, Cattaruzzi C, Troncon MG, Agostinis L, Wallander MA, Johansson S. Use of cimetidine, omeprazole, and ranitidine in pregnant women and pregnancy outcomes. Am J Epidemiol 1999;150:476–81.
23. Dehlink E, Yen E, Leichtner AM, Hait EJ, Fiebiger E. First evidence of a possible association between gastric acid suppression during pregnancy and childhood asthma: a population-based register study. Clin Exp Allergy 2009;39:246–53.

R

24. Greer IA, Fellows K. Anaphalactoid reaction to ranitidine in labour. Br J Clin Pract 1990;44:78.
25. Barry JE, Madan R, Hewitt PB. Anaphylactoid reaction to ranitidine in an obstetric patient. Anaesthesia 1992;47:360–1.
26. Powell JA, Maycock EJ. Anaphylactoid reaction to ranitidine in an obstetric patient. Anaesth Intensive Care 1993;21:702–3.
27. Kaneko K, Maruta H. Severe anaphylactoid reaction to ranitidine in a parturient with subsequent fetal distress. J Anesth 2003;17:199–200.
28. Garbis H, Elefant E, Diav-Citrin O, Mastroiacovo P, Schaefer C, Vial T, Clementi M, Valti E, McElhatton P, Smorlesij C, Rodriguez EP, Robert-Gnansia E, Merlob P, Peiker G, Pexieder T, Schueler L, Ritvanen A, Mathieu-Nolf M. Pregnancy outcome after exposure to ranitidine and other H_2-blockers—a collaborative study of the European Network of Teratology Information Services. Reprod Toxicol 2005;453–8.
29. Broussard CN, Richter JE. Treating gasto-oesophageal reflux disease during pregnancy and lactation. What are the safest therapy options? Drug Saf 1998;19:325–37.
30. Katz PO, Castell DO. Gastroesophageal reflux disease during pregnancy. Gastroenterol Clin N Am 1998;27:153–67.
31. Richter JE. Gastroesophageal reflux disease during pregnancy. Gastroenterol Clin N Am 2003;32:235–61.
32. Richter JE. Review article: the management of heartburn in pregnancy. Aliment Pharmacol Ther 2005;22:749–57.
33. Gill SK, O'Brien L, Koren G. The safety of histamine 2 (H2) blockers in pregnancy: a meta-analysis. Dig Dis Sci 2009;54:1835–8.
34. Matok I, Gorodischer R, Koren G, Sheiner E, Wiznitzer A, Uziel E, Levy A. The safety of H_2-blockers use during pregnancy. J Clin Pharmacol 2010;50:81–7.
35. Riley AJ, Crowley P, Harrison C. Transfer of ranitidine to biological fluids: milk and semen. In: Misiewicz JJ, Wormsley KG, eds. *Proceedings of the 2nd International Symposium on Ranitidine*. London, England: Medicine Publishing Foundation, 1981:78–81.
36. Kearns GL, McConnell RF Jr, Trang JM, Kluza RB. Appearance of ranitidine in breast milk following multiple dosing. Clin Pharm 1985;4:322–4.

RANOLAZINE

Antianginal Agent

PREGNANCY RECOMMENDATION: No Human Data—Animal Data Suggest Risk
BREASTFEEDING RECOMMENDATION: No Human Data—Potential Toxicity

PREGNANCY SUMMARY

No reports describing the use of ranolazine in human pregnancy have been located. The animal data suggest risk, but the absence of human pregnancy experience prevents a complete assessment of the embryo–fetal risk.

FETAL RISK SUMMARY

Ranolazine is an oral racemic mixture that has anti-ischemic and antianginal effects but is not a vasodilator. It is indicated for the treatment of chronic angina. There are no other agents in the cardiovascular subclass. The drug undergoes extensive metabolism. The activity of the metabolites has not been well characterized. Ranolazine is moderately bound (about 62%) to plasma proteins. The apparent terminal half-life is 7 hours (1).

Reproduction studies have been conducted in rats and rabbits. In pregnant rats, a dose 2 times the maximum recommended human dose based on BSA (MRHD) caused an increased incidence of misshapen sternebrae and reduced ossification of pelvic and cranial bones. In pregnant rabbits, a dose 1.5 times the MRHD was associated with reduced ossification of sternebrae. The doses in both species were associated with an increased maternal mortality rate (1).

No evidence of carcinogenic potential was found with long-term studies in mice and rats. The maximally tolerated doses in these species were 0.1 and 0.8 times the MRHD. There also was no evidence of genotoxicity in multiple assays (1). (*No information was provided regarding effects on fertility.*)

It is not known if ranolazine crosses the human placenta. The molecular weight (about 428), moderate plasma protein binding, and terminal half-life suggest that exposure of the embryo–fetus is likely.

BREASTFEEDING SUMMARY

No reports describing the use of ranolazine during human lactation have been located. The molecular weight (about 428), moderate (about 62%) plasma protein binding, and terminal half-life (7 hours) suggest that the drug will be excreted into breast milk. The effect of this exposure on a nursing infant is unknown. In adults, the drug is extensively metabolized in the intestine and liver, but this may not occur in infants because of the relative immaturity of metabolizing systems. In adults, the most common (>4%) adverse effects were dizziness, headache, constipation, and nausea (1).

Reference

1. Product information. Ranexa. Gilead Sciences, 2009.

RASAGILINE

Antiparkinson Agent

PREGNANCY RECOMMENDATION: No Human Data—Animal Data Suggest Risk
BREASTFEEDING RECOMMENDATION: No Human Data—Potential Toxicity

R

PREGNANCY SUMMARY

No reports describing the use of rasagiline in human pregnancy have been located. The animal reproduction data when rasagiline was used alone or in combination with levodopa/carbidopa suggest risk, but the absence of human pregnancy experience prevents an assessment of the embryo–fetal risk. However, monoamine oxidase (MAO) inhibitors are characterized by interactions with several drugs, including some agents used for general anesthesia, and tyramine-rich foods, beverages, dietary supplements, or amines from over-the-counter medications. These interactions can result in severe, sometimes fatal, hypertension. Because this toxicity would have severe consequences for a woman and her pregnancy, rasagiline is best avoided during gestation.

FETAL RISK SUMMARY

Rasagiline is an oral irreversible MAO type B (MAO-B) inhibitor. Inhibition of MAO-B lasts at least 1 week after the last dose. Rasagiline is indicated for treatment of the signs and symptoms of idiopathic Parkinson's disease as initial monotherapy and as adjunctive therapy to levodopa. (See also Levodopa.) It is in the same class as selegiline. (See Selegiline.) The mean elimination half-life at steady state is 3 hours but there is no correlation between the half-life and pharmacologic effect as inhibition of MAO-B is irreversible. Plasma protein binding, primarily to albumin, is 88%–94%. Rasagiline undergoes nearly complete metabolism in the liver before excretion (1).

Reproduction studies with rasagiline, either alone or in combination with levodopa/carbidopa, have been conducted in rats and rabbits. Pregnant rats given daily doses from the beginning of organogenesis to day 20 postpartum that produced plasma concentrations 10 and 16 times the maximum recommended human dose (MRHD) based on AUC (MRHD-AUC) caused decreased offspring survival and body weight. The plasma concentration for the no-effect dose was not determined, but it was one-third the lowest dose causing fetal toxicity and was equal to the MRHD based on BSA (MRHD-BSA). In another study, pregnant rats were given the same doses as above combined with levodopa/carbidopa throughout organogenesis. An increased incidence of wavy ribs in fetuses was observed at a dose producing exposures that were 8 times the MRHD-AUC for rasagiline and equal to the MRHD-BSA for levodopa/carbidopa (1).

Pregnant rabbits given daily doses producing exposures that were about ≥7 times the MRHD-AUC throughout organogenesis in combination with levodopa/carbidopa had an increase in fetal death. There was an increase in cardiovascular defects when levodopa/carbidopa was given alone at daily doses that were equal to the MRHD-BSA. This teratogenicity occurred to a greater extent when rasagiline, at exposures that were 1–13 times the MRHD-AUC, was given in combination with levodopa/carbidopa (1).

Carcinogenicity studies were conducted for 2 years in mice and rats. In mice, there was an increase in lung tumors (combined adenomas/carcinomas). The no-effect dose was about 5 times the MRHD-AUC. In rats, there was no increase in tumors at any dose tested. The highest doses tested in male and female rats were about 33 and 260 times, respectively, the MRHD-AUC. Rasagiline was mutagenic and/or clastogenic in some assays but negative in others. No effect was observed on mating performance or fertility in male and female rats with doses producing exposures that were ≤30 times the MRHD-AUC.

It is not known if rasagiline crosses the human placenta. The molecular weight (about 267 for the mesylate salt), protein binding, and elimination half-life suggest that the drug will cross to the embryo–fetus.

BREASTFEEDING SUMMARY

No reports describing the use of rasagiline during human lactation have been located. The molecular weight (about 267 for the mesylate salt), protein binding (88%–94%), and elimination half-life (3 hours) suggest that the drug will be excreted into breast milk. Rasagiline inhibits prolactin and may inhibit milk secretion (1). Nevertheless, the potential for severe adverse effects in a nursing infant suggest that women taking rasagiline should not breastfeed.

R

Reference

1. Product information. Azilect. Teva Neuroscience, 2006.

RASBURICASE

Antineoplastic

PREGNANCY RECOMMENDATION: No Human Data—Animal Data Suggest Moderate Risk
BREASTFEEDING RECOMMENDATION: Contraindicated

PREGNANCY SUMMARY

No reports describing the use of rasburicase in human pregnancy have been located. The agent caused significant developmental toxicity in one animal species at a dose that was ≥10 times the recommended human dose (RHD) and in a second species at a much higher dose, but both comparisons to the human dose appeared to be based on body weight.

Moreover, a no-observed-effect-level (NOEL) for such toxicity was not established in either species. The absence of human data prevents a complete assessment of the embryo–fetal risk but, if indicated, the maternal benefit appears to outweigh the unknown risk. If possible, avoiding the 1st trimester use would be preferred.

FETAL RISK SUMMARY

Rasburicase, a tetrameric protein with identical subunits, is a recombinant urate-oxidase produced from a *Saccharomyces cerevisiae* strain. It is in the same antineoplastic subclass of antimetabolites that reduce uric acid levels as allopurinol. Rasburicase is indicated for the initial management of plasma uric acid levels in pediatric and adult patients with leukemia, lymphoma, and solid tumor malignancies who are receiving anti-cancer therapy expected to result in tumor lysis and subsequent elevation of plasma uric acid. The drug is given as a 30-minute IV infusion daily for up to 5 days. The mean terminal half-life is 15.7–22.5 hours (1).

Reproduction studies have been conducted in rats and rabbits. In rats, doses that were about 250 times the RHD (*assumed to be based on body weight*) were associated with multiple heart and great vessel malformations. In rabbits during organogenesis, doses that were about 10–100 times the RHD resulted in maternal toxicity (weight loss and mortality), decreases in uterine weights and viable fetuses, and increased fetal resorptions, preimplantation and postimplantation losses, and abortions. Decreased fetal body weights and malformations involving the heart and great vessel malformations also were observed at all dose levels (1).

Studies for carcinogenicity potential have not been conducted, but the drug was not mutagenic in multiple assays. No effects on reproductive performance were observed in male and female rats at a dose 50 times the RHD (1).

It is not known if rasburicase crosses the human placenta. The molecular weight (about 34,000) suggests that clinically significant amounts will not cross, but the dosing regimen and the long terminal half-life will place the agent at the maternal–fetal interface for prolonged periods.

BREASTFEEDING SUMMARY

No reports describing the use of rasburicase during human lactation have been located. The molecular weight (about 34,000) suggests that clinically significant amounts will not be excreted into breast milk. However, the dosing regimen (daily IV infusions for 5 days) and the long terminal half-life (15.7–22.5 hours) indicate that the drug will be in the maternal plasma and available for excretion for prolonged periods. The effects of this potential exposure on a nursing infant, as well as the amount of systemic absorption, are unknown. Serious toxicities, such as anaphylaxis, hemolysis, and methemoglobinemia have been reported in patients treated with rasburicase.

Reference

1. Product information. Elitek. Sanofi-Aventis, 2010.

RASPBERRY LEAF

Herb

PREGNANCY RECOMMENDATION: Compatible
BREASTFEEDING RECOMMENDATION: Compatible

R

PREGNANCY SUMMARY

Raspberry leaf tea is one of the most common tonics used by pregnant women. Although it appears to have little if any toxicity, its efficacy as a uterine tonic to shorten labor is questionable. One source recommended that pregnant women should not use the tea without guidance of a health care professional because it can cause uterine contractions and might have estrogenic effects (1). However, because of the absence of reports of embryo, fetal, or newborn harm, if a woman chooses to use it in pregnancy, there is no reason to counsel against it.

FETAL RISK SUMMARY

Raspberry leaf, also known as red raspberry, is derived from the plant, *Rubus idaeus* (Eurasian) or *R. strigosus* (North American). The principal compounds isolated from the leaves are tannins and flavonoids. Raspberry leaf tea has been used for diarrhea and as mouthwash because of its astringent properties. It also is used as a uterine tonic to stimulate labor. The typical doses taken as a tea are 1.5–2.4 g/day. Although the information is nearly nonexistent, there is no evidence that raspberry tea is toxic (2). One review considered the chemicals in raspberry to be so common that the need for caution was no different from that of foods consumed in pregnancy (3).

Raspberry tea is used by thousands of women during pregnancy (3–6). Raspberry leaf also is combined with other herbs to make teas promoted for pregnancy (7). One popular product recommends it for a "healthy" pregnancy and to "tone the uterine muscles and prepare the womb for childbirth." The manufacturer of the product recommends its use throughout pregnancy and in first few postpartum weeks.

The tea is a combination of the leaves of raspberry, spearmint, strawberry, lemongrass, alfalfa, lemon verbena, rose hip, and fennel seed (7).

Raspberry tea is often prescribed by nurse-midwives. The most common uses of the tea during gestation are to treat nausea and vomiting (3–5) and to stimulate labor (5,6). A national survey found that among nurse-midwives who used herbal preparations to stimulate labor, 45% used black cohosh, 60% used evening primrose oil, 63% used raspberry leaf, and 90% used castor oil (6). No pregnancy complications were reported with the free use of raspberry leaf tea in late pregnancy. Although the dose recommended by the nurse-midwives was not cited, the authors cited a common dosage of 2 g dried leaves steeped in 240 mL boiling water for 5 minutes (6).

A 2001 report described a double-blind, randomized, placebo-controlled trial conducted to determine if raspberry leaf tablets (1.2 g/tablet) were effective and safe in terms of labor and birth outcomes (8). Subjects (*N* = 96) and controls (*N* = 96) were given 2 tablets/day of either raspberry leaf or placebo from 32 weeks' gestation until labor. There were no significant differences between the groups in the length of labor or the stages of labor, the mode of delivery, admissions to the neonatal intensive care unit, or birth outcomes, including Apgar scores and birth weight (8).

BREASTFEEDING SUMMARY

There are no reports describing the use of raspberry leaf during lactation. The near absence of reported toxicity with raspberry leaf tea suggests that the tea can be safely consumed during lactation. The risk to a nursing infant appears to be nil.

References

1. Raspberry Leaf. In: *Natural Medicines Comprehensive Database*. 5th ed. Stockton, CA: Therapeutic Research Faculty, 2003:1105–6.
2. Raspberry. In: *The Review of Natural Products*. St. Louis, MO: Wolters Kluwer Health, 2004.
3. Johns T, Sibeko L. Pregnancy outcomes in women using herbal therapies. Birth Defects Res B Dev Reprod Toxicol 2003;68:501–4.
4. Wilkinson JM. What do we know about herbal morning sickness treatments? A literature survey. Midwifery 2000;16:224–8.
5. Allaire AD, Moos MK, Wells SR. Complementary and alternative medicine in pregnancy: a survey of North Carolina certified nurse-midwives. Obstet Gynecol 2000;95:19–23.
6. McFarlin BL, Gibson MH, O'Rear J, Harman P. A national survey of herbal preparation use by nurse-midwives for labor stimulation. Review of the literature and recommendations for practice. J Nurse-Midwifery 1999;44:205–16.
7. Tsui B, Dennehy D, Tsourounis C. A survey of dietary supplement use during pregnancy at an academic medical center. Am J Obstet Gynecol 2001;185:433–7.
8. Simpson M, Parsons M, Greenwood J, Wade K. Raspberry leaf in pregnancy: its safety and efficacy in labor. J Midwifery Women's Health 2001;46:51–9.

REGORAFENIB

Antineoplastic (Multikinase Inhibitor)

PREGNANCY RECOMMENDATION: Contraindicated
BREASTFEEDING RECOMMENDATION: Contraindicated

PREGNANCY SUMMARY

No reports describing the use of regorafenib in human pregnancy have been located. The animal data suggest but the absence of human pregnancy experience prevents a more complete assessment of the embryo–fetal risk. However, the mechanism of action suggests that the drug can cause fetal harm. The manufacturer recommends that women of reproductive potential should take effective contraception during treatment and up to 2 months after completion of therapy (1). If a woman takes this drug during pregnancy, she should be informed of the potential harm to her embryo and/or fetus.

R

FETAL RISK SUMMARY

Regorafenib is an inhibitor of multiple membrane-bound and intracellular kinases involved in normal cellular functions and in pathologic processes such as oncogenesis, tumor angiogenesis, and maintenance of the tumor microenvironment. There are several other agents in the same subclass (see Appendix). Regorafenib is indicated for the treatment of patients with metastatic colorectal cancer who have been previously treated with fluoropyrimidine-, oxaliplatin-, and irinotecan-based chemotherapy. Regorafenib has two major active metabolites, M-2 and M-5. The parent drug and its two active metabolites are highly bound (>99%) to human plasma proteins, whereas the mean elimination half-lives and ranges are 28 hours (14–58 hours), 25 hours (14–32 hours), and 51 hours (32–70 hours), respectively (1).

Reproduction studies have been conducted in rats and rabbits. In rats, 100% resorption of the litter was observed at about 6% of the recommended human dose (RHD) based on BSA (RHD-BSA) and in rabbits, at about 25% of the RHD based on AUC (RHD-AUC). In rats during organogenesis, doses that were about 5%–11% of the RHD-BSA or about 10% of the RHD-AUC caused dose-dependent delayed ossification, skeletal malformations, cleft palate, enlarged fontanelle, cardiovascular malformations, external abnormalities, diaphragmatic hernia, and dilation of the renal pelvis. In rabbits during organogenesis, doses that were about 7%–15% of the RHD-AUC caused ventricular septal defects and dose-dependent increases in the incidence of additional cardiovascular malformations, skeletal anomalies, and urinary system adverse effects (missing kidney/ureter; small, deformed and malpositioned kidney; and hydronephrosis). In two rabbit embryo–fetal toxicity studies, there was a dose-dependent decrease in the number of viable male fetuses (1).

Carcinogenicity studies with regorafenib have not been conducted. The parent drug was not genotoxic in assays but the metabolite, M-2, was positive for clastogenicity, causing chromosome aberration in Chinese hamster cells. Fertility studies have not been conducted but the toxicity observed in male and female rats and dogs, at doses similar to or less than the RHD-AUC, suggest that the drug will adversely affect human fertility. In male rats and dogs, the toxic effects included tubular atrophy and degeneration in the testes, atrophy in the seminal vesicle, and cellular debris and oligospermia in the epididymides. In female rats and dogs, necrotic corpora lutea in the ovaries was observed (1).

It is not known if regorafenib or its two active metabolites cross the human placenta. The molecular weight of the parent drug (about 483 for the nonhydrated molecule) and the long elimination half-lives for the parent drug and active metabolites suggest that they will cross to the embryo–fetus, but the high plasma protein binding might limit the exposure.

BREASTFEEDING SUMMARY

No reports describing the use of regorafenib during human lactation have been located. The molecular weight of the parent drug (about 483 for the nonhydrated molecule) and the long elimination half-lives for the parent drug (28 hours) and two active metabolites (25 and 51 hours) suggest that they will be excreted into breast milk. However, the high plasma protein binding for the three agents (all >99%) might limit the amount in milk. Nevertheless, the severe toxicity that has been observed with regorafenib in adults suggest that a woman taking this drug should not breastfeed.

Reference

1. Product information. Stivarga. Bayer HealthCare Pharmaceuticals, 2013.

REMIFENTANIL

Narcotic Agonist Analgesic

PREGNANCY RECOMMENDATION: Human Data Suggest Risk in 3rd Trimester
BREASTFEEDING RECOMMENDATION: No Human Data—Probably Compatible

PREGNANCY SUMMARY

Remifentanil was not teratogenic or toxic in animals, but the absence of reports in early gestation prevents an assessment of its risk to the human fetus. However, narcotic analgesics are not considered to be human teratogens. Neonatal respiratory depression and sedation immediately after birth are potential complications of all narcotics when administered to a woman during labor. The short duration of remifentanil and its apparent rapid metabolism by the fetus may lessen these potential effects, but additional studies are needed to demonstrate this benefit. If remifentanil is used in pregnancy, health care professionals are encouraged to call the toll free number 800-670-6126 for information about patient enrollment in the Motherisk study.

FETAL RISK SUMMARY

Remifentanil is a rapid-onset, short-acting, synthetic mu-opioid agonist analgesic that is administered IV, in combination with other agents, for the induction and maintenance of general anesthesia. The elimination half-life is approximately 3–10 minutes. Because remifentanil is extensively metabolized by nonspecific esterases, not plasma cholinesterase (pseudocholinesterase), a normal duration of action is expected in patients with atypical cholinesterase. Further, remifentanil is not appreciably metabolized by the liver or lung (1), as are other opioid analgesics.

Fertility studies in male and female rats were conducted with IV doses 40 and 80 times, respectively, the maximum recommended human dose based on BSA (MRHD) (1). Reduced fertility was observed in male rats when the dose was administered daily for more than 70 days. In contrast, no effect was observed on the fertility of female rats dosed daily for at least 15 days before mating. Reproduction studies conducted in pregnant rats and rabbits at doses up to 400 and 125 times, respectively, the MRHD revealed no evidence of teratogenicity (1). The timing of the exposures was not specified. When remifentanil was given to rats throughout late gestation and lactation at a dose about 400 times the MRHD, no significant effect on the survival, development, or reproductive performance was observed in the exposed offspring. The drug crosses the placenta in pregnant rats and rabbits (1).

Consistent with its molecular weight (about 413) and high lipid solubility, remifentanil crosses the human placenta (1–3). The manufacturer reported that in human clinical trials, the average maternal concentration was approximately twice the levels observed in the fetus (1). However, in some cases, the maternal:fetal ratios were similar. The umbilical artery:umbilical vein (UA:UV) ratio, however, was approximately 0.30 suggesting metabolism of the drug in the fetus (1).

In an abstract (2) and a full report (3), information was presented on the placental transfer of remifentanil in 16 healthy women who were delivered by nonemergent cesarean section. Anesthesia appropriate for cesarean section was established with a lidocaine/epinephrine epidural before starting an IV infusion of remifentanil (0.1 mcg/kg/minute) that was continued until skin closure. The mean umbilical vein:maternal artery (UV:MA) and UA:UV ratios for remifentanil were 0.88 and 0.29, respectively (3). For remifentanil acid, the inactive primary metabolite, the mean UV:MA and UA:UV ratios were 0.56 and 1.23, respectively (3). These results suggested to the investigators that the narcotic rapidly crossed the placenta and was metabolized and redistributed in the fetus. The mean Apgar scores (ranges in parentheses) at 1, 5, 10, and 20 minutes were 8 (4–9), 9 (8–9), 9 (9–10), and 9 (9–10), respectively. Neurobehavioral and Adaptive Capacity Scores noted at 30 and 60 minutes were 37 (range 35–39) and 35 (range 34–39), respectively, all within normal limits. Although there were no adverse effects in the newborns, sedative and respiratory depressant effects were noted in the mothers (3).

A 1998 report described the case of a woman at term with mixed mitral valve disease, marked obesity, asthma, and preeclampsia (4). After receiving a bupivacaine/fentanyl epidural, she was delivered by an emergency cesarean section under general anesthesia. Rapid-sequence induction was conducted with remifentanil (2 mcg/kg), etomidate (20 mg), and succinylcholine (100 mg). A male infant (birth weight not given) was delivered 3 minutes after induction of anesthesia. The Apgar scores were 6, 8, and 8 at 1, 5, and 10 minutes, respectively. No signs of respiratory depression were observed (4).

A 30-year-old woman was delivered by cesarean section at 36 weeks' because of the need for surgical resection of a right acoustic neuroma (5). Remifentanil (0.1–0.2 mcg/kg/minute) was infused for induction of general anesthesia followed by propofol and succinylcholine. A healthy 2970-g female infant was delivered 7 minutes after the start of remifentanil. Apgar scores were 7 and 8 at 1 and 5 minutes, respectively. Although there were no clinical signs of respiratory distress, her initial room air oxygen saturation was 85%–91% and she was placed in a 40% oxygen tent for 1 hour. She was discharged home at 3 days of age (5).

A 23-year-old woman at 37 weeks' gestation whose condition was complicated by a recurrent aortic coarctation with 50% narrowing of the aortic arch was delivered by an elective cesarean section (6). Remifentanil infusion up to 0.2 mcg/kg/minute was combined with etomidate, succinylcholine, and isoflurane. Delivery took place 7 minutes after induction of anesthesia. The newborn (sex and weight not specified) had Apgar scores of 6 and 9 at 1 and 5 minutes, respectively. The infant did well after birth with no need for naloxone or evidence of respiratory distress (6).

Three studies have been located that describe the use of remifentanil for labor pain (7–9). In one study, four laboring women with singleton term pregnancies were treated with remifentanil either from a patient-controlled analgesia (PCA) pump (0.25 mcg/kg, 5-minute lockout duration) or with IV bolus doses (0.25–0.50 mcg/kg every 2 minutes as needed) (7). Failure of the pain to respond to increased doses and adverse effects (sedation, oxygen desaturation episodes, respiratory depression, nausea and vomiting, and pruritus) resulted in removal of the patients from the study. Healthy newborns (sex and weight not specified) were delivered 4–6 hours after discontinuance of remifentanil. All had Apgar scores of 9 or 10 (7). A study published in 2000 described two women in labor who were treated with remifentanil administered by a PCA pump (8). The on-demand dose was 20 mcg with a 3-minute lockout duration (no basal infusion). The total doses administered during labor were 740 and 940 mcg. No adverse effects attributable to the analgesic were observed in the newborns. The effects of remifentanil PCA on 42 laboring women were described in a 2001 abstract (9). The technique used was thought to be safe for the mother and newborn (9).

A 1999 study concluded that remifentanil-based general anesthesia (combined with propofol or isoflurane but without nitrous oxide) was a suitable alternative to sedation (induced by midazolam, diazepam, or propofol) for oocyte retrieval in an in vitro fertilization program (10). In a comparison between the general anesthesia and sedation groups, no significant differences were observed in the number of fertilized oocytes, or in the cleavage and pregnancy rates. However, the number of collected oocytes was significantly higher in the general anesthesia group (10).

BREASTFEEDING SUMMARY

No reports describing the use of remifentanil in a lactating woman have been located. The molecular weight (about 413) and high lipid solubility suggest that it will be excreted into breast milk. Other narcotic agents (e.g., codeine, fentanyl, and morphine) are excreted into breast milk but are classified as compatible with breastfeeding by the American Academy of Pediatrics (see specific agents). The very short elimination time suggests that use of remifentanil during cesarean section or other surgery would not represent a significant risk to a newborn that started or continued breastfeeding a few hours later.

References

1. Product information. Ultiva. Abbott Laboratories, 2001.
2. Hughes SC, Kan RE, Rosen MA, Kessin C, Preston PG, Lobo EP, Johnson LR, Johnson JL. Remifentanil: ultra-short acting opioid for obstetric anesthesia (abstract). Anesthesiology 1996;85:A894.
3. Kan RE, Hughes SC, Rosen MA, Kessin C, Preston PG, Lobo EP. Intravenous remifentanil. Placental transfer, maternal and neonatal effects. Anesthesiology 1998;88:1467–74.
4. Scott H, Bateman C, Price M. The use of remifentanil in general anaesthesia for caesarean section in a patient with mitral value disease. Anaesthesia 1998;53:691–701.
5. Bedard JM, Richardson MG, Wissler RN. General anesthesia with remifentanil for cesarean section in a parturient with an acoustic neuroma. Can J Anesth 1999;46:576–80.
6. Manullang TR, Chun K, Egan TD. The use of remifentanil for cesarean section in a parturient with recurrent aortic coarctation. Can J Anesth 2000;47:454–9.
7. Olufolabi AJ, Booth JV, Wakeling HG, Glass PS, Penning DH, Reynolds JD. A preliminary investigation of remifentanil as a labor analgesic. Anesth Analg 2000;91:606–8.
8. Thurlow JA, Waterhouse P. Patient-controlled analgesia in labour using remifentanil in two parturients with platelet abnormalities. Br J Anaesth 2000;84:411–3.
9. Evron S, Sadan O, Ezri T, Boaz M, Glezerman M. Remifentanil: a new systemic analgesic for labor pain and an alternative to dolestine (abstract). Am J Obstet Gynecol 2001;185:S210.
10. Hammadeh ME, Wilhelm W, Huppert A, Rosenbaum P, Schmidt W. Effects of general anaesthesia vs. sedation on fertilization, cleavage and pregnancy rates in an IVF program. Arch Gynecol Obstet 1999;263:56–9.

REPAGLINIDE

Antidiabetic

PREGNANCY RECOMMENDATION: Limited Human Data—Animal Data Suggest Moderate Risk
BREASTFEEDING RECOMMENDATION: No Human Data—Potential Toxicity

PREGNANCY SUMMARY

The published human pregnancy experience is limited. No teratogenicity was observed in two animal species but, in one species, exposure during late pregnancy through lactation resulted in adverse effects on long-bone growth. The embryo–fetal risk from exposure to repaglinide cannot be fully assessed but, based on the animal and limited human data, inadvertent exposure early in gestation does not appear to represent a major risk. However, insulin is the treatment of choice for pregestational and gestational control of maternal hyperglycemia because, in general, most hypoglycemic agents do not provide adequate glycemic control. Moreover, insulin, unlike oral agents, does not cross the placenta to the fetus, thus eliminating the additional concern that the drug therapy itself will adversely affect the fetus. Carefully prescribed insulin therapy provides better control of the mother's glucose, thereby preventing the fetal and neonatal complications that occur with this disease. High maternal glucose levels, as may occur in diabetes mellitus, are closely associated with a number of maternal and fetal adverse effects, including fetal structural anomalies if the hyperglycemia occurs early in gestation. To prevent this toxicity, the American College of Obstetricians and Gynecologists recommends that insulin be used for types 1 and 2 diabetes occurring during pregnancy and, if diet and exercise alone are not successful, for gestational diabetes (1,2).

FETAL RISK SUMMARY

Repaglinide is an oral blood glucose–lowering agent that is chemically unrelated to the sulfonylurea insulin secretagogues. It is in the same antidiabetic subclass of meglitinides as nateglinide. Repaglinide is indicated as an adjunct to diet and exercise to improve glycemic control in adults with type 2 diabetes mellitus. The drug is completely metabolized to inactive metabolites. Plasma protein binding to albumin is >98% and the mean half-life is 1.0–1.4 hours (range 0.4–8 hours) (3). It is often combined with metformin.

Reproduction studies have been conducted in rats and rabbits. Repaglinide was not teratogenic in these species when given throughout pregnancy at doses that were about 40 and 0.8 times, respectively, the human clinical exposure based on BSA (HCE). When a dose that was 15 times the HCE was given to rats during gestational days 17–22 and during lactation, offspring developed nonteratogenic skeletal deformities consisting of shortening, thickening, and bending of the humerus during the postnatal period. This effect was not seen at doses up to 2.5 times the HCE given on gestational days 1–22 or at higher doses on gestational days 1–16 (3).

Another study found effects similar to those above in pregnant rats (4). Because the toxic effects on long bone development were observed only after organogenesis and only with high doses, the investigators concluded that the toxicity was limited to effects on growth and that repaglinide was not teratogenic (4).

No evidence of carcinogenicity was found in long-term studies in mice and female rats. In male rats there was an increased incidence of benign adenomas of the thyroid and liver. Multiple tests for genotoxicity were negative. No effects on fertility of male and female rats were observed with doses >40 times the HCE (3).

It is not known if repaglinide crosses the human placenta. The molecular weight (about 453) suggests that it will cross, but the extensive metabolism, high plasma protein binding, and short half-life suggest that the embryo–fetal exposure may be limited.

A 2006 report from Italy described the outcomes of two pregnancies treated with repaglinide for type 2 diabetes early in gestation (5). In both patients, the gestational age was confirmed by ultrasound and their therapy was changed to insulin. The first case involved a 38-year-old woman (pregestational body mass index [BMI] 26.2 kg/m^2) who had been on long-term repaglinide 1.5 mg/day and metformin 3 g/day when she presented in the 7th week of pregnancy. Her HbA_{1c} values were 6.8% (preconception), 7% (conception), and 5.6% (3rd trimester). Gestational hypertension developed at 29 weeks' gestation and was treated with methyldopa. At 40 weeks', she gave birth to a healthy 3690-g female infant with Apgar scores of 9 and 10. The infant developed jaundice that needed phototherapy for 1 day. The second case was a nulliparous 34-year-old woman (pregestational BMI 21.3 kg/m^2) who had been taking repaglinide 2.5 mg/day for 2 years when she presented in the 6th gestational week. Her HbA_{1c} values at conception and in the 3rd trimester were 6.4% and 5.1%, respectively. At 39 weeks', she gave birth by cesarean section to a 2650-g male infant with Apgar scores 9 and 10. The birth weights for both infants were appropriate for gestational age, and no minor or major malformations were noted. Both infants were doing well at 6 weeks of age (5).

A report from England on the safety profile of repaglinide briefly mentioned five pregnancies exposed to the drug during pregnancy (6). The outcomes of the pregnancies were three infants with no abnormalities reported, one stillborn at 26 weeks' (mother had Fraser syndrome), and one outcome was unknown (no other details provided).

A brief 2007 report described the pregnancy outcome of a 38-year-old woman with type 2 diabetes who was exposed to repaglinide up to the 7th week (7). At that time her therapy was changed to insulin. In the 39th week, she delivered a normal 3350-g infant (sex not specified). The newborn had no evidence of hypoglycemia.

BREASTFEEDING SUMMARY

No reports describing the use of repaglinide during lactation have been located. The molecular weight (about 453) suggests that it will be excreted into breast milk, but the extensive metabolism and high plasma protein binding (>98%) suggest that the amount in milk will be limited. Although the mean half-life (1.0–1.4 hours) also suggests limited exposure, the range might be as great as 8 hours and suggests otherwise. The effect of this exposure on a nursing infant is unknown, but hypoglycemia is a potential complication. Thus, if a woman plans to breastfeed, changing her therapy to other agents, such as insulin or a second-generation sulfonylurea (see Glipizide and Glyburide) might be appropriate. In any case, monitoring the infant's blood glucose concentrations should be conducted.

References

1. American College of Obstetricians and Gynecologists. Pregestational diabetes mellitus. *ACOG Practice Bulletin.* No. 60, March 2005.
2. American College of Obstetricians and Gynecologists. Gestational diabetes. *ACOG Practice Bulletin.* No. 30, September 2001.
3. Product information. Prandin. Novo Nordisk, 2009.
4. Viertel B, Guttner J. Effects of the oral antidiabetic repaglinide on the reproduction of rats. Arzneim-Forsch/Drug Res 2000;50:425–40.
5. Napoli A, Ciampa F, Colatrella A, Fallucca F. Use of repaglinide during the first weeks of pregnancy in two type 2 diabetic women. Diabetes Care 2006;29:2326–7.
6. Marshall V, Wilton L, Shakir S. Safety profile of repaglinide as used in general practice in England: results of a prescription-event monitoring study. Acta Diabetol 2006;43:6–13.
7. Mollar-Puchades MA, Martin-Cortes A, Perez-Calvo A, Diaz-Garcia C. Use of repaglinide on a pregnant woman during embryogenesis. Diabetes Obes Metab 2007;9:146–7.

RESERPINE

Antihypertensive

PREGNANCY RECOMMENDATION: Limited Human Data—No Relevant Animal Data
BREASTFEEDING RECOMMENDATION: Limited Human Data—Probably Compatible

PREGNANCY SUMMARY

The limited human pregnancy experience and the absence of animal reproduction data prevent an assessment of the embryo–fetal risk. The data from one source suggest that avoiding exposure in the 1st trimester would be a wise choice.

FETAL RISK SUMMARY

The Collaborative Perinatal Project monitored 50,282 mother–child pairs, 48 of whom had 1st trimester exposure to reserpine (1, p. 376). There were four defects with 1st trimester use. Although this incidence (8%) is greater than the expected frequency of occurrence, no major category or individual malformations were identified. For use anytime in pregnancy, 475 exposures were recorded (1, p. 441). Malformations included the following: microcephaly (7 cases); hydronephrosis (3 cases); hydroureter (3 cases); and inguinal hernia (12 cases) (1, p. 495).

Reserpine crosses the placenta. Use of reserpine near term has resulted in nasal discharge, retraction, lethargy, and anorexia in the newborn (2). Concern over the ability of reserpine to deplete catecholamine levels has appeared (3). The significance of this is not known.

In a surveillance study of Michigan Medicaid recipients involving 229,101 completed pregnancies conducted between 1985 and 1992, 15 newborns had been exposed to reserpine during the 1st trimester (F. Rosa, personal communication, FDA, 1993). No major birth defects were observed (one expected).

BREASTFEEDING SUMMARY

Reserpine is excreted into breast milk (4). No reports of adverse effects in a nursing infant have been located.

References

1. Heinonen OP, Slone D, Shapiro S. *Birth Defects and Drugs in Pregnancy.* Littleton, MA: Publishing Sciences Group, 1977.
2. Budnick IS, Leikin S, Hoeck LE. Effect in the newborn infant to reserpine administration ante partum. Am J Dis Child 1955;90:286–9.
3. Towell ME, Hyman AI. Catecholamine depletion in pregnancy. J Obstet Gynaecol Br Commonw 1966;73:431–8.
4. Product information. Serpasil. Ciba Pharmaceutical, 1993.

R

RETAPAMULIN

Antibiotic

PREGNANCY RECOMMENDATION: No Human Data—Probably Compatible
BREASTFEEDING RECOMMENDATION: No Human Data—Probably Compatible

PREGNANCY SUMMARY

No reports describing the use of retapamulin in human pregnancy have been located. The animal reproduction data are not relevant because, although there was developmental toxicity (death and restricted weight), these effects occurred with maternal toxicity. The absence of human pregnancy experience prevents a complete assessment of the embryo–fetal risk. However, the very low plasma concentrations suggest that there is little or no risk when the antibiotic is used topically in pregnancy.

FETAL RISK SUMMARY

Retapamulin is a semisynthetic pleuromutilin antibiotic that is available as a 1% ointment. The antibiotic is isolated through fermentation from *Clitopilus passeckerianus* (formerly *Pleurotus passeckerianus*). It is indicated for the topical treatment of impetigo due to *Staphylococcus aureus* (methicillin-susceptible isolates only) or *Streptococcus pyogenes*. Small amounts of retapamulin are absorbed into the systemic circulation.

In 380 adult and 136 pediatric (age 2–17 years) patients undergoing treatment with twice daily applications, 11% had measurable plasma concentrations (lower limit of quantitation 0.5 ng/mL), of which the median concentration was 0.8 ng/mL. The maximum measured concentrations in adult and pediatric patients were 10.7 and 18.5 ng/mL, respectively. The antibiotic is about 94% bound to plasma proteins, but the elimination half-life has not been determined due to the very low plasma concentrations. Retapamulin is metabolized by the liver to numerous metabolites (1).

Reproduction studies have been conducted in rats and rabbits. In rats, oral doses of ≥150 mg/kg/day (relationship to the human exposure not stated) caused maternal toxicity (decreased body weight and food consumption), decreased fetal weight, and delayed skeletal ossification. No treatment-related malformations were observed in the offspring. In rabbits, continuous IV infusions with doses producing exposures that were 8 times the estimated maximum achievable human exposure based on AUC were associated with maternal toxicity (decreased body weight and food consumption) and abortions. There were no other treatment-related effects on embryo–fetal development (1).

Carcinogenicity studies have not been conducted with retapamulin, but the drug was not genotoxic in multiple assays. No effects on fertility were noted in male and female rats given oral doses up to 450 mg/kg/day (1).

It is not known if retapamulin crosses the human placenta. The molecular weight (about 518) is low enough, but the very low plasma concentrations suggest that clinically significant exposure of the embryo and/or fetus is unlikely.

BREASTFEEDING SUMMARY

No reports describing the use of retapamulin during human lactation have been located. The molecular weight (about 518) is low enough for excretion into breast milk, but the very low plasma concentrations suggest that clinically significant exposure of a nursing infant is unlikely. Use of the antibiotic during breastfeeding probably is safe.

Reference

1. Product information. Altabax. GlaxoSmithKline, 2007.

RETEPLASE

Thrombolytic

PREGNANCY RECOMMENDATION: Compatible—Maternal Benefit >> Embryo–Fetal Risk
BREASTFEEDING RECOMMENDATION: No Human Data—Probably Compatible

PREGNANCY SUMMARY

One report described the use of reteplase in human pregnancy. Bleeding appears to be the potential risk but was not observed in this case. Pregnancy may increase this risk (1). However, if indicated, the maternal benefit appears to outweigh the potential risk to the embryo–fetus.

FETAL RISK SUMMARY

The enzyme reteplase is a nonglycosylated deletion mutein of tissue plasminogen activator (tPA; see also Alteplase and Tenecteplase) produced by recombinant technology in *Escherichia coli*. It contains 355 of the 527 amino acids of natural human tPA. Reteplase is indicated for use in the management of acute myocardial infarction for the improvement of ventricular function, the reduction in the incidence of congestive heart failure, and the reduction of mortality. The effective half-life of reteplase is 13–16 minutes, based on the measurement of thrombolytic activity (1).

Reproduction studies have been conducted in rats and rabbits. In rats, doses up to 15 times the human dose (HD) revealed no evidence of impaired fertility or teratogenicity. In rabbits, a dose 3 times the HD administered in mid-gestation resulted in genital bleeding and abortions (1).

It is not known if reteplase crosses the human placenta. The molecular weight (39,571) and very short effective half-life suggest that clinically significant amounts of the protein will not cross to the embryo–fetus.

A 2002 report described the use of reteplase for acute massive pulmonary embolism in a pregnant woman at 30 weeks' gestation (2). The patient was given a 10 mg IV bolus followed by 90 mg IV over 2 hours with marked improvement in her condition. Heparin was given for remainder of the pregnancy. At 36 weeks' she gave birth to a healthy male infant (no other details were provided) (2).

BREASTFEEDING SUMMARY

No reports describing the use of reteplase during human lactation have been located. However, the indication for reteplase suggests that such reports will not be forthcoming. In addition, the molecular weight (39,571) and very short effective half-life (13–16 minutes) suggest that the protein will not be excreted in clinically significant amounts into breast milk. Therefore, breastfeeding should be initiated or resumed based on the mother's condition and not the drug therapy.

References

1. Product information. Retavase. Centocor, 2004.
2. Yap LB, Alp NJ, Forfar JC. Thrombolysis for acute massive pulmonary embolism during pregnancy. Int J Cardiol 2002;82:193–4.

REVIPARIN

Anticoagulant

PREGNANCY RECOMMENDATION: Compatible
BREASTFEEDING RECOMMENDATION: No Human Data—Probably Compatible

PREGNANCY SUMMARY

Reviparin is a low-molecular-weight heparin prepared by depolymerization of heparin obtained from porcine intestinal mucosa (1). It is not available in the United States (see also Dalteparin and Enoxaparin). Reviparin has an average molecular weight of 3500–4500 (range 2000–8000) (1). Because this is a relatively large molecule, it probably does not cross the placenta and presents a low risk to the embryo–fetus.

FETAL RISK SUMMARY

An abstract published in 1997 described the use of reviparin and aspirin (100 mg/day) in 50 women with unexplained recurrent fetal loss and autoantibodies (2). Reviparin was administered either as 4900 units SC once daily or as 2800 units SC twice daily. The once-daily injection produced comparable plasma anti-factor Xa levels to the twice-daily regimen. No maternal bleeding, thrombocytopenia, or decreased bone density was noted and no placental pathology was found in the 43 women who had completed their pregnancies (7 pregnancies were still in progress). The outcomes of the 43 completed pregnancies were 35 normal newborns (no premature deliveries), 7 spontaneous abortions, and 1 ectopic pregnancy. No congenital malformations or low-birth-weight newborns were observed.

BREASTFEEDING SUMMARY

No reports describing the use of reviparin during human lactation have been located. Reviparin, a low-molecular-weight heparin, still has a high molecular weight (average 3500–4500) and, as such, should not be expected to be excreted into human milk. Because reviparin would be inactivated in the gastrointestinal tract, the risk to a nursing infant from ingesting the drug is probably nil.

References

1. Reynold JEF, ed. *Martindale. The Extra Pharmacopoeia*. 30th ed. London, UK: The Pharmaceutical Press, 1993:232.
2. Laskin C, Ginsberg J, Farine D, Crowther M, Spitzer K, Soloninka C, Ryan G, Seaward G, Ritchie K. Low molecular weight heparin and ASA therapy in women with autoantibodies and unexplained recurrent fetal loss (U-RFL). Society of Perinatal Obstetricians abstracts. Am J Obstet Gynecol 1997;176:S125.

RIBAVIRIN

Antiviral

PREGNANCY RECOMMENDATION: Contraindicated
BREASTFEEDING RECOMMENDATION: No Human Data—Potential Toxicity

PREGNANCY SUMMARY

The animal data suggest high risk, but the limited human pregnancy experience has not reported developmental toxicity attributable to ribavirin. However, only one case involved exposure during organogenesis. There also is no evidence of embryo–fetal harm when men were treated with ribavirin before fathering an infant. Although the data are very limited, this argues against a mutagenic effect of the drug and/or the transfer of clinically significant amounts of ribavirin in sperm. Nevertheless, if ribavirin is indicated, pregnancy should be avoided in female patients and in female partners of male patients for at least 6 months after the end of therapy (1,2).

FETAL RISK SUMMARY

Ribavirin is available in oral, IV, and inhalation formulations. The plasma elimination half-life is 12 days, but may persist in nonplasma compartments (e.g., red blood cells) for as long as 6 months.

Ribavirin has demonstrated dose-related teratogenicity or embryolethality at doses well below the recommended human dose in all animal species tested (1–3). Malformations observed in the offspring of hamsters, rats, and rabbits included defects of the skull, palate, eye, jaw, limbs, skeleton, and gastrointestinal tract. The manufacturers of oral ribavirin warn that the drug should not be used by men with female partners of reproductive age unless effective contraception (two reliable forms) is used or if their female partner is pregnant (1,2). Effective contraception should be continued for 6 months after ribavirin therapy has been stopped.

A 34-year-old woman, at 33 weeks' gestation, was treated with ribavirin inhalation therapy for influenza pneumonia complicated by respiratory failure (4). Shortly after treatment, a cesarean section was performed because of worsening maternal cardiopulmonary function. A normal female infant was delivered, who was alive and well at 1 year of age (4).

R

In 1988, the CDC stated that the use of ribavirin during pregnancy is contraindicated (5). In a statement addressing the issue of inhaled ribavirin exposure among health care personnel, the CDC commented: "... health care workers who are pregnant, or may become pregnant should be advised of the potential risks of exposure during direct patient care when patients are receiving ribavirin through oxygen tent or mist mask and should be counseled about risk-reduction strategies, including alternative job responsibilities" (5).

In 13 pregnant or postpartum women hospitalized because of measles, 10 were treated for pneumonitis and/or severe disease in the 2nd or 3rd trimesters with ribavirin aerosol therapy (6). One woman was treated for 5 days before an elective abortion for worsening pulmonary status at 21 weeks' gestation. The remaining nine women had normal newborns with Apgar scores of 7–9 and 8–10 at 1 and 5 minutes, respectively (6).

A 36-year-old woman with an unknown pregnancy at 7 weeks received three ribavirin 200 mg injections over a 3-day period for suspected severe acute respiratory syndrome (SARS) (7). SARS was ruled out and she completed an uneventful pregnancy, delivering at term a 3.35-kg female infant with normal Apgar scores. At 8 months of age, the child was developing normally with normal growth and no evidence of major or minor malformations (7).

A 2001 case report described two men with chronic hepatitis C who were treated with a combination of ribavirin (800 and 1200 mg/day) and interferon alfa-2a (6 million units every other day) (8). After about 5 months of therapy, their wives became pregnant and both delivered healthy infants at term. The infants were developing normally at 4 months of age (8).

A second case report described a pregnancy outcome in which the father was treated with interferon alfa-2b (3 million units 3 times per week) and ribavirin (1000 mg/day) for 4 weeks before the last menstrual cycle and continued during the pregnancy of the patient's partner (9). A healthy 3380-g male infant was delivered at term with no evidence of malformations. The authors noted the lack of information relating the amount of ribavirin in sperm and the lack of experimental or clinical evidence for birth defects after paternal exposure (9).

A 2003 review summarized the developmental toxicity of ribavirin and interferon alfa-2b, a combination used for the treatment of hepatitis C (10). The authors lamented the lack of reported human pregnancy experience and the possibility that the labels overstated the risks of men passing a potentially toxic amount of ribavirin in their sperm to a pregnant woman.

BREASTFEEDING SUMMARY

No reports describing the use of ribavirin during human lactation have been located. The molecular weight (about 244) and prolong plasma elimination half-life (12 days) suggest that the drug will be excreted into breast milk. The effects of this exposure on a nursing infant are unknown.

References

1. Product information. Copegus. Roche Laboratories, 2007.
2. Product information. Rebetol. Schering, 2007.
3. Product information. Virazole. Valeant North America, 2007.

4. Kirshon B, Faro S, Zurawin RK, Samo TC, Carpenter RJ. Favorable outcome after treatment with amantadine and ribavirin in a pregnancy complicated by influenza pneumonia: a case report. J Reprod Med 1988;33:399–401.
5. CDC. Assessing exposures of health care personnel to aerosols of ribavirin—California. MMWR 1988;37:560–3.
6. Atmar RL, Englund JA, Hammill H. Complications of measles during pregnancy. Clin Infect Dis 1992;14:217–26.
7. Rezvani M, Koren G. Pregnancy outcome after exposure to injectable ribavirin during embryogenesis. Reprod Toxicol 2006;21:113–5.
8. Hegenbarth K, Maurer U, Kroisel PM, Fickert P, Trauner M, Stauber RE. No evidence for mutagenic effects of ribavirin: report of two normal pregnancies. Am J Gastroenterol 2001;96:2286–7.
9. Biana S, Ettore G. Male periconceptional ribavirin—interferon alpha-2B exposure with no adverse fetal effects. Birth Defects Res A Clin Mol Teratol 2003;67:77–8.
10. Polifka JE, Friedman JM. Developmental toxicity of ribarvirin/IFα combination therapy: is the label more dangerous than the drugs? Birth Defects Res A Clin Mol Teratol 2003;67:8–12.

RIBOFLAVIN

Vitamin

PREGNANCY RECOMMENDATION: Compatible
BREASTFEEDING RECOMMENDATION: Compatible

PREGNANCY SUMMARY

Riboflavin (vitamin B_2), a water-soluble B-complex vitamin, acts as a coenzyme in humans and is essential for tissue respiration systems. The National Academy of Sciences' recommended dietary allowance (RDA) for riboflavin in pregnancy is 1.6 mg (1).

FETAL RISK SUMMARY

Riboflavin is actively transferred to the fetus resulting in higher concentrations of the vitamin in the newborn than in the mother (2–12). The placenta converts flavin adenine dinucleotide existing in the maternal serum to free riboflavin found in the fetal circulation (5,6). This allows retention of the vitamin by the fetus because the transfer of free riboflavin back to the mother is inhibited (6,12). At term, the mean riboflavin values in 174 mothers was 184 ng/mL (range 80–390 ng/mL) and in their newborns was 318 ng/mL (range 136–665 ng/mL) (7). In a more recent study, the cord serum concentration was 158 nmol/L compared with 113 nmol/L in the maternal serum (11).

The incidence of riboflavin deficiency in pregnancy is low (7,13). In two studies, no correlation was discovered between the riboflavin status of the mother and the outcome of pregnancy even when riboflavin deficiency was present (14,15). A 1977 study found no difference in riboflavin levels between infants of low and normal birth weight (10).

Riboflavin deficiency is teratogenic in animals (16). Although human teratogenicity has not been reported, low riboflavin levels were found in six mothers who had given birth to infants with neural tube defects (17). Other vitamin deficiencies present in these women were thought to be of more significance (see Folic Acid and Vitamin B_{12}).

A mother has been described with multiple acylcoenzyme A dehydrogenase deficiency probably related to riboflavin metabolism (18). The mother had given birth to a healthy child followed by one stillbirth and six infants who had been breastfed and died in early infancy after exhibiting a strong sweaty foot odor. In her 9th and 10th pregnancies, she was treated with 20 mg/day of riboflavin during the 3rd trimesters and delivered healthy infants. The authors thought the maternal symptoms were consistent with a mild form of acute fatty liver of pregnancy.

BREASTFEEDING SUMMARY

Riboflavin (vitamin B_2) is excreted into breast milk (19–23). Well-nourished lactating women were given supplements of a multivitamin preparation containing 2.0 mg of riboflavin (19). At 6 months postpartum, milk concentrations of riboflavin did not differ significantly from those in control patients not receiving supplements. In a study of lactating women with low nutritional status, supplementation with riboflavin in doses of 0.10–10.0 mg/day resulted in mean milk concentrations of 200–740 ng/mL (20). Milk concentrations were directly proportional to dietary intake. A 1983 English study measured riboflavin levels in pooled human milk obtained from preterm (26 mothers: 29–34 weeks) and term (35 mothers: ≥39 weeks) patients (21). Milk obtained from preterm mothers rose from 276 ng/mL (colostrum) to 360 ng/mL (6–15 days) and then fell to 266 ng/mL (16–196 days). During approximately the same time frame, milk levels from term mothers were 288, 279, and 310 ng/mL. In a Finnish study, premature infants (mean gestational age 30.1 weeks) fed human milk, but without riboflavin supplementation, became riboflavin deficient by 6 weeks of age (24).

The National Academy of Sciences' RDA for riboflavin during lactation is 1.8 mg (1). If the diet of the lactating woman adequately supplies this amount, supplementation with riboflavin is not needed (22). Maternal supplementation with the RDA for riboflavin is recommended for those women with inadequate nutritional intake. The American Academy of Pediatrics classifies riboflavin as compatible with breastfeeding (25).

References

1. American Hospital Formulary Service. *Drug Information 1997*. Bethesda, MD: American Society of Health-System Pharmacists, 1997:2817–8.
2. Hill EP, Longo LD. Dynamics of maternal–fetal nutrient transfer. Fed Proc 1980;39:239–44.

3. Lust JE, Hagerman DD, Villee CA. The transport of riboflavin by human placenta. J Clin Invest 1954;33:38–40.
4. Frank O, Walbroehl G, Thomason A, Kaminetzky H, Kubes Z, Baker H. Placental transfer: fetal retention of some vitamins. Am J Clin Nutr 1970;23:662–3.
5. Kaminetzky HA, Baker H, Frank O, Langer A. The effects of intravenously administered water-soluble vitamins during labor in normovitaminemic and hypovitaminemic gravidas on maternal and neonatal blood vitamin levels at delivery. Am J Obstet Gynecol 1974;120:697–703.
6. Kaminetzky HA, Baker H. Micronutrients in pregnancy. Clin Obstet Gynecol 1977;20:363–80.
7. Baker H, Frank O, Thomason AD, Langer A, Munves ED, De Angelis B, Kaminetzky HA. Vitamin profile of 174 mothers and newborns at parturition. Am J Clin Nutr 1975;28:59–65.
8. Baker H, Frank O, Deangelis B, Feingold S, Kaminetzky HA. Role of placenta in maternal–fetal vitamin transfer in humans. Am J Obstet Gynecol 1981;141:792–6.
9. Bamji MS. Enzymic evaluation of thiamin, riboflavin and pyridoxine status of parturient women and their newborn infants. Br J Nutr 1976;35:259–65.
10. Baker H, Thind IS, Frank O, DeAngelis B, Caterini H, Louria DB. Vitamin levels in low-birth-weight newborn infants and their mothers. Am J Obstet Gynecol 1977;129:521–4.
11. Kirshenbaum NW, Dancis J, Levitz M, Lehanka J, Young BK. Riboflavin concentration in maternal and cord blood in human pregnancy. Am J Obstet Gynecol 1987;157:748–52.
12. Dancis J, Lehanka J, Levitz M. Placental transport of riboflavin: differential rates of uptake at the maternal and fetal surfaces of the perfused human placenta. Am J Obstet Gynecol 1988;158:204–10.
13. Dostalova L. Correlation of the vitamin status between mother and newborn during delivery. Dev Pharmacol Ther 1982;4(Suppl 1):45–57.
14. Vir SC, Love AHG, Thompson W. Riboflavin status during pregnancy. Am J Clin Nutr 1981;34:2699–705.
15. Heller S, Salkeld RM, Korner WF. Riboflavin status in pregnancy. Am J Clin Nutr 1974;27:1225–30.
16. Shepard TH. *Catalog of Teratogenic Agents*. 6th ed. Baltimore, MD: The Johns Hopkins University Press, 1989:557–8.
17. Smithells RW, Sheppard S, Schorah CJ. Vitamin deficiencies and neural tube defects. Arch Dis Child 1976;51:944–50.
18. Harpey JP, Charpentier C. Acute fatty liver of pregnancy. Lancet 1983;1:586–7.
19. Thomas MR, Sneed SM, Wei C, Nail PA, Wilson M, Sprinkle EE III. The effects of vitamin C, vitamin B_6, vitamin B_{12}, folic acid, riboflavin, and thiamin on the breast milk and maternal status of well-nourished women at 6 months postpartum. Am J Clin Nutr 1980;33:2151–6.
20. Deodhar AD, Rajalakshmi R, Ramakrishnan CV. Studies on human lactation. Part III. Effect of dietary vitamin supplementation on vitamin contents of breast milk. Acta Paediatr Scand 1964;53:42–8.
21. Ford JE, Zechalko A, Murphy J, Brooke OG. Comparison of the B vitamin composition of milk from mothers of preterm and term babies. Arch Dis Child 1983;58:367–72.
22. Nail PA, Thomas MR, Eakin R. The effect of thiamin and riboflavin supplementation on the level of those vitamins in human breast milk and urine. Am J Clin Nutr 1980;33:198–204.
23. Gunther M. Diet and milk secretion in women. Proc Nutr Soc 1968;27:77–82.
24. Ronnholm KAR. Need for riboflavin supplementation in small prematures fed human milk. Am J Clin Nutr 1986;43:1–6.
25. Committee on Drugs, American Academy of Pediatrics. The transfer of drugs and other chemicals into human milk. Pediatrics 2001;108:776–89.

RIFABUTIN

Antituberculosis Agent

PREGNANCY RECOMMENDATION: No Human Data—Animal Data Suggest Low Risk
BREASTFEEDING RECOMMENDATION: No Human Data—Potential Toxicity Contraindicated (Patients with HIV Infection)

PREGNANCY SUMMARY

No reports describing the use of rifabutin in human pregnancy have been located. The animal data are suggestive of low risk, but the absence of human pregnancy experience prevents an assessment of the embryo–fetal risk. However, the maternal benefit appears to outweigh the unknown risk to the embryo or fetus, so therapy should not be withheld because of pregnancy.

FETAL RISK SUMMARY

Rifabutin is an oral semi-synthetic ansamycin antibiotic that is derived from rifamycin S. It is indicated for the prevention of disseminated *Mycobacterium avium* complex (includes *M. avium* and *M. intracellulare*) disease in patients with advanced human HIV infection. Five metabolites have been identified, one of which is active (contributes up to 10% of the antimicrobial activity). Rifabutin is moderately (about 85%) bound to plasma proteins and has a mean terminal half-life of 45 hours (1).

Rifabutin was not carcinogenic in mice and rats at doses about 32 and 12 times, respectively, the recommended human daily dose (RHDD). In addition, no mutagenicity was observed in several assays (1).

Reproduction tests have been conducted in rats and rabbits. In rats, doses up to 40 times the RHDD were not teratogenic, but the highest dose caused a decrease in fetal viability. At 8 times the RHDD, an increase in fetal skeletal variants was observed. In rabbits, no teratogenic effects were observed with doses up to 40 times the RHDD. A dose 16 times the RHDD was maternal toxic and resulted in an increase in fetal skeletal anomalies (1).

It is not known if rifabutin or its active metabolite crosses the human placenta. The molecular weight of the parent compound (about 847), moderate plasma protein binding, high lipid solubility, and prolonged terminal half-life suggest that passage to the embryo–fetus will occur.

Rifabutin induces the metabolism of ethinyl estradiol and norethindrone, thereby decreasing the efficacy of oral contraceptives (1). Therefore, additional, nonhormonal methods of birth control should be used during treatment with this antibiotic.

BREASTFEEDING SUMMARY

No reports describing the use of rifabutin during human lactation have been located. The molecular weight (about 847), moderate plasma protein binding, and prolonged terminal half-life suggest that excretion into milk should be expected. Milk may be stained a brown-orange color. The effect of this exposure on a nursing infant is unknown but serious toxicity (e.g., leukopenia, neutropenia, rash) is a potential complication. If the drug is used during breastfeeding, monitoring for these toxicities should be considered. Moreover, rifabutin is indicated for the prevention of disseminated *M. avium* complex in patients with advanced HIV infection, and women with HIV should not breastfeed.

Reference

1. Product information. Mycobutin. Pharmacia & Upjohn, 2004.

RIFAMPIN

Antituberculosis Agent

PREGNANCY RECOMMENDATION: Compatible
BREASTFEEDING RECOMMENDATION: Compatible

PREGNANCY SUMMARY

Several reviews have evaluated the available treatment of tuberculosis during pregnancy (1–3). All concluded that rifampin was not a proven teratogen and recommended use of the drug with isoniazid and ethambutol if necessary. Other reports on the use of the agent in pregnancy have observed no fetal harm (4,5). Prophylactic vitamin K_1 has been recommended to prevent hemorrhagic disease of the newborn (6).

FETAL RISK SUMMARY

Reproduction studies with rifampin in mice and rats at doses >150 mg/kg produced spina bifida in both species and cleft palates in the mouse fetuses (7). Teratogenicity in rodents has been reported with oral doses 15–25 times the human dose (8). Studies with pregnant rabbits revealed no evidence of teratogenicity (7).

In a surveillance study of Michigan Medicaid recipients involving 229,101 completed pregnancies conducted between 1985 and 1992, 20 newborns had been exposed to rifampin during the 1st trimester (F. Rosa, personal communication, FDA, 1993). No major birth defects were observed (one expected).

No controlled studies have linked the use of rifampin with congenital defects (9,10). One report described nine malformations in 204 pregnancies that went to term (11). This incidence, 4.4%, is similar to the expected frequency of defects in a healthy nonexposed population but higher than the 1.8% rate noted in other tuberculosis patients. The malformations were anencephaly (one case), hydrocephalus (two cases), limb malformations (four cases), renal tract defects (one case), and congenital hip dislocation (one case) (11).

Rifampin crosses the placenta to the fetus (12–14). At term, the cord:maternal serum ratio ranged 0.12–0.33 (13). In a second report involving pregnancy termination at 13 weeks' gestation, the fetal:maternal ratio 4 hours after a 300-mg dose was 0.23 (12).

Rifampin has been implicated as one of the agents responsible for hemorrhagic disease of the newborn (6). In one of the three infants affected, only laboratory evidence of hemorrhagic disease of the newborn was present, but in the other two, clinically evident bleeding was observed. Prophylactic vitamin K_1 is recommended to prevent this serious complication (see Phytonadione).

Rifampin may interfere with oral contraceptives, resulting in unplanned pregnancies (see Oral Contraceptives) (15).

BREASTFEEDING SUMMARY

Rifampin is excreted into human milk. In one report, the concentrations were 1–3 mcg/mL with about 0.05% of the daily dose appearing in the milk (16). In another study, milk levels were 3.4–4.9 mcg/mL, 12 hours after a single 450-mg oral dose (17). Maternal plasma samples averaged 21.3 mcg/mL, indicating a milk:plasma ratio of about 0.20. These amounts were thought to represent a very low risk to the nursing infant (18). No reports describing adverse effects in nursing infants have been located. The American Academy of Pediatrics classifies rifampin as compatible with breastfeeding (19).

References

1. Snider DE, Layde PM, Johnson MW, Lyle MA. Treatment of tuberculosis during pregnancy. Am Rev Respir Dis 1980;122:65–79.
2. American Thoracic Society. Treatment of tuberculosis and tuberculosis infection in adults and children. Am Rev Respir Dis 1986;134:355–63.
3. Medchill MT, Gillum M. Diagnosis and management of tuberculosis during pregnancy. Obstet Gynecol Surv 1989;44:81–4.
4. Shneerson JM, Frances RS. Ethambutol in pregnancy: foetal exposure. Tubercle 1979;60:167–9.
5. Kingdon JCP, Kennedy DH. Tuberculosis meningitis in pregnancy. Br J Obstet Gynaecol 1989;96:233–5.
6. Eggermont E, Logghe N, Van De Casseye W, Casteels-Van Daele M, Jaeken J, Cosemans J, Verstraete M, Renaer M. Haemorrhagic disease of the newborn in the offspring of rifampicin and isoniazid treated mothers. Acta Paediatr Belg 1976;29:87–90.
7. Tuchmann-Duplessis H, Mercier-Parot L. Influence d'un antibiotique, la rifampicine, sur le developpement prenatal des rongeurs. C R Acad Sci (d)

R

(Paris) 1969;269:2147–9. As cited in Shepard TH. *Catalog of Teratogenic Agents*. 6th ed. Baltimore, MD: The Johns Hopkins University Press, 1989:558–9.
8. Product information. Rifadin. Hoechst Marion Roussel, 2000.
9. Reimers D. Missbildungen durch Rifampicin. Bericht ueber 2 faelle von normaler fetaler entwicklung nach rifampicin therapie in der fruehsch wangerschaft. Munchen Med Wochenschr 1971;113:1690.
10. Warkany J. Antituberculous drugs. Teratology 1979;20:133–8.
11. Steen JSM, Stainton-Ellis DM. Rifampicin in pregnancy. Lancet 1977;2:604–5.
12. Rocker I. Rifampicin in early pregnancy. Lancet 1977;2:48.
13. Kenny MT, Strates B. Metabolism and pharmacokinetics of the antibiotic rifampin. Drug Metab Rev 1981;12:159–218.
14. Holdiness MR. Transplacental pharmacokinetics of the antituberculosis drugs. Clin Pharmacokinet 1987;13:125–9.
15. Gupta KC, Ali MY. Failure of oral contraceptives with rifampicin. Med J Zambia 1980;15:23.
16. Vorherr H. Drug excretion in breast milk. Postgrad Med J 1974;56:97–104.
17. Lenzi E, Santuari S. Preliminary observations on the use of a new semi-synthetic rifamycin derivative in gynecology and obstetrics. Atti Accad Lancisiana Roma 1969;13(Suppl 1):87–94. As cited in Snider DE Jr, Powell KE. Should women taking antituberculosis drugs breastfeed? Arch Intern Med 1984;144:589–90.
18. Snider DE Jr, Powell KE. Should women taking antituberculosis drugs breastfeed? Arch Intern Med 1984;144:589–90.
19. Committee on Drugs, American Academy of Pediatrics. The transfer of drugs and other chemicals into human milk. Pediatrics 2001;108:776–89.

RIFAPENTINE

Antituberculosis Agent

PREGNANCY RECOMMENDATION: Limited Human Data—Animal Data Suggest Risk
BREASTFEEDING RECOMMENDATION: No Human Data—Probably Compatible

PREGNANCY SUMMARY

Rifapentine induced toxicity and teratogenicity in two experimental animal species at doses close to those used in humans. Human pregnancy experience is limited to three cases, two of which ended in 1st trimester spontaneous abortions. Although comorbid conditions were present and may have caused the losses, the outcomes are sufficiently concerning to warrant caution in prescribing rifapentine early in pregnancy. Until additional data are forthcoming, rifapentine is best avoided during the 1st trimester.

FETAL RISK SUMMARY

The antibiotic rifapentine is a semi-synthetic cyclopentyl derivative of rifamycin and has a similar profile of microbiologic activity to rifampin. It is indicated for the treatment of pulmonary tuberculosis. The antibiotic inhibits DNA-dependent RNA polymerase in *Mycobacterium tuberculosis*, but this effect does not occur in mammalian cells. The elimination half-lives of rifapentine and its active metabolite are each about 13 hours (1).

Reproduction studies with rifapentine in rats and rabbits produced teratogenic and toxic effects in both species. In rats, doses 0.6 times the human dose based on BSA (HD) administered during organogenesis resulted in cleft palates, right aortic arch, an increased incidence of delayed ossification, and an increased number of ribs. Embryo and fetal toxic effects included increases in resorption rates, postimplantation losses, and stillbirths, and decreased fetal weight. Administration of doses 0.3 times the HD from day 15 of gestation through postpartum day 21 was associated with decreased pup weights and stillbirths. Major anomalies observed in the offspring of pregnant rabbits administered doses 0.3–1.3 times the HD included ovarian agenesis, pes varus (i.e., talipes varus), arhinia, microphthalmia, and irregularities of the ossified facial tissues. When doses 1.3 times the HD were given, increased incidences of postimplantation losses and stillbirths were observed (1).

It is not known if rifapentine crosses the human placenta. The molecular weight (about 877) is low enough that exposure of the embryo and fetus probably occurs. In addition, the prolonged elimination half-lives of the parent compound and its active metabolite increase the opportunity for passage of the agents into the fetal compartment.

In a clinical study by the manufacturer, three women became pregnant while receiving rifapentine, 600 mg twice weekly (combined with isoniazid, ethambutol, pyrazinamide, and pyridoxine) and three became pregnant during follow-up (1,2). The first patient had a positive serum pregnancy test at baseline and subsequently received a single 600-mg dose of rifapentine before being dropped from the study. An elective abortion was conducted to terminate the pregnancy. The second patient, with a history of alcohol abuse, received 10 doses of rifapentine 600 mg over 42 days before exclusion from the study. She had a 1st trimester spontaneous abortion 9 days after the last dose. The third woman had an HIV infection as well as tuberculosis. She was treated over 85 days with 22 rifapentine 600-mg doses and had a 1st trimester spontaneous abortion 16 days after the last dose. The investigator concluded that the abortion was secondary to the HIV infection. The outcomes of the three pregnancies in the follow-up stage of the study, which were not thought to have been exposed to the drug during gestation, were two normal deliveries and one lost to follow-up (1,2).

When taken in the last few weeks of pregnancy, rifapentine may cause hemorrhage in both the mother and newborn secondary to vitamin K deficiency (1). This effect is similar to that observed with rifampin. Prophylactic vitamin K_1 is recommended to prevent hemorrhage. (See also Phytonadione.)

Rifapentine may increase the metabolism and reduce the activity of oral or other systemic hormonal contraceptives (1).

Unplanned pregnancies may result from this interaction. Patients receiving rifapentine should be advised to change to nonhormonal methods of birth control (1).

Because active untreated tuberculosis represents a greater risk to the fetus than does treatment, immediate initiation of drug therapy is usually recommended, regardless of the gestational stage (3–6). The CDC recommends a combination of isoniazid (plus pyridoxine), rifampin, and ethambutol as the treatment of choice for pulmonary tuberculosis during pregnancy and breastfeeding (5). An earlier statement by the World Health Organization recommended a 6-month regimen of isoniazid (plus pyridoxine), rifampin, and pyrazinamide as first-line treatment in pregnancy (6). Ethambutol was recommended if a fourth drug was needed during the initial phase. Although the CDC did not recommend pyrazinamide, it classified this agent as probably safe in pregnancy (5). Moreover, the CDC stated that if pyrazinamide was not included in the initial treatment regimen, the minimum duration of therapy should be 9 months (39 weeks) instead of 6 months (26 weeks). Importantly, the CDC did not recommend rifapentine in pregnancy because of insufficient information (5).

BREASTFEEDING SUMMARY

No reports describing the use of rifapentine during lactation have been located. The molecular weight of rifapentine (about 877) and the prolonged half-lives of the parent compound and the active metabolite (both about 13 hours) suggest that these agents will be excreted into milk. Breast milk may be discolored because rifapentine produces a red-orange discoloration of body fluids. The effects of this exposure, if any, on a nursing infant are unknown. Rifampin, a closely related antibiotic with a similar molecular weight (about 823), is excreted in low amounts into breast milk. The American Academy of Pediatrics classifies rifampin as compatible with breastfeeding (see Rifampin).

References

1. Product information. Priftin. Aventis Pharmaceuticals, 2004.
2. Center for Drug Evaluation and Research. FDA. Approval package: Priftin (Rifapentine) 150 mg tablets. Hoechst Marion Roussel, June 22, 1998.
3. Medchill MT, Gillum M. Diagnosis and management of tuberculosis during pregnancy. Obstet Gynecol Surv 1989;44:81–4.
4. American Thoracic Society. Treatment of tuberculosis and tuberculosis infection in adults and children. Am J Respir Crit Care Med 1994;149:1359–74.
5. CDC. Treatment of tuberculosis. MMWR 2003;52(RR11):1–77.
6. World Health Organization. *Treatment of Tuberculosis: Guidelines for National Programs*. 2nd ed. Geneva, Switzerland, 1997.

RIFAXIMIN

Antibiotic

PREGNANCY RECOMMENDATION: No Human Data—Animal Data Suggest Risk
BREASTFEEDING RECOMMENDATION: No Human Data—Probably Compatible

PREGNANCY SUMMARY

No reports describing the use of rifaximin in human pregnancy have been located. The animal reproduction data suggest risk, but the amount absorbed from the gastrointestinal tract was not quantified. In humans, the very small amounts absorbed systemically suggest that the embryo–fetal risk is low, if it exists at all. Although inadvertent exposure early in gestation appears to represent a low risk, the safest course, because of the animal data, is to avoid the antibiotic in the 1st trimester. Until human pregnancy data are available, women should be counseled that the absence of human pregnancy experience prevents an accurate assessment of the embryo–fetal risk.

FETAL RISK SUMMARY

Rifaximin is a semi-synthetic antibiotic that is poorly absorbed after oral administration. Following oral dosing, a mean 0.32% of the dose was recovered in the urine. The remainder was found in the feces as unchanged drug. Rifaximin is indicated for the treatment of patients with travelers' diarrhea caused by noninvasive strains of *Escherichia coli* (1). It is a derivative of rifamycin that has antibacterial activity against a broad spectrum of gram-positive and gram-negative bacteria, including aerobic, anaerobic, and enteropathogens (2,3). In addition to an oral formulation, it is available outside of the United States as a 5% cream for topical application (3).

Reproduction studies have been conducted in rats and rabbits. In pregnant rats, doses about 2.5–5 times the human clinical dose adjusted for BSA (HCD) were teratogenic, as were doses in pregnant rabbits about 2–33 times the HCD. The effects included cleft palate, agnathia, jaw shortening, hemorrhage, partially open eye, small eyes, brachygnathia, incomplete ossification, and increased thoracolumbar vertebrae. There was no effect on fertility in male or female rats given doses up to about 5 times the HCD. Carcinogenicity studies with rifaximin have not been conducted. Assays for genotoxicity were negative (1).

It is not known if rifaximin crosses the human placenta. The molecular weight (about 786) is low enough for passive transfer, but only a very small amount of the antibiotic is absorbed into the systemic circulation. After a 400-mg dose in healthy nonpregnant subjects, the mean maximum plasma concentrations were in the range of 4–10 ng/mL (1). The elimination half-life was about 6 hours.

A 2005 review concluded that the lack of absorption and the safety profile in nonpregnant adults suggested that rifaximin was safe in pregnancy for the treatment of infectious diarrhea (2). A second 2005 reference reviewed the use of rifaximin for infections other than diarrhea, such as skin infections, bacterial vaginosis (BV), and periodontal disease (3). The authors of this review concluded that for these uses, only the efficacy of rifaximin in skin infections had been documented, but that further study for BV and periodontal disease was warranted.

Pregnant women may be at higher risk for "traveler's diarrhea" because of the lowered gastric acidity and increased transient time through the gastrointestinal tract that is characteristic of pregnancy (4). Although rifaximin is effective and minimally absorbed, the effects of the antibiotic in human pregnancy have not been studied.

BREASTFEEDING SUMMARY

No reports describing the use of rifaximin during lactation have been located. The molecular weight (about 786) is low enough for excretion into breast milk, but only very small amounts of the antibiotic are absorbed into the systemic circulation. The effects of this exposure on a nursing infant are unknown, but appear to be negligible.

References

1. Product information. Xifaxan. Salix Pharmaceuticals, 2005.
2. Ericsson CD, DuPont HL. Rifaximin in the treatment of infectious diarrhea. Chemotherapy 2005;51(Suppl 1):73–80.
3. Pelosini I, Scarpignato C. Rifaximin, a peculiar rifamycin derivative: established and potential clinical use outside the gastrointestinal tract. Chemotherapy 2005;51(Suppl 1):122–30.
4. Yates J. Traveler's diarrhea. Am Fam Physician 2005;71:2095–100.

RILONACEPT

Immunologic Agent (Immunomodulator)

PREGNANCY RECOMMENDATION: No Human Data—Animal Data Suggest Risk
BREASTFEEDING RECOMMENDATION: No Human Data—Potential Toxicity

PREGNANCY SUMMARY

No reports describing the use of rilonacept in human pregnancy have been located. The protein caused developmental toxicity (structural anomalies and death) in two animal species. If the agent is given shortly before or during pregnancy, the woman should be counseled as to the potential embryo–fetal risk.

FETAL RISK SUMMARY

Rilonacept is a dimeric fusion protein that acts as an interleukin-1 blocker. It is indicated for the treatment of cryopyrin-associated periodic syndromes, including familial cold auto-inflammatory syndrome and Muckle-Wells syndrome in adults and children ≥12 years of age. Pharmacokinetic data are not available from the manufacturer, but after weekly SC doses, steady-state concentrations were reached at 6 weeks (1). In a 2009 reference, the circulation half-life was cited as 8.6 days (2).

Reproduction studies have been conducted in cynomolgus monkeys and mice. In monkeys given doses up to about 3.7 times the human doses of 160 mg based on BSA (HD), all doses reduced serum levels of estradiol up to 64% compared with controls. In addition, all doses increased the incidence of lumbar ribs compared with both control animals and historical control incidences. The fetus of the only monkey exposed during the later period of gestation showed multiple fusion and absence of the ribs and thoracic vertebral bodies and arches. In this monkey, the exposure was below that expected clinically. A murine analog of rilonacept was used in mice. The highest dose, about 6 times higher than the HD, resulted in threefold increase in the number of stillbirths. In a perinatal and postnatal mouse study with the murine analog, all doses up to about 6 times the HD caused an increased incidence of unscheduled death in the offspring.

Neither carcinogenic nor mutagenic studies have been conducted with rilonacept. No adverse effects on fertility parameters were observed in male and female mice given multiple doses of the murine analog up to about 6 times the HD (1).

It is not known if rilonacept crosses the human placenta. The molecular weight (about 251,000) suggests that passive transfer will not occur, but the long circulation half-life will place the protein at the maternal–fetal interface for a prolonged period. Moreover, other proteins (e.g., see Immune Globulin Intravenous) cross the placenta. If the toxicity observed in the two animal species were direct effects (i.e., effects on the embryo and/or fetus and not caused by maternal effects), this would be evidence that the protein can cross hemochorial placentas.

BREASTFEEDING SUMMARY

No reports describing the use of rilonacept during human lactation have been located. The high molecular weight of this protein (about 251,000) suggests that excretion into mature breast milk will be inhibited. Because immunoglobulins and other high-molecular-weight substances are excreted into colostrum, exposure of the nursing infant to rilonacept might occur during the first few days after birth. The effect of this exposure on a nursing infant is unknown. However, in children and adult patients treated with this drug, an increase in infections is a common complication due to interference with the immune response. Nursing infants of women receiving the drug should be monitored for this effect.

References

1. Product information. Arcalyst. Regeneron Pharmaceuticals, 2009.
2. Kapur S, Bonk ME. Rilonacept (Arcalyst), an interleukin-1 trap for the treatment of cryopyrin-associated periodic syndromes. P&T 2009;34:138–41.

RILPIVIRINE

Antiviral

PREGNANCY RECOMMENDATION: Compatible—Maternal Benefit >> Embryo–Fetal Risk
BREASTFEEDING RECOMMENDATION: Contraindicated

PREGNANCY SUMMARY

No reports describing the use of rilpivirine in human pregnancy have been located. The animal reproduction data suggest low risk but the absence of human pregnancy experience prevents a complete assessment of the embryo–fetal risk. Nevertheless, because HIV is a potentially fatal disease, the drug if indicated should not be withheld because of pregnancy.

FETAL RISK SUMMARY

Rilpivirine is an HIV type1 specific, nonnucleoside reverse transcriptase inhibitor (NNRTI) that is given orally. It is in the same NNRTI class as delavirdine, efavirenz, etravirine, and nevirapine. Rilpivirine is indicated to be used in combination with other antiretroviral agents for the treatment of HIV-1 infection in treatment-naïve adult patients. The drug undergoes oxidative metabolism, apparently to inactive metabolites. Plasma protein binding, primarily to albumin, is about 99.7% and the terminal elimination half-life is about 50 hours (1).

Reproduction studies have been conducted in rats and rabbits. In these species during pregnancy and lactation, no evidence of embryo or fetal toxicity, or effect on reproductive function was observed at exposures that were 15 and 70 times higher, respectively, than the exposure in humans at the recommended dose of 25 mg once daily (RHD) (1).

In 2-year studies, no carcinogenic effects were observed in rats, but in mice hepatocellular neoplasms occurred in both males and females. The observed hepatocellular findings in mice may be rodent-specific. Assays for mutagenicity were negative. In fertility studies with rats, rilpivirine had no effect on mating or fertility with exposures up to about 40 times the RHD (1).

It is not known if rilpivirine crosses the human placenta. The molecular weight (about 367 for the free base) and long elimination terminal half-life suggest that the drug will cross to the embryo–fetus. However, the high plasma protein binding might limit the exposure.

Although the use of rilpivirine for the treatment of HIV was discussed in three recent publications, no information was given about its use in pregnancy (2–4).

BREASTFEEDING SUMMARY

No reports describing the use of rilpivirine during lactation have been located. The molecular weight (about 367 for the free base) and long terminal elimination half-life (about 50 hours) suggest that the drug will be excreted into breast milk. The effect of this exposure on a nursing infant is unknown.

Reports on the use of rilpivirine during human lactation are unlikely because the antiviral agent is used in the treatment of HIV infections. HIV-1 is transmitted in milk, and in developed countries, breastfeeding is not recommended (5–10). In developing countries, breastfeeding is undertaken, despite the risk, because there are no affordable milk substitutes available. Until 1999, no studies had been published that examined the effect of any antiretroviral therapy on HIV-1 transmission in milk. In that year, a study involving zidovudine was published that measured a 38% reduction in vertical transmission of HIV-1 infection despite breastfeeding when compared with controls (see Zidovudine).

References

1. Product information. Edurant. Tibotec Pharmaceuticals, 2011.
2. Ford N, Calmy A. Improving first-line antiretroviral therapy in resource-limited settings. Curr Opin HIV AIDS 2010;5:38–47.
3. Editorial. HIV/AIDS and the road to Rome. Lancet 2011;378:199.
4. Penazzato M, Giaquinto C. Role of non-nucleoside reverse transcriptase inhibitors in treating HIV-infected children. Drugs 2011;71:2131–49.
5. Carpenter CCJ, Fischi MA, Hammer SM, Hirsch MS, Jacobsen DM, Katzenstein DA, Montaner JSG, Richman DD, Saag MS, Schooley RT, Thompson MA, Vella S, Yeni PG, Volberding PA. Antiretroviral therapy for HIV infection in 1996. JAMA 1996;276;146–54.
6. Minkoff H, Augenbraun M. Antiretroviral therapy for pregnant women. Am J Obstet Gynecol 1997;176:478–89.
7. Panel on Antiretroviral Guidelines for Adults and Adolescents. *Guidelines for the Use of Antiretroviral Agents in HIV-1-infected Adults and Adolescents*. Department of Health and Human Services. March 27, 2012:1–161. Available at http://www.aidsinfo.nih.gov/ContentFiles/AdultandAdolescentGL.pdf. Accessed January 13, 2013:I–20.
8. Brown ZA, Watts DH. Antiviral therapy in pregnancy. Clin Obstet Gynecol 1990;33:276–89.
9. De Martino M, Tovo P-A, Pezzotti P, Galli L, Massironi E, Ruga E, Floreea F, Plebani A, Gabiano C, Zuccotti GV. HIV-1 transmission through breast-milk: appraisal of risk according to duration of feeding. AIDS 1992;6:991–7.
10. Van de Perre P. Postnatal transmission of human immunodeficiency virus type 1: the breast feeding dilemma. Am J Obstet Gynecol 1995;173: 483–7.

RILUZOLE

Central Nervous System (Miscellaneous)

PREGNANCY RECOMMENDATION: Compatible—Maternal Benefit >> Embryo–Fetal Risk
BREASTFEEDING RECOMMENDATION: No Human Data—Potential Toxicity

PREGNANCY SUMMARY

Although the animal data suggest risk, the very limited human pregnancy experience does not allow an accurate assessment of the human embryo–fetal risk. Nevertheless, amyotrophic lateral sclerosis (ALS) is a severe progressive disease with marked morbidity resulting in eventual death. Consequently, the maternal benefit appears to be much greater than the unknown embryo–fetal risk.

FETAL RISK SUMMARY

Riluzole is indicated for the treatment of patients with ALS to extend survival and/or time to tracheostomy. It is a member of the benzothiazole class. The agent is extensively metabolized and some of the metabolites are pharmacologically active. Riluzole is 96% bound to plasma proteins, mainly to albumin and lipoproteins. The mean elimination half-life is 12 hours (1).

Reproduction studies have been conducted in rats and rabbits. In these species, doses that were 2.6 and 11.5 times, respectively, the maximum recommended daily dose based on BSA (MRDD) caused embryotoxicity. Maternal toxicity also was observed at these doses. When rats received a dose that was 1.5 times the MRDD before and during mating (males and females) and throughout pregnancy and lactation, decreased implantations, increased intrauterine death, and adverse effects in offspring viability and growth were observed (1).

Riluzole was not carcinogenic in mice and rats, and there was no evidence of mutagenic or clastogenic potential in multiple assays. The major active metabolite, *N*-hydroxyriluzole, did cause chromosomal damage in two tests, but negative results were observed in other assays. As discussed above, Riluzole impaired fertility when administered to male and female rats (1).

It is not known if riluzole or its metabolites cross the human placenta. The molecular weight of the parent drug (about 234) and long elimination half-life suggest that riluzole and its metabolite will cross to the embryo–fetus.

The first report of riluzole use in human pregnancy appeared in 2009 (2). A 28-year-old woman was diagnosed with ALS and treated with riluzole (dose not specified). When her pregnancy was discovered at 9 weeks' gestation, riluzole was discontinued. She had a normal pregnancy and gave birth vaginally at 40 weeks' to a healthy male infant. No other information about the infant was given other than that he was in good health at the time of this report. The woman eventually had a second pregnancy, apparently without riluzole (2).

A 2010 case report described the pregnancy outcome of a 34-year-old primigravida Japanese woman with ALS (3). The woman had been taking riluzole (100 mg/day) for 2 years. Her pregnancy was diagnosed at 30 weeks' gestation and riluzole was continued. She gave birth vaginally at 38 weeks' to a 2280-g growth-restricted female infant with Apgar scores of 8 and 8 at 1 and 5 minutes, respectively. The growth restriction may have been wholly or partially due to cigarette smoking. The infant was developing normally at 1 year of age. In addition to this case, the authors reviewed the pregnancy outcomes of 11 women with ALS (all occurring before the availability of riluzole) (3).

BREASTFEEDING SUMMARY

No reports describing the use of riluzole during human lactation have been located. The molecular weight (about 234) and long elimination half-life (12 hours) suggest that the drug, and possibly its metabolites, will be excreted into breast milk. The effect of this exposure on a nursing infant is unknown. However, the drug caused marked toxicity in adults with about 14% of patients in clinical trials discontinuing riluzole because of adverse effects (1).

References

1. Product information. Rilutek. Sanofi-Aventis, 2009.
2. Sarafov S, Doitchinova M, Karagiozova Z, Slancheva B, Dengler R, Petri S, Kollewe K. Two consecutive pregnancies in early and late stage of amyotrophic lateral sclerosis. Amyotroph Lateral Scler 2009;10:483–6.
3. Kawamichi Y, Makino Y, Matsuda Y, Miyazaki K, Uchiyama S, Ohta H. Riluzole use during pregnancy in a patient with amyotrophic lateral sclerosis: a case report. J Int Med Res 2010;38:720–6.

RIMANTADINE

Antiviral

PREGNANCY RECOMMENDATION: No Human Data—Animal Data Suggest Moderate Risk
BREASTFEEDING RECOMMENDATION: No Human Data—Potential Toxicity

PREGNANCY SUMMARY

The human pregnancy experience with rimantadine is limited. As of late 1996, the FDA had not received any reports of pregnancy exposure to rimantadine (F. Rosa, personal communication, FDA, 1996). Although the lack of human data does not allow an assessment of fetal risk, the absence of significant animal teratogenicity may indicate that rimantadine is a lower risk during pregnancy than the closely related drug, amantadine.

FETAL RISK SUMMARY

Rimantadine is a synthetic antiviral agent used in the prophylaxis and treatment of influenza A virus infections. In nonpregnant patients, rimantadine shares the toxic profile of a similar antiviral agent, amantadine, which is also used for influenza A virus infections (see Amantadine) (1).

It is not known if rimantadine crosses the human placenta, but the relatively low molecular weight (about 216) suggests that exposure of the embryo–fetus probably occurs.

Rimantadine was embryotoxic (increased fetal resorption) in rats at a dose 11 times the recommended human dose based on BSA (RHD) (2). This dose also produced maternal toxicity. No embryotoxicity was observed in rabbits given up to 5 times the RHD, but a developmental abnormality was observed as evidenced by an increase in the ratio of fetuses with 12–13 ribs from the normal litter distribution of 50:50 to 80:20 (2).

A retrospective cohort study, covering the period 2003–2008, described 239 pregnancies that were treated with antiviral agents during pregnancy (3). Of these, 104 women received M2 ion channel inhibitors (rimantadine, amantadine, or both) and 135 received oseltamivir. The pregnancy outcomes of these patients were compared with 82,097 controls from the site's overall obstetric patient population. The exposure timing for the combined treated groups was 13% in 1st trimester, 32% in 2nd trimester, and 55% in 3rd trimester. There were no significant differences between the treated groups and controls in terms of maternal and delivery characteristics except that M2 inhibitors had more multiple gestations. For M2 inhibitors, oseltamivir vs. controls, there also were no differences in stillbirths (0%, 0% vs. 1%), major defects (1% [trisomy 21], 0% vs. 2%), and minor defects (19%, 15% vs. 22%). The only significant finding in the characteristics of liveborn, singleton neonates, after exclusion of twins and major anomalies, was a higher risk of necrotizing enterocolitis in both treatment groups compared with controls—1.0%, 0.8% vs. 0.02%. (3).

BREASTFEEDING SUMMARY

No reports describing the use of rimantadine during human lactation have been located. The molecular weight (about 216) is low enough that excretion into breast milk should be expected. The effect of this exposure on a nursing infant is unknown. The manufacturer recommends the drug not be administered to nursing women (2).

References

1. Morris DJ. Adverse effects and drug interactions of clinical importance with antiviral drugs. Drug Safety 1994;10:281–91.
2. Product information. Flumadine. Forest Pharmaceuticals, 2000.
3. Greer LG, Sheffield JS, Rogers VL, Roberts SW, McIntire DD, Wendel GD Jr. Maternal and neonatal outcomes after antepartum treatment of influenza with antiviral medications. Obstet Gynecol 2010;115:711–6.

RISEDRONATE

Bisphosphonate

PREGNANCY RECOMMENDATION: Limited Human Data—Animal Data Suggest Risk
BREASTFEEDING RECOMMENDATION: No Human Data—Probably Compatible

PREGNANCY SUMMARY

The use of risedronate before or during pregnancy has been described, but the data are very limited. No drug-induced toxicity was seen in the offspring. Although the animal data suggest risk of developmental toxicity, the near absence of human pregnancy experience prevents an assessment of the embryo–fetal risk. However, the very long elimination half-life from bone indicates that women treated with risedronate will have detectable concentrations of the drug for a prolonged interval. The amount of drug retained in bone and eventually released back into the systemic circulation is directly related to the dose and duration of treatment. Thus, administration before pregnancy may result in low-level, continuous exposure throughout gestation. The use of etidronate in women who may become pregnant or during pregnancy is not recommended. However, based on the animal and limited human data, inadvertent exposure during early pregnancy does not appear to represent a major risk to the embryo–fetus.

FETAL RISK SUMMARY

Bisphosphonates are synthetic analogs of pyrophosphate that bind to the hydroxyapatite found in bone. Other agents in this class include alendronate, etidronate, ibandronate, pamidronate, tiludronate, and zoledronic acid. Risedronate, a specific inhibitor of osteoclast-mediated bone resorption, is indicated for the treatment and prevention of osteoporosis in postmenopausal women. It also is indicated for the prevention and treatment of glucocorticoid-induced osteoporosis in men and women, and in the treatment of Paget's disease of bone (osteitis deformans). Risedronate is not metabolized, and plasma protein binding is minimal (about 24%). The elimination half-life is biphasic with an initial serum half-life of about 1.5 hours. The very long terminal half-life (480 hours) is thought to be secondary to its slow dissociation from the surface of bone. The mean absolute oral bioavailability is 0.63% and is reduced even further by meals. Steady state serum drug concentrations are obtained within 57 days of daily dosing (1).

Reproduction studies have been conducted in rats and rabbits. Treatment during mating and gestation with doses as low as the maximum recommended human dose of 30 mg/day based on BSA (MRHD) resulted in periparturient hypocalcemia and mortality in pregnant rats. This same dose was associated with a low incidence of cleft palate in fetuses. During gestation, doses as low as about 5.2 times the MRHD resulted in decreased survival of neonates. At 26 times the MRHD, the body weight of surviving neonates decreased. A significant increase in the number of fetuses with incomplete ossification of sternebrae or skull was observed at about 2.3 times the MRHD, and both incomplete ossification and unossified sternebrae were increased at about 5.2 times the MRHD. In rabbits, no significant fetal ossification effects were observed at doses up to 6.7 times the MRHD. At this dose, however, 1 of 14 litters was aborted and 1 litter delivered prematurely (1).

Long-term studies in rats revealed no evidence of carcinogenesis. In addition, various assays have found no evidence of mutagenesis when nontoxic doses were used. Risedronate, however, did impair fertility in male rats and dogs at doses as low as about 5.2 and 8 times the MRHD, respectively. In female rats, ovulation was inhibited at a dose about 5.2 times the MRHD, and decreased implantation was noted at a dose about 2.3 times the MRHD (1).

It is not known if risedronate crosses the human placenta. The molecular weight (about 350 for the hemi-pentahydrate form), low protein binding, and lack of metabolism suggest that the drug will cross to the embryo–fetus. The amount available for diffusion across the placenta during treatment should be minimal because of the low oral bioavailability and short serum elimination half-life. When treatment has been discontinued, the amount of drug available for diffusion during the prolonged bone elimination should be even lower, but the drug will be present at the maternal–fetal interface for months or longer.

A 2008 review described 51 cases of exposure to bisphosphonates before or during pregnancy: alendronate (*N* = 32), pamidronate (*N* = 11), etidronate (*N* = 5), risedronate (*N* = 2), and zoledronic acid (*N* = 1) (2). The authors concluded that although these drugs may affect bone modeling and development in the fetus, no such toxicity has yet been reported.

BREASTFEEDING SUMMARY

No reports describing the use of risedronate during human lactation have been located. The molecular weight (about 350 for the hemi-pentahydrate form), low protein binding (about 24%), lack of metabolism, and very long bone elimination half-life (480 hours) suggest that some drug will be excreted into milk. However, the amount excreted into milk during human treatment should be minimal because of the low oral bioavailability (0.63%) and short serum elimination half-life (about 1.5 hours). When treatment has been discontinued, the amount of drug available for excretion during the prolonged bone elimination should be even lower, although excretion into milk could occur for several months. The effect of this exposure on a nursing infant is unknown but is probably negligible.

References

1. Product information. Actonel. Procter & Gamble Pharmaceuticals, 2005.
2. Djokanovic N, Klieger-Grossmann C, Koren G. Does treatment with bisphosphonates endanger the human pregnancy? J Obstet Gynaecol Can 2008;30:1146–8.

R

RISPERIDONE

Antipsychotic

PREGNANCY RECOMMENDATION: Compatible—Maternal Benefit >> Embryo–Fetal Risk
BREASTFEEDING RECOMMENDATION: Limited Human Data—Potential Toxicity

PREGNANCY SUMMARY

Although no structural malformations attributable to risperidone have been reported, the number of exposures is too low to fully assess the embryo–fetal risk. In addition, there is a risk of extrapyramidal and/or withdrawal symptoms in the newborn if the drug is used in the 3rd trimester. Nevertheless, risperidone is indicated for severe debilitating mental disease and the benefits to the mother appear to outweigh the potential embryo–fetal risks. Folic acid 4 mg/day has been recommended for women taking atypical antipsychotics because they may have a higher risk of neural tube defects due to inadequate folate intake and obesity (1).

FETAL RISK SUMMARY

Risperidone, an atypical antipsychotic, is indicated for the management of the manifestations of psychotic disorders, such as schizophrenia. Risperidone is metabolized to an active metabolite, 9-hydroxyrisperidone (see Paliperidone), that has similar pharmacological activity as risperidone. Plasma protein binding is 90% and the mean elimination half-life of the parent drug and metabolite combined in extensive and poor metabolizers is about 20 hours (2). Risperidone is a benzisoxazole derivative in the same antipsychotic subclass as iloperidone, paliperidone, and ziprasidone. Although not approved for this indication by the FDA, it is also used for the management of bipolar disorder and in patients with dementia-related psychotic symptoms.

Reproduction studies have been conducted in pregnant rats and rabbits. No increase in the incidence of congenital malformations was observed in either species at doses 0.4–6 times the human dose based on BSA (HD). At 1.5 times the HD, however, an increase in stillbirths was noted in rats. In addition, increased pup mortality during the first 4 days of lactation occurred at 0.1–3 times the HD. There was no no-effect dose for this toxicity. It was not known if the deaths were due to a direct effect on the pups or toxicity in the dams. Risperidone caused a dose-related decrease in serum testosterone in Beagle dogs, as well as a decrease in sperm motility and concentration, at doses 0.6–10 times the HD (2).

Consistent with the molecular weight (about 410), risperidone crosses the human placenta.

In a 2007 study, six women taking a staple dose (mean 3 mg/day) of quetiapine for a mean 25.9 weeks before delivery had maternal and cord concentrations of the drug determined at birth (3). The cord blood concentration was 49.2% of the maternal concentration. The pregnancy outcomes included one growth-restricted infant (<2500 g). The mean Apgar scores were 8.7 and 9.2 at 1 and 5 minutes, respectively. There were no neonatal complications and no infants were admitted to the neonatal intensive care unit (3).

The outcomes of 10 pregnancies involving 9 women were described in a large postmarketing study involving 7684 patients treated with risperidone (4). The outcomes were three elective terminations and seven live births. No congenital malformations were reported among the live births (4). The manufacturer has also reported an unpublished case of agenesis of the corpus callosum in an infant exposed to risperidone during gestation (2). The relationship between the drug and the defect is unknown.

A 1997 review of antipsychotic use in pregnancy concluded that the safety of risperidone in human pregnancy had not been established (5). The reviewers commented that although no teratogenicity or direct toxicity had been shown in animal studies, some indirect, prolactin- and CNS-mediated effects had been observed.

A brief 2002 report described the pregnancy outcomes of two women with schizophrenia who were treated with risperidone throughout gestation (6). Both women delivered apparently healthy infants at term. The weight of the male infant was 8 pounds (about 3.63 kg), whereas the female infant weighed 5.81 pounds (about 2.64 kg). Risperidone was continued after birth and during nursing. No developmental abnormalities were noted in the infants at 9 months and over 1 year, respectively (6).

A 36-year-old pregnant woman was treated with multiple medications for schizophrenia and other conditions (7). Risperidone 4 mg/day was taken in gestational weeks 6–7. Other psychotropic agents were (daily dose and gestational weeks in parentheses): mirtazapine (30 mg; 1–5), thioridazine (300 mg; 1–5), diazepam (10 mg; 4–5), hydroxyzine (12.5 mg; 4–7), clomipramine (150 mg; 6–7), fluvoxamine (100 mg; 8–21), alprazolam (0.5 mg; 8–21), quetiapine (500–600 mg; 8–37), carbamazepine (600 mg; 8–21), and haloperidol (10 mg; 31–36). She gave birth at 37 weeks' to a healthy 3000-g female infant with Apgar scores of 8 and 9, who was developing normally after 4 months (7).

A 2005 study, involving women from Canada, Israeli, and England, described 151 pregnancy outcomes in women using atypical antipsychotic drugs (8). The exposed group was matched with a comparison group ($N = 151$) who had not been exposed to these agents. The drugs and number of pregnancies were olanzapine ($N = 60$), risperidone ($N = 49$), quetiapine ($N = 36$), and clozapine ($N = 6$). In those exposed, there were 110 live births (72.8%), 22 spontaneous abortions (14.6%), 15 elective abortions (9.9%), and 4 stillbirths (2.6%). Among the live births, one infant exposed in utero to olanzapine had multiple anomalies including midline defects (cleft lip, encephalocele, and aqueductal stenosis). The mean birth weight was 3341 g. There were no statistically significant differences, including rates of neonatal complications, between the cases and controls, with the exceptions of low birth weight (10% vs. 2%, $p = 0.05$) and elective abortions (9.9% vs. 1.3%, $p = 0.003$). The low birth weight may have been caused by the increased rate of cigarette smoking (38% vs. 13%, $p \leq 0.001$) and heavy/binge alcohol use (5 vs. 1) in the exposed group (8).

In a comparison of drugs used in the treatment of schizophrenia during pregnancy, the American Academy of Pediatrics (AAP) classified risperidone as high potency (9). The classification was based on the potential for extrapyramidal reactions (e.g., acute dystonia, akathisia, parkinsonism, and tardive dyskinesia). The AAP cautioned that large maternal doses of high-potency drugs could produce these effects in newborns. However, it did note that high-potency antipsychotics were preferred to minimize maternal anticholinergic, hypotensive, and antihistamine effects. No recommendation concerning the use of risperidone during pregnancy was made because of the lack of data (9).

The manufacturer reported a case of agenesis of the corpus callosum in an infant exposed to risperidone during pregnancy (2). No further details were provided.

A 2006 case report described a woman with a long history of paranoid schizophrenia who was treated with oral risperidone (10). Early in an unknown pregnancy she was started on IM risperidone 25 mg every 2 weeks; the therapy was stopped when she was found pregnant in the 20th week. At 38 weeks, she was hospitalized because of psychotic decompensation with malnutrition (weight 59 kg). She gave birth spontaneously about 2 weeks later to a healthy but small-for-date 2900-g female infant without malformations. At 2.5 years of age, no major health problems had occurred. A minor retardation in her motor development was described but still within the normal range (10).

A 35-year-old woman with a 7-year history of schizophrenia was treated before and throughout pregnancy with long-acting IM risperidone 25 mg every 2 weeks (11). At 37 weeks, her membranes ruptured and she delivered vaginally a 2230-g female infant with Apgar scores of 9 at 1 and 5 minutes. No congenital anomalies were found and the infant was developing normally at 8 months of age (11).

In an extensive literature search, representatives of a manufacturer identified 713 pregnancies in which the mothers were treated with risperidone (12). The reported data were prospective in 516 cases and retrospective in the remaining 197 cases. Adverse pregnancy outcomes were more frequently reported in the retrospective cases. In the 68 prospectively reported pregnancies with a known outcome and after exclusion of 13 elective abortions, structural anomalies and spontaneous abortions occurred in 3.8% and 16.9%, respectively. These results were thought to be consistent with the background rates in the general population. In the retrospective cases, major structural anomalies were observed in 12 pregnancies. The defects most frequently reported involved the heart, brain, and lip and/or palate. In addition, there were 37 outcomes involving perinatal syndromes, of which 21 involved behavioral or motor disorders. The authors concluded that the results do not appear to show an increased risk of congenital anomalies or SABs, but limited extrapyramidal effects in the neonate did occur when risperidone was used in the 3rd trimester (12).

BREASTFEEDING SUMMARY

Risperidone and its active metabolite, 9-hydroxyrisperidone, are excreted into breast milk (13–15). A 21-year-old mother with a 2-year history of bipolar disorder stopped all medication when her pregnancy was diagnosed (13). She did well during pregnancy and delivered a healthy infant at 38 weeks' gestation. When her disease relapsed, she was admitted to the hospital 2.5 months after birth of her infant, stopped breastfeeding, and started on risperidone, eventually reaching a steady-state dose of 6 mg/day. Concentrations of risperidone and the active metabolite were determined in the plasma and milk. The milk:plasma ratios for the parent drug and metabolite, based on AUC, were 0.42 and 0.24, respectively. Based on a daily milk intake of 150 mL/kg, the nursing infant would have received 0.84% of the mother's risperidone dose (mg/kg/day) and an additional 3.46% from the metabolite (as risperidone equivalents), or about 4.3% of the weight-adjusted maternal dose. Although the combined amounts of risperidone and metabolite in breast milk appear to be too low to cause extrapyramidal effects, concern was expressed for other effects, such as neuroleptic malignant syndrome, and effects on cognitive development (13).

A 2004 study measured the steady-state plasma and milk concentrations of risperidone and 9-hydroxyrisperidone in two breastfeeding women and one woman with risperidone-induced galactorrhea (14). The 29-year-old woman with galactorrhea was taking risperidone 3 mg at night (37.5 mcg/kg/day) for schizophrenia. The galactorrhea was attributed to elevated prolactin concentrations due to the D_2 antagonist effects of risperidone. Milk and plasma samples were collected 20 hours postdose, and then milk only on days 2 and 3, each at 21 hours postdose. The plasma concentrations of risperidone and the metabolite were <1 and 14 mcg/L, respectively. All milk risperidone concentrations were <1 mcg/L, whereas the mean concentration of the metabolite was 5.1 mcg/L (range 4.4–5.6 mcg/L). Although the woman was not nursing, the absolute and relative infant doses were 0.88 mcg/kg/day or 2.3% (as risperidone equivalents) (14).

The two women who were breastfeeding were treated for psychosis with risperidone doses of 42.1 mcg/kg/day (2 mg every 12 hours) and 23.1 mcg/kg/day (0.5 mg in the morning and 1 mg at night), respectively (14). The nursing infants were a 3.3-month-old female and a 6-week-old male, respectively. In the first woman, milk concentrations of the parent drug and metabolite were 49 and 142 mcg•hr/L (AUC), respectively, whereas the average concentrations were 2.1 and 6 mcg/L, respectively. The absolute infant doses were 0.32 and 0.9 mcg/kg/day, respectively. In the second woman, milk concentrations were 3.1 and 56.5 mcg•hr/L (AUC), respectively, whereas the average concentrations over 24 hours were 0.39 and 7.06 mcg/L, respectively. The absolute infant doses were 0.06 and 1.06 mcg/kg/day, respectively. The milk:plasma ratios were 0.1 and 0.5, respectively. Neither risperidone nor the metabolite was detected in the plasma of the infants and both were developing normally at 9 and 12 months, respectively (14).

No developmental abnormalities were observed in two infants of mothers treated with risperidone throughout gestation and during breastfeeding (6) (see Fetal Risk Summary).

A 23-year-old woman, nursing a 4.2-kg male infant, was diagnosed with paranoid schizophrenia 1 week after birth (15). She was hospitalized and started on risperidone 1 mg twice daily. The dose was changed to 2 mg every evening on day 7, and then to 3 mg every evening on day 10. Milk (fore and hind) and maternal plasma concentrations of risperidone and paliperidone were determined on days 6, 10, and 20. No drug accumulation was observed and the concentrations of paliperidone always exceeded those of risperidone. The ranges of risperidone and paliperidone milk concentrations were 0–3 and 1.2–11 ng/mL, respectively, whereas the plasma concentrations were 0.4–10 and 4–43 ng/mL, respectively. Moreover, the concentrations in fore- and hind-milk were comparable. On day 10, 15 hours after a 2 mg dose, the concentrations of risperidone and paliperidone in infant plasma were 0 and 0.1 ng/mL, respectively. The mother was discharged home on risperidone after 5 weeks. The psychomotor development of the infant during the mother's hospitalization was normal and no adverse effects or sedation in the infant were observed. The mother and infant were doing well 2 months after discharge (15).

The AAP classifies other antipsychotic drugs as agents for which the effect on nursing infants is unknown but may be of concern, especially when given for long periods (16). Although risperidone was not mentioned, the AAP noted that antipsychotics are excreted into breast milk and could conceivably alter both short-term and long-term central nervous system function. Although no adverse effects from exposure to risperidone have been observed, studies have not been conducted to determine if there are long-term effects.

References

1. Koren G, Cohn T, Chitayat D, Kapur B, Remington G, Myles-Reid D, Zipursky RB. Use of atypical antipsychotics during pregnancy and the risk of neural tube defects in infants. Am J Psychiatry 2002;159:136–7.
2. Product information. Risperdal. Janssen Pharmaceuticals, 2011.
3. Newport DJ, Calamaras MR, DeVane CL, Donovan J, Beach AJ, Winn S, Knight BT, Gibson BB, Viguera AC, Owens MJ, Nemeroff CB, Stowe ZN.

R

Atypical antipsychotic administration during late pregnancy: placental passage and obstetrical outcomes. Am J Psychiatry 2007;164:1214–20.
4. Mackay FJ, Wilton LV, Pearce GL, Freemantle SN, Mann RD. The safety of risperidone: a post-marketing study on 7684 patients. Hum Psychopharmacol Clin Exp 1998;13:413–8.
5. Trixler M, Tenyi T. Antipsychotic use in pregnancy. What are the best treatment options? Drug Safety 1997;16:403–10.
6. Ratnayake T, Libretto SE. No complications with risperidone treatment before and throughout pregnancy and during the nursing period. J Clin Psychiatry 2002;63:76–7.
7. Yaris F, Yaris E, Kadioglu M, Ulku C, Kesim M, Kalyoncu NI. Use of polypharmacotherapy in pregnancy: a prospective outcome in a case. Prog Neuropsychopharmacol Biol Psychiatry 2004;28:603–5.
8. McKenna K, Koren G, Tetelbaum M, Wilton L, Shakir S, Diav-Citrin O, Levinson A, Zipursky RB, Einarson A. Pregnancy outcome of women using atypical antipsychotic drugs: a prospective comparative study. J Clin Psychiatry 2005;66:444–9.
9. Committee on Drugs, American Academy of Pediatrics. Use of psychoactive medication during pregnancy and possible effects on the fetus and newborn. Pediatrics 2000;105:880–7.
10. Dabbert D, Heinze M. Follow-up of a pregnancy with risperidone microspheres. Pharmacopsychiatry 2006;39:235.
11. Kim SW, Kim KM, Kim JM, Shin IS, Shin HY, Yang SJ, Yoon JS. Use of long-acting injectable risperidone before and throughout pregnancy in schizophrenia. Prog Neuropsychopharmacol Biol Psychiatry 2007;31:543–5.
12. Coppola D, Russo LJ, Kwarta RF Jr, Varughese R, Schmider J. Evaluating the postmarketing experience of risperidone use during pregnancy—pregnancy and neonatal outcomes. Drug Saf 2007;30:247–64.
13. Hill RC, McIvor RJ, Wojnar-Horton RE, Hackett LP, Ilett KF. Risperidone distribution and excretion into human milk: case report and estimated infant exposure during breast-feeding. J Clin Psychopharmacol 2000;20:285–6.
14. Ilett KF, Hackett LP, Kristensen JH, Vaddadi KS, Gardiner SJ, Begg EJ. Transfer of risperidone and 9-hydroxyrisperidone into human milk. Ann Pharmacother 2004;38:273–6.
15. Aichhorn W, Stuppaeck C, Whitworth AB. Risperidone and breast-feeding. J Psychopharmacol 2005;19:211–3.
16. Committee on Drugs, American Academy of Pediatrics. The transfer of drugs and other chemicals into human milk. Pediatrics 2001;108:776–89.

RITODRINE

[Withdrawn from the market. See 9th edition.]

RITONAVIR

Antiviral

PREGNANCY RECOMMENDATION: Compatible—Maternal Benefit >> Embryo–Fetal Risk
BREASTFEEDING RECOMMENDATION: Contraindicated

PREGNANCY SUMMARY

Although the limited human data do not allow an assessment of the risk of ritonavir during pregnancy, the animal data suggest that the drug may represent a low risk to the developing fetus. If indicated, the drug should not be withheld because of pregnancy.

FETAL RISK SUMMARY

Ritonavir is an inhibitor of protease in HIV types 1 and 2 (HIV-1 and HIV-2). Protease is an enzyme that is required for the cleavage of viral polyprotein precursors into active functional proteins found in infectious HIV. The mechanism of action is similar to four other protease inhibitors: amprenavir, indinavir, nelfinavir, and saquinavir (1).

Reproduction studies have been conducted in pregnant rats and rabbits. Maternal toxicity and fetal toxicity, but not teratogenicity, were observed in rats at dose exposures equivalent to approximately 30% of that achieved with the human dose. Fetal toxicity consisted of early resorptions, decreased body weight, ossification delays, and developmental variations. At a dose exposure equivalent to 22% of that achieved with the human dose, a slight increase in cryptorchidism was observed. Fetal toxicity (resorptions, decreased litter size, and decreased weights) and maternal toxicity were observed in rabbits at a dose 1.8 times the human dose based on BSA (1).

A 1998 in vitro experiment using term perfused human placentas demonstrated that the placental transfer of ritonavir was concentration dependent and that the clearance index, at both maternal trough and peak concentrations, was very low (2). The investigators attributed the low transfer to the molecular weight (about 721) and solubility characteristics of ritonavir (2). In another report, the drug was detected in cord blood samples (577 and 1020 ng/mL) of twins born at 34 weeks from a woman treated with ritonavir 100 mg twice daily from 25 to 34 weeks (3).

The Antiretroviral Pregnancy Registry reported, for the period January 1989 through July 2009, prospective data (reported before the outcomes were known) involving 4702 live births that had been exposed during the 1st trimester to one or more antiretroviral agents (4). Congenital defects were noted in 134, a prevalence of 2.8% (95% confidence interval [CI] 2.4–3.4). In the 6100 live births with earliest exposure in the 2nd/3rd trimesters, there were 153 infants with defects (2.5%, 95% CI 2.1–2.9). The prevalence rates for the two periods did not differ significantly. There were 288 infants with birth defects among 10,803 live births with exposure anytime during pregnancy (2.7%, 95% CI 2.4–3.0). The prevalence rate did not differ significantly from the rate expected in a nonexposed population.

There were 2552 outcomes exposed to ritonavir (1000 in the 1st trimester and 1552 in the 2nd/3rd trimesters) in combination with other antiretroviral agents. There were 61 birth defects (22 in the 1st trimester and 39 in the 2nd/3rd trimesters). In reviewing the birth defects of prospective and retrospective (pregnancies reported after the outcomes were known) registered cases, the Registry concluded that, except for isolated cases of neural tube defects with efavirenz exposure in retrospective reports, there was no other pattern of anomalies (isolated or syndromic) (4). (See Lamivudine for required statement.)

The experience of one perinatal center with the treatment of HIV-infected pregnant women was summarized in a 1999 abstract (5). Of 55 women receiving 3 or more antiviral drugs, 39 were treated with a protease inhibitor (6 with ritonavir). The outcomes included 2 spontaneous abortions, 5 elective abortions, 27 newborns, and 5 ongoing pregnancies. One woman was taken off indinavir because of ureteral obstruction and another (drug therapy not specified) developed gestational diabetes. None of the newborns tested positive for HIV, and none had major congenital anomalies or complications (5).

A public health advisory has been issued by the FDA on the association between protease inhibitors and diabetes mellitus (6). Because pregnancy is a risk factor for hyperglycemia, there was concern that these antiviral agents would exacerbate this risk. An abstract published in 2000 described the results of a study involving 34 pregnant women treated with protease inhibitors (5 with ritonavir) compared with 41 controls that evaluated the association with diabetes (7). No association between protease inhibitors and an increased incidence of gestational diabetes was found.

A case of combined transient mitochondrial and peroxisomal β-oxidation dysfunction after exposure to nucleoside analog reverse transcriptase inhibitors (NRTIs) (lamivudine and zidovudine) combined with protease inhibitors (ritonavir and saquinavir) throughout gestation was reported in 2000 (8). A male infant was delivered at 38 weeks' gestation. He received postnatal prophylaxis with lamivudine and zidovudine for 4 weeks until the agents were discontinued because of anemia. Other adverse effects that were observed in the infant (age at onset) were hypocalcemia (shortly after birth), Group B streptococcal sepsis, ventricular extrasystoles, prolonged metabolic acidosis, and lactic acidemia (8 weeks), a mild elevation of long chain fatty acids (9 weeks), and neutropenia (3 months). The metabolic acidosis required treatment until 7 months of age, whereas the elevated plasma lactate resolved over 4 weeks. Cerebrospinal fluid lactate was not determined nor was a muscle biopsy conducted. Both the neutropenia and the cardiac dysfunction had resolved by 1 year of age. The elevated plasma fatty acid level was confirmed in cultured fibroblasts, but other peroxisomal functions (plasmalogen biosynthesis and catalase staining) were normal. Although mitochondrial dysfunction has been linked to NRTI agents, the authors were unable to identify the cause of the combined abnormalities in this case. The child was reported to be healthy and developing normally at 26 months of age (8).

A multicenter, retrospective survey of pregnancies exposed to protease inhibitors was published in 2000 (9). There were 92 liveborn infants delivered from 89 women (3 sets of twins) at 6 health care centers. One nonviable infant, born at 22 weeks' gestation, died. The surviving 91 infants were evaluated in terms of adverse effects, prematurity rate, and frequency of HIV-1 transmission. Most of the infants were exposed in utero to a single protease inhibitor, but a few were exposed to more than one because of sequential or double combined therapy. The number of newborns exposed to each protease inhibitor was indinavir ($N = 23$), nelfinavir ($N = 39$), ritonavir ($N = 5$), and saquinavir ($N = 34$). Protease inhibitors were started before conception in 18, and during the 1st, 2nd, or 3rd trimesters in 12, 44, and 14, respectively, and not reported in 1. Other antiretrovirals used with the protease inhibitors included four NRTIs (didanosine, lamivudine, stavudine, and zidovudine). The most common NRTI regimen was a combination of zidovudine and lamivudine (65% of women). In addition, seven women were enrolled in the AIDS Clinical Trials Group Protocol 316 and, at the start of labor, received a single dose of either the non-NRTI nevirapine or placebo. Maternal conditions, thought possibly or likely to be related to therapy, were mild anemia in eight, severe anemia in one (probably secondary to zidovudine), and thrombocytopenia in one. Gestational diabetes mellitus was observed in three women (3.3%), a rate similar to the expected prevalence of 2.6% in a nonexposed population. One mother developed postpartum cardiomyopathy and died 2 months after birth of twins, but the cause of death was not known. For the surviving newborns, there was no increase in adverse effects over that observed in previous clinical trials of HIV-positive women, including the prevalence of anemia (12%), hyperbilirubinemia (6%; none exposed to indinavir), and low birth weight (20.6%). Premature delivery occurred in 19.1% of the pregnancies (close to the expected rate). The percentage of infants infected with HIV was 0 (95% CI 0%–3%) (9).

Two reviews, one in 1996 and the other in 1997, concluded that all women currently receiving antiretroviral therapy should continue to receive therapy during pregnancy and that treatment of the mother with monotherapy should be considered inadequate therapy (10,11). The same conclusion was reached in a 2003 review with the added admonishment that therapy must be continuous to prevent emergence of resistant viral strains (12). In 2009, the updated United States Department of Health and Human Services guidelines for the use of antiretroviral agents in HIV-1-infected patients continued the recommendation that therapy, with the exception of efavirenz, should be continued during pregnancy (13). If indicated, therefore, protease inhibitors, including ritonavir, should not be withheld in pregnancy because the expected benefit to the HIV-positive mother outweighs the unknown risk to the fetus. Pregnant women taking protease inhibitors should be monitored for hyperglycemia. The updated guidelines for the use of antiretroviral drugs to reduce perinatal HIV-1 transmission also were released in 2010 (14). Women receiving antiretroviral therapy during pregnancy should continue the therapy but, regardless of the regimen, zidovudine administration is recommended during the intrapartum period to prevent vertical transmission of HIV to the newborn (14).

BREASTFEEDING SUMMARY

No reports describing the use of ritonavir during lactation have been located. The molecular weight (about 721) is low enough that excretion into breast milk should be expected. The effect on a nursing infant is unknown.

Reports on the use of ritonavir during human lactation are unlikely because the antiviral agent is used in the treatment of HIV infection. HIV-1 is transmitted in milk, and in developed countries, breastfeeding is not recommended (10,11,13,15–17). In developing countries, breastfeeding is undertaken, despite the risk, because there are no affordable milk substitutes available. Until 1999, no studies had been published that examined the effect of any antiretroviral therapy on HIV-1 transmission in milk. In that year, a study involving zidovudine was published that measured a 38% reduction in vertical transmission of HIV-1 infection despite breastfeeding when compared with controls (see Zidovudine).

References

1. Product information. Norvir. Abbott Laboratories, 2001.
2. Casey BM, Bawdon RE. Placental transfer of ritonavir with zidovudine in the ex vivo placental perfusion model. Am J Obstet Gynecol 1998;179:758–61.
3. Furco A, Gosrani B, Nicholas S, Williams A, Braithwaite W, Pozniak A, Taylor G, Asboe D, Lyall H, Shaw A, Kapembwa M. Successful use of darunavir, etravirine, enfuvirtide and tenofovir/emtricitabine in pregnant woman with multiclass HIV resistance. AIDS 2009;23:434–5.
4. Antiretroviral Pregnancy Registry Steering Committee. *Antiretroviral Pregnancy Registry International Interim Report for 1 January 1989 through 31 July 2009*. Wilmington, NC: Registry Coordinating Center; 2009. Available at www.apregistry.com. Accessed May 29, 2010.
5. Stek A, Kramer F, Fassett M, Khoury M. The safety and efficacy of protease inhibitor therapy for HIV infection during pregnancy (abstract). Am J Obstet Gynecol 1999;180:S7.
6. CDC. Public Health Service Task Force recommendations for the use of antiretroviral drugs in pregnant women infected with HIV-1 for maternal health and for reducing perinatal HIV-1 transmission in the United States. MMWR 1998;47:No. RR-2.
7. Fassett M, Kramer F, Stek A. Treatment with protease inhibitors in pregnancy is not associated with an increased incidence of gestational diabetes (abstract). Am J Obstet Gynecol 2000;182:S97.
8. Stojanov S, Wintergerst U, Belohradsky BH, Rolinski B. Mitochondrial and peroxisomal dysfunction following perinatal exposure to antiretroviral drugs. AIDS 2000;14:1669.
9. Morris AB, Cu-Uvin S, Harwell JI, Garb J, Zorrilla C, Vajaranant M, Dobles AR, Jones TB, Carlan S, Allen DY. Multicenter review of protease inhibitors in 89 pregnancies. J Acquir Immune Defic Syndr 2000;25:306–11.
10. Carpenter CCJ, Fischi MA, Hammer SM, Hirsch MS, Jacobsen DM, Katzenstein DA, Montaner JSG, Richman DD, Saag MS, Schooley RT, Thompson MA, Vella S, Yeni PG, Volberding PA. Antiretroviral therapy for HIV infection in 1996. JAMA 1996;276;146–54.
11. Minkoff H, Augenbraun M. Antiretroviral therapy for pregnant women. Am J Obstet Gynecol 1997;176:478–89.
12. Minkoff H. Human immunodeficiency virus infection in pregnancy. Obstet Gynecol 2003;101:797–810.
13. Panel on Antiretroviral Guidelines for Adults and Adolescents. *Guidelines for the Use of Antiretroviral Agents in HIV-1-Infected Adults and Adolescents*. Department of Health and Human Services. December 1, 2009:1–161. Available at http://www.aidsinfo.nih.gov/ContentFiles/AdultandAdolescentGL.pdf. Accessed September 17, 2010:60, 96–8.
14. Panel on Treatment of HIV-Infected Pregnant Women and Prevention of Perinatal Transmission. *Recommendations for Use of Antiretroviral Drugs in Pregnant HIV-1-Infected Women for Maternal Health and Interventions to Reduce Perinatal HIV Transmission in the United States*. May 24, 2010:1–117. Available at http://aidsinfo.nih.gov/ContentFiles/PerinatalGL.pdf. Accessed September 17, 2010:30 (Table 5).
15. Brown ZA, Watts DH. Antiviral therapy in pregnancy. Clin Obstet Gynecol 1990;33:276–89.
16. De Martino M, Tovo P-A, Pezzotti P, Galli L, Massironi E, Ruga E, Floreea F, Plebani A, Gabiano C, Zuccotti GV. HIV-1 transmission through breast-milk: appraisal of risk according to duration of feeding. AIDS 1992;6:991–7.
17. Van de Perre P. Postnatal transmission of human immunodeficiency virus type 1: the breast feeding dilemma. Am J Obstet Gynecol 1995;173: 483–7.

RITUXIMAB

Antineoplastic/Immunologic Agent (Antirheumatic)

PREGNANCY RECOMMENDATION: Human Data Suggest Low Risk
BREASTFEEDING RECOMMENDATION: No Human Data—Potential Toxicity

PREGNANCY SUMMARY

The use of rituximab in human pregnancy has been described in more than 200 cases. All of the live births were healthy, and none had structural anomalies that were thought to be related to rituximab. These outcomes are consistent with the reproduction studies with monkeys in which exposures that were nearly equivalent to human exposures were not associated with congenital defects. However, a functional deficit (depletion of B lymphocytes) was observed in monkey offspring and has occurred in at least two human newborns. The immunosuppression was reversible, with normal B-cell counts measured in monkey offspring by 6 months and in the infants. No increase in infectious disease was seen in any of the in utero exposed infants. Nevertheless, there is a risk for severe infections in immunosuppressed individuals, and this should be considered in all infants exposed in utero to rituximab.

FETAL RISK SUMMARY

Rituximab is a genetically engineered chimeric murine/human monoclonal immunoglobulin G1 (IgG1) kappa antibody that is directed against the CD20 antigen found on the surface of normal and malignant B lymphocytes. It has three indications: (a) for the treatment of patients with relapsed or refractory, low-grade or follicular, CD20-positive, B-cell, non-Hodgkin's lymphoma (NHL); (b) for the first-line treatment of diffuse large B-cell, CD20-positive, non-Hodgkin's lymphoma in combination with CHOP or other anthracycline-based chemotherapy regimens; and (c) in combination with methotrexate to reduce signs and symptoms in adult patients with moderately to severely active rheumatoid arthritis who have had an inadequate response to one or more TNF antagonist therapies. The elimination half-life of rituximab is dose-related. In patients with NHL, the mean serum half-life after the first of four weekly infusions was 76.3 hours (range 31.5–152.6 hours), whereas the mean half-life after the fourth infusion was

205.8 hours (range 83.9–407.0 hours). In patients with rheumatoid arthritis, the mean terminal elimination half-life after two doses, 2 weeks apart, was 19 days (1).

Rituximab may cause severe infusion-related toxicity, including hypotension and other adverse effects. Premedication with acetaminophen and an antihistamine is recommended before each infusion (1). Hypotension in a pregnant woman could have deleterious effects on placental perfusion, resulting in embryo or fetal harm.

Reproduction studies have been conducted in cynomolgus monkeys. During organogenesis, monkeys were given three daily IV loading doses, then four weekly doses. The highest weekly dose resulted in exposures that were 0.8 times the human exposure from a 2-g dose based on AUC. There was no evidence of teratogenicity. However, the antibody did produce a decrease in B cells in the offspring. Subsequent studies showed that the decreased B cells and immunosuppression noted in the offspring returned to normal levels and functions within 6 months of birth. Long-term studies for carcinogenicity, mutagenicity, or effects on fertility have not been conducted (1).

Even though the molecular weight is high (about 145,000), the antibody crosses the monkey placenta (1). Rituximab also crosses the human placenta, at least near term. Very high levels of the antibody have been measured in cord blood and the young infant (2).

A 35-year-old woman was diagnosed with Burkitt's lymphoma of the left breast at 15 weeks' gestation (2). Starting at week 16, she was treated with four weekly infusions of rituximab 375 mg/m^2. Then at 3-week intervals, she was treated with four courses of the R-CHOP regimen followed by two courses of CHOP. The patient was in complete remission at 37 weeks. At 41 weeks', a healthy female infant was delivered via cesarean section. At birth, rituximab serum levels in the cord blood and mother were 32,095 and 9750 ng/mL (cord blood:mother ratio 3.3), respectively. Serum levels in the infant at 4 and 18 weeks of age were 5399 and 700 ng/mL, respectively, whereas the mother's serum level at 18 weeks was 500 ng/mL (infant:mother ratio 1.4). No CD19 B-cells were found in the mother or newborn. In the infant at 4 and 18 weeks of age, B-cell counts were 70 and 1460 cells/micro-L) (normal range for infants 3–6 months: 200–1100 cells/micro-L), respectively. At 20 months of age, the infant's B-cell count was normal and no infectious complications, malformations, or other immune dysfunction have been observed in the now 26-month-old child (2).

A brief 2001 correspondence described the use of rituximab in the 2nd trimester (3). The 29-year-old woman, with diffuse large B-cell NHL, in her 21st week of pregnancy was treated with rituximab 375 mg/m^2 on day 1, doxorubicin 50 mg/m^2 on day 3, vincristine 2 mg on day 3, and prednisolone 100 mg on days 3–7, given in 4-week cycles. At 35 weeks' gestation, 2 weeks after the last of four cycles, she delivered a healthy female infant (birth weight or other details not given) via cesarean section. The child was developing normally and a normal peripheral B-cell population was noted at 4 months of age (3).

A 37-year-old woman with an 8-year history of follicular NHL was treated with weekly infusions (375 mg/m^2) of rituximab for 4 weeks (4). Pregnancy was detected 1 week after the last dose with conception occurring between the first and second infusions. No further rituximab treatment was given. The woman delivered a normal, healthy 3610-g female infant at 40 weeks' gestation. No hematological or immunological adverse effects were detected in the infant. At 18 months of age, the child has normal immunity and has had no major infections (4).

A 31-year-old woman at 15 weeks' gestation was diagnosed with B-cell NHL (5). She was treated with six cycles of R-CHOP on a 14-day schedule (rituximab 375 mg/m^2, cyclophosphamide 750 mg/m^2, doxorubicin 50 mg/m^2, vincristine 1.4 mg/m^2, and prednisone 100 mg/day on days 1–5). Filgrastim 300 mcg/day was given on days 6–11. At 33 weeks' gestation, 2 months after the last cycle, the woman spontaneously delivered a healthy female infant (weight and size within the 50th–90th percentiles) with Apgar scores of 8, 10, and 10 at 1, 5, and 10 minutes, respectively. The 16-month-old child has been closely evaluated every 3 months since birth and has had no infections or evidence of physiological or developmental abnormalities (5).

A 2006 report briefly mentioned the use of weekly infusions of rituximab (375 mg/m^2) for severe thrombotic thrombocytopenic purpura (TTP) (6). The woman had a left-sided stroke and seizure at 16 weeks' gestation and was diagnosed with acute TTP. Rituximab infusions were started at 27 weeks' to reduce the risk of further complications by reducing IgG antibodies. The woman suffered another seizure in the 30th week of pregnancy and an emergency cesarean section delivered a 1045-g male infant. The infant has had no infectious complications (6).

A 41-year-old woman, with a history of cardiac valvulopathy responsible for left ventricular failure, was treated for recurrent autoimmune hemolytic anemia with four weekly IV doses of rituximab (375 mg/m^2) and daily corticosteroids (7). Unbeknownst to her physicians, the patient also was pregnant, receiving the four rituximab doses between 7 and 10 weeks of gestation. No other exposures occurred during the remainder of a normal pregnancy and she delivered a normal, 3060-g female infant at 38 weeks' gestation. Apgar scores were 10 at 1, 5, and 10 minutes. Mature B-cells and B-cell precursors were present at birth, as well as during the first 55 days after birth. A mild bone depression at the sacrum–coccyx level was noted, but an evaluation completely excluded spina bifida occulta. Other than a possible mild infection at 24 hours of age, and a transient and slight lymphopenia on days 2 and 3, no other alterations in the infant were detected (7).

Treatment during pregnancy of a 36-year-old woman with long-standing immune-mediated thrombocytopenia was discussed in a 2008 report (8). Her initial treatment during pregnancy consisted of corticosteroids and IV immunoglobulins, but only a small rise was noted in the platelet count and she had persisting hemorrhagic diathesis. Treatment was changed to prednisone 60 mg/day and continued to 36 weeks'. At week 30, she was given rituximab weekly for 4 consecutive weeks followed by additional IV immunoglobulins. At 38 weeks', 4 weeks after the last dose of rituximab, labor was induced and a 3780-g female infant was born with Apgar scores of 7, 8, and 8 at 1, 5, and 10 minutes, respectively. The rituximab concentration in the newborn was 6.7 mg/L. The number of B-cells in the neonate was 0, but a rise was detected at 3 months of age so that at 6 months they were in the normal range. At 10 months of age, growth and development were normal. She did not have any infections and the vaccination titers were normal (8).

A 2011 study, authored by investigators from Stanford University School of Medicine and the manufacturer, described 231 pregnancies gathered worldwide that were exposed to rituximab in the 1st and 2nd trimesters (9). More than half of the pregnancies were also exposed to other potentially teratogenic agents. Of the 231 pregnancies, 67 outcomes were unknown, 11 were ongoing, and 153 outcomes were known. In the latter group, there were 90 live births, 1 maternal death (cerebral hemorrhage from preexisting autoimmune thrombocytopenia), 1 stillbirth (20 weeks' due to fetal hypoxemia from umbilical card knot), 33 spontaneous abortions (all in 1st trimester), and 28 elective abortions (1 for trisomy 13). Among the live births, there were 22 premature infants, 1 neonatal death at 6 weeks, and 11 neonates with hematologic abnormalities, but none had corresponding infections. Four neonates had infection (fever, bronchlolitis, cytomegalovirus hepatitis, and chorioamnionitis). Two infants had a structural anomaly, clubfoot in one twin, and a cardiac malformation in a singleton birth (9).

A brief 2011 report described the outcome of a pregnancy that was exposed to rituximab given 6 weeks before conception (10). The 32-year-old woman was treated with rituximab for long-standing rheumatoid arthritis resistant to other therapies. After an uncomplicated pregnancy, she gave birth to twin females at 37 weeks', one with a clubfoot and the other with transient erythema toxicum neonatorum. Normal B-cell counts and normal immunoglobulin levels were measured during 8 months of follow-up, but one girl had transient mild leucocytosis without signs of infection. Both were developing normally, without serious infectious complications, although one had mild asthma (10).

A 2012 case report described the pregnancy of a 34-year-old woman at 27 weeks' with systemic lupus erythematosus who developed severe thrombocytopenia (11). She was treated with high-dose corticosteroids, IV immunoglobulin, rituximab (weekly for 4 doses starting at about 27 weeks'), one dose of cyclophosphamide, eltrombopag, and anti-D immunoglobulin, but the thrombocytopenia was resistant to these agents. Romiplostim (weekly for 3 doses) was then given and the platelet count rose from 4×10^9/L to 91×10^9/L. Because her platelet count began to fall, she was given the third dose of romiplostim 1 day before induction of labor at 34 weeks'. A healthy normal female baby was born with a normal platelet count (*no additional details provided*) (11).

In a second 2012 case report, a 22-year-old woman during the 12th week of pregnancy was diagnosed with primary mediastinal large B-cell lymphoma (12). In the 13th week, she was started on standard doses of R-CHOP regimen (rituximab, cyclophosphamide, doxorubicin, vincristine, and prednisone) given every 3 weeks for six cycles. Her last cycle was at her 31st week of pregnancy. At 34 weeks', she underwent labor induction and gave birth to a healthy male baby with Apgar scores of 9 and 9 (*no other details given*). At 1 year of age, the infant has shown no developmental delays or physical abnormalities (12).

A 2013 case report described the outcomes of two pregnancies exposed to rituximab in the 1st trimester (13). In the first case, a 25-year-old woman with rheumatoid arthritis conceived while receiving rituximab (500 mg on days 1 and 15 of each cycle) and methotrexate (10 mg/week). Rituximab was given at weeks 2 and 4. Both drugs were then stopped. The previous cycle had been given 6 months before the current cycle. A cesarean section was performed at week 37 to give birth to a healthy 3110-g neonate (sex not specified) with Apgar scores of 10 and 10 at 5 and 10 minutes, respectively. The child was doing well at 4.5 years follow-up. The second case involved a 31-year-old woman with multiple relapsing TTP. Her last dose of rituximab occurred 9 weeks before conception. Serum concentrations of rituximab at 11 and 31 weeks' were 0.11 mcg/mL and undetected, respectively. Based on the pharmacokinetics, the theoretical concentration at conception was estimated to be 1 mcg/mL. At 39 weeks', a healthy 3024-g neonate (sex not specified) was born vaginally with Apgar scores of 10 and 10 at 5 and 10 minutes, respectively. The infant was doing well at 1.5 years of age (13).

A 2013 review summarized seven reports on the use of rituximab in pregnancy (14). The seven studies (2,5–9,11) are discussed above. The authors concluded that, although the drug could not be considered completely safe, it could be given if the maternal benefit outweighed the potential embryo–fetal risk (14). Another 2013 review examined the available evidence on drugs used for dermatologic diseases in pregnancy (15). Based on case reports or clinical experience, the authors classified rituximab as safe in pregnancy.

BREASTFEEDING SUMMARY

No reports describing the use of rituximab during human lactation have been located. The molecular weight (about 145,000) is very high, but human IgG is excreted into milk, and therefore, rituximab also may be excreted. The effects of this potential exposure on a nursing infant are unknown, but immunosuppression and other severe adverse effects are potential complications.

References

1. Product information. Rituxan. Genentech, 2007.
2. Friedrichs B, Tiemann M, Salwender H, Verpoort K, Wenger MK, Schmitz N. The effects of rituximab treatment during pregnancy on a neonate. Haematologica 2006;91:1426–7.
3. Herold M, Schnohr S, Bittrich H. Efficacy and safety of combined rituximab chemotherapy during pregnancy. J Clin Oncol 2001;19:3439.
4. Kimby E, Sverrisdottir A, Elinder G. Safety of rituximab therapy during the first trimester of pregnancy: a case history. Eur J Haematol 2004;72:292–3.
5. Decker M, Rothermundt C, Hollander G, Rochlitz C. Rituximab plus CHOP for treatment of diffuse large B-cell lymphoma during second trimester of pregnancy. Lancet Oncol 2006;7:693–4.
6. Scully M, Starke R, Lee R, Mackie I, Machin S, Cohen H. Successful management of pregnancy in women with a history of thrombotic thrombocytopaenic purpura. Blood Coagul Fibrinolysis 2006;17:459–63.
7. Ojeda-Uribe M, Gilliot C, Jung G, Drenou B, Brunot A. Administration of rituximab during the first trimester of pregnancy without consequences for the newborn. J Perinatol 2006;26:252–5.
8. Klink DT, van Elburg RM, Schreurs MWJ, van Well TJ. Rituximab administration in third trimester of pregnancy suppresses neonatal B-cell development. Clin Dev Immunol 2008;2008:271363.
9. Chakravarty EF, Murray ER, Kelman A, Farmer P. Pregnancy outcomes after maternal exposure to rituximab. Blood 2011;117:1499–1506.
10. Ton E, Tekstra J, Hellmann PM, Nuver-Zwart IHH, Bijlsma WJ. Safety of rituximab therapy during twins' pregnancy. Rheumatology 2011;50:806–8.
11. Alkaabi J, Alkindi S, Riyami N, Zia F, Balla L, Balla S. Successful treatment of severe thrombocytopenia with romiplostim in a pregnant patient with systemic lupus erythematosus. Lupus 2012;21:1571–4.
12. Perez CA, Amin J, Aguina L, Cioffi-Lavina M, Santos ES. Primary mediastinal large B-cell lymphoma during pregnancy. Case Rep Hematol 2012;2012:197347.
13. Ojeda-Uribe M, Afif N, Dahan E, Sparsa L, Haby C, Sibilia J, Ternant D, Ardizzone M. Exposure to abatacept or rituximab in the first trimester of pregnancy of three women with autoimmune diseases. Clin Rheumatol 2013;32:695–700.

R

14. Sarno MA, Mancari R, Azim HA, Colombo N, Peccatori FA. Are monoclonal antibodies a safe treatment for cancer during pregnancy. Immunotherapy 2013;5:733–41.

15. Braunstein I, Werth V. Treatment of dermatologic connective tissue disease and autoimmune blistering disorders in pregnancy. Dermatol Ther 2013;26:354–63.

RIVAROXABAN

Anticoagulant

PREGNANCY RECOMMENDATION: No Human Data—Animal Data Suggest Moderate Risk
BREASTFEEDING RECOMMENDATION: No Human Data—Potential Toxicity

PREGNANCY SUMMARY

No reports describing the use of rivaroxaban during human pregnancy have been located. The animal data in one species suggest risk but the adverse embryo–fetal outcomes may have been caused by maternal hemorrhage. Structural malformations were not observed in the animals. Pregnancy-related hemorrhage and/or emergent delivery is a concern because the drug cannot be reliably monitored with standard laboratory testing, and the anticoagulant effect is not readily reversible other than waiting about 24 hours (1). For these reasons, the drug should be avoided in pregnancy (2). In addition, the treatments of deep venous thrombosis or pulmonary embolism are not approved indications and rivaroxaban should not be used as heparin is the treatment of choice for these indications (3). However, if rivaroxaban is the treatment of choice for its approved indications, it should not be withheld because of pregnancy.

FETAL RISK SUMMARY

Rivaroxaban is an oral factor Xa inhibitor in the same pharmacologic class as apixaban. It is indicated to reduce the risk of stroke and systemic embolism in patients with nonvalvular atrial fibrillation and for the prophylaxis of deep vein thrombosis which may lead to pulmonary embolism in patients undergoing knee or hip replacement surgery. Rivaroxaban undergoes partial metabolism to inactive metabolites; the parent drug is the predominant moiety in plasma with no major or active circulating metabolites. Plasma protein binding, primarily to albumin, is 92%–95% and the terminal elimination half-life is 5–9 hours in healthy subjects (1).

Reproduction studies with oral rivaroxaban have been conducted in rats and rabbits. Pronounced maternal hemorrhage occurred in rats but the dose was not specified. Decreased fetal body weights were observed with doses that were about 14 times the human exposure of unbound drug based on AUC at the highest recommended dose of 20 mg/day (HE). Maternal hemorrhage also occurred in rabbits given a dose that produced exposures during organogenesis that were about 4 times the HE. At this dose, embryo–fetal toxicity in rabbits included increased resorptions, decreased number of live fetuses, and decreased fetal body weight. Without mentioning the animal species, the manufacturer reported that during labor and delivery a dose about 6 times the HE resulted in maternal bleeding and maternal and fetal death. Rivaroxaban crossed the placenta in both rats and rabbits (1).

Two-year studies for carcinogenesis were negative in mice and rats. Studies for mutagenicity also were negative, as were studies for impaired fertility in male and female rats (1).

As demonstrated by autoradiography, moderate amounts of rivaroxaban cross the human placenta (4). The transfer is consistent with the molecular weight (about 436), limited metabolism, and moderately long elimination half-life. Although the amount crossing has not been determined, it may be limited by the high plasma protein binding.

BREASTFEEDING SUMMARY

No reports describing the use of rivaroxaban during human lactation have been located. A 2012 reference on the treatment of pulmonary embolism in pregnancy, however, stated without further details that the drug is excreted into breast milk (2). This would be consistent with the molecular weight (about 436), limited metabolism, and moderately long elimination half-life (5–9 hours), but the moderately high plasma protein binding (92%–95%) might limit the excretion. The effect of this exposure on a nursing infant is unknown, but hemorrhage is a potential complication. Until additional data on the amount in breast milk are available, the safest course is to not breastfeed when taking this drug.

References

1. Product information. Xarelto. Janssen Pharmaceuticals, 2011.
2. Cutts BA, Dasgupta D, Hunt BJ. New directions in the diagnosis and treatment of pulmonary embolism in pregnancy. Am J Obstet Gynecol 2013;208:102–8.
3. Greer IA. Thrombosis in pregnancy: updates in diagnosis and management. Hematology Am Soc Hematol Educ Program 2012;2012:203–7. doi: 10.1182/asheducation-2012.1.203.
4. Rivaroxaban FDA DDAC document. Available at www.fda.gov. As cited by Huisman MV. Further issues with new oral anticoagulants. Curr Pharm Des 2010;16:3487–9.

R

RIVASTIGMINE

Cholinesterase Inhibitor (CNS Agent)

PREGNANCY RECOMMENDATION: No Human Data—Animal Data Suggest Low Risk
BREASTFEEDING RECOMMENDATION: No Human Data—Potential Toxicity

PREGNANCY SUMMARY

No reports describing the use of rivastigmine in human pregnancy have been located. Because of its indication, such reports would be rare. Moreover, the animal data suggest that the risk to the embryo–fetus is low. Therefore, inadvertent exposure to rivastigmine during pregnancy should not be a reason for pregnancy termination.

FETAL RISK SUMMARY

Rivastigmine is a reversible cholinesterase inhibitor that is indicated for the treatment of mild to moderate dementia of the Alzheimer's type. Rivastigmine penetrates the blood–brain barrier with drug concentrations in the cerebral spinal fluid about 40% of those in the plasma. It is extensively metabolized to inactive metabolites. Protein binding is moderate (about 40%) and the plasma elimination half-life is about 1.5 hours (1).

Reproduction studies have been conducted in rats and rabbits. In rats, doses up to about 2 times the maximum recommended human dose based on BSA (MRHD) were not teratogenic. Decreased fetal/pup weights were observed in rats at doses several-fold lower than the MRHD, usually at doses causing some maternal toxicity. No effects on fertility or reproductive performance were observed at doses about 0.9 times the MRHD. No evidence of teratogenicity was noted in rabbits given doses up to about 4 times the MRHD (1). Rivastigmine and/or its metabolites cross the rabbit placenta producing an average fetal-to-placenta tissue ratio of 0.5 (2).

It is not known if rivastigmine or its metabolites cross the human placenta. The molecular weight of the parent compound (about 250 for the free base), moderate protein binding, and the ability to cross the blood–brain barrier suggest that the drug will cross to the fetal compartment. The very short elimination half-life should decrease the amount of drug available for transfer.

BREASTFEEDING SUMMARY

No reports describing the use of rivastigmine during human lactation have been located.

Because of its indication, such reports should be rare. The molecular weight (about 250 for the free base), moderate protein binding, and the ability to cross the blood–brain barrier suggest that the drug will be excreted into breast milk. The very short elimination half-life should decrease the amount of drug available for excretion. The effect of this exposure on a nursing infant is unknown.

References

1. Product information. Exelon. Novartis Pharmaceuticals, 2004.
2. Habucky K, Tse FLS. Disposition of SDZ ENA 713, an acetylcholinesterase inhibitor, in the rabbit. Biopharm Drug Dispos 1998;19:285–90.

RIZATRIPTAN

Antimigraine

PREGNANCY RECOMMENDATION: Limited Human Data—Animal Data Suggest Moderate Risk
BREASTFEEDING RECOMMENDATION: No Human Data—Probably Compatible

PREGNANCY SUMMARY

Although no adverse outcomes were observed in liveborn offspring in the Merck Prospective Registry or clinical trials, the limited number of exposures studied is not sufficient to detect a risk of rare disorders such as individual birth defects (1). However, a 2008 review of triptans in pregnancy found no evidence for teratogenicity, but the data did suggest a possible increase in the rate of preterm birth (2).

R

FETAL RISK SUMMARY

Rizatriptan, an oral, selective 5-hydroxytryptamine$_{1B/1D}$ receptor agonist, is indicated for the treatment of acute migraine attacks with or without aura in adults. The drug is metabolized to inactive metabolites. Plasma protein binding is low (14%) and the average plasma half-life is 2–3 hours (3).

Reproduction studies have been conducted in rats and rabbits. Female rats were treated before and during mating, and throughout gestation and lactation with doses that produced maternal exposures (AUC) 15 and 225 times, respectively, the exposure in humans from the maximum recommended human dose of 30 mg (MRHD). These doses were not maternal toxic, but did cause decreased birth weight and reduced preweaning and postweaning weight gain in offspring. In a prenatal and postnatal development toxicity study in rats, doses producing maternal exposures 225 to more than 500 times the MRHD caused toxicity in the offspring as shown by increased mortality at birth and for the first 3 days after birth, reduced preweaning and postweaning weight gain, and decreased learning capacity. The no-effect dose for all of these effects was approximately 7.5 times the MRHD. In embryo and fetal development studies, no teratogenic effects were observed in rats and rabbits given doses during organogenesis producing maternal exposures 225 and 115 times, respectively, the MRHD. Fetal weights were decreased at these doses, but maternal weight gain was also reduced. The developmental no-effect doses, in both species, were approximately 15 times the MRHD. Rizatriptan crosses the placentas of rats and rabbits (3).

It is not known if rizatriptan crosses the human placenta. The molecular weight of the free base (about 269), low plasma protein binding, and moderate plasma half-life suggest that exposure of the embryo–fetus should be expected.

In the Merck Pregnancy Registry program, 81 women were prospectively enrolled after exposure to rizatriptan (1). The outcomes of these pregnancies were 26 lost to follow-up, 3 spontaneous abortions (SABs), 1 elective abortion (EAB) (chromosomal anomaly—partial replication of chromosome 3 in a 39-year-old woman), 2 fetal deaths (1 cord accident; twin B), 1 neonatal death (due to prematurity), and 50 live births. The 3 SABs occurred in the 1st trimester. In addition to the chromosomal anomaly noted above, three outcomes involved congenital defects: juxtaposition of the arteries (exposure timing unknown), bladder outlet obstruction in twin B (mother with gestational diabetes and hypertension; twin A live birth, twin B died at 23 weeks), and hypospadias of the glans (surgical correction required). Of nine retrospective reports, three involved outcomes with congenital anomalies: two cases of chromosomal abnormalities (one a de novo duplication of chromosome 2 and one with Turner syndrome) and one case of anencephaly (EAB at 16 weeks).

In international prospective reports, three cases of congenital anomalies were described (trimester of exposure): (a) premature infant with growth restriction, subependymal cyst, interatrial communication, and mild persistent ductus arteriosus (1st trimester); (b) hemangioma of unreported size of the head and neck (1st trimester); and (c) trisomy 21, died in utero at 20 weeks. International retrospective reports involved two cases of defects: a baby born with cataracts and the other with an unspecified fetal anomaly. In clinical trials, there were no known adverse effects among live births (1).

The manufacturer maintains a pregnancy registry for women exposed to rizatriptan. Health care professionals are encouraged to report pregnancy exposures to the registry by calling the toll-free number 800-986-8999.

BREASTFEEDING SUMMARY

No reports describing the use of rizatriptan in human lactation have been located. The molecular weight of the free base (about 269), low plasma protein binding (14%), and moderate plasma half-life (2–3 hours) suggest that the drug will be excreted into breast milk. The effect of this exposure on a nursing infant is unknown.

References

1. Eleventh annual report from the Merck Pregnancy Registry for Maxalt (rizatriptan benzoate) covering the period from approval (June 1998) through July 31, 2009.
2. Soldin OP, Dahlin J, O'Mara DM. Triptans in pregnancy. Ther Drug Monit 2008;30:5–9.
3. Product information. Maxalt. Merck, 2008.

R

ROCURONIUM

Skeletal Muscle Relaxant

PREGNANCY RECOMMENDATION: Limited Human Data—Animal Data Suggest Low Risk
BREASTFEEDING RECOMMENDATION: No Human Data—Probably Compatible

PREGNANCY SUMMARY

Human pregnancy experience with rocuronium is limited to the 2nd and 3rd trimesters. Although the absence of exposures during organogenesis prevents a more thorough assessment, neuromuscular blocking agents generally do not appear to represent a significant risk for an embryo or fetus. The animal data for rocuronium suggest low embryo–fetal risk. Moreover, the agent contains a quaternary ammonium site in its structure that will limit its placental transfer. One review predicted that the maternal drug concentrations would always exceed fetal levels (1). Neuromuscular blockade in a newborn is probably a rare but potential toxicity (2). If indicated, rocuronium should not be withheld because of pregnancy.

FETAL RISK SUMMARY

Rocuronium (rocuronium bromide) is a competitive (nondepolarizing) neuromuscular blocking agent. Structurally, it is a quaternary ammonium compound that is an analog of vecuronium. Rocuronium is indicated as an IV adjunct to general anesthesia to provide skeletal muscle relaxation during surgery or mechanical ventilation. In normal adult patients, the elimination half-life is about 2.4 hours. Approximately 30% is bound to plasma proteins (3).

Reproduction studies have been conducted in rats and rabbits. In these species, the maximum tolerated IV dose administered 3 times daily during organogenesis was not teratogenic. The doses were 15%–30% and 25%, respectively, of the human intubation dose of 0.6–1.2 mg/kg based on BSA. In rats, the incidence of fetal death was increased, an effect that was thought to be due to oxygen deficiency that resulted from acute symptoms of respiratory dysfunction in the dams (3).

Consistent with the molecular weight (about 610 for rocuronium bromide) and the limitation placed on placental passage by ionization at physiologic pH, small amounts of rocuronium cross the placenta. In 32 patients from the study below, the mean maternal venous (MV) and umbilical venous (UV) blood was about 2412 and 390 ng/mL, respectively. The UV:MV ratio was 0.16. In 12 patients, the mean drug concentration in umbilical arterial (UA) plasma was about 271 ng/mL, resulting in a UA:UV ratio of 0.62 (4).

In a 1994 prospective, nonrandomized, multicenter study, 40 women undergoing cesarean section at term received anesthesia induction with rocuronium and thiopental, followed by isoflurane and nitrous oxide maintenance (4). No adverse effects on the newborns attributable to rocuronium were observed as evaluated by Apgar scores, time to sustained respiration, total and muscular neuroadaptive capacity scores, acid–base status, and blood–gas tensions in umbilical arterial and venous blood (4). This study generated a number of letters referring either to the doses used or to what was considered the drug of choice (succinylcholine) (5–9).

A 1996 report described the use of rocuronium in a 31-year-old patient at 28 weeks' gestation who presented with a penetrating injury of her left eye secondary to a motor vehicle accident (10). Prior to induction of anesthesia, she was started on IV magnesium sulfate to treat newly onset uterine contractions. Anesthesia was induced with rocuronium (0.9 mg/kg), fentanyl (200 mcg), and sodium thiopental (400 mg). The fetal heart rate (140–150 beats/minute) was monitored throughout the 6-hour surgical procedure. Except for a decrease in short-term variability attributable to anesthesia of the fetus, no other effects on the fetal heart rate were observed. Although the authors were aware of the interaction with magnesium, they choose a higher dose (usual dose is 0.6 mg/kg) to allow for more rapid intubation. As expected, the duration of paralysis was prolonged secondary to the high dose and interaction with magnesium, but the authors thought that this was acceptable given the patient's condition. The woman was discharged from the hospital 6 days after surgery with an apparently normal ongoing pregnancy (10). Information on the pregnancy outcome was not provided. Later correspondence regarding this case report discussed the benefits and risks of the therapy and dose (11,12).

Rocuronium was used in a 35-year-old patient undergoing a combined cesarean section delivery and posterior fossa craniotomy at 37 weeks' gestation (13). The patient had von Hippel-Lindau disease and surgery was required for an enlarged hemangioblastoma. General anesthesia was induced with rocuronium (50 mg), fentanyl (200 mcg), and sodium thiopental (300 mg). A male infant (weight not specified) was delivered with Apgar scores of 5, 7, and 9 at 1, 5, and 10 minutes, respectively. Naloxone was required because of weak respiratory efforts 2 minutes after delivery (13).

A 1997 study compared thiopental–rocuronium with ketamine–rocuronium (20 in each group) for rapid sequence intubation in women undergoing cesarean section (14). The authors concluded that either drug combination was suitable. Based on 1- and 5-minute Apgar scores, no significant differences in neonatal condition were found between the two groups.

BREASTFEEDING SUMMARY

No reports describing the use of rocuronium in a lactating woman have been located. Because of the indications for this agent, it is doubtful if such reports will be forthcoming. The molecular weight (about 610 for rocuronium bromide) is low enough for excretion into breast milk, but the amount excreted will be limited because the drug is ionized at physiologic pH. The effects of this exposure on a nursing infant are unknown, but are probably not clinically significant.

References

1. Guay J, Grenier Y, Varin F. Clinical pharmacokinetics of neuromuscular relaxants in pregnancy. Clin Pharmacokinet 1998;34:483–96.
2. Atherton DP, Hunter JM. Clinical pharmacokinetics of the newer neuromuscular blocking drugs. Clin Pharmacokinet 1999;36:169–89.
3. Product information. Zemuron. Organon USA, 2004.
4. Abouleish E, Abboud T, Lechevalier T, Zhu J, Chalian A, Alford K. Rocuronium (Org 9426) for caesarean section. Br J Anaesth 1994;73:336–41.
5. Kwan WF, Chen BJ, Liao KT. Rocuronium for caesarean section. Br J Anaesth 1995;74:347.
6. Abouleish E, Abboud T. Rocuronium for caesarean section. Br J Anaesth 1995;74:347–8.
7. McSiney M, Edwards C, Wilkins A. Rocuronium for caesarean section. Br J Anaesth 1995;74:348.
8. Swales HA, Gaylord DG. Rocuronium for caesarean section. Br J Anaesth 1995;74:348.
9. Abouleish E, Abboud T. Rocuronium for caesarean section. Br J Anaesth 1995;74:348.
10. Gaiser RR, Seem EH. Use of rocuronium in a pregnant patient with an open eye injury, receiving magnesium medication, for preterm labour. Br J Anaesth 1996;77:669–71.
11. James MFM. Use of rocuronium in a pregnant patient receiving magnesium medication. Br J Anaesth 1997;78:772.
12. Gaiser K. Use of rocuronium in a pregnant patient receiving magnesium medication (Reply). Br J Anaesth 1997;78:772.
13. Boker A, Ong BY. Anesthesia for cesarean section and posterior fossa craniotomy in a patient with von Hippel-Lindau disease. Can J Anesth 2001;48:387–90.
14. Baraka AS, Sayyid SS, Assaf BA. Thiopental-rocuronium versus ketamine-rocuronium for rapid-sequence intubation in parturients undergoing cesarean section. Anesth Analg 1997;84:1104–7.

ROFECOXIB

[Withdrawn from the market. See 9th edition.]

ROFLUMILAST

Respiratory (Selective Phosphodiesterase 4 Inhibitor)

PREGNANCY RECOMMENDATION: No Human Data—Animal Data Suggest Moderate Risk
BREASTFEEDING RECOMMENDATION: No Human Data—Potential Toxicity

PREGNANCY SUMMARY

No reports describing the use of roflumilast in human pregnancy have been located. Developmental toxicity, at doses that were ≤10 or less than the human dose, occurred in only one of three species tested, but teratogenicity was not observed. However, the lack of human pregnancy experience prevents a more complete assessment of the embryo–fetal risk. If the maternal benefit clearly outweighs the unknown risk, the drug should not be withheld but the woman should be informed of the unknown risk.

FETAL RISK SUMMARY

Roflumilast is an oral selective inhibitor of phosphodiesterase 4. It is indicated as a treatment to reduce the risk of chronic obstructive pulmonary disease (COPD) exacerbations in patients with severe COPD associated with chronic bronchitis and a history of exacerbations. The drug is metabolized to an active metabolite. Plasma protein binding of roflumilast and its active metabolite is about 99% and 97%, respectively. For the two agents, the median plasma effective half-life is about 17 and 30 hours, respectively (1).

Animal reproduction studies have been conducted in mice, rats, and rabbits. In mice, stillbirth and decreased pup viability occurred at doses that were about ≥16 times the maximum recommended human dose based on BSA (MRHD). Postimplantation loss was induced in rats at doses that were ≥10 times the MRHD. No treatment-related effects on embryo–fetal development were noted in mice, rats, and rabbits at doses that were about 12, 3, and 26 times the MRHD, respectively. However, the drug did adversely affect postnatal development of mice pups when dams were given the drug during pregnancy and lactation. At about 49 times the MRHD, pup rearing frequencies were decreased and, at about 97 times the MRHD, decreased survival and forelimb grip reflex and delayed pinna detachment were noted. Moreover, at about 16 times the MRHD, the drug disrupted the labor and delivery process in mice (1).

In long-term studies, roflumilast was carcinogenic in hamsters but not in mice. The drug was mutagenic in one assay but negative in multiple other assays. In a 3-month human study, roflumilast had no effects on semen parameters or reproductive hormones. In contrast, a dose-related effect on male rat fertility was noted with increases in the incidence of tubular atrophy, degeneration in the testis and spermiogenic granulation in the epididymides. No effect on female fertility was observed at the highest dose tested (1).

It is not known if roflumilast or its active metabolite cross the human placenta. The molecular weight of the parent drug (about 403), and the long effective half-lives of the parent drug and active metabolite suggest that both will cross to the embryo–fetus. However, the high plasma protein binding may limit the exposure.

BREASTFEEDING SUMMARY

No reports describing the use of roflumilast during human lactation have been located. The molecular weight of the parent drug (about 403), and the long effective half-lives (17 and 30 hours, respectively) of the parent drug and active metabolite suggest that both will be excreted into breast milk. However, the high plasma protein binding (99% and 97%, respectively) may limit the excretion. The effect of this exposure on a nursing infant is unknown. If a mother chooses to breastfeed while taking roflumilast, her nursing infant should be monitored for the most common (≥2%) adverse reactions observed in adults (diarrhea, weight decrease, nausea, headache, back pain, insomnia, dizziness, and decreased appetite) (1).

Reference

1. Product information. Daliresp. Forest Pharmaceuticals, 2011.

R

ROMIDEPSIN

Antineoplastic

PREGNANCY RECOMMENDATION: Contraindicated
BREASTFEEDING RECOMMENDATION: No Human Data—Potential Toxicity

PREGNANCY SUMMARY

No reports describing the use of romidepsin in human pregnancy have been located. Only one animal species was tested and a slight decrease in fetal weight was observed. The study did not expose pregnant rats to enough of the drug to evaluate adverse outcomes fully (1). Romidepsin competes with β-estradiol for binding to estrogen receptors. Because estrogen is required to maintain pregnancy throughout gestation, the competition between romidepsin and β-estradiol could cause pregnancy loss. Moreover, romidepsin may reduce the effectiveness of estrogen-containing contraceptives.

FETAL RISK SUMMARY

The antineoplastic romidepsin, a histone deacetylase inhibitor, is administered as an IV infusion on days 1, 8, and 15 of a 28-day cycle. It is in the same subclass as vorinostat. Romidepsin is indicated for the treatment of cutaneous T-cell lymphoma in patients who have received at least one prior systemic therapy. The drug competes with β-estradiol for binding to estrogen receptors and may reduce the effectiveness of estrogen-containing contraceptives. Romidepsin undergoes extensive metabolism. Plasma protein binding is high (92%–94%), primarily to α_1-acid-glycoprotein, and the terminal half-life is about 3 hours. No accumulation in the plasma was observed after repeated dosing (1).

A reproduction study was conducted in rats. During organogenesis, rats were given daily IV doses up to about 18% of the estimated human daily dose based on BSA. This dose resulted in a 5% reduction in fetal weight. However, embryo–fetal toxicities and other adverse developmental outcomes were not adequately assessed in this study (1).

Carcinogenicity studies have not been conducted. The drug was not mutagenic or clastogenic in various assays. Romidepsin caused impaired fertility in rats and mice. In male rats and mice, at exposures much less than those obtained in humans, the drug caused testicular degeneration. In addition, seminal vesicle and prostate organ weights were decreased in male rats. In female rats, atrophy was observed in the ovary, uterus, vagina, and mammary gland, as well as maturation arrest of ovarian follicles and decreased weight of ovaries. These toxicities occurred at doses and systemic exposures that were a small fraction of the human dose and exposure and probably resulted from the drug's high affinity for binding to estrogen receptors (1).

It is not known if romidepsin crosses the human placenta. The molecular weight (about 541) and the elimination half-life suggest that the drug will cross, but the high plasma protein binding may limit the exposure.

BREASTFEEDING SUMMARY

No reports describing the use of romidepsin during human lactation have been located. The molecular weight (about 541) and the elimination half-life (3 hours) suggest that the drug will be excreted into breast milk, but the high plasma protein binding (92%–94%) might limit the amount excreted. The effect of this exposure on a nursing infant is unknown but the potential for severe toxicity is a concern. Because the drug caused a wide-range of toxicity in adults that involved many systems (e.g., gastrointestinal, CNS, hematologic) and competes with β-estradiol for binding to estrogen receptors, mothers should not breastfeed while receiving this drug. However, the elimination half-life and the dosing schedule (IV infusion over 4 hours on days 1, 8, and 15 of a 28-day cycle) might allow breastfeeding on the days a dose is not given. If this strategy is chosen, the mother should "pump and dump" to maintain milk production and decrease discomfort from engorgement for at least 15 hours (i.e., five half-lives would allow about 97% of the drug to be eliminated from her blood) after the end of the infusion.

Reference

1. Product information. Istodax. Gloucester Pharmaceuticals, 2009.

ROMIPLOSTIM

Hematopoietic

PREGNANCY RECOMMENDATION: Limited Human Data—Animal Data Suggest Low Risk
BREASTFEEDING RECOMMENDATION: No Human Data—Probably Compatible

PREGNANCY SUMMARY

Only two reports describing the use of romiplostim in human pregnancy have been located. Although fetal toxicity was observed in one of three animal species, maternal toxicity also occurred making the result uninterpretable. However, use of the protein in human pregnancy might cause increased fetal platelet counts, a potential complication. If romiplostim is used in pregnancy, health care providers are encouraged to enroll pregnant patients in the Nplate Pregnancy Registry by calling 1-877-Nplate 1 (1-877-675-2831). Pregnant patients also can enroll themselves by calling the same number.

FETAL RISK SUMMARY

Romiplostim is an Fc-peptide fusion protein. It is indicated for the treatment of thrombocytopenia in patients with chronic immune (idiopathic) thrombocytopenia purpura (ITP) who have had an insufficient response to corticosteroids, immunoglobulins, or splenectomy. It is given as weekly SC injections. The half-life is a median 3.5 days (range 1–34 days) (1).

Reproduction studies have been conducted in rats, rabbits, and mice. In pregnant rats and rabbits, no evidence of fetal harm was observed with doses up to 11 and 83 times, respectively, the maximum human dose based on systemic exposure (MHD). In rats, a dose 11 times the MHD caused an increase in perinatal pup mortality. Romiplostim crossed the rat placenta and increased fetal platelet counts at clinically equivalent and higher doses. In mice, a dose 5 times the MHD resulted in maternal toxicity (reduced body weight) and increased postimplantation loss (1).

Neither studies for carcinogenicity nor mutagenesis have been conducted with romiplostim. There was no effect on fertility with doses up to 37 times the RHD (1).

It is not known if romiplostim crosses the human placenta. The molecular weight (59,000) (2) is high enough to limit transfer, but the long half-life may assist transfer, especially in the 2nd and 3rd trimesters.

A 2012 case report described the pregnancy of a 34-year-old woman at 27 weeks' with systemic lupus erythematosus who developed severe thrombocytopenia (3). She was treated with high-dose corticosteroids, IV immunoglobulin, rituximab (weekly for 4 doses), one dose of cyclophosphamide, eltrombopag, and anti-D immunoglobulin, but the thrombocytopenia was resistant to these agents. Romiplostim (weekly for 3 doses) was then given and the platelet count rose from 4×10^9/L to 91×10^9/L. Because her platelet count began to fall, she was given the third dose of romiplostim 1 day before induction of labor at 34 weeks'. A healthy normal female baby was born with a normal platelet count (*no additional details were provided*) (3).

In a 2013 case report, a 28-year-old primigravid with chronic immune thrombocytopenic purpura conceived while receiving romiplostim (4). During the 1st trimester, her platelets were stable on 3 mcg/kg/week but, at week 14, thrombocytopenia associated with epistaxis developed. Dexamethasone and IV immunoglobulin were added to supplement romiplostim in response to thrombocytopenic episodes. Alternating periods of profound thrombocytopenia and thrombocytosis occurred during the remainder of pregnancy. At about 34 weeks' labor was induced to deliver a 1910-g male infant with Apgar scores of 8 and 8 at 1 and 5 minutes, respectively. The neonate's platelets decreased markedly within 8 hours of birth and treated with IV immunoglobulin and a platelet transfusion. Other problems in the infant, in addition to thrombocytopenia, were a grade III intraventricular hemorrhage, adrenal insufficiency, and phimosis. However, at 10 months, the infant was developmentally normal (4).

BREASTFEEDING SUMMARY

No reports describing the use of romiplostim during human lactation have been located. The molecular weight (59,000) (2) is high enough to limit excretion, but the long half-life (3.5 days) may assist excretion. The effect on a nursing infant is unknown. However, if excretion does occur, the protein might be digested in the infant's gut.

References

1. Product Information. Nplate. Amgen, 2008.
2. Romiplostim. Available at http://en.wikipedia.org/wiki/Romiplostim. Accessed February 1, 2011.
3. Alkaabi J, Alkindi S, Riyami N, Zia F, Balla L, Balla S. Successful treatment of severe thrombocytopenia with romiplostim in a pregnant patient with systemic lupus erythematosus. Lupus 2012;21:1571–4.
4. Patil AS, Dotters-Katz SK, Metjian AD, James AH, Swamy GK. Use of thrombopoietin mimetic for chronic immune thrombocytopenic purpura in pregnancy. Obstet Gynecol 2013;122:483–5.

ROPINIROLE

Antiparkinson Agent

PREGNANCY RECOMMENDATION: No Human Data—Animal Data Suggest Risk
BREASTFEEDING RECOMMENDATION: No Human Data—Potential Toxicity

R

PREGNANCY SUMMARY

No reports describing the use of ropinirole in human pregnancy have been located. The agent, when given alone, produced digital malformations in rats at embryo–fetal toxic doses. In rabbits, an increased incidence and severity of digital anomalies also were observed when ropinirole, at a dose 8 times the human dose, was combined with levodopa. The complete absence of human pregnancy experience, however, prevents an assessment of the human risk. Since Parkinson's disease is relatively uncommon during the childbearing years, the use of ropinirole during pregnancy also will be uncommon. Until data on such use are available, the safest course is to avoid, if possible, the use of ropinirole during the 1st trimester.

FETAL RISK SUMMARY

Ropinirole is a nonergoline dopamine agonist that is indicated for the treatment of the signs and symptoms of idiopathic Parkinson's disease. The drug has high specificity for the D_2 and D_3 dopamine receptor subtypes. Ropinirole is metabolized to inactive compounds and eliminated renally with a half-life of about 6 hours. Up to 40% is bound to plasma proteins (1). The agent is commonly used in combination with levodopa.

Reproduction studies in pregnant rats and rabbits have revealed embryo–fetal toxicity and teratogenicity (1). In rats, decreased fetal weight, increased fetal deaths, and digital malformations were observed with doses 24, 36, and 60 times, respectively, the maximum recommended human clinical dose based on BSA administered during organogenesis and later. In pregnant rabbits during organogenesis, no harmful fetal effects were observed when ropinirole was given at a maternally toxic dose 16 times the maximum recommended human dose based on BSA (MRHD). However, when ropinirole (8 times the MRHD) was combined with levodopa (250 mg/kg/day), a greater incidence and severity of fetal malformations (primarily digit defects) occurred than when levodopa was used alone. In a 2-year carcinogenicity study in mice, ropinirole was associated with an increase in benign uterine endometrial polyps at a dose 10 times the MRHD (1).

It is not known if ropinirole can cross the placenta. The molecular weight (about 260 for the free base) and the moderate degree of protein binding suggest that the drug will cross to the embryo–fetus.

BREASTFEEDING SUMMARY

No reports describing the use of ropinirole during human lactation have been located (1). The molecular weight (about 260 for the free base) and its moderate degree of protein binding (up to 40%) suggest that it will be excreted into breast milk. Because milk is slightly acidic compared with the plasma, accumulation (ion trapping) in milk may occur. The effect of this exposure on a nursing infant is unknown. Infants should be monitored for adverse events commonly observed in adults, such as fatigue, syncope, somnolence, dizziness, dyspepsia, and nausea and vomiting. Ropinirole inhibits prolactin secretion and may inhibit lactation. Until data are available, the best course is to not breastfeed if ropinirole is being taken.

Reference

1. Product information. Requip. GlaxoSmithKline, 2003.

ROPIVACAINE

Local Anesthetic

PREGNANCY RECOMMENDATION: Compatible
BREASTFEEDING RECOMMENDATION: No Human Data—Probably Compatible

R

PREGNANCY SUMMARY

The human and animal data suggest that the risk to a human fetus from the use of ropivacaine in pregnancy is very low or nonexistent. However, there is no human pregnancy experience in the 1st trimester. The amounts measured in the maternal circulation are very low and do not appear to represent a significant embryo–fetal risk.

FETAL RISK SUMMARY

Ropivacaine is a member of the amino amide class of local anesthetics. It is indicated for local or regional anesthesia for surgery and for acute pain management. Ropivacaine is a pure S-enantiomer that is structurally similar to bupivacaine. It has been used for local and regional anesthesia before cesarean section and during labor. Plasma protein binding (94%) is primarily to α_1-glycoprotein. The mean terminal half-life is 4.2 hours after epidural administration (1).

Reproduction studies have been conducted in rats and rabbits. In rats, daily SC doses up to about 0.33 times the maximum recommended human dose (epidural, 770 mg/24 hours) based on BSA (MRHD) during organogenesis revealed no teratogenic effects. When rats were given daily SC doses from gestational day 15 through postpartum day 20, there were no treatment-related effects on late fetal development, parturition, lactation, neonatal viability, or growth of the offspring. In another study, female rats were given daily SC doses that were about 0.3 times the MRHD for 2 weeks before mating, then during mating, pregnancy, and lactation, up to day 42 post-coitus. There was an increased loss of pups during the first 3 days postpartum, an effect thought to have occurred because of reduced maternal care due to maternal toxicity. In rabbits, SC doses up to about 0.33 times the MRHD during organogenesis revealed no teratogenicity (1).

Pregnant sheep were given a 60-minute IV infusion of a local anesthetic (ropivacaine, bupivacaine, or levobupivacaine) at a rate that obtained a maternal serum concentration equivalent to that obtained during routine epidural anesthesia for cesarean delivery (2). No significant changes (heart rate, mean arterial blood pressure, arterial blood pH, and arterial oxygenation) in the fetuses were observed. Maternal hemodynamic parameters also were not affected. All three anesthetics crossed the placenta to the fetus with varying concentrations measured in all fetal tissues tested (heart, brain, liver, lung, kidney, and adrenals). The ropivacaine fetal:maternal serum ratio was approximately 0.3 (2).

A 1999 study used a dual perfused, single cotyledon human placental model to compare the placental transfer of ropivacaine and bupivacaine (3). Simulation of the actual in vivo plasma protein concentration (using a 4% albumin solution) resulted in a 50% decrease in the amounts transferred compared with a 2% albumin solution. In addition, decreasing the pH on the fetal side resulted in a significant increase in placental transfer. The investigators concluded that the placental transfer of both anesthetics was highly influenced by the amount of maternal and fetal protein binding and fetal pH (3).

In another study, epidural ropivacaine was given to women for cesarean section (4). The umbilical:maternal (U:M) veins ratio of unbound drug at delivery was 0.72 (4). A 1997 report measured mean U:M vein ratios for total and unbound ropivacaine after epidural of 0.31 and 0.74, respectively (5). In a third study, total ropivacaine concentrations in the umbilical vein and artery were 0.13–0.52 and 0.12–0.41 mg/L, respectively, whereas the concentrations of unbound drug were 0.027–0.063 and 0.027–0.058 mg/L, respectively (6).

A number of studies have reported normal Apgar scores, umbilical acid–base values, and neurobehavioral assessments when ropivacaine epidurals were used in women in labor (4–11). In one study conducted at six different centers, fewer infants delivered vaginally from mothers receiving ropivacaine had abnormal neurological and adaptive capacity scores at 24 hours compared with those delivered vaginally from mothers receiving bupivacaine (11).

R

BREASTFEEDING SUMMARY

No reports describing the use of ropivacaine during human lactation have been located. As noted above, the primary use in pregnancy of this local anesthetic occurs during labor. Only very small amounts appear in the maternal circulation after epidural use and these concentrations would be cleared within 24 hours. Therefore, there appears to be no risk for a nursing infant.

References

1. Product information. Naropin. AstraZeneca, 2001.
2. Santos AC, Karpel B, Noble G. The placental transfer and fetal effects of levobupivacaine, racemic bupivacaine, and ropivacaine. Anesthesiology 1999;90:1698–703.
3. Johnson RF, Cahana A, Olenick M, Herman N, Paschall RL, Minzter B, Ramasubramanian R, Gonzalez H, Downing JW. A comparison of the placental transfer of ropivacaine versus bupivacaine. Anesth Analg 1999;89:703–8.
4. Datta S, Camann W, Bader A, VanderBurgh L. Clinical effects and maternal and fetal plasma concentrations of epidural ropivacaine versus bupivacaine for cesarean section. Anesthesiology 1995;82:1346–52.
5. Morton CPJ, Bloomfield S, Magnusson A, Jozwiak H, McClure JH. Ropivacaine 0.75% for extradural anaesthesia in elective caesarean section: an open clinical and pharmacokinetic study in mother and neonate. Br J Anaesth 1997;79:3–8.
6. Irestedt L, Ekblom A, Olofsson C, Dahlstrom AC, Emanuelsson BM. Pharmacokinetics and clinical effect during continuous epidural infusion with ropivacaine 2.5 mg/ml or bupivacaine 2.5 mg/ml for labour pain relief. Acta Anaesthesiol Scand 1998;42:890–6.
7. Gaiser RR, Venkateswaren P, Cheek TG, Persiley E, Buxbaum J, Hedge J, Joyce TH, Gutsche BB. Comparison of 0.25% ropivacaine and bupivacaine for epidural analgesia for labor and vaginal delivery. J Clin Anesthesia 1997;9:564–8.
8. McCrae AF, Jozwiak H, McClure JH. Comparison of ropivacaine and bupivacaine in extradural analgesia for the relief of pain in labour. Br J Anaesth 1995;74:261–5.
9. Eddleston JM, Holland JJ, Griffin RP, Corbett A, Horsman EL, Reynolds F. A double-blind comparison of 0.25% ropivacaine and 0.25% bupivacaine for extradural analgesia in labour. Br J Anaesth 1996;76:66–71.
10. Irestedt L, Emanuelsson BM, Ekblom A, Olofsson C, Reventlid H. Ropivacaine 7.5 mg/ml for elective caesarean section. A clinical and pharmacokinetic comparison of 150 mg and 187.5 mg. Acta Anaesthesiol Scand 1997;41:1149–56.
11. Writer WDR, Stienstra R, Eddleston JM, Gatt SP, Griffin R, Gutsche BB, Joyce TH, Hedlund C, Heeroma K, Selander D. Neonatal outcome and mode of delivery after epidural analgesia for labour with ropivacaine and bupivacaine: a prospective meta-analysis. Br J Anaesth 1998;81:713–7.

ROSIGLITAZONE

Antidiabetic Agent

PREGNANCY RECOMMENDATION: Limited Human Data—Animal Data Suggest Risk
BREASTFEEDING RECOMMENDATION: No Human Data—Probably Compatible

PREGNANCY SUMMARY

Two cases of rosiglitazone use in pregnancy have been located and neither was associated with developmental toxicity. Insulin is the treatment of choice for pregnant diabetic patients because, in general, other hypoglycemic agents do not provide adequate glycemic control. Moreover, insulin, unlike most oral agents, does not cross the placenta to the fetus, thus eliminating the additional concern that the drug therapy itself will adversely affect the fetus. Carefully prescribed insulin therapy provides better control of the mother's glucose, thereby preventing the fetal and neonatal complications that occur with this disease. High maternal glucose levels, as may occur in diabetes mellitus, are closely associated with a number of maternal and fetal adverse effects, including fetal structural anomalies if the hyperglycemia occurs early in gestation. To prevent this toxicity, the American College of Obstetricians and Gynecologists recommends that insulin be used for types I and II diabetes occurring during pregnancy and, if diet therapy alone is not successful, for gestational diabetes (1,2).

FETAL RISK SUMMARY

Rosiglitazone, a thiazolidinedione antidiabetic agent, is used as an adjunct to diet and exercise to improve glycemic control in patients with type II diabetes (noninsulin-dependent diabetes mellitus). It is used either alone or in combination with metformin. Rosiglitazone is not an insulin secretagogue, but acts to decrease insulin resistance in the periphery and in the liver (i.e., decreases insulin requirements). Rosiglitazone undergoes extensive metabolism to inactive metabolites. The plasma half-life of rosiglitazone-related materials (parent drug and inactive metabolites) ranges from 103 to 158 hours and the binding to plasma proteins, primarily albumin, is high (99.8%) (3).

Reproduction studies with rosiglitazone have been conducted in rats and rabbits at doses up to 20 and 75 times, respectively, the AUC at the maximum recommended human daily dose (MRHDD). No teratogenicity or adverse effect on implantation or the embryos were observed in either species, but placental pathology was noted in rats. Moreover, dosing during midgestation to late gestation was associated with fetal death and growth restriction in both rats and rabbits. Treatment extending through the lactation period in rats was associated with reduced litter size and decreased neonatal viability and postnatal growth. Growth restriction was reversible after puberty. For effects on the placenta, embryo, fetus, and offspring, the no-effect dose levels were approximately 4 times the MRHDD for both species (3).

Consistent with the molecular weight of the free base (about 357) and prolonged elimination half-life of the parent drug and/or inactive metabolites, rosiglitazone crosses the human placenta. In 31 women undergoing an elective abortion at 8–12 weeks' gestation and given two 4 mg doses before the procedure, rosiglitazone was detected in 19 fetuses (4). The mean fetal tissue concentration was about 53 ng/g. The drug was more likely to be detected at 10 or more weeks' gestation (4). Using the technique of dual perfusion of placental lobule, rosiglitazone, in the presence of human serum albumin, readily crossed the placenta (5). In contrast, a study using 10 near-term placentas in an ex vivo human perfusion model found minimal transfer and fetal accumulation of rosiglitazone (6).

A 2002 report described the use of rosiglitazone in early pregnancy (7). A 35-year-old woman with several diseases (hypertension, diabetes mellitus, hypercholesterolemia, anxiety disorder, epilepsia, and morbid obesity) who conceived while being treated with multiple drugs: rosiglitazone (4 mg/day), gliclazide (a sulfonylurea), atorvastatin, acarbose, spironolactone, hydrochlorothiazide, carbamazepine, thioridazine, amitriptyline, chlordiazepoxide, and pipenzolate bromide (an antispasmodic). Pregnancy was diagnosed in the 8th week of gestation and all medications were stopped. She was treated with methyldopa and insulin for the remainder of her pregnancy. At 36 weeks' gestation, a repeat cesarean section delivered a healthy, 3.5-kg female infant with Apgar scores of 7 and 8 at 1 and 5 minutes, respectively. The infant was developing normally after 4 months (7).

A 2005 case report described the use rosiglitazone between the 13th and 17th week of gestation in a woman with type 2 diabetes (8). Before the 13th week, the woman's diabetes had been managed with diet and exercise. Insulin was started after rosiglitazone was stopped and the woman delivered a healthy, 4.5-kg male infant at 37 weeks' gestation. No major or minor malformations were observed (8).

Rosiglitazone is sometimes used for the treatment of insulin resistance in women with polycystic ovarian syndrome. Spontaneous ovulation and enhancement of clomiphene-induced ovulation resulting in conception has been reported after the use of rosiglitazone (9–11). Because this treatment may result in pregnancy, appropriate contraception is advised (12).

BREASTFEEDING SUMMARY

No reports describing the use of rosiglitazone during human lactation have been located. The molecular weight of the free base (about 357) and long elimination half-life (103–158 hours) suggest that excretion into breast milk should be expected. The effect of this exposure on a nursing infant is unknown. However, weak bases are known to accumulate in milk with concentrations higher than those in maternal plasma.

References

1. American College of Obstetricians and Gynecologists. Pregestational diabetes mellitus. *ACOG Practice Bulletin*. No. 60. March 2005. Obstet Gynecol 2005;105:675–85.
2. American College of Obstetricians and Gynecologists. Gestational diabetes. *ACOG Practice Bulletin*. No. 30. September 2001. Obstet Gynecol 2001;98:525–38.
3. Product information. Avandia. SmithKline Beecham Pharmaceuticals, 2000.
4. Chan LYS, Yeung JHK, Lau TK. Placental transfer of rosiglitazone in the first trimester of human pregnancy. Fertil Steril 2005;83:955–8.
5. Patrikeeva S, Hemauer S, Nanovskaya T, Hankins G, Ahmed M. Transplacental transfer and distribution of rosiglitazone (abstract). Am J Obstet Gynecol 2006;195:S128.

R

6. Holmes HJ, Casey BM, Bawdon RE. Placental transfer of rosiglitazone in the ex vivo human perfusion model. Am J Obstet Gynecol 2006;195:1715–9.
7. Yaris F, Yaris E, Kadioglu M, Ulku C, Kesim M, Kalyoncu NI. Normal pregnancy outcome following inadvertent exposure to rosiglitazone, gliclazide, and atorvastatin in a diabetic and hypertensive woman. Reprod Toxicol 2004;18:619–21.
8. Kalyoncu NI, Yaris F, Ulku C, Kadioglu M, Kesim M, Unsal M, Dikici M, Yaris E. A case of rosiglitazone exposure in the second trimester of pregnancy. Reprod Toxicol 2005;19:563–4.
9. Cataldo NA, Abbasi F, McLaughlin TL, Lamendola C, Reaven GM. Improvement in insulin sensitivity followed by ovulation and pregnancy in a woman with polycystic ovary syndrome who was treated with rosiglitazone. Fertil Steril 2001;76:1057–9.
10. Belli SH, Graffigna MN, Oneto A, Otero P, Schurman L, Levalle OA. Effect of rosiglitazone on insulin resistance, growth factors, and reproductive disturbances in women with polycystic ovary syndrome. Fertil Steril 2004;81:624–9.
11. Ghazeeri G, Kutteh WH, Bryer-Ash M, Haas D, Ke RK. Effect of rosiglitazone on spontaneous and clomiphene citrate-induced ovulation in women with polycystic ovary syndrome. Fertil Steril 2003;79:562–6.
12. O'Moore-Sullivan TM, Prins JB. Thiazolidinediones and type 2 diabetes: new drugs for an old disease. Med J Aust 2002;176:381–6.

ROSUVASTATIN

Antilipemic Agent

PREGNANCY RECOMMENDATION: Contraindicated
BREASTFEEDING RECOMMENDATION: Contraindicated

PREGNANCY SUMMARY

No reports describing the use of rosuvastatin in human pregnancy have been located. There was developmental toxicity (growth restriction and/or death) in two animal species at exposures that were close to those obtained in humans, but maternal toxicity also was observed in one of the species. The absence of human pregnancy experience prevents a more complete assessment of the embryo–fetal risk. Because the interruption of cholesterol-lowering therapy during pregnancy should have no apparent effect on the long-term treatment of hyperlipidemia, rosuvastatin should not be used during pregnancy. Moreover, cholesterol and other products of cholesterol biosynthesis are essential components for fetal development (1). Women taking this agent before conception should stop the therapy before becoming pregnant and certainly on recognition of pregnancy. Accidental use of the drug during gestation, though, apparently has no proven consequences for the fetus.

FETAL RISK SUMMARY

Rosuvastatin (a statin) is a lipophilic agent that is used to lower elevated levels of cholesterol. It has the same cholesterol-lowering mechanism (i.e., inhibition of hepatic 3-hydroxy-3-methylglutaryl-coenzyme A [HMG-CoA] reductase) as other agents available in this class: atorvastatin, fluvastatin, lovastatin, pitavastatin, pravastatin, and simvastatin (cerivastatin was withdrawn from the market in 2001). Rosuvastatin undergoes little metabolism (about 19%). The main metabolite has some activity but ≤50% than that of the parent compound. Protein binding, mostly to albumin, is about 88%. The primary route of elimination is in the feces with an elimination half-life of about 19 hours (1).

Reproduction studies have been conducted in rats and rabbits. Decreased fetal body weight (female pups) and delayed ossification were observed in the offspring when female rats were given a dose before mating and continuing through day 7 postcoitus that resulted in exposures 10 times the human exposure from 40 mg/day based on AUC (HE-AUC). Decreased pup survival was observed with continuous dosing from day 7 of gestation through lactation day 21 (weaning) at 10 times the HE-AUC or ≥12 times the human exposure based on BSA (HE-BSA). In pregnant rabbits given a dose equivalent to the HE-BSA from gestation day 6 through lactation day 18 (weaning), decreased fetal viability and maternal mortality were observed. Rosuvastatin was not teratogenic in rats or rabbits at systemic exposures equivalent to the HE-AUC or HE-BSA (1).

In 2-year carcinogenicity studies in rats and mice, increased incidences of uterine stromal polyps and hepatocellular adenoma/carcinoma, respectively, were observed at a dose 20 times the HE-AUC. No mutagenic or clastogenic effects were noted in a variety of tests. There also were no effects on fertility in male or female rats at doses up to 10 times the HE-AUC. However, in male dogs and monkeys, doses that were 20 and 10 times, respectively, the HE-BSA caused spermatidic giant cells. In addition, vacuolation seminiferous tubular epithelium was observed in male monkeys (1).

It is not known if rosuvastatin crosses the human placenta. The molecular weight is moderately high (about 966 for the free acid) as is protein binding, but the low metabolism and prolonged elimination half-life suggest that exposure of the embryo–fetus should be expected.

Pregnancy exposures to this class of drugs that had been reported to the FDA were described in 2004 (2). (See Lovastatin.) Twenty of the 178 reported cases involved major congenital malformations. Although none of the cases involved exposure to rosuvastatin (approved by the FDA in August 2003), and the sample was biased because of its voluntary nature and the likely reporting of severe outcomes, some of the defects might be consistent with the inhibition of cholesterol biosynthesis (2). In another 2004 report, among 214 exposures reported to the FDA (none involving rosuvastatin), there were 22 birth defects, 4 infants with intrauterine growth restriction, and 5 cases of fetal death (3). (See Lovastatin.) As in the first report, it was thought that some of the defects might be consistent with inhibition of cholesterol biosynthesis (3).

BREASTFEEDING SUMMARY

No reports describing the use of rosuvastatin during lactation have been located. The excretion of rosuvastatin into breast milk should be expected because of the molecular weight (about 966 for the free acid), low metabolism (10%), and long elimination half-life (about 19 hours). At least two similar agents (fluvastatin and pravastatin) appear in human milk. Because of the potential for adverse effects in the nursing infant, the drug should not be used during lactation.

References

1. Product information. Crestor. AstraZeneca, 2005.
2. Edison RJ, Muenke M. Central nervous system and limb anomalies in case-reports of first trimester statin exposure. New Engl J Med 2004;350: 1579–82.
3. Edison RJ, Muenke M. Mechanistic and epidemiologic considerations in the evaluation of adverse birth outcomes following gestational exposure to statins. Am J Med Genet 2004;131A:287–98.

RUFINAMIDE

Anticonvulsant

PREGNANCY RECOMMENDATION: No Human Data—Animal Data Suggest Risk
BREASTFEEDING RECOMMENDATION: No Human Data—Potential Toxicity

PREGNANCY SUMMARY

No reports describing the use of rufinamide in human pregnancy have been located. The drug caused embryo–fetal toxicity in two animal species at systemic exposures less than the human exposure. If a pregnant woman is exposed to this drug, she should be informed of the absence of human pregnancy experience and the potential for embryo–fetal risk.

FETAL RISK SUMMARY

Rufinamide is an oral triazole derivative that is unrelated to other anticonvulsants. It is indicated for adjunctive treatment of seizures associated with Lennox-Gastaut syndrome in children ≥4 years of age and adults. Rufinamide is extensively metabolized to inactive metabolites. Only 34% of the drug is bound to plasma proteins, mostly to albumin, and the plasma half-life is about 6–10 hours (1).

Reproduction studies have been conducted in rats and rabbits. In rats, daily oral doses during organogenesis resulting in plasma exposures (AUC) that were 2 times the plasma exposure (AUC) from the maximum recommended human dose of 3200 mg/day (MRHD) caused decreased fetal weights and increased incidences of skeletal abnormalities, but maternal toxicity also was evident. In rabbits, daily oral doses during organogenesis resulting in exposures that were >0.2 times the MRHD resulted in embryo–fetal death, decreased fetal body weights, and increased incidences of visceral and skeletal abnormalities. A dose 2 times the MRHD caused abortions. In both species, the no-observed-effect-level (NOEL) for adverse effects on embryo–fetal development was 0.2 times the MRHD. In prenatal and postnatal studies with rats, daily oral doses given from implantation through weaning resulting plasma exposures that were <0.1–1.5 times the MRHD caused decreased offspring growth and survival at all doses. A NOEL was not established in these studies (1).

Long-term exposures to rufinamide in mice and rats were carcinogenic, but the drug was not mutagenic or clastogenic in multiple assays. In male and female rats daily doses that were ≥0.2 times than the MRHD before and throughout mating, and continued in females up to gestational day 6, were associated with impaired fertility including decreased sperm count and motility, decreased conception rates, mating, and fertility indices, decreased numbers of corpora lutea, implantations, and live embryos, and increased preimplantation loss. A NOEL for impaired fertility was not established (1).

It is not known if rufinamide crosses the human placenta. The low molecular weight (about 238), lipophilic nature, and long plasma half-life suggest that exposure of the embryo–fetus will occur. However, the extensive metabolism to inactive compounds might limit the exposure.

BREASTFEEDING SUMMARY

No reports describing the use of rufinamide during human lactation have been located. The low molecular weight (about 238), lipophilic nature, and long plasma half-life suggest that the drug will be excreted into breast milk, but the extensive metabolism should limit the amount. The effect of this exposure on a nursing infant is unknown. If mother chooses to nurse her infant while taking rufinamide, the infant should be closely observed for changes in behavior and other signs of toxicity. Somnolence, vomiting, and headache were the three most frequent adverse reactions observed in pediatric patients treated with the drug (1).

Reference

1. Product information. Banzel. Eisai, 2008.

R

RUXOLITINIB

Antineoplastic (Janus Associated Kinase Inhibitor)

PREGNANCY RECOMMENDATION: Contraindicated
BREASTFEEDING RECOMMENDATION: Contraindicated

PREGNANCY SUMMARY

No reports describing the use of ruxolitinib in human pregnancy have been located. The animal data suggested risk (reduced fetal weights and late resorptions in two species) but these effects occurred with doses that were maternally toxic. However, lower nonmaternal toxic doses in rats were associated with postimplantation losses. Although the drug's mechanism of action suggests that use in pregnancy could cause fetal harm, the absence of human pregnancy experience prevents a better assessment of the embryo–fetal risk. If the drug is indicated in a pregnant woman, she should be informed of the potential risk to her embryo–fetus.

FETAL RISK SUMMARY

Ruxolitinib is an oral inhibitor of janus associated kinases which mediate the signaling of a number of cytokines and growth factors that are important for hematopoiesis and immune function. It is indicated for the treatment of patients with intermediate- or high-risk myelofibrosis, including primary myelofibrosis, postpolycythemia vera myelofibrosis, and postessential thrombocythemia myelofibrosis. Ruxolitinib is partially metabolized to two active metabolites. Plasma protein binding is about 97%, primarily to albumin. The mean elimination half-life for ruxolitinib alone is about 3 hours, whereas it is about 5.8 hours for the parent drug plus active metabolites (1).

Reproduction studies have been conducted in rats and rabbits. In these species, no teratogenic effects were observed at the highest doses tested resulting in exposures (AUC) that were about 2 times and 7%, respectively, of the clinical exposure at the maximum recommended dose of 25 mg twice daily (CEMRD). At these doses, reduced fetal weights were noted in rats and rabbits, and increased late resorptions in rabbits, but maternal toxicity occurred in both species. In a predevelopment and postnatal development study in rats, doses up to 34% of the CEMRD given from implantation through lactation resulted in no drug-related adverse effects in pups for fertility indices or for maternal or embryo–fetal survival, growth, and developmental parameters (1).

Ruxolitinib was not carcinogenic in long-term studies in mice and rats, and was not mutagenic or clastogenic in multiple assays. In male and female rats, no effects were observed on fertility or reproductive performance, but increased postimplantation loss was noted at exposures that were about 34% of the CEMRD (1).

It is not known if ruxolitinib or its two active metabolites cross the human placenta. The molecular weight of the parent drug (about 404) suggests that the drug will cross, but the high plasma protein binding and relatively short mean elimination half-lives should limit the exposure.

BREASTFEEDING SUMMARY

No reports describing the use of ruxolitinib during human lactation have been located. The molecular weight of the parent drug (about 404) suggests that the drug, and possibly its two active metabolites, will be excreted into breast milk, but the high (97%) plasma protein binding and relatively short mean elimination half-lives (3 hours for the parent drug and 5.8 hours for the parent drug plus active metabolites) should limit the amount excreted. The effect of any exposure on a nursing infant is unknown. However, thrombocytopenia and anemia occurred in >20% of patients treated with the drug and >10% experienced bruising, dizziness, and headache (1). Thus, if the drug is given during breastfeeding, a nursing infant should be monitored for these adverse effects.

Reference

1. Product information. Jakafi. Incyte, 2012.

R

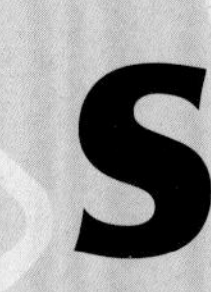

SACCHARIN

Artificial Sweetener

PREGNANCY RECOMMENDATION: Limited Human Data—Animal Data Suggest Low Risk
BREASTFEEDING RECOMMENDATION: Compatible

PREGNANCY SUMMARY

There is limited information available on the risk for humans following in utero exposure to saccharin. The Calorie Control Council believes that the agent can be safely used by pregnant women (1). However, others recommended avoidance of saccharin or, at least, cautious use of it in pregnancy (2–4).

FETAL RISK SUMMARY

Saccharin is a nonnutritive sweetening agent discovered accidentally in 1879; it has been used in the United States since 1901. The agent is approximately 300 times sweeter than sucrose. Saccharin, a derivative of naphthalene, is absorbed slowly after oral ingestion and is rapidly and completely excreted, as the unmetabolized compound, by the kidneys. Although a large amount of medical research has been generated concerning saccharin, very little of this information pertains to its use by pregnant women or to its effect on the fetus (2,3).

In pregnant rhesus monkeys administered IV saccharin, fetal accumulation of the sweetener occurred after rapid, but limited, transfer across the placenta (5). Saccharin appeared to be uniformly distributed to all fetal tissues except the CNS. Fetal levels were still present 5 hours after the end of the infusion and 2 hours after maternal concentrations were undetectable. A study, published in 1986, documented that saccharin also crosses the placenta to the human fetus (6). Six diabetic women, consuming 25–100 mg/day of saccharin by history, were delivered at 36–42 weeks. Maternal serum saccharin concentrations, measured between 0.5 hour before to 2 hours after delivery, ranged from 20 to 263 ng/mL. Cord blood samples varied from 20 to 160 ng/mL (6).

Saccharin is not an animal teratogen (5,7,8). No increase in the incidence of spontaneous abortions among women consuming saccharin has been found (9). Concerns for human use focus on the potential carcinogenicity of the agent. In some animal species, particularly after second-generation studies, an increased incidence of bladder tumors was observed (3). However, epidemiologic studies have failed to associate the human use of saccharin with bladder cancer (3). Similarly, no evidence was found in a study of the Danish population that in utero saccharin exposure was associated with an increased risk of bladder cancer during the first 30–35 years of life (3,10). However, at least one investigator believes that these studies must be extended much further before they are meaningful, because bladder cancer is usually diagnosed in the elderly (4).

BREASTFEEDING SUMMARY

Saccharin is excreted into human milk (11). In six healthy women, saccharin, 126 mg/12 fluid ounces, contained in two commercially available soft drinks, was given every 6 hours for nine doses. After single or multiple doses, median peak concentrations of saccharin occurred at 0.75 hour in plasma and at 2.0 hours in milk. Milk concentrations ranged from <200–1056 ng/mL after one dose to 1765 ng/mL after nine doses. The AUC ratios for milk and plasma averaged 0.542 on day 1 and 0.715 on day 3, indicating that accumulation in the milk occurred with time. The amounts of saccharin a nursing infant could consume from milk were predicted to be much less than the usual intakes of children <2 years old (11).

References

1. Nabors LO. Letter to the editors. J Reprod Med 1988;33(8):102.
2. London RS. Saccharin and aspartame: are they safe to consume during pregnancy? J Reprod Med 1988;33:17–21.
3. Council on Scientific Affairs, American Medical Association. Saccharin: review of safety issues. JAMA 1985;254:2622–4.
4. London RS. Letter to the editors. J Reprod Med 1988;33(8):102.
5. Pitkin RM, Reynolds WA, Filer LJ Jr, Kling TG. Placental transmission and fetal distribution of saccharin. Am J Obstet Gynecol 1971;111:280–6.
6. Cohen-Addad N, Chatterjee M, Bekersky I, Blumenthal HP. In utero exposure to saccharin: a threat? Cancer Lett 1986;32:151–4.
7. Fritz H, Hess R. Prenatal development in the rat following administration of cyclamate, saccharin and sucrose. Experientia 1968;24:1140–1.
8. Shepard TH. *Catalog of Teratogenic Agents*. 6th ed. Baltimore, MD: The Johns Hopkins University Press, 1989:566–7.
9. Kline J, Stein ZA, Susser M, Warburton D. Spontaneous abortion and the use of sugar substitutes. Am J Obstet Gynecol 1978;130:708–11.
10. Jensen OM, Kamby C. Intra-uterine exposure to saccharin and risk of bladder cancer in man. Int J Cancer 1982;15:507–9.
11. Collins Egan P, Marx CM, Heyl PS, Popick A, Bekersky I. Saccharin excretion in mature human milk (abstract). Drug Intell Clin Pharm 1984; 18:511.

SAFFLOWER

Herb

PREGNANCY RECOMMENDATION: Compatible (as a Food)
BREASTFEEDING RECOMMENDATION: Compatible (as a Food)

PREGNANCY SUMMARY

No reports describing the use of safflower in pregnancy have been located. However, safflower oil is widely used in cooking. It is doubtful that such use would have any adverse effect on a pregnancy. Abortifacient and emmenagogue effects have been suggested (1,2), but there apparently is no clinical evidence to support these effects when safflower oil is used as a food. Other uses or high doses of safflower should be avoided in pregnancy.

FETAL RISK SUMMARY

The seeds of safflower (*Carthamus tinctorius*), a plant widely cultivated throughout Europe and the United States, are primarily used as a source of edible oil. The oil contains a high concentration of n-6 polyunsaturated fatty acids, including the essential linoleic acid. In addition, the seeds contain tracheloside (a lignan glycoside) and serotonin derivatives. The oil is used in cooking and has been given for its laxative action. In addition, capsules containing safflower oil have sometimes served as controls in clinical trials. A tea prepared from safflower has been used to treat fever by inducing sweating. The flowers have been used as yellow and red dyes since ancient times, as well as a flavoring agent in foods (1,2).

An aqueous extract of the flowers was studied in pregnant mice (3). At doses of ≥1.6 mg/kg/day, embryo death was observed, whereas a lower dose (1.2 mg/kg/day) was teratogenic. An in vitro assay found a concentration-dependent cytotoxic effect (3).

BREASTFEEDING SUMMARY

No reports describing the use of safflower during human lactation have been located. However, safflower oil is widely used in cooking. Although mature human milk contains n-3 fatty acids (4), the probable small amounts of n-6 fatty acids excreted into milk when safflower oil is used as a food should not adversely affect a nursing infant. Other uses or high doses of safflower should be avoided during breastfeeding.

References

1. Safflower. In: *The Review of Natural Products*. St. Louis, MO: Wolters Kluwer Health, March 2009.
2. Safflower. In: *Natural Medicines Comprehensive Database*. Stockton, CA: Therapeutic Research Faculty, 2008:1290–1.
3. Nobakht M, Fattahi M, Hoormand M, Milanian I, Rahbar N, Mahmoudian M. A study on the teratogenic and cytotoxic effects of safflower extract. J Ethnopharmacol 2000;73:453–9.
4. Biochemistry of human milk. In: Lawrence RA, Lawrence RM. *Breastfeeding—A Guide for the Medical Profession*. 5th ed. St. Louis, MO: Mosby, 1999:115.

SALMETEROL

Respiratory Drug (Bronchodilator)

PREGNANCY RECOMMENDATION: Limited Human Data—Probably Compatible
BREASTFEEDING RECOMMENDATION: No Human Data—Probably Compatible

PREGNANCY SUMMARY

One review concluded that salmeterol was safe during human pregnancy (1), but others thought it should not be a first-line drug because of the lack of published human experience (2,3). Although human data have been published and no congenital malformations attributable to salmeterol were observed, the data are too limited to assess the safety of salmeterol. Moreover, the above study lacked the sensitivity to identify minor anomalies because of the absence of standardized examinations. Late-appearing major defects may also have been missed because of the timing of the questionnaires. However, if a patient with moderate or severe asthma had demonstrated a good therapeutic response before conception, this may favor the drug's continuation during pregnancy (2). Moreover, salmeterol is more effective than doubling the dose of inhaled corticosteroids and may have advantages over theophylline in terms of effectiveness and tolerability (2). In addition, the very low or undetectable maternal plasma levels that occur with therapeutic inhaled doses suggest that the risk to the fetus from the drug is probably minimal or nonexistent. If salmeterol is used in pregnancy, healthcare professionals are encouraged to call the toll-free number (877-311-8972) for information about patient enrollment in an Organization of Teratology Information Specialists (OTIS) study.

FETAL RISK SUMMARY

Salmeterol is a selective β_2-adrenergic bronchodilator that is indicated in the management of asthma. It is administered as an aerosol or powder for oral inhalation. Because the drug acts locally in the lung, plasma levels are very low or undetectable and are a result of swallowed salmeterol.

Animal reproduction studies have been conducted in the rat and rabbit (4). In the rat, oral doses up to approximately 160 times the maximum recommended daily human inhalation dose based on BSA (MRDHID-BSA) produced no evidence of impaired fertility or teratogenic effects. In pregnant Dutch rabbits, an oral dose about 10 times the maximum recommended daily human inhalation dose based on AUC (MRDHID-AUC) produced no fetal toxicity. When the dose was increased to about 20 times the MRDHID-AUC, fetal toxicity secondary to β-adrenoceptor stimulation was observed (precocious eyelid openings, cleft palate, sternebral fusion, limb and paw flexures, and delayed ossification of the frontal cranial bones). However, New Zealand White rabbits were much less sensitive—exhibiting only delayed ossification of the frontal cranial bones at oral doses 1600 times the MRDIHD-BSA. The fetal toxicity noted in rabbits was not thought to be relevant to humans because β-agonists characteristically induce these effects in animals (4).

In a study with pregnant rats, salmeterol concentrations in mammary tissue, placenta, and fetus after oral administration were comparable to those in maternal blood up to 6 hours after a dose (5). At 24 hours, the disposition of the drug in the fetus was primarily in the gastrointestinal tract.

It is not known if salmeterol crosses the placenta to the fetus. Although the molecular weight (about 604 for salmeterol xinafoate) is low enough, plasma levels after an inhaled therapeutic dose are very low or undetectable.

A 1998 noninterventional observational cohort study described the outcomes of pregnancies in women who had been prescribed ≥1 of 34 newly marketed drugs by general practitioners in England (6). Data were obtained by questionnaires sent to the prescribing physicians 1 month after the expected or possible date of delivery. In 831 (78%) of the pregnancies, a newly marketed drug was thought to have been taken during the 1st trimester, with birth defects noted in 14 (2.5%) singleton births of the 557 newborns (10 sets of twins). In addition, two birth defects were observed in aborted fetuses. However, few of the aborted fetuses were examined. Salmeterol was taken during the 1st trimester in 65 pregnancies. The outcomes of these pregnancies included 7 spontaneous abortions, 2 ectopic pregnancies, 4 elective abortions, 5 unknown outcomes, and 47 live births (3 premature). One full-term newborn was diagnosed with Aarskog's syndrome (a male child with short stature, and facial, digital, and genital malformations; pectus excavatum, metatarsus adductus, and joint laxity are frequent skeletal features [7]) (6). The syndrome is thought to be secondary to X-linked recessive inheritance (7).

BREASTFEEDING SUMMARY

No reports describing the use of salmeterol during human lactation have been located. The molecular weight (about 604 for salmeterol xinafoate) is low enough for excretion into breast milk, but maternal plasma levels after an inhaled therapeutic dose are very low or undetectable. Thus, it is unlikely that clinically significant amounts would be found in milk.

References

1. Anonymous. Drugs for asthma. Med Letter Drugs Ther 2000;42:19–24.
2. The American College of Obstetricians and Gynecologists (ACOG) and the American College of Allergy, Asthma and Immunology (ACAAI). The use of newer asthma and allergy medications during pregnancy. Position statement. Ann Allergy Asthma Immunol 2000;84:475–80.
3. Tan KS, Thomson NC. Asthma in pregnancy. Am J Med 2000;109:727–33.
4. Product information. Serevent. Glaxo Wellcome, 2002.
5. Manchee GR, Barrow A, Kulkarni S, Palmer E, Oxford J, Colthup PV, Maconochie JG, Tarbit MH. Disposition of salmeterol xinafoate in laboratory animals and humans. Drug Metab Dispos 1993;21:1022–8.
6. Wilton LV, Pearce GL, Martin RM, Mackay FJ, Mann RD. The outcomes of pregnancy in women exposed to newly marketed drugs in general practice in England. Br J Obstet Gynaecol 1998;105:882–9.
7. Buyse ML, editor. *Birth Defects Encyclopedia*. Volume 1. Cambridge, MA: Blackwell Scientific Publications, 1990:1–2.

SALVIA DIVINORUM

Herb/Hallucinogen

PREGNANCY RECOMMENDATION: No Human Data—No Relevant Animal Data
BREASTFEEDING RECOMMENDATION: No Human Data—Potential Toxicity

S

PREGNANCY SUMMARY

No reports describing the use of *Salvia divinorum* or its active ingredient, salvinorin A, in human pregnancy have been located. The herb is used by some cultures in Mexico and exposure during gestation may have occurred. However, because smoking the herb has caused toxic, persistent psychosis in an 18-year-old female and a 21-year-old male (1–3), it is best avoided in pregnancy.

FETAL RISK SUMMARY

Salvia divinorum is a perennial herb that is a species of sage cultivated in certain regions of Mexico. The hallucinogenic substances from the leaves and juices of the herb have been used by some groups in Mexico for healing and divinatory rituals. In addition, it is thought to have antidiarrheal properties. The hallucinogenic effects are produced by smoking or chewing the leaves or drinking the juices. When taken orally, systemic effects are dependent upon absorption across the oral mucosa, as the active agent is deactivated in the gastrointestinal tract (1,4). The active psychotropic agent is the diterpene salvinorin A, also referred to as divinorin A, a nonalkaloid hallucinogen. It acts as kappa opioid receptor agonist. The major metabolite is salvinorin B (1), but it is not known if it is active. The substance crosses the blood–brain barrier, resulting in a rapid onset of effects but of short duration (1,5). In female monkeys, the elimination half-life of salvinorin A is 80 minutes (6).

Animal reproduction studies have not been conducted with *S. divinorum* or its active ingredient, salvinorin A.

BREASTFEEDING SUMMARY

No reports describing the use of *S. divinorum* or its active ingredient, salvinorin A, during human lactation have been located. The herb is used by some cultures in Mexico and exposure during breastfeeding may have occurred. However, because smoking the herb has caused toxic, persistent psychosis in two persons (1–3), it is best avoided.

References

1. Salvia divinorum. In *The Review of Natural Products*. St. Louis, MO: Wolters Kluwer Health, June 2010.
2. Paulzen M, Grunder G. Toxic psychosis after intake of the hallucinogen salvinorin A. J Clin Psychiatry 2008;69:1501–2.
3. Prezekop P, Lee T. Persistent psychosis associated with *Salvia divinorum* use. Am J Psychiatry 2009;166:832.
4. Siebert DJ. *Salvia divinorum* and salvinorin A: a new pharmacologic findings. J Ethnopharmacol 1994;43:53–6.
5. Butelman ER, Prisinzano TE, Deng H, Rus S, Kreek MJ. Unconditioned behavioral effects of the powerful k-opioid hallucinogen salvinorin A in nonhuman primates: fast onset and entry into cerebrospinal fluid. J Pharmacol Exp Ther 2009;328:588–97.
6. Schmidt MD, Schmidt MS, Butelman ER, Harding WW, Tidgewell K, Murry DJ, Kreek MJ, Prisinzano TE. Pharmacokinetics of the plant-derived k-opioid hallucinogen salvinorin A in nonhuman primates. Synapse 2005;58:208–10.

SAPROPTERIN

Antidote (Phenylketonuria)

PREGNANCY RECOMMENDATION: No Human Data—Animal Data Suggest Moderate Risk
BREASTFEEDING RECOMMENDATION: No Human Data—Probably Compatible

PREGNANCY SUMMARY

No reports describing the use of sapropterin in human pregnancy have been located. Phenylketonuria (PKU) can cause significant developmental toxicity (low birth weight, microcephaly, congenital heart disease, and mental retardation). (See Aspartame.) Although the animal data suggest moderate risk, the risk of uncontrolled PKU to the embryo and/or fetus probably is much greater. If diet alone is not adequate to control maternal phenylalanine concentrations, the use of sapropterin appears to be reasonable. However, in clinical trials with nonpregnant adults, only 20%–56% of PKU patients responded to treatment with sapropterin. The manufacturer plans to establish a pregnancy registry for women who are pregnant while receiving Kuvan treatment (details not available).

FETAL RISK SUMMARY

Sapropterin dihydrochloride is a synthetic preparation of naturally occurring tetrahydrobiopterin (BH4), the cofactor for the enzyme phenylalanine hydroxylase (PAH). The enzyme hydroxylates phenylalanine to form tyrosine. In patients with PKU, PAH activity is absent or deficient. Treatment with sapropterin activates residual PAH, resulting in improved oxidative metabolism of phenylalanine, thereby decreasing the blood concentrations of phenylalanine in some, but not all, patients (1). Sapropterin is indicated to reduce blood phenylalanine levels in patients with hyperphenylalaninemia due to BH4-responsive PKU. It is used in conjunction with a phenylalanine-restricted diet. Sapropterin tablets are dissolved in water or apple juice and taken once daily. The mean elimination half-life is about 6.7 hours (range 3.9–17 hours) (1).

Reproduction studies have been conducted in rats and rabbits. In pregnant rats, oral doses up to about 3 times the maximum recommended human dose of 20 mg/kg/day based on BSA (MRHD) produced no clear evidence of teratogenicity. Similar findings were observed in pregnant rabbits at doses up to about 10 times the MRHD, but a nonsignificant increase in the incidence of holoprosencephaly was noted. No effect on fertility or reproductive function was observed in male and female rats at doses up to about 3 times the MRHD (1).

Carcinogenicity studies have been conducted in mice and rats with doses up to about 2 times the MRHD. In a 104-week study in rats, a significant increase in the incidence of benign adrenal pheochromocytoma was observed in male rats at the maximum dose. No evidence of carcinogenicity was observed in mice, but the study was conducted for only 78 weeks. Genotoxicity was observed in some in vitro and in vivo studies but not in others (1).

It is not known if sapropterin crosses the human placenta. The molecular weight (about 241 for the free base) and moderately long elimination half-life suggest that the drug will cross to the embryo and fetus.

BREASTFEEDING SUMMARY

No reports describing the use of sapropterin during human lactation have been located. The molecular weight (about 241 for the free base) and moderately long elimination half-life (6.7 hours; range 3.9–17 hours) suggest that the drug will be excreted into breast milk. The effect of this exposure on a nursing infant is unknown. Although the drug probably is compatible with breastfeeding, infants should be monitored for adverse effects commonly seen in adults, such as headache, rhinorrhea, diarrhea, and pharyngolaryngeal pain.

Reference

1. Product information. Kuvan. BioMartin Pharmaceutical, 2008.

SAQUINAVIR

Antiviral

PREGNANCY RECOMMENDATION: Compatible—Maternal Benefit >> Embryo/Fetal Risk
BREASTFEEDING RECOMMENDATION: Contraindicated

PREGNANCY SUMMARY

Although the limited human data do not allow an assessment of the risk of saquinavir during pregnancy, the animal data suggests that the embryo–fetal risk is low. If indicated, the drug should not be withheld because of pregnancy.

FETAL RISK SUMMARY

Saquinavir, a synthetic peptide-like substrate analog, inhibits the activity of HIV protease, thus preventing the cleavage of viral polyproteins and the maturation of infectious virus. The mechanism of action is similar to four other protease inhibitors: amprenavir, indinavir, nelfinavir, and ritonavir (1).

In reproduction studies in rats and rabbits, embryotoxicity and teratogenicity were not observed at plasma concentrations up to approximately 50% and 40%, respectively, of the human exposure based on AUC achieved from the recommended clinical dose. There was also no evidence that at this dose the drug affected fertility or reproductive performance in rats. A similar lack of toxicity, as measured by survival, growth, and development of offspring to weaning, was found in rats treated during late pregnancy through lactation with doses producing the same plasma concentrations as those above (1).

It is not known if saquinavir crosses the human placenta. The molecular weight of the free base (about 671) is low enough that some degree of transfer should be anticipated. In rats and rabbits, placental transfer of saquinavir is low (<5% of maternal plasma concentrations) (1).

The Antiretroviral Pregnancy Registry reported, for the period January 1989 through July 2009, prospective data (reported before the outcomes were known) involving 4702 live births that had been exposed during the 1st trimester to one or more antiretroviral agents (2). Congenital defects were noted in 134, a prevalence of 2.8% (95% confidence interval [CI] 2.4–3.4). In the 6100 live births with earliest exposure in the 2nd/3rd trimesters, there were 153 infants with defects (2.5%, 95% CI 2.1–2.9). The prevalence rates for the two periods did not differ significantly. There were 288 infants with birth defects among 10,803 live births with exposure anytime during pregnancy (2.7%, 95% CI 2.4–3.0). The prevalence rate did not differ significantly from the rate expected in a nonexposed population. There were 354 outcomes exposed to saquinavir (158 in the 1st trimester and 196 in the 2nd/3rd trimesters) in combination with other antiretroviral agents. There were 14 birth defects (6 in the 1st trimester and 8 in the 2nd/3rd trimesters). In reviewing the birth defects of prospective and retrospective (pregnancies reported after the outcomes were known) registered cases, the Registry concluded that, except for isolated cases of neural tube defects with efavirenz exposure in retrospective reports, there was no other pattern of anomalies (isolated or syndromic) (2). (See Lamivudine for required statement.)

A study published in 1999 evaluated the safety, efficacy, and perinatal transmission rates of HIV in 30 pregnant women receiving various combinations of antiretroviral agents (3). Many of the women were substance abusers. Protease inhibitors (nelfinavir [*N* = 7], indinavir [*N* = 6], and saquinavir [*N* = 1] in combination with nelfinavir) were used in 13 of the women. Antiretroviral therapy was initiated at a median of 14 weeks' gestation (range preconception to 32 weeks). Despite previous histories of extensive antiretroviral experience and of vertical transmission of HIV, combination therapy was effective in treating maternal disease and in preventing transmission to the current newborns. The outcomes of the pregnancies treated with protease inhibitors appeared to be similar to the 17 cases that did not receive these agents, except that the birth weights were lower (3).

The experience of one perinatal center with the treatment of HIV-infected pregnant women was summarized in a 1999 abstract (4). Of 55 women receiving more than three antiviral drugs, 39 were treated with a protease inhibitor (11 with saquinavir). The outcomes included 2 spontaneous abortions, 5 elective abortions, 27 newborns, and 5 ongoing pregnancies. One woman was taken off indinavir because of ureteral obstruction and another (drug therapy not specified) developed gestational diabetes. None of the newborns tested positive for HIV, had major congenital anomalies, or complications (4).

A public health advisory was issued by the FDA on the association between protease inhibitors and diabetes mellitus (5). Because pregnancy is a risk factor for hyperglycemia, there was concern that these antiviral agents would exacerbate this risk. The manufacturer's product information also notes the potential risk for new-onset diabetes, exacerbation of preexisting diabetes, and hyperglycemia in HIV-infected patients receiving protease inhibitor therapy (1). An abstract published in 2000 described the results of a study involving 34 pregnant women treated with protease inhibitors (7 with saquinavir) compared with 41 controls that evaluated the association with diabetes (6). No relationship between protease inhibitors and an increased incidence of gestational diabetes was found.

A case of combined transient mitochondrial and peroxisomal β-oxidation dysfunction after exposure to nucleoside analog reverse transcriptase inhibitors (NRTIs) (lamivudine and zidovudine) combined with protease inhibitors (ritonavir and saquinavir) throughout gestation was reported in 2000 (7). A male infant was delivered at 38 weeks' gestation. He received postnatal prophylaxis with lamivudine and zidovudine for 4 weeks until the agents were discontinued because of anemia. Other adverse effects that were observed in the infant (age at onset) were hypocalcemia (shortly after birth), group B streptococcal sepsis, ventricular extrasystoles, prolonged metabolic acidosis, and lactic acidemia (8 weeks), a mild elevation of long-chain fatty acids (9 weeks), and neutropenia (3 months). The metabolic acidosis required treatment until 7 months of age, whereas the elevated plasma lactate resolved over 4 weeks. Cerebrospinal fluid lactate was not determined nor was a muscle biopsy conducted. Both the neutropenia and the cardiac dysfunction had resolved by 1 year of age. The elevated plasma fatty acid level was confirmed in cultured fibroblasts, but other peroxisomal functions (plasmalogen biosynthesis and catalase staining) were normal. Although mitochondrial dysfunction has been linked to NRTI agents, the authors were unable to identify the cause of the combined abnormalities in this case (7). The child was reported to be healthy and developing normally at 26 months of age.

A multicenter, retrospective survey of pregnancies exposed to protease inhibitors was published in 2000 (8). There were 92 liveborn infants delivered from 89 women (3 sets of twins) at six healthcare centers. One nonviable infant, born at 22 weeks' gestation, died. The surviving 91 infants were evaluated in terms of adverse effects, prematurity rate, and frequency of HIV type 1 (HIV-1) transmission. Most of the infants were exposed in utero to a single protease inhibitor, but a few were exposed to more than one because of sequential or double combined therapy. The number of newborns exposed to each protease inhibitor was indinavir (N = 23), nelfinavir (N = 39), ritonavir (N = 5), and saquinavir (N = 34). Protease inhibitors were started before conception in 18, and during the 1st, 2nd, or 3rd trimester in 12, 44, and 14, respectively, and not reported in one. Other antiretrovirals used with the protease inhibitors included four NRTIs (didanosine, lamivudine, stavudine, and zidovudine). The most common NRTI regimen was a combination of zidovudine and lamivudine (65% of women). In addition, seven women were enrolled in the AIDS Clinical Trials Group Protocol 316 and, at the start of labor, received a single dose either of the nonnucleoside reverse transcriptase inhibitor, nevirapine, or placebo. Maternal conditions, thought possibly or likely to be related to therapy, were mild anemia in eight, severe anemia in one (probably secondary to zidovudine), and thrombocytopenia in one. Gestational diabetes mellitus was observed in three women (3.3%), a rate similar to the expected prevalence of 2.6% in a nonexposed population (8). One mother developed postpartum cardiomyopathy and died 2 months after birth of twins, but the cause of death was not known. For the surviving newborns, there was no increase in adverse effects over that observed in previous clinical trials of HIV-positive women, including the prevalence of anemia (12%), hyperbilirubinemia (6%; none exposed to indinavir), and low birth weight (20.6%). Premature delivery occurred in 19.1% of the pregnancies (close to the expected rate). The percentage of infants infected with HIV was 0 (95% CI 0%–3%) (8).

Two reviews, one in 1996 and the other in 1997, concluded that all women currently receiving antiretroviral therapy should continue to receive therapy during pregnancy and that treatment of the mother with monotherapy was inadequate therapy (9,10). The same conclusion was reached in a 2003 review with the added admonishment that therapy must be continuous to prevent emergence of resistant viral strains (11). In 2009, the updated U.S. Department of Health and Human Services guidelines for the use of antiretroviral agents in HIV-1-infected patients continued the recommendation that therapy, with the exception of efavirenz, should be continued during pregnancy (12). If indicated, therefore, protease inhibitors, including saquinavir, should not be withheld in pregnancy because the expected benefit to the HIV-positive mother outweighs the unknown risk to the fetus. Pregnant women taking protease inhibitors should be monitored for hyperglycemia. Updated guidelines for the use of antiretroviral drugs to reduce perinatal HIV-1 transmission also were released in 2010 (13). Women receiving antiretroviral therapy during pregnancy should continue the therapy but, regardless of the regimen, zidovudine administration is recommended during the intrapartum period to prevent vertical transmission of HIV to the newborn (13).

BREASTFEEDING SUMMARY

No reports describing the use of saquinavir during lactation have been located. The molecular weight of the free base (about 671) is low enough that excretion into breast milk should be expected. The effect on a nursing infant is unknown.

Reports on the use of saquinavir during lactation are unlikely because the drug is indicated in the treatment of patients with HIV. HIV type 1 (HIV-1) is transmitted in milk, and in developed countries, breastfeeding is not recommended (9,10,12,14–16). In developing countries, breastfeeding is undertaken, despite the risk, because there are no affordable milk substitutes available. Until 1999, no studies had been published that examined the effect of any antiviral therapy on HIV-1 transmission in milk. In that year, a study involving zidovudine was published that measured a 38% reduction in vertical transmission of HIV-1 infection despite breastfeeding when compared with controls (see Zidovudine).

References

1. Product information. Invirase. Roche Laboratories, 2005.
2. Antiretroviral Pregnancy Registry Steering Committee. *Antiretroviral Pregnancy Registry International Interim Report for 1 January 1989 through 31 July 2009.* Wilmington, NC: Registry Coordinating Center; 2009. Available at www.apregistry.com. Accessed May 29, 2010.
3. McGowan JP, Crane M, Wiznia AA, Blum S. Combination antiretroviral therapy in human immunodeficiency virus-infected pregnant women. Obstet Gynecol 1999;94:641–6.
4. Stek A, Kramer F, Fassett M, Khoury M. The safety and efficacy of protease inhibitor therapy for HIV infection during pregnancy (abstract). Am J Obstet Gynecol 1999;180:S7.
5. CDC. Public Health Service Task Force recommendations for the use of antiretroviral drugs in pregnant women infected with HIV-1 for maternal health and for reducing perinatal HIV-1 transmission in the United States. MMWR 1998;47:No. RR-2.
6. Fassett M, Kramer F, Stek A. Treatment with protease inhibitors in pregnancy is not associated with an increased incidence of gestational diabetes (abstract). Am J Obstet Gynecol 2000;182:S97.
7. Stojanov S, Wintergerst U, Belohradsky BH, Rolinski B. Mitochondrial and peroxisomal dysfunction following perinatal exposure to antiretroviral drugs. AIDS 2000;14:1669.
8. Morris AB, Cu-Uvin S, Harwell JI, Garb J, Zorrilla C, Vajaranant M, Dobles AR, Jones TB, Carlan S, Allen DY. Multicenter review of protease inhibitors in 89 pregnancies. J Acquir Immune Defic Syndr 2000;25:306–11.
9. Carpenter CCJ, Fischi MA, Hammer SM, Hirsch MS, Jacobsen DM, Katzenstein DA, Montaner JSG, Richman DD, Saag MS, Schooley RT, Thompson MA, Vella S, Yeni PG, Volberding PA. Antiretroviral therapy for HIV infection in 1996. JAMA 1996;276:146–54.
10. Minkoff H, Augenbraun M. Antiretroviral therapy for pregnant women. Am J Obstet Gynecol 1997;176:478–89.
11. Minkoff H. Human immunodeficiency virus infection in pregnancy. Obstet Gynecol 2003;101:797–810.
12. Panel on Antiretroviral Guidelines for Adults and Adolescents. *Guidelines for the Use of Antiretroviral Agents in HIV-1-Infected Adults and Adolescents.* Department of Health and Human Services. December 1, 2009;1–161. Available at http://www.aidsinfo.nih.gov/ContentFiles/AdultandAdolescentGL.pdf. Accessed September 17, 2010: 60, 96–8.
13. Panel on Treatment of HIV-Infected Pregnant Women and Prevention of Perinatal Transmission. *Recommendations for Use of Antiretroviral Drugs in Pregnant HIV-1-Infected Women for Maternal Health and Interventions to Reduce Perinatal HIV Transmission in the United States.* May 24, 2010: 1–117. Available at http://aidsinfo.nih.gov/ContentFiles/PerinatalGL.pdf. Accessed September 17, 2010: 30, Table 5.
14. Brown ZA, Watts DH. Antiviral therapy in pregnancy. Clin Obstet Gynecol 1990;33:276–89.
15. De Martino M, Tovo P-A, Pezzotti P, Galli L, Massironi E, Ruga E, Floreea F, Plebani A, Gabiano C, Zuccotti GV. HIV-1 transmission through breast-milk: appraisal of risk according to duration of feeding. AIDS 1992;6:991–7.
16. Van de Perre P. Postnatal transmission of human immunodeficiency virus type 1: the breast feeding dilemma. Am J Obstet Gynecol 1995;173:483–7.

SARGRAMOSTIM

Hematopoietic

PREGNANCY RECOMMENDATION: No Human Data—No Relevant Animal Data
BREASTFEEDING RECOMMENDATION: No Human Data—Probably Compatible

PREGNANCY SUMMARY

No reports describing the use of sargramostim in human pregnancy have been located. The absence of animal and human pregnancy data prevents an assessment of the risk from maternal administration that this cytokine presents to a human embryo or fetus.

However, sargramostim differs only slightly from endogenous granulocyte-macrophage colony stimulating factor (GM-CSF). In addition, maternal serum concentrations of natural GM-CSF increase throughout pregnancy with the highest levels occurring during term labor (1). Therefore, it is doubtful if recommended doses of sargramostim will cause direct toxicity to the embryo or fetus. Until human pregnancy data are available, however, the safest course is to avoid sargramostim during gestation. Planned or inadvertent pregnancy exposure appears to represent a low risk for the embryo and fetus.

FETAL RISK SUMMARY

The human GM-CSF sargramostim is produced by recombinant DNA technology. Sargramostim differs slightly from the natural human GM-CSF. It has several specific indications: (a) following induction chemotherapy in acute myelogenous leukemia; (b) for mobilization and following transplantation of autologous peripheral blood progenitor cells; (c) for myeloid reconstitution after allogeneic bone marrow transplantation; and (d) for bone marrow transplantation failure or engraftment delay. The mean beta half-lives after IV and SC administration were 60 and 162 minutes, respectively. Animal reproduction studies have not been conducted with sargramostim (2).

Sargramostim is a 127-amino-acid glycoprotein that is characterized by three primary molecular species with molecular weights of 19,500, 16,800, and 15,500, respectively. Although studies involving placental passage of sargramostim have not been conducted, endogenous GM-CSF does cross the human placenta. In an in vitro experiment using term placentas, small amounts (about 2.4%) of GM-CSF crossed to the fetal side (3). Therefore, sargramostim also probably crosses the placenta, at least at term.

Endogenous GM-CSF promotes the growth and development of preimplantation embryos (4). GM-CSF is synthesized in the uterus with the highest concentrations occurring around the interval when implantation would occur (5).

In a 2003 study, levels of endogenous free GM-CSF were measured in peripheral blood in pregnant and nonpregnant women and in women with recurrent spontaneous abortions (RSAs) (6). In healthy women, a significant increase in GM-CSF levels was measured during pregnancy, but there was no increase in women with RSA. After an IV infusion of immunoglobulin, however, the GM-CSF levels almost doubled in women with RSA (6).

Other investigators have reached conflicting conclusions on the presence of endogenous GM-CSF in maternal blood and amniotic fluid. One study was unable to detect GM-CSF expression (using mRNA coding) in maternal serum at any stage of pregnancy or in nonpregnant women (7). Similarly, amniotic fluid GM-CSF was undetectable in laboring and non-laboring women at term in another study (8). In contrast, a third study found that amniotic fluid GM-CSF concentrations increased as a function of gestational age, the status of the membranes (intact or ruptured), and the presence of labor (9). In addition, a fourth study found a significant increase in placental and peripheral blood levels of GM-CSF in women with preeclampsia (10).

BREASTFEEDING SUMMARY

No reports describing the use of sargramostim during human lactation have been located. Endogenous granulocyte-macrophage GM-CSF is excreted into breast milk (11). Based on an immunoradiometric assay, milk concentrations of GM-CSF (100 pg/mL) were much higher than the levels in the cord blood or maternal and infant serums. At 5 days of age, breastfed infants had higher serum GM-CSF concentrations than formula-fed infants, but the difference was not significant. However, there was no difference in neutrophil chemotaxis between the groups, suggesting that either GM-CSF was inactivated or not absorbed from the milk (11). In contrast, a study using an enzyme-linked immunosorbent assay (ELISA) was unable to detect GM-CSF (<10 pg/mL) in breast milk (12).

Whether sargramostim, a glycoprotein that is slightly different from the natural protein, is excreted into milk is not known, but its close similarity to native GM-CSF suggests that it also will be excreted into milk. The effect on a nursing infant from this exposure is unknown, but because endogenous GM-CSF is present in milk and appears to be inactivated or not absorbed, the risk from sargramostim is probably very low or nonexistent.

References

1. Vassiliadis S, Ranella A, Papadimitriou L, Makrygiannakis A, Athanassakis I. Serum levels of pro- and anti-inflammatory cytokines in non-pregnant women, during pregnancy, labour and abortion. Mediators Inflamm 1998;7:69–72.
2. Product information. Leukine. Berlex Laboratories, 2004.
3. Gregor H, Egarter C, Levin D, Sternberger B, Heinze G, Leitich H, Reisenberger K. The passage of granulocyte-macrophage colony-stimulating factor across the human placenta perfused in vitro. J Soc Gynecol Investig 1999;6:307–10.
4. Sjöblom C, Wikland M, Robertson SA. Granulocyte-macrophage colony-stimulating factor (GM-CSF) acts independently of the beta common subunit of the GM-CSF receptor to prevent inner cell mass apoptosis in human embryos. Biol Reprod 2002;67:1817–23.
5. Salamonsen LA, Dimitriadis E, Robb L. Cytokines in implantation. Semin Reprod Med 2000;18:299–310.
6. Perricone R, De Carolis C, Giacomelli R, Guarino MD, De Sanctis G, Fontana L. GM-CSF and pregnancy: evidence of significantly reduced blood concentrations in unexplained recurrent abortion efficiently reverted by intravenous immunoglobulin treatment. Am J Reprod Immunol 2003;50:232–7.
7. Tranchot-Diallo J, Gras G, Parnet-Mathieu F, Benveniste O, Marcé D, Roques P, Milliez J, Chaquat G, Dormont D. Modulations of cytokine expression in pregnant women. Am J Reprod Immunol 1997;37:215–26.
8. Oláh KS, Vince GS, Neilson JP, Deniz G, Johnson PM. Interleukin-6, interferon-γ, interleukin-8, and granulocyte-macrophage colony-stimulating factor levels in human amniotic fluid at term. J Reprod Immunol 1996;32:89–98.
9. Bry K, Hallman M, Teramo K, Waffarn F, Lappalainen U. Granulocyte-macrophage colony-stimulating factor in amniotic fluid and in airway specimens of newborn infants. Pediatr Res 1997;41:105–9.
10. Hayashi M, Hamada Y, Ohkura T. Elevation of granulocyte-macrophage colony-stimulating factor in the placenta and blood in preeclampsia. Am J Obstet Gynecol 2004;190:456–61.
11. Gasparoni A, Chirico G, Ciardelli L, Marchesi ME, Rondini G. Granulocyte-macrophage colony-stimulating factor in human milk. Eur J Pediatr 1996;155:69.
12. Srivastave MD, Srivastava A, Brouhard B, Saneto R, Groh-Wargo S, Kubit J. Cytokines in human milk. Res Commun Mol Pathol Pharmacol 1996;93:263–87.

SAXAGLIPTIN

Antidiabetic Agent

PREGNANCY RECOMMENDATION: No Human Data—Animal Data Suggest Low Risk
BREASTFEEDING RECOMMENDATION: No Human Data—Probably Compatible

S

PREGNANCY SUMMARY

No reports describing the use of saxagliptin in human pregnancy have been located.The animal reproduction data suggest low risk, but the absence of human pregnancy experience prevents a complete assessment of the embryo–fetal risk. Although the use of saxagliptin may help decrease the incidence of fetal and newborn morbidity and mortality in developing countries where the proper use of insulin is problematic, insulin still is the treatment of choice for this disease during pregnancy. Moreover, insulin does not cross the placenta, which eliminates the additional concern that the drug therapy is adversely affecting the fetus. Carefully prescribed insulin therapy will provide better control of the mother's blood glucose, thereby preventing the fetal and neonatal complications that occur with this disease. High maternal glucose levels, as might occur in diabetes mellitus, are associated with a number of maternal and fetal adverse effects, including fetal structural anomalies if the hyperglycemia occurs early in gestation. To prevent this toxicity, the American College of Obstetricians and Gynecologists recommends that insulin be used for types 1 and 2 diabetes occurring during pregnancy and, if diet therapy alone is not successful, for gestational diabetes (1,2). If a woman becomes pregnant while taking saxagliptin, changing the therapy to insulin should be considered.

FETAL RISK SUMMARY

Saxagliptin is an oral inhibitor of the dipeptidyl peptidase-4 (DPP4) enzyme. It is in the same antidiabetic subclass as linagliptin and sitagliptin. Saxagliptin is indicated as an adjunct to diet and exercise to improve glycemic control in adults with type 2 diabetes mellitus. The lipophilic drug is metabolized to an active metabolite, which is one-half as potent as saxagliptin. The plasma protein binding of the parent drug and the active metabolite are negligible, and the mean terminal half-life of the two compounds is 2.5 and 3.1 hours, respectively (3,4).

Reproduction studies have been conducted in rats and rabbits. In these species, no teratogenic effects were observed at any dose given during organogenesis. The drug did cross the rat placenta (not specified for the rabbit). In rats, incomplete ossification of the pelvis, a form of developmental delay, was observed at a dose that was about 1503 and 66 times the human exposure to saxagliptin and the active metabolite, respectively, at the maximum recommended human dose of 5 mg (MRHD). At 7986 and 328 times, respectively, the MRHD, maternal toxicity and reduced fetal body weights were observed. When saxagliptin was combined with metformin (metformin exposure 4 times the human exposure of 2000 mg/day), no teratogenic or embryolethal effects were observed at saxagliptin exposures that were 21 times the MRHD. At 109 times the saxagliptin MRHD, the combination was associated with craniorachischisis (a rare neural tube defect characterized by incomplete closure of the skull and spinal column) in two fetuses from a single dam. When given to rats from gestation day 6 to lactation day 20, decreased body weights in male and female offspring were observed only at maternally toxic doses that were ≥1629 and 53 times, respectively, the MRHD. No functional or behavioral toxicity was observed in rat offspring at any dose. In rabbits, minor skeletal variations were observed at a maternally toxic dose that was about 1432 and 992 times, respectively, the MRHD (3,4).

Saxagliptin did not induce tumors in mice or rats. The parent drug (with or without metabolic activation) was not mutagenic or clastogenic in multiple assays and, in a separate assay, the active metabolite was not mutagenic. In a study with rats, the drug did not affect male or female fertility at exposures that were 603 and 776 times, respectively, the MRHD. Much higher doses that caused maternal toxicity were associated with increased fetal resorptions and effects on estrous cycling, fertility, ovulation, and implantation (3,4).

It is not known if saxagliptin or its active metabolite crosses the human placenta. The molecular weight of the parent compound (about 315 for the nonhydrated form), lipophilic properties, lack of plasma protein binding, and terminal half-lives suggest that exposure of the embryo–fetus is likely.

BREASTFEEDING SUMMARY

No reports describing the use of saxagliptin during human lactation have been located. The molecular weight of the parent compound (about 315 for the nonhydrated form), lipophilic properties, lack of plasma protein binding, and terminal half-lives (2.5 hours for saxagliptin and 3.1 hours for the active metabolite) suggest that saxagliptin and its metabolite will be excreted into breast milk. The effect of this exposure on a nursing infant is unknown. Saxagliptin overdose (80 times the maximum recommended human dose for 2 weeks) in healthy adults caused no dose-related adverse reactions (3,4). Thus, hypoglycemia in a nursing infant appears to be unlikely but should be monitored. The most common (≥5%) adverse reaction in adults was headache (3,4).

References

1. American College of Obstetricians and Gynecologists. Pregestational diabetes mellitus. *ACOG Practice Bulletin*. No. 60, March 2005. Obstet Gynecol 2005;105:675–85.
2. American College of Obstetricians and Gynecologists. Gestational diabetes. *ACOG Practice Bulletin*. No. 30. September 2001. Obstet Gynecol 2001;98:525–38.
3. Product information. Onglyza. Bristol-Myers Squibb, 2009.
4. Product information. Onglyza. AstraZeneca Pharmaceuticals, 2009.

SCOPOLAMINE

Parasympatholytic (Anticholinergic)

PREGNANCY RECOMMENDATION: Human Data Suggest Low Risk
BREASTFEEDING RECOMMENDATION: Limited Human Data—Probably Compatible

PREGNANCY SUMMARY

Except for a single case of overdose during labor, there is no evidence of embryo–fetal harm when scopolamine is used in pregnancy.

FETAL RISK SUMMARY

Scopolamine is an anticholinergic agent. A scopolamine transdermal system is used to prevent nausea and vomiting associated with motion sickness and recovery from anesthesia and surgery.

Reproduction studies in rats with daily IV doses did not observe fetal harm. A marginal embryotoxic effect was seen in rabbits at daily IV doses that produced plasma concentrations approximately 100 times the level achieved in humans with the transdermal system (1).

The Collaborative Perinatal Project monitored 50,282 mother–child pairs, 309 of whom used scopolamine in the 1st trimester (2, pp. 346–353). For anytime use, 881 exposures were recorded (2, p. 439). In neither case was evidence found for an association with malformations. However, when the group of parasympatholytics was taken as a whole (2323 exposures), a possible association with minor malformations was found (2, pp. 346–353).

In a surveillance study of Michigan Medicaid recipients involving 229,101 completed pregnancies conducted between 1985 and 1992, 27 newborns had been exposed to scopolamine during the 1st trimester (F. Rosa, personal communication, FDA, 1993). One (3.7%) major birth defect was observed (one expected), but specific information on the malformation is not available. No anomalies were observed in six categories of defects, including cardiovascular defects, oral clefts, spina bifida, polydactyly, limb reduction defects, and hypospadias.

Scopolamine readily crosses the placenta (3). When administered to the mother at term, fetal effects include tachycardia, decreased heart rate variability, and decreased heart rate deceleration (4–6). Maternal tachycardia was comparable to that with other anticholinergic agents, such as atropine or glycopyrrolate (7).

Scopolamine toxicity in a newborn has been described (8). The mother had received six doses of scopolamine (1.8 mg total) with several other drugs during labor. Symptoms in the female infant consisted of fever, tachycardia, and lethargy; she was also "barrel chested" without respiratory depression. Therapy with physostigmine reversed the condition.

In a clinical study in women undergoing cesarean section, a scopolamine transdermal system was used with epidural anesthesia and opiate analgesia and no evidence of CNS depression was observed in the newborns (1).

BREASTFEEDING SUMMARY

No reports of adverse effects secondary to scopolamine in breast milk have been located. The drug is excreted into breast milk (1). The American Academy of Pediatrics classifies scopolamine as compatible with breastfeeding (9).

References

1. Product information. Transderm Scop. Novartis Consumer Health, 2000.
2. Heinonen OP, Slone D, Shapiro S. *Birth Defects and Drugs in Pregnancy*. Littleton, MA: Publishing Sciences Group, 1977.
3. Moya F, Thorndike V. The effects of drugs used in labor on the fetus and newborn. Clin Pharmacol Ther 1963;4:628–53.
4. Shenker L. Clinical experiences with fetal heart rate monitoring of one thousand patients in labor. Am J Obstet Gynecol 1973;115:1111–6.
5. Boehm FH, Growdon JH Jr. The effect of scopolamine on fetal heart rate baseline variability. Am J Obstet Gynecol 1974;120:1099–104.
6. Ayromlooi J, Tobias M, Berg P. The effects of scopolamine and ancillary analgesics upon the fetal heart rate recording. J Reprod Med 1980;25:323–6.
7. Diaz DM, Diaz SF, Marx GF. Cardiovascular effects of glycopyrrolate and belladonna derivatives in obstetric patients. Bull NY Acad Med 1980;56: 245–8.
8. Evens RP, Leopold JC. Scopolamine toxicity in a newborn. Pediatrics 1980;66:329–30.
9. Committee on Drugs, American Academy of Pediatrics. The transfer of drugs and other chemicals into human milk. Pediatrics 2001; 108:776–89.

SECOBARBITAL

Sedative/Hypnotic

PREGNANCY RECOMMENDATION: Limited Human Data—Probably Compatible
BREASTFEEDING RECOMMENDATION: Limited Human Data—Probably Compatible

PREGNANCY SUMMARY

No reports linking the use of secobarbital with congenital defects have been located.

FETAL RISK SUMMARY

The Collaborative Perinatal Project monitored 50,282 mother–child pairs, 378 of whom had 1st trimester exposure to secobarbital (1). No evidence was found to suggest a relationship to large categories of major or minor malformations or to individual defects. Hemorrhagic disease of the newborn and barbiturate withdrawal are theoretical possibilities (see also Phenobarbital).

An in utero study found no evidence of chromosomal changes on exposure to secobarbital (2).

BREASTFEEDING SUMMARY

Secobarbital is excreted into breast milk (3). The amount and effects on the nursing infant are not known. The American Academy of Pediatrics classifies secobarbital as compatible with breastfeeding (4).

References

1. Heinonen OP, Slone D, Shapiro S. *Birth Defects and Drugs in Pregnancy*. Littleton, MA: Publishing Sciences Group, 1977:336–7.
2. Stenchever MA, Jarvis JA. Effect of barbiturates on the chromosomes of human cells in vitro—a negative report. J Reprod Med 1970; 5:69–71.
3. Wilson JT, Brown RD, Cherek DR, Dailey JW, Hilman B, Jobe PC, Manno BR, Manno JE, Redetzki HM, Stewart JJ. Drug excretion in human breast milk: principles, pharmacokinetics and projected consequences. Clin Pharmacokinet 1980;5:1–66.
4. Committee on Drugs, American Academy of Pediatrics. The transfer of drugs and other chemicals into human milk. Pediatrics 2001; 108:776–89.

SELEGILINE

Antiparkinson Agent

PREGNANCY RECOMMENDATION: Limited Human Data—Animal Data Suggest Low Risk
BREASTFEEDING RECOMMENDATION: Limited Human Data—Potential Toxicity

PREGNANCY SUMMARY

Only two cases of exposure to selegiline during human pregnancy have been located, and only one of them involved exposure throughout gestation. Although there is no indication of physical teratogenicity in animal studies or the two human cases, selegiline did result in significant neurochanges in rats when combined with another monoamine oxidase (MAO) inhibitor. Until additional human data are available, the use of selegiline during pregnancy should be avoided if possible (1,2).

FETAL RISK SUMMARY

Selegiline (*l*-deprenyl), a selective irreversible inhibitor of MAO type B (MAO-B), is used as an adjunct in the management of parkinsonian patients being treated with levodopa/carbidopa. The drug has no beneficial effect when used alone (3,4).

Reproduction studies in pregnant rats and rabbits at doses up to 35 and 95 times the human therapeutic dose based on BSA (HTD), respectively, did not reveal any evidence of teratogenicity. At the highest doses tested, however, rat fetal body weight was decreased, and the number of resorptions and postimplantation losses in rabbits increased, resulting in fewer live fetuses. An increase in the number of stillbirths and decreases in pup survival and body weight (at birth and throughout the lactation period) were observed when rats were given doses up to 15 and 62 times the HTD during late gestation and throughout lactation. At 62 times the HTD, no pups born alive survived to day 4 postpartum (3,4)

In a 1994 study, rats were treated daily throughout gestation with a combination of SC selegiline (3 mg/kg) and clorgyline, an MAO type A (MAO-A) inhibitor (3 mg/kg) (5). In another treatment group, the same doses of the drugs were administered to pregnant females throughout gestation but, at birth, the daily injections of the drugs were administered to the pups until sacrifice. Saline control groups were used for comparison. Pregnancy duration was significantly longer in the treated groups than in controls, but the litter sizes were the same. Other developmental milestones (eye opening, incisor eruption, or olfactory responses) were similar to that of controls. Pup weight gain in both treatment groups was significantly slower than that in controls. The decreased weight gain may have been due to less frequent nursing, a condition that was not resolved even when the pups were cross-fostered with control dams. None of the exposed offspring had changes in the development of the dopamine system (as indicated by dopamine terminal density). Moreover, MAO activity in the brain tissue of pups exposed to the drugs only during gestation was not significantly different from that of controls at 5 days of age. In contrast, MAO activity in pups continually exposed to the drugs was significantly less than that of controls. Compared with controls, the treatment groups were very aggressive, frequently biting the investigators. In addition, significant deficits in passive avoidance were observed at 24 days of age, and open field activity was significantly increased at 30 days of age. These two results were thought to be a measure of impulsivity. Major alterations of the serotonin system were also observed (as indicated by serotonin terminal density) in the hippocampus (higher density), caudate (higher density), and cortex (less density at 5 and 30 days, but increased at 15 days). Seizures and visual impairment were noted in pups that received the drugs during pregnancy and after birth, but not in those exposed only in utero (5).

It is not known if selegiline crosses the human placenta. The low molecular weight (about 188 for the free base) suggests that passage to the embryo–fetus should be expected.

Human pregnancy experience with selegiline is limited. A 1998 report described a case involving a 34-year-old woman with an 8-year history of Parkinson's disease, who became pregnant while under treatment with selegiline (10 mg/day), levodopa (450 mg/day), and benserazide (128.25 mg/day) (1). Because of insufficient pregnancy safety information, selegiline was discontinued (gestational time not specified). A normal healthy, 3050-g, 49-cm-long male infant was delivered at term with Apgar scores of 9, 10, and 10 at 1, 5, and 10 minutes, respectively (1).

In a second case, a 39-year-old woman with a 5-year history of Parkinson's disease took selegiline (10 mg/day), levodopa (400–600 mg/day), and benserazide (100–150 mg/day) throughout gestation (2). She was advised to stop selegiline but continued it against medical advice. She delivered a healthy 3800-g male infant at term with Apgar scores of 10 at 1 and 10 minutes. She breastfed the infant for 3 days and then changed to bottle feeding out of concern over drug transfer into her breast milk. The boy, monitored closely by a pediatrician and a neurologist, was doing very well at 10 years of age with normal somatic and mental development, and was excelling at school and in sports (2).

BREASTFEEDING SUMMARY

Except for the one case above (breastfeeding for 3 days), no reports have described the use of selegiline during human lactation. The low molecular weight (about 188 for the free base) suggests that excretion into breast milk will occur. The effect of this exposure on a nursing infant is unknown. Because of significant neurotoxicity observed in animals (see above), the safest course is to avoid selegiline during nursing until data are available.

References

1. Hagell P, Odin P, Vinge E. Pregnancy in Parkinson's disease: a review of the literature and a case report. Mov Disord 1998;13:34–8.
2. Kupsch A, Oertel WH. Selegiline, pregnancy, and Parkinson' disease. Mov Disord 1998;13:175–94.
3. Product information. Carbex. Endo Pharmaceuticals, 2000.
4. Product information. Eldepryl. Somerset Pharmaceuticals, 2000.
5. Whitaker-Azmitia PM, Zhang X, Clarke C. Effects of gestational exposure to monoamine oxidase inhibitors in rats: preliminary behavioral and neurochemical studies. Neuropsychopharmacology 1994; 11:125–32.

SENNA

Laxative

PREGNANCY RECOMMENDATION: Compatible
BREASTFEEDING RECOMMENDATION: Compatible

PREGNANCY SUMMARY

Senna, a naturally occurring laxative, contains the stereoisomeric glucosides, sennosides A and B. No reports of human teratogenicity or other fetal toxicity have been located.

FETAL RISK SUMMARY

Senna contains prodrug anthraquinone glucosides that are converted by bacterial enzymes in the colon to rhein-9-anthrone. This metabolite is then oxidized to rhein, the active cathartic agent of senna (1). Senna is not teratogenic in animals (2).

A 2009 population-based, case–control study examined the association of senna exposure during pregnancy with congenital anomalies (3). The population-based large data set of the Hungarian Case-Control Surveillance System of Congenital Abnormalities was used for the study. Most women were taking daily doses of 20 mg (range 10–30 mg). There were 22,843 cases with and 38,151 cases without congenital anomalies. In these groups, senna was used by 506 (2.2%) vs. 937 (2.5%), respectively, of the mothers. Compared with 500 matched controls, there was no higher risk for 23 different congenital anomalies groups in the 260 study mothers who were treated with senna during the second and/or third gestational months. The results indicated that senna treatment was not associated with a higher risk of congenital anomalies in offspring (3).

BREASTFEEDING SUMMARY

Sennosides A and B are not excreted into breast milk. A 1973 study using colorimetric analysis (sensitivity limit 0.34 mcg/mL) failed to detect the natural agents (4). The active metabolite, rhein, however, is excreted into milk in very small amounts (1). Lactating women administered 5 g of senna daily for 3 days excreted a mean 0.007% of the dose in their milk and no adverse effects were observed in the nursing infants. This is compatible with the fact that the anthraquinone laxatives are absorbed only slightly after oral administration (5).

In addition to the study above (1), use of the laxative during lactation has been reported in three other studies (4,6,7). Although diarrhea occurred in some of the infants, this was probably related to other causes, not to senna. In one study, mothers who ingested a single 100-mg dose of senna (containing 8.6 mg of sennosides A and B) and whose infants developed diarrhea were later given a double dose of the laxative (4). No diarrhea was observed in the infants after the higher dose. The American Academy of Pediatrics classifies senna as compatible with breastfeeding (8).

References

1. Faber P, Strenge-Hesse A. Relevance of rhein excretion into breast milk. Pharmacology 1988;36(Suppl 1):212–20.
2. Shepard TH. *Catalog of Teratogenic Agents*. 6th ed. Baltimore, MD: The Johns Hopkins University Press, 1989:574–5.
3. Acs N, Banhidy F, Puho EH, Czeizel AE. Senna treatment in pregnant women and congenital abnormalities in their offspring—a population-based case-control study. Reprod Toxicol 2009;28:100–4.
4. Werthmann MW Jr, Krees SV. Quantitative excretion of Senokot in human breast milk. Med Ann Dist Col 1973;42:4–5.
5. American Hospital Formulary Service. *Drug Information 1997*. Bethesda, MD: American Society of Health-System Pharmacists, 1997:2236–8.
6. Baldwin WF. Clinical study of senna administration to nursing mothers: assessment of effects on infant bowel habits. Can Med Assoc J 1963;89:566–8.
7. Greenhalf JO, Leonard HSD. Laxatives in the treatment of constipation in pregnant and breast-feeding mothers. Practitioner 1973; 210:259–63.
8. Committee on Drugs, American Academy of Pediatrics. The transfer of drugs and other chemicals into human milk. Pediatrics 2001; 108:776–89.

SERTACONAZOLE

Antifungal

PREGNANCY RECOMMENDATION: No Human Data—Probably Compatible
BREASTFEEDING RECOMMENDATION: No Human Data—Probably Compatible

PREGNANCY SUMMARY

No reports describing the use of sertaconazole in human pregnancy have been located. The lack of animal developmental toxicity and the failure to detect the drug in the plasma after multiple applications to diseased skin suggest that risk to the human embryo–fetus is negligible. If indicated, the topical antifungal appears to be compatible with pregnancy.

FETAL RISK SUMMARY

Sertaconazole is available as a topical cream. It is in the same antifungal class of imidazole derivatives as butoconazole, clotrimazole, econazole, ketoconazole, miconazole, oxiconazole, sulconazole, and tioconazole. Sertaconazole is indicated for the treatment of interdigital tinea pedis caused by *Trichophyton rubrum, T. mentagrophytes,* and *Epidermophyton floccosum* in immunocompetent patients. Systemic absorption of sertaconazole from diseased skin after multiple applications is negligible as plasma concentrations were below the level of detection (2.5 ng/mL) (1).

Reproduction studies have been conducted with sertaconazole in rats and rabbits. No evidence of maternal toxicity, embryo toxicity, or teratogenesis was observed in pregnant rats and rabbits given oral doses 40 and 80 times, respectively, the maximum recommended human dose based on BSA (MRHD). In a peri-postnatal study in rats, doses 20–40 times the MRHD caused a decrease in live birth indices and an increase in the number of stillborn pups. The antifungal agent had no effect on fertility in male and female rats at doses 16 times the MRHD. Although long-term studies for carcinogenicity have not been conducted, tests for mutagenicity or clastogenicity were negative (1).

It is not known if sertaconazole crosses the human placenta. Since systemic absorption after topical application was not detected in one study, it appears that exposure of the embryo and/or fetus does not occur.

BREASTFEEDING SUMMARY

No reports describing the use sertaconazole during human lactation have been located. The drug does not produce detectable plasma concentrations after multiple applications to diseased skin. Therefore, the risk to a nursing infant can be considered negligible, and the antifungal agent is probably compatible with breastfeeding.

Reference

1. Product information. Ertaczo. OrthoNeutrogena Division of Ortho-McNeil Pharmaceuticals, 2006.

SERTRALINE

Antidepressant

PREGNANCY RECOMMENDATION: Human Data Suggest Risk in 3rd Trimester
BREASTFEEDING RECOMMENDATION: Limited Human Data—Potential Toxicity

S

PREGNANCY SUMMARY

The limited animal and human data suggest that sertraline is not a major teratogen. Two large case–control studies did find increased risks for some birth defects, but the absolute risk appears to be small (1,2). However, selective serotonin reuptake inhibitor (SSRI) antidepressants, including sertraline, have been associated with several developmental toxicities, including spontaneous abortions, low birth weight, preterm delivery, neonatal serotonin syndrome, neonatal behavioral syndrome (withdrawal), possible sustained abnormal neurobehavior beyond the neonatal period, respiratory distress, and persistent pulmonary hypertension of the newborn (PPHN).

FETAL RISK SUMMARY

Although the mechanism of action of the antidepressant, sertraline, is unknown, it is an SSRI similar to other drugs in this class. This effect of sertraline results in the potentiation of serotonin activity in the brain. The chemical structure of sertraline is unrelated to other antidepressants.

All the antidepressant agents in the SSRI class (citalopram, escitalopram, fluoxetine, fluvoxamine, paroxetine, and sertraline) are thought to share a similar mechanism of action, although they have different chemical structures. These differences could be construed as evidence against any conclusion that they share similar effects on the embryo, fetus, or newborn. In the mouse embryo, however, craniofacial morphogenesis appears to be regulated, at least in part, by serotonin. Interference with serotonin regulation by chemically different inhibitors produces similar craniofacial defects (3). Regardless of the structural differences, therefore, some of the potential adverse effects on pregnancy outcome may also be similar.

Reproductive studies in rats and rabbits, conducted with doses up to approximately 4 times the maximum recommended human dose based on BSA (MRHD), did not reveal evidence of teratogenicity. Delayed ossification of rat and rabbit fetuses, however, occurred at doses during organogenesis that were half and four times the MRHD, respectively. When female rats received a dose equal to the MRHD during the last third of gestation and throughout lactation, an increased number of stillbirths, decreased pup survival, and decreased pup weights were observed. The decreased pup survival was shown to be due to in utero exposure to sertraline. The no-effect dose for rat pup mortality was half the MRHD (4).

Consistent with the molecular weight of the free base (about 307), sertraline crosses the human placenta. A 2003 study of the placental transfer of antidepressants found cord blood:maternal serum ratios for sertraline and its metabolite that were 0.14–0.66 and 0.14–0.77, respectively (5). The dose-to-delivery interval was 7–35 hours, with the highest ratio for the parent drug and metabolite occurring at 24 hours.

A 24-year-old woman was treated before and during the first few weeks of gestation with sertraline for depression and bulimia (K. Murray and D. Jackson, personal communication, Eugene, Oregon, 1994). Ultrasound revealed a single fetus with anencephaly and an abdominal wall defect. Chromosomal analysis performed after termination indicated that the fetus had trisomy 18 (47,XX+18). Because trisomy 18 is a naturally occurring mutation, in the absence of any animal or other evidence for a causal relationship, it is doubtful that the drug therapy was related to the outcome of this pregnancy.

Fifteen diverse birth defects from sertraline-exposed pregnancies were reported to the FDA as of December 1995 (F. Rosa, personal communication, FDA, 1996).

A 1995 report described the use of sertraline 100 mg/day and nortriptyline 125 mg/day in a woman with recurrent major depression (6). The patient was treated before and throughout gestation. Attempts to discontinue the agents in the 1st and 2nd trimesters were unsuccessful. She eventually gave birth at term to a healthy infant (sex and weight not specified) who, at age 3 months, was doing well and achieving the appropriate developmental milestones (see also Breastfeeding Summary below) (6).

A brief 1995 report described a case of a 32-year-old woman who took sertraline 200 mg/day throughout pregnancy (7). Lithium and thioridazine were also taken during the first 6 weeks of gestation. She continued the same dose of sertraline for 3 weeks after delivery of a healthy, full-term male infant. During this period, she breastfed the infant, who was feeding and developing normally. One day after she stopped sertraline, the infant developed agitation, restlessness, poor feeding, constant crying, insomnia, and enhanced startle reaction. The infant's symptoms continued for another 48 hours before gradually resolving over several days. Similar symptoms were not observed in the mother. Because the same types of symptoms have been observed in adults after discontinuing sertraline (1), the authors attributed them to withdrawal (7).

A 1998 noninterventional observational cohort study described the outcomes of pregnancies in women who had been prescribed ≥1 of 34 newly marketed drugs by general practitioners in England (8). Data were obtained by questionnaires sent to the prescribing physicians 1 month after the expected or possible date of delivery. In 831 (78%) of the pregnancies, a newly marketed drug was thought to have been taken during the 1st trimester with birth defects noted in 14 (2.5%) singleton births of the 557 newborns (10 sets of twins). In addition, two birth defects were observed in aborted fetuses. However, few of the aborted fetuses were examined. Sertraline was taken during the 1st trimester in 51 pregnancies. The outcomes of these pregnancies included 1 ectopic pregnancy, 2 spontaneous abortions, 11 elective abortions, 1 intrauterine death, 26 normal full-term newborns, 2 infants with birth defects, and 8 pregnancies lost to follow-up. The congenital malformations were one case each of congenital laryngeal stridor and a duplication cyst (gastrointestinal) (8).

A prospective, multicenter, controlled cohort study published in 1998 evaluated the pregnancy outcomes of 267 women exposed to ≥1 SSRI antidepressants during the 1st trimester: fluvoxamine (*N* = 26); paroxetine (*N* = 97); and sertraline (*N* = 147) (9). The women were combined into a study group without differentiation as to the drug they had consumed. A randomly selected control group (*N* = 267) was formed comprising women who had exposures to nonteratogenic agents. In most cases, the pregnancy outcomes were determined 6–9 months after delivery. No significant differences were observed in the number of live births, spontaneous or elective abortions, stillbirths, major malformations, birth weight, or gestational age at birth. Nine major malformations were observed in each group. The relative risk (RR) for major anomalies was 1.06 (*ns*). No clustering of defects was apparent. The outcomes of women who took an antidepressant throughout gestation were similar to those who took an antidepressant only during the 1st trimester (9). All of the women in the study group had taken an antidepressant during embryogenesis (10).

A 1999 abstract detailed the prospectively ascertained outcomes of 112 pregnant women taking sertraline compared with 191 controls (11). The rate of major congenital defects did not differ significantly between subjects and controls (3.8% vs. 1.9%). Infants exposed to sertraline in the 3rd trimester were more likely to be premature, to have neonatal transition difficulty, or to be admitted to a special care nursery. A dose–response relation was noted for the latter two complications (11).

The effect of SSRIs on birth outcomes and postnatal neurodevelopment of children exposed prenatally was reported in 2003 (12). Thirty-one children (mean age 12.9 months) exposed during pregnancy to SSRIs (15 sertraline, 8 paroxetine, 7 fluoxetine, and 1 fluvoxamine) were compared with 13 children (mean age 17.7 months) of mothers with depression who elected not to take medications during pregnancy. All of the mothers had healthy lifestyles. The timing of the exposures was 71% in the 1st trimester, 74% in the 3rd trimester, and 45% throughout. The average duration of breastfeeding in the subjects and controls was 6.4 and 8.5 months. Twenty-eight (90%) subjects nursed their infants, 17 of whom took an SSRI (10 sertraline, 4 paroxetine, and 3 fluoxetine) compared with 11 (85%) controls, 3 of whom took sertraline. There were no significant differences between the groups in terms of gestational age at birth, premature births, birth weight and length or, at follow-up, in sex distribution or gain in weight and length. Seven (23%) of the exposed infants were admitted to a neonatal intensive care unit (six respiratory distress, four meconium aspiration, and one cardiac murmur) compared with none of the controls (*ns*). Follow-up examinations were conducted by a pediatric neurologist, a psychologist, and a dysmorphologist who were blinded to the mother's mediations status. The mean Apgar scores at 1 and 5 minutes were lower in the exposed group than in controls, 7.0 vs. 8.2, and 8.4 vs. 9.0, respectively. There was one major defect in each group: small asymptomatic ventricular septal defect (exposed) and bilateral lacrimal duct stenosis that required surgery (control). The test outcomes for mental development were similar in the groups, but significant differences in the subjects included a slight delay in psychomotor development and lower behavior motor quality (tremulousness and fine motor movements) (12).

A 2004 prospective study examined the effect of four SSRIs (citalopram, fluoxetine, paroxetine, and sertraline) on newborn neurobehavior, including behavioral state, sleep organization, motor activity, heart rate variability, tremulousness, and startles (13). Seventeen SSRI-exposed, healthy, full-birth-weight newborns and 17 nonexposed, matched controls were studied. A wide range of disrupted neurobehavioral outcomes were shown in the subject infants. After adjustment for gestational age, the exposed infants were found to differ significantly from controls in terms of tremulousness, behavioral states, and sleep organization. The effects observed on motor activity, startles, and heart rate variability were not significant after adjustment (13).

A 2003 prospective study evaluated the pregnancy outcomes of 138 women treated with SSRI antidepressants during gestation (14). Women using each agent were 73 fluoxetine, 36 sertraline, 19 paroxetine, 7 citalopram, and 3 fluvoxamine. Most (62%) took an SSRI throughout pregnancy and 95% were taking an SSRI at delivery. Birth complications were observed in 28 infants, including preterm birth (9 cases), meconium aspiration, nuchal cord, floppy at birth, and low birth weight. Four infants (2.9%) had low birth weight, all exposed to fluoxetine (40–80 mg/day) throughout pregnancy, including two of the three infants of mothers taking 80 mg/day. One infant had Hirschsprung disease, a major defect, and another had cavum septi pellucidi (neither the size of the cavum nor the SSRI agents were specified) (14). The clinical significance of the cavum septi pellucidi is doubtful as it is nearly always present at birth but resolves in the first several months (15).

A 2005 meta-analysis of seven prospective comparative cohort studies involving 1774 patients was conducted to quantify the relationship between seven newer antidepressants and major malformations (16). The antidepressants were bupropion, fluoxetine, fluvoxamine, nefazodone, paroxetine, sertraline, and trazodone. There was no statistical increase in the risk of major birth defects above the baseline of 1%–3% in the general population for the individual or combined studies (16).

The database of the World Health Organization (WHO) was used in a 2005 report on neonatal SSRI withdrawal syndrome (17). Ninety-three suspected cases with either neonatal convulsions or withdrawal syndrome were identified in the WHO database. The agents were 64 paroxetine, 14 fluoxetine, 9 sertraline, and 7 citalopram. The analysis suggested that paroxetine might have an increased risk of convulsions or withdrawal compared with other SSRIs (17).

Evidence for the neonatal behavioral syndrome that is associated with in utero exposure to SSRIs and serotonin and norepinephrine reuptake inhibitors (SNRIs) (collectively referred to as serotonin reuptake inhibitors [SRIs]) in late pregnancy was reviewed in a 2005 reference (18). The report followed a recent agreement by the FDA and manufacturers for a class labeling change about the neonatal syndrome. Analysis of case reports, case series, and cohort studies revealed that late exposure to SRIs carried an overall risk ratio of 3.0 (95% confidence interval [CI] 2.0–4.4) for the syndrome compared with early exposure. The case reports ($N = 18$) and case series ($N = 131$) involved 97 cases of paroxetine, 18 of fluoxetine, 16 of sertraline, 12 of citalopram, 4 of venlafaxine, and 2 of fluvoxamine. There were nine cohort studies analyzed. The typical neonatal syndrome consisted of CNS, motor, respiratory, and gastrointestinal signs that were mild and usually resolved within 2 weeks. Only one of 313 quantifiable cases involved a severe syndrome consisting of seizures, dehydration, excessive weight loss, hyperpyrexia, and intubation. There were no neonatal deaths attributable to the syndrome (18).

Possible sustained neurobehavioral outcomes beyond the neonatal period were reported in 2005 (19). Based on the previous findings that prenatally exposed newborns had reduced pain responses, biobehavioral responses to acute pain (heel lance) were prospectively studied in 2-month-old infants. The responses included facial action (Neonatal Facial Coding System) and cardiac autonomic reactivity (derived from respiratory activity and heart rate variability). Three groups of infants were formed: 11 infants with prenatal SSRI exposure alone (2 fluoxetine and 9 paroxetine); 30 infants with prenatal and postnatal (from breast milk) SSRI exposure (6 fluoxetine, 20 paroxetine, and 4 sertraline); and 22 nonexposed controls (mothers not depressed). The exposure during breastfeeding was considered to be very low. Heel lance-induced facial action increased in all three groups but was significantly lowered (blunted) in the first group. Heart rate was significantly lower in the exposed infants during recovery. Moreover, exposed infants had a greater return of parasympathetic cardiac modulation, whereas controls had a sustained sympathetic response. The findings were consistent with the patterns of pain reactivity observed in exposed newborns and suggested sustained neurobehavioral outcomes (19).

A significant increase in the risk of low birth weight (<10th percentile) and respiratory distress after prenatal exposure to SSRIs was reported in 2006 (20). The population-based study, representing all live births (*N* = 119,547) during a 39-month period in British Columbia, Canada, compared pregnancy outcomes of depressed mothers treated with SSRIs with outcomes in depressed mothers not treated with medication and in nonexposed controls. The severity of depression in the depressed groups was accounted for by propensity score matching (20).

A 30% incidence of SSRI-induced neonatal abstinence syndrome was found in a 2006 cohort study (21). Sixty neonates with prolonged in utero exposure to SSRIs were compared with nonexposed controls. The agents used were paroxetine (62%), fluoxetine (20%), citalopram (13%), venlafaxine (3%), and sertraline (2%). Assessment was conducted by the Finnegan score. Ten of the infants had mild and eight had severe symptoms of the syndrome. The maximum mean score in infants with severe symptoms occurred within 2 days of birth, but some occurred as long as 4 days after birth. Because of the small numbers, a dose–response study could only be conducted with paroxetine. Infants exposed to mean maternal doses that were <19 mg/day had no symptoms, <23 mg/day had mild symptoms, and 27 mg/day had severe symptoms (21).

A meta-analysis of clinical trials (1990–2005) with SSRIs was reported in 2006 (22). The SSRI agents included were citalopram, fluoxetine, fluvoxamine, paroxetine, and sertraline. The specific outcomes analyzed were major, minor, and cardiac malformations, and spontaneous abortions. The odds ratio (OR) with 95% CI (in parentheses) for the four outcomes were 1.394 (0.906–2.145), 0.97 (0.13–6.93), 1.193 (0.531–2.677), and 1.70 (1.28–2.25), respectively. Only the risk of spontaneous abortions was significantly increased (22).

A brief 2005 report described significant associations between the use of SSRIs in the 1st trimester and congenital defects (23). The data were collected by the CDC-sponsored National Birth Defects Prevention Study in an on-going case–control study of birth defect risk factors. Case infants (*N* = 5357) with major birth defects were compared with 3366 normal controls. A positive association was found with omphalocele (*N* = 161; OR 3.0, 95% CI 1.4–6.1). Paroxetine, which accounted for 36% of all SSRI exposures, had the strongest association with the defect (OR 6.3, 95% CI 2.0–19.6). The study also found a significant association between the use of any SSRI and craniosynostosis (*N* = 372; OR 1.8, 95% CI 1.0–3.2) (23). An expanded report from this group was published in 2007 (1).

In 1999, the Swedish Medical Birth Registry compared the use of antidepressants in early pregnancy and delivery outcomes for the years 1995–1997 (24). There were no significant differences for birth defects, infant survival, or risk of low birth weight (<2500 g) among singletons between those exposed to any depressant, SSRIs only, or non-SSRIs only, but a shorter gestational duration (<37 weeks) was observed for any antidepressant exposure (OR 1.43, 95% CI 1.14–1.80) (24). A second Registry report, published in 2006 and covering the years 1995–2003, analyzed the relationship between antidepressants and major malformations or cardiac defects (25). There was no significant increase in the risk of major malformations with any antidepressant. The strongest effect among cardiac defects was with ventricular or atrial septum defects (VSDs-ASDs). Significant increases were found with paroxetine (OR 2.22, 95% CI 1.39–3.55) and clomipramine (OR 1.87, 95% CI 1.16–2.99 (25). In 2007, the analysis was expanded to include the years 1995–2004 (26). There were 6481 women (6555 infants) who had reported the use of SSRIs in early pregnancy. The number of women using a single SSRI during the 1st trimester was 2579 citalopram, 1807 sertraline, 908 paroxetine, 860 fluoxetine, 66 escitalopram, and 36 fluvoxamine. After adjustment, only paroxetine was significantly associated with an increased risk of cardiac defects (*N* = 13, RR 2.62, 95% CI 1.40–4.50) or VSDs-ASDs (*N* = 8, RR 3.07, 95% CI 1.32–6.04). Analysis of the combined SSRI group, excluding paroxetine, revealed no associations with these defects. The study found no association with omphalocele or craniostenosis (26).

A 2007 study evaluated the association between 1st trimester exposure to paroxetine and cardiac defects by quantifying the dose–response relationship (27). A population-based pregnancy registry was used by linking three administrative databases so that it included all pregnancies in Quebec between 1997 and 2003. There were 101 infants with major congenital defects, 24 involving the heart, among the 1403 women using only one type of antidepressant during the 1st trimester. The use of paroxetine or other SSRIs did not significantly increase the risk of major defects or cardiac defects compared with non-SSRI antidepressants. However, a paroxetine dose >25 mg/day during the 1st trimester was significantly associated with an increased risk of major defects (OR 2.23, 95% CI 1.19–4.17) and of cardiac defects (OR 3.07, 95% CI 1.00–9.42) (27).

A 2007 retrospective cohort study examined the effects of exposure to SSRIs or venlafaxine in the 3rd trimester on 21 premature and 55 term newborns (28). The randomly selected unexposed control group consisted of 90 neonates of mothers not taking antidepressants, psychotropic agents, or benzodiazepines at the time of delivery. There were significantly more premature infants among the subjects (27.6%) than in controls (8.9%), but the groups were not matched. The antidepressants, and number of subjects and daily doses (in parentheses) in the exposed group were paroxetine (46; 5–40 mg), fluoxetine (10; 10–40 mg), venlafaxine (9; 74–150 mg), citalopram (6; 10–30 mg), sertraline (3; 125–150 mg), and fluvoxamine (2; 50–150 mg). The behavioral signs that were significantly increased in exposed compared with nonexposed infants were CNS: abnormal movements, shaking, spasms, agitation, hypotonia, hypertonia, irritability, and insomnia; respiratory system: indrawing, apnea/bradycardia, and tachypnea; and other: vomiting, tachycardia, and jaundice. In exposed infants, CNS (63.2%) and respiratory system (40.8%) signs were most common, appearing during the first day of life and lasting for a median duration of 3 days. All of the exposed premature infants exhibited behavioral signs compared with 69.1% of exposed term infants. The duration of hospitalization was significantly longer in exposed premature compared with nonexposed premature infants, 14.5 days vs. 3.7 days, respectively. In 75% of the term and premature infants, the signs resolved within 3 and 5 days, respectively. There were six infants in each group with congenital malformations, but the drugs involved were not specified (28).

A 2007 review conducted a literature search to determine the risk of major congenital malformations after 1st trimester exposure to SSRIs and SNRIs (29). Fifteen controlled studies were analyzed. The data were adequate to suggest that citalopram, fluoxetine, sertraline, and venlafaxine were not associated with an increased risk of congenital defects.In contrast, the analysis did suggest an increased risk with paroxetine. The data were inadequate to determine the risk for the other SSRIs and SNRIs (29).

A case–control study, published in 2006, was conducted to test the hypothesis that exposure to SSRIs in late pregnancy was associated with PPHN (30). A total of 1213 women were enrolled in the study, 377 cases whose infants had PPHN and 836 matched controls and their infants. Mothers were interviewed by nurses who were blinded to the hypothesis. Fourteen case infants had been exposed to an SSRI after the 20th week of gestation compared with six control infants (OR 6.1, 95% CI 2.2–16.8). The numbers were too small to analyze the effects of dose, SSRI used, or reduction of the length of exposure before delivery. No increased risk of PPHN was found with the use of SSRIs before the 20th week or with the use of non-SSRI antidepressants at any time during pregnancy. If the relationship was causal, the absolute risk was estimated to be about 1% (30).

Two large case–control studies assessing associations between SSRIs and major birth defects were published in 2007 (1,2). The findings related to SSRIs as a group, as well as to four specific agents: citalopram, fluoxetine, paroxetine, and sertraline. An accompanying editorial discussed the findings and limitations of these and other related studies (31). Details of the studies and the editorial are described in the paroxetine review (see Paroxetine).

A prospective cohort study evaluated a large group of pregnancies exposed to antidepressants in the 1st trimester to determine if there was an association with major malformations (32). The patient population came from the Motherisk database and involved 928 cases that met their criteria. The 928 matched (for age, smoking, and alcohol use) controls were pregnancies not exposed to antidepressants or known teratogens. In addition to the 61 sertraline cases, the other cases were 113 bupropion, 184 citalopram, 21 escitalopram, 61 fluoxetine, 52 fluvoxamine, 68 mirtazapine, 39 nefazodone, 148 paroxetine, 17 trazodone, and 154 venlafaxine. In the antidepressant group, there were 24 (2.5%) major defects compared with 25 (2.6%) in controls (odds ratio 0.9, 95% CI 0.5–1.61). There was one major anomaly, a hiatus hernia, in the sertraline group. There were no major defects in the pregnancies exposed to bupropion, escitalopram, or trazodone (32).

BREASTFEEDING SUMMARY

Eight reports describing the use of sertraline during lactation have been located (6,33–39). In a 1995 case (described above), a woman with recurrent major depression consumed sertraline 100 mg/day and nortriptyline 125 mg/day throughout gestation and while exclusively breastfeeding her term infant (6). Milk levels (over a 24-hour period) were obtained at 3 weeks, and maternal and infant serum levels were measured at 3 and 7 weeks. Milk levels were 8.8–43 ng/mL, with the highest concentrations at 5 and 9 hours postdose. Maternal serum levels at 3 and 7 weeks were 48 and 47 ng/mL, respectively, but were undetectable in the infant. At the 3-week sampling, serum levels of nortriptyline in the mother and child were 120 ng/mL and undetectable, respectively. The infant was doing well at 3 months of age with normal weight gain and development (6).

A brief 1995 correspondence described a 32-year-old woman who was treated with sertraline 150 mg/day during the second half of gestation and while breastfeeding (33). She stopped nursing after 11 days. No adverse effects were noted in the healthy infant either during or after breastfeeding.

Four lactating women were treated for postpartum depression with sertraline 50 mg/day ($N = 2$) or 100 mg/day ($N = 2$) (34). Whole blood 5-hydroxytryptamine (serotonin; 5-HT) levels in the mothers and infants were determined before and after 9–12 weeks of therapy. Sertraline and desmethylsertraline plasma levels were also measured at the time of postexposure sampling. One infant in each dose group was fully breastfed and the other two infants were breastfed 3 or 4 times daily. The ages of the infants at the start of maternal treatment were 15 days, 26 days, 6 months, and 12 months. Sertraline and metabolite plasma levels in the infants were <2.5 and 5 ng/mL, respectively, compared with maternal plasma levels 10.3–48.2 and 19.7–64.5 ng/mL, respectively. Little to no change was observed in the platelet (equivalent to whole-blood) levels of serotonin in the infants, in contrast to the marked decreases measured in the mothers (34).

Milk samples were collected from 12 women after a sertraline dose at 4–6 hours for 24 hours (35). Additionally, maternal (24 hours after a dose) and infant serum levels (2–4 hours after nursing) were also determined in 11 mother–infant pairs. All of the subjects had been taking a fixed dose (25–200 mg/day) for 14–21 days. Sertraline (range 17–173 ng/mL) and the relatively inactive metabolite, desmethylsertraline (range 22–294 ng/mL), were present in all milk samples. The first 10–20 mL of milk (foremilk) had approximately one-half of the drug concentrations of sertraline and metabolite as did the hindmilk. The mean milk:serum ratios for the parent drug and metabolite were 2.3 and 1.4, respectively. In maternal serum (doses 25–150 mg/day), the concentrations of sertraline and metabolite ranged from 9 to 92 and from 15 to 212 ng/mL, respectively. In contrast, only three infants had measurable serum sertraline levels (2.7–3.0 ng/mL), whereas six had measurable metabolite levels (1.6–10.0 ng/mL). The calculated sertraline and metabolite doses received by the infants from milk were 0.019–0.124 and 0.023–0.181 mg/day, respectively (35).

In a 1998 study, the mean milk:plasma ratios of sertraline and the metabolite in eight lactating women (mean dose 1.05 mg/kg/day) were 1.93 and 1.64, respectively (36). The estimated infant doses were 0.2% and 0.3%, respectively, of the weight-adjusted maternal dose. Neither sertraline nor desmethylsertraline was detected in the plasma samples obtained from four infants. No adverse effects from the drug exposure were noted in the infants. All had achieved normal development milestones (36).

In another 1998 study, serum levels of sertraline and desmethylsertraline were measured in nine nursing mother:infant pairs (37). The maternal serum levels were 12–134 and 28–285 ng/mL, respectively. In six infants, the serum concentration of sertraline was below the quantification limit (<2 ng/mL), undetectable in one, and 3 ng/mL in another. The metabolite serum levels in these eight infants ranged from nonquantifiable to 24 ng/mL. In the ninth infant, however, the serum sertraline concentration was 64 ng/mL, 55% of the mother's serum level (117 ng/mL). The metabolite serum concentrations in the infant and mother were 68 and 117 ng/mL,

S

respectively. The mother's dose in this case was 100 mg/day. The serum samples from the mother and infant were drawn 2 hours after a dose. Because the levels were so unusual, the investigators checked the values twice. Although they speculated as to possible cause(s), they were unable to determine why the levels in this particular case were so high (37).

The effect of sertraline on 5-HT reuptake in nursing infants was studied in 14 mother–infant pairs in a 2001 report (38). Preexposure levels of 5-HT were drawn from the infants at a mean age of 17.3 weeks, whereas postexposure levels were drawn at a mean age of 26.3 weeks. The mean maternal plasma levels of sertraline and the metabolite, desmethylsertraline, were 30.7 ng/mL and 45.3 ng/mL, respectively. In the mothers, sertraline (25–200 mg/day) caused marked declines (70%–96%) in whole blood 5-HT levels. In contrast, 5-HT levels in whole blood of the nursing infants were not affected (preexposure 223.7 vs. postexposure 227.0 ng/mL). Infant plasma levels of sertraline and the metabolite were undetectable. The results suggested that treatment of the mother with sertraline would not affect peripheral or central 5-HT transport in their nursing infants (38).

A 2004 study was conducted in 25 women (nursing 26 infants) to quantify the concentration of the SSRI or SNRI in their breast milk (39). The antidepressants taken by the women were citalopram (nine), paroxetine (six), sertraline (six), fluoxetine (one), and venlafaxine (three). The maternal mean dose of sertraline was 64 mg/day (50–100 mg/day). The mean milk concentration was 151 nmol/L (97–230 nmol/L), resulting in a theoretical maximum infant dose that was 0.9% of the mother's weight-adjusted dose. Sertraline was not detected in the serum of the infants. There was no evidence of adverse effects in the breastfeeding infants (39).

A 1999 review of SSRI agents concluded that if there were compelling reasons to treat a mother for postpartum depression, a condition in which a rapid antidepressant effect is important, the benefits of therapy with SSRIs would most likely outweigh the risks (40). However, because the long-term effects of exposure to SSRI antidepressants in breast milk on the infant's neurobehavioral development are unknown (no such adverse effects have been identified to date, but research is needed), stopping or reducing the frequency of breastfeeding should be considered if therapy with these agents is required. Avoiding nursing around the time of peak maternal concentration (about 4 hours after a dose) may limit infant exposure. However, the long elimination half-lives of all SSRIs and their weakly basic properties, which are conducive to ion trapping in the relatively acidic milk, probably will lessen the effectiveness of this strategy. The American Academy of Pediatrics classifies sertraline as a drug for which the effect on nursing infants is unknown but may be of concern (41).

A 2010 study using human and animal models found that drugs that disturb serotonin balance such as SSRIs and SNRIs can impair lactation (42). The authors concluded that mothers taking these drugs may need additional support to achieve breastfeeding goals.

References

1. Alwan S, Reefhuis J, Rasmussen SA, Olney RS, Friedman JM, for the National Birth Defects Prevention Study. Use of selective serotonin-reuptake inhibitors in pregnancy and the risk of birth defects. N Engl J Med 2007;356:2684–92.
2. Louik C, Lin AE, Werler MM, Hernandez-Diaz S, Mitchell AA. First-trimester use of selective serotonin-reuptake inhibitors and the risk of birth defects. N Engl J Med 2007;356:2675–83.
3. Shuey DL, Sadler TW, Lauder JM. Serotonin as a regulator of craniofacial morphogenesis: site-specific malformations following exposure to serotonin uptake inhibitors. Teratology 1992;46:367–78.
4. Product information. Zoloft. Pfizer, 2000.
5. Hendrick V, Stowe ZN, Altshuler LL, Hwang S, Lee E, Haynes D. Placental passage of antidepressant medications. Am J Psychiatry 2003;160:993–6.
6. Altshuler LL, Burt VK, McMullen M, Hendrick V. Breastfeeding and sertraline: a 24-hour analysis. J Clin Psychiatry 1995;56:243–5.
7. Kent LSW, Laidlaw JDD. Suspected congenital sertraline dependence. Br J Psychiatry 1995;167:412–3.
8. Wilton LV, Pearce GL, Martin RM, Mackay FJ, Mann RD. The outcomes of pregnancy in women exposed to newly marketed drugs in general practice in England. Br J Obstet Gynaecol 1998;105:882–9.
9. Kulin NA, Pastuszak A, Sage SR, Schick-Boschetto B, Spivey G, Feldkamp M, Ormond K, Matsui D, Stein-Schechman AK, Cook L, Brochu J, Rieder M, Koren G. Pregnancy outcome following maternal use of the new selective serotonin reuptake inhibitors. A prospective controlled multicenter study. JAMA 1998;279:609–10.
10. Koren G. In reply. Risk of fetal anomalies with exposure to selective serotonin reuptake inhibitors. JAMA 1998;279:1873–4.
11. Chambers CD, Dick LM, Felix RJ, Johnson KA, Jones KL. Pregnancy outcome in women who use sertraline (abstract). Teratology 1999;59:376.
12. Casper RC, Fleisher BE, Lee-Ancajas JC, Gilles A, Gaylor E, DeBattista A, Hoyme HE. Follow-up of children of depressed mothers exposed or not exposed to antidepressant drugs during pregnancy. J Pediatr 2003;142:402–8.
13. Zeskind PS, Stephens LE. Maternal selective serotonin reuptake inhibitor use during pregnancy and newborn neurobehavior. Pediatrics 2004;113: 368–75.
14. Hendrick V, Smith LM, Suri R, Hwang S, Haynes D, Altshuler L. Birth outcomes after prenatal exposure to antidepressant medication. Am J Obstet Gynecol 2003;188:812–5.
15. DeMyer W. Brain. Midline caves. In: Buyse ML, ed. *Birth Defects Encyclopedia*. Cambridge, MA: Blackwell Scientific Publications, 1990:238.
16. Einarson TR, Einarson A. Newer antidepressants in pregnancy and rates of major malformations: a meta-analysis of prospective comparative studies. Pharmacoepidemiol Drug Saf 2005;14:823–7.
17. Sanz EJ, De-las-Cuevas C, Kiuru A, Edwards R. Selective serotonin reuptake inhibitors in pregnant women and neonatal withdrawal syndrome: a database analysis. Lancet 2005;365:482–7.
18. Moses-Kolko EL, Bogen D, Perel J, Bregar A, Uhl K, Levin B, Wisner KL. Neonatal signs after late in utero exposure to serotonin reuptake inhibitors. JAMA 2005;293:2372–83.
19. Oberlander TF, Grunau RE, Fitzgerald C, Papsdorf M, Rurak D, Riggs W. Pain reactivity in 2-month-old infants after prenatal and postnatal selective serotonin reuptake inhibitor medication exposure. Pediatrics 2005;115:411–25.
20. Oberlander TF, Warburton W, Misri S, Aghajanian J, Hertzman C. Neonatal outcomes after prenatal exposure to selective serotonin reuptake inhibitor antidepressants and maternal depression using population-based linked health data. Arch Gen Psychiatry 2006;63:898–906.
21. Levinson-Castiel R, Merlob P, Linder N, Sirota L, Klinger G. Neonatal abstinence syndrome after in utero exposure to selective serotonin reuptake inhibitors in term infants. Arch Pediatr Adoles Med 2006;160:173–6.
22. Rahimi R, Nikfar S, Abdollahi M. Pregnancy outcomes following exposure to serotonin reuptake inhibitors: a meta-analysis of clinical trials. Reprod Toxicol 2006;22:571–5.
23. Alwan S, Reefhuis J, Rasmussen S, Olney R, Friedman JM. Maternal use of selective serotonin reuptake inhibitors and risk for birth defects (abstract). Birth Defects Res (Part A) 2005;73:291.
24. Ericson A, Kallen B, Wiholm BE. Delivery outcome after the use of antidepressants in early pregnancy. Eur J Clin Pharmacol 1999;55:503–8.
25. Kallen B, Olausson PO. Antidepressant drugs during pregnancy and infant congenital heart defect. Reprod Toxicol 2006;21:221–2.
26. Kallen BAJ, Olausson PO. Maternal use of selective serotonin re-uptake inhibitors in early pregnancy and infant congenital malformations. Birth Defects Res A Clin Mol Teratol 2007;79:301–8.
27. Berard A, Ramos E, Rey E, Blais L, St.-Andre M, Oraichi D. First trimester exposure to paroxetine and risk of cardiac malformations in infants: the importance of dosage. Birth Defects Res B Dev Reprod Toxicol 2007;80:18–27.

28. Ferreira E, Carceller AM, Agogue C, Martin BZ, St-Andre M, Francoeur D, Berard A. Effects of selective serotonin reuptake inhibitors and venlafaxine during pregnancy in term and preterm neonates. Pediatrics 2007; 119:52–9.
29. Bellantuono C, Migliarese G, Gentile S. Serotonin reuptake inhibitors in pregnancy and the risk of major malformations: a systematic review. Hum Psychopharmacol Clin Exp 2007;22:121–8.
30. Chambers CD, Hernandez-Diaz S, Van Marter LJ, Werler MM, Louik C, Jones KL, Mitchell AA. Selective serotonin-reuptake inhibitors and risk of persistent pulmonary hypertension of the newborn. N Engl J Med 2006;354:579–87.
31. Greene MF. Teratogenicity of SSRIs—Serious concern or much ado about little? N Engl J Med 2007;356:2732–3
32. Einarson A, Choi J, Einarson TR, Koren G. Incidence of major malformations in infants following antidepressant exposure in pregnancy: results of a large prospective cohort study. Can J Psychiatry 2009;54:242–6.
33. Ratan DA, Friedman T. Antidepressants in pregnancy and breast-feeding. Br J Psychiatry 1995;167:824.
34. Epperson CN, Anerson GM, McDougle CJ. Sertraline and breast-feeding. N Engl J Med 1997;336:1189–90.
35. Stowe ZN, Owens MJ, Landry JC, Kilts CD, Ely T, Llewellyn A, Nemeroff CB. Sertraline and desmethylsertraline in human breast milk and nursing infants. Am J Psychiatry 1997;154:1255–60.
36. Kristensen JH, Ilett KF, Dusci LJ, Hackett LP, Yapp P, Wojnar-Horton RE, Roberts MJ, Paech M. Distribution and excretion of sertraline and *N*-desmethylsertraline in human milk. Br J Clin Pharmacol 1998;45:453–7.
37. Wisner KL, Perel JM, Blumer J. Serum sertraline and *N*-desmethylsertraline levels in breastfeeding mother–infant pairs. Am J Psychiatry 1998;155: 690–2.
38. Epperson N, Czarkowski KA, Ward-O'Brien D, Weiss E, Gueorguieva R, Jatlow P, Anderson GM. Maternal sertraline treatment and serotonin transport in breast-feeding mother–infant pairs. Am J Psychiatry 2001;158: 1631–7.
39. Berle JO, Steen VM, Aamo TO, Breilid H, Zahlsen K, Spigset O. Breastfeeding during maternal antidepressant treatment with serotonin reuptake inhibitors: infant exposure, clinical symptoms, and cytochrome P450 genotypes. J Clin Psychiatry 2004;65:1228–34.
40. Edwards JG, Anerson I. Systematic review and guide to selection of selective serotonin reuptake inhibitors. Drugs 1999; 57:507–33.
41. Committee on Drugs, American Academy of Pediatrics. The transfer of drugs and other chemicals into human milk. Pediatrics 2001;108:776–89.
42. Marshall AM, Nommsen-Rivers LA, Hernandez LI, Dewey KG, Chantry CJ, Gregerson KA, Horseman ND. Serotonin transport and metabolism in the mammary gland modulates secretory activation and involution. J Clin Endocrin Metab 2010;95:837–46.

SEVELAMER

Antidote (Phosphate Binder)

PREGNANCY RECOMMENDATION: No Human Data—Animal Data Suggest Moderate Risk
BREASTFEEDING RECOMMENDATION: No Human Data—Probably Compatible

PREGNANCY SUMMARY

No reports describing the use of sevelamer in human pregnancy have been located. The limited animal data suggest a moderate risk of toxicity that may be partially due to a deficiency of fat-soluble vitamins, such as vitamin D. The effect of sevelamer on the absorption of vitamins in pregnant women has not been studied (1). However, supplementation with higher oral doses of vitamins, especially fat-soluble vitamins (except vitamin A), might be required or IV vitamins should be considered.

FETAL RISK SUMMARY

Sevelamer is a polymeric phosphate binder that is administered orally. It is used in patients with end-stage renal disease for the reduction of serum phosphorus. The drug inhibits intestinal phosphate absorption by binding phosphorus. Sevelamer is not absorbed into the systemic circulation (1).

Reproduction studies have been conducted in rats and rabbits. No evidence of impaired fertility was observed in male and female rats. In pregnant rats, doses about 15 times the human dose (HD) or higher caused reduced or irregular ossification of fetal bones. The toxicity was thought to be due to reduced absorption of vitamin D. In rabbits, a dose about 10 times the HD caused an increased incidence of early resorptions, resulting in a slight increase in prenatal mortality (1).

BREASTFEEDING SUMMARY

No reports describing the use of sevelamer during human lactation have been located. The drug is not absorbed into the systemic circulation, but it may cause vitamin deficiencies in the mother by preventing intestinal vitamin absorption, especially of fat-soluble vitamins. Because vitamins are excreted into breast milk, thereby further reducing maternal vitamin concentrations, women who are taking sevelamer might have to take higher oral doses of vitamins, especially fat-soluble vitamins (except vitamin A), or IV vitamin administration should be considered.

Reference

1. Product information. Renagel. Genzyme, 2004.

SEVOFLURANE

General Anesthetic

PREGNANCY RECOMMENDATION: Limited Human Data—Animal Data Suggest Low Risk
BREASTFEEDING RECOMMENDATION: No Human Data—Probably Compatible

PREGNANCY SUMMARY

Sevoflurane is teratogenic in mice, but no reports of its use in early human gestation have been located. The absence of human experience during organogenesis prevents an assessment of the risk for structural anomalies. In addition, general anesthesia usually involves the use of multiple pharmacological agents. Although no teratogenicity has been observed with other halogenated general anesthetic agents, only halothane has 1st trimester human exposure data (see Halothane). Sevoflurane has been used immediately prior to delivery, but its effect on the newborn has not been studied. However, its effect on the newborn is probably no different from other general anesthetic agents. The uterine effects of sevoflurane (relaxation and increased blood loss) also appear to be similar to other agents in this class, but the low concentrations used clinically minimize these actions (see Enflurane). All anesthetic agents can cause depression in the newborn that may last for 24 hours or more but, again, this is lessened by the low doses. The potential reproductive toxicity (spontaneous abortion and infertility) of occupational exposure to halogenated general anesthetic agents has not been adequately studied.

FETAL RISK SUMMARY

Sevoflurane, a noninflammable general anesthetic agent administered via vaporizer, is indicated for the induction and/or maintenance of anesthesia during surgery. Sevoflurane is in the same class of volatile liquid halogenated agents as desflurane, enflurane, halothane, isoflurane, and methoxyflurane. It has a lower solubility in lipids (oil:gas partition coefficient about 47–53) and blood (blood:gas partition coefficient 0.68) than halothane or isoflurane, but higher than desflurane (1). The anesthetic potency, based on the minimum alveolar anesthetic concentration (MAC), is about 50% less than that of isoflurane but about 30% more than that of desflurane (1). (*Note: MAC is the concentration that causes immobility in 50% of patients exposed to a noxious stimulus such as a surgical incision; it represents the* ED_{50} *[2]*).

In an animal reproduction study, mice were exposed for 8 hours to sevoflurane and enflurane combined with three different concentrations of oxygen (3). Both anesthetic agents caused cleft palate, but the incidence was lower than that observed with halothane. Increasing the concentrations of oxygen lowered the incidence of the defect (3).

The teratogenic potential of sevoflurane, enflurane, and isoflurane was studied by evaluating the effect of each agent on the proliferation and differentiation of cells exiting from the G1-phase of the cell cycle (4). The theory behind the study was that normal development during embryogenesis, organogenesis, and histogenesis depended upon the proliferation and differentiative processes of cell migration (4). For example, valproate, a known human teratogen, is a potent G1-phase inhibitor of the in vitro proliferation rate at concentrations less than two times the therapeutic plasma concentration. At anesthetic concentrations less than two times the MAC, the antiproliferative potency of the three agents was isoflurane = enflurane >> sevoflurane. However, in the growth-arrested cell population, there was no specific accumulation of any cell-cycle phase and no specific effect on the G1 phase. The investigators concluded that the three agents lacked the specific in vitro characteristics of valproate (4).

In an in vitro experiment with pregnant rats, sevoflurane, halothane, and isoflurane significantly inhibited oxytocin-induced contractions of uterine smooth muscle (5).

Two reviews have concluded that, in general, inhalational anesthetics are freely transferred to fetal tissues (6,7) and, in most cases, the maternal and fetal concentrations are equivalent (7). The low molecular weight (about 200) and the presence of sevoflurane in the maternal brain support this assertion.

A 1999 case report described the use of sevoflurane for maintenance of general anesthesia during a nonobstetric surgery in a 25-year-old woman at 13 weeks' gestation (8). Six months later, a cesarean section delivered a 2820-g female infant without abnormalities.

Two reports described the use of sevoflurane for emergency cesarean section (9,10). Although successful outcomes occurred in both cases, the former report generated several letters and a reply (11–16).

Chronic occupational exposure to anesthetic gases in operating rooms during pregnancy has raised concerns that such exposure could cause birth defects and spontaneous abortions (17). A 1988 review cited a number of studies investigating the possible association between occupational exposure to anesthetic gases and adverse pregnancy outcomes (6). The reviewer concluded that serious methodological weaknesses in these studies precluded arriving at a firm conclusion, but a slightly increased risk of miscarriage was a possibility. However, there was no evidence of an association between occupational exposure and congenital anomalies (6).

A 2004 study, however, found a significant association between maternal occupational exposure to waste anesthetic gases during pregnancy and developmental deficits in their children, including gross and fine motor ability, inattention/hyperactivity, and IQ performance (see Nitrous Oxide).

BREASTFEEDING SUMMARY

Although sevoflurane has been administered during delivery, the effects of this exposure on the infant who begins nursing immediately after birth have not been described. Sevoflurane is probably excreted into colostrum and milk as suggested by its presence in the maternal blood and its low molecular weight (about 200), but the toxic potential of this exposure for the infant is unknown. However, the risk to a nursing infant from exposure to sevoflurane via milk is probably very low (18). Halothane, another halogenated inhalation anesthetic, is classified as compatible with breastfeeding by the American Academy of Pediatrics (see Halothane).

References

1. Patel SS, Goa KL. Sevoflurane. A review of its pharmacodynamic and pharmacokinetic properties and its clinical use in general anaesthesia. Drugs 1996;51:658–700.
2. Trevor AJ, Miller RD. General anesthetics. In: Katzung BG, ed. *Basic and Clinical Pharmacology*. 8th ed. New York, NY: McGraw-Hill, 2001:426.

S

3. Natsume N, Miura S, Sugimoto S, Nakamura T, Horiuchi R, Kondo S, Furukawa H, Inagaki S, Kawai T, Yamada M, Arai T, Hosoda R. Teratogenicity caused by halothane, enflurane, and sevoflurane, and changes depending on O_2 concentration (abstract). Teratology 1990;42:30A.
4. O'Leary G, Bacon CL, Odumeru O, Fagan C, Fitzpatrick T, Gallagher HC, Moriarty DC, Regan CM. Antiproliferative actions of inhalational anesthetics: comparisons to the valproate teratogen. Int J Devl Neurosci 2000;18:39–45.
5. Yamakage M, Tsujiguchi N, Chen X, Kamada Y, Namiki A. Sevoflurane inhibits contraction of uterine smooth muscle from pregnant rats similarly to halothane and isoflurane. Can J Anesth 2002;49:62–6.
6. Friedman JM. Teratogen update: anesthetic agents. Teratology 1988;37: 69–77.
7. Kanto J. Risk–benefit assessment of anaesthetic agents in the puerperium. Drug Saf 1991;6:285–301.
8. Kanazawa M, Kinefuchi Y, Suzuki T, Fukuyama H, Takiguchi M. The use of sevoflurane anesthesia during early pregnancy. Tokai J Exp Clin Med 1999;24:53–5.
9. Schaut DJ, Khona R, Gross JB. Sevoflurane inhalation induction for emergency cesarean section in a parturient with no intravenous access. Anesthesiology 1997;86:1392–4.
10. Que JC, Lusaya VO. Sevoflurane induction for emergency cesarean section in a parturient in status asthmaticus. Anesthesiology 1999;90:1475–6.
11. Klafta JM. The practice of using sevoflurane inhalation induction for emergency cesarean section and a parturient with no intravenous access. Anesthesiology 1998;88:275.
12. Bhavani-Shankar K, Camann WR. The practice of using sevoflurane inhalation induction for emergency cesarean section and a parturient with no intravenous access. Anesthesiology 1998;88:275–6.
13. Sitzman BT. The practice of using sevoflurane inhalation induction for emergency cesarean section and a parturient with no intravenous access. Anesthesiology 1998;88:276.
14. Gambling DR, Reisner LS. The practice of using sevoflurane inhalation induction for emergency cesarean section and a parturient with no intravenous access. Anesthesiology 1998;88:276–7.
15. Maltby JR. The practice of using sevoflurane inhalation induction for emergency cesarean section and a parturient with no intravenous access. Anesthesiology 1998;88:277–8.
16. Gross JB. The practice of using sevoflurane inhalation induction for emergency cesarean section and a parturient with no intravenous access. Anesthesiology 1998;88:278.
17. Corbett TH. Cancer and congenital anomalies associated with anesthetics. Ann NY Acad Sciences 1976;271:58–66.
18. Spigset O. Anaesthetic agents and excretion in breast milk. Acta Anaesthesiol Scand 1994;38:94–103.

SIBUTRAMINE

[Removed from the market. See 9th edition.]

SILDENAFIL

Vasodilator/Impotence Agent

PREGNANCY RECOMMENDATION: Limited Human Data—Animal Data Suggest Low Risk
BREASTFEEDING RECOMMENDATION: No Human Data—Potential Toxicity

PREGNANCY SUMMARY

Pregnancy is not advised in women with pulmonary arterial hypertension because of the high risk of morbidity and death. However, pregnancies have continued because of the mother's wishes and have been treated successfully with sildenafil. Although the data are very limited, no embryo–fetal harm has been observed. The drug has not caused developmental toxicity in animals. Because pulmonary arterial hypertension is a high-risk condition, the drug should not be withheld because of pregnancy.

FETAL RISK SUMMARY

Sildenafil is an inhibitor of cyclic guanosine monophosphate-specific phosphodiesterase type-5 in the smooth muscle of the pulmonary vasculature and in the corpus cavernosum of the penis. It is indicated for the treatment of pulmonary arterial hypertension (WHO Group 1) to improve exercise ability and delay clinical worsening (1). It is also indicated for the treatment of erectile dysfunction (2). The drug is available in formulations for oral and IV use. Sildenafil has an active metabolite and both are about 96% bound to plasma proteins. The terminal half-life of sildenafil and its active metabolite are about 4 hours (1,2).

Reproduction studies have been conducted in rats and rabbits. In these species, doses up to 20–32 and 40–68 times, respectively, the recommended human dose based on BSA (RHD) revealed no evidence of teratogenicity, embryotoxicity, or fetotoxicity (1,2). In the rat prenatal and postnatal development study, the no-observed-adverse-effect-level (NOAEL) was 5 times the RHD (1) or about 20 times human exposure based on AUC (2).

Studies for carcinogenicity, mutagenicity, and clastogenicity were negative. In addition, the drug did not impair the fertility of male and female rats (1,2).

It is not known if sildenafil crosses the human placenta. The molecular weight (about 667) and terminal half-life suggest that the drug and its active metabolite will cross to the embryo–fetus, but the high plasma protein binding should limit the exposure.

A 22-year-old woman with Eisenmenger's syndrome that was managed with sildenafil 50 mg/day was diagnosed with an atrial septal defect that was closed surgically (3). Eight days after surgery, the patient reported 7 weeks of amenorrhea and a pregnancy test was positive. Sildenafil 150 mg/day and diltiazem 60 mg/day were started. Two weeks later, sildenafil was discontinued because of its high cost and the dose of diltiazem was increased to 180 mg/day. Because of worsening pulmonary hypertension at 31 weeks, sildenafil 150 mg/day was restarted and diltiazem was discontinued. The fetal weight was estimated to be in the 15th percentile. At 32 weeks, L-arginine (a nitric oxide donor) 3 g/day was started. During the next 2 weeks, the estimated fetal weight increased to the 35th percentile. Because of superimposed preeclampsia, a cesarean section was performed at 36 weeks' to deliver a 2.290-kg male infant with Apgar scores of 9 and 9. No additional information on the infant was provided (3).

A 2005 case report described the use of bosentan throughout pregnancy in a woman with Eisenmenger's syndrome due to pulmonary hypertension (4). Sildenafil was added at 27 weeks' gestation. At 30 weeks, a planned cesarean section delivered a healthy 1.41-kg female infant. Postoperatively, the mother was treated with bosentan, sildenafil, and warfarin. Her infant was nursed in the hospital for 11 weeks without problems, but died at 26 weeks of age from a respiratory infection (4).

Sildenafil (150 mg/day), bosentan (250/day), hydroxychloroquine (200 mg/day), azathioprine (100 mg/day), and phenprocoumon were used up to 5 weeks' gestation in a 29-year-old woman with systemic lupus erythematosus-associated pulmonary arterial hypertension (5). At that time, bosentan and phenprocoumon were discontinued and the other three agents were continued along with low-molecular-weight heparin. At 35 weeks, inhaled iloprost was added. At 37 weeks', a planned cesarean section delivered a healthy 2.760-kg female infant with Apgar scores of 8, 9, and 10. Breastfeeding was declined. At the time of the report, the child was doing well (5).

BREASTFEEDING SUMMARY

No reports describing the use of sildenafil during human lactation have been located. The molecular weight (about 667) and terminal half-life (about 4 hours) suggest that the drug and its active metabolite will be excreted into breast milk, but the high plasma protein binding should limit the amount excreted. The effect of this exposure on a nursing infant is unknown. In clinical trials in adults, the three most common adverse effects were headache, flushing, and dyspepsia (1,2).

References

1. Product information. Revatio. Pfizer Labs, 2009.
2. Product information. Viagra. Pfizer Labs, 2010.
3. Lacassie HJ, Germain AM, Valdes G, Fernandez MS, Allamand F, Lopez H. Management of Eisenmenger syndrome in pregnancy with sildenafil and L-arginine. Obstet Gynecol 2004;103:1118–20.
4. Molelekwa V, Akhter P, McKenna P, Bowen M, Walsh K. Eisenmenger's syndrome in a 27 week pregnancy—management with bosentan and sildenafil. Ir Med J 2005;98:87–8.
5. Streit M, Speich R, Fischler M, Ulrich S. Successful pregnancy in pulmonary arterial hypertension associated with systemic lupus erythematosus: a case report. J Med Case Reports 2009;3:7255.

SILICONE BREAST IMPLANTS

Miscellaneous

PREGNANCY RECOMMENDATION: Compatible
BREASTFEEDING RECOMMENDATION: Compatible

PREGNANCY SUMMARY

Approximately 2 million women in the United States alone have received silicone implants (1), but no estimation of the number of pregnant women exposed to these devices has been located. The passage of polydimethylsiloxane (PDMS) to the fetus should not occur because of the high molecular weight of this polymer, and no evidence has been published that any of its multiple breakdown products cross the placenta. However, silicon, the second most abundant element in the earth's crust and a major component of biologic systems including the human skeleton (2), crosses to the fetus with concentrations in the amniotic fluid ranging from 34 to 800 ng/mL (mean 154.7 ng/mL) at 16–19 weeks' gestation (3). Transplacental passage of maternal immunoglobulin antibodies (IgG, IgA, or IgM) from silicone-induced immune disease is potentially possible, but this was not found in the study cited below. Moreover, some data presented in the Breastfeeding Summary argue against the clinical significance of this occurrence. Furthermore, a meta-analysis found no evidence that silicone implants are associated with connective-tissue or autoimmune diseases.

FETAL RISK SUMMARY

Silicone breast implants are composed of a shell of high-molecular-weight PDMS (dimethicone) gum (i.e., elastomer or rubber) containing either saline, a silicone "oil" composed of unlinked polymers, or a lower-viscosity PDMS gel (2,4). The difference in the viscosity of the organosiloxane shell and filler is dependent on the average molecular weight and molecular number distribution of the polymer (4). Leakage (bleeding) of the filler onto the surface of the shell may occur by simple diffusion and is associated with contracture of fibrous tissue around the implant, a foreign body response, or both. Gel bleeding may decrease the tensile strength of the shell and, by implication, may increase the incidence of implant rupture. The prevalence of implant rupture has been estimated to be 4%–6% (4).

Silicone breast implants have been generally available since the early 1980s, although they were first used experimentally in the 1940s (2). Several serious health concerns have been raised in relation to these implants, including silicone gel implant bleed, contracture (moderate degrees of contracture may be beneficial), implant rupture, carcinogenesis, immune disorders, and impaired breast cancer detection (1,2,4). However, a causal relationship between breast implants and connective-tissue and autoimmune disease seems unlikely based on the results of a meta-analysis described below.

A 2000 study conducted a meta-analysis of 20 studies (9 cohort, 9 case–control, and 2 cross-sectional) to determine if breast implants were associated with an increased risk of connective-tissue and autoimmune diseases (5). The study was part of a report prepared by a scientific panel formed to advise the federal judiciary on silicone breast implants (6). No evidence of an increase in individual connective-tissue diseases (rheumatoid arthritis, systemic lupus erythematosus, scleroderma or systemic sclerosis, and Sjogren's syndrome), all connective-tissue diseases combined, or other autoimmune or rheumatic conditions was found. Similarly, no evidence of a significantly increased risk was found specifically for silicone-gel-filled implants (5).

A study published in 1996 found no significant difference in the prevalence of autoantibodies between children ($N = 80$) born to mothers with silicone breast implants and control children ($N = 42$) born to mothers without implants (7). Moreover, no association between the clinical symptoms in the children and the presence of autoantibodies was found. Control children had been referred to the authors because of irritable bowel syndrome or lactose intolerance ($N = 21$) or fibromyalgia ($N = 21$), whereas the children in the study group had been referred because of concerns about adverse effects from the mother's implants. The authors concluded that determination of the antibodies was of limited clinical value in this patient population (7).

In a three-part study, investigators studied whether the immunogenicity of silicone, which appears to have been confirmed in humans and in at least one animal model, could be transferred from the mother to her offspring (8). In part 1 of the study, using silicon dioxide (silica), T lymphocyte cell-mediated immune responses were elicited in 21 of 24 children from 15 women with silicone breast implants. Subjects in part 2 of the study were the offspring of three women who gave birth to four children before they received their implants and to seven children after the implants. Five of the postimplant offspring were found to be positive to T-cell memory for silica compared with none of the preimplant offspring. Part 3 was a blinded study that evaluated 30 children of mothers with silicone implants compared with 10 control children of mothers without implants. A significant increase in T-cell stimulation was measured in the exposed children in comparison to the controls. Because not all of the above offspring were breastfed, the investigators concluded that the results indicated either the transplacental passage of immunogens from silicone or the transfer by maternal–fetal cellular exchange (8).

A 1998 epidemiologic cohort study conducted in Denmark examined the occurrence of esophageal disorders, connective tissue diseases, and congenital malformations in children (born during 1977–1992) of mothers with breast implants (9). A total of 939 children born from mothers with breast implants for cosmetic reasons (660 before the implant surgery and 279 after) were compared with 3906 children born from mothers who had undergone breast reduction surgery (1739 before surgery and 2167 after). The mean times from surgery to delivery for the two groups were 5.0 and 5.5 years, respectively. In the implant group, the observed/expected ratios (95% confidence intervals in parentheses) for various offspring outcomes before and after implants were as follows: esophageal disorders 2.7 (1.4–4.7) and 2.9 (0.8–7.4); rheumatic diseases 0.7 (0.0–4.1) and 0.0 (0.0–12.9); all types of congenital malformations 1.2 (0.9–1.5) and 1.3 (0.8–2.0); and defects of the digestive organs 1.4 (0.5–3.0) and 1.3 (0.2–4.6). Among the four children with an esophageal disorder who were born after the implants, three were hospitalized because of mild regurgitation that resolved without treatment. The fourth case involved a child with microcephaly, which was diagnosed as part of a genetic syndrome, and cerebral palsy. The results provided no evidence that silicone breast implants were associated with an increased risk of connective tissue diseases or malformations. Similar, nonsignificant differences for each of the categories were also found in the breast reduction group. The investigators concluded that women in both groups were more likely to seek professional medical care for problems normally solved outside the hospital (9).

BREASTFEEDING SUMMARY

Studies concerning the excretion of PDMS (see above) or the breakdown products of this macromolecule into milk have not been located, but two reports discussed below have described unusual disease symptoms in breastfed infants of mothers with silicone breast implants (10,11). For the present, any association between the symptoms and the organosiloxane components of the implants is speculative and further studies are needed to establish a causal relationship.

A 1994 report described 67 (56 breastfed, 11 bottle-fed) children born to mothers with silicone breast implants, who had been self-referred because of concerns relating to implant-induced toxicity (10). Forty-three (35 breastfed, 8 bottle-fed) of the children had complaints of recurrent abdominal pain, and 26 (20 breastfed, 6 bottle-fed) of this group had additional symptoms, such as recurrent vomiting, dysphagia, decreased weight:height ratio, or a sibling with these complaints. Of these latter 26 children, 11 (8 breastfed, 3 bottle-fed; mean age 6.0 years, range 1.5–13 years; 6 boys and 5 girls) agreed to undergo further evaluation. A group composed of 17 subjects (mean age 10.7 years; range 2–18 years; 11 boys and 6 girls) with abdominal pain who had not been exposed to silicone breast implants served as controls. No significant differences were found between the implant-exposed breastfed and bottle-fed subjects or between the total exposed group and controls (7 of the 17 were tested) in autoantibodies to eight antigens (nuclear, Sci-70, centromere, ribonucleoprotein, Sm, Ro, La, and phospholipid). Endoscopy was performed on all subjects, and no gross visual abnormalities were observed. Chronic esophagitis was discovered on biopsy specimens in 8 exposed (6 breastfed, 2 bottle-fed) children (all graded as mild) and in 13 of 16 controls (1 not tested) (mild-to-moderate in 7, severe in 6). No granulomas or crystals were identified in the biopsy specimens. The histology of the specimens did not differ between the exposed children or between the exposed children and controls. When esophageal manometry was used to test the esophageal motility of the subjects, six of the eight breastfed exposed children were found to have significantly abnormal motility with nearly absent peristalsis in the distal two-thirds of the esophagus. Esophageal sphincter pressure, esophageal wave propagation, and wave amplitude were measured and compared in the breastfed exposed, bottle-fed exposed, and control groups by an investigator blinded to the clinical status of the children. The following results were obtained in the three groups: 13.1 (*ns* compared with controls), 22.7, and 24.8 mmHg, respectively; 14.7% (*ns* compared with controls), 64.3%, and 53.0%, respectively; and 42.3, 60.3, and 50.6 mmHg, respectively. No improvement in the motility abnormalities was found in three of the breastfed exposed subjects who were retested 10 months later after long-term ranitidine therapy had reduced the episodes of abdominal pain (10).

The symptoms present in the breastfed exposed children were considered to be characteristic of systemic sclerosis, although the children did not meet the clinical criteria for the disease (10). Moreover, the investigators excluded the possibility that the abnormal motility was a consequence of chronic esophagitis. The blinded manometric findings suggested that the esophageal disorder might have been related to exposure to substances in breast milk because the bottle-fed exposed children had values similar to those of controls. The nature of these substances, if any, could not be determined by this study, but the investigators considered the possibilities to include silicone and other breakdown products of the implants that could be transferred across the immature intestinal barrier of the nursing infant and eventually lead to immunologically mediated damage (10).

In an accompanying editorial to the above report, several possible mechanisms for silicone-induced toxicity were explored (12). These included mother-to-child transmission of silicone products or maternal autoantibodies across the placenta or through breast milk. However, an argument against the latter mechanism is the usually short-term effects of passively acquired antibodies compared with the prolonged nature of the disorders in the affected children (12).

The second study, also published in 1994, described two female children, ages 2.67 and 9 years of age, who had long-standing, unusual, diffuse myalgias and arthralgias, not consistent with juvenile arthritis, and positive antinuclear antibodies (1:80 and 1:160, respectively; both speckled pattern) (11). The 9-year-old girl had a markedly elevated titer of antibodies against denatured human type II collagen. Both girls had been breastfed, the youngest for 3 months and the other for 6 months, by mothers with silicone breast implants. The right implant in the mother of the youngest girl had ruptured during pregnancy, and a recent breast ultrasound of the other mother was suggestive for implant rupture, but the timing was unknown (11).

A number of comments were published in response to the above two studies (13–25). In one of the comments, the authors described the results of a study in which no silicone was detected (detection level 0.5 mcg/mL) in two women with silicone breast implants (17). Two of the references stated that without more evidence, breastfeeding by women with silicone breast implants should not be contraindicated (22) or should be recommended (23).

Macrophage activation was suggested from the results of a case–control study of 38 breastfed children from mothers with silicone breast implants compared with 30 controls (healthy children $N = 10$, children with gastrointestinal symptoms similar to study patients $N = 10$, children with benign urinary abnormalities $N = 7$, and children with joint symptoms similar to study patients $N = 3$) (26). Researchers measured the urinary excretion of stable nitric oxide (NO) metabolites (NO_3^- plus NO_2^-) and neopterin, inflammatory mediators released by phagocytosis of foreign material by macrophages. Mean levels of NO metabolites in the study patients were higher than those in controls, but significantly higher only when compared with levels in the subgroup of healthy children. Mean neopterin excretion in study patients was higher than each of the four control subgroups, but significantly so only in comparison to the healthy, gastrointestinal, and joint symptom subgroups. The investigators speculated that macrophage activation by silicone results in the release of NO and other substances with subsequent inhibition of esophageal peristalsis (26).

At follow-up (mean 2.1 years) of 11 children with esophageal dysmotility who had been breastfed by mothers with silicone breast implants, 7 had subjective clinical improvement in their symptoms (27). Esophageal sphincter pressures (both lower and upper) and percent of wave propagation into the distal esophagus following swallowing were statistically similar to the values obtained at initial manometric testing. Wave amplitude in the distal esophagus, however, did increase significantly. Urinary neopterin decreased significantly, whereas urinary nitrates (NO_3^- plus NO_2^-) decreased but not significantly. The data suggested that the dysmotility had become a chronic condition in this group of children (27).

In a 1998 study, silicon concentrations in milk and blood of 15 women with bilateral silicone gel-filled implants were compared with similar samples in 34 women with no implants, store-bought cow's milk, and 26 brands of commercially available infant formula (28). Silicon was used as a "proxy" measure for silicone. Mean milk and blood silicon levels were statistically similar in the implant group compared with women without implants: 55.45 and 79.29 ng/mL vs. 51.05 and 103.76 ng/mL, respectively. Much higher mean silicon concentrations were found in cow's milk (708.94 ng/mL) and commercial infant formula (4402.5 ng/mL) (28).

Two studies have described unusual signs and symptoms in children who had been breastfed by mothers with silicone breast implants. Follow-up studies by the same investigators suggested that these effects may have been caused by the transfer of maternal mutagenicity to silicone to the fetuses or infants during pregnancy or breastfeeding and that the pathogenesis in the offspring might be caused by macrophage activation. However, these conclusions are controversial (29–31) and have not been confirmed. Many experts recommend that women with silicone breast implants should be encouraged to breastfeed because the benefits of breastfeeding appear to far outweigh the potential, if any, risk to the nursing infant. Mothers with silicone breast implants should be fully informed of the current state of knowledge so that they are actively involved in the decision whether to breastfeed. The American Academy of Pediatrics concluded that the available evidence does not justify classifying silicone implants as a contraindication to breastfeeding (32).

References

1. Kessler DA, Merkatz RB, Schapiro R. A call for higher standards for breast implants. JAMA 1993;270:2607–8.
2. Yoshida SH, Chang CC, Teuber SS, Gershwin ME. Silicon and silicone: theoretical and clinical implications of breast implants. Regul Toxicol Pharmacol 1993;17:3–18.
3. Hall GS, Carr MJ, Cummings E, Lee M-L. Aluminum, barium, silicon, and strontium in amniotic fluid by emission spectrometry. Clin Chem 1983;29:1318.
4. Council on Scientific Affairs, American Medical Association. Silicone gel breast implants. JAMA 1993;270:2602–6.
5. Janowsky EC, Kupper LL, Hulka BS. Meta-analyses of the relation between silicone breast implants and the risk of connective-tissue diseases. N Engl J Med 2000;342:781–90.
6. Hulka BS, Kerkvliet NL, Tugwell P. Experience of a scientific panel formed to advise the federal judiciary on silicone breast implants. N Engl J Med 2000;342:812–5.
7. Levine JJ, Lin H-C, Rowley M, Cook A, Teuber SS, Ilowite NT. Lack of autoantibody expression in children born to mothers with silicone breast implants. Pediatrics 1996;97:243–5.
8. Smalley DL, Levine JJ, Shanklin DR, Hall MF, Stevens MV. Lymphocyte response to silica among offspring of silicone breast implant recipients. Immunobiol 1996/1997;196:567–74.
9. Kjoller K, McLaughlin JK, Friis S, Blot WJ, Mellemkjaer L, Hogsted C, Winther JF, Olsen JH. Health outcomes in offspring of mothers with breast implants. Pediatrics 1998;102:1112–5.
10. Levine JJ, Ilowite NT. Sclerodermalike esophageal disease in children breast-fed by mothers with silicone breast implants. JAMA 1994; 271:213–6.
11. Teuber SS, Gershwin ME. Autoantibodies and clinical rheumatic complaints in two children of women with silicone gel breast implants. Int Arch Allergy Immunol 1994;103:105–8.
12. Flick JA. Silicone implants and esophageal dysmotility. Are breast-fed infants at risk? JAMA 1994;271:240–1.
13. Bartel DR. Sclerodermalike esophageal disease in children of mothers with silicone breast implants. JAMA 1994;272:767.
14. Cook RR. Sclerodermalike esophageal disease in children of mothers with silicone breast implants. JAMA 1994;272:767–8.
15. Epstein WA. Sclerodermalike esophageal disease in children of mothers with silicone breast implants. JAMA 1994;272:768.
16. Placik OJ. Sclerodermalike esophageal disease in children of mothers with silicone breast implants. JAMA 1994;272:768–9.
17. Liau M, Ito S, Koren G. Sclerodermalike esophageal disease in children of mothers with silicone breast implants. JAMA 1994;272:769.
18. Levine JJ, Ilowite NT. Sclerodermalike esophageal disease in children of mothers with silicone breast implants. In reply. JAMA 1994;272:769–70.
19. Brody GS. Sclerodermalike esophageal disease in children of mothers with silicone breast implants. JAMA 1994;272:770.
20. Flick JA. Sclerodermalike esophageal disease in children of mothers with silicone breast implants. In reply. JAMA 1994;272:770.
21. Williams AF. Silicone breast implants, breastfeeding, and scleroderma. Lancet 1994;343:1043–4.
22. Berlin CM Jr. Silicone breast implants and breast-feeding. Pediatrics 1994;94:547–9.
23. Jordan ME, Blum RWM. Should breast-feeding by women with silicone implants be recommended? Arch Pediatr Adolesc Med 1996;150:880–1.
24. Epstein WA. Silicone breast implants and sclerodermalike esophageal disease in breast-fed infants. JAMA 1996;275:184.
25. Levine JJ, Ilowite NT. Silicone breast implants and sclerodermalike esophageal disease in breast-fed infants. JAMA 1996;275:184–5.
26. Levine JJ, Ilowite NT, Pettei MJ, Trachtman H. Increased urinary NO_3^- + NO_2^- and neopterin excretion in children breast fed by mothers with silicone breast implants: evidence for macrophage activation. J Rheumatol 1996;23:1083–7.
27. Levine JJ, Trachtman H, Gold DM, Pettei MJ. Esophageal dysmotility in children breast-fed by mothers with silicone breast implants. Long-term follow-up and response to treatment. Dig Dis Sci 1996;41:1600–3.
28. Semple JL, Lugowski SJ, Baines CJ, Smith DC, McHugh A. Breast milk contamination and silicone implants: preliminary results using silicon as a proxy measurement for silicone. Plast Reconstr Surg 1998; 102:528–33.
29. Epstein WA. Silicone breast implants and breast feeding. J Rheumatol 1997;24:1013.
30. Hoshaw SJ, Klykken PC, Abbott JP. Silicone breast implants and breast feeding. J Rheumatol 1997;24:1014.
31. Levine JL, Ilowite NT, Pettei MJ, Trachtman H. Silicone breast implants and breast feeding. J Rheumatol 1997;24:1014–5.
32. Committee on Drugs, American Academy of Pediatrics. The transfer of drugs and other chemicals into human milk. Pediatrics 2001; 108:776–89.

SIMETHICONE

Antiflatulent/Defoaming Agent

PREGNANCY RECOMMENDATION: Compatible
BREASTFEEDING RECOMMENDATION: No Human Data—Compatible

PREGNANCY SUMMARY

Simethicone is an over-the-counter nonabsorbable silicone product that is used as an antiflatulent. No published reports linking the use of this agent with congenital defects have been located.

FETAL RISK SUMMARY

In a surveillance study of Michigan Medicaid recipients involving 229,101 completed pregnancies conducted between 1985 and 1992, 248 newborns had been exposed to simethicone during the 1st trimester (F. Rosa, personal communication, FDA, 1993). A total of 14 (5.6%) major birth defects were observed (11 expected). Specific data were available for six defect categories, including (observed/expected) 6/2 cardiovascular defects, 0/0.5 oral clefts, 0/0 spina bifida, 2/1 polydactyly, 0/.5 limb reduction defects, and 1/0.5 hypospadias. Although the number of cardiovascular defects was more than expected, simethicone could not have caused them because the drug is not absorbed into the systemic circulation. Other factors, such as the mother's disease, concurrent drug use, and chance, are most likely involved. Thus, the drug can be classified as compatible in pregnancy.

BREASTFEEDING SUMMARY

No reports describing the use of simethicone during human lactation have been located. There is no risk to a nursing infant from maternal use of the drug as it is not absorbed.

S

SIMVASTATIN

Antilipemic Agent

PREGNANCY RECOMMENDATION: Contraindicated
BREASTFEEDING RECOMMENDATION: Contraindicated

PREGNANCY SUMMARY

Based on the animal data and limited human experience, exposure to simvastatin during early pregnancy does not appear to present a significant risk to the fetus. However, because the interruption of cholesterol-lowering therapy during pregnancy should have no apparent effect on the long-term treatment of hyperlipidemia, simvastatin should not be used during pregnancy. Women taking this agent before conception should ideally stop the therapy before becoming pregnant and certainly on recognition of pregnancy. Accidental use of the drug during gestation, though, apparently has no known consequences for the fetus.

FETAL RISK SUMMARY

Simvastatin (a statin) is a lipophilic agent that is used to lower elevated levels of cholesterol. It has the same cholesterol-lowering mechanism (i.e., inhibition of hepatic 3-hydroxy-3-methylglutaryl-coenzyme A [HMG-CoA] reductase) as other agents available in this class, atorvastatin, fluvastatin, lovastatin, pitavastatin, pravastatin, and rosuvastatin (cerivastatin was withdrawn from the market in 2001). It is structurally similar to lovastatin and pravastatin.

Simvastatin was not teratogenic in rats and rabbits at doses up to three times the human exposure based on BSA (1). A decrease in fertility was observed in male rats dosed for 34 weeks at four times the maximum human exposure level based on AUC, but this effect was not observed when the study was repeated for 11 weeks (1). Male dogs given 10 mg/kg/day (about twice the human exposure based on AUC at 80 mg/day) demonstrated a drug-related testicular atrophy, decreased spermatogenesis, spermatocytic degeneration, and giant cell formation (1).

Shepard reviewed four studies involving the administration of simvastatin to pregnant rats and rabbits (2–5). Although maternal weight was reduced compared with controls, no teratogenicity, adverse effects on fertility, or interference with postnatal behavior or fertility were observed.

Five cases of fetal loss were reported to the FDA in 1995, but additional data on these cases are not available (F. Rosa, personal communication, FDA, 1995).

A surveillance study of simvastatin and lovastatin exposures during pregnancy, conducted by the manufacturer, was reported in 1996 (6) and updated in 2005 (7). Of the 477 reports, all involving 1st trimester exposure, 386 were prospective (319 simvastatin, 67 lovastatin) and 91 were retrospective (53 simvastatin, 38 lovastatin). The pregnancy outcomes were known for 225 (58%) of the prospective reports. There were congenital defects in five liveborn and one stillborn, all involving simvastatin. The outcomes with defects were as follows (maternal dose and exposure in weeks from last menstrual period shown in parentheses): (i) postaxial polydactyly with small, boneless, outgrowth from hand (10 mg/day, 3–4 weeks); (ii) cleft lip (20 mg/ day, 0–12 weeks); (iii) balanic hypospadias (10 mg/ day, 2–6 weeks); (iv) trisomy 18, multiple malformations in a dead fetus, other twin normal (10 mg/day, 0–7 weeks); (v) duodenal atresia (20 mg/day, 0–8 weeks); and (vi) balanced translocation chromosomes I and II, baby reported to look and behave normally, mother also treated for hypertension (20 mg/day, 3–5 weeks). The cases of postaxial polydactyly, cleft lip, and hypospadias are relatively common birth defects. Only postaxial polydactyly has been associated with inborn errors of cholesterol metabolism. The trisomy and chromosomal abnormality were also dismissed as drug induced because there is no evidence that these defects could be caused by drugs. Other outcomes were 18 spontaneous abortions (SABs), 49 elective abortions (EABs), 4 fetal deaths, and 148 live births without defects. All of the outcomes, with the exception of fetal deaths, were similar to the population background rate. Although the number of fetal deaths was increased, there was no specific pattern to suggest a common cause. One death involved a nuchal cord and another was a trisomy 18. No congenital defects were reported in the SABs or EABs (7).

There were 13 cases of congenital defects in retrospective reports; 6 involving simvastatin and 7 with lovastatin (7). The details of the congenital defects after exposure to simvastatin were (daily dose and exposure in weeks from last menstrual period) as follows:

(a) "major anomalies," EAB (dose not reported, 1st trimester);
(b) suspected triploidy, SAB (20 mg, 0–9 weeks);
(c) unilateral cleft lip (10 mg, 2–6 weeks);
(d) right lower limb aplasia of one tarsal bone, foot hypoplasia, equal shortening of the fibula and tibia (intercalary deficiency (20 mg, 0–4 weeks);
(e) clubfoot (10 mg, 1st trimester);
(f) features of VATER association (vertebral defects, anal atresia, tracheoesophageal fistula, esophageal atresia, radial limb reduction, and renal defect) with other abnormalities, EAB (10 mg, 2–12 weeks).

There were no specific patterns observed in the prospective or retrospective reports (7).

A 2004 report described the outcomes of pregnancy that had been exposed to statins and reported to the FDA (see Lovastatin).

Among 19 cases followed by a teratology information service in England, seven involved 1st trimester exposure to simvastatin (8). The pregnancy outcomes included two

SAbs; three healthy newborns; and two infants with congenital defects: sacral pit, intrauterine growth restriction (also exposed to enalapril, labetalol, and nifedipine); and mild positional talipes (8).

A 2005 case report described the pregnancy outcome of a 33-year-old woman treated with simvastatin in the first 8 weeks of an unplanned pregnancy (9). Diseases in the patient included hypercholesterolemia, hypertension, morbid obesity, and type 2 diabetes mellitus. Other drugs used by the woman were glimepiride, orlistat, ramipril, thiocolchicoside (a muscle relaxant), metformin, ciprofloxacin, and aspirin. When pregnancy was diagnosed at 8 weeks, all medications were stopped, and she was started on methyldopa and insulin. She gave birth at 38 weeks to a 3.470-kg female infant with Apgar scores of 5 and 7 at 1 and 5 minutes, respectively. No minor or major malformations were observed in the infant (9).

BREASTFEEDING SUMMARY

No published reports describing the use of simvastatin during lactation have been located. However, the passage of simvastatin into milk should be expected because at least two other similar agents (fluvastatin and pravastatin) appear in human milk. Because of the potential for adverse effects in the nursing infant, the drug should not be used during lactation.

References

1. Product information. Zocor. Merck, 2000.
2. Wise LD, Minsker DH, Robertson RT, Bokelman DL, Akutsu S, Fujii T. Simvastatin (mk-0733): oral fertility study in rats. Oyo Yakuri 1990;39:127–41. As cited in Shepard TH. *Catalog of Teratogenic Agents*. 7th ed. Baltimore, MD: The Johns Hopkins University Press, 1992:359–60.
3. Wise LD, Majka JA, Robertson RT, Bokelman DL. Simvastatin (mk-0733): oral teratogenicity study in rats pre- and postnatal observation. Oyo Yakuri 1990;39:143–58. As cited in Shepard TH. *Catalog of Teratogenic Agents*. 7th ed. Baltimore, MD: The Johns Hopkins University Press, 1992:359–60.
4. Wise LD, Prahalada S, Robertson RT, Bokelman DL, Akutsu S, Fujii T. Simvastatin (mk-0733): oral teratogenicity study in rabbits. Oyo Yakuri 1990;39:159–67. As cited in Shepard TH. *Catalog of Teratogenic Agents*. 7th ed. Baltimore, MD: The Johns Hopkins University Press, 1992: 359–60.
5. Minsker DH, Robertson RT, Bokelman DL. Simvastatin (mk-0733): oral late gestation and lactation study in rats. Oyo Yakuri 1990;39:169–79. As cited in Shepard TH. *Catalog of Teratogenic Agents*. 7th ed. Baltimore, MD: The Johns Hopkins University Press, 1992:359–60.
6. Manson JM, Freyssinges C, Ducrocq MB, Stephenson WP. Postmarketing surveillance of lovastatin and simvastatin exposure during pregnancy. Reprod Toxicol 1996;10:439–46.
7. Pollack PS, Shields KE, Burnett DM, Osborne MJ, Cunningham ML, Stepanavage ME. Pregnancy outcomes after maternal exposure to simvastatin and lovastatin. Birth Defects Res A Clin Mol Teratol 2005;73:888–96.
8. McElhatton P. Preliminary data on exposure to statins during pregnancy (abstract). Reprod Toxicol 2005;20:471–2.
9. Kalyoncu NI, Yaris F, Kadioglu M, Kesim M, Ulku C, Yaris E, Unsal M, Dikici M. Pregnancy outcome following exposure to orlistat, ramipril, glimepiride in a woman with metabolic syndrome. Saudi Med J 2005;26:497–9.

SIROLIMUS

Immunologic Agent (Immunosuppressant)

PREGNANCY RECOMMENDATION: Limited Human Data—Animal Data Suggest Moderate Risk
BREASTFEEDING RECOMMENDATION: No Human Data—Potential Toxicity

PREGNANCY SUMMARY

Only a few reports of exposure to sirolimus in human pregnancy have been located. The animal reproduction data suggest a potential for toxicity, but not for teratogenicity. The in vitro study described suggests that sirolimus could affect growth of the fetal and neonatal heart. Although the clinical significance of the concentrations used in that study is unknown, there was no attempt to determine the no-effect concentration. The very limited human pregnancy experience prevents a full assessment of the risk. Reviews discussing transplantation in pregnancy are ambivalent regarding the use of sirolimus; with some not recommending its use (1) and others implying that it may be continued in pregnancy (2). Until human data are available, however, the safest course is to avoid the drug in pregnancy. If sirolimus is used in pregnancy, or in the event of inadvertent exposure, close monitoring of the embryo–fetus for developmental toxicity is warranted. The manufacturer recommends that women of childbearing potential use effective contraception before and during therapy, and for 12 weeks after therapy is stopped (3).

FETAL RISK SUMMARY

Sirolimus (rapamycin) is a distinct, oral immunosuppressant that is indicated for the prophylaxis of organ rejection in patients receiving renal transplants. It is recommended that it initially be used in combination with cyclosporine and corticosteroids. Chemically, the drug is a macrocyclic lactone produced by *Streptomyces hygroscopicus*. Sirolimus inhibits T-lymphocyte activation and proliferation induced by antigenic and cytokine (interleukin-2 [IL-2], IL-4, and IL-15) stimulation. Sirolimus is classified as a small-molecule immunosuppressant agent (4). It is highly protein bound to plasma albumin and other proteins (about 92%) and has a mean terminal half-life in renal transplant patients of about 62 hours (3).

Reproduction studies have been conducted in rats and rabbits. In rats, doses about 0.2–0.5 times the human clinical dose based on BSA (HCD) were embryo–fetal toxic (death;

reduced fetal weights with associated delays in skeletal ossification). However, structural defects were not observed. No effect on female rat fertility was observed at doses about 1–3 times the HCD. When combined with cyclosporine, increased embryo–fetal death compared with sirolimus alone was observed in rats. In pregnant rabbits, there were no effects on development at a maternal toxic dose about 0.3–0.8 times the HCD (3).

In carcinogenesis studies in mice and rats, there was a significant increase in malignant lymphoma at all doses tested (about 16–135 times the HCD). In mice, a lower dose (about 3–16 times the HCD) was associated with hepatocellular adenoma and carcinoma (males). In rats, a dose approximately equivalent to the HCD significantly increased the incidence of testicular adenoma. Sirolimus was not genotoxic in a variety of assays (3).

A 1998 in vitro study examined the effect of sirolimus on heart cell growth (5). Cardiac myocytes were isolated from 15-day-old fetal rats and exposed for 5 days in culture medium to various concentrations of sirolimus. (*Note: The lowest concentration tested [0.5 ng/mL] was about 1.3% of the adult mean maximum concentration [37.4 ng/mL] obtained with a 5 mg/day dose*). The exposed cells were then washed and grown in culture medium without sirolimus for an additional 5 days. Sirolimus inhibited both short-term and subsequent proliferation of cardiac myocytes. The investigators noted that fetal and neonatal heart growth occurs predominantly through myocyte proliferation (5).

It is not known if sirolimus crosses the human placenta. The molecular weight (about 914) is within the range for passive diffusion, and the elimination half-life will allow the drug to be present at the maternal:fetal interface for a long interval. However, the high protein binding should limit the amount of drug available to cross the placenta.

A 2003 report from the National Transplantation Pregnancy Registry briefly described four female kidney recipients who were treated during pregnancy with sirolimus and other immunosuppressants (6). The outcomes of the pregnancies were three live births (at 31, 36, and 38 weeks' gestation) and one spontaneous abortion (at 8 weeks' gestation). The only structural defect observed in the four cases was a cleft lip/palate and an ear deformity in a 1531-g infant delivered at 31 weeks' gestation. Immunosuppression during the first 24 weeks consisted of mycophenolate mofetil, tacrolimus, and prednisone (6). Sirolimus, added at 24 weeks' gestation for biopsy-proven acute rejection, was not related to the anomalies.

A 2004 case report described the use of sirolimus in a 21-year-old woman who became pregnant 3 years after liver transplantation (7). At the time of conception, immunosuppression was maintained with sirolimus, tacrolimus, and corticosteroids (doses not specified). Pregnancy was diagnosed at 6 weeks' gestation and sirolimus was discontinued, but corticosteroids and tacrolimus were continued throughout pregnancy. At 39 weeks' gestation, a healthy, 2950-g female infant was delivered by cesarean section. The infant's physical development has been normal, and no unusual infections have been observed (7).

BREASTFEEDING SUMMARY

No reports describing the use of sirolimus during human lactation have been located. The molecular weight (about 914) and the prolonged half-life (about 62 hours) suggest that the drug will be excreted into breast milk. The effect of this potential exposure on a nursing infant is unknown, but consideration should be given to the carcinogenic properties of sirolimus, especially with long-term exposures. A 2002 review concluded that because of possible drug transfer into milk, women taking sirolimus should not breastfeed (1).

References

1. EBPG Expert Group on Renal Transplantation. European best practice guidelines for renal transplantation. Section IV: long-term management of the transplant recipient. IV.10. Pregnancy in renal transplant recipients. Nephrol Dial Transplant 2002;17 (Suppl 4):50–5.
2. Danesi R, Del Tacca M. Teratogenesis and immunosuppressive treatment. Transplant Proc 2004;36:705–7
3. Product information. Rapamune. Wyeth Pharmaceuticals, 2005.
4. Halloran PF. Immunosuppressive drugs for kidney transplantation. N Engl J Med 2004;351:2715–29.
5. Burton PBJ, Yacoub MH, Barton PJR. Rapamycin (sirolimus) inhibits heart cell growth in vitro. Pediatr Cardiol 1998;19:468–70.
6. Armenti VT, Radomski JS, Moritz MJ, Gaughan WJ, McGrory CH, Coscia LA. Report from the National Transplantation Pregnancy Registry (NTPR): outcomes of pregnancy after transplantation. Clin Transpl 2003;131–41.
7. Jankowska I, Oldakowska-Jedynak U, Jabiry-Zieniewicz Z, Cyganek A, Pawlowska J, Teisseyre M, Kalicinski P, Markiewicz M, Paczek L, Socha J. Absence of teratogenicity of sirolimus used during early pregnancy in a liver transplant recipient. Transplant Proc 2004;36:3232–3.

SITAGLIPTIN

Antidiabetic Agent

PREGNANCY RECOMMENDATION: Limited Human Data—Animal Data Suggest Low Risk
BREASTFEEDING RECOMMENDATION: No Human Data—Probably Compatible

PREGNANCY SUMMARY

The animal reproduction data suggest low risk, but the very limited human pregnancy experience prevents a complete assessment of the embryo–fetal risk. No congenital anomalies attributable to sitagliptin (either alone or combined with metformin) have been reported.

Although the use of sitagliptin may help decrease the incidence of fetal and newborn morbidity and mortality in developing countries where the proper use of insulin is problematic, insulin still is the treatment of choice for this disease during pregnancy. Moreover, insulin does not cross the placenta and, this eliminates the additional concern that the drug therapy itself is adversely affecting the fetus. Carefully prescribed insulin therapy will provide better control of the mother's blood glucose, thereby preventing the fetal and neonatal complications that occur with this disease. High maternal glucose levels, as might occur in diabetes mellitus, are associated with a number of maternal and fetal adverse effects, including fetal structural anomalies if the hyperglycemia occurs early in gestation. To prevent this toxicity, the American College of Obstetricians and Gynecologists recommends that insulin be used for types 1 and 2 diabetes occurring during pregnancy and, if diet therapy alone is not successful, for gestational diabetes (1,2). If a woman becomes pregnant while taking sitagliptin, changing the therapy to insulin should be considered.

The manufacturer maintains a pregnancy registry for women exposed to sitagliptin. Healthcare professionals are encouraged to report pregnancy exposures to the registry by calling the toll-free number 800-986-8999.

FETAL RISK SUMMARY

Sitagliptin is an orally active inhibitor of the dipeptidyl peptidase-4 (DPP4) enzyme. It is in the same antidiabetic subclass as linagliptin and saxagliptin. Sitagliptin is indicated as monotherapy as an adjunct to diet and exercise to improve glycemic control in patients with type 2 diabetes mellitus. It also is indicated in patients with type 2 diabetes mellitus to improve glycemic control in combination with metformin or a thiazolidinedione when the single agent alone, with diet and exercise, does not provide adequate glycemic control. In studies in healthy and diabetic subjects, sitagliptin did not lower blood glucose or cause hypoglycemia. Sitagliptin is partially metabolized with about 79% excreted in the urine as unchanged drug. The elimination half-life after a single dose was 12.4 hours. Plasma protein binding is low (38%) (3).

Reproduction studies have been conducted in rats and rabbits. In pregnant rats and rabbits, doses given during organogenesis that resulted in exposures about ≤30 and ≤20 times, respectively, the human exposure at the maximum recommended dose of 100 mg/day based on AUC (MRHD) were not teratogenic. At about 100 times the MRHD, an increased incidence of rib malformations was observed in offspring. A dose given to rats from gestation day 6 through lactation day 21 that resulted in exposures about 100 times the MRHD caused decreased body weight in offspring. No functional or behavioral toxicity was observed in the offspring (3).

Two-year carcinogenicity studies were conducted in male and female rats. An increased incidence of combined liver adenoma/carcinoma in males and females and of liver carcinoma in females was observed at an exposure about 60 times the MRHD. Liver tumors were not observed at about 20 times the MRHD. A similar study, performed in male and female mice with doses ≤70 times the MRHD, found no increase in the incidence of tumors in any organ. Sitagliptin was not mutagenic or clastogenic with or without metabolic activation in multiple assays. No impairment of fertility or fetal harm was observed in rats and rabbits given doses resulting in exposures that were about ≤12 times the MRHD (3).

Sitagliptin crosses the rat and rabbit placentas (3). Although it has not been studied, the drug probably crosses the human placenta. The molecular weight (about 505 for the phosphate salt), low metabolism and plasma protein binding, and prolonged elimination half-life suggest that the drug will cross to the embryo–fetus. However, the low lipid solubility might limit the exposure.

The Merck Pregnancy Registry for Januvia (sitagliptin) and Janumet (sitagliptin/metformin) covered the period August 4, 2006 through August 3, 2009 (4). During clinical trials, eight women were exposed to sitagliptin or sitagliptin/metformin during the 1st trimester. The outcomes of these pregnancies were five healthy liveborn infants, two spontaneous abortions (SABs), and one fetal death (at 34 weeks' in a mother who took sitagliptin and metformin separately for the first 5 weeks of pregnancy). The outcomes of 16 prospectively enrolled pregnancies (exposures in the Registry are combined and do not distinguish between the two drugs) were nine live births (one set of twins), one SAB, five lost to follow-up, and two pregnancies pending. There were no congenital anomalies reported. There were six retrospectively enrolled pregnancies: two live births, three SABs, and one elective abortion at 19 weeks for encephalocele and intrauterine growth restriction (exposed to sitagliptin/metformin for 7 weeks during 1st trimester). In an internationally reported case, a woman took sitagliptin, insulin, metformin, and rosiglitazone for about 5 weeks in the 1st trimester. She gave birth at 33 weeks to a male infant with dysplastic left kidney, a missing kidney, severe hypospadias, a missing right testicle, and a poorly descended left testicle. The anomalies were consistent with diabetic embryopathy. A right inguinal hernia also was noted (4).

BREASTFEEDING SUMMARY

No reports describing the use of sitagliptin during human lactation have been located. The molecular weight (about 505 for the phosphate salt), low metabolism (about 21%) and plasma protein binding (about 38%), and prolonged elimination half-life (12.4 hours) suggest that the drug will be excreted into breast milk. The low lipid solubility might limit the exposure. The effect of this exposure on a nursing infant is unknown. Sitagliptin overdose (six times the maximum recommended human dose for 10 days) in healthy adults caused no dose-related adverse reactions (3). Thus, hypoglycemia in a nursing infant appears to be unlikely but should be monitored. The most common (≥5%) adverse reaction in adults receiving monotherapy was nasopharyngitis (3).

S

References

1. American College of Obstetricians and Gynecologists. Pregestational diabetes mellitus. *ACOG Practice Bulletin*. No. 60. March 2005. Obstet Gynecol 2005;105:675–85.

2. American College of Obstetricians and Gynecologists. Gestational diabetes. *ACOG Practice Bulletin*. No. 30. September 2001. Obstet Gynecol 2001;98:525–38.
3. Product information. Januvia. Merck, 2007.
4. Third Annual Report on exposure during pregnancy from the Merck Pregnancy Registry for Januvia (sitagliptin phosphate) and Janumet (sitagliptin phosphate/metformin hydrochloride) August 4, 2006 through August 3, 2009.

SODIUM BICARBONATE

Nutrient/Antacid

PREGNANCY RECOMMENDATION: Limited Human Data—Animal Data Suggest Low Risk
BREASTFEEDING RECOMMENDATION: No Human Data—Potential Toxicity

PREGNANCY SUMMARY

No reports of human 1st trimester use of sodium bicarbonate in pregnancy have been located. Animal studies have not suggested an increased risk for structural anomalies (1–5). Use of sodium bicarbonate (baking soda) for routine gastrointestinal ailments of pregnancy such as heartburn is typically not recommended due to the potential for fluid retention in pregnancy and subsequent complications and because alternatives are available (1). IV sodium bicarbonate therapy may be indicated for acute treatment of metabolic acidosis, certain drug intoxications, and severe diarrhea.

FETAL RISK SUMMARY

Sodium bicarbonate is an alkalinizing agent composed of sodium and bicarbonate ions. It is given as an IV solution to treat electrolyte disturbances resulting from severe metabolic acidosis that can occur in renal disease, uncontrolled diabetes, or severe dehydration. It also is used to treat overdoses of certain drugs such as barbiturates or salicylates. Sodium bicarbonate is used orally as an antacid to relieve symptoms of heartburn, indigestion, or stomach upset.

In animal studies, no teratogenic effect was noted among the offspring of rats given 40 to more than 4000 mg/kg/day of sodium bicarbonate during pregnancy (2–4). Similarly, no teratogenic effect was seen among the offspring of mice given 500 mg/kg/day of sodium bicarbonate during pregnancy (5).

Bicarbonate is a normal constituent of body fluids and plasma concentration is regulated by the kidney through acidification of the urine when there is a deficit or by alkalinization of the urine when there is an excess. In a healthy adult with normal kidney function, practically all the glomerular filtered bicarbonate ion is reabsorbed; less than 1% is excreted in the urine. Treatment with exogenous sodium bicarbonate increases plasma bicarbonate, buffers excess hydrogen ion concentration, and raises blood pH (1).

Oral sodium bicarbonate is not recommended for the treatment of common complaints of heartburn and indigestion during pregnancy because of the potential for sodium-related fluid retention and edema that could contribute to other complications of pregnancy such as hypertension. Alternative treatments for chronic gastrointestinal complications of pregnancy that do not lead to fluid retention are preferred (1).

One human case report has been located (6). A woman who ingested 454 g of sodium bicarbonate a day between 29 and 31 weeks of pregnancy developed hypokalemic alkalosis, rhabdomyolysis, and hypertension. She subsequently gave birth to an apparently normal infant.

No studies of sodium bicarbonate and human fertility have been located. However, bicarbonate and carbon dioxide are common components in the secretions of the female reproductive tract, especially the oviduct (7). At physiologic concentrations, they are believed to play an important role in sperm hyperactivation and capacitation (8). An improvement of cervical mucus viscoelasticity and sperm penetration following vaginal douching with sodium bicarbonate has been reported (9).

BREASTFEEDING SUMMARY

Although sodium bicarbonate is known to be excreted into breast milk (1), no reports describing its use during human lactation have been located. However, chronic or indiscriminate use of the product as an antacid is not recommended during breastfeeding (1).

References

1. Clinical Pharmacology. Sodium bicarbonate. http://www.clinicalpharmacology-ip.com accessed, November 5, 2012.
2. Khera KS. Chemically induced alterations in maternal homeostasis and histology of conceptus: their etiologic significance in rat fetal anomalies. Teratology 1991;44:259–97.
3. Mayura K, Hayes AW, Berndt WO. Teratogenicity of secalonic acid D in rats. Toxicology 1982;25:311–22.
4. Nakatsuka T, Fujikake N, Hasebe M, Ikeda H. Effects of sodium bicarbonate and ammonium chloride on the incidence of furosemide-induced fetal skeletal anomaly, wavy rib, in rats. Teratology 1993;48:139–47.
5. Reddy CS, Reddy RV, Hayes AW. Teratogenicity of secalonic acid D in mice. J Toxicol Environ Health 1981;7:445–55.
6. Grotegut CA, Dandolu V, Katari S, Whiteman VE, Geifman-Holtzman O, Teitelman M. Baking soda pica: a case of hypokalemic metabolic alkalosis and rhabdomyolysis in pregnancy. Obstet Gynecol 2006;107:484–6.
7. Brackett BG, Mastroianni I. Composition of oviductal fluid. In: Johnson AD, Foley CW, eds. *The Oviduct and its Functions*. New York, NY: Academic Press, Inc. 1974:135–99.
8. Boatman DE, Robbins RS. Bicarbonate: carbon-dioxide regulation of sperm capacitation, hyperactivated motility, and acrosome reactions. Biol Reprod 1991;44: 806–13.
9. Everhardt E, Dony JM, Jansen H, Lemmens WA, Doesburg WH. Improvement of cervical mucus viscoelasticity and sperm penetration with sodium bicarbonate douching. Hum Reprod 1990;5:133–7.

S

SODIUM IODIDE

Respiratory Drug (Expectorant)

See Potassium Iodide.

SODIUM IODIDE ^{125}I

Radiopharmaceutical

See Sodium Iodide ^{131}I.

SODIUM IODIDE ^{131}I

Radiopharmaceutical/Antithyroid

PREGNANCY RECOMMENDATION: Contraindicated
BREASTFEEDING RECOMMENDATION: Hold Breastfeeding

PREGNANCY SUMMARY

Iodine-131-labeled sodium iodide ($Na^{131}I$) is a proven human teratogen. Because the effects of even small doses are not predictable, the use of the drug for diagnostic and therapeutic purposes should be avoided during pregnancy. A 1999 reference reviewed the effects of ^{131}I on the fetal thyroid after administration to the mother in early gestation (1).

FETAL RISK SUMMARY

$Na^{131}I$ is a radiopharmaceutical agent used for diagnostic procedures and for therapeutic destruction of thyroid tissue. The diagnostic dose is approximately one-thousandth of the therapeutic dose. Like all iodides, the drug concentrates in the thyroid gland. ^{131}I readily crosses the placenta. The fetal thyroid is able to accumulate ^{131}I until after about 10–12 weeks of gestation (1–4). At term, the maternal serum:cord blood ratio is 1 (5).

As suggested by the above studies on the uptake of ^{131}I in fetal thyroids, maternal treatment with radioiodine early in the 1st trimester should not pose a significant danger to the fetus. Two reports describing $Na^{131}I$ therapy at 4 and 8 weeks' gestation resulting in normal infants seemingly confirmed the lack of risk (6,7). However, a newborn, who was exposed to $Na^{131}I$ at about 2 weeks' gestation, has been described as having a large head, exophthalmia, and thick, myxedematous-like skin (8). The infant died shortly after birth. In another early report, exposure to a diagnostic dose of $Na^{131}I$ during the middle of the 1st trimester was considered the cause of anomalies observed in the newborn, including microcephaly, hydrocephaly, dysplasia of the hip joints, and clubfoot (9). Finally, $Na^{131}I$ administered 1–3 days before conception was suggested as the cause of a spontaneous abortion at the end of the 1st trimester (10). All three of these latter reports must be viewed with caution because of the uniqueness of the effects and the timing of the exposure. Factors other than radioiodine may have been involved.

Therapeutic doses of radioiodine administered near the end of the 1st trimester (12 weeks) or beyond usually result in partial or complete abolition of the fetal thyroid gland (11–21). This effect is dose-dependent, however, as one mother was treated at 19 weeks' gestation with 6.1 mCi of $Na^{131}I$ apparently without causing fetal harm (2). In the pregnancies terminating with a hypothyroid infant, $Na^{131}I$ doses ranged from 10 to 225 mCi (11–21). Clinical features observed at or shortly after birth in 10 of the 12 newborns were consistent with congenital hypothyroidism. One of these infants was also discovered to have hypoparathyroidism (21). In one child, exposed in utero to repeated small doses during a 5-week period (total dose 12.2 mCi), hypothyroidism did not become evident until 4 years of age (18). Unusual anomalies observed in another infant included hydrocephaly, cardiopathy, genital hypotrophy, and a limb deformity (16).

In a 1998 case report, a woman received 500 MBq of ^{131}I in the 20th gestational week (22). Based on gamma camera examinations, the fetal thyroid gland uptake at 24 hours was estimated to be 10 MBq (2% of the dose) or an absorbed dose to the gland of 600 Gy (an ablative dose). The absorbed dose to the fetal body and brain was approximately 100 mGy, whereas the fetal gonads received about 40 mGy. At term, a hypothyroid, but otherwise healthy 3150-g male infant was delivered. Treatment with thyroxine was begun at 14 days of age. A neuropsychological examination at 8 years of age revealed normal mental performance, but with a low attention score and subnormal capacity regarding figurative memory. Plans were made for long-term surveillance of the infant because of the potential for thyroid cancer (22).

BREASTFEEDING SUMMARY

$Na^{131}I$ is concentrated in breast milk (23–26). $Na^{125}I$ also appears in milk in significant quantities (27,28). Uptake of ^{131}I contained in milk by an infant's thyroid gland has been observed (23). The time required for elimination of radioiodine from the milk may be as long as 14 days. For iodine-123 (^{123}I) and iodine-125 (^{125}I), radioactivity may be present in milk for up to 36 hours and 12 days, respectively (29). Since exposure to radioactive iodine may result in damage to the nursing infant's thyroid, including an increased risk of thyroid cancer, breastfeeding should be stopped until radioactivity is no longer present in the milk (29).

References

1. Pauwels EKJ, Thomson WH, Blokland JAK, Schmidt ME, Bourguignon M, El-Maghraby TAF, Broerse JJ, Harding LK. Aspects of fetal thyroid dose following iodine-131 administration during early stages of pregnancy in patients suffering from benign thyroid disorders. Eur J Nucl Med 1999;26:1453–7.
2. Chapman EM, Corner GW Jr, Robinson D, Evans RD. The collection of radioactive iodine by the human fetal thyroid. J Clin Endocrinol Metab 1948;8:717–20.
3. Hodges RE, Evans TC, Bradbury JT, Keettel WC. The accumulation of radioactive iodine by human fetal thyroids. J Clin Endocrinol Metab 1955;15:661–7.
4. Shepard TH. Onset of function in the human fetal thyroid: biochemical and radioautographic studies from organ culture. J Clin Endocrinol Metab 1967;27:945–58.
5. Kearns JE, Hutson W. Tagged isomers and analogues of thyroxine (their transmission across the human placenta and other studies). J Nucl Med 1963;4:453–61.
6. Hollingsworth DR, Austin E. Observations following I^{131} for Graves' disease during first trimester of pregnancy. South Med J 1969;62:1555–6.
7. Talbert LM, Thomas CG Jr, Holt WA, Rankin P. Hyperthyroidism during pregnancy. Obstet Gynecol 1970;36:779–85.
8. Valensi G, Nahum A. Action de l'iode radio-actif sur le foetus humain. Tunisie med 1958;36:69. As cited in Nishimura H, Tanimura T. *Clinical Aspects of the Teratogenicity of Drugs*. New York, NY: American Elsevier, 1976:260.
9. Falk W. Beitrag zur Frage der menschlichen Fruchtschadigung durch kunstliche radioaktive Isotope. Medizinische 1959;22:1480. As cited in Nishimura H, Tanimura T. *Clinical Aspects of the Teratogenicity of Drugs*. New York, NY: American Elsevier, 1976:260.
10. Berger M, Briere J. Les dangers de la therapeutique par l'iode radioactif au debut d'une grossesse ignoree. Bull Med leg Toxicol Med 1967;10:37. As cited in Nishimura H, Tanimura T. *Clinical Aspects of the Teratogenicity of Drugs*. New York, NY: American Elsevier, 1976:260.
11. Russell KP, Rose H, Starr P. The effects of radioactive iodine on maternal and fetal thyroid function during pregnancy. Surg Gynecol Obstet 1957;104:560–4.
12. Ray EW, Sterling K, Gardner LI. Congenital cretinism associated with I^{131} therapy of the mother. Am J Dis Child 1959;98:506–7.
13. Hamill GC, Jarman JA, Wynne MD. Fetal effects of radioactive iodine therapy in a pregnant woman with thyroid cancer. Am J Obstet Gynecol 1961;81:1018–23.
14. Fisher WD, Voorhess ML, Gardner LI. Congenital hypothyroidism in infant following maternal I^{131} therapy. J Pediatr 1963;62:132–46.
15. Pfannenstiel P, Andrews GA, Brown DW. Congenital hypothyroidism from intrauterine ^{131}I damage. In: Cassalino C, Andreoli M, eds. *Current Topics in Thyroid Research*. New York, NY: Academic Press, 1965:749. As cited in Nishimura H, Tanimura T. *Clinical Aspects of the Teratogenicity of Drugs*. New York, NY: American Elsevier, 1976:260.
16. Sirbu P, Macarie E, Isaia V, Zugravesco A. L'influence de l'iode radio-actif sur le foetus. Bull Fed Soc Gynecol Obstet Franc 1968;20: Suppl 314. As cited in Nishimura H, Tanimura T. *Clinical Aspects of the Teratogenicity of Drugs*. New York, NY: American Elsevier, 1976:260.
17. Hollingsworth DR, Austin E. Thyroxine derivatives in amniotic fluid. J Pediatr 1971;79:923–9.
18. Green HG, Gareis FJ, Shepard TH, Kelley VC. Cretinism associated with maternal sodium iodide I 131 therapy during pregnancy. Am J Dis Child 1971;122:247–9.
19. Jafek BW, Small R, Lillian DL. Congenital radioactive iodine-induced stridor and hypothyroidism. Arch Otolaryngol 1974;99:369–71.
20. Exss R, Graewe B. Congenital athyroidism in the newborn infant from intrauterine radioiodine action. Biol Neonate 1974;24:289–91.
21. Richards GE, Brewer ED, Conley SB, Saldana LR. Combined hypothyroidism and hypoparathyroidism in an infant after maternal ^{131}I administration. J Pediatr 1981;99:141–43.
22. Berg GEB, Nystrom EH, Jacobsson L, Lindberg S, Lindstedt RG, Mattsson S, Niklasson CA, Noren AH, Westphal OGA. Radioiodine treatment of hyperthyroidism in a pregnant woman. J Nucl Med 1998;39:357–61.
23. Nurnberger CE, Lipscomb A. Transmission of radioiodine (I^{131}) to infants through human maternal milk. JAMA 1952;150:1398–1400.
24. Miller H, Weetch RS. The excretion of radioactive iodine in human milk. Lancet 1955;2:1013.
25. Weaver JC, Kamm ML, Dobson RL. Excretion of radioiodine in human milk. JAMA 1960;173:872–5.
26. Karjalainen P, Penttila IM, Pystynen P. The amount and form of radioactivity in human milk after lung scanning, renography and placental localization by ^{131}I labelled tracers. Acta Obstet Gynecol Scand 1971;50:357–61.
27. Bland EP, Crawford JS, Docker MF, Farr RF. Radioactive iodine uptake by thyroid of breastfed infants after maternal blood-volume measurements. Lancet 1969;2:1039–41.
28. Palmer KE. Excretion of ^{125}I in breast milk following administration of labelled fibrinogen. Br J Radiol 1979;52:672–3.
29. Committee on Drugs, American Academy of Pediatrics. The transfer of drugs and other chemicals into human milk. Pediatrics 2001;108: 776–89.

SODIUM OXYBATE

Psychotherapeutic (Miscellaneous)

PREGNANCY RECOMMENDATION: Limited Human Data—Animal Data Suggest Low Risk
BREASTFEEDING RECOMMENDATION: No Human Data—Potential Toxicity

PREGNANCY SUMMARY

One report describing the use of sodium oxybate in human pregnancy has been located. The animal data suggest low risk, but the near absence of human pregnancy experience prevents a more complete assessment of the embryo–fetal risk. However, the indication suggests that the maternal benefit, under close medical supervision, may outweigh the unknown risk to the embryo–fetus.

FETAL RISK SUMMARY

Sodium oxybate, gamma hydroxybutyrate (GHB), is a CNS depressant that is available as an oral solution. It is indicated for the treatment of excessive daytime sleepiness and cataplexy in patients with narcolepsy. Because it is a known drug of abuse, sodium oxybate is only available through the Xyrem Success Program, using a centralized pharmacy. The drug is mainly eliminated by metabolism with <5% of unchanged drug appearing in the urine within 6–8 hours after dosing. Plasma protein binding is <1% and the half-life is 0.5–1 hour (1).

Reproduction studies have been conducted in rats and rabbits. Doses in these species that were about equal to and three times, respectively, the maximum recommended human dose based on BSA (MRHD) revealed no evidence of teratogenicity. In rats, a dose that was about equal to the MRHD given from day 6 of gestation through day 21 postpartum caused slight decreases in pup and maternal weight gains. No other drug effects on development were observed (1).

Sodium oxybate was not carcinogenic in long-term studies in male and female rats. A test for mutagenicity and a chromosomal aberration assay were negative. Doses that were about equal to the MRHD did not impair fertility in rats (1).

It is not known if sodium oxybate, or its acid, cross the human placenta. The molecular weight of 4-hydroxybutyric acid (about 104) and the minimal plasma protein binding suggest that it will cross to the embryo–fetus, but the extensive, rapid metabolism and short half-life should limit the exposure.

A brief 2004 case report described a woman in labor who developed mild respiratory depression (2). The event was initially thought to be due to the opioid used for spinal–epidural analgesia. The depression was treated with face mask oxygen and 2 hours later she delivered a healthy newborn with a good Apgar score (scores not specified). Routine toxicology screening revealed the presence of GHB, also known as liquid ecstasy, and the mother admitted that she had used the drug (2).

BREASTFEEDING SUMMARY

No reports describing the use of sodium oxybate (GBH) during human lactation have been located, but such use is unlikely because of the drug's rapid action. The molecular weight of the acid form (4-hydroxybutyric acid) (about 104) and the minimal plasma protein binding (<1%) suggest that it will be excreted into breast milk, but the extensive, rapid metabolism and short half-life (0.5–1 hour) should limit the amount excreted. The effect of this exposure on a nursing infant is unknown, but sedation and confusion are potential complications. However, because the drug is taken immediately before bedtime, nursing no sooner than 5 hours after a dose to just before the next dose should prevent clinically significant exposure of an infant.

References

1. Product information. Xyrem. Jazz Pharmaceuticals, 2009
2. Kuczkowski KM. Liquid ecstasy during pregnancy. Anaesthesia 2004;59:926.

SOLIFENACIN

Urinary Tract Agent (Antispasmodic)

PREGNANCY RECOMMENDATION: No Human Data—Animal Data Suggest Moderate Risk
BREASTFEEDING RECOMMENDATION: No Human Data—Probably Compatible

PREGNANCY SUMMARY

No reports describing the use of solifenacin in human pregnancy have been located. The animal data suggest moderate risk, but the absence of human pregnancy experience prevents a complete assessment of the embryo–fetal risk. However, there is no evidence that other anticholinergic drugs or agents in the subclass of urinary antispasmodics cause developmental toxicity. Nevertheless, until human pregnancy data are available, the safest course is to avoid solifenacin during pregnancy, especially in the 1st trimester. If inadvertent exposure in pregnancy does occur, the embryo–fetal risks probably are low.

S

FETAL RISK SUMMARY

The anticholinergic, solifenacin is a competitive antagonist of muscarinic receptors that are involved in cholinergic functions such as contractions of urinary bladder smooth muscle and stimulation of salivary secretion. Solifenacin is indicated for the treatment of overactive bladder with symptoms of urge urinary incontinence, urgency, and urinary frequency. It is in the same subclass as darifenacin, flavoxate, oxybutynin, and tolterodine, and trospium. Solifenacin is extensively metabolized by hepatic enzymes (mainly CYP3A4), but other metabolic pathways exist. One of the metabolites is active, but the concentration is low and is not thought to contribute significantly to clinical activity. Plasma protein binding is about 98%, primarily by α_1-acid glycoprotein. The plasma elimination half-life with chronic dosing is 45–68 hours (1).

Reproduction studies have been conducted in mice, rats, and rabbits. In pregnant mice, doses ≥3.6 times the exposure at the maximum recommended human dose (MRHD) during organogenesis resulted in reduced fetal body weights. When this dose was continued in pregnancy and during lactation, reduced peripartum and postnatal survival, reductions in body weight gain, and delayed physical development (eye opening and vaginal patency) were observed. A dose 7.9 times the MRHD during organogenesis was associated with increased incidences of cleft palate and a greater percentage of male offspring. No embryotoxicity was observed at 1.2 times the MRHD. No embryotoxicity was observed in rats and rabbits at doses that were <1 and 1.8 times the MRHD, respectively (1).

Solifenacin was not carcinogenic in mice and assays for mutagenicity were negative. The drug also had no effect on male and female fertility, reproductive performance, or early embryonic development in mice at a dose 13 times the MRHD, or in male and female rats at <1 and 1.7 times the MRHD, respectively (1).

It is not known if the solifenacin crosses the human placenta. The molecular weight (about 363 for the free base) and prolonged plasma elimination half-life suggest that the drug and/or its metabolites will cross to the embryo–fetus.

BREASTFEEDING SUMMARY

No reports describing the use of solifenacin during human lactation have been located. The molecular weight (about 363 for the free base) and prolonged plasma elimination half-life suggest that the drug and/or its metabolites will be excreted into breast milk. Although neonates are particularly sensitive to anticholinergics, two other agents in the anticholinergic class are classified by the American Academy of Pediatrics as compatible with breastfeeding (see Atropine and Scopolamine). The effect of solifenacin exposure in a nursing infant is unknown, but the risk of toxicity probably is low.

Reference

1. Product information. Vesicare. Astellas Pharma US, 2007.

SOMATOSTATIN

Pituitary Hormone

PREGNANCY RECOMMENDATION: No Human Data—Probably Compatible
BREASTFEEDING RECOMMENDATION: No Human Data—Probably Compatible

PREGNANCY SUMMARY

No reports describing the use of somatostatin during human pregnancy have been located. (See also Octreotide.)

BREASTFEEDING SUMMARY

No reports describing the use of somatostatin during human lactation have been located. (See also Octreotide.)

SORAFENIB

Antineoplastic (Kinase Inhibitor)

PREGNANCY RECOMMENDATION: Contraindicated
BREASTFEEDING RECOMMENDATION: Contraindicated

S

PREGNANCY SUMMARY

No reports describing the use of sorafenib in human pregnancy have been located. The animal reproduction data suggest risk, but the absence of human pregnancy experience prevents a more complete assessment of embryo–fetal risk. It should be noted, though, that sorafenib inhibits angiogenesis, a critical component of embryonic and fetal development. The manufacturer recommends that adequate contraception should be used during therapy and for at 2 weeks after completing therapy (1). However, renal cell carcinoma can be fatal, so if a woman requires sorafenib and informed consent is obtained, treatment should not be withheld because of pregnancy. If an inadvertent pregnancy occurs, the woman should be advised of the potential risk for severe adverse effects in the embryo and fetus.

FETAL RISK SUMMARY

Sorafenib is an oral multikinase inhibitor that decreases tumor cell proliferation, probably by reducing angiogenesis. There are several other antineoplastics in the same subclass (see Appendix). Sorafenib is indicated for the treatment of patients with advanced renal cell carcinoma. The mean plasma elimination half-life is 25–48 hours. After hepatic metabolism, at least eight metabolites have been identified, one of which has activity similar to the parent compound. Plasma protein binding is 99.5% (1).

Reproduction studies have been conducted in rats and rabbits. In these species, doses that were about 0.008 times the AUC in cancer patients taking the recommended human daily dose (RHDD) resulted in postimplantation loss, resorptions, skeletal retardations, and restricted fetal weight. A no-observed-adverse-effect-level (NOAEL) was not determined (1).

Studies for carcinogenicity have not been conducted with sorafenib. The drug was clastogenic, in the presence of metabolic activation, in one test but was not mutagenic or clastogenic in other tests. An intermediate in the manufacturing process that also is present in the final product (<0.15%) was mutagenic when tested independently (1). Specific studies for fertility impairment have not been conducted, but sorafenib does adversely affect male and female reproductive organs. These effects, more pronounced in rats than in mice or dogs, included testicular atrophy and degeneration, oligospermia, degeneration of epididymis, prostate, and seminal vesicles, central necrosis of the corpora lutea, and arrested follicular development at doses that were about 0.3–0.5 times the RHDD (1).

It is not known if sorafenib crosses the human placenta. The molecular weight (433 for the free acid) and the long elimination half-life suggest that the drug will cross to the embryo and/or fetus.

BREASTFEEDING SUMMARY

No reports describing the use of sorafenib during human lactation have been located.

The molecular weight (433 for the free acid) and the long elimination half-life suggest that the drug will be excreted into breast milk. Because it is an acid, if excreted, the milk:plasma ratio should be <1. The effects of this exposure on a nursing infant are unknown, but severe toxicity may occur. In adults, hand–foot skin reaction and rash were the most common adverse events, but diarrhea, hemorrhage, and hypertension were also common.

Reference

1. Product information. Nexavar. Bayer Pharmaceuticals, 2007.

SOTALOL

Antiarrhythmic

PREGNANCY RECOMMENDATION: Human Data Suggest Risk in 2nd and 3rd Trimesters
BREASTFEEDING RECOMMENDATION: Limited Human Data—Potential Toxicity

PREGNANCY SUMMARY

The use of sotalol in gestation appears to be low risk, but the pregnancy experience, especially in the 1st trimester, is limited. Several reviews have examined the use of β-adrenergic blockers in human pregnancy, concluding that these agents are relatively safe for the fetus (1–4). However, some β-blockers may cause intrauterine growth restriction (IUGR) and reduced placental weight, especially those lacking intrinsic sympathomimetic activity (ISA) (i.e., partial agonist). Sotalol has no ISA, but fetal growth restriction has not been reported. Typically, for β-blockers without ISA, continuous treatment beginning early in the 2nd trimester results in the greatest weight reductions, whereas treatment restricted to the 3rd trimester primarily affects only placental weight. IUGR and reduced placental weight may potentially occur with all agents within this class. Although IUGR is a serious concern, the benefits of maternal therapy with β-blockers, in some cases, might outweigh the risks to the fetus and must be judged on a case-by-case basis. Newborns exposed near delivery should be closely observed during the first 24–48 hours for signs and symptoms of β-blockade. Long-term effects of in utero exposure to this class of drugs have not been studied but warrant evaluation.

FETAL RISK SUMMARY

Sotalol is a sympatholytic agent indicated for the treatment of cardiac arrhythmias. The antiarrhythmic action of the drug includes both class II (β-adrenoreceptor blocking) and class III (cardiac action potential duration prolongation) properties. It has also been used for hypertension. Sotalol is a racemic mixture of the *d*- and *l*-isomers. Only the *l*-isomer exhibits β-adrenergic blocking activity (without intrinsic sympathomimetic activity), but both isomers have Class III antiarrhythmic properties (5).

Sotalol was not teratogenic in rats and rabbits given doses 9 and 7 times the maximum recommended human dose based on BSA (MRHD), respectively, during organogenesis. In rabbits, a dose 16 times the MRHD, but not 8 times, resulted in a slight increase in fetal death that was thought to be related to maternal toxicity. Fetal resorptions were observed in rats at 18 times the MRHD, but not at 2.5 times (6).

In a 1996 study, the embryotoxicity of *d*-sotalol in rats was shown to be related to gestational age and resulted from dose-dependent bradycardia in in vitro (rat embryo culture) and in vivo (pregnant rat) experiments (7). In embryo cultures, the minimum effective concentration (15 mcg/mL) for causing significant bradycardia was about five times the human therapeutic plasma concentration (3 mcg/mL) achieved in pregnant women after a 400-mg oral dose. In nine pregnant rats, a single oral dose (1000 mg/kg) was administered on gestational day 13. No malformations were observed, but a resorption rate of almost 14% was noted (7).

The pharmacokinetics of sotalol in the 3rd trimester (32–36 weeks' gestation) of pregnancy and in the postpartum (at 6 weeks) period was reported in 1983 (8).

Sotalol crosses the placenta to the fetus (9–13). Twelve hypertensive pregnant women were prescribed sotalol (final daily dose 200–800 mg) beginning at 10–31 weeks' gestation (9). The mean gestational age at delivery was 37.7 weeks (range 32–40 weeks). The mean maternal plasma concentration of sotalol at delivery was 1.8 mcg/mL, nearly identical to the mean umbilical cord plasma level of 1.7 mcg/mL. In six women, the mean amniotic fluid concentration of sotalol was 7.0 mcg/mL. No data were provided on the time interval between the last sotalol dose and the collection of plasma samples (9). In a second study, eight women scheduled for elective cesarean section were given 80 mg of the drug orally 3 hours before the procedure (10). The mean maternal concentration of sotalol at surgery was 0.68 mcg/mL, compared with the mean umbilical vein concentration of 0.32 mcg/mL, a fetal:maternal ratio of 0.47 (10). A 1990 report described the use of sotalol, 80 mg twice daily, in one woman throughout gestation (11). A cesarean section was performed at approximately 37 weeks' gestation, 11 hours after the last dose. Maternal plasma and umbilical cord sotalol concentrations were 0.95 and 1.35 mcg/mL, respectively, a ratio of 1.42 (11). Maternal and cord serum concentrations of sotalol at delivery from a woman treated with 80 mg three times daily throughout a 42 weeks' gestation were 0.77 and 0.65 mcg/mL (fetal:maternal ratio 0.84), respectively (12).

A 2003 study reported the use of sotalol in 18 pregnancies with fetal arrhythmias (9 with atrial flutter and 9 with supraventricular tachycardia [SVT]) (13). In the 17 surviving fetuses, one died, the mean birth weight was 3266 g. The mean fetal:maternal sotalol plasma concentration ratio was 1.1, and the mean amniotic fluid:fetal blood ratio was 3.2. These results suggested that sotalol accumulated in the amniotic fluid, but not in the fetus. In addition, there was no correlation between the effectiveness of sotalol therapy and maternal blood levels (13).

Sotalol was used in 12 pregnant women for the treatment of hypertension (details above) (9). No fetal adverse effects attributable to the drug were observed, but bradycardia (90–110 beats/minute), lasting up to 24 hours, was discovered in five of the six newborns with continuous heart rate monitoring (9). In a 1987 report, sotalol, in increasing doses up to 480 mg/day during a 12-day period, was combined with digoxin beginning at 31 weeks' gestation in an unsuccessful attempt to treat a hydropic fetus with SVT (14). Therapy was eventually changed to amiodarone plus digoxin with return of a normal fetal heart rate and resolution of the fetal edema. A normal infant was delivered at 38 weeks' gestation who was alive and well at 10 months of age (14).

A 23-year-old woman was treated throughout gestation with sotalol and flecainide for bursts of ventricular tachycardia (VT) and polymorphous ventricular premature complexes associated with an aneurysm of the left ventricle (11). A normal infant was delivered at approximately 37 weeks' gestation by cesarean section. No adverse effects of drug exposure, including bradycardia, were noted in the newborn, which was growing normally at 1 year of age (11).

A 1998 retrospective study reported the use of oral sotalol after the use of digoxin in 14 cases of fetal SVT (15). Treatment occurred at a median 28 weeks' gestation (range 24–36 weeks) with a median duration of 5 weeks (range 2–11 weeks). Two fetuses did not respond and two severely hydropic fetuses died 1 and 10 days, respectively, after starting sotalol. Of the surviving infants, 11 were doing well and 1 had cerebral atrophy, hypotonia, and developmental delay thought to be due to the arrhythmia and a thromboembolism (15).

A 2000 retrospective study evaluated the use of sotalol for fetal tachycardia in 21 pregnant women (16). The fetal arrhythmias were atrial flutter (AF) (N = 10), SVT (N = 10), and VT (N = 1). Hydrops fetalis was present in nine fetuses. Sinus rhythm was established in eight fetuses with AF and six with SVT, but four deaths (19%) occurred (one with AF and three with SVT). Two newborns (one each with AF and SVT), both successfully converted to a sinus rhythm in utero, had significant neurological morbidity consisting of intracranial hemorrhage in one and cerebral hypoxic ischemia in the other. The authors concluded that sotalol was effective in AF, but the mortality and low conversion rate in fetuses with SVT indicated that the risks of sotalol outweighed the benefits in this group (16).

BREASTFEEDING SUMMARY

Sotalol is concentrated in human milk with milk levels three to five times those in the mother's plasma (9,11,12). Twenty paired samples of breast milk and maternal blood were obtained from 5 of the 12 women treated during and after pregnancy with sotalol for hypertension (dosage detailed above) (9). Specific details of dosage and the timing of sample collection in relationship to the last dose were not given. The mean concentrations in milk and plasma were 10.5 mcg/mL (range 4.8–20.2 mcg/mL) and 2.3 mcg/mL (range 0.8–5.0 mcg/mL), respectively. The mean milk:plasma ratio was 5.4 (range 2.2–8.8). No β-blockade effects were observed in the five nursing infants, including the one infant who had bradycardia at birth. The mother of this infant produced the highest concentrations of sotalol in milk (20.2 mcg/ mL) observed in the study (9).

A woman treated throughout gestation with sotalol (80 mg twice daily) and flecainide was continued on these drugs during the postpartum period (11). The infant was not breastfed. Simultaneous milk and plasma samples were drawn 3 hours after the second dose of the day on the 5th and 7th postpartum days. The milk and plasma concentrations on day 5 were 5 and 1.4 mcg/mL, respectively, compared with 4.4 and 1.60 mcg/mL, respectively, on day 7. The two milk:plasma ratios were 3.57 and 2.75, respectively (11).

Sotalol, 80 mg three times daily, was taken by a woman throughout a 42 weeks' gestation and during the first 14 days of the postpartum period, at which time the dose was reduced to 80 mg twice daily (12). On the 5th postpartum day, milk and serum levels, approximately 6.5 hours after a dose (prefeeding), were 4.06 and 0.72 mcg/mL, respectively, a ratio of 5.6. A postfeeding milk sample collected 0.7 hour later yielded a concentration of 3.65 mcg/mL. The study was repeated on the 105th postpartum day, yielding prefeeding milk and serum concentrations 2.8 hours after the last dose of 2.36 and 0.97 mcg/mL (ratio 2.4), respectively. A postfeeding milk level 0.5 hour later was 3.16 mcg/mL. The infant was consuming about 20%–23% of the maternal dose. No adverse effects were observed in the infant, who continued to develop normally throughout the study period (12).

Although symptoms of β-blockade, such as bradycardia and hypotension, were not observed in the nursing infants described above, these effects have been noted with other β-adrenergic blockers (see also Acebutolol, Atenolol, and Nadolol) and may occur with sotalol. Long-term effects of exposure to β-blockers from milk have not been studied but warrant evaluation. The American Academy of Pediatrics classifies sotalol as compatible with breastfeeding (17).

References

1. Tamari I, Eldar M, Rabinowitz B, Neufeld HN. Medical treatment of cardiovascular disorders during pregnancy. Am Heart J 1982;104:1357–63.
2. Rotmensch HH, Elkayam U, Frishman W. Antiarrhythmic drug therapy during pregnancy. Ann Intern Med 1983;98:487–97.
3. Sandstrom B. Clinical trials of adrenergic antagonists in pregnancy hypertension. Acta Obstet Gynecol Scand 1984;Suppl 118:57–60.
4. Lubbe WF. Treatment of hypertension in pregnancy. J Cardiovasc Pharmacol 1990;16(Suppl 7):S110–3.
5. American Hospital Formulary Service. *Drug Information 2000*. Bethesda, MD: American Society of Health-System Pharmacists, 2000:1596–600.
6. Product information. Betapace. Berlex Laboratories, 2001.
7. Webster WS, Brown-Woodman PDC, Snow MD, Danielsson BRG. Teratogenic potential of almokalant, dofetilide, and d-sotalol: drugs with potassium channel blocking activity. Teratology 1996;53:168–75.
8. O'Hare MF, Leahey W, Murnaghan GA, McDevitt DG. Pharmacokinetics of sotalol during pregnancy. Eur J Clin Pharmacol 1983;24:521–4.
9. O'Hare MF, Murnaghan GA, Russell CJ, Leahey WJ, Varma MPS, McDevitt DG. Sotalol as a hypotensive agent in pregnancy. Br J Obstet Gynaecol 1980;87:814–20.
10. Erkkola R, Lammintausta R, Liukko P, Anttila M. Transfer of propranolol and sotalol across the human placenta. Their effect on maternal and fetal plasma renin activity. Acta Obstet Gynecol Scand 1982;61:31–4.
11. Wagner X, Jouglard J, Moulin M, Miller AM, Petitjean J, Pisapia A. Coadministration of flecainide acetate and sotalol during pregnancy: lack of teratogenic effects, passage across the placenta, and excretion in human breast milk. Am Heart J 1990;119:700–2.
12. Hackett LP, Wojnar-Horton RE, Dusci LJ, Ilett KF, Roberts MJ. Excretion of sotalol in breast milk. Br J Clin Pharmacol 1990;29:277–8.
13. Oudijk MA, Ruskamp JM, Ververs FFT, Ambachtsheer EB, Stoutenbeek P, Visser GHA, Meijboom EJ. Treatment of fetal tachycardia with sotalol: transplacental pharmacokinetics and pharmacodynamics. J Am Coll Cardiol 2003;42:765–70.
14. Arnoux P, Seyral P, Llurens M, Djiane P, Potier A, Unal D, Cano JP, Serradimigni A, Rouault F. Amiodarone and digoxin for refractory fetal tachycardia. Am J Cardiol 1987;59:166–7.
15. Sonesson SE, Fouron JC, Wesslen-Eriksson E, Jaeggi E, Winberg P. Foetal supraventricular tachycardia treated with sotalol. Acta Paediatr 1998;87:584–7.
16. Oudijk MA, Michon MM, Kleinman CS, Kapusta L, Stoutenbeek P, Visser GHA, Meijboom EJ. Sotalol in the treatment of fetal dysrhythmias. Circulation 2000;101:2721–6.
17. Committee on Drugs, American Academy of Pediatrics. The transfer of drugs and other chemicals into human milk. Pediatrics 2001;108:776–89.

SPARFLOXACIN

[Withdrawn from the market. See 9th edition.]

SPECTINOMYCIN

[Withdrawn from the market. See 9th edition.]

SPINOSAD

Dermatological (Pediculicide)

PREGNANCY RECOMMENDATION: No Human Data—Probably Compatible
BREASTFEEDING RECOMMENDATION: No Human Data—Probably Compatible

PREGNANCY SUMMARY

No reports describing the use of spinosad in human pregnancy have been located. The animal reproduction is not relevant because oral doses were used and the drug is given topically in humans. Moreover, topical use of the drug suspension does not produce quantifiable amounts of spinosad in human plasma. Although the suspension contains an unspecified amount of benzyl alcohol, it is doubtful if sufficient amounts of the additive would be absorbed to cause embryo–fetal toxicity.

FETAL RISK SUMMARY

Spinosad is a pediculicide that is available as a suspension. It is indicated for the topical treatment of head lice infestations in patients 4 years or age or older. The drug has not been detected in the plasma (limit of quantitation 3 ng/mL) after topical use. The suspension contains a nonspecified amount of benzyl alcohol; plasma concentrations of this agent from use of the suspension have not been determined (1). (See also Benzyl Alcohol.)

Reproduction studies have been conducted in rats and rabbits. In these species, oral doses of 10–200 mg/kg/day given during organogenesis resulted in no teratogenic effects, but maternal toxicity was noted in rats at 200 mg/kg/day and, in rabbits, at 50 mg/kg/day. A two-generation dietary reproduction studied was performed in male and female rats with oral doses of 3–100 mg/kg/day from 10 to 12 weeks before mating and throughout mating, parturition, and lactation. No reproductive or developmental toxicity was observed up to 10 mg/kg/day. The 100 mg/kg/day dose was maternal toxic and adverse effects noted were increased dystocia in parturition, decreased gestation survival, litter size, pup body weight, and neonatal survival (1). Comparisons with the human dose were not specified in any of these studies probably because plasma concentrations after topical use are below the level of quantification.

Two other published studies examining the effects in rats and rabbits from oral spinosad found results similar to those noted above (2,3).

Long-term carcinogenesis studies in mice and rats with oral spinosad were negative. Various assays for mutagenic or clastogenic potential also were negative. No effects of fertility were noted in rats (1).

It is not known if spinosad crosses the human placenta. Clinically significant exposure of the embryo–fetus is not expected because plasma concentrations of the drug after topical use are below the level of quantification.

BREASTFEEDING SUMMARY

No reports describing the use of spinosad during human lactation have been located. However, excretion of clinically significant amounts of the drug into breast milk is unlikely because plasma concentrations of the drug after topical use are below the level of quantification. Although an unspecified amount of benzyl alcohol also is present in the circulation, it is doubtful if sufficient amounts of the additive would be absorbed to cause toxicity in a nursing infant. Thus, use of the drug during breastfeeding appears to be compatible.

References

1. Product information. Natroba. ParaPRO and Pernix Therapeutics, 2011.
2. Breslin WJ, Marty MS, Vedula U, Liberacki AB, Yano BL. Developmental toxicity of spinosad administered by gavage to CD® rats and New Zealand white rabbits. Food Chem Toxicol 2000;38:1103–12.
3. Hanley Jr TR, Breslin WJ, Quast JF, Carney EW. Evaluation of spinosad in a two-generation dietary reproduction study using Sprague-Dawley rats. Toxicol Sci 2002;67:144–52.

SPIRAMYCIN

[Withdrawn from the market. See 9th edition.]

SPIRONOLACTONE

Diuretic

PREGNANCY RECOMMENDATION: Limited Human Data—Animal Data Suggest Risk
BREASTFEEDING RECOMMENDATION: Limited Human Data—Probably Compatible

PREGNANCY SUMMARY

No reports linking spironolactone with human congenital defects have been located. Some have commented, however, that spironolactone may be contraindicated during pregnancy based on the known anti-androgenic effects in humans and the feminization observed in male rat fetuses (1). Other investigators consider diuretics in general to be contraindicated in pregnancy, except for patients with cardiovascular disorders, because they do not prevent or alter the course of toxemia and they may decrease placental perfusion (2–4). In general, diuretics are not recommended for the treatment of gestational hypertension because of the maternal hypovolemia characteristic of this disease.

FETAL RISK SUMMARY

Spironolactone is a potassium-conserving diuretic, an action that results from its antagonism of aldosterone in the distal convoluted renal tubule. The diuretic action results in an antihypertensive effect. Spironolactone also has progestational and anti-androgenic activity. The latter activity may result in apparent estrogenic adverse effects in humans (5).

Reproduction studies in mice at 20 mg/kg/day, a dose substantially below the maximum recommended human dose based on BSA (MRHD), revealed no embryo or fetal adverse effects. In rabbits dosed at 20 mg/kg/day (approximately the MRHD), an increased number of resorptions and lower number of live fetuses was observed. Because of spironolactone's anti-androgenic activity, feminization of male rat fetuses occurred at a dose of 200 mg/kg/day administered to the mothers during late embryogenesis and fetal development. In addition, rat offspring of both sexes exposed in utero in late gestation to 50 or 100 mg/kg/day exhibited permanent dose-related changes in their reproductive tracts. It was also noted that spironolactone was tumorigenic in rats (5).

In a surveillance study of Michigan Medicaid recipients involving 229,101 completed pregnancies conducted between 1985 and 1992, 31 newborns had been exposed to spironolactone during the 1st trimester (F. Rosa, personal communication, FDA, 1993). Two (6.5%) major birth defects were observed (one expected), one of which was an oral cleft (none expected). No anomalies were observed in five other categories of defects (cardiovascular defects, spina bifida, polydactyly, limb reduction defects, and hypospadias) for which specific data were available.

BREASTFEEDING SUMMARY

It is not known whether unmetabolized spironolactone is excreted in breast milk. Canrenone, the principal and active metabolite, was excreted with milk:plasma ratios of 0.72 at 2 hours and 0.51 at 14.5 hours (6). These amounts would provide an estimated maximum of 0.2% of the mother's daily dose to the infant (6). The effect on the infant from this ingestion is unknown, but the amounts appear to be clinically insignificant. The American Academy of Pediatrics classifies spironolactone as compatible with breastfeeding (7).

References

1. Messina M, Biffignandi P, Ghiga E, Jeantet MG, Molinatti GM. Possible contraindication of spironolactone during pregnancy. J Endocrinol Invest 1979;2:222.
2. Pitkin RM, Kaminetzky HA, Newton M, Pritchard JA. Maternal nutrition: a selective review of clinical topics. Obstet Gynecol 1972;40:773–85.
3. Lindheimer MD, Katz AI. Sodium and diuretics in pregnancy. N Engl J Med 1973;288:891–4.
4. Christianson R, Page EW. Diuretic drugs and pregnancy. Obstet Gynecol 1976;48:647–52.
5. Product information. Aldactone. G.D. Searle, 2000.
6. Phelps DL, Karim A. Spironolactone: relationship between concentrations of dethioacetylated metabolite in human serum and milk. J Pharm Sci 1977;66:1203.
7. Committee on Drugs, American Academy of Pediatrics. The transfer of drugs and other chemicals into human milk. Pediatrics 2001;108:776–89.

STAVUDINE

Antiviral

PREGNANCY RECOMMENDATION: Compatible—Maternal Benefit >> Embryo/Fetal Risk
BREASTFEEDING RECOMMENDATION: Contraindicated

PREGNANCY SUMMARY

The animal and human data suggest that stavudine represents a low risk to the embryo–fetus. Theoretically, exposure to stavudine at the time of implantation could result in impaired fertility because of embryonic cytotoxicity, but this has not been studied in humans. Stavudine peak serum concentrations achievable in humans with therapeutic doses, however, are in the same range that has been found to inhibit postblastocyst development in mice. Mitochondrial dysfunction in offspring exposed in utero or postnatally to nucleoside reverse transcriptase inhibitors (NRTIs) has been reported (see Lamivudine and Zidovudine), but these findings are controversial and require confirmation. If indicated, the drug should not be withheld because of pregnancy.

FETAL RISK SUMMARY

Stavudine (2′,3′-didehydro-3′-deoxythymidine; d4T) inhibits viral reverse transcriptase and DNA synthesis. It is classified as an NRTI used for the treatment of HIV infection. Its mechanism of action is similar to that of five other nucleoside analogs: abacavir, didanosine, lamivudine, zalcitabine, and zidovudine. Stavudine is converted by intracellular enzymes to the active metabolite, stavudine triphosphate (1).

No evidence of teratogenicity was observed in pregnant rats and rabbits exposed to maximum plasma concentrations up to 399 and 183 times, respectively, of those produced by a human dose of 1 mg/kg/day. A dose-related increase in common skeletal variations, postimplantation loss, and early neonatal mortality was observed in one or both species (1).

Antiretroviral nucleosides have been shown to have a direct dose-related cytotoxic effect on preimplantation mouse embryos. A 1994 report compared this toxicity among zidovudine and three newer compounds, stavudine, didanosine, and zalcitabine (2). Whereas significant inhibition of blastocyst formation occurred with a 1 μmol/L concentration of zidovudine, stavudine and zalcitabine toxicity was not detected until 100 μmol/L, and no toxicity was observed with didanosine up to 100 μmol/L. Moreover, postblastocyst development was severely inhibited in those embryos that did survive exposure to 1 μmol/L zidovudine. As for the other compounds, stavudine, at a concentration of 10 μmol/L (2.24 mcg/mL), inhibited postblastocyst development, but no effect was observed with concentrations up to 100 μmol/L of didanosine or zalcitabine. Although there are no human data, the authors of this study concluded that the three newer agents may be safer than zidovudine to use in early pregnancy.

Similar to other nucleoside analogues, stavudine appears to cross the human placenta by simple diffusion (3). The relatively low molecular weight (about 224) is in agreement with this. Stavudine also crosses the placenta in rats, resulting in a fetal:maternal ratio of approximately 0.5 (1). In near-term macaques, the steady-state fetal:maternal plasma ratio was approximately 0.8 (4). A related study found that zidovudine did not affect the placental transfer of stavudine in macaques (5). However, no reports in animals or humans have been located relating to the placental transfer of stavudine triphosphate (the active metabolite) or to the capability of the placenta or the fetus to metabolize stavudine.

Three experimental in vitro models using perfused human placentas to predict the placental transfer of NRTIs (didanosine, stavudine, zalcitabine, and zidovudine) were described in a 1999 publication (6). For each drug, the predicted fetal:maternal plasma drug concentration ratios at steady state with each of the three models were close to those actually observed in pregnant macaques. Based on these results, the authors concluded that their models would accurately predict the mechanism, relative rate, and the extent of in vivo human placental transfer of NRTIs (6).

The Antiretroviral Pregnancy Registry reported, for the period January 1989 through July 2009, prospective data (reported before the outcomes were known) involving 4702 live births that had been exposed during the 1st trimester to one or more antiretroviral agents (7). Congenital defects were noted in 134, a prevalence of 2.8% (95% confidence interval [CI] 2.4–3.4). In the 6100 live births with earliest exposure in the 2nd/3rd trimesters, there were 153 infants with defects (2.5%, 95% CI 2.1–2.9). The prevalence rates for the two periods did not differ significantly. There were 288 infants with birth defects among 10,803 live births with exposure anytime during pregnancy (2.7%, 95% CI 2.4–3.0). The prevalence rate did not differ significantly from the rate expected in a nonexposed population. There were 962 outcomes exposed to stavudine (771 in the 1st trimester and 191 in the 2nd/3rd trimesters) in combination with other antiretroviral agents. There were 25 birth defects (19 in the 1st trimester and 6 in the 2nd/3rd trimesters). In reviewing the birth defects of prospective and retrospective (pregnancies reported after the outcomes were known) registered cases, the Registry concluded that, except for isolated cases of neural tube defects (NTDs) with efavirenz exposure in retrospective reports, there was no other pattern of anomalies (isolated or syndromic) (7). (See Lamivudine for required statement.)

A 2000 case report described the adverse pregnancy outcomes, including NTDs, of two pregnant women with HIV infection who were treated with the anti-infective combination, trimethoprim/sulfamethoxazole, for prophylaxis against *Pneumocystis carinii*, concurrently with antiretroviral agents (8). Exposure to stavudine occurred in one of these cases. A 31-year-old woman presented at 15 weeks' gestation. She was receiving trimethoprim/sulfamethoxazole, didanosine, stavudine, nevirapine, and vitamin B supplements (specific vitamins and dosage not given) that had been started before conception. A fetal ultrasound at 19 weeks' gestation revealed spina bifida and ventriculomegaly. The patient elected to terminate her pregnancy. The fetus did not have HIV infection. Defects observed at autopsy included ventriculomegaly, an Arnold-Chiari malformation, sacral spina bifida, and a lumbo-sacral meningomyelocele. The authors attributed the NTDs in both cases to the antifolate activity of trimethoprim (8).

A 1999 case report described a 26-year-old woman with a 5-year history of HIV infection (9). Two years before her current pregnancy, she had received monotherapy with zidovudine for 19 months, followed by 6 months of monotherapy with zalcitabine. She stopped therapy during the first 19 gestational weeks, then started stavudine and lamivudine that were continued until vaginal delivery at term of a healthy 3560-g female infant. The infant was not infected with HIV and was doing well at 9 months of age.

No data are available on the advisability of treating pregnant women who have been exposed to HIV via occupational exposure, but one author discourages this use (10).

Two reviews, one in 1996 and the other in 1997, concluded that all women currently receiving antiretroviral therapy should continue to receive therapy during pregnancy and that treatment of the mother with monotherapy should be considered inadequate therapy (11,12). The same conclusion was reached in a 2003 review with the added admonishment that therapy must be continuous to prevent emergence of resistant viral strains (13). In 2009, the updated U.S. Department of Health and Human Services guidelines for the use of antiretroviral agents in HIV type 1 (HIV-1)-infected patients continued the recommendation that therapy, with the exception of efavirenz, should be continued during pregnancy (14). If indicated, stavudine should not be withheld in pregnancy because the expected benefit to the HIV-positive mother outweighs the unknown risk to the fetus. Updated guidelines for the use of antiretroviral drugs to reduce perinatal HIV-1 transmission also were released in 2010 (15). Women receiving antiretroviral therapy during pregnancy should continue the therapy but, regardless of the regimen, zidovudine administration is recommended during the intrapartum period to prevent vertical transmission of HIV to the newborn (15).

BREASTFEEDING SUMMARY

No reports describing the use of stavudine during lactation have been located. The molecular weight (about 224) suggests that stavudine will be excreted into breast milk. The effect of this exposure on a nursing infant is unknown.

Reports on the use of stavudine during human lactation are unlikely because the antiviral agent is used in the treatment of HIV infection. HIV-1 is transmitted in milk, and in developed countries, breastfeeding is not recommended (11,12,14,16–18). In developing countries, breastfeeding is undertaken, despite the risk, because there are no affordable milk substitutes available. Until 1999, no studies had been published that examined the effect of any antiretroviral therapy on HIV-1 transmission in milk. In that year, a study involving zidovudine was published that measured a 38% reduction in vertical transmission of HIV-1 infection despite breastfeeding when compared with controls (see Zidovudine).

References

1. Product Information. Zerit. Bristol-Myers Squibb, 2001.
2. Toltzis P, Mourton T, Magnuson T. Comparative embryonic cytotoxicity of antiretroviral nucleosides. J Infect Dis 1994;169:1100–2.
3. Bawdon RE, Kaul S, Sobhi S. The ex vivo transfer of the anti-HIV nucleoside compound d4T in the human placenta. Gynecol Obstet Invest 1994;38:1–4.
4. Odinecs A, Nosbisch C, Keller RD, Baughman WL, Unadkat JD. In vivo maternal-fetal pharmacokinetics of stavudine (2′,3′-didehydro-3′-deoxythymidine) in pigtailed macaques (*Macaca nemestrina*). Antimicrob Agents Chemother 1996;40:196–202.
5. Odinecs A, Nosbisch C, Unadkat JD. Zidovudine does not affect transplacental transfer or systemic clearance of stavudine (2′,3′-didehydro-3′-doxythymidine) in the pigtailed macaque (*Macaca nemestrina*). Antimicrob Agents Chemother 1996;40:1569–71.
6. Tuntland T, Odinecs A, Pereira CM, Nosbisch C, Unadkat JD. In vitro models to predict the in vivo mechanism, rate, and extent of placental transfer of dideoxynucleoside drugs against human immunodeficiency virus. Am J Obstet Gynecol 1999;180:198–206.
7. Antiretroviral Pregnancy Registry Steering Committee. *Antiretroviral Pregnancy Registry International Interim Report for 1 January 1989 through 31 July 2009.* Wilmington, NC: Registry Coordinating Center; 2009. Available at www.apregistry.com. Accessed May 29, 2010.
8. Richardson MP, Osrin D, Donaghy S, Brown NA, Hay, Sharland M. Spinal malformations in the fetuses of HIV infected women receiving combination antiretroviral therapy and co-trimoxazole. Eur J Obstet Gynecol Reprod Biol 2000;93:215–7.

9. Ristola M, Salo E, Ammala P, Suni J. Combined stavudine and lamivudine during pregnancy. AIDS 1999;13:285.
10. Gerberding JL. Management of occupational exposures to blood-borne viruses. N Engl J Med 1995;332:444–51.
11. Carpenter CCJ, Fischi MA, Hammer SM, Hirsch MS, Jacobsen DM, Katzenstein DA, Montaner JSG, Richman DD, Saag MS, Schooley RT, Thompson MA, Vella S, Yeni PG, Volberding PA. Antiretroviral therapy for HIV infection in 1996. JAMA 1996;276;146–54.
12. Minkoff H, Augenbraun M. Antiretroviral therapy for pregnant women. Am J Obstet Gynecol 1997;176:478–89.
13. Minkoff H. Human immunodeficiency virus infection in pregnancy. Obstet Gynecol 2003;101:797–810.
14. Panel on Antiretroviral Guidelines for Adults and Adolescents. *Guidelines for the Use of Antiretroviral Agents in HIV-1-Infected Adults and Adolescents.* Department of Health and Human Services. December 1, 2009;1–161. Available at http://www.aidsinfo.nih.gov/ContentFiles/AdultandAdolescentGL.pdf. Accessed September 17, 2010:60, 96–8.
15. Panel on Treatment of HIV-Infected Pregnant Women and Prevention of Perinatal Transmission. *Recommendations for Use of Antiretroviral Drugs in Pregnant HIV-1-Infected Women for Maternal Health and Interventions to Reduce Perinatal HIV Transmission in the United States.* May 24, 2010:1–117. Available at http://aidsinfo.nih.gov/ContentFiles/PerinatalGL pdf. Accessed September 17, 2010:30, Table 5.
16. Brown ZA, Watts DH. Antiviral therapy in pregnancy. Clin Obstet Gynecol 1990;33:276–89.
17. De Martino M, Tovo P-A, Tozzi AE, Pezzotti P, Galli L, Livadiotti S, Caselli D, Massironi E, Ruga E, Fioredda F, Plebani A, Gabiano C, Zuccotti GV. HIV-1 transmission through breast-milk: appraisal of risk according to duration of feeding. AIDS 1992;6:991–7.
18. Van de Perre P. Postnatal transmission of human immunodeficiency virus type 1: the breast-feeding dilemma. Am J Obstet Gynecol 1995;173: 483–7.

STEVIA

Dietary Supplement

PREGNANCY RECOMMENDATION: No Human Data—Probably Compatible
BREASTFEEDING RECOMMENDATION: No Human Data—Probably Compatible

PREGNANCY SUMMARY

Although no reports describing the use of stevia during human pregnancy have been located, this dietary supplement is consumed extensively throughout the world. Exposure in pregnancy is inevitable, but the lack of reports prevents a thorough assessment of the embryo–fetal risk. In Brazil, South Korea, and Japan, stevioside and highly refined extracts are routinely used as a low-calorie sweetener (1). Such use in the United States started in 1995 (1). Animal reproduction studies have not shown evidence of developmental toxicity except at very high doses. The benefits of stevioside as a dietary supplement have been listed as its being a stable, noncaloric product that maintains good dental health by reducing the intake of sugar, and can be used by diabetic and phenylketonuria patients (1). Moreover, stevioside, the major sweetening compound in stevia, either is not absorbed into the systemic circulation or the absorption is very low. Information on the other compounds such as the rebaudiosides is lacking. Nevertheless, the moderate use of stevia or stevioside as sweeteners appears to represent a low risk to the embryo–fetus, if it exists at all.

FETAL RISK SUMMARY

The perennial shrub *Stevia rebaudiana* Bertoni (stevia) is indigenous to South America but is grown commercially in areas such as Central America, Israel, Thailand, and China. The leaves have been used as a low-calorie sweetener for hundreds of years. The largest use of stevia appears to be in Japan where it is used to replace aspartame and saccharin (2). Oral stevia is also used as a weight-loss aid; for contraception and lowering uric acid levels; for the treatment of diabetes, hypertension, and heartburn; and as a cardiotonic and diuretic (3).

The sweetness of stevia is mainly due to stevioside, a sweet ent-kaurene glycoside that is 300 times sweeter than sucrose (0.4% solution). There also are several variants of rebaudioside, another ent-kaurene glycoside that is present in lower concentrations. Stevia leaves contain 6%–18% of stevioside. In addition to the glycosides, the leaves contain minor amounts of nonsweet sterols (stigmasterol, beta-sitosterol, and campesterol), vitamins (A, B, and C), electrolytes, minerals, and protein (1,2).

Reproduction and growth studies have been conducted with stevioside in male and female hamsters with daily oral doses up to 2.5 g/kg (4). No abnormalities in growth, fertility, or reproduction performance were observed through three generations. Moreover, histological examination of reproductive tissues revealed no evidence of stevia-induced abnormalities. The investigators briefly cited other studies that observed no toxic effects in mice and rats (4).

In a 2006 study, female rats before mating were given an aqueous extract of various mixtures of *Aegle marmelos* (6%), a Thai medicinal plant popularly consumed as a herbal tea, and stevia (0%–10%) (5). The rats then were mated with untreated males, and the effects on reproduction were examined at day 14 of pregnancy. Compared with untreated controls, there were no significant differences in terms of number of corpus lutea, implanted and dead fetuses, or fetal growth (5).

A 2003 review cited several other animal reproduction studies using stevia extracts that observed no developmental toxicity in chicken embryos, mice, rats, and hamsters (1). There also was no adverse effect on spermatogenesis or interstitial cell proliferation in male rats, except at very high doses.

A 1985 study found that stevioside was not mutagenic in *Salmonella typhimurium*, but that steviol, an aglycone metabolite of stevioside, was mutagenic when it was further

S

metabolized (6). The clinical significance of this toxicity was unknown because the complete metabolic disposition of stevioside in humans had not been fully characterized. A review cited four studies that confirmed the mutagenicity but noted that the mutagenicity activity was low (1). In addition, the presence in blood of the steviol metabolites after feeding of stevioside has not been proven. Moreover, there is no evidence in animals or humans that stevioside is carcinogenic (1).

The pharmacology of stevia in animals and humans has been reviewed (1). The author concluded that the dietary supplement is safe when used as a sweetener. In humans, oral stevioside either is not absorbed or the uptake is extremely low. Even so, the European Commission refused to accept stevia or stevioside as a novel food because of inadequate or controversial studies on its safety (1). For the same reason, the FDA classifies stevia as an "unsafe food additive" (3).

BREASTFEEDING SUMMARY

Although the dietary supplement stevia is used extensively as a natural, low-calorie sweetener, no reports describing its use during lactation have been located. Stevioside, the major sweetening compound in stevia, is either not absorbed into the systemic circulation or the absorption is very low. However, information on the other compounds, such as the rebaudiosides, is lacking. Nevertheless, the risk to the nursing infant from maternal intake of stevia, if it exists, appears to be low.

References

1. Geuns JMC. Stevioside. Phytochemistry 2003;64:913–21.
2. Stevia. In: DerMarderosian A, Beutler JA, eds. *The Review of Natural Products*. St. Louis, MO: Wolters Kluwer Health. July, 2004.
3. Stevia. In: Jellin JM, ed. *Natural Medicines Comprehensive Database*. 10th ed. Stockton, CA: Therapeutic Research Faculty, 2008:1387–8.
4. Yodyingyuad V, Bunyawong S. Effect of stevioside on growth and reproduction. Hum Reprod 1991;6:158–65.
5. Saenphet K, Aritajat S, Saenphet S, Manosroi J, Manosroi A. Safety evaluation of aqueous extracts from *Aegle marmelos* and *Stevia rebaudiana* on reproduction of female rats. Southeast Asian J Trop Med Public Health 2006;37 Suppl 3:203–5.
6. Pezzuto JM, Compadre CM, Swanson SM, Nanayakkara NPD, Kinghorn AD. Metabolically activated steviol, the aglycone of stevioside, is mutagenic. Proc Natl Acad Sci USA 1985;82:2478–82.

ST. JOHN'S WORT

Herb

PREGNANCY RECOMMENDATION: Limited Human Data—Probably Compatible
BREASTFEEDING RECOMMENDATION: Limited Human Data—Potential Toxicity

PREGNANCY SUMMARY

Two reports describing the use of St. John's wort (*Hypericum perforatum*) during human pregnancy have been located. Some of the animal studies apparently did not look for structural defects, but did not observe neurobehavioral deficits. Moreover, no mutagenicity was found with various tests involving mammalian cells. Hypericum has demonstrated human sperm toxicity in vitro, but no reports describing this adverse effect after ingestion of the drug have been located. Similarly, the uterotonic action observed in an in vitro animal experiment has not been reported in animals or humans following consumption. This lack of reported toxicity is reassuring. Moreover, because the use of St. John's wort is widespread and dates back thousands of years, it is doubtful that a major teratogenic action or other developmental toxicity would have escaped notice. More subtle or low-incidence effects, however, including structural and neurobehavioral toxicity, the induction of abortions, and infertility may have escaped detection, and further study is warranted.

FETAL RISK SUMMARY

Hypericum perforatum (St. John's wort) is an aromatic, aggressive perennial weed that is native to Europe but also grows throughout the United States and parts of Canada (1). The plant is harvested for medicinal purposes during July and August (1). A large number of chemical constituents have been isolated from the plant, including hypericin, pseudohypericin, flavonoids, glycosides, phenols, tannins, volatile oils, and other compounds (1–8). Hypericin and pseudohypericin are considered to be the primary orally active ingredients (1,5–8).

Preparations made from *H. perforatum* have been used for medicinal purposes for thousands of years. These uses have included the management of anxiety, depression, insomnia, inflammation, and gastritis. They have also been used as a diuretic and, topically, for the treatment of hemorrhoids and to enhance wound healing (1–5). More recently, hypericin has been investigated for activity against the HIV and other viruses (1,5,8). In addition, extracts and tinctures of hypericum have shown activity against gram-negative and gram-positive bacteria (1).

No data are available on the animal or human placental transfer of hypericin, pseudohypericin, or other constituents of St. John's wort.

The mechanism of antidepressant action is thought to be related to selected serotonin-reuptake inhibition, monoamine oxidase inhibitors, a combination of both, or other mechanisms (1–4,6–9). Adverse effects induced by hypericum preparations, relatively infrequent in nonpregnant humans but not studied in pregnant women, include gastrointestinal upset and constipation, allergic reactions, fatigue, dry mouth, dizziness, and confusion (1–10). Rare photosensitivity in fair-skinned individuals has also been observed.

Surprisingly, for a product that has been in use since ancient Greek and Roman times, only two reports have been located that described its consumption during human pregnancy (see below). Moreover, there are few animal reproductive studies available for evaluation of its embryo and fetal safety. Aqueous extractions of *H. perforatum* demonstrated weak uterine tonus-enhancing activity in experiments using isolated rabbit and guinea pig uterine horns (11). Uterotonic activity or abortions, however, have apparently not been reported after consumption of the herb by animals or humans.

In a randomized, placebo-controlled reproductive study, adult female mice were fed either hypericum (180 mg/kg/day) or placebo for 2 weeks before mating and then throughout gestation (12). The dose, which has antidepressant efficacy in adult mice, was equivalent to the human dose on a kg/ m^2 basis (12,13). The birth weights of all exposed pups were smaller than controls, but only the reduced birth weights of male pups reached statistical significance in comparison to controls (1.68 vs. 1.75 g, $p < 0.01$) (13). Moreover, successful performance on the negative geotaxis task, a measure of behavior during early development, was significantly lower in the exposed male pups (but not the female pups) on postnatal day 3 (13). Both the body weight and the negative geotaxis task performance were comparable to controls by postnatal day 5 (13). No differences, regardless of gender, were observed between the exposed and nonexposed pups in body length, head circumference, sexual maturation, or the attainment of developmental milestones up to adulthood (12). Similarly, no differences were observed between the groups in pup–dam interactions, performance of locomotor, depression, and anxiety tasks during juvenile and adult periods, or in male sexual behavior and aggression. An evaluation of second-generation offspring found no differences between the groups in any measurement (12,13).

An aqueous ethanolic extract of hypericum was tested for mutagenic activity in a study published in 1990 (14). Using both in vitro and in vivo test systems (mice, hamsters, etc.), no evidence of mutagenic effects was observed.

In a sperm penetration assay, zona-free hamster oocytes were incubated for 1 hour with two concentrations of *H. perforatum*, 0.06 and 0.6 mg/mL, dissolved in HEPES-buffered synthetic human tubal fluid (modified HTF) (15). Fresh human donor sperm was suspended in the modified HTF and then mixed with the oocytes for 3 hours. Modified HTF served as the control. At the 0.06 mg/mL concentration, all the oocytes were penetrated, whereas at 0.6 mg/mL, zero penetration occurred. The decrease in penetration was not associated with a decrease in sperm motility (15). In the second part of the study, sperms were incubated with the herbal solutions for 7 days (15). Both concentrations caused significant sperm DNA denaturation concomitant with decreases in sperm viability compared with controls. The higher concentration showed point mutation of a selected sperm sentinel gene, the BRCA1 exon 11 gene (15). Extrapolation of these data to the reproductive risk of hypericum in males is difficult, in part because the concentration of hypericum in semen or sperm has not been studied (15). Moreover, although the doses used in this study are small fractions of the actual recommended human dose, usually expressed in grams of hypericin, there is no published evidence that the adverse effects observed have occurred in vivo.

Hypericum or placebo was given to mice 2 weeks before mating and throughout gestation (16). No differences between the groups were noted in gestational ages at birth and litter sizes. Offspring were followed from postnatal day 3 to adulthood. No differences between the groups were found in the increases of body weight and length, and head circumference, or in the times to reach physical milestones. There also was no effect on reproductive capability, perinatal outcomes, and growth and development of the second-generation offspring (16).

A brief 1998 case report described the use of St. John's wort by two pregnant women, but only one of the cases has outcome data (17). In the first case, a 38-year-old woman began taking St. John's wort, 900 mg/day, at 24 weeks' gestation for a major depressive disorder that had recurred during the 1st trimester. She continued the herbal medicine throughout the remainder of her pregnancy, taking her last dose 24 hours before delivery (gestational age not specified). Other than late-onset thrombocytopenia (platelet count 88,000), the pregnancy was unremarkable. The woman delivered a healthy, about 3400-g female infant with Apgar scores of 9 and 9 at 1 and 5 minutes. The physical examination and laboratory results were normal. Neonatal jaundice developed on day 5 but responded to brief phototherapy. Behavioral assessment at 4 and 33 days of age was normal. The second case involved a 43-year-old woman who had been taking fluoxetine and methylphenidate for a recurrent major depressive disorder (16). After an unexpected conception, she discontinued these medications because of concerns about potential adverse fetal effects and began self-medicating with St. John's wort, 900 mg/day. Apparently, this pregnancy was ongoing, because no outcome data were presented (17).

A 2009 study assessed the effects of the herb in pregnancy using a prospective, observational, controlled cohort design (18). Samples and controls were women who had contacted the Motherisk Program, a teratogen information service in Canada. The study group was 54 St. John's wort–exposed pregnancies, 39 (72%) of whom were taking the herb for depression. The two matched control groups included 56 women taking other agents for depression (disease comparator) and 56 healthy women not exposed to any known teratogens (healthy group). There was no statistical difference in the rates of major malformations in the three groups, 5%, 4%, and 0%, respectively. None of the other pregnancy outcomes differed statistically among the three groups. Although both the subject and disease comparator groups had higher rates of spontaneous abortions (SABs) than healthy controls (20.3% vs 12.5% vs 8.9% [*ns*], respectively) the authors cited references that women with depression had increased rates of SABs. Because the authors did not examine the offspring, the study could not determine if minor malformations were present (18).

Because standardization of any herbal product as to its constituents, concentrations, and the presence of contaminants is generally lacking, consumption of these preparations during pregnancy may result in fetal exposure to unintended chemicals and doses. Furthermore, pregnant women should be counseled on the risks to themselves and their pregnancies that may result from self-medication or discontinuing prescribed therapy without first consulting their healthcare provider.

BREASTFEEDING SUMMARY

One report describing the use of St. John's wort during human lactation has been located. A 38-year-old mother had taken 900 mg/day of St. John's wort from 24 weeks' gestation until delivery (16). (See case above.) She began breastfeeding her female infant after delivery and then resumed taking the herbal product 20 days after delivery. Neonatal jaundice was noted at 5 days of age but responded to brief phototherapy. Behavioral assessments of the nursing infant at 4 and 33 days of age were normal.

It is not known if any of the constituents and possible contaminants that may be found in preparations of St. John's wort are excreted into human milk or if exposure to them via the milk represents a risk to a nursing infant.

References

1. St. John's Wort. In: *The Review of Natural Products*. St. Louis, MO: Facts and Comparisons, November 1997.
2. Chavez ML, Chavez PI. Saint John's' wort. Hosp Pharm 1997;32:1621–32.
3. Miller LG. Herbal medicinals. Selected clinical considerations focusing on known or potential drug–herb interactions. Arch Intern Med 1998;158:2200–11.
4. Klepser TB, Klepser ME. Unsafe and potentially safe herbal therapies. Am J Health-Syst Pharm 1999;56:125–38.
5. Pepping J. St. Alternative therapies. St. John's wort: *Hypericum perforatum*. Am J Health-Syst Pharm 1999;56:329.
6. Wong AHC, Smith M, Boon HS. Herbal remedies in psychiatric practice. Arch Gen Psychiatry 1998;55:1033–44.
7. Bennett DA Jr, Phun L, Polk JF, Voglino SA, Zlotnik V, Raffa RB. Neuropharmacology of St. John's wort (*Hypericum*). Ann Pharmacother 1998;32:1201–8.
8. Cupp MJ. Herbal remedies: adverse effects and drug interactions. Am Fam Physician 1999;59:1239–44.
9. Zink T, Chaffin J. Herbal 'health' products: what family physicians need to know. Am Fam Physician 1998;58:1133–40.
10. Linde K, Ramirez G, Mulrow CD, Pauls A, Weidenhammer W, Melchart D. St. John's wort for depression—an overview and meta-analysis of randomised clinical trials. Br Med J 1996;313:253–8.
11. Shipochliev T. Uterotonic action of extracts from a group of medicinal plants. Vet Med Nauki. 1981;18:94–8.
12. Christensen HD, Rayburn WF, Coleman FH, Gonzalez CL. Effect of antenatal hypericum (St. John's wort) on growth and physical development of mice offspring (abstract). Teratology 1999;59:411.
13. Rayburn WF, Christensen HD, Gonzalez CL. Effect of antenatal exposure to Saint John's wort (*Hypericum*) on neurobehavior of developing mice. Am J Obstet Gynecol 2000;183:1225–31.
14. Okpanyi SN, Lidsba H, Scholl BC, Miltenburger HG. Genotoxicity of a standardized hypericum extract. Arzneimittel-Forschung 1990;40:851–5.
15. Ondrizek RR, Chan PJ, Patton WC, King A. An alternative medicine study of herbal effects on the penetration of zona-free hamster oocytes and the integrity of sperm deoxyribonucleic acid. Fertil Steril 1999; 71:517–22.
16. Rayburn WF, Gonzalez CL, Christensen HD, Stewart JD. Effect of prenatally administered hypericum (St John's wort) on growth and physical maturation of mouse offspring. Am J Obstet Gynecol 2001; 184:191–5.
17. Grush LR, Nierenberg A, Keefe B, Cohen LS. St. John's wort during pregnancy. JAMA 1998;280:1566.
18. Moretti ME, Maxson A, Hanna F, Koren G. Evaluating the safety of St. John's wort in human pregnancy. Reprod Toxicol 2009;28:96–9.

STREPTOKINASE

[Withdrawn from the market. See 9th edition.]

STREPTOMYCIN

Antibiotic (Aminoglycoside)

PREGNANCY RECOMMENDATION: Human Data Suggest Risk
BREASTFEEDING RECOMMENDATION: Compatible

PREGNANCY SUMMARY

Streptomycin may cause fetal ototoxicity, resulting in deafness in newborns. The risk of this toxicity is low if there is appropriate dose monitoring and the duration of fetal exposure is limited.

FETAL RISK SUMMARY

Streptomycin is an aminoglycoside antibiotic. The drug rapidly crosses the placenta into the fetal circulation and amniotic fluid, obtaining concentrations that are usually less than 50% of the maternal serum level (1,2). Early investigators, well aware of streptomycin-induced ototoxicity, were unable to observe this defect in infants exposed in utero to the agent (3–5). Eventually, ototoxicity was described in a 2-1/2-month-old infant whose mother had been treated for tuberculosis with 30 g of streptomycin during the last month of pregnancy (6). The infant was deaf with a negative cochleopalpebral reflex. Several other case reports and small surveys describing similar toxicity followed this initial report (7,8). In general, however, the incidence of congenital ototoxicity, cochlear or vestibular, from streptomycin is low, especially with careful dosage calculations and if the duration of fetal exposure is limited (9).

Except for eighth cranial nerve damage, no reports of congenital defects caused by streptomycin have been located. The Collaborative Perinatal Project monitored 50,282 mother–child pairs, 135 of whom had 1st trimester exposure to streptomycin (10, pp. 297–301). For use anytime during pregnancy, 355 exposures were recorded (10, p. 435). In neither group was evidence found to suggest a relationship to large categories of major or minor malformations or to individual defects.

In a group of 1619 newborns whose mothers were treated for tuberculosis during pregnancy with multiple drugs, including streptomycin, the incidence of congenital defects was the same as in a healthy control group (2.34% vs. 2.56%) (11). Other investigators had previously concluded that the use of streptomycin in pregnant tuberculosis patients was not teratogenic (12).

The population-based data set of the Hungarian Case-Control Surveillance of Congenital Abnormalities, covering the period of 1980–1996, was used to evaluate the teratogenicity of aminoglycoside antibiotics (parenteral gentamicin, streptomycin, tobramycin, and oral neomycin) in a study published in 2000 (13). A case group of 22,865 women who had fetuses or newborns with congenital malformations were compared with 38,151 women who had no newborns with structural defects. A total of 38 cases and 42 controls were treated with the aminoglycosides. There was one case, but no controls, treated with streptomycin (odds ratio 5.0, 95% confidence interval 0.2–122.9). The investigators concluded that there was no detectable teratogenic risk for structural defects for any of the aminoglycoside antibiotics (13). They also concluded, although it was not investigated in this study, that the risk of deafness after in utero aminoglycoside exposure was small.

BREASTFEEDING SUMMARY

Streptomycin is excreted into breast milk. Milk:plasma ratios of 0.5–1.0 have been reported (14). Because the oral absorption of this antibiotic is poor, ototoxicity in the infant would not be expected. However, three potential problems exist for the nursing infant: modification of bowel flora, direct effects on the infant, and interference with the interpretation of culture results if a fever workup is required. The American Academy of Pediatrics classifies streptomycin as compatible with breastfeeding (15).

References

1. Woltz J, Wiley M. Transmission of streptomycin from maternal blood to the fetal circulation and the amniotic fluid. Proc Soc Exp Biol Med 1945;60:106–7.
2. Heilman D, Heilman F, Hinshaw H, Nichols D, Herrell W. Streptomycin: absorption, diffusion, excretion and toxicity. Am J Med Sci 1945;210: 576–84.
3. Watson E, Stow R. Streptomycin therapy: effects on fetus. JAMA 1948;137:1599–1600.
4. Rubin A, Winston J, Rutledge M. Effects of streptomycin upon the human fetus. Am J Dis Child 1951;82:14–6.
5. Kistner R. The use of streptomycin during pregnancy. Am J Obstet Gynecol 1950;60:422–6.
6. Leroux M. Existe-t-il une surdité congénitale acquise due à la streptomycine? Ann Otolaryngol 1950;67:194–6.
7. Nishimura H, Tanimura T. *Clinical Aspects of the Teratogenicity of Drugs*. New York, NY: Excerpta Medica, 1976:130.
8. Donald PR, Sellars SL. Streptomycin ototoxicity in the unborn child. S Afr Med J 1981;60:316–8.
9. Mann J, Moskowitz R. Plaque and pregnancy. A case report. JAMA 1977;237:1854–5.
10. Heinonen OP, Slone D, Shapiro S. *Birth Defects and Drugs in Pregnancy*. Littleton, MA:Publishing Sciences Group, 1977.
11. Marynowski A, Sianozecka E. Comparison of the incidence of congenital malformations in neonates from healthy mothers and from patients treated because of tuberculosis. Ginekol Pol 1972;43:713–5.
12. Lowe C. Congenital defects among children born under supervision or treatment for pulmonary tuberculosis. Br J Prev Soc Med 1964;18:14–6.
13. Czeizel AE, Rockenbauer M, Olsen J, Sorensen HT. A teratological study of aminoglycoside antibiotic treatment during pregnancy. Scand J Infect Dis 2000;32:309–13.
14. Wilson JT. Milk/plasma ratios and contraindicated drugs. In: Wilson JT, ed. *Drugs in Breast Milk*. Balgowlah, Australia: ADIS Press, 1981:79.
15. Committee on Drugs, American Academy of Pediatrics. The transfer of drugs and other chemicals into human milk. Pediatrics 2001;108:776–89.

STREPTOZOCIN

Antineoplastic

PREGNANCY RECOMMENDATION: Limited Human Data—Animal Data Suggest Risk
BREASTFEEDING RECOMMENDATION: Contraindicated

PREGNANCY SUMMARY

Streptozocin is teratogenic or embryotoxic in several animal species and possesses mutagenic and carcinogenic effects. The potential for human embryo–fetal injury is a concern, but because the animal reproduction data lacks dosage and time of exposure information and other data, the degree of risk is unknown. One report has described the use of this drug during the latter half of gestation without apparent fetal harm. Until additional data are forthcoming, streptozocin should be considered a potential human teratogen if exposure occurs during organogenesis.

FETAL RISK SUMMARY

Streptozocin (streptozotocin) is an alkylating antineoplastic that is obtained from *Streptomyces achromogenes*. This nitrosourea agent belongs to the same group as carmustine (BCNU) and lomustine (CCNU). Streptozocin is indicated for the treatment of metastatic islet cell carcinoma of the pancreas and also is used in other cancers. It is rapidly cleared from the plasma and is distributed to tissues, primarily the kidneys, liver, intestines, and pancreas (1,2). Streptozocin undergoes extensive metabolism and, although it does not cross the blood–brain barrier, its metabolites are found in the cerebrospinal fluid (CSF) (1).

Streptozocin is mutagenic in bacteria, plants, and mammalian cells and is carcinogenic (renal, hepatic, stomach, and pancreatic tumors) in various animal species such as mice, rats, and hamsters (2). The drug also is diabetogenic in laboratory animals (3).

Reproduction studies with streptozocin have been conducted in pregnant rats and rabbits. Although the doses and administration times were not specified, streptozocin was teratogenic (types of defects not specified) in rats and had abortifacient effects in rabbits (2). No mention was made of maternal toxicity in these studies.

Studies investigating the passage of streptozocin across the human placenta have not been located. The molecular weight (about 265) is low enough that exposure of the embryo or fetus should be expected. Moreover, in pregnant monkeys administered IV streptozocin, the agent appeared rapidly in the fetal circulation (2). However, the rapid clearance from the blood and the absence of the parent drug in the CSF suggest that the amount crossing the placenta, at least of unmetabolized drug, will be limited.

A 1984 report described a 21-year-old woman with diffuse histiocytic lymphoma treated before pregnancy with multiple courses of chemotherapy including cyclophosphamide, doxorubicin, vincristine, bleomycin, methotrexate, cytarabine, and etoposide, in addition to radiation therapy to the neck (4). Because of the failure of that therapy, she was changed to carmustine and procarbazine for 5 months before conception. The patient refused to terminate her pregnancy, and treatment with carmustine and procarbazine was continued during the first 24 weeks of pregnancy. Because of disease progression, her therapy was changed at 24 weeks' gestation to three courses of streptozocin, 800 mg IV/day for 3 days every 4 weeks. The last course was administered 2 weeks before delivery at 35 weeks' gestation. The normal-appearing male infant weighed 2.34 kg with a head circumference of 32.5 cm and a length of 51.5 cm. The Apgar scores were 7 and 9 at 1 and 5 minutes, respectively. Initial tests revealed normal hemoglobin, and white blood cell and platelet counts. All other clinical tests were within normal limits, including electrolytes, multiple chemistry, urinalysis, renal ultrasound, and chromosome studies (2).

BREASTFEEDING SUMMARY

No reports describing the use of streptozocin during human lactation have been located. The molecular weight (about 265) suggests that the drug will be excreted in breast milk. The effects of this exposure on a nursing infant are unknown. Because of the potential for serious toxicity, women receiving streptozocin should not nurse.

References

1. Parfitt K, ed. *Martindale: The Complete Drug Reference*. 32nd ed. London, UK: Pharmaceutical Press, 1999:562.
2. Product information. Zanosar. Pharmacia & Upjohn, 2000.
3. Schein PS, Winokur SH. Immunosuppressive and cytotoxic chemotherapy: long-term complications. Ann Intern Med 1975;82:84–95.
4. Schapira DV, Chudley AE. Successful pregnancy following continuous treatment with combination chemotherapy before conception and throughout pregnancy. Cancer 1984;54:800–3.

SUCCIMER

Antidote/Chelating Agent

PREGNANCY RECOMMENDATION: Limited Human Data—Animal Data Suggest Risk
BREASTFEEDING RECOMMENDATION: Contraindicated

PREGNANCY SUMMARY

Two reports have described the use of succimer during human pregnancy. The chelating agent has produced fetotoxicity and teratogenicity in mice and fetotoxicity in rats. These toxic effects often occurred at oral doses ≤10 times the human dose (weight basis). In addition, succimer-induced modulation of adult female rat immune function has been demonstrated. The exact mechanism of the animal developmental toxicity is unknown but appears to result from disturbances in mineral metabolism, especially that of zinc and copper. Therefore, if succimer is used in human pregnancy, the effects on maternal and fetal mineral metabolism—in particular, of zinc and copper—should be evaluated (1).

S

FETAL RISK SUMMARY

The heavy metal chelating agent succimer (*meso*-2,3-dimercaptosuccinic acid [DMSA]) is indicated for the treatment and prophylaxis of lead poisoning in pediatric patients (2). The drug has also been used as an antidote for the treatment of arsenic, mercury, and cadmium poisoning (3). Succimer has no significant effect on the urinary elimination of iron, calcium, or magnesium but doubles the excretion of zinc (2). After oral administration, approximately 60% is absorbed systemically from an initial dose of 30 mg/kg/day (1050 mg/m²/day) with an apparent elimination half-life of approximately 2 days.

In addition to the animal reproductive data provided by the manufacturer (2), a number of published animal studies have described the effect of succimer on the fetus (3–12). In pregnant rats, doses of 100–1000 mg/kg/day administered orally on gestational days 6–15 were not teratogenic but did produce maternal toxicity (decreased weight gain) (3). At pregnancy termination on day 20, fetal toxicity, characterized by increased early resorptions, postimplantation losses, and reduced fetal body weight per litter, was evident at all doses. The no-observable-effect level (NOEL) was <100 mg/kg/day (3).

In another portion of the above study, the concentrations of five minerals (calcium, magnesium, zinc, copper, and iron) were measured in maternal and fetal tissues (4). Marked alterations were observed on the mineral concentrations in the fetuses. These effects suggested that the fetal toxicity noted was partially due to changes in mineral metabolism (4).

Succimer was teratogenic and fetotoxic when SC doses were given to pregnant mice during organogenesis (days

6–15 of gestation) at doses of 410–1640 mg/kg/day (2,5). At the maximum dose, maternal toxicity (reduced weight gain) was evident (5). Significant embryo and fetal toxicity, as evidenced by an increased incidence of resorptions and stunting, and a decrease in the number of live fetuses per litter, were observed at 1640 mg/kg/day. At 820 mg/kg/day, significant decreases in fetal weight and length were noted. A dose relationship was found for structural defects, including significant increases (compared with controls) in gross external defects (hematomas in the facial area, exencephaly, and micrognathia), internal soft tissue defects (hydrocephaly, small thoracic cavities, and brain defects), and skeletal variations (decreased ossification, hypoplasia of the mandible, and irregular-shaped ribs). The no-effect dose for defects was 410 mg/kg/day (5).

In continuation of the above study, pregnant mice were given oral succimer (200–800 mg/kg/day) from gestational day 14 through postnatal day 21 (weaning) (6). No maternal toxicity was observed at any dose. Adverse effects were observed only in the offspring exposed during lactation to the highest maternal dose. The effects observed in the nursing pups included significant decreases in body weight and a corresponding increase in relative brain weight (brain weight/body weight). The NOEL for adverse effects in the nursing pups was >400 mg/kg/day (6).

The type of developmental toxicity observed in mice suggested to some investigators that the toxicity may have been related to an interaction between succimer and zinc (5). However, in a subsequent report, no consistent changes could be demonstrated in mice fetal tissue levels of zinc, iron, calcium, or magnesium (7). Moreover, supplemental zinc did not protect the fetuses. Disturbance of maternal–fetal copper metabolism may have been related to the developmental toxicity because dose-dependent decreases in fetal liver copper levels were observed (7).

A 1991 report examined the efficacy of succimer to protect mice fetuses from the toxicity and teratogenicity of an intraperitoneal (IP) dose (12 mg/kg) of sodium arsenite administered to pregnant mice on day 10 of gestation (8). In the dose-finding portion of the study, succimer SC doses of 80, 160, and 320 mg/kg were given immediately after sodium arsenite injection. An increasing protective effect was noted with an increasing succimer dose. The effect of the time interval between IP injection of sodium arsenite and injection of succimer was then studied. A single SC dose of succimer (320 mg/kg) was given to pregnant mice at various times up to 12 hours after a dose of sodium arsenite. Significant reductions in arsenite-induced embryo toxicity and teratogenicity were achieved only when succimer was administered within 1 hour of the arsenite dose (8).

Using a similar study design, the above investigators examined the effect of succimer in protecting fetal mice from the toxicity and teratogenicity of dibasic sodium arsenate (9). Sodium arsenate is the most common form of inorganic arsenic in the environment and is less fetotoxic than sodium arsenite (8,9). As in the above study, the investigators demonstrated a dose-related protective effect of succimer at SC doses of 37.5, 75, and 150 mg/kg administered at four successive time intervals (2, 24, 48, and 72 hours) after IP injection of dibasic sodium arsenate (45 mg/kg) (9).

A 1978 study in pregnant rats demonstrated that daily administration of succimer was effective in reducing methylmercury concentrations in neonatal rat brains (10). A 40-mg oral dose was more effective (70% reduction in methylmercury) than a 20-mg dose (50% reduction). In a later study with pregnant mice, a dose-related protective effect from methylmercury-induced embryolethality and teratogenicity was demonstrated with the maximum protection achieved with an SC dose of 320 mg/kg/day (11).

The effect on the immune function of female rats exposed to succimer in utero was described in a 1999 report (12). Pregnant rats were administered lead acetate (250 ppm) in drinking water from 2 weeks before mating until parturition. Succimer (60 mg/kg/day), given orally from days 6–21 of gestation, significantly lowered the blood lead levels in both the dams and embryos. Several lead-induced changes in 13-week-old female offspring were reversed by the chelating agent (succimer-induced changes in parentheses), including body weight (increased), relative spleen weight (decreased), interferon γ (increased), and interleukin-4 (decreased). However, succimer alone affected immune function in the female offspring by decreasing the delayed-type hypersensitivity response and increasing interleukin-2 production. Therefore, succimer treatment during gestation did reverse some of the lead-induced immunotoxicity but also caused subsequent adult immunomodulation (12).

It is not known if succimer crosses the human placenta. The molecular weight (about 182) is low enough that fetal exposure should be expected. The studies cited above suggest that succimer crosses the placenta in mice and rats.

A 2001 case report described an 18-day course of oral succimer for lead poisoning at about 29–32 weeks' gestation (13). There was no effect on the woman's blood lead concentrations (44.0 mcg/dL before chelation and 43.9 mcg/ dL after treatment). She gave birth at 37 weeks' to a 3.04-kg, female infant with Apgar scores of 8 and 9. At birth, the mother's blood lead level was 57.6 mcg/dL, whereas the cord blood lead concentration was 126 mcg/dL. The source of the lead in the mother was not found, even though an extensive search for the source was conducted. The infant was treated with chelation therapy and, although the concentrations remained elevated, her appearance and behavior were normal at 6.5 months of age (13).

One pregnant woman, in a series of seven, was treated with succimer for lead poisoning in a 2003 report (14). The source of the lead in most cases was the ingestion of pica (soil/clay-based substances). No lead-induced congenital defects were noted in the infants, but all received chelation therapy in the neonatal period (14).

S

BREASTFEEDING SUMMARY

No studies describing the use of succimer during lactation have been located. The molecular weight (about 182) suggests that the drug will be excreted into milk. The effects of this exposure on a nursing infant are unknown. However, because the use of succimer implies poisoning with lead, or other heavy metals, these substances might also be excreted into milk and cause toxicity in a nursing infant. Therefore, breastfeeding is contraindicated in women receiving succimer.

References

1. Domingo JL. Developmental toxicity of metal chelating agents. Reprod Toxicol 1998;12:499–510.
2. Product information. Chemet. Sanofi-Synthelabo, 2002.
3. Domingo JL, Ortega A, Paternain JL, Llobet JM. Oral *meso*-2,3-dimercaptosuccinic acid in pregnant Sprague-Dawley rats: teratogenicity

and alterations in mineral metabolism. I. Teratological evaluation. J Toxicol Environ Health 1990;30:181–90.

4. Paternain JL, Ortega A, Domingo JL, Llobet JM. Oral *meso*-2, 3-dimercaptosuccinic acid in pregnant Sprague-Dawley rats: teratogenicity and alterations in mineral metabolism. II. Effect on mineral metabolism. J Toxicol Environ Health 1990;30:191–7.
5. Domingo JL, Paternain JL, Llobet JM, Corbella J. Developmental toxicity of subcutaneously administered *meso*-2,3-dimercaptosuccinic acid in mice. Fundam Appl Toxicol 1988;11:715–22.
6. Domingo JL, Bosque MA, Corbella J. Effects of oral *meso*-2, 3-dimercaptosucinic acid (DMSA) administration on late gestation and postnatal development in the mouse. Life Sci 1990;47:1745–50.
7. Taubeneck MW, Domingo JL, Llobet JM, Keen CL. *Meso*-2, 3-dimercaptosuccinic acid (DMSA) affects maternal and fetal copper metabolism in Swiss mice. Toxicology 1992;72:27–40.
8. Domingo JL, Bosque MA, Piera V. *meso*-2,3-dimercaptosuccinic acid and prevention of arsenite embryotoxicity and teratogenicity in the mouse. Fundam Appl Toxicol 1991;17:314–20.
9. Bosque MA, Domingo JL, Llobet JM, Corbella J. Effects of *Meso*-2, 3-dimercaptosuccinic acid (DMSA) on the teratogenicity of sodium arsenate in mice. Bull Environ Contam Toxicol 1991;47:682–8.
10. Hughes JA, Sparber SB. Reduction of methylmercury concentration in neonatal rat brains after administration of dimercaptosuccinic acid to dams while pregnant. Res Commun Chem Pathol Pharmacol 1978;22:357–63.
11. Sanchez DJ, Gomez M, Llobet JM, Domingo JL. Effects of *meso*-2,3-dimercaptosuccinic acid (DMSA) on methyl mercury-induced teratogenesis in mice. Ecotoxicol Environ Saf 1993;26:33–9.
12. Chen S, Golemboski KA, Sander FS, Dietert RR. Persistent effect of in utero meso-2,3-dimercaptosuccinic acid (DMSA) on immune function and lead-induced immunotoxicity. Toxicology 1999;132:67–79.
13. Horowitz BZ, Mirkin DB. Lead poisoning and chelation in a mother–neonate pair. J Toxicol Clin Toxicol 2001;39:727–31.
14. Shannon M. Severe lead poisoning in pregnancy. Ambul Pediatr 2003;3: 37–9.

SUCCINYLCHOLINE

Skeletal Muscle Relaxant

PREGNANCY RECOMMENDATION: Compatible
BREASTFEEDING RECOMMENDATION: No Human Data—Probably Compatible

PREGNANCY SUMMARY

Succinylcholine is not embryotoxic or teratogenic in two animal species or, although the data are very limited, in humans. Succinylcholine has been routinely used in obstetric patients prior to delivery since the 1950s and no reports of fetal toxicity have been located. Partial or complete newborn paralysis, with resulting respiratory depression, has been reported when the drug was administered to women with the genetic trait for atypical cholinesterase. Prolonged newborn respiratory depression may occur when this trait has been inherited by the infant. The level of cholinesterase activity in the infant will determine the duration of paralysis. Women without the genetic trait for atypical cholinesterase rapidly metabolize the drug and, because clinically significant placental transfer is dependent on concentration, prevent toxicity in the newborn.

FETAL RISK SUMMARY

Succinylcholine is a depolarizing neuromuscular blocking agent that is used as an adjunct to general anesthesia, to facilitate tracheal intubation, and to provide skeletal muscle relaxation during surgery or mechanical ventilation. Approximately 90% of the drug is rapidly hydrolyzed by plasma cholinesterase to succinylmonocholine, a metabolite that is clinically inactive, and then more slowly to succinic acid and choline. The remaining 10% is excreted unchanged in the urine (1).

According to the manufacturer, reproduction studies in animals with succinylcholine have not been conducted (1). A 1984 source, however, stated that studies conducted in the 1950s in rabbits and dogs did not observe embryo or fetal toxicity or teratogenicity (2). Succinylcholine has no direct action on the uterus or other smooth muscles and, because it is highly ionized and has low lipid solubility, does not readily cross the placenta (1).

A study published in 1961 noted the lack of quantitative data on the placental transfer of succinylcholine in animals and humans (3). Although published reports involving more than 1800 deliveries had shown the drug to be safe for the fetus and newborn, there were anecdotal reports of flaccid, apneic infants whose condition was attributed to succinylcholine (3). The authors cited two studies in which doses <100 mg in pregnant rabbits had no adverse effect on the newborns, but in dogs, paralysis was demonstrated in pups when a 400-mg dose was administered to the mother immediately before delivery (3). They then studied 14 patients delivered by cesarean section under general anesthesia, in which a single 100-mg IV dose of succinylcholine was followed by a continuous infusion of a 0.2% succinylcholine solution (3). The patients received a total dose (IV plus infusion) of 100–600 mg. Three of the newborn infants had Apgar scores <7 (time when determined was not specified). In an additional eight patients undergoing vaginal delivery, a single 100-mg IV dose was given within 4 minutes of birth. None of these infants had a depressed Apgar score. Of the total 22 newborns, no paralysis was observed. Placental transfer of succinylcholine as determined by a biologic test, however, could not be demonstrated in any of the cases (3).

In a second study by these same authors, pregnant rabbits at term were treated with a single IV dose of succinylcholine (0.25–570 mg/kg) with delivery of the fetuses 3–6 minutes later (4). A difference in vigor compared with that in controls was observed when the mother had received 340 mg/kg, about 600 times the human clinical dose based on weight. (The human clinical dose to facilitate tracheal intubation is 0.6 mg/kg IV, range 0.3–1.1 mg/kg [1]). At 540 mg/kg, all rabbit fetuses were alive but paralyzed. In the human part of this study, 13 women at term who were about to undergo vaginal delivery were given a single 200- to 500-mg rapid IV dose, 1–5.25 minutes before delivery (4). Maternal blood levels varied from 0 to 11.6 mcg/mL, whereas cord blood concentrations varied from 0 to 2.0 mcg/mL. Cord blood levels of 1.1–2.0 mcg/mL occurred in six of eight fetuses whose mothers had received doses of ≥300 mg/kg. No drug was found in the cord blood of five newborns after a 200-mg/kg maternal dose. None of the newborns appeared to be affected by succinylcholine, but all of the mothers were apneic at delivery and for periods up to 16 minutes.

The placental transfer of succinylcholine using radioactive tracers was studied in near-term monkeys, using IV doses of 2–3 mg/kg followed by repeated doses of 1.2 and 2 mg/kg (5). Rapid placental transfer occurred, reaching a peak fetal plasma concentration approximately 30% of the maternal plasma level 5–10 minutes after the dose. Fetal metabolism of succinylcholine to inactive succinylmonocholine was demonstrated, albeit at a slower rate than that which occurred in the mother, an indication that fetal cholinesterase (pseudocholinesterase) activity was lower than that in the mother (5). The authors concluded that the amount of active drug transferred to the fetus produced a slight effect on skeletal muscle activity and was unlikely to depress respiration in the newborn (5).

Atypical cholinesterase is an autosomal dominant inherited condition with prevalence, for the dibucaine-resistant form, of 1:2000–1:4000 in various populations (6). The homozygote state is diagnosed by the onset of prolonged apnea (>10 minutes), in the absence of excessive amounts of other depressants, after succinylcholine (1–3 mg/kg) administration (6). Some of the anecdotal reports, mentioned in reference 3 of flaccid, apneic infants after succinylcholine administration may represent cases of this genetic trait. Four maternal cases of atypical cholinesterase, with probable atypical homozygote infants in three, are discussed below.

A study published in 1975 described respiratory depression and decreased muscular activity in a newborn whose mother had received succinylcholine, 80 mg IV followed by an IV infusion that delivered an additional 60 mg of drug, for cesarean section at term (7). Newborn ventilation support was required for 10 minutes after birth. Neuromuscular block in the mother continued for approximately 5.5 hours. Because the cholinesterase activity in the mother and that in the 2-day-old infant were 10% of normal, neither was able to rapidly metabolize the succinylcholine (7).

Low concentrations of plasma cholinesterase were thought to be responsible for transient respiratory depression in a newborn following the use of succinylcholine for cesarean section (8). The mother had received 200 mg thiamylal (a barbiturate similar to thiopental that is not currently available) and 100 mg succinylcholine IV for induction of general anesthesia 3 minutes prior to delivery. The onset of respiration and the development of an acceptable respiratory pattern in the newborn were slightly delayed with Apgar scores of 5 and 8 at 1 and 5 minutes, respectively. After recovery, the newborn did well. The mother required mechanical ventilation for 4 hours before return of spontaneous muscular activity and respiration (8). Cholinesterase activity in the mother was below the level of test sensitivity. Enzyme activity in the newborn was 410 U/L (normal 2436–4872 U/L) (8). Three months later, the infant's pseudocholinesterase activity had risen to 910 U/L. Enzyme concentrations in the father (2420 U/L) were slightly low, normal in one sibling (2480 U/L), and markedly depressed in five other siblings (range 150–760 U/L).

A description of two mothers at term with atypical cholinesterase who were administered succinylcholine prior to elective cesarean section was reported in 1975 (9). The first mother received 100 mg of IV succinylcholine 5 minutes before delivery of a male infant. Apnea in the mother persisted for 2.5 hours after delivery before return of spontaneous respirations. Her infant was flaccid, apneic, and unresponsive to stimulation. Respiratory assistance was required for 6 hours before occurrence of full recovery. In the second mother, who also received succinylcholine 100 mg IV, recovery from paralysis required 2 hours. Her infant, delivered 10 minutes after the dose, cried immediately and had Apgar scores of 8 and 10 at 1 and 5 minutes, respectively. Analysis of serum cholinesterase activity and dibucaine numbers in the mothers and infants revealed that the mothers and the affected infant were atypical homozygotes, whereas the unaffected infant was a heterozygote (9).

The Collaborative Perinatal Project monitored 50,282 mother–child pairs, 26 of whom had 1st trimester exposure to succinylcholine (10). No congenital malformations were observed in any of the newborns.

BREASTFEEDING SUMMARY

The passage of succinylcholine into breast milk has not been studied. Because the drug is rapidly hydrolyzed by plasma cholinesterase (pseudocholinesterase) to an inactive metabolite, it is doubtful that clinically significant amounts of active drug are transferred into milk (11). Women with the genetic trait for atypical cholinesterase will have high concentrations of succinylcholine, but the effects of the drug on the mother will preclude nursing.

References

1. Product information. Anectine. Glaxo Wellcome, 1998.
2. Onnis A, Grella P. *The Biochemical Effects of Drugs in Pregnancy*. Vol 1. West Sussex, England: Ellis Horwood Limited, 1984:230–1.
3. Moya F, Kvisselgaard N. The placental transmission of succinylcholine. Anesthesiology 1961;22:1–6.
4. Kvisselgaard N, Moya F. Investigation of placental thresholds to succinylcholine. Anesthesiology 1961;22:7–10.
5. Drabkova J, Crul JF, van der Kleijn E. Placental transfer of ^{14}C labelled succinylcholine in near-term Macaca mulatta monkeys. Br J Anaesthesia 1973;45:1087–96.
6. Donnell GN. Cholinesterase, atypical. In: Buyse ML. Editor-in-Chief. *Birth Defects Encyclopedia*. Vol 1. Cambridge, MA: Blackwell Scientific Publications, 1990:316–7.
7. Owens WD, Zeitlin GL. Hypoventilation in a newborn following administration of succinylcholine to the mother: a case report. Anesth Analg 1975;54:38–40.
8. Cherala SR, Eddoe DN, Sechzer PH. Placental transfer of succinylcholine causing transient respiratory depression in the newborn. Anaesthesia Intensive Care 1989;17:202–4.
9. Baraka A, Haroun S, Bassili M, Abu-Haider G. Response of the newborn to succinylcholine injection in homozygotic atypical mothers. Anesthesiology 1975;43:115–6.
10. Heinonen OP, Slone D, Shapiro S. *Birth Defects and Drugs in Pregnancy*. Littleton, MA: Publishing Sciences Group, 1977:358–60.
11. Spigset O. Anaesthetic agents and excretion in breast milk. Acta Anaesthesiol Scand 1994;38:94–103.

SUCRALFATE

Gastrointestinal Agent (Antisecretory)

PREGNANCY RECOMMENDATION: Compatible
BREASTFEEDING RECOMMENDATION: No Human Data—Probably Compatible

PREGNANCY SUMMARY

Although the toxicity of aluminum has been well documented, there is no evidence that normal doses of aluminum-containing medications, such as sucralfate, present a risk to the fetuses of pregnant women with normal renal function. A study showing an association between in utero exposure to gastric acid-suppressing drugs and childhood allergy and asthma requires confirmation. Oral absorption of aluminum is poor, with only an average of 12% retained in one study of six normal subjects ingesting 1–3 g/day of aluminum (1). Moreover, no evidence has been found to suggest that aluminum is actively absorbed from the gastrointestinal tract (1). Because of these characteristics and the lack of reports of adverse fetal effects in humans or animals attributable to sucralfate, the risk to the fetus is probably nil. A 1985 review on the use of gastrointestinal drugs during pregnancy and lactation by the American College of Gastroenterology classified sucralfate as an agent whose potential benefits outweighed any potential risks (2).

FETAL RISK SUMMARY

Sucralfate is an aluminum salt of a sulfated disaccharide that inhibits pepsin activity and protects against ulceration. The drug is a highly polar anion when solubilized in strong acid solutions, which probably accounts for its poor gastrointestinal absorption. Its ulcer protectant and healing effects are exerted through local, rather than systemic, action (3). The small amounts that are absorbed, up to 2.2% of a dose in one study using healthy males (4), are excreted in the urine (3,4).

In mice, rats, and rabbits, sucralfate had no effect on fertility and was not teratogenic with doses up to 50 times those used in humans (3). Sucralfate is a source of bioavailable aluminum (1,5). Each 1-g tablet of sucralfate contains 207 mg of aluminum (1). The potential fetal toxicity of this drug relates to its aluminum content.

When administered parenterally to pregnant animals, aluminum accumulated in the fetus, causing an increased perinatal mortality and impaired learning and memory (6,7). Teratogenic effects, however, were not observed (7). Prolonged exposure to the metal has caused neurobehavioral and skeletal toxicity (8). A 1985 review of aluminum described these toxic effects on the brain and bone tissue as dialysis encephalopathy in patients with renal failure and a unique form of osteodystrophy in uremic patients (1). Aluminum received from IV fluids may also be related to osteopenia in premature infants (9). A 1991 report described the results of a study of 88 pregnancies in women exposed to high amounts of aluminum sulfate that had been accidentally added to the city's water supply (10). Except for an increased rate of talipes (clubfoot) (four cases, one control; $p = 0.01$), there was no evidence that the exposure was harmful to the fetuses. Several theoretical explanations for the four cases of clubfoot were offered by the investigators, including the possibility that the observed incidence occurred by chance (10).

In patients with end-stage chronic renal failure, the use of sucralfate to bind phosphate resulted in serum aluminum levels comparable to those obtained from the antacid aluminum hydroxide (5). Administration of sucralfate to normal subjects did not increase plasma aluminum concentrations, but evidence of tissue aluminum loading was found in experiments with animals (1).

Analysis of 97 amniotic fluid samples, mostly from women undergoing amniocentesis for advanced maternal age, found a mean aluminum concentration of 93.4 mcg/L (range 37–149 mcg/L) (11). The authors of this study did not mention whether the women were consuming aluminum-containing medications, and the measured levels are apparently the normal baseline for the patient population studied.

In a surveillance study of Michigan Medicaid recipients involving 229,101 completed pregnancies conducted between 1985 and 1992, 183 newborns had been exposed to sucralfate during the 1st trimester (F. Rosa, personal communication, FDA, 1993). A total of five (2.7%) major birth defects were observed (eight expected). Specific data were available for six defect categories, including (observed/expected) 1/2 cardiovascular defects, 1/0 oral clefts, 0/0 spina bifida, 1/0.5 polydactyly, 0/0.5 limb reduction defects, and 1/0.5 hypospadias. These data do not support an association between the drug and congenital defects.

A population-based observational cohort study formed by linking data from three Swedish national healthcare registers over a 10-year period (1995–2004) was reported in 2009 (12). The main outcome measures were a diagnosis of allergic disease or a prescription for asthma or allergy medications. The drug types included in the study were gastric acid suppressors, including H2-receptor antagonists, prostaglandins, proton pump inhibitors, combinations for eradication of *Helicobacter pylori*, and drugs for peptic ulcer and gastroesophageal reflux disease, such as sucralfate. Of 585,716 children, 29,490 (5.0%) met the diagnosis and 5645 (1%) had been exposed to gastric acid suppression therapy in pregnancy. Of these children, 405 (0.07%) were treated for allergic disease. For developing allergy, the odds ratio (OR) was 1.43 and the 98% confidence interval (CI) was 1.29–1.59, irrespective of the drug, time of exposure during pregnancy, and maternal history of allergy. For developing childhood asthma, but not other allergic diseases, the OR was 1.51 and the 95% CI was 1.35–1.69, irrespective of the type of acid-suppressive drug and the time of exposure in pregnancy. The authors proposed three possible mechanisms for their findings: (a) exposure to increased amounts of allergens could cause sensitization to digestion labile antigens in the fetus; (b) maternal Th2 cytokine pattern could promote an allergy-prone phenotype in the fetus; and (c) maternal allergen-specific immunoglobulin E could cross the placenta and sensitize fetal immune cells to food and airborne allergens. Several limitations of the study that might have affected their findings were identified, including a general increase in childhood asthma but not necessarily an increase in allergic asthma (12). The study requires confirmation.

BREASTFEEDING SUMMARY

Minimal, if any, excretion of sucralfate into milk should be expected because only small amounts of this drug are absorbed systemically.

References

1. Lione A. Aluminum toxicology and the aluminum-containing medications. Pharmacol Ther 1985;29:255–85.
2. Lewis JH, Weingold AB. The use of gastrointestinal drugs during pregnancy and lactation. Am J Gastroenterol 1985;80:912–23.
3. Product information. Carafate. Hoechst Marion Roussel, 2000.
4. Giesing D, Lanman R, Runser D. Absorption of sucralfate in man (abstract). Gastroenterology 1982;82:1066.
5. Leung ACT, Henderson IS, Halls DJ, Dobbie JW. Aluminum hydroxide versus sucralfate as a phosphate binder in uraemia. Br Med J 1983;286:1379–81.
6. Yokel RA. Toxicity of gestational aluminum exposure to the maternal rabbit and offspring. Toxicol Appl Pharmacol 1985;79:121–33.
7. McCormack KM, Ottosen LD, Sanger VL, Sprague S, Major GH, Hook JB. Effect of prenatal administration of aluminum and parathyroid hormone on fetal development in the rat (40493). Proc Soc Exp Biol Med 1979;161:74–7.
8. Yokel RA, McNamara PJ. Aluminum bioavailability and disposition in adult and immature rabbits. Toxicol Appl Pharmacol 1985;77:344–52.
9. Sedman AB, Klein GL, Merritt RJ, Miller NL, Weber KO, Gill WL, Anand H, Alfrey AC. Evidence of aluminum loading in infants receiving intravenous therapy. N Engl J Med 1985;312:1337–43.
10. Golding J, Rowland A, Greenwood R, Lunt P. Aluminum sulphate in water in north Cornwall and outcome of pregnancy. Br Med J 1991;302:1175–7.
11. Hall GS, Carr MJ, Cummings E, Lee M. Aluminum, barium, silicon, and strontium in amniotic fluid by emission spectrometry. Clin Chem 1983;29:1318.
12. Dehlink E, Yen E, Leichtner AM, Hait EJ, Fiebiger E. First evidence of a possible association between gastric acid suppression during pregnancy and childhood asthma: a population-based register study. Clin Exp Allergy 2009;39:246–53.

SUFENTANIL

Narcotic Agonist Analgesic

PREGNANCY RECOMMENDATION: Human Data Suggest Risk in 3rd Trimester
BREASTFEEDING RECOMMENDATION: No Human Data—Probably Compatible

PREGNANCY SUMMARY

The use of sufentanil during pregnancy with clinically used doses does not appear to present a significant risk to the fetus or newborn. Although no reports describing the use of the narcotic during the 1st trimester have been located, the lack of teratogenicity in animals and the general opinion that narcotic agents, in general, pose little risk of congenital malformations are reassuring. Sufentanil rapidly crosses the placenta to the fetus, even more so in the presence of fetal acidosis, and similar to all narcotics, dose-related depression of the fetus and newborn may occur. Both respiratory depression and adverse effects on neonatal neurobehavior are potential problems in the newborn. If sufentanil is used in pregnancy, healthcare professionals are encouraged to call the toll-free number (800-670-6126) for information about patient enrollment in the Motherisk study.

S

FETAL RISK SUMMARY

Sufentanil is a potent narcotic drug that is used as an analgesic adjunct to, or primary anesthetic agent during, general anesthesia and in combination with bupivacaine for epidural anesthesia during labor and vaginal delivery.

No evidence of teratogenicity has been observed in rats and rabbits, but the drug was embryocidal (most likely due to maternal toxicity) in both species when it was given for 10–30 days in a dose 2.5 times the upper human IV dose (1). No adverse reproductive (number of implantations and live fetuses, percent fetal wastage per litter, or mean fetal weight) or teratogenic effects (major or minor malformations) were observed in rats administered continuous infusions of sufentanil at doses of 10, 50, or 100 mcg/kg/day from day 5 through day 20 of pregnancy (2).

The placental transfer of sufentanil was studied in an experiment using the dual-perfused, single-cotyledon human placental model at doses of 1, 10, 20, and 100 ng/mL (3). Sufentanil was shown to rapidly cross the placenta by passive diffusion, but high maternal protein binding significantly reduced this transfer, whereas progressive fetal acidemia (reduction in pH from 7.4 to 6.8 in 0.2 increments) significantly increased transfer. Placental tissues appeared to bind sufentanil, but this accumulation apparently did not affect the overall net drug transfer to the fetus (i.e., the placenta accumulated sufentanil during periods of increasing maternal concentrations and then functioned as a source to sustain fetal drug levels when maternal concentrations declined) (3).

In another in vitro study, a single-pass (open) placental perfusion model was used to assess the placental transfer of sufentanil (1 and 100 ng/mL) and the effect of maternal plasma proteins, placental metabolism, and fetal pH (7.4–6.8) on the transfer (4). The conclusions of this study were identical to those of the study above, in that sufentanil rapidly crossed the placenta by passive diffusion, the placenta acted as a depot for the narcotic, maternal protein binding (not albumin) decreased transfer, and fetal acidosis increased the amount reaching the fetus (4). The authors also concluded that because of its low initial transfer (umbilical vein concentration only 2% of maternal concentration at 5 minutes), sufentanil may be the narcotic of choice if delivery is imminent (<45 minutes) (4).

Sufentanil crosses the placenta to the fetal circulation following maternal epidural anesthesia (5,6). In a 1991 double-blind study, 60 women undergoing elective cesarean section at term were randomized to receive epidural anesthesia consisting of 0.5% bupivacaine with epinephrine (1:200,000) alone (*N* = 20), sufentanil 20 mcg plus bupivacaine with epinephrine (*N* = 20), or sufentanil 30 mcg plus bupivacaine with epinephrine (*N* = 20) (6). The mean plasma concentrations of sufentanil in the mother and newborn in the 20-mcg group (14 subjects) were 0.030 and 0.025 ng/mL, respectively, whereas those in the 30-mcg group (15 subjects) were 0.056 and 0.042 ng/mL, respectively. The fetal:maternal ratios in the two groups were 0.83 and 0.75, respectively. To evaluate the safety of the epidural solutions for the newborn, the Neurological and Adaptive Capacity Score (NACS) was used to evaluate the infants at birth and between 1 and 2 hours. In each of the three groups, the percentage of neonates with a perfect score in each category of the NACS was statistically similar (6).

The placental transfer of sufentanil, fentanyl, and bupivacaine was studied in a double-blind, randomized trial involving 36 women at term who received epidural anesthesia during labor prior to vaginal delivery (6). Patients received a 12-mL bolus of (a) bupivacaine 0.25% alone (*N* = 13), (b) bupivacaine 0.125% plus sufentanil 15 mcg (*N* = 9), or (c) bupivacaine 0.125% plus fentanyl 75 mcg (*N* = 14), followed by a 10 mL/hr infusion of bupivacaine 0.125% alone, bupivacaine 0.125% plus sufentanil 0.25 mcg/mL, or bupivacaine 0.125% plus fentanyl 1.5 mcg/mL. The mean umbilical vein:maternal vein (UV:MV) ratios for bupivacaine in the three groups were 0.29, 0.43, and 0.33, respectively. The mean UV concentrations of the narcotics for sufentanil and fentanyl were 0.016 and 0.18 ng/mL, respectively, whereas the mean MV concentrations were 0.019 and 0.52 ng/mL, respectively. The UV:MV ratios for sufentanil and fentanyl were 0.81 and 0.37, respectively. The NACS was used to assess the newborns in each group at delivery, 2 hours of age, and 24 hours of age (6). No statistical differences among the three groups were observed at delivery or at 2 hours of age, but at 24 hours, the bupivacaine-fentanyl group's NACS was significantly lower than that of the bupivacaine-sufentanil group, a result thought to reflect the continued presence of fentanyl in the neonate (6).

Intrathecal sufentanil (10 mcg), followed at least 1 hour later with bupivacaine epidural analgesia (*N* = 65), was compared with bupivacaine epidural analgesia alone (*N* = 64) in a 1996 report comparing the effects of the two analgesic regimens on fetal heart rate changes during labor (7). No statistical differences were observed between the groups in the incidence of clinically significant fetal heart rate tracing abnormalities (recurrent late decelerations and/or bradycardia) or in maternal hypotension within the 1st hour of administration (7). In addition, there were no differences between the groups in arterial or venous cord pH or the number of 5-minute Apgar scores <7. No abnormal fetal heart rate patterns were observed in an earlier study that compared intrathecal sufentanil (10 mcg) either alone (*N* = 20) or with 0.2 mg epinephrine (*N* = 20) (8). Epinephrine did not prolong analgesia but did increase the incidence of vomiting while decreasing the incidence and severity of pruritus. In a 1993 report, abnormal fetal heart rate changes were observed in 15% (11 of 73 tracings that were acceptable for analysis) among 108 women who received intrathecal sufentanil (10 mcg) during active labor (9). Of the 11 abnormal tracings, 5 were of moderate but transient variable decelerations, 4 were of mild nonrepetitive late decelerations, 1 was of a single episode of bradycardia, and 1 was of an episode of decreased variability. None of the 11 affected pregnancies required intervention for fetal compromise.

A number of studies have reported the successful use of sufentanil to produce adequate labor analgesia without fetal or newborn harm (10–19). A 1992 reference concluded that 10 mcg of sufentanil administered intrathecally produced faster and superior analgesia to that observed with epidural or IV administration of the same dose (10). Intermittent injections of intrathecal sufentanil (5 mcg) were compared with intermittent injections of intrathecal fentanyl (10 mcg) or meperidine (10 mg) in another 1992 report (11). In this study, meperidine provided better maternal analgesia once cervical dilation had progressed beyond 6 cm (11). No intergroup differences were observed in umbilical cord blood gases and none of the newborns had a 5-minute Apgar score <7. No significant differences were observed in Apgar scores, umbilical cord blood pH levels, or NACS at 2 and 24 hours in a study comparing epidural sufentanil plus bupivacaine (*N* = 30) to epidural fentanyl plus bupivacaine (*N* = 30) (12). During labor, the patients received epidural infusions at 12 mL/hr of either sufentanil (0.25 mcg/mL) or fentanyl (2.5 mcg/mL), both in 0.0625% bupivacaine. The total narcotic doses of sufentanil or fentanyl were 15.9 and 139.8 mcg, respectively. In seven other studies, spinal sufentanil either alone or combined with other various agents compared favorably with controls in efficacy and fetal and newborn safety (13–19).

A case of maternal respiratory depression following a 15-mcg dose of intrathecal sufentanil during labor was described in 1994 (20). A marked decrease (to 89%) in the patient's hemoglobin oxygen saturation was noted that was treated with tactile stimulation and oxygen via face mask. A healthy, 3905-g male infant was delivered 2.5 hours later with Apgar scores of 7 and 8 at 1 and 5 minutes, respectively. No adverse effects were observed in the neonate during routine hospital follow-up.

BREASTFEEDING SUMMARY

The use of sufentanil during lactation is unlikely because of its clinical indications. It is not surprising, therefore, that no reports describing the use of this agent during lactation have been located. The molecular weight (about 579) of sufentanil citrate, the commercial form of the drug, is low enough that passage into milk should be expected. The effects, if any, of this exposure on a nursing infant are unknown.

S

References

1. Product information. Sufenta. Janssen Pharmaceutica, 1998.
2. Fujinaga M, Mazze RI, Jackson EC, Baden JM. Reproductive and teratogenic effects of sufentanil and alfentanil in Sprague-Dawley rats. Anesth Analg 1988;67:166–9.
3. Johnson RF, Herman N, Arney TL, Johnson HV, Paschall RL, Downing JW. The placental transfer of sufentanil: effects of fetal pH, protein binding, and sufentanil concentration. Anesth Analg 1997;84:1262–8.
4. Krishna BR, Zakowski MI, Grant GJ. Sufentanil transfer in the human placenta during in vitro perfusion. Can J Anaesth 1997;44:996–1001.
5. Vertommen JD, Van Aken H, Vandermeulen E, Vangerven M, Devlieger H, Van Assche AF, Shnider SM. Maternal and neonatal effects of adding epidural sufentanil to 0.5% bupivacaine for cesarean delivery. J Clin Anesth 1991;3:371–6.
6. Loftus JR, Hill H, Cohen SE. Placental transfer and neonatal effects of epidural sufentanil and fentanyl administered with bupivacaine during labor. Anesthesiology 1995;83:300–8.
7. Nielsen PE, Erickson JR, Abouleish EI, Perriatt S, Sheppard C. Fetal heart rate changes after intrathecal sufentanil or epidural bupivicaine *[sic]* for labor analgesia: incidence and clinical significance. Anesth Analg 1996;83:742–60.
8. Camann WR, Minzter BH, Denney RA, Datta S. Intrathecal sufentanil for labor analgesia. Effects of added epinephrine. Anesthesiology 1993;78:870–4.
9. Cohen SE, Cherry CM, Holbrook RH Jr, El-Sayed YY, Gibson RN, Jaffe RA. Intrathecal sufentanil for labor analgesia—sensory changes, side effects, and fetal heart rate changes. Anesth Analg 1993;77:1155–60.
10. Camann WR, Denney RA, Holby ED, Datta S. A comparison of intrathecal, epidural, and intravenous sufentanil for labor analgesia. Anesthesiology 1992;77:884–7.
11. Honet JE, Arkoosh VA, Norris MC, Huffnagle HJ, Silverman NS, Leighton BL. Comparison among intrathecal fentanyl, meperidine, and sufentanil for labor analgesia. Anesth Analg 1992;75:734–9.
12. Russell R, Reynolds F. Epidural infusions for nulliparous women in labour. A randomised double-blind comparison of fentanyl/bupivacaine and sufentanil/bupivacaine. Anaesthesia 1993;48:856–61.
13. Phillips GH. Epidural sufentanil/bupivacaine combinations for analgesia during labor: effect of varying sufentanil doses. Anesthesiology 1987;67:835–8.
14. Van Steenberge A, Debroux HC, Noorduin H. Extradural bupivacaine with sufentanil for vaginal delivery. A double-blind trial. Br J Anaesth 1987;59:1518–22.
15. Le Polain B, De Kock M, Scholtes JL, Van Lierde M. Clonidine combined with sufentanil and bupivacaine with adrenaline for obstetric analgesia. Br J Anaesth 1993;71:657–60.
16. Grieco WM, Norris MC, Leighton BL, Arkoosh VA, Huffnagle HJ, Honet JE, Costello D. Intrathecal sufentanil labor analgesia: the effects of adding morphine or epinephrine. Anesth Anal 1993;77:1149–54.
17. D'Angelo R, Anderson MT, Philip J, Eisenach JC. Intrathecal sufentanil compared to epidural bupivacaine for labor analgesia. Anesthesiology 1994;80:1209–15.
18. Vertommen JD, Lemmens E, Van Aken H. Comparison of the addition of three different doses of sufentanil to 0.125% bupivacaine given epidurally during labour. Anaesthesia 1994;49:678–81.
19. Dahlgren G, Hultstrand C, Jakobsson J, Norman M, Eriksson EW, Martin H. Intrathecal sufentanil, fentanyl, or placebo added to bupivacaine for cesarean section. Anesth Analg 1997;85:1288–93.
20. Hays RL, Palmer CM. Respiratory depression after intrathecal sufentanil during labor. Anesthesiology 1994;81:511–2.

SULBACTAM

Anti-infective

PREGNANCY RECOMMENDATION: Compatible
BREASTFEEDING RECOMMENDATION: Compatible

PREGNANCY SUMMARY

Sulbactam is always given in combination with ampicillin. It has caused no harm in animal reproduction studies, but reports of human exposure in early gestation are lacking. However, none of the penicillins has been shown to be teratogenic. Sulbactam readily crosses the human placenta to the fetus. Although no direct adverse effects of this exposure on the fetus or newborn have been reported, use of the antibiotic combination near delivery may result in superinfection with resistant bacteria in the newborn.

FETAL RISK SUMMARY

Sulbactam is a semisynthetic beta-lactamase irreversible inhibitor that is derived from the basic penicillin nucleus. When used alone, sulbactam does not have effective anti-infective activity (accept against the *Neisseriaceae*). However, sulbactam extends the activity of ampicillin when given in combination with this antibiotic (1).

Reproduction studies reported by the manufacturer involved mice, rats, and rabbits, but only with the combination of sulbactam and ampicillin (1). There was no evidence of impaired fertility or fetal harm in each species at doses up to 10 times the human dose. Pregnant rats given IV sulbactam at doses up to 500 mg/kg/day at various times, including before mating and throughout gestation, showed no evidence of adverse reproductive effects (2).

Sulbactam crosses the human placenta to the fetus at term (3,4). Placental transfer studies early in gestation have not been located. An abstract from a 1983 symposium reported a linear relationship between fetal and maternal serum sulbactam concentrations when sulbactam/ampicillin was given as a single dose (either 0.5 g/1 g or 1 g/1 g) just before cesarean section. The mean peak fetal serum level of sulbactam was <20 mcg/mL (3). In an in vitro experiment with bidirectional perfused human placental lobules, sulbactam was demonstrated to cross by simple diffusion (4). The placental transfer is consistent with its low molecular weight (about 255).

A 1992 study compared the concentration of three antibiotics (sulbactam/ampicillin, ticarcillin/clavulanic acid, and cefotaxime) in maternal blood, placental tissue, and cord blood in 15 laboring women with chorioamnionitis at ≥37 weeks' gestation (5). Five of the women received the sulbactam/ampicillin combination. The mean concentrations of sulbactam in maternal blood, placental tissue, and cord blood were 7.25, 3.75, and 9.68 mcg/mL. The cord:maternal ratio was 1.3. The time interval between dosing and delivery and the dose used were not specified (5).

The pharmacokinetics of sulbactam at term were described in a 1993 study (6). The kinetics (area under drug vs. time curve, elimination rate constant, half-life, volume of distribution, and clearance) of a 0.5-g dose of sulbactam (combined with 1 g ampicillin) administered IV at cord clamping were not significantly different from those in nonpregnant patients. Changes were noted but did not reach statistical significance (6).

The combination of sulbactam and ampicillin has been used frequently in the 2nd and 3rd trimesters of pregnancy (7–15). These studies involved prophylaxis, as in cases of preterm premature rupture of the membranes, and therapy for established infections. No cases of fetal or newborn direct harm from exposure to the combination were reported. However, indirect harm to the newborn from antibiotic-related superinfection with resistant bacteria is a concern (15).

Inadvertent intrauterine infusion of sulbactam (1 g) plus ampicillin (2 g) was reported in a brief 2000 communication (16). The antibiotic combination was being given for prophylaxis of preterm premature rupture of the membranes at 30 weeks' gestation. Apparently the error occurred when the antibiotic was infused into an intrauterine catheter instead of the intended IV catheter. A 1690-g infant (sex not specified) was delivered by cesarean section the next day. No adverse effects of the error were observed.

BREASTFEEDING SUMMARY

Sulbactam is excreted into human breast milk. Sulbactam (0.5 or 1.0 g) was infused either with cephalothin or ampicillin in four postpartum women 2 days after cesarean section (17). The milk concentrations obtained 10–21 hours after a dose ranged from 0.13 to 1.2 mcg/mL (mean 0.52 mcg/mL). No sulbactam was found in one sample obtained at 49 hours. The investigators did not state whether the infants were allowed to nurse. The potential effects of exposure to sulbactam on a nursing infant is unknown, but are probably similar to those that might occur with other antibiotics: modification of bowel flora, direct effects on the infant (e.g., allergy or sensitization), and interference with the interpretation of culture results if a fever workup is required. The American Academy of Pediatrics classifies sulbactam as compatible with breastfeeding (18).

S

References

1. Product information. Unasyn. Pfizer, 2002.
2. Horimoto M, Sakai T, Ohtsuki I, Noguchi Y. Reproduction studies with sulbactam and combinations of sulbactam and cefoperazone in rats. Chemotherapy 1984;32:108–15. As cited in Shepard TH. *Catalog of Teratogenic Agents*. 10th ed. Baltimore, MD: The Johns Hopkins University Press, 2001:469.
3. Dubois M, Coibion M, Deco J, Delapierre D, Lambotte R, Dresse A. The transplacental transfer of sulbactam sodium when co-administered with ampicillin to healthy pregnant women in labor (abstract). In: Spitzy KH, Karrer K, Breyer S, Lenzhofer R, Moser K, Pichler H, Rainer H, eds. 13th International Congress of Chemotherapy: Vienna, 28th August to 2 September, 1983. TOM 1, Antimicrobial Symposia. Verlag H. Egermann, Publ. Vienna, 1983.
4. Fortunato SJ, Bawdon RE, Baum M. Placental transfer of cefoperazone and sulbactam in the isolated in vitro perfused human placenta. Am J Obstet Gynecol 1988;159:1002–6.
5. Maberry MC, Trimmer KJ, Bawdon RE, Sobhi S, Dax JB, Gilstrap LC III. Antibiotic concentration in maternal blood, cord blood and placental tissue in women with chorioamnionitis. Gynecol Obstet Invest 1992;33:185–6.
6. Chamberlain A, White S, Bawdon R, Thomas S, Larsen B. Pharmacokinetics of ampicillin and sulbactam in pregnancy. Am J Obstet Gynecol 1993;168:667–73.
7. Smith LG Jr, Summers PR, Miles RW, Biswas MK, Pernoll ML. Gonococcal chorioamnionitis associated with sepsis: a case report. Am J Obstet Gynecol 1989;160:573–4.
8. Newton ER, Shields L, Ridgway LE III, Berkus MD, Elliott BD. Combination antibiotics and indomethacin in idiopathic preterm labor: a randomized double-blind clinical trial. Am J Obstet Gynecol 1991; 165:1753–9.
9. Lewis DF, Fontenot MT, Brooks GG, Wise R, Perkins MB, Heyman AR. Latency period after preterm premature rupture of membranes: a comparison of ampicillin with and without sulbactam. Obstet Gynecol 1995;86:392–5.
10. Adair CD, Ernest JM, Sanchez-Ramos L, Burrus DR, Boles ML, Veille JC. Meconium-stained amniotic fluid-associated infectious morbidity: a randomized, double-blind trial of ampicillin-sulbactam prophylaxis. Obstet Gynecol 1996;88:216–20.
11. Lewis DF, Brody K, Edwards MS, Brouillette RM, Burlison S, London SN. Preterm premature ruptured membranes: a randomized trial of steroids after treatment with antibiotics. Obstet Gynecol 1996; 88:801–5.
12. Cox SM, Bohman VR, Sherman ML, Leveno KJ. Randomized investigation of antimicrobials for the prevention of preterm birth. Am J Obstet Gynecol 1996;174:206–10.
13. Lovett SM, Weiss JD, Diogo MJ, Williams PT, Garite TJ. A prospective, double-blind, randomized, controlled clinical trial of ampicillin-sulbactam for preterm premature rupture of membranes in women receiving antenatal corticosteroid therapy. Am J Obstet Gynecol 1997;176:1030–8.
14. Perry KG Jr, Gebhart LD III, Turner KY, Martin RW. Ampicillin/sulbactam and corticosteroids in the management of preterm premature rupture of membranes (abstract). Am J Obstet Gynecol 1998; 178:S201.
15. Carroll EM, Heywood PA, Besinger RE, Muraskas JK, Fisher SG, Gianopoulos JG. A prospective randomized double-blind trial of ampicillin with and without sulbactam in preterm premature rupture of the membranes (abstract). Am J Obstet Gynecol 2000;182:S61.
16. Sigg TR, Kuhn BR. Inadvertent intrauterine infusion of ampicillin-sulbactam. Am J Health-Syst Pharm 2000;57:215.
17. Foulds G, Miller RD, Knirsch AK, Thrupp LD. Sulbactam kinetics and excretion into breast milk in postpartum women. Clin Pharmacol Ther 1985;38:692–6.
18. Committee on Drugs, American Academy of Pediatrics. The transfer of drugs and other chemicals into human milk. Pediatrics 2001; 108:776–89.

SULCONAZOLE

Antifungal

PREGNANCY RECOMMENDATION: No Human Data—Potential Toxicity
BREASTFEEDING RECOMMENDATION: No Human Data—Probably Compatible

PREGNANCY SUMMARY

No reports describing the use of sulconazole in human pregnancy have been located. When given orally, sulconazole was embryotoxic and prolonged gestation in one animal species, but the systemic exposures appeared to be far higher than those that could possibly be obtained after topical use. Sulconazole is partially absorbed with the amount reaching the plasma dependent on the dose and application site. The effects of this exposure are unknown. One study did find a significant increase (relative risk 1.4) in the risk of spontaneous abortion after vaginitis therapy with imidazole antifungals, clotrimazole and miconazole (1). A later study speculated that this effect might have been due to inhibition of the critical placental enzyme aromatase (2). There is no other evidence suggesting that similar topical imidazole-derivative antifungal agents cause embryo–fetal harm. However, sulconazole was a more potent inhibitor of aromatase than either of the two agents associated with the abortions (2). Until additional data are available, the best course is to avoid the use of sulconazole in the 1st trimester or the application of the antifungal to large areas of skin at any time in pregnancy.

FETAL RISK SUMMARY

Sulconazole is available as a 1% cream for topical application. It is in the same antifungal class of imidazole derivatives as butoconazole, clotrimazole, econazole, ketoconazole, miconazole, oxiconazole, sertaconazole, and tioconazole. Sulconazole is indicated for the treatment of tinea pedis (athlete's foot), tinea cruris, and tinea corporis caused by *Trichophyton rubrum, T. mentagrophytes, Epidermophyton floccosum, Microsporum canis*, and tinea versicolor (3).

In a 1988 study with seven adults, two applications (4.5 g/each) of the radiolabeled 1% cream were made on the abdominal skin at 0 and 12 hours (4). The site was then washed at 24 hours and then every 24 hours for 3 days. Radioactivity was detectable in the plasma from 8 to 96 hours, with a peak at 24 hours. The total percutaneous absorption was estimated to be 8.7%–11.3% of the total dose, the highest reported among imidazole derivatives (4).

Reproduction studies have been conducted in rats and rabbits. In rats, an oral dose 125 times the adult human dose based on body weight was embryotoxic. This dose also resulted in prolonged gestation and dystocia. No teratogenicity was observed in rats and rabbits given oral doses of 50 mg/kg/day (comparison to human dose not specified) (3).

It is not known if sulconazole crosses the human placenta. The molecular weight (about 461) suggests that exposure of the embryo–fetus will occur. However, the dose and application site will have a major role in determining the amount of drug available to cross the placenta.

A 2002 study evaluated azole antifungals commonly used in pregnancy for their potential to inhibit aromatase, a placental enzyme that is critical for the production of estrogen and for the maintenance of pregnancy (2). The authors speculated that the embryotoxicity observed in animals and humans (see also Clotrimazole and Miconazole) might be explained by inhibition of aromatase. They found that the most potent inhibitors of aromatase were (shown in order of decreasing potency) econazole, bifonazole (not available in the United States), sulconazole, clotrimazole, and miconazole. The potential plasma concentrations of sulconazole in humans were thought to be high enough to partially inhibit the enzyme (2). However, an earlier study reported a pregnancy that was maintained even when there was severe fetal and placental aromatase deficiency (<0.3% of that of controls) caused by a rare genetic defect (5). In this case, both the fetus and mother were virilized because of diminished conversion of androgens to estrogen. Because the pregnancy was maintained and the virilization, the case suggested that the main function of placental aromatase was to protect the mother and fetus from exposure to adrenal androgens (5).

BREASTFEEDING SUMMARY

No reports describing the use of sulconazole during human lactation have been located. The molecular weight (about 461) suggests that the drug will be excreted into breast milk. The drug is absorbed systemically (see above). The effect of this exposure on a nursing infant is unknown. Because the systemic absorption was the highest known among similar agents, other imidazole antifungals might be more appropriate if a nursing woman requires topical antifungal therapy.

References

1. Rosa FW, Baum C, Shaw M. Pregnancy outcomes after first-trimester vaginitis drug therapy. Obstet Gynecol 1987;69:751–5.
2. Kragie L, Turner SD, Patten CJ, Crespi CL, Stresser DM. Assessing pregnancy risks of azole antifungals using a high throughput aromatase inhibition assay. Endocr Res 2002;28:129–40.
3. Product information. Exelderm. Bristol-Myers Squibb, 2007.
4. Franz TJ, Lehman P. Percutaneous absorption of sulconazole nitrate in humans. J Pharm Sci 1988;77:489–91.
5. Harada N. Genetic analysis of human placental aromatase deficiency. J Steroid Biochem Mol Biol 1993;44:331–40.

S

SULFASALAZINE

Gastrointestinal Agent/Immunologic Agent (Antirheumatic)

PREGNANCY RECOMMENDATION: Human Data Suggest Low Risk
BREASTFEEDING RECOMMENDATION: Limited Human Data—Potential Toxicity

PREGNANCY SUMMARY

Sulfasalazine is a compound composed of 5-aminosalicylic acid (5-ASA) joined to sulfapyridine by an azo-linkage (refer to Sulfonamides for a complete review of this class of agents). No evidence of developmental toxicity has been located. Although it has not been reported, there is a potential risk of neonatal jaundice if the drug is administered close to delivery. If sulfasalazine is used in pregnancy for the treatment of rheumatoid arthritis, healthcare professionals are encouraged to call the toll-free number (877-311-8972) for information about patient enrollment in the Organization of Teratology Information Specialists (OTIS) Rheumatoid Arthritis study.

FETAL RISK SUMMARY

Sulfasalazine is used for the treatment of ulcerative colitis, Crohn's disease, and rheumatoid arthritis. Reproduction studies in rats and rabbits at doses up to 6 times the human dose revealed no impairment of fertility or fetal harm (1).

No increase in human congenital defects or newborn toxicity has been observed from its use in pregnancy (2–12). However, three reports, involving five infants (two stillborn), have described congenital malformations after exposure to this drug (13–15). It cannot be determined whether the observed defects were related to the therapy, the disease, or a combination of these or other factors: bilateral cleft lip/palate, severe hydrocephalus, death (13); ventricular septal defect, coarctation of aorta (14); Potter-type IIa polycystic kidney, rudimentary left uterine cornu, stillborn (first twin) (14); Potter's facies, hypoplastic lungs, absent kidneys and ureters, talipes equinovarus, stillborn (second twin) (14); ventricular septal defect, coarctation of aorta, macrocephaly; gingival hyperplasia, small ears (both thought to be inherited) (15).

Sulfasalazine and its metabolite, sulfapyridine, readily cross the placenta to the fetal circulation (6,7). Fetal concentrations are approximately the same as maternal concentrations. Placental transfer of 5-ASA is limited because only negligible amounts are absorbed from the cecum and colon, and these are rapidly excreted in the urine (16).

At birth, concentrations of sulfasalazine and sulfapyridine in 11 infants were 4.6 and 18.2 mcg/mL, respectively (7). Neither of these levels was sufficient to cause significant displacement of bilirubin from albumin (7). Kernicterus and severe neonatal jaundice have not been reported following maternal use of sulfasalazine, even when the drug was given up to the time of delivery (7,8). Caution is advised, however, because other sulfonamides have caused jaundice in the newborn when given near term (see Sulfonamides).

Sulfasalazine is a folic acid antagonist (dihydrofolate reductase inhibitor). In a 2000 case–control study, the effect of folic acid supplementation on the risks for certain congenital defects were examined (17). Supplementation reduced the teratogenic risk from sulfasalazine and similar acting folic acid antagonists. See Trimethoprim for details of this study.

Sulfasalazine may adversely affect spermatogenesis in male patients with inflammatory bowel disease (18,19). Sperm counts and motility are both reduced and require ≥2 months after the drug is stopped to return to normal levels (18).

BREASTFEEDING SUMMARY

Sulfapyridine is excreted into breast milk (6,16,20) (see also Sulfonamides). Milk concentrations were approximately 40%–60% of maternal serum levels. One infant's urine contained 3–4 mcg/mL of the drug (1.2–1.6 mg/24 hours), representing about 30%–40% of the total dose excreted in the milk. Unmetabolized sulfasalazine was detected in only one of the studies (milk:plasma ratio of 0.3) (6). Levels of 5-ASA were undetectable. No adverse effects were observed in the 16 nursing infants exposed in these reports (6,16,20). However, bloody diarrhea in an infant exclusively breastfed, occurring first at 2 months of age and then recurring 2 weeks later and persisting until 3 months of age, was attributed to the mother's sulfasalazine therapy (3 g/day) (21). The mother was a slow acetylator with a blood concentration of sulfapyridine of 42.4 mcg/mL (therapeutic range 20–50 mcg/mL). The acetylation phenotype of the infant was not determined, but his blood level of sulfapyridine was 5.3 mcg/mL. A diagnostic workup of the infant was negative. The bloody diarrhea did stop, however, 48–72 hours after discontinuance of the mother's therapy. A repeat colonoscopy of the infant 1.5 months later was normal (21).

Based on the above report, the American Academy of Pediatrics classifies sulfasalazine as a drug that has been associated with significant effects in some nursing infants and should be given to nursing mothers with caution (22).

References

1. Product information. Azulfidine EN-tabs. Pharmacia & Upjohn, 2000.
2. McEwan HP. Anorectal conditions in obstetric practice. Proc R Soc Med 1972;65:279–81.
3. Willoughby CP, Truelove SC. Ulcerative colitis and pregnancy. Gut 1980;21:469–74.
4. Levy N, Roisman I, Teodor I. Ulcerative colitis in pregnancy in Israel. Dis Colon Rectum 1981;24:351–4.
5. Mogadam M, Dobbins WO III, Korelitz BI, Ahmed SW. Pregnancy in inflammatory bowel disease: effect of sulfasalazine and corticosteroids on fetal outcome. Gastroenterology 1981;80:72–6.
6. Azad Khan AK, Truelove SC. Placental and mammary transfer of sulphasalazine. Br Med J 1979;2:1553.
7. Jarnerot G, Into-Malmberg MB, Esbjorner E. Placental transfer of sulphasalazine and sulphapyridine and some of its metabolites. Scand J Gastroenterol 1981;16:693–7.
8. Mogadam M. Sulfasalazine, IBD, and pregnancy (reply). Gastroenterology 1981;81:194.
9. Fielding JF. Pregnancy and inflammatory bowel disease. J Clin Gastroenterol 1983;5:107–8.

S

10. Sorokin JJ, Levine SM. Pregnancy and inflammatory bowel disease: a review of the literature. Obstet Gynecol 1983;62:247–52.
11. Baiocco PJ, Korelitz BI. The influence of inflammatory bowel disease and its treatment on pregnancy and fetal outcome. J Clin Gastroenterol 1984;6:211–6.
12. Fedorkow DM, Persaud D, Nimrod CA. Inflammatory bowel disease: a controlled study of late pregnancy outcome. Am J Obstet Gynecol 1989;160:998–1001.
13. Craxi A, Pagliarello F. Possible embryotoxicity of sulfasalazine. Arch Intern Med 1980;140:1674.
14. Newman NM, Correy JF. Possible teratogenicity of sulphasalazine. Med J Aust 1983;1:528–9.
15. Hoo JJ, Hadro TA, Von Behren P. Possible teratogenicity of sulfasalazine. N Engl J Med 1988;318:1128.
16. Berlin CM Jr, Yaffe SJ. Disposition of salicylazosulfapyridine (Azulfidine) and metabolites in human breast milk. Dev Pharmacol Ther 1980;1:31–9.
17. Hernandez-Diaz S, Werler MM, Walker AM, Mitchell AA. Folic acid antagonists during pregnancy and the risk of birth defects. N Engl J Med 2000;343:1608–14.
18. Toovey S, Hudson E, Hendry WF, Levi AJ. Sulphasalazine and male infertility: reversibility and possible mechanism. Gut 1981;22:445–51.
19. Freeman JG, Reece VAC, Venables CW. Sulphasalazine and spermatogenesis. Digestion 1982;23:68–71.
20. Jarnerot G, Into-Malmberg MB. Sulphasalazine treatment during breast feeding. Scand J Gastroenterol 1979;14:869–71.
21. Branski D, Kerem E, Gross-Kieselstein E, Hurvitz H, Litt R, Abrahamov A. Bloody diarrhea-a possible complication of sulfasalazine transferred through human breast milk. J Pediatr Gastroenterol Nutr 1986;5:316–7.
22. Committee on Drugs, American Academy of Pediatrics. The transfer of drugs and other chemicals into human milk. Pediatrics 2001;108: 776–89.

SULFONAMIDES

Anti-infective

PREGNANCY RECOMMENDATION: Human Data Suggest Risk in 3rd Trimester
BREASTFEEDING RECOMMENDATION: Limited Human Data—Potential Toxicity

PREGNANCY SUMMARY

Taken in sum, sulfonamides, as single agents, do not appear to pose a significant teratogenic risk. One study has found associations with birth defects, but a causative association cannot be determined with this type of study and they may have been due to other factors, particularly if trimethoprim was combined with the sulfonamide. Confirmation is required. Because of the potential toxicity to the newborn, these agents should be avoided near term.

FETAL RISK SUMMARY

Sulfonamides are a large class of antibacterial agents. Although there are differences in their bioavailability, all share similar actions in the fetal and newborn periods, and they will be considered as a single group.

Sulfamethoxazole was teratogenic (primarily cleft palates) in rats given oral doses of 533 mg/kg (1). The highest dose that did not produce cleft palates was 512 mg/kg.

The sulfonamides readily cross the placenta to the fetus during all stages of gestation (2–10). Equilibrium with maternal blood is usually established after 2–3 hours, with fetal levels averaging 70%–90% of maternal levels. Significant levels may persist in the newborn for several days after birth when given near term. The primary danger of sulfonamide administration during pregnancy is manifested when these agents are given close to delivery. Toxicities that may be observed in the newborn include jaundice, hemolytic anemia, and, theoretically, kernicterus. Severe jaundice in the newborn has been related by several authors to maternal sulfonamide ingestion at term(11–16). Premature infants seem especially prone to development of hyperbilirubinemia (15). However, a study of 94 infants exposed to sulfadiazine in utero for maternal prophylaxis of rheumatic fever failed to show an increase in prematurity, hyperbilirubinemia, or kernicterus (17). Hemolytic anemia has been reported in two newborns and in a fetus following in utero exposure to sulfonamides (11,12,16). Both newborns survived. In the case involving the fetus, the mother had homozygous glucose-6-phosphate dehydrogenase deficiency (16). She was treated with sulfisoxazole for a urinary tract infection 2 weeks before delivery of a stillborn male infant. Autopsy revealed an infant at 36 weeks' gestation with maceration, severe anemia, and hydrops fetalis.

Sulfonamides compete with bilirubin for binding to plasma albumin. In utero, the fetus clears free bilirubin by the placental circulation; however, after birth, this mechanism is no longer available. Unbound bilirubin is free to cross the blood–brain barrier and may result in kernicterus. Although this toxicity is well known when sulfonamides are administered directly to the neonate, kernicterus in the newborn following in utero exposure has not been reported. Most reports of sulfonamide exposure during gestation have failed to demonstrate an association with congenital malformations (10,11,18–24). Offspring of patients treated throughout pregnancy with sulfasalazine (sulfapyridine plus 5-aminosalicylic acid) for ulcerative colitis or Crohn's disease have not shown an increase in adverse effects (10,21,23) (see also Sulfasalazine). In contrast, a retrospective study of 1369 patients found that significantly more mothers of 458 infants with congenital malformations took sulfonamides than did mothers in the control group (25). A 1975 study examined the in utero drug exposures of 599 children born with oral clefts (26). A significant difference ($p < 0.05$), as compared with matched controls, was found with 1st and 2nd trimester sulfonamide use only when other defects, in addition to the clefts, were present.

S

As noted above, some sulfonamides are animal teratogens. Because of this, warnings of human teratogenicity have been published (27,28). In two reports, investigators associated in utero sulfonamide exposure with tracheoesophageal fistula and cataracts, but additional descriptions of these effects have not appeared (29,30). A mother treated for food poisoning with sulfaguanidine in early pregnancy delivered a child with multiple anomalies (31). The author attributed the defects to use of the drug, but a relationship is doubtful.

The Collaborative Perinatal Project monitored 50,282 mother–child pairs, 1455 of whom had 1st trimester exposure to sulfonamides (32, pp. 296–313). For use anytime during pregnancy, 5689 exposures were reported (32, p. 435). In neither group was evidence found to suggest a relationship to large categories of major or minor malformations. Several possible associations were found with individual defects after anytime use, but independent confirmation is required: ductus arteriosus persistens (8 cases), coloboma (4 cases), hypoplasia of limb or part thereof (7 cases), miscellaneous foot defects (4 cases), urethral obstruction (13 cases), hypoplasia or atrophy of adrenals (6 cases), and benign tumors (12 cases) (32, pp. 485–486).

In a surveillance study of Michigan Medicaid recipients involving 229,101 completed pregnancies conducted between 1985 and 1992, 131 newborns had been exposed to sulfisoxazole, 1138 to sulfabenzamide vaginal cream, and 2296 to the combination of sulfamethoxazole-trimethoprim during the 1st trimester (F. Rosa, personal communication, FDA, 1993). For sulfisoxazole, eight (6.1%) major birth defects were observed (six expected), two cardiovascular defects (one expected), and one oral cleft (none expected). No anomalies were observed in four other categories of defects (spina bifida, polydactyly, limb reduction defects, and hypospadias) for which data were available. For sulfabenzamide, 43 (3.8%) major birth defects were found (44 expected), including (observed/expected) 11/10 cardiovascular defects, 0/2 oral clefts, 0/0.5 spina bifida, 2/3 polydactyly, 1/2 limb reduction defects, and 1/3 hypospadias. The data for sulfisoxazole and sulfabenzamide do not support an association between the drug and congenital defects. In contrast, a possible association was found between sulfamethoxazole-trimethoprim and congenital defects (126 observed/98 expected; 5.5%) in general and for cardiovascular defects (37/23) in particular (see Trimethoprim for details).

A 2009 report from the National Birth Defects Prevention Study estimated the association between antibacterial agents and >30 selected birth defects (33). The authors conducted a population-based, multiple site, case–control study of women who gave birth to an infant with 1 of >30 selected defects. The outcomes were identified in a 10-state birth defect surveillance program and involved 13,155 cases and 4941 controls selected from the same geographical regions. Exposure to an antibacterial was determined by a detailed telephone interview conducted within 24 months after the estimated date of delivery. Women were considered exposed if they had used an antibacterial drug during the month before the estimated date of conception through the end of the 1st trimester (defined as the end of the 3rd month of pregnancy). Significant associations with multiple selected birth defects were found (total number of exposed cases/controls) with sulfonamides (145/42) (probably combined with trimethoprim) and nitrofurantoin (150/42). The adjusted odds ratios and 95% confidence intervals (in parentheses) for sulfonamides were anencephaly 3.4 (1.3–8.8), hypoplastic left heart syndrome 3.2 (1.3–7.6), coarctation of the aorta 2.7 (1.3–5.6), choanal atresia 8.0 (2.7–23.5), transverse limb deficiency 2.5 (1.0–5.9), and diaphragmatic hernia 2.4 (1.1–5.4). Significant associations (total number of exposed cases/controls; number of associations) also were found for penicillins (716/293; 1), erythromycins (202/78; 2), cephalosporins (128/47; 1), quinolones (42/14; 1), and tetracyclines (36/6; 1). The results for quinolones and tetracyclines, however, were based on small numbers of exposed cases and controls (33).

As with all retrospective case–control studies, the data can determine associations, but not causative associations (33). Moreover, several limitations were identified by the authors, including spurious associations caused by the large number of analyses, interviews conducted 6 weeks to 2 years after the pregnancy making recall difficult for cases and controls, recall bias, and inability to distinguish between drug-induced defects and defects resulting from the infection (33).

BREASTFEEDING SUMMARY

Sulfonamides are excreted into breast milk in low concentrations. Milk levels of sulfanilamide (free and conjugated) are reported to range from 6 to 94 mcg/mL (4,34–39). Up to 1.6% of the total dose could be recovered from the milk (34,37). Milk levels often exceeded serum levels and persisted for several days after maternal consumption of the drug was stopped. Milk:plasma ratios during therapy with sulfanilamide were 0.5–0.6 (38). Reports of adverse effects in nursing infants are rare. One author found reports of diarrhea and rash in breastfed infants whose mothers were receiving sulfapyridine or sulfathiazole (7). (See Sulfasalazine for another report of bloody diarrhea.) Milk levels of sulfapyridine, the active metabolite of sulfasalazine, were 10.3 mcg/mL, a milk:plasma ratio of 0.5 (10). Based on these data, the nursing infant would receive approximately 3–4 mg/kg/day of sulfapyridine, an apparently nontoxic amount for a healthy neonate (17). Sulfisoxazole, a very water-soluble drug, was reported to produce a low milk:plasma ratio of 0.06 (40). The conjugated form achieved a ratio of 0.22. The total amount of sulfisoxazole recovered in milk during 48 hours after a 4-g divided dose was only 0.45%. Although controversial, breastfeeding during maternal administration of sulfisoxazole seems to represent a very low risk for the healthy neonate (41,42).

In a 1993 cohort study, diarrhea was reported in 32 (19.3%) nursing infants of 166 breastfeeding mothers who were taking antibiotics (43). For the 12 women taking sulfamethoxazole-trimethoprim, no diarrhea was observed but 2 (17%) had poor feeding, an effect that was considered minor because it did not require medical attention (43).

Sulfonamide excretion into breast milk apparently does not pose a significant risk for the healthy, full-term neonate. Exposure to sulfonamides via breast milk should be avoided in ill, stressed, or premature infants and in infants with hyperbilirubinemia or glucose-6-phosphate dehydrogenase deficiency. With these latter precautions, the American Academy of Pediatrics classifies sulfapyridine, sulfisoxazole, and sulfamethoxazole (when combined with trimethoprim) as compatible with breastfeeding (44).

References

1. Product information. Bactrim. Roche Laboratories, 2000.
2. Barker RH. The placental transfer of sulfanilamide. N Engl J Med 1938;219:41.
3. Speert H. The passage of sulfanilamide through the human placenta. Bull Johns Hopkins Hosp 1938;63:337–9.
4. Stewart HL Jr, Pratt JP. Sulfanilamide excretion in human breast milk and effect on breastfed babies. JAMA 1938;111:1456–8.
5. Speert H. The placental transmission of sulfanilamide and its effects upon the fetus and newborn. Bull Johns Hopkins Hosp 1940;66:139–55.
6. Speert H. Placental transmission of sulfathiazole and sulfadiazine and its significance for fetal chemotherapy. Am J Obstet Gynecol 1943;45:200–7.
7. Von Freisen B. A study of small dose sulphamerazine prophylaxis in obstetrics. Acta Obstet Gynecol Scand 1951;31(Suppl):75–116.
8. Sparr RA, Pritchard JA. Maternal and newborn distribution and excretion of sulfamethoxypyridazine (Kynex). Obstet Gynecol 1958;12:131–4.
9. Nishimura H, Tanimura T. *Clinical Aspects of the Teratogenicity of Drugs*. New York, NY: Excerpta Medica, 1976:88.
10. Azad Khan AK, Truelove SC. Placental and mammary transfer of sulphasalazine. Br Med J 1979;2:1553.
11. Heckel GP. Chemotherapy during pregnancy. Danger of fetal injury from sulfanilamide and its derivatives. JAMA 1941;117:1314–6.
12. Ginzler AM, Cherner C. Toxic manifestations in the newborn infant following placental transmission of sulfanilamide. With a report of 2 cases simulating erythroblastosis fetalis. Am J Obstet Gynecol 1942;44:46–55.
13. Lucey JF, Driscoll TJ Jr. Hazard to newborn infants of administration of long-acting sulfonamides to pregnant women. Pediatrics 1959;24:498–9.
14. Kantor HI, Sutherland DA, Leonard JT, Kamholz FH, Fry ND, White WL. Effect on bilirubin metabolism in the newborn of sulfisoxazole administration to the mother. Obstet Gynecol 1961;17:494–500.
15. Dunn PM. The possible relationship between the maternal administration of sulphamethoxypyridazine and hyperbilirubinaemia in the newborn. J Obstet Gynaecol Br Commonw 1964;71:128–31.
16. Perkins RP. Hydrops fetalis and stillbirth in a male glucose-6-phosphate dehydrogenase-deficient fetus possibly due to maternal ingestion of sulfisoxazole. Am J Obstet Gynecol 1971;111:379–81.
17. Baskin CG, Law S, Wenger NK. Sulfadiazine rheumatic fever prophylaxis during pregnancy: does it increase the risk of kernicterus in the newborn? Cardiology 1980;65:222–5.
18. Bonze EJ, Fuerstner PG, Falls FH. Use of sulfanilamide derivative in treatment of gonorrhea in pregnant and nonpregnant women. Am J Obstet Gynecol 1939;38:73–9.
19. Carter MP, Wilson F. Antibiotics and congenital malformations. Lancet 1963;1:1267–8.
20. Little PJ. The incidence of urinary infection in 5000 pregnant women. Lancet 1966;2:925–8.
21. McEwan HP. Anorectal conditions in obstetric patients. Proc R Soc Med 1972;65:279–81.
22. Williams JD, Smith EK. Single-dose therapy with streptomycin and sulfametopyrazine for bacteriuria during pregnancy. Br Med J 1970;4:651–3.
23. Mogadam M, Dobbins WO III, Korelitz BI, Ahmed SW. Pregnancy in inflammatory bowel disease: effect of sulfasalazine and corticosteroids on fetal outcome. Gastroenterology 1981;80:72–6.
24. Richards IDG. A retrospective inquiry into possible teratogenic effects of drugs in pregnancy. Adv Exp Med Biol 1972;27:441–55.
25. Nelson MM, Forfar JO. Association between drugs administered during pregnancy and congenital abnormalities of the fetus. Br Med J 1971;1:523–7.
26. Saxen I. Associations between oral clefts and drugs taken during pregnancy. Int J Epidemiol 1975;4:37–44.
27. Anonymous. Teratogenic effects of sulphonamides. Br Med J 1965;1:142.
28. Green KG. "Bimez" and teratogenic action. Br Med J 1963;2:56.
29. Ingalls TH, Prindle RA. Esophageal atresia with tracheoesophageal fistula. Epidemiologic and teratologic implications. N Engl J Med 1949;240:987–95.
30. Harly JD, Farrar JF, Gray JB, Dunlop IC. Aromatic drugs and congenital cataracts. Lancet 1964;1:472–3.
31. Pogorzelska E. A case of multiple congenital anomalies in a child of a mother treated with sulfaguanidine. Patol Pol 1966;17:383–6.
32. Heinonen OP, Slone D, Shapiro S. *Birth Defects and Drugs in Pregnancy*. Littleton, MA: Publishing Sciences Group, 1977.
33. Crider KS, Cleves MA, Reefhuis J, Berry RJ, Hobbs CA, Hu DJ. Antibacterial medication use during pregnancy and risk of birth defects. Arch Pediatr Adolesc Med 2009;163:978–85.
34. Adair FL, Hesseltine HC, Hac LR. Experimental study of the behavior of sulfanilamide. JAMA 1938;111:766–70.
35. Hepburn JS, Paxson NF, Rogers AN. Secretion of ingested sulfanilamide in breast milk and in the urine of the infant. J Biol Chem 1938;123:liv–v.
36. Pinto SS. Excretion of sulfanilamide and acetylsulfanilamide in human milk. JAMA 1938;111:1914–6.
37. Hac LR, Adair FL, Hesseltine HC. Excretion of sulfanilamide and acetylsulfanilamide in human breast milk. Am J Obstet Gynecol 1939;38:57–66.
38. Foster FP. Sulfanilamide excretion in breast milk: report of a case. Proc Staff Meet Mayo Clin 1939;14:153–5.
39. Hepburn JS, Paxson NF, Rogers AN. Secretion of ingested sulfanilamide in human milk and in the urine of the nursing infant. Arch Pediatr 1942;59:413–8.
40. Kauffman RE, O'Brien C, Gilford P. Sulfisoxazole secretion into human milk. J Pediatr 1980;97:839–41.
41. Elliott GT, Quinn SI. Sulfisoxazole in human milk. J Pediatr 1981;99:171–2.
42. Kauffman RE. Sulfisoxazole in human milk (reply). J Pediatr 1981;99:172.
43. Ito S, Blajchman A, Stephenson M, Eliopoulos C, Koren G. Prospective follow-up of adverse reactions in breast-fed infants exposed to maternal medication. Am J Obstet Gynecol 1993;168:1393–9.
44. Committee on Drugs, American Academy of Pediatrics. The transfer of drugs and other chemicals into human milk. Pediatrics 2001;108:776–89.

SULINDAC

Nonsteroidal Anti-inflammatory

PREGNANCY RECOMMENDATION: Human Data Suggest Risk in 1st and 3rd Trimesters
BREASTFEEDING RECOMMENDATION: No Human Data—Potential Toxicity

S

PREGNANCY SUMMARY

Sulindac, a prostaglandin synthesis inhibitor, potentially could cause constriction of the ductus arteriosus in utero, as well as inhibition of labor, prolongation of pregnancy, and suppression of fetal renal function (1,2). Persistent pulmonary hypertension of the newborn should also be considered (3). Women attempting to conceive should not use any prostaglandin synthesis inhibitor, including sulindac, because of the findings in a variety of animal models that indicate these agents block blastocyst implantation (4,5). Moreover, as noted below, nonsteroidal anti-inflammatory drugs (NSAIDs) have been associated with spontaneous abortions (SABs) and congenital malformations. The absolute risk for these defects, however, appears to be low.

FETAL RISK SUMMARY

Sulindac is an NSAID prodrug that is converted in vivo to the biologically active sulfide metabolite. It is used for the relief of the signs and symptoms of rheumatoid arthritis, osteoarthritis, gouty arthritis, ankylosing spondylitis, and acute painful shoulder (6). Sulindac is in the same NSAID subclass (acetic acids) as diclofenac, indomethacin, and tolmetin. However, sulindac, a derivative of indomethacin, is seven times more cyclooxygenase (COX)-2 selective than indomethacin and is sometimes referred to as a COX-2 selective agent (7).

When administered to pregnant rats, similar to other NSAIDs, sulindac reduces fetal weight and pup survival (at doses ≥2.5 times than the usual maximum human daily dose), prolongs the duration of gestation, and may cause dystocia (6,8).

Consistent with the molecular weight (about 356), sulindac and its active metabolite cross the human placenta to the fetus. Nine women at a mean gestational age of 31.8 weeks (24.3–36.4 weeks) were given a single 200-mg oral dose of the drug a mean 5.5 hours (4.4–6.7 hours) before cordocentesis (9,10). Maternal serum was obtained at a mean 5.8 hours (3.5–7.3 hours) after the dose. The mean concentrations of sulindac in the mothers and fetuses were 0.59 and 0.98 mcg/mL, respectively, and of the sulfide metabolite 1.42 and 0.68 mcg/mL, respectively. The corresponding sulfide:sulindac ratios in the mother and fetal compartments were 2.32 and 0.53, respectively. The reduced amounts of metabolite in the fetus, compared with those in the mother, were thought to be caused by decreased placental transfer of the metabolite and slower metabolism of sulindac in the fetus (10). Because of these findings, the investigators theorized that, as a tocolytic, sulindac would be expected to cause less fetal toxicity than indomethacin.

Using a human term placental perfusion model, a 1999 study demonstrated that the sulfide metabolite reaches the fetus in higher concentrations than does sulindac or indomethacin (11). The fetal:maternal ratios after 2-hour perfusions were 0.34 (sulindac), 0.54 (sulfide metabolite), and 0.45 (indomethacin). Neither sulindac nor indomethacin was metabolized by the placenta (11).

In a surveillance study of Michigan Medicaid recipients involving 229,101 completed pregnancies conducted between 1985 and 1992, 69 newborns had been exposed to sulindac during the 1st trimester (F. Rosa, personal communication, FDA, 1995). Three (4.3%) major birth defects were observed (three expected), including one cardiovascular defect (one expected). No anomalies were observed in five other categories of defects (oral clefts, spina bifida, polydactyly, limb reduction defects, and hypospadias) for which specific data were available. For exposure during any trimester (102 newborns), two malformations of the eyeball (excluding oculomotor and ptosis) were observed (none expected), but no brain defects were recorded.

A combined 2001 population-based, observational cohort study and a case–control study estimated the risk of adverse pregnancy outcome from the use of NSAIDs (12). The use of NSAIDs during pregnancy was not associated with congenital malformations, preterm delivery, or low birth weight, but a positive association was discovered with SABs. A similar study, also published in 2001, failed to find a relationship, in general, between NSAIDs and congenital malformations, but did find a significant association with cardiac defects and orofacial clefts (13). In addition, a 2003 study found a significant association between exposure to NSAIDs in early pregnancy and SABs (14). (See Ibuprofen for details on these three studies.)

A brief 2003 editorial on the potential for NSAID-induced developmental toxicity concluded that NSAIDs, specifically those with greater COX-2 affinity, had a lower risk of this toxicity in humans than aspirin (15).

An abstract and a full report, both published in 1992, described the use of sulindac in the treatment of preterm labor in comparison with indomethacin (16,17). The gestational ages at treatment for the groups were 29 and 30 weeks, respectively. The sulindac group (N = 18) received 200 mg orally every 12 hours for 48 hours, whereas those receiving indomethacin (N = 18) were given 100 mg orally once followed by 25 mg orally every 4 hours for 48 hours. Both groups received IV magnesium sulfate and some in both groups received SC terbutaline. The response to tocolysis was statistically similar for sulindac and indomethacin. However, the sulindac-treated women had significantly greater hourly fetal urine output, the deepest amniotic fluid pocket, and the largest amniotic fluid index. Patent ductus arteriosus (PDA) was observed in 11% vs. 22%, respectively, and intraventricular hemorrhage (IVH) in the newborn occurred in 11% of both groups. These differences were not significant. No cases of primary pulmonary hypertension in the newborns were observed (16,17).

A comparison between sulindac (200 mg orally every 12 hours for 4 days) and indomethacin (100 mg rectally on the 1st day, then 50 mg orally every 8 hours for 3 days) on fetal cardiac function was published in 1995 (18). Each group was composed of 10 patients with threatened premature labor at 28–32 weeks' gestation. Significant reductions in the mean pulsatility index of the fetal ductus arteriosus began 4 hours after the first indomethacin dose. The reduction increased with time and resolved 24 hours after the last dose. Other secondary changes in fetal cardiac function resulting from ductal constriction were also noted. In the sulindac group, a significant decrease in the mean pulsatility index, without secondary changes, was observed only at 24 hours (18).

A study comparing the fetal cardiovascular effects of sulindac (200 mg orally every 12 hours) and terbutaline (5 mg orally every 4 hours) for 68 hours at an approximate mean gestational age of 32 weeks was published in an abstract form in 1996 (19) and in a full report in 1999 (20). Significant ductal constriction was noted only in the sulindac group. In contrast to the study cited above, therapy was stopped because of severe constriction in 2 (one at 12 hours and the other at 24 hours) of the 10 patients. The constriction of the fetal ductus arteriosus occurred within 5 hours of receiving sulindac and resolved within 48 hours of discontinuing the drug (19,20).

A 1994 abstract reported that the tocolytic effect of a 7-day course of sulindac, 200 mg orally every 12 hours, following arrest of labor with IV magnesium sulfate, was no different from placebo and observation (21). The difference in prolongation of pregnancy between the sulindac (N = 13) and placebo (N = 15) groups (33 vs. 26 days, respectively) was not significant. No differences between the groups on days 0, 7, and 14 were found for hourly fetal urine production, amniotic fluid index, or ductus arteriosus velocity (21).

Two 1995 references from the same group of investigators, using a similar study design, concluded that sulindac did not reduce the rate of premature birth but did lengthen the interval to retocolysis in those patients who required retocolysis (22,23). No difference was found between sulindac and placebo in prolongation of pregnancy, delivery at >35 weeks' gestation, recurrent preterm labor, birth weight, or time spent in the neonatal intensive care unit. No adverse effects were observed in the exposed fetuses (22,23).

As demonstrated with other NSAIDs (see also Indomethacin), sulindac reduces amniotic fluid volume by decreasing fetal urine output in a dose-related manner (24). Sulindac, 200 mg twice daily, was given to the mothers of three sets of monoamniotic twins, diagnosed as having cord entanglement, beginning at 24, 27, and 29 weeks, respectively, and continued until elective cesarean section at 32 weeks' gestation. One of the twins had a preexisting heart defect (transposition of the great vessels and a ventricular septal defect). The dose was reduced in one patient to 200 mg/day to maintain an adequate amniotic fluid index. No significant changes in the umbilical artery or the ductus arteriosus Doppler waveforms were observed. All of the newborns had appropriate weights for gestation and normal renal function during the first week of life, and none required ventilation (24).

A 2000 abstract described a retrospective case–cohort study that compared the neonatal effects of sulindac with indomethacin (25). The infants (born between 1994 and 1999) had been exposed to antenatal sulindac (N = 25) or indomethacin (N = 66) and weighed <1500 g. Those exposed to both drugs or with congenital abnormalities were excluded. There were no significant differences between the indomethacin and sulindac groups in IVH (32% vs. 36%), grades III-IV IVH (14% vs. 12%), necrotizing enterocolitis (8% vs. 8%), serum creatinine >1.4 mg/dL (19% vs. 15%), PDA (17% vs. 28%), and mortality (12% vs. 12%), respectively. However, there was a significant increase in the risk for bronchopulmonary dysplasia after exposure to indomethacin (adjusted odds ratio 4.9, 95% confidence interval 1.01–23.44) (25).

A 2003 review concluded that COX-2 selective drugs, such as sulindac, should only be used as tocolytics in randomized controlled trials (7). This conclusion was based on the uncertainty over whether the fetal toxicity observed with sulindac resulted from COX-2-dependent effects, or from fetal accumulation of drug levels sufficient to cause COX-1 inhibition (7).

BREASTFEEDING SUMMARY

No reports describing the use of sulindac during lactation have been located. The mean adult serum half-life of the biologically active sulfide metabolite is 16.4 hours (6). One reviewer concluded that because of the prolonged half-life, other agents in this class (diclofenac, fenoprofen, flurbiprofen, ibuprofen, ketoprofen, ketorolac, and tolmetin) were safer alternatives if an NSAID was required during nursing (26).

References

1. Levin DL. Effects of inhibition of prostaglandin synthesis on fetal development, oxygenation, and the fetal circulation. Semin Perinatol 1980;4:35–44.
2. Fuchs F. Prevention of prematurity. Am J Obstet Gynecol 1976;126:809–20.
3. Van Marter LJ, Leviton A, Allred EN, Pagano M, Sullivan KF, Cohen A, Epstein MF. Persistent pulmonary hypertension of the newborn and smoking and aspirin and nonsteroidal antiinflammatory drug consumption during pregnancy. Pediatrics 1996;97:658–63.
4. Matt DW, Borzelleca JF. Toxic effects on the female reproductive system during pregnancy, parturition, and lactation. In: Witorsch RJ, ed. *Reproductive Toxicology*. 2nd ed. New York, NY: Raven Press, 1995:175–93.
5. Dawood MY. Nonsteroidal antiinflammatory drugs and reproduction. Am J Obstet Gynecol 1993;169:1255–65.
6. Product information. Clinoril. Merck, 2001.
7. Loudon JAZ, Groom KM, Bennett PR. Prostaglandin inhibitors in preterm labour. Best Pract Res Clin Obstet Gynaecol 2003;17:731–44.
8. Lione A, Scialli AR. The developmental toxicity of indomethacin and sulindac. Reprod Toxicol 1995;9:7–20.
9. Kramer W, Saade G, Belfort M, Ou C-N, Rognerud C, Knudsen L, Moise K Jr. Placental transfer of sulindac and its active metabolite in humans (abstract). Am J Obstet Gynecol 1994;170:389.
10. Kramer WB, Saade G, Ou C-N, Rognerud C, Dorman K, Mayes M, Moise KJ Jr. Placental transfer of sulindac and its active sulfide metabolite in humans. Am J Obstet Gynecol 1995;172:886–90.
11. Lampela ES, Nuutinen LH, Ala-Kkokko TL, Parikka RM, Laitinen RS, Jouppila PI, Vahakangas KH. Placental transfer of sulindac, sulindac sulfide, and indomethacin in a human placental perfusion model. Am J Obstet Gynecol 1999;180:174–80.
12. Nielsen GL, Sorensen HT, Larsen H, Pedersen L. Risk of adverse birth outcome and miscarriage in pregnant users of non-steroidal anti-inflammatory drugs: population-based observational study and case–control study. Br Med J 2001;322:266–70.
13. Ericson A, Kallen BAJ. Nonsteroidal anti-inflammatory drugs in early pregnancy. Reprod Toxicol 2001;15:371–5.
14. Li DK, Liu L, Odouli R. Exposure to non-steroidal anti-inflammatory drugs during pregnancy and risk of miscarriage: population based cohort study. Br Med J 2003;327:368–71.
15. Tassinari MS, Cook JC, Hurtt ME. NSAIDs and developmental toxicity. Birth Defects Res B Dev Reprod Toxicol 2003;68:3–4.
16. Carlan SJ, O'Brien WF, O'Leary TD, Mastrogiannis DS. A randomized comparative trial of indomethacin and sulindac for the treatment of refractory preterm labor (abstract). Am J Obstet Gynecol 1992;166:361.
17. Carlan SJ, O'Brien WF, O'Leary TD, Mastrogiannis D. Randomized comparative trial of indomethacin and sulindac for the treatment of refractory preterm labor. Obstet Gynecol 1992;79:223–8.
18. Rasanen J, Jouppila P. Fetal cardiac function and ductus arteriosus during indomethacin and sulindac therapy for threatened preterm labor: a randomized study. Am J Obstet Gynecol 1995;173:20–5.
19. Kramer W, Saade G, Belfort M, Dorman K, Mayes M, Moise K Jr. Randomized double-blind study comparing sulindac to terbutaline: fetal cardiovascular effects (abstract). Am J Obstet Gynecol 1996;174:326.
20. Kramer WB, Saade GR, Belfort M, Dorman K, Mayes M, Moise KJ Jr. A randomized double-blind study comparing the fetal effects of sulindac to terbutaline during the management of preterm labor. Am J Obstet Gynecol 1999;180:396–401.
21. Carlan S, Jones M, Schorr S, McNeill T, Rawji H, Clark K. Oral sulindac to prevent recurrence of preterm labor (abstract). Am J Obstet Gynecol 1994;170:381.
22. Jones M, Carlan S, Schorr S, McNeill T, Rawji R, Clark K, Fuentes A. Oral sulindac to prevent recurrence of preterm labor (abstract). Am J Obstet Gynecol 1995;172:416.
23. Carlan SJ, O'Brien WF, Jones MH, O'Leary TD, Roth L. Outpatient oral sulindac to prevent recurrence of preterm labor. Obstet Gynecol 1995;85:769–74.
24. Peek MJ, McCarthy A, Kyle P, Sepulveda W, Fisk NM. Medical amnioreduction with sulindac to reduce cord complications in monoamniotic twins. Am J Obstet Gynecol 1997;176:334–6.
25. Sciscione A, Leef K, Vakili B, Paul D. Neonatal effects after antenatal treatment with indomethacin vs. sulindac (abstract). Am J Obstet Gynecol 2000;182:S66.
26. Anderson PO. Medication use while breast feeding a neonate. Neonatal Pharmacol Q 1993;2:3–14.

SUMATRIPTAN

Antimigraine

PREGNANCY RECOMMENDATION: Limited Human Data—Animal Data Suggest Moderate Risk
BREASTFEEDING RECOMMENDATION: Limited Human Data—Probably Compatible

PREGNANCY SUMMARY

Sumatriptan has caused toxicity and malformations in one animal species, but the drug does not appear to present a major teratogenic risk in humans. There was no consistent pattern among the reported birth defects to suggest a common cause. The studies, however, lack the sensitivity to identify minor anomalies because of the absence of standardized examinations. In one study, late-appearing major defects may also have been missed due to the timing of the questionnaires. Thus, although the data are generally reassuring, the number and follow-up of exposed pregnancies are still too limited to assess, with confidence, the safety of the agent or its teratogenic potential. However, a 2008 review of triptans in pregnancy found no evidence for teratogenicity, but the data did suggest a possible increase in the rate of preterm birth (1).

FETAL RISK SUMMARY

Sumatriptan (GR 43175) is a selective serotonin (5-hydroxytryptamine 1 [5-HT]) receptor subtype agonist used for the acute treatment of migraine headaches. It is available in oral tablets and as an SC injection. Sumatriptan has also been used for the treatment of cluster headaches. The drug is closely related to almotriptan, eletriptan, frovatriptan, naratriptan, rizatriptan, and zolmitriptan.

It is metabolized to inactive metabolites. Plasma protein binding is low (14%–21%) and the elimination half-life is about 2.5 hours (2).

Sumatriptan was embryolethal in rabbits when given in daily IV doses approximately equivalent to the maximum recommended single human SC dose of 6 mg based on BSA (MRHD). The doses were at or close to those producing maternal toxicity. Fetuses of rabbits administered oral sumatriptan (at doses >50 times the MRHD) during organogenesis had an increased incidence of cervicothoracic vascular and skeletal anomalies. In contrast, embryo or fetal lethality was not observed in pregnant rats treated throughout organogenesis with IV doses approximately 20 times the MRHD. Moreover, no rat embryo–fetal lethality or teratogenicity was observed with daily SC doses before and throughout gestation (2). Shepard (3) described a study in which no fetal adverse effects were observed in rats given up to 1000 mg/kg orally during organogenesis.

No studies examining the placental transfer of sumatriptan in animals or humans have been located. The molecular weight (about 414), low plasma protein binding, and the elimination half-life suggest that exposure of the embryo and fetus should be expected.

Individual reports and data from Medicaid studies totaled 14 spontaneous abortions (SABs) with the use of sumatriptan during early pregnancy (F. Rosa, personal communication, FDA, 1996). Seven birth defect case reports received by the FDA included two chromosomal anomalies (both of which could have been exposed before conception), one infant with an ear tag, one case of a phocomelia, a reduction defect of the lower limbs (tibial aplasia), a case of developmental retardation, and one unspecified defect (some of these defects appear to be also included in data from the pregnancy registry cited below).

An interim report of the Sumatriptan/Naratriptan/Treximet Pregnancy Registry, covering the period January 1, 1996 through April 30, 2009, described the outcomes of 761 prospectively enrolled pregnancies exposed to sumatriptan: 578 outcomes (including 6 sets of twins and 1 set of triplets), 170 lost to follow-up, and 21 pending (4). Some of the data were also reported in a 1997 abstract (5). There were 494 outcomes with earliest exposure in the 1st trimester, 66 with earliest exposure in the 2nd trimester, 14 in the 3rd trimester, and 4 exposed at an unspecified time. In the 1st trimester group, there were 20 birth defects (16 live births, 1 fetal death, and 3 elective abortions [EABs]), whereas in the group with no birth defects reported, there were 427 live births, 4 fetal deaths, and 11 EABs. In the combined 1st trimester group, there were 32 SABs (<20 weeks' gestation). In the 66 outcomes with earliest exposure in the 2nd trimester, there were 3 live births with birth defects and 63 live births without defects. The 3rd trimester group had 14 live births without defects, and the unspecified group had 1 EAB with a birth defect and 3 live births without defects. Excluding fetal deaths and EABs without reported birth defects and all SABs, the observed proportion of birth defects in the 1st trimester group was 4.5% (95% confidence interval [CI] 2.8%–6.9%). For any trimester exposure, the proportion (with the same exclusions) was 4.5% (95% CI 3.0%–6.7%). The prevalence of birth defects in women with migraine has been estimated at 3.4%. The Registry noted the occurrence of ventricular septal defects in 4 of the 447 (0.89%) prospective 1st trimester exposures, 2 of which were clinically insignificant. There were three pregnancies exposed to Treximet (sumatriptan plus naproxen) prospectively enrolled and all are pending outcome (4).

Although retrospective reports (reported after the pregnancy outcome was known) are often biased (only adverse outcomes are reported), there were 26 birth defects reported to the Registry, 23 with earliest exposure in the 1st trimester, 1 with earliest exposure in the 2nd trimester, and 2 with unspecified trimester. Review of all birth defects from prospective and retrospective reports revealed no signal or consistent pattern to suggest a common etiology (4).

A 1998 report (first published in 1997 as an abstract [6]) described the prospectively determined pregnancy outcomes of 96 women exposed to sumatriptan (95 exposed during

S

1st trimester) (7). No difference in the rate of major birth defects was found between the study patients and nonteratogen-exposed controls or disease-matched controls. One major birth defect was reported in a sumatriptan-exposed infant: vesicoureteral reflux requiring bilateral reimplant (7).

A 1998 noninterventional observational cohort study described the outcomes of pregnancies in women who had been prescribed ≥1 of 34 newly marketed drugs by general practitioners in England (8). Data were obtained by questionnaires sent to the prescribing physicians one month after the expected or possible date of delivery. In 831 (78%) of the pregnancies, a newly marketed drug was thought to have been taken during the 1st trimester with birth defects noted in 14 (2.5%) singleton births of the 557 newborns (10 sets of twins). In addition, two birth defects were observed in aborted fetuses. However, few of the aborted fetuses were examined. Sumatriptan was taken during the 1st trimester in 35 pregnancies. The outcomes of these pregnancies included 4 SABs, 3 EABs, 5 pregnancies lost to follow-up, and 23 normal infants (2 premature) (8).

A 2004 case report described a 24-year-old woman who took sumatriptan (100 mg about once a week), naproxen (550 mg about twice a week), and bisoprolol (5 mg/day) for migraine headaches during the first 5 weeks of pregnancy (9). An elective cesarean section was performed at 37 weeks' for breech presentation to deliver a 3125-g male infant. The infant had a wide bilateral cleft lip/palate, marked hypertelorism, a broad nose, and bilateral but asymmetric toe abnormalities (missing and hypoplastic phalanges) (9).

In an in vitro study, only high concentrations of sumatriptan were capable of increasing uterine contractions (10). The findings suggested that therapeutic concentrations of the drug would not induce preterm labor.

A second 2008 review of triptans in pregnancy concluded that sumatriptan appeared to be safe for use in the 1st trimester for the treatment of new-onset or worsened migraines (11). However, the data were insufficient to similarly classify other triptans.

Required statement (4): Sumatriptan: The number of exposed pregnancy outcomes accumulated to date represents a sample of insufficient size for reaching definitive conclusions regarding the possible teratogenic risk of sumatriptan. Specifically, the sample size to date remains too small for formal comparisons of the frequency of specific birth defects. If the baseline frequency of total birth defects is 3 in 100 live births, a sample size of 324 for 1st trimester exposure has an 80 percent chance (80% power) of correctly detecting at least a 1.9-fold increase from baseline in the frequency of birth defects. If the baseline frequency of specific birth defects is 1 in 1000 live births, a sample size of 324 for 1st trimester exposure has an 80 percent (80% power) of correctly detecting at least an 8.1-fold increase from baseline in the frequency of a specific birth defect.

Naratriptan: The data represent a sample of insufficient size for reaching definitive conclusions regarding the possible teratogenic risk of naratriptan. If the baseline frequency of total birth defects is 3 in 100 live births, a sample size of 31 for the 1st trimester exposure has an 80 percent chance (80% power) of correctly detecting at least a 4.6-fold increase from baseline in the frequency of total birth defects. If the baseline frequency for a specific birth defect is 1 in 1000 live births, a sample size of 31 for 1st trimester exposure has an 80 percent chance (80% power) of correctly detecting at least a 40.9-fold increase from baseline in the frequency of a specific birth defect.

The number of exposed pregnancy outcomes accumulated to date represents a sample of insufficient size for reaching definitive conclusions regarding the possible teratogenic risk of sumatriptan or naratriptan. It is expected that a teratogenic exposure in the 1st trimester would result in an increased frequency of one or a combination of individual defects or types of defects, but not necessarily in all defects.

As reporting of pregnancies to the Sumatriptan and Naratriptan Registry is voluntary, it is possible that even in prospectively reported pregnancies there could be bias in type of pregnancies reported. For example, differential reporting of low-risk or high-risk pregnancies may be a potential limitation to this type of registry. In addition, reporting of defects from maternal health care providers may limit detection of detects not immediately apparent at birth. Despite this, the Registry is intended both to supplement animal toxicology studies and other structured epidemiologic studies and clinical trial data, and to assist clinicians in weighing the risks and benefits of treatment for individual patients and circumstances.

BREASTFEEDING SUMMARY

Sumatriptan is excreted into human milk. Five women with a mean duration of lactation of 22.2 weeks (range 10.8–28.4 weeks) were administered a 6-mg SC dose of sumatriptan (12). Milk samples were obtained hourly for 8 hours by emptying both breasts of each subject with a breast pump. Frequent blood samples were also obtained from the women. The mean milk:plasma ratio was 4.9. The mean cumulative excretion of drug in milk during the 8-hour sampling period was 12.6 mcg and, by extrapolation, a total recovery of only 14.4 mcg after a 6-mg dose. Using this latter value, the authors estimated that the mean weight-adjusted dose (mcg sumatriptan/kg of infant body weight as a percentage of the mother's dose in mcg/kg) for the infants would have been 3.5%. The investigators considered the risk to a nursing infant from this exposure to be not significant (12).

In adults, the mean oral bioavailability of sumatriptan is 14%–15% (range 10%–26%) (2,13), suggesting that absorption from the gastrointestinal tract is inhibited. Thus, although the oral absorption in infants may be markedly different from adults, the amount of sumatriptan reaching the systemic circulation of a breastfeeding infant is probably negligible. Discarding the milk for 8 hours after a dose, an interval during which about 88% of the amount excreted into milk can be recovered, would reduce even more the small amounts present in milk. The American Academy of Pediatrics classifies sumatriptan as compatible with breastfeeding (14).

References

1. Soldin OP, Dahlin J, O'Mara DM. Triptans in pregnancy. Ther Drug Monit 2008;30:5–9.
2. Product information. Imitrex. GlaxoSmithKline, 2007.

3. Shepard TH. *Catalog of Teratogenic Agents*. 8th ed. Baltimore, MD: The Johns Hopkins University Press, 1995:397.
4. The Sumatriptan/Naratriptan/Treximet Pregnancy Registry. Interim Report. 1 January 1996 through 30 April 2009. GlaxoSmithKline, August 2009.
5. Eldridge RE, Ephross SA. Monitoring birth outcomes in the sumatriptan pregnancy registry (abstract). Teratology 1997;55:48.
6. Shuhaiber S, Pastuszak A, Schick B, Koren G. Pregnancy outcome following gestational exposure to sumatriptan (Imitrex) (abstract). Teratology 1997;55:103.
7. Shuhaiber S, Pastuszak A, Schick B, Matsui D, Spivey G, Brochu J, Koren G. Pregnancy outcome following first trimester exposure to sumatriptan. Neurology 1998;51:581–3.
8. Wilton LV, Pearce GL, Martin RM, Mackay FJ, Mann RD. The outcomes of pregnancy in women exposed to newly marketed drugs in general practice in England. Br J Obstet Gynaecol 1998;105:882–9.
9. Kajantie E, Somer M. Bilateral cleft lip and palate, hypertelorism and hypoplastic toes. Clin Dysmorphol 2004;13:195–6.
10. Gei A, Longo M, Vedernikov Y, Saade G, Garfield R. The effect of sumatriptan on the uterine contractility of human myometrium (abstract). Am J Obstet Gynecol 2001;184:S193.
11. Evans EW, Lorber KC. Use of 5-HT_1 agonists in pregnancy. Ann Pharmacother 2008;42:543–9.
12. Wojnar-Horton RE, Hackett LP, Yapp P, Dusci LJ, Paech M, Ilett KF. Distribution and excretion of sumatriptan in human milk. Br J Clin Pharmacol 1996;41:217–21.
13. Fullerton T, Gengo FM. Sumatriptan: a selective 5-hydroxytryptamine receptor agonist for the acute treatment of migraine. Ann Pharmacother 1992;26:800–8.
14. Committee on Drugs, American Academy of Pediatrics. The transfer of drugs and other chemicals into human milk. Pediatrics 2001;108:776–89.

SUNITINIB

Antineoplastic (Tyrosine Kinase Inhibitor)

PREGNANCY RECOMMENDATION: Contraindicated
BREASTFEEDING RECOMMENDATION: Contraindicated

PREGNANCY SUMMARY

No reports describing the use of sunitinib in human pregnancy have been located. The animal reproduction data suggest risk, but the absence of human pregnancy experience prevents a more complete assessment. However, there are limited human pregnancy data for imatinib, a drug in the same subclass and with same mechanism of action as dasatinib. (See Imatinib.) Nevertheless, agents in this subclass inhibit angiogenesis, a critical component of embryonic and fetal development. Women of reproductive age should use effective contraception. However, gastrointestinal cancers can be fatal, so if a woman requires imatinib and informed consent is obtained, treatment should not be withheld because of pregnancy. If an inadvertent pregnancy occurs, the woman should be advised of the potential risk for severe adverse effects in the embryo and fetus.

FETAL RISK SUMMARY

Sunitinib is an oral tyrosine kinase inhibitor that inhibits tumor growth, pathologic angiogenesis, and metastatic progression of cancer. There are several other agents in this subclass (see Appendix). Sunitinib is indicated for the treatment of gastrointestinal stromal tumor after disease progression on or intolerance to imatinib. It is extensively metabolized by the liver. One of the metabolites is active and comprises 23%–37% of the total exposure. The terminal elimination half-lives of sunitinib and the active metabolite are 40–60 and 80–110 hours, respectively, whereas the binding to human plasma proteins is 95% and 90%, respectively. Elimination is primarily in the feces (1).

Reproduction studies have been conducted in rats and rabbits. In pregnant rats, doses producing systemic exposures that were about 5.5 times than the systemic exposure in humans from the recommended daily dose of 50 mg based on AUC (SE-RDD) caused significant increases in the incidences of embryo death and structural anomalies (malformations of the ribs and vertebrae). The no-effect exposure in rats was 2.3 times the SE-RDD. In pregnant rabbits, an exposure about 2.7 times the SE-RDD caused a significant increase in embryo death and in cleft lips and palates. A lower exposure, about 0.3 times the SE-RDD, caused cleft lip only (1).

Studies for carcinogenicity have not been conducted with sunitinib. The drug did not cause genotoxicity in multiple tests. In a 3-month study in monkeys, with a dose producing systemic exposures that were about 5.1 times the SE-RDD, ovarian changes (decreased follicular development) were noted, while an exposure about 0.4 times the SE-RDD caused uterine changes (endometrial atrophy). When the study period was lengthened to 9 months, an exposure 0.8 times the SE-RDD caused vaginal atrophy, as well as the ovarian and uterine changes. A no-effect dose was not determined in the 3-month study but, in the 9-month study, it was about 0.2 times the SE-RDD. No effects on fertility were observed in male and female rats (1).

It is not known if sunitinib or its active metabolite crosses the human placenta. The molecular weight (about 399 for the free base) of the parent compound and the long elimination half-lives for sunitinib and the metabolite suggest that the agents will cross to the embryo–fetus.

BREASTFEEDING SUMMARY

No reports describing the use of sunitinib during human lactation have been located. The molecular weight (about 399 for the free base) of the parent compound and the long elimination half-lives for sunitinib and its active metabolite suggest that the agents will be excreted into breast milk. The risk to a nursing infant is unknown, but there is potential for severe toxicity affecting multiple systems.

Reference

1. Product information. Sutent. Pfizer, 2007.

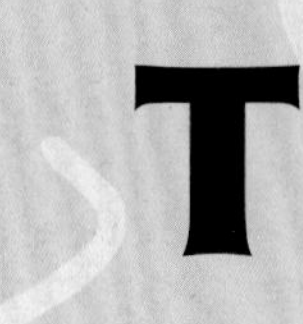

TACROLIMUS

Immunologic Agent (Immunosuppressant)

PREGNANCY RECOMMENDATION: Human Data Suggest Low Risk
BREASTFEEDING RECOMMENDATION: Limited Human Data—Probably Compatible

PREGNANCY SUMMARY

Tacrolimus has demonstrated abortifacient properties in three animal species and dose-related teratogenicity in one, but the use of this agent during human pregnancy has not been associated with either of these outcomes. The available human pregnancy experience continues to suggest that the embryo–fetal risk for congenital malformations is low. Common complications in infants, however, are hyperkalemia, which usually resolves untreated within 24–48 hours, renal toxicity, intrauterine growth restriction (IUGR), and premature delivery (because of hypertension, preeclampsia, and premature rupture of membranes). Based on one report, renal dysfunction is more common with cyclosporine than it is with tacrolimus. Moreover, IUGR and premature delivery are associated with the use of all immunosuppressant agents in pregnant transplant recipients. Because of the risk of cytomegalovirus infection in the mother and fetus, two reviews advised waiting at least 6 months before conception is attempted following transplantation and during periods of rejection when high doses of immunosuppressant agents may be used (i.e., the periods when infection with the virus is most likely) (1,2). Another report suggested waiting for 1 year to lower the risk of low birth weight and prematurity (3). Nevertheless, recent data suggest that the overall risk to the embryo–fetus is low. However, the long-term consequences of in utero exposure to tacrolimus, such as functional and/or neurobehavioral deficits, have not been studied.

FETAL FISK SUMMARY

Tacrolimus (FK506) is a macrolide immunosuppressant agent produced by *Streptomyces tsukubaensis* that acts similar to cyclosporine but is a more potent immunosuppressant. It is used either orally or IV for the prophylaxis of organ rejection in patients receiving various allogeneic organ transplants, such as kidney, liver, heart, and pancreas. The ointment is used for atopic dermatitis (4).

Reproduction studies have been reported in rats, rabbits, and mice (5,6). In pregnant rabbits, tacrolimus given in oral doses about 0.5–1 and 1.6–3.3 times the recommended human dose based on BSA (RHD) during organogenesis was associated with maternal toxicity and an increased incidence of abortions (5). At the higher dose, an increased incidence of malformations and developmental variations was also observed (type of defects was not specified). Pregnant rats dosed at 2.3–4.6 times the RHD exhibited maternal toxicity and an increase in late resorptions, decreased numbers of live births, and decreased pup weight and viability. Oral doses 0.7–1.4 and 2.3–4.6 times the RHD given after organogenesis and during lactation were associated with reduced pup weight (5).

Mice were treated with IM tacrolimus (0.17 or 1.37 mg/kg/day; relationship to human dose not specified), from day 1 through day 16 of gestation (6). No effects on maternal weight gain were observed in the low-dose group, but the number of resorptions was significantly increased over the number observed in controls. In contrast, none of the 13 pregnancies treated with high-dose tacrolimus was carried to term, and maternal weight gain was significantly less than that of controls. Except for the embryocidal action, low-dose tacrolimus, compared with untreated and saline controls, had no effect on mean placental or fetal weight and was not associated with an increase in malformations (6).

The molecular weight of tacrolimus (about 804) is low enough that the drug crosses the human placenta (5,7–9). In 12 pregnant women with liver transplants who were treated with tacrolimus (mean dose in 11 patients was about 10 mg/day; 1 patient treated with 48–64 mg/day), the mean cord:maternal plasma ratio was 0.49 (7). The placentas contained higher drug amounts (mean 4.30 ng/g) than that measured in maternal plasma (about 4 times) or cord plasma (2–56 times) and were thought to indicate a partial placental barrier to passage of the drug (7). A cord:maternal plasma ratio of 0.49 also was reported in another case (see below) (8). In two pregnancies (described below) under tacrolimus immunosuppression, the mothers were taking 15 and 10 mg/day, respectively (9). At delivery, umbilical cord blood concentrations were 13.2 and 5.9 ng/mL, respectively, whereas the maternal venous blood concentrations were 11.8 and 31.2 ng/mL, respectively. The cord:maternal blood ratios were 1.12 and 0.19, respectively.

A number of reports have described the use of tacrolimus during human pregnancy. A 1993 letter reported a case of a woman with a liver transplant who was receiving tacrolimus (0.1 mg/kg/day with a target plasma level of <1.0 ng/mL) and who conceived about a year after her second transplant (8). At 28 weeks' gestation, a threatened acute graft rejection (tacrolimus plasma level <0.05 ng/mL) was successfully treated with bolus corticosteroids and an increase in the tacrolimus dose to 0.15 mg/kg/day. She delivered a healthy 2860-g male infant at 36 weeks' gestation that was doing well at 12 months of age. The tacrolimus cord blood and maternal plasma concentrations at birth were 0.24 and 0.49 ng/mL, respectively, a ratio of 0.49 (8).

A woman who had received a combined kidney and pancreaticoduodenal graft conceived while receiving tacrolimus (12 mg/day) and prednisolone (7.5 mg/day) (9). She also received furosemide and methyldopa for hypertension that was well controlled throughout gestation. Her pregnancy was complicated by hyperemesis gravidarum, septicemia (*Escherichia coli*), endocarditis, and esophagitis. At 38 weeks' gestation, she delivered a normal, 3410-g female infant with Apgar scores of 9 and 9 at 1 and 5 minutes, respectively. At delivery, the tacrolimus cord:maternal blood ratio was 1.12. In a second case, a woman conceived approximately 22 months after her second renal transplant. She received tacrolimus (10 mg/day), azathioprine (75 mg/day), and prednisolone (5 mg/day) for immunosuppression. Nifedipine and methyldopa were used to control her hypertension. Because of a possible placental abruption at 36 weeks' gestation, a normal 2400-g female infant was delivered by cesarean section. Her Apgar scores were 9 and 9 at 1 and 5 minutes, respectively. The tacrolimus cord:maternal blood ratio was 0.19. Both of the above infants were doing well at 3 months of age (9).

In a 1993 letter, the pregnancy outcomes of nine liver transplant recipients who had received tacrolimus (2–64 mg/day) immunosuppression throughout their gestation were detailed (10). Five of the women had also received corticosteroid therapy during pregnancy. None of the newborns was small for gestational age. Complications observed in the newborns included hyperkalemia in five (range 6.1–10.9 mEq/L; potassium levels measured in seven of the nine newborns), hypoxia in one who tested positive for cocaine (mother was taking cocaine), and anuria for 36 hours in one (thought to be secondary to high tacrolimus concentrations in the cord blood due to the mother's renal impairment) who regained normal renal function in 1 week; death after delivery occurred in one at 22 weeks' gestation. In this latter case, the mother had conceived 1 month after transplantation and had cytomegalovirus in her blood and gastrointestinal tract that was being treated with ganciclovir. Of the eight surviving infants, all were alive and developing normally (10).

Some of the cases described in reference 10 above may have been included in a 1997 abstract that reported the outcomes of 14 pregnancies in 13 liver transplant recipients receiving various immunosuppressant agents, including tacrolimus (11). Although the agent used in each of the pregnancies was not specified, the complications included maternal renal insufficiency ($N = 8$), early hypertension ($N = 5$), preeclampsia ($N = 4$), worsening hypertension ($N = 2$), pyelonephritis ($N = 2$), anemia ($N = 4$), prolonged premature rupture of the membranes ($N = 3$), and cytomegalovirus infection ($N = 3$). The mean gestational age at delivery was 32.6 weeks, and the mean birth weight was 1913 g. Three newborns died; all three deaths were associated with cytomegalovirus infection and prematurity. No structural birth defects were mentioned (11).

A 1997 report detailed the outcomes of 27 pregnancies of 21 liver recipients who were treated with tacrolimus before and throughout gestation (7). The mean gestational age at delivery was 36.6 weeks, and the mean birth weight was 2638 g (50.2 percentile). Two infants died from prematurity after delivery at 23 and 24 weeks, respectively. The mean follow-up time of the infants was 39 months, and their mean growth weight percentile was 62. Unilateral nonfunctional cystic renal disease in one newborn was the only congenital anomaly observed in this series. In addition to the restricted growth and premature births in the total series, two other transient complications, noted among the first 13 infants born, were hyperkalemia in 10 and renal impairment in 7. Both adverse effects were thought to be caused by the drug (7).

Successful immunosuppression with tacrolimus following heart transplantation had been maintained for 2 years before conception occurred in a 39-year-old woman (12). She also took prophylactic trimethoprim–sulfamethoxazole before and throughout gestation, and her chronic hypertension was controlled with a long-acting calcium channel blocker (name not specified). Preeclampsia (rising blood pressure, proteinuria, and worsening renal impairment) was manifested between 26 and 31 weeks' gestation. An apparently normal, 2093-g female infant, who had Apgar scores of 9 and 9 at 1 and 5 minutes, respectively, was delivered by cesarean section at 33 weeks (12).

A 26-year-old renal transplant recipient was treated with tacrolimus (10 mg/day) and prednisolone (10 mg/day) throughout a 33.5-week pregnancy (13). Conception had occurred about 25 months after transplantation. The target blood concentration was 10 ng/mL. Symmetrical IUGR was discovered after 20 weeks' gestation. Because of spontaneous rupture of the membranes and breech presentation, a 1312-g female infant was delivered by cesarean section. A physical and ultrasonic examination found no congenital malformations. Complications other than IUGR noted in the newborn included mild hyperkalemia and a prolonged course of hyperbilirubinemia. Although not stated, the latter complication may have been secondary to prematurity (13).

A 1998 case report described the course and outcome of a pregnancy in a 32-year-old woman after renal transplantation (14). Tacrolimus, with a target plasma level of 5.0–11.5 ng/mL, was used alone throughout gestation after discontinuance of prednisolone (5 mg/day) early in gestation. Hypertension developed in the 22nd week of gestation which was treated with isradipine. A cesarean section was performed at 31 weeks' gestation because of severe hypertension, a progressive decline in graft function, and an abnormal Doppler assessment of blood velocity in the umbilical artery. No congenital malformations were noted in the 1140-g (3rd percentile) male infant who had Apgar scores of 8, 9, and 9 at 1, 5, and 10 minutes, respectively. The tacrolimus concentration in the umbilical vein was 8.1 ng/mL (maternal level at the time of delivery was not reported). At 2 days of age, the plasma drug level had decreased to 6.4 ng/mL, and at 8 days, the level was <5.0 ng/mL. Complications in the infant included mild hyperkalemia (6.4 mmol/L) on the 2nd day and transient renal impairment (serum creatinine 3.0 mg/dL at birth) that resolved completely over the next few weeks. A renal ultrasound examination was normal. Respiratory distress syndrome and a patent ductus arteriosus were successfully treated, and at a corrected age of 4 months, the healthy infant was developing normally (14).

A 1998 study examined the relationship between antenatal complications and various maternal factors in women who had undergone orthotopic liver transplantation (15). Of the 14 pregnancies studied, tacrolimus had been used in 5 (combined with prednisone in 3; with azathioprine and prednisone in 1), cyclosporine in 8 (combined with prednisone in 6; with azathioprine and prednisone in 2), and prednisone only in 1. Three of the complications—preeclampsia, worsening hypertension, and small for gestational age—occurred only in women with renal dysfunction (creatinine ≥1.3 mg/dL) at conception. Cyclosporine was more commonly associated ($p = 0.03$) with renal dysfunction than was tacrolimus (15).

A review of pregnancy outcomes after renal transplant was published in 1998 (16). The liveborn incidence among seven cases treated with tacrolimus was 71% (16).

In a 1998 report from the National Transplantation Pregnancy Registry (NTPR), the pregnancy outcomes of six women who were recipients of a lung transplant were described, one of whom was treated with tacrolimus (13–15 mg/day) throughout gestation (17). Her pregnancy was complicated by preterm labor at 24 weeks' gestation and a 1616-g infant (sex not specified) was delivered by cesarean section at 30 weeks'. The infant was successfully treated for respiratory distress syndrome and was healthy and doing well at 15 months of age (17). An updated report from the NTPR was published in 2005 (18). A total of 18 pregnancy outcomes were described from women who were recipients of kidney, liver, or heart transplants. In addition, two 2008 references (19,20) described the pregnancy outcomes of transplant recipients receiving tacrolimus in combination with mycophenolate (see Mycophenolate for details, in references 18–20).

In a 1999 case report, a woman who had a renal transplant was treated throughout gestation with tacrolimus (10–12 mg/day), prednisone, amlodipine, and labetalol (21). Azathioprine was also used during the first 10 weeks. At 32 weeks' gestation, she delivered twin male infants who developed severe respiratory distress syndrome and congestive heart failure. Echocardiograms showed dilated heart chambers in both infants and only twin B survived. Autopsy of twin A revealed thrombotic cardiomyopathy with degeneration of cardiac muscle. Because animal studies had shown that tacrolimus could cause vasculitis in the cardiac muscle of baboons and dogs, the authors concluded that the cardiomyopathy seen in the twins might have been caused by tacrolimus (21).

A 2000 reference described the outcomes of 100 pregnancies in 84 women who were receiving tacrolimus for autoimmune disease (Behcet's disease) ($N = 1$) or solid organ transplants (liver [$N = 55$], kidney [$N = 22$], heart [$N = 3$], kidney–pancreas [$N = 1$], pancreas [$N = 1$], and lung [$N = 1$]) (22). During pregnancy, the mean daily tacrolimus dose was 12.1–12.8 mg/day (range 1.0–64 mg/day). The outcomes of the pregnancies were 70 live births (2 neonates died in the perinatal period), 12 spontaneous abortions (SABs), 12 elective abortions (EABs), 1 stillbirth, 2 pregnancies ongoing, and 3 lost to follow-up. Gestational age at birth was known in 63 neonates, 37 (59%) of whom were premature. The birth weight was known in 64 cases with a mean weight of 2573 g (range 886–4346 g). The weight was appropriate for gestational age in 58 cases (90%). There were no malformations observed in the 24 aborted fetuses. However, four of the live births, all exposed to tacrolimus throughout the 1st trimester, had structural anomalies, one of which was alcoholic embryopathy. There was no pattern among the remaining three anomalies that suggested a single cause. The defects were meningocele, urogenital defects, and umbilical hernia; ear defect, cleft palate, and hypospadia; and multicystic dysplastic kidney and dimple without areola. The most common complications in the infants at birth were hypoxia, hyperkalemia, and renal dysfunction (22).

Two case reports, one in 2001 and the other in 2004, detailed the use of tacrolimus and mycophenolate during pregnancies that involved adverse outcomes (see Mycophenolate). A 2003 retrospective review detailed the outcomes of 38 pregnancies in 29 women who had undergone liver transplantation before pregnancy (23). Sixteen pregnancies (nine live births, seven elective abortions) had been exposed to tacrolimus combined with other agents. There were no fetal or neonatal deaths. Two tacrolimus-exposed infants had small membranous ventricular septal defects (23).

Another 2003 report described the pregnancy outcomes of 37 women, all after liver transplantation, who delivered 49 infants (all single gestations) (24). All mothers were treated with tacrolimus that was, in some cases, combined with other agents. In 47 infants, the mean gestational age was 36.4 weeks, but 2 infants were born at 23 and 24 weeks' gestation, respectively. Both of the very premature infants died, as did one infant from a mother with Alagille syndrome. The latter infant had a tracheoesophageal fistula and valvular heart disease. One of the surviving infants had a nonfunctional unilateral cystic kidney. The mean birth weight was 2797 g, with 78% of the infants weighing more than 2000 g (24).

The pregnancies of 38 renal allograft recipients were reported in a 2003 study (25). Four of the patients were treated with tacrolimus in combination with other agents. The outcomes of 73 pregnancies (48 live births) in the group were compared with 59 pregnancies (41 women; 48 live births) with primary renal disease not treated with immunosuppressive drugs. The study group had significantly more preterm deliveries, infants with intrauterine growth restriction, and infants requiring hospitalization in neonatal intensive care units. However, there was no statistical difference in the incidence of major (4.2% vs. 4.2%) and minor malformations (20.8% vs. 16.6%) (25).

In a 2004 report, the pregnancy outcomes of 13 mothers (19 babies) after kidney transplantation and 2 mothers (3 babies) after kidney–pancreas implantation, all under tacrolimus immunosuppression, were described (26). One mother had a stillborn secondary to amniotic fluid leak and a small, ischemic placenta. The mean gestational age of the infants and their birth weight were 34.4 weeks and 2373 g, respectively. No congenital defects were detected (26).

A brief 2005 communication reported 16 women with 19 pregnancies after renal transplantation under tacrolimus (27). Appropriate birth weights and no malformations were observed in 10 successful pregnancies. The outcomes of the other nine cases were four SABs and five (EABs) (27).

There were 71 pregnancies among 45 women with liver transplantation in a 2006 report (3). Tacrolimus and cyclosporine were used in 42 and 29 of the pregnancies, respectively. The outcomes of the pregnancies were live births (29 vs. 21), SABs (7 vs. 6), EABs (5 vs. 1), molar pregnancy (1 vs. 0), and intrauterine death (0 vs. 1) (all *ns*). The median gestational age and birth weight were 37.5 vs. 37 weeks and 2660 vs. 2951 g, respectively (all *ns*). Pregnancies occurring within 1 year of transplantation had the highest incidence of prematurity and lowest birth weight. No congenital anomalies were observed (3).

Four successful pregnancies under tacrolimus in women with liver transplants were described in 2006 (28). The mean gestational age and birth weight were 34.4 weeks and 2302 g, respectively. No birth defects were detected in the infants.

A 2005 case report described the use of tacrolimus throughout pregnancy in a woman with refractory ulcerative colitis (29). She delivered a healthy 3500-g, height 51 cm, baby girl at 40 weeks' gestation with Apgar scores of 9, 10, and 10.

A 2007 short communication described the pregnancy outcome of a 35-year-old woman treated with tacrolimus after a liver transplant (30). The woman conceived 5 years after the transplant and remained on tacrolimus throughout the pregnancy. Except for hypertension (treated with methyldopa) and suspected chorioamnionitis, the pregnancy was uncomplicated. A cesarean section in the 38th week delivered a healthy 2780-g female infant. No additional information on the infant was provided (30).

Another 2007 reference described the outcomes of 16 pregnancies in renal transplant recipients that were exposed to tacrolimus combined with other immunosuppressive agents (13 with azathioprine and prednisone, 1 with azathioprine, and 2 with prednisone) (31). An additional 33 pregnancies (all in women after renal transplants) were treated with cyclosporine with azathioprine and/or prednisone and 3 pregnancies were treated with azathioprine and prednisone alone. The mean patient age was 26.5 years (range 17–38 years). In the 52 pregnancies, preterm delivery occurred in 20 (38%) and fetal growth restriction in 16 (31%) (outcomes by specific drug exposure not provided). There was one fetal death due to extreme prematurity (26 weeks'). No congenital malformations in the offspring were observed (31).

In a 2007 case report, a 28-year-old woman became pregnant while taking tacrolimus (5 mg/day) and prednisolone (15 mg/day), 1.5 years after her second renal transplant (32). The pregnancy was uneventful and she gave birth vaginally to a healthy 3535-g male infant at term with Apgar scores of 9 and 10.

A 2012 case report described the use of tacrolimus (12 mg/day) throughout pregnancy in a woman with an intestinal transplant (33). Other medications used were prednisone (5 mg/day), esomeprazole (40 mg/day), diphenoxylate-atropine (2 tablets/day), tacrolimus (12 mg/day), ferrous sulfate (650 mg/day), ascorbic acid (1 g/day), prenatal vitamins (1/day), and magnesium supplementation. At 39 3/7 weeks, labor was induced and she had a spontaneous vaginal delivery of a healthy female infant (33).

BREASTFEEDING SUMMARY

Tacrolimus is excreted into breast milk. Ten colostrum samples were obtained from six women in the immediate postpartum period (0–3 days) with a mean drug concentration of 0.79 ng/mL (range 0.3–1.9 ng/mL) (7). The median milk:maternal plasma ratio was 0.5. The authors of this study did not mention if the women breastfed their infants.

In a 2003 report, a mother who had taken tacrolimus (0.1 mg/kg/day) throughout pregnancy because of liver transplantation continued the drug while breastfeeding her infant (34). From manually expressed samples, the highest and mean drug concentrations were 0.57 and 0.429 ng/mL, respectively. The milk:blood ratios before a dose and 1-hour postdose were 0.08 and 0.9, respectively. The estimated half-life, calculated on limited data, in milk was 12.85 hours. The estimated maximum dose the infant would absorb was 0.02% of the mother's weight-adjusted dose. The infant was developing normally at 2.5 months of age (34).

In a second case, a mother with a renal transplant was taking tacrolimus (4 mg/day) while exclusively breastfeeding her 3-month-old infant (35). The milk:blood ratio was 0.23, whereas the average tacrolimus milk concentration was 1.8 mcg/L (1.8 ng/mL). The estimated infant dose was 0.5% of the mother's weight-adjusted dose (35).

In a case described above, a mother took tacrolimus throughout pregnancy and continued the drug while breastfeeding her infant (33). The infant's tacrolimus level was <1.0 ng/mL at 1 week of age.

The absolute oral bioavailability of tacrolimus in healthy adults is 18%, but food, especially fat, markedly decreases the bioavailability (5). Based on the two cases above, breastfeeding during tacrolimus therapy does not appear to represent a significant risk to the infant. However, monitoring infant plasma levels is an option.

References

1. Laifer SA, Guido RS. Reproductive function and outcome of pregnancy after liver transplantation in women. Mayo Clin Proc 1995;70:388–94.
2. Casele HL, Laifer SA. Pregnancy after liver transplantation. Sem Perinatol 1998;22:149–55.
3. Christopher V, Al-Chalabi T, Richardson PD, Muiesan P, Rela M, Heaton ND, O'Grady JG, Heneghan MA. Pregnancy outcome after liver transplantation: a single-center experience of 71 pregnancies in 45 recipients. Liver Transpl 2006;12:1138–43.
4. Peters DH, Fitton A, Plosker GL, Faulds D. Tacrolimus. A Review of its pharmacology, and therapeutic potential in hepatic and renal transplantation. Drugs 1993;46:746–94.
5. Product information. Prograf. Astellas Pharma US, 2007.
6. Farley DE, Shelby J, Alexander D, Scott JR. The effect of two new immunosuppressive agents, FK506 and didemnin B, in murine pregnancy. Transplantation 1991;52:106–10.
7. Jain A, Venkataramanan R, Fung JJ, Gartner JC, Lever J, Balan V, Warty V, Starzl TE. Pregnancy after liver transplantation under tacrolimus. Transplantation 1997;64:559–65.
8. Winkler ME, Niesert S, Ringe B, Pichlmayr R. Successful pregnancy in a patient after liver transplantation maintained on FK 506. Transplantation 1993;56:751–3.
9. Midtvedt K, Hartmann A, Brekke IB, Lyngdal PT, Bentdal O, Haugen G. Successful pregnancies in a combined pancreas and renal allograft recipient and in a renal graft recipient on tacrolimus treatment. Nephrol Dial Transplant 1997;12:2764–5.
10. Jain A, Venkataramanan R, Lever J, Warty V, Fung J, Todo S, Starzl T. FK506 and pregnancy in liver transplant patients. Transplantation 1993;56:751.
11. Casele H, Woelkers D, Laifer S. Pregnancy outcome after liver transplantation (abstract). Am J Obstet Gynecol 1997;176:S23.
12. Laifer SA, Yeagley CJ, Armitage JM. Pregnancy after cardiac transplantation. Am J Perinatol 1994;11:217–9.
13. Yoshimura N, Oka T, Fujiwara Y, Ohmori Y, Yasumura T, Honjo H. A case report of pregnancy in a renal transplant recipient treated with FK506 (tacrolimus). Transplantation 1996;61:1552–3.
14. Resch B, Mache CJ, Windhager T, Holzer H, Leitner G, Muller W. FK 506 and successful pregnancy in a patient after renal transplantation. Transplant Proc 1998;30:163–4.

T

15. Casele HL, Laifer SA. Association of pregnancy complications and choice of immunosuppressant in liver transplant patients. Transplantation 1998;65:581–3.
16. Armenti VT, McGrory CH, Carter JR, Radomski JS, Moritz MJ. Pregnancy outcomes in female renal transplant recipients. Transplant Proc 1998;30:1732–4.
17. Armenti VT, Gertner GS, Eisenberg JA, McGrory CH, Moritz MJ. National Transplantation Pregnancy Registry: outcomes of pregnancies in lung recipients. Transplant Proc 1998;30:1528–30.
18. Armenti VT, Radomski JS, Moritz MJ, Gaughan WJ, Gulati R, McGrory CH, Coscia LA. Report from the National Transplantation Pregnancy Registry (NTPR): outcomes of pregnancy after transplantation. Clin Transpl 2005:69–83.
19. Perez-Aytes A, Ledo A, Boso V, Saenz P, Roma E, Poveda JL, Vento M. In utero exposure to mycophenolate mofetil: a characteristic phenotype? Am J Med Genet A 2008;146A:1–7.
20. Pisoni CN, D'Cruz DP. The safety of mycophenolate mofetil in pregnancy. Expert Opin Drug Saf 2008;7:219–22.
21. Vyas S, Kumar A, Piecuch S, Hidalgo G, Singh A, Anderson V, Markell MS, Baqi N. Outcome of twin pregnancy in a renal transplant recipient treated with tacrolimus. Transplantation 1999;67:490–2.
22. Kainz A, Harabacz I, Cowlrick IS, Gadgil SD, Hagiwara D. Review of the course and outcome of 100 pregnancies in 84 women treated with tacrolimus. Transplantation 2000;70:1718–21.
23. Nagy S, Bush MC, Berkowitz R, Fishbein TM, Gomez-Lobo V. Pregnancy outcome in liver transplant recipients. Obstet Gynecol 2003;102:121–8.
24. Jain AB, Reyes J, Marcos A, Mazariegos G, Eghtesad B, Fontes PA, Cacciarelli TV, Marsh JW, De Vera ME, Rafail A, Starzl TE, Fung JJ. Pregnancy after liver transplantation with tacrolimus immunosuppression: a single center's experience update at 13 years. Transplantation 2003;76:827–32.
25. Bar J, Stahl B, Hod M, Wittenberg C, Pardo J, Merlob P. Is immunosuppression therapy in renal allograft recipients teratogenic? A single-center experience. Am J Med Genet 2003;116A:31–6.
26. Jain AB, Shapiro R, Scantlebury VP, Potdar S, Jordan ML, Flohr J, Marcos A, Fung JJ. Pregnancy after kidney and kidney-pancreas transplantation under tacrolimus: a single center's experience. Transplantation 2004;77:897–902.
27. Garcia-Donaire JA, Acevedo M, Gutierrez MJ, Manzanera MJ, Oliva E, Gutierrez E, Andres A, Morales JM. Tacrolimus as basic immunosuppression in pregnancy after renal transplantation. A single-center experience. Transplant Proc 2005;37:3754–5.
28. Jabiry-Zieniewicz Z, Kaminski P, Pietrzak B, Cyganek A, Bobrowska K, Ziotkowski J, Otdakowska-Jedynak U, Zieniewicz K, Paczek L, Jankowska I, Wielgos M, Krawczyk M. Outcome of four high-risk pregnancies in female liver transplant recipients on tacrolimus immunosuppression. Transplant Proc 2006;38:255–7.
29. Baumgart DC, Sturm A, Wiedenmann B, Dignass AU. Uneventful pregnancy and neonatal outcome with tacrolimus in refractory ulcerative colitis. Gut 2005;54:1822–3.
30. Ducarme G, Theron-Gerard L, Duvoux C, Uzan M, Poncelet C. Pregnancy after liver transplantation with tacrolimus. Eur J Obstet Gynecol Reprod Biol 2007;133:249–50.
31. Olivelra LG, Sass N, Sato JL, Ozaki KS, Medina-Pastana JO. Pregnancy after renal transplantation—a five-yr single-center experience. Clin Transplant 2007;21:301–4.
32. Midtvedt K, Bjorang O, Letting AS. Successful pregnancy in renal transplant recipient with previous known polyomavirus nephropathy. Clin Transplant 2007;21:571–3.
33. Gomez-Lobo V, Landy HJ, Matsumoto C, Fishbein TM. Pregnancy in an intestinal transplant recipient. Obstet Gynecol 2012;120:497–500.
34. French AE, Soldin SJ, Soldin OP, Koren G. Milk transfer and neonatal safety of tacrolimus. Ann Pharmacother 2003;37:815–8.
35. Gardiner SJ, Begg EJ. Breastfeeding during tacrolimus therapy. Obstet Gynecol 2006;107:453–5.

TAFLUPROST

Ophthalmic (Prostaglandin Agonist)

PREGNANCY RECOMMENDATION: **No Human Data—Probably Compatible**
BREASTFEEDING RECOMMENDATION: **No Human Data—Probably Compatible**

PREGNANCY SUMMARY

No reports describing the use of tafluprost in human pregnancy have been located. The animal data suggest moderate risk, but the amount appearing in the systemic circulation is very low. Moreover, the elimination half-life from plasma appears to be very fast. Although the absence of human pregnancy experience prevents a more complete assessment of embryo–fetal risk, the risk of harm appears to be low. Nevertheless, because the drug will be given daily for long periods, it may be best to use other antiglaucoma agents that have some human data (e.g., Latanoprost).

FETAL RISK SUMMARY

Tafluprost, a fluorinated analog of prostaglandin F2α, is available as a 0.0015% ophthalmic solution that is given as single drop in the conjunctival sac of the affected eye(s) once daily. It is in the same class of prostaglandin agonists as bimatoprost, latanoprost, and travoprost. Tafluprost is indicated for reducing elevated intraocular pressure in patients with open-angle glaucoma or ocular hypertension. It is hydrolyzed within the eye to an active metabolite, tafluprost acid, that undergoes further metabolism to inactive metabolites. Very small amounts of tafluprost acid are absorbed into the systemic circulation. At a median 10 minutes postinstillation in each eye of healthy adults, mean plasma concentrations were 26–27 pg/mL. At 30 minutes postinstillation, mean plasma concentrations were below the limit of quantification (10 pg/mL) (1). This suggests an elimination half-life of about <17 minutes.

Reproduction studies have been conducted in rats and rabbits. When IV doses of tafluprost were given, increased postimplantation losses were observed in rats and rabbits and reduced fetal body weights in rats. The drug also increased the incidence of vertebral skeletal defects in rats. In rats, the no-effect dose corresponded to maternal plasma levels of tafluprost acid that were 343 times the maximum clinical exposure based on the maximum plasma concentration (C_{max}). In a prenatal and postnatal study in rats, increased mortality of newborns, decreased body weights, and delayed pinna unfolding were noted in offspring. The no observed adverse effect level for these effects was at a tafluprost IV dose that was >3 times the maximum recommended clinical

T

dose based on BSA. In rabbits, an increased incidence of skull, brain, and spine malformations was observed at maternal plasma levels of tafluprost acid during organogenesis that were about 5 times higher than the clinical exposure based on C_{max}. At the no-effect dose in rabbits, maternal plasma levels of tafluprost acid were below the level of quantification (20 pg/mL) (1).

In long-term studies, tafluprost was not carcinogenic in mice and rats, nor was it mutagenic or clastogenic in multiple assays. No adverse effects on mating performance or fertility were observed in given high IV doses of the drug (1).

It is not known if tafluprost acid crosses the human placenta. The molecular weight (about 453) is low enough, but the very small plasma concentrations of the drug are below the limit of quantification (10 pg/mL) 30 minutes postinstillation.

Prostaglandin F2α has been used for pregnancy termination in humans via intrauterine extra-amniotic infusion to treat missed abortion or intrauterine death. However, there is no evidence that at doses given to reduce elevated ophthalmic pressure, an increased risk for uterine contractions would be seen (see Latanoprost).

BREASTFEEDING SUMMARY

No reports describing the use of tafluprost during human lactation have been located. The molecular weight (about 453) is low enough for excretion, but the very small plasma concentrations (26–27 pg/mL) of the drug are below the limit of quantification (10 pg/mL) 30 minutes postinstillation. It is unlikely that these brief concentrations would have any effect on a nursing infant.

Reference

1. Product information. Zioptan. Merck, 2013.

TALIGLUCERASE ALFA

Endocrine/Metabolic Agent (Gaucher Disease)

PREGNANCY RECOMMENDATION: No Human Data—Probably Compatible
BREASTFEEDING RECOMMENDATION: No Human Data—Probably Compatible

PREGNANCY SUMMARY

No reports describing the use of taliglucerase alfa in human pregnancy have been located. The animal data suggest low risk, but the absence of human pregnancy experience prevents a more complete assessment of embryo–fetal risk. Although pregnancy may exacerbate existing Gaucher disease or result in new disease manifestations, the data for other agents in this subclass (e.g., see Imiglucerase) suggest that treatment may reduce the risk of spontaneous abortion and bleeding complications. If indicated, the drug should not be withheld because of pregnancy.

FETAL RISK SUMMARY

Taliglucerase alfa, given as an IV infusion, is a recombinant active form of the lysosomal enzyme, β-glucocerebrosidase, that differs from the human enzyme by nine amino acids. It is a hydrolytic lysosomal glucocerebroside-specific enzyme produced by recombinant DNA technology using plant cell culture (carrot). Taliglucerase alfa is indicated for long-term enzyme replacement therapy for patients with a confirmed diagnosis of type 1 Gaucher disease. It is in the same pharmacologic subclass as alglucerase, imiglucerase, and velaglucerase alfa. The median terminal half-life is about 19–29 minutes (1).

Reproduction studies have been conducted in rats and rabbits. In these species, an IV dose that was about 5 times the recommended human dose of 60 units/kg based on BSA (RHD) in both species revealed no evidence of impaired fertility or fetal harm (1).

Studies to evaluate carcinogenic or mutagenic potential have not been conducted. In male and female rats, doses that were about 5 times the RHD did not cause any significant adverse effects on fertility parameters (1).

It is not known if taliglucerase alfa, a glycoprotein, crosses the human placenta. The high molecular weight (56,640) and short terminal half-life suggest that it will not cross to the embryo–fetus, at least early in pregnancy.

BREASTFEEDING SUMMARY

No reports describing the use of taliglucerase alfa during human lactation have been located. The molecular weight (56,640) and the short terminal half-life (19–29 minutes) suggest that clinically significant amounts of the drug will not be excreted into breast milk. In addition, there are limited data for two other agents in this class that support the use of the drug during breastfeeding (see Alglucerase and Imiglucerase). Moreover, if excretion does occur, the drug would most likely be digested in the infant's gut and not absorbed systemically.

Reference

1. Product information. Elelyso. Pfizer Labs, 2012.

TAMOXIFEN

Antineoplastic/Antiestrogen

PREGNANCY RECOMMENDATION: Contraindicated
BREASTFEEDING RECOMMENDATION: Contraindicated

PREGNANCY SUMMARY

Tamoxifen is an antiestrogen that has weak estrogenic activity in some tissues. Although tamoxifen is not considered an animal teratogen, it is carcinogenic in rodents and has been associated with intrauterine growth restriction, abortions, and premature delivery in some species. Uterine cancer has been reported in human adults treated with tamoxifen. Moreover, tamoxifen has produced toxic changes in the reproductive tracts of animals. Some of these changes were similar to those observed in humans exposed in utero to diethylstilbestrol (DES), but the risk of tamoxifen-induced clear cell adenocarcinoma of the vagina or cervix in exposed offspring is unknown because too few humans have been exposed during pregnancy or followed up long enough. Two adverse outcomes following inadvertent exposure to tamoxifen during gestation have been described. The relationship between tamoxifen and Goldenhar's syndrome in the first case is unknown, but, in the second case, a causal association between the drug and the ambiguous genitalia noted in the female infant appears to be more certain. In addition, several fetal and neonatal disorders and defects have been reported to the manufacturer, but it is not known whether this is the result of retrospective reporting. Because of the various toxicities noted in animals, the increased incidence of abortions noted in some patients when the drug was used for ovulation induction, and the possible human teratogenicity, the best course is to avoid use of tamoxifen during pregnancy. Moreover, because both the parent compound and the major metabolite have prolonged half-lives that may require ≤8 weeks to eliminate, women of childbearing age should be informed that a pregnancy occurring within 2 months of tamoxifen therapy may expose the embryo and/or fetus to the drug. If an inadvertent pregnancy does occur, the potential fetal and newborn risks must be discussed with the patient. Offspring who have been exposed to tamoxifen during pregnancy require long-term (≤20 years) follow-up to access the risk of carcinogenicity.

FETAL RISK SUMMARY

Tamoxifen, a triphenylethylene derivative that is structurally related to clomiphene, is a nonsteroidal, antiestrogen agent used in the treatment of breast cancer (1,2). In addition to its antiestrogen properties, it may also produce weak estrogenic and estrogenic-like activity at some sites. Unlabeled uses have included induction of ovulation and treatment of idiopathic oligospermia. Tamoxifen is thought to act by competing with estrogen for binding sites in target tissues (2). The parent drug has an elimination half-life of about 5–7 days (range 3–21 days) (1,2), whereas the elimination half-life of the major metabolite, *N*-desmethyltamoxifen, is approximately 9–14 days (1). Following prolonged treatment (e.g., 2–3 months), clearance of tamoxifen and its metabolites from the system may require 6–8 weeks (3).

Tamoxifen is carcinogenic, producing ovarian and testicular tumors in immature and mature mice and hepatocellular carcinoma in rats, at all doses tested (5, 20, and 35 mg/kg/day for up to 2 years) (2). The drug is also genotoxic in rat liver cells and in the human lymphoblastoid cell line. Tamoxifen, at a dose of 0.04 mg/kg/day (approximately 1/10th the human dose) for 2 weeks before conception through day 7 of pregnancy, impaired the fertility of female rats causing a decreased number of implantations and 100% fetal mortality (2).

In reproductive studies reported by the manufacturer, no teratogenicity was observed with rats, rabbits, and marmosets, but fetal toxicity was common (2). In rats, however, reversible, nonteratogenic developmental skeletal changes were observed at doses equal to or below the human dose (2). An increased fetal death rate occurred in pregnant rats when tamoxifen (0.16 mg/kg/day; human dose about 0.4–0.8 mg/kg/day) was administered from day 7 to day 17 (2). When this dose was given from day 17 of pregnancy to 1 day before weaning, an increased number of dead pups were noted and some of the surviving pups demonstrated slower learning behavior. Moreover, in utero growth restriction was evident in some of the pups (2). Tamoxifen (0.125 mg/kg/day) administered to pregnant rabbits during days 6 through 18 of pregnancy caused abortions and premature delivery (2). Higher doses produced fetal deaths. Abortions were observed in pregnant marmosets given 10 mg/kg/day either during organogenesis or in the last half of pregnancy (2).

A 1976 study administered oral tamoxifen (2 mg/kg/day) to rabbits starting at either day 10 or day 20 of pregnancy (4). A significant increase in embryonic loss occurred in the first group, whereas treatment later in gestation resulted in premature delivery or abortion.

Several studies have described the effectiveness of tamoxifen as a postcoital contraceptive in animals (5–11). The action of tamoxifen as an antifertility agent appears to be a dose-related, antiestrogen effect that prevents implantation in the uterus. In one report, however, a single 5-mg/kg dose on day 4 after ovulation in macaques had no effect on fertility (12). No reports describing the use of tamoxifen as a contraceptive in humans have been located.

In rats and guinea pigs, tamoxifen produced significant, dose-related changes in the reproductive tract of the fetus and newborn (13–17). These changes, most pronounced in the guinea pig, involved trophic effects on the uterus and vagina similar to those produced by estrogens. Abnormalities in sexual differentiation of female offspring of guinea pigs have also been observed (18).

In a study published in 1987, the estrogenicity and potential teratogenicity of tamoxifen were demonstrated in genital tracts isolated from aborted 4- to 19-week-old human female fetuses grown for 1–2 months in mice (19). Some mice were used as controls, and others were treated with tamoxifen, clomiphene, or DES. In comparison with controls, abnormalities observed in the drug-treated mice included proliferation and maturation of the squamous vaginal epithelium; a decrease in the number of endometrial and cervical glands; impaired condensation and segregation of the uterine mesenchyme; and hyperplastic, disorganized epithelium and distorted mucosal plications in the fallopian tube. The abnormalities induced by tamoxifen and clomiphene were, in most instances, comparable to those of DES (19). A study published in 1979 examined the effects of tamoxifen administration on newborn female rats (5 mcg on days 1, 3, and 5), observing several abnormalities of reproductive development, including early vaginal opening, absence of cycles, atrophic ovaries and uteri, vaginal adenosis, and severe squamous metaplasia of the oviducts (20). Gonad and genitourinary tract abnormalities, including uterine hypoplasia and vaginal adenosis, were also observed in newborn female mice given tamoxifen for 5 days (21). A 1997 report compared the uterotrophic effects of tamoxifen (100 mcg), DES (1 mcg), or placebo administered SC daily to newborn female rat pups for 5 days (22). At postnatal day 6, both tamoxifen and DES produced significant epithelial hypertrophy and myometrial thickening, as well as other uterine changes that led the investigators to conclude that tamoxifen's estrogenic action on the developing uterus was similar to that produced by DES (22).

The clinical significance of the above studies demonstrating developmental changes in animals, three of which involved neonatal exposure to tamoxifen, is presently unknown, but some of the alterations observed in experiments, especially vaginal adenosis, are similar to those observed in young women following in utero exposure to DES (2). Moreover, too few women have been exposed in utero to tamoxifen and followed sufficiently long (≤20 years) to determine whether the drug presents a risk of clear-cell adenocarcinoma of the vagina or cervix similar to DES (about 1 in 1000) (2) (see also Diethylstilbestrol). It should also be noted that long-term exposure of nonpregnant, adult humans to tamoxifen has been associated with an increased incidence of endometrial cancer (2).

Data pertaining to human fetal exposure to tamoxifen are limited. A 1993 letter cited a statement made by tamoxifen researchers that 85 women had become pregnant while receiving the drug and that no fetal abnormalities had been reported (23). A 1994 letter, however, citing data (oral and written) reported to the manufacturer, described the outcomes of 50 pregnancies associated with tamoxifen therapy (24). Of the total, there were 19 normal births, 8 elective abortions, 10 with a fetal or neonatal disorder (2 of which were congenital craniofacial defects), and 13 unknown outcomes. Although the number of adverse outcomes is suggestive of human teratogenicity, no mention was made whether the above cases represented prospective or retrospective reporting. The latter type frequently involves biased reporting in that adverse outcomes are much more likely to be communicated. Also included in this letter was the description of a case in which a 35-year-old woman, following breast cancer surgery, took tamoxifen (20 mg/day) throughout an approximately 27-week pregnancy (24). Because of premature labor, chorioamnionitis, and an abnormal lie, a cesarean section was performed to deliver an 896-g, karyotypically normal infant (sex not specified). Malformations noted in the infant, consistent with a diagnosis of Goldenhar's syndrome, included right-sided microtia, preauricular skin tags, and hemifacial microsomia (24). Other exposures, in addition to tamoxifen, were cocaine and marijuana smoking (1 or 2 times/week) during the first 6 weeks of gestation and a bone scan performed using technetium-99m medronate. The causal relationship between tamoxifen and the defects in the infant was unknown (24), but in some reports of familial cases, the patterns of inheritance of Goldenhar's syndrome (oculoauriculovertebral anomaly) have been described as consistent with an autosomal dominant, autosomal recessive, and multifactorial inheritance (25).

Ambiguous genitalia in a female newborn exposed in utero to tamoxifen during the first 20 weeks of pregnancy was reported in 1997 (26). The 35-year-old mother had been treated with tamoxifen (20 mg daily) for about 1 year for metastatic breast cancer. Because of the mother's deteriorating condition, the normal 46,XX karyotype, 1360-g infant was delivered at 29 weeks' gestation. Reproductive malformations included an enlarged, phallic-like clitoris (1.4 × 0.6 cm), a single perineal opening for the urethra and vagina, and fusion of the posterior portion of the rugated labioscrotal folds without palpable glands. An ultrasound examination revealed a normal uterus and ovaries without identifiable male structures. Congenital adrenal hyperplasia was excluded and a serum testosterone level was normal for a female infant. At 6 months of age, a reduction phalloplasty and vaginal reconstruction were performed without complications (26).

Two reports have described three successful pregnancies following chemotherapy with tamoxifen (27,28). In one of two cases described in a 1986 reference, a 26-year-old woman with a pituitary microadenoma and primary infertility was successfully treated with tamoxifen (20 mg/day) and bromocriptine (10 mg/day) (27). Combination therapy was used because she could not tolerate high-dose bromocriptine monotherapy. She ovulated and conceived approximately 7.5 months after combination therapy was begun. Tamoxifen was discontinued when pregnancy was confirmed (exact timing not specified), but bromocriptine was continued until 8 weeks' gestation. She delivered a normal 3240-g female infant at term. In the second case, a 25-year-old woman with a pituitary macroadenoma and primary infertility was treated for about 3 months with the same combination therapy as in the first case, again because of intolerance to monotherapy (27). Combination therapy was stopped when pregnancy was confirmed (exact timing not specified) and she delivered a normal 2600-g female infant at 37 weeks' gestation. The third pregnancy involved a 31-year-old woman with a diagnosis of well-differentiated adenocarcinoma of the endometrium who elected to receive 6 months of hormonal therapy with tamoxifen (30 mg/day) and megestrol acetate (160 mg/day) combined with repeated hysteroscopy and uterine curettage rather than undergo a hysterectomy (28). She was then placed on combination oral contraceptives for 3 months and conceived 1 month after they were discontinued. She eventually delivered a normal 3340-g male infant at term. In addition, two case reports have described the use of tamoxifen in combination with trastuzumab in pregnant women with breast cancer (see Trastuzumab).

Several studies have examined the efficacy of tamoxifen, often in direct comparison with clomiphene, for ovulation induction in infertile women (29–35). Although no fetal anomalies were reported in these pregnancies following tamoxifen induction, a higher than expected occurrence of spontaneous abortion was noted in two studies (29,33). In contrast to clomiphene, however, tamoxifen induction did not appear to increase the frequency of multiple gestations (34).

In males, tamoxifen, like clomiphene, has been used for the treatment of idiopathic oligospermia (36–41). Tamoxifen appears to improve sperm density and the number of live spermatozoa, but conflicting results have been reported concerning the effect on sperm motility or morphology (37,40,41). A 1987 review, moreover, concluded that there was no convincing evidence that tamoxifen was effective in increasing the conception rate (41).

BREASTFEEDING SUMMARY

Tamoxifen has been shown to inhibit lactation (42,43). In a double-blind, placebo-controlled trial, tamoxifen started within 2 hours after delivery was effective in preventing milk secretion and breast engorgement (42). Two treatment courses were studied: 30 mg twice daily for 2 days, then 20 mg twice daily for 2 days, then 10 mg twice daily for 2 days (N = 50); and 10 mg twice daily for 14 days (N = 42). Two groups of control patients (N = 25 and N = 23) received similar placebo tablets. The 6-day treatment course was "superior" (statistical analysis was not done) to the 14-day treatment course with 43 (86%) vs. 31 (74%) of the women having a "good" response (i.e., either no milk in their breasts or only slight to moderate milk secretion) (42). Only six (13%) of the control patients had a "good" response. No adverse effects or rebound engorgement were observed in the women who had received tamoxifen.

In a second, placebo-controlled, single-blinded study, tamoxifen (N = 60, 10 mg 4 times daily) or placebo (N = 20) was started within 24 hours of delivery and continued for 5 days (43). Breast stimulation using a mechanical breast pump was used before the first dose, and then on days 3 and 5, followed by blood sampling for serum prolactin. By the 5th day, a significant decrease (compared with baseline) in serum prolactin concentration occurred in the tamoxifen group, but not in controls. Moreover, tamoxifen was effective in inhibiting lactation and preventing breast engorgement, and no rebound lactation was observed (43).

Because tamoxifen inhibits lactation and because of the adverse effects noted in newborn animals and human adults (see Fetal Risk Summary above) given the drug directly, the drug is contraindicated during nursing.

References

1. American Hospital Formulary Service. *Drug Information 1997*. Bethesda, MD: American Society of Health-System Pharmacists, 1997:861–6.
2. Product information. Nolvadex. Zeneca Pharmaceuticals, 1997.
3. Jordan VC. The role of tamoxifen in the treatment and prevention of breast cancer. Curr Probl Cancer 1992;16:129–76.
4. Furr BJA, Valcaccia B, Challis JRG. The effects of Nolvadex (tamoxifen citrate; ICI 46,474) on pregnancy in rabbits. J Reprod Fertil 1976;48:367–9.
5. Bloxham PA, Pugh DM, Sharma SC. An effect of tamoxifen (I.C.I. 46,474) on the surface coat of the late preimplantation mouse blastocyst. J Reprod Fertil 1975;45:181–3.
6. Watson J, Anderson FB, Alam M, O'Grady JE, Heald PJ. Plasma hormones and pituitary luteinizing hormone in the rat during the early stages of pregnancy and after post-coital treatment with tamoxifen (ICI 46,474). J Endocrinol 1975;65:7–17.
7. Pugh DM, Sumano HS. The anti-implantation action of tamoxifen in mice. Arch Toxicol 1982;5(Suppl):209–13.
8. Ravindranath N, Moudgal NR. Use of tamoxifen, an antioestrogen, in establishing a need for oestrogen in early pregnancy in the bonnet monkey (*Macaca radiata)*. J Reprod Fertil 1987;81:327–36.
9. Bowen RA, Olson PN, Young S, Withrow SJ. Efficacy and toxicity of tamoxifen citrate for prevention and termination of pregnancy in bitches. Am J Vet Res 1988;49:27–31.
10. Majumdar M, Datta JK. Contraceptive efficacy of tamoxifen in female hamsters. Contraception 1990;41:93–103.
11. Hodgson BJ. Effects of indomethacin and ICI 46,474 administered during ovum transport on fertility in rabbits. Biol Reprod 1976;14:451–7.
12. Tarantal AF, Hendrickx AG, Matlin SA, Lasley BL, Gu Q-Q, Thomas CAA, Vince PM, Van Look PFA. Tamoxifen as an antifertility agent in the long-tailed macaque (*Macaca fascicularis*). Contraception 1993;47:307–16.
13. Clark JH, McCormack SA. The effect of clomid and other triphenylethylene derivatives during pregnancy and the neonatal period. J Steroid Biochem 1980;12:47–53.
14. Pasqualini JR, Gulino A, Sumida C, Screpanti I. Anti-estrogens in fetal and newborn target tissues. J Steroid Biochem 1984;20:121–8.
15. Gulino A, Screpanti I, Pasqualini JR. Differential estrogen and antiestrogen responsiveness of the uterus during development in the fetal, neonatal and immature guinea pig. Biol Reprod 1984;31:371–81.
16. Nguyen BL, Giambiagi N, Mayrand C, Lecerf F, Pasqualini JR. Estrogen and progesterone receptors in the fetal and newborn vagina of guinea pig: biological, morphological, and ultrastructural responses to tamoxifen and estradiol. Endocrinology 1986;119:978–88.
17. Pasqualini JR, Giambiagi N, Sumida C, Nguyen BL, Gelly C, Mayrand C, Lecerf F. Biological responses of tamoxifen in the fetal and newborn vagina and uterus of the guinea-pig and in the R-27 mammary cancer cell line. J Steroid Biochem 1986;24:99–108.
18. Hines M, Alsum P, Roy M, Gorski RA, Goy RW. Estrogenic contributions to sexual differentiation in the female guinea pig: influences of diethylstilbestrol and tamoxifen on neural, behavioral, and ovarian development. Horm Behav 1987;21:402–17.
19. Cunha GR, Taguchi O, Namikawa R, Nishizuka Y, Robboy SJ. Teratogenic effects of clomiphene, tamoxifen, and diethylstilbestrol on the developing human female genital tract. Hum Pathol 1987;18:1132–43.
20. Chamness GC, Bannayan GA, Landry LA Jr, Sheridan PJ, McGuire WL. Abnormal reproductive development in rats after neonatally administered antiestrogen (tamoxifen). Biol Reprod 1979;21:1087–90.
21. Iguchi T, Hirokawa M, Takasugi N. Occurrence of genital tract abnormalities and bladder hernia in female mice exposed neonatally to tamoxifen. Toxicology 1986;42:1–11.
22. Poulet FM, Roessler ML, Vancutsem PM. Initial uterine alterations caused by developmental exposure to tamoxifen. Reprod Toxicol 1997;11:815–22.
23. Clark S. Prophylactic tamoxifen. Lancet 1993;342:168.
24. Cullins SL, Pridjian G, Sutherland CM. Goldenhar's syndrome associated with tamoxifen given to the mother during gestation. JAMA 1994;271:1905–6.
25. Rollnick BR, Kaye CI. Oculo-auriculo-vertebral anomaly. In: Buyse ML, ed. *Birth Defects Encyclopedia*. Volume II. Cambridge, MA: Blackwell Scientific Publications, 1990:1272–4.
26. Tewari K, Bonebrake RG, Asrat T, Shanberg AM. Ambiguous genitalia in infant exposed to tamoxifen in utero. Lancet 1997;350:183.
27. Koizumi K, Aono T. Pregnancy after combined treatment with bromocriptine and tamoxifen in two patients with pituitary prolactinomas. Fert Steril 1986;46:312–4.

T

28. Lai C-H, Hsueh S, Chao A-S, Soong Y-K. Successful pregnancy after tamoxifen and megestrol acetate therapy for endometrial carcinoma. Br J Obstet Gynaecol 1994;101:547–9.
29. Ruiz-Velasco V, Rosas-Arceo J, Matute MM. Chemical inducers of ovulation: comparative results. Int J Fertil 1979;24:61–4.
30. Messinis IE, Nillius SJ. Comparison between tamoxifen and clomiphene for induction of ovulation. Acta Obstet Gynecol Scand 1982;61:377–9.
31. Fukushima T, Tajima C, Fukuma K, Maeyama M. Tamoxifen in the treatment of infertility associated with luteal phase deficiency. Fertil Steril 1982;37:755–61.
32. Tajima C, Fukushima T. Endocrine profiles in tamoxifen-induced ovulatory cycles. Fertil Steril 1983;40:23–30.
33. Tsuiki A, Uehara S, Kyono K, Saito A, Hoshi K, Hoshiai H, Hirano M, Suzuki M. Induction of ovulation with an estrogen antagonist, tamoxifen. Tohoku J Exp Med 1984;144:21–31.
34. Weseley AC, Melnick H. Tamoxifen in clomiphene-resistant hypothalamic anovulation. Int J Fertil 1987;32:226–8.
35. Suginami H, Yano K, Kitagawa H, Matsubara K, Nakahashi N. A clomiphene citrate and tamoxifen citrate combination therapy: a novel therapy for ovulation induction. Fertil Steril 1993;59:976–9.
36. Lunglmayr G. Potentialities and limitations of endocrine treatment in idiopathic oligozoospermia. Acta Eur Fertil 1983;14:401–4.
37. Schill WB, Schillinger R. Selection of oligozoospermic men for tamoxifen treatment by an antiestrogen test. Andrologia 1987;19:266–72.
38. Brake A, Krause W. Treatment of idiopathic oligozoospermia with tamoxifen—a follow-up report. Int J Androl 1992;15:507–8.
39. Breznik R, Borko E. Effectiveness of antiestrogens in infertile men. Arch Androl 1993;31:43–8.
40. Kotoulas I-G, Mitropoulos D, Cardamakis E, Dounis A, Michopoulos J. Tamoxifen treatment in male infertility. I. Effect on spermatozoa. Fertil Steril 1994;61:911–4.
41. Sigman M, Vance ML. Medical treatment of idiopathic infertility. Urol Clin North Am 1987;14:459–69.
42. Shaaban MM. Suppression of lactation by an antiestrogen, tamoxifen. Eur J Obstet Gynecol Reprod Biol 1975;4:167–9.
43. Masala A, Delitala G, Lo Dico G, Stoppelli I, Alagna S, Devilla L. Inhibition of lactation and inhibition of prolactin release after mechanical breast stimulation in puerperal women given tamoxifen or placebo. Br J Obstet Gynecol 1978;85:134–7.

TAMSULOSIN

Sympatholytic

PREGNANCY RECOMMENDATION: No Human Data—Animal Data Suggest Low Risk
BREASTFEEDING RECOMMENDATION: No Human Data—Potential Toxicity

PREGNANCY SUMMARY

No reports describing the use of tamsulosin in human pregnancy have been located. The animal data suggest low risk, but the absence of human pregnancy experience prevents a more complete assessment of the embryo–fetal risk. Until such data are available, the safest course is to avoid use in pregnancy.

FETAL RISK SUMMARY

Tamsulosin is an antagonist of α_{1A}-adrenoceptors in the prostate. It is available as oral capsules and is indicated for the treatment of the signs and symptoms of benign prostatic hyperplasia (1). The drug is used off-label as adjunctive therapy in the management of ureteral stones (2,3). Tamsulosin is extensively metabolized and has an elimination half-life in the range of 9–15 hours. Plasma protein binding is 94%–99%, primarily to α_1-acid glycoprotein (1).

Reproduction studies have been conducted in rats and rabbits. In pregnant rats, doses up to about 50 times the human therapeutic AUC exposure revealed no evidence of fetal harm. Similar results were observed in pregnant rabbits (1).

In carcinogenicity studies with male and female rats, no increase in tumor incidence was noted with the exception of a modest increase in the frequency of mammary gland fibroadenomas in female rats. In mice, there were no significant findings in males, but females had significant increases in the incidence of mammary gland fibroadenomas and adenocarcinomas. In both rats and mice, the increased incidences of mammary gland neoplasms were considered secondary to drug-induced hyperprolactinemia. Tamsulosin was not mutagenic in multiple assays. High doses of the drug resulted in reversible male and female rat infertility (1).

It is not known if tamsulosin crosses the human placenta. The molecular weight (about 445) and moderately long elimination half-life suggest that the drug will cross to the embryo and/or fetus, but the extensive plasma protein binding should limit the amount crossing the placenta.

BREASTFEEDING SUMMARY

No reports describing the use of tamsulosin during human lactation have been located. The molecular weight (about 445) and moderately long elimination half-life (9–15 hours) suggest that the drug will be excreted into breast milk, but the extensive plasma protein binding (94%–99%) should limit the amount excreted. However, because antiadrenergic agents can cause hypotension, the safest course is to not breastfeed.

References

1. Product information. Flomax. Boehringer Ingelheim Pharmaceuticals and Astellas Pharma US, 2009.
2. *Drug Facts and Comparisons Tamsulosin Hydrochloride*. St. Louis, MO: Wolters Kluwer Health, 2007:501.
3. Porena M, Guiggi P, Balestra A, Micheli C. Pain killers and antibacterial therapy for kidney colic and stones. Urol Int 2004;72(Suppl 1):34–9.

T

TAPENTADOL

Narcotic Agonist Analgesic

PREGNANCY RECOMMENDATION: No Human Data—Probably Compatible
BREASTFEEDING RECOMMENDATION: No Human Data—Potential Toxicity

PREGNANCY SUMMARY

No reports describing the use of tapentadol in human pregnancy have been located. The drug caused significant embryo–fetal developmental toxicity in two animal species but always in the presence of maternal toxicity. In general, occasional use of narcotic agonist analgesics in pregnancy is considered low risk. However, tapentadol, as with other agents in this class, has the potential for abuse and such use could cause embryo–fetal harm. Respiratory depression of the newborn is a potential complication if the drug is used close to birth. A narcotic antagonist, such as naloxone, should be readily available to reverse neonatal respiratory depression if present.

FETAL RISK SUMMARY

Tapentadol is an oral centrally acting synthetic analgesic. It is indicated for the relief of moderate to severe acute pain in patients 18 years of age or older. Similar to other mu-opioid agonists, tapentadol has addictive properties and may be sought by drug abusers. The drug is extensively metabolized to inactive metabolites. Plasma protein binding is low (about 20%), whereas the average terminal half-life is 4 hours (1).

Reproduction studies have been conducted in rats and rabbits. No teratogenic effects were observed during organogenesis in rats given SC doses resulting in plasma exposures up to the plasma exposure at the maximum recommended human dose of 700 mg/day based on AUC (MRHD). The highest dose caused significant maternal toxicity and was associated with embryo–fetal toxicity that included transient delays in skeletal maturation (i.e., reduced ossification). Exposures up to 1.7 times the MRHD during late gestation and early postnatal period did not influence physical or reflex development, the outcome of neurobehavioral tests or reproductive parameters. However, at maternal toxic exposures, treatment-related developmental delay was observed, including incomplete ossification, significant reductions in pup body weights and weight gains, and increased pup mortality (1).

During organogenesis, rabbits received SC doses resulting in plasma exposures that were 0.2–1.85 times the MRHD. At exposures ≥0.6 times the MRHD, embryo–fetal toxicity was observed that consisted of reduced fetal viability, skeletal delays and other variations, and multiple malformations (gastroschisis/thoracogastroschisis, amelia/phocomelia, and cleft palate). Malformations observed at exposures that were 1.85 times the MRHD were ablepharia, encephalopathy, and spina bifida. However, the exposures caused significant maternal toxicity and this may have caused the embryo–fetal toxicities, including malformations (1).

In 2-year studies for carcinogenicity, no increase in tumor incidence was observed in mice and rats. The drug was not mutagenic in several assays. A clastogenic effect was noted in one assay but was not confirmed in a repeat test or in vivo. In fertility tests in rats, plasma exposures up to 0.4 times the MRHD did not alter fertility at any dose level. However, maternal toxicity was observed at plasma exposures <0.4 times the MRHD that resulted in a decreased number of implantations and live conceptuses, and increased preimplantation and postimplantation losses (1).

It is not known if tapentadol crosses the human placenta. The molecular weight (about 222 for the free base), low plasma protein binding, and the terminal half-life suggest that the drug will reach the embryo–fetus.

BREASTFEEDING SUMMARY

No reports describing the use of tapentadol during human lactation have been located. The molecular weight (about 222 for the free base), low plasma protein binding (about 20%), and the average terminal half-life (4 hours) suggest that the drug will be excreted into breast milk. As with all basic drugs, accumulation in the more acidic milk, as compared with plasma, should occur with continuous dosing and result in milk:plasma ratios >1. The effect of this exposure on a nursing infant is unknown, but respiratory depression and other narcotic effects are a potential complication.

Reference

1. Product information. Nucynta. PriCara (Division of Ortho-McNeil-Janssen Pharmaceuticals), 2009.

TAZAROTENE

Dermatologic Agent

PREGNANCY RECOMMENDATION: Contraindicated
BREASTFEEDING RECOMMENDATION: Limited Human Data—Potential Toxicity

PREGNANCY SUMMARY

Tazarotene is a retinoid that causes retinoid-like malformations in experimental animals. Because of this and the experience with other retinoids (e.g., see Isotretinoin), the drug is contraindicated in women who are or who may become pregnant. A negative pregnancy test should be obtained within 2 weeks before starting therapy with this agent, which should begin during a normal menstrual period (1).

FETAL RISK SUMMARY

Tazarotene is a retinoid prodrug that is rapidly converted in vivo to the active form, the cognate carboxylic acid of tazarotene (tazarotenic acid). The drug is indicated for the topical treatment of acne vulgaris and plaque psoriasis. The active drug is absorbed into the systemic circulation producing peak plasma levels up to approximately 2 ng/mL. In females treated for acne, doses applied to 15% of the BSA produced peak plasma levels 12 times higher than those from applications to only the face (1.2 vs. 0.1 ng/mL). Peak plasma levels occurred on day 15 of treatment and the highest observed level was 1.91 ng/mL (1).

Reproduction studies have been conducted in rats and rabbits (1). Topical doses resulted in reduced fetal body weights and reduced skeletal ossification in rats and single incidents of retinoid malformations, including spina bifida, hydrocephaly, and heart defects in rabbits. The systemic exposures resulting from the doses used in rats and rabbits were 1.2 and 13 times, respectively, the exposure resulting from treating a psoriatic patient with 0.1% cream over 35% of the BSA, and 4.0 and 44 times, respectively, the maximum systemic exposure of acne patients treated with 0.1% cream over 15% of the BSA (1). Oral administration of tazarotene caused developmental delays in rats, and teratogenicity and resorptions in rats and rabbits at doses 1.1 and 26 times, respectively, the systemic exposure of a psoriatic patient and 3.5 and 85 times, respectively, the maximum systemic exposure of acne patients.

It is not known whether tazarotene or its active metabolite crosses the placenta to the fetus. The molecular weight (about 351) is low enough that transfer usually would be expected. However, the drug is highly bound to plasma protein (>99%) and maternal plasma concentrations are very low. Both of these factors should inhibit placental transfer.

The manufacturer has reports on nine pregnant women who were inadvertently exposed to tazarotene during clinical trials, two during studies involving acne patients and seven in other trials (1). One woman terminated her pregnancy, and healthy infants were delivered in the other eight cases. The timing of the exposures and the dosage used were not certain, so the significance of these findings is unknown (1).

BREASTFEEDING SUMMARY

Trace amounts of tazarotene are excreted into human milk (1). The risk to a nursing infant from this exposure is unknown.

Reference

1. Product information. Tazorac. Allergan, 2003.

TAZOBACTAM

Anti-infective

PREGNANCY RECOMMENDATION: Limited Human Data—Animal Data Suggest Low Risk
BREASTFEEDING RECOMMENDATION: Limited Human Data—Probably Compatible

PREGNANCY SUMMARY

Although the human data are very limited, the tazobactam–piperacillin combination appears to be relatively safe in pregnancy. No fetal harm in animals was observed at doses very close to those used in humans. Moreover, there is substantial experience with penicillins in human pregnancy that has shown this class of anti-infectives to be safe for the embryo–fetus. Because tazobactam is a derivative of the penicillin nucleus, it also probably is safe in pregnancy.

FETAL RISK SUMMARY

Tazobactam, a β-lactamase inhibitor, is combined with piperacillin to increase its antibacterial spectrum. It is not available as a single agent. Structurally, tazobactam is a derivative of the penicillin nucleus and is metabolized to an inactive metabolite. The plasma half-life ranges from 0.7 to 1.2 hours. Only 30% of tazobactam (and none of the metabolite) is bound to plasma proteins.

Reproduction studies with tazobactam have been conducted in mice and rats. No evidence of fetal harm was observed in these species at doses ≤6 and 14 times, respectively, the human dose based on BSA (HD). In rats, no effects on fertility were observed with doses 3 or fewer times the HD.

Consistent with its molecular weight (about 322) and its low protein binding, tazobactam crosses the human placenta. A 1998 report described the pharmacokinetics of piperacillin–tazobactam in six women with gestations of 25–32 weeks (2). Because of the increase in renal clearance and other factors, a marked decrease in maternal serum concentrations of both agents was observed. In one of the women (samples were inadequate in the other five), the fetal:maternal serum ratio of tazobactam was 2 approximately 3 hours after a dose. In two other women, low concentrations of tazobactam, 2.3 and 3.7 mcg/mL, respectively, were measured in the amniotic fluid and, in two others, low concentrations in fetal urine, 8.2 and 12.4 mcg/mL, respectively.

BREASTFEEDING SUMMARY

Although specific details were lacking, the manufacturer states that tazobactam is excreted into breast milk in low concentrations (1). This is consistent with its molecular weight (about 322) and low protein binding (30%). Piperacillin also is excreted into milk (see Piperacillin). The effects of this low exposure on a nursing infant probably are not clinically significant, but three potential problems exist for the nursing infant: modification of bowel flora, direct effects on the infant, and interference with the interpretation of culture results if a fever workup is required.

References

1. Product information. Zosyn. Wyeth Pharmaceuticals, 2004.
2. Bourget P, Sertin A, Lesne-Hulin A, Fernandez H, Ville Y, Van Peborgh P. Influence of pregnancy on the pharmacokinetic behaviour and the transplacental transfer of the piperacillin-tazobactam combination. Eur J Obstet Gynecol Reprod Biol 1998;76:21–7.

TECHNETIUM Tc-99m

Diagnostic Agent

PREGNANCY RECOMMENDATION: **Limited Human Data—Probably Compatible**
BREASTFEEDING RECOMMENDATION: **Limited Human Data—Probably Compatible**

PREGNANCY SUMMARY

Limited data from two studies of technetium Tc-99m (Tc-99m) exposure in human pregnancy have not suggested an increased risk for the embryo or fetus. Although it is desirable to minimize ionizing radiation exposure during pregnancy, a radiopharmaceutical may be administered either in an unrecognized pregnancy or for urgent diagnostic reasons. In these situations, the radiation dose to the embryo–fetus is estimated to be well below the 5Gy limit of concern.

FETAL RISK SUMMARY

Tc-99m is a gamma-emitting metastable nuclear isomer of technetium-99. It is the most common radioisotope used in medical diagnostic procedures. It is available either in the pertechnetate soluble salt form or in complex with various other agents. These radiopharmaceuticals are administered orally, IV, or by inhalation to aid in diagnostic imaging and functional studies of the brain, myocardium, thyroid, lungs, liver, gallbladder, kidneys, skeleton, blood, and tumors. The physical half-life (decay through gamma emission) of Tc-99m is approximately 6 hours, and the biological half-life is approximately 24 hours (1).

Animal reproduction studies with Tc-99m have not been conducted. Studies for carcinogenicity or mutagenic potential have not been conducted for most Tc-99m products. No genotoxic activity was observed for the active metabolite of Tc-99m sestamibi in various tests. At cytotoxic concentrations (>20 mcg/mL), an increase in cells with chromosome aberrations was observed in the human lymphocyte assay. No genotoxic effects in the in vivo mouse micronucleus test were observed at a dose that caused systemic and bone marrow toxicity (9 mg/kg, >600 times the maximum human dose). Fertility studies have not been conducted with Tc-99m (1).

Tc-99m is known to cross the placenta in animals and it is presumed that the same is true for the human placenta.

High-dose radiation exposure to the embryo or fetus is known to be associated with risks for intrauterine growth restriction, embryo–fetal loss, mental deficiency, and cancer. However, it is generally accepted that doses <5Gy to the embryo or fetus are not teratogenic. To evaluate potential risks for diagnostic procedures that utilize Tc-99m radiopharmaceuticals, estimates of the radiation dose available to the human embryo or fetus have been calculated under various scenarios, and these estimates are under the 5Gy limit. This suggests a low level of concern in situations where the diagnostic procedure is necessary in pregnancy or has been inadvertently performed in an unrecognized pregnancy (2–4).

In a 2009 study conducted by a German teratogen information service, 122 pregnancies were prospectively followed up in which the mothers were exposed sometime between the 2nd and 17th weeks of gestation to one of five Tc-99m radiopharmaceuticals for diagnosis of bone, thyroid, kidney, or lung conditions (5). Outcomes were compared with 366 unexposed pregnancies. No increased risks for growth deficiency, pregnancy loss, or major birth defects were noted in the exposed infants (5).

In a 1997 British study, data were abstracted from medical records for 82 pregnant women who had been evaluated for pulmonary embolism with either a Tc-99m perfusion or ventilation scan or both. Most scans were conducted late in pregnancy. No adverse pregnancy outcomes were reported, although no details were provided (6).

BREASTFEEDING SUMMARY

Tc-99m is excreted into breast milk. In a 1994 study, breast milk samples were obtained from 60 women who had been exposed to Tc-99m radiopharmaceuticals (7). Analysis found generally low radiation doses in breast milk across the samples, but there was distinct variability by specific radiopharmaceutical. Based on estimated dose, the recommendation for those products that produce the highest concentrations, such as Tc-99m pertechnetate, is to interrupt breastfeeding until activity in milk samples reaches a threshold concentration. For other products, no interruption in breastfeeding was considered necessary (8–10).

References

1. Product information. Technetium Tc 99m Sestamibi Injection, 2008.
2. Adelstein SJ. Administered radionuclides in pregnancy. Teratology 1999;59:236–9.
3. International Commission on Radiological Protection Pregnancy and Medical Radiation. Ann ICRP 2000;30:1–43.
4. Taskar-Pandit N, Dauer LT, Montgomery L, St. Germain J, Zanzonico PB, Divgi CR. Organ and fetal absorbed dose estimates from ^{99m}tc-sulfur colloid lymphoscintigraphy and sentinel node localization in breast cancer patients. J Nucl Med 2006;47:1202–8.
5. Schaefer C, Meister R, Wentzeck R, Weber-Schoendorfer C. Fetal outcome after technetium scintigraphy in early pregnancy. Reprod Toxicol 2009;28:161–6.
6. Balan KK, Critchley M, Vedavathy KK, Smith ML, Vinjamuri S. The value of ventilation-perfusion imaging in pregnancy. Br J Radiol 1997;70:338–40.
7. Rubow S, Klopper J, Wasserman H, Baard B, van Niekerk M. The excretion of radiopharmaceuticals in human breast milk: additional data and dosimetry. Eur J Nucl Med 1994;21:144–53.
8. Rose MR, Prescott MC, Herman KJ. Excretion of iodine-123-hippuran, technetium-99m-red blood cells, and technetium-99m-macroaggregated albumin into breast milk. J Nucl Med 1990;31:978–84.
9. Marshall DS, Newberry NR, Ryan PJ. Measurement of the secretion of technetium-99m hexamethylpropylene amine oxime into breast milk. Eur J Nucl Med 1996;23:1634–5.
10. McCauley E, Mackie A. Breast milk activity during early lactation following maternal $^{99}Tc^{m}$ macroaggregated albumin lung perfusion scan. Br J of Radiol 2002;75:464–6.

TEDUGLUTIDE

Gastrointestinal Agent (Glucagon-Like Peptide-2 Analog)

PREGNANCY RECOMMENDATION: No Human Data—Probably Compatible
BREASTFEEDING RECOMMENDATION: No Human Data—Potential Toxicity

PREGNANCY SUMMARY

No reports describing the use of teduglutide in human pregnancy have been located. In the animal data, comparisons to the human dose were based on body weight. Even though such comparisons usually cannot be interpreted, the doses were up to 1000 times the human dose and might suggest low risk. Moreover, the drug is an analog of a naturally occurring peptide secreted by L-cells of the distal intestine (1). Consequently, if indicated the drug should not be withheld because of pregnancy.

FETAL RISK SUMMARY

Teduglutide, given as a daily SC injection, is a 33 amino acid analog of naturally occurring human glucagon-like peptide-2 that is known to increase intestinal and portal blood flow and inhibit gastric acid secretion. It is indicated for the treatment of adult patients with short bowel syndrome (SBS) who are dependent on parenteral support. It is metabolized to inactive components. The mean terminal half-life is about 2 hours in healthy subjects and 1.3 hours in SBS patients (1). However, information regarding plasma protein binding is apparently unknown.

Reproduction studies have been conducted in rats and rabbits. In these species, SC doses up to 1000 times the recommended human daily dose based on body weight (RHDD) did not reveal any evidence of fetal harm or impaired fertility. In addition, no evidence of adverse effects were observed in predevelopment and postdevelopment studies in rats with SC doses up to 1000 times the RHDD (1).

In a 2-year carcinogenicity rat study, teduglutide caused significant increases in the incidence of adenomas in the bile duct and jejunum of male rats. Studies for mutagenicity were negative, as were studies of impaired fertility and reproductive performance in male and female rats (1).

It is not known if teduglutide crosses the human placenta. The molecular weight (about 3752) and the relatively short mean terminal half-life suggest that clinically significant amounts of the drug probably will not reach the embryo or fetus, at least early in gestation.

BREASTFEEDING SUMMARY

No reports describing the use of teduglutide during human lactation have been located. The molecular weight (about 3752) and the relatively short (1.3 hours) mean terminal half-life in SBS patients suggest that the drug will probably not be excreted into breast milk, at least in clinically significant amounts. Even if some excretion did occur, the peptide would probably be digested in the infant's gut. However, teduglutide is given as a daily SC injection and the manufacturer states that women receiving teduglutide should not breastfeed because of the tumorigenicity shown in rats (1).

Reference

1. Product information. Gattex. NPS Pharmaceuticals, 2013.

T

TEGASEROD

[Withdrawn from the market. See 9th edition.]

TELAPREVIR

Antiviral Agent

PREGNANCY RECOMMENDATION: No Human Data—Animal Data Suggest Low Risk (Contraindicated—3-Drug Combination)
BREASTFEEDING RECOMMENDATION: No Human Data—Potential Toxicity (3-Drug Combination)

PREGNANCY SUMMARY

No reports describing the use of telaprevir in human pregnancy have been located. The animal data suggest low risk. However, the indication for telaprevir involves the combined use with ribavirin and peginterferon alfa. Although peginterferon alfa is probably compatible with pregnancy (see Interferon, Alfa), ribavirin is contraindicated because it has caused developmental toxicity in all animal species tested (see Ribavirin). The 3-drug combination should be avoided in pregnancy.

FETAL RISK SUMMARY

Telaprevir, a protease inhibitor, is a direct-acting antiviral agent against the hepatitis C virus. It is indicated, in combination with peginterferon alfa and ribavirin, for the treatment of genotype 1 chronic hepatitis C in adult patients with compensated liver disease, including cirrhosis, who are treatment-naive or who have previously been treated with interferon-based treatment, including prior null responders, and relapsers. Telaprevir is extensively metabolized to inactive metabolites. Plasma protein binding, primarily to α_1-acid glycoprotein and albumin, is moderate (59%–76%). The mean elimination half-life after a single dose was 4.0–4.7 hours and 9–11 hours at steady state (1).

Reproduction studies with telaprevir alone have been conducted in mice and rats. The highest doses tested produced exposures that were 1.84 and 0.60 times, respectively, the human exposure at the recommended clinical dose (HERCD). No harm to the fetuses were observed at these exposures (1). However, ribavirin causes dose-related teratogenicity or embryo lethality in animals (see Ribavirin) and peginterferon alfa causes dose-related abortions in animals (see Interferon, Alfa).

The carcinogenic potential of telaprevir has not been studied. Multiple assays for genotoxicity were negative. However, the drug did have adverse effects on fertility parameters in rats. The no-observed-adverse-effect level for testicular toxicity was an exposure 0.17 times the HERCD. At exposures 0.30 times the HERCD, potential effects were decreased motile sperm and increased nonmotile sperm count. In female rats, there were minor increases in preimplantation loss in percent of dams with nonviable embryos, and percent of nonviable conceptuses per litter. These effects were probably related to testicular toxicity in males, but contributions of the female could not be ruled out (1).

It is not known if telaprevir crosses the human placenta. The molecular weight (about 680), moderate plasma protein binding, and long elimination half-life suggest that the drug will cross to the embryo–fetus.

BREASTFEEDING SUMMARY

No reports describing the use of telaprevir during human lactation have been located. The molecular weight (about 680), moderate plasma protein binding (59%–76%), and long elimination half-life (9–11 hours at steady state) suggest that the drug will be excreted into breast milk. The effect of this exposure on a nursing infant is unknown. However, telaprevir is always combined with ribavirin and peginterferon alfa (see Ribavirin and Interferon, Alfa). The latter agent is known to be excreted into breast milk and ribavirin is probably excreted. If a woman taking this therapy is breastfeeding, her nursing infant could be exposed to all three agents. Thus, the best course of action is to not breastfeed.

Reference

1. Product information. Incivek. Vertex Pharmaceuticals, 2012.

T

TELAVANCIN

Antibiotic

PREGNANCY RECOMMENDATION: No Human Data—Animal Data Suggest Low Risk
BREASTFEEDING RECOMMENDATION: No Human Data—Potential Toxicity

PREGNANCY SUMMARY

No reports describing the use of telavancin, a synthetic derivative of vancomycin, in human pregnancy have been located. The manufacturer interpreted the animal reproduction data as showing risk of limb and skeletal malformations. However, a presentation by Anthony Scialli, MD, Tetra Tech Sciences, at a public meeting of the FDA Advisory Committee on Antimicrobial Drugs, November 2008, did not support that interpretation. Among 654 rat and 156 rabbit fetuses, shortened limbs were observed in only three fetuses: two rats (one of which was not confirmed) and a rabbit. In minipigs, polydactyly was observed in controls and in all drug groups except the high-dose group, so inclusion of these results is questionable. Nevertheless, a better reason for not using this drug, at least until human pregnancy data are available, is that it does not appear to offer a clear advantage for its indication over other available antibiotics that do have pregnancy experience. A pregnancy registry has been established by the manufacturer to monitor pregnancy outcomes in women exposed to telavancin. Either the physician or the patient herself can register by calling 1-888-658-4228 (1).

FETAL RISK SUMMARY

Telavancin is a lipoglycopeptide antibacterial that is a synthetic derivative of vancomycin. It is given as an IV infusion. Telavancin is indicated for the treatment of adult patients with complicated skin and skin structure infections caused by susceptible isolates of the following gram-positive microorganisms: *Staphylococcus aureus* (including methicillin-susceptible and -resistant isolates), *Streptococcus pyogenes*, *Streptococcus agalactiae*, *Streptococcus anginosus* group (includes *Streptococcus anginosus*, *Staphylococcus intermedius*, and *Streptococcus constellatus*), or *Enterococcus faecalis* (vancomycin-susceptible isolates only). The drug is partially metabolized. Binding to plasma proteins, primarily to albumin, is about 90%, and the elimination half-life is about 8 hours. The drug is highly lipophilic (1).

Reproduction studies have been conducted in rats, rabbits, and minipigs. In these species, IV doses resulting in exposures that were about 1–2 times the human exposure (AUC) at the maximum recommended clinical dose showed a potential to cause limb and skeletal malformations that included brachymelia (rats, rabbits), syndactyly (rats, minipigs), adactyly (rabbits), and polydactyly (minipigs) (*see also above Summary*). Other findings were flexed front paw and absent ulna (rabbits), misshapen digits and deformed front leg (minipigs), and an increase in the number of stillborn pups and decreased fetal body weights (rats) (1).

Long-term carcinogenicity studies have not been conducted. The drug was not mutagenic or clastogenic in multiple assays. Telavancin did not impair fertility or reproductive performance in male and female rats. When the drug was given for longer periods in male rats at doses resulting in exposures similar to those in humans, reversible altered sperm parameters were observed (1).

It is not known if telavancin crosses the human placenta. The molecular weight (about 1756 for the free base) and moderately high plasma protein binding may partially inhibit placental crossing, but the high fat solubility and long elimination half-life suggest that the drug will cross to the embryo–fetus.

BREASTFEEDING SUMMARY

No reports describing the use of telavancin during human lactation have been located. The molecular weight (about 1756 for the free base) and moderately high plasma protein binding (about 90%) may partially inhibit excretion into breast milk, but the high fat solubility and long elimination half-life (8 hours) suggest that some drug will cross into milk. Because telavancin is a weak base, ion trapping in the more acidic milk may occur that results in a milk:plasma ratio >1. The effect of this exposure on a nursing infant is unknown, but three potential problems exist: modification of bowel flora, direct effects on the infant (e.g., allergic response), and interference with the interpretation of culture results if a fever workup is required.

Reference

1. Product information. Vibativ. Astellas Pharma US, 2009.

T

TELBIVUDINE

Antiviral

PREGNANCY RECOMMENDATION: Limited Human Data—Animal Data Suggest Low Risk
BREASTFEEDING RECOMMENDATION: No Human Data—Potential Toxicity

PREGNANCY SUMMARY

The human pregnancy experience with telbivudine is very limited. Although the animal reproduction data are encouraging, additional human pregnancy experience is required for a full assessment of the embryo–fetal risk. Theoretically, exposure to agents in this class at the time of implantation could impair fertility as a result of embryonic cytotoxicity. This toxicity was not observed with telbivudine in animal studies but has not been studied in humans. Mitochondrial dysfunction has been reported with two nucleoside reverse transcriptase inhibitors (see Lamivudine and Zidovudine). However, no appreciable mitochondrial toxicity was observed with telbivudine at concentrations much higher than those required to inhibit hepatitis B viral DNA synthesis (1). If indicated, the drug should not be withheld because of pregnancy. Physicians are encouraged to register exposed patients in the Antiretroviral Pregnancy Registry by calling 1-800-258-4263 (1).

FETAL RISK SUMMARY

Telbivudine is an oral synthetic thymidine nucleoside analog with antiviral activity against hepatitis B virus DNA polymerase. It has no activity against the HIV. It is phosphorylated to the active metabolite by cellular kinases. Telbivudine is indicated for the treatment of chronic hepatitis B in adult patients with evidence of viral replication and either evidence of persistent elevations in serum aminotransferases (alanine aminotransferase [ALT] or aspartate aminotransferase [AST]) or histologically active disease. The agent is in the same class of nucleoside reverse transcriptase inhibitors as abacavir, didanosine, emtricitabine, lamivudine, stavudine, tenofovir, and zidovudine. Plasma protein binding is very low (3%). The plasma terminal elimination half-life is 40–49 hours and the drug is eliminated primarily by urinary excretion of unchanged drug (1).

Reproduction studies have been conducted in rats and rabbits. No evidence of fetal harm was observed in these species at exposures up to 6 and 37 times, respectively, the exposure levels from the human therapeutic dose of 600 mg/day (HTD). The drug crossed the placentas of both species (1).

Studies with telbivudine have found no evidence of carcinogenicity in mice and rats or genotoxicity in multiple assays (1,2). No evidence of impaired fertility was seen in male and female rats given doses that produced systemic exposures about 14 times the HTD (1).

It is not known if telbivudine crosses the human placenta. The low molecular weight (about 242) and plasma protein binding, and long elimination half-life suggest that the drug will reach the embryo and fetus.

The Antiretroviral Pregnancy Registry reported, for the period January 1989 through July 2009, prospective data (reported before the outcomes were known) involving 4702 live births that had been exposed during the 1st trimester to one or more antiretroviral agents (3). Congenital defects were noted in 134, a prevalence of 2.8% (95% confidence interval [CI] 2.4–3.4). In the 6100 live births with earliest exposure in the 2nd/3rd trimesters, there were 153 infants with defects (prevalence 2.5%, 95% CI 2.1–2.9). The prevalence rates for the two periods did not differ significantly. There were 288 infants with birth defects among 10,803 live births with exposure anytime during pregnancy (prevalence 2.7%, 95% CI 2.4–3.0). The prevalence rate did not differ significantly from the rate expected in a nonexposed population. There were six outcomes exposed to telbivudine (five in the 1st trimester and one in the 2nd/3rd trimesters) in combination with other antiretroviral agents. There were no birth defects. In reviewing the birth defects of prospective and retrospective (pregnancies reported after the outcomes were known) registered cases, the Registry concluded that, except for isolated cases of neural tube defects with efavirenz exposure in retrospective reports, there was no other pattern of anomalies (isolated or syndromic) (3) (see Lamivudine for required statement).

BREASTFEEDING SUMMARY

No reports describing the use of telbivudine during human lactation have been located. The molecular weight (about 242), plasma protein binding (3%), and long elimination half-life (40–49 hours) suggest that the drug will be excreted into breast milk. The effect of this exposure on a nursing infant is unknown. Infants of mothers with hepatitis B are at high risk of chronic hepatitis B virus infection when the maternal infection occurs perinatally or in early infancy (4). Hepatitis B immune globulin and hepatitis B virus vaccine given simultaneously to the infant at birth will prevent chronic infection in nearly all cases, regardless of whether the infant is breastfed (4). If the mother elects to breastfeed, the infant should be monitored closely for the most common telbivudine-induced toxicities observed in adults, such as upper respiratory infection, fatigue, malaise, abdominal pain, cough, fever, insomnia, rash, nausea, vomiting, diarrhea, and loose stools.

References

1. Product information. Tyzeka. Novartis Pharmaceuticals, 2007.
2. Bridges EG, Selden JR, Luo S. Nonclinical safety profile of telbivudine, a novel potent antiviral agent for treatment of hepatitis B. Antimicrob Agents Chemother 2008;52:2521–8.
3. Antiretroviral Pregnancy Registry Steering Committee. *Antiretroviral Pregnancy Registry International Interim Report for 1 January 1989 through 31 July 2009*. Wilmington, NC: Registry Coordinating Center; 2009. Available at www.apregistry.com. Accessed May 29, 2010.
4. Lawrence RM, Lawrence RA. The breast and the physiology of lactation. In: Creasy RK, Resnik R. eds. *Maternal and Fetal Medicine*. 5th ed. Philadelphia, PA: WB Saunders, 2004:146, 148.

TELITHROMYCIN

Antibiotic

PREGNANCY RECOMMENDATION: No Human Data—Animal Data Suggest Low Risk
BREASTFEEDING RECOMMENDATION: No Human Data—Probably Compatible

PREGNANCY SUMMARY

No reports describing the use of telithromycin in human pregnancy have been located. The animal reproduction data suggest low risk, but the absence of human pregnancy experience prevents a more complete assessment. Although there are no other agents in the ketolide class, telithromycin is a chemical derivative of erythromycin, a macrolide anti-infective that is considered compatible in pregnancy. There is currently no evidence that macrolides are associated with developmental toxicity. However, telithromycin may cause severe hepatocellular hepatitis that can be fatal (1). The hepatotoxicity has special significance for pregnant women because liver toxicity sometimes occurs in pregnancy (e.g., viral hepatitis, fatty liver of pregnancy, preeclampsia, and HELLP [**h**emolysis, **e**levated **l**iver enzymes, and **l**ow **p**latelets] syndrome). Therefore, until there are human pregnancy data, the best course is to avoid the use of telithromycin in pregnancy.

FETAL RISK SUMMARY

Telithromycin, a ketolide, is a semisynthetic antibacterial agent that is a derivative of erythromycin. The chemical structure of telithromycin differs from the macrolide group.

The antibacterial is indicated for the treatment of community-acquired pneumonia (mild to moderate severity). Telithromycin is partially metabolized to inactive metabolites. Plasma protein binding is 60%–70%, primarily to albumin. The terminal elimination half-lives after single and multiple doses are about 7 and 10 hours, respectively (2).

Reproduction studies have been conducted in rats and rabbits. No evidence of structural defects was found when doses that were about 1.8 and 0.49 times, respectively, the daily human dose based on BSA (DHD) were given to these species. No adverse effects on prenatal or postnatal development on rat pups were observed at 1.5 times the DHD. However, doses higher than 1.8 and 0.49 times, respectively, the DHD in rats and rabbits were associated with maternal toxicity and delayed fetal maturation (2).

Carcinogenicity studies have not been conducted, but tests for genotoxicity were negative. Doses that were about 0.61 times the DHD had no effect on fertility in rats. Higher doses, 1.8–3.6 times the DHD, did impair fertility but also caused toxicity in both male and female rats (2).

It is not known if telithromycin crosses the human placenta. The molecular weight (about 812), moderate plasma protein binding, and the long elimination half-life suggest that the antibacterial agent will cross to the embryo–fetus.

BREASTFEEDING SUMMARY

No reports describing the use of telithromycin during human lactation have been located.

The molecular weight (about 812), moderate plasma protein binding (60%–70%), and long elimination half-life (≤10 hours) suggest that telithromycin will be excreted into breast milk. The effect of this exposure on a nursing infant is unknown. Although modification of the bowel flora, direct effects, and interference with the interpretation of culture results if a fever workup is required are potential effects, a closely related antibacterial, erythromycin is considered compatible with nursing. When taking this drug and nursing, a mother should observe her infant for the most common adverse effects reported in adults, such as diarrhea, nausea, vomiting, headache, and dizziness.

References

1. Ross DB. The FDA and the case of Ketek. N Engl J Med 2007;356:1601–4.
2. Product information. Ketek. Sanofi-Aventis U.S., 2007.

TELMISARTAN

Antihypertensive

PREGNANCY RECOMMENDATION: Human Data Suggest Risk in 2nd and 3rd Trimesters
BREASTFEEDING RECOMMENDATION: No Human Data—Probably Compatible

T

PREGNANCY SUMMARY

The antihypertensive mechanisms of action of telmisartan and angiotensin-converting enzyme (ACE) inhibitors are very close. That is, the former selectively blocks the binding of angiotensin II to AT_1 receptors, whereas the latter prevents the formation of angiotensin II itself. Therefore, use of this drug during the 2nd and 3rd trimesters may cause teratogenicity and severe fetal and neonatal toxicity that is identical to that seen with ACE inhibitors (e.g., see Captopril or Enalapril). Fetal toxic effects may include anuria, oligohydramnios, fetal hypocalvaria, intrauterine growth restriction, prematurity, and patent ductus arteriosus. Anuria-associated oligohydramnios may produce fetal limb contractures, craniofacial deformation, and pulmonary hypoplasia. Severe anuria and hypotension that are resistant to both pressor agents and volume expansion may occur in the newborn following in utero exposure to telmisartan. Newborn renal function and blood pressure should be closely monitored.

FETAL RISK SUMMARY

Telmisartan is a selective angiotensin II receptor blocker (ARB) that is used, either alone or in combination with other antihypertensive agents, for the treatment of hypertension. Telmisartan blocks the vasoconstrictor and aldosterone-secreting effects of angiotensin II by preventing angiotensin II from binding to AT_1 receptors (1).

Reproduction studies have been conducted in pregnant rats and rabbits. No teratogenicity was observed in either species at oral doses up to about 6.3 and 6.4 times the maximum recommended human dose of 80 mg based on BSA (MRHD), respectively, but embryolethality was noted at the highest dose in rabbits. The highest doses were maternally toxic (reduced body weight gain and food consumption) in both species. In rats, an oral dose approximately 1.9 times the MRHD (also maternal toxic) during late gestation and lactation resulted in neonatal adverse effects, including reduced viability, low birth weight, delayed maturation, and decreased weight gain. The no-observed-effect doses for developmental toxicity in rats and rabbits were 0.64 and 3.7 times the MRHD, respectively. No adverse effects on reproductive performance were noted in male and female rats at a dose about 13 times the MRHD (1).

It is not known if telmisartan crosses the human placenta to the fetus. The drug is found in rat fetuses in late gestation (1). The molecular weight (about 515) is low enough that passage to the human fetus should be expected.

A 2003 case report described transient renal failure in a newborn secondary to maternal use of telmisartan (2). A 35-year-old woman with hypertension was treated with telmisartan throughout pregnancy. Oligohydramnios was diagnosed at 34 weeks' gestation and a 2.2-kg female infant was delivered by cesarean section. Apgar scores were 9, 10, and 10 at 1, 5, and 10 minutes, respectively. The infant was anuric until the third day of life, but renal function improved thereafter. Telmisartan plasma levels on day 10 and 13 were 20 and 13 ng/L, respectively. The infant's renal function had normalized by 1.5 months of age (2).

A 2012 review of the use of ACE inhibitors and ARBs in the 1st trimester concluded that there may be an elevated teratogenic risk, but the risk appeared to be related to other factors (3). The factors, that typically coexist with hypertension in pregnancy, included diabetes, advanced maternal age, and obesity.

BREASTFEEDING SUMMARY

No reports describing the use of telmisartan during human lactation have been located. The molecular weight (515) is low enough that excretion into human breast milk should be expected. The effect of this exposure on a nursing infant is unknown. The American Academy of Pediatrics, however, classifies ACE inhibitors, a closely related group of antihypertensive agents, as compatible with breastfeeding (see Captopril or Enalapril).

References

1. Product information. Micardis. Boehringer Ingelheim Pharmaceuticals, 2000.
2. Pietrement C, Malot L, Santerne B, Roussel B, Motte J, Morville P. Neonatal acute renal failure secondary to maternal exposure to telmisartan, angiotensin II receptor antagonist. J Perinatol 2003;23:254–5.
3. Polifka JE. Is there an embryopathy associated with first-trimester exposure to angiotensin-converting enzyme inhibitors and angiotensin receptor antagonists? A critical review of the evidence. Birth Defects Res (Part A) 2012;94:576–98.

TEMAZEPAM

Hypnotic

PREGNANCY RECOMMENDATION: Limited Human Data—Animal Data Suggest Risk
BREASTFEEDING RECOMMENDATION: Limited Human Data—Potential Toxicity

PREGNANCY SUMMARY

Temazepam is a benzodiazepine that is used as a hypnotic for the short-term management of insomnia. Limited human data suggest an association between the drug and oral clefts, but confirming studies are required. Fetal death, possibly related to an interaction between temazepam and diphenhydramine, has been reported. The lethal interaction was apparently confirmed in an animal study.

FETAL RISK SUMMARY

Reproductive studies in rats revealed increased resorptions and an increased incidence of rudimentary ribs, which were considered skeletal variants (1). Exencephaly and fusion or asymmetry of ribs were observed in rabbits (1).

In a surveillance study of Michigan Medicaid recipients involving 229,101 completed pregnancies conducted between 1985 and 1992, 146 newborns had been exposed to temazepam during the 1st trimester (F. Rosa, personal communication, FDA, 1993). Six (4.1%) major birth defects were observed (six expected), including one cardiovascular defect (one expected) and two oral clefts (none expected). No anomalies were observed in four other categories of defects (spina bifida, polydactyly, limb reduction defects, and hypospadias) for which specific data were available. Although the two oral clefts suggest a relationship with the drug, other factors, such as the mother's disease, concurrent drug use, and chance, may be involved.

A potential drug interaction between temazepam and diphenhydramine, resulting in the stillbirth of a term female

T

infant, has been reported (2). The mother had taken diphenhydramine 50 mg for mild itching of the skin and approximately 1.5 hours later took 30 mg of temazepam for sleep. Three hours later, she awoke with violent intrauterine fetal movements, which lasted several minutes and then abruptly stopped. The stillborn infant was delivered approximately 4 hours later. Autopsy revealed no gross or microscopic anomalies. In an experiment with pregnant rabbits, neither of the drugs alone caused fetal mortality but when combined, 51 (81%) of 63 fetuses were stillborn or died shortly after birth (2). No definite mechanism could be established for the apparent interaction.

BREASTFEEDING SUMMARY

Temazepam is excreted into breast milk. Ten mothers, within 15 days of delivery, were administered 10–20 mg of temazepam for at least 2 days as a bedtime hypnotic (3). Milk and plasma samples were obtained about 15 hours later corresponding to an infant feeding. Temazepam was detected (limit of detection 5 ng/mL) in the milk of only one woman with before- and after-feed levels of 28 and 26 ng/mL, respectively. The milk:plasma ratio in this patient was 0.12. Although no adverse effects were observed in the nursling, nursing infants of mothers consuming temazepam should be closely observed for sedation and poor feeding. The American Academy of Pediatrics classifies temazepam as a drug for which the effect on nursing infants is unknown but may be of concern (4).

References

1. Product information. Restoril. Sandoz Pharmaceuticals Corp., 1993.
2. Kargas GA, Kargas SA, Bruyere HJ Jr, Gilbert EF, Opitz JM. Perinatal mortality due to interaction of diphenhydramine and temazepam. N Engl J Med 1985;313:1417.
3. Lepedevs TH, Wojnar-Horton RE, Yapp P, Roberts MJ, Dusci LJ, Hackett LP, Ilett KF. Excretion of temazepam in breast milk. Br J Clin Pharmacol 1992;33:204–6.
4. Committee on Drugs, American Academy of Pediatrics. The transfer of drugs and other chemicals into human milk. Pediatrics 2001;108:776–89.

TEMOZOLOMIDE

Antineoplastic

PREGNANCY RECOMMENDATION: No Human Data—Animal Data Suggest Risk
BREASTFEEDING RECOMMENDATION: Contraindicated

PREGNANCY SUMMARY

No reports describing the use of temozolomide in human pregnancy have been located. The animal reproduction data suggest risk, but the absence of human pregnancy experience prevents a more complete assessment of embryo–fetal risk. The recommended first cycle of temozolomide is 42 days of consecutive therapy, followed by an increased dose for six cycles (5 consecutive days of therapy in each 4-week cycle). Thus, exposure could potentially occur throughout most of gestation. Women of childbearing age should employ adequate contraceptive methods to prevent pregnancy. However, if a woman requires temozolomide and informed consent is obtained, therapy should not be withheld because of pregnancy. If an inadvertent pregnancy occurs during therapy, the woman should be advised of the unknown, but potentially severe, risk for her embryo and/or fetus.

FETAL RISK SUMMARY

Temozolomide, an imidazotetrazine derivative, is an oral prodrug that undergoes rapid nonenzymatic conversion at physiologic pH to the reactive compound MTIC. The cytotoxic effect of MTIC is thought to be mainly due to alkylation of DNA. There are no other agents in this antineoplastic subclass. Temozolomide is indicated for the treatment of adult patients with newly diagnosed glioblastoma multiforme concomitantly with radiotherapy and then as maintenance treatment. It also is indicated for the treatment of adult patients with refractory anaplastic astrocytoma. Plasma protein binding of temozolomide is minimal (about 15%) and its elimination half-life is short (1.8 hours) (1).

Reproduction studies have been conducted in rats and rabbits. During organogenesis, rats and rabbits were given daily oral doses that were 0.375 and 0.75 times, respectively, the maximum recommended human dose based on BSA (MRHD) for 5 consecutive days. Numerous malformations were observed in both species, including defects of the external organs, soft tissues, and skeletons. Daily doses that were 0.75 times the MRHD also caused embryolethality (resorptions) (1).

Short-term studies for carcinogenicity have been conducted in rats. When rats were given a dose of temozolomide that was equal to the MRHD for 5 consecutive days every 28 days for three cycles, mammary carcinomas were found in males and females. When six cycles were given with doses that were 0.125, 0.25, or 0.625 times the MRHD, mammary carcinomas were observed at all doses. In addition, the highest dose was associated with multiple other tumors (1).

It is not known if temozolomide crosses the human placenta. The molecular weight of the parent compound (about 194) and the minimal plasma protein binding suggest that the drug will cross to the embryo and fetus. However, after absorption, temozolomide undergoes rapid hydrolysis to MTIC, and this compound also may cross the placenta.

BREASTFEEDING SUMMARY

No reports describing the use of temozolomide during human lactation have been located.

The molecular weight of the parent compound (about 194) and the minimal plasma protein binding (about 15%) suggest that the drug will be excreted into breast milk. Moreover, after absorption, temozolomide undergoes rapid hydrolysis to the active agent MTIC, so this compound also may be excreted into milk. The effect of these exposures on a nursing infant is unknown. In adults, the drug is rapidly and completely absorbed and may also be absorbed by a nursing infant. Thus, it is best that a woman receiving this agent does not breastfeed. If she chooses to do so, the infant should be closely monitored for the most common or serious adverse effects observed in adults. These effects include alopecia, nausea, vomiting, anorexia, headache, constipation, fatigue, thrombocytopenia, and convulsions (1).

Reference

1. Product information. Temodar. Schering, 2007.

TEMSIROLIMUS

Antineoplastic (Kinase Inhibitor)

PREGNANCY RECOMMENDATION: Contraindicated
BREASTFEEDING RECOMMENDATION: Contraindicated

PREGNANCY SUMMARY

No reports describing the use of temsirolimus in human pregnancy have been located. The animal reproduction studies suggest risk, but the absence of human pregnancy experience prevents a full assessment of the embryo–fetal risk. The manufacturer recommends advising women of childbearing potential to avoid becoming pregnant during treatment and for 3 months after the last dose (1). The manufacturer also recommends that men be counseled on the potential effects of the drug on the fetus and sperm, and, if their partner is of childbearing potential, should use reliable contraception during treatment and for 3 months after the last dose (1). (See also Sirolimus.)

FETAL RISK SUMMARY

Temsirolimus is an antineoplastic agent indicated for the treatment of advanced renal cell carcinoma. It is a mTOR inhibitor (mammalian target of rapamycin) that is the same subclass as everolimus. Temsirolimus is given as an IV infusion over 30–60 minutes once weekly. The drug is metabolized to five metabolites. Sirolimus is the principal metabolite in humans. Plasma protein binding of sirolimus is about 92% but apparently is not known for the parent compound. The mean half-lives of temsirolimus and sirolimus are about 17 and 55 hours, respectively (1).

Reproduction studies have been conducted in rats and rabbits. Exposures after daily oral doses that produced embryo–fetal toxicity in rats and rabbits were about 0.04 and 0.12 times the AUC in cancer patients at the human recommended dose, respectively. Toxicity in the rat consisted of reduced fetal weight and reduced ossification, whereas in the rabbit it was reduced fetal weight, omphalocele, bifurcated sternebrae, notched ribs, and incomplete ossifications (1).

Carcinogenic studies have not been conducted with temsirolimus, but sirolimus was carcinogenic in mice and rats (see Sirolimus). Temsirolimus was not genotoxic in multiple assays. Fertility was impaired in male rats at doses that were about 0.2 times the human recommended IV dose (RHID). The effects observed were decreased number of pregnancies, decreased sperm concentration and motility, decreased reproductive organ weights, and testicular tubular degeneration. At about 2 times the RHID, fertility was absent. In female rats, an increased incidence of pre- and postimplantation losses was noted at an oral dose about 0.3 times the RHID (1).

It is not known if temsirolimus or sirolimus crosses the human placenta. The molecular weights of the two compounds, about 1030 and 914, respectively, are within the range for passive diffusion. In addition, the elimination half-lives will place the drug at the maternal–fetal interface for long periods.

BREASTFEEDING SUMMARY

No reports describing the use of temsirolimus during human lactation have been located. There also are no reports of the use of sirolimus, the active metabolite, during lactation (see Sirolimus). The molecular weights of the two compounds, about 1030 and 914, respectively, are low enough for excretion into breast milk. Moreover, the elimination half-lives, about 17 and 55 hours, respectively, suggest that both temsirolimus and sirolimus will be excreted. The effect of this exposure on a nursing infant is unknown. However, serious toxicity has been observed in adults, such as hypersensitivity reactions, including anaphylaxis, infections, interstitial lung disease, bowel perforation, renal failure, and abnormal wound healing.

Reference

1. Product information. Torisel. Wyeth Pharmaceuticals, 2007.

TENECTEPLASE

Thrombolytic

PREGNANCY RECOMMENDATION: Compatible—Maternal Benefit >> Embryo–Fetal Risk
BREASTFEEDING RECOMMENDATION: Hold Breastfeeding

PREGNANCY SUMMARY

No reports describing the use of tenecteplase in human pregnancy have been located. The limited animal data do not suggest a direct risk. Moreover, fetal toxicity has not been observed with limited pregnancy exposure to another, similar glycoprotein enzyme, alteplase. Although maternal hemorrhage is a major risk, tenecteplase should not be withheld because of pregnancy if the maternal condition requires such therapy.

FETAL RISK SUMMARY

Tenecteplase is a modified form of human tissue plasminogen activator (tPA) that is produced by recombinant DNA technology using Chinese hamster ovary cells. It is a 527 amino acid glycoprotein that is indicated to reduce the mortality associated with acute myocardial infarction. Tenecteplase is cleared from the plasma with a half-life of 20–24 minutes, but the terminal phase half-life is 90–130 minutes (1).

In pregnant rabbits given multiple IV daily doses of 0.5, 1.5, and 5.0 mg/kg/day, vaginal hemorrhage resulted in maternal deaths. No fetal anomalies were observed. Single IV doses (the recommended human dose is a single bolus injection) in rabbits did not cause maternal or embryo toxicity. The no-observable-effect-level (NOEL) of a single IV dose was 5 mg/kg (about 8–10 times the human dose) (1).

It is not known if tenecteplase crosses the human placenta. Tenecteplase is a glycoprotein and, although some proteins do cross, the short plasma half-life will limit the exposure of the embryo–fetus to the enzyme.

BREASTFEEDING SUMMARY

No reports describing the use of tenecteplase during human lactation have been located. It is not known whether the glycoprotein is excreted into human milk. Because of the nature of the indication for this agent and its very short plasma and terminal half-life, the opportunities for its use during lactation or the possible exposure of a nursing infant are minimal.

Reference

1. Product information. TNKase. Genentech, 2004.

TENIPOSIDE

Antineoplastic

PREGNANCY RECOMMENDATION: Contraindicated—1st Trimester
BREASTFEEDING RECOMMENDATION: No Human Data—Potential Toxicity

PREGNANCY SUMMARY

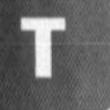

Teniposide, a podophyllin derivative, has been used in the 2nd and 3rd trimesters of one pregnancy (1). An apparently normal infant was delivered at 37 weeks' gestation.

FETAL RISK SUMMARY

Reproduction studies in rats given IV doses of 0.1–3 mg/kg (0.6–18 mg/m^2) every second day from day 6 to day 16 postcoital revealed dose-related embryotoxicity and teratogenicity (2). Congenital malformations consisted of spinal and rib defects, deformed extremities, anophthalmia, and celosomia.

Long-term studies of growth and mental development in offspring exposed to antineoplastic agents during the 2nd trimester, the period of neuroblast multiplication, have not been conducted (3).

Occupational exposure of the mother to antineoplastic agents during pregnancy may present a risk to the fetus. A position statement from the National Study Commission on Cytotoxic Exposure and a research article involving some antineoplastic agents are presented in the monograph for cyclophosphamide (see Cyclophosphamide).

BREASTFEEDING SUMMARY

No reports describing the use of teniposide during human lactation have been located. Because of the potential for toxicity in a nursing infant, the safest course is not to breastfeed if this drug is administered.

References

1. Lowenthal RM, Funnell CF, Hope DM, Stewart IG, Humphrey DC. Normal infant after combination chemotherapy including teniposide for Burkitt's lymphoma in pregnancy. Med Pediatr Oncol 1982;10:165–9.
2. Product information. Vumon. Bristol-Myers Squibb, 2000.
3. Dobbing J. Pregnancy and leukaemia. Lancet 1977;1:1155.

TENOFOVIR

Antiviral

PREGNANCY RECOMMENDATION: Compatible—Maternal Benefit >> Embryo–Fetal Risk
BREASTFEEDING RECOMMENDATION: Contraindicated

PREGNANCY SUMMARY

Although the animal data are suggestive of risk (decreased growth), the limited human experience suggests that the embryo–fetal risk is low, at least for structural anomalies. If indicated, the drug should not be withheld because of pregnancy.

FETAL RISK SUMMARY

Tenofovir is available as a prodrug, tenofovir disoproxil fumarate (PMPA), a fumaric acid salt of the ester derivative that is converted to tenofovir after oral administration. Tenofovir is an acyclic nucleoside analog reverse transcriptase inhibitor in the same antiviral class as abacavir, didanosine, emtricitabine, lamivudine, stavudine, zalcitabine, and zidovudine. It has activity against HIV types 1 and 2. Tenofovir is indicated in combination with other antiretroviral agents for the treatment of HIV-1. Less than 0.7% and 7% of tenofovir are bound to human plasma or serum proteins, respectively (1).

Reproduction studies have been conducted in rats and rabbits. In these species, doses up to 14 and 19 times the human dose based on BSA (HD), respectively, revealed no evidence of impaired fertility or fetal harm. There were no effects on fertility or mating performance, or early embryonic development in male and female rats given doses up to 10 times the HD for several weeks prior to mating and, in female rats, through the first 7 days of gestation (1).

Tenofovir crosses the placentas of gravid rhesus monkeys (2). Tenofovir was given to the monkeys at a dose of 30 mg/kg SC once daily starting early in the 2nd trimester (gestational day 80) and continuing until delivery at term (gestational day 157). The fetal:maternal blood levels (based on AUC mcg/hr) were 49.2/117.3 (ratio 0.42; gestational day 120) and 39.1/87.0 (ratio 0.45; gestational day 140). Although normal fetal growth patterns were observed, the mean birth weight of tenofovir-exposed newborns was significantly less (about 381 vs. 467 g) than nonexposed controls. In addition, the crown-rump, humerus, and femur lengths were significantly reduced (2).

In a follow-up to the above study, investigators gave rhesus monkeys tenofovir (30 mg/kg) SC once daily from gestation days 20 to 150 (3). As in the study above, fetal development was normal but body weights and crown-rump lengths were significantly less than age-matched controls. In addition, fetal insulin-like growth factor was significantly reduced, as was fetal bone porosity, but alkaline phosphatase levels were increased. Transient alterations in maternal body weights and bone-related biomarkers and elevated alkaline phosphatase were observed during treatment (3).

The passage of tenofovir across the human placenta apparently has not been studied. The molecular weight (about 636 for the prodrug), and low plasma and serum protein binding, combined with the data from monkeys, suggest that the drug will cross to the human embryo–fetus.

The Antiretroviral Pregnancy Registry reported, for the period January 1989 through July 2009, prospective data (reported before the outcomes were known) involving 4702 live births that had been exposed during the 1st trimester to one or more antiretroviral agents (4). Congenital defects were noted in 134, a prevalence of 2.8% (95% confidence interval [CI] 2.4–3.4). In the 6100 live births with earliest exposure in the 2nd/3rd trimesters, there were 153 infants with defects (prevalence 2.5%, 95% CI 2.1–2.9). The prevalence rates for the two periods did not differ significantly. There were 288 infants with birth defects among 10,803 live births with exposure anytime during pregnancy (prevalence 2.7%, 95% CI 2.4–3.0). The prevalence rate did not differ significantly from the rate expected in a nonexposed population. There were 1217 outcomes exposed to tenofovir (756 in the 1st trimester and 461 in the 2nd/3rd trimesters) in combination with other antiretroviral agents. There were 26 birth defects (18 in the 1st trimester and 8 in the 2nd/3rd trimesters). In reviewing the birth defects of prospective and retrospective (pregnancies reported after the outcomes were known) registered cases, the Registry concluded that, except for isolated cases of neural tube defects with efavirenz exposure in retrospective reports, there was no other pattern of anomalies (isolated or syndromic) (4) (see Lamivudine for required statement).

Two reviews, one in 1996 and the other in 1997, concluded that all women currently receiving antiretroviral therapy should continue to receive therapy during pregnancy and that treatment of the mother with monotherapy should be considered inadequate therapy (5,6). The same conclusion was reached in a 2003 review with the added admonishment that therapy must be continuous to prevent emergence of resistant viral strains (7). In 2009, the updated U.S. Department of Health and Human Services guidelines for the use of antiretroviral agents in patients infected with HIV-1 continued the recommendation that therapy, with the exception of efavirenz, should be continued during pregnancy (8). If indicated, tenofovir should not be withheld in pregnancy because the expected benefit to the HIV-positive mother outweighs the unknown risk to the fetus. Updated guidelines for the use of antiretroviral drugs to reduce perinatal HIV-1 transmission also were released in 2010 (9). Women receiving antiretroviral therapy during pregnancy should continue the therapy but, regardless of the regimen, zidovudine administration is recommended during the intrapartum period to prevent vertical transmission of HIV to the newborn (9).

BREASTFEEDING SUMMARY

No reports describing the use of tenofovir during human lactation have been located. The molecular weight (about 636 for the prodrug) and low plasma (about 1%) and serum (about 7%) protein binding suggest that the drug will be excreted into human breast milk. The effect of this exposure on a nursing infant is unknown.

Reports on the use of tenofovir during lactation are unlikely because the drug is indicated in the treatment of patients with HIV. HIV-1 is transmitted in milk, and in developed countries, breastfeeding is not recommended (5,6,8,10–12). In developing countries, breastfeeding is undertaken, despite the risk, because there are no affordable milk substitutes available.

References

1. Product information. Viread. Gilead Sciences, 2006.
2. Tarantal AF, Marthas ML, Shaw JP, Cundy K, Bischofberger N. Administration of 9-[2-(R)-(phosphonomethoxy)propyl]adenine (PMPA) to gravid and infant rhesus macaques (*Macaca mulatta*): safety and efficacy studies. J Acquir Immune Defic Syndr Hum Retroviral 1999;20:323–33.
3. Tarantal AF, Castillo A, Ekert JE, Bischofberger N, Martin RB. Fetal and maternal outcome after administration of tenofovir to gravid rhesus monkeys (*Macaca mulatta*). J Acquir Immune Defic Syndrome 2002;29:207–20.
4. Antiretroviral Pregnancy Registry Steering Committee. *Antiretroviral Pregnancy Registry International Interim Report for 1 January 1989 through 31 July 2009*. Wilmington, NC: Registry Coordinating Center; 2009. Available at www.apregistry.com. Accessed May 29, 2010.
5. Carpenter CCJ, Fischi MA, Hammer SM, Hirsch MS, Jacobsen DM, Katzenstein DA, Montaner JSG, Richman DD, Saag MS, Schooley RT, Thompson MA, Vella S, Yeni PG, Volberding PA. Antiretroviral therapy for HIV infection in 1996. JAMA 1996;276:146–54.
6. Minkoff H, Augenbraun M. Antiretroviral therapy for pregnant women. Am J Obstet Gynecol 1997;176:478–89.
7. Minkoff H. Human immunodeficiency virus infection in pregnancy. Obstet Gynecol 2003;101:797–810.
8. Panel on Antiretroviral Guidelines for Adults and Adolescents. *Guidelines for the Use of Antiretroviral Agents in HIV-1-Infected Adults and Adolescents*. Department of Health and Human Services. December 1, 2009:1–161. Available at http://www.aidsinfo.nih.gov/ContentFiles/AdultandAdolescentGL.pdf. Accessed September 17, 2010:60, 96–8.
9. Panel on Treatment of HIV-Infected Pregnant Women and Prevention of Perinatal Transmission. *Recommendations for Use of Antiretroviral Drugs in Pregnant HIV-1-Infected Women for Maternal Health and Interventions to Reduce Perinatal HIV Transmission in the United States*. May 24, 2010:1–117. Available at http://aidsinfo.nih.gov/ContentFiles/PerinatalGL.pdf. Accessed September 17, 2010:30 (Table 5).
10. Brown ZA, Watts DH. Antiviral therapy in pregnancy. Clin Obstet Gynecol 1990;33:276–89.
11. De Martino M, Tovo P-A, Pezzotti P, Galli L, Massironi E, Ruga E, Floreea F, Plebani A, Gabiano C, Zuccotti GV. HIV-1 transmission through breast-milk: appraisal of risk according to duration of feeding. AIDS 1992;6:991–7.
12. Van de Perre P. Postnatal transmission of human immunodeficiency virus type 1: the breast-feeding dilemma. Am J Obstet Gynecol 1995;173:483–7.

TERAZOSIN

Sympatholytic (Antiadrenergic)

PREGNANCY RECOMMENDATION: No Human Data—Animal Data Suggest Low Risk
BREASTFEEDING RECOMMENDATION: No Human Data—Probably Compatible

T

PREGNANCY SUMMARY

Terazosin is a peripherally acting α_1-adrenergic blocking agent used in the treatment of hypertension and symptomatic benign prostatic hyperplasia. No reports describing the use of terazosin in human pregnancy have been located.

FETAL RISK SUMMARY

Reproduction studies in rats and rabbits at doses 280 and 60 times the recommended maximum human dose (RMHD), respectively, revealed no teratogenic effects, but an increased incidence of fetal resorptions occurred in both species (1). In addition, decreased fetal weight and an increased number of supernumerary ribs were observed in rabbit offspring. The embryo–fetal toxicity in both species was attributed to maternal toxicity (1). A significant increase in rat pup mortality was also seen at doses more than 75 times the RMHD in peri- and postnatal studies (1).

It is not known if terazosin crosses the human placenta. The molecular weight (about 388 for the nonhydrated free base) is low enough that exposure of the embryo–fetus should be expected.

BREASTFEEDING SUMMARY

No reports describing the use of terazosin during lactation have been located. The molecular weight (about 388 for the nonhydrated free base) is low enough that excretion into breast milk should be expected. The effect of this exposure on a nursing infant is unknown.

Reference

1. Product information. Hytrin. Abbott Laboratories, 2000.

TERBINAFINE

Antifungal

PREGNANCY RECOMMENDATION: No Human Data—Animal Data Suggest Low Risk
BREASTFEEDING RECOMMENDATION: Limited Human Data—Potential Toxicity

PREGNANCY SUMMARY

Although the animal reproduction data are encouraging, the lack of human pregnancy experience does not allow a full assessment of the fetal risk from terbinafine. If possible, therefore, waiting to begin treatment until after a pregnancy has been concluded would be the safest course. If terbinafine is used in pregnancy, health care professionals are encouraged to call the toll free number 800-670-6126 for information about patient enrollment in the Motherisk study.

FETAL RISK SUMMARY

Terbinafine is a synthetic allylamine antifungal agent that is indicated for the treatment of onychomycosis of the toenail or fingernail due to dermatophytes (tinea unguium) (1). No studies evaluating the placental transfer of terbinafine in humans have been located. The molecular weight (about 328) is low enough that transfer to the embryo–fetus should be expected.

Reproduction studies have been conducted in rats and rabbits (1). Oral doses in rats up to about 12 times the maximum recommended human dose based on BSA (MRHD) had no effect on fertility or other reproductive parameters. In pregnant rabbits, intravaginal administration of terbinafine did not cause abortions, premature delivery, or affect fetal parameters. In pregnant rats and rabbits, no evidence of impaired fertility or fetal harm was seen with oral doses up to 12 and 9 times the MRHD, respectively (1).

BREASTFEEDING SUMMARY

Terbinafine is excreted into human milk. No specific details were given, but the milk:plasma ratio in nursing women was 7:1 (1). The effect of this exposure on a nursing infant is unknown. Because the duration of therapy is usually prolonged (6 or 12 weeks for patients with fingernail or toenail onychomycosis, respectively), the potential for serious toxicity in a nursing infant may be increased. Based on the accumulation in milk and the prolonged exposure, women taking terbinafine probably should not breastfeed.

Reference

1. Product information. Lamisil. Novartis Pharmaceuticals, 2001.

TERBUTALINE

Sympathomimetic/Bronchodilator

PREGNANCY RECOMMENDATION: Limited Human Data—Animal Data Suggest Low Risk
BREASTFEEDING RECOMMENDATION: Limited Human Data—Probably Compatible

PREGNANCY SUMMARY

Terbutaline is used as a tocolytic and as a bronchodilator in asthma and such use has been considered low risk. However, new data have suggested an association exists between continuous use (≥2 weeks) of terbutaline by any route and autism spectrum disorders. Short-term use, such as 48–72 hours to allow for corticosteroid use to improve fetal lung maturation, is probably safe, but there may be a subpopulation of mothers and fetuses at increased risk secondary to genetic predisposition. In addition, there is a report of an association between 1st trimester terbutaline exposure for

T

asthma and cardiac defects. The risk magnitude for these toxicities requires confirmation. Because of these reports, avoiding β_2-adrenergics early in gestation, except for quick relief of asthmatic symptoms with low inhaled doses, and continuous use in the 2nd/3rd trimesters appear to be warranted. If terbutaline is used in pregnancy for the treatment of asthma, health care professionals are encouraged to call the toll-free number 877-311-8972 for information about patient enrollment in an Organization of Teratology Information Specialists (OTIS) study.

FETAL RISK SUMMARY

Terbutaline is a β_2-sympathomimetic indicated for the prevention and reversal of bronchospasm. During pregnancy, it is primarily used as a tocolytic agent in the late 2nd and early 3rd trimesters.

Reproduction studies in mice, rats, and rabbits at doses ≤1500 times the SC maximum recommended human daily dose of 0.1 mg/kg have revealed no evidence of impaired fertility or fetal harm (1).

A 2003 report described the effects of terbutaline given to rat pups (2). Because rats are altricial, the investigators gave the pups SC terbutaline 10 mg/kg/day in two different periods, one during the early postnatal period (days 2–5) and the other second spanning the time of eye opening (days 11–14). Hearts were examined for cardiac damage 24 hours after the last dose and on postnatal day 30. Compared with controls, neither treatment caused an increase in cardiac anomalies. However, there was a significant decrease in the number of cardiac nuclei in female pups (2).

In a surveillance study of Michigan Medicaid recipients involving 229,101 completed pregnancies conducted between 1985 and 1992, 149 newborns had been exposed to terbutaline during the 1st trimester (F. Rosa, personal communication, FDA, 1993). Seven (4.7%) major birth defects were observed (six expected), including three cardiovascular defects (two expected) and one oral cleft (none expected). No anomalies were observed in four other categories of defects (spina bifida, polydactyly, limb reduction defects, and hypospadias) for which specific data were available. These data do not support an association between the drug and congenital defects.

Terbutaline rapidly crosses the placenta to the fetus (3). In seven women given 0.25 mg IV during the second stage of labor, cord blood levels 7–60 minutes after the dose ranged from 12% to 55% (mean 36%) of maternal serum.

Terbutaline has been used as a tocolytic agent since the early 1970s (4,5). The incidence of maternal side effects is usually low (e.g., ≤5%) but may be severe (4,6–10). A 1983 review listed the more serious side effects of parenteral β_2-sympathomimetic therapy (e.g., terbutaline, ritodrine) as pulmonary edema, myocardial ischemia, cardiac arrhythmias, cerebral vasospasm, hypotension, hyperglycemia, and miscellaneous metabolic alterations (hypokalemia, increased serum lactate, and a decrease in measured hemoglobin concentration) (11). The more serious adverse effects are seen with continuous infusions of these drugs. Avoidance of this route of administration as well as careful selection of patients, appropriate dosing, and close monitoring of patient status may help to prevent serious maternal effects.

Terbutaline may cause fetal and maternal tachycardia (4,6–8). Fetal rates are usually <175 beats/minute (7). As mentioned previously, maternal hypotension may occur, especially in the bleeding patient (11). More commonly, increases in systolic pressure and decreases in diastolic pressure occur with no reduction in mean arterial pressure and, thus, do not adversely affect the fetus (8,11,12).

As with all β-mimetics, terbutaline may cause transient maternal hyperglycemia followed by an increase in serum insulin levels (4,13,14). Sustained neonatal hypoglycemia may be observed if maternal effects have not terminated before delivery (13). Maternal glucose intolerance was observed at 1 hour in 19 of 30 patients receiving oral terbutaline for at least 1 week (15). Although macrosomia was not observed, the birth weights (after adjustment for gestational age) of infants from terbutaline-treated mothers had a tendency to be greater than those of babies from comparable controls (15).

Sudden, unexplained intrapartum death in a fetus at 30 weeks' gestation occurred 5 hours after the start of an IV infusion of terbutaline for premature labor (16). No evidence of uterine, placental, or fetal anomalies was discovered.

Myocardial necrosis in a newborn was reported in 1991 (17). A continuous SC infusion of terbutaline (initial dose 0.5 mg/hr) was started at 25 weeks' gestation for premature labor in a 22-year-old woman with gestational diabetes. Therapy was continued until delivery at 37 weeks' of a 2850-g male infant. Tachypnea (80–100 breaths/minute) developed shortly after birth and chest radiography demonstrated mild cardiomegaly with increased pulmonary vascularity. A right ventricular biopsy obtained during cardiac catheterization showed marked myocardial fiber degeneration and focal bizarre nuclear dysmorphism. These findings were believed to be caused by catecholamine excess. Normal electrocardiogram and echocardiogram were found on examination at 1 month of age (17).

In a 1996 epidemiologic study that looked for correlations between drug exposure and major malformations, 1472 births with defects (cases) were compared with 9682 births without major or minor malformations (controls) (18). Overall, there was no significant association between β_2-sympathomimetics (bronchodilators) and major malformations. When the malformations were divided into 10 organ categories, an association with cardiac defects (types not specified) was significant (odds ratio 5.8, 95% confidence interval 1.4–24) ($p = 0.05$) (18).

Maternal liver impairment was reported in a patient after 1 week of continuous IV administration of terbutaline (19). Therapy was stopped and 1 week later, a healthy newborn was delivered without signs of liver toxicity.

A paradoxical reaction to terbutaline was observed in a patient after 0.25 mg IV produced marked uterine hypertonus and subsequent severe fetal bradycardia (<50 beats/minute) (20). A healthy baby was delivered by emergency cesarean section.

Terbutaline has been used frequently to treat intrapartum fetal distress (21–25). The mechanism of the beneficial effects on fetal pH and heart rate are thought to be caused by relief of the ischemia produced by uterine contractions on the placental circulation.

Although maternal complications may occur, few direct adverse effects, other than transient tachycardia and hypoglycemia, and the single report of myocardial necrosis, have been observed in the fetus or newborn. In many studies, neonatal complications are minimal or nonexistent (26–30). Compared with controls, prophylactic terbutaline in low-risk patients with twin gestations has produced significant gains in birth weights caused by longer gestational times (29). In addition, terbutaline decreases the incidence of neonatal respiratory distress syndrome in a manner similar to other β-mimetics (31). Long-term evaluation of infants exposed to terbutaline in utero has been reported (32–34). No harmful effects in the infants (2–24 months) have been found.

A 26-year-old woman became pregnant with quadruplets after a gamete intrafallopian transfer procedure (35). Preterm labor began at 18 weeks' gestation and treatment was started with IV ritodrine for 2 weeks and then changed to SC terbutaline. She was maintained on terbutaline, except for a "24-hour rest period" every week, for 51 days. During this period, she received 200 mg of terbutaline. Labor progressed and a cesarean section was performed in the 28th week of gestation. Between 28 and 32 hours after birth, three of the four infants developed cardiovascular decompensation with bradycardia, metabolic acidosis, poor tissue perfusion, and decreased urine output. The conditions were resistant to standard interventions but responded to dobutamine. The infants required dobutamine for 3–9 days. The authors speculated that the prolonged β-sympathomimetic therapy led to downregulation of fetal β-receptors (35).

A study published in 2005 reported an association between continuous use of terbutaline for ≥2 weeks and increased concordance for autism spectrum disorders in dizygotic twins (36). The investigators concluded that genetic factors and over stimulation of β_2-adrenergic receptors by terbutaline could affect developmental programs in the fetal brain leading to autism.

A 2009 report examined the evidence for the use and toxicity of β_2-agonists in pregnancy, particularly for terbutaline and ritodrine as tocolytic agents and albuterol for asthma (37). Based on animal and human reports, the authors concluded that there was a biological plausible basis for associating prolonged in utero exposure to β_2-agonists with functional and behavioral teratogenesis, such as increased risks for autism spectrum disorders, psychiatric disorders, and poor cognitive, motor function, and school performance. There also were increased risks for elevated heart rate and hypertension. The mechanisms for these effects appeared to be a decrease in parasympathetic activity resulting in an increase in sympathetic activity. A genetic predisposition for the toxicity was supported by data. The available data suggested that short-term terbutaline use (2–3 days) was not associated with these toxicities, but prolonged use (≥2 weeks) was associated (37).

BREASTFEEDING SUMMARY

Terbutaline is excreted into breast milk. In two mothers with chronic asthma about 6–8 weeks postpartum, 5 mg 3 times daily produced mean maternal plasma levels of 1.9–4.8 ng/mL, whereas milk concentrations ranged between 2.5 and 3.8 ng/mL (38). The nursing infants ingested approximately 0.2% of the maternal dose, and the drug could not be detected in their plasma. In the second report, two mothers, both at 3 weeks postpartum and both with chronic asthma, were treated with 2.5 mg 3 times a day (39). Plasma levels varied between 0.97 and 3.07 ng/mL, whereas mean milk levels were 2.76–3.91 ng/mL. Peak milk concentrations occurred at about 4 hours. The milk:plasma ratios of 1.4–2.9 are indicative of ionic trapping in the milk. Concentrations of terbutaline were highest in the fat fraction of the milk. Based on calculations, the infants were ingesting approximately 0.7% of the maternal dose (39).

No symptoms of adrenergic stimulation were observed in the four infants and all exhibited normal development. Long-term effects of this exposure, however, have not been studied. The American Academy of Pediatrics classifies terbutaline as compatible with breastfeeding (40).

References

1. Product information. Brethine. Novartis Pharmaceuticals, 2000.
2. Rhodes MC, Nyska A, Seidler FJ, Slotkin TA. Does terbutaline damage the developing heart? Birth Defects Res B 2003;68:449–55.
3. Ingemarsson I, Westgren M, Lindberg C, Ahren B, Lundquist I, Carlsson C. Single injection of terbutaline in term labor: placental transfer and effects on maternal and fetal carbohydrate metabolism. Am J Obstet Gynecol 1981;139:697–701.
4. Haller DL. The use of terbutaline for premature labor. Drug Intell Clin Pharm 1980;14:757–64.
5. Ingemarsson I. Cardiovascular complications of terbutaline for preterm labor. Am J Obstet Gynecol 1982;142:117.
6. Andersson KE, Bengtsson LP, Gustafson I, Ingermarsson I. The relaxing effect of terbutaline on the human uterus during term labor. Am J Obstet Gynecol 1975;121:602–9.
7. Ingermarrson I. Effect of terbutaline on premature labor. A double-blind placebo-controlled study. Am J Obstet Gynecol 1976;125:520–4.
8. Ravindran R, Viegas OJ, Padilla LM, LaBlonde P. Anesthetic considerations in pregnant patients receiving terbutaline therapy. Anesth Analg (Cleve) 1980;59:391–2.
9. Katz M, Robertson PA, Creasy RK. Cardiovascular complications associated with terbutaline treatment for preterm labor. Am J Obstet Gynecol 1981;139:605–8.
10. Ingemarsson I, Bengtsson B. A five-year experience with terbutaline for preterm labor: low rate of severe side effects. Obstet Gynecol 1985;66:176–80.
11. Benedetti TJ. Maternal complications of parenteral β-sympathomimetic therapy for premature labor. Am J Obstet Gynecol 1983;145:1–6.
12. Vargas GC, Macedo GJ, Amved AR, Lowenberg FE. Terbutaline, a new uterine inhibitor. Ginecol Obstet Mex 1974;36:75–88.
13. Epstein MF, Nicholls RN, Stubblefield PG. Neonatal hypoglycemia after beta-sympathomimetic tocolytic therapy. J Pediatr 1979;94:449–53.
14. Westgren M, Carlsson C, Lindholm T, Thysell H, Ingemarsson I. Continuous maternal glucose measurements and fetal glucose and insulin levels after administration of terbutaline in term labor. Acta Obstet Gynecol Scand 1982;(Suppl 108):63–5.
15. Main EK, Main DM, Gabbe SG. Chronic oral terbutaline tocolytic therapy is associated with maternal glucose intolerance. Am J Obstet Gynecol 1987;157:644–7.
16. Lenke RR, Trupin S. Sudden, unforeseen fetal death in a woman being treated for premature labor: a case report. J Reprod Med 1984;29:872–4.
17. Fletcher SE, Fyfe DA, Case CL, Wiles HB, Upshur JK, Newman RB. Myocardial necrosis in a newborn after long-term maternal subcutaneous terbutaline infusion for suppression of preterm labor. Am J Obstet Gynecol 1991;165:1401–4.
18. Queisser-Luft A, Eggers I, Stolz G, Kieninger-Baum D, Schlaefer K. Serial examination of 20,248 newborn fetuses and infants: correlations between drug exposure and major malformations. Am J Med Genet 1996;63:268–76.
19. Suzuki M, Inagaki K, Kihira M, Matsuzawa K, Ishikawa K, Ishizuka T. Maternal liver impairment associated with prolonged high-dose administration of terbutaline for premature labor. Obstet Gynecol 1985;66:14S–15S.
20. Bhat N, Seifer D, Hensleigh P. Paradoxical response to intravenous terbutaline. Am J Obstet Gynecol 1985;153:310–1.
21. Tejani NA, Verma UL, Chatterjee S, Mittelmann S. Terbutaline in the management of acute intrapartum fetal acidosis. J Reprod Med 1983;28:857–61.

T

22. Barrett JM. Fetal resuscitation with terbutaline during eclampsia-induced uterine hypertonus. Am J Obstet Gynecol 1984;150:895.
23. Ingemarsson I, Arulkumaran S, Ratnam SS. Single injection of terbutaline in term labor. I. Effect on fetal pH in cases with prolonged bradycardia. Am J Obstet Gynecol 1985;153:859–65.
24. Ingemarsson I, Arulkumaran S, Ratnam SS. Single injection of terbutaline in term labor. II. Effect on uterine activity. Am J Obstet Gynecol 1985;153:865–9.
25. Mendez-Bauer C, Shekarloo A, Cook V, Freese U. Treatment of acute intrapartum fetal distress by β2-sympathomimetics. Am J Obstet Gynecol 1987;156:638–42.
26. Stubblefield PG, Heyl PS. Treatment of premature labor with subcutaneous terbutaline. Obstet Gynecol 1982;59:457–62.
27. Caritis SN, Carson D, Greebon D, McCormick M, Edelstone DI, Mueller-Heubach E. A comparison of terbutaline and ethanol in the treatment of preterm labor. Am J Obstet Gynecol 1982;142:183–90.
28. Kaul AF, Osathanondy R, Safon LE, Frigoletto FD Jr, Friedman PA. The management of preterm labor with the calcium channel-blocking agent nifedipine combined with the β-mimetic terbutaline. Drug Intell Clin Pharm 1985;19:369–71.
29. O'Leary JA. Prophylactic tocolysis of twins. Am J Obstet Gynecol 1986;154:904–5.
30. Arias F, Knight AB, Tomich PB. A retrospective study on the effects of steroid administration and prolongation of the latent phase in patients with preterm premature rupture of the membranes. Am J Obstet Gynecol 1986;154:1059–63.
31. Bergman B, Hedner T. Antepartum administration of terbutaline and the incidence of hyaline membrane disease in preterm infants. Acta Obstet Gynecol Scand 1978;57:217–21.
32. Wallace R, Caldwell D, Ansbacher R, Otterson W. Inhibition of premature labor by terbutaline. Obstet Gynecol 1978;51:387–93.
33. Svenningsen NW. Follow-up studies on preterm infants after maternal β-receptor agonist treatment. Acta Obstet Gynecol Scand 1982;(Suppl 108):67–70.
34. Karlsson K, Krantz M, Hamberger L. Comparison of various β-mimetics on preterm labor, survival and development of the child. J Perinat Med 1980;8:19–26.
35. Thorkelsson T, Loughead JL. Long-term subcutaneous terbutaline tocolysis: report of possible neonatal toxicity. J Perinatol 1991;11:235–8.
36. Connors SL, Crowell DE, Eberhart CG, Copeland J, Newschaffer CJ, Spence SJ, Zimmerman AW. B_2-adrenergic receptor activation and genetic polymorphisms in autism: data from dizygotic twins. J Clin Neurol 2005;20:876–84.
37. Witter FR, Zimmerman AW, Reichmann JP, Connors SL. In utero beta 2 adrenergic agonist exposure and adverse neurophysiologic and behavioral outcomes. Am J Obstet Gynecol 2009;210:553–9.
38. Lonnerholm G, Lindstrom B. Terbutaline excretion into breast milk. Br J Clin Pharmacol 1982;13:729–30.
39. Boreus LO, de Chateau P, Lindberg C, Nyberg L. Terbutaline in breast milk. Br J Clin Pharmacol 1982;13:731–2.
40. Committee on Drugs, American Academy of Pediatrics. The transfer of drugs and other chemicals into human milk. Pediatrics 2001;108:776–89.

TERCONAZOLE

Antifungal

PREGNANCY RECOMMENDATION: Human Data Suggest Low Risk
BREASTFEEDING RECOMMENDATION: No Human Data—Probably Compatible

PREGNANCY SUMMARY

Although no published reports describing the use of terconazole in human pregnancy have been located, the FDA database provided information on a large number of exposures. This pregnancy experience, combined with the animal data, suggest that the embryo–fetal risk is low. However, additional human studies are required for confirmation.

FETAL RISK SUMMARY

Terconazole is available as either a vaginal cream or suppositories. The antifungal agent is absorbed into the systemic circulation in humans after vaginal administration. Fetal exposure to the drug is also possible by direct transfer of terconazole across the amniotic membranes after vaginal administration (1). Terconazole is a triazole antifungal agent in the same class as fluconazole, itraconazole, posaconazole, and voriconazole.

No evidence of teratogenicity was found after oral and SC administration of terconazole to rats and rabbits, but some embryotoxicity was observed at high doses (1).

In a surveillance study of Michigan Medicaid recipients involving 229,101 completed pregnancies conducted between 1985 and 1992, 1167 newborns had been exposed to terconazole during the 1st trimester (F. Rosa, personal communication, FDA, 1993). A total of 34 (2.9%) major birth defects were observed (48 expected). Specific data were available for six defect categories, including (observed/expected) 14/12 cardiovascular defects, 0/2 oral clefts, 0/0.5 spina bifida, 3/3 polydactyly, 1/2 limb reduction defects, and 1/3 hypospadias. These data do not support an association between the drug and congenital defects.

BREASTFEEDING SUMMARY

No reports describing the use of terconazole during lactation have been located.

Reference

1. Product information. Terazol. Ortho Pharmaceutical, 1993.

TERFENADINE

[Withdrawn from the market. See 9th edition.]

TERIFLUNOMIDE

Immunologic Agent (Immunomodulator)

PREGNANCY RECOMMENDATION: Contraindicated
BREASTFEEDING RECOMMENDATION: No Human Data—Potential Toxicity

PREGNANCY SUMMARY

One report cited a clinical trial that involved 43 pregnancies (1). Although no details of the exposures were provided, the report stated that there was no increased risk of spontaneous abortions, lower birth weights, lower gestational ages, or congenital malformations. The animal reproduction data suggest risk, including embryo malformations and fetal death. The manufacturer classifies the drug as contraindicated in pregnancy. If a woman conceives while taking this drug, or a woman a childbearing potential stops the drug, the 11-day procedure for accelerated elimination of teriflunomide is recommended because it takes on average 8 months, but possibly as long as 2 years, to reach plasma concentrations (<0.02 mg/mL) that are considered minimal risk (see package insert for procedure) (2). If exposure does occur in pregnancy, physicians are encouraged to enroll their patient in the manufacturer's pregnancy registry, or women can enroll themselves, by calling 1-800-745-4447, option 2.

FETAL RISK SUMMARY

Teriflunomide, an oral immunomodulator with anti-inflammatory properties, inhibits a mitochondrial enzyme involved in de novo pyrimidine synthesis. It is the principal active metabolite of leflunomide and is responsible for leflunomide's activity (see also Leflunomide). Teriflunomide is indicated for the treatment of patients with relapsing forms of multiple sclerosis. The drug is mainly distributed in plasma. It is metabolized to inactive metabolites. Plasma protein binding is high (>99%), and the dose-dependent elimination half-life is very long (18–19 days). The drug has been detected in human semen (2).

Reproduction studies with teriflunomide have been conducted in rats and rabbits. In rats given oral doses during organogenesis that were not maternal toxic, high incidences of fetal defects, mainly craniofacial, and axial and appendicular skeletal defects, as well as embryo–fetal death were observed. The no-effect maternal plasma exposure for embryo–fetal developmental toxicity was less than that in humans at the maximum recommended human dose (MRHD). When nonmaternal toxic doses were administered during gestation and lactation, decreased growth, eye and skin abnormalities, and high incidences of limb defects and postnatal death were observed in the offspring. The no-effect maternal plasma exposure for prenatal and postnatal developmental toxicity in rats was less than that in humans at the MRHD. In rabbits given oral doses that caused minimal maternal toxicity, high incidences of defects (similar to those seen in rats) and embryo–fetal death, were observed. The maternal plasma exposure at the no-effect dose for prenatal and postnatal developmental toxicity in rabbits was less than that in humans at the MRHD (2).

No evidence of carcinogenicity was observed in mice and rats in lifetime studies. Both positive and negative results for mutagenic and clastogenic effects were noted in various assays. In studies with male rats, no adverse effect on fertility was noted, but a dose-related decrease in epididymal sperm count did occur. In female rats, oral doses before and during mating resulted in embryolethality, reduced fetal body weight, and malformations at all doses tested (2).

It is not known if teriflunomide crosses the human placenta. The molecular weight (about 270) and very long elimination half-life suggest that the drug will cross to the embryo–fetus, but the high plasma protein binding might limit the exposure.

A 2013 reference cited data from a clinical trial database that involved 43 pregnancies exposed to teriflunomide (1). Although no information was provided on the dose, timing of the exposures, or specific data on outcomes, the citation stated that no increased risk of spontaneous abortions, lower birth weights, lower gestational ages, or congenital malformations were observed (1).

BREASTFEEDING SUMMARY

No reports describing the use of teriflunomide during human lactation have been located. The molecular weight (about 270) and very long elimination half-life (about 18–19 days) suggest that the drug will be excreted into breast milk, but the high plasma protein binding (>99%) might limit the amount excreted. Because of the severe toxicity that has occurred in adults taking the drug (e.g., severe hepatotoxicity, bone marrow depression, immunosuppression), the drug is best not used in women who are nursing an infant.

References

1. Kieseier B, Benamor M, Benzerdjeb H, Stuve O. Pregnancy outcomes from the teriflunomide clinical development programme: retrospective analysis of the teriflunomide clinical trial database. Multi Scler 2012;18 (Suppl 4):P737. As cited by Lu E, Wang BW, Guimond C, Synnes A, Sadovnick AD, Dahlgren L, Traboulsee A, Tremlett H. Safety of disease-modifying drugs for multiple sclerosis in pregnancy: current challenges and future considerations for effective pharmacovigilance. Expert Rev Neurother 2013;13:251–61.
2. Product information. Aubagio. Genzyme, 2012.

TERPIN HYDRATE

Respiratory Drug (Expectorant)

PREGNANCY RECOMMENDATION: Contraindicated (Significant Alcohol Content)
BREASTFEEDING RECOMMENDATION: Contraindicated (Significant Alcohol Content)

PREGNANCY SUMMARY

Terpin hydrate is available as a liquid preparation that contains a significant amount (about 42%) of ethanol. It should not be used in pregnancy.

FETAL RISK SUMMARY

Although no longer approved as an expectorant, this agent has been used for a number of years and may still be available for this indication. At one time it was combined with codeine as an expectorant–antitussive proprietary mixture. No animal reproductive studies of terpin hydrate have been located.

The Collaborative Perinatal Project monitored 50,282 mother–child pairs, 146 of whom had 1st trimester exposure to terpin hydrate (1, pp. 378–89). Congenital malformations were observed in 13 (standardized relative risk [SRR] 1.29) of the newborns. For use anytime in pregnancy, 1762 mother–child pairs were exposed (1, p. 442). Twenty-nine (30.6 expected) of the newborns had anomalies (SRR 0.95). Neither of the exposure periods indicates an increased fetal risk from the drug. Specific malformations or conditions identified following use of terpin hydrate anytime in pregnancy were any benign tumors 9 (SRR 1.9), clubfoot 11 (SRR 1.2), and inguinal hernia 34 (SRR 1.4) (1, p. 496). However, these data are uninterruptible without independent confirmation from other studies. Any positive or negative associations may have occurred by chance (1, p. 481). A 1964 study found no abnormalities in six infants exposed in utero to terpin hydrate (with or without codeine) during the 1st trimester (2). Neither of the above studies specified the doses consumed by the patients.

The recommended dose of terpin hydrate, which contains approximately 42% ethanol, is 5–10 mL 3–4 times daily. The maximum daily dose would therefore contain about 17 mL of absolute ethanol or about one-half of the amount that has been shown to produce mild fetal alcohol syndrome (see Ethanol). Because the minimum amount of ethanol exposure required to produce fetal developmental toxicity is unknown, this product should be avoided during pregnancy.

BREASTFEEDING SUMMARY

No reports describing the use of terpin hydrate during lactation have been located. Because of the high ethanol content (about 42%) of terpin hydrate, frequent use of this product should be avoided during lactation (see also Ethanol).

References

1. Heinonen OP, Slone D, Shapiro S. *Birth Defects and Drugs in Pregnancy*. Littleton, MA: Publishing Sciences Group, 1977.
2. Mellin GW. Drugs in the first trimester of pregnancy and the fetal life of *Homo sapiens*. Am J Obstet Gynecol 1964;90:1169–80.

TESAMORELIN

Growth Hormone Releasing Factor

PREGNANCY RECOMMENDATION: Contraindicated
BREASTFEEDING RECOMMENDATION: Contraindicated

T

PREGNANCY SUMMARY

No reports describing the use of tesamorelin acetate in human pregnancy have been located. Animal data suggest risk, but the absence of human pregnancy experience prevents an assessment of the embryo–fetal risk. However, during human pregnancy, visceral adipose tissue increases due to normal hormonal and metabolic changes. Altering these changes with tesamorelin offers no known benefit and could result in fetal harm. Therefore, tesamorelin is contraindicated in pregnancy.

FETAL RISK SUMMARY

Tesamorelin is given as a daily SC injection. It is a growth hormone releasing factor (GRF) analog indicated for the reduction of excess abdominal fat in HIV-infected patients with lipodystrophy. Tesamorelin binds and stimulates human GRF receptors with potency similar to endogenous GRF. Metabolism in humans has not been studied. The mean elimination half-life is 26 minutes in healthy subjects and 38 minutes in HIV-infected patients (1).

Reproduction studies have been conducted in rats and rabbits. In rats during organogenesis, doses that were about 2 and 4 times the human clinical dose based on AUC (HCD) resulted in hydrocephaly in offspring. Lower doses that were about 0.1–1 times the HCD during organogenesis caused delayed skull ossification. No adverse developmental effects were observed in rabbits at doses up to 500 times the HCD (1).

Carcinogenicity studies in rodents have not been conducted with tesamorelin. The drug was not genotoxic in multiple assays. There was no effect on fertility in male or female rats after doses approximately equal to the HCD for 28 days in males or 14 days in females. In a 26-week study, female rats given 16 and 25 times the HCD were more likely to be in diestrus (1).

It is not known if tesamorelin crosses the human placenta. The molecular weight (about 5136 for the free base) and the short elimination half-life suggest that exposure of the embryo–fetus will be limited.

BREASTFEEDING SUMMARY

No reports describing the use of tesamorelin during human lactation have been located. The molecular weight (about 5136 for the free base) and the short elimination half-life (38 minutes for HIV-infected patients) suggest that excretion into milk will be limited. Moreover, any drug in breast milk would most likely be digested in the infant's gut. However, tesamorelin is a weak base, and when used during lactation, accumulation in the milk may occur with concentrations significantly greater than corresponding plasma levels. Nevertheless, it is unlikely that tesamorelin will be used during breastfeeding because the drug is indicated for use in HIV-infected patients and breastfeeding is not recommended in this patient population.

Reference

1. Product information. Egrifta. EMD Serono, 2012.

TESTOSTERONE

Androgenic Hormone

PREGNANCY RECOMMENDATION: Contraindicated
BREASTFEEDING RECOMMENDATION: Contraindicated

PREGNANCY SUMMARY

First trimester in utero exposure of female fetuses to exogenous testosterone or its derivatives causes clitoral hypertrophy, fused or partial fused labia, and, possibly, absent vagina. These varying degrees of masculinization are referred to as nonadrenal female pseudohermaphroditism. Exposure to testosterone hormones at any gestational age is associated with clitoral hypertrophy (1). However, to cause labial–scrotal fusion, exposure must occur before the 10th or 11th fetal week when female differentiation of external genitalia is complete (1). Other than the genital abnormalities, testosterone and its derivatives do not appear to cause structural defects. Only one report of nongenital malformations after testosterone exposure has been published, but this association lacks confirmation. However, a study in monkeys has suggested that long-term potentially permanent changes in the central nervous system of female offspring may result from in utero testosterone exposure. Apparently, this has not been studied in humans. Testosterone and its derivatives are contraindicated at any time during pregnancy.

FETAL RISK SUMMARY

Testosterone is a natural hormone with androgenic and anabolic properties. Testosterone and its derivatives (e.g., methyltestosterone) are primarily indicated as replacement therapy in male hypogonadal disorders secondary to various causes. Preparations of testosterone products are available for oral, buccal, topical, and IM administration. About 80% of testosterone is bound to sex-hormone-binding globulin. Several metabolic pathways of testosterone have been identified, including aromatization to form estrogenic derivatives. The plasma elimination half-life of testosterone is in the range of 10–100 minutes (2). Testosterone rapidly crosses the human placenta to the embryo or fetus (3).

In a 1987 study, testosterone exposure of female rhesus monkeys in utero appeared to have induced irreversible changes in the pattern of luteinizing hormone secretion in adult life (4). Seventeen female monkey pseudohermaphrodites (exposed in utero) and 24 normal females were studied at about 13–14 years of age. All subject and control animals demonstrated evidence of ovulatory menstrual cycles. The 17 monkeys with pseudohermaphroditism had been exposed in utero to testosterone that had resulted in external genital masculinization/obliteration of the external vaginal orifice or clitoromegally alone (degree of genital masculinization was dependent on the timing of exposure). Compared with controls, significant increases in the ratio of luteinizing hormone to follicle-stimulating hormone in the luteal and follicular phases of the ovulatory menstrual cycles were measured in the pseudohermaphrodites (4).

A 1957 report cited several animal studies published in the late 1940s and early 1950s that had demonstrated that administration of testosterone or its derivatives to pregnant animals resulted in masculinization of female fetuses (5). A later report also reviewed the animal data and specifically evaluated the dose and fetal age associated with masculinization of female fetuses (3).

Testosterone and its derivates are contraindicated in pregnancy because they cause virilization of female fetuses (5–16). Two case reports, one in 1953 and another in 1955 (both in German), were the first to describe female pseudohermaphroditism in human infants after exposure to a testosterone derivative (methylandrostenediol; methandriol) (6) or testosterone/methyltestosterone/estradiol (7).

The first English language cases of nonadrenal human female pseudohermaphroditism secondary to maternal use of testosterone were published in 1957. A woman was treated with oral methyltestosterone 20 mg/day for alopecia starting in the 7th week of pregnancy and continuing irregularly until term (total dose 1.5 g) (5). During treatment, the woman noted a deepening voice, hirsutism, and a male-pattern of body hair, as well as partial resolution of her alopecia. Sex of the newborn, which initially appeared to be male, was not established until 7 months of age when the diagnosis of female pseudohermaphroditism was made (5). In the second case, a woman at 10 weeks' gestation was treated with two doses of testosterone (100 mg IM on day 1 and 3) and 51 days of oral methyltestosterone (30 mg/day) for nausea and vomiting of pregnancy (8). The therapy was discontinued because of the woman's deepening voice. A 3.4-kg infant was delivered at term who had cyanosis and bradycardia of short duration. Although the sex was ambiguous (small penis, undescended testes), the infant was raised as a male. Detailed examination at 6 months of age revealed the infant to be a female (8).

Other cases have described nonadrenal female pseudohermaphroditism secondary to exposures to methyltestosterone or testosterone, sometimes in combination with estradiol or other estrogens, in the 1st trimester (9–16). In each of these cases, examination of the newborn infant usually revealed a hypoplastic penis, cryptorchidism, and hypospadias. The actual diagnosis of female sex with clitoral hypertrophy, with or without fused labia, and an occasionally absent vagina, was made weeks to months after birth. Surgery was usually required to correct the genital abnormalities. In two cases, the infants had been exposed to methyltestosterone or testosterone during the first 12 or 16 weeks of pregnancy (13,14). They were later diagnosed as females and the genital abnormalities were corrected surgically. In their early 20s, both had normal pregnancies and gave birth to healthy infants (14,15). In another case, the mother received daily oral methyltestosterone from the 14th week until term for breast engorgement (3). In addition, she was given four IM doses of testosterone (total dose 115 mg) between the 14th and 35th weeks of gestation. Except for clitoral hypertrophy, no other signs of virilization were observed in the infant or the mother (3).

The only report of structural defects, other than genital, associated with the use of testosterone appeared in a 1953 article (17). Three infants with limb anomalies had been exposed during the 1st trimester to a combination of testosterone and progesterone.

The Collaborative Perinatal Project monitored 50,282 mother–child pairs, 26 of whom were exposed to a group of miscellaneous hormones during the 1st trimester (18). Among the 26 cases, 3 were exposed to testosterone, 4 to methandrostenolone, and 1 each to methyltestosterone, fluoxymesterone, and an unspecified male hormone. There were no congenital malformations observed in the 26 exposures (18).

BREASTFEEDING SUMMARY

Testosterone, usually combined with an estrogen, has been used to suppress lactation and to treat postpartum breast pain and engorgement (19–29). Testosterone suppresses lactation apparently by prolactin inhibition (29). Although the amount of testosterone administered was very large, no cases of virilization or other adverse effects attributable to the androgen have been reported. The combination, however, is no longer used because the estrogen–testosterone combination was associated with frequent rebound lactation and an increased incidence of postpartum thromboembolic disease (29).

Although testosterone inhibits prolactin, suckling or any breast manipulation may antagonize the inhibitory effect (21). This has been shown in cases where a mother has received the testosterone–estrogen combination, then changed her mind and breastfed her infant. The amounts of testosterone excreted into milk have apparently not been determined. The absence of reports of adverse effects in nursing infants probably indicates that the short-term exposure is benign. However, the effects from long-term maternal use of testosterone or its derivatives on a nursing infant have not been studied. Therefore, breastfeeding should be halted if these agents are required.

References

1. Reilly WA. Hormone therapy during pregnancy: effects on the fetus and newborn. Q Rev Pediatr 1958;13:198–202.
2. Parfitt K, ed. *Martindale. The Complete Drug Reference*. 32nd ed. London, UK: Pharmaceutical Press, 1999:1464–6.
3. Grumbach MM, Ducharme JR. The effects of androgens on fetal sexual development. Fert Steril 1960;11:157–80.
4. Dumesic DA, Abbott DH, Eisner JR, Goy RW. Prenatal exposure of female rhesus monkeys to testosterone propionate increases serum luteinizing hormone levels in adulthood. Fertil Steril 1997;67:155–63.
5. Hayles AB, Nolan RB. Female pseudohermaphroditism: report of case in an infant born of a mother receiving methyltestosterone during pregnancy. Proc Staff Meet Mayo Clin 1957;32:41–4.
6. Zander J, Muller HA. Uber die methylandrosteniolbehandlung wahrend emer schwangerschaft. Geburtschilfe Frauenheilkd 1953;13:216–4. As cited by Schardein JL. *Chemically Induced Birth Defects*. 3rd ed. New York, NY: Marcel Dekker, 2000:286.
7. Hoffman F, Overzier C, Uhde G. Zur frage der hormonanlen frzeugung fataler zwittenbildungen beim menschen. Geburtschilfe Frauenheilkd 1955;15:1061–70. As cited by Schardein JL. *Chemically Induced Birth Defects*. 3rd ed. New York, NY: Marcel Dekker, 2000:286.
8. Grunwaldt E, Bates T. Nonadrenal female pseudrohermaphrodism after administration of testosterone to mother during pregnancy. Pediatrics 1957;20:503–5.
9. Nellhaus G. Artificially induced female pseudohermaphroditism. N Engl J Med 1958;258:935–8.
10. Gold AP, Michael AF Jr. Testosterone-induced female pseudrohermaphrodism. J Pediatr 1958;52:279–83.
11. Moncrieff A. Non-adrenal female pseudohermaphroditism associated with hormone administration in pregnancy. Lancet 1958;2:267–8.
12. Black JA, Bentley JFR. Effect on the foetus of androgens given during pregnancy. Lancet 1959;1:21–4.
13. Dewhurst CJ, Gordon RR. Change of sex. Lancet 1963;2:1213–6.
14. Reschini E, Giustina G, D'Alberton A, Candiani GB. Female pseudohermaphroditism due to maternal androgen administration: 25-year follow-up. Lancet 1985;1:1226.
15. Dewhurst J, Gordon RR. Fertility following change of sex: a follow-up. Lancet 1984;2:1461–2.
16. Bisset WH, Bain AD, Gauld IK. Female pseudo-hermaphrodite presenting with bilateral cryptorchidism. Br Med J 1966;1:279–80.
17. Martinie-Dubousquet J. Embryopathy entailed by administration of sex hormones to the mother. Rev Pathol Gen Comp 1953;53:1065–76. As cited by Schardein JL. *Chemically Induced Birth Defects*. 3rd ed. New York, NY: Marcel Dekker, 2000:289.

18. Heinonen OP, Slone D, Shapiro S. *Birth Defects and Drugs in Pregnancy*. Littleton, MA: Publishing Sciences Group, 1977:389–90.
19. Iliya FA, Safon L, O'Leary JA. Testosterone enanthate (180 mg.) and estradiol valerate (8 mg.) for suppression of lactation: a double-blind evaluation. Obstet Gynecol 1966;27:643–5.
20. Morris JA, Creasy RK, Hohe PT. Inhibition of puerperal lactation. Double-blind comparison of chlorothianesene, testosterone enanthate and estradiol valerate and placebo. Obstet Gynecol 1970;36:107–14.
21. Vorherr H. Suppression of postpartum lactation. Postgrad Med 1972; 52:145–52.
22. Ng KH, Lee KH. Inhibition of postpartum lactation with single-dose drugs. Aust N Z J Obstet Gynaecol 1972;12:59–61.
23. McNicol E, Struthers JO. A combined/oestrogen/progestogen/testosterone agent for the inhibition of lactation. Br J Clin Pract 1972;26:567–8.
24. Llewellyn-Jones D, Lawrenson K. A new method of inhibition of lactation. Med J Aust 1973;2:780–1.
25. Schwartz DJ, Evans PC, Garcia CR, Rickels K, Fisher E. A clinical study of lactation suppression. Obstet Gynecol 1973;42:599–606.
26. Louviere RL, Upton RT. Evaluation of Deladumone OB in the suppression of postpartum lactation. Am J Obstet Gynecol 1975;121:641–2.
27. Biggs JSG, Hacker N, Andrews E, Munro C. Bromocriptine, methyltestosterone and placebo for inhibition of physiologic lactation. Med J Aust 1978;2(3 Suppl):23–5.
28. Welti H, Paiva F, Felber JP. Prevention and interruption of postpartum lactation with bromocriptine (Parlodel) and effect on plasma prolactin, compared with a hormonal preparation (Ablacton). Eur J Obstet Gynecol Reprod Biol 1979;9:35–9.
29. Kochenour NK. Lactation suppression. Clin Obstet Gynecol 1980;23:1045–59.

TETANUS/DIPHTHERIA TOXOIDS (ADULT)

Toxoid

See Diphtheria/Tetanus Toxoids (Adult).

TETANUS TOXOID/REDUCED DIPHTHERIA TOXOID/ACELLULAR PERTUSSIS VACCINE ADSORBED

Vaccine/Toxoid

See Vaccine, Pertussis (Acellular).

TETRABENAZINE

Antichorea

PREGNANCY RECOMMENDATION: Limited Human Data—Animal Data Suggest Moderate Risk
BREASTFEEDING RECOMMENDATION: No Human Data—Potential Toxicity

PREGNANCY SUMMARY

The very limited human pregnancy experience prevents an assessment of the embryo–fetal risk. However, tetrabenazine caused stillbirths and pup mortality in one animal species. Moreover, the drug rapidly distributes into the brain and reversibly depletes monoamines, such as dopamine, serotonin, norepinephrine, and histamine (1). Thus, it is best avoided in pregnancy.

FETAL RISK SUMMARY

Tetrabenazine, a reversible monoamine depletory, is indicated for the treatment of chorea associated with Huntington's disease. The drug undergoes rapid and extensive hepatic metabolism to two active metabolites resulting in plasma concentrations of the parent drug that are generally below the limit of detection. Plasma protein binding of the two metabolites is moderate, in the range of 59%–68%, and their half-lives are 4–8 hours and 2–4 hours, respectively (1).

Reproduction studies have been conducted in rats and rabbits. In rats, doses up to 3 times the maximum recommended human dose of 100 mg/day based on BSA (MRHD) from the beginning or organogenesis through the lactation period had no clear effects on embryo–fetal development. However, increases in stillbirths and postnatal mortality were observed at doses 1.5–3 times the MRHD, as well as delayed pup maturation at doses 0.5–3 times the MRHD. The no-effect dose for stillbirths and postnatal mortality was 0.5 times the MRHD. In rabbits, dose up to 12 times the MRHD during organogenesis had no effect on embryo–fetal development (1).

Neither carcinogenicity nor fertility impairment studies have been conducted. The parent drug and the active metabolites were negative in mutagenic studies, but were clastogenic in two assays (1).

It is not known if tetrabenazine or its two active metabolites cross the human placenta. The molecular weight of the

T

parent compound (about 317), and the plasma protein binding and half-lives of the metabolites suggest that all three compounds will cross to the embryo–fetus.

A woman with chorea gravidarum was treated with tetrabenazine starting late in the 2nd trimester (2). No drug-induced fetal or newborn effects were observed. The small ventricular septal defect in the infant was probably not related to tetrabenazine exposure (2).

BREASTFEEDING SUMMARY

No reports describing the use of tetrabenazine during lactation have been located. The molecular weight of the parent compound (about 317), and the plasma protein binding and half-lives of the two metabolites (see above) suggest that at least the metabolites will be excreted into breast milk. The effect of this exposure on a nursing infant is unknown. However, common adverse effects observed in adults, such as sedation, somnolence, insomnia, depression, akathisia, and other toxicities, are potential complications.

References

1. Product information. Xenazine. Lundbeck, 2009.
2. Lubbe WF, Walker EB. Chorea gravidarum associated with circulating lupus anticoagulant: Successful outcome of pregnancy with prednisone and aspirin therapy. Case report. Br J Obstet Gynaecol 1983;90:487–90.

TETRACAINE

Local Anesthetic

PREGNANCY RECOMMENDATION: Limited Human Data—Probably Compatible
BREASTFEEDING RECOMMENDATION: No Human Data—Probably Compatible

PREGNANCY SUMMARY

A 1988 review concluded that the available human pregnancy data for tetracaine were inadequate to estimate the embryo–fetal risk from use of the local anesthetic in pregnancy (1). Animal reproduction data also are very limited but did not indicate risk. However, the highest dose used was equal to the human dermal dose based on BSA. In addition, there are no studies regarding the amount of tetracaine reaching the systemic circulation after topical (other than the skin patch) or spinal administration. Nevertheless, based on very small numbers, tetracaine does not appear to represent a risk of embryo and/or fetal harm any greater than that of other local anesthetics (see also Lidocaine, Pramoxine, and Ropivacaine). Thus, although the combined data are inadequate, the risk of embryo–fetal harm from tetracaine is probably low.

FETAL RISK SUMMARY

Tetracaine is an ester type local anesthetic agent. Because of the potential for severe systemic toxicity, its use is restricted to topical anesthesia and spinal block. For some procedures, injectable lidocaine is considered to be a safer alternative (2). Tetracaine is available as topical preparations (concentrations) that include solutions (2%), gels (2%), creams (1% and 2%), and ointments (1%), ophthalmic solutions (0.5%), and formulations for spinal anesthesia (0.2%, 0.3%, and 1%). It is also available in equal combination (70 mg each) with lidocaine as a skin patch that is indicated for use on intact skin to provide local dermal anesthesia for superficial venous access and superficial dermatological procedures such as excision, electrodessication, and shave biopsy of skin lesions (3). Little, if any, tetracaine is absorbed from the skin patch. Plasma levels of the anesthetic were not detectable (<0.9 ng/mL) at 30 and 60 minutes, whereas lidocaine was detectable in the plasma (<5 ng/mL) (3).

Reproduction studies have been conducted in rats and rabbits. In these species, SC doses up to the single dermal administration dose based on BSA (SDAD) were not teratogenic. In addition, no other reproductive or developmental toxicity was observed when tetracaine was given during gestation and lactation at a SC dose that was equal to the SDAD. Tetracaine has not been studied for carcinogenicity, but tests for mutagenicity were negative. The anesthetic agent had no effect on male and female rat fertility at SC doses up to the SDAD (3).

The low molecular weight (about 264) suggests that tetracaine crosses the human placenta, as does lidocaine and other local anesthetics (see Lidocaine). However, the amounts in the systemic circulation appear to be very low, at least from the skin patch, so the amount reaching the embryo and/or fetus will also be very low. Although the absorption of tetracaine into the blood from other formulations is unknown, it also is probably low.

The Collaborative Perinatal Project monitored 50,282 mother–child pairs, 23 of whom had exposure to tetracaine during the 1st trimester (4, pp. 358, 360). No evidence of an association with malformations was found.

A 1981 report described 53 women who received spinal anesthesia with tetracaine diluted to 0.5% (5). Prolongation of the induction-to-delivery interval had no effect on the Apgar scores or the neonatal acid-base values. However, when the uterine incision-to-delivery interval was more than 3 minutes, there were significantly lower mean pH and pO_2 values in the umbilical vein and artery, and significantly higher mean pCO_2 and base deficit results in the umbilical artery. Moreover, the prolonged interval was also associated with significantly more Apgar scores less than 7 at 1 and 5 minutes (5).

BREASTFEEDING SUMMARY

No reports describing the use of tetracaine during human lactation have been located. The low molecular weight (about 264) suggests that tetracaine will be excreted into human breast milk, as does lidocaine. (See Lidocaine.) However, the amount of tetracaine in the systemic circulation appears to be very low, at least from the skin patch, so the amount excreted into breast milk will also be very low. Although the absorption of tetracaine into the blood from other formulations is unknown, it also is probably low. Based on these estimates, the risk to a nursing infant from tetracaine given to the mother appears to be nil.

References

1. Friedman JM. Teratogen update: anesthetic agents. Teratology 1988;37:69–77.
2. Sweetman SC, ed. Tetracaine. *Martindale: The Complete Drug Reference.* 34th ed. London: Pharmaceutical Press, 2005:1385.
3. Product information. Synera. Endo Pharmaceuticals, 2007.
4. Heinonen OP, Slone D, Shapiro S. *Birth Defects and Drugs in Pregnancy.* Littleton, MA: Publishing Sciences Group, 1977.
5. Datta S, Ostheimer GW, Weiss JB, Brown WU Jr, Alper MH. Neonatal effect of prolonged anesthetic induction for cesarean section. Obstet Gynecol 1981;58:331–5.

TETRACYCLINE

Antibiotic (Tetracycline)

PREGNANCY RECOMMENDATION: Contraindicated—2nd and 3rd Trimesters
BREASTFEEDING RECOMMENDATION: Compatible

PREGNANCY SUMMARY

Tetracyclines are a class of antibiotics that should be used with extreme caution, if at all, in pregnancy. These agents can cause significant maternal and fetal toxicity. The discussion below, unless otherwise noted, applies to all members of this class.

FETAL RISK SUMMARY

Problems attributable to the use of the tetracyclines during or around the gestational period can be classified into four areas:

Adverse effects on fetal teeth and bones
Maternal liver toxicity
Congenital defects
Miscellaneous effects

Placental transfer of a tetracycline was first demonstrated in 1950 (1). The tetracyclines were considered safe for the mother and fetus and were routinely used for maternal infections during the following decade (2–5). It was not until 1961 that an intense yellow-gold fluorescence was observed in the mineralized structures of a fetal skeleton whose mother had taken tetracycline just before delivery (6). Following this report, a 2-year-old child was described whose erupted deciduous teeth formed normally but were stained a bright yellow because of tetracycline exposure in utero (7). Fluorescence under ultraviolet light and yellow-colored deciduous teeth that eventually changed to yellow-brown were associated with maternal tetracycline ingestion during pregnancy by several other investigators (8–22). An increase in enamel hypoplasia and caries was initially suspected but later shown not to be related to in utero tetracycline exposure (14,15,22). Newborn growth and development were normal in all of these reports, although tetracycline has been shown to cause inhibition of fibula growth in premature infants (6). The mechanism for the characteristic dental defect produced by tetracycline is related to the potent chelating ability of the drug (13). Tetracycline forms a complex with calcium orthophosphate and becomes incorporated into bones and teeth undergoing calcification. In the latter structure, this complex causes a permanent discoloration, because remodeling and calcium exchange do not occur after calcification is completed. Because the deciduous teeth begin to calcify at around 5 or 6 months in utero, use of tetracycline after this time will result in staining.

The first case linking tetracycline with acute fatty metamorphosis of the liver in a pregnant woman was described in 1963 (23), although two earlier papers reported the disease without associating it with the drug (24,25). This rare but often fatal syndrome usually follows IV dosing of >2 g/day. Many of the pregnant patients were being treated for pyelonephritis (24–37). Tetracycline-induced hepatotoxicity differs from acute fatty liver of pregnancy in that it is not unique to pregnant women and reversal of the disease does not occur with pregnancy termination (38). The symptoms include jaundice, azotemia, acidosis, and terminal irreversible shock. Pancreatitis and nonoliguric renal failure are often related findings. The fetus may not be affected directly, but as a result of the maternal pathology, stillborns and premature births are common. In an experimental study, increasing doses of tetracycline caused increasing fatty metamorphosis of the liver (39). The possibility that chronic maternal use of tetracycline before conception could result in fatal hepatotoxicity of pregnancy has been raised (36). The authors speculated that tetracycline deposited in the bone of a 21-year-old patient was released during pregnancy, resulting in liver damage.

In a surveillance study of Michigan Medicaid recipients involving 229,101 completed pregnancies conducted between 1985 and 1992, a large number of newborns had been exposed to the tetracycline group of antibiotics during the 1st trimester (F. Rosa, personal communication, FDA, 1993). For four tetracyclines (T, tetracycline; D, doxycycline; O, oxytetracycline; M, minocycline), specific data were available for six defect categories, including (observed/expected):

	T	D	O	M
Number of exposures	1795	1795	26	181
Number of major defects	47	78	1	8
Percent	4.7%	4.3%	3.8%	4.4%
Number of major defects expected	46	76	1	7
Cardiovascular defects	12/10	20/18	0/0.3	2/2
Oral clefts	1/2	0/3	0/0	1/0.5
Spina bifida	0/0.5	2/1	0/0	0/0
Polydactyly	5/3	7/5	0/0	0/0.5
Limb reduction defects	1/2	0/3	0/0	0/0.5
Hypospadias	1/2	4/4	0/0	0/0.5

These data do not support an association between the drugs and the specific malformations evaluated.

The Collaborative Perinatal Project monitored 50,282 mother–child pairs, 341 of whom had 1st trimester exposure to tetracycline, 14 to chlortetracycline, 90 to demeclocycline, and 119 to oxytetracycline (40, pp. 297–313). For use anytime in pregnancy, 1336 exposures were recorded for tetracycline, 0 for chlortetracycline, 280 for demeclocycline, and 328 for oxytetracycline (40, p. 435). The findings of this study were as follows:

Tetracycline: Evidence was found to suggest a relationship to minor, but not major, malformations. Three possible associations were found with individual defects, but independent confirmation is required: hypospadias (1st trimester only) (5 cases); inguinal hernia (25 cases); and hypoplasia of limb or part thereof (6 cases) (40, pp. 472, 485).

Chlortetracycline: No evidence was found to suggest a relationship to large categories of major or minor malformations or to individual defects. However, the sample size is extremely small, and safety should not be inferred from these negative results.

Demeclocycline: No evidence was found to suggest a relationship to large categories of major or minor malformations, but the sample size is small (40, pp. 297–313). Two possible associations were found with individual defects, but independent confirmation is required: clubfoot (1st trimester only) (3 cases); and inguinal hernia (8 cases) (40, pp. 472, 485).

Oxytetracycline: Evidence was found to suggest a relationship to large categories of major and minor malformations (40, pp. 297–313). One possible association was found with individual defects, but independent confirmation is required: inguinal hernia (14 cases) (40, pp. 472, 485).

In 1962, a woman treated with tetracycline in the 1st trimester for acute bronchitis delivered an infant with congenital defects of both hands (41,42). The mother had a history of minor congenital defects on her side of the family and doubt was cast on the role of the drug in this anomaly (43). A possible association between the use of tetracyclines in pregnancy or during lactation and congenital cataracts has been reported in four patients (44). The effects of other drugs, including several antibiotics, and maternal infection could not be determined, and a causal relationship to the tetracyclines seems remote. An infant with multiple anomalies whose mother had been treated for acne with clomocycline daily during the first 8 weeks of pregnancy has been described (45). Some of the defects, particularly the incomplete fibrous ankylosis and bone changes, made the authors suspect this tetracycline as the likely cause.

Doxycycline has been used for 10 days very early in the 1st trimester for the treatment of *Mycoplasma* infection in a group of previously infertile women (46). Dosage was based on the patient's weight, varying from 100 to 300 mg/day. All 43 of the exposed liveborn were normal at 1 year of age. Bubonic plague occurring in a woman at 22 weeks' gestation was successfully treated with tetracycline and streptomycin (47). Long-term evaluation of the infant was not reported.

A 1997 report examined the question of doxycycline-induced teratogenicity in the large population-based dataset of the Hungarian Case–Control Surveillance of Congenital Abnormalities, 1980–1992 (48). Some mild defects were excluded, including hemangiomas and minor malformations. Moreover, although an extensive retrospective assessment of drug use during pregnancy was performed, a history of tobacco and alcohol exposure was not obtained because the accuracy of these data was believed to have low validity. Among the 32,804 women who had normal infants (controls), 63 (0.19%) had taken doxycycline, whereas 56 (0.30%) of the 18,515 women who delivered infants with congenital anomalies had taken the antibiotic ($p = 0.01$). A case–control pair analysis of exposures during the 2nd and 3rd months of gestation, however, did not show a significant difference among the groups in any of the malformation types (48).

A retrospective cohort study using data from Tennessee Medicaid included 30,049 infants born in 1985–2000 was published in 2009 (49). Infants with fetal exposures in the 1st trimester to four antibiotics recommended for potential bioterrorism attacks (doxycycline, amoxicillin, ciprofloxacin, and azithromycin) were compared to infants with no fetal exposure to any antibiotic. Erythromycin was included as a positive control. In the 1691 infants exposed to doxycycline and no other antibiotics, the number of cases, risk ratios, and 95% confidence interval [CI] were: any malformation (42, 0.85, 0.59–1.23); cardiac (15, 0.86, 0.47–1.57); musculoskeletal (12, 0.94, 0.47–1.88); genitourinary (4, 0.45, 0.15–1.34); gastrointestinal (3, 0.35, 0.10–1.20); CNS (4, 0.87, 0.27–2.78); and orofacial (5, 2.96, 0.75–11.67). The authors concluded that the four antibiotics should not result in a greater incidence of overall major malformations (see also Amoxicillin, Azithromycin, and Ciprofloxacin) (49).

A 2000 report, using the same database as above, but now for the years 1980–1996, examined the relationship between oral oxytetracycline and congenital malformations (50). Of 22,865 women who had offspring with a congenital defect, 216 (0.9%) had been treated with oxytetracycline, whereas of 38,151 women with offspring without defects, 214 (0.6%) had been treated (odds ratio [OR] 1.7, 95% CI 1.4–2.0). Analysis of medically documented treatment in the 2nd/3rd months of gestation revealed significant associations with

T

neural tube defects (NTD) (OR 9.7, 95% CI 2.0–47.1), cleft palate (OR 17.2, 95% CI 3.5–83.5), and multiple defects (mainly neural tube defects and cardiovascular malformations) (OR 12.9, 95% CI 3.8–44.3). However, these results were based on a very small number of cases: two NTD, two cleft palates, and four multiple defects. The number of cases, OR, and 95% CI occurring in the entire pregnancy for these outcomes were NTDs (7, 5.4, 2.4–12.1), cleft palate (3, 4.6, 1.4–15.0), and multiple defects (6, 3.3, 1.4–7.9) (50).

Under miscellaneous effects, two reports have appeared that, although they do not directly relate to effects on the fetus, do directly affect pregnancy. In 1974, a researcher observed that a 1-week administration of 500 mg/day of chlortetracycline to male subjects was sufficient to produce semen levels of the drug averaging 4.5 mcg/mL (51). He theorized that tetracycline overdose could modify the fertilizing capacity of human sperm by inhibiting capacitation. Finally, a possible interaction between oral contraceptives and tetracycline resulting in pregnancy has been reported (52). The mechanism for this interaction may involve the interruption of enterohepatic circulation of contraceptive steroids by inhibiting gut bacterial hydrolysis of steroid conjugates, resulting in a lower concentration of circulating steroids.

BREASTFEEDING SUMMARY

Tetracycline is excreted into breast milk in low concentrations. Milk:plasma ratios vary between 0.25 and 1.5 (4,53,54). In a 1996 case, black breast milk was reported in a woman taking minocycline, a semisynthetic derivative of tetracycline (55). She had stopped breastfeeding 18 months before she was treated with minocycline 150 mg/day and topical clindamycin for acne. Within 4 weeks of starting minocycline, milk expressed from her breasts was black. No other abnormalities were found on a diagnostic workup. Analysis of the milk demonstrated black pigment particles within macrophages, as well as extracellular, that stained positive for iron. The milk contained a high iron concentration (11.9 μmol/g wet weight) (55).

Theoretically, dental staining and inhibition of bone growth could occur in breastfed infants whose mothers were consuming tetracycline. However, this theoretical possibility seems remote, because tetracycline serum levels in infants exposed in such a manner were undetectable (<0.05 mcg/mL) (4). Three potential problems may exist for the nursing infant even though there are no reports in this regard: modification of bowel flora, direct effects on the infant, and interference with the interpretation of culture results if a fever workup is required. The American Academy of Pediatrics classifies tetracycline as compatible with breastfeeding (56).

References

1. Guilbeau JA, Schoenbach EG, Schaub IG, Latham DV. Aureomycin in obstetrics: therapy and prophylaxis. JAMA 1950;143:520–6.
2. Charles D. Placental transmission of antibiotics. J Obstet Gynaecol Br Emp 1954;61:750–7.
3. Gibbons RJ, Reichelderfer TE. Transplacental transmission of demethylchlortetracycline and toxicity studies in premature and full term, newly born infants. Antibiot Med Clin Ther 1960;7:618–22.
4. Posner AC, Prigot A, Konicoff NG. Further observations on the use of tetracycline hydrochloride in prophylaxis and treatment of obstetric infections. In: *Antibiotics Annual, 1954-55*. New York, NY: Medical Encyclopedia, 1955:594–8.
5. Posner AC, Konicoff NG, Prigot A. Tetracycline in obstetric infections. In: *Antibiotics Annual, 1955-56*. New York, NY: Medical Encyclopedia, 1956: 345–8.
6. Cohlan SQ, Bevelander G, Bross S. Effect of tetracycline on bone growth in the premature infant. Antimicrob Agents Chemother 1961:340–7.
7. Harcourt JK, Johnson NW, Storey E. In vivo incorporation of tetracycline in the teeth of man. Arch Oral Biol 1962;7:431–7.
8. Rendle-Short TJ. Tetracycline in teeth and bone. Lancet 1962;1:1188.
9. Douglas AC. The deposition of tetracycline in human nails and teeth: a complication of long term treatment. Br J Dis Chest 1963;57:44–7.
10. Kutscher AH, Zegarelli EV, Tovell HM, Hochberg B. Discoloration of teeth induced by tetracycline. JAMA 1963;184:586–7.
11. Kline AH, Blattner RJ, Lunin M. Transplacental effect of tetracyclines on teeth. JAMA 1964;188:178–80.
12. Macaulay JC, Leistyna JA. Preliminary observations on the prenatal administration of demethylchlortetracycline HCl. Pediatrics 1964;34:423–4.
13. Stewart DJ. The effects of tetracyclines upon the dentition. Br J Dermatol 1964;76:374–8.
14. Swallow JN. Discoloration of primary dentition after maternal tetracycline ingestion in pregnancy. Lancet 1964;2:611–2.
15. Porter PJ, Sweeney EA, Golan H, Kass EH. Controlled study of the effect of prenatal tetracycline on primary dentition. Antimicrob Agents Chemother 1965:668–71.
16. Toaff R, Ravid R. Tetracyclines and the teeth. Lancet 1966;2:281–2.
17. Kutscher AH, Zegarelli EV, Tovell HM, Hochberg B, Hauptman J. Discoloration of deciduous teeth induced by administrations of tetracycline antepartum. Am J Obstet Gynecol 1966;96:291–2.
18. Brearley LJ, Stragis AA, Storey E. Tetracycline-induced tooth changes. Part 1. Prevalence in pre-school children. Med J Aust 1968;2:653–8.
19. Brearley LJ, Storey E. Tetracycline-induced tooth changes. Part 2. Prevalence, localization and nature of staining in extracted deciduous teeth. Med J Aust 1968;2:714–9.
20. Baker KL, Storey E. Tetracycline-induced tooth changes. Part 3. Incidence in extracted first permanent molar teeth. Med J Aust 1970;1:109–13.
21. Anthony JR. Effect on deciduous and permanent teeth of tetracycline deposition in utero. Postgrad Med 1970;48:165–8.
22. Genot MT, Golan HP, Porter PJ, Kass EH. Effect of administration of tetracycline in pregnancy on the primary dentition of the offspring. J Oral Med 1970;25:75–9.
23. Schultz JC, Adamson JS Jr, Workman WW, Normal TD. Fatal liver disease after intravenous administration of tetracycline in high dosage. N Engl J Med 1963;269:999–1004.
24. Bruno M, Ober WB. Clinicopathologic conference: jaundice at the end of pregnancy. NY State J Med 1962;62:3792–800.
25. Lewis PL, Takeda M, Warren MJ. Obstetric acute yellow atrophy. Report of a case. Obstet Gynecol 1963;22:121–7.
26. Briggs RC. Tetracycline and liver disease. N Engl J Med 1963;269:1386.
27. Leonard GL. Tetracycline and liver disease. N Engl J Med 1963;269:1386.
28. Gough GS, Searcy RL. Additional case of fatal liver disease with tetracycline therapy. N Engl J Med 1964;270:157–8.
29. Whalley PJ, Adams RH, Combes B. Tetracycline toxicity in pregnancy. JAMA 1964;189:357–62.
30. Kunelis CT, Peters JL, Edmondson HA. Fatty liver of pregnancy and its relationship to tetracycline therapy. Am J Med 1965;38:359–77.
31. Lew HT, French SW. Tetracycline nephrotoxicity and nonoliguric acute renal failure. Arch Intern Med 1966;118:123–8.
32. Meihoff WE, Pasquale DN, Jacoby WJ Jr. Tetracycline-induced hepatic coma, with recovery. A report of a case. Obstet Gynecol 1967;29:260–5.
33. Aach R, Kissane J. Clinicopathologic conference: a seventeen year old girl with fatty liver of pregnancy following tetracycline therapy. Am J Med 1967;43:274–83.
34. Whalley PJ, Martin FG, Adams RH, Combes B. Disposition of tetracycline by pregnant women with acute pyelonephritis. Obstet Gynecol 1970;36:821–6.
35. Pride GL, Cleary RE, Hamburger RJ. Disseminated intravascular coagulation associated with tetracycline-induced hepatorenal failure during pregnancy. Am J Obstet Gynecol 1973;115:585–6.
36. Wenk RE, Gebhardt FC, Behagavan BS, Lustgarten JA, McCarthy EF. Tetracycline-associated fatty liver of pregnancy, including possible pregnancy risk after chronic dermatologic use of tetracycline. J Reprod Med 1981;26:135–41.
37. King TM, Bowe ET, D'Esopo DA. Toxic effects of the tetracyclines. Bull Sloane Hosp Women 1964;10:35–41.
38. Kaplan MM. Acute fatty liver of pregnancy. N Engl J Med 1985;313:367–70.
39. Allen ES, Brown WE. Hepatic toxicity of tetracycline in pregnancy. Am J Obstet Gynecol 1966;95:12–8.

T

40. Heinonen O, Slone D, Shapiro S. *Birth Defects and Drugs in Pregnancy*. Littleton, MA: Publishing Sciences Group, 1977.
41. Wilson F. Congenital defects in the newborn. Br Med J 1962;2:255.
42. Carter MP, Wilson F. Tetracycline and congenital limb abnormalities. Br Med J 1962;2:407–8.
43. Mennie AT. Tetracycline and congenital limb abnormalities. Br Med J 1962;2:480.
44. Harley JD, Farrar JF, Gray JB, Dunlop IC. Aromatic drugs and congenital cataracts. Lancet 1964;1:472.
45. Corcoran R, Castles JM. Tetracycline for acne vulgaris and possible teratogenesis. Br Med J 1977;2:807–8.
46. Horne HW Jr, Kundsin RB. The role of mycoplasma among 81 consecutive pregnancies: a prospective study. Int J Fertil 1980;25:315–7.
47. Coppes JB. Bubonic plague in pregnancy. J Reprod Med 1980;25:91–5.
48. Czeizel AE, Rockenbauer M. Teratogenic study of doxycycline. Obstet Gynecol 1997;89:524–8.
49. Cooper WO, Hernandez-Diaz S, Arbogast PG, Dudley JA, Dyer SM, Gideon PS, Hall KS, Kaltenbach LA, Ray WA. Antibiotics potentially used in response to bioterrorism and the risk of major congenital malformations. Paediatr Perinat Epidemiol 2009;23:18–28.
50. Czeizel AE, Rockenbauer M. A population-based case-control teratologic study of oral oxytetracycline treatment during pregnancy. Eur J Obstet Gynecol Reprod Biol 2000;88:27–33.
51. Briggs M. Tetracycline and steroid hormone binding to human spermatozoa. Acta Endocrinol 1974;75:785–92.
52. Bacon JF, Shenfield GM. Pregnancy attributable to interaction between tetracycline and oral contraceptives. Br Med J 1980;1:283.
53. Knowles JA. Drugs in milk. Pediatr Curr 1972;21:28–32.
54. Graf VH, Reimann S. Untersuchungen uber die Konzentration von Pyrrolidino-methyl-tetracycline in der Muttermilch. Dtsch Med Wochenschr 1959;84:1694.
55. Hunt MJ, Salisbury ELC, Grace J, Armati R. Black breast milk due to minocycline therapy. Br J Dermatol 1996;134:943–4.
56. Committee on Drugs, American Academy of Pediatrics. The transfer of drugs and other chemicals into human milk. Pediatrics 2001;108:776–89.

THALIDOMIDE

Immunologic Agent (Immunomodulator)

PREGNANCY RECOMMENDATION: Contraindicated
BREASTFEEDING RECOMMENDATION: No Human Data—Potential Toxicity

PREGNANCY SUMMARY

Thalidomide is a potent human teratogen. The severe malformations induced by thalidomide may involve defects of the limbs, axial skeleton, head and face, eyes, ears, tongue, teeth, central nervous, respiratory, cardiovascular, and genitourinary systems, and the gastrointestinal tract. The neurological complications may include severe mental retardation secondary to sensory deprivation. The critical period of exposure is 34–50 days after the first day of the last menstrual period (LMP) (20–36 days after conception). The drug is contraindicated in pregnancy.

FETAL RISK SUMMARY

Thalidomide is an immunomodulatory agent used for the acute treatment of erythema nodosum leprosum, a cutaneous manifestation of Hansen's disease (leprosy) (1). The agent was recently approved for use in the United States for the first time, making its debut in 1999. Thalidomide was one of the first drugs that was clearly shown to be a human teratogen and probably has caused more known severe malformations in humans than any other drug.

A large number (>30) of animal (mice, rats, rabbits, and monkeys) reproduction studies conducted with thalidomide were reviewed in a 1976 reference (2). Embryolethality and teratogenicity (structural and/or functional abnormalities) were noted commonly in some species. Evidence of significant thalidomide teratogenicity was found in monkeys, but in mice and rats, limb reduction defects were not observed and, in some cases, there was no evidence of teratogenicity. Amelia and micromelia were noted in two mouse fetuses and a limb defect in another that closely resembled the defects observed in humans, but these reports were considered inconclusive (2). In a 1983 study with rats, however, increased rates of both embryolethality and congenital defects involving the skeleton (ribs and spine) and eyes (ophthalmorrhexis and microphthalmia) were observed (3). The authors speculated that the difference in outcome between their study and previous experimental work with rats was possibly due to hydrolysis of the drug before administration, the use of toxic solvents that masked the teratogenic effect of thalidomide, or the low solubility of thalidomide in the solvent that prevented delivery of an effective dose to the target site (3). Experiments in rabbits have consistently revealed fetal limb malformations that are very similar to those seen in human infants exposed in utero to thalidomide (4–8). Other anomalies noted in rabbit fetuses included hemangioma of the nose and defects of the skull, nostril, external genitalia, and tail (6). Another study with rabbits observed limb anomalies, arthrogryposis, dysplasia of the kidneys and gallbladder, cleft palate, hernia, and gastric hypoplasia (8). Experiments with chick embryos demonstrated that thalidomide induced cardiovascular anomalies in this species (9).

Several reviews have described the various human systems affected by thalidomide-induced embryopathy (10–19). One of these reviews presented the pregnancy history of two children (twins), born in the United States, who had very different severity of thalidomide embryopathy (10). The first twin, 2211-g female, was born with duodenal atresia, a rectoperineal fistula, and hypoplastic, dislocated thumbs (right thumb worse than left). The other twin, a 2240-g male, had phocomelia of both upper extremities and a midline hemangioma on the forehead. Missing or hypoplastic digits were noted on both hands (10).

The critical period of fetal exposure to thalidomide is 34–50 days after the first day of the LMP (20–36 days after conception) (13,16–18). Congenital malformations that have been associated with approximate time periods within this 17-day interval include (days after LMP; when two ranges are shown, the references cited disagreed): anotia (34–38 days), microtia (39–43 days), thumb duplication (35–38 days), thumb aplasia (35–43 days), thumb hypoplasia (38–40 days), thumb triphalangism (46–50 days), eye defects (35–42 days), cardiovascular defects (ductus, conotruncal defects, and septal defects) (36–45 days), duplication of the vagina (35–39 days), cranial nerve palsy (35–37 days), amelia of the arms (38–43 days), phocomelia of the arms (38–47 or 49 days), dislocation of the hip (38–48 days), amelia of the legs (41–45 days), phocomelia of the legs (40 or 42–47 days), choanal atresia (43–46 days), duodenal atresia (40–47 days), anal atresia (41–43 days), aplasia of gallbladder (42–43 days), pyloric stenosis (40–47 days), duodenal stenosis (41–48 days), rectal stenosis (49–50 days), ectopic kidney and hydronephrosis (38–43 days), other genitourinary defects (45–47 days), and abnormal lobulation of lungs (43–46 days) (13,17).

Perhaps the best description of the spectrum of congenital defects caused by thalidomide was written by Newman (16,17). The limb reduction defects are bilateral, usually grossly symmetric, and upper limb anomalies are commonly associated with lower limb defects. Shoulder and hip malformations occur with increasing severity of upper limb defects. Vertebral defects include an increased incidence of progressive ossification of the anterior spinal ligaments that converts the sacral and lumbar vertebral bodies into one bone mass, loss of distal segment of the sacrum, and spondylolisthesis. Spina bifida occulta and meningomyelocele occur with increased frequency. A nonspecific facial asymmetry may occur, as well as tooth hypoplasia and a deficiency in the number of teeth. There may be a hypoplastic nasal bridge with an expanded nasal tip, and choanal atresia can affect one or both nostrils. Laryngeal and tracheal anomalies and abnormal lobulation of the lungs have been observed. Ocular defects include refractive errors, pupillary abnormalities, muscle dysfunction, coloboma, microphthalmos, cataracts, and abnormalities of all three components of the oculomotor nerve. Ear defects are frequently associated with ocular malformations, as is facial nerve palsy. The defects of the ears include external, middle, and internal anomalies which are frequently associated with deafness (either conductive, neural, or both). A midline capillary hemangioma or nevus of the nose and philtrum have been described, but may fade as the child grows older. Cardiac defects, commonly of the conotruncal region, occur frequently and are a major cause of early death (30% at birth, 6% in survivors). Gastrointestinal tract defects include atresia and stenosis, and absence of the gallbladder and appendix. Inguinal hernias may be observed. Genitourinary malformations involve the kidneys (ectopic, horseshoe, hydronephrosis, and double ureter), double vagina, and cryptorchism (16,17).

Thalidomide was introduced into clinical medicine in West Germany in 1956 (20). Although a wide range of indications was promoted for the drug, it was primarily used as a sedative and tranquilizer. Because of the concern over birth defects, thalidomide was withdrawn from the market in most countries in late 1961 (21).

In 1961, two cases of congenital defects of the limbs were presented at a German pediatric meeting (22). At the meeting, Lenz (23) proposed that thalidomide was the cause of the defects. A brief 1961 correspondence, however, was the first published English language article to describe birth defects that were suspected as being induced by thalidomide (24). McBride (24) had noted an approximate 20% incidence of polydactyly, syndactyly, and limb reduction defects consisting of abnormally short femora and radii in infants exposed in utero to thalidomide. In early 1962, Lenz (23) estimated that 2000–3000 thalidomide-exposed babies had been born in West Germany since 1959.

A number of communications have been published that describe the types of congenital malformations caused by thalidomide (10,15–19,23–81):

Thalidomide Embryopathy

Limb Defects

- **Upper and lower limbs** (bilateral amelia or phocomelia; absence or hypoplasia of radius/ulna and/or tibia/fibula; femoral hypoplasia; preaxial aplasia of upper and lower limbs; absence of the fingers and/or toes; thumb defects such as duplication, hypoplasia, and triphalangism; duplication of big toe and triphalangism) (10,15–19,23–38,40,41, 45–47,49–51,54–59,61–66,68,70,71,74–81)
- **Osteochondritis of femoral head** (Legg-Calve-Perthes disease) (possibly a late complication that results from growth disturbance of the upper end of the femur; appeared in early childhood) (51)
- **Knee joints** (laxity of cruciate ligaments) (16,17,61)

Other Skeletal Defects

- **Spine** (ossification of sacral and lumbar vertebrae, loss of distal segment of sacrum, spondylolisthesis, scoliosis) (15–18,35–37,40,43,49,50,58,61,66,71,78,79)
- **Shoulder** (hypoplasia/dysplasia of glenoid cavity, dysplasia of neck of scapula, altered humeral head) (16,17,19,61)
- **Hip/pelvis** (dislocation, pelvic girdle hypoplasia) (16,17,19,35,51,59,61,66,78,79)
- Jaw (69,74)

Craniofacial

- **Eye** (refractive errors, pupil, motility, coloboma of the iris, uvea, lens, and choroid, microphthalmos, cataracts, glaucoma, crocodile-tear syndrome) (15–19,25,30,33,36,37,40, 45–47,49,50,62,63,65,66,68,70–77)
- **Ear** (anotia, microtia, low set, middle and internal ear, deafness) (15–19,23,25–27,29,30,33,35, 37,39,41,43–45,48,53,56–58,61–68,70,73–77)
- **Face/skull** (face—asymmetrical; skull—rhomboid shape) (16,17,58,69)
- **Tongue** (dysplasias of lingual frenulum in the form of an ankyloglossia [tongue-tie] or a shortened, sinew-shaped frenulum; grooved point of tongue [bifid tongue]) (16,69)
- **Nose** (hypoplastic nasal bridge with expanded nasal tip) (16,17,19,58,66)
- **Choanal atresia** (16–19,29,37,62,65,70,71,75)
- **Teeth** (hypodontia, hyperdontia, malformed crown, enamel hypoplasia, discoloring, malocclusion, missing teeth) (16–18,58,60,69,75)
- **Midline hemangioma or nevus** (nose, upper lip, frontal area) (10,16,17,23,25,30,33,35,45,46,57,58,60,65,66,71)

T

Central Nervous System

Facial nerve palsy (often associated with eye and ear anomalies) (15–19,35,39,43,61,63,68,71,73,75–77)

Hydrocephalus (37,57,65,73)

Spina bifida occulta (16,17,78,79)

Meningomyelocele (16,17,35)

Autism (18,77)

Epilepsy (15,16,76,77)

Marcus Gunn phenomenon or jaw winking syndrome (16,19)

Crocodile-tear syndrome (see **Eye**)

Major Organ Systems

Respiratory system (laryngeal and tracheal abnormalities, abnormal lobulation of lungs) (16,17,19,29,33,36,37,49,62,65,66,74,75)

Cardiovascular (ventricular septal defect, atrial septal defect, tetralogy of Fallot, cor triloculare, pericardial effusion, hypertrophy of atrium and ventricle, coarctation of aorta, systolic murmurs) (16–19,23,25,30,33,35–37,39,40,42,43,45,57,61,62,65,66,70,73,75,76)

Gastrointestinal tract

Esophageal atresia (23,29,30,37,74)

Duodenal atresia (10,16,19,23,29,30,33,35,37,49,61,62,66,70)

Common bileduct atresia (33,66)

Anal atresia (16,18,19,23,29,30,33,35,37,44,61,62,66,75)

Rectoperineal fistula (10)

Malrotation (25,30,33,35,66)

Stenosis (16–19,25,30,37,40,45,46,53,61,62,65,66,70,76)

Abnormal lobulation of liver (33,37)

Aplasia of appendix (16,17,19,23,29,30,33,37,40,46,52,53,59,65,66)

Aplasia of cecum (33)

Aplasia of gallbladder (16,17,19,23,30,33,36,49,57,65,66)

Rectoperineal fistula (10)

Genitourinary system

Unspecified (25,30,33,37,75)

Renal abnormalities (16–19,29,35–37,46,57,59,61,62,65,66,70,74,75,81)

Defects and duplication of ureters (16,17,19,37,81)

Aplasia of fallopian tube (62)

Defects of uterus and/or vagina (16,17,19,33,37,55,62,65,66,80)

Penile maldevelopment (65)

Cryptorchism (16,17,19,25,36,61,65,66)

Other

Excessive sweating (52,54)

Inguinal hernias (16,17,19,61,66)

Cleft lip with or without cleft palate has occasionally been observed in newborns with thalidomide embryopathy (35,44,48,49,65,66,69–71), but it is not thought to be related to thalidomide exposure (19).

In 1962, Lenz and Knapp (62) reviewed the fetal effects of thalidomide that were known at the time. Of 293 cases known to the authors or from published reports, the approximate percentage of each defect was arms only (52%); arms and legs (28%); arms, legs, and ears (3%); arms and ears (6%); ears only (7%); legs only (2%); and other malformations (3%). The anomalies observed in the eight infants grouped as "other malformations" included one case each of a right polycystic kidney with aplasia of the left kidney, aplasia of left fallopian tube and left cornu of the uterus, multicystic kidneys, anal stenosis with hydronephrosis, fistula of the neck, congenital heart disease, choanal atresia, and anal atresia (62). In addition, malformations that accompanied those of the limbs and ears were pyloric stenosis, duodenal stenosis, duodenal atresia, cardiac defect, microphthalmos, anophthalmia, imperforate anus, and choanal atresia (62). Two additional review articles by Lenz, focusing on thalidomide-induced defects, appeared in 1966 (63) and 1971 (64), one with a commentary by Warkany (82).

In 1963, Japanese investigators reported phocomelia and other malformations in 10 cases (5 live infants and 5 stillbirths or early neonatal deaths) (65). Another investigator evaluated 160 cases of thalidomide embryopathy that occurred in Japan (66). Of the 160 cases, 99 had a well-documented history of thalidomide intake in early pregnancy. Of these, 70% had defects of the arms only; 14% of arms and legs; 5% of the arms, legs, and ears; 5% of the ears only; 3% of the arms and ears; and 3% of other organs (66). In 41 of the cases with malformations of the limbs and ears, an autopsy found multiple other defects of various organ systems that were similar to those reported by Lenz and Knapp (see reference 62) (66).

The importance of early examinations for ear anomalies, especially for resulting hearing impairment, was emphasized in a study published in 1965 (67). The author had observed 14 cases of bilateral congenital meatal atresia in thalidomide-exposed infants at his center, but he was aware of 50 such cases throughout England. Eleven of the cases (three were unsuitable for operation) underwent either bilateral or unilateral surgery to construct a sound conducting mechanism. Gross malformations determined by x-ray and tomographic examinations in the 14 cases (28 ears) involved the ossicles (32%), middle ear (21%), and labyrinth (25%) (67).

A later study, published in 1976, evaluated the ear anomalies in 18 children, ages 12–16 years, who had thalidomide-induced malformations (68). Hearing impairment and vestibular hypofunction or absence of function were each found in 15 (83%) of the children. External and middle ear anomalies found in 11 of the 18 children included bilateral microtia ($N = 5$), bilateral microtia and bilateral atresia of the auditory canal ($N = 5$), and bilateral microtia and unilateral atresia of the auditory canal ($N = 1$). In one 13-year-old girl, surgical exploration revealed that the stapes and the oval and round windows had not developed, the long process of the incus was shaped like a string, and there was a nearly normal malleus. X-ray examination revealed inner ear malformations in 15 cases (83%) consisting of bilateral inner ear aplasia ($N = 9$), cystic deformity with the shape of the anterior semicircular canal ($N = 4$), large cystic defect of the inner ear ($N = 1$), and a narrow, internal auditory canal bilaterally ($N = 1$) (68). In addition to the ear defects, 12 children had eye-movement disturbances consisting of bilateral abducens palsy ($N = 5$), bilateral abducens palsy and bilateral adduction disturbance ($N = 6$), and unilateral abducens palsy

T

($N = 1$). Bilateral ($N = 3$) or unilateral ($N = 3$) facial palsy, and "crocodile-tear" syndrome (i.e., abnormal lacrimation that accompanies eating) ($N = 7$) were also observed (68).

A 1968 reference described the findings that resulted from clinical, orthodontic, and radiologic examinations of the face and jaws of children with thalidomide embryopathy (69). The findings in 127 children (approximate ages 4–6 years) with thalidomide embryopathy (group 1) were compared with 57 children with nonthalidomide-induced dysmelia (group 2), and 120 children without malformation of the limbs (group 3). Thalidomide exposure did not disturb either the shape or number of the deciduous or permanent teeth (69). However, in the 103 children of group 1 with complete deciduous dentition, there was an increase in the frequency of abnormalities of the maxilla and/or mandible. The other important findings were malformation at the base of the skull, asymmetry of the skull, and dysplasia of the point of the tongue and the frenum (69).

One investigator categorized the malformations found in 154 children with thalidomide embryopathy using a classification system of principal defects that he had designed (70). The type of defects were the same as those listed above for thalidomide embryopathy. In eight groups, limb defects were dominant but other defects were often present, whereas in two groups, limb defects were absent or minimal. The defect classifications and the number and approximate percentage of children in each group were as follows: upper limb amelia or phocomelia with normal legs ($N = 60$, 39%); upper limb amelia or phocomelia with other leg defects ($N = 18$, 12%); forearm defects with normal legs ($N = 17$, 11%); four limb phocomelia ($N = 15$, 10%); anomalies of the ears ($N = 16$, 10%); severe lower limb defects with less severe upper limb defects ($N = 10$, 6%); other limb defects ($N = 9$, 6%); forearm defects with defects of the lower limbs ($N = 5$, 3%); lower limb defects with normal upper limbs ($N = 3$, 2%); and other anomalies ($N = 1$, <1%). A discussion of the disabilities caused by the defects in each group was also included in the text (70).

The focus of eight studies was on thalidomide-induced ocular malformations (18,46,47,71–75). Four children with ocular defects and typical thalidomide embryopathy were described in a 1964 report (46). The eye defects thought to be thalidomide related were as follows: left optic disc with a very deep physiologic cup; bilateral coloboma of the iris, unilateral coloboma of the choroid and retina involving the optic disc, and unilateral microphthalmos; unilateral coloboma of the choroid and retina; and bilateral coloboma of the iris, choroid, and retina, involving the optic disc on one side, and unilateral microphthalmos (46). At one ophthalmology center, minor ocular abnormalities were found in some children consisting of pigmentary retinopathy, a high refractive error, and reduced visual acuity (47). A 1963 study evaluated 20 children with known or suspected thalidomide-induced limb malformations for ocular anomalies (71). Of the children, 13 had anatomically normal eyes with apparently normal function and 7 (35%) had visual defects. Five of the seven had structural defects consisting of either unilateral or bilateral coloboma of the iris, choroid, or lens, sometimes involving the macular areas or the disc, and microphthalmos. The other two had anatomically normal eyes but abnormalities in visual function. The visual prognosis was rated as good in three cases, poor in two, and uncertain in two (71). A 1966 study from Sweden examined 38 children for ocular malformations who had thalidomide-induced defects (72). Abducens paralysis was found in 17 children, bilateral in 13, and unilateral in 4. Bilateral oculomotor paralysis was present in two of these cases and unilateral in one (72). Other conditions, often concomitant with additional defects, included strabismus, unequal pupils (both reactive to light), nonreactive pupil, microphthalmos (both bilateral and unilateral), anophthalmos on one side and severe microphthalmos on the other, coloboma of the choroid, bilateral aplasia of macula with nystagmus, and bilateral epiphora (with free tear ducts and grossly normal drainage system) (72). Of note, more than half of the children had hearing impairment of varying severity. A 1967 report reviewed the previously published cases of ocular abnormalities induced by thalidomide and presented additional data on 21 Canadian children (ages 3–4.5 years) exposed in utero to the drug (73). Only four of these children had ocular malformations and none had a coloboma.

Ocular abnormalities associated with thalidomide embryopathy were reported in a 1991 study of 21 Swedish patients, ages 28–29 years (74). Horizontal incomitant strabismus, usually of the Duane syndrome type, was the most common ocular motility abnormality, but other motility abnormalities were also noted (74). Abnormal tearing, facial nerve (7th cranial nerve) palsy, and ear anomalies were also present in some cases. Citing previous studies, facial nerve palsy and ear anomalies were thought to have occurred from thalidomide exposure on days 20–29 after conception (74). This time period is consistent with the time intervals (34–43 days after LMP) given earlier. Two years later, these same authors reported the results of an ophthalmological study conducted in 86 of 100 Swedes with documented thalidomide embryopathy (75). The subjects, 49 males and 37 females, ranged in age from 27 to 30 years. Forty-six (54%) had one or more abnormal eye signs. The ocular abnormalities included the following: (a) motility defects ($N = 43$, 50%), including 37 with horizontal incomitant strabismus (26 with Duane syndrome, 4 with marked limitation of abduction, and 7 with gaze paresis), and 6 with horizontal comitant strabismus (all esotropia); (b) facial nerve palsy ($N = 17$, 20%); (c) abnormal lacrimation ($N = 17$, 20%); (d) coloboma of uvea and optic disc ($N = 1$, 1%) or optic disc only ($N = 2$, 2%); (e) microphthalmos ($N = 2$, 2%); and (f) one each of congenital glaucoma, conjunctival lipodermoid, and hypertelorism (75).

In a subsequent paper, the authors again reviewed the above ocular findings but also included the multiple other thalidomide-induced defects that were found in the 86 subjects (18). The defects and the number of cases for each were (note that all cases had more than one defect): thumbs (triphalangeal, absent, misplaced, hypoplastic, or extra digit) $N = 70$ (81%), upper limb excluding thumb $N = 59$ (69%), lower limb $N = 21$ (24%), ears/hearing $N = 33$ (38%), facial nerve palsy $N = 17$ (20%), kidney (absent, horseshoe, hydronephrosis, dysfunctional) $N = 12$ (14%), cardiovascular (ventricular septal defect [VSD], arrhythmia, ductus botalli, murmur) $N = 7$ (8%), chest/lung (cardiovascular defects, pulmonary atresia, enlarged chest wall or structural anomaly) $N = 4$ (5%), genitalia (absent uterus and vagina, double vagina) $N = 3$ (3%), anal atresia $N = 4$ (5%), choanal atresia $N = 2$ (2%), dental anomalies $N = 4$ (5%), mental retardation (moderate to severe) $N = 5$ (6%), and autism (all had mental retardation) $N = 4$ (5%) (18). The authors also expanded the type of ocular malformations listed in their previous study (reference 73) to include two cases of myelinated nerve fiber, two cases of ptosis, and one additional case each of coloboma (uveal or optic disc) and microphthalmos (18).

Neurologic complications of thalidomide embryopathy include epilepsy. In a study that appeared in 1976, the incidence of epilepsy was determined from a database that included all surviving children ($N = 408$) with documented thalidomide embryopathy in the United Kingdom (76). Seven children (1.7%) met established criteria for the diagnosis of epilepsy and were classified into two groups: (a) children with normal ears (four had upper limb defects, two had mental impairment, and one had ocular anomalies, facial palsy, and "high intelligence") ($N = 4$); and (b) children with abnormal ears (in addition, one had ocular defects and facial palsy, one had defects of the thumbs, and one had facial palsy and bilateral sixth nerve palsies) ($N = 3$) (76). In a third group, those with cardiac abnormalities, the diagnosis of epilepsy was uncertain. The two children in this group also had other defects consisting of amelia of the upper limbs, pyloric stenosis, and ocular and ear defects in one, and upper limb defects in the other. These two cases were apparently excluded from the prevalence rate calculations below. The prevalence rates of epilepsy calculated for various ages were significant when compared with published rates in the population as a whole: active epilepsy—5 cases, 12.5/1000 vs. 2.7/1000 ($p < 0.01$); epilepsy between birth and 9 years of age—7 cases, 17.2/1000 vs. 2.42/1000 ($p < 0.0001$); and new cases in first 7 years of life—6 cases, 2.1/1000 vs. 0.43/1000 ($p < 0.01$) (76). The types of epilepsy in the first group (normal ears) were thought to be consistent with structural defects of the cerebral cortex (76). Moreover, two of the children in this group had severe refractory epilepsy, a prevalence of 5/1000 vs. 0.5/1000 in the general population. The unlocalized or generalized seizures in the second group (abnormal ears) suggested abnormalities in the brain stem (76).

Five subjects, suspected of having a severe learning disorder (IQ scores <20 to 70–84), were identified from a group of 100 patients previously studied for ocular malformations (77). The five cases were then evaluated for the presence of autism. The ages of the subjects (three males, two females) ranged from 30 to 31 years. All had physical stigmata (i.e., ocular motility defects, other cranial nerve disorders, ear and upper-limb anomalies) characteristic of thalidomide embryopathy that had occurred from drug exposure approximately 20–24 days after conception (34–38 days after LMP). Four of the cases (two males, two females) met the criteria for autism. Based on an incidence of 4%, compared with a prevalence of about 0.08% in the general population, the investigators estimated that there was a 50 times higher rate of autism in those with thalidomide embryopathy (77).

A 1977 report evaluated the spinal deformities in 28 children, ages 10–14 years, who had thalidomide embryopathy (78). The children's spinal defects had been first studied at 4–8 years of age (79), and the current study was part of a continuing evaluation of their status. The initial group contained 32 cases, but 4 were either lost to follow-up or had died. All of the subjects had characteristic limb defects. In both studies, the spinal abnormalities were classified into five types. The initial and current (shown in *italics*) findings for each group were: (a) local anomalies of bone development (spina bifida, $N = 3$; fusion of adjacent spinous processes, $N = 2$), *neural arch defect more obvious, increased number of minor changes*; (b) scoliosis ($N = 18$), *20 children now had scoliosis*; (c) wedge deformity of solitary vertebral bodies ($N = 4$), *worsened in four cases*; (d) disc space calcification ($N = 3$); and (e) end-plate and disc defects ($N = 16$), *two additional cases of vertebral fusion, extension of fusion in two others, reduction in lumbar lordosis in 10 cases* (78).

The pregnancy outcomes of women with thalidomide embryopathy were presented in a 1988 publication (80), and also discussed in 1989 (83). The pregnancy of one woman was described in detail (80). This case involved a 24-year-old primigravida with upper limb amelia and lower limb phocomelia. Although there were many technical difficulties (e.g., blood pressure determination, blood sampling, and obesity), she eventually delivered a term, 3.4-kg healthy female infant without any apparent abnormalities. The baby was doing well at the first postnatal check. During the cesarean section, a left rudimentary uterine horn was noted that did not communicate with the uterine cavity (80). Supplementing their case history, the authors described the outcomes of 70 pregnancies in 35 women (includes the case history) who were living in England and who had thalidomide embryopathy (8 with absent upper and/or lower limbs; 27 with minor disabilities of the upper limbs and ears). Six miscarriages (9%) had occurred, but there were no congenital malformations in the 64 live births (80).

Renal failure complicated the fifth pregnancy of a 26-year-old woman with upper limb phocomelia and kidney and ureter malformations secondary to thalidomide (81). At 11 years of age, bilateral refluxing megaureters with dilated calices and thinning of the renal cortex were diagnosed because of chronic urinary tract infections and she underwent a bilateral antireflux procedure. Her first pregnancy, at 19 years of age, had been normotensive but complicated by proteinuria, hematuria, and premature labor thought to have been precipitated by a urinary tract infection. She had delivered a 660-g female infant who was currently alive and well. Her next three pregnancies resulted in a spontaneous abortion and two elective terminations. At 24 weeks' gestation in the index pregnancy, complications included normochromic normocytic anemia, hypertension, proteinuria, hematuria, urinary tract infection, and renal failure (creatinine clearance 11 mL/minute). A renal ultrasound revealed small kidneys with diffuse caliceal clubbing, a very thin parenchyma, and dilated ureters to the bladder (81). Peritoneal dialysis, in addition to antihypertensive, antibiotic, and iron therapy, was initiated with ritodrine tocolysis. Two weeks later, however, ultrasound confirmed that no fetal growth had occurred and her hypertension and renal failure had worsened. A cesarean section was performed to deliver a 460-g male infant who died 6 hours after birth. Because of her continued renal failure, the patient eventually received a kidney transplant (81).

The mechanism of thalidomide-induced malformations is unknown. The findings of many investigations have been discussed in reviews published in 1988 (84) and 2000 (85,86). Four other references (87–90) have developed additional hypotheses to explain how thalidomide causes structural defects.

A review published in 1988 listed 24 proposed mechanisms for thalidomide teratogenesis (84). Eight of the proposals were rejected by the author for various reasons.

The remaining 16 proposed mechanisms were classified as those involving biochemical or molecular mechanisms ($N = 9$), cellular mechanisms ($N = 2$), or tissue-level mechanisms ($N = 5$) (84). The absence of solid experimental evidence for the proposed mechanisms, however, led the author to the conclusion that none of the proposals could adequately account for thalidomide teratogenicity (84).

The role of a toxic arene oxide metabolite was thought to be involved in thalidomide teratogenicity according to a 1981 study (87). In an in vitro experiment, the human lymphocyte toxicity of a thalidomide metabolite was enhanced in the presence of epoxide hydrolase inhibitors and abolished by addition of the pure enzyme. The toxic thalidomide metabolite was not produced by rat liver microsomes, but was produced in hepatic preparations from maternal rabbits, and fetal rabbits, monkeys, and humans. These results were consistent with the lack of sensitivity to thalidomide teratogenesis in the rat vs. the sensitivity of rabbits, monkeys, and humans (87). A decrease in ascorbic acid (vitamin C) levels has been suggested as a mechanism of thalidomide teratogenesis (88). Two important consequences of ascorbic acid deficiency in the fetus would be inhibition of collagen synthesis and disruption of the development of nerve ganglia innervating limb buds (88).

A 1996 research study used developing chick embryos to test the hypothesis that elimination of the mesonephros, in the absence of scarring, would produce limb abnormalities similar to those observed with thalidomide (89). Tantalum foil barriers were used at various levels of the intermediate mesoderm to prevent caudal elongation of the mesonephros. Limb reduction defects were produced when the mesonephros was prevented from forming caudal to somite 14. The types and percentage of limb defects in the chick embryos were: upper limb only (57%), upper and lower limb (31%), and lower limb only (12%). In comparison, the corresponding percentages of limb reduction defects in 1252 human cases of thalidomide embryopathy were 64%, 34%, and 2%, respectively (89). Based on these results and previous studies, the investigators concluded that disruption of the mesonephros (or factors produced in the mesonephros) results in limb reduction defects and that the mechanism of thalidomide-induced limb anomalies probably also involves disruption of the mesonephros (89).

Whole embryo culture was used in a study directly comparing thalidomide-resistant rats and thalidomide-sensitive rabbits (90). Various concentrations of thalidomide were shown to significantly decrease the concentration of glutathione in rabbit visceral yolk sacs, but not in the rat. Cysteine concentrations were not affected in either species, but the cysteine levels in control rabbits were 65% lower than those in control rats. Thus, a possible role for glutathione was suggested by the results (90).

In a study published in 1996, a highly teratogenic derivative of thalidomide (EM12) was used in an experiment with nonhuman primates (marmosets) (91). EM12 was chosen because it is a more potent teratogen than thalidomide; it is more stable to hydrolysis and produces a teratogenic incidence close to 100% in the marmoset. Moreover, the pattern of malformations produced in the marmoset is identical to those seen in humans after in utero exposure to thalidomide (91). The data indicated that thalidomide produced a statistically significant downregulation (in some cases, complete disappearance) of several surface adhesion receptors found on early limb bud cells and other organs. The adhesion receptors identified were receptors of the integrin family (β_1-integrins, β_2-integrins, and β_3-integrins), the immunoglobulin family, and the selectin family. These receptors are involved in the development of the limbs, heart, head, and body. The downregulation of these receptors, which was most pronounced in those involved with limb development, was expected to alter cell–cell and cell–extracellular matrix interactions (91).

A 1998 communication proposed that the mechanism of limb reduction anomalies induced by thalidomide was related to the inhibition of mesenchymal proliferation in the limb bud (92). In the progress-zone model, the proximal and distal structures of the limb are specified sequentially by a continuous signal (thought to be fibroblast growth factor [FGF]) from the apical ectodermal ridge (92). The mesenchyme at the tip of the limb bud is respecified by FGF to produce distal structures, whereas those not receiving a continuous FGF signal develop into proximal structures. If thalidomide blocks mesenchymal cell growth, all of the progress-zone cells remain under the influence of FGF and are programmed to form the only distal most elements (i.e., a phocomelia) (92).

Two 2000 reviews by the same group of investigators evaluated 30 mechanistic hypotheses of thalidomide embryopathy (85,86). Of the proposals, 14 were rejected because they were either unsubstantiated or had not been proved to be viable. The 16 remaining hypotheses were grouped into 6 categories with thalidomide affecting: (a) DNA synthesis or transcription, synthesis and/or function of (b) growth factors (insulin-like growth factor and FGF); or (c) integrins (α subunit type v and β subunit type 3); (d) angiogenesis; (e) chondrogenesis; or (f) cell death or injury (85,86). The hypotheses were not thought to be necessarily mutually exclusive, but could eventually be fitted into a unified model (85,86). Citing evidence from the literature, they proposed that thalidomide, or a metabolite, intercalates into the DNA of specific promoter regions of genes that code for proteins involved in normal limb development. The binding of thalidomide would inhibit the transcription of these genes, resulting in interference with the development of new blood vessels and leading to truncation of the limb (85,86).

Although thalidomide was withdrawn from England and the European markets in late 1961, the agent has continued to be available in 8 of 10 South American countries for the treatment of leprosy (56,93). Thalidomide is manufactured in Argentina and Brazil and is available either through pharmacies (Brazil) or government health agencies (Brazil and Argentina) (93). A 1987 case report from Brazil described a 17-week-old fetus that was diagnosed by prenatal ultrasound with malformations secondary to thalidomide (56). After pregnancy termination, an autopsy revealed upper limb phocomelia, absent tibiae and fibulae (both feet connected directly to the femora), missing toes on both feet, and absent external ears (56). This case was apparently the first to report a prenatal diagnosis of thalidomide syndrome (56). In a second report, 34 children with thalidomide embryopathy who were born in South America after 1965 were identified by the Latin American Collaborative Study of Congenital Malformations (ECLAMC) in endemic areas for leprosy (93). Specific details of the typical thalidomide-induced malformations in 11 of these cases (including the case in reference 56) were presented.

A study published in 1988 reviewed the history of thalidomide embryopathy and cited 4336 cases that had been identified in various countries (20). The number of cases was considered a minimal estimate, however, because stillborns and early deaths were underrepresented and the ascertainment of surviving cases in many countries was thought to be incomplete (20). The countries and the number of affected fetuses/infants are shown below. Note that none of the cases from the United States (resulting from thalidomide obtained elsewhere) were included.

Country	Number of Affected Fetuses/Infants
Australia	26
Austria	7
Belgium	35
Brazil	99
Canada	122
Denmark	20
Finland	8
Ireland	51
Italy	86
Japan	299
Mexico	4
Netherlands	34
Norway	11
Portugal	8
Spain	5
Sweden	153
Switzerland	12
Taiwan	36
United Kingdom	271
West Germany	3049

Seventeen years before the above report, a review on the medicolegal implications of the thalidomide tragedy estimated that a total of 5000–6000 babies had been affected, about 4000 of these in West Germany (94).

The critical maternal dose is at least 100 mg (95). However, normal pregnancy outcomes have occurred, even when thalidomide was taken during the critical period (45,96). In addition, other causes of limb reduction defects and heart defects, such as Holt-Oram syndrome, may mimic thalidomide-induced malformations (19).

The risk of congenital malformations after exposure during the critical period has been estimated to be between 20% and 50% (17). The large degree of uncertainty in the estimated risk is a result of the lack of epidemiologic studies and any organized attempt to determine the number of normal, yet exposed children (17). Just as uncertain, because it is based on only four reports, the frequency of specific malformations is thought to be in the following order: arms only > arms and legs > ears only > arms and ears ≥ arms, legs, and ears > legs only (62,66,70,89). The frequencies of the other malformations associated with thalidomide are unknown, partially because many of them were determined at autopsy, were only recognized later in life or in specialized groups, or have not been fully analyzed.

Although thalidomide had not been approved for use in the United States when thalidomide embryopathy was discovered, at least 17 such cases were delivered in this country, apparently from women who had received the drug elsewhere (10,94). Fortunately, thalidomide did not receive approval in the United States because of the alertness of the FDA (94,97). Thalidomide is indicated (FDA approved) for the treatment of a leprosy skin complication (erythema nodosum leprosum) (1), but it may also have eventual application in other serious conditions, such as chronic graft-versus-host disease, rash due to systemic lupus erythematosus, Behcet's syndrome, inflammatory bowel disease, prostate cancer, metastatic breast cancer, rheumatoid arthritis, uremic pruritus, severe atopic erythroderma, weight loss in tuberculosis, and in the complications of acquired immunodeficiency syndrome (aphthous ulcers, microsporidioses diarrhea, macular degeneration, wasting, Kaposi's sarcoma, and HIV replication) (85,98,99). The mechanism of action of thalidomide teratogenesis is unknown, but recent investigations have suggested that it involves disruption of specific genes involved in normal limb development. If the mechanism can be fully understood, development of nonteratogenic derivatives, that retain the ability to treat disease, may be possible (85,86).

Thalidomide is contraindicated during pregnancy and in women of childbearing age who are not receiving two reliable methods of contraception for 1 month prior to starting therapy, during therapy, and for 1 month after stopping therapy (1). In addition, it is contraindicated in women who do not meet the specific requirements of the STEPS program (System for Thalidomide Education and Prescribing Safety). The STEPS program was developed by the manufacturer to limit the prescribing and use of thalidomide to tightly controlled situations and to prevent inadvertent exposure of pregnant women (1,99). Any suspected fetal exposure to thalidomide should be reported to the FDA (Medwatch Program at 1-800-FDA-1088) and/or to the manufacturer (1).

BREASTFEEDING SUMMARY

No reports describing the use of thalidomide during lactation have been located. The molecular weight (about 258) is low enough that excretion into milk should be expected. Moreover, nothing is known about the excretion of thalidomide metabolites into breast milk. Women who are taking thalidomide should not nurse because the effect on an infant from exposure to thalidomide and its metabolites in breast milk is unknown.

References

1. Product information. Thalomid. Celgene Corporation, 2000.
2. Nishimura H, Tanimura T. *Clinical Aspects of The Teratogenicity of Drugs*. New York, NY: American Elsevier Publishing Company, 1976:292–7.
3. Parkhie M, Webb M. Embryotoxicity and teratogenicity of thalidomide in rats. Teratology 1983;27:327–32.
4. Somers GF. Thalidomide and congenital abnormalities. Lancet 1962;1: 912–3.
5. Spencer KEV. Thalidomide and congenital abnormalities. Lancet 1962;2:100.
6. Dekker A, Mehrizi A. The use of thalidomide as a teratogenic agent in rabbits. Bull Johns Hopkins Hosp 1964;115:223–30.

T

7. Vickers TH. Concerning the morphogenesis of thalidomide dysmelia in rabbits. Br J Exp Pathol 1967;48:579–92.
8. Sterz H, Nothdurft H, Lexa P, Ockenfels H. Teratologic studies on the Himalayan rabbit: new aspects of thalidomide-induced teratogenesis. Arch Toxicol 1987;60:376–81.
9. Gilani SH. Cardiovascular malformations in the chick embryo induced by thalidomide. Toxicol Appl Pharmacol 1973;25:77–83.
10. Mellin GW, Katzenstein M. The saga of thalidomide. Neuropathy to embryopathy, with case reports of congenital anomalies. N Engl J Med 1962;267:1184–93.
11. Mellin GW, Katzenstein M. The saga of thalidomide (concluded). Neuropathy to embryopathy, with case reports of congenital anomalies. N Engl J Med 1962;267:1238–44.
12. Taussig HB. A study of the German outbreak of phocomelia. JAMA 1962;180:1106–14.
13. Nowack E. The sensitive period of thalidomide embryopathy (in German). Humangenetik 1965;1:516–36.
14. Smithells RW. The thalidomide legacy. Proc R Soc Med 1965;58:491–2.
15. Newman CGH. Clinical observations on the thalidomide syndrome. Proc R Soc Med 1977;70:225–7.
16. Newman CGH. Teratogen update: clinical aspects of thalidomide embryopathy—a continuing preoccupation. Teratology 1985;32:133–44.
17. Newman CGH. The thalidomide syndrome: risks of exposure and spectrum of malformations. Clin Perinatol 1986;13:555–73.
18. Miller MT, Stromland K. Teratogen update: thalidomide: a review, with focus on ocular findings and new potential uses. Teratology 1999;60:306–21.
19. Brent RL, Holmes LB. Clinical and basic science lessons from the thalidomide tragedy: what have we learned about the causes of limb defects? Teratology 1988;38:241–51.
20. Lenz W. A short history of thalidomide embryopathy. Teratology 1988;38:203–15.
21. Hayman DJ. Distaval. Lancet 1961;2:1262.
22. Kosenow W, Pfeiffer RA. *Micromelia, Haemangioma und Duodenal Stenosis Exhibit*. Kassel: German Pediatric Society, 1960. As cited by Taussig HB. A study of the German outbreak of phocomelia. JAMA 1962;180:1106–14.
23. Lenz W. Thalidomide and congenital abnormalities. Lancet 1962;1:45.
24. McBride WG. Thalidomide and congenital abnormalities. Lancet 1961;2:1358.
25. Pfeiffer RA, Kosenow W. Thalidomide and congenital abnormalities. Lancet 1962;1:45–6.
26. Jones EE, Williamson DAJ. Thalidomide and congenital abnormalities. Lancet 1962;1:222.
27. Burley DM. Thalidomide and congenital abnormalities. Lancet 1962;1:271.
28. Lenz W. Thalidomide and congenital abnormalities. Lancet 1962;1:271–2.
29. Speirs AL. Thalidomide and congenital abnormalities. Lancet 1962;1:303–5.
30. Anonymous. Thalidomide and congenital malformations. Lancet 1962;1:307–8.
31. Kohler HG, Fisher AM, Dunn PM. Thalidomide and congenital abnormalities. Lancet 1962;1:326.
32. Willman A, Dumoulin JG. Thalidomide ("Distaval") and foetal abnormalities. Br Med J 1962;1:477.
33. Pliess G. Thalidomide and congenital abnormalities. Lancet 1962;1:1128–9.
34. Rodin AE, Koller LA, Taylor JD. Association of thalidomide (Kevadon) with congenital anomalies. Can Med Assoc J 1962;86:744–6.
35. Smithells RW. Thalidomide and malformations in Liverpool. Lancet 1962;1:1270–3.
36. Kajii T. Thalidomide and congenital deformities. Lancet 1962;2:151.
37. Leck IM, Millar ELM. Incidence of malformations since the introduction of thalidomide. Br Med J 1962;2:16–20.
38. Jacobs J. Drugs and foetal abnormalities. Br Med J 1962;2:407.
39. Pfeiffer RA, Nessel E. Multiple congenital abnormalities. Lancet 1962;2:349–50.
40. Ward SP. Thalidomide and congenital abnormalities. Br Med J 1962;2:646–7.
41. Knapp K, Lenz W, Nowack E. Multiple congenital abnormalities. Lancet 1962;2:725.
42. Owen R, Smith A. Cor triloculare and thalidomide. Lancet 1962;2:836.
43. Rosendal T. Thalidomide and aplasia-hypoplasia of the otic labyrinth. Lancet 1963;1:724–5.
44. Kajii T, Goto M. Cleft lip and palate after thalidomide. Lancet 1963;2:151–2.
45. McBride WG. The teratogenic action of drugs. Med J Aust 1963;2:689–93.
46. Cullen JF. Ocular defects in thalidomide babies. Br J Ophthalmol 1964;48:151–3.
47. Cant JS. Minor ocular abnormalities associated with thalidomide. Lancet 1966;1:1134.
48. Fogh-Andersen P. Thalidomide and congenital cleft deformities. Acta Chir Scand 1966;131:197–200.
49. Kajii T, Kida M, Takahashi K. The effect of thalidomide intake during 113 human pregnancies. Teratology 1973;8:163–6.
50. Murphy R, Mohr P. Two congenital neurological abnormalities caused by thalidomide. Br Med J 1977;2:1191.
51. Stainsby GD, Quibell EP. Perthes-like changes in the hips of children with thalidomide deformities. Lancet 1967;2:242–3.
52. Smithells RW. Thalidomide, absent appendix, and sweating. Lancet 1978;1:1042.
53. Bremner DN, Mooney G. Agenesis of appendix: a further thalidomide anomaly. Lancet 1978;1:826.
54. McBride WG. Excessive sweating and reduction deformities. Lancet 1978;1:826.
55. McBride WG. Another, late thalidomide abnormality. Lancet 1981;2:368.
56. Gollop TR, Eigier A, Guidugli-Neto J. Prenatal diagnosis of thalidomide syndrome. Prenat Diag 1987;7:295–8.
57. Hagen EO. Congenital malformations in a thalidomide baby: a postmortem anatomical study. Can Med Assoc J 1965;92:283–6.
58. Hammarstrom L, Henrikson CO, Larsson KS. Anomalies of the teeth in a child with upper phocomelia. Report of a case. Oral Surg 1970;29:191–6.
59. Shand JEG, Bremner DN. Agenesis of the vermiform appendix in a thalidomide child. Br J Surg 1977;64:203–4.
60. Axrup K, d'Avignon M, Hellgren K, Henrikson C-O, Juhlin I-M, Larsson KS, Persson GE, Welander E. Children with thalidomide embryopathy: odontologic observations and aspects. Dental Digest 1966;72:403–5425.
61. Ruffing L. Evaluation of thalidomide children. Birth Defects Orig Article Ser 1977;13:287–300.
62. Lenz W, Knapp K. Thalidomide embryopathy. Arch Environ Health 1962;5:100–5.
63. Lenz W. Malformations caused by drugs in pregnancy. Am J Dis Child 1966;112:99–106.
64. Lenz W. How can the teratogenic action of a factor be established in man? South Med J 1971;64(Suppl 1):41–7.
65. Tabuchi A, Yamada A, Umisa H, Shintani T, Horikawa M, Shirasuna K, Sawasaki M. Phocomelia-like deformity and thalidomide preparations. Hiroshima J Med Sci 1963;12:11–35.
66. Kajii T. Thalidomide experience in Japan. Ann Paediatr 1965;205:341–54.
67. Livingstone G. Congenital ear abnormalities due to thalidomide. Proc R Soc Med 1965;58:493–7.
68. Takemori S, Tanaka Y, Suzuki J-I. Thalidomide anomalies of the ear. Arch Otolaryngol 1976;102:425–7.
69. Stahl A. Clinical, orthodontic, and radiological findings in the jaws and face of children with dysmelia associated with thalidomide-embryopathy. Inter Dental J 1968;18:631–8.
70. Smithells RW. Defects and disabilities of thalidomide children. Br Med J 1973;1:269–72.
71. Gilkes MJ, Strode M. Ocular anomalies in association with developmental limb abnormalities of drug origin. Lancet 1963;1:1026–7.
72. Zetterstrom B. Ocular malformations caused by thalidomide. Acta Ophthalmol 1966;44:391–5.
73. Rafuse EV, Arstikaitis M, Brent HP. Ocular findings in thalidomide children. Can J Ophthalmol 1967;2:222–5.
74. Miller MT, Stromland K. Ocular motility in thalidomide embryopathy. J Pediatr Ophthalmol Strab 1991;28:47–54.
75. Stromland K, Miller MT. Thalidomide embryopathy: revisited 27 years later. Acta Ophthalmol 1993;71:238–45.
76. Stephenson JBP. Epilepsy: a neurological complication of thalidomide embryopathy. Dev Med Child Neurol 1976;18:189–97.
77. Stromland K, Nordin V, Miller M, Akerstrom B, Gillberg C. Autism in thalidomide embryopathy: a population study. Dev Med Child Neurol 1994;36:351–6.
78. Edwards DH, Nichols PJR. The spinal abnormalities in thalidomide embryopathy. Acta Orthop Scand 1977;48:273–6.
79. Nichols PJR, Boldero JL, Goodfellow JW, Hamilton A. Abnormalities of the vertebral column associated with thalidomide-induced limb deformities. Orthop (Oxford) 1968;1:71–90. As cited by Edwards DH, Nichols PJR. The spinal abnormalities in thalidomide embryopathy. Acta Orthop Scand 1977;48:273–6.
80. Maouris PG, Hirsch PJ. Pregnancy in women with thalidomide-induced disabilities. Case report and a questionnaire study. Br J Obstet Gynecol 1988;95:717–9.
81. Brown MA, Farrell C, Newton P, Child RP. Thalidomide, pregnancy and renal failure. Med J Aust 1990;152:148–9.
82. Warkany J. How can the teratogenic action of a factor be established in man? Comments. South Med J 1971;64(Suppl 1):48–50.

83. Chamberlain G. The obstetric problems of the thalidomide children. Br Med J 1989;298:6.
84. Stephens TD. Proposed mechanisms of action in thalidomide embryopathy. Teratology 1988;38:229–39.
85. Stephens TD, Fillmore BJ. Hypothesis: thalidomide embryopathy-proposed mechanism of action. Teratology 2000;61:189–95.
86. Stephens TD, Bunde CJW, Fillmore BJ. Mechanism of action in thalidomide teratogenesis. Biochem Pharmacol 2000;59:1489–99.
87. Gordon GB, Spielberg SP, Blake DA, Balasubramanian V. Thalidomide teratogenesis: evidence for a toxic arene oxide metabolite. Proc Natl Acad Sci USA 1981;78:2545–8.
88. Vaisman B. To the editor. Teratology 1996;53:283–4.
89. Smith DM, Torres RD, Stephens TD. Mesonephros has a role in limb development and is related to thalidomide embryopathy. Teratology 1996;54:126–34.
90. Hansen JM, Carney EW, Harris C. Differential alteration by thalidomide of the glutathione content of rat vs. rabbit conceptuses in vitro. Reprod Toxicol 1999;13:547–54.
91. Neubert R, Hinz N, Thiel R, Neubert D. Down-regulation of adhesion receptors on cells of primate embryos as a probable mechanism of the teratogenic action of thalidomide. Life Sci 1996;58:295–316.
92. Tabin CJ. A developmental model for thalidomide defects. Nature 1998;396:322–3.
93. Castilla EE, Ashton-Prolla P, Barreda-Mejia E, Brunoni D, Cavalcanti DP, Correa-Neto J, Delgadillo JL, Dutra MG, Felix T, Giraldo A, Juarez N, Lopez-Camelo JS, Nazer J, Orioli IM, Paz JE, Pessoto MA, Pina-Neto JM, Quadrelli R, Rittler M, Rueda S, Saltos M, Sanchez O, Schuler L. Thalidomide, a current teratogen in South America. Teratology 1996;54:273–7.
94. Curran WJ. The thalidomide tragedy in Germany: the end of a historic medicolegal trial. N Engl J Med 1971;284:481–2.
95. Buyse ML, ed. *Birth Defects Encyclopedia*. Volume 1. Dover, MA: Center for Birth Defects Information Services, 1990:726–7.
96. Pembrey ME, Clarke CA. Normal child after maternal thalidomide ingestion in critical period of pregnancy. Lancet 1970;1:275–7.
97. McFadyen RE. Thalidomide in America: a brush with tragedy. Clin Medica 1976;11:79–93.
98. Friedman JM, Kimmel CA. Teratology Society 1988 Public Affairs Committee symposium: the new thalidomide era: dealing with the risks. Teratology 1999;59:120–3.
99. Public Affairs Committee, Teratology Society. Teratology Society Public Affairs Committee position paper: thalidomide. Teratology 2000;62: 172–3.

THEOPHYLLINE

Respiratory Drug (Bronchodilator)

PREGNANCY RECOMMENDATION: Compatible
BREASTFEEDING RECOMMENDATION: Compatible

PREGNANCY SUMMARY

Theophylline is the bronchodilator of choice for asthma and chronic obstructive pulmonary disease in the pregnant patient (1–6). No published reports linking the use of theophylline with congenital defects have been located.

FETAL RISK SUMMARY

Reproduction studies in mice and rats at oral doses up to about 2 and 3 times, respectively, the recommended human dose based on BSA (RHD) revealed no evidence of teratogenicity (7). At a slightly lower dose (about 2.5 times the RHD) in rats, embryo toxicity, but not maternal toxicity, was observed.

In a surveillance study of Michigan Medicaid recipients involving 229,101 completed pregnancies conducted between 1985 and 1992, 1240 newborns had been exposed to theophylline and 36 to aminophylline during the 1st trimester (F. Rosa, personal communication, FDA, 1993). A total of 68 (5.5%) major birth defects were observed (53 expected) with theophylline and 1 (2.8%) major defect (2 expected) with aminophylline. For theophylline, specific data were available for six defect categories, including (observed/expected) 20/12 cardiovascular defects, 5/1 oral clefts, 2/0.5 spina bifida, 5/4 polydactyly, 0/2 limb reduction defects, and 2/3 hypospadias. Three of the defect categories, cardiovascular, oral clefts, and spina bifida, suggest an association with the drug, but other factors, such as the mother's disease, concurrent drug use, and chance, may be involved. For aminophylline, the single defect was a polydactyly.

The Collaborative Perinatal Project monitored 193 mother–child pairs with 1st trimester exposure to theophylline or aminophylline (8). No evidence was found for an association with malformations.

Theophylline crosses the placenta, and newborn infants may have therapeutic serum levels (9–13). Transient tachycardia, irritability, and vomiting have been reported in newborns delivered from mothers consuming theophylline (9,10). These effects are more likely to occur when maternal serum levels at term are in the high therapeutic range or above (therapeutic range 8–20 mcg/mL) (11). Cord blood levels are approximately 100% of the maternal serum concentration (12,13).

In patients at risk for premature delivery, aminophylline (theophylline ethylenediamine) was found to exert a beneficial effect by reducing the perinatal death rate and the frequency of respiratory distress syndrome (14,15). In a nonrandomized study, aminophylline 250 mg IM every 12 hours up to a maximum of 3 days was compared with betamethasone, 4 mg IM every 8 hours for 2 days (15). Patients in the aminophylline group were excluded from receiving corticosteroids because of diabetes (4 patients), hypertension (10 patients), and ruptured membranes for more than 24 hours (4 patients). The aminophylline and steroid groups were comparable in length of gestation (32.5 vs. 32.1 weeks), male:female infant sex ratio (10:8 vs. 8:8), Apgar score (7.6 vs. 7.7), birth weight (1720 vs. 1690 g), and hours between treatment and delivery (73 vs. 68). Respiratory distress syndrome occurred in 11% (2 of 18) of the aminophylline group compared with 0% (0 of 16) of the corticosteroid group (*ns*). A significant difference ($p = 0.01$) was found in the incidence of neonatal infection with 8 of 16 (50%) of the betamethasone group having signs of infection and none in the aminophylline group. The mechanism proposed for aminophylline-induced fetal lung maturation is similar to that observed with betamethasone: enhancement of tissue cyclic adenosine monophosphate (AMP) by inhibition of cyclic AMP phosphodiesterase and a corresponding increased production and/or release of phosphatidylcholine (15).

An IV infusion of aminophylline has been tested for its tocolytic effects on oxytocin-induced uterine contractions (16). A slight decrease in uterine activity occurred in the first 15 minutes, but this was related to the effect on contraction intensity, not frequency. The author concluded that aminophylline was a poor tocolytic agent. However, a more recent in vitro study examined the effect of increasing concentrations of aminophylline on pregnant human myometrium (17). Aminophylline produced a dose-related decrease in contraction strength and a nondose-dependent lengthening of the period of contraction. In this study, the authors concluded that aminophylline may be a clinically useful tocolytic agent (17).

A reduction in the occurrence of preeclampsia among pregnant asthmatic women treated with theophylline has been reported (18). Preeclampsia occurred in 1.2% (1 of 85) of patients treated with theophylline compared with 8.8% (6/68) ($p < 0.05$) of asthmatic patients not treated with the drug. Although the results were significant, the small numbers indicate that the results must be interpreted cautiously (18). The authors proposed a possible mechanism for the protective effect, if indeed it does occur, involving the inhibition of platelet aggregation and the altering of vascular tone, two known effects of theophylline (18).

Concern over the depressant effects of methylxanthines on lipid synthesis in developing neural systems has been reported (19). Recent observations that infants treated for apnea with theophylline exhibit no overt neurologic deficits at 9–27 months of age are encouraging (20,21). However, the long-term effects of these drugs on human brain development are not known (19).

Frequent, high-dose asthmatic medication containing theophylline, ephedrine, phenobarbital, and diphenhydramine was used throughout pregnancy by one woman who delivered a stillborn girl with complete triploidy (22). Although drug-induced chromosomal damage could not be proven, theophylline has been shown in in vitro tests to cause breakage of chromosomes in human lymphocytes (23). However, the clinical significance of this breakage is doubtful.

Theophylline withdrawal in a newborn exposed throughout gestation has been reported (12). Apneic spells developed at 28 hours after delivery and they became progressively worse over the next 4 days. Therapy with theophylline resolved the spells.

The pharmacokinetics of theophylline during pregnancy has been studied (24,25). One report suggested that plasma concentrations of theophylline fall during the 3rd trimester because of an increased maternal volume of distribution (24). However, a more recent study found a significantly lower clearance of theophylline during the 3rd trimester, ranging in some cases between 20% and 53% (25). Two women had symptoms of toxicity requiring a dosage reduction.

BREASTFEEDING SUMMARY

Theophylline is excreted into breast milk (26,27). A milk:plasma ratio of 0.7 has been measured (27). Estimates indicate that <1% of the maternal dose is excreted into breast milk (26,27). However, one infant became irritable secondary to a rapidly absorbed oral solution of aminophylline taken by the mother (26). Because very young infants may be more sensitive to levels that would be nontoxic in older infants, less rapidly absorbed theophylline preparations may be advisable for nursing mothers (10,28). Except for the precaution that theophylline may cause irritability in the nursing infant, the American Academy of Pediatrics classifies the drug as compatible with breastfeeding (29).

References

1. Greenberger P, Patterson R. Safety of therapy for allergic symptoms during pregnancy. Ann Intern Med 1978;89:234–7.
2. Weinstein AM, Dubin BD, Podleski WK, Spector SL, Farr RS. Asthma and pregnancy. JAMA 1979;241:1161–5.
3. Hernandez E, Angell CS, Johnson JWC. Asthma in pregnancy: current concepts. Obstet Gynecol 1980;55:739–43.
4. Turner ES, Greenberger PA, Patterson R. Management of the pregnant asthmatic patient. Ann Intern Med 1980;93:905–18.
5. Pratt WR. Allergic diseases in pregnancy and breast feeding. Ann Allergy 1981;47:355–60.
6. Lalli CM, Raju L. Pregnancy and chronic obstructive pulmonary disease. Chest 1981;80:759–61.
7. Product information. Theo-Dur. Key Pharmaceuticals, 2000.
8. Heinonen OP, Slone D, Shapiro S. *Birth Defects and Drugs in Pregnancy*. Littleton, MA: Publishing Sciences Group, 1977:367, 370.
9. Arwood LL, Dasta JF, Friedman C. Placental transfer of theophylline: two case reports. Pediatrics 1979;63:844–6.
10. Yeh TF, Pildes RS. Transplacental aminophylline toxicity in a neonate. Lancet 1977;1:910.
11. Labovitz E, Spector S. Placental theophylline transfer in pregnant asthmatics. JAMA 1982;247:786–8.
12. Horowitz DA, Jablonski W, Mehta KA. Apnea associated with theophylline withdrawal in a term neonate. Am J Dis Child 1982;136:73–4.
13. Ron M, Hochner-Celnikier D, Menczel J, Palti Z, Kidroni G. Maternal–fetal transfer of aminophylline. Acta Obstet Gynecol Scand 1984;63:217–8.
14. Hadjigeorgiou E, Kitsiou S, Psaroudakis A, Segos C, Nicolopoulos D, Kaskarelis D. Antepartum aminophylline treatment for prevention of the respiratory distress syndrome in premature infants. Am J Obstet Gynecol 1979;135:257–60.
15. Granati B, Grella PV, Pettenazzo A, Di Lenardo L, Rubaltelli FF. The prevention of respiratory distress syndrome in premature infants: efficacy of antenatal aminophylline treatment versus prenatal glucocorticoid administration. Pediatr Pharmacol (New York) 1984;4:21–4.
16. Lipshitz J. Uterine and cardiovascular effects of aminophylline. Am J Obstet Gynecol 1978;131:716–8.
17. Bird LM, Anderson NC Jr, Chandler ML, Young RC. The effects of aminophylline and nifedipine on contractility of isolated pregnant human myometrium. Am J Obstet Gynecol 1987;157:171–7.
18. Dombrowski MP, Bottoms SF, Boike GM, Wald J. Incidence of preeclampsia among asthmatic patients lower with theophylline. Am J Obstet Gynecol 1986;155:265–7.
19. Volpe JJ. Effects of methylxanthines on lipid synthesis in developing neural systems. Semin Perinatol 1981;5:395–405.
20. Aranda JV, Dupont C. Metabolic effects of methylxanthines in premature infants. J Pediatr 1976;89:833–4.
21. Nelson RM, Resnick MB, Holstrum WJ, Eitzman DV. Development outcome of premature infants treated with theophylline. Dev Pharmacol Ther 1980;1:274–80.
22. Halbrecht I, Komlos L, Shabtay F, Solomon M, Book JA. Triploidy 69, XXX in a stillborn girl. Clin Genet 1973;4:210–2.
23. Weinstein D, Mauer I, Katz ML, Kazmer S. The effect of methylxanthines on chromosomes of human lymphocytes in culture. Mutat Res 1975;31:57–61.
24. Sutton PL, Koup JR, Rose JQ, Middleton E. The pharmacokinetics of theophylline in pregnancy. J Allergy Clin Immunol 1978;61:174.
25. Carter BL, Driscoll CE, Smith GD. Theophylline clearance during pregnancy. Obstet Gynecol 1986;68:555–9.
26. Yurchak AM, Jusko WJ. Theophylline secretion into breast milk. Pediatrics 1976;57:518–25.
27. Stec GP, Greenberger P, Ruo TI, Henthorn T, Morita Y, Atkinson AJ Jr, Patterson R. Kinetics of theophylline transfer to breast milk. Clin Pharmacol Ther 1980;28:404–8.
28. Berlin CM. Excretion of methylxanthines in human milk. Semin Perinatol 1981;5:389–94.
29. Committee on Drugs, American Academy of Pediatrics. The transfer of drugs and other chemicals into human milk. Pediatrics 2001;108:776–89.

THIABENDAZOLE

[Withdrawn from the market. See 9th edition.]

THIAMINE

Vitamin

PREGNANCY RECOMMENDATION: Compatible
BREASTFEEDING RECOMMENDATION: Compatible

PREGNANCY SUMMARY

Thiamine is compatible with pregnancy, but doses above the RDA should be avoided.

FETAL RISK SUMMARY

Thiamine (vitamin B_1), a water-soluble B-complex vitamin, is an essential nutrient required for carbohydrate metabolism (1). The National Academy of Sciences' recommended dietary allowance (RDA) for thiamine in pregnancy is 1.5 mg (1).

Thiamine is actively transported to the fetus (2–5). As with other B-complex vitamins, concentrations of thiamine in the fetus and newborn are higher than in the mother (4–11).

Maternal thiamine deficiency is common during pregnancy (11,12). Supplementation with multivitamin products reduces the thiamine hypovitaminemia only slightly (9). Since 1938, several authors have attempted to link this deficiency to toxemia of pregnancy (13–16). A 1945 paper summarized the early work published in this area (14). All of the reported cases, however, involved patients with poor nutrition and pregnancy care in general. More recent investigations have failed to find any relationship between maternal thiamine deficiency and toxemia, fetal defects, or other outcomes of pregnancy (8,17).

No association was found between low birth weight and thiamine levels in a 1977 report (7). One group has shown experimentally, however, that the characteristic intrauterine growth restriction of the fetal alcohol syndrome may be caused by ethanol-induced thiamine deficiency (18).

Thiamine has been used to treat hyperemesis gravidarum, although pyridoxine (vitamin B_6) was found to be more effective (see Pyridoxine) (19–21). In one early report, thiamine was effective in reversing severe neurologic complications associated with hyperemesis (19). A mother treated with frequent injections of thiamine and pyridoxine, 50 mg each/dose, for hyperemesis during the first half of two pregnancies delivered two infants with severe convulsions, one of whom died within 30 hours of birth (21). The convulsions in the mentally slow second infant were eventually controlled with pyridoxine. Pyridoxine dependency–induced convulsions are rare. The authors speculated that the defect was caused by in utero exposure to high circulating levels of the vitamin. Thiamine was not thought to be involved (see Pyridoxine).

An isolated case report described an anencephalic fetus whose mother was under psychiatric care (22). She had been treated with very high doses of vitamins B_1, B_6, C, and folic acid. The relationship between the vitamins and the defect is unknown. Also unproven is the speculation by one researcher that an association exists between thiamine deficiency and Down's syndrome (trisomy 21) or preleukemic bone marrow changes (23).

BREASTFEEDING SUMMARY

Thiamine (vitamin B_1) is excreted into breast milk (24–27). One group of investigators supplemented well-nourished lactating women with a multivitamin preparation containing 1.7 mg of thiamine (24). At 6 months postpartum, milk concentrations of thiamine did not differ significantly from those of control patients not receiving supplements. In a study of lactating women with low nutritional status, supplementation with thiamine (0.2–20.0 mg/day) resulted in mean milk concentrations of 125–268 ng/mL (25). Milk concentrations were directly proportional to dietary intake. A 1983 English study measured thiamine levels in pooled human milk obtained from preterm (26 mothers: 29–34 weeks) and term (35 mothers: 39 weeks or longer) patients (26). Milk obtained from preterm mothers rose from 23.7 ng/mL (colostrum) to 89.3 ng/mL (16–196 days), whereas milk from term mothers increased during the same period from a level of 28.4 to 183 ng/mL.

In Asian mothers with severe thiamine deficiency, including some with beriberi, infants have become acutely ill after breastfeeding, leading in some cases to convulsions and sudden death (28–31). Pneumonia was usually a characteristic finding. One author thought the condition was related to toxic intermediary metabolites, such as methylglyoxal, passing to the infant via the milk (28). Although a cause-and-effect relationship has not been proven, one report suggested that thiamine deficiency may aggravate the condition (29). Indian investigators measured very low thiamine milk levels in mothers of children with convulsions of unknown cause (32). Mean milk thiamine concentrations in mothers of healthy children were 111 ng/mL, whereas those in mothers of children with convulsions were 29 ng/mL. The authors were unable to establish an association between the low thiamine content in milk and infantile convulsions (see Pyridoxine for correlation between low levels of vitamin B_6 and convulsions).

A 1992 case described the features of "Shoshin beriberi" in a 3-month-old breastfed infant (33). Both the infant and the mother had biochemical evidence of thiamine deficiency. Clinical features in the infant included cardiac failure with vasoconstriction, hypotension, severe metabolic acidosis, and atypical grand-mal seizures. He responded quickly to thiamine and made an unremarkable recovery.

The National Academy of Sciences' RDA for thiamine during lactation is 1.6 mg (1). If the diet of the lactating woman adequately supplies this amount, maternal supplementation with thiamine is not needed (27). Supplementation with the RDA for thiamine is recommended for those women with inadequate nutritional intake. The American Academy of Pediatrics classifies thiamine as compatible with breastfeeding (34).

References

1. American Hospital Formulary Service. *Drug Information 1997*. Bethesda, MD: American Society of Health-System Pharmacists, 1997:2818–20.
2. Frank O, Walbroehl G, Thomson A, Kaminetzky H, Kubes Z, Baker H. Placental transfer: fetal retention of some vitamins. Am J Clin Nutr 1970;23:662–3.
3. Hill EP, Longo LD. Dynamics of maternal–fetal nutrient transfer. Fed Proc 1980;39:239–44.
4. Kaminetzky HA, Baker H, Frank O, Langer A. The effects of intravenously administered water-soluble vitamins during labor in normovitaminemic and hypovitaminemic gravidas on maternal and neonatal blood vitamin levels at delivery. Am J Obstet Gynecol 1974;120:697–703.
5. Baker H, Frank O, Deangelis B, Feingold S, Kaminetzky HA. Role of placenta in maternal–fetal vitamin transfer in humans. Am J Obstet Gynecol 1981;141:792–6.
6. Slobody LB, Willner MM, Mestern J. Comparison of vitamin B_1 levels in mothers and their newborn infants. Am J Dis Child 1949;77:736–9.
7. Baker H, Thind IS, Frank O, DeAngelis B, Caterini H, Lquria DB. Vitamin levels in low-birth-weight newborn infants and their mothers. Am J Obstet Gynecol 1977;129:521–4.
8. Heller S, Salkeld RM, Korner WF. Vitamin B_1 status in pregnancy. Am J Clin Nutr 1974;27:1221–4.
9. Baker H, Frank O, Thomson AD, Langer A, Munves ED, De Angelis B, Kaminetzky HA. Vitamin profile of 174 mothers and newborns at parturition. Am J Clin Nutr 1975;28:59–65.
10. Tripathy K. Erythrocyte transketolase activity and thiamine transfer across human placenta. Am J Clin Nutr 1968;21:739–42.
11. Bamji MS. Enzymic evaluation of thiamin, riboflavin and pyridoxine status of parturient women and their newborn infants. Br J Nutr 1976;35:259–65.
12. Dostalova L. Correlation of the vitamin status between mother and newborn during delivery. Dev Pharmacol Ther 1982;4(Suppl 1):45–57.
13. Siddall AC. Vitamin B_1 deficiency as an etiologic factor in pregnancy toxemias. Am J Obstet Gynecol 1938;35:662–7.
14. King G, Ride LT. The relation of vitamin B_1 deficiency to the pregnancy toxaemias: a study of 371 cases of beri-beri complicating pregnancy. J Obstet Gynaecol Br Emp 1945;52:130–47.
15. Chaudhuri SK, Halder K, Chowdhury SR, Bagchi K. Relationship between toxaemia of pregnancy and thiamine deficiency. J Obstet Gynaecol Br Commonw 1969;76:123–6.
16. Chaudhuri SK. Role of nutrition in the etiology of toxemia of pregnancy. Am J Obstet Gynecol 1971;110:46–8.
17. Thomson AM. Diet in pregnancy. 3. Diet in relation to the course and outcome of pregnancy. Br J Nutr 1959;13:509–25.
18. Roecklein B, Levin SW, Comly M, Mukherjee AB. Intrauterine growth retardation induced by thiamine deficiency and pyrithiamine during pregnancy in the rat. Am J Obstet Gynecol 1985;151:455–60.
19. Fouts PJ, Gustafson GW, Zerfas LG. Successful treatment of a case of polyneuritis of pregnancy. Am J Obstet Gynecol 1934;28:902–7.
20. Willis RS, Winn WW, Morris AT, Newsom AA, Massey WE. Clinical observations in treatment of nausea and vomiting in pregnancy with vitamins B_1 and B_6: a preliminary report. Am J Obstet Gynecol 1942;44:265–71.
21. Hunt AD Jr, Stokes J Jr, McCrory WW, Stroud HH. Pyridoxine dependency: report of a case of intractable convulsions in an infant controlled by pyridoxine. Pediatrics 1954;13:140–5.
22. Averback P. Anencephaly associated with megavitamin therapy. Can Med Assoc J 1976;114:995.
23. Reading C. Down's syndrome, leukaemia and maternal thiamine deficiency. Med J Aust 1976;1:505.
24. Thomas MR, Sneed SM, Wei C, Nail P, Wilson M, Sprinkle EE III. The effects of vitamin C, vitamin B_6, vitamin B_{12}, folic acid, riboflavin, and thiamin on the breast milk and maternal status of well-nourished women at 6 months postpartum. Am J Clin Nutr 1980;33:2151–6.
25. Deodhar AD, Rajalakshmi R, Ramakrishnan CV. Studies on human lactation. Part III. Effect of dietary vitamin supplementation on vitamin contents of breast milk. Acta Paediatr Scand 1964;53:42–8.
26. Ford JE, Zechalko A, Murphy J, Brooke OG. Comparison of the B vitamin composition of milk from mothers of preterm and term babies. Arch Dis Child 1983;58:367–72.
27. Nail PA, Thomas MR, Eakin R. The effect of thiamin and riboflavin supplementation on the level of those vitamins in human breast milk and urine. Am J Clin Nutr 1980;33:198–204.
28. Fehily L. Human-milk intoxication due to B_1 avitaminosis. Br Med J 1944;2:590–2.
29. Cruickshank JD, Trimble AP, Brown JAH. Interstitial mononuclear pneumonia: a cause of sudden death in Gurkha infants in the Far East. Arch Dis Child 1957;32:279–84.
30. Mayer J. Nutrition and lactation. Postgrad Med 1963;33:380–5.
31. Gunther M. Diet and milk secretion in women. Proc Nutr Soc 1968;27:77–82.
32. Rao RR, Subrahmanyam I. An investigation on the thiamine content of mother's milk in relation to infantile convulsions. Indian J Med Res 1964;52:1198–201.
33. Debuse PJ. Shoshin beriberi in an infant of a thiamine-deficient mother. Acta Paediatr 1992;81:723–4.
34. Committee on Drugs, American Academy of Pediatrics. The transfer of drugs and other chemicals into human milk. Pediatrics 2001;108:776–89.

THIETHYLPERAZINE

[Withdrawn from the market. See 9th edition.]

THIOGUANINE

Antineoplastic

PREGNANCY RECOMMENDATION: Human and Animal Data Suggest Risk
BREASTFEEDING RECOMMENDATION: Contraindicated

PREGNANCY SUMMARY

Thioguanine is a purine analog that interferes with nucleic acid biosynthesis. It is classified as an antimetabolite in the same antineoplastic subclass of purine analogs and related agents as cladribine, clofarabine, fludarabine, pentostatin, and mercaptopurine. The drug is potentially mutagenic, carcinogenic, and teratogenic (1).

FETAL RISK SUMMARY

Reproduction studies in rats at a dose 5 times the human dose caused resorptions and malformed or stunted offspring (1). Malformations observed included generalized edema, cranial defects, general skeletal hypoplasia, hydrocephalus, ventral hernia, situs inversus, and limb defects (1).

The use of thioguanine in pregnancy has been reported in 26 patients, 4 during the 1st trimester (2–19). An elective abortion, resulting in a normal fetus, was performed at 21 weeks' gestation in one pregnancy after 4 weeks of chemotherapy (17). Use in the 1st and 2nd trimesters has been associated with chromosomal abnormalities in one infant (relationship to antineoplastic therapy unknown), trisomy group C autosomes with mosaicism (2), and congenital malformations in another, two medial digits of both feet missing and distal phalanges of both thumbs missing with hypoplastic remnant of right thumb (3). In a third case, a fetus, who was not exposed to antineoplastic agents until the 23rd week, long after development of the affected extremity, was delivered at 42 weeks' gestation with polydactyly (six toes on the right foot), a condition that had occurred previously in this family (18).

Two cases of intrauterine fetal death have occurred after antineoplastic therapy with thioguanine and other agents (15,18). In one case, a mother, whose antileukemic chemotherapy was initiated at 15 weeks' gestation, developed severe pregnancy-induced hypertension in the 29th week of pregnancy (15). Before this time, fetal well-being had been continuously documented. One week after onset of the preeclampsia, intrauterine fetal death was confirmed by ultrasound. In the second case, a woman, with a history of two previous 1st trimester spontaneous abortions, was treated for acute myeloblastic leukemia and ulcerative colitis beginning at 15 weeks' gestation (18). Intrauterine fetal death occurred at 20 weeks. No congenital abnormalities were found at autopsy in either of the fetuses.

Data from one review indicated that 40% of the infants exposed to anticancer drugs were of low birth weight (20). This finding was not related to the timing of exposure. Long-term studies of growth and mental development in offspring exposed to thioguanine during the 2nd trimester, the period of neuroblast multiplication, have not been conducted (21). However, individual children have been followed for periods ranging from a few months to 5 years and, in each case, normal development was documented (14,15,17,18).

Although abnormal chromosomal changes were observed in one aborted fetus, the clinical significance of this observation and the relationship to antineoplastic therapy are unknown. In two other newborns, karyotyping of cultured cells did not show anomalies (2,5). Paternal use of thioguanine with other antineoplastic agents before conception has been suggested as a cause of congenital defects observed in three infants: anencephalic stillborn (22), tetralogy of Fallot with syndactyly of the first and second toes (22), and multiple anomalies (23). However, confirmation of these data has not been forthcoming, and any such relationship is probably tenuous at best. Exposed men have also fathered normal children (23,24).

Occupational exposure of the mother to antineoplastic agents during pregnancy may present a risk to the fetus. A position statement from the National Study Commission on Cytotoxic Exposure and a research article involving some antineoplastic agents are presented in the monograph for cyclophosphamide (see Cyclophosphamide).

BREASTFEEDING SUMMARY

No reports describing the use of thioguanine during human lactation have been located. It is not known if the drug is excreted into breast milk. Because of the potential for severe toxicity, including tumors, in a nursing infant, women receiving thioguanine should not breastfeed.

References

1. Product information. Thioguanine. Glaxo Wellcome, 2000.
2. Maurer LH, Forcier RJ, McIntyre OR, Benirschke K. Fetal group C trisomy after cytosine arabinoside and thioguanine. Ann Intern Med 1971;75:809–10.
3. Schafer AI. Teratogenic effects of antileukemic chemotherapy. Arch Intern Med 1981;141:514–5.
4. Au-Yong R, Collins P, Young JA. Acute myeloblastic leukaemia during pregnancy. Br Med J 1972;4:493–4.
5. Raich PC, Curet LB. Treatment of acute leukemia during pregnancy. Cancer 1975;36:861–2.
6. Gokal R, Durrant J, Baum JD, Bennett MJ. Successful pregnancy in acute monocytic leukaemia. Br J Cancer 1976;34:299–302.
7. Lilleyman JS, Hill AS, Anderton KJ. Consequences of acute myelogenous leukemia in early pregnancy. Cancer 1977;40:1300–3.
8. Moreno H, Castleberry RP, McCann WP. Cytosine arabinoside and 6-thioguanine in the treatment of childhood acute myeloblastic leukemia. Cancer 1977;40:998–1004.
9. Manoharan A, Leyden MJ. Acute nonlymphocytic leukaemia in the third trimester of pregnancy. Aust NZ J Med 1979;9:71–4.
10. Taylor G, Blom J. Acute leukemia during pregnancy. South Med J 1980;73:1314–5.
11. Tobias JS, Bloom HJG. Doxorubicin in pregnancy. Lancet 1980;1:776.
12. Pawliger DF, McLean FW, Noyes WD. Normal fetus after cytosine arabinoside therapy. Ann Intern Med 1971;74:1012.
13. Plows CW. Acute myelomonocytic leukemia in pregnancy: report of a case. Am J Obstet Gynecol 1982;143:41–3.
14. Lowenthal RM, Marsden KA, Newman NM, Baikie MJ, Campbell SN. Normal infant after treatment of acute myeloid leukaemia in pregnancy with daunorubicin. Aust NZ J Med 1978;8:431–2.
15. O'Donnell R, Costigan C, O'Connell LG. Two cases of acute leukaemia in pregnancy. Acta Haematol 1979;61:298–300.
16. Hamer JW, Beard MEJ, Duff GB. Pregnancy complicated by acute myeloid leukaemia. NZ Med J 1979;89:212–3.
17. Doney KC, Kraemer KG, Shepard TH. Combination chemotherapy for acute myelocytic leukemia during pregnancy: three case reports. Cancer Treat Rep 1979;63:369–71.
18. Volkenandt M, Buchner T, Hiddemann W, Van De Loo J. Acute leukaemia during pregnancy. Lancet 1987;2:1521–2.
19. Feliu J, Juarez S, Ordonez A, Garcia-Paredes ML, Gonzalez-Baron M, Montero JM. Acute leukemia and pregnancy. Cancer 1988;61:580–4.
20. Nicholson HO. Cytotoxic drugs in pregnancy: review of reported cases. J Obstet Gynaecol Br Commonw 1968;75:307–12.

T

21. Dobbing J. Pregnancy and leukaemia. Lancet 1977;1:1155.
22. Russell JA, Powles RL, Oliver RTD. Conception and congenital abnormalities after chemotherapy of acute myelogenous leukaemia in two men. Br Med J 1976;1:1508.
23. Evenson DP, Arlin Z, Welt S, Claps ML, Melamed MR. Male reproductive capacity may recover following drug treatment with the L-10 protocol for acute lymphocytic leukemia. Cancer 1984;53:30–6.
24. Matthews JH, Wood JK. Male fertility during chemotherapy for acute leukemia. N Engl J Med 1980;303:1235.

THIORIDAZINE

Antipsychotic

PREGNANCY RECOMMENDATION: Limited Human Data—No Relevant Animal Data
BREASTFEEDING RECOMMENDATION: No Human Data—Potential Toxicity

PREGNANCY SUMMARY

Although occasional reports have attempted to link various phenothiazine agents with congenital malformations, most of the evidence suggests that these drugs are low risk for the embryo–fetus (see Chlorpromazine).

FETAL RISK SUMMARY

Thioridazine is a piperidyl phenothiazine. The drug is not teratogenic in animals (species not specified) (1).

Phenothiazines readily cross the placenta (2). Extrapyramidal symptoms were seen in a newborn exposed to thioridazine in utero, but the reaction was probably caused by chlorpromazine (3).

In a surveillance study of Michigan Medicaid recipients involving 229,101 completed pregnancies conducted between 1985 and 1992, 63 newborns had been exposed to thioridazine during the 1st trimester (F. Rosa, personal communication, FDA, 1993). Two (3.2%) major birth defects were observed (three expected), one of which was a cardiovascular defect (one expected). No anomalies were observed in five other categories of defects (oral clefts, spina bifida, polydactyly, limb reduction defects, and hypospadias) for which specific data were available.

A case of a congenital heart defect was described in 1969 (4). However, one investigator found no anomalies in the offspring of 23 patients exposed throughout gestation to thioridazine (5). Twenty of the infants were evaluated for up to 13 years.

A brief 1993 report described a 31-year-old woman with depression, panic disorder, and migraine headaches who was exposed to a number of drugs in the first 6 weeks of pregnancy, including thioridazine, dihydroergotamine, citalopram, buspirone, and etilefrin (a sympathomimetic agent) (6). An elective abortion at 12 weeks' gestation revealed a normal fetus.

BREASTFEEDING SUMMARY

No reports describing the use of thioridazine during human lactation have been located. It is not known if the drug is excreted into breast milk. However, other phenothiazines are present in milk and have caused toxicity (see Chlorpromazine). Sedation is a possible effect in nursing infants.

References

1. Product information. Mellaril. Sandoz Pharmaceutical Corporation, 1993.
2. Moya F, Thorndike V. Passage of drugs across the placenta. Am J Obstet Gynecol 1962;84:1778–98.
3. Hill RM, Desmond MM, Kay JL. Extrapyramidal dysfunction in an infant of a schizophrenic mother. J Pediatr 1966;69:589–95.
4. Vince DJ. Congenital malformations following phenothiazine administration during pregnancy. Can Med Assoc J 1969;100:223.
5. Scanlan FJ. The use of thioridazine (Mellaril) during the first trimester. Med J Aust 1972;1:1271–2.
6. Seifritz E, Holsboer-Trachsler E, Haberthur F, Hemmeter U, Poldinger W. Unrecognized pregnancy during citalopram treatment. Am J Psychiatry 1993;150:1428–9.

THIOTEPA

Antineoplastic

PREGNANCY RECOMMENDATION: Contraindicated—1st Trimester
BREASTFEEDING RECOMMENDATION: Contraindicated

PREGNANCY SUMMARY

No reports describing embryo–fetal harm caused by thiotepa have been located. However, the drug is a polyfunctional cytotoxic agent that is related chemically and pharmacologically to nitrogen mustard (mechlorethamine), an alkylating antineoplastic. Moreover, the animal reproduction data suggest risk.

FETAL RISK SUMMARY

Thiotepa impairs fertility and is carcinogenic, mutagenic, and teratogenic in animals (1). Reproduction studies in mice and rats at intraperitoneal doses one-eighth and one times, respectively, the maximum recommended human dose based on BSA (MRHD) revealed teratogenicity in both species. Embryolethality was noted in rabbits at a dose twice the MRHD (1).

It is not known if thiotepa crosses the human placenta. The molecular weight (about 189) is low enough that passage to the embryo–fetus should be expected.

Thiotepa has been used during the 2nd and 3rd trimesters in one patient without apparent fetal harm (2). Long-term studies of growth and mental development in offspring exposed to antineoplastic agents during the 2nd trimester, the period of neuroblast multiplication, have not been conducted (3).

Occupational exposure of the mother to antineoplastic agents during pregnancy may present a risk to the fetus. A position statement from the National Study Commission on Cytotoxic Exposure and a research article involving some antineoplastic agents are presented in the monograph for cyclophosphamide (see Cyclophosphamide).

BREASTFEEDING SUMMARY

No reports describing the use of thiotepa during lactation have been located. The molecular weight (about 189) is low enough that excretion into breast milk should be expected. Because of the potential for severe toxicity, including tumors, in a nursing infant, women receiving thiotepa should not breastfeed.

References

1. Product information. Thioplex. Immunex, 2000.
2. Gililland J, Weinstein L. The effects of cancer chemotherapeutic agents on the developing fetus. Obstet Gynecol Surv 1983;38:6–13.
3. Dobbing J. Pregnancy and leukaemia. Lancet 1977;1:1155.

THIOTHIXENE

Antipsychotic

PREGNANCY RECOMMENDATION: Limited Human Data—Animal Data Suggest Low Risk
BREASTFEEDING RECOMMENDATION: No Human Data—Potential Toxicity

PREGNANCY SUMMARY

Thiothixene, a phenothiazine derivative, is structurally and pharmacologically related to trifluoperazine and chlorprothixene (see Trifluoperazine). Although occasional reports have attempted to link various phenothiazines with congenital malformations, most of the evidence suggests that these drugs are low risk for the embryo–fetus.

FETAL RISK SUMMARY

No published reports, other than the one study below, describing the use of the drug in human pregnancy have been located. The drug is not teratogenic in mice, rats, rabbits, and monkeys (1–3).

It is not known if thiothixene crosses the human placenta. The molecular weight (about 444) is low enough that passage to the embryo–fetus should be expected.

In a surveillance study of Michigan Medicaid recipients involving 229,101 completed pregnancies conducted between 1985 and 1992, 38 newborns had been exposed to thiothixene during the 1st trimester (F. Rosa, personal communication, FDA, 1993). One (2.6%) major birth defect (two expected), a cardiovascular defect (0.5 expected), was observed. No anomalies were observed in five other categories of defects (oral clefts, spina bifida, polydactyly, limb reduction defects, and hypospadias) for which specific data were available.

BREASTFEEDING SUMMARY

No reports describing the use of thiothixene during lactation have been located. The molecular weight (about 444) is low enough that excretion into breast milk should be expected. The effect on a nursing infant from exposure to the drug in milk is unknown. However, other phenothiazines are present in milk and have caused toxicity (see Chlorpromazine). Sedation is a possible effect in nursing infants.

References

1. Owaki Y, Momiyama H, Yokoi Y. Teratological studies on thiothixene in mice. (Japanese) Oyo Yakuri 1969;3:315–20. As cited in Shepard TH. *Catalog of Teratogenic Agents*. 6th ed. Baltimore, MD: The Johns Hopkins University Press, 1989:618.
2. Owaki Y, Momiyama H, Yokoi Y. Teratological studies on thiothixene (Navane) in rabbits. (Japanese) Oyo Yakuri 1969;3:321–4. As cited in Shepard TH. *Catalog of Teratogenic Agents*. 6th ed. Baltimore, MD: The Johns Hopkins University Press, 1989;618.
3. Product information. Navane. Pfizer, 2000.

THIPHENAMIL

[Withdrawn from the market. See 8th edition.]

THIPROPAZATE

[Withdrawn from the market. See 8th edition.]

THYROGLOBULIN

Thyroid

See Thyroid.

THYROID

Thyroid

PREGNANCY RECOMMENDATION: Compatible
BREASTFEEDING RECOMMENDATION: Compatible

PREGNANCY SUMMARY

Thyroid contains the two thyroid hormones levothyroxine (T4) and liothyronine (T3) plus other materials peculiar to the thyroid gland. It is used during pregnancy for the treatment of hypothyroidism. Congenital defects have been reported with the use of thyroid but they are thought to be caused by maternal hypothyroidism or other factors (see Levothyroxine and Liothyronine).

FETAL RISK SUMMARY

Neither T4 nor T3 crosses the placenta when physiologic serum concentrations are present in the mother (see Levothyroxine and Liothyronine). In one report, however, two patients, each of whom had produced two cretins in previous pregnancies, were given huge amounts of thyroid, up to 1600 mg/day or more (1). Both newborns were normal at birth even though one was found to be athyroid. The authors concluded that sufficient hormone was transported to the fetuses to prevent hypothyroidism.

In a surveillance study of Michigan Medicaid recipients involving 229,101 completed pregnancies conducted between 1985 and 1992, 44 newborns had been exposed to thyroid during the 1st trimester (F. Rosa, personal communication, FDA, 1993). One (2.3%) major birth defect (two expected), a cardiovascular defect (0.5 expected), was observed.

Combination therapy with thyroid–antithyroid drugs was advocated at one time for the treatment of hyperthyroidism but is now considered inappropriate (see Propylthiouracil).

BREASTFEEDING SUMMARY

See Levothyroxine and Liothyronine.

Reference

1. Carr EA Jr, Beierwaltes WH, Raman G, Dodson VN, Tanton J, Betts JS, Stambaugh RA. The effect of maternal thyroid function on fetal thyroid function and development. J Clin Endocrinol Metab 1959;19:1–18.

T

THYROTROPIN

Thyroid

PREGNANCY RECOMMENDATION: Compatible
BREASTFEEDING RECOMMENDATION: Compatible

PREGNANCY SUMMARY

Thyrotropin (thyroid-stimulating hormone; TSH) does not cross the placenta (1). No correlation exists between maternal and fetal concentrations of TSH at any time during gestation (2).

BREASTFEEDING SUMMARY

No reports describing the excretion of thyrotropin in human milk have been located. Serum levels of this hormone have been measured and compared in breastfed and bottlefed infants (3–7). Breast milk does not provide sufficient levothyroxine (T4) or liothyronine (T3) to prevent the effects of congenital hypothyroidism (see Levothyroxine and Liothyronine). As a consequence, serum levels of TSH in breastfed hypothyroid infants are markedly elevated (3,4). In euthyroid babies, no differences in TSH levels have been discovered between breastfed and bottlefed groups (5–7).

References

1. Cohlan SQ. Fetal and neonatal hazards from drugs administered during pregnancy. NY State J Med 1964;64:493–9.
2. Feely J. The physiology of thyroid function in pregnancy. Postgrad Med J 1979;55:336–9.
3. Abbassi V, Steinour TA. Successful diagnosis of congenital hypothyroidism in four breastfed neonates. J Pediatr 1980;97:259–61.
4. Letarte J, Guyda H, Dussault JH, Glorieux J. Lack of protective effect of breastfeeding in congenital hypothyroidism: report of 12 cases. Pediatrics 1980;65:703–5.
5. Mizuta H, Amino N, Ichihara K, Harada T, Nose O, Tanizawa O, Miyai K. Thyroid hormones in human milk and their influence on thyroid function of breastfed babies. Pediatr Res 1983;17:468–71.
6. Hahn HB Jr, Spiekerman M, Otto WR, Hossalla DE. Thyroid function tests in neonates fed human milk. Am J Dis Child 1983;137:220–2.
7. Franklin R, O'Grady C, Carpenter L. Neonatal thyroid function: comparison between breastfed and bottlefed infants. J Pediatr 1985;106:124–6.

TIAGABINE

Anticonvulsant

PREGNANCY RECOMMENDATION: Limited Human Data—Animal Data Suggest Risk
BREASTFEEDING RECOMMENDATION: No Human Data—Probably Compatible

PREGNANCY SUMMARY

Tiagabine was not teratogenic or embryo–fetal toxic in experimental animals at doses that did not cause maternal toxicity. However, the no–observed-effect levels were much <10 times the MRHD. The human data are too limited to determine the risk magnitude this agent represents to the embryo–fetus. Of concern, however, metabolism of tiagabine results in epoxide metabolites. As noted above, these intermediate arene oxide metabolites from other anticonvulsants have been associated with human teratogenicity. Therefore, the safest course is to avoid tiagabine, if possible, during the 1st trimester, but there is no evidence that exposure during organogenesis or at any other time during gestation will result in fetal harm. If tiagabine is required, monotherapy using the lowest effective dose is preferred, but because of its status as adjunctive therapy, this may not be possible. In addition, folic acid 4–5 mg/day should be taken with tiagabine.

FETAL RISK SUMMARY

The oral anticonvulsant tiagabine enhances the activity of γ-aminobutyric acid, the major inhibitory neurotransmitter, in the central nervous system. It is not known if this relates to its anticonvulsant activity. Tiagabine is indicated as adjunctive therapy in the treatment of partial seizures. Its elimination half-life is 7–9 hours, but is decreased to 4–7 hours in patients who are concurrently receiving hepatic enzyme-inducing anticonvulsants (e.g., carbamazepine, phenytoin, primidone, and phenobarbital). A 1996 review stated that the elimination half-life was 4–13 hours (mean 7 hours) and decreased to 2–3 hours when combined with enzyme-inducing anticonvulsants (2). In plasma, 96% is bound to albumin and α_1-acid glycoprotein (1,2). Although not all of the metabolites have been identified, at least one is inactive (1). Of particular interest, a 1996 review stated that metabolism of tiagabine (based on data from a manufacturer) results in arene oxide metabolites (3). These intermediate free radicals have been associated with human teratogenicity (see Carbamazepine, Phenytoin, and Valproic Acid).

Reproduction studies with tiagabine have been conducted in rats and rabbits. In pregnant rats treated during organogenesis, maternal toxic (weight loss/reduced weight gain) doses approximately 16 times the maximum recommended human dose based on BSA (MRHD) were associated with an increased incidence of fetal malformations (craniofacial, appendicular, and visceral defects) and growth restriction. When this dose was given during late gestation and throughout parturition and lactation, maternal toxicity (decreased weight gain), stillbirths, and decreased postnatal offspring viability and growth were observed. No maternal or fetal adverse effects were observed at 3 times the MRHD. In pregnant rabbits, a dose 8 times the MRHD caused maternal toxicity (decreased weight gain), embryo death, and fetal variations. The no-effect dose for maternal, embryo, and fetal toxicity was approximately equivalent to the MRHD (1).

In rats, high doses (36–100 times the plasma exposure [AUC] obtained with the maximum recommended human dose of 56 mg/day) for 2 years were carcinogenic (hepatocellular adenomas in females and Leydig cell tumors of the testis in males). In an in vitro test, tiagabine, in the absence of metabolic activation, caused increased structural chromosome aberration frequency in human lymphocytes. This toxicity, however, was not observed in the assay in the presence of metabolic activation. Similarly, no genetic toxicity was observed in several other in vitro or in vivo assays (1).

It is not known if tiagabine crosses the human placenta. The molecular weight (376 for the free base) is low enough that exposure of the embryo–fetus should be

T

expected. The moderately long elimination half-life will result in prolonged concentrations of the drug at the maternal blood–placenta interface, thus increasing the opportunity for embryo–fetal exposure.

A 1996 report described the outcomes of 23 human pregnancies exposed to tiagabine (3). Among the pregnancies exposed in a preclinical trial, there was one maternal death (unrelated to therapy), four spontaneous abortions (SABs), eight elective abortions (EABs) (including one blighted ovum and one ectopic pregnancy), eight normal outcomes, and one infant with unspecified malformations (also receiving other unspecified anticonvulsants). Specific data relating to the exposures (e.g., dose, duration, timing) were not provided.

In a 1999 analysis of 53 clinical trials involving tiagabine, 2531 epileptic patients were treated, including 22 pregnancies (4). Some data from this report also might have been reported in the above reference. The pregnancy outcomes were: four SABs, seven EABs (includes one blighted ovum and one ectopic pregnancy), eight normal outcomes, one infant with hip displacement related to a breech presentation, and one ongoing pregnancy. In the last case, the mother, who had taken tiagabine only during the first 2 months of pregnancy, had a seizure and drowned in her bathtub. Autopsy revealed a normal fetus with growth consistent to the gestational age (4).

The Lamotrigine Pregnancy Registry, an ongoing project conducted by the manufacturer, was first published in January 1997. The final report was published in July 2010 (5). The Registry is now closed. In five prospectively enrolled pregnancies exposed in the 1st trimester to tiagabine and lamotrigine, with or without other anticonvulsants, the outcomes were four live births without birth defects and one SAB (5).

The effect of tiagabine on folic acid levels and metabolism is unknown (3). Although not specifically referring to tiagabine, a 2003 review recommended that to reduce the risk of birth defects from anticonvulsants, women should start multivitamins with folic acid before conception (6). Although the recommendation did not specify the amount of folic acid, a recent study found that multivitamin supplements with folic acid (typically 0.4 mg) did not reduce the risk of congenital malformations from four first-generation anticonvulsants (see Carbamazepine, Phenytoin, Phenobarbital, or Primidone). Therefore, until further information is available, the best course is to start folic acid supplementation before conception. Although a specific dosage recommendation has not been determined for patients receiving anticonvulsants, 4 mg/day appears to be reasonable.

BREASTFEEDING SUMMARY

No studies describing the use of tiagabine during human lactation have been located. The molecular weight (about 376 for the free base) and the moderately long elimination half-life (as long as 13 hours) suggest that excretion into breast milk should be expected. The effect on the nursing infant from exposure to tiagabine in milk is unknown.

References

1. Product information. Gabitril. Cephalon, 2003.
2. Perucca E, Bialer M. The clinical pharmacokinetics of the newer antiepileptic drugs. Clin Pharmacokinet 1996;31:29–46.
3. Morrell MJ. The new antiepileptic drugs and women: efficacy, reproductive health, pregnancy, and fetal outcome. Epilepsia 1996;37(Suppl 6):S34–44.
4. Leppik IE, Gram L, Deaton R, Sommerville KW. Safety of tiagabine: summary of 53 trials. Epilepsy Res 1999;33:235–46.
5. The Lamotrigine Pregnancy Registry. Final Report. September 1, 1992 through March 31, 2010. GlaxoSmithKline, July 2010.
6. Yerby MS. Clinical care of pregnant women with epilepsy: neural tube defects and folic acid supplementation. Epilepsia 2003;44(Suppl 3):33–40.

TICAGRELOR

Hematologic (Antiplatelet)

PREGNANCY RECOMMENDATION: No Human Data—Animal Data Suggest Risk
BREASTFEEDING RECOMMENDATION: No Human Data—Potential Toxicity

PREGNANCY SUMMARY

No reports describing the use of ticagrelor in human pregnancy have been located. The animal data suggest risk, but the absence of human pregnancy experience prevents a more complete assessment of the embryo–fetal risk. However, if indicated, the benefits to the mother might be greater than the risks to the embryo–fetus and must be evaluated on a case-by-case basis.

FETAL RISK SUMMARY

Ticagrelor is an oral reversible inhibitor of platelet activation and aggregation. It is indicated to reduce the rate of thrombotic cardiovascular events in patients with acute coronary syndrome (unstable angina, non-ST elevation myocardial infarction, or ST elevation myocardial infarction). Ticagrelor is metabolized to an approximately equipotent metabolite. Both the parent drug and metabolite are highly bound (>99%) to plasma proteins and mean half-lives are about 7 and 9 hours, respectively (1).

Reproduction studies have been conducted in rats and rabbits. Rats were given oral doses that were about 1–16.5 times the maximum recommended human dose of 90 mg twice daily for a 60-kg human (MRHD) based on BSA (MRHD-BSA) during organogenesis. Adverse outcomes in the offspring caused by the highest dose were supernumerary liver lobe and ribs, incomplete ossification of sternebrae, displaced articulation of pelvis, and misshapen misaligned sternebrae. When rats were given a dose that was about 10 times the MRHD-BSA during late gestation and lactation, pup deaths and effects on pup growth were observed. Minor effects such as delays in pinna unfolding and eye opening occurred at doses that were about 0.5–3.2 times the MRHD-BSA. In rabbits, an oral dose that was 6.8 times the MRHD-BSA given during organogenesis resulted in delayed gall bladder development and incomplete ossification of the hyoid, pubis, and sternebrae (1).

In studies in mice and rats, no carcinogenic effects were noted in mice or male rats. In female rats, doses that were 29 times the MRHD based on AUC (BSA-AUC) were associated with uterine carcinomas, uterine adenocarcinomas, and hepatocellular adenomas. A lower dose that was about 8 times the MRHD-AUC was not carcinogenic. Neither the parent drug nor active metabolite were mutagenic in multiple assays. In fertility studies, ticagrelor had no effect on male rats, but an increased incidence of irregular duration of estrus cycles was observed in female rats (1).

It is not known if ticagrelor or its active metabolite cross the human placenta. The molecular weight (about 523) of the parent drug and moderately long half-lives suggest that both agents will cross to the embryo–fetus. However, the high plasma protein binding should limit the exposure.

BREASTFEEDING SUMMARY

No reports describing the use of ticagrelor during human lactation have been located. The molecular weight (about 523) of the parent drug and moderately long half-lives of the parent drug (7 hours) and its approximately equipotent metabolite (9 hours) suggest that both agents will be excreted into breast milk. However, the high (>99%) plasma protein binding of both agents should limit the exposure. The effects of the exposure on a nursing infant are unknown. If the drug is used during breastfeeding, the infant should be monitored for the most common adverse reactions observed in adults (bleeding and dyspnea).

Reference

1. Product information. Brilinta. AstraZeneca, 2011.

TICARCILLIN

Antibiotic (Penicillin)

PREGNANCY RECOMMENDATION: Compatible
BREASTFEEDING RECOMMENDATION: Compatible

PREGNANCY SUMMARY

No reports linking the use of ticarcillin with congenital defects have been located. Although the reported pregnancy experience is limited, all penicillins are considered low risk in pregnancy.

FETAL RISK SUMMARY

Ticarcillin is a penicillin antibiotic. Reproduction studies in mice and rats have revealed no evidence of impaired fertility or fetal harm (1).

Ticarcillin rapidly crosses the placenta to the fetal circulation and amniotic fluid (2). Following a 1-g IV dose, single determinations of the amniotic fluid from six patients, 15–76 minutes after injection, yielded levels of 1.0–3.3 mcg/mL. Similar measurements of ticarcillin in cord serum ranged from 12.6 to 19.2 mcg/mL. In a study using in vitro perfused human placentas, the fetal:maternal ratio of ticarcillin was 0.91 (3).

The Collaborative Perinatal Project monitored 50,282 mother–child pairs, 3546 of whom had 1st trimester exposure to penicillin derivatives (4, pp. 297–313). For use anytime during pregnancy, 7171 exposures were recorded (4, p. 435). In neither group was evidence found to suggest a relationship to large categories of major or minor malformations or to individual defects.

BREASTFEEDING SUMMARY

Ticarcillin is excreted into breast milk in low concentrations. After a 1-g IV dose given to five patients, only trace amounts of drug were measured at intervals up to 6 hours (2). Although these amounts are probably not significant, three potential problems exist for the nursing infant: modification of bowel flora, direct effects on the infant (e.g., allergic response), and interference with the interpretation of culture results if a fever workup is required. The American Academy of Pediatrics classifies ticarcillin as compatible with breastfeeding (5).

References

1. Product information. Ticar. SmithKline Beecham Pharmaceuticals, 2000.
2. Cho N, Nakayama T, Vehara K, Kunii K. Laboratory and clinical evaluation of ticarcillin in the field of obstetrics and gynecology. Chemotherapy (Tokyo) 1977;25:2911–23.
3. Fortunato SJ, Bawdon RE, Swan KF, Bryant EC, Sobhi S. Transfer of Timentin (ticarcillin and clavulanic acid) across the in vitro perfused human placenta: comparison with other agents. Am J Obstet Gynecol 1992;167:1595–9.
4. Heinonen OP, Slone, D, Shapiro S. *Birth Defects and Drugs in Pregnancy*. Littleton, MA: Publishing Sciences Group, 1977.
5. Committee on Drugs, American Academy of Pediatrics. The transfer of drugs and other chemicals into human milk. Pediatrics 2001;108:776–89.

TICLOPIDINE

Hematological Agent (Antiplatelet)

PREGNANCY RECOMMENDATION: Limited Human Data—Animal Data Suggest Low Risk
BREASTFEEDING RECOMMENDATION: No Human Data—Potential Toxicity

PREGNANCY SUMMARY

Ticlopidine is not teratogenic in experimental animals, but the human pregnancy experience is too limited to assess the potential risk to the embryo or fetus. Three case reports have described the use of ticlopidine in human pregnancy, one of which ended in a spontaneous abortion (SAB). Ticlopidine may cause life-threatening blood dyscrasias, including neutropenia/agranulocytosis, thrombotic thrombocytopenia purpura, and aplastic anemia (1). The peak incidence for these disorders is in the first 3 months of therapy. The adverse effects are not predictable by any known demographic or clinical characteristics (1). Theoretically, if ticlopidine crossed the placenta, the fetus or newborn could also be at risk, as well as the mother. Therefore, because other antiplatelet agents are available, ticlopidine should be used during pregnancy only if other agents are judged to be less effective for the mother's condition.

FETAL RISK SUMMARY

Ticlopidine is a direct, irreversible inhibitor of adenosine diphosphate (ADP)–induced platelet aggregation. The drug has at least 20 metabolites, all of which appear to be inactive. Reversible protein binding is extensive (98%), primarily to albumin and lipoproteins, but some (15%) also is bound to α_1-acid glycoprotein. Ticlopidine is indicated to reduce the risk of thrombotic stroke in patients who have stroke precursors and in patients who have had a completed thrombotic stroke (1).

Reproduction studies have been conducted in mice, rats, and rabbits at doses up to 200, 400, and 200 mg/kg/day, respectively (1). There was no evidence of teratogenicity at these doses, but maternal and fetal toxicity was observed at 200, 400, and 100 mg/kg/day, respectively. In male and female rats, however, no effects on fertility were observed at the highest dose. The maximum doses in mice and rats were approximately 29 and 56 times, respectively, the human clinical dose (HCD), or 3 and 8 times, respectively, the HCD on a BSA basis. Ticlopidine was not carcinogenic in mice or rats, or mutagenic in in vitro or in vivo assays (1).

Whether ticlopidine crosses the placenta is not known, but the molecular weight (about 300) is low enough that transfer to the fetus should be expected. Of interest, a platelet aggregation study was conducted on cord blood from a term pregnancy of a woman who had been receiving ticlopidine and aspirin for 2 weeks (2). Complete inhibition of platelet aggregation to 20 micromoles of ADP was demonstrated.

A 1998 case report described the treatment of an acute myocardial infarction in a 30-year-old woman at 38 weeks' gestation (2). Her condition did not improve with aspirin, heparin, nitrates, or balloon angioplasty, so a stent was placed in the partially occluded left anterior descending coronary artery during abciximab (an antiplatelet agent) infusion. Adequate flow was re-established in the artery. Postoperatively, she was treated with ticlopidine, aspirin, and an unspecified β-blocker. Two weeks later, she delivered vaginally a healthy baby boy with a normal ductus arteriosus (no other details were provided). No excessive maternal bleeding was observed (2).

A woman with a history of essential thrombocytopenia and an anterior wall myocardial infarction was treated with chemotherapy (details not specified) to normalize her platelet count (3). After cardiac bypass surgery, she conceived while taking ticlopidine (500 mg/day) and aspirin (300 mg/day). An SAB occurred in the 2nd trimester, 6 months after surgery. The woman's therapy was changed to clopidogrel and intermittent low-molecular-weight heparin, and she eventually had a normal pregnancy. The relationship between the abortion and the ticlopidine/aspirin combination is unknown (3).

A 24-year-old woman with a history of aortic valve replacement with a 21-mm St. Jude Medical mechanical valve and two SABs was treated before and through the 36th week of pregnancy with ticlopidine (300 mg/day), dipyridamole (300 mg/day), and aspirin (81 mg/day) (4). At that time, oral therapy was replaced with continuous IV heparin until delivery of a healthy baby (sex not specified) by an elective cesarean section at 38 weeks' gestation. No maternal or fetal thrombotic or bleeding complications were observed. Other than being healthy, no other information was given about the newborn (4).

BREASTFEEDING SUMMARY

No reports describing the use of ticlopidine during human lactation have been located. The molecular weight (about 300) is low enough that excretion into breast milk should be expected. The effect of this exposure on a nursing infant is unknown. However, the life-threatening hematological adverse reactions that have been reported with this drug (see above), especially in the first 3 months of therapy, suggest that ticlopidine should not be used by the lactating woman.

T

References

1. Product information. Ticlid. Roche Pharmaceuticals, 2002.
2. Sebastian C, Scherlag M, Kugelmass A, Schechter E. Primary stent implantation for acute myocardial infarction during pregnancy: use of abciximab, ticlopidine, and aspirin. Cathet Cardiovasc Diagn 1998;45:275–9.
3. Klinzing P, Markert UR, Liesaus K, Peiker G. Case report: successful pregnancy and delivery after myocardial infarction and essential thrombocythemia treated with clopidogrel. Clin Exp Obstet Gynecol 2001;28:215–6.
4. Ueno M, Masuda H, Nakamura K, Sakata R. Antiplatelet therapy for a pregnant woman with a mechanical aortic valve: report of a case. Surg Today 2001;31:1002–4.

TIGECYCLINE

Antibiotic (Tetracycline)

PREGNANCY RECOMMENDATION: Human Data Suggest Risk in 2nd and 3rd Trimesters
BREASTFEEDING RECOMMENDATION: No Human Data—Potential Toxicity

PREGNANCY SUMMARY

No reports describing the use of tigecycline in human pregnancy have been located. In one animal species, exposures close to those obtained in humans that did not cause maternal toxicity did result in reduced fetal weight and minor skeletal anomalies. Moreover, tigecycline crosses the placentas of rats and rabbits and enters fetal tissues, including fetal bony structures (1). Similar to tetracyclines, tigecycline can permanently discolor the teeth if used in the second half of pregnancy (1). Inadvertent or planned use in the 1st trimester probably does not represent a major risk to the embryo or fetus, but use in later trimesters should be avoided.

FETAL RISK SUMMARY

Tigecycline is a glycylcycline, broad-spectrum antibacterial agent with bacteriostatic activity that is given by IV infusion. It is structurally related to the tetracycline class of antibiotics and may have similar adverse effects. Tigecycline undergoes partial metabolism. The elimination half-life after a single IV dose is about 27 hours, whereas after multiple dosing the half-life is about 42 hours. The primary route of elimination is by biliary excretion. The in vitro plasma protein binding ranges from about 71% to 89% (1).

Reproduction studies have been conducted in rats and rabbits. No teratogenic effects were observed in either species at exposures about 5 times and equal to, respectively, the human daily dose based on AUC (HDD). However, these exposures were associated with slight reductions in fetal weights and an increased incidence of minor skeletal anomalies (delays in bone ossification). The exposure in rabbits was maternally toxic and was associated with an increased incidence of fetal loss (1).

Studies for carcinogenicity have not been conducted with tigecycline, but tests for mutagenicity and clastogenicity were negative. No effects on reproductive performance or fertility were observed in male and female rats given doses resulting in exposures that were 5 times the HDD (1).

Tigecycline crosses the placentas of animals (1). However, it is not known if the drug crosses the human placenta. The molecular weight (about 586), prolonged elimination half-life, and wide distribution in tissues suggest that the antibiotic will cross to the embryo–fetus. Moreover, tetracycline is known to cross the human placenta resulting in fetal toxicity.

BREASTFEEDING SUMMARY

No reports describing the use of tigecycline during human lactation have been located. The molecular weight (about 586), prolonged elimination half-life, and wide distribution in tissues suggest that the antibiotic will be excreted into breast milk. However, the oral bioavailability of tigecycline is such that there might be little or no systemic exposure. Even if the oral bioavailability in infants is negligible, the presence of the antibiotic in milk could cause three potential problems: modification of bowel flora, direct effects on the infant's gut, and interference with the interpretation of culture results if a fever workup is required.

Reference

1. Product information. Tygacil. Wyeth Pharmaceuticals, 2005.

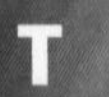

TILUDRONATE

Bisphosphonate

PREGNANCY RECOMMENDATION: No Human Data—Animal Data Suggest Moderate Risk
BREASTFEEDING RECOMMENDATION: No Human Data—Probably Compatible

PREGNANCY SUMMARY

No reports describing the use of tiludronate in human pregnancy have been located. Developmental toxicity (growth restriction, structural anomalies, and death) at doses close to those used in humans was observed in three animal species, but the maternal toxicity evident in two of the species prevents a better assessment of the animal embryo–fetal toxicity. The complete lack of human pregnancy experience with tiludronate and the very limited human data for the bisphosphonate class prevent further assessment of the risk. The amount of drug retained in bone and eventually released back into the systemic circulation is directly related to the dose and duration of treatment. Because tiludronate probably crosses the placenta, treatment of the mother before conception could result in continuous exposure of the embryo and fetus to an unknown amount of drug. Therefore, the use of tiludronate is not recommended in women who may become pregnant or during pregnancy. There is a theoretical risk of fetal harm (e.g., skeletal and other abnormalities) (1), but the magnitude of this risk cannot be estimated at the present time. Infants exposed in utero to tiludronate should be monitored for hypocalcemia during the first few days after birth.

FETAL RISK SUMMARY

Tiludronate is a bisphosphonate in the same class as alendronate, etidronate, ibandronate, pamidronate, risedronate, and zoledronic acid. It is indicated for the treatment of Paget's disease of bone (osteitis deformans). Tiludronate undergoes little, if any, metabolism. The plasma elimination half-life is about 150 hours, but the elimination rate from bone is unknown (1).

Reproduction studies have been conducted in mice, rats, and rabbits. In mice during organogenesis, a dose 7 times the 400 mg/day human dose based on BSA (HD) caused maternal toxicity (decreased body weight gain) and embryo–fetal developmental toxicity (increased postimplantation loss, decreased number of fetuses per dam, and decreased fetal body weight). A low incidence of malformations of the paw (shortened or missing digits, blood blisters between or in place of digits) was seen in one litter. Similar effects, including maternal toxicity but not fetal malformations, were observed in rats dosed at 10 times the HD. When rats were given doses 2 times the HD from day 15 of gestation to day 26 postpartum, protracted parturition and maternal death, presumably due to hypocalcemia, were observed. In rabbits during organogenesis, doses 2 and 5 times the HD caused dose-related scoliosis that was thought to be attributable to the pharmacologic properties of the drug (1).

Tiludronate was not genotoxic in several assays. The drug also had no effect on male or female rat fertility at doses up to twice the HD (1).

It is not known if tiludronate crosses the human placenta. The molecular weight (about 326 for the free acid), prolonged plasma elimination half-life (150 hours), and lack of metabolism suggest that active drug will cross to the embryo–fetus.

A 2008 review described 51 cases of exposure to bisphosphonates before or during pregnancy: alendronate (N = 32), pamidronate (N = 11), etidronate (N = 5), risedronate (N = 2), and zoledronic acid (N = 1) (2). The authors concluded that although these drugs may affect bone modeling and development in the fetus, no such toxicity has yet been reported.

BREASTFEEDING SUMMARY

No reports describing the use of tiludronate during lactation have been located. The molecular weight (about 326 for the free acid), prolonged plasma elimination half-life (150 hours), and lack of metabolism suggest that active drug will be excreted into breast milk. Although the oral bioavailability in infants differs from that of adults, the very low adult oral bioavailability (<1% with food) and the binding of tiludronate by the calcium in milk suggest that the amount absorbed by the infant will be clinically insignificant. Thus, breastfeeding is probably compatible with tiludronate treatment.

References

1. Product information. Skelid. Sanofi-Synthelabo, 2003.
2. Djokanovic N, Klieger-Grossmann C, Koren G. Does treatment with bisphosphonates endanger the human pregnancy? J Obstet Gynaecol Can 2008;30:1146–8.

TIMOLOL

Sympatholytic (Antihypertensive)

PREGNANCY RECOMMENDATION: Human Data Suggest Risk in 2nd and 3rd Trimesters
BREASTFEEDING RECOMMENDATION: Limited Human Data—Probably Compatible

T

PREGNANCY SUMMARY

Systemic use of some β-blockers may cause intrauterine growth restriction (IUGR) and reduced placental weight, especially those lacking intrinsic sympathomimetic activity (ISA) (i.e., partial agonist). Treatment beginning early in the 2nd trimester results in the greatest weight reductions, whereas treatment restricted to the 3rd trimester primarily affects only placental weight. Timolol does not possess ISA. However, IUGR and reduced placental weight may potentially occur with all agents within this class. Although IUGR is a serious concern, the benefits of maternal therapy with β-blockers, in some cases, might outweigh the risks to the fetus and must be judged on a case-by-case basis.

The systemic use near delivery of some agents in this class has resulted in persistent β-blockade in the newborn (see Acebutolol, Atenolol, and Nadolol). Thus, newborns exposed in utero to timolol should be closely observed during the first 24–48 hours after birth for bradycardia and other symptoms. The long-term effects of in utero exposure to β-blockers have not been studied but warrant evaluation.

FETAL RISK SUMMARY

Timolol is a nonselective β-adrenergic blocking agent used for the treatment of hypertension, after myocardial infarction, for the prophylaxis of migraine headache, and topically for the treatment of glaucoma.

Reproductive studies in mice, rats, and rabbits at doses up to about 40 times the maximum recommended daily human dose based on patient weight of 50 kg (MRHD) found no evidence of teratogenicity (1). However, fetotoxicity (resorptions) was observed in rabbits at this dose and in mice exposed to 830 times the MRHD (a maternal toxic dose).

A study using an in vitro perfusion system of human placental tissue demonstrated that timolol crossed to the fetal side of the preparation (2). The placental transfer is consistent with the molecular weight of the compound (about 433 for timolol maleate).

A woman with glaucoma was treated throughout gestation with topical timolol (0.5%) two drops in each eye, pilocarpine, and oral acetazolamide (3). Within 48 hours of delivery at 36 weeks' gestation, the infant developed hyperbilirubinemia, hypocalcemia, hypomagnesemia, and metabolic acidosis. The toxic effects, attributed to the carbonic anhydrase inhibitor, acetazolamide (see Acetazolamide), quickly resolved on treatment. Mild hypertonicity was observed on examinations at 1, 3, and 8 months of age (3).

In a 1998 case report, a 37-year-old woman at 21 weeks' gestation was referred because of fetal bradycardia (74 beats/minute [bpm]) with irregularity (4). There were no cardiac structural anomalies and no fetal hydrops. The mother had been taking timolol eye drops 0.5%, one drop in each eye once daily, for glaucoma for 3 years. Because no other cause of the bradycardia could be found, the dose was reduced to 0.25% in each eye once daily at about 25 weeks' gestation. Three days later, the fetal heart rate increased to 96 bpm, and then to 120 bpm 1 week later. After consulting with an ophthalmologist, timolol was stopped completely at about 30 weeks, and 3 days later the fetal heart rate was around 130 bpm. At term, a 3025-g female infant was delivered with Apgar scores of 8 and 10 at 1 and 5 minutes, respectively. After birth, a cardiac arrhythmia developed that was diagnosed as right ventricle tachycardia (200 bpm) with atrial extra systole. The condition required digitalization. The baby was doing well at 2 months of age (4).

A case report published in 1986 described the pregnancy of a 24-year-old woman at 30 weeks' gestation who was treated for recurrent pheochromocytoma with a combination of timolol, prazosin (an α_1-adrenergic blocker), and metyrosine (a tyrosine hydroxylase inhibitor) (5). Hypertension had been noted at her first prenatal visit at 12 weeks' gestation. Because of declines in fetal breathing, body movements, and amniotic fluid volume that began 2 weeks after the start of therapy, a cesarean section was conducted at 33 weeks. The 1450-g female infant had Apgar scores of 3 and 5 at 1 and 5 minutes, respectively. Mild metabolic acidosis was found on analysis of umbilical cord blood gases. Multiple infarcts were noted in the placenta but no evidence of metastatic tumor. The growth-restricted infant did well and was discharged home on day 53 of life (5).

BREASTFEEDING SUMMARY

Timolol is excreted into breast milk (6,7). In nine lactating women given 5 mg orally 3 times daily, the mean milk concentration of timolol 105–135 minutes after a dose was 15.9 ng/mL (6). When a dose of 10 mg 3 times daily was given to four patients, mean milk levels of 41 ng/mL were measured. The milk:plasma ratios for the two regimens were 0.80 and 0.83, respectively.

A woman with elevated intraocular pressure applied ophthalmic 0.5% timolol drops to the right eye twice daily, resulting in excretion of the drug in her breast milk (7). Maternal timolol levels in milk and plasma were 5.6 and 0.93 ng/mL, respectively, about 1.5 hours after a dose. A milk sample taken 12 hours after the last dose contained 0.5 ng/mL of timolol. Assuming that the infant nursed every 4 hours and received 75 mL at each feeding, the daily dose would be below that expected to produce cardiac effects in the infant (7).

In a 2008 report, milk concentrations of timolol were measured from a woman with open-angle glaucoma who had been administering timolol 0.5% eye drops twice daily to her right eye for 6 months (8). Four milk samples were collected over 6 days. The mean timolol concentration in milk was 0.12 ng/mL (range 0–0.37 ng/mL). The theoretical maximum relative infant dose expressed as a percentage of the mother's weight-adjusted dose was 0.012%. Even doubling the dose to reflect the standard practice of treating both eyes would only have raised the relative dose to 0.024%. These infant exposures were thought to be clinically insignificant (8). Comments on this study and a reply also have been published (9,10).

No adverse reactions were noted in the nursing infants described in the above reports. However, infants exposed to timolol via breast milk should be closely observed for bradycardia and other signs or symptoms of β-blockade. Long-term effects of exposure to β-blockers from milk have not been studied but warrant evaluation. The American Academy of Pediatrics classifies timolol as compatible with breastfeeding (11).

References

1. Product information. Blocadren. Merck, 2000.
2. Schneider H, Proegler M. Placental transfer of β-adrenergic antagonists studied in an in vitro perfusion system of human placental tissue. Am J Obstet Gynecol 1988;159:42–7.
3. Merlob P, Litwin A, Mor N. Possible association between acetazolamide administration during pregnancy and metabolic disorders in the newborn. Eur J Obstet Gynecol Reprod Biol 1990;35:85–8.
4. Wagenvoort AM, Van Vugt JMG, Sobotka M, Van Geijn HP. Topical timolol therapy in pregnancy: is it safe for the fetus? Teratology 1998;58:258–62.
5. Devoe LD, O'Dell BE, Castillo RA, Hadi HA, Searle N. Metastatic pheochromocytoma in pregnancy and fetal biophysical assessment after maternal administration of alpha-adrenergic, beta-adrenergic, and dopamine antagonists. Obstet Gynecol 1986;68:15S–18S.
6. Fidler J, Smith V, DeSwiet M. Excretion of oxprenolol and timolol in breast milk. Br J Obstet Gynaecol 1983;90:961–5.
7. Lustgarten JS, Podos SM. Topical timolol and the nursing mother. Arch Ophthalmol 1983;101:1381–2.
8. Madadi P, Koren G, Freeman DJ, Oertel R, Campbell RJ, Trope GE. Timolol concentrations in breast milk of a woman treated for glaucoma: calculation of neonatal exposure. J Glaucoma 2008;17:329–31.
9. Novack GD. Timolol concentrations in breast milk of a woman treated for glaucoma: calculation of neonatal exposure. J Glaucoma 2008;17:510.
10. Madadi P, Koren G, Campbell RJ, Trope GE. Timolol concentrations in breast milk of a woman treated for glaucoma: calculation of neonatal exposure. J Glaucoma 2008;17:511.
11. Committee on Drugs, American Academy of Pediatrics. The transfer of drugs and other chemicals into human milk. Pediatrics 2001;108:776–89.

T

TINIDAZOLE

Anti-infective (Antiprotozoal)

PREGNANCY RECOMMENDATION: Limited Human Data—Animal Data Suggest Moderate Risk
BREASTFEEDING RECOMMENDATION: Hold Breastfeeding (Single Dose)
Limited Human Data—Potential Toxicity (Divided Dose)

PREGNANCY SUMMARY

The human pregnancy experience with tinidazole is very limited. Although there was a slight increase in fetal deaths in one animal species at a dose close to that used in humans, no other evidence of developmental toxicity was noted in animal studies. Tinidazole is chemically related to metronidazole, and there is no convincing evidence of embryo or fetal harm with that anti-infective. Nevertheless, it would be prudent to choose metronidazole for those infections where both agents are recommended. Tinidazole could be used in cases where metronidazole therapy has failed to eradicate the infection. However, until more human data are available, avoidance of the 1st trimester should be considered.

FETAL RISK SUMMARY

Tinidazole is an oral synthetic antiprotozoal agent that chemically is a second-generation 5-nitroimidazole. It is closely related structurally to metronidazole. Tinidazole is indicated for the treatment of trichomoniasis caused by *Trichomonas vaginalis*, giardiasis caused by *Giardia duoenalis*, and amebiasis caused by *Entamoeba histolytica*. Oral bioavailability is 100%. It is partially metabolized and has a plasma half-life of about 12–14 hours. Plasma protein binding of tinidazole is about 12% (1).

Reproduction studies have been conducted in mice and rats. In pregnant mice, no evidence of embryo or fetal harm was observed with doses up to about 6.3 times the maximum human therapeutic dose based on BSA (MHTD). In pregnant rats, a slightly higher incidence of fetal death was noted with a dose 2.5 times the MHTD. No biologically relevant neonatal developmental effects were noted in rat pups after maternal doses as high as 3 times the MHTD (1).

Long-term studies for carcinogenic effects have not been conducted with tinidazole. A closely related agent, metronidazole, has been studied and found to be associated with tumors in mice and rats (1) (see also Metronidazole). Assays for mutagenicity with tinidazole have resulted in both positive and negative results (1).

Decreased fertility and testicular histopathology occurred in male rats given doses that were about 3 times the MHTD for 60 days. Spermatogenic effects were noted at doses that were about ≥1.5 times the MHTD. The no-observed-adverse-effect level for testicular and spermatogenic effects was about half the MHTD. These findings are characteristic of agents in the 5-nitroimidazole class (1).

Tinidazole crosses the human placenta. A single 500-mg IV infusion was given over 20 minutes to 11 women undergoing a 1st trimester abortion (2). Sixty minutes after the start of the infusion, the uterus was evacuated. The mean concentrations of tinidazole in the maternal serum, fetal tissue, and placental tissue were 13.2 mcg/mL, 7.6 mcg/g, and 4.9 mg/g, respectively. The fetal tissue level was 58% of the maternal serum concentration (2).

The large population-based dataset of the Hungarian Case–Control Surveillance of Congenital Abnormalities was used to evaluate the effect of oral tinidazole (1–2 g/day for 6–7 days) on pregnancy outcomes in terms of congenital defects (3). Among the 22,843 cases with congenital anomalies, 10 (0.04%) had taken tinidazole, whereas in 38,151 controls, 16 (0.04%) had been exposed to the drug. The exposures had occurred in the 1st trimester in six cases and six controls. Although the data are very limited, there was no suggestion that tinidazole exposures resulted in a higher rate of congenital anomalies (3).

A 2006 review of the treatment of trichomoniasis concluded that single, 2-g oral dose of either metronidazole or tinidazole were first-line therapy (4). If a decision was made to treat a pregnant woman, metronidazole was preferred because of the greater amount of data related to pregnancy.

According to the CDC's 2006 Sexually Transmitted Diseases Treatment guidelines, recurrent and persistent urethritis was best treated with single, 2-g oral dose of either metronidazole or tinidazole (5). No special consideration was made for pregnancy. A similar recommendation was made for trichomoniasis. In this case, however, the limited human pregnancy experience with tinidazole was mentioned (5).

BREASTFEEDING SUMMARY

Tinidazole is excreted into breast milk. In a 1972 report, four women had milk:serum ratios as high as 1.62 after 7 days of treatment with tinidazole (6). A 1983 investigation studied the milk excretion of the drug in 24 women (7). After cord clamping, an IV infusion of tinidazole 500 mg was given to the mother over 20 minutes. Milk (colostrum) and blood samples were collected at 12, 24, 48, 72, and 96 hours after the end of the infusion. Mean maternal serum concentrations (mcg/mL) in the five samples were 6.1, 3.7, 1.2, 0.1, and 0, respectively. Milk samples at 12 and 24 hours were mixed samples, whereas the samples at 48, 72, and 96 hours were collected as fore- and hind-milk. The mixed milk concentrations were 5.8 and 3.5 mcg/mL, respectively. At the three other times, the concentrations (fore-milk/hind-milk) were

T

1.28/1.20, 0.32/0.30, and trace/trace, respectively. It was not stated if the infants were allowed to breastfeed (7).

In a 1985 study, five women undergoing a cesarean section received a single IV dose of tinidazole 1600 mg infused within 1.5 hours immediately after cord clamping (8). Blood and milk samples were collected at 8- and 4-hour intervals, respectively, for 96 hours. The average half-life of tinidazole in serum was 11.4 hours. The milk:serum ratios ranged from 0.62 to 1.39 with milk concentrations highly related to serum concentrations ($r = 0.969$). By 72 hours, only one woman had a milk concentration greater than 0.5 mcg/mL. The infants were not allowed to breastfeed. It was estimated that at 72 hours, the maximum daily dose for a nursing infant would be 0.1 mg/kg (assuming 3.5 kg body weight and 400 mL of milk consumed), and that breastfeeding then could commence (8).

The effect of exposure to tinidazole in breast milk is unknown because none of the above mothers breastfed their infants. Because of the close similarity between tinidazole and metronidazole, the American Academy of Pediatrics classifies both drugs as agents whose effect on nursing infants is unknown but may be of concern (9). If single-dose therapy is given, discontinuing breastfeeding for 12–24 hours to allow excretion of the drug was recommended.

References

1. Product information. Tindamaz. Presutti Laboratories, 2004.
2. Karhunen M. Placental transfer of metronidazole and tinidazole in early human pregnancy after a single infusion. Br J Clin Pharmacol 1984;18:254–7.
3. Czeizel AE, Kazy Z, Vargha P. Oral tinidazole treatment during pregnancy and teratogenesis. Int J Gynecol Obstet 2003;83:305–6.
4. Nanda N, Michel RG, Kurdgelashvili G, Wendel KA. Trichomoniasis and its treatment. Expert Rev Anti Infect Ther 2006;4:125–35.
5. CDC. Sexually transmitted diseases treatment guidelines, 2006. MMWR 2006;55(RR11):1–94.
6. Welling PG, Monro AM. The pharmacokinetics of metronidazole and tinidazole in man. Arzneimittelforsch 1972;22:2128–32. As cited in Mannisto PT, Karhunen M, Koskela O, Suikkari AM, Mattila J, Haataja H. Concentrations of tinidazole in breast milk. Acta Pharmacol Toxicol (Copenh) 1983;53:254–6.
7. Mannisto PT, Karhunen M, Koskela O, Suikkari AM, Mattila J, Haataja H. Concentrations of tinidazole in breast milk. Acta Pharmacol Toxicol (Copenh) 1983;53:254–6.
8. Evaldson GR, Lindgren S, Nord CE, Rane AT. Tinidazole milk excretion and pharmacokinetics in lactating women. Br J Clin Pharmacol 1985;19:503–7.
9. Committee on Drugs, American Academy of Pediatrics. The transfer of drugs and other chemicals into human milk. Pediatrics 2001;108:776–89.

TINZAPARIN

[Withdrawn from the market. See 9th edition.]

TIOCONAZOLE

Antifungal

PREGNANCY RECOMMENDATION: Limited Human Data—Animal Data Suggest Low Risk
BREASTFEEDING RECOMMENDATION: No Human Data—Probably Compatible

PREGNANCY SUMMARY

Although the animal reproduction data suggest low risk, there was no comparison with the recommended human dose. Only very small amounts of tioconazole are absorbed systemically from the human vagina and comparison with the oral doses used in the animal studies would have little meaning. The limited human data also suggest low risk, but the failure to specify the gestational ages and other data limits the assessment of embryo–fetal risk. The use of intravaginal tioconazole during pregnancy does not appear to represent a major risk, but more commonly used agents such as clotrimazole, miconazole, or nystatin should be considered the antifungals of choice during pregnancy.

FETAL RISK SUMMARY

Tioconazole is a topical antifungal agent that is indicated for the local treatment of vulvovaginal candidiasis (moniliasis). In the United States, it is available only as a single-dose, 300-mg (6.5% ointment) for intravaginal administration. Systemic absorption of tioconazole after intravaginal administration of a 300-mg dose is negligible (1–3). Six women with vaginal candidosis were treated with intravaginal 2% tioconazole cream (100 mg tioconazole in 5 g) for 14 consecutive days. The drug was not detected in blood samples drawn before and 2, 4, and 8 hours after the first and last doses (2). In another study, a 300-mg dose was given to 10 nonpregnant women. The mean plasma concentration was 21.2 ng/mL 8 hours after a dose and was undetectable (detection limit 10 ng/mL) at 24 hours in 9 of the 10 women. In contrast, the mean concentration in vaginal fluid was 21,400 ng/mL (3).

Reproduction studies have been performed in rats and rabbits. No adverse effects on fetal viability or growth and no major structural anomalies were observed in pregnant rats given 55–165 mg/kg/day orally during organogenesis. An increase in the incidence of dilated ureters, hydroureters, and hydronephrosis in fetuses was not evident in pups raised to 21 days of age. These effects were not observed when a 2% tioconazole cream (about 10 mg/kg/day) was given intravaginally. Similar to other azole antimycotic agents, when treatment was extended through parturition in rats, tioconazole caused dystocia, prolongation of pregnancy, embryo–fetal deaths, and impaired pup survival. The no-effect dose for this toxicity was about 20 mg/kg/day orally and about 9 mg/kg/day intravaginally. In pregnant rabbits, there was no evidence of embryo toxicity or teratogenicity with oral doses ≤165 mg/kg/day or daily intravaginal application of about 2–3 mg/kg from a 2% cream during organogenesis. No effects on parturition occurred in rabbits at 50 mg/kg/day orally (1).

It is not known if tioconazole crosses the human placenta. The molecular weight (about 388) is low enough, but systemic absorption of the drug from the vagina is negligible. Thus, exposure of the embryo–fetus to clinically significant concentrations is unlikely.

In an open 1987 study, 45 pregnant women with intractable vaginal candidosis were treated with a single-dose 300-mg tioconazole vaginal ovule (4). In addition, they applied a tioconazole 1% cream intra-anally, and rubbed the cream onto the perianal and vulva regions once daily for 7 days. The gestational ages of the women were not specified. All 45 women had spontaneous vaginal deliveries of normal healthy infants (gestational age at delivery and status of the newborn not specified). At 6-week follow-up, the infants were in satisfactory condition (4).

BREASTFEEDING SUMMARY

No reports describing the use of tioconazole during human lactation have been located. The molecular weight (about 388) is low enough for excretion into breast milk. However, systemic absorption of the drug from the vagina is negligible and detectable concentrations in milk are unlikely. Moreover, a 1% tioconazole cream has been used safely in neonates and infants to treat candidal diaper rash (5). Thus, the effect of maternal use of intravaginal tioconazole on a nursing infant appears to be nil.

References

1. Product information. Vagistat-1. Bristol-Myers Squibb. Available at http://www.rxlist.com/cgi/generic/tioconaz.htm. Accessed January 21, 2008.
2. Gjonnaess H, Jerve F, Bergen T. Tioconazole 2% cream in vaginal candidosis: systemic absorption and results of three days treatment compared to clotrimazole vaginal tablets. Cur Therap Res 1981;30:995–1004.
3. Houang ET, Lawrence AG. Systemic absorption and persistence of tioconazole in vaginal fluid after insertion of a single 300-mg tioconazole ovule. Antimicrob Agents Chemother June 1985:964–5.
4. Adetoro OO. Tioconazole in the management of recurrent vaginal candidosis during pregnancy in Ilorin, Nigeria. Cur Therap Res 1987;41:647–50.
5. Gibbs DL, Kashin P, Jevons S. Comparative and non-comparative studies on the efficacy and tolerance of tioconazole cream 1% versus another imidazole and/or placebo in neonates and infants with candidal diaper rash and/or impetigo. J Inter Med Res 1987;15:23–31.

TIOTROPIUM

Respiratory Drug (Bronchodilator)

PREGNANCY RECOMMENDATION: **No Human Data—Animal Data Suggest Low Risk**
BREASTFEEDING RECOMMENDATION: **No Human Data—Probably Compatible**

PREGNANCY SUMMARY

No reports describing the use of tiotropium during human pregnancy have been located. The approved indication for the drug suggests that such experience will be rare, but its use in asthmatic patients is possible. Although the animal data suggest low risk, the absence of pregnancy data prevents a full assessment of human risk. There are human pregnancy data for ipratropium, which is the preferred inhaled anticholinergic bronchodilator in pregnancy. However, because its long elimination half-life, use of tiotropium immediately before the diagnosis of an inadvertent pregnancy would most likely result in the exposure of a portion of organogenesis. Therefore, if a nonpregnant woman has shown a good response to inhaled tiotropium, it would be reasonable to continue her on this drug during pregnancy. If the maternal condition warrants starting tiotropium in pregnancy, avoidance of the 1st trimester should be considered.

FETAL RISK SUMMARY

Tiotropium is a parasympatholytic (anticholinergic), quarternary ammonium compound that has specificity for muscarinic receptors. It is formulated as capsules that contain a powder given by oral inhalation. Tiotropium is indicated for the long-term maintenance treatment of bronchospasm associated with chronic obstructive pulmonary disease (COPD), including chronic bronchitis and emphysema. As expected, the majority of the dose is deposited in the gastrointestinal tract, but oral bioavailability is poor (2%–3%). The absolute bioavailability of an inhaled dose, primarily from the lung, is about 20%. The terminal elimination half-life after inhalation is 5–6 days (1,2).

Reproduction studies have been conducted with tiotropium in experimental animals. Long-term studies in rats revealed no evidence of tumorigenicity, mutagenicity, or clastogenicity. In pregnant rats and rabbits, inhalation doses up to about 660 and 6 times, respectively, the maximum recommended human daily dose based on BSA (MRHD) revealed no evidence of structural anomalies. In rats, however, a dose about 35 times the MRHD resulted in fetal toxicity (resorptions, litter loss, decreased number of live pups at birth, decreased mean birth weight, and a delayed pup sexual maturation) and, in a fertility study, decreased number of corpora lutea and percentage of implants. In rabbits an increase in postimplantation loss was noted at about 360 times the MRHD. The no-observed-effect level (NOEL) for these toxicities in rats and rabbits was about 4 and 80 times the MRHD, respectively. However, these dose multiples may be over-estimated because of the difficulties in measuring deposited doses in animal inhalation studies (1,2).

It is not known if tiotropium crosses the placenta. The drug's molecular weight (about 490 for the bromide monohydrate salt) is low enough to cross. The peak plasma concentrations at steady state are very low (17–19 pg/mL), thus limiting the amount of drug at the maternal–fetal interface.

BREASTFEEDING SUMMARY

No reports describing the use of tiotropium during human lactation have been located. Because of the very low amounts in plasma (steady state peak plasma levels of 17–19 pg/mL) and the poor oral bioavailability (about 2%–3%), maternal use of the drug during lactation probably would have no effect on a nursing infant. However, close monitoring of the infant for anticholinergic effects (e.g., dry mouth, constipation, urinary retention, and increased heart rate) is warranted.

References

1. Product information. Spiriva. Boehringer Ingelheim Pharmaceuticals, 2005.
2. Product information. Spiriva. Pfizer, 2005.

TIPRANAVIR

Antiviral

PREGNANCY RECOMMENDATION: Compatible—Maternal Benefit >> Embryo–Fetal Risk
BREASTFEEDING RECOMMENDATION: Contraindicated

PREGNANCY SUMMARY

The very limited human pregnancy experience during the 1st trimester does not allow a prediction as to the risk of tipranavir during gestation. The animal data suggest low risk, but the obtainable systemic exposures were very low. If indicated, the drug should not be withheld because of pregnancy.

FETAL RISK SUMMARY

Tipranavir is a nonpeptide inhibitor of HIV type 1 (HIV-1) protease. Tipranavir is indicated, in combination with ritonavir 200 mg, for combination antiretroviral treatment of adults infected with HIV-1 with evidence of viral replication, who are highly treatment-experienced or have HIV-1 strains resistant to multiple protease inhibitors. Tipranavir and ritonavir are combined because tipranavir is primarily metabolized by CYP3A and ritonavir inhibits CYP3A, thereby markedly increasing the plasma concentrations of tipranavir (darunavir and lopinavir also are combined with ritonavir for the same reason). Metabolism in the presence of ritonavir is minimal. Tipranavir is extensively bound to plasma proteins (>99.9%), both albumin and α_1-acid-glycoprotein. In HIV-infected adults, the mean terminal elimination half-life is about 6 hours when combined with ritonavir (1).

Reproduction studies have been conducted in rats and rabbits. In pregnant rats, no effect on early embryonic development was observed at tipranavir exposures about equal to the human exposure from the recommended dose of 500/200 mg tipranavir/ritonavir given twice daily. No teratogenicity was observed in rats or rabbits with tipranavir doses up to 1.1 and 0.1 times, respectively, the human exposure (AUC) of tipranavir at the recommended dose (HE). At about 0.8 times the HE or higher in rats, fetal toxicity (decreased sternebrae ossification and body weights) was observed. In rats and rabbits, fetal toxicity was not observed at exposures (AUC) that were about 0.2 and 0.1 times, respectively, the HE. In pre- and postdevelopment studies in rats, dose levels about 0.8 times the HE caused growth inhibition in pups and maternal toxicity. The no-adverse-effect level was about 0.2 times the HE (1).

Long-term carcinogenicity studies have not been completed with tipranavir and tipranavir/ritonavir. No evidence of mutagenicity or clastogenicity was observed in a variety of assays. There also was no evidence of impaired fertility in rats at tipranavir exposures about equal to the human exposure from the recommended dose of 500/200 mg tipranavir/ritonavir given twice daily (1).

It is not known if tipranavir crosses the human placenta. The molecular weight (about 603), minimal metabolism, and elimination half-life suggest that the drug will cross, but the high plasma protein binding will be limiting factor.

A 33-year-old woman with drug-resistant HIV presented to a treatment center at 27 weeks' gestation (2). The woman's current therapy was stavudine, tenofovir, and lopinavir/ritonavir, but the response to this combination had been poor, as had been her compliance. Her therapy was changed to zidovudine, lamivudine, abacavir, tenofovir, enfuvirtide, and tipranavir/ritonavir. The patient was hospitalized. High-dose zidovudine was given at 34 weeks' gestation and a cesarean section delivered a healthy infant (sex not specified). No evidence of HIV was found in the infant on the day of birth and at 6 and 26 weeks of age (2).

In 1998, a public health advisory was issued by the FDA on the association between protease inhibitors and diabetes mellitus (3). Because pregnancy is a risk factor for hyperglycemia, there was concern that these antiretroviral agents would exacerbate this risk. The manufacturer's product information also notes the potential risk for new-onset diabetes, exacerbation of preexisting diabetes, and hyperglycemia in HIV-infected patients receiving protease inhibitor therapy (1). An abstract published in 2000 described the results of a study involving 34 pregnant women treated with protease inhibitors compared with 41 controls that evaluated the association with diabetes (4). No association between protease inhibitors and an increased incidence of gestational diabetes was found.

The Antiretroviral Pregnancy Registry reported, for the period January 1989 through July 2009, prospective data (reported before the outcomes were known) involving 4702 live births that had been exposed during the 1st trimester to one or more antiretroviral agents (5). Congenital defects were noted in 134, a prevalence of 2.8% (95% confidence interval [CI] 2.4–3.4). In the 6100 live births with earliest exposure in the 2nd/3rd trimesters, there were 153 infants with defects (prevalence 2.5%, 95% CI 2.1–2.9). The prevalence rates for the two periods did not differ significantly. There were 288 infants with birth defects among 10,803 live births with exposure anytime during pregnancy (prevalence 2.7%, 95% CI 2.4–3.0). The prevalence rate did not differ significantly from the rate expected in a nonexposed population. There were five outcomes exposed to tipranavir (four in the 1st trimester and one in the 2nd/3rd trimesters) in combination with other antiretroviral agents. There were no birth defects. In reviewing the birth defects of prospective and retrospective (pregnancies reported after the outcomes were known) registered cases, the Registry concluded that, except for isolated cases of neural tube defects with efavirenz exposure in retrospective reports, there was no other pattern of anomalies (isolated or syndromic) (5) (see Lamivudine for required statement).

Two reviews, one in 1996 and the other in 1997, concluded that all women currently receiving antiretroviral therapy should continue to receive therapy during pregnancy and that treatment of the mother with monotherapy should be considered inadequate therapy (6,7). The same conclusion was reached in a 2003 review with the added admonishment that therapy must be continuous to prevent emergence of resistant viral strains (8). In 2009, the updated U.S. Department of Health and Human Services guidelines for the use of antiretroviral agents in HIV-1-infected patients continued the recommendation that the therapy, with the exception of efavirenz, should be continued during pregnancy (9). If indicated, therefore, protease inhibitors, including tipranavir, should not be withheld in pregnancy because the expected benefit to the HIV-positive mother outweighs the unknown risk to the fetus. Pregnant women taking protease inhibitors should be monitored for hyperglycemia. Updated guidelines for the use of antiretroviral drugs to reduce perinatal HIV-1 transmission also were released in 2010 (10). Women receiving antiretroviral therapy during pregnancy should continue the therapy but, regardless of the regimen, zidovudine administration is recommended during the intrapartum period to prevent vertical transmission of HIV to the newborn (10).

BREASTFEEDING SUMMARY

No reports describing the use of tipranavir during lactation have been located. The molecular weight (about 603), minimal metabolism, an elimination half-life (6 hours) suggest that the drug will be excreted into breast milk. The effect of this exposure on a nursing infant is unknown.

Reports on the use of tipranavir during human lactation are unlikely because the antiviral agent is used in the treatment of HIV infection. HIV-1 is transmitted in milk, and in developed countries, breastfeeding is not recommended (6,7,9,11–13). In developing countries, breastfeeding is undertaken, despite the risk, because there are no affordable milk substitutes available. Until 1999, no studies had been published that examined the effect of any antiretroviral therapy on HIV-1 transmission in milk. In that year, a study involving zidovudine was published that measured a 38% reduction in vertical transmission of HIV-1 infection despite breastfeeding when compared with controls (see Zidovudine).

References

1. Product information. Aptivus. Boehringer Ingelheim Pharmaceuticals, 2007.
2. Wensing AMJ, Boucher CAB, van Kasteren M, van Dijken PJ, Geelen SP, Juttmann JR. Prevention of mother-to-child transmission of multi-drug-resistant HIV-1 using maternal therapy with both enfuvirtide and tipranavir. AIDS 2006;20:1465–7.
3. CDC. Public Health Service Task Force recommendations for the use of antiretroviral drugs in pregnant women infected with HIV-1 for maternal health and for reducing perinatal HIV-1 transmission in the United States. MMWR 1998;47:No. RR-2.
4. Fassett M, Kramer F, Stek A. Treatment with protease inhibitors in pregnancy is not associated with an increased incidence of gestational diabetes (abstract). Am J Obstet Gynecol 2000;182:S97.
5. Antiretroviral Pregnancy Registry Steering Committee. *Antiretroviral Pregnancy Registry International Interim Report for 1 January 1989 through 31 July 2009*. Wilmington, NC: Registry Coordinating Center; 2009. Available at www.APRegistry.com. Accessed May 29, 2010.
6. Carpenter CCJ, Fischi MA, Hammer SM, Hirsch MS, Jacobsen DM, Katzenstein DA, Montaner JSG, Richman DD, Saag MS, Schooley RT, Thompson MA, Vella S, Yeni PG, Volberding PA. Antiretroviral therapy for HIV infection in 1996. JAMA 1996;276;146–54.
7. Minkoff H, Augenbraun M. Antiretroviral therapy for pregnant women. Am J Obstet Gynecol 1997;176:478–89.
8. Minkoff H. Human immunodeficiency virus infection in pregnancy. Obstet Gynecol·2003;101:797–810.
9. Panel on Antiretroviral Guidelines for Adults and Adolescents. *Guidelines for the Use of Antiretroviral Agents in HIV-1-Infected Adults and Adolescents*. Department of Health and Human Services. December 1, 2009:1–161. Available at http://www.aidsinfo.nih.gov/ContentFiles/AdultandAdolescentGL.pdf. Accessed September 17, 2010:60, 96–8.
10. Panel on Treatment of HIV-Infected Pregnant Women and Prevention of Perinatal Transmission. *Recommendations for Use of Antiretroviral Drugs in Pregnant HIV-1-Infected Women for Maternal Health and Interventions to Reduce Perinatal HIV Transmission in the United States*. May 24, 2010:1–117. Available at http://aidsinfo.nih.gov/ContentFiles/PerinatalGL.pdf. Accessed September 17, 2010:30 (Table 5).
11. Brown ZA, Watts DH. Antiviral therapy in pregnancy. Clin Obstet Gynecol 1990;33:276–89.
12. De Martino M, Tovo P-A, Pezzotti P, Galli L, Massironi E, Ruga E, Floreea F, Plebani A, Gabiano C, Zuccotti GV. HIV-1 transmission through breast-milk: appraisal of risk according to duration of feeding. AIDS 1992;6:991–7.
13. Van de Perre P. Postnatal transmission of human immunodeficiency virus type 1: the breastfeeding dilemma. Am J Obstet Gynecol 1995;173:483–7.

T

TIROFIBAN

Antiplatelet Agent

PREGNANCY RECOMMENDATION: Compatible—Maternal Benefit >> Embryo–Fetal Risk
BREASTFEEDING RECOMMENDATION: Hold Breastfeeding

PREGNANCY SUMMARY

Only one report describing the use of tirofiban in human pregnancy has been located. The pregnancy was still ongoing at the time of the report. The animal data are reassuring but human pregnancy experience is required to assess the risk this agent presents to the embryo–fetus. The primary risk, however, appears to be from maternal hemorrhage during drug administration. If this is adequately controlled, the benefits of the drug to the mother appear to far outweigh the unknown risks to the fetus.

FETAL RISK SUMMARY

Tirofiban, a nonpeptide antagonist of the platelet glycoprotein IIb/IIIa receptor, is an inhibitor of platelet aggregation. It is given by continuous IV infusion for up to 108 hours depending on the indication. Tirofiban is in the same subclass of antiplatelet agents as abciximab and eptifibatide. It is indicated, in combination with heparin, for the treatment of acute coronary syndrome, including patients who are to be managed medically and those undergoing percutaneous transluminal coronary angioplasty (PTCA) or atherectomy. The metabolism of the agent is limited and about 65% is bound to plasma proteins. The half-life is about 2 hours (1).

Reproduction studies have been conducted in rats and rabbits. In these species, IV doses up to 5 and 13 times, respectively, the maximum recommended human dose based on BSA (MRHD) revealed no harm to the fetus (1).

Studies evaluating the carcinogenic potential of tirofiban have not been conducted. Multiple assays for mutagenicity and chromosomal aberration were negative. Fertility and reproductive performance were not affected in male and female rats given IV doses up to about 5 times the MRHD (1).

It is not known if tirofiban crosses the human placenta. The drug does cross the placenta in rats and rabbits. The molecular weight (about 441 for the nonhydrated free base), limited metabolism, and moderate plasma protein binding suggest that the drug will cross to the embryo–fetus. Moreover, the drug is given as a continuous IV infusion for periods up to 108 hours, thus allowing for prolonged contact at the maternal–fetal interface.

A 43-year-old woman, with a history of diabetes and hypertension, was in her sixth pregnancy when she had an acute myocardial infarction at 20 weeks' gestation (2). She was treated with aspirin, nitroglycerin, and then tirofiban with heparin for PTCA and intracoronary stenting. She was discharged home, 5 days after the procedure, on aspirin, clopidogrel, and metoprolol (doses not specified). The pregnancy was ongoing at the time of the report (2).

BREASTFEEDING SUMMARY

No reports describing the use of tirofiban during human lactation have been located. The molecular weight (about 441 for the nonhydrated free base), limited metabolism, and moderate plasma protein binding (65%) suggest that the drug will be excreted into breast milk. Moreover, the drug is given as a continuous IV infusion for periods up to 108 hours. The drug is commonly combined with heparin and sometimes with aspirin. The effect of this exposure on a nursing infant is unknown, as is its oral bioavailability. However, the safest course is to hold breastfeeding during the infusion.

References

1. Product information. Aggrastat. Medicure International, 2007.
2. Boztosun B, Olcay A, Avci A, Kirma C. Treatment of acute myocardial infarction in pregnancy with coronary artery balloon angioplasty and stenting: use of tirofiban and clopidogrel. Int J Cardiol 2008;127:413–6.

TIZANIDINE

Skeletal Muscle Relaxant

PREGNANCY RECOMMENDATION: No Human Data—Animal Data Suggest Risk
BREASTFEEDING RECOMMENDATION: No Human Data—Potential Toxicity

PREGNANCY SUMMARY

No reports describing the use of tizanidine in human pregnancy have been located. The animal data suggest toxicity but not congenital defects. The absence of human pregnancy experience prevents an assessment of the embryo–fetal risk. However, dose-related hypotension has been observed in humans and this could be a potentially serious adverse effect in pregnant women. Single doses of the recommended dose (8 mg) have caused a 20% reduction in either the systolic or the diastolic blood pressure in two-thirds of patients. This effect may be minimized by titration of the dose, but close monitoring of the maternal blood pressure is required. In addition, if the drug must be used in pregnancy, avoidance in the 1st trimester is recommended.

FETAL RISK SUMMARY

Tizanidine is a centrally acting α_2-adrenergic agonist structurally related to clonidine that is used for the management of spasticity. Based on animal studies, tizanidine has no direct effect on skeletal muscle fibers or the neuromuscular junction. Although, in animals the drug has a small fraction (2%–10%) of the potency of clonidine in lowering blood pressure, dose-related hypotension has been observed in humans. The terminal elimination half-life is about 2.5 hours (1).

Reproduction studies have been conducted in rats and rabbits. In rats, a dose equal to the maximum recommended human dose based on BSA (MRHD) revealed no evidence of teratogenicity. At doses up to 8 times the MRHD, increased duration of gestation, increased prenatal and postnatal pup mortality and slow development were noted. In rabbits, no evidence of structural defects was evident at a dose 16 times the MRHD. However, postimplantation loss was increased at a dose equal to or greater than 0.5 times the MRHD (1).

It is not known if tizanidine crosses the human placenta. The relatively low molecular weight (about 254 for the free base) and lipid solubility suggest that passage to the embryo or fetus should be expected.

BREASTFEEDING SUMMARY

No reports describing the use of tizanidine during human lactation have been located. The molecular weight (about 254 for the free base) and lipid solubility suggest that excretion into breast milk will occur. The effect of this exposure on a nursing infant is unknown, but serious toxicity (e.g., sedation, hypotension, liver injury, and hallucinations/psychotic-like symptoms as seen in adults) is a potential complication. Because of these potential adverse effects, breastfeeding is not recommended.

Reference

1. Product information. Zanaflex. Elan Biopharmaceuticals, 2004.

TOBRAMYCIN

Antibiotic (Aminoglycoside)

PREGNANCY RECOMMENDATION: Human Data Suggest Low Risk
BREASTFEEDING RECOMMENDATION: Compatible

PREGNANCY SUMMARY

No reports linking the use of tobramycin with congenital defects have been located. The antibiotic is not teratogenic in two animal species (1). Ototoxicity, which is known to occur after tobramycin therapy, has not been reported as an effect of in utero exposure. However, eighth cranial nerve toxicity in the fetus is well known following exposure to other aminoglycosides (see Kanamycin and Streptomycin) and may potentially occur with tobramycin.

FETAL RISK SUMMARY

Tobramycin is an aminoglycoside antibiotic. Renal toxicity was observed in pregnant rats and their fetuses after maternal administration of high doses of tobramycin (30 or 60 mg/kg/day) for 10 days, during organogenesis. The dose-related fetal renal toxicity consisted of granularity and swelling of proximal tubule cells, poor glomerular differentiation, and increased glomerular density (2).

Tobramycin crosses the placenta into the fetal circulation and amniotic fluid (3,4). Studies in patients undergoing elective abortions in the 1st and 2nd trimesters indicate that tobramycin distributes to most fetal tissues except the brain and cerebrospinal fluid (3). Amniotic fluid levels generally did not occur until the 2nd trimester. The highest fetal concentrations were found in the kidneys and urine (3). In a woman undergoing surgical termination of an ovarian gestation in a 22-week heterotopic pregnancy (intrauterine and ovarian), a single 2 mg/kg IV dose of tobramycin was administered for 10 minutes, 5.6 hours before cesarean section (4). Tobramycin was found in all fluids and tissues of the 260-g ovarian fetus, with the highest concentrations occurring in the fetal spleen (1.53 mcg/mL) and kidney (2.98 mcg/mL). The intrauterine fetus developed normally and a healthy 2900-g girl was eventually delivered at 38 weeks' gestation. Reports measuring the passage of tobramycin in the 3rd trimester or at term are lacking.

In a surveillance study of Michigan Medicaid recipients involving 229,101 completed pregnancies conducted between 1985 and 1992, 81 newborns had been exposed to tobramycin during the 1st trimester (F. Rosa, personal communication, FDA, 1993). A total of three (3.7%) major birth defects were observed (three expected), one of which was a cardiovascular defect (one expected). No anomalies were observed in five other categories of defects (oral clefts, spina bifida, polydactyly, limb reduction defects, and hypospadias) for which specific data were available.

The population-based dataset of the Hungarian Case–Control Surveillance of Congenital Abnormalities, covering the period of 1980–1996, was used to evaluate the teratogenicity of aminoglycoside antibiotics (parenteral gentamicin, streptomycin, tobramycin, and oral neomycin) in a study published in 2000 (5). A case group of 22,865 women who had fetuses or newborns with congenital malformations were compared with 38,151 women who had newborns with no structural defects. A total of 38 cases and 42 controls were treated with aminoglycosides. There were two cases and four controls treated with tobramycin (odds ratio 0.8, 95% confidence interval 0.2–3.9). The investigators concluded that there was no detectable teratogenic risk for structural defects for any of the aminoglycoside antibiotics. They also concluded, although it was not investigated in this study, that the risk of deafness after in utero aminoglycoside exposure was small (5).

A potentially serious drug interaction may occur in newborns treated with aminoglycosides who were also exposed in utero to magnesium sulfate (see Gentamicin).

BREASTFEEDING SUMMARY

Tobramycin is excreted into breast milk. Following an 80-mg IM dose given to five patients, milk levels varied from a trace to 0.52 mcg/mL over 8 hours (6). Peak levels occurred at 4 hours after injection. Because oral absorption of this antibiotic is poor, ototoxicity in the infant would not be expected. However, three potential problems exist for the nursing infant: modification of bowel flora, direct effects on the infant, and interference with the interpretation of culture results if a fever workup is required.

References

1. Welles JS, Emmerson JL, Gibson WR, Nickander R, Owen NV, Anderson RC. Preclinical toxicology studies of tobramycin. Toxicol Appl Pharmacol 1973;25: 398–409. As cited in Shepard TH. *Catalog of Teratogenic Agents*. 6th ed. Baltimore, MD: The Johns Hopkins University Press, 1989;623.
2. Mantovani A, Macri C, Stazi AV, Ricciardi C, Guastadisegni C, Maranghi F. Tobramycin-induced changes in renal histology of fetal and newborn Sprague-Dawley rats. Teratogenesis Carcinog Mutagen 1992;12:19–30.
3. Bernard B, Garcia-Cazares S, Ballard C, Thrupp L, Mathies A, Wehrle P. Tobramycin: maternal–fetal pharmacology. Antimicrob Agents Chemother 1977;11:688–94.
4. Fernandez H, Bourget P, Delouis C. Fetal levels of tobramycin following maternal administration. Obstet Gynecol 1990;76:992–4.
5. Czeizel AE, Rockenbauer M, Olsen J, Sorensen HT. A teratological study of aminoglycoside antibiotic treatment during pregnancy. Scand J Infect Dis 2000;32:309–13.
6. Takase Z. Laboratory and clinical studies on tobramycin in the field of obstetrics and gynecology. Chemotherapy (Tokyo) 1975;23:1402.

TOCAINIDE

[Withdrawn from the market. See 9th edition.]

TOCILIZUMAB

Immunologic Agent (Immunomodulator)

PREGNANCY RECOMMENDATION: Limited Human Data—Probably Compatible
BREASTFEEDING RECOMMENDATION: No Human Data—Probably Compatible

PREGNANCY SUMMARY

Outcomes in 31 human pregnancies including 10 live births and 1 newborn death have been reported with no teratogenic effects noted. Teratogenicity was not observed in cynomolgus monkeys, but compared with controls, an increased risk of fetal death was observed at the two highest doses. No other forms of developmental toxicity were observed in the monkey model or in a mouse analog. If tocilizumab is used in pregnancy, patients should be informed of the lack of adequate human pregnancy experience. The manufacturer maintains a pregnancy registry (1). Physicians are encouraged to register patients and patients can register themselves by calling 1-877-311-8972.

T

FETAL RISK SUMMARY

Tocilizumab is a recombinant humanized IgG1κ monoclonal antibody against the human interleukin-6 receptor (IL-6). It is indicated for the treatment of adult patients with moderately to severely active rheumatoid arthritis who have had inadequate response to other therapies, and for the treatment of patients with juvenile idiopathic arthritis who are 2 years of age or older. The terminal elimination half-life in adult patients is up to 11 days for doses of 4 mg/kg and up to 13 days for doses of 8 mg/kg given by IV infusion every 4 weeks (1).

Reproduction studies have been conducted in pregnant cynomolgus monkeys who received daily doses of 0 (control), 2, 10, and 50 mg/kg given by IV infusion from gestation day 20 to 50. The comparability of these doses to the human dose of 8 mg/kg given every 2 to 4 weeks is unclear; however, there was no evidence of teratogenicity at any dose. An increase in embryo–fetal deaths was observed at the 10 and 50 mg/kg doses (embryo–fetal losses of 10%, 10%, 20%, and 30%, respectively, for the 0, 2, 10, and 50 mg/kg/day groups) (1,2).

In other studies in rats, rabbits, and mice no evidence of teratogenicity was noted. In addition, no effects on postnatal development including functional performance or immune competence were observed in mice. In rabbits, at the intermediate dose of 5 mg/kg, an increase in fetal mortality was noted, but effects were thought to be secondary to maternal toxicity (1,2).

The carcinogenic potential of tocilizumab has not been evaluated. Tocilizumab was negative for mutagenicity in two assays. No impairment of fertility was noted in male or female mice analog studies (1).

It is not known if tocilizumab crosses the human placenta, but the antibody does cross the cynomolgus monkey placenta (1,2). Although the molecular weight is high (about 148,000), the prolonged elimination half-life (up to 13 days) may allow the protein to cross the human placenta. Similar to other immune globulin antibodies, placental transfer should be expected late in gestation (1,2).

Thirty-three human pregnancies with known outcomes occurring in 32 patients with rheumatoid arthritis have been reported in abstract (3). Thirteen pregnancies ended in elective termination; 7 spontaneously aborted (5 of whom were also exposed to methotrexate); and 10 pregnancies resulted in healthy newborns. One additional liveborn infant died of respiratory distress after intrapartum feto-maternal hemorrhage due to placenta previa. No congenital malformations were reported (3).

In another study of 10 pregnant patients with preterm premature rupture of the membranes, the regulation of matrix metalloproteinase (MMP) expression by inflammatory cytokines in human amnion cells was investigated. Treatment with IL-6 increased secretion of selected MMPs, whereas treatment with 1 mcg/mL tocilizumab inhibited the IL-6-induced secretion (4).

BREASTFEEDING SUMMARY

No reports describing the use tocilizumab during human lactation have been located. The high molecular weight (about 148,000) suggests that the antibody will not be excreted into breast milk, but the prolonged elimination half-life (up to 13 days) may allow some excretion.

Because maternal antibodies are excreted into breast milk, especially early in lactation, the presence of tocilizumab in milk should be expected. The effect of this exposure on a nursing infant is unknown.

References

1. Product information. Actemra, Genentech, 2011.
2. Health Canada. Summary Basis of Decision (SBD) Actemra, 2010.
3. Rubbert-Roth A, Goupile PM, Moosavi S, Hou A. First experiences with pregnancies in RA patients receiving tocilizumab therapy (abstract). Arthritis Rheum 2010;(Suppl):384.
4. Mano Y, Shibata K, Sumigama S, Hayakawa H, Ino K, Yamamoto E, Kajiyama H, Nawa A, Kikkawa F. Tocilizumab inhibits interleukin-6-mediated matrix metalloproteinase-2 and -9 secretions from human amnion cells in preterm premature rupture of membranes. Gynecol Obstet Invest 2009; 68:145–53.

TOFACITINIB

Immunologic Agent (Antirheumatic)

PREGNANCY RECOMMENDATION: No Human Data—Animal Data Suggest Risk (Contraindicated if Combined with Methotrexate)

BREASTFEEDING RECOMMENDATION: No Human Data—Potential Toxicity (Contraindicated if Combined with Methotrexate)

PREGNANCY SUMMARY

No reports describing the use of tofacitinib in human pregnancy have been located. Animal reproduction data suggest risk, but the absence of human pregnancy experience prevents a more complete assessment of the embryo–fetal risk. The drug should not be used in pregnancy if combined with methotrexate. Women who are either pregnant or of reproductive age should be informed of the potential risk of this drug if taken in pregnancy. Either physicians or pregnant women themselves are encouraged to register in the manufacturer's pregnancy registry for tofacitinib by calling 1-877-311-8972.

FETAL RISK SUMMARY

Tofacitinib is an inhibitor of Janus kinases that are intracellular enzymes. It is indicated for the treatment of adult patients with moderately to severely active rheumatoid arthritis who have had an inadequate response or intolerance to methotrexate. The drug may be used as monotherapy or in combination with methotrexate or other nonbiologic disease-modifying antirheumatic drugs. Tofacitinib is partially metabolized to inactive metabolites. Plasma protein binding to albumin is about 40% and the elimination half-life is about 3 hours (1).

Reproduction studies have been conducted in rats and rabbits. In rats, the drug was teratogenic at exposure levels about 146 times the maximum recommended human dose based on AUC (MRHD) at oral doses of 100 mg/kg/day (MRHD-100). Defects included external and soft-tissue malformations of anasarca and membranous ventricular septal defects, respectively, and skeletal malformations or variations (absent cervical arch; bent femur, fibula, humerus, radius, scapula, tibia, and ulna; sternoschisis; absent rib; misshapen femur; branched rib; fused rib; fused sternebra; and hemicentric thoracic centrum). Early and late abortions also were observed as was decreased fetal weight and postnatal survival. The no-observed-effect exposure level (NOEL) for developmental toxicity was about 58 times the MRHD at oral doses of 30 mg/kg/day (MRHD-30). In rabbits, exposure levels about 13 times the MRHD-30 caused teratogenic effects consisting of thoracogastroschisis, omphalocele, membranous ventricular septal defects, and cranial/skeletal malformations (microstomia, microphthalmia), mid-line and tail defects. An increase in abortions also was observed. No developmental toxicity was observed at exposure levels about 3 times the MRHD at oral doses of 10 mg/kg/day (1).

In long-term studies, tofacitinib was not carcinogenic in mice but was carcinogenic in monkeys (lymphomas) and in rats (benign Leydig cell tumors, hibernomas, and benign thymomas). The drug was not mutagenic in multiple assays but was clastogenic in one assay. Reduced fertility due to increased postimplantation loss was seen in some rat studies but this effect was not observed when lower doses were used. Doses that were about 133 times the MRHD-100 had no effect on male fertility, sperm motility, or sperm concentrations (1).

It is not known if tofacitinib crosses the human placenta. The molecular weight (about 312 for the free base), moderate plasma protein binding, and elimination half-life suggest that the drug will cross to the embryo–fetus.

BREASTFEEDING SUMMARY

No reports describing the use of tofacitinib during human lactation have been located. The molecular weight (about 312 for the free base), moderate plasma protein binding (about 40%), and elimination half-life (about 3 hours) suggest that the drug will be excreted into breast milk. The effect of this exposure on a nursing infant is unknown. However, because tofacitinib has been associated with severe adverse effects in adults, including infections that have resulted in death, the drug is best avoided during breastfeeding.

Reference

1. Product information. Xeljanz. Pfizer Laboratories, 2012.

TOLAZAMIDE

Antidiabetic Agent

PREGNANCY RECOMMENDATION: Human Data Suggest Risk in 3rd Trimester
BREASTFEEDING RECOMMENDATION: No Human Data—Potential Toxicity

PREGNANCY SUMMARY

Although the use of tolazamide during human gestation does not appear to be related to structural anomalies, insulin is still the treatment of choice for this disease. Oral hypoglycemics might not be indicated for the pregnant diabetic. Moreover, insulin, unlike tolazamide, does not cross the placenta and, thus, eliminates the additional concern that the drug therapy is adversely affecting the fetus. Carefully prescribed insulin therapy will provide better control of the mother's blood glucose, thereby preventing the fetal and neonatal complications that occur with this disease. High maternal glucose levels, as may occur in diabetes mellitus, are closely associated with a number of maternal and fetal adverse effects, including structural anomalies if the hyperglycemia occurs early in gestation. To prevent this toxicity, the American College of Obstetricians and Gynecologists recommends that insulin be used for types 1 and 2 diabetes occurring during pregnancy and, if diet therapy alone is not successful, for gestational diabetes (1,2). If tolazamide is used during pregnancy, therapy should be changed to insulin and tolazamide discontinued before delivery (the exact time before delivery is unknown) to lessen the possibility of prolonged hypoglycemia in the newborn.

FETAL RISK SUMMARY

Tolazamide is a sulfonylurea used for the treatment of adult-onset diabetes mellitus. It is not indicated for the pregnant diabetic.

No reports describing the placental transfer of tolazamide have been located. The molecular weight (about 311) suggests that transfer to the fetus probably occurs (see Chlorpropamide).

A 1991 report described the outcomes of pregnancies in 21 noninsulin-dependent diabetic women who were treated with oral hypoglycemic agents (17 sulfonylureas, 3 biguanides, and 1 unknown type) during the 1st trimester (3). The duration of exposure ranged from 3 to 28 weeks, but all patients were changed to insulin therapy at the first prenatal visit. Forty noninsulin-dependent diabetic women matched for age, race, parity, and glycemic control served as a control group. Eleven (52%) of the exposed infants had major or minor congenital malformations compared with six (15%) of the controls. Moreover, ear defects, a malformation that is observed, but uncommonly, in diabetic embryopathy, occurred in six of the exposed infants and in none of the controls (1). One of the infants with an ear defect (thickened curved pinnae and malformed superior helices) was exposed in utero to tolazamide during the first 12 weeks of gestation. Sixteen live births occurred in the exposed group compared with 36 in controls. The groups did not differ in the incidence of hypoglycemia at birth (53% vs. 53%), but three of the exposed newborns had severe hypoglycemia lasting 2, 4, and 7 days even though the mothers had not used oral hypoglycemics (none of the three was exposed to tolazamide) close to delivery. The authors attributed this to irreversible β-cell hyperplasia that may have been increased by exposure to oral hypoglycemics. Hyperbilirubinemia was noted in 10 (67%) of 15 exposed newborns compared with 13 (36%) controls ($p < 0.04$), and polycythemia and hyperviscosity requiring partial exchange transfusions were observed in 4 (27%) of 15 exposed vs. 1 (3.0%) control ($p < 0.03$) (1 exposed infant was not included in these data because the infant was delivered after completion of the study) (3).

BREASTFEEDING SUMMARY

No reports describing the use of tolazamide during human lactation have been located. The molecular weight (about 311) is low enough that excretion in milk should be expected (see Chlorpropamide). The effect of exposure to the drug in milk on the nursing infant is unknown, but hypoglycemia is a potential toxicity.

References

1. American College of Obstetricians and Gynecologists. Pregestational diabetes mellitus. *ACOG Practice Bulletin*. No. 60. March 2005. Obstet Gynecol 2005;105:675–85.
2. American College of Obstetricians and Gynecologists. Gestational diabetes. *ACOG Practice Bulletin*. No. 30. September 2001. Obstet Gynecol 2001;98:525–38.
3. Piacquadio K, Hollingsworth DR, Murphy H. Effects of in-utero exposure to oral hypoglycaemic drugs. Lancet 1991;338:866–9.

TOLAZOLINE

[Withdrawn from the market. See 9th edition.]

TOLBUTAMIDE

Antidiabetic Agent

PREGNANCY RECOMMENDATION: Human Data Suggest Risk in 3rd Trimester
BREASTFEEDING RECOMMENDATION: Limited Human Data—Potential Toxicity

PREGNANCY SUMMARY

Although the use of tolbutamide during human gestation does not appear to be related to structural anomalies, insulin is still the treatment of choice for diabetes. Oral hypoglycemics might not be indicated for the pregnant diabetic. Moreover, insulin, unlike tolbutamide, does not cross the placenta and, thus, eliminates the additional concern that the drug therapy itself is adversely affecting the fetus. Because tolbutamide crossed the placenta, prolonged hypoglycemia occurred in a premature infant. Carefully prescribed insulin therapy will provide better control of the mother's blood glucose, thereby preventing the fetal and neonatal complications that occur with this disease. High maternal glucose levels, as may occur in diabetes mellitus, are closely associated with a number of maternal and fetal adverse effects, including fetal structural anomalies if the hyperglycemia occurs early in gestation. To prevent this toxicity, the American College of Obstetricians and Gynecologists recommends that insulin be used for types 1 and 2 diabetes occurring during pregnancy and, if diet therapy alone is not successful, for gestational diabetes (1,2). If tolbutamide is used during pregnancy, therapy should be changed to insulin and tolbutamide discontinued before delivery to lessen the possibility of prolonged hypoglycemia in the newborn. The timing when therapy should be changed to insulin is not certain but at least 4 days before delivery appears reasonable based on one case.

FETAL RISK SUMMARY

Tolbutamide is a sulfonylurea used for the treatment of adult-onset diabetes mellitus. It is not the treatment of choice for the pregnant diabetic patient.

Shepard (3) reviewed four studies that had reported teratogenicity in mice and rats, but not in rabbits. In a study using early-somite mouse embryos in whole-embryo culture, tolbutamide produced malformations and growth restriction at concentrations similar to therapeutic levels in humans (4). The defects were not a result of hypoglycemia. In a similar experiment, but using tolbutamide concentrations 2–4 times the human therapeutic level, investigators concluded that tolbutamide had a direct embryotoxic effect on the rat embryos (5).

When administered near term, the drug crosses the placenta (6,7). Neonatal serum levels are higher than corresponding maternal concentrations. In one infant whose mother took 500 mg/day, serum levels at 27 hours were 7.2 mg/dL (maternal 2.7 mg/dL) (7).

An abstract (8), and later full report (9), described the in vitro placental transfer, using a single-cotyledon human placenta, of four oral hypoglycemic agents. As expected, molecular weight was the most significant factor for drug transfer, with dissociation constant (pK_a) and lipid solubility providing significant additive effect. The cumulative percent placental transfer at 3 hours of the four agents and their approximate molecular weight (shown in parenthesis) were tolbutamide (270) 21.5%, chlorpropamide (277) 11.0%, glipizide (446) 6.6%, and glyburide (494) 3.9%.

Although teratogenic in animals, an increased incidence of congenital defects, other than those expected in diabetes mellitus, has not been found with tolbutamide in a number of studies (10–20). Four malformed infants have been attributed to tolbutamide but the relationship is unclear: right-sided preauricular skin tag, accessory right thumb, thrombocytopenia (nadir 19,000/mm^3 on fourth day) (7); hand and foot anomalies, finger and toe syndactyly, external ear defect, atresia of external auditory canal, gastrointestinal, heart, and renal anomalies (21); grossly malformed (22); and severe talipes, absent left toe (23). The neonatal thrombocytopenia, persisting for about 2 weeks, was thought to have been induced by tolbutamide (7).

In a surveillance study of Michigan Medicaid recipients involving 229,101 completed pregnancies conducted between 1985 and 1992, 4 newborns had been exposed to tolbutamide during the 1st trimester (F. Rosa, personal communication, FDA, 1993). One (25%) major birth defect was observed (none expected), but specific information on the defect is not available. No anomalies were observed in six categories of defects (cardiovascular defects, oral clefts, spina bifida, polydactyly, limb reduction defects, and hypospadias).

A 1991 report described the outcomes of pregnancies in 21 noninsulin-dependent diabetic women who were treated with oral hypoglycemic agents (17 sulfonylureas, 3 biguanides, and 1 unknown type) during the 1st trimester (24). The duration of exposure ranged from 3 to 28 weeks, but all patients were changed to insulin therapy at the first prenatal visit. Forty noninsulin-dependent diabetic women matched for age, race, parity, and glycemic control served as a control group. Eleven (52%) of the exposed infants had major or minor congenital malformations compared with six (15%) of the controls. Moreover, ear defects, a malformation that is observed, but uncommonly, in diabetic embryopathy, occurred in six of the exposed infants and in none of the controls. None of the infants with defects was exposed to tolbutamide. Sixteen live births occurred in the exposed group compared with 36 in controls. The groups did not differ in the incidence of hypoglycemia at birth (53% vs. 53%), but three of the exposed newborns had severe hypoglycemia lasting 2, 4, and 7 days even though the mothers had not used oral hypoglycemics (none of the three was exposed to tolbutamide) close to delivery. The authors attributed this to irreversible β-cell hyperplasia that may have been increased by exposure to oral hypoglycemics. Hyperbilirubinemia was noted in 10 (67%) of 15 exposed newborns compared with 13 (36%) of controls ($p < 0.04$), and polycythemia and hyperviscosity requiring partial exchange transfusions were observed in 4 (27%) of 15 exposed vs. 1 (3.0%) control ($p < 0.03$) (1 exposed infant was not included in these data because the infant was delivered after completion of the study) (24).

A case of prolonged hypoglycemia in a premature infant whose mother was treated with tolbutamide for gestational diabetes was reported in 1998 (25). The mother was treated with tolbutamide starting from 23 weeks' gestation until delivery at 34 weeks. The male infant's weight and length were 3200 g and 49 cm, respectively, both values above 1 standard deviation of the mean for gestational age. Hypoglycemia was diagnosed 1 hour after birth and IV 20% glucose was required for the first 3 days of life. Subcutaneous octreotide was also administered for first 9 days of life. Serum tolbutamide concentrations decreased from 38 mcg/mL (140.6 µmol/L) at 3 hours after birth to 2 mcg/mL (7.4 µmol/L) at 90 hours. The decline in serum concentration showed zero-order kinetics with an initial half-life of 46 hours that declined to 6 hours. The change in tolbutamide elimination suggested immaturity of hepatic elimination during the first 2 days of life. The infant displayed normal psychomotor development without seizures and normal glucose values at 3 months of age (25).

BREASTFEEDING SUMMARY

Tolbutamide is excreted into breast milk. Following long-term dosing with 500 mg orally twice daily, milk levels in two patients averaged 3 and 18 mcg/mL 4 hours after a dose (26). Milk:plasma ratios were 0.09 and 0.40, respectively. The effect on an infant from these levels is unknown, but hypoglycemia is a potential toxicity. The American Academy of Pediatrics, although noting the possibility of jaundice in the nursing infant, classifies tolbutamide as compatible with breastfeeding (27).

References

1. American College of Obstetricians and Gynecologists. Pregestational diabetes mellitus. *ACOG Practice Bulletin*. No. 60. March 2005. Obstet Gynecol 2005;105:675–85.
2. American College of Obstetricians and Gynecologists. Gestational diabetes. *ACOG Practice Bulletin*. No. 30. September 2001. Obstet Gynecol 2001;98:525–38.
3. Shepard TH. *Catalog of Teratogenic Agents*. 8th ed. Baltimore, MD: The Johns Hopkins University Press, 1995:417.
4. Smoak IW. Teratogenic effects of tolbutamide on early-somite mouse embryos in vitro. Diabetes Res Clin Pract 1992;17:161–7.
5. Ziegler MH, Grafton TF, Hansen DK. The effect of tolbutamide on rat embryonic development in vitro. Teratology 1993;48:45–51.
6. Miller DI, Wishinsky H, Thompson G. Transfer of tolbutamide across the human placenta. Diabetes 1962;11(Suppl):93–7.
7. Schiff D, Aranda J, Stern L. Neonatal thrombocytopenia and congenital malformation associated with administration of tolbutamide to the mother. J Pediatr 1970;77:457–8.
8. Elliott B, Schenker S, Langer O, Johnson R, Prihoda T. Oral hypoglycemic agents: profound variation exists in their rate of human placental transfer. Society of Perinatal Obstetricians Abstract. Am J Obstet Gynecol 1992;166:368.
9. Elliott BD, Schenker S, Langer O, Johnson R, Prihoda T. Comparative placental transport of oral hypoglycemic agents in humans: a model of human placental drug transfer. Am J Obstet Gynecol 1994;171:653–60.
10. Ghanem MH. Possible teratogenic effect of tolbutamide in the pregnant prediabetic. Lancet 1961;1:1227.
11. Dolger H, Bookman JJ, Nechemias C. The diagnostic and therapeutic value of tolbutamide in pregnant diabetics. Diabetes 1962;11(Suppl):97–8.
12. Jackson WPU, Campbell GD, Notelovitz M, Blumsohn D. Tolbutamide and chlorpropamide during pregnancy in human diabetes. Diabetes 1962;11(Suppl):98–101.
13. Campbell GD. Chlorpropamide and foetal damage. Br Med J 1963;1:59–60.
14. Macphail I. Chlorpropamide and foetal damage. Br Med J 1963;1:192.
15. Jackson WPU, Campbell GD. Chlorpropamide and perinatal mortality. Br Med J 1963;2:1652.
16. Malins JM, Cooke AM, Pyke DA, Fitzgerald MG. Sulphonylurea drugs in pregnancy. Br Med J 1964;2:187.
17. Moss JM, Connor EJ. Pregnancy complicated by diabetes. Report of 102 pregnancies including eleven treated with oral hypoglycemic drugs. Med Ann Dist Col 1965;34:253–60.
18. Adam PAJ, Schwartz R. Diagnosis and treatment: should oral hypoglycemic agents be used in pediatric and pregnant patients? Pediatrics 1968;42:819–23.
19. Dignan PSJ. Teratogenic risk and counseling in diabetes. Clin Obstet Gynecol 1981;24:149–59.
20. Burt RL. Reactivity to tolbutamide in normal pregnancy. Obstet Gynecol 1958;12:447–53.
21. Larsson Y, Sterky G. Possible teratogenic effect of tolbutamide in a pregnant prediabetic. Lancet 1960;2:1424–6.
22. Campbell GD. Possible teratogenic effect of tolbutamide in pregnancy. Lancet 1961;1:891–2.
23. Soler NG, Walsh CH, Malins JM. Congenital malformations in infants of diabetic mothers. Q J Med 1976;45:303–13.
24. Piacquadio K, Hollingsworth DR, Murphy H. Effects of in-utero exposure to oral hypoglycaemic drugs. Lancet 1991;338:866–9.
25. Christesen HBT, Melander A. Prolonged elimination of tolbutamide in a premature newborn with hyperinsulinaemic hypoglycaemia. Eur J Endocrinol 1998;138:698–701.
26. Moiel RH, Ryan JR. Tolbutamide (Orinase) in human breast milk. Clin Pediatr 1967;6:480.
27. Committee on Drugs, American Academy of Pediatrics. The transfer of drugs and other chemicals into human milk. Pediatrics 2001;108:776–89.

TOLCAPONE

Antiparkinson Agent

PREGNANCY RECOMMENDATION: No Human Data—Animal Data Suggest Risk
BREASTFEEDING RECOMMENDATION: No Human Data—Potential Toxicity

PREGNANCY SUMMARY

No reports describing the use of tolcapone in human pregnancy have been located. Because the drug is always used concomitantly with levodopa/carbidopa, the increased incidence of fetal anomalies and reduced fetal weight observed in rats treated with combination therapy resulting in plasma exposures of tolcapone only one-half of the expected human exposure is noteworthy. Embryo and/or fetal toxicity were also observed in rats and rabbits with tolcapone doses ranging from less than to slightly above the typical human dose. The complete lack of human pregnancy experience, however, prevents an assessment of the potential embryo and fetal risk from tolcapone. The low incidence of Parkinson's disease in women of reproductive age and the risk of potentially fatal, acute fulminant liver failure should markedly limit the use of tolcapone in this patient population.

FETAL RISK SUMMARY

Tolcapone is used as an adjunct to levodopa/carbidopa for the treatment of Parkinson's disease. The agent is a selective and reversible inhibitor of catechol-O-methyltransferase (COMT), an enzyme involved in the metabolism of levodopa. Inhibition of COMT by tolcapone allows for more sustained plasma levels of levodopa resulting in greater beneficial effects on the signs and symptoms of Parkinson's disease. Because the drug may cause potentially fatal, acute fulminant liver failure, it is recommended that it should be used only in patients who are not appropriate candidates for other adjunctive therapies (1). Tolcapone is nearly completely metabolized to inactive metabolites before excretion in the urine. It has an elimination half-life of 2–3 hours with no evidence of accumulation after repeat dosing (1).

Reproduction studies with tolcapone alone have been conducted in rats and rabbits. In rats, doses up to 5.7 times the recommended human clinical dose of 600 mg/day based on BSA (RHCD) had no effect on fertility or general reproductive performance. There was no evidence of teratogenicity with these doses during organogenesis, but the highest dose was associated with maternal toxicity (decreased weight gain, death). When tolcapone was given to rats in late gestation and throughout lactation, decreased litter size, and impaired growth and learning performance were observed in female pups. Because the initial dose (4.8 times the RHCD) was associated with a high rate of maternal mortality, the dose was reduced during late gestation to 2.9 times the RHCD (1).

Treatment of rabbits during organogenesis with doses up to 15 times the RHCD revealed no evidence of teratogenicity, but an increased rate of abortion was observed at 3.7 times the RHCD (plasma exposure half the expected human exposure based on AUC). Maternal toxicity was evident at the highest dose (15 times the RHCD) (1). Pregnant rabbits were also treated with a combination of tolcapone (half the expected human exposure based on AUC) and levodopa/carbidopa (6 times the expected human therapeutic exposure of levodopa based on AUC) during organogenesis. The three-drug regimen (tolcapone, levodopa, and carbidopa) resulted in an increased incidence of fetal anomalies, primarily external and skeletal digit defects, compared with levodopa/carbidopa alone. The combination of levodopa–carbidopa is known to cause visceral and skeletal malformations in rabbits. The three-drug regimen in pregnant rats with tolcapone (0.5 times the expected human exposure or higher based on AUC) and levodopa/carbidopa (levodopa exposures 21 times the human exposure or higher) was associated with reduced fetal body weights. However, no effect on fetal body weight was observed when tolcapone (1.4 times the expected human exposure based on AUC) was used alone (1).

It is not known if tolcapone crosses the human placenta. The molecular weight (about 273) is low enough that embryo–fetal exposure should be expected. The nearly complete metabolism and relatively short elimination half-life should limit the amount of active parent drug available for distribution to the fetus.

BREASTFEEDING SUMMARY

No reports describing the use of tolcapone during human lactation have been located. The molecular weight (about 273) is low enough that excretion into breast milk should be expected. The nearly complete metabolism and relatively short elimination half-life should limit the amount of active drug available for passage into milk. The effect on a nursing infant from exposure to tolcapone from milk is unknown. Because of the potential for severe toxicity (e.g., potentially fatal, acute fulminant liver failure as seen in adults), lactating women who are taking tolcapone should not breastfeed.

Reference

1. Product information. Tasmar. Roche Pharmaceuticals, 2003.

TOLMETIN

Nonsteroidal Anti-inflammatory

PREGNANCY RECOMMENDATION: Human Data Suggest Risk in 1st and 3rd Trimesters
BREASTFEEDING RECOMMENDATION: Limited Human Data—Probably Compatible

PREGNANCY SUMMARY

Constriction of the ductus arteriosus in utero is a pharmacologic consequence arising from the use of prostaglandin synthesis inhibitors during pregnancy (see also Indomethacin) (1). Persistent pulmonary hypertension of the newborn may occur if these agents are used in the 3rd trimester close to delivery (1,2). These drugs also have been shown to inhibit labor and prolong pregnancy, both in humans (3) (see also Indomethacin) and in animals (4). Women attempting to conceive should not use any prostaglandin synthesis inhibitor, including tolmetin, because of the findings in a variety of animal models that indicate these agents block blastocyst implantation (5,6). Moreover, as noted above, nonsteroidal anti-inflammatory drugs (NSAIDs) have been associated with spontaneous abortions (SABs) and congenital malformations. The absolute risk for these defects, however, appears to be low.

FETAL RISK SUMMARY

Tolmetin is an NSAID used for the relief of the signs and symptoms of rheumatoid arthritis, juvenile arthritis, and osteoarthritis. It is in the same subclass (acetic acids) as three other NSAIDs (diclofenac, indomethacin, and sulindac).

Tolmetin is not teratogenic in rats and rabbits (7,8). The doses used in some of the studies were up to 1.5 times the maximum clinical dose based on a body weight of 60 kg (8).

It is not known if tolmetin crosses the human placenta. The molecular weight of the sodium salt (about 315) is low enough that passage to the fetus should be expected.

In a surveillance study of Michigan Medicaid recipients involving 229,101 completed pregnancies conducted between 1985 and 1992, 99 newborns had been exposed to tolmetin during the 1st trimester (F. Rosa, personal communication, FDA, 1993). One (1.0%) infant had a major birth defect (four expected) consisting of a cardiovascular defect (one expected) and polydactyly (none expected).

A combined 2001 population-based observational cohort study and a case–control study estimated the risk of adverse pregnancy outcome from the use of NSAIDs (9). The use of NSAIDs during pregnancy was not associated with congenital malformations, preterm delivery, or low birth weight, but a positive association was discovered with SABs. A similar study, also published in 2001, failed to find a relationship, in general, between NSAIDs and congenital malformations, but did find a significant association with cardiac defects and orofacial clefts (10). In addition, a 2003 study found a significant association between exposure to NSAIDs in early pregnancy and SABs (11). (See Ibuprofen for details on these three studies.)

A brief 2003 editorial on the potential for NSAID-induced developmental toxicity concluded that NSAIDs, and specifically those with greater COX-2 affinity, had a lower risk of this toxicity in humans than aspirin (12).

BREASTFEEDING SUMMARY

Tolmetin is excreted into breast milk (8,13). In the 4 hours following a single 400-mg oral dose, milk levels varied from 0.06 to 0.18 mcg/mL with the highest concentration occurring at 0.67 hour. Milk:plasma ratios were 0.005–0.007. The clinical significance of these levels to the nursing infant is unknown. The American Academy of Pediatrics classifies tolmetin as compatible with breastfeeding (14).

References

1. Levin DL. Effects of inhibition of prostaglandin synthesis on fetal development, oxygenation, and the fetal circulation. Semin Perinatol 1980;4:35–44.
2. Van Marter LJ, Leviton A, Allred EN, Pagano M, Sullivan KF, Cohen A, Epstein MF. Persistent pulmonary hypertension of the newborn and smoking and aspirin and nonsteroidal antiinflammatory drug consumption during pregnancy. Pediatrics 1996;97:658–63.
3. Fuchs F. Prevention of prematurity. Am J Obstet Gynecol 1976;126: 809–20.
4. Powell JG, Cochrane RL. The effects of a number of non-steroidal anti-inflammatory compounds on parturition in the rat. Prostaglandins 1982;23:469–88.
5. Matt DW, Borzelleca JF. Toxic effects on the female reproductive system during pregnancy, parturition, and lactation. In: Witorsch RJ, ed. *Reproductive Toxicology*. 2nd ed. New York, NY: Raven Press, 1995: 175–93.
6. Dawood MY. Nonsteroidal antiinflammatory drugs and reproduction. Am J Obstet Gynecol 1993;169:1255–65.
7. Nishimura K, Fukagawa S, Shigematsu K, Makumoto K, Terada Y, Sasaki H, Nanto T, Tatsumi H. Teratogenicity study of tolmetin sodium in rabbits. (Japanese) Iyakuhin Kenkyu 1977;8:158–64. As cited in Shepard TH. *Catalog of Teratogenic Agents*. 6th ed. Baltimore, MD: The Johns Hopkins University Press, 1989:625.
8. Product information. Tolectin. Ortho-McNeil Pharmaceutical, 2001.
9. Nielsen GL, Sorensen HT, Larsen H, Pedersen L. Risk of adverse birth outcome and miscarriage in pregnant users of non-steroidal anti-inflammatory drugs: population based observational study and case–control study. Br Med J 2001;322:266–70.
10. Ericson A, Kallen BAJ. Nonsteroidal anti-inflammatory drugs in early pregnancy. Reprod Toxicol 2001;15:371–5.
11. Li DK, Liu L, Odouli R. Exposure to non-steroidal anti-inflammatory drugs during pregnancy and risk of miscarriage: population based cohort study. Br Med J 2003;327:368–71.
12. Tassinari MS, Cook JC, Hurtt ME. NSAIDs and developmental toxicity. Birth Defects Res (Part B) 2003;68:3–4.
13. Sagraves R, Waller ES, Goehrs HR. Tolmetin in breast milk. Drug Intell Clin Pharm 1985;19:55–6.
14. Committee on Drugs, American Academy of Pediatrics. The transfer of drugs and other chemicals into breast milk. Pediatrics 2001;108: 776–89.

T

TOLTERODINE

Urinary Tract Agent (Antispasmodic)

PREGNANCY RECOMMENDATION: No Human Data—Animal Data Suggest Low Risk
BREASTFEEDING RECOMMENDATION: No Human Data—Potential Toxicity

PREGNANCY SUMMARY

No reports describing the use of tolterodine in human pregnancy have been located. The limited animal data suggest low risk, but the complete lack of human pregnancy experience prevents an assessment of embryo–fetal risk. The safest course is to avoid the 1st trimester, but inadvertent exposure in early pregnancy does not appear to represent a major risk.

FETAL RISK SUMMARY

Tolterodine is a competitive muscarinic receptor antagonist that is indicated for the treatment of overactive bladder with symptoms of urge urinary incontinence, urgency, and frequency. It is in the same subclass as darifenacin, flavoxate, oxybutynin, solifenacin, and trospium. Tolterodine is metabolized in the liver to a major active metabolite that has the same potency as tolterodine. Metabolism is mediated by the cytochrome P450 2D6 (CYP2D6). After multiple dosing, the elimination half-life is 2.2 hours in extensive metabolizers. In those lacking CYP2D6 (poor metabolizers; about 7% of the population), metabolism (to an inactive metabolite) is mediated by CYP3A4 and the elimination half-life of tolterodine is 9.6 hours. About 96% of tolterodine is bound in the plasma, primarily to α_1-glycoprotein, but the binding of the active metabolite is only 64% (1).

Reproduction studies have been conducted in mice and rabbits. In pregnant mice, oral doses producing systemic exposures about 14 times the human exposure (HE) revealed no evidence of teratogenicity. At doses 20–25 times the HE, embryolethality, reduced fetal weight, and increased incidences of intra-abdominal hemorrhage and malformations (cleft palate and digital and various skeletal abnormalities) were seen. In pregnant rabbits, SC doses producing systemic exposures about 3 times the HE did not cause embryotoxicity or teratogenicity. Tolterodine is neither carcinogenic nor mutagenic in experimental systems (1).

Tolterodine crosses the placenta in mice (2). It is not known if tolterodine or its active metabolite crosses the human placenta. The molecular weight of tolterodine tartrate (about 476) is low enough that exposure of the embryo–fetus should be expected.

BREASTFEEDING SUMMARY

No reports describing the use of tolterodine during human lactation have been located. The molecular weight of the parent compound (about 476) is low enough that excretion into breast milk should be expected. Moreover, tolterodine has an equipotent metabolite that also might be excreted into milk. The effect of this exposure in a nursing infant is unknown.

References

1. Product information. Detrol. Pharmacia & Upjohn, 2004.
2. Pahlman I, d'Argy R, Nilvebrant L. Tissue distribution of tolterodine, a muscarinic receptor antagonist, and transfer into fetus and milk in mice. Arzneimittelforschung 2001;51:125–33.

TOLVAPTAN

Vasopressin Receptor Antagonist

PREGNANCY RECOMMENDATION: No Human Data—Animal Data Suggest Low Risk
BREASTFEEDING RECOMMENDATION: No Human Data—Potential Toxicity

PREGNANCY SUMMARY

No reports describing the use of tolvaptan in human pregnancy have been located. The animal reproduction data suggests low risk because all of the toxic effects occurred in the presence of maternal toxicity and at doses that were much greater than 10 times the human dose. Although human pregnancy experience is needed for a better risk assessment, there does not appear to be a reason to withhold the drug in pregnancy if indicated.

FETAL RISK SUMMARY

Tolvaptan is an oral selective vasopressin receptor antagonist. It is in the same class as conivaptan. Tolvaptan is indicated for the treatment of clinically significant hypervolemic and euvolemic hyponatremia (serum sodium <125 mEq/L or less marked hyponatremia that is symptomatic and resisted correction with fluid restriction), including patients with heart failure, cirrhosis, and syndrome of in appropriate antidiuretic hormone. The drug is metabolized to inactive metabolites. Tolvaptan is highly plasma protein bound (99%) and has a terminal phase half-life of about 12 hours (1).

Reproduction studies have been conducted in rats and rabbits. In rats during organogenesis, decreased fetal body weights and delayed ossification were observed at the highest dose that was 162 times the maximum recommended human dose based on BSA (MRHD). Maternal toxicity (reduced body weight gain and food consumption) were noted at ≥16 times the MRHD. In rabbits during organogenesis, maternal toxicity (reduced body weight and food consumption) occurred with doses that were ≥32 times the MRHD and abortions at ≥97 times the MRHD. Increased rates of embryo–fetal death, microphthalmia, open eyelids, cleft palate, brachymelia and skeletal malformations occurred at doses that were 324 times the MRHD (1).

Tolvaptan was not carcinogenic in 2-year studies in rats and mice. Tests also were negative for genotoxicity. No effect on fertility was noted in male rats but, in female rats a dose that was 162 times the MRHD caused significantly fewer corpora lutea and implants than controls (1).

It is not known if tolvaptan crosses the human placenta. The molecular weight (about 449) and long terminal phase half-life suggest that the drug will cross, but the high plasma protein binding should limit the embryo–fetal exposure.

BREASTFEEDING SUMMARY

No reports describing the use of tolvaptan during human lactation have been located. The molecular weight (about 449) and long terminal phase half-life (about 12 hours) suggest that it will be excreted into breast milk, but the high plasma protein binding (99%) should limit the amount. The effect of this exposure on a nursing infant is unknown. However, because the drug promotes urinary water excretion, dehydration and hypovolemia are potential complications.

Reference

1. Product information. Samsca. Otsuka America Pharmaceutical, 2009.

TOPIRAMATE

Anticonvulsant

PREGNANCY RECOMMENDATION: Human and Animal Data Suggest Risk
BREASTFEEDING RECOMMENDATION: Limited Human Data—Potential Toxicity

PREGNANCY SUMMARY

A 2012 review concluded that the use of topiramate during pregnancy was associated with a two- to threefold increased risk of malformations, largely due to an increased risk for cleft lip with or without cleft palate (1). Another 2012 study found significant effects on cognitive functions and other matters (see below) (2). Consistent with previous anticonvulsants studies, the risk of birth defects appears to be increased when topiramate is combined with other antiepileptics. Topiramate does not produce epoxide metabolites (3). Because these intermediate arene oxide metabolites have been associated with teratogenicity (see Carbamazepine, Phenytoin, and Valproic Acid), this may indicate a lower risk of teratogenicity compared with other agents. The effect of topiramate on folic acid levels or metabolism is unknown (3). Until this information is available, the safest course is to start folic acid supplementation (4–5 mg/day) before conception, as is done with other antiepileptic agents. Topiramate should be avoided, if possible, during the 1st trimester but, if required, monotherapy with the lowest effective dose is preferred. The risk for neonatal hypocalcemic seizures following in utero exposure to topiramate requires further study.

T

FETAL RISK SUMMARY

Topiramate, a sulfamate-substituted monosaccharide, is an antiepileptic agent indicated as adjunctive therapy in patients with partial onset seizures, primary generalized tonic-clonic seizures, and seizures associated with Lennox-Gastaut syndrome. The drug undergoes partial metabolism to six metabolites, none of which constitutes more than 5% of the dose, with approximately 70% of the dose eliminated unchanged in the urine. Only 13%–17% is bound to human plasma proteins and the mean plasma elimination half-life is 21 hours. Topiramate is a weak carbonic anhydrase inhibitor, but this activity is not thought to be a major contributing factor to its antiepileptic action (4).

Reproduction studies with topiramate have been conducted in mice, rats, and rabbits. In pregnant mice, oral doses, 0.2–5 times the recommended human dose (400 mg/day) based on BSA (RHD), administered during organogenesis increased the incidence of fetal malformations at all doses. The primary anomalies were craniofacial defects. At the highest dose (5 times the RHD), reduced fetal body weights and ossification were evident, but this dose also caused maternal toxicity (decreased body weight gain) (4).

Topiramate at doses of 0.005–12.5 times the RHD was administered to pregnant rats during organogenesis. At ≥10 times the RHD, the frequency of limb malformations (ectrodactyly, micromelia, and amelia) was increased. In addition, in the postnatal portion of the study, pups exposed to topiramate during organogenesis exhibited delayed physical development (doses 10 times the RHD) and persistent reductions in body weight gain (doses ≥1 times the RHD). The teratogenic dose (≥10 times the RHD) produced clinical signs of maternal toxicity. At ≥2.5 times the RHD, reduced maternal weight gain was evident. However, fetotoxicity (reduced fetal body weight and increased incidence of structural variations) was observed at half the RHD. Pregnant rats also were treated during the latter part of gestation and throughout lactation with doses ranging from 0.005 to 5 times the RHD. No drug-related effects on gestation length or parturition were observed at any studied dose. At ≥0.05 times the RHD, reductions in pre- and/or postweaning body weight gain were observed. At 5 times the RHD, offspring exhibited decreased viability and delayed physical development (4).

Pregnant rabbits were administered oral doses during organogenesis that were approximately 0.6–11 times the RHD. At ≥2 times the RHD, embryo and fetal mortality was observed, but maternal toxicity (decreased body weight gain, clinical signs, and/or mortality) also were evident. At 6 times the RHD, teratogenic effects, primarily rib and vertebral malformations, were observed (4).

Topiramate crosses the placenta to the fetus with cord and maternal plasma drug levels approximately equivalent at term (5,6). Diffusion across the placenta to the embryo early in gestation has not been studied. The molecular weight (about 339), the relatively lack of protein binding and low metabolism, and the prolonged plasma elimination half-life favor transfer of the drug to the embryo and fetus.

Postmarketing experience has been reported by the manufacturer (4). Without providing specific details, the manufacturer stated that cases of hypospadias had been observed in male infants exposed in utero to the drug, with or without other anticonvulsants. A causal relationship with topiramate has not been established (4).

A 2003 reference cited details from pregnancy exposure during clinical trials (5). Among 28 pregnancies, all involving polytherapy (other anticonvulsants not specified), there was "one malformation and two children with anomalies." In addition, the outcomes of 139 pregnancies identified during postmarketing surveillance were 87 live births, 23 elective abortions, and 29 lost to follow-up. The patient's anticonvulsant therapy was not specified. Five cases of hypospadias were observed, presumably in the live births (5).

In cases reported in a 2002 publication, five women were treated with topiramate (100–400 mg/day) combined with either carbamazepine (four cases) or valproic acid (one case) throughout gestation (6). All five newborns were healthy, normal infants. Birth weights of three infants ranged from 3520 to 3855 g, whereas the other two, both delivered from smoking mothers, had lower weights: 3160 g (6 cigarettes/day) and 2720 g (10 cigarettes/day), respectively. Cord blood levels of topiramate (average 8.1 microM) were nearly equivalent to the maternal plasma concentration at delivery (average 8.4 microM) (6).

A 2002 review cited a case of a pregnant patient who had been treated with topiramate (1400 mg/day) monotherapy throughout gestation (7). The growth-restricted newborn had several minor anomalies, including generalized hirsutism, a third fontanelle, short nose with anteverted nares, blunted distal phalanges and nails, and fifth nail hypoplasia. The similarity of some of these anomalies to those observed with other anticonvulsants suggested to the authors that genetic factors might have been involved (7).

A 2006 report from the United Kingdom Epilepsy and Pregnancy Register provided information on 35 pregnancies treated with topiramate for epilepsy, 28 of which involved monotherapy (8). Two newborns, both exposed to monotherapy, had major congenital malformations (rate 7.1%, 95% confidence interval [CI] 2.0%–22.6%); one with cleft lip–palate and the other with hypospadias.

A second report from the above Register described the outcomes of 203 pregnancies exposed to topiramate (70 monotherapy and 133 polytherapy) (9). The outcomes of this prospective (enrolled before the outcome was known) observational study were 18 spontaneous abortions (SABs), 5 elective abortions, 2 stillbirths, and 178 live births (62 monotherapy and 116 polytherapy). The mean topiramate dose in the two groups was 245 mg (range 50–800 mg) and 299 mg (range 25–1000 mg), respectively, whereas the mean gestational age at delivery and the birth weight was 39.2 and 38.8 weeks, and 3168 and 3062 g, respectively. Three (4.8%, 95% CI 1.7%–18.2%) major anomalies were observed in the monotherapy group (daily dose): cleft lip and bilateral cleft palate (200 mg); hypospadias (400 mg); and cleft lip and palate (600 mg). There also were five (8.1%) infants with minor malformations who had been exposed to doses of 50–750 mg/day. Among the 116 live births exposed to polytherapy, 13 (11.2%, 95% CI 6.7%–18.2%) had major defects (daily dose): left hydronephrosis, dysmorphic (800 mg); pyloric stenosis (3 cases) (75, 150, 800 mg); hernia and hydrocele (250 mg); anal atresia (175 mg); tracheoesophageal fistula (150 mg); hypospadias (50 mg); cleft palate, crossed toes (500 mg); bilateral dislocated hips (400 mg); Harold type II talipes, plagiocephaly (350 mg); congenital dislocated hip (500 mg); and left cleft lip and palate (250 mg). The other anticonvulsants were carbamazepine, clobazam, ethosuximide, lamotrigine, levetiracetam, phenobarbital, sodium valproate, and vigabitrin. Minor defects, including two infants with glandular or mild hypospadias, were observed in 10 (8.6%) infants exposed to polytherapy. In the combined groups, four oral clefts (2.2%, 95% 0.9%–5.6%) were observed, and among 78 male infants, 4 had hypospadias (5.1%, 95% CI 0.2%–10.1%). The rate of oral clefts was 11 times the background rate (9).

A teratogen information service (TIS) in Israel reported the outcomes of 52 pregnancies that were exposed to topiramate including in the 1st trimester (10). Compared with 212 controls not exposed to teratogens, there were statistically significant differences in SABs (11.3% vs. 2.8%, $p = 0.017$), birth weight (2932 vs. 3300 g, $p = 0.024$), and birth weight of single term infants (3084 vs. 3356 g, $p = 0.001$). After adjustment of the abortion data for gestational age when the TIS was called, maternal age, previous miscarriages, and smoking, regression analysis revealed that gestational age at initial TIS contact was a significant predictor and did not support a drug effect. The total number of major birth defects (4/41, 9.8%) was not statistically different from controls (7/206, 3.4%) ($p = 0.090$), but the possibility of a small increased risk could not be excluded because of the sample size. However, two of the anomalies were genetic in origin and were not caused by drugs. The other cases were pulmonary artery stenosis (topiramate 475 mg/day) and multiple brain cysts with neonatal seizures (topiramate 50 mg/day plus valproic acid 800 mg/day and clonazepam 1 mg/day). The reason for the low birth weight was unknown (10).

In the 2007 report from the Australian Registry of Antiepileptic Drugs in Pregnancy, no malformations were observed in the offspring of 15 pregnancies treated with topiramate monotherapy in the 1st trimester (11).

The Lamotrigine Pregnancy Registry, an ongoing project conducted by the manufacturer, was first published in January 1997. The final report was published in July 2010 (12). The Registry is now closed. Among 54 prospectively enrolled pregnancies exposed to topiramate and lamotrigine, with or without other anticonvulsants, 48 were exposed in the 1st trimester resulting in 40 live births, 2 birth defects, 3 SABs, and 3 EABs. There were six exposures in the 2nd/3rd trimesters resulting in five live births and one birth defect (12).

A 2007 report described two siblings that developed hypocalcemic seizures shortly after birth from a mother taking topiramate throughout pregnancy (13). The mother had developed seizures during her first pregnancy at age 20 and had been treated with valproic acid. Following that pregnancy, her anticonvulsant therapy had been changed to topiramate, 200 mg twice daily. Seven years later she became pregnant a second time and gave birth to a normal appearing, 3153-g male infant that was formula fed. Seizures began on day 3 of life and were associated with hypocalcemia, hypomagnesemia, and hyperphosphatemia but normal parathyroid hormone concentrations. Other laboratory parameters were within normal limits. He was treated with IV calcium and a low-phosphorus formula, and was discharged home at age 14 days on phenobarbital. At age 6 months, phenobarbital was discontinued. His development and neurologic examination were normal at 1 year of age. The mother subsequently delivered a normal baby girl (weight not specified) at term that was formula fed. During this pregnancy, her third, she had taken topiramate 100 mg twice daily. Seizures were noted at age 7 days and were associated with the same electrolyte and hormone abnormalities as in the first case. The infant was treated with IV calcium, magnesium, phenobarbital, and a change in the formula. No further seizures occurred after age 8 days, and she was discharged home on short-term courses of oral calcium and phenobarbital. Her neurological examination was normal at 2 months of age. Because there was no identifiable biochemical etiology for the seizures in the two infants, the seizures were attributed to hypocalcemia caused by hypoparathyroidism. It was proposed that in utero exposure to topiramate led to hypoparathyroidism and subsequent hypocalcemia via effects on protein kinase A signaling (13).

In a 2012 study, 9 children of preschool age (3–7 years) exposed during pregnancy to topiramate were compared with 18 children not exposed (2). The two groups were compared on developmental measures of visual, fine and gross motor function, and behavior and cognitive functions. The exposed group performed significantly worse than controls in almost all measures, including verbal, nonverbal, and general IQ scores (2).

A dose-related interaction between topiramate and a combined oral contraceptive (ethinylestradiol 35 mcg/northethindrone 1 mg) has been reported (4,14). At a dose of 400 mg/day, peak levels of the estrogen were decreased. At 800 mg/day, estrogen bioavailability was reduced and clearance increased. Norethindrone clearance was also increased at 800 mg/day. The concurrent use of these agents could reduce the efficacy of the contraceptive, possibly requiring a higher-dose contraceptive combination (14).

Topiramate is known to induce hepatic enzymes and may increase the incidence of early hemorrhagic disease of the newborn by depleting fetal vitamin K stores. Although vitamin K_1 (see Phytonadione) does not readily cross the placenta, 10 mg/day of the vitamin may be given orally to the mother in the last 4 weeks of pregnancy. In addition, 1 mg of vitamin K_1 should be given IV or IM to the infant at birth (15).

BREASTFEEDING SUMMARY

Topiramate is excreted into breast milk. This is consistent with the low molecular weight (about 339), protein binding (13%–17%), and metabolism (about 30%), and the prolonged plasma elimination half-life (21 hours).

Three women who had been treated with topiramate throughout pregnancy (see above) and continued during nursing were studied (6). The daily doses were 150, 200, and 200 mg/day. The mean milk:plasma ratio 3 weeks after delivery was 0.86 (range 0.67–1.1). In one case, 3 months after delivery, the ratio was 0.69. The minimum weight-adjusted infant doses, based on 150 mL/kg of milk per day, were about 0.1–0.7 mg/kg/day or 3%–23% of the maternal doses. Plasma concentrations of topiramate in two infants at 3 weeks of age, before and after nursing, were 1.4 and 1.3 microM, and 1.6 and 1.9 microM, respectively. The latter infant had a topiramate plasma concentration of 2.1 microM at 3 months of age. (*Note: Possible antiepileptic effects of topiramate on cultured neurons are concentration-dependent within the range of 1 to 200 microM* [*3*]). Plasma levels in the third infant were undetectable at 2 and 4 weeks postdelivery. The elimination half-life in the infants was estimated to be about 24 hours compared with 20–30 hours among healthy adult controls. No adverse effects of the exposure were observed (6).

In pediatric patients (ages 2–16 years), common adverse effects (most occurred twice as often or more than those in placebo-treated patients) associated with topiramate were fatigue, somnolence, difficulty with concentration/attention, aggressive reaction, confusion, difficulty with memory, ataxia, purpura, epistaxis, infections (viral and pneumonia), and anorexia and weight decrease (4). (Patients also were receiving one or two other anticonvulsants.) The potential for these or other adverse effects in a nursing infant cannot be assessed with the available data. Therefore, nursing women who are being treated with topiramate, particularly those receiving high doses, should be advised to monitor their infants for signs of toxicity and for changes in alertness, behavior, and feeding habits.

References

1. Holmes LB, Hernandez-Diaz S. Newer anticonvulsants: lamotrigine, topiramate, and gabapentin. Birth Defects Res A Clin Mol Teratol 2012;94:599–606.
2. Rihtman T, Parush S, Ornoy A. Preliminary findings of the developmental effects of *in utero* exposure to topiramate. Reprod Toxicol 2012;34:308–11.
3. Morrell MJ. The new antiepileptic drugs and women: efficacy, reproductive health, pregnancy, and fetal outcome. Epilepsia 1996;37(Suppl 6):S34–44.
4. Product information. Topamax. Ortho-McNeil Pharmaceutical, 2003.
5. Yerby MS. Clinical care of pregnant women with epilepsy: neural tube defects and folic acid supplements. Epilepsia 2003;44(Suppl 3):33–40.
6. Ohman I, Vitols S, Luef G, Soderfeldt B, Tomson T. Topiramate kinetics during delivery, lactation, and in the neonate: preliminary observations. Epilepsia 2002;43:1157–60.
7. Palmieri C, Canger R. Teratogenic potential of the newer antiepileptic drugs. What is known and how should this influence prescribing? CNS Drugs 2002;16:755–64.

T

8. Morrow J, Russell A, Guthrie E, Parsons L, Robertson I, Waddell R, Irwin B, McGivern RC, Morrison PJ, Craig J. Malformation risks of antiepileptic drugs in pregnancy: a prospective study from the UK Epilepsy and Pregnancy Register. J Neurol Neurosurg Psychiatry 2006;77:193–8.
9. Hunt S, Russell A, Smithson WH, Parsons L, Robertson I, Waddell R, Irwin B, Morrison PJ, Morrow J, Craig J. Topiramate in pregnancy: preliminary experience from the UK Epilepsy and Pregnancy Register. Neurology 2008;71:272–6.
10. Ornoy A, Zvi N, Arnon J, Wajnberg R, Shechtman S, Diav-Citrin O. The outcome of pregnancy following topiramate treatment: a study on 52 pregnancies. Reprod Toxicol 2008;25:388–9.
11. Vajda FJE, Hitchcock A, Graham J, O'Brien T, Lander C, Eadie M. The Australian Register of Antiepileptic Drugs in Pregnancy: the first 1002 pregnancies. Aust N Z J Obstet Gynaecol 2007;47:468–74.
12. The Lamotrigine Pregnancy Registry. Final Report. September 1, 1992 through March 31, 2010. GlaxoSmithKline, July 2010.
13. Gorman MP, Soul JS. Neonatal hypocalcemic seizures in siblings exposed to topiramate in utero. Pediatr Neurol 2007;36:274–6.
14. Crawford P. Interactions between antiepileptic drugs and hormonal contraception. CNS Drugs 2002;16:263–72.
15. Bruno MK, Harden CL. Epilepsy in pregnancy women. Curr Treat Options Neurol 2002;4:31–40.

TOPOTECAN

Antineoplastic

PREGNANCY RECOMMENDATION: No Human Data—Animal Data Suggest Risk
BREASTFEEDING RECOMMENDATION: Contraindicated

PREGNANCY SUMMARY

No reports describing the use of topotecan in human pregnancy have been located. The animal reproduction data suggest risk, but the absence of human pregnancy experience prevents a more thorough assessment of the embryo–fetal risk. Because of the potential for embryo and fetal harm, women of childbearing potential should employ adequate contraceptive methods to prevent pregnancy. However, all of the indications for topotecan involve potentially fatal cancers, so if informed consent is obtained, treatment should not be withheld because of pregnancy. If an inadvertent pregnancy occurs during therapy, the woman should be advised of the unknown, but potentially severe risk for her embryo–fetus.

FETAL RISK SUMMARY

The DNA topoisomerase I-inhibitor, topotecan, is a semi-synthetic derivative of camptothecin that is given as an IV infusion. It is in the same antineoplastic subclass as irinotecan. Topotecan is indicated as secondary therapy for metastatic carcinoma of the ovary, small-cell lung cancer, and, in combination with cisplatin, recurrent or persistent carcinoma of the cervix. The cytotoxicity of topotecan is thought to involve the inhibition of the enzyme responsible for the repair of normally occurring single-strand breaks in DNA. Topotecan undergoes partial metabolism in the liver. Binding to plasma proteins is about 35% and the terminal elimination half-life is 2–3 hours (1).

Reproduction studies have been conducted in the rat and rabbit. In rats, a daily dose about equal to the clinical dose based on BSA (CD) given for 14 days before mating through gestation day 6 caused preimplant loss, fetal resorption, and microphthalmia. The dose also produced mild maternal toxicity. A lower daily dose, about 0.5 times the CD, given on gestation days 6–17 caused increased postimplantation mortality and fetal malformations. The most frequent malformations involved the eye (microphthalmia, anophthalmia, rosette formation of the retina, coloboma of the retina, and ectopic orbit), brain (dilated lateral and third ventricles), skull, and vertebrae. In pregnant rabbits, a daily dose about equal to the CD given on gestation days 6–20 caused maternal toxicity, embryo death, and decreased fetal body weight (1). The route of drug administration in the above animal studies was not specified.

Studies for carcinogenicity have not been conducted. However, topotecan is known to be genotoxic in mammalian cells and is probably a carcinogen (1). The drug also is mutagenic and clastogenic, with or without metabolic activation (1).

It is not known if topotecan crosses the human placenta. The molecular weight (about 422 for the free base), low metabolism and plasma protein binding suggest that the drug will cross to the embryo–fetus.

BREASTFEEDING SUMMARY

No reports describing the use of topotecan during human lactation have been located.

The molecular weight (about 422 for the free base), low metabolism and plasma protein binding (35%) suggest that the drug will be excreted into breast milk. The effect of this exposure on a nursing infant is unknown, but may be severe. It is best that a woman receiving this agent does not breastfeed. However, if she chooses to do so, the infant should be closely monitored for the most common or serious adverse effects observed in adults. These effects include bone marrow suppression (primarily neutropenia), headache, nausea, vomiting, diarrhea or constipation, abdominal pain, alopecia, and hepatic toxicity (1).

Reference

1. Product information. Hycamtin. GlaxoSmithKline, 2007.

TORSEMIDE

Diuretic

PREGNANCY RECOMMENDATION: No Human Data—Probably Compatible
BREASTFEEDING RECOMMENDATION: No Human Data—Probably Compatible

PREGNANCY SUMMARY

No reports describing the use of torsemide in human pregnancy have been located. Fetotoxicity was observed in animal studies but only with maternal toxic doses. In general, exposure to diuretics in early pregnancy has not been associated with structural anomalies, but the lack of human pregnancy experience with torsemide prevents a better assessment of the embryo–fetal risk. Diuretics do not prevent or alter the course of toxemia but may decrease placental perfusion (see also Chlorothiazide) because of maternal hypovolemia characteristic of this disease.

FETAL RISK SUMMARY

Torsemide is a loop diuretic in the same pharmacologic class as bumetanide, ethacrynic acid, and furosemide. The drug can be given orally or IV. Torsemide is indicated for the treatment of edema associated with congestive heart failure, renal disease, or hepatic disease. It is also indicated for the treatment of hypertension alone or in combination with other antihypertensive agents. Torsemide undergoes hepatic metabolism to primarily inactive metabolites. Plasma protein binding is >99% and the elimination half-life is about 3.5 hours (1).

Reproduction studies have been conducted in rats and rabbits. In these species, doses up to 10 and 1.7 times, respectively, the human dose of 20 mg/day based on BSA caused no fetotoxicity or teratogenicity. Doses that were 5 (rats) and 4 (rabbits) times larger caused maternal toxicity (decreased average body weight) and fetal toxicity (increased resorptions and delayed ossification) (1).

No overall increase in tumor incidence was noted when torsemide was given to rats and mice throughout their lives. In addition, no mutagenic activity was noted in a variety of assays and no adverse effects were noted on the reproductive performance of male and female rats (1).

It is not known if torsemide crosses the human placenta. The molecular weight (about 348) and moderate elimination half-life suggest that the drug will cross, but the high plasma protein binding may limit the amount available for transfer.

BREASTFEEDING SUMMARY

No reports describing the use of torsemide during human lactation have been located. The molecular weight (about 348) and moderate elimination half-life (about 3.5 hours) suggest that the drug will be excreted into breast milk, but the high plasma protein binding (>99%) should limit the amount in milk. The effect of this exposure on a nursing infant is unknown, but no adverse effects in nursing infants exposed to diuretics in milk have been reported. Of note, however, thiazide diuretics have been used to suppress lactation (see Chlorothiazide).

Reference

1. Product information. Demadex. Roche Pharmaceuticals, 2003.

TRAMADOL

Central Analgesic

PREGNANCY RECOMMENDATION: Human Data Suggest Risk
BREASTFEEDING RECOMMENDATION: Limited Human Data—Potential Toxicity

PREGNANCY SUMMARY

The National Birth Defects Prevention Study discussed below found evidence that opioid use during organogenesis is associated with a low absolute risk of congenital birth defects. Neonatal withdrawal is a potential complication after continuous use in the mother. The long-term effects on the neurobehavior of offspring are unknown but warrant study.

FETAL RISK SUMMARY

Tramadol is a synthetic, centrally acting, analgesic analog of codeine that has the potential to cause physical dependence similar to, but much less than, that produced by opiates. Because of its low addiction potential, tramadol is not classified as a controlled substance. The drug is available only as an oral tablet in the United States but has been used both parenterally and rectally in other countries. The drug is extensively metabolized to active and inactive metabolites. The active metabolite (M1) is a more potent analgesic than the parent drug. Plasma protein binding of tramadol is about 20%. The plasma elimination half-lives of tramadol and M1 are about 6–7 hours (1).

Reproduction studies in mice, rats, and rabbits at doses that were 1.4, ≥0.6, and ≥3.6 times the maximum daily human dose based on BSA (MDHD) were embryotoxic, fetotoxic, and maternally toxic, but not teratogenic. Embryo and fetal toxicity consisted of decreased fetal weights, skeletal ossification, and increased supernumerary ribs. In perinatal and postnatal studies in rats, doses that were ≥1.2 times the MDHD resulted in decreased pup weights and survival. Transient delays in developmental or behavioral parameters were seen in rat pups (1). Shepard described a reproductive study using oral and SC tramadol in mice and rats with no observed teratogenic effects (2).

Tramadol has a molecular weight of about 300 and crosses the placenta to the fetus. In 40 women given 100 mg of tramadol during labor, the mean ratio of drug concentrations in the umbilical cord and maternal serum was 0.83 (3).

Several studies outside of the United States, some of which were reviewed in 1993 (4) and 1997 publications (3), have compared the use of tramadol with meperidine or morphine for labor analgesia (5–13). In five of these studies (5–9), the use of tramadol was associated with less neonatal respiratory depression than meperidine, but no difference was observed in four studies in comparison with meperidine or morphine (10–13). Tramadol also has been combined with bupivacaine for epidural during labor (14).

The effects of tramadol and meperidine (100 mg IV), for each drug, were compared in laboring patients in a study conducted in Thailand (8). A second or third dose of 50 mg IV was given at 30-minute intervals if requested. A significant increase in the incidence of neonatal respiratory depression was observed in the offspring of the meperidine group, if delivery occurred 2–4 hours after the last dose. The respiratory depressant effects of meperidine are known to be time- and dose-related, increasing markedly after 60 minutes (see Meperidine).

A study from Singapore found that 100 mg IM of tramadol was equivalent in analgesic effect to 75 mg IM of meperidine for the control of labor pain (9). Meperidine was associated with a significantly higher frequency of adverse effects (nausea, vomiting, fatigue, drowsiness, and dizziness) in the mothers and a significantly lower respiratory rate in the newborns. However, the injection–delivery interval in the patients was 7–8 hours.

In a 1997 case report, a male infant developed withdrawal symptoms between 24 and 48 hours after birth (15). Symptoms consisted of trembling, tachypnea, tachycardia, hypertonic muscle tone, signs of tetany when touched, and a single mild convulsion. The mother admitted to taking tramadol 300 mg/day for 4 years. The infant was treated with diazepam and/or phenobarbital for 13 days until the symptoms had fully resolved. No long-term follow-up of the infant was reported. The authors concluded that the drug's estimated elimination half-life of 36 hours in the infant was consistent with the course of the withdrawal syndrome (15).

Four other reports, involving seven infants, have described neonatal abstinence syndrome after long-term use of tramadol (200–800 mg/day) in pregnancy (16–19). Withdrawal symptoms in the infants occurred on the second day of life and persisted for up to about 2 weeks.

Results of a National Birth Defects Prevention Study (1997–2005) were published in 2011 (20). This population-based case–control study examined the association between maternal use of opioid analgesics and >30 types of major structural birth defects. In 17,449 case mothers, therapeutic opioid use was reported by 454 (2.6%) compared with 134 (2.0%) of 6701 control mothers. Indications for use of opioid analgesics were surgical procedures (41%), infections (34%), chronic diseases (20%), and injuries (18%). Dose, duration, or frequency were not evaluated. The exposure period evaluated was from 1 month before to 3 months after conception. Limiting the exposure period to the first 2 months after conception produced similar results. Infants with >1 defect were included in multiple birth defect categories. The following opioids were included (number of cases for each agent not specified): codeine, hydrocodone, hydromorphone, fentanyl, meperidine, methadone, morphine, oxycodone, pentazocine, propoxyphene, and tramadol. The birth defect, total number, number exposed, and the adjusted odds ratio (aOR) with 95% confidence interval (CI) were as follows:

Birth Defect	Total	Cases	aOR (95% CI)
Spina bifida	718	26	2.0 (1.3–3.2)
Any heart defect (20 types)	7724	211	1.4 (1.1–1.7)
Atrioventricular septal defect	175	9	2.4 (1.2–4.8)
Teratology of Fallot	672	21	1.7 (1.1–2.8)
Conotruncal defect	1481	41	1.5 (1.0–2.1)
Conoventricular septal defect	110	6	2.7 (1.1–6.3)
Left ventricular outflow tract obstruction defect	1195	36	1.5 (1.0–2.2)
Hypoplastic left heart syndrome	357	17	2.4 (1.4–4.1)
Right ventricular outflow tract obstruction defect	1175	40	1.6 (1.1–2.3)
Pulmonary valve stenosis	867	34	1.7 (1.2–2.6)
Atrial septal defect (ASD)	511	17	2.0 (1.2–3.6)
Ventricular septal defect + ASD	528	17	1.7 (1.0–2.9)
Hydrocephaly	301	11	2.0 (1.0–3.7)
Glaucoma/anterior chamber defects	103	5	2.6 (1.0–6.6)
Gastroschisis	726	26	1.8 (1.1–2.9)

The authors speculated that the activity of opioids and their receptors as growth regulators during development of the embryo might be a mechanism to explain the above findings. The exposure data were obtained by retrospective maternal self-report; the authors acknowledged that recall bias and misclassification might have affected their results. They concluded that the absolute risk was a modest absolute increase above the baseline risk for birth defects (20).

A 2012 review of tramadol in pregnancy and lactation found no clear evidence of fetal or neonatal harm, but concluded that the drug should be avoided during conception and the 1st trimester because of lack of data during these periods (21). The above study was not cited in the review.

BREASTFEEDING SUMMARY

Both tramadol and its pharmacologic active metabolite (M1) are excreted into human milk (1). After a single 100-mg IV dose, the cumulative amounts of the parent drug and M1 excreted into milk within 16 hours were 100 and 27 mcg, respectively (1). The recommended dose of tramadol is 50–100 mg every 4–6 hours up to a maximum of 400 mg/day. Moreover, the mean absolute bioavailability of a 100-mg oral dose is 75%. Thus, ingestion of the recommended dose may produce drug amounts in breast milk that could exceed those reported above. The effect of this exposure on a nursing infant is unknown.

In a 2008 study, 75 breastfeeding mothers were taking tramadol (100 mg every 6 hours) on days 2–4 after cesarean section (22). Samples were collected after four or more doses. On the study date, 49% of the subjects and 100% of the controls also took other opiate analgesics (mostly oxycodone) while 61% of the subjects and 58% of the controls also took nonsteroidal anti-inflammatory agents (mostly diclofenac). The mean milk:plasma ratio was 2.2 for tramadol and 2.8 for M1. For tramadol, the estimated absolute and relative infant doses were 112 mcg/kg/day and 0.64%, respectively, whereas for M1 the doses were 30 mcg/kg/day and 2.24%, respectively. Compared with controls not taking tramadol, there were no significant behavioral adverse effects (22).

A 2012 review of tramadol in pregnancy and lactation concluded that the use of tramadol during early breastfeeding was unlikely to cause harm in healthy term infants (21).

References

1. Product information. Ultram. Janssen Pharmaceuticals, 2013.
2. Yamamoto H, Kuchii M, Hayano T, Nishino H. A study on teratogenicity of both CG-315 and morphine in mice and rats. Oyo Yakuri 1972;6:1055–69. As cited in Shepard TH. *Catalog of Teratogenic Agents*. 8th ed. Baltimore, MD: The Johns Hopkins University Press, 1995:420.
3. Lewis KS, Han NH. Tramadol: a new centrally acting analgesic. Am J Health-Syst Pharm 1997;54:643–52.
4. Lee CR, McTavish D, Sorkin EM. Tramadol: a preliminary review of its pharmacodynamic and pharmacokinetic properties, and therapeutic potential in acute and chronic pain states. Drugs 1993;46:313–40.
5. Husslein P, Kubista E, Egarter C. Obstetrical analgesia with tramadol-results of a prospective randomized comparative study with pethidine. Z Geburtshilfe Perinatol 1987;191:234–7.
6. Bitsch M, Emmrich J, Hary J, Lippach G, Rindt W. Obstetrical analgesia with tramadol. Fortschr Med 1980;98:632–4.
7. Bredow V. Use of tramadol versus pethidine versus denaverine suppositories in labor—a contribution to noninvasive therapy of labor pain. Zentralbl Gynakol 1992;114:551–4.
8. Suvonnakote T, Thitadilok W, Atisook R. Pain relief during labour. J Med Assoc Thailand 1986;69:575–80.
9. Viegas OAC, Khaw B, Ratnam SS. Tramadol in labour pain in primiparous patients. A prospective comparative clinical trial. Eur J Obstet Gynecol Reprod Biol 1993;49:131–5.
10. Prasertsawat PO, Herabutya Y, Chaturachinda K. Obstetric analgesia: comparison between tramadol, morphine, and pethidine. Curr Ther Res Clin Exp 1986;40:1022–8.
11. Kainz C, Joura E, Obwegeser R, Plockinger B, Gruber W. Effectiveness and tolerance of tramadol with or without an antiemetic and pethidine in obstetric analgesia. Z Geburtshilfe Perinatol 1992;196:78–82.
12. Keskin HL, Keskin EA, Avsar AF, Tabuk M, Caglar GS. Pethidine versus tramadol for pain relief during labor. Int J Gynaecol Obstet 2003; 82:11–6.
13. Khooshideh M, Shahriari A. A comparison of tramadol and pethidine analgesia on the duration of labour: a randomised clinical trial. Aust N Z J Obstet Gynaecol 2009;49:59–63.
14. Rao ZA, Choudhri A, Naqvi S, Ehsan-ul-Haq. Walking epidural with low dose bupivacaine plus tramadol on normal labour in primipara. J Coll Physicians Surg Pak 2010;20:295–8.
15. Meyer FP, Rimasch H, Blaha B, Banditt P. Tramadol withdrawal in a neonate. Eur J Clin Pharmacol 1997;53:159–60.
16. Willaschek C, Wolter E, Buchhorn R. Tramadol withdrawal in a neonate after long-term analgesic treatment of the mother. Eur J Clin Pharmacol 2009;65:429–30.
17. Hartenstein S, Proquitte H, Bauer S, Bamberg C, Rochr CC. Neonatal abstinence syndrome (NAS) after intrauterine exposure to tramadol. J Perinat Med 2010;38:695–6.
18. O'Mara K, Gal P, DaVanzo C. Treatment of neonatal withdrawal with clonidine after long-term, high-dose maternal use of tramadol. Ann Pharmacother 2010;44:1342–4.
19. Anonymous. Tramadol withdrawal symptoms in infants exposed in utero. Prescribe Int 2012;21:71–2.
20. Broussard CS, Rasmussen SA, Reefhuis J, Friedman JM, Jann MW, Riehle-Colarusso T, Honein MA, for the National Birth Defects Prevention Study. Maternal treatment with opioid analgesics and risk for birth defects. Am J Obstet Gynecol 2011;204:314–7.
21. Bloor M, Paech MJ, Kaye R. Tramadol in pregnancy and lactation. Int J Obstet Anesth 2012;21:163–7.
22. Ilett KF, Paech MJ, Page-Sharp M, Sy SK, Kristensen JH, Goy R, Chua S, Christmas T, Scott KL. Use of a sparse sampling study design to assess transfer of tramadol and its O-desmethyl metabolite into transitional breast milk. Br J Clin Pharmacol 2008;65:661–6.

TRANDOLAPRIL

Antihypertensive

PREGNANCY RECOMMENDATION: Human Data Suggest Risk in 2nd and 3rd Trimesters
BREASTFEEDING RECOMMENDATION: No Human Data—Probably Compatible

PREGNANCY SUMMARY

The fetal toxicity of trandolapril in the 2nd and 3rd trimesters is similar to other angiotensin-converting enzyme (ACE) inhibitors. The use of this drug during the 2nd and 3rd trimesters may cause teratogenicity and severe fetal and neonatal toxicity. Fetal toxic effects may include anuria, oligohydramnios, fetal hypocalvaria, intrauterine growth restriction (IUGR), prematurity, and patent ductus arteriosus. Stillbirth or neonatal death may occur. Anuria-associated oligohydramnios may produce fetal limb contractures, craniofacial deformation, and pulmonary hypoplasia. Severe anuria and hypotension, which is resistant to both pressor agents and volume expansion, may occur in the newborn following in utero exposure. Newborn renal function and blood pressure should be closely monitored.

FETAL RISK SUMMARY

The prodrug, trandolapril, is rapidly metabolized to the active drug, trandolaprilat. It is indicated in the management of hypertension either alone, or in combination with other antihypertensives (e.g., hydrochlorothiazide). Trandolapril is also indicated in the management of stable patients with heart failure or left-ventricular dysfunction after myocardial infarction. The active metabolite, trandolaprilat, is an ACE inhibitor, thus preventing the conversion of angiotensin I to angiotensin II (1).

Reproduction studies have been conducted in rats, rabbits, and cynomolgus monkeys. No teratogenicity was observed in the three species at doses that were 2564, 3, and 108 times, respectively, the maximum projected human dose based on BSA (1).

It is not known if trandolapril or trandolaprilat cross the human placenta. The molecular weights (about 431 for trandolapril; about 403 for trandolaprilat) are low enough that transfer to the fetus should be expected.

A retrospective study using pharmacy-based data from the Tennessee Medicaid program identified 209 infants, born between 1985 and 2000, who had 1st trimester exposure to ACE inhibitors (2). Infants of mothers with evidence of diabetes, either before or during pregnancy, were excluded, as were those exposed to angiotensin-receptor antagonists (ARBs), ACE inhibitors, or other antihypertensives beyond the 1st trimester, and exposure to known teratogens. Two comparison groups, other antihypertensives (N = 202) and no antihypertensives (N = 29,096), were formed. The number of major birth defects in each of the three groups was 18 (8.6%), 4 (2%), and 834 (2.9%), respectively. Compared with the no antihypertensives group, exposure to ACE inhibitors was associated with a significantly increased risk of major defects (relative risk [RR] 2.71, 95% confidence interval [CI] 1.72–4.27). When the analysis was conducted by the type of defect, the highest rates were with cardiovascular defects, 9, 2, and 294, respectively, RR 3.72, 95% CI 1.89–7.30, and with CNS defects, 3, 0, and 80, respectively, RR 4.39, 95% CI 1.37–14.02. The major defects observed in the subject group were: atrial septal defect (N = 6) (includes three with pulmonic stenosis and/or three with patent ductus arteriosus [PDA]), renal dysplasia (N = 2), PDA alone (N = 2), and one each of ventricular septal defect, spina bifida, microcephaly with eye anomaly, coloboma, hypospadias, intestinal and choanal atresia, Hirschsprung disease, and diaphragmatic hernia (2). In an accompanying editorial, it was noted that neither previous reports of 1st trimester exposure to ACE inhibitors nor the animal studies had observed an increased risk of birth defects (3). It also was noted that no mechanism for ACE inhibitor-induced teratogenicity was known. A subsequent communication raising concerns about the validity of the study in terms of adequate exclusion of diabetes, charting and coding errors in busy medical practices, and the effects of maternal obesity (4) was addressed by the investigators (5).

Trandolapril and other ACE inhibitors are human teratogens when used in the 2nd and 3rd trimesters, producing fetal hypocalvaria and renal defects. The cause of the defects and other toxicity is probably related to fetal hypotension and decreased renal blood flow. The compromise of the fetal renal system may result in severe, and at times fatal, anuria, both in the fetus and in the newborn. Anuria-associated oligohydramnios may produce pulmonary hypoplasia, limb contractures, persistent PDA, craniofacial deformation, and neonatal death (6,7). IUGR, prematurity, and severe neonatal hypotension may also be observed. Two reviews of fetal and newborn renal function indicated that both renal perfusion and glomerular plasma flow are low during gestation and that high levels of angiotensin II may be physiologically necessary to maintain glomerular filtration at low perfusion pressures (8,9). Trandolapril prevents the conversion of angiotensin I to angiotensin II and, thus, may lead to in utero renal failure. Because the primary means of removal of the drug is renal, the impairment of this system in the newborn prevents elimination of the drug resulting in prolonged hypotension. Newborn renal function and blood pressure should be closely monitored. If oligohydramnios occurs, stopping trandolapril may resolve the problem but may not improve infant outcome because of irreversible fetal damage (6). In those cases in which trandolapril must be used to treat the mother's disease, the lowest possible dose should be used combined with close monitoring of amniotic fluid levels and fetal well-being. Guidelines for counseling exposed pregnant patients have been published and should be of benefit to health professionals faced with this task (6,10).

The observation in Tennessee Medicaid data of an increased risk of major congenital defects after 1st trimester exposure to ACE inhibitors raises concerns about teratogenicity that have not been seen in other studies (3). Medicaid data are a valuable tool for identifying early signals of teratogenicity, but are subject to a number of shortcomings and their findings must be considered hypotheses until confirmed by independent studies.

A 2012 review of the use of ACE inhibitors and ARBs in the 1st trimester concluded that there may be an elevated teratogenic risk, but the risk appeared to be related to other factors (11). The factors, that typically coexist with hypertension in pregnancy, included diabetes, advanced maternal age, and obesity.

BREASTFEEDING SUMMARY

No reports describing the use of trandolapril in human lactation have been located. The molecular weights (about 431 for trandolapril; about 403 for trandolaprilat) suggest that excretion into breast milk should be expected. The effect of this exposure on a nursing infant is unknown. However, other ACE inhibitors are excreted into breast milk and are considered compatible with breastfeeding by the American Academy of Pediatrics (see Captopril and Enalapril).

References

1. Product information. Mavik. Knoll Pharmaceutical, 2001.
2. Cooper WO, Hernandez-Diaz S, Arbogast PG, Dudley JA, Dyer S, Gideon PS, Hall K, Ray WA. Major congenital malformations after first-trimester exposure to ACE inhibitors. N Engl J Med 2006;354:2443–51.
3. Friedman JM. ACE inhibitors and congenital anomalies. N Engl J Med 2006;354:2498–500.
4. Scialli AR, Lione A. ACE inhibitors and major congenital malformations. N Engl J Med 2006;355:1280.
5. Cooper WO, Ray WA. Reply—ACE inhibitors and major congenital malformations. N Engl J Med 2006;355:1281.
6. Barr M Jr. Teratogen update: angiotensin-converting enzyme inhibitors. Teratology 1994;50:399–409.
7. Shotan A, Widerhorn J, Hurst A, Elkayam U. Risks of angiotensin-converting enzyme inhibition during pregnancy: experimental and clinical evidence, potential mechanisms, and recommendations for use. Am J Med 1994;96:451–6.
8. Robillard JE, Nakamura KT, Matherne GP, Jose PA. Renal hemodynamics and functional adjustments to postnatal life. Semin Perinatol 1988;12:143–50.
9. Guignard J-P, Gouyon J-B. Adverse effects of drugs on the immature kidney. Biol Neonate 1988;53:243–52.
10. Brent RL, Beckman DA. Angiotensin-converting enzyme inhibitors, an embryopathic class of drugs with unique properties: information for clinical teratology counselors. Teratology 1991;43:543–6.
11. Polifka JE. Is there an embryopathy associated with first-trimester exposure to angiotensin-converting enzyme inhibitors and angiotensin receptor antagonists? A critical review of the evidence. Birth Defects Res (Part A) 2012;94:576–98.

TRANEXAMIC ACID

Hemostatic

PREGNANCY RECOMMENDATION: Limited Human Data—Animal Data Suggest Low Risk
BREASTFEEDING RECOMMENDATION: Limited Human Data—Probably Compatible

PREGNANCY SUMMARY

No adverse effects attributable to use of tranexamic acid during pregnancy, in either animals or humans, have been reported in the fetus or newborn. The drug crosses the placenta to the fetus, but its reported lack of effect on plasminogen activator activity in the vascular wall (1,2) (vs. its known effect in the peripheral circulation) may protect the fetus and newborn from potential thromboembolic complications.

FETAL RISK SUMMARY

This hemostatic agent, a competitive inhibitor of plasminogen activation, is used to reduce or prevent hemorrhage in hemophilia and in other bleeding disorders. The drug blocks the action of plasminogen activators (e.g., tissue plasminogen activator [alteplase; t-PA], streptokinase, and urokinase) by inhibiting the conversion of plasminogen to plasmin (3).

No adverse fetal effects were observed in reproductive toxicity testing in mice, rats, and rabbits (3,4). Both Schardein (5) and Shepard (6) cited a 1971 study in which doses up to 1500 mg/kg/day were given to mice and rats during organogenesis without causing adverse fetal effects.

Tranexamic acid crosses the human placenta to the fetus (7). Twelve women were given an IV dose of 10 mg/kg just before cesarean section. Cord serum and maternal blood samples were drawn immediately following delivery, a mean of 13 minutes after the dose of tranexamic acid. The mean drug concentrations in the cord and maternal serum were 19 mcg/mL (range <4–31 mcg/mL) and 26 mcg/mL (range 10–53 mcg/mL), respectively, a ratio of 0.7 (7).

Twelve women with vaginal bleeding between 24 and 36 weeks' gestation were treated with 7-day courses of tranexamic acid, 1 g orally every 8 hours (8). Additional courses were given if bleeding continued (number of patients with repeat courses not specified). Four women underwent cesarean section (placenta previa in three, breech in one) and the remainder had vaginal deliveries. One of the newborns was delivered at 30 weeks' gestation, but the gestational ages of the other newborns were not specified. All of the newborns were alive and well. Two of the mothers were receiving treatment at the time of delivery, and the drug concentrations in the cord blood were 9 and 12 mcg/mL (8).

A pregnant woman with fibrinolysis was treated with tranexamic acid and fibrinogen for 64 days until spontaneous delivery of a normal 1400-g girl at 30 weeks' gestation (9). No adverse fetal or newborn effects attributable to the drug were reported. Tranexamic acid was used in a woman with abruptio placentae during her third pregnancy (10). She had a history of two previous pregnancy losses because of the disorder. Treatment with tranexamic acid (1 g IV every 4 hours for 3 days, then 1 g orally 4 times daily) was begun at 26 weeks' gestation and continued until 33 weeks' gestation, at which time a cesarean section was performed because of the risk of heavier bleeding. A healthy 1430 g male infant was delivered (10).

The use of tranexamic acid in a woman with Glanzmann's thrombasthenia disease was described in an abstract published in 1981 (11). Treatment was started at 24 weeks' gestation and continued until spontaneous delivery at 42 weeks' gestation of a healthy boy. A study published in 1980 described the use of tranexamic acid in 73 consecutive cases of abruptio placentae, 6 of which were treated for 1–12 weeks (1). Six (8.2%) of the newborns were either stillbirths ($N = 4$) or died shortly after delivery ($N = 2$), a markedly reduced mortality rate compared with the expected 33%–37% at that time (10). None of the deaths was attributed to the drug. No cases of increased hemorrhage, thromboses, or maternal deaths were observed (1).

Tranexamic acid (4 g/day) was used in a 21-year-old primigravida at 26 weeks' gestation for the treatment of vaginal bleeding (12). She also received terbutaline and

T

betamethasone for premature labor. Tranexamic acid was administered as a single dose on admission, and 6 days later a 10-day course was initiated for continued bleeding. Acute massive pulmonary embolism occurred at the termination of tranexamic acid, and following 2–3 days of treatment with heparin and streptokinase, a preterm 1140-g male infant was spontaneously delivered. No adverse effects in the fetus or newborn attributable to the drug therapy were noted (12).

A retrospective study published in 1993 examined the question of whether tranexamic acid was thrombogenic when administered during pregnancy (2). In the period 1979–1988 in Sweden, among pregnant women with various bleeding disorders, 256 had been treated with tranexamic acid (mean duration 46 days), whereas 1846 had not been treated (controls). Two patients (0.78%) in the treated group had pulmonary embolism compared with four (0.22%) (three deep vein thromboses, one pulmonary embolism) (odds ratio 3.6, 95% confidence interval [CI] 0.7–17.8) in the control group. In the subgroups of those patients who were delivered by cesarean section (168 treated, 439 controls), the rates of thromboembolism were 1 (0.60%) and 4 (0.91%) (odds ratio 0.65, 95% CI 0.1–5.8), respectively. Thus, no evidence was found indicating that the use of tranexamic acid during gestation was thrombogenic. Although the purpose of this study did not include examining the effects of the therapy on the fetus or newborn, the authors concluded that in the absence of a thrombogenic risk, there was no reason to change the indications for its use during pregnancy (2).

BREASTFEEDING SUMMARY

Tranexamic acid is excreted into human milk. One hour after the last dose following a 2-day treatment course in lactating women, the milk concentration of the agent was 1% of the peak serum concentration (13). In adults, approximately 30%–50% of an oral dose is absorbed (1). The amount a nursing infant would absorb is unknown, as is the effect of the small amount of drug present in milk.

References

1. Svanberg L, Åstedt B, Nilsson IM. Abruptio placentae—treatment with the fibrinolytic inhibitor tranexamic acid. Acta Obstet Gynecol Scand 1980;59:127–30.
2. Lindoff C, Rybo G, Åstedt B. Treatment with tranexamic acid during pregnancy and the risk of thrombo-embolic complications. Thromb Haemost 1993;70:238–40.
3. Product information. Cyklokapron. Pharmacia, 1996.
4. Onnis A, Grella P, Lewis PJ. *The Biochemical Effects of Drugs in Pregnancy*. Volume 1. Chichester, England: Ellis Horwood, 1984:385.
5. Schardein JL. *Chemically Induced Birth Defects*. 2nd ed. New York, NY: Marcel Dekker, 1993:107.
6. Shepard TH. *Catalog of Teratogenic Agents*. 8th ed. Baltimore, MD: The Johns Hopkins University Press, 1995:420.
7. Kullander S, Nilsson IM. Human placental transfer of an antifibrinolytic agent (AMCA). Acta Obstet Gynecol Scand 1970;49:241–2.
8. Walzman M, Bonnar J. Effects of tranexamic acid on the coagulation and fibrinolytic systems in pregnancy complicated by placental bleeding. Arch Toxicol 1982;(Suppl 5):214–20.
9. Storm O, Weber J. Prolonged treatment with tranexamic acid (Cyklokapron) during pregnancy. Ugeskr Laeg 1976;138:1781–2.
10. Åstedt B, Nilsson IM. Recurrent abruptio placentae treated with the fibrinolytic inhibitor tranexamic acid. Br Med J 1978;1:756–7.
11. Sundqvist S-B, Nilsson IM, Svanberg L, Cronberg S. Glanzmann's thrombasthenia: pregnancy and parturition (abstract). Thromb Haemost 1981;46:225.
12. Fagher B, Ahlgren M, Åstedt B. Acute massive pulmonary embolism treated with streptokinase during labor and the early puerperium. Acta Obstet Gynecol Scand 1990;69:659–62.
13. Eriksson O, Kjellman H, Nilsson L. *Tranexamic Acid in Human Milk after Oral Administration of Cyklokapron to Lactating Women*. Data on file, KabiVitrum AB, Stockholm, Sweden. (Data supplied by R.G. Leonardi, Ph.D., KabiVitrum, 1987).

TRANYLCYPROMINE

Antidepressant

PREGNANCY RECOMMENDATION: Limited Human Data—No Relevant Animal Data
BREASTFEEDING RECOMMENDATION: No Human Data—Potential Toxicity

PREGNANCY SUMMARY

Tranylcypromine is a monoamine oxidase inhibitor used in the treatment of major depressive episode without melancholia. Other agents in this subclass are iproniazid, isocarboxazid, nialamide, and phenelzine. Although risk was suggested in consecutive pregnancies from one woman, the human pregnancy experience is too limited to assess adequately the embryo–fetal risk.

FETAL RISK SUMMARY

Relevant animal reproduction data have not been located. However, the drug crosses the rat placenta (1).

The Collaborative Perinatal Project monitored 21 mother–child pairs exposed to monoamine oxidase inhibitors during the 1st trimester, 13 of whom were exposed to tranylcypromine (2). Three of the 21 infants had malformations (relative risk 2.26). Details of the 13 cases with exposure to tranylcypromine were not specified.

A brief 2000 abstract described two consecutive adverse pregnancy outcomes in a woman treated with tranylcypromine (3). In the first pregnancy, the 41-year-old woman with severe depression was treated with tranylcypromine (100 mg/day), pimozide (1 mg/day), and diazepam (5–10 mg/day). The woman delivered a stillborn fetus at 31 weeks' gestation. Examination of the macerated female fetus revealed hypertelorism, a large atrioventricular septal defect, single coronary ostium, and right pulmonary isomerism. The placenta had multiple infarcts that were considered significant factors in the fetal death. In her second pregnancy (other drugs and doses not specified), an ultrasound at 19 weeks' revealed a fetus with a head described as "lemon-shaped." A female infant (normal karyotype) was delivered at 38 weeks' because of poor growth (weight not specified). The infant had multiple defects, including hypertelorism, low-set overfolded ears, cleft palate, micrognathia, marked distal phalangeal hypoplasia, agenesis of the corpus callosum, and an atrioventricular septal defect (first detected at 26 weeks'). The outcomes of both pregnancies were attributed to tranylcypromine, possibly due to reduced uterine and placental blood flow (3).

It is not known if tranylcypromine crosses the human placenta. The molecular weight (about 365) is low enough that exposure of the embryo–fetus should be expected.

BREASTFEEDING SUMMARY

No reports describing the use of tranylcypromine during lactation have been located. The molecular weight (about 365) is low enough that excretion into breast milk should be expected. The effect of this exposure on a nursing infant is unknown.

References

1. Product information. Parnate. SmithKline Beecham Pharmaceuticals, 2000.
2. Heinonen OP, Slone D, Shapiro S. *Birth Defects and Drugs in Pregnancy*. Littleton, MA: Publishing Sciences Group, 1977:336–7.
3. Kennedy DS, Evans N, Wang I, Webster WS. Fetal abnormalities associated with high-dose tranylcypromine in two consecutive pregnancies (abstract). Teratology 2000;61:441.

TRASTUZUMAB

Antineoplastic

PREGNANCY RECOMMENDATION: Limited Human Data—Animal Data Suggest Low Risk
BREASTFEEDING RECOMMENDATION: No Human Data—Potential Toxicity

PREGNANCY SUMMARY

The human pregnancy experience with trastuzumab is limited to six cases, three of which involved 1st trimester exposure. No congenital malformations were noted in the infants and all were developing normally. However, fetal renal toxicity, as evidenced by oligohydramnios or anhydramnios, was observed in four cases. The toxicity might have been secondary to inhibition of epidermal growth factor receptor 2 (HER2) in the fetal kidneys but additional study is required. The toxicity appears to be reversible when trastuzumab is stopped. Although the action of this receptor in human fetal development requires study, HER2 protein expression is high in many embryonic tissues, such as cardiac and neural tissues, and blocking this expression may be harmful. Trastuzumab has a very long elimination half-life and could be present in the maternal system for ≤5 months after the last dose.

FETAL RISK SUMMARY

Trastuzumab, a recombinant DNA-derived humanized monoclonal antibody (an IgG_1 kappa), selectively binds with high affinity to the extracellular domain of the human epidermal growth factor receptor 2 (HER2) protein. It is indicated, either alone or in combination with paclitaxel, for the treatment of patients with metastatic breast cancer whose tumors overexpress the HER2 protein. Trastuzumab is administered as an IV infusion. The mean elimination half-life, after a 4 mg/kg loading dose followed by a weekly maintenance dose of 2 mg/kg, was 5.8 days (range 1–32 days) (1).

No evidence of impaired fertility or fetal harm were observed in female cynomolgus monkeys administered doses up to 25 times the weekly human dose of 2 mg/kg. However, HER2 protein expression is high in many embryonic tissues, such as cardiac and neural tissues. Early death was observed in embryos of mutant mice that lacked this protein. Trastuzumab was not mutagenic in multiple assays or clastogenic in one test (1).

It is not known if trastuzumab crosses the human placenta. The antibody does cross the placentas of cynomolgus monkeys in both early (gestational days 20 and 50) and late (gestational days 120 and 150) pregnancy. The presence of trastuzumab in the serum of infant monkeys had no adverse effect on growth or development from birth to 3 months of age (1).

Six case reports have described the use of trastuzumab during pregnancy (2–7). A 28-year-old woman had undergone bilateral mastectomy for breast cancer, followed by chemotherapy with cyclophosphamide, doxorubicin and paclitaxel, and then radiation therapy (2). She then received trastuzumab 580 mg every 3 weeks. Pregnancy was diagnosed at 23 weeks' gestation, 3 weeks after the last dose of trastuzumab. Anhydramnios was present with normal appearing fetal kidneys and an estimated fetal weight of 475 g. The anhydramnios slowly resolved and a normal 2950-g female infant was delivered vaginally at 37.5 weeks' with Apgar scores of 8 and 9, at 1 and 5 minutes, respectively. The placenta pathology was unremarkable with normal fetal membranes. The infant had normal renal function at birth and no evidence of pulmonary hypoplasia. The 6-month-old child was doing well with growth at the 75th percentile (2).

In another 2005 case report, a 26-year-old woman with breast cancer was treated with trastuzumab, paclitaxel, fluorouracil, epirubicin, and cyclophosphamide, followed by a left mastectomy and radiation therapy (3). Fourteen months later,

T

in the 27th week of pregnancy, multiple hepatic metastases were detected. She was treated with trastuzumab (4 mg/kg loading dose, then 2 mg/kg every week) and vinorelbine (25 mg/m^2 weekly for 3 weeks followed by a week of rest) until 34 weeks' gestation. Oligohydramnios was noted during therapy. Because of decreased fetal movement, labor was induced at 34 weeks' gestation and a healthy 2.6-kg male infant was delivered vaginally with Apgar scores of 9, 9, and 10 at 1, 5, and 10 minutes, respectively. At 6 months of age, the infant was healthy and developing normally (3).

A 30-year-old woman with breast cancer was treated with epirubicin, cyclophosphamide, fluorouracil, a bilateral mastectomy, and radiation therapy (4). She was enrolled in a clinical trial and was randomized to receive trastuzumab 736 mg as a loading dose and then 523 mg every 3 weeks for the first year. Conception occurred 3 days after her second cycle. A third cycle was apparently given before she was withdrawn from the study. She delivered a normal female infant at term (no other details provided) (4).

A 38-year-old woman at 17 weeks' in her second pregnancy had spinal-cord compression secondary to metastatic disease 7 years after undergoing treatment for breast cancer (5). Treatment had consisted of surgery, six cycles of fluorouracil, methotrexate, and cyclophosphamide, radiotherapy, and then 5 years of tamoxifen. She was given radiotherapy to the cervical vertebrae, with lead shielding of the uterus to protect the fetus. At about 26 weeks' gestation, she received trastuzumab 8 mg/kg and paclitaxel 175 mg/m^2. A second cycle of trastuzumab (6 mg/kg) and paclitaxel was given 3 weeks later. At 26–32 weeks', fetal abdominal circumference stopped growing and amniotic fluid decreased to near anhydramnios. At the end of this period, the volume of both fetal kidneys was below the 5th percentile and the fetal bladder was barely visible. Corticosteroids were given for fetal lung maturity and a cesarean section delivered a growth-restricted 1.460-kg (10th percentile) male infant. Complications in the newborn included bacterial sepsis with hypotension, transient renal failure, and respiratory failure. The renal impairment resolved within 14 days. The infant was discharged home at 6 weeks weighing 2.335 kg and was developing normally at 12 weeks of age. Although the cause of the fetal renal impairment was not known with certainty, it was noted that epidermal growth factor receptors are expressed in the kidney during fetal development and blocking these receptors may have prevented normal kidney growth and development (5).

A 2007 case report described a woman treated during the first 24 weeks of pregnancy with trastuzumab (6). The patient had a history of breast cancer with multiple metastases that had been treated with surgery, paclitaxel, carboplatin, trastuzumab, and radiation. She had been on trastuzumab exclusively for a year when pregnancy was diagnosed at 5 weeks' gestation. Trastuzumab was continued until 24 weeks' at which time it was stopped because of reversible, asymptomatic maternal heart failure (low ejection fraction). At 37 weeks', a healthy 2.6-kg female infant was delivered by cesarean section with Apgar scores of 9 and 10 at 1 and 5 minutes, respectively. At 2 months of age, the infant's weight, height, and head circumference were 4.4 kg (25th percentile), 55 cm (25th percentile), and 40 cm (50th percentile), respectively. No abnormalities were found on physical and neurological examination and her development was within normal limits for age (6).

Another 2007 case report described a 28-year-old woman with a history of radical mastectomy, chemotherapy, and radiotherapy 1 year before pregnancy (7). Because of metastases, she was treated with docetaxel and trastuzumab at 23 and 26 weeks' gestation, trastuzumab alone at 27 weeks', and docetaxel alone at 30 weeks'. Trastuzumab was omitted at 30 weeks' because an ultrasound revealed anhydramnios and fetal growth at the 5th percentile. The anhydramnios was thought to be due to trastuzumab. At 33 weeks', oligohydramnios was noted. An elective cesarean section was conducted at 36 weeks' to deliver a 2.23-kg male infant with Apgar scores of 7 and 9 at 1 and 5 minutes, respectively. No evidence of positional deformations or respiratory abnormalities from the prolonged low amniotic fluid was noted and the neonatal urine output was normal. The development of the infant also was normal (7).

Because of the unknown potential for embryo–fetal harm, two reviews recommended that the use of trastuzumab in pregnancy should be avoided or limited until adequate human pregnancy experience is available (8,9). However, as noted in one review, compared with standard chemotherapy, the use of trastuzumab could improve the pregnancy outcome for both the mother and her fetus (8).

BREASTFEEDING SUMMARY

No reports describing the use of trastuzumab during human lactation have been located.

Human immunoglobulin G also is excreted into breast milk (1,7). The effect of this exposure on a nursing infant is unknown. In adults, adverse effects include left ventricular dysfunction and congestive failure, anemia, leucopenia, diarrhea, and an increased incidence of infection. The manufacturer recommends that women should not breastfeed while receiving trastuzumab and for 6 months after the last dose (1).

References

1. Product information. Herceptin. Genentech, 2007.
2. Watson WJ. Herceptin (trastuzumab) therapy during pregnancy: association with reversible anhydramnios. Obstet Gynecol 2005;105:642–3.
3. Fanale MA, Uyei AR, Therialult RL, Adam K, Thompson RA. Treatment of metastatic breast cancer with trastuzumab and vinorelbine during pregnancy. Clin Breast Cancer 2005;6:354–6.
4. Waterston AM, Graham J. Effect of adjuvant trastuzumab on pregnancy. J Clin Oncol 2006;24:321–2.
5. Bader AA, Schiembach D, Tamussino KF, Pristauz G, Petru E. Anhydramnios associated with administration of trastuzumab and paclitaxel for metastatic breast cancer during pregnancy. Lancet Oncol 2007;8:79–81.
6. Shrim A, Garcia-Bournissen F, Maxwell C, Farine D, Koren G. Favorable pregnancy outcome following trastuzumab (Herceptin®) use during pregnancy—case report and updated literature review. Reprod Toxicol 2007;23:611–13.
7. Sekar R, Stone PR. Trastuzumab use for metastatic breast cancer in pregnancy. Obstet Gynecol 2007;110:507–10.
8. Leslie KK. Chemotherapy and pregnancy. Clin Obstet Gynecol 2002;45:153–64.
9. Kelly HL, Collichio FA, Dees EC. Concomitant pregnancy and breast cancer: options for systemic therapy. Breast Dis 2005–2006;23:95–101.

TRAVOPROST

Ophthalmic (Prostaglandin Agonist)

PREGNANCY RECOMMENDATION: No Human Data—Probably Compatible
BREASTFEEDING RECOMMENDATION: No Human Data—Probably Compatible

PREGNANCY SUMMARY

No reports describing the use of travoprost in human pregnancy have been located. The animal data suggest moderate risk, but the amount appearing in the systemic circulation is very low. Moreover, the elimination half-life from plasma is very fast. Although the absence of human pregnancy experience prevents a more complete assessment of embryo–fetal risk, the risk of harm appears to be low. Nevertheless, because the drug will be given daily for long periods, it may be best to use other anti-glaucoma agents that have some human data (e.g., Latanoprost).

FETAL RISK SUMMARY

Travoprost is a synthetic prostaglandin F analog that acts as a selective FP prostanoid receptor agonist to reduce intraocular pressure by increasing uveoscleral outflow. It is available as an 0.004% ophthalmic solution that is given as one drop in the affected eye(s) once daily. It is in the same class of prostaglandin agonists as bimatoprost, latanoprost, and tafluprost. Travoprost is indicated for the reduction of elevated intraocular pressure in patients with open-angle glaucoma or ocular hypertension. It is hydrolyzed in the eye to the active free acid and systemically to inactive metabolites. In most nonpregnant subjects, plasma concentrations were below the quantification limit (0.01 ng/mL) of the assay. In subjects with quantifiable plasma levels, the mean plasma maximum concentration was 0.018 ng/mL and the elimination half-life was estimated to be 45 minutes (range 17–86 minutes) (1).

Reproduction studies have been conducted in mice and rats. In rats, a daily IV dose up to 250 times the maximum recommended human ocular dose (MRHOD) was associated with an increase in the incidence of skeletal malformations and external and visceral defects (fused sternebrae, domed head, and hydrocephaly). Teratogenicity was not observed with daily IV doses up to 75 times the MRHOD in rats or in mice with daily SC doses up to 25 times the MRHOD. Travoprost caused an increase in postimplantation loses and a decrease in fetal viability in rats at daily IV doses up to 75 times the MRHOD or in mice with daily SC doses up to 7.5 times the MRHOD. When rats received a daily SC dose that was 3 times the MRHOD from day 7 of pregnancy to lactation day 21 there was an increased incidence of postnatal mortality and decreased neonatal body weight gain. Neonatal development also was affected as evidenced by delayed eye opening, pinna detachment, preputial separation, and decreased motor activity (1).

No evidence of carcinogenicity was observed in 2-year studies in mice and rats with SC doses. Most assays for mutagenicity were negative but a slight increase in mutant frequency was observed in one assay. No effect on mating or fertility was observed in male or female rats, but at the highest dose (250 times the MRHOD), the mean number of corpora lutea was reduced and postimplantation losses were increased (1).

It is not known if travoprost free acid crosses the human placenta. The molecular weight of the parent drug (about 501) is low enough but the short elimination half-life and very low plasma concentrations suggest that clinically significant amounts of the drug will not cross to the embryo–fetus.

Prostaglandin F2α has been used for pregnancy termination in humans via intrauterine extra-amniotic infusion to treat missed abortion or intrauterine death. However, there is no evidence that at doses given to reduce elevated ophthalmic pressure, an increased risk for uterine contractions would be seen (see Latanoprost).

BREASTFEEDING SUMMARY

No reports describing the use of travoprost during human lactation have been located. The molecular weight of the parent drug (about 501) is low enough but the short elimination half-life (45 minutes) and very low plasma concentrations suggest that clinically significant amounts of the drug will not be excreted into breast milk.

Reference

1. Product information. Travatanz. Alcon Laboratories, 2011.

TRAZODONE

Antidepressant

PREGNANCY RECOMMENDATION: Limited Human Data—Animal Data Suggest Low Risk
BREASTFEEDING RECOMMENDATION: Limited Human Data—Potential Toxicity

PREGNANCY SUMMARY

The animal and limited human data suggest that the risk for major malformations in the embryo is low. Studies for other aspects of developmental toxicity in the embryo–fetus, however, have not been conducted.

FETAL RISK SUMMARY

Trazodone is an antidepressant. At high doses in some animal species, trazodone is fetal toxic and teratogenic. However, others have reported no teratogenicity in rats and rabbits (1).

One manufacturer has received several anecdotal descriptions concerning the use of trazodone in pregnancy (T. Donosky, personal communication, Mead Johnson Pharmaceutical Division, 1987). Included in these was a report of an infant born with an undefined birth defect after in utero exposure to the antidepressant. Another report described a normal infant exposed throughout gestation beginning with the 5th week. No confirmatory follow-up information was available for either of these cases. A third case from the manufacturer's files involved a woman who took trazodone, 50–100 mg/day, during the first 3 weeks of pregnancy and eventually delivered a normal infant. Finally, a woman was treated with trazodone for 8 days, at which time the drug was discontinued because of a positive pregnancy test. A spontaneous abortion occurred approximately 1.5 months later. No cause and effect relationship can be inferred between trazodone and any of the above adverse outcomes.

In a surveillance study of Michigan Medicaid recipients involving 229,101 completed pregnancies conducted between 1985 and 1992, 100 newborns had been exposed to trazodone during the 1st trimester (F. Rosa, personal communication, FDA, 1993). One (1%) major birth defect was observed (four expected), but details are not available. No anomalies were observed in six defect categories (cardiovascular defects, oral clefts, spina bifida, polydactyly, limb reduction defects, and hypospadias) for which specific data were available.

A prospective multicenter study evaluated the effects of lithium exposure during the 1st trimester in 148 women (2). One of the pregnancies was terminated at 16 weeks' gestation because of a fetus with the rare congenital heart defect, Ebstein's anomaly. The fetus had been exposed to lithium, trazodone, fluoxetine, and L-thyroxine during the 1st trimester. The defect was attributed to lithium exposure.

In a 1996 descriptive case series, the European Network of the Teratology Information Services (ENTIS) prospectively examined the outcomes of 689 pregnancies exposed to antidepressants (3). Multiple drug therapy occurred in about two-thirds of the mothers. Trazodone was used in 13 pregnancies. The outcomes of these pregnancies were two elective abortions, eight normal newborns (includes one premature infant), and three normal infants who died after birth (after difficult delivery; twins delivered at 27 weeks'; multiple other drugs) (3).

A 2003 prospective controlled study described the outcomes of 147 pregnancies exposed in the 1st trimester (52 used the drugs throughout gestation) to either trazodone or nefazodone, a closely related antidepressant (4). The data were gathered from five teratology information services in Canada (two sites), the United States (two sites), and Italy. The outcomes were compared with two control groups (one exposed to other antidepressants and one exposed to nonteratogens). There were no significant differences between the three groups in terms of spontaneous abortions, elective abortions, stillbirths, major malformations, gestational age at birth, or birth weights. In the study group, there were two (1.4%) major malformations: neural tube defect and Hirschsprung disease (4).

A 2005 meta-analysis of seven prospective comparative cohort studies involving 1774 patients was conducted to quantify the relationship between 7 newer antidepressants and major malformations (5). The antidepressants were bupropion, fluoxetine, fluvoxamine, nefazodone, paroxetine, sertraline, and trazodone. There was no statistical increase in the risk of major birth defects above the baseline of 1%–3% in the general population for the individual or combined studies (5).

A prospective cohort study evaluated a large group of pregnancies exposed to antidepressants in the 1st trimester to determine if there was an association with major malformations (6). The patient population came from the Motherisk database and involved 928 cases that met their criteria. The 928 matched (for age, smoking, and alcohol use) controls were pregnancies not exposed to antidepressants or known teratogens. In addition to the 17 trazodone cases, the other cases were 113 bupropion, 184 citalopram, 21 escitalopram, 61 fluoxetine, 52 fluvoxamine, 68 mirtazapine, 49 nefazodone, 148 paroxetine, 61 sertraline, and 154 venlafaxine. In the antidepressant group, there were 24 (2.5%) major defects compared with 25 (2.6%) in controls (odds ratio 0.9, 95% CI 0.5–1.61). There were no major defects in the pregnancies exposed to bupropion, escitalopram, or trazodone (6).

BREASTFEEDING SUMMARY

Trazodone is excreted into human milk. Six healthy lactating women, 3–8 months postpartum, were given a single 50-mg oral dose of trazodone after an overnight fast (7). Simultaneous serum and milk samples were collected at various times ≤30 hours after ingestion. The infants of the mothers were not allowed to breastfeed during the first 4 hours after the dose. The mean milk:plasma ratio, based on AUC for the two fluids, was 0.142. Based on 500 mL of milk consumed during a 12-hour interval, the infants would have received a trazodone dose of 0.005 mg/kg. This study was unable to include a potentially active metabolite, 1-*m*-chlorophenylpiperazine, in the analysis (7).

A 2006 report described six women taking quetiapine and other psychotropic agents during breastfeeding (8). One woman was treated with trazodone, quetiapine, and venlafaxine throughout gestation. Details of the pregnancy or its outcome were not provided. At 6.5 weeks postpartum, milk samples were obtained for analysis after doses of 75 mg

T

for each drug (timing of samples and daily doses were not specified). Quetiapine was not detected (<30 nmol/L), but the milk levels of trazodone and venlafaxine were 108 and 371 nmol/L, respectively. The estimated infant daily doses for all three drugs were <0.01 mg/kg/day. In addition, the infant's behavior was assessed using the Bayley Scales of Infant Development, Second Edition, that suggested normal development (8).

Although the amount of trazodone in milk is very small, the American Academy of Pediatrics classifies trazodone as a drug for which the effect on nursing infants is unknown but may be of concern (9).

References

1. Schardein JL. Psychotropic drugs. *Chemically Induced Birth Defects*. 3rd ed. New York, NY: Marcel Dekker, 2000:252.
2. Jacobson SJ, Jones K, Johnson K, Ceolin L, Kaur P, Sahn D, Donnenfeld AE, Rieder M, Santelli R, Smythe J, Pastuszak A, Einarson T, Koren G. Prospective multicentre study of pregnancy outcome after lithium exposure during first trimester. Lancet 1992;339:530–3.
3. McElhatton PR, Garbis HM, Elefant E, Vial T, Bellemin B, Mastroiacovo P, Arnon J, Rodriguez-Pinilla E, Schaefer C, Pexieder T, Merlob P, Dal Verme S. The outcome of pregnancy in 689 women exposed to therapeutic doses of antidepressants. A collaborative study of the European Network of Teratology Information Services (ENTIS). Reprod Toxicol 1996;10:285–94.
4. Einarson A, Bonari L, Voyer-Lavigne S, Addis A, Matsui D, Johnson Y, Koren G. A multicentre prospective controlled study to determine the safety of trazodone and nefazodone use during pregnancy. Can J Psychiatry 2003;48:106–9.
5. Einarson TR, Einarson A. Newer antidepressants in pregnancy and rates of major malformations: a meta-analysis of prospective comparative studies. Pharmacoepidemiol Drug Saf 2005;14:823–7.
6. Einarson A, Choi J, Einarson TR, Koren G. Incidence of major malformations in infants following antidepressant exposure in pregnancy: results of a large prospective cohort study. Can J Psychiatry 2009;54:242–6.
7. Verbeeck RK, Ross SG, McKenna EA. Excretion of trazodone in breast milk. Br J Clin Pharmacol 1986;22:367–70.
8. Misri S, Corral M, Wardrop AA, Kendrick K. Quetiapine augmentation in lactation. A series of case reports. J Clin Psychopharm 2006;26:508–11.
9. Committee on Drugs, American Academy of Pediatrics. The transfer of drugs and other chemicals into human milk. Pediatrics 2001;108:776–89.

TREPROSTINIL

Hematologic Agent (Antiplatelet)

PREGNANCY RECOMMENDATION: No Human Data—Animal Data Suggest Low Risk
BREASTFEEDING RECOMMENDATION: No Human Data—Potential Toxicity

PREGNANCY SUMMARY

No reports describing the use of treprostinil during human pregnancy have been located. The animal data suggest low risk, but the lack of human pregnancy experience prevents an assessment of the embryo–fetal risk. However, maternal hypotension, resulting in decreased placental perfusion and fetal hypoxia, is a potential risk.

FETAL RISK SUMMARY

Treprostinil is an inhibitor of platelet aggregation. Its action includes direct vasodilation of pulmonary and systemic arterial vascular beds. Treprostinil is administered by continuous SC infusion for the treatment of pulmonary arterial hypertension. The terminal elimination half-life is about 2–4 hours. Treprostinil is extensively metabolized in the liver but the biological activity of the metabolites is unknown (1).

Reproduction studies have been conducted in rats and rabbits. In pregnant rats during organogenesis, continuous SC infusions of doses up to about 117 times the recommended starting rate in humans based on BSA (HD) and about 16 times the average rate achieved in clinical trials (AR) revealed no evidence of fetal harm. At doses up to about 8 times the AR, continuous SC infusions administered from implantation to the end of lactation had no effect on growth or development of offspring. In pregnant rabbits during organogenesis, a continuous SC infusion at 41 times the HD and about 5 times the AR produced fetal skeletal variations. However, maternal toxicity (decreased body weight and food consumption) was evident at this dose (1).

It is not known if treprostinil crosses the human placenta. The molecular weight (about 412) is low enough that passage to the fetus should be expected. Moreover, the drug is administered as a continuous SC infusion that should result in relatively constant plasma drug concentrations at the placental maternal–fetal interface.

BREASTFEEDING SUMMARY

No reports describing the use of treprostinil during lactation have been located. The molecular weight (about 412) and method of administration (continuous SC infusion) suggest that the drug will be excreted into breast milk. In adults, treprostinil undergoes extensive hepatic metabolism, but the biological activity of the metabolites has not been characterized. However, even if the metabolites are inactive, the neonatal immature hepatic function could allow systemic levels of the parent drug. Although the effect of this exposure on a nursing infant is unknown, treprostinil has caused clinically significant adverse effects in adults (e.g., headache, nausea/vomiting, restlessness, and anxiety). A nursing infant should be closely observed for these effects if a woman receiving treprostinil elects to breastfeed.

Reference

1. Product information. Remodulin. United Therapeutics, 2002.

T

TRETINOIN (SYSTEMIC)

Antineoplastic/Vitamin

PREGNANCY RECOMMENDATION: Contraindicated—1st Trimester
BREASTFEEDING RECOMMENDATION: No Human Data—Probably Compatible

PREGNANCY SUMMARY

Tretinoin (all-*trans* retinoic acid; retinoic acid; vitamin A acid) is a retinoid and vitamin A (retinol) metabolite that is available both as a topical formulation (see Tretinoin [Topical]) and as an oral antineoplastic for the treatment of acute promyelocytic leukemia. As with other retinoids, all-*trans* retinoic acid is a potent teratogen when taken systemically during early pregnancy (see Etretinate, Isotretinoin, and Vitamin A), producing a pattern of birth defects termed retinoic acid embryopathy (CNS, craniofacial, cardiovascular, and thymic anomalies). The teratogenic effect of all-*trans* retinoic acid is dose-dependent because an endogenous supply of the vitamin is required for normal morphogenesis and differentiation of the embryo, including a role in physiologic developmental gene expression (1). A low serum concentrations or frank deficiency of vitamin A and all-*trans* retinoic acid is also teratogenic (see Tretinoin [Topical]).

FETAL RISK SUMMARY

The teratogenicity of all-*trans* retinoic acid in animals is summarized under the topical formulation as is the reported human pregnancy experience following topical use.

A number of reports have described the use of systemic tretinoin (45 mg/m^2/day in 10 cases, 70 mg/day in 1) for the treatment of acute promyelocytic leukemia during pregnancy (2–12). In one case treatment was started during the sixth week of gestation (about 36 days from the last menstruation) (2); in six cases (one set of twins), treatment was started during the 2nd trimester (3–8); and in four cases, treatment was started during the 3rd trimester (9–12). No congenital abnormalities were observed in the 12 newborns, although 10 were premature. The growth and development in nine of the infants (postnatal examinations not reported in two cases) were normal in the follow-up periods ranging up to 4 years.

BREASTFEEDING SUMMARY

Vitamin A and, presumably, tretinoin (all-*trans* retinoic acid) are natural constituents of human milk. There are no data available on the amount of all-*trans* retinoic acid excreted into breast milk following the doses used for the treatment of promyelocytic leukemia or the risk, if any, this may present to a nursing infant.

References

1. Morriss-Kay G. Retinoic acid and development. Pathobiology 1992;60:264–70.
2. Simone MD, Stasi R, Venditti A, Del Poeta G, Aronica G, Bruno A, Masi M, Tribalto M, Papa G, Amadori S. All-*trans* retinoic acid (ATRA) administration during pregnancy in relapsed acute promyelocytic leukemia. Leukemia 1995;9:1412–3.
3. Stentoft J, Lanng Nielsen J, Hvidman LE. All-*trans* retinoic acid in acute promyelocytic leukemia in late pregnancy. Leukemia 1994;8(Suppl 2):S77–80.
4. Harrison P, Chipping P, Fothergill GA. Successful use of all-trans retinoic acid in acute promyelocytic leukaemia presenting during the second trimester of pregnancy. Br J Haematol 1994;86:681–2.
5. Lin C-P, Huang M-J, Liu H-J, Chang IY, Tsai C-H. Successful treatment of acute promyelocytic leukemia in a pregnant Jehovah's Witness with all-trans retinoic acid, rhG-CSF, and erythropoietin. Am J Hematol 1996;51:251–2.
6. Incerpi MH, Miller DA, Posen R, Byrne JD. All-trans retinoic acid for the treatment of acute promyelocytic leukemia in pregnancy. Obstet Gynecol 1997;89:826–8.
7. Morton J, Taylor K, Wright S, Pitcher L, Wilson E, Tudehope D, Savage J, Williams B, Taylor D, Wiley J, Tsoris D, O'Donnell A. Successful maternal and fetal outcome following the use of ATRA for the induction APML late in the first trimester (abstract). Blood 1995;86(Suppl 1):772a.
8. Giagounidis AAN, Beckman MW, Giagoundis AS, Aivado M, Emde T, Germing U, Riehs T, Heyll A, Aul C. Acute promyelocytic leukemia and pregnancy. Eur J Haematol 2000;64:267–71.
9. Watanabe R, Okamoto S, Moriki T, Kizaki M, Kawai Y, Ikeda Y. Treatment of acute promyelocytic leukemia with all-*trans* retinoic acid during the third trimester of pregnancy. Am J Hematol 1995;48:210–1.
10. Nakamura K, Dan K, Iwakiri R, Gomi S, Nomura T. Successful treatment of acute promyelocytic leukemia in pregnancy with all-*trans* retinoic acid. Ann Hematol 1995;71:263–4.
11. Lipovsky MM, Biesma DH, Christiaens GCML, Petersen EJ. Successful treatment of acute promyelocytic leukaemia with all-*trans*-retinoic-acid during late pregnancy. Br J Haematol 1996;94:699–701.
12. Consoli U, Figuera A, Milone G, Meli CR, Guido G, Indelicato F, Moschetti G, Leotta S, Tornello A, Poidomani M, Murgano P, Pinto V, Giustolisi R. Acute promyelocytic leukemia during pregnancy: report of 3 cases. Int J Hematol 2004;79:31–6.

T

TRETINOIN (TOPICAL)

Dermatologic Agent

PREGNANCY RECOMMENDATION: Human Data Suggest Low Risk
BREASTFEEDING RECOMMENDATION: No Human Data—Probably Compatible

PREGNANCY SUMMARY

Elevated serum concentrations of all-*trans* retinoic acid in early gestation are considered teratogenic in humans. Because of its relatively poor systemic absorption (if occlusive dressings are not used) after topical administration, tretinoin is not thought to present a significant fetal risk. Because some absorption does occur, however, it is not possible to exclude a teratogenic risk (1). Congenital malformations, some of which are consistent with those observed in retinoic acid embryopathy, have been reported after topical use, but a causal association has yet to be established. The reports may reflect (a) greater-than-normal fetal exposure from higher-than-usual maternal doses or enhanced systemic absorption, or (b) selective reporting of adverse outcomes that are not caused by tretinoin. Until more data are available, however, the safest course is to avoid the use of tretinoin during pregnancy, especially in the 1st trimester. But if inadvertent exposure does occur during early pregnancy, the fetal risk, if any, appears to be very low.

FETAL RISK SUMMARY

Tretinoin (all-*trans* retinoic acid; retinoic acid; vitamin A acid) is a retinoid and vitamin A (retinol) metabolite used topically for the treatment of acne vulgaris and other skin disorders and systemically in the treatment of acute promyelocytic leukemia (see Tretinoin [Systemic]). As with other retinoids, the drug is a potent teratogen after exposure in early pregnancy (see also Etretinate, Isotretinoin, and Vitamin A), producing a pattern of birth defects termed retinoic acid embryopathy (CNS, craniofacial, cardiovascular, and thymic anomalies). However, an endogenous supply of retinoic acid is required for normal morphogenesis and differentiation of the embryo, including a role in physiologic developmental gene expression. The teratogenic effect of retinoic acid is manifested when the levels are excessive (2).

Low serum concentration or frank deficiency of vitamin A and all-*trans* retinoic acid is also teratogenic. Recent studies have shown that inhibition of the conversion of retinol to retinoic acid or depletion of retinol may be involved in the teratogenic mechanisms of such agents as ethanol (3–7) and some anticonvulsants (8).

Two manufacturers have stated that reproduction studies with topical tretinoin in animals are equivocal. In pregnant rats, daily doses >200 times the recommended human topical dose (RHTD) were associated with shortened or kinked tail. At 2000 times the RHTD, skeletal anomalies (humerus: short, bent; os parietale incompletely ossified) were observed. In rabbits, fetotoxicity was observed with doses 100 times the RHTD. Doses approximately 80 times the RHTD in pregnant rabbits were associated with domed head and hydrocephaly, anomalies that are typical of retinoid-induced malformations in this species. In addition, a dose 91 times the RHTD was also associated with an increased incidence of cleft palate (9). In contrast, other studies with topical tretinoin in rats and rabbits at doses 100–200 times the RHTD have not demonstrated a teratogenic effect (9,10).

A 1997 report described the developmental toxicity of topical and oral tretinoin in pregnant rats (11). Topical doses of ≥10 mg/kg/day (approximately 2000 times the RHTD) were not tolerated, causing severe local and systemic maternal toxicity. Maternal toxicity (reduced weight gain and food consumption) was also evident at doses of 2.5 mg/kg/day (approximately 500 times the RHTD) or more. A significant increase in the occurrence of supernumerary ribs was observed at this dose, a result thought to be nonspecific or maternally mediated. In contrast, oral tretinoin doses of 5 and 10 mg/kg/day were not maternally toxic, but were associated with an increased incidence of supernumerary ribs (5 mg/kg/day) and cleft palate (10 mg/kg/day). Based on these results, the investigators concluded that only the highest oral dose was teratogenic (11).

Dose-related maternal toxicity was observed in rabbits treated topically with tretinoin cream at dosages of 10 and 100 times the human clinical dose (500 mg of 0.05% cream in a 50-kg adult equals 0.005 mg/kg/day) based on body weight (12). Maternal endogenous plasma tretinoin levels were below the detection level (5 ng/mL) in all animals. After treatment, however, a few rabbits had detectable concentrations of retinoic acid, 13-*cis*-retinoic acid, or their metabolites. The maternal toxicity was associated with an increased incidence of abortions, resorptions, and reduced fetal body weight. Some significant ($p \leq 0.01$) increases in malformations (open eyelids and cleft palate) and variations (nasal ossification, fused sternebrae, and irregular-shaped scapular alae) were observed. However, these were not considered to be tretinoin-related because they were not dose-related, and the litter incidences either did not differ significantly from those of controls or were within expected ranges for the species (12).

Additional literature on the teratogenicity of both systemic and topical tretinoin in various animal species has been summarized in several sources (13–17). The latter reference has particular application to the study of the teratogenic effects of tretinoin because it examined the toxicity of very small oral doses of this compound at presomite stages in mouse embryos, thought to be the most sensitive period for retinoid-induced teratogenesis (17). An increasing incidence of severe microphthalmia, anophthalmia, and iridial colobomata was produced as the dose was increased from 0 to 1.25 mg/kg. These doses were much less than those typically used for reproductive toxicity testing at later gestational periods. Slightly higher threshold doses produced exencephaly (2.5 mg/kg) and marked craniofacial defects (7.5 mg/kg) representative of the holoprosencephaly–aprosencephaly spectrum (17).

When tretinoin is used topically, its teratogenic risk had been thought to be close to 0 (18). According to one source, no cases of toxicity had been reported after nearly 20 years of use (18). In support of this, it has been estimated that even if maximal absorption (approximately 33%) occurred from a 1-g daily application of a 0.1% preparation, this would result in only about one-seventh of the vitamin A activity received from a typical prenatal vitamin supplement (19). One source stated that 80% of a 0.1% formulation in alcohol remained on the skin's surface, but when a 0.1% ointment was applied to the back with a 16-hour occlusive dressing, only 50% of the drug remained on the skin surface and 6% was excreted in the urine within 56 hours (20).

Authors of a 1992 reference reviewed the teratogenicity of vitamin A and its congeners, including tretinoin, but did not derive a conclusion on the safety of the drug after topical use (21), most likely because of the lack of studies with the drug in pregnancy.

Five reports of congenital malformations in newborns whose mother's were using tretinoin during the 1st trimester have been located (22–26). The first case involved a woman who had used tretinoin cream 0.05% during the month before her last menstruation and during the first 11 weeks of pregnancy (22). Her term, growth-restricted (weight 2620 g, <3rd percentile; length 49 cm, 25th percentile; head circumference 32.5 cm, 3rd percentile) female infant had a crumpled right hypoplastic ear and atresia of the right external auditory meatus, a pattern of ear malformation identical with that observed with vitamin A congeners. The remainder of the examination was normal, including the eyes, cerebral computed tomography, and chromosomal analysis (22).

The second report described the female infant of a woman who had used an over-the-counter alcohol-based liquid preparation of 0.05% tretinoin for severe facial acne (23). The infant had multiple congenital defects consisting of supra-umbilical exomphalos, a diaphragmatic hernia, a pericardial defect, dextroposition of the heart, and a right-sided upper limb reduction defect.

A 1998 case report described the pregnancy outcome of a woman who had used, before conception and during the first 2 months of gestation, a topical alcohol-based preparation of tretinoin 0.05% combined with benzoyl peroxide 2.5% for facial acne (24). Except for doxycycline (200 mg/ day) that had been taken for an unknown duration, she had no other exposures to medications or vitamins. An ultrasound examination at 5 months' gestation detected hand and heart malformations. The female infant (2800 g; length 48 cm; normal karyotype 46,XX) was delivered at term with coarctation of the aorta, hypoplastic left hand, and small ear canals. The authors noted the similarity of some of the anomalies to those observed in retinoic acid embryopathy and speculated that the keratolytic action of benzoyl peroxide may have enhanced the cutaneous absorption of tretinoin. However, they also noted that any association between tretinoin and the birth defects may have been fortuitous (24).

Severe malformations were reported in a term, female infant whose mother had used tretinoin (0.05%) twice daily for facial acne before and throughout gestation (25). The defects were thought to be consistent with abnormal cranial neural crest cell migration. They included craniofacial defects (cleft palate and harelip, fused palpebral fissures, hypertelorism, a depressed nasal bridge, and deficient left naris) and CNS anomalies (disorganized rudimentary optic cup derivatives with optic tract dysgenesis, arrhinencephaly, agenesis of the corpus callosum, fornices and cingulate gyri, cerebellar hypoplasia, and aqueduct stenosis with hydrocephalus) (25).

The fifth case report involved a 4090-g term male infant who was born with absence of the right ear and external auditory canal (26). The mother had used tretinoin 0.025% topically on her face and over a large area of her back before conception and during the first 2–3 months of gestation. She took prenatal vitamins during pregnancy. The father was using isotretinoin before conception. Examinations at 16 and 20 months of age revealed a nonverbal infant with poor receptive language consistent with cognitive impairment. He had age-appropriate muscle strength, tone and bulk. There was a diminished optokinetic response and no oculovertibular response when rotating toward the right. Extensive examinations revealed cerebral calcification of the right posterior hemisphere, an overall reduction in the volume of the right cerebral hemisphere, a remote infarct in the deep basal ganglia, focal atrophy and encephalomalacia of the right parieto-occipital lobe. Marked abnormalities were noted in the posterior cerebral artery and some of its branches. Hypometabolism, sometimes severe, was observed in several regions of the brain, including the thalamus (26).

The results of a prospective survey involving 60 completed pregnancies exposed to tretinoin early in pregnancy were presented in a 1994 abstract (27). From these pregnancies there were 53 liveborns (1 set of twins), 3 lost to follow-up, 4 spontaneous abortions, and 1 elective termination. No major malformations characteristic of retinoic acid embryopathy were observed except for one case in which the mother had also taken isotretinoin (27).

Among 25 birth defect cases with 1st trimester exposure to tretinoin reported to the FDA from 1969 to 1993, 5 were cases of holoprosencephaly (28). Six other cases of holoprosencephaly involved other vitamin A derivatives: isotretinoin ($N = 4$), etretinate ($N = 1$), and megadose vitamin A ($N = 1$). In contrast, among 8700 nonretinoid-exposed birth defect reports to the FDA, only 19 involved suspected holoprosencephalies (28). Pregnancy outcomes from 1120 apparent 1st trimester tretinoin exposures were also examined. Among the 49 birth defects observed (the expected incidence), no cases of holoprosencephaly were seen. Although it is speculation, the contrasting findings in the above two reports (27,28) on early pregnancy tretinoin exposure may reflect (a) fetal exposure to different doses of tretinoin at the critical times from the use of higher maternal doses or from enhanced systemic absorption, or (b) selective (biased) reporting of adverse pregnancy outcomes to the FDA.

A 1993 report summarized data gathered from the Group Health Cooperative of Puget Sound, Washington, involving 1st trimester exposure to topical tretinoin and congenital malformations (29). A total of 215 women who had delivered live or stillborn infants and were presumed to have been exposed to the drug in early pregnancy were compared with 430 age-matched nonexposed controls of women whose live or stillborn infants were delivered at the same hospitals. A total of 4 (1.9%) infants in the exposed group had major anomalies compared with 11 (2.6%) among the controls, a relative risk of 0.7 (95% confidence interval 0.2–2.3). The defects observed in the exposed infants were hypospadias, undescended or absent testicles, metatarsus adductus, and esophageal reflux. The three stillborn infants in the exposed group were all associated with umbilical cord accidents. The authors concluded that these data provided no evidence for a relationship between topical tretinoin and the congenital abnormalities normally observed with other vitamin A congeners or for an increased incidence of defects compared with data from women not using tretinoin (29). The findings of this study were summarized in a review article on retinoids and teratogenicity (30).

A brief 1997 report described a prospective, observational, controlled study that compared the pregnancy outcomes of 94 women who had used topical tretinoin during pregnancy with 133 women not exposed to topical tretinoin or other known human teratogens (31). Both groups were composed of pregnant women who had contacted a teratology information service in the years from 1988 to 1996. No differences between the groups were found for the number of live births, miscarriages, elective terminations, major malformations, duration of pregnancy, cesarean sections, birth weight (after exclusion of one baby weighing 5396 g in the control group), and low birth weight. Two liveborn infants from the tretinoin-exposed group had major birth defects: a bicuspid aortic valve in one and dysplastic kidneys in one. Neither defect is consistent with retinoic acid embryopathy. Malformations in the four infants from the control group were congenitally dislocated hip in two, aortic valvular stenosis in one, and imperforate anus in one (31).

Several comments concerning the above study were made in a 1999 letter (32). The primary concern expressed was that the number of subjects enrolled in the study was too small to derive any conclusions as to the safety of tretinoin in the 1st trimester. The authors thought that the risk of certain birth defects, specifically cardiac anomalies and microtia, could not be excluded, and that the use of tretinoin in pregnancy was contraindicated (32).

BREASTFEEDING SUMMARY

Vitamin A and, presumably, tretinoin (all-*trans* retinoic acid) are natural constituents of human milk. There are no data available on the amount of all-*trans* retinoic acid excreted into milk after topical use. Although other retinoids are excreted (see Vitamin A), the minimal absorption that occurs after topical application of tretinoin probably precludes the detection of clinically significant amounts in breast milk from this source. Thus, use of tretinoin while breastfeeding does not appear to represent a significant risk to a nursing infant.

References

1. Rothman KF, Pochi PE. Use of oral and topical agents for acne in pregnancy. J Am Acad Dermatol 1988;19:431–42.
2. Morriss-Kay G. Retinoic acid and development. Pathobiology 1992;60: 264–70.
3. Keir WJ. Inhibition of retinoic acid synthesis and its implications in fetal alcohol syndrome. Alcohol Clin Exp Res 1991;15:560–4.
4. Pullarkat RK. Hypothesis: prenatal ethanol-induced birth defects and retinoic acid. Alcohol Clin Exp Res 1991;15:565–7.
5. Duester G. A hypothetical mechanism for fetal alcohol syndrome involving ethanol inhibition of retinoic acid synthesis at the alcohol dehydrogenase step. Alcohol Clin Exp Res 1991;15:568–72.
6. Dreosti IE. Nutritional factors underlying the expression of the fetal alcohol syndrome. Ann NT Acad Sci 1993;678:193–204.
7. DeJonge MH, Zachman RD. The effect of maternal ethanol ingestion on fetal rat heart vitamin A: a model for fetal alcohol syndrome. Pediatr Res 1995;37:418–23.
8. Fex G, Larsson K, Andersson A, Berggren-Söderlund M. Low serum concentration of *all-trans* and *13-cis* retinoic acids in patients treated with phenytoin, carbamazepine and valproate. Possible relation to teratogenicity. Arch Toxicol 1995;69:572–4.
9. Product information. Avita. Bertek Pharmaceuticals, 2002.
10. Product information. Renova, Retin-A. Ortho Dermatological, 2002.
11. Seegmiller RE, Ford WH, Carter MW, Mitala JJ, Powers WJ Jr. A developmental toxicity study of tretinoin administered topically and orally to pregnant Wistar rats. J Am Acad Dermatol 1997;36:S60–6.
12. Christian MS, Mitala JJ, Powers WJ Jr, McKenzie BE, Latriano L. A developmental toxicity study of tretinoin emollient cream (Renova) applied topically to New Zealand white rabbits. J Am Acad Dermatol 1997;36:S67–76.
13. Schardein JL. *Chemically Induced Birth Defects*. 2nd ed. New York, NY: Marcel Dekker, 1993:555–62.
14. Shepard TH. *Catalog of Teratogenic Agents*. 8th ed. Baltimore, MD: The Johns Hopkins University Press, 1995:370–3.
15. Sanders DD, Stephens TD. Review of drug-induced limb defects in mammals. Teratology 1991;44:335–54.
16. Apgar J, Kramer T, Smith JC. Retinoic acid and vitamin A: effect of low levels on outcome of pregnancy in guinea pigs. Nutr Res 1994;14:741–51.
17. Sulik KK, Dehart DB, Rogers JM, Chernoff N. Teratogenicity of low doses of all-trans retinoic acid in presomite mouse embryos. Teratology 1995;51:398–403.
18. Kligman AM. Question and answers: is topical tretinoin teratogenic? JAMA 1988;259:2918.
19. Zbinden G. Investigations on the toxicity of tretinoin administered systemically to animals. Acta Derm Venereol (Stockh) 1975;(Suppl 74):36–40.
20. American Hospital Formula Service. *Drug Information 1996*. Bethesda, MD: American Society of Health-System Pharmacists, 1996:2608–10.
21. Pinnock CB, Alderman CP. The potential for teratogenicity of vitamin A and its congeners. Med J Aust 1992;157:804–9.
22. Camera G, Pregliasco P. Ear malformation in baby born to mother using tretinoin cream. Lancet 1992;339:687.
23. Lipson AH, Collins F, Webster WS. Multiple congenital defects associated with maternal use of topical tretinoin. Lancet 1993;341:1352–3.
24. Navarre-Belhassen C, Blanchet P, Hillaire-Buys D, Sarda P, Blayac JP. Multiple congenital malformations associated with topical tretinoin. Ann Pharmacother 1998;32:505–6.
25. Colley SMJ, Walpole I, Fabian VA, Kakulas BA. Topical tretinoin and fetal malformations. Med J Aust 1998;168:467.
26. Selcen D, Seidman S, Nigro MA. Otocerebral anomalies associated with topical tretinoin use. Brain Dev 2000;22:218–20.
27. Johnson KA, Chambers CD, Felix R, Dick L, Jones KL. Pregnancy outcome in women prospectively ascertained with Retin-A exposures: an ongoing study (abstract). Teratology 1994;49:375.
28. Rosa F, Piazza-Hepp T, Goetsch R. Holoprosencephaly with 1st trimester topical tretinoin (abstract). Teratology 1994;49:418–9.
29. Jick SS, Terris BZ, Jick H. First trimester topical tretinoin and congenital disorders. Lancet 1993;341:1181–2.
30. Jick H. Retinoids and teratogenicity. J Am Acad Dermatol 1998;39:S118–22.
31. Shapiro L, Pastuszak A, Curto G, Koren G. Safety of first-trimester exposure to topical tretinoin: prospective cohort study. Lancet 1997;350:1143–4.
32. Martinez-Frias ML, Rodriguez-Pinilla E. First-trimester exposure to topical tretinoin: its safety is not warranted. Teratology 1999;60:5.

TRIAMCINOLONE

Corticosteroid

PREGNANCY RECOMMENDATION: Compatible (Inhaled)
Human and Animal Data Suggest Risk (Oral/Parenteral)
BREASTFEEDING RECOMMENDATION: No Human Data—Probably Compatible

PREGNANCY SUMMARY

Triamcinolone is a corticosteroid with potency slightly greater than prednisone. Use in the 1st trimester has a small absolute risk of oral clefts. Continuous use during pregnancy has also caused fetal growth restriction. However, inhaled triamcinolone does not appear to cause embryo–fetal harm. Depending on the indication, the benefit of therapy may outweigh these risks.

FETAL RISK SUMMARY

Triamcinolone is a synthetic fluorinated corticosteroid that can be administered, depending on the preparation selected, orally, parenterally, topically, or by oral inhalation. In animal models of inflammation, triamcinolone is approximately 1–2 times as potent as prednisone, whereas triamcinolone acetonide is about 8 times more potent (1). Oral inhalation of usual therapeutic doses of the latter agent does not appear to suppress the hypothalamic–pituitary–adrenal axis (2).

Triamcinolone is teratogenic in animals. Cleft palate was induced in fetal mice and rats exposed in utero to triamcinolone, triamcinolone acetonide, or triamcinolone diacetate (3–5). In one study with mice, high dietary fat intake (48% compared with a low-fat diet of 5.6%) increased the frequency and severity of cleft palate (5). IM administration of nonlethal maternal doses (0.125–0.5 mg/kg/day) of triamcinolone acetonide in pregnant rats at various gestational ages produced fetal growth restriction at all doses tested (6). Higher doses were associated with resorption, cleft palate, umbilical hernias, undescended testes, and reduced ossification (6). A second report by these latter investigators compared the teratogenic potency, as measured by the induction of cleft palate, of triamcinolone, triamcinolone acetonide, and cortisol in rats (7). Triamcinolone acetonide was 59 times more potent than triamcinolone, which, in turn, was more potent than cortisol. Other anomalies observed with triamcinolone acetonide were umbilical hernias, resorption, and fetal death. All three agents produced fetal growth restriction.

Morphologically abnormal lungs and increased epithelial maturation were found in fetal rat whole organ lung cultures exposed to triamcinolone acetonide (8). Similarly, accelerated fetal lung maturation was observed following administration of IM triamcinolone acetonide to pregnant rhesus macaques at various stages of gestation (9). However, treatment earlier in gestation produced growth restriction of some of the lung septa, as well as decreased body weight and length (9).

A series of studies described the teratogenic effects of single and multiple doses of IM triamcinolone acetonide administered early in gestation to nonhuman primates (bonnet monkeys, rhesus monkeys, and baboons) at doses ranging from approximately equivalent to the human dose up to 300 times the human dose (10–13). Resorption; intrauterine death; orocraniofacial anomalies; and defects of the thorax, hind limbs, thymus, adrenal glands, and kidney were observed. The most common malformations involved the central nervous system and cranium in all three species (11); growth restriction was also common in all species (10).

Published human pregnancy experience with triamcinolone is limited to 16 cases. The Collaborative Perinatal Project monitored 50,282 mother–child pairs, 56 of whom were exposed during the 1st trimester to a category of miscellaneous corticosteroids (14). Included in this group were eight triamcinolone-exposed mother–child pairs. Two (3.6%; relative risk 0.47) newborns with malformations were observed in the total group, suggesting a lack of any relationship to large categories of major or minor malformations or to individual defects.

A 1966 reference described a woman with benign adrenogenital syndrome who took 4–8 mg of triamcinolone orally throughout gestation (15). She delivered a normal 2.61-kg male infant at 38 weeks without evidence of hypoadrenalism. A 1975 report included 5 patients treated with triamcinolone acetonide, presumably by oral inhalation, among 70 women with asthma who were treated with various corticosteroids throughout gestation (16). No adverse fetal outcomes were observed in the five triamcinolone-exposed cases, although one of the mothers delivered prematurely. None of the 70 newborns had evidence of adrenal insufficiency.

Symmetric growth restriction was observed in a 700-g, small-for-gestational-age newborn delivered via cesarean section at 31 weeks' gestation because of fetal distress, diminished amniotic fluid, and lack of growth (17). The Dubowitz evaluation was compatible with the menstrual dates. The normotensive, nonsmoking mother had applied 0.05% triamcinolone acetonide cream to her legs, abdomen, and extremities for atopic dermatitis from 12 to 29 weeks' gestation. The authors estimated her daily dose to be approximately 40 mg, but she had no signs or symptoms of adrenal insufficiency. The newborn was breathing room air within 12 hours without evidence of respiratory distress. Although not discussed, the apparent fetal lung maturity in a 31-week fetus may have been the result of chronic corticosteroid exposure. At 14 days of age, necrotizing enterocolitis occurred and, following multiple surgeries, the infant was alive at 10 months of age on total parenteral nutrition. In an addendum to their report, the authors noted that the mother had had a second pregnancy, this time without the use of triamcinolone, and delivered a 1660-g (10th percentile for gestational age) male infant at 34 weeks' gestation. The authors attributed the growth restriction in the first infant to triamcinolone because no other cause was discovered. The result of the second pregnancy, however, probably indicates that other factors were involved in addition to any effect of the corticosteroid.

Four large epidemiologic studies have associated the use of corticosteroids during the 1st trimester with orofacial clefts. The specific corticosteroid was not identified in three of these studies (see Hydrocortisone for details), but in a 1999 study described below, the corticosteroids were listed.

In a case–control study, the California Birth Defects Monitoring Program evaluated the association between selected congenital anomalies and the use of corticosteroids 1 month before to 3 months after conception (periconceptional period) (18). Case infants or fetal deaths diagnosed with orofacial clefts, conotruncal defects, neural tubal defects (NTD), and limb anomalies were identified from a total of 552,601 births that occurred from 1987 through the end of 1989. Controls, without birth defects, were selected from the same database. Following exclusion of known genetic syndromes, mothers of case and control infants were interviewed by telephone, an average of 3.7 years (cases) or 3.8 years (controls) after delivery, to determine various exposures during the periconceptional period. The number of interviews completed were orofacial cleft case mothers (*N* = 662, 85% of eligible), conotruncal case mothers (*N* = 207, 87%), NTD case mothers (*N* = 265, 84%), limb anomaly case mothers (*N* = 165, 82%), and control mothers (*N* = 734, 78%) (18). Orofacial clefts were classified into four phenotypic groups: isolated cleft lip with or without cleft palate (ICLP, *N* = 348), isolated cleft palate (ICP, *N* = 141), multiple cleft lip with or without cleft palate (MCLP, *N* = 99), and multiple cleft palate (MCP, *N* = 74). A total of 13 mothers reported using corticosteroids during the periconceptional period for a wide variety of indications. Six case mothers of infants with ICLP and three of infants with ICP used corticosteroids (unspecified corticosteroid *N* = 1, prednisone *N* = 2, cortisone *N* = 3, triamcinolone acetonide *N* = 1, dexamethasone *N* = 1, and cortisone plus prednisone *N* = 1). One case mother of an infant with NTD used cortisone and an injectable unspecified corticosteroid, and three controls used corticosteroids (hydrocortisone *N* = 1 and prednisone *N* = 2). The odds ratio for corticosteroid use and ICLP was 4.3 (95% confidence interval [CI] 1.1–17.2), whereas the odds ratio for ICP and corticosteroid use was 5.3 (95% CI 1.1–26.5). No increased risks were observed for the other anomaly groups. Commenting on their results, the investigators thought that recall bias was unlikely because they did not observe increased risks for other malformations, and it was also unlikely that the mothers would have known of the suspected association between corticosteroids and orofacial clefts (18).

A 2004 study examined the effect of inhaled corticosteroids on low birth weight, preterm births, and congenital malformations in pregnant asthmatic patients (19). The inhaled steroids and the number of patients were beclomethasone (*N* = 277), fluticasone (*N* = 132), triamcinolone (*N* = 81), budesonide (*N* = 43), and flunisolide (*N* = 25). Compared with the general population, the study found no increased incidence of small-for-gestational-age infants (less than 10th percentile for gestational age), low birth weight (<2500 g), preterm births, and congenital malformations (19).

A 2006 meta-analysis on the use of inhaled corticosteroids during pregnancy was published in 2006 (20). The analysis included five agents: beclomethasone, budesonide, flunisolide, fluticasone, and triamcinolone. The results showed that these agents do not increase the risk of major congenital defects, preterm delivery, low birth weight, and pregnancy-induced hypertension. Thus, they could be used during pregnancy (20).

T

BREASTFEEDING SUMMARY

No reports describing the use of triamcinolone during lactation have been located. The molecular weight (about 394) is low enough that excretion into breast milk should be expected. Small amounts of other corticosteroids (see Hydrocortisone and Prednisone) are excreted into milk and do not appear to present a risk to a nursing infant. Similar excretion probably occurs following inhaled triamcinolone. At least one source states that inhaled corticosteroids used for asthma are not contraindicated during breastfeeding (21).

References

1. Product information. Azmacort. Rhône-Poulenc Rorer Pharmaceuticals, Inc., 1994.
2. American Hospital Formulary Service. *Drug Information 1997*. Bethesda, MD: American Society of Health-System Pharmacists, 1997:2368–70.
3. Walker BE. Cleft palate produced in mice by human-equivalent dosage with triamcinolone. Science 1965;149:862–3.
4. Walker BE. Induction of cleft palate in rats with antiinflammatory drugs. Teratology 1971;4:39–42.
5. Zhou M, Walker BE. Potentiation of triamcinolone-induced cleft palate in mice by maternal high dietary fat. Teratology 1993;48:53–7.
6. Rowland JM, Hendrickx AG. Teratogenicity of triamcinolone acetonide in rats. Teratology 1983;27:13–8.
7. Rowland JM, Hendrickx AG. Comparative teratogenicity of triamcinolone acetonide, triamcinolone, and cortisol in the rat. Teratogenesis Carcinog Mutagen 1983;3:313–9.
8. Massoud EAS, Sekhon HS, Rotschild A, Thurlbeck WM. The in vitro effect of triamcinolone acetonide on branching morphogenesis in the fetal rat lung. Pediatr Pulmonol 1992;14:28–36.
9. Bunton TE, Plopper CG. Triamcinolone-induced structural alterations in the development of the lung of the fetal rhesus macaque. Am J Obstet Gynecol 1984;148:203–15.
10. Hendrickx AG, Sawyer RH, Terrell TG, Osburn BI, Hendrickson RV, Steffek AJ. Teratogenic effects of triamcinolone on the skeletal and lymphoid systems in nonhuman primates. Fed Proc 1975;34:1661–5.
11. Hendrickx AG, Pellegrini M, Tarara R, Parker R, Silverman S, Steffek AJ. Craniofacial and central nervous system malformations induced by triamcinolone acetonide in nonhuman primates: I. General teratogenicity. Teratology 1980;22:103–14.
12. Parker RM, Hendrickx AG. Craniofacial and central nervous system malformations induced by triamcinolone acetonide in nonhuman primates: II. Craniofacial pathogenesis. Teratology 1983;28:35–44.
13. Tarara RP, Cordy DR, Hendrickx AG. Central nervous system malformations induced by triamcinolone acetonide in nonhuman primates: pathology. Teratology 1989;39:75–84.
14. Heinonen OP, Slone D, Shapiro S. *Birth Defects and Drugs in Pregnancy*. Littleton, MA: Publishing Sciences Group, 1977:388–400.
15. Rolf BB. Corticosteroids and pregnancy. Am J Obstet Gynecol 1966;95: 339–44.
16. Schatz M, Patterson R, Zeitz S, O'Rourke J, Melam H. Corticosteroid therapy for the pregnant asthmatic patient. JAMA 1975;233:804–7.
17. Katz VL, Thorp JM Jr, Bowes WA Jr. Severe symmetric intrauterine growth retardation associated with the topical use of triamcinolone. Am J Obstet Gynecol 1990;162:396–7.
18. Carmichael SL, Shaw GM. Maternal corticosteroid use and risk of selected congenital anomalies. Am J Med Genet 1999;86:242–4.
19. Namazy J, Schatz M, Long L, Lipkowitz M, Lillie M, Voss M, Deitz RJ, Petitti D. Use of inhaled steroids by pregnant asthmatic women does not reduce intrauterine growth. J Allergy Clin Immunol 2004;113:427–32.
20. Rahimi R, Nikfar S, Abdollahi M. Meta-analysis finds use of inhaled corticosteroids during pregnancy safe: a systematic meta-analysis review. Hum Exp Toxicol 2006;25:447–52.
21. Report of the Working Group on Asthma and Pregnancy. *Management of Asthma during Pregnancy*. U.S. Department of Health and Human Services, NIH Publication No. 93-3279, 1993:19.

TRIAMTERENE

Diuretic

PREGNANCY RECOMMENDATION: Human Data Suggest Risk
BREASTFEEDING RECOMMENDATION: No Human Data—Probably Compatible

PREGNANCY SUMMARY

Many investigators consider diuretics to be contraindicated in pregnancy, except for patients with heart disease, because they do not prevent or alter the course of toxemia, and they may decrease placental perfusion (1–3). In general, diuretics are not recommended for the treatment of gestational hypertension because of the maternal hypovolemia characteristic of this disease. Folic acid, at least 0.4 mg/day, should be taken before and during gestation because triamcinolone is a weak folic acid inhibitor.

FETAL RISK SUMMARY

Triamterene is a potassium-conserving diuretic. It is a weak folic acid antagonist. Reproduction studies in rats at doses up to 6 times the maximum recommended human dose based on BSA found no evidence of fetal harm (4).

It is not known if triamterene crosses the human placenta. The molecular weight (about 253) is low enough that exposure of the embryo–fetus should be expected.

No defects were observed in five infants exposed to triamterene in the 1st trimester (5, p. 372). For use anytime during pregnancy, 271 exposures were recorded without an increase in malformations (5, p. 441).

In a surveillance study of Michigan Medicaid recipients involving 229,101 completed pregnancies conducted between 1985 and 1992, 318 newborns had been exposed to triamterene during the 1st trimester (F. Rosa, personal communication, FDA, 1993). A total of 15 (4.7%) major birth defects were observed (13 expected). Three cases of cardiovascular defects (three expected) and one case of polydactyly (one expected) were observed, but specific information was not available for the other defects. No anomalies were observed in four other categories of defects (oral clefts, spina bifida, limb reduction defects, and hypospadias) for which data were available. These data do not support an association between the drug and congenital defects.

The effects of exposure (at any time during the 2nd or 3rd month after the last menstrual period) to folic acid antagonists on embryo–fetal development were evaluated in a large, multicenter, case–control surveillance study published in 2000 (6). The report was based on data collected between 1976 and 1998 by the Slone Epidemiology Unit Birth Defects Study from 80 maternity or tertiary care hospitals in Boston, Philadelphia, Toronto, and Iowa. Mothers were interviewed within 6 months of delivery about their use of drugs during pregnancy. Folic acid antagonists were categorized into two groups: group I—dihydrofolate reductase inhibitors (aminopterin, methotrexate, sulfasalazine, pyrimethamine, triamterene, and trimethoprim); group II—agents that affect other enzymes in folate metabolism, impair the absorption of folate, or increase the metabolic breakdown of folate (carbamazepine, phenytoin, primidone, and phenobarbital) (3). The case subjects were 3870 infants with cardiovascular defects, 1962 with oral clefts, and 1100 with urinary tract malformations. Infants with defects associated with a syndrome were excluded, as were infants with coexisting neural tube defects (NTDs; known to be reduced by maternal folic acid supplementation). Too few infants with limb reduction defects were identified to be analyzed. Controls (N = 8387) were infants with malformations other than oral clefts and cardiovascular, urinary tract, and limb reduction defects, and NTDs, but included infants with chromosomal and genetic defects. The risk of malformations in control infants would not have been reduced by vitamin supplementation, and none of the controls used folic acid antagonists (3). For group I cases, the relative risks (RRs) of cardiovascular defects and oral clefts were 3.4 (95% confidence interval [CI] 1.8–6.4) and 2.6 (95% CI 1.1–6.1), respectively. For group II cases, the RRs of cardiovascular and urinary tract defects, and oral clefts were 2.2 (95% CI 1.4–3.5), 2.5 (95% CI 1.2–5.0), and 2.5 (95% CI 1.5–4.2), respectively. Maternal use of multivitamin supplements with folic acid (typically 0.4 mg) reduced the risks in group I cases, but not in group II cases (6).

BREASTFEEDING SUMMARY

No reports describing the use of triamterene during lactation have been located. The molecular weight (about 253) is low enough that excretion into breast milk should be expected. The effect of this exposure on a nursing infant is unknown.

References

1. Pitkin RM, Kaminetzky HA, Newton M, Pritchard JA. Maternal nutrition: a selective review of clinical topics. Obstet Gynecol 1972;40:773–85.
2. Lindheimer MD, Katz AI. Sodium and diuretics in pregnancy. N Engl J Med 1973;288:891–4.
3. Christianson R, Page EW. Diuretic drugs and pregnancy. Obstet Gynecol 1976;48:647–52.
4. Product information. Dyrenium. WellSpring Pharmaceuticals, 2001.
5. Heinonen OP, Slone D, Shapiro S. *Birth Defects and Drugs in Pregnancy*. Littleton, MA: Publishing Sciences Group, 1977.
6. Hernandez-Diaz S, Werler MM, Walker AM, Mitchell AA. Folic acid antagonists during pregnancy and the risk of birth defects. N Engl J Med 2000;343:1608–14.

T

TRIAZOLAM

Hypnotic

PREGNANCY RECOMMENDATION: Limited Human Data—Animal Data Suggest Low Risk
BREASTFEEDING RECOMMENDATION: No Human Data—Potential Toxicity

PREGNANCY SUMMARY

A 1990 report evaluated the available published data to determine the fetal risk that occurs from exposure to various drugs (1). The risk for triazolam, based on poor data, was determined to be "none minimal." This risk assignment was defined as "...a magnitude that patients and physicians would generally consider to be too small to influence the management of an exposed pregnancy" (1).

FETAL RISK SUMMARY

Triazolam, a short-acting benzodiazepine, is used as a hypnotic for the treatment of insomnia. Although no congenital anomalies have been attributed to the use of triazolam during human pregnancies, other benzodiazepines (e.g., see Chlordiazepoxide and Diazepam) have been suspected of producing fetal malformations after 1st trimester exposure. Because of this association, the manufacturer classifies the drug as contraindicated in pregnancy (2). In one report, the drug was not teratogenic in pregnant animals when administered in large oral doses (3).

It is not known if triazolam crosses the human placenta. However, other benzodiazepines, such as diazepam, freely cross the placenta and accumulate in the fetus (see Diazepam). A similar distribution pattern should be expected for triazolam.

By the middle of 1988, the manufacturer had received >100 reports of in utero exposure to triazolam (J.H. Markillie, personal communication, Upjohn, 1989). Approximately one-seventh of these women were either lost to follow-up or further information was not available. Of the cases in which the outcome was known, more than one-half of the completed pregnancies ended with the delivery of a normal infant. Some of these exposures were reported in a 1987 correspondence that also included experience with alprazolam, another short-acting benzodiazepine (4). From these two sources, a total of five infants with congenital malformations have been described after in utero exposure to triazolam: extra digit on left foot and cleft uvula; incomplete closure of the foramen ovale (resolved spontaneously); small-for-gestational-age infant with left pelvic ectopic kidney; ventricular septal defect and possible coarctation of aorta (exposed to multiple drugs including triazolam); and premature, low-birth-weight infant with ventricular septal defect, pulmonary stenosis, intraventricular hemorrhage, hydrocephalus, apnea, bradycardia, anemia, jaundice, and seizure disorder (exposed to single 0.125-mg tablet at 1–2 weeks' gestation).

Single reports received by the manufacturer of defects in infants exposed in utero to either triazolam or alprazolam include pyloric stenosis, moderate tongue-tie, umbilical hernia and ankle inversion, and clubfoot (4).

Three cases of nonmalformation toxicities have been observed in infants exposed during gestation to triazolam: tachycardia, bradycardia, respiratory pauses, hypotonia and axial hypotony, impaired arachnoid reflexes, hypothermia, sleepiness and lifeless (symptoms resolved after infant received supportive care for several days; mother took multiple medications during pregnancy); fetal distress requiring emergency cesarean section and infant resuscitation, umbilical cord wrapped around neck, seizure activity, and generalized cortical atrophy (exposed to triazolam and a second [not identified] benzodiazepine early in pregnancy and during the last week of gestation; apparent recovery with no permanent disability by 6 months of age); bradycardia, malaise, cyanosis, leukopenia, and chewing movements at 4 days of age (exposed during 3rd trimester; symptoms resolved by 1 week of age) (4).

Based on the available information, a causal relationship between triazolam and the various infant outcomes does not appear to exist. Moreover, these cases cannot be used to derive rate or incidence data, because of the probable bias involved in the reporting of pregnancy exposures to the manufacturer (4).

In a surveillance study of Michigan Medicaid recipients involving 229,101 completed pregnancies conducted between 1985 and 1992, 138 newborns were exposed to triazolam during the 1st trimester (F. Rosa, personal communication, FDA, 1993). A total of seven (5.1%) major birth defects were observed (six expected). One cardiovascular defect (one expected) and one case of polydactyly (0.5 expected) were observed, but specific information on the other defects was not available. No anomalies were observed in four other categories of defects (oral clefts, spina bifida, limb reduction defects, and hypospadias) for which specific data were available. These data do not support an association between the drug and congenital defects.

BREASTFEEDING SUMMARY

No reports describing the use of triazolam during human lactation or measuring the amount excreted into milk have been located. The molecular weight (about 343) is low enough that passage into human milk should be expected. The effect of this exposure on a nursing infant is unknown, but closely related drugs are classified by the American Academy of Pediatrics as agents that may be of concern during breastfeeding (e.g., see Diazepam).

References

1. Friedman JM, Little BB, Brent RL, Cordero JF, Hanson JW, Shepard TH. Potential human teratogenicity of frequently prescribed drugs. Obstet Gynecol 1990;75:594–9.
2. Product information. Halcion. Pharmacia & Upjohn, 2008.
3. Matsuo A, Kast A, Tsunenari Y. Reproduction studies of triazolam in rats and rabbits. Iyakuhin Kenkyu 1979;10:52–67. As cited in Shepard TH. *Catalog of Teratogenic Agents*. 6th ed. Baltimore, MD: The Johns Hopkins University Press, 1989:630.
4. Barry WS, St. Clair SM. Exposure to benzodiazepines in utero. Lancet 1987;1:1436–7.

TRICHLORMETHIAZIDE

Diuretic

See Chlorothiazide.

TRIDIHEXETHYL

[Withdrawn from the market. See 9th edition.]

TRIENTINE

Chelating Agent

PREGNANCY RECOMMENDATION: Limited Human Data—Animal Data Suggest Moderate Risk
BREASTFEEDING RECOMMENDATION: No Human Data—Potential Toxicity

PREGNANCY SUMMARY

Although the animal data suggest moderate risk, no developmental toxicity has been observed in the limited human pregnancy data. Copper deficiency is thought to be teratogenic, but evidence was found in one study that fetuses exposed to trientine are not copper deficient.

FETAL RISK SUMMARY

Trientine is a chelating agent used for the removal of excess copper from the systems of patients with Wilson's disease who either cannot tolerate penicillamine or who have developed penicillamine resistance. The drug is available in the United States only as an orphan drug.

In studies with pregnant rats, trientine was teratogenic in doses similar to those used in humans (1–6). The frequency of fetal resorptions and malformations, including hemorrhage and edema, was directly related to the decrease in fetal copper concentrations.

It is not known if trientine crosses the human placenta. The molecular weight (about 147 for the free base) suggests that exposure of the embryo–fetus should be expected.

A 1996 report described the use of trientine in seven human pregnancies (7). The women were treated for Wilson's disease through 11 pregnancies. At the time of conception, the average duration of trientine therapy had been 5 years (range 2–3 weeks to 9 years). Therapy was continued throughout pregnancy in seven cases, interrupted in the 2nd trimester of one because of inability to obtain the drug, and apparently was discontinued in the final few weeks of still another because of nausea not related to trientine (7). One woman underwent a therapeutic abortion at 10 weeks' gestation and one spontaneously aborted a normal male fetus, together with a copper contraceptive coil, at 14 weeks' gestation. Of the pregnancies ending with a live infant, there were four males, four females, and one infant whose sex was not specified. The mean birth weight of the full-term infants was 3263 g. Two of the infants were delivered prematurely, one male at 36 weeks (2400 g) and one female at 31 weeks (800 g). The latter infant had an isochromosome X, but both parents had normal X chromosomes. No other abnormalities were observed in the infants at the time of birth.

Because copper deficiency is thought to be teratogenic, the results led to the conclusion that the fetuses had not become copper depleted (7). Evidence supporting this conclusion was obtained from the mean ceruloplasmin concentration of cord blood, 9.9 mg/dL, which was nearly identical to nontreated controls (10 mg/dL) (7). Additional studies, however, are needed before this conclusion can be accepted with confidence. Except for slow progress at 3 months in the infant with the isochromosome X, development in the other children was normal during follow-up evaluations ranging from 2 months to 9 years.

In a 1998 case report, a 20-year-old woman with Wilson's disease took trientine (900 mg/day) throughout pregnancy (8). At 42 weeks', she vaginally delivered a normal 3280-g female infant with Apgar scores of 10, 10, and 10 at 1, 5, and 10 minutes, respectively. No complications were observed in the mother or infant during the postpartum period (8).

BREASTFEEDING SUMMARY

No reports describing the use of trientine during lactation have been located. The molecular weight (about 147 for the free base) is low enough that excretion into breast milk should be expected. The effect of this exposure on a nursing infant is unknown. Copper deficiency, however, is a potential toxicity.

References

1. March L, Fraser FC. Chelating agents and teratogenesis. Lancet 1973;2:846.
2. Keen CL, Mark-Savage P, Lonnerdal B, Hurley LS. Low tissue copper and teratogenesis in rats resulting from D-penicillamine (abstract). Fed Proc 1981;40:917.
3. Keen CL, Cohen NL, Lonnerdal B, Hurley LS. Low tissue copper and teratogenesis in trientine-treated rats. Lancet 1982;1:1127.
4. Keen CL, Lonnerdal B, Cohen NL, Hurley LS. Drug-induced Cu deficiency: a model for Cu deficiency teratogenicity (abstract). Fed Proc 1982;41:944.
5. Cohen NL, Keen CL, Lonnerdal B, Hurley LS. Low tissue copper and teratogenesis in triethylenetetramine-treated rats (abstract). Fed Proc 1982;41:944.
6. Product information. Syprine. Merck, 2000.
7. Walshe JM. The management of pregnancy in Wilson's disease treated with trientine. Q J Med 1986;58;81–7.
8. Desbriere R, Roquelaure B, Sarles J, Boubli L. Pregnancy in a patient treated with trientine dihydrochloride for Wilson's disease. Presse Med 1998;27:806.

TRIFLUOPERAZINE

Antipsychotic

PREGNANCY RECOMMENDATION: Limited Human Data—Animal Data Suggest Low Risk
BREASTFEEDING RECOMMENDATION: No Human Data—Potential Toxicity

PREGNANCY SUMMARY

Although some reports have attempted to link trifluoperazine with congenital defects, most evidence suggests that the drug is safe for the mother and low risk for the embryo–fetus.

FETAL RISK SUMMARY

Trifluoperazine is a piperazine phenothiazine. The drug readily crosses the placenta (1). It has been used for the treatment of nausea and vomiting of pregnancy, but it is primarily used as a psychotropic agent.

Reproduction studies with trifluoperazine have been conducted in rats, rabbits, and monkeys (2). In rats, doses >600 times the human dose revealed an increased incidence of malformations and reduced litter size and weight associated with maternal toxicity. These effects were not observed when the dose was reduced to half (2). No fetal adverse effects were observed in rabbits or monkeys at doses of 700 and 25 times the human dose, respectively.

In 1962, the Canadian Food and Drug Directorate released a warning that eight cases of congenital defects had been associated with trifluoperazine therapy (3). This correlation was refuted in a series of articles from the medical staff of the manufacturer of the drug (4–6). In 480 trifluoperazine-treated pregnant women, the incidence of liveborn infants with congenital malformations was 1.1%, as compared with 8472 nontreated controls with an incidence of 1.5% (5). Two reports of phocomelia appeared in 1962–1963 and a case of a congenital heart defect in 1969 (7–9): twins, both with phocomelia of all four limbs (7); phocomelia of upper limbs (8); and complete transposition of great vessels in the heart (9). In none of these cases is there a clear relationship between use of the drug and the defect.

Extrapyramidal symptoms have been described in a newborn exposed to trifluoperazine in utero, but the reaction was probably caused by chlorpromazine (see Chlorpromazine) (10).

The Collaborative Perinatal Project monitored 50282 mother–child pairs, 42 of whom had 1st trimester exposure to trifluoperazine (11). No evidence was found to suggest a relationship to malformations or an effect on perinatal mortality rate, birth weight, or IQ scores at 4 years of age.

In a surveillance study of Michigan Medicaid recipients involving 229,101 completed pregnancies conducted between 1985 and 1992, 29 newborns had been exposed to trifluoperazine during the 1st trimester (F. Rosa, personal communication, FDA, 1993). One (3.4%) major birth defect (one expected), a cardiovascular malformation (0.5 expected), was observed.

Attempted maternal suicide at 31 weeks' gestation with trifluoperazine and misoprostol resulting in fetal death has been described (12). The adverse fetal outcome was attributed to tetanic uterine contractions caused by misoprostol (see Misoprostol).

Reviewers have concluded that phenothiazines are not teratogenic (13,14).

BREASTFEEDING SUMMARY

No reports describing the use of trifluoperazine during lactation have been located. The molecular weight (about 408 for the free base) is low enough that passage into milk should be expected. The American Academy of Pediatrics classifies trifluoperazine as a drug for which the effect on nursing infants is unknown but may be of concern (15).

References

1. Moya F, Thorndike V. Passage of drugs across the placenta. Am J Obstet Gynecol 1962;84:1778–98.
2. Product information. Stelazine. SmithKline Beecham Pharmaceuticals, 2000.
3. Canadian Department of National Health and Welfare, Food and Drug Directorate. *Letter of Notification to Canadian Physicians*. Ottawa, December 7, 1962.
4. Moriarity AJ. Trifluoperazine and congenital malformations. Can Med Assoc J 1963;88:97.
5. Moriarty AJ, Nance MR. Trifluoperazine and pregnancy. Can Med Assoc J 1963;88:375–6.
6. Schrire I. Trifluoperazine and foetal abnormalities. Lancet 1963;1:174.
7. Corner BD. Congenital malformations. Clinical considerations. Med J Southwest 1962;77:46–52.
8. Hall G. A case of phocomelia of the upper limbs. Med J Aust 1963;1:449–50.
9. Vince DJ. Congenital malformations following phenothiazine administration during pregnancy. Can Med Assoc J 1969;100:223.
10. Hill RM, Desmond MM, Kay JL. Extrapyramidal dysfunction in an infant of a schizophrenic mother. J Pediatr 1966;69:589–95.
11. Slone D, Siskind V, Heinonen OP, Monson RR, Kaufman DW, Shapiro S. Antenatal exposure to the phenothiazines in relation to congenital malformations, perinatal mortality rate, birth weight, and intelligence quotient score. Am J Obstet Gynecol 1977;128:486–8.
12. Bond GR, Zee AV. Overdosage of misoprostol in pregnancy. Am J Obstet Gynecol 1994;171:561–2.
13. Ayd FJ Jr. Children born of mothers treated with chlorpromazine during pregnancy. Clin Med 1964;71:1758–63.
14. Ananth J. Congenital malformations with psychopharmacologic agents. Compr Psychiatry 1975;16:437–45.
15. Committee on Drugs, American Academy of Pediatrics. The transfer of drugs and other chemicals into human milk. Pediatrics 2001;108:776–89.

TRIFLUPROMAZINE

[Withdrawn from the market. See 9th edition.]

TRIHEXYPHENIDYL

Parasympatholytic (Anticholinergic)

PREGNANCY RECOMMENDATION: Limited Human Data—No Relevant Animal Data
BREASTFEEDING RECOMMENDATION: No Human Data—Probably Compatible

PREGNANCY SUMMARY

The absence of animal reproduction data and the very limited human pregnancy experience prevents an assessment of the embryo–fetal risk. However, in general, anticholinergics are considered low risk in pregnancy.

FETAL RISK SUMMARY

Trihexyphenidyl is an anticholinergic agent used in the treatment of parkinsonism. In a large prospective study, 2323 patients were exposed to this class of drugs during the 1st trimester, 9 of whom took trihexyphenidyl (1). A possible association was found between the total group and minor malformations.

BREASTFEEDING SUMMARY

No reports describing the use of trihexyphenidyl during human lactation have been located.

Reference

1. Heinonen OP, Slone D, Shapiro S. *Birth Defects and Drugs in Pregnancy*. Littleton, MA: Publishing Sciences Group, 1977:346–53.

TRIMEPRAZINE

[Withdrawn from the market. See 9th edition.]

TRIMETHADIONE

[Withdrawn from the market. See 9th edition.]

TRIMETHAPHAN

[Withdrawn from the market. See 9th edition.]

TRIMETHOBENZAMIDE

Antiemetic

PREGNANCY RECOMMENDATION: Human Data Suggest Low Risk
BREASTFEEDING RECOMMENDATION: No Human Data—Probably Compatible

PREGNANCY SUMMARY

The animal reproduction data and the limited human pregnancy experience suggest that the embryo–fetal risk with this drug is low.

FETAL RISK SUMMARY

Trimethobenzamide is an antiemetic agent. Reproduction studies have been conducted in rats and rabbits and revealed no evidence of teratogenicity (1). An increased incidence of resorptions and stillborn pups was noted in rats (at 20 and 100 mg/kg) and an increased number of resorptions in rabbits (at 100 mg/kg), but these adverse effects occurred in only one or two dams in both species (1).

It is not known if trimethobenzamide crosses the human placenta. The molecular weight (about 389 for the free base) suggests that exposure of the embryo–fetus should be expected.

Trimethobenzamide has been used in pregnancy to treat nausea and vomiting (2,3). No adverse effects in the fetuses were observed. In a third study, 193 patients were treated with trimethobenzamide in the 1st trimester (4). The incidences of severe congenital defects at 1 month, 1 year, and 5 years were 2.6%, 2.6%, and 5.8%, respectively. The 5.8% incidence was increased compared with nontreated controls (3.2%) ($p < 0.05$), but other factors, including the use of other antiemetics in some patients, may have contributed to the results. The authors concluded that the risk of congenital malformations with trimethobenzamide was low.

BREASTFEEDING SUMMARY

No reports describing the use of trimethobenzamide during lactation have been located. The molecular weight (about 389 for the free base) is low enough that excretion into breast milk should be expected. The effect of this exposure on a nursing infant is unknown.

References

1. Product information. Tigan. Roberts Pharmaceutical, 2000.
2. Breslow S, Belafsky HA, Shangold JE, Hirsch LM, Stahl MB. Antiemetic effect of trimethobenzamide in pregnant patients. Clin Med 1961;8:2153–5.
3. Winters HS. Antiemetics in nausea and vomiting of pregnancy. Obstet Gynecol 1961;18:753–6.
4. Milkovich L, van den Berg BJ. An evaluation of the teratogenicity of certain antinauseant drugs. Am J Obstet Gynecol 1976;125:244–8.

TRIMETHOPRIM

Anti-infective

PREGNANCY RECOMMENDATION: Human and Animal Data Suggest Risk
BREASTFEEDING RECOMMENDATION: Compatible

PREGNANCY SUMMARY

Trimethoprim is a dihydrofolate reductase inhibitor that is teratogenic in animals and humans. Defects that have been associated with trimethoprim include cardiovascular defects and neural tube defects (NTDs), and possibly oral clefts. Folic acid supplementation, at least 0.4 mg/day, started before conception or concurrently with trimethoprim may reduce the risk of these congenital defects.

FETAL RISK SUMMARY

Trimethoprim is available as a single agent and in combination with various sulfonamides (see Sulfonamides). Because trimethoprim is a folate antagonist, caution has been advocated for its use in pregnancy (1–3). Published case reports and placebo-controlled trials involving several hundred patients, during all phases of gestation, have failed to demonstrate an increase in fetal abnormalities (4–13). However, other reports (14–20) and the unpublished data cited below are suggestive that trimethoprim use during the 1st trimester may result in structural defects. Maternal supplementation with multivitamins that contain folic acid may reduce this risk (16).

Trimethoprim (200 mg/kg) given to pregnant rats resulted in cleft palates (21). The no-effect dose was 192 mg/kg. When trimethoprim (88 mg/kg) was combined with sulfamethoxazole (355 mg/kg), cleft palates were observed in one of nine litters. In two other rat studies, however, no teratogenic effects were seen at a combined dose of 128 and 512 mg/kg, respectively. In some studies with pregnant rabbits, a trimethoprim dose 6 times the human therapeutic dose was associated with resorptions, fetal death, and malformations (21).

Trimethoprim (molecular weight about 290) crosses the placenta, producing similar levels in fetal and maternal serum and in amniotic fluid (22–25). Using an in vitro perfused human cotyledon, both trimethoprim and sulfamethoxazole were shown to cross the placenta (25). After 1 hour in a closed system at maternal trimethoprim concentrations of 7.2 and 1.0 mcg/mL, concentrations on the fetal side were 1.4 (19%) and 0.08 mcg/mL (8%), respectively. Under similar conditions, maternal sulfamethoxazole levels of 29.6, 112.6, and 127.7 mcg/mL produced fetal levels of 5.1 (17%), 9.6 (9%), and 14.8 mcg/mL (12%). (*Note: The mean steady state serum levels following 160 mg/800 mg trimethoprim–sulfamethoxazole orally twice daily are 1.72 and 68 mcg/mL, respectively* [*21*].)

A 27-year-old woman consumed a low-calorie (Nutra System) diet 10 months before conception through the 4th gestational week (14). Her pregnancy was complicated by otitis, treated with a combination of trimethoprim–sulfamethoxazole for 10 days beginning in the 3rd week, and the onset of hyperemesis gravidarum at 5–6 weeks' gestation that lasted until the 8th month. Dimenhydrinate was taken intermittently as an antiemetic from the 7th week through the 8th month. She gave birth at 38 weeks' gestation to a 3225-g female infant with a lobar holoprosencephaly. The malformations included a median cleft lip and palate, a flat nose without nostrils, hypoplasia of the optic discs, and a single ventricle and midline fused thalami. The infant developed progressive hydrocephalus, myoclonic jerks, intractable seizures, and muscle tone that changed from hypotonic to hypertonic at 2 months of age. Although the critical period for development of holoprosencephaly was thought to be during the period of gastrulation (i.e., the 3rd week of pregnancy), the cause of the defects was unknown (14).

In a surveillance study of Michigan Medicaid recipients involving 229,101 completed pregnancies conducted between 1985 and 1992, 2296 newborns had been exposed to the combination of trimethoprim–sulfamethoxazole during the 1st trimester (F. Rosa, personal communication, FDA, 1993). A total of 126 (5.5%) major birth defects were observed (98 expected). This incidence is suggestive of an association between the drug combination and congenital defects. Specific data were available for 6 defect categories, including (observed/expected) 37/23 cardiovascular defects, 3/4 oral clefts, 1/1 spina bifida, 7/7 polydactyly, 3/4 limb reduction defects, and 7/5 hypospadias. Only the cardiovascular defects are suggestive of an association among the six specific malformations, but other factors such as the mother's disease, concurrent drug use, and chance may be involved.

A 2000 case report described the adverse pregnancy outcomes, including NTDs, of two pregnant women with HIV infection who were treated with the anti-infective combination, trimethoprim–sulfamethoxazole, for prophylaxis against *Pneumocystsis carinii*, concurrently with antiretroviral agents (15). In the first case, a 32-year-old woman with a 3-year history of HIV and recent diagnosis of acquired immunodeficiency syndrome was treated before and throughout gestation with the anti-infective combination plus zidovudine and zalcitabine. Folic acid, 10 mg/day, was added after the diagnosis of pregnancy (gestational age not specified). At term, a female infant without HIV infection was delivered by cesarean section, but she had a bony mass in the lumbar spine (identified by ultrasound at 32 weeks' gestation). A diagnostic evaluation revealed that the second lumbar vertebra consisted of hemivertebrae and projected posteriorly into the spinal canal. A malformed and displaced first lumbar vertebra was also noted. Surgery was planned to correct the defect. The second case involved a 31-year-old woman who presented at 15 weeks' gestation. She was receiving trimethoprim–sulfamethoxazole, didanosine, stavudine, nevirapine, and vitamin B supplements (specific vitamins and dosage not given) that had been started before conception. A fetal ultrasound at 19 weeks' gestation revealed spina bifida and ventriculomegaly. The patient elected to terminate her pregnancy. The fetus did not have HIV infection. Defects observed at autopsy included ventriculomegaly, an Arnold-Chiari malformation, sacral spina bifida, and a lumbo-sacral meningomyelocele. The authors attributed the NTDs in both cases to the antifolate activity of trimethoprim (15).

The effects of exposure (at any time during the 2nd or 3rd month after the last menstrual period) to folic acid antagonists on embryo–fetal development were evaluated in a large, multicenter, case–control surveillance study published in 2000 (16). The report was based on data collected between 1976 and 1998 by the Slone Epidemiology Unit Birth Defects Study from 80 maternity or tertiary care hospitals in Boston, Philadelphia, Toronto, and Iowa. Mothers were interviewed within 6 months of delivery about their use of drugs during pregnancy. Folic acid antagonists were categorized into two groups: group I—dihydrofolate reductase inhibitors (aminopterin, methotrexate, sulfasalazine, pyrimethamine, triamterene, and trimethoprim); group II—agents that affect other enzymes in folate metabolism, impair the absorption of folate, or increase the metabolic breakdown of folate (carbamazepine, phenytoin, primidone, and phenobarbital). The case subjects were 3870 infants with cardiovascular defects, 1962 with oral clefts, and 1100 with urinary tract malformations. Infants with defects associated with a syndrome were excluded, as were infants with coexisting NTDs (known to be reduced by maternal folic acid supplementation). Too few infants with limb reduction defects were identified to be analyzed. Controls (*N* = 8387) were infants with malformations other than oral clefts and cardiovascular, urinary tract, and limb reduction defects and NTDs, but included infants with chromosomal and genetic defects. The risk of malformations in control infants would not have been reduced by vitamin supplementation, and none of the controls used folic acid antagonists (16). For group I cases, the relative risks (RRs) of cardiovascular defects and oral clefts were 3.4 (95% confidence interval [CI] 1.8–6.4) and 2.6 (95% CI 1.1–6.1), respectively. For group II cases, the RRs of cardiovascular and urinary tract defects, and oral clefts were 2.2 (95% CI 1.4–3.5), 2.5 (95% CI 1.2–5.0), and 2.5 (95% CI 1.5–4.2), respectively. Maternal use of multivitamin supplements with folic acid (typically 0.4 mg) reduced the risks in group I cases. For cardiovascular defects, the RR and 95% CI without or with folic acid were 7.7 (2.8–21.7) and 1.5 (0.6–3.8), respectively. The same comparison for oral clefts could not be completed because only three case infants were exposed to folic acid during the second and third month. However, there were six (0.3%) cases of oral clefts without folic acid and three (0.2%) with folic acid. In contrast, in group II cases, folic acid did not reduce the risks of cardiovascular defects, oral clefts, or urinary tract defects (16).

Additional data related to the above study appeared in a reply to correspondence (17). Analysis for trimethoprim exposure resulted in an RR of 4.2 (95% CI 1.5–11.5) for cardiovascular defects based on 12 cases. Additional analysis for oral clefts (three cases) and urinary tract defects (one case) was not conducted because of the small number of exposures (17).

A 2001 case–control study, using the same database as in the above study, compared data on 1242 infants with NTDs (spina bifida, anencephaly, and encephalocele) with a control group of 6660 infants with congenital defects not related to vitamin supplementation (18). Based on five exposed cases, the adjusted odds ratio (OR) for trimethoprim was 4.8, 95% CI 1.5–16.1. For all folic acid antagonists (carbamazepine, phenobarbital, phenytoin, primidone, sulfasalazine, triamterene, and trimethoprim), based on 27 cases, the adjusted OR was 2.9, 95% CI 1.7–4.6 (18).

A 2002 review, briefly citing the above two studies, stated that the results were consistent with previous studies that folic acid supplementation early in pregnancy reduces the risk of cardiac defects, oral clefts, and NTDs (19). However, additional studies are needed to determine if early folic acid supplementation would also reduce the risk of these anomalies from trimethoprim (19).

A 2001 case–control study used the population-based dataset of the Hungarian Case–Control Surveillance of Congenital Abnormalities, 1980–1996, to examine the teratogenic risk of trimethoprim in combination with either sulfamethoxazole or sulfamethazine (20). There were 22,865 case women who had delivered an infant with congenital malformations and 38,151 controls who had infants without malformations. In the cases and controls, 351 (1.5%) and 443 (1.2%) were treated with trimethoprim–sulfamethoxazole, respectively, in the 2nd/3rd months of pregnancy. For trimethoprim–sulfamethazine, 45 (0.2%) cases and 39 (0.1%) controls were treated, respectively, in the 2nd/3rd months of pregnancy. Because both combinations contained trimethoprim, the drugs were combined in the case–control pair analysis. Two congenital abnormalities had higher use of drug treatments: cardiovascular anomalies (29 vs. 10; adjusted OR 2.9, 95% CI 1.4–6.0) and multiple anomalies (mainly urinary tract and cardiovascular) (9 vs. 1; adjusted OR 9.0, 95% CI 1.1–71.0). For NTDs, analysis of trimethoprim–sulfamethoxazole in the 1st month revealed nine cases (adjusted OR 4.3, 95% CI 2.1–8.6) and seven cases in the 2nd/3rd months (adjusted OR 2.2, 95% CI 1.0–4.8) (20).

A case of Niikawa-Kuroki syndrome (i.e., Kabuki make-up syndrome) has been described in a non-Japanese girl whose mother had a viral and bacterial infection during the 2nd month of pregnancy (26). The bacterial infection was treated with trimethoprim–sulfamethoxazole. The syndrome is characterized by mental and growth restriction and craniofacial malformations (26). The cause of the defects in this patient, as in all cases of this syndrome, was unknown. Some have speculated, however, that the syndrome is caused by autosomal dominant inheritance (27).

Sulfonamide–trimethoprim combinations have been shown to cause a drop in the sperm count after 1 month of continuous treatment in males (28). Decreases varied between 7% and 88%. The authors theorized that trimethoprim deprived the spermatogenetic cells of active folate by inhibiting dihydrofolate reductase.

No interaction between trimethoprim–sulfamethoxazole and oral contraceptives was found in one study (29). Short courses of the anti-infective combination are unlikely to affect contraceptive control.

BREASTFEEDING SUMMARY

Trimethoprim is excreted into breast milk in low concentrations. Following 160 mg twice daily for 5 days, milk concentrations varied between 1.2 and 2.4 mcg/mL (average 1.8 mcg/mL) with peak levels occurring at 2–3 hours (30). No adverse effects were reported in the infants. Nearly identical results were found in a study with 50 patients (31). Mean milk levels were 2.0 mcg/mL, representing a milk:plasma ratio of 1.25. The authors concluded that these levels represented a negligible risk to the suckling infant.

In a 1993 cohort study, diarrhea was reported in 32 (19.3%) nursing infants of 166 breastfeeding mothers who were taking antibiotics (32). For the 12 women taking trimethoprim–sulfamethoxazole, no diarrhea was observed in the infants but 2 (17%) had poor feeding, an effect that was considered minor because it did not require medical attention (32).

The American Academy of Pediatrics classifies the combination of trimethoprim–sulfamethoxazole as compatible with breastfeeding (33).

References

1. McEwen LM. Trimethoprim/sulphamethoxazole mixture in pregnancy. Br Med J 1971;4:490–1.
2. Smithells RW. Co-trimoxazole in pregnancy. Lancet 1983;2:1142.
3. Tan JS, File TM Jr. Treatment of bacteriuria in pregnancy. Drugs 1992;44:972–80.

T

4. Williams JD, Condie AP, Brumfitt W, Reeves DS. The treatment of bacteriuria in pregnant women with sulphamethoxazole and trimethoprim. Postgrad Med J 1969;45(Suppl):71–6.
5. Ochoa AG. Trimethoprim and sulfamethoxazole in pregnancy. JAMA 1971;217:1244.
6. Brumfitt W, Pursell R. Double-blind trial to compare ampicillin, cephalexin, co-trimoxazole, and trimethoprim in treatment of urinary infection. Br Med J 1972;2:673–6.
7. Brumfitt W, Pursell R. Trimethoprim/sulfamethoxazole in the treatment of bacteriuria in women. J Infect Dis 1973;128(Suppl):S657–63.
8. Brumfitt W, Pursell R. Trimethoprim/sulfamethoxazole in the treatment of urinary infection. Med J Aust 1973;1(Suppl):44–8.
9. Bailey RR. Single-dose antibacterial treatment for bacteriuria in pregnancy. Drugs 1984;27:183–6.
10. Soper DE, Merrill-Nach S. Successful therapy of penicillinase-producing *Neisseria gonorrhoeae* pharyngeal infection during pregnancy. Obstet Gynecol 1986;68:290–1.
11. Cruikshank DP, Warenski JC. First-trimester maternal *Listeria monocytogenes* sepsis and chorioamnionitis with normal neonatal outcome. Obstet Gynecol 1989;73:469–71.
12. Seoud M, Saade G, Awar G, Uwaydah M. Brucellosis in pregnancy. J Reprod Med 1991;36:441–5.
13. Frederiksen B. Maternal septicemia with *Listeria monocytogenes* in second trimester without infection of the fetus. Acta Obstet Gynecol Scand 1992;71:313–5.
14. Ronen GM. Holoprosencephaly and maternal low-calorie weight-reducing diet. Am J Med Genet 1992;42:139.
15. Richardson MP, Osrin D, Donaghy S, Brown NA, Hay P, Sharland M. Spinal malformations in the fetuses of HIV infected women receiving combination antiretroviral therapy and co-trimoxazole. Eur J Obstet Gynecol Reprod Biol 2000;93:215–7.
16. Hernandez-Diaz S, Werler MM, Walker AM, Mitchell AA. Folic acid antagonists during pregnancy and the risk of birth defects. N Engl J Med 2000;343:1608–14.
17. Hernandez-Diaz S, Mitchell AA. Folic acid antagonists during pregnancy and risk of birth defects. N Engl J Med 2001;344:934–5.
18. Hernandez-Diaz S, Werler MM, Walker AM, Mitchell AA. Neural tube defects in relation to use of folic acid antagonists during pregnancy. Am J Epidemiol 2001;153:961–8.
19. Shepard TH, Brent RL, Friedman JM, Jones KL, Miller RK, Moore CA, Polifka JE. Update on new developments in the study of human teratogens. Teratology 2002;65:153–61.
20. Czeizel AE, Rockenbauer M, Sorensen HT, Olsen J. The teratogenic risk of trimethoprim-sulfonamides: a population based case-control study. Reprod Toxicol 2001;15:637–46.
21. Product information. Septra. Monarch Pharmaceuticals, 2001.
22. Ylikorkala O, Sjostedt E, Jarvinen PA, Tikkanen R, Raines T. Trimethoprim-sulfonamide combination administered orally and intravaginally in the 1st trimester of pregnancy: its absorption into serum and transfer to amniotic fluid. Acta Obstet Gynecol Scand 1973;52:229–34.
23. Reid DWJ, Caille G, Kaufmann NR. Maternal and transplacental kinetics of trimethoprim and sulfamethoxazole, separately and in combination. Can Med Assoc J 1975;112:67s–72s.
24. Reeves DS, Wilkinson PJ. The pharmacokinetics of trimethoprim and trimethoprim/sulfonamide combinations, including penetration into body tissues. Infection 1979;7(Suppl 4):S330–41.
25. Bawdon RE, Maberry MC, Fortunato SJ, Gilstrap LC, Kim S. Trimethoprim and sulfamethoxazole transfer in the in vitro perfused human cotyledon. Gynecol Obstet Invest 1991;31:240–2.
26. Koutras A, Fisher S. Niikawa-Kuroki syndrome: a new malformation syndrome of postnatal dwarfism, mental retardation, unusual face, and protruding ears. J Pediatr 1982;101:417–9.
27. Niikawa N. Kabuki make-up syndrome. In: Buyse ML, ed. *Birth Defects Encyclopedia*. Volume 2. Dover, MA: Center for Birth Defects Information Services, 1990:998–9.
28. Murdia A, Mathur V, Kothari LK, Singh KP. Sulpha-trimethoprim combinations and male fertility. Lancet 1978;2:375–6.
29. Grimmer SFM, Allen WL, Back DJ, Breckenridge AM, Orme M, Tjia J. The effect of cotrimoxazole on oral contraceptive steroids in women. Contraception 1983;28:53–9.
30. Arnauld R, Soutoul JH, Gallier J, Borderon JC, Borderon E. A study of the passage of trimethoprim into the maternal milk. Quest Med 1972;25:959–64.
31. Miller RD, Salter AJ. The passage of trimethoprim/sulphamethoxazole into breast milk and its significance. In: Daikos GK, ed. *Progress in Chemotherapy*, Proceedings of the Eighth International Congress of Chemotherapy, Athens, 1973. Athens: Hellenic Society for Chemotherapy, 1974:687–91.
32. Ito S, Blajchman A, Stephenson M, Eliopoulos C, Koren G. Prospective follow-up of adverse reactions in breast-fed infants exposed to maternal medication. Am J Obstet Gynecol 1993;168:1393–9.
33. Committee of Drugs, American Academy of Pediatrics. The transfer of drugs and other chemicals into human milk. Pediatrics 2001;108:776–89.

TRIMETREXATE

[Withdrawn from the market. See 9th edition.]

TRIMIPRAMINE

Antidepressant

PREGNANCY RECOMMENDATION: Human Data Suggest Low Risk
BREASTFEEDING RECOMMENDATION: No Human Data—Potential Toxicity

PREGNANCY SUMMARY

The animal data suggest low risk but, if the comparison to the human dose had been based on BSA, the toxic dose would have been close to the human dose. The human data are too limited to assess the risk to the embryo–fetus. In general, though, most tricyclic antidepressants do not have a known teratogenic effect in humans (1). In addition, of the tricyclic antidepressants, nortriptyline and desipramine are preferred during pregnancy because they have the least sedative action and maternal adverse effects (1).

FETAL RISK SUMMARY

Trimipramine is a tricyclic antidepressant in the same class as amitriptyline, clomipramine, doxepin, and imipramine. It is indicated for the relief of symptoms of depression (2). Trimipramine has an elimination half-life of 9–11 hours and it is metabolized in the liver to an active metabolite (3).

Reproduction studies have been conducted in rats, rabbits, and mice. In rats and rabbits, evidence of embryotoxicity and/or increased incidence of major anomalies (type not specified) were observed at doses 20 times the human dose (2). A single SC dose given to mice on day 9 of gestation resulted in exencephaly and other defects of the central nervous system (4). In the isolated rat uterus, trimipramine had greater antihistamine H_2 activity than cimetidine, amitriptyline, or imipramine (5).

It is not known if trimipramine or its active metabolite crosses the human placenta. The molecular weight of the free base (about 294) and the long elimination half-life suggest that both compounds will cross to the embryo–fetus.

In a 1996 descriptive case series, the European Network of the Teratology Information Services (ENTIS) prospectively examined the outcomes of 689 pregnancies exposed to antidepressants (6). Multiple drug therapy occurred in about two-thirds of the mothers. There were nine exposures to trimipramine. The outcomes of these pregnancies were eight normal newborns (including three premature infants) and one normal infant with a neonatal disorder (bilateral metatarsus varus [possibly positional]) (6).

BREASTFEEDING SUMMARY

No reports describing the use of trimipramine during human lactation have been located. The molecular weight of the free base (about 294) and the long elimination half-life (9–11 hours) suggest that both compounds will be excreted into milk. The effect of this exposure on a nursing infant is unknown. However, the American Academy of Pediatrics classifies other tricyclic antidepressants as drugs whose effect on the nursing infant is unknown but may be of concern (see Amitriptyline).

References

1. Committee on Drugs, American Academy of Pediatrics. Use of psychoactive medication during pregnancy and possible effects on the fetus and newborn. Pediatrics 2000;105:880–7.
2. Product information. Surmontil. Odyssey Pharmaceuticals, 2004.
3. Parfitt K, ed. *Martindale: The Complete Drug Reference*. 32nd ed. London, UK: Pharmaceutical Press, 1999:310.
4. Jurand A. Malformations of the central nervous system induced by neurotropic drugs in mouse embryos. Develop Growth Differ 1980;22:61–78. As cited by Shepard TH. *Catalog of Teratogenic Agents*. 10th ed. Baltimore, MD: The Johns Hopkins University Press, 2001:510.
5. Alvarez FJ, Casas E, Franganillo A, Velasco A. Effects of antidepressants on histamine H^2 receptors in rat isolated uterus. J Pharmacol (Paris) 1986;17:351–4.
6. McElhatton PR, Garbis HM, Elefant E, Vial T, Bellemin B, Mastroiacovo P, Arnon J, Rodriguez-Pinilla E, Schaefer C, Pexieder T, Merlob P, Dal Verme S. The outcome of pregnancy in 689 women exposed to therapeutic doses of antidepressants. A collaborative study of the European Network of Teratology Information Services (ENTIS). Reprod Toxicol 1996;10:285–94.

TRIPELENNAMINE

[Withdrawn from the market. See 9th edition.]

TRIPROLIDINE

Antihistamine

PREGNANCY RECOMMENDATION: Compatible
BREASTFEEDING RECOMMENDATION: Limited Human Data—Probably Compatible

PREGNANCY SUMMARY

The human pregnancy experience with triprolidine suggests low risk. In general, antihistamines are considered low risk in pregnancy. However, exposure near birth of premature infants has been associated with an increased risk of retrolental fibroplasia.

FETAL RISK SUMMARY

Triprolidine is an antihistamine in the same class as brompheniramine, chlorpheniramine, and dexchlorpheniramine. The drug is used in a number of proprietary decongestant–antihistamine mixtures.

It is not known if triprolidine crosses the human placenta. The molecular weight (about 279 for the nonhydrated free base) suggests that exposure of the embryo–fetus should be expected.

The Collaborative Perinatal Project monitored 50,282 mother–child pairs, 16 of whom had 1st trimester exposure to triprolidine (1). From this small sample, no evidence was found to suggest a relationship to large categories of major or minor malformations or to individual malformations.

In a 1971 study, infants and mothers who had ingested antihistamines during the 1st trimester actually had fewer abnormalities when compared with controls (2). Triprolidine was the third most commonly used antihistamine.

The manufacturer claims that in more than 20 years of marketing the drug, no reports of triprolidine teratogenicity have been received (M.F. Frosolono, personal communication, Burroughs Wellcome, 1980). Their animal studies have also been negative.

Two studies, one appearing in 1981 (3) and the second in 1985 (4), described the 1st trimester drug exposures of 6837 and 6509 mothers, respectively, treated by the Group Health Cooperative of Puget Sound and whose pregnancies terminated in a live birth. Both studies covered 30-month periods, 1977–1979 and 1980–1982, respectively. From the total of 13,346 mothers, 628 (4.7%) consumed during the 1st trimester (based on the filling of a prescription) a proprietary product containing triprolidine and pseudoephedrine (Actifed). Nine (1.4%) of the exposed infants had a major congenital abnormality (type not specified). Spontaneous or induced abortions, stillbirths, and many minor anomalies, such as clubfoot, syndactyly, polydactyly, clinodactyly, minor ear defects, coronal or first-degree hypospadias, and hernia, were excluded from the data.

In two surveillance studies of Michigan Medicaid recipients involving 333,440 completed pregnancies conducted between 1980 and 1983, and 1985 and 1992, 910 newborns had been exposed to triprolidine during the 1st trimester (F. Rosa, personal communication, FDA, 1994). Of the 900 exposed newborns identified in the 1980–1983 group, 65 (7.2%) had major birth defects (59 expected), 10 of which were cardiovascular defects (8 expected). No cases of cleft lip and/or palate were observed. None of the 10 newborns included in the 1985–1992 data had congenital malformations.

BREASTFEEDING SUMMARY

Triprolidine is excreted into breast milk (5). Three mothers, who were nursing healthy infants, were given an antihistamine–decongestant preparation containing 2.5 mg of triprolidine and 60 mg of pseudoephedrine. The women had been nursing their infants for 14 weeks, 14 weeks, and 18 months, respectively. Triprolidine was found in the milk of all three subjects, with milk:plasma ratios in one woman at 1, 3, and 12 hours of 0.5, 1.2, and 0.7, respectively. Using AUCs in the other two women gave more reliable results of 0.56 and 0.50 (5). The authors calculated that a milk production of 1000 mL/24 hours would contain 0.001–0.004 mg of triprolidine base, or about 0.06%–0.2% of the maternal dose. The American Academy of Pediatrics classifies triprolidine as compatible with breastfeeding (6).

References

1. Heinonen OP, Slone D, Shapiro S. *Birth Defects and Drugs in Pregnancy*. Littleton, MA: Publishing Sciences Group, 1977:323.
2. Nelson MM, Forfar JO. Associations between drugs administered during pregnancy and congenital abnormalities of the fetus. Br Med J 1971;1:523–7.
3. Jick H, Holmes LB, Hunter JR, Madsen S, Stergachis A. First-trimester drug use and congenital disorders. JAMA 1981;246:343–6.
4. Aselton P, Jick H, Milunsky A, Hunter JR, Stergachis A. First-trimester drug use and congenital disorders. Obstet Gynecol 1985;65:451–5.
5. Findlay JWA, Butz RF, Sailstad JM, Warren JT, Welch RM. Pseudoephedrine and triprolidine in plasma and breast milk of nursing mothers. Br J Clin Pharmacol 1984;18:901–6.
6. Committee on Drugs, American Academy of Pediatrics. The transfer of drugs and other chemicals into human milk. Pediatrics 2001;108:776–89.

TROGLITAZONE

[Withdrawn from the market. See 9th edition.]

TROLEANDOMYCIN

[Withdrawn from the market. See 9th edition.]

TROSPIUM

Urinary Tract Agent (Antispasmodic)

PREGNANCY RECOMMENDATION: No Human Data—Animal Data Suggest Low Risk
BREASTFEEDING RECOMMENDATION: No Human Data—Probably Compatible

PREGNANCY SUMMARY

No reports describing the use of trospium in human pregnancy have been located. The drug caused fetal death in two animal species but maternal toxicity was also evident. There was no evidence of malformations or developmental delays in surviving offspring. Although the absence of human pregnancy experience prevents a full assessment of the embryo–fetal risk, there is no evidence that other parasympatholytics (e.g., see Atropine), in the absence of maternal toxicity, cause developmental toxicity. Until human experience is available, the safest course is to avoid trospium in pregnancy. However, if inadvertent exposure in pregnancy does occur, the embryo–fetal risk is probably low.

FETAL RISK SUMMARY

Trospium, a quaternary ammonium compound, is an antispasmodic, antimuscarinic agent indicated for the treatment of overactive bladder with symptoms or urge urinary incontinence, urgency, and urinary frequency. The drug has negligible affinity for nicotinic receptors compared with muscarinic receptors. Trospium is in the same subclass as darifenacin, flavoxate, oxybutynin, solifenacin, and tolterodine. A mean 9.6% of an oral dose is absorbed under fasting conditions, but when ingested with a high fat meal, this limited systemic bioavailability is reduced by 70%–80%. Protein binding in serum ranges from 50% to 85% at therapeutic concentrations. The plasma elimination half-life is about 20 hours (1).

Reproduction studies have been conducted in rats and rabbits. In rats, a dose producing exposure about 10 times the human exposure (HE) caused maternal toxicity and a decrease in fetal survival. However, no impaired fertility, malformations, or developmental delays were observed. The no-effect levels for maternal and fetal toxicity were approximately equivalent to the HE. Neither malformations nor developmental delays were observed in pregnant rabbits. The no-effect levels for maternal and fetal toxicity were 5–6 times the HE. Trospium was not carcinogenic in long-term studies conducted in mice and rats and was not mutagenic in various assays (1).

It is not known if trospium crosses the human placenta. The molecular weight (about 428) and elimination half-life suggest that the drug will cross. However, trospium is a water-soluble quaternary ammonium compound that is ionized at physiologic pH. These characteristics should limit the amount of drug reaching the embryo–fetal compartment.

BREASTFEEDING SUMMARY

No reports describing the use of trospium during human lactation have been located. The molecular weight (about 428) and elimination half-life (about 20 hours) suggest that the drug will be excreted, especially into colostrum during the first 2–3 days after birth. Trospium is a water-soluble quaternary ammonium compound that is ionized at physiologic pH. This should limit the amount of drug reaching mature milk. Although neonates are particularly sensitive to anticholinergics, two other agents in this class (both tertiary amine compounds) are classified by the American Academy of Pediatrics as compatible with breastfeeding (see Atropine and Scopolamine). The effect of exposure to trospium on a nursing infant is unknown, but the risk of toxicity is probably low.

Reference

1. Product information. Sanctura. Odyssey Pharmaceuticals, 2005.

TROVAFLOXACIN

[Withdrawn from the market. See 9th edition.]

TYROPANOATE

[Withdrawn from the market. See 9th edition.]

T

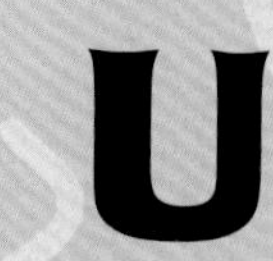

ULIPRISTAL

Emergency Contraceptive

PREGNANCY RECOMMENDATION: Contraindicated
BREASTFEEDING RECOMMENDATION: Contraindicated

PREGNANCY SUMMARY

No reports describing the use of ulipristal in human pregnancy have been located. As an emergency contraceptive, the main action is delaying or inhibiting ovulation (1–5). Animal studies suggest that pregnancy loss is a risk, but the absence of human pregnancy experience prevents a more complete assessment of this effect. The drug is contraindicated in pregnancy.

FETAL RISK SUMMARY

Ulipristal is an oral selective progesterone receptor modulator with potent antagonist/partial agonist properties that is used as an emergency contraceptive. It is indicated for prevention of pregnancy within 120 hours (5 days) after unprotected intercourse or a known or suspected contraceptive failure. The pharmacodynamic effects of ulipristal depend on the phase of the menstrual cycle when it is administered. Administration in the mid-follicular phase results in the inhibition of folliculogenesis and a reduction in estradiol concentration. When given at the time of the luteinizing hormone peak, follicular rupture is delayed by 5–9 days. Dosing in the early luteal phase does not significantly delay endometrial maturation but does decrease endometrial thickness, thereby interfering with implantation. Ulipristal is metabolized to its active metabolite, monodemethyl-ulipristal. Ulipristal is highly bound (>94%) to plasma proteins, including lipoproteins, α-1-acid glycoprotein, and albumin. The terminal half-lives of ulipristal and monodemethyl-ulipristal are about 32 and 27 hours, respectively (1).

Reproduction studies have been conducted in rats, rabbits, and monkeys. In rats and rabbits, doses during organogenesis at daily exposures that were 0.33 and 0.5 times, respectively, the human exposure based on BSA (HE-BSA) resulted in embryo–fetal loss in all of the pregnant rats and in half of the pregnant rabbits. No malformations were noted in the surviving fetuses. Adverse effects were not observed in rat offspring when the dose was about 0.04 times the HE based on AUC during organogenesis through lactation. In pregnant monkeys, daily doses for 4 days during the 1st trimester that were about 4 times the HE-BSA caused pregnancy termination in two of five animals (1).

Carcinogenicity studies have not been conducted with ulipristal. The drug was not genotoxic in multiple assays. In rats, single doses at 2 times the HE-BSA prevented ovulation in 50% of the animals. When given on postcoital days 4 or 5, single doses that were 4–12 times the HE-BSA prevented pregnancy in 80%–100% of the rats. Similar doses in rabbits on postcoital days 5 or 6 prevented pregnancy in 50% of the animals. Lower doses for 4 days in rats and rabbits were also effective in preventing ovulation and pregnancy (1).

It is not known if ulipristal or its active metabolite crosses the human placenta. The molecular weights (about 476 for ulipristal acetate; lower for the active metabolite) and the long elimination half-lives of both agents suggest that they will cross to the embryo–fetus, but the high plasma protein binding may limit the exposure.

BREASTFEEDING SUMMARY

No reports describing the use of ulipristal during human lactation have been located. The molecular weights (about 476 for ulipristal acetate; lower for the active metabolite) and the long elimination half-lives (32 and 27 hours) of the parent drug and active metabolite suggest that both will be excreted into breast milk, but the high plasma protein binding may limit the amount excreted. The effect on a nursing infant from short-term exposure to a potent progesterone antagonist/partial agonist is unknown. However, not breastfeeding is the best course.

References

1. Product information. Ella. Watson Pharma, 2010.
2. Benagiano G, Bastianelli, Farris M. Selective progesterone receptor modulators 1: use during pregnancy. Expert Opin Pharmacother 2008;9:2459–72.
3. Gemzell-Danielsson K, Meng CX. Emergency contraception: potential role of ulipristal acetate. Int J Womens Health 2010;2:53–61.
4. Fine PM. Ulipristal acetate: a new emergency contraceptive that is safe and more effective than levonorgestrel. Women's Health (Long Engl) 2011;7:9–17.
5. Fine PM. Update on emergency contraception. Adv Ther 2011;28:87–90.

UREA

Diuretic

PREGNANCY RECOMMENDATION: No Human Data—No Relevant Animal Data
BREASTFEEDING RECOMMENDATION: No Human Data—Probably Compatible

PREGNANCY SUMMARY

Urea is an osmotic diuretic that is used primarily to treat cerebral edema. Topical formulations for skin disorders are also available. No reports of its use in pregnancy following IV, oral, or topical administration have been located. Urea, given by intra-amniotic injection, has been used for the induction of abortion (1).

BREASTFEEDING SUMMARY

No reports describing the use of urea during human lactation have been located.

Reference

1. Ware A, ed. *Martindale: The Extra Pharmacopoeia*. 27th ed. London: The Pharmaceutical Press, 1977:572.

UROKINASE

Thrombolytic

PREGNANCY RECOMMENDATION: Limited Human Data—Animal Data Suggest Low Risk
BREASTFEEDING RECOMMENDATION: No Human Data—Probably Compatible

PREGNANCY SUMMARY

The use of urokinase during pregnancy does not appear to represent a major risk to the fetus. The drug is not fetotoxic or teratogenic in rodents. However, only two human cases treated with this thrombolytic agent during the 1st trimester (one at 14 weeks and the other at 3 months) have been reported. It is not known whether the drug crosses the placenta to the fetus, but placental tissue contains proteinase inhibitors that inactivate urokinase (1,2). Placental separation and hemorrhage is a potential complication and has been reported in one case.

FETAL RISK SUMMARY

Urokinase, 100,000 IU/kg intraperitoneal, was not teratogenic in rats or mice (3). The manufacturer cites studies in which doses up to 1000 times the human dose did not impair fertility or produce fetal harm in rats and mice (4). Six reports of its use in human pregnancy have been located.

A woman at 28 weeks' gestation was treated with urokinase, 4400 IU/kg for 10 minutes followed by 4400 IU/kg/hr for 12 hours, for pulmonary embolism (5). Heparin therapy was then administered, first IV and then SC, for the remainder of the pregnancy. A healthy term infant was delivered 2 months after initiation of therapy (5).

A 1995 review briefly cited two reports of patients treated with urokinase, apparently without fetal or neonatal complications, for thrombosed prosthetic heart valves (6). A 36-year-old woman was treated at 14 and 32 weeks' gestation and had an uncomplicated cesarean delivery at 34 weeks (6,7). The other patient, a 32-year-old woman, was treated twice with different thrombolytics: first at 3 months' gestation with urokinase and second at 6 months' gestation with streptokinase (6,8). Minor uterine hemorrhage because of placental separation occurred at 3 months and a cesarean section was performed at 7 months' gestation. Maternal transfusion and surgical drainage were required following the delivery.

A 27-year-old woman in premature labor developed a massive pulmonary embolism at 31 weeks' gestation (9). She was initially treated with a bolus dose of urokinase (200,000 IU) and heparin. Dobutamine was also administered to maintain a stable hemodynamic state. Because her condition continued to deteriorate, she was treated with low-dose alteplase with eventual successful resolution of the embolism. A healthy preterm 2100-g male infant was delivered about 3 days after urokinase administration (9).

A 1994 report described a woman at 26 weeks' gestation who suffered a myocardial infarction (10). Following stabilization, she underwent cardiac catheterization 9 days after the initial infarction, which revealed 90% occlusion of the proximal right coronary artery and mild narrowing of other cardiac arteries. A prolonged intracoronary infusion of urokinase, in preparation for a planned angioplasty, failed to improve the right coronary occlusion, and coronary stents were subsequently placed. A healthy female infant was eventually delivered at 39 weeks (10).

The treatment of massive pulmonary embolism, diagnosed in a 20-year-old woman at 21 weeks' gestation, with urokinase and heparin was described in a 1995 case report (11). The patient markedly improved after receiving two courses of urokinase, 4400 IU/kg for 10 minutes followed by 4400 IU/kg/hr continuous infusion for 12 hours, approximately 6 hours apart, followed by continuous heparin. No complications of therapy were observed in the fetus, and she eventually delivered a healthy 3122-g male infant at term (11).

BREASTFEEDING SUMMARY

No reports describing the use of urokinase during lactation have been located. Because of the nature of the indications for urokinase and its very short half-life (≤20 minutes), the opportunities for its use during lactation and the potential exposure of the nursing infant are minimal.

References

1. Holmberg L, Lecander I, Persson B, Åstedt B. An inhibitor from placenta specifically binds urokinase and inhibits plasminogen activator released from ovarian carcinoma in tissue culture. Biochem Biophys Acta 1978;544:128–37.
2. Walker JE, Gow L, Campbell DM, Ogston D. The inhibition by plasma of urokinase and tissue activator-induced fibrinolysis in pregnancy and the puerperium. Thromb Haemost 1983;49:21–3.
3. Shepard TH. *Catalog of Teratogenic Agents*. 8th ed. Baltimore, MD: The Johns Hopkins University Press, 1995:437–8.
4. Product information. Abbokinase. Abbott Laboratories, 2000.
5. Delclos GL, Davila F. Thrombolytic therapy for pulmonary embolism in pregnancy: a case report. Am J Obstet Gynecol 1986;155:375–6.
6. Turrentine MA, Braems G, Ramirez MM. Use of thrombolytics for the treatment of thromboembolic disease during pregnancy. Obstet Gynecol Survey 1995;50:534–41.
7. Jimenez M, Vergnes C, Brottier L, Dequeker JL, Billes MA, Lorient Roudaut MF, Choussat A, Boisseau MR. Thrombose récidivante d'une prothèse valvulaire aortique chez une femme enceinte. Traitement par urokinase. J Mal Vasc 1988;13:46–9.
8. Tissot H, Vergnes C, Rougier P, Bricaud H, Dallay D. Traitement fibrinolytique par urokinase et streptokinase d'une thrombose récidivante sur double prothèse valvulaire aortique mitrale au cours de la grossesse. J Gynecol Obstet Biol Reprod (Paris) 1991;20:1093–6.
9. Flossdorf TH, Breulmann M, Hopf HB. Successful treatment of massive pulmonary embolism with recombinant tissue type plasminogen activator (rt-PA) in a pregnant woman with intact gravidity and preterm labour. Intensive Care Med 1990;16:454–6.
10. Sanchez-Ramos L, Chami YG, Bass TA, DelValle GO, Adair CD. Myocardial infarction during pregnancy: management with transluminal coronary angioplasty and metallic intracoronary stents. Am J Obstet Gynecol 1994;171:1392–3.
11. Kramer WB, Belfort M, Saade GR, Surani S, Moise KJ Jr. Successful urokinase treatment of massive pulmonary embolism in pregnancy. Obstet Gynecol 1995;86:660–2.

URSODIOL

Gastrointestinal Agent (Gallstone Solubilizing Agent)

PREGNANCY RECOMMENDATION: Compatible
BREASTFEEDING RECOMMENDATION: No Human Data—Probably Compatible

PREGNANCY SUMMARY

Ursodiol is effective in the treatment of intrahepatic cholestasis of pregnancy and its use for this purpose appears to be low risk for the fetus. Studies have shown a significant decrease in maternal morbidity and fetal mortality. No explanation could be found for the case of stillbirth, but these outcomes in untreated cholestasis have been reported.

FETAL RISK SUMMARY

Ursodiol (ursodeoxycholic acid) is a naturally occurring bile acid used orally to dissolve gallstones. The drug has been used for the treatment of intrahepatic cholestasis of pregnancy.

No fetal adverse effects were observed when ursodiol (up to 200 mg/kg/day) was fed to pregnant rats (1). Embryotoxicity was observed in another rat study, but this was less than with another closely related bile acid, chenodiol, and no evidence of hepatotoxicity was observed at three dose levels (2). Reproduction studies in rats with doses up to 22 times the recommended maximum human dose based on BSA (RMHD) and in rabbits with doses up to 7 times the RMHD revealed no evidence of impaired fertility or fetal harm (3).

Ursodiol is absorbed from the small intestine and is extracted and conjugated by the liver. Although 30%–50% of a dose may enter the systemic circulation, continuous hepatic uptake keeps ursodiol blood levels low and uptake by tissues other than the liver is considered nil (4). These factors combined with tight binding to albumin probably indicate that placental passage to the fetus does not occur.

During clinical trials, inadvertent exposure during the 1st trimester to therapeutic doses of ursodiol in four women had no effect on their fetuses or newborns (3). Several reports, summarized below, described the apparent safe use of ursodiol in the latter portion of human pregnancy for the treatment of intrahepatic cholestasis.

A brief 1991 report described the use of ursodiol in the treatment of late-onset intrahepatic cholestasis during pregnancy (5). A 30-year-old primigravida was given ursodiol 600 mg/day in two divided doses for 20 days starting at 34 weeks' gestation. No signs of fetal distress were observed during treatment. Labor was induced at 37 weeks' gestation and a healthy 2670-g female infant was delivered with Apgar scores of 9 and 10 at 1 and 5 minutes, respectively (5).

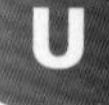

A second report, published in 1992, briefly described the successful outcome of eight pregnant women with intrahepatic cholestasis treated with ursodiol, 1 g/day for 3 weeks (6). The full report of this study was also published in 1992 (7). Treatment began after 25 weeks' gestation in the eight women, five receiving 1 g/day in divided dose for 20 consecutive days and the other three receiving the same dose for two 20-day treatment courses, separated by a 14-day drug-free interval (7). The mean dose was 14 mg/kg/day (range 12–17 mg/kg/day). All of the newborns had Apgar scores >7 at 1 and 5 minutes and all were progressing normally at a 5-month follow-up (7).

A 1994 report described the use of ursodiol, 450 mg/day, in three pregnancies (singleton, twin, and quintuplet) for intrahepatic cholestasis (8). Ursodiol was started because of unsuccessful attempts to control the disease with cholestyramine or ademetionine (S-adenosyl-L-methionine [SAMe]). The singleton pregnancy was treated from 29 weeks' gestation to delivery at 37 weeks' gestation, the twin pregnancy from 27 to 33 weeks' gestation, and the woman with quintuplets from 21 weeks' gestation to delivery at 30 weeks' gestation. No adverse effects were observed in the eight newborns (8).

A significant reduction in the perinatal mortality and morbidity associated with cholestasis of pregnancy following the use of ursodiol was described in a study published in 1995 (9). Eight women with a history of 13 pregnancies affected by the disease were referred to a specialty clinic before conception. Expectant management had been used in 12 of the 13 pregnancies, with 11 experiencing adverse outcomes: 8 stillbirths, 2 premature deliveries with 1 death in the perinatal period, and 1 emergency cesarean section for fetal distress. Subsequently, three of the women became pregnant again and each suffered a recurrence of cholestasis. Therapy with ursodiol, 750 mg/day in two and 1000 mg/day in one, was initiated at 31, 33, and 37 weeks' gestation, respectively. The first patient had been pretreated with ademetionine from 16 to 31 weeks in an unsuccessful attempt to prevent cholestasis. Each of the three women showed rapid clinical improvement and resolution of abnormal liver tests following initiation of ursodiol. Normal infants, who were doing well, were delivered at 35, 35, and 38 weeks, respectively (9).

A double-blind, placebo-controlled trial in women with intrahepatic cholestasis of pregnancy compared the effect of ursodiol treatment ($N = 8$) with placebo ($N = 8$) (10). Significant decreases in the pruritus score and all liver biochemical parameters occurred in the ursodiol group, but only the pruritus score and alanine aminotransferase were significantly improved in controls. Moreover, the gestational age at delivery in the treated group was 38 weeks compared with 34 weeks in controls ($p < 0.01$), resulting in higher mean birth weights (2935 vs. 2025 g). Apgar scores were also higher in the treated group. Fetal distress was observed in four of the control pregnancies (none in the study group) and these were delivered by cesarean section. In the treated group, six of the eight newborns were delivered vaginally. At a 5-month follow-up, all infants were developing normally (10). A number of other reports have found that ursodiol is safe and effective for the treatment of cholestasis of pregnancy (11–15).

A 2006 case report described a woman at 28 weeks' gestation who presented with intrahepatic cholestasis of pregnancy (16). She was initially treated with cholestyramine and then changed to two separate courses of ursodiol with resulting decreased transaminases and bile acids. Although the patient's course was followed closely, death of a 3400-g female fetus occurred at 39 3/7 weeks. At autopsy, meconium was noted in the bronchioles and alveoli, but no other abnormalities were found. The cause of the fetal death was unknown (16).

BREASTFEEDING SUMMARY

No reports have been located that described the use of ursodiol during lactation. Because only small amounts of ursodiol appear in the systemic circulation, which are tightly bound to albumin, it is doubtful that clinically significant amounts are excreted into breast milk.

References

1. Toyoshima S, Fujita H, Sakurai T, Sato R, Kashima M. Reproduction studies of ursodeoxycholic acid in rats. II. Teratogenicity study. Oyo Yakuri 1978;15:931–45. As cited in Shepard TH. *Catalog of Teratogenic Agents*. 8th ed. Baltimore, MD: The Johns Hopkins University Press, 1995:438.
2. Celle G, Cavanna M, Bocchini R, Robbiano L. Chenodeoxycholic acid (CDCA) versus ursodeoxycholic acid (UDCA): a comparison of their effects in pregnant rats. Arch Int Pharmacodyn Ther 1980;246:149–58.
3. Product information. Urso. Axcan Pharma U.S., 2000.
4. Bachrach WH, Hofmann AF. Ursodeoxycholic acid in the treatment of cholesterol cholelithiasis. Part I. Dig Dis Sci 1982;27:737–61.
5. Mazzella G, Rizzo N, Salzetta A, Iampieri R, Bovicelli L, Roda E. Management of intrahepatic cholestasis in pregnancy. Lancet 1991;338:1594–5.
6. Palma J, Reyes H, Ribalta J, Iglesias J, Gonzalez M. Management of intrahepatic cholestasis in pregnancy. Lancet 1992;339:1478.
7. Palma J, Reyes H, Ribalta J, Iglesias J, Gonzalez MC, Hernandez I, Alvarez C, Molina C, Danitz AM. Effects of ursodeoxycholic acid in patients with intrahepatic cholestasis of pregnancy. Hepatology 1992;15:1043–7.
8. Floreani A, Paternoster D, Grella V, Sacco S, Gangemi M, Chiaramonte M. Ursodeoxycholic acid in intrahepatic cholestasis of pregnancy. Br J Obstet Gynaecol 1994;101:64–5.
9. Davies MH, da Silva RCMA, Jones SR, Weaver JB, Elias E. Fetal mortality associated with cholestasis of pregnancy and the potential benefit of therapy with ursodeoxycholic acid. Gut 1995;37:580–4.
10. Diaferia A, Nicastri PL, Tartagni M, Loizzi P, Iacovizzi C, Di Leo A. Ursodeoxycholic acid therapy in pregnant women with cholestasis. Int J Gynecol Obstet 1996;52:133–40.
11. Floreani A, Paternoster D, Melis A, Grella PV. S-adenosylmethionine versus ursodeoxycholic acid in the treatment of intrahepatic cholestasis of pregnancy: preliminary results of a controlled trial. Eur J Obstet Gynecol Reprod Biol 1996;67:109–13.
12. Palma J, Reyes H, Ribalta J, Hernandez I, Sandoval L, Almuna R, Liepins J, Lira F, Sedano M, Silva O, Toha D, Silva JJ. Ursodeoxycholic acid in the treatment of cholestasis of pregnancy: a randomized, double-blind study controlled with placebo. J Hepatol 1997;27:1022–8.
13. Brites D, Rodrigues CMP, Oliveira N, Cardoso MC, Graca LM. Correction of maternal serum bile acid profile during ursodeoxycholic acid therapy in cholestasis of pregnancy. J Hepatol 1998;28:91–8.
14. Brites D, Rodrigues CMP, Cardoso MC, Graca LM. Unusual case of severe cholestasis of pregnancy with early onset, improved by ursodeoxycholic acid administration. Eur J Obstet Gynecol Reprod Biol 1998;76:165–8.
15. Nicastri PL, Diaferia A, Taartagni M, Loizzi P, Fanelli M. A randomized placebo-controlled trial of ursodeoxycholic acid and S-adenosylmethionine in the treatment of intrahepatic cholestasis of pregnancy. Br J Obstet Gynaecol 1998;105:1205–7.
16. Sentilhes L, Verspyck E, Pia P, Marpeau L. Fetal death in a patient with intrahepatic cholestasis of pregnancy. Obstet Gynecol 2006;107:458–60.

USTEKINUMAB

Immunologic Agent (Immunomodulator)

PREGNANCY RECOMMENDATION: Limited Human Data—Animal Data Suggest Low Risk
BREASTFEEDING RECOMMENDATION: No Human Data—Potential Toxicity

PREGNANCY SUMMARY

No published reports describing the use of ustekinumab in human pregnancy have been located. Thirteen pregnancies (protocol deviations) were identified during clinical studies, but specific details of the outcomes are very limited. Although the animal data suggest low risk, the limited human pregnancy experience prevents a more complete assessment of the embryo–fetal risk.

FETAL RISK SUMMARY

Ustekinumab is a human immunoglobulin GI_k ($IgG1_k$) monoclonal antibody against the P40 subunit of the interleukin (IL)-12 and IL-23 cytokines. It is given as an SC injection that is repeated at 4 weeks and then every 12 weeks. There are no other agents in this subclass. Ustekinumab is indicated for the treatment of patients with moderate to severe plaque psoriasis who are candidates for phototherapy or systemic therapy. Although the metabolism has not been fully characterized, the antibody is expected to be degraded into small peptides and amino acids similar to endogenous IgG. The mean half-life is about 15–46 days, but ranges are very long (1).

Reproduction studies were conducted in pregnant monkeys with doses up to 45 times the human dose based on body weight (HD) given either SC twice weekly or IV once weekly during organogenesis. No significant adverse developmental effects were observed. In a separate study, monkeys were given SC doses twice weekly up to 45 times the HD from the beginning of organogenesis to day 33 after delivery. In dams, there were no treatment-related effects on mortality, clinical signs, body weight, food consumption, hematology, or serum biochemistry. There were two neonatal deaths: one at 22.5 times the HD and one at 45 times the HD. No drug-related abnormalities were observed in the offspring from birth through 6 months of age in clinical signs, body weight, hematology, serum biochemistry, functional development before and after weaning, morphologic and immunologic development, and gross and histopathologic examinations (1).

Studies evaluating the carcinogenic or mutagenic potential of ustekinumab have not been conducted. However, in mice, inhibition of IL-12/IL-23p40 increased the risk of malignancy, but the relevance of these findings for malignancy risk in humans is unknown. The antibody did not cause toxicity or affect fertility parameters in male monkeys. An analogous antibody did not cause toxicity or affect fertility parameters in female mice that were given SC doses of the agent twice weekly beginning 15 days before cohabitation and continuing through gestational day 7 (1).

It is not known if ustekinumab crosses the human placenta before term. The molecular weight (range 148,079–149,690) is high, but IgG crosses the placenta late in pregnancy (see Immune Globulin Intravenous). Placental transfer of IgG was a function of dose, as well as gestational age. Moreover, the long half-life will place the protein at the maternal–fetal interface for prolonged periods. In unpublished data, ustekinumab crossed the placenta at the time of cesarean section (2).

During clinical studies, 30 pregnancies occurred (protocol deviations), 13 involved exposures in pregnant women and 17 were the result of paternal exposure (2). The drug was discontinued at the time of pregnancy diagnosis in all women. The outcome of the 13 cases were 2 live births with no defect or other adverse effect, 1 spontaneous abortion (SAB), 5 elective abortions (EABs) (all within 12 weeks of pregnancy), 3 ongoing pregnancies, and 2 unknown outcomes. The SAB occurred at 12 weeks' in a 42-year-old woman. No information was available on the presence or absence of fetal abnormalities in the EABs (2).

BREASTFEEDING SUMMARY

No reports describing the use of ustekinumab during human lactation have been located. The molecular weight (range 148,079–149,690) is high, but immunoglobulins and other large proteins are excreted into colostrum during the first 48 hours after birth. Moreover, the long half-life (15–46 days) will assure that the antibody is in the maternal plasma for long periods. In addition, ustekinumab is excreted into the milk of lactating monkeys (1). These data suggest that the antibody will be excreted into breast milk. The effect of this exposure on a nursing infant is unknown, but there may be an increased risk of infections and malignancies.

References

1. Product information. Stelara. Centocor Ortho Biotech, 2009.
2. Dermatologic and Ophthalmic Drugs Advisory Committee. Briefing document for ustekinumab (CNTO 1275). Available at http://www.fda.gov. Accessed May 4, 2010.

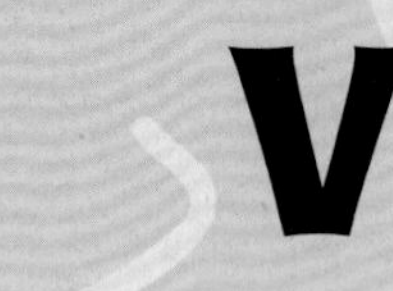

VACCINE, ADENOVIRUS TYPE 4 AND TYPE 7, LIVE

Vaccine

PREGNANCY RECOMMENDATION: Contraindicated
BREASTFEEDING RECOMMENDATION: No Human Data—Potential Toxicity

PREGNANCY SUMMARY

No apparent embryo or fetal harm was observed in four pregnancies inadvertently exposed to the vaccine. However, because naturally occurring infections with adenoviruses have been associated with fetal harm, the vaccine is contraindicated in pregnancy. Animal reproduction studies have not been conducted. If a pregnant woman receives the vaccine or becomes pregnant within 6 weeks following vaccination, clinicians are encouraged to report the exposure to the Adenovirus Pregnancy Registry by calling 1-866-790-4549 (1).

FETAL RISK SUMMARY

Adenovirus Type 4 and Type 7 vaccine, live, consists of nonattenuated, selected strains of human adenovirus Type 4 and human adenovirus Type 7. The vaccine is given as a single oral dose of two enteric coated tablets, one containing adenovirus Type 4 and the other adenovirus Type 7. The tablets are designed to pass intact through the stomach and release the live virus in the intestine. The vaccine is indicated for active immunization for the prevention of febrile acute respiratory disease caused by the two types of virus and is approved for use in military populations 17 through 50 years of age. Virus shedding in the stool following vaccination occurs over 28 days (1).

Animal studies for effects on reproduction and fertility have not been conducted, nor have studies for carcinogenicity or mutagenicity (1).

The manufacturer reported the pregnancy outcomes of four women enrolled in clinical trials who were given the vaccine. In three cases, the subjects were estimated to have conceived 2–13 days before vaccination, whereas the fourth subject conceived about 21 weeks after vaccination. In all four cases, healthy infants were born at estimated gestational ages of 36–40 weeks (1).

The effects of fetal infection with adenovirus were described in two case reports (2,3). In the first case, a 26-year-old woman presented at 29 weeks' gestation with a 1-week history of pedal and facial edema and polyhydramnios (2). Two weeks earlier, the woman had an upper respiratory tract infection characterized by low grade fever, conjunctivitis, rhinorrhea, and general malaise. At presentation, the fetal heart rate was 140–200 beats/minute. An ultrasound examination revealed fetal anasarca, massive ascites, scalp and skin edema, and pericardial and pleural effusions secondary to myocarditis presenting as nonimmune hydrops fetalis. A 2670-g female infant was born at 34 weeks' with an Apgar scores of 4 and 8 at 1 and 5 minutes, respectively. The infant had poor respiratory function and low heart rate that improved with treatment, scattered facial and truncal petechiae, periorbital edema, prominent right ventricular impulse without murmur, and hepatomegaly. An infection with adenovirus type 2 was diagnosed by polymerase chain reaction (PCR). The infant was discharged home at 2 weeks of age and was doing well 8 months later (2). The second case involved a 25-year-old woman with twins at 20 weeks' gestation (3). An ultrasound screen had noted hydrops fetalis in twin B. The mother had experienced upper airway congestion, myalgias, and malaise beginning 2 weeks before the screen. PCR analysis of the amniotic fluid revealed adenovirus (type not specified) in twin B but not in twin A. Polyhydramnios developed in twin B at 24 weeks'. Intrauterine fetal death of both twins occurred at 26 weeks'. Twin A weighed 615 g and twin B weighed 1685 g. No congenital anomalies were noted at autopsy (3).

BREASTFEEDING SUMMARY

No reports describing the exposure to the vaccine during lactation have been located. The live, nonattenuated viruses are shed in the stool over 28 days. The potential for febrile respiratory disease in a nursing infant from exposure is unknown. Nevertheless, the safest course is to avoid the vaccine during breastfeeding and for at least 28 days after vaccination.

References

1. Product information. Adenovirus Type 4 and Type 7 vaccine, Live. Teva Pharmaceuticals, 2011.
2. Towbin JA, Griffin LD, Martin AB, Nelson S, Moise KJ Jr, Zhang YH. Intrauterine adenoviral myocarditis presenting as nonimmune hydrops fetalis: diagnosis by polymerase chain reaction. Pediatr Infect Dis J 1994;13:144–50.
3. Forsnes EV, Eggleston MK, Wax JR. Differential transmission of adenovirus in a twin pregnancy. Obstet Gynecol 1998;91:817–8.

VACCINE, ANTHRAX

Vaccine

PREGNANCY RECOMMENDATION: Compatible
BREASTFEEDING RECOMMENDATION: Compatible

PREGNANCY SUMMARY

Although animal reproduction studies with anthrax vaccine adsorbed (AVA) have not been conducted, there appears to be no plausible biological mechanism for adverse pregnancy effects. Because of the absence of human pregnancy experience, however, the use of AVA during gestation is not recommended. The human reproduction data, limited to vaccination before conception, do not appear to suggest a risk from vaccination to either a woman's subsequent fertility or a subsequent pregnancy outcome. However, the published study cited below lacked sufficient power to detect adverse birth outcomes (1). Until more data are available, the recommendation made by the CDC in 2000 and 2008 (2,3) that "pregnant women should be vaccinated against anthrax only if the potential benefits outweigh the potential risks to the fetus" is still relevant.

FETAL RISK SUMMARY

Anthrax vaccine adsorbed is prepared from a cell-free, noninfectious filtrate of *Bacillus anthracis* that contains a mix of cellular products adsorbed to aluminum hydroxide (2). This vaccine has replaced a previously available alum-precipitated vaccine. An avirulent, nonencapsulated strain (V770-NP10R) of *B. anthracis* is used in the production of the vaccine, which contains no dead or live bacteria (1,2). The cellular products in the vaccine include, in unknown amounts, three proteins known as protective antigen (PA), lethal factor (LF), and edema factor (EF). Live *B. anthracis* forms combinations of these proteins resulting in two exotoxins known as lethal toxin (PA and LF) and edema toxin (PA and EF). The recommended vaccination schedule is 0.5 mL at 0, 2, and 4 weeks; three booster vaccinations at 6, 12, and 18 months; and then an annual booster injection (2).

Reproduction studies with anthrax vaccine have not been conducted in animals (4). However, no plausible biological mechanism for an adverse effect on an embryo or fetus has been proposed (1).

The placental transfer of the three proteins contained in the vaccine has not been studied. Because of the very high molecular weight, simple diffusion does not appear to be possible for transfer.

Only one study has been located that examined the effects of anthrax vaccine, administered before conception, on pregnancy outcome (1). Women, aged 17–44 years, assigned to two U.S. Army installations formed the study population. During the study period from January 1999 to March 2000, 3136 women received at least one dose of the vaccine (most received two or three doses), whereas 962 women were not vaccinated. Departure from the study sites was the most common reason for not receiving the vaccine. The only acceptable medical indications to defer or refuse the vaccine were pregnancy or immunity-compromising disease. There were 385 pregnancies after at least one dose of the vaccine. The annualized pregnancy rates in those vaccinated and not vaccinated were 159.5 and 160.0 per 1000 person-years, respectively. These rates were nearly identical to the pregnancy rates before the study. Compared with unvaccinated women, vaccinated women were 1.2 times as likely to give birth (95% confidence interval [CI] 0.8–1.8). Adjustment for marital status, race, and age did not change the odds ratio (OR). A total of 327 births (vaccinated and unvaccinated) were available for outcome analysis. Low birth weight (<2500 g) occurred in 11 cases (3.4%). After adjustment, the OR for vaccination and low birth weight was 1.3, 95% CI 0.2–6.4. Congenital malformations (specific details not provided) were observed in 15 cases, but no unusual patterns or clusters were noted. Only one malformation (polydactyly of the fingers) had multiple occurrences (three cases: two vaccinated, one unvaccinated). After adjustment, the OR for vaccination and structural anomalies was 0.7, 95% CI 0.2–2.3. The adjusted OR for vaccination and any adverse birth outcome was 0.9, 95% CI 0.4–2.4 (1).

BREASTFEEDING SUMMARY

No reports describing the use of anthrax vaccine in lactating women have been located. Because of the nature of anthrax vaccine, the potential for adverse effects in a nursing infant appear to be nil. The CDC states that there is no evidence to suggest a risk to the mother or nursing infant, and the administration of the vaccine during breastfeeding is not medically contraindicated (2,3).

References

1. Wiesen AR, Little CT. Relationship between prepregnancy anthrax vaccination and pregnancy and birth outcomes among US Army women. JAMA 2002;287:1556–60.
2. CDC. Use of anthrax vaccine in the United States. Recommendations of the Advisory Committee on Immunization Practices (ACIP). MMWR 2000;49(No. RR15):11.
3. CDC. *Guidelines for Vaccinating Pregnant Women*. Available at http://www.cdc.gov/vaccines/pubs/preg-guide.htm. Accessed May 16, 2010.
4. CDC. Notice to readers: Status of U.S. Department of Defense preliminary evaluation of the association of anthrax vaccination and congenital anomalies. MMWR 2002;51(6):127.

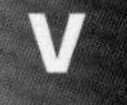

VACCINE, BCG

Vaccine

PREGNANCY RECOMMENDATION: Compatible—Maternal Benefit >> Embryo–Fetal Risk
BREASTFEEDING RECOMMENDATION: No Human Data—Probably Compatible

PREGNANCY SUMMARY

BCG vaccine is a live, attenuated bacteria vaccine used to provide immunity to tuberculosis (1). Animal reproduction studies have not been conducted with the vaccine. The risk to the fetus from maternal vaccination is unknown. Because it is a live preparation, the CDC recommends that it not be used in pregnancy (2).

BREASTFEEDING SUMMARY

No reports describing the use of BCG vaccine in human lactation have been located. However, there does not appear to be any risk to a nursing infant if the mother receives the vaccine (2).

References

1. American Hospital Formulary Service. *Drug Information 1997*. Bethesda, MD: American Society of Health-System Pharmacists, 1997:2569–72.
2. CDC. *Guidelines for Vaccinating Pregnant Women*. Available at http://www.cdc.gov/vaccines/pubs/preg-guide.htm. Accessed May 16, 2010.

VACCINE, CHOLERA

Vaccine

PREGNANCY RECOMMENDATION: Compatible
BREASTFEEDING RECOMMENDATION: Compatible

PREGNANCY SUMMARY

Cholera vaccine is a killed bacteria vaccine (1). Cholera during pregnancy may result in significant morbidity and mortality to the mother and the fetus, particularly during the 3rd trimester. The risk to the fetus from maternal vaccination is unknown because there is no specific information on the safety of the vaccine during pregnancy (2).

BREASTFEEDING SUMMARY

Maternal vaccination with cholera vaccine has increased specific IgA antibody titers in breast milk (3). In a second study, cholera vaccine (whole cell plus toxoid) was administered to six lactating mothers, resulting in a significant rise in milk anti-cholera toxin IgA titers in five of the patients (4). Milk from three of these five mothers also had a significant increase in anti-cholera toxin IgG titers.

References

1. Amstey MS. Vaccination in pregnancy. Clin Obstet Gynaecol 1983;10:13–22.
2. CDC. Recommendations of the Immunization Practices Advisory Committee. Cholera Vaccine. MMWR 1988;37 (No. 40):617–24.
3. Svennerholm AM, Holmgren J, Hanson LA, Lindblad BS, Quereshi F, Rahimtoola RJ. Boosting of secretory IgA antibody responses in man by parenteral cholera vaccination. Scand J Immunol 1977;6:1345–49.
4. Merson MH, Black RE, Sack DA, Svennerholm AM, Holmgren J. Maternal cholera immunisation and secretory IgA in breast milk. Lancet 1980;1:931–2.

VACCINE, *ESCHERICHIA COLI*

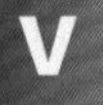

Vaccine

PREGNANCY RECOMMENDATION: Limited Human Data—Probably Compatible
BREASTFEEDING RECOMMENDATION: Compatible

PREGNANCY SUMMARY

Escherichia coli (*E. coli*) vaccine is a nonpathogenic strain of bacteria used experimentally as a vaccine. Two reports of its use (strains O111 and 083) in pregnant women in labor or waiting for the onset of labor have been located (1,2). The vaccines were given to these patients in an attempt to produce antimicrobial activity in their colostrum. No adverse effects in the newborns were noted.

BREASTFEEDING SUMMARY

Escherichia coli (*E. coli* strains O111 and 083) vaccines were given to mothers in labor or waiting for the onset of labor (1,2). Antibodies against *E. coli* were found in the colostrum of 7 of 47 (strain 0111) and 3 of 3 (strain 083) treated mothers but in only 1 of 101 controls. No adverse effects were noted in the nursing infants.

References

1. Dluholucky S, Siragy P, Dolezel P, Svac J, Bolgac A. Antimicrobial activity of colostrum after administering killed Escherichia coli O111 vaccine orally to expectant mothers. Arch Dis Child 1980;55:558–60.
2. Goldblum RM, Ahlstedt S, Carlsson B, Hanson LA, Jodal U, Lidin-Janson G, Sohl-Akerlund A. Antibody-forming cells in human colostrum after oral immunisation. Nature 1975;257:797–9.

VACCINE, GROUP B STREPTOCOCCAL

Vaccine

PREGNANCY RECOMMENDATION: Compatible
BREASTFEEDING RECOMMENDATION: Compatible

PREGNANCY SUMMARY

Group B Streptococcus (GBS) capsular polysaccharides (CPS) vaccine has been used in pregnancy in an attempt to prevent infection in the newborn (1). The vaccine is considered safe in pregnancy.

FETAL RISK SUMMARY

Forty women at a mean gestational age of 31 weeks (range 26–36 weeks) were administered a single 50-mcg dose of type III CPS of GBS (1). No adverse effects were observed in the 40 newborns. The overall response rate to the vaccine, which is not commercially available, was 63%. Of the 25 infants born to mothers who had responded to the vaccine, at 1 and 3 months of age, 80% and 64%, respectively, continued to have protective levels of antibody (1). Although the vaccine is considered safe (2), as are other bacterial vaccines (3), the clinical effectiveness of the vaccine has not been determined and its use remains controversial (4–7).

In an attempt to improve on the immunogenic response in adults, researchers designed a GBS type III CPS–tetanus toxoid conjugate vaccine (8). Although administered to nonpregnant women, vaccination with the CPS–protein conjugate preparation resulted in enhanced immunogenicity compared with uncoupled vaccine. Although the results are encouraging, it is not known at the present time whether this vaccine will produce a similar response in pregnant women or whether it will prevent perinatal infection.

BREASTFEEDING SUMMARY

Although there are no reports describing the use of Group B streptococcal vaccine during lactation, the agent should represent no risk to a nursing infant.

References

1. Baker CJ, Rench MA, Edwards MS, Carpenter RJ, Hays BM, Kasper DL. Immunization of pregnant women with a polysaccharide vaccine of Group B streptococcus. N Engl J Med 1988;319:1180–5.
2. Faix RG. Maternal immunization to prevent fetal and neonatal infection. Clin Obstet Gynecol 1991;34:277–87.
3. CDC. Immunization Practices Advisory Committee. General recommendations on immunization. MMWR 1989;38:205–27.
4. Franciosi RA. Group B streptococcal vaccine in pregnant women. N Engl J Med 1989;320:807–8.
5. Baker CJ, Edwards MS. Group B streptococcal vaccine in pregnant women. N Engl J Med 1989;320:808.
6. Insel RA. Group B streptococcal vaccine in pregnant women. N Engl J Med 1989;320:808–9.
7. Linder N, Ohel G. In utero vaccination. Clin Perinatol 1994;21:663–74.
8. Kasper DL, Paoletti LC, Wessels MR, Guttormsen H-K, Carey VJ, Jennings HJ, Baker CJ. Immune response to type III Group B streptococcal polysaccharide-tetanus toxoid conjugate vaccine. J Clin Invest 1996;98:2308–14.

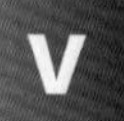

VACCINE, HAEMOPHILUS B CONJUGATE

Vaccine

PREGNANCY RECOMMENDATION: Compatible
BREASTFEEDING RECOMMENDATION: Compatible

PREGNANCY SUMMARY

Commercially available Haemophilus b conjugate vaccine is a combination of the capsular polysaccharides or oligosaccharides purified from *Haemophilus influenzae* type b bound with various proteins including tetanus toxoid, diphtheria toxoid, meningococcal protein, or diphtheria CRM_{197} (1). The human pregnancy experience is very limited, but the vaccine is probably compatible in pregnancy.

FETAL RISK SUMMARY

Two reports (2,3) and a review (4) have described the maternal immunization with the capsular polysaccharide vaccine of *H. influenzae* type b during the 3rd trimester of pregnancy to achieve passive immunity in the fetus and newborn. No adverse effects were observed in the newborns.

BREASTFEEDING SUMMARY

Women who were vaccinated with Haemophilus b conjugate vaccine at 34–36 weeks' gestation had significantly higher antibody titers (>20 times) in their colostrum than either nonimmunized women or those who were vaccinated before pregnancy (5). Breast milk antibody titers were also significantly higher (>20 times) than the comparison groups at 3 and 6 months after delivery.

References

1. American Hospital Formulary Service. *Drug Information 1997*. Bethesda, MD: American Society of Health-System Pharmacists, 1997:2574–81.
2. Amstey MS, Insel R, Munoz J, Pichichero M. Fetal-neonatal passive immunization against *Hemophilus influenzae*, type b. Am J Obstet Gynecol 1985;153:607–11.
3. Glezen WP, Englund JA, Siber GR, Six HR, Turner C, Shriver D, Hinkley CM, Falcao O. Maternal immunization with the capsular polysaccharide vaccine for *Haemophilus influenzae* type b. J Infect Dis 1992;165(Suppl 1):S134–6.
4. Linder N, Ohel G. In utero vaccination. Clin Perinatol 1994;21:663–74.
5. Insel RA, Amstey M, Pichichero ME. Postimmunization antibody to the *Haemophilus influenzae* type B capsule in breast milk. J Infect Dis 1985;152:407–8.

VACCINE, HEPATITIS A

Vaccine

PREGNANCY RECOMMENDATION: No Human Data—Probably Compatible
BREASTFEEDING RECOMMENDATION: No Human Data—Probably Compatible

PREGNANCY SUMMARY

Hepatitis A virus vaccine inactivated is a noninfectious vaccine (1,2). No reports describing the use of the vaccine in pregnant humans have been located, but based on similar vaccines, the risk to the fetus from maternal vaccination appears to be minimal.

FETAL RISK SUMMARY

Animal reproduction studies have not been conducted with the vaccine.

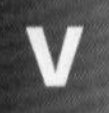

The CDC considers the theoretical risk to the developing fetus to be low (3,4). The CDC and others state that hepatitis A vaccine can be given to pregnant women at high risk of exposure (3–5).

BREASTFEEDING SUMMARY

No data are available, but based on other inactivated viral vaccines, hepatitis A vaccine does not appear to be contraindicated during nursing.

References

1. Product information. Havrix (Hepatitis A Vaccine, Inactivated). SmithKline Beecham, 2001.
2. Product information. Vaqta (Hepatitis A Vaccine, Inactivated). Merck, 2001.
3. CDC. Prevention of hepatitis A through active or passive immunization: recommendations of the Advisory Committee on Immunization Practices (ACIP). MMWR 1996;46 (No. RR-15):1–30.
4. CDC. *Guidelines for Vaccinating Pregnant Women*. Available at http://www.cdc.gov/vaccines/pubs/preg-guide.htm. Accessed May 16, 2010.
5. Duff B, Duff P. Hepatitis A vaccine: ready for prime time. Obstet Gynecol 1998;91:468–71.

VACCINE, HEPATITIS B

Vaccine

PREGNANCY RECOMMENDATION: Compatible
BREASTFEEDING RECOMMENDATION: No Human Data—Probably Compatible

PREGNANCY SUMMARY

Hepatitis B virus vaccine inactivated (recombinant) is a noninfectious surface antigen (HBsAg) vaccine. Animal reproduction studies have not been conducted with the vaccine. No risks to the fetus from maternal vaccination have been reported (1,2).

FETAL RISK SUMMARY

One source recommends administration after the 1st trimester, because of a theoretical risk of teratogenicity (3). However, the CDC states that there is no apparent risk of fetal adverse effects (based on unpublished CDC data) and that pregnancy is not a contraindication to vaccination in women (1,2). Preexposure and postexposure prophylaxis is indicated in pregnant women at high risk of infection (2,4) (see also Immune Globulin, Hepatitis B).

BREASTFEEDING SUMMARY

No data are available, but the vaccine can be used during lactation (1).

References

1. CDC. Hepatitis B virus: a comprehensive strategy for eliminating transmission in the United States through universal childhood vaccination. Recommendations of the Immunization Practices Advisory Committee (ACIP). MMWR 1991;40(No. RR-13):1–25.
2. CDC. *Guidelines for Vaccinating Pregnant Women*. Available at http://www.cdc.gov/vaccines/pubs/preg-guide.htm. Accessed May 16, 2010.
3. Linder N, Ohel G. In utero vaccination. Clin Perinatol 1994;21:663–74.
4. Faix RG. Maternal immunization to prevent fetal and neonatal infection. Clin Obstet Gynecol 1991;34:277–87.

VACCINE, HUMAN PAPILLOMAVIRUS BIVALENT (TYPES 16 AND 18), RECOMBINANT

Vaccine

PREGNANCY RECOMMENDATION: Limited Human Data—Probably Compatible
BREASTFEEDING RECOMMENDATION: No Human Data—Probably Compatible

PREGNANCY SUMMARY

Animal studies in one species found no evidence of reproductive or developmental toxicity at doses based on body weight that were much higher than those used in humans (1). The human experience supports the lack of embryo–fetal toxicity from vaccination received around the time of conception. Moreover, the vaccine is noninfectious and preservative free. As of 2010, the CDC recommends avoiding the vaccine in pregnant women (2). If the vaccine is given in pregnancy, health care professionals are encouraged to call the toll-free number 877-311-8972 for information about patient enrollment in the Organization of Teratology Information Specialists (OTIS) study.

FETAL RISK SUMMARY

Human papillomavirus bivalent (HPV-B) is a noninfectious, recombinant, AS04-adjuvanted vaccine that contains the major antigenic protein of the capsid of HPV types 16 and 18. It contains no preservatives. HPV-B is indicated for the prevention of the following diseases caused by oncogenic HPV types 16 and 18: cervical cancer, cervical intraepithelial neoplasia (CIN) grade 2 or worse and adenocarcinoma in situ, and CIN grade 1. It is approved for use in females 10 through 25 years of age. It is administered as an IM injection (1).

Reproduction studies have been conducted in rats. Doses that were about 47 times the human dose based on body weight revealed no evidence of impaired fertility or fetal harm. When given before conception and during organogenesis, no adverse effects on mating, fertility, pregnancy, parturition, lactation, or prenatal or postnatal development were observed. The vaccine did not cause teratogenicity. The vaccine has not been evaluated for carcinogenic or mutagenic potential (1).

In clinical studies, pregnancy was excluded before administration of each dose of the vaccine and patients were instructed to avoid pregnancy until 2 months after the last vaccination (1). Before licensure, 7276 pregnancies were reported among 3696 women who had received the vaccine and 3580 women who had received the control dose (hepatitis A vaccine or placebo). The pregnancy outcomes for the subjects and controls were similar in terms of normal infants, spontaneous abortions (SABs), elective abortions, abnormal infants other than congenital anomaly, and premature birth. There also were no differences between the groups in the rate of congenital anomaly, stillbirth, and ectopic pregnancy. In a sub-analysis, the pregnancy outcomes were examined in 761 women (396 subjects and 365 controls) who had their last menstrual period within 30 days before, or 45 days after a vaccine dose. The same outcomes noted above were again similar, but more SABs had occurred in subjects (13.6% vs. 9.6%). It was not known if the increased numbers of SABs was a vaccine-related effect (1).

A 2010 study examined the possible association of HPV-B vaccine with SABs (3). Women who received three doses of the vaccine (N = 13,075) were compared with controls given hepatitis A vaccine (N = 13,055). The estimated rate of SABs in the two groups was 11.5% and 10.2%, respectively. In secondary descriptive analyses of pregnancies that began within 3 months of the latest vaccination, the SAB rates were 14.7% and 9.1%. The authors concluded that there was no evidence for an association between HPV-B and SAB (3).

BREASTFEEDING SUMMARY

It is not known if anti-HPV-16 and anti-HPV-18 antibodies are excreted into breast milk (1). If they are, the effect on a nursing infant is unknown. However, based on the human experience with the quadrivalent vaccine, the bivalent vaccine is probably compatible with breastfeeding.

References

1. Product information. Cervarix. GlaxoSmithKline Biologicals, 2009.
2. CDC. *Guidelines for Vaccinating Pregnant Women*. Available at http://www.cdc.gov/vaccines/pubs/preg-guide.htm. Accessed June 5, 2010.
3. Wacholder S, Chen BE, Wilcox A, Macones G, Gonzalez P, Befano B, Hildesheim A, Rodrigues AC, Solomon D, Herrero R, Schiffman M. Risk of miscarriage with bivalent vaccine against human papillomavirus (HPV) types 16 and 18: pooled analysis of two randomized controlled trials. BMJ 2020;340:c712. doi:10.1136/bmj.c712.

VACCINE, HUMAN PAPILLOMAVIRUS QUADRIVALENT, RECOMBINANT

Vaccine

PREGNANCY RECOMMENDATION: Limited Human Data—Probably Compatible
BREASTFEEDING RECOMMENDATION: Compatible

PREGNANCY SUMMARY

Animal studies in one species found no evidence of reproductive or developmental toxicity at doses, based on body weight, that were much higher than those used in humans. The human pregnancy experience supports the lack of toxicity for the embryo and/or fetus. Moreover, the vaccine is noninfectious and preservative- and antibiotic-free. If the vaccine is given in pregnancy, health care professionals are encouraged to call the toll-free number 877-311-8972 for information about patient enrollment in the Organization of Teratology Information Specialists (OTIS) study.

FETAL RISK SUMMARY

Human papillomavirus (HPV) quadrivalent vaccine is prepared by recombinant technology to contain virus-like particles of the major capsid protein of HPV types 6, 11, 16, and 18. It is administered as an IM injection. The vaccine is not infectious and does not contain preservatives or antibiotics. HPV vaccine is indicated in girls and women 9–26 years of age for prevention of the following diseases caused by HPV: cervical cancer, genital warts (condyloma acuminata), cervical adenocarcinoma in situ, and intraepithelial neoplasia of the cervix (grades 1, 2 and 3), vulva (grades 2 and 3), and vagina (grades 2 and 3) (1).

Reproduction studies have been conducted in rats. In pregnant rats, doses up to 300 times the human dose revealed no effects on fertility, pregnancy, parturition, lactation, or embryo or fetal pre- or postweaning development. No vaccine-related structural malformations were observed. In addition, there were no effects on the development, behavior, reproductive performance, or fertility of the offspring (1).

In the third annual report from the Merck Pregnancy Registry covering the period June 2006–May 2009, there were 1636 prospective reported pregnancies, but 396 were lost to follow-up and 132 outcomes were pending. Of the remaining 1108 pregnancies, there were 968 live births (974 newborns includes 1 surviving twin), 64 spontaneous abortions (SABs), 65 elective abortions (EABs), 10 fetal deaths (1 of twins), and 2 ectopic pregnancies (2). The reasons for the EABs were usually unknown, but one termination involved a fetus with anencephaly and a hypoplastic heart defect. Of the 974 newborns, 926 (95%) were normal, 21 had major defects, 26 had minor defects, and there was 1 early neonatal death of an infant born at about 30 weeks with intrauterine growth restriction (mother had antiphospholipid syndrome and was homozygous for methylene-tetra-hydro-folate reductase mutation). The prevalence of major structural anomalies recognized at birth was 2.4 cases per 100 live births. Among 261 retrospective (reported after the outcome was known) cases, there were 12 major defects. The Registry stated that the limited number of reports with known outcomes prevented any definite conclusions about the potential effects of exposure to the vaccine in pregnancy. However, the rates of SABs and major defects, and the fact that the anomalies were varied, suggested that the outcomes were related to the background risk rather than to the vaccine (2).

A 2009 study reported the pregnancy and infant outcomes during phase III clinical trials with quadrivalent HPV vaccine (*Note: The Registry data presented above updates the number of exposures*) (3). Women aged 15–45 years received the vaccine or placebo on day 1 and months 2 and 6. If a pregnancy test immediately before a dose was positive they were excluded from further doses. During the study, the number of pregnancies with known outcomes in the vaccinated and placebo groups was 1796 and 1824, respectively. There were no significant differences in the proportion of pregnancies resulting in live births, fetal loss, or spontaneous abortion. Congenital anomalies were noted in 40 and 30 neonates, respectively (*ns*). The anomalies were diverse and consistent with those commonly seen in the general population (3). Two comments on this study were published in 2009 and 2010 (4,5). Because the vaccine and placebo groups did not represent comparable randomized populations, and because some pregnancies were still ongoing, the author recommended that avoiding the vaccine in pregnancy or near the time of conception was still warranted (5).

The American College of Obstetricians and Gynecologists recommends avoiding HPV vaccine in pregnancy. If a woman becomes pregnant before completion of the three-dose schedule, completion of the series should be delayed until the pregnancy is completed (6). As of 2010, the CDC also recommends avoiding the vaccine in pregnant women (7).

BREASTFEEDING SUMMARY

It is not known if the HPV antigens or the antibodies induced by the vaccine are excreted into human breast milk. Five hundred nursing mothers were given the vaccine during clinical trials, compared with 495 women who received a placebo vaccine. The number of nursing infants experiencing a serious adverse experience was higher in the mothers receiving the vaccine than in those receiving a placebo, 4.2% ($N = 21$) vs. 2.0% ($N = 10$), respectively. However, none of the adverse experiences were judged to be related to the vaccine. In clinical studies, more nursing infants with acute respiratory illnesses were found in the group of mothers who had received the vaccine within 30 days ($N = 6$), than in the control group ($N = 2$) (1,2).

The American College of Obstetricians and Gynecologists states that the vaccine can be given to lactating women because it is safe for the mother and the nursing infant (6). Until further studies demonstrate otherwise, the use of HPV vaccine can be classified as compatible with breastfeeding.

References

1. Product information. Gardasil. Merck and Company, 2006.
2. Third Annual Report on Exposure during Pregnancy from the Merck Pregnancy Registry for Quadrivalent Human Papillomavirus (types 6, 11, 16, 18) Recombinant Vaccine (Gardasil/Silgard). Covering the period from first approval (June 1, 2006) through May 31, 2009.
3. Garland SM, Ault KA, Gall SA, Paavonen J, Sings HL, Ciprero KL, Saah A, Marino D, Ryan D, Radley D, Zhou H, Haupt RM, Garner SM, on behalf of the Quadrivalent Human Papillomavirus Vaccine Phase III Investigators. Pregnancy and infant outcomes in the clinical trials of a human papillomavirus type 6/11/16/18 vaccine—a combined analysis of five randomized controlled trials. Obstet Gynecol 2009;114:1179–88.
4. Smith-McCune K, Sawaya GF. Update on quadrivalent human papillomavirus vaccination and pregnancy outcomes. Obstet Gynecol 2009;114:1168–9.
5. Smith-McCune K. Quadrivalent HPV vaccine administered to women who became pregnant during trials did not appear to adversely affect pregnancy outcome; however, use during pregnancy is not recommended. Evid Based Med 2010;15:80–1.
6. American College of Obstetricians and Gynecology. Human papillomavirus vaccination. *Committee Opinion*. No. 467, September 2010. Obstet Gynecol 2010;116:800–3.
7. CDC. *Guidelines for Vaccinating Pregnant Women*. Available at http://www.cdc.gov/vaccines/pubs/preg-guide.htm. Accessed May 16, 2010.

VACCINE, INFLUENZA

Vaccine

PREGNANCY RECOMMENDATION: Compatible
BREASTFEEDING RECOMMENDATION: Compatible

PREGNANCY SUMMARY

Influenza vaccine is an inactivated virus vaccine (1). The vaccine is considered safe during all stages of pregnancy (2–7). However, the intranasal vaccine spray contains a live, attenuated virus and should not be used in pregnancy (1). Animal reproduction studies have not been conducted with the vaccine. If influenza vaccine is used in pregnancy, health care professionals are encouraged to call the toll-free number 877-311-8972 for information about patient enrollment in the Organization of Teratology Information Specialists (OTIS) study.

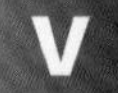

FETAL RISK SUMMARY

Neonatal passive immunization of short duration has been documented in some studies (4). The American College of Obstetricians and Gynecologists recommends that the vaccine be given to women who will be pregnant during the flu season (October–mid May) and to those at high risk for pulmonary complications regardless of trimester (1).

The CDC recommends the inactivated vaccine for women who will be pregnant during the influenza season (5). In addition, pregnant women who have medical conditions that increase their risk for complications from influenza should receive the vaccine (5).

A 2005 study used an electronic database to identify 252 pregnant women who had received influenza vaccine between 1998 and 2003 (8). Vaccination occurred at a mean gestational age of 26.1 weeks (range 4–39 weeks). There were no serious adverse events within 42 days of vaccination. Compared with controls who were not vaccinated, there were no differences between the groups in terms of pregnancy outcomes and infant medical conditions from birth to 6 months of age (8).

BREASTFEEDING SUMMARY

Maternal vaccination is compatible with breastfeeding and presents no risk to the nursing infant (5).

References

1. American College of Obstetricians and Gynecologists. Influenza vaccination during pregnancy. *Committee Opinion*. No. 468, October 2010. Obstet Gynecol 2010;116:1006–7.
2. Philit F, Cordier J-F. Therapeutic approaches of clinicians to influenza pandemic. Eur J Epidemiol 1994;10:491–2.
3. Bandy U. Influenza: prevention and control. R I Med 1994;77:393–4.
4. Linder N, Ohel G. In utero vaccination. Clin Perinatol 1994;21:663–74.
5. CDC. *Guidelines for Vaccinating Pregnant Women*. Available at http://www.cdc.gov/vaccines/pubs/preg-guide.htm. Accessed May 16, 2010.
6. Yeager DP, Toy EC, Baker B III. Influenza vaccination in pregnancy. Am J Perinatol 1999;16:283–6.
7. Kashyap S, Gruslin A. Influenza vaccination during pregnancy. Prim Care Update Ob/Gyns 2000;7:7–11.
8. Munoz FM, Greisinger AJ, Wehmanen OA, Mouzoon ME, Hoyle JC, Smith FA, Glezen WP. Safety of influenza vaccination during pregnancy. Am J Obstet Gynecol 2005;192:1098–106.

VACCINE, INFLUENZA A (H1N1)

Vaccine

PREGNANCY RECOMMENDATION: Compatible (Inactivated Vaccine)
No Human Data—Probably Compatible (Live Virus Vaccine and Adjuvanted Vaccine)
BREASTFEEDING RECOMMENDATION: Compatible

PREGNANCY SUMMARY

Because the H1N1 vaccines were released late in 2009, there are no reports describing their use in pregnancy. However, pregnant women are a priority population to receive the inactivated H1N1 vaccine because they are at high risk for morbidity and mortality. There is no evidence that influenza virus types A and B vaccines caused embryo or fetal harm (see Vaccine, Influenza). There is, however, a possible increased rate of spontaneous abortions from disease caused by these viruses (1). Inactivated virus vaccines are preferred over vaccines containing live viruses. The American College of Obstetricians and Gynecologists classifies live virus vaccines as usually contraindicated (1). The potential for developmental toxicity from the adjuvants, added to one of the H1N1 vaccines to enhance the immune response to the antigen (i.e., the virus), is not known. In rats, however, developmental toxicity was observed in two studies with AS03-adjuvanted H5N1 antigen. Neither of the vaccines available in the United States contains an adjuvant. If H1N1 vaccine is used in pregnancy, health care professionals are encouraged to call the toll-free number 877-311-8972 for information about patient enrollment in the Organization of Teratology Information Specialists (OTIS) study.

FETAL RISK SUMMARY

Three vaccines, two with inactivated virus and one with live virus, are available to prevent infection with novel influenza A (H1N1) (previously known as swine flu). The vaccines are indicated for the active immunization against influenza disease caused by pandemic (H1N1) 2009 virus (2–4). Influenza A (H1N1) 2009 monovalent vaccine, given by IM injection, is an inactivated vaccine indicated for persons 6 months of age and older (2). Influenza A (H1N1) 2009 monovalent vaccine live, given intranasally, is indicated for individuals 2–49 years of age (3). Arepanrix H1N1 inactivated virus vaccine, available in Canada, is indicated in an officially declared pandemic situation (4). The adjuvants in Arepanrix are DL-α-tocopherol, squalene, and polysorbate 80.

Animal reproduction studies with H1N1 vaccines have not been conducted (2–4). Neither have studies been conducted for carcinogenesis, mutagenesis, or impairment of fertility. Two reproductive studies in rats with AS03-adjuvanted H5N1 antigen (doses not specified) have been conducted to evaluate the embryo–fetal and postnatal toxicity up to the end of the lactation period (4). The findings in the two studies were an increased incidence of postimplantation loss, fetal malformations (markedly medially thickened/kinked ribs and bent scapula), dilated ureter, and delayed neurobehavioral maturation. However, the significance of the outcomes was uncertain because not all findings were observed in both studies (4).

BREASTFEEDING SUMMARY

Because the H1N1 vaccines were released late in 2009, there are no reports describing their use during breastfeeding. Nevertheless, maternal vaccination with any of these vaccines is compatible with breastfeeding and presents no risk to a nursing infant.

References

1. American College of Obstetricians and Gynecologists. Influenza vaccination during pregnancy. *Committee Opinion*. No. 468, October 2010. Obstet Gynecol 2010;116:1006–7.
2. Product information. Influenza A (H1N1) 2009 Monovalent Vaccine. Sanofi Pasteur, 2009.
3. Product information. Influenza A (H1N1) 2009 Monovalent Vaccine Live, Intranasal. MedImmune, 2009.
4. Product information. Arepanrix H1N1 AS03-Adjuvanted H1N1 Pandemic Influenza Vaccine. GlaxoSmithKline, 2009.

VACCINE, LYME DISEASE

Vaccine

PREGNANCY RECOMMENDATION: No Human Data—Probably Compatible
BREASTFEEDING RECOMMENDATION: No Human Data—Probably Compatible

PREGNANCY SUMMARY

The occurrence of Lyme disease during pregnancy presents a serious but apparently small risk to the fetus. The greatest fetal risk may be in cases where the mother does not receive appropriate antibiotic treatment. The data to support this conclusion are limited and controversial. Because there have been no reports on the use of Lyme disease vaccine during gestation, the fetal risk from the vaccine is unknown. However, because Lyme disease itself may cause fetal harm and the vaccine is noninfectious, vaccination of women of childbearing age who are at risk for acquiring the disease may be the safest course. Although the direct risk to a fetus appears to be low, the Advisory Committee on Immunization Practices recommends that pregnant women not receive the vaccine because its safety during pregnancy has not been established (1).

FETAL RISK SUMMARY

Lyme disease vaccine (recombinant OspA) contains an outer surface protein of *Borrelia burgdorferi* sensu stricto (lipoprotein OspA) that is noninfectious (1,2). The recombinant OspA protein is expressed in *Escherichia coli* and then purified. Only the LYMErix vaccine is licensed for use in the United States (1). The vaccine (30 mcg/0.5 mL) is administered IM on a three-dose schedule of 0, 1, and 12 months.

Lyme disease is a tickborne infection caused by the spirochete *B. burgdorferi*, with an incubation period from infection to onset of rash (erythema migrans) of 7–14 days (range 3–30 days). The disease is characterized by rash, fever, malaise, fatigue, headache, myalgia, and arthralgia. Without adequate antibiotic treatment, chronic disease of the nervous system, musculoskeletal system, or the heart may occur (1).

No cases describing the use of Lyme disease vaccine in pregnancy have been located. Moreover, animal reproductive tests have not been conducted with the vaccine.

A 1985 case report described a woman who developed Lyme disease during the 1st trimester of pregnancy (3). She received no antibiotic therapy for her disease. She delivered a 3000-g male infant at an estimated 35 weeks' gestation who developed respiratory distress shortly after birth. Studies revealed a dilated, poorly contractile left ventricle, aortic valvular stenosis, patent ductus arteriosus, and coarctation of the aorta. The infant died at age 39 hours. Cardiovascular malformations found at autopsy were tubular hypoplasia of the ascending aorta and aortic arch, marked endocardial fibroelastosis, and a persistent left superior vena cava draining into the coronary sinus. No signs of infection, such as inflammation, necrosis, or granuloma formation, were found in the heart or other organs, but a few spirochetes similar to the Lyme disease spirochete were found in the spleen, renal tubules, and bone marrow. Evaluation of the mother was consistent with Lyme disease, and she was successfully treated with tetracycline therapy (3).

A second case of fetal death associated with Lyme disease was published in 1987 (4). A 24-year-old woman with an apparent onset of infection (annular erythematous patch noted near her left knee followed by pain and swelling in the knee) near the time of conception delivered a 2500-g stillborn infant at term. Serologic studies of maternal blood were positive for *B. burgdorferi* in two of three samples. At autopsy, the only malformation found was an atrioventricular canal ventricular septal defect. Spirochetes immunologically consistent with *B. burgdorferi* were recovered from the fetal liver, myocardium, adrenal gland, and subarachnoid space of the midbrain. The authors concluded that the fetus had died near term of overwhelming spirochetosis (4).

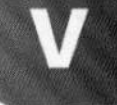

The outcomes of 19 pregnancies of women with documented Lyme disease were described in 1986 (5). Eight of the pregnancies were followed prospectively, and 11 were identified retrospectively. Among the 17 women with erythema chronicum migrans (ECM), 8 had the onset of disease in the 1st trimester, 7 in the 2nd trimester, and 2 in the 3rd trimester. The onset of infection could not be determined in the remaining two, but one developed facial palsy in the 1st trimester and the other developed arthritis in the 3rd trimester.

Normal outcomes occurred in 14 pregnancies, 7 with onset of illness in the 1st trimester, 4 in the 2nd trimester, 2 in the 3rd trimester, and 1 with unknown time of onset. Five of the women (three in 1st trimester; one in 2nd trimester; one in 3rd trimester) did not receive antibiotic therapy, but all delivered apparently normal infants, although two had transient problems. One of these, a 2100-g infant delivered prematurely, developed hyperbilirubinemia at 4 days of age but has had otherwise normal development through 9 years of age. Another, delivered 7 days after onset of maternal ECM and meningitis, had hyperbilirubinemia and a generalized, petechial, vesicular rash at 5 days of age. Viral and bacterial blood and skin cultures were negative; tests for *B. burgdorferi* were not available at that time. The rash faded within 1 week during treatment with penicillin. The remaining three pregnancies had abnormal outcomes as described below (time of onset of maternal illness shown in parentheses):

(1st trimester) intrauterine fetal death at 16 weeks'; no congenital abnormalities; no inflammation noted in fetal tissues; culture and indirect immunofluorescence assay of placenta and fetal tissues were negative

(2nd trimester) syndactyly (type 1) of second and third toes

(2nd trimester) full-term, healthy male infant at birth, developed cortical blindness and developmental delay at 8 months of age; diagnostic studies were negative; no serum antibodies to *B. burgdorferi* found at 1 year of age; mother had a previous child with trisomy 18

None of the five adverse outcomes described above can be directly attributed to maternal Lyme disease (5). At least one is known to be a fairly common genetic defect (i.e., syndactyly), and two were minor, transient adverse effects. Moreover, no cardiovascular anomalies were observed, but because only eight cases with ECM occurred in the 1st trimester, the power of this study to detect such defects is limited (5).

Two reports from the same group of investigators, one published in 1993 and the other in 1995, examined the effects of maternal exposure to Lyme disease and pregnancy outcome (6,7). A total of 2014 women were enrolled in the first study at their first prenatal visit (6). Of these, 11 were seropositive for Lyme disease, but information on the presence of congenital malformations was available for only 10 of their infants. Among these 10 newborns, 1 infant had a major defect (multiple major anomalies with VATER association [vertebral defects, imperforate anus, tracheoesophageal fistula, and radial and renal dysplasia]). Two other infants had minor malformations: metatarsus adductus and stomach reflux. Other outcome data included no spontaneous abortions and a mean birth weight of 3650 g. None of these outcomes differed significantly from the group without Lyme disease exposure (i.e., with no significant titer and negative clinical history) (6).

In the second study, no difference in the incidence of total congenital malformations (odds ratio [OR] 0.87; 95% confidence interval [CI] 0.70–1.06) was observed in the infants of mothers in an endemic hospital cohort (N = 2504) compared with the infants of mothers in a control hospital (N = 2507) (7). The total number represented 81% of all eligible infants. However, the rate of cardiac malformations (most commonly ventricular septal defect [VSD]) was significantly higher in the endemic cohort (OR 2.40; 95% CI 1.25–4.59). Although the incidence of total minor malformations was no different between the groups, three minor defects (hemangiomas, polydactyly, and hydrocele) were significantly higher ($p < 0.05$) in the control group. Only the difference in polydactyly could be explained by demographic variations. Comparisons of mean birth weights between the cohorts found no significant differences (7).

In the endemic cohort, 22 of the mothers had Lyme disease before pregnancy (7). Among their 23 offspring (1 set of twins), there were 2 major malformations: multiple heart defects (infant died), and hydrocele and laryngomalacia. Six mothers contracted the disease during pregnancy and one of their infants had a major defect (hypospadias). Three infants with major malformations (VSD, vesicoureteral block with reflux, and hypospadias) and five with minor defects (inguinal hernia, laryngomalacia, hemangioma, genu varum, and metatarsus adductus) were observed in the mothers (N = 67) who had reported a tick bite during pregnancy. Of the 20 infants born from mothers who had immunoglobulin G anti-*B. burgdorferi* antibodies in their cord blood (all infants were tested), 1 had a minor defect (cryptorchidism). Within the endemic cohort, there were no differences between those who had possible exposure to Lyme disease or who had positive cord serology compared with those who were not exposed and had negative serology in terms of mean birth weight or the rate of major or minor abnormalities (7).

A 1999 retrospective case–control study compared 796 children with a diagnosis of congenital cardiac anomaly with 704 children from the same region without cardiac defects (8). Records of all of the children were obtained from a medical center in a suburban area where Lyme disease is endemic. All had been born in the study area. No statistical differences in the frequencies of maternal conditions and exposures between the two groups were found for cigarette smoking, alcohol use, conception while using contraceptives, the use of fertility drugs, the use of electric blankets or heated waterbeds, vaginal bleeding during pregnancy, occupational exposure to video display terminals, asthma, upper respiratory tract infections, or thyroid disorders. More study mothers had high blood pressure (6.7% vs. 3.5%, p = 0.007), whereas more controls had occupational exposure to x-ray films or anesthesia (6.1% vs. 9.1%, p = 0.03). There were no statistical differences between the groups in Lyme disease during pregnancy (or 3 months, 1 year, or at anytime before conception) or in those who had received a tick bite during pregnancy (or 3 months, 1 year, or at anytime before conception). The authors concluded that there was no increased risk of congenital heart defects when maternal Lyme disease was contacted before or during pregnancy. However, their study could not exclude a risk to a fetus from undiagnosed and untreated Lyme disease (8).

Although there is concern that maternal Lyme disease may infect the fetus as do other spirochetal infections (e.g., syphilis) (5,9), the risk for this, based on the above studies, appears to be low. In addition, a survey published in 1994 found no cases of clinically significant nervous system disease attributable to transplacentally acquired Lyme disease that had been recognized among pediatric neurologists in regions of the United States in which Lyme disease was endemic (10). The regions surveyed included all or portions of Connecticut, Massachusetts, Minnesota, New Jersey,

New York, Rhode Island, and Wisconsin. Some adult neurologists were also contacted in Connecticut. One pediatric neurologist was following three children with "congenital Lyme disease," but none of the mothers of these children met the CDC's diagnostic criteria for Lyme disease (10). The authors concluded that either congenital neuroborreliosis was not occurring or that the incidence was extremely low in endemic areas (10).

BREASTFEEDING SUMMARY

No reports describing the use of Lyme disease vaccine during lactation have been located. DNA of the spirochete *B. burgdorferi* has been detected in the breast milk of two women by polymerase chain reaction (PCR) (11). Breast milk samples from three healthy controls were nonreactive. Both women with reactive samples had Lyme disease as characterized by the presence of erythema migrans, and both had PCR-positive urine samples. One of the nursing infants was hospitalized at 6 months of age because of fever and vomiting. The cause of the symptoms was undetermined, but they resolved spontaneously after a few days. The urine of the infant and mother were tested 1 year later, and both were nonreactive.

References

1. CDC. Recommendations for the use of Lyme disease vaccine. Recommendations of the Advisory Committee on Immunization Practices (ACIP). MMWR 1999;48(RR-7):1–17.
2. Product information. LYMErix. SmithKline Beecham Pharmaceuticals, 2001.
3. Schlesinger PA, Duray PH, Burke BA, Steere AC, Stillman T. Maternal-fetal transmission of the Lyme disease spirochete, *Borrelia burgdorferi*. Ann Intern Med 1985;103:67–8.
4. MacDonald AB, Benach JL, Burgdorfer W. Stillbirth following maternal Lyme disease. NY State J Med 1987;87:615–6.
5. Markowitz LE, Steere AC, Benach JL, Slade JD, Broome CV. Lyme disease during pregnancy. JAMA 1986;255:3394–6.
6. Strobino BA, Williams CL, Abid S, Chalson R, Spierling P. Lyme disease and pregnancy outcome: a prospective study of two thousand prenatal patients. Am J Obstet Gynecol 1993;169:367–74.
7. Williams CL, Strobino B, Weinstein A, Spierling P, Medici F. Maternal Lyme disease and congenital malformations: a cord blood serosurvey in endemic and control areas. Paediatr Perinat Epidemiol 1995;9:320–30.
8. Strobino B, Abid S, Gewitz M. Maternal Lyme disease and congenital heart disease: a case–control study in an endemic area. Am J Obstet Gynecol 1999;180:711–6.
9. Shapiro ED. Lyme disease in children. Am J Med 1995;98(Suppl 4A):69S–73S.
10. Gerber MA, Zalneraitis EL. Childhood neurologic disorders and Lyme disease during pregnancy. Pediatr Neurol 1994;11:41–3.
11. Schmidt BL, Aberer E, Stockenhuber C, Klade H, Breier F, Luger A. Detection of *Borrelia burgdorferi* DNA by polymerase chain reaction in the urine and breast milk of patients with Lyme borreliosis. Diagn Microbiol Infect Dis 1995;21:121–8.

VACCINE, MEASLES

Vaccine

PREGNANCY RECOMMENDATION: Contraindicated
BREASTFEEDING RECOMMENDATION: No Human Data—Probably Compatible

PREGNANCY SUMMARY

Measles (rubeola) vaccine is a live, attenuated virus vaccine (1,2). It should not be given in pregnancy. Animal reproduction studies have not been conducted with the vaccine.

FETAL RISK SUMMARY

Measles occurring during pregnancy may result in significant maternal morbidity, an increased abortion rate, stillbirth, prematurity, and congenital malformations (1). Although a fetal risk from the vaccine has not been confirmed, the vaccine should not be used during pregnancy because fetal infection with the attenuated viruses may occur (1–3). The manufacturer lists pregnancy as a contraindication to its use and states that pregnancy should be avoided for 3 months following vaccination (1). A shorter interval is recommended by the CDC (4). They recommend that women avoid becoming pregnant for 28 days after vaccination, but no cases of congenital malformations attributable to measles vaccine virus have been reported (4).

BREASTFEEDING SUMMARY

No reports describing the use of measles vaccine during lactation have been located. However, the vaccine is probably compatible with breastfeeding.

References

1. Product information. Attenuvax. Merck, 2004.
2. Amstey MS. Vaccination in pregnancy. Clin Obstet Gynaecol 1983;10:13–22.
3. Linder N, Ohel G. In utero vaccination. Clin Perinatol 1994;21:663–74.
4. CDC. *Guidelines for Vaccinating Pregnant Women*. Available at http://www.cdc.gov/vaccines/pubs/preg-guide.htm. Accessed May 16, 2010.

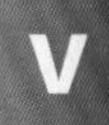

VACCINE, MENINGOCOCCAL

Vaccine

PREGNANCY RECOMMENDATION: Compatible
BREASTFEEDING RECOMMENDATION: No Human Data—Probably Compatible

PREGNANCY SUMMARY

The risk to the fetus from vaccination during pregnancy is unknown. The CDC recommends that if it is given during pregnancy, the woman should consult her health care provider or the vaccine manufacturer, because there are no data available on the safety of the vaccine during pregnancy (1). In one study, vaccination resulted in transfer of maternal antibodies to the fetus, but the transfer was irregular and was not dependent on maternal titer or the period in pregnancy when vaccination occurred (2). If meningococcal vaccine is given in pregnancy, health care professionals are encouraged to call the toll-free number 877-311-8972 for information about patient enrollment in the Organization of Teratology Information Specialists (OTIS) study.

FETAL RISK SUMMARY

Meningococcal vaccine is available in two formulations: meningococcal polysaccharide vaccine, groups A, C, Y, and W-135 combined (Menomune—A/C/Y/W-135), a freeze-dried product requiring reconstitution; and meningococcal (groups A, C, Y, and W-135) polysaccharide diphtheria toxoid conjugate vaccine (Menactra), a fluid product ready for administration. Either formulation is a killed bacteria (cell wall) vaccine (3,4).

Animal reproduction studies have not been conducted with Menomune (3). Reproduction studies have been conducted in mice with Menactra (4). A dose 900 times the human dose (based on body weight) had no effect on fertility, maternal health, embryo–fetal survival, or postnatal development (4). One of the 234 fetal skeletons examined had a cleft palate compared with none in the control group. This was the only skeletal and organ anomaly observed and was not thought to be related to the vaccine.

A 1998 study evaluated the pregnancy outcomes of 34 women who received meningococcal vaccine during pregnancy (5). The trimesters of exposures were 4 (11.8%) in the 1st, 17 (50.0%) in the 2nd, and 13 (38.2%) in the 3rd. There were 34 singleton deliveries with a mean follow-up of the offspring of 13.2 months (range 1–24 months). Excluding one congenital malformation, there was no increase in the observed unusual birth events compared with the expected rates. In fact, there were significantly fewer cases of newborn cardiac murmurs and physiologic jaundice in offspring of vaccinated mothers. One birth defect observed in an infant of a mother vaccinated at 33 weeks' gestation was consistent with the oromandibular limb hypogenesis spectrum (Charlie M syndrome) (expected frequency <0.00002%). This pattern of defects would probably have occurred very early in gestation. The cause of Charlie M syndrome is unknown; it has not yet been identified as a genetic defect and it has not been associated with teratogens. All of the infants had normal growth and development in the follow-up period (5).

A 1994 review stated that the use of the vaccine during pregnancy is controversial (6). However, in a 1996 study, 75 mothers received meningococcal vaccine in the last trimester of pregnancy (7). No adverse effects in the newborns attributable to the vaccine were observed.

BREASTFEEDING SUMMARY

No reports describing the administration of meningococcal vaccine during human lactation have been located.

References

1. CDC. *Guidelines for Vaccinating Pregnant Women*. Available at http://www.cdc.gov/vaccines/pubs/preg-guide.htm. Accessed May 16, 2010.
2. Carvalho ADA, Giampaglia CMS, Kimura H, Pereira OADC, Farhat CK, Neves JC, Prandini R, Carvalho EDS, Zarvos AM. Maternal and infant antibody response to meningococcal vaccination in pregnancy. Lancet 1977;2:809–11.
3. Product information. Menomune—A/C/Y/W-135. Sanofi Pasteur, 2005.
4. Product information. Menactra. Sanofi Pasteur, 2007.
5. Letson GW, Little JR, Ottman J, Miller GL. Meningococcal vaccine in pregnancy: an assessment of infant risk. Pediatr Infect Dis 1998;17:261–3.
6. Linder N, Ohel G. In utero vaccination. Clin Perinatol 1994;21:663–74.
7. O'Dempsey TJD, McArdle T, Ceesay SJ, Banya WAS, Demba E, Secka O, Leinonen M, Kayhty H, Francis N, Greenwood BM. Immunization with a pneumococcal capsular polysaccharide vaccine during pregnancy. Vaccine 1996;14:963–70.

VACCINE, MUMPS

Vaccine

PREGNANCY RECOMMENDATION: Contraindicated
BREASTFEEDING RECOMMENDATION: No Human Data—Probably Compatible

PREGNANCY SUMMARY

Mumps vaccine is a live attenuated virus vaccine (1,2). It should not be given in pregnancy. Animal reproduction studies have not been conducted with the vaccine.

FETAL RISK SUMMARY

Mumps occurring during pregnancy may result in an increased rate of 1st trimester spontaneous abortion (2). Although a fetal risk from the vaccine has not been confirmed, the vaccine should not be used during pregnancy because fetal infection with the attenuated viruses may occur (1–3). The manufacturer (2). In addition, the manufacturer recommends avoiding pregnancy for 3 months following vaccination (2). A shorter interval is recommended by the CDC (4), which recommends that women who receive the mumps vaccine should avoid becoming pregnant for 28 days. However, no cases of congenital malformations attributable to infection with mumps vaccine virus have been reported and having been vaccinated with the vaccine should not be a reason to terminate a pregnancy (5).

BREASTFEEDING SUMMARY

No reports describing the administration of mumps vaccine during human lactation have been located.

References

1. Amstey MS. Vaccination in pregnancy. Clin Obstet Gynaecol 1983;10: 13–22.
2. Product information. Mumpsvax. Merck, 2001.
3. Linder N, Ohel G. In utero vaccination. Clin Perinatol 1994;21:663–74.
4. CDC. *Guidelines for Vaccinating Pregnant Women*. Available at http://www.cdc.gov/vaccines/pubs/preg-guide.htm. Accessed May 16, 2010.
5. CDC. Measles, mumps, and rubella-vaccine use and strategies for elimination of measles, rubella, and congenital rubella syndrome and control of mumps. Recommendations of the Advisory Committee on Immunization Practices (ACIP). MMWR 1998;47(No. RR-8):1–57.

VACCINE, PERTUSSIS (ACELLULAR)

Vaccine/Toxoid

PREGNANCY RECOMMENDATION: Compatible—Maternal Benefit >> Embryo–Fetal Risk
BREASTFEEDING RECOMMENDATION: Compatible

PREGNANCY SUMMARY

Although no reports describing the use of tetanus toxoid/reduced diphtheria toxoid/acellular pertussis vaccine adsorbed (Tdap) or diphtheria/tetanus toxoids/acellular pertussis vaccine adsorbed (DTaP) in human pregnancy have been located, one report did describe the inadvertent administration of acellular pertussis vaccine without toxoids in early gestation. Diphtheria/tetanus toxoids are recommended in pregnancy under certain conditions (see Diphtheria/Tetanus Toxoids [Adult]) and whole cell pertussis vaccine (no longer available) has been used in late pregnancy. Studies in which Tdap is given in the 2nd and 3rd trimesters have been proposed to determine if higher titers of pertussis antibodies can be obtained in the newborn (1–4). Currently, if tetanus or diphtheria protection is needed during pregnancy, the CDC and the American College of Obstetricians and Gynecologists (ACOG) recommend that Tdap be considered in the 2nd or 3rd trimesters, or earlier if protection is needed urgently (5–7). Tdap should only be given once during a lifetime.

Pertussis antibodies are known to cross the placenta and could potentially provide infants greater protection until they reach the age for active immunization. The American Academy of Pediatrics has recommended that pregnant adolescents should be given the same consideration for immunization as nonpregnant adolescents, and that the vaccine should be given before 36 weeks' gestation (4). However, the CDC concluded that it was not clear if the increased titers of pertussis antibodies would be adequate to protect the infant from pertussis, nor was it known if the increased titers would interfere with later active immunization of the infant (6). If Tdap is used in pregnancy, health care professionals are encouraged to call the toll-free number 877-311-8972 for information about patient enrollment in the Organization of Teratology Information Specialists (OTIS) Pertussis Vaccines study.

FETAL RISK SUMMARY

Acellular pertussis vaccine is available in five formulations: Tdap (for adolescents/adults) (Adacel, Boostrix); and DTaP (for infants/children) (Daptacel, Infanrix, Tripedia). Pertussis vaccine is a combination, noninfectious product containing the two toxoids and inactivated pertussis vaccine (8–12) (see also Tetanus/Diphtheria Toxoids [Adult]). Compared with DTaP, Tdap has reduced diphtheria toxoid. All five of the vaccines are given as an IM injection. The acellular vaccine replaced the whole cell vaccine in 1997 (13). In addition to the two toxoids, the vaccines contain three pertussis antigens (inactivated pertussis toxin [PT], formaldehyde-treated filamentous hemagglutinin [FHA], and pertactin) adsorbed onto aluminum hydroxide. The pertussis antigens are isolated from *Bordetella pertussis*, the cause of whopping cough. The adolescent/adult formulations are indicated for active booster immunization to prevent tetanus, diphtheria, and pertussis as a single dose in persons 10–18 years of age (Boostrix) and 11–64 years of age (Adacel) (8,9). The infant/children products are indicated for the active immunization of infants and children 6 weeks to 7 years of age (before the seventh birthday) (10–12). The information presented here applies to all of the formulations.

Reproduction studies have been conducted in rats and rabbits. DTaP (Infanrix) was given IM to rats prior to gestation and Tdap (Boostrix) was administered IM during organogenesis (days 6, 8, and 11) and later in pregnancy (day 15) (8). Each dose of Boostrix was about 45 times the human dose based on body weight (HD). No adverse effects were observed on pregnancy, lactation, or embryo–fetal or preweaning development, and there was no evidence of teratogenic effects. Studies have not been conducted for carcinogenicity, mutagenicity, or effects on fertility (8).

In rabbits, Adacel was administered IM twice before conception, during organogenesis (day 6), and later in pregnancy (day 29). Each dose was 17 times the HD. No adverse effects were observed on pregnancy, parturition, lactation, embryo–fetal or preweaning development, and there was no evidence of teratogenic effects (9).

A 1986 review on the epidemiology of pertussis cited a 1943 reference in which pertussis vaccine was given to 29 women during the sixth and seventh month of pregnancy (14). High protective antibody titers were found in mothers and their newborns. Because of the date, the product used was probably the whole cell pertussis vaccine (14).

A 2003 article reviewed the current prevalence of pertussis in the United States including its morbidity and mortality in different age groups (13). The author also discussed a 1990 serologic study conducted in her institution in which the placental transfer of maternal antibodies to pertussis was evaluated (the mothers had not received a pertussis vaccine during pregnancy) (15). Antibodies to PT in cord sera were 2.9 times higher than those in maternal sera, suggesting active transport to the embryo–fetus. In contrast, cord sera titers of antibodies to FHA and agglutinin did not differ significantly from maternal sera. Because cord blood concentrations of anti-pertussis immunoglobulin G (IgG) were nearly comparable to maternal titers, the author concluded that maternal immunization would be effective in providing infants with protection until they reached the age for active immunization (13).

A 1999 study evaluated the safety and efficacy of an acellular pertussis vaccine, which did not contain diphtheria or tetanus toxoids, in healthy men and women 18 years of age or older (16). Although pregnant women were excluded, 2 of the 200 female subjects conceived. The first woman conceived about 8 days after immunization. A spontaneous abortion occurred on gestational day 34. The second woman became pregnant within 0–4 weeks of immunization. She underwent an elective abortion at about 1 month of gestation. The investigators concluded that neither outcome was related to the vaccine (16).

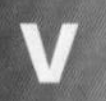

BREASTFEEDING SUMMARY

No reports describing the administration of any of the four formulations of pertussis vaccine during human lactation have been located. Tdap should present no risk to a nursing infant because antibodies to pertussis, tetanus, and diphtheria should be present in both the mother and the infant. Moreover, DTaP is indicated for infants and children 6 weeks through 6 years of age (before seventh birthday). The CDC and ACOG recommend Tdap in breastfeeding women who have not received the vaccine previously or 2 years or more have elapsed since the most recent Td administration (5,6).

References

1. McIntyre P. Vaccines for other neonatal infections. Expert Rev Vaccines 2004;3:375–8.
2. Van Rie A, Wendelboe AM, Englund JA. Role of maternal pertussis antibodies in infants. Pediatr Infect Dis J 2005;24(Suppl):S62–5.
3. Forsyth K, Tan T, von Konig CHW, Caro JJ, Plotkin S. Potential strategies to reduce the burden of pertussis. Pediatr Infect Dis J 2005;(Suppl):S69–74.
4. Committee on Infectious Diseases. American Academy of Pediatrics. Prevention of pertussis among adolescents: recommendations for use of tetanus toxoid, reduced diphtheria toxoid, and acellular pertussis (Tdap) vaccine. Pediatrics 2006;117:965–78.
5. American College of Obstetricians and Gynecologists. Update on immunization and pregnancy: tetanus, diphtheria, and pertussis vaccination. *Committee Opinion*, No. 438, August 2009.
6. Advisory Committee on Immunization Practices (ACIP). Prevention of pertussis, tetanus, and diphtheria among pregnant and postpartum women and their infants. MMWR 2008;57(RR4):1–51. Available at http://www.cdc.gov/mmwr/PDF/rr/n5704.pdf. Accessed December 28, 2009.
7. CDC. *Guidelines for Vaccinating Pregnant Women*. Available at http://www.cdc.gov/vaccines/pubs/preg-guide.htm. Accessed May 16, 2010.
8. Product information. Boostrix. GlaxoSmithKline, 2007.
9. Product information. Adacel. Sanofi Pasteur, 2007.
10. Product information. Infanrix. GlaxoSmithKline, 2007.
11. Product information. Daptacel. Sanofi Pasteur, 2007.
12. Product information. Tripedia. Sanofi Pasteur, 2007.
13. Edwards KM. Pertussis: an important target for maternal immunization. Vaccine 2003;21:3483–6.
14. Muller AS, Leeuwenburg J, Pratt DS. Pertussis: epidemiology and control. Bull World Health Organ 1986;64:321–31.
15. Van Savage J, Decker MD, Edwards KM, Sell SH, Karzon DT. Natural history of pertussis antibody in the infant and effect on vaccine response. J Infect Dis 1990;161:487–92.
16. Rothstein EP, Pennridge Pediatric Associates, Anderson EL, Decker MD, Poland GA, Reisinger KS, Blatter MM, Jacobson RM, Mink CM, Gennevois D, Izu AE, Sinangil F, Langenberg AGM. An acellular pertussis vaccine in healthy adults: safety and immunogenicity. Vaccine 1999;17:2999–3006.

VACCINE, PLAGUE

Vaccine

PREGNANCY RECOMMENDATION: No Human Data—Probably Compatible
BREASTFEEDING RECOMMENDATION: No Human Data—Probably Compatible

PREGNANCY SUMMARY

Plague vaccine is a killed bacteria vaccine (1). No risk to the fetus from vaccination during pregnancy has been reported. Animal reproduction studies have not been conducted with the vaccine.

BREASTFEEDING SUMMARY

No reports describing the administration of plague vaccine during human lactation have been located.

Reference

1. Amstey MS. Vaccination in pregnancy. Clin Obstet Gynaecol 1983;10: 13–22.

VACCINE, PNEUMOCOCCAL POLYVALENT

Vaccine

PREGNANCY RECOMMENDATION: Compatible
BREASTFEEDING RECOMMENDATION: No Human Data—Probably Compatible

PREGNANCY SUMMARY

The risk to the fetus from pneumococcal polysaccharide vaccine during the 1st trimester of pregnancy is unknown (1–3). However, the Advisory Committee on Immunization Practices (ACIP) states that there are no reports of adverse consequences in newborns whose mothers were inadvertently vaccinated during pregnancy (3,4).

FETAL RISK SUMMARY

Pneumococcal vaccine polyvalent is a killed bacteria vaccine that contains a mixture of purified capsular polysaccharides from 23 types of *Streptococcus pneumoniae* (1,2). Animal reproduction studies have not been conducted with the vaccine (1,2). A 1991 review stated that maternal antibodies induced by pneumococcal polyvalent vaccine cross the placenta and may offer significant protection to the newborn (5).

A study conducted in Bangladesh and published in 1995 described the administration of pneumococcal polyvalent vaccine to healthy women at 30–34 weeks' gestation (6). Meningococcal vaccine was administered to a control group. The immunologic response of the infants resulting from the maternal immunization was monitored from birth to 5 months of age. The results indicated that sufficient amounts of specific immunoglobulin G serum antibody passed to the fetus to provide passive immunity to invasive pneumococcal infection in early infancy. The authors concluded that, in geographic regions where such infections are a serious public health problem, maternal immunization would be a safe and inexpensive method to reduce the incidence of the disease, if subsequent studies did not show that passive immunity of the infants interfered with active immunization later in life (6).

In a 1996 study, pneumococcal polyvalent vaccine was administered in the 3rd trimester in an attempt to protect against pneumococcal disease in the infant during the first few months of life (7). The degree and duration of protection was uncertain because the pneumococcal antibodies in the infants disappeared rapidly. A 1998 reference noted that large studies are needed to determine if maternal administration of the vaccine can decrease infant mortality and morbidity (8).

Because of the high cost of vaccinations with newly developed conjugate vaccines, one author thought that vaccination of pregnant women with the polysaccharide vaccine might be the most practical method for preventing pneumococcal sepsis in young infants in developing countries (9).

BREASTFEEDING SUMMARY

In a study conducted in Bangladesh (described above), marked increases of specific immunoglobulin A (IgA) antibody titers were measured in the colostrum of mothers who had received pneumococcal polyvalent vaccine at 30–34 weeks' gestation (6). Antibody titers remained higher than controls up to 5 months after delivery.

References

1. Product information. Pneumovax. Merck, 2001.
2. Product information. PNU-Mune. Lederle Pharmaceutical, 2001.
3. CDC. Prevention of pneumococcal disease: recommendations of the Advisory Committee on Immunization Practices (ACIP). MMWR 1997;46:(No. RR-8):1–24.
4. CDC. *Guidelines for Vaccinating Pregnant Women*. Available at http://www.cdc.gov/vaccines/pubs/preg-guide.htm. Accessed May 16, 2010.
5. Faix RG. Maternal immunization to prevent fetal and neonatal infection. Clin Obstet Gynecol 1991;34:277–87.
6. Shahid NS, Steinhoff MC, Hoque SS, Begum T, Thompson C, Siber GR. Serum, breast milk, and infant antibody after maternal immunisation with pneumococcal vaccine. Lancet 1995;346:1252–7.
7. O'Dempsey TJD, McArdle T, Ceesay SJ, Banya WAS, Demba E, Secka O, Leinonen M, Kayhty H, Francis N, Greenwood BM. Immunization with a pneumococcal capsular polysaccharide vaccine during pregnancy. Vaccine 1996;14:963–70.
8. Mulholland K. Maternal immunization for the prevention of bacterial infection in young infants. Vaccine 1998;16:1464–6.
9. Glezen WP. Pneumococcal polysaccharide vaccine in pregnancy. Pediatrics 1999;104:1417–8.

VACCINE, POLIOVIRUS INACTIVATED

Vaccine

PREGNANCY RECOMMENDATION: Compatible
BREASTFEEDING RECOMMENDATION: No Human Data—Probably Compatible

PREGNANCY SUMMARY

Poliovirus vaccine inactivated (Salk vaccine, IPV) is an inactivated virus vaccine administered by injection (1). Animal reproductions studies have not been conducted with the vaccine. Although fetal damage may occur when the mother contracts the disease during pregnancy, the risk to the embryo–fetus from the vaccine appears to be low if at all.

FETAL RISK SUMMARY

No adverse effects attributable to the use of the inactivated vaccine have been reported (1,2). The CDC recommends use of the vaccine during pregnancy only if an increased risk of exposure exists (2). If immediate protection against poliomyelitis is needed, the Advisory Committee on Immunization Practices (ACIP) states that the IVP may be used in accordance with the recommended schedules for adults (see reference for specific details) (2).

The Collaborative Perinatal Project monitored 50,282 mother–child pairs, 6774 of whom had 1st trimester exposure to the vaccine (3, p. 315). Congenital malformations were observed in 461 (standardized relative risk [SRR] 1.03). In general, no associations (SRR >1.5) were found (3, p. 318). Specific malformations with SRR >1.5 were: craniosynostosis, 6 (SRR 2.1); atrial septal defect, 6 (SRR 4.0); cleft lip with or without cleft palate, 9 (SRR 1.6); omphalocele, 5 (SRR 2.4); and any malignant tumors, 7 (SRR 3.3) (3, pp. 473–4). For use anytime in pregnancy, 18,219 mother–child pairs were exposed (3, p. 436). A total of 374 newborns had anomalies (SRR 1.08). Specific malformations with SRR >1.5 were: hypoplasia of limb or part thereof, 24 (SRR 1.6); malformations of thoracic wall, 9 (SRR 2.4); anomalies of the teeth, 8 (SRR 2.0); corneal opacity, 5 (SRR 3.5); and CNS tumors, 7 (SRR 17.9) (3, pp. 486–7). The authors of this study cautioned that these data cannot be interpreted without independent confirmation from other studies and that any positive or negative association may have occurred by chance (3).

BREASTFEEDING SUMMARY

No reports describing the administration of poliovirus inactivated vaccine during human lactation have been located (see also Vaccine, Poliovirus Live).

References

1. Linder N, Ohel G. In utero vaccination. Clin Perinatol 1994;21:663–74.
2. CDC. *Guidelines for Vaccinating Pregnant Women*. Available at http://www.cdc.gov/vaccines/pubs/preg-guide.htm. Accessed May 16, 2010.
3. Heinonen OP, Slone D, Shapiro S. *Birth Defects and Drugs in Pregnancy*. Littleton, MA: Publishing Sciences Group, 1977.

VACCINE, POLIOVIRUS LIVE

Vaccine

PREGNANCY RECOMMENDATION: Compatible
BREASTFEEDING RECOMMENDATION: Compatible

PREGNANCY SUMMARY

Poliovirus vaccine live (Sabin vaccine; OPV; TOPV) is a live, trivalent (types 1, 2, and 3) attenuated virus strain vaccine administered orally. Animal reproductions studies have not been conducted with the vaccine. Although fetal damage may occur when the mother contracts the disease during pregnancy, the risk to the embryo–fetus from the vaccine appears to be low if at all. (*Withdrawn from the United States market.*)

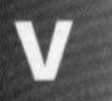

FETAL RISK SUMMARY

A brief 1990 report found no increase in spontaneous abortions or adverse effect on the placenta or embryo following 1st trimester use of oral poliovirus vaccine (1).

The Advisory Committee on Immunization Practices (ACIP) recommends use of the vaccine during pregnancy only if an increased risk of exposure exists (2). If immediate protection against poliomyelitis is needed, the ACIP states that either the inactivated or the oral vaccine may be used in accordance with the recommended schedules for adults (see reference for specific details) (2). The inactivated vaccine, however, was preferred over the oral form because of a lower risk of vaccine-associated paralysis.

The Collaborative Perinatal Project monitored 50,282 mother–child pairs, 1628 of whom had 1st trimester exposure to oral live poliovirus vaccine (3, p. 315). Congenital malformations were observed in 114 (standardized relative risk [SRR] 1.11) of the newborns. Malformations identified with SRR >1.5 were gastrointestinal (GI) defects (SRR 1.67) and Downs' syndrome (SRR 1.60) (3, p. 319). Specific malformations with SRR >1.5 were omphalocele, 3 (SRR 5.4); malrotation of the GI tract, 5 (SRR 7.9); and any benign tumors, 7 (SRR 1.8) (3, p. 474). For use anytime in pregnancy, 3059 mother–child pairs were exposed (3, p. 436). In this group, there were 44 malformed children (SRR 0.81) with the following specific malformations having SRR >1.5: Hirschsprung's disease, 4 (SRR 8.8); any benign tumors, 12 (SRR 1.7); and pectus excavatum, 8 (SRR 2.0) (3, p. 487). The authors of this study cautioned that these data cannot be interpreted without independent confirmation from other studies and that any positive or negative association may have occurred by chance (3).

The death of a 3-month old male infant because of complications arising from bilateral renal dysplasia affecting predominantly the glomeruli was thought possibly to be caused by maternal vaccination with oral poliovirus vaccine during the 1st or 2nd month of pregnancy (4). A causal relationship, however, could not be established based on the pathologic findings.

A 19-year-old previously immune woman inadvertently received oral poliovirus vaccine at 18 weeks' gestation (5). For other reasons, she requested termination of the pregnancy at 21 weeks' gestation. Polio-like changes were noted in the small-for-dates female fetus (crown–rump and foot length compatible with 17.5–19 weeks' gestation) consisting of damage to the anterior horn cells of the cervical and thoracic spinal cord with more limited secondary skeletal muscle degenerative changes in the arm (5). Poliovirus could not be isolated from the placenta or fetal brain, lung, or liver. Specific fluorescent antibody tests for poliovirus types 2 and 3 were positive in the dorsal spinal cord but not at other sites.

In response to an outbreak of wild-type 3 poliovirus in Finland, a mass vaccination program of adults was initiated with trivalent oral poliovirus vaccine in 1985, with 94% receiving the vaccine during about a 1-month period (6). Because Finland has compulsory notification of all congenital malformations detected during the first year of life, a study was conducted to determine the effect, if any, on the incidence of birth defects from the vaccine. In addition to all defects, two indicator groups were chosen because of their high detection and reporting rates: central nervous system defects and orofacial clefts. No significant changes from the baseline prevalence were noted in the three groups, but the data could not exclude an increase in less common types of congenital defects (6).

A follow-up to the above report was published in 1993 that included all structural malformations occurring during the 1st trimester (7). The outcomes of approximately 9000 pregnancies were studied, divided nearly equally between those occurring before, during, or after (i.e., one study and two reference cohorts) the vaccination program. Women in the study group had been vaccinated during the 1st trimester (defined as from conception through 15 weeks). A total of 209 cases (2.3%) were identified from liveborns, stillborns, and known abortions. There was no difference in outcomes between the cohorts (the study had a statistical power estimate to detect an increase greater than 0.5%) (7).

The analysis of Finnish women receiving the oral poliovirus vaccine during gestation was expanded to anytime during pregnancy in a 1994 report (8). The outcomes of three study groups (about 3000 pregnant women vaccinated in each of the three trimesters of pregnancy) were compared with two reference cohorts (about 6000 pregnant women who delivered before the vaccination program and about 6000 who conceived and delivered afterward). No differences were found between the study and reference groups in terms of intrauterine growth or in the prevalence of stillbirth, neonatal death, congenital anomalies, premature birth, perinatal infection, and neurologic abnormalities (8). The authors concluded that the vaccination of pregnant women with the oral poliovirus vaccine, as conducted in Finland, appeared to be safe.

A 1993 report described the use of oral poliovirus vaccine in a nationwide (Israel) vaccination campaign, including pregnant women, after the occurrence of 15 cases of polio in the summer of 1988 (9). The investigators compared the frequency of anomalies and premature births in their area in 1988 (controls) with those in 1989 (exposed). In 1988, 15,021 live births occurred, with 204 malformed newborns (1.4%) and 999 (6.7%) premature infants. These numbers did not differ statistically from those in 1989; 15,696, 243 (1.5%), and 1083 (6.9%), respectively. The authors concluded that oral poliovirus vaccine was preferred to the inactivated vaccine if vaccination was required during pregnancy (9).

In a follow-up of the Israel vaccination campaign, investigators measured the presence of neutralizing antibodies to the three poliovirus types in the sera of infants whose mothers had been vaccinated 2–7 weeks before delivery (10). In newborns, higher levels of protecting antibodies were found for poliovirus types 1 and 2 than for type 3, indicating less placental transfer and a greater risk of infection with poliovirus type 3.

BREASTFEEDING SUMMARY

Human milk contains poliovirus antibodies in direct relation to titers found in the mother's serum. When oral poliovirus vaccine (Sabin vaccine, OPV) is administered to the breastfed infant in the immediate neonatal period, these antibodies, which are highest in colostrum, may prevent infection and development of subsequent immunity to wild poliovirus (11–22). To prevent inhibition of the vaccine, breastfeeding should be withheld 6 hours before and after administration of the vaccine, although some authors recommend shorter times (17–21).

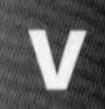

In the United States, the ACIP and the Committee on Infectious Diseases of the American Academy of Pediatrics do not recommend vaccination before 6 weeks of age (3,23). At this age or older, the effect of the oral vaccine is not inhibited by breastfeeding and no special instructions or planned feeding schedules are required (3,23–27).

References

1. Ornoy A, Arnon J, Feingold M, Ben Ishai P. Spontaneous abortions following oral poliovirus vaccination in first trimester. Lancet 1990;335:800.
2. CDC. Poliomyelitis prevention in the United States: introduction of a sequential vaccination schedule of inactivated poliovirus vaccine followed by oral poliovirus vaccine. Recommendations of the Advisory Committee on Immunization Practices (ACIP). MMWR 1997;46(No. RR-3):1–25.
3. Heinonen OP, Slone D, Shapiro S. *Birth Defects and Drugs in Pregnancy*. Littleton, MA: Publishing Sciences Group, 1977.
4. Castleman B, McNeely BU. Case records of the Massachusetts General Hospital. Case 47-1964. Presentation of Case. N Engl J Med 1964;271: 676–82.
5. Burton AE, Robinson ET, Harper WF, Bell EJ, Boyd JF. Fetal damage after accidental polio vaccination of an immune mother. J R Coll Gen Pract 1984;34:390–4.
6. Harjulehto T, Aro T, Hovi T, Saxen L. Congenital malformations and oral poliovirus vaccination during pregnancy. Lancet 1989;1:771–2.
7. Harjulehto-Mervaala T, Aro T, Hiilesmaa VK, Saxen H, Hovi T, Saxen L. Oral polio vaccination during pregnancy: no increase in the occurrence of congenital malformations. Am J Epidemiol 1993;138:407–14.
8. Harjulehto-Mervaala T, Aro T, Hiilesmaa VK, Hovi T, Saxen H, Saxen L. Oral polio vaccination during pregnancy: lack of impact on fetal development and perinatal outcome. Clin Infect Dis 1994;18:414–20.
9. Ornoy A, Ben Ishai PB. Congenital anomalies after oral poliovirus vaccination during pregnancy. Lancet 1993;341:1162.
10. Linder N, Handsher R, Fruman O, Shiff E, Ohel G, Reichman B, Dagan R. Effect of maternal immunization with oral poliovirus vaccine on neonatal immunity. Pediatr Infect Dis J 1994;13:959–62.
11. Lepow ML, Warren RJ, Gray N, Ingram VG, Robbins FC. Effect of Sabin type I poliomyelitis vaccine administered by mouth to newborn infants. N Engl J Med 1961;264:1071–8.
12. Holguin AH, Reeves JS, Gelfand HM. Immunization of infants with the Sabin oral poliovirus vaccine. Am J Public Health 1962;52:600–10.
13. Sabin AB, Fieldsteel AH. Antipoliomyelitic activity of human and bovine colostrum and milk. Pediatrics 1962;29:105–15.
14. Sabin AB, Michaels RH, Krugman S, Eiger ME, Berman PH, Warren J. Effect of oral poliovirus vaccine in newborn children. I. Excretion of virus after ingestion of large doses of type I or of mixture of all three types, in relation to level of placentally transmitted antibody. Pediatrics 1963;31:623–40.
15. Warren RJ, Lepow ML, Bartsch GE, Robbins FC. The relationship of maternal antibody, breast feeding, and age to the susceptibility of newborn infants to infection with attenuated polioviruses. Pediatrics 1964;34:4–13.
16. Plotkin SA, Katz M, Brown RE, Pagano JS. Oral poliovirus vaccination in newborn African infants. The inhibitory effect of breast feeding. Am J Dis Child 1966;111:27–30.
17. Katz M, Plotkin SA. Oral polio immunization of the newborn infant; a possible method for overcoming interference by ingested antibodies. J Pediatr 1968;73:267–70.
18. Adcock E, Greene H. Poliovirus antibodies in breastfed infants. Lancet 1971;2:662–3.
19. Anonymous. Sabin vaccine in breastfed infants. Med J Aust 1972;2:175.
20. John TJ. The effect of breastfeeding on the antibody response of infants to trivalent oral poliovirus vaccine. J Pediatr 1974;84:307.
21. Plotkin SA, Katz M. Administration of oral polio vaccine in relation to time of breast feeding. J Pediatr 1974;84:309.
22. Deforest A, Smith DS. The effect of breast-feeding on the antibody response of infants to trivalent oral poliovirus vaccine (reply). J Pediatr 1974;84:308.
23. Kelein JO, Brunell PA, Cherry JD, Fulginiti VA, eds. *Report of the Committee on Infectious Diseases*. 19th ed. Evanston, IL: American Academy of Pediatrics, 1982:208.
24. Kim-Farley R, Brink E, Orenstein W, Bart K. Vaccination and breastfeeding. JAMA 1982;248:2451–2.
25. Deforest A, Parker PB, DiLiberti JH, Yates HT Jr, Sibinga MS, Smith DS. The effect of breastfeeding on the antibody response of infants to trivalent oral poliovirus vaccine. J Pediatr 1973;83:93–5.
26. John TJ, Devarajan LV, Luther L, Vijayarathnam P. Effect of breastfeeding on seroresponse of infants to oral poliovirus vaccination. Pediatrics 1976;57:47–53.
27. Welsh J, May JT. Breastfeeding and trivalent oral polio vaccine. J Pediatr 1979;95:333.

VACCINE, RABIES (HUMAN)

Vaccine

PREGNANCY RECOMMENDATION: Compatible—Maternal Benefit >> Embryo–Fetal Risk
BREASTFEEDING RECOMMENDATION: No Human Data—Probably Compatible

PREGNANCY SUMMARY

Rabies vaccine (human) is an inactivated virus vaccine (1). Animal reproduction studies have not been conducted with the vaccine. Because rabies is nearly 100% fatal if contracted, the vaccine should be given for postexposure prophylaxis (1,2).

FETAL RISK SUMMARY

The CDC states that indications for prophylaxis are not altered by pregnancy (1). Three reports described the use of rabies vaccine (human) during pregnancy (3–5). Passive immunity was found in one newborn (titer >1:50) but was lost by 1 year of age (3). No adverse effects from the vaccine were noted in the newborn. The mother had not delivered at the time of the report in the second case (4).

A 1990 brief report described the use of rabies vaccine in 16 pregnant women, 15 using the human diploid cell vaccine and 1 receiving the purified chick embryo cell product (5). In 15 cases, the stage of pregnancy was known: nine 1st trimester, three 2nd trimester, and three 3rd trimester. Two women had spontaneous abortions, but the causes were probably not vaccine related. The remaining pregnancy outcomes were 12 full-term healthy newborns, 1 premature delivery at 36 weeks' gestation, and 1 newborn with grand-mal seizures on the 2nd day. In the latter case, no anti-rabies antibodies were detectable in the infant's serum, indicating that the condition was not vaccine related (5).

In two reports, duck embryo-cultured vaccine was used during pregnancy (6,7). In 1974, a report appeared describing the use of rabies vaccine (duck embryo) in a woman in her 7th month of pregnancy (6). She was given a 21-day treatment course of the vaccine. She subsequently delivered a healthy term male infant who was developing normally at 9 months of age. The second case was described in 1975 involving a woman exposed to rabies at 35 weeks' gestation (7). She was treated with a 14-day course of vaccine (duck embryo) followed by three booster injections. She gave birth at 39 weeks' gestation to a healthy male infant. Cord blood rabies neutralizing antibody titer was 1:30, indicative of passive immunity, compared with a titer of 1:70 in maternal serum. Titers in the infant fell to 1:5 at 3 weeks of age, then to <1:5 at 6 weeks. Development was normal at 9 months of age (7).

A 1989 report from Thailand described the use of purified Vero cell rabies vaccine for postexposure vaccination in 21 pregnant women (8). Equine rabies immune globulin was also administered to 12 of the women with severe exposures. One patient aborted 3 days after her first rabies vaccination, but she had noted vaginal bleeding on the day of rabies exposure. No congenital malformations were observed and none of the mothers or their infants developed rabies after a 1-year follow-up (8).

In a subsequent prospective study, the above researchers administered the purified Vero cell rabies vaccine (five-dose regimen) after exposure to 202 pregnant women (9). Some of these women also received a single dose of rabies immune globulin (human or equine). Follow-up of 1 year or greater was conducted in 190 patients; 12 patients were lost to follow-up following postexposure treatment. No increase in maternal (spontaneous abortion, hypertension, placenta previa, or gestational diabetes) or fetal (stillbirth, minor birth defect, or low birth weight) complications was observed in comparison with a control group of nonvaccinated, nonexposed women. The one minor congenital defect observed in the treated group was a type of clubfoot (talipes equinovalgus) (9).

BREASTFEEDING SUMMARY

No reports describing the administration of rabies (human) vaccine during human lactation have been located.

References

1. CDC. *Guidelines for Vaccinating Pregnant Women*. Available at http://www.cdc.gov/vaccines/pubs/preg-guide.htm. Accessed May 16, 2010.
2. Amstey MS. Vaccination in pregnancy. Clin Obstet Gynaecol 1983;10:13–22.
3. Varner MW, McGuinness GA, Galask RP. Rabies vaccination in pregnancy. Am J Obstet Gynecol 1982;143:717–8.
4. Klietmann W, Domres B, Cox JH. Rabies postexposure treatment and side effects in man using HDC (MRC 5) vaccine. Dev Biol Stand 1978;40:109–13.
5. Fescharek R, Quast U, Dechert G. Postexposure rabies vaccination during pregnancy: experience from post-marketing surveillance with 16 patients. Vaccine 1990;8:409–10.
6. Cates W Jr. Treatment of rabies exposure during pregnancy. Obstet Gynecol 1974;44:893–6.
7. Spence MR, Davidson DE, Dill GS Jr, Boonthai P, Sagartz JW. Rabies exposure during pregnancy. Am J Obstet Gynecol 1975;123:655–6.
8. Chutivongse S, Wilde H. Postexposure rabies vaccination during pregnancy: experience with 21 patients. Vaccine 1989;7:546–8.
9. Chutivongse S, Wilde H, Benjavongkulchai M, Chomchey P, Punthawong S. Postexposure rabies vaccination during pregnancy: effect on 202 women and their infants. Clin Infect Dis 1995;20:818–20.

VACCINE, RUBELLA

Vaccine

PREGNANCY RECOMMENDATION: Contraindicated
BREASTFEEDING RECOMMENDATION: Compatible

PREGNANCY SUMMARY

Although no defects attributable to rubella vaccine have been reported, the CDC calculates the theoretical risk of congenital rubella syndrome (CRS) following vaccination with the RA 27/3 vaccine to range from 0% to 1.6%, or from 0% to 1.2%, if data from all rubella vaccines are included (1). These risks are considerably lower than the ≥20% risk associated with wild rubella virus infection during the 1st trimester (2). Because a theoretical risk does exist, the use of the vaccine in pregnancy is contraindicated (1–6). Moreover, both the manufacturer and the CDC recommend that women should avoid becoming pregnant for 3 months after receiving the vaccine (1,4). However, if vaccination does occur within 3 months (now 4 weeks [3]) of conception or during pregnancy, the actual risk, as stated above, is considered to be negligible and, in itself, should not be an indication to terminate the pregnancy (2,3,5–8).

FETAL RISK SUMMARY

Rubella (German measles) vaccine is a live, attenuated virus vaccine (4). Animal reproduction studies have not been conducted with the vaccine.

Rubella occurring during pregnancy may result in the CRS. The greatest risk period for viremia and congenital defects is 1 week before to 4 weeks after conception (5). Moreover, rubella reinfection, most often presenting as a subclinical infection that can be detected by a rise in antibody titers, may occur in previously vaccinated patients and in those who are naturally immune (9,10). The fetal risk of infection in these cases is low but has not yet been quantified.

The CDC defines CRS as any two complications from list A or one complication from list A plus one from list B (5):

List A

Cataracts or congenital glaucoma
Congenital heart disease
Loss of hearing
Pigmentary retinopathy

List B

Purpura
Splenomegaly
Jaundice (onset within 24 hours of birth)
Microcephaly
Mental retardation
Meningoencephalitis
Radiolucent bone disease

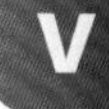

Before April 1979, the CDC collected data on 538 women vaccinated within 3 months before or after conception with either the Cendehill or HPV-77 vaccines (5). A total of 149 of these women were known to be susceptible at the time of vaccination and the outcome of pregnancy was known for 143 (96%). No evidence of CRS or other maternal or fetal complication was found in any of these cases or in an additional 196 infants exposed during pregnancy. Eight infants had serologic evidence of intrauterine infection after maternal vaccination, but follow-up for 2–7 years revealed no problems attributable to CRS (5).

Since January 1979, only RA 27/3 rubella vaccine has been available in the United States. In the United States between January 1979 and December 1988, a total of 683 women vaccinated with RA 27/3 have been reported to the CDC (2). The outcomes of these pregnancies were as follows:

Total vaccinated (1/79–12/88)	*683*
Susceptible at vaccination	*272*
Live births	212 (2 sets of twins)
Spontaneous abortions or stillbirths	13
Induced abortions	31
Outcome unknown	18
Immune or unknown at vaccination	*411*
Live births	350 (1 set of twins)
Spontaneous abortions or stillbirths	9
Induced abortions	24
Outcome unknown	29

Evidence of subclinical infection was found in 3 (2%) of the 154 liveborn infants from susceptible mothers who were serologically evaluated (2). However, no evidence of defects compatible with CRS was found in the total sample of 212 liveborn infants. Two infants did have asymptomatic glandular hypospadias, but both mothers had negative rubella-specific immunoglobulin M (IgM) titers in the cord blood at birth (2). In a 1985 evaluation of earlier CDC data, no defects compatible with CRS were found in any of the fetuses or infants in whom the outcome was known (6). Examinations up to 29 months after birth have revealed normal growth and development (2,6).

A 2000 report described six women who received rubella vaccine (live, attenuated vaccine strain RA27/3) either in the pre- or periconceptional periods (11). No evidence of fetal infection was observed in five of the women. In one case, however, vertical transmission of the virus was documented that resulted in persistent fetal infection. The 25-year-old woman, unaware of her pregnancy, received the vaccine 3 weeks after conception. Virus isolation and polymerase chain reaction (PCR) of amniotic fluid obtained by amniocentesis at 16 weeks' gestation confirmed the vertical transmission. Multiple maternal and fetal serologic and virologic testings were done throughout the pregnancy. Rising IgG titers and persistent IgM levels were measured in the fetus. At 39 weeks' gestation, a cord blood sample was positive for virus isolation and PCR. Although a persistent rubella viral infection was documented, frequent monitoring of the pregnancy revealed no pathologic findings or complications and a healthy 3450-g male infant was delivered at 40 weeks' gestation. Apgar scores were 9, 9, and 10 at 1, 5, and 10 minutes, respectively. At 23 weeks of age, IgM, PCR, and virus isolation in his peripheral blood were negative. His growth and development have been normal up to 14 months of age (11).

BREASTFEEDING SUMMARY

The CDC recommends vaccination of susceptible women with rubella vaccine in the immediate postpartum period (1). Many of these women will breastfeed their newborns. Although two studies failed to find evidence of the attenuated virus in milk, subsequent reports have demonstrated transfer (12–16).

In one case, the mother noted rash and adenopathy 12 days after vaccination with the HPV-77 vaccine on the 1st postpartum day (14). Rubella virus was isolated from her breast milk and from the infant's throat (14). A significant level of rubella-specific cell-mediated immunity was found in the infant, but there was no detectable serologic response as measured by rubella hemagglutination inhibition antibody titers (14). No adverse effects were noted in the infant. In a second case report, a 13-day-old breastfed infant developed rubella about 11 days after maternal vaccination with HPV-77 (17). It could not be determined whether the infant was infected by virus transmission via the milk (18,19). Nine (69%) of 13 lactating women given either HPV-77 or RA 27/3 vaccine in the immediate postpartum period shed virus in their milk (15). In another report by these same researchers, 11 (69%) of 16 vaccinated women shed rubella virus or virus antigen in their milk (16). No adverse effects or symptoms of clinical disease were observed in the infants.

References

1. CDC. Measles, mumps, and rubella—vaccine use and strategies for elimination of measles, rubella, and congenital rubella syndrome and control of mumps: recommendations of the Advisory Committee on Immunization Practices (ACIP). MMWR 1998;47(No. RR-8):1–57.
2. CDC. Rubella vaccination during pregnancy—United States, 1971–1988. MMWR 1989;38:289–93.
3. CDC. *Guidelines for Vaccinating Pregnant Women*. Available at http://www.cdc.gov/vaccines/pubs/preg-guide.htm. Accessed May 16, 2010.
4. Product information. Meruvax. Merck, 2001.
5. CDC. Rubella vaccination during pregnancy—United States, 1971–1982. MMWR 1983;32:429–32.
6. Preblud SR, Williams NM. Fetal risk associated with rubella vaccine: implications for vaccination of susceptible women. Obstet Gynecol 1985;66:121–3.
7. Burgess MA. Rubella vaccination just before or during pregnancy. Med J Aust 1990;152:507–8.
8. Linder N, Ohel G. In utero vaccination. Clin Perinatol 1994;21:663–74.
9. Burgess MA. Rubella reinfection—what risk to the fetus? Med J Aust 1992;156:824–5.
10. Condon R, Bower C. Congenital rubella after previous maternal vaccination. Med J Aust 1992;156:882.
11. Hofmann J, Kortung M, Pustowoit B, Faber R, Piskazeck U, Liebert UG. Persistent fetal rubella vaccine virus infection following inadvertent vaccination during early pregnancy. J Med Virol 2000;61:155–8.
12. Isacson P, Kehrer AF, Wilson H, Williams S. Comparative study of live, attenuated rubella virus vaccines during the immediate puerperium. Obstet Gynecol 1971;37:332–7.
13. Grillner L, Hedstrom CE, Bergstrom H, Forssman L, Rigner A, Lycke E. Vaccination against rubella of newly delivered women. Scand J Infect Dis 1973;5:237–41.
14. Buimovici-Klein E, Hite RL, Byrne T, Cooper LZ. Isolation of rubella virus in milk after postpartum immunization. J Pediatr 1977;91:939–41.
15. Losonsky GA, Fishaut JM, Strussenberg J, Ogra PL. Effect of immunization against rubella on lactation products. I. Development and characterization of specific immunologic reactivity in breast milk. J Infect Dis 1982;145:654–60.
16. Losonsky GA, Fishaut JM, Strussenberg J, Ogra PL. Effect of immunization against rubella on lactation products. II. Maternal-neonatal interactions. J Infect Dis 1982;145:661–6.
17. Landes RD, Bass JW, Millunchick EW, Oetgen WJ. Neonatal rubella following postpartum maternal immunization. J Pediatr 1980;97:465–7.
18. Lerman SJ. Neonatal rubella following maternal immunization. J Pediatr 1981;98:668.
19. Bass JW, Landes RD. Neonatal rubella following maternal immunization (reply). J Pediatr 1981;98:668–9.

VACCINE, SMALLPOX

Vaccine

PREGNANCY RECOMMENDATION: Human Data Suggest Risk
BREASTFEEDING RECOMMENDATION: Contraindicated

PREGNANCY SUMMARY

The CDC classifies smallpox vaccine as contraindicated during pregnancy, within 28 days of conception, and in persons who might have close contact with pregnant women within 28 days of their vaccination (1,2). Other sources also consider smallpox vaccine to be contraindicated during pregnancy (3–6). However, the vaccine should be given to pregnant women who have been exposed to smallpox or monkeypox (1,2,7). Because the risk for fetal vaccinia is low, inadvertent exposure to the vaccine during or before pregnancy should not be a reason for pregnancy termination (1).

FETAL RISK SUMMARY

Smallpox vaccine is a live, attenuated virus vaccine (3,4). Although smallpox infection had a high mortality rate, the disease has been largely eradicated from the world (3,5). Vaccination during pregnancy between 3 and 24 weeks has resulted in fetal death (4,5). A 1974 reference reviewed the published reports of smallpox vaccination during pregnancy and found 20 cases of fetal vaccinia among more than 8500 maternal vaccinations (8). Of the 21 exposed fetuses (1 set of twins), only 3 of the 10 liveborns survived. There was only weak evidence, however, that vaccination during the 1st trimester increased fetal wastage compared with that occurring later in gestation (8).

In a 2004 review that documented the rarity of fetal vaccinia, only about 50 cases were found of fetal infection after smallpox vaccination during pregnancy or shortly before conception (9). Although the exact number of women given the vaccine during pregnancy was unknown, the number is probably large because, in past years, pregnant women were routinely vaccinated during outbreaks of smallpox. The 50 cases were documented in women who had received the vaccine at anytime in pregnancy, after primary vaccination and revaccination, and in nonvaccinated women who had contact with vaccines. The authors concluded that there was insufficient evidence to recommend prophylactic treatment with vaccinia immune globulin if the woman was pregnant or shortly before conception when she received the vaccine (9).

The CDC announced the establishment of the National Smallpox Vaccine in Pregnancy Registry in 2003 (10). The Registry was established to monitor pregnancy outcomes of women who had received the vaccine during pregnancy, or who became pregnant or were in close contact with a vaccinee within 28 days after vaccination. Health care providers and public health staff were encouraged to report cases by calling 877-554-4625 or 404-639-8253 (10).

Two months after the above announcement, the CDC reported, for the period of November 2001–April 2003, that 103 women had received the vaccine either during pregnancy or within 4 weeks of conception (1). The exposures occurred in military personnel, civilian health care and public health workers, and clinical studies. In the civilian group, two women conceived within 1 week before vaccination and four conceived within 28 days after vaccination. Two (timing of vaccination not specified) of the six women had early spontaneous abortions (1). Other pregnancy outcomes, other than these two, have apparently not yet been reported.

BREASTFEEDING SUMMARY

No reports of nursing women receiving smallpox vaccine have been located. In an unusual report, however, tertiary contact vaccinia transmission from a mother to her nursing infant through direct skin-to-skin and skin-to-mucous membrane contact was documented (11). The father, a soldier in the United States Army, had received smallpox vaccination, but had reportedly taken standard precautions to avoid spread to his family. Approximately 1–2 weeks later, his wife developed vesicles on both areolas. About 2 weeks later, a papule developed on the philtrum of the breastfeeding infant. Polymerase chain reaction and culture for vaccinia of the mother and infant confirmed contact vaccinia (11).

Because of the risk of contact vaccinia in a nursing infant, the CDC recommends that breastfeeding mothers should not be routinely vaccinated (11). However, based on the recommendations during pregnancy, if a nursing woman is exposed to smallpox or monkeypox, she should receive the vaccine but should probably stop breastfeeding.

References

1. CDC. Women with smallpox vaccine exposure during pregnancy reported to the National Smallpox Vaccine in Pregnancy Registry—United States, 2003. MMWR 2003;52:386–88.
2. CDC. *Guidelines for Vaccinating Pregnant Women*. Available at http://www.cdc.gov/vaccines/pubs/preg-guide.htm. Accessed May 16, 2010.
3. Amstey MS. Vaccination in pregnancy. Clin Obstet Gynaecol 1983;10:13–22.
4. American Hospital Formulary Service. *Drug Information 1997*. Bethesda, MD: American Society of Health-System Pharmacists, 1997:2646–9.
5. Hart RJC. Immunization. Clin Obstet Gynaecol 1981;8:421–30.
6. Linder N, Ohel G. In utero vaccination. Clin Perinatol 1994;21:663–74.
7. Jamieson DJ, Cono J, Richards CL, Treadwell TA. The role of the obstetrician-gynecologist in emerging infectious diseases: monkeypox and pregnancy. Obstet Gynecol 2004;103:754–6.
8. Levine MM. Live-virus vaccines in pregnancy. Risks and recommendations. Lancet 1974;2:34–8.
9. Napolitano PG, Ryan MAK, Grabenstein JD. Pregnancy discovered after smallpox vaccination: is vaccinia immune globulin appropriate? Am J Obstet Gynecol 2004;191:1863–7.
10. CDC. Notice to readers: National Smallpox Vaccine in Pregnancy Registry. MMWR 2003;52:256.
11. Garde V, Harper D, Fairchok MP. Tertiary contact vaccinia in a breastfeeding infant. JAMA 2004;291:725–7.

VACCINE, TC-83 VENEZUELAN EQUINE ENCEPHALITIS

Vaccine

PREGNANCY RECOMMENDATION: Contraindicated
BREASTFEEDING RECOMMENDATION: No Human Data—Probably Compatible

PREGNANCY SUMMARY

One case of human pregnancy exposure to TC-83 Venezuelan equine encephalitis vaccine has been reported, but the adverse fetal outcome combined with the animal data indicate that the vaccine should not be given to pregnant women. In the United States, routine immunization is not practiced, but some laboratory workers may require the vaccine because of potential exposure to the virus in their work (1). Based on the available data, pregnancy should be excluded before administration of the vaccine, and the woman warned against conception in the immediate future (in the case above, the woman was advised not to become pregnant for 1 month after vaccination, but references confirming this as a safe interval for this vaccine have not been located).

FETAL RISK SUMMARY

A live, attenuated strain of Venezuelan equine encephalitis (VEE) virus, TC-83, is used as a vaccine (1). VEE, transmitted by mosquitoes, is primarily found in South America and Central America, but cases have occurred in Texas (1). Although many human cases of VEE are asymptomatic, some patients may have severe symptoms, including confusion, seizures, and nuchal rigidity (1).

VEE was embryo- and fetotoxic and teratogenic in rats inoculated with the virulent Guajira strain during the first 2 weeks of pregnancy (2). All embryos died within 3–4 days with evidence of necrosis and hemorrhage. Inoculation later in pregnancy resulted in similar outcomes, including infarcts of the placenta.

Fetal rhesus monkeys were administered TC-83 VEE virus vaccine via the intracerebral route at 100 days' gestation and then were allowed to proceed to term (159–161 days' gestation) (3). All of the infected fetuses were born alive. Some of the newborns were killed and examined within 24 hours of birth, others at 1 month, and the remainder at 3 months. Malformations evident in all of the offspring were microencephaly, hydrocephaly, and cataracts, and two-thirds had porencephaly.

A 1977 brief accounting of the 1962 outbreak of VEE in Venezuela cited the frequent abortion of women who were infected during the 1st trimester (4). In addition, the infection of seven pregnant women, between the 13th and 36th weeks of gestation, and the subsequent fatal fetal and newborn outcomes were discussed (4). All of the fetuses and newborns had destruction of the fetal cerebral cortex, the degree of which was determined by the interval between infection and delivery. In one of the cases, the mother had severe encephalitis at 13 weeks and eventually gave birth at 33 weeks' gestation. Microcephaly, microphthalmia, luxation of the hips, severe medulla hypoplasia, and the near absence of neural tissue in the cranium were evident in the stillborn fetus (4).

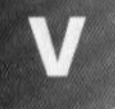

The fatal outcome of a case in which a 21-year-old laboratory worker became pregnant (against medical advice) after receiving the TC-83 vaccine was described in a 1987 report (1). The mother's VEE virus titers were 1:20 at 17 weeks' gestation and 1:10, 3 months later. Maternal serum α-fetoprotein and an ultrasound examination were normal at 17 weeks, but a lack of fetal movement was noted at 26 weeks. One week later, a stillborn, hydropic female fetus was delivered. Generalized edema, ascites, hydrothorax, and a large multilobulated cystic hygroma were noted on examination. Mononuclear infiltrate was found in the myocardium and pulmonary arterioles and an inflammatory cell infiltrate was noted in the trachea, intestinal adventitia, brain, uterus, and fallopian tubes (1). Marked autolysis of the brain had occurred. Abnormalities in the placenta included calcifications, infarcts, petechiae, and thrombosis in the decidua (1).

BREASTFEEDING SUMMARY

No reports describing the administration of TC-83 Venezuelan equine encephalitis vaccine during human lactation have been located.

References

1. Casamassima AC, Hess LW, Marty A. TC-83 Venezuelan equine encephalitis vaccine exposure during pregnancy. Teratology 1987;36:287–9.
2. Garcia-Tamayo J, Esparza J, Martinez AJ. Placental and fetal alterations due to Venezuelan equine encephalitis virus in rats. Infect Immun 1981;32:813–21.
3. London WT, Levitt NH, Kent SG, Wong VG, Sever JL. Congenital cerebral and ocular malformations induced in rhesus monkeys by Venezuelan equine encephalitis virus. Teratology 1977;16:285–96.
4. Wenger F. Venezuelan equine encephalitis. Teratology 1977;16:359–62.

VACCINE, TULAREMIA

Vaccine

PREGNANCY RECOMMENDATION: Compatible—Maternal Benefit >> Embryo–Fetal Risk
BREASTFEEDING RECOMMENDATION: No Human Data—Probably Compatible

PREGNANCY SUMMARY

Tularemia vaccine is a live, attenuated bacteria vaccine (1,2). Because tularemia is a severe disease, preexposure prophylaxis of indicated persons should occur regardless of pregnancy (1).

FETAL RISK SUMMARY

Tularemia is a serious infectious disease occurring primarily in laboratory personnel, rabbit handlers, and forest workers (1). The risk to the fetus from the vaccine is unknown. One report described vaccination in a woman early in the 1st trimester with transplacental passage of antibodies (2,3). No adverse effects were observed in the term infant or at 1-year follow-up.

BREASTFEEDING SUMMARY

No reports describing the administration of tularemia vaccine during human lactation have been located.

References

1. Amstey MS. Vaccination in pregnancy. Clin Obstet Gynaecol 1983;10:13–22.
2. Albrecht RC, Cefalo RC, O'Brien WF. Tularemia immunization in early pregnancy. Am J Obstet Gynecol 1980;138:1226–7.
3. Linder N, Ohel G. In utero vaccination. Clin Perinatol 1994;21:663–74.

VACCINE, TYPHOID

Vaccine

PREGNANCY RECOMMENDATION: Compatible—Maternal Benefit >> Embryo–Fetal Risk
BREASTFEEDING RECOMMENDATION: No Human Data—Probably Compatible

PREGNANCY SUMMARY

Typhoid is a serious infectious disease with high morbidity and mortality. The risk to the fetus from the vaccine is unknown (1).

FETAL RISK SUMMARY

Three typhoid vaccines are available: typhoid Vi polysaccharide vaccine that is given IM (2); typhoid vaccine live attenuated oral Ty21a (3); and typhoid vaccine of inactivated (killed) bacteria that is given SC (4). No animal reproduction studies have been conducted with any of the vaccine types.

BREASTFEEDING SUMMARY

No reports describing the administration of typhoid vaccine during human lactation have been located.

References

1. CDC. Typhoid immunization. Recommendations of the Advisory Committee on Immunization Practices (ACIP). MMWR 1994;43 (No. RR-14):1–7.
2. Product information. Typhim VI. Aventis Pasteur, 2001.
3. Product information. Vivotif Berna Vaccine. Berna Products, 2001.
4. Product information. Typhoid Vaccine. Wyeth-Ayerst Pharmaceuticals, 2001.

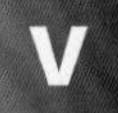

VACCINE, VARICELLA VIRUS

Vaccine

PREGNANCY RECOMMENDATION: Contraindicated
BREASTFEEDING RECOMMENDATION: Compatible

PREGNANCY SUMMARY

The risk of congenital varicella syndrome with natural (wild) varicella virus is approximately 1%–2% during the first 20 weeks of gestation. Moreover, there is significant risk for infectious morbidity and possible mortality in the neonate and young child when maternal varicella infection occurs after the 1st trimester. The risk from the vaccine is thought to be much less, because the virulence of the attenuated virus used in the vaccine is less than that of the natural virus. Although varicella virus vaccine is contraindicated immediately before and during pregnancy because of unknown fetal effects, the potential for harmful fetal effects appears to be very low as estimated below. No cases of varicella vaccine-induced fetal harm have been identified to date. Because of this, the Advisory Committee on Immunization Practices (ACIP) recommends that a decision to terminate a pregnancy should not be based on whether the vaccine was given during pregnancy (1). Health care professionals are encouraged to report patients who receive the vaccine 3 months before or at any time during pregnancy to the Varivax Pregnancy Registry by calling 800-986-8999.

FETAL RISK SUMMARY

Varicella virus vaccine is prepared from the Oka/Merck strain of live, attenuated varicella-zoster virus (1,2). The vaccine became commercially available in May 1995. Animal reproductive studies have not been conducted with the vaccine.

The manufacturer considers vaccination of a woman within 3 months of conception and during pregnancy to be contraindicated because the effects of the vaccine on the fetus are unknown (2). Both the ACIP and the American Academy of Pediatrics, however, recommend avoiding pregnancy for only 1 month following an immunization injection (1,3). Vaccination of a child is not contraindicated if the child's nonimmune mother or other nonimmune household member is pregnant (1,3).

Many references have described the effects of natural (wild) varicella infection during pregnancy on the fetus and newborn (3,4–39). Infection with wild varicella-zoster virus during the first 20 weeks of pregnancy is associated with a risk of congenital varicella syndrome (1,4–6). The syndrome is commonly characterized by low birth weight. Other clinical features, not all of which may be apparent in each case, are shown below (1,4–6):

Cutaneous: cicatricial skin lesions, denuded skin
Neurologic: microcephaly, cortical atrophy, myoclonic seizures, hypotonia, hyporeflexia, encephalomyelitis, dorsal radiculitis, Horner's syndrome, bulbar dysphagia, deafness, mental retardation
Ophthalmic: microphthalmia, chorioretinitis, cataracts, nystagmus, anisocoria, enophthalmos, hypoplasia of the optic discs, optic atrophy, squint
Skeletal: limb hypoplasia of bone and muscle (usually on same side as scarring), hypoplasia of mandible, clavicle, scapula, ribs, fingers and toes, club foot
Gastrointestinal: gastroesophageal reflux, duodenal stenosis, jejunal dilatation, microcolon, atresia of sigmoid colon, malfunction of anal sphincter
Genitourinary: neurogenic bladder

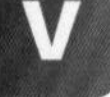

In addition, infection in the 2nd and 3rd trimesters (13 weeks' gestation to term) is associated with a risk of clinical varicella infection during the newborn period or with clinical zoster during infancy and early childhood (1). Severe neonatal varicella may occur in 17%–30% of newborns if the onset of maternal varicella infection is 5 days before to 2 days after delivery. Although based on small numbers, possibly affected by reporting bias and not reflective of modern treatment models (data reported in 1974), the death rate in neonates whose mothers had an onset of rash 0–4 days before delivery was 31% (1).

Data from five prospective studies indicate the risk of congenital varicella syndrome during the 1st trimester was 1.0% (6 of 617 infants) (range 0%–9.1%) (4,7–10). A higher risk, 2.0% (7 of 351 infants), was found if the infection occurred during 13–20 weeks' gestation (10). Based on these five studies, the overall incidence of congenital varicella syndrome from maternal infection during the first 20 weeks' gestation was 1.3% (13 of 968).

In addition to children 12 months of age or older who have not had varicella, the ACIP recommends vaccination for nonimmune adults because of the severity of chickenpox in this population (1,3). Vaccination is contraindicated in pregnancy because of the unknown effects of the vaccine on the fetus and because of the known fetal adverse effects of the natural (wild) varicella-zoster virus (1–3).

A 1996 report from the manufacturer's pregnancy registry for Varivax described seven pregnant women who had received the vaccine between June 1995 and late 1996 (40,41). The women, thought to be nonimmune, had been exposed to varicella and were inadvertently given the vaccine instead of the indicated varicella-zoster immune globulin (see also Immune Globulin, Varicella-Zoster [Human]). Moreover, one of the women received 5 times the recommended dose of the vaccine (40,41). None of the women had histories of varicella infection, but their immune status prior to the vaccine was not reported. Four of the seven women had a gestational age at vaccination of <20 weeks, and three had pregnancy durations in the range of >20 weeks to 31 weeks. Two women had delivered healthy children but the outcomes of the other five pregnancies were pending at the time of this report.

The annual report from the Merck/CDC Pregnancy Registry covered the period from March 17, 1995, through March 16, 2009 (42). These data, which include the first seven pregnancy exposures discussed above, involved 1255 women vaccinated 3 months prior to or at any time during pregnancy and who met the enrollment criteria, but does not include 33 women who had due dates after March 16, 2009. The number of enrolled women included 1190 prospective cases (reported before the outcome was known) and 65 retrospective exposures (reported after the outcome was known). Among the prospective cases, 399 were lost to follow-up, 52 had elective abortions (EABs), and 2 pregnancies were pending. The outcomes for the remaining 737 pregnancies were 72 spontaneous abortions (SABs), 1 late fetal death (at 23 weeks, cause unknown), and 674 live births (includes 8 twins and 1 set of triplets). There were 18 prospective reports and 8 retrospective reports of major birth defects, but none had features consistent with congenital varicella syndrome. Also, there were no birth defects consistent with congenital varicella syndrome in the reports that ended with an SAB or EAB. There were 14 birth defects reported in pregnancy outcomes ≥20 weeks from the last menstrual period among 674 prospectively reported live births, a rate of 2.1%. These results do not support a relationship between congenital varicella syndrome or other birth defects and vaccine exposure during pregnancy. However, the Registry does not have sufficient statistical power to rule out a very low risk (42).

A 1997 report described a well-documented case of child-to-mother transmission of varicella vaccine virus (43). A 12-month-old boy received varicella vaccine and about 3 weeks later had approximately 30 generalized lesions without fever or feeling ill. The lesions were thought to be mild varicella. The 30-year-old mother had a serologic titer negative for varicella and a negative urine pregnancy test at that time. Neither the mother nor her child had any evidence (clinical or laboratory) of immunodeficiency. Sixteen days after appearance of the lesions on her child, she developed a papulovesicular rash diagnosed as varicella. A repeat urine pregnancy test was now positive with an estimated gestational age of 5–6 weeks. Five days later, approximately 100 lesions were counted on the mother, who remained afebrile. On repeat test, seroconversion was documented with a positive varicella titer. Virus was isolated from three of the mother's lesions and identified as Oka strain varicella-zoster virus by polymerase chain reaction test, indicating that her lesions resulted from the vaccine administered to her child. She had an elective abortion during the 7th gestational week because of her concerns that the fetus could acquire the congenital varicella syndrome or other malformations. No varicella-zoster virus DNA was isolated from the fetal tissue. The authors, using a transmission rate of 17% reported for vaccinees with leukemia, estimated the risk of virus transmission from a healthy vaccinee with rash to a nonimmune household member to be about 0.85% (43).

In an editorial comment on the above case, the child's medical history before vaccination was thought to be compatible with a significant allergic diathesis (44). Moreover, at the time of the vaccination his eczema was being treated with the topical corticosteroid, desonide 0.05% (45). A combination of factors, including the number of postvaccination lesions on the child, the contribution of the child's eczema to viral expression, the immunosuppression produced by the corticosteroid, the close contact of the mother to the child resulting from the child's age and the application of the topical corticosteroid, and her pregnancy, were believed to account for the abundance of lesions on the mother. The author estimated the maximum theoretical risk for congenital varicella syndrome resulting from the transmission of varicella vaccine virus to a nonimmune pregnant woman to be <1 in 10,000 (<0.01%). The actual risk, however, was thought to be "exponentially lower," possibly 0, because of the rarity of documented viremia in children after vaccination and the absence of reported embryopathy with attenuated varicella-zoster virus (44). Neither the author of the editorial (44) nor another correspondent (45) thought that vaccination of a child should be postponed if a nonimmune mother was pregnant or attempting to conceive.

BREASTFEEDING SUMMARY

In a 1986 study, no viruses were cultured from the breast milk of two women with varicella-zoster virus infections (46). One of the women had herpes zoster dermatitis 6 months postpartum and was nursing. Direct lesion contact was prevented, and she continued to breastfeed. In the other case, the woman developed varicella pneumonia at 40 weeks' gestation and her infant was delivered by emergency cesarean section. The infant did not become infected after prophylactic treatment with immune globulin varicella-zoster (human) and parenteral acyclovir. Despite the mother's serious postpartum condition, she maintained lactation with a breast pump. Although a varicella virus culture of the milk was negative, the milk was not given to her infant, nor was the infant allowed to breastfeed (46).

A 2003 study reported that varicella DNA was not detected in 217 postvaccination samples of breast milk from 12 women who had received 2 doses of vaccine (47). Because there was no evidence of varicella vaccine virus excretion into milk, the investigators concluded that there was no need to delay vaccination in breastfeeding women (47).

Both the CDC and the American Academy of Pediatrics consider the vaccination of a varicella-zoster virus-susceptible nursing mother to be appropriate if the risk of exposure to the natural virus is high (1,3).

References

1. CDC. Prevention of varicella. MMWR 1996;45(RR-11):1–36.
2. Product information. Varivax. Merck, 2000.
3. Committee on Infectious Diseases, American Academy of Pediatrics. Recommendations for the use of live attenuated varicella vaccine. Pediatrics 1995;95:791–6.
4. Pastuszak AL, Levy M, Schick B, Zuber C, Feldkamp M, Gladstone J, Bar-Levy F, Jackson E, Donnenfeld A, Meschino W, Koren G. Outcome after maternal varicella infection in the first 20 weeks of pregnancy. N Engl J Med 1994;330:901–5.
5. Dickinson J, Gonik B. Teratogenic viral infections. Clin Obstet Gynecol 1990;33:242–52.
6. Birthistle K, Carrington D. Fetal varicella syndrome—a reappraisal of the literature. J Infect 1998;36(Suppl 1):25–9.
7. Siegel M. Congenital malformations following chickenpox, measles, mumps, and hepatitis. Results of a cohort study. JAMA 1973;226:1521–4.

V

8. Paryani SG, Arvin AM. Intrauterine infection with varicella-zoster virus after maternal varicella. N Engl J Med 1986;314:1542–6.
9. Balducci J, Rodis JF, Rosengren S, Vintzileos AM, Spivey G, Vosseller C. Pregnancy outcome following first-trimester varicella infection. Obstet Gynecol 1992;79:5–6.
10. Enders G, Miller E, Cradock-Watson J, Bolley I, Ridehalgh M. Consequences of varicella and herpes zoster in pregnancy: prospective study of 1739 cases. Lancet 1994;343:1547–50.
11. Laforet EG, Lynch CL Jr. Multiple congenital defects following maternal varicella. Report of a case. N Engl J Med 1947;236:534–7.
12. Harris RE, Rhoades ER. Varicella pneumonia complicating pregnancy. Report of a case and review of literature. Obstet Gynecol 1965;25:734–40.
13. Sever J, White LR. Intrauterine viral infections. Annu Rev Med 1968;19:471–86.
14. McKendry JBJ, Bailey JD. Congenital varicella associated with multiple defects. Can Med Assoc J 1973;108:66–8.
15. Savage MO, Moosa A, Gordon RR. Maternal varicella infection as a cause of fetal malformations. Lancet 1973;1:352–4.
16. Srabstein JC, Morris N, Larke RPB, DeSa DJ, Castelino BB, Sum E. Is there a congenital varicella syndrome? J Pediatr 1974;84:239–43.
17. Frey HM, Bialkin G, Gershon AA. Congenital varicella: case report of a serologically proved long-term survivor. Pediatrics 1977;59:110–2.
18. Bai PVA, John TJ. Congenital skin ulcers following varicella in late pregnancy. J Pediatr 1979;94:65–7.
19. Enders G. Varicella-zoster virus infection in pregnancy. Prog Med Virol 1984;29:166–96.
20. Landsberger EJ, Hager WD, Grossman JH III. Successful management of varicella pneumonia complicating pregnancy. A report of three cases. J Reprod Med 1986;31:311–4.
21. Hockberger RS, Rothstein RJ. Varicella pneumonia in adults: a spectrum of disease. Ann Emerg Med 1986;15:931–4.
22. Glaser JB, Loftus J, Ferragamo V, Mootabar H, Castellano M. Varicella-zoster infection in pregnancy. N Engl J Med 1986;315:1416.
23. Preblud SR, Cochi SL, Orenstein WA. Varicella-zoster infection in pregnancy. N Engl J Med 1986;315:1416–7.
24. Trlifajova J, Benda R, Benes C. Effect of maternal varicella-zoster virus infection on the outcome of pregnancy and the analysis of transplacental virus transmission. Acta Virol 1986;30:249–55.
25. Alkalay AL, Pomerance JJ, Rimoin DL. Fetal varicella syndrome. J Pediatr 1987;111:320–3.
26. Higa K, Dan K, Manabe H. Varicella-zoster virus infections during pregnancy: hypothesis concerning the mechanisms of congenital malformations. Obstet Gynecol 1987;69:214–22.
27. Hankins GDV, Gilstrap LC III, Patterson AR. Acyclovir treatment of varicella pneumonia in pregnancy. Crit Care Med 1987;15:336–7.
28. Eder SE, Apuzzio JJ, Weiss G. Varicella pneumonia during pregnancy. Treatment of two cases with acyclovir. Am J Perinatol 1988;5:16–8.
29. Boyd K, Walder E. Use of acyclovir to treat chickenpox in pregnancy. Br Med J 1988;296:393–4.
30. Smego RA Jr, Asperilla MO. Use of acyclovir for varicella pneumonia during pregnancy. Obstet Gynecol 1991;78:1112–6.
31. Broussard RC, Payne K, George RB. Treatment with acyclovir of varicella pneumonia in pregnancy. Chest 1991;99:1045–7.
32. Michie CA, Acolet D, Charlton R, Stevens JP, Happerfield LC, Bobrow LG, Kangro H, Gau G, Modi N. Varicella-zoster contracted in the second trimester of pregnancy. Pediatr Infect Dis J 1992;11:1050–3.
33. Pretorius DH, Hayward I, Jones KL, Stamm E. Sonographic evaluation of pregnancies with maternal varicella infection. J Ultrasound Med 1992;11:459–63.
34. Whitty JE, Renfroe YR, Bottoms SF, Isada NB, Iverson R, Cotton DB. Varicella pneumonia in pregnancy: clinical experience (abstract). Am J Obstet Gynecol 1993;168:427.
35. Martin KA, Junker AK, Thomas EE, Van Allen MI, Friedman JM. Occurrence of chickenpox during pregnancy in women seropositive for varicella-zoster virus. J Infect Dis 1994;170:991–5.
36. Jones KL, Johnson KA, Chambers CD. Offspring of women infected with varicella during pregnancy: a prospective study. Teratology 1994;49:29–32.
37. Andreou A, Basiakos H, Hatzikoumi I, Lazarides A. Fetal varicella syndrome with manifestations limited to the eye. Am J Perinatol 1995;12:347–8.
38. Figueroa-Damian R, Arredondo-Garcia JL. Perinatal outcome of pregnancies complicated with varicella infection during the first 20 weeks of gestation. Am J Perinatol 1997;14:411–4.
39. Nathwani D, Maclean A, Conway S, Carrington D. Varicella infections in pregnancy and the newborn. A review prepared for the UK Advisory Group on Chickenpox on behalf of the British Society for the Study of Infection. J Infect 1998;36(Suppl 1):59–71.
40. CDC. Unintentional administration of varicella virus vaccine—United States, 1996. MMWR 1996;45:1017–8.
41. CDC. Unintentional administration of varicella virus vaccine—United States, 1996. MMWR 1996;45:1017–8 as cited in JAMA 1996;276:1792.
42. Merck/CDC Pregnancy Registry for varicella-containing vaccines (Varivax, Proquad, & Zostavax). The 14th annual report: 2009. Covering the period from approval of Varivax (March 17, 1995) through March 16, 2009.
43. Salzman MB, Sharrar RG, Steinberg S, LaRussa P. Transmission of varicella-vaccine virus from a healthy 12-month-old child to his pregnant mother. J Pediatr 1997;131:151–4.
44. Long SS. Toddler-to-mother transmission of varicella-vaccine virus: how bad is that? J Pediatr 1997;131:10–2.
45. Wald ER. Transmission of varicella-vaccine virus: what is the risk? J Pediatr 1998;133:310.
46. Frederick IB, White RJ, Braddock SW. Excretion of varicella-herpes zoster virus in breast milk. Am J Obstet Gynecol 1986;154:1116–7.
47. Bohlke K, Galil K, Jackson LA, Schmid DS, Starkovich P, Loparev VN, Seward JF. Postpartum varicella vaccination: is the vaccine virus excreted in breast milk? Obstet Gynecol 2003;102:970–7.

VACCINE, YELLOW FEVER

Vaccine

PREGNANCY RECOMMENDATION: Compatible—Maternal Benefit >> Embryo–Fetal Risk
BREASTFEEDING RECOMMENDATION: No Human Data—Probably Compatible

V

PREGNANCY SUMMARY

Yellow fever vaccine is a live, attenuated virus vaccine (1). Yellow fever is a serious infectious disease with high morbidity and mortality. The risk to the fetus from the vaccine is unknown (1,2). The CDC states that the vaccine should not be used in pregnancy except if exposure to yellow fever was unavoidable (2).

FETAL RISK SUMMARY

The Collaborative Perinatal Project monitored 50,282 mother–child pairs, 3 of whom had 1st trimester exposure to yellow fever vaccine (3). There were no birth defects.

A 1993 report described the use of yellow fever vaccine (vaccine strain 17D) in 101 women at various stages of pregnancy during the 1986 outbreak of yellow fever in Nigeria (4). The women received the vaccine during gestation either because of an unknown pregnancy or because they feared acquiring the disease. The vaccine was administered to 4 women in the 1st trimester, 8 in the 2nd trimester, and 89 in the 3rd trimester, with the gestational ages ranging from 6 to 38 weeks. Serum samples were obtained before and after vaccination from the women as well as from 115 vaccinated, nonpregnant controls. Measurements of immunoglobulin M (IgM) antibody and neutralizing antibody in these samples revealed that the immune response of pregnant women was significantly lower than that of controls. One woman, with symptoms of acute yellow fever during the week before vaccination, suffered a spontaneous abortion 8 weeks after vaccination. Although the cause of the abortion was unknown, the investigators concluded that it was not caused by the vaccine. No evidence was found for transplacental passage of the attenuated virus. Nine of the mothers produced IgM antibody after vaccination, but the antibody was not detected in their newborns. Neutralizing antibody either crossed the placenta or was transferred via colostrum in 14 of 16 newborns delivered from mothers with this antibody. No adverse effects on physical or mental development were observed in the offspring during a 3- to 4-year follow-up period (4).

The first reported case of congenital infection following vaccination was described in a study in which attenuated yellow fever vaccine, in response to a threat of epidemic yellow fever, was administered to 400,000 people in Trinidad (5). Pregnant women, all of whom received the vaccine during the 1st trimester of pregnancies unrecognized at the time of vaccination, were identified retrospectively. Serum samples were collected from 47 women and 41 term infants, including 35 mother–child pairs. Women who delivered prematurely and those suffering spontaneous abortions were not sampled. One of the 41 infants had IgM and elevated neutralizing antibodies to yellow fever, indicating congenital infection. Natural exposure to the virus was thought to be unlikely because virus transmission during that period was limited to forest monkeys with no human cases reported. The infected 2920-g infant, the product of a normal full-term pregnancy, appeared healthy on examination and without observable effect on morphogenesis. However, because the neurotropism of yellow fever virus for the developing nervous system has been well documented (e.g., vaccine-induced encephalitis occurs almost exclusively in infants and young children), the authors considered this case as further evidence that the vaccine should be avoided during pregnancy (5).

A 1999 report from the European Network of Teratology Information Services described the prospectively ascertained outcomes in 58 of 74 pregnancies exposed to yellow fever vaccine (6). Timing of exposure was before the last menstrual period (LMP), in the 1st trimester, or in the 2nd trimester in 3, 69, and 2, respectively. Sixteen of the cases did not have complete follow-up data and were excluded from the analysis. The pregnancy outcomes included 7 spontaneous abortions, 5 induced abortions, and 46 live births. In the newborns, there were two major malformations: ureteral stenosis and triphalangeal hallux. There were also three cases of minor anomalies: bilateral pes varus, slight deviation of the nasal wall, and mild ventricular septal defect. Vaccination in all of these five cases occurred early in gestation. The rates of abortion and congenital malformations are within expected ranges. The investigators also found 4 cases exposed in utero to yellow fever vaccine among 23,925 cases of birth defects reported between 1980 and 1995 to the France/Central-East Registry of Malformations. The defects in these cases were (timing of exposure in parentheses) right ectromelia of upper limb (1st trimester), a VATER (vertebral defects, anal atresia, tracheoesophageal fistula with esophageal atresia, and radial and renal anomalies) association (2nd trimester), stenosis of the aortic orificium (1st trimester), and hydrocephalus in an infant stillborn near term (2nd trimester). Two other cases of spontaneous abortion (respectively at 6 and 13 weeks after the LMP) were reported by a French manufacturer to the investigators. The authors concluded that although their sample was far too small to rule out a moderately increased risk of adverse outcome, their data do not support such an association and could be used to reassure pregnant women who have inadvertently received the vaccine (6).

A 1994 review concluded that pregnant women should be vaccinated, preferably after the 1st trimester, if exposure to a yellow fever epidemic is unavoidable (7).

BREASTFEEDING SUMMARY

No reports describing the administration of yellow fever vaccine during human lactation have been located.

References

1. Amstey MS. Vaccination in pregnancy. Clin Obstet Gynaecol 1983;10:13–22.
2. CDC. *Guidelines for Vaccinating Pregnant Women*. Available at http://www.cdc.gov/vaccines/pubs/preg-guide.htm. Accessed May 16, 2010.
3. Heinonen OP, Slone D, Shapiro S. *Birth Defects and Drugs in Pregnancy*. Littleton, MA: Publishing Sciences Group, 1977:315.
4. Nasidi A, Monath TP, Vandenberg J, Tomori O, Calisher CH, Hurtgen X, Munube GRR, Sorungbe AOO, Okafor GC, Wali S. Yellow fever vaccination and pregnancy: a four-year prospective study. Trans R Soc Trop Med Hyg 1993;87:337–9.
5. Tsai TF, Paul R, Lynberg MC, Letson GW. Congenital yellow fever virus infection after immunization in pregnancy. J Infect Dis 1993;168:1520–3.
6. Robert E, Vial T, Schaefer C, Arnon J, Reuvers M. Exposure to yellow fever vaccine in early pregnancy. Vaccine 1999;17:283–5.
7. Linder N, Ohel G. In utero vaccination. Clin Perinatol 1994;21:663–74.

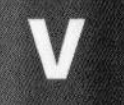

VALACYCLOVIR

Antiviral

PREGNANCY RECOMMENDATION: Compatible
BREASTFEEDING RECOMMENDATION: Compatible

PREGNANCY SUMMARY

For the management of herpes in pregnancy, either valacyclovir or acyclovir are recommended for primary or first-episode infection (for 7–10 days), symptomatic recurrent episode (for 5 days), and daily suppression (from 36 weeks' gestation until delivery), but only acyclovir is recommended for severe or disseminated disease (1). Although the experience with valacyclovir in early pregnancy is limited, many studies have reported the use of acyclovir during all stages of pregnancy (see also Acyclovir). Based on the combined data, there is no evidence of a major risk to the human fetus from valacyclovir or acyclovir. Long-term follow-up of children exposed in utero to these agents is warranted.

FETAL RISK SUMMARY

Valacyclovir is biotransformed to acyclovir and *L*-valine by first-pass intestinal and/or hepatic metabolism. The drug is active against herpes simplex virus (HSV) types 1 and 2 and varicella-zoster virus. It is used in the treatment of herpes zoster (shingles) and recurrent genital herpes simplex.

Reproduction studies were conducted in rats and rabbits during organogenesis with doses producing concentrations 10 and 7 times human plasma levels, respectively (2). No teratogenic effects were observed with these doses.

The active metabolite, acyclovir, readily crosses the human placenta (see Acyclovir). An abstract and study, both published in 1998, compared the pharmacokinetics of valacyclovir and acyclovir in late pregnancy (3,4). Acyclovir accumulated in the amniotic fluid but not in the fetus. The mean maternal/umbilical vein plasma ratio at delivery was 1.7.

The Valacyclovir Pregnancy Registry listed 157 prospective reports of women exposed to the oral antiviral drug during gestation covering the period from January 1, 1995, through April 30, 1999 (5). Of the total, 47 (30%) pregnancies were lost to follow-up. Among the 111 (1 set of twins) known outcomes, 29 had earliest exposure in the 1st trimester and their outcomes were 5 spontaneous abortions, 2 induced abortions, 1 infant with a birth defect (talipes), and 21 infants (including the twins) without birth defects. When the earliest exposure was in the 2nd trimester, 31 pregnancies were enrolled and their outcomes were 2 stillbirths, 2 infants with birth defects (fingers and toes fused—extensive webbing; small cleft in front gum), and 27 without birth defects. In the remaining 51, the earliest exposure occurred in the 3rd trimester, with 1 infant with a dermal sinus tract and 50 without birth defects (5).

A total of 34 retrospective reports of valacyclovir exposure during pregnancy were submitted to the Registry (5). Two of the exposures occurred during an unspecified gestational time and both resulted in live births without defects. In 14 pregnancies, the earliest exposure occurred during the 1st trimester. The outcomes of these pregnancies were three spontaneous losses, eight induced abortions, and three infants without birth defects. For the pregnancies whose earliest exposure was in the 2nd trimester ($N = 4$) or 3rd trimester ($N = 14$), there was 1 birth defect (2nd trimester exposure) and 17 infants without defects (5).

A 1999 case report described a woman at 20 weeks' gestation who had a generalized HSV infection that was treated with IV acyclovir for about 2 weeks followed by valacyclovir for the remainder of the pregnancy (6). She delivered a full-term, healthy female infant who was treated prophylactically with oral acyclovir for 1 month. No abnormalities were detected during a neurologic examination at 8 months of age (6).

A prospective, double-blind, placebo controlled trial was conducted to estimate the efficacy of valacyclovir to reduce HSV infection at delivery (7). Valacyclovir 500 mg twice daily ($N = 170$) or placebo ($N = 168$) was given from 36 weeks' gestation until delivery. Compared with controls, valacyclovir significantly reduced HSV shedding and need for cesarean section. There were no differences between the groups in terms of delivery and neonatal outcomes (7).

A 2009 review of genital herpes concluded that the benefits from the use of acyclovir or valacyclovir for the treatment of the virus in pregnancy far outweighed the potential fetal risks (8). Because there was no evidence to suggest a risk of major defects with acyclovir, the reviewers also concluded that the pro-drug valacyclovir, even though the pregnancy experience was limited, could be viewed similarly.

A 2010 study used a population-based historical cohort of 837,795 liveborn infants in Denmark to determine if there were associations between 1st trimester exposure to acyclovir, valacyclovir, and famciclovir and major birth defects (9). Subjects were excluded if they had chromosomal abnormalities, genetic syndromes, birth defect syndromes, or congenital viral infections. Among 1804 pregnancies exposed to one of the antivirals, there were 40 (2.2%) infants with a major birth defect compared with 19,920 (2.4%) among those unexposed (adjusted prevalence odds ratio [POR] 0.89, 95% confidence interval [CI] 0.65–1.22). In the valacyclovir group, 7 (3.1%) infants had a major defect from the 229 with 1st trimester exposure (POR 1.21, 95% CI 0.56–2.62). The prevalence of major defects with acyclovir and famciclovir were 2.0% (POR 0.82, 95% CI 0.57–1.17) and 3.8%, respectively, but only 26 pregnancies (1 infant with a defect) were exposed to famciclovir. The study limited the evaluation to 13 major birth defect types by organ system. For any antiviral drug, POR >1 were found for defects of the nervous system, eye, abdominal wall, urinary tract, and a miscellaneous group of defects; none reached statistical significance. The authors concluded that 1st trimester exposure to valacyclovir and acyclovir was not associated with an increased risk of major birth defects (9). The authors of an accompanying editorial thought that the large number of exposures during organogenesis without an overall increased risk of major defects was reassuring, especially for acyclovir. However, more data were needed to examine the associations with individual defects (10).

BREASTFEEDING SUMMARY

Valacyclovir is rapidly and nearly completely converted to acyclovir and the amino acid, *L*-valine. Acyclovir is concentrated in human milk with milk:plasma ratios in the range 3–4 (see Acyclovir).

In a 2002 study, five healthy postpartum women who were breastfeeding were given valacyclovir (500 mg) twice daily for 7 days (11). Maternal serum and milk samples were collected after the first dose, on day 5, and 24 hours after the last dose. Infant urine samples were collected on day 5. All samples were analyzed for acyclovir. The peak milk concentration occurred 4 hours after the first dose (milk:serum ratio 3.4), whereas the peak serum level occurred at 2 hours. At steady state, the milk:serum ratio was about 1.9. The median infant urine acyclovir concentration was 0.74 mcg/mL. Twenty-four hours after the last dose, the milk:serum ratio was 0.25. The estimated infant dose (based on a consumption of 750 mL/day of milk by a 2.75-kg infant) would be about 0.2% of the therapeutic dose for neonates (11).

Because acyclovir has been used to treat herpesvirus infections in the neonate, and because of the lack of adverse effects in reported cases in which acyclovir was used during breastfeeding, the American Academy of Pediatrics classifies acyclovir as compatible with breastfeeding (see Acyclovir). Valacyclovir also appears to be compatible with breastfeeding.

References

1. American College of Obstetricians and Gynecologists. Management of herpes in pregnancy. *ACOG Practice Bulletin*. No. 82, June 2007.
2. Product information. Valtrex. Glaxo Wellcome, 1997.
3. Kimberlin DF, Weller S, Andrews WW, Hauth JC, Whitley RJ, Lakeman F, Miller G, Lee C, Goldenberg RL. Valaciclovir pharmacokinetics in late pregnancy (abstract). Am J Obstet Gynecol 1998;178:S12.
4. Kimberlin DF, Weller S, Whitley RJ, Andrews WW, Hauth JC, Lakeman F, Miller G. Pharmacokinetics of oral valacyclovir and acyclovir in late pregnancy. Am J Obstet Gynecol 1998;179:846–51.
5. Acyclovir Pregnancy Registry and Valacyclovir Pregnancy Registry. Final study report. 1 June 1984 through 30 April 1999. Glaxo Wellcome, 1999.
6. Anderson R, Lundqvist A, Bergstrom T. Successful treatment of generalized primary herpes simplex type 2 infection during pregnancy. Scand J Infect Dis 1999;31:201–2.
7. Sheffield JS, Hill JB, Hollier LM, Laibl VR, Roberts SW, Sanchez PJ, Wendel GD Jr. Valacyclovir prophylaxis to prevent recurrent herpes at delivery. Obstet Gynecol 2006;108:141–7.
8. Nath AK, Thappa DM. Newer trends in the management of genital herpes. Indian J Dermatol Venereol Leprol 2009;75:566–74.
9. Pasternak B, Hviid A. Use of acyclovir, valacyclovir, and famciclovir in the first trimester of pregnancy and the risk of birth defects. JAMA 2010;304:859–66.
10. Mills JL, Carter TC. Acyclovir exposure and birth defects—an important advance, but more are needed. JAMA 2010;304:905–6.
11. Sheffield JS, Fish DN, Hollier LM, Cadematori S, Nobles BJ, Wendel GD Jr. Acyclovir concentrations in human breast milk after valaciclovir administration. Am J Obstet Gynecol 2002;186:100–2.

VALDECOXIB

[Withdrawn from the market. See 9th edition.]

VALERIAN

Herb

PREGNANCY RECOMMENDATION: Limited Human Data—No Relevant Animal Data
BREASTFEEDING RECOMMENDATION: No Human Data—Potential Toxicity

PREGNANCY SUMMARY

The very limited animal and human data do not allow a conclusion as to the safety of valerian during pregnancy. Moreover, as a natural, unregulated product, the concentration, contents, and presence of contaminants in valerian preparations cannot be easily determined. Because of this uncertainty and the potential for cytotoxicity in the fetus and hepatotoxicity in the mother, the product should be avoided during pregnancy. Other authors have arrived at the same conclusion (1,2). The risk to a fetus from short-term or inadvertent use during any part of gestation, however, is probably low, if it exists at all.

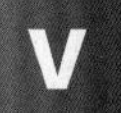

FETAL RISK SUMMARY

Valeriana officinalis, the plant most often used for medicinal purposes, is 1 species of approximately 200 of the genus *Valeriana*, an herbaceous perennial that grows widely in the temperate regions of North America, Europe, and Asia (4). A large number of preparations containing valerian are commercially available (4). The herb is used as a sedative and hypnotic for anxiety, restlessness, and sleep disturbances (1–5). Other pharmacologic claims that have been made for valerian include antispasmodic, anticonvulsive, antidepressant, and antihypertensive properties (2–4). The extracts and root oil have also been used as flavorings for foods and beverages (3).

Although the specific agents responsible for the effects of valerian are unknown, as is the mechanism of action, three classes of compounds have been identified: a volatile oil that contains sesquiterpenes; nonglycosidic iridoid esters (known as valepotriates); and alkaloids (3,4). Of these, the valepotriates, found primarily in the roots, are most likely responsible for the sedative action, but components from the other two classes probably contribute as well (3,4). Because these compounds produce central nervous system depression, they should not be used with other depressants, such as alcohol, benzodiazepines, barbiturates, or opiates (1,2,5). Moreover, nonpregnant adult human hepatotoxicity has been associated with short-term use (i.e., a few days to several months) of herbal preparations containing valerian (6). Long-term use in a male has also been associated with benzodiazepine-like withdrawal symptoms resulting in cardiac complications and delirium (7).

Reproductive studies in animals with valerian have not shown antiovulation, antifertilization, or embryotoxic effects (8). Further, the valepotriates exhibit low toxicity in mice, producing no deaths in doses of up to 1600 mg/kg IP or 4600 mg/kg orally (3). Toxicity in mice was characterized by ataxia, hypothermia, and increased muscle relaxation.

The cytotoxic activities of three valepotriate compounds, valtrate, didrovaltrate, and baldrinal (a degradation product of valtrate), in cultured rat hepatoma cells were described in a 1981 reference (9). Both valtrate and didrovaltrate demonstrated much greater cytotoxic activity than did baldrinal, with rapid and irreversible toxicity. In addition, the antitumor activity of didrovaltrate was demonstrated in vivo on female mice KREBS II ascitic tumors (9). Five surviving mice were then bred with normal male mice 50 days after treatment with didrovaltrate. Each had a normal pregnancy and produced normal offspring.

In a 1988 report, two cases of attempted suicide with valerian dry extract plus other drugs were described (10). In one case, a woman at 10 weeks' gestation ingested 2.5 g of valerian dry extract and 0.5 g of phenobarbital. An apparently normal, 4350-g female infant was delivered at 42 weeks' gestation. Examination of the child (age not specified) indicated an IQ in the range of 111–120. In the second case, the mother ingested a combination of valerian dry extract (3.0 g), phenobarbital (0.6 g), glutethimide (5.0 g), amobarbital (5.0 g), and promethazine (0.3 g) at 20 weeks' gestation. A mentally slow, 2650-g male infant was born at 36 weeks' gestation. About 2 years later in her next pregnancy, this woman again attempted suicide at 20 weeks' gestation, by ingesting glutethimide (3.75 g), amobarbital (3.75 g), and promethazine (0.23 g). She delivered another mentally slow, 2650-g male infant at 43 weeks'. The infant also had a unilateral undescended testicle. Of interest, none of the woman's other 10 children is mentally slow.

Two additional cases of self-poisoning with valerian were described in 1987 by the same group responsible for the above report (11). In both cases exposure occurred early in gestation, with ingestion of 5 and 2 g of valerian at 3 and 4 weeks of fetal development, respectively. No congenital abnormalities were observed in the offspring.

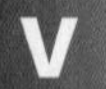

BREASTFEEDING SUMMARY

No reports describing the use of valerian during lactation have been located. For the reasons cited above, the use of this herbal product should be avoided during breastfeeding.

References

1. Klepser TB, Klepser ME. Unsafe and potentially safe herbal therapies. Am J Health-Syst Pharm 1999;56:125–38.
2. Wong AHC, Smith M, Boon HS. Herbal remedies in psychiatric practice. Arch Gen Psychiatry 1998;55:1033–44.
3. Valerian. *The Lawrence Review of Natural Products: Facts and Comparisons*. St. Louis, MO: J.B. Lippincott, October 1991.
4. Reynolds JEF, ed. *Martindale. The Extra Pharmacopoeia*. 31st ed. London, England: Royal Pharmaceutical Society, 1996:1765–6.
5. Miller LG. Herbal medicines. Selected clinical considerations focusing on known or potential drug-herb interactions. Arch Intern Med 1998;158:2200–11.
6. MacGregor FB, Abernethy VE, Dahabra S, Cobden I, Hayes PC. Hepatotoxicity of herbal remedies. Br Med J 1989;299:1156–7.
7. Garges HP, Varia I, Doraiswamy PM. Cardiac complications and delirium associated with valerian root withdrawal. JAMA 1998;280:1566–7.
8. Randor S, Einarson TR, Pastuszak A, Koren G. Maternal-fetal toxicology of medicinal plants: a clinician's guide. In: Koren G, ed. *Maternal-Fetal Toxicology: A Clinician's Guide*. 2nd ed. New York, NY: Marcel Dekker, 1994:495–6.
9. Bounthanh C, Bergmann C, Beck JP, Haag-Berrurier M, Anton R. Valepotriates, a new class of cytotoxic and antitumor agents. Planta Med 1981;41:21–8.
10. Czeizel A, Szentesi I, Szekeres H, Molnar G, Glauber A, Bucski P. A study of adverse effects on the progeny after intoxication during pregnancy. Arch Toxicol 1988;62:1–7.
11. Czeizel AE, Tomcsik M, Timar L. Teratologic evaluation of 178 infants born to mothers who attempted suicide by drugs during pregnancy. Obstet Gynecol 1997;90:195–201.

VALGANCICLOVIR

Antiviral

PREGNANCY RECOMMENDATION: Compatible—Maternal Benefit >> Embryo–Fetal Risk
BREASTFEEDING RECOMMENDATION: Contraindicated

PREGNANCY SUMMARY

No reports describing the use of valganciclovir in human pregnancy have been located. For ganciclovir, human pregnancy experience has not shown toxicity, but the number of cases is very limited. The animal data for ganciclovir are suggestive of high embryo–fetal risk because carcinogenic, mutagenic, teratogenic, and embryotoxic effects have been observed. Primary cytomegalovirus (CMV) infections occurring in pregnancy have a high risk of transplacental passage of the virus to the fetus. Some of the embryos or fetuses exposed to the virus will be damaged and the development of later toxicity in childhood is an additional concern. However, the prevention of these in utero infections by ganciclovir has not been proven (see Ganciclovir).

FETAL RISK SUMMARY

After oral administration, the prodrug valganciclovir is rapidly converted to ganciclovir by intestinal and hepatic enzymes. The antiviral effect, therefore, is identical to ganciclovir (see Ganciclovir). Valganciclovir is indicated for the treatment of CMV retinitis in patients with AIDS. Plasma protein binding of valganciclovir is not relevant because of its rapid metabolism to ganciclovir, but binding of ganciclovir is very low (1%–2%). The elimination half-life of ganciclovir after valganciclovir administration is about 4.1 hours, compared with 3.8 hours when IV ganciclovir is administered (1). Ganciclovir crosses the human placenta (see Ganciclovir).

Reproduction studies in animals have been conducted with the active metabolite ganciclovir (1) (see Ganciclovir).

BREASTFEEDING SUMMARY

No reports describing the use of valganciclovir during human lactation have been located. Because the active metabolite, ganciclovir, has the potential to cause serious toxicity in a nursing infant, mothers taking this drug should not breastfeed. Further, breastfeeding is contraindicated if the mother is infected with HIV.

Reference

1. Product information. Valcyte. Roche Pharmaceuticals, 2004.

VALPROIC ACID

Anticonvulsant

PREGNANCY RECOMMENDATION: Human Data Suggest Risk
BREASTFEEDING RECOMMENDATION: Limited Human Data—Potential Toxicity

PREGNANCY SUMMARY

Valproic acid and the salt form, sodium valproate, are human teratogens. The absolute risk of producing a child with neural tube defects (NTDs) when these agents are used between the 17th and 30th days after fertilization is 1%–2%. A characteristic pattern of minor facial defects is apparently also associated with valproic acid. Studies have suggested that a distinct constellation of defects and fetal growth restriction may exist for infants exposed in utero to the anticonvulsant. These defects involve the head and face, digits, urogenital tract, and mental and physical growth. A correlation between maternal dose and major and minor anomalies has been reported. There also are reports of a significant association with autism. Other problems, such as hyperbilirubinemia, hepatotoxicity, and fetal or newborn distress, need additional investigation.

FETAL RISK SUMMARY

Valproic acid and its salt form, sodium valproate, are anticonvulsants used in the treatment of seizure disorders. The drugs readily cross the placenta to the fetus. At term, the range of cord blood:maternal serum ratios of total valproic acid (protein bound and unbound) has been reported to be 0.52–4.6 (1–13). Studies that are more recent have reported mean ratios of 1.4–2.4 (4,7,9–13). In contrast, the mean cord blood:maternal serum ratio of free (unbound) valproic acid was 0.82 (10). Two mechanisms have been proposed to account for the accumulation of total valproic acid in the fetus: partial displacement of the drug from maternal binding sites by increased free fatty acid concentrations in maternal blood at the time of birth (10) and increased protein binding of valproic acid in fetal serum (11). Increased unbound valproic acid in the maternal serum may also be partially a result of decreased serum albumin (14). Although one study measured a mean serum half-life for valproic acid in the newborn of 28.3 hours (9), other studies have reported values of 43–47 hours, approximately 4 times the adult value (2,4,8,10,13). In agreement with these data, valproic acid has been shown to lack fetal hepatic enzyme induction activity when used alone and will block the enzyme induction activity of primidone when the two anticonvulsants are combined during pregnancy (15).

In published reports, doses of valproic acid in pregnancy have ranged from 300 to 3000 mg (1–3,8,12,16–28). Although a good correlation between serum levels and seizure control is not always observed, most patients will respond when levels are in the range of 50–100 mcg/mL (29). In early pregnancy, high (i.e., >1000 mg) daily doses of valproic acid may produce maternal serum concentrations that are >100 mcg/mL (8). However, as pregnancy progresses and without dosage adjustment, valproic acid levels fall steadily so that in the 3rd trimester, maternal levels are often <50 mcg/mL (8). One study concluded that the decreased serum concentrations were a result of increased hepatic clearance and an increased apparent volume of distribution (8).

Fetal or newborn consequences resulting from the use of valproic acid and sodium valproate during pregnancy have been reported to include major and minor congenital abnormalities, intrauterine growth restriction, hyperbilirubinemia, hepatotoxicity (which may be fatal), transient hyperglycinemia, afibrinogenemia (one case), and fetal or neonatal withdrawal.

Before 1981, the maternal use of valproic acid was not thought to present a risk to the fetus. A 1981 editorial recommended sodium valproate or carbamazepine as anticonvulsants of choice in appropriate types of epilepsy for women who may become pregnant (30). Although the drug was known to be a potent animal teratogen (31), more potent than phenytoin and at least as potent as trimethadione (32), only a single unconfirmed case of human teratogenicity (in a fetus exposed to at least two other anticonvulsants) had been published between 1969 and 1976 (33). (An editorial comment in that report noted that subsequent investigation had failed to confirm the defect.) In other published cases, both before and after 1980, healthy term infants resulted after in utero exposure to valproic acid (1–3,12,19,27,28,32,34–38). Moreover, a committee of the American Academy of Pediatrics stated in 1982 that the data for a teratogenic potential in humans for valproic acid were inadequate and that recommendations for or against its use in pregnancy could not be given (39).

The first confirmed report of an infant with congenital defects after valproic acid exposure during pregnancy appeared in 1980 (16). The mother, who took 1000 mg of valproic acid daily throughout gestation, delivered a growth-restricted infant with facial dysmorphism and heart and limb defects. The infant died at 19 days of age. Since this initial report, a number of studies and case reports have described newborns with malformations after in utero exposure to either valproic acid monotherapy or combination therapy (4,17–26,36,40–60).

The most serious abnormalities observed with valproic acid (or sodium valproate) exposure are defects in neural tube closure. The absolute risk of this defect is approximately 1%–2%, about the same risk for a familial occurrence of this anomaly (37,40,61,62). No cases of anencephaly have been associated with valproic acid (21,62,63). Exposure to valproic acid between the 17th and 30th day after fertilization must occur before the drug can be considered a cause of NTDs (64). Other predominant defects involve the heart, face, and limbs. A characteristic pattern of minor facial abnormalities has been attributed to valproic acid (61). Cardiac anomalies and cleft lip and palate occur with most anticonvulsants and a causal relationship with valproic acid has not been established (37,46). In addition, almost all types of congenital malformations have been observed after treatment of epilepsy during pregnancy (see Janz 1982, Phenytoin). Consequently, the list below, although abstracting the cited references, is not meant to be inclusive and, at times, reflects multiple anticonvulsant therapy.

NEURAL TUBE DEFECTS

Defects in neural tube closure (includes entire spectrum from spina bifida occulta to meningomyelocele) (17,19,21,22,24,26,40–42,44–46,53–58)

CARDIAC DEFECTS

Multiple (not specified) (21,24,26,37,42,44,51)
Levocardia (16)
Anomalies of great vessels (51)
Patent ductus arteriosus (4,26,48,50,52)
Valvular aortic stenosis (23,48)
Ventricular septal defect (4,20,48)
Tetralogy of Fallot (18,51)
Partial right bundle branch block (16)

FACIAL DEFECTS

Facial dysmorphism (4,26,42,46,50,53,59)
Small nose (16,20,24,26,50,53,59)
Small nose (16,20,24,26,50,53,59)
Depressed nasal bridge (18,20,26,50,59)
Epicanthal folds (4,26,50,53,59)
Protruding eyes (16)
Hypertelorism (4,26)
Low-set/rotated ears (4,16,24,26,50)
Micrognathia/retrognathia (16,23,26)
Depigmentation of eyelashes and brow (16,25)
Thin upper vermilion border (24,26,48,50,53)
Down-turned angles of mouth (50,59)
High forehead (24,26)
Bulging frontal eminences (16,20)
Strabismus (50)
Nystagmus (50)
Flat orbits (26)
Coarsened facies (20)
Cleft lip/palate (18,37,42,44,51)
Microstomia (24,26,48,50)
Esotropia (50)
Long upper lip (26,50,59)
Short palpebral fissure (26,48,50)
Agenesis of lacrimal ducts (51)

HEAD/NECK DEFECTS

Brachycephaly (24,26)
Hydrocephaly (19,21,42,46)
Short neck (20)
Abnormal or premature stenosis of metopic suture (24,26,50)
Microcephaly (4,21,24,38,50,64,65)
Wide anterior fontanelle (18)
Craniostenosis (26)
Aplasia cutis (60)

UROGENITAL DEFECTS

Bilateral duplication of caliceal collecting systems (25)
Bilateral undescended testes (23)
Nonspecified (26)
Hypospadias (21,23,26,46,50)
Bilateral renal hypoplasia (23)

SKELETAL/LIMB DEFECTS

Aplasia of radius (23,26)
Dislocated hip (16,26,35)
Hypoplastic thumb (20)
Hemifusion of second and third lumbar vertebrae (25)
Arachnodactyly (24,26)
Overlapping fingers/toes (24,26)
Broad or asymmetric chest (16,26)
Multiple (not specified) (24)
Reduced head circumference (85)
Rib defects (24,26)
Foot deformity (17,23,24,50)
Abnormal digits (23,26,37,42)
Shortened fingers and toes (4,20)
Abnormal sternum (16,26)
Scoliosis (25)
Clinodactyly of fingers (26)
Tracheomalacia (53)
Talipes equinovarus (53)

SKIN/MUSCLE DEFECTS

Accessory, wide-spaced, or inverted nipples (20,26)
Diastasis recti abdominis (4,25)
Syndactyly of toes (16,23,50)
Hyperconvex fingernails (24,26)
Hemangioma (4,25,26,50)
Sacral dimple (43)
Telangiectasia (4)
Omphalocele (59)
Cutis aplasia of scalp (50)
Weak abdominal walls (4)
Hirsutism (26)
Abnormal palmar creases (16,18,50)
Hypoplastic nails (4,18)
Umbilical hernias (4,26)
Linea alba hernia (47)
Inguinal hernia (4,26,50)

OTHER DEFECTS

Multiple defects (not specified) (24,51)
Duodenal atresia (25)
Single umbilical artery (50)
Withdrawal or irritation (4,50)
Mental retardation (4,20,50,51,53)

A 2010 study combined data from 8 published cohort studies (1565 pregnancies exposed to valproic acid monotherapy in the 1st trimester) to identify 118 major malformations, 14 of which were significantly more common in the offspring (66). Using these 14 malformations, they then conducted a case–control study using data from the European Surveillance of Congenital Anomalies (EUROCAT) antiepileptic study database that is derived from population-based registries that contained data for 3.8 million births (1995–2005) in 14 European countries. A total of 37,154 cases were compared with 39,472 controls without chromosomal abnormalities (group 1), and 11,763 controls with chromosomal abnormalities (group 2). First trimester exposure to valproic acid monotherapy occurred in 122, 45, and 13, respectively, of the cases and two control groups. As compared with no use of an anticonvulsant during the 1st trimester (control group 1), significantly increased risks were found for 6 of the 14 malformations under consideration (adjusted odds ratio [OR], 95% confidence interval [CI]): spina bifida 12.7 (7.7–20.7); atrial septal defect 2.5 (1.4–4.4); cleft palate 5.2 (2.8–9.9); hypospadias 4.8 (2.9–8.1); polydactyly 2.2 (1.0–4.5); and craniosynostosis 6.8 (1.8–18.8). Except for polydactyly, significant associations also were found for these malformations when compared with the control group 2 (66).

Although a wide variety of minor anomalies, many of which are similar in nature, occurs in infants of epileptic mothers, three groups of investigators have concluded that the deformities associated with valproic acid are distinctly different from those associated with other anticonvulsants and may constitute a fetal valproate syndrome (FVS) (26,50,53). The combined features cited in the three reports were (a) NTDs; (b) craniofacial: brachycephaly, high forehead, epicanthal folds, strabismus, nystagmus, shallow orbits, flat nasal bridge, small up-turned nose, hypertelorism, long upper lip, thin upper vermillion border, microstomia, down-turned angles of mouth, low-set/rotated ears; (c) digits: long, thin, partly overlapping fingers and toes, hyperconvex nails; (d) urogenital: hypospadias (in about 50% of males); and (e) other: slow psychomotor development, low birth weight. Normal psychomotor development has been observed, however, in follow-up studies of children up to 4 years of age after in utero exposure to either mono- or combination therapy with valproic acid (3,34,65,67).

A 1995 review listed the facial features seen in the FVS as trigonocephaly, tall forehead with bifrontal narrowing, epicanthic folds, medial deficiency of eyebrows, flat nasal bridge, broad nasal root anteverted nares, shallow philtrum, long upper lip with thin vermilion border, thick upper lip, and small, downturned mouth (68). The most common major congenital defects observed were NTDs, congenital heart disease, cleft lip and palate, genital anomalies, and limb defects. Other, less common abnormalities were tracheomalacia, abdominal wall defects, and strabismus. Dose-related withdrawal symptoms (irritability, jitteriness, hypotonia, and seizures) were considered to be very common, typically occurring 12–48 hours after birth (68).

A correlation between valproic acid dosage and the number of minor anomalies in an infant has been proposed (26). Such a correlation has not been observed with other anticonvulsants (26). The conclusion was based on the high concentrations of valproic acid that occur in the 1st trimester after large doses (i.e., 1500–2000 mg/day).

In a surveillance study of Michigan Medicaid recipients involving 229,101 completed pregnancies conducted between 1985 and 1992, 26 newborns had been exposed to valproic acid during the 1st trimester (F. Rosa, personal communication, FDA, 1993). Five (19.2%) major birth defects were observed (one expected), one of which was a hypospadias. No anomalies were observed in five other categories of defects (cardiovascular, oral clefts, spina bifida, polydactyly, and limb reduction defects) for which specific data were available. Hypospadias has been associated with 1st trimester valproic acid exposure (see above).

A 2000 study, using data from the MADRE (**MA**lformation and **DR**ug **E**xposure) surveillance project, assessed the human teratogenicity of anticonvulsants (69). Among 8005 malformed infants, the cases included infants with a specific malformation, whereas controls were infants with other anomalies. Of the total group, 299 were exposed in the 1st trimester to anticonvulsants. Among these, exposure to monotherapy occurred in the following: valproic acid (N = 80), phenobarbital (N = 65), mephobarbital (N = 10), carbamazepine (N = 46), phenytoin (N = 24), and other agents (N = 16). Statistically significant associations (CI not overlapping 1 and $p \leq 0.05$) were found between valproic acid monotherapy and spina bifida (N = 12); hypospadias (N = 10); porencephaly/multiple cerebral cysts and other specified anomalies of brain (N = 2); microstomia, microcheilia, and other anomalies of face (N = 2); coarctation of aorta (N = 2); and limb reduction defects (N = 5). When all 1st trimester exposures (mono- and polytherapy) were evaluated, significant associations were found between valproic acid and spina bifida (N = 14), cardiac defects (N = 26), hypospadias (N = 14), porencephaly/multiple cerebral cysts and other specific anomalies of brain (N = 2), limb reduction defects (N = 5), and hypertelorism, localized skull defects (N = 2). Although the study confirmed some previously known associations, several new associations with anticonvulsants were discovered which require independent confirmation (see also Carbamazepine, Mephobarbital, Phenobarbital, and Phenytoin) (69).

The risk of valproic acid–induced limb deficiencies was estimated in a 2000 study that used data from the Spanish Collaborative Study of Congenital Malformations (ECEMC) collected between 1976 and 1997 (70). A total of 22,294 consecutive malformed infants (excluding genetic syndromes) were compared with 21,937 control infants. A total of 57 malformed infants and 10 controls were exposed to valproic acid during the 1st trimester (OR 5.62, 95% CI 2.78–11.71, $p < 0.0000001$). Among the 57 infants, 21 (36.8%) had congenital limb defects of different types (overlapping digits, talipes, clinodactyly, arachnodactyly, hip dislocation, pre- and postaxial polydactyly, and limb deficiencies). Five of the 21 cases, however, were thought to have resulted from immobility (e.g., talipes equinovarus) caused by spina bifida. After exclusion of these cases and their respective controls, the OR for congenital limb defects was 3.95, 95% CI 1.24–13.94, $p = 0.01$. Three of the malformed infants had limb deficiencies: hypoplasia of the left hand; unilateral forearm defect and hypoplastic first metacarpal bone in the left hand; and short hands with hypoplastic first metacarpal bone absent and hypoplastic phalanges (this case also had retrognathia, facial asymmetry, hypospadias, telangiectatic angioma in the skull, and hypotonia). The case–control analysis showed a risk for limb deficiencies of OR 6.17, 95% CI 1.28–29.66, $p = 0.023$. In their population, the prevalence at birth of limb deficiencies was 6.88 per 10,000 live births. Based on this, the risk of limb deficiencies after exposure to valproic acid in the 1st trimester was estimated to be about 0.42% (70).

A prospective study published in 1999 described the outcomes of 517 pregnancies of epileptic mothers identified at one Italian center from 1977 (71). Excluding genetic and chromosomal defects, malformations were classified as severe structural defects, mild structural defects, and deformations. Minor anomalies were not considered. Spontaneous (N = 38) and early (N = 20) voluntary abortions were excluded from the analysis, as were 7 pregnancies that delivered at other hospitals. Of the remaining 452 outcomes, 427 were exposed to anticonvulsants of which 313 involved monotherapy: valproate (N = 44), carbamazepine (N = 113), phenobarbital (N = 83), primidone (N = 35), phenytoin (N = 31), clonazepam (N = 6), and other (N = 1). There were no defects in the 25 pregnancies not exposed to anticonvulsants. Of the 42 (9.3%) outcomes with malformations, 24 (5.3%) were severe, 10 (2.2%) were mild, and 8 (1.8%) were deformities. There were eight malformations with valproic acid monotherapy: six (13.6%) were severe (spina bifida, hydrocephalus, pyloric stenosis, and cardiac defect), one (2.3%) was mild (inguinal hernia), and one was a deformation (arthrogryposis). The investigators concluded that the anticonvulsants were the primary risk factor for an increased incidence of congenital malformations (see also Carbamazepine, Clonazepam, Phenobarbital, Phenytoin, and Primidone) (71).

The Lamotrigine Pregnancy Registry, an ongoing project conducted by the manufacturer, was first published in January 1997. The final report was published in July 2010 (72). The Registry is now closed. Among 181 prospectively enrolled pregnancies exposed to valproate and lamotrigine, with or without other anticonvulsants, 169 were exposed in the 1st trimester resulting in 140 live births, 17 birth defects, 2 fetal deaths, 6 spontaneous abortions, and 4 elective abortions. There were 11 exposures in the 2nd/3rd trimesters resulting in 9 live births, 1 birth defect, and 1 fetal death. One live birth was exposed in an unspecified trimester (72).

A 1997 case report described autism diagnosed in a 5.5-year-old boy who had typical clinical features of the FVS (73). The mother had taken valproic acid (2000 mg/day) during the first 5 months of pregnancy for the treatment of dizzy spells, possible absence seizures, and an abnormal electroencephalogram (EEG). Although his gross motor milestones were normal, both his speech and language development were delayed. Based on their review of the literature, the authors concluded that a possible relationship between autism and FVS existed (73).

A population-based study of all children born alive in Denmark during 1996–2006 was published in 2013 (74). Of 655,615 children, 5437 had autism spectrum disorder, including 2067 with childhood autism. The estimated absolute risk was 1.53% (95% CI 1.47–1.58) for autism spectrum disorder and 0.48% (95% CI 0.46–0.51) for childhood autism. For the 508 children exposed in utero to valproate, the absolute risk was 4.4% (95% CI 2.59–1.46) for autism spectrum disorder (adjusted hazard ratio [AHR] 2.9) (95% CI 1.7–4.9), whereas for childhood autism the absolute risk was 2.50% (95% CI 1.30–4.81), AHR 5.2 (95% CI 2.7–10.0). When the analysis was restricted to the 6584 children born to mothers with epilepsy, the absolute risk of autism spectrum disorder among 432 exposed to valproate was 4.15% (95% CI 2.20–7.81), AHR 1.7 (95% CI 0.9–3.2) and for childhood autism 2.95% (95% CI 1.42–6.11), AHR 2.9 (95% CI 1.4–6.0) vs. the two outcomes for 6152 children not exposed to valproate 2.44% (95% CI 1.88–3.16) and 1.02% (95% CI 0.70–1.49). The data indicated that in utero exposure to valproate was associated with a significantly increased risk of autism spectrum disorder and childhood autism even after adjusting for maternal epilepsy (74). Other studies and reviews have reported the association between fetal valproate exposure and autism (75–77).

The relationship between maternal anticonvulsant therapy, neonatal behavior, and neurological function in children was reported in a 1996 study (78). Among newborns exposed to maternal monotherapy, 18 were exposed to phenobarbital (including primidone), 13 to phenytoin, and 8 to valproic acid. Compared with controls, neonates exposed to phenobarbital had significantly higher mean apathy and optimality scores. Phenytoin-exposed neonates also had a significantly higher mean apathy score. However, the neonatal optimality and apathy scores did not correlate with neurological outcome of the children at 6 years of age. In contrast, those exposed to valproic acid had optimality and apathy scores statistically similar to controls but a significantly higher hyperexcitability score. Moreover, the hyperexcitability score correlated with minor and major neurological dysfunction at age 6 years (78).

A 2013 study reported dose-dependent associations with reduced cognitive abilities across a range of domains at 6 years of age after fetal valproate exposure (79). Analysis showed that IQ was significantly lower for valproate (mean 97, 95% CI 94–101) than for carbamazepine (mean 105, 95% CI 102–108; $p = 0.0015$), lamotrigine (mean 108, 95% CI 105–110; $p = 0.0003$), or phenytoin (mean 108, 95% CI 104–112; $p = 0.0006$). Mean IQs were higher in children whose mothers had taken folic acid (mean 108, 95% CI 106–111) compared with children whose mothers had not taken the vitamin (mean 101, 95% CI 98–104; $p = 0.0009$) (79).

A valproate dose relationship with major fetal malformations has been reported (80–82). In these studies, doses >1100 mg/day were associated with a higher incidence of major defects. However, a 2013 review stated that daily doses of ≥1000 mg, as well as polytherapy, were associated with a higher teratogenic risk (77).

Intrauterine growth restriction (IUGR) or small-for-gestational-age infants have been noted in several reports (4,16,19,23,24,47,48,50,65,84,85). Both monotherapy and combination therapy with valproic acid were involved in these cases. However, normal birth weights, heights, and head circumferences have been reported with valproic acid monotherapy (25,50,53,65). Growth impairment is a common problem with some anticonvulsant therapy (e.g., see Phenytoin), but the relationship between this problem and valproic acid needs further clarification.

A study published in 2009 examined the effect of AEDs on the head circumference in newborns (85). Significant reductions in mean birth-weight-adjusted mean head circumference (bw-adj-HC) was noted for monotherapy with carbamazepine and valproic acid. No effect on bw-adj-HC was observed with gabapentin, phenytoin, clonazepam, and lamotrigine. A significant increase in the occurrence of microcephaly (bw-adj-HC smaller than 2 standard deviations below the mean) was noted after any AED polytherapy but not after any monotherapy, including carbamazepine and valproic acid. The potential effects of these findings on child development warrant study (85).

A 1983 letter proposed that the mechanism for valproic acid–induced teratogenicity involved zinc deficiency (84). From in utero studies, the authors had previously shown that valproic acid readily binds zinc. Low zinc serum levels potentiated the teratogenicity of certain drugs in animals and produced adverse effects similar to valproic acid–induced human toxicity (84). Another proposed mechanism, especially when valproic acid is combined with other anticonvulsants, involves the inhibition of liver microsomal epoxide hydrolase, the enzyme responsible for the biotransformation of reactive epoxide metabolites (86). The inhibition of the detoxifying enzyme could result in enhanced fetal exposure to reactive epoxide metabolites, such as carbamazepine epoxide, by preventing its biotransformation to a *trans*-dihydrodiol metabolite. Based on these findings, the authors recommended that combination drug therapy with valproic acid be avoided during pregnancy (86).

Three reports have observed hyperbilirubinemia in nine newborns exposed in utero to valproic acid monotherapy and in one infant exposed to combination therapy (4,25,48). A causal relationship is uncertain because other studies have not reported this problem.

Liver toxicity has been observed in three infants after in utero exposure to valproic acid (47,48). In the first report, a growth-restricted female infant, exposed to valproic acid and phenytoin, had a linea alba hernia noted at birth but her liver function tests were normal (47). The mother breastfed the child for the first several weeks. At 2.5 months of age, the infant presented with an enlarged liver, slight icterus, vomiting, and failure to thrive. Liver function tests indicated a cholestatic type of hyperbilirubinemia, and liver biopsy specimen demonstrated fibrosis with ongoing necrosis of liver cells. Although they were unable to determine which anticonvulsant caused the injury, the authors concluded that valproic acid was the more likely offending agent. The second report described two siblings born of a mother treated with valproic acid monotherapy during two pregnancies (48). A male infant, exposed in utero to 300 mg/day, was normal at birth but died at age 5 months of liver failure. Autopsy revealed liver atrophy, necrosis, and cholestasis. The female infant, exposed in utero to 500 mg/day, died at age 6 weeks of liver failure. At birth, the infant was noted to have defects characteristic of valproic acid exposure (defects described in the list above), IUGR, hyperbilirubinemia, hypoglycemia, hypocalcemia, and seizures. Liver atrophy and cholestasis were noted at autopsy (48).

Undetectable fibrinogen levels resulting in fatal hemorrhage in a full-term 2-day-old infant were attributed to in utero sodium valproate exposure (87). The mother had taken daily doses of sodium valproate 600 mg, phenytoin 375 mg, and lorazepam 1 mg throughout pregnancy. In a subsequent pregnancy, the measurement of slightly decreased maternal fibrinogen levels in late gestation caused the authors to discontinue the sodium valproate while continuing the other two agents. Oral vitamin K was also administered to the mother and she delivered a healthy infant without bleeding problems (87).

Transient hyperglycinemia has been observed in two newborns exposed in utero to sodium valproate combination therapy (combined with phenytoin in one and phenytoin, carbamazepine, and clonazepam in the other) (3). Similar increases of glycine have been observed in epileptic adults treated with valproic acid. No adverse effects in the newborns resulted from the amino acid alteration (3).

Fetal distress during labor (late decelerations, silent or accelerated beat-to-beat variations) was observed in 6 (43%) of 14 cases exposed to valproic acid monotherapy (26). Two of the newborns with fetal distress plus two others had low Apgar scores (0–3 after 1 minute or 0–6 after 5 minutes). Maternal doses were 1500–1800 mg/day in three cases and 600 mg/day in one case. Low Apgar scores were not observed in 12 infants whose mothers had been treated with valproic acid combination therapy. Other studies and case reports have not mentioned this complication. The fetal and newborn depression was thought to have resulted from a threefold increase in the maternal serum of valproic acid free fraction (26). A similar increase had been measured in an earlier study (10).

No decreases in adrenocorticotropic hormone or cortisol levels were measured in a mother or her newborn after the use of valproic acid 3000 mg/day during the last 3 months of pregnancy (28). The mother had received combination anticonvulsant therapy during the first 6 months of gestation.

Valproic acid has been measured in the semen of two healthy males (88). Following oral doses of 500 mg, semen levels ranged from 0.53 to 3.26 mcg/mL up to 39 hours after the dose. Simultaneous serum levels were 11–17 times those measured in the semen. No effect on sperm motility was suggested based on animal experiments (88).

Because of the risk for NTDs, women exposed during the critical period of gestation should consult their physician about prenatal testing (37,89,90).

BREASTFEEDING SUMMARY

Valproic acid and its salt, sodium valproate, are excreted into human milk in low concentrations (1,2,4,5,8,10,12,91,92). Milk concentrations up to 15% of the corresponding level in the mother's serum have been measured. In two infants, serum levels of valproate were 1.5% and 6.0% of maternal values (92).

Only one report of adverse effects in a nursing infant attributable to valproate in breast milk has been located. Thrombocytopenia purpura, anemia, and reticulocytosis were observed in a 3-month-old male breastfed infant whose mother was taking sodium valproate (monotherapy; 1200 mg/day) for epilepsy (93). The infant had a 2-week history of increasing petechiae and minor hematoma on the lower part of the legs. The infant's serum valproate level was 6.6 mcg/mL. Breastfeeding was discontinued for 5 days but had no effect on the infant's low platelet count. The mother continued to nurse for another 2 weeks and again stopped. Twelve days later, valproate was undetectable in the infant's serum and 7 days later (19 days after nursing was stopped), the platelet count began to rise, reaching normal values sometime after 35 days. At about this same time, the petechiae had resolved. The blood hemoglobin and the reticulocytes normalized between 12 and 19 days after breastfeeding was stopped (93).

In a 2010 study, 199 children who had been breastfed while their mothers were taking a single antiepileptic drug (carbamazepine, lamotrigine, phenytoin, or valproate) were evaluated at 3 years of age cognitive outcome (94). Mean adjusted IQ scores for exposed children were 99 (95% CI 96–103), whereas the mean adjusted IQ scores of nonbreastfed infants were 98 (95% CI 95–101).

The American Academy of Pediatrics classifies valproic acid as compatible with breastfeeding (95).

References

1. Alexander FW. Sodium valproate and pregnancy. Arch Dis Child 1979;54:240.
2. Dickinson RG, Harland RC, Lynn RK, Smith WB, Gerber N. Transmission of valproic acid (Depakene) across the placenta: half-life of the drug in mother and baby. J Pediatr 1979;94:832–5.
3. Simila S, von Wendt L, Hartikainen-Sorri A-L, Kaapa P, Saukkonen A-L. Sodium valproate, pregnancy, and neonatal hyperglycinaemia. Arch Dis Child 1979;54:985–6.
4. Nau H, Rating D, Koch S, Hauser I, Helge H. Valproic acid and its metabolites: placental transfer, neonatal pharmacokinetics, transfer via mother's milk and clinical status in neonates of epileptic mothers. J Pharmacol Exp Ther 1981;219:768–77.
5. Froescher W, Eichelbaum M, Niesen M, Altmann D, von Unruh GE. Antiepileptic therapy with carbamazepine and valproic acid during pregnancy and lactation period. In: Dam M, Gram L, Penry JK, eds. *Advances in Epileptology: the XIIth Epilepsy International Symposium*. New York, NY: Raven Press, 1981;581–8. As cited in Froescher W, Gugler R, Niesen M, Hoffmann F. Protein binding of valproic acid in maternal and umbilical cord serum. Epilepsia 1984;25:244–9.
6. Froescher W, Niesen M, Altmann D, Eichelbaum M, Gugler R, Hoffmann F, Penin H. Antiepileptika-Therapie wahrend Schwangerschaft und Geburt. In: Remschmidt H, Rentz R, Jungmann J, eds. *Epilepsie 1980*. Stuttgart: Georg Thieme Publishers, 1981:152–63. As cited in Froescher W, Gugler R, Niesen M, Hoffman F. Protein binding of valproic acid in maternal and umbilical cord serum. Epilepsia 1984;25:244–9.

7. Iskizaki T, Yokochi K, Chiba K, Tabuchi T, Wagatsuma T. Placental transfer of anticonvulsants (phenobarbital, phenytoin, valproic acid) and the elimination from neonates. Pediatr Pharmacol 1981;1:291–303.
8. Nau H, Kuhnz W, Egger H-J, Rating D, Helge H. Anticonvulsants during pregnancy and lactation: transplacental, maternal and neonatal pharmacokinetics. Clin Pharmacokinet 1982;7:508–43.
9. Kaneko S, Otani K, Fukushima Y, Sato T, Nomura Y, Ogawa Y. Transplacental passage and half-life of sodium valproate in infants born to epileptic mothers. Br J Clin Pharmacol 1983;15:503–6.
10. Nau H, Helge H, Luck W. Valproic acid in the perinatal period: decreased maternal serum protein binding results in fetal accumulation and neonatal displacement of the drug and some metabolites. J Pediatr 1984;104: 627–34.
11. Froescher W, Gugler R, Niesen M, Hoffmann F. Protein binding of valproic acid in maternal and umbilical cord serum. Epilepsia 1984;25:244–9.
12. Philbert A, Pedersen B, Dam M. Concentration of valproate during pregnancy, in the newborn and in breast milk. Acta Neurol Scand 1985;72: 460–3.
13. Nau H, Schafer H, Rating D, Jakobs C, Helge H. Placental transfer and neonatal pharmacokinetics of valproic acid and some of its metabolites. In: Janz D, Bossi L, Dam M, Helge H, Richens A, Schmidt D, eds. *Epilepsy, Pregnancy, and the Child*. New York, NY: Raven Press, 1982:367–72.
14. Perucca E, Ruprah M, Richens A. Altered drug binding to serum proteins in pregnant women: therapeutic relevance. J R Soc Med 1981;74:422–6.
15. Rating D, Jager-Roman E, Koch S, Nau H, Klein PD, Helge H. Enzyme induction in neonates due to antiepileptic therapy during pregnancy. In: Janz D, Bossi L, Dam M, Helge H, Richens A, Schmidt D, eds. *Epilepsy, Pregnancy, and the Child*. New York, NY: Raven Press, 1982:349–55.
16. Dalens B, Raynaud E-J, Gaulme J. Teratogenicity of valproic acid. J Pediatr 1980;97:332–3.
17. Gomez MR. Possible teratogenicity of valproic acid. J Pediatr 1981;98:508–9.
18. Thomas D, Buchanan N. Teratogenic effects of anticonvulsants. J Pediatr 1981;99:163.
19. Weinbaum PJ, Cassidy SB, Vintzileos AM, Campbell WA, Ciarleglio L, Nochimson DJ. Prenatal detection of a neural tube defect after fetal exposure to valproic acid. Obstet Gynecol 1986;67:31S–3S.
20. Clay SA, McVie R, Chen H. Possible teratogenic effect of valproic acid. J Pediatr 1981;99:828.
21. Robert E, Guibaud P. Maternal valproic acid and congenital neural tube defects. Lancet 1982;2:937.
22. Blaw ME, Woody RC. Valproic acid embryopathy? Neurology 1983;33:255.
23. Bailey CJ, Pool RW, Poskitt EME, Harris F. Valproic acid and fetal abnormality. Br Med J 1983;286:190.
24. Koch S, Jager-Roman E, Rating D, Helge H. Possible teratogenic effect of valproate during pregnancy. J Pediatr 1983;103:1007–8.
25. Bantz EW. Valproic acid and congenital malformations: a case report. Clin Pediatr 1984;23:353–4.
26. Jager-Roman E, Deichi A, Jakob S, Hartmann A-M, Koch S, Rating D, Steldinger R, Nau H, Helge H. Fetal growth, major malformations, and minor anomalies in infants born to women receiving valproic acid. J Pediatr 1986;108:997–1004.
27. Shakir RA, Johnson RH, Lambie DG, Melville ID, Nanda RN. Comparison of sodium valproate and phenytoin as single drug treatment in epilepsy. Epilepsia 1981;22:27–33.
28. Hatjis CG, Rose JC, Pippitt C, Swain M. Effect of treatment with sodium valproate on plasma adrenocorticotropic hormone and cortisol concentrations in pregnancy. Am J Obstet Gynecol 1985;152:315–6.
29. Product information. Depakene. Abbott Laboratories, 2000.
30. Anonymous. Teratogenic risks of antiepileptic drugs. Br Med J 1981;283; 515–6.
31. Paulson GW, Paulson RR. Teratogenic effects of anticonvulsants. Arch Neurol 1981;38:140–3.
32. Brown NA, Kao J, Fabro S. Teratogenic potential of valproic acid. Lancet 1980;1:660–1.
33. Whittle BA. Pre-clinical teratological studies on sodium valproate (Epilim) and other anticonvulsants. In: Legg NJ, ed. *Clinical and Pharmacological Aspects of Sodium Valproate (Epilim) in the Treatment of Epilepsy*. Tunbridge Wells, England: MCS Consultants, 1976:105–11.
34. Hiilesmaa VK, Bardy AH, Granstrom M-L, Teramo KAW. Valproic acid during pregnancy. Lancet 1980;1:883.
35. Nakane Y, Okuma T, Takahashi R, Sato Y, Wada T, Sato T, Fukushima Y, Kumashiro H, Ono T, Takahashi T, Aoki Y, Kazamatsuri H, Inami M, Komai S, Seino M, Miyakoshi M, Tanimura T, Hazama H, Kawahara R, Otsuki S, Hosokawa K, Inanaga K, Nakazawa Y, Yamamoto K. Multi-institutional study on the teratogenicity and fetal toxicity of antiepileptic drugs: a report of a collaborative study group in Japan. Epilepsia 1980;21:663–80.
36. Jeavons PM. Non-dose-related side effects of valproate. Epilepsia 1984;25(Suppl 1):S50–5.
37. CDC. Valproate: a new cause of birth defects report from Italy and follow-up from France. MMWR 1983;32:438–9.
38. Bossi L, Battino D, Boldi B, Caccamo ML, Ferraris, G, Latis GO, Simionato L. Anthropometric data and minor malformations in newborns of epileptic mothers. In: Janz D, Bossi L, Dam M, Helge H, Richens A, Schmidt D, eds. *Epilepsy, Pregnancy, and the Child*. New York, NY: Raven Press, 1982: 299–301.
39. Committee on Drugs, American Academy of Pediatrics. Valproic acid: benefits and risks. Pediatrics 1982;70:316–9.
40. Bjerkedal T, Czeizel A, Goujard J, Kallen B, Mastroiacova P, Nevin N, Oakley G Jr, Robert E. Valproic acid and spina bifida. Lancet 1982;2: 1096, 1172.
41. Stanely OH, Chambers TL. Sodium valproate and neural tube defects. Lancet 1982;2:1282.
42. Jeavons PM. Sodium valproate and neural tube defects. Lancet 1982;2:1282–3.
43. Castilla E. Valproic acid and spina bifida. Lancet 1983;2:683.
44. Robert E, Rosa F. Valproate and birth defects. Lancet 1983;2:1142.
45. Mastroiacovo P, Bertollini R, Morandini S, Segni G. Maternal epilepsy, valproate exposure, and birth defects. Lancet 1983;2:1499.
46. Lindhout D, Meinardi H. Spina bifida and in utero exposure to valproate. Lancet 1984;2:396.
47. Felding I, Rane A. Congenital liver damage after treatment of mother with valproic acid and phenytoin? Acta Paediatr Scand 1984;73:565–8.
48. Legius E, Jaeken J, Eggermont E. Sodium valproate, pregnancy, and infantile fatal liver failure. Lancet 1987;2:1518–9.
49. Rating D, Jager-Roman E, Koch S, Gopfert-Geyer I, Helge H. Minor anomalies in the offspring of epileptic parents. In: Janz D, Bossi L, Dam M, Helge H, Richens A, Schmidt D, eds. *Epilepsy, Pregnancy, and the Child*. New York, NY: Raven Press, 1982:283–8.
50. DiLiberti JH, Farndon PA, Dennis NR, Curry CJR. The fetal valproate syndrome. Am J Med Genet 1984;19:473–81.
51. Lindhout D, Meinardi H, Barth PG. Hazards of fetal exposure to drug combinations. In: Janz D, Bossi L, Dam M, Helge H, Richens A, Schmidt D, eds. *Epilepsy, Pregnancy, and the Child*. New York, NY: Raven Press, 1982: 275–81.
52. Koch S, Hartmann A, Jager-Roman E, Rating D, Helge H. Major malformations in children of epileptic parents due to epilepsy or its therapy? In: Janz D, Bossi L, Dam M, Helge H, Richens A, Schmidt D, eds. *Epilepsy, Pregnancy, and the Child*. New York, NY: Raven Press, 1982:313–5.
53. Ardinger HH, Atkin JF, Blackston RD, Elsas LJ, Clarren SK, Livingstone S, Flannery DB, Pellock JM, Harrod MJ, Lammer EJ, Majewski F, Schinzel A, Toriello HV, Hanson JW. Verification of the fetal valproate syndrome phenotype. Am J Med Genet 1988;29:171–85.
54. Staunton H. Valproate, spina bifida, and birth defect registries. Lancet 1989;1:381.
55. Oakeshott P, Hunt GM. Valproate and spina bifida. Br Med J 1989;298: 1300–1.
56. Oakeshott P, Hunt G. Valproate and spina bifida. Lancet 1989;1:611.
57. Martinez-Frias ML, Rodriguez-Pinilla E, Salvador J. Valproate and spina bifida. Lancet 1989;1:611–2.
58. Carter BS, Stewart JM. Valproic acid prenatal exposure: association with lipomyelomeningocele. Clin Pediatr 1989;28:81–5.
59. Boussemart T, Bonneau D, Levard G, Berthier M, Oriot D. Omphalocele in a newborn baby exposed to sodium valproate in utero. Eur J Pediatr 1995;154:220–1.
60. Hubert A, Bonneau D, Couet D, Berthier M, Oriot D, Larregue M. Aplasia cutis congenita of the scalp in an infant exposed to valproic acid in utero. Acta Paediatr 1994;83:789–90.
61. CDC. Valproic acid and spina bifida: a preliminary report—France. MMWR 1982;31:565–6.
62. Lammer EJ, Sever LE, Oakley GP Jr. Teratogen update: valproic acid. Teratology 1987;35:465–73.
63. Anonymous. Valproate and malformations. Lancet 1982;2:1313–4.
64. Lemire RJ. Neural tube defects. JAMA 1988;259:558–62.
65. Jager-Roman E, Rating D, Koch S, Gopfert-Geyer I, Jacob S, Helge H. Somatic parameters, diseases, and psychomotor development in the offspring of epileptic parents. In: Janz D, Bossi L, Dam M, Helge H, Richens A, Schmidt D, eds. *Epilepsy, Pregnancy, and the Child*. New York, NY: Raven Press, 1982:425–32.
66. Jentink J, Loane MA, Dolk H, Barisic I, Garne E, Morris JK, de jong-van den Berg LTW, for the EUROCAT Antiepileptic Study Working Group. Valproic acid monotherapy in pregnancy and major congenital malformations. N Engl J Med 2010;362:2185–93.

67. Granstrom M-L. Development of the children of epileptic mothers: preliminary results from the prospective Helsinki study. In: Janz D, Bossi L, Dam M, Helge H, Richens A, Schmidt D, eds. *Epilepsy, Pregnancy, and the Child.* New York, NY: Raven Press, 1982;403–8.
68. Clayton-Smith J, Donnai D. Fetal valproate syndrome. J Med Genet 1995;32:724–7.
69. Arpino C, Brescianini S, Robert E, Castilla EE, Cocchi G, Cornel MC, de Vigan C, Lancaster PAL, Merlob P, Sumiyoshi Y, Zampino G, Renzi C, Rosano A, Mastroiacovo P. Teratogenic effects of antiepileptic drugs: use of an international database on malformations and drug exposure (MADRE). Epilepsia 2000;41:1436–43.
70. Rodriguez-Pinilla E, Arroyo I, Fondevilla J, Garcia MJ, Martinez-Frias ML. Prenatal exposure to valproic acid during pregnancy and limb deficiencies: a case–control study. Am J Med Genet 2000;90:376–81.
71. Canger R, Battino D, Canevini MP, Fumarola C, Guidolin L, Vignoli A, Mamoli D, Palmieri C, Molteni F, Granata T, Hassibi P, Zamperini P, Pardi G, Avanzini G. Malformations in offspring of women with epilepsy: a prospective study. Epilepsia 1999;40:1231–6.
72. The Lamotrigine Pregnancy Registry. Final Report. September 1, 1992 through March 31, 2010. GlaxcoSmithKline, July 2010.
73. Williams PG, Hersh JH. A male with fetal valproate syndrome and autism. Dev Med Child Neurol 1997;39:632–4.
74. Christensen, J, Gronborg TK, Sorensen MJ, Schendel D, Parner ET, Pedersen LH, Vestergaard M. Prenatal valproate exposure and risk of autism spectrum disorders and childhood autism. JAMA 2013;309:1696–703.
75. Moore SJ, Turnpenny P, Quinn A, Glover S, Lloyd DJ, Montgomery T, Dean JCS. A clinical study of 57 children with fetal anticonvulsant syndromes. J Med Genet 2000;37:489–97.
76. Williams G, King J, Cunningham M, Stephan M, Kerr B, Hersh JH. Fetal valproate syndrome and autism: additional evidence of an association. Dev Med Child Neurol 2001;43:202–6.
77. Ornoy A. Valproic acid in pregnancy: how much are we endangering the embryo and fetus? Reprod Toxicol 2009;28:1–10.
78. Koch S, Jager-Roman E, Losche G, Nau H, Rating D, Helge H. Antiepileptic drug treatment in pregnancy: drug side effects in the neonate and neurological outcome. Acta Paediatr 1996;84:739–46.
79. Meador KJ, Baker GA, Browning N, Cohen MJ, Bromley RL, Clayton-Smith J, Kalayjian LA, Kanner A, Liporace JD, Pennell PB, Privitera M, Loring DW, for the NEAD Study Group. Fetal antiepileptic drug exposure and cognitive outcomes at age 6 years (NEAD study): a prospective observational study. Lancet Neurol 2013;12:244–52.
80. Vajda FJ, O'Brien TJ, Hitchcock A, Graham J, Cook M, Lander C. Critical relationship between sodium valproate dose and human teratogenicity: results of the Australian register of anti-epileptic drugs in pregnancy. J Clin Neurosci 2004;11:854–8.
81. Vajda FJE, Eadie MJ. Maternal valproate dosage and foetal malformations. Acta Neurol Scand 2005;112:137–43.
82. Vajda FJE, Hitchcock A, Graham J, Solinas C, O'Brien TJ, Lander CM, Fadie MJ. Foetal malformations and seizure control: 52 months data of the Australian Pregnancy Registry. Eur J Neurol 2006;13:645–54.
83. Granstrom M-L, Hiilesmaa VK. Physical growth of the children of epileptic mothers: preliminary results from the prospective Helsinki study. In: Janz D, Bossi L, Dam M, Helge H, Richens A, Schmidt D, eds. *Epilepsy, Pregnancy, and the Child.* New York, NY: Raven Press, 1982:397–401.
84. Hurd RW, Wilder BJ, Van Rinsvelt HA. Valproate, birth defects, and zinc. Lancet 1983;1:181.
85. Almgren M, Kallen B, Lavebratt C. Population-based study of antiepileptic drug exposure *in utero*—influence on head circumference in newborns. Seizure 2009;18:672–5.
86. Kerr BM, Levy RH. Inhibition of epoxide hydrolase by anticonvulsants and risk of teratogenicity. Lancet 1989;1:610–1.
87. Majer RV, Green PJ. Neonatal afibrinogenaemia due to sodium valproate. Lancet 1987;2:740–1.
88. Swanson BN, Harland RC, Dickinson RG, Gerber N. Excretion of valproic acid into semen of rabbits and man. Epilepsia 1978;19:541–6.
89. Frew J. Valproate link to spina bifida. Med J Aust 1983;1:150.
90. Committee on Drugs, American Academy of Pediatrics. Valproate teratogenicity. Pediatrics 1983;71:980.
91. Bardy AH, Granstrom M-L, Hiilesmaa VK. Valproic acid and breastfeeding. In: Janz D, Bossi L, Dam M, Helge H, Richens A, Schmidt D, eds. *Epilepsy, Pregnancy, and the Child.* New York, NY: Raven Press, 1982:359–60.
92. Wisner KL, Perel JM. Serum levels of valproate and carbamazepine in breastfeeding mother–infant pairs. J Clin Psychopharmacol 1998;18:167–9.
93. Stahl MMS, Neiderud J, Vinge E. Thrombocytopenic purpura and anemia in a breast-fed infant whose mother was treated with valproic acid. J Pediatr 1997;130:1001–3.
94. Meador KJ, Baker GA, Browning N, Clayton-Smith J, Combs-Cantrell DT, Cohen M, Kalayjian LA, Kanner A, Liporace JD, Pennell PB, Privitera M, Loring DW, for the NEAD Study Group. Effects of breastfeeding in children of women taking antiepileptic drugs. Neurology 2010;75:1954–60.
95. Committee on Drugs, American Academy of Pediatrics. The transfer of drugs and other chemicals into human milk. Pediatrics 2001;108:776–89.

VALRUBICIN

Antineoplastic

PREGNANCY RECOMMENDATION: No Human Data—Probably Compatible (Intact Bladder)
BREASTFEEDING RECOMMENDATION: No Human Data—Probably Compatible (Intact Bladder)

PREGNANCY SUMMARY

No reports describing the use of valrubicin in human pregnancy have been located. The animal data suggest risk, but the drug was given IV on a daily basis and neither systemic concentrations nor a no-observed-effect level (NOEL) was reported. However, the systemic levels in the animals must have been much higher than those seen in humans with intact urinary bladders. Thus, these results are not relevant to the human exposure unless perforation of the bladder has occurred. Although the lack of human pregnancy experience prevents a more complete assessment of the embryo–fetal risk, the drug should not be withheld, if indicated and the bladder is intact, because of pregnancy.

FETAL RISK SUMMARY

Valrubicin, an anthracycline antibiotic, is a semisynthetic analog of doxorubicin. It is in the same antineoplastic subclass of anthracyclines as daunorubicin, doxorubicin, epirubicin, and idarubicin. Valrubicin is indicated for intravesical therapy of BCG-refractory carcinoma in situ of the urinary bladder in patients for whom immediate cystectomy would be associated with unacceptable morbidity or mortality. The drug should not be given to patients with a perforated bladder or if the bladder mucosa has been compromised. Only nanogram quantities of valrubicin are absorbed into the systemic circulation, and valrubicin metabolites have been measured in blood. If urinary bladder perforation has occurred, much higher concentrations are absorbed which can cause systemic hematologic toxicity (1).

Reproduction studies have been conducted in rats. Daily IV doses that were one-sixth or one-third the recommended human intravesical dose based on BSA caused fetal malformations. At the higher dose, numerous, severe alterations in the fetal skull and skeleton were observed, as well as an increase in fetal resorptions and a decrease in viable fetuses (1).

Studies for carcinogenicity and fertility have not been conducted. Valrubicin does cause damage to DNA in vitro and was mutagenic and clastogenic in assays (1).

It is not known if valrubicin crosses the human placenta. The molecular weight (about 724) and high lipophilic property suggest that the drug, if it reaches the systemic circulation, would cross to the embryo–fetus. However, in the presence of an intact urinary bladder, only nanogram amounts appear in the blood suggesting that such exposure would not be clinically significant.

BREASTFEEDING SUMMARY

No reports describing the use of valrubicin during human lactation have been located. The molecular weight (about 724) and high lipophilic property suggest that the drug, if it reaches the systemic circulation, will be excreted into breast milk. However, in the presence of an intact urinary bladder, only nanogram amounts appear in the blood and excretion of these amounts into milk probably is not clinically significant.

Reference

1. Product information. Valstar. Endo Pharmaceuticals, 2009.

VALSARTAN

Antihypertensive

PREGNANCY RECOMMENDATION: Human Data Suggest Risk in 2nd and 3rd Trimesters

BREASTFEEDING RECOMMENDATION: No Human Data—Probably Compatible

PREGNANCY SUMMARY

The antihypertensive mechanisms of action of valsartan and angiotensin-converting enzyme (ACE) inhibitors are very close. That is, the former selectively blocks the binding of angiotensin II to AT_1 receptors, whereas the latter prevents the formation of angiotensin II itself. Therefore, use of this drug during the 2nd and 3rd trimesters may cause teratogenicity and severe fetal and neonatal toxicity identical to that seen with ACE inhibitors (e.g., see Captopril or Enalapril). Fetal toxic effects may include anuria, oligohydramnios, fetal hypocalvaria, intrauterine growth restriction, prematurity, and patent ductus arteriosus. Anuria-associated anhydramnios/oligohydramnios may produce fetal limb contractures, craniofacial deformation, and pulmonary hypoplasia. Severe anuria and hypotension, resistant to both pressor agents and volume expansion, may occur in the newborn following in utero exposure to valsartan. Newborn renal function and blood pressure should be closely monitored.

FETAL RISK SUMMARY

Valsartan is a selective angiotensin II receptor blocker (ARB) that is used, either alone or in combination with other antihypertensive agents, for the treatment of hypertension. Valsartan blocks the vasoconstrictor and aldosterone-secreting effects of angiotensin II by preventing angiotensin II from binding to AT_1 receptors (1).

Reproduction studies have been conducted in pregnant mice, rats, and rabbits (1). No teratogenic effects were observed in these species at oral doses up to 9, 18, and 0.5 times the maximum recommended human dose of 320 mg/day based on BSA (MRHD), respectively. The highest dose caused rat maternal toxicity (reduction in body weight gain and food consumption). At this dose, administration during organogenesis or late gestation and lactation resulted in significant decreases in fetal weight, pup birth weight, and pup survival rate, and slight delays in developmental milestones (1). In rabbits, maternal toxic doses (0.25 and 0.5 times the MRHD) resulted in fetal resorptions, litter loss, abortions, and low fetal body weight as well as maternal mortality. The no-observed-adverse-effect doses in mice, rats, and rabbits were 9, 6, and 0.1 times the MRHD, respectively (1). No adverse effects on reproductive performance of male and female rats were noted at oral doses up to 6 times the MRHD (1).

It is not known if valsartan crosses the human placenta to the fetus. The molecular weight (about 436) is low enough that passage to the fetus should be expected.

A 2001 case report described the pregnancy outcome of a 40-year-old woman with well-controlled chronic hypertension and diet-controlled type 2 diabetes mellitus that was treated with valsartan (80 mg/day) and atenolol (75 mg/day) until presentation at 24 weeks' gestation (2). Anhydramnios (amniotic fluid index zero), most likely due to valsartan, was diagnosed by ultrasound, but fetal growth was appropriate for gestational age. Valsartan was stopped and atenolol was continued at the same dose. The amniotic fluid volume normalized within 2 weeks. The blood pressure and the diabetes remained under adequate control and there was no evidence of toxemia. Intrauterine fetal death was diagnosed at 31 weeks' gestation. At autopsy, very small, hypoplastic lungs were found (weight 18 g/expected 44 g), as were heavy kidneys (31 g/expected 18 g). The placenta was below the 10th percentile for gestational age (148 g/expected 311 g for gestational age at the 10th percentile). No other anomalies were detected. The very small placenta was thought to be primarily due to atenolol, but valsartan may have contributed to the condition. Death of the female fetus probably resulted from chronic placental insufficiency induced by the combination of valsartan and atenolol (2).

Three other case reports described the effects of valsartan on six pregnancy outcomes (3–5). In a 2001 report, three women were taking valsartan (80 mg/day) for hypertension at the time of conception (3). The drug therapy was stopped at 7, 10, and 18 weeks' gestation, respectively. No congenital defects or evidence of renal dysfunction were observed in the newborns delivered at 38, 38, and 32 weeks', respectively. However, growth restriction attributed to hypertension was observed in one infant (3). In the another 2001 case report, two women (one with type 2 diabetes) were taking valsartan (80 mg/day in one, dose not specified in the other) in combination with hydrochlorothiazide during pregnancy (4). Anhydramnios was noted at 24 and 28 weeks', respectively. Although the anhydramnios resolved in both cases when valsartan was discontinued, the pregnancies were terminated. Both fetuses had foot and face deformities, hypoplastic skull bones with widely open sutures, and large kidneys that were microscopically abnormal. Neither fetus had pulmonary hypoplasia (4). In 2004, anhydramnios was observed in a woman at 20 weeks' gestation (5). She had been taking valsartan for chronic hypertension. The drug was stopped and complete recovery of the amniotic fluid was noted at 23.5 weeks'. A healthy 3050-g female infant was delivered at term and was developing normally at 6 months of age.

In a 2003 report, the outcomes of 42 pregnancies exposed to ARBs were described (6). The outcomes of 37 pregnancies (1 set of twins) exposed in the 1st trimester were 3 spontaneous abortions (drugs not specified), 4 elective abortions (one for exencephaly; candesartan until 4 3/7 weeks, carbimazole, hydrochlorothiazide, maternal obesity), 1 stillbirth (no anomalies; valsartan until week 4, cigarette smoking, other antihypertensives), 1 minor malformation (undescended testicles; therapy not specified), and 28 healthy newborns. There was one major malformation (cleft palate, patent ductus arteriosus, modest coarctation of the aorta, growth restriction; valsartan until week 13, hydrochlorothiazide, metoprolol, cigarette smoking). Five cases involved late exposure to ARBs and their outcomes involved one or more of the following: oligohydramnios/anhydramnios, anuria, hypoplastic skull bones, limb contractions, lung hypoplasia, and neonatal death (6).

A 2005 case report and review described a pregnancy complicated by chronic hypertension that was treated with valsartan (80 mg/day), hydrochlorothiazide (12.5 mg/day), prazosin (10 mg/day), and methyldopa (750 mg/day) (7). Anhydramnios was diagnosed at 24 weeks' gestation and ultrasound of the fetus revealed bilateral hyperechoic kidneys. Valsartan and hydrochlorothiazide were stopped 1 week later. Amniotic fluid volume normalized by 31 weeks'. A cesarean section at 38 weeks' delivered a 3060-g male infant with Apgar scores of 6 and 7 at 1 and 5 minutes, respectively. Mild skull bone hypoplasia (wide cranial suture), limb deformation (mild varus of the right foot), and abnormally large, hyperechogenic kidneys with decreased blood perfusion were observed in the infant. The infant's blood pressure was normal and he first passed urine at 6 hours. At 30 months of age, the child has had normal growth and development but mild chronic renal insufficiency (creatinine 1.1–1.4) (7).

In another 2005 case report, a 40-year-old woman took throughout pregnancy four daily medications for chronic hypertension: valsartan (8 mg), hydrochlorothiazide (0.15 mg), lecardinipine (20 mg) (a calcium channel blocker), and clonidine (0.15 mg) (8). At 36 weeks' gestation, oligohydramnios was diagnosed and a 2680-g female infant was delivered vaginally. The infant had a Potter's syndrome facies, hypocalvaria, and limb deformities consisting of bilateral talus valgus and fixed internal rotation of the right hand. Shortly after birth, the infant developed respiratory distress, acute rental failure (hyperechogenic kidneys with absent Cortico-medullary differentiation), and severe hypotension. However, the infant survived and renal function was normal at 8 months of age with substantial growth of the skull bones (8).

A 2007 review cited 64 published cases of pregnancies exposed to ARBs, 42.2% of which had unfavorable outcomes (9). The duration of ARB exposure was longer in the cases with poor outcomes compared with those with good outcomes, 26.3 ± 10.5 vs. 17.3 ± 11.6 weeks.

A 2012 review of the use of ACE inhibitors and ARBs in the 1st trimester concluded that there may be an elevated teratogenic risk, but the risk appeared to be related to other factors (10). The factors, that typically coexist with hypertension in pregnancy, included diabetes, advanced maternal age, and obesity.

BREASTFEEDING SUMMARY

No reports describing the use of valsartan during human lactation have been located. The molecular weight (about 436) is low enough that excretion into breast milk should be expected. The effect of this exposure on a nursing infant is unknown. The American Academy of Pediatrics classifies ACE inhibitors, a closely related group of antihypertensive agents, as compatible with breastfeeding (see Captopril or Enalapril).

References

1. Product information. Diovan. Novartis Pharmaceuticals, 2001.
2. Briggs GG, Nageotte MP. Fatal fetal outcome with the combined use of valsartan and atenolol. Ann Pharmacother 2001;35:859–61.
3. Chung NA, Lip GYH, Beevers M, Beevers DG. Angiotensin-II-receptor inhibitors in pregnancy. Lancet 2001;357:1620–1.
4. Martinovic J, Benachi A, Laurent N, Daikha-Dahmane F, Gubler MC. Fetal toxic effects and angiotensin-II-receptor antagonists. Lancet 2001;358:241–2.
5. Berkane N, Carlier P, Verstraete L, Mathieu E, Heim N, Uzan S. Fetal toxicity of valsartan and possible reversible adverse side effects. Birth Defects Res (Part A) 2004;70:547–9.
6. Schaefer C. Angiotensin II-receptor-antagonists: further evidence of fetotoxicity but not teratogenicity. Birth Defects Res (Part A) 2003;67:591–4.
7. Bos-Thompson MA, Hillaire-Buys D, Muller F, Dechaud H, Mazurier E, Boulot P, Morin D. Fetal toxic effects of angiotensin II receptor antagonists: case report and follow-up after birth. Ann Pharmacother 2005;39:157–61.
8. Vendemmia M, Garcia-Meric P, Rizzotti A, Boubred F, Lacroze V, Liprandi A, Simeoni U. Fetal and neonatal consequences of antenatal exposure to type 1 angiotensin II receptor-antagonists. J Matern Fetal Neonatal Med 2005;19:137–40.
9. Velazquez-Armenta EY, Han JY, Choi JS, Yang KM, Nava-Ocampo AA. Angiotensin II receptor blockers in pregnancy: a case report and systematic review of the literature. Hypertens Pregnancy 2007;26:51–66.
10. Polifka JE. Is there an embryopathy associated with first-trimester exposure to angiotensin-converting enzyme inhibitors and angiotensin receptor antagonists? A critical review of the evidence. Birth Defects Res (Part A) 2012;94:576–98.

VANCOMYCIN

Antibiotic

PREGNANCY RECOMMENDATION: Compatible
BREASTFEEDING RECOMMENDATION: Limited Human Data—Probably Compatible

PREGNANCY SUMMARY

Vancomycin is an antibiotic that is used for gram-positive bacteria when either the organisms are resistant to less toxic anti-infectives (e.g., penicillins and cephalosporins) or the patient is sensitive to these agents. No cases of congenital defects attributable to vancomycin have been located. The manufacturer has received reports on the use of vancomycin in pregnancy without adverse fetal effects (A.F. Crumley, personal communication, Eli Lilly, 1983).

FETAL RISK SUMMARY

Reproduction studies in rats and rabbits at doses up to 1 and 1.1 times the maximum recommended human dose based on BSA (MRHD), respectively, have revealed no teratogenic effects. No effects on fetal weight or development were seen with the same doses in rats or slightly lower doses in rabbits (0.74 times the MRHD) (1).

The pharmacokinetics of vancomycin in a woman at 26.5 weeks' gestation was described in a 1991 reference (2). Accumulation of the antibiotic, administered as 1 g IV every 12 hours (15 mg/kg/dose), was demonstrated in amniotic fluid (1.02 mcg/mL on day 1; 9.2 mcg/mL on day 13). At delivery at 28 weeks' gestation, cord blood levels were 3.65 mcg/mL (6 hours after the mother's maximum serum concentration), 76% of the mother's serum level. The newborn's serum level, 3.25 hours after birth, was 2.45 mcg/mL, indicating a half-life in the infant of 10 hours (2).

In a 2007 report, 13 nonlaboring, noninfected women at term, scheduled for cesarean section, were given a single 1-g IV dose of vancomycin (3). The full 1-g dose could be given to only six women, because four of five women given a 60-minute infusion and three of eight given a 90-minute infusion experienced a reaction to the antibiotic ("red man syndrome": pruritus, shortness of breath, flushing, headache, and one case of hypotension). All seven infants had normal Apgar scores and blood gasses. Scheduling complications also prevented giving the vancomycin at the planned intervals before delivery. The actual time intervals from the end of the infusion to maternal sample were 26–509 minutes, and there was a strong correlation between cord and maternal concentrations. Regardless of the interval, all 13 cord serum samples contained low amounts of vancomycin (3–9.4 mcg/mL), but these amounts were considered to be above the minimal inhibitory concentration for group B streptococcus (3).

Vancomycin was used for subacute bacterial endocarditis prophylaxis in a penicillin-allergic woman at term with mitral valve prolapse (4). One hour before vaginal delivery, a 1-g IV dose was given during 3 minutes (recommended infusion time is 60 minutes [1,5]). Immediately after the dose, maternal blood pressure fell from 130/74 to 80/40 mmHg and then recovered in 3 minutes. Fetal bradycardia, 90 beats/minute, persisted for 4 minutes. No adverse effects of the hypotension-induced fetal distress were observed in the newborn. The Apgar scores were 9 and 10 at 1 and 5 minutes, respectively (4).

A 1989 report examined the effects of multiple-dose vancomycin on newborn hearing and renal function (6). Ten pregnant, drug-dependent women were treated with IV vancomycin (1 g every 12 hours for at least 1 week) for suspected or documented infections caused by methicillin-resistant *Staphylococcus aureus*. Of the 10 women, 4 also received concomitant gentamicin. Two control groups, neither of which received antibiotics, were formed: 10 infants from nondrug-dependent mothers (group 2), and 10 infants from drug-dependent mothers (group 3). Auditory brainstem response testing was conducted on the infants at birth and at 3 months of age, and blood urea nitrogen and serum creatinine were measured at birth. The placental transfer of vancomycin was measured in two patients with cord blood levels of 16.7 and 13.2 mcg/mL, 6 and 2.5 hours after infusion, respectively. At birth, abnormal auditory brainstem responses were measured in a total of six infants: two infants from the study group (neither exposed to gentamicin), three from control group 2, and one from control group 3. The hearing defect in all six infants was an absent wave V at 40 dB (the average behavioral threshold of adult listeners) in one or both ears. Repeat testing at 3 months in five infants was normal, indicating that the initial tests were falsely positive. In the sixth infant (in the study group), the tests at 3 months again showed no response in either ear at 40 dB. This infant's mother had received a 2-g vancomycin dose after initial dosing had produced low serum levels (<20 mcg/mL) of the antibiotic. The peak serum level obtained following the double dose was 65.7 mcg/mL, a potentially toxic level if it was maintained. Following this, the mother was treated with the same regimen as the other women. On further examination, however, reduced compliance was discovered in both ears and the loss of hearing was diagnosed as a conduction defect, rather than sensorineural. Tests at 12 months, following improved compliance in both ears, were normal. Renal function studies in all 30 infants were also normal, although this latter conclusion has been challenged (7) and defended (8).

BREASTFEEDING SUMMARY

Vancomycin is excreted into breast milk. In one woman treated with IV vancomycin (1 g every 12 hours for at least 1 week), a milk level 4 hours after a dose was 12.7 mcg/mL (6). This value was nearly identical to the serum trough concentration measured at 12 hours in the mother during pregnancy. The effect on the nursing infant of vancomycin in milk is unknown. Vancomycin is poorly absorbed from the normal, intact gastrointestinal tract, and thus, systemic absorption would not be expected (5). However, three potential problems exist for the nursing infant: modification of bowel flora, direct effects on the infant (e.g., allergic response or sensitization), and interference with the interpretation of culture results if a fever workup is required.

References

1. Product information. Vancocin. Eli Lilly, 2000.
2. Bourget P, Fernandez H, Delouis C, Ribou F. Transplacental passage of vancomycin during the second trimester of pregnancy. Obstet Gynecol 1991;78:908–11.
3. Laiprasert J, Klein K, Mueller BA, Pearlman MD. Transplacental passage of vancomycin in noninfected term pregnant women. Obstet Gynecol 2007;109:1105–10.
4. Hill LM. Fetal distress secondary to vancomycin-induced maternal hypotension. Am J Obstet Gynecol 1985;153:74–5.
5. American Hospital Formulary Service. *Drug Information 1997*. Bethesda, MD: American Society of Health-System Pharmacists, 1997:403–8.
6. Reyes MP, Ostrea EM Jr, Cabinian AE, Schmitt C, Rintelmann W. Vancomycin during pregnancy: does it cause hearing loss or nephrotoxicity in the infant? Am J Obstet Gynecol 1989;161:977–81.
7. Gouyon JB, Petion AM. Toxicity of vancomycin during pregnancy. Am J Obstet Gynecol 1990;163:1375–6.
8. Reyes MP, Ostrea EM Jr. Toxicity of vancomycin during pregnancy. Reply. Am J Obstet Gynecol 1990;163:1376.

VANDETANIB

Antineoplastic (Tyrosine Kinase Inhibitor)

PREGNANCY RECOMMENDATION: Contraindicated
BREASTFEEDING RECOMMENDATION: Conraindicated

PREGNANCY SUMMARY

No reports describing the use of vandetanib in human pregnancy have been located. In the only animal species studied, the drug was embryotoxic, fetotoxic, and teratogenic at exposures close to or less than the human exposure. However, the absence of human pregnancy experience prevents a complete assessment of the embryo–fetal risk. Because of the risk of fetal harm, the manufacturer recommends that women of reproductive potential use effective contraception to prevent pregnancy during treatment and for at least 4 months following the last dose.

FETAL RISK SUMMARY

Vandetanib is an oral inhibitor of tyrosine kinase. There are several other agents in this subclass (see Appendix). It is indicated for the treatment of symptomatic or progressive medullary thyroid cancer in patients with unresectable locally advance or metastatic disease. Vandetanib is metabolized to apparently inactive metabolites. The mean plasma protein binding to albumin and α_1-acid-glycoprotein is 93.7% and the median plasma half-life is 19 days (1).

Reproduction studies have been conducted in rats. In rats before mating and through the 1st week of pregnancy, exposures that were equal to or less than the exposure expected from the recommended human dose of 300 mg/day (HE) resulted in increases in preimplantation and postimplantation loss, including embryo–fetal death, and a significant decrease in the number of live embryos. Total litter loss occurred when the drug was given during organogenesis until expected parturition. All doses (about 0.03–1.0 times the maximum concentration [C_{max}] in humans with cancer at the recommended dose) given during organogenesis caused both malformations of heart vessels and skeletal variations (delayed ossification of the skull, vertebrae, and sternum) that indicated delayed fetal development. A no-effect level for malformations was not identified in this study. In a separate study, doses identical to those used above caused maternal toxicity and, when given during gestation and/or lactation, resulted in decreased pup survival and/or reduced postnatal pup growth (1).

Carcinogenicity studies have not been conducted. Various assays for mutagenic and clastogenic effects were negative. Fertility in male rats was not impaired but, in female rats, there was a slight decrease in the number of live embryos. There also was a trend toward increased estrus cycle irregularity and a decrease in the number of corpora lutea in the ovaries (1).

It is not known if vandetanib crosses the human placenta. The molecular weight (about 475) and the long plasma half-life suggest that the drug will cross to the embryo–fetus, but high plasma protein binding might lessen the exposure.

BREASTFEEDING SUMMARY

No reports describing the use of vandetanib during human lactation have been located. The molecular weight (about 475) and the long plasma half-life (19 days) suggest that the drug will be excreted into breast milk, but high plasma protein binding (93.7%) might lessen the exposure. The effect of this exposure on a nursing infant is unknown. However, the drug has caused serious toxicity in adults, such as skin reactions and Stevens-Johnson syndrome, pneumonitis, ischemic cerebrovascular events, and hemorrhage. The most common adverse reactions (>20%) in adults were diarrhea, rash, acne, nausea, hypertension, headache, fatigue, upper respiratory tract infections, decreased appetite, and abdominal pain. If a woman receiving the drug chooses to breastfeed, her infant should be closely monitored for these effects.

Reference

1. Product information. Caprelsa. AstraZeneca Pharmaceuticals, 2012.

V

VARENICLINE

Central Nervous System Agent (Smoking Deterrent)

PREGNANCY RECOMMENDATION: No Human Data—Animal Data Suggest Low Risk
BREASTFEEDING RECOMMENDATION: No Human Data—Potential Toxicity

PREGNANCY SUMMARY

No reports describing the use of varenicline in human pregnancy have been located. The animal data suggest low risk, but the absence of human pregnancy experience prevents a more complete assessment of embryo–fetal risk. However, smoking is known to cause significant developmental toxicity (as well as toxicity in the smoker) (see Cigarette Smoking). Thus, the benefit to the woman and her pregnancy appears to outweigh the unknown risk to the embryo and/or fetus. If nonpharmacologic methods to stop smoking have failed, and the use of varenicline is indicated, it should not be withheld because of pregnancy.

FETAL RISK SUMMARY

Varenicline is a partial agonist selective for $\alpha_4\beta_2$ nicotinic acetylcholine receptor subtypes. This binding is thought to prevent nicotine from binding to these receptors. Varenicline is indicated as an aid in smoking cessation treatment. Oral bioavailability is nearly complete and metabolism of a dose is about 8%. Binding to plasma proteins also is low (≤20%), but the elimination half-life is long (about 24 hours) (1).

Reproduction studies have been conducted in rats and rabbits. In these species, no teratogenicity was observed with daily oral doses ≤36 and 50 times the maximum recommended human daily exposure based on AUC at 1 mg twice daily (MRHDE), respectively. However, in the offspring of pregnant rats given the highest dose there was an increased incidence of auditory startle response. In pregnant rabbits, the highest dose resulted in decreased fetal weights. The no-effect dose in rabbits was 23 times the MRHDE (1).

In 2-year carcinogenicity studies, there was no evidence of carcinogenic effects in mice given daily doses up to 47 times the MRHDE. In male rats, but not females, tumors of the brown fat (hibernoma) were observed at daily doses that were 23 and 67 times, respectively, the MRHDE. Various studies for mutagenicity were negative. No effects on fertility were observed in male and female rats given daily doses up to 67 and 36 times, respectively, the MRHDE. However, a decrease in fertility was noted in the offspring of pregnant rats given a daily dose that was 36 times, but not at 9 times, the MRHDE (1).

It is not known if varenicline crosses the human placenta. The molecular weight (about 361), high oral bioavailability, low metabolism and plasma protein binding, and the long elimination half-life suggest that the drug will pass to the embryo and fetus.

BREASTFEEDING SUMMARY

No reports describing the use of varenicline during human lactation have been located. The molecular weight (about 361), high oral bioavailability, low metabolism (about 8%) and plasma protein binding (≤20%), and the long elimination half-life (about 24 hours) suggest that the drug will be excreted into breast milk. The effects of this exposure on a nursing infant are unknown. However, smoking during breastfeeding is known to represent a significant risk to the nursing infant, as well as to the mother. (See Cigarette Smoking.) Thus, the benefit to the woman and her infant appears to outweigh the unknown risk to the infant. If a woman uses this drug while breastfeeding, she should closely monitor her infant for the adverse effects commonly observed in adults: nausea and vomiting, sleep disturbance, constipation, and flatulence.

Reference

1. Product information. Chantix. Pfizer, 2007.

VASOPRESSIN

Pituitary Hormone

PREGNANCY RECOMMENDATION: Compatible
BREASTFEEDING RECOMMENDATION: Compatible

PREGNANCY SUMMARY

No reports linking the use of vasopressin with congenital defects have been located. Vasopressin and the structurally related synthetic polypeptides desmopressin and lypressin have been used during pregnancy to treat diabetes insipidus, a rare disorder (1–11). Desmopressin has also been used at delivery in three women for the management of von Willebrand's disease (12). No adverse effects on the newborns were reported.

FETAL RISK SUMMARY

A threefold increase of circulating levels of endogenous vasopressin has been reported for women in the last trimester and in labor as compared with nonpregnant women (13). Although infrequent, the induction of uterine activity in the 3rd trimester has been reported after IM and intranasal vasopressin use (14). The IV use of desmopressin, which is normally given intranasally, has also been reported to cause uterine contractions (4).

Two investigators speculated that raised levels of vasopressin resulted from hypoxemia and acidosis and could produce signs of fetal distress (bradycardia and meconium staining) (15).

A 1995 reference described the use of desmopressin during pregnancy in 42 women with diabetes insipidus, 29 of whom received the drug throughout the whole pregnancy (16). One patient, treated with vasopressin during the first 6 months and then changed to desmopressin, delivered an infant who had a ventricular septal defect, a patent ductus arteriosus, and simian lines. The child died at age 14 years because of hypophyseal disease. Three of the infants exposed throughout gestation to desmopressin had birth weights close to or outside of the 99% confidence interval (two low and one high). The authors concluded that the use of desmopressin throughout pregnancy did not constitute a major fetal risk (16).

Diabetes insipidus developed in a 14-year-old girl at 33 weeks' gestation with resulting oligohydramnios and an amniotic fluid index of 0 (17). She was treated with intranasal desmopressin (10 mcg twice daily) with rapid resolution of the oligohydramnios and eventual, spontaneous delivery of a healthy 2700-g male infant at 38 weeks.

BREASTFEEDING SUMMARY

Patients receiving vasopressin, desmopressin, or lypressin for diabetes insipidus have been reported to breastfeed without apparent problems in the infant (1,2). Experimental work in lactating women suggests that suckling almost doubles the maternal blood concentration of vasopressin (13).

References

1. Hime MC, Richardson JA. Diabetes insipidus and pregnancy. Obstet Gynecol Surv 1978;33:375–9.
2. Hadi HA, Mashini IS, Devoe LD. Diabetes insipidus during pregnancy complicated by preeclampsia. A case report. J Reprod Med 1985;30:206–8.
3. Phelan JP, Guay AT, Newman C. Diabetes insipidus in pregnancy: a case review. Am J Obstet Gynecol 1978;130:365–6.
4. van der Wildt B, Drayer JIM, Eske TKAB. Diabetes insipidus in pregnancy as a first sign of a craniopharyngioma. Eur J Obstet Gynecol Reprod Biol 1980;10:269–74.
5. Ford SM Jr. Transient vasopressin-resistant diabetes insipidus of pregnancy. Obstet Gynecol 1986;68:288–9.
6. Ford SM Jr, Lumpkin HL III. Transient vasopressin-resistant diabetes insipidus of pregnancy. Obstet Gynecol 1986;68:726–8.
7. Rubens R, Thiery M. Case report: diabetes insipidus and pregnancy. Eur J Obstet Gynecol Reprod Biol 1987;26:265–70.
8. Hughes JM, Barron WM, Vance ML. Recurrent diabetes insipidus associated with pregnancy: pathophysiology and therapy. Obstet Gynecol 1989;73:462–4.
9. Goolsby L, Harlass F. Central diabetes insipidus: a complication of ventriculoperitoneal shunt malfunction during pregnancy. Am J Obstet Gynecol 1996;174:1655–7.
10. Stubbe E. Pregnancies in diabetes insipidus. Geburtsh und Frauenheilk 1994;54:111–3.
11. Ray JG. DDAVP use during pregnancy: an analysis of its safety for mother and child. Obstet Gynecol Surv 1998;53:450–5.
12. Swanbeck J, Baxi L, Hurlet AM. DDAVP in the management of Von Willebrand's disease in pregnancy (abstract). Am J Obstet Gynecol 1992;166:427.
13. Robinson KW, Hawker RW, Robertson PA. Antidiuretic hormone (ADH) in the human female. J Clin Endocrinol Metab 1957;17:320–2.
14. Oravec D, Lichardus B. Management of diabetes insipidus in pregnancy. Br Med J 1972;4:114–5.
15. Gaffney PR, Jenkins DM. Vasopressin: mediator of the clinical signs of fetal distress. Br J Obstet Gynaecol 1983;90:987.
16. Kallen BA, Carlsson SS, Bengtsson BKA. Diabetes insipidus and use of desmopressin (Minirin) during pregnancy. Eur J Endocrinol 1995;132:144–6.
17. Hanson RS, Powrie RO, Larson L. Diabetes insipidus in pregnancy: a treatable cause of oligohydramnios. Obstet Gynecol 1997;89:816–7.

VECURONIUM

Autonomic (Skeletal Muscle Relaxant)

PREGNANCY RECOMMENDATION: Limited Human Data—No Relevant Animal Data
BREASTFEEDING RECOMMENDATION: No Human Data—Probably Compatible

PREGNANCY SUMMARY

Vecuronium has been used as an adjunct to general anesthesia during gamete intrafallopian transfer (GIFT) procedures and cesarean sections. It has also been used in the 2nd and 3rd trimesters by direct IV and IM fetal dosing to produce paralysis during various procedures. No adverse effects attributable to vecuronium on pregnancy rates, the fetus, or the newborn have been reported in these studies. Small amounts of vecuronium cross the placenta, even though this transfer is inhibited by the drug's low lipid solubility and ionization at physiologic pH. Animal reproduction studies have not been conducted with vecuronium, and no studies, animal or human, have reported its use during organogenesis. Based on this lack of information, the embryo risk from exposure to vecuronium during organogenesis cannot be determined. Use in later times of gestation, however, appears to carry little, if any, risk to the fetus or newborn.

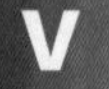

FETAL RISK SUMMARY

The muscle relaxant vecuronium bromide is a nondepolarizing neuromuscular blocking agent that acts by competing for cholinergic receptors at the motor end plate (1). This quaternary ammonium compound belongs to the same general subclass (aminosteroidal) of neuromuscular blockers as pancuronium, pipecuronium, rapacuronium, and rocuronium (2). Vecuronium is indicated as an adjunct to general anesthesia, to facilitate endotracheal intubation, and to provide skeletal muscle relaxation during surgery or mechanical ventilation (1). Reproduction studies of vecuronium in experimental animals have not been located.

The pharmacokinetics of vecuronium in pregnancy was summarized in a 1998 review (3). At term, the elimination half-life of a 0.04 mg/kg dose was 36 minutes, approximately twice as long as atracurium but half the time of pancuronium (3).

The molecular weight (about 638) suggests that vecuronium will cross the placenta, but the ionization and low lipid solubility should limit the exposure of the embryo and fetus. Small amounts of vecuronium do cross the human placenta at term (4–8). In 20 women undergoing general anesthesia for cesarean section, vecuronium (60–80 mcg/kg) was administered between 5 and 21 minutes before delivery (4). The venous cord:maternal ratio averaged 0.11. No neonatal adverse effect was noted as evidenced by normal 1- and 5-minute Apgar scores (4). Others have reported an identical (0.11) umbilical vein:maternal vein ratio (5,6). In these studies, the mean vecuronium-to-delivery interval was 6–7 minutes. No adverse effects on the newborns were observed, as noted by the Apgar scores at 1 and 5 minutes, and the Neurologic and Adaptive Capacity Scores (NACS) determined at 15 minutes, 2, and 24 hours after birth (6).

A 1990 report described the use of vecuronium in 21 patients who were delivered at 36–41 weeks' gestation by elective cesarean section (7). In one group, 11 women received a 0.01 mg/kg IV priming dose, followed 4–6 minutes later by a 0.1 mg/kg IV dose. The second group of 10 women received a single IV dose of 0.2 mg/kg. The mean induction to delivery time intervals in the two groups was 9 and 11 minutes, respectively. The mean umbilical (UV) and maternal (MV) venous plasma concentrations of vecuronium in group 1 were 73 and 515 ng/mL, respectively, a UV/MV ratio of 0.14, whereas in group 2 the values were 107 and 838 ng/mL, respectively, a ratio of 0.13. The mean birth weights in the two groups were 3443 and 3405 g, respectively. The percentage of newborns having Apgar scores <7 in groups 1 and 2 at 1 minute were 70% and 50%, respectively, and at 5 minutes 100% and 90%, respectively. There were no significant differences between the two groups in the 1- and 24-hour NACS, or in individual tests of passive and active tone within the overall NACS profile. However, the data suggested that vecuronium caused residual effects in the infants (7). A number of other reports have discussed the safe use of vecuronium during cesarean section (8–12).

In a 1999 report, investigators concluded that a more accurate estimation of vecuronium placental transfer during cesarean section would be shown by the ratio of umbilical vein (UV) to maternal artery (MA) concentrations (13). Following an intubation dose of 0.11 mg/kg, the mean UV/MA ratio was 0.056 at an intubation-to-umbilical-cord clamping (I-D) interval of 280 seconds. As expected, the ratio decreased as the I-D interval shortened.

Vecuronium (1–10 mg) has been used as an adjunct to general anesthesia in GIFT procedures (14). No effect on the pregnancy rate following GIFT was noted.

In a 1983 study, 19 newborns of mothers who had received vecuronium before delivery by cesarean section were compared with 9 newborns whose mothers had not received the agent (15). No significant difference in the Apgar scores at 1 and 5 minutes were observed between the two groups. In addition, vecuronium had no effect on maternal plasma cholinesterase activity (15).

A 1988 case study described the direct fetal administration of vecuronium under ultrasound guidance for fetal magnetic resonance imaging at 33 weeks' gestation of a brain defect (16). The dose used was 0.2 mg (0.1 mg/kg). A 3540-g male infant was delivered at 39 weeks' with Apgar scores of 10 and 10 at 1 and 5 minutes, respectively. Examination at 9 days of age confirmed the defect (16).

The successful anesthetic management of a woman at 32 weeks' gestation with dextrocardia, situs inversus, a double-outlet right ventricle, ventricular septal defect, and severe pulmonary stenosis was described in a 1994 report (17). No adverse effects attributable to vecuronium (0.1 mg/kg) were observed in the growth-restricted (0.94 kg) infant, who was doing well at 2 weeks of age. Vecuronium (10 mg) was used to assist mechanical ventilation in another case involving a woman at 36 weeks' gestation in labor who had developed severe respiratory distress secondary to myocardial infarction related to cocaine use (18). The mother also received fentanyl and midazolam. Four hours later, the woman delivered a live female infant. Specific information on the infant's condition was not given.

A 1998 case report described respiratory muscle rigidity in a newborn that was attributed to fentanyl (see Fentanyl) (19). In addition to other drugs, the mother had received vecuronium (7 mg) at 31 weeks' gestation.

Vecuronium was used to paralyze 14 fetuses during 17 intrauterine intravascular exchange transfusions (20). The mean gestational age was 29.2 weeks (range 22–35 weeks) and the mean estimated fetal weight was 1610 g (range 500–2500 g). The dose used (0.1 mg/kg) resulted in a mean onset of paralysis of 97.6 seconds (range 45–150 seconds) with a mean duration, as determined by maternal perception of fetal movements, of 122 minutes. The duration of paralysis was not correlated with gestational age. No maternal or fetal adverse effects were noted. All fetuses were delivered alive at a mean 35.8 weeks' gestation (20). In another 1992 report, vecuronium (0.15 mg/kg IV or IM) was used in nine intrauterine procedures involving five fetuses (21). The authors noted that whereas vecuronium caused no fetal heart rate changes, pancuronium caused increased fetal heart rates and decreased beat-to-beat variability for 2.5 hours postdose.

Two pregnant women undergoing general anesthesia for cesarean section developed difficulty with breathing after receiving IV priming doses of vecuronium (10 and 13.7 mcg/kg) (22). Rapid sequence induction was initiated and healthy infants with normal Apgar scores were delivered.

BREASTFEEDING SUMMARY

No reports describing the use of vecuronium during lactation have been located. However, even if such use was reported, it is doubtful if clinically significant amounts of vecuronium would be excreted into breast milk. The molecular weight (about 638) is low enough, but the low lipid solubility and ionization at physiologic pH would inhibit its excretion into milk. These factors suggest that vecuronium represents no risk to a breastfeeding infant.

References

1. Product information. Norcuron. Organon, 2002.
2. Muscle relaxants. In: Parfitt K, ed. *Martindale*. 32nd ed. London: Pharmaceutical Press, 1999:1302.
3. Guay J, Grenier Y, Varin F. Clinical pharmacokinetics of neuromuscular relaxants in pregnancy. Clin Pharmacokinet 1998;483–96.
4. Demetriou M, Depoix JP, Diakite B, Fromentin M, Duvaldestin P. Placental transfer of ORG NC45 in women undergoing caesarean section. Br J Anaesth 1982;54:643–5.
5. Dailey PA, Fisher DM, Shnider SM, Baysinger CL, Shinohara Y, Miller RD, Abboud TK, Kim KC. Pharmacokinetics, placental transfer, and neonatal effects of vecuronium (ORG NC45) administered prior to delivery (abstract). Anesthesiology 1982;57:A391.
6. Dailey PA, Fisher DM, Shnider SM, Baysinger CL, Shinohara Y, Miller RD, Abboud TK, Kim KC. Pharmacokinetics, placental transfer, and neonatal effects of vecuronium and pancuronium administered during Cesarean section. Anesthesiology 1984;60:569–74.
7. Hawkins JL, Johnson TD, Kubicek MA, Skjonsby BS, Morrow DH, Joyce TH III. Vecuronium for rapid-sequence intubation for Cesarean section. Anesth Analg 1990;71:185–90.
8. Baraka A, Jabbour S, Tabboush Z, Sibai A, Bijjani A, Karam K. Onset of vecuronium neuromuscular block is more rapid in patients undergoing caesarean section. Can J Anaesth 1992;39:135–8.
9. Teviotdale BM. Vecuronium-thiopentone induction for emergency caesarean section under general anaesthesia. Anaesth Intensive Care 1993;21:288–91.
10. Brimacombe J, Berry A. Vecuronium for emergency caesarean section. Anaesth Intens Care 1994;22:119.
11. Teviotdate B. Vecuronium for emergency caesarean section. Reply. Anaesth Intens Care 1994;22:119–20.
12. Das S, Bhattacharjee M, Maitra S. Study of neonatal status after use of vecuronium as a muscle relaxant in caesarean section. J Indian Med Assoc 1993;91:54–6.
13. Iwama H, Kaneko T, Tobishima S, Komatsu T, Watanabe K, Akutsu H. Time dependency of the ratio of umbilical vein/maternal artery concentrations of vecuronium in Caesarean section. Acta Anaesthesiol Scand 1999; 43:9–12.
14. Pierce ET, Smalky M, Alper MM, Hunter JA, Amrhein RL, Pierce EC Jr. Comparison of pregnancy rates following gamete intrafallopian transfer (GIFT) under general anesthesia with thiopental sodium or propofol. J Clin Anesth 1992;4:394–8.
15. Baraka A, Noueihed R, Sinno H, Wakid N, Agoston S. Succinylcholine-vecuronium (ORG NC 45) sequence for Cesarean section. Anesth Analg 1983;62:909–13.
16. Daffos F, Forestier F, MacAleese J, Aufrant C, Mandelbrot L, Cabanis EA, Iba-Zizen MT, Alfonso JM, Tamraz J. Fetal curarization for prenatal magnetic resonance imaging. Prenat Diagn 1988;8:312–4.
17. Rowbottom SJ, Gin T, Cheung LP. General anaesthesia for Caesarean section in a patient with uncorrected complex cyanotic heart disease. Anaesth Intens Care 1994;22:74–8.
18. Liu SS, Forrester RM, Murphy GS, Chen K, Glassenberg R. Anaesthetic management of a parturient with myocardial infarction related to cocaine use. Can J Anaesth 1992;39:858–61.
19. Lindemann R. Respiratory muscle rigidity in a preterm infant after use of fentanyl during Caesarean section. Eur J Pediatr 1998;157:1012–3.
20. Leveque C, Murat I, Toubas F, Poissonnier MH, Brossard Y, Saint-Maurice C. Fetal neuromuscular blockade with vecuronium bromide: studies during intravascular intrauterine transfusion in isoimmunized pregnancies. Anesthesiology 1992;76:642–4.
21. Watson WJ, Atchison SR, Harlass FE. Comparison of pancuronium and vecuronium for fetal neuromuscular blockade during invasive procedures. J Matern Fetal Med 1996;5:151–4.
22. Cherala S, Eddie D, Halpern M, Shevdi K. Priming with vecuronium in obstetrics. Anaesthesia 1987;42:1021.

VELAGLUCERASE ALFA

Endocrine/Metabolic Agent (Gaucher Disease)

PREGNANCY RECOMMENDATION: No Human Data—Probably Compatible
BREASTFEEDING RECOMMENDATION: No Human Data—Probably Compatible

PREGNANCY SUMMARY

No reports of human pregnancy exposure to velaglucerase alfa have been located. Animal studies have not suggested risk. Limited information is available on pregnancies complicated by type I Gaucher disease and treated with similar enzyme-replacement therapies, alglucerase or imiglucerase, and these data have not suggested fetal risk. Pregnancy may exacerbate existing disease or result in new disease manifestations, but the limited human data for alglucerase and imiglucerase suggest that treatment during pregnancy may reduce risks for spontaneous abortion and bleeding complications.

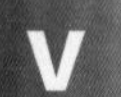

FETAL RISK SUMMARY

Velaglucerase alfa, an enzyme given by IV infusion, is used in the treatment of patients with type I Gaucher disease. Velaglucerase alfa replaces the endogenous enzyme β-glucocerebrosidase with a product produced by gene activation technology in a human cell line. The enzyme has the same amino acid sequence as the naturally occurring human enzyme. After infusion, the terminal elimination half-life ranges between 5 and 12 minutes (1).

Developmental and reproductive toxicology studies have been conducted in rats and rabbits at doses of 17 and 20 mg/kg, respectively. It is unclear how these compare with recommended human doses but they appear to be substantially higher than the maximum recommended human dose of 60 U/kg on a mg/kg basis. No maternal or developmental treatment-related effects were demonstrated in either species (1).

The carcinogenic and mutagenic potential of velaglucerase alfa has not been studied. Reproductive toxicity studies in male and female rats revealed no evidence of impaired fertility (1).

It is not known if velaglucerase alfa crosses the human placenta. The high molecular weight (about 63,000) and the short terminal half-life suggest that placental transfer may be limited.

Outcomes of exposed pregnancies treated with other similar enzyme therapies, alglucerase or imiglucerase, have been summarized from surveys gathered from international treatment centers, from reports in the literature, and the manufacturer's pharmacovigilance database (see Alglucerase and Imiglucerase) (2,3).

BREASTFEEDING SUMMARY

No reports of velaglucerase alfa in human lactation have been located. The high molecular weight (about 63,000) and the short terminal half-life suggest that excretion into milk will be limited. Moreover, the glycoprotein probably is destroyed in the digestive tract and even if small amounts are transferred into breast milk, the enzyme is unlikely to reach the systemic circulation of a breastfed infant.

References

1. Product information. VPRIV, Shire, 2010.
2. Zimran A, Morris E, Mengel E, Kaplan P, Belmatoug N, Hughes DA, Malinova V, Heitner R, Sobreira E, Mrsic M, Granovsky-Frisaru S, Amato D, vom Dahl S. The female Gaucher patient: the impact of enzyme replacement therapy around key reproductive events (menstruation, pregnancy and menopause). Blood Cells Mol Dis 2009;43:264–88.
3. Granovsky-Grisaru S, Belmatoug N, vom Dahl S, Mengel E, Morris E, Zimran A. The management of pregnancy in Gaucher disease. Eur J Obstet Gynecol Reprod Biol 2011;156:3–8.

VEMURAFENIB

Antineoplastic (Kinase Inhibitor)

PREGNANCY RECOMMENDATION: Contraindicated
BREASTFEEDING RECOMMENDATION: Contraindicated

PREGNANCY SUMMARY

Only one report describing the use of vemurafenib in human pregnancy has been located. The fetus had growth restriction, but the reduced growth had began a week before treatment was started. Although the drug crossed the placenta, the infant eventually did well. The animal data suggest low risk, but the exposures were around the clinical exposure. Higher doses may have not been possible because of maternal toxicity. Because of the drug's mechanism of action, the manufacturer states that it may cause fetal harm (1). If the drug is used in pregnancy, the patient should be informed of the potential risk to the fetus.

FETAL RISK SUMMARY

Vemurafenib is an inhibitor of some mutated forms of BRAF serine-threonine kinase and other kinases that are given orally. It is indicated for the treatment of patients with unresectable or metastatic melanoma with BRAFV600E mutation as detected by an FDA-approved test. Metabolism is very limited. Following a single oral dose, mean data from plasma samples analyzed over a 48-hour period found that vemurafenib and its metabolites represented 95% and 5%, respectively, of the components in plasma. Vemurafenib is highly (>99%) bound to plasma albumin and α_1-acid-glycoprotein. The median elimination half-life is about 57 hours (range about 30–120 hours) (1).

Animal reproduction studies have been conducted in rats and rabbits. In these species, no evidence of teratogenicity was observed at doses resulting in exposures up to about 1.3 and 0.6 times, respectively, the human clinical exposure based on AUC (HCE). Fetal levels of vemurafenib were 3%–5% of the maternal levels (1).

The carcinogenic potential of vemurafenib has not been studied. However, the drug increased the development of cutaneous squamous cell carcinomas in patients in clinical trials. Various assays for genetic damage were negative. Although vemurafenib-induced impairment of fertility in animals has not been studied, no histopathological findings were observed in the reproductive organs of male and female rats and dogs during repeat-dose toxicological studies (1).

Vemurafenib crosses the human placenta. In the report below, infant levels were about 45% of the maternal concentration at birth. The molecular weight (about 490), minimal metabolism, and long elimination half-life are consistent with this report, but the high plasma protein binding might have limited the exposure.

A 2013 case report described the use of vemurafenib in a pregnant woman with malignant melanoma (2). After corticosteroids for fetal lung maturity, the standard dose of 960 mg twice daily was started at 25 weeks' gestation. The patient rapidly responded to the treatment with a decrease in pain and new metastasis disappeared. Fetal growth restriction (of the body, not the head) that had started a week before initiation of vemurafenib continued and a cesarean section was performed in the 30th week of gestation. Blood concentrations of vemurafenib at birth in the mother, umbilical cord, and 1028-g infant were 24.3, 10.9, and 10.9 mcg/mL, respectively. The infant had uncomplicated stay in the neonatal ward and was eventually discharged home in good condition. The mother died 3.5 months after initiation of vemurafenib therapy (2).

BREASTFEEDING SUMMARY

No reports describing the use of vemurafenib during human lactation have been located. The molecular weight (about 490), minimal metabolism, and long elimination half-life suggest that the drug will be excreted into breast milk, but the high plasma protein binding might limit the exposure. The effect of this exposure on a nursing infant is unknown. The most common adverse reactions in adults (≥30%) treated with the drug are arthralgia, rash, alopecia, fatigue, photosensitivity reaction, nausea, pruritus, and skin papilloma (1). Moreover, there was a 24% incidence of cutaneous squamous cell carcinoma in clinical trials (1). Thus, there is potential risk to a nursing infant and, if the mother requires the drug, the best course would be to not breastfeed.

References

1. Product information. Zelboraf. Genentech, 2011.
2. Maleka A, Enblad G, Sjörs G, Lindqvist A, Ullenhag GJ. Treatment of metastatic malignant melanoma with vemurafenib during pregnancy. J Clin Oncol 2013;31:e192–3.

VENLAFAXINE

Antidepressant

PREGNANCY RECOMMENDATION: Human Data Suggest Risk in 3rd Trimester
BREASTFEEDING RECOMMENDATION: Limited Human Data—Potential Toxicity

PREGNANCY SUMMARY

Neither the animal reproduction data nor the human pregnancy experience suggests that venlafaxine is a major risk for structural anomalies. However, venlafaxine, as well as selective serotonin reuptake inhibitors (SSRIs), have been associated with developmental toxicity, including spontaneous abortions (SABs), low birth weight, prematurity, neonatal serotonin syndrome, neonatal behavioral syndrome (withdrawal including seizures), possibly sustained abnormal neurobehavior beyond the neonatal period, and respiratory distress. Persistent pulmonary hypertension of the newborn (PPHN) is an additional potential risk, but confirmation is needed.

FETAL RISK SUMMARY

Venlafaxine is an antidepressant structurally unrelated to other available antidepressants. It is in the same serotonin-norepinephrine reuptake inhibitors (SNRIs) antidepressant subclass as desvenlafaxine, duloxetine, and milnacipran. Venlafaxine is indicated for the treatment of major depressive disorder. Venlafaxine is metabolized to an active metabolite, O-desmethylvenlafaxine (ODV). Oral venlafaxine is well absorbed (at least 92%). Plasma protein binding of venlafaxine and ODV are minimal (27% and 30%, respectively), but the elimination half-lives are 5 and 11 hours, respectively (1).

Reproduction studies in rats and rabbits at doses ≤2.5 and 4 times the maximum recommended human daily dose based on BSA (MRHD), respectively, did not reveal teratogenicity (1). When rats were given the same maximum dose during pregnancy through weaning, however, there was a decrease in pup weight and an increased number of stillbirths and pup deaths during the first 5 days of lactation. The no-effect dose for pup mortality was 0.25 times the MRHD (1).

Both venlafaxine and ODV cross the human placenta (2). In 11 women taking a median 225 mg/day (range 150–300 mg/day), the cord blood concentrations at birth of venlafaxine and ODV were 20 mcg/L (9–53 mcg/L) and 184 mcg/L (123–348 mcg/L), respectively. These results are consistent with the molecular weight of venlafaxine (about 314), the minimal protein binding, and the moderately long elimination half-lives. The median cord:maternal ratio for the parent drug and metabolite were 0.72 and 1.08, respectively (2).

A 1994 review of venlafaxine included citations of data from the clinical trials of this drug involving its use during gestation in 10 women for periods ranging from 10 to 60 days (3), apparently during the 1st trimester. No adverse effects of the exposure were observed in four of the infants (information not provided for the other six exposed pregnancies).

In a 2001 prospective controlled study, the pregnancy outcomes of 150 women exposed to venlafaxine were compared with those of 150 women exposed to other SSRI antidepressants and 150 women exposed to nonteratogenic agents (4). There were no significant differences in the outcomes in the three groups in terms of SABs, elective abortions, gestational age at birth, live births, birth weights, and major malformations. In the cases exposed to venlafaxine, there were two infants with birth defects (hypospadias; neural tube defect and clubfoot). In the control groups, there were three defects in the other-SSRI group (ventricular septal defect; pyloric stenosis; and absent corpus callosum) and one in the nonteratogen group (congenital heart defect). The results suggested that venlafaxine does not increase the rates of major congenital defects over that expected in a nonexposed population (4).

A 2010 review evaluated 15 prospective studies involving antidepressants that had been published in 1975–2009 to determine if there was an association between specific agents and SABs (5). Most of the studies involved tricyclic antidepressants or SSRIs. After adjustment, only paroxetine (odds ratio [OR] 1.7, 95% confidence interval [CI] 1.3–2.3) and venlafaxine (OR 2.1, 95% CI 1.3–3.3) were significantly associated with the risk of SABs (5).

The use of venlafaxine late in the 3rd trimester may result in functional and behavioral deficits in the newborn infant. The product information was changed by the manufacturer in 2004 to reflect this potential developmental toxicity (1).

The observed toxicities include respiratory distress, cyanosis, apnea, seizures, temperature instability, feeding difficulty, vomiting, hypoglycemia, hypotonia, hypertonia, hyperreflexia, tremor, jitteriness, irritability, and constant crying. The clinical features are consistent with either a direct toxic effect or drug discontinuation syndrome and, occasionally, may resemble a serotonin syndrome. The complications may require prolonged hospitalization, respiratory support, and tube feeding (1).

Evidence for the neonatal behavioral syndrome that is associated with in utero exposure to SSRIs and SNRIs (collectively called serotonin reuptake inhibitors [SRIs]) in late pregnancy was reviewed in a 2005 reference (6). The report followed a recent agreement by the FDA and manufacturers for a class labeling change about the neonatal syndrome. Analysis of case reports, case series, and cohort studies revealed that late exposure to SRIs carried an overall risk ratio of 3.0 (95% confidence interval [CI] 2.0–4.4) for the syndrome compared with early exposure. The case reports (*N* = 18) and case series (*N* = 131) involved 97 cases of paroxetine, 18 fluoxetine, 16 sertraline, 12 citalopram, 4 venlafaxine, and 2 fluvoxamine. Nine cohort studies were analyzed. The typical neonatal syndrome consisted of central nervous system, motor, respiratory, and gastrointestinal signs that were mild and usually resolved within 2 weeks. Only 1 of 313 quantifiable cases involved a severe syndrome consisting of seizures, dehydration, excessive weight loss, hyperpyrexia, and intubation. There were no neonatal deaths attributable to the syndrome (6).

A 30% incidence of SSRI-induced neonatal abstinence syndrome was found in a 2006 cohort study (7). Sixty neonates with prolonged in utero exposure to SSRIs were compared with nonexposed controls. The agents used were paroxetine (62%), fluoxetine (20%), citalopram (13%), venlafaxine (3%), and sertraline (2%). Assessment was conducted by the Finnegan score. Ten of the infants had mild and eight had severe symptoms of the syndrome. The maximum mean score in infants with severe symptoms occurred within 2 days of birth, but some occurred as long as 4 days after birth. Because of the small numbers, a dose–response analysis could only be conducted with paroxetine (7) (see Paroxetine).

A 2004 report described the pregnancy outcomes of 11 women who had taken venlafaxine (doses 75–225 mg/day) during the 1st trimester (8). One patient also took venlafaxine for 3 weeks in the 2nd trimester, but none of the women were exposed in the second half of pregnancy. The outcomes included two induced abortions and nine healthy infants that were doing well at 12 months of age (8).

In a 2006 case, a 2-day-old infant, exposed throughout pregnancy to venlafaxine (375 mg/day), exhibited signs and symptoms of lethargy, jitteriness, rapid breathing, poor suck, and dehydration. The symptoms in the breastfed infant slowly resolved over 1 week (9).

Another 2006 report described seizures in two infants after in utero exposure to venlafaxine (10). The first newborn, exposed to 150 mg/day, was delivered at 37 weeks' with Apgar scores of 1 and 6 at 1 and 5 minutes, respectively. At 30 minutes, the otherwise normal but depressed infant exhibited lip smacking and extensor limb posturing associated with bradycardia and hypertension. The generalized hypertonia and hyperreflexia was treated with phenobarbital for 2 weeks. The infant started breastfeeding on the day after birth. At 1 year of age, her growth and neurodevelopment were normal. The second infant was born at 39 weeks' with an Apgar score of 9 at 5 minutes. The mother was taking venlafaxine 225 mg/day. Breastfeeding was started but the infant had bilious vomiting and, at 24 hours of age, developed multifocal myoclonic seizures involving all limbs. He was treated with phenobarbital for 5 days. The child was doing well at 1 year of age (10).

A 2007 retrospective cohort study examined the effects of exposure to SSRIs or venlafaxine in the 3rd trimester on 21 premature and 55 term newborns (11). The randomly selected unexposed control group consisted of 90 neonates of mothers not taking antidepressants, psychotropic agents, or benzodiazepines at the time of delivery. There were significantly more premature infants among the subjects (27.6%) than among controls (8.9%), but the groups were not matched. The antidepressants, number of subjects, and daily doses in the exposed group were paroxetine (46; 5–40 mg), fluoxetine (10; 10–40 mg), venlafaxine (9; 74–150 mg), citalopram (6; 10–30 mg), sertraline (3; 125–150 mg), and fluvoxamine (2; 50–150 mg). The behavioral signs that were significantly increased in exposed compared with nonexposed infants were: CNS—abnormal movements, shaking, spasms, agitation, hypotonia, hypertonia, irritability, and insomnia; respiratory system—indrawing, apnea/bradycardia, and tachypnea; and other—vomiting, tachycardia, and jaundice. In exposed infants, CNS (63.2%) and respiratory system (40.8%) signs were most common, appearing during the first day of life and lasting for a median duration of 3 days. All of the exposed premature infants exhibited behavioral signs compared with 69.1% of exposed term infants. The duration of hospitalization was significantly longer in exposed premature compared with nonexposed premature infants, 14.5 days vs. 3.7 days, respectively. In 75% of the term and premature infants, the signs resolved within 3 and 5 days, respectively. There were six infants in each group with congenital malformations, but the drugs involved were not specified (11).

A 2007 review conducted a literature search to determine the risk of major congenital malformations after 1st trimester exposure to SSRIs and SNRIs (12). Fifteen controlled studies were analyzed. The data were adequate to suggest that citalopram, fluoxetine, sertraline, and venlafaxine were not associated with an increased risk of congenital defects. In contrast, the analysis did suggest an increased risk with paroxetine. The data were inadequate to determine the risk for the other SSRIs and SNRIs (12).

A case–control study, published in 2006, found that exposure to SSRIs in late pregnancy was associated with PPHN (13) (see Paroxetine or other SSRIs). Although exposure to venlafaxine (number of exposures not specified) was correctly classified as a non-SSRI antidepressant, the action of venlafaxine is similar enough to the SSRIs that it might cause the same effect (see references 1 and 6).

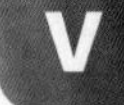

Using data from the Swedish Medical Birth Registry, 732 women who had used SNRIs or noradrenergic reuptake inhibitors during gestation were identified (14). Venlafaxine was the only antidepressant used in 501 pregnancies (505 infants), whereas 12 other pregnancies (12 infants) were exposed to a combination of venlafaxine plus another antidepressant (mianserin, mirtazapine, or reboxetine). Although there was no increased risk of structural anomalies, the rate of preterm births was significantly increased (OR 1.6, CI 1.19–2.15). Compared with exposure to SSRIs during gestation, a similar pattern of neonatal symptoms was observed that included respiratory problems, low Apgar scores, hypoglycemia, and neonatal convulsions. The authors concluded that the symptoms in neonates exposed to SNRIs closely resemble those observed in infants exposed to SSRIs (14).

A 2009 prospective observational study examined the neonatal effects of venlafaxine (N = 11) and SSRIs (N = 27) in pregnancy (2). The neurobehavior of the exposed neonates (N = 38) was compared with a nonexposed, matched control group (N = 18) in six areas: habituation, social-interactive, motor, range, regulation, autonomic. Exposed cases had significantly lower scores ($p <0.05$) than controls in habituation, social-interactive, motor, and autonomic functions. However, when the cases were divided into SSRI and venlafaxine groups, only motor (maturity, pull-to-sit, and activity level) and autonomic (tremors and startles) functions were significantly lower than controls. There were no significant differences in neurobehavior between the two antidepressant groups (2).

A prospective cohort study evaluated a large group of pregnancies exposed to antidepressants in the 1st trimester to determine if there was an association with major malformations (15). The patient population came from the Motherisk database and involved 928 cases that met their criteria. The 928 matched (for age, smoking, and alcohol use) controls were pregnancies not exposed to antidepressants or known teratogens. In addition to the 154 venlafaxine cases, the other cases were 113 bupropion, 184 citalopram, 21 escitalopram, 61 fluoxetine, 52 fluvoxamine, 68 mirtazapine, 39 nefazodone, 148 paroxetine, 61 sertraline, and 17 trazodone. In the antidepressant group, there were 24 (2.5%) major defects compared with 25 (2.6%) in controls (OR 0.9, 95% CI 0.5–1.61). There were two major anomalies in the venlafaxine group: hypospadias and a club foot. There were no major defects in the pregnancies exposed to bupropion, escitalopram, or trazodone (15).

BREASTFEEDING SUMMARY

Venlafaxine is excreted into breast milk. A 1998 study measured the excretion of venlafaxine and its active metabolite ODV in the milk of three breastfeeding women (16). The three mothers, started on the antidepressant after delivery, had been taking a stable dose (3.04–8.18 mg/kg/day) for 0.23–5 months. The ages of the infants were 0.37–6 months. The mean milk:plasma (M:P) ratio (in two cases based on AUC and in one on a single point) for the parent drug was 4.14 (range 3.26–5.18), whereas it was 3.06 (range 2.93–3.19) for ODV. The mean infant doses for venlafaxine and ODV were 3.49% and 4.08% of the mother's weight-adjusted dose, respectively. Venlafaxine was not detected in infant's plasma, but the median infant ODV plasma concentration was 100 mcg/L (range 23–225 mcg/L). The mean total infant dose was 7.57% (range 4.74%–9.23%). No adverse effects in the suckling infants were noted. Because of the relatively high infant dose in comparison with other antidepressants, it was recommended that close observation of the infant for short-term adverse effects (e.g., agitation, insomnia, poor feeding, or failure to thrive) was required (16).

A brief 2001 report described two postpartum women who were taking venlafaxine and exclusively breastfeeding their infants (17). One mother had started the drug (75 mg/day) at delivery, whereas the other had taken the antidepressant throughout pregnancy (150 mg/day). At 3–4 weeks of age, maternal and infant samples were drawn 2–3 hours after a dose. The concentrations of parent drug and ODV in the two women were 31 and 148 ng/mL and 38 and 230 ng/mL, respectively. Parent drug was not detected in the infants, but ODV levels were 16 and 21 ng/mL, respectively. No adverse effects were observed in the infants (17).

A 2004 study was conducted in 25 women (nursing 26 infants) to quantify the concentration of the SSRI or SNRI in their breast milk (18). The antidepressants taken by the women were citalopram (nine), paroxetine (six), sertraline (six), fluoxetine (one), and venlafaxine (three). The maternal mean dose of venlafaxine was 131 mg/day (75–225 mg/day). The mean milk concentration was 2314 nmol/L (1012–3203 nmol/L), resulting in a theoretical maximum infant dose that was 5.2% of the mother's weight-adjusted dose. Venlafaxine was detected in the serum of one infant, but the metabolite was detected in the serum of three infants (mean infant serum level 91 nmol/L, range 31–128 nmol/L [sum of parent drug plus metabolite]). There was no evidence of adverse effects in the breastfeeding infants (18).

A 2002 study determined the milk:plasma ratios (M:P) based on AUC and infant doses of venlafaxine and its metabolite desvenlafaxine in six mothers (mean age 34.5 years and weight 84.3 kg) and their seven nursing infants (mean age 7.0 months and weight 7.3 kg) (19). The median venlafaxine dose was 244 mg/day. The mean M:P ratios for the drug and its metabolite were 2.5 (range 2.0–3.2) and 2.7 (range 2.3–3.2), whereas the mean maximum milk concentrations were 1161 and 796 mcg/L. Using an estimated milk production rate of 150 mL/kg/day, the mean infant exposure expressed as a percentage of the weight-adjusted maternal dose was 3.2% (95% confidence interval [CI] 1.7%–4.7%) for venlafaxine and 3.2% (95% CI 1.9%–4.9%) for desvenlafaxine. Venlafaxine was detected in the plasma of one infant (5 mcg/L), whereas desvenlafaxine was detected in four infants (range 3–38 mcg/L). All of the infants were healthy (19).

In a 2009 report, 13 women taking venlafaxine (mean dose 194.3 mg/day) and their nursing infants (mean age about 21 weeks) were studied (20). The highest venlafaxine and desvenlafaxine concentrations in milk occurred 8 hours after maternal ingestion. For combined venlafaxine plus desvenlafaxine, the mean M:P ratio was 2.75, and the theoretical infant dose was 0.208 mg/kg/day. The relative infant dose as a percentage of the mother's weight-adjusted dose was 8.1%. The theoretical and relative infant doses for desvenlafaxine were 1.97 and 2.24 times higher than those for venlafaxine. No adverse effects were observed or reported in the infants (20).

Maternal plasma concentrations of desvenlafaxine and venlafaxine determine the amount of drug excreted into milk. In this regard, a 2009 study appears to have important implications for choosing which agent to use in a lactating woman (21). The study evaluated the effect of cytochrome P450 2D6 extensive metabolizer (EM) or poor metabolizer (PM) status on the pharmacokinetics of single doses of venlafaxine extended release and desvenlafaxine in healthy adults. The maximum plasma concentrations and AUC of desvenlafaxine were statistically similar in the two groups. In contrast, venlafaxine concentrations and AUC were significantly higher in the PM phenotype compared with the EM phenotype, whereas the desvenlafaxine concentrations and AUC were significantly lower in the PM group (21).

The long-term effects on neurobehavior and cognitive development from exposure to SNRIs and SSRIs during a period of rapid CNS development have not been adequately studied. The American Academy of Pediatrics classifies other antidepressants as drugs for which the effect on nursing infants is unknown but may be of concern (22).

References

1. Product information. Effexor. Wyeth Pharmaceuticals, 2006.
2. Rampono J, Simmer K, Ilett KF, Hackett LP, Doherty DA, Elliot R, Kok CH, Coenen A, Forman T. Placental transfer of SSRI and SNRI antidepressants and effects on the neonate. Pharmacopsychiatry 2009;42:95–100.
3. Ellingrod VL, Perry PJ. Venlafaxine: a heterocyclic antidepressant. Am J Hosp Pharm 1994;51:3033–46.
4. Einarson A, Fatoye B, Sarkar M, Voyer-Lavigne S, Brochu J, Chambers C, Mastroiacovo P, Addis A, Matsui D, Schuler L, Einarson TR, Koren G. Pregnancy outcome following gestational exposure to venlafaxine: a multicenter prospective controlled study. Am J Psychiatry 2001;158:1728–30.
5. Broy P, Berard A. Gestational exposure to antidepressants and the risk of spontaneous abortion: a review. Curr Drug Deliv 2010;7:76–92.
6. Moses-Kolko EL, Bogen D, Perel J, Bregar A, Uhl K, Levin B, Wisner KL. Neonatal signs after late in utero exposure to serotonin reuptake inhibitors. Literature review and implications for clinical applications. JAMA 2005;293:2372–83.
7. Levinson-Castiel R, Merlob P, Linder N, Sirota L, Klinger G. Neonatal abstinence syndrome after in utero exposure to selective serotonin reuptake inhibitors in term infants. Arch Pediatr Adoles Med 2006;160:173–6.
8. Yaris F, Kadioglu M, Kesim M, Ulku C, Yaris E, Kalyoncu NI, Unsal M. Newer antidepressants in pregnancy: prospective outcome of a case series. Reprod Toxicol 2004;19:235–8.
9. Koren G, Moretti M, Kapur B. Can venlafaxine in breast milk attenuate the norepinephrine and serotonin reuptake neonatal withdrawal syndrome? J Obstet Gynaecol Can 2006;28:299–302.
10. Pakalapati RK, Bolisetty S, Austin MP, Oei J. Neonatal seizures from in utero venlafaxine exposure. J Paediatr Child Health 2006;42:737–8.
11. Ferreira E, Carceller AM, Agogue C, Martin BZ, St-Andre M, Francoeur D, Berard A. Effects of selective serotonin reuptake inhibitors and venlafaxine during pregnancy in term and preterm neonates. Pediatrics 2007;119:52–9.
12. Bellantuono C, Migliarese G, Gentile S. Serotonin reuptake inhibitors in pregnancy and the risk of major malformations: a systematic review. Hum Psychopharmacol Clin Exp 2007;22:121–8.
13. Chambers CD, Hernandez-Diaz S, Van Marter LJ, Werler MM, Louik C, Jones KL, Mitchell AA. Selective serotonin-reuptake inhibitors and risk of persistent pulmonary hypertension of the newborn. N Engl J Med 2006;354:579–87.
14. Lennestal R, Kallen B. Delivery outcome in relation to maternal use of some recently introduced antidepressants. J Clin Psychopharmacol 2007;27:607–13.
15. Einarson A, Choi J, Einarson TR, Koren G. Incidence of major malformations in infants following antidepressant exposure in pregnancy: results of a large prospective cohort study. Can J Psychiatry 2009;54:242–6.
16. Ilett KF, Hackett LP, Dusci LJ, Roberts MJ, Kristensen JH, Paech M, Groves A, Yapp P. Distribution and excretion of venlafaxine and *O*-desmethylvenlafaxine in human milk. Br J Clin Pharmacol 1998;45:459–62.
17. Hendrick V, Altshuler L, Wertheimer A, Dunn WA. Venlafaxine and breast-feeding. Am J Psychiatry 2001;158:2089–90.
18. Berle JO, Steen VM, Aamo TO, Breilid H, Zahlsen K, Spigset O. Breastfeeding during maternal antidepressant treatment with serotonin reuptake inhibitors: infant exposure, clinical symptoms, and cytochrome P450 genotypes. J Clin Psychiatry 2004;65:1228–34.
19. Ilett KF, Kristensen JH, Hackett LP, Paech M, Kohan R, Rampono J. Distribution of venlafaxine and its O-desmethyl metabolite in human milk and their effects in breastfed infants. Br J Clin Pharmacol 2002;53:17–22.
20. Newport DJ, Ritchie JC, Knight BT, Glover BA, Zach EB, Stowe ZN. Venlafaxine in human breast milk and nursing infant plasma: determination of exposure. J Clin Psychiatry 2009;70:1304–10.
21. Preskorn S, Patroneva A, Silman H, Jiang Q, Isler JA, Burczynski ME, Ahmed S, Paul J, Nichols AI. Comparison of the pharmacokinetics of venlafaxine extended release and desvenlafaxine in extensive and poor cytochrome P450 2D6 metabolizers. J Clin Psychopharmacol 2009;29:39–43.
22. Committee on Drugs, American Academy of Pediatrics. The transfer of drugs and other chemicals into human milk. Pediatrics 2001;108:776–89.

VERAPAMIL

Calcium Channel Blocker

PREGNANCY RECOMMENDATION: Compatible

BREASTFEEDING RECOMMENDATION: Limited Human Data—Probably Compatible

PREGNANCY SUMMARY

Verapamil is a calcium channel inhibitor used as an antiarrhythmic agent. The use of this drug in any stage of pregnancy appears to be low risk.

FETAL RISK SUMMARY

Reproductive studies in rats and rabbits at oral doses up to 60 mg/kg/day (6 times the human oral dose) and 15 mg/kg/day (1.5 times the human oral dose) found no evidence of teratogenicity (1). In rats, however, this dose was embryocidal, and it restricted fetal growth and development, probably because of maternal toxicity (1).

Placental passage of verapamil has been demonstrated in two of six patients given 80 mg orally at term (2). Cord levels were 15.4 and 24.5 ng/mL (17% and 26% of maternal serum) in two newborns delivered at 49 and 109 minutes after verapamil administration, respectively. Verapamil could not be detected in the cord blood of four infants delivered 173–564 minutes after the dose. IV verapamil was administered to patients in labor at a rate of 2 mcg/kg/minute for 60–110 minutes (3). The serum concentrations of the infants averaged 8.5 ng/mL (44% of maternal serum).

A 33-week fetus with a tachycardia of 240–280 beats/minute was treated in utero for 6 weeks with β-acetyldigoxin and verapamil (80 mg 3 times daily) (2). The fetal heart rate returned to normal 5 days after initiation of therapy, but the authors could not determine whether verapamil had produced the beneficial effect. At birth, no signs of cardiac hypertrophy or disturbances in repolarization were observed. Several other reports have described successful in utero treatment of supraventricular tachycardia with verapamil in combination with other agents (4–6). In one case, indirect therapy via the mother with verapamil, digoxin, and procainamide failed to control the fetal arrhythmia and direct fetal digitalization was required (7). In another case, verapamil (120 mg 3 times daily) and digoxin were used successfully to control a fetal supraventricular tachycardia at 32 weeks' gestation (8). At 36 weeks' gestation, after 4 weeks of therapy, ultrasound examination showed complete resolution of both the hydropic changes and polyhydramnios, but the fetus died within 2 days. No autopsy was permitted. The authors speculated that the drug combination may have caused complete heart block (8). Maternal supraventricular tachycardia occurring in the 3rd trimester has been treated with a single 5-mg IV dose of verapamil (9). Other than the single case of fetal death in which the cause is not certain, no adverse fetal or newborn effects attributable to verapamil have been noted in the above reports.

Verapamil was used to lower blood pressure in a woman in labor with severe gestational hypertension (10). A 15-mg dose was given by rapid IV injection followed by an infusion of 185 mg during 6 hours. Fetal heart rate increased from 60 to 110 beats/minute, and a normal infant was delivered without signs or symptoms of toxicity. Tocolysis with verapamil, either alone or in combination with β-mimetics, has also been described (11–13).

In a surveillance study of Michigan Medicaid recipients involving 229,101 completed pregnancies conducted between 1985 and 1992, 76 newborns had been exposed to verapamil during the 1st trimester (F. Rosa, personal communication, FDA, 1993). One (1.3%) major birth defect was observed (three expected), a cardiovascular defect. These data do not support an association between the drug and congenital defects.

A 1995 case report described the pregnancy outcome of a woman treated with two doses of IV verapamil for supraventricular tachycardia at about 30 and 32 weeks' gestation (14). The remainder of the pregnancy was uneventful and an apparently normal infant was delivered (birth details not provided). At 5 days of age, an echocardiogram revealed obstructive biventricular hypertrophic cardiomyopathy. The cause of the defect could not be determined, but it was noted that congenital hypertrophic cardiomyopathy in rat offspring had been associated with high doses of verapamil during gestation (14).

A brief 1993 study reported three women treated for bipolar disorder with verapamil through most of their pregnancies (15). Normal pregnancy outcomes were observed in the women.

A prospective, multicenter cohort study of 78 women (81 outcomes; 3 sets of twins) who had 1st trimester exposure to calcium channel blockers, including 41% to verapamil, was reported in 1996 (16). Compared with controls, no increase in the risk of major congenital malformations was found. Moreover, the manufacturer has reports of patients treated with verapamil during the 1st trimester without production of fetal problems (M.S. Anderson, personal communication, GD Searle & Co., 1981). However, hypotension (systolic and diastolic) has been observed in patients after rapid IV bolus (17), and reduced uterine blood flow with fetal hypoxia is a potential risk.

BREASTFEEDING SUMMARY

Verapamil is excreted into breast milk (18–20). A daily dose of 240 mg produced milk levels that were approximately 23% of maternal serum (18). Serum levels in the infant were 2.1 ng/mL but could not be detected (<1 ng/mL) 38 hours after treatment was stopped. No effects of this exposure were observed in the infant (18). In a second lactating woman, verapamil 80 mg 4 times daily was started 9 days after delivery for recurrent supraventricular tachycardia (19). The infant was not given the mother's milk. Five days later, verapamil milk levels ranged from about 100 to 300 ng/mL, much higher than expected (19).

A mother was treated with 80 mg 3 times daily for 4 weeks before serum and milk samples were obtained for analysis (20). Steady-state concentrations of verapamil and the metabolite, norverapamil, in milk were 25.8 and 8.8 ng/mL, respectively. These values were 60% and 16% of the concentrations in plasma. The investigators estimated that the breastfed child received less than 0.01% of the mother's dose. Neither verapamil nor the metabolite could be detected in the plasma of the child (20).

The American Academy of Pediatrics classifies verapamil as compatible with breastfeeding (21).

References

1. Product information. Calan. G.D. G.D. Searle, 2000.
2. Wolff F, Breuker KH, Schlensker KH, Bolte A. Prenatal diagnosis and therapy of fetal heart rate anomalies: with a contribution on the placental transfer of verapamil. J Perinat Med 1980;8:203–8.
3. Strigl R, Gastroph G, Hege HG, Döring P, Mehring W. Nachweis von Verapamil in Mutterlichen und fetalen Blut des Menschen. Geburtshilfe Frauenheilkd 1980;40:496–9.
4. Lilja H, Karlsson K, Lindecrantz K, Sabel KG. Treatment of intrauterine supraventricular tachycardia with digoxin and verapamil. J Perinat Med 1984;12:151–4.
5. Rey E, Duperron L, Gauthier R, Lemay M, Grignon A, LeLorier J. Transplacental treatment of tachycardia-induced fetal heart failure with verapamil and amiodarone: a case report. Am J Obstet Gynecol 1985;153:311–2.
6. Maxwell DJ, Crawford DC, Curry PVM, Tynan MJ, Allan LD. Obstetric importance, diagnosis, and management of fetal tachycardias. Br Med J 1988;297:107–10.
7. Weiner CP, Thompson MIB. Direct treatment of fetal supraventricular tachycardia after failed transplacental therapy. Am J Obstet Gynecol 1988;158:570–3.
8. Owen J, Colvin EV, Davis RO. Fetal death after successful conversion of fetal supraventricular tachycardia with digoxin and verapamil. Am J Obstet Gynecol 1988;158:1169–70.
9. Klein V, Repke JT. Supraventricular tachycardia in pregnancy: cardioversion with verapamil. Obstet Gynecol 1984;63:16S–8S.
10. Brittinger WD, Schwarzbeck A, Wittenmeier KW, et al. Klinisch Experimentelle Untersuchungen uber die Blutdruckendende Wirkung von Verapamil. Dtsch Med Wochenschr 1970;95:1871–7.
11. Mosler KH, Rosenboom HG. Neuere Moglichkeiten einer tokolytischen Behandlung in de Geburtschilfe. Z Geburtshilfe Perinatol 1972;176: 85–96.
12. Gummerus M. Prevention of premature birth with nylidrin and verapamil. Z Geburtshilfe Perinatol 1975;179:261–6.
13. Gummerus M. Treatment of premature labor and antagonization of the side effects of tocolytic therapy with verapamil. Z Geburtshilfe Perinatol 1977;181:334–40.
14. Shen O, Entebi E, Yagel S. Congenital hypertrophic cardiomyopathy associated with in utero verapamil exposure. Prenat Diagn 1995;15: 1088–9.
15. Goodnick PJ. Verapamil prophylaxis in pregnant women with bipolar disorder. Am J Psychiatry 1993;150:1560.

16. Magee LA, Schick B, Donnenfeld AE, Sage SR, Conover B, Cook L, McElhatton PR, Schmidt MA, Koren G. The safety of calcium channel blockers in human pregnancy: a prospective, multicenter cohort study. Am J Obstet Gynecol 1996;174:823–8.
17. Rotmensch HH, Rotmensch S, Elkayam U. Management of cardiac arrhythmias during pregnancy: current concepts. Drugs 1987;33:623–33.
18. Andersen HJ. Excretion of verapamil in human milk. Eur J Clin Pharmacol 1983;25:279–80.
19. Inoue H, Unno N, Ou MC, Iwama Y, Sugimoto T. Level of verapamil in human milk. Eur J Clin Pharmacol 1984;26:657–8.
20. Anderson P, Bondesson U, Mattiasson I, Johansson BW. Verapamil and norverapamil in plasma and breast milk during breast feeding. Eur J Clin Pharmacol 1987;31:625–7.
21. Committee on Drugs, American Academy of Pediatrics. The transfer of drugs and other chemicals into human milk. Pediatrics 2001;108: 776–89.

VERTEPORFIN

Ophthalmic Phototherapy

PREGNANCY RECOMMENDATION: Limited Human Data—Animal Data Suggest Low Risk
BREASTFEEDING RECOMMENDATION: Limited Human Data—Potential Toxicity

PREGNANCY SUMMARY

Although the animal reproduction data suggest low risk, the near absence of human pregnancy experience prevents an assessment of the embryo–fetal risk. The human pregnancy experience is limited to three cases. Nevertheless, verteporfin is indicated for severe eye disease that might cause blindness if not treated. Therefore, if a pregnant woman requires verteporfin and she consents, treatment should not be withheld because of her pregnancy. Avoiding the period of organogenesis should be considered.

FETAL RISK SUMMARY

Verteporfin is a light-activated drug used in photodynamic therapy that is given by IV infusion. The drug then is activated in the eye with light from a nonthermal diode laser. Once activated in the presence of oxygen, highly reactive, short-lived singlet oxygen and reactive oxygen radicals are generated. Verteporfin is indicated for the treatment of patients with predominantly classic subfoveal choroidal neovascularization due to age-related macular degeneration, pathologic myopia, or presumed ocular histoplasmosis. Verteporfin undergoes limited metabolism by liver and plasma esterases. Excretion is by the fecal route. The elimination half-life of verteporfin is about 5–6 hours (1).

Reproduction studies have been performed in rats and rabbits. In pregnant rats during organogenesis, a dose resulting in exposures that were about 40 times the human exposure based on AUC (HE-AUC) caused an increased incidence of anophthalmia/microphthalmia in fetuses. At 125 times the HE-AUC, rat fetuses had an increased incidence of wavy ribs and anophthalmia/microphthalmia. In pregnant rabbits, no teratogenic effects were observed with doses that were not maternally toxic (1). Light activation was not mentioned in any of the above studies.

Carcinogenicity studies have not been conducted with verteporfin. Photodynamic therapy as a class has been reported to cause DNA damage that might result in chromosomal aberrations and mutations. It is not known how these effects translate into human risk (1). No effects on fertility were observed in male and female rats with doses that were about ≤60 and ≤40 times the HE-AUC, respectively (1).

It is not known if verteporfin crosses the human placenta. The molecular weight (about 719), limited metabolism, and the elimination half-life suggest that exposure of the embryo–fetus will occur.

A 2004 case report described the administration of verteporfin to a 35-year-old woman in the first week after conception of her first pregnancy (2). After counseling, the woman continued her pregnancy and delivered a healthy 2750-g female infant by cesarean section at 38 weeks' gestation. Apgar scores were 9 and 10 at 1 and 5 minutes, respectively. The child was developing normally at 26 months of age (2).

A brief 2009 report described the use of verteporfin and bevacizumab in a pregnant woman treated for choroidal neovascularization secondary to punctate inner choroidopathy (3). She received photodynamic therapy with IV verteporfin about 1–2 weeks postconception. At 3 months postconception, she underwent intravitreal injection of 1.25 mg bevacizumab. The patient delivered a healthy infant at term with no evidence of congenital anomalies at birth or at 3 months of age (3).

In another 2009 report, a 45-year-old woman with choroidal neovascularization and an unknown pregnancy received fluorescein angiography at 9 weeks and verteporfin at 12 weeks (4). Pregnancy was diagnosed at about 25 weeks. At about 37 weeks, she gave birth spontaneously to a healthy 2410-g female infant without congenital anomalies and with Apgar scores of 9 and 10. The normal infant was doing well at 16 months of age (4).

BREASTFEEDING SUMMARY

Verteporfin and its diacid metabolite are excreted into human breast milk (1). After a 6 mg/m^2 infusion, milk concentrations of the drug were 66% of the corresponding plasma concentration. Verteporfin was undetectable in milk after 12 hours, but the metabolite was measured in milk up to at least 48 hours (1). The excretion into milk is consistent with the molecular weight (about 719), limited metabolism, and elimination half-life (5–6 hours). The effect of this exposure on a nursing infant is unknown, but adverse effects affecting many organ systems are common in adults treated with IV infusions of the drug. Withholding breastfeeding for about 48 hours should lessen the exposure and potential risk of toxicity in the infant.

References

1. Product information. Visudyne. Novartis Pharmaceuticals, 2007.
2. De Santis M, Carducci B, De Santis L, Lucchese A, Straface G. First case of post-conception verteporfin exposure: pregnancy and neonatal outcome. Acta Ophthalmol Scand 2004;82:623–4.
3. Rosen E, Rubowitz A, Ferencz JR. Exposure to verteporfin and bevacizumab therapy for choroidal neovascularization secondary to punctate inner choroidopathy during pregnancy. Eye (Lond) 2009;23:1479.
4. Rodrigues M, Meira D, Batista S, Carrilho MM. Accidental pregnancy exposure to verteporfin: obstetrical and neonatal outcomes: a case report. Aust NZ J Obstet Gynaecol 2009;49:236–7.

VIDARABINE

Antiviral (Ophthalmic)

PREGNANCY RECOMMENDATION: Limited Human Data—Probably Compatible
BREASTFEEDING RECOMMENDATION: No Human Data—Probably Compatible

PREGNANCY SUMMARY

Vidarabine is only available as an ophthalmic ointment. Systemic concentrations do not occur after swallowing lacrimal secretions because the drug is rapidly deaminated in the gastrointestinal tract.

FETAL RISK SUMMARY

Vidarabine is a potent teratogen in mice, rats, and rabbits after topical and IM administration (1,2). Daily instillations of a 10% solution into the vaginas of pregnant rats in late gestation had no effect on the offspring (2).

Vidarabine was used for disseminated herpes simplex in one woman at about 28 weeks' gestation (3,4). Spontaneous rupture of the membranes occurred 48 hours after initiation of therapy, and a premature infant was delivered. The infant died on the 13th day of life of complications of prematurity. In a second case, a woman at 32 weeks' gestation with herpes simplex type II encephalitis was treated with vidarabine (10 mg/kg/day) and acyclovir (5). A female infant with culture-documented herpes neonatorum was delivered by cesarean section 13 days later. The infant responded to further treatment with acyclovir and is alive and well at 2 months of age, but the mother died 2 days after delivery.

Vidarabine, 10 mg/kg/day (800 mg/day), was administered to a woman at 26 weeks' gestation with varicella pneumonitis (6). Peak and trough levels of the agent were 12.8 and 2.7 mcg/mL, respectively. She delivered a healthy female infant at 38 weeks' gestation that is developing normally at 12 months of age. In a similar case, another woman with varicella pneumonitis at 27 weeks' gestation was treated with vidarabine (6). Except for a delay in speech at age 3 years that responded to special education, the child has done well and was considered normal at 5 years of age.

BREASTFEEDING SUMMARY

No reports involving the use of vidarabine in lactating women have been located. The drug is only available as an ophthalmic ointment. Systemic concentrations do not occur after swallowing lacrimal secretions because the drug is rapidly deaminated in the gastrointestinal tract.

References

1. Pavan-Langston D, Buchanan RA, Alford CA Jr, eds. *Adenine Arabinoside: An Antiviral Agent*. New York, NY: Raven Press, 1975:153.
2. Schardein JL, Hertz DL, Petretre JA, Fitzgerald JE, Kurtz SM. The effect of vidarabine on the development of the offspring of rats, rabbits and monkeys. Teratology 1977;15:213–42.
3. Hillard P, Seeds J, Cefalo R. Disseminated herpes simplex in pregnancy: two cases and a review. Obstet Gynecol Surv 1982;37:449–53.
4. Peacock JE Jr, Sarubbi FA. Disseminated herpes simplex virus infection during pregnancy. Obstet Gynecol 1983;61:13S–8S.
5. Berger SA, Weinberg M, Treves T, Sorkin P, Geller E, Yedwab G, Tomer A, Rabey M, Michaeli D. Herpes encephalitis during pregnancy: failure of acyclovir and adenine arabinoside to prevent neonatal herpes. Isr J Med Sci 1986;22:41–4.
6. Landsberger EJ, Hager WD, Grossman JH III. Successful management of varicella pneumonia complicating pregnancy: a report of three cases. J Reprod Med 1986;31:311–4.

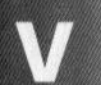

VIGABATRIN

Anticonvulsant

PREGNANCY RECOMMENDATION: Limited Human Data—Animal Data Suggest Risk
BREASTFEEDING RECOMMENDATION: Limited Human Data—Probably Compatible

PREGNANCY SUMMARY

The human pregnancy experience with vigabatrin is limited. Although adverse outcomes have been described, the drug was always combined with first-generation antiepileptic drugs known to cause structural anomalies and other forms of developmental toxicity. The contribution of vigabatrin to this toxicity has not been determined. Because the drug can cause vision loss that may be permanent in a high percentage of patients, it should be reserved for resistant cases. Vision abnormalities were not found in six children exposed in utero who were examined for this toxicity. If a woman becomes pregnant while receiving vigabatrin or is given the drug during pregnancy, she should be informed of the risks of developmental toxicity. Moreover, based on an animal study, women taking the drug during pregnancy should be supplemented with folic acid, as is done with other anticonvulsants.

FETAL RISK SUMMARY

Vigabatrin is an oral anticonvulsant indicated as adjunctive therapy for adult patients with refractory complex partial seizures who have inadequately responded to several alternative treatments and for whom the potential benefits outweigh the risk of vision loss. The drug is a racemate consisting of two enantiomers, one active and one inactive. The drug is hydrophilic, is not significantly metabolized, and does not bind to plasma proteins. The half-life is about 7.5 hours (1).

Reproduction studies have been conducted in rats, rabbits, and mice. In rats given the drug throughout organogenesis, the no-effect dose for embryo–fetal toxicity was about 0.2 times the maximum recommended human dose of 3 g/day based on BSA (MRHD). Higher doses resulted in decreased fetal body weights and increased incidences of fetal anatomic variations. When given from the latter part of pregnancy through weaning, doses that were about ≥0.2 times the MRHD produced long-term neurohistopathologic (hippocampal vacuolation) and neurobehavioral (convulsions) abnormalities in the offspring. A no-effect dose for developmental neurotoxicity was not determined. In rabbits during organogenesis, doses greater than the no-effect dose of about 0.5 times the MRHD were associated with an increased incidence of malformations (oral clefts) and embryo–fetal death (1).

In a study that administered a single intraperitoneal (IP) dose to mice during organogenesis, an increase in malformations (including cleft palate) was observed. Another study gave the drug during the early postnatal period (4–65 days) to young rats which produced neurobehavioral (convulsions, neuromotor impairment, learning deficits) and neurohistopathological (brain vacuolation, decreased myelination, retinal dysplasia) abnormalities. The early postnatal period in rats is thought to correspond to late pregnancy in humans in terms of brain development. The no-effect dose for developmental neurotoxicity in juvenile rats was associated with plasma exposures (AUC) <1/30th of those measured in pediatric patients receiving an oral dose of 50 mg/kg (1).

In a 2001 study, mice were given a single IP dose during organogenesis and amino acid concentrations were measured (2). Compared with controls, methionine concentration was most severely affected in the mother, placenta, and fetus. The authors speculated that methionine deficiency could be a possible teratogenic mechanism (2).

A 2010 study in mice examined the effect of vigabatrin on pregnancy outcomes and maternal plasma folate and vitamin B_{12} concentrations (3). Mice were given a single dose of 450 mg/kg in late gestation. Within 12 hours, maternal levels of the two vitamins were markedly reduced. Fetuses were examined 1–3 days after the dose and found to have a significant incidence of fetal death, abortion, intrauterine growth restriction (IUGR), and skeletal hypoplasia. When mice were given folic acid before vigabatrin, no abortions occurred and the fetuses had better body weight and a lower rate of IUGR. Because the above vigabatrin dose was maternal toxic, the study was repeated with a nonmaternal toxic dose of 350 mg/kg. This dose also caused significant fetal loss and IUGR (3).

Studies for carcinogenesis and mutagenesis were negative. No effects on fertility were observed in male and female rats (1).

Four properties of vigabatrin suggest that it crosses the human placenta, but one suggests that the transfer will be limited. The properties suggesting placental passage are the low molecular weight (about 129), low metabolism, nonbinding by plasma proteins, and moderately long half-life, but the hydrophilic property will inhibit transfer. A 1992 study with human isolated perfused placenta found that the maternal to fetal transfer was low (4). The low transfer was confirmed in a 1998 study in two patients (5). The umbilical vein:maternal plasma concentration ratio was less than 1 for the active enantiomer.

A 1994 report described the outcome of 13 pregnancies treated with anticonvulsants, 1 of which received vigabatrin (3500 mg/day) and carbamazepine (800 mg/day) (*also listed as oxcarbazepine 1500 mg/day in a table*) (6). The newborn male infant had coronal hypospadias, broad depressed nasal bridge, telecanthus, high-arched palate, prominent ear shelves and lobes, upward slanting but apparently small palpebral fissures, diastasis musculus recti abdominis, slightly deep palmar flexion creases, bilateral clinodactyly of fourth toes, and apparently wide internipple distance. The contribution of vigabatrin to any of the defects was unknown. However, in her first pregnancy, the mother had taken carbamazepine and also gave birth to an infant with hypospadias (6).

A 1996 review listed the number of pregnancies, from postmarketing experience, exposed to vigabatrin as >80 (7). The outcomes of these pregnancies, excluding five elective abortions, were spontaneous abortions (SABs) (10%), normal (72%), and abnormal (18%) (specific details not provided). All of the exposures involved polytherapy, and there was no pattern among the malformations (7).

A 1998 noninterventional observational cohort study described the outcomes of pregnancies in women who had been prescribed ≥1 of 34 newly marketed drugs by general practitioners in England (8). Data were obtained by questionnaires sent to the prescribing physicians 1 month after the expected or possible date of delivery. In 831 (78%) of the pregnancies, a newly marketed drug was thought to have been taken during the 1st trimester with birth defects noted in 14 (2.5%) singleton births of the 557 newborns (10 sets of twins). In addition, two birth defects were observed in aborted fetuses. However, few of the aborted fetuses were examined. Vigabatrin was taken during the 1st trimester in 76 pregnancies. The outcomes of these pregnancies included 18 SABs, 11 elective abortions (EABs), and 45 normal newborns (8 premature). Congenital anomalies were observed in two full-term infants: bowed tibiae, increased tone (also exposed to valproate, carbamazepine, and clobazam); occipital plagiocephaly, premature fusion of lambdoid suture, and clicky hips (also exposed to phenytoin and folic acid) (8). The study lacked the sensitivity to identify minor anomalies and late-appearing major defects may have been missed due to the timing of the questionnaires.

Bilateral anophthalmia, situs viscerum inversus, levoisomerism, single ventricle, infundibular stenosis, agenesis of corpus callosum, enlargement of the third ventricle, and bilateral clubfoot in a male infant exposed to vigabatrin was reported in a 1997 abstract (9). The nulliparous 23-year-old woman had severe mental retardation. She took (daily dose) vigabatrin (1000 mg), carbamazepine (800 mg), and dexamethasone (0.75 mg) throughout gestation. The birth weight was 2360 g, length 44 cm, and the karyotype was normal (46,XY). The cause of the defects was unknown, but a genetic defect or multifactorial inheritance could not be excluded (9).

A brief 2003 report described the pregnancy outcome of a 32-year-old woman with a history of epilepsy and a combined liver and renal transplant for primary hyperoxaluria Type 1 (10). She took (daily dose) prednisolone (5 mg), vigabatrin (1000 mg), sodium valproate (2000 mg), and folic acid (5 mg) throughout pregnancy. At 20 weeks' gestation, an ultrasound of the fetus revealed a two-vessel cord and talipes. Labetalol was added at 22 weeks' gestation for hypertension. Because of fetal growth restriction and worsening preeclampsia, a 1280-g female infant was delivered by cesarean section at 34 weeks' gestation. Apgar scores were 5, 6, and 9 at 1, 5, and 10 minutes, respectively. In addition to bilateral talipes, the infant had mild dysmorphic features suggestive of valproate embryopathy (details not provided). At 5 weeks corrected age, poor visual fixation was suspected and a cerebral ultrasound revealed mild ventricular dilatation, but her development was normal at 5.5 months corrected age. The authors speculated that the delayed visual maturation may have been due to vigabatrin (10).

Because vigabatrin-induced visual field defect is an important safety issue with the drug, a 2005 report examined two children who had been exposed during pregnancy (11). In the first case, the mother had taken vigabatrin 1 g/day and carbamazepine until 22 weeks' gestation, at which time the vigabatrin was slowly tapered (total dose during pregnancy 190 g). Examination at 7.75 years of age revealed retrognathia, irregular placement of teeth in the lower jaw, and large prominent ears. However, the boy's visual and ophthalmic examinations were normal. In the second case, the mother had received carbamazepine and valproate until 16 weeks' gestation at which time vigabatrin was added because of resistant seizures (total dose during pregnancy 370 g). The boy had a seizure at 4.67 years of age. At 5 years of age, his psychomotor development was deemed to be slow and he was thought to have mild mental retardation. At 6.83 years of age, multiple major and minor malformations probably due to carbamazepine and valproate were apparent, but no evidence of visual or eye abnormalities was found (11).

In another study, published in 2009, four children from three mothers, two of whom exhibited vigabatrin-attributed visual field loss, had been exposed to vigabatrin in utero (12). The children, ages ranging from about 7 to 16 years, had normal visual fields and retinal nerve fiber layer thickness.

The Lamotrigine Pregnancy Registry, an ongoing project conducted by the manufacturer, was first published in January 1997. The final report was published in July 2010 (13). The Registry is now closed. Among 12 prospectively enrolled pregnancies exposed to vigabatrin and lamotrigine, with or without other anticonvulsants, 11 were exposed in the 1st trimester resulting in 10 live births without defects and 1 EAB. There was one exposure in the 2nd/3rd trimesters resulting in a live birth without defects (13).

BREASTFEEDING SUMMARY

Vigabatrin is excreted into breast milk (5). In two women, 7 days postpartum and both taking vigabatrin (1000 mg twice daily), the predose M:P ratio was <1. The ratio was also <1 in the one woman tested at 3 and 6 hours postdose. The estimated daily maximum doses that a nursing infant would receive as a percentage of the mother's daily weight-adjusted dose was 1% for the active enantiomer and 3.6% for the inactive enantiomer (5). These exposures, if confirmed by other reports, appear to be clinically insignificant (14). However, milk samples may have been obtained before the greatest amount of mature milk production (about 14 days) had been reached.

References

1. Product information. Sabril. Lundbeck, 2009.
2. Abdulrazzaq YM, Padmanabhan R, Bastaki SMA, Ibrahim A, Bener A. Placental transfer of vigabatrin (γ-vinyl GABA) and its effect on concentration of amino acids in the embryo of TO mice. Teratology 2001;63:127–33.
3. Padmanabhan R, Abdulrazzaq YM, Bastaki SMA, Nurulain M, Shafiullah M. Vigabatrin (VGB) administered during late gestation lowers maternal folate concentration and causes pregnancy loss, fetal growth restriction and skeletal hypoplasia in the mouse. Reprod Toxicol 2010;29:366–77.
4. Challier JC, Rey E, Bintein T, Olive G. Passage of S(+) and R(−) γ-vinyl-GABA across the human isolated perfused placenta. Br J Clin Pharmacol 1992;34:139–43.
5. Tran A, O'Mahoney T, Rey E, Mai J, Mumford JP, Olive G. Vigabatrin: placental transfer in vivo and excretion into breast milk of the enantiomers. Br J Clin Pharmacol 1998;45:409–11.
6. Lindhout D, Omtzigt JGC. Teratogenic effects of antiepileptic drugs: implications for the management of epilepsy in women of childbearing age. Epilepsia 1994;35(Suppl4):S19–28.
7. Morrell MJ. The new antiepileptic drugs and women: efficacy, reproductive health, pregnancy, and fetal outcome. Epilepsia 1996;37(Suppl 6):S34–44.
8. Wilton LV, Pearce GL, Martin RM, Mackay FJ, Mann RD. The outcomes of pregnancy in women exposed to newly marketed drugs in general practice in England. Br J Obstet Gynaecol 1998;105:882–9.
9. Calzolari E, Calabrese O, Cocchi G, Gualandi F, Milan M, Morini MS. Anophthalmia and situs viscerum inversus in an infant exposed to vigabatrin. Teratology 1997;56:397.
10. Gosakan R, von Knorring N, Stewart P. Successful pregnancy in a patient with hyperoxaluria and combined liver and renal transplant. J Obstet Gynaecol 2003;23:434–5.
11. Sorri I, Herrgard E, Viinikainen K, Paakkonen A, Heinonen S, Kalviainen R. Ophthalmologic and neurologic findings in two children exposed to vigabatrin in utero. Epilepsy Res 2005;65:117–20.
12. Lawthom C, Smith PEM, Wild JM. In utero exposure to vigabatrin: no indication of visual field loss. Epilepsia 2009;50:318–21.
13. The Lamotrigine Pregnancy Registry. Final Report. September 1, 1992 through March 31, 2010. GlaxoSmithKline, July 2010.
14. Bar-Oz B, Nulman I, Koren G, Ito S. Anticonvulsants and breast feeding—a critical review. Paediatr Drugs 2000;2:113–26.

VILAZODONE

Antidepressant

PREGNANCY RECOMMENDATION: Human Data Suggest Risk in 3rd Trimester
BREASTFEEDING RECOMMENDATION: No Human Data—Potential Toxicity

PREGNANCY SUMMARY

No reports describing the use of vilazodone, a selective serotonin reuptake inhibitor (SSRI), in human pregnancy have been located. Although the animal data suggest low risk, SSRI antidepressants have been associated with developmental toxicities, including spontaneous abortions, low birth weight, preterm delivery, neonatal serotonin syndrome, neonatal behavioral syndrome (withdrawal), possible sustained abnormal neurobehavior beyond the neonatal period, respiratory distress, and persistent pulmonary hypertension of the newborn (PPHN). The risk:benefit ratio for using any SSRI in pregnancy must be determined on a case-by-case basis.

FETAL RISK SUMMARY

In addition to its action as an SSRI antidepressant, vilazodone hydrochloride also is a partial agonist at serotonergic 5-HT_{1A} receptors. It is indicated for the treatment of major depressive disorder. Vilazodone is in the same class of SSRIs as citalopram, escitalopram, fluoxetine, fluvoxamine, paroxetine, and sertraline. Vilazodone is extensively metabolized to inactive metabolites. Plasma protein binding is about 96%–99% and the terminal half-life is about 25 hours (1).

Reproduction studies have been conducted in rats and rabbits. No teratogenic effects were observed in either species at oral doses that were 48 and 17 times, respectively, the maximum recommended human dose of 40 mg based on BSA (MRHD). However, at these doses, fetal body weight gain was reduced and skeletal ossification was delayed in both rats and rabbits. These effects were not observed at doses up to 10 and 4 times, respectively, the MRHD. Some maternal toxicity (*not otherwise specified*) was noted in rats given a dose that was 30 times the MRHD during organogenesis and throughout pregnancy and lactation. Fetal effects observed at this dose included decreased number of live pups and increased early postnatal pup mortality. Among surviving pups there was decreased body weight, delayed maturation, and decreased fertility in adulthood. These effects were not observed at dose 6 times MRHD (1).

Two-year carcinogenicity studies have been conducted in mice and rats. In mice, dose-related hepatocellular carcinomas were observed in males and malignant mammary gland tumors in females. Elevated levels of prolactin also were observed and are known to cause mammary tumors in rodents. No carcinogenic effects were seen in male and female rats. Vilazodone was not mutagenic in various assays. It was clastogenic in some assays but not in others. Dose-related impairment of male fertility was observed in rats but there was no effect on female fertility (1).

It is not known if vilazodone crosses the human placenta. The molecular weight (about 478) and long terminal half-life suggest that the drug will cross to the embryo–fetus. However, the high plasma protein binding may limit the amount of transfer.

BREASTFEEDING SUMMARY

No reports describing the use of vilazodone during human lactation have been located. The molecular weight (about 478) and long terminal half-life (about 25 hours) suggest that the drug will be excreted into breast milk. Although the high plasma protein binding (96%–99%) may limit the amount excreted, vilazodone is a weak base and because the pH of milk is usually lower than that of plasma, milk concentrations may be higher than plasma levels due to "ion trapping."

The effect of exposure to the drug in milk by a nursing infant is unknown. However, excessive somnolence, decreased feeding, and weight loss have been observed in infants exposed to another SSRI (see Citalopram). Thus, nursing infants should be closely monitored for evidence of toxicity. The American Academy of Pediatrics classifies other SSRI antidepressants as drugs for which the effect on nursing infants is unknown but may be of concern (e.g., see Fluoxetine).

A 2010 study using human and animal models found that drugs that disturb serotonin balance such as SSRIs and serotonin norepinephrine reuptake inhibitors (SNRIs) can impair lactation (2). The authors concluded that mothers taking these drugs may need additional support to achieve breastfeeding goals.

References

1. Product information. Viibryd. Forest Pharmaceuticals, 2011.
2. Marshall AM, Nommsen-Rivers LA, Hernandez LI, Dewey KG, Chantry CJ, Gregerson KA, Horseman ND. Serotonin transport and metabolism in the mammary gland modulates secretory activation and involution. J Clin Endocrin Metab 2010;95:837–46.

VINBLASTINE

Antineoplastic

PREGNANCY RECOMMENDATION: Limited Human Data—Animal Data Suggest High Risk
BREASTFEEDING RECOMMENDATION: Contraindicated

PREGNANCY SUMMARY

Vinblastine is an antimitotic antineoplastic agent. Although the drug is embryocidal and teratogenic in laboratory animals (no details provided) (1), the limited human data do not support a significant association with developmental toxicity.

FETAL RISK SUMMARY

Vinblastine has been used in pregnancy, including the 1st trimester, without producing malformations (2–10). However, two cases of malformed infants have been reported following 1st trimester exposure to vinblastine (10,11). In 1974, a case of a 27-year-old woman with Hodgkin's disease who was given vinblastine, mechlorethamine, and procarbazine during the 1st trimester was described (11). At 24 weeks' gestation, she spontaneously aborted a male fetus with oligodactyly of both feet with webbing of the third and fourth toes. These defects were attributed to mechlorethamine therapy. A mother with Hodgkin's disease treated with vinblastine, vincristine, and procarbazine in the 1st trimester (3 weeks after the last menstrual period) delivered a 1900-g male infant at about 37 weeks of gestation (12). The newborn developed fatal respiratory distress syndrome. At autopsy, a small secundum atrial septal defect was found.

Vinblastine in combination with other antineoplastic agents may produce gonadal dysfunction in men and women (13–16). Alkylating agents are the most frequent cause of this problem (15). Although total aspermia may result, return of fertility has apparently been documented in at least two cases (16). Ovarian function may return to normal with successful pregnancies possible, depending on the patient's age at the time of therapy and the total dose of chemotherapy received (14,17). The long-term effects of combination chemotherapy on menstrual and reproductive function were described in a 1988 report (18). Only 5 of 40 women treated for malignant ovarian germ cell tumors received vinblastine. The results of this study are discussed in the monograph for cyclophosphamide (see Cyclophosphamide).

In 436 long-term survivors treated with chemotherapy for gestational trophoblastic tumors between 1958 and 1978, 11 (2.5%) received vinblastine as part of their treatment regimens (19). Of the 11 women, 2 (18%) had at least one live birth (mean and maximum vinblastine dose 20 mg), and 9 (82%) did not try to conceive (mean dose 37 mg, maximum dose 80 mg). Additional details, including congenital anomalies observed, are described in the monograph for vincristine (see Vincristine).

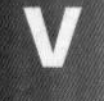

Data from one review indicated that 40% of infants exposed to anticancer drugs were of low birth weight (20). This finding was not related to the timing of exposure. Long-term studies of growth and mental development in offspring exposed to vinblastine during the 2nd trimester, the period of neuroblast multiplication, have not been conducted (21). However, two children, exposed throughout gestation, beginning with the 3rd to 4th week of gestation, were normal at 2 and 5 years of age, respectively (10).

Occupational exposure of the mother to antineoplastic agents during pregnancy may present a risk to the fetus. A position statement from the National Study Commission on Cytotoxic Exposure and a research article involving some antineoplastic agents are presented in the monograph for cyclophosphamide (see Cyclophosphamide).

BREASTFEEDING SUMMARY

No reports describing the use of vinblastine during lactation have been located. Because of the potential for severe toxicity in a nursing infant, women who require this agent should not breastfeed.

References

1. Product information. Velban. Eli Lilly, 2000.
2. Armstrong JG, Dyke RW, Fouts PJ, Jansen CJ. Delivery of a normal infant during the course of oral vinblastine sulfate therapy for Hodgkin's disease. Ann Intern Med 1964;61:106–7.
3. Rosenzweig AI, Crews QE Jr, Hopwood HG. Vinblastine sulfate in Hodgkin's disease in pregnancy. Ann Intern Med 1964;61:108–12.
4. Lacher MJ. Use of vinblastine sulfate to treat Hodgkin's disease during pregnancy. Ann Intern Med 1964;61:113–5.
5. Lacher MJ, Geller W. Cyclophosphamide and vinblastine sulfate in Hodgkin's disease during pregnancy. JAMA 1966;195:192–4.
6. Nordlund JJ, DeVita VT Jr, Carbone PP. Severe vinblastine-induced leukopenia during late pregnancy with delivery of a normal infant. Ann Intern Med 1968;69:581–2.
7. Goguei A. Hodgkin's disease and pregnancy. Nouv Presse Med 1970;78:1507–10.
8. Johnson IR, Filshie GM. Hodgkin's disease diagnosed in pregnancy: case report. Br J Obstet Gynaecol 1977;84:791–2.
9. Nisce LZ, Tome MA, He S, Lee BJ III, Kutcher GJ. Management of coexisting Hodgkin's disease and pregnancy. Am J Clin Oncol 1986;9:146–51.
10. Malone JM, Gershenson DM, Creasy RK, Kavanagh JJ, Silva EG, Stringer CA. Endodermal sinus tumor of the ovary associated with pregnancy. Obstet Gynecol 1986;68(Suppl):86S–9S.
11. Garrett MJ. Teratogenic effects of combination chemotherapy. Ann Intern Med 1974;80:667.
12. Thomas RPM, Peckham MJ. The investigation and management of Hodgkin's disease in the pregnant patient. Cancer 1976;38:1443–51.
13. Morgenfeld MC, Goldberg V, Parisier H, Bugnard SC, Bur GE. Ovarian lesions due to cytostatic agents during the treatment of Hodgkin's disease. Surg Gynecol Obstet 1972;134:826–8.
14. Ross GT. Congenital anomalies among children born of mothers receiving chemotherapy for gestational trophoblastic neoplasms. Cancer 1976;37:1043–7.
15. Schilsky RL, Lewis BJ, Sherins RJ, Young RC. Gonadal dysfunction in patients receiving chemotherapy for cancer. Ann Intern Med 1980;93:109–14.

16. Rubery ED. Return of fertility after curative chemotherapy for disseminated teratoma of testis. Lancet 1983;1:186.
17. Shalet SM, Vaughan Williams CA, Whitehead E. Pregnancy after chemotherapy induced ovarian failure. Br Med J 1985;290:898.
18. Gershenson DM. Menstrual and reproductive function after treatment with combination chemotherapy for malignant ovarian germ cell tumors. J Clin Oncol 1988;6:270–5.
19. Rustin GJS, Booth M, Dent J, Salt S, Rustin F, Bagshawe KD. Pregnancy after cytotoxic chemotherapy for gestational trophoblastic tumours. Br Med J 1984;288:103–6.
20. Nicholson HO. Cytotoxic drugs in pregnancy: review of reported cases. J Obstet Gynaecol Br Commonw 1968;75:307–12.
21. Dobbing J. Pregnancy and leukaemia. Lancet 1977;1:1155.

VINCRISTINE

Antineoplastic

PREGNANCY RECOMMENDATION: Limited Human Data—Animal Data Suggest High Risk
BREASTFEEDING RECOMMENDATION: Contraindicated

PREGNANCY SUMMARY

Vincristine is an antimitotic antineoplastic agent. The drug is embryocidal and teratogenic in mice, hamsters, and monkeys at doses that did not cause maternal toxicity (1). The use of vincristine, always in combination with other antineoplastics, has been described in at least 36 pregnancies (1 with twins), 9 during the 1st trimester (2–31). Developmental toxicity was observed in some of these pregnancies, but the relationship to vincristine is unknown. (*See Rituximab for additional data.*)

FETAL RISK SUMMARY

A mother with Hodgkin's disease treated with vincristine, vinblastine, and procarbazine in the 1st trimester (3 weeks after the last menstrual period) delivered a 1900-g male infant at about 37 weeks' gestation (10). Neonatal death occurred because of respiratory distress syndrome. At autopsy, a small secundum atrial septal defect was found. In a patient with Hodgkin's disease who was treated with vincristine, mechlorethamine, and procarbazine during the 1st trimester, the electively aborted fetus had malformed kidneys (markedly reduced size and malpositioned) (16). Other adverse fetal outcomes observed following vincristine use include a 1000-g male infant born with pancytopenia who was exposed to six different antineoplastic agents in the 3rd trimester (2) and transient severe bone marrow hypoplasia in another newborn that was most likely caused by mercaptopurine (19). Intrauterine fetal death occurred in a 1200-g female fetus 36 hours after maternal treatment with vincristine, doxorubicin, and prednisone for diffuse, undifferentiated lymphoma of T-cell origin at 31 weeks' gestation (22). The fetus was macerated, but no other abnormalities were observed at autopsy. In another case, a 34-year-old woman with acute lymphoblastic leukemia was treated with multiple antineoplastic agents from 22 weeks' gestation until delivery of a healthy female infant 18 weeks later (25). Vincristine was administered 4 times between 22 and 25 weeks' gestation. Chromosomal analysis of the newborn revealed a normal karyotype (46,XX) but with gaps and a ring chromosome. The clinical significance of these findings is unknown, but because these abnormalities may persist for several years, the potential existed for an increased risk of cancer, as well as for a risk of genetic damage in the next generation (25).

A 1999 report from France described the outcomes of pregnancies in 20 women with breast cancer who were treated with antineoplastic agents (31). The first cycle of chemotherapy occurred at a mean gestational age of 26 weeks with delivery occurring at a mean 34.7 weeks. A total of 38 cycles were administered during pregnancy with a median of two cycles per woman. None of the women received radiation therapy during pregnancy. The pregnancy outcomes included two spontaneous abortions (SABs) (both exposed in the 1st trimester), one intrauterine death (exposed in the 2nd trimester), and 17 live births, one of whom died at 8 days of age without apparent cause. The 16 surviving children were developing normally at a mean follow-up of 42.3 months (31). Vincristine (V), in combination with doxorubicin (D), epirubicin (E), and/or methotrexate (M), was administered to two women at a mean dose of 2 mg/m^2. The outcomes were one SAB (VEM; exposed at 6 weeks' gestation) and one surviving liveborn infant (exposed to VD in the 2nd trimester) (31).

Data from one review indicated that 40% of the infants exposed to anticancer drugs were of low birth weight (32). This finding was not related to the timing of exposure. Long-term studies of growth and mental development in offspring exposed to these drugs during the 2nd trimester, the period of neuroblast multiplication, have not been conducted (33). However, individual infants have been evaluated for periods ranging from a few weeks up to 7 years and all have had normal growth and development (17–20,22–24,26,27,29).

Vincristine, in combination with other antineoplastic agents, may produce gonadal dysfunction in men and women (34–41). Alkylating agents are the most frequent cause of this problem (38). Ovarian and testicular function may return to normal with successful pregnancies possible, depending on the patient's age at time of treatment and the total dose of chemotherapy received (34). In a 1989 case report, a woman with an immature teratoma of the ovary was treated with conservative surgery and chemotherapy consisting of six

V

courses of vincristine, dactinomycin, and cyclophosphamide (42). She conceived 20 months after her last chemotherapy and eventually delivered a normal 3340-g male infant. The long-term effects of combination chemotherapy on menstrual and reproductive function have been described in a 1988 report (43). Of 40 women treated for malignant ovarian germ cell tumors, 29 received vincristine. The results of this study are discussed in the monograph for cyclophosphamide (see Cyclophosphamide).

In 436 long-term survivors treated with chemotherapy between 1958 and 1978 for gestational trophoblastic tumors, 132 (30%) received vincristine in combination with other antineoplastic agents (44). The mean duration of chemotherapy was 4 months with a mean interval from completion of therapy to the first pregnancy of 2.7 years. Conception occurred within 1 year of therapy completion in 45 women (antineoplastic agents used in these women were not specified), resulting in 31 live births, 1 anencephalic stillbirth, 7 SABs, and 6 elective abortions. Of the 132 women treated with vincristine, 37 (28%) had at least one live birth (numbers in parentheses refer to mean/maximum vincristine dose in milligrams) (7.4/17.0), 8 (6%) had no live births (7.1/22.0), 4 (3%) failed to conceive (7.3/18.0), and 83 (63%) did not try to conceive (11.3/46.0). The average ages at the end of treatment in the four groups were 24.9, 24.4, 24.4, and 31.5 years, respectively. Congenital abnormalities noted in the total group (368 conceptions) were two cases of anencephaly, and one case each of spina bifida, tetralogy of Fallot, talipes equinovarus, collapsed lung, umbilical hernia, desquamative fibrosing alveolitis, asymptomatic heart murmur, and mental retardation. Another child had tachycardia but developed normally after treatment. One case of sudden infant death syndrome occurred in a female infant at 4 weeks of age. None of these outcomes differed statistically from that expected in a normal population (44).

Occupational exposure of the mother to antineoplastic agents during pregnancy may present a risk to the fetus. A position statement from the National Study Commission on Cytotoxic Exposure and a research article involving some antineoplastic agents are presented in the monograph for cyclophosphamide (see Cyclophosphamide).

BREASTFEEDING SUMMARY

No reports describing the use of vincristine during lactation have been located. Because of the potential for severe toxicity in a nursing infant, women who require this agent should not breastfeed.

References

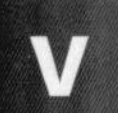

1. Product information. Oncovin. Eli Lilly, 2000.
2. Pizzuto J, Aviles A, Noriega L, Niz J, Morales M, Romero F. Treatment of acute, leukemia during pregnancy: presentation of nine cases. Cancer Treat Rep 1980;64:679–83.
3. Colbert N, Najman A, Gorin NC, Blum F, Treisser A, Lasfargues G, Cloup M, Barrat H, Duhamel G. Acute leukaemia during pregnancy: favourable course of pregnancy in two patients treated with cytosine arabinoside and anthracyclines. Nouv Presse Med 1980;9:175–8.
4. Daly H, McCann SR, Hanratty TD, Temperley IJ. Successful pregnancy during combination chemotherapy for Hodgkin's disease. Acta Haematol (Basel) 1980;64:154–6.
5. Tobias JS, Bloom HJG. Doxorubicin in pregnancy. Lancet 1980;1:776.
6. Garcia V, San Miguel J, Borrasea AL. Doxorubicin in the first trimester of pregnancy. Ann Intern Med 1981;94:547.
7. Dara P, Slater LM, Armentrout SA. Successful pregnancy during chemotherapy for acute leukemia. Cancer 1981;47:845–6.
8. Burnier AM. Discussion. In: Plows CW. *Acute Myelomonocytic Leukemia in Pregnancy: Report of a Case*. Am J Obstet Gynecol 1982;143:41–3.
9. Lilleyman JS, Hill AS, Anderton KJ. Consequences of acute myelogenous leukemia in early pregnancy. Cancer 1977;40:1300–3.
10. Thomas PRM, Peckham MJ. The investigation and management of Hodgkin's disease in the pregnant patient. Cancer 1976;38:1443–51.
11. Pawliger DF, McLean FW, Noyes WD. Normal fetus after cytosine arabinoside therapy. Ann Intern Med 1971;74:1012.
12. Lowenthal RM, Funnell CF, Hope DM, Stewart IG, Humphrey DC. Normal infant after combination chemotherapy including teniposide for Burkitt's lymphoma in pregnancy. Med Pediatr Oncol 1982;10:165–9.
13. Sears HF, Reid J. Granulocytic sarcoma: local presentation of a systemic disease. Cancer 1976;37:1808–13.
14. Durie BGM, Giles HR. Successful treatment of acute leukemia during pregnancy: combination therapy in the third trimester. Arch Intern Med 1977;137:90–1.
15. Newcomb M, Balducci L, Thigpen JT, Morrison FS. Acute leukemia in pregnancy: successful delivery after cytarabine and doxorubicin. JAMA 1978;239:2691–2.
16. Mennuti MT, Shepard TH, Mellman WJ. Fetal renal malformation following treatment of Hodgkin's disease during pregnancy. Obstet Gynecol 1975;46:194–6.
17. Coopland AT, Friesen WJ, Galbraith PA. Acute leukemia in pregnancy. Am J Obstet Gynecol 1969;105:1288–9.
18. Doney KC, Kraemer KG, Shepard TH. Combination chemotherapy for acute myelocytic leukemia during pregnancy: three case reports. Cancer Treat Rep 1979;63:369–71.
19. Okun DB, Groncy PK, Sieger L, Tanaka KR. Acute leukemia in pregnancy: transient neonatal myelosuppression after combination chemotherapy in the mother. Med Pediatr Oncol 1979;7:315–9.
20. Weed JC Jr, Roh RA, Mendenhall HW. Recurrent endodermal sinus tumor during pregnancy. Obstet Gynecol 1979;54:653–6.
21. Kim DS, Park MI. Maternal and fetal survival following surgery and chemotherapy of endodermal sinus tumor of the ovary during pregnancy: a case report. Obstet Gynecol 1989;73:503–7.
22. Karp GI, von Oeyen P, Valone F, Khetarpal VK, Israel M, Mayer RJ, Frigoletto FD, Garnick MB. Doxorubicin in pregnancy: possible transplacental passage. Cancer Treat Rep 1983;67:773–7.
23. Haerr RW, Pratt AT. Multiagent chemotherapy for sarcoma diagnosed during pregnancy. Cancer 1985;56:1028–33.
24. Volkenandt M, Buchner T, Hiddemann W, Van De Loo J. Acute leukaemia during pregnancy. Lancet 1987;2:1521–2.
25. Schleuning M, Clemm C. Chromosomal aberrations in a newborn whose mother received cytotoxic treatment during pregnancy. N Engl J Med 1987;317:1666–7.
26. Feliu J, Juarez S, Ordonez A, Garcia-Paredes ML, Gonzalez-Baron M, Montero JM. Acute leukemia and pregnancy. Cancer 1988;61:580–4.
27. Turchi JJ, Villasis C. Anthracyclines in the treatment of malignancy in pregnancy. Cancer 1988;61:435–40.
28. Weinrach RS. Leukemia in pregnancy. Ariz Med 1972;29:326–9.
29. Ortega J. Multiple agent chemotherapy including bleomycin of non-Hodgkin's lymphoma during pregnancy. Cancer 1977;40:2829–35.
30. Jones RT, Weinerman ER. MOPP (nitrogen mustard, vincristine, procarbazine, and prednisone) given during pregnancy. Obstet Gynecol 1979;54:477–8.
31. Giacalone PL, Laffargue F, Benos P. Chemotherapy for breast carcinoma during pregnancy. Cancer 1999;86:2266–72.
32. Nicholson HO. Cytotoxic drugs in pregnancy: review of reported cases. J Obstet Gynaecol Br Commonw 1968;75:307–12.
33. Dobbing J. Pregnancy and leukaemia. Lancet 1977;1:1155.
34. Schilsky RL, Sherins RJ, Hubbard SM, Wesley MN, Young RC, DeVita VT Jr. Long-term follow-up of ovarian function in women treated with MOPP chemotherapy for Hodgkin's disease. Am J Med 1981;71:552–6.
35. Schwartz PE, Vidone RA. Pregnancy following combination chemotherapy for a mixed germ cell tumor of the ovary. Gynecol Oncol 1981;12:373–8.
36. Estiu M. Successful pregnancy in leukaemia. Lancet 1977;1:433.
37. Johnson SA, Goldman JM, Hawkins DF. Pregnancy after chemotherapy for Hodgkin's disease. Lancet 1979;2:93.

38. Schilsky RL, Lewis BJ, Sherins RJ, Young RC. Gonadal dysfunction in patients receiving chemotherapy for cancer. Ann Intern Med 1980;93:109–14.
39. Sherins RJ, DeVita VT Jr. Effect of drug treatment for lymphoma on male reproductive capacity. Ann Intern Med 1973;79:216–20.
40. Sherins RJ, Olweny CLM, Ziegler JL. Gynecomastia and gonadal dysfunction in adolescent boys treated with combination chemotherapy for Hodgkin's disease. N Engl J Med 1978;299:12–6.
41. Lendon PRM, Peckham MJ. The investigation and management of Hodgkin's disease in the pregnant patient. Cancer 1976;38:1944–51.
42. Lee RB, Kelly J, Elg SA, Benson WL. Pregnancy following conservative surgery and adjunctive chemotherapy for stage III immature teratoma of the ovary. Obstet Gynecol 1989;73:853–5.
43. Gershenson DM. Menstrual and reproductive function after treatment with combination chemotherapy for malignant ovarian germ cell tumors. J Clin Oncol 1988;6:270–5.
44. Rustin GJS, Booth M, Dent J, Salt S, Rustin F, Bagshawe KD. Pregnancy after cytotoxic chemotherapy for gestational trophoblastic tumours. Br Med J 1984;288:103–6.

VINORELBINE

Antineoplastic

PREGNANCY RECOMMENDATION: Limited Human Data—Animal Data Suggest Risk
BREASTFEEDING RECOMMENDATION: Contraindicated

PREGNANCY SUMMARY

Although the animal reproduction data suggest risk during organogenesis, the human pregnancy experience with vinorelbine is limited to 10 cases, all in the 2nd and 3rd trimesters. Transient anemia was observed in one infant and another had mild leukopenia and thrombocytopenia, but other antineoplastic agents were used in each case. The limited human data prevent a more complete assessment of the embryo–fetal risk. Avoiding the use of this agent in gestation, especially in the 1st trimester and/or close to delivery, is reasonable. However, if the mother's condition requires this therapy and consent is given, vinorelbine should not be withheld because of pregnancy.

FETAL RISK SUMMARY

Vinorelbine is a semisynthetic vinca alkaloid that is used in the treatment of cancer. It is related to two other vinca alkaloids, vinblastine and vincristine.

Reproduction studies in mice at one-third the human dose (HD) and in rabbits at one-fourth the HD have shown embryo and/or fetal toxicity (1). At maternal nontoxic doses, intrauterine growth restriction and delayed ossification were observed. Vinorelbine did not affect fertility when administered to rats at weekly doses that were one-third the HD or alternate-day doses that were one-seventh the HD before and during mating (1). The agent did reduce spermatogenesis and prostate/seminal vesicle secretion in male rats given biweekly doses about 1/15th and 1/4th the HD, respectively, for 13 or 26 weeks (1).

It is not known if vinorelbine crosses the placenta to the fetus. The molecular weight (about 1079) suggests that placental transfer of the drug to the embryo or fetus would be inhibited, but probably not prevented.

In a brief 1997 report, three pregnant women with breast cancer were successfully treated with two or three courses of vinorelbine (20–30 mg/m^2) and fluorouracil (500–750 mg/m^2) at 24, 28, and 29 weeks' gestation, respectively (2). Delivery occurred at 34, 41, and 37 weeks' gestation, respectively. One patient also required six courses of epidoxorubicin and cyclophosphamide. Her infant developed transient anemia at 21 days of age that resolved spontaneously. No adverse effects were observed in the other two newborns. All three infants were developing normally at about 2–3 years of age (2).

A 1999 report from France described the outcomes of pregnancies in 20 women with breast cancer who were treated with antineoplastic agents (3). The first cycle of chemotherapy occurred at a mean gestational age of 26 weeks with delivery occurring at a mean 34.7 weeks. A total of 38 cycles were administered during pregnancy with a median of two cycles per woman. None of the women received radiation therapy during pregnancy. The pregnancy outcomes included two spontaneous abortions (both exposed in the 1st trimester), one intrauterine death (exposed in the 2nd trimester), and 17 live births, 1 of whom died at 8 days of age without apparent cause. The 16 surviving children were developing normally at a mean follow-up of 42.3 months. Vinorelbine, in combination with fluorouracil, was administered to four women at a mean dose of 37 mg/m^2 (range 20–50 mg/m^2) during the 2nd or 3rd trimesters. The outcomes were four surviving liveborn infants (3).

A 34-year-old woman with a history of breast cancer presented at 15 weeks' gestation with metastases to the spine, pelvis, and hips (4). She refused all antineoplastic therapy until about 19 weeks'. At that time, she was started on vinorelbine (25 mg/m^2) but her condition continued to deteriorate. Therapy was changed to docetaxel (100 mg/m^2) and methylprednisolone every 3 weeks. After three cycles, a planned cesarean section at 32 weeks' delivered a normal, 1620-g female infant with Apgar scores of 8 and 9. The child was developing normally at 20 months of age (4).

Rapidly progressing nonsmall-cell lung cancer was diagnosed in a 31-year-old woman at 25 weeks' gestation (5). One week later, she received vinorelbine (25 mg/m^2) and cisplatin (100 mg/m^2), but because her condition continued to worsen, a cesarean section was performed 4 days later to deliver a healthy male infant with Apgar scores of 7 and 8 at 1 and 5 minutes, respectively. Ten days after chemotherapy, a transient decrease in the infant's white blood cell and platelet counts was observed but both resolved 3 weeks after birth (5).

A 26-year-old woman with breast cancer was treated with trastuzumab, paclitaxel, fluorouracil, epirubicin, and cyclophosphamide, followed by a left mastectomy and radiation therapy (6). Fourteen months later, in the 27th week of pregnancy, multiple hepatic metastases were detected. She was treated with trastuzumab (one dose of 4mg/kg, then 2 mg/kg every week) and vinorelbine (25 mg/m^2 weekly for 3 weeks followed by a week of rest) until 34 weeks' gestation. Oligohydramnios occurred during therapy that was most likely secondary to trastuzumab (see Trastuzumab). Because of decreased fetal movement, labor was induced at 34 weeks' gestation and a healthy 2.6-kg male infant was delivered vaginally with Apgar scores of 9, 9, and 10. At 6 months of age, the infant was healthy and developing normally (6).

BREASTFEEDING SUMMARY

No reports describing the use of vinorelbine during lactation have been located. Because of the potential for severe toxicity (e.g., bone marrow depression as seen in adults) in a nursing infant, women who require this agent should not breastfeed.

References

1. Product information. Navelbine. Glaxo Wellcome, 1999.
2. Cuvier C, Espie M, Extra JM, Marty M. Vinorelbine in pregnancy. Eur J Cancer 1997;33:168–9.
3. Giacalone PL, Laffargue F, Benos P. Chemotherapy for breast carcinoma during pregnancy. Cancer 1999;86:2266–72.
4. De Santos M, Lucchese A, De Carolis S, Ferrazzani S, Caruso A. Metastatic breast cancer in pregnancy: first case of chemotherapy with docetaxel. Eur J Cancer Care (Engl) 2000;9:235–7.
5. Jänne PA, Rodriguez-Thompson D, Metcalf DR, Swanson SJ, Greisman HA, Wilkins-Haug L, Johnson BE. Chemotherapy for a patient with advanced nonsmall-cell lung cancer during pregnancy: a case report and a review of chemotherapy treatment during pregnancy. Oncology 2001;61:175–83.
6. Fanale MA, Uyei AR, Therialult RL, Adam K, Thompson RA. Treatment of metastatic breast cancer with trastuzumab and vinorelbine during pregnancy. Clin Breast Cancer 2005;6:354–6.

VISMODEGIB

Antineoplastic (Miscellaneous)

PREGNANCY RECOMMENDATION: Contraindicated
BREASTFEEDING RECOMMENDATION: No Human Data—Potential Toxicity

PREGNANCY SUMMARY

No reports describing the use of vismodegib in human pregnancy have been located. In the one animal species studied, the drug caused embryo and fetal death, as well as structural anomalies at systemic exposures that were close to or below the predicted human exposure. The absence of human pregnancy experience prevents a more complete assessment of the embryo–fetal risk. In clinical trials in women of reproductive potential, amenorrhea has been observed (1). The manufacturer recommends a negative pregnancy test within 7 days before starting therapy and a highly effective form of contraception before the first dose and for 7 months after the last dose.

FETAL RISK SUMMARY

Vismodegib is an inhibitor of the Hedgehog pathway that is given orally. It is indicated for the treatment of adults with metastatic basal cell carcinoma, or with locally advance basal cell carcinoma that has recurred following surgery or who are not candidates for surgery, and who are not candidates for radiation. The drug undergoes limited metabolism with >98% of the total circulating drug-related components being the parent drug. Plasma protein binding to albumin and α_1-acid-glycoprotein is high (>99%) and the elimination half-life is 4 days (1).

Reproduction studies have been conducted in rats. In this species, oral doses that resulted in exposures that were about ≥2 times the systemic exposure at the recommended dose based on AUC (SERD) caused preimplantation and postimplantation losses, which included early resorption of 100% of the fetuses. Exposures that were about 0.2 times the RD resulted in malformations (including missing and/or fused digits, open perineum and craniofacial anomalies) and retardations or variations (including dilated renal pelvis, dilated ureter, and incompletely or unossified sternal elements, centra of vertebrae, or proximal phalanges and claws).

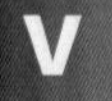

Carcinogenicity studies have not been conducted. Vismodegib was not mutagenic or clastogenic in multiple assays. Fertility impairment studies have not been done. However, data from repeat-dose toxicology studies in rats and dogs indicated that the drug may impair male and female reproductive function and fertility (1).

It is not known if vismodegib crosses the human placenta. The molecular weight (about 421) and long elimination half-life suggest that the drug will cross to the embryo–fetus, but the high plasma protein binding might limit the exposure.

BREASTFEEDING SUMMARY

No reports describing the use of vismodegib during human lactation have been located. The molecular weight (about 421) and long elimination half-life (4 days) suggest that the drug will be excreted into breast milk, but the high plasma protein binding (>99%) might limit the exposure. The effect of the exposure on a nursing infant is unknown. Some of the most common adverse reactions (≥10%) in adults were muscle spasms, alopecia, diarrhea or constipation, nausea, vomiting, weight loss, decreased appetite, and fatigue. If a woman receiving the drug chooses to breastfeed, her infant should be closely monitored for these effects.

Reference

1. Product information. Erivedge. Genentech USA, 2012.

VITAMIN A

Vitamin

PREGNANCY RECOMMENDATION: Compatible
Contraindicated (Doses above U.S. RDA)
BREASTFEEDING RECOMMENDATION: Compatible

PREGNANCY SUMMARY

Excessive doses of preformed vitamin A are teratogenic, as may be marked maternal deficiency. In addition, recent evidence has demonstrated that severe maternal vitamin A deficiency may increase the risk of mother-to-child HIV transmission and reduced infant growth during the first year. β-Carotene, a vitamin A precursor, has not been associated with either human or animal toxicity (see β-Carotene). Doses exceeding the recommended daily allowance (RDA) (8000 IU/day) should be avoided by women who are pregnant or who may become pregnant. Moreover, the RDA established by the FDA should be considered the maximum dose (1).

FETAL RISK SUMMARY

Vitamin A (retinol; vitamin A_1) is a fat-soluble essential nutrient that occurs naturally in various foods. Vitamin A is required for the maintenance of normal epithelial tissue and for growth and bone development, vision, and reproduction (2). Two different daily intake recommendations for pregnant women in the United States have been made for vitamin A. The National Academy of Sciences' RDA for normal pregnant women, published in 1989, is 800 retinol equivalents/day (about 2700 IU per day of vitamin A) (2,3). The FDA's RDA (i.e., U.S. RDA) for pregnant women, a recommendation made in 1976, is 8000 IU/day (1,4). The U.S. RDA of 8000 IU/day should be considered the maximum dose (1), although the difference between the two recommendations is probably not clinically significant.

The teratogenicity of vitamin A in animals is well known. Both high levels and deficiency of the vitamin have resulted in defects (5–13). In the past, various authors have speculated on the teratogenic effect of the vitamin in humans (5,14–16). A 1983 case report suggested that the vitamin A contained in a multivitamin product may have caused a cleft palate in one infant; however, the mother had a family history of cleft palate and had produced a previous infant with a malformation (16). Another case report, this one published in 1987, described an infant with multiple defects whose mother had consumed a vitamin preparation containing 2000 IU/day of vitamin A (17). The authors thought the phenotype of their patient was similar to the one observed with isotretinoin, but they could not exclude other causes of the defect, including a phenocopy of the isotretinoin syndrome (17). Therefore, in both cases, no definite association between the defects and vitamin A can be established, and the possibility that other causes were involved is high.

In response to the 1983 case report cited above, one investigator wrote in 1983 that there was no acceptable evidence of human vitamin A teratogenicity and none at all with doses <10,000 IU/day (18). Since that time, however, two synthetic isomers of vitamin A, isotretinoin and etretinate, have been shown to be potent human teratogens (see Isotretinoin and Etretinate). In addition, recent studies have revealed that high doses of preformed vitamin A are human teratogens. These and the other reports are summarized below. Because of the combined animal and human data for vitamin A, and because of the human experience with isotretinoin and etretinate, large doses or severe deficiency of vitamin A must be viewed as harmful to the human fetus.

Severe human vitamin A deficiency has been cited as the cause of three malformed infants (19–21). In the first case, a mother with multiple vitamin deficiencies produced a baby with congenital xerophthalmia and bilateral cleft lip (19). The defects may have been caused by vitamin A deficiency because of their similarity to anomalies seen in animals deprived of this nutrient. The second report involved a malnourished pregnant woman with recent onset of blindness whose symptoms were the result of vitamin A deficiency (20). The mother gave birth to a premature male child with microcephaly and what appeared to be anophthalmia. The final case described a blind, mentally slow girl with bilateral microphthalmia, coloboma of the iris and choroid, and retinal aplasia (21). During pregnancy, the mother was suspected of having vitamin A deficiency manifested by night blindness.

In 1986, investigators from the FDA reviewed 18 cases of suspected vitamin A-induced teratogenicity (22). Some of these cases had been reviewed in previous communications by an FDA epidemiologist (23,24). Six of the cases (25–30) had been published previously and 12 represented unpublished reports. All of the cases, except one, involved long-term, high-dose (>25,000 IU/day) consumption continuing past conception. The exception involved a woman who accidentally consumed 500,000 IU, as a single dose, during the 2nd month of pregnancy (29). Twelve of the infants had malformations similar to those seen in animal and human retinoid syndromes (i.e., central nervous system and cardiovascular anomalies, microtia, and clefts) (22). The defects observed in the 18 infants were microtia ($N = 4$), craniofacial ($N = 4$), brain ($N = 4$), facial palsy ($N = 1$), micro/anophthalmia ($N = 2$), facial clefts ($N = 4$), cardio-aortic ($N = 2$), limb reduction ($N = 4$), gastrointestinal atresia ($N = 1$), and urinary ($N = 4$) (22).

The CDC reported in 1987 the results of an epidemiologic study conducted by the New York State Department of Health from April 1983 through February 1984 (4). The mothers of 492 liveborn infants without congenital defects were interviewed to obtain their drug histories. Vitamin A supplements were taken by 81.1% (399 of 492) of the women. Of this

V

group, 0.6% (3 of 492) took ≥25,000 IU/day and 2.6% (13 of 492) consumed 15,000–24,999 IU/day. In an editorial comment, the CDC noted that the excessive vitamin A consumption by some of the women was a public health concern (4).

Results of an epidemiologic case–control study conducted in Spain between 1976 and 1987 were reported in preliminary form in 1988 (31) and as a full report in 1990 (32). A total of 11,293 cases of malformed infants were compared with 11,193 normal controls. Sixteen of the case mothers (1.4/1000) used high doses of vitamin A either alone or in combination with other vitamins during their pregnancies, compared with 14 (1.3/1000) of the controls, an odds ratio (OR) of 1.1 (*ns*). Five of the case infants and 10 of the controls were exposed to doses <40,000 IU/day (OR 0.5, $p = 0.15$). In contrast, 11 of the case infants and 4 controls were exposed to ≥40,000 IU (OR 2.7, $p = 0.06$). The risk of congenital anomalies, although not significant, appeared to be related to gestational age because the highest risk in those pregnancies exposed to ≥40,000 IU/day occurred during the first 2 months (32). The data suggested a dose–effect relationship and provided support for earlier statements that doses lower than 10,000 IU were not teratogenic (31,32).

Data from a case–control study were used to assess the effects of vitamin A supplements (daily use for at least 7 days of vitamin A either alone or with vitamin D, or of fish oils) and vitamin A-containing multivitamin supplements (33). Cases were 2658 infants with malformations derived, at least in part, from cranial neural crest cells (primarily craniofacial and cardiac anomalies). Controls were 2609 infants with other malformations. Case mothers used vitamin A supplements in 15, 14, and 10 pregnancies during lunar months 1, 2, and 3, respectively, compared with 6 control mothers in each period (33). Although not significant, the OR in each period was 2.5 (95% confidence interval [CI] 1.0–6.2), 2.3 (95% CI 0.9–5.8), and 1.6 (95% CI 0.6–4.5), respectively. The authors cautioned that their data should be considered tentative because of the small numbers and lack of dosage and nutrition information (33). Even a small increased risk was excluded for vitamin A-containing multivitamins (33).

A congenital malformation of the left eye was attributed to excessive vitamin A exposure during the 1st trimester in a 1991 report (34). The mother had ingested a combination of liver and vitamin supplements that provided an estimated 25,000 IU/day of vitamin A. The unusual eye defect consisted of an "hourglass" cornea and iris with a reduplicated lens (34).

A brief 1992 correspondence cited the experience in the Hungarian Family Planning Program with a prenatal vitamin preparation containing 6000 IU of vitamin A (35). Evaluating their 1989 database, the authors found no relationship, in comparison with a nonexposed control group, between the daily intake of the multivitamin at least 1 month before conception through the 12th week of gestation and any congenital malformation.

A study published in 1995 examined the effect of preformed vitamin A, consumed from vitamin supplements and food, on pregnancy outcomes (36). Vitamin A ingestion, from 3 months before through 12 weeks from the last menstrual period, was determined for 22,748 women. Most of the women were enrolled in the study between week 15 and week 20 of pregnancy. From the total group, 339 babies met the criteria for congenital anomalies established by the investigators. These criteria included malformations in four categories (number of defects of each type shown): cranial-neural-crest defects (craniofacial, central nervous system, and thymic $N = 69$; heart defects $N = 52$); neural tube defects (NTDs) (spina bifida, anencephaly, and encephalocele $N = 48$); musculoskeletal ($N = 58$) and urogenital ($N = 42$) defects; and other defects (gastrointestinal defects $N = 24$; agenesis or hypoplasia of the lungs, single umbilical artery, anomalies of the spleen, and cystic hygroma $N = 46$) (36). The 22,748 women were divided into four groups based on their total (supplement plus food) daily intake of vitamin A: 0–5000 IU ($N = 6410$), 5001–10,000 IU ($N = 12,688$), 10,001–15,000 IU ($N = 3150$), and ≥15,001 IU ($N = 500$). Analysis of this grouping revealed that the women who took ≥15,001 IU/day had a higher prevalence ratio for defects associated with cranial-neural-crest tissue compared with those in the lowest group, 3.5 (95% CI 1.7–7.3). A slightly higher ratio was found for musculoskeletal and urogenital defects, no increase for neural tube defects or other defects, and for all birth defects combined, a ratio of 2.2 (95% CI 1.3–3.8). Analysis of three groups (0–5000, 5001–10,000, and ≥10,001 IU) of vitamin A ingestion levels from food alone was hampered by the small number of women and, although some increased prevalence ratios were found in the highest groups, the small numbers made the estimates imprecise. A third analysis was then conducted based on four groups (0–5000, 5001–8000, 8001–10,000, and ≥10,001 IU) of vitamin A ingestion levels from supplements. Compared with the lowest group, the prevalence ratio for all birth defects in the highest group was 2.4 (95% CI 1.3–4.4) and for defects involving the cranial-neural-crest tissue, the ratio was 4.8 (95% CI 2.2–10.5). Of interest, the mean vitamin A intake in the highest group was 21,675 IU. Based on these data, the investigators concluded that following in utero exposure to more than 10,000 IU of vitamin A from supplements, about 1 infant in 57 (1.75%) had a vitamin A-induced malformation (36).

In response to the above study, a note of caution was sounded by two authors from the CDC (37). Citing results from previous studies, these authors concluded that without more data, they could not recommend use of the dose–response curve developed in the above study for advising pregnant women of the specific risk of anomalies that might arise from the ingestion of excessive vitamin A. Although they agreed that very large doses of vitamin A might be teratogenic, the question of how large a dose remained (37). A number of correspondences followed publication of the above study, all describing perceived methodologic discrepancies that may have affected the conclusions (38–42) with a reply by the authors supporting their findings (43).

Using case–control study data from California, a paper published in 1997 examined the relationship between maternal vitamin A ingestion and the risk of NTDs in singleton liveborn infants and aborted fetuses (44). Although the number of cases was small, only 16 exposed to ≥10,000 IU/day and 6 to ≥15,000 IU/day, the investigators did not find a relationship between these levels of exposure and NTDs.

Referring to the question on the teratogenic level of vitamin A, a 1997 abstract reported the effects of increasing doses of the vitamin in the cynomolgus monkey, a species that is a well-documented model for isotretinoin-induced

V

teratogenicity (45). Four groups of monkeys were administered increasing doses of vitamin A (7500–80,000 IU/kg) in early gestation (day 16–27). A dose-related increase in abortions and typical congenital malformations was observed in the offspring. The NOAEL (no-observed-adverse-effect level) was 7500 IU/kg, or 30,000 IU/day based on an average 4-kg animal. A human NOAEL extrapolated from the monkey NOAEL would correspond to >300,000 IU/day (45).

A brief 1995 report described the outcomes of 7 of 22 women who had taken very large doses of vitamin A during pregnancy, 20 of whom had taken the vitamin during the 1st trimester (46). The mean daily dose was 70,000 IU (range 25,000–90,000 IU) for a mean of 44 days (range 7–180 days). None of the offspring of the seven patients available at follow-up had congenital malformations. Data on the other 15 women were not available (46).

Two abstracts published in 1996 examined the issue of vitamin A supplementation in women enrolled in studies in Atlanta, Georgia, and in California, both during the 1980s (47,48). In the first abstract, no increase in the incidence of all congenital defects or those classified as involving cranial-neural-crest-derived was found for doses <8000 IU/day, or for those who took both a multivitamin and a vitamin A supplement (47). In the other abstract, subjects took amounts thought likely to exceed 10,000 IU/day and, again, no association with the major anomalies derived from cranial-neural-crest cells (cleft lip, cleft palate, and conotruncal heart defects) was discovered (48).

Using data collected between 1985 and 1987 in California and Illinois by the National Institute of Child Health and Human Development Neural Tube Defects Study, a case–control study published in 1997 examined whether periconceptional vitamin A exposure was related to NTDs or other major congenital malformations (49). Three study groups of offspring were formed shortly after the pregnancy outcome was known (prenatally and postnatally): those with NTDs (N = 548), those with other major malformations (N = 387), and normal controls (N = 573). The latter two groups were matched to the NTDs group. A subgroup, formed from those with other major malformations, involved those with cranial-neural-crest malformations (N = 89), consisting mainly of conotruncal defects of the heart and great vessels, including ventricular septal defects, and defects of the ear and face (49). The vitamin A (supplements and fortified cereals) exposure rates by group for those ingesting a mean >8000 IU/day or >10,000 IU/day were: NTDs (3.3% and 2.0%), other major malformations (3.6% and 1.6%), cranial-neural-crest malformations (3.4% and 2.2%), and controls (4.5% and 2.1%), respectively. None of the values were statistically significant, thus, no association between moderate consumption of vitamin A and the defect groups was found (49).

Several investigators have studied maternal and fetal vitamin A levels during various stages of gestation (5,50–61). Transport to the fetus is by passive diffusion (61). Maternal vitamin A concentrations are slightly greater than those found in either premature or term infants (50–52). In women with normal levels of vitamin A, maternal and newborn levels were 270 and 220 ng/mL, respectively (51). In 41 women not given supplements of vitamin A, a third of whom had laboratory evidence of hypovitaminemia A, mean maternal levels exceeded those in the newborn by almost a 2:1 ratio (51). In two reports, maternal serum levels were dependent on the length of gestation with concentrations decreasing during the 1st trimester, then increasing during the remainder of pregnancy until about the 38th week when they began to decrease again (5,53). A more recent study found no difference in serum levels between 10 and 33 weeks' gestation, even though amniotic fluid vitamin A levels at 20 weeks onward were significantly greater than at 16–18 weeks (54). Premature infants (36 weeks or less) have significantly lower serum retinol and retinol-binding protein concentrations than do term neonates (50,55–57).

Mild to moderate deficiency is common during pregnancy (51,58). A 1984 report concluded that vitamin A deficiency in poorly nourished mothers was one of the features associated with an increased incidence of prematurity and intrauterine growth restriction (50). An earlier study, however, found no difference in vitamin A levels between low-birth-weight (<2500 g) and normal-birth-weight (>2500 g) infants (52). Maternal vitamin A concentrations of the low-birth-weight group were lower than those of normals, 211 vs. 273 ng/mL, but not significantly. An investigation in premature infants revealed that infants developing bronchopulmonary dysplasia had significantly lower serum retinol levels as compared with infants who did not develop this disease (57).

Relatively high liver vitamin A stores were found in the fetuses of women younger than 18 and older than 40 years of age, two groups that produce a high incidence of fetal anomalies (5). Low fetal liver concentrations were measured in 2 infants with hydrocephalus and high levels in 14 infants with NTDs (5). In another report relating to NTDs, a high liver concentration occurred in an anencephalic infant (59). Significantly, higher vitamin A amniotic fluid concentrations were discovered in 12 pregnancies from which infants with NTDs were delivered as compared with 94 normal pregnancies (60). However, attempts to use this measurement as an indicator of anencephaly or other fetal anomalies failed because the values for abnormal and normal fetuses overlapped (54,60).

The effect of stopping oral contraceptives shortly before conception on vitamin A levels has been studied (62). Because oral contraceptives had been shown to increase serum levels of vitamin A, it was postulated that early conception might involve a risk of teratogenicity. However, no difference was found in early pregnancy vitamin A levels between users and nonusers. The results of this study have been challenged based on the methods used to measure vitamin A (63).

Vitamin A is known to affect the immune system (64). Three recent studies (65–67) and an editorial (68) have described or commented on the effect that maternal vitamin A deficiency has on the maternal–fetal transmission of HIV. In each of the studies, a low maternal level of vitamin A was associated with HIV transmission to the infant. In the one study conducted in the United States, severe maternal vitamin A deficiency (<0.70 μmol/L) was associated with HIV transmission with an adjusted OR of 5.05 (95% CI 1.20–21.24) (67). In a related study, maternal vitamin A deficiency during pregnancy in women infected with HIV was significantly related to growth failure (height and weight) during the 1st year of life in their children, after adjustment for the effects of body mass index, child gender, and child HIV status (69).

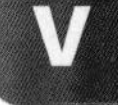

Although the minimum teratogenic dose has not yet been defined, doses of 25,000 IU/day or more, in the form of retinol or retinyl esters, should be considered potentially teratogenic (1,3,22), but based on one study, smaller doses than this may be teratogenic (36). One of the recommendations of the Teratology Society, published in a 1987 position paper, states: "Women in their reproductive years should be informed that the excessive use of vitamin A shortly before and during pregnancy could be harmful to their babies" (1). The Teratology Society also noted that the average balanced diet contains approximately 7000–8000 IU of vitamin A from various sources, and this should be considered prior to additional supplementation (1).

BREASTFEEDING SUMMARY

Vitamin A is a natural constituent of breast milk. Deficiency of this vitamin in breastfed infants is rare (70). The RDA of vitamin A during lactation is approximately 4000 IU (2). It is not known whether high maternal doses of vitamin A represent a danger to the nursing infant or whether they reduce HIV transmission via the milk.

References

1. Public Affairs Committee, Teratology Society. Position paper: recommendations for vitamin A use during pregnancy. Teratology 1987;35:269–75.
2. American Hospital Formulary Service. *Drug Information 1997*. Bethesda, MD: American Society of Health-System Pharmacists, 1997:2806–9.
3. National Research Council. *Recommended Dietary Allowances*, 10th ed. Washington, DC: National Academy Press, 1989.
4. CDC. Use of supplements containing high-dose vitamin A—New York State, 1983–1984. MMWR 1987;36:80–2.
5. Gal I, Sharman IM, Pryse-Davies J. Vitamin A in relation to human congenital malformations. Adv Teratol 1972;5:143–59.
6. Cohlan SQ. Excessive intake of vitamin A as a cause of congenital anomalies in the rat. Science 1953;117:535–6.
7. Muenter MD. Hypervitaminosis A. Ann Intern Med 1974;80:105–6.
8. Morriss GM. Vitamin A and congenital malformations. Int J Vitam Nutr Res 1976;46:220–2.
9. Fantel AG, Shepard TH, Newell-Morris LL, Moffett BC. Teratogenic effects of retinoic acid in pigtail monkeys (*Macaca nemestrina*). Teratology 1977;15:65–72.
10. Vorhees CV, Brunner RL, McDaniel CR, Butcher RE. The relationship of gestational age to vitamin A induced postnatal dysfunction. Teratology 1978;17:271–6.
11. Ferm VH, Ferm RR. Teratogenic interaction of hyperthermia and vitamin A. Biol Neonate 1979;36:168–72.
12. Geelen JAG. Hypervitaminosis A induced teratogenesis. CRC Crit Rev Toxicol 1979;6:351–75.
13. Kamm JJ. Toxicology, carcinogenicity, and teratogenicity of some orally administered retinoids. J Am Acad Dermatol 1982;6:652–9.
14. Muenter MD. Hypervitaminosis A. Ann Intern Med 1974;80:105–6.
15. Read AP, Harris R. Spina bifida and vitamins. Br Med J 1983;286:560–1.
16. Bound JP. Spina bifida and vitamins. Br Med J 1983;286:147.
17. Lungarotti MS, Marinelli D, Mariani T, Calabro A. Multiple congenital anomalies associated with apparently normal maternal intake of vitamin A: a phenocopy of the isotretinoin syndrome? Am J Med Genet 1987;27:245–8.
18. Smithells RW. Spina bifida and vitamins. Br Med J 1983;286:388–9.
19. Houet R, Ramioul-Lecomte S. Repercussions sur l'enfant des avitaminoses de la mere pendant la grossesse. Ann Paediatr 1950;175:378. As cited in Warkany J. *Congenital Malformations: Notes and Comments*. Chicago, IL: Year Book Medical Publishers, 1971:127–8.
20. Sarma V. Maternal vitamin A deficiency and fetal microcephaly and anophthalmia. Obstet Gynecol 1959;13:299–301.
21. Lamba PA, Sood NN. Congenital microphthalmos and colobomata in maternal vitamin A deficiency. J Pediatr Ophthalmol 1968;115–7. As cited in Warkany J. *Congenital Malformation: Notes and Comments*. Chicago, IL: Year Book Medical Publishers, 1971:127–8.
22. Rosa FW, Wilk AL, Kelsey FO. Teratogen update: vitamin A congeners. Teratology 1986;33:355–64.
23. Rosa FW. Teratogenicity of isotretinoin. Lancet 1983;2:513.
24. Rosa FW. Retinoic acid embryopathy. N Engl J Med 1986;315:262.
25. Pilotti G, Scorta A. Ipervitaminosi A gravidica e malformazioni neonatali dell'apparato urinaria. Minerva Ginecol 1965;17:1103–8. As cited in Nishimura H, Tanimura T. *Clinical Aspects of the Teratogenicity of Drugs*. New York, NY: American Elsevier, 1976:251–2.
26. Bernhardt IB, Dorsey DJ. Hypervitaminosis A and congenital renal anomalies in a human infant. Obstet Gynecol 1974;43:750–5.
27. Stange L, Carlstrom K, Eriksson M. Hypervitaminosis A in early human pregnancy and malformations of the central nervous system. Acta Obstet Gynecol Scand 1978;57:289–91.
28. Morriss GM, Thomson AD. Vitamin A and rat embryos. Lancet 1974;2:899–900.
29. Mounoud RL, Klein D, Weber F. A propos d'un cas de syndrome de Goldenhar: intoxication aigue a la vitamine A chez la mere pendant la grossesse. J Genet Hum 1975;23:135–54.
30. Von Lennep E, El Khazen N, De Pierreux G, Amy JJ, Rodesch F, Van Regemorter N. A case of partial sirenomelia and possible vitamin A teratogenesis. Prenat Diagn 1985;5:35–40.
31. Martinez-Frias ML, Salvador J. Megadose vitamin A and teratogenicity. Lancet 1988;1:236.
32. Martinez-Frias ML, Salvador J. Epidemiological aspects of prenatal exposure to high doses of vitamin A in Spain. Eur J Epidemiol 1990;6:118–23.
33. Werler MM, Lammer EJ, Rosenberg L, Mitchell AA. Maternal vitamin A supplementation in relation to selected birth defects. Teratology 1990;42:497–503.
34. Evans K, Hickey-Dwyer MU. Cleft anterior segment with maternal hypervitaminosis A. Br J Ophthalmol 1991;75:691–2.
35. Dudas I, Czeizel AE. Use of 6,000 IU vitamin A during early pregnancy without teratogenic effect. Teratology 1992;45:335–6.
36. Rothman KJ, Moore LL, Singer MR, Nguyen U-SDT, Mannino S, Milunsky A. Teratogenicity of high vitamin A intake. N Engl J Med 1995;333:1369–73.
37. Oakley GP Jr, Erickson JD. Vitamin A and birth defects. Continuing caution is needed. N Engl J Med 1995;333:1414–5.
38. Werler M, Lammer EJ, Mitchell AA. Teratogenicity of high vitamin A intake. N Engl J Med 1996;334:1195.
39. Brent RL, Hendrickx AG, Holmes LB, Miller RK. Teratogenicity of high vitamin A intake. N Engl J Med 1996;334:1196.
40. Watkins M, Moore C, Mulinare J. Teratogenicity of high vitamin A intake. N Engl J Med 1996;334:1196.
41. Challem JJ. Teratogenicity of high vitamin A intake. N Engl J Med 1996;334:1196–7.
42. Hunt JR. Teratogenicity of high vitamin A intake. N Engl J Med 1996;334:1197.
43. Rothman KJ, Moore LL, Singer MR, Milunsky A. Teratogenicity of high vitamin A intake. N Engl J Med 1996;334:1197.
44. Shaw GM, Velie EM, Schaffer D, Lammer EJ. Periconceptional intake of vitamin A among women and risk of neural tube defect-affected pregnancies. Teratology 1997;55:132–3.
45. Hendrickx AG, Hummler H, Oneda S. Vitamin A teratogenicity and risk assessment in the cynomolgus monkey (abstract). Teratology 1997;55:68.
46. Bonati M, Nannini S, Addis A. Vitamin A supplementation during pregnancy in developed countries. Lancet 1995;345:736–7.
47. Khoury MJ, Moore CA, Mulinare J. Do vitamin A supplements in early pregnancy increase the risk of birth defects in the offspring? A population-based case–control study (abstract). Teratology 1996;53:91.
48. Lammer EJ, Shaw GM, Wasserman CR, Block G. High vitamin A intake and risk for major anomalies involving structures with an embryological cranial neural crest cell component (abstract). Teratology 1996;53:91–2.
49. Mills JL, Simpson JL, Cunningham GC, Conley MR, Rhoads GG. Vitamin A and birth defects. Am J Obstet Gynecol 1997;177:31–6.
50. Shah RS, Rajalakshmi R. Vitamin A status of the newborn in relation to gestational age, body weight, and maternal nutritional status. Am J Clin Nutr 1984;40:794–800.
51. Baker H, Frank O, Thomson AD, Langer A, Munves ED, De Angelis B, Kaminetzky HA. Vitamin profile of 174 mothers and newborns at parturition. Am J Clin Nutr 1975;28:59–65.
52. Baker H, Thind IS, Frank O, DeAngelis B, Caterini H, Lquria DB. Vitamin levels in low-birth-weight newborn infants and their mothers. Am J Obstet Gynecol 1977;129:521–4.
53. Gal I, Parkinson CE. Effects of nutrition and other factors on pregnant women's serum vitamin A levels. Am J Clin Nutr 1974;27:688–95.

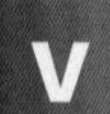

54. Wallingford JC, Milunsky A, Underwood BA. Vitamin A and retinol-binding protein in amniotic fluid. Am J Clin Nutr 1983;38:377–81.
55. Brandt RB, Mueller DG, Schroeder JR, Guyer KE, Kirkpatrick BV, Hutcher NE, Ehrlich FE. Serum vitamin A in premature and term neonates. J Pediatr 1978;92:101–4.
56. Shenai JP, Chytil F, Jhaveri A, Stahlman MT. Plasma vitamin A and retinol-binding protein in premature and term neonates. J Pediatr 1981:99:302–5.
57. Hustead VA, Gutcher GR, Anderson SA, Zachman RD. Relationship of vitamin A (retinol) status to lung disease in the preterm infant. J Pediatr 1984;105:610–5.
58. Kaminetzky HA, Langer A, Baker H, Frank O, Thomson AD, Munves ED, Opper A, Behrle FC, Glista B. The effect of nutrition in teen-age gravidas on pregnancy and the status of the neonate. I. A nutritional profile. Am J Obstet Gynecol 1973;115:639–46.
59. Gal I, Sharman IM, Pryse-Davies J, Moore T. Vitamin A as a possible factor in human teratology. Proc Nutr Soc 1969;28:9A–10A.
60. Parkinson CE, Tan JCY. Vitamin A concentrations in amniotic fluid and maternal serum related to neural-tube defects. Br J Obstet Gynaecol 1982;89:935–9.
61. Hill EP, Longo LD. Dynamics of maternal–fetal nutrient transfer. Fed Proc 1980;39:239–44.
62. Wild J, Schorah CJ, Smithells RW. Vitamin A, pregnancy, and oral contraceptives. Br Med J 1974;1:57–9.
63. Bubb FA. Vitamin A, pregnancy, and oral contraceptives. Br Med J 1974;1:391–2.
64. Bates C. Vitamin A and infant immunity. Lancet 1993;341:28.
65. Semba RD, Miotti PG, Chiphangwi JD, Saah AJ, Canner JK, Dallabetta GA, Hoover DR. Maternal vitamin A deficiency and mother-to-child transmission of HIV-1. Lancet 1994;343:1593–7.
66. Semba RD, Miotti PG, Chiphangwi JD, Liomba G, Yang L-P, Saah AJ, Dallabetta GA, Hoover DR. Infant mortality and maternal vitamin A deficiency during human immunodeficiency virus infection. Clin Infect Dis 1995;21:966–72.
67. Greenberg BL, Semba RD, Vink PE, Farley JJ, Sivapalasingam M, Steketee RW, Thea DM, Schoenbaum EE. Vitamin A deficiency and maternal-infant transmission of HIV in two metropolitan areas in the United States. AIDS 1997;11:325–32.
68. Bridbord K, Willoughby A. Vitamin A and mother-to-child HIV-1 transmission. Lancet 1994;343:1585–6.
69. Semba RD, Miotti P, Chiphangwi JD, Henderson R, Dallabetta G, Yang L-P, Hoover D. Maternal vitamin A deficiency and child growth failure during human immunodeficiency virus infection. J Acqir Immune Defic Syndr Human Retrovirol 1997;14:219–22.
70. Committee on Nutrition, American Academy of Pediatrics. Vitamin and mineral supplement needs in normal children in the United States. Pediatrics 1980;66:1015–21.

VITAMIN B_{12}

Vitamin

PREGNANCY RECOMMENDATION: Compatible
BREASTFEEDING RECOMMENDATION: Compatible

PREGNANCY SUMMARY

Severe maternal vitamin B_{12} deficiency may result in megaloblastic anemia with subsequent infertility and poor pregnancy outcome. Less severe maternal deficiency apparently is common and does not pose a significant risk to the mother or fetus. Ingestion of vitamin B_{12} during pregnancy up to the recommended daily allowance (RDA) either via the diet or by supplementation is recommended.

FETAL RISK SUMMARY

Vitamin B_{12} (cyanocobalamin), a water-soluble B-complex vitamin, is an essential nutrient required for nucleoprotein and myelin synthesis, cell reproduction, normal growth, and the maintenance of normal erythropoiesis (1). The National Academy of Sciences' RDA for vitamin B_{12} in pregnancy is 2.2 mcg (1).

Vitamin B_{12} is actively transported to the fetus (2–6). This process is responsible for the progressive decline of maternal levels that occurs during pregnancy (6–14). Fetal demands for the vitamin have been estimated to be approximately 0.3 mcg/day (0.2 nmol/day) (15). Similar to other B-complex vitamins, higher concentrations of B_{12} are found in the fetus and newborn than in the mother (5–9,16–24). At term, mean vitamin B_{12} levels in 174 mothers were 115 pg/mL and in their newborns 500 pg/mL, a newborn:maternal ratio of 4.3 (16). Comparable values have been observed by others (5,7,21–23). Mean levels in 51 Brazilian women, in their newborns, and in the intervillous space of their placentas were approximately 340, 797, and 1074 pg/mL, respectively (24). The newborn:maternal ratio in this report was 2.3. The high levels in the placenta may indicate a mechanism by which the fetus can accumulate the vitamin against a concentration gradient. This study also found a highly significant correlation between vitamin B_{12} and folate concentrations. This is in contrast to an earlier report that did not find such a correlation in women with megaloblastic anemia (25).

Maternal deficiency of vitamin B_{12} is common during pregnancy (16,17,26,27). Tobacco smoking reduces maternal levels of the vitamin even further (28). Megaloblastic anemia may result when the deficiency is severe, but it responds readily to therapy (29–32). On the other hand, tropical macrocytic anemia during pregnancy responds erratically to vitamin B_{12} therapy and is better treated with folic acid (32,33).

Megaloblastic (pernicious) anemia may be a cause of infertility (30,31,34). One report described a mother with undiagnosed pernicious anemia who had lost her 3rd, 9th, and 10th pregnancies (30). A healthy child resulted from her 11th pregnancy following treatment with vitamin B_{12}. In another study, eight infertile women with pernicious anemia were treated with vitamin B_{12} and seven became pregnant within 1 year of therapy (31). One of three patients in still another report may have had infertility associated with very low vitamin B_{12} levels (34).

Vitamin B_{12} deficiency was associated with prematurity (as defined by a birth weight $\leq$2500 g) in a 1968 paper (9). However, many of the patients who delivered prematurely had normal or elevated vitamin B_{12} levels. No correlation between vitamin B_{12} deficiency and abruptio placentae was found in two studies published in the 1960s (35,36). Two reports found a positive association between low birth weight and low vitamin B_{12} levels (21,37). In both instances, however, folate levels were also low and iron was deficient in one. Others could not correlate low vitamin B_{12} concentrations with the weight at delivery (11,26). Based on these reports, it is doubtful whether vitamin B_{12} deficiency is associated with any of the conditions.

In experimental animals, vitamin B_{12} deficiency is teratogenic (7,38). Investigators studying the cause of neural tube defects measured very low vitamin B_{12} levels in three of four mothers of anencephalic fetuses (39). Additional evidence led them to conclude that the low vitamin B_{12} resulted in depletion of maternal folic acid and involvement in the origin of the defects. In contrast, two other reports have shown no relationship between low levels of vitamin B_{12} and congenital malformations (9,19).

No reports linking high doses of vitamin B_{12} with maternal or fetal complications have been located. Vitamin B_{12} administration at term has produced maternal levels approaching 50,000 pg/mL with corresponding cord blood levels of approximately 15,000 pg/mL (4,5). In fetal methylmalonic acidemia, large doses of vitamin B_{12}, 10 mg orally initially then changed to 5 mg IM, were administered daily to a mother to treat the affected fetus (40). On this dosage regimen, maternal levels rose as high as 18,000 pg/mL shortly after a dose. This metabolic disorder is not always treatable with vitamin B_{12}: one study reported a newborn with the vitamin B_{12}-unresponsive form of methylmalonic acidemia (41).

BREASTFEEDING SUMMARY

Vitamin B_{12} is excreted into breast milk. In the first 48 hours after delivery, mean colostrum levels were 2431 pg/mL and then fell rapidly to concentrations comparable with those of normal serum (42). One group of investigators also observed very high colostrum levels ranging from 6 to 17.5 times that of milk (2). Milk:plasma ratios are approximately 1.0 during lactation (19). Reported milk concentrations of vitamin B_{12} vary widely (43–46). Mothers supplemented with daily doses of 1–200 mcg had milk levels increase from a level of 79 to a level of 100 pg/mL (43). Milk concentrations were directly proportional to dietary intake. In a study using 8-mcg/day supplements, mean milk levels of 1650 pg/mL at 1 week and 1100 pg/mL at 6 weeks were measured (44). Corresponding levels in nonsupplemented mothers were significantly different at 1220 and 610 pg/mL, respectively. Other investigators also used 8-mcg/day supplements and found significantly different levels compared with women not receiving supplements: 910 vs. 700 pg/mL at 1 week and 790 vs. 550 pg/mL at 6 weeks (45). In contrast, others found no difference between supplemented and nonsupplemented well-nourished women with 5–100 mcg/day (46). The mean vitamin B_{12} concentration in these latter patients was 970 pg/mL. A 1983 English study measured vitamin B_{12} levels in pooled human milk obtained from preterm (26 mothers: 29–34 weeks) and term (35 mothers: 39 weeks or longer) patients (47). Milk from preterm mothers decreased from a level of 920 pg/mL (colostrum) to a level of 220 pg/mL (16–196 days), whereas milk from term mothers decreased over the same period from a level of 490 to a level of 230 pg/mL.

Vitamin B_{12} deficiency in the lactating mother may cause severe consequences in the nursing infant. Several reports have described megaloblastic anemia in infants exclusively breastfed by vitamin B_{12}-deficient mothers (48–52). Many of these mothers were vegetarians whose diets provided low amounts of the vitamin (49–52). The adequacy of vegetarian diets in providing sufficient vitamin B_{12} has been debated (53–55). However, a recent report measured only 1.4 mcg of vitamin B_{12} intake/day in lactovegetarians (56). This amount is approximately 54% of the RDA for lactating women in the United States (1). Moreover, a 1986 case of vitamin B_{12}-induced anemia supports the argument that the low vitamin B_{12} intake of some vegetarian diets is inadequate to meet the total needs of a nursing infant for this vitamin (57). The case involved a 7-month-old male infant, exclusively breastfed by a strict vegetarian mother, who was diagnosed as suffering from macrocytic anemia. The infant was lethargic, irritable, and failing to thrive. His vitamin B_{12} level was less than 100 pg/mL (normal 180–960 pg/mL), but iron and folate levels were both within normal limits. The anemia responded rapidly to administration of the vitamin, and he was developing normally at 11 months of age (57).

The National Academy of Sciences' RDA for vitamin B_{12} during lactation is 2.6 mcg (1). If the diet of the lactating woman adequately supplies this amount, maternal supplementation with vitamin B_{12} is not needed. Supplementation with the RDA for vitamin B_{12} is recommended for those women with inadequate nutritional intake. The American Academy of Pediatrics classifies vitamin B_{12} as compatible with breastfeeding (58).

References

1. American Hospital Formulary Service. *Drug Information 1997*. Bethesda, MD: American Society of Health-System Pharmacists, 1997:2820–3.
2. Luhby AL, Cooperman JM, Donnenfeld AM, Herrero JM, Teller DN, Wenig JB. Observations on transfer of vitamin B_{12} from mother to fetus and newborn. Am J Dis Child 1958;96:532–3.
3. Hill EP, Longo LD. Dynamics of maternal–fetal nutrient transfer. Fed Proc 1980;39:239–44.
4. Kaminetzky HA, Baker H, Frank O, Langer A. The effects of intravenously administered water-soluble vitamins during labor in normovitaminemic and hypovitaminemic gravidas on maternal and neonatal blood vitamin levels at delivery. Am J Obstet Gynecol 1974;120:697–703.
5. Frank O, Walbroehl G, Thomson A, Kaminetzky H, Kubes Z, Baker H. Placental transfer: fetal retention of some vitamins. Am J Clin Nutr 1970;23:662–3.
6. Luhby AL, Cooperman JM, Stone ML, Slobody LB. Physiology of vitamin B_{12} in pregnancy, the placenta, and the newborn. Am J Dis Child 1961;102:753–4.
7. Baker H, Ziffer H, Pasher I, Sobotka H. A Comparison of maternal and foetal folic acid and vitamin B_{12} at parturition. Br Med J 1958;1:978–9.
8. Boger WP, Bayne GM, Wright LD, Beck GD. Differential serum vitamin B_{12} concentrations in mothers and infants. N Engl J Med 1957;256:1085–7.
9. Temperley IJ, Meehan MJM, Gatenby PBB. Serum vitamin B12 levels in pregnant women. J Obstet Gynaecol Br Commonw 1968;75:511–6.
10. Boger WP, Wright LD, Beck GD, Bayne GM. Vitamin B_{12}: correlation of serum concentrations and pregnancy. Proc Soc Exp Biol Med 1956;92:140–3.
11. Martin JD, Davis RE, Stenhouse N. Serum folate and vitamin B12 levels in pregnancy with particular reference to uterine bleeding and bacteriuria. J Obstet Gynaecol Br Commonw 1967;74:697–701.
12. Ball EW, Giles C. Folic acid and vitamin B_{12} levels in pregnancy and their relation to megaloblastic anaemia. J Clin Pathol 1964;17:165–74.
13. Izak G, Rachmilewitz M, Stein Y, Berkovici B, Sadovsky A, Aronovitch Y, Grossowicz N. Vitamin B_{12} and iron deficiencies in anemia of pregnancy and puerperium. Arch Intern Med 1957;99:346–55.

14. Edelstein T, Metz J. Correlation between vitamin B12 concentration in serum and muscle in late pregnancy. J Obstet Gynaecol Br Commonw 1969;76:545–8.
15. Herbert V. Recommended dietary intakes (RDI) of vitamin B_{12} in humans. Am J Clin Nutr 1987;45:671–8.
16. Baker H, Frank O, Thomson AD, Langer A, Munves ED, De Angelis B, Kaminetzky HA. Vitamin profile of 174 mothers and newborns at parturition. Am J Clin Nutr 1975;28:59–65.
17. Kaminetzky HA, Baker H. Micronutrients in pregnancy. Clin Obstet Gynecol 1977;20:363–80.
18. Lowenstein L, Lalonde M, Deschenes EB, Shapiro L. Vitamin B_{12} in pregnancy and the puerperium. Am J Clin Nutr 1960;8:265–75.
19. Baker SJ, Jacob E, Rajan KT, Swaminathan SP. Vitamin B_{12} deficiency in pregnancy and the puerperium. Br Med J 1962;1:1658–61.
20. Killander A, Vahlquist B. The vitamin B_{12} concentration in serum from term and premature infants. Nord Med 1954;51:777–9.
21. Baker H, Thind IS, Frank O, DeAngelis B, Caterini H, Lquria DB. Vitamin levels in low-birth-weight newborn infants and their mothers. Am J Obstet Gynecol 1977;129:521–4.
22. Okuda K, Helliger AE, Chow BF. Vitamin B_{12} serum level and pregnancy. Am J Clin Nutr 1956;4:440–3.
23. Baker H, Frank O, Deangelis B, Feingold S, Kaminetzky HA. Role of placenta in maternal–fetal vitamin transfer in humans. Am J Obstet Gynecol 1981;141:792–6.
24. Giugliani ERJ, Jorge SM, Goncalves AL. Serum vitamin B_{12} levels in parturients, in the intervillous space of the placenta and in full-term newborns and their interrelationships with folate levels. Am J Clin Nutr 1985;41:330–5.
25. Giles C. An account of 335 cases of megaloblastic anaemia of pregnancy and the puerperium. J Clin Pathol 1966;19:1–11.
26. Roberts PD, James H, Petrie A, Morgan JO, Hoffbrand AV. Vitamin B_{12} status in pregnancy among immigrants to Britain. Br Med J 1973;3:67–72.
27. Dostalọva L. Correlation of the vitamin status between mother and newborn during delivery. Dev Pharmacol Ther 1982;4(Suppl 1):45–57.
28. McGarry JM, Andrews J. Smoking in pregnancy and vitamin B_{12} metabolism. Br Med J 1972;2:74–7.
29. Heaton D. Another case of megaloblastic anemia of infancy due to maternal pernicious anemia. N Engl J Med 1979;300:202–3.
30. Varadi S. Pernicious anaemia and infertility. Lancet 1967;2:1305.
31. Jackson IMD, Doig WB, McDonald G. Pernicious anaemia as a cause of infertility. Lancet 1967;2:1059–60.
32. Chaudhuri S. Vitamin B_{12} in megaloblastic anaemia of pregnancy and tropical nutritional macrocytic anaemia. Br Med J 1951;2:825–8.
33. Patel JC, Kocher BR. Vitamin B_{12} in macrocytic anaemia of pregnancy and the puerperium. Br Med J 1950;1:924–7.
34. Parr JH, Ramsay I. The presentation of osteomalacia in pregnancy. Case report. Br J Obstet Gynaecol 1984;91:816–8.
35. Streiff RR, Little AB. Folic acid deficiency as a cause of uterine hemorrhage in pregnancy. J Clin Invest 1965;44:1102.
36. Streiff RR, Little AB. Folic acid deficiency in pregnancy. N Engl J Med 1967;276:776–9.
37. Whiteside MG, Ungar B, Cowling DC. Iron, folic acid and vitamin B_{12} levels in normal pregnancy, and their influence on birth weight and the duration of pregnancy. Med J Aust 1968;1:338–42.
38. Shepard TH. *Catalog of Teratogenic Agents*. 3rd ed. Baltimore, MD: The Johns Hopkins University Press, 1980:348–9.
39. Schorah CJ, Smithells RW, Scott J. Vitamin B_{12} and anencephaly. Lancet 1980;1:880.
40. Ampola MG, Mahoney MJ, Nakamura E, Tanaka K. Prenatal therapy of a patient with vitamin B_{12}-responsive methylmalonic acidemia. N Engl J Med 1975;293:313–7.
41. Morrow G III, Schwarz RH, Hallock JA, Barness LA. Prenatal detection of methylmalonic acidemia. J Pediatr 1970;77:120–3.
42. Samson RR, McClelland DBL. Vitamin B_{12} in human colostrum and milk. Acta Paediatr Scand 1980;69:93–9.
43. Deodhar AD, Rajalakshmi R, Ramakrishnan CV. Studies on human lactation. Part III. Effect of dietary vitamin supplementation on vitamin contents of breast milk. Acta Paediatr Scand 1964;53:42–8.
44. Thomas MR, Kawamoto J, Sneed SM, Eakin R. The effects of vitamin C, vitamin B_6, and vitamin B_{12} supplementation on the breast milk and maternal status of well-nourished women. Am J Clin Nutr 1979;32:1679–85.
45. Sneed SM, Zane C, Thomas MR. The effects of ascorbic acid, vitamin B_6, vitamin B_{12}, and folic acid supplementation on the breast milk and maternal nutritional status of low socioeconomic lactating women. Am J Clin Nutr 1981;34:1338–46.
46. Sandberg DP, Begley JA, Hall CA. The content, binding, and forms of vitamin B_{12} in milk. Am J Clin Nutr 1981;34:1717–24.
47. Ford JE, Zechalko A, Murphy J, Brooke OG. Comparison of the B vitamin composition of milk from mothers of preterm and term babies. Arch Dis Child 1983;58:367–72.
48. Lampkin BC, Shore NA, Chadwick D. Megaloblastic anemia of infancy secondary to maternal pernicious anemia. N Engl J Med 1966;274:1168–71.
49. Jadhav M, Webb JKG, Vaishnava S, Baker SJ. Vitamin B_{12} deficiency in Indian infants: a clinical syndrome. Lancet 1962;2:903–7.
50. Lampkin BC, Saunders EF. Nutritional vitamin B_{12} deficiency in an infant. J Pediatr 1969;75:1053–5.
51. Higginbottom MC, Sweetman L, Nyhan WL. A syndrome of methylmalonic aciduria, homocystinuria, megaloblastic anemia and neurologic abnormalities in a vitamin B_{12}-deficient breastfed infant of a strict vegetarian. N Engl J Med 1978;299:317–23.
52. Frader J, Reibman B, Turkewitz D. Vitamin B_{12} deficiency in strict vegetarians. N Engl J Med 1978;299:1319.
53. Fleiss PM, Douglass JM, Wolfe L. Vitamin B_{12} deficiency in strict vegetarians. N Engl J Med 1978;299:1319.
54. Hershaft A. Vitamin B_{12} deficiency in strict vegetarians. N Engl J Med 1978;299:1319–20.
55. Nyhan WL. Vitamin B_{12} deficiency in strict vegetarians. N Engl J Med 1978;299:1320.
56. Abdulla M, Aly KO, Andersson I, Asp NG, Birkhed D, Denker I, Johansson CG, Jagerstad M, Kolar K, Nair BM, Nilsson-Ehle P, Norden A, Rassner S, Svensson S, Akesson B, Ockerman PA. Nutrient intake and health status of lactovegetarians: chemical analyses of diets using the duplicate portion sampling technique. Am J Clin Nutr 1984;40:325–38.
57. Sklar R. Nutritional vitamin B12 deficiency in a breastfed infant of a vegan-diet mother. Clin Pediatr 1986;25:219–21.
58. Committee on Drugs, American Academy of Pediatrics. The transfer of drugs and other chemicals into human milk. Pediatrics 2001;108:776–89.

VITAMIN C

Vitamin

PREGNANCY RECOMMENDATION: Compatible
BREASTFEEDING RECOMMENDATION: Compatible

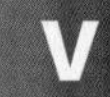

PREGNANCY SUMMARY

Mild to moderate vitamin C deficiency or excessive doses do not seem to pose a major risk to the mother or fetus. Because vitamin C is required for good maternal and fetal health and an increased demand for the vitamin occurs during pregnancy, intake up to the recommended daily allowance (RDA) is recommended.

FETAL RISK SUMMARY

Vitamin C (ascorbic acid) is a water-soluble essential nutrient required for collagen formation, tissue repair, and numerous metabolic processes including the conversion of folic acid to folinic acid and iron metabolism (1). The National Academy of Sciences' RDA for vitamin C in pregnancy is 70 mg (1).

Vitamin C is actively transported to the fetus (2–5). When maternal serum levels are high, placental transfer changes to simple diffusion (5). During gestation, maternal serum vitamin C progressively declines (6,7). As a consequence of this process, newborn serum vitamin C (9–22 mcg/mL) is approximately 2–4 times that of the mother (4–10 mcg/mL) (4–19).

Maternal deficiency of vitamin C without clinical symptoms is common during pregnancy (18–20). Most studies have found no association between this deficiency and maternal or fetal complications, including congenital malformations (11,12,21–24). When low vitamin C levels were found in women or fetuses with complications, it was a consequence of the condition and not a cause. However, a 1971 retrospective study of 1369 mothers found that deficiency of vitamin C may have a teratogenic effect, although the authors advised caution in the interpretation of their results (25). In a later investigation, low 1st trimester white blood cell vitamin C levels were discovered in six mothers giving birth to infants with neural tube defects (26). Folic acid, vitamin B_{12}, and riboflavin were also low in serum or red blood cells. The low folic acid and vitamin B_{12} levels were thought to be involved in the etiology of the defects (see also Folic Acid, Vitamin B_{12}, and Riboflavin).

A 1965 report suggested that high daily doses of vitamin C during pregnancy might have produced a "conditioned" scurvy in two infants (27). The mothers had apparent daily intakes of vitamin C in the 400-mg range throughout pregnancy, but both of their offspring had infantile scurvy. To study this condition, laboratory animals were given various doses of vitamin C throughout gestation. Of the 10 offspring exposed to the highest doses, 2 developed symptoms and histologic changes compatible with scurvy (27). The investigators concluded that the high in utero exposure may have induced ascorbic acid dependency. More recent reports of this condition have not been located; thus, the clinical significance is unknown.

Only one report has been found that potentially relates high doses of vitamin C with fetal anomalies. This was in a brief 1976 case report describing an anencephalic fetus delivered from a woman treated with high doses of vitamin C and other water-soluble vitamins and nutrients for psychiatric reasons (28). The relationship between the defect and the vitamins is unknown. In another study, no evidence of adverse effects was found with doses up to 2000 mg/day (29).

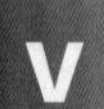

BREASTFEEDING SUMMARY

Vitamin C (ascorbic acid) is excreted into breast milk. Reported concentrations in milk vary from 24 to 158 mcg/mL (30–38). In lactating women with low nutritional status, milk vitamin C is directly proportional to intake (31,32). Supplementation with 4–200 mg/day of vitamin C produced milk levels of 24–61 mcg/mL (31). Similarly, in another group of women with poor vitamin C intake, supplementation with 34–103 mg/day resulted in levels of 34–55 mcg/mL (32). In contrast, studies in well-nourished women consuming the RDA or more of vitamin C in their diets indicate that ingestion of greater amounts does not significantly increase levels of the vitamin in their milk (33–34). Even consumption of total vitamin C exceeding 1000 mg/day, 10 times the RDA, did not significantly increase milk concentrations or vitamin C intake of the infants (36). However, maternal urinary excretion of the vitamin did increase significantly. These studies indicate that vitamin C excretion into milk is regulated to prevent exceeding a saturation level (36).

Storage of human milk in the freezer for up to 3 months did not affect vitamin C concentrations of milk obtained from preterm mothers but resulted in a significant decrease in vitamin C concentrations in milk from term mothers (39). Both types of milk, however, maintained sufficient vitamin C to meet the RDA for infants.

The RDA for vitamin C during lactation is 95 mg (1). Well-nourished lactating women consuming the RDA of vitamin C in their diets normally excrete sufficient vitamin C in their milk to reach a saturation level and additional supplementation is not required. Maternal supplementation up to the RDA is needed only in those women with poor nutritional status.

References

1. American Hospital Formulary Service. *Drug Information 1997*. Bethesda, MD: American Society of Health-System Pharmacists, 1997:2823–5.
2. Hill EP, Longo LD. Dynamics of maternal–fetal nutrient transfer. Fed Proc 1980;39:239–44.
3. Streeter ML, Rosso P. Transport mechanisms for ascorbic acid in the human placenta. Am J Clin Nutr 1981;34:1706–11.
4. Hamil BM, Munks B, Moyer EZ, Kaucher M, Williams HH. Vitamin C in the blood and urine of the newborn and in the cord and maternal blood. Am J Dis Child 1947;74:417–33.
5. Kaminetzky HA, Baker H, Frank O, Langer A. The effects of intravenously administered water-soluble vitamins during labor in normovitaminemic and hypovitaminemic gravidas on maternal and neonatal blood vitamin levels at delivery. Am J Obstet Gynecol 1974;120:697–703.
6. Snelling CE, Jackson SH. Blood studies of vitamin C during pregnancy, birth, and early infancy. J Pediatr 1939;14:447–51.
7. Adlard BPF, De Souza SW, Moon S. Ascorbic acid in fetal human brain. Arch Dis Child 1974;49:278–82.
8. Braestrup PW. Studies of latent scurvy in infants. II. Content of ascorbic (cevitamic) acid in the blood-serum of women in labour and in children at birth. Acta Paediatr 1937;19:328–34.
9. Braestrup PW. The content of reduced ascorbic acid in blood plasma in infants, especially at birth and in the first days of life. J Nutr 1938;16: 363–73.
10. Slobody LB, Benson RA, Mestern J. A comparison of the vitamin C in mothers and their newborn infants. J Pediatr 1946;29:41–4.
11. Teel HM, Burke BS, Draper R. Vitamin C in human pregnancy and lactation. I. Studies during pregnancy. Am J Dis Child 1938;56:1004–10.
12. Lund CJ, Kimble MS. Some determinants of maternal and plasma vitamin C levels. Am J Obstet Gynecol 1943;46:635–47.
13. Manahan CP, Eastman NJ. The cevitamic acid content of fetal blood. Bulletin Johns Hopkins Hospital 1938;62:478–81.
14. Raiha N. On the placental transfer of vitamin C. An experimental study on guinea pigs and human subjects. Acta Physiol Scand 1958;45(Suppl):155.
15. Khattab AK, Al Nagdy SA, Mourad KAH, El Azghal HI. Foetal maternal ascorbic acid gradient in normal Egyptian subjects. J Trop Pediatr 1970;16:112–5.
16. McDevitt E, Dove MA, Dove RF, Wright IS. Selective filtration of vitamin C by the placenta. Proc Soc Exp Biol Med 1942;51:289–90.
17. Sharma SC. Levels of total ascorbic acid, histamine and prostaglandins E_2 and $F_2\alpha$ in the maternal antecubital and foetal umbilical vein blood immediately following the normal human delivery. Int J Vitam Nutr Res 1982;52:320–5.
18. Dostalova L. Correlation of the vitamin status between mother and newborn during delivery. Dev Pharmacol Ther 1982;4(Suppl 1):45–57.

19. Baker H, Frank O, Thomson AD, Langer A, Munves ED, De Angelis B, Kaminetzky HA. Vitamin profile of 174 mothers and newborns at parturition. Am J Clin Nutr 1975;28:59–65.
20. Kaminetzky HA, Langer A, Baker H, Frank O, Thomson AD, Munves ED, Opper A, Behrle FC, Glista B. The effect of nutrition in teenage gravidas on pregnancy and the status of the neonate. I. A nutritional profile. Am J Obstet Gynecol 1973;115:639–46.
21. Martin MP, Bridgforth E, McGanity WJ, Darby WJ. The Vanderbilt cooperative study of maternal and infant nutrition. X. Ascorbic acid. J Nutr 1957;62:201–24.
22. Chaudhuri SK. Role of nutrition in the etiology of toxemia of pregnancy. Am J Obstet Gynecol 1971;110:46–8.
23. Wilson CWM, Loh HS. Vitamin C and fertility. Lancet 1973;2:859–60.
24. Vobecky JS, Vobecky J, Shapcott D, Munan L. Vitamin C and outcome of pregnancy. Lancet 1974;1:630.
25. Nelson MM, Forfar JO. Associations between drugs administered during pregnancy and congenital abnormalities of the fetus. Br Med J 1971;1:523–7.
26. Smithells RW, Sheppard S, Schorah CJ. Vitamin deficiencies and neural tube defects. Arch Dis Child 1976;51:944–50.
27. Cochrane WA. Overnutrition in prenatal and neonatal life: a problem? Can Med Assoc J 1965;93:893–9.
28. Averback P. Anencephaly associated with megavitamin therapy. Can Med Assoc J 1976;114:995.
29. Korner WF, Weber F. Zur toleranz hoher Ascorbinsauredosen. Int J Vitam Nutr Res 1972;42:528–44.
30. Ingalls TH, Draper R, Teel HM. Vitamin C in human pregnancy and lactation. II. Studies during lactation. Am J Dis Child 1938;56:1011–9.
31. Deodhar AD, Rajalakshmi R, Ramakrishnan CV. Studies on human lactation. Part III. Effect of dietary vitamin supplementation on vitamin contents of breast milk. Acta Paediatr 1964;53:42–8.
32. Bates CJ, Prentice AM, Prentice A, Lamb WH, Whitehead RG. The effect of vitamin C supplementation on lactating women in Keneba, a West African rural community. Int J Vitam Nutr Res 1983;53:68–76.
33. Thomas MR, Kawamoto J, Sneed SM, Eakin R. The effects of vitamin C, vitamin B_6, and vitamin B_{12} supplementation on the breast milk and maternal status of well-nourished women. Am J Clin Nutr 1979;32:1679–85.
34. Thomas MR, Sneed SM, Wei C, Nail PA, Wilson M, Sprinkle EE III. The effects of vitamin C, vitamin B_6, vitamin B_{12}, folic acid, riboflavin, and thiamin on the breast milk and maternal status of well-nourished women at 6 months postpartum. Am J Clin Nutr 1980;33:2151–6.
35. Sneed SM, Zane C, Thomas MR. The effects of ascorbic acid, vitamin B_6, vitamin B_{12}, and folic acid supplementation on the breast milk and maternal nutritional status of low socioeconomic lactating women. Am J Clin Nutr 1981;34:1338–46.
36. Byerley LO, Kirksey A. Effects of different levels of vitamin C intake on the vitamin C concentration in human milk and the vitamin C intakes of breast-fed infants. Am J Clin Nutr 1985;41:665–71.
37. Salmenpera L. Vitamin C nutrition during prolonged lactation: optimal in infants while marginal in some mothers. Am J Clin Nutr 1984;40:1050–6.
38. Grewar D. Infantile scurvy. Clin Pediatr 1965;4:82–9.
39. Bank MR, Kirksey A, West K, Giacoia G. Effect of storage time and temperature on folacin and vitamin C levels in term and preterm human milk. Am J Clin Nutr 1985;41:235–42.

VITAMIN D

Vitamin

PREGNANCY RECOMMENDATION: Compatible
BREASTFEEDING RECOMMENDATION: Compatible

PREGNANCY SUMMARY

Vitamin D analogs are a group of fat-soluble nutrients essential for human life with antirachitic and hypercalcemic activity (1). The National Academy of Sciences' recommended dietary allowance (RDA) for normal pregnant women in the United States is 400 IU (1). However, based on evidence that vitamin D deficiency is very common in pregnancy, a much higher dose is required to prevent and treat the deficiency. Although the required pregnancy dose is still under investigation, it may be in the range of 1000–2000 IU of vitamin D_3/day or 50,000 IU of vitamin D_2 every 2 weeks (see reference 37).

FETAL RISK SUMMARY

The two natural biologically active forms of vitamin D are 1,25-dihydroxyergocalciferol and calcitriol (1,25-dihydroxyvitamin D_3) (1). A third active compound, 25-hydroxydihydrotachysterol, is produced in the liver from the synthetic vitamin D analog, dihydrotachysterol.

Ergosterol (provitamin D_2) and 7-dehydrocholesterol (provitamin D_3) are activated by ultraviolet light to form ergocalciferol (vitamin D_2) and cholecalciferol (vitamin D_3), respectively. These, in turn, are converted in the liver to 25-hydroxyergocalciferol and calcifediol (25-hydroxyvitamin D_3), the major transport forms of vitamin D in the body. Activation of the transport compounds by enzymes in the kidneys results in the two natural active forms of vitamin D.

The commercially available forms of vitamin D are ergocalciferol, cholecalciferol, calcifediol, calcitriol, and dihydrotachysterol. Although differing in potency, all of these products have the same result in the mother and fetus. Thus, only the term *vitamin D*, unless otherwise noted, will be used in this monograph.

High doses of vitamin D are known to be teratogenic in experimental animals, but direct evidence for this is lacking in humans. Because of its action to raise calcium levels, vitamin D has been suspected in the pathogenesis of the supravalvular aortic stenosis syndrome, which is often associated with idiopathic hypercalcemia of infancy (2–4). The full features of this rare condition are characteristic elfin facies, mental and growth restriction, strabismus, enamel defects, craniosynostosis, supravalvular aortic and pulmonary stenosis, inguinal hernia, cryptorchidism in males, and early development of secondary sexual characteristics in females (2). Excessive intake or retention of vitamin D during pregnancy by mothers of infants who develop supravalvular aortic stenosis (SAS) syndrome has not been consistently found (2,3,5). However, it is now known that SAS syndrome is a feature of a severe genetic affliction, Williams syndrome, and is not caused by vitamin D (see reference 36).

Very high levels of vitamin D have been used to treat maternal hypoparathyroidism during pregnancy (6–9). In two studies, 15 mothers were treated with doses averaging 107,000 IU/day throughout their pregnancies to maintain maternal calcium levels within the normal range (6,7). All of the 27 children were normal at birth and during follow-up examinations ranging up to 16 years. Calcitriol, in doses ≤3 mcg/day, was used to treat another mother with hypoparathyroidism (8). The high dose was required in the latter half of pregnancy to prevent hypocalcemia. The infant had no apparent adverse effects from this exposure. In a similar case, a mother received 100,000 IU/day throughout gestation, resulting in a healthy, term infant (9). In contrast, a 1965 case report described a woman who received 600,000 IU of vitamin D and 40,000 IU of vitamin A daily for 1 month early in pregnancy (10). The resulting infant had a defect of the urogenital system, but this was probably caused by ingestion of excessive vitamin A (see Vitamin A).

Vitamin D deficiency can be induced by decreased dietary intake or lack of exposure to sunlight. The conversion of provitamin D_3 to vitamin D_3 is catalyzed by ultraviolet light striking the skin (1). Severe deficiency during pregnancy, resulting in maternal osteomalacia, leads to significant morbidity in the mother and fetus (11–21). Pitkin (22), in a 1985 article, reviewed the relationship between vitamin D and calcium metabolism in pregnancy.

The peak incidence of vitamin D deficiency occurs in the winter and early spring when exposure to sunlight is at a minimum. Certain ethnic groups, such as Asians, seem to be at greater risk for developing this deficiency because of their dietary and sun exposure habits (11–21). In the pregnant woman, osteomalacia may cause, among other effects, decreased weight gain and pelvic deformities that prevent normal vaginal delivery (11,12). For the fetus, vitamin D deficiency has been associated with the following:

- Reduced fetal growth (11,12)
- Neonatal hypocalcemia without convulsions (12–14,20)
- Neonatal hypocalcemia with convulsions (tetany) (15–17)
- Neonatal rickets (18,19)
- Defective tooth enamel (21,23)

Long-term use of heparin may induce osteopenia by inhibiting renal activation of calcifediol to the active form of vitamin D_3 (calcitriol or 1,25-dihydroxyvitamin D_3) (22). The decreased levels of calcitriol prevent calcium uptake by bone and result in osteopenia (see reference 23 for detailed review of calcium metabolism in pregnancy). One investigator suggests that these patients may benefit from treatment with supplemental calcitriol (22).

Numerous investigators have measured vitamin D levels in the mother during pregnancy and in the newborn (24–34). Although not universal, most studies have found a significant correlation between maternal serum and cord blood levels (24–28). In one study, a close association between both of the transport vitamin D forms in maternal and cord serum was discovered (29). No significant correlation could be demonstrated, however, between the two biologically active forms in maternal and cord blood.

Using a perfused human placenta, a 1984 report confirmed that calcifediol and calcitriol were transferred from the mother to the fetus, although at a very slow rate (35). Binding to vitamin D_3-binding protein was a major rate-limiting factor, especially for calcifediol, the transport form of vitamin D_3. The researchers concluded that placental metabolism of calcifediol was not a major source of fetal calcitriol (35).

Maternal levels of vitamin D at term are usually higher than those in the newborn because the fetus has no need for intestinal calcium absorption (24–30). Maternal levels are elevated in early pregnancy and continue to increase throughout pregnancy (32). During the winter months a weak correlation may exist between maternal vitamin D intake and serum levels, with exposure to ultraviolet light the main determinant of maternal concentrations (33,34). A Norwegian study, however, was able to increase maternal concentrations of active vitamin D significantly during all seasons with daily supplementation of 400 IU (29).

A 2004 review discussed vitamin D requirements during pregnancy and lactation (36). The daily recommended dose of 200–400 IU was based on erroneous data and was thought to be too low, especially for persons with darkly pigmented skin. Although the appropriate dose in pregnancy and lactation as a function of latitude and race is unknown, the authors thought that daily doses exceeding 1000 IU vitamin D, such as 2000–10,000 IU, were required to overcome vitamin D deficiency and/or to maintain normal blood concentrations of vitamin D. They also cited published evidence showing that the cause of supravalvular aortic stenosis syndrome was actually a severe genetic disorder, Williams syndrome, and was not associated with high concentrations of vitamin D (36).

In a 2007 review of vitamin D deficiency, the recommended doses of vitamin D to prevent and maintain vitamin D concentrations to avoid deficiency in pregnancy or lactation caused by fetal utilization, inadequate sun exposure, or supplementation were vitamin D_3: 1000–2000 IU/day, up to 4000 IU/day is safe for 5 months; vitamin D_2: 50,000 IU every 2 or 4 weeks (37). To treat deficiency caused by the above three conditions, the recommended dose of vitamin D_2 was 50,000 IU every week for 8 weeks and, if the 25-hydroxyvitamin D concentration was <30 ng/mL, repeated for another 8 weeks (37).

In a study reported in 2010, vitamin D levels were measured in 928 pregnant women and 5173 nonpregnant women (38). The mean concentrations in the two groups were 65 and 59 nmol/L (26 and 24 ng/mL), respectively, with a prevalence of <75 nmol/L (<30 ng/mL) in 69% and 78%, respectively. Based on recent evidence, the investigators considered 75 or 100 nmol/L (30 or 40 ng/mL) to be required for optimal health. The clinical implications from this research were: (a) current recommendations for vitamin D supplementation of 200–400 IU/day are inadequate for many women and their infants; (b) vitamin D supplementation should begin a few months before pregnancy; and (c) further studies are required to determine the dose for vitamin D supplementation (38).

A 2010 report noted that vitamin D deficiency was estimated to occur in up to 50% of pregnant women and, compared with other groups African American women had a much higher risk (39). The authors described the effects of vitamin D deficiency on the mother and newborn based on serum concentrations of vitamin D. The maternal effects of severe deficiency (defined as <10 ng/mL) were an increased risk of preeclampsia, calcium malabsorption, bone loss, poor weight gain, myopathy, and higher parathyroid hormone levels, whereas those in the newborn included small for gestational age, hypocalcemia with possible seizures, heart failure, enamel defects, large fontanelle, congenital rickets, and rickets of infancy if breastfed. For serum concentrations (11–32 ng/mL) considered insufficient, the maternal effects were bone loss and subclinical myopathy, whereas those in the newborn were hypocalcemia, decreased bone mineral activity, and rickets if breastfed. There were no maternal or newborn adverse effects if the vitamin D concentration was 32–100 ng/mL, but levels >100 ng/mL could cause maternal hypercalcemia and increased urine calcium loss, and hypercalcemia in the newborn (39).

BREASTFEEDING SUMMARY

Vitamin D is excreted into breast milk in limited amounts (40). A direct relationship exists between maternal serum levels of vitamin D and the concentration in breast milk (41). Chronic maternal ingestion of large doses may lead to greater than normal vitamin D activity in the milk and resulting hypercalcemia in the infant (42). In the lactating woman who was not receiving supplements, controversy exists about whether her milk contained sufficient vitamin D to protect the infant from vitamin deficiency. Several studies had supported the need for infant supplementation during breastfeeding (12,40,43–45). Other investigators had concluded that supplementation is not necessary if maternal vitamin D stores are adequate (28,46–48).

The National Academy of Sciences' RDA for vitamin D in the lactating woman is 400 IU (1). However, recent evidence suggests that vitamin D supplementation of lactating women with much higher doses is necessary to increase the nutritional vitamin D status of the mother and her breastfeeding infant (36,37). This is especially true for darkly pigmented individuals and those having limited exposure to ultraviolet light. Although the required dose has not been adequately studied, doses identical to those described for pregnancy (see Fetal Risk Summary section) have been suggested (37).

A study published in 1977 measured high levels of a vitamin D metabolite in the aqueous phase of milk (49). Although two other studies supported these findings, the conclusions were in direct opposition to previous measurements and have been vigorously disputed (50,51). The argument that human milk is low in vitamin D is supported by clinical reports of vitamin D deficiency-induced rickets and decreased bone mineralization in breastfed infants (44,45,52–54). Moreover, one investigation measured the vitamin D activity of human milk and failed to find any evidence for significant activity of water-soluble vitamin D metabolites (55). Vitamin D activity in the milk was 40–50 IU/L, with 90% of this accounted for by the usual fat-soluble components.

The Committee on Nutrition, American Academy of Pediatrics, recommends vitamin D supplements for breastfed infants if maternal vitamin D nutrition is inadequate or if the infant lacks sufficient exposure to UV light (56). A second committee of the American Academy of Pediatrics classifies vitamin D as compatible with breastfeeding, but recommends monitoring the serum calcium levels of the infant if the mother is receiving pharmacologic doses (57).

References

1. American Hospital Formulary Service. *Drug Information 1997*. Bethesda, MD: American Society of Health-System Pharmacists, 1997:2826–8.
2. Friedman WF, Mills LF. The relationship between vitamin D and the craniofacial and dental anomalies of the supravalvular aortic stenosis syndrome. Pediatrics 1969;43:12–8.
3. Rowe, RD, Cooke RE. Vitamin D and craniofacial and dental anomalies of supravalvular stenosis. Pediatrics 1969;43:1–2.
4. Taussig HB. Possible injury to the cardiovascular system from vitamin D. Ann Intern Med 1966;65:1195–1200.
5. Anita AU, Wiltse HE, Rowe RD, Pitt EL, Levin S, Ottesen OE, Cooke RE. Pathogenesis of the supravalvular aortic stenosis syndrome. J Pediatr 1967;71:431–41.
6. Goodenday LS, Gordan GS. Fetal safety of vitamin D during pregnancy. Clin Res 1971;19:200.
7. Goodenday LS, Gordan GS. No risk from vitamin D in pregnancy. Ann Intern Med 1971;75:807–8.
8. Sadeghi-Nejad A, Wolfsdorf JI, Senior B. Hypoparathyroidism and pregnancy: treatment with calcitriol. JAMA 1980;243:254–5.
9. Greer FR, Hollis BW, Napoli JL. High concentrations of vitamin D_2 in human milk associated with pharmacologic doses of vitamin D_2. J Pediatr 1984;105:61–4.
10. Pilotti G, Scorta A. Ipervitaminosi A gravidica e malformazioni neonatali dell'apparato urinaria. Minerva Ginecol 1965;17:1103–8. As cited in Nishimura H, Tanimura T. *Clinical Aspects of the Teratogenicity of Drugs*. New York, NY: American Elsevier, 1976:251–2.
11. Parr JH, Ramsay I. The presentation of osteomalacia in pregnancy. Case report. Br J Obstet Gynaecol 1984;91:816–8.
12. Brooke OG, Brown IRF, Bone CDM, Carter ND, Cleeve HJW, Maxwell JD, Robinson VP, Winder SM. Vitamin D supplements in pregnant Asian women: effects on calcium status and fetal growth. Br Med J 1980;280:751–4.
13. Rosen JF, Roginsky M, Nathenson G, Finberg L. 25-Hydroxyvitamin D: plasma levels in mothers and their premature infants with neonatal hypocalcemia. Am J Dis Child 1974;127:220–3.
14. Watney PJM, Chance GW, Scott P, Thompson JM. Maternal factors in neonatal hypocalcaemia: a study in three ethnic groups. Br Med J 1971;2:432–6.
15. Heckmatt JZ, Peacock M, Davies AEJ, McMurray J, Isherwood DM. Plasma 25-hydroxyvitamin D in pregnant Asian women and their babies. Lancet 1979;2:546–9.
16. Roberts SA, Cohen MD, Forfar JO. Antenatal factors associated with neonatal hypocalcaemic convulsions. Lancet 1973;2:809–11.
17. Purvis RJ, Barrie WJM, MacKay GS, Wilkinson EM, Cockburn F, Belton NR, Forfar JO. Enamel hypoplasia of the teeth associated with neonatal tetany: a manifestation of maternal vitamin D deficiency. Lancet 1973;2:811–4.
18. Ford JA, Davidson DC, McIntosh WB, Fyfe WM, Dunnigan MG. Neonatal rickets in Asian immigrant population. Br Med J 1973;3:211–2.
19. Moncrieff M, Fadahunsi TO. Congenital rickets due to maternal vitamin D deficiency. Arch Dis Child 1974;49:810–1.
20. Watney PJM. Maternal factors in the aetiology of neonatal hypocalcaemia. Postgrad Med J 1975;51(Suppl 3):14–7.
21. Cockburn F, Belton NR, Purvis RJ, Giles MM, Brown JK, Turner TL, Wilkinson EM, Forfar JO, Barrie WJM, McKay GS, Pocock SJ. Maternal vitamin D intake and mineral metabolism in mothers and their newborn infants. Br Med J 1980;2:11–4.
22. Pitkin RM. Calcium metabolism in pregnancy and the perinatal period: a review. Am J Obstet Gynecol 1985;151:99–109.
23. Stimmler L, Snodgrass GJAI, Jaffe E. Dental defects associated with neonatal symptomatic hypocalcaemia. Arch Dis Child 1973;48:217–20.
24. Hillman LS, Haddad JG. Human perinatal vitamin D metabolism. I: 25-hydroxyvitamin D in maternal and cord blood. J Pediatr 1974;84:742–9.
25. Dent CE, Gupta MM. Plasma 25-hydroxyvitamin D levels during pregnancy in Caucasians and in vegetarian and nonvegetarian Asians. Lancet 1975;2:1057–60.
26. Weisman Y, Occhipinti M, Knox G, Reiter E, Root A. Concentrations of 24,25-dihydroxyvitamin D and 25-hydroxyvitamin D in paired maternal-cord sera. Am J Obstet Gynecol 1978;130:704–7.
27. Steichen JJ, Tsang RC, Gratton TL, Hamstra A, DeLuca HF. Vitamin D homeostasis in the perinatal period: 1,25-dihydroxyvitamin D in maternal, cord, and neonatal blood. N Engl J Med 1980;302:315–9.
28. Birkbeck JA, Scott HF. 25-Hydroxycholecalciferol serum levels in breastfed infants. Arch Dis Child 1980;55:691–5.
29. Markestad T, Aksnes L, Ulstein M, Aarskog D. 25-Hydroxyvitamin D and 1,25-dihydroxyvitamin D of D_2 and D_3 origin in maternal and umbilical cord serum after vitamin D_2 supplementation in human pregnancy. Am J Clin Nutr 1984;40:1057–63.
30. Kumar R, Cohen WR, Epstein FH. Vitamin D and calcium hormones in pregnancy. N Engl J Med 1980;302:1143–5.

V

31. Hillman LS, Haddad JG. Perinatal vitamin D metabolism. II. Serial 25-hydroxyvitamin D concentrations in sera of term and premature infants. J Pediatr 1975;86:928–35.
32. Kumar R, Cohen WR, Silva P, Epstein FH. Elevated 1,25-dihydroxyvitamin D plasma levels in normal human pregnancy and lactation. J Clin Invest 1979;63:342–4.
33. Hillman LS, Haddad JG. Perinatal vitamin D metabolism. III. Factors influencing late gestational human serum 25-hydroxyvitamin D. Am J Obstet Gynecol 1976;125:196–200.
34. Turton CWG, Stanley P, Stamp TCB, Maxwell JD. Altered vitamin D metabolism in pregnancy. Lancet 1977;1:222–5.
35. Ron M, Levitz M, Chuba J, Dancis J. Transfer of 25-hydroxyvitamin D_3 and 1,25-dihydroxyvitamin D_3 across the perfused human placenta. Am J Obstet Gynecol 1984;148:370–4.
36. Hollis BW, Wagner CL. Assessment of dietary vitamin D requirements during pregnancy and lactation. Am J Clin Nutr 2004;79:717–26.
37. Holick MF. Vitamin D deficiency. N Engl J Med 2007;357:266–81.
38. Ginde AA, Sullivan AF, Mansbach JM, Camargo CA Jr. Vitamin D insufficiency in pregnant and nonpregnant women of childbearing age in the United States. Am J Obstet Gynecol 2010;202:436.e1–8.
39. Mulligan ML, Felton SK, Riek AE, Bernal-Mizrachi C. Implications of vitamin D deficiency in pregnancy and lactation. Am J Obstet Gynecol 2010;202:429.e1–9.
40. Greer FR, Hollis BW, Cripps DJ, Tsang RC. Effects of maternal ultraviolet B irradiation on vitamin D content of human milk. J Pediatr 1984;105:431–3.
41. Rothberg AD, Pettifor JM, Cohen DF, Sonnendecker EWW, Ross FP. Maternal-infant vitamin D relationships during breastfeeding. J Pediatr 1982;101:500–3.
42. Goldberg LD. Transmission of a vitamin D metabolite in breast milk. Lancet 1972;2:1258–9.
43. Greer FR, Ho M, Dodson D, Tsang RC. Lack of 25-hydroxyvitamin D and 1,25-dihydroxyvitamin D in human milk. J Pediatr 1981;99:233–5.
44. Greer FR, Searcy JE, Levin RS, Steichen JJ, Steichen-Asch PS, Tsang RC. Bone mineral content and serum 25-hydroxyvitamin D concentration in breastfed infants with and without supplemental vitamin D. J Pediatr 1981;98:696–701.
45. Greer FR, Searcy JE, Levin RS, Steichen JJ, Steichen-Asche PS, Tsang RC. Bone mineral content and serum 25-hydroxyvitamin D concentrations in breastfed infants with and without supplemental vitamin D: one-year follow-up. J Pediatr 1982;100:919–22.
46. Fairney A, Naughten E, Oppe TE. Vitamin D and human lactation. Lancet 1977;2:739–41.
47. Roberts CC, Chan GM, Folland D, Rayburn C, Jackson R. Adequate bone mineralization in breastfed infants. J Pediatr 1981;99:192–6.
48. Chadwick DW. Commentary. Water-soluble vitamin D in human milk: a myth. Pediatrics 1982;70:499.
49. Lakdawala DR, Widdowson EM. Vitamin D in human milk. Lancet 1977;1:167–8.
50. Greer FR, Reeve LE, Chesney RW, DeLuca HF. Water-soluble vitamin D in human milk: a myth. Pediatrics 1982;69:238.
51. Greer FR, Reeve LE, Chesney RW, DeLuca HF. Commentary. Water-soluble vitamin D in human milk: a myth. Pediatrics 1982;70:499–500.
52. Bunker JWM, Harris RS, Eustis RS. The antirachitic potency of the milk of human mothers fed previously on "vitamin D milk" of the cow. N Engl J Med 1933;208:313–5.
53. O'Connor P. Vitamin D-deficiency rickets in two breastfed infants who were not receiving vitamin D supplementation. Clin Pediatr (Phila) 1977;16:361–3.
54. Little JA. Commentary. Water-soluble vitamin D in human milk: a myth. Pediatrics 1982;70:499.
55. Reeve LE, Chesney RW, DeLuca HF. Vitamin D of human milk: identification of biologically active forms. Am J Clin Nutr 1982;36:122–6.
56. Committee on Nutrition, American Academy of Pediatrics. Vitamin and mineral supplement needs in normal children in the United States. Pediatrics 1980;66:1015.
57. Committee on Drugs, American Academy of Pediatrics. The transfer of drugs and other chemicals into human milk. Pediatrics 2001;108:776–89.

VITAMIN E

Vitamin

PREGNANCY RECOMMENDATION: Compatible
BREASTFEEDING RECOMMENDATION: Compatible

PREGNANCY SUMMARY

Neither deficiency nor excess of vitamin E has been associated with maternal or fetal complications during pregnancy. One study did find a lower birth weight in infants of women taking high doses of vitamin E during pregnancy, but the reduced weight was not thought to be clinically significant and may have been due to other factors. However, in well-nourished women, adequate vitamin E is consumed in the diet and supplementation is not required. If dietary intake is poor, supplementation up to the recommended daily allowance (RDA) for pregnancy is recommended.

FETAL RISK SUMMARY

Vitamin E (tocopherols) is comprised of a group of fat-soluble vitamins that are essential for human health, although their exact biologic function is unknown (1). The National Academy of Sciences' RDA for vitamin E in pregnancy is 10 mg (1).

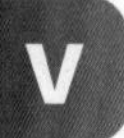

Vitamin E concentrations in mothers at term are approximately 4–5 times that of the newborn (2–8). Levels in the mother rise throughout pregnancy (3). Maternal blood vitamin E level usually ranges between 9 and 19 mcg/mL with corresponding newborn levels varying from 2 to 6 mcg/mL (2–9). Supplementation of the mother with 15–30 mg/day had no effect on either maternal or newborn vitamin E concentrations at term (4). Use of 600 mg/day in the last 2 months of pregnancy produced about a 50% rise in maternal serum vitamin E (+8 mcg/mL) but a much smaller increase in the cord blood (+1 mcg/mL) (7). Although placental transfer is by passive diffusion, passage of vitamin E to the fetus is dependent on plasma lipid concentrations (8–10). At term, cord blood is low in β-lipoproteins, the major carriers of vitamin E, in comparison with maternal blood; as a consequence, it is able to transport less of the vitamin (8). Because vitamin E is transported in the plasma by these lipids, recent investigations have focused on the ratio of vitamin E (in milligrams) to total lipids (in grams) rather than on blood vitamin E concentrations alone (9). Ratios above about 0.6–0.8 are considered normal depending on the author cited and the age of the patients (9,11,12).

A 2005 prospective, observational study reported the pregnancy outcomes of 82 women who had taken high-dose vitamin E (≥400 IU/day) in the 1st trimester and compared them with 130 matched controls exposed to agents not known to cause embryo–fetal harm (13). The reason given by the women for taking high doses was that large amounts of vitamins were part of a healthy lifestyle, but none took large doses of vitamins A and D. The two groups were enrolled in the study at a mean gestational age of 13.1 and 6.2 weeks', respectively. In the subject group, doses of 400, 800, or 1200 IU/day were taken by 74, 7, and 1 women, respectively. The mean duration was 6 months and 44 (54%) took a high dose throughout gestation. There were no differences in the outcomes between the groups in terms of live births, spontaneous abortions, elective abortions, stillbirths, gestational age at delivery, prematurity, and malformations. The mean birth weight, however, was lower in subjects than in controls, 3173 vs. 3417 g, respectively ($p = 0.0015$). Because only two infants had a birth weight <2500 g, the difference was thought to have a questionable clinical significance. Moreover, vigorous exercise was thought to be part of a "healthy lifestyle" and it might also reduce birth weight (13).

Vitamin E deficiency is relatively uncommon in pregnancy, occurring in less than 10% of all patients (3,4,14). No maternal or fetal complications from deficiency or excess of the vitamin have been identified. Doses far exceeding the RDA have not proved to be harmful (7,15,16). Early studies used vitamin E in conjunction with other therapy in attempts to prevent abortion and premature labor, but no effect of the vitamin therapy was demonstrated (17,18). Premature infants born with low vitamin E stores may develop hemolytic anemia, edema, reticulocytosis, and thrombocytosis if not given adequate vitamin E in the first months following birth (16,19,20). In two studies, supplementation of mothers with 500–600 mg of vitamin E during the last 1–2 months of pregnancy did not produce values significantly different from controls in the erythrocyte hemolysis test with hydrogen peroxide, a test used to determine adequate levels of vitamin E (7,16).

BREASTFEEDING SUMMARY

Vitamin E is excreted into breast milk (11,12,21,22). Human milk is more than 5 times richer in vitamin E than cow's milk and is more effective in maintaining adequate serum vitamin E and vitamin E:total lipid ratio in infants up to 1 year of age (11,22). A 1985 study measured 2.3 mcg/mL of the vitamin in mature milk (21). Milk obtained from preterm mothers (gestational age 27–33 weeks) was significantly higher (8.5 mcg/mL) during the first week and then decreased progressively over the next 6 weeks to 3.7 mcg/mL (21). The authors concluded that milk from preterm mothers plus multivitamin supplements would provide adequate levels of vitamin E for very low-birth-weight infants (<1500 g and appropriate for gestational age).

Japanese researchers examined the pattern of vitamin E analogs (α-, γ-, δ-, and β-tocopherols) in plasma and red blood cells from breastfed and bottle-fed infants (23). Several differences were noted, but the significance of these findings to human health is unknown.

Vitamin E applied for 6 days to the nipples of breastfeeding women resulted in a significant rise in infant serum levels of the vitamin (24). The study group, composed of 10 women, applied the contents of one 400-IU vitamin E capsule to both areolae and nipples after each nursing. Serum concentrations of the vitamin rose from 4 to 17.5 mcg/mL and those in a similar group of untreated controls rose from 3.4 to 12.2 mcg/mL. The difference between the two groups was statistically significant ($p < 0.025$). Although no adverse effects were observed, the authors cautioned that the long-term effects were unknown.

The National Academy of Sciences' RDA of vitamin E during lactation is 12 mg (1). Maternal supplementation is recommended only if the diet does not provide sufficient vitamin E to meet the RDA.

References

1. American Hospital Formulary Service. *Drug Information 1997*. Bethesda, MD: American Society of Health-System Pharmacists, 1997:2832–3.
2. Moyer WT. Vitamin E levels in term and premature newborn infants. Pediatrics 1950;6:893–6.
3. Leonard PJ, Doyle E, Harrington W. Levels of vitamin E in the plasma of newborn infants and of the mothers. Am J Clin Nutr 1972;25:480–4.
4. Baker H, Frank O, Thomson AD, Langer A, Munves ED, De Angelis B, Kaminetzky HA. Vitamin profile of 174 mothers and newborns at parturition. Am J Clin Nutr 1975;28:59–65.
5. Dostalova L. Correlation of the vitamin status between mother and newborn during delivery. Dev Pharmacol Ther 1982;4(Suppl I):45–57.
6. Kaminetzky HA, Baker H. Micronutrients in pregnancy. Clin Obstet Gynecol 1977;20:363–80.
7. Mino M, Nishino H. Fetal and maternal relationship in serum vitamin E level. J Nutr Sci Vitaminol 1973;19:475–82.
8. Haga P, Ek J, Kran S. Plasma tocopherol levels and vitamin E/B-lipoprotein relationships during pregnancy and in cord blood. Am J Clin Nutr 1982;36:1200–4.
9. Martinez FE, Goncalves AL, Jorge SM, Desai ID. Vitamin E in placental blood and its interrelationship to maternal and newborn levels of vitamin E. J Pediatr 1981;99:298–300.
10. Hill EP, Longo LD. Dynamics of maternal-fetal nutrient transfer. Fed Proc 1980;39:239–44.
11. Martinez FE, Jorge SM, Goncalves AL, Desai ID. Evaluation of plasma tocopherols in relation to hematological indices of Brazilian infants on human milk and cows' milk regime from birth to 1 year of age. Am J Clin Nutr 1984;39:969–74.
12. Mino M, Kitagawa M, Nakagawa S. Red blood cell tocopherol concentrations in a normal population of Japanese children and premature infants in relation to the assessment of vitamin E status. Am J Clin Nutr 1985;41:631–8.
13. Boskovic R, Gargaun L, Oren D, Djulus J, Koren G. Pregnancy outcome following high doses of vitamin E supplementation. Reprod Toxicol 2005;20:85–8.
14. Kaminetzky HA, Langer A, Baker O, Frank O, Thomson AD, Munves ED, Opper A, Behrle FC, Glista B. The effect of nutrition in teenage gravidas on pregnancy and the status of the neonate. I. A nutritional profile. Am J Obstet Gynecol 1973;115:639–46.
15. Hook EB, Healy KM, Niles AM, Skalko RG. Vitamin E: teratogen or anti-teratogen? Lancet 1974;1:809.
16. Gyorgy P, Cogan G, Rose CS. Availability of vitamin E in the newborn infant. Proc Soc Exp Biol Med 1952;81:536–8.
17. Kotz J, Parker E, Kaufman MS. Treatment of recurrent and threatened abortion. Report of two hundred and twenty-six cases. J Clin Endocrinol 1941;1:838–49.
18. Shute E. Vitamin E and premature labor. Am J Obstet Gynecol 1942;44:271–9.
19. Oski FA, Barness LA. Vitamin E deficiency: a previously unrecognized cause of hemolytic anemia in the premature infant. J Pediatr 1967;70:211–20.
20. Ritchie JH, Fish MB, McMasters V, Grossman M. Edema and hemolytic anemia in premature infants. A vitamin E deficiency syndrome. N Engl J Med 1968;279:1185–90.
21. Gross SJ, Gabriel E. Vitamin E status in preterm infants fed human milk or infant formula. J Pediatr 1985;106:635–9.
22. Friedman Z. Essential fatty acids revisited. Am J Dis Child 1980;134:397–408.
23. Mino M, Kijima Y, Nishida Y, Nakagawa S. Difference in plasma- and red blood cell-tocopherols in breastfed and bottle-fed infants. J Nutr Sci Vitaminol 1980;26:103–12.
24. Marx CM, Izquierdo A, Driscoll JW, Murray MA, Epstein MF. Vitamin E concentrations in serum of newborn infants after topical use of vitamin E by nursing mothers. Am J Obstet Gynecol 1985;152:668–70.

VITAMINS, MULTIPLE

Vitamins

PREGNANCY RECOMMENDATION: Compatible
BREASTFEEDING RECOMMENDATION: Compatible

PREGNANCY SUMMARY

The use of multivitamins up to the recommended daily allowance (RDA) for pregnancy is recommended for the general good health of the mother and the fetus. There is no strong evidence to suggest that vitamin supplementation can prevent cleft lip and/or palate (CLP). However, a body of evidence has accumulated that supplementation during the first few weeks of gestation, especially with folic acid, may reduce the risk of neural tube defects (NTDs) (see Folic Acid). The evidence appears particularly strong for the prevention of NTD recurrences in England. Additional studies will be needed to establish whether the protective effect includes only certain types of patients. Until that time, it seems prudent to recommend that folate-containing multivitamin preparations should be used immediately before and during at least the first few months of pregnancy. Women who have had gastric bypass surgery for obesity may be at increased risk for delivering offspring with NTDs, and pregnancy counseling to ensure adequate nutritional intake may be of benefit.

FETAL RISK SUMMARY

Vitamins are essential for human life. Preparations containing multiple vitamins (multivitamins) are routinely given to pregnant women. A typical product will contain the vitamins A, D, E, and C, plus the B-complex vitamins thiamine (B_1), riboflavin (B_2), niacin (B_3), pantothenic acid (B_5), pyridoxine (B_6), B_{12}, and folic acid. Miscellaneous substances that may be included are iron, calcium, and other minerals. The practice of supplementation during pregnancy with multivitamins varies from country to country but is common in the United States. The National Academy of Sciences' RDA for pregnant women, as of 1989, is as follows (1):

Vitamin A	800 RE	Niacin (B_3)	17 mg
Vitamin D	400 IU	Pyridoxine (B_6)	2.2 mg
Vitamin C	70 mg	Folic acid	0.4 mg
Thiamine (B_1)	1.5 mg	Vitamin B_{12}	2.2 mcg
Riboflavin (B_2)	1.6 mg	Vitamin E	10 mg

Although essential for health, vitamin K is normally not included in multivitamin preparations because it is adequately supplied from natural sources. The fat-soluble vitamins, A, D, and E, may be toxic or teratogenic in high doses. The water-soluble vitamins, C and the B-complex group, are generally considered safe in amounts above the RDA, but there are exceptions. Deficiencies of vitamins may also be teratogenic (see individual vitamin monographs for further details).

The role of vitamins in the prevention of certain congenital defects continues to be a major area of controversy. Two classes of anomalies, CLP and NTDs, have been the focus of numerous investigations with multivitamins. An investigation into a third class of anomalies, limb reduction defects, has also appeared. The following sections will summarize the published work on these topics.

Animal research in the 1930s and 1940s had shown that both deficiencies and excesses of selected vitamins could result in fetal anomalies, but it was not until two papers in 1958 (2,3) that attention was turned to humans. These investigations examined the role of environmental factors, in particular the B-complex vitamins, as agents for preventing the recurrence of CLP. In that same year, a study was published that involved 87 women who had previously given birth to infants with CLP (4). Although the series was too small to draw statistical conclusions, 48 women given no vitamin supplements had 78 pregnancies, resulting in 4 infants with CLP. The treated group, composed of 39 women, received multivitamins plus injectable B-complex vitamins during the 1st trimester. This group had 59 pregnancies with none of the infants having CLP. A similar study found a CLP incidence of 1.9% (3 of 156) in treated pregnancies compared with 5.7% (22 of 383) in controls (5). The difference was not statistically significant. However, other researchers, in a 1964 survey, found no evidence that vitamins offered protection against CLP (6). Also in 1964, research was published involving 594 pregnant women who had previously given birth to an infant with CLP (7). This work was further expanded, and the total group involving 645 pregnancies was presented in a 1976 paper (8). Of the total group, 417 women were not given supplements during pregnancy, and they gave birth to 20 infants (4.8%) with CLP. In the treated group, 228 women were given B-complex vitamins plus vitamin C before or during the 1st trimester. From this latter group, seven infants (3.1%) with CLP resulted. Although suggestive of a positive effect, the difference between the two groups was not significant. Another investigator found only one instance of CLP in his group of 85 supplemented pregnancies (9). These patients were given daily multivitamins plus 10 mg of folic acid. In 206 pregnancies in women not given supplements in which the infants or fetuses were examined, 15 instances of CLP resulted. The difference between the two groups was significant ($p = 0.023$). In contrast, one author suggested that the vitamin A in the supplements caused a cleft palate in his patient (10). However, the conclusion of this report has been disputed (11). Thus, the published studies involving the role of multivitamins in the prevention of cleft lip and/or palate are inconclusive. No decisive benefit (or risk) of multivitamin supplementation has emerged from any of the studies.

The second part of the controversy surrounding multivitamins and the prevention of congenital defects involves their role in preventing NTDs. (Three excellent reviews on the pathophysiology and various other aspects of NTDs, including discussions on the role that multivitamins might play in the cause and prevention of these defects, have been recently published [12–14].) In a series of articles from 1976 to 1983, British investigators examined the effect of multivitamin supplements on a group of women who had previously given birth to one or more children with NTDs (15–19). For the purpose of their study, they defined NTDs to include anencephaly, encephalocele, cranial meningocele, iniencephaly, myelocele, myelomeningocele, and meningocele but excluded isolated hydrocephalus and spina bifida occulta (17). In their initial publication, they found that, in six mothers who had given birth to infants with NTDs, there were lower 1st trimester levels of serum folate, red blood cell folate, white blood cell vitamin C, and riboflavin saturation index (15). The differences between the case mothers and the controls were significant for red blood cell folate ($p < 0.001$) and white blood cell vitamin C ($p < 0.05$). Serum vitamin A levels were comparable with those of controls. Based on this experience, a multicenter study was launched to compare mothers receiving full supplements with control patients not receiving supplements (16–19). The supplemented group received a multivitamin–iron–calcium preparation from 28 days before conception to the date of the second missed menstrual period, which is after the time of neural tube closure. The daily vitamin supplement provided:

Vitamin A	4000 IU	Nicotinamide	15 mg
Vitamin D	400 IU	Pyridoxine	1 mg
Vitamin C	40 mg	Folic acid	0.36 mg
Thiamine	1.5 mg	Ferrous sulfate	75.6 mg (as Fe)
Riboflavin	1.5 mg	Calcium phosphate	480 mg

Their findings, summarized in 1983, are shown below for the infants and fetuses who were examined (19):

One Previous NTD	
Supplemented	385
Recurrences	2* (0.5%)
Not supplemented	458
Recurrences	19* (4.1%) *$p = 0.0004$
Two or More Previous NTDs	
Supplemented	44
Recurrences	1* (2.3%)
Not supplemented	52
Recurrences	5* (9.6%) *$p = 0.145$
Total	
Supplemented	429
Recurrences	3 (0.7%)
Not supplemented	510
Recurrences	24 (4.7%)

Although the numbers were suggestive of a protective effect offered by multivitamins, at least three other explanations were offered by the investigators (16):

1. A low-risk group had selected itself for supplementation.
2. The study group aborted more NTD fetuses than did controls.
3. Other factors were responsible for the reduction in NTDs.

A 1980 report found that women receiving well-balanced diets had a lower incidence and recurrence rate of infants with NTDs than did women receiving poor diets (20). Although multivitamin supplements were not studied, it was assumed that those patients who consumed adequate diets also consumed more vitamins from their food compared with those with poor diets. This study, then, added credibility to the thesis that good nutrition can prevent some NTDs. Other researchers, using Smithells' protocol, observed that fully supplemented mothers ($N = 83$) had no recurrences, whereas a nonsupplemented group ($N = 141$) had four recurrences of NTDs (21,22). Interestingly, a short report that appeared 6 years before Smithells' work found that both vitamins and iron were consumed more by mothers who gave birth to infants with anencephalus and spina bifida (23).

The above investigations have generated many discussions, criticisms, and defenses (24–57). The primary criticism centered on the fact that the groups were not randomly assigned but were self-selected for supplementation or no supplementation. A follow-up study, in response to some of these objections, was published in 1986 (58). This study examined six factors that may have influenced the earlier results by increasing the risk of recurrence of NTDs: (a) two or more previous NTDs, (b) residence in Northern Ireland, (c) spontaneous abortions immediately before the studied pregnancy, (d) <12 months between studied pregnancy and abortion, (e) social class, and (f) therapeutic abortion immediately before the studied pregnancy. The relative risk was increased only for the first four factors, and only in those cases with two or more previous NTDs was the increase significant. In addition, none of the four factors would have predicted more than a 4% increase in the recurrence rate in nonsupplemented mothers compared with those supplemented. The results indicated that none of these factors contributed significantly to the differential risk between supplemented and nonsupplemented mothers, thus leading to the conclusion that the difference in recurrence rates was caused by the multivitamin (58).

Several recent studies examining the effect of multivitamins on NTDs have been published. A case–control, population-based study evaluated the association between periconceptional (3 months before and after conception) multivitamin use and the occurrence of NTDs (59). The case group involved either liveborn or stillborn infants with anencephaly or spina bifida born during the years 1968–1980 in the Atlanta area. A total of 347 infants with NTDs were eligible for enrollment and became the case group, whereas 2829 infants without birth defects served as controls. Multivitamin usage and other factors were ascertained by interview 2–16 years after the pregnancies. This long time interval might have induced a recall problem into the study, even though the authors did take steps to minimize any potential bias (59). A protective effect of periconceptional multivitamin usage against having an infant with an NTD was found in comparison with controls with an estimated relative risk for all NTDs of 0.41 (95% confidence interval [CI] 0.26–0.66); anencephaly 0.47 (95% CI 0.25–0.91); and spina bifida 0.37 (95% CI 0.19–0.70). The odds ratios for whites, but not for other races, were statistically significant. Except for anencephaly among whites (odds ratio [OR] 0.68, 95% CI 0.35–1.34), similar results were obtained when infants with congenital defects other than NTDs were used as controls. Although the results indicated that periconceptional use of multivitamins did protect against NTDs, the authors could not determine whether the effect was related to vitamins or to some unknown characteristic of vitamin users (59). In commenting on this study, one investigator speculated that if the lack of a statistical effect observed in black women was confirmed, it may be related to a different genetic makeup of the population (60). In other words, the gene(s) that cause NTDs are responsive to periconceptional multivitamins only in whites (60).

Three brief letter communications examined the effects of gastric or intestinal bypass surgery, performed for obesity, on the incidence of NTDs (61–63). The first report appeared in 1986 and described three births with NTDs occurring in Maine (61). During the interval 1980–1984, 261 gastric bypass procedures were performed in Maine, but only 133 were in women under the age of 35. One woman delivered an anencephalic fetus 2 years after her surgery. A second suffered a spontaneous abortion at 16 weeks' gestation, 6 years after a gastrojejunostomy. Her serum α-fetoprotein level 10 days before the abortion was 4.8 times the median. She became pregnant again 2 years later and eventually delivered a stillborn infant in the 3rd trimester. The infant had a midthoracic meningomyelocele, iniencephaly, absence of diaphragms, and hypoplastic lungs. During this latter pregnancy, she had intermittent heavy alcohol intake. In the third case, a woman, whose surgery had been done 7 years earlier, had an anencephalic fetus associated with a lumbar rachischisis diagnosed at 6 months' gestation. In response to this report, investigators in Denmark and Sweden could find no cases of NTDs in 77 infants born after their mothers had bypass operations for obesity (62). However, the procedures in these cases involved intestinal bypass, not gastric. Low birth weight and growth restriction were increased in 64 liveborn infants. Gastric bypass surgery is known to place recipients at risk for nutritional deficiencies, especially for iron, calcium, vitamin B_{12}, and folate (61,63). In the third report, of a total of 908 women who underwent the procedure, 511 (56%) responded to a questionnaire (63). Of these, 87 (17%) had been pregnant at least once after the surgery. The 87 women had 73 pregnancies (more than 20 weeks' gestation) before the operation with no cases of NTDs. After the surgery, these women had 110 pregnancies with two cases of NTDs. This represented a 12 times increase in the risk for NTDs compared with the general population (incidence 0.15%) (63). A third case of an infant with an NTD born from a mother who had undergone the operation was identified later, but the mother was not part of the original group. In each of the three cases, the birth of the infant with an NTD had occurred $>$4 years after the bypass surgery. Moreover, the three mothers had not consumed vitamin supplements as prescribed by their physicians. Because of these findings, the authors recommended pregnancy counseling for any woman who has undergone this procedure and who then desires to become pregnant (63).

In another brief reference, the final results of a British clinical trial were presented in 1989 (64). Women who resided in the Yorkshire region were enrolled in the study if (a) they had one or more previous NTD infants, (b) they were not pregnant at the time of enrollment, and (c) they were considering another pregnancy. Mothers were requested to take the vitamin formulation described above for at least 4 weeks before conception and until they had missed two menstrual periods (i.e., same as previously). The results of the study included three reporting intervals: 1977–1980, 1981–1984, and 1985–1987. The 148 fully supplemented mothers (those who took vitamins as prescribed or missed taking vitamins on only 1 day) had 150 infants or fetuses, only 1 (0.7%) of whom had an NTD. In contrast, 315 nonsupplemented mothers had 320 infants or fetuses among which there were 18 (5.6%) cases of NTDs. The difference between the groups was significant (p = 0.006). In addition, 37 partially supplemented (defined as mothers who took the prescribed vitamin for a shorter period of time than the fully supplemented group) women had 37 pregnancies with no cases of NTDs. The investigators concluded that the difference between the groups could not be attributed to declining NTD recurrence rates or to selection bias. Summarizing these and previously published results, only 1 NTD recurrence had been observed in 315 infants or fetuses born to 274 fully supplemented mothers, and no recurrences had been observed among 57 examined infants or fetuses born to 58 partially supplemented women (64).

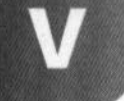

A 1989 study conducted in California and Illinois examined three groups of patients to determine whether multivitamins had a protective effect against NTDs (65). The groups were composed of women who had a conceptus with an NTD (N = 571) and two control groups: those who had a stillbirth or other defect (N = 546), and women who had delivered a normal child (N = 573). In this study, NTDs included anencephaly, meningocele, myelomeningocele, encephalocele, rachischisis, iniencephaly, and lipomeningocele. The periconceptional use of multivitamins, both in terms of vitamin supplements only and when combined with fortified cereals, was then evaluated for each of the groups. The outcome of this study, after appropriate adjustment for potential confounding factors, revealed an OR of 0.95 (95% CI 0.78–1.14) for NTD-supplemented mothers (i.e., those who received the RDA of vitamins or more) compared with nonsupplemented mothers of abnormal infants, and an OR of 1.00 (95% CI 0.83–1.20) when the NTD group was compared with unsupplemented mothers of normal infants. Only slight differences from these values occurred when the data were evaluated by considering vitamin supplements only (no fortified cereals) or vitamin supplements of any amount (i.e., less than the RDA). Similarly, examination of the data for an effect of folate supplementation on the occurrence of NTDs did not change the results. Thus, this study could not show that the use of either multivitamin or folate supplements reduced the frequency of NTDs. However, the investigators cautioned that their results could not exclude the possibility that vitamins might be of benefit in a high-risk population. Several reasons were proposed by the authors to explain why their results differed from those obtained in the Atlanta study cited above: (a) recall bias, (b) a declining incidence of NTDs, (c) geographic differences such that a subset of vitamin-preventable NTDs was in the Atlanta region but not in the areas of the current study, and (d) the Atlanta study did not consider the vitamins contained in fortified cereals (65). However, others concluded that this study lead to a null result because: (a) the vitamin consumption history was obtained after delivery, (b) the history was obtained after the defect was identified, or (c) the study excluded those women taking vitamins after they knew they were pregnant (66).

In contrast to the above report, a Boston study published in 1989 found a significant effect of folic acid–containing multivitamins on the occurrence of NTDs (66). The study population was comprised of 22,715 women for whom complete information on vitamin consumption and pregnancy outcomes was available. Women were interviewed at the time of a maternal serum α-fetoprotein screen or an amniocentesis. Thus, in most cases, the interview was conducted before the results of the tests were known to either the patient or the interviewer. A total of 49 women had an NTD outcome (2.2/1000). Among these, 3 cases occurred in 107 women with a history of previous NTDs (28.0/1000), and 2 in 489 women with a family history of NTDs in someone other than an offspring (4.1/1000). After excluding the 87 women whose family history of NTDs was unknown, the incidence of NTDs in the remaining women was 44 cases in 22,093 (2.0/1000). Among the 3157 women who did not use a folic acid–containing multivitamin, 11 cases of NTD occurred, a prevalence of 3.5/1000. For those using the preparation during the first 6 weeks of pregnancy, 10 cases occurred from a total of 10,713 women (prevalence 0.9/1000). The prevalence ratio estimate for these two groups was 0.27 (95% CI 0.12–0.59). For mothers who used vitamins during the first 6 weeks that did not contain folic acid, the prevalence was 3 cases in 926, a ratio of 3.2. The ratio, when compared with that of nonusers, was 0.93 (95% CI 0.26–3.3). When vitamin use was started in the 7th week of gestation, there were 25 cases of NTD from 7795 mothers using the folic acid–multivitamin supplements (prevalence 3.2/1000; prevalence ratio 0.92) and no cases in the 66 women who started consuming multivitamins without folate. This study, then, observed a markedly reduced risk of NTDs when folic acid–containing multivitamin preparations were consumed in the first 6 weeks of gestation.

An investigation into a third class of anomalies, limb reduction defects, was opened by a report that multivitamins may have caused this malformation in an otherwise healthy boy (52). The mother was taking the preparation because of a previous birth of a child with an NTD. A retrospective analysis of Finnish records, however, failed to show any association between 1st trimester use of multivitamins and limb reduction defects (67).

BREASTFEEDING SUMMARY

Vitamins are naturally present in breast milk (see individual vitamins). The recommended dietary allowance of vitamins and minerals during lactation (first 6 months) are as follows (1):

Vitamin A	1300 RE	Vitamin B_{12}	2.6 mcg
Vitamin D	400 IU	Calcium	1200 mg
Vitamin E	12 mg	Phosphorus	1200 mg
Vitamin C	95 mg	Iodine	200 mcg
Folic acid	280 mcg	Iron	15 mg
Thiamine (B_1)	1.6 mg	Magnesium	355 mg
Riboflavin (B_2)	1.8 mg	Zinc	19 mg
Niacin (B_3)	20 mg	Selenium	75 mcg
Pyridoxine (B_6)	2.1 mg		

References

1. American Hospital Formulary Service. *Drug Information 1997*. Bethesda, MD: American Society of Health-System Pharmacists, 1997:2805.
2. Douglas B. The role of environmental factors in the etiology of "so-called" congenital malformations. I. Deductions from the presence of cleft lip and palate in one of identical twins, from embryology and from animal experiments. Plast Reconstr Surg 1958;22:94–108.
3. Douglas B. The role of environmental factors in the etiology of "so-called" congenital malformations. II. Approaches in humans; study of various extragenital factors, "theory of compensatory nutrients," development of regime for first trimester. Plast Reconstr Surg 1958;22:214–29.
4. Conway H. Effect of supplemental vitamin therapy on the limitation of incidence of cleft lip and cleft palate in humans. Plast Reconstr Surg 1958;22:450–3.
5. Peer LA, Gordon HW, Bernhard WG. Experimental production of congenital deformities and their possible prevention in man. J Int Coll Surg 1963;39:23–35.
6. Fraser FC, Warburton D. No association of emotional stress or vitamin supplement during pregnancy to cleft lip or palate in man. Plast Reconstr Surg 1964;33:395–9.
7. Peer LA, Gordon HW, Bernhard WG. Effect of vitamins on human teratology. Plast Reconstr Surg 1964;34:358–62.
8. Briggs RM. Vitamin supplementation as a possible factor in the incidence of cleft lip/palate deformities in humans. Clin Plast Surg 1976;3:647–52.
9. Tolarova M. Periconceptional supplementation with vitamins and folic acid to prevent recurrence of cleft lip. Lancet 1982;2:217.
10. Bound JP. Spina bifida and vitamins. Br Med J 1983;286:147.
11. Smithells RW. Spina bifida and vitamins. Br Med J 1983;286:388–9.
12. Main DM, Mennuti MT. Neural tube defects: issues in prenatal diagnosis and counseling. Obstet Gynecol 1986;67:1–16.
13. Rhoads GG, Mills JL. Can vitamin supplements prevent neural tube defects? Current evidence and ongoing investigations. Clin Obstet Gynecol 1986;29:569–79.
14. Lemire RJ. Neural tube defects. JAMA 1988;259:558–62.
15. Smithells RW, Sheppard S, Schorah CJ. Vitamin deficiencies and neural tube defects. Arch Dis Child 1976;51:944–50.
16. Smithells RW, Sheppard S, Schorah CJ, Seller MJ, Nevin NC, Harris R, Read AP, Fielding DW. Possible prevention of neural-tube defects by periconceptional vitamin supplementation. Lancet 1980;1:339–40.
17. Smithells RW, Sheppard S, Schorah CJ, Seller MJ, Nevin NC, Harris R, Read AP, Fielding DW. Apparent prevention of neural tube defects by periconceptional vitamin supplementation. Arch Dis Child 1981;56:911–8.
18. Smithells RW, Sheppard S, Schorah CJ, Seller MJ, Nevin NC, Harris R, Read AP, Fielding DW, Walker S. Vitamin supplementation and neural tube defects. Lancet 1981;2:1425.
19. Smithells RW, Nevin NC, Seller MJ, Sheppard S, Harris R, Read AP, Fielding DW, Walker S, Schorah CJ, Wild J. Further experience of vitamin supplementation for prevention of neural tube defect recurrences. Lancet 1983;1:1027–31.
20. Laurence KM, James N, Miller M, Campbell H. Increased risk of recurrence of pregnancies complicated by fetal neural tube defects in mothers receiving poor diets, and possible benefit of dietary counselling. Br Med J 1980;281:1592–4.
21. Holmes-Siedle M, Lindenbaum RH, Galliard A, Bobrow M. Vitamin supplementation and neural tube defects. Lancet 1982;1:276.
22. Holmes-Siedle M. Vitamin supplementation and neural tube defects. Lancet 1983;2:41.
23. Choi NW, Klaponski FA. On neural-tube defects: an epidemiological elicitation of etiological factors. Neurology 1970;20:399–400.
24. Stone DH. Possible prevention of neural-tube defects by periconceptional vitamin supplementation. Lancet 1980;1:647.
25. Smithells RW, Sheppard S. Possible prevention of neural-tube defects by periconceptional vitamin supplementation. Lancet 1980;1:647.
26. Fernhoff PM. Possible prevention of neural-tube defects by periconceptional vitamin supplementation. Lancet 1980;1:648.
27. Elwood JH. Possible prevention of neural-tube defects by periconceptional vitamin supplementation. Lancet 1980;1:648.
28. Anonymous. Vitamins, neural-tube defects, and ethics committees. Lancet 1980;1:1061–2.
29. Kirke PN. Vitamins, neural tube defects, and ethics committees. Lancet 1980;1:1300–1.
30. Freed DLJ. Vitamins, neural tube defects, and ethics committees. Lancet 1980;1:1301.
31. Raab GM, Gore SM. Vitamins, neural tube defects, and ethics committees. Lancet 1980;1:1301.
32. Hume K. Fetal defects and multivitamin therapy. Med J Aust 1980;2:731–2.
33. Edwards JH. Vitamin supplementation and neural tube defects. Lancet 1982;1:275–6.
34. Renwick JH. Vitamin supplementation and neural tube defects. Lancet 1982;1:748.
35. Chalmers TC, Sacks H. Vitamin supplements to prevent neural tube defects. Lancet 1982;1:748.
36. Stirrat GM. Vitamin supplementation and neural tube defects. Lancet 1982;1:625–6.
37. Kanofsky JD. Vitamin supplements to prevent neural tube defects. Lancet 1982;1:1075.
38. Walsh DE. Vitamin supplements to prevent neural tube defects. Lancet 1982;1:1075.
39. Meier P. Vitamins to prevent neural tube defects. Lancet 1982;1:859.
40. Smith DE, Haddow JE. Vitamins to prevent neural tube defects. Lancet 1982;1:859–60.

41. Smithells RW, Sheppard S, Schorah CJ, Seller MJ, Nevin NC, Harris R, Read AP, Fielding DW. Vitamin supplements and neural tube defects. Lancet 1982;1:1186.
42. Anonymous. Vitamins to prevent neural tube defects. Lancet 1982;2: 1255–6.
43. Lorber J. Vitamins to prevent neural tube defects. Lancet 1982;2:1458–9.
44. Read AP, Harris R. Spina bifida and vitamins. Br Med J 1983;286:560–1.
45. Rose G, Cooke ID, Polani PE, Wald NJ. Vitamin supplementation for prevention of neural tube defect recurrences. Lancet 1983;1:1164–5.
46. Knox EG. Vitamin supplementation and neural tube defects. Lancet 1983;2:39.
47. Emanuel I. Vitamin supplementation and neural tube defects. Lancet 1983;2:39–40.
48. Smithells RW, Seller MJ, Harris R, Fielding DW, Schorah CJ, Nevin NC, Sheppard S, Read AP, Walker S, Wild J. Vitamin supplementation and neural tube defects. Lancet 1983;2:40.
49. Oakley GP Jr, Adams MJ Jr, James LM. Vitamins and neural tube defects. Lancet 1983;2:798–9.
50. Smithells RW, Seller MJ, Harris R, Fielding DW, Schorah CJ, Nevin NC, Sheppard S, Read AP, Walker S, Wild J. Vitamins and neural tube defects. Lancet 1983;2:799.
51. Elwood JM. Can vitamins prevent neural tube defects? Can Med Assoc J 1983;129:1088–92.
52. David TJ. Unusual limb reduction defect in infant born to mother taking periconceptional multivitamin supplement. Lancet 1984;1:507–8.
53. Blank CE, Kumar D, Johnson M. Multivitamins and prevention of neural tube defects: a need for detailed counselling. Lancet 1984;1:291.
54. Smithells RW. Can vitamins prevent neural tube defects? Can Med Assoc J 1984;131:273–6.
55. Wald NJ, Polani PE. Neural-tube defects and vitamins: the need for a randomized clinical trial. Br J Obstet Gynecol 1984;91:516–23.
56. Seller MJ. Unanswered questions on neural tube defects. Br Med J 1987;294:1–2.
57. Harris R. Vitamins and neural tube defects. Br Med J 1988;296:80–1.
58. Wild J, Read AP, Sheppard S, Seller MJ, Smithells RW, Nevin NC, Schorah CJ, Fielding DW, Walker S, Harris R. Recurrent neural tube defects, risk factors and vitamins. Arch Dis Child 1986;61:440–4.
59. Mulinare J, Cordero JF, Erickson JD, Berry RJ. Periconceptional use of multivitamins and the occurrence of neural tube defects. JAMA 1988;260: 3141–5.
60. Holmes LB. Does taking vitamins at the time of conception prevent neural tube defects? JAMA 1988;260:3181.
61. Haddow JE, Hill LE, Kloza EM, Thanhauser D. Neural tube defects after gastric bypass. Lancet 1986;1:1330.
62. Knudsen LB, Kallen B. Gastric bypass, pregnancy, and neural tube defects. Lancet 1986;2:227.
63. Martin L, Chavez GF, Adams MJ Jr, Mason EE, Hanson JW, Haddow JE, Currier RW. Gastric bypass surgery as maternal risk factor for neural tube defects. Lancet 1988;1:640–1.
64. Smithells RW, Sheppard S, Wild J, Schorah CJ. Prevention of neural tube defect recurrences in Yorkshire: final report. Lancet 1989;2:498–9.
65. Mills JL, Rhoads GG, Simpson JL, Cunningham GC, Conley MR, Lassman MR, Walden ME, Depp OR, Hoffman HJ. The absence of a relation between the periconceptional use of vitamins and neural-tube defects. N Engl J Med 1989;321:430–5.
66. Milunsky A, Jick H, Jick SS, Bruell CL, MacLaughlin DS, Rothman KJ, Willett W. Multivitamin/folic acid supplementation in early pregnancy reduces the prevalence of neural tube defects. JAMA 1989;262:2847–52.
67. Aro T, Haapakoski J, Heinonen OP, Saxen L. Lack of association between vitamin intake during early pregnancy and reduction limb defects. Am J Obstet Gynecol 1984;150:433.

VORICONAZOLE

Antifungal

PREGNANCY RECOMMENDATION: No Human Data—Animal Data Suggest Risk
BREASTFEEDING RECOMMENDATION: No Human Data—Potential Toxicity

PREGNANCY SUMMARY

No reports describing the use of voriconazole in human pregnancy have been located. The animal data are suggestive for a risk of toxicity and teratogenicity. However, inhibition of estrogen synthesis was observed in rats. This effect also has been noted in rats treated with another triazole agent, fluconazole. In those studies, the anti-estrogen action was thought to be responsible for the observed cleft palate and bone abnormalities (see Fluconazole). Whether this mechanism also applies to voriconazole is unknown. Nevertheless, based only on the animal data, one review concluded that voriconazole should be avoided in pregnancy (1). Although there are currently no human data, the close relationship with fluconazole, a suspected teratogen in high doses, is reason enough to avoid voriconazole in the 1st trimester. If advertent exposure has occurred, the patient should be advised of the potential but unknown risk to the embryo.

FETAL RISK SUMMARY

The antifungal drug voriconazole is indicated for the treatment of various systemic fungal infections (2). It is a triazole antifungal in the same class as fluconazole, itraconazole, posaconazole, and terconazole.

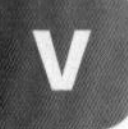

Reproduction studies have been conducted in rats and rabbits. In pregnant rats, a dose 0.3 times the recommended human maintenance dose or higher based on BSA (RHMD) was teratogenic (cleft palates, hydronephrosis, and hydroureter). Toxic effects observed at this dose were reduced ossification of sacral and caudal vertebrae, skull, and pubic and hyoid bones, super numerary ribs, anomalies of the sternebrae, and dilatation of the ureter/renal pelvis. Treatment later in gestation resulted in increased gestational length and dystocia with a subsequent increase in perinatal pup mortality. Plasma estradiol in pregnant rats was reduced at all dose levels. In pregnant rabbits, toxic effects, noted at 6 times the RHMD, consisted of increased embryo mortality, reduced fetal weight, and increased incidences of skeletal variations, cervical ribs, and extra sternebrae ossification sites (2).

In 2-year studies, hepatocellular adenomas were observed in female rats at an oral dose 1.6 times the RHMD, and hepatocellular carcinomas were seen in male rats at oral doses 0.2 and 1.6 times the RHMD. In mice, hepatocellular adenomas were observed in male and female mice and hepatocellular carcinomas in male mice at oral doses that were 1.4 times the RHMD. Voriconazole was clastogenic in an in vitro assay with human lymphocytes, but was not genotoxic in four other assays (2).

It is not known if voriconazole crosses the placenta to the fetus. The molecular weight (about 349) is low enough that exposure of the embryo and/or fetus should be expected.

BREASTFEEDING SUMMARY

No reports describing the use of voriconazole during lactation have been located. The molecular weight (about 349) suggests that the agent will be excreted into breast milk. There is potential for toxicity in nursing infants, especially during the neonatal period when hepatic function is immature. Therefore, women taking this drug should not breastfeed.

References

1. Moudgal VV, Sobel JD. Antifungal drugs in pregnancy: a review. Expert Opin Drug Saf 2003;2:475–83.
2. Product information. Vfend. Pfizer, 2004.

VORINOSTAT

Antineoplastic

PREGNANCY RECOMMENDATION: No Human Data—Animal Data Suggest Risk
BREASTFEEDING RECOMMENDATION: Contraindicated

PREGNANCY SUMMARY

No reports describing the use of vorinostat in human pregnancy have been located. The animal reproductive data suggest risk, but the absence of human pregnancy experience prevents a more complete assessment of embryo–fetal risk. However, the drug probably crosses the placenta and exposure of the embryo and/or fetus should be expected. In addition, although there are no other agents in this antineoplastic subclass, there are other histone deacetylase inhibitors (e.g., valproic acid [1]). If a pregnant woman requires vorinostat, avoiding the 1st trimester and obtaining informed consent are recommended. In case of an inadvertent pregnancy, the woman should be advised of the potential risk for severe adverse effects in the embryo and fetus.

FETAL RISK SUMMARY

Vorinostat is an oral histone deacetylase inhibitor that is indicated for the treatment of cutaneous manifestations in patients with cutaneous T-cell lymphoma who have progressive, persistent, or recurrent disease on or following two systemic therapies. It is given as a daily oral dose. Vorinostat is in the same antineoplastic subclass as romidepsin. The drug is extensively metabolized to two inactive metabolites. Plasma protein binding (71%) is moderate. The mean terminal elimination half-life of vorinostat and one metabolite is about 2 hours, but the half-life of the other inactive metabolite is about 11 hours (1).

Reproductive studies have been conducted in rats and rabbits. The highest dose tested in rats, exposures about half the human exposure based on AUC (HE), caused developmental toxicity consisting of decreased mean live fetal weights; incomplete ossifications of the fetal skull, thoracic vertebra, and sternebrae; and skeletal variations (cervical ribs, supernumerary ribs, vertebral count, and sacral arch variations). The highest dose tested in rabbits, also about half the HE, was associated with reductions in mean live fetal weight and an increased incidence of incomplete ossification of the metacarpals. The no-observed-effect level in rats and rabbits was <0.1 times the HE. However, a dose-related increase in the incidence of gall bladder malformations was observed in rabbits (1,2).

Studies for carcinogenicity have not been conducted with vorinostat, but the drug was mutagenic and clastogenic in tests. No effects on reproductive performance were noted in male rats given doses resulting in exposures up to about 0.70 times the HE for 70 days before mating. Female rats were given doses resulting in exposures up to about 0.70 times the HE for 14 days before mating and through day 7 of gestation. Dose-related increases in corpora lutea, peri-implantation losses, and incidences of dead fetuses and in resorptions were observed at exposures that were ≥0.15, ≥0.36, and 0.70 times the HE, respectively (1).

It is not known if vorinostat crosses the human placenta. The molecular weight (about 264) and moderate plasma protein binding suggest that the drug will cross the human placenta, but the short elimination half-life should decrease the exposure.

BREASTFEEDING SUMMARY

No reports describing the use of vorinostat during human lactation have been located. The molecular weight (about 264) and moderate plasma protein binding (about 71%) suggest that the drug will be excreted into breast milk. However, the short elimination half-life (about 2 hours) should decrease the amount excreted. The potential effects on a nursing infant are unknown, but toxicity is possible. In adults, the most common adverse effects were gastrointestinal (diarrhea, nausea/vomiting, anorexia, weight decrease, constipation), fatigue, chills, hematologic (thrombocytopenia, anemia), and taste disorders (dysgeusia, dry mouth) (1).

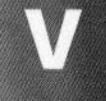

References

1. Product information. Zolinza. Merck, 2006.
2. Wise LD, Turner KJ, Kerr JS. Assessment of developmental toxicity of vorinostat, a histone deacetylase inhibitor, in Sprague-Dawley rats and Dutch belted rabbits. Birth Defects Res (Part B) 2007;80:57–68.

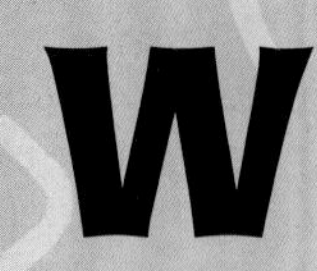

WARFARIN

Anticoagulant

See Coumarin Derivatives.

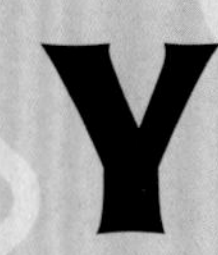

YOHIMBINE

Herb/Sympatholytic/Impotence Agent

PREGNANCY RECOMMENDATION: No Human Data—No Relevant Animal Data
BREASTFEEDING RECOMMENDATION: No Human Data—Probably Compatible

PREGNANCY SUMMARY

No reports describing the use of yohimbine or yohimbe in human pregnancy have been located. The one animal reproduction study located was not relevant for the reasons cited. Yohimbe is available over the counter as a herbal supplement and has been used as an aphrodisiac and for weight loss and sexual dysfunction. Although it has no FDA-sanctioned indications, yohimbine is available by prescription for male erectile dysfunction. It has also been used for treatment of orthostatic hypotension.

FETAL RISK SUMMARY

Yohimbine is an extract of the bark of the *Pausinystalia yohimbe* tree and chemically related to reserpine. The term "yohimbe" refers to the bark extract, which is available in many health stores as a supplement, while "yohimbine" refers to the pharmaceutical pure extract. Both yohimbine and yohimbe are administered orally. Yohimbine is available only by prescription. Yohimbine and yohimbe have been used as aphrodisiacs, for weight loss, and for sexual dysfunction. The primary off-label indication for yohimbine is sexual dysfunction, particularly for the treatment of male erectile dysfunction. This action may be secondary to its blockage of α_2-adrenergic receptors. A second off-label indication is for orthostatic hypotension. Yohimbine is metabolized to apparently inactive metabolites. Plasma protein binding is 82% and the elimination half-life is about 36 minutes (1,2).

In a reproduction study with rats, a single IM injection (20 mg/kg) of yohimbine on day 5 of gestation did not alter the course of pregnancy or affect litter size (3). However, the dose was given before the period of organogenesis (days 9–17 in rats) and thus missed the period of greatest vulnerability for structural anomalies. Moreover, the dose was not compared with the human dose based on BSA or AUC, so the results are not interpretable for estimating human risk.

No studies on the carcinogenicity, mutagenicity, or effects on fertility of yohimbine have been located. In male Swiss albino mice, oral doses of yohimbe for 90 days resulted in significant increases in sperm abnormalities and the weight of seminal vesicles, and a decrease in sperm motility and count. A nonsignificant decrease in pre- and postimplants also was observed (4).

It is not known if yohimbine crosses the human placenta. The molecular weight (about 355) suggests that exposure of the embryo–fetus will occur. However, the very short elimination half-life should limit the amount crossing the placenta.

BREASTFEEDING SUMMARY

No reports describing the use of yohimbine or yohimbe during human lactation have been located. In rats, the sympatholytic (blockage of presynaptic α_2-adrenergic receptors) action of the herb was shown to increase prolactin levels (5). This effect has not been studied in humans. Nevertheless, the relatively low molecular weight (about 355) suggests that the herb will be excreted into breast milk. Moreover, both formulations of the herb are basic and accumulation in breast milk may occur. The effect of this exposure on a nursing infant is unknown.

References

1. DerMarderosian A, Beutler JA, eds. Yohimbe. *The Review of Natural Products*. St. Louis, MO: Wolters Kluwer Health, 2009.
2. Tam SW, Worcel M, Wyllie M. Yohimbine: a clinical review. Pharmacol Ther 2001;91:215–43.
3. Bovet-Nitti F, Bovet D. Action of some sympatholytic agents on pregnancy in the rat. Proc Soc Exp Biol Med 1959;100:555–7.
4. Al-Majed AA, Al-Yahya AA, Al-Bekairi AM, Al-Shabanah OA, Qureshi S. Reproductive, cytological and biochemical toxicity of yohimbe in male Swiss albino mice. Asian J Androl 2006;8:469–76.
5. Lien EL, Morrison A, Kassarich J, Sullivan D. Alpha-2-adrenergic control of prolactin. Neuroendocrinology 1986;44:184–9.

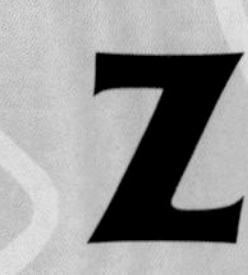

ZAFIRLUKAST

Respiratory Agent

PREGNANCY RECOMMENDATION: Limited Human Data—Animal Data Suggest Low Risk
BREASTFEEDING RECOMMENDATION: Limited Human Data—Potential Toxicity

PREGNANCY SUMMARY

Zafirlukast is not teratogenic in animals, and the few adverse outcomes in humans do not demonstrate a pattern that suggests a common cause. However, the human data are limited. One source stated that zafirlukast may be safe to use during pregnancy, but this conclusion was based solely on animal studies (1). A 2000 position statement of the American College of Obstetricians and Gynecologists (ACOG) and the American College of Allergy, Asthma and Immunology (ACAAI) recommended that zafirlukast could be considered in patients with recalcitrant asthma who had shown a uniquely favorable response to the drug prior to becoming pregnant (2).

FETAL RISK SUMMARY

Zafirlukast is an oral selective peptide leukotriene receptor antagonist that is indicated for the prophylaxis and chronic treatment of asthma. It is extensively metabolized to inactive compounds that are primarily eliminated in the feces. Plasma protein binding is >99%. The mean terminal half-life is about 10 hours, but other studies have reported the plasma half-lives in the 8- to 16-hour range (3).

Reproduction studies conducted in mice and rats with oral doses ≤160 and 410 times the maximum recommended human dose based on BSA (MRHD-BSA), respectively, and in monkeys with doses resulting in exposures up to about 20 times the MRHD based on AUC of the drug plus metabolites (MRHD-AUC), did not observe any evidence of teratogenicity. The maximum doses in rats and monkeys were maternally toxic, resulting in maternal deaths in some cases (rats), fetal resorptions (rats), and spontaneous abortions (SABs) (monkeys) (3).

Zafirlukast was carcinogenic (hepatocellular adenomas) in male mice at a dose about 30 times the MRHD-BSA. Female mice at this dose had a greater incidence of whole-body histocytic sarcomas. Male and female rats at an exposure about 160 times the MRHD-AUC had an increased incidence of urinary bladder transitional cell papillomas. The no-effect doses in mice and rats were 10 times the MRHD-BSA and 140 times the MRHD-AUC, respectively. Assays for mutagenic and clastogenic effects were negative. In addition, no evidence of impaired fertility or reproduction was observed in male and female rats with doses up to about 410 times the MRHD-BSA (3).

It is not known if zafirlukast crosses the human placenta. The molecular weight (about 576) and long elimination half-life suggest that passage to the embryo and fetus should be expected. However, the extensive metabolism and protein binding should limit the exposure.

A 2007 report described the pregnancy outcomes of 96 women exposed to leukotriene receptor antagonists (montelukast and zafirlukast) (4). The women were enrolled in the Organization of Teratology Information Specialists (OTIS) Asthma Medications in Pregnancy study. Two comparison groups were formed consisting of 122 pregnant women who exclusively took short-acting β_2-sympathomimetics or 346 pregnant women without asthma (control group). Among the 96 subjects, 72 took montelukast, 22 took zafirlukast, and 2 took both drugs. Most subjects (89.6%) were exposed in the 1st trimester and 50% were exposed throughout gestation. There were no differences among the three groups in terms of preterm delivery, Apgar scores at 1 and 5 minutes, birth weight and height ≤10th percentile, or ponderal index <2.2. The adjusted mean birth weight in subject infants was significantly lower than that in infants from controls without asthma (3384 vs. 3529 g) ($p < 0.05$). There were no significant differences in pregnancy loss (SABs, ectopic pregnancies, and stillbirths), gestational diabetes, preeclampsia, and maternal weight gain. There were significantly ($p < 0.05$) more birth defects in subjects (5.95%) compared with the control group (0.3%), but the prevalence in the control group was abnormally low. There was no significant difference in the prevalence of defects between subjects and those treated with β_2-agonists (3.9%). No birth defects were reported in stillbirths, SABs, or elective abortions. Birth defects in liveborn infants of subjects (specific exposure not given) were Sturge–Weber sequence, congenital hip dislocation, bilateral club foot, neurofibromatosis type 1 (an autosomal-dominant inheritance pattern); and imperforate anus. The causes of the other four defects are either unknown or multifactorial, but no specific pattern of defects is evident (4).

BREASTFEEDING SUMMARY

The manufacturer reports that zafirlukast is excreted into breast milk (3). In healthy women taking 40 mg orally twice daily, the average steady-state concentration of zafirlukast in milk was 50 ng/mL compared with 255 ng/mL in the plasma (milk:plasma ratio 0.2). The effects in a nursing infant from exposure to the drug in milk are unknown. The manufacturer recommends against breastfeeding because of the potential for tumorigenicity noted in mice and rats, as well as the enhanced sensitivity to the adverse effects of the drug in neonatal rats and dogs (3).

References

1. Anonymous. Drugs for asthma. Med Lett Drugs Ther 2000;42:19–24.
2. Joint Committee of the American College of Obstetricians and Gynecologists (ACOG) and the American College of Allergy, Asthma and Immunology (ACAAI). The use of newer asthma and allergy medications during pregnancy. Ann Allergy Asthma Immunol 2000;84:475–80.
3. Product information. Accolate. AstraZeneca Pharmaceuticals, 2004.
4. Bakhireva LN, Jones KL, Schatz M, Klonoff-Cohen HS, Johnson D, Slymen DJ, Chambers CD., and the Organization of Teratology Information Specialists Collaborative Research Group. Safety of leukotriene receptor antagonists in pregnancy. J Allergy Clin Immunol 2007;119:618–25.

ZALCITABINE

[Withdrawn from the market. See 9th edition.]

ZALEPLON

Hypnotic

PREGNANCY RECOMMENDATION: Human Data Suggest Low Risk
BREASTFEEDING RECOMMENDATION: Limited Human Data—Probably Compatible

PREGNANCY SUMMARY

No reports describing the use of zaleplon in human pregnancy have been located. The agent does compare favorably to other hypnotic benzodiazepine receptor agonists due to its rapid onset (15 minutes), short elimination half-life, and the absence of active metabolites (1). The drug is not an animal teratogen and the risk of human teratogenicity is probably low. However, information from studies in one of the animal species suggests that long-term use could potentially result in human embryo–fetal toxicity. Therefore, the use of zaleplon in pregnancy should be restricted to occasional, short-term treatment (e.g., 7–10 days).

FETAL RISK SUMMARY

The oral hypnotic, zaleplon, is chemically unrelated to benzodiazepines, barbiturates, and other known hypnotic agents, but it is a benzodiazepine receptor agonist. It is indicated for the short-term (e.g., 7–10 days) treatment of insomnia. Zaleplon undergoes substantial presystemic metabolism that significantly reduces its absolute bioavailability. Nearly all of zaleplon is metabolized to inactive metabolites. Plasma protein binding is moderate (about 60%) and the terminal-phase elimination half-life is short (about 1 hour). Zaleplon has an abuse potential similar to benzodiazepines and benzodiazepine-like hypnotics (2).

Reproduction studies have been conducted in rats and rabbits. No evidence of teratogenicity was observed in rats treated throughout organogenesis with doses up to about 49 times the maximum recommended human dose of 20 mg based on BSA (MRHD). At the maximum dose, pre- and postnatal growth was decreased in rat offspring, but this dose was also maternally toxic (clinical signs and reduced body weight). Fertility and reproductive performance in female rats was also impaired at the maximum dose. The no-effect dose during organogenesis for reduced growth in offspring was 5 times the MRHD. However, treatment of pregnant rats in late gestation and during lactation, with a dose that did not cause maternal toxicity (about 3.4 times the MRHD or greater), did result in an increased incidence of stillbirth and postnatal death, as well as decreased growth and physical development. The toxicity was thought to have resulted from both in utero and lactational exposure to the drug. For exposure in late gestation and during lactation, the no-effect dose was about half the MRHD. In rabbits, no evidence of teratogenicity or embryo/fetal toxicity was observed at doses up to 48 times the MRHD given throughout organogenesis (2).

It is not known if zaleplon crosses the human placenta. The molecular weight (about 305) is low enough, but the short elimination half-life will limit the amount of drug available at the maternal:fetal interface.

In a study published in 2011, data from the Swedish Medical Birth Registry, covering the period 1995–2007, identified 1318 women who gave birth to 1341 infants and who reported the use of a hypnotic benzodiazepine receptor agonist at the first prenatal visit (3). The three most commonly reported agents and the number of exposed infants were zopiclone ($N = 692$) (*not available in USA*), zolpidem ($N = 603$), and zaleplon ($N = 32$). The reference group during the study period was 1,106,001 women who gave birth to 1,125,734 infants. The rate of congenital malformations was similar in the exposed and nonexposed groups, 4.3% ($N = 58$) and 4.7% ($N = 52,773$), adjusted odds ratio (aOR) 0.89, 95% confidence interval (CI) 0.68–1.16. One mother who had two infants with probably unrelated malformations (cleft lip and hypospadias) had used zopiclone in both pregnancies. For relatively severe defects, there were 42 exposed infants (3.1%) compared with 36,321 nonexposed infants (3.2%), aOR 0.95, 95% CI 0.0.69–1.30. The authors concluded that use of these agents did not appear to increase the risk of malformations (3).

BREASTFEEDING SUMMARY

Small amounts of zaleplon are excreted into breast milk (2,4). In a study by the manufacturer, the peak drug concentrations in milk occurred about 1 hour after a 10-mg dose. The mean plasma elimination half-life in five lactating women (mean weight 65.1 kg) was about 1 hour, similar to nonlactating women (2,4). The average milk:plasma ratio was 0.5 (4). The investigators estimated the maximum infant exposure during a feeding at peak milk concentrations to be in the range of 1.28–1.66 mcg (4). As the women did not breastfeed during the study, the effects of this exposure on a nursing infant are unknown. For a 65.1-kg woman nursing a 4-kg infant, the maximum estimated infant dose, as a percentage of the mother's dose, is 0.27%. It is doubtful if this amount from a 10-mg dose would have a clinically significant effect on a nursing infant. In addition, within 5 hours of a dose, about 97% of the drug will be eliminated from the maternal plasma and milk.

References

1. Hunt CE, ed. Sleep problems and sleep disorders. As cited in *Clinical Updates in Women's Health Care*. Washington, DC: American College of Obstetricians and Gynecologists, 2004;3 (April):66–7.
2. Product information. Sonata. Monarch Pharmaceuticals, 2004.
3. Wikner BN, Kallen B. Are hypnotic benzodiazepine receptor agonists teratogenic in humans? J Clin Psychopharmacol 2011;31:356–9.
4. Darwish M, Martin PT, Cevallos WH, Tse S, Wheeler S, Troy SM. Rapid disappearance of zaleplon from breast milk after oral administration to lactating women. J Clin Pharmacol 1999;39:670–4.

ZANAMIVIR

Antiviral

PREGNANCY RECOMMENDATION: Compatible—Maternal Benefit >>Embryo/Fetal Risk
BREASTFEEDING RECOMMENDATION: No Human Data—Probably Compatible

PREGNANCY SUMMARY

Reports describing the use of zanamivir during five human pregnancies have been located. Although the animal data suggest low risk, the near absence of human pregnancy experience prevents an assessment of the risk to the embryo–fetus. Nevertheless, if the drug is indicated in a pregnant woman, the maternal benefit outweighs the unknown embryo–fetal risk.

FETAL RISK SUMMARY

Zanamivir is formulated as a powder to be administered by oral inhalation. The agent is thought to act by inhibiting influenza virus neuraminidase with the possibility of alteration of virus particle aggregation and release. Zanamivir is indicated for the treatment of uncomplicated acute illness due to influenza A and B virus in patients who have been symptomatic for no more than 2 days. It is also indicated for prophylaxis of influenza in patients aged 5 years and older. The systemic bioavailability of the drug is approximately 4%–17%, plasma protein binding is <10%, and it is excreted unchanged (no metabolites have been detected) in the urine with a serum elimination half-life of 2.5–5.1 hours (1). In April, 2009, the FDA issued an Emergency Use Authorization to allow zanamivir to be used to treat and prevent influenza in children under 1 year of age, and to provide alternate dosing recommendations for children older than 1 year (2).

Reproduction studies with IV or SC zanamivir have been conducted in rats and rabbits. In pregnant rats, the highest IV daily doses administered produced exposures that were >300 times the human exposure from the clinical dose based on AUC (HE). Drug administration, during gestational days 6–15 or during gestational day 16 until litter day 21–23, revealed no evidence of malformations, embryotoxicity, or maternal toxicity. In a different strain of rats administered SC zanamivir 3 times daily during gestational days 7–17, the highest SC dose produced exposures that were >1000 times the HE. In this study, minor skeletal alterations and variations were observed in the exposed offspring, but the incidence of these effects was within the background rates for the strain studied. In pregnant rabbits, IV doses (identical to the rat doses, but relationship to human dose not specified) administered during gestational days 7–19 revealed no evidence of malformations, embryotoxicity, or maternal toxicity (1).

Zanamivir was not carcinogenic in 2-year studies in mice and rats, was not mutagenic in multiple assays, and did not impair fertility or mating in male and female rats (1).

It is not known if zanamivir crosses the human placenta. The molecular weight (about 332), combined with the lack of metabolism and plasma protein binding, and the moderately long elimination half-life, suggest that the drug will cross to the embryo–fetus. However, the low systemic bioavailability after oral inhalation should limit the amount of drug available for crossing at the maternal:fetal interface.

A 1999 review on the safety of zanamivir briefly described three pregnancies inadvertently exposed during clinical trials (3). The pregnancy outcomes were one spontaneous abortion, one elective abortion, and one healthy baby born 2 weeks early. These results were similar to four pregnancies exposed to placebo in the same clinical trials. A 2009 review concluded that unvaccinated women who come in contact with the H1N1 virus should receive prophylactic antiviral therapy and, although the pregnancy data are limited, it was reassuring (4).

Another 2009 review mentioned a woman in Japan who had taken zanamivir at 4 weeks' gestation and gave birth to a healthy baby at term (no other details provided) (5).

A 2010 case report from Thailand described the fatal outcome of a pregnancy treated with nebulized zanamivir (6). The 25-year-old woman at 26 weeks' gestation presented with influenza A (H1N1) pneumonia. Treatment with oral oseltamivir, nebulized zanamivir, and IV dexamethasone was started. The patient was ventilated but the ventilator constantly malfunctioned, eventually leading to the patient's death. The problem was traced to filter blockade caused by the lactose in the double doses of zanamivir (20 mg) commonly used in Thailand at the time (6).

BREASTFEEDING SUMMARY

No reports describing the use of zanamivir during human lactation have been located, but two 2009 reviews consider the drug to be compatible with breastfeeding (4,5). The molecular weight (about 332), moderately long elimination half-life, and the lack of metabolism and plasma protein binding suggest that the drug will be excreted into breast milk. However, the low systemic bioavailability after oral inhalation should limit the amount of drug excreted into breast milk. The effect, if any, of this exposure on a nursing infant is unknown, but the risk of harm appears to be low.

References

1. Product information. Relenza. GlaxoSmithKline, 2013.
2. FDA News Release. FDA authorizes emergency use of influenza medicines, diagnostic test in response to swine flu outbreak in humans. Available at http://www.fda.gov/NewsEvents/Newsroom/PressAnnouncements/ucm149571.htm. Accessed October 30, 2013.
3. Freund B, Gravenstein S, Elliott M, Miller I. Zanamivir—a review of clinical safety. Drug Saf 1999;21:267–81.
4. Bozzo P, Djokanovic N, Koren G. H1N1 influenza in pregnancy: risks, vaccines, and antivirals. J Obstet Gynaecol Can 2009;31:1172–5.
5. Tanaka T, Nakajima K, Murashima A, Garcia-Bournissen F, Koren G, Ito S. Safety of neuraminidase inhibitors against novel influenza A (H1N1) in pregnant and breastfeeding women. CMAJ 2009;181:55–8.
6. Kiatboonsri S, Kiatboonsri C, Theerawit P. Fatal respiratory events caused by zanamivir nebulization. Clin Infect Dis 2010;50:620.

ZICONOTIDE

Analgesic

PREGNANCY RECOMMENDATION: No Human Data—Animal Data Suggest Low Risk
BREASTFEEDING RECOMMENDATION: No Human Data—Probably Compatible

PREGNANCY SUMMARY

No reports describing the use of ziconotide in human pregnancy have been located. Ziconotide is indicated for long-term intrathecal (IT) therapy and, as such, any exposure would occur throughout gestation. However, clinically significant amounts do not appear to reach the plasma during continuous IT infusions. The small amounts that are in the systemic circulation are metabolized in organ tissues to peptide fragments and free amino acids. Moreover, animal reproduction studies in two species suggest that the risk to the human embryo or fetus is low. Although the absence of human pregnancy experience prevents a more complete assessment, the risk to the embryo–fetus appears to be low. If a woman requires IT therapy with ziconotide, the benefit to her appears to far outweigh the unknown risk to her developing baby.

FETAL RISK SUMMARY

Ziconotide, a 25-amino-acid polypeptide, is a synthetic equivalent of a naturally occurring conopeptide found in the piscivorous marine snail, *Conus magus*. The hydrophilic peptide is given as an IT infusion for the management of severe chronic pain in patients for whom IT therapy is warranted, and who are intolerant of or refractory to other treatment, such as systemic analgesics, adjunctive therapy, or IT morphine (1). The terminal half-life in the cerebrospinal fluid (CSF) is about 4.5 hours (range 2.9–6.5 hours). About 50% of ziconotide is bound to plasma proteins, but metabolism to peptide fragments and individual free amino acids occurs in organs, such as the kidney, liver, lung, and muscle, not in the CSF or blood. The biologic activity of the metabolic products has not been determined. Although ziconotide should not be given IV, minimal amounts of the drug (<1%) were recovered from the urine after an IV infusion (1).

During constant IT infusions at rates ranging from 0.1 to 7 mcg/hr, plasma concentrations were below the level of detection (0.04 ng/mL) in slightly more than half of the patients. More patients had detectable plasma concentrations when higher doses were used (1).

Reproduction studies have been conducted in rats and rabbits. Ziconotide caused embryo death in pregnant rats given continuous IV infusions about 700 times higher than the expected plasma exposure resulting from the maximum recommended human daily IT dose of 0.8 mcg/hr (19.2 mcg/day) (MRHD). No structural defects were observed in rats and rabbits given continuous IV infusions during organogenesis that were up to about 26,000 and 940 times higher, respectively, than the expected plasma exposure resulting from the MRHD. Maternal toxicity (decreased body weight gain and food consumption) was observed at all dose levels. In rats, maternal toxicity, at doses about ≥8900 times higher than the expected plasma exposure resulting from the MRHD, resulted in reduced fetal weight and delayed ossification of the pubic bones. The no-observed-adverse-effect level (NOAEL) for embryo–fetal development in rats and rabbits was about 400 and 940 times higher, respectively, than the expected plasma exposure from the MRHD.

In prenatal and postnatal studies in rats, continuous IV infusions up to about 3800 times higher than the expected plasma exposure resulting from the MRHD had no effect on pup development or reproductive performance. Maternal toxicity, as noted above, was observed at all dose levels.

It is not known if ziconotide crosses the human placenta. The molecular weight (2639) and the very low plasma concentrations suggest that little, if any, drug will reach the embryo or fetus.

BREASTFEEDING SUMMARY

No reports describing the use of ziconotide during human lactation have been located. Ziconotide is a 25-amino-acid polypeptide with a molecular weight of 2639. Although excretion into milk is possible, only small, probably clinically insignificant amounts of ziconotide appear in the plasma during IT infusions. It is not known if the drug would be detectable in breast milk. The risk to a nursing infant appears to be negligible.

Reference

1. Product information. Prialt. Elan Pharmaceuticals, 2005.

ZIDOVUDINE

Antiviral

PREGNANCY RECOMMENDATION: Compatible—Maternal Benefit >> Embryo/Fetal Risk
BREASTFEEDING RECOMMENDATION: Contraindicated

PREGNANCY SUMMARY

Zidovudine (AZT) is effective for the reduction of maternal–fetal transmission of HIV type 1 (HIV-1) infection with few, if any, adverse effects in the newborns. However, neonatal anemia, a known toxic effect of AZT, may occur and requires monitoring. Although yet unproven, AZT may be effective in reducing the transmission of HIV-1 from semen, thereby lessening the chance of infection in a woman who, when pregnant, could transmit the virus to her offspring. The drug is not teratogenic in animals, except at very high doses, and the experience in humans shows no pattern of birth defects. Experimental evidence, however, indicates that AZT is toxic to rodent embryos, preventing blastocyst development when administered before implantation. In addition, evidence has also been published that AZT may affect human trophoblast cell growth and function in a dose-related manner. This cytotoxicity may have resulted in the reduced fertility observed in nonhuman primates. Thus, impaired human fertility is a concern if AZT is administered in high therapeutic doses during early pregnancy. Additionally, there are unanswered questions relating to the potential for long-term toxicity, such as mutagenesis, carcinogenesis, liver disease, heart disease, and reproductive system effects. One study cited, however, found no cancer in AZT-exposed children, some of whom were followed up to 6 years of age. Mitochondrial dysfunction in offspring exposed in utero to AZT and other nucleoside reverse transcriptase inhibitors (NRTIs) has been reported. Moreover, evidence of dose-dependent mitochondrial dysfunction was demonstrated in monkey fetuses whose mothers were given a human-equivalent AZT dose. However, a recent study did not find cardiac toxicity in a small sample of children exposed to AZT during the perinatal period. The incidence and clinical significance of mitochondrial dysfunction after in utero exposure to AZT is therefore still unknown and requires further study. If indicated, the drug should not be withheld because of pregnancy.

FETAL RISK SUMMARY

The thymidine analog zidovudine is an NRTI that is used for the treatment of HIV infection. Other drugs in this class are abacavir, didanosine, lamivudine, stavudine, and zalcitabine.

AZT was not teratogenic in pregnant rats or rabbits at oral doses up to 500 mg/kg/day (1). These doses resulted in peak plasma concentrations in rats 66–226 times, and in rabbits 12–87 times, the mean steady-state peak human plasma levels obtained with the recommended human dose (100 mg every 4 hours). At 150 or 450 mg/kg/day (rats) and 500 mg/kg/day (rabbits), embryo/fetal toxicity was observed as evidenced by an increased incidence of fetal resorptions (1). At a dose of 3000 mg/kg/day in rats (near the median lethal dose), marked maternal toxicity and an increased incidence of fetal malformations were observed (1). This dose produced peak plasma concentrations 350 times the peak human plasma levels (1). In an in vitro study, a dose-related reduction in blastocyst formation was noted in fertilized mouse oocytes (1).

A 1991 study in rats compared the in vitro and in vivo toxicity of five virustatic nucleoside analogs in whole-embryo cultures and on the 10th day of gestation (2). Among the agents tested (vidarabine, ganciclovir, zalcitabine, 2′3′-dideoxyadenosine [ddA], and AZT), AZT had the lowest teratogenic potential.

In an investigation conducted by the manufacturer, a split-dose regimen of 300 mg/kg on gestational day 10 in rats had no adverse effect on the mothers or offspring (3). The AZT concentration in the embryos was approximately one-third of that in the mother, 21.1 vs. 62.6 mcg/g, respectively. However, another study administered AZT to pregnant mice from days 1 to 13 of gestation and observed dose-related fetal toxicity (decrease in the number of fetuses and fetal growth) (4). Concomitant treatment with erythropoietin, vitamin E, or interleukin-3 lessened the fetal toxicity. The adverse effects were thought most likely to be caused by a direct toxic effect on fetal cells, although a partial effect of maternal bone marrow depression could not be excluded.

Four studies have confirmed a direct dose-related toxic effect of AZT on preimplantation mouse embryos (5–8). The doses tested ranged from 1 to 20 times the concentrations obtainable with therapeutic human doses. Using an in vitro model, investigators demonstrated that exposure to AZT was highly correlated with failure to develop to the blastocyst stage (5). Similar developmental arrest, possibly caused by inhibition of DNA synthesis in blastomeres, was observed in a second study of preimplantation mouse embryos exposed in vitro to AZT (6). During the postimplantation portion of this investigation, no adverse fetal effects were observed with doses up to 300 mg/kg/day through all or part of gestation. A third study demonstrated that, when preimplantation mouse embryos were exposed to AZT either in vivo or in vitro, development was unable to proceed beyond the blastocyst stage (7). Exposure at the blastocyst and postblastocyst stages resulted in a lower degree of retarded cell division, indicating that the critical period of toxicity in mouse embryos is between ovulation and implantation. The comparative mouse embryo cytotoxicity of four antiretroviral nucleosides (AZT, didanosine, stavudine, and zalcitabine) was reported in a 1994 study (8). All of the agents showed dose-related inhibition of blastocyst formation, but AZT was the most toxic of the drugs. Cytotoxicity of the other agents was only evident at concentrations equal to the highest obtainable after therapeutic human doses (stavudine) or much higher (didanosine and zalcitabine).

AZT (1.5 mg/kg/dose every 4 hours) was administered via gastric catheter at least 10 days before and throughout gestation to pigtailed macaques (9,10). Mean plasma concentrations (AUC) of the drug were comparable to those obtained in human studies. Twelve pregnancies were brought to term (six AZT, six controls), but significantly more matings (17 vs. 9, $p = 0.007$) were required to achieve pregnancy in the AZT-treated primates. A significant decrease in maternal hemoglobin was observed in the AZT-treated animals, but no differences in the mean hematocrit of the drug-exposed newborns or in fetal growth were found in comparison with controls. Moreover, no adverse effects were discovered in neurologic, perceptual, or motor development during a 9- to 10-month follow-up.

The authors of the above investigation speculated that the retarded macaque fertility might have been related to AZT blockage of progesterone synthesis. However, the following two studies on human trophoblast growth and function indicate that inhibition of cell division before blastocyst formation, as demonstrated in the previously described murine studies (5–8), must also be considered (11,12). Human trophoblasts were isolated from 1st trimester and term pregnancies and maintained in culture (11). Using relatively high drug concentrations (20 μmol/L vs. recommended therapeutic concentrations of 3–5 μmol/L) for prolonged periods (2–11 days), no significant effects on trophoblast function, as measured by human chorionic gonadotropin (hCG) secretion, protein synthesis, and glucose consumption, were observed. In one of the five term placentas, AZT exposure resulted in a significant decrease (20% of the control value) in progesterone secretion, but the secretion rate (17.2 ng/hr/10^6 cells) was still much higher than the control values of the other placentas (3.26–15.63 ng/hr/10^6 cells).

A 1999 study investigated the effects of a single 24-hour exposure of AZT or didanosine (ddI) on human trophoblast cells using a human choriocarcinoma cell line that exhibited many characteristics of the early placenta (12). Two drug concentrations (7.6 mM or 0.076 mM) were studied for their effects on trophoblast cell proliferation and hormone production (hCG, estradiol [E_2], and progesterone [P_4]). The higher concentrations of AZT or ddI resulted in significant decreases in cell numbers and growth rate (38% and 51% of control values, respectively), but increased production of hCG, E_2, and P_4. The decrease in trophoblast cell proliferation may have been the mechanism for the increased incidence of rodent embryo loss observed with AZT (12). In contrast, the lower concentrations of AZT and ddI did not cause changes in cell numbers, producing only significant increases in E_2 production. Because of these findings, the researchers concluded that high therapeutic doses of either AZT or ddI during early human gestation were potentially embryotoxic (12).

Adverse effects on neurobehavior development in mice offspring resulting from a combination of AZT and lamivudine were described in a 2001 study (13). Pregnant mice received both drugs from day 10 of gestation to delivery. The effects on somatic and sensorimotor development were minor but more marked in exposed offspring than when either drug was given alone (13). Both development endpoints were delayed with respect to control animals. Further, alterations of social behavior were observed in both sexes of exposed offspring (13).

AZT crosses the placenta to the fetus, both in animals (14–16) and in humans (1,17–27). Placental transfer of the drug is rapid and is by simple diffusion (17–19). Seven pregnant HIV-seropositive women with gestational lengths between 14 and 26 weeks were scheduled for therapeutic abortions (20). The women were given AZT, 200 mg orally every 4 hours for five doses, 1–2.75 hours before pregnancy termination. Fetal blood concentrations of the parent compound and its inactive glucuronide metabolite ranged from 100 to 287 ng/mL and from 346 to 963.5 ng/mL, respectively. In six patients (one woman had blood levels below the level of detection), mean AZT concentrations in the maternal blood, amniotic fluid, and fetal blood were 143, 168, and 205 ng/mL, respectively.

In a 1990 study, the pregnancy of an HIV-seropositive woman was terminated at 13 weeks' gestation (21). She had been taking AZT, 100 mg four times daily, for 6 weeks, with her last dose consumed approximately 4 hours before the abortion. Both AZT and the glucuronide metabolite were found in the amniotic fluid and various fetal tissues. The lower limit of detection for the assay was 0.01 μmol/L (0.01 nmol/g). The concentrations of the parent compound and the metabolite in maternal plasma were 0.35 and 0.90 μmol/L, respectively. In comparison, the fetal concentrations of AZT (corresponding levels of the metabolite are shown in parentheses) were amniotic fluid, 0.31 μmol/L (1.16 μmol/L); liver, 0.14 nmol/g (0.16 nmol/g); muscle, 0.26 nmol/g (0.50 nmol/g); and CNS, 0.01 nmol/g (0.05 nmol/g). The low levels of AZT in the latter system probably indicate that transplacental passage of the drug, at this dose, may be insufficient to treat HIV infection of the fetal CNS (21). The significance of this result is increased by the finding that neurologic and neuropsychologic morbidity in infants exposed to HIV in utero is high (21,28).

A 1989 report described the treatment of a 30-year-old HIV-seropositive woman who was treated before and throughout gestation with AZT, 1200 mg/day (22). IV AZT, 0.12 mg/kg/hr, was infused 24 hours before labor induction at 39 weeks' gestation. An uncomplicated vaginal delivery occurred, resulting in the birth of a normal male infant weighing 3110 g, with a height and head circumference of 48.5 and 35 cm, respectively. The newborn's renal and hepatic functions were normal, and no other toxicity, such as anemia or macrocytosis, was noted. At birth, concentrations of AZT in the maternal blood, amniotic fluid, and cord blood were 0.28, 3.82, and 0.47 mcg/mL, respectively. AZT concentrations in the infant's blood at 6, 24, 36, and 48 hours were 0.46, 0.51, 0.44, and 0.27 mcg/mL, respectively, indicating that in the first 24 hours elimination of the drug from the newborn was negligible (22). Levels of the inactive metabolite were also determined concurrently; in each sample, the metabolite concentration was higher than that of the parent compound. The infant was doing well and growing normally at 6 months of age.

Two HIV-positive women at 18 and 21 weeks' gestation were treated with AZT (1000 mg/day) for 3 days before elective abortion (23). The final 200-mg dose was consumed 2–3 hours before abortion. Both AZT and its metabolite were found in the two women and in amniotic fluid and fetal blood, with fetal:maternal ratios for AZT of 1.10 and 6.00, respectively, and for the metabolite of 0.84 and 3.75, respectively.

Three experimental in vitro models using perfused human placentas to predict the placental transfer of NRTIs (didanosine, stavudine, zalcitabine, and AZT) were described in a 1999 publication (29). For each drug, the predicted fetal:maternal plasma drug concentration ratios at steady state with each of the three models were close to those actually observed in pregnant macaques. Based on these results, the authors concluded that their models would accurately predict the mechanism, relative rate, and extent of in vivo human placental transfer of NRTIs (29).

The pharmacokinetics of AZT during human and nonhuman primate pregnancies have been determined in a number of studies (24,26,27,30–33). AZT was administered to seven HIV-positive women beginning at 28–35 weeks' gestation with a 200-mg IV dose on day 1, followed by 200 mg orally 5 times a day from day 2 until labor (24). The mean maternal plasma concentrations of AZT and its inactive glucuronide metabolite at delivery were 0.29 and 0.87 mcg/mL, respectively. Similar amounts were measured in umbilical cord venous blood, with mean concentrations of 0.28 and 1.01 mcg/mL, respectively, suggesting that the fetuses and newborns were unable to metabolize AZT (24). No significant drug-induced adverse effects were observed in the women or their newborns and no congenital malformations were noted. Fetal growth was normal in six and accelerated in one, and the slightly lower than normal hemoglobin values were not considered clinically significant (24).

In pregnant macaques or humans, the pharmacokinetics of AZT were not affected by pregnancy (macaques) (30), nor did AZT affect the transplacental pharmacokinetics of didanosine (macaques) (31), lamivudine (humans) (32), or stavudine (macaques) (33). Two other studies involving four women infected with HIV measured peak AZT maternal serum levels and elimination half-lives that were statistically similar to those of nonpregnant adults (26,27). However, in three women, the AUC during pregnancy was significantly less than after pregnancy (4.5 μmol/L vs. 6.8 μmol/L, $p = 0.02$), and the apparent total body clearance was significantly greater (2.5 L/hr/kg vs. 1.7 L/hr/kg, $p = 0.05$) (26). Moreover, the difference in the apparent volume of distribution during and after pregnancy reached near significance (3.9 L/kg vs. 2.6 L/kg, $p = 0.07$) (26).

The effect of AZT on the transplacental passage of HIV is unknown. A 1990 review of AZT in pregnancy focused on the issue of whether the drug prevented HIV passage to the fetus and concluded that available data were insufficient to provide an answer to this question (22). However, a 1993 study observed that, although AZT is transferred to the fetus relatively intact, the approximately 50% retained by the placenta is extensively metabolized, with one of the metabolites being zidovudine triphosphate, the product responsible for the antiviral activity of the parent drug (34). The effect of this may be a reduction in the risk of HIV transmission to the fetus (34).

Brief descriptions of the treatment and pregnancy outcome of 12 HIV-seropositive women were provided in a 1991 abstract (35). AZT therapy was started before conception in 4 women and between 21 and 34 weeks' (mean 25 weeks) gestation in 8. The mean duration of therapy was 8 weeks (range 1–24 weeks). Three of the women who had conceived while taking AZT underwent therapeutic abortions of grossly normal fetuses between 10 and 12 weeks' gestation. Five women had delivered grossly normal infants with a mean birth weight of 2900 g, and the infants of the remaining four women were undelivered between 24 and 36 weeks. Three other abstracts that appeared in 1992 and 1993 described 46 pregnant women treated with AZT without producing toxic effects or anomalies in their fetuses (36–38).

In a surveillance study of Michigan Medicaid recipients involving 229,101 completed pregnancies conducted between 1985 and 1992, two newborns had been exposed to AZT during the 1st trimester (F. Rosa, personal communication, FDA, 1993). No major birth defects were observed.

Data on 45 newborns (2 sets of twins) of 43 pregnant women, enrolled in studies conducted by 17 institutions participating in AIDS Clinical Trial Units and who had been treated with AZT, were described in 1992 (39). AZT dosage ranged from 300 to 1200 mg/day, with 24 of the women taking the drug during at least two trimesters. All the infants were born alive. No congenital abnormalities were observed in 12 infants who had been exposed in utero to AZT during the 1st trimester, although 1 newborn with elevated 17α-hydroxyprogesterone levels had clitoral enlargement. Normal levels of the hormone were measured in this infant at 4 months of age. Two term infants were growth restricted, but 38 other singleton term infants had a mean birth weight of 3287 g. Seven infants had hemoglobin values less than 13.5 g/dL; three of these were delivered prematurely. The authors concluded that the few cases of anemia and growth restriction might have been, at least partially, caused by maternal AZT therapy (39). Another report involving 29 pregnant patients treated with AZT at government-sponsored AIDS clinical trial centers appeared in 1992, but no data on the outcome of these pregnancies were given (40).

The outcomes of 104 pregnancies in which AZT was used were described in a 1994 report (41). Sixteen of the pregnancies terminated during the 1st trimester—eight spontaneous and eight elective abortions. Among the remaining 88 cases, 8 infants had birth defects, 4 after 1st trimester exposure, and 4 after exposure during the 2nd or 3rd trimesters. None of the defects could be attributed to AZT exposure (41): multiple minor anomalies (low-set ears, retrognathia, hirsutism, triangular face, blue sclera, prominent sacral dimple)*; multiple minor anomalies (type not specified)*; extra digits on both hands, hare lip (central), cleft palate; fetal alcohol syndrome; atrial septal defect (asymptomatic) with pectus excavatum*; microcephaly, chorioretinitis (*Toxoplasma gondii* infection); pectus excavatum*; and albinism with congenital ptosis, growth restriction, and oligohydramnios (* indicates chromosomal analysis normal) (41).

The Antiretroviral Pregnancy Registry reported, for the period January 1989 through July 2009, prospective data (reported before the outcomes were known) involving 4702 live births that had been exposed during the 1st trimester to one or more antiretroviral agents (42). Congenital defects were noted in 134, a prevalence of 2.8% (95% confidence interval [CI] 2.4–3.4). In the 6100 live births with earliest exposure in the 2nd/3rd trimesters, there were 153 infants with defects (2.5%, 95% CI 2.1–2.9). The prevalence rates for the two periods did not differ significantly. There were 288 infants with birth defects among 10,803 live births with exposure anytime during pregnancy (2.7%, 95% CI 2.4–3.0). The prevalence rate did not differ significantly from the rate expected in a nonexposed population. There were 9735 outcomes exposed to AZT (3167 in the 1st trimester and 6568 in the 2nd/3rd trimesters) in combination with other antiretroviral agents. There were 264 birth defects (97 in the 1st trimester and 167 in the 2nd/3rd trimesters). In reviewing the birth defects of prospective and retrospective (pregnancies reported after the outcomes were known) registered cases, the Registry concluded that, except for isolated cases of NTDs with efavirenz exposure in retrospective reports, there was no other pattern of anomalies (isolated or syndromic) (42). (See Lamivudine for required statement.)

The failure of maternal AZT therapy to prevent the transmission of HIV-1 infection to one of the mother's female twins was described in a 1990 report (43). The woman was treated with AZT, 400 mg/day, from 18 weeks' gestation until delivery. A cesarean section was performed at 27 weeks' gestation because of premature labor that was not responsive to tocolytic therapy. Twin A was diagnosed with culture-proven HIV-1 and cytomegalovirus infection. At the time of the report, the child was 9 months old with limited sight, severe failure to thrive, and encephalopathy. An HIV-1 culture in twin B was negative, but analysis for HIV-1 antigens continued to be positive through 20 weeks of age. A number of possible explanations were proposed by the authors concerning the failure of AZT to protect twin A from infection. Included among these were passage of the virus before the onset of treatment at 18 weeks' gestation, intrauterine transfer of the virus via an amniocentesis performed at 14 weeks' gestation, viral resistance to the drug, low fetal tissue drug levels, maternal noncompliance (doubtful), and acquisition of the virus during birth (43).

A 1992 review on the treatment of HIV-infected pregnant women stated that most obstetric experts offered AZT therapy in cases of AIDS, AIDS-related complex, or when the CD4+ cell counts were below 200 cells/micro-L (44). Although no fetal toxicity secondary to AZT had been reported, the author recommended caution with 1st trimester use of the agent and noted the potential for fetal bone marrow depression and resulting anemia.

A clinical trial, the subject of several reviews and editorials (45–51), conducted from 1991 to 1993 and published in 1994, found that the risk of maternal–infant transmission of HIV disease could be decreased by 67.5% by treatment of pregnant women (who had mildly symptomatic HIV disease) with AZT (52). The randomized, double-blind, placebo-controlled trial enrolled untreated HIV-infected pregnant women, at 14–34 weeks' gestation, which had CD4+ T-lymphocyte counts above 200 cells/mm^3 and no clinical indications for antenatal antiretroviral therapy. The maternal AZT treatment regimen consisted of antepartum oral therapy (100 mg orally five times daily) and intrapartum IV dosing (2 mg/kg for 1 hour, then 1 mg/kg/hr until delivery). The newborns were treated with oral AZT (2 mg/kg every 6 hours) for 6 weeks. A total of 477 women were enrolled, 409 of whom delivered 415 liveborn infants during the study period. Among those with known HIV-infection status were 180 infants from the AZT-treated group and 183 placebo-treated controls. The authors of this study used statistical methods to predict the number of infants who would be HIV-infected at 18 months of age, thus allowing a faster analysis of their data. They estimated that the number of HIV-infected children would be 8.3% (95% CI 3.9%–12.8%) in the AZT group and 25.5% (95% CI 18.4%–32.5%) in the placebo group (52). This was a 67.5% (95% CI 40.7%–82.1%) reduction in the risk of HIV transmission (p = 0.00006). No differences in growth, prematurity, or the number and patterns of major or minor congenital abnormalities were observed between the two groups. Thirty-three liveborn infants had congenital defects, 17 of 206 (8.3%) in the treatment group and 16 of 209 (7.7%) in the nontreated controls. Cardiac malformations were observed in 10 infants (5 in each group), CNS defects in 5 (3 in the AZT group, 2 in controls), and 9 unspecified defects in each group. The total incidence of congenital malformations is higher than expected in the general population, but this probably reflects the population studied. The only drug-related adverse effect observed in the newborns was a decrease in hemoglobin concentration in those exposed to AZT in utero. The maximum difference in hemoglobin concentration between the groups, 1 g/dL, occurred at 3 weeks of age, but by 12 weeks of age, the hemoglobin values were similar (52).

Although AZT appeared to be effective in reducing transmission of HIV-1 to the fetus, some infants became infected despite treatment. Possible reasons proposed for these failures included (a) virus transmission before treatment began, (b) ineffective suppression of maternal viral replication, (c) poor maternal compliance with the drug regimen, and (d) virus resistance to AZT (52).

A series of studies and editorials appeared in 1998–2000 that evaluated or discussed the effect of short courses of AZT on the perinatal transmission of HIV in various populations (53–59). The most effective therapy, however, involved starting treatment of the mother at 28 weeks' gestation, with 6 weeks of treatment in the infant (58,59).

A 2000 review described seven clinical trials that have been effective in reducing perinatal transmission, five with

AZT alone, one with AZT plus lamivudine, and one with nevirapine (60). Six of the trials were in less-developed countries. Prolonged use of AZT in the mother and infant was the most effective for preventing vertical transmission of HIV, but also was the most expensive. The combination of AZT and lamivudine, consisting of antepartum, intrapartum, and postpartum maternal therapy with continued therapy in the infant for 1 week, may have been as effective as prolonged AZT (60).

A study published in 1999 evaluated the safety, efficacy, and perinatal transmission rates of HIV in 30 pregnant women receiving various combinations of antiretroviral agents (61). Many of the women were substance abusers. AZT was used by 26 women in various combinations that included didanosine, lamivudine, indinavir, nelfinavir, nevirapine, saquinavir, and delavirdine. Antiretroviral therapy was initiated at a median of 14 weeks' gestation (range preconception to 32 weeks). Despite previous histories of extensive antiretroviral experience and of vertical transmission of HIV, combination therapy was effective in treating maternal disease and in preventing transmission to the current newborns. The outcomes of the pregnancies included one stillbirth, one case of microcephaly, and five infants with birth weights <2500 g, two of which were premature (61).

In another 1999 study, the safety and efficacy of a short course of nevirapine was compared with AZT for the prevention of perinatal transmission of HIV-1 (62). At the onset of labor, women were randomly assigned to receive either a single dose of nevirapine (200 mg) plus a single dose (2 mg/kg) to their infants within 72 hours of birth ($N = 310$) or AZT (600 mg then 300 mg every 3 hours until delivery) plus 4 mg/kg twice daily for 7 days to their infants ($N = 308$). Nearly all (98.8%) of the women breastfed their infants immediately after birth. Up to age 14–16 weeks, significantly fewer infants in the nevirapine group were HIV-1 infected, lowering the risk of infection or death, compared with AZT, by 48% (95% CI 24%–65%) (62). The prevalence of maternal and infant adverse effects were similar in the two groups. In an accompanying study, the nevirapine regimen was shown to be cost-effective in various seroprevalence settings (63).

In an unusual case, a woman was exposed to HIV through self-insemination with fresh semen obtained from a man with a high HIV ribonucleic acid viral load (>750,000 copies/mL plasma) (64). Ten days later, she was started on a prophylactic regimen of AZT (600 mg/day), lamivudine (300 mg/day), and indinavir (2400 mg/day). Pregnancy was confirmed 14 days after insemination. The indinavir dose was reduced to 1800 mg/day 4 weeks after the start of therapy because of the development of renal calculi. All antiretroviral therapy was stopped after 9 weeks because of negative tests for HIV. She gave birth at 40 weeks' gestation to a healthy 3490-g male infant, without evidence of HIV disease, who was developing normally at 2 years of age (64).

A case of life-threatening anemia following in utero exposure to antiretroviral agents was described in 1998 (65). A 30-year-old woman with HIV infection was treated with AZT, didanosine, and trimethoprim/sulfamethoxazole (three times weekly) during the 1st trimester. Vitamin supplementation was also given. Because of an inadequate response, didanosine was discontinued and lamivudine and zalcitabine were started in the 3rd trimester. Two weeks before delivery, the HIV viral load was undetectable. At term, a pale, male infant was delivered who developed respiratory distress shortly after birth. Examination revealed a hyperactive precordium and hepatomegaly without evidence of hydrops. The hematocrit was 11% with a reticulocyte count of zero. An extensive work-up of the mother and infant failed to determine the cause of the anemia. Bacterial and viral infections, including HIV, parvovirus B19, cytomegalovirus, and others, were excluded. The infant received a transfusion and was apparently doing well at 10 weeks of age. Because no other cause of the anemia could be found, the authors attributed the condition to bone marrow suppression, most likely to AZT. A contribution of the other agents to the condition, however, could not be excluded (65).

A study of the inhibitory effects of AZT on hematopoiesis was published in 1996 (66). The researchers compared the effect of increasing concentrations of AZT on hematopoietic progenitors from women of childbearing age (from bone marrow aspirates), mid-trimester aborted fetuses (from bone marrow and liver), and term newborns (from cord blood). The inhibitory effect of AZT was more pronounced on fetal and neonatal erythroid progenitors than those from the bone marrow of the women. AZT had no effect on granulocyte colony-stimulating factor or erythropoietin. The authors concluded that neonatal anemia after in utero exposure to AZT was due to reduced clonal maturation of erythroid progenitors (66).

A 1999 report from France described the possible association of AZT and lamivudine (NRTIs) use in pregnancy with mitochondrial dysfunction in the offspring (67). Mitochondrial disease is relatively rare in France (estimated prevalence is 1 in 5000–20,000 children). From an ongoing epidemiological survey of 1754 mother–child pairs exposed to AZT and other agents during pregnancy, however, eight children with possible mitochondrial dysfunction were identified. None of the eight infants were infected with HIV, but all received prophylaxis for up to 6 weeks after birth with the same antiretroviral regimen as given during pregnancy. Four of the cases were exposed to AZT alone and four to a combination of AZT and lamivudine. Two from the combination group died at about 1 year of age. All eight cases had abnormally low respiratory-chain enzyme activities. The authors concluded that their results supported the hypothesis of a causative association between mitochondrial respiratory-chain dysfunction and NRTIs. Moreover, the toxicity may have been potentiated by a combination of these agents (67).

In a paper following the above study, investigators noted that NRTIs inhibit DNA polymerase γ, the enzyme responsible for mitochondrial DNA replication (68). They then hypothesized that this inhibition would induce depletion of mitochondrial DNA and mitochondrial DNA-encoded mitochondrial enzymes, thus resulting in mitochondrial dysfunction (69). Moreover, they stated that support for their hypothesis was suggested by the closeness of the clinical manifestations of inherited mitochondrial diseases with the adverse effects attributed to NRTIs. These adverse effects included polyneuropathy, myopathy, cardiomyopathy, pancreatitis, bone marrow suppression, and lactic acidosis. They also postulated that this mechanism was involved in the development of a lipodystrophy syndrome of peripheral fat wasting and central adiposity, a condition that has been thought to be related to protease inhibitors (68).

A commentary on the above two studies concluded that the evidence for NRTI-induced mitochondrial dysfunction was equivocal (69). First, the clinical presentations in the infants were varied and not suggestive of a single cause; indeed, three of the infants were symptom-free and one had Leigh's syndrome, a classic mitochondrial disease (69). Second, the clinical features, in some cases, were not suggestive of mitochondrial dysfunction. Although three had neurologic symptoms, none had raised levels of lactate in the cerebrospinal fluid. Moreover, histologic or histochemical features of mitochondrial disease were only found in two cases. Finally, low mitochondrial DNA, which would have been a direct evidence of NRTI toxicity, was not found in the three cases in which it was measured (69).

A case of combined transient mitochondrial and peroxisomal β-oxidation dysfunction after exposure to NRTIs (AZT and lamivudine) combined with protease inhibitors (ritonavir and saquinavir) throughout gestation was reported in 2000 (70). A male infant was delivered at 38 weeks' gestation. He received postnatal prophylaxis with AZT and lamivudine for 4 weeks until the drugs were discontinued because of anemia. Other adverse effects that were observed in the infant (age at onset) were hypocalcemia (shortly after birth); group B streptococcal sepsis, ventricular extrasystoles, prolonged metabolic acidosis, and lactic acidemia (8 weeks); a mild elevation of long-chain fatty acids (9 weeks); and neutropenia (3 months). The metabolic acidosis required treatment until 7 months of age, whereas the elevated plasma lactate resolved over 4 weeks. Cerebrospinal fluid lactate was not determined nor was a muscle biopsy conducted. Both the neutropenia and the cardiac dysfunction had resolved by 1 year of age. The elevated plasma fatty acid level was confirmed in cultured fibroblasts, but other peroxisomal functions (plasmalogen biosynthesis and catalase staining) were normal. Although mitochondrial dysfunction has been linked to NRTI agents, the authors were unable to identify the cause of the combined abnormalities in this case. The child was reported to be healthy and developing normally at 26 months of age (70).

A study involving *Erythrocebus patas* monkeys exposed in utero to AZT was thought to be relevant to the reports of mitochondrial dysfunction in humans (71). Ten pregnant monkeys in the last half of gestation were given daily oral doses of AZT (1.5 mg/kg/day [$N = 3$] or 6 mg/kg/day [$N = 3$]) or no AZT (controls [$N = 4$]). The doses of AZT were 21% and 86% of the human dose, respectively, based on body weight for a 70-kg pregnant woman. All fetuses were delivered by cesarean section 24 hours after the last AZT dose and 3–5 days before term. No gross defects were evident in the heart left ventricle tissue or skeletal muscle tissue from AZT-exposed or control fetuses. Mitochondria observed by electron microscopy in the two tissue sites were similar in the AZT low-dose and control groups. In contrast, numerous abnormalities were observed in both heart and muscle tissue mitochondria from fetuses exposed to the AZT high-dose group. Moreover, there were dose-dependent alterations in oxidative phosphorylation enzyme assays, in the specific activities of NADH dehydrogenase (complex I), succinate dehydrogenase (complex II), and cytochrome-c oxidase (complex IV), and a dose-dependent depletion of mitochondrial DNA levels. The data were consistent with AZT-induced cardiac and skeletal muscle mitochondrial myopathy (71).

Based on the findings of the above research, a prospective study of the left ventricular structure and function of 382 noninfected (36 exposed to AZT) and 58 HIV-infected (12 exposed to AZT) infants born to HIV-infected women was published in 2000 (72). The median length of in utero exposure to AZT was 103 days (105 days for those not infected and 68 days for those infected at birth). Echocardiographic studies (mean left ventricular fractional shortening, contractility, end-diastolic dimension, and left ventricular mass) were conducted every 4–6 months during the first 14 months of life. All echocardiograms were examined without knowledge of the child's clinical status or medications. No statistical differences were found among the four echocardiographic measures in the four groups of children. The investigators identified at least four limitations of their study, including a small sample size that was unable to estimate the frequency of an uncommon toxic effect, the lack of an assessment of a possible dose effect, the possibility that the sickest children were missed because they were unable to attend follow-up visits, and the effects of other drug therapy in the HIV-infected subgroup that could obscure the effects of AZT. Nonetheless, they concluded that perinatal exposure to AZT was not associated with acute or chronic abnormalities in left ventricular structure or function (72).

A 2000 case report described the adverse pregnancy outcomes, including NTDs, of two pregnant women with HIV infection who were treated with the anti-infective combination trimethoprim/sulfamethoxazole for prophylaxis against *Pneumocystis carinii*, concurrently with antiretroviral agents (73). Exposure to AZT occurred in one of these cases. A 32-year-old woman with a 3-year history of HIV and recent diagnosis of AIDS was treated before and throughout gestation with the anti-infective combination plus AZT and zalcitabine. Folic acid 10 mg/day was added after the diagnosis of pregnancy (gestational age not specified). At term, a female infant was delivered by cesarean section without HIV infection, but with a bony mass in the lumbar spine (identified by ultrasound at 32 weeks' gestation). A diagnostic evaluation revealed that the second lumbar vertebra consisted of hemivertebrae and projected posteriorly into the spinal canal. A malformed and displaced first lumbar vertebra was also noted. Surgery was planned to correct the defect. The authors attributed the NTDs in both cases to the antifolate activity of trimethoprim (73).

The case of a 6-month-old male infant who was diagnosed with acute lymphoblastic leukemia (ALL) was described in a 2000 case report (74). His mother had been diagnosed with HIV infection during the 5th month of gestation. She had been treated with oral AZT for the last 3 months of pregnancy. The 3.5-kg infant had been delivered by cesarean section and treated with AZT prophylaxis (2 mg/kg 4 times a day) for 6 weeks. All tests for HIV in the infant were negative. He achieved complete remission after chemotherapy for the ALL and was currently receiving the maintenance phase of chemotherapy at age 16 months. The relationship between AZT exposure and the ALL was unknown (74).

Because of the AZT-induced carcinogenicity observed in animal studies, a 1999 study evaluated the short-term risk for tumors in a total of 727 children who had been exposed in utero (antepartum) and/or during the neonatal period to HIV and AZT (75). The children were participants in one of two multicenter clinical studies: Pediatric AIDS Clinical Trials Group (PACTG) 076/219 ($N = 115$) or the Women and Infants Transmission Study (WITS) ($N = 612$). The mean infant follow-up in the PACTG 076/219 group was 38.3 months

(366.9 person-years follow-up), whereas it was 14.5 months (743.7 person-years follow-up) for WITS participants. The range for all children was 1 month to 6 years. No tumors of any nature were reported in the children (relative risk 0, 95% CI 0–17.6) (75).

The long-term effects of in utero exposure to AZT were the subject of a study published in 1999 (76). HIV-uninfected children (*N* = 234) born to 231 HIV-infected women enrolled in the PACTG 076 were evaluated under the PACTG 219 protocol (122 exposed to AZT, 112 in the placebo group). The main outcome measures included physical growth, immunologic parameters, cognitive/developmental function, tumors, and mortality data. Children were evaluated every 6 months up to 24 months, then yearly thereafter or as clinically indicated. The median age at the time of last follow-up was 4.2 years (range 3.2–5.6 years). There were no significant differences between those exposed to AZT and those not exposed in terms of the sequential outcome measurements. In addition, there were no deaths or malignancies. In the 137 (59%) children who had at least one ophthalmologic examination, 72 were in the AZT group and 65 were in the placebo group. Although there was no significant difference (p = 0.99) between the groups in abnormal ophthalmic findings, astigmatism was noted in two (AZT group), ptosis in one (AZT group), and epicanthal folds in one (placebo group). Two other AZT-exposed children had ophthalmic abnormalities: (a) bilateral "thinned vessels; discs look slightly pale" in one with normal vision; and (b) one with a fundus reported as "copper beaten look" that was not thought to be related to metabolic disease. One other asymptomatic, healthy 4-year-old child in the AZT group had a mild cardiomyopathy on echocardiogram (76).

New York Medicaid data were used in a study published in 2000 to determine if there was an association between prenatal AZT use and congenital anomalies (77). The study cohort included 1932 liveborn infants delivered from 1993 to 1996 to HIV-infected women in the state of New York, 29.5% of whom were exposed in utero to AZT. The prevalence of any anomaly in the study cohort was 2.76 (95% CI 2.36–3.17) compared with the general New York State population. When AZT-exposed outcomes were compared with those not exposed, the adjusted odds ratios (aORs) for major congenital malformations by trimester of first prescription were as follows: 1.20 (95% CI 0.58–2.51) (1st trimester), 1.47 (95% CI 0.85–2.55) (2nd trimester), and 1.84 (95% CI 1.04–3.25) (3rd trimester). There was an increased unadjusted OR for CNS defects when compared with those not exposed to AZT (7.98 [95% CI 1.56–37.46]). However, this finding was based on only four such defects and must be interpreted cautiously (77).

High semen levels of AZT have been reported (78). Six males with HIV disease were treated with 200 mg of the antiviral agent orally every 4–6 hours. AZT concentrations in semen 3.0–4.5 hours after a dose ranged from 1.68 to 6.43 μmol/L, representing semen:serum ratios of 1.3–20.4. The semen levels were above the in vitro minimum inhibitory concentration for HIV-1. A 1994 study reported that AZT reversed the effects of HIV-1 disease progression on semen quality, including ejaculate volume, sperm concentration and total count, and the number of abnormal sperm forms (79). Moreover, AZT therapy significantly reduced the semen white blood cell count, the principal HIV-1 host cells in ejaculates of HIV-1-infected males. The researchers concluded that this might explain why infected males treated with AZT have a reduced viral load in their semen and a lower rate of sexual transmission (79).

Two reviews, one in 1996 and the other in 1997, concluded that all women currently receiving antiretroviral therapy should continue to receive therapy during pregnancy and that treatment of the mother with monotherapy should be considered inadequate therapy (80,81). The same conclusion was reached in a 2003 review with the added admonishment that therapy must be continuous to prevent emergence of resistant viral strains (82). In 2009, the updated U.S. Department of Health and Human Services guidelines for the use of antiretroviral agents in HIV-1-infected patients continued the recommendation that therapy, with the exception of efavirenz, should be continued during pregnancy (83). If indicated, AZT should not be withheld in pregnancy because the expected benefit to the HIV-positive mother outweighs the unknown risk to the fetus. Updated guidelines for the use of antiretroviral drugs to reduce perinatal HIV-1 transmission also were released in 2010 (84). Women receiving antiretroviral therapy during pregnancy should continue the therapy but, regardless of the regimen, AZT administration is recommended during the intrapartum period to prevent vertical transmission of HIV to the newborn (84).

BREASTFEEDING SUMMARY

Only one report describing the excretion of AZT in breast milk has been located (85). Six HIV-seropositive women were given a single 200-mg dose of AZT, and serum and breast milk samples were collected 1, 2, 4, and 6 hours later. Peak serum and milk concentrations, ranging between 422.1 and 1019.3 ng/mL and 472.1 and 1043.0 ng/mL, respectively, were measured at approximately 1–2 hours after the dose. The milk:serum ratio (based on AUC) ranged between 1.11 and 1.78. The authors speculated that the milk concentrations were sufficiently high to decrease the viral load in milk, thereby reducing the potential for maternal–infant HIV transmission (85).

Breastfeeding is not recommended in women with HIV infection because HIV-1 is transmitted in milk (80,81,83,86–88). Until 1999, no studies had been published that examined the effect of any antiretroviral therapy on HIV-1 transmission in milk. In that year, a double-blind, placebo-controlled trial investigated the effect of oral AZT in the postpartum period on the transmission of HIV-1 to the breastfeeding infant (56). Infants (at 6 months of age) of women who had received an oral AZT regimen of 300 mg twice daily until labor, 600 mg at beginning of labor, then 300 mg twice daily for 7 days postpartum, had a 38% reduction (relative efficacy 0.38, 95% CI 0.05–0.60; p = 0.027) in vertical transmission of HIV-1 infection despite breastfeeding when compared with controls. Furthermore, no excess of major adverse biological or clinical events were observed in the AZT group compared with controls (56).

References

1. Product information. Retrovir. Glaxo Wellcome, 2001.
2. Klug S, Lewandowski C, Merker H-J, Stahlmann R, Wildi L, Neubert D. In vitro and in vivo studies on the prenatal toxicity of five virustatic nucleoside analogues in comparison to aciclovir. Arch Toxicol 1991;65:283–91.

3. Greene JA, Ayers KM, De Miranda P, Tucker WE Jr. Postnatal survival in Wistar rats following oral dosage with zidovudine on gestation day 10. Fund Appl Toxicol 1990;15:201–6.
4. Gogu SR, Beckman BS, Agrawal KC. Amelioration of zidovudine-induced fetal toxicity in pregnant mice. Antimicrob Agents Chemother 1992;36:2370–4.
5. Toltzis P, Marx CM, Kleinman N, Levine EM, Schmidt EV. Zidovudine-associated embryonic toxicity in mice. J Infect Dis 1991;1212–8.
6. Sieh E, Coluzzi ML, Cusella de Angelis MG, Mezzogiorno A, Floridia M, Canipari R, Cossu G, Vella S. The effects of AZT and DDI on pre- and post-implantation mammalian embryos: an in vivo and in vitro study. AIDS Res Hum Retroviruses 1992;8:639–49.
7. Toltzis P, Mourton T, Magnuson T. Effect of zidovudine on preimplantation murine embryos. Antimicrob Agents Chemother 1993;37:1610–3.
8. Toltzis P, Mourton T, Magnuson T. Comparative embryonic cytotoxicity of antiretroviral nucleosides. J Infect Dis 1994;169:1100–2.
9. Nosbisch C, Ha JC, Sackett GP, Conrad SH, Ruppenthal GC, Unadkat JD. Fetal and infant toxicity of zidovudine in *Macaca nemestrina* (abstract). Teratology 1994;49:415.
10. Ha JC, Nosbisch C, Conrad SH, Ruppenthal GC, Sackett GP, Abkowitz J, Unadkat JD. Fetal toxicity of zidovudine (azidothymidine) in *Macaca nemestrina*: preliminary observations. J Acquir Immune Defic Synd 1994;7:154–7.
11. Esterman AL, Rosenberg C, Brown T, Dancis J. The effect of zidovudine and 2′3′-dideoxyinosine on human trophoblast in culture. Pharmacol Toxicol 1995;76:89–92.
12. Plessinger MA, Miller RK. Effects of zidovudine (AZT) and dideoxyinosine (ddI) on human trophoblast cells. Reprod Toxicol 1999;13:537–46.
13. Venerosi A, Valanzano A, Alleva E, Calamandrei G. Prenatal exposure to anti-HIV drugs: neurobehavioral effects of zidovudine (AZT) + lamivudine (3TC) treatment in mice. Teratology 2001;63:26–37.
14. Unadkat JD, Lopez AA, Schuman L. Transplacental transfer and the pharmacokinetics of zidovudine (ZDV) in the near term pregnant macaque. In: *Program and Abstracts of the Twenty-eighth Interscience Conference on Antimicrobial Agents and Chemotherapy, Los Angeles, October 1988*. Los Angeles, CA: American Society for Microbiology, 1988:372. As cited in Hankins GDV, Lowery CL, Scott RT, Morrow WR, Carey KD, Leland MM, Colvin EV. Transplacental transfer of zidovudine in the near-term pregnant baboon. Am J Obstet Gynecol 1990;163:728–32.
15. Lopez-Anaya A, Unadkat JD, Schumann LA, Smith AL. Pharmacokinetics of zidovudine (azidothymidine). I. Transplacental transfer. J Acquir Immune Defic Synd 1990;3:959–64.
16. Hankins GDV, Lowery CL Jr, Scott RT, Morrow WR, Carey KD, Leland MM, Colvin EV. Transplacental transfer of zidovudine in the near-term pregnant baboon. Am J Obstet Gynecol 1990;163:728–32.
17. Liebes L, Mendoza S, Wilson D, Dancis J. Transfer of zidovudine (AZT) by human placenta. J Infect Dis 1990;161:203–7.
18. Bawdon RE, Sobhi S, Dax J. The transfer of anti-human immunodeficiency virus nucleoside compounds by the term human placenta. Am J Obstet Gynecol 1992;167:1570–4.
19. Schenker S, Johnson RF, King TS, Schenken RS, Henderson GI. Azidothymidine (zidovudine) transport by the human placenta. Am J Med Sci 1990;299:16–20.
20. Gillet JY, Garraffo R, Abrar D, Bongain A, Lapalus P, Dellamonica P. Fetoplacental passage of zidovudine. Lancet 1989;2:269–70.
21. Lyman WD, Tanaka KE, Kress Y, Rashbaum WK, Rubinstein A, Soeiro R. Zidovudine concentrations in human fetal tissue: implications for perinatal AIDS. Lancet 1990;335:1280–1.
22. Chavanet P, Diquet B, Waldner A, Portier H. Perinatal pharmacokinetics of zidovudine. N Engl J Med 1989;321:1548–9.
23. Pons JC, Taburet AM, Singlas E, Delfraissy JF, Papiernik E. Placental passage of azathiothymidine (AZT) during the second trimester of pregnancy: study by direct fetal blood sampling under ultrasound. Eur J Obstet Gynecol Reprod Biol 1991;40:229–31.
24. O'Sullivan MJ, Boyer PJJ, Scott GB, Parks WP, Weller S, Blum MR, Balsley J, Bryson YJ, Zidovudine Collaborative Working Group. The pharmacokinetics and safety of zidovudine in the third trimester of pregnancy for women infected with human immunodeficiency virus and their infants: Phase I Acquired Immunodeficiency Syndrome Clinical Trials group study (protocol 082). Am J Obstet Gynecol 1993;168:1510–6.
25. Unadkat JD, Pereira CM. Maternal-fetal transfer and fetal toxicity of anti-HIV drugs. A review. Trophoblast Res 1994;8:67–82.
26. Watts DH, Brown ZA, Tartaglione T, Burchett SK, Opheim K, Coombs R, Corey L. Pharmacokinetic disposition of zidovudine during pregnancy. J Infect Dis 1991;163:226–32.
27. Sperling RS, Roboz J, Dische R, Silides D, Holzman I, Jew E. Zidovudine pharmacokinetics during pregnancy. Am J Perinatol 1992;9:247–9.
28. Tindall B, Cotton R, Swanson C, Perdices M, Bodsworth N, Imrie A, Cooper DA. Fifth International Conference on the acquired immunodeficiency syndrome. Med J Aust 1990;152:204–14.
29. Tuntland T, Odinecs A, Pereira CM, Nosbisch C, Unadkat JD. In vitro models to predict the in vivo mechanism, rate, and extent of placental transfer of dideoxynucleoside drugs against human immunodeficiency virus. Am J Obstet Gynecol 1999;180:198–206.
30. Lopez-Anaya A, Unadkat JD, Schumann LA, Smith AL. Pharmacokinetics of zidovudine (azidothymidine). III. Effect of pregnancy. J Acquir Immune Defic Synd 1991;4:64–8.
31. Pereira CM, Nosbisch C, Baughman WL, Unadkat JD. Effect of zidovudine on transplacental pharmacokinetics of ddI in the pigtailed macaque (*Macaca nemestrina*). Antimicrob Agents Chemother 1995;39:343–5.
32. Moodley J, Moodley D, Pillay K, Coovadia H, Saba J, van Leeuwen R, Goodwin C, Harrigan PR, Moore KHP, Stone C, Plumb R, Johnson MA. Pharmacokinetics and antiretroviral activity of lamivudine alone or when coadministered with zidovudine in human immunodeficiency virus type 1-infected pregnant women and their offspring. J Infect Dis 1998;178:1327–33.
33. Odinecs A, Nosbisch C, Unadkat JD. Zidovudine does not affect transplacental transfer or systemic clearance of stavudine (2′,3′-didehydro-3′-deoxythymidine) in the pigtailed macaque (*Macaca nemestrina*), Antimicrob Agents Chemother 1996;40:1569–71.
34. Liebes L, Mendoza S, Lee JD, Dancis J. Further observations on zidovudine transfer and metabolism by human placenta. AIDS 1993;7:590–2.
35. Viscarello RR, DeGennaro NJ, Hobbins JC. Preliminary experience with the use of zidovudine (AZT) during pregnancy. Society of Perinatal Obstetricians Abstracts. Am J Obstet Gynecol 1991;164:248.
36. Cullen MT, Delke I, Greenhaw J, Viscarello RR, Paryani S, Sanchez-Ramos L. HIV in pregnancy: factors predictive of maternal and fetal outcome. Society of Perinatal Obstetricians Abstracts. Am J Obstet Gynecol 1992;166:386.
37. Taylor U, Bardeguez A. Antiretroviral therapy during pregnancy and post-partum. Society of Perinatal Obstetricians Abstracts. Am J Obstet Gynecol 1992;166:390.
38. Delke I, Greenhaw J, Sanchez-Ramos L, Roberts W. Antiretroviral therapy during pregnancy. Society of Perinatal Obstetricians Abstracts. Am J Obstet Gynecol 1993;168:424.
39. Sperling RS, Stratton P, O'Sullivan MJ, Boyer P, Watts DH, Lambert JS, Hammill H, Livingston EG, Gloeb DJ, Minkoff H, Fox HE. A survey of zidovudine use in pregnant women with human immunodeficiency virus infection. N Engl J Med 1992;326:857–61.
40. Stratton P, Mofenson LM, Willoughby AD. Human immunodeficiency virus infection in pregnant women under care at AIDS Clinical Trials centers in the United States. Obstet Gynecol 1992;79:364–8.
41. Kumar RM, Hughes PF, Khurranna A. Zidovudine use in pregnancy: a report of 104 cases and the occurrence of birth defects. J Acquir Immune Defic Synd 1994;7:1034–9.
42. Antiretroviral Pregnancy Registry Steering Committee. *Antiretroviral Pregnancy Registry International Interim Report for 1 January 1989 through 31 July 2009*. Wilmington, NC: Registry Coordinating Center; 2009. Available at www.apregistry.com. Accessed May 29, 2010.
43. Barzilai A, Sperling RS, Hyatt AC, Wedgwood JF, Reidenberg BE, Hodes DS. Mother to child transmission of human immunodeficiency virus 1 infection despite zidovudine therapy from 18 weeks of gestation. Pediatr Infect Dis J 1990;9:931–3.
44. Sperling RS, Stratton P, Obstetric-Gynecologic Working Group of the AIDS Clinical Trials Group of the National Institute of Allergy and Infectious Diseases. Treatment options for human immunodeficiency virus-infected pregnant women. Obstet Gynecol 1992;79:443–8.
45. Rogers MF, Jaffe HW. Reducing the risk of maternal-infant transmission of HIV: a door is opened. N Engl J Med 1994;331:1222–3.
46. CDC. Zidovudine for the prevention of HIV transmission from mother to infant. MMWR 1994;43:285–7.
47. CDC. Zidovudine for the prevention of HIV transmission from mother to infant. JAMA 1994;271:1567, 1570.
48. Cotton P. Trial halted after drug cuts maternal HIV transmission rate by two thirds. JAMA 1994;271:807.
49. Anonymous. Zidovudine for mother, fetus, and child: hope or poison? Lancet 1994;344:207–9.

50. Spector SA. Pediatric antiretroviral choices. AIDS 1994;4(Suppl 3):S15–8.
51. Murphy R. Clinical aspects of human immunodeficiency virus disease: clinical rationale for treatment. J Infect Dis 1995;171(Suppl 2):S81–7.
52. Connor EM, Sperling RS, Gelber R, Kiselev P, Scott G, O'Sullivan MJ, VanDyke R, Bey M, Shearer W, Jacobson RL, Jimenez E, O'Neill E, Bazin B, Delfraissy J-F, Culnane M, Coombs R, Elkins M, Moye J, Stratton P, Balsley J, for the Pediatric AIDS Clinical Trials Group Protocol 076 Study Group. Reduction of maternal-infant transmission of human immunodeficiency virus type 1 with zidovudine treatment. N Engl J Med 1994;331:1173–80.
53. Wade NA, Birkhead GS, Warren BL, Charbonneau TT, French PT, Wang L, Baum JB, Tesoriero JM, Savicki R. Abbreviated regimens of zidovudine prophylaxis and perinatal transmission of the human immunodeficiency virus. N Engl J Med 1998;339:1409–14.
54. Shaffer N, Chuachoowong R, Mock PA, Bhadrakom C, Siriwasin W, Young NL, Chotpitayasunondh T, Chearskul S, Roongpisuthipong A, Chinayon P, Karon J, Mastro TD, Simonds RJ, on behalf of the Bangkok Collaborative Perinatal HIV Transmission Study Group. Short-course zidovudine for perinatal HIV-1 transmission in Bangkok, Thailand: a randomised controlled trial. Lancet 1999;353:773–80.
55. Wiktor SZ, Ekpini E, Karon JM, Nkengasong J, Maurice C, Severin ST, Roels TH, Kouassi MK, Lackritz EM, Coulibaly IM, Greenberg AE. Short-course oral zidovudine for prevention of mother-to-child transmission of HIV-1 in Abidjan, Côte d'Ivoire: a randomised trial. Lancet 1999;353:781–5.
56. Dabis F, Msellati P, Meda N, Welffens-Ekra C, You B, Manigart O, Leroy V, Simonon A, Cartoux M, Combe P, Ouangre A, Ramon R, Ky-Zerbo O, Montcho C, Salamon R, Rouzioux C, Van de Perre P, Mandelbrot L, for the DITRAME Study Group. 6-month efficacy, tolerance, and acceptability of a short regimen of oral zidovudine to reduce vertical transmission of HIV in breastfed children in Côte d'Ivoire and Burkina Faso: a double-blind placebo-controlled multicentre trial. Lancet 1999;353:786–92.
57. Mofenson LM. Short-course zidovudine for prevention of perinatal infection. Lancet 1999;353:766–7.
58. Lallemant M, Jourdain G, Le Coeur S, Kim S, Koetsawang S, Comeau AM, Phoolcharoen W, Essex M, McIntosh K, Vithayasai V, for the Perinatal HIV Prevention Trial (Thialand) investigators. A trial of shortened zidovudine regimens to prevent mother-to-child transmission of human immunodeficiency virus type 1. N Engl J Med 2000;343:982–91.
59. Peckham C, Newell ML. Preventing vertical transmission of HIV infection. N Engl J Med 2000;343:1036–7.
60. Mofenson LM, McIntyre JA. Advances and research directions in the prevention of mother-to-child HIV-1 transmission. Lancet 2000;355:2237–44.
61. McGowan JP, Crane M, Wiznia AA, Blum S. Combination antiretroviral therapy in human immunodeficiency virus-infected pregnant women. Obstet Gynecol 1999;94:641–6.
62. Guay LA, Musoke P, Fleming T, Bagenda D, Allen M, Nakabiito C, Sherman J, Bakaki P, Ducar C, Deseyve M, Emel L, Mirochnick M, Fowler MG, Mofenson L, Miotti P, Dransfield K, Bray D, Mmiro F, Jackson JB. Intrapartum and neonatal single-dose nevirapine compared with zidovudine for prevention of mother-to-child transmission of HIV-1 in Kampala, Uganda: HIVNET 012 randomised trial. Lancet 1999;354:795–802.
63. Marseille E, Kahn JG, Mmiro F, Guay L, Musoke P, Fowler MG, Jackson JB. Cost effectiveness of single-dose nevirapine regimen for mothers and babies to decrease vertical HIV-1 transmission in sub-Saharan Africa. Lancet 1999;354:803–9.
64. Loch M, Carr A, Vasak E, Cunningham P, Smith D. The use of human immunodeficiency virus postexposure prophylaxis after successful artificial insemination. Am J Obstet Gynecol 1999;181:760–1.
65. Watson WJ, Stevens TP, Weinberg GA. Profound anemia in a newborn infant of a mother receiving antiretroviral therapy. Pediatr Infect Dis J 1998;17:435–6.
66. Shah MM, Li Y, Christensen RD. Effects of perinatal zidovudine on hematopoiesis: a comparison of effects on progenitors from human fetuses versus mothers. AIDS 1996;10:1239–47.
67. Blanche S, Tardieu M, Rustin P, Slama A, Barret B, Firtion G, Ciraru-Vigneron N, Lacroix C, Rouzioux C, Mandelbrot L, Desguerre I, Rotig A, Mayaux MJ, Delfraissy JF. Persistent mitochondrial dysfunction and perinatal exposure to antiretroviral nucleoside analogues. Lancet 1999;354:1084–9.
68. Brinkman K, Smeitink JA, Romijn JA, Reiss P. Mitochondrial toxicity induced by nucleoside-analogue reverse-transcriptase inhibitors is a key factor in the pathogenesis of antiretroviral-therapy-related lipodystrophy. Lancet 1999;354:1112–5.
69. Morris AAM, Carr A. HIV nucleoside analogues: new adverse effects on mitochondria? Lancet 1999;354:1046–7.
70. Stojanov S, Wintergerst U, Belohradsky BH, Rolinski B. Mitochondrial and peroxisomal dysfunction following perinatal exposure to antiretroviral drugs. AIDS 2000;14:1669.
71. Gerschenson M, Erhart SW, Paik CY, St.Claire MC, Nagashima K, Skopets B, Harbaugh SW, Harbaugh JW, Quan W, Poirier MC. Fetal mitochondrial heart and skeletal muscle damage in *Erythrocebus patas* monkeys exposed in utero to 3′-azido-3′-deoxythymidine. AIDS Res Hum Retroviruses 2000;16:635–44.
72. Lipshultz SE, Easley KA, Orav EJ, Kaplan S, Starc TJ, Bricker JT, Lai WW, Moodie DS, Sopko G, McIntosh K, Colan SD, for the Pediatric Pulmonary and Cardiac Complications of Vertically Transmitted HIV Infection Study Group. Absence of cardiac toxicity of zidovudine in infants. N Engl J Med 2000;343:759–66.
73. Richardson MP, Osrin D, Donaghy S, Brown NA, Hay P, Sharland M. Spinal malformations in the fetuses of HIV infected women receiving combination antiretroviral therapy and co-trimoxazole. Eur J Obstet Gynecol Reprod Biol 2000;93:215–7.
74. Moschovi M, Theodoridou M, Papaevangelou V, Tzortzatou-Stathopoulou F. Acute lymphoblastic leukaemia in an infant exposed to zidovudine in utero and early infancy. AIDS 2000;14:2410–1.
75. Hanson IC, Antonelli TA, Sperling RS, Oleske JM, Cooper E, Culnane M, Fowler MG, Kalish LA, Lee SS, McSherry G, Mofenson L, Shapiro DE. Lack of tumors in infants with perinatal HIV-1 exposure and fetal/neonatal exposure to zidovudine. J Acquir Immune Defic Syndr Hum Retrovirol 1999;20: 463–7.
76. Culnane M, Fowler MG, Lee SS, McSherry G, Brady M, O'Donnell K, Mofenson L, Gortmaker SL, Shapiro DE, Scott G, Jimenez E, Moore EC, Diaz C, Flynn P, Cunningham B, Oleske J, for the Pediatric AIDS Clinical Trials Group Protocol 219/076 Teams. Lack of long-term effects of in utero exposure to zidovudine among uninfected children born to HIV-infected women. JAMA 1999;281:151–7.
77. Newschaffer CJ, Cocroft J, Anderson CE, Hauck WW, Turner BJ. Prenatal zidovudine use and congenital anomalies in a Medicaid population. J Acquir Immune Defic Syndr 2000;24:249–56.
78. Henry K, Chinnock BJ, Quinn RP, Fletcher CV, de Miranda P, Balfour HH Jr. Concurrent zidovudine levels in semen and serum determined by radioimmunoassay in patients with AIDS or AIDS-related complex. JAMA 1988;259:3023–6.
79. Politch JA, Mayer KH, Abbott AF, Anderson DJ. The effects of disease progression and zidovudine therapy on semen quality in human immunodeficiency virus type 1 seropositive men. Fertil Steril 1994;61;922–8.
80. Carpenter CCJ, Fischi MA, Hammer SM, Hirsch MS, Jacobsen DM, Katzenstein DA, Montaner JSG, Richman DD, Saag MS, Schooley RT, Thompson MA, Vella S, Yeni PG, Volberding PA. Antiretroviral therapy for HIV infection in 1996. JAMA 1996;276:145–54.
81. Minkoff H, Augenbraun M. Antiretroviral therapy for pregnant women. Am J Obstet Gynecol 1997;176:478–89.
82. Minkoff H. Human immunodeficiency virus infection in pregnancy. Obstet Gynecol 2003;101:797–810.
83. Panel on Antiretroviral Guidelines for Adults and Adolescents. *Guidelines for the Use of Antiretroviral Agents in HIV-1-Infected Adults and Adolescents.* Department of Health and Human Services. December 1, 2009:1–161. Available at http://www.aidsinfo.nih.gov/ContentFiles/AdultandAdolescentGL.pdf. Accessed September 17, 2010:60, 96–8.
84. Panel on Treatment of HIV-Infected Pregnant Women and Prevention of Perinatal Transmission. *Recommendations for Use of Antiretroviral Drugs in Pregnant HIV-1-Infected Women for Maternal Health and Interventions to Reduce Perinatal HIV Transmission in the United States.* May 24, 2010:1–117. Available at http://aidsinfo.nih.gov/ContentFiles/PerinatalGL.pdf. Accessed September 17, 2010:30 (Table 5).
85. Ruff A, Hamzeh, Lietman P, Siberry G, Boulos R, Bell K, McBrien M, Davis H, Coberly J, Joseph D, Halsey N. *Excretion of Zidovudine (ZDV) in Human Breast Milk* (Abstract). Presented at the 34th Interscience Conference on Antimicrobial Agents and Chemotherapy, American Society for Microbiology, Orlando, FL, October, 1994.
86. Brown ZA, Watts DH. Antiviral therapy in pregnancy. Clin Obstet Gynecol 1990;33:276–89.
87. De Martino M, Tovo P-A, Tozzi AE, Pezzotti P, Galli L, Livadiotti S, Caselli D, Massironi E, Ruga E, Fioredda F, Plebani A, Gabiano C, Zuccotti GV. HIV-1 transmission through breast-milk: appraisal of risk according to duration of feeding. AIDS 1992;6:991–7.
88. Van de Perre P. Postnatal transmission of human immunodeficiency virus type 1: the breast-feeding dilemma. Am J Obstet Gynecol 1995;173:483–7.

ZILEUTON

Respiratory Agent

PREGNANCY RECOMMENDATION: No Human Data—Animal Data Suggest Risk
BREASTFEEDING RECOMMENDATION: No Human Data—Probably Compatible

PREGNANCY SUMMARY

No reports on the use of zileuton in human pregnancy have been found. One source, based solely on animal data, recommends that the drug be avoided during gestation (1).

FETAL RISK SUMMARY

Zileuton, a specific inhibitor of the enzyme (5-lipoxygenase) that catalyzes the formation of leukotrienes (LTB_4, LTC_4, LTD_4, and LTE_4) from arachidonic acid, is given orally for the prophylaxis and chronic treatment of asthma (2).

Reproduction studies have been conducted in rats and rabbits. No effects on fertility were observed in male and female rats given oral doses approximately 8 and 18 times the systemic exposure (AUC) achieved at the maximum recommended human daily oral dose (MRHD), respectively. However, at doses ≥9 times the MRHD-AUC, a reduction in fetal implants was observed. At ≥4 times the MRHD-AUC, increases in gestation length and the number of stillbirths were noted. In addition, offspring of pregnant rats given 18 times the MRHD-AUC had reduced body weight and increased skeletal variations. A decrease in rat pup survival and growth occurred at this same dose in perinatal and postnatal studies. In pregnant rabbits given oral doses equivalent to the MRHD (based on BSA), 3 (2.5%) of 118 fetuses had cleft palates (2).

It is not known if zileuton crosses the human placenta to the fetus, but the molecular weight (about 236) is low enough that transfer should be expected. The drug and/or its metabolites cross the rat placenta (2).

BREASTFEEDING SUMMARY

No reports describing the use of zileuton during human lactation have been located. The molecular weight (about 236) is low enough that passage into human breast milk should be expected. The effects on a nursing infant from this exposure are unknown.

References

1. Anonymous. Drugs for asthma. Med Lett Drugs Ther 2000;42:19–24.
2. Product information. Zyflo. Abbott Laboratories, 2000.

ZIPRASIDONE

Antipsychotic

PREGNANCY RECOMMENDATION: Limited Human Data—Animal Data Suggest Risk
BREASTFEEDING RECOMMENDATION: Limited Human Data—Potential Toxicity

PREGNANCY SUMMARY

Two reports describing the use of ziprasidone in human pregnancy have been located, one of which described an infant with a cleft palate. The animal reproduction data suggests risk as all aspects of developmental toxicity were observed. However, the limited human pregnancy experience prevents a more complete assessment of embryo–fetal risk. Although none of the antipsychotic class of agents has been proven to cause structural anomalies, there is a concern for long-term neurobehavioral deficits. Therefore, until human pregnancy data are available, the safest course is to avoid ziprasidone in pregnancy. However, if a woman requires treatment and informed consent is obtained, ziprasidone should not be withheld because of pregnancy. If an inadvertent pregnancy does occur during treatment, the woman should be advised of the unknown risks to her embryo–fetus. If ziprasidone is used in pregnancy, healthcare professionals are encouraged to call the toll-free number 800-670-6126 for information about patient enrollment in the Motherisk study.

FETAL RISK SUMMARY

The atypical antipsychotic ziprasidone is a benzisoxazole derivative in the same subclass of antipsychotic agents as iloperidone, paliperidone, and risperidone. Ziprasidone is indicated for the treatment of schizophrenia, including acute agitation in schizophrenic patients. It also is indicated for the treatment of acute manic or mixed episodes associated with bipolar disorder. Elimination is mostly by hepatic metabolism to inactive metabolites. After oral administration, the mean terminal elimination half-life is about 7 hours, but a mean 2–5 hours after a single IM dose. Plasma protein binding to albumin and α_1-acid glycoprotein is >99% (1).

Reproduction studies have been conducted in rats and rabbits. In rats, oral doses that were 0.5–8 times the maximum recommended human dose of 200 mg/day based on BSA (MRHD) given during organogenesis or throughout gestation caused embryo–fetal toxicity consisting of decreased fetal weights and delayed skeletal ossification. There was no evidence of structural anomalies. Doses that were 2 and 8 times the MRHD were maternally toxic. The developmental no-effect dose for embryo–fetal toxicity was 0.2 times the MRHD. When rats were treated throughout gestation and lactation with a dose that was half the MRHD, there was an increase in the number of pups born dead and decreased postnatal survival during the first 4 days of lactation. Developmental delays and impaired neurobehavioral function were observed in offspring with doses ≥0.2 times the MRHD. A no-effect dose for these effects was not established (1).

In pregnant rabbits during organogenesis, a dose 3 times the MRHD was associated with an increased incidence of ventricular septal defects, other cardiovascular malformations, and kidney alterations. There was no maternal toxicity at this dose. The developmental no-effect dose was equivalent to the MRHD (1).

Two-year studies for carcinogenicity were conducted in rats and mice with doses that were 0.1–0.6 and 1–5 times, respectively, the MRHD. In rats and male mice, there was no evidence of an increased incidence of tumors. However, in female mice, there were dose-related increases in the incidences of pituitary gland adenoma and carcinoma, and mammary gland adenocarcinoma at all doses tested. These effects have been observed in rodents with other antipsychotic agents and were thought to be prolactin-mediated. Ziprasidone was mutagenic in some tests (1).

In fertility tests with rats, doses that were 0.5–8 times the MRHD increased the time to copulation. Fertility was decreased at 8 times the MRHD, but there was no effect on fertility at 2 times the MRHD. The effect appeared to be confined to female rats as fertility was not impaired in male rats given a dose that was 8 times the MRHD and mated with untreated females. In addition, there were no treatment-related effects in the testes in a study with male rats at 10 times the MRHD for 6 months (1).

It is not known if ziprasidone crosses the human placenta. The molecular weight of the free base (about 413) and the elimination half-life suggest that the drug will cross to the embryo and/or fetus. However, the very high plasma protein binding should limit the amount crossing to the embryo/fetus.

A 2009 case report described the pregnancy of a 26-year-old woman with severe psychotic depression (2). She was treated with ziprasidone 40 mg/day and citalopram 60 mg/day throughout pregnancy. At 39 weeks' gestation, she gave birth to a healthy, 2.64-kg male infant with Apgar scores of 8 and 9 at 1 and 5 minutes, respectively. No anomalies, drug-related adverse effects, or withdrawal were observed in the infant who was doing well at 6 months of age (2).

In a 2010 case report, a 33-year-old woman with paranoid schizophrenia was treated throughout pregnancy with ziprasidone (daily doses of 120 mg during first 3 months, then 80 mg for 2 months, then 40 mg until birth), fluvoxamine and diazepam (doses not specified) (3). She gave birth at term to a 3.070-kg female infant with a cleft palate. The infant's karyotype was normal, and the mother denied smoking, drinking coffee or alcohol, taking other drugs during pregnancy (3).

BREASTFEEDING SUMMARY

A woman with schizophrenia who was breastfeeding her infant was started on ziprasidone on postpartum day 9 (4). Breastfeeding was stopped because of concerns of toxicity in the infant. Ziprasidone was not detected (limit of quantification was 10 ng/mL) until day 10 of treatment. At that time, the milk and maternal plasma concentrations were 11 and 170 ng/mL (milk:plasma ratio 0.06). The theoretical relative dose received by the infant per kg body weight based on the weight-adjusted maternal dose was 1.2% (4).

In a 2009 case (see Fetal Risk Summary), a mother taking ziprasidone and citalopram breastfed her full-term infant for 6 months. No adverse effects were noted and the infant was deemed healthy by his pediatrician (2).

Consistent with the molecular weight of the free base (about 413) and the elimination half-life (up to 7 hours), ziprasidone is excreted into breast milk but, as suggested by the very high plasma protein binding (>99%), only low levels were excreted. However, the absorption of ziprasidone in adults is increased twofold in the presence of food (1).

Although no adverse effects were observed in one case, additional data are needed before a better assessment of risk can be made. Moreover, because treatment with ziprasidone will usually be long term, there is concern for potential adverse effects involving the neurobehavior of an infant.

References

1. Product information. Geodon. Pfizer, 2007.
2. Werremeyer A. Ziprasidone and citalopram use in pregnancy and lactation in a woman with psychotic depression. Am J Psychiatry 2009;166:1298.
3. Peitl MV, Petric D, Peitl V. Ziprasidone as a possible cause of cleft palate in a newborn. Psychiatr Danub 2010;22:117–9.
4. Schlotterbeck P, Saur R, Hiemke C, Grunder G, Vehren T, Kircher T, Leube D. Low concentration of ziprasidone in human milk: a case report. Int J Neuropsychopharmacol 2009;12:437–8.

ZIV-AFLIBERCEPT

Antineoplastic (Tyrosine Kinase Inhibitor)

PREGNANCY RECOMMENDATION: Contraindicated
BREASTFEEDING RECOMMENDATION: Contraindicated

PREGNANCY SUMMARY

No reports describing the use of ziv-aflibercept in human pregnancy have been located. Animal reproduction data suggest risk, but the absence of human pregnancy experience prevents a more complete assessment of embryo–fetal risk. However, ziv-aflibercept is given in combination with two other antineoplastics and the three agents potentially could cause embryo–fetal harm. In addition, ziv-aflibercept has caused reversible impaired fertility in male and female cynomolgus monkeys at systemic exposures that were less than those obtained in humans. Taken in sum, the drug should be considered contraindicated in pregnancy. Moreover, the manufacturer recommends that females and males of reproductive potential should use highly effective contraception during treatment and up to a minimum of 3 months after the last dose (1).

FETAL RISK SUMMARY

Ziv-aflibercept, a dimeric glycoprotein, is a recombinant fusion protein that binds to vascular endothelial growth factor-A (VEGF-A). It is indicated, in combination with 5-fluorouracil, leuvovorin, and irinotecan, for patients with metastatic colorectal cancer that is resistant to or has progressed following an oxaliplatin-containing regimen (see also Fluorouracil, Irinotecan, and Leuvovorin). The metabolism and plasma protein binding were not specified, but the elimination half-life of free ziv-aflibercept was about 6 days (range 4–7 days) (1).

Reproduction studies have been conducted in rabbits. In this species, IV doses that resulted in systemic exposures that were about ≥30% of the AUC in patients at the recommended dose, given every 3 days during organogenesis resulted in adverse embryo–fetal effects. These effects included increased incidences of postimplantation losses and external (anasarca, umbilical hernia, diaphragmatic hernia and gastroschisis, cleft palate, ectrodactyly, and atresia), visceral (great vessels and arteries in the heart), and skeletal fetal anomalies (fused vertebrae, sternebrae, and ribs; supernumerary arches and ribs, and incomplete ossification). The incidence and severity of fetal anomalies increased with increasing dose (1).

Studies for carcinogenicity and mutagenicity have not been conducted. In sexually mature young cynomolgus monkeys given IV doses that were about ≥60% of the AUC in patients at the recommended dose every 2 weeks for 6 months, impaired reproductive function was noted at all doses tested. In females, the drug inhibited ovarian function and follicular development as shown by decreased ovary weight, amount of luteal tissue, and number of maturing follicles; atrophy of uterine endometrium and myometrium, vaginal atrophy, abrogation of progesterone peaks and menstrual bleeding. In males, alterations in sperm morphology and decreased sperm motility were noted. All of these effects were reversible within 18 weeks after cessation of therapy (1).

It is not known if free ziv-aflibercept crosses the human placenta. The molecular weight (about 115,000) suggests that it will not cross, at least early in gestation, but the elimination half-life is very long. Moreover, the drug did cause embryo–fetal toxicity in rabbits during organogenesis.

BREASTFEEDING SUMMARY

No reports describing the use of ziv-aflibercept during human lactation have been reported. The molecular weight (about 115,000) suggests that it will not be excreted into mature milk, but it probably will be excreted during the colostral period. However, the drug is given in combination with 5-fluorouracil, leuvovorin, and irinotecan (see also these three agents) and the two antineoplastic agents are probably excreted into breast milk. Consequently, breastfeeding should be considered contraindicated if a woman is receiving this combined therapy.

Reference

1. Product information. Zaltrap. Regeneron Pharmaceuticals, 2012.

ZOLEDRONIC ACID

Bisphosphonate

PREGNANCY RECOMMENDATION: Limited Human Data—Animal Data Suggest Moderate Risk
BREASTFEEDING RECOMMENDATION: No Human Data—Potential Toxicity

PREGNANCY SUMMARY

One report has described the use of zoledronic acid use in human pregnancy. The animal data suggest risk, but the limited human pregnancy experience prevents a complete assessment of the embryo–fetal risk. The amount of zoledronic acid incorporated into bone and eventually released back into the systemic circulation is directly related to the total dose and duration of treatment. Because zoledronic acid probably crosses the placenta, the use of the drug shortly before or during gestation could expose the embryo and/or fetus to a potentially toxic agent. Thus, administration before pregnancy may result in low-level, continuous exposure throughout gestation. The use of zoledronic acid in women who may become pregnant or during pregnancy is not recommended. However, based on the animal and limited human data, inadvertent exposure during early pregnancy does not appear to represent a major risk to the embryo–fetus.

FETAL RISK SUMMARY

Zoledronic acid is given by IV infusion. It is indicated for the treatment of hypercalcemia of malignancy. Other agents in this pharmacologic class are alendronate, etidronate, ibandronate, pamidronate, risedronate, and tiludronate. Only about 3% of an oral dose is absorbed into the systemic circulation. Zoledronic acid is not metabolized, and plasma protein binding is only 22%. The postinfusion half-life in the plasma is 1.87 hours, whereas the terminal elimination half-life is 146 hours, correlating with the low concentrations in the plasma observed up to 28 days postdose (1).

Reproduction studies have been conducted in rats and rabbits. In pregnant rats, daily SC doses producing exposures 1.2, 2.4, and 4.8 times the human systemic exposure after an IV dose of 4 mg based on AUC (HSE) were associated with adverse fetal effects. At 1.2 times the HSE, fetal skeletal variations were noted. Doses producing exposures 2.4 and 4.8 times the HSE caused pre- and postimplantation losses; decreases in viable fetuses; and fetal skeletal, visceral, and external malformations. The fetal skeletal effects observed at 4.8 times the HSE were unossified or incompletely ossified bones; thickened, curved, or shortened bones; wavy ribs, and shortened jaw. Other adverse fetal effects observed in the high-dose group were reduced lens, rudimentary cerebellum, reduction or absence of liver lobes, reduction or absence of lung lobes, vessel dilation, cleft palate, and edema, but maternal toxicity (reduced body weight and food consumption) also was observed (1).

In female rats given SC doses producing exposures ≥ 0.2 times the HSE for 15 days before mating and continuing through gestation, the number of stillbirths was increased and survival of neonates was decreased. Higher exposure (1.2 times the HSE) inhibited ovulation, resulting in a decrease in the number of pregnant rats. Maternal toxicity (dystocia and periparturient mortality) was observed at all exposures ≥ 0.7 times the HSE. This toxicity was thought to be secondary to drug-induced inhibition of skeletal calcium mobilization, resulting in hypocalcemia, a bisphosphonate class effect (1).

In pregnant rabbits, SC doses resulting in exposures ≤ 0.5 times the HSE did not cause fetal harm. However, exposures >0.05 times the HSE were associated with maternal mortality and abortion in all treatment groups. The maternal toxicity may have been caused by drug-induced hypocalcemia (1).

Long-term carcinogenicity studies with oral zoledronic acid were positive in male and female mice but not in rats. Various assays for mutagenicity were negative (1).

It is not known if zoledronic acid crosses the human placenta. The molecular weight (about 290 for the hydrated form), lack of metabolism, low plasma protein binding, plasma half-life, and the prolonged terminal elimination half-life all suggest that exposure of the embryo and/or fetus will occur. Moreover, detectable amounts of the drug can be measured in plasma for up to 28 days postdose (1).

A 33-year-old woman with metastatic breast cancer was treated with zoledronic acid (two IV courses 28 days apart; dose not specified) and tamoxifen in the 2nd and 3rd trimesters (2). She also received five cycles of 5-fluorouracil, epirubicin, and cyclophosphamide before conception and during the 1st trimester, as well as radiotherapy at 17 weeks' gestation. Her pregnancy was diagnosed at 28 weeks. A cesarean section at 35 weeks' delivered a 2070-g female infant with Apgar scores of 10 at 1 and 5 minutes, respectively. All hematologic and biochemistry parameters were normal for age. The healthy infant apparently was developing normally at 12 months of age (2).

A 2008 review described 51 cases of exposure to bisphosphonates before or during pregnancy: alendronate (*N* = 32) pamidronate (*N* = 11), etidronate (*N* = 5), risedronate (*N* = 2), and zoledronic acid (*N* = 1) (3). They concluded that although these drugs may affect bone modeling and development in the fetus, no such toxicity has yet been reported.

BREASTFEEDING SUMMARY

No reports describing the use of zoledronic acid during human lactation have been located. The molecular weight (about 290 for the hydrated form), lack of metabolism, low plasma protein binding, plasma half-life, and the prolonged terminal elimination half-life suggest that the drug will be excreted into breast milk. Detectable amounts of the drug are measured in adult plasma for up to 28 days postdose (1). Although the low lipid solubility of zoledronic acid may limit the amount present in milk, and maternal treatment may be compatible with nursing, the best course is to not breastfeed until data are available.

References

1. Product information. Zometa. Novartis Pharmaceuticals, 2006.
2. Andreadis C, Charalampidou M, Diamantopoulos N, Chouchos N, Mouratidou D. Combined chemotherapy and radiotherapy during conception and first two trimesters of gestation in a woman with metastatic breast cancer. Gynecol Oncol 2004;95:252–5.
3. Djokanovic N, Klieger-Grossmann C, Koren G. Does treatment with bisphosphonates endanger the human pregnancy? J Obstet Gynaecol Can 2008;30:1146–8.

ZOLMITRIPTAN

Antimigraine

PREGNANCY RECOMMENDATION: No Human Data—Animal Data Suggest Low Risk
BREASTFEEDING RECOMMENDATION: No Human Data—Probably Compatible

PREGNANCY SUMMARY

No reports describing the use of zolmitriptan in human pregnancy have been located. The animal data suggest low risk, but an assessment of the actual risk cannot be determined until human pregnancy experience is available. Although a 2008 review of triptans in pregnancy found no evidence for teratogenicity, the data did suggest a possible increase in the rate of preterm birth (1).

FETAL RISK SUMMARY

Zolmitriptan is an oral selective serotonin (5-hydroxytryptamine; 5HT) receptor agonist that has high affinity for $5HT_{1B}$ and $5HT_{1D}$ receptors. The drug is closely related to almotriptan, eletriptan, frovatriptan, naratriptan, rizatriptan, and sumatriptan. It is indicated for the acute treatment of migraine with or without aura in adults. Protein binding is low (about 25%). Zolmitriptan has a several metabolites, one of which is 2–6 times more potent for the $5HT_{1B/1D}$ receptors than is the parent compound. The active metabolite contributes a substantial portion of the pharmacologic effect because its concentrations are about two-thirds that of zolmitriptan (2). The elimination half-life of zolmitriptan is apparently unknown.

Reproduction studies have been conducted in rats and rabbits. In rats, zolmitriptan was given during organogenesis at oral doses resulting in maternal exposures ranging from 280 to 5000 times the exposure in humans receiving the maximum recommended total daily dose of 10 mg (MRHD). A dose-related increase in embryolethality was observed, which became statistically significant at the high dose, but maternal toxicity (decreased weight gain during gestation) was also noted. When pregnant rats were treated throughout gestation and lactation, an increased incidence of hydronephrosis was seen in the offspring at a dose 1100 times the MRHD. This dose was also maternally toxic. In pregnant rabbits treated during organogenesis, an increased incidence of embryolethality was observed at maternally toxic doses ≥11 times the MRHD. At 42 times the MRHD, increased incidences of fetal malformations (fused sternebrae, rib anomalies) and variations (blood vessels, rib ossification) were observed. The no-effect dose was equivalent to the MRHD (2).

It is not known if zolmitriptan or its active metabolite crosses the human placenta to the fetus. The molecular weight of the parent compound (about 287) and the minimal plasma protein binding suggest that the drug will cross to the embryo–fetus.

BREASTFEEDING SUMMARY

No reports describing the use of zolmitriptan during human lactation have been located. The molecular weight (about 287) and low plasma protein binding (25%) suggest that the drug, and possibly its active metabolite, will be excreted into breast milk. The effect of this exposure on a nursing infant is unknown.

References

1. Soldin OP, Dahlin J, O'Mara DM. Triptans in pregnancy. Ther Drug Monit 2008;30:5–9.
2. Product information. Zomig. Astrazeneca, 2004.

ZOLPIDEM

Hypnotic

PREGNANCY RECOMMENDATION: Human Data Suggest Risk
BREASTFEEDING RECOMMENDATION: Limited Human Data—Probably Compatible

PREGNANCY SUMMARY

Although no increased risk of congenital malformations has been observed, two studies did find increased risks for preterm birth, low birth weights, small for gestational age (SGA) infants, and cesarean birth. Although the drug has addiction potential, withdrawal symptoms have not been reported in exposed newborns.

FETAL RISK SUMMARY

Zolpidem is a nonbenzodiazepine hypnotic of the imidazopyridine class. In subjects with normal liver function, a single 5-mg dose of zolpidem had a relatively short elimination half-life (2.6 hours; range 1.4–4.5 hours) (1).

In reproductive studies in rats, no teratogenic effects were observed, but dose-related toxicity was observed in the fetuses (delayed maturation as characterized by incomplete ossification of the skull) at doses about 25 and 125 times the maximum human dose based on BSA (MHD) (1). The no-effect dose was 5 times the MHD. In rabbits, increased postimplantation fetal loss and incomplete ossification of the sternum in surviving fetuses were observed at about 28 times the MHD, both possibly related to maternal toxicity (decreased weight gain) (1). The no-effect dose in rabbits was 7 times the MHD. No teratogenic effects of the drug were observed. Shepard (2) reviewed a reproductive toxicity study in rats during organogenesis that found no teratogenicity, but did observe a decrease in fetal weight at doses ranging from 5 to 125 mg/kg and an increase in wavy ribs at the highest dose.

The FDA had not received any reports of adverse fetal or newborn outcomes from pregnancy exposures to zolpidem between its approval in December 1992 and 1996 (F. Rosa, personal communication, FDA, 1996).

Consistent with the molecular weight (about 765 for the tartrate salt), zolpidem crosses the placenta, at least at term. A 2007 report described the pregnancy outcome of a woman apparently addicted to zolpidem (3). The woman experienced vaginal bleeding and abdominal pain, diagnosed as placental abruption, at about 27 weeks' gestation. She had been taking 10–15 zolpidem tablets/night (strength not specified). Within 24 hours of hospitalization, the patient had withdrawal-like symptoms (nervousness and anxiety) that were thought to be due to zolpidem withdrawal. She was prescribed zolpidem 15 mg/night and was discharged home on hospital day 7.

Polyhydramnios was diagnosed at 35 weeks but had resolved by 37 weeks. At 38 weeks, she delivered vaginally a healthy 3.9-kg female infant with Apgar scores of 8 and 9. No withdrawal signs were observed in the neonate or the mother over a 48-hour interval until discharge. The cord blood concentration of zolpidem was 41 ng/mL. In adults, the mean peak plasma levels after 5- and 10-mg doses are 29–113 ng/mL (mean 59 ng/mL) and 58–272 ng/mL (mean 121 ng/mL), respectively. Although the interval between the mother's last dose and delivery was not known, the interval from admission and the cord blood sample was about 14.33 hours (3). No follow-up on the infant was reported.

A 2009 study evaluated the placental passage of zolpidem at term and infant outcomes in 45 women with psychiatric illness who had taken the drug during pregnancy compared with 45 matched pregnant women who had not (4). Exposures to zolpidem occurred in 17 (38%) women in the 1st trimester, 25 (56%) in the 2nd trimester, and 35 (78%) in the 3rd trimester. The drug was taken throughout pregnancy in 11 (24%). The mean dose was 8.8±3.9 mg/day and the mean duration of exposure was 13.8±12.9 weeks. In comparisons between those exposed and those not exposed, there were higher rates of preterm birth (26.7% vs. 13.3%) and low birth weight (15.6% vs. 4.4%) in those exposed, but the differences were not statistically significant. In six subjects, the mean zolpidem concentrations in cord and maternal blood were 8.2 and 17.3. The mean cord:maternal ratio was 1.34. No major malformations were noted in any of the infants of the 90 women (4).

A 1998 noninterventional, observational cohort study described the outcomes of pregnancies in women who had been prescribed ≥1 of 34 newly marketed drugs by general practitioners in England (5). Data were obtained by questionnaires sent to the prescribing physicians 1 month after the expected or possible date of delivery. In 831 (78%) of the pregnancies, a newly marketed drug was thought to have been taken during the 1st trimester with birth defects noted in 14 (2.5%) singleton births of the 557 newborns (10 sets of twins). In addition, two birth defects were observed in aborted fetuses. However, few of the aborted fetuses were examined. Zolpidem was taken during the 1st trimester in 18 pregnancies. The outcomes of these pregnancies included 2 spontaneous abortions, 6 elective abortions, and 11 normal, term infants (1 set of twins) (5).

A 2010 study from Taiwan compared the outcomes of 2497 women who had used zolpidem during pregnancy with 12,485 randomly selected mothers who had not received the drug (6). In four outcomes, the adjusted odds ratios (aORs) were higher in exposed pregnancies: preterm birth (1.49, 95% confidence interval [CI] 1.28–1.74; $p < 0.001$), low birth weight (1.39, 95% CI 1.17–1.64; $p < 0.001$), small for gestational age (1.34, 95% CI 1.20–1.49; $p < 0.001$), and cesarean section (1.74, 95% CI 1.59–1.90; $p < 0.001$). Congenital anomalies were observed in 12 (0.48%) infants exposed in utero compared with 81 (0.65%) infants not exposed (0.70, 95% CI 0.38–1.28) (6).

In a study published in 2011, data from the Swedish Medical Birth Registry, covering the period 1995–2007, identified 1318 women who gave birth to 1341 infants and who reported the use of a hypnotic benzodiazepine receptor agonist at the first prenatal visit (7). The three most commonly reported agents and the number of exposed infants were zopiclone (N = 692) (*not available in USA*), zolpidem (N = 603), and zaleplon (N = 32). The reference group during the study period was 1,106,001 women who gave birth to 1,125,734 infants. The rate of congenital malformations was similar in the exposed and nonexposed groups, 4.3% (N = 58) and 4.7% (N = 52,773), aOR 0.89, 95% CI 0.68–1.16. One mother who had two infants with probably unrelated malformations (cleft lip and hypospadias) had used zopiclone in both pregnancies. For relatively severe defects, there were 42 exposed infants (3.1%) compared with 36,321 nonexposed infants (3.2%), aOR 0.95, 95% CI 0.0.69–1.30. The authors concluded that use of these agents did not appear to increase the risk of malformations (7).

BREASTFEEDING SUMMARY

Zolpidem is excreted into breast milk, but the effects, if any, on a nursing infant have not been studied. In a 1989 report, five lactating women were administered a single 20-mg dose 3–4 days after delivery of a full-term infant (8). Breastfeeding was halted for 24 hours after drug administration. Milk and serum samples were collected before and 1.5 (serum only), 3, 13, and 16 hours after the dose. The total amount of zolpidem in milk at 3 hours (both breasts emptied with an electric breast pump and the milk pooled for each woman) ranged from 0.76 to 3.88 mcg, representing 0.004%–0.019% of the dose. The drug was not detected in milk (detection level 0.5 ng/mL) at the other sampling times (8). The dose used in this study was twice the current maximum recommended human hypnotic dose.

In healthy adult patients, zolpidem has a relatively short serum half-life (about 2.6 hours) and accumulation is not expected to occur. The small amount of drug measured in milk after a dose that was twice the recommended human dose probably indicates that few, if any, adverse effects would occur in a nursing infant whose mother was consuming this hypnotic. In those instances in which the mother is taking zolpidem, however, she should observe her nursing infant for increased sedation, lethargy, and changes in feeding habits. Based on the one study above, the American Academy of Pediatrics classifies zolpidem as compatible with breastfeeding (9).

References

1. Product information. Ambien. G.D. Searle, 2000.
2. Shepard TH. *Catalog of Teratogenic Agents*. 8th ed. Baltimore, MD: The Johns Hopkins University Press, 1995:231.
3. Askew JP. Zolpidem addiction in a pregnant woman with a history of second-trimester bleeding. Pharmacotherapy 2007;27:306–8.
4. Juric S, Newport J, Ritchie JC, Galanti M, Stowe ZN. Zolpidem (Ambien®) in pregnancy: placental passage and outcome. Arch Womens Ment Health 2009;12:441–6.
5. Wilton LV, Pearce GL, Martin RM, Mackay FJ, Mann RD. The outcomes of pregnancy in women exposed to newly marketed drugs in general practice in England. Br J Obstet Gynaecol 1998;105:882–9.
6. Wang LH, Lin HC, Lin CC, Chen YH, Lin HC. Increased risk of adverse pregnancy outcomes in women receiving zolpidem during pregnancy. Clin Pharmacol Ther 2010;88:369–74.
7. Wikner BN, Kallen B. Are hypnotic benzodiazepine receptor agonists teratogenic in humans? J Clin Psychopharmacol 2011;31:356–9.
8. Pons G, Francoual C, Guillet PH, Moran C, Hermann PH, Bianchetti G, Thiercelin J-F, Thenot J-P, Olive G. Zolpidem excretion in breast milk. Eur J Clin Pharmacol 1989;37:245–8.
9. Committee on Drugs, American Academy of Pediatrics. The transfer of drugs and other chemicals into human milk. Pediatrics 2001;108:776–89.

ZONISAMIDE

Anticonvulsant

PREGNANCY RECOMMENDATION: Limited Human Data—Animal Data Suggest High Risk
BREASTFEEDING RECOMMENDATION: Limited Human Data—Potential Toxicity

PREGNANCY SUMMARY

Zonisamide is teratogenic in three animal species and embryolethal in a fourth at doses or exposures very near or less than doses and systemic concentrations used or obtained clinically. Human pregnancy experience is limited. Two infants with congenital anomalies have been observed, but in both cases, other anticonvulsants known to be human teratogens also were used. If treatment with zonisamide in pregnancy is required, monotherapy using the lowest effective dose is preferred, but because of its status as adjunctive therapy, this may not be possible.

FETAL RISK SUMMARY

Zonisamide, a sulfonamide derivative, is indicated as adjunctive therapy in the treatment of partial seizures. Its anticonvulsant mechanism of action is unknown. The drug is bound extensively to erythrocytes with concentrations in red blood cells eight times higher than in plasma. Approximately 40%–60% is bound to plasma proteins, mainly albumin (1,2). After single oral doses, the elimination half-lives from erythrocytes and from plasma are 105 and 50–68 hours, respectively (1,2). The plasma elimination half-life is decreased to about 25–35 hours if the patient is receiving concurrent treatment with hepatic enzyme-inducing anticonvulsants (carbamazepine, phenytoin, phenobarbital, or primidone) (2).

Reproduction studies with zonisamide have been conducted during organogenesis in mice, rats, dogs, and cynomolgus monkeys. In pregnant mice, doses approximately 1.5–6.0 times the maximum recommended human dose of 400 mg/day based on BSA (MRHD-BSA) were associated with increased rates of fetal malformations (skeletal and/or craniofacial defects). In rats, increased frequencies of malformations (cardiovascular defects) and variations (persistent cords of thymic tissue and decreased skeletal ossification) were observed at all doses tested (0.5–5.0 times the MRHD-BSA). Perinatal deaths resulted when a dose 1.4 times the MRHD-BSA was given in the latter part of gestation up to weaning. The no-effect level for this toxicity was 0.7 times the MRHD-BSA (1).

In pregnant dogs, doses that produced peak maternal plasma levels (25 mcg/mL) about 0.5 times the highest plasma levels measured in humans receiving the maximum recommended human dose of 400 mg/day (MRHD-PL) resulted in an increased incidence of fetal cardiovascular defects (ventricular septal defects, cardiomegaly, and valvular and arterial anomalies). At doses that produced plasma levels (44 mcg/mL) approximately equal to the MRHD-PL, about 50% of the fetuses had cardiovascular malformations as well as increased incidences of skeletal malformations. Fetal growth restriction and increased rates of skeletal variations were observed with peak maternal dog plasma levels produced by all doses tested (0.25–1.0 times the MRHD-PL). When zonisamide was given to pregnant monkeys at doses approximately 0.1 times the MRHD-PL or higher, embryo–fetal deaths were observed. The cause of the deaths was unknown, but the possibility that they were due to malformations could not be excluded (1).

Zonisamide was not carcinogenic in mice and rats after 2 years of dietary administration. The agent was mutagenic in one test but not mutagenic or clastogenic in other tests (1).

No reports describing the placental crossing of zonisamide early in gestation have been located. At term delivery of one newborn, the cord blood and maternal blood concentrations were 14.4 and 15.7 mcg/mL (ratio 0.92), respectively (3). A comparable amount of drug was found in a second full-term newborn, but specific data were not given. Zonisamide probably also crosses the placenta early in gestation because of its low molecular weight (about 212). In addition, the long elimination half-life from red blood cells and plasma will result in prolonged concentrations of the drug at the maternal blood:placenta interface, thus increasing the opportunity for embryo/fetal exposure.

A 1996 report described the outcomes of 26 offspring whose mothers had been treated with zonisamide during pregnancy (22 women; 25 pregnancies; 1 set of twins). The offspring were exposed to zonisamide either alone (4 cases) or combined with other anticonvulsants (22 cases) (4). Doses ranged from 100 to 600 mg/day. There were 2 elective abortions and 24 liveborn infants (1 set of twins). Two offspring (7.7%), both exposed to combination anticonvulsants, had major malformations. Neither of the mothers experienced seizures during pregnancy. The first case, electively terminated at 16 weeks' gestation, involved an anencephalic fetus (sex unknown) exposed to zonisamide (100 mg/day) and phenytoin (275 mg/day) throughout gestation. The second infant, a 2022-g female, was delivered by cesarean section at 37 weeks' gestation. She had an atrial septal defect. Combination therapy throughout gestation included zonisamide (200 mg/day), phenytoin (200 mg/day), and valproic acid (400 mg/day) (4).

In a 2002 case report, two women took multiple anticonvulsants throughout gestation and delivered apparently normal infants at about 40 weeks' gestation (3). One of the women took zonisamide (400 mg/day), carbamazepine (1000 mg/day) and clonazepam (1 mg/day), whereas the other took zonisamide (400 mg/day) and carbamazepine

(800 mg/day). Both newborns had Apgar scores at 1 and 5 minutes of 8 and 9, respectively. Birth weights were 3094 g and 3164 g, respectively (3).

The Lamotrigine Pregnancy Registry, an ongoing project conducted by the manufacturer, was first published in January 1997. The final report was published in July 2010 (5). The Registry is now closed. There were 12 prospectively enrolled pregnancies exposed to zonisamide and lamotrigine, with or without other anticonvulsants in the 1st trimester, resulting in 12 live births without birth defects (5).

The effect of zonisamide on folic acid levels and metabolism is unknown. A 2003 review recommended that to reduce the risk of birth defects from anticonvulsants, women should start multivitamins with folic acid before conception (6). Although the recommendation did not specify the amount of folic acid, a recent study found that multivitamin supplements with folic acid (typically 0.4 mg) did not reduce the risk of congenital malformations from four first-generation anticonvulsants (see Carbamazepine, Phenytoin, Phenobarbital, or Primidone). Therefore, until further information is available, the best course is to start folic acid supplementation before conception. Although a specific dosage has not been recommended for patients receiving anticonvulsants, 4 mg/day appears to be reasonable.

BREASTFEEDING SUMMARY

Zonisamide is excreted into breast milk. A woman took 300 mg/day (100 mg three times daily) during pregnancy and continued the anticonvulsant while breastfeeding (7). The cord plasma drug concentration at delivery was 6.72 mcg/mL, 2.5 hours after a dose. Milk and maternal plasma levels were determined on postpartum days 3, 6, 14, and 30 (1.5–2.5 hours after a dose). Milk concentrations ranged from 8.25 (day 3) to 10.5 mcg/mL (day 30), whereas maternal plasma levels ranged from 9.52 (day 14) to 10.6 mcg/mL (day 3). The milk:plasma (M:P) ratio consistently increased at each sampling. The average milk:plasma ratio was 0.93 (range 0.81–1.03). No neonatal behavior problems were observed (7).

In another report, two mothers receiving zonisamide (400 mg/day) and other anticonvulsants (mother no. 1: carbamazepine and clonazepam; mother no. 2: carbamazepine) throughout gestation as well as postpartum breastfed their apparently normal infants (see above) (3). Zonisamide concentrations were determined in the breast milk of mother no. 1. From delivery to postpartum day 9, the unbound maternal plasma zonisamide concentration ranged from 10.7 to 13.3 mcg/mL, whereas the total zonisamide level ranged from 17.5 to 25.2 mcg/mL. During the same interval, the drug concentrations in the watery portion of the milk (i.e., whey) ranged from 8.9 to 10.9 mcg/mL. The breast milk transfer rate was 41%–57%. The plasma zonisamide level in the infant on day 24 was 3.9 mcg/mL (15% of the mother's level on postpartum day 9). No adverse effects in either nursing infant were mentioned (3).

No adverse effects were noted in four nursing infants, but the milk concentrations were high enough that clinically significant doses appear to have been ingested. The relatively high plasma level found in one infant supports this assessment. Therefore, if a woman under treatment with zonisamide chooses to breastfeed, close clinical monitoring of her infant is recommended as well as the measurement of infant plasma drug levels. The long-term effects on nursing infants from this exposure are unknown but warrant investigation.

References

1. Product information. Zonegran. Elan Biopharmaceuticals, 2003.
2. Percucca E, Bialer M. The clinical pharmacokinetics of the newer antiepileptic drugs. Clin Pharmacokinet 1996;31:29–46.
3. Kawada K, Itoh S, Kusaka T, Isobe K, Ishii M. Pharmacokinetics of zonisamide in perinatal period. Brain Dev 2002;24:95–7.
4. Kondo T, Kaneko S, Amano Y, Egawa I. Preliminary report on teratogenic effects of zonisamide in the offspring of treated women with epilepsy. Epilepsia 1996;37:1242–4.
5. The Lamotrigine Pregnancy Registry. Final Report. 1 September 1992 through 31 March 2010. GlaxoSmithKline, July 2010.
6. Yerby MS. Clinical care of pregnant women with epilepsy: neural tube defects and folic acid supplementation. Epilepsia 2003;44 (Suppl 3):33–40.
7. Shimoyama R, Ohkubo T, Sugawara K. Monitoring of zonisamide in human breast milk and maternal plasma by solid-phase extraction HPLC method. Biomed Chromatogr 1999;13:370–2.

ZUCLOPENTHIXOL

[Withdrawn from the market. See 9th edition.]

APPENDIX

Classification of Drugs by Pharmacologic Category

[See drug's generic name in Index for location of drug in this Appendix.]

1. ANESTHETICS

A. Local

Benzocaine
Camphor
Lidocaine
Pramoxine
Ropivacaine
Tetracaine

B. General

Desflurane
Enflurane
Halothane
Isoflurane
Ketamine
Methohexital Sodium
Nitrous Oxide
Sevoflurane

2. ANTIDOTES

Acetylcysteine
Black Widow Spider Antivenin
Centruroides Immune (Scorpion) $F(ab')_2$ (Equine)
Deferasirox
Deferoxamine
Digoxin Immune FAB (Ovine)
Dimercaprol
Edetate Calcium Disodium
Flumazenil
Fomepizole
Glucagon
Glucarpidase
Lanthanum Carbonate
Pralidoxime
Sapropterin
Sevelamer
Succimer

3. ANTIHISTAMINES

Azelastine
Brompheniramine
Carbinoxamine
Cetirizine
Chlorcyclizine
Chlorpheniramine
Clemastine
Cyclizine
Cyproheptadine
Desloratadine
Dexbrompheniramine
Dexchlorpheniramine
Dimenhydrinate
Diphenhydramine
Doxylamine
Epinastine
Fexofenadine
Hydroxyzine
Levocetirizine
Loratadine
Meclizine
Olopatadine
Pheniramine
Phenyltoloxamine
Promethazine
Pyrilamine
Triprolidine

4. ANTI-INFECTIVES

A. Amebicide

Iodoquinol
Metronidazole
Paromomycin

B. Aminoglycosides

Amikacin
Gentamicin
Kanamycin
Neomycin
Paromomycin
Streptomycin
Tobramycin

C. Anthelmintics

Albendazole
Gentian Violet
Ivermectin
Mebendazole
Piperazine
Praziquantel
Pyrantel Pamoate

D. Antibiotics/Anti-infectives

Azithromycin
Aztreonam
Bacitracin
Benzyl Alcohol
Chloramphenicol
Chlorhexidine
Clarithromycin
Clavulanate Potassium
Clindamycin
Colistimethate
Daptomycin
Doripenem
Ertapenem
Erythromycin
Fidaxomicin
Fosfomycin
Furazolidone
Hexachlorophene
Imipenem-Cilastatin Sodium
Lincomycin
Linezolid
Mafenide
Meropenem
Metronidazole
Mupirocin
Nitrofurazone
Polymyxin B
Quinupristin/Dalfopristin
Retapamulin
Rifaximin
Sulbactam
Tazobactam
Telithromycin
Telavancin
Tinidazole
Trimethoprim
Vancomycin

E. Antifungals

i. Allylamines

Terbinafine

ii. Benzylamines

Butenafine

iii. Imidazoles

Butoconazole
Clotrimazole
Econazole
Ketoconazole
Miconazole
Oxiconazole
Sertaconazole
Sulconazole
Tioconazole

iv. Lipopeptides

Anidulafungin
Caspofungin
Micafungin

v. Polyenes

Amphotericin B
Nystatin

vi. Pyrimidines

Flucytosine

vii. Triazoles

Fluconazole
Itraconazole
Posaconazole
Terconazole
Voriconazole

viii. Miscellaneous
Ciclopirox
Griseofulvin
Naftifine

F. Antimalarials
Chloroquine
Dapsone
Hydroxychloroquine
Mefloquine
Primaquine
Proguanil
Pyrimethamine
Quinacrine
Quinidine
Quinine

G. Antiprotozoal
Atovaquone
Metronidazole
Nitazoxanide
Pentamidine
Tinidazole

H. Antituberculosis
para-Aminosalicylic Acid
Bedaquiline
Capreomycin
Cycloserine
Ethambutol
Ethionamide
Isoniazid
Pyrazinamide
Rifabutin
Rifampin
Rifapentine

I. Antiretroviral Agents
i. Integrase Strand Transfer Inhibitor
Raltegravir
ii. Nucleoside Reverse Transcriptase Inhibitors
Abacavir
Adefovir
Didanosine
Emtricitabine
Lamivudine
Stavudine
Telbivudine
Tenofovir
Zidovudine
iii. Nonnucleoside Reverse Transcriptase Inhibitors
Delavirdine
Efavirenz
Etravirine
Nevirapine
Rilpivirine
iv. Protease Inhibitors
Amprenavir
Atazanavir
Darunavir
Fosamprenavir
Indinavir
Lopinavir
Nelfinavir
Ritonavir
Saquinavir
Tipranavir
v. Entry Inhibitors
Enfuvirtide
Maraviroc

J. Other Antivirals
Acyclovir
Adefovir
Amantadine
Boceprevir
Cidofovir
Entecavir
Famciclovir
Foscarnet
Ganciclovir
Idoxuridine
Oseltamivir
Penciclovir
Ribavirin
Rimantadine
Telaprevir
Valacyclovir
Valganciclovir
Vidarabine
Zanamivir

K. Cephalosporins
Cefaclor
Cefadroxil
Cefazolin
Cefdinir
Cefditoren
Cefepime
Cefixime
Cefotaxime
Cefotetan
Cefoxitin
Cefpodoxime
Cefprozil
Ceftaroline
Ceftazidime
Ceftibuten
Ceftizoxime
Ceftriaxone
Cefuroxime
Cephalexin

L. Iodine
Iodine
Povidone-Iodine

M. Leprostatics
Clofazimine
Dapsone

N. Macrolides
Azithromycin
Clarithromycin
Erythromycin

O. Penicillins
Amoxicillin
Ampicillin
Carbenicillin
Dicloxacillin
Nafcillin
Oxacillin
Penicillin G
Penicillin G, Benzathine
Penicillin G, Procaine
Penicillin V
Piperacillin
Ticarcillin

P. Quinolones
Cinoxacin
Ciprofloxacin
Gemifloxacin
Levofloxacin
Lomefloxacin
Moxifloxacin
Nalidixic Acid
Norfloxacin
Ofloxacin

Q. Scabicide/Pediculicide
Benzyl Alcohol
Lindane
Permethrin
Pyrethrins with Piperonyl Butoxide

R. Sulfonamides
Sulfonamides

S.Tetracyclines
Chlortetracycline
Clomocycline
Demeclocycline
Doxycycline
Minocycline
Oxytetracycline
Tetracycline
Tigecycline

T. Trichomonacides
Metronidazole

U. Urinary Germicides
Cinoxacin
Methenamine
Methylene Blue
Nalidixic Acid
Nitrofurantoin

5. ANTILIPEMIC AGENTS

A. Bile Acid Sequestrants
Cholestyramine
Colesevelam
Colestipol

B. Fibric Acid Derivatives
Gemfibrozil
Fenofibrate

C. HMG–CoA Inhibitors (statins)
Atorvastatin
Fluvastatin
Lovastatin
Pitavastatin
Pravastatin
Rosuvastatin
Simvastatin

D. Thyroid
Dextrothyroxine

E. Vitamin
Niacin

F. Miscellaneous
Ezetimibe
Lomitapide

6. ANTINEOPLASTICS
Cytoprotectants
Amifostine
Dexrazoxane
Mesna

A. Alkylating Agents
Bendamustine
Busulfan
Carmustine
Chlorambucil
Cyclophosphamide
Dacarbazine
Ifosfamide
Mechlorethamine
Melphalan
Streptozocin

B. Anthracenedione
Mitoxantrone

C. Anthracycline Antibiotics
Daunorubicin
Doxorubicin
Epirubicin
Idarubicin
Valrubicin

D. Antiandrogen
Enzalutamide

E. Antibody-Drug Conjugate
Brentuximab Vedotin

F. Antibiotics
Bleomycin
Dactinomycin
Mitomycin

G. Antimetabolites
i. Folic Acid Antagonists
Methotrexate
Pemetrexed
Pralatrexate
ii. Purine Analogs
Cladribine
Clofarabine
Fludarabine phosphate
Mercaptopurine
Pentostatin
Thioguanine
iii. Pyrimidine Analogs
Capecitabine
Cytarabine
Floxuridine
Fluorouracil
Gemcitabine
iv. Agents That Reduce Uric Acid Levels
Allopurinol
Rasburicase

H. Antimitotics
i. Epothilones
Ixabepilone
ii. Taxoids
Cabazitaxel
Docetaxel
Paclitaxel
iii. Vinca Alkaloids
Vinblastine
Vincristine
Vinorelbine

I. Aromatase inhibitors
Letrozole

J. Biological Response Modifiers
Aldesleukin
Denileukin Diftitox

K. DNA Demethylation Agents
Azacitidine
Decitabine
Nelarabine

L. DNA Topoisomerase Inhibitors
Irinotecan
Topotecan

M. Enzymes
Asparaginase

N. Epipodophyllotoxins
Etoposide
Teniposide

O. Histone Deacetylase Inhibitors
Romidepsin
Vorinostat

P. Hormones
Abiraterone Acetate
Exemestane
Leuprolide
Tamoxifen

Q. Imidazotetrazine Derivatives
Temozolomide

R. Kinase Inhibitors
i. BRAF Inhibitor
Vemurafenib
ii. Janus Associated Kinase Inhibitor
Ruxolitinib
iii. mTOR Inhibitors
Everolimus
Temsirolimus
iv. Multikinase Inhibitors
Sorafenib
Regorafenib
v. Tyrosine Kinase Inhibitors
Axitinib
Bosutinib
Cabozantinib
Crizotinib
Dasatinib
Erlotinib
Gefitinib
Imatinib
Lapatinib
Nilotinib
Pazopanib
Ponatinib
Sunitinib
Vandetanib
Ziv-Aflibercept

S. Methylhydrazine Derivatives
Procarbazine

T. Monoclonal Antibodies
Alemtuzumab
Bevacizumab
Cetuximab
Ipilimumab
Ibritumomab Tiuxetan
Ofatumumab
Panitumumab
Pertuzumab
Rituximab
Trastuzumab

U. Nontaxane Microtubule Dynamic Inhibitor
Eribulin

V. Platinum Coordination Complex
Carboplatin
Cisplatin
Oxaliplatin

W. Protein Synthesis Inhibitor
Omacetaxine

X. Proteasome Inhibitor
Bortezomib
Carfilzomib

Y. Retinoids
Bexarotene
Tretinoin (Systemic)

Z. Substituted Ureas
Hydroxyurea

ZZ. Miscellaneous
Interferon Alfa

(includes Interferon Alfa -n3, -NL, -2a, and -2b)
Porfimer
Thiotepa
Trimetrexate
Vismodegib

7. ARTIFICIAL SWEETENERS

Aspartame
Cyclamate
Saccharin

8. AUTONOMICS

A. Parasympathomimetics (Cholinergics)

Bethanechol
Carbachol
Cevimeline
Echothiophate
Edrophonium
Neostigmine
Physostigmine
Pilocarpine
Pyridostigmine

B. Parasympatholytics (Anticholinergics)

Atropine
Belladonna
Benztropine
Clidinium
Dicyclomine
Glycopyrrolate
Homatropine
l-Hyoscyamine
Mepenzolate
Methscopolamine
Propantheline
Scopolamine
Trihexyphenidyl

C. Sympatholytics

Acebutolol
Atenolol
Betaxolol
Bisoprolol
Carteolol
Carvedilol
Dihydroergotamine
Doxazosin
Ergotamine
Esmolol
Guanethidine
Guanfacine
Labetalol
Metoprolol
Nadolol
Nebivolol
Penbutolol
Pindolol
Prazosin
Propranolol
Sotalol
Tamsulosin
Terazosin
Timolol

D. Sympathomimetics (Adrenergics)

Albuterol
Cocaine
Dobutamine
Dopamine
Ephedrine
Epinephrine
Isometheptene
Isoproterenol
Isoxsuprine
Midodrine
Norepinephrine
Oxymetazoline
Phenylephrine
Pseudoephedrine
Terbutaline

9. BISPHOSPHONATES

Alendronate
Etidronate
Ibandronate
Pamidronate
Risedronate
Tiludronate
Zoledronic Acid

10. CALCIUM RECEPTOR AGONIST

Cinacalcet

11. CARDIOVASCULAR DRUGS

A. Antihypertensives

i. Angiotensin Converting Enzyme Inhibitors

Benazepril
Captopril
Enalapril
Fosinopril
Lisinopril
Moexipril
Perindopril
Quinapril
Ramipril
Trandolapril

ii. Angiotensin II Receptor Antagonists

Azilsartan
Candesartan Cilexetil
Eprosartan
Irbesartan
Losartan
Olmesartan
Telmisartan
Valsartan

iii. Renin Inhibitor

Aliskiren

iv. Other Antihypertensives

Acebutolol
Atenolol
Betaxolol
Bisoprolol
Carteolol
Carvedilol
Clonidine
Diazoxide
Doxazosin
Epoprostenol
Esmolol
Fenoldopam
Guanabenz
Guanadrel
Guanethidine
Guanfacine
Hydralazine
Labetalol
Mepindolol
Methyldopa
Metoprolol
Metyrosine
Minoxidil
Nadolol
Nebivolol
Nitroprusside
Oxprenolol
Penbutolol
Phenoxybenzamine
Phentolamine
Pindolol
Prazosin
Propranolol
Reserpine
Terazosin
Sotalol
Timolol

B. Calcium Channel Blockers

Amlodipine
Clevidipine
Diltiazem
Felodipine
Isradipine
Nicardipine
Nifedipine
Nimodipine
Nisoldipine
Verapamil

C. Cardiac Drugs

Acetyldigitoxin
Adenosine
Amiodarone
Deslanoside
Digitalis
Digitoxin
Digoxin
Disopyramide
Dofetilide
Dronedarone
Flecainide
Ibutilide

Lanatoside C
Lidocaine
Mexiletine
Milrinone
Moricizine
Procainamide
Propafenone
Quinidine
Sotalol

D. Vasodilators
Ambrisentan
Amyl Nitrite
Bosentan
Epoprostenol
Erythrityl Tetranitrate
Hydralazine
Iloprost
Isosorbide Dinitrate
Isosorbide Mononitrate
Isoxsuprine
Minoxidil
Nesiritide
Nitroglycerin
Sildenafil

E. Sclerosing Agents
Polidocanol

F. Miscellaneous Antianginal Agents
Ranolazine

12. CENTRAL NERVOUS SYSTEM DRUGS

A. Analgesics and Antipyretics
Acetaminophen
Antipyrine
Ziconotide

B. Antialcoholic Agents
Acamprosate
Disulfiram

C. Antichorea
Tetrabenazine

D. Anticonvulsants
Bromides
Carbamazepine
Clobazam
Clonazepam
Clorazepate
Ethosuximide
Ethotoin
Ezogabine
Felbamate
Gabapentin
Gabapentin Enacarbil
Lacosamide
Lamotrigine
Levetiracetam
Magnesium Sulfate
Methsuximide
Oxcarbazepine
Perampanel
Phenobarbital
Phenytoin
Pregabalin
Primidone
Rufinamide
Tiagabine
Topiramate
Valproic Acid
Zonisamide

E. Antidepressants
i. Aminoketone
Bupropion
ii. Monoamine Oxidase Inhibitors
Isocarboxazid
Phenelzine
Tranylcypromine
iii. Phenylpiperazine
Nefazodone
iv. Selective Serotonin Reuptake Inhibitors
Citalopram
Escitalopram
Fluoxetine
Fluvoxamine
Paroxetine
Sertraline
Vilazodone
v. Serotonin and Norepinephrine Reuptake Inhibitors
Duloxetine
Desvenlafaxine
Milnacipran
Venlafaxine
vi. Tetracyclics
Maprotiline
Mirtazapine
vii. Tricyclics
Amitriptyline
Amoxapine
Clomipramine
Desipramine
Doxepin
Imipramine
Nortriptyline
Protriptyline
Trimipramine
viii. Triazolopyridine
Trazodone

F. Antimigraine Agents
Almotriptan
Dihydroergotamine
Eletriptan
Ergotamine
Frovatriptan
Naratriptan
Rizatriptan
Sumatriptan
Zolmitriptan

G. Antiparkinson Agents
Amantadine
Carbidopa
Entacapone
Levodopa
Pramipexole
Rasagiline
Ropinirole
Selegiline
Tolcapone

H. Antipsychotics
Typical Antipsychotics
i. Phenylbutylpiperadines
Butyrophenones
Droperidol
Haloperidol
Diphenylbutypiperadines
Pimozide
ii. Phenothiazines
Chlorpromazine
Fluphenazine
Perphenazine
Prochlorperazine
Thioridazine
Trifluoperazine
iii. Thioxanthenes
Thiothixene

Atypical Antipsychotics
i. Benzoisothiazol
Lurasidone
ii. Benzisoxazoles
Iloperidone
Paliperidone
Risperidone
Ziprasidone
iii. Dibenzapines
Asenapine
Clozapine
Loxapine
Olanzapine
Quetiapine
iv. Quinolinones
Aripiprazole

Miscellaneous Antipsychotics
Lithium

I. Central Analgesics
Clonidine

J. Cholinesterase Inhibitors
Donepezil
Galantamine
Rivastigmine

K. Hallucinogens
Lysergic Acid Diethylamide
Marijuana
Mescaline
Peyote

Phencyclidine
Salvia Divinorum

L. Narcotic Agonist Analgesics

Alfentanil
Codeine
Dihydrocodeine
Fentanyl
Heroin
Hydrocodone
Hydromorphone
Levorphanol
Meperidine
Methadone
Morphine
Oxycodone
Oxymorphone
Remifentanil
Sufentanil
Tapentadol
Tramadol

M. Narcotic Agonist–Antagonist Analgesics

Buprenorphine
Butorphanol
Nalbuphine
Pentazocine

N. Narcotic Antagonists

Methylnaltrexone
Naloxone
Naltrexone

O. Nonsteroidal Anti-inflammatory Drugs

Aspirin
Celecoxib
Diclofenac
Diflunisal
Etodolac
Fenoprofen
Flurbiprofen
Ibuprofen
Indomethacin
Ketoprofen
Ketorolac
Meclofenamate
Mefenamic Acid
Meloxicam
Nabumetone
Naproxen
Oxaprozin
Oxyphenbutazone
Piroxicam
Sulindac
Tolmetin

P. Physical Adjunct

Botulinum Toxin Type A

Q. Potassium Channel Blocker

Dalfampridine

R. Psychotherapeutics (Miscellaneous)

Atomoxetine
Sodium Oxybate

S. Sedatives and Hypnotics

Alprazolam
Amobarbital
Bromides
Buspirone
Butalbital
Chloral Hydrate
Chlordiazepoxide
Clorazepate
Dexmedetomidine
Diazepam
Dichloralphenazone
Estazolam
Eszopiclone
Ethanol
Ethchlorvynol
Etomidate
Flurazepam
Fospropofol
Lorazepam
Mephobarbital
Meprobamate
Methotrimeprazine
Midazolam
Oxazepam
Pentobarbital
Phenobarbital
Propofol
Quazepam
Ramelteon
Secobarbital
Temazepam
Triazolam
Zaleplon
Zolpidem

T. Skeletal Muscle Relaxants

Atracurium
Baclofen
Carisoprodol
Chlorzoxazone
Cyclobenzaprine
Dantrolene
Metaxalone
Methocarbamol
Orphenadrine
Pancuronium
Rocuronium
Succinylcholine
Tizanidine
Vecuronium

U. Smoking Deterrents

Bupropion
Clonidine
Nicotine Replacement Therapy
Nortriptyline
Varenicline

V. Stimulants and/or Anorexiants

Amphetamine
Armodafinil
Benzphetamine
Caffeine
Cigarette Smoking
Dexmethylphenidate
Dextroamphetamine
Diethylpropion
Doxapram
Ecstasy
Lisdexamfetamine
Lorcaserin
Methamphetamine
Methylphenidate
Modafinil
Phendimetrazine
Phentermine

W. Miscellaneous

Riluzole

13. CHELATING AGENTS

Deferoxamine
Deferasirox
Penicillamine
Succimer
Trientine

14. DERMATOLOGIC AGENTS

Acitretin
Adapalene
Anthralin
Azficel-T
Butenafine
Calcipotriene
Calcitriol
Collagenase Clostridium
Histolyticum
Etretinate
Fluocinolone
Fluocinonide
Hydroquinone
Ingenol Mebutate
Isotretinoin
Kunecatechins
Methoxsalen
Spinosad
Tazarotene
Tretinoin (Topical)

15. DIAGNOSTIC AGENTS

Diatrizoate
Ethiodized Oil
Evans Blue
Fluorescein Sodium
Gadobenate Dimeglumine
Gadobutrol
Gadodiamide
Gadofosveset
Gadopentetate Dimeglumine

Gadoteridol
Gadoversetamide
Indigo Carmine
Iocetamic Acid
Iodipamide
Iodoxamate
Ioflupane I^{123}
Iohexol
Iopamidol
Iopanoic Acid
Iothalamate
Ipodate
Methylene Blue
Technetium Tc-99m

16. DIETARY SUPPLEMENTS

Chondroitin
Glucosamine
Omega-3 Fatty Acid Supplements
Stevia

17. DIURETICS

Acetazolamide
Amiloride
Bendroflumethiazide
Benzthiazide
Bumetanide
Chlorothiazide
Chlorthalidone
Dehydroepiandrosterone
Dichlorphenamide
Ethacrynic Acid
Furosemide
Hydrochlorothiazide
Hydroflumethiazide
Indapamide
Isosorbide
Mannitol
Methazolamide
Methyclothiazide
Metolazone
Polythiazide
Spironolactone
Torsemide
Triamterene
Trichlormethiazide
Urea

18. ELECTROLYTES

Potassium Chloride
Potassium Citrate
Potassium Gluconate

19. ENDOCRINE/METABOLIC AGENTS

A. Adrenal
Beclomethasone
Betamethasone
Budesonide
Cortisone
Dexamethasone
Hydrocortisone
Prednisolone
Prednisone
Triamcinolone

B. Androgens
Danazol
Fluoxymesterone
Methyltestosterone
Testosterone

C. Antiadrenal
Aminoglutethimide

D. Antidiabetic Agents
i. Alpha-Glucosidase Inhibitors
Acarbose
Miglitol
ii. Amylin Analog
Pramlintide
iii. Biguanides
Metformin
iv. Dipeptidyl Peptidase-4 Inhibitors
Linagliptin
Saxagliptin
Sitagliptin
v. Glucagon-like Peptide 1 Receptor Agonists
Exenatide
Liraglutide
vi. Insulins
Insulin
Insulin Aspart
Insulin Detemir
Insulin Glargine
Insulin Glulisine
Insulin Lispro
vii. Meglitinides
Nateglinide
Repaglinide
viii. Sulfonylureas
Chlorpropamide
Glimepiride
Glipizide
Glyburide
Tolazamide
Tolbutamide
ix. Thiazolidinediones
Pioglitazone
Rosiglitazone

E. Antiestrogens
Tamoxifen

F. Antigout
i. Uricosurics
Allopurinol
Febuxostat
Pegloticase
Probenecid
ii. Miscellaneous
Colchicine

G. Antiprogestogen
Mifepristone

H. Antithyroid
Carbimazole
Methimazole
Propylthiouracil
Sodium Iodide ^{131}I

I. Calcium Regulation Hormone
Calcitonin-Salmon

J. Emergency Contraceptive
Ulipristal

K. Enzymes
Agalsidase Alfa
Agalsidase Beta
Alglucosidase Alfa
Alpha-Galactosidase A
Galsulfase
Laronidase

L. Estrogens
Clomiphene
Diethylstilbestrol
Estradiol
Estrogens, Conjugated
Estrone
Ethinyl Estradiol
Mestranol
Oral Contraceptives

M. Gaucher Disease
Alglucerase
Imiglucerase
Miglustat
Taliglucerase Alfa
Velaglucerase Alfa

N. Growth Hormone Receptor Antagonist
Pegvisomant

O. Growth Hormone Releasing Factor
Tesamorelin

P. Hyperammonemia
Carglumic Acid

Q. Pineal Gland
Melatonin

R. Pituitary
Corticotropin/Cosyntropin
Desmopressin
Leuprolide
Somatostatin
Vasopressin

S. Progestogens
Ethynodiol
17 Alpha-Hydroxyprogesterone
Medroxyprogesterone
Norethindrone
Norgestrel
Oral Contraceptives

T. Prostaglandins
Carboprost
Dinoprostone

U. Selective Estrogen Receptor Modulator
Raloxifene

V. Somatostatin Analogs
Octreotide
Pasireotide

W. Thyroid Agents
Levothyroxine
Liothyronine
Liotrix
Thyroglobulin
Thyroid
Thyrotropin

X. Vasopressin Receptor Antagonists
Conivaptan
Tolvaptan

Y. Miscellaneous Agents
Bromocriptine
Cabergoline
Ivacaftor

20. GASTROINTESTINAL AGENTS

A. Antacids
Calcium Carbonate
Sodium Bicarbonate

B. Antidiarrheals
Alosetron
Bismuth Subsalicylate
Crofelemer
Diphenoxylate
Kaolin/Pectin
Loperamide
Opium

C. Antiemetics
Alosetron
Aprepitant
Cyclizine
Dimenhydrinate
Dolasetron
Doxylamine
Dronabinol
Droperidol
Granisetron
Meclizine
Metoclopramide
Nabilone
Ondansetron
Palonosetron
Prochlorperazine
Promethazine
Trimethobenzamide

D. Antiflatulents
Simethicone

E. Anti-inflammatory Bowel Disease Agents
Balsalazide
Infliximab
Mesalamine
Olsalazine
Sulfasalazine

F. Antisecretory Agents
i. H_2-Receptor Antagonists
Cimetidine
Famotidine
Nizatidine
Ranitidine
ii. Proton Pump Inhibitors
Dexlansoprazole
Esomeprazole
Lansoprazole
Omeprazole
Pantoprazole
Rabeprazole
iii. Miscellaneous
Misoprostol
Sucralfate

G. Gallstone Solubilizing Agents
Chenodiol
Ursodiol

H. Glucagon-Like Peptide-2 Analog
Teduglutide

I. Laxatives/Purgatives
Bisacodyl
Casanthranol
Cascara Sagrada
Castor Oil
Docusate Calcium
Docusate Potassium
Docusate Sodium
Glycerin
Lactulose
Linaclotide
Lubiprostone
Magnesium Sulfate
Mineral Oil
Polyethylene Glycol (3350 & 4000)
Senna

J. Lipase Inhibitors
Orlistat

K. Peripheral Opioid Antagonist
Alvimopan

L. Stimulants
Dexpanthenol
Metoclopramide

21. HEMATOLOGIC AGENTS

A. Anticoagulants
Apixaban
Coumarin Derivatives
Dalteparin
Dabigatran Etexilate
Enoxaparin
Ethyl Biscoumacetate
Fondaparinux
Heparin
Nicoumalone
Phenindione
Phenprocoumon
Reviparin
Rivaroxaban
Warfarin

B. Antiheparin
Protamine

C. Antihemophilic
Factor XIII Concentrate (Human)

D. Antiplatelet
i. Aggregation Inhibitors
Cilostazol
Clopidogrel
Prasugrel
Ticagrelor
Ticlopidine
Treprostinil
ii. Glycoprotein IIb/IIIa Inhibitors
Abciximab
Eptifibatide
Tirofiban
iii. Miscellaneous
Anagrelide
Dipyridamole

E. Bradykinin Inhibitor
Icatibant

F. Hematopoietic
Darbepoetin Alfa
Eltrombopag
Epoetin Alfa
Filgrastim
Hemin
Oprelvekin
Pegfilgrastim
Peginesatide
Plerixafor
Romiplostim
Sargramostim

G. Hemorrheologic
Pentoxifylline

H. Hemostatics
Aminocaproic Acid
Aprotinin
Tranexamic Acid

I. Kallikrein Inhibitor
Ecallantide

J. Thrombin Inhibitor
Antithrombin III (Human)

Argatroban
Bivalirudin
Desirudin
Lepirudin

K. Thrombolytics
Alteplase
Drotrecogin Alfa (Activated)
Reteplase
Tenecteplase
Urokinase

22. HERBS
Arnica
Black Seed/Kalanji
Blue Cohosh
Chamomile
Echinacea
Evening Primrose Oil
Feverfew
Garlic
Ginger
Ginkgo Biloba
Ginseng
Kudzu
Nutmeg
Passion Flower
Peppermint
Pumpkin Seed
Raspberry Leaf
Safflower
Salvia Divinorum
St.John's Wort
Valerian
Yohimbine

23. IMMUNOLOGIC AGENTS

A. Antihemolysis
Eculizumab

B. Antiosteoporosis
Denosumab

C. Antirheumatic Agents
Abatacept
Auranofin
Gold Sodium Thiomalate
Hydroxychloroquine
Infliximab
Leflunomide
Methotrexate
Sulfasalazine
Tofacitinib

D. Immunomodulators
Adalimumab
Anakinra
Belimumab
Canakinumab
Certolizumab Pegol
Etanercept
Fingolimod
Golimumab
Imiquimod
Infliximab
Interferon Alfa (includes Interferon Alfa-n3, -NL, -2a, and -2b)
Interferon Beta-1b
Interferon Gamma-1b
Lenalidomide
Natalizumab
Pimecrolimus
Rilonacept
Teriflunomide
Thalidomide
Tocilizumab
Ustekinumab

E. Immunosuppressants
Alefacept
Azathioprine
Basiliximab
Belatacept
Cyclosporine
Daclizumab
Efalizumab
Glatiramer
Muromonab-CD3
Mycophenolate
Rituximab
Sirolimus
Tacrolimus

24. IMPOTENCE AGENTS
Avanafil
Sildenafil
Yohimbine

25. KERATOLYTIC AGENTS
Podofilox
Podophyllum

26. KERATINOCYTE GROWTH FACTOR
Palifermin

27. NUTRIENTS/NUTRITIONAL SUPPLEMENTS
Calcium Carbonate
Hyperalimentation, Parenteral
Lipids
L-Lysine
Melatonin

28. OPHTHALMICS

A. Antihistamine
Alcaftadine
Bepotastine

B. Anti-infective
Besifloxacin
Gatifloxacin

C. Corticosteroid
Fluocinolone

D. Mast Cell Stabilizer
Lodoxamide

D. Nonsteroidal Anti-inflammatory
Bromfenac
Nepafenac

E. Phototherapy
Verteporfin

F. Prostaglandin Agonist
Bimatoprost
Latanoprost
Tafluprost
Travoprost

G. Selective Vascular Endothelial Growth Factor Antagonist
Pegaptanib
Ranibizumab

H. Sympathomimetic (Adrenergic)
Naphazoline

I. Miscellaneous
Ocriplasmin

29. OXYTOCICS
Castor Oil
Methylergonovine Maleate
Misoprostol

30. RADIOPHARMACEUTICALS
Sodium Iodide ^{125}I
Sodium Iodide ^{131}I

31. RESPIRATORY DRUGS

A. Anti-inflammatory (Inhaled)
Cromolyn Sodium
Nedocromil Sodium

B. Antitussives
Codeine
Dextromethorphan
Hydrocodone

C. Bronchodilators
i. β_2-Adrenergic Agents
Albuterol
Arformoterol
Formoterol
Indacaterol
Levalbuterol
Metaproterenol
Pirbuterol
Salmeterol
Terbutaline
ii. Other Sympathomimetics
Ephedrine

Epinephrine
Isoproterenol

iii. Xanthine Derivatives

Aminophylline
Dyphylline
Theophylline

iv. Anticholinergics

Aclidinium
Ipratropium
Tiotropium

D. Corticosteroids (Inhaled)

Beclomethasone
Budesonide
Ciclesonide
Flunisolide
Fluticasone
Mometasone
Triamcinolone

E. Expectorants

Ammonium Chloride
Guaifenesin
Iodinated Glycerol
Potassium Iodide
Sodium Iodide
Terpin Hydrate

F. Leukotriene Receptor Antagonists

Montelukast
Zafirlukast

G. Leukotriene Formation Inhibitor

Zileuton

H. Monoclonal Antibody

Omalizumab
Palivizumab

I. Mucolytic

Acetylcysteine
Dornase Alfa

J. Phosphodiesterase Inhibitor

Roflumilast

32. SERUMS AND TOXOIDS

A.Serums

Immune Globulin, Hepatitis B
Immune Globulin Intramuscular
Immune Globulin Intravenous
Immune Globulin, Rabies
Immune Globulin, Tetanus
Immune Globulin, Varicella Zoster (Human)

B. Toxoids

Tetanus/Diphtheria Toxoids (Adult)

33. TOXINS

Ciguatoxin

34. URINARY TRACT AGENTS

A. Analgesic

Pentosan
Phenazopyridine

B. Antispasmodics

Darifenacin
Fesoterodine
Flavoxate
Mirabegron
Oxybutynin
Solifenacin
Tolterodine
Trospium

C. Urinary Acidifier

Ammonium Chloride

D. Urinary Alkalinizers

Potassium Citrate

E. Urinary Germicides

(see Anti-infectives, Section T)

35. VACCINES

Adenovirus Type 4 and Type 7, Live
Anthrax
BCG
Cholera
Escherichia coli
Group B Streptococcal
Haemophilus b Conjugate
Hepatitis A
Hepatitis B
Human Papillomavirus Bivalent
Human Papillomavirus Quadrivalent
Influenza
Influenza A (H1N1)
Lyme Disease
Measles
Meningococcal
Mumps
Plague
Pneumococcal Polyvalent
Poliovirus Inactivated
Poliovirus Live
Rabies (Human)
Rubella
Smallpox
TC-83 Venezuelan Equine Encephalitis
Tetanus/Diphtheria Toxoids & Acellular Pertussis
Tularemia
Typhoid
Varicella Virus
Yellow Fever

36. VAGINAL SPERMICIDES

Nonoxynol-9/Octoxynol-9

37. VITAMINS

Acitretin
β-Carotene
Calcifediol
Calcitriol
Cholecalciferol
Dexpanthenol
Dihydrotachysterol
Ergocalciferol
Etretinate
Folic Acid
Isotretinoin
Leucovorin
Niacin
Niacinamide
Pantothenic Acid
Paricalcitol
Phytonadione
Pyridoxine
Riboflavin
Thiamine
Tretinoin (Systemic)
Vitamin A
Vitamin B_{12}
Vitamin C
Vitamin D
Vitamin E
Vitamins, Multiple

38. MISCELLANEOUS

Electricity
Silicone Breast Implants

Index

Generic names are shown in **bold** with two sets of page numbers. The first set, also shown in **bold**, refers to the page number in the text where the monograph is located. The second set, shown in parentheses, refers to the page number in the Appendix where the drug is located by pharmacologic class. The trade names and synonyms are shown with one set of page numbers. These refer to their location in the text.

A

E

F

G

H

I

J

K

L

M

N

O

P

Q

R

S

U

V

W

X

Y

Z